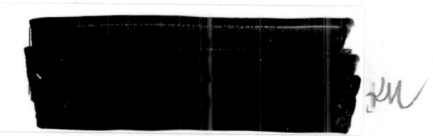
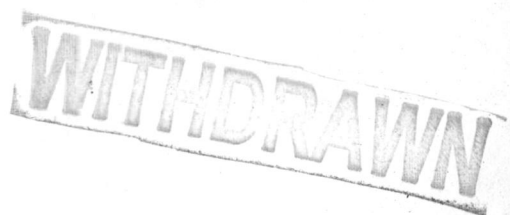

W9-AGK-666

WITHDRAWN

VIRAL
IMMUNITY

VIRAL IMMUNITY

A 10-Step Plan to Enhance Your Immunity Against Viral Disease Using Natural Medicines

J. E. Williams, O.M.D.

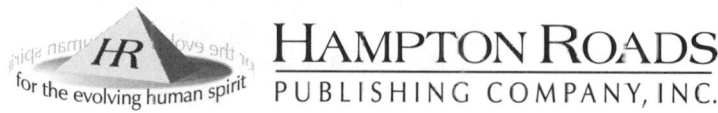

HAMPTON ROADS
PUBLISHING COMPANY, INC.

for the evolving human spirit

Interior illustrations by Anne L. Louque
Cover design by Marjoram Productions
Cover image ©2002 Corbis Images/Picture Quest
About the cover image: Tobacco mosaic virus;
the first virus to be isolated and also the first virus
to be photographed by electronmicroscopy.
Interior photograph of influenza virus
©2002 Corbis Images/Picture Quest

Hampton Roads Publishing Company, Inc.
1125 Stoney Ridge Road
Charlottesville, VA 22902

434-296-2772
fax: 434-296-5096
e-mail: hrpc@hrpub.com
www.hrpub.com

If you are unable to order this book from your local
bookseller, you may order directly from the publisher.
Call 1-800-766-8009, toll-free.

Library of Congress Catalog Card Number: 2002100967
ISBN 1-57174-265-4
10 9 8 7 6 5 4 3 2 1
Printed on acid-free paper in Canada

Disclaimer

This book is written as a source of information to educate the reader. It is not intended to replace medical advice or care, whether provided by a primary care physician, a specialist, or a licensed alternative medical professional. Please consult your doctor before beginning any new medications, diet, nutrients, or any form of health program. Dosages are given in ranges for the average adult and are to be used as guidelines only. Effects from any medication can vary a great deal from person to person, and applications must be adjusted to meet individual requirements. The author has spent a great deal of time and energy supporting the information contained in this book with published documentation; however, this research is not meant to be used as justification for any of the recommendations contained in the book.

Neither the author nor the publisher shall be liable or responsible for any adverse effects arising from the use or application of any of the information contained herein, nor do they guarantee that everyone will benefit or be healed by these techniques, and are not responsible if they are not. The author has no financial ties to any of the products, clinics, services, or medications cited in the text.

Table of Contents

Preface

I grew up in a small New England farming community in the 1950s and 1960s. Second- and third-growth forests of birch, maple, and white pine blanketed a landscape dotted with green patches of pasture, orchards, and only an occasional front lawn. Streams were full of trout, deer roamed the forests, and beavers built dams and flooded hollows, creating ponds where migrating mallards rested on their way to Canada. However, all was not completely pastoral.

On the viral scene, smallpox had yet to be eradicated; the new "kissing disease" emerged at a time when French-kissing before marriage was still taboo. Paranoia over viruses was common. Rabies, for example, was a serious issue among farming folk, and even the favorite dog was put down if there was the slightest hint of foaming at the mouth or strange behavior. Children were forbidden to play with wild animals, and bats—common in attics and barns—also conjured up dark fears of rabies. During the hot, humid summers, swimming in the local watering holes was a pleasure; however, on several occasions these ponds were off limits. They were called "polio pits," and parents scared children into avoiding them with stories of the crippling effects of poliomyelitis.

Ironically, at the same time we were allowed to swim in a river that had been chemically "purified" by run-off from a factory just upstream. The water was so clean that no fish, algae, or any life at all grew in it. No one questioned the effects of swimming there, not realizing that it was sterile due to toxic chemical runoff. Another river was so polluted that it turned an opaque green, and at times, small bursts of fire flickered on its surface.

Luckily, in the countryside, serious contagious infections were almost non-existent. The worst-case scenarios and parental fears never materialized, and I never caught anything more than a seasonal cold or mild flu. Those times were the beginning of the age of vaccinations that were given to all children by the local country doctor in the school gymnasium. Things have changed dramatically since then, yet the notion of viral plagues is still an ingrained part of the psyche.

It seems every generation has had its viral epidemic: in those times it was polio, while the decades between 1980–2000 belonged to AIDS. Now, chronic hepatitis may prove to be the virus of our times, and the next after that may belong to stealth viruses, a new super-flu, a previously unknown virus, or the re-emergence of smallpox through an act of bioterrorism.

My professional interest in viral diseases began early in my career. In the early 1980s I worked with AIDS support groups in San Diego, as well as with chronic Epstein-Barr virus and cytomegalovirus cases at the California Clinic of Preventive Medicine in Del Mar. My work with these viral illnesses lead me to look at other viruses, including hepatitis C in the late 1980s and later at human herpes virus-6.

In 1997, my own near-death encounter with an infectious illness brought the frightening reality of emerging disease to my doorstep. Most likely contracted during a trip to Peru where I conduct ethnomedical research, studying the medical systems of indigenous peoples, I experienced an acute episode of high fever, severe headache, and the loss of my color vision (it returned after two weeks), followed by rheumatoid arthritis three months after my return from the Amazon.

Though numerous blood tests were ordered, all attempts to determine a diagnosis were futile, leaving the most likely diagnosis to be a rare form of delayed-onset dengue. A mosquito-born virus that mimics the symptoms of malaria, it had caused an autoimmune reaction in which my body's defense system attacked itself.

Conventional medicine was useless for my condition. Since all the blood tests were inconclusive, and a name could not be assigned to my case, it was considered untreatable. I even went to the world famous Scripps Clinic in La Jolla, California to consult the most prestigious infectious disease specialists—all to no avail. It was as if my illness did not exist. So when the internists, infectious disease specialists, pathologists, and immunologists threw up their hands, I became impatient with modern medicine and began treating myself with natural medicine.

For treatment, I drew upon my considerable knowledge of traditional Chinese medicine, homotoxicology (a modern form of medical homeopathy discussed in part 2), and nutritional medicine, as well as with Taoist breathing exercises, meditation, and shamanic techniques.

In the process of recovery, I became determined to find out more about such conditions, so as to help others with viral diseases. This lead me to intensive study and to interviewing immunologists and virologists, as well as naturopathic physicians and doctors of Oriental medicine who had experience in treating viral diseases. I subsequently published several academic papers on the integrated management of hepatitis C, and out of all this developed the practical ideas for this book.

In the twenty-first century the specter of a viral epidemic looms over us, and in many ways our fears are justified. A brief review of the history of infectious disease and modern viral illnesses will set the stage for this book.

I find it enlightening to listen to doctors and nurses of the older generations speak about their experiences prior to World War II. At that time, infectious diseases were still common in the United States, and doctors were trained in medical school to routinely recognize and rapidly diagnosis tuberculosis, smallpox, yellow fever, malaria, scarlet fever, diphtheria, typhoid fever, and even cholera.

In fact, serious infectious diseases were among the most common of problems for which a physician was tasked in those days of house calls. Children still died of diarrheal diseases. Syphilis was incurable before the advent of penicillin, and among the elderly, influenza was a dreaded and often deadly disease. Patients with tuberculosis were housed to overflowing in special sanatoriums because before antibiotics, there was no specific treatment for this disease other than bed rest, fresh air, fluids, time, and prayer.

We have come a long way since then—technologically speaking—but, ironically, the more we improve, the more vulnerable we become to other diseases, especially viruses.

When, then-U.S. Surgeon General William H. Stewart,[1] announced that the "war" on infectious disease was "won" in 1969, the medical profession and the general public applauded, genuinely believing that humans had indeed permanently triumphed over nature. Stewart's pronouncements promoted a sense of false security that created a policy de-emphasizing infectious disease as a major public health issue for two decades, and as a consequence people in America and the industrialized world quickly forgot that deadly infections ever existed.

How far from the truth they were was unimaginable until only very recently.

A little more then a decade later, "new" threats began emerging, one after the other: AIDS, caused by the human immunodeficiency virus; genital herpes, caused by a virus in the herpes family; hepatitis C and other viral diseases, including a new strain of influenza A; and deadly hemorrhagic fevers like Ebola and hantavirus.

Other nonviral infectious agents were not sitting around quietly either. The medical world was shocked at the re-emergence of a drug-resistant form of tuberculosis; cholera epidemics in Peru killed thousands; and deadly outbreaks of food-borne *Escherichia coli* were found in fast-food hamburgers. Lyme disease, a spirochete bacterial infection that is still baffling doctors, has become endemic in some parts of the United States, and antibiotic-resistant infections threaten hospitalized patients with flesh-eating bacteria. Anthrax, a deadly bacterial disease once rare in the United States, re-emerged in 2001 as a consequence of bioterrorism.

Many questions arise from these facts, which I address in the first part of this book. Are these "new" illnesses or are they diseases that have always existed and only now are manifesting through a natural evolutionary process of which we are unaware? One of the most important questions is this: are these new illnesses strictly medical issues solvable by stronger pharmaceutical drugs and better vaccines, or are they environmental, ecological, and largely social issues of public health?

We are inclined to think of modern medicine as one unified army of gallant and heroic medical doctors and nurses marching toward a clear and steady victory over the common enemy of disease. The reality of both war and medicine is strikingly different from this romantic scenario. War moves over a terrain of rugged hills and steep valleys, though bitter, icy winters and unbearably hot, sweltering summers, it's about getting stuck in the mud, getting lost and having to retrace your steps, being wounded and sometimes losing the battle—or your life.

Our social myth of ever-victorious and all-knowing modern medicine persisted well into the 1980s, even when the mystique was fading. A brief historical sketch will help to illustrate this.

By the 1950s and early 1960s, the age of optimism in medicine had peaked. Doctors were firmly entrenched in linear, cause-and-effect thinking, riding high on earlier successes that included the first use of penicillin and the development of other, even more powerful antibiotics, the use of cortisone to treat inflammatory diseases, drugs for psychiatric illnesses, open-heart surgery, and the beginning of the smallpox eradication program that began in 1953 and ended in 1977 with the last reported case in Somalia.

By the end of the 1960s, the progress of previous decades was reaching a climax even though the decline of modern medicine was beginning. In the 1970s, the age of the specialists came into being, and by the early 1980s medicine had turned into a highly sophisticated and extremely profitable enterprise. The light of medicine that shone so brightly early in the twentieth century was growing dim. The era of medicine as big business had begun.

Ironically, during the age of the specialists and at a time when the newly emerging infectious diseases were first starting to appear, the medical specialty of infectious disease was in decline. Viewed more as an academic pursuit or a matter that affected the Third World than as an important field for modern doctors—certainly not one in which glory and money could be had—very few medical students embarked upon a career in this field. Bacteriology was considered out of date, a subject in which all the major questions had already been addressed. Antibiotics killed bacteria; end of story.

The fate of a sub-specialty such as virology was even bleaker. As recently as the 1970s, the study of viruses mainly was confined to analyzing the clinical presentation of virally caused diseases and determining symptoms. Though at one time most cancers were thought to be caused by an unknown virus, not until the AIDS crisis gripped public attention was there much interest in viruses, and even then relatively few scientists became interested in viral biology until the late 1990s.

Despite such criticism, the progress made in medicine in the last hundred years has marked one of the most impressive epochs in the history of medicine. Yet paradoxically, as we come to the end of this period, it is also now almost universally accepted that medical technology is out of hand and dangerous, health care is too expensive, public health is at risk, and incidences of infectious diseases are *increasing* despite the use of antibiotics and vaccines. So we are at a crossroads in modern medicine, or perhaps it is better to describe it as a standoff with the victor yet to be decided.

In a medical system that viewed itself as infallible and all-powerful, there was no motive to use any but the tried and presumed true methods. However, with the advent of antibiotic-resistant strains of bacteria, vaccine-resistant viruses, drug-resistant parasitic diseases like malaria, and the increasing strength of viral illnesses, the conventional methods are being questioned and the accepted thinking challenged.

Antibiotic-resistant bacteria are so common that 10 percent of all patients hospitalized overnight, two million each year, acquire a nonviral, nosocomial (hospital-acquired) infection. In intensive care, the statistics are even higher: 50 percent of patients acquire a nosocomial infection. Drugs themselves are potentially dangerous, with an estimated 100,000 deaths in the United States alone due to medications. Vaccines, once believed to be the ultimate answer for the prevention and eradication of many common viral illnesses, have their own set of problems and have been known to cause cancer, neurological disease, and even death from contaminated supplies.

How did we end up in such a frightful situation?

In a medical system that viewed itself as infallible and all-powerful, there was no motive to use any but the tried and presumed true methods. Natural methods were ridiculed as old-fashioned and worthless. However, with the advent of antibiotic-resistant strains of bacteria, vaccine-resistant viruses, drug-resistant parasitic diseases like malaria, and the increasing strength of viral illnesses, the conventional methods are being questioned and the accepted thinking challenged.

A clear example of this outmoded thinking comes from the research and treatment of human immunodeficiency virus, the presumed cause of AIDS. Despite nearly twenty years of research and treatment, until the year 2000 the global AIDS epidemic had not made us more aware of viral diseases in all their varieties. It did not highlight the need for more effective and safer antiviral medications; nor did it stimulate more vigilance against the powerful, deadly, emerging viruses. Call it complacency, misguided use of research funds, or ignorance of deeper issues, the end results have been the same: the prospect for even good symptomatic treatment of viral diseases remains grim.

When the AIDS epidemic caught us by surprise in the late 1970s, the experts immediately followed the old model they had used for smallpox and polio: they focused on how the disease manifested in patients and began what has become an empty search for a vaccine. Dramatizing the issue, the uninformed and vicious among the medical establishment, along with conservative politicians, immediately called for more strident measures, a repetition of the combative old ways involving quarantine, high dosages of powerful toxic drugs, and blaming those who indulged in forbidden sexual practices, the blacks in Africa and Haiti, and intravenous drug users. It was a witch hunt. All of these measures and attitudes eventually proved ineffective and morally wrong.

Though researchers gathered vast amounts of information over the last two decades of the twentieth century on how AIDS manifests, they still debate its cause and they have still not provided a clue for a cure. Despite the enormous sums of money spent on AIDS research, we still have not found a vaccine that works for HIV infection, and have only partially effective drug treatments to manage viral activity, and these have a high side effect profile.

To make matters more complicated, when high dosages of the few antiviral drugs that we have are used on HIV patients, the virus mutates. The rapid turnover of HIV-1 generates extraordinary genetic diversity within the virus population, thereby rendering the drug ineffective.

Not to be outdone by AIDS, we were again caught by surprise when a previously unknown liver inflammation mysteriously appeared. At first labeled non-A, non-B type hepatitis, because neither known type of hepatitis was detectable in patients, hepatitis C virus originally appeared in individual patients in Japan in the 1970s and then was discovered in the blood supply in the United States in the late 1980s. A potentially fatal viral disease that has no effective treatment and no cure was lurking undetected in blood banks until it infected tens of thousands of victims who now have passed on the infection to thousands of others, many still not diagnosed.

In addition, ongoing outbreaks of fatal viruses such as Ebola in Africa in 1976, hantavirus in New Mexico in 1993, increasing fatalities caused by hemorrhagic dengue fever in Southeast Asia, and West Nile fever in New York in 1999, startled the medical profession and shocked the world.

Somehow we forgot that new viral strains surface *regularly* and that science and modern medicine are not infallible all of the time.

To make matters worse, evidence mounted and suggested that viruses were causing other diseases. At first thought to be the underlying cause of all cancers, certain viruses are now clearly linked with some types of cancer, as well as diabetes, heart disease, chronic fatigue, Alzheimer's, and certain forms of arthritis. Also, during the same time period when AIDS and hepatitis C were first discovered and initial research into them was instigated from the early 1980s to the mid-1990s, patients began complaining about conditions for which there were no medical diagnoses. Doctors were stumped and suggested to these patients that their condition did not exist, since there was no name for what they complained about, and routinely referred them for psychological therapy.

Needless to say, the profession of private practice clinical psychology boomed. Unfortunately, talk therapy did not work for the majority of these patients since they were not neurotic, but had legitimate physical conditions that defied conventional diagnoses but which did include as part of their symptom profiles mood changes and fatigue—symptoms commonly associated with depression, according to accepted medical standards.

Then a new phenomenon appeared on the medical front. With the advent of newer and safer antidepressants, doctors referred fewer patients to psychologists and began the wholesale prescribing of Prozac and other selective serotonin re-uptake inhibitors (SSRIs) under the false assumption that these patients were not merely neurotic, but clinically depressed—which of course the majority were not.[2]

These new illnesses included chronic fatigue, depression-like mood disorders, and unexplained, continuous muscle pain—all of which may be linked eventually to viral causes and immune system disruption. Over time, it became evident that neither psychotherapy nor psychoactive drugs were the answer for these patients, so doctors then mysteriously suggested that the cause of these new conditions could be a virus for which there was no treatment and therefore no culpability, which meant that there was nothing medicine could do.

In addition, increasing incidences of allergy-like symptoms and environmental sensitivity, menstrual complaints and menopausal symptoms, an increasing infertility rate among white women, and increasing adult onset diabetes, glucose intolerance, and obesity further confused a conventional medical profession that relied solely on a single cause-and-effect model.[3] Gulf War Syndrome added another dimension and was perhaps the first medical condition taken to the floor of Congress for discussion as to whether it *existed*.

Then, in one of the great medical paradoxes of the twentieth century, individual patients began a gradual and silent defection that often involved a heroic quest to search for alternative solutions to their infirmities. By the late 1980s, alternative medical therapies were well established, and by the 1990s, more than two-thirds of all Americans had used some form of alternative medicine.

However, alternative practitioners, those to whom the public turns when conventional medicine fails, were in an even worse state of affairs as far as viral disease was concerned than their conventional counterparts. Nearly no one in these fields had a specific interest in viral diseases, nor had anyone studied viral illnesses in any depth or detail. Likewise, there was no organized body of information available to those few who practiced in this area.

Though patients experienced a hit-or-miss approach with alternative practitioners, they often were provided some symptomatic relief from their complaints. Such results, though not completely curative, encouraged both patients and practitioners to continue therapy. Conventional doctors were put on notice.

Thankfully, things are now starting to change on both fronts. Conventional medical practitioners recognize the benefits of alternative therapies and research is mounting on effective natural antiviral therapies.

At the beginning of the twenty-first century, humanity seems caught between its own creative destructiveness on the one hand, and nature's deadly equalizers on the other, and the possibilities of nuclear destruction, unbridled pollution, and the greenhouse effect may soon be outweighed by infectious illnesses—especially by emerging viral diseases. Could it also be that these newly emerged viral diseases are not only a serious health threat to individual humans but also a harbinger of new disease patterns in a world out of balance?

This bigger picture has been largely ignored except by a few of the more enlightened researchers and alternative medicine practitioners who have dared to suggest that the new viruses might be the result of trans-species migration, microbial mutations, immune suppression, chemical toxic overload, and environmental destruction (especially in the tropical rain forests). All these concepts contradict current medical thinking and political interests. Robin Hening, the author of *A Dancing Matrix* says, "The intrusion of humankind into the natural order of things seems to be the single most important factor in the emergence of new viruses" (Henning 1994).

The good news is that though a lot of mistakes have been made, we are continuously improving our knowledge in an attempt to understand our world and the many diseases we must deal with, and we actively keep searching for alternative ways to improve our health.

While those in conventional medicine were ignoring the epidemic rise of emerging infectious disease and novel chronic illnesses, others were investigating evolutionary links to disease. Referred to as the new science of evolutionary, or Darwinian, medicine, with theories highly compatible with natural and functional medicine, this system presents a complete way of viewing disease where *patterns* have as much validity as cause and effect. In addition, research in nutrition, herbal medicines, and nutraceuticals—natural, standardized, nonprescription medications—has led to outstanding clinical results and numerous products that have great potential in treating the new diseases, many of which are discussed in part 2.

Though one must be wary of solutions that seem too easy, could it be that there are straightforward answers to the many complex questions that arise when we consider the importance of these new diseases in human suffering, lost productivity, and reduced quality of life?

A very real threat from emerging viruses does exist and must be taken with the utmost seriousness. The issue is of such gravity that alternative practitioners and natural healthcare consumers must not fall into the same trap as did conventional medicine, which was to become smug in its accomplishments. The possibility that the world could be thrown into a crisis of unprecedented proportions is real. The convergence of increasing immune compromise, an increasing population of older people with chronic disease, increasing antibiotic and antiviral resistance, burgeoning third world population with endemic infectious disease, and increasing environmental population and rain forest devastation—it all takes the "ground zero" scenario and the theorized coming biological apocalypse from the realm of fiction to that of possibility.

The main question is not if we will have a viral epidemic, but what direction is the current epidemic of microbial illnesses taking? In answering this, keep the broader view in mind, and realize that the scenario of epidemic chronic and acute infectious diseases, many of which are virally induced, is already upon us. Though no one can predict the future with absolute certainty, there are three possible scenarios.

The first is of an increasing incidence of acute plagues, either drug-resistant old ones, newly emerged ones, or a combination of both.

The second is the increasing incidence of endemic chronic infections. Of these two, the most likely scenario for the wealthy countries is that of endemic chronic illness combined with immune suppression, rather than the wide-sweeping plagues of past centuries.

This, however, is not the case for the over-crowded, poorer countries in the southern hemisphere. They will likely continue to suffer from acute infections as well as the effects of environmental degradation on their homelands by their wealthy neighbors to the north. Malnutrition, the result of widening and deepening poverty in these countries, causes immune weakness and dramatically increases susceptibility to infection, setting up a vicious cycle that makes an efficient breeding ground for all forms of microbial infectious organisms, including viruses.

The third scenario is viral bioterrorism—unleashing a virus, like smallpox, for which we no longer have immunity, a limited supply of vaccine, and no effective drug with which to treat it.

From a global perspective, the most likely scenario is a combination of all three: an increasing incidence of chronic degenerative disease and infectious epidemics combined with the sporadic release of infectious microbes by agents of international terrorism. Currently this is already happening in the world's large cities, in rich and poor countries alike, where a combination of rich and poor commingle, where stress and environmental pollution are highest, and where poor

A very real threat from emerging viruses does exist and must be taken with the utmost seriousness. The possibility that the world could be thrown into a crisis of unprecedented proportions is real. The main question is not if we will have a viral epidemic, but what direction is the current epidemic of microbial illnesses taking?

and nutritionally impaired immigrants harboring viral illnesses arrive daily from China, Mexico, South America, Africa, and the Caribbean.

One question remains: will viruses finally wipe out human life on this planet?

In the early years of the AIDS epidemic, the media capitalized on sensational projections indicating that if unstopped, AIDS would eventually infect every person alive within one lifetime. It did not happen and will not happen, but how the bigger scenario of viruses and humans will play out is still anyone's guess. I am not betting on the germs, but neither am I waiting for science to catch up to the bugs and deliver a safe and effective cure.

In writing this book, my agenda has been straightforward and clear: to help people understand the seriousness of viral illnesses and to place at their disposal (and their doctor's) evidence-based tools for prevention and safe treatment. These methods are not infallible, but there are currently no specific or reasonably safe and effective antiviral drugs, so the medical situation is obvious. We have no choice but to use natural alternatives in the interim while the research continues. Perhaps in the process we may find them to be the best primary choice after all.

Acknowledgments

A book with the scope of this one is never the work of one person. First, clinical and laboratory researchers, as well as other authors whose work and ideas support the principles of this book, are acknowledged in the notes and listed in the bibliography. Second, I thank my editor, Richard Leviton, a medical writer himself, for his confidence, encouragement, support, and for helping me craft this work into a polished book.

Then, there are those whose energies as mentors, friends, and supportive family members lent help in a multitude of nontechnical ways: foremost among them is my companion over the years that this book was in progress, the Mexican painter, Norma Michel, for her infinite patience and depth of understanding of the creative process; and Bill Galt and Gail Weaver of *LifeTime Health and Nutrition, Inc.* My special thanks goes to Don Bodenbach, the host of the radio program *The Nature of Health*, who supported the idea of this book from its inception and encouraged my clinical work for a number of years.

Several writers gave unselfishly from their experiences, and without them the writing process would have remained a hidden mystery to me. I would especially like to thank the author Gerald Hausman for his many years of mentorship and for the quality of his friendship. Other writers who have encouraged and offered me their support and help along the way include the Ayurvedic physician Robert Svoboda;

Judy Goldstein, M.D.; Michael Murray, N.D.; Arnie Lade, L.Ac.; Ralph Alan Dale, Ph.D.; and Cory J. Meachum.

A number of doctors and scientists took time from their busy schedules to review parts of the manuscript or provide inspiration along the way. Among these are James Murphy, D.O.; William Pollack, M.D., Ph.D.; Thierry Hertoghe, M.D.; Brett Jacques, N.D.; and Robert Bradford, D.Sc.

I would never have gained the experience and knowledge to write this book without having learned from my patients and from the work of those pioneers in the fields of natural and integrated medicine who have been my teachers, guides, instructors, and betters. I thank you all.

Introduction

What Viral Immunity Is, How You Can Achieve It, and Why It's So Important

Viral immunity is the ability of the immune system to prevent, defend against, neutralize, and eliminate viruses from the body. You can achieve it by following the 10-step viral immunity plan outlined in this book.

The 10 steps to viral immunity are:

- Build a strong immune foundation with lifestyle, diet, and nutritional supplements.

- Defend your immune system with antioxidants and oxidative therapies.

- Rejuvenate your immune system with phytonutrient-rich foods and enzymes.

- Renew your cells and cleanse your liver and lymphatic system through detoxification.

- Restore the innate immune response and manage inflammation.

- Boost your immunity with natural immune enhancers.

- Target viruses with natural antiviral alternatives.

- Empower your viral immunity program with Chinese medicine.

- Optimize immune performance with hormonal balance.

- Implement the viral immunity program.

Viral immunity is without question one of the most important health issues of this century. The erosion and impending failure of our natural immunity due to ecological alterations of the environment and the consequences of viral infection will affect nearly everyone. Immune system failure also plays a leading role in all major modern diseases including cancer, heart disease, diabetes, rheumatoid arthritis, multiple sclerosis, thyroid conditions, fungal infections, chronic bacterial infections, and chronic fatigue syndrome. Most of these conditions are also triggered by viruses.

What You Will Learn in this Book

The message of this book is clear. You can improve your immune system in general with diet, lifestyle, and natural medicines. We need viral immunity in particular because of the dramatically increasing incidence of powerful new viral infections such as human herpes virus-6, human immunodeficiency viruses, hepatitis C, dengue hemorrhagic fever, West Nile virus, new and stronger strains of influenza, the newly discovered TT virus,[1] and the possibility of the epidemics of rare viruses or re-emergence of those once thought eliminated, through acts of bioterroism.

There are 170 million cases of hepatitis C and 350 million cases of hepatitis B worldwide. More than 50 million people are infected with the AIDS virus, most in sub-Saharan Africa where one in five have AIDS. In comparison, the virus that causes dengue fever infects more than fifty million people annually, and in the United States alone 25 percent of the population will suffer from influenza-associated illnesses, which cause more than 20,000 deaths each year.

Drugs do not improve our immune systems. In fact, they often disrupt their normal functioning, and they are not the way to viral immunity. Though antiviral drugs help reduce symptoms early on in their use, eventually they cause drug resistance in the viruses. According to Sally Blower, Ph.D., an evolutionary biologist, renowned biomathematician, and professor at the University of California, Los Angeles, HIV resistance to antiviral drugs will increase from 3 percent in 1997 to 42 percent by the year 2005.

Alternative solutions for the treatment of viral illnesses are available, and we can take preventive steps today by following the health-promoting and immune-enhancing measures presented in steps 1 through 4. If you already have a condition caused by a virus, you may use the specialized natural antiviral and immune-enhancing medications described in this book to strengthen your immune system.

In this book you will learn about viruses, the basic principles of immunology, and the reasons why our immune systems are breaking down. You will also learn how to prevent infection, strengthen your immune system, and manage chronic viral illness with the most effective natural medicines available. The information contained in this book is useful for all types of people, for the caregivers of viral infection victims, and for health care workers.

Some of the viruses discussed include:

- Human immunodeficiency virus (HIV)

- Hepatitis B (HBV)

- Hepatitis C (HCV)

- Influenza

- Viruses that cause the common cold

- Dengue

- Herpes viruses, including human herpes virus-6 (HHV-6)

In *Viral Immunity* you will find natural ways of improving immune function, remedies to treat viral infections, and suggestions on how to reframe outdated concepts that could otherwise prevent you from obtaining effective treatment. The book discusses alternative therapies and looks at the new evolutionary model of medicine as well as the view of Chinese medicine on viral illnesses. I discuss pathology as well as a more holistic and integrated view of how lifestyle, habitual thought patterns, spiritual beliefs (or lack of them), and the environment in which we live all contribute to our health, well being, and the integrity of our immune systems.

Along the way in *Viral Immunity,* you will learn why these statements are true:

- The experts are not completely in agreement about the most important health concerns of the twenty-first century. They disagree about the underlying cause of AIDS, and while doing this, HCV will kill more people in the United States than HIV.

- Though chronic fatigue syndrome may not be due directly to a specific virus, this devastating illness is certainly related to immune dysfunction and is similar in many ways to AIDS and other chronic viral diseases.

- Due to environmental toxins, stress, and modern lifestyle, our immune systems are becoming dysfunctional.

- Fatigue is replacing fever and inflammation as the first line of immune defense.

- In terms of health, the global environment is much more important than we ever imagined. Unfortunately, we may have realized this too late.

- Contrary to popular fear-based fiction, viruses will not destroy the human race. However, epidemic diseases for which there are no cures will destabilize national economies and even whole continents; this has already begun in Africa and threatens to spread to India, China, Southeast Asia, and the Caribbean.

- "Stealth" and chronic viral diseases coupled with immune dysfunction will cost the wealthy countries tens of billions of dollars in ineffective medical care and will rob many people of their energy and health.

- Neurological diseases, like multiple sclerosis and Alzheimer's, as well as most forms of cancer, are increasing, and many may have causes associated with immune system dysfunction and viruses.

- Conventional medicine's "magic bullet" model of one cause, one cure is not working for the new illnesses of chronic fatigue, immune dysfunction, and viral diseases.

- Hope for a vaccine for HIV is receding into the distance, while expensive antiviral drug therapy is causing devastating side effects and the rapid emergence of drug-resistant strains.

The Viral Immunity Program

The 10-step program outlined in *Viral Immunity* is a comprehensive method that helps build a strong immune system, and it is a guide for preventing and treating viral diseases with natural medicines. It is unique to this book and is based on a multidisciplinary approach to mind-body healing that I have developed and used successfully with patients in my own practice for nearly twenty years. The natural medications and lifestyle approaches discussed in the book are supported by scientific research and extensive clinical evidence, and prove that natural medicines can and will play an increasing role in the treatment of viral illnesses.

As conventional medicine falters, is dragged down by over-reliance on antibiotics and other powerful drugs that cause microbial-resistant strains, and becomes preoccupied with the spiraling cost of hospitalization and medical care, the key to successfully building viral immunity is an educated public actively involved in preventing disease and managing their own health in ways such as the 10 steps to viral immunity presented in this book.

The 10-step program outlined in Viral Immunity *is a comprehensive method that helps build a strong immune system, and it is a guide for preventing and treating viral diseases with natural medicines. It is unique to this book and is based on a multidisciplinary approach to mind-body healing that I have developed and used successfully with patients in my own practice for nearly twenty years.*

Viral Immunity is divided into two parts. Part 1 discusses how we become ill and how we heal. It describes how the immune system functions and it introduces some of the viral agents that make us sick. I explain how a toxic environment and continuing stress contribute to the downward spiral of our immune deficiency. Part 2 presents a detailed step-by-step program to fortify your immune system and to assist it in fighting off viral infections. Following is a brief description of the 10 steps:

- In the first step you will learn the elements of an immune-enhancing lifestyle including dietary suggestions that build the foundation for deeper healing, ways to reduce and manage stress, and discussion of the best dietary supplements.

- In the second step you will learn the critical role of oxygen in viral immunity, and how to use immune-strengthening antioxidants like vitamin C, zinc, selenium, and the amino acid arginine. It describes in detail the evidence for their use and which dosages work best. As in all the steps, safety issues and contraindications are explained. You will also learn about medical bio-oxidation therapies like ozone, and when and how to use them to treat viral infections.

- Enzymes and phytonutrient-rich foods enhance the diet, improve digestion, add specialized nutrients like carotenoids and other antioxidants, improve natural detoxification, and reduce inflammation. The third step tells you which phytonutrient-rich foods are the best for viral immunity and how to use enzymes to improve your health.

- Detoxification regimes and cleansing strategies are essential and important to prevent disease and improve immune function. The fourth step emphasizes the important role of natural medications in cleansing the lymphatic system and the liver—both systems are critical for viral immunity. You will learn how to safely conduct your own viral immunity detoxification program and which natural medications and nutrients promote tissue and cellular cleansing.

- Natural anti-inflammatory agents are important in building viral immunity, as is managing autoimmune-induced tissue inflammation in chronic viral diseases. In the fifth step, you will learn how to use natural anti-inflammatory medicines like curcumin extract and quercetin to reduce tissue damage caused by inflammation occurring in your tissues and organs.

- The sixth step explains how to use immune-modulating substances to boost your immunity. These products are considerably more powerful than herbs and vitamins, and include beta glucan, transfer factor, and lactoferrin. Dosages are provided for each medication as well as contraindications for their use.

- Natural antiviral medicines are critical for successfully treating viral illness. In the seventh step, you will learn how to use nature's most effective antivirals such as olive leaf extract and echinacea. Dosages and directions on how to use them safely and effectively are presented in detail.

- Using Chinese herbal remedies can considerably increase the effectiveness of your program. No other culture provides such a rich source of knowledge about viral infections and the methods and medicines that treat them than the Chinese. In step 8, you will learn how to use powerful and effective Chinese antivirals like isatis, immune modulators including the ganoderma mushroom, energy enhancers like ginseng, and anti-inflammatory medicines like bupleurum.

- Hormones play an integral role in maintaining a strong immune system. Step 9 shows you how to use natural hormonal therapies including DHEA, thymic hormones, human growth hormone, and thyroid hormone to increase your health, energy, mood, and to enhance your immunity.

- In the last step, you will learn how to design your own viral immunity program and how to work with natural medicines. In this step, you will also learn how to pick the right doctor and understand which laboratory tests are most useful for viral immunity. Safe and effective treatments for selected viruses such as for the common cold, influenza, and hepatitis C are presented.

Additional Material to Help You Achieve Viral Immunity

In the appendices you will find a comprehensive list of resources, including recommended laboratories and doctors to facilitate your viral immunity goals. Notes are provided at the end of the book for each section for those wishing more explanations on certain technical points. There is a glossary of terms, and an extensive bibliography is provided as documentation for the material presented in the book.

Viruses, Immunity, and Evolution

1

The Virus at Our Doorstep

Viruses recognize no international borders or time zones. They have no obligations to country, race, social status, or gender. Rich and poor alike are victims of viral infections. If given the opportunity, viruses do not stay in any one place and may travel over extraordinarily long distances. In 1983, the Asian tiger mosquito, *Ades albopictus,* a relative of *A. aegypti,* the mosquito that transmits dengue fever virus, was found in the United States for the first time. The mosquito larvae, stowaways in accumulated rainwater inside automobile tires, were transported on a cargo ship from Southeast Asia.

In our modern world, viruses and other infectious microbes can easily hitch rides on international flights to and from any major city. A European tourist visiting Thailand can bring home a strain of immunodeficiency virus from a sexual encounter in Bangkok; a Cantonese grandmother visiting her family in San Francisco can harbor a potent influenza virus in her lungs and carry it all the way from China and pass it to her grandchildren who transmit it to other children in preschool.

Viruses do not leave fossil remains or other archeological clues. They leave only what we have found, for example, in frozen tissue samples of their victims, such as from the remains of Eskimos in the

Arctic tundra, or victims of the influenza epidemic of 1918. Though there are a variety of theories, there is no way of completely knowing the origin, natural history, or evolution of viruses. Yet what we do know is fascinating.

For one, we know that viruses have been with us a long time. Archeological evidence indicates that smallpox developed along with civilization in the river basin agricultural settlements of Asia and the Middle East as early as 10,000 years ago. We also know that viral epidemic diseases were unheard of in the New World before the arrival of the Spanish. Viruses are not only the cause of many infectious diseases, ranging from the common cold to slow death of AIDS and the frightening hemorrhagic fevers, but they have dramatically influenced history as well.

Why Have Viral Infections Become So Devastating in Recent Years?

As agents of change, they have toppled dynasties, changed the outcomes of wars, and altered populations. In the twentieth century, smallpox alone killed an estimated 300 million people. In the sixteenth and seventeenth centuries, smallpox killed the emperors of Japan and Burma, as well as kings and queens of Europe. Queen Mary of England died of smallpox in 1694; Louis XV of France, Joseph I of Germany, and Peter II of Russia also died from the same disease.

The Aztec emperor and many in his immediate household were killed by smallpox. It is a matter of historical record that the successful conquest of the Aztec empire in Mexico by Hernando Cortez and the Incan empire by Francisco Pizarro in Peru were ultimately achieved more by the enormous deaths from fatal epidemics of smallpox and measles than by superior military strategy or overwhelming firepower.

The 1918–19 epidemic of Spanish influenza killed 20–40 million people in less than a year, causing more deaths than all the massive military casualties of World War I. In the spring of 1918, the German Army's assault on Paris was halted by this flu. It not only affected Europeans, but an unbelievable 80 percent of the United States Army's death toll was from the Spanish flu that killed 43,000 American soldiers between 1917 and 1919—nearly as many as died in combat in the Korean War some thirty years later.

Viruses not only infect humans but all living things including plants, animals, birds, and sea creatures. In 1988, seal plague virus killed 2,800 seals in the United Kingdom; a similar disease had already devastated the rare freshwater seals of Lake Baikal in Siberia in 1987. Canine distemper and other common animal viruses kill our pets as well as livestock. Rinderpest, or cattle plague, killed an estimated 2 million cattle annually in South Africa during the 1920s. The virus responsible was introduced into South Africa in 1889, and within the first ten years there it spread northward, killing an estimated 90 percent of the wild buffalo population in Kenya.

Viruses are everywhere, and due to their microscopic size they also infect the invisible world, including bacteria, fungi, and protozoa. If viruses are ubiquitous in nature and have intimately accompanied us in the human evolutionary journey, why have viral infections become so devastating in *recent years*?

This question is as yet unanswered even by the experts. My hypothesis, which I develop throughout this book, is that it is because of widespread immunological breakdown caused by the stress of modern living, environmental destruction, and toxic chemical pollution—nature out of balance. The experts are starting to catch up with this possibility.

What Is a Virus?

The most frequently quoted popular definition of a virus belongs to Sir Peter Medawar (1983): "A virus is a piece of bad news wrapped up in protein." However succinct and graphic this definition is, it does not describe a virus in sufficient detail, nor does it answer any of the evolutionary and ecological questions concerning the nature of viruses. The word "virus," coming from the Latin meaning "poisonous fluid," also does not reveal what a virus is. Here are three things that a virus is: small, parasitic, and genetically lean.

Viruses Are Very Small: Viruses are referred to as subcellular organisms, meaning they are smaller than cells, smaller than bacteria, and certainly smaller than most human host cells. Bacteria are measured in micrometers (10^{-6} meters) and viruses in nanometers (10^{-9}), which is a thousand times smaller. Viruses are so minute they can maintain their ability to infect even after passing through filters small enough to strain out all bacteria. In fact, they are so small that they can only be seen by the most powerful of electron microscopes.

Viruses were long thought of as the smallest infectious agent, yet we now know of two other pathogens that are even smaller: prions, the suspected cause of Mad Cow Disease, discovered only recently by the 1997 Nobel Laureate in medicine, Stanely Prusiner; and viroids, organisms that only affect plants.

Viruses Are Parasites: Viruses are intracellular molecular parasites. They enter the body silently, and in the case of HIV and hepatitis C viruses, they often do so without notice. Then they use our cells to manufacture substances needed for their own replication and life cycle. They have no metabolic life of their own outside a host cell, which makes them dependent on living cells for their existence. Viruses have a receptor binding protein that allows them to attach to other cells and convert them into virus-producing mini-factories. They do not make their own energy or proteins for survival and cannot reproduce without the assistance of cellular material from other living cells. Viruses grow and multiply only within other living cells—human, animal, plant, bacteria. Outside the host cell, a virus is not alive and exists in a world between the living and nonliving.

Viruses Are Genetically Lean: The basic viral particle or single virus is called a virion. It consists of a nucleic acid genome, in which the virus's hereditary information is stored, surrounded by a shell of protein. Unlike most living cells, viruses do not have cell walls composed of a plasma membrane. Instead, a protein coat called a capsid, which may also contain lipids and sugars, protects the viral genome.

All living cells contain both known types of genetic material, RNA and DNA, but viruses possess only one type, either RNA or DNA. They also have a very small number of genes compared to other cells. For comparison: the human immunodeficiency virus (HIV) has fewer than ten genes; a larger virus like smallpox contains between 200 and 400 genes, but even the smallest bacteria contains 5,000 to 10,000 genes, and a human cell has 80,000 to 100,000 genes (see figure 1-1).

While at first it seems like a reproductive disadvantage compared to other life forms, minuteness and limited genetic material become an advantage for the virus. These characteristics make it easier for a virus to jump from one host to another, and at times from one species to another, rearranging and reengineering the host's genetic material to suit its needs. Dorothy Crawford, Ph.D., in *The Invisible Energy* (2000) describes viruses as "rogue pieces of genetic material," as if they were accidents waiting to happen.

Nothing could be further from the truth. Viruses exhibit a remarkable intelligence and a superb ability to survive and adapt to new environments, but Western science has only recently focused its attention on the viral world.

Advances in microbiology and bacteriology were at least a century ahead of those in virology, which is a relatively new science with its beginnings only in the twentieth century. Though there were many microbe hunters in the early 1800s, the first virus discovered is credited to the Russian scientist, Dimitri Ivanowsky. In 1892, while studying tobacco mosaic disease, he found that the agent that caused the disease was small enough to pass through a filter known to trap all bacteria.

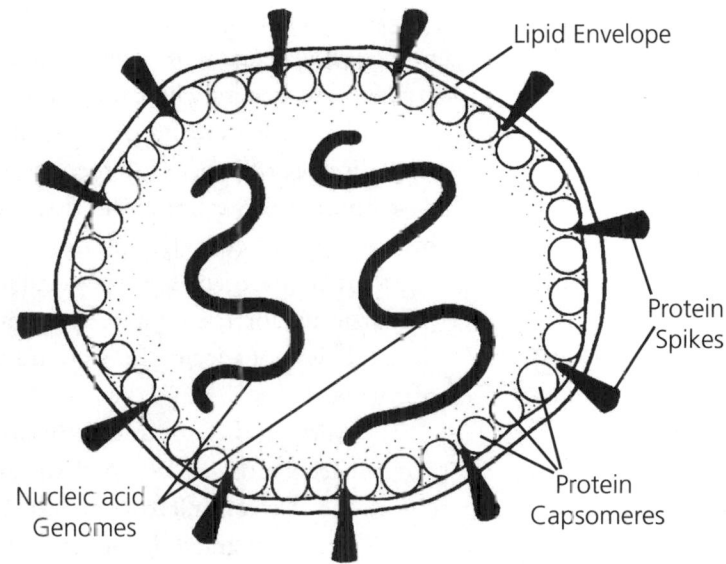

Figure 1-1: Representation of a Basic Viral Unit

The virion is a subcellular particle with a shell or envelope of protein and lipids called a capsid. The capsid may contain protein spikes or round capsomeres that serve to help penetration of a host cell. Inside the shell is the functional portion containing the virus's genetic material, referred to as the nucleic acid genome, which directs the activity and function of the virus.

Yellow fever was the first human virus identified. One of the most devastating plagues of past centuries, and a re-emerging infectious disease of the twenty-first century, yellow fever has been responsible for tens of millions of deaths. Although Carlos Juan Finlay, a Cuban physician practicing in Havana in 1880, proposed that yellow fever, then epidemic in Cuba, was a mosquito-borne infection, it was not until 1901 that Walter Reed, a physician and colonel in the United States Army, identified the causative source as a virus. Once mosquitoes were identified as the disease vector (the method of how the virus is carried from human to human), the introduction of aggressive mosquito control dramatically reduced the incidence of yellow fever within a few years.

Antibiotic drugs were developed far in advance of drugs to treat viruses. Penicillin, the first antibiotic, was discovered in 1928 by

Alexander Fleming and introduced for clinical use in 1941. However, no antiviral drugs were developed until the late 1950s and were not available for general clinical use until two decades later.

Since there were no drugs until recently that treated infectious viral disease, the focus of medical research for viruses was on the development of vaccines. The first vaccine developed in the West was by Edward Jenner in 1796[1] against smallpox. Though controversy and different opinions plague it, vaccination continues to be one of the cornerstones for the treatment of viruses in modern medicine. (The use and risks of vaccinations are discussed in appendix D at the end of this book.)

However, it was not until 1930 that the first virus was actually *seen*. The tobacco mosaic virus had the honors here (as pictured on the cover); the electron microscope brought the vague viral symmetry into view. Detailed characterization of viruses only began in the later part of the twentieth century with the advent of better techniques for studying viruses, including more advanced electron microscopy, cell culture, high-speed centrifugation, electrophoresis of RNA and DNA genomes, and nucleotide sequencing.

The Evolutionary Perspective— Long-Term Coexistence?

Before discussing viruses and the diseases they cause, let's establish a point of view that suggests a relationship between the co-evolution of viruses and other species. The conventional, current model looks at a virus as a unique entity separate from the host, with a linear relationship between them: the virus infects the host, the host gets sick and develops symptoms; gets well, dies, or carries the virus which eventually infects others to continue its life cycle. This linear model is useful in analyzing basic viral characteristics and in quickly assessing and treating symptoms. However, it does not penetrate deep enough into the viral world and is not solving the problem of the current viral disease paradigm.

The evolutionary model questions this hypothesis and suggests that it may be more of a two-way street with virus and host *exchanging* genetic material. This idea presents more of an interdependent picture than is currently postulated, and allows for an understanding of how humans and viruses *coexist* and have done so for hundreds of thousands of years.

Though simple compared to the complexity of a human being, viruses are elegantly constructed organisms exhibiting remarkable bioarchitecture, beautiful design, and precision functioning. They play a significant role in the life cycles of all living organisms and are rightfully imbedded in the ecological infrastructure. From this evolutionary and ecological point of view, viruses have a place in assisting human evolution by assuring the survival of the species through natural selection. By exchanging genetic material from host to host, they influence the heredity of cells. As evolutionary messengers, viruses have effectively colonized nearly every living thing on this planet, from bacteria to humans. That is why viral disease will remain among us and why it can never eliminate the human race: we depend on each other.

The evolutionary model presents more of an interdependent picture than is currently postulated, and allows for an understanding of how humans and viruses coexist and have done so for hundreds of thousands of years.

There is an ancient Chinese saying, "Pure water has no fish" (Zhang 2000). For some things to live, other things must die, and nothing lives in a completely purified environment. Ultimately it may be a great mistake of modern medicine to attempt to sterilize the planet of viruses.

Interdependence among all living things is a rule of nature. We live in a biological world populated by billions of microscopic organisms that are friendly, neutral, and lethal. Biological life is a continuum, and there is less separation between independent organisms than previously thought. In fact, there may be no separation at all; viruses are not "us," yet their DNA has been worked into our genes, and therefore is a part of what we are as biological beings.

Four Thousand Types of Viruses— Welcome to the Viral Realm

There are 4,000 known types of viruses, but less than 4 percent are well characterized, and new viruses are discovered regularly. Indeed, at least fifty have been identified since 1988. Classification of viruses is based on several criteria, mainly by the type of nucleic acid (DNA or RNA) and by whether the genome contains a single strand (ss) or double strand (ds) of genetic material.

For example, smallpox is a dsDNA virus and HIV has an ssRNA genome. Among the DNA type are viruses that cause hepatitis B infections, herpes simplex blisters, and warts. In the RNA family, there are viruses that cause yellow fever, measles, polio, bronchitis, AIDS, and hepatitis C (see table 1).

Besides being based on the type of genetic material, classification of viruses is also made on structural characteristics that include: size (ranging from 20 to 450 nanometers in diameter); symmetry (helical, icosahedral, or complex); and presence of an envelope membrane.

Classification of Viruses: Viruses are classified into seventy-one families (distinct groups) with names ending in "-viridae," and 164 genera (subgroups that share similar characteristics) with endings of "virus." Further classification into individual species is not used for viruses.[2]

The specific identification of virally produced illnesses is based on clinical or immunological means, such as the symptoms and clinical signs presented by the patient. For example, in measles, the patient develops Koplik spots, small spots that resemble white grains of sand

Table 1: Important Viruses and Associated Diseases

Family Name	Representative Viruses	Example of Human Disease
DNA VIRUSES (DS)		
Adenoviridae	Adenoviruses	Common cold
Hepadnaviridae	Hepatitis virus	Hepatitis B
Herpesviridae	Herpes simplex virus	Herpes, chickenpox, shingles
Papovaviridae	Papillomavirus	Warts
Poxviridae	Vaccinia virus, Variola virus	Smallpox
RNA viruses (ss)		
Coronaviridae	Infectious bronchitis viruses	Bronchitis, common cold
Flaviviridae	Yellow fever virus, Hepatitis C virus	Yellow fever, Hepatitis C
Orthomyxoviridae	Influenza viruses	Flu
Paramyxoviridae	Measles virus	Measles, mumps
Picornaviridae	Poliovirus, Rhinovirus	Polio, common cold
Togaviridae	Rubella virus, Alphavirus	German measles, encephalitis

on the inside of the mouth opposite the first and second upper molar teeth. They also develop the characteristic measles rash that starts on the neck and spreads to the trunk, arms, and legs. For hepatitis C virus, diagnosis is made by a positive test for antibodies to the virus and for an elevated alanine aminotransferase (ALT level, which is a test for liver function.

Naming new viruses is an interesting exercise. Some are named after the type of disease they cause, such as poxviruses (i.e., smallpox). Others are named for the location where they were first isolated, such as the Spanish flu from Spain, or the Marburg virus from a town in Germany. Others are given numerical designations like HHV-4 for Epstein-Barr virus, which, as it was originally named after its discoverers, has two names. Some viruses are named after their structure or morphological features, such as corona viruses for the halo of spikes projecting from the virion.

Viral Carriers and Natural Hosts: To understand how viruses cause disease, it is important to discuss a few additional concepts and define some commonly used terms. Although the specific origin of viruses is unknown, it is accepted that they usually descend from a parent source that already exists in nature and then spread from animal to animal and then from animals to humans. The infected animal or person is referred to as the host

Since viral infections are often transmitted by an intermediary, such as a mosquito or tick bite, the mode of disease transmission is referred to as a vector. Viruses can inhabit as well as infect virtually any living organism, so relationships often develop between the virus and living host allowing both to coexist. The host acts as a carrier, such as occurs with herpes or hepatitis viruses, assuring the survival of the virus by spreading it from one person to another.

Viruses have a high mutation rate and produce great diversity among the different possible types or subtypes. This adaptive characteristic not only assures survival for viruses but also makes it easier for them to avoid a potential host's defenses. It also makes them a difficult foe to treat successfully. Viruses mutate readily when exposed to antiviral drugs; however, they have a difficult time adapting to the broad *spectrum* of active components in botanical medicines. This is one of the reasons why herbal antivirals are effective in treating viral illnesses and why working with natural processes works better than artificial chemical drugs.

Still, the role that viral mutation plays in disease is poorly understood. However, evolution occurs in three forms, independently or in combination, creating new or emerging viruses: (1) they evolve as a newly appearing variant; (2) they are introduced from another species; and (3) they disseminate from a smaller population and spread into a larger population, changing form as they do so. Mutation, as a form of rapid environmental adaptation, benefits the evolutionary needs of the virus but makes it difficult to understand and treat effectively. That is why it is important to work with the natural processes of your body by enhancing health and immunity.

Although the individual person is understandably concerned only with his own ailment, what many people are unaware of is that even the most common of viral diseases originate in animal hosts. For example, though influenza virus causes common respiratory infections worldwide, most strains of it originate in China where the natural hosts are livestock, especially pigs, chickens, and ducks. Other animal hosts that carry viruses infecting humans are migratory waterfowl, birds, rodents, and monkeys.

Humans can also carry viral disease, and certain human groups are more likely to carry viruses than others. Interestingly, children are the most common hosts and carriers for many viruses such as the common cold and measles. Due to their high exposure to sickness, healthcare workers are also frequent carriers for viruses. The most seriously affected, and the groups in which the most mortality are seen are the very young and the very old; this is why public health measures concentrate on vaccinations for children and flu shots for seniors. Since healthcare workers like doctors and nurses are particularly at risk due to their daily exposure to sick people, they are also encouraged to be vaccinated against influenza virus.

Viruses have a unique way of promoting their own life cycle. First they infect the host, often causing sickness in the process, and then they pass out of the host, usually in body fluids. For example, rotaviruses that cause traveler's diarrhea (or more serious and even lethal illnesses) pass from the body of the host in the feces. In every gram of infected feces reside about one billion rotaviruses. If sanitation measures are not in place, these active viruses readily enter the water or food supply to infect many others. People spread influenza by coughing and sneezing virus-laden particles of saliva and mucus into the air, which are then inhaled by every person in the vicinity.

How Viruses Enter the Body: There are three locations where viruses typically enter the human body: the respiratory tract (nose, throat, and lungs); the gastrointestinal tract (mouth, stomach, and intestines); and the genitourinary tract (the sex organs and urinary area). Viruses gain entry into the body via the respiratory tract by inhaled air that people sick with a virus have coughed or sneezed into, such as with the flu; or via the gastrointestinal tract through contaminated food, as in hepatitis A. Sexual intercourse can also cause the passing of viruses, as with HIV and herpes through the genitourinary tract.

Though these three routes are the main ways viruses enter the body, the skin is another way in which viruses can infect us (such as through warts), by kissing (mononucleosis), or hand contact. From a simple handshake, one can rub a virus into one's eyes or nose or mouth. One of my acupuncture colleagues developed a serious herpes infection in his eye after inadvertently rubbing an itch in his eye immediately after treating a patient for herpes simplex virus.

Perhaps appropriately, in Asia, hand-shaking is not the custom as it is in the West, and intimate touching of people in public is discouraged—perhaps for good health reasons. A polite or formal bow is preferred. If one has had the experience of traveling in Asia, the dense congestion of people and tightly packed crowds can be overwhelming. It is no wonder that such a custom developed: it is a practical way of reducing the passing of germs. Perhaps in our modern, population-dense world with our ever-increasing viral concerns, some thought should be given to alternative public ways of showing affection.

Viruses also have been quick to exploit modern medical practices. The normal portals of entry now include direct blood-to-blood transmission, such as found in blood transfusions. Though unintentionally, blood transfusions greatly contributed to the spread of HIV and hepatitis B and C. Shared hypodermic needle use in the case of hepatitis C also caused widespread viral transmission among drug users. When viruses are introduced directly into the blood stream, they bypass natural immune defenses (the respiratory mucosa or hydrochloric acid in the stomach) that might have screened them out.

In effect, the immune system receives a surprise attack and its response must be appropriately strong enough to eliminate the virus. Often, as in HIV and HCV, there is no immediate immune response, as the virus has stealth mechanisms to outsmart the body's natural defenses. Only after the virus is well-established in the liver or nervous system does the immune system react, and even then it may be in a manner that is more destructive to the host than to the virus. Something very strange is occurring with the spread of these diseases, and it may take generations for the human immune system to adapt to them.

Some viruses, like German measles and HIV, can spread from mother to child, passing through the placenta during pregnancy. In the case of herpes simplex virus, a baby can be infected from the mother's blood when passing through the birth canal. Some viruses can also be passed along in breast milk, such as cytomegalovirus (CMV) and HIV.

The Mechanics of Viral Infection: Viral infection can lead to a variety of effects. However, first the virus must invade the host, travel in the blood or other body fluids, identify an organ or tissue that it has affinity with, attach itself to a target cell, and then get inside the susceptible cell. To enter an individual target cell the virus must cross the cell membrane and enter its cytoplasm. Sometimes the cell invites the virus in by a process of translocation across the cell membrane. Why this happens is still unknown. Other types of viruses fuse with the target cell's outer membrane and inject their own protein directly into the cytoplasm of the target cell.

Once the viral protein is within the target cell it places its genes into that cell's nucleus (where the genetic material is) and begins to make substances to create the next generation of itself. This process is not happening to only one or two cells at a time, but to millions of cells concurrently.

The virus then replicates itself quickly enough to overcome the body's local defenses, and it does this at an alarming rate. A complete viral cycle takes an average of only six to eight hours, and in the course of that time each single infected cell can release an additional 10,000 copies of the virus. Once this bridgehead has been breeched, the viral infection can spread from the site of inoculation to other areas, called secondary sites, via the bloodstream or lymph. Once reaching its target area, such as the liver in hepatitis or the spinal nerves in herpes zoster (shingles), it replicates further, and eventually the specific symptoms of infection appear, such as jaundice in hepatitis or pain and blistering with shingles.

These events establish the beginning of the infectious stage. After the virus has infected the host's cells, cell death usually follows with the bursting of the infected cell. Finally, the virus exits its former host, usually in body fluids, to directly infect others through this same process. Some viruses are very tough and can survive outside the host almost indefinitely. Many can endure temperature extremes, strong acids or alkalis, and drying, while others are more sensitive and die with exposure to air.

Clinical Manifestations of Viral Infection: Doctors are trained that viral infections follow characteristic stages. An incubation period of several days to a few weeks occurs before symptoms of the initial infection begin to appear. In chronic viral infections, like HCV or CMV, the incubation period is extended and the virus can remain dormant or silent for years before symptoms appear.

In acute viral infections, the first set of symptoms are called pro-dromal and manifest as fever, fatigue, and malaise, followed by the specific characteristics of the disease like the red rash from chicken-pox. For acute viral illnesses like measles, there is also a peak when the illness reaches its worst stage during which time the patient is the sick-est. Several days later, the symptoms begin to diminish and the patient recovers, thanks to their immune system's ability to control the viral invader.

Types of Viral Infections: The list of diseases caused by viruses is immense and ranges from the common cold to cancer. Viruses not only cause specific diseases with clear diagnostic symptoms, but they can also cause a constellation of symptoms that can defy diagnosis. Some viral diseases mimic other illnesses, like the fatigue caused by anemia, or cause secondary inflammation, like the joint pain associ-ated with arthritis. Certain viruses have specific affinity for only one type of tissue, such as the liver or skin, while others range among many body organs and systems. Viruses can cause localized infections such as warts or a sore throat, or a generalized infection such as in influenza, in which your whole body feels sick.

The patterns of disease caused by viruses are classified into several groups. Acute infections were originally thought to be the only man-ner in which viruses caused illnesses: you got sick and then you either got better or died. However, it is now well known that acute infections come in many forms. Therefore, viral illnesses are now classified as acute, chronic, latent, reactivated, and transforming (see figure 1-2).

The advantage of acute infections is that they cause rapid cell death, which results in active and aggressive management by the immune

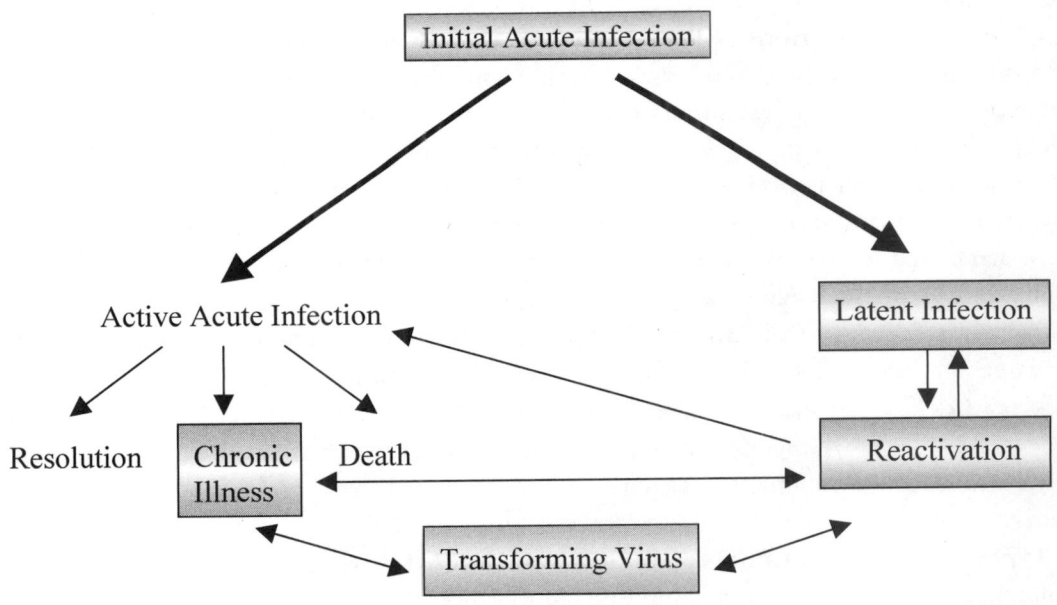

Figure 1-2: Patterns of Viral Disease

After initial infection, the virus can cause an active acute infection or a latent infection. Reactivation of a latent infection can return to latency, cause an acute response, or cause chronic illness, as in the case of Epstein-Barr virus and chronic fatigue.

system. On the other hand, a chronic or low-grade infection kills a smaller number of cells than in an acute infection. In this type of infection, the person may feel constantly or episodically ill, as in chronic Epstein-Barr virus (EBV), or they may have no symptoms at all, as in the early stages of HCV. The immune response develops a tolerance to the virus, and the host lives on, but with reduced energy and wellness.

Some viruses can become completely latent or exist in a dormant state, such as herpes simplex virus (HVS), only maintaining sufficient activity to sustain themselves. When circumstances are right, the virus can reactivate itself, causing symptoms. Viruses can also transform the infected cell in such a way as to cause cancer in a process called onco-genesis. Both herpes and hepatitis viruses are associated with the trans-formation of normal cells to cancerous ones (see discussion to follow).

Clinical Classification of Viral Infections: Viral infections are also further classified as persistent or non-persistent. Acute non-persistent infections are generally short-lived and have no other con-sequences than the immediate symptoms during the infection. You get sick, your immune system goes to work, and you get better within a week or two. Examples include the common cold or a mild flu. Persistent infections with acute onset are often due to a latent infec-tion, or a virus that persists in the cell host, and may activate or reac-tivate on more than one occasion, causing episodes of illness. Examples include herpes simplex and cytomegalovirus.

In the case of recurring illness, you feel repeatedly sick. Often, just when you start to feel better, you get sick again, as is the case with repetitive colds. Chronic, persistent infections are those in which the viral agent is being continually produced to cause a viral load suffi-cient to produce ongoing symptoms, such as in some types of Epstein-Barr virus (EBV) and the retroviruses, like HIV.

Additionally, viral co-infections can occur such as when AIDS and HCV appear together; or a satellite virus may assist another virus, each using the other to replicate. Opportunistic bacterial infections are also commonly seen with viral infections, such as in cases of influenza co-infected by staphylococcus or streptococcus, causing a bacterial bron-chitis, or when a viral rhinitis or common cold turns into bacterial sinusitis.

Stealth Infections: Those viruses associated with long incuba-tion periods during which time there may be no symptoms or signs of infection at all are often referred to as slow viruses. Examples of insidious viral infections include the "slow" or "stealth" viruses that often cause no apparent acute or chronic symptoms until the organ-ism is well invaded and the tissue cells are compromised by a fully entrenched virus, as in the cases of HCV and HHV-6.

The slow virus concept first appeared in 1957 with the work of a National Institute of Health scientist, Carleton Gajdusek, who was in New Guinea investigating kuru, a fatal type of spongiform encephalopathy that attacked the victim's brain, leading to paralysis and death. Upon uncovering the grizzly details, which suggested that a virus was responsible, and was transmitted when New Guinea tribesmen cannibalized their victims and ate the brain, Gajdusek proceeded to infect lab monkeys with brain tissue from kuru victims. In time, the monkeys developed neurological symptoms and eventually died. When the government of New Guinea enforced sanctions against cannibalism, kuru was eliminated.

The term "stealth infection" was coined by Paul W. Ewald, Ph.D., an evolutionary biologist at Amherst College in Massachusetts, to refer to microbial infections that cause other seemingly unrelated illnesses. The stealth concept has been expanded to include difficult-to-diagnose neurological conditions like some forms of multiple sclerosis (MS), in which a virus is suspected.

The terminology is not very specific and sometimes the concepts of a slow virus and a stealth infection are combined and referred to as stealth virus. This term seems appropriate, since not only do they seem to invade the host tissues slowly, causing no symptoms, but they sneak up on the infected individual and only give warning when it is too late, like the stealth fighter bomber or the cloaking devices used by alien vessels in the *Star Trek* science fiction series.

The most notorious stealth virus is human immunodeficiency virus (HIV), the currently accepted cause of AIDS. HIV belongs to a family of viruses called lentivirus that mostly produce diseases in domestic livestock, though some affect primates. Two other stealth viruses are hepatitis C and HHV-6. For the virus, this is an ideal situation: a nearly symptomless infection, with the host's immune system unable to clearly detect or destroy the virus so it lives for decades within the host, which provides it comfortable and safe accommodations and then transmits it to others through reproductive activity.

The Virus and Cancer Connection: Cancer remains one of the leading causes of death in the developed countries. One out of every three (and it's rapidly approaching one out of two) individuals will develop some form of cancer. Despite efforts made in conventional medicine and science, and even alternative therapies, most people who develop cancer will die from it. Contrary to previous opinion, cancer is not merely a localized disease with a single cause, but it derives from a multitude of factors. Immune suppression by drugs used to control the rejection of transplanted organs, many commonly used pharmaceutical drugs, environmental toxins, tobacco smoking, diets high in fat, family genetics, stress, and others conditions all work as cofactors in contributing to cancer risk.

Oncogenesis, the term used to describe the development of cancer, has long been associated with viruses. Since viruses directly interact with genetic material, and due to their small size can potentially gain access to any site and cell in the body, it is no surprise that they can also cause cancer.

The first proven human cancer caused by a virus, human T-cell leukemia virus-1 (HTLV1), was identified in 1981. Though rare in North America and Europe, Burkitt's lymphoma, another virally induced cancer, caused by Epstein-Barr virus (EBV) is the most common cancer in children in tropical Africa. Anthony Epstein, the primary researcher (after whom the virus is named), was later to find several other tumors induced by EBV, including nasopharyngeal carcinoma and cancers of the lymph glands.

Other virally induced cancers include cervical cancer, one of the most common cancers in women, caused by the papillomavirus, a member of the same viral family that causes warts; hepatocellular carcinoma caused by hepatitis B and C; and Kaposi's sarcoma, caused by a newly discovered herpes virus, HHV-8, which occurs in AIDS.

Though the idea that viruses cause cancer seems to go in and out of favor, finding specific viral causes of cancer is a relatively new field of research, and an extremely important one. Before the 1970s, a considerable amount of research effort was directed towards finding a viral cause of cancer. Failing that, scientists abandoned the theory and moved on to genetic causes. Current statistics show that around 15 percent of all cancers worldwide are linked to viral infections.

One of the unanswered questions about virally induced cancers is why more cancers are developing from common viruses that have coexisted with humans for thousands of years. Why does the immune system let the virus get in at all and, once there, why does it let it get away with inducing cancerous changes in the infected cells?

No one yet has the answers to these questions, but it is known that there is a long interval between the original infection and the onset of cancer; in the case of hepatitis C, it may take thirty years or longer to induce cellular changes in the liver that cause cancer. Since the incidence of cancer is so high, and viruses are becoming more accepted as potential causative factors, it is important for each of us to prevent viral infections, effectively treat existing or suspected infections, and improve immune function. (I discuss how to accomplish this in part 2.)

Looking for a Viral Cause to Syndromes: It has become all too common for a medical doctor to blame the cause of a patient's complaints on a nonspecific virus when he does not know what the cause is. We used to call this type of diagnosis a "wastebasket diagnosis," one that the physician just throws out. Though it may be the current trend to blame things on a virus, there may be some truth behind it. Many of the new illnesses are poorly defined and take on the characteristics of other diseases. They also display a constellation of symptoms, often unrelated, and situated in different parts of the body. This type of condition is called a syndrome, and many may have a viral cause, such as chronic fatigue syndrome, which has been blamed on EBV, chronic influenza A, and other viruses.

Even some forms of heart disease are linked to common viruses. Evidence that cytomegalovirus (CMV), found in nearly half of all American men over the age of 40, may be involved in atherosclerosis was only discovered in 1999. CMV and other chronic sub-clinical infections like the bacteria chlamydia can stimulate an immune response that causes inflammation in the heart and coronary blood vessels, and can even lead to fatal heart attacks.

Viral illnesses can also cause damage to the nervous system leading to paralysis, as is the case in transverse myelitis, a neurological syndrome caused by inflammation of the spinal cord and characterized by progressive demyelination (loss of the fatty tissue around the nerves). Its cause is often attributed to herpes simplex virus or Epstein-Barr virus. Both Parkinson's and Alzheimer's have been theoretically linked to a viral trigger or viral causative component.

Emerging Viruses: The AIDS pandemic is viewed as the paradigm for the emergence of new viral diseases. Though still hotly debated by some scientists (notably Donald Carrigan of the Wisconsin Viral Research Group and Peter Duesberg of the University of California in Berkeley, both discussed in more detail in chapter 2), by 1983 the cause of AIDS was identified as HIV, now divided into two types: HIV-1 and HIV-2. The source of the AIDS pandemic appears to have been Africa, with the first identified cases simultaneously occurring in the United States and Africa in 1981, though doctors were treating strange fatal infections in homosexual men in the late 1970s without knowing the cause of these deaths.

HIV is a retrovirus closely related to a virus that infects chimpanzees, and it appears to have first originated from a primate pool and then spread to humans. Among the many unanswered questions of the AIDS epidemic is why did a virus in monkeys spread to humans in the middle of the twentieth century when primates and humans have lived in close proximity in the same geographical regions for more than a hundred thousand years?

AIDS is a severe chronic viral infection. Statistics indicate that 50 million people worldwide are HIV-positive or have AIDS, and many of them—24.5 million—live in Africa. AIDS, like other viral diseases, spreads by infection, causing severe illness and eventual death in nearly all cases. Since it weakens the immune system by infecting and depleting CD4 helper T-lymphocytes (a type of white blood cell), AIDS patients can develop life-threatening co-infections such as pneumonia and fungal conditions.

There is no doubt that we are experiencing illnesses caused by viral infections that were either once rare or unheard of, or are new infections that were not involved in human illness in the past. The alarming rate at which they are occurring is of considerable concern.

However, new fatal infections or previously unrecognized diseases are familiar to human history. After all, smallpox was new to the Aztecs and Incas, but not to the Spanish. Another example is HHV-6, a recently identified herpes virus, which was first identified in 1988 by Japanese scientists as the cause of roseola, a common childhood disease. Though first scientifically discovered in 1920, roseola has been with us for a long time; therefore HHV-6 is also likely to have been around for at least as long. It is only our *identification* of it as the specific cause of roseola that is new. More importantly, why have some children in recent times who have contracted roseola developed severe neurological disease, damage to their kidneys and liver, and even died from it?

There is no doubt that we are experiencing illnesses caused by viral infections that were either once rare or unheard of, or are new infections that were not involved in human illness in the past. The alarming rate at which they are occurring is of considerable concern.

Linked to the increasing incidence of emerging infections is a mutation in the microbe and/or a change in the immune status of the host. A number of environmental and ecological factors are implicated here, such as changes in agriculture and wildlife habitats, new dams and irrigation systems, large-scale cutting of tropical rain forests, increasing human population density, rapid mass-transport systems (such as airplanes) allowing for infected humans to move from one location to another, the large number of wars in the twentieth century, and medical technology (transfusions, drug resistance, and immune suppressing drugs).

Other new viral infections include hepatitis C virus and the feared hemorrhagic fevers. Viral hemorrhagic fevers include yellow fever, dengue, hanta, Junin, Machupo, Lassa, Marburg, and the alarming Ebola viruses. In addition, known viruses like West Nile Fever are appearing in parts of the world where they were unheard of before. This mosquito-borne virus, a member of the viral family that causes encephalitis, was first isolated in Uganda in 1937. It has since appeared throughout Africa, India, China, and parts of Europe. However, West Nile virus (WNV) was never seen in the Western Hemisphere until late 1999 when its appearance in New York City caused eight deaths.

It seems there is no end to new and dangerous viruses. Among the most recent is TT virus (TTV). Like HCV, this new mystery virus was first discovered by the Japanese. It was at first thought a hepatitis virus since it produces a similar symptom presentation. But, according to Isa Mushahwar, the main researcher on the TTV trail, sufficient evidence shows that it is not related to the hepatitis virus families, and is structurally distinct enough to have a family of its own, the Circinoviridae.

Mushahwar speculates that TTV is present in 33–92 percent of the healthy population, and questions what these viruses are doing in humans and why they are not causing disease. However, immune dysfunction and mutation of a TTV subspecies can still cause disease in humans, as is the case with TTV-caused hepatitis.

Other new infections not caused by viruses are also appearing, including Lyme disease, the re-emergence of bubonic plague, and drug-resistant strains of tuberculosis (TB), all caused by bacteria. One third of the world's population is infected with TB, and there are 16 million active cases, 95 percent in developing nations—an astonishing figure.

Complications surrounding TB are frightening. The AIDS virus can activate dormant TB, leading to a lethal combination of a bacterial and viral infection. Unbeknownst to most people, TB is still the greatest single infectious cause of death worldwide, killing two million people each year. The re-emergence of malaria, compounded by drug resistance, is another serious concern with 300-500 million cases worldwide and one to two million deaths each year.

A New Viral Plague? Historically, it appears that diseases go into latent or dormant phases and then re-emerge when conditions are favorable for their spread—just as they do in our bodies. What is of concern now is the increasing *variety* of new viruses and other infectious diseases, the weakening of natural immunity from toxic pollutants and stress, and the spread of potent viruses into areas of dense human population. Every element is in place for a new plague.

In the past, when population density was considerably smaller and the balanced laws of nature still ruled the plains, savannas, forests, and mountains, human viral diseases were rare and appeared primarily in the overcrowded and filthy cities. After the great smallpox epidemics that occurred during the clash of cultures when Europeans colonized the rest of the planet, viral diseases were relatively quiescent. The new viral diseases described in this chapter (discussed in more detail in subsequent chapters) are a phenomenon of the late twentieth century, and they will be of great concern to us in the twenty-first century.

Since the linear scientific paradigm is having considerable difficulty in understanding and effectively managing these new diseases, especially viruses, it is important that we explore and try to understand other ways of viewing and treating disease. The evolutionary model is a good step, but it is still bound up with logical Western thinking. Not that logical thinking is the problem. The problem is that this one way of thinking occupies all our time and resources; if it is not working, repeating it endlessly will not work and will waste time. One option is to explore alternative models of disease causation and to develop a deeper insight into how we interact with viral illnesses.

Our world and the universe are complex. In order to advance civilization and understand the changing nature of disease, we must acknowledge that our contribution to modern disease has been the polluting of the environment with toxins and destroying the ecological balance that nature created. Alternative ways of conceptualizing medical care are therefore required.

To accomplish this we could usefully explore the ancient systems of energy medicine of the Chinese and Ayurvedic medicine from India. In these, we will find a way of thinking that fulfills the basic requirements to complement Western thinking. They are less linear, balance logic with intuition, work with the changing nature of biology rather than attempt to dominate it, and emphasize the health of the individual rather than concentrating excessively on disease. Today, as a culture, we are also beginning to re-examine our view of the beliefs of indigenous peoples, like shamanic practices and their attunement with natural forces. Evolutionary biology and quantum physics are only the beginning of this new way of thinking.

My own background demonstrates this new way of thinking in medicine which is supported by an increasing volume of research data and the conversion of many medical doctors to the practice of alternative therapies. A brief review of this background will make my point clear.

During my undergraduate studies in biology and anthropology, I became involved in native cultures, and in 1968 was "adopted" by a Siberian Eskimo family on St. Lawrence Island in the Bering Sea. After that I made numerous excursions, learning from indigenous cultures in North America, Mexico, and South America. Those experiences developed into my interest in enthomedical practices and ethnobotany, the study of medical plants used for healing by native peoples. I also extensively explored Chinese culture, philosophy, and health practices like qi gong and tai chi. In 1974, I started the study of acupuncture and Chinese medicine, receiving my first diploma in acupuncture in 1983 from the California Acupuncture College in San Diego and my doctor of Oriental medicine (O.M.D.) in 1985 from Sino-American University of Oriental Medicine in Los Angeles.

I completed my hospital rotations at the Shanghai College of Chinese Medicine in China. Study in naturopathic medicine followed my course of oriental medicine, and I received national board certification as a naturopathic physician (N.D.) in 1997 from the American Naturopathic Medicine Certification and Accreditation Board in Washington, D.C. Among my other credentials include a fellowship with the American Association of Integrative Medicine, and a diplomate certified in Integrative Medicine, and diplomate in Chinese Herbology.

I have sat at the feet of Chinese Taoist and Buddhist masters, and studied under Chinese, Ayurvedic, naturopathic, and medical doctors. I have hunted seal and walrus with Eskimo hunters, lived in remote jungle areas in Central and South America, and participated in indigenous healing ceremonies. These experiences, along with an open scientific mind, equipped me to explore other areas of consciousness; prompted me to think outside the conventional medical box, and to reconceptualize the causes of disease and how we heal.

Among these causes are the individual's inherent and created immune status, and the susceptibility to not only infectious disease but chronic disease and age-related disease as well. Subtle energy and balance between organ function, body chemistry, and the body's relationship to the immediate and greater environment play significant roles in health and disease, and I explain these ideas in more detail in chapter 5 and step 10.

The Energy Model of Viral Disease

So far in this chapter I have discussed viruses based on Western models of modern allopathic medicine and I have introduced current evolutionary theory, as rooted in Western thought. However, traditional forms of medicine, notably what is called Traditional Chinese Medicine, the source of acupuncture, has a different and, I contend, a viable alternative model for understanding and treating illness. That model is based not so much on biochemistry and physiology, but on the *energy* underlying both.

The Organization of Energy: The Chinese model of health is based upon balance and harmony within the individual and between the individual, society, and nature. According to Chinese medicine, there are four essential substances that rule this balance: qi (pronounced "chee"), blood, yin, and yang. Chinese scholars debate to this day about the nature of these substances, so it is not surprising if the concepts are difficult for a Westerner to understand. Let me try to explain them in a way that will help make further reading of the book much easier.

The force called qi is the vital intrinsic energy of all living things. Qi has five attributes: defense mechanisms, constant movement, transformation, warmth and the maintenance of body temperature, and holding things in place by resisting gravity. If the qi is strong, the body can defend itself against pestilence and disease. Emotional states also affect the qi. If the emotions are harmonious, then qi flows effortlessly and its defense mechanisms work well to guard one against infection.

In Chinese medicine, the blood is thought to be more than a fluid that carries oxygen, cells, and nutrients. It is one of the major media for the concentration of the life force, the qi. The other media for qi are the sexual secretions (semen), spinal fluid, and most importantly, the acupuncture meridians, which are conduits or channels where refined qi flows. If the blood is abundant, vital, and healthy, the qi is also strong and vital. The qi and blood are two sides of the same coin: the qi is invisible energy and the blood is energy made visible.

The Chinese insist, and I agree, that if you improve the quality of your blood through correct diet, herbal medicines, and acupuncture, the blood will purify itself and become vital and healthy. The same is true for the qi: you can enhance your body's qi by practicing slow moving exercises like tai chi (pronounced "tie chee") and breathing exercises called qi gong (pronounced "chee gung"), by receiving acupuncture, and by doing meditation practices.

In addition, the constitution of the person is important. Some people have an innately stronger immunity than others; they require less attention to strengthening their system and may only need to prevent illness. Others who are weaker need to actively cultivate balance and inner strength through qi gong, the use of tonic herbs, and a balanced lifestyle. Herbs for cultivating qi and blood are discussed in part 2.

Qi and blood are among the most important aspects of the body but are governed by a yet deeper principle of mutually dependent opposites. According to Chinese cosmology, yin and yang are the underlying universal principles that make up the structure and character of all things on this planet. Yang is the male force and is aggressive, quick-acting, fiery, and symbolized by the sun. Yin is the feminine principle and is passive, more patient, cooler, and symbolized by the moon. Since one cannot exist without the other, the variety of relationships between yin and yang is endless. In the body yin and yang forces are called *yin qi* and *yang qi*, and when these are harmonious and in a balanced relationship, the individual is healthy. You might call this interplay "the dance of health." However, when the yin qi and yang qi fall into conflict, the dance is disharmonious, the individual is more susceptible to infection, and illness arises.

In modern society, stress, overwork, the fast pace of living, and overuse of prescription drugs, especially antibiotics, causes a gradual reduction in the amount of yin qi, which predisposes the body to chronic viral diseases like AIDS and HCV.[3] This concept will be discussed in more detail in chapter 5 and step 8. As you will see in the next section, the Chinese knew the concepts and clinical presentations of both acute and chronic viral diseases long before the West discovered viruses.

The Chinese View of Viral Disease

The Chinese have an unbroken history of keeping detailed medical records. As early as several thousand years ago Chinese doctors were well aware of epidemic diseases and categorized them as "pestilent" factors. Based upon a complex codex of the nature and treatment of disease, they developed a comprehensive system of medicine that encompassed all types of illnesses, as well as health and preventive medicine. They were also adept at treating what we now know are viral diseases. According to the Chinese, pestilent factors were associated with the wind and changed from season to season.

In the *The Yellow Emperor's Classic on Internal Medicine,* a translation of *Huang Ti Nei Ching* (Veth 1949), the Yellow Emperor mused: "I should like to hear why it is that in certain years everyone is struck by a similar illness." Shao-shih, a physician-sage of the second century B.C., answered: "This is the result of a manifestation of the winds of the eight seasonal turning points."*

In traditional Chinese medicine, "wind" meant both the physical wind and a subtle wind that was similar to qi, invisible and active in the body. The Chinese concept of wind also carried the connotation of "bad air" or "evil wind" as a carrier of disease. One was "attached by wind" or became ill from the influence of an unfavorable circumstance carried upon the wind. This is not as simplistic as it might seem.

It is well known that viral particles of influenza spread through the atmosphere. The Chinese also believed that people were susceptible to seasonal differences in illnesses. The most vulnerable time was when one season transitioned to the next, like when summer is turning to fall, and at each of the solstices and equinoxes—making a total of eight turning points.

Though the ancient Chinese did not identify or name "viruses" as the direct cause of specific infectious diseases, they developed extraordinarily detailed empirical knowledge about the occurrence and treatment of what we now call viral diseases, including yellow fever, hepatitis, and influenza. In fact, since China is the homeland for many of these viruses, it is not surprising to find that Chinese practitioners have an extensive *materia medica* of antiviral herbal medications, many which are discussed in detail in part 2 of this book.

Modern doctors of Chinese medicine recognize viruses and viral diseases, while retaining the traditional knowledge of how the body's energy systems function and respond to viral infections. In fact, since the 1980s, intense research has been carried out on the identification of herbs with the most potential as antivirals. Both Chinese and Western scientists are investigating a new class of substances called immune modulators which enhance and normalize immune activity.

The Energy Model, Ecology, and Evolutionary Medicine: The energy model looks closely at the relationships of the outer environments, such as the workplace and home, and inner environments, such as the health of the large intestine and liver, and works towards improving their relationships and functions. It does not focus exclusively on pathology and the symptoms of disease.

The energy model is comprehensive and provides a holistic understanding of disease, supports health and focuses on prevention, including immune-enhancing medications, and it teaches exercises and lifestyle recommendations that improve immune function.

Therefore, the energy model is comprehensive and provides a holistic understanding of disease, supports health and focuses on prevention, including immune-enhancing medications, and it teaches exercises and lifestyle recommendations that improve immune function. It offers functional support for organs, such as the liver, that are critical in the process of removing viruses from our bodies, and prescribes potent antiviral herbs that reduce the overall viral load (discussed in later chapters).

The Chinese model of energy medicine dovetails with evolutionary medicine. Both look at a broader picture of disease placing it within *ecological* contexts and taking into consideration the specific individual's symptoms and condition. More importantly, though Chinese medicine may take longer to have a symptomatic effect, it poses little environmental impact by using low-tech methods and nontoxic medicines, and leaves the patient with few or no side effects. Often Chinese medical therapies strengthen the individual, leaving one in better condition than before the disease occurred, and they provide a curative effect unavailable with the use of chemical drugs.

CHAPTER SUMMARY

Viruses are intracellular parasites.

They imbed themselves within our genome, and we interact with them immunologically and genetically.

Though viral diseases have been with humanity at least from the time of domesticated animals, we are just beginning to understand viruses.

We know of several thousand different types of viruses, but only a small fraction of those are well-characterized, and even these are not yet completely understood.

Viruses cause many human illnesses and range from the common cold to epidemic diseases like smallpox.

Many new or emerging viruses are appearing at an alarming rate.

The current medical paradigm appears too linear and cumbersome to effectively deal with these new viral and other infectious diseases. The seriousness of this situation makes it mandatory to look at other models of medicine and to explore new therapeutic approaches.

The evolutionary medical model is a necessary balance to the current allopathic approach. However, though theoretically valuable, it may not be practical enough to deal with the emerging viral crisis and a possible imminent plague scenario.

It is wise to consider the energy model of Chinese medicine, and to integrate it and other useful natural forms of therapy into a new system of medicine that treats the person as well as the disease.

It is not enough to look at individual viruses, energy and evolutionary models of medicine, and alternative therapies. A broader ecological viewpoint may be our only hope in finally understanding emerging viral illnesses and in meeting the challenge of impending plagues.

2

Viruses: Common and Exotic—
A Review of the Key Viral Agents

In order to better understand the principles used to renew the immune system and how to use natural antiviral medications effectively, it helps to have some knowledge about the key agents on the viral playing field. In this chapter, I present the most common and most important of current viruses. Some are only mentioned, while those that have more importance in chronic and serious disease, such as hepatitis C and herpes, are discussed in more detail.

Since there are many authoritative books on HIV and AIDS, this subject is covered only briefly; however some important issues surrounding its origin are presented to illustrate how differing opinions of the experts in the field of virology confuse the issues. Many viruses have been omitted here because they are not specifically pertinent to the theme of this book, although that does not make them less serious or dangerous.

We know so little about viruses and how and when new infections might emerge that the specter of a viral plague looms as a threatening backdrop to modern civilization. Among the viruses presented in this chapter (see table 2), the one most likely to cause a pandemic (a worldwide epidemic) is the flu, perhaps the most common and widely known of all viral diseases. Indeed, it is a real threat, and one that has a high likelihood of occurring within the next decade or so, if micro-biologists' predictions are correct.[1]

From the standpoint of the evolutionary model, we have as much or more to worry about from chronic viruses and depressed immune system states than we do from an influenza pandemic. Prior to the mid-twentieth century, poor sanitation and crowded cities facilitated the transmission of viral infections from person to person. In modern times, chronic viral illnesses occur due to hosts with compromised immunity, and in some parts of the world, nineteenth-century condi-tions still exist alongside widespread immune system weakness.

The worse case scenario for viral problems is if an outbreak of an extremely lethal, acute viral infection, combined with spreading chronic infections that debilitate and kill slowly were to occur at the same time. In fact, such situations already exist in Africa and parts of India. In these countries, millions are affected by horrible living con-ditions, and tens of thousands of people die every day from the effects of malnutrition and suppressed immune systems.

While AIDS and common infections take their toll, these unfor-tunate souls are also under the constant threat of serious viral disease such as yellow fever, dengue fever, and nonviral infectious diseases like malaria and cholera. So far, these conditions have not spread into the developed countries, except in poverty-stricken sections of many of the larger industrial cities, where deepening third-worldlike condi-tions facilitate the spread of AIDS, tuberculosis, and transplanted infectious disease.

The Common Cold

Respiratory tract infections (those that affect the nose, throat, and lungs) are the most common of acute viral illnesses and include the common cold and flu. However, what most people, and even many doctors call "the flu" is actually caused by adenoviruses and paramyx-oviruses, and is not "true flu," which is caused by a different family of viruses (discussed in more detail below).

In the Northern Hemisphere, common respiratory tract infections generally occur seasonally, primarily in the late fall and winter and into the early spring. They can, however, occur at any time of the year in tropical countries, and even in the southern parts of the United States,

Disease	Viral Families and Causes	Table 2: Summary of Vector
Common Cold	Picornaviridae family, Rhinovirus: seasonal changes	Humans, especially children
Gastroenteritis	Reoviridae family, rotavirus: spread through diarrhea in fecal matter	Humans
Flu	Orthomyxoviridae family influenza: livestock to human contact	Ducks, pigs, chickens
Herpes	Herpesviridae family: human activities	Humans
AIDS	Lentivirus, HIV infection: lifestyle and environmental factors that suppress immunity	Humans, primates
Hepatitis B	Hepadnaviridae family: human fluids and secretions	Humans
Hepatitis C	Flaviviridae family: blood supply and transfusion practices	Humans
Dengue	Flaviviridae virus family: increased urbanization in tropics	Mosquitoes
Ebola	Filoviridae: cause still unknown	Unknown
Hantavirus	Bunyaviridae family: animal to human contact	Rodents
Yellow Fever	Flaviviridae: poor sanitation, and standing water	Mosquitoes

Selected Viral Infections

Mode of Transmission	Symptoms	Treatment and Prevention
Infected mucus particles by coughing, sneezing, and touching	Head congestion, sneezing, discharge of phlegm	Rest, inhaling steam, herbal remedies, vitamin C
Contact with infected food, water, handshaking	Diarrhea, vomiting, dehydration, low-grade fever	Rest, fluid replacement, Chinese herbs
Airborne from coughing	Sore throat, fever, achiness	Rest and fluids, herbal remedies, vitamin C, immunization, antiviral drugs
Kissing, sexual contact, birth	Wide range from cold sores to fatal infection and cancer	Acyclovir, nutrition, herbal medications, diet
Sexual contact, blood transfusions, mother to child	Severe immune deficiency; opportunistic infections	Antiviral drugs; nutrition, natural immune-modulating substances. No known cure
Contact with saliva, semen, blood	Nausea, vomiting, jaundice	Vaccination, interferon; Chinese herbal medicine, nutrition
Contact with infected blood	Usually silent	Interferon alpha with Ribavarin, Chinese herbs, nutrition
Bite from infected mosquito	High fever and severe joint pain, hemorrhaging	Analgesics, anti-inflammatories, herbal medicines
Direct contact with infected blood, secretions, semen	Sudden fever, diarrhea, vomiting and massive hemorrhaging	No known cure
Inhaling aerosolized rodents' urine and feces	Abdominal pain, fever, kidney failure, hemorrhage	No known cure
Bite from infected mosquito	Fever, headache, muscle pain, vomiting	Analgesics for pain, rest, fluids, electrolyte replacement, herbal remedies

including Southern California and Florida. Why certain viruses appear at different times of the year is still a mystery, but one explanation may be found in the theory of temperature selectivity of viruses.

Many viruses, such as those that cause the common cold, reproduce better in cooler temperatures and are inhibited by heat. Your immune system exploits this characteristic to your benefit by raising the body's temperature with a fever to control viral spread in the early stages of infection. In the fall and winter, the body's natural immunity is more stressed by inclement weather, exacerbated by radical temperature changes from a warm house to the colder outside, and in summer in moving from air-conditioned buildings to a hot outer environment.

From the viewpoint of Chinese medicine, autumn is the season of the lungs, and a time when the respiratory tract becomes more vulnerable. From an evolutionary point of view, winter is the time when natural selection takes place. Trees are pruned by winter storms and toppled from the wind, wild animals hibernate or die off from starvation, and humans are prone to viral infections that in the past killed the elderly and the very young, allowing only the strongest to survive and mate in the spring.

How Colds Are Spread: Respiratory viruses spread from person to person by sneezing, coughing, or hand contact, and from touching objects like cups, phone handsets, keyboards, and doorknobs contaminated by the person suffering from a cold. As I mentioned in chapter 1, the customary Asian greeting of bowing instead of shaking hands is an excellent means of preventing the spread of viruses. In Asia, people greet each other at arms length and bow to each other without hand contact, or even face-to-face exposure, thereby minimizing the chance that the other person might breathe or sneeze directly into your face.

Viral particles from a human sneeze can travel at 40 mph and reach a distance of 30 feet from the infected person, easily covering a normal-size room. These viral particles then launch their attack on the lining of the nose or throat, or even from direct access to the lung tissue, if they are inhaled directly. Small children are the perfect carriers for colds, flu, and other common viruses. As children play and move around a room, they sneeze and cough without covering their mouths, and they constantly wipe their hands across dripping and draining noses, thereby spreading virus-laden mucus by touching objects and other people.

The Viruses Responsible for Colds: The majority of common colds are caused by a group of viruses called rhinoviruses, of which there are more than 150 types. All rhinoviruses are members of the Picornaviridae family. Two to ten percent of colds are caused by coronaviruses, another common respiratory tract virus. In addition to rhinoviruses and coronaviruses, two other viral groups cause common respiratory tract infections including symptoms identical to the common cold; these involve members of the Adenoviridae and Paramyxoviridae families.

Adenoviruses cause about 5–10 percent of coldlike infections and are one of the most common infections in young children, causing coughs and stuffy or runny noses. Older children and adults infected with adenoviruses mainly experience sore throat (pharyngitis) and mild nasal symptoms. Adenoviruses also cause other infections, such as redness and swelling of the eyes (conjunctivitis), urinary tract infections (cystitis and urethritis), and infections in the intestinal tract (gastroenteritis). In immunosuppressed people, including AIDS patients, adenoviruses can cause life-threatening pneumonia.

The paramyxoviruses cause croup, bronchitis, pneumonia, middle-ear infections (otitis media), and measles and mumps. One member of this family, parainfluenzavirus, causes up to one-half of all respiratory infections in young children. Like other common viruses, there is no pharmaceutical cure, and natural remedies are the best treatment option.

The Course, Symptoms, and Treatment of the Common Cold: After an incubation period of two to three days, typical acute cold symptoms begin. Usually starting with a sore throat, head congestion, stuffiness of the nose, and frontal headache or pain in the back of the neck and upper shoulders, a cold can progress rapidly to coughing and sneezing with copious discharge of mucus from the nose. If a fever is present at all, it is mild and may be accompanied by chills.

As a rule, colds resolve by themselves in a week or two and leave no other diseases in their wake. A common medical school saying wryly illustrates this: "An untreated cold lasts one week, and a treated one lasts seven days." Interestingly, since I was in medical training, the timing has changed from seven days to twenty-one. Does this mean that colds are stronger than in the past and run a longer course, or that people have weaker immune systems?

Serious secondary infections with colds are rare, but it is not uncommon for a cold to turn into a bacterial sinus infection or bronchitis in the elderly or immune-compromised patients of any age.

Western medical doctors are taught that there is no cure for the common cold. The standard recommended treatment includes bed rest, fluids, and waiting. Symptomatic over-the-counter medicines such as cough suppressants, acetaminophen or aspirin for headache, decongestants, and antihistamines to dry up nasal drainage are recommended. Despite wide use by doctors and as over-the-counter remedies, none of these have any proven effectiveness.

Patients often have their own favorite way of managing colds and most medical doctors tolerate these "folk remedies," including old-fashioned chicken soup. It turns out this remedy has been shown by research studies to have value in reducing inflammation and the symptoms attributed to the common cold. A vaporizer or the inhalation of steam is also useful in breaking up chest congestion.

In traditional Chinese medicine, the symptoms of common respiratory tract illnesses are classified under the term *biao zheng,* which denotes an illness of the exterior, as compared to an illness of the organs and interior part of the body, called *li zheng.* Specifically, viral induced conditions of the upper respiratory tract are called *biao han,* or "wind-cold" illness, and the common cold is referred to as *gan mao.*

Despite the difference in terminology, the symptomology of the common cold in Chinese medicine and Western medicine is identical, with the exception that in traditional Chinese medicine, determining a pulse pattern and examining the tongue coating are added as part of the diagnosis. Doctors of traditional Chinese medicine routinely examine the patient's pulse at the radial artery on the wrist of both hands to evaluate the qi. A pulse that is stronger near the surface of the wrist is called a superficial pulse and indicates an active defense response against *biao han,* or acute illness caused by an attack of wind and cold. There are numerous different pulse qualities that the Chinese doctor uses to determine the state of the patient's health, the location of the illness, the strength of the defensive response, and the quality of yin and yang.

Tongue diagnosis is the other main method of assessment used in Chinese medicine. The body of the tongue is evaluated for color, thinness or thickness, dryness or moisture, and to see if there are ridges, teeth marks, or other geographic abnormalities. The coating is also considered, and is more important than the body of the tongue in assessing acute conditions like the common cold. The tongue of a healthy person is of average size, without teeth marks along the edges, is neither too dry nor too moist, is of a fresh pink color, and has a thin white coat. With a cold, the pulse is superficial and the tongue coating is a thicker white than normal.

In naturopathic medicine, diagnosis for the common cold is exactly the same as that of a conventional medical doctor, though treatment is different. There is a telling joke told by naturopaths about the difference between the two systems of medicine. It goes like this:

Question: "What is the difference between an M.D. and an N.D. (naturopathic doctor)?"

Answer: "When a patient calls in the middle of the night with a runny nose, sore throat, and headache, the M.D. says, 'Take two aspirin and call me in the morning.' The N.D. says, 'Take 20 drops of echinacea and call me in the morning.'"

All three schools of medicine (Western, Chinese, and naturopathic) acknowledge the same symptoms; however, each system has a different perspective concerning the cause.

In Chinese medicine, it is the changing seasons and the colder winds that cause an imbalance in the person's energy state, leading to the activation of defensive mechanisms that attempt to expel the pathogenic influence from the surface of the body. The most common treatment is to cause sweating (diaphoresis), take herbs that expel the pathogenic wind and cold from the surface of the body, and treat accompanying symptoms like headache and cough.

If the body is weak, Chinese doctors also recommend nourishing its intrinsic energy (qi) with chicken soup combined with herbs, or taking tonic herbs like astragalus *(Astragalus membranaceus)*. In fact, there are many excellent traditional Chinese remedies for cold symptoms. One of the most widely used is *gan mao ling*. It comes in tablets, tea, and instant granules (called *ganmao tuire chongji* or *gan mao char*). These remedies can be easily obtained in any Chinese herb store, from most acupuncturists' offices, or by mail from one of the resources listed in appendix E. Their use is explained in detail in part 2.

Naturopaths agree with traditional medical doctors (as do modern Chinese medicine doctors) that the cause of a cold is a virus, and that the symptoms are largely the results of the body's natural defense mechanisms working to neutralize the virus. However, the similarity ends there, as naturopathic philosophy contends that the doctor should *assist* these natural mechanisms and not suppress symptoms, especially by the use of antihistamines that reduce nasal secretions which are part of the body's mechanical means of expelling virus particles. Naturopathic doctors state it is important to allow the body to discharge the virus, and that suppressing symptoms makes the individual more prone to other illnesses.

Many natural remedies are effective for managing a cold, including high doses of vitamin C. A review of twenty-one placebo-controlled studies on vitamin C indicated that between 1,000 to 8,000 mg daily reduces the duration and severity of symptoms (Hemila, et al. 1995) . Zinc lozenges and oral zinc tablets or capsules are also very effective in managing a cold.

Many natural remedies are effective for managing a cold, including high doses of vitamin C. A review of twenty-one placebo-controlled studies on vitamin C indicated that between 1,000 to 8,000 mg daily reduces the duration and severity of symptoms.

A number of common herbal teas and tinctures are helpful and include elder flowers, echinacea, yarrow, sage, fresh ginger, and boneset. The therapeutic use of these herbs is explained in part 2.

Viral Gastroenteritis

Viral gastroenteritis, also called the stomach flu, the intestinal flu, or grippe, can be caused by adenoviruses, rotaviruses, caliciviruses, or astroviruses. Symptoms appear suddenly after a very brief incubation period, and include abdominal cramping, mild fever, diarrhea, and vomiting. Because these illnesses are frequently contracted from contaminated food or water, people often think they have food poisoning when in fact they have a case of viral gastroenteritis. However, clinically, both illnesses are often indistinguishable and both resolve in 24–48 hours. In young children or susceptible individuals, dehydration can occur from vomiting and diarrhea, so adequate fluid intake is necessary to prevent dehydration.

Prevention and Treatment of Gastroenteritis: Conventional medical treatment includes mostly supportive care such as bed rest and easy access to a toilet. Typically, fluids like sweetened warm tea, ginger ale, and bland foods like broths or cooked cereal are recommended, since it is difficult to eat without feeling nauseous, vomiting, or having diarrhea. Low blood sugar can occur from lack of food, and drinking fruit juice or fluids sweetened with honey can help prevent hypoglycemic symptoms of weakness and shakiness. Intravenous electrolytes are given if dehydration is severe; however, this is rarely necessary in the average case of gastroenteritis.

Natural medicine views common gastroenteritis similarly as does conventional medicine, but it adds additional remedies like acidophilus to replenish lost "friendly" bacteria and to control unfriendly species in the intestines. High dosages of vitamin C should be avoided since they can cause more diarrhea.[2] Although it is generally considered good practice to allow the body to cleanse the offending agent out of the system by not suppressing diarrhea, if the diarrhea is persistent (but not severe enough to require intravenous electrolyte and glucose replacement) mild astringent herbs like blackberry *(Rubus fruticosus)*, blueberry *(Vaccinium spp.)*, or raspberry leaves *(Rubus idaeus)* can be helpful. You can sweeten herbal teas with honey to keep the blood sugar level normal and prevent fatigue.

Supplements or vegetable broths can provide minerals and electrolytes such as sodium and potassium that are depleted by diarrhea. Chamomile tea *(Matricaria recutita)* is very useful in reducing cramping and gastrointestinal upset. Berberine,[3] a yellow alkaloid and the active ingredient in goldenseal *(Hydrastis canadensis)*, barberry *(Berberis vulgaris)*, and Oregon grape root *(Berberis aquifolium)* have antimicrobial properties and can help reduce the viral activity in the intestines.

Chinese medicine has several excellent remedies for gastroenteritis. Most contain *huang lian (Coptis snaensis)*, a berberine-containing herb like goldenseal, only stronger. Chinese medicine also recommends not suppressing diarrhea caused by acute mild gastroenteritis, and encourages managing nausea and fever with herbal medicines. Other remedies for diarrhea and gastrointestinal viruses are discussed in detail in part 2.

Influenza

Influenza is called the "last of the great uncontrolled plagues," and some epidemiologists believe that we are imminently due for an influenza epidemic of plague proportions like that of 1918. Evolutionary biologists disagree, arguing that conditions for transmission and rapid viral spread are very different now from the Europe during World War I. They also point out that antibiotics are readily available to treat secondary bacterial infections like pneumonia, infections that were fatal in 1918; they contend that reasonably safe and successful vaccines are more widely used now. They also hypothesize that a combination of the two known influenza pandemic strains (hemagglutin type 1 and neuraminidase type 1) does not inevitably lead to a deadly strain similar to that of 1918, as is suggested by conventional virologists (see figure 2-1).

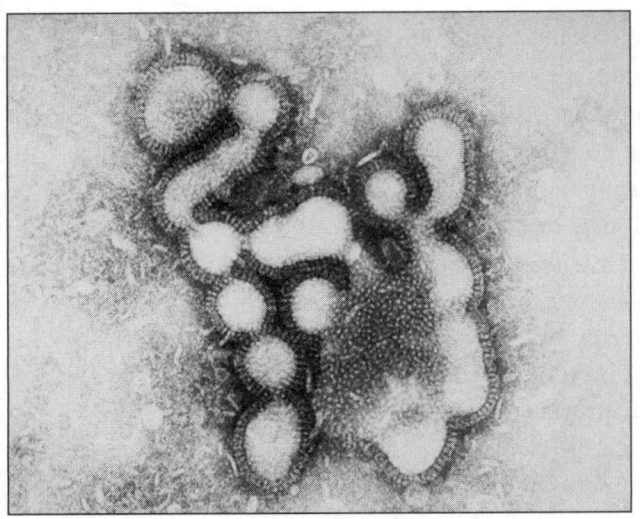

Figure 2-1: Structure of Influenza Virus

This electron micrograph of a cluster of influenza virions shows the typical spherical shape and closely packed spikes that create the characteristic halo around individual influenza virions.

Such discussion seems more like the splitting of hairs because viral reality is completely different from and independent of human opinion. Viruses have their own agenda. Influenza is a potentially fatal disease that is still very much among us. It is just a matter of when, how many people will be infected, and how many deaths will occur. Given the increasing virulence and frequency of other viruses, it seems certain that a more potent influenza virus will appear.

In the temperate regions, like North America and Europe, flu outbreaks occur every winter and epidemics approximately every eight to ten years. Worldwide influenza pandemics occur every ten to forty years, and in the last century the world experienced three: the Spanish flu of 1918; the Asian flu in 1957; and the Hong Kong flu in 1968.

Pandemics occur when there is a major change in the genetic material of the virus, creating an entirely new strain and one against which the world's population has no immunity. Given these parameters, and if the conventional experts are correct in their calculations, we could experience another sweeping influenza outbreak some time in the first decade of the twenty-first century. As one British researcher chillingly remarked, "Put simply, each year brings us closer to the next pandemic" (Shortridge 1995).

The Cause and Types of Influenza: True flu, or influenza virus, is caused by a member of the Orthomyxoviridae family. There are three known types of flu that infect humans: influenza viruses A, B, and C. The most important of these is influenza A, which has over thirty known subtypes. One of the unique characteristics of influenza A is its ability to cause infections in a wide range of animals, including humans, pigs, horses, aquatic mammals like seals, and birds. This ability to infect a broad spectrum of different species effectively ensures its survival.

In humans, influenza virus causes acute outbreaks of severe respiratory tract infection. It has a remarkable ability to evade individual host defenses and to undergo massive genetic changes that prevent human populations from acquiring permanent immunity against it—a trait that contributes to its characteristic rapid spread and ability to cause pandemics.

Influenza A can also change by gene swapping. In an infected cell, different virus particles can share genes. As a shared disease of both humans and livestock, influenza A can rearrange itself in unpredictable intervals, forming new strains in rapid succession. RNA viruses, of which influenza is a member (as is hepatitis C), have extraordinary rates of mutation—estimated at one million times higher than human DNA—producing one mutation for every ten thousand viral replications and taking less than an hour to achieve.

Vectors: Domesticated poultry, primarily ducks and chickens. are the primary vectors for influenza A. From there it spreads to pigs, thereby accounting for the name of one type of influenza A virus, "swine flu." While rooting around the farmyard, pigs inhale and ingest infected poultry droppings, causing the pigs to catch the flu; from them the virus is passed to humans working and living around the pigs; the virus then travels from human to human.

In a country with very high population density based mostly on rural, self-sufficient farms raising ducks, chickens, and pigs (where the virus keeps continuously circulating), the disease has a chance to jump back and forth between animal species and humans, gene-swapping and mutating to its advantage (see figure 2-2).

Influenza was not known in the New World prior to colonization by Europeans. One explanation is that American indigenous cultures did not have domesticated pigs, cows, or horses, and only in tropical Central and South America were wild birds like parrots, turkeys, and ducks kept as pets, but not in farmyards as they are in Europe or China. Influenza proved to be a particularly severe and mostly fatal disease among American Indians in both North and South America.

Ducks in particular are thought to be the main reservoir of flu viruses. Though not affected themselves, they act as carriers and spread the virus in their droppings. Wild migratory ducks also spread influenza viral particles by dropping feces as they fly, and when they stop over in ponds and lakes they contaminant the water with their feces, which are then taken up by other ducks that fly long distances themselves further spreading the disease.

Origins of Influenza: Historically, southern China is considered the place of origin for most influenza A pandemics. From China they

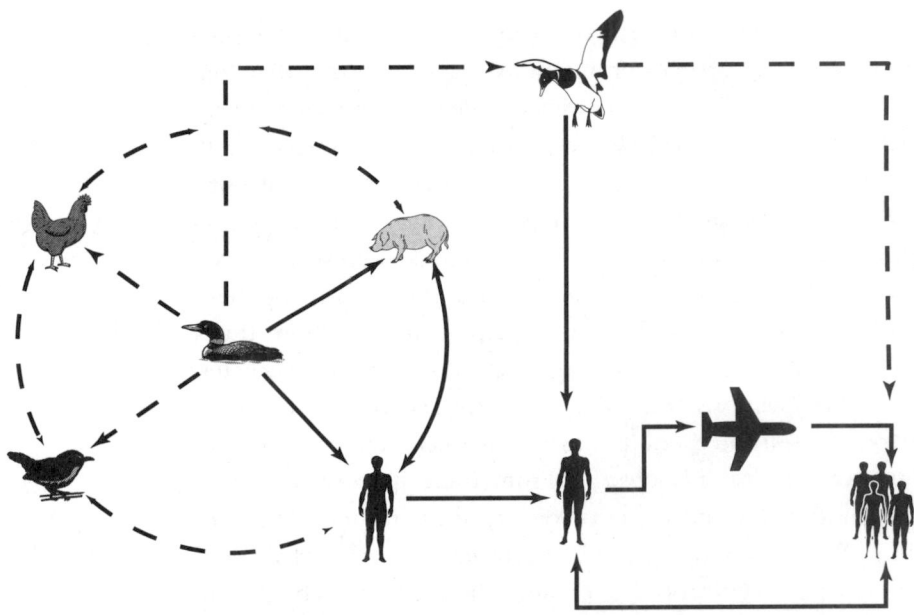

Figure 2-2: How the Flu Is Spread

Influenza virus has an animal reservoir and vector, primarily ducks and pigs. Humans inhale viral particles released from the breakdown of fecal matter from ducks or from exposure to pigs. Human-to-human transmission takes place through droplets of air when an infected person coughs or sneezes. A single infected person can carry the flu over thousands of miles in an airplane, and infect an entire population of people.

spread through Russia into Europe, and then to the Americas. In centuries past, when land travel was slow, a viral epidemic might run its course, spending itself before spreading too far. However, with the advent of increased world trade and faster means of transportation, a powerful strain of influenza virus could easily reach Europe and America in a matter of days; and with jet travel, and Chinese flying to the West and Westerners traveling to China, viral spread is all the more global and rapid, and could, conceivably, occur in a matter of hours.

When I was first in China in the early 1980s, long before most Westerners were allowed to enter this closed society, one expected to catch a severe respiratory infection caused by influenza virus within the first two weeks. Westerners had no immunity to the Chinese influenza strains and became very sick and bedridden for up to three weeks with symptoms of fatigue, headache, coughing, and high fever. As China opened her doors and trade goods flowed in both directions along with businesspeople, students, and tourists, Chinese strains of influenza have spread from country to country with ease. It is conceivable that a potential strong virus could easily arrive in the United States in this fashion.[4]

Virulence: Virulence refers to the degree of damage an infectious organism can inflict on its host. The amount of damage is influenced by several factors that include the activity of the organism and the strength of the host's immune system. Influenza has a wide range of virulence, and though it can be a fatal disease, it is generally considered a comparatively short-lived infection of the upper respiratory tract, affecting the nose, throat, and lungs.

The severity of a bout of flu is usually related to the immune function of the host, such that those with weakened immune responses, such as older people, the chronically ill, and those with compromised immune systems, suffer the most. It can also be a fatal illness in these groups of people. In the United States alone, influenza kills more then twenty thousand people each year, most of them elderly.

Secondary complications, like bacterial bronchitis and viral pneumonia, are intertwined with severe flu and are considered the probable cause of most of the deaths from the 1918 Spanish flu epidemic, a time when antibiotics were still undiscovered. In the one year that the Spanish flu was at its peak, one in every one hundred people died from influenza or complications. If such an outbreak were to occur today, a one percent death rate would mean that 60 million people, more than the population of France, would die in one year.

Contagion and Symptoms: Infection from influenza virus is simple, extremely effective, and universal. It occurs from breathing contaminated air containing viral particles spread by coughing and sneezing. After an incubation period of two to three days, symptoms start abruptly with shivering, malaise, fatigue, headache, and aching of the limbs and back. Fever is often present and can be as high as 102° to 104° F. When you are sick with the flu you can feel so ill that you have to stay in bed. A typical flu generally runs its course in seven to ten days, but generalized symptoms can linger longer with malaise and fatigue lasting up to three to four weeks.

Pandemic influenza tends to be extremely virulent, much more so then regular flu, and progresses very rapidly. It can cause primary viral pneumonia and death can follow as soon as forty-eight hours or less after primary infection. For the average person and even most doctors, influenza is largely ignored for most of the year, but between

December and the end of February large numbers of workers and school children are home sick with the flu. In recent years with the introduction of new strains from China, there have been stronger flu outbreaks, but no major epidemic and as yet no pandemic.

Most medical experts consider influenza, even in its most severe forms, an acute but short-lived infection without any complications or residual effects, however, bacterial secondary infections are common during the course of the illness. Middle ear infection, or otitis media, is a frequent complication of influenza infection in children and causes considerable discomfort for the child and has the potential to cause permanent hearing loss. Influenza virus can also invade the cells of the central nervous system or muscles and cause chronic infections in each called encephalopathy and myositis, respectively.

Fibromyalgia, one of the new diseases and a condition similar to myositis (though more systemic in its effects, including insomnia, fatigue, and irritable bowel complaints) still defies medicine's attempts to assign a definitive cause. There are several theories about the cause of fibromyalgia, including a virally induced cause blamed mostly on herpes viruses. Though little attention is paid to a possible connection between fibromyalgia and influenza A, some experts suggest it is an overlooked syndrome.

In one research paper, Allen Tyler, a medical doctor and naturopathic physician, reports that fibromyalgia was not seen before the 1918 flu pandemic. In his research, he found that 90 percent of fibromyalgia patients tested positive for influenza A antibodies. Tyler postulates that since not all people who contract influenza A come down with fibromyalgia, and though it may be the primary precipitating event, it may be only one factor among many, including stress, altered immunity, and low serotonin levels, that contribute to the full syndrome (Tyler 1997).

Though the conventional medical establishment has not endorsed this theory, Dr. Tyler is not alone in his thinking about chronic influenza infections. German homeopaths have long considered the connection between immune impairment and chronic viral infection to be one of the main causes of modern diseases,[5] such as fibromyalgia, and British and Australian physicians are aware of influenza virus-induced myalgias and fatigue.

In these days of complicated viral illnesses, it is prudent to know what flu symptoms are and how to differentiate them from the common cold or other respiratory viral infections. With careful observation you can easily tell the difference between a cold and the flu. At the outset, influenza does not have the characteristic symptoms of a cold like runny nose, sore throat, and sneezing. Flu starts with fever, achy joints, and sore muscles while a cold starts with headache, stuffiness in the head, and congested sinus passages. Fatigue and malaise are present in both the flu and a cold, but with the flu the fatigue is stronger.

Diagnosis and Treatment: There are no commonly used clinical lab tests to diagnose the flu. Rather the diagnosis is based upon the characteristic presentation of symptoms and the knowledge that an outbreak is occurring in the general population. Antibody studies (blood tests that measure levels of immune substances) to influenza virus are available but are used mainly by researchers and not clinically by your typical family physician. A new 30-minute test involving a throat swab, like the ones used to test for strep throat, is available but it does not yet have wide clinical acceptance.

German homeopaths have long considered the connection between immune impairment and chronic viral infection to be one of the main causes of modern diseases, such as fibromyalgia, and British and Australian physicians are aware of influenza virus-induced myalgias and fatigue.

Though there is no medical treatment for the flu, most doctors routinely prescribe antibiotics as prevention or treatment for secondary bacterial infections—a practice that is causing concern over the development of antibiotic-resistant bacterial strains. With the advent of newer antivirals, some experts are suggesting wider use of antiviral drugs to obviate antibiotic use in viral infections, and thus cut down on antibioticresistant bacteria. Such a practice appears to be replacing one problem with a potentially greater one—viruses can develop drug resistance at an alarming rate, one that is often, in fact, faster than bacteria.

Common over-the-counter medicines are sometimes recommended by doctors to treat the symptoms caused by the flu, such as Tylenol (acetaminophen) for fever, Advil (ibuprofen) for joint pain, or nasal decongestants like Sudafed (pseudoephedrine hydrochloride). Sometimes antihistamines are recommended to dry up runny mucus, or a combination of the above is used, such as in commercial flu remedies (for example, TheraFlu).

Even though aspirin is commonly used for the symptoms of flu, in some cases, if taken by children or teenagers, it can cause a rare but potentially fatal complication of influenza called Reye's Syndrome, so it is not routinely recommended for younger patients. However, the aspirin connection is not well understood and since Reye's Syndrome is so rare, there has been no motivation to investigate it further. Until we know more about aspirin-induced syndromes, it is best not to give aspirin to young children when they have the flu.

The "flu shot" is the accepted form of prevention and is mainly taken by high-risk groups such as medical workers, police and fire departments, teachers, and the elderly. The 2001–2002 influenza vaccine guidelines from the Centers for Disease Control and Prevention (CDC) include three categories: those over sixty-five; people fifty to sixty-four years old who have chronic medical conditions (weakening their immune system and making them more susceptible to severe complications); and high-risk people such as health care workers and their families.

Flu vaccines are safer now than in earlier years, but the chances of the vaccine containing the specific antigen, or immune-triggering agent, that matches the *current* virus is estimated at a success rate of only fifty percent.

Influenza vaccines have a checkered history. In 1976, the swine flu created a national scare as experts predicted an influenza epidemic. Though it never materialized, a mass immunization program was initiated by the federal government under the order of President Gerald Ford. The experts acted aggressively and some forty million Americans were vaccinated. Ironically, the virus, unaffected by the vaccine, ran a benign and short-lived course on its own.

Critics say that the government reacted too strongly and the vaccine, untested at the time, caused about five hundred people to contract Guillain-Barré Syndrome (GBS), a sometimes fatal condition characterized by rapid onset of symptoms with inflammation of the peripheral nerves, those outside the brain and spinal cord, leading to debility and paralysis. About 50 percent of GBS victims report their condition started immediately after a case of influenza. Many recover, but the process can take several years with most patients never returning to normal strength and energy.

Influenza A is inhibited by a class of antiviral drugs called neuraminidase inhibitors, though they are not widely used by doctors because they are relatively new, not well understood, and there is concern about adverse effects. Amantadine hydrochloride and rimantadine hydrochloride are the two most common of these drugs and have been in use for a number of years. Two newer ones, zanamivir and oseltamivir, were approved in 1999 for the treatment of uncomplicated influenza A and B. Amantadine has a high degree of effectiveness in reducing the severity and duration of a flu but all these drugs have side effects that include nervousness, anxiety, lightheadedness, nausea, and vomiting. There is also concern about overuse causing the emergence of drug-resistant viruses that could make the drugs eventually ineffective.

Since vitamin C and other natural remedies also have been shown to reduce the severity and duration of the flu, and do not cause drug-resistance, it seems prudent to try natural medicines first. Natural medicines for the flu include Oscillococcinum, a French homeopathic medication prepared from the livers of Mallard ducks *(Anac barbariae)*. Many common herbal remedies are used for influenza including echinacea *(Echinacea purpurea* and *angustifolia)*; elder flowers *(Sambucus nigra)*; wild indigo *(Baptista tinctoria)*; boneset *(Eupatorium perfoliatum)*; and goldenseal *(Hydrastis canadensis)*. Strengthening the immune system with beta-1,3 glucan; zinc; other antioxidants in addition to vitamin C; and the Chinese herb astragalus *(Astragalus membranaceus)*; and other adaptogens, is helpful as a preventive measure. These measures are discussed in part 2.

Since China is the origin of most influenza virus strains, it is not surprising that Chinese doctors have developed many effective herbal medications for the treatment of the flu. Like the common cold, traditional Chinese medicine classifies influenza symptoms in the external disease category of *wen bing* and *biao zheng,* as discussed in the previous chapter. However, based upon symptoms, flu has a category of its own called *biao re,* or "wind-heat." The Chinese make a distinction between herbs that treat symptoms of the common cold and those that treat influenza and more virulent respiratory tract viral infections.

You may recall that "wind-cold" or *gan mao* was the Chinese diagnosis of the common cold. You may also remember that one of the distinctions between a cold and the flu is that during a case of the flu, the fever is much higher. The heat generated by the fever and accompanying inflammation is simply called "wind-heat," or *biao re* in Chinese, referring to an externally caused illness characterized by fever and inflammation. Herbs that treat wind-heat are febrifuges that help to lower fever and are considered cool in nature. Herbs that treat wind-cold are warming in nature and cause sweating. Many of the herbs used for the flu have been scientifically shown to contain antiviral, anti-inflammatory, and antifebrile properties. Many of these are discussed in part 2.

Individual Chinese herbs used for influenza include isatis *(Isatis tinctoria)*; andrographis *(Andrographis paniculata)*; bupleurum root *(Bupleurum falcatum)*; wild chrysanthemum flowers *(Chrysanthemum indicum)*; honeysuckle flowers *(Lonicera japonica)*; and houttuynia *(Houttuynia cordata)*. Unlike Western herbology, which uses individual herbs or a mixture of herbs with similar functions, in Chinese medicine herbs are combined into formulas that exert synergistic effects.[7] Two commonly used formulas for influenza are *yin chao san* and *zhong gan ling* (discussed in part 2).

Influenza Summary: Influenza appears to be a disease that will remain with us as long as pigs, ducks, chickens, and humans intermix. However, it is a disease that we can become more familiar with, and against which we can develop better and safer methods of prevention and treatment. As mentioned earlier, there is a high probability that another influenza pandemic will occur within the next ten years. Being prepared, by understanding the way influenza spreads and having a medicine chest of natural flu remedies, is wise. Exercise good judgment when considering use of the flu vaccine, and use antiviral drugs only as the medication of last resort. Prepare for seasonal illnesses and a possible flu pandemic by using natural remedies, especially Chinese medicine, to shorten its duration and intensity.

Warts

Human papilloma viruses (HPV) belong to the Papovaviridae family and cause common warts, plantar warts, and genital warts. There are over 80 known different types of HPV, and though most are benign, some types can develop into cancer. The most important of the potentially malignant type are those that occur in the female cervix, especially HPV types 16 and 18. These are found by a physician performing routine pelvic examinations and are often easily seen by eye or with a colposcope. An annual Papanicolaou staining smear (Pap test) is taken and sent to a pathology lab where the pathologist looks at the slide under a microscope to determine if any irregular cells are present. Cervical lesions are treated by freezing or cone biopsy.

Natural remedies for HPV include antioxidants, herbal medicines, homeopathic remedies, and antiviral suppositories that are inserted against the cervix. Though the natural medications used to treat HPV are safe, the proper application and correct dosages, as well as appropriate follow-up Pap smears, require the supervision of a naturopathic physician. Such care is outside the scope of this book, and I suggest you consult with a doctor skilled in natural gynecology.

Herpes Virus

Herpes viruses cause a variety of infections in humans, including cold sores, sexually transmitted infections, and neurological diseases, and they are also implicated in certain forms of cancer and chronic disease states like chronic fatigue immune deficiency syndrome (CFIDS). What makes herpes viruses such a potential problem is that 95 percent of the world's population harbors some form of herpes virus, and after initial exposure and primary infection, all of these viruses enter a dormant state within different tissues or cells, such as skin or cells of the nervous system. Infection is therefore permanent, and latency of the virus is lifelong.

Under most circumstances, the immune system is able to contain the virus or maintain it in a latent state. However, when the immune system is weakened, the virus may awaken and reactivate, causing disease. This characteristic makes the herpes viral family one of the most insidious of all the viruses, and is the reason some researchers think herpes viruses are responsible for many of the modern chronic ailments, such as CFIDS, multiple sclerosis, and even Alzheimer's.

If the concept that the stress of modern living and the exposure to environmental toxins contribute to immune deficiency is valid, then the potential for herpes viruses to remain latent in infected cells for years and even decades is cause for considerable concern for two reasons. First, because it is so common; and second, because of its effects, such as the central nervous system damage found in multiple sclerosis.

The virus can stay in a dormant state inside the nucleus of a cell without detection from the normal immune system, and because the viral genome is not being expressed the immune system is not even alerted to its presence. When the circumstances are ripe for reactivation—such as the use of immunosuppressive drugs, the development of AIDS or other infections, age-related immune decline, hormonal changes as accompany menstruation, or other causes—the viral genome begins to replicate.

The immune system reacts, but it may not be in time to control the infection caused by the reactivated virus, or it may not be sufficiently

Table 3: Herpes Viruses

Name	Numerical designation	Common name or abbreviation
Herpes simplex type 1	HHV-1	HSV-1, oral herpes
Herpes simplex type 2	HHV-2	HSV-2, genital herpes
Varicella-zoster	HHV-3	VZV, chicken pox, shingles
Epstein-Barr virus	HHV-4	EBV
Cytomegalovirus	HHV-5	CMV
Human herpesvirus 6	HHV-6	HHV-6
Human herpesvirus 7	HHV-7	HHV-7
Kaposi's sarcoma-associated herpesvirus	HHV-8	KSHV, Kaposi's sarcoma

effective. Severe, debilitating disease and even death can result from herpes viruses. In addition, since the virus is within the cells that make up body tissue, the immune system can react against itself and inappropriately start attacking the body's joints and muscles, causing a rheumatoid-like autoimmune inflammation.

There are eight known types of herpes virus that infect humans and all of them belong to the Herpesviridae family. Herpes viruses have been extensively studied and much is known about their structure. They are large viruses containing up to 150,000 nucleotide molecules, the smallest unit of information stored in the chromosome, in much the same way as data stored on a computer disc. The herpes genome is highly effective, and the viruses have an impressive array of biomolecular techniques to infect a host, invade the immune system, and survive. A numerical system is used to differentiate the types (see table 3).

Herpes Simplex: Herpes simplex (HSV-1 and -2) viruses are similar but cause different infections in humans. HSV-1 affects the upper part of the body, mostly the lips and gums, causing the familiar "cold sore," whereas HSV-2 primarily affects the lower part of the body, usually in the genital region. Both are spread by human contact: HSV-1 by kissing and HSV-2 by genital sex. Infection is divided into initial and latent infections, and since one person can be infected with both types, the first infection is called the primary infection.

If repeated outbreaks occur, which is common in both types of herpes simplex infections, they are called reactivations of the latent infection. Both types have outbreaks characterized by blisters that occur in the same area each time, and these can be very sore, uncomfortable, and unsightly. Mild systemic symptoms like fatigue and general malaise, or a mild "flu-like" feeling can also occur. The social stigma of genital herpes, though less now than in the 1980s, can still be the cause of considerable emotional stress.

Both HSV types appear on a cyclical basis. They reactivate when the immune system is at a lower ebb or are triggered by a variety of other causes. Many people know what conditions trigger their own outbreaks, such as a cold or flu, stress, or even menstruation. Interestingly, different types of light affect HSV viruses. Ultraviolet light can set off an occurrence in some people, reactivating cold sores from sun exposure. People who are sensitive to sunlight should use sun block or zinc oxide applied to the skin before exposure to the sun. Infrared light has the opposite effect; it can prevent or shorten outbreaks.

HSV-1 infection can also invade the eye (herpetic keratoconjunctivitis) and can lead to permanent damage of the eye and even loss of vision. Other complications of herpes simplex infection include meningitis and fatal encephalitis.

Acyclovir (acycloguanosine) is the drug of choice for treatment and prevention of both HSV-1 and -2 by conventional medical doctors. However, to be fully effective it must be given at the early stages of an outbreak. No treatment other than topical acyclovir is generally prescribed for local lesions (or boric acid washes for the eyes).

Studies have shown, and patient results have confirmed that supplementing with the amino acid lysine and reducing dietary intake of arginine-containing foods are helpful in preventing and managing outbreaks of herpes simplex. Arginine-containing foods include nuts, peanuts, and chocolate.

Physicians practicing natural therapies know from repeated clinical experience that herpes simplex can be controlled, sometimes completely, by enhancing the immune system and using natural antivirals such as olive leaf extract and plant tannins. Immune-enhancing nutrients like vitamin C, vitamin A, zinc, and selenium are also effective. Topical application of lemon balm *(Melissa officinalis)* extract has been shown to be helpful for cold sores (Wohlbling 1994).

Studies have shown, and patient results have confirmed that supplementing with the amino acid lysine and reducing dietary intake of arginine-containing foods are helpful in preventing and managing outbreaks of herpes simplex (Albert 1987). Arginine-containing foods include nuts, peanuts, and chocolate. Though lysine can be obtained from nonfat dairy products, it is best used as a supplement in dosages between 1,000 to 3,000 mg. (For detailed use of all of these nutrients and antiviral herbs, see part 2.)

Chinese herbal medicines can be very effective in the treatment of severe oral blisters and genital herpes. Formulas containing gentiana *(Gentiana macrophylla),* such as *long dan xia gan tang,* are particularly useful. For viral infections in the eye, the coptis-containing formula *nu huang jie du pian* (Bovine Bezoar Toxin-Resolving Pill) is effective. The use of these medications is discussed in part 2.

Varicella-Zoster Virus: Primary infection with varicella-zoster virus (VZV) causes chickenpox, a common childhood infection with an incubation period of about two weeks and resulting in the characteristic rash on the trunk of the body. Adults with chickenpox may have severe systemic symptoms affecting their whole body along with a widespread rash. Most cases of chickenpox run a benign course and conventional treatment is usually limited to bed rest and applying calamine lotion to control the itching. Natural medicine also recommends resting and application of calamine lotion, baking soda, or oatmeal baths to reduce itching, but also prescribes vitamin C, vitamin A, and echinacea to manage the virus.

Complications are rare in simple cases of chickenpox, but in immune-compromised patients, chickenpox can lead to pneumonia (varicella pneumonitis) and brain infections (post-infection encephalitis). Individuals with cancer, children with leukemia, AIDS patients, and those on immunosuppressing drugs, should be particularly careful if they are exposed to chickenpox.

Generally, after the primary infection, natural immunity takes place and the individual cannot be re-infected; however, like all herpes viruses, this virus goes into hiding. VZV remains latent for life, hiding in the nerve cells in the dorsal root ganglion along the spine. Facial nerves, like the trigeminal nerve, can also be affected. When the immune system is weakened, as when under stress, in older people, or when the immune system is compromised by another disease or drugs, the virus reactivates and causes a new condition called herpes zoster, or shingles, causing the skin to break out in painful blisters.

Shingles usually occur on the trunk of the body, but can also be in the lower back and waist, or on the face and head, including entry into the eye. The infected nerve itself can be damaged by the virus, leading to a condition called post-herpetic neuralgia, one of the most painful conditions known.

In the early 1980s, when I was first practicing, shingles was considered a disease of the elderly. At that time, most of the patients I saw for this condition were well into their eighties, with the youngest around sixty-five. Then, as environmental conditions changed and natural immunity became challenged, people started to have shingles at earlier and earlier ages, including children of five years old. In addition, with the advent of AIDS, shingles became a common secondary illness due to immune deficiency.

One of the most tragic cases of my career was that of a twenty-six-year-old man who developed herpes zoster in his right eye. This very handsome and athletic young man was one of the kindest patients I had met. He was very health-conscious and kept extremely fit with regular exercise as well as maintaining his professional dance career. His diet was largely vegetarian and he took adequate dosages of supplements, including extra antioxidants.

However, he was HIV-positive, and during a drawn-out stressful crisis involving his work, his immune system weakened and the herpes zoster virus reactivated. Due to the severity of the pain, he was admitted to the hospital, and once there declined very rapidly, dying of secondary infections within a month. It happened so fast, there was very little I was able to do for him.

Conventional treatment for shingles is limited to time, application of Zostrix, a cream containing extract of cayenne pepper, and the antiviral drug acylcovir or related drugs like famvir. However, these measures are mostly ineffective and the patients often suffer needlessly when there are good natural remedies available. Surgery is resorted to in severe cases, and I have seen patients with eyes removed in attempts to control herpetic-induced pain.

Luckily, if caught in time, there are alternatives for shingles and post-herpetic neuralgia. Acupuncture is effective in reducing the pain and shortens the duration of the attacks. Vitamin C, vitamin A, selenium, and zinc, along with olive leaf extract, are very helpful.

Two other cases illustrate how natural methods can help. Several years ago, two women, both in their thirties, came to my office in the same week with the same complaint: an itchy painful rash about the size of a half dollar on the cheek. Both had a case of herpes zoster.

The first had already been to her conventional medical doctor and the drugs prescribed did not work. When she came to my office, the pain was severe and the woman was in tears because of the unsightliness of the lesion.

I treated her daily with acupuncture and prescribed natural medications. Before the week was over, the pain was gone, she felt normal, and the rash was in retreat. By the end of eight days, it was completely gone. The other woman did not have much pain and was not inclined to use conventional medicine. She came to see me first. I treated her in the same way and the results were just as good as the first patient.

Epstein-Barr Virus: Epstein-Barr virus (EBV) has been called the most sinister of the herpes virus family because of its association with certain forms of cancer and its ability to reappear in chronic and reactivated forms. Remarkably, 80 to 95 percent of all adults worldwide have antibodies to EBV, which means that it is a common—almost ubiquitous—infection.

Primary infection occurs mainly in children or young adults and can cause no symptoms at all, mild flu-like symptoms, or infectious mononucleosis (the "kissing disease"), with symptoms of fever, sore and swollen throat, fatigue, and enlargement of the lymph nodes and spleen. Recovery from mononucleosis takes three to four weeks, but in severe cases, lassitude and fatigue can linger for months. However, complete return to normal is the rule. Like other herpes viruses, it then remains latent for life.

There are two types of EBV, the A and B forms. Type A is the most common form, but in equatorial Africa and with AIDS patients, type B can predominate. Both types can coexist in the same person and according to current knowledge, both types cause similar infections. EBV causes infection of the B-lymphocytes, important cells in second-line defense, and induces more than eighty known virus-specific antigens in the B cells. These antigens are important for the laboratory diagnosis of EBV, from which your doctor can tell if you have an active or chronic infection or if you merely have the immune markers from a previous, normal exposure without evidence of current or chronic infection.

EBV is also implicated in several forms of cancer: Burkitt's lymphoma, nasopharyngeal cancer, and B-cell lymphoma, and it has been linked to T-cell lymphomas and Hodgkin's disease. To date, most of these EBV-induced cancers occur in the Third World. However there is concern that in the developed countries, EBV causes other non-cancerous chronic diseases that may have connections to other cancers.

Epstein-Barr virus is implicated in numerous chronic diseases including fatigue syndromes. In the late 1970s and early 1980s, people started to complain of vague but persistent and often debilitating symptoms of fatigue and flu-like sensations. At first, doctors thought these symptoms were caused by ordinary neuroses or mild depression masquerading as tiredness. Since the victims were mostly women in their late twenties to mid-thirties who were often high achievers and overworked in professional jobs, the syndrome was dubbed the "yuppie flu."

However, in 1984 an outbreak of strange symptoms with a common fatigue profile among the patients took place in Incline Village, a small town on the Nevada side of Lake Tahoe. Symptoms included severe and persistent fatigue, "brain fog," and mildly swollen lymph glands—a condition very much like mononucleosis. However, the symptoms did not go away or resolve over a period of time, as mononucleosis would.

Even more strangely, when the individual started to feel better and exerted any amount of energy, such as trying to exercise, their symptoms worsened for two to three weeks afterwards. These relapses were a complete mystery to medical doctors and a source of considerable anxiety for the patients.

Paul Cheney, a family practice physician in Incline Village, was among the first to suggest that the cause for this pattern was EBV. The syndrome became referred to as chronic Epstein-Barr virus (CEBV). However since then, researchers have failed to conclusively prove that all cases of chronic fatigue, now called Chronic Fatigue Syndrome (CFS) or Chronic Fatigue Immune Deficiency Syndrome (CFIDS), have positive laboratory evidence of active or chronic active EBV infection. Cheney, pursuing the disease further, found that a majority of blood samples of CFIDS patients tested positive for HTLV-1 and HTLV-2, a retrovirus related to HIV, and discussed in the next section. However, he was unable to conclusively prove that this virus was the specific cause rather than EBV.

While more and more patients turned up at doctors' offices with the same pattern of symptoms, the controversy whether chronic fatigue was an organic disease caused by a virus or a stress-related psychological disease akin to depression continues to this day. Most conventional doctors were completely baffled by CFIDS, as they still are, having no training in medical school on how to diagnosis or manage such an illness. Eventually complications to CFIDS started to appear: fibromyalgia, irritable bowel syndrome, leaky gut syndrome, and cognitive disorders like poor memory and reduced ability to concentrate.

For CFIDS, some of the typical presentations are psychological symptoms; it is therefore not surprising that medical doctors, who diagnose largely by the presenting symptoms, would think that the cause was depression. Patients with this condition often feel hopeless and become depressed, and experience mood changes that include irritability and bouts of unexplained anger.

In the early and mid-1980s, I treated scores of such patients. One in particular comes to mind: a medical professional herself and an athlete, this woman suffered from recurrent sore throats, debilitating fatigue, and significant mood changes which included depression, irritability, and hopelessness. For several years she was unable to work at her own clinical practice. She traveled extensively in an unsuccessful search for a definitive diagnosis and effective treatment, including trips to several of the top university research centers in the country. In the end, what seemed to work best was simply time, rest, and vitamins and minerals. She gradually improved enough to return to her work, but never recovered completely and never obtained a definitive diagnosis.

A profound lack of will is an interesting aspect of chronic Epstein-Barr virus infection, but it is distinctively different from common or classical depression. However, many medical doctors, not understanding chronic fatigue or the difference in mood between clinical depression and fatigue states, continue to diagnosis chronic fatigue patients with depression.

When the selective serotonin re-uptake inhibitor (SSRI) antidepressants (like Prozac) came out, conventional medicine thought these drugs were the solution to the chronic fatigue problem. The reasoning went something like this: if the condition was a biochemically induced depression related to serotonin, this class of drugs should work—another case of the "magic bullet" mentality, and one that completely ignored social, psychological, and environmental conditions.

However, in my clinical experience I have seen patient after patient with fatigue syndromes try Prozac or Paxil and later tell me they had no improvement or that their mood was slightly better but they still were just as fatigued as ever. Though antidepressants can sometimes play a complementary role in the treatment of this condition, SSRIs do not cure chronic fatigue syndrome and are not very effective in the treatment of depression related to EBV infection.

In his groundbreaking book *Chronic Fatigue Syndrome: The Hidden Epidemic*, Jesse Stoff, M.D., one of the original proponents of the chronic EBV theory,[7] stated that EBV can cause a transient state of immune deficiency (different from acquired immune deficiency syndrome, AIDS) leading to chronic disease which is CFIDS in its mild form. In its severe form, EBV can penetrate the nervous system, causing encephalitis, Guillain-Barré syndrome, and a condition called transverse myelitis, a neurological syndrome characterized by the rapid development of leg weakness.

Transverse myelitis is a condition similar to multiple sclerosis (MS), and though little is known about its cause, most evidence indicates that it is triggered by an infection, such as from viruses in the herpes family. This condition is most likely a repercussion of the immune system attacking the whole nervous system trying to get at the virus lodged in the nerve cells. It's like a pack of dogs tearing up your yard to get at a few gophers.

In addition, according to Dr. Stoff, chronic EBV can contribute to numerous other inflammatory conditions like myocarditis, pneumonitis, and pancreatitis, as well as metabolic disorders like diabetes and hypothyroidism.

Besides affecting the nervous system, one of the primary targets of EBV is the liver. A liver chronically affected by a low-grade viral infection may not show signs of cellular damage for twenty or more years, if ever. However, its function will be impaired, consequently affecting metabolism and many other processes in the body, all of which can impair one's health.

Cytomegalovirus and Stealth Viruses: Cytomegalovirus (CMV), another member of the herpes family, can be passed from mother to fetus during pregnancy, while breast-feeding, or from the urine or saliva of other infants if they lay together, such as in childcare. Adolescents and young adults can acquire it from kissing and sex. It can also be contracted from contaminated blood during a transfusion, and from infected donated organs. Like other herpes viruses, once CMV is acquired it lasts for life, lying dormant in the body with the capacity for reactivation. At least 50 percent of Americans over forty years old test positive for exposure to CMV.

Active CMV infection is similar to mononucleosis without the sore throat and swollen lymph glands. AIDS patients are particularly at risk for serious CMV infection, as are those undergoing organ transplant using immune-suppressing drugs.

CMV appears to be the perfect virus. Often first contracted in infancy, its transmission is usually unnoticed. In later years, its transmission is usually through sexual activity, and if any symptoms arise, and often they do not, it only causes an illness similar to mononucleosis. Diagnosis is therefore often missed. Then, undetected by the immune system, it remains latent until the situation is right for reactivation. In an immune-compromised individual, its reactivation can cause severe illness with secondary, and sometimes fatal, infection of the lungs.

CMV is involved in chronic disease and causes a wide range of neurological and autoimmune illnesses while remaining undetected by the immune system and undiagnosed by medical professionals. Therefore, it often goes untreated. Inflammation caused by CMV infection is also thought to contribute to heart disease by exacerbating atherogenic lesions, or plaques, that form in the blood vessels of the heart.[8] Perhaps the most devious design of CMV is its possible role in hidden brain infections.

W. John Martin, M.D., Ph.D., director of the Center for Complex Infectious Disease in Rosemead, California, investigates complex neurological disease and CFIDS and believes he has identified a new class of cytopathic (cell killing) viruses, which he calls "stealth viruses" (Martin 1994). In his studies, he has found that there is considerable laboratory and clinical evidence to suggest that patients with CFIDS and neurological diseases like MS and transverse myelitis are suffering from an atypical viral infection, most likely caused by a form of CMV, but he also has found positive evidence for other herpes viruses like EBV, HSV, and HHV-6.

Dr. Martin's clinical research has lead him to hypothesize that a new class of virus, derived from herpes virus and capable of evading detection from the immune system, is a possible cause for the wide range of new complex diseases, including CFIDS, fibromyalgia, the increasing incidences of MS, and some forms of psychosis.

Like Dr. Stoff, Dr. Martin has also found viral evidence in other tissue. Liver, thyroid, muscle, skin, salivary glands, urinary tract, and intestinal tract, and diseases related to these organs and tissues all interplay in his stealth virus paradigm. In this paradigm, he suggests that these viruses use cytokines (immune system proteins that affect the behavior of other cells) as a growth factor.

Dr. Martin's treatment strategies make sense in light of this idea. Primary treatment is aimed at regulating cytokine activity. Suppression of viral activation and replication by antibiotics and antivirals is reserved for severe cases only. Relying mainly on natural medications, primarily quercitin, a flavonoid antioxidant with anti-reverse transcriptase (an enzyme that is an essential component of retroviruses) activity, Dr. Martin employs a wide range of natural substances and practices, dietary recommendations, and nutritional supplements that support cellular metabolism, such as antioxidants, amino acids, and essential fatty acids.

In addition, he suggests stress reduction, behavior modification, and other strategies including antidepressants and nootrophics (brain-enhancing medications) to improve neurological function. Finally, he recommends evaluation and treatment for secondary conditions such as hypothyroidism, correction of bowel ecology, adrenal enhancement, allergy testing, and improvement of blood circulation—treatments that are very much in accordance with the way a naturopathic physician would treat.

Dr. Martin's clinical research has lead him to hypothesize that a new class of virus, derived from herpes virus and capable of evading detection from the immune system, is a possible cause for the wide range of new complex diseases, including CFIDS, fibromyalgia, the increasing incidences of MS, and some forms of psychosis.

Though Dr. Martin's work is not finished, the direction of his research is correct and fits all the criteria that I present in this book. First, it comes out of a thought process that allows for complex disease patterns caused by evolutionarily adapted infectious organisms, in this case, a stealth virus. Second, it does not attempt to eradicate the virus with a treatment that may be worse than the cure; instead it neutralizes its growth factors. Third, he uses supportive natural medications to improve the function of other vital systems of the body, allowing for greater immune strength and organ reserve (the term used to describe the normal tissue health and immune status of an organ). We need more physicians like Dr. Martin.

Human Herpesvirus 6: One of the newest members of the herpes family, human herpesvirus-6 (HHV-6), was discovered by Robert Gallo, M.D., in 1986. Like its cousins EBV and CMV, HHV-6 is usually acquired early in life. In children, it causes roseola, a common childhood infection with symptoms of fever, sometimes convulsions suggesting central nervous system involvement, and a characteristic rash on the trunk of the child's body. When contracted later in life, it may cause a mono-like illness. After the initial infection, which can be silent in both children and adults, the virus goes into latency. Also like the other two herpes viruses, when reactivation of HHV-6 occurs, it can cause CFIDS and other chronic neurological diseases, including MS. Unbelievably, an estimated 90 percent of adult Americans have antibodies to HHV-6, meaning they have been exposed to it.

There are two known variations: HHV-6A and HHV-6B. Another form, HHV-7, has also been identified causing illnesses similar to HHV-6. This virus infects the T lymphocytes, a type of white blood cell, and researchers believe that it is capable of disabling key components of the immune system, especially the CD4+ T lymphocytes. HHV-6 can also destroy natural killer (NK) cells, part of the first line defense against viral infection and cancer.

Coincidentally, NK cells are also disabled in both CFIDS patients and AIDS victims. Donald Carrigan, Ph.D., the foremost American HHV-6 researcher, believes HHV-6 can be a co-infection contributing to the immune deficiency associated problems in both diseases. Carrigan's colleague, Konnie Knox, Ph.D., has conclusively found evidence from autopsy tissue samples that HHV-6 is extremely active at the time of death in AIDS patients, suggestive that it, and not HIV, is the viral killing factor in AIDS. Her doctoral dissertation, "Human Herpesvirus Six (HHV-6): Evidence for Its Role as a Cofactor in the Pathogenesis of AIDS" (Carrigan et al. 1996), further supports Carrigan's theory (Regush 2000).

Herpes Virus Summary: Nearly every adult is infected by one or more members of the herpes virus family. Usually acquired in childhood or infancy, herpes viruses are latent for life. Though they are common in humans and generally are considered to be more inconvenient than life-threatening, in a world of increasing immune incompetence, herpes viruses can become lethal causing severe and debilitating symptoms. At least one member of this family, HHV-6, is linked to AIDS either as a cofactor or as the cause of death. HHV-6 is an extremely potent and dangerous virus, one that most people have been exposed to and now carry in their bodies.

As immune dysfunction is becoming increasingly more common,

it seems prudent that more research be focused on it. In the meantime, I suggest doctors familiarize themselves with the consequences of chronic herpes infections and the effective natural ways to treat them.

EBV is one of the most insidious of all the herpes viruses and can cause or participate in a wide range of illnesses. Conventional medical doctors, who diagnose from symptoms and standard blood tests, will most likely miss a diagnosis of CEBV, CMV, or HIV-6. Specialized blood tests are required (see the appendix).

There is no one-shot drug for herpes viruses. Most viral diseases are ineffectively controlled by drugs and only HSV-1 responds well to pharmaceutical antiviral drugs. However, keep in mind that if you have a life-threatening viral infection, drug therapy might save your life, but a better approach is to prevent viral infection and to strengthen the immune system with the natural therapies listed in part 2. Many of these natural medications effectively treat herpes infections.

Retroviruses and HIV

Though the overwhelming majority of AIDS researchers support the theory that human immunodeficiency virus (HIV) causes AIDS, the HHV-6 controversy of a stealth virus or deadly cofactor and other equally confusing issues continue to overlap with AIDS research, causing considerable concern. This issue of what actually are the real viral dynamics in immunodeficiency states is extremely important for individual and global future health. If the dominant consensus is wrong, then government and research establishments have wasted tens of billions of dollars and years of time going in the wrong direction. Even if they are correct, the final chapter on AIDS is far from being written, and certainly the nineteenth-century infectious model based on Koch's postulate is not working well enough in the twenty-first century. A more comprehensive evolutionary approach would be helpful.

Since 1884, when Robert Koch (1843–1910), a German physician who won the Nobel Prize for medicine in 1905, presented his theory, the idea that infectious microbes like bacteria and viruses cause disease has been one of the cornerstones of Western medicine. However, it has become more accepted that the immune status of the host contributes to resistance to infection and influences virulence.

The evolutionary model suggests that disease is the result of *inter-action* between the host and the microbe, and is not simply based upon the strength of the infectious agent.[9] The model of Chinese medicine takes it a step further: the *strength* of the host's immune system is the primary factor in *preventing* infectious disease.

A Brief History of HIV: The retrovirus family, of which HIV is a member, is not new to virologists, and was first identified in the early years of virology. In 1910, Peyton Rous, M.D., working with the Rockefeller Institute for Medical Research in New York, discovered a virus (avian sarcoma virus) that caused tumors in chickens; for his research he was awarded a Nobel Prize. In 1930, other tumor-causing retroviruses were discovered in mice and other animals, including feline leukemia virus—a disease that causes immune deficiency and death in cats. In 1978, the first human retrovirus, human T-cell leukemia virus type 1 (HTLV-1), was discovered by Robert Gallo, the same scientist who discovered HHV-6.

During the late 1970s and early 1980s, while laboratory scientists were laboring over individual viruses, clinicians were trying to unravel the causes of a new fatigue syndrome with life-threatening respiratory infectious complications. Paul Cheney, still on the trail of CFIDS, moved on from thinking of EBV as the sole cause and developed a theory, based on the available lab tests of the time, that HTLV was the possible causative agent for CFIDS. Then a new and more severe form of fatigue syndrome developed, casting an even more somber tone on both the clinical and laboratory scene.

Joseph Sonnabend, a New York medical doctor, reported numerous cases of gay men with unusual and complicated illnesses characterized by profound immunodeficiency with a common element, the development of fatal *Pneumocystis carinii* pneumonia (PCP). In 1981, the condition was named acquired immune deficiency syndrome (AIDS).

A virus was suspected and reactivated CMV was first considered the most likely candidate because it often occurred in the later stages of the illness. In 1983, Luc Montagnier, a cancer researcher at the Pasteur Institute in Paris, uncovered a new retrovirus in the *Lentivirus* genus: human immunodeficiency virus (HIV). The Latin root, *lentus,* means "slow." Gallo and his coworkers later confirmed HIV's involvement by independent research, and eventually two types were identified: HIV-1 and HIV-2. However, Sonnabend and other practicing physicians still argued that AIDS was a syndrome, or constellation of many factors, including various possible viruses, that together contributed to the disease rather than it being caused by only one infectious agent.

In fact, questions still circulate concerning both Montagnier's and Gallo's research about a positively identified, unique HIV genome. Debate continues to this day whether a unique AIDS virus in fact exists, if HIV is the sole cause or an opportunistic virus, and what the role of other immune factors in the progression of the disease is.

Essentially, the confusion arises from a difference of paradigms. The "old school" of medical science still favors the single-agent, or one-cause, theory. Researchers look for one infectious organism and then attempt to develop a vaccine or drug to kill it. Koch's Postulate of 1884 is still used, which states that the infectious organism must be found in all patients with the same disease; that the organism can be isolated and cultivated in the laboratory outside of the infected host; that a similar disease should develop when infecting animals with the laboratory organism; and that the same organism should be recovered from the inoculated experimental animals.

Old-school practitioners do not favor theories based on lifestyle or a broader view of disease, which is the realm of evolutionary thinkers who view AIDS as a product of our times, related to environment, lifestyle, and perhaps reconstituted viruses—but not to a single causative agent.

Further AIDS Controversy: Even though the Durban Declaration, delivered at the Thirteenth International AIDS Conference in Durban, South Africa, in May and June of 2000, tried to put the AIDS controversy to rest by affirming Koch's Postulate stating that all patients with AIDS are infected with HIV and that HIV is the causative agent of AIDS, numerous influential scientists continue to disagree. Among the dissenters are Peter Duesberg, Ph.D., a microbiologist at the University of California at Berkeley, and Eleni Papadopulos-Eleopulos, Ph.D., a researcher from the Royal Perth Hospital in Australia and head of the Perth Group.

Papadopulos-Eleopulos is convinced that the decrease in CD4+ T cells seen in AIDS is not due to destruction by HIV but is caused by lifestyle-induced immune deterioration. In one paper, she proposed that oxidative cellular damage, the negative effects of oxygen activity on cellular molecules, is one of the critical steps in the progression of immune deficiency.

Not ending her case there, she has published numerous other articles defending her group's theory, and has offered an explanation for the African AIDS epidemic. She contends that HIV-positive blood tests do not prove it is the cause of AIDS since the symptoms and diseases African victims experience are identical to tuberculosis, diarrheal diseases, parasitic infections, and other diseases that have existed in Africa since Egyptian times.

Duesberg also questions the proposition that the cause of AIDS is the retrovirus HIV. He has referred to the AIDS virus as a harmless "passenger" virus, just another virus among many living parasitically in the human body, and he claims that a positive HIV test is merely a viral marker (and not indicative of the cause) indicating immune system damage.

In his opinion, based upon exhaustive research, AIDS is an immune deficiency disorder caused by overuse of recreational drugs and a lifestyle that burns the candle at both ends, including promiscuous sex. Eventually, the immune system collapses. Then pre-existing latent viruses reactivate: some cause illness like CMV and others, like HIV, proliferate but are only along for the ride. Finally, other opportunistic infections take over, like candidiasis *(Candida albicans)* and *Pneumocystis pneumonia,* which eventually kill the patient.

The debate continues: the majority still favor the one-cause-fits-all theory and the dissidents support an evolutionary theory that makes sense but that cannot yet be conclusively proven. From my clinical perspective, if Duesberg and Papadolpulos-Eleopulos were correct, AIDS patients would recover with rest, change of lifestyle, and nutritional supportive medications. If infectious symptoms are managed with antibiotics, antifungals, and antivirals, patients should improve and recover. But they do not.

Nutritional support and natural therapies do make a substantial difference in how AIDS patients feel by reducing their symptoms, but in themselves they have not been found to be curative. So what is happening with the immune function of these patients?

According to some experts, such as Papadolpulos-Eleopulos, the answer lies not in how the body recovers, but in how gradual, irreparable cellular damage occurs, caused by environmental toxins, drugs, and stress. Like the saying, "You can make a pickle out of a cucumber, but not a cucumber out of a pickle," once a certain cellular line has been crossed, the tissues are incapable of returning to a completely normal state. However, this is not the end of the story.

To further complicate matters, Howard B. Urnovitz, Ph.D., a microbiologist with Calypte Biomedical in Berkeley, California, has challenged the notions of the monkey origin of AIDS. According to Dr. Urnovitz (elegantly documented in *The River* [1999] by Edward Hooper), AIDS was caused by oral polio vaccine contaminated with monkey virus causing a recombined hybrid virus, HIV-1. If this is the case, given the right circumstances, then additional millions of people worldwide will start showing symptoms of immune deficiency. Further, in those people who have suffered genetic damage, this damage will be passed on to their children and their children's children.

Hooper's book caused enough controversy to stimulate some researchers into action, and three short papers were published in the journal *Nature* in 2001 exonerating polio vaccines (Weiss 2001). Still, Hooper and others are unsatisfied and continue to press the contamination theory. It may be a long time before we ever know the real origins of human immunodeficiency disease.

An even more sinister scenario was proposed and documented by Leonard Horowitz, a Tufts- and Harvard-educated dentist with a Master's degree in public health, in his controversial book, *Emerging Viruses: AIDS & Ebola, Nature, Accident, or Intentional* (1996). Horowitz's worst-case scenario, his primary theory, is of a CIA-conducted biological weapons experiment gone wild. His alternative theory is similar to Hooper's: the accidental outbreak from contaminated vaccines. Neither of Horowitz's theories have been conclusively proven, but due to the seriousness of his accusations, both deserve further investigation.

Not only are the causative factors questioned, but the progression of AIDS is also disputed. Louis J. Picker, M.D., associate director of the Vaccine and Gene Therapy Institute at Oregon Health and Sciences University in Portland, Oregon, argues that there is no direct association between levels of HIV-specific CD4+ T cells and disease progression, and suggests that lowered levels of these cells in AIDS patients could be a countermeasure by the immune system to reduce target cell levels so the virus has fewer activated cells to attack.

Not all HIV-positive patients progress to full AIDS. I have encountered many of these individuals in my own practice. By practicing a healthy lifestyle that includes nutritional supplements, antioxidants, antiviral herbal medications, and immune-enhancing substances, they remain active and lead normal lives. Many, like basketball star Magic Johnson, are able to lead high-performance, athletic lifestyles.

A few HIV-positive patients, over time and after up to ten years of treatment with natural therapies and lifestyle changes, have tested negative for the virus. Though very few researchers are investigating the role of natural immunity in minimizing or preventing AIDS, some believe that the immune system has the ability to contain and even eliminate the virus completely.

Urnovitz reports that in a study of seven patients, at least five with confirmed exposure to HIV, none of the seven subjects had any symptoms of AIDS, and two of the patients who previously tested positive for HIV by urine samples later tested negative (Barnum 1993). In an interview with a British medical journal, Urnovitz is quoted as saying, "What this tells me is that there is hope in reversing HIV infection if we pay attention to how to do it" (Stolberg 1993).

This study suggests that immunity may play a larger role in preventing and eventually halting the spread of AIDS. Though documentation for these cases is still lacking and more research and publications are needed, our immune systems may win the race between science and nature.

This study suggests that immunity may play a larger role in preventing and eventually halting the spread of AIDS. Though documentation for these cases is still lacking and more research and publications are needed, our immune systems may win the race between science and nature.

Is There a CFIDS-AIDS Continuum? Though each condition is still looked at as an independent disease, after I carefully sifted through all the differences of opinion, one common thread emerged and one immense question remained unanswered. Are CFIDS (chronic fatigue complicated by immune deficiency)[10] and AIDS related conditions on a continuum of immune system breakdown, rather than different conditions with specific viral infections?

As I will describe in a later chapter, though a viral trigger is suspected in about 80 percent of CFIDS cases, the syndrome does not have a single obvious viral cause that can be substantiated by lab tests. Therefore, from the point of view of the conventional biomedical model, both are distinct disease entities: HIV causes AIDS while CFIDS has not been linked to a virus.

Though research has found that both conditions display immune deficiency patterns, to my knowledge, few researchers are pursuing this line of thought. Nancy Klimas M.D., of the University of Miami School of Medicine in Florida, is one of those investigating the immunological abnormalities in chronic fatigue patients. Her work suggests a gradual progression of the illness, starting with a genetic predisposition and a triggering event or series of events, such as a viral infection complicated by immune system weakening as occurs in stress or from toxic exposure (Klimas 1990).

In a world out of balance with environmental pollution at unprecedented levels, ecological disruption, overwhelming psychological stress, repeated wars and violent civil strife tearing individual lives and entire countries apart, abuse of stimulant drugs, sexual promiscuity, and over-use of pharmaceutical drugs causing microbial drug-resistance, immune system disruption may be the root cause of a variety of apparently different but actually similar diseases.

Treatment Options: Despite the fact that HIV has become the most medicated viral disease in medical history, there still is no cure. In a stunning article published in *The Scientist*, Myrna Watanabe writes (2001): "Despite billions of dollars spent in research funding and a brief reprieve in Western nations after the introduction of multidrug therapy, AIDS continues to win its battle against humankind."

In the face of such evidence, the current treatment remains the use of several drugs at the same time—multidrug therapy. Initially heralded as a possible cure because patients showed early improvement, this aggressive "cocktail therapy" appears to cause more harm than good, and creates drug-resistant viral strains at an alarming rate. The side effects are severe, including liver damage.

Even when symptomatically effective, it does not kill all of the virus, which has developed ways of hiding out in the memory cells of the immune system, a strategy similar to latency. In this case, however, the dormancy is a response to pharmaceutical medications. When the drugs are discontinued, the virus emerges from these temporary reservoirs and rebounds, causing renewed infection—the drugs having only masked the symptoms without effectively treating the underlying cause.

Until recently, people with AIDS in Africa, India, and the world's poor countries could not afford drugs. However, pirated patents are now available at a fraction of the cost in the United States and Europe, and some drug companies bowing to international pressure have made generic drugs available. In the next few years, drug treatment for HIV will skyrocket. Even at reduced costs, poorer nations will not be able to afford medications without bankrupting their already strained economies.

In the developed nations, AIDS has become a severe chronic disease that one lives with for years under the management of extensive drugs, before eventually succumbing to an opportunistic infection. Considerable evidence suggests that natural and alternative therapies can have significant influence on managing the infection in the early stages and in slowing progression over the course of the disease. Rather than a single factor, such as a virus, influencing outcome, HIV infection is influenced by many different factors including genetic susceptibility, response to therapy, nutritional status, immune status at the time of infection, metabolic and hormonal changes, and previous infections such as latent CMV.

An AIDS vaccine, if an effective one is found, is still at least another ten years away. Seth Berkley, M.D., an epidemiologist and head of the International AIDS Vaccine Initiative, a global call for action launched at the United Nations General Assembly special session on HIV/AIDS, June 2000, contends that a vaccine is our last and best hope of halting the AIDS epidemic. I agree that searching for a vaccine is important, but without radically altering how we *live* in this world, deadly viral diseases will continue to defy the notion that we have superiority over nature.

The Perfect Virus: HIV may be nature's perfect virus. It spreads by an act common to almost all humans, sexual activity, and infection progresses slowly, allowing for a host carrier to spread it to other individuals before full symptoms appear. It invades specific cells of the immune system causing increased vulnerability to a wide variety of fatal infections. It has proven impossible to eradicate; mutates rapidly, defying antiviral drugs; and when suppressed by drugs, it is capable of lying latent indefinitely.

It is challenging modern medicine's superiority complex and altering economies and the politics of nations, especially in Africa and Asia. In a matter of two decades it shattered conventional medical opinion from one of arrogance and complacency about infectious diseases to a more realistic awareness that new diseases continuously emerge. The AIDS pandemic has defied our notion of superiority and shocked infectious disease theorists at their roots because HIV infection does not follow Koch's Postulate.

AIDS also forced social changes by opening the closet doors on homosexuality; it altered people's sex lives and birthed a new genre of literature, theatre, film, and painting. It brought increased awareness of the global disparity between the rich and poor, and by entrenching itself in the most vulnerable communities and countries: mostly poor, uneducated, and people of color. It has called our attention to the greatest moral issue of our time. AIDS also served to accelerate the acceptance of alternative medicine and stimulated new research into the areas of nutrition and natural antivirals.

Hepatitis

Hepatitis, a general medical term for liver inflammation, is not caused by only one virus. Though many different viruses cause infections in the liver, including Epstein-Barr virus, three main viruses cause damage to human liver cells, the hepatocytes, resulting in true hepatitis (see table 4).

Hepatitis A: Infectious hepatitis, or hepatitis A (HAV), is caused by an RNA virus of the Picornaviridae family, the same group that includes poliovirus and rhinovirus, that causes the common cold, and HAV is contracted through feces containing viral particles that then contaminate water or food consumed by humans. It can also be transmitted through blood transfusions, shared needles, and sexual contact. Minor HAV outbreaks occur regularly in the United States but as it is still a common disease in third world countries, and care should be taken when traveling overseas to have only well-cooked food and bottled water.

Table 4: Common Hepatitis Viruses

Name	Numerical designation	Route of transmission	Family name	Genetic type
Hepatitis A	HAV	oral-fecal	Picornaviridae	RNA
Hepatitis B	HBV	blood and body fluids	Hepadnaviridae	DNA
Hepatitis C	HCV	blood, other	Flaviviridae	RNA

After an incubation period of two to six weeks, symptoms of fatigue, vague abdominal discomfort, and fever occur. Jaundice, the classic sign of hepatitis (yellowing of the skin and whites of the eyes), follows. Generally HAV is a short-lived acute infection that passes without complications. However, if the immune system is run down, it can cause severe fatigue and illness enough to make you bedridden for a month. Though prevention is the main way of avoiding infection, there is an effective inactivated vaccine available and human immunoglobulin shots give temporary natural immunity for people traveling in endemic areas, such as India. Herbal remedies are used in India, Nepal, and China to treat HAV.

Hepatitis B: Hepatitis B (HBV), sometimes referred to as serum hepatitis, is a serious blood-borne viral illness that can lead to chronic liver disease, liver cancer, or in the case of severe rapid infection (a condition called fulminate hepatitis) it can cause death. It is a member of the Hepadnaviridae family and is transmitted in blood and other body fluids, like semen and breast milk.

A highly contagious disease, HBV can be contracted through sexual intercourse, the use of contaminated needles (including unsterilized hypodermic and acupuncture needles, tattoo needles, and needles shared by drug addicts), and through blood transfusions. It is endemic in China and other parts of Asia where up to 20 percent of the general population is infected; it is less common in Europe and North America. There are an estimated 350 million HBV carriers worldwide.

HBV has been studied extensively both in the laboratory and clinic, so today there are several accurate laboratory tests to show if you have ever been exposed to HBV and if you have developed effective immunity against it. Despite the extensive knowledge about HBV, there is no effective treatment available in Western medicine. First generation live vaccines, introduced in the late 1900s, caused several deaths and considerable controversy. Though a genetically engineered vaccine has been developed and is reported to be safe (it requires a series of shots with a booster every five years), until the vaccine is proven to be completely safe and effective, caution is strongly advised in its use.

Since the incidence of infection is so high in China, HBV has been recognized for centuries and many traditional herbal medicines are used to treat its acute and chronic states. Several of these herbal formals, such as *sho-saiko-to* (Japanese for *xiao chai hu tang*, or minor bupleurum decoction), have also been shown by modern scientific studies to be effective in the management of HBV (see part 2).

Hepatitis C: In the mid-1970s, around the same time AIDS and CFIDS symptoms first appeared, another new infection was emerging. Originally called non-A, non-B hepatitis, it was first found in blood transfusion patients. Named hepatitis C (HCV) in 1989, it was first described as a new virus in *Science* (Choo et al. 1989) and has since become the most prevalent infectious disease and the most important liver condition in the United States and Canada, with an estimated four million Americans infected. Currently 8,000 to 10,000 deaths occur each year in the United States alone due to HCV. Worldwide, 170 million people are infected—more than four times as many as HIV.

ORIGINS AND TRANSMISSION: Like HIV, the origins of the hepatitis C epidemic remain obscure and speculative. An RNA virus, HCV belongs to the Flaviviridae family, the same group of viruses that includes yellow fever and dengue. There are currently one hundred identified strains of HCV.

HCV is considered a blood-borne virus, but many cases report no contact with any possible source of contaminated blood. This mystery has yet to be solved; however, it appears there are modes of transmission other than blood. Known sources of infection include injection drug use, needle-stick accidents by health workers, contact with infected blood products, sexual contact with menstrual blood in infected persons, infants born to infected women, tattoos, and shared toothbrushes and razors. Though a mosquito vector was ruled out by researchers in the late 1990s, preliminary studies by French scientists at the Hospital Pasteur in Paris strongly suggest that some HCV cases may be mosquito-transmitted.

THE COURSE OF HCV INFECTION: Though acute HCV infection can sometimes lead to death, the majority of cases develop silent and slow-progressing infections, called chronic hepatitis C. In these cases, cirrhosis and hepatocelluar carcinoma are the predominant causes of death. However, at least 15 percent of cases resolve completely without complications, and even many cases of chronic infection remain stable and do not develop into cirrhosis. In the majority of cases, symptoms only appear when advanced liver disease has already developed, although some individuals complain of fatigue, joint pain, and itching during the early course of the disease.

Disease progression appears to be more rapid in elderly and immune-compromised individuals. In addition, slow progressive liver disease causes fibrosis—or hardening of the liver tissue—which greatly impairs liver function. Alcohol consumption and HIV infection accelerate the progression of HCV.

When this impairment is severe enough, even without cirrhosis—the end stage of liver fibrosis—a variety of systemic conditions can develop: ascites (a buildup of fluid in the abdomen); esophageal varices (bleeding from varicose veins); stagnation of blood in the veins of the legs complicated by edema; reduced immune function; fatigue; and mental confusion. Hepatocellular carcinoma, or cancer of the liver cells, is the worst-case scenario and generally leads to death (see figure 2-3).

TREATMENT OPTIONS: Medications of choice include interferon alpha—a chemical messenger produced naturally by the immune system—administered by injection, and the oral antiviral agent Ribavirin, a nucleoside analog. Even so, they are ineffective, cause considerable side effects, and this therapy is very expensive. Meta-analysis has shown that interferon alpha, when given for one year, has an effective rate of only 16–23 percent, and the cost for forty-eight weeks of combined treatment is around $20,000. As in AIDS, combination therapy has become popular, although interferon plus Ribavirin produce a sustained response in only 40 percent of patients. (See table 5 for a summary of drug approaches to viruses.)

However, once the drugs are discontinued, most patients relapse and only 50 percent of patients who relapse and are treated with a second course respond favorably. This is a dismal clinical picture. Liver transplant, a life-saving measure, is reserved for patients with end-stage liver disease, though mild HCV infection to the transplanted liver occurs in most of these patients.

SIDE EFFECTS: Side effects of therapy are common and frequently debilitating, with the majority of patients experiencing severe flu-like symptoms. Tachycardia (rapid heart rate), restlessness, irritability, depression, and insomnia may also occur. Bone marrow suppression and severe neuropsychiatric disorders, including suicidal depression, may occur later in therapy. Conventional treatment of side effects is based on symptoms and includes the use of acetaminophen, electrolyte management, and selective serotonin re-uptake inhibiting antidepressants. Alternative treatments for side effects, which include

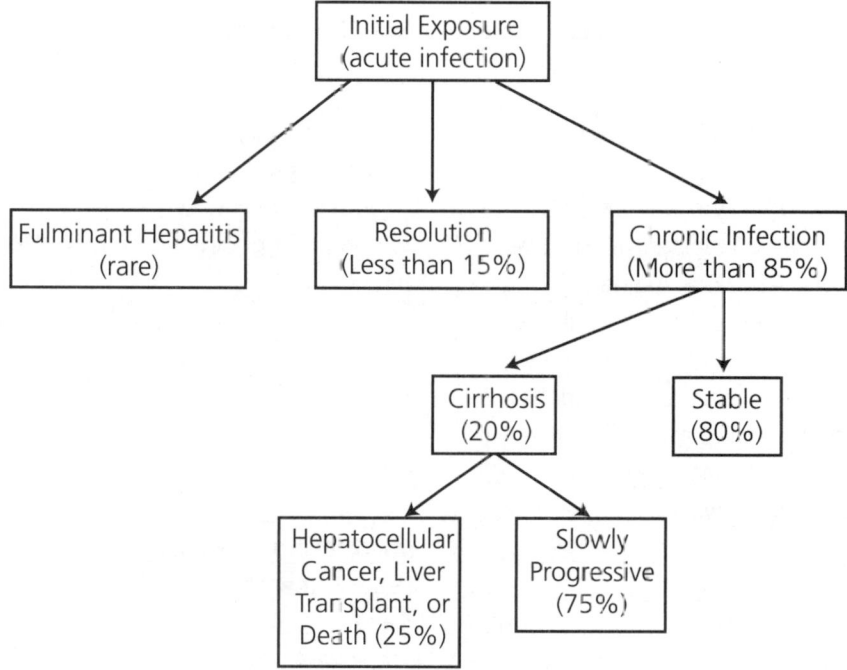

Figure 2-3: Course of Hepatitis C Infection

Approximately 15 percent of people infected with HCV completely clear the virus from their systems. The other 85 percent develop chronic HCV. The majority (80 percent of people with the chronic form) do not develop serious complications, and of the remaining (20 percent) who develop cirrhosis, most (75 percent of those with cirrhosis) slowly progress, and only a minority (25 percent) actually develop hepatocellular cancer or require a liver transplant.

acupuncture, herbs, and nutritional supplements, are very effective and safe.

One of my patients, a professional in his late forties, experienced severe and nearly intolerable side effects of combination therapy, including nausea and vomiting, headaches, debilitating fatigue, insomnia, and depression and mood changes. Within two treatments of acupuncture and herbal remedies, the nausea and headaches were completely gone; he was sleeping better and had more energy. By the end of six weeks, the side effects were controlled enough for him to return to work.

This patient continued on the interferon and ribaviran therapy. In fact, he did two complete courses. In the process, his viral count

Table 5: Selected Antiviral Drugs

Drug	Viruses Treated
Vidarabine (adenine arabinoside)	Herpes simplex (HSV-1 and -2)
Zovirax (acyclovir sodium)	Herpes simplex (HSV)
Ganciclovir and Valcyte (valganciclovir)	Cytomegalovirus (CMV)
Nucleoside analog reverse transcriptase inhibitors: AZT (Zidovudine), ddI (Didanosine), ddC (Zalcitabine), d4T (Stavudine), 3TC (Lamivudine)	Human Immunodeficiency Virus (HIV)
Non-nucleoside reverse transcriptase inhibitors: Nevirapine, Delavirdine	HIV
Protease Inhibitors: Saquinavir, Ritonavir, Indinavir, Nelfinavir	HIV
Virazole (ribavirin)	Broad spectrum: Hepatitis C (HCV), HSV, measles, mumps, Lassa fever
Amantadine (amantadine hydrochloride), Flumadine (rimantadine hydrochloride)	Influenza A strains
Relenza (zanamivir) and Tamiflu (oseltamavir)	Influenza strains A and B
Picovir (pleconaril)	Picorna viruses: common cold
Interferons (interferon alpha-2a, -2b, and alphacon-1)	Hepatitis B and HCV

reduced considerably, but once he discontinued the treatments the virus rebounded and his counts went back up to pre-treatment levels. He has now accepted that natural therapies are best, and that through them he can improve his immune status and his body can learn to coexist with the virus without damaging itself.

ALTERNATIVE APPROACHES: A number of alternative therapies have been suggested for the treatment and management of HCV. Alcohol is a well known liver toxin and must be eliminated completely in order to effectively manage liver inflammation and the progression of hepatitis C.

Excess tissue iron can damage the liver and promote the growth of bacteria that cause secondary infections. If you have hepatitis C, avoid taking an iron supplement and use a multivitamin and mineral that is iron-free. Also eliminate red meat and egg yolks, though keep your protein intake adequate by eating fish and poultry. If your blood levels of iron are too high from your blood test, you may benefit from old-fashioned blood-letting by having your physician draw off a small amount of blood in a procedure called venesection, as is used to take blood when you have a blood test.

Bile salts reduce liver injury by lowering bile acid levels in the liver and gallbladder, and they also have immune-enhancing properties and as yet unknown activity that protect the liver cells. Bile salts are often found in digestive enzyme formulas or can be prescribed by your medical doctor or naturopathic physician.

Supplemental use of antioxidants (vitamins C and E, and lipoic acid); oral N-acetyl cysteine (NAC) combined with interferon alpha, aspirin and other nonsteroidal anti-inflammatory drugs; and the use of thymosin with interferon alpha are helpful.[11]

Schisandrin C, derived from the Chinese herb *Schisandra chinensis* (*wu wei zi*), and silymarin (the active flavonoid component of milk thistle, *Silybum marianum*) have been shown to have liver protective action. Licorice extract *(Glycyrrhiza glabra)* is effective when combined with interferon alpha. Many of these substances are discussed in part 2.

Due to the high incidence of viral hepatitis B in China, traditional Chinese medicine has had a long history of treating chronic hepatitis utilizing a systematic and comprehensive methodology underlying its principles of treatment. Although hepatitis is not specifically mentioned in *The Yellow Emperor's Classic,* it did describe syndromes that closely resemble the symptom profile of hepatitis in the acute and chronic stages.

Though most research in China on herbal treatment for hepatitis has been on hepatitis B, recent studies demonstrate equal effectiveness against HCV. One double-blind study in Australia utilizing a new Chinese formula called CH-100 for HCV indicated significant reduction in ALT, an enzyme used to measure liver function and whose elevated levels are not desirable. Another study in Japan on minor bupleurum decoction *(sho-saiko-to)* showed it to have activity against HCV. This formula is one of the most researched formulas for hepatitis in China and Japan, and is commonly used by North American practitioners for all types of liver disorders.

Though researchers are not entirely clear how this formula works, it is suggested that it may activate macrophages, increase cytokine production, and promote natural killer cell activity.[12] A promising preliminary study on a new combination of Chinese herbs named "Eurocel," containing extracts of *Patrinia villosa,* was performed at the Institute of Life Sciences at Chungbuk National University in Korea and showed a decrease in viral markers.

The most promising work with Chinese herbs and HCV is by Qingcai Zhang who was trained as a medical doctor in China and who now practices traditional Chinese medicine and acupuncture, along with extensive clinical research, in New York City. Dr. Zhang's work with AIDS and HCV patients over a period of fifteen years clearly indicates that Chinese herbs, if properly prescribed and in concentrated preparations taken over a long period of time, can control viral spread and even reduce the viral load to such a degree that a few cases of his have subsequently tested negative for viral markers (Zhang 2001).

Due to the high incidence of viral hepatitis B in China, traditional Chinese medicine has had a long history of treating chronic hepatitis utilizing a systematic and comprehensive methodology underlying its principles of treatment.

Complications or side effects of these herbs appear to be rare. If they do occur, they are usually minor gastrointestinal upset or diarrhea, which are self-limiting upon reduction of the dose or discontinuance of the medication. There is evidence that minor bupleurum decoction may cause interstitial pneumonitis, a form of pneumonia, when used in combination with interferon alpha.[13]

Licorice root and glycyrrhizin (licorice extract) are common additions in Chinese herbal formulas. It is generally considered safe to use, however in high dosages or in susceptible individuals, it can cause fluid retention and lower potassium levels causing fatigue and high blood pressure. Considered a harmonizing tonic herb in traditional Chinese pharmacology, it is processed by steaming to remove any toxic effects and when taken in the usual prescribed amounts it generally does not cause any side effects. To be safe, people with hypertension should not use it.

HEPATITIS C SUMMARY: Serious liver disease constitutes a chronic uncontrollable stress resulting in physical, emotional, and immune disruption. Integrated therapy—conventional allopathic methods combined with alternative therapies, lifestyle modification, and psychological counseling—appears to offer great promise.

Though the ultimate therapeutic goal is the eradication of all detectable viruses, in many patients with chronic HCV this outcome is very difficult or impossible to achieve. One of the reasons HCV has become so common is that natural immunity to HCV infection appears to be weak or absent—yet another sign that the increasing incidence of viral diseases is equally a problem due to emerging species, heightened virulence of known viruses, and a possible immune deficiency in the general population.

Mosquito, Tick, and Rodent-Spread Viruses

The viruses in this group include a wide range of viral diseases from several different viral families. Among them are well known diseases like yellow fever and dengue, as well as newly emerging ones like Ebola and hanta viruses. Insects spread most of these viruses—one in particular: the *Aedes aegypti* mosquito. This species of mosquito is responsible for dengue and yellow fever viruses.

Dengue: Another of the old world diseases brought to the Americas, dengue—also called "break-bone fever"—was once common in North America at least as far north as Philadelphia. It reached a high point after World War II and then declined to a point where it was considered an uncommon and benign disease causing little more than flu-like symptoms. But since 1980, dengue has revived to epidemic proportions, and a newer deadly form, dengue hemorrhagic fever, has emerged.

Though mostly concentrated in Southeast Asia, where thousands of cases are reported annually, dengue hemorrhagic fever shock syndrome (DHFS)—a condition once found only in children—is now also found in the Caribbean and South America. Dengue has also returned to the United States. In the mid-1980s, the Asian tiger mosquito (*Aedes albopictus*, a close relative of *A. aegypti*) arrived in a freighter load of tires containing standing water. Worldwide, dengue infects between fifty and a hundred million people each year and is considered the most common mosquito-borne virus.

Dengue belongs to the Flaviviridae family which also includes yellow fever and hepatitis C, and there are four known sub-types: dengues 1–4. Symptoms appear rapidly after an average incubation period of five to eight days and include severe joint and muscle pain—thus the name "break-bone fever" because of the severe bone pain. Alternating severe chills and high fever are common, severe headache, pain behind the eyes, and the patient is so sick he can hardly move.

Though there are few fatalities from typical dengue, the illness can be so severe the patient feels as if he is dying. In severe cases the patient feels exhausted and remains debilitated for weeks or months, or longer. There is no medical treatment other than bed rest, replacement of fluids, and transfusions of whole blood in hemorrhagic cases. Aspirin or Tylenol is recommended to help relieve pain. This is an appalling situation given the frequency of dengue and its increasing severity, and more effort should be given to mosquito control in third world countries in addition to finding better treatments.

In colonial America, the specific herb for break-bone fever was boneset *(Eupatorium perfoliatum)*, a member of the daisy family (Astericae) to which echinacea also belongs. It is prepared as a strong infusion and drunk as a tea; it may also be used as a tincture combined with echinacea, and homeopathic preparations are also available.

Yellow Fever and Other Viral Disasters: Arthropod-borne viruses, diseases caused by "blood-sucking" insects, produce an array of viral illnesses that range from mild flu-like symptoms to death. Of these, yellow fever, carried by the same mosquito as dengue, is the most severe. It arrived in the Americas by slave ships from West Africa and became one of the most feared of diseases up until the early part of the twentieth century. Yellow fever is a hemorrhagic disease that attacks the liver causing jaundice, necrosis (death of cells), and death. It is still common in tropical Africa, Latin America, and Asia. An effective vaccine is available, but there is no specific treatment other than management of symptoms and blood transfusion.

A number of other insect-borne viral illnesses that cause illnesses in America include Venezuelan equine encephalitis, Colorado tick fever, Eastern equine encephalitis, Western equine encephalitis, St. Louis encephalitis, California encephalitis, and West Nile Fever. Most of these viruses cause (or can lead to) inflammation of the central nervous system. Other viruses that also cause central nervous system damage include the herpes viruses, HIV, poliovirus, and the mumps; however, these are not insect-borne illnesses.

Rodents, such as squirrels, mice, and rats, spread viruses in their droppings when they forage for food. The contaminated food is then eaten, or dried fecal matter contaminates the air and is then inhaled. The most notorious of rodent-related viruses is hanta. First identified in 1954 during the Korean War, the virus was isolated from samples found near the Hantaan River in 1978. This disease, originally called Korean Hemorrhagic Fever, belongs to the Bunyavirus family and has a genus of its own, *Hantavirus,* with three types identified. In 1993, an emerging hantavirus was identified in New Mexico, which caused headline news over an emerging viral threat. It attacks the kidneys and can cause lung inflammation, internal bleeding, and death.

Next to AIDS, Ebola virus—because of its terrifying consequences—has become the virus most imprinted on contemporary consciousness. There are three types of Ebola, which is also a bleeding fever like Hanta and dengue, but only two types affect humans; the other known type infects only monkeys. It is endemic in parts of Africa, but Ebola has "cousins," all members of the Filovirus family, that occur in other parts of the world including Europe, South America, and Asia. The most notorious of these is the Marburg virus, first identified in South Africa. Other fatal hemorrhagic viral diseases include Lassa, Argentine, and Bolivian fevers.

With increasing human population density, less funding for public health measures in third world countries and Eastern Europe, uncontrolled rodent and insect populations, increasing genetic diversity among viruses, and increasing destruction of natural biodiversity and habitat, it is likely that we will see more incidences of these diseases, especially of dengue fever, in the future.

Inorganic Infections

One of the strangest things about viruses is that they are often described as being both dead and alive—or neither dead nor alive—a paradox that scientists have yet to solve and medical philosophers continue to puzzle over. Looking at the triangular, hexagonal, and spiral structures of viruses, I am amazed at their beauty and symmetry, which more resemble that of minerals and crystals than animal or plant cells.

Prions and the BSE Crisis: A number of diseases have appeared that are not identifiable according to any of the known microbial categories: they are neither a virus, a bacteria, a protozoa, nor a parasite. A new category, proteinaceous infectious particles (PrPs), or prions, the cause of mad cow disease, or bovine spongiform encephalopathy (BSE), are rogue proteins that convert normal protein into misshapen and deadly forms. What makes these diseases threatening is their ability to jump species and easily penetrate brain tissue.

Prion diseases are unique from other infectious illnesses in that they are both an infectious and hereditary disease, and occur in animals and humans. Humans can become infected from contaminated beef, as a result of general surgery, by hormone injections from contaminated products, in corneal transplants in eye surgery, and by genetic transmission. The chief human prion disease is Creutzfeld-Jacob Disease (CJD), a condition that causes loss of motor control, dementia, paralysis, and death. How prion diseases progress is still unknown and there is no effective treatment.

Pleomorphism: The phenomenon of microbial pleomorphism, that infectious agents can have more than one shape, was documented as early as 1881 in Sweden by Ernst Almquist, a student of Robert Koch (of Koch's Postulate). Since then, pleomorphic forms have been identified for fungal and bacterial species and are one of the suspected causes of stealth infections. It would not be surprising if viruses also displayed the ability to "morph."

The ability of microorganisms to change forms like the shape-shifters of science fiction may eventually add another dimension to our understanding of evolution. Humans, like all vertebrates, require many thousands and even millions of years to evolve even the simplest of changes. Microorganisms, on the other hand, can see generations come and go in a matter of minutes, and they are able to evolve more quickly than we are, as evidenced in drug-resistant forms of bacteria and viruses. Therefore, treatment strategies that work with nature to achieve environmental balance within the body are required to either complement existing or developing pharmaceutical drug treatments, or in some cases to replace them entirely.

Plants have very complex structures and their immune mechanisms work to inhibit viruses from several different avenues at the same time, making it difficult for the viruses to develop resistance to natural compounds. Evidenced by the increased interest by scientist worldwide in antiviral and immunomodulating natural compounds, herbal medication can play a significant role in the treatment of viruses, especially in light of drug-resistant and pleomorphic forms of those viruses.

Extraterrestrial Origins: Sir Fred Hoyle (1915–2001), an outstanding British astronomer and professor at Cambridge University, and the most visible proponent of the theory that life on this planet was seeded from outer space, believed that extraterrestrial events and forces influenced viral pandemics. Viruses, in his theory, are charged particles that penetrate the Earth's atmosphere and genetically intermingle with existing viruses causing new strains. Though his theories are impossible to prove and have vexed scientists for decades, the premise underlying Hoyle's unusual theories is that the universe is interconnected and displays intelligence. It is this concept of the intelligence of all things that makes his ideas so fascinating, and not too far from those of modern evolutionary biology, shamanism, and Eastern cosmology.

If all life and events are animated by a universal intelligence, and I tend to think they are, understanding how this intelligence operates and attuning to its principles will promote health and prevent disease. Natural medicines inherently contain more of this intelligence than chemical drugs, and if applied correctly have a remarkable ability to promote recovery and cure, even from viral diseases.

CHAPTER SUMMARY

Viruses have always been and will always be among us.

They vary and mutate at rates we can barely imagine and cannot contain.

Nature has methods and means of controlling viral rates of replication, and even the most virulent and deadly of viral outbreaks tend to run a course and recede—that is, if natural laws are respected and disease resistance is not created by manmade pharmaceutical drugs.

Of equal or perhaps more concern than viral plagues are the effects of chronic viruses such as HIV, HHV-6, and HCV. All of these viral diseases are related to lifestyles that promote viral spread (shared hypodermic needles, promiscuous unprotected sex, crowded cities, unsanitary living conditions) and cause immune deficiency.

Natural medicines are effective for reducing the symptoms and shortening the duration of the common cold, flu, gastroenteritis, and herpes virus.

Natural medicines can also serve as both primary and complementary treatment for more serious viral infections including HIV, HCV, HHV-6, and CMV.

3

Immunity and Viral Disease

Viruses display remarkable biological intelligence. They not only cause health conditions and diseases resulting in tissue and organ damage, but as AIDS has shown us, they can disable the immune system itself. Why this happens is still unknown. However, when explored from the evolutionary perspective and the standpoint of energy medicine, answers begin to fall into place and a larger picture emerges that makes more sense than any simplistic germ theory.

This book is not only about viral illnesses but is also about a new paradigm in medical thinking. Therefore in this chapter, alongside the basic, important traditional immunology principles, are the latest concepts about immune function, coupled with evolutionary ideas and principles of energey medicine. These new ideas provide a better theoretical framework in which to understand the principles behind natural alternative antiviral therapies.

Traditional Concepts of Immunity and New Reinterpretations

The Earth is far from sterile. In fact, we live in a thick biological soup of highly active, aggressive, competitive, and potentially life-threatening microorganisms and chemical substances. Most are naturally occurring and others are manmade. These recently manmade substances are disrupting and challenging a human immune system that has adapted over hundreds of thousands of years to only naturally occurring compounds and organisms. Yet, in only a few hundred years' time, chemical toxic substances have permeated the Earth's atmosphere, crust, ice caps, and water systems, and entered into the food chain to such a degree that some researchers and clinicians, including myself, believe these substances are, to a large degree part of the cause of the current immune deficiency crisis.

If immune dysfunction is caused by modern living, then we must also change the way we live and work. I suggest that we gradually begin to make improvements in the way we live, while enhancing our immune systems with natural substances in the meantime.

So we are faced with a dilemma. There is no doubt that viral diseases are increasing, but do we try to kill the viral invaders or enhance our immunity? If immune dysfunction is caused by modern living, then we must also change the way we live and work—a proposition that is much more difficult to accomplish than to talk about. As the Chinese saying goes, "A journey of a thousand miles begins with a single step," so I suggest that we gradually begin to make improvements in the way we live, while enhancing our immune systems with natural substances in the meantime.

For those with active viral disease, it is important to manage or reduce the viral load in the body using natural antiviral medications and perhaps even through the wise use of pharmaceutical antivirals. In the end, if we proceed intelligently, diligently, and with significant care, we will arrive at our destination: improved health for ourselves, families, loved ones, and society.

A healthy, well-functioning immune system is a marvel of natural microbiology, physics, and biochemistry (see figure 3-1). Without it, we could not survive for even the shortest period of time on this planet. Every living organism, from animals to plants, has an immune system—each with differences that promote individual survival and health.

Conventional medical immunology identifies several organs that play important roles in the immune system. These are the thymus gland, lymph nodes, spleen, and Peyer's patches in the intestine. Newer models expand this view and include the gut-associated lymphoid tissue (GALT), which includes the appendix as well as the Peyer's patches. Similar groups of tissue protect the lungs and are called bronchial-associated lymphoid tissue (BALT), and the lungs' mucus lining called mucosal-associated lymphoid tissue (MALT). Since all immune cells originate in the bone marrow, it is also considered an immune tissue.

From the viewpoint of functional medicine and naturopathy, insofar as these glands and tissues contribute to the origin and development of mature immune cells, their function is regarded as vital for immune enhancement and general health. Liver detoxification to assist in the removal of toxins from the body, colon cleansing to improve GALT function, lymphatic cleansing, and thymus support are necessary elements of a complete immune-enhancing program.

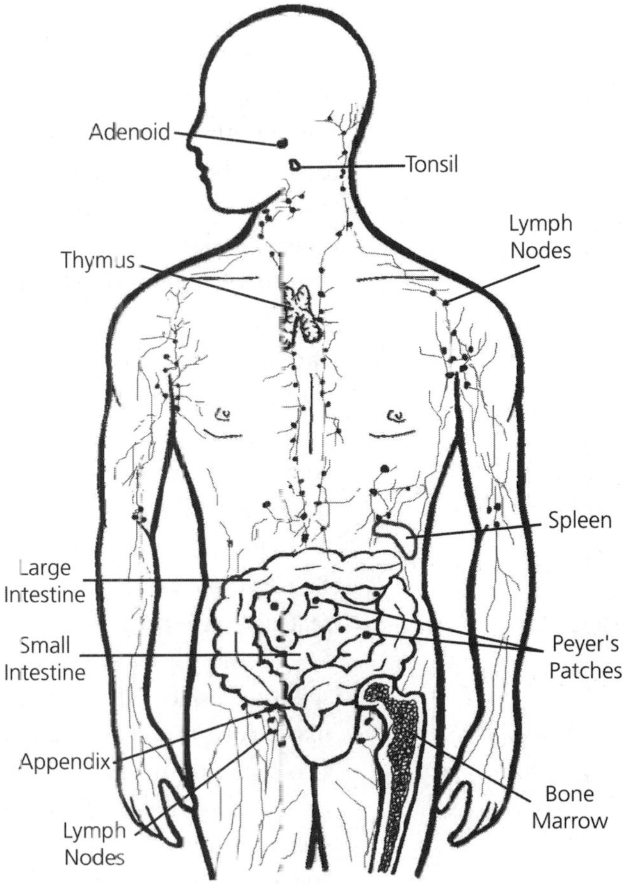

Immunology is the scientific study of the immune system, and entails the mechanisms by which the body maintains its biochemical identity and defends itself and survives against infectious agents, including viruses, and other foreign substances like toxic chemicals. Medical immunology is concerned with immune-related diseases and with substances that affect the immune system and treat the body against infectious microorganisms.

Like most of modern science, those who study immunology do not focus on the whole system, but on the ways in which particular types of cells defend the body by means of recognition and elimination of foreign microbes and other substances. It is a brilliant science of microscopic parts, but it tends to proceed without any sense of how the immune system works as a unified whole.

Traditional immunology is based on a mechanistic model developed in the 1930s and '40s, which originated from studies by Ilya

Figure 3-1: The Human Immune System
Organs, glands, tissues, and vessels of the human immune system.

Ilyich Metchnikoff (1845–1916), the Russian who shared the Nobel Prize in Physiology and Medicine in 1908 with Paul Ehrlich for their work on how the body rids itself of foreign particles. According to this model, the immune system is a *reactive* mechanism designed to defend the body against invading microorganisms, foreign materials, and objects that include pollens, chemicals, dust, animal dander, particles of soot or sand, and toxic chemicals.

In 1960, the Nobel Prize in Physiology and Medicine was jointly awarded to Sir Frank Macfarlane Burnet and Peter Brian Medawar for the discovery of acquired immunological tolerance, a discovery which set the tone for modern immunology. For several decades, their conclusions that there were two immune systems—one innate, the other acquired, and that newborns had immature immunity—remained unchallenged.

Then, in the late 1990s, Marcella Sarzotti-Kelsoe, Ph.D., of the Baltimore Veterans Affairs Medical Center found that newborns in fact did have fully competent immune systems. These findings called for a reinterpretation of the Burnet and Medawar theories, and other scientists followed the call. The immune system began to look more like a continuum with multiple interconnections than a system with two separate mechanical parts.

Another principle of traditional immunology is that the immune system is able to maintain a distinct division between individuals and species, between the individual organism and the environment by distinguishing self from non-self. This recognition ability was considered a key concept in immunology for nearly a century. Not any longer.

Polly Matzinger, Ph.D., of the National Institute of Allergy and Infectious Diseases, found that this kind of classification was limiting and did not fully describe how the immune system worked. Matzinger said that the old theory of a clear division between self and non-self "made it virtually impossible to uncover the rule by which the immune system could make the necessary distinctions" (Matzinger 2001) to function properly. In her view, the immune system is much more complicated. It responds to the vast array of infectious agents, chemicals, and the changing nature of the environment through equal complexity.

Like clinical medicine, traditional immunologists used war analogies to explain their theories: the immune system is like a "double-edged sword"; it maintains "first- and second-line defenses"; it is a surveillance system that "guards" and "fights" against "invading" germs; it either "wins" or is "defeated."

This linear, battle-based way of thinking produces a limited model, in which individual parts are first discovered and studied, then theories are invented afterwards in an attempt to figure out how the parts work. Linear models can never fully explain how a complex system operates and cannot completely accommodate nuances, individual differences, variety, or evolutionary changes that take place continuously in all living systems.

Nature, on the other hand, favors balance rather than superior "firepower." Careful observation reveals that the body dislikes extremes and that pushing it beyond its limits results in ill health. Disrupting the immune system with unnatural toxic chemicals and the exhaustion of vital metabolic and hormonal reserves due to stress and aging further deplete our immune systems' ability to function.

Charles A. Janeway, M.D., of Yale University School of Medicine, suggests that the immune system is more of a "sensory system." He effectively challenges the idea that the innate immune response is limited to inflammation and simple cellular "search and destroy operations," like a war machine. In his model, the old idea that innate immunity is nothing more than a rudimentary, evolutionary, knee-jerk reaction to an invading non-self organism gives way to the idea that the immune response is a powerful *screening* mechanism that includes intricate cellular communications, more like a powerful computer antivirus program that continuously monitors your system for abnormal changes and alerts you when things go wrong.

However, to be fair, no matter how linear the current model is, we have learned much about immunity through the study of cellular microbiology. In fact, the more we learn, the more complex it all seems and the more the immune system is appreciated as an integrated, intelligent biosystem. Most contemporary immunology researchers are now well aware of and accept the paradoxical tendencies the immune system demonstrates. For example: immunity is influenced by mood as well as infections; it can display hyperimmune states at the same time as immune-deficient ones. We truly exist in a biochemically interconnected ecological matrix where complexity is the norm rather than the exception.

In light of this discussion, one of my patients comes to mind. A young woman in her late twenties, Beth had advanced rheumatoid arthritis. Besides severe crippling joint pain and swelling, she had allergies and recurrent infections. Her inflammatory symptoms were suppressed with steroid drugs, which depressed her immune system and led to chronic bacterial sinusitis, recurrent colds, and viral infections. When I first saw her, Beth was continuously on antibiotics to treat the sinus infections, which caused constant vaginal yeast infections. Still, her body adapted, and she heroically survived. Though the drugs did not cure her condition or reduce the daily experience of constant pain, they helped her live a relatively normal life that included a marriage and job.

When she first came to see me, Beth immediately asked if stress had anything to do with her condition because she noticed that the symptoms waxed and waned based on her stress levels. I explained that the immune system responds to changes in hormone and neurotransmitter levels due to stress, which can vary with menstrual rhythms. Beth was amazed at how complex her body was.

By applying techniques to regulate the immune system, many of which are described in part 2, Beth was able to reduce her use of steroids to a minimum and eventually to eliminate them altogether, allowing her natural immunity to recover. Her sinus infections cleared completely and she stopped getting colds every few weeks. Antibiotics became unnecessary, and consequently her yeast infections disappeared. Acupuncture treatments and herbal medicines helped to manage her pain and joint inflammation and she was eventually able to eliminate all anti-rheumatic drugs as well. Beth had an autoimmune condition complicated by immune deficiency, but natural therapies helped restore balance to her immune system.

Nonspecific or Innate Immunity

The classical view of immunity divides the immune system into two parts with different lines of defense: nonspecific or innate immunity, and specific or adaptive immunity. Each part has various components and characteristics that contribute to its effectiveness. Since the conventional model still serves as a good starting point in understanding the basic function of the immune system, in this section I will explain the most important components of innate immunity. In the next chapter, I will discuss the innate immune response in more detail and why I consider it one of the most important, and most overlooked, aspects of the current immune crisis. Later in this chapter I discuss specific immunity.

According to the traditional model, the body's first line of defense is the innate immune response. Its essential characteristic is to distinguish between self and non-self, to protect us ("self") from microbes ("non-self"). Its principle challenge is to detect and then mount a rapid and effective defense against any invading pathogen (microorganisms such as bacteria, parasites, or viruses that cause disease) or antigen (any foreign substance, like pollen, that causes allergies, or otherwise stimulates an immune response).[1]

Innate immunity (also called natural or native) is what we are born with. In the newborn, it is augmented by its mother's mature immunity and is conferred in the colostrum of the first breast milk. That is why breast-feeding for at least a few months is so important to an infant's natural immunity and, sometimes, survival.

The components of innate immunity include physical and chemical barriers that prevent microorganisms from entering the body, as well as specific cells that are on the prowl to eliminate them if they gain access to the body, or so to speak, if they get under your skin. Let's examine these barriers and cells.

The skin is the first barrier against microorganisms, and most types cannot enter healthy unbroken skin. That is one of the reasons why it is important to keep even minor wounds clean and covered, especially when in contact with others who harbor infections.

Physical and Chemical Barriers: The skin is the first barrier against microorganisms, and most types cannot enter healthy *unbroken* skin. That is one of the reasons why it is important to keep even minor wounds clean and covered, especially when in contact with others who harbor infections; some microbes can enter directly into the bloodstream through broken skin.

Not only does the skin act as a physical barrier, its secretions serve as a chemical deterrent to pathogens as well. The acidic pH of sweat, unsaturated fatty acid secretions of the sebaceous glands, and enzymes called lysozymes that occur in tears and sweat are natural antiseptics that help to keep the skin free of pathogenic organisms. Even the salt in sweat is mildly antibacterial.

Regular bathing and routine hand washing remove dirt and bacteria from our bodies. However, overly washing one's hands with strong antibacterial soaps may produce more trouble than benefit. Sterilizing everything in sight and trying to get rid of all bacteria is not necessary, and may eliminate some helpful germs in the process.

Ordinary soap and regular hand washing before preparing food and after using the restroom are adequate.

Other common areas by which germs, allergens, and pollutants enter the body are the nose, throat, and lungs, through the mouth and the digestive tract, and through the rectum, urinary tract, and sex organs. Natural methods of protection operate in all of these areas of the body. For example, the mucous lining of the respiratory and gastrointestinal tracts trap and remove microorganisms and are expelled in phlegm. One public health measure of earlier days used to be the prohibition of spitting and the removal of spittoons from public buildings. Many microorganisms are also caught on their way to the lungs in the nose and throat by the adenoids and tonsils, both of which are lymphatic glands important to first-line immunity.

The indiscriminate, and often unnecessary, surgical removal of these glands does not solve the underlying immunological problem that caused them to be swollen and diseased in the first place. Often, after a short period of improvement, it leads to chronic allergy problems. If the microorganisms get past the tonsils and adenoids, ciliated microfilaments lining the upper passages of the lungs remove them in secreted phlegm; they do this in a wavelike fashion, much like firemen of an earlier time on a bucket brigade.

Enzymes in the saliva, stomach, and small intestine, along with the acidic pH of the stomach, manage to kill most microbes upon contact. Friendly bacteria, like *Staphylococcus albus* on the skin, *Streptococcus viridans* in the throat, and numerous naturally occurring bacteria in the colon, like *Lactobacillus acidophilus*,[2] have a powerful effect on maintaining healthy immune status. In fact, the lower gastrointestinal tract contains the greatest number of immune cells in the body. Urination causes regular flushing of bacteria from the urinary tract, and the acidic pH of the vagina prevents colonization of it by yeast and fungi, as well as by bacteria and viruses.

Phagocytosis: Besides physical, mechanical, and chemical means of preventing microorganisms from entering the body, innate immunity also has cellular defenses. This next line of defense consists of specialized immune cells that destroy the invader once it has entered the body. The destruction of foreign cells inside the body is called phagocytosis, which means the "eating of cells."

All the immune cells spend at least some part or all of their lives in the bloodstream, but before they enter the blood they are created in

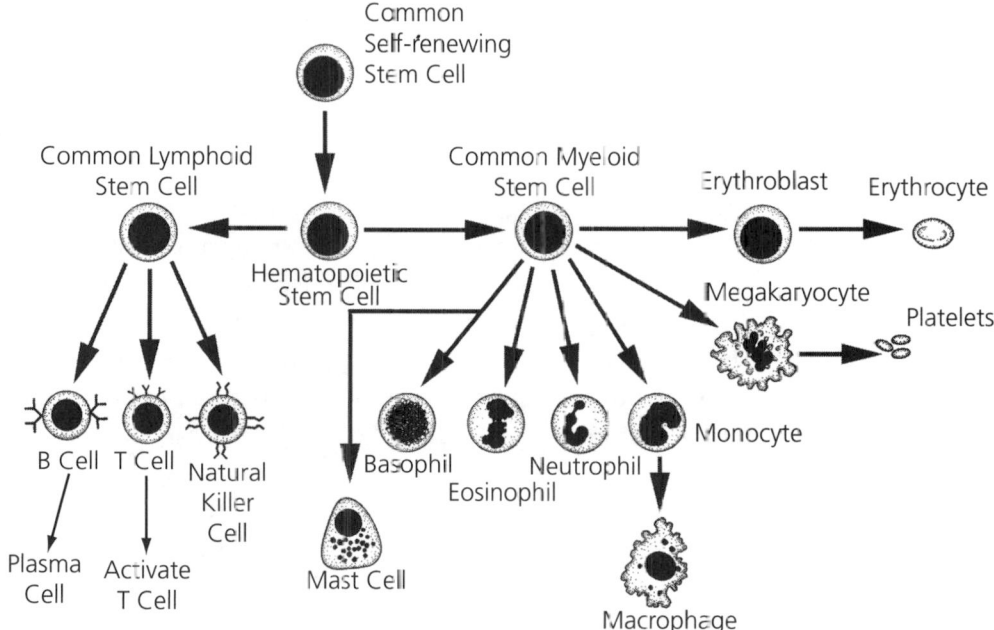

Figure 3-2: Cells of the Immune System

All cells of the immune system originate in the bone marrow from one hematopoietic stem cell, a self-renewing parent cell involved in the generation of blood cells. This cell divides to produce two specialize types of stem cells: a lymphoid stem cell, which creates T and B lymphocytes and natural killer cells, and a myeloid stem cell. From the common myeloid stem cell arise white blood cells (basophils, eosinophils, neutrophils, and monocytes), red blood cells (erythrocytes), and platelets, which are important in blood clotting. Mast cells are important in allergic responses and macrophages are involved in tissue defense.

References: Janeway, Charles A., et al. *Immunobiology*; Roitt, Ivan, et al. *Immunology*; Benjamini, Eli, et al. *Immunology, A Short Course*.

the bone marrow, which also produces red cells (erythrocytes, cells that carry oxygen), platelets (cells that control bleeding), and the white cells (leukocytes). It is the white cells and their secretions that make up the main components of the immune system. The importance of the white cells may be seen in the diversity of types compared to that of red cells and platelets. There is only one type of red cell and one type of platelet, but more than eight types (or subtypes) of white cells (see figure 3-2).

White cells, or leukocytes, consist of neutrophils, basophils, eosinophils, monocytes, and lymphocytes. Two of these are phagocytic cells: neutrophils and monocytes, which in their mature form are called macrophages. Neutrophils are also called segmented neutrophils or segs. They belong to a group called polymorphonucelar leukocytes, or polys, or simply PMNs, a group that also includes basophils and eosinophils. Phagocytic cells engulf and ingest foreign particles and microorganisms. Once they are ingested, the phagocytes secrete powerful enzymes to digest these particles, and metabolize and remove them from the system, essentially cleaning up after themselves.

These first-line phagocytic cells effectively identify and neutralize the invading particle without overly disturbing the host, your body. They are positioned strategically in areas of the body where they encounter the greatest numbers of microbes and offer the most protection for organs, such as the liver, vulnerable to infection. Besides removing microbes and their toxins, macrophages continuously scavenge dead or worn-out cells. The main sites in the body where macrophages are found in abundance are the Kupffer cells in the liver, the red pulp of the spleen, and the airways of the lungs.

Besides phagocytosis, infection also triggers macrophages to release cytokines. These increase the permeability of blood vessels, allowing fluids, proteins, and immune cells to pass into the damaged tissue area. This process is part of the inflammatory aspect of immunity (discussed in more detail in the next chapter).

Neutrophils are like the pawns on a chessboard. They are so numerous that nearly 60 percent of bone marrow activity is spent producing them, and they make up 50 to 70 percent of all white cells. Once manufactured by the bone marrow, neutrophils continuously circulate in the blood on the lookout for foreign particles.

Neutrophils are short-lived cells that engulf substances, destroy them, and then die. Besides participating in phagocytosis, neutrophils perform a variety of biochemical activities against microorganisms, including production of peroxide and superoxide radicals that act as germ-killing toxic oxidants and the manufacture of lactoferrin, that inhibits bacterial growth by binding up (chelating) iron, thereby withholding it from iron-hungry bacteria. They also contribute to the destruction of microbes through the production of nitric oxide (a free radical gas). This is a cellular metabolic process also important in many chronic degenerative diseases, so defects in neutrophil function or production often manifest as chronic or recurrent infections.

Monocytes are also phagocytic, but unlike the free-swimming neutrophils, these cells reside in organs, tissues, and specialized cavities in the body, waiting for action there. Their numbers are much smaller than neutrophils, comprising 2–8 percent of white cells. After being produced in the marrow they circulate in the bloodstream for about a day and then settle in their chosen "lairs." Once there, they differentiate further into specific forms called tissue macrophages or histiocytes. Immunologists give these cells specialized names depending on their site of activity, such as Kupffer cells in the liver, alveolar macrophages in the lungs, microphial cells in the central nervous system, and splenic macrophages in the spleen.

Macrophages lie in wait until activated by any of a variety of physical and biochemical stimuli. Like neutrophils, activated macrophages release an immense range of biologically active chemicals as the immune response. Macrophages are part of the reticuloendothelial system, a group of tissue-based cells that filter and remove debris from the blood, and make up an important part of the first line defense strategy of the immune system in eliminating bacteria and parasites. Macrophages also prepare and mark partially digested cells for further destruction, a process called antigen-presenting.

Natural Killer Cells: Natural killer (NK) cells, a type of cytotoxic cell (toxic to other cells), are a specialized group of lymphocytes responsible for destroying virus-infected cells and cancer cells, as well as cells infected with bacteria and protozoa. NK cells compose between 5–16 percent of the total number of lymphocytes. Very little is known about exactly how NK cells work, but we do know they play an important role in recognizing and eliminating cancer cells in the early stages of cancer growth and in killing viruses. They also contribute to immune activity by secreting various cytokines, primarily interferon.

Since viruses invade and take up residence inside cells, the regular phagocytic cells (neutrophils and macrophages) are unable to get at the viral particle, so the immune system provides an alternative method: NK cells. These release biological weapons against the parasitic virion. They bind to the infected cell and release chemicals that destroy the cellular membrane, causing the target cell to burst. Other immune cells then clean up the cellular debris.

NK cells are particularly important in controlling recurrent herpes viral infections, such as EBV, CMV, and VZV. Natural killer cell numbers tend to be low in chronic viral disease, such as herpes, and in many cancers. This may suggest either that they are being used up in the immune system's attempt to manage the condition, or that lower than normal levels allowed the condition in the first place. We still do not know enough about how the immune system works to interpret much of the clinical information we are able to collect.

NK cell levels and function are affected by a variety of nutritional deficiencies, including protein and overall caloric deficiencies, low levels of vitamins C, E, and D, and of trace minerals such as zinc and magnesium. Toxic metals, like lead, and other noxious environmental substances can depress NK cell levels. Numerous natural immune-modulating substances, such as transfer factor and the mushroom glucans, can increase the number of NK cells. These (and other substances discussed in part 2) are important medications that improve immune function and should play a central role in any plan to rid the body of viral disease.

Biologically Active Immune Substances: Current research has shown that many tissues and immune cells produce a large variety of biochemical substances harmful to microorganisms. These include enzymes, free radicals,[3] acids, growth inhibitors, fever-producing pyrogens, tumor necrosis factor, interleukins, and interferons. Macrophages produce interleukin-1 (IL-1) that stimulates helper T lymphocytes. Macrophages also produce tumor necrosis factor that kills cancer cells and helps regulate other immune functions. Alpha interferon is produced by lymphocytes and it also increases NK cell activity.

Circulating Protein Substances: Protein substances circulating in the blood form the complement system[4] that recognizes microbes and is involved in the development of inflammation. Paul Ehrlich, winner of the Nobel Prize in Medicine in 1908, described an activity in the blood that assisted, or complemented, the ability of other immune components to destroy bacteria. He was the first to use the term "complement" in this context. The activity of the complement system promotes the killing of microbes, facilitates the clearing of immune complexes that have become unnecessary, and enhances antibody responses. Like many immune complexes, complement can also cause harm if it is activated by an autoimmune response to act against normal body tissues.

Immunologists describe two pathways, classical and alternative, by which the complement system works. The classification of the many components of the complement system is complex and beyond the scope of this book; however, it is important to keep in mind that this system is very influential on innate immune function, and, as with low numbers of NK cells, complement deficiency is associated with increased infections.

Adaptive or Acquired Immunity

We now turn to the second pole of the immune system. Adaptive, also called specific or acquired, immunity is characterized by recognition and *memory* of an encounter with a foreign pathogen. This ability of the immune system to *remember* is considered the second main principle of traditional immunology. The initial encounter between an invading pathogen and cells of the adaptive immune system produces a delayed immune response that is specific against a particular infectious microorganism. Therefore adaptive immunity is developed only after exposure resulting in natural immunization.

Since the 1950s, microbiologists and immunologists have focused almost entirely on the cellular and chemical components of the adaptive immune response, yielding a wealth of information. However, as mentioned, the immune system is far more elaborate than researchers had previously thought.

Lymphocytes, the principle cells involved in adaptive immunity, come in two major types: T lymphocytes (originating in the thymus gland) and B lymphocytes (the B is for bone marrow, their place of origin). There are two aspects of adaptive immunity: humoral immunity (involving B cells) and cell-mediated immunity (involving T cells).

Humoral Immunity: Humoral immunity is mediated by antibodies, protein substances that help to protect against foreign material,[5] produced by B lymphocytes. These cells originate in the bone marrow where they mature, enter the blood circulation, and, over a lengthy process of differentiation, culminate in two types of cells: plasma cells and memory cells. Plasma cells produce antibodies that circulate in the serum and result in humoral or antibody-mediated immunity. B cells make up about 5 to 15 percent of circulating lymphocytes.

Antibodies detect and bind to specific antigens and then activate the complement system and its enzymes to destroy the marked cells or stimulate phagocytes to eliminate the antibody-flagged foreign cells.

There are five types of human antibodies, collectively known as immunoglobulins, which are protein substances secreted by B cells that circulate in the blood and help the immune system recognize foreign substances.[6] Each immunoglobulin (Ig) is given a letter to differentiate it: IgA, IgM, IgG, IgD, and IgE, and each immunoglobulin has its own set of biological functions and properties.

- IgA is mainly found in the gastrointestinal tract, saliva, tears, other body secretions, and in the linings of the lungs and urinary tract.

- IgM is the first antibody produced after immunization or infection.

- IgG antibodies can cross the placenta barrier and confer immunity to the fetus from the mother. IgG antibodies are also part of the secondary immune response and are important in the neutralization of animal venoms and viruses.

- IgD immunoglobulins are not well understood, but are thought to play a role with IgM antibodies.

- IgE antibodies are associated with allergies and parasitic infections.

Cell-Mediated Immunity: The T lymphocytes are the main cellular component of cell-mediated immunity of the adaptive immune response, and help control intracellular pathogens like viruses. Like all other immune cells, these cells originate in the bone marrow but then migrate to the thymus gland (behind the sternum in the chest) where they mature and are then called thymocytes, or T cells. T cells fight cancer cells and some types of bacterial and fungal infections as well as certain viruses. They circulate freely, like NK cells and neutrophils, and are available for immune defense when needed. Unlike NK cells and neutrophils, they do not destroy antigens at will, but require a specific marker on a cell tagged with an antibody before they start to neutralize the target cell.

T cells do not produce antibodies, but many of their immune functions are interrelated with B cells, which do secrete antibodies. For example, B cells make the antibodies necessary for T cells to kill most viruses. T cell and B cell cooperation involves a subclass of T lymphocytes called T-helper cells that trigger B cells to make antibodies. T-helper cells stimulate the maturation of B cells, cooperate with B cells to promote the production of antibodies, enhance the function of cytotoxic T cells (the second main type of T cell, and an essential cellular component in defense against viruses), and assist in the production of immune chemicals like interleukin 2 (IL-2) and gamma interferon.

T-lymphocyte cells were once divided into just two types: T-helper and T-suppressor cells, but the quantity of new information on T cells has made their classification complex. In recent years, more sophisticated knowledge of how immune cells function has lead to changes in terminology. Immunologists now use the Cluster Designation (CD) system to differentiate different types of immune cells.

Lymphocytes and other white blood cells have different molecules on their surface (called surface markers), which are used to identify subsets of cells. For example, T cells are divided into many different subtypes based upon the different type of surface markers.

CD3 is the general designation for T cells. CD4 cells are a type of T-helper cell that promotes or induces the immune response. In AIDS patients, CD4+ T cells are very low and this deficiency state contributes to increased infections (Lappé 1997).

CD8 cells are cytotoxic cells and also function as suppressor T cells. Less is known about them than CD4 cells, but recent research suggests that CD8 cells are able to kill virus-infected cells. They also inhibit the function of the B cells when sufficient amounts of antibodies have been produced, and suppress the function of cytotoxic T cells when their job has been completed. Cells with the CD56 marker are NK cells.

Measuring the levels by blood testing of the different immune cells following the CD designation provides useful clinical information for the identification of chronic viral infection, cancer, and immune deficiency. Natural immune-enhancing therapies can raise levels of both CD4 and CD8 cells, thereby promoting immune function and preventing viral illness.

Cytotoxic T cells, a third subset of T lymphocytes, attach themselves to a tagged antigen and immediately destroy the target cell. NK cells and cytotoxic T cells are similar as they are both killer cells, but NK cells are nonspecific and can attack a foreign antigen directly upon contact, whereas the cytotoxic T cell is part of acquired immunity and destroys only previously tagged cells.

Chemicals That Communicate: Aside from physical barriers, the inflammatory response (an aspect of immunity involving swelling in response to tissue damage or infection), and cellular components of the immune system, scientists have discovered a vast array of immune modulators that interface with all aspects of immunity and even directly destroy invading pathogens. Immune modulators are substances that modulate, regulate, or influence the immune system (see part 2).

T lymphocytes, macrophages, and other immune cells release substances called cytokines, which are small proteins that function as chemical mediators within the immune system. They are thought to determine whether an immune response will be predominantly cell-mediated or antibody-mediated. Cytokines also communicate with cells from other systems, such as the nervous system and probably with the endocrine system as well, helping to preserve and restore homeostasis—the physiologically balanced state of a healthy body.

Scientists have discovered a vast array of immune modulators that interface with all aspects of immunity and even directly destroy invading pathogens. Immune modulators are substances that modulate, regulate, or influence the immune system.

Cytokines have a variety of functions. Besides regulating the specific immune response, they are involved in the innate immune response to viruses and other microorganisms, and produce inflammation and fever. They also produce delayed hypersensitivity associated with allergic reactions and they affect the movement of leukocytes (white blood cells). There are many known cytokines, such as interleukins (IL 1–18), interferons (INF), tumor necrosis factors (TNF), and immune cell growth factors.

Chemokines, a class of cytokines referred to as chemoattractants, have been called immunology's "high impact factors." First discovered in relationship to inflammatory responses, there are now over forty known types. Chemokines are mainly responsible for the movement and positioning of immune cells.

This *orchestration* of immune cells is one of the most important functions of the immune system. Without it, the immune cells cannot interact with one another and are unable to mount an immune response. Ironically, some viruses and other microbes (HIV-1, CMV, and the malaria parasite) have learned to use chemokine receptors to gain entry into the body.

Of particular importance is the therapeutic use of chemokine receptor antagonists. These are drugs currently in development which block chemokine activity. These substances are considered a new generation of anti-inflammatory medications. The chemokine story gets more interesting when we add to it the fact that viruses also appear to use naturally occurring chemokine antagonists to block inflammatory immune responses. This may explain how stealth viruses get past the immune system.

By inhibiting the initial inflammatory mechanisms, the viruses can then enter the bloodstream and circulate through the body, eventually arriving at their chosen site of infection—often the brain and central nervous system in the case of stealth viruses like CMV. In addition, stealth viruses may use chemokines as growth factors. In this case, the virus bypasses the inflammatory response thereby not alerting the specific immune cells; once in the body, it uses chemokines to replicate and produce more viruses.

The research of Dr. Martin, cited earlier, suggests that a number of the newer antibiotics, notably clarithromycin (Biaxin), that cross the blood-brain barrier are capable of suppressing chemokines. The blood-brain barrier is a term used in medicine to describe the protective ability of the brain and surrounding tissue to keep out toxins and microorganisms. Several natural medications and nutritional products also suppress chemokines and are useful in the treatment of stealth viral infections. These include vitamins B3, B6, B12, and vitamin D. The female sex hormones progesterone and estrogen also have chemokine antagonist properties. The flavonoid antioxidant quercitin has potent activity against chemokines and enzymes that favor viral replication, and it is an important part of the antiviral protocols described in part 2 of this book. Herbal medicines, especially Chinese herbs, may also have activity against unfavorable chemokines (discussed in part 2).

Other Immune Cells: Eosinophils compose 2–5 percent of total white blood cells and are capable of acting as phagocytes to kill microorganisms. They are believed to have a specific role in immunity against parasites. Levels of eosinophils become elevated during parasitic infection. They also deactivate histamine and often are found in increased levels in people with allergies.

Basophils and mast cells are very similar to each other in function and are found in very small numbers in the blood. Mast cells are associated with mucous membranes and connective tissue, and are found in greater profusion during allergic reactions. Platelets, cells usually associated with blood clotting but also involved in immune responses, are important in inflammation and healing after injury. They also release serotonin, a neurotransmitter associated with normal brain and nervous system function.

The Evolving Immune System

Advancing knowledge of how the immune system functions has contributed to a greater understanding of its biological complexity. What was once thought of as a system based on two distinct and separate aspects, a nonspecific attack response (innate immunity) and a specific learned response (adaptive immunity), is now known to be an intricate web of interrelated chemical and cellular activity intimately connected to the brain and neuroendocrine system. In *The Tao of Immunity*, Marc Lappé, Ph.D., an internationally known toxicologist, public health specialist, and the director of the Center for Ethics and Toxics (CETOS) in Gualala, California, says, "The immune system is a kind of modern-day cybernetic machine that fluctuates between stimulating and suppressing, eradicating and enriching, annihilating and restoring" (Lappé 1997).

Though we are just beginning to understand the complexities of the immune system and its evolving nature, there are four characteristics of the immune system that are important to discuss before we go further: redundancy, polymorphism, synergy, and mutual antagonism.

1) Redundancy describes many overlapping systems and repetitious functions of the immune system. To the human mind, this seems inefficient at first glance. However, inefficiency is a human concept, and particularly a Western one, and the immune system is not bound by language, culture, or belief. Its purpose is to work well enough for the survival of the individual, and more importantly, the species.

It is like an ant colony: To obtain a crumb of bread, thousands of ants are sent out from the colony, even if only ten ants can or will actually do the job. On the way, some are killed but others may find the morsel to take back. This is how our immune systems function: Tens of thousands of immune cells are employed to deal with every infection.

Cloning is a characteristic of immune cells that relates to redundancy and is an efficient way of preparing sufficient numbers of cells to neutralize an infection. Identical cells are produced daily, each an exact replica of the other. Immunology is largely a numbers game, so if there are enough active cells, the immune system is constantly prepared for possible penetration by microorganisms. Generally we think of clones as replicas with limited programmed functions; however, the immune system takes cloning a step further. Immune cells display a trait called polymorphism that allows them to meet new and changing circumstances.

2) Polymorphism means something can have more than one

shape or function. We are beginning to understand that immune cells can have more than one function and can change their chemical shapes as needed. This trait allows for superb adaptability, especially against super microorganisms that have the ability to mutate their forms, a trait called pleomorphism.

The next two characteristics, synergism and mutual antagonism, imply relationships. All natural things exist in relationship to something, and usually to numerous things.

3) Synergism suggests that one plus one does not simply equal two, but could also equal three, four, or five hundred. Synergism describes a situation in which the whole is greater than the sum of the parts and is also an important therapeutic principle, especially in natural medicine. To many conventional physicians natural medicines are considered weak compared to pharmaceutical drugs; however, when applied correctly using a variety of medications in a synergistic manner, powerful results appear. In part 2, you will learn to use therapeutic synergism to effectively stimulate the immune system.

4) In nature, many things coexist, some that are actually antagonistic or even poisonous to each other. For example: lions live side-by-side with gazelles while other creatures like crocodiles wait unsuspected in the watering holes. In your immune system, there are cells that reduce or trigger inflammation, but these same cells can cause damage to each other. This paradoxical activity is referred to as mutual antagonism.

As mentioned earlier, we live in a biological stew comprised of a staggering array of microorganisms and compounds, including pathogens such as viruses that have no "respect" for age, wealth, or social status. If you were to lie on a lawn, within minutes, ants and numerous other insects will find you and start biting your flesh, crawling into your orifices. To the denizens of the lawn, you are just another organic substance. Nature is neutral, and operates on principles that foster long-term balance in biological systems; such a system does not favor individuals, even though modern humans are obsessed with understanding and controlling these principles.

These principles are intricate and extraordinarily complex, and they are in constant transition, so it is difficult to understand changing phenomena, especially when they involve substances and pathogens at the submolecular level. Many of these are infectious microorganisms with rules of their own, and pay no heed to the workings of Man—or laboratory scientists.

The immune system, as an integral part of the organic natural matrix, continuously attempts to keep up with advancing infections and emerging new diseases, as well as with the "standard" ones. The immune system is considerably more dynamic and adaptive than is conventionally understood. Think of it as a web of interconnectedness that can simultaneously recognize and interface with many different microbes and immune challenges. It manages these challenges selectively, allowing certain infections to exist in our bodies while preventing others from taking root in our cells. Continuously transforming and adapting to circumstances, it brilliantly adjusts to the profile of the invading organism; all of this amazing operation is done without our awareness. However, there are times when the immune system fails.

When Things Go Wrong Immunologically

I am continuously impressed by the beauty and effectiveness of the immune system and its innate ability to protect us from illness. When we are healthy, we take it for granted, but there are many ways in which the immune system can become compromised and dysfunctional. Chief among them are autoimmune disease and immune deficiency.

Immune Malfunction: As mentioned earlier, the biochemical recognition of self from non-self is a key principle of immunity. A healthy immune system displays tolerance of self and does not stage immune responses against its own normal tissue and cells. If the immune system does attack normal tissue, immunologists call this an *auto*immune response—against the self—such as what happens in systemic lupus erythematosus (SLE), rheumatoid arthritis, and multiple sclerosis (MS).

Autoimmune reactions can also come as part of the normal immune response to an infection or other disease, such as arthritis with hepatitis B, or MS after CMV infection. Conventional immunology assumes that autoimmune responses are the operation of a malfunctioning or misguided immune system, and this abnormal response must be suppressed with drugs. However, it is possible that in some cases the immune system is attempting to remove damaged or diseased tissue, some virally infected, at the apparent expense of the host.

Autoimmune responses may be part of the normal process of "house-cleaning" by the immune system, meant to be only short-lived, acute, inflammatory episodes. Due to numerous factors including a toxic internal environment, weakened organ function, diminished detoxification pathways, poor nutrition, and stress, the autoimmune response can become chronically active, resulting in connective tissue diseases.

Immune Compromise: There are times when the immune system cannot keep up with the job of processing every foreign substance and organism, especially if they are novel or exotic chemicals and microbes. Viruses in particular can be difficult to eradicate. Once inside the body, they enter individual cells and may even pocket themselves away into recesses of organs and tissues. The drain on immune capacity can be severe resulting in weakened immune reserves. Many other conditions that adversely affect the immune system include:

Malnutrition and dietary stressors

Infections

Chronic stress

Chemical toxins

Aging

Chronic pain

Overexposure to ultraviolet light

MALNUTRITION AND DIETARY STRESSORS: Worldwide, malnutrition, dietary stress, and starvation cause more deaths and indirectly more fatal and chronic disease than any other one cause. It's estimated that a billion people are malnourished or undernourished in the world today. Protein-energy malnutrition (PEM) is a form of chronic macronutrient (protein, carbohydrate, and fat) starvation and results in anemia, retarded growth, weakness, and edema; it is what you usually see in the horrific photographs of African children reduced to skin and bones. In less severe forms it can affect elderly people, anorexics, lower-income people, and those on protein-restricted diets. Macronutrient starvation has a severe impact on the immune system, so starving and weakened individuals are more susceptible to infections.

Vitamin-deficiency diseases like scurvy and beriberi are now rare in the wealthier countries, but chronic poor or insufficient nutrition is very common, even in the midst of plenty. Also called micronutrient starvation, this condition gradually leads to reduced immune system function. In this case, the diet does not provide sufficient amounts of essential immune nutrients like vitamin A, zinc, and beta-carotene. Teenagers eating a diet of predominantly junk foods, as well as marginalized low-income people eating excess refined carbohydrates, are chronically undernourished in this manner. And, over time, they may develop a chronic low-level immune deficiency.

In industrialized nations, overeating and consuming excess amounts of the wrong foods cause the most problems. Dietary stressors cause disease and can negatively affect the immune system. Ironically, people can be overweight and undernourished.

One reason is that they consume large amounts of refined carbohydrates or hydrogenated fats and not enough fresh fruits and vegetables. This way of eating provides an excess of calories that the body cannot use, and it stores the excess as adipose tissue, or body fat. At the same time, these foods are notoriously low in nutrients, especially the trace elements vital for a healthy immune system.

Nutritional influences on illness and immune strength are more far-reaching than once thought by Western physicians. Think of nutritional deficiency midway on a continuum, with the severe forms of PEM and vitamin deficiency diseases on one end, and optimal nutrition, which can be defined as a diet rich in nutrient-dense foods, on the other (see figure 3-3).

These include fresh seasonal organic fruits and vegetables; dairy products (for those not allergic to them or who do not have lactose intolerance, a condition characterized by the absence of the enzyme lactase that digests milk proteins); seeds and nuts; vegetable oils like olive and safflower oils; condiments and spices like oregano, cumin, basil, and other culinary herbs; as well as adequate amounts of complete protein from plant and animal sources; and complex carbohydrates such as whole wheat (for those not allergic to gluten), rice, corn, potatoes, winter squash, and other sources of energy like the South American grain quinoa.

Optimal nutrition also means avoiding foods that have detrimental effects on health, such as refined carbohydrates like white sugar and white flour, products containing these ingredients such as commercial cookies and pastries, overly processed foods and foods containing toxic preservatives, additives, and dyes. It also means avoiding the excess use of alcohol and the unnecessary use of pharmaceutical drugs. These foods and substances promote obesity and degenerative diseases like

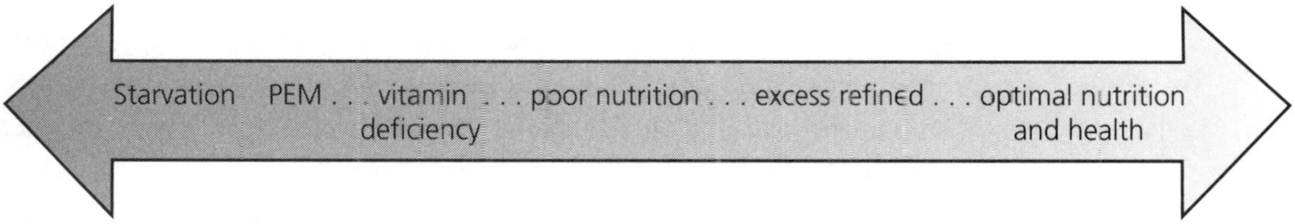

Starvation   PEM . . . vitamin . . . poor nutrition . . . excess refined . . . optimal nutrition
deficiency   and health

Figure 3-3: The Dietary Continuum

At one end of the dietary continuum are starvation and death, and at the other end are optimal nutrition and health. In the middle are sub-optimal nutritional states resulting from vitamin deficiencies, foods of poor nutritional quality, and excess amounts of foods that are high in refined carbohydrates and low in nutritional value.

diabetes. In addition to correct food choices, optimal nutrition includes supplementing the diet with vitamins and minerals (see part 2).

Optimal nutrition promotes a healthy immune system and prevents disease. Unfortunately, most people in the West consume far too much animal protein, fat, and refined sugar. Patrick Quillin, Ph.D., the author of *Beating Cancer With Nutrition,* estimates that only about 10 percent of Americans are optimally nourished, a situation that leads to sub-optimal nutrition (Quillin 1994). In these cases, for the majority of people a gradual erosion of immune status takes place allowing for disease processes to occur including cancer, autoimmune diseases, and increased susceptibility to viruses.

INFECTIONS: Not only do certain viruses weaken specific immune cells (HIV and CD4+ T cells),[7] but many chronic infections cause poor immune system function and predispose the body to other infections, fatigue syndromes, and possible tissue and organ failure including cancer. This can be seen with HCV and hepatocellular carcinoma.

Chronic and hidden bacterial infections also weaken the immune system. Chronic sinusitis, dental abscesses, chronic prostate infection, chronic appendicitis, diverticulosis (a condition of small pockets forming in the colon), gall bladder infections, and other conditions can weaken the body systems and fatigue our natural immunity.

Parasitic infections can be worse. Excess populations of normal gut bacteria, like klebsiella (a gram-negative bacteria in the Enterobacteriaceae family), can lead to rheumatic joint inflammation; malaria is notoriously immunosuppressant; and the Lyme spirochete not only causes damage to the nervous system but also weakens the immune system. Fungal infections are becoming more common and are equally a sign that the immune system is weakened. For example, chronic candida yeast infection causes a wide array of symptoms very similar to allergies and chronic viral infection, including fatigue, cloudy thinking, and gastrointestinal bloating.

CHRONIC STRESS: There is considerable scientific evidence that stress weakens the immune system. There are several models of how stress affects the immune system, and each has a common component: stress triggers a nervous system response, causing a brain response, which in turn affects glandular, and thus hormonal, function. Stress hormones then affect the hypothalamus, the region of the brain responsible for maintaining normal physiological functions like heart rate, temperature, hunger, weight control, and sleep.

Three interrelated glands—hypothalamus, pituitary, adrenals—interact with the nervous system and affect the immune system. As part of what's called the hypothalamic-pituitary-adrenal axis (HPA), cortisol is released by the adrenal gland in response to signals from the pituitary. High levels of cortisol suppress lymphocyte production and inhibit the release of IL-2 (Interleukin-2, an immune-enhancing cytokine).[8] In addition, epinephrine and norepinephrine—commonly called adrenaline, the chemicals that produce the "fight-or-flight" response—become elevated under stress. This can reduce the levels of CD4 helper T lymphocytes.

People with clinical depression have been shown to have more outbreaks of cold sores, genital herpes, and more frequent symptoms of the common cold. They also have poorer outcomes from cancer and degenerative diseases. Surprisingly, overly strenuous exercise causes increased numbers of free radicals from the burning of more oxygen demanded by intense activity. This results in depletion of antioxidants,[9] one of the key components of optimal immune function.

There is now an epidemic of sleep disorders in the United States. In our fast-paced society, it is a luxury to spend a day in bed. One of my Chinese medical colleagues said to me that in America we treat our bodies like machines, expecting them to run at high efficiency whenever we want, just like our cars. However, the body is not a machine. It needs adequate rest and sleep as part of its restorative cycle in order to function effectively.

Several studies have shown that going without sleep and enduring chronic sleep deprivation are harmful to immunity. In one study, sleep deprivation reduced natural killer cell levels. Carol Everson,

Ph.D., a neurobiology researcher at the University of Chicago, found startling evidence here. In chronic progressive loss of sleep a "negative energy" balance resulted in reduced immunity, and it allowed normally occurring gut bacteria to migrate to otherwise healthy tissue sites, resulting in infection (Everson 1993).

Dr. Everson also found that this deep negative energy balance caused by chronic sleep deprivation reduced the normal inflammatory response, allowing abnormal levels of bacteria to survive unmolested by the immune system. Negative energy balance is a state where more energy is expended than is replenished in the normal restorative cycle of sleep, rest, and eating. A host of symptoms appear when sleep deprivation occurs including fatigue, increased appetite (the body's way of attempting to make up for lost energy by eating more), weight loss, increased susceptibility to common infections like colds and sinusitis, and hormonal changes such as low levels of thyroid hormone and growth hormone.

During times of stress, getting enough sleep and being able to sleep deeply and uninterruptedly greatly improves immune function.

CHEMICAL TOXINS: Excessive toxic load from environmental chemical exposure caused one of the most significant adverse effects on health in the twentieth century. It is accelerating into this century as well, and will continue to unless we make significant changes in the way we live. The liver, the most important detoxification organ, has evolved extraordinarily effective mechanisms to detoxify normal levels of naturally occurring toxins, such as plant toxins in foods. However, it becomes incapable of dealing with or keeping up with the immense amount of novel chemical toxins from over-the-counter and prescription drugs, preservatives in foods, insecticides, fungicides, hydrocarbons, and other environmental poisons in the air, food, and water we consume.

There are several classes of chemicals that cause disease in humans. These are mutagens, teratogens, and immunosuppressants. Mutagens are chemicals that cause abnormal cell changes (or mutations) that lead to cancer. If these mutagenic changes occur in the genetic material, altered genes can pass from parent to child, causing disease for generations

> *Dr. Everson also found that this deep negative energy balance caused by chronic sleep deprivation reduced the normal inflammatory response, allowing abnormal levels of bacteria to survive unmolested by the immune system. Negative energy balance is a state where more energy is expended than is replenished in the normal restorative cycle of sleep, rest, and eating.*

Teratogens are chemicals that cause abnormal tissue changes in the fetus, leading to birth defects. Since the immune system is unable to successfully deal with these chemicals once they have gained entry into the body and have caused irreparable cellular damage, the body may put other systems into play to keep us from exposure. One researcher found that the increasing incidence of morning sickness, which is now called nausea of pregnancy or pregnancy sickness, may be a natural way of preventing the mother from eating, thereby reducing her exposure to birth-defect-causing chemicals in foods.

The field of toxicology has mainly focused on cancer-causing agents and less on the immune system. However, immunotoxicology—the study of how toxic chemicals damage immune function—describes not only carcinogenic, or cancer-causing, agents, but also the mechanics of reduced general immunity and increased susceptibility to infection.

Immunosuppressants are toxic environmental chemicals that cause suppression of the immune system, thereby allowing for increased vulnerability to infection or causing direct acute toxicity and even death. Long-term, low-level exposure to these substances can insidiously alter immune response, a condition which might first manifest as more frequent cold-like or allergic symptoms or asthma, but which can eventually lead to more complex degenerative illness. It may even participate in destabilizing the immune system, allowing reactivated herpes viruses infections, or it may reduce resistance to common bacterial, viral, or fungal infections. Xenobiotics—foreign chemicals that interact with living systems and even mimic hormones and other naturally occurring substances—are considered the most dangerous of environmental toxins.

The list of these toxic substances is long and includes the polychlorinated biphenyls (PCBs) and related substances such as polychlorinated dibenzofurans (PCDFs) and polychlorinated dibenzodioxins (PCDDs)—a group that includes the toxic agent dioxin. As PCBs concentrate in the food chain, people who eat fatty meats and large amounts of fish are particularly at risk. Organophosphate pesticides (diazinon, malathion) residues on foods, heavy metals (iron, lead, mercury, zinc), and scores of other environmental toxins also cause immune damage.

In addition, many prescription drugs—ironically even some, like AZT, used to treat immunodeficiency—and the abuse of recreational drugs and alcohol also cause significant immune damage. Chemical substances and drugs like acetaminophen cause liver toxicity, indirectly fostering illness and immune system compromise. Steroid drugs, like Prednisone, routinely used for only minor respiratory tract inflammations, are powerful immune suppressants.

AGING: Aging, or senescence, is the gradual wearing out of living organisms, and it is one of medicine's greatest mysteries. Though we may not know exactly why we age, we do know some of the effects of aging. Among the many aspects of aging is a decline in immune function and an increased predisposition to chronic inflammation. Persistent inflammation can damage important tissues such as the coronary arteries of the heart, and inflict the joint pain of arthritis. Ironically, this inflammation can be triggered by immune reactions. The same system that works to promote our survival may also participate in our aging.

During our lives, we are exposed to an increasing toxic chemical load and this causes tissue and cellular damage from free radicals associated with or produced by the toxic substances. This damage, referred to as free radical pathology, also weakens our immune status (see part 2).

Hormonal decline also occurs with age. Steroid, sex, and stress hormones help to manage inflammation and tissue damage, but if they are deficient, as happens in aging, the tissue damage can become chronic, leading to a predisposition to disease and the reactivation of viral infections. On the other hand, using steroid hormone drugs like Prednisone reduces inflammation but causes significant immune suppression.

The thymus gland in the chest is of particular importance to immune senescence. It tends to atrophy with age, and this shrinking-gland phenomenon causes reduced immune function and increased susceptibility to infection. The function of hormones and immunity is discussed in part 2, including ways to supplement hormonal deficiency.

CHRONIC PAIN: Ongoing pain, in the low back or neck and as found in arthritis, is one of the most common complaints reported to doctors, and it can weaken your immunity. Pain causes the release of inflammatory chemicals that suppress immunity. The stress of chronic pain and the sleep disruption that pain creates also reduce your immune system's ability to fight infections. The immune-suppressing trio of stress, sleep deprivation, and pain over an extended period of time can weaken your health and make you more susceptible to cancer and viral disease.

Overexposure to Ultraviolet Light: Repeated or long exposure to ultraviolet radiation can suppress the immune system. Research has shown that activation of chemicals in the skin and the secretion of interleukin-10 (IL-10, a cytokine) reduces resistance to tumor formation and infections.

Outbreaks of oral herpes simplex virus can be triggered by sunlight. People in tropical countries, where there are more hours of daylight per year and where the highest levels of solar radiation occur, experience the highest incidence of infectious disease, including oral herpes virus. Of course, there are other factors that cause more infections in tropical countries than in temperate regions, such as poor diet due to poverty. Besides the sun, other sources of ultraviolet light include indoor lighting, growth lamps for plants, and tanning beds.

Purposeful Immunosuppression: Modern medicine uses drugs and radiation to suppress the immune system. In the case of rheumatoid arthritis, an autoimmune disease characterized by aggressive joint inflammation, drugs such as methotrexate and cortisone are used. In organ transplant patients, the immune system must be continually suppressed for the transplanted organ to be retained and accepted. Radiation, a common therapy in cancer, suppresses production of white cells in the bone marrow.

In all these cases, increasingly large numbers of people in the general population are artificially immunosuppressed by drugs. These patients are more prone to simple infections and are often on multiple courses of antibiotics to treat and prevent opportunistic bacterial infections. This may result in these individuals harboring drug-resistant species of viruses, bacteria, and fungi—essentially becoming living, walking test tubes for super bugs.

Symptoms of a Compromised Immunity: The immune system is extraordinarily resilient. Under normal circumstances of regular exposure to infectious illnesses, the immune system manages quite well. However, under siege by toxins, stress, complicated with adaptation to new viruses and antibiotic-resistant bacteria, and combined with age, sleep deprivation, and other physiological stressors, it gradually becomes compromised. Once the immune system reaches a point where deficiencies and imbalances occur, symptoms show themselves. When immune compromise is severe, life-threatening conditions occur, usually caused by opportunistic infections like CMV and pneumonia.

Deficiency of specific components of the immune system results in

Table 6: Immune Deficiency Disorders

Deficiency	Associated Disease
B-cell deficiency	Recurrent bacterial infections (i.e., otitis media)
T-cell deficiency	Increased susceptibility to viral and fungal infections
T- and B-cell deficiency	Increased susceptibility to all types of infections
Phagocytic-cell deficiency	Low-grade systemic bacteria infections
NK-cell deficiency	Increased susceptibility to viral infections and cancer
Complement deficiency	Bacterial infections

primary immune deficiency syndromes (see table 6), considered rare clinical diseases. However, larger numbers of people seem to be exhibiting signs of immune deficiency patterns Perhaps, as I previously mentioned, there is a continuum of disease states related to immune deficiency with early signs and symptoms that might go unnoticed.

Fortunately, most early immune deficiencies do not develop into much more than frequent colds or recurrent bacterial infections. However, at the extreme end we find CFIDS and AIDS. In the case of AIDS, the immune system becomes so compromised that immune-deficiency diseases, such as chronic skin and mucous membrane infection by the fungus *Candida albicans,* once thought rare, occur with significant frequency.

Many common viruses become lethal in patients who are immunocompromised due to chemotherapy (cytotoxic treatments) and drugs used to suppress the immune system in transplants. They include herpes simplex and zoster that can cause severe local infections, and cytomegalovirus that can cause pneumonitis (a lung infection), which can lead to death.

Immune Response to Viral Infection

The immune system's response to viruses is complex. There are thousands of viruses, and each infects the host in a different way and elicits a different immune response. There is not one specific immune component, chemical, or cell that specifically reacts to a virally infected cell; rather, many different immune cells and processes work together to neutralize a viral insult. In addition, due to the small size of viruses and their ability to lie dormant within individual cells, the immune

Stages of Immune Compromise

After more than twenty years of clinical practice, a large part of it spent treating patients with an immunological aspect of their condition including allergies, CFIDS, fibromyalgia, chronic hepatitis, and cancer, I have come to think of immune compromise and resultant deficiency states in levels.

First Level: Episodal fatigue, recurrent headaches, generalized low-level aches and pains, recurrent colds and catching colds easily, and frequent allergies.

Second Level: All of level one symptoms increase in severity and frequency, plus fatigue becomes a constant concern. Memory and cognition are also affected; sleep disturbance is present.

Third Level: Appearance of shingles and other herpes virus infections, and the appearance of recurrent co-infections like fungal and bacterial infections (*Candida albicans*, sinusitis). Nervous system symptoms appear, including MS-like conditions (weakness in the extremities and loss of balance), severe memory impairment, depression and anxiety disorders, inability to cope with stress.

Fourth Level: Disease states are now clearly manifest (MS, CFIDS, and AIDS). All symptoms of levels 1 through 3 worsen. Fatigue states can be profound.

Fifth Level: Complete immune failure resulting in death from opportunistic infections or cancer.

system may attack the whole cell, tissues, or entire organs containing the virus in order to destroy it. In the process an autoimmune reaction may be triggered, disabling or killing not just the cell but the host as well, as in hemorrhagic fevers and dengue shock syndrome.

Viruses are not passive organisms. They have evolved highly sophisticated strategies for avoiding recognition by the immune system of the host, including the production of decoy proteins that interfere with antiviral defenses and the utilization of the host's own chemokines to support their proliferation.

Before they can replicate, viruses must infect a living cell. To do so, they must enter the body. After the virus gains entry into the body, it attaches itself to a target cell and penetrates the cell membrane. Once inside the host cell, it replicates and reassembles into unique virion particles, which burst the host cell and escape (see figure 3-4).

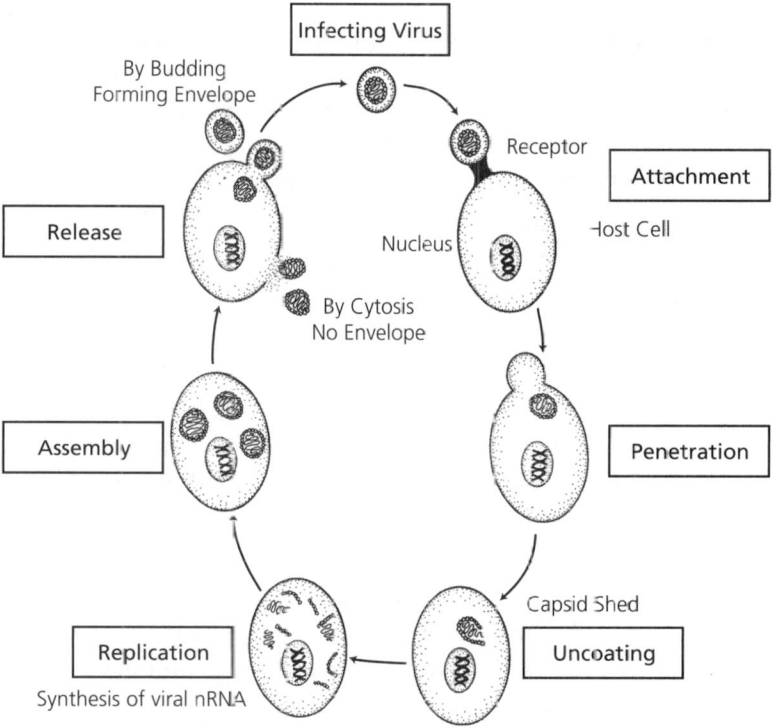

Figure 3-4: Stages of Cell Infection

After entry into the body, viruses infect individual cells by (1) attaching themselves to a target cell (host) and then (2) penetrating its cell membrane thereby gaining entry into the host cell. Before beginning the replication process, the virus (3) uncoats its own membrane and then (4) replicates itself using the genetic material of the host cell. The virions then (5) reassemble and escape the former host (now dead) cell through a process of (6) release by budding (forming a new envelope) or by dissolving the former host's cell membrane (cytolysis without an envelope). Each new virus is capable of re-infecting additional target cells.

Key Immune Components Active Against Viruses: The main immune system components specific to viral immunity are antibodies, produced by the B lymphocytes in cooperation with T lymphocytes, and components of cell-mediated immunity, especially NK cells, and helper and suppressor T lymphocytes. Interferons and interleukins are an early protective mechanism and also play a role in response to viruses. The complement system provides some protection against viruses by damaging their envelopes.

Newly discovered immune enzymes also play a role. Robert J. Suhadolnik, Ph.D., of Temple University School of Medicine in

Immune Components Involved in Viral Immunity:

Antibodies	Interferons
Complement	Interleukins
Cytotoxic and Helper T cells	Macrophages
Immune Enzymes	NK cells

Philadelphia has defined a specific enzymatic pathway (2′, 5′-oligoad-enylate trimer 5′-triphosphate, 2-5A), which involves a molecule that activates an enzyme, RNase L, which in turn degrades viral RNA. Though Suhadolnik's research is predominantly on HIV, he found that this enzyme was significantly active in CFIDS patients.

Innate Immune Response: The early immune protective phase against viral infection is seen in nonspecific mechanical events of the innate immune system, such as increased amounts of mucus with respiratory infections and diarrhea in gastrointestinal viruses. Once the virus has entered the body and infected the cells, the innate immune systems responds with activity by NK cells and macrophages.

At this stage, interferons and interleukins also play a role. Interferon alerts neighboring cells of imminent infection, enabling them to prepare a defense. In an active early-stage immune response, fever and inflammation occur (see next chapter). Interferon also activates NK cells, which are active within two days after initial infection and go to work to attack and mop up viruses (see figure 3-5).

Adaptive Response: As the infection spreads, cytotoxic T cells, helper T cells, and antiviral antibodies appear to continue the work started by the innate response. IgA production is increased in the mucosal tissue to prevent reinfection. Other antibodies also arrive on the scene, including IgM and IgG molecules. Though antibodies block viruses from attaching to and entering host cells, they are only effective against free viruses, those that have not yet entered a cell. Once a virus has entered a cell, it is considerably more difficult to eradicate without damaging the host cell. Complement may work along with antibodies to damage the virion envelope and neutralize free viruses.

The body's T-cell system is highly specific and very efficient against viruses. Both CD4 (helper) and CD8 (cytotoxic) T cells play

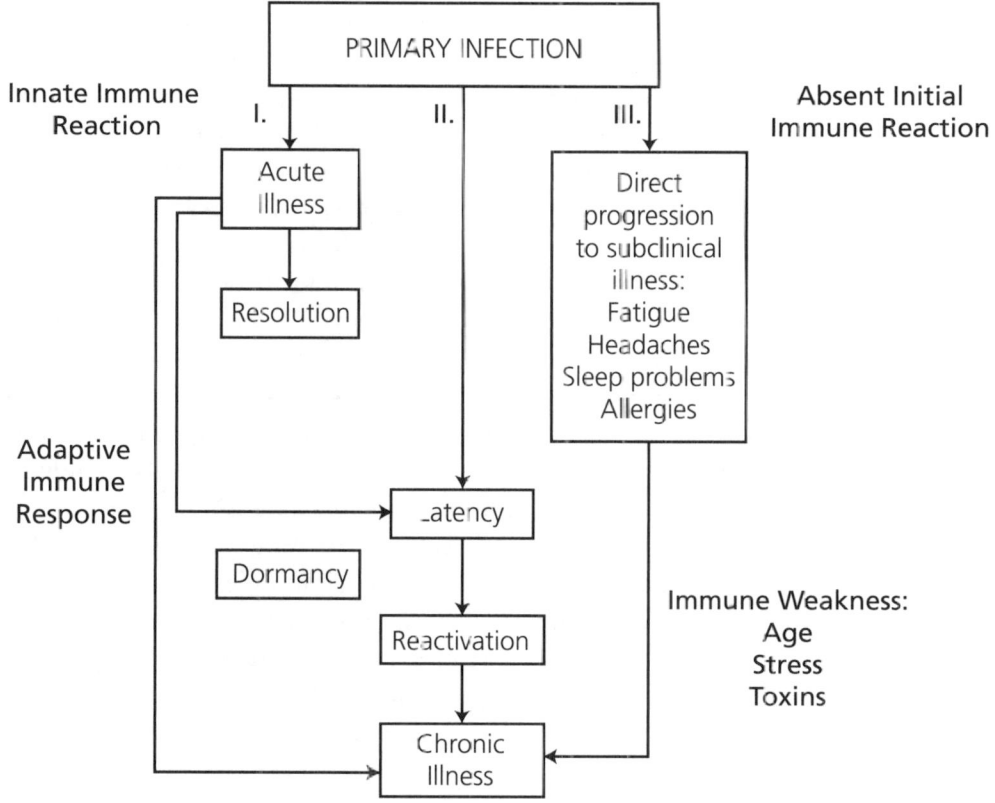

Figure 3-5: Viral Pathways and Immune Response

Primary viral infection can generate three types of immune responses. (1) A typical infection proceeds to the acute stage (influenza or cold) and is acted upon by the innate and adaptive immune system and then usually resolves (goes away without consequences). However, acute primary infections can also lead to latency or chronic illness (as with some herpes viruses). In the absence of an adequate immune response, a primary viral infection can proceed directly to (2) latency, or (3) chronic illness (as in chronic hepatitis C).

major roles in the immune response against viral infection. Interferon and tumor necrosis factor are key cytokines in the adaptive response against viruses.

Resolution of Infection and Return to Normal: As the immune system is responding to viral infection, the virus goes through its own process and eventually is shed from the body. Once outside the body, it remains active and may infect other people, thereby continuing the cycle of immune response and viral replication. The best-case scenario is when the immune system *completely* eliminates all viral residue so that no viral particles remain dormant inside the body. The worst-case scenario is if the virus takes up permanent residency in the body's tissues. However, if all goes well, the infected individual returns to normal and the immune system is readied for the next challenge.

Absence of the Immune Response: As you have seen in this chapter, under normal and reasonable circumstances, the immune system is more than capable of neutralizing viral infections. However, due to the overwhelming amounts of environmental toxins, the effects of stress, improper diet, and other factors that suppress immune function, the immune response is sometimes unable to effectively deal with the challenge of infection. In these cases, complete resolution does not occur and the virus either enters a latent stage or produces a chronic infection, causing increasing symptoms.

Often the manifestation of these symptoms is completely different from an active infection. For example, multiple sclerosis can be caused by an autoimmune response, which could have been triggered by a viral infection. Looking at the symptomatic presentation alone and giving immune suppressing drugs can temporarily reduce symptoms but further weaken the immune system's ability to neutralize the virus.

CHAPTER SUMMARY

The Earth is far from sterile. Microorganisms coexist with us in a world of extraordinary biodiversity.

Viruses display remarkable biological intelligence.

A healthy immune system is equal to this challenge and is prepared to interface with infectious microorganisms to promote our survival in a manner whose complexity defies explanation.

Traditional immunology offers a wealth of detailed information but does not provide the bigger picture of evolutionary and energy medicine. Integrating these views may be beneficial and practical in understanding how to treat individual patients with viral infections.

There are two main divisions of the immune system: innate, or nonspecific immunity and adaptive, or acquired immunity.

The innate immune response is composed of physical barriers, mechanical processes, and cellular defenses.

Adaptive immunity is made up of a vast array of cellular and chemical components.

Immune compromise may be more prevalent that previously thought, and not only affects HIV and CFIDS patients, but may play a role in the increasing incidence of autoimmune diseases as well.

Viral immunity requires the coordination of many different components from both branches of the immune system.

If any of these components are missing, combined with the overwhelming number of viruses and their evolutionary adaptability, the probability of a chronic viral infection is increased.

4

Fever and Fatigue

In this chapter, we come to one of the major cruxes of modern immunity. We are experiencing a global immune crisis of unprecedented proportions, one accompanied by serious consequences as seen in AIDS, CFIDS, HCV, and other viral pandemics; increasing incidences of other infectious diseases, many types of cancer, and an epidemic of allergic diseases. Unfortunately for the average patient, it is a situation that has been paid little attention to by most clinicians, and until only very recently by most researchers.

I propose that an increasingly dysfunctional natural immunity, combined with increasing virulence of infectious disease are simultaneous causes of the current health crisis. If this hypothesis is correct, then we should expect to see *more* problems, not only with new viral diseases but with autoimmune diseases, fatigue states, allergies, asthma, and disorders related to chronic inflammation.

However, many of these conditions overlap, often making it difficult to categorize specific diseases into set categories and for a doctor to recognize an underlying immune problem. For example: a case of multiple sclerosis could be triggered by a virus and also be an autoimmune problem, while at the same time present with fatigue as well as inflammation of the nervous system.

Such cases are difficult to treat. Drugs are powerful agents that exert marked effects on only a few aspects of the body's chemistry and physiology, but in doing so may significantly imbalance other aspects, making the patient much worse from the therapy. Natural therapies and more comprehensive approaches to these new conditions are needed.

In this chapter, I explore this hypothesis further and explain why prevention and correction of *underlying* immune weakness is more important than treatment of acute symptoms. I focus on the first-line defense mechanisms of inflammation and fever and show how they are disrupted, suppressed, and blunted. I discuss the importance of fatigue and how it is replacing inflammation and fever as the most predominant symptom of the new chronic diseases, and I explain why it's important to understand this aberration from normal immunity. Since treatment is necessary for those with viral illness, later in part 2 I discuss and outline methods of using natural medicines to treat viral diseases and provide specific immune-enhancing techniques.

Understanding the Immune-Viral Disease Crisis

Put simply, it is as follows:

- There is a breakdown in our normal innate immune response mechanisms.

- Fever and acute inflammation normally associated with infection are often blunted, and even absent, while fatigue is more prevalent.

- This reversal of the natural immune mechanisms allows for viruses to bypass the nonspecific phases of the innate immune response.

- Once past the front line immune barriers and into the bloodstream, viruses are able to go directly to a target organ or tissue, including immune cells, and cause considerable damage.

- This results in a variety of chronic diseases, the worst being AIDS, CFIDS, chronic hepatitis C, and nervous system diseases such as multiple sclerosis.

The cause of this breakdown of the natural immune cycle is multifactorial and therefore it is not easy to pinpoint one particular cause.

Unlike the proverbial single rotten apple, it seems that all the "apples" in the immune barrel are spoiling at different stages. However, as the data comes in, researchers seem certain that the causes include environmental toxins, confusion in gene expression by hormone disrupters,[1] stress-triggered dysfunction of hormone regulation between the pituitary gland and adrenals (HPA axis), chronic sleep disturbance, increased microbial virulence combined with drug resistance, immune suppressive drugs, and lifestyle-related factors (discussed in previous chapters) such as a nutrient-deficient diet.

The cause of this breakdown of the natural immune cycle is multifactorial and therefore it is not easy to pinpoint one particular cause. Unlike the proverbial single rotten apple, it seems that all the "apples" in the immune barrel are spoiling at different stages.

The increasing prevalence of allergic disorders like asthma, atopic dermatitis (skin rashes), rhinitis (hay fever), and sinusitis is also an indication of an immune imbalance. In the United States, the incidence of asthma has increased by 75 percent between 1980 and 1994 (Wills-Karp 2001). Certainly, worsening indoor and outdoor air quality play a significant role in causing asthma and triggering allergic symptoms, but a more important factor may be the lower incidence of childhood infections, vaccinations, and overuse of antibiotics.

In the absence of minor infections that children in the past were routinely exposed to, which they contracted from other children or from playing in the dirt (a practice that is not condoned by advocates of modern, overly hygienic child-rearing practices), the adaptive immune system does not build up antibodies in preparation for future infections. This lack of adaptive immunity, combined with an artificially manipulated immune response from vaccines, can tip the balance of the helper T cells, allowing for increased reactivity to allergic antigens. Allergic diseases can cause chronic inflammation, setting the stage for autoimmune diseases like rheumatoid arthritis.

It is becoming more common to see cases of chronic low-grade inflammation, as in irritable bowel syndrome (IBS), even though, paradoxically, the innate inflammatory response is blunted or absent in the face of infection. Chronic inflammation has been associated with increased risk for heart disease, Alzheimer's, and it often accompanies chronic fatigue.

Another factor disrupting immunity and contributing to increased allergies and inflammation is the disruption of intestinal flora from antibiotic use and the consumption of refined foods. Antibiotics destroy normal bacteria, like *Lactobacillus* species, as well as harmful bacteria. A normal intestinal environment is essential for a strong immune system, and appears to also play a role in reducing allergic reactivity. Refined foods do not provide the proper medium for friendly intestinal bacteria to thrive. Foods that promote a healthy intestinal environment are fermented products like miso and yogurt (see part 2).

Illustrative Case: Martha: A case study helps us understand this issue. Martha was a brilliant woman in her mid-thirties who first came to see me with multiple complaints that centered on chronic fatigue. In addition to her low energy, she had allergies, chemical and food sensitivities, recurrent colds, sinus congestion with repeated bouts of sinus infections, and yeast infections. When she first saw me, her medical doctors were treating her with an antidepressant and a drug to kill fungus, and she was self-medicating with an assortment of vitamins and herbs. Interestingly, Martha also was very sensitive to many vitamins (or the binders used to hold the tablets together or fill the capsules), so she ended up with many unusable bottles of supplements.

Reviewing her medical history, I found Martha was previously employed in a job that involved a high degree of toxic exposure to pesticides. Prior to that, she had been very active and healthy, except for childhood allergies for which she had had her tonsils and adenoids removed, both of which are lymphatic tissue and part of the immune system. She had been under high pressure and stress for many years.

Martha traced her problems to what she originally thought was a cold that would not go away. She had been severely ill for about four months, though she pushed herself to continue working, until she sought medical advice. Her conventional doctor gave her an antibiotic for sinusitis and recommended rest; however, she only experienced mild relief and pursued further diagnostic studies.

These revealed that she had been exposed to cytomegalovirus and had an elevated antinuclear antibody (ANA). This is a blood marker found in patients whose immune system is predisposed to or already causing inflammation against their own connective tissue. ANA can be elevated in viral or bacterial infections, cancer, autoimmune hormonal diseases, systemic lupus erythematosus, rheumatoid arthritis, and Sjörgen's syndrome. Martha next went to several specialists including a rheumatologist who prescribed nonsteroidal anti-inflammatory drugs.

In Martha's case, we can see that she had a lifelong allergic condition, which was not addressed properly and for which she had to have her tonsils and adenoids removed as a child because they became so swollen due to inflammation and infection. As a person goes through puberty and adolescence, the increased levels of sex and steroid hormones secreted by the glands responsible for these changes often cause symptoms of allergy and asthma to disappear, and these can re-emerge later in life.

Several years of ongoing stress combined with occupational exposure to toxic chemicals further weakened Martha's immune system, and her allergies not only resurfaced but worsened and were complicated by sinus infections. This was most likely followed by reactivation of a latent cytomegaloviral infection; her immune system was able to contain the virus, yet this condition caused an increase in immune chemicals that promote inflammation and helped cause her fatigue.

After her first visit, I referred her to an allergist specializing in disorders with environmental causes. This doctor was able to pinpoint specific allergens and start her on weekly desensitization allergy injections. I treated Martha with acupuncture, nutrients, and herbal medications, and she improved considerably over the first six weeks of treatment. Her fatigue lessened considerably, the sinus symptoms of congestion and pressure disappeared, and she was able to exercise without fatigue or shortness of breath. Over time, her predisposition to catching colds and flu vanished, she had no yeast problems, and she experienced improved tolerance to chemicals, foods, and was able to use most of her vitamins.

Since the cause of her problem was not depression, and as she felt better, she was able to eliminate her antidepressant drugs. Though she still harbored the virus, Martha's body had managed to reestablish immunological equilibrium between itself and the virus.

This case is typical of hundreds of patients that I have seen and highlights several important points. Underlying allergies or immune and endocrine imbalances are not recognized in childhood; often, only symptoms are treated or surgery is used to remove the inflamed tissue, such as tonsils and adenoids. This does nothing for the underlying cause and generally results in lifelong allergy problems. As stress further weakens the immune system and as symptoms of minor infections such as sinusitis occur, the person is treated with more antibiotics. Antibiotics generally fail to work over time, and often cause fungal infections due to the disruption of the internal ecology between friendly bacteria and yeast.

Next, allergies increase and asthma may develop, which is treated with steroids that further disrupt the immune system and further encourage fungal and yeast growth. The resultant vaginal yeast or nail fungal infections are then treated with an anti-fungal drug. By that time, the patient is also often worried, stressed, anxious, not sleeping well, and very tired. They are then treated with a mild antidepressant. Usually, it is about that time that they start to seek alternative treatment. Often, these same patients will also have fibromyalgia or another condition of chronic pain or inflammation like irritable bowel syndrome.

By themselves, alternative therapies generally are palliative for these conditions, though if applied in a comprehensive manner and if they include diet, exercise, lifestyle changes, and stress management, they help many patients to improve significantly. A better model as I used in Martha's case, uses an integrative approach that evaluates many factors including allergies, gastrointestinal function, detoxification pathways, antioxidant status, inflammatory status, viral activity, and immunological function, and applies multiple therapies appropriate to the individual case to restore immune balance and normal homeostasis, the body's self-regulating mechanisms.

The Immunological Function of Inflammation

Inflammation is part of the healing response, and it is a complex process involving nonspecific and specific immunological mechanisms designed to protect our bodies from pathogens and to assist in repairing damaged tissue. Healthy, normal tissue is not inflamed. Since inflammation is a protective response, once the offending agent has been removed and the damaged or diseased tissue healed, the body automatically returns to a normal quiescent state.

Inflammation is not only part of the healing response, it is also a symptom that something is wrong: you limp or stay off a sprained ankle; call the doctor if your tonsils are swollen; or apply ice to a twisted knee. Inflammation is a common occurrence of daily living, everyone has experienced pain and swelling from a twisted ankle, sore and enlarged tonsils, a stomachache after eating too much spicy or acidic food, a headache, a blister from tight shoes, a cut from working in the garden, or a sunburn. All are examples of inflammation.

The understanding of inflammation is part of the study of medicine and its characteristics have been known in Western medicine since the time of the Greeks. The main hallmarks of inflammation are redness, swelling, heat, and pain, and all four usually, but not always, occur together. In medical terminology, the suffix "itis" in a word means inflammation. Some examples include tendonitis (inflammation of a tendon); arthritis (joint inflammation); hepatitis (liver inflammation); and gastroenteritis (inflammation of the stomach and intestines).

Inflammatory activity is initiated when injury occurs from an external trauma (cuts or burns) or internal deterioration of tissue (cancer, liver disease, or arthritis). Activation of the inflammatory response also takes place from biological insults, such as infection by microorganisms, including viruses.

Inflammation is divided by location into two types, localized and systemic, and by activity into acute or chronic. Localized inflammation occurs when you bang your thumb or have an eye infection like conjunctivitis. Systemic inflammation affects the whole body, as happens in influenza. When you catch the flu, your joints and muscles ache and fever develops; you feel tired and want to stay in bed. Systemic inflammation also occurs in more serious viral infections and other diseases like pneumonitis (inflammation of the lungs) and hepatitis.

Acute Inflammation: In acute inflammation, several processes occur in a complex chain of events. White blood cell production immediately increases and the number of white cells grows. White blood cells, or leukocytes, make up the immune cells or immunocytes, so once leukocytes arrive at the site of infection they release chemicals that control activities of other cells including secretion of inflammatory mediators. These include histamine, serotonin, interleukin, complement, and prostaglandin, among others. Plasma molecules and antigens are also released. Swelling occurs, accompanied by redness and warmth in the local tissue that increases blood supply to the area, and pus may develop.

For minor acute inflammation the treatment is time, rest, and the application of ice. Elevation of an inflamed appendage reduces some of the pressure caused by the swelling. For inflammation with infection, antibiotics or antimicrobial natural medications are necessary if severe bacterial infection occurs. Occasionally, surgical drainage is necessary to remove pus and infected material.

Stress Response to Inflammation: Inflammation is a stressor on the body so the hypothalamic-pituitary-adrenal (HPA) axis responds by increasing the synthesis of cortisol, a hormone from the adrenal gland. Cortisol has natural anti-inflammatory effects. An increased production of acute-phase proteins occurs, like C-reactive protein (CRP). This binds to the membranes of microorganisms, activating the complement system in order to increase phagocytosis, the nonspecific destruction of invading antigens. CRP has other important biological functions in noninfectious inflammatory processes, most notably in heart disease where an elevated CRP level, as determined by lab test, can serve as a predictor of possible heart attack

Autoimmune-Induced Inflammation: Autoimmune responses can cause serious and painful progressive inflammation. This type of inflammation does not resolve in a normal fashion, but persists and can lead to further tissue damage, as in the joint destruction of rheumatoid arthritis or the kidney damage of lupus. In these cases, the normally protective and beneficial inflammatory mechanism—usually our ally in healing—becomes our nemesis.

Therapeutically, autoimmune-mediated inflammation must be reduced and neutralized. In conventional medicine the treatment of choice is steroid drugs like prednisone and nonsteroidal anti-inflammatory drugs (NSAIDs) like aspirin and ibuprofen. Though steroid drugs are effective in controlling symptoms caused by inflammation, they also powerfully suppress immune function.

Recall the case of the young woman with rheumatoid arthritis who had been on prednisone for several years (discussed earlier in the book). Though the drug helped reduce some of the inflammation, she developed repeated sinus infections. Once I stabilized her condition with natural medications, she was able to reduce and then eliminate the steroid. Her immune system recovered enough so that she did not have any more sinus problems.

Caution: In autoimmune or pro-inflammatory states, it is important not to take substances that might promote or accelerate inflammation. These conditions include rheumatoid arthritis, lupus, scleroderma, and Sjögren's Syndrome. Even minor inflammatory states such as eczema, hives, and irritable bowel syndrome can sometimes be aggravated by immune-enhancing natural medications like echinacea or dairy-based products like colostrum. For more on the potential pro-inflammatory nature of some natural supplements see part 2.

Chronic Inflammation: Another area of major concern, particularly in many of the modern illnesses, is chronic low-grade inflammation. Aging, chronic viral illnesses, irritable bowel syndrome, atherosclerosis, fibromyalgia, low back pain, cardiovascular disease, and many other chronic conditions all have inflammatory characteristics. Chronic inflammation is abnormal and is not a part of healthy tissue or normal aging. In these cases, pain—often constant and debilitating—is usually present as a symptom and a low-grade inflammation persists.

We are just beginning to understand the mechanisms and consequences of chronic inflammation. Though chronic inflammation may be considered a state of imbalance between anti-inflammatory and pro-inflammatory immune modulators, such as cytokines like interleukin-1β and various chemokines, it is more insidious than that and involves multiple events.

Environmental toxins, free radical pathology, abnormal gut ecology, bacterial and viral infections, and naturally occurring metabolic toxins trigger immunological responses that can cause chronic inflammation. Stress also plays a significant role.

An increase in other pro-inflammatory chemicals also occurs: first come prostaglandins, commonly occurring substances derived from arachidonic acid (a fatty acid and key player in the inflammation cycle), involved in many biological processes including roles in the mediation of inflammation; second is Nuclear Factor kappa B (NF-kappa B, a protein that regulates gene expression inside cells). NF-kappa B actually is part of a family of factors that influence immunity, promote the cell proliferation involved in cancer growth, and that induce inflammation. In addition, metabolic and endocrine changes take place concurrently with chronic inflammation, causing fatigue and generalized low-grade malaise.

Normally, the body has several means to resolve recurring inflammation. It may increase inflammatory activity, temporarily causing more swelling and pain, in an attempt to stimulate the tissue response to pass through an acute crisis and heal the diseased area. The body can also automatically neutralize pro-inflammatory immune mediators, like NF-kappa B, and their byproducts by using naturally occurring

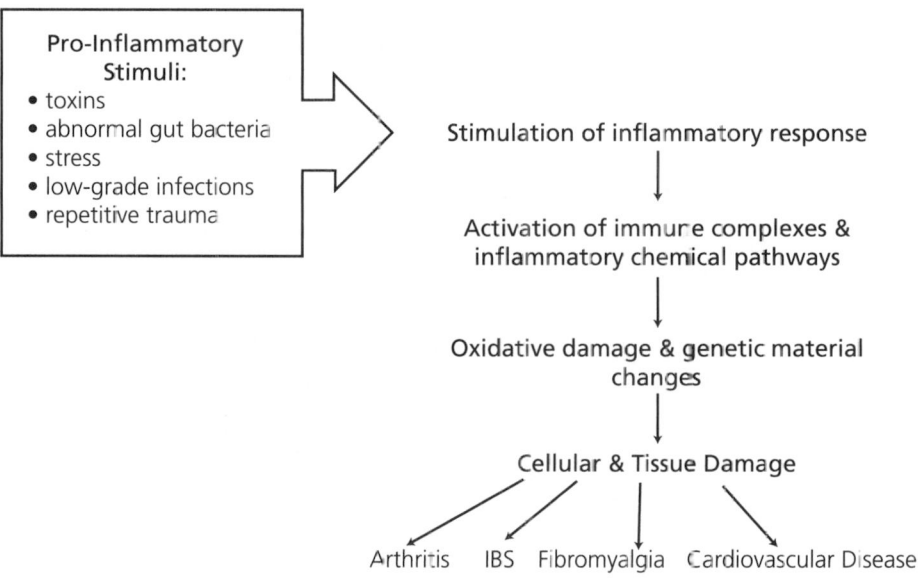

**Figure 4-1: Effects of Pro-Inflammatory
Stimuli on Chronic Inflammation**

Repeated stimuli from environmental toxins, chronic viral and bacterial infections, repetitive trauma, the effects of stress, and abnormal intestinal bacteria trigger a cascade of biochemical events that result in diseases with chronic inflammation as a common characteristic.

anti-inflammatory chemicals. For yet unknown reasons, in many of the modern illnesses these naturally occurring mechanisms do not function properly.

The resulting state of chronic low-grade inflammation is characterized by pain, increased tissue breakdown, and accelerated aging. Though slowly progressing—and usually not differentiating into a specific disease—the consequences of these conditions are low-grade illness, fatigue, and reduced quality of life. Examples of conditions where chronic inflammation plays a significant role include irritable bowel syndrome (IBS), fibromyalgia, myositis, interstitial cystitis, nonspecific autoimmune disorders, skin diseases like psoriasis, as well as chronic viral illnesses like hepatitis C or herpes virus.

Environmental toxins, free radical pathology, abnormal gut ecology, bacterial and viral infections, and naturally occurring metabolic toxins trigger immunological responses that can cause chronic inflammation (see figure 4-1). Stress also plays a significant role. It can not only trigger inflammation, but can disrupt the hypothalamic-pituitary-adrenal (HPA) axis to such a degree that the naturally occurring anti-inflammatory hormones, such as cortisol, cannot function properly.

As we have seen in previous chapters, stress-induced HPA insufficiency, as this condition is sometimes called, not only weakens the immune system but causes endocrine imbalances that contribute to chronic inflammation, which further weakens the immune system.

Pain Response to Inflammation: The inflammatory process begins with an initiating stimulus, which can be chemical, microbial, or physical. The immune system responds by activating a series of biochemical events, referred to as a cascade because it is like one drop of water on the mountainside that eventually turns into a waterfall. It is not the drop of water that causes the eventual effects; it is the power of the water falling over the waterfall that exerts the most damaging effects on our health.

As the cascade of inflammatory chemicals progresses, prostaglandins, hormone-like substances that contribute to pain and inflammation, produce increased sensitivity of nerve tissue in the locally inflamed area causing diffuse muscle and joint pain. In response to pain and inflammation, interleukin-1 levels increase dramatically in the spinal fluid and travel to the brain. Interleukin-1β leads to production of cyclooxygenose-2 (COX-2) and increased synthesis of prostaglandins, especially prostaglandin E2, a potent inflammatory mediator. COX-2 is an enzyme that acts with arachadonic acid, a lipid substance found in the membranes of all cells in the body, to form prostaglandins. Hypersensitivity to pain results, along with the systemic symptoms of inflammation, such as fever, fatigue, malaise, and anorexia.

Laboratory Tests to Evaluate Inflammation

There are three blood tests that serve as indicators of inflammation in the body. These are the erythrocyte sedimentation rate (ESR or sed rate); C-reactive protein (CRP); and the antinuclear antibody test (ANA).

ESR: This is the traditional test used to measure generalized inflammatory activity. This test measures how fast the red blood cells (erythrocytes) settle to form a sediment in a test tube. There are different methods of measurement. The Westergren method is one of the most commonly used and normal values are less than 20 millimeters per hour (mm/hr). However, the lower the value the better. ESR is elevated in rheumatoid arthritis and other autoimmune diseases and it is also elevated in a wide range of other inflammatory conditions and infectious illnesses such as tuberculosis and severe cases of influenza.

CRP: This is a protein produced by the liver that interacts with the complement system and is only present during acute inflammation produced by the innate immune response, especially in bacterial infections. Like the ESR, it is not specific for any disease; however, elevation can occur in autoimmune conditions and heart disease. Recent research indicates that elevated CRP may also be associated with Alzheimer's disease, arthritis, and metastatic cancer. CRP it is an invaluable marker for evaluating inflammation.

ANA: This is also referred to as the fluorescent antinuclear antibody test (FANA). It is a sensitive screening test to evaluate the presence of autoimmune-induced inflammation. ANA is elevated in systemic lupus erthematosus, Sjörgen's syndrome, rheumatoid arthritis, polymyositis, and other connective tissue diseases, but it is not generally elevated in fibromyalgia. ANA can also be elevated when the kidneys or the lungs are inflamed in viral or bacterial infections, and in colitis and liver inflammation.

During a first visit with a new patient complaining of chronic pain, inflammation, chronic viral illness, other infections, or any disease associated with poor immune function, I order these tests along with other lab studies. Patients with chronic illness in the absence of clearly defined pathology often show a moderately elevated ESR in the range of 20–30 mm/hr. Conventional medical doctors are often at a loss to explain to the patient why their sedimentation rate is slightly elevated, and they frequently dismiss it as irrelevant to the case, or as a transient elevation due to a virus. I think this is a serious clinical mistake.

In my opinion, any elevation above 10 mm/hr is suspect for inflammation, and though an elevation around 30 mm/hr may not make you deathly ill, it is still an indication of chronic active inflammation. I always recommend that the cause be found and treated appropriately. As the patient improves, the ESR returns to normal levels.

A similar scenario often occurs with ANA. Patients with chronic illness may have a slightly elevated ANA, and though most conventional medical doctors discount this, I believe that healthy people do not have such elevations, even if nominal.

Blood, saliva, and urinary pH can also serve as indicators of a predisposition to inflammation. The pH scale goes from 0 to 14, with 7 being neutral, between 0 and 6.9 acidic, and from 7.1 to 14 alkaline. The body holds tightly to a very narrow pH range, especially in the blood with a pH of between 7.35 and 7.45. Saliva is also slightly alkaline with an average of 7.4, while urine ranges from slightly acidic in the morning (6.5–7.0) to alkaline in the evening (7.5–8.0). If the blood or saliva indicates an acidic condition, neutralizing the body towards a slightly alkaline state by a change in diet can help manage chronic inflammation (see part 2).

Inflammation and Viral Illnesses

The inflammatory response in viral infection is essential in initiating immune defenses, and it plays a role in controlling the spread of infection. Immunologists believe that early immune reactions to a primary viral infection, though poorly understood, can profoundly influence the final outcome. I agree completely. Some viruses, like influenza, trigger strong inflammatory responses, while others, such as hepatitis C, may not cause any response though those initially infected with hepatitis C who experience an acute inflammatory reaction have a better chance of completely clearing the virus.

Inflammation is essentially positive and protective, yet its consequences in the tissues are part of what makes us feel achy and sick. The severity of how sick we feel depends on the virulence of the virus, how actively our immune systems respond, and the site of infection. The brain and central nervous system are critical areas, and in viral encephalitis, infection can cause extreme symptoms from inflammation of the membranes that surround the brain and spinal cord. The skin is a less critical area, and extreme systemic reactions are rare, as with herpes virus or inflammatory skin disorders like psoriasis.

Systemic Effects of Inflammation: Viral infections can produce localized inflammation. However, most produce systemic symptoms affecting the whole body. Immune cells release inflammatory cytokines that produce fatigue, lethargy, sleepiness, and lack of appetite. Fever is also a common symptom of the immune system's inflammatory reaction to infection. These symptoms are an adaptive mechanism urging the patient to rest so that the normal healing process can take place without interference from daily activity. It also is a method of natural quarantine: you are too sick and tired to go to work or to a movie, therefore you do not infect other people.

In contrast, when you take anti-inflammatory medications, you not only temporarily mask symptoms, but by continuing to engage in daily activities, you inhibit your body's normal healing mechanisms and restorative cycle. You also infect others.

Treatment of Inflammation: Western medicine typically relies on synthetic adrenal cortical steroids (prednisone and topical hydrocortisone) and non-steroidal anti-inflammatory drugs (NSAIDs), such as aspirin, ibuprofen, ketoprofen, naproxen, or piroxicam to treat inflammation. COX-2 inhibitors (celecoxib), a newer class of NSAIDs, have recently been developed and are currently in use. Though steroids have wide use in modern medicine and can be lifesaving, they also exert profound counter-wellness effects on the immune system. In chronic viral infections their use should be avoided with the exception of the most serious of cases.

By reducing inflammation, steroids *mask* symptoms of infection. They suppress immune resistance allowing for increased microbial activity, and they exacerbate latent amebic infections, latent viruses, and fungal infections. They should never be used casually, as they often are in the general medicine practice; they are best reserved for life-threatening situations or conditions uncontrollable by other methods. Hydrocortisone, a short-acting synthetic version of the naturally occurring cortisol, is used in low doses to treat chronic fatigue; it may be a safer alternative in mild forms of chronic inflammation. Its use is discussed later in this chapter.

Besides their anti-inflammatory effects, NSAIDs also reduce pain and fever. Though they are widely used in over-the-counter and prescription forms, the exact way NSAIDs work is still unknown. They are commonly used for the symptomatic relief of pain, inflammation, and fever associated with conditions ranging from the common cold to arthritis. However, at least 25 percent of those using NSAIDs develop side effects.

These include damage to the stomach lining, the liver, and kidneys, and minor stomachaches are common side effects of these medications. In some cases, serious gastrointestinal toxicity can occur, with bleeding and even perforation of the lining of the stomach or intestines. Sometimes the consequences of NSAID use are fatal.

NSAIDs do not cure, and I do not recommend them for long-term use in patients with inflammation associated with chronic viral illness or in chronic nonspecific inflammatory conditions like fibromyalgia.

Many NSAIDs, like ibuprofen and aspirin, are effective COX-2 inhibitors, medications that stop the activity of this inflammation-inducing enzyme. Due to the high side-effect profile of long-term NSAID use, newer, or second-generation, COX-2 inhibitors have been developed, such as celecoxib (Celebrex). Though effective for suppressing inflammation and controlling pain, these drugs also have side effects, and since long-term use may create other immune system imbalances, I recommend their use only for short-term symptom management.

For chronic inflammation, natural anti-inflammatory medications are a better first choice and can be readily incorporated into a treatment plan. Naturally occurring antagonists that can block cyclooxygenase isozymes (COX) are the most effective. These are the key enzymes involved in the synthesis of prostaglandins, particularly COX-2 (the "bad" COX) inhibitors. One example is the common ginger root *(Zingiber officinale)*. The active ingredients in ginger affect the production of eicosanoids, a group of biological response substances, which includes prostaglandins, that mediate healing mechanisms and immune function. Rosemary oil and the resin from frankincense *(Boswellia serrata),* both rich in ursolic and oleanoic acid, also have COX-2 inhibiting activity.

Chronic inflammation can accelerate cellular damage caused by use of oxygen that generates free radicals. Protection from oxidative damage to tissues and cells is helped by a process called redox, involving antioxidants. Vitamin C, lipoic acid, N-acetyle cysteine, coenzyme CoQ10, and the flavonoids in green tea are antioxidants that protect against inflammation. Curcumin, the active ingredient in medicinal turmeric *(Curcuma longa),* is both a powerful antioxidant and anti-inflammatory and is useful for the control of pain associated with inflammation.

The Immunological Function of Fever

As in the case of inflammation, the physiological phenomenon of fever was well known to the Greek physicians more than two thousand years ago. Hippocrates wrote extensively on its causes and manifestations. Even earlier than the Greeks, the Chinese observed the manifestation of fever in disease and developed extensive theories and ideas, some which are still in use today.

Fever is one of the most common manifestations of infection and inflammation. It is so common and universal that even non-medically trained people know that fever is associated with illness. Nearly everyone has experienced a fever with symptoms of elevated temperature, chills, and sweating, and every mother has spent at least one sleepless night sponging down a small child in fever.

Normal healthy people do not have fever. The body maintains a very tightly regulated temperature through the hypothalamus, a gland within the brain. There is no exact "normal" temperature; the "average" body temperature of 98.6° F (37° C) varies considerably from person to person, and even at different times of the day. The fever response to infection is triggered by pyrogens, cytokines that act on the hypothalamus to raise body temperature. Once the temperature rises close to or over 100° F, feverish sensations usually appear, and include warmth or flushing, chills, sweating, and aching joints and muscles.

Generally, high fever (102°–104° F, or even as high as 106° F) indicates acute infectious illness and is accompanied by severe chills, profuse sweating, and even hallucinations. In chronic disease, patients can have a low-grade fever that lingers between 99° F and 100° F and may appear periodically at certain times of the day, usually in the late afternoon; this is called tidal fever.

Fever in Viral Illness: Fever is present in nearly every case of local and systemic infections including viral illnesses. The fever response to viral infection is not well understood, but immunologists think it involves interleukin-1 and interleukin-6, produced by macrophages arriving at the scene of infection. Evolutionary biologists and naturopathic doctors contend that fever is an adaptive mechanism to help the body fight infection, and therefore should not be suppressed. Human viruses are generally intolerant of heat and even a slight elevation in temperature inhibits replication of viruses, making fever an ally in fighting disease, rather than an enemy.

The intensity of fever in viral infections can vary from barely any elevation (the common cold) to very high temperatures (dengue). In acute infections like dengue fever, febrile symptoms can be very severe, with bone-shaking chills and high fever coming in waves.

Benefits of Fever and Risks of Suppressing Mild Fevers: Naturopathic physicians and Oriental medicine practitioners contend that suppressing fever with acetaminophen or aspirin thwarts the natural immune function and predisposes one to further illness or allows deeper penetration of the viral agent into the body. Fever, we say, is an unpleasant and even painful, but *useful* process; assisting the body's natural defense mechanisms is a wiser way of preventing chronic and degenerative diseases than relying on drugs for every symptom. Evolutionary biologists and some medical researchers tend to agree. However, there are very few scientific studies done on the benefits of the febrile response, so conventional medical doctors are not ready to embrace these theories.

Naturopathic physicians and Oriental medicine practitioners contend that suppressing fever with acetaminophen or aspirin thwarts the natural immune function and predisposes one to further illness or allows deeper penetration of the viral agent into the body.

Fever as an adaptive mechanism has evolved among humans and other mammals over more than a hundred million years.[3] Fever's presence is not only a cardinal manifestation or sign of disease, but it is an integral part of the healing process. Its purpose is still not fully understood, yet modern medicine somehow considers it a condition to be suppressed. Using drugs to suppress fever interferes with evolutionary mechanisms and may set the stage for further disease.

Of course, this does not happen in every person who uses an over-the-counter medication to suppress a fever from the common cold or average flu, but over time, people who repeatedly use these medications may develop dysfunctional immune responses. The key point is this: If the inflammatory and febrile responses are blunted, you are more susceptible to chronic infection.

Repeatedly suppressing a fever may affect the immune response of future generations. Many children now do not manifest systemic febrile responses, but harbor recurrent infections with localized inflammation. Antibiotics are commonly prescribed, and as the gut flora is wiped out by these drugs, stronger pathogenic microorganisms resistant to antibiotics take their place. The result is that the entire internal ecosystem of the child is unbalanced, which predisposes the child to further infections. Suppressing the fever and the inflammatory response may also reduce the antibody response, allowing for increased vulnerability to future infections. So it is not surprising that repeated ear infections, recurrent colds, and viral infections are on the rise.

In the meantime, viruses are not idle. They are actively evolving organisms that take advantage of those with weakened immunity. It would not surprise me if they also were encoding messages into the nuclear material of the cells announcing an "easy ride" to other viruses. This is not unlike a story my great aunt told me. She said that during the Great Depression of the 1930s, hobos would mark telephone poles with chalk to indicate houses that provided easy handouts.

Treating Fever: I have always believed, and taught my students, that one of the hallmarks of the good doctor is his skill in managing fever. In years past, this seemed a straightforward process. Before the modern drug era, the art of medicine was about deciding when to let a fever run its course and when to suppress it. In serious illnesses, the doctor was often helpless to alter the course of an acute disease, so treatment was limited to monitoring the patient and providing fluids and comfort. Now, a variety of over-the-counter medications are available to treat minor inflammations and fever, as well as many prescription strength drugs. Unfortunately, these are highly overused by the general public and doctors.

Since acute fever is a sign of an infection, the swift diagnosis and successful treatment of the underlying cause to eliminate the fever is appropriate. However, universal suppression of all fevers is not only unnecessary, but could be dangerous to your health. According to naturopathy, mild fevers between 99–101° F should be allowed to run their course since they are considered part of the body's natural protective processes.

In fevers over 101° F, tepid baths or sponge baths with cool water are necessary to manage a fever and keep it from further elevation. In some cases, especially with children, high fever can cause delirium, seizures, and brain injury, so body temperatures above 102° F should be aggressively managed. In children, mild fevers can be managed with homeopathic remedies and herbs; liquid Tylenol may be necessary if the natural remedies do not work within a few hours.

The acute high fevers associated with malaria, dengue, encephalitis, and other serious infectious diseases require aggressive and effective medical management. Do not attempt to manage these on your own. High fever accompanied by sweating can cause loss of fluids and electrolytes; therefore, additional water, juices, and vegetable broths are necessary. Fluid loss to the point of dehydration may require hospitalization for intravenous fluid and electrolyte replacement.

Fevers associated with common infections like colds or flu can be managed at home. Dr. N. C. A. Vogel, and other "Nature cure" doctors of previous decades, advocated a natural comprehensive management of fever. In his book, *The Nature Doctor,* Dr. Vogel (1952) emphasizes that the body will manage the fever itself if given the opportunity.

However, he stresses the importance of keeping the eliminative organs functioning by using an enema, sponging down the skin, or using diaphoretic (sweat-promoting) herbs to open the pores, and even drinking mild diuretic (urine-promoting) teas. Dr. Vogel also recommends reducing solid food intake during the fever and while there is no appetite. Diluted juices or honey and water keep the blood sugar levels up and prevent hypoglycemia and exhaustion. Additional fluids in the form of pure water, non-acidic fruit juices, and vegetable broths and mixed vegetable juices are also necessary.

Common herbal remedies for managing fever include elder flowers *(Sambucus nigra)* or yarrow flower *(Achillea millefolium).* Drink one cup, taken as an infusion, until mild sweating occurs. Chinese herbs are excellent for managing fever; they are used as teas, instant granules, tablets, powders, or capsules containing concentrated extracts (see part 2).

Homeopaths are legendary for the number of remedies they use for managing febrile illnesses. The most useful are *Aconite, Belladonna,* and *Gelsemium.* These are taken in low potency (6 to 30 X)[6] frequently until the fever subsides. There are also several excellent combination remedies for inflammation and fever. A detailed discussion on homeopathy is beyond the scope of this book; however, for more information on the specialized use of homeopathic medicines for viral illnesses see part 2.

Caution: Homeopathy is the study and practice of specially prepared remedies. The dispensing of these remedies follows specific guidelines, so consult a homeopath or carefully read a homeopathic home treatment guide before using homeopathic remedies.

Management strategies are different for chronic low grade or intermittent fevers. With the new chronic diseases, it is difficult to tell if the fever is part of the healing process or a sign of deterioration in the patient's condition. Usually it is a sign of poor immune function, generalized poor health, the body's inability to neutralize toxins, and chronic infection. In these cases, traditional nature cure doctors who practice "by the book" might encourage promoting the fever. However, in my experience, it is a mistake to attempt to promote a fever associated with chronic disease.

Increased inflammation may result, not only causing the patient more discomfort, but more tissue damage may occur. The course of action for these conditions is to find the underlying cause through accurate diagnosis and remove the cause to eliminate the fever. Obviously, this requires the expertise of a skilled physician.

Hyperthermia, raising the body temperature over a sustained period of time, is another way of using the febrile response therapeutically. This form of therapy is mainly used for cancer patients, but it might have a role in the treatment of other chronic diseases including viral illnesses. Exercise, saunas, steam baths, and sweat lodge ceremonies are also ways to raise body temperature to manage chronic inflammation, though some conditions, such as multiple sclerosis, are also worsened by heat.

Has Something Gone Wrong with the Human Inflammatory and Fever Response?

The answer is yes. However, it is such a complicated and poorly understood issue that an explanation is difficult to find. Certainly there appears to be something awry with the immune response in an increasing number of people, especially the initial non-specific inflammatory process. We are blunted by stress, drugs, and overwork, so viruses now have easy access to our bodies. Once in the bloodstream, they are able to penetrate to deep regions of the body like the liver or brain where they are difficult, if not impossible, to eradicate. In addition to this, the normal cellular immune responses appear to be dysfunctional.

I have seen patient after patient report essentially the same thing. They do not know how they ended up in their conditions. When I question them, invariably they tell me that they do not remember a serious infection or a particularly stressful event that caused their symptoms. At times, I can trace their history back to recurrent throat infections or overuse of antibiotics for childhood ear infections, but more often, it is difficult to isolate a specific cause. This leads me to believe that either their inflammatory immune responses were already blunted and they were unaware of an infection, or an accumulation of environmental, psychological, and infectious stressors gradually eroded their health.

There are two different explanations for this increasingly common condition: either the immune system did not recognize the virus as a pathogenic agent or the virus evolved strategies that helped it evade the immune response. As mentioned already, the two most common reactions of the immune system to infection are fever and inflammation. Without these symptoms, you cannot tell that you were infected.

Once the virus bypasses the immune response and enters the body, it lodges in the cells of its target organ. Gradual tissue injury occurs, along with low-grade inflammation, accumulations of toxic byproducts of viral damage to the host cells, and impaired function of the target organ. This is clearly seen in chronic hepatitis C.

In the absence of any initial immune response of fever and inflammation, the infected individual is completely unaware that infection by the virus took place. It is often only until years later when symptoms appear that the person realizes they are infected. Chronic hepatitis C infection causes liver tissue damage resulting in inflammation and impaired liver function. The patient may feel fatigued for no apparent reason as a result of the inflammation and reduced organ function. If the fatigue is severe enough, the patient will eventually seek a doctor's advice, but usually not until after trying many over-the-counter remedies, increasing the intake of stimulants like coffee, and taking a variety of herbs and vitamin supplements.

The scenario for epidemics of chronic viral disease is set. Due to environmental changes and ecological pressure, new viruses are

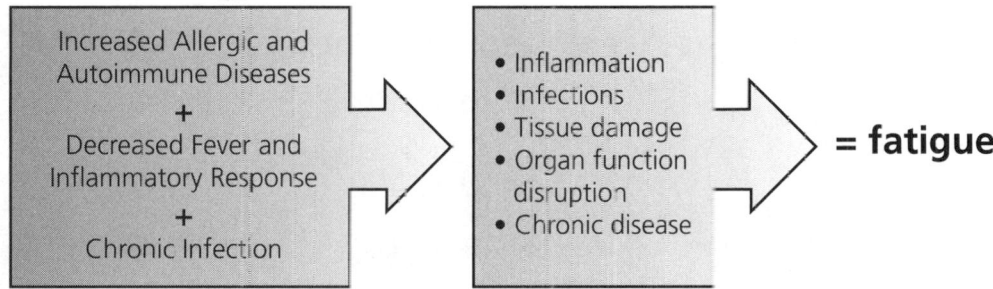

Figure 4-2: Conditions Causing Fatigue States

The results of disrupted immunity (increased allergic and autoimmune diseases plus decreased fever and inflammatory response), in combination, predispose one to a variety of conditions including chronic inflammation, chronic opportunistic infections, tissue damage, disturbance of normal organ and endocrine function, and chronic disease states. All have fatigue as a leading symptom.

emerging and old viruses are becoming more virulent. The human immune system is in a state of imbalance with an impaired innate response (absence of fever and initial inflammation), and at the same time there is an increase in allergic and autoimmune diseases. Opportunistic bacterial, parasitic, and fungal infections occur more easily. These are treated with antibiotics, antiparasitic, and antifungal drugs, which cause further disruption of homeostasis and immunity.

This immune-disrupting cycle becomes self-perpetuating, and in the next section, I discuss why fatigue plays such an important role (see figure 4-2).

Fatigue and Malaise Instead of Fever: It is my clinical observation that in the absence of the normal inflammatory process and with a blunted febrile response, the most prevalent symptom in chronic disease has become fatigue rather than fever. Fatigue is even less understood than fever. Interestingly, in researching material for this book I regularly consulted several textbooks on medical immunology and not one of them had fatigue as an entry in their indices.

Fatigue and malaise are part of the general process of inflammation. Characterized by a sense of weakness, loss of energy, sleepiness, and a generalized sense of feeling sick, one has the desire to lie down. This is a natural response. The body requires rest to fight off the illness and recuperate, and it automatically withdraws energy, causing tiredness. We all have had this experience when sick with the flu. We feel exhausted and need to stay in bed for a few days or longer to

Selected Conditions Associated with Fatigue

Anemia	Adrenal insufficiency
Hypothyroidism	Depression
Diabetes	Anxiety
Congestive heart failure	Kidney failure
Obstructive lung conditions like emphysema or chronic bronchitis	Advanced liver disease
	Cancer
Parasitic conditions	Toxicity from overuse of prescription drugs (tranquilizers, hypnotic antihistamines, hypertension drugs, antidepressants)
Viral infections like mononucleosis and hepatitis	
Pituitary insufficiency	Autoimmune diseases

recover. In the case of mononucleosis or hepatitis, one can feel profoundly weak, and often a month of bed rest is required.

However, in our modern, super-rushed, high-tech, information-overloaded culture, we push this natural process aside and force ourselves to continue working. This behavior deprives our bodies of rest, uses up more energy, and furthers weakens our organs, leading to more fatigue, and increased susceptibility to viral infection and illness.

The body is not only tired from the effects of the illness, but it is fatigued from fighting it without all of its healing mechanisms in full operation. As mentioned in the previous chapter, there are numerous environmental chemicals and drugs that are immunosuppressive. Of course, this only worsens the scenario.

Fatigue may occur from many causes. The obvious ones are overexertion, poor nutrition or lack of energy-providing foods, generally poor fitness, inadequate sleep, obesity, and illness. The list of diseases that cause fatigue is long, and includes anemia, cancer, and rheumatoid arthritis and other autoimmune diseases. Endocrine conditions such as hypothyroidism, low testosterone, and reduced adrenal function also cause fatigue.

As I have suggested, fatigue is a symptom, but it is not appreciated sufficiently as such by most doctors. Though it is true that fatigue and the feeling of not wanting to do anything are associated with depression and chronic pain, medical doctors routinely misdiagnose fatigued patients as being depressed. The most common form of treatment is an antidepressant drug which, of course, does nothing for the fatigue unless it is directly associated with clinical depression.

There is an easy way to assess fatigue. In depressed patients, if they push themselves to exercise, they feel not only less depressed but also have more energy. On the other hand, when the pathologically-fatigued patient tries to exercise, even slight exertion worsens the exhaustion, often putting them to bed for days.

Do not accept a diagnosis of depression and treatment with drugs to treat a mood disorder if your complaint is chronic fatigue Of course, there may be times when your fatigue may indeed be associated with depression, and you should discuss and review this carefully with your doctor.

Fatigue and Viral Illness: Though patients with chronic viral illnesses commonly experience fatigue, there is surprisingly little information about this condition, even for such a universally occurring illness as hepatitis. According to Mark Swain, M.D., assistant professor of medicine at the University of Calgary in Edmonton, Canada, "The rigorous examination of fatigue as a symptom in viral hepatitis has only recently received scientific scrutiny" (Swain 1998).

Perhaps this lack of information is due to the fact that fatigue has been long considered a symptom rather than a condition, and there are no specific medications in Western pharmacology to specifically treat fatigue. This is not the case in Chinese medicine, where numerous herbs, such as ginseng, are used to prevent and treat fatigued states.

Even so, fatigue is mysterious and paradoxical, and therefore difficult to understand. For example, it is not routinely present in all cases of chronic hepatitis C, HIV positive, and other chronic viral illnesses such as Epstein-Barr virus. On the other hand, fatigue can be a profound symptom in some of these cases. It is universal in mononucleosis and other acute viruses but absent in others. To complicate things further, despite much clinical investigation, there has been no conclusive evidence that chronic fatigue syndrome is caused by a specific virus.

In viral illnesses, fatigue and sleepiness are associated with the acute phase of the inflammatory response. You feel tired and have the

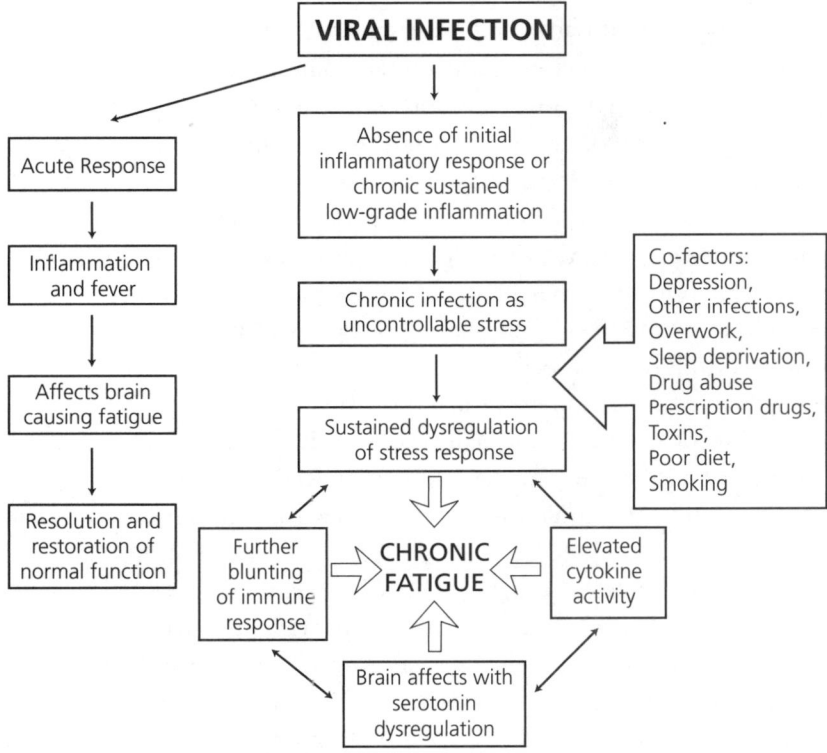

Figure 4-3: Viral Infection and Fatigue Mechanisms

Acute viral infection, in a healthy person with a well-functioning immune system, generates a febrile and inflammatory response causing temporary fatigue and then resolves without complications. In the presence of a dysfunctional immune system, the acute phase may not reach resolution and pass directly to the chronic stage. In a person with a blunted initial immune response, the virus bypasses the initial response entirely and proceeds to the chronic stage. Fatigue becomes the main symptom of the chronic stage.

desire to lie down or sleep when you have the flu, mono, or hepatitis A (the food-borne type). The fatigue effect is thought to be caused by the action of inflammatory cytokines on the brain and central nervous system. The stress of an infection also affects the HPA axis, and changes in adrenal and other hormones occur that also cause fatigue. Since this type of fatigue passes, and the individual returns to normal after recovering from an acute viral infection, no further clinical questions are usually asked.

However, less is known about the causes of fatigue in chronic viral infections or why some people experience more tiredness than others. Instead of one cause, there seems to be a series of events that trigger a sustained fatigue response. In this case, fatigue becomes central in the symptom profile and less of a transient, minor occurrence as in acute infections; it involves sustained imbalances in the stress response and blunting of the immune system (see figure 4-3).

The Real Issue with Chronic Fatigue: As mentioned in Western medicine fatigue is considered a symptom of underlying disease and not a condition in and of itself. It was not until more than a decade after chronic fatigue cases first appeared that it was given a disease category of its own. In 1988, chronic fatigue syndrome (CFS), referred to as chronic fatigue immunodeficiency syndrome (CFIDS) in its severe form, was officially recognized as a disease condition. Though many years have passed since then, the real cause of this condition remains unknown, although several theories have been put forward, some sounder then others.

In general, they all agree that the cause of CFIDS is associated with stress disruption of the HPA axis that result in adrenal dysfunction, changes in such immune parameters with a reduced number of natural killer cells and abnormal levels of cytokines, the activity of environmental toxins that interrupt mitochondrial function (the energy producing part of cells), the presence of viral infections, and co-infections by parasites, fungal organisms, bacteria, and other viruses.

Even with these explanations, many questions remain unanswered. One of the main ones is whether CFIDS is an immune deficiency syndrome or a virally-induced condition. Though the potential of a viral cause has been well researched, there is still no agreement as to what virus it may be. The possible players include any of the herpes virus family, most notably EBV, CMV, or HHV-6. Other possible viruses include HIV subtypes, polio mutants and other vaccination-borne viruses, undiagnosed chronic HCV, and perhaps an as yet unidentified emerging virus.

The proponents of the conventional medical paradigm insist on finding one specific infectious agent for chronic fatigue. Certainly many cases of fatigue have a viral or bacterial cause, and it is well known that fatigue accompanies chronic viral infections like chronic hepatitis, but it is likely that more than one virus may be involved, working synergistically to enhance the effects of the others. However, if the majority of clinicians and researchers are looking for a single infectious agent that does not exist, years will be wasted on dead-ends, prolonging the suffering of patients.

It is difficult for the proponents of the old paradigm to look at CFIDS from either an evolutionary or multifactorial point of view, but unless we are able to make the transition from linear thinking to more complex thinking in which purposefulness, though not immediately evident, is accepted as integral to the web of life, there is little chance of understanding chronic fatigue.

It is difficult for the proponents of the old paradigm to look at CFIDS from either an evolutionary or multifactorial point of view, but unless we are able to make the transition from linear thinking to more complex thinking, there is little chance of understanding chronic fatigue.

Even so, chronic fatigue is still a spreading epidemic. In 1991, *Science* put the estimated number of cases in the United States at 100,000, but a recent study at DePaul University indicates that there are as many as 800,000 Americans with CFIDS, and that the majority of these are still undiagnosed and many that have been diagnosed with CFIDS are not receiving effective medical care.

Majid Ali, M.D., president of Capital University of Integrated Medicine in Washington, D.C., in his *The Canary and Chronic Fatigue* (1995) says, "Chronic fatigue will be the dominant chronic health disorder of the next century." Dr. Ali contends that CFIDS is a disease of accelerated oxidative molecular damage caused by modern living. He says it is both preventable and curable.

Dr. Ali's three main points of clinical strategy are to catch it in the early stages, avoid drugs for treatment, and prevent relapses. His treatments include increasing antioxidant nutrients to normalize the effects of dysfunctional oxygen metabolism in the cells. Antioxidants include vitamin C, zinc, selenium, and other vitamins, minerals, and amino acids (discussed in part 2).

Jeffrey Bland, Ph.D., a nutritional biochemist and founder of HealthComm International and the Functional Medicine Research Center in Gig Harbor, Washington, promotes a similar theory. However, Dr. Bland emphasizes defects in cellular metabolism and a biochemical energy crisis that cause dysfunction in genomic expression (Bland 2000). In this model of chronic fatigue, hereditary predispositions for certain diseases are encoded into the individual's genome. Environmental toxins, an unhealthy lifestyle, and poor diet contribute to biochemical disturbances in cellular metabolism, where all of the body's energy is manufactured. The combination of environmental and lifestyle factors on genetic defects result in a deficiency of the production of energy, in effect a biochemical energy crisis—the cells run out of usable material to generate energy.

According to Dr. Bland, chronic fatigue is the result. The underlying cause for this crisis is abnormal immune system activation, tissue oxidative stress, and imbalanced HPA axis function. His treatment protocol uses diet, antioxidants, nutritional supplements, and low-dose hydrocortisone.

As mentioned earlier, hydrocortisone is the synthetic version of cortisol—a naturally occurring adrenal hormone. An interesting historical note here is that some doctors were already treating fatigued states in patients in the 1960s. They termed the condition hypoadrenia, adrenal insufficiency, adrenal exhaustion, or "a bite of Addison's" disease—a condition of adrenal hypofunction characterized by weakness, fatigue, low blood pressure, and increased skin pigmentation. Since the normal adrenal gland produces 20 to 30 mg of cortisol daily, based upon the work of William Jefferies, M.D., in *Safe Uses of Cortisol* (1981), some doctors recommend between 5 and 20 mg of hydrocortisone daily.

Recently several articles were published on hydrocortisone use in the British journal *Lancet* (Jeffcoate 1999) and one in the *Journal of the American Medical Association* in 1998 (McKenzie 1998). Clinically, physicians who use this therapy for CFIDS report that some patients respond dramatically. However, in my clinical opinion, successes are exaggerated because the approach still follows the old "one disease, one drug" paradigm, and it is not a comprehensive strategy—the evolutionary and energetic components are missing.

Testing for CFIDS: It is vital that you and your doctor understand what type of fatigue you are experiencing. If you have the

CFIDS Symptom Complex

Incapacitating fatigue longer than six months

Severe fatigue after exertion that does not improve with rest

Poor concentration and memory

Flu-like symptoms

Joint and muscle pains

Nonrestorative sleep

Tender or swollen lymph nodes

Recurrent or chronic sore throat

Recurrent or chronic headaches

Steps in Diagnosing Chronic Fatigue:

Rule out common causes of fatigue

Rule out infectious causes

Evaluate immune status

Add functional studies

complex of symptoms that constitute CFIDS, your condition must be ultimately diagnosed from a functional medicine point of view. There is no specific laboratory test that defines the diagnosis of CFIDS. Rather, a combination of clinical history, results of the examination and questionnaire, and a variety of lab tests suggest a state of chronic fatigue. However, since fatigue may be caused by many conditions, you should first be tested to rule out or eliminate common conditions, such as anemia or low thyroid function.

If you do not have any of the common causes of fatigue, then proceed with tests to rule out viral infections such as HIV, HHIV-6, EBV, CMV, and chronic HBV and HCV. Consider screening for influenza-A virus antibodies if your condition started after a flu-like illness. Antibody testing for other chronic infectious such as the yeast *Candida albicans,* parasites, Lyme disease, and chlamydia, a sexually transmitted bacteria (trachomatis), should also be considered.

The next step is a functional diagnosis of the immune system with a blood panel including natural killer cell activity and counts of the different lymphocytes. Another functional test is the Comprehensive Digestive Stool Analysis (CDSA) to evaluate gut bacteria and parasites. (See part 2 for information on lab tests.)

Caution: It is unlikely that you will be able to manage the conditions discussed in this chapter on your own. You need to find a naturopathic physician (N.D.), a doctor of Oriental Medicine (O.M.D.), a skilled homeopath or acupuncturist, or an osteopath (D.O.) or medical doctor (M.D.) trained in functional medicine to assist you in understanding how to manage febrile illness and treat chronic inflammation with natural medicines.

CHAPTER SUMMARY

There are several types of inflammation: some protect our bodies and others have adverse effects.

Inflammation may be mild or severe, acute or chronic, involving a normal response mechanism or an abnormal and destructive process. Acute inflammation generally runs its course in three days to a week and then normalizes. Severe acute inflammation, as seen in the early stages of hepatitis infection, requires medical attention. Aggressive inflammation as seen in rheumatoid arthritis may also require drugs to reduce tissue destruction.

Treating autoimmune disease requires an integrated approach of conventional Western and alternative medicine.

If chronic inflammation is present, reducing it and the management of the inflammatory process are important features in the viral immunity treatment plan.

Immune dysfunction plays a role in the epidemic of allergic diseases, activating autoimmune inflammatory responses, and it is implicated in chronic inflammatory disorders.

An elevated body temperature is one of the nonspecific mechanisms of the immune system. Under normal circumstances, a fever disappears when your immune system eliminates the offending microorganisms. However, in increasing frequency, the normal inflammatory immune and febrile responses seem to be blunted and dysfunctional.

In the new illnesses, including many viral diseases, the first symptom to appear is fatigue rather than fever or acute inflammation.

Chronic fatigue seems to be the most common predictor of functional illness and is becoming the most common disease of this century, in which fatigue replaces fever with the result of slow, debilitating illness over a long period of time, rather than rapid resolution or death.

Chronic fatigue and chronic inflammation are part of the symptom pattern of chronic viral illness.

Because it is a complex disease, there is no specific lab test for CFIDS.

The diagnosis of CFIDS requires a knowledgeable clinician who combines the medical history, symptoms, a physical examination, and a variety of lab tests to determine the status of the immune system, influence of chronic infections, and other laboratory information to assess the condition.

5

Why We Get Sick and How to Get Better

So far in this book we've discussed the problem of viral disease and immune deficiency by reviewing the scope of the viral crisis, what viruses are, some of the most important viruses involved in this crisis, how the immune system functions, and how immune dysfunction contributes to viral illness. We've seen how these are all related and how environmental toxins and pharmaceutical drugs contribute to the problem. Now it is time to discuss the solutions, to consider the treatments, and to understand how they affect the body.

To set the stage for the discussion on treatments, the 10 steps to viral immunity, let's first explore why we get sick and how we get better, and define what viral immunity is and how we can achieve it.

The Mystery of Disease

Over several millennia of recorded history, humans have accumulated considerable experience concerning health and disease, and we have gleaned from this vast pool of information some very valuable knowledge.[1] Still, the ultimate answers to life's fundamental questions remain elusive even in this age of modern science. How do we grow and age, and why do we die? Why is the body designed to be so vulnerable to disease? Why do we get sick, how are we healed, and how do we recover and thrive again?

These are the questions that doctors and philosophers have pondered, struggled with, and strived to answer since the beginning of self-conscious thought in our species, and they still do so to this day. In this section, we will explore some of these questions and how their answers relate to viral immunity.

Different medical systems explain disease according to their own theories. Examples from two of the approaches discussed in this book help to illustrate this. According to traditional Western medicine, diseases are caused by microbial infections, trauma, toxic chemicals, and genetic abnormalities. Chinese medicine says that diseases are caused by an imbalance in invisible cosmological forces, yin and yang, that govern all phenomena on Earth, and by environmental factors that weaken the natural health of the body.

Though at first glance these two systems appear to be in direct opposition to each other, upon closer examination they are at opposite ends of the same spectrum. Western medicine focuses on the end product of the disease and treats it with dangerous drugs. Chinese medicine emphasizes health and prevention and provides natural medications to strengthen the individual's system against disease. My clinical experience is that the methods of both systems are applicable for viral illnesses and many other diseases.

Western medicine focuses on the end product of the disease and treats it with dangerous drugs. Chinese medicine emphasizes health and prevention and provides natural medications to strengthen the individual's system against disease. My clinical experience is that the methods of both systems are applicable for viral illnesses and many other diseases.

Illness is multifactoral. Disease is simply a part of living, and no matter how hard we try to eliminate all illness, it does not go away forever. Whether we get sick or not depends on several factors. These include infectious agents, our immune mechanisms, toxic environmental factors, and stress. They also include the effects of previous treatments, our predisposition to certain diseases, and our beliefs and attitudes. The age of the patient also plays a significant role in the type of illness and its virulence.

Our Inherent and Acquired Disease Vulnerability: Vulnerability to disease offers a part of the explanation of why we get sick. It is easy to understand that if you were under a tree when a branch broke, the bump and accompanying pain you have are the results of it hitting your head. This is the manner in which allopathic thinking proceeds. There is one cause, the branch hitting your head, and one result, a large bump or concussion. If you had worn a hard-hat, you would have been less vulnerable to the bump. However, vulnerability becomes more complex when we consider the risk of infection and immunity.

First, there are inherited factors that accompany you from birth. Genetic defects in the immune system are predisposing factors to whether you become infected or not. Second, you can acquire immune deficiency later in life, and when your immune system is weakened, your vulnerability to viral infection increases. If you are frequently exposed to infectious agents, your vulnerability increases as it does by the virulence of the disease factor.

Virulence of the Disease Agent: The strength or potential of a disease agent to infect and cause disease is another factor in why we get sick. Some diseases are more powerful than others, that is, they have the ability to more easily cause infections to those exposed. Cholera, for example, is very virulent, while the common cold is of mild virulence. The combination of virulence and vulnerability influence the incidence of infection and the outcome.

Stress: Emotion and physical stress play a significant role in why we get sick. One misconception my patients often have concerning the role of stress in their illness is they believe stress is the sole cause, and blame it on others or outside influences. It is true that severe shock, such as experiencing bombing during wartime or a serious car accident, can cause permanent changes to our health. However, most modern Americans do not experience this type of acute and overwhelming stress. Rather, they live under chronic, repetitive, relentless pressure and duress for years at a time with the result that this type of stress, combined with other factors, gradually erodes one's immune foundation.

Toxins and Novel Environments: Environmental toxins are also important disruptors of natural physiological processes, and play a considerable role as immune system disrupters that contribute to making us more vulnerable to disease. Poor adaptability to novel environments challenges our immune functions and is a significant source of stress to our systems; this also contributes to increased vulnerability and disease risk.

Different Medical Approaches to Healing

It seems that we cannot escape illness and that there are no panaceas. Life remains a great mystery, and disease an unwanted and sometimes feared part of living. We have theories, vast experience, and knowledge, yet disease is as puzzling as how the body heals itself, how a cure works, or why some approaches work better for certain conditions and different people at different times. Before we pursue the question of how we get better, let's look at the difference between healing and cure more closely, and then at a few of the different healing systems. All of this will better equip us to appreciate and apply the 10 steps to viral immunity in part 2.

There are many different styles of medicine, but some characteristics are common to all of them. Each begins with experience and the accumulation of knowledge, and then organizes that body of knowledge into a formal practice administered to the patient. One possessing skill and knowledge in applying the medical techniques of that system, a nurse, provides patient care. The doctor is the one who intercedes between the disease and the patient with his or her knowledge and "power."

Once a treatment is administered, success or failure to cure or improve the patient's condition is evaluated and the results added to the ever-expanding pool of medical experience and knowledge, which is then passed on to other doctors and medical students. Each medical system has a different way of attaining its medical knowledge.

Western Models of Medical Thinking: In the West, medical knowledge is based upon the scientific method.[2] This method first gathers specialized information about individual aspects or parts of something, establishes a theory, attempting to prove or disprove it using a rigorous methodology that is repeatable by another person independent of the beliefs and subjective manipulations of the first person.

For modern medicine, the highest standard of proof is based on the double-blind, placebo-controlled study. In this type of research, neither the patient nor the dispensing researcher knows which medicine is the real one and which is the placebo, the one devoid of medical activity. Western doctors and scientists believe that an ultimate understanding of all phenomena is possible through scientific investigation; from their point of view, in time, the human brain can work out all the details. To these scientists, there is no Mystery, only unsolved riddles.

This is the biomedical model, and its strong point is its ever-increasing body of information about biological systems. Its weak point is that much of this information lacks any knowledge of how the *individual* patient feels, experiences her illness, or gets better. Instead, in practice, it emphasizes generalities and averages.

Allopathic Medicine: There are two major scientific schools of thought in Western medicine. The first is the allopathic form that dominates modern medicine. It classifies disease into what can be seen and tested in the laboratory and it bases diagnoses on symptoms and observable signs. You feel hot when you have a fever, and this can be verified by an elevated temperature as taken by a thermometer and perhaps an elevated white blood cell count from the lab test. These are symptoms and signs of an infection.

Conventional allopathic medicine is based on a theory that assigns external causes to disease, principally two: microbial infection (referred to as the "germ theory") and physical injury. It seeks to answer questions about what happens and how things work, and it revolves around the study of structure and mechanisms, offering straightforward explanations about physically observable things. It is a useful system for formulating easily-grasped concepts of health and disease, but its great weakness is that only one hypothesis can be right at one time. This limits new thinking and precludes any other theories that might fall outside the proscribed system. It has led itself down the road towards entrenched and dogmatic thinking.

Evolutionary Medicine: The second school within the Western model looks at evolutionary causes. This evolutionary school is very recent and is an outcome of new advances in biology and physics; it has been deeply influenced by ecology and increasing scientific evidence on natural therapies and the role of functional medicine. Evolutionary medicine answers questions about origins and function; it looks at six categories of explanation for the cause of disease: defenses, infection, environment, genetics, design, and evolution.

Doctors and scientists of evolutionary medicine say there is something inherently wrong with allopathic medicine's linear view of cause and effect, but caution us not to throw out the progress made in science. They would look at the evolutionary nature of things, come to terms with the incongruities at the core of the conventional system, and slow down enough to grasp the deeper nature of living things.

Wenda Trevathan, Ph.D., a professor of biological anthropology at New Mexico State University, says. "Evolutionary medicine takes the view that many contemporary social, psychological, and physical ills are related to incompatibility between the lifestyle and the environments in which humans currently live and the conditions under which biology evolved" (Trevathan 1999).

This relatively new system of medical thought is critically important in understanding and managing infectious disease, especially viruses. It is concerned, among other things, with co-evolutionary history, the relationships between humans and pathogens, and between humans and curative factors in plants and other natural substances.

Evolutionary biologists suggest that disease-causing microorganisms like viruses may have benefits we do not know about. Many viruses are benign and coexist in plants or humans, while others only trigger disease when they, or the host organism, interact with new environments or toxic environmental factors. From the evolutionary viewpoint, *coexistence* is as equally legitimate to natural systems as competition and dominance. However, ecological thinking like this is very new to the Western scientific mind, and much remains to be known about how biological systems work and how disease shapes evolution.

What we are certain about is that instances of viral diseases increase when environmental systems are disrupted. Here are typical examples: the building of a large dam that prevents fish from swimming upstream, diverts water for commercial agriculture, and pollutes ground water; rainforest destruction that disrupts the evolution of biodiversity and lowers the oxygen content in our air; mass migration of humans from one cultural and geographical region to another, sometimes in a matter of only days; the movement of animals from one bioregion to another precipitated by rapid environmental devastation or civil wars. Scores of other, similar environmental factors cause global changes that profoundly influence the immunity of individuals and therefore their susceptibility to disease.

The evolutionary nature of illness, and viral diseases in particular, is an important theme in this book. It is my prediction that the principles of evolutionary medicine will shape the course of both conventional and alternative medicine for centuries to come.

Functional Medicine: Though the modern allopathic form is the dominant system of Western medicine, there are many variations in styles of practice and therapies, including naturopathy, osteopathy, chiropractic, homeopathy, quantum medicine, integrative medicine, and functional medicine. It is well beyond the scope and purpose of this book to describe all of these systems, and therefore I have chosen those that best fit the principles necessary to understand how the immune system works and how to treat viral conditions. One of the most promising of these is functional medicine, a system based on evidence of outcomes—also referred to as clinical outcome studies.

Jeffrey Bland, Ph.D., the system's main spokesman, notes, "Practitioners who follow the prevailing philosophy often prescribe specific medications for specific symptoms. The medications typically work by blocking particular biochemical/physiological processes associated with cellular communication. Uncoupling (i.e., blocking) the intercellular message with a medication may, in some cases, be like shooting the messenger" (Bland 1999).

Very similar to modern naturopathic medicine, functional medicine utilizes herbal medications and nutrients to improve the body's natural ability to heal itself. This system is valuable for the treatment of chronic degenerative diseases, such as rheumatoid arthritis, Type II diabetes, the new diseases like chronic fatigue syndrome, for strengthening the immune system, and can be used as part of an integrated treatment approach to chronic viral diseases.

The Medical Insights of Chinese Medicine

Until now, we have mostly looked at Western medical models. Now we will learn about the important role Chinese medicine plays in viral immunity. Chinese medicine works in distinct contrast to the Western medical model. The Chinese developed a system of thought just as complex as their Western counterpart, but their approach is fundamentally different. The Western model is based on material science, but the Eastern is founded on a spiritual cosmology.

In this model, observation of the whole and the attempt to understand the interrelatedness of natural phenomena take precedence over detailed scrutiny of individual parts. The Chinese do not have exag-

gerated expectations of discovering the end of knowledge or an ultimate understanding of the universe, as do Westerners. They accept
that all things are constantly changing and that therefore the results,
as well as the rules of therapy, must adapt to these changes.

Their model describes all natural processes and all the possibilities and combinations of natural events. The Chinese method accepts
that change is inherent in the original design of the universe, but that
the underlying principles remain the same. There is one moon and
one sun in the sky; water is always wet; snow is always cold. In its
essence, it is a practical, empirical, and philosophical system based
upon the direct observation of natural phenomena.[3]

This methodology makes Chinese medicine preeminent in evaluating complex disease conditions in a comprehensive manner and in
providing effective and safe treatments for a wide variety of conditions, viral diseases among them. It also has considerable benefits in
treating chronic degenerative diseases, chronic infections, and the new
environmentally and stress-induced illnesses.

For viral illnesses in particular, the Chinese model has much to
offer, for as a nation, China has a long history of analyzing and treating virally induced diseases. As mentioned earlier, most influenza
strains originate in China, and one third of all hepatitis cases in the
world occur in China. This has enabled the Chinese to form a comprehensive understanding of how the body manages viruses and how
clinicians can treat viral diseases using natural and effective remedies.

One of the most useful characteristics of the Chinese system is its
emphasis on causes of disease that involve the health status of the
host. Among the conditions that affect the host are weakness of the
qi and blood, poor defense mechanisms, aging, stress, and emotional
factors. This model presents an analysis in terms of patterns of disharmony, which in themselves are not the cause of the disease, but an
expression of the presenting imbalance.

The cause will be found at a deeper level in the patient's lifestyle,
exposure to the elements (wind, cold, etc.) or other disease, diet, daily
habits, environment, and sexual habits. The cause is determined by
examining the complete *pattern* of how the patient lives and how the
illness manifests in the individual, not merely by studying the symptoms, as in Western medicine. The pattern of the manifestation of illness is composed of the inherited strengths and weaknesses of the
patient, symptoms or the subjective complaints, observable signs like

sweating or fever, and additional symptoms and signs like headaches, difficulty urinating, or dry skin.

For the treatment of viral disease and immune enhancement, Chinese medicine is invaluable. In part 2, you will learn to apply effective Chinese medicines as part of the 10-step viral immunity program.

Integration of Effective Medical Approaches

I have intensively studied and applied many different systems of healing for more than twenty-five years, but my preferred approach is simple: do what works best for the patient. The approach I propose is the integrated model that combines the most useful theories, methods, and treatments from different medical systems (see table 7). It may be wise at this point to look at the strengths and weaknesses of each system and see how an individual patient may benefit from the use of an integrated approach, or by using one or the other of the main systems. One of the training techniques in medicine is called the case study, a narrative description of a patient's condition, treatment, and outcome. Several such cases are presented in this book, as well as short clinical anecdotes, to illustrate concepts and principles of immunity and the treatment of viral conditions.

Case Study in Allergies and Immune Dysfunction: George was a fifty-nine-year-old retired man with a life-long history of sinus congestion and allergies. As an executive for a large corporation, he popped over-the-counter antihistamine capsules almost every day to relieve his runny nose and other allergy symptoms so he could function. To treat his recurrent sinus infections, he was on one round of antibiotics after the other, none of which worked.

His symptoms worsened and he finally consented to surgery to "put a drain into it"; this was performed on the right maxillary sinus, the sinus cavity under the eye. The procedure helped his breathing some but did nothing to cure the allergic condition and sinus infections.

More antibiotics and antihistamines, nasal sprays, and decongestants were prescribed. Eventually, George gave up on the conventional medical route, and tried its other, usually final, option: "Learn to live with it." This failed miserably as well, though he was at least free of aggressive and ineffective interventions, and his body adapted to a continuous level of low-grade infections. He was drug free, but miserable.

Table 7: Comparison of Different Medical Models Discussed in This Book

Conventional	Evolutionary	Functional	Chinese
Body as machine: "clock"	Body as dynamic machine: "computer"	Body as biodynamic: "interactive computer"	Body as a biodynamic whole, related to the complete environment
Reductionistic: parts are all-important	Comprehensive: parts and their design are important	Integrated: parts, design, and function are important	Wholistic: the whole is as important as the parts
Mind and body are distinctively separated	Mind and body are separated, but influence each other	An attempt is made at re-integration of mind and body	Mind and body clearly influence each other because they are inseparable
Focus on eliminating disease	Focuses on understanding symptoms and removing the causes of disease	Emphasizes achieving health	Emphasizes return to balance
External causes: germs and trauma	External and internal: germs, trauma, genetics	Internal: biochemical imbalances, immune weakness, hormonal imbalances, stress	Internal, external, and other: disharmonic energy
Treatments mainly suppress symptoms	Treatments control symptoms and address causes	Treatments address underlying cause	Treatments attempt to re-establish harmony
Focus on intervention: highly specialized experts using high-tech life-saving measures	Focuses on predisposition, genetics, and assisting the body's natural defenses	Individualized focus on nutrition, biochemistry, prevention	Focus on less technology: using sustainable methods like herbs and acupuncture
Interested in objective signs: lab tests and statistics	Interested in explanations: evaluates symptoms and signs as well as vulnerabilities and host defense	Interested in evidence-based research	Interested in a complete array of evidence: how the patient feels, lifestyle, etc.
Physician as all-knowing and emotionally detached	Physician as biologist and ecologist	Physician as caring, empathetic provider	Physician as keen observer of patterns of disharmony
Patient is passive receiver of services	Patient is studied	Patient is proactive participant, often managing his own care	Patient both passively receives and participates
Use of expensive, non-renewable methods	Uses all methods that work and cause the least ecological disruption	Use of less expensive methods like diet and vitamins	Use of renewable methods

George was gradually able to be free of even over-the-counter anti-histamines and nasal sprays, yet he continued to suffer from daily congestion, breathing through his mouth because of it. He had difficulty sleeping due to breathing problems at night, bouts of infection several times a month, facial pressure, and daily headaches. The long-term drain on his system eventually led to immune weakness, and he began experiencing frequent colds and flu, low energy, and a general sense of "feeling lousy."

Influenced by the increasing flood of information about alternative medicine, George started to take a vitamin and mineral complex, garlic capsules, and an herbal mixture designed for the respiratory system, along with an immune-enhancing substance called beta glucan. He told me that his sinus symptoms were about the same after starting this health regimen, but he did not have the repeated severe colds that he had had for years, and his sinus condition did not have the awful aggravations he often experienced. He considered himself "lucky" and did not want to return to a conventional medical doctor, and he wanted to see if a more specific natural medicine plan would work for him since he had seen some results with the remedies from the health foods store. That is when he came to see me.

My work-up began with a detailed history of his condition and symptoms. I made a list of all George's drugs and over-the-counter medications, including vitamins and minerals and any natural medication self-prescribed or recommended by an alternative heath care provider. I investigated his allergic condition by reviewing the results of his previous allergy testing, and ordered some new tests; I also ordered a comprehensive chemistry panel and complete blood count. Then, after an examination of his throat, ears, and lymph nodes, and taking his temperature, I formulated my conclusions on his case.

George suffered from a common condition: chronically inflamed sinus passages that deteriorated into frequent bouts of a low-grade bacterial sinusitis. He developed a nonspecific immune weakness, allowing for recurrent upper respiratory viral infections and an increased allergic profile. Basically, he had a complicated version of old fashioned sinusitis, a condition that affects as many as 31–35 million Americans each year.

In George's case, once I had determined the diagnosis, I prescribed an herbal antimicrobial, natural antiviral medications, and nutrients to support his immune system. I gave him acupuncture sessions to eliminate the headaches, facial pressure, and neck pain. Within two weeks, all of his generalized symptoms were completely gone and they had not returned after a routine six-month follow-up. His nasal congestion was reduced by at least fifty percent, and his energy improved along with his general sense of wellness.

The Allopathic View of George's Condition: From the perspective of conventional medicine, in a patient with bacterial sinusitis, the cause is a bacterial infectious microorganism and the treatment is a 10- to 14-day course of antibiotics. Acute bacterial sinusitis is such a common condition that it is the fifth most common diagnosis for which antibiotics are prescribed.

According to this view, if the right antibiotic is prescribed, and if there are no side effects from the antibiotic that would cause the patient to discontinue the treatment, the infection should theoretically subside. However, this was not the case with George, nor has it been with many of my patients with chronic sinusitis.

In this approach, other drugs may be used in combination with the antibiotics: decongestants may be given to help open the air passages, analgesics (pain killers) may also be used to help manage facial pain or headache caused by the swollen sinuses, antihistamines may be used to reduce nasal drainage, and systemic or nasal steroid sprays are sometimes used to reduce inflammation. For none of these are there definitive studies that show their effectiveness.

In the case of a viral infection, which is how most sinus conditions start out, conventional medicine has no effective treatment. Even though studies show that only 0.5–2.0 percent of adults with viral sinusitis progress to a bacterial infection, the patient is often prescribed an antibiotic even if it is ineffective against viral agents (Berg 1986). Of course it does not work at all, and the inappropriate use of an antibiotic for a viral condition may lead to antibiotic resistance and cause the antibiotic to become ineffective for future use, as seen in George's case. As is commonly the case in chronic sinusitis, the bacteria learn how to outsmart, and thereby resist, the drug.

Though antibiotics are a mainstay of conventional medicine and are often the drug of first choice for sinusitis, this model does not take into account the relationships between the different microbial infections that can occur in chronic sinusitis (bacterial, viral, fungal), and it only rarely recognizes the allergic aspects. It does not take into account toxic environmental exposure that might have inflamed the sinus membranes in the first place, contributing to easier infection, and it does nothing to improve the patient's immune status or prevent further infections. It only treats *current* symptoms as they present each time. To be fair, antibiotics do help in many cases of bacterial sinusitis and should definitely be considered for certain, but not all, cases.

The Evolutionary View of George's Case: In the evolutionary model, our patient with bacterial sinusitis may still be prescribed an antibiotic if necessary, but additional questions are asked and the probable outcome of the use of an antibiotic is considered. The doctor evaluates the patient's defense system and considers the past history of antibiotic use. In recurrent or chronic cases like George's, the evolutionary medicine doctor will consider if the illness is now in an adaptive state with the host and if there are co-evolving pathogens or other illnesses. This doctor will also consider other factors, such as occasional irritation by smoke from cigarettes, stress issues that may further weaken the immune system, and hereditary predisposition.

Retracing the medical history, the physician will find stress, environmental factors (such as long hours spent in an office building with recycled air), and the mismanagement of pharmaceutical drugs. George's immune system will be carefully evaluated and allergy tests performed. Since there is considerable viral involvement, antibiotics would not be used because they are ineffective for viruses.

The Functional Medicine View of George's Case: The doctor practicing functional medicine will look at the patient's immune function, nutritional status, age, and hormonal balance. He will suggest different nutrients and herbal medications to strengthen immunity, reduce inflammation and tissue damage produced by the infection, minimize the consequences of antibiotic therapy, and improve general health. If the functional medicine practitioner is not a medical doctor and an obvious acute bacterial infection is present and the body's immune system is not capable of controlling it, he would refer the patient to a medical doctor for evaluation and possible antibiotics.

The Chinese Medicine View of George's Case: Diagnosed in Chinese medicine, the same patient with bacterial sinusitis may fall under a variety of rubrics such as "wind-heat," or "wind-cold transforming to heat," or "hot-phlegm," and be prescribed a complex combination of herbs. Within the same formula are herbs with antimicrobial activity, mucolytics (mucus-dissolving agents), decongestants, and toxin-relieving substances. Viral sinusitis would be treated with a combination of herbs used for "wind-cold" or "cold-phlegm." Simultaneously, George's immune and general health status would be treated with strengthening qi tonics.

The benefit of this type of treatment is that its comprehensiveness and multi-faceted approach does not interfere with the body's own healing potential. It is most useful for viral infections. The disadvantage is that it is time consuming. The herbs must be taken four or five times daily, and it may take several days or a week before results are evident. In the process, the patient's condition could worsen. The herbs may not be sufficiently powerful to manage a very aggressive bacterial infection.

The Integrated Approach to George's Case: A doctor practicing integrated medicine may combine aspects of allopathic, evolutionary, and functional medicine and may refer the patient for acupuncture, Chinese medicine, or nutritional supplementation. She may consider the use of an antibiotic, but would first carefully evaluate the patient and perform a nasal or sputum culture to find out which specific organism was the most likely cause of the infectious aspect. Then she would decide which antibiotic would be most effective.

If it is a viral sinusitis, she will not use an antibiotic as the first measure, but she might prescribe a nutraceutical antiviral medication like echinacea, along with a natural decongestant, dietary restrictions, and an immune-enhancing regimen of vitamins, minerals, and herbs. She might also refer George for nonspecific therapies that promote health and are not focused on the treatment of a specific disease, such as treatment with Chinese medicine to strengthen the body's energy, or prescription of stress reduction therapies like yoga or meditation.

She would look in depth at the possible allergic triggers for sinusitis and suggest that they be removed from the patient's immediate environment. Acupuncture might be recommended to relieve headache, neck pain, and facial pressure that often accompany sinus conditions.

The doctor practicing this new style of medicine must take into consideration *all* of these factors and more, when evaluating a patient like George. It is not enough to simply diagnose the disease or condition. The disease state and stage should be evaluated along with the underlying constitution of the patient, his age and general health, combined with an estimation of his immune status Each disease must be looked at individually, and far more completely than most doctors are used to.

The Purpose of Medical Practice

What then is the purpose of medical practice? From the Western allopathic model, it is to treat the disease, but not necessarily to make the patient feel better. This model breeds a cold and emotionally isolated system in which the doctor becomes a distant provider of medical techniques, estranged from the patient who is expected to be a passive receiver of medical services. In this system, the doctor often treats the lab results and not the person, and patients often complain that, though their lab numbers are improved, they still feel sick.

Modern medicine in itself is not wrong, but it operates in a socioeconomic system that places profit first. For all of its good points, it functions in a very constricted manner, limited in its viewpoint, confining allopathic doctors to an outmoded paradigm.

Though still within the Western model, evolutionary and functional medicine attempt to improve this situation by focusing more on the broad view, examining why we get sick and how we heal. These approaches consider multiple causative factors, they improve the patient's lifestyle, and they foster faith in the possibilities of healing.

If the goal of medicine is not only to treat the disease but to help the patient, then the Chinese model is the better system as it focuses on enhancing the physical constitution, preventing disease, and restoring health. However, the Chinese model also has its weaknesses. It is a difficult system to grasp in its entirety, even for the Chinese who have been experimenting with these ideas for several thousand years. Yet, they do seem to be ahead of the West in integrated medicine.

Starting in 1949, with the Communist revolution, traditional Chinese medicine was reinstated as a system equal to Western medicine, and in modern China there are now three systems of medicine: Western allopathic medicine and surgery, traditional Chinese medicine and acupuncture, and integrated Western and Chinese medicine.

There is no doubt that we can learn much from the Chinese medical experience. However, on a global scale, especially in light of increasing viral diseases, what is required is a new paradigm in the way people think about disease. We need to move from a linear view of humanity's ever-increasing conquest of nature to a nonlinear model that considers inner and outer causes and sees how these fit into the bigger picture of nature and humankind. This new model of medicine sees individual physical components fully linked with functional body systems in a dynamic web of energy.

In this way, we come closer to a complete system of medicine, one that will serve us in the new viral plague times we are already in. The purpose of medical practice becomes treating the patient in the context of his specific, individual environment and personal spiritual and psychological needs, with the goal of effectively reestablishing systemic balance through safe, natural therapeutics whenever possible.

On a global scale, especially in light of increasing viral diseases, what is required is a new paradigm in the way people think about disease. This new model of medicine sees individual physical components fully linked with functional body systems in a dynamic web of energy.

The Difference between Healing and Cure: If that's how we practice, how do we heal? Healing is different from curing. The word "heal" comes from the old English *halen,* and carries the concept of wholeness, or as the saying goes, "hale and hearty." The words "holy" and "holistic" come from the same linguistic root. To cure means to restore to health, with the connotation that a method or course of medical treatment is involved. It comes from the Latin, *cura,* "to take care of," and from the same root found in the Spanish word for a traditional healer, *curandero.*

True healing comes from within and results in a state of health, wholeness, and complete well-being. In a sense, we heal ourselves. Healing invokes the spark of life that originally made us, a restoration of energetic balance, a harmony of mind and body, and the sense of being touched by the Great Spirit who created all things.

But to heal, a variety of factors have to come into play, and, in some cases, this may involve the necessity of a cure. A cure might require an antibiotic to kill excessive bacterial growth that our immune systems cannot fight off on their own, nutritional supplements to improve our immune status, antiviral herbs, or other treatments and therapies.

Curing is what is done to us when we are sick, while healing is stimulated from within our bodies, minds, and spirits. You can both heal and cure yourself by following the ten steps to viral immunity outlined in part 2. By using safe, proven remedies, practicing a healthy lifestyle, restoring organ function, and following the ways of nature and natural medicine, and by the grace of God, you can restore and sustain your good health.

CHAPTER SUMMARY

The cause of modern chronic viral diseases involves many factors.

There are many different systems of medicine and each has distinct benefits and disadvantages.

To treat the newly emerging diseases, especially viruses, an integrated approach appears to offer the most advantages, rather than an approach focused exclusively on one system.

Primary treatment, when at all possible, should be based upon medicines from naturally occurring products.

Treatment principles might be served best when, as in naturopathy, they are rooted in evolutionary biology and Chinese philosophy, combined with the latest in immunological research, modern medicine, and physiologically based medicine.

The mystery of disease can only be solved by mastering health.

Ten Steps to Viral Immunity

Introduction to Part Two

The material in part 1 addressed viruses, immunity, how viruses cause illness, and why we are facing an immune crisis and experiencing viral plagues. At this point, let's summarize the most important areas that influence viral immunity

Susceptibility

Virulence

Immune status

Immune stressors

Inflammation

Fatigue

Susceptibility is the degree to which you are vulnerable to infection. Virulence describes how potent the virus is. If your immune status is strong, your susceptibility is less, even if the virus is very virulent. However, the immune system can be weakened by many factors that are common in modern life, such as psychological stress and environmental toxins, thereby reducing your immune status. Due to these and other factors we have discussed, chronic infection is becoming more common than acute infectious illness, resulting in chronic inflammation, which damages tissues and causes discomfort, pain, and fatigue.

Now that we have identified the problems, let's look at the solutions.

Viral immunity is composed of two aspects and ten steps. The two aspects are prevention and treatment. Preventing viral infections involves avoiding viral diseases and conditions that are conducive to infection while strengthening the immune system. Treatment involves the management of existing viral illness, reducing the viral load in the body with natural antivirals, and strengthening the immune system. Before going further, let's define viral load and review the definition of viral immunity.

Viral Load: Technically speaking, viral load is the number of viruses per milliliter of blood, measured by a special laboratory test. This test gives an approximation of the amount of specific viruses in the body. There are three viral load tests used: the PCR (polymerase chain reaction), dDNA (branched chain DNA assay), and the NASBA (nucleic acid sequence-based amplification) tests. The PCR test is the most widely used of the three. "Viral burden" is a better, nontechnical, way of describing the impact viral disease has on the body. Effective therapy should reduce both the detectable viral load and symptomatic effects caused by the viral burden.

Viral Immunity: Viral immunity is the ability of the body's immune system to effectively resist viral infection, neutralize viruses in the body, remove viral toxins from the body, and normalize inflammation and autoimmune processes caused by viral disease. The 10-step viral immunity program of this book tells you how to achieve optimal viral immunity. The goal of the 10-step viral immunity plan is to help you *prevent* viral infections, *strengthen* your natural immunity, and to effectively *treat* viral infections with safe, natural medicines.

Now, let's review and outline all of the important components of the 10-step viral immunity plan. The steps are organized into prevention, treatment, and application:

- Steps 1–4 are largely preventive.

- Steps 5–9 focus on treatment.

- Step 10 explains how to design your own viral immunity plan.

Remember that each step is related to every other step. For example, if you follow step 1 and build a strong immune foundation, it will not only help you prevent viral disease and strengthen your immunity, but will help the treatments in step 7 work better.

Here is a brief outline of each step and what you can expect from reading them.

1. **Build a Strong Immune Foundation with an Immune-Enhancing Lifestyle:** In the first step you will learn the elements of an immune-enhancing lifestyle, including dietary suggestions that constitute the foundation for deeper healing. You will learn how to reduce and manage stress, and what dietary supplements are best to support your foundation. A strong will and a positive attitude are essential in winning the struggle with any illness—viral diseases included—and are critical factors in keeping the immune system strong and responsive. Mental and psychological strategies are also discussed in step 1.

2. **Defend and Strengthen Your Immune System with Antioxidants and Oxidative Therapies:** In this step you will learn the critical role of oxygen in viral immunity, and how to use immune-strengthening antioxidants. It describes the evidence for their use and explains which dosages work best. As in all the steps, safety issues and contraindications are explained. You will also learn what medical oxygenation therapies are and when and how to use them to treat viral infections.

3. **Rejuvenate Your Immune System with Enzymes:** Enzymes and phytonutrient-rich foods enhance the diet, improve digestion, add specialized nutrients like carotenoids and other naturally occurring antioxidants to the diet, improve natural detoxification, and reduce inflammation. This step tells you which phytonutrient-rich foods are the best for viral immunity and how to use enzymes to improve your health.

4. **Renew Your Cells through Detoxification:** Detoxification regimens and cleansing strategies are essential and important to prevent disease and improve immune function. This step emphasizes the important role of natural medications in cleansing the lymphatic system and the liver, both critical for viral immunity. You will learn how to safely conduct your own viral immunity

detoxification program, which natural medications and nutrients promote tissue and cellular cleansing, and which remove the toxins produced by viruses from your body.

5. **Restore Your Innate Immune Response and Manage Inflammation:** Natural anti-inflammatory agents are important in building viral immunity as is managing autoimmune-induced tissue inflammation in chronic viral diseases. In this step, you will learn how to use natural anti-inflammatory medicines to reduce tissue damage from inflammation occurring in your tissues and organs, caused by viral disease or autoimmune activity.

6. **Boost Your Immunity with Natural Immune-Enhancers:** Natural immune-building medications are a key component in the treatment of immune dysfunction and viral infections. This step explains how to use immune-enhancing substances, or immunomodulators, to boost your immunity. These products are considerably more powerful than herbs and vitamins, and include mushroom glucans, transfer factor, and lactoferrin. Dosages are provided for each medication, along with contraindications for their use.

7. **Target Viruses with Natural Antiviral Alternatives:** Natural antiviral medicines are critical for successfully treating viral illness. In this step you will learn how to use nature's most effective antiviral medicines. Dosages and direction on how to use them safely and effectively are presented in detail.

8. **Empower Your Viral Immunity Program with Chinese Medicines:** Using Chinese herbal remedies can considerably increase the effectiveness of your program. No other culture provides such a rich source of knowledge about viral infections and the methods and medicines that treat them than the Chinese. In this step you will learn how to use powerful and effective Chinese antivirals, immune modulators, energy enhancers, and anti-inflammatory medicines.

9. **Optimize Immune Performance with Hormonal Balance:** Hormones play an integral role in maintaining a strong immune

system. This step shows you how to use natural hormonal therapies including DHEA, thymic hormones, human growth hormone, and thyroid hormone to increase your health, energy, and mood, and enhance your immunity.

10. **Implement Your Viral Immunity Plan:** The last step teaches you how to design your own viral immunity program, work effectively with natural medications, measure success and teaches you which lab tests are most helpful. It presents treatment recommendations for selected viruses such as for the common cold, the flu, and hepatitis C.

Caution: **Note on Dosages in Part 2:** The material in this book is written for adults. The author understands that senior adults and children have special requirements; however, these are not specifically addressed in this book. For seniors, dosages should be reduced by at least one half, and for children by at least one quarter of the lowest recommended dosage. Dosages are given in ranges for the *average* adult to be used as *guidelines* only. Effects from remedies can vary a great deal from person to person, and applications must be adjusted to meet *individual* requirements. Consult your doctor or pharmacist if you have any questions about interactions between natural medicines and prescription or over-the-counter drugs

6

STEP ONE

Build a Strong Immune Foundation with an Immune-Enhancing Lifestyle

It is well known that if the foundation of a building is sound, the structure built upon it will be strong and long-lasting. Consider the great pyramids of Egypt. They have a deep and broad base and have lasted for thousands of years. We also know, from organic and biodynamic gardening, that if the soil is rich and well cared for, the root systems of the plants will be deep, strong, and vital, and the plant itself will be healthy and able to resist pests and disease. Natural medicine can produce a similar foundation. It aims at establishing a solid foundation of mental and physical health to prevent disease, resist infection, and to enable the organism to live for a long time.

To build an immune-enhancing lifestyle, it is best to start young and when you are not sick. However, the body is very resilient; it cooperates with the right cures and works toward healing itself. In fact, in some instances, it can spontaneously heal itself. Of course, if you are sick, you need appropriate and effective treatment, but the principles of health still apply. Mastering them is the first step toward viral immunity and healing.

In this chapter we look at the building blocks of health, how they influence immunity, and how they make an immune-enhancing lifestyle. Since the connection between mind, body, and immune system is so important for healthy immunity, we look closely at the science of psychoneuroimmunology (PNI), the scientific discipline that attempts to understand the interactions between the immune system, the nervous system, and the psyche—the realm of mind, mood, and emotions, and the influences of the body and mind on viral immunity.

The Body-Mind Connection and Viral Immunity

Your body-mind has an extraordinary power to defend itself against even the most virulent of viruses and to heal and regenerate even when disease occurs. Of course, to be realistic about viral disease, there is more to it than that, but an integrated body-mind has an exquisite sense of timing and expresses immunity exactly when you most need it.

Think of the immune system as an employee: If he arrives too early or too late, his unreliability disrupts the entire department We do not want him working more than necessary, as a hyperactive immune system can lead to inflammation and autoimmune disease; nor do we want him to be lazy, as an under-functioning immune system lets in any virus that comes along.

Many complex processes regulate this body-mind connection, including brain function, the nervous system, the endocrine glands (those that secrete hormones), and the activity of the physical body. Both physical and psychological stress influence these processes and can disturb the immune system leaving us more vulnerable to viral diseases. Exercise, diet, nutritional supplements, stress reduction, and other factors improve these processes and promote a healthy immune system. For the present, let's look at each part of the body-mind unit, and review the science behind it.

The human body is a remarkable creation and it is often referred to as the temple of the soul. It contains almost every known chemical on Earth and has the ability to manufacture its own healing substances. Your body contains the most sophisticated pharmacy imaginable: it creates custom drugs to order and, given the right stimulus and chemical building blocks, it will manufacture the exact healing substance on demand. However, to support the healing process and to build a strong immune system, the body requires adequate exercise, rest, deep sleep, pure water, clean air, and proper nutrition. Often, you need dietary and nutritional supplements as well.

Exercise and Immunity: Most people do not exercise enough. The obvious consequences are lack of fitness and weight gain, but not getting enough exercise also impairs immunity. For example, the number of natural killer cells and their function is improved with exercise. Physical exercise also restores hormone balance, such as the levels of growth hormone and cortisol, which play a significant role in immunity.

The exercise effect is mediated by interactions between the somatic nervous system, the autonomic nervous system, and the endocrine system. Regular exercise coordinates these different systems in a manner that makes their response more organized, thus more effective, resulting in better immunity. The somatic nervous system controls voluntary movement of the muscles. The autonomic nervous system maintains homeostasis by regulating organ functions like heart rate and digestion without your awareness. There are two parts of the autonomic nervous system: the sympathetic and parasympathetic systems. The sympathetic part helps the body during crisis and stress while the parasympathetic helps to conserve energy and controls many specific functions in the body like slowing down heart rate.

There is no question that exercise improves health and natural immunity. What many people do not know is that overdoing it through intense, repetitive exercise does more harm than good. Excessive stress-producing exercise stimulates the sympathetic nervous system and decreases immunity. Too much exercise also increases oxidative damage to cells, causing tissue damage and accelerating aging. It also produces a higher risk of respiratory infections and can trigger latent viruses. A Danish study showed that intense exercise lowers levels of natural killer (NK) cells and lymphokine-activated killer (LAK) cells (Peterson 2001). Research shows that the immune system is overwhelmed by the trauma of excessive exercise, so too much exercise can be as injurious to your health as too little.

One of my patients, a world-class female athlete, came to see me for recurrent injuries and debilitating fatigue. Despite her problems, Sarah continued to train because, like many athletes, she thought the answer to her condition was more training. She pushed herself beyond her body's limits. Eventually she sought medical help, and her doctors told her if she rested she would be fine, but by that time she had caused immune deficiency and even with more rest her condition did not improve.

During my first interview with Sarah, I found that her condition started with flu-like symptoms that occurred immediately after a competitive event (which she won); since then, her condition had cycled between periods of weakness and times when she felt better. During the good times, Sarah would train heavily and then suffer the consequences of more fatigue. My diagnosis, confirmed by specialized blood studies, was a chronic virus and immune deficiency caused by excessive physical training and the depletion of tissue and organ reserve of vital nutrients.

Sarah's treatments included diet, nutritional supplements, rest, and deep sleep to restore organ reserve, as well as antiviral herbs, acupuncture, and massage. Over time, she regained her health, though because of the damage caused by over-training while ill, she was not able to reenter the competitive world of professional athletics until several years later.

This case illustrates how excessive exercise, even by a professional athlete, seriously impairs immune function. The same consequences can happen to you, so be careful not to overexercise.

We know that lack of exercise leads to poor health and that too much exercise is bad for the immune system, so what is the best type and amount of exercise? Keep in mind that you should begin any exercise by gradually getting fit, to reduce injury, and then continue regular training to maintain that fitness. In this manner, you increase your exercise tolerance, retrain your neuromuscular system, and improve the coordination between the somatic and autonomic nervous systems.

Gradually, you adapt to higher levels of well-being. It is not wise to practice intense exercise when you're not fit or only once every week or so. The "weekend warrior" syndrome only leads to more fatigue and potential injuries, and it causes a cyclical pattern of avoidance of exercise alternated with infrequent bouts of too much exercise.

Besides improving immunity, regular exercise provides the following benefits:

- Normalizes blood pressure

- Increases muscle mass and reduces body fat

- Lowers total cholesterol and increases high-density lipoprotein cholesterol, the "good" type

- Improves cardiovascular function

- Increases energy and improves resistance to fatigue

- Decreases cravings for sweets and normalizes appetite

- Improves mood and sense of well-being

- Reduces need for sleep

- Lengthens the life span

In my clinical opinion, the best exercises ever designed for humans are those from the East: hatha yoga and tai chi. They are not just exercises, but complete systems of physical and mental health that train mind, body, and spirit. Hatha yoga is the master exercise system for the body and mind, while tai chi is the best exercise for the nervous system and mental-emotional state, and it also has profound positive effects on the body.

A number of research studies on hatha yoga (Bickel 2000) and tai chi (Husted 1999) testify in a scientific manner to the benefits of these systems.[1] If qualified teachers for hatha yoga or tai chi are available in your area, I recommend that you try these exercises and experience the benefits. There are no age limits, but speak with the instructor before you begin if you are older or have an injury so they can safely guide you.

Second best, and perhaps more easily available for many Americans, is a combination or variety of exercises, often referred to as "cross-training," in which different parts of your body are worked out, not only one system or area; this form of exercise combines aerobic and light weight training. It improves fitness, increases muscle mass and strength, promotes weight loss, and improves immunity. Alternating swimming, bicycling, or walking (aerobic exercises), with isometrics and weight training (anaerobic), produces the best results and the least

> *In my clinical opinion, the best exercises ever designed for humans are those from the East: hatha yoga and tai chi. They are not just exercises, but complete systems of physical and mental health that train mind, body, and spirit.*

injuries. Don't forget to include stretching in your exercise plan to promote flexibility.

If you are not currently exercising regularly, first think about how much time each week you can devote to physical exercise and schedule it into your calendar. If you are unsure of how to start an exercise program, find a fitness instructor and work with her to design an exercise program that fits your needs. If you are not able to do any of the exercise forms mentioned in this chapter, start walking outdoors at least three times per week for a minimum of 20 minutes.

My recommendation is to vary your program to include 2–3 days of weight training, alternated with 2–3 days of aerobic activity each week. These should be your main exercises; allow 60–90 minutes for each workout. Include stretching and some isometric exercises with these as warm-ups and on off days perform a minimum of 20 minutes of isometrics and stretching at home. Take one or two rest days each week when you do not exercise. Research has shown that recuperation between exercising is as important to the immune system as the exercise.

The Anti-Stress Benefits of Rest: Rest counters the effects of stress and improves immunity. Herbert Benson, M.D., of the Mind/Body Medical Institute in Boston, and the author of *The Relaxation Response* (1975), has studied the effects of rest on the body since the 1970s. Benson found the body has a counterbalancing mechanism that neutralizes the negative effects of stress. The relaxation response decreases blood pressure, lowers heart rate, and relaxes muscle tension. When practiced regularly, your health and immune system improve.

Rest and repose are crucial aspects of your viral immunity plan. This includes, for example, adequate rest between repetitions of weightlifting or stretching, and during the day or evening (after dinner) when the body is allowed to unwind and recover. When possible, an afternoon siesta will help to calm your nerves and recharge your mind and body so you can finish your day in a better mood, with more energy for the evening with your family or friends. Rest also includes vacation time away from work schedules and routines; social time with friends, walks on the beach or in the woods, gardening, visits to art museums, or listening to music.

Judeo-Christian religions set aside one day each week—a Sabbath—for rest and worship. This is a custom that perhaps we should consider returning to. Meditation provides deep rest and is highly recommended for people suffering from stress, chronic disease, viral illness, or mood disorders. Therapeutic massage and acupuncture treatments, by promoting the release of relaxation-inducing chemicals called endorphins (substances that alter mood), induce deep rest and provide a sense of wellness.

In my clinical opinion, if you have a viral illness, regular rest periods during the day and at least one full day per week are necessary for the body to regenerate itself. Twice a day, take a 30–60-minute rest to reduce the effects of stress and improve your immunity.

How Sleep Helps Immunity: Sleep is not only important for feeling recharged in the morning, but it promotes proper body functioning, helps the organs regenerate, relaxes the mind, and restores the spirit. It enhances and regulates the immune system, aiding in the recovery from illness, including viral disease, and in the prevention of disease. Humans, like all animals, require a restorative cycle each day, and without adequate sleep you will find it difficult to recover from any illness.

Numerous scientific studies support the profound effect sleep has on our well-being. Disrupted sleep, an increasingly common condition among modern urban people, decreases the level of natural killer (NK) cells (Irwin 1996). Lack of sleep causes increased susceptibility to infections, such as colds and influenza. Stress, lack of rest between periods of work or activity, and disruption of the regular deep sleep cycle make us more vulnerable to infections. Long, sound sleep, even in the daytime, is one of the best remedies for the flu. J. Allan Hobson, a professor of sleep science at Harvard University, argues that the universal exhortation of mothers to their children to "get a good night's sleep," may be one of the best natural remedies available to ward off infections (Hobson 1994).

The need for sleep in a healthy person ranges from 6–10 hours each night, the average being 8. However, when one is ill or the immune system is fighting off a virus, the requirement moves towards the higher end of the range. Get 9–10 hours of good sleep each night, and up to 12 hours if you have an active infection.

The Importance of Pure Water and Clean Air in Immune Health: Air and water are essential to life. Polluted air and contaminated water contribute to illness. The human body requires adequate hydration regularly throughout the day to function properly. The recommendation of six to eight, 8-ounce glasses of water each day is the standard rule; however, when you are ill, exercising vigorously, or exposed to higher temperatures, your need for water increases. Therefore, using eight glasses (64 fluid ounces) of water each day as a starting point, increase by two glasses for each additional hour of activity, and another one or two glasses if the weather is hot or you are exercising in a heated room. This can bring the total up to sixteen glasses (1 gallon) of pure water daily. While herbal teas, soups, juices, coffee, sodas, and the fluid contained in foods help to hydrate the tissues, they should not be considered as a replacement for pure water. Some beverages, like black tea and coffee, are diuretics and will cause your body to lose water.

If you have a viral illness, it is essential that you avoid tap water and use only purified water or spring water in glass or hard plastic bottles. Polystyrene, the soft plastic used in most commercial water bottling, contains hormone-disrupting substances like nonylpherol, a synthetic chemical that mimics estrogen, and the synthetic chemicals found in tap water do not promote healing, weaken your immunity, and can promote cancer.

Clean air is also important for healing. Avoid buildings that do not have windows that open to the outside air and that recirculate air. These places are traps for all types of allergens, especially molds and chemicals, as well as viruses.

Besides avoiding unhealthy indoor environments, you can enhance the air your take into your body with special exercises. The best forms were developed in the East and are called *pranayama* in the yogic traditions and qi gong in the Chinese traditions. If classes in these are not available in your area, you can practice deep breathing by inhaling and exhaling deeply in front of an open window (away from traffic and pollution, of course) or outdoors, preferably in the early morning and while standing next to green plants or trees. Stand straight and relaxed with your chest out and stomach in, and inhale, bringing your arms out to your sides at the same time. Hold for a second or two, and exhale deeply while bringing your arms towards your front and hands together. Repeat three times in sets of three, and breathe slowly and rhythmically.

In the early 1990s, I worked at Scripps Memorial Hospital in La Jolla, California, where I was a member of the system-wide advisory rehabilitation board, and taught stroke victims modifications of

Eastern breathing exercises. All of the attendees reported improved stamina, a greater sense of well-being, increased mental clarity, and several dramatically improved their motor skills. Practicing regular breathing exercises can dramatically improve your health and appearance.

Proper Nourishment Promotes Immunity: Kenneth Bock, M.D., who practices natural immune-enhancing methods, says in his book *The Road To Immunity,* "The immune system is extremely sensitive to nutritional deficiencies and is more easily damaged by under-nutrition than any other system" (Bock 1997). Poor eating habits, under-nutrition of important immune-enhancing trace minerals, and eating refined carbohydrates (like white bread), sugar, and processed foods weaken immunity and inhibit healing.

To strengthen your immune system, eat healthy, natural foods. Eating a natural diet does not come easily; it requires a new understanding of how important foods are to your health and immunity. It is not the purpose of this book to go into diet in detail, only to point out the *importance* of a healthy diet and the different styles of good diets that promote a strong immune system. Now, let's look at some healthy diets.

Everyone wants to know what is the best diet. Honestly, it is not an easy question to answer. The flood of diet books on the market today is an indication of the diversity of ideas; rather than helping us, they often confuse the issue. We live in a global society powered by information, and we can get information on how other people eat, what their traditional diet is, and compare it to others and evaluate the health of the different groups. Researchers have found that some diets are healthier than others. As one sorts through all the information, we can see a common thread. In the following examples, we will look at several different diets to find what they have in common:

- The Mediterranean diet appears to be very good for maintaining general health and preventing heart disease. However, because about 40 percent of calories in this diet come from fats, mostly olive oil; the higher fat content along with overuse of pasta, as many Americans are prone to do, may lead to obesity.

- The traditional Chinese diet, high in phytoestrogenic foods and fresh vegetables, promotes proper hormone metabolism and contributes to a youthful appearance. We have learned much from the

Chinese diet, including the benefits of green tea, steaming vegetables and fish instead of pan-frying, the use of medicinal soups, and the importance of always using garden-fresh vegetables.

• The macrobiotic diet, high in alkaline grains and root vegetables, and low in fluid intake, is similar to the traditional Japanese diet and is reported to lower the risk for certain cancers. It emphasizes the use of seasonally fresh and locally grown fruits and vegetables, but it may be too high in carbohydrates, even in their complex form, and does not allow for enough fluids.

• The vegetarian and low calorie diet of India and China fosters longevity. However, when applied to the American way of life—active, aggressive, busy, and extreme—pure vegetarianism does not provide enough protein and may cause iron and vitamin B12 deficiency. Also, a vegetarian diet that includes dairy products and is high in carbohydrates from wheat may cause problems for Americans who have allergies to milk proteins and inflammatory substances in wheat.

To complicate matters, even when we find the right diet, our vegetables are full of pesticides, our meats are loaded with hormones and antibiotics, our fish may have high levels of toxic mercury, our store-bought fruits are often unripe. No wonder Americans continue to suffer from chronic disease and obesity, are prone to heart disease, and have dysfunctional immune systems.

There is a way around these concerns. Start with the basics: overeating is not good for your health and predisposes you to all types of disease, including heart attacks. Not eating enough is also bad for your health, though short periods dedicated to fasting or cleansing are okay (see step 4). Extremes are not good—balance is better.

Every individual has different and specific nutritional needs. Eastern medical and philosophical systems, like Ayurveda, base dietary requirements on constitutional types. For the average person, unless you have expert guidance, it is difficult to formulate the exact diet for your type, or even to know your type. Let's review some *general* guidelines, the common threads among the different health-oriented diets that I have found to work for most people, most of the time, and which are accepted by nutritionists and doctors as sound approaches to diet. Avoid any extreme diet unless you're under the guidance of a qualified medical or nutritional professional.

A healthy diet, one that empowers your immune system, is high in naturally occurring antioxidants, low in the "bad" fats (animal grease and margarines), and high in the "good" fats (vegetable oils, especially olive oil). It has adequate complete protein from fish, poultry, meats, eggs, and milk products, is low or absent in refined sugars, and has a reasonable amount of complex carbohydrates (whole wheat pasta, potatoes, dried legumes, and winter squash). If you have a chronic disease, viral illness, hormonal imbalances, or cancer, I recommend avoiding dairy products altogether. If you have allergies, avoid foods that you know cause allergies, and also avoid dairy products, eggs, and wheat, which are generally allergenic.

Further, have three regular meals each day, except when fasting or if you're on a hypoglycemic diet (which recommends four equal meals), composed of a variety of fresh vegetables, some meats, fish, and poultry, seasonal fresh ripe fruits, an assortment of seeds and nuts, and small amounts of spices and herbs. All foods should be fresh and organically raised whenever possible.

In my clinical practice, I use two dietary models that I modify for the individual patient. Both advocate the avoidance of refined sugars and the minimal intake of natural sugars from honey, fruit juices, and maple syrup. Both emphasize alkaline foods over acid-forming foods,[2] and both call for adequate fluid intake. Acid-forming foods include sugar, meat, sour fruits like lemons and pineapple, and tomatoes. Alkaline foods include most vegetables and natural sweeteners like honey.

Another element of my recommended diet is food rotation: the same food should not be eaten more than two times per week, with at least three days between. Otherwise food intolerance or allergies may develop.

Food should be alive and full of energy. In the 1970s I learned much about natural diet from my mentors, notably the naturopath Dr. Bernard Jensen, who taught that food is our best medicine. One of his most important lessons was that when food is served it should retain its vital energy, or life force—called *prana* in yoga philosophy and *qi* by the Chinese.

To measure this, look at the color of food after cooking. If the food retains its natural color and the vegetables are bright and vibrant, vital energy is still present; if vitality is present, health will follow. The Chinese are experts at retaining the *qi* in foods, and only eat freshly picked vegetables. For them, even when fish is eaten, it must be alive and still flopping just before it is prepared for cooking. They also cook the whole fish—head and all! They believe this preserves the *qi*, which can then be absorbed when the fish is eaten.

The basic dietary program I recommend is suitable for most people. It contains moderate amounts of complex carbohydrates (primarily brown or basmati rice), adequate fats and proteins,[3] and abundant fresh fruits and vegetables. The emphasis is always on vegetables. This diet comprises 50–55 percent complex carbohydrates; 15–20 percent high quality protein; and 20–25 percent healthy fats and oils.

The other diet I recommend is a low-carbohydrate diet, and for short periods of time (up to one month) I may advise a no-carbohydrate diet. This type of diet is similar to that advocated by Barry Sears and is known as the 30-30-40 Zone diet (Sears 1995). This diet is essential for people who have trouble metabolizing carbohydrates, such as people with diabetes, hypoglycemia, or insulin-resistance or dysglycemia, a sub-clinical condition of disrupted blood-sugar metabolism that is called Syndrome X.

It also benefits people with yeast infections and is very useful for losing weight and gaining muscle. It is an important diet to use when recovering from all types of diseases. If a viral disease is present, the protein intake remains high but should be composed of mostly plant protein foods such as seeds, nuts, and legumes, with less protein from animal sources.

I rarely recommend complete vegetarian diets, though occasionally I will recommend them for short periods of time (up to three months) or for certain individuals who function better on a vegetarian diet.

In both diets, the food sources are critical: carbohydrates should be unrefined, high-fiber, with a low glycemic index;[4] proteins should be principally from vegetable sources, such as seeds, nuts, and legumes, but organically raised lean meats and poultry, as well as fish and shellfish are allowed. Fats should be unsaturated oils, rich in omega-3 oils such as from flax seeds and fish. In both diets, I emphasize the importance of plenty of vegetables as a source of vitamins, minerals, and natural fiber. Along with meats, they are the most nutrient-dense of foods. Four to six servings of vegetables a day is a minimum, and they may be prepared as vegetable soups, salads, raw fresh juice, steamed, baked, or sautéed.

Dietary and Nutritional Supplements: Supplementation is an essential part of modern nutrition, and it becomes even more critical as people age and the immune system naturally declines. Adding vitamins and minerals to the diet is not a replacement for food, but is meant to be *supplemental* to a good diet. One mistake many of my patients make is taking too many supplements, often skipping meals in the process; this results in imbalanced nutrition and the wrong mixture of proteins, carbohydrates, and fats.

Supplementation is essential to building a strong immune foundation by increasing the micronutrient saturation of the tissues. According to Robert Rountree, M.D., in *Immunotics* (2000), micronutrient starvation is: "the number one cause of poor immune function and, therefore, disease." Micronutrients include trace minerals and vitamins that we need in small amounts, such as selenium and folic acid. A diet composed mainly of processed foods, low in fresh fruits and vegetables but high in calories, is deficient in these essential micronutrients.

Most Americans have access to lots of food, in fact, too much food of the wrong kinds. Fast-food restaurants are on nearly every corner and supermarkets are in every shopping center. However, the standard American diet (SAD) is actually deficient in many essential nutrients and is low in nutrient density. Our stressful modern lifestyle and its high exposure to toxic environmental pollutants and an ever-increasing variety of microbial agents requires of us even more optimal nutrition, and that can only be obtained by supplementation.

My general recommendations for daily supplementation are:

- Take a broad spectrum, high quality hypoallergenic multivitamin and mineral daily with food.

- Include an essential fatty acid supplement, like flaxseed oil or fish oil.

- Provide sufficient antioxidants, especially vitamins C and E, and the minerals zinc and selenium.

Now that we have reviewed the body part of the body-mind unit, let's look at how the mind and emotions influence immunity and what we can do to improve the integration of body and mind and reduce the effects of stress.

Caution: When you have a viral illness, avoid taking multivitamin and mineral preparations that contain iron. Do not take a separate iron supplement unless recommended by a doctor knowledgeable in the treatment of viral diseases. During infection, the body withholds iron from the tissues because pathogenic microorganisms use iron to promote their spread. Sources of supplemental iron include: ferrous sulfate, ferrous gluconate, ferrous asparatate, ferrous fumarate, and others.

Bringing the Mind into the Immune Picture

The mind is an important part in healing and plays a significant role in immunity. The mind can be your best friend or worst enemy. It can distract you from following your purpose in life, lead you astray once you have become successful, and figure out where the closest convenience store is to buy cigarettes even when you have vowed to stop smoking. On the other hand, it can help you organize your life to work towards better health, help you find the right information to improve your understanding of health, and provide you with discrimination when the three doctors that you consult each have different opinions. For a cure to take place, your mind must become an ally in the healing process.

We have seen how stress can make you sick and how the body affects the immune system. Now we will discover how the mind communicates with the immune system.

How the Mind Talks to the Immune System: Actually, the communication is more of a dialogue between the nervous system (the brain), the endocrine system (the adrenal and other glands), chemical mediators (cytokines, chemokines, and neurotransmitters like serotonin), and cells of the immune system.

Stress, physical trauma, and infection activate a coordinated response between the innate immune system and the endocrine system. Chemicals released by these two systems activate the brain to send signals back to the immune system. The chemical messengers between the brain and immune system include cortisol (an adrenal hormone), and a variety of cytokines, primarily interleukin-1, interleukin-6, and tumor necrosis factor. In addition, nerve impulses between the brain and immune organs, like the spleen and the lymph nodes, signal changes in the activity and production of immune cells.

In chronic viral infection, a continuous exchange between these different systems occurs, resulting in an accumulation of cytokines and an imbalance of adrenal and other hormones. Normally, regulating mechanisms of the immune system prevent uncontrolled or continuous activation of these immune chemicals. However, when a breakdown of the normal communication between these systems takes place, changes in behavior occur, including fatigue, the feeling of sleepiness, loss of appetite, reduced interest in sex, and muscle and joint pain.

These are the same symptoms I described in chapter 5 about chronic fatigue and chronic inflammation. So you can see that a strong immune system depends on effective normal communications between the mind and the immune system, and integration of the body and mind. Otherwise, what we know as sickness behavior develops.

Most patients with the new disease (CFIDS, fibromyalgia, and irritable bowel syndrome) display this type of behavior. Often, patients may have a milder form of one of these conditions but still also have many of the symptoms of a dysfunctional nervous system and immune system. Doctors often refer to these patients as the "walking unwell" to describe a person who is functioning on a daily basis, but who feels sick most of the time. In the past, these people were called hypochondriacs. We now know that sickness behavior is triggered by both emotional and chemical changes in the body.

Unfortunately, if this type of patient does not get the medical care that addresses the cause of the problem rather than only its symptoms, she could eventually develop a combination of fatigue and chronic inflammation syndromes (like irritable bowel syndrome with fibromyalgia), or multiple sclerosis.

The proof that communication occurs between the mind and the immune system comes from the field of psychoneuroimmunology (PNI).

Hans Selye, M.D., a Canadian researcher, was the first Western scientist to take stress seriously. When he published the results of his work in the journal *Nature* in 1935, he was immediately criticized by his colleagues for suggesting that emotional stress affected the body's physiology. It was not until 1956, when he published *The Stress of Life* for the general public, that his ideas were accepted. Since then, thousands of research papers have been published on the effects of stress on the immune system.

PNI researchers have found that stress causes alterations in the way the secondary lymphoid tissues (spleen, lymph nodes, and mucosal tissue) function. It is thought that stress induces activity in the brain, which causes imbalances between the endocrine system and the lymphoid tissue, resulting in abnormal amounts and activity of the immune cells.

Within the brain, the hypothalamus is directly affected by stress. The hypothalamus is a small gland (situated in the center of the brain and above the brain stem) that is responsible for regulating blood pressure, body temperature, fluid balance, body weight, and many other functions directly related to homeostasis. Activation of the hypothalamus activates the autonomic nervous system, the same system we saw that was influenced by exercise and rest, and plays a role in immunity.

Mood and Emotion—Another Key Immune Factor: The ability to feel deeply and powerfully makes us human, and compassion and the ability to express impersonal love make us more than human—saintly. Albert Schweitzer and Mother Theresa were such people. A study with medical students at Harvard found that immunity was improved simply by watching a video of Mother Theresa. On the other hand, unbalanced emotions, lack of purpose, depression, apathy, harboring anger or guilt or shame, are negative emotions that destroy the immune system. Positive feelings and the belief in a higher power that knows what it is doing enhance our immunity.

Norman Cousins became famous for the "laughing cure." Humor—not taking life or yourself too seriously—is very important in being able to enjoy life and let the small things roll off your back. Some people think the worst is happening even when their health condition is mild or easily curable. Fear takes over and makes them expect the worst, causing their emotions to spiral downward in anticipation of catastrophe. A black cloud hangs over their heads and follows them wherever they go. These patients need constant reassurance that the worst is not going to happen and that they have the ability to recover and lead normal lives.

In the early years of my practice, I treated a young, up-and-coming Broadway actress named Ellen who suffered from repeated respiratory viral infections. She was deathly afraid of ruining her career from her constant illnesses. She had one cold after another, with an average of two a month, and she had frequent bouts of sinusitis and bronchitis.

When I first saw Ellen, she burst into tears in my office, emotionally overwhelmed by each illness episode and afraid of the next. I smiled and said, "You realize that these are only mild viral infections, symptoms of a poorly functioning immune system, and not serious illness. With some education about how your body works and some immune-enhancing nutrition you are going to be fine."

She was incredulous for a moment. Then, Ellen started to present me with one reason after the other why she was always sick. I listened attentively but then politely told her that everything she described might be emotionally real, but she was concentrating all of her energy on the problem and not on a solution. She described in detail all of her medications, including the repeated courses of antibiotics, and all the doctors she had seen.

Again, I listened carefully, and then asked her if her mother was overly protective and if she catastrophized every minor illness into a medical emergency when Ellen was a child. Her eyes widened and she told me that her mother was exactly that way, that when she was a little girl, her mother turned every childhood sniffle into a potentially life-threatening situation. Within a few minutes, we had gotten to the root of her problem, cleared her mind of irrational memories, established a new positive emotional base, and started her on a regime of immune-enhancing natural medications.

I saw Ellen a few more times before she returned to New York. She had no more colds or flu. Several months later she called me and thanked me for restoring her health and her faith in the ability to be well. In Ellen's case, the immune-enhancing supplements helped to restore her natural immunity, but reducing stress and helping her restructure conditioned thinking and emotional patterns allowed her immune system to maintain a healthy status.

Physical diseases have specific symptoms and are easy to locate. We can point to the place where an injury occurred and see swelling and bruising, or we can say arthritis produces pain, swelling, and an enlarged joint. It is much more difficult to point to a specific symptom of immune dysfunction or to say that emotional stress is the cause. However, researchers are finding underlying connections between the body, mind, and immune system. Many anti-stress hormones, like DHEA and prolactin, and neurotransmitters like gamma-aminobutyric acid (GABA) and serotonin, enhance mood and improve immune function. For example, prolactin, the hormone that controls the secretion of milk production in the breast, produces a peaceful state of mind in nursing mothers. DHEA, an adrenal hormone, protects the hypothalamus from the negative effects of stress and elevates mood.

Though PNI is a relatively new field of scientific investigation, in Chinese medicine, emotional states have long been considered one of the three main causes of illness, the others being environmental factors and accidents. According to Chinese medical theory, harmonious emotional states promote health, strengthen immunity, and prevent disease, while imbalanced and excessive emotional states promote disease.

In our world today we have less positive human contact than our forebears, though even something as simple as human touch can improve our mood and immune system. No wonder therapeutic massage and healing touch have become so popular. One study with nurses showed that therapeutic touch of the style first developed by Dolores Krieger, R.N. (1979), improves T-lymphocyte function (Olson 1997).

In Chinese medicine, emotional states have long been considered one of the three main causes of illness. According to Chinese medical theory, harmonious emotional states promote health, strengthen immunity, and prevent disease, while imbalanced and excessive emotional states promote disease.

Having something to do, having a circle of supportive friends and family, or helping in the community takes our attention away from ourselves, improves mood, gives a sense of belonging, and improves immune function. A 1997 study in the *Journal of the American Medical Association* showed that social ties reduce the susceptibility to the common cold (Cohen 1997).

We have seen how stress weakens immunity and how the mind and immune system talk to each other. Now we will look at some ways to help the body-mind connection function better. According to Leo Galland, M.D., "cognitive restructuring" is the psychological strategy used to gain perspective on our lives and the disease that has become a part of that life (Galland 1997). Cognitive changes begin with clearing unnecessary mental debris from the mind, keeping a firm faith in the healing potential, and having the willpower to do what is necessary to get well.

Right Thinking Fosters Healing: Willpower, a positive mental outlook, and mind control are essential in creating and maintaining a healthy lifestyle and in recovering from disease. Anxious behavior, negative thinking, and making wrong choices about your health based on culturally accepted but incorrect ideas destroy health and contribute to immune dysfunction. Irrational ways of thinking, fostered by wrong ideas about the limitations of medicine and how the body heals, can create monumental detours on your road to health.

In my clinical practice, most of my patients have chronic diseases and infections that have been difficult to diagnose by conventional methods, that were poorly treated with drugs, or that have already failed to respond to drug therapies. Sadly, many of these patients still believe in the magic bullet theory of medicine. They assume someone or some pill will miraculously cure their ailment, and they expect natural therapies to do the same job that the conventional model could not do, but even better, faster, less painfully, and cheaper. They put enormous, unrealistic expectations on themselves and their doctors. These patients need help in gaining a better understanding of their conditions.

To do this, I first assist them in accepting the diagnosis and then getting down to business of getting better, which often starts with cognitive restructuring.

For viral illnesses, sorting fact from fiction may be what separates you from wellness or disease. Here are a few of the medical myths that I have found to be the greatest obstacles in healing:

- *Killing all the germs is the only way to get well.* In the case of viruses, not only is that usually impossible, but to emphasize complete sterilization of microorganisms in the body causes other imbalances in the immune system, often resulting in a worse condition than the one you began with. Since viruses are part of our own cellular material, we can never completely destroy them without eliminating ourselves in the process. To heal, emphasis should be placed more on immune enhancement and less on killing germs. We have lived with viruses in our bodies for a long time and can relearn to live with them again.

- *Healing requires sophisticated modern technology.* The fact is that healing is not a complicated process requiring highly specialized health professionals who charge exorbitant amounts of money and provide sophisticated technological services. Many people believe that they can only get better with expensive technological treatments. In fact, the opposite often happens. Patients get worse from these forms of medical care. Natural remedies can cure. You have the healing power already within you.

- *Only drugs can cure.* Drugs are not the answer to every ailment. In fact, they often do not work in the manner for which they are designed and often cause serious side effects. They are not all-powerful, and do not provide any advantage when treating most of the modern diseases, including chronic fatigue. Majid Ali, M.D., succinctly states that "chronic fatigue states cannot be understood through simplistic one disease–one drug thinking" (Ali 1995). Exclusive drug therapy for chronic viruses does not work. Many natural therapies are very effective for viruses, especially when they are combined in a comprehensive program like this book's 10-step viral immunity plan.

- *Seeing doctors is the only way to get better.* Medical treatments, including alternative therapies, are endless. You can go from doctor to doctor, as many patients do, receiving every kind of treatment imaginable. There are times when you may need a doctor's services to assist you in healing, but healing is a process that begins and ends within your own body.

Noncognitive Ways of Improving the Body-Mind Connection: Many noncognitive methods activate the mind and improve the immune response. We have already seen how physical exercise and the relaxation response improve immunity. Now let's look at some less orthodox ways to enhance the immune system, such as healing rituals, prayer, mantras, and meditation.

Humans have used healing rituals since prehistoric times, so a positive response to rituals is embedded in our consciousness. Even today we continue to use rituals in political and military ceremonies, every Sunday when we go to church, and even in the doctor's office. The white coat worn by most physicians is more of a ritual garment than a necessity, establishing the wearer as a high priest of healing, as one separate and different from the patient who does not own such a vestment. However, in modern times this ritual often has the opposite effect.

In the so-called "white coat syndrome," patients feel worse when they go to the doctor. Their blood pressure goes up; they become anxious and scared, anticipating the diagnosis or the toxic drug the doctor might prescribe. They may even feel humiliated or outraged at the impersonal and arrogant manner of many doctors. None of this helps immune function at all. Wiser doctors have realized this effect and no longer wear the white coat in their offices. In our emotionally stressed and fragmented society, we need more positive healing rituals that take us out of our everyday mindset and allow us to heal.

Another noncognitive way to enhance immunity is through prayer. Prayer is nothing new to the West. In the East, prayer is also used, but in the form of a mantra, or the repetition of one of the holy names of God, such as Rama or Krishna in Hinduism, or the *Om Mani Padme Om* chant of Buddhism. After decades of medical dogma that severed the mind from the body and the spirit from medical practice, prayer has recently become more available to patients.

Larry Dossey, M.D., the founder of the journal *Alternative Therapies in Health and Disease* and the author of several books, is one of the strongest supporters of prayer as an integral part of healing (Dossey 1997). Dr. Dossey and other prominent medical figures, such as Roger Sperry, Ph.D., who won the Nobel prize in medicine in 1981, believe that mind and spirit must be returned to their rightful place at the top of the hierarchy of human endeavors, including medicine, and that prayer must be a part of the paradigm of mind-body therapies. Only in that way can healing be reintegrated into the practice of medicine.

Research has shown that intercessory prayer, done for you by another, influences the outcome of disease. In a 1988 study, under the direction of Randolph Byrd, M.D., 400 heart patients participated in a double-blind randomized controlled study in the Coronary Care Unit at San Francisco General Hospital in San Francisco, California. The patients who received prayer experienced better health and required less use of antibiotics (Byrd 1998). Another study reviewed twenty-three trials involving nearly 3,000 patients on distant healing as medical treatment and concluded that prayer helped in 57 percent of the cases (Austin 2000).

More research is required to scientifically prove the power of prayer in healing, but its potential immune benefits and long history among the world's religions recommend it. If you have an affinity to prayer, develop the habit of praying according to your chosen religious system or style. If you are more attuned to Eastern methods, practice a mantra. You may also intuitively find ways to enter into a dialogue with your soul, the universal spirit, or God in a way that suits your needs and personality. Regardless of what way you choose, allow time to regularly connect with spirit.

The Immune-Enhancing Lifestyle

A well-balanced and regulated lifestyle promotes health and longevity, enhancing the immune system in the process. Yoga teaches it, tai chi and qi gong masters are examples of it in practice, and science is now getting around to confirming it. Radically restructuring the lifestyle is nearly impossible for the average American; however, even small changes will produce great benefits.

Will these changes make you immune to infections and "bullet-proof" to disease? Not completely. Life's design is an evolving matrix of constant change, and we still live in bodies that are vulnerable to unpredictable biological events; therefore, even the healthiest get sick from time to time. But you can increase the odds of being well and reduce your risks of illness by following the principles outlined in this chapter.

Keep in mind that results are achieved by a synthesis of all aspects, rather than through one isolated aspect, and remember that a health-oriented lifestyle is the beginning of a strong immune system.

Conditioning the Immune System: Just as stress reduction is a part of the body-mind paradigm and can be pivotal in enhancing the immune system, the body and the immune system also need challenges to thrive and evolve. Evolutionary immunologists have found that the immune system functions best when exposed to small amounts of infectious agents during childhood when adaptive immunity is forming. If you are never exposed to antigens, your immune system does not develop and you are more vulnerable to viruses, cancer formation, and allergic diseases like asthma.

The immune-enhancing lifestyle conditions the immune system, just as regular exercise conditions the muscles, making it stronger and more responsive. It is the foundation for all of the viral immunity treatments discussed in this book. For people who are already healthy, the immune-enhancing lifestyle may be enough. However, for those with weakened immunity or who already have a viral condition, it is just the beginning. In the next chapters, we will discuss the most important methods of conditioning and strengthening the immune system.

CHAPTER SUMMARY

Exercise is a natural immunomodulating activity, essential to the viral immunity program. Exercise regularly and, if you can find a qualified teacher, practice yoga or tai chi.

Do not over-exercise; physical stress is just as devastating to the immune system as psychological stress.

Get adequate rest between work, activity, and exercise.

Get at least 9–10 hours of sleep each night if you have a viral illness.

Drink eight glasses of pure water daily, in addition to other fluids in teas, soups, or juices. After strenuous physical exercise, drink one glass for each additional hour of activity.

Practice relaxed deep breathing, outdoors if possible, and get at least 2–4 hours of daylight exposure every day.

Eat a healthy and nutritious diet that is right for your constitution, age, and level of activity. Do not take diets to extremes.

Take a multivitamin and mineral supplement daily with meals. In addition, take extra vitamin C, E, and other antioxidants like zinc and selenium.

Maintain a positive attitude and have faith in the healing powers of your body and mind.

Practice a healing ritual or prayer to restore your peace of mind and improve your immune system.

Balance your emotions by practicing meditation and stress-reducing techniques, listening to music, taking walks in nature, and seeking the company of supportive friends.

7

STEP TWO

Defend and Strengthen Your Immune System with Antioxidants and Oxidative Therapies

In the previous chapter, I discussed how diet and the habits of daily living influence immunity. Once an immune-enhancing lifestyle is in place as a foundation, you can begin to build upon it. In this second step, you start the process of strengthening your immunity by reducing oxidative stress to the immune cells with antioxidants and by incorporating bio-oxidative therapies into your viral immunity plan.

Oxidative stress, also referred to as free radical damage, is the product of the natural process of using oxygen for metabolism. Antioxidants, substances that neutralize oxidative stress, are necessary to defend your body against cellular damage and to strengthen the immune system. In our highly polluted world, we can easily become oxygen-deficient, and in some cases of viral illness, improving oxygen utilization or even adding oxygen by using oxidative therapies such as ozone, can help your immune system defend the body against viruses.

In this chapter, I explain how oxygen, one of the fundamental elements for life, helps and hinders natural immunity. I show how antioxidant adaptation (the way cells cope with the consequences of oxygen metabolism) is one of the most important biochemical components in the treatment of chronic and degenerative diseases, aging, and viral illnesses.

You can improve your oxidative adaptation by adding antioxidants to your nutritional supplement plan. Additionally, you can complement your dietary protein intake with a full-spectrum amino acid supplement along with specific single amino acids with antioxidant activity. This is recommended for immune enhancement and viral protection. Further recommendations include the use of second-generation antioxidants, specialized powerful nutritional substances, and glutathione, crucial to health and immunity.

Oxygen: Nature's Great Paradox

Oxygen is the most important element on Earth, required for life by all higher organisms. Paradoxically, even though we cannot live without oxygen, the same cellular processes that utilize oxygen produce destructive byproducts. Let's look at why oxygen is so necessary, how it is utilized, the problems that arise when our cells metabolize oxygen, and what happens when we are oxygen deficient.

Biologists divide living organisms into two basic groups depending on how they utilize sunlight and air: aerobic, or oxygen-using organisms, and anaerobic, those that can live in low-oxygen or oxygen-free environments. Anaerobic organisms are primarily microbes that include pathogens such as viruses, while among the aerobic types are animals, plants, and humans.

The air we breathe is composed of mostly nitrogen, hydrogen, and oxygen. The human body contains these same elements plus carbon, and these four primary elements make up about 95 percent of our bodies' mass; trace elements make up the remainder. Oxygen, the most abundant element on this planet, composes 50 percent by weight of the Earth's crust; it's found in water as H_2O (hydrogen plus oxygen), and in the atmosphere, of which 20 percent is oxygen. It is also the most abundant element in the human body: We breathe in an average of 150 cubic feet of pure oxygen each day.

Oxygen supports all the biochemical activity in our organs, tissues, and cells. It is the primary fuel that makes energy to support life. Scientists who study oxygen report that by measuring air samples and oxygen levels from bubbles trapped in amber and polar ice, they have determined that two million years ago the oxygen content of Earth's atmosphere was between 35 and 44 percent. Today's oxygen air content is now about 20 percent, and in cities with excessive pollution, the oxygen content can be as low as 9 percent.

It may be that one of the causes of immune dysfunction is both antioxidant maladaptation and decreased oxygen intake. Also, if we breathe rapidly and shallowly due to stress, as is very common with urban dwellers, we take in less oxygen and retain more carbon dioxide. Not only does this type of respiration reduce our oxygen levels, but it causes acid buildup in the blood, further predisposing us to illness and increasing our susceptibility to viral infection.

The process of converting air to energy is nothing short of miraculous, but at the same time, it is very simple. We take in oxygen through our lungs when we breathe; then the oxygen and other elements are separated out, the oxygen is retained, carbon dioxide and other wastes are exhaled. Oxygen is then mixed into the blood and pumped throughout the body by the heart. The oxygen-enriched blood is carried in the hemoglobin, an iron-containing molecule within individual red blood cells, to every cell in the body. A fully oxygenated system is required for health and natural immunity; poor oxygen intake or improper utilization of oxygen can lead to brain fog, fatigue, and increased susceptibility to infections and degenerative chronic conditions like heart disease.

Smoking, exposure to indoor and outdoor air pollution, poor diet, inadequate water intake, anemia, allergy and respiratory infections, and lack of fitness all reduce oxygen levels in our bodies. On the other hand, general fitness and regular aerobic exercise—walking, running, jumping rope, chopping wood, bicycling, or swimming—all promote and improve respiration and better oxygenation. Breathing exercises like *pranayama* or *qi gong* (mentioned earlier) are excellent for getting more oxygen to the tissues and cells without stressing the body. However, during aggressive exercise, although more oxygen is utilized, it can increase oxidative stress and cellular damage, making one more vulnerable to viral infections.

As mentioned earlier, most pathogens (including viruses and bacteria) are anaerobic—they do not require oxygen to live and reproduce. They also do not have strong natural protective defenses against oxygen-containing molecules such as superoxides and peroxides (like hydrogen peroxide, discussed below). Therefore, viruses and other anaerobic microorganisms cannot survive in richly oxygenated tissues; this means the greater the oxygen level in our bodies, the more resistant our cells are to invasion and infection by viruses and bacteria. Here again we see the oxygen paradox: more oxygen helps protect us *and* it also produces increased oxidative stress.

We should never minimize the importance of air quality, oxygen content, and proper breathing. If air pollution is high, oxygen content will be low, and in addition, you will take all the toxic chemicals in the polluted air into your body through the natural process of respiration. These chemicals contribute to immune dysfunction and increase your risk for cancer and other degenerative diseases.

> *Viruses and other anaerobic microorganisms cannot survive in richly oxygenated tissues; this means the greater the oxygen level in our bodies, the more resistant our cells are to invasion and infection by viruses and bacteria. We should never minimize the importance of air quality, oxygen content, and proper breathing.*

Low oxygen levels cause fatigue, increased susceptibility to infection, and metabolic imbalances that can lead to low thyroid function and other conditions. Among other things, that is why it is so important to practice deep-breathing exercises (as discussed in chapter 6). Keep in mind that deeply inhaling polluted air only increases the concentration of toxic chemicals in your body, so practice deep breathing in as pure an environment as possible.

The Chinese say that the best time to practice is in the very early morning hours between five and seven when the air pollution is lower and the oxygen content is higher after a night of photosynthesis by local plants. You can also temporarily increase the oxygen content in your body through specialized treatments that supply oxygenated substances, which we'll consider next.

Increase Your Oxygen Levels through Bio-Oxidative Therapies

Bio-oxidative therapies involve oxygenating substances, such as hydrogen peroxide, dioxychlor, and ozone, that increase the oxygen levels in the body. These are used to treat diseases including cancer, heart disease, and active chronic viral infections like hepatitis. A physician trained in bio-oxidative medicine administers ozone therapy and intravenous hydrogen peroxide. Oral methods of enhancing oxygen are also available, and include taking hydrogen peroxide and dioxy-chlor, both of which have been shown to neutralize viruses. Hyperbaric oxygen is another form of oxygen therapy in which pure oxygen is administered to the patient who lies in a pressurized chamber. Hyperbaric oxygen is used to improve wound healing from crush injuries, burns, and radiation injuries. It reduces swelling and edema and is being researched for use in heart disease, after stroke, chronic fatigue, and multiple sclerosis.

Let's look at three bio-oxidative therapies useful in the treatment of chronic viral infections.

Ozone: Ozone (O_3) may be thought of as an energized form of simple oxygen, O_2. It is a pale blue gas that naturally occurs in the Earth's atmosphere, formed when oxygen interacts with ultraviolet radiation from the sun. It is produced commercially for industrial and medical purposes. Before the antibiotic era, ozone was used to treat a variety of infections including wounds: it was a disinfectant in dentistry and used to treat colitis through rectal insufflation. In 1945, the German surgeon, Erwin Payr, M.D., was among the first to use ozone intravenously to treat disease.

Ozone therapy has developed considerably since then and it is now used to treat a wide variety of conditions including viruses such as hepatitis and herpes. Ozone therapy is administered by removing 50 to 100 milliliters of the patient's blood, enriching it with ozone, and then reinfusing it intravenously. Some doctors also irradiate the blood with ultraviolet light before reinfusing it into the patients.

Besides medical ozone therapies, there are other ways to enhance the levels of ozone in your body. Ozone generators increase the ozone content of the air in a room. Treating water with ozone causes the oxidization of a wide range of chemicals and also kills bacteria, fungi, parasites, and viruses. Though ozone generators help purify air and ozonated water is a proven disinfectant, both of which improve general health, they do not directly affect viruses in your body.

Because of its antimicrobial effects and oxidative properties, ozone therapy is useful for viral immunity. If you have a chronic viral disease, consider medical ozone therapy to reduce the viral burden in the tissues. Keep in mind that intravenous ozone is not an approved therapy for chronic viral disease and though it may be helpful, it does not completely eradicate all viruses in your body. Only use a physician certified in the use of medical ozone therapies.

Hydrogen Peroxide: Hydrogen peroxide (H_2O_2) production is a naturally occurring process in the body. Cells of the innate immune system produce hydrogen peroxide in response to microbial infection; it is also involved in other cellular processes including hormone regulation and the metabolism of protein, carbohydrates, fats, vitamins, and minerals.

H_2O_2 is a clear, colorless liquid that mixes readily with water and is widely used as a topical disinfectant in a 3 percent solution commonly sold in pharmacies and grocery stores. A 30 percent reagent grade is diluted in sterile distilled water and used in bio-oxidative medicine. Though this form of hydrogen peroxide can be helpful in chronic viral diseases, it can cause serious burns to the skin and inside the blood vessels and must be administered with the utmost caution.

Oral ingestion of 35 percent "food grade" hydrogen peroxide is recommended by some doctors when intravenous therapy is unavailable. A few drops of the solution are added to water and consumed on an empty stomach three times daily. It is important to avoid eating food or taking vitamins and minerals at the same time because the hydrogen peroxide can cause rapid oxidation of these substances resulting in stomach irritation. However, I do not recommend either intravenous or oral hydrogen peroxide to my patients since it is such a highly caustic substance, and if handled improperly can cause permanent tissue damage.

A safer method is the use of hydrogen peroxide as a detoxifying bath. Add one pint of 35 percent food-grade hydrogen peroxide to a full bathtub of warm water. If you have sensitive skin begin by adding a quarter of a cup of hydrogen peroxide and gradually increase the amount each day until you achieve at least one cup per bathtub. Soak for at least 20 to 30 minutes. Although this way of using hydrogen peroxide does not get it directly into the body, it assists in detoxifying the skin, thereby improving health.

Dioxychlor: Dioxychlor is an oral product developed by Professor Robert W. Bradford of American Biologics and Medical Center, and used extensively in his clinic in Tijuana, Mexico. It is composed of chlorine and two atoms of oxygen, prepared in a homeopathic form called Dioxychlor D3 for oral use by patients. According to Dr. Bradford, who reports having used it extensively with patients over the last decade, Dioxychlor is safe and effective for adjunctive treatment of fungal infections and viruses.

Table 8: Bio-oxidative Therapies for Viral Immunity

In my clinical experience, the following therapies are most useful in treating viral diseases.

Therapy	How Administered	Route of Entry	Physician Required
Ozone	Intravenous	Blood	Yes
Hydrogen Peroxide	Detoxifying Bath	Skin	No
Dioxychlor	Oral	Gastrointestinal	No

The Health Consequences of Oxidative Stress

Oxygen is important to life and essential to good health, yet living in an oxygen-rich environment generates negative consequences. This is referred to as the oxygen paradox. As mentioned earlier, oxygenation is the process of introducing oxygen to a system. By breathing (respiration), we inhale oxygen-containing air and thereby oxygenate our tissues and individual cells, which need oxygen for their metabolism. Oxidation, the energy-releasing process in which oxygen combines with other chemicals, is a result of oxygen metabolism. Oxidation removes an electron, resulting in a release of stored chemical energy.

Normal oxidation happens within the body and in all natural things. You can see it in the rusting of iron or the browning of an apple when cut in half and left uneaten on the table. Oxygen fuels combustion; without O_2, fires don't burn at all, and in a similar manner it stimulates cellular metabolism. Unless tissue levels of oxygen remain within appropriate ranges, excess spontaneous oxygen activity (oxidation) occurs and can lead to cellular and tissue damage, called oxidative stress. This can produce damage to DNA, resulting in increased risk of disease, including cancer, and eventually the complete degeneration of tissue and death of the organism. Oxidative stress is one of the causes of disease and aging, but at the same time it is an essential part of life.

Oxidation is a spontaneous and irreversible chemical process—a match does not un-burn, a brown apple does not become white and crisp again. However, our bodies are neither a match nor an apple, and though some oxidative processes exhaust important chemicals in our bodies, we have the ability to regenerate our cells and tissues by providing nutrients, especially antioxidants.

Free Radicals and Antioxidant Maladaptation: Due to stress, aging, infection, and other factors, chemical bonds become split in such a way that a molecule is left with an unpaired electron, making it very reactive and unstable. This is called a free radical. Free radical molecules react with the first compatible molecule to restore their stability, altering the structure of both in the process. Normally the body has adaptive mechanisms that automatically restore metabolic stability by providing extra molecules to neutralize free radicals. This neutralization process, the adding of electrons by taking one from another molecule, is called reduction, and is the natural opposite pole to oxidation. The entire process is referred to as the oxidation-reduction cycle.

However, a chain reaction can occur when there is an excess of free radicals. As mentioned earlier, free radical accumulation can be caused by exposure to pollution, radiation, smoke, stress, lack of exercise, or repetitively overexercising. The normal reduction process cannot keep pace with the increased level of oxidation, and this imbalance in the oxidation-reduction cycle is referred to as antioxidant maladaptation. Tissue and cellular damage, called free radical pathology, result because antioxidant activity is insufficient.

At this point, even though tissue damage has started, no specific disease may manifest. The person with active free radical pathology may only feel tired or vaguely not well. However, the stage is set for illness as a wide range of diseases are associated with the damage caused by free radical pathology, including cancer, heart disease, allergies, cataracts, macular degeneration, mental impairment and Alzheimer's disease, diabetes, and nearly all of the other chronic degenerative diseases.

Antioxidant maladaptation and free radical pathology can significantly affect the immune system, which can result in increased vulnerability to viral infections. Immune dysfunction from antioxidant maladaptation can occur in many components of the immune system, and include:

- Natural Killer (NK) cell deficiency and reduced functional activity

- Depressed specific immunity with inability of immune cells to respond to an infection

- Reduced numbers and function of other lymphocytes

- Changes in humoral response, including deficiency of IgA and imbalances in other antibodies, such as increased IgE

- Elevated levels of chemokines

- Increased levels of autoimmune antibodies, such as rheumatoic factor (RF) and antinuclear antibodies (ANA), both of which are now often seen elevated in so-called normal patients.

Drugs cannot treat the causes or results of oxidative stress. In fact, many drugs deplete the very substances that repair oxidative damage. Only naturally occurring substances can help the body overcome antioxidant maladaptation, rebuild immunity, and restore health.

The Balancing Role of Antioxidants

Antioxidants are substances that are naturally manufactured in our bodies and provided in the diet that help to neutralize free radical damage. Antioxidants work *against oxidation*. As we age, deal with a chronic disease, live in urban areas high in pollution, or live under psychological stress, free radical damage occurs, and we require more antioxidant protection. In other words, more free radicals get generated than our bodies can normally handle or adapt to. Under normal conditions, antioxidant adaptation naturally occurs within our bodies and includes the activities of enzymes, glutathione, and uric acid. Though these substances are very powerful and essential antioxidants, most must be obtained from food.

Naturally occurring antioxidants are found in brightly colored fruits and vegetables, as well as dark green, leafy vegetables, green tea, and herbs. Though most antioxidants can be obtained from food, in people living under environmental and psychological stress, those with viral infections or cancer, and those eating a poor diet, the need for antioxidants is higher and supplements are required.

The most common nutritional antioxidants include vitamins C, E, B2, B6, B12, carotenoids (beta carotene), the minerals zinc and selenium, and the amino acids arginine, lysine, cysteine, and glutamine. Second-level antioxidants include co-enzyme Q10, lipoic acid, flavonoids, and proanthocyanidins such as are found in grape seeds.

Vitamin C: The foundation of any antioxidant program is vitamin C, the single most important antioxidant. It is useful in preventing premature aging and cell death, and it protects us against cancer and other diseases, including those caused by viruses

Vitamin C, also known as ascorbic acid, is a water-soluble vitamin and is an essential nutrient for normal body function. The nine water-soluble vitamins in our bodies (vitamins B1, B2, B3, B5, B6, B12, biotin folate, and vitamin C) are essential nutrients that readily dissolve in water. They are not stored well in body tissue, so must be continuously supplied through the diet or by supplementation. Most animal species can synthesize vitamin C from glucose and other sugars, but humans, monkeys, guinea pigs, and a few other animals need to obtain it in their diet. It is required for the synthesis of collagen, a structural, glue-like component of nearly all tissues, especially blood vessels, tendons, ligaments, bone, and the joints. It also has numerous other functions, including an immune-enhancing activity.

Though the exact details of how vitamin C works to enhance immune activity are still unknown, research indicates that it improves the activity of disease-fighting white blood cells; increases interferon levels; modifies antibody responses; increases IgA, IgG, and IgG antibody levels; and supports thymus gland function. In one study, buffered vitamin C was found to raise NK cell function tenfold in 78 percent of patients.

Vitamin C is found in nearly all foods, but is highest in fruits and vegetables. Some tropical sources, like camu camu *(Myrciaria dubia),* an Amazonian fruit containing thirty times more vitamin C than citrus, make excellent supplemental sources. Broccoli, Brussels sprouts, cabbage, sweet red peppers, parsley, currants, acerola berries, rose hips, all citrus fruits, strawberries, and even potatoes are good sources of vitamin C. However, the amounts of vitamin C in these foods are not sufficient to treat diseases other than scurvy, the classical vitamin C deficiency disease and the cause of many deaths in previous centuries. To maximize the immune system and antioxidant properties of vitamin C, or treat viral illnesses, supplemental dosages of vitamin C are required in addition to dietary sources.

How to Take Vitamin C: Vitamin C is usually taken orally, although it is also used intravenously by physicians for acute and chronic viral infections. It comes in a variety of forms, the least expensive and most widely being pure ascorbic acid crystals; this is a mild acid usually well tolerated by most people taking average dosages of vitamin C. However, when using very large dosages to treat infections, I recommend the buffered form, which is gentler on the stomach and does not over-acidify the system.

To buffer ascorbic acid, sodium, potassium, calcium, magnesium, or combinations of these minerals are combined with ascorbic acid. Avoid the sodium form of buffered vitamin C as it may contribute to water retention and high blood pressure. When higher dosages are indicated, I recommend powdered calcium-magnesium-potassium ascorbate, which provides about 2,500 mg of vitamin C per rounded teaspoon.

Though two-time Nobel prize winner Linus Pauling popularized high dosages of vitamin C in the early 1970s for everything from the common cold to cancer, it had extensive clinical use as early as the 1950s, notably by Frederick Klenner, M.D. who practiced in North Carolina. He advocated the "100 gram cold": 100 grams (1,000mg = 1 gram) of pure ascorbic acid powder in water taken over a twenty-four-hour period to treat the common cold (Klenner 1971). Though no doctor today would recommend such a high dose to treat a cold, vitamin C is still used for its many benefits in dosages that far exceed the recommended dietary allowance (RDA) of 60 milligrams per day.

Numerous studies done on vitamin C for the common cold have shown that it has limited effect on directly preventing a cold, but that taking vitamin C does reduce the severity and shorten the duration of the cold by about one third. Vitamin C has been used effectively to treat numerous viral illnesses including mononucleosis, chicken pox, hepatitis, herpes simplex and herpes zoster, viral encephalitis, viral pneumonia, and the flu.

It is now accepted that moderate daily dosages of vitamin C in the ranges from 200 mg to 500 mg are sufficient for daily supplementation. However, most naturopathic physicians, as well as medical doctors practicing natural therapies, recommend higher dosages in the range of 500–2,000 mg daily. Since optimal blood levels of vitamin C are reached easily with 200 mg, and amounts over that are excreted in the urine, I recommend taking vitamin C in frequent but lower dosages: 200–500 mg two to four times per day, providing a daily total up to 1,000–2,000 mg.

However, there are times when larger dosages are necessary, such as in the treatment of chronic viruses. In these cases it is usually recommended to take the highest dose that the body will tolerate—called bowel tolerance—over a course of several days or even weeks; this may be as high as 10–30 g per day (1 g = 1,000 mg).

The term "bowel tolerance" was coined by Robert Cathcart, M.D., of Los Altos, California, in 1981 to indicate that when the body has reached a level of tissue saturation, a temporary, acute gastrointestinal intolerance to vitamin C occurs, causing urgent watery diarrhea (Cathcart 1981). Uncomfortable gas and bloating may also occur. Interestingly, though average bowel tolerance is reached in most people between 2,000–5,000 mg, in cases of infection, patients can tolerate 20,000 mg (20 g), or more, of vitamin C taken by mouth over the course of a day without any signs of diarrhea.

Bowel tolerance is still used as a method of monitoring the body's need for vitamin C when using higher dosages. Here's how: take 1,000 mg of vitamin C in divided dosages (the total dose divided into smaller amounts) every one to two hours until diarrhea appears, then reduce by 1,000 mg until it stops. Stay on the tolerated amount (the therapeutic dose) until your condition resolves. Then decrease it slowly to avoid "rebound scurvy," a temporary condition thought to occur when high dosages of vitamin C are abruptly discontinued, and move toward a daily maintenance dose of 500 to 2,000 mg.

VITAMIN C SAFETY AND INTERACTIONS: Though vitamin C is very safe, it has recently been called a "pro-oxidant," which means the opposite of an antioxidant, because it is thought to cause oxidative damage to blood vessels leading to atherosclerosis. Pro-oxidants are substances that accelerate oxidative stress. One of the main pro-oxidants in the body is iron, and some scientists have expressed concern that vitamin C, when taken in high dosages, can increase the pro-oxidative damage caused by iron. Other safety concerns have been raised about taking high doses of vitamin C, and include the possibility of increased risk for calcium oxalate kidney stones, vitamin B-12 depletion leading to pernicious anemia, increased iron absorption, depletion of copper, and increased urinary excretion of uric acid.

None of these concerns have been conclusively proven. However, dialysis patients, those with chronic kidney disease, patients with hemochromatosis (an iron-overload disease), gout, and those with a history of forming kidney stones should avoid taking vitamin C in the higher ranges unless under the direct supervision of a physician. Keep in mind that regardless of the outcome of the above concerns, when taken in high dosages, vitamin C can cause uncomfortable gastrointestinal gas, bloating, and diarrhea.

Several drugs deplete vitamin C levels, including estrogen-containing birth control pills, corticosteroids like prednisone, and frequent use of aspirin. The reverse is less significant; vitamin C has a limited or no effect on any drugs. However, those on anticoagulants, like Coumadin (warfarin sodium), should limit their use of vitamin C, as high dosages may interfere with the blood thinning activity of these drugs.

VITAMIN C SUMMARY: Vitamin C is essential in any supplement plan, and for general health, taking 75–200 mg in a daily multivitamin is adequate to prevent heart disease and achieve basic benefits. The Linus Pauling Institute at Oregon State University in Cornelius, Oregon, recommends 120 mg daily, double the RDA but lower than therapeutic levels. For optimum risk reduction of heart disease, stroke, and cancer, certain people may require substantially larger amounts of vitamin C for optimal physical health and to achieve therapeutic benefits.

To obtain maximum antioxidant benefits, most doctors practicing natural medicine recommend daily dosages in the range of 500–2,000 mg. When taking vitamin C in dosages above 500 mg, take it in *divided* dosages spread out throughout the day. For the treatment of viral illness, very high dosages are required, taken orally (6,000–30,000 mg) to bowel tolerance or used intravenously (30,000 mg or higher) in a physician's office. Though some studies indicate toxicity in high dosages, none of these adverse reactions have been confirmed in the laboratory or in human subjects. Indeed, many thousands of people take very high dosages of vitamin C daily without any ill effects.

Vitamin E: The second most important antioxidant is vitamin E. It is the premier fat-soluble antioxidant (as vitamin C is the most important water-soluble antioxidant). Fat-soluble vitamins (vitamins E, D, A, and K) dissolve in the presence of fats and oils, and are stored in the body's fatty tissues and the liver. Vitamin E is not a single substance, but a group of compounds called tocopherols and tocotrienols.

Alpha-tocopherol is the most abundant and most biologically active form. Vitamins C and E work synergistically in the body, such that vitamin E partners with vitamin C, helping to reduce any pro-oxidant effects of vitamin C, while vitamin C assists in regenerating used (oxidized) vitamin E, thus increasing the antioxidant effects of vitamin E.[1] It also works synergistically with selenium and vitamin A.

Though vitamin E does not have specific effects on the immune system, it is so highly protective against oxidative damage that it is important to an immune-enhancing program. It protects the thymus gland and white blood cells from chronic viral disease, such as in AIDS or chronic HCV, during times of tissue stress. Vitamin E slows down the aging process, protects against cancer, improves circulation, speeds wound healing, and reduces inflammation caused by prostaglandin activity (body chemicals involved in inflammation). All of these properties indirectly bolster immune function. Vitamin E is particularly helpful in the elderly and is so important an antioxidant that all multivitamin supplements contain it.

How to Take Vitamin E: Food sources include polyunsaturated vegetable oils (like canola and safflower oil), seeds, nuts, whole grains, wheat germ oil, and soybeans. Leafy greens, like spinach, also contain small amounts of vitamin E. Like vitamin C, sufficient amounts of vitamin E can be obtained from dietary sources for general health, but for optimal health and disease-prevention benefits, supplemental vitamin E is required.

Vitamin E comes in many forms but is available in two basic forms: the synthetic alpha-tocopherol acetate and the all-natural d-alpha-tocopherol, which can be found with other naturally occurring tocopherols such as gamma- and delta-tocopherols. The natural forms are considered more absorbable, so I recommend all-natural, fat-soluble vitamin E succinate (a weak acid used in cellular metabolism) containing mixed tocopherols. It is best taken with a meal or with some oily food, like avocado or nuts, to assist absorption. Water-soluble forms of vitamin E are also available, and though more expensive than fat-soluble forms, they may be useful in patients who have poor absorption of fats and oils.

Though the RDA is less than 30 IU, the generally recommended foundational dose is 200–500 IU. Occasionally up to 800–1,600 IU is required for heart disease patients, or for post-mastectomy patients and those with fibrocystic breast disease. However, when taking vitamin E to bolster immune function, such high dosages are not necessary. In my practice, I generally recommend dosages between 400–800 IU.

Safety and Interactions: Vitamin E is well tolerated and is safe even in the higher ranges, though some people have reported headaches and nausea when taking over 1,000 IU at one time. Since vitamin E can affect blood clotting, patients on blood thinners, like Coumadin or even aspirin, should take only the lower dosages unless under the supervision of a physician. In these cases, vitamin E may interfere with platelet aggregation (clumping of the blood-clotting cells), causing an increased bleeding tendency. Cholesterol-lowering drugs like cholestryramine resin (Prevalite and Questran) and colestipol (Colestid) can deplete vitamin E in the body.

Vitamin A and the Carotenoid Family: Though not classified as an antioxidant, vitamin A deserves mention in this section because it is a fat-soluble substance essential for proper immune function. Vitamin A maintains healthy epithelial tissue, such as the skin and the outer lining and mucous membranes of the respiratory tract. Since these tissues serve as the first line of nonspecific, defense-inhibiting viral organisms to lodge on the surface of your lungs, throat, and nasal passages, it is important to keep them strong and vital. By maintaining healthy epithelia, vitamin A helps in creating a strong barrier against infection.

Vitamin A also improves white blood cell function and increases antibody responses to infections. For viral infections, this vitamin is one of the most important nutritional factors, and it is well known that a vitamin A deficiency contributes to increased susceptibility to infection.

Vitamin A also improves white blood cell function and increases antibody responses to infections. For viral infections, this vitamin is one of the most important nutritional factors, and it is well known that a vitamin A deficiency contributes to increased susceptibility to infection. A number of studies have shown that vitamin A supplementation reduces morbidity (the relative incidence of disease) and death from measles; it has also been used to reduce morbidity in AIDS patients.

Vitamin A is taken orally in a preventive range of 5,000–25,000 IU, and clinically is used as high as 150,000 IU or more for short-term therapeutic purposes under the supervision of a physician. For proper absorption, vitamin A requires fat and minerals and is synergistic with vitamin E, vitamin C, lipoic acid, zinc, and all of the carotenoids. Therefore, it is best taken with food and a multivitamin and mineral supplement.

Vitamin A belongs to a class of substances called retinoids, which are found only in animal products. Dietary sources of vitamin A include animal liver, butter, milk, egg yolks, salmon, shellfish, and fish liver oils. Vitamin A precursors are found in chili peppers and carotene-containing fruits and vegetables. Commercially, it is obtained from fish liver oil and is available in inexpensive softgel capsules.

Since vitamin A is stored in the liver, high therapeutic dosages, if taken over a period of several months, can cause liver damage in humans. For this reason, the more expensive water-soluble, or mycelized form—which is less hard on the liver since it absorbs more readily into the bloodstream and bypasses the liver—is recommended in viral hepatitis or any condition where liver damage is present, such as cirrhosis. Since safety can be an issue when using vitamin A, it is contraindicated in pregnancy, during nursing, or for women attempting pregnancy. Children are particularly susceptible to vitamin A toxicity, so all bottles should be keep out of their reach.

In adults, large dosages in the range of 50,000 IU or higher, if taken for long periods of time (at least several months or longer) can produce symptoms of hypervitaminosis A, which include headache, fatigue, emotional instability, nausea, and muscle and joint pain; followed by dry, cracked skin, brittle nails, hair loss, and irritability. If you are taking vitamin A and are experiencing any of these symptoms, discontinue your intake until all the symptoms clear.

CAROTENOIDS: Vitamin A is a family of nutrients composed of retinal (preformed A) and carotenoid (provitamin A) groups. Carotenoids are called provitamins since they are converted to vitamin A in the body; this takes place by the action of enzymes in the intestinal tract that split the carotene molecule in half. The conversion process to make retinal from carotenoids depends on hormones and other nutrients, such as thyroid hormone, zinc, and vitamin C.

Besides being converted to vitamin A, carotenoids have useful properties of their own. Though they do not have the same antiviral effect as vitamin A, they exert a powerful antioxidant action on cancer activity, are associated with a lower risk of cardiovascular disease, and have immune-enhancing capabilities. One study demonstrated an increase of CD4+ T lymphocytes with supplements of beta-carotene. Numerous studies have shown that beta-carotene reduces oxidative stress in HIV and AIDS, and can assist in endothelial tissue preservation.

Carotenoids are found only in plants, and the intense red, blue, purple, yellow, and orange colors in fruits and vegetables are due to plant pigments that have high carotenoid content. There are over 600 known carotenoids in nature, though only about 30 to 50 have vitamin A activity.

Carotenes, a group of carotenoids, are found in all dark green, leafy vegetables (spinach, collards), yellow- and orange-colored fruits and vegetables (apricots, peaches, carrots, yams, squash), and red fruits and vegetables (strawberries, tomatoes). Beta-carotene is the most abundant of the carotenoids found in human food and is named after the orange color in carrots, a food high in beta-carotene.

HOW TO TAKE CAROTENES: Though a diet rich in vegetables and fruits can supply the basic carotenes, extra supplementation of the full spectrum of carotenoids is often necessary to obtain optimal immune function and antioxidant protection. Carrot juice, vegetable juice made from dark, leafy greens, and many of the "green" health drinks from freshwater or sea algae (spirulina, chlorella) are rich in mixed carotenes. Indeed, they are so rich in carotenes that if carrot juice or mixed green vegetable juice is included in the diet several times per week, additional supplementation of beta-carotene is rarely needed.

Carotenes are available commercially in synthetic or natural forms, but they are best taken in the natural form derived from palm oil or the algae species of the *Dunaliella* genus. Most commercial beta-carotene supplements are the synthetic form, so read labels carefully. The supplemental range is from 25,000 IU up to 300,000 IU (100,000 IU = 60 mg).

CAROTENE SAFETY AND INTERACTIONS: Carotenes are considered very safe but should be used with caution in patients with existing liver damage. When taking high dosages or drinking carrot juice daily, the palms of the hands and soles of the feet can take on a distinctive yellow-orange hue. This condition, called carotenosis or carotemia, is harmless and clears up completely once the supplementation or juice is discontinued. The same cholesterol-lowering drugs that deplete vitamin A can reduce beta-carotene absorption.

OTHER CAROTENOIDS: Besides beta-carotene, other carotenoids are also important in disease prevention. These include alpha-carotene, gamma-carotene, beta-zeacarotene, cryptoxanthine, zeaxanthine, lutein, and lycopene. The red color in tomatoes and watermelon is due to pigmentation from lycopene, which has been shown to reduce the risk of prostate cancer. Lutein, found in cool-weather, green, leafy vegetables like kale, collards, peas, and romaine lettuce, may help to prevent macular degeneration in the eyes.

B-Vitamin Antioxidants: Nearly all members of the B-complex family are water-soluble, including B2, B6, and B12, and are not stored in the body in appreciable amounts, so they must be provided daily in the diet. Vitamins B2, B6, and B12 have important antioxidant activity and are necessary for normal immune function. Since B vitamins are synergistic with each other, it is generally advised to take a B-complex or a multivitamin when using additional B vitamin supplementation.

VITAMIN B2: Vitamin B2, or riboflavin, is a member of a group of fluorescent yellow pigments called flavins. It is the substance that turns the urine bright yellow when you take extra B2. It acts as a coenzyme necessary for normal energy metabolism of carbohydrates, fats, and proteins, and it helps to activate vitamin B6 and convert niacin (B3) into a form more easily utilized by the body.

Among its numerous other functions, vitamin B2 has antioxidant activity and assists the function of vitamin E. Low levels of riboflavin can result in reduced antibody production, leading to reduced immunity. It is found in organ meats, like liver, and in all red meat, eggs, and dairy products. Unless there are specific symptoms of deficiency, dietary sources and a multivitamin provide adequate levels. However, numerous drugs cause depletion of riboflavin, including thorazine, tricyclic antidepressants (Elavil, Tofranil), oral contraceptives, and many antibiotics (minocycline, the penicillins, tetracycline, and sulfonamides).

VITAMIN B6: B6, or pyridoxine, is one of the most important vitamins, functioning in the formation of proteins and as a coenzyme in more than one hundred different metabolic processes in the body. Among its many functions, it has antioxidant capabilities, and, as is the case with riboflavin, a deficiency of pyridoxine can lead to fewer antibodies, a reduction in lymphocytes, and thymus gland atrophy.

It is found in organ meats, red meat, milk, eggs, seafood, whole grains, bananas, avocados, soybeans, nuts, seeds, and brewer's yeast. Additional supplementation of B6 is useful, and is available in two forms: pyridoxine hydrochloride and pyridoxal-5-phosphate, which is the more active form and the form into which the liver converts pyridoxine in the body.

General dosage is between 50–100 mg, with a therapeutic range of up to 500 mg. B6 works synergistically with other B vitamins and magnesium, but it is best absorbed when taken alone, with an additional B-complex or multivitamin taken at a different time. Dosages in excess of 2,000 mg, or long-term use of dosages of 500 mg, can lead to nerve damage, with symptoms of numbness and tingling in the hands and feet and a stumbling gait. Once discontinued, all symptoms clear without any lasting effects. Many of the same drugs that deplete B2 also lower B6 levels: conjugated estrogens (Premarin) and esterified estrogens (Estratab) deplete B6.

VITAMIN B12: Like B6, vitamin B12, or cyanocobalamin, is necessary for the metabolism of proteins, carbohydrates, and fats, and it prevents pernicious anemia, a condition of the red blood cells that occurs most often in the elderly. Vitamin B12 is also necessary for the maturation of the white blood cells. Like B2 and B6, vitamin B12 plays a role in the immune function such that low levels can impair natural immunity. This vitamin may also have activity against viruses; in one laboratory study, B12 inhibited HIV viral replication in human monocytes and lymphocytes (Weinberg 1995).

The best dietary sources are liver, red meat, eggs, dairy products, and seafood, but B12 is available in a wide range of pills, tablets, sublingual and nasal sprays, and can be taken by injection or intravenously. Unless there is medical evidence of severe B12 deficiency or a condition that would benefit from the injectable form, oral administration is effective over time for healthy adults.

There are two coenzyme forms of B12: methylcobalamin and adenosylcobalamin; since methylcobalamin is more efficiently utilized, it is the preferred form for oral supplementation. Coenzymes are nonprotein substances, including many vitamins and minerals, that act as enzymes in the body. A basic oral dosage is between 1,000–2,000 micrograms (mcg) with a therapeutic upper range of 6,000 mcg.

For the elderly and patients with chronic disease or viral illness, most natural-medicine oriented doctors still prefer intramuscular injections or intravenously administered B12 over oral forms. Injections of 1,000–3,000 mcg are given in the hip or buttock muscle 1–3 times each week.

Many drugs inhibit B12 absorption, including oral contraceptives, time-released potassium, histamine-2 blockers used for gastritis and ulcers (Axid, Pepsin, Tagamet, Zantac), proton pump inhibitors (Prevacid, Prilosec), antibiotics, and cholesterol-lowering drugs. There is virtually no known toxicity to B12, even in high dosages.

Antioxidant Minerals: Several common trace minerals such as selenium and zinc are critical for proper immune function. There is concern over agricultural practices that deplete soil (and therefore the foods grown on the depleted soil) of essential trace elements, particularly those that affect immunity. This makes supplementation mandatory in immune deficiency states or when fighting an infection.

SELENIUM: Selenium, considered one of the most important trace minerals in the body, is necessary for the production of the antioxidant enzyme system called glutathione peroxidase, a substance that works with vitamin E and helps to convert harmful oxidized fats into less harmful substances. Selenium also has antioxidant roles of its own and is one of the most potent anticancer nutrients. Richard A. Passwater, Ph.D., who has researched selenium since 1959, contends that it not only prevents cancer, but may cure some of its types. In addition, selenium helps thyroid hormone function, protects against heart attack and stroke, and helps to remove mercury and cadmium from the system.

Its immune system activities include stimulating phagocyte activity (the white cells that destroy invading microorganisms), increasing T lymphocytes, and improving thymus function. Supplementation with only 200 mcg of selenium has been shown to increase NK cell activity. Because of its immune-stimulating function and antiviral activity, selenium supplementation is recommended by many health authorities as a supportive therapy in both the early and advanced stages of AIDS.

The RDA for selenium is 55 mcg per day, though optimal protection is achieved at 200 mcg daily. Selenium is synergistic with vitamin E, helping to enhance its antioxidant effect. Therapeutic dosages can range from 400–1,200 mcg, though these higher dosages should not be used for longer than one month without professional supervision. The preferred oral forms are selenium picolinate or selenomethionine, and the best food sources are Brazil nuts, yeast, whole grains, garlic, eggs, liver, and seafood.

Dietary selenium deficiency has a direct effect on lowering immune activity, while selenium toxicity, which includes symptoms of depression, nervousness, nausea and vomiting, is rare. It can occur when supplemental intake reaches 3,500–5,000 mcg, but in some people, as little as 900 mcg can result in toxicity. Selenium is depleted by corticosteroids, such as Prednisone, and has been shown to reduce the toxicity of the anticancer drug Adriamycin without reducing its therapeutic effects.

ZINC: Zinc has antioxidant effects and works with superoxide dismutase (SOD), one of three naturally occurring enzymes in the body that has antioxidant properties, to neutralize oxidative damage to the cell's genetic material. Zinc is found in every cell of the body and is a component of more than 300 known enzymes and involved in more than 100 metabolic processes, including nearly every aspect of immune function and wound healing. It plays a significant role in immunity and healing.

Adequate levels of zinc maintain T-cell function, assist thymus hormone function, and white cell activity. Zinc supplementation improves age-related low immune status, restores thymus hormone levels, and has antiviral activity. Zinc and copper work synergistically as passive viral inhibitors, and they can help prevent autoimmune diseases, allergies, and cancer.

A typical daily dosage for zinc is between 15–25 mg, with an upper limit for therapeutic purposes at 150 mg. I recommend the picolinate form, which is zinc bound with picolinic acid. Sucking on 15–25 mg zinc gluconate lozenges can shorten a common cold. Zinc is found naturally in oysters and shellfish, red meat, liver, black-eyed peas, eggs, wheat germ, tofu, and pumpkin seeds.

Zinc is considered nontoxic, but long-term use above 300 mg can cause copper depletion, resulting in anemia and reduced HDL-cholesterol. When taking extra zinc in the higher dosages, consider adding 1 mg of copper (best taken in a multimineral), as zinc competes with copper, iron, calcium, and magnesium absorption. In high dosages, zinc may depress immune function, and numerous drugs deplete zinc, including corticosteroids, oral contraceptives, and diuretics used to treat high blood pressure.

Second-Line Antioxidants: Referred to as second-line antioxidants, several classes of very potent antioxidant substances have been discovered in the last few decades. Ongoing research indicates very promising results for some of them including coenzyme Q10, lipoic acid, and flavonoids.

COENZYME Q10: Coenzyme Q10 (CoQ10), or ubiquinone, is densely concentrated within the mitochondria, the energy-producing sites within cells. It is a powerful antioxidant and prevents tissue damage throughout the body. CoQ10 is found in all plant and animals cells; however, dietary sources are insufficient to produce the effects attributed to it in lab studies, so supplementation is necessary. Food sources include organ meats, red meat, fish, nuts, vegetable oils, cereal bran, and dark green, leafy vegetables.

Though CoQ10 is principally known as a nutrient for heart disease, it has also been found to improve the body's energy reserves and enhance general immunity in older people and those with chronic illness. Since tissues and cells involved in immune function have a high requirement for energy, CoQ10 may be an important adjunct in maintaining normal immune integrity and in supporting the immune system when weakened by viral disease.

It has been shown to normalize immunoglobulin G (IgG), an antibody that is part of the humoral immune response and often is elevated in chronic viral disease; to increase phagocytic activity of macrophages; and to reduce morbidity from infections. Studies suggest that CoQ10 may help to reverse immunosuppression related to aging or in chronic disease.

Most of the CoQ10 in the body is biosynthesized within the cells in a complex process involving other nutrients, particularly the B vitamins, vitamin C, and trace minerals. Therefore, a healthy diet and a multivitamin and mineral supplement are important in maintaining sufficient levels of this important antioxidant. A foundational dosage of CoQ10 is 30–90 mg, and the therapeutic range is between 100–300 mg.

CoQ10 is a pharmaceutically-produced substance and comes as a tablet or capsule. Since it is fat soluble, it absorbs best when taken with a fatty meal or with a little oil. Some manufacturers offer it in a softgel caplet combined in soybean or palm oil. It works synergistically with vitamin E to prevent damage to lipid membranes and plasma lipids, and also with carnitine, lipoic acid, lycopene, magnesium, and B vitamins. Idebenone, a synthetic analog and newer form of CoQ10, is considered more easily absorbed than ubiquinone, making it more useful for older people; it is taken in the same dosages. However, it is difficult to obtain in the United States.

There are no reported adverse effects of CoQ10 supplementation, though some people find it too energizing and should not take it in the evening before bedtime as it may cause difficulty in falling asleep. CoQ10 helps to protect against the side effects of several drugs, including Adriamycin. It is depleted by many drugs, including diuretics, some antidepressants, and blood pressure lowering medications.

Lipoic Acid: Alpha-lipoic acid (ALA), also called thioctic acid, is found in small amounts in the body and in a variety of foods, especially red meat and organ meats. In the body, it is important for energy production as it helps to convert carbohydrates into usable energy. For this reason, it is often used as an adjunctive treatment for diabetes. ALA is a powerful antioxidant and helps to recycle other antioxidants, principally vitamins C and E. However, it may replace vitamin E when it is in short supply in the body, since it is both water- and fat-soluble and has a broader range of antioxidant activity than either vitamins C or E. It also functions as a chelating agent in the removal of excess iron, copper, and toxic metals like mercury, lead, and cadmium.

Lipoic acid has been shown to be an effective antioxidant in the treatment of AIDS due to its ability to raise plasma levels of vitamin C and glutathione, and to improve immune function by raising the number of T-helper cells. It has also been shown to inhibit viral replication in AIDS. The preventative dosage range is between 25–100 mg, an average treatment range is 300–600 mg, and the therapeutic range is as high as 600–1,000 mg. There are no known toxic effects with these higher dosages, but as with all nutrients, I recommend taking lipoic acid in therapeutic-range doses only under the supervision of a health professional.

FLAVONOIDS: Flavonoids are a group of polyphenolic compounds commonly found in nearly all plants, in which they are concentrated in the seeds, bark, flowers, peel, or skin. There are over 4,000 known flavonoids and many occur in common beverages like tea, coffee, beer, wine, and fruit juices. These include red- and blue-pigmented anthocyanidins; the white and pale-yellow compounds rutin, quercetin, and kaempferol; citrus bioflavonoids; and green tea polyphenols.

Most medicinal herbs are also rich in flavonoids, such as ginkgo *(Ginkgo biloba)* and milk thistle *(Silybum marianum)*. These compounds have considerable health benefits including anti-inflammatory, anti-allergic, antiviral, antibacterial, anticarcinogenic, and antioxidant activity.

- Quercetin: Quercetin is one of the most common flavonoids in the human diet and one of the most important in an antiviral program. It is found in apples, onions, black tea, leafy green vegetables, beans, and other fruits, vegetables, and herbs. It has been studied for its anticancer activity in breast, colon, lung, ovarian, prostate, and other cancers. Quercetin has been shown to affect natural killer cell function, and it is thought to have activity that protects cells (cytoprotective) from oxidative damage. Perhaps its most interesting uses are as a chemokine and cytokine inhibitor in the treatment of chronic viral illnesses and as an antimicrobial against antibiotic-resistant bacteria.

  Quercetin is recommended by naturopathic physicians as a natural antihistamine for allergies, and it is useful in treating hay fever and asthma. It is also useful in the treatment of interstitial cystitis, a chronic urinary tract inflammatory syndrome characterized by severe pelvic pain. The recommended dosage of quercetin is 400 mg, 2 to 3 times daily. To treat chronic viral infections, the dosage is 1,000 mg, 3 times daily. There have been no proven cases of toxicity with quercetin supplementation, and though there is some concern that quercetin may pose a cancer risk, no human studies or clinical evidence have confirmed this.

- Proanthocyanidin: Originally called pycnogenol by its discoverer, Jacques Masquelier, a professor at the University of Bordeaux, France, oligomeric proanthrocyanidin complexes (OPCs), also called procyanidolic oligomers (PCOs), were first extracted from pine bark in 1951 and later from grape seeds in 1970. They have powerful antioxidant activity. In fact, grape seed extracts have stronger antioxidant effects than vitamins C and E, or beta-carotene. PCOs also exert antibacterial, antiviral, anticarcinogenic, anti-inflammatory, and anti-allergic effects.

  Proanthocyanidins are found in pine bark, grape seeds and grape skin (and therefore in red wine), tea (green and black), and many herbs, notably bilberry *(Vaccinium myrtillus)*, cranberry *(Vaccinium macrocarpon)*, black currants *(Ribes nigrum)*, and elderberry *(Sambucus nigra)*. Antiviral effects have been shown with elderberry extracts against influenza virus. Another herb, hamamelis bark (*Hamamelis virginiana*, also known as witch hazel), has activity against human herpes virus 1; the Amazonian herb, *Sangre de Drago (Croton lechleri)*, containing several flavonols including proanthocyanidins, has also been shown to be effective against viral infections. Daily dosage recommendations range between 50–100 mg. No side effects or interactions are attributed to proanthocyanidin supplementation.

Antioxidant Amino Acids and Whey Protein

Amino acids are the building blocks of proteins and enzymes and are necessary for the structural components of the body and the maintenance of life. Proteins make our muscles, tissues, and organs, and even compose part of our bones. The immune system is also largely made from proteins, including the immunoglobulins (one of the main components of first-line defense), and is directly affected by

Table 9: Recommended Dosages of Antioxidants

Antioxidant	Recommended Form	RDA	Basic Dosage	Therapeutic Range
Vitamin C	ascorbic acid; calcium, magnesium, or potassium ascorbate	35–95 mg	200–2,000 mg	6,000–20,000 mg; up to 100,000 mg
Vitamin E	d-alpha tocopherol	15–30 IU	200–500 IU	800–1,600 IU
Carotenes	beta-carotene as natural mixture of all-trans and cis forms; mixed carotinoids	none	25,000–100,000 U	up to 300,000 IU
Selenium	selenium picolinate; selenomethionine	10–75 mg	200 mcg	400–1,200 mcg
Zinc	zinc picolinate; zinc gulconate (lozenges)	5–19 mg	15–25 mg	45–150 mg
CoQ10	Ubiquinone; Idebenone	none	30–90 mg	100–300 mg
Lipoic Acid	Alpha-lipoic acid	none	25–100 mg	300–600 mg
Vitamin B2	Riboflavin Hydrochloride; Riboflavin-5-Phosphate	1.7 mg	10–100 mg	up to 400 mg
Vitamin B6	Pyridoxine Hydrochloride, Pyridoxal Hydrochloride, Pyridoxal-5-Phosphate	2 mg	50–100 mg	150–500 mg
Vitamin B12	Cyanocobalamin, Methylocablanin, Adenosylcobalamin (Coenzyme B12)	0.3–2.6 mcg	1,000–2,000 mcg	2,000–6,000 mcg

References: The Linus Pauling Institute, *The New Recommendations for Dietary Antioxidants;* Pelton, R., et al. *Drug-Induced Nutrient Depletion Handbook;* Designs for Health, *Supplement Monograph Manual;* Roberts, AJ, et al. *Nutraceuticals, the Complete Encyclopedia;* Gaby, AR and Wright, JV, *Nutritional Therapy in Medical Practice.*

how proteins are utilized in the body, how much protein we eat, and the quality of protein we take in. A full complement of amino acids is found in high-quality protein from seeds and nuts, legumes, whole grains, eggs, fish, poultry, and organic meats.

An amino acid is a compound containing an amino group and an acidic function. This acidic function makes proteins from meat more acidic in the body, so it is recommended that the majority of dietary protein come from plant sources. If one is eating large amounts of animal protein—as one does in bodybuilding—the flushing out of accumulated acids with plenty of water is essential, along with abundant intake of alkaline vegetables to balance acid buildup from eating meat.

Twenty specific amino acids make up all the proteins in the human body: alanine, arginine, asparagine, aspartic acid, cysteine, glutamic acid, glutamine, glycine, histidine, isoleucine, leucine, lysine, methionine, phenylalanine, proline, serine, threonine, tryptophan, tyrosine, and valine. There are other amino acids in the body, such as taurine and ornithine, that have functions not directly related to building protein. These twenty amino acids are divided into two groups, called essential and nonessential.

This terminology is somewhat misleading, as all the amino acids are crucial to life; however, what biologists refer to as the essential group are those that cannot be synthesized in the body and must be obtained through the diet. There are eight essential amino acids: isoleucine, methionine, leucine, lysine, phenylalanine, threonine, tryptophan, and valine.

In chronic disease, aging, and chronic viral illness, adequate dietary protein is critical, as was outlined in step 1. However, people with these conditions often are not able to digest and absorb all the amino acids they need for tissue repair and healing. To enhance protein intake, an amino acid supplement is recommended, and is best taken in the form of a protein powder drink.

Supplemental amino acids come in many varieties, and certain forms are much better for immune-enhancing than others. Due to possible gastrointestinal allergic reactions, like cramping or gas for people with chronic disease, I suggest avoiding amino acid products made from soy, milk casein, gluten (or wheat proteins), and eggs. Proteins consumed should also have a high biological value, as measured by the nitrogen retained for growth (expressed as a percentage of absorbed nitrogen), and be lactose free.

Like many nutritionists and naturopathic physicians, I specifically recommend hydrolyzed, or pure, dairy or goat whey because it is made up of smaller, more easily digested particles that have less allergic reactivity than conventional whey products. Some products combine hypoallergenic rice protein to complement the whey; many of these products are classified as medical foods and are not available in health stores. To obtain them, consult your doctor or see the resource section at the end of this book.

Whey protein includes many subfractions besides amino acids, including beta-lactoglobulin, immunoglobulins, bovine (cow) serum albumin, lactoperoxidases, lysozyme, and lactoferrin—a potent immunomodulating substance discussed in step 6.

Some whey products contain very high levels of immunoglobulin complexes, substances necessary for rebuilding the immune system, and in certain cases they may be more beneficial than pure whey. However, it is extremely important not to take whey protein products, especially the immunoglobulin-enhanced products, if you have an autoimmune condition like lupus or rheumatoid arthritis, or any chronic inflammatory condition. In these cases, adding immunoglobulins from milk-based products could cause the immune system to overreact to the foreign proteins, causing increased inflammation.

People who benefit most from whey protein supplementation are those with weakened constitutions, age-related immune decline, who are in recovery from a long illness, or have general immune weakness.

The recommended supplemental dosage is between 15–20 g per day. Of course, whey is also beneficial for healthy people who want to improve their protein status and increase their muscle mass. Hydrolyzed whey protein has been shown to effectively boost levels of glutathione, the powerful, naturally occurring antioxidant (discussed in the previous section on antioxidants). In addition to a whey protein supplement, specific amino acids have been shown to improve immune status and enhance glutathione levels, so additional supplementation with these substances can further enhance immunity.

People who benefit most from whey protein supplementation are those with weakened constitutions, age-related immune decline, who are in recovery from a long illness, or have general immune weakness. The recommended supplemental dosage is between 15–20 g per day.

Arginine: This amino acid is sometime referred to as a growth hormone enhancer and muscle builder. It is important for cell growth, wound healing, recovery from illness, and during times of stress. It strengthens the immune system by increasing NK cell activity, increasing white cell production, and stimulating white cell response. It promotes resistance against infection and stimulates the thymus gland. It is useful in chronic fatigue syndrome and immune dysfunction. I recommend a foundational dose of 500–1,000 mg daily, with a therapeutic range of 1,500–6,000 mg, and sometimes as high as 30 g.

However, high sustained dosages have been shown to activate herpes simplex virus, acting as an antagonist to lysine, an amino acid that helps to reduce herpes virus activity. In these cases, arginine supplementation should not be used and one should even avoid arginine-containing foods such as nuts, cheeses, and chocolate.

Otherwise, arginine is a safe substance, free from side effects; however, since arginine works synergistically with ornithine to stimulate growth hormone, some doctors warn against its use in diabetes, as the growth hormone increase it can cause may overwork the pancreas. Arginine should also be avoided in cancer patients, as high dosages have been shown to increase cancer cell growth.

Lysine: Lysine is an essential amino acid necessary for growth and needed to maintain nitrogen balance. It helps in the absorption of calcium and reduces its excretion, maintains healthy blood vessels, and reduces activity of sexually transmitted herpes viruses and cold sores. Food sources include brewer's yeast, legumes, dairy, wheat germ, fish, turkey, and meat. Generally, supplementation of lysine is not needed; however, to treat an active herpes condition 1,500–3,000 mg of lysine twice daily is required.

Lysine is considered safe; however, when taking high dosages (15–40 g) abdominal cramping and diarrhea have been reported. Also, high dosages may increase the risk of gallstones and raise cholesterol. I generally recommend using lysine only during the duration of a herpes outbreak, though some doctors suggest a maintenance dosage of 1,000 mg daily to prevent recurrences.

Cysteine: Cysteine is an important amino acid due to its antioxidant activity. It is a nonessential amino acid and is one of only a few that contains the sulfur component thiol. Cysteine is involved in many of the body's detoxification pathways; it helps eliminate toxins, drugs, and heavy metals that have a destructive effect on the immune system. It also increases the formation of glutathione. Research has shown that cysteine increases white blood cell numbers, activates cytotoxic T cells, and improves immunomodulation.

The recommended supplemental form is as N-acetyl cysteine (NAC) in dosages of 200–500 mg per day, with a therapeutic range of between 1,500–5,000 mg. NAC is an important therapeutic nutrient in its own right, and is used as a mucolytic (a substance that reduces phlegm). It is also beneficial in the treatment of respiratory conditions such as bronchitis. Since cysteine can leach out metals, it is best to take it along with a multiple vitamin and mineral supplement with additional zinc and copper. Vitamin C prevents cysteine from oxidizing into cystine, another amino acid that can lead to kidney stones when elevated in the body.

Glutamine: Glutamine is the most abundant amino acid in the body and is important in building muscle and speeding wound healing. It is also used by the brain as an alternative fuel when glucose levels are low, and serves as an energy source for the cells of the gastrointestinal tract and is useful in "leaky gut" syndrome and irritable bowel syndrome (IBS).

Glutamine has immune-enhancing functions that include increasing white cell proliferation, and it is used by the white cells and macrophages as a source of energy. It combines with NAC to promote glutathione synthesis and is synergistic with vitamin B6 and magnesium. Though healthy people do not need glutamine supplementation, it is useful for general immune weakness and for those losing muscle mass due to illness.

Therapeutic dosages can be as high as 40 g per day, but a basic range is from 500–2,000 mg. During periods of stress, when you are engaging in heavy exercise, and/or treating bowel disease, the dosage can climb upward to 4,000–8,000 mg (4–8 g). The optimal dosage is not yet known, but there are no toxic side effects. It is best taken in the powdered form, mixed directly into water or juice. Glutamine should not be taken by those with kidney failure or cirrhosis of the liver.

Food sources include all meats, fish, and eggs; however, overcooking animal protein foods destroys much of the available glutamine. Slow cooking, pressure cooking, or steaming help preserve glutamine and other important vitamins and minerals.

Glutathione and Its Restoration: Glutathione, referred to as GHS in its reduced form, is a naturally occurring protein composed of three amino acids: cysteine, glutamic acid, and glycine. Due to its powerful antioxidant activity, it has been referred to as the master antioxidant.

According to Parris Kidd, Ph.D., a cellular biologist, co-author of *Antioxidant Adaptation*, and former professor at the University of California at Berkley, it can "fine-tune" the oxidative state of cells, helping to maintain a cellular environment conducive to antioxidant activity, and thereby protecting cells from oxidative damage. It is associated with protection from cancer and a wide variety of degenerative diseases. Research has also found that higher levels of glutathione in

Table 10: Dosages for Amino Acids

Amino Acid	Recommended Form	RDA	Basic Dosage	Therapeutic Range
Arginine	L-arginine	none	500–1,000 mg	1,500–6,000 mg; up to 30,000 mg
Lysine	L-lysine	none	500–1,000 mg	1,500–3,000 mg
Cysteine	N-acetyl-l-cysteine (NAC)	none	200–500 mg	1,500–5,000 mg
Glutamine	L-glutamine	none	500–2,000 mg	up to 4,000–8,000 mg
Glutathione	reduced L-glutathione	none	50–100 mg	150–300 mg

References: The Linus Pauling Institute, *The New Recommendations for Dietary Antioxidants;* Pelton, R., et al. *Drug-Induced Nutrient Depletion Handbook;* Designs for Health, *Supplement Monograph Manual;* Roberts, AJ, et al. *Nutraceuticals, the Complete Encyclopedia;* Gaby, AR and Wright, JV, *Nutritional Therapy in Medical Practice.*

older adults is associated with better health, which has led to the idea that low levels of glutathione in white cells is a predictor of premature aging and poor immune status.

Glutathione is mainly stored and metabolized in the liver, the organ most involved in detoxification processes. The liver is also one of the principle sites of common viral infections such as hepatitis B and C, as well as several of the Epstein-Barr viruses. Liver protection with natural medications and glutathione restoration becomes critically important in a viral immunity program.

Glutathione deficiency inhibits the natural immune response. It is thought to have potent antiviral activity, and low glutathione levels may cause a "pro-viral" effect. Adequate levels in the cells are necessary for T-cell proliferative response, activation of cytotoxic T cells, and other T-lymphocyte functions. Numerous studies have shown significant glutathione depletion in AIDS and HCV patients.

Effective glutathione restoration involves avoidance of substances that cause depletion, practicing detoxification regimens, and deliberate supplementation. Though low glutathione levels are associated with poor health and immune status, it is still unclear if oral supplementation is of any direct benefit to humans, even though some studies in mice indicate it has effectiveness in increasing natural killer cell activity.

Many of the antioxidants and amino acids discussed in this section increase glutathione levels, including vitamin C, NAC, and glutamine. Vitamin C supplementation (as little as 500 mg) in particular appears to significantly raise glutathione levels. Michael Murray, N.D., a naturopathic physician and a leading authority on natural medicine, strongly agrees and recommends that doctors avoid the use of the expensive glutathione supplements, suggesting that patients stay with vitamin C. The amino acid L-methionine and its activated form, S-adenosylmethionine (SAM), also raise glutathione levels.

Many toxic substances deplete glutathione including common over-the-counter drugs, especially acetaminophen (Tylenol). Meanwhile, NAC protects the liver against acetaminophen toxicity and is often recommended to be taken with acetaminophen in patients with compromised liver function. Other factors that cause glutathione deficiency include dietary methionine deficiency, ultraviolet exposure from sunlight, iron overload, tissue damage from injury or burns, and bacterial and viral infection. Patients with compromised immunity and chronic viral diseases should not take iron or iron-containing multivitamins; they should also avoid the use of acetaminophen and shun direct sun exposure.

Table 11: Quick Guide to Antioxidants and Nutrients Used for Viruses

Nutrient	Use	DOSAGE Acute Infection	Chronic Infection
Vitamin C	All viral conditions	500–1,000 mg every few hours	1,000–2,500 mg, 3–4 times per day
Vitamin A	Common cold and flu	25,000 IU, 2–6 times per day	25,000 IU, 2 times per day
Selenium	All viral conditions	400 mcg, 3 times daily	200 mcg, 2–4 times daily
Zinc	All viral conditions	30–50 mg, 2–3 times daily	30–45 mg, 2 times daily
L-Lysine	Herpes Simplex 1 and 2	1,500 mg, 3–4 times daily	500–1,000 mg, 2–3 times daily
NAC	AIDS and hepatitis C	1500 mg, 2–3 times daily	500–1000 mg, 2 times daily

CHAPTER SUMMARY

Eat an oxygen-rich diet of natural foods high in fresh fruits and vegetables, including one or two 6–8 ounce glasses of carrot and mixed green vegetable juice each week.

In addition to improving general fitness, practice oxygen-enhancing exercises like Chinese qi gong or yoga pranayama.

Improve indoor air quality with an ozone generator.

If you have an active viral disease, consider using bio-oxidative therapies.

Make sure your multivitamin and mineral supplement has all of the antioxidants discussed in this section and in adequate basic dosages; then supplement with extra antioxidants.

Take extra vitamin C—it's the most important antioxidant and the cornerstone to glutathione restoration. If you have a viral illness, take at least 2,000 mg of vitamin C daily, and increase your dosage up to bowel tolerance.

Take a total of at least 400 IU of natural vitamin E; if your immune system is weakened or you have heart disease, take an additional 400–500 IU.

Eat adequate amounts of complete, high-quality proteins and complement this with another 10–20 g of protein from a hydrolyzed pure whey protein drink.

Consider individual amino acid supplements for immune enhancement, especially NAC for glutathione restoration.

Glutathione restoration is critical in reestablishing healthy antioxidant activity. However, since there is currently no perfect supplemental GHS source, avoid the factors that cause glutathione depletion.

8

STEP THREE

Rejuvenate Your Immune System with Enzymes

In step 2, I discussed the oxidative process and antioxidants, and in step 1, I introduced the basics of diet and the importance of foundational vitamin and mineral supplements. In this chapter, you will learn about the importance of digestion and how to use dietary and supplemental enzymes for the rejuvenation of the immune system.

Steps 1–3 equip you for the fundamental construction of natural health and are a cornerstone of your viral immunity plan. The information contained in these steps is an essential requirement for healing degenerative chronic disease conditions and viral illnesses.

Enzymes—Nature's Reactive Factors

Life as we know it could not function without enzymes, referred to in medicine as the "sparks of life." We produce thousands of different enzymes in our bodies every day. Enzymes are critical catalysts involved in every chemical reaction in our bodies including cell metabolism, hormone metabolism, and digestion. Without these substances to enhance cell metabolism, the immune system could not function.

The pancreas manufactures digestive enzymes that facilitate the breakdown of food into particles small enough to be absorbed. In addition, metabolic enzymes are produced in our cells and are responsible for all biological and chemical processes from reproduction to movement, vision, hearing, breathing, and very importantly, for immunity.

Enzymes are also commercially produced from animal pancreas tissue, concentrated out of enzyme-rich fruits, and grown on special microorganisms. The most commonly used plant sources for commercial enzymes are papaya and pineapple. Supplemental enzymes are provided in specialized products sold in health stores or prescribed by doctors as tablets or capsules. Enzymes also have medical uses for specific conditions and are administered intravenously or by injection, but those uses, though clinically important and interesting, are not part of the scope of this book.

Enzyme Sources: Enzymes are found throughout nature, especially in plants. Plants process sunlight and air in their leaves through a process called photosynthesis, and that creates energy which is converted into plant products such as starch. In this process, mainly occurring at night, plants use carbon dioxide and give off oxygen—another reason to keep green living things in your personal environment. Plants also produce pigments that include green chlorophyll; polyphenols including flavonoids; carotenoids; lignins; fiber; and thousands of other substances including hormones, vitamins, protective substances, as well as enzymes.

Dietary enzymes are found only in fermented foods, and raw fruits, vegetables, and herbs. Though all foods contain natural enzymes, some are richer in enzymes than others. Those with the highest amounts of enzymes include apples, papayas, pineapples, melons, sprouted grains and beans, fermented foods (like tamari, tempeh, yogurt, buttermilk, pickles, and olives), brewed beer, wine, the fresh green shoots of grasses (barley and wheat grass), and various salt- and freshwater green and blue-green algae.

Cooked foods do not contain active enzymes. The pasteurization process, heating foods to destroy microorganisms, also destroys enzymes in beer, milk, and other food products. This is not to say that a diet of completely raw foods with raw milk and dairy products is the best diet. In fact, such a diet can be very unhealthy over a period of time, weakening the body and depriving it of proteins for muscle, carbohydrates for energy, and cholesterol to make hormone precursors. Raw foods also harbor bacteria and mold that, over time, may accumulate in the intestinal tract and make you more susceptible to disease.

The daily diet should be balanced between cooked and raw foods; it should be pleasing to look at, good tasting, and matched to your individual body type, temperament, age, and lifestyle. It should be supplemented with vitamins and minerals, especially antioxidants, and complemented with raw foods and juices and other enzyme-rich foods in small amounts, included in the daily fare to make it more appetizing and varied.

What Are Enzymes? Enzymes make chemical reactions proceed more efficiently. They are catalysts and support life by making all biochemical processes possible at body temperature. A catalyst is a substance that triggers chemical reactions without itself being consumed in the reactive process. Enzymes are used in very small amounts, and can be reused again and again; however, they are very specific and have affinity for a single reaction only.

Like proteins, enzymes are composed of two parts: the protein component, called an apoenzyme, and a non-protein part. This "non-protein" part is called a coenzyme if organic elements, such as vitamins, are involved, or a cofactor if it is made up of inorganic minerals such as magnesium. Since many enzymatic reactions require both coenzymes and cofactors, you can again see how important it is to have a good diet and supplemental vitamins and minerals.

Types of Enzymes: There are six main types of enzymes: oxidoreductases, transferases, hydrolases, lyases, isomerases, and ligases. The oxidoreductases are made up of two groups of enzymes that assist oxygenation processes, discussed in the preceding chapter on antioxidants. One group, oxidizing enzymes, speed up oxidation by adding one oxygen atom or removing two hydrogen atoms from a molecule; the other, reducing enzymes, help in removing oxygen. Hydrolases, or hydrolytic enzymes, require water to catalyze reactions, and are the main type of enzymes discussed in this chapter.

For practical purposes, enzymes can be divided into three groups: metabolic enzymes, food enzymes, and digestive enzymes. We can influence metabolic enzymes by providing sufficient coenzymes and cofactors in the diet, through vitamin and mineral supplementation, and by reducing metabolic stress from toxic exposure, overwork or excessive exercise, and psychological stress.

Other factors that influence metabolic enzyme processes are temperature and pH. Enzymatic activity increases with warmer temperatures and slows down in colder temperatures. There is also an optimal acid-alkaline balance at which enzymatic reactions occur. In general, the body functions best in a slightly alkaline environment.

Food enzymes are provided in plant foods, and their levels can be effectively increased by using concentrated juices, green drinks, and phytonutrient-enzyme-rich foods. Digestive enzyme function can be improved by eating a healthy diet (or worsened by an unhealthy one of refined foods and high fats), along with exercise, hatha yoga, and stress reduction.

Digestive enzymes are mainly secreted by the pancreas but also in the mouth, and by the stomach and small intestine. This group includes amylase, disaccharidases, trypsin, chymotrypsin, protease, lipase, and cellulase. Amylase digests carbohydrates—like those found in potatoes, bread, and pasta—breaking them down to smaller molecules, all the way down to glucose, the simplest form of sugar and the energy fuel of the cells of our bodies and brains.

Disaccharidases assist the processes of reducing disaccharides, substances composed of two sugar molecules, like sucrose (cane sugar) and lactose (milk sugar), into glucose. Trypsin is one of the principle enzymes that break down proteins, and is often found with chymotrypsin. Proteases also digest proteins, breaking them down into amino acids. Lipase digests fat and cellulase breaks down fiber. Cellulase is not manufactured in the body and must be supplied in the diet or by enzyme supplements.

Enzymes and Immunity

Enzymes play vital supporting roles in maintaining strong immune function. By themselves, enzymes do not directly attack viruses, but their indirect role in natural immunity is substantial and they perform many roles in a comprehensive viral immunity plan.

Enzymes work in oxidative processes to reduce the effects of harmful pollutants and assist in the management of cancer. They are very important in controlling excessive inflammation and are necessary in tissue repair and for fighting infections. Enzyme preparations have been shown to increase the cytotoxic activity of macrophages, influence interleukins, remove excessive immune complexes in tissues, and many other immune mechanisms. Twenty-two enzymes are known to be involved in the immunological complement system.

Microorganisms also produce enzymes, especially proteases involved in cellular metabolic processes, including viral replication. Protease inhibitors, a class of antiviral drugs used to treat HIV infection (and being researched for HCV), inhibit viral proteases and thereby reduce their replication. The structure of proteases for cytomegalovirus and other herpes viruses is also known, and scientists may develop protease inhibitors for these viruses as well. Unfortunately, protease inhibitors not only affect the viral protease but also the metabolism of normal cells. Thus this class of drugs does not cure AIDS and is in fact associated with numerous side effects due to their toxicity.

One side effect, called lipodystrophy, is a syndrome similar to Syndrome X, an insulin resistant related metabolic disorder. Both are characterized by an accumulation of fat around the central part of the body (abdomen and trunk) and a withdrawal of fat from the face, arms, legs, and buttocks. Triglyceride and cholesterol levels are elevated and insulin resistance is present; 8–10 percent of lipodystrophy cases progress to Type 2 diabetes.

These viral proteases are not to be confused with naturally occurring human protease, a hydrolytic enzyme produced in the body that circulates in the serum and is secreted in the digestive tract to break down protein foods. Taking oral proteolytic enzymes does not interfere with these drugs. In fact, numerous scientific studies have shown the effectiveness of oral proteolytic enzymes in cancer, acute and chronic inflammation, chronic prostatitis caused by chlamydial infection, and antibiotic-resistant bacteria. Proteolytic enzymes have also been used to treat herpes zoster (shingles), hepatitis C virus, and HIV infection. European studies by the Medical Enzyme Research Institute in Germany have shown that the progression of AIDS is slowed and symptoms are considerably improved with oral enzyme therapy.

The Energy View of Digestion and Enzymes

Though the Chinese did not describe specific enzymes in the manner of modern Western medical science, they were well aware of the importance of enzyme-rich foods and condiments. Soy sauce, miso, tofu, Japanese-style pickles, and many other fermented products are common to the average Oriental diet. Other enzyme-rich foods used by the Chinese include bird's nests made from the salivary secretion of swallows, varieties of fungi, and seaweeds.

The Chinese also used enzyme-containing herbs to treat illnesses of the digestive system as well as deficiencies of energy states. For example, herbs that enhance digestive function such as *mu xiang (Saussurea lappa)* are frequently added to herbal formulas that tonify the *qi* and benefit the stomach and spleen to improve digestive power and create more energy. Several other herbal medicinals rich in naturally occurring enzymes, like sprouted rice *nuo dao gen xu (Oryza sativa)* and *shen qu (Massa fermentata),* made from fermenting a mixture of wheat and several herbs, are used to improve digestion and treat gastrointestinal disorders like gastritis and liver disease.

Central to the Chinese concept of health is *huo qi* or "fire energy." Ayurvedic medicine has a similar concept called *agni.* In both systems, this fire energy is said to be responsible for digestive power and it also influences temperament. If a person has too much *huo qi,* he will be restless and hotheaded; too little and the person becomes lethargic, passive, and has poor resistance to disease. The most desirable state of *huo qi* is one of moderation and balance. The person's temperament is not too aggressive, yet they have plenty of energy. They do not tire easily, do not easily get sick, and they have a good appetite and enjoy eating.

Huo qi is said to come from the heart and is influenced by *pi qi,* or "spleen energy." Interestingly, in Chinese medicine, the heart is paired in a yin/yang relationship with the small intestine, and along with the spleen is associated with pancreatic function—both organs (spleen and pancreas) that are predominantly responsible for the manufacture and secretion of digestive enzymes. Therefore, keeping the digestive organs, especially the pancreas and small intestine (both enzyme-secreting organs), healthy is necessary for adequate enzyme production.

Phytonutrient-Rich Foods and Juices

The Chinese consider good digestion to be crucial to health, saying that without good digestive power, one is listless, weak, and in poor health. Western functional and naturopathic medicine also value the importance of good digestive function. A healthy digestive tract begins with sound teeth and good dental hygiene, and includes proper gastric and small intestine function, along with a healthy liver and pancreas.

Eating easy-to-digest natural foods, combined correctly and prepared properly, facilitates digestive function. Eating too quickly, eating when stressed, overeating, and eating highly processed and fried foods, all greatly disrupt digestive function. Providing the body with adequate fluids, but not over consuming iced water during meals, also aids digestion. Culinary herbs like basil, coriander, and ginger help digestive function; herbal bitters like gentian root can improve appetite. Exercise in general, and yoga postures in particular, enhance digestive function. Let's turn now to specific plant foods high in nutrients and enzymes.

The Chinese consider good digestion to be crucial to health, saying that without good digestive power, one is listless, weak, and in poor health. Western functional and naturopathic medicine also value the importance of good digestive function.

Phytonutrient-rich foods include the cabbage family (cruciferous vegetables including all cabbages, broccoli, brussels sprouts, cauliflower, collards, and kale); soyfoods (tofu, tamari, soy sauce, tempeh, *edamame* [green soybeans in the pod], soybean sprouts);[1] sulfur-containing thiol substances (garlic, ginger, citrus, bioflavonoids); carotene-containing foods like carrots; quercetin-containing onions; lycopene-containing tomatoes; and chlorophyll-containing alfalfa and sunflower seed sprouts. All these are among a long list of commonly available, naturally occurring enzyme sources.

All of these foods can be added to the diet and many can be mixed into your juices or blended drinks. Blends of phytonutrients, green foods, and soy isoflavone-containing concentrates are also available commercially. Small amounts of fermented foods and condiments add significant amounts of enzymes to the diet; therefore, you do not need to use large amounts, but rather, you can add them to your diet as condiments.

For example, soy sauce, prepared from fermenting soybean flour and roasted wheat or barley (using the fungus *Aspergillus oryzae*), is a phytonutrient- and enzyme-rich liquid; it contains highly active enzymes called pronases that help in the breakdown of meat protein. Many culinary herbs and condiments also contain enzymes, including mustard, basil, rosemary, and coriander seeds. The use of small amounts of fresh salsa made from tomatoes and green chili peppers is also a phytonutrient-rich condiment loaded with natural enzymes.

Vegetable Juice Base

4–6 medium carrots
1 small to medium beet
10–12 sprigs of fresh parsley
2 sticks of celery
Add any of the following to your drink:
Fresh gota kola leaves
Wheat or barley grass
A few sprigs of cilantro
One or two cloves of fresh garlic
A small piece of fresh ginger root
Several pieces of fresh nopale cactus
A small amount of fresh aloe vera gel
Other vegetables such as spinach, tomatoes, or cabbage to create your own version of V-8

The Value of Fresh Juices: Around the turn of the twentieth century, nature cure doctors[2] advocated the use of hand-cranked juice machines to extract the liquid from various fruits, vegetables, spices, and herbs for health. In the 1950s, Bernard Jensen, an American naturopathic doctor of international reputation, similarly promoted the health benefits of raw foods and juices. Dr. Jensen advised people to "use more foods from nature's garden." He practiced what he preached at his Hidden Valley Ranch in Escondido, California, where he maintained a healing center and organic garden above the Southern California hills.

When I started in natural health more than thirty years ago, nature cure doctors were still called "quacks," and juicing was considered part of the fringe counter culture. How times have changed! Now juice bars are found in nearly every shopping mall and many airports, and lots of people have juicers or high-speed blenders at home.

Traditionally, people have eaten fruits and vegetables as they come off the tree or vine—fresh and ripe. Then they learned to press out the juice and make wine, cider, and other fermented alcoholic beverages. This was followed by mechanical, hand-turned juice extractors, and then by electrical juicers. Next came concentrated green drinks made from wheat grass, followed by other green products made from algae or the young shoots of barley. The latest developments are highly concentrated plant mixtures from phytonutrient-rich foods. These phytonutrient-rich food supplements are not to be confused with medical foods marketed as liquid or powder products and used in weight-loss programs.

However, we cannot continue to eat only refined and highly processed foods, nor can we rely completely on these new medical foods for our health. To recover our health and prevent disease, we must utilize all the available nutrient-dense methods of providing concentrated dietary complements and supplements, especially in the form of raw juices.

The value of juicing is twofold. First, juices supply abundant flavonoid antioxidants like vitamin C and beta-carotene; second, they are full of live enzymes. Juices can be made from fresh (organic, if at all possible) vegetables, fruits, and herbs, and should be drunk immediately after juicing. However, if you cannot drink all of your juice just after it is made, fresh juices can be kept in a tightly closed container in the refrigerator for twenty-four hours.

Still, I highly recommend that you take your juice straight from the juicer directly to your mouth. The nature cure doctors said, "Chew your juices and drink your foods." This meant that one should masticate well all solid and liquid foods so as to add salivary enzymes before swallowing. A good rule of thumb is to chew each mouthful of food at least thirty times, and to mix your vegetable juice with your saliva by swirling it around your mouth a few times before swallowing.

Mixed Vegetable Drinks: My recommendation for general health is 1 to 2 medium (4–6 ounces) glasses of fresh (organic, if possible) mixed vegetable juice each week. If you have an illness, I suggest a glass of fresh juice daily; during a cleansing program, you may drink fresh juices several times per day. Some ideas for healthy mixtures are given in the sidebar, but remember that each person has different tastes, so adapt the mixture to suit your taste.

Blended Mixed Vegetable Drinks: Blended vegetable drinks are made into an electrolyte-rich broth, rich in minerals like potassium, by combining different partially cooked vegetables in an electric blender. You may drink blended vegetable juice warm or cooled in the refrigerator. One advantage of a blended drink is that you can use other vegetables that do not juice well, such as zucchini or other squashes. Another is that since they are partially cooked, blended broths are easier to digest and are more beneficial for older people or those who are very sick and confined to bed.

For prevention and health maintenance, if you alternate fresh juice on one day and a blended broth on another, you will enrich your diet immensely, and save money on vitamin supplements.

Fruit Drinks: Many fruits (especially papayas and pineapples) contain high amounts of enzymes and are

Blended Vegetable Base

Slightly blanch or steam:
1–2 chopped carrots
1/2–1 small zucchini
1–2 stalks of celery
4–6 leaves of spinach
1/2–1 whole roma tomato
Suggested Additions:
1–2 tablespoons of flaxseed or olive oil
1/2 teaspoon of fresh lemon or lime juice
1/2 cup of cabbage, broccoli, or other cruciferous vegetable
2–4 stalks of celery
1 parsnip, rutabaga, or turnip
1/4 part of fennel root
Fresh oregano or other culinary herbs

Blended Fruit Drink

1 cup of papaya
1/2 cup ripe pineapple
1/2 ripe banana
1 whole chopped apple
Suggested Additions:
1–2 tablespoons of whey protein
1/4–1/2 cup of plain nonfat yogurt
1/2 teaspoon of flaxseed oil
soy or rice milk

Blended Green Drink

Combine the following ingredients in a blender with 2 cups of filtered or spring water. Blend at medium or high speed until thoroughly liquefied, then strain and serve.

Several handfuls of fresh young wheat or barley grass shoots, or 1 teaspoon of barley grass or algae powder

1/4 cup of alfalfa sprouts

1/2 cup of spinach, chard, kale, beet greens, or a mixture of them all

Suggested Additions:

2 leaves of fresh comfrey (remove the center rib)

4–6 pieces of fresh rosemary

1–2 stems of fresh basil

Several stems of fresh mint

A few sprigs of fresh cilantro

important additions to a healthy diet. However, since fruits (and fruit drinks) are high in natural fruit sugars (fructose), they should not be consumed frequently. One or two times per week is more than sufficient. Fruit drinks can be made with any type of fruit, either juiced in the same way as vegetables, or blended with water, yogurt, or low-fat milk. Whey powder can be added to make a nutritious, high-protein drink.

Green Drinks: Chlorophyll is the pigment that gives plants their beautiful green color. The word *chloros* is from the Greek meaning "yellowish green." Chlorophyll has been called "plant blood," and indeed it is similar in its chemistry to human blood, with the exception of one molecule. Blood contains iron in hemoglobin which gives it the red color, whereas chlorophyll has a central magnesium molecule. With the exception of those who have green eyes, the only place in the human body that is green is the bile manufactured in the liver and stored in the gall bladder.

Chlorophyll has a long history in natural medicine. Nature cure doctors touted chlorophyll as a blood cleanser. Along with herbs such as red clover, herbal blood cleansers were supposed to purify the blood and cure whatever ailed you. In the 1970s, Ann Wigmore popularized the use of wheat grass juice as a cure for cancer; she wrote: "It acts to strengthen the cells, detoxify the liver and blood stream, and chemically neutralize the polluting elements themselves" (Wigmore 1985). Of course, none of these claims were based on scientific evidence; however, intuitively, nature cure practitioners knew the importance of chlorophyll in healing.

We now know that chlorophyll contains several important nutrients for health, including vitamin K (for clotting and bleeding problems), and is rich in antioxidant carotenoids. It is reputed to have anti-inflammatory properties, is useful as a disinfectant for wounds and in gum disease, and eliminates bad breath and body odor.

Good sources of chlorophyll include green tea; all leafy green vegetables like spinach and chard; leafy green herbs like comfrey, dandelion, borage, and lemon grass; the young shoots of wheat, rye, and barley grasses; and many green and blue-green algae. Many aquatic algae, like chlorella and spirulina, provide chlorophyll and other important nutrients necessary for health. Commercially, chlorophyll comes as a concentrated liquid, in pressed tablets, capsules, lipid-bound concentrates in softgel capsules, and powders that are to be mixed with water. However, with a little creativity you can also make your own green drinks at home.

Sea Vegetables: Sea vegetables, commonly called seaweeds, have been used for centuries in the daily diets of the Japanese, Chinese, and traditional societies in the North Atlantic. There are over 2,500 different varieties of seaweed, and more than a few of them qualify as super healing foods.

Among the most commonly used are kombu or kelp *(Laminaria japonica)*; nori (a processed form of red marine algae made into flat, dark-colored sheets used to wrap sushi rolls); wakame *(Undaria pinnatifida)*; and seaweeds from the red marine algae family Dumontiaceae. In the 1970s, researchers investigated red marine algae for antiviral activity and found several varieties that inhibited herpes simplex virus. Though in 1990, Michael Neushul, Ph.D., of the University of California, Santa Barbara, updated and validated the earlier research (Neushul 1990), there has not been too much interest in further studies on the antiviral affects of seaweeds.

As the healthiest people in the world favor the use of small amounts of seaweeds in the daily diet, it makes sense for us to use them. Kelp can be found as a dry powder and sprinkled on vegetables or added to vegetable drinks. Nori can be cut into small squares and added to soups, salads, or main dishes as a garnish. Red marine algae is available in capsules or can be sparingly added to soups.

Enzyme Supplementation

Obtaining enzymes from plant food sources is important for the prevention of disease and the promotion of optimal health. However, when disease is present, food sources may not be adequate, and supplementing the diet with oral enzymes becomes very beneficial. There are two kinds of supplemental enzymes available: digestive enzymes and systemic proteolytic enzymes.

Digestive Enzymes: I often recommend pancreatic enzymes for elderly patients with chronically poor digestion and for other patients with poor carbohydrate or fat digestion with symptoms of abdominal distention, constipation, and belly pain more than twenty minutes after eating. Patients with food allergies also benefit from pancreatic enzymes, as do those with chronic inflammatory bowel disorders like Crohn's disease and irritable bowel syndrome Pancreatic enzymes are made from pig (porcine) pancreases. Plant-derived digestive enzymes are also available for those who would rather use a vegetarian source.

Digestive enzymes are rated by strength as established by the United States Pharmacopeia (USP). Each standard "X" contains not less than 25 USP units of amylase, 2 USP units of lipase, and 25 USP units of protease. Most digestive enzyme supplements are supplied as 4X pancreatin per 500 mg tablet or capsule. The recommended dosage is 1–3 capsules with or immediately after meals, though some nutritionally oriented physicians recommend 10X pancreatin.

Pancreatic enzymes are generally well tolerated and have no side effects or interactions in the recommended dosages. However, if you have difficulty digesting fats, proteins, and have a malabsorption syndrome, discuss taking enzymes with your doctor since, in general, pancreatin contains all three enzymes and they may compete with one another, aggravating your condition.

Systemic Proteolytic Enzymes: Proteolytic enzymes help digest protein in food, and are found in pancreatic enzymes (trypsin and chymotrypsin), papaya (papain), and pineapple (bromelain). Concentrated proteolytic enzymes are used to treat cancer and medical conditions, including acute and chronic inflammation.

European scientists were the first to develop commercial methods and the technology to manufacture and use enzymes for the treatment of disease. Wobenzyme, for example, is made by the German company MUCOS Pharma, the largest company of its kind in the world. Wobenzyme contains the proteolytic systemic enzymes bromelain, papain, plus pancreatin in concentrated dosages. These absorb well into the bloodstream and reach systemic saturation after several days of continued use. Numerous studies have shown them to be effective for the treatment of inflammatory diseases like rheumatoid arthritis, for the management of acute inflammation from trauma and sports injuries, in sinusitis and bronchitis, in urinary tract infections, and in cardiovascular disease.

Proteolytic enzymes may also improve immune function and are useful in all viral diseases. Though more clinical studies and research need to be conducted on the use of enzymes in viral diseases, they are considered useful as adjunctive therapy in any chronic viral condition, especially those associated with inflammation, like hepatitis.

In high dosages, concentrated proteolytic enzymes have been used effectively in thousands of cases of cancer. The idea of treating cancer with proteolytic enzymes was first put forth by John Beard, a physician practicing in the early part of twentieth century. Then William Donald Kelley, a Texas dentist reported that he cured himself of pancreatic cancer using enzymes, and he went on to treat tens of thousands of cancer patients with nutritional therapies and enzymes.

In the 1980s, Kelley's results were reviewed by Nicholas Gonzalez, M.D., an oncologist trained at Cornell University Medical College, and were found to have merit. Dr. Gonzalez currently practices in New York City where he employs enzyme therapy for his cancer patients; he is also conducting a research study of enzyme therapy and cancer sponsored by the National Institutes of Health.

Proteolytic enzymes are safe to take over long periods of time and have no reported side effects. Bromelain can increase antibiotic concentration, and may increase an antibiotic's effect when they are taken together. This may make the antibiotic more effective, as in cases of staphylococcus infections. Unless supervised by a physician, however, do not take enzymes and antibiotics at the same time; space them out by at least two hours. Papain has anticlotting activity, and should not be taken with blood-thinning drugs like Coumadin. Proteolytic enzymes, like Wobenzyme, come in easily swallowed flat tablets and are taken by mouth 1–1 1/2 hours before food. The generally recommended dosage is four tablets, three times daily.

Chapter Summary

To prevent disease and optimize recovery from the modern illnesses of CFIDS, AIDS, HCV, and other chronic viral illness, Lyme disease, autoimmune conditions, cancer, and cardiovascular disease, you must provide your diet with higher than average or RDA amounts of nutrients, antioxidants, and enzyme-rich foods.

Avoid concentrated, commercial, tableted, or encapsulated vegetable concentrates unless you are sure of their potency and contents.

Avoid refined and overly processed commercial medical food drinks.

Drink 1–2 cups of freshly made mixed vegetable juice each week.

If you have a viral infection, drink 1–2 cups of this juice daily.

Avoid sweetened and concentrated commercial fruit juices. Drink 1–2 glasses of fresh, nonacidic fruit juice each week.

Supplement your diet with enzyme-containing, phytonutrient-rich foods.

Papayas and ripe pineapples are the best sources of enzymes.

Supplement your diet with concentrated green powders from wheat or barley grass, alfalfa, or algae like spirulina or chlorella.

Consider adding sea vegetables to your diet in small amounts, especially red marine algae like nori.

If you have digestive problems, are elderly, or suffer from any chronic health condition, take a pancreatic digestive enzyme daily with meals.

If you have a condition involving inflammation, take 4–6 tablets of a proteolytic enzyme like Wobenzyme 3–4 times daily, 1–1 1/2 hours before meals.

9

STEP FOUR

Renew Your Cells through Detoxification

There was never a more perfect metaphor for detoxification than the ancient and wise Arabian Night's tale of Aladdin and the magic lamp. The lamp seller wanders the streets at night crying, "New lamps for old." In the same fashion, one of my mentors, Dr. Bernard Jensen, taught that one is not cured until "old diseased cells are replaced by new healthy cells."

Put another way, we could say medicines do not cure. They only create the opportunity for your immune system and natural detoxification pathways to do *their* job of regeneration and healing. Similarly, the saying "What's old is new" might also have been custom-made for this chapter. Though fasting and detoxification are *en vogue* today, to experienced naturopathic physicians and doctors of Oriental medicine there is nothing new about these practices. They are a cornerstone of natural healing approaches.

To be well, we need to renew ourselves from the *inside* out, exchange old cells for new. When individual cells are renewed, tissues are improved and organ function can be restored—only then does a cure take place. The curative process begins with detoxification, a cornerstone of natural health and the key to cellular renewal—which is to say, the beginning of a lasting cure.

Strangely, in this modern age, our technological advancements exist side by side with the waste from excess consumption. We pollute the air we breathe, the water we drink, and the food we eat. The accumulation of toxic chemicals greatly weakens our immune systems and undermines not only our health but also undermines the treatments designed to rid us of disease. Fortunately, we are becoming more aware of the necessity to use detoxification and cleansing therapies as part of a total health plan.

Detoxification therapies, like fasting and hygienic diets, have been used since the time of Hippocrates. Indian Ayurvedic medicine has well-developed and extensive systems of detoxification called *panchakarma* that are thousands of years old. Nature cure practitioners like Benedict Lust, Bernard Jensen, and John Bastyr (the founder of Bastyr University of Naturopathic Medicine in Seattle, Washington), healed people in America and Canada with detoxification regimens in the early and mid-1900s.

Now in the twenty-first century, we know more about detoxification from a scientific point of view than before, and we're able to put this new knowledge to work in assisting the body in its job of cleansing and purification. Modern practitioners of scientific natural detoxification include Walter Crinnion, N.D., who specializes in environmental medicine in Bellevue, Washington, and David W. Quig, Ph.D., a research scientist in the field of nutrition and heavy metal detoxification at Cornell University in Ithaca, New York.

Many medical doctors, notably Leo Galland, David Perlmutter, Majid Ali, and Sandra Cabot, are convinced that modern chronic illnesses cannot be cured with drugs alone. That is why these enlightened physicians have incorporated natural therapeutic detoxification therapies—also referred to as tissue cleansing—into their practices.

For detoxification therapy to be effective, it is necessary to reduce the toxic burden on the body's organs, tissues, and cells. Every second of every day, toxic substances are ravaging our planet's environment and the consequences of chemical wastes and the way they combine with other molecules predispose us to all types of disease, including increased susceptibility to viral infection. Evidence keeps mounting on how toxic environmental substances reduce our immune capacity by as much as 50 percent.

Toxic substances in the environment have three primary targets: (1) the immune system, primarily affecting cell-mediated immunity and leading to an increase in humoral immune components like inflammatory cytokines; (2) the nervous system, leading to diseases like multiple sclerosis; and (3) the endocrine system, causing infertility, menstrual disorders, birth defects, and menopausal symptoms.

In more than twenty years of clinical practice, I have taught and supervised detoxification programs with several thousand patients, and from these patients I have learned what the nature cure doctors, Oriental healers, and yoga masters already know: detoxification *works* and will improve your health.

> ## Partial List of Toxic Chemicals and Drugs
>
> Simple aromatic organic compounds: benzene (in gasoline), styrene (in styrofoam disposable cups), toluene (also in gasoline), and others
>
> Pesticides: DDT, 1,4-dichlorobenzene (in mothballs and household deodorizers), and others
>
> Chlorinated organic chemicals: PCBs, tetrachloroethane, and others
>
> Phenols: ethylphenol (in drinking water), butylbenylphtale (in plastics), and others
>
> Toxic heavy metals: mercury, lead, uranium, cadmium, arsenic
>
> Recreational drugs: cocaine, amphetamines, heroin, etc.

My system of detoxification for viral immunity is based upon a synthesis of the best from the Eastern energy models, modern naturopathic medicine, outcome-oriented functional medicine, and the latest scientific research—all placed upon the shoulders of earlier nature cure giants like Jensen and the others mentioned.

Two case studies come to mind, and both clearly illustrate how effective these methods are. The first I wrote up and published in the *American Journal of Acupuncture* in 1992. With this patient, I successfully applied detoxification therapies, along with Chinese herbs and acupuncture, to normalize the patient's liver function (as indicated by her blood studies), and improved her overall health and sense of well being. In fact, she was so impressed with the results that she enrolled in an acupuncture college shortly afterwards and is practicing natural therapies today (Williams 1992).

The second case also involved a patient who had abnormal liver enzymes, as revealed by his blood tests. Since he had no apparent disease according to his medical doctors, even though he did not feel well, he was told there was nothing wrong with him. In his late fifties, this

Table 12: Normalized Liver Enzyme AST with Detoxification and Natural Therapies

Elevation of the liver enzyme aspartate amino-transferase (AST), formerly called serum glutamic-oxaloacetic transaminase (SGOT), is seen in many conditions involving liver cell (hepatocyte) damage. Though not an exact test for any specific liver condition, it is a good laboratory test to monitor the course of liver disease. Lowering the levels of AST with natural medicines may indicate improvement in the condition of the liver.

Patient	AST (SGOT) Normal Range 0-35 u/L	
	Before	After
Case 1	39	33
Case 2	71	26

man complained of headaches, abdominal pains, and digestive difficulty; he had high cholesterol and suffered from constipation. After detoxification therapies that included intravenous DMPS (discussed below) for mercury toxicity along with natural therapies, his liver enzymes normalized (see table 12), the cholesterol levels declined into the normal range, his abdominal pain completely disappeared, his digestive problems and constipation cleared up, and he felt great.

The present book is not a detoxification manual. It is about the immune system and viral disease. However, because of the vital importance of detoxification for health, in this chapter you will learn about the necessity of cleansing diets, how to promote natural detoxification, and how to conduct a specialized detoxification regimen safely and effectively to enhance your natural immunity.

Detoxification helps your body overcome viral illness. If you are healthy now and without a viral illness, or if you are generally well but catch colds and the flu frequently, application of the information in this chapter can help prevent infections from taking root in your body.

An Overview of Detoxification Therapy

Detoxification therapy is the process of cleansing the body from the inside out using natural methods like herbs and nutritional supplements, combined with nutraceutical and even pharmaceutical medications when necessary. There are many other descriptive terms used for general detoxification, including tissue cleansing, internal cleansing, and detox. This term refers to many different processes such as drug and alcohol detox; removal of industrial chemical byproducts, and environmental cleanup.

In the context of this book, I use the term therapeutic detoxification therapy to indicate the removal of the disease-promoting toxic burden from the cells, tissues, and organs for the purpose of improving health, normalizing immunity, and the complementary treatment of chronic disease. The toxic burden of the body is the total load of accumulated environmental toxic substances from inhalation and contact exposure, use of drugs, toxic chemicals ingested in the diet, and naturally occurring toxins generated by metabolic processes within the body.

Detoxification Pathways: The body is designed by nature to regulate and repair itself. As part of this design, inherent mechanisms exist for the removal of wastes and toxins. Referred to as detoxification pathways, these processes are largely carried out by the liver and involve a two-step process called Phase I and II detoxification. Both phases work synergistically and are codependent on many endogenous molecules (ones already in the body), such as steroid hormones, fatty acids, and amino acids, to complete their function.

Phase I involves activation of a series of enzymes called the cytochrome P450 mixed-function oxidases. These have oxidation, reduction, hydrolysis, hydration, and dehalogenation activities.[1] Jeffrey Bland, Ph.D., and Stephen Barrie, N.D., director of Great Smokies Laboratory in North Carolina, have written extensively on the importance of the cytochrome P450 cycle (Bland 1997; Bennett 1999). In this stage, P450 enzymes break down toxins into intermediate forms called biotransformed intermediates. Some of the biotransformed toxins are ready for elimination at this stage but others require more processing.

I use the term therapeutic detoxification therapy to indicate the removal of the disease-promoting toxic burden from the cells, tissues, and organs for the purpose of improving health, normalizing immunity, and the complementary treatment of chronic disease.

In Phase II, these new forms, unlike the original toxin yet still toxic—some may even be more toxic than their original forms—are eventually converted into non-toxic, water-soluble molecules through a series of different pathways. These nontoxic waste products are eventually excreted by the kidneys in the urine or are conjugated in the bile by the liver and excreted via the gallbladder into the intestines and then eliminated in the stool.

I find it amazing that the body detoxifies and neutralizes toxins *before* eliminating and passing them into the environment. Industrial corporations might copy this example of environmental responsibility from how the body works, and process their own chemical wastes into

Phase II Detoxification Pathways

Glutathione conjugation
Sulfation
Peptide conjugation
Glucuronidation
Acetylation
Methylation

safe organic substances *before* they are released into the environment.

Depending on the authority, there are between six and eight different detoxification routes that biotransformed toxins follow before final elimination from the body. Among the Phase II pathways, one of the most important routes in eliminating toxins is the glutathione conjugation pathway. This pathway is also responsible for eliminating many pharmaceutical drugs, environmental toxins, and alcohol.

However, if liver function is compromised by viral disease, drinking alcohol, or medical or recreational drug use, or if one has had excessive exposure to chemicals or environmental toxins, or is under severe emotional stress, the body will not be able to keep up with detoxification. It is as if you were cleaning your house while the kids were still messing it up. If the body is overwhelmed with toxins, it cannot keep up. To reduce the toxic load, first you must remove the offending toxins, reduce stress, and take only essential pharmaceutical drugs. In this way, the incoming burden on the body is reduced and detoxification can more effectively take place.

Such situations, especially the accumulation of heavy metals like mercury, can exhaust glutathione reserves. Chronic viral infections, as in HIV and HCV, as well as in cirrhosis, tax the liver's detoxification potential and use up glutathione in the process. Now you can see another reason why I emphasize restoring glutathione reserves in step 2. Without adequate glutathione, you are at risk for toxemia, chronic disease, premature aging, and increased susceptibility to viral infection. Detoxification processes also depend on glutathione to function properly.

The Organs of Detoxification

All living things have mechanisms for detoxification, even the smallest of cells. Bodily processes fluctuate between life-supporting growth activities and those that de-animate, tear down, detoxify, and remove. When this balance is unfavorably tipped due to accumulation of toxins, along with the direct damage they cause, disease gradually develops. Though many of the body's internal organs, tissues, and cells contribute to detoxification and the removal of wastes, certain organs are more responsible than others for carrying out the detoxification processes. Ultimately, of course, it is the cells within the tissue of these

organs that perform the bulk of the detoxification processes.

Liver: The liver is the primary organ
of detoxification, filtering viruses and bacteria from the bloodstream. It is the most
metabolically active organ in the body and
performs an estimated 500 functions.
These are too numerous to list here, but
among the most important are: assisting
in carbohydrate, fat, and protein metabolism; maintaining blood sugar levels; producing bile to break down dietary fats;
storing vitamins D, A, and B12; and regu-

> # The Main Organs and Systems Involved in Detoxification
>
> Liver
> Large Intestine
> Blood and Lymphatic System
> Connective Tissue
> Kidneys
> Lungs
> Skin

lating the body's use of iron. The liver is also involved in cholesterol
metabolism and its conversion into steroid hormones such as estrogen
and testosterone, as well as in the removal of used estrogen and other
hormones from the bloodstream.

The liver is the primary focus in all detoxification regimens.
Besides nutrients from the diet and antioxidants, a number of substances improve liver function, promote detoxification, and protect
the liver cells from damage by toxins and alcohol. Liver-protective
herbs, such as milk thistle *(Silybum marianum)*, celandine *(Chelidonium
majus)*, and dandelion *(Taxaxacum officinale)*, and lipotrophic nutrients
(substances that break down fat in the liver) such as the amino acid
methionine, as well as choline, betaine, folic acid, and vitamin B12, are
essential for restoring liver function. Many foods improve liver function, including beets, radishes, radish seed spouts, dandelion greens,
and all green leafy vegetables.

These are the typical signs of a sluggish liver:

- Digestive problems: heartburn, abdominal pain, bloating and discomfort after eating, difficulty digesting fats, intolerance to alcohol,
  nausea, floating stools, constipation, bitter taste in the mouth, and
  a thick, yellow tongue coating.

- Skin problems: acne, rosacea, poor skin tone, swelling and edema,
  brown spots on the skin ("liver spots"), increased numbers of visible
  small red blood vessels (spider nevi), and lipomas or lumps of fat
  under the skin.

- Menstrual and hormonal problems: premenstrual tension, painful periods, diarrhea during the period, and reactions to hormone replacement.

- Neurological and psychological problems: headaches, irritability, insomnia, depression, poor concentration, overheating of the face and upper torso.

- Immune problems: allergies, food and chemical sensitivities, chronic fatigue, fibromyalgia and joint inflammation, systemic infections, and viral hepatitis.

- Appearance: sallow or yellowish complexion, yellowing or dullness of the whites of the eyes, dark circles under the eyes, protruding lower abdomen (pot belly), cellulite, accumulation of fat around the upper abdomen under the ribs (liver roll), and being overweight.

Large Intestine: I have always found it interesting that each country has a certain organ on which their folk medicine historically blames everything. What is more fascinating is that these are always the main organs of detoxification and elimination. To the Chinese it is the kidney; in France and Germany, it is the liver; for the British and United States, it is the large intestine.

This is not surprising because the lining of the gastrointestinal tract is the body's first site of contact with toxins ingested with food or medications, and with a wide array of infectious microorganisms. Also, part of the first line of immune defense is in the gastrointestinal tract. The gut lining provides a physical barrier, keeping toxic substances and organisms from entering the body, and the mucosal membrane inhibits and removes toxins and microorganism.

The second most important organ of detoxification (after the liver) is the large intestine. Contrary to popular notions, the large intestine or colon is more than a mechanical tube for the passage of feces, ending in defecation. Within it exists a living environment densely packed with anaerobic bacteria (called intestinal microflora), some "friendly" and some possibly pathogenic, crowded together with parasites, yeast and molds, tissue cells of various kinds, bile salts, excreted hormones, toxins, drug residues, water, and digested food material. Microflora are as integral to effective cleansing and health as is a good diet; microflora supplementation with acidophilus bacteria is often a part of a detoxification and rejuvenation program.

Blood and Lymphatic System: Traditional nature cure doctors knew that "cure" meant the complete replacement of diseased cells with healthy ones. To achieve this, they emphasized that cleansing the blood was the first goal of detoxification therapy. Without healthy and clean blood, the cells can never be renewed.

These are the typical signs of toxic blood:

- One easily has adverse reactions to most drugs, including opposite effects or effects with only small dosages.

- Adverse reactions to caffeine, including difficulty falling asleep even from coffee consumed in the morning.

- Pimples, red welts, or boils, and easily infected hair follicles.

Another vital body system for detoxification is the lymphatic channels, which are of particular importance for clearing out viruses. The lymphatic system is a network of tiny tubules running through all tissues in the body. Lymph, a clear fluid filtered from blood, circulates in these tubules. The lymph nodes are filtering stations positioned along these channels and are mostly found on the front and back of the neck, in the armpit, along the groin, and in the abdomen. White blood cells are very active inside the lymph nodes, clearing out viruses, bacteria, other infectious microorganisms, and allergens.

For detoxification therapy to be successful, it must improve lymph circulation, cleanse the lymph fluid and nodes, and improve liver and bowel function. Naturopaths and medical doctors who are adopting the naturopathic model believe that the three main goals of detoxification are to detoxify the liver, cleanse the colon and restore the microflora environment, and clean the blood. For viral immunity, this list should also include a fourth goal—to purify the lymph.

Exercise helps to move the lymph, especially aerobic types such as using a mini-trampoline, jumping rope, or old-fashioned calisthenics. Aerobic types of yoga are perhaps the best exercises to move the lymph. Inversion of the body, as done in many yoga postures, is very beneficial for improving lymph circulation and providing great benefit for general health. I cannot overemphasize the importance of correct physical activity for health, because without exercise, you cannot be completely physically healthy.

Antimicrobial and blood-cleansing herbs are essential in clearing the lymph vessels from toxic overload in chronic viral disease. These herbs include red clover *(Trifolium pratense)*, yellow dock *(Rumex crispus)*, and echinacea *(Echinacea purpurea, E. angustifolia)*. Mixtures of these herbs along with other blood purifiers have a long history of use in natural medicine, including the famous Hoxsey and Essiac cancer formulas. Though these formulas may not be cures for cancer, they are both excellent detoxification formulas, and I often recommend them to my patients as part of a cleansing program.

Connective Tissue: According to the late Dr. Hans-Heinrich Recheweg, a German medical doctor and the founder of homotoxicology (a system of medicine using homeopathic combinations to remove toxins and stimulate natural immunity), the connective tissue is one of the branches of what he called "the great defense system."

The connective tissue, and the thick extracellular collagen fluids that embed the connective tissue fibers, are easily damaged by toxins, disease, infection, inflammation, and excessive bacterial die-off from antibiotic use. Connective tissue is responsible for maintaining the form of the body, as well as for cushioning and support, and includes adipose fatty tissue, cartilage, ligaments, tendons, and the bones. These tissues are also directly affected by stress by the adrenal hormone cortisol. All of these influences increase inflammation and contribute to chronic pain and abnormal immune response.

The web of the connective tissues, a viscous group of protein fibers and a transparent substance composed of glycoproteins and glycosaminoglycans (long chains of polysaccharides), exchanges fluid and molecular compounds with the blood and lymph. This relationship between the connective tissue, the substances that compose them, and the circulating blood and lymph is critical to health. If the lymph is not draining properly due to sluggishness, is loaded with infection, or the nodes are swollen with antigens and allergens; and if the blood is clogged with fat (as in those with high cholesterol and triglyceride levels), or full of circulating toxins and antibodies to infectious microorganisms, then the connective tissue will become loaded with toxins and become blocked with mucus and fat.

Therefore, cleansing the connective tissue is imperative for effective detoxification to take place. Exercise, especially graceful types that activate the limbic or "ancestral" brain such as tai chi, dancing, swimming, and yoga, are helpful in improving lymphatic circulation. Also connective tissue massage, acupuncture, and trigger point therapy are helpful. General detoxification measures are useful, and once the blood and liver are freer of toxins, the connective tissue can often resume cleansing itself if the toxic burden is not too great. To support the connective tissue repair process, specialized biological medications called drainage remedies, composed of cellular enzymes and herbs, are used.

Drainage remedies are natural herbal medicines or homeopathic preparations that assist in the removal of toxins and promote the function of the organs and substances of detoxification, primarily the liver, blood, lymph, and the connective tissue. Antimicrobial, anti-inflammatory medications, and others dedicated to cellular detoxification, may be combined with organ drainage remedies to destroy bacteria and viruses circulating in the blood and lymph.

Cellular detoxification is part of the body's defense mechanisms and is the process by which the cells themselves release toxins, as well as viruses and viral particles, into the bloodstream for elimination from the body. Since viruses are intercellular parasites, gradual cellular detoxification is necessary to eventually rid yourself of the virus or to establish a symbiotic balance of coexistence between your immunity and the virus.

Professional drainage and cellular immunity products can be obtained through a physician practicing detoxification therapies. There are several homotoxicology drainage remedies that I routinely use in my practice, which I'll list here:

- Pascoe Lymphdiaral cream: applied topically in the area of the lymph glands in order to promote lymph drainage; apply two times daily.

- Heel Lymphomyosot sub-lingual vials: to clear the lymph and reduce edema and swollen glands; dissolve the contents of one vial under your tongue two times daily, at least twenty minutes away from food in the morning and evening.

- Heel Ubichinon sub-lingual oral vials: to stimulate defense mechanisms against toxins in order to reactivate blocked enzymatic pathways; take in the same manner as Lymphomyosot.

- Heel Chelidonium-Homaccord oral drops: to clear the liver and treat hepatic inflammation; take in the same manner as Lymphomyosot.

How to Make a Homemade Antiviral Drainage Remedy

Simmer 2 quarts of distilled or filtered water for 20 minutes with 2–3 teaspoons (10–12 grams) of the following herbs:

- Red clover flowers (*Trifolium pratense*)
- Lonicera flowers (*Lonicera japonica*, the Chinese herb *jin yin hua*)
- Cut and sifted yellow dock root (*Rumex crispus*)
- Andrographis herb (*Andrographis paniculata*, the Chinese herb *chuan xin lian*)
- Isatis root (*Isatis tinctoria*, the Chinese herb *ban lang gan*)

After simmering, let the mixture stand with a tight lid for another 20 minutes, then strain into a large glass jar. Discard the herbs. Add 1 bottle of echinacea tincture and 1 bottle of goldenseal root tincture to the tea. Take 1/4 cup of the mixture 4 times daily during the cleansing process.

- Heel Coenzyme Compositum oral sub-lingual vials: to stimulate blocked enzymatic systems in degenerative disease; take in the same manner as Lymphomyosot.

- HVS Biosode and Detoxosode oral liquids: for organ system support and cellular regeneration and repair; place one teaspoon of each under your tongue in the same manner as Lymphomyosot.

Drainage remedies can also be prepared at home by mixing herbal tinctures or teas. You can make an effective drainage remedy by combining tinctures of echinacea and goldenseal into a tea of red clover, yellow dock root, and other herbs.

Other Organs Involved in Detoxification and Elimination: Included in this group are the kidneys, lungs, and skin. The kidneys are not primary detoxification organs like the liver and large intestine, but they are important in helping to maintain normal fluid levels and facilitate the exchange of fresh fluids in body tissues. They also filter the blood and excrete urine, through which a number of toxins, hormones, and immune substances are eliminated. Drinking copious amounts of pure water, fresh juices, and herbal teas is an important feature of a cleansing program. However, it is important not to overconsume fluids on a regular basis, since they can cause excessive excretion of minerals.

The lungs are responsible for respiration. They are the site in your body where air from the outside atmosphere interacts with the internal environment. Through a process involving specialized lung tissue, an exchange of gases occurs in the lungs and eventually oxygen circulates in the blood. Due to the direct contact with outside air, the lungs are influenced directly by environmental toxins and allergens. Since air must first pass through the nose and then to the lungs via the sinuses, it is not surprising that there is an epidemic of allergic rhinitis (inflammation of the nasal passages) and chronic sinusitis due to increasing exposure to toxins and irritants.

Gargling with salt water and using saline rinses or sprays in the nose are necessary to cleanse and heal the mucous membranes of the upper respiratory passages. Qi gong breathing exercises and yogic alternate-nostril breathing are helpful in cleansing the lungs. Most importantly, one has to stop smoking and avoid indoor air contamination and outdoor pollution. The habit of jogging during lunch hour in urban environments should be strictly avoided, as the pollution levels are highest around midday due to increased automobile exhaust and heat from solar radiation; this causes increased release of toxins from plastics and synthetic building materials.

As I have previously mentioned, when you exercise outdoors it is always best to perform your routine early in the morning when the air is freshest, the oxygen content richer, and the outdoor pollutant levels lower.

The skin is the last organ of elimination I'll mention in this discussion. Toxins are eliminated in the sweat and in secreted oils from the sebaceous glands distributed all over the body's outer protective sheath, the skin (the intestinal lining is the other, inner, sheath). I recommend showering at least twice daily during a cleansing regimen and taking at least one hot bath in Epsom salt, or a detoxifying bath composed of hydrogen peroxide and sea salt. Dry skin-brushing is also very helpful, as are saunas, steam baths, or soaking in hot mineral water.

Detoxifying Baths

- Epsom salt: add 1–2 cups per tub full of warm water; soak up to 20 minutes.

- Peroxide and Sea Salt: add 1 quart of 3 percent hydrogen peroxide and 1/2 teaspoon of sea salt to a tub full of warm water; soak for 20 minutes.

Skin Brushing

Before your shower or bathe: using a dry lufa sponge, a coarse all-natural cotton wash cloth, or a dry vegetable bristle brush, gently but briskly rub your entire body. Shower off immediately after. Perform dry skin brushing once a day.

Therapeutic Detoxification and Immunity

I have already discussed how detoxification improves general health by removing wastes and stagnated toxins from the connective tissue, how it improves sluggish lymph, enhances liver function, promotes the return of normal gut ecology, and improves many other physiological and biochemical processes. Detoxification improves overall health, and by doing so indirectly engenders a positive effect on the immune system.

The specialized viral immunity cleanse is somewhat different from typical detoxification regimens because it focuses on improving immune function and the removal of viruses and their wastes from your system. It uses drainage medications to discharge cellular toxins, cleanse the blood, and defeat infectious microorganisms at the cellular level. Keep in mind that this program will not directly kill viruses, nor is it meant to do so. It is designed to be a complementary part of the complete 10-step viral immunity program. Results occur gradually, so patience and perseverance are required to achieve the best results.

Detoxification improves general health by removing wastes and stagnated toxins from the connective tissue, improves sluggish lymph, enhances liver function, promotes the return of normal gut ecology, and improves many other physiological and biochemical processes.

Is It Safe to Use Detoxification Therapies for Viral Illnesses? In my experience, it is not only safe, but *mandatory* to practice detoxification if you have a chronic viral disease. Remember, it is not a fast. During the three-day viral immunity cleanse, described later, you eat whole foods and take supplements and herbs. I do not recommend complete fasting for patients with a viral illness, and I never recommend active cleansing during the acute phases of illness when inflammation and fever are present, or at the end stages of viral infections when the patient is extremely weakened by the disease process.

During acute phases, the body's inflammatory and febrile processes must be supported and managed (discussed in step 5), and during end-stage disease, the body must be supported and nourished. Detoxification plays a role in both these cases, but it is beyond the scope of this book to explain it here. I suggest you seek the help of a licensed naturopathic physician or other doctor skilled in these methods if you have an advanced viral disease and want to detoxify.

In viral illness, the body is already weakened by at least three things. The first is the original immune deficiency that allowed the virus to enter and remain in your body. Factors that negatively influence immunity include environmental toxins, stress, unhealthy aging, or all the other contributors discussed in part 1. The second is the damage to tissue and organs caused by the virus itself, and the third is immune elements from your own body that build up in response to the virus but may cause more harm than good and result in chronic inflammation.

It is important not to stress your system further and never to push it beyond its capacity to regenerate. Remember, the goal is improved health. The steps to good health begin with a healthy diet and balanced lifestyle, supplementation of micronutrients, detoxification, and regeneration therapies to restore organ reserve and promote normal physiological and biological body function.

Fasting on water or juices for too long may further weaken your body, allowing the virus to dig in deeper and perhaps even replicate further. With that said, let me say that this is a generalization. Some people may benefit from short fasting (1–3 days). However in my opinion, fasting any longer than a few days should *only* be done with the approval of and under the supervision of a qualified professional and in a facility with twenty-four-hour care.

In addition, people with inflammatory skin disorders like psoriasis, or with rheumatoid arthritis, may experience severe exacerbations of their conditions and should never undergo a fast or lengthy detoxification regimen. If you have these conditions, you should be able to safely undergo the three-day viral immunity cleanse presented below; however, if your symptoms worsen during the program, discontinue it immediately.

Who Will Benefit Most? Nearly everyone in our stress-filled, toxic world will benefit from natural detoxification methods. For many health conditions, detoxification is a mandatory part of a comprehensive healing program. Patients with chronic fatigue, fibromyalgia, irritable bowel syndrome, and degenerative neurological conditions can benefit most from detoxification.

Healthy people can promote wellness and prevent disease by using detoxification therapies. Those with minor recurrent problems like headaches, joint pains, stiffness, constipation, edema, and who are overweight can also greatly benefit from detoxification. The methods in this chapter are specifically designed for people with immune challenges and chronic viral disease, so they will receive the most benefit.

Detoxify When and for How Long? You might be wondering if detoxification is so important why isn't it step 1 or 2 instead of step 4. The reason is simple. You should never detoxify unless you are strong enough to handle the release of toxins from your body. Detoxification is not a benign process. My clinical mentors referred to detoxification and fasting as "nature's operating table."

It puts great demands on your body's reserves and stresses metabolic processes. In addition, chemical toxins and residues are released into the bloodstream, causing the liver to function at an increased level during the cleansing process. As mentioned, some of these released chemicals are even more toxic than their original forms. Sometimes this leads to a detoxification crisis with severe headaches and nausea. Generally, these crises last only a few hours or no more than a day; however, occasionally, they are so severe you will have to discontinue the detoxification process and start again later when your body is better prepared. Do not be discouraged. As long as you persistently move forward, even with a few false starts, you will eventually succeed.

Therefore, you have to first eliminate harmful substances, improve your diet, and strengthen your body with health-giving nutrients and enzymes. Then, by optimizing nutritional factors, your body will automatically begin its own intracellular detoxification. It will restore glutathione reserves, improve organ function and restore organ energy reserve, improve the management of oxidative stress from free radicals, improve gut ecology, build mineral reserves, and improve your strength and endurance.

How Can You Tell When You Are Strong Enough to Detoxify? If you are acutely ill, you are probably not ready for detoxification and should stay with steps 1–3 for an extended period of time, even up to one to two years, before you attempt detoxification. For the most part, it is relatively easy to tell when you are ready for detoxification.

If you are not overly weak, are gaining strength, feeling much better than before you started the first three steps, and have been on steps 1–3 for at least three months, then you are ready. If your exercise tolerance has improved, your appetite is better, and you are able to eat more foods and tolerate more different foods, you are most likely ready.

When Is the Best Time to Start? There are many cleansing styles and different types of detoxification regimens, so the answer to this question is that the best time is individualized. However, for those with viral disease, my recommendation is for a mild three-day detoxification program repeated once each month for up to one year. Take a month off if you are feeling very tired or have an active exacerbation of an infection. Set aside a weekend, begin on a Thursday night, and go through to Sunday afternoon.

In general, for longer cleansing diets and detoxification programs, begin any time and go from seven to twenty-one days. For more intensive detoxification, you need at least seven to nine days set aside,

Nine Important Therapeutic Detoxification Strategies

Strategy #1. Remove toxic lifestyle factors

Strategy #2. Emphasize phytonutrient- and enzyme-rich foods, juices, and amino-acid-rich whey protein

Strategy #3. Increase redox (oxidation-reduction capacity) with antioxidants

Strategy #4. Improve blood and lymph circulation

Strategy #5. Promote elimination

Strategy #6. Improve liver function

Strategy #7. Promote kidney function

Strategy #8. Use drainage remedies

Strategy #9. Rest and recharge

preferably without working too hard and with no social functions to attend. For those with serious viral illness, I recommend that you only do the longer and more serious detoxification programs under the direct supervision of a qualified health care practitioner or in a facility that specializes in detoxification therapies and provides twenty-four-hour care. Several such facilities are listed in the back of this book. Regardless of how long or when you plan to start your detoxification program, it is important to plan ahead and make it a priority that you schedule into your busy life.

In this section, the nine most important strategies for detoxification are outlined. Each is mandatory and contains important clues to successfully carrying out your detoxification plan. In the next section, I give a sample program. Review each strategy and program carefully, and read them several times to be sure you understand every point.

Strategy #1. Remove toxic lifestyle factors: You begin a detoxification regimen by removing, gradually, and over time if necessary, all dietary and lifestyle habits that are not health-promoting. This includes reducing, or stopping altogether, smoking, alcohol consumption, the use of coffee, caffeinated soft drinks, and recreational drugs including marijuana, as cannabinoids may be liver-toxic. It is not wise to start a detoxification program until the negative influences on your health are permanently removed.

Prescription drugs pose a problem. Some drugs are critical for controlling symptoms while at the same time they place a high toxic load on the liver. If you are taking prescription medications, review each one with a pharmacist and discuss their necessity with a medical doctor or osteopathic physician who supports your choice of following a detoxification regimen. You can still do the three-day viral immunity cleansing program if you are taking prescription drugs; however, under these conditions, I recommend supervision by a physician for your own safety.

Limit or completely avoid the use of refined sugar in any form, such as commercial fruit juices, candy, pastries, and sweetened cereals. The consumption of all other refined or processed foods, fried and preserved foods (including chips and commercial pickles), and processed fats and oils, like margarines including soy spreads, should be discontinued. Avoid all cow's milk and milk products such as yogurt and cheese, since dairy products increase intestinal fermentation and yeast activity, are highly allergenic, and may contain hormones and antibiotics.

Strategy #2. Emphasize phytonutrient- and enzyme-rich foods, juices, and amino-acid-rich whey protein: To support natural detoxification and maximize Phase I and II liver detoxification pathways, enhance your diet by eating only fresh, seasonal, (organic, if possible) vegetables and whole fruits. Rice is allowed, but all wheat products are out; animal meats, fish, and poultry are not allowed. Drink 1–2 glasses of fresh vegetable juice or a green drink every day.

According to David W. Quig, Ph.D., a specialist in detoxification processes, cold-processed, hydrolyzed whey protein is one of the most important supplements for cleansing. Whey protein increases glutathione levels, adds important amino acids that support liver detoxification pathways, and is high in cysteine and branched-chain amino acids (BCCAs). These prevent the heavy metals that move into the bloodstream during detoxification from entering the brain. The following is a list of generally allowed foods during a detoxification program:

- Carbohydrates: rice (organic white, jasmine or Thai, basmati, brown).

- Legumes: soy products (tofu, miso, tempeh), mung bean sprouts, aduki beans.

- Vegetables: all leafy green vegetables (red leaf, romaine, and other garden lettuces; spinach, endive, kale, Swiss chard, beet greens, bok choy and Chinese broccoli, arugula, mustard green, dandelion greens); all root vegetables (carrots, beets, parsnips, radishes, fennel root, yams, potatoes [also a carbohydrate], turnips, daikon, gobo, yucca, rutabaga); cruciferous vegetables (cabbage, cauliflower, broccoli, brussels sprouts, collards); cucumbers; squashes; onion family (shallots, red and white onions, green onions, leeks, garlic); asparagus; okra; celery; sweet and hot peppers; tomatoes.

- Fruits: eat all fruits, except grapefruit (since it contains substances that inhibit liver detoxification); keep acidic citrus to a minimum. However, do not over-do the fruits since they are high in natural fruit sugar and low in vitamins and minerals compared to vegetables.

- Seeds and nuts: small amounts of raw organic seeds and nuts are acceptable if you get hungry between meals; grind and mix with juice or make as nut butters to ease digestion.

- Oils: cold-pressed olive oil is allowed and can be added to cooked vegetables or on salads; evening primrose and organic flaxseed oil are also recommended to support omega 3 and 6 fatty acid balance.

- Seaweeds: all sea vegetables are allowed and recommended.

- Spices and condiments: use vegetable salts, naturally fermented soy sauce or tamari (wheat-free soy sauce), Bragg's liquid aminos, and all culinary spices (sage, thyme, basil, cilantro, cardamom, cumin, oregano, marjoram, rosemary, and others), and small amounts of vinegar of all types.

- Teas and herbs: all herbal teas (mints, chamomile, raspberry), chrysanthemum tea, green tea, and jasmine tea are allowed.

- Water: distilled, filtered, or spring water.

Strategy #3. Increase redox with antioxidants: Increasing supplemental antioxidants is essential, and vitamin C is again the main building block. Take 500–1,000 mg of pure or buffered vitamin C powder frequently throughout the day, up to bowel tolerance. Take the recommended dosages given in step 2.

Additionally, antioxidant amino acids and specialty antioxidants that facilitate detoxification pathways are necessary, such as: L-glycine, L-glutamine, taurine, N-acetyl cysteine (NAC), and methionine. Here is a detoxification nutrient schedule:

Two Chelating Agents

Keep in mind that if you are chelating heavy metals from your body either by oral DMSA or intravenous DMPS, it is best to avoid supplemental minerals twenty-four hours before and three days during or after chelation, as these minerals will also be chelated out of your system. However, it is critical to add them back in, along with molybdenum and copper, immediately following the chelation period to replace those lost in the process.

DMSA, or dimercaptosuccinic acid (Captomer), and DMPS, or sodium dimercaptopropanesulfonate (Dimaval), are chemical substances that bind to mercury and lead and remove them from the body. DMSA is a nontoxic, water-soluble oral medication that is capable of removing heavy metals, including mercury, from brain and other difficult-to-access body tissues.

DMPS is administered intravenously or by injection, and once in the bloodstream binds with mercury and is excreted in the urine. It is used as a challenge test to evaluate mercury toxicity by collecting a sample of overnight urine, administering 300 mg of DMPS, and then collecting another urine sample 6 hours later. If mercury levels are elevated, indicating mercury toxicity, another chelator, EDTA, is used to chelate the mercury from the system. EDTA, ethylenediaminetetra-acetic acid, is a weak acid used to remove heavy metals and it is considered beneficial in reversing atherosclerosis.

- Vitamin C: 500–1,000 mg, every two hours, up to 10–20 g or to bowel tolerance

- Vitamin E: 400–500 IU, two times daily with meals

- Selenium: 400 mcg, two times daily between meals

- Zinc: 50 mg, daily between meals

- Lipoic acid: 600 mg, two times daily between meals

- NAC: 500 mg, two times daily between meals

- L-glycine: 1,500–3,000 mg, once daily between meals

- Methionine: 1,000 mg, two times daily between meals

- Taurine: 500 mg, two times daily between meals

- L-glutamine: 500–1,000 mg, two times daily between meals

- Choline: 500 mg, two times daily with meals

- Calcium d-glucarate: 500 mg, two times daily between meals

- Magnesium: 250–500 mg, two times daily between meals

- Niacinaminde (non-flushing form of vitamin B3, niacin): 500 mg, two times daily between meals

- Methylsulfonylmethane (MSM) or organic sulfur: 500 mg, once daily

You can obtain each of these supplements separately, or use a commercial detoxification products such as UltraClear Plus or MediClear. These products are composed of all of the supplements listed above along with vitamins and minerals in a hypoallergenic rice base; I regularly recommend them for my patients.

Strategy #4. Improve blood and lymph circulation: Circulation of blood and lymph is essential. Light, non-strenuous exercise such as tai chi, swimming, walking, mild cardiovascular work-outs on the treadmill, and calisthenics is helpful. Strenuous exercise like martial arts, jogging, tennis, and heavy weight training are too enervating and you should not do these during a cleanse. Never exert yourself to the point of exhaustion.

Sweating in a sauna is very helpful to improve lymph drainage and eliminate toxins in the body fluids, but do not stay in for longer than twenty minutes. Drink at least three liters (3.15 quarts) of distilled water daily to replace the fluid lost in sweating and urination, and an extra liter (1.05 quarts) if you sweat heavily. Bikram's (or "hot yoga") is a style of intensive yoga practice done in a room heated to 105° F and is an excellent way to cleanse and strengthen the body as it causes copious sweating during practice; it can be exhausting for some people, so take it easy if you attend a class. These practices can be performed daily during the cleanse regimen.

Swedish or lymphatic massage can be helpful, but remind your massage therapist that you are undergoing a detoxification regimen and ask him to do a thorough but light massage so as not to release too many toxins from the connective tissue. You can have a light massage daily if you wish, but be sure to drink at least a quart of water immediately afterward to facilitate the cleansing of acids released from your tissues as a result of the massage.

Skin brushing is also helpful. Use a dry luffa or vegetable-bristle brush and lightly stimulate the skin over all of your body until it seems to glow. A dry, coarse washcloth will also work. Do not rub or brush yourself too hard. Immediately afterwards, take a warm shower and rinse, but without using any soap.

Strategy #5. Promote elimination: Never allow yourself to become constipated during the detoxification process. Take extra fiber, such as 1–2 teaspoons of psyllium powder with bentonite clay, 1–2 times daily. If you experience constipation, first try increasing your dosage of vitamin C; as mentioned, high dosages of vitamin C

Liver-Protective Herbs

Milk thistle *(Silybum marianum)*
Dandelion *(Taxaxacum officinale)*
Celandine *(Chelidonium majus)*

Liver-Supportive Foods

Beets
Radishes, radish sprouts, daikon
Dandelion greens
Endive

have a laxative effect. If necessary, use an herbal laxative containing cape aloe *(Aloe socotrina),* cascara *(Rhamnus purshiana),* or senna *(Cassia senna).* Commercial products containing these herbs are available from health food stores.

Coffee enemas have a long history of use in detoxification therapies. They activate the liver pathways, stimulate the gallbladder to release bile, and act as a laxative. However, I do not recommend enemas unless you are experienced in the correct manner of delivery or are under the supervision of a health care practitioner. Likewise, colonic irrigation can be helpful; however, limit its use to one colonic per cleanse and use only as necessary, as they can be enervating. Older, weaker, and frail patients should not use colonics.

Probiotic supplements of acidophilus should be taken during the cleansing process. I generally recommend 5–10 billion units two times daily of a combination of *Lactobacillus acidophilus* and *Bifidobacterium infantis;* both are readily available in combination from health food stores.[2]

Strategy #6. Improve liver function: Many of the nutrients listed and the cleansing diet in general facilitate liver function. Several herbs in particular greatly improve the outcome of the detoxification process and protect the liver from excessive overload by free radicals and toxins activated by the cleanse. Combinations of these herbs are obtainable from health stores or from your naturopathic doctor.

Strategy #7. Promote kidney function: Natural diuretics are found in carrots, parsley, watermelon, peaches, and peach leaf tea, and should be used during your cleanse to promote urination. Water itself is also a diuretic, leading to increased urination. Kidney-supportive herbs include uva ursi *(Arctostaphylos uva ursi),* stinging nettle *(Urtica dioica),* and cleavers *(Galium aparine).* Carrot juice, especially with added parsley, and watermelon juice work well as mild diuretics. During the summer peach season, ripe peaches can prove effective in promoting urination; green tea is also a diuretic if taken in large amounts.

Urine that's dark yellow (not bright yellow, which is from B vitamins), cloudy, or frothy indicates excessive concentration and insufficient fluid. If you experience this during your detoxification, increase your water intake. If the urine continues to be a dark brownish-yellow color or has a strong odor, try the juices. If that is not enough to turn the urine to a clear color, add the diuretic herbal teas while increasing water intake until your urine becomes clear or a very light yellow and without any odor.

Strategy #8. Use drainage remedies: Drainage remedies are important additions to the viral immunity detox program, assisting and protecting the liver, improving kidney function, activating cellular response, and cleaning the lymphatic vessels. If you have access to the homeopathic medications previously mentioned, use them as indicated. Otherwise use the homemade tea and tincture combination explained earlier. If none are available, use echinacea tincture by itself; empty a two-ounce bottle into a quart of water and drink a quarter of a cup four times each day. As a reminder, the homotoxicology drainage remedies for the three-day viral immunity detox are:

- Heel Lymphomyosot

- Heel Chelidonium-Homaccord

- Heel Ubichinon

- Heel Coenzyme Compositum

Strategy #9. Rest and recharge: Get as much rest, stress reduction, peace, and quiet as you can. Allow your body to experience the natural cleansing process and give it the opportunity to heal itself. See step 10 for more advice on how the mind and spirit can heal the body. The three days of the cleanse program is your time to rest and recover.

Special Guidelines for Three-Day Viral Immunity Detoxification Regimen: Even though the detoxification method I have outlined is very safe, there are several special circumstances of which you need to be aware.

Heavy metal toxicity: If you have mercury amalgam dental filings, have worked in a dental office, or have tested positive for accumulation of environmental mercury, you will have to undergo intravenous or oral chelation therapy. The most effective form is EDTA given in a series of intravenous sessions and administered by a licensed physician. Oral DMSA is somewhat effective for mercury and is equally effective as DMPS or EDTA for other heavy metals like lead and cadmium. These therapies should only be administered by a qualified health care professional.

Three-Day Viral Immunity Detoxification Regimen

Thursday: Prepare body, mind, and spirit

1. Conduct your normal daily routine, though slow down and mentally prepare.

2. *Follow strategy #1:* Remove alcohol, unnecessary medications, sugar, sodas, and processed foods. Eliminate milk products.

3. Prepare the cleansing products.

4. Eat normally in the morning and afternoon, but do not eat after dinner.

5. Take a detoxifying bath and retire to bed early.

Friday: Day 1

1. *Morning:* Upon waking, drink one ounce of aloe vera juice with two ounces of the homemade antiviral drainage tea, along with liver-protective herbs.
   a. Meditate or pray for 10–20 minutes
   b. Practice breathing exercises for 10 minutes
   c. Drink 6–8 ounces of water
   d. Exercise for 10–20 minutes
   e. Rest if you can, or go to work

2. *Mid-morning:* Around ten, take the first dose of supplements (listed in strategy #3) with 6–8 ounces of water and 2 tablespoons of whey powder, which you can blend with fruit, a teaspoon of flaxseed oil, or diluted fruit juice. If you are able to obtain UltraClear Plus or MediClear, mix one scoop in a cup of water and drink it completely.

3. An hour later drink 6–8 ounces of mixed vegetable juice, or a green drink.

4. *Lunch:* Eat a mixed vegetable salad seasoned with olive oil, lemon or lime juice or vinegar for dressing.
   a. Take vitamin E with your meal

5. *Mid-afternoon:* Take the second dose of supplements, without food, along with a second glass of vegetable juice, and a second cup of UltraClear Plus or MediClear.

   a. Exercise for 10–20 minutes, or take a yoga class of 1–2 hours if you can

6. *Dinner:* Eat a full dinner, but only from the allowed food groups (see the list of allowed foods in strategy #2):

   a. Carbohydrate (choose one): rice, baked or boiled potato, baked yam, tofu

   b. Steamed vegetables or vegetable soup

   c. Mixed green salad

7. *After dinner:* Take the homotoxicological medications from strategy #8 (choose one from the group or take another cup of drainage tea).

   a. Take 1 teaspoon of a probiotic powder or 2 capsules with warm water

   b. Take a cleansing bath

Saturday: Day 2

1. Repeat Friday's schedule.

2. Have a massage or acupuncture treatment.

3. Take a yoga class or exercise lightly.

Sunday: Day 3

1. Repeat Saturday's schedule for the morning.

2. At noon, have a lunch of vegetable soup and a mixed salad.

3. Repeat the afternoon schedule.

4. Have a normal meal in the evening and return to your normal routine on Monday.

Very weak or elderly patients: People who are frail, very elderly, or weakened from disease may undergo cleansing therapies and even fasting, but only under the supervision of a qualified health care professional.

Patients with serious infections: Those with serious viral infections, like HIV and HCV, should only undergo aggressive detoxification under the supervision of a qualified healthcare professional. The Three-Day Viral Immunity Detoxification Regimen should pose no problem; however, if you have a concern, consult a professional experienced in detoxification *before* you begin.

Patients with other microbial infections: Patients with yeast, fungal, bacterial, or parasitic infections need specialized medications to combat these infections, and this is beyond the scope of this book. However, if you have other microbial infections, you can use the basic three-day detox plan, adding to it antimicrobial and antiparasitic herbs.

Herxheimer and other reactions: First noticed with the early use of antibiotics, if excessive die-off of microorganisms occurs, flulike achiness and malaise or a worsening of symptoms can occur. This is known to medicine as the Herxheimer reaction. For a short time, you feel worse than before as your system struggles to eliminate a great deal of toxic substances. With natural remedies, massive die-off with Herxheimer reactions does not usually occur, but is possible. The best way to deal with microbial die-off is to increase vitamin C by taking 500 mg of buffered C every half hour until the symptoms disappear. Because many viruses are expelled in the stool, colonic irrigation can also be extremely useful to limit these reactions.

If the liver is excessively burdened or unprepared for detoxification, you may experience severe headaches and fatigue, perhaps even dizziness. If this happens, increase your fluid intake, reduce solid food, and increase vitamin C. Usually headaches clear in a matter of hours; however, if they persist or are severe, you will have to discontinue the cleanse and start again next month.

Energy Medicine and Detoxification

Systems of cleansing and detoxification are also integral to both Chinese and Ayurvedic medicine. Ayurvedic physicians use complex regimens of fasting, steaming the body, cleaning out the orifices (like the sinus cavities), purging the colon of fecal matter, using retained oil enemas (which means the oil is retained in the lower large intestine for a short while), and taking cleansing herbs. Called *panchakarma*, these programs have been used for thousands of years in India and are now practiced in specialized centers in the West. Traditional yoga practices also have numerous cleansing regimens and rituals, many of which, such as nasal washing with a saline solution, are practiced daily; they can be learned from an advanced yoga teacher.

Chinese medicine, mainly practiced in cooler, more temperate climates than India, advises against harsh cleansing regimens. Instead, it focuses on improving the energy flow within the body, thereby indirectly enhancing the body's own natural detoxification mechanisms. Enemas, colonics, and emetics have a potential to weaken the body, so are used only when necessary. However, energy clearing and rebalancing—recharging one's batteries—are essential during a cleansing regimen.

The ancient Chinese concept of *ping gan*, or "settling down" the liver, would greatly improve the quality of health in the West if we were to apply it. According to this concept, rest, extra sleep, and general peace and quiet provide the opportunity for the liver to harmonize itself. Metaphorically, the white caps on the waves of a choppy sea settle down on their own when the wind stops. It's the same with the liver.

Exercises that activate the limbic brain, such as tai chi or qi gong, are excellent ways to clear the acupuncture energy meridians or channels during a cleanse. Energy balancing therapies, like acupuncture and acupressure, are very useful also and may be included as part of a detoxification and regeneration process.

CHAPTER SUMMARY

Detoxification is a crucial cornerstone of natural healing.

Everyone can benefit from detoxification, and for most people suffering from chronic disease, including viral illness, it is mandatory.

It is best to start slowly and with short detoxification programs of no more than three days, done one weekend per month for six months to a year.

Always include drainage remedies when detoxifying.

Always increase your redox potential with extra vitamin C and other antioxidants.

Add specialized amino acids and other nutrients that facilitate detoxification.

Drink plenty of filtered, distilled, or pure spring water.

Do not fast completely on water or juices; instead, use a vegetable-based cleansing diet.

Avoid becoming constipated by eating high-fiber vegetable foods before and during your cleanse, and use herbal laxatives only as a last measure.

Headaches and fatigue are normal during detoxification; however, they should not last any longer than 24–36 hours. If they last longer than that, terminate your cleanse and restart when you feel stronger.

Herxheimer die-off reactions may occur. It you experience flu-like symptoms that are severe or persist for more than six hours, this may be from microorganism die-off. Have a session of colonic irrigation, make sure you are drinking plenty of water, and increase your vitamin C intake. If symptoms persist, discontinue the cleanse.

Get plenty of rest.

10

STEP FIVE

Restore Your Innate Immune Response and Manage Inflammation

The cornerstones for viral immunity were laid in steps 1 through 4. In this fifth step, you will learn how to restore the normal innate immune response and how to manage inflammation and chronic pain associated with degenerative disease and chronic viral infection.

An Illustrative Case

Valerie, a young, energetic, bright, and ambitious woman, went into the business world right after college. To get well positioned in her company as soon as possible, she worked long hours and took work home on the weekends. No stranger to a sampling of marijuana in college, more aggressive drugs at parties in the corporate world, and the social cocktail or glass of wine, she couldn't see the harm in the occasional use of drugs or alcohol. Work came before boyfriends, so her relationships were transitory, though she recently had met an attorney who she thought had potential for her. To keep fit, Valerie exercised regularly at a gym and also ran several times weekly.

Four Good Reasons to Use the Strategies Outlined in This Chapter

If you have chronic fatigue associated with a viral illness.

If the first symptom of a common viral infection is fatigue rather than fever.

If you frequently experience chills with fatigue at the first sign of a cold.

If you have inflammation associated with a chronic viral disease.

There are several steps involved in restoring normal inflammatory responses, some that you may do on your own and some that will require the supervision of a physician. Please review the following lists carefully before you continue:

What You Can Do

Reduce stress.

Get regular rest.

Replace strenuous exercise with slow, limbic-system stimulating movements like tai chi, yoga, or swimming and walking.

Replace pharmaceutical NSAIDs and COX-2 inhibitors with natural anti-inflammatory medications, acupuncture, massage, and chiropractic.

What Your Doctor Can Help You With

Prescribe a sleeping medication to assist in improving your sleep cycle.

Help you taper off steroid drugs, and replace them with hydrocortisone or natural cortisol, if necessary, and manage rebound inflammatory conditions as the dosage is reduced.

Prescribe short-term antibiotics to manage bacterial infections, but with the goal of *eliminating* antibiotics.

Prescribe and manage NSAIDs, with the goal of replacing them with natural alternatives or eliminating their need.

Precautionary Note: *If you are taking steroid drugs like prednisone to manage an autoimmune condition, under no circumstances should you or any unqualified person, reduce or stop using steroid drugs without medical supervision.*

Her daily routine went something like this: she got up at 6:15, showered, checked e-mail while the coffee was brewing, drank a glass of packaged orange juice, and poured the coffee to drink in the car. She applied her makeup and brushed her teeth while driving, as well as answering her cell phone's voicemail and calling her girlfriend to set up a dinner date for that evening. When she arrived at work, she bought a bagel in the deli on the ground floor of her office building and ate it while standing in the hall taking to coworkers. For snacks, she nibbled all morning on candy at her desk and drank a second cup of coffee around mid-morning; then more candy, a break outside, and an occasional cigarette, depending on the stress of the day.

She ate lunch at her desk, and this frequently consisted of a commercially pre-packaged chicken Caesar salad and two glasses of ice tea with sugar. Her afternoon business schedule included reviewing reports, calls, meetings, coffee, and candy. At the end of the day, she worked an extra forty minutes to straighten her desk and finish e-mails, then she rushed to get home, only to end up stuck in traffic; she turned the radio on loudly to control her frustration. In fact, she wanted to scream most times, but instead reached for breath mints and downed five or six sugar-and-menthol tabs.

At home, Valerie would check her voice messages while changing into her jogging outfit, and immediately take off on a four-mile run to burn off stress and extra pounds. When she returned home, she showered and then drove to meet her friend for seafood pasta and salad, two glasses of white wine, a cup of decaf coffee, and a small dessert. Typically, she had a great time. At home, she would realize she forgot to take her vitamins, so she'd pop a handful of pills and capsules. She didn't know why she took them, but said she was told they are good for energy, weight control, and general health. They energized her, so she often found it hard to fall asleep afterward.

Then, one weekend, she ran a half-marathon sponsored by her company for needy, crippled children. Afterwards she hugged some of the kids wearing t-shirts with her company logo. One of them had the sniffles; the next day Valerie was sneezing and had a running nose. She thought it was an allergy. By the end of the day, she had a headache and felt achy all over. On the way home she stopped at the drugstore and bought an over-the-counter cold medicine. She stayed up late working on a document due the next morning. In the morning, when she woke up she felt feverish and her head was pounding.

She took more cold medications and two aspirins. At work, she gave the presentation, and went home sick in the afternoon.

At home, just as she was trying to rest, Valerie's sister called. One of her kids fell down and has to go to the emergency room for stitches. Could she come right over and watch the baby for a few hours? Valerie grabbed some paperwork and a box of Kleenex, and drove a few miles to her sister's place. The baby also had a cold, and Valerie had to hold it the entire time she was there to keep it comforted. When she got home, she took more aspirin, finished another report, then fell into bed.

The next day, Valerie felt tired and her head was congested, but she went to work anyway. Her cold lingered through the week, and on Friday her affair with the attorney took a turn for the worse. She stressed and worried over it on the weekend. On Monday, half of the employees of the company were coughing and sneezing. In fact, she had noticed that people were frequently sick with colds or had allergies in her building.

Just before her menstruation, Valerie had an outbreak of herpes, something she contracted in her wilder days before college. She started on the Acyclovir her physician prescribed for her last year. The next week, she had pressure in her head and felt tired and saw her physician, who spent a few minutes with her and diagnosed sinusitis. He prescribed antibiotics and decongestants.

Valerie developed a vaginal yeast infection the third day into the antibiotics and also had diarrhea. To reduce her stress, she took an extra-long run, even though she was feeling poorly. Rather than the energized sensation she usually had after a run, she felt exhausted. The next week she had no sinus symptoms but was still tired.

Since the relationship was finished, Valerie stopped taking her birth control pills and the irregular menstruation and cramping that she had before her use of the pill returned. Stress mounted in her company due to labor cutbacks, and though she did not lose her job, the worry and anxiety of the other employees affected her. More people seemed to have colds and flu, and she caught two in three months. The third cold caused symptoms of wheezing and chest pressure, and her doctor prescribed medications and steroid inhalers for asthma.

In the fall, Valerie had another sinus infection, and in the winter she had another bout of asthma and got more prescription drugs for treatment. Her PMS increased, and she comforted herself during her period with candy. Valerie's weight gradually went up and she was unhappy with how she looked, so she started dieting. Her weight went down but so did her energy. Work was as stressful as ever. Her new boyfriend was nice but lived in another city, and they only saw each other once or twice a month.

In the winter, Valerie had yet another cold that led to sinusitis. This time, she had no fever and experienced head pain and pressure on the left side of her face. The asthma returned, and she was using the inhalers every day. The sinus infection was treated with another round of antibiotics, which did not work at all this time. The doctor tried a different antibiotic, which also did not work, so he sent her to an eye, ear, nose, and throat specialist, who prescribed a stronger antibiotic, which caused a rash all over her body.

By this time, Valerie was able to continue to work and function socially, but she did not feel well. She had recurrent diarrhea, episodes of vaginal yeast infections, frequent herpes outbreaks, PMS and cramps, irregular periods, sinusitis and asthma, and she routinely took several prescription medications. When she got a cold, which is every few months, she felt tired but kept working. She did not have a fever and the doctor never asked her about how her colds started or presented, but only treated her symptoms.

You can see that Valerie had a weakened innate immune response. She did not get a fever when she caught cold or flu or had a sinus infection. Stress was disrupting her hormonal rhythms and poor diet exacerbated problems with her periods. Her metabolism had trouble regulating her blood sugar, so she craved sugar, and stress disrupted her adrenal function, resulting in insufficiency of cortisol. This added to the sugar metabolism problem. She had minor chronic inflammation in the intestines and in her respiratory tract. The drugs were not curing her condition, but only treating some of the symptoms, while creating other problems directly due to continued use.

When Valerie came to see me she had chronic fatigue, chronic herpes reactivation, increasing incidence of allergic-like reactions, food intolerance, irritable bowel syndrome, and was on an antidepressant. She was an excellent candidate for the strategies outlined in this book, and her case and lifestyle illustrate many of the points I've made about immunological fitness and how we lose it.

You can learn several things from Valerie's case. First, her condition was largely self-inflected due to a stressful lifestyle. Second, toxic environmental conditions contributed to her immune disruption. Third, prescription drugs complicated her clinical picture as the different aspects of her initial complaints were not differentiated from those that were actually a result of an infection and those that were part of her immune response (or lack of it).

Simply put, you cannot get completely better if the normal febrile and inflammatory responses of your innate immune system are blunted or if you have chronic inflammation. Certainly, if you have a serious autoimmune disease it may be possible to reduce your symptoms and improve your quality of life by using anti-inflammatory drugs. Indeed, sometimes this is the best option one can use *temporarily*, but it is not possible to attain a complete cure without normalizing pro-inflammatory immune chemicals and restoring the innate immune response.

You cannot get completely better if the normal febrile and inflammatory responses of your innate immune system are blunted or if you have chronic inflammation. It is not possible to attain a complete cure without normalizing pro-inflammatory immune chemicals and restoring the innate immune response.

Restoring the Febrile Response

As discussed in chapter 4, fever is a naturally occurring response of the innate immune system to infection. It triggers changes in brain chemistry, local tissue and cell activity, and the release of cytokines, resulting in an elevated temperature. However, in repeated infections (perhaps coupled with frequent use of aspirin or acetaminophen to suppress mild fevers), the febrile immune response becomes blunted or absent. Why this happens is not well understood. The results of this blunting effect is that fever, the universal sign that humans know as the first clue of illness and infection, is missing. Instead the first symptom of an infection becomes fatigue.

The Significance of Rest: The restoration of the febrile response takes time and patience, and once again we come back to the basics of diet, exercise (or when not to exercise), and, all-importantly, rest. For those with a blunted febrile response replaced by fatigue, the first thing to do is to develop the awareness of when your body is sick and tired.

Rest when you feel tired and at the first signs of a cold or flu, such as a stuffy nose, sneezing, headache, or pain in the back of the neck or head. At this time, you are more vulnerable to other infections, allergens, antigens, and indoor air pollution, so stay home and avoid further exposure. This may be a foreign idea to many Americans who are used to rushing home from work, taking the kids to soccer practice, and visiting an aging mother in the nursing home. However, if we do not change our life- and work-styles, we will become a nation of ever sicker individuals.

Rest means that you cease activity and work. When attempting to rebuild your innate immune system, allow your body the space and time to slowly and progressively work its miracles. Stay home from work and cease any activity around the house; do not watch television, read for long periods of time, or listen to loud music, as the nervous system and sensory organs must also rest. Instead, listen to soothing music while resting in bed or sitting comfortably in your favorite chair. Shut the phones off or screen your calls.

Keep the shades drawn and avoid bright sunlight, as excessive sunlight disrupts the immune system. Ultraviolet radiation can affect the severity of infectious disease; worsening skin diseases like herpes and smallpox. Bright sunlight also lowers melatonin levels, a hormone of the pineal gland that not only helps you sleep but is a powerful antioxidant. A shaded room is more conducive to rest and recovery during illness. Practice quietness and stillness. Repeat healing affirmations, like "My cells are growing stronger and I am getting healthier minute by minute." Meditate, if you like.

If you work for a large company, ask your doctor for a note explaining your condition and recommending that over the next three months, if you feel ill, you will have to stay at home. A short-term leave of absence of a week or two may be necessary if your condition persists or is severe. Disability should be reserved for only the severest cases. Your doctor can advise and help you with these issues.

The Necessity of Sleep: Sleep is critical in cases of both blunted febrile response and chronic inflammation. While resting, allow yourself to sleep if you feel sleepy. In general, you need 9–12 hours of sound sleep each night to restore immune reserves. During periods of active infection, your body may require up to 14 hours or more of sleep.

In the early years of my practice, I was amazed by a phenomenon that occurred regularly among my patients. When healing responses were activated either by acupuncture, hands-on energy work, or cranial therapy, patients often became very drowsy and routinely fell asleep on the treatment table. In fact, it was not uncommon for some to go home, even in the afternoon, feeling so overwhelmingly sleepy (not simply tired) that they would lie down and sleep for 14–20 hours straight. When they woke, they felt great.

This type of response is the body's instinctive mechanism taking over to restore and heal through sleep. In the ancient Greek temples dedicated to Asklepios, the god of healing, patients went there to sleep and dream, allowing their bodies' healing power to work a cure.

Sleep is so important that having insomnia is one of the few instances in which I allow a short-term prescription of pharmaceutical sleeping medications. If you have a sleep disorder, try the natural remedies listed in step 1, but if these do not help improve the quality and patterns of your sleep, you may need to consult with your doctor for the temporary use of sleeping medications.[1]

Managing Fever: As you follow the viral immunity principles in this book, your health will gradually return, as will your febrile response. Your first fever may be mild and fluctuate during the day, worsening at night. Fever is a sign of infection, but not all infections are bad. This next point is very important. When your next fever or infection develops, work with a naturopathic physician or other doctor experienced in managing fever. Do not attempt to treat the first fever on your own. This first fever may require several different treatments and medications to assist your body in restoring a normal immune response.

Useful treatments include acupuncture, homeopathy, and herbal medicines. Immune-modulating medications, such as lactoferrin or transfer factor, may be also required. Your immune system may still be too weak to fight off a bacterial co-infection. Access to a physician who uses intravenous vitamin C or concentrated allicin (a medical garlic extract) may be necessary to control an opportunistic bacterial infection.

If the infection cannot be controlled with natural medicines, you may need to take an antibiotic or use steroid drugs again. However, this should be viewed as a *temporary* crutch only, and do not allow a temporary setback to discourage your will to continue. If you persist on the path towards rebuilding your immune system, eventually you will succeed and your immune function will be restored.

Temperature Fluctuations: Symptoms of fever include an overall warm body sensation, flushed cheeks, a forehead warmer than the body, a warm or sweaty feeling, and sometimes chills. You can take your temperature with a mercury thermometer, an oral digital thermometer, or the newer ones that insert in the ear.

The average normal body temperature is 98.6° F, but at about 99.0–99.5° F, you may only feel slightly flushed and experience only a mild fever. This is considered a low-grade fever. If it persists more than a few days or longer, you may have a smoldering internal infection and require medical evaluation. Even then, it is often difficult to determine the cause of persistent low-grade fevers. Regardless, a fever induced by the innate immune response will rise and then decline as the illness wanes; generally, it does not persist over ten days.

Above 100° F, you will have the classic symptoms of fever and systemic inflammation, including loss of appetite, general malaise, stiffness and aching, weakness, and sleepiness. A fever above 101° F in an adult or 102° F in an infant or child requires active management and even medical intervention.

What to Do About a Fever: A low-grade fever is managed with rest, increased fluid intake, and natural remedies. Remember, fever is a sign of infection and even a low-grade fever persisting more than two weeks requires a consultation with your doctor to determine the cause. For mild infections, use echinacea, boneset, or elderberry tea.

The long-held notion of "starving a fever" is supported by naturopathic physicians and doctors who uphold evolutionary medical principles. Eric R. Yarnell, N.D., president of the Botanical Medical Academy in Sisters, Oregon, says that substances called dietary lectins can increase the likelihood of infection from viruses and other pathogenic microorganisms, and they can also induce autoimmune diseases (Yarnell 2001). Lectins are proteins that bind with sugars, and are found in many common foods including milk, wheat, legumes, and the nightshade family (potato, tomato, eggplant, and peppers). Fasting when you have a fever, or at least completely avoiding all dairy and wheat products, helps to prevent the risk of more serious illness.

Active fevers under 102° F can also be managed with rest, increased fluid intake, and natural remedies. Increased body temperature exerts stress on metabolic functions and reduces appetite, but not eating may lower your blood sugar levels, making you feel very weak. To avoid this possibility, add honey to the herbal teas to keep your blood sugar levels stable.

You will need to take natural antimicrobial medications, such as garlic and grapefruit seed extracts, to manage the infection. (These medications are explained in detail in step 7.) Cool baths or sponge baths can control mild fevers by keeping your overall body temperature lowered. In high fevers, Tylenol, or children's Tylenol for those sensitive

Factors that Increase Inflammation

Abnormal fatty acid metabolism

Acidosis

Allergies

Cortisol imbalances

Buildup of pro-inflammatory cytokines

Excessive and prolonged stress

Excessive or overstrenuous exercise

Glucose dysregulation

Gut dysbiosis

Increased sympathetic dominance

Increased oxidative stress

Poor blood and lymph circulation

Tissue breakdown

Tissue damage from repetitive use, or trauma of muscles and tissues

Toxins

Steps that Will Decrease Inflammation

Improve fatty acid metabolism

Increase alkalinity and reduce acidity

Remove and avoid allergens, and improve allergic tolerance

Normalize cortisol

Reduce cytokine and chemokine activity

Reduce stress

Balance your exercise with rest and recovery time

Eliminate refined sugar and improve glucose tolerance

Improve intestinal symbiosis

Increase parasympathetic activity

Reduce oxidative stress

Improve blood, lymph, and connective tissue fluid circulation

Increase anabolic metabolism and reduce catabolism

Change your work or exercise routine to minimize repetitive trauma

Detoxification

to medication, may be necessary to manage an active fever.

Managing Inflammation with Natural Remedies

The inflammatory response is intimately connected with immunity, degenerative processes, and healing. Usually, if chronic inflammation is present, no true cure takes place until the inflammatory process is under control and the underlying causes eliminated. Normal inflammation occurs when there is tissue damage from trauma or infection as part of the natural inflammatory immune response. Chronic inflammation is also part of the body's way of attempting to keep an abnormal condition under control. However, in the process, it can cause harm to other tissues and lead to organ degeneration and even organ failure, as is the case with advanced chronic hepatitis C virus.

There are three types of imbalanced inflammatory responses: 1) chronic low-grade inflammation; 2) absent or blunted response; and 3) heightened response. As discussed in chapter 4, many factors increase abnormal inflammation and because of their significance, they are worth reviewing. Avoid or remove as many of these factors as you can.

Strategy #1. Rest and improve sleep: It may come as no surprise to you by now that the first step involves rest and appropriate sleep. Looking at the list of biological factors that decrease inflammation, several are affected by rest: balancing acidosis and increasing alkalinity; improving allergic tolerance; normalizing cortisol; reducing stress; enhancing recovery; improving autonomic nervous system balance and increasing parasympathetic activity; and reducing repetitive trauma. Deep sleep normalizes body rhythms, relieves stress, restores hormone balance, promotes the body's healing capacity, and helps to reduce inflammation.

Strategy #2: Balance diet and ratio of omega-6 to omega-3 fatty acids: Nutritional influences play a significant role in reducing inflammation. Protein and carbohydrate deficiencies, and low levels of vitamins A, C, D, E, B-complex, and trace minerals can exacerbate inflammation. Steps 1 and 2 provide information on dietary and supplemental nutrition to help manage inflammation. Additionally, improving the intake ratio of fatty acids by ensuring adequate omega-3 fatty acids will help reduce inflammation.

Eicosapentaenoic acid (EPA), gamma linolenic acid (GLA), linoleic acid (LA), and docosahexaenoic acid (DHA) are referred to as essential fatty acids (EFAs), and adding them to your diet can reduce inflammation and influence immunity. However, the balance between the different types of oils is crucial.

EPA comes from cold-water fish like salmon and is an omega-3 fatty acid. It is useful for managing inflammation and treating depression. GLA and LA belong to the omega-6 fatty acid family. GLA sources include borage, black currant, and evening primrose oils. These are referred to as the "good" omega-6 fatty acids and are used to reduce inflammatory abdominal pain and improve the mood fluctuations associated with premenstrual syndrome.

Linoleic acids are also found in plants and include the oils of sesame, safflower, sunflower, flax, pumpkin, and walnut seeds. Omega-6 fatty

9 Strategies to Help You Manage Chronic Inflammation

Strategy #1. Rest and improve sleep

Strategy #2. Balance diet and ratio of omega-6 to omega-3 fatty acids

Strategy #3. Exercise

Strategy #4. Avoid allergenic foods

Strategy #5. Reduce acidosis

Strategy #6. Regulate cortisol

Strategy #7. Take proteolytic enzymes

Strategy #8. Manage pro-inflammatory cytokines and chemokines

Strategy #9. Use anti-inflammatory herbs and nutrients

acids are necessary for healthy skin and hair growth and help to regulate metabolism, among their many functions in the body.

DHA, another omega-3 fatty acid from fish oil is important for the normal functioning of the nervous, immune, and cardiovascular systems, and helps regulate inflammation during infection. It is used to treat a wide range of diseases including arthritis and psoriasis, and can help reduce blood pressure. Using excessive amounts of olive oil can decrease DHA's anti-inflammatory properties. Omega-6 fatty acids, found in both olive and corn oil, when consumed in excess amounts, can produce inflammation.

Omega-3 and omega-6 fatty acids follow similar metabolic pathways in the body, but if the ratio between the two favors omega-6 fatty acids, inflammation can develop. The recommended ratio is 1 to 1; however, in the Western diet, the ratio is unbalanced with an excess of omega-6 fatty acids.

Reduce olive oil consumption and use safflower seed and sunflower seed oils. Supplement with a tablespoon of flaxseed or pumpkin seed oil instead; take 2–4 grams of EPA and DHA in capsules from fish oil. Eliminate corn oil and all fried foods.

Strategy #3. Exercise: Strenuous exercise increases inflammation, tissue damage, and oxidation, so avoid strenuous exercise and change to slow, rhythmic movements. Balance rest with exercise. It is not healthy to remain stationary or sedentary for long periods; movement is essential. Swim, practice hatha yoga or tai chi, or walk. Take saunas; as described in step 4, they improve lymph and blood circulation and help to reduce inflammation.

Strategy #4. Avoid allergenic foods: Certain foods have greater potential to cause allergies than others, and allergies can trigger inflammation in susceptible individuals. The most reactive foods are wheat and products like bread and pasta made from wheat, and cow's milk and products like cheese and yogurt. Other common allergenic foods are soy, eggs, yeast, and peanuts.

If you have chronic inflammation or a viral illness, do not eat these foods for one month. Once you introduce them back into your diet, follow a rotation diet and do not eat the same food more than two times per week and allow two days between each time you have them. If you suspect allergies are part of the cause of your illness, consider allergy testing for food hypersensitivity by a laboratory blood test called the enzyme-linked immunosorbent assay (ELISA).

Strategy #5. Reduce acidosis: Acidosis, an abnormal increase in the acidity of bodily fluids, generally accompanies inflammation. If you have inflammation, change your vitamin C from pure ascorbic acid to a calcium-magnesium buffered form. Additionally, take a quarter teaspoon or two 250 mg capsules of sodium and potassium bicarbonate every one or two hours during active inflammation and then reduce to a maintenance dose two to three times daily for one to two weeks. Sodium and potassium bicarbonates are highly alkaline, and when taken as nutritional supplements rapidly reduce acidosis in the body. Other, though slower, ways to reduce acidosis are by drinking green vegetable juices and adding more vegetables in your diet.

Caution: Do not take bicarbonates for longer than two weeks, as you can over-alkalinize your system. Though excess alkalinity is not associated with inflammation in the same way acidosis is, it can cause other symptoms, including a sensation of excess energy and insomnia that could indirectly make your condition worse by robbing you of rest or sleep.

Strategy #6. Regulate cortisol: Excessive or deficient levels of cortisol, an important adrenal hormone, are often involved in inflammatory conditions. Resting, following the diet outlined in previous chapters, managing blood sugar levels, getting appropriate exercise, and reducing stress all help to restore normal cortisol activity. However, for some people with adrenal insufficiency, either genetic or as the result of excessive stress, supplementing with adrenal cortical extracts or hydrocortisone may be necessary. (For more details on hormone balancing see step 9.)

Strategy #7. Take proteolytic enzymes: Proteolytic enzymes, introduced and discussed in step 3, have potent anti-inflammatory activity. Take four to six tablets of Wobenzyme three to four times daily between meals or one hour before eating. Proteolytic enzymes are safe and have no adverse effects other than causing occasional indigestion. If that occurs reduce your dosage until your system adapts to them and the indigestion ceases.

Strategy #8. Manage pro-inflammatory cytokines and chemokines: Use quercetin, a flavonoid discussed in step 2, to manage pro-inflammatory cytokines, the immune molecules associated with inflammation

Table 13: Natural Medicines for Inflammation

Medication	Action	Dosage
Curcumin	Inhibits COX-2 enzymes and prostaglandins	500 mg 3 times daily away from food
Quercetin	Inhibits pro-inflammatory chemokines	500–1,000 mg 3 times daily away from food
EPA/DHA	Balances omega-3 essential fatty acids	Up to 10 g with food
Lipoic Acid	Inhibits NF-κB	300 mg 2 times daily away from food
Selenium	Improves immune function and works as an antioxidant	400 mcg 2–3 times daily away from food
Moducare	Reduces inflammation by promoting interleukin-2 and inhibiting interleukin-6	2 capsules 3 times daily for the first week, then reduce to 1 capsule 3

(interleukin-1β, interleukin 6, and nuclear factor Kappa B). Many other substances, including B-vitamins, inhibit cytokines and chemokines, so by taking the supplement program outlined in step 1 and the phytonutrient-rich foods in step 3, your program will have sufficient amounts of these substances. Take 1,000 mg of quercetin three times per day.

Strategy #9. Use anti-inflammatory herbs and nutrients: There are a number of natural herbal preparations for managing chronic inflammation, such as the extract of curcumin/turmeric *(Curcumin longa)*. Selenium and lipoic acid also help to reduce inflammation. Take 500 mg of curcumin three times daily, increase your selenium to 400 mcg three times daily, and lipoic acid to 300 mg twice daily. Ginger root *(Zingiber officinale)* is also a very useful natural anti-inflammatory and can be used as a tea made from the fresh or dry powdered root (use 1–4 g per cup).

Plant sterols, or phytosterols, are a group of fat compounds found in all plants, but mostly in unprocessed seeds, nuts, legumes, and grains. The most active phytosterols are beta-sitosterol and beta-sitosterolin; these function as immune modulators by enhancing the secretion of interleukin-2 and gamma-interferon, but without promoting pro-inflammatory cytokines such as interleukin-6. They also improve natural killer cell function.

Phytosterol concentrates are useful in the treatment of autoimmune diseases like rheumatoid arthritis and managing inflammation due to the effects of chronic viral infections such as HCV. They are useful in treating chronic prostatitis, allergies, hives, and the management of inflammation due to chronic infection. Plant sterols are commercially produced under the trademarked name of Moducare (Sterinol) in a standardized form (20 mg of total plant sterols and 200 mcg of sterolins); the recommended dose is 2 capsules, three times daily for one week, and then 1 capsule, three times per day thereafter.

Nourishing Energy Deficiency

Many recurrent and chronic illnesses are associated with weakness in one or more important energy systems of your body. Once again, fatigue is the common symptom among them all. If important vital organs, such as the kidney or spleen, are very deficient, they will require long-term supplementation with adaptogenic (stress protective) substances.

The Chinese medical model clearly defines deficiency patterns in ways that allopathic and even naturopathic medicine do not. According to traditional Chinese medicine, the organs that most easily become deficient are the kidneys (and adrenal glands) and the spleen (and pancreas). In addition, the energy substrates of qi and blood may become deficient.

> ## Conditions Associated with Energy Deficiency
>
> Catching cold and flu easily
> Chilly feelings, or sensitive to wind, air conditioning, or cold weather
> Chronic fatigue
> Chronic viral illness
> Colds that last more than two weeks
> Difficulty recovering from exercise or after staying up past midnight
> Easily fatigued after mild exertion
> Recurrent herpes outbreaks
> Recurrent or chronic bacterial or fungal infections

Each organ, as well as the qi and blood, has yin or yang qualities. Yin is more passive, feminine, and cool in temperature. Yang is hot, fiery, aggressive, and masculine. For example, when the kidney yin is deficient there is less coolness and more fire, causing headaches and hot flashes. When the qi and yang energy are deficient, you feel tired, chilled, and have an aversion to cold; your complexion is pale, as is the body of your tongue. You easily catch cold and have a tendency to feel much more tired than usual when ill. The innate defense system, the *wei qi*, is deficient.

The herb of first choice for qi and yang deficiency is *huang chi*, also known as astragalus *(Astragalus membranaceus)*. Astragalus contains

Table 14: Chinese Herbs to Restore Innate Immunity and Manage Inflammation

Herb	Indications	Forms and Dosage
Astragalus	Restoration of the innate immune system (wei chi deficiency)	Tea: 9–15 g, Tablet or capsule: 500 mg, 3 times daily
Ligustrum	Treatment of inflammation in chronic viral disease (with yin deficiency)	Tablet or capsule: 250–300 mg of the extract, 3 times daily

flavonoids, and the triterpene glycosides astragaloside I-VII, the main immune-modulating substrates in this herb. It is available in health stores or from your acupuncturist, and is taken as a tablet, capsule, or tea. If you have the deficiency symptoms listed above, take this herb daily as part of your natural supplement program. There are no known side effects or interactions; however, astragalus is traditionally contraindicated during fever, inflammation, or in yin deficiency (described below; see step 8 for more details on this herb).

Your yin systems are deficient if you have chronic inflammation and pain, organ inflammation or enlargement, low-grade fever, a tendency to have excessive yellow or greenish phlegm, hot flashes or night sweats; or if your tongue is red or you experience fatigue. In this case, you can use the Chinese yin tonic herb, *nu zhen zi,* or ligustrum *(Ligustrum lucidum).*

Like astragalus, ligustrum has been extensively studied in the laboratory and in clinical research. Its active ingredient is oleanolic acid, or ligustrin, and it is used to treat inflammation in immune-deficient patients. It has been shown to reduce alanine aminotransferase (ALT) levels and cirrhosis in chronic hepatitis, promote phagocytosis by macrophages, and improve white blood cell count in cancer patients whose immune function has been suppressed by radiation or chemotherapy. Ligustrum is taken in tablet or capsule form and has no known toxicity or interactions.

CHAPTER SUMMARY

Rest and restoration of the normal sleep cycle are the most important factors in reducing inflammation and restoring innate immunity.

Avoiding and eliminating causative factors should come before using supplements or natural medications.

Treat bacterial co-infections with natural antibiotic alternatives.

Add selected natural anti-inflammatory and chemokine-inhibiting medicines.

Nourish energy-deficiency states with Chinese herbs.

As your health improves, gradually taper off NSAIDs, COX-2 inhibitors, steroids, antibiotics, and over-the-counter cold medicines with help from a supportive allopathic physician and naturopath.

11

STEP SIX

Boost Your Immunity with Natural Immune Enhancers

Can we program or stimulate the immune system to perform better? If we could, it would solve many of the problems caused by viruses, other infections, and cancer. Unfortunately, though we can condition the immune system, stimulating it is not like training a watchdog. It is much more complex: There is no simple "on" or "off" button.

To protect us and keep us alive, our immunity adapts to constantly changing environmental influences and evolves in a manner based upon principles we are only just beginning to understand. Though we cannot yet program the immune system, there are ways to manage and enhance its functions. This chapter will discuss natural immune modulators and how to use them, including information on clinical advances that might in time help us enhance immunity against the modern viral plagues.

What Are Immune Modulators?

Immune modulators (immunomodulators) are substances that have regulating effects on the immune system. Researchers often use the term biological response modifiers interchangeably with immunomodulators. To allopathic medicine, immunomodulators include a variety of drugs that either down-regulate (suppress) or up-regulate (increase) immune activity. These include steroids, interferon, and inosine, a substance that increases the effect of interferon and which has been studied in the treatment of herpes simplex virus.

From the alternative medicine perspective, natural immune modulators are thought to tune up the immune system and to reverse or prevent illnesses related to immunity, aging, and chronic infection.

Immune modulators have also been called immunostimulatants, immunoceuticals, and immunotics. This is a term with a familiar ring to its suffix in that it refers to pharmacologically produced substances like pharmaceu*tics* (drugs) and nutraceu*tics* (pharmacologically manufactured nutritional or herbal substances in more concentrated amounts than occur naturally). Immunotics, a term coined by Robert Rountree, M.D., is also semantically connected to probiotics (substances like acidophilus that support natural microflora) and antibiotics (medications that destroy bacteria including microflora) (Rountree 2000). Regardless of what term is used, the substances and medications in this chapter are immune-*enhancing*—stimulating—and boosting agents.

What Do Immune Modulators Boost? Until the 1990s, most of the research on natural immune-enhancing agents has focused on the treatment of cancer. From the results of this research, many of these agents were found to affect the immune system in a manner that also improved antiviral activity. The majority of the early research in the viral area was for the treatment of AIDS, later for herpes viruses and HBV, and now HCV. However, some of the knowledge gained from cancer and AIDS investigations can be applied to other viruses.

We know that immunomodulators increase NK cell activity, enhance B-cell and T-cell function, increase production of various cytokines, reduce pro-inflammatory cytokines, and promote macrophage activity. For the most part, they benefit all aspects of innate immunity. Some are also powerful antioxidants that scavenge cellular debris left by radiation and infection.

Keep in mind that though there are thousands of scientific studies on immune-modulating agents, and that a significant amount of clinical evidence indicates they improve immune activity, they are not sufficiently powerful to work alone in improving immune function.

However, a synergy occurs when they are combined with other immune-enhancing agents, such as antioxidants, stress reduction techniques, and phytonutrients. Follow the entire viral immunity program in order to achieve the most benefits along these lines.

Who Needs an Immune Boost? This is easy to answer: in our postindustrial toxic world, *everyone* needs immune-enhancing. Those with chronic fatigue, all forms of chronic microbial infections including viruses, recurrent colds and flu, cancer, or allergies and asthma, all require immune modulation and most will benefit from these substances. Certain precautions may apply, so read about each immune modulator before you choose which one is best for your condition.

> *In our postindustrial toxic world, everyone needs immune-enhancing. Those with chronic fatigue, all forms of chronic microbial infections including viruses, recurrent colds and flu, cancer, or allergies and asthma, all require immune modulation and most will benefit from these substances.*

From my clinical experience, all my patients with cancer, chronic fatigue syndrome, autoimmune disorders, recurrent infections, and chronic infections (including viral disease) have a disrupted immune system and benefit from immune enhancement. Additionally, immunological concerns are not only involved in diseased states, but are important to everyone exposed to the modern toxic environment—particularly urban dwellers. Given the number of factors that can disrupt the immune system, medicines that have the power to normalize it have enormous potential. To meet this need, many new immune-enhancing medications have been produced from naturally occurring substances, most of them previously used in traditional medicine.

In my clinical opinion, immune dysfunction is becoming increasingly common and may become one of our most serious health concerns. To meet this challenge, evaluating immune status should be a standard part of a regular physical examination. Currently only a complete blood count (CBC) is routinely taken, and only if significant deviations from normal are seen does a medical doctor even take notice. However, with the increasing incidence of immune system disorders and chronic infectious illnesses, as well as cancer, white blood cells should be looked at more closely.

If imbalances are present, or if the patient has symptoms indicating immune dysfunction (such as chronic fatigue or recurrent respiratory tract infections), then a comprehensive T-lymphocyte panel should be performed. By tracking abnormal immune cell levels or activity, such as is done with NK cells, you can judge the effectiveness of your immune enhancement regimen.

A Review of the Best Immune Modulators

The following immune-modulating substances are those that have the best substantiating research behind them and a history of wide clinical use. However, no one knows exactly how they work in the body or the best way to take them to obtain the maximum results. Some companies have put several immune modulators together in one product, as there is some evidence that a synergistic affect occurs. They are all generally safe and there are no known contraindications for mixing them, except where noted.

Acemannan: Indigenous to Africa, but now found globally, there are over 200 known species of aloe. The best known is true or common aloe *(Aloe vera, Aloe barbadensis)*. The raw gel has been used since the time of the Egyptians for the treatment of burns and cuts, and in India for intestinal infections and constipation. It is also considered to have anti-inflammatory properties.

Acemannan, an immune-enhancing mucopolysaccharide (a carbohydrate), is an extracted component found in the gel of the aloe vera leaf. Research has shown it to increase cytotoxic T-cell activity, stimulate macrophage function, and to release interleukin-1 from monocytes. Two prescription drugs have been developed from acemannan by Carrington Labs. Carrisyn, used as an immune stimulating adjunct with antiretroviral therapy in AIDS, has been shown to improve CD-4 counts. Carravet, a veterinary preparation, is used for the treatment of feline leukemia virus and fibrosarcoma (a connective tissue cancer of the bone or around muscles or nerves).

Manapol, also manufactured by Carrington, is a nonprescription oral acemannan concentrate that is used as an immune enhancer. A dose of 40 mg of Manapol is equivalent to 1 ounce of the fresh aloe gel and is taken by mouth in dosages from 80–240 mg daily. Aloe gel, if taken in high dosages, can cause loss of potassium due to diarrhea, but Manapol is considered safe to take in the recommended dosages and apparently does not have the laxative effect of the gel or dried pure concentrate. There are no known drug interactions with acemannan. It is a general immune system booster and is frequently found in combination formulas containing glucans and transfer factor, or with antioxidant vitamins and minerals.

Arabinogalactan: Another polysaccharide, arabinogalactan, is commonly found in nature in carrots, radishes, pears, black beans, corn, wheat, red wine, tomatoes, and coconuts. Several herbs already mentioned in this book also contain arabinogalactans, such as *Echinacea purpurea, Baptista tinctoria,* and *Curcuma longa.* The wood of the Western larch tree *(Larix occidentalis),* native to the Pacific Northwest, provides the raw material for the extraction of medicinal arabinogalactan.

Pharmaceutical-grade larch arabinogalactan is a fine, dry, white powder that readily dissolves in water; it has a slightly sweet taste due to the presence of two sugar molecules: galactose and arabinose. It is considered extremely safe and may even be given to children. There are no known side effects in the recommended dosages other than occasional intestinal gas and bloating due to fermentation by gut flora, and there are no known drug interactions.

Like acemannan, arabinogalactan has been primarily studied as a possible adjunctive anticancer agent. In laboratory studies it was shown to stimulate NK cell and macrophage activity. Larch arabinogalactan can be used as an immune modulator in acute and chronic viral diseases, chronic fatigue, and multiple sclerosis. Peter D'Adamo, N.D., naturopath and the author of *Eat Right 4 Your Type,* suggests that arabinogalactan acts synergistically with vitamin C (D'Adamo 1996). This combination makes sense because vitamin C appears to enhance the immune-stimulating function of polysaccharides by making them easier to absorb.

The dosage is 1–3 tablespoons (1 tablespoon equals 4–5 g) of the powder per day, mixed in juice or water, and buffered vitamin C may be added. Since it is a good source of fiber and exerts vigorous activity on intestinal flora, the "friendly" bacteria *Bifidobacterium bifidum* and *Lactobacillus acidophilus* may be mixed with larch arabinogalactan powder. In one study, these probiotic substances together caused an increase in B cells. For children, the dose of larch arabinogalactan is 1 teaspoon in juice, given in divided dosages 2–3 times per day.

Beta 1, 3-D Glucan: Beta-glucans are components of fungal cell walls and are commercially derived from mushroom species and common baker's yeast. Glucans and proteoglycans isolated from mushrooms also have promising immunoceutical potential. Extracts of cordyceps, a glucan-containing Chinese medicinal fungus, are one of the best of the immune-modulating substances for viral infections. Beta-glucans have been widely studied as biological response modifiers since the 1940s. They have considerable broad spectrum immune-enhancing effects, including tumor rejection, prevention of bacterial infection in postoperative cases, modification functions against certain fungal and parasitic infections, improved immunity in older people, and the treatment of viral diseases.

Beta 1, 3-D Glucan is a pure isolated polysaccharide compound extracted from the cell walls of baker's yeast *(Saccharomyces cerevisiae)*. Like many of the other immune modulators discussed in this section, it stimulates innate immunity and is a powerful antioxidant. Its main activity is as a potent macrophage stimulant; its maximum peak of macrophage activity occurs 72 hours after ingestion. It is prepared as an intramuscular or intravenous medication, and can also be taken orally. The oral dosage range is from 100 mg daily for prevention up to 20 g (20,000 mg) during active infection.

It is considered safe and nontoxic; not only does it have no known drug interactions, beta glucan may help antimicrobial drugs work better. Since it is a pure compound, even though it is extracted from yeast, there are no reported allergic reactions among users with yeast or mold sensitivities.

Mushroom Immunoceuticals: A considerable amount of research has been done on more than fifty different mushroom species with potential immune-modulating properties. They have been known for their medicinal benefits in Asia for thousands of years. However, researchers only discovered the active beta-D-glucan component recently.

Of the many mushrooms studied, five chemicals have shown activity against human cancers: lentinan from the shiitake mushroom *(Lentinus edodes);* active hexose correlated compound (AHCC), also from shiitake; maitake D-fraction from the maitake mushroom *(Grifola frondosa)*; schizophyllan from *Schizophyllum commune;* and various proteoglycans (PSK and PSP) from *Coriolus versicolor.*

The ones most commonly available on the American market are the trade combinations AHCC and MGM-3 (discussed below). Other mushroom extract combinations are also available, and research continues on new promising species. Though few have been researched for their effects on viruses, the significant enhancement of innate immune function they create warrants inclusion in an immune system rebuilding program.

MGM-3: Originally developed in Japan and researched by the internationally recognized immunologist Mamdooh Ghoneum, Ph.D., an expert on how the body's immune system fights cancer, MGM-3 is a patented blend of rice-bran hemicellulose B (a carbohydrate) and three different mushroom extracts including shiitake. This compound has been found to dramatically increase NK cell activity. Besides his work with cancer, Dr. Ghoneum, currently chief of research at Charles Drew University of Medicine and Science in Los Angeles, has also tested MGM-3 on HIV-1 and found it inhibits replication of the virus.

The recommended dosage is 3–4 g, three times daily for two weeks as a loading dose, and then 1–2 g, two times daily thereafter. A "loading dose" is a higher amount of a medication in the beginning of therapy in order to saturate the tissues and achieve adequate therapeutic blood levels of the medication. Once saturation levels are reached, a lower dosage is prescribed to maintain them.

AHCC: A cultured substance from hybridyzed mushrooms, AHCC contains hemicellulose, alpha 1, 4-glucan, and other substances. Like MGM-3, it is used extensively in Japan and Korea as a nutritional cancer preventative, and it is undergoing research as an adjunctive cancer medicine. The recommended daily dose is 6 g divided during the day.

Several anecdotal case reports on chronic hepatitis C involving these mushroom products are circulating on the Internet and indicate liver-protective effects and a reduction in viral load. There seem to be no scientific studies or clinical documentation to verify these claims, yet for those with HCV, including these products into your regimen may be of benefit, especially as there are no known side effects or toxicity associated with them.

GANODERMA: *Ganoderma lucidum,* the Chinese "mushroom of immortality" called *ling zhi* (in Japan, *reishi*) has been extensively studied in the laboratory for antiviral activity and is well known for its immune-modulating activity. My teacher of Chinese medicine, the late Dr. York Why Loo,[1] kept a specimen of dried wild Chinese *ling zhi* in a jar for use in his old age. So revered by Chinese doctors is *ling zhi* that it is frequently pictured on their business cards or displayed in their shop windows as a sign of respect for its importance.

Several Japanese and Chinese studies indicate that the polysaccharide compounds found in ganoderma have antiviral activity against herpes simplex types 1 and 2. In traditional Chinese medicine, ganoderma is used for weakness and deficiency of the entire system and is thought to be a cardiotonic. It is safe to take, without any known contraindications.

CORDYCEPS: *Dong chong xia cao* ("winter worm, summer plant") is a highly valued traditional Chinese medicine composed of the entire fungus, *Cordyceps sinensis,* and the dried body of the larvae of the moth on which it grows. It tonifies both yin and yang, thereby balancing the body, and it has anti-cancer, antimicrobial, sedative, anti-asthmatic, and adrenal gland-improving effects.

It has been studied extensively in China for its medicinal properties, and though once very expensive, commercial production has lowered its price dramatically. The Beijing Institute of Materia Medica of the Chinese Medical Academy in Beijing, China, found that the cultivated type has the same chemical constituents and is as effective as the naturally occurring form. In addition to its uses listed above, the Beijing researchers found cordyceps to have immune-modulating and anti-inflammatory activity.

Cordyceps increases interferon levels, tumor necrosis factor-alpha, and interleukin-1 and 2. It increases helper T cell counts, improves the helper-to-suppressor ratio, and stimulates NK-cell activity. In viral hepatitis it lowers ALT, increases albumin (a water-soluble protein), improves liver function, and reduces enlargement of the spleen and liver. This action reduces pressure on the portal vein, improves subjective symptoms, and dramatically improves stamina.

With these properties, cordyceps appears to be the ideal natural immune modulator for chronic viral disease. The dosage is 6–15 g of the dried herb made into a tea or 500–1,000 mg of the extract, three times daily, taken 10–20 minutes before food. It is safe even in very high dosages.

Caution: In traditional Chinese medicine, cordyceps is considered safe and may be taken over a long period of time. However, it is contraindicated in external conditions, i.e., it should not be used if fever is present, during an active cold or flu, or the acute phases of a reactivated virus.

Immune Products from Mother's Milk: Colostrum, a thin yellowish fluid, is the first pre-milk substance produced by the mammary glands of female mammals during the few days just after giving birth.

It is through the colostrum that the mother passively donates her immunity to the newborn child. Not surprisingly, colostrum contains several immune-modulating products including immunoglobulins, lactoferrin, transfer factor, fibronectin, and growth factors.

Three of these are available commercially and are promising components in a viral immunity program: immunoglobulins, lactoferrin, and transfer factor. I have already discussed whey immunoglobulins, and recommended that you include cold-processed whey powder in your general dietary plan, for detoxification, and for general immune enhancement.

COLOSTRUM: Commercially prepared from dairy cattle, whole purified bovine colostrum can be added to the category of a supportive dietary supplement for an aging immune system and general immune deficiency. It is very safe to use and is taken in dosages ranging from 1–4 g daily on an empty stomach.

LACTOFERRIN: Lactoferrin, an abundant protein component of human colostrum, binds to iron. By binding to iron, lactoferrin makes iron less available for use by bacteria and other pathogenic microorganisms, including fungi and viruses, which use iron to promote their own growth. Lactoferrin's ability to regulate iron also influences T-cell, neutrophil, and monocyte proliferation, all essential components of the immune response. Iron-regulating strategies are also essential to normal growth and the control of the advancement of disease processes in the body.

Several studies support the premise that lactoferrin acts as a natural antibiotic and antifungal agent and that it has anti-cancer activity. Though lactoferrin is found in high amounts in human colostrum, its concentration in bovine colostrum is low, so a separate supplement of lactoferrin should be used. Lactoferrin is useful for fungal and bacterial co-infections in those with chronic viral diseases and to manage iron regulation in hepatitis. Dosages range from 250–750 mg, taken before bed, nightly.

TRANSFER FACTOR: Immunological information is passed from the mother to her child in the colostrum through the action of transfer factor. William Hennen, Ph.D., the father of the modern use of oral transfer factor, refers to it as "graduate level training for the immune system" (Hennen 2000). Transfer factor, along with antibodies in the colostrum and breast milk, passively confers some of the mother's cell-mediated immunity to the infant until it acquires its own. Infants have a very responsive innate immune system; they quickly react to foreign substances with high fever, for example.

But since they have not been exposed to environmental antigens, their adaptive immune responses to foreign substances are less reactive, making them highly susceptible to microbial infection. Mortality among infants and children under five years of age used to account for the greatest number of deaths in the pre-industrial era in the United States and Europe, and it continues to be today in the impoverished third world countries.

Originally discovered in the late 1940s, transfer factor has been the subject of intense investigation for its use as an immune stimulant. It is considered an essential component of the immune system. Most of the current transfer factor research has been conducted in Italy by Giancarlo Pizza, M.D., president of the International Transfer Factor Society. Dr. Pizza and his colleagues investigated treatments with HIV patients, chronic fatigue syndrome, prostate and bladder cancers, HHV-6, herpes simplex, and other viral conditions.

So far in this chapter I have discussed non-specific immune modulators that mainly stimulate innate immunity. Transfer factor (TF), to my knowledge, is the only naturally occurring immune modulator that can affect cell-mediated immunity. Steven J. Bock, M.D., says, "Transfer factor probably produces a trigger for T-cell recognition of antigen" (Bock 2000). He has found TF useful in allergic conditions, autoimmune disorders, and chronic viruses. TF also affects innate immunity by enhancing NK cell activity.

There are two types of transfer factor, unspecific and antigen-specific. Dr. Pizza's work is with antigen-specific transfer factor as prepared from extracts from white blood cells. Commercial antigen-specific transfer factor can be prepared in the laboratory and has activity against specific viruses, fungi, and other infectious microorganisms. Chisolm Biological Laboratories in South Carolina produces antigen-specific transfer factor products from the white blood cells of chickens for a variety of diseases, including hepatitis B and C, HHV-6 and other herpes viruses, as well as *Candida* and other fungal organisms.

Though there is no conclusive evidence that antigen-specific TF is better than unspecific transfer factor, this conclusion makes sense and I have recommended its use in patients with HCV, Lyme disease, and other infections. Antigen-specific transfer factor can be taken orally or by injection and is administered by a medical doctor or naturopathic physician.

Unspecific transfer factor is prepared from bovine colostrum and is available without a prescription or doctor's recommendation. It is

Functions of Transfer Factor

Trains the immune system and improves immune memory function

Inhibits macrophage migration, thereby keeping them in the area where they are needed

Increases number of natural killer cells and greatly enhances their activity

Antigen-specific transfer factor increases secretion of gamma-interferon without increasing the number of pro-inflammatory cytokines.

taken orally and is considered very safe, even when taken over long periods of time, and it can be taken by elderly patients and infants as well. For viral infections, the recommended dose is three to five 200 mg capsules taken three times daily with water and away from food.

Caution: Though commercial colostrum, transfer factor, and lactoferrin are made from milk, they are highly purified and contain only small amounts of allergic milk proteins (albumin and gamma globulin) and lactose. Even if you are allergic to dairy or are lactose intolerant, you should be able to take these products. However, start very slowly with a fraction of the recommended dosage and gradually increase the dose. Whole colostrum contains more milk allergens than lactoferrin or transfer factor, so if you notice any allergic symptoms, discontinue immediately.

Nutrients and Herbs As Immune Modulators: Many herbs have immune-modulating effects. For viral conditions, the best known and most effective include echinacea and cat's claw. These herbs also have antiviral activity and are discussed in step 7, the chapter on natural antiviral medications. Many Chinese herbs have immune-enhancing and adaptogenic properties, such as astragalus and ginseng, and are included in step 8, the chapter on Chinese medicine.

Many nutrients also have immune-modulating effects, such as co-enzyme Q10, selenium, zinc, and vitamin B6, and have already been discussed in the chapter on antioxidants. However, one vitamin, folic acid, and a trace mineral, germanium, that I have not discussed, are worth mentioning here for their immune-enhancing properties.

FOLIC ACID: Folic acid, or folate, is necessary for DNA synthesis. It keeps homocysteine levels within normal range, and is used to make

SAMe (S-adenosyl-L-methionine). The RDA for folic acid is 200 mcg daily and 800 mcg daily during pregnancy to prevent neural tube defects in the developing fetus. A foundational multivitamin formula and a diet rich in green leafy vegetables, mixed vegetable juices, and green drinks generally supply adequate folate. However, in cases of chronic viral infection, take 1–5 mg daily (1 mg = 1,000 mcg).

GERMANIUM: Germanium is a trace mineral that has been found to improve immunity. The main research was performed in Japan by Kazuhiko Asai, Ph.D., at the Germanium Research Institute in Tokyo; its use as a powerful antioxidant was later promoted by Stephen Levine, Ph.D., an international expert on free radical pathology and founder of Allergy Research Group in Hayward, California. Interestingly, germanium is found in shiitake mushrooms, so I generally prefer to use mushrooms rather than prescribing the mineral itself since it is very expensive. Organic germanium is available from Allergy Research as bis-carboxyethyl germanium sesquioxide; the recommended dosage is 275 mg, three times daily.

CAT'S CLAW: Cat's claw or *Uña de Gato (Uncaria tomentosa)* has anti-inflammatory properties and has been investigated for immunomodulating activity. Professor Hildebert Wagner of the University of Munich, one of the world's authorities on immune-modulating agents from plants such as echinacea, has found substantial immunomodulating activity in cat's claw.

Though research on cat's claw is still in the preliminary stages, one or two promising products based on it have recently entered the market. For one, C-Med-100 is a patented cat's claw extract standardized to 8 percent carboxyl-alkyl-esters with a recommended dose of 300 mg daily. The other, Saventaro, is an extract of the root standardized to contain 1.3 percent pentacyclic oxindole alkaloids. The recommended dosage is one 20 mg capsule, three times daily as a loading dose for the first ten days, then one capsule daily.

How to Use Immune Modulators

In general, those with any chronic illness or impaired immunity may benefit from immune modulators. One or more of the substances discussed in this chapter may be added to your daily supplement regimen and can be taken often with other vitamins or antioxidants, though they are best taken apart from food. Do not take

Table 15: Recommended Dosages for Selected Immune Modulators

Substance	Form and Amount	Dosage
Acemannan	Oral powder or capsule: 80 mg	1–3 times daily
Larch Arabinogalactan	Powder: 2 g (may be combined with 500–1,000 mg of vitamin C)	2 times daily
Beta 1, 3-D Glucan	Capsules: 100–300 mg	3–4 times daily
Ganoderma mushroom combination	Capsules: 750 mg	1–2 times daily, up to 4 times daily
Cordyceps	Capsules: 500–1,000 mg	3 times daily
Transfer Factor	Capsules: 200–1,000 mg	3 times daily

all of them at one time. Experimenting on your own using immune-modulating medications is safe, but if you have a serious condition, you may find it better to consult a doctor who has experience in immunological disorders and the use of immune modulators.

In my clinical practice, I order a comprehensive lymphocyte panel that includes NK-cell counts and activity for all patients with chronic infections and any immunologically related disorder. I evaluate the number and activity of natural killer cells and the balance between helper and suppressor T cells. I then establish a regimen of immune modulators, along with other natural medications. Besides following improvement in symptoms, it is a good idea to have your NK-cell activity checked every three to six months until it returns to normal, then once a year thereafter until you are completely recovered.

CHAPTER SUMMARY

Use immune modulators if your immune function is low. Evaluate your need by evaluating symptoms, the nature of your condition, and by measuring NK-cell activity and lymphocyte counts.

Acemannan, arabinogalactan, beta-glucan, and colostrum are general immune modulators that can be taken in low dosages for symptom prevention, by those with allergies, recurrent colds and flu, and other minor immunological conditions, including age-related immune deficiency.

Mushroom extracts offer valuable immune-enhancing support. For viral conditions, a formulation of ganoderma, shiitake, and maitake extracts combined with cordyceps is effective.

Transfer factor (TF) offers substantial immune benefits. Unspecific TF can be used in lower dosages to benefit the immune system, and in higher dosages to complement a treatment program for viral infections. Antigen-specific TF can be a powerful agent in the treatment of viral disease; however, a physician should supervise its use.

Rotate the immune modulators you're using every three to six months.

If you have an autoimmune condition, avoid colostrum and whey protein, due to their high antibody content. For conditions like rheumatoid arthritis, use immune modulators with anti-inflammatory activity, and which include phytosterols.

If you are lactose intolerant or allergic to dairy protein, avoid all products derived from colostrum if you notice allergenic sensitivity.

Consult a physician experienced in the use of immune modulators for more specific information. (See the resource section.)

12

STEP SEVEN

Target Viruses with Natural Antiviral Alternatives

Among the greatest threats to humans and wild and domesticated animals in our age of environmental destruction are viral infections and immune disorders and their consequences such as cancer, chronic fatigue syndrome, and liver damage. Under the best of conditions, our immune systems are completely capable of preventing viral infection, ridding the body of viruses once our cells become infected, or arriving at a symbiotic balance in which the virus lives in our bodies but does little or no harm.

However, in some cases, as discussed in part 1, our immune systems are unable to prevent, eradicate, or keep the virus under control. In this scenario, the virus takes over and kills us, as in rampant cytomegalovirus infection; or it gets the upper hand and makes us gradually sicker and sicker, as in chronic hepatitis C or HIV infections. In the latter cases, we do not die as a direct cause of the virus but of its long-term effects on other organs and systems.

If you have an active, chronic, or recurrent viral infection that your immune system is unable to control, you need to reduce the viral burden on your system with antiviral medicines. The material in this chapter provides information on proven antiviral alternatives and their use to accomplish that goal.

What Are Antivirals?

Antiviral medications are substances that destroy viruses or prevent their replication. As I described in part 1, pharmaceutical antiviral drugs are relatively new on the clinical front. This is because, in the past, bacterial infections were a larger threat to infants and young children, from infections in mothers after delivery, after surgery, and from wounds caused by war injuries. In all of these cases, bacterial infections often lead to death. Therefore, the belief among medical scientists of the time was that antibiotics treat bacterial infections and viral infections are best prevented with vaccines.

Viruses were once thought to be on their way out of human life, and vaccination was for a time seen as the universal answer to viral infections. Little attention was paid to researching antiviral drugs until the advent of AIDS in the 1980s. We know now in hindsight that this was the wrong strategy, or at least an insufficient approach.

Though a number of antiviral drugs are now available, most are not effective, have significant side effects, and rapidly cause antiviral resistance. Another problem with powerful antiviral drugs is collateral damage. Recall that viruses reside within the cells; attempting to kill a virus directly also destroys some of our own cells. Fortunately, nature has provided us with a considerable array of antiviral plants and other natural substances that can deal with the viruses without destroying our cells.

Since plants are rooted in the soil and cannot move, they have developed powerful biochemical arsenals to defend themselves against viruses, fungi, bacteria, and insects. Natural antiviral medications may be used to complement other therapies, or in many cases they can make up the first line of therapy, reserving drugs for an as-needed basis only. The natural antiviral alternatives discussed in this chapter have all shown antiviral activity in the research lab and in clinical use. Doctors have successfully used many of them for decades, or longer, and several were discovered from ethnobotanical studies of indigenous healing practices.

Once you have established the foundational plan outlined in steps 1 through 4, have addressed inflammation (step 5), and are working

9 Antiviral Herbs

Boneset
Echinacea
Elderberry
Witch hazel
Lomatium
Lemon balm
Phyllanthus
Sangre de drago
St. John's wort

with immune modulators (step 6), the next step is to directly target viral infection in your body. The medications involved may be taken short-term for active, chronic infections (a herpes outbreak) or for acute viral infections (a cold or flu). Some may be used long-term for chronic viral conditions, such as HCV. Study the information on each medication carefully before use; if you have questions, consult a physician who has knowledge of the use of natural antiviral alternatives.

Natural antiviral alternatives are found in many plants, seaweeds, mushrooms, mother's milk, and in plant components such as alkaloids, tannins, essential oils, sesquiterpenes, and limonene. Due to side effects and viral resistance of pharmaceutical antivirals, pharmaceutical researchers have investigated hundreds of natural substances for potential antiviral activity. Nature has not disappointed them, and many effective antiviral alternatives are available.

For the purpose of this book, I have categorized them into herbal antiviral medicines, homeopathic antiviral remedies, and antiviral nutraceuticals (pharmacological concentrates and extracts from natural products). As you read about these medications you will find that many have been mentioned in other chapters. This is because natural products contain complex compounds that may have a wide array of uses, for example: echinacea stimulates the immune system, has antiviral properties, and has antibacterial actions.

Natural Herbal Antiviral Medicines

Herbs make up the majority of antiviral alternatives. They include a wide range of different plant families and come from locations around the world. Some of the most interesting to me are those from the upper Amazon in South America, an area that we have only just explored around the fringes and where I conduct annual field research. Chinese antiviral herbs, another area that I specialize in, are among the most powerful and are discussed in the next chapter.

Boneset (*Eupatorium perfoliatum*): Boneset is a member of the Compositae family, which contains a number of commonly used herbal plant remedies including echinacea. It contains the sesquiterpene lactones euperfolin, euperfolitin, and eufoliatin; polysaccharides, pyrrolizidine alkaloids, essential oils, many flavonoids including rutin and quercetin, and plant sterols. Research has shown it to stimulate white blood cells and increase phagocytosis four times better than echinacea.

The flowering plant is collected in the late summer or fall, dried, cut, and then usually prepared into an alcohol tincture, though the dried herb can also be made into a tea. It was once used to treat fever resulting from malaria, as well as dengue, common cold, or influenza viruses. It is very bitter, and as a tea can cause nausea or vomiting. Boneset should not be used during pregnancy. Due to the presence of pyrrolizidine alkaloids, which can cause liver toxicity, it also should not be used if you have liver disease. There are no known drug interactions with boneset.

For the reasons described above, boneset is used short-term for no more than 5–7 days to treat acute viral infections like the common cold and respiratory tract infections caused by influenza. Take 20–30 drops (1/3 teaspoon) of the tincture every few hours until symptoms subside. To make a tea: steep 1 ounce (25 g) of the dried herb in 1 quart of boiled water for 10–15 minutes; drink 1 cup of hot herb tea three to four times per day.

Echinacea (*Echinacea purpurea, E. angustifolia, E. pallida*): Echinacea has become the best-selling herbal medication in recent years, despite a considerable amount of controversy over how it works. It contains caffeic acid derivatives, polysaccharides including arabinogalactan, and the lipophilic components polyacetylenes, and alkylamides. It is a low-growing wildflower native to the American West and, like boneset, it is a member of the Compositae family.

Echinacea is extremely popular in Europe, especially Germany and Switzerland, where it is commercially grown. It is prepared as a tincture, a dry or liquid extract, and is also available in injectable forms. The most-researched forms are oral liquid extract preparations made from the fresh plant; however, dry extracts are also available. Alcohol tinctures are also useful, but more tincture has to be taken to achieve a dose equivalent to that of a concentrate. Injectables are very effective, but have limited availability in the United States. Teas are not very effective, as most of the active ingredients in echinacea are alcohol-soluble and therefore do not readily dissolve in water.

Though there is no doubt in the scientific community that echinacea works, there is still controversy about how it works and whether echinacea is primarily an immune stimulant or an antimicrobial. For viral infections, it would seem that it makes little difference, since an ideal antiviral agent would have both properties. However, as you have learned from earlier chapters, the wrong type of stimulation can lead to undesirable pro-inflammatory conditions. The final word is not yet out on echinacea, but I will attempt to explain some of the issues this controversial herb has created and how it is best used.

There have been at least fifteen randomized, double-blind, placebo-controlled trials (the "gold standard" of medical research) testing echinacea's effectiveness for viral upper-respiratory tract infections. An excellent review article of these trials was written by Bruce Barrett, M.D., Ph.D., Assistant Professor of Medicine at the University of Wisconsin Medical School in Madison, Wisconsin, and nationally known researcher in alternative medicine. He reported that, based on the studies, echinacea is useful in shortening the duration of common respiratory tract infections, including the common cold, but not in preventing colds. Dr. Barrett points out that though echinacea is effective, it is not extremely effective (Barrett 2000). This has also been my clinical experience.

As an immune stimulant, echinacea is also still not well understood, but studies indicate that it increases phagocytosis by 20–30 percent. Though it has a high degree of safety, controversy also surrounds contraindications for the use of echinacea. The German Commission E,[1] the world's leading authority on herbal medicines, states that due to its immune stimulatory mechanisms, echinacea should not be used in progressive conditions like autoimmune diseases and chronic viruses.

In two papers published in *Alternative Medicine Review*, Kerry Bone, N.D., reviews all the existing literature and clinical studies, as well as traditional uses, and concludes that: "Limitations on the use of echinacea have resulted from preconceived and somewhat simplistic concepts of echinacea's influence on the immune system" (Bone 1997). He concludes that echinacea is safe for long-term use and suggests an extensive list of conditions it can be used for. In addition, echinacea has recently been approved for use during pregnancy based on a Canadian research study involving 412 women (Gallo 2000).

The German combination remedy Esberitox N, containing echinacea, thuja (*Thujae occidentalis*) and wild indigo root (*Baptista tinctoria*), has shown effectiveness in the treatment of bacterial and viral upper respiratory tract infections. It is manufactured by Schaper &

Brümmer and imported into the United States by Enzymatic Therapy, and is available in drops or tablets. Take three tablets, or 10–20 drops, three times daily for ten days.

Another German product, Pascotox Forte-injectopas is a prescription injectable medication containing 500 mg of *Echinacea pallida* extract. This remedy is not available in the United States; however, if you travel to Europe you can obtain it for personal use. I highly recommend this medication for those with recurrent colds and flu and as a complement to other treatments for acute or chronic infections. The dosage is 1 ampoule (2ml) injected intramuscularly every other day for acute conditions and once a week for chronic cases.

Like boneset, echinacea is best used in the short term for minor respiratory tract infections caused by viruses and bacteria. Though I have not seen any side effects in either progressive illnesses like multiple sclerosis or chronic viruses, I generally recommend taking echinacea for three to five days only, and not as a long-term treatment or as prevention. Take 3–4 ml (about 1 teaspoon) of the tincture or 300 mg of the dry extract three to four times daily.

Elderberry *(Sambucus nigra)*: Elderberry is another useful remedy for minor upper respiratory tract viruses. It has a long history of use in Europe and North America, and has been studied for effectiveness against influenza type A and B viruses, including the Beijing, Shandong, and Singapore flu strains. It contains a newly discovered substance (novel type 2 ribosome-inactivating protein) that appears to have an inhibiting effect on certain viruses.

For home use, the flowers are used as a tea for the treatment of the symptoms of the flu by steeping 3–5 g per 1 cup of boiled water for 10–15 minutes. It is drunk warm with honey three times daily. The tincture is also available, taken at a dosage of 1/2 to 1 teaspoon in water three to four times per day during an acute respiratory infection.

Witch hazel *(Hamamelis virginiana)*: Like the three herbal medicines discussed above, witch hazel is a remedy we learned from the Native Americans. It is mostly known as a mild alcohol distillate for insect bites and swelling. However, it is also an effective, though mild, antiviral and has been studied for its anti-inflammatory and antiviral effects in the treatment of herpes simplex virus. The bark and leaves contain tannins and volatile oils that have astringent properties. Small amounts of the tincture or ointment may be applied to herpes lesions. Do not drink witch hazel.

Lomatium *(Lomatium dissectum)*: This herb received considerable attention as an antiviral in the mid-1980s, but has since fallen out of favor except among the most avid herbalists. It grows in the Western United States and is a member of the carrot family (Umbelliferae), and during the spring when the shoots are tender, it can be eaten. The root is the medicinal part and contains tetronic acids, luteolin, and resins.

It has not been studied to any degree. However, one Canadian team screened over one hundred plants for antiviral activity and found that lomatium completely inhibited the cytopathic effects of rotavirus (common diarrhea-causing viruses). Lomatium is used as a tincture: 1–3 ml taken three times daily. The resin fraction can cause a whole-body rash even in moderate amounts, so if you use this herb, discontinue it immediately if you feel any itching or notice a rash.

Lemon balm *(Melissa officinalis)*: Lemon balm is a member of the mint family (Labiatae) and contains tannins, volatile oils, flavonoids, rosmarinic acid, and other compounds. It has been studied for its antiviral properties since the 1960s and is used as a topical ointment for herpes virus blisters on the lips. The German commercial preparation, Herpilyn contains a 70:1 concentration of lemon balm extract with 1 percent allantoin from the comfrey plant. It is safe to use long-term and is applied to the lips two to four times daily.

Phyllanthus *(Phyllanthus niruri, P. amarus, P. urinaria)*: Phyllanthus is a member of the Euphorbiaceae family and is found in tropical South America and Asia. It is one of the most effective herbal antivirals. The Indian variety, *Phyllanthus niruri,* used in Ayurvedic medicine for thousands of years, has been extensively studied for the treatment of hepatitis B. Other varieties *(Phyllanthus myrtifolius and P. urinaria)* have also been studied and found to have antiviral effects against Epstein-Barr and other viruses.

The compounds in phyllanthus include tannins, alkaloids, flavonoids, lignans, phenols, and terpenes. In addition to antiviral activity, they have a considerable liver-protective function, giving this herb great therapeutic potential in the treatment of chronic hepatitis and hepatocellular (liver) cancer. The majority of patients with chronic hepatitis B show improvement in their blood tests within one month of treatment. Though studies are just beginning for the use of phyllanthus in chronic HCV, many clinicians (including myself) have used this herb for several years to help successfully manage liver inflammation in HCV patients.

There are no known contraindications, drug interactions or harmful effects. Phyllanthus is taken as a powdered extract in dosages ranging from 900 to 2,500 mg daily for three months or longer. In my practice, when using phyllanthus in chronic hepatitis, I generally alternate it every three months with the Chinese herbal formula Minor Bupleurum Decoction, or *xiao chai hu tang (sho-saiko-to:* discussed in the next chapter). *Chanca piedra,* an Amazonian variety of *Phyllanthus niruri,* is traditionally used to treat kidney stones but may also have antiviral activity. It is worth trying for chronic hepatitis.

Sangre de drago *(Croton lechleri)*: Sangre de drago, meaning "dragon's blood" in Spanish, is also a member of the Euphorbiaceae family (like phyllanthus) and grows along the slopes of the Andes into the Amazonian rainforests of Peru, Brazil, and Ecuador. Its name is derived from the red latex extracted from the tree. The resin and bark are used medicinally and contain proanthocyanidins, flavonoids, phenols, lignans, and plant sterols.

Sangre de drago is used as an anti-inflammatory, antiseptic, antifungal, and antiviral against herpes and upper respiratory tract viruses. It is also used for the treatment of diarrhea, and for this purpose has been developed into a patented standardized extract by Shaman Pharmaceuticals of San Francisco, and manufactured as Normal Stool Formula (NSF). The active ingredient in NSF is an oligomeric proanthocyanidin compound called SP-303. Research studies show that this medication successfully treats HIV-associated diarrhea (Carlson 2000). NSF comes in 350 mg tablets; the recommended dosage for chronic diarrhea is one tablet, two to four times daily.

Though many Amazonian herbs, including sangre de drago, have been studied for their active constituents and though the therapeutic potential is great, there are few scientific publications on their use and safety. However, in my clinical experience, it is a safe and useful herb, although it has a bitter taste.

Sangre de drago can be taken as a tincture (20–30 drops, three times daily) or as a powdered extract (1/2 teaspoon dissolved in water, taken one to three times daily). Liquid extracts and tinctures can be obtained from Rainforest Bio-Energetics. Powdered extracts have limited availability in the United States.

St. John's wort *(Hypericum perforatum)*: St. John's wort is best known as a natural antidepressant and is widely used for that purpose. However, it also has antiviral properties, and was at one time investigated

4 Homotoxicology Antiviral Alternatives

Echinacea compositum S

Engystol N

Gripp-Heel

Pascotox

for use in HIV. Though a common flowering herb, its chemical nature is very complex, and contains hypericin, hyperforin, flavonoids, and xanthones. Some doctors like the combination of an antidepressant with an antiviral and recommend it for patients with chronic viral conditions who also have depression or whose moods are low due to their illness.

Though there is no scientific or clinical evidence to support this rationale, St. John's wort is a safe herb with few side effects. If you have a chronic viral condition and depression, try it for four to six weeks, which is how long it typically takes to show benefits.

German studies indicate that 2.4 percent of patients develop adverse effects within four weeks of using of St. John's wort, which include stomach upset, dizziness, headache, dry mouth, and restlessness. Sensitivity to sunlight is also a reported reaction to this herb. Drug interactions to one of the active components, hypericin, have been reported. If you are taking other antidepressants, anticoagulants, and/or digoxin for your heart, do not use St. John's wort while you are on these drugs. The standard dosage is 300 mg of the extract, taken three times daily.

Homeopathic Antiviral Remedies

In the homeopathic *materia medica,* dozens of remedies are listed for use in viral conditions, and since classical homeopathic prescribing focuses on the constitution of the patient and not the pathology of the disease, the repertory of possible remedies is immense. In this next section, I will mention only those remedies that I have clinical experience with and whose use is supported by the scientific literature. If you have an interest in pursuing this approach further, consult with a physician skilled in homeopathy who has experience in treating viral diseases.

The remedies listed below are composite medications containing several homeopathic substances. They are described as homotoxicologics and are all manufactured by the German companies Heel Biotherapeutics and Pasco. I routinely use all of these medications as supportive therapy in acute and chronic viral conditions, especially for influenza.

Echinacea compositum S: This is a Heel product, packaged in oral or injectable vials. It contains *Echinacea angustifolia* D3, Aconitum D3,

Sanguinaria D4, and several other homeopathic substances. It is very useful for influenza and minor bacterial infections. The dosage is one oral vial three times daily for acute conditions, and one vial daily for ten days for chronic conditions. Injectables need to be administered by your doctor and are generally given by intramuscular injection three times per week.

Engystol N: This is another Heel product, specific for influenza and acute or chronic viral diseases. It contains *Vincetoxicum* (swallow wort) and homeopathic sulfur in graduated potencies. In one study, a total of 1479 cases were treated with Engystol by 154 physicians from three European countries. The study reported that 85–90 percent of patients with flu symptoms reported improvement within one week of treatment; the treatment was only completely unsuccessful in 4 percent of cases.

Engystol is very useful as supportive therapy in all viral conditions and taken alone for symptoms of the flu or common cold. The dosage is one tablet dissolved in the mouth three times daily, or more frequently in acute infections; do not take with food. It also comes in an injectable form that is available only by prescription from your doctor. Here, one ampoule is administered intramuscularly three times weekly for one week.

Gripp-Heel: Also from Heel Biotherapeutics, this contains Aconitum D4 120 mg, Bryonia D4, Lachesis D12, *Eupatorium perfoliatum* (boneset) D3, and Phosphorus D5. It is used alone or with other natural medications for the treatment of influenza. The dosage is one tablet (allowed to dissolve in the mouth) three to five times daily for a course of seven days. In acute stages, take one tablet every 15 minutes.

Pascotox: This is a remedy similar in composition to Heel's Echinacea compositum and Esberitox N, with the exception that it contains a concentrated dry extract of *Echinacea pallida* root combined with homeopathics. Pascotox is also used for symptoms of the flu. It comes in tablets and drops and the dosage is 4–6 tablets or 40 drops every hour for acute conditions, or 2 tablets/20 drops, three times a day for chronic cases. It is also manufactured as an injectable medication but is not available in this form in the United States.

Additional Homeopathic Influenza Remedies: A modern homeopathic remedy for flu, and available over the counter in most health stores, is Oscillococcinum *(Ana barbariae)*. It is prepared from duck livers by the French homeopathic company Boiron. The dosage is three pellets dissolved in the mouth three times daily (not taken with food) at the first signs of flu symptoms.

Eupatorium, prepared from boneset, described above, is used to treat chills and fever accompanied by deep aching pain. Gelsemium is used when flu is accompanied by fatigue and body aches that comes on gradually. Aconitum is used to treat flu symptoms that come on suddenly and intensely.

> ## A Note on Homeopathic Potencies:
>
> Homeopathic medications are prepared according to strict standards and come in potencies based on increasing dilutions of 10, 100, or 1000. Dilutions of 10 are written as 1X, 6X, 30X, etc. (or in Europe as D). Dilutions of 100 are written as 1C, 2C, etc., and those of 1000 as 1M, 10M, etc. Homeopaths vary in their system and style of prescribing. I generally recommend the lower dilutions between 1X(D) to 6X(D).

Antiviral Nutraceuticals

Antiviral nutraceuticals are substances extracted from naturally occurring products prepared pharmacologically as concentrates. They are standardized to guarantee that each unit dose has a specified amount of the active ingredient. The use of these medications is also supported by scientific research. Though there are more known herbal antivirals, the greatest therapeutic potential lies in these new nutraceutical agents.

Olive Leaf Extract: Extracts from the leaves of the common Mediterranean olive tree *(Olea europaea)* have become the leading natural antiviral available. Though researched since the 1960s by leading pharmaceutical companies, the nutraceutical version was first available in the United States in 1995.

Many physicians practicing natural medicine use olive leaf extract for a wide range of viral illness ranging from respiratory tract infections and chronic hepatitis, to herpes zoster. Besides its potent antimicrobial activity against viruses, bacteria, and fungal organisms, olive leaf is an antioxidant, has immune-stimulating properties, and creates positive effects on the cardiovascular system.

Unfortunately, like many commercial natural products, it is marketed heavily to the public without substantial proof of the effectiveness of different products, making it difficult to judge which of these is the most effective.

Of the more than ninety-eight known compounds found in olive leaf, oleuropein (the phenolic glycoside compound elenoic acid) is considered to be the biological active component against viruses. A synthetic derivative of the calcium salt of elenoic acid, calcium elenolate (originally researched by Upjohn and abandoned as an antiviral in the mid-1970s), was later independently developed by East Park Research. It is thought to have broad-spectrum activity against a number of viruses and bacteria.

In my clinical practice, I use the standardized extract containing 17–23 percent oleuropein (85–115 mg per 500 mg capsule) for acute respiratory tract infections, as an antiviral therapy for hepatitis and other chronic viral infections, and to treat bacterial co-infections in patients with chronic viral diseases.

It is a safe medication with no known contraindications or side effects; however, due to its potent antimicrobial activity, you may experience a Herxheimer reaction, or die-off effect. Combining olive leaf with drainage remedies, taking vitamin C to bowel tolerance, and supporting your system with other antioxidants will minimize this effect if it occurs.

Plant Tannins: Plant tannins are naturally occurring, water-soluble polyphenols and are found only in plants. Also collectively referred to as tannic acid, tannins are yellowish-white to brown in color and are found in many common foods and beverages consumed by humans. These include grapes, legumes, red wine, tea, coffee, and chocolate, as well as commonly used herbs like black cohosh, red raspberry, ginkgo, and chamomile.

Though people have used tannins in foods and drinks (we seem to find the tannic taste pleasing) since the time of our ancestors, the scientific study of tannins as nutraceutical medicines is very new. Researchers at the University of Okayama in Japan have investigated tannins and suggest that they are a new class of bioactive substances worth serious study.

Tannins have powerful antioxidant properties and are toxic to a wide range of microorganisms, including yeast, fungi, bacteria, and viruses. They have been studied for activity against HIV-1, herpes virus, and other viruses. Though there is great potential for tannins as antiviral medicines, few have been developed for clinical use. This may be due to their ability to impair carbohydrate and protein digestibility, causing reduced nutrition, and they have other potential side effects as well, including gastrointestinal irritation.

Tannins can trigger migraines in susceptible individuals, and concentrated herbal tannins should not be used over the long term. My suggestion is to confine their use to four weeks or less per course of

---

4 Antiviral Nutraceuticals

Olive Leaf Extract
Plant Tannins
Monolaurin
RC-183

---

treatment. You may repeat courses of treatment after a break of one month, but do not repeat more than three courses without consulting a knowledgeable physician.

The tannin product I use in my practice is Viracin, a combination of herbal tannins and zinc developed by Scientific Consulting Services. This product is primarily used for the treatment of gastrointestinal viruses and may be combined with natural antifungal or anti-bacterial substances to treat *Candida* and other pathogenic microorganisms in the gastrointestinal tract. The standard dosage is one capsule, two times daily, not to be taken with food or before meals.

Monolaurin: Monolaurin is a medium chain saturated fatty-acid compound (from monoglycerides of lauric acid) naturally occurring in mother's milk and commercially prepared from coconut oil. It is effective against lipid-coated viruses, including HIV, CMV, HSV-1, and influenza virus; it is also active against a wide range of opportunistic fungal and bacterial infections. Lauric acid has been used as a food preservative since 1964, though only recently has it been studied for its use as an antiviral medication in humans. Lauricidin, available from Ecological Formulas, contains 300 mg of monolaurin and is taken in dosages ranging from 1,800–3,600 mg daily. It is considered entirely safe for long term consumption.

RC-183: A new class of antiviral compounds called RC-183 discovered by researchers at the University of Wisconsin in 1999 has shown effectiveness against influenza A virus, chickenpox, and herpes (Piraino 1999). The active ubiquitin-containing component, RC-183, is found in the gypsy mushroom *(Rozites caperata)* and blocks viral replication. It is being tested by pharmaceutical companies for the treatment of viral infections and is not available to the consumer. However, you may look for other antiviral mushroom products from Fungi Perfecti.

How to Use Natural Antivirals

Since prescribing natural medicines is matched to a composite of the individual patient's symptoms, their immune strengths and weaknesses, as well as the pathological condition, there is no specific protocol that I can outline to make this section easier for you to understand. However, there are a number of guiding therapeutic principles that experienced naturopathic clinicians generally follow. These are:

- Natural medicines are not as powerful as pharmaceutical drugs.

- Herbs and other natural medicines tend to work slowly.

- Natural medicines tend to work synergistically.

- Natural medicines are dose-dependent.

Natural medicines, including antiviral and antibiotic alternatives, are not as powerful as pharmaceutical drugs. That is not to say that they are ineffective, which they certainly are not, because for chronic infections they may be our first choice for therapy. However, they tend to work more slowly and results come gradually.

On the other hand, they do not cause disruption of other biological systems in your body and they tend to enhance life processes, resulting in deeper healing and more complete recovery. They also tend to work synergistically with other natural remedies, along with diet and nutritional supplements. The art, of course, is knowing how to combine them effectively; that discussion is beyond the purpose and scope of this book.

You also have to take sufficient amounts of natural antivirals frequently at regular intervals during the day to achieve effectiveness. For

Table 16: Antiviral Alternatives Arranged by Condition

Condition	Herbs	Homeopathics	Nutraceuticals
Influenza virus	Echinacea, Elderberry, Boneset	Echinacea compositum, Engystol, Gripp-Heel, Pascotox, Oscillococcinum	Olive leaf extract, grapefruit seed extract
Gastrointestinal viruses and virus-associated diarrhea	Sangre de drago, Lomatium	Plant tannins	
Herpes viruses	Lemon balm (Melissa) and Witch Hazel (Hamamelis) for topical application		Olive leaf extract, grapefruit seed extract, monolaurin RC-183
Hepatitis B and C viruses	Phyllanthus	Olive leaf extract	
Nonspecific viral conditions	Echinacea	Engystol	Olive leaf extract, grapefruit seed extract, monolaurin

acute viral infections, use herbal antivirals taken in high dosages for a few days to a few weeks. For chronic viruses, take herbal combinations in moderate dosages over several months' duration. Refer to the tables in this chapter for recommendations on how and when to use natural antiviral alternatives (see table 16).

Nutraceutical Antibiotic Alternatives: In chronic viral disease and immune deficiency conditions, it is rare that one would only have a virus and no other microbial infections. Usually bacterial, fungal, parasitical, and protozoal co-infections occur at the same time or appear cyclically during the course of the viral illness. Managing bacterial and other co-infections with natural antibiotic alternatives is essential in successfully treating viral illnesses. While this book is not intended to cover herbal antimicrobial agents in any detail, it is important to mention a few of the best of them.

Berberine: This is a naturally occurring, yellow-colored bitter alkaloid found in many important medicinal plants like goldenseal *(Hydrastis canadensis)*, the Chinese herb coptis/*huang lian (Coptidis chinensis)*, and Oregon grape root *(Berberis aquifolium)*. It is prepared as a concentrated standardized extract for medicinal purposes, and is effective against both gram-negative and gram-positive bacteria, fungi, protozoa, and viruses.

I use it for gastrointestinal and urinary tract infections typically in dosages ranging from 200–400 mg, two to four times daily. It is generally considered safe for short-term use, but should not be used during pregnancy, by children, or if it causes any gastrointestinal discomfort.

Allicin: This is the antimicrobial active component of garlic *(Allium sativa)* and is effective against bacteria, fungi, protozoa, and some viruses. I use it in concentrated form (20 mg of allicin per capsule) for upper respiratory tract infections like sinusitis and bronchial infections, and for deep fungal infections. It is safe to take, even over a long period of time. However, eventually you will exude the typical garlic odor, and for some people it causes mild nausea and abdominal gas. A typical dosage is two capsules, two to three times daily with food.

Grapefruit Seed Extract (GSE): Also known as citrus seed extract, it is processed from the seeds of *Citrus paradisi.* Though all of the chemical components of this natural antibiotic are not yet known,

Nutraceutical Antibiotic Alternatives

Berberine

Allicin

Grapefruit Seed Extract

researchers have isolated phenolic compounds that are active against a wide variety of fungi, bacteria, and also some viruses. It has been studied by the world-famous Pasteur Institute in Paris and is endorsed as an antiseptic by WHO (World Health Organization); it is used as a hospital disinfectant against antibiotic-resistant germs and as a veterinary medicine.

It is commercially available in liquid concentrate or as a dry extract. The dosage for the liquid is from two to five (and up to 15) drops in 6–8 ounces of water one to three times daily. I use the dry extract in my practice, recommending 50–250 mg, three times daily to treat an active respiratory or gastrointestinal tract infection. GSE is generally safe, but the liquid can cause skin and mucous membrane irritation, so it should always be diluted in water or juice.

Herbal Antibiotic Alternatives: Fresh garlic or garlic capsules can be used for nearly any type of bacterial infection. The down side is the strong odor and the difficulty in eating enough of the cloves without causing stomach cramps. I prefer the concentrated allicin mentioned earlier.

Goldenseal is a common antimicrobial herb, but due to possible side effects that include abdominal cramping, it should only be used for one to two weeks at a time. It is also contraindicated in pregnancy or while nursing. Goldenseal is frequently combined with echinacea for upper respiratory tract infections. I do not use it much in practice, preferring the concentrated berberine extract, because of goldenseal's extreme bitterness.

Sage tea is an effective natural antibiotic alternative for throat and respiratory tract infections. Steep 2 teaspoons of the powdered leaf in 1 cup of hot water for 10 minutes and drink warm. You can use it as a gargle for sore throat.

Usnea, a common gray-green lichen that grows on the bark of trees worldwide, has been shown to be effective against gram-positive bacteria and is useful in treating pneumonia and other difficult-to-eradicate respiratory tract infections. Use it in tincture form, 1 teaspoon 4–6 times daily. Since it can cause mucous membrane irritation, always dilute it in water before drinking.

Common Herbal Antibiotic Alternatives

Garlic

Goldenseal

Sage

Usnea

Note on Dosages:

Some dosages are given in ranges. As a rule, for chronic conditions start with the lower dosage and gradually work towards the higher dosage, monitoring your response for possible adverse effects. For acute conditions, start with the higher dosages but only for a maximum of seven to ten days, and then discontinue.

Table 17: Natural Alternatives for Common Viral Conditions

Herbal Antiviral Alternatives

Medication	Use	Form	Dosage
Boneset	Influenza, dengue	Tea	3–5 g per cup, drink 3 times daily
Echinacea	Influenza, common cold	Tincture, dry or liquid extract	1/3 teaspoon, 3–4 times daily; 300 mg 3–4 times daily
Elderberry	Influenza	Tea	3–5 g per cup, drink 3 times daily
Esberitox	Influenza, common cold	Liquid extract	10–12 drops, 3 times daily
Witch hazel (Hamamelis)	Herpes	Liquid extract, ointment	Apply to local area, 2–4 times daily
Lemon Balm (Melissa)	Herpes	Ointment (Herpilyn)	Apply locally, 2–4 times daily
Lomatium	Rotavirus	Tincture	1/3 teaspoon, 3–4 times daily
Pascotox Forte	Influenza, common cold	Injection (Rx)	1 ampoule, 3–5 times weekly
Phyllanthus	Hepatitis B and C	Dry extract	300–800 mg, 3 times daily
Sangre de drago	HIV-associated diarrhea	Dry extract (NSF)	1 tablet, 2–4 times daily
St. John's wort	Depression associated with viral illness	Dry extract	300 mg, 3 times daily

Homeopathic Antiviral Alternatives

Medication	Use	Form	Dosage
Echinacea Compositum S	Influenza, common cold	Liquid	1 ampoule under the tongue, 1–3 times daily for a course of 10 days, repeat as needed
Engystol N	Influenza, common cold, nonspecific viral infections	Tablets, injection (Rx)	1 tablet, 3 times daily, or every hour for acute infections
Gripp-Heel	Influenza, common cold	Tablets, injection (Rx)	1 tablet, 3 times daily, or every 15 minutes for acute infections
Pascotox	Influenza, common cold	Liquid or tablets	20–40 drops or 4–6 tablets, 3–6 times daily
Oscillococcinum	Influenza	Pellets	3 pellets, 3 times daily
Eupatorium	Influenza, common cold	Tablets, drops	3 tablets or 10 drops, every two hours
Gelsemium	Influenza, common cold	Tablets, drops	3 tablets, every two hours
Aconitum	Influenza, common cold	Tablets, drops	3 tablets, every two hours

Nutraceutical Antiviral Alternatives

Olive leaf extract	Herpes, Hepatitis	Dry extract	500–1,000 mg, 3–4 times daily
Plant tannins	Gastrointestinal viruses	Dry extract (Viracin)	1 capsule, 2 times daily
Monolaurin	Herpes, HIV, CMV	Extract (Lauricidin)	600–1,200 mg, 3 times daily
RC-183	Herpes	Extract	unknown

Nutraceutical Antibiotic Alternatives

Berberine	Gastrointestinal and urinary tract infections	Dry extract	200–400 mg, 2–4 times daily
Allicin	Respiratory infections and deep fungal infections	Dry extract	20–40 mg, 2–3 times daily
Grapefruit seed extract	Respiratory infections	Dry extract or liquid extract	50–250 mg, 3 times daily; 2–15 drops, 3 times daily

CHAPTER SUMMARY

Many natural antiviral alternatives are available, and though they are necessary in your viral immunity program, they do not cure illnesses or heal tissues and cells. Diet and the other natural regimens described in steps 1 through 4 assist in deeper healing; the antivirals keep the viral load down so your system can recover.

Most antiviral alternatives are herbal. Though teas can be used for minor, uncomplicated viral illnesses like the common cold or flu, standardized extracts or tinctures provide the greatest therapeutic advantage in chronic conditions.

Nutraceutical antiviral substances are more concentrated than herbs and can have greater antiviral activity than even herbal extracts; they should be considered the first line of treatment.

Homeopathic antiviral remedies can be used to complement herbal or nutraceutical antiviral medications.

Co-infections are common in serious chronic viral infections such as HIV and HCV. Combine natural antibiotic alternatives with antiviral medications to treat bacterial and fungal co-infections.

Dosages vary according to the size, age, and general health of the person.

13

STEP EIGHT

Empower Your Viral Immunity Program with Chinese Medicines

Though this book has presented many references to Chinese medical philosophy, acupuncture energy systems, and Chinese herbs, it is not intended to be a text on Chinese medicine nor does it have an agenda to advocate Chinese medicine over any other system. However, in my clinical view, no treatment of viruses is complete without the use of Chinese medicine.

In this chapter I discuss several Chinese herbal medicines that are essential inclusions in your viral immunity program. Chinese medicines will not only make your plan more effective, but they will provide additional health benefits, like improved cardiovascular function, and they may even reduce the effects of aging.

Let's look at some of the reasons why Chinese medicine is so important in the treatment of viral conditions.

Eight Advantages to Chinese Medicine

1. The Chinese have vast experience with viruses: most influenza outbreaks originate in China; herpes virus is thought to have originated in Southeast Asia and Southern China; and hepatitis B is endemic in China.

2. Chinese doctors treat hundreds of millions of people every year, and have done so for a considerable length of time. These astounding numbers of patients provide a great pool of empirical knowledge unmatched anywhere else in the world.

3. The Chinese are a practical people. Unlike the United States where marketing practices drive sales and drug prescriptions, the Chinese tend to focus on what works and believe that clinical success motivates people to "buy." Of course, this does not completely ensure that all Chinese medicines are effective or safe, but as a general rule if a medication does not work, the Chinese practitioners won't use it.

4. China has an extensive infrastructure for the cultivation, harvesting, storage, and processing of herbs, including the preparation of extracts. Outside China, a worldwide distribution network is already in place making herbal products readily available.

5. The Chinese have the will, facilities, and manpower to conduct extensive clinical and scientific research; they are doing so in several research facilities in China. (Japan, Korea, Taiwan, Hong Kong, and Singapore, all countries more modernized than China, and advanced European countries like Germany, are also conducting scientific research on Chinese herbs.)

6. The Chinese are great record keepers and have documented their clinical experience over several thousand years, in tens of thousands of written texts. This immense library of Chinese medical knowledge constitutes a wealth of information on healthcare and disease, much of it still untapped.

7. They have developed two therapeutic methods mostly unknown to either allopathic or alternative medicine in the West, and both exert significant influence on the immune system: (1) the use of adaptogens (ginseng and astragalus) that nourish and rebuild organ, glandular, and nervous system energy reserves; and (2) "harmonizing formulas" (Minor Bupleurum Decoction) that rebalance disharmonic energy by reducing inflammation, stimulating the immune system at the same time.

8. There are more than 400 individual herbs routinely used by doctors of traditional Chinese medicine; more than 600 are in general use; and there are several thousand additional Chinese herbs that have known therapeutic benefits, many with potential antiviral and immune-enhancing properties.

Potential Uses and Benefits of Chinese Herbs in Viral Illnesses

They can reduce the side effects of drug therapy.
They can act as powerful immune modulators.
Many have significant antiviral activity.
Many reduce inflammation.
They have liver-protecting properties.
They can restore organ energy reserves.

This information may seem daunting, but let me assure you that it is not necessary for you to be an expert in Chinese medicine to put these therapies to use in your program, any more than you have to be a nutritionist to eat properly. However, if you have questions or desire a more detailed approach to the use of Chinese medicine for viral conditions, read further from the books in the recommended reading list or seek the services of an experienced acupuncturist or doctor of Oriental medicine. A skilled Chinese medicine professional can perform a detailed diagnostic workup for you, and will recommend a treatment plan that may include acupuncture as well as herbs matched to your individual situation.

Chinese herbal medicines cover all the aspects of immune protection discussed in this book, along with some additional benefits. Therefore, they can enhance and improve every step of your viral immunity program.

If you use steroids, antiviral drugs, or pharmaceutical interferon, certain Chinese herbs may be used concurrently to reduce the side effects of those drugs. For example, ginseng and *wu jia pi*/radix acanthopanax *(Acanthopanax senticosus)* have been used to protect against damage to the immune system caused by radiation treatments during cancer therapy. Formulas containing *Chai Hu*/radix bupleuri *(Bupleurum falcatum)* have been used to enhance the effects of steroids and at the same time reduce the immune-damaging side effects of these drugs. Keep in mind that combining herbs with drugs may cause complications and should be only done by a knowledgeable physician, especially in the case of bupleurum-containing formulas (see the section on bupleurum in this chapter for more details).

Many Chinese herbs, such as ginseng and astragalus, have powerful immune-modulating effects. A considerable number of them have been shown to induce production of natural interferons, including bupleurum, astragalus, and lithospermum *(Lithospermum crythrorhizon)*. Additionally, in our age of rampant cancers, AIDS, and worldwide chronic hepatitis, extensive screening of Chinese herbs has taken place for their immune-modulating effects and antiviral activity.

A recent *Cochrane Review,* an authoritative collection of scientific evidence for the presumed efficacy of medical therapies from Oxford University in England, assessed nine randomized trials of 936 patients and concluded that some Chinese herbs have effectiveness against hepatitis B virus (Liu 2001). The authors recommended further research to evaluate the potential clinical use for these herbs in conventional therapy. In another study, 1,000 Chinese herbs were screened for antiviral activity and 127 were found to be effective, and 28 were classified as highly inhibitory (Zheng 1992).

Chinese herbs exert anti-inflammatory effects and are useful in inflammatory conditions induced by cell-mediated immunity, irritable bowel syndrome, pneumonitis (a respiratory tract inflammation), and tissue inflammation caused by viruses (like herpes blisters or liver inflammation from hepatitis virus). The flavonoids in *huang qin*/radix scutellaria *(Scutellaria baicalensis)* and other Chinese herbs act as modulators of the inflammatory response. Many Chinese herbs have liver-protective properties and are useful in managing the liver-damaging effects of chronic hepatitis B and C.

One of the most important contributions of Chinese herbs to world medicine is the use of adaptogens—substances (like ginseng) that improve homeostasis, reduce the effects of stress, restore organ energy reserves, and enhance hormone balance. In dysfunctional immunological states, chronic underlying homeostatic disturbances occur, and no drug can put all the pieces of the immunological system back together again. In such cases, the long-term ingestion of traditional Chinese tonic remedies with adaptogenic properties is not only helpful, but may be essential to complete recovery.

In the following sections, you will learn about the most important Chinese herbs in these categories. I focus on those individual herbs and formulas that have antiviral activity and that are the best-known immune enhancers.

Immune-Empowering Herbs from the Chinese Medicine Chest

I have already introduced several Chinese herbs with antiviral activity, including phyllanthus, cordyceps, and ganoderma. In this section, I will discuss several more important antiviral and immune-modulating Chinese herbs.

Andrographis: *Chuan xin lian*/herba andrographis *(Andrographis paniculata)* has great therapeutic potential in the treatment of infections. It is a member of the Acanthaceae family and grows wild or under cultivation in China, India, and Southeast Asia. It contains the lactone compound, andrographolide, and has been studied in the treatment of HIV, bacterial infections, and the common cold.

> ### Selected Antiviral and Immune-Enhancing Chinese Herbs
>
> Andrographis
> Astragalus
> Bupleurum
> Coptis
> Ginseng
> Isatis
> Licorice
> Ligustrum
> Schizandra

Traditionally, andrographis is used in Chinese medicine to treat respiratory, throat, urinary tract, and skin infections. I have used andrographis successfully for several decades in my practice for the treatment of bacterial and viral upper respiratory tract infections like sinusitis, for tonsillitis and pharyngitis (sore throat), and as a detoxifying agent in cancer treatments.

It is generally considered safe, but in high dosages or with extended use it may cause allergic reactions, so its use is best limited to 1–2 weeks at a time. It is available in tinctured form, dry extracts, and can be found packaged in capsules under the name Andrographis Formula, a 90 percent andrographis extract with 10 percent *yan hu suo*/rhizoma corydalis *(Corydalis yanhusuo)*; this is a Chinese medicine to activate blood circulation and relieve pain. The dosage of Andrographis Formula is two capsules three to four times daily, or 10–20 drops of the tincture three to four times daily. It can be used to treat influenza, the common cold, or opportunistic bacterial co-infections in chronic viral illnesses or deficient immunity.

Astragalus: Like ginseng, *huang qi*/radix astragali *(Astragalus membranaceus)* is considered an adaptogenic tonic that regulates the body's physiology and helps to restore normal homeostasis. Also like ginseng, astragalus is valued in traditional Chinese medicine for its ability to improve digestion and rebuild the body's energy, referred to as the spleen qi and yang.

Its particular characteristic of stabilizing the immune system's defensive energy *(wei qi)* makes astragalus the ideal herb for immune enhancement. In Chinese medicine, the three energy functions of strong spleen qi (digestive and nutritive function), yang energy (aggressive energy), and *wei qi* (immune resistance), are the most important factors for a healthy immune system that can defend the body against infections.

Astragalus is a polysaccharide-rich plant that has a marked effect on the human immune system. It stimulates interferon production, enhances immune cell activity, and stimulates the destruction of cancer cells. Though astragalus has no direct antiviral activity, it is important as an adaptogen (an immunomodulator) in a viral immunity program. It is usually taken as a tea by simmering 9–30 g of the dried sliced root per cup of water. Astragalus is safe to take in dosages up to 60 g or even more, and there are no reported side effects for long-term daily use of dosages in the 9–30 g range. It is also available in capsules: take two to three 500 mg capsules two times daily.

Bupleurum: *Chai hu*/radix bupleuri *(Bupleurum falcatum)* belongs to the Apiaceae family which has sixty-five different bupleurum species in temperate climate zones worldwide. It is a perennial herb native to northern China, across northern Asia, and parts of Europe. Bupleurum contains several saponin compounds (saikosaponin c, a, and d), triterpene glycosides (saikosides), the essential oils furfural and bupleurumol, and flavonoids. It is reported to have anti-inflammatory properties, to activate phagocytosis, and be liver protective; it stimulates T and B cells, and inhibits herpes simplex and other viruses. In Chinese medicine, the root is used medicinally to treat unresolved respiratory tract infections and hepatitis. However, it is not used alone, but combined with other herbs.

The most well-known bupleurum-containing formula is Minor Bupleurum Decoction, which is used for the treatment of chronic hepatitis (see below). Though scientific data on this herb is limited, bupleurum is considered nontoxic and safe for short-term use in treating acute viral illnesses like influenza. However, serious interactions between this herb and some drugs have been seen. Refer to the precautionary note on bupleurum-containing formulas further on in this chapter.

Coptis: *Huang lian*/rhizoma coptidis *(Coptis chinensis)* is used in traditional Chinese medicine to clear "damp heat" syndromes; conditions characterized by inflammation, tissue swelling and edema, and discharge of body fluids like diarrhea or mucus drainage. Coptis is used in the treatment of bacterial infections of the gastrointestinal and respiratory tracts like abscesses, dysentery, gastritis, and sinusitis. It is also a very useful remedy for conjunctivitis, or "pink eye," an inflammation of the white part of the eye caused by bacteria or viruses. Coptis contains the isoquinoline berberine chlorides, sulfates, and coptisine; berberine is the bright yellow, bitter antimicrobial alkaloid discussed in the previous chapter. Coptis berberines have been extensively studied in Asia for their anti-inflammatory effects; coptis also has liver-protective properties and anti-cancer activity.

Coptis can be used by itself or in combination with other berberine-containing compounds and along with other antimicrobial herbs to treat systemic bacterial co-infections. It is a very powerful herb, and I have found it to be as effective as or more effective than standardized mixed berberine extracts. However, since individual patients respond differently to various formulations, even of similar compounds, I use both the European standardized berberine extract and Chinese coptis. The herb is considered safe and without toxicity, and may be used long term without side effects.

In my clinical practice, I use two forms of coptis. The traditional form is called *Huang Lian Su Pian*, and consists of the extract coptin; it is packaged in glass vials containing twelve small tablets per vial. I use this form for minor food poisoning, gastritis, and traveler's diarrhea. Typically, I recommend two tablets two to four times daily until symptoms improve. For liver and gallbladder inflammation, and systemic bacterial and yeast infections accompanying chronic viruses, I use a standardized extract of coptis. Each tablet contains 100 mg of coptin and is available from HepaPro. The typical dosage is two tablets taken three to four times daily, 10–20 minutes before ingesting food.

Ginseng: *Ren shen*/radix ginseng *(Panax ginseng)* is the most studied of Chinese herbs. The Chinese revere ginseng for its use as a longevity medicine, and the highest quality ginseng is worth more than its weight in gold. Traditionally it is considered the premier energy tonic and is used to treat weakness and deficiency of the spleen and kidney qi. In 1986, immunostimulating polysaccharides were isolated from ginseng; research since has shown that ginseng improves cell-mediated immunity. An Italian study in 1996 with 227 subjects showed that ginseng had preventive effects on the common cold and influenza. The main therapeutic components of ginseng are ginsenosides; several recent studies have shown that the ginsenosides Rb1 and Rb2 inhibit cancer progression, and another study discovered a new protein from ginseng called panaxagin, which has both antifungal and antiviral activity.

Ginseng improves stamina, reduces the effects of stress, has anti-inflammatory activity, elevates mood and energy, and when taken consistently over a period of time can give a sense of well being, benefit blood sugar control, and improve liver function. It is usually taken in capsules, 100–300 mg, yielding approximately 5–15 mg of ginsenosides, daily.

Ginseng improves stamina, reduces the effects of stress, has anti-inflammatory activity, elevates mood and energy, and when taken consistently over a period of time can give a sense of well being, benefit blood sugar control, and improve liver function. For therapeutic purposes, I recommend the standardized extract rather than the tea form. It is usually taken in capsules, 100–300 mg, yielding approximately 5–15 mg of ginsenosides, daily. The tea is used as an energy tonic, but not as a stimulant or replacement for coffee. Korean red ginseng extracts are also very effective and are available in most Korean markets. A decoction is made from the root by slowly boiling 3–10 g of the dried and sliced root for about one hour. This method can yield up to 100 mg of ginsenosides per day.

Though ginseng is considered safe for long-term use, there are several contraindications. It should not be taken if you have high blood pressure, have an active infection, fever, or inflammatory condition, and you should not take ginseng if you are taking monoamine oxidase (MAO) inhibiting antidepressants (Nardil, Parnate) or anti-Parkinson drugs like selegiline (Deprenyl) that have MAO inhibiting activity. Do not take ginseng during pregnancy or give it to children.

Isatis: *Ban lan gen*/radix isatidis *(Isatis tinctoria)* is another powerful antimicrobial Chinese herb. It is a member of the mustard family and is the source of a natural indigo dye. In Chinese medicine it is used to clear "internal heat," inflammation and infection in the organs, and can treat bacterial, parasitic, and viral infections. I use it for influenza and combine it with antimicrobial herbs, like andrographis, to lower viral load in chronic viral illnesses.

Licorice: *Gan cao*/radix glycyrrhizae *(Glycyrrhiza uralensis)* is Chinese licorice and is the most frequently used of all Chinese herbs.

Traditionally, it is combined in formulas to enhance the activity of the other herbs and is thought to nourish the spleen, expel phlegm, and clear "latent heat"—the unresolved conditions of chronic viral infections like herpes and hepatitis C. In these latent heat cases, low-grade inflammation and infection linger in the tissues and are difficult to eradicate.

In modern Chinese medicine, the concentrated extract glycyrrhizine (often given intravenously) is used as a powerful anti-inflammatory medication. It also has antiviral activity and used as a detoxifying agent and for peptic ulcers in a form with the glycyrrhizine removed.

Glycyrrhizine is also considered an immunomodulating drug and mimics naturally-produced steroid hormones. It contains the triterpenes glycyrrhizin and glycyrrhetinic acid and has been studied extensively for the treatment of hepatitis. The mechanisms by which glycyrrhizin works for hepatitis are still unknown and the pharmaceutical form is not an approved drug in the United States. In my practice, I use an oral extract form for active liver inflammation in patients with HCV. It is available in capsules; however, due to its potential serious side effects, I do not recommend you use concentrated glycyrrhizine without the supervision of a doctor.

Caution: In traditional Chinese medicine, licorice root is only used in very small amounts as a complement to other formulas. Since the side effects were known by the ancient Chinese, precautions were taken to remove some of the active component by steaming and drying to reduce the toxic effects. This purified form can be used in small dosages safely without concern of side effects.

Concentrated glycyrrhizine, on the other hand, can cause swelling, high blood pressure, and fatigue in about 20 percent of patients due to its effects on mineralocorticoid hormones. Do not use glycyrrhizine if you have edema, hypertension, kidney disease, or arrhythmia (heartbeat irregularity), or if you are taking prescription diuretics or Digoxin.

Ligustrum: *Nu zhen zi*/fructus ligustri *(Ligustrum lucidum)* is used traditionally as a liver yin tonic to treat dizziness, tinnitus, and eye problems. Ligustrin, the concentrated extract, contains oleanolic acid and other substances and is used as a liver-protective medication. Ligustrin has been shown to inhibit liver degeneration, protect against liver damage from hepatitis and liver cancer, and exert immune-modulating effects. It is a safe herb and can be taken over a long period of time. The therapeutic dosage of ligustrin is 300 mg, taken three times daily 10–20 minutes before meals. A tea can also be prepared from the roasted seeds; however, it is time-consuming to make and is not as effective as the extract.

Schizandra: *Wu wei zi*/fructus schizandrae *(Schizandra chinensis)* is a member of the magnolia family and is traditionally used to control "leakage of vital essence" from the body. The Chinese believe that the body produces a vital essence, *jing*. This is different from yet similar to and just as important to health as the qi; it is present in semen, saliva, and other body fluids. Schizandra treats cough, wheezing, asthma, noninfectious frequent urination, and spontaneous sweating. Extensive research in Asia has been conducted on schizandra for its liver-protective effects and seven liver-enzyme lowering substances have been found including schizandrin B and C. Schizandrin has powerful antioxidant properties and can significantly improve glutathione status.

Extracts of schizandra are generally not used alone, but are commonly found as a primary ingredient in formulas for HCV, such as Hepala or Eurocell, both discussed in the next section. Generally considered safe, schizandrin is contraindicated in pregnancy, in patients with epilepsy, or if you have a peptic ulcer.

Chinese Herbal Formulas

Though several of the herbs discussed in the previous section (ginseng, astragalus, and coptis) can be used alone, Chinese medicine usually applies formulas containing several ingredients, using a family of different herbs, as it were, each with its own characteristics and personalities.

The wisdom of the Chinese doctors is that individual herbs work *synergistically* to increase the overall effect of a formula while also decreasing toxicity. Combination therapy also greatly increases the number of active component interactions and thereby reduces the chance of microorganisms developing resistance—an important concept in working with viral infections.

In my clinical practice, I mainly use formulas that are based upon traditional principles of prescribing. I also follow the modern Chinese research and will experiment with new or adapted formulas or individual herbs. However, in respect for a system that has thousands of years of continuous use, I always remain rooted in traditional Chinese methods.

Minor Bupleurum Decoction: Minor Bupleurum Decoction (MBD) is the formula of our times. In my practice I routinely prescribe this formula for a variety of conditions including lingering or recurrent influenza and chronic HCV. It is so versatile that many modern American practitioners of Chinese medicine rank it among their favorite formulas. This one formula addresses many of the immune conditions affecting modern people: it increases energy, controls infections, clears phlegm, and detoxifies.

Traditionally, MBD is the premier formula for *shaoyang* stage illnesses, that is, those conditions characterized by lingering symptoms that are stuck between the interior regions of the body and the surface. Located principally between the diaphragm and the throat, especially around the liver area on the right side under the rib cage, *shaoyang* conditions manifest as chronic viral disease chronic inflammatory conditions, and chronic fatigue—all the conditions discussed in this book.

The individual herbs in the formula are thought to harmonize the defensive and constructive energies simultaneously, allowing the body to remove pathogenic influences and rebuild energy and strength. MBD is composed of six Chinese herbs with several slices of fresh ginger added. Bupleurum root clears stagnation from the liver and supports detoxification functions; it also has antiviral and immune-modulating activity as mentioned earlier, and clears pathogenic influences from the surface of the body.

It is paired in the decoction with Chinese skullcap or scutellaria root *(Scutellariae baicalensis)*, which clears dampness and heat from the liver, gallbladder, stomach, and large intestine; it also removes pathogenic influences from the interior of the body. Scutellaria is a flavonoid-rich plant with anti-inflammatory, antiviral, antiretroviral, antitumor, and antibacterial properties.

Together, bupleurum and scutellaria synergistically regulate the *shaoyang,* and by doing so, help to reduce inflammation. A small amount of ginseng is added, complemented by red dates *(Zizyphi*

Ingredients of Minor Bupleurum Decoction

12 g bupleurum root *(chai hu)*

9 g scutellaria rhizome *(huang qin)*

9 g pinellia rhizome *(ban xia)*

6 g ginseng root *(ren shen)*

3 g licorice root *(gan cao)*

3–5 pieces jujube red date *(da zao)*

3–5 pieces fresh ginger root slices *(sheng jiang)*

jujubae) and honey-fried licorice, to improve digestive function, enhance the constructive energies, supplement and fortify the spleen, and "nourish" the spirit *(shen)* residing in the heart. In Chinese medicine, the therapeutic method of "nourishing the spirit" refers to herbal or acupuncture treatments that calm the nerves, lessen anxiety, improve the mood, and clear the mind.

Pinellia *(Pinelliae ternatae)* in this decoction removes stagnant phlegm from the chest and stomach. The fresh ginger supports the stomach and enhances the activity of the entire formula as latent pathogens rise to the surface for removal from the system.

MBD *(xiao chai hu tang* in Chinese; *sho-saiko-to* in Japanese) is the best selling traditional Chinese herbal formula in Japan and one of the most widely used in the world. It was originally recorded in the herbal classic *Shan Han Lun* more than a thousand years ago. Consider this: A medication in continuous use for thousands of years is not only still in use, but more widely used now than it ever has been. Can you imagine a Western drug that will be in use one thousand years from now?

Ginseng is the most researched of all individual Chinese herbs (and one of the ingredients in the formula), and MBD is the most researched herbal formula, extensively studied in Japan, Korea, and China for its use in hepatitis. Pharmacologically, it has immune-modulating activity, reduces inflammation, is antiviral and antibacterial, and exerts liver-protective effects. MBD is used to treat bronchial asthma, influenza, common cold, sinusitis, and chronic hepatitis B and C.

It is available in concentrated extract form from several Taiwanese manufacturers. In my practice, I use Brion (Sun Ten) Herbs. For lingering influenza or colds, the dosage is typically three to four capsules, three times daily, away from food, for 5–10 days. For chronic viral diseases, I typically recommend two capsules, three times daily for 1–3 months. I generally alternate the next 1–3 months with phyllanthus or a different Chinese antiviral formula as a method of preventing the possibility of side effects occurring from continuous use of any one herb or herbal formula. Three months is also a sufficient amount of time to achieve therapeutic benefits.

Though Minor Bupleurum Decoction is considered safe and nontoxic for short-term use, when given concurrently with interferon for the treatment of hepatitis C it has been associated with increased incidence of acute pneumonitis (inflammation of the lungs) and interstitial pneumonia, having produced sixteen fatal cases in Japan.

Since the herbal formula alone does not cause lung inflammation and interstitial pneumonia can occur with interferon therapy alone, researchers suspect that it is the combination of the two that causes the increased incidence of this serious side effect rather than herbs in the formula. Though the exact interaction is still unknown, researchers suggest the herbs may increase pro-inflammatory interleukin levels, while the interferon may cause neutrophils to accumulate in the lungs triggering an immune reaction. Never take this formula if you are taking interferon.

Additionally, Minor Bupleurum Decoction is known to inhibit prednisolone (a common steroid drug) metabolism. This can result in higher levels of the drug in the body, leading to increased possibility of steroid-induced side effects, such as immune suppression. Do not take this formula while on any type of steroid medication without the supervision of a doctor. As it also can up-regulate the immune system, it should not be used by people with rheumatoid arthritis, transplant patients, or for any condition in which over-active immunity is undesirable.

> **Modern Chinese Antiviral Formulas for Chronic Hepatitis**
> CH-100
> Euroce
> HEPA 1A Formula
> Qing Tui Tang

Modern Chinese Antiviral Formulas

Due to the increasing incidence of HIV and HCV infection, Chinese doctors have researched individual herbs and formulas from their traditional *materia medica* and have created new formulas, or modifications of existing formulas, to meet the demands generated by emerging viral diseases. In one study, 472 herbs were screened for antiviral activity against herpes simplex virus; after repeated testing, ten new herbs were found to have antiviral activity, among them *Patrinia villosa*, one of the active herbs in Eurocel, a formula discussed below.

CH-100: This was tested on HCV patients in a study performed in John Hunter Hospital of Newcastle, Australia, by Professor R. G. Batey of Newcastle University. Like most of the formulas discussed in this chapter, CH-100 proved to be effective in normalizing levels of ALT (alanine aminotransferase), but not in reducing the overall viral load. Because ALT is usually elevated in hepatitis C patients, it is used as a sensitive indicator of injury to liver cells. During the course of treatment, ALT levels are often tracked by doctors to determine improvement or worsening of liver inflammation. CH-100 is imported from China by Cathay Herbal Laboratories.

Eurocel: This is a Korean product distributed by Allergy Research Group in the U.S. It is composed of *Patrinia villosa, Artemisia capillaries,* and schizandra. Patrinia, or *bai hua bai jiang cao,* is a wild perennial plant used in Japan and Korea to reduce liver toxicity. What makes this formula attractive for HCV treatment is that a small pilot study carried out over a two-year period in Korea showed dramatic reduction in ALT levels, as well as viral load.

Keep in mind that one study of ten patients does not mean that this formula will work for you, but it may be worth a trial of four to six months with a liver function panel taken before and after. One of my HCV patients added this formula to his regimen of natural medicines, and after four months of treatment, his ALT levels dropped by 50 percent—a significant change. The typical recommended dosage is two to three capsules, two times per day.

HEPA 1A Formula: Developed by Dr. Zhang, one of the leading authorities on the treatment of HCV with Chinese medicine, this remedy contains several Chinese herbs with broad-spectrum antiviral and liver-protective effects, including radix scutellaria/*huang qin (Scutellariae baicalensis)* and fructus schizandra/*wu wei zhi (Schizandrae chinensis).* Scutellaria has broad-spectrum antimicrobial effects and anti-inflammatory activity useful in treating viral hepatitis. Schizandra has been studied extensively in liver diseases and hepatitis. It lowers ALT levels, improves liver function, and aids in regeneration of liver tissue.

This formula is used to reduce liver inflammation and lower the viral load in HCV patients. A typical dosage is to take two 500 mg capsules, three times daily on an empty stomach, about 10–20 minutes before meals.

Qing Tui Tang: Developed in China and available in the United States from the Institute for Traditional Medicine in Portland,

Oregon, this antiviral formula has been shown to improve liver function and reduce inflammation in HCV patients. The formula contains several herbs including bupleurum, polygonum, and astragalus. It is taken as a 5:1 concentrate in granule form, 6–9 g, three times daily without food. It is considered safe and non-toxic.

> ## Effective Chinese Flu and Cold Remedies
>
> Gan Mao preparations
>
> Yin Qiao San
>
> Zhong Gan Ling

Chinese Medicines for Flu and the Common Cold

Although echinacea and other North American and European herbs are commonly used to treat the common cold and influenza, I highly recommend that you learn how to use Chinese prepared medicines for these illnesses. I have discussed the reasons elsewhere in the book, but because of their importance, it is worthwhile mentioning them again.

Foremost is that influenza virus strains originate in China and the Chinese have several thousands of years of experience treating these illnesses with sophisticated herbal formulas. If you use echinacea frequently, you may have noticed that its effectiveness ebbs over time. No one knows why this happens, but researchers and clinicians suggest that either the body adapts to the herb, becoming less responsive, or that the infectious organisms develop resistance to the herbal ingredients.

Since Chinese formulas for influenza are composed of at least eight to twelve herbs from different therapeutic classes, there is less chance of either the body or the microorganisms adapting. Regardless of the reasons why an herb may lose effectiveness, it is a good idea to have four to six *different* herbal flu remedies in your cupboard, and to alternate them every few months during flu season to prevent adaptation.

Gan Mao: This is the Chinese term for the common cold. There are several different forms of the prepared medicine Gan Mao, but one of my clinical favorites for mild cases of the common cold or flu is *Gan Mao Tui Re Chun Ji,* an instant granule preparation containing isatis; it is mixed directly into hot water. It also works well as a preventative. Take one package three to four times daily for treatment of a cold or one to two packages daily for prevention. It also comes as a tablet or capsule and is called *Gan Mao Ling.* Though the herbal ingredients of the tablet are somewhat different from the granules, they both can be used for fever due to the common cold or flu. Typically, I advise people to take four to five tablets three times daily, or every hour in the acute stages.

Yin Qiao San: This is a formula from the Qing Dynasty (1644–1911) and very popular in China. Its action is similar to *Gan Mao Ling,* and they may be used interchangeably. Yin Qiao has been adapted into a new formula that suits modern febrile illnesses. Called *Yin Qiao Jie Du Pian,* this formula has immune-stimulating properties, is antiviral, and reduces fever and inflammation; it is stronger than regular Yin Qiao. A recommended dose is two to three tablets, three times a day or more frequently for acute symptoms.

Zhong Gan Ling: The third remedy for seasonal viral infections is Zhong Gan Ling. It is used primarily for influenza with symptoms of fever and achiness, and is stronger than regular Gan Mao Ling or Yin Qiao San. A recommended dose is four to six tablets, three times a day.

Herbs for Restoring the Yin

Our environment and fast-paced lifestyle deplete deep reserves of our energy and exhaust the essence—the *yin* and *jing qi*—of our vital organs. According to doctors of traditional Chinese medicine, this severe depletion is one of the underlying causes of the breakdown of our immune function. Chinese doctors have always been masters of the knowledge of replenishment (the opposite of depletion): the preservation, cultivation, and restoration of intrinsic energy, vital resources, and the tonification of healing potential within the body. This system of therapy of restoration, called *fushen,* is needed now more than ever.

Knowledge of replenishment therapies is critical in managing serious viral diseases like HIV and HCV, and it can help to prevent immune dysfunction and retard aging. I have already discussed several Chinese herbs in this category, chief among them ginseng. Others include ganoderma and astragalus, each notable for its ability to restore qi and yang.

Another herb, equally important, but one that restores the body's yin essences and builds the blood is *Ho Shou Wu (Polygonum multiflorum).* In use for thousands of years, its properties were first recorded in the Tang Dynasty nearly two thousand years ago. Ho Shou Wu is carefully prepared by soaking the root of the polygonum plant with black soybeans; then it is dried and sliced into very thin, dark red wafers.

Traditionally, polygonum is used as a tonic for the yin and blood, to nourish the hair, strengthen the bones and muscles, and for the treatment of dizziness, tinnitus, weakness in the loins and knees, and numbness in the extremities. It also is useful for abnormal uterine bleeding, and is noted for its recuperative powers for the treatment of weakness after illness or for lingering diseases like malaria. It is an immune modulator and improves cell-mediated immunity, it slows down the degeneration of glands, and it improves cardiovascular function.

Chinese medical theory teaches that if the kidney essence (yin) is depleted by excessive sex, overwork, stress, drugs, or lack of sleep, the body's immune system is unable to defend against all the myriad microorganisms to which we are exposed.

From the energetic point of view, Chinese medical theory teaches that if the kidney essence (yin) is depleted by excessive sex, overwork, stress, drugs, or lack of sleep, the body's immune system is unable to defend against all the myriad microorganisms to which we are exposed. When this happens, we either become sick with a chronic active disease, like hepatitis C, or if we are still somewhat strong, the pathogenic factor, often a virus or other infectious organism, becomes latent, producing slow, lingering effects. The immune system, unable to eliminate the illness with the normal innate response in the early stages of infection, is also unable, due to faulty adaptive mechanisms, to fully eradicate the condition.

If the pathogenic factor is a virus, it then gravitates to certain organs or tissues that it has an affinity for, usually the liver or the nervous system. In either case, unless the yin essence is restored, the body's immune response is inadequate to expel latent or chronic active viruses, and you gradually become sicker.

To assess your yin status, answer the questionnaire in the Yin Deficiency Self-Test. If you answer "yes" to more than three questions, most likely you have some stage of yin deficiency and should consider adding polygonum into your viral immunity program. The typical dosage is 9–15 g of the root, prepared as a tea by simmering the herb in one quart of water for 30–45 minutes. Drink one cup, two times daily, away from food.

Polygonum also comes as a prepared medicine from China. Called *Shuo Wu Pian* and produced by the Shanghai Medicine Works, it comes

Yin Deficiency Self-Test

Do you have night sweats?

Do you have hot flushing or tend to feel warmer than normal?

Is your tongue bright red?

Do you have tinnitus (ear ringing) and/or dizziness?

Are you consistently fatigued?

Do you have insomnia, with either difficulty falling asleep or waking up where you cannot go back to sleep?

Do (did) you have prematurely gray hair?

Do you have numbness of the feet or lower legs?

in a bottle of 100 easy-to-swallow coated tablets. The recommended dose is five to ten pills, three times daily on an empty stomach. You can also buy it combined with other tonic herbs in a liquid extract called *Shou Wu Chih.* This preparation is taken in 1-ounce doses, one time daily in the evening, or it can be added to hot water to make a tea. Polygonum is a safe and non-toxic herb and can be taken over a long period of time without side effects.

How to Use Chinese Herbs in Your Viral Immunity Plan: Chinese herbs are used in two main ways: as adaptogens to improve energy status and organ reserve and as antimicrobials to treat viral illnesses and bacterial co-infections. If you have a chronic viral disease and are fatigued, add ginseng, cordyceps, ganoderma, astragalus, or polygonum to your program. Cordyceps and ganoderma may be combined with other immune-modulating mushroom extracts for general immune enhancement. Ginseng is used if you are very fatigued, feel cold, and have weakened digestion. Astragalus is used if there are recurrent colds, repeated minor infections, muscle weakness, poor healing or recovery, and mild fatigue. Polygonum, as described above, is for symptoms of yin deficiency.

Chinese antimicrobial herbs are essential in any plan that treats chronic viral disorders. Choose one of the formulas discussed in this chapter and take it as directed for three months. If you have an acute infection or a bacterial co-infection, choose one of the individual herbs, like coptin or andrographis, and combine it into your program along with the formula. If you have concerns or questions, be sure to discuss them with a specialist in Chinese medicine.

Caution: Here is a summary of precautions to take when using Chinese herbs.

When selecting Chinese herbs, choose only one or two individual herbs, and only one formula at a time.

Just as well-organized groups of herbs can be synergistic and beneficial when used together, taking multiple herbs at the same time can cause interactions to take place that can either cancel out their positive effects or cause unexpected side effects. Luckily, with natural medicine any negative effects are usually limited to gastrointestinal upset.

If you experience nausea, abdominal bloating or discomfort, or diarrhea when taking Chinese herbs, discontinue immediately.

Consult a specialist in Chinese medicine to help tailor herbs to your specific condition and individual needs.

Acupuncture and Bioenergetic Balancing

Acupuncture is a therapeutic system that uses thin stainless steel or other metallic needles inserted lightly into the skin and underlying soft tissue (muscle, ligament, and adipose) at the sites of specific acupuncture points. This is done to manipulate energy currents that flow in the body and to promote healing, reduce pain and inflammation, and harmonize the body's intrinsic energy.

Though there is little conclusive scientific evidence that acupuncture increases specific immune activity, there is considerable *empirical* evidence that acupuncture treatments strengthen and normalize immunity. Acupuncturists and their patients repeatedly report that treatments confer immune benefits. For example: patients report considerably fewer colds and incidences of influenza, more energy, sleep improvement, less pain, uplifted moods—all conditions that influence the immune system in a positive manner.

For the treatment of viral illnesses, the acupuncturist selects points that promote the dispersal of pathogenic energy from within the body. It moves to the surface where it is met, acted upon, and transformed by the defensive energy, the *wei chi.* The transformed pathogenic energy is dispersed into the body fluids and is then removed from the body in the sweat, respiration, stool, urine, or mucus.

In Chinese medicine, viral illnesses fall under several different classifications, and each is treated differently. For example, a "wind-cold" pattern, characterized by headache and chills, may be caused by viruses or bacteria, resulting in the common cold, influenza, measles, sinusitis, or conjunctivitis. A "wind-heat" pattern, characterized by fever, sweating, and malaise, may cause all the same viral or bacterial infections, as well as bronchitis and conditions characterized by high fever. A "damp-heat" pattern, associated with inflammation and swelling, can be associated with hepatitis as well as gastritis, an inflammation of the stomach. The acupuncturist selects points that match the Chinese diagnosis for the treatment of the imbalanced energy.

The energy of the disease and its manifestation in the body constitute the pathogenic pattern. The acupuncturist further takes into consideration the level at which the disease is lodged and the strength of the patient. For example, in AIDS, the disease affects the deepest levels, those of the blood and bone marrow. On the other extreme, a minor bout of the common cold, which is only on the surface of the body, affecting the respiratory passages like the sinuses, is classified as a superficial "wind-cold" attack with or without hot or cold phlegm retention.

In my clinical experience, acupuncture best serves as an adjunctive therapy in the treatment and management of viral disease. It can shorten the length of a cold or flu; it can reduce the side effects of interferon treatment in patients with HCV, promote internal peace and balance, manage inflammation and reduce pain, improve the quality of sleep, and reduce the incidence of infections.

Phlegm is a common sign in respiratory infections, like a runny nose during a cold or the spitting-up (expectoration) of phlegm with bronchitis. In Chinese medicine, "cold phlegm" is clear or white in color and is not associated with serious infection. On the other hand, "hot phlegm" is yellow, green, or brown and is associated with active infection and is therefore more serious. Needle technique, choice of points, and style of manipulation of the needle are different for each condition, the individual's constitution, the state of the body's energy, and the disease.

From the perspective of Chinese medicine, everything in the body is in a constant state of flux that ebbs and flows between health and disease, excess and deficiency, strength and weakness, heat and cold. A skilled acupuncturist seeks to balance disharmony in your body with needles, harmonizing this fluid state of energy, skillfully tonifying weaknesses and smoothing out stagnation, strengthening deficiency, and removing excess—using a variety of techniques to activate your body's healing power.

Though acupuncture can serve as an immune-modulating technique, there are no specific acupuncture points for viruses. That is not to say that acupuncture does not work as an adjunct in the treatment of viral diseases, as it can improve the flow of qi in the liver meridian and into other corresponding physical organs, thereby improving liver function. However, it cannot directly eliminate RNA viruses that cause hepatitis C. But, if in improving liver qi, acupuncture treatments cause effects that enhance the immune response and manage inflammation, then the liver cells themselves could potentially expel the virus.

In my clinical experience, acupuncture best serves as an adjunctive therapy in the treatment and management of viral disease. It can shorten the length of a cold or flu; it can reduce the side effects of interferon treatment in patients with HCV, promote internal peace and balance, manage inflammation and reduce pain, improve the quality of sleep, and reduce the incidence of infections. For an acute viral illness like the common cold, you may need only two to three acupuncture treatments over a period of one to two weeks to get deep relief. For chronic sinusitis, you may need treatment two times weekly for three to six weeks or longer; and for chronic hepatitis, weekly treatments of several months or even a year or two may be required.

CHAPTER SUMMARY

Chinese herbs and energy-balancing strategies play a pivotal role in a viral immunity plan.

The simplest approach is to add one or two immune-modulating or antimicrobial Chinese herbs to your plan.

A more comprehensive approach is to add one Chinese formula to your plan along with several individual herbs.

For chronic viral diseases, especially hepatitis B and C, Minor Bupleurum Decoction is the formula of choice. Review precautions carefully before taking this medication.

For effective relief from seasonal viral illnesses like the common cold or flu, try Chinese prepared medicines such as the Gan Mao formulas.

The most important immune-modulating Chinese herb is astragalus, useful in all types of immune-deficiency conditions, cancer, and chronic viral infections.

Ginseng, ganoderma, and cordyceps are important immune-modulating herbs, and like astragalus, they are mainly for qi and yang deficiency.

If you have yin deficiency, you need a yin tonic like polygonum.

14

STEP NINE

Optimize Immune Performance with Hormonal Balance

Correcting hormonal imbalances can greatly improve your immune function. In this chapter, we study the link between hormones and the immune system. With all that we know about hormones and disease, it is unfortunate that most conventional physicians rarely look at hormone levels when evaluating immune-related conditions, whether they are allergies, autoimmune diseases, inflammatory conditions, chronic fatigue syndrome, or chronic viral illness.

From my clinical experience in the anti-aging field and the treatment of immune-related disorders, I know that without evaluating hormone status an important piece of the diagnostic picture is missing. The following sections explain how you can optimize your immune performance with natural hormones, but first let's review how hormones interact with your immune system.

Hormones and the Immune System

Hormones play vital roles in maintaining immunity, especially during severe long-term stress and in chronic illness. In step 1, I discussed the deleterious effects of our modern lifestyles, stress, and aging on immunity and showed how these factors negatively influence hormone production and disturb hormonal balance. In addition to causing anxiety and depression, stress interferes with hormone regulation, one influence triggering another, perpetuating illness in a vicious cycle.

Though doctors and scientists have accepted the connection between hormones and immunity for more than a hundred years, it is still far from clear how this connection works. For example, when the stress hormones adrenaline and cortisol increase, T-lymphocyte and cytokine function is altered, but we are unclear which cells are inhibited and which ones are activated. We only know the function is *altered*.

On the other hand, we know that steroid drugs suppress immune reactions and that due to this effect, corticosteroid drugs like prednisone, prednisolone, and methylprednisolone are used to treat conditions characterized by aggressive inflammation and autoimmune reactivity, such as multiple sclerosis and rheumatoid arthritis. However, when steroids are used in very high dosages, they suppress immune reactions and in turn create severe side effects that eventually can be worse than the disease—but we don't know *why*.

Another example is growth hormone. We know that natural immunity tends to decline with age, and that lower growth hormone levels are associated with aging. Though little immune research has been done on human growth hormone (HGH), it is known that increasing HGH levels improves lymphocyte function, but exactly what the connection is between aging, immunity, and HGH is uncertain.

An immune challenge, such as an infection, triggers activity in the cells of the innate immune system, causing the release of cytokines, primarily interleukin-1 ß. This dynamic process proceeds at a rapid pace, critical for survival. In a normally functioning immune system, inflammation starts almost immediately, causing the release of additional cytokines. Many of these chemicals serve as messengers that influence the brain, the liver, and the endocrine system—including the adrenal, thymus, thyroid, hypothalamus, and pituitary glands.

Immune-Modulating Hormones

The hormones discussed in this next section have immune-modulating effects. There are many other hormones, such as estrogen and progesterone, that influence immune activity, but the ones discussed here are the most important for a well-functioning immune system.

Though most doctors do not test for hormone function in chronic viral disease or autoimmune conditions, accurate testing is readily available to evaluate the function of all of the hormones discussed below. If hormonal deficiencies are identified by clinical evaluation and lab testing, it is relatively easy to improve their function with natural hormone replacement or nutritional supplementation. If replacement is necessary, each of the hormones has a naturally occurring form, so you can avoid the use of foreign synthetic molecules such as prednisone.

> ## 6 Important Immune-Modulating Hormones
>
> Cortisol
> DHEA
> Growth Hormone
> Melatonin
> Thymic Hormones
> Thyroid Hormones

In some cases, substances called secretagogues can stimulate hormonal secretion, or hormonal precursors (the chemical building blocks from which hormones are constructed) can be added to your nutritional supplement program to improve hormonal status. In addition, if hormonal activity is very low, each hormone has a bio-identical pharmaceutical counterpart that can be prescribed, if necessary, by a medical or osteopathic doctor.

Therefore, if you have hormone imbalances, there is no need to go untreated. You may gain relief either by careful self-treatment or under the supervision of a knowledgeable doctor.

The Adrenal Hormone Cortisol: Stress and immune challenges trigger a cascade of hormones that eventually affects immune function. One of the first responses by the endocrine system to an immune challenge is the release of cortisol and other adrenal steroid hormones. Therefore, for the immune system to be in optimal condition, the adrenal glands must also be functioning properly.

In addition to cortisol, adrenaline (epinephrine), excreted by the adrenal medulla, is also activated by a stressful situation and causes the "fight-or-flight" response, turning on the sympathetic nervous system. This system is also referred to as the arousal system, the opposite of the parasympathetic system that conserves energy and promotes harmonic balance. In an arousal response, our heart rate speeds up and we feel sweaty.

However, when adrenaline is in excess, the hormones and brain communicate in a way that tells the pituitary gland in the brain to down-regulate adrenal activity to control excess adrenaline, in other words, to shut down production.

Features of Cortisol Deficiency

Flu-like fatigue

Exhaustion after and slow recovery from exertion

Poor resistance to infections

Difficulty handling stress

Anxiety

Chronic inflammation

Hypoglycemia and sugar craving

Allergies

Thin body frame, underweight, difficulty gaining weight

Joint pains

In this way our stress hormone levels and autonomic nervous systems stay in balance. However, with chronic inflammation, ongoing or repeated infection, and unrelenting stress, the adrenal gland becomes worn down. Fatigue sets in and production of both cortisol and DHEA, another adrenal cortical hormone, can be severely affected, even diminished, causing symptoms of adrenal insufficiency.

Cortisol is the most potent of the glucocorticoid steroid hormones. Following daily cycles, it is naturally secreted in the body with the highest production in the morning and the lowest in the afternoon. At about one in the morning, your cortisol levels begin to rise; followed by a progressive increase during sleep until maximum levels are reached between seven and nine in the morning. The lowest levels of the day are around four in the afternoon.

Cortisol's role is to help maintain appropriate levels of glucose in the blood, thereby ensuring energy production for metabolic activity. Cortisol also helps our bodies fight off infections and manage inflammation, and it has profound effects on the immune system. It influences cytokines and immune cells at the site of infection and inflammation, but when elevated, it suppresses immune activity and inflammation. However, if cortisol levels are low, you will feel very tired with a profound flu-like fatigue and be prone to infections. William Jefferies, M.D., in his book, *Safe Uses of Cortisol* (1996) documents numerous clinical cases of low cortisol levels in cases of influenza and other viral infections, and the rapid improvement in those cases when cortisol was taken.

Like adrenaline, cortisol (hydrocortisone) is also produced in response to stress, though it is made in a different part of the adrenal gland—the adrenal cortex, or exterior portion. Hydrocortisone, available as an over-the-counter cream, is commonly used for skin rashes and swellings. It is effective because it reduces inflammation, and in our bodies, cortisol works in a similar way to help manage inflammatory reactions.

Stress or massive infection stimulate the release of larger amounts of cortisol which in turn activates the immune system. After the infection is resolved or the stressful event is over, the cortisol level returns to normal. If you have a chronic infection or inflammation, or are under constant stress, the adrenal glands will produce cortisol over an extended period of time and may eventually become exhausted. Cortisol levels will then become lower than normal. Chronic fatigue patients tend to have low cortisol levels, which causes them to feel tired all the time and to have a tendency to have minor recurrent viral, bacterial, and fungal infections.

The Adrenal Hormone DHEA: DHEA (dehydroepiandrosterone) is an androgenic hormone (one that causes masculine features like facial hair growth) secreted by the adrenal cortex. It is the most abundant androgen in the body. Its production declines with age, in response to long-term stress, in autoimmune conditions like rheumatoid arthritis, and it is frequently low in patients with chronic infections and viral diseases. DHEA helps to manage inflammation and has been shown to inhibit interleukin 6 (IL-6), a pro-inflammatory cytokine whose levels tend to increase with age and in people with chronic inflammatory diseases.

The effects of DHEA supplementation include improvement of mood and energy, deepening of sleep, increases in bone mineral density, improvements in muscle mass and strength, and promotion of hair growth. DHEA supplementation has been shown to improve immune function. This hormone has become widely popularized in the last few years, and though it is a prescription drug in most European countries, it is available in the United States as an over-the-counter nutritional supplement. I frequently recommend it as a hormonal optimizer, along with other specific natural hormones, in the treatment of menopausal symptoms, in anti-aging programs, and for chronic fatigue and chronic viral diseases.

Evaluating Adrenal Function: Conventional medical doctors rarely test for adrenal function in patients with chronic fatigue or chronic infections. The reason for this is that they are not taught functional or physiological approaches in medical school and do not look for conditions like adrenal insufficiency in their patients. Though you can order some tests on your own, for the accurate determination of adrenal function a naturopathic physician or a medical doctor who

---

Features of DHEA Deficiency

Dry skin and eyes

Lack of pubic and underarm hair

Low energy (not as profound as in cortisol deficiency)

Low mood with mild anxiety or depression

Weak or poorly developed muscles

respects the importance of adrenal function and its role in chronic disease will best serve you.

DHEA and cortisol can be measured in blood, saliva, or urine. In my clinical practice, I use all three forms for testing adrenal function, but you will find that the easiest is salivary testing. Saliva testing is quite reliable, and measures the free, or bio-available hormone, making this test valuable in assessing adrenal function. Since the adrenal gland secretes hormones on a rhythmical basis each day (called the diurnal cycle), the patient takes four samples of saliva at regular intervals throughout the day and night. The DHEA and cortisol results are plotted on a chart and the doctor evaluates their relationships. (There are several reliable labs that offer salivary testing; the ones I recommend are listed in the resource section.)

Urinary tests are valuable in a comprehensive evaluation of adrenal activity. For these studies, the patient collects all of his urine over a twenty-four-hour period and the sum total of hormones detected is reported as a daily average. I use these tests often if I want a comprehensive view of adrenal activity, testosterone, estrogens, and progesterone levels, along with other adrenal hormones. This test requires interpretation from your doctor. In general, for evaluating DHEA and cortisol only, the salivary method is preferable.

Blood testing is also available, but it measures only the total circulating levels, and these are rarely abnormal except in adrenal diseases like Cushing's syndrome, a condition of persistently elevated cortisol levels. Blood tests are also not sensitive enough to evaluate borderline adrenal insufficiency because of the wide range of values in normal people. I use them only in patients in which I suspect excess levels of cortisol, such as in Syndrome X, a condition characterized by abdominal obesity, insulin resistance, high triglycerides, and high blood pressure.

For blood testing, cortisol levels are measured around eight in the morning (the time of highest secretion activity) and again around four in the afternoon (the lowest). For increased accuracy and to see how poor adrenal function is affecting blood sugar metabolism, I suggest the morning level be taken before eating breakfast (between 7 A.M. and 9 A.M.) and that an insulin level also be taken, followed by a 2-hour glucose tolerance test. A 2-hour glucose tolerance test (GTT) is performed by first drawing blood from a patient who has fasted for at least 12 hours, usually in the morning before breakfast. Glucose levels are measured, and the patient is given 75 g of a glucose solution to drink. Blood is drawn again after two hours, and glucose levels are measured for a second time. The results before drinking the glucose solution and two hours after are then compared.

Normal values for blood glucose when fasting are between 70 and 110 milligrams/deciliter (mg/dL). Higher or lower glucose levels after drinking the solution indicate abnormal glucose metabolism. Concentrations lower than 70 mg/dL indicate hypoglycemia, and values higher than 200 are indicative of diabetes. Adrenal insufficiency is suspected if either cortisol or blood sugar levels are low (before or after the glucose drink). If insulin levels are high and blood sugar levels are also elevated, then Syndrome X (insulin resistance) is suspected.

Low fasting blood cortisol levels can be found sometimes in patients with truly underactive adrenal function, but the most accurate way to test for low adrenal function is to have your doctor perform an ACTH challenge test. ACTH (adrenal corticotropic hormone) is the pituitary hormone that controls the release of hormones (such as cortisol) produced by the adrenal cortex. To perform this test, your blood cortisol levels are measured and then you are injected with a dose of synthetic ACTH. Blood is then checked after the challenge test, and these should at least double in response to the stimulation by the ACTH. If the cortisol level remains low, you most likely have adrenal insufficiency.

As blood tests for DHEA are accurate, I often use this method to establish a baseline in a comprehensive evaluation of adrenal function. The consensus among doctors practicing functional medicine and hormone balancing is that the best test for the evaluation of DHEA status is the sulfate form, DHEA-S. Conventional medical doctors use DHEA-S primarily to evaluate cases of hirsutism (women displaying excessive facial hair growth). However, according to Thierry Hertoghe, M.D., of Brussels, Belgium, and an authority on hormone therapies, DHEA-S provides a better picture of functional activity (Hertoghe 2000).[1]

DHEA-S levels are measured in micrograms per deciliter (mcg/dL). The so-called "youthful" ranges are from 400–560 mcg/dL for men, and 350–430 mcg/dL for women. As people age or when they are suffering from chronic disease, their levels may be well below 150 mcg/dL. In my clinical practice, I never push for the optimal "youthful" levels, because I believe that the amount of hormone this requires places additional stress on other systems of the body—principally the liver since it has to process all steroid hormones. I am satisfied with attaining levels above 250 mcg/dL for both men and women.

If either DHEA-S or cortisol levels are low, and you have the correct symptom profile, replacement may be necessary. If levels of either of these hormones are elevated, this may indicate excessive adrenal stimulation often due to high stress; in such cases, serious stress reduction is necessary. Elevated levels in the absence of previous supplementation may also indicate a disease pattern, and you should discuss this promptly with your doctor.

How to Correctly Supplement Adrenal Hormones: You can supplement cortisol and DHEA by taking adrenal glandular extracts, natural hydrocortisone (a synthetic prescription), or pharmaceutical grade DHEA. Only supplement these hormones if your levels are low.

Glandular extracts are made from the adrenal glands of livestock such as cows or pigs, and contain low dosages of all the adrenal hormones, including cortisol, adrenaline, and DHEA. Though glandular extracts are the treatment of choice for supplementing borderline low adrenal activity, there are advantages and disadvantages to their use.

The advantage of using glandular extracts is that they are natural and provide low dosages of adrenal hormones as a corrective medication, rather than as a drug. This ensures that you are not over-dosing steroid hormones, since often only very small amounts are needed to re-establish normal adrenal function. Too much can suppress adrenal function. However, there are several disadvantages.

The first is that glandular substances may not contain any hormones at all or the amounts may be too low to do any good. Another disadvantage is that most of these products are made from whole tissue, containing both adrenaline and cortisol. Since adrenaline can cause hyperactivity and insomnia, I do not recommend whole adrenal extracts. Use only a product that is made from the adrenal cortex, the part that contains cortisol and DHEA.

The third disadvantage is that the amount of cortisol in extracts is not always the same. Most adrenal extracts available at health stores are not adequate for supplementation; however, your doctor can provide you with concentrated cortical extracts containing standardized amounts of naturally occurring cortisol. The typical dosage is between 1.25 and 2.5 mg of cortisol equivalent in divided dosages daily, usually taken in the morning, at noon, and in the later afternoon. Do not take them before bed, as your sleep could be affected.

Nutritional supplements and herbs are also helpful in restoring adrenal reserves. In most cases of borderline low adrenal function, stress reduction, rest, and improving your dietary habits will correct the problem. Pantothenic acid (vitamin B5), vitamin C, and ginseng are most commonly used. If you have followed steps 1 through 4, it is likely that you are already getting adequate vitamin C and some pantothenic acid in your multivitamin supplements. For adrenal nutrition, I generally recommend taking a total of 500 mg of pantothenic acid 2-3 times daily.

Doctors of Chinese medicine and acupuncturists are experts in improving adrenal function by natural methods. In their view, ginseng is an excellent medicine for enhancing and balancing adrenal function. You may already be using ginseng, and if you stay with the recommended dosage (described in the previous chapter), you will be taking enough to improve your adrenal function. Licorice root extracts are also considered helpful in improving adrenal activity. However, do not take ginseng or licorice if you have high blood pressure. In general, only use these two herbs if your cortisol levels are low.

If your cortisol levels are very low or you are not improving over a period of four to six months with the all-natural approach, you may need a prescription of hydrocortisone, a synthetic drug whose molecular structure is identical to human cortisol. The typical recommended dosage is 5-10 mg, two to four times daily. I recommend that you start with a low dose and gradually increase until you feel an increase in energy. For example, you could begin with 2.5 mg, two times daily, then increase this by 2.5 mg weekly and take the new dose four times daily.

For replacement therapy, 20 mg of cortisol daily should be the maximum dosage, divided into four equal dosages taken morning, mid-morning, noon, and late afternoon. If your adrenal function is very low, your doctor may want to put you on even higher dosages; however, keep in mind that more than 30-40 mg daily will cause suppression of your own adrenal hormone production.

DHEA is available over the counter, by prescription, or in a micronized form, which is the form I recommend. Since its particle size is smaller, the micronized form is easily absorbed and more efficient for the body to utilize. Though most doctors recommend dosages ranging from 25-50 mg for women and from 50-100 mg for men, I have found these to be too high for people with chronic disease and those who are very weak. Instead, I often recommend 5–10 mg for both men and women, and only under a doctor's supervision may you increase the dosage up to 20–30 mg.

A newer form of DHEA is 7-Keto DHEA, reported to have many of DHEA's benefits but none of the side effects. Though many doctors are recommending 7-Keto DHEA, I do not use it in my practice. It is much more expensive than regular DHEA and in my experience, it does not have the same hormonal benefits.

DHEA is best taken with food in the morning, at noon, and around four in the afternoon. Do not take cortisol-containing compounds in the evening or before bed, as they can cause insomnia. DHEA is considered safe in low dosages and is not associated with increased risk for disease. On the contrary, research indicates that it may be protective against cancer and cardiovascular disease.

However, as with all steroid hormones, there is some concern that extended use may cause liver damage. Patients with liver disease should take a sublingual form of DHEA or use a transdermal cream applied to the skin. This will prevent the first bypass effect in the liver; normally, when oral preparations are absorbed through the intestines, they pass directly to the liver through the portal vein. By avoiding this direct route, less stress is placed on liver.

Caution: Both DHEA and cortisol are steroid hormones and have considerable physiological activity in the body. In general, low dosages of cortisol are safe and without side effects, but do not use it for more than six months without re-testing your hormone levels. Since DHEA is an androgenic hormone, it can convert in the body to testosterone. In some cases this may be beneficial; however, it can also cause facial hair growth in women, and acne in both men and women. It has also been associated with high blood pressure.

Men should have their PSA (prostate-specific antigen) tested regularly if they are using DHEA. Do not use DHEA, except under medical supervision, if you have an enlarged prostate gland. Do not use DHEA if you have hypertension or are concerned about acne, and discontinue immediately if any of these occur. Too high a dose of hydrocortisone, above 30 mg for more than a few weeks, can suppress immune function. Do not take dosages of cortisol above 10 mg per day unless you are supervised by a physician.

Low adrenal function, also referred to as adrenal insufficiency, can cause chronic fatigue, low blood sugar, and a host of other symptoms as well as difficulty recuperating from colds and flu, lack of stamina, lowered immune function, and premature aging. If you have chronic fatigue, chronic viral infections, a bacterial infection that is difficult to eradicate, recurrent colds and flu, slow recovery from an illness, or immune deficiency, taking natural cortisol or DHEA may improve your condition.

Human Growth Hormone: Sorting through the Controversy

Human growth hormone (HGH) plays a role in immunity, and if you are elderly, using it as part of your viral immunity program may benefit your ability to resist infection. However, it is still not known how HGH supplementation works. There are also potential risks with long-term use, such as irreversible acromegaly (abnormal enlargement of the bones), diabetes, edema, and the cancer risk from HGH has not yet been fully defined.

Low adrenal function, also referred to as adrenal insufficiency, can cause chronic fatigue, low blood sugar, and a host of other symptoms as well as difficulty recuperating from colds and flu, lack of stamina, lowered immune function, and premature aging.

The abnormal fluid retention that HGH can cause in some people may result in carpal tunnel symptoms (severe tingling of the forearms, inside of the wrists, and palms of the hands). Both psychological stress and the distress associated with chronic viral disease affect water balance in the body and kidney function, and both physical and psychological stress increase HGH production.

Therefore, HGH supplementation has the potential to aggravate fluid metabolism and should be used with care in patients with kidney disease. However, in the short term and when using lower doses, HGH gives an increased sense of well being, improves energy, increases sexual vitality, and is used as an anti-aging hormone.

Testing for HGH: HGH levels are evaluated indirectly by testing for insulin-like growth factor (IGF-1), also called somatomedin C, in blood. Urinary tests that measure growth hormone are available, but are not in common use yet. IGF-1 is a hormone produced primarily in the liver in response to growth hormone, and its concentration range in blood varies depending on a person's age and gender, decreasing gradually by about 14 percent every ten years after the age of thirty. There is no universal standard for optimal IGF-1 levels; however, most anti-aging physicians believe that levels approximating those of a healthy twenty-nine- to thirty-two-year-old are a reasonable goal. The range for a male of this age is 114–492 nanograms per milliliter (ng/mL).[2]

For those suffering from chronic viral diseases and for middle-aged adults (those between roughly forty-eight and sixty-five years of age) aiming for levels of a thirty-year-old may be too high and the therapy to attain them too aggressive. I suggest more moderate goals. Two national experts, James Jamieson, Ph.D., a pharmacologist involved in growth hormone secretagogue research, and Allan Broughton, M.D., who developed the first commercial IGF-1 laboratory test, agree. In an article published in 1998, Jamieson suggests an upper limit of 250 ng/dL. In my practice, I have found that patients receive benefits from HGH enhancement if their levels are functionally low (less than 110–145 ng/dL), and then increased to 165–250 ng/dL.

How to Safely Supplement HGH: There are three ways to increase IGF-1 levels and enhance HGH: lifestyle and diet, oral secretagogues, and injections of synthetic HGH. A healthy diet, adequate exposure to sunlight, strenuous exercise, and plenty of deep sleep support the natural release of growth hormone, and detoxification and fasting also improve HGH levels. The amino acid arginine (discussed in step 2 as an immune-enhancing agent) assists growth hormone production.

Oral HGH secretagogues have become popular in the last few years. Unfortunately, very few of the hundreds sold on the market have any value in consistently raising IGF-1 levels, and many do not work at all. The one that I recommend is MediTropin. Research and clinical data have shown that MediTropin significantly raises IGF-1 levels. It is available through a physician's office or a pharmacy. Dissolve one to two tablets in one glass of water and drink before bed nightly, two hours after eating.

In some cases, such as in the very elderly, when IGF-1 levels are very low (less than 110 ng/dL), nutrition and oral secretagogues may not be enough to raise levels above 165 ng/dL. In this case, you may wish to use synthetic recombinant human growth hormone, also called somatropin, taken by injection. This is a prescription substance in the U.S., though it may be obtained in Mexico and other countries without a prescription.

Recombinant HGH is produced by a special purified strain of *E. coli* bacteria and contains the same 119 amino acids that constitute naturally occurring pituitary human growth hormone. I usually recommend Humatrope, manufactured by the French pharmaceutical company Eli Lilly, but there are other excellent brands such as Norditropin, made by Novo Nordisk in Denmark. The typical dosage for adults is by body weight, with an average replacement range from 0.5–1.0 IU per day. However, when applying all of the dietary, lifestyle, nutritional, and herbal recommendations in this book, you can achieve effective results with considerably lower dosages.

Thierry Hertoghe, M.D., one of the world's experts on hormone balancing and HGH replacement, promotes the concept that when balancing other hormones, a synergistic affect occurs. In these cases, daily dosages of 0.25 to 0.5 IU are often sufficient to achieve symptom improvement, enhance immunity, and raise IFG-1 levels. Often, a combination of daily use of an oral secretagogue combined with low-dose biweekly injections provide significant benefits at less cost and with less risk.

Caution: A prescription is required for recombinant HGH and you will also need instructions from your doctor on how to do the injections yourself. In the dosage I have recommended, HGH enhancement is safe and without side effects. However, like all of the stronger medications listed in this book, if you notice any unusual symptoms, discontinue immediately and discuss them with your doctor.

Although low-dose recombinant HGH injections or oral secretagogues are without significant risk, long-term use can cause receptor resistance making. This is a condition in which hormone receptors in the cells do not allow the hormone molecule to attach to them or in which they become immune to the effects of the hormone, requiring higher and higher levels (as in insulin resistance and Syndrome X) to achieve effects. Your doctor should monitor long-term use (more than one year) of HGH-enhancing substances, even in low dosages.

Melatonin: Super Hormone and Rhythmic Modulator

Melatonin is a substance produced by the pineal gland, situated deep within the brain, and in other tissues such as bone marrow cells. Suppressed by light and increased in darkness, it is associated with sleep induction, sexuality, longevity, the balancing of thyroid and other hormones, powerful antioxidant protection, viral replication inhibition, and immune system enhancement.

Researchers are not clear if melatonin is a hormone in the sense that cortisol or estrogen are, or if it is in a separate class of its own. William Regelson, M.D., in *The Super-Hormone Promise,* refers to it as a "buffer" hormone because unlike other hormones that have specific target sites, melatonin *indirectly* influences *all* organ systems, exerting a synergistic effect on many different hormones at the same time (Regelson 1996). Walter Pierpaoli, M.D., Ph.D., of the Italian National Research Center on Aging in Ancuna, Italy, and the world's leading authority on melatonin research, suggests that melatonin is not a hormone in the classic sense, but is rather a mediator of the biological clock, and as such directly influences health, aging, and immunity (Pierpaoli 1995).

Investigation of receptor sites on lymphocytes suggests that melatonin is a powerful immune-modulating substance (Rabin 1999). Inhibition of normal pineal gland activity due to stress, long hours under artificial light, lack of daylight exposure, and use of drugs that deplete melatonin (indomethacin, beta-blockers, steroids, and many antidepressant and anti-anxiety drugs) contribute to serious imbalances in melatonin. Pierpaoli has shown that inhibition of melatonin synthesis suppresses normal immune response.

Other researchers have found that melatonin has anti-inflammatory effects and is capable of reducing tissue damage during inflammatory reactions. Could it be that another link in the immune deficiency puzzle is abnormal melatonin synthesis, and thus another consequence of modern living?

Testing Melatonin Levels: Since all people living in modern urban areas are exposed to stress, unnatural lighting, and the other causes of the inhibition of melatonin synthesis, it is generally not necessary to test for melatonin levels in order to supplement this important anti-aging and immune-enhancing substance. Also, the laboratory tests for melatonin are not highly sensitive to its circadian secretion variations. Blood tests are available, but the best way to test for melatonin is by salivary studies; at least three samples are taken over a twenty-four-hour period and then plotted on a graph.

How to Supplement Melatonin: Melatonin is a prescription medication in many European countries, but is available over the counter as a nutritional supplement in the United States. I recommend melatonin supplements to all of my patients over sixty years of age, those on estrogen replacement therapy, and those with chronic hypothyroidism, breast cancer, and chronic viral infections. Pineal glandular extracts are available, but either contain only trace amounts of melatonin or none at all, so I do not recommend glandular substances for melatonin replacement.

In my clinical practice, I use synthetic melatonin in a sublingual form or in oral capsules in the range of 0.5–3.0 mg directly before sleep. The most common dosage and form that I use is a 1 mg sublingual preparation. Sublingual melatonin gets into your bloodstream very quickly, creating higher levels of melatonin in a short period.

I do not consider melatonin a sleep aid and only use it in higher dosages to reduce the effects of jet lag. A typical dose is 5–10 mg three days before your flight, during the flight, and three days after arrival. Doubling your cortisol dose during and immediately after a long flight also reduces jet lag; repeat the same schedule for the return trip.

For immune stimulation and the treatment of chronic viral diseases, dosages up to 20–50 mg may be taken on a cyclic basis (three weeks on, one week off). Since these dosages are considerably higher than those generally taken, I recommend that you evaluate melatonin levels before and during treatment, and that you be supervised by a doctor. If you choose to take melatonin in a higher dosage without supervision, start slowly, beginning with 1 mg nightly and gradually increasing 1 mg at a time, every three days until you are at 5 mg. From there, you can increase by 5 mg weekly until you reach 20 mg.

Melatonin is completely safe and non-toxic even in the higher dosage ranges. However, it can cause strange effects in some people, including vivid dreaming or nightmares. Some people taking melatonin experience stimulating effects and are unable to sleep—exactly the opposite effect that most people experience. Melatonin is a close cousin to the neurotransmitter serotonin, a substance that profoundly influences mood, so people sensitive to serotonin or those taking selective serotonin re-uptake inhibiting (SSRI) antidepressants (Prozac and Paxil) can experience exacerbations of depression and mental illness when taking melatonin. Therefore, I do not recommend taking melatonin while you are using antidepressant drugs.

The Thymus Gland: Essential for Immune Function

Lymphocytes, one of the most important immune cell types, mature in the thymus gland (behind the sternum) through a complex molecular process involving thymic hormones. These hormones also circulate in the blood, and though little is known about how thymic hormones influence immunity, researchers consider them to be important for a well-functioning immune system.

Lifestyle, diet, and nutrition are the first line of therapy to improve thymus function. By following all the steps outlined in this book, including balancing all the hormones as discussed in this chapter, the activity of your thymus gland will naturally improve. Stress and increased levels of cortisol cause a marked decrease in the size of the thymus gland. A shrinking thymus is also associated with the aging process, as is declining immunity. Therefore, stress reduction and lifestyle changes that foster health and longevity also improve thymic function and benefit immunity.

Studies have shown that zinc supplementation restores thymic function in older experimental animals, as does melatonin. Since the thymus is innervated by both sympathetic and parasympathetic nerve connections, regulating the autonomic nervous system through acupuncture, yoga, and tai chi, can also rejuvenated the thymus.

Although there are blood tests that measure thymic hormones, these are used primarily for research purposes and not for clinical evaluation of thymic function. To evaluate thymus function, I order a comprehensive lymphocyte panel.

How to Use Thymic Extracts: Whole thymus glandular extracts for immune stimulation have been in use for decades. Made from bovine thymus glands, they are processed to produce a dry powder which is made into tablets or capsules. Though these products may contain trace amounts of thymic hormones and are commonly used by alternative health practitioners, I have not found them to be strong enough to produce any noticeable clinical results in viral conditions.

Other options for the enhancement of thymus function are concentrated thymic extracts, thymic protein, and synthetic thymosin. Thanks to modern pharmaceutical practices, we now have these potent thymic preparations, and I routinely recommend these for my patients with chronic viral diseases to improve immune status, prevent infections, and reverse immunosenescence. Thymic hormones are considered by some anti-aging experts to be the missing link in preventing age-related diseases.

Numerous research studies have been conducted on these products, and the general professional consensus is that they appear to work as immune modulators by improving cell-mediated immunity. They have been shown to be useful as adjunctive therapy in hepatitis B and C, in the treatment of AIDS, and in other viral infections. Several thymus medications are available, including oral and injectable preparations.

One of the new immunoceutical medications, Thymic Protein A, developed by Terry Beardsley, Ph.D., an immunologist and eminent researcher on the thymus gland, is endorsed by many physicians as one of the leading oral thymic immune-supporting medications. Thymic protein A has been shown to stimulate helper T-4 cell function. I use this product in my practice and have found it effective and safe. It is manufactured by BioPro and is sold as ProBoost in individual packets containing a white freeze-dried powder. I often advise taking one packet one to three times daily, emptied directly into the mouth and dissolved under the tongue.

The Canadian company, Atrium Biotechnologies, produces whole, live-cell tissue extracts from bovine thymus glands. Live cell therapy extracts, glandular injections from sheep or cow glands, have been popular in Europe for decades as a rejuvenation therapy. NatCell Thymus is an oral liquid that arrives frozen and must be kept frozen until just before use.

Though there is no question that live cell therapy is valuable in restoring organ energy reserves, these products are very expensive making them nearly prohibitive for the average patient. Still, I consider them important adjunctive therapy for immune enhancement and rebuilding the thymus gland. For treatment of viral infections, one to three vials are taken daily for a course of ten to twelve vials, which may be repeated monthly for several months. For maintenance, one to two vials per week are necessary.

Several high-quality, prescription-strength thymic extracts are produced in Germany. Thymomodulin, also known as Leucotrofina (an Italian version), is made by Ellen Pharmaceuticals, and research suggests it is useful in preventing recurrent respiratory infections, improving T-cell defects in AIDS patients, in treating chronic hepatitis B and C, relieving allergies, and restoring white blood cells in cancer patients after chemotherapy and radiation treatments.

A similar product, Thym-Uvocal (produced by Mulli in Germany), is a safe medicine of good quality and comes in both injectable ampoules or oral tablets. Though other oral preparations are available, including Thymomodulin and Thymus Mucos, injectables are the preferred form because the medication gets directly into the bloodstream. Since these substances are not licensed drugs in the United States, injectable medications are available only through alternative avenues such as buyers' clubs or International Anti-aging Systems over the Internet. The dosage is one ampoule injected intramuscularly every other day, and for oral forms two (240 mg) tablets taken on an empty stomach three times daily.

The synthetic immunomodulating drug Thymosin alpha-1 is used for the same purposes: as an immune modulator for adjunctive therapy in hepatitis B and C, AIDS, and cancer. Zaduxin, a proprietary form, is licensed in twenty countries worldwide (except the United States where it is classified as an "orphan drug" for the treatment of hepatitis B) for the treatment and prevention of influenza.

Several studies have shown that thymosin improves the outcome of HCV patients when given with interferon. HIV/AIDS patients have also reported benefits from taking thymosin. It increases the activity of interleukin-2 receptors on T cells, increases maturation of T cells, and increases the production of gamma and alpha interferon. Although it is an injectable drug and requires a prescription, some AIDS health groups import it from Italy or other countries. It may also be possible to obtain it over the Internet.

Safety Information on Thymus and Other Glandular Extracts Derived from Cows: Oral thymic extracts are considered safe and non-toxic and may be used for chronic viral conditions. However, there are several conditions in which their use is contraindicated: thymus tumors, myasthenia gravis, multiple sclerosis, untreated hypothyroidism, during pregnancy, and for people on immune-suppressive therapy to prevent organ transplant rejection.

With the exception of synthetic thymosin, thymic extracts are made from the thymus glands of calves, mainly in European countries. There is currently no evidence of contagion of BSE (bovine spongiform encephalopathy), or mad cow disease, pathogens through the use of bovine extracts for medicinal purposes. However, the German government issued a warning in 1994 stating the possibility of transmission of this disease through glandular tissue products. Before you use any glandular product, consult your doctor, the manufacturer, or a governmental agency that reports on current safety issues related to BSE.

The Thyroid Gland: The Great Imitator

Hypothyroidism, or underactive thyroid gland function, is the most common thyroid disorder and one of the most common of all endocrine conditions. It is characterized by a well-recognized set of symptoms and very specific abnormalities in lab testing. The gold standard is an elevated level of thyroid-stimulating hormone (TSH). Hyperthyroidism, or overactive thyroid function, is becoming more common, as are autoimmune-related thyroid conditions like Hashimoto's disease (thyroiditis resulting in thyroid hormone deficiency) and Grave's disease (also known as thyrotoxicosis).

The thyroid gland, located in the middle of the lower neck just above the collarbone (clavicle), is actually composed of two halves (lobes): the right and left lobes lying on either side of the trachea, which are joined together in the middle by a narrow segment called the isthmus. The thyroid gland secretes the hormones thyroxine (T_4) and triiodothyronine (T_3) that help the brain regulate many bodily functions including metabolism (including weight loss and gain), brain development, normal growth and development, heart function, temperature regulation (helps heat production), and nervous system function.

Most likely linked to immune dysfunction, thyroid imbalances are becoming increasingly common. Weakened hormone function, causing subclinical slow progression that does not reveal classic symptoms of hypothyroidism or show abnormal blood test results, and other hormonal imbalances are showing up at an increasing rate. Richard Shames, M.D., a primary care doctor, observes in *Thyroid Power: 10 Steps to Total Health* (2001): "Although extremely common, low thyroid is largely an unsuspected illness."

Medical doctors practicing conventional allopathic medicine are unprepared for this epidemic. In my practice, I have worked with cases of low thyroid and autoimmune thyroid conditions since the early 1980s. As a rule of thumb, I have found that in most people with chronic fatigue, those who catch frequent colds and flu, who have female hormonal imbalances, allergies, and environmental sensitivities all have a thyroid component to their problems. They may not have hypothyroidism, but the function of their thyroid gland is below par, and when treated with natural medicine, the majority of these patients experience pronounced symptomatic improvement.

Since thyroid hormones control virtually every chemical reaction in your body, if your thyroid function is even slightly out of the normal functioning range, it will cause your metabolism to waver and your immunity to falter.

Thyroid Case Study: A case in point is Beverly, a thirty-two-year-old single woman without any children who formerly led an active professional life. When I first saw her she was on disability due to chronic environmental sensitivities, recurrent respiratory tract infections, severe menstrual problems, chronic unexplained pain, and multiple allergies. She had already tried conventional medicine, and her doctors could not find anything wrong with her other than a slightly low thyroid function, for which synthetic thyroxin was prescribed. She had also experimented with various alternative therapies.

Although she repeatedly told her primary care doctor that sometimes her symptoms improved markedly for a few hours when she took her synthetic thyroid medication, he dismissed it as a placebo effect. He was convinced that the majority of her problems were "all in her head."

I worked with Beverly over several months to stabilize her response to the thyroid medication and improve her own natural thyroid function with acupuncture and nutrition. At the end of three months she began to show improvement. When I divided her thyroid dose into three equal parts, spread out during the day rather than all at once in the morning, her symptoms improved enough so that she was able to return to work.

Since thyroid hormones control virtually every chemical reaction in your body, if your thyroid function is even slightly out of the normal functioning range, it will cause your metabolism to waver and your immunity to falter. Frequent bacterial, yeast, or viral infections can be the result of low thyroid function. Here is the irony: low thyroid function may have a cause rooted in the immune system and low thyroid function causes lowered immunity.

The most likely causes in the hypothyroid epidemic are rampant environmental toxins, stress, poor diet, and infectious microorganisms including viruses. These are the same causes that appear to trigger immune deficiency crises as well. The clinical challenge is that if the homeostatic mechanisms of the brain shut the immunity down in order to protect the thyroid glandular tissue, will stimulating thyroid function improve or worsen immune reactions?

This is an unanswered question. However, if you approach the matter of improving your thyroid function carefully and gradually, you should not experience any harm or worsening of your symptoms. Working with a medical professional skilled and experienced in managing borderline thyroid dysfunction may be useful. I highly recommend this option if you have known thyroid disease, or under- or overactive thyroid function.

How to Evaluate Low Thyroid Function: The most common symptom of an underactive thyroid is fatigue. However, it is not the typical feeling of being just tired. Fatigue caused by low thyroid function creates a sense of utter exhaustion, both mentally and physically. Additionally, an underactive thyroid can cause many other complaints, such as anemia, heavier-than-normal menstrual bleeding, constipation, dry skin, hair loss, and cold in the extremities.

Begin evaluating your thyroid function by carefully reviewing your symptoms. Take the Low Thyroid Self-Test, and if you answer "yes" to any three of the questions, in addition to exhaustion, you may have low thyroid.

If you answered "yes" to at least three or four of these questions, the next thing to do is to check your body's basal metabolic temperature. To do this you will need a special thermometer called a basal thermometer, which you can readily buy in any drug store or pharmacy. Set a notebook and pen or pencil along with the thermometer next to your bed before sleep.

In the morning, when you awaken but before getting out of bed even to use the toilet, place the mercury bulb of the thermometer directly under your bare armpit. Rest comfortably in bed, not moving the covers, allowing the thermometer to stay snugly under your arm for several minutes. Read it directly upon removing it from your

Low Thyroid Self-Test

I have . . .

- exhausted feelings that are not related to stress or amount of work or exercise
- morning tiredness, even after a full night's sleep
- depression that does not respond to antidepressants, diet, or exercise
- unexplained anxiety and panic attacks
- been told that I move as if in slow motion, and take too long to respond to questions
- a frequently low or hoarse voice (for a woman)
- mental sluggishness and difficulty focusing
- low sex drive and do not experience significant sexual arousal
- high cholesterol that has been unresponsive to diet or medications
- a tendency to feel cold, even in warm weather
- chronic aches and pains that are not due to accidents or exercise
- problems with allergies
- difficulty losing weight and keeping it off
- very dry skin, and have acne or eczema
- diabetes, anemia, rheumatoid arthritis, or other autoimmune condition
- problem with periods, including abnormal menstrual bleeding
- infertility or a history of miscarriages
- significant menopausal symptoms
- a tendency to have chronic constipation even with a high-fiber diet
- lots of hair falling out or brittle hair
- vitiligo (a skin discoloration problem)
- trembling of the hands or stumbling for no reason

armpit and record the number in your diary. Repeat the same procedure for at least seven days.

I ask my patients to perform this test daily for one month to get a better average. Menstruating women should start on the first day of their periods. The average, "normal," under-arm temperature is about 98° F first thing in the morning. If your temperature averages less than 97.6 degrees (and you have symptoms), you may have low thyroid. The next step is to find a doctor with experience in evaluating and treating sub-clinical hypothyroidism.

As a confirmation of low thyroid you will need a group of laboratory tests. In my clinical practice I use blood and urine testing to evaluate thyroid function. Of course, I order individual tests based upon the patient's specific history and symptoms, but if you or your doctor suspect low thyroid, I highly recommend that you have at least one comprehensive panel of tests performed. This is because the standard tests, usually limited to measuring thyroid-stimulating hormone by most HMOs, often miss borderline cases of low thyroid.

> ## Recommended Thyroid Blood Tests
> TSH (thyroid-stimulating hormone)
> Total T-4 (thyroxine)
> Free T-4 (available thyroxine)
> Total T-3 (triiodothyronine)
> Free T-3 (available triiodothyronine)
> Antiperoxidase antibody (antimicrosomal antibody)

Your doctor may want to include one or more additional tests, and though they add more information, they are not substitutes for these tests. Additional tests include T-3U (T-3 resin uptake), FTI (free thyroxine index), RT-3 (reverse T-3), TRH (thyrotropin releasing hormone), and TBG (thyroid binding globulin).

Long used in Europe, urinary thyroid tests are only just becoming available in the United States. They are easy to use, relatively inexpensive, and are useful if levels must be monitored frequently. Urinary studies measure free T-3 and free T-4, and kits are available through your doctor from AAL Reference Laboratories.

If you have symptoms of low thyroid function, have an under-arm temperature that is consistently lower than normal, and have shown positive laboratory results for low thyroid function, you need to correct your thyroid imbalance *before* you can be well and enjoy optimal energy and immunity. Depending on the case, of course, I generally recommend beginning with a corrective approach using natural medications and alternative therapies.

How to Correct Low Thyroid with Natural Medicines: Review steps 1 through 4: lifestyle, antioxidants, detoxification, and a phytonutrient-rich diet. If environmental toxins are part of the problem, it makes sense to begin with detoxification. The same anti-inflammatory, anti-autoimmune, balanced diet outlined earlier in the book also works for correcting thyroid problems.

In addition, avoid foods (even though some are phytonutrient-rich) that inhibit thyroid function. These include large amounts of soy, cabbage-family vegetables (cabbage, broccoli, cauliflower, and mustard greens), rutabaga, turnips, walnuts, almonds, peanuts, pine nuts, millet, sorghum, and cassava (tapioca).

A low-carbohydrate diet and low calorie diets for weight loss can also inhibit thyroid function, resulting in the opposite affect, namely,

Nutritional Supplements for Thyroid Support

Tyrosine
Organic iodine
Selenium
Copper
Zinc
Thyroid glandular extracts

difficulty in losing weight due to poor thyroid performance. Therefore, if you have low thyroid function, eat equally proportioned meals four to five times daily and include carbohydrates, such as rice or fruits, in each meal.

According to Ridha Arem, M.D., an endocrinologist and Associate Professor of Medicine at Baylor College of Medicine in Houston, Texas, stress can play a significant role in thyroid disorders (Arem 1999). If you are under serious stress and have a thyroid disease, I strongly suggest you start a stress reduction program, including lifestyle changes, meditation, yoga, massage, and other calming and unwinding activities.

Tyrosine, an amino acid, is the basic building block for thyroid hormone. You may safely take 500–1,000 mg, two to three times daily as a typical dosage. It is a safe supplement without side effects. Though adequate amounts of iodine, selenium, copper, and zinc are required for proper thyroid function, if you are following the recommended dosages in steps 1 and 2, you will be taking more than adequate amounts of these trace minerals.

Many alternative practitioners suggest extra iodine is needed, but most Americans have sufficient amounts in their diets and from multivitamin and mineral supplements, and too much iodine can suppress thyroid function. Remember that most modern thyroid conditions are caused from immune-related problems and not a deficiency of iodine as in times past.

Caution: Adding extra iodine or overdoing your intake of iodine-containing kelp and other seaweeds can cause an increase of dietary or supplemental iodine. Artificially increasing iodine levels can trigger autoimmune reactions, thereby worsening a thyroid condition. Do not take iodine supplements *except* under the advice of a qualified health professional and then only for short periods of time lasting no longer than two to four weeks.

After trying the nutritional approach for six to eight weeks, if your thyroid function still remains low, add a whole thyroid glandular supplement. Natural thyroid glandulars provide bio-available thyroid hormone and a range of intermediary substances that work similarly to the way your own thyroid hormones work; they can be very effective in normalizing thyroid function.

Most glandular products sold in health foods stores do not contain active thyroxine, and although some might contain trace amounts, preparations with active amounts of thyroxine (T_4) and triiodothyronine (T_3) can be obtained through a health professional or on the Internet. If you are taking an active form, start with 1/4 grain (usually equivalent to one 250 mg capsule) and gradually increase up to 1 grain of thyroxine equivalence (two capsules, two times daily). Be sure to ask your doctor if the glandular you are taking has active thyroid hormone or if it is thyroxine-free.

Acupuncture and yoga postures are also useful in correcting thyroid weakness. I generally recommend twice-weekly acupuncture sessions over a course of six weeks. At the end of the course of treatments, have your blood studies rechecked. Generally, cases improve with one or two courses of treatment (twelve to twenty-four acupuncture sessions) and many improve in as few as six sessions.

If You Need Thyroid Hormone Replacement: The current standard for the treatment of hypothyroidism in the United States is replacement with synthetic T_4 (commercially available as Synthroid, Levothroid, and Levoxyl), synthetic T_3 (Cytomel), or a synthetic combination of T_4 and T_3 (Thyrolar). For most medical doctors there is no other option. However, natural prescription thyroid is available and should be the medication of choice for most people with borderline immune-related low thyroid.

Like whole glandulars, prescription natural thyroid is prepared from desiccated beef or pork thyroid glands. However, these glandulars contain standardized amounts of T_4 and T_3, and are highly purified and safe to use. The most commonly used brand is Armour Thyroid, but two other forms are also available: thyroid USP (generic desiccated thyroid) and Bio-Throid from Bio-Tech. Both use glands from animals raised without synthetic dietary hormones, and these may be a healthier choice in this age of feed contaminants. Have your pharmacist order these specially, or you can order them yourself from an Internet pharmacy or a compounding pharmacy as long as you have a prescription from your doctor.

Prescription natural thyroid is provided in tablets or very small capsules. For hormone balancing, different from hormone replacement which requires higher dosages, I recommend that you start with 15 mg (1/4 grain) in the morning before ten and gradually increase every week until you are taking 60 mg (1 grain) daily in the morning on an empty stomach. You may find that you get more benefit by dividing the dosage between morning and noon.

Generally you will not need more than 1 grain to feel improvement in energy and to see many of the symptoms highlighted in the Low Thyroid Self-Test disappear. If you do not find that you are improving, your problem may not be thyroid-related or you may require a higher dosage. Consult your doctor if feel you need more than 1 grain of natural thyroid daily, and discontinue immediately if you experience insomnia, headaches, or rapid heart beat. People with low thyroid as a result of autoimmune problems often have poor conversion from T_4, the form that the thyroid gland secrets directly and that circulates in the blood, to T_3, the active form that directly affects the tissues. In these cases, higher dosages of T_3 are required and must be prescribed by a physician.

Thyroid Balancing Involves Other Hormones: Thyroid hormone function is synergistic with the activities of other hormones discussed in this section, including HGH, cortisol, and especially melatonin. To benefit and balance hormone activity in the entire body, all of my patients with low thyroid take 0.5–1.0 mg of melatonin nightly, directly before bed, even if they do not have sleep problems.

Women with menstrual abnormalities like PMS or irregular cycles, infertility, and those experiencing the symptoms of perimenopause may to need balance their estrogens and progesterone before their thyroid functions normally; that subject is beyond the focus of this book. If you suspect other hormonal imbalances, consult a doctor qualified to evaluate your condition.

Hormones and Immunosenescence

Both men and women over the age of fifty-five have lowered sex hormone levels. For men, testosterone deficiency predominates, and for women it is estrogen and progesterone, though many women also have lower levels of testosterone. Other hormones decline in aging as well. For many people, the levels of these hormones can be low enough to affect their energy, mood, sleep, and memory, and they may also impair immunity, creating a condition called immunosenescence, or age-related immune system deficiency.

Researchers have shown that aging causes a shift in subsets of T-helper cells, creating an imbalance between these immune cells. This imbalance results in fewer NK cells, fewer T cells, and changes in the types of interleukins that are secreted. A Japanese research team headed by Keizo Deguchi, M.D., at the University of Tokushima in Japan, has confirmed that estrogen replacement therapy in post-menopausal women may prevent some of these age-related immune declines (Deguchi 2001). If you are between the ages of forty-eight and fifty-two, it may be advisable to have your doctor check your levels of these important hormones. If they are low, consider natural hormone replacement or supplementation.

Hormones work synergistically with each other in a harmonious interplay of molecules. That is exactly the reason that doctors practicing functional medicine with natural biological medications can get better results with lower dosages. Hormones work well *together*.

Some examples of this are the following: Melatonin helps both thymus and thyroid function, HGH and thyroid help each other's function, DHEA can raise HGH levels. The reverse can be equally true: an excess of the adrenal hormone cortisol can cause the thymus to shrink, resulting in under-functioning immune activity. Therefore, I generally prescribe at least two hormones, and sometimes more, but never in high dosages.

How to Start Incorporating Hormones into Your Viral Immunity Plan

Start by adding DHEA (5–10 mg) and melatonin (0.5–1.0 mg) into your viral immunity program. If your thyroid is underactive, add whole natural thyroid (1/4–1 grain). If you are still fatigued and your cortisol is low, add natural adrenal cortex extract (1.25–2.5 mg).

At this point you should notice a considerable improvement in your energy, vitality, and general well-being. However, if you are not experiencing these positive changes, if you are over sixty years of age, and if you have tested low for IFG-1, try one of the HGH secretagogues. If the oral form does not improve your symptoms or raise your IGF-1 levels after three months, discuss a trial of injectable HGH with your doctor.

Finally, if you have HCV, are HIV positive or have AIDS, or if you have recurrent upper respiratory tract infections, add thymus extract. Start with Thymic Protein A; if this is not improving symptoms after several months, try a different form of thymus extract.

CHAPTER SUMMARY

Hormones play a significant role as immune modulators in your viral immunity program. They regulate endocrine function, moderate the effects of stress, improve energy, promote sleep, and serve as anti-aging factors.

The six most important hormones for immunity are cortisol, DHEA, HGH, melatonin, thymic hormones, and thyroid hormones.

Cortisol is a double-edged sword: if it is too low, you will feel tired; if too high, it can cause the thymus gland to atrophy and imbalance other hormones.

DHEA is the most common steroid hormone in your body and is frequently low in chronic disease, autoimmune disease, aging, and when under long-term stress. Begin supplementation with low dosages of DHEA.

HGH supplementation is controversial. Do not jump into taking advertised substances that claim to raise IGF-1 levels. Only use medically recognized products and only take them if you have clearly demonstrated a need based on symptoms, age, clinical profile, disease condition, and blood tests.

Melatonin is an important regulator of other hormones. Along with DHEA, it can buffer negative effects of stress hormones and enhance the activity of HGH, and the thyroid and thymus glands.

The thymus is the most important immune gland; enhancement of thymic hormones may be the linchpin in your viral immunity program.

Improving thyroid function can improve your entire hormonal system.

Hormones work synergistically. Do not supplement one without another, but only work with those you need. To work best, hormone therapy should be tailored to your individual metabolism.

15

STEP TEN

Implement Your Viral Immunity Plan

In this final step, you'll see how you can use this information to correctly treat, restore, and heal yourself of viral illness. I discuss how to design your *individualized* viral immunity program, which laboratory tests are most useful, and how to evaluate the results of your program and make modifications for better results. Serious viral illness requires good medical care, so I discuss how you can find the right doctor.

However, before we launch into the discussion on treatment, it is important to begin with a review of the main points from this book that influence and guide treatment.

There are seven key points about viral illness we need to keep in mind:

1. Viruses are parasitic organisms entirely dependent on your tissues, cells, and genetic material to survive and reproduce. They are so small that many can live inside a single cell's nucleus.[1]

2. Due to these characteristics, antiviral drugs are unable to target individual viruses; they cannot get into an infected cell without

causing damage to that individual cell or extensive collateral damage to normal tissue.

3. Vaccines have a better record of success than antiviral drugs, but there is concern about their long-term genetic effects and the spread of other viruses through contaminated vaccines or unsanitary vaccination techniques. There is no evidence that vaccines work against the new and emerging viruses. If they do, it is not known how long it will take the virus to develop resistant strains, rendering the vaccines ineffective.

4. Only the healthy immune system has the potential to neutralize a virus, allowing the body to live normally with a dormant virus.

5. Since viruses can cause extensive tissue damage to vital tissues such as the liver, the brain, and other aspects of the nervous system, a comprehensive approach to treatment that includes antioxidant therapy and management of inflammation is necessary for effective treatment of viral diseases.

6. Natural medicines support the function of the immune system and promote cellular, tissue, and organ adaptation to viral infection, yet as a rule they are not powerful enough when used alone to eradicate a serious viral infection.

7. An integrated approach works best for the treatment of viral illness.

The Importance of Preventing Viral Infection

Perhaps even more basic than the points listed above is prevention. Obviously, if you do not become infected there is no need for treatment. However, when it comes to viruses, prevention is not as easy as it sounds.

First, many people are already infected with viruses and do not know it. For them, it is too late for prevention. Hepatitis C can be harbored in your liver for thirty or forty years before tissue damage shows up on blood tests, and even then no symptoms may be present at all. Many of those already infected can be active carriers and spread infection to others unknowingly.

Second, there are many routes of transmission that are beyond our control. Take mosquitoes: even with effective public health controls, mosquitoes still breed and will bite and infect unsuspecting individuals given the opportunity. Also consider influenza; it can be spread by waterfowl flying in the sky above your home and is easily transmitted by children and even a person coughing in a crowded room.

Third, viruses are passed from person to person through normal human functions like giving birth, breast-feeding, eating, and sex. Giving birth and breast-feeding are functions that we cannot change, but by encouraging healthy lifestyle practices, prenatal and postpartum care, we can reduce the incidence of viral disease spread in this manner. Care can be taken for sanitary preparation of food. Sexually transmitted viruses can be controlled by "safe sex" and abstinence. However, humans are highly sexual creatures and safety and abstinence in all cases all of the time is improbable.

Humans cannot stop eating, forego making love, or stop breathing. However, we can change the manner in which we obtain our food, we can stop polluting our air, alter our personal habits, and maximize our health and healing potential with natural medicines. In both the short and long run, prevention is the means of *diminishing* the spread of viral infections.

Here are some preventive measures to keep in mind:

- If you are sexually active, practice safe sex and avoid sexually promiscuous behavior.

- If you have a cold or the flu, stay home so as not to infect others, and avoid people who are sneezing or coughing in public places. Sneeze or cough into a tissue that you dispose of in a covered container.

- Do not spit in public places.

- When you have a cold or the flu, or are introduced to someone who is sick, avoid shaking hands.

- Since many common viruses are spread when children touch things while sick, keep their hands and faces wiped with plain water and a clean, soft washcloth. Do not use strong antiseptic soaps or cleansing agents.

• If you are in the high-risk group for influenza, consider taking a flu shot.

Epidemics and the effects of bioterrorism constitute a special circumstance. If we were to experience a rapidly spreading viral epidemic from either a natural source or from an act of terrorism, survival would still depend upon the strength of your immune system, your body's reserves of energy, your age, and the other factors that influence health and immunity. Therefore, following the viral immunity principles and steps increases your chances of resisting such developments. Measures to prevent contamination would be more aggressive than outlined above, including quarantine of infected individuals, wearing rubber gloves when caring for the sick, and using surgical or gauze masks to reduce inhalation exposure.

Now that we have reviewed prevention, let's look at the treatment aspect of viral immunity.

Designing Your Viral Immunity Program

Your viral immunity program begins and ends with your lifestyle. Natural medicines work best when applied to a person who eats well, exercises regularly, and takes care of his body. The medications discussed in part 2 are important, but ultimately their role is secondary to having a healthy body and mind. By building your viral immunity program step by step, you will achieve the best results, including permanent healing and lasting health.

Building the Foundation: The foundation of your viral immunity program is composed of steps 1 through 4. These are the cornerstones of viral immunity (see figure 15-1). The most important parts are diet, exercise, detoxification, and antioxidants. Here are some reminders to help you get started:

• Avoid sugar and all refined, packaged, and processed foods; keep your salt intake down.

• Drink plenty of fresh, pure water. Avoid sodas, carbonated water, alcohol, coffee, and commercial fruit drinks.

• Eat a healthy diet based on natural whole foods; buy organically grown products whenever possible.

- Find the diet that works best for you; do not follow every fad diet that you read about.

- Include essential fatty acids from plants, like flaxseed oil (omega-6), and from cold-water fish (omega-3) in your diet.

- Eat adequate amounts of complete protein. Take a whey protein supplement.

- Enhance your diet with phytonutrient-rich foods.

- Exercise regularly and develop a fitness mentality along with a daily regimen that fits your physical and mental state. Set exercise goals.

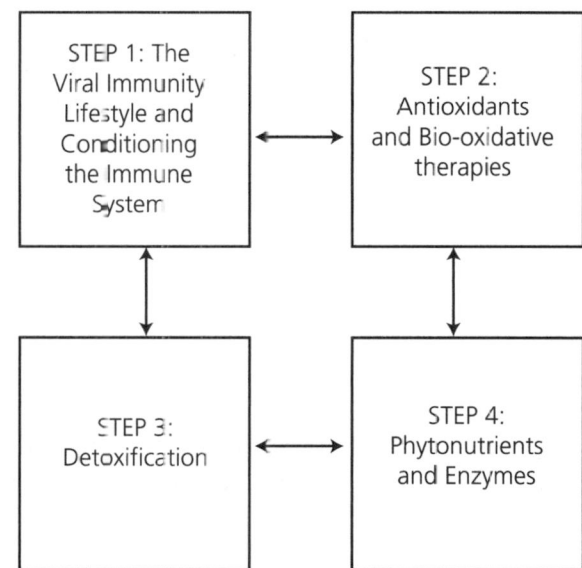

Figure 15-1: Cornerstones of Viral Immunity

- Practice detoxification therapies at least once a year.

- Take a digestive enzyme with meals; use proteolytic enzymes between meals.

- Take antioxidants along with a multivitamin and mineral supplement.

Managing Inflammation: Viruses stimulate immune activity and activate systemic inflammation. Viruses also cause localized tissue damage and inflammation. As it is so difficult to eradicate viruses once they take hold in the body, if you have an active viral infection, inflammation management is critical. When treating viral illness, the most important part of your program after lifestyle is managing inflammation. Here's how in review:

- Get adequate rest, but do not become lazy.

- Remove or avoid those factors that contribute to inflammation.

- Take omega 3 fatty acids (EPA/DHA) and reduce your consumption of all fried foods.

- Evaluate your cortisol levels.

- Use a few natural anti-inflammatory medications.

Enhance Your Natural Immunity: Use adaptogenic and immune-modulating natural medicines to enhance your immune system. In steps 6 and 8, several such agents are discussed, so study these chapters and choose one or two medicines, or a combination immune-enhancing medication.

For general enhancement and prevention, select one of the following:

- Acemannan

- Arabinogalactan

- Astragalus

If you have frequent colds and flu, or repeated mild infections, select one of the following:

- Beta 1, 3-D Glucan

- Echinacea extract

- Transfer Factor

If you have a chronic viral condition, take:

- A mushroom complex with ganoderma and cordyceps, in addition to those listed above.

Select Natural Antivirals: Carefully review the chapters on natural antiviral and antimicrobial alternatives and Chinese herbs. If you have an active or chronic viral illness, choose several agents or an herbal combination from this category.

Mild antivirals useful for colds, flu, and general viral conditions include:

- Echinacea

- Boneset

- Elderberry flowers

- Lemon Balm

- Lomatium

Stronger natural antivirals include:

- Phyllanthus

- Olive leaf extract

For those with HCV or more severe viral illness, add a Chinese herbal formula:

- Minor Bupleurum Decoction

- Hepa 1A Formula

Caution: As long as your system tolerates the herbs in a Chinese formula, stay with it for three months then evaluate your progress. You can add individual herbs or nutrients to your program, but it is better not to add additional complex herbal formulas.

Evaluate and Balance Hormones: If you are over fifty and suffer from chronic fatigue or are thirty-five or older and have a chronic illness, you may have one or more hormonal imbalances. Correct hormone activity is crucial for all stages of immunity and influences all the steps in your viral immunity program. Read step 9 on optimizing hormones and take the self-questionnaire. If you suspect a hormonal deficiency, ask your doctor to perform the recommended tests to evaluate your hormonal function. If the lab tests reveal values outside the range or within the range but less than optimal, consider hormone supplementation. Here are some hormone tips:

- The two most important hormones for immune enhancement are thyroid hormone and cortisol.

- If you are over age 60, human growth hormone may be helpful.

- Use thymus extracts for all chronic, severe, and long-term immune-related illnesses.

- Nearly everyone with an immune deficiency condition or autoimmune disorder can benefit from DHEA and melatonin; keep your dosage very low unless you have a lab test first to determine how much you need.

Working with Natural Medications

It is not easy to pick which medications will be the most effective, even for an experienced doctor who has considerable knowledge of natural medicine. Individual responses vary, and the effectiveness of any particular medication is influenced by many different factors. Though there is now more science in alternative medicine than there was twenty years ago, in the clinical practice of alternative medicine we are largely dependent on what a particular doctor's experience is or what patients report. Unfortunately, this style of practice does not tell you exactly how a particular medicine will work in your body. You will have to take the medicine to know that. In this next section, I discuss several clinical factors that influence the effectiveness and safety of taking medications.

Safety: The number one rule is to never take any medication, natural or chemical, when you do not know its safety. I have made every attempt to present only safe remedies that have proven effectiveness. Some of the proof is from laboratory or clinical studies; some medicines are also empirically proven from my own and other doctors' experiences. As with any substance you take into your body, individual reactions, allergies, and other unpredictable problems can occur.

Table 18: Selected Natural Substances with Overlapping Immunological Actions

Substance	Antioxidant	Anti-Inflammatory	Immunomodulating	Antiviral
Acemannan	X	X	X	X
Arabinogalactan			X	X
Astragalus		X	X	X
Beta 1, 3-D glucan			X	X
Bupleurum	X	X	X	X
Cordyceps	X	X	X	X
Curcumin	X	X		
Echinacea			X	X
Ganoderma	X	X	X	X
Ligustrum		X	X	X
Monolaurin			X	X
Olive Leaf			X	X
Proteolytic enzymes		X	X	
Quercetin	X	X	X	
Selenium	X	X	X	X
Vitamin C	X	X	X	X
Zinc	X	X	X	X

Substances Can Have Multiple Immunological Actions. Those marked under the substance's function indicate areas of overlapping activity.

If you experience any uncomfortable reaction with any of these medications, discontinue its use immediately.

Overlaps: Most medicines have more than one use. The general rule of thumb is that the more complex the medicine is, the more potential uses it is likely to have. This is especially true for natural medications. Due to their highly complex molecular structures and the many different chemical substances they contain, natural substances possess a variety of therapeutic actions (see table 18). To make use of this characteristic, I usually choose as first-line medications those that have the broadest pharmacological range.

Specificity: Once you have incorporated nutrients into a healthy lifestyle and have chosen one or two broad-spectrum immune-enhancing medications, I suggest you next select those that have the most specificity to your condition. Though most natural products are considered nonspecific in their mode of action (meaning they influence function rather than directly manipulating specific biochemical, metabolic, or immunological activities), many display remarkable specificity.

In comparison, pharmaceutical drugs are designed to absorb well into the body and have specific activity, such as the use of prednisone for its anti-inflammatory effects. However, even with drug specificity, these are foreign chemicals and cause other effects that often result in harm to the body.

Dosages, Timing, and Interactions: For most of the substances listed in this book, I have given a dosage range from a low starting dose to an upper limit. Begin with the lower dosage listed, and gradually increase to the higher dosage if you are male or a woman over 150 pounds. For women and those men under 150 pounds, start at the lower dosage and gradually increase to mid-range. Reduce the dosage by half if you experience any uncomfortable effects—usually stomach upset, diarrhea, or bloating. Discontinue if such symptoms persist. Children require dosages that are generally one quarter to one half of the suggested lower dosage.

When you take medications it is important to maximize their absorption and utilization. Review the instructions for each and take them according to the recommended timing, such as with or without meals, in the morning or evening.

Serious interactions with drugs rarely occur with natural substances, but the possibility does exist. Read about each nutrient, herb, or nutraceutical substance in detail *before* you start taking it. If you are taking prescription drugs, read the insert that comes with the medication, ask your pharmacist, or speak with your doctor about possible interactions. In the recommended reading list, you will find books that discuss possible interactions between pharmaceutical drugs and natural substances.

When you take multiple natural medications, as many people do, interactions among the various substances are likely to occur, but it is not well known what their consequences are. For best results, I suggest you take only the minimum *amount of natural medications at any one time, but optimize the dosage.*

In Chinese medicine, the study of interactions among herbal ingredients in a formula is an exacting discipline. Strict rules define which herbs combine best with others. When you take multiple natural medications, as many people do, interactions among the various substances are likely to occur, but it is not well known what their consequences are. It is naïve to believe that since they are natural they are completely benign and that you can mix everything together. For best results, I suggest you take only the *minimum* amount of natural medications at any one time, but optimize the dosage.

Your Age: Though this book is written primarily for adults between the ages of twenty-five and sixty-five, mothers wanting to optimize their family's health and immune status can apply the principles outlined in the book. Keep in mind that infants and children have specific requirements, including much lower dosages than those recommended. They will be unable to tolerate many different medications at the same time, and are more likely to have gastrointestinal upset from herbs and nutrients than adults. The same applies for the elderly. Use lower dosages and fewer medicines. Consult an experienced physician before self-prescribing for infants, children under fifteen years old, or for seniors over sixty-five. However, the general rule is to reduce the dosage to 1/4 to 1/2 of the lowest recommended amount for these age groups.

Measuring Your Viral Immunity Success

For chronic viral conditions, evaluate your progress after three months of treatment, whether self-directed or physician-assisted. To measure your success, first assess any side effects of the treatment. If there were no complications, then you are on a safe regimen. However, to be sure, review the information on each medication you are taking to see if there are any restrictions for continuing past three months. If there are, change that medication; if there are none, continue the evaluation process.

Next, redo the self-questionnaire in step 9 and compare the new results to your original answers. If you answered, "yes" to fewer of the questions this time, you may be improving. Take a mental inventory of your systems. Are you less tired? Do you have more energy? Do you sleep better? Is there less inflammation or less pain? Are bacterial and yeast infections fading? If your symptoms are lessening or disappearing one by one and your energy is increasing, you are making progress.

You may also retest your earlier abnormal laboratory results. I generally retest in increments of 90 days, or in 180 or 360 days. Only retest if necessary. Tests will not affect the course of your therapy and testing too much may cause anxiety. Don't watch lab tests too closely, as they are only part of a complete evaluation. Unnecessarily retesting is also time consuming and costly. Ask yourself if the results of the lab tests, whether positive or negative, will change what you are doing. If the answer is no, then wait to retest.

Natural medicines work more slowly than drugs. In treating chronic illness, you may not notice any progress on a daily or even weekly basis. Once your viral immunity program starts, you may not notice any improvement for three to four weeks, and in some cases for as long as four to six months, or more. Restoring your immunity and organ function takes time. Exercise patience and follow the procedures outlined above for evaluating your progress.

Modifying Your Program: If you are showing improvement and your lab values are normalizing, continue on the same program for another three to six months before re-evaluating. After the six-month evaluation, if you continue to improve, remain on the same program or make a few modest additions and continue to the end of the first year and continue for up to two years.

If you are not improving by the time of your first self-evaluation, change or modify your program by adding or replacing medications. If you still are not improving after six months, you may need professional advice; I suggest you seek the services of a physician skilled in this type of care. If you are worsening at any time in your program, either with worsening symptoms or returning abnormal lab values, find a good doctor.

In closing this section, I offer advice from my clinical experience. Consider the following five treatment principles. They will provide you with a yardstick to measure your program and results:

- In treating human disease, all the different medical systems work some of the time, but none of them work all of the time in all cases. Use what works best.

- Each individual is different and different individuals can express considerable variation in the same disease. Treatment should be individualized.

- Natural medicine works best when applied in a milieu of several different, complementary therapies. Natural therapies and treatments must work synergistically to be effective.

- Lifestyle, diet, and nutrition are the foundation of any natural medicine treatment program. Build a lasting immune foundation with a healthier lifestyle.

- Only take medications, natural or chemical, when you know they are safe and have a reasonable chance of helping you. Do not do yourself harm, even when using natural substances.

As you proceed with your viral immunity program, you will gain experience and sufficient insight to heal yourself. Keep in mind that your experiences relate particularly and specifically to you, and no one else. A mistake many people make is that once they improve, they immediately imagine that they have found a cure for disease. They have: they cured *their* condition. But it does not mean they have found the cure for everyone else.

Keep in mind these five healing principles:

- Only nature can create and re-create living things.

- True healing comes from within and is not dependent on drugs. Healing results in a state of health and wellness.

- The mystery of disease can only be solved by the mastery of health.

- All things, animate and inanimate, have an energetic or spiritual essence; the disturbance in the balance between this essence and life processes is at the root of all disease.

- In Chinese philosophy, the Tao is self-regenerating and constantly self-becoming, therefore the self-healing potential is real and ever-present within you, just as you are an integral part of the Tao.

Finally, I will guide you through different viral illnesses so you can see what I might prescribe for a patient with each different virus. You can use this review as an exercise in how a viral immunity plan might be organized for yourself. This information is not meant to replace good medical care or to serve as a manual on self-care. For more information, consult the recommended reading list.

Common Cold

Diagnosis: This is based upon symptoms and signs of cough, sore throat, headache, sinus and ear congestion, runny nose, and general malaise.

Diet and Fluids: Increase fluids; eat lightly of only chicken or vegetable soups.

Lifestyle and Activity: Rest and reduce activity; inhaling steam from a warm vaporizer can be helpful.

Natural Medications: There are numerous natural remedies, including vitamin C and zinc, that significantly improve cold symptoms and reduce the severity and duration of a cold; none actually cure this common viral condition. Ginger or cinnamon tea with honey is helpful; or choose herbal remedies from chapters 12 and 13. Also helpful are:

- Echinacea preparations

- Elderberry

- Boneset

- Larch Arabinogalactan

- Chinese patent medicine—*gan mao*

Drugs: Antihistamines help dry up nasal secretions; decongestants help improve breathing and clear up congestion in the nose and ears; aspirin can help relieve a headache and body aches. However, most of these over-the-counter drugs are not necessary for the treatment of a cold. Use them only if necessary to control symptoms. Antibiotics or antivirals should not be used to treat the common cold.

Influenza

Diagnosis: This is based upon symptoms and signs of fever, cough, headache, malaise, and systemic body aches. Symptoms can be mild or severe, and even life-threatening in elderly people. Respiratory symptoms can be severe. Complications include bronchitis, pneumonia, asthma, and encephalitis.

Diet and Fluids: Eat lightly, use chicken or vegetable soups, drink plenty of fluids.

Lifestyle and Activity: Bed rest and avoid exertion. Use steam or a vaporizer to improve respiration and keep the mucous membranes moistened. Gargle with salt water for sore throat.

Natural Medications: You may use the same herbal medications as for the common cold, but increase the dosage and take them for 10–14 days, even after symptoms subside. Gargle with myrrh tincture for sore throat. Stronger natural medications include:

- Echinacea extract or injectable (Pascotox forte or Heel Echinacea compositum)

- Oscillococcinum

- Olive leaf extract

- Allicin

- Grapefruit seed extract

- Chinese patent medicines: *yin chao san* or *zhong gan ling*

Drugs: Aspirin or acetaminophen can be used to manage fever and to reduce head and body aches when severe; the antiviral drugs Amantadine and Ribavirin can be helpful when used in the early stages and for uncomplicated influenza. Opportunistic bacterial infections frequently accompany the flu; however, unless they are severe or compromise an already weak patient, antibiotics are rarely needed.

Herpes Simplex Virus

Diagnosis: This is based upon symptoms and signs of recurrent clear fluid-filled blisters that occur on the lips in HSV-I, and in the genital region in the case of HSV-II. A positive antibody test confirms the diagnosis.

Diet and Fluids: Increase fluids and avoid arginine-containing foods.

Lifestyle and Activity: Rest when lesions are active and avoid direct sunlight.

Natural Medications: Many natural antiviral agents are effective against both types of herpes, as well as for shingles (HZV). Natural topical medications are also helpful. Take 1,500–3,000 mg of L-lysine daily.

- Echinacea extract and injectables

- Lemon balm extract (Herpilyn) applied topically

- Monolaurin

- Olive leaf extract

- Sangre de drago extract (SB-300) applied topically

Drugs: Acyclovir and some of the newer antivirals can be helpful in some cases.

Hepatitis C

The treatment of chronic hepatitis is considerably more complicated than the previous three viral illnesses. For HCV and other serious viral diseases, carefully re-read chapters 10–14 and read several of the recommended books on hepatitis. For the purposes of this discussion, I will focus on a case of HCV in which active inflammation is present but has not deteriorated to cirrhosis or liver failure.

Diagnosis: This is based on a positive antibody test, an elevated viral load measured by PCR (polymerase chain reaction) test, and an elevated ALT (alanine aminotransferase) level. In advanced stages, other abnormal lab test results may appear such as decreased albumin, and elevated AST (aspartate aminotransferase). Diagnosis is also based on liver biopsy, a procedure in which a small piece of tissue is taken from the liver and examined under a microscope to check for cirrhosis. In the early stages, HCV often does not display any obvious symptoms or signs of illness.

Diet and Fluids: Have a normal fluid intake but avoid dehydration. Avoid excess iron-containing foods and use iron-free nutritional supplements. Have a moderate to low animal protein, and a higher vegetable protein intake. Possibly supplement with branched-chain amino acids (leucine, valine, and isoleucine). Increase calcium intake and restrict sodium use. Avoid cold foods and foods that are difficult to digest, such as fatty foods. Eliminate alcohol and coffee; reduce or eliminate all refined sugar. Eat frequent (four to six times daily), smaller meals to reduce hypoglycemic tendencies.

Lifestyle and Activity: Maintain normal activity and never exercise to exhaustion. Maintain a positive attitude and guard against the emotional ups and downs you may experience from routine fluctuations of lab test results. It is mandatory that you follow the principles of chapters 6–10 to establish a healthy lifestyle and one that promotes optimal immune function and reduces inflammatory activity in the body.

Natural Medications: There are many natural medications that work with HCV, and most are reasonably successful in managing liver inflammation and lowering ALT levels. Over time, some have the potential to lower the viral load. My first choice for HCV is to make sure you are taking adequate amounts of antioxidants, especially vitamin C and selenium (see chapter 7 for antioxidants).

I suggest a three- to six-month course of a combination of ganoderma with other mushroom glucans and cordyceps (see chapter 11). Next, you need a natural antiviral such as phyllanthus or olive leaf extract (chapter 12). Finally, I recommend a Chinese herbal formula (chapter 13):

- Eurocel

- HEPA 1A Formula

- Minor Bupleurum Decoction

- *Qing Tui Tang*

Drugs: Conventional medicine relies on interferon and Ribaviron and other antiviral drugs, as well as liver transplant as the mainstay of current therapy for HCV.

How the Prescriptions Work in Actual Cases

At this point it is helpful to conclude our discussions with two case studies to illustrate what complete treatment and follow-up plans look like. Also, it is instructive to discuss a case in which complete resolution was not possible.

The first case is interesting in many ways. First, I have been treating this patient for about eight years, and during that time, though I do not see him socially outside of the office, we have come to know each other as supportive friends. By becoming friends, I not only take more interest in his case, but his successes and setbacks affect not only him but touch me as well.

Second, though he came to me in an advanced stage of his illness, many of his complaints have been significantly improved or eliminated and his viral condition stabilized to a great degree. This is important because it shows that alternative therapies have a place in the integrated management of patients with chronic disease, and provides patients with effective and safe methods of treating parallel illnesses without resorting to additional drugs.

Third, we achieved some degree of clinical success, yet his underlying condition remains unchanged. The final outcome, though still unpredictable and less bleak than when he first came to see me, is that he is not completely well and may never be. This case shows how conventional medicine, alternative medicine, and self-care work together.

Case Study on Hepatitis: Phil is a middle-aged man of good bearing and character who raised two children and put them through college; he has been in a stable second marriage for twenty years. During his youth, he experimented with recreational drugs and alternative lifestyles, but by his later twenties he settled into his chosen profession and developed his own business. It was very successful, affording him a comfortable lifestyle with plenty of time to pursue his other interests in art and world cultures.

His youthful experimentation, though more than thirty years before I first saw him, exposed Phil to the hepatitis C virus. By the time he was diagnosed with HCV, he was overweight, had Type-II diabetes, high blood pressure, and a host of other symptoms including fatigue and joint pains. His medical doctors treated each of his complaints as *different* diseases, according to the allopathic model: hypoglycemic agents for the diabetes, blood pressure-lowering drugs for the hypertension, non-steroidal anti-inflammatory medications for pain, and antidepressants and sleeping pills for his fatigue.

The results were as could only be expected. His blood pressure was improved but not normal, glucose levels were lower but not normal, he was drowsy from the psychoactive drugs, he had to be taken off the anti-inflammatory and cholesterol-lowering drugs when his liver enzymes increased, and still he did not feel any better.

Realizing he was not improving, and was even gradually worsening, Phil spoke with his family and friends about their experiences with alternative medicine. A few had some good experiences but none knew much about alternative options for chronic hepatitis. His wife suggested he speak with his general physician about it. Though Phil expected his conventional medical doctor would not only know nothing about alternative medicine, but might be antagonistic toward it, Phil was surprised to find that his doctor was open to having him try this option and referred Phil to me. He told Phil that other patients of his had worked with me on various health problems and that most had improved or at least felt better. Phil called me the next day.

I carefully evaluated his case, including his prescription drugs. I ordered a new set of blood tests, sent for old medical records, and mailed the referring doctor a summary of my findings.

Phil's case was advanced hepatitis C virus with moderate cirrhosis, complicated by diabetes and hypertension. He was particularly interested in the Chinese medicinal approach, so I started treatment with Chinese herbs to remove accumulated pathogenic "dampness" and to tonify his underlying deficiency of organ energy reserves, using yin tonics for the liver and kidney. I corrected his diet and encouraged Phil to lose weight and start exercising moderately. Since his iron levels were elevated, he was to avoid red meat and all supplements with iron. I started him on extra vitamin C, an antioxidant combination, and milk thistle extract.

Within three months, his glucose levels were falling below normal and his doctor gradually took him off all anti-diabetic medications. His blood pressure also normalized and he was able to reduce his anti-hypertension drugs to a very minimal dose. Acupuncture effectively controlled all of his pain complaints and his energy and mood improved to the point where he no longer needed sleeping aids or antidepressant drugs.

His previously elevated test results for liver function lowered, but never fully normalized; and his viral load remained over one million. When the viral load, or number of viruses, is over one million, active viral disease is present. A person without viral disease should have no viruses present. The goals of therapy in chronic hepatitis are to reduce inflammation, treat co-infections, improve liver function, prevent cirrhosis and hepatocellular cancer, and to ultimately reduce or eliminate the viral load.

Phil, who continues to see me regularly, is on a regimen of anti-inflammatory and antiviral Chinese herbs along with nutritional supplementations. He is cured of diabetes and his blood pressure is normalized. His cholesterol has also lowered considerably, but is still above normal values. His energy and mood are good. He reads and regularly browses the Internet for information on hepatitis C; after culling what he finds, he shows me what he thinks is promising, and I approve or disapprove of adding it to his regimen.

His general practitioner has been cooperative during the time I have been treating Phil; and his hepatologist, though pessimistic about the outcome of any chronic hepatitis case, has had to admit that Phil is holding his own and that his liver, though not "cured," has been stable for nearly a decade.

Second Case Study on Hepatitis: Elizabeth also came to see me for hepatitis C. She is over fifty but looks and acts much younger than her age. Ironically, as with many patients with HCV, fatigue was not a significant symptom of her condition, which concealed the seriousness of her case until it was already well advanced. I reviewed her medical history and lab studies, then took a detailed account of her symptoms and complaints. She reported hot flashes, that her period was becoming very irregular, that she was finding it difficult to fall asleep, and that she was often woken up by night sweats. Her memory was declining, her mood ebbed low at times, and she had neck pain. She had a history of chronic vaginal yeast infections, chemical sensitivity, abdominal bloating, intolerance to fatty foods, constipation, and dry, itchy skin.

Her previous lab tests revealed extremely elevated ALT and AST levels, a very high viral load, higher-than-average thyroid stimulating hormone (TSH), and slightly lower levels of the thyroid hormone free T_4. A liver biopsy confirmed cirrhosis, and a bone density study revealed the early stages of osteoporosis. An MRI of her neck showed a mild disc protrusion. Since many of Elizabeth's symptoms, as well as her age, suggested she was experiencing menopausal changes. I ordered follicle stimulating hormone (FSH), estradiol, progesterone, and DHEA-S tests.

The function of the ovaries decline with age and when measured by a blood test, the levels of ovarian hormones, estrogens (estradiol being the most active) and progesterone are low. At the same time, FSH (a pituitary hormone that influences the secretion of estrogen) becomes very elevated. The combination of elevated FSH and low estradiol indicates menopause.

As expected, Elizabeth's FSH was elevated in the menopausal range; the estradiol was very low, as was the DHEA-S; and the progesterone was in the normal range, as she was self-medicating with an over-the-counter cream.

WESTERN MEDICINE INTERPRETATION: Elizabeth was diagnosed by her internist as having chronic hepatitis C virus, early stage cirrhosis consistent with hepatitis infection, osteopenia, menopausal syndrome, and neck pain caused by degenerative disc disease of the cervical spine. I thought her case was thoroughly worked up from the allopathic point of view. However, her doctors offered few solutions to her problems other than interferon therapy (she was very afraid of this) and an estrogen patch.

ENERGETIC MEDICINE INTERPRETATION: Though Elizabeth had been an energetic and robust woman, her energy was beginning to decline. Her yin was not depleted, yet the beginnings of age-related yin and blood deficiency were showing up in the degeneration of her bones, liver, and in the hot flashes and night sweats. Stagnation of liver qi was present, as evidenced by the abdominal bloating and difficulty digesting fatty foods. The virus was chronically active within her liver, and had already penetrated to the deeper energetic layers even though her basic energy was still relatively alive and active.

INTEGRATIVE MEDICINE INTERPRETATION: Though the Western medicine diagnoses were correct, they were incomplete. Elizabeth had borderline thyroid insufficiency, recurrent fungal infections, and was heading full-force into menopause. Her ovarian hormones were very low and her adrenal function was also stressed. Her liver was inflamed, and degeneration of liver tissue and cells was advancing. Still, her general constitution was strong and she was not overwhelmed physically or mentally by her symptoms. She was a firm believer in natural medicine and told me several previous stories of "cures" she had enjoyed with homeopathy and herbal therapies.

TREATMENT: The immediate goal of therapy was to manage Elizabeth's inflammation and to lower the ALT and AST levels. For this, I gave her a blend of Chinese herbs including cordyceps, the liver-protecting herb milk thistle *(Silybum marianum)*; L-tyrosin to promote thyroid function; sublingual DHEA; and a low-dose topical natural estrogen and progesterone cream. To treat the fungal problem, I prescribed allicin and other natural antifungals. For her neck pain, I advised acupuncture.

Elizabeth already had eliminated alcohol and most of her daily coffee and caffeinated sodas. However, I advised her to eliminate all caffeine except that in green tea, to avoid eating red meat, eliminate sugar, and eat more vegetables and fresh whole fruits. She started with a monthly mild detoxification program using UltraClear Plus, and resumed her yoga practice. Elizabeth was already on a good multivitamin and mineral supplement, but I asked her to change to one that contained no iron, and to take additional vitamin C in a buffered form, extra selenium, quercetin, and a calcium and magnesium supplement.

Elizabeth established a daily prayer routine and attended a weekly meditation group. Her psychologist encouraged her renewed interest in spirituality, and she attended two shamanic ceremonies and felt a connection with nature. She renewed her commitment to her relationships with family and friends. She is interested in following these new spiritual awakenings and we have discussed her participation in a tour to the Amazon to take an herbal cleansing program in the rainforest and undergo an authentic shamanic experience in an *ayahuasca* ceremony.

CLINICAL EVALUATION: By the end of one month on the program, her ALT levels had dropped by 50 percent. Her menopausal symptoms were considerably lessened, her skin was less dry, her fungal infection cleared nicely, and she had lost a few pounds. Her mood was positive and hopeful, and she was enthusiastic and fully participating in her treatment plan.

Three months later, her ALT levels were approaching the normal range. Her hot flashes and night sweats were completely gone, her neck was considerably better with acupuncture, and her skin was clearing without itching or further vaginal yeast infections. Her newfound spiritual growth through yoga, prayer, meditation, and shamanic rituals had given her a new view of life's transitions and uncertainties. Her disease was no longer a burden. The shamanic ceremonies helped to free her from the overwhelming fear of a horrible life and a painful death.

Perhaps the virus was something of an ally in helping her reach into herself and to the universal spirit to which we are all connected.

What the Cases Mean: Both Phil's and Elizabeth's cases remind us that the path of healing can be long and arduous. But we can also heed the wise saying, "An ounce of prevention is worth a pound of cure" and avoid illness and disease by creating a positive and healthy lifestyle. In treating chronic viral illness, we must be patient and work towards healing over time. We should not overdo medications, even natural ones, and we need to allow time for them to work before changing the program.

In the face of serious viral illness, I recommend you to seek the advise of a wise and knowledgeable doctor whenever possible. Chronic illness can be painful, physically and emotionally, and it can be very lonely. It is a blessing to have the companionship of a caring physician in your journey to recovery and healing.

Yet, no matter how important taking personal preventive steps may be, a significant proportion of the current immune dilemma is due to environmental problems beyond our individual control. As long as continued large-scale destruction of virgin forests, the pollution of water systems, and other ecologically unsound practices continue, viruses and other infectious diseases will spread in a massive and unpredictable manner. Wars and rapid global transportation assist the spread of viruses worldwide.

Keep in mind that it not simply a viral problem, but an immune system issue. Without stronger environmental laws, increased ecological consciousness, and more ethical and morally sound political strategies, the air you breathe, the water you drink, and the food you eat, will continue to contain chemical toxins that disrupt your immunity, making you increasingly vulnerable to ubiquitous viruses.

In the face of serious viral illness, I recommend you to seek the advise of a wise and knowledgeable doctor whenever possible. Chronic illness can be painful, physically and emotionally, and it can be very lonely. It is a blessing to have the companionship of a caring physician in your journey to recovery and healing.

In the process of restoring our health, we must eventually return to the source of our creation: the healing power in our bodies, the intelligence of our cells, and our purpose for being—our personal destiny. Go deep within and allow yourself to feel the wellspring of life.

Appendix A

Finding the Right Doctor to Oversee Your Viral Immunity Program

It is difficult to say what makes the "right" doctor, but squarely put, the right doctor is the one who helps you get better. The second best doctor is one who does not make you worse, and refers you to the right doctor; and the third best doctor is one who makes you feel better by managing your symptoms, but is not able to actually resolve your condition.

I have often seen patients virtually in love with their physician, acupuncturist, or alternative practitioner, and stay with them year after year yet not improve at all. In fact, many worsen. In these cases, perhaps the doctor is kind and personable, but is not the "right" doctor to help them actually get better. I have also heard patients complain about this or that doctor who treated them poorly, but when I asked if they were helped or if the surgeon did a good job, they answered affirmatively.

Ironic, isn't it, that patients are often the worst judge of who is the right doctor? Though there is no guarantee that you will chose the right doctor on the first try, here are a few guidelines you can apply when you start looking.

Interview Carefully: If you are reasonably healthy and are going for an annual physical exam, need an acupuncturist to treat a knee strain or a chiropractor to work on a stiff neck, you need only find the doctor who provides you with the best service for the most reasonable fee. This is largely a matter of shopping the phone book, your insurance company's physician directory, or calling a referral service.

However, if you have a serious chronic condition, that is the wrong approach. For such a condition, you need the best doctor available, one who is knowledgeable about *your* condition, who has the time and willingness to work with *you*—a person you can trust and develop a professional rapport with over a period of years.

Since chronic viral conditions take time to undo and you may be seeing the same doctor every few months, consider asking a few questions at the time of your first visit or interview. Ask if the doctor has had a similar condition. What made her choose this area to specialize in? Doctors see many patients day after day, and an astute physician knows who gets better and what medications and therapies tend to work better than others. Ask what her cure rates are.

Remember you want to know what *her* professional success rate is and not the general statistics—after all, the research studies were not performed on *you.*

Keep in mind the healing profession is stressful. Do not be overly demanding or confrontational with your doctor. If she turns out to be the right doctor, you will want her to think of you as an intelligent, informed, and concerned patient who will cooperate, rather than as a difficult and stubborn patient who asks endless questions that waste both of your time.

Don't Assume Your Doctor Knows Everything: Many people make the mistake (based upon another medical myth that doctors are akin to deities) that your doctor knows everything. In truth, the doctor is another person like yourself who also may have experienced an illness, who will age, and who has to pay bills and taxes. If you feel you might get nervous and only later remember questions you wanted to ask the doctor, prepare a list before your visit. Do not bring in a page full of questions or make it a habit of calling after your visit to ask more questions that would have been better answered in person. Speaking from experience, I can say these approaches annoy and frustrate doctors.

Listen to your doctor's answers carefully. Ask him to write down instructions for you if you have a hard time remembering details. In my practice, being used to the memory loss and concentration difficulties many patients with chronic illness have, I explain the reasons for my treatments, summarize them, and write them down for the patient. Sometimes in a complex case, I also type out a summary and mail it to the patient.

It is acceptable to provide your doctor with literature and information, but do not overwhelm him with books and especially do not confront him with marketing pieces from nutritional companies advertising the latest cure for whatever ails you. Select sources related to your condition and make copies of parts of articles or highlight a paragraph or two that you think he might find interesting or that you would like his comments on. Remember, you are there to access the doctor's expertise and not to confuse the issues of your case with potentially extraneous information.

Revealing Information: It is important to have a relationship with your doctor that is open and frank, though with respect on your end and empathy on hers. Do not withhold information about other treatments or self-prescribed medications you are taking. If your medical doctor is opposed to alternative therapies, inquire on what grounds she bases her opinion. If her answer does not satisfy you, look for another primary care doctor.

The same is true for any alternative medicine practitioners. If they are against allopathic medicine, you will find it difficult to communicate effectively on issues that involve medical intervention and drug therapy. If you need a referral or are faced with a medical emergency, you will be unsupported.

Keep your doctor informed, but don't overwhelm her with every detail about every acupuncture session you've had or what the clerk in the health foods store told you last week. Write a list of all the supplements you are taking so there is a copy in your file. Update it periodically. Keep your alternative practitioner advised on what drugs you are taking, but don't expect her to answer questions on prescription medications that your medical doctor has ordered.

Ask the nurse, the prescribing medical doctor, or the dispensing pharmacist your questions concerning pharmaceutical drugs. Don't expect your medical doctor to know everything about vitamins; save those questions for your naturopath or nutritionist.

If stress plays a key role in your illness, make sure you reveal this to your doctors, but don't expect them to listen to your personal problems for all of your scheduled visit. Save that for your therapist or psychologist.

On Self-Care and Second Opinions: In this book, you have been introduced to several methods of treatment, different conventional and alternative medicine styles, and energetic medicine. There is competition among these methods for the same health care dollar. Unless you have a referral from a trusted source, approach your medical care as you would any other business arrangement: adequately prepared and with care.

This book provides you with information for self-care, which is different from care provided by a medical practitioner. Be responsible for reading the material carefully, consulting the additional recommended literature, asking questions of your health care providers, making decisions on what natural medications might best suit your condition, obtaining these medications, and then adding them into you treatment schedule.

You may want to consider the option of "guided self-care" where you work with a natural-medicine oriented physician to order lab tests and monitor your progress. This alternative opinion can be invaluable in a long-term program. Do not hesitate to seek a second, or even third, opinion if you or your doctor are confused or you do not think you are making sufficient progress.

A Note to Your Doctor: Your patient has read my book on viral immunity. In it, I discuss immunity concepts from an evolutionary point of view and present self-directed strategies using natural medicines for the prevention, care, and management of viral diseases, including influenza, herpes simplex virus, chronic hepatitis C, and several other common viral illnesses.

The information contained in this book is garnered from nearly twenty years of clinical practice, and knowing that my audience may include not only lay readers, but professionals like yourself, I have extensively investigated and documented the material in this book with research from authoritative books and prestigious medical journals. Indeed, I have left out hundreds of other articles solely for the sake of space and time.

Though this book is meant to help patients with viral ailments which prove to be difficult to cure, it is not meant to replace the advice, guidance, and medical abilities of a physician. Nor is the material contained in this book meant to be used by your patient to challenge your practice of medicine. It is solely intended to help your patients improve their chances of restoring their health.

Appendix B

Useful Laboratory Tests that Support Your Viral Immunity Program

There are numerous lab tests that can help your doctor evaluate and diagnose your condition. In fact, there are far too many to discuss in this book. The purpose of this book has been to educate you about how the immune system works, what viruses are and how they cause disease, and to outline a method of designing a safe and effective self-directed plan to enhance your immunity and treat the consequences of your viral illness with natural medications.

Thus, the lab studies reviewed here are not meant to deliver a specific diagnosis, which is the work of a licensed doctor, but to assist you and your doctor in understanding the function of your body and immunity and to provide objective markers with which to evaluate improvement. Medical diagnosis is between you and your doctor.

Interpretation of blood or urine tests involves a considerable amount of training and experience, and should be left to a competent naturopathic physician, medical doctor, or doctor of osteopathic medicine. No test replaces a complete review of your medical history, a detailed list of your symptoms, and a thorough physical examination by a skilled and astute clinician.

Selected Useful Laboratory Tests

For general health evaluation in patients with viral disease:

- Blood Chemistry Panel: Previously called a SMAC 20 and also referred to as a metabolic panel, this involves a wide range of tests. The most common are protein, albumin, globulin, calcium, phosphorous, chloride, sodium, glucose, blood urea nitrogen (BUN), uric acid, bilirubin, alkaline phosphatase, aspartate aminotransferase (AST), and alanine aminotransferase (ALT).

- Complete Blood Count (CBC): This evaluates the number of both red and white cells and consists of red blood cell (RBC) count, hematocrit (Hct), hemoglobin (Hgb), red cell indices, white blood cell (WBC) count, and differential count of white cell count including lymphocytes, neutrophils, monocytes, basophils, and eosinophils.

- Lipid Profile: This tests total cholesterol: triglycerides, low density lipoproteins (LDL), and high density lipoprotein (HDL). You or your doctor may wish to add other tests for a more comprehensive cardiovascular evaluation including Apolipoprotein A1, lipoprotein(a), fibrinogen, homocysteine, and HDL subtypes.

To evaluate for inflammation:

- ANA (chapter 5)

- C-Reactive Protein (chapter 5)

- ESR (chapter 5)

- Protein Electrophoresis (optional): This measures proteins to evaluate acute and chronic inflammatory activity.

To evaluate immune status:

- Activated Complete Lymphocyte Panel: This is a comprehensive evaluation of T and B lymphocytes, cytotoxic T cells, and ratios of helper and suppressor cells. Some cytokines may also be included, such as interleukin (IL) 2 and tumor necrosis factor (TNF)-alpha.

- Natural Killer Cell Total and Function

- Total IgG, IgA, IgM, IgE Antibodies (optional)

- Antioxidant Status (optional): This screens for antioxidant levels in blood or urine and to evaluate status after taking supplemental antioxidants after at least six to twelve months. This test is useful in patients with compromised immunity, chronic viral disease, and cancer. There are different methods for measuring antioxidant levels and determining oxidative status, but all generally include vitamin C, zinc, selenium, beta carotene and other carotenoids, and perhaps coenzyme Q10 and other antioxidant substances.

Toxic chemicals:

- Screening for heavy metals by hair analysis or by twenty-four-hour urine analysis: This is a useful tool for evaluating toxic status by measuring levels of mercury and other toxic minerals that weaken immunity.

Hormones:

- Cortisol

- DHEA

- Human Growth Hormone (for those over 60)

- Melatonin (optional)

- Thyroid Function

My Recommended Panel of Laboratory Tests

For patients with chronic viral disease or other illness in which immune function is impaired, have the tests listed below to establish a baseline. If your doctor suspects a virus, he will order a screening panel for several viruses or will check antibody levels for a specific virus.

Complete Blood Chemistry and Lipid Profile

Blood Count with differential

ESR

ANA

TSH, total T_4, free T_3

DHEA-S

Activated Complete Lymphocyte Panel with NK cell count and function

Other Methods of Testing

Blood testing is not the only method of evaluating health and immune status. Several useful alternative methods are available, though keep in mind that there are often no well-established standards for these tests and interpretation may vary greatly among practitioners.

Bio-energetic Techniques: Electro-acupuncture according to Voll (EAV), also called electrodermal screening (EDS), is a bio-energetic method developed in Germany performed by using a small probe along the sides of the fingers to measure very small amounts of electrical current in the acupuncture meridian system. This form of testing is often applied when other diagnostic results are inconclusive or difficult to evaluate; it can have a wide range of clinical uses including evaluation of different types of latent viral infection.

Dark Field Microscopy: This method is performed by taking a drop of blood from the patient's finger and placing it on a slide that is then viewed under a special "dark field" microscope. The advantage of this system is that you are looking directly at *living* blood cells. It can evaluate some aspects of general health status but it is not as conclusive a diagnostic method as some proponents believe.

High Resolution Microscopy: This method, designed by Robert Bradford of American Biologics in Mexico, is considered highly accurate for evaluating live blood and other tissue in ways that dark field microscopy cannot. Bradford, once a leading figure in dark field analysis, uses high resolution microscopy to detect subtle biochemical changes at the tissue level in order to evaluate the patient's health status and monitor progress of therapy.

Clinical Microscopy: A skilled immunologist or pathologist will often look at your blood, urine, or other live tissue under a normal light microscope in his office. William Hitt, M.D., Ph.D., also in Mexico, is famous for his ability to evaluate slides prepared from a patient's nasal swab to assess immune reactivity including allergy, virally induced, or other inflammation. Clinical microscopy can be an invaluable addition to laboratory diagnosis and a good medical history and exam.

Chinese and Ayurvedic Pulse Reading: This method is used by Oriental medicine practitioners to evaluate the body's energetic status, including the energy flow in the individual meridians and channels.

Tongue Diagnosis: Both Chinese and Ayurvedic practitioners use tongue diagnosis, but it is more emphasized by the Chinese. The practitioner evaluates the state of your body fluids, digestive function, and other aspects of the body's internal function by examining the condition of your tongue.

Facial Diagnosis and Body Morphology: Through examining the face and body constitution, skin and hair quality, and other bodily features, a skilled practitioner can gather information on your character, stress reactions, constitutional tendencies, hormonal deficiencies, and energy balance.

Physician-Administered and -Prescribed Therapies

This book provides self-directed care in using natural medicine for viral illnesses, such as for hepatitis C, AIDS, Epstein-Barr virus and other viruses that are serious or difficult to eradicate. Yet you will need the assistance of a medical doctor (M.D.) or doctor of osteopathy (D.O.) who offers more intensive therapies that require prescribing privileges. The following list includes the physician-administered therapies mentioned in part 2.

Antibiotics

Antiviral drugs

Armour Thyroid

Human growth hormone

Hydrocortisone

Injectable echinacea and homo-toxicology medications

Injectable thymus extract

Intravenous hydrogen peroxide

Intravenous vitamins, minerals, and amino acids

Ozone

Ultraviolet Therapy

Appendix D

A Note On Vaccinations

My patients frequently ask my opinion on vaccination and because the question of vaccination will come up while or after you have read this book, I include this short commentary here on the vaccination controversy. I do not advocate for or against vaccines. Though such a position does not ultimately resolve the difficult dilemma of whether to use vaccinations or not, the following information may help you make wiser decisions.

Routine medical vaccination has been performed for more than half a century, during which time standards and safety have improved immensely. Principles of immunization through vaccines have been known for hundreds of years, or longer, but even so, controversy remains active to this day.

In light of the material contained in this book, the most pressing questions related to vaccination are these: Have the mass vaccination programs of previous decades contributed to the AIDS epidemic and other diseases? Though safer vaccines are now available, do they contribute to neurological damage and immune system dysfunction? Does the use of live-virus vaccines cause yet-to-be determined biological alterations of the genetic material?

There is clear scientific evidence validating the effectiveness of immunization through vaccination, but there is also a growing body of evidence challenging its safety. It is not my intention to go into this issue in detail, but it is my clinical opinion that the disruption of the immune system is potentially a very serious problem, one which could affect every individual on this planet, and until clear, unbiased, and well-documented data is available, individuals and parents should approach the vaccination issue with caution.

Further Reading

Buttram, H. "Vaccine scene 2001—update and overview." *Townsend Letter for Doctors and Patients*. June 2001: 70–79.

Coulter, Harris with Barbara Fisher. *DPT: A Shot in the Dark*. New York: Penguin, 1991.

Coulter, Harris. *Vaccination, Social Violence, and Criminality*. Berkley, Calif.: North Atlantic Books, 1990.

Neustaeder, Randall. *The Vaccine Guide, Making an Informed Consent*. Berkley, Calif.: North Atlantic Books, 1996.

O'Shea, Tim. "Vaccination is not immunization." *Alternative Medicine*. July 2001: 70–89.

Appendix E

Resources

Doctors and Clinics: All the doctors listed have extensive experience in the viral and related conditions listed in this book. In addition, they have either written books on the subject or published scientific research and academic papers.

Kenneth Bock, M.D.
108 Montgomery Street
Rhinebeck, NY 12572
845-876-7082
www.rhinebeckhealth.com

Misha Cohen, O.M.D., L.Ac.
3128 16th Street
San Francisco, CA 94103
415-864-7234
www.docmisha.com

Jesse Stoff, M.D.
3402 East Broadway Boulevard
Tucson, AZ 85716
520-319-9074
www.drstoff.com

W. John Martin, M.D., Ph.D.
Center for Complex Infectious Diseases
3328 Stevens Avenue, 2nd Floor
Rosemead, CA 91770
626-572-7288
www.ccid.org

Qingcai Zhang, M.D. (China), L.Ac.
420 Lexington Avenue,
Greybar Building, Suite 631
New York, NY 10170
212-573-9584
www.dr-zhang.com

Paul Cheney, M.D.
86 Keelson Row
Bald Head Island, NC 28461
910-457-7133
www.fnmedcenter.com

Clinics outside the U.S.: Due to expense, medical politics, and availability of different medications and therapies, it is becoming more common for patients with serious illnesses to seek medical care outside the United States. Depending on the medical boards of the individual countries, you might be able to obtain high quality services and medications that, though "illegal" in one country, are available in another.

However, before you decide on such a venture, I strongly advise you to research the clinic and its medical director in as much detail as possible before proceeding to invest your time and money. There are good doctors and those that are less skilled, so ask the same questions before going to a clinic outside the U.S. as you would in the United States. I have listed several clinics in Mexico with which I am familiar and that have a good reputation—they are not included here as endorsements of their medical philosophy or style of care.

William Hitt, M.D., Ph.D.
William Hitt Center
Ave Paseo, Tijuana 406, Suite 403
Tijuana, B.C., Mexico
888-671-9849

Professor Robert Bradford
American Biologics Integrated Medical
    Center
Playas, Tijuana, Mexico
American mailing address:
1180 Walnut Avenue
Chula Vista, CA 91911
800-227-4458
www.als-cancer-fibromyalgia-ms.com

Rodrigo Rodriquez, M.D.
International BioCare Hospital
Azucenas No. 15, Frace. Del Prado
Tijuana, B.C., Mexico 22440
800-785-0490
www.ibchospital.com

Drs. Jorge Vazquez, M.D. and
    Filiberto Muñoz, M.D.
San Diego Clinic
Circuito Bursatil #9031, Edificio Terra,
Zona Rio, Suite 306
C.P. 22320, Tijuana, B.C., Mexico
011-52-6-683-1398
www.sdclinic.com

Medical Associations: If you are unable to find a practitioner, you can contact a regional or national medical association for a referral.

Chinese Medicine and Acupuncture
Association of Canada
154 Wellington Street
London, Ontario, Canada, N6B 2K8
519-642-1970
www.cmaac.ca

American Association of Integrative
Medicine
2750 E. Sunshine
Springfield, MO 65804
417-881-9995
www.aaimedicine.com

American Association of Naturopathic
Physicians
8201 Greensboro Drive, Suite 300
McLean, VA 22102
703-610-9037
www.naturopathic.org

American Association of Oriental Medicine
433 Front Street
Catasauqua, PA 18032
610-266-1433
www.aaom.org

American Holistic Medical Association
6728 McLean Village Drive
McLean, VA 22101-8729
703-556-8729
www.holisticmedicine.org

American Osteopathic Association
142 East Ontario Street
Chicago, IL 60611
800-6211-1773
www.aoa-net.org

British Association of Oriental Medicine
206-208 Latimer Road, Suite D
London, England, W10 6RE
0181-968-3469
www.demon.co.uk/acupuncture/baab.html

California State Oriental Medical Association
2710 X Street, Suite 2A
Sacramento, CA 95818
www.csomaonline.org

International Oxidative Medicine
Association
P.O. Box 891954
Oklahoma City, OK 73109
405-634-7855

National Center for Homeopathy
801 North Fairfax Street, Suite 306
Alexandria, VA 22314
703-548-7790
www.healthy.net/nch

Specialty Laboratories

Antioxidant Profiles:

Genox Corporation
1414 Key Highway
Baltimore, M.D. 21230
410-347-7616
www.genox.com

Pantox Laboratories
4622 Sante Fe Street
San Diego, CA 92109
888-726-8698
www.pantox.com

Hormone Panels:

AAL Reference Laboratories
1715 E. Wilshire, #715
Santa Ana, CA 92705
800-522-2621
www.aalrl.com

Genox Corporation
1414 Key Highway
Baltimore, M.D. 21230
410-347-7616
www.genox.com

Meridian Valley Laboratory
515 West Harrison Street, Suite 9
Kent, Washington 98032
253-859-8700

Immunological Profiles:

AAL Reference Laboratories
1715 E. Wilshire, #715
Santa Ana, CA 92705
800-522-2621
www.aalrl.com

Virus Testing:

ViraCor
1210 NE Windsor Drive
Lee's Summit, MO 64086
800-305-5198
www.viracor.com

AAL Reference Laboratories
1715 E. Wilshire, #715
Santa Ana, CA 92705
800-522-2621
www.aalrl.com

Vitamin and Natural Supplements and Supplies

Willner Chemists
100 Park Avenue
New York, NY 10017
800-633-1106
www.willner.com

Professional Quality Vitamins and Minerals

Life Factor Research
315 South Coast Highway 101, Suite U-6
Encinitas, CA 92024
877-668-5983
www.lifefactorresearch.com

Beta-glucan and Transfer Factor

Chisolm Biological Laboratory
542 Legion Road
Warrenville, SC 29851-9362
800-664-1333
www.chisolmbio.com

Physician-Dispensed Medications: These companies distribute nutraceutical medications that your doctor will have to order for you. You cannot buy direct unless you are a health care professional. I have found that these companies produce or import excellent products of very high quality.

Allergy Research carries organic germanium and other immune products: 1-800-545-9960

Bezwecken manufacturers and suppliers of natural hormones to doctors: 1-800-743-2256

Heel homotoxicology medications are imported from Germany by Heel/BHI: 1-800-621-7644

HVS Laboratories manufactures homeopathic detoxification products: 1-800-521-7722

Integrative Therapeutics distributes *PhytoPharmic* line and *NF Formulas,* both excellent clinical-quality natural products: 1-800-931-1709

Metagenics distributes *UltraClear Plus* and other detoxification products designed by Jeffrey Bland: 1-800-692-9400

Nutraceutic carries the growth hormone secretagogue *Meditropin*: 1-877-664-6684

Pure Encapsulations: DHEA and professional quality nutrients: 1-800-753-2277

Scientific Consulting Service carries herbal tannins: 1-800-333-7417

SISU Natural Products imports *Pascoe* homotoxicology medications from Germany: 877-747-8872

Thorne Research produces some of the purest natural medicines available including MediClear:
1-800-228-1966

Chinese Herbs

Sun Ten Laboratories, Inc.
9250 Jeronimo Road
Irvine, CA 92618
800-715-7846
www.sunten.com

Hepapro International (Dr. Zhang's herbal
formulas)
P.O. Box 7442
Laguana Niguel, CA 92677-7442
888-788-4372
www.hepapro.com

Institute for Traditional Medicine
2017 Southeast Hawthorne Boulevard
Portland, OR 97214
503-233-4907
www.itmonline.org

Mayway Corp
1338 Mandela Parkway
Oakland, CA 94607
800-262-9929
www.mayway.com

Websites

Acupuncture:
Acupuncture.com
www.acupunture.com

Alternative Medicine:
Institute for Traditional Medicine
www.itmonline.org

Alternative Medicine.Com
www.alternativemedicine.com

National Center for Complementary and
Alternative Medicine
www.nccam.org

Hepatitis C:
www.hepatitis-central.com
www.hepnet.com
www.hepc-connection.org
www.hepcfoundation.org

Chronic Fatigue:
The CFIDS Association of America
www.cfids.org

Other Helpful Sites:
Centers for Disease Control and Prevention
www.cdc.gov

Think Like A Doctor
www.thinklikeadoctor.com

The Official Mad Cow Disease Home Page
www.mad-cow.org

Appendix F

Additional Reading

Bock, Kenneth, and Nellie Sabin. 1997. *The Road to Immunity; How To Survive and Thrive in a Toxic World.* New York: Pocket Books.

Cohen, Misha, and Robert G. Gish. 2000. *The Hepatitis C Help Book.* New York: St. Martin's Press.

Diamond, Jared. 1997. *Guns, Germs, and Steel.* New York: W.W. Norton & Co.

Dolan, Matthew. 1999. *The Hepatitis C Handbook.* Berkeley: North Atlantic Books.

Ewald, Paul W. 2000. *Plague Time: How Stealth Infections Cause Cancers, Heart Disease, and Other Deadly Ailments.* New York: The Free Press.

Hening, Robin Marantz. 1994. *A Dancing Matrix, How Science Confronts Emerging Viruses.* New York: Vintage.

Lininger, Schuyler W., ed. 1999. *The Natural Pharmacy.* Roseville, Calif.: Prima Publishing.

Murray, Michael. 1996. *Encyclopedia of Nutritional Supplements.* Rocklin, Calif.: Prima Publishing.

Pelton, Ross, et al. 2000. *Drug-Induced Nutrient Depletion Handbook.* Hudson, Ohio: Lexi-Comp.

Glossary

Adaptive Immunity: Also called acquired or specific immunity, adaptive immunity is the immune system's response by antigen-specific lymphocytes to an antigen.

Antibody: A protein found in the serum that binds with an antigen and that is formed in response to an infection or immunization.

Antigen: A foreign molecule that generates antibody formation.

Autoimmune response: An autoimmune response is when the adaptive immune system attacks your own body's tissue and causes autoimmune disease.

BALT: The bronchial-associated lymphoid tissue (BALT) is composed of lymph cells in the respiratory tract and is important in immune responses to respiratory tract infections.

B cells: B cells are one of the two major types of lymphocytes, the other being T cells. B cells develop in the bone marrow and produce antibodies.

Bio-oxidative therapies: The term for medical therapies that use oxygen, such as ozonization, to treat disease.

Capsid: The term for the protective coat of a virus.

CD (Cluster Designation) markers: Molecules on the surface of white blood cells and platelets that are used to assess the status of different types of immune cells.

CD3 cells: The Cluster Designation for the complex of different T cells.

CD4 cells: The designation for helper T lymphocyte subsets.

CD8 cells: The designation for cytotoxic T lymphocytes whose major function is to kill cells infected by pathogens.

Chemokines: These are small cytokines involved in the movement and activation of immune cells and have an important role in inflammatory responses.

Complement: The complement system is composed of plasma proteins that work together to attack pathogens outside the cells.

Complementary medicine: A term used to describe the use of alternative therapies to complement conventional medical practices.

Cytokines: A generic term for the proteins produced by immune cells that influence the behavior and activity of other cells.

Endemic: A pattern of disease that commonly occurs in a particular geographical region.

Energy medicine: The general term used to describe alternative therapies, like acupuncture, that work with the body's subtle energy systems.

Epidemic: A pattern of disease involving rapid spread, large numbers of victims, and that occurs over a wide geographical area.

Evolutionary medicine: The term for a philosophy of medical practice that allows for the wisdom of nature and the body, and that not only treats symptoms, as does conventional medicine, but looks for the underlying cause of the illness.

Free radicals: Molecules with an unpaired electron causing chemical instability. This results in the robbing of an electron from another molecule, which sets into motion a chain reaction of unstable molecules leading to large numbers of free radicals, each of which causes cellular and tissue damage.

Functional medicine: A type of medicine that uses natural therapies to normalize physiological function in the body in order to eliminate disease.

GALT: Gut-associated lymphoid tissues (GALT) are lymphatic tissues in the gastrointestinal tract that protect the body against foreign antigens in food, and is also involved in normalization of the intestinal micro flora.

Genome: One set of chromosomes, found in the nucleus of a cell, that contains all the genetic information for the cell or organism.

Homeopathy: A system of medicine that uses minute dosages of a substance to treat disease and restore homeostasis.

Homeostasis: A general term used to describe the state of balance in the body or between different physiological systems.

Homotoxicology: A system of medicine that utilizes specialized homeopathic preparations to treat disease by removing toxins from the body's tissues.

Host: The term for the organism that is infected by a pathogen.

Immunoglobulins (Ig): The term used for all antibody molecules belonging to a family of plasma proteins.

Inflammation: This general term is used to describe the characteristic events following an inflammatory response, including accumulation of fluid, plasma proteins, and white blood cells in and around damaged tissue. Warmth and pain are also associated with inflammation.

Innate immunity: Refers to the innate immune response and is the first line of defense against infection.

Integrative medicine: A way of medical practice that equally includes conventional and alternative therapies.

Interferon (INF): A group of cytokines, involved in communication between different immune cells, which are particularly important for protection against viruses.

Interleukin (IL): A group of cytokines produced by white blood cells which are involved in immune responses between cells.

Leukocytes: The term for white blood cells, which are the collective cells of the immune system.

MALT: Mucosa-associated lymphoid tissue (MALT) are lymphatic tissues associated with immunity involving the mucosal lining of the gastrointestinal and respiratory tracts.

Natural killer (NK) cells: These lymphocytes recognize and kill cells infected by viruses and also destroy some tumor cells.

Naturopathy: A system of medicine that utilizes a wide variety of natural therapies and medications to treat disease and restore health.

Organ reserve: An important concept in natural therapies, organ reserve is the term used to describe the normal tissue health and immune status of an organ. Age, disease, infection, abusive lifestyle all deplete organ reserve. Natural medicines and a healthy lifestyle replenish organ reserve.

Oxidation: The chemical reaction occurs when oxygen is combined with another substance.

Oxidative damage: This is the result of oxidation when free radicals produce destructive cellular changes.

Oxygenation: The process by which oxygen enters the blood and cells.

Pandemic: A worldwide epidemic.

Pathogen: The term used to describe a disease-causing microorganism.

Phagocytosis: The process where immune cells engulf and destroy infected cells.

Prion: Very small infectious particles composed of protein and believed to be the cause of bovine spongiform encephalopathy (BSE), or mad cow disease.

Probiotics: Substances that promote the growth of normal intestinal flora, like *Lactobacillus acidophilus*, and by doing so, improve health.

Prostaglandins: Molecules derived from arachidonic acid and that are involved in inflammation.

Reservoirs: Places within body tissues that can indefinitely harbor latent viruses.

Retrovirus: A family of viruses, including HIV, that is capable of using RNA (ribonucleic acid) as genetic information and transcribing it into DNA (deoxyribonucleic acid).

Synergy: The term used to describe cooperative interaction between cells, and also to explain interactions between more than one medication where the total effect is greater than the healing response expected of their sums.

Systemic infection: An infection that involves more than one system of the body and may cause symptoms that affect the whole body.

T cells: Also called T lymphocytes, T cells are immune cells that develop in the thymus and are designated among the CD3 complex.

Thymus: The thymus gland is situated in the center of the chest behind the breast bone and is involved in the development of T cells.

Traditional Chinese medicine: The system of medicine developed in China that includes acupuncture, Chinese herbs, and a variety of other therapies and techniques to treat disease by restoring the balance of yin and yang.

Tumor necrosis factor (TNF): A term used to define a family of cytokines that are produced by macrophages and are involved in attracting immune cells to sites of infection and then activating those cells to destroy microbes. When released in large amounts, TNF can cause inflammation.

Vaccine: A medically prepared microbial antigen used to induce protective immunity against infection.

Variolation: The method employed in previous centuries of using cowpox to protect against smallpox infection.

Vector: Something that transports an infectious microorganism from one host to another. Common vectors include mosquitoes, fleas, and ticks.

Viron: A term used to describe a single mature infectious virus.

Virulence: The degree of illness an infectious organism is capable of producing in the host.

Virus: An intracellular parasitic organism involved in a wide range of diseases.

Notes

Preface

1. William H. Stewart, M.D., served as U.S. Surgeon General in the Johnson administration from 1965–69. His speeches, most notably December 4, 1967's "A Mandate for State Action," presented at the Association of State and Territorial Health Offices, in Washington, D.C., are frequently quoted in infectious disease books.

2. SSRI is a term that refers to a class of antidepressant drugs called selective serotonin reuptake inhibitors. They are considered safer than and equally effective as the old tricyclics such as Elavil (amitriptyline HCI). More than half of all new antidepressant prescriptions in the United States are for SSRIs and include: Prozac (fluoxetine), Zoloft (sertraline), Paxil (paroxetine), Luvox (fluvoxamine), and Celexa (citalopram). There are natural methods of improving mood, including extracts of the herb St. John's wort, vitamins, omega-3 fatty acids, and amino acids.

3. A presupposition of this book is that modern medical practice demonstrates a remarkable indifference toward and misunderstanding of the complex nature of disease and has been particularly unprepared to understand and treat emerging infectious diseases. By viewing all disease as external and by only looking for one specific cause, modern medicine developed a professional myopia. With the advent of drug-resistant infections, increasing incidence of cancer and chronic disease, and the onset of the previously unheard-of ailments—red flags that went up all over the place—modern medicine became viewed as not only ineffective but potentially dangerous, causing serious side effects and even death in the process of providing medical care.

Modern medicine is an extension of European medical thought first developed in the nineteenth century. It is often referred to as "reductionistic," a system that focuses on reducing diseases into specific categories and then labeling them with technical names. Only when a title is given can investigation for an effective treatment begin. This system creates an impasse for doctors confronted with patients complaining about conditions that did not appear in medical school textbooks.

It has been reported that approximately 75–85 percent of all regular doctor visits are either for conditions that have a cause rooted in lifestyle or are not possible to treat effectively and safely with drugs or surgery, the main tools of modern medicine. One physician that I shared a desk with for two years in a large cooperative medical group often told me that 80 percent of her patients' complaints were non-medical problems—in other words, conditions that medical doctors were not trained to diagnose or deal with.

From my clinical experience, which includes twenty years of extensive practice working with medical doctors, psychologists, and a full array of alternative practitioners, I never thought this class of patients were the "worried well" as James Le Fanu, M.D., phrases it (Le Fanu 1999), but more of the "walking unwell," as some physicians like to call them.

Due to the large number of increasing non-medical complaints by patients, an explosion of alternative therapies practitioners has emerged to meet the demands of these patients, and more openness on the part of conventional medicine to these new conditions results in more of them being defined, and many have been legitimized by official names and ICD-9 (International Classification of Diseases, ninth revision) codes for diagnostic purposes and insurance billing.

Condition	New Diagnosis	ICD Code Number
Chronic fatigue	CFS—Chronic Fatigue Syndrome	780.71
Unexplained muscle pain	Fibromyalgia	729.1
Menstrual mood swings	PMS—Premenstrual Syndrome	625.4
Menopausal symptoms	Menopausal Syndrome	627.9
Insulin resistance	Syndrome X	413.9

Introduction

1. TT virus is a new virus discovered by a group of Japanese scientists in hospitalized patients that causes an acute illness similar to hepatitis. Though it has been found in the blood of 2 to 3 percent of the general population, where it appears to be harmless, the significance of TTV remains unclear (Mushahwar 1999).

Chapter 1

1. Variolation, the transfer of smallpox material from one person to the other for the purpose of inoculation, is now believed to have originated in China in the first century. Documentation records such practices in the Sung Dynasty from 960 to 1280; however, it is not clear whether such practices actually originated in China or in India where variolation was also performed. The practice traveled to Persia and Turkey, and the Royal Society of London was first informed of such practices around 1700.

2. Viruses, like all living things, are given specialized names by scientists in order classify them into an organized system called taxonomy. This taxonomic method of biological classification was developed by Carl Linnaeus in 1758 and is still used today. Organisms are usually referred to by their genus and species names. However, the official nomenclature for viruses uses only families, subfamilies, and genera. Unlike other organisms, viruses have not been yet studied enough for scientists to have found unique individual species, so viruses do not have a species name. Latinized endings are used for family groups such as Herpesviridae and Adenoviridae.

3. Unlike modern Western science, which is only a few hundred years old and is devoid of spiritual implications, Chinese medicine is based upon a cosmology that is thousands of years old. However, the Chinese did not produce any definitive laws of nature as Western physicists did, and are still trying to do. Instead they discovered underlying *forces of activity* such as qi and yin and yang, that govern the laws of the physical world. Attunement with these principles, rather than manipulation of laws, generates harmony and balance and promotes natural health.

Western medicine, confined to the rules of biomechanics and biochemistry, produces results that tend to end in imbalance, disrupt peace and harmony, and do not promote health. The organizing principle behind the manifestations of qi and yin and yang, is called the *dao*. The dao is not the equivalent to what Westerners call God, but might be understood as the creative spiritual energy of the universe. Its particular manifestations on the Earth are animated by the qi, which can exist in two states: yin and yang. Therefore when referring to the qi in the body, the Chinese often call it yin qi or yang qi.

Chapter 2

1. I remain continually puzzled by the way medical and scientific "experts" predict the future. Unknown diseases seem to always be five to eight years away and vaccines are always five to ten years away. In another five years, they repeat the same rhetoric. Similarly, the five-year survival rate for cancer survivors only says that with the drug and other conventional cancer therapies, the treated patients live longer within the five-year framework than do the untreated patients. It says nothing about their quality of life, their degree or lack of suffering, and nothing at all about the period after the first five years. There are also no studies comparing alternative methods to conventional methods for the same disease.

2. Vitamin C is considered a nontoxic substance even in high dosages and is well-tolerated by the gastrointestinal tract. Small amounts, ranging from a few hundred milligrams to a thousand milligrams, are readily absorbed from the small intestine. However, due to vitamin C's (ascorbic acid) acidic content, after saturation is reached in the gut irritation and osmotic effects can occur. Fluid is drawn into the intestine through osmosis and watery diarrhea can occur.

In general, this type of diarrhea is harmless. In fact many doctors use it as a sign that maximum absorption, called "bowel tolerance," has been achieved. However, in cases of acute diarrhea during gastroenteritis, further fluid loss may lead to dehydration and worsening of the ailment.

3. Berberine ($C_{20}H_{19}NO_5$) is a water-soluble isoquinoline alkaloid and acts as an astringent in inflammation of the mucous membranes. Other similar alkaloids, found in goldenseal *(Hydrastis canadensis)*, are hydrastine and canadine. Berberine is considered a tonic alkaloid for the intestinal tract and is often found in combinations of herbs for constipation, diarrhea, irritable bowel syndrome, and gastritis. Berberine also has antimicrobial and immunostimulatory effects. It can be used to treat respiratory, urogenital, and gastrointestinal infections, secretory diarrhea, fungal infections, and can be used as a natural broad-spectrum antibiotic.

Though it is considered nontoxic, high, sustained dosages can cause lowering of blood pressure, difficulty breathing, flu-like symptoms, intestinal discomfort, and possible heart damage. The average recommended dose of the extract is 200 mg, two to four times daily. The bright yellow color of berberine was favored in ancient Asian for religious paintings and manuscripts such as the Dunhuang Diamond Sutra.

4. The information on the Chinese origin of influenza contained in this and other sections of the book is based upon accepted scientific knowledge and personal experience. It is not meant as a commentary on Chinese culture or individuals. In fact, due to the high incidence of influenza viruses in China many effective natural medications were developed and are just as useful for treating Westerners as they are for Chinese.

5. In the German discipline of homotoxicology's view, immune impairment can occur from pharmaceutical drugs, environmental toxins, and chemical toxins released in the body. An immune-impaired body is vulnerable to new or reactivated viral infections, and conversely, a virus can increase the body's own toxic load as well as promote inflammation, both further damaging the immune system.

6. Though individual Chinese herbal names are given, unlike in Western herbology where individual herbs or herbs with similar functions are grouped together, in Chinese medicine herbs are nearly always combined in formulas. The combining of herbs requires extensive knowledge in herbal pharmacology and clinical symptomology. Herbs are combined for synergistic effects, to reduce toxicity of one or more herbs in the formula, and to make the formula more palatable to drink.

7. Dr. Stoff practices in Tucson, Arizona. Contact information can be found in the resource section.

8. Heart attacks and stroke are considered the end result of atherogenic disease, also called atherosclerosis or hardening of the arteries, involving the development of plaques in the blood vessels of the heart, the coronary vessels. Current medical wisdom states that the most commonly associated risk factors with cardiovascular disease are age and high cholesterol. However, numerous other factors play an equally, if not more important role in the development of lesions. These other factors include cytomegalovirus, *Chlamydia pneumoniae,* homocysteine, and lipoprotein(a).

9. Koch's postulate has four main points, summarized as follows:

a. A microbial organism can be isolated from a host suffering from a disease and found in all patients with the same disease.

b. The infectious organism can be cultured in a laboratory outside the host.

c. The isolated organism causes the same disease when introduced into another host, either animal or human.

d. The same organism can be re-isolated from the experimentally infected host.

If all of these four criteria are met, the postulate is considered to be met and the isolated organism is considered the cause of the infection. As science progressed in the latter part of the twentieth century, and as more infectious diseases were discovered and studied, it became more difficult to meet Koch's postulate in all cases of infectious diseases. Some diseases, such as leprosy, were found not to meet Koch's postulate at all. Emerging antibiotic-resistant bacterial infections and the new viral diseases challenged the conventional and overly simplistic model of Koch's postulate.

Rethinking such assumptions is important in the assessment and treatment of the new infectious diseases like AIDS—to evaluate which symptoms are directly caused by the infecting organism and which are due to host immune dysfunction.

10. As explained earlier in this chapter, there is still no consensus on the cause, development, or spread of chronic fatigue. This confusion is exacerbated by a lack of definition, including what to call this syndrome. The two most common terms and acronyms are chronic fatigue syndrome (CFS) and chronic fatigue immune deficiency syndrome (CFIDS). The only distinction between the two is that CFIDS implies a connection with immune deficiency disorders.

11. Thymosin is a synthetic thymus extract used to improve immune function. Several scientific studies found it useful in both AIDS and HIV patients.

12. Macrophages are large white blood cells that destroy foreign organisms in the body. Cytokines are a class of chemical substances secreted by cells and have a variety of effects upon other cells and organisms. Natural killer (NK) cells are large immune cells that actively kill cancer and viruses. Immune-enhancing substances often stimulate the function and activity of macrophages and NK cells, and regulate cytokine production to promote defense against viruses and tumor cells.

13. Several cases of fatal interstitial pneumonitis were associated with minor bupleurum decoction in Japan. The exact cause or mechanism, if the deaths were directly related to the herb formula, remains unclear, but the suspicion is that excessive stimulation of neutrophil activity caused unusual peroxide-induced lung tissue damage. In patients with compromised immune systems with a chronic virus, it is conceivable that such a condition could occur.

Chapter 3

1. Antigens are large molecules composed of proteins combined with long chains of glucose, called polysaccharides, which trigger the immune response. Antigens, like cat dander or flower pollen, can be inhaled; or eaten, such as shellfish or milk products. All antigens can generate an allergic response in a susceptible individual. Antigens can also be introduced under the skin, as is done during vaccination, and they can be generated within cells such as during a viral infection or from cancer cells. The initial immune response to an antigen requires recognition by a T lymphocyte.

2. The body harbors a vast array of both friendly (beneficial) and pathogenic (harmful) bacteria. Friendly bacteria include *Lactobacillus acidophilus* and *Bifidobacterium*, found in yogurt and naturally occurring in the human intestine. These beneficial bacterial organisms, often collectively referred to as probiotics, function as health promoters, improving gastrointestinal function by lowering pH, protecting against harmful microorganisms like yeasts and parasites, assisting in the synthesis of vitamin K and many of the B vitamins, and influencing immunity. Probiotics are the opposite of antibiotics, artificial substances that destroy both friendly and harmful bacteria.

3. See step 1: A free radical is an unstable molecule containing an unpaired electron. Among health enthusiasts, reducing the number of free oxygen radicals in the body approaches the realm of an obsession, based on the fact that free radical molecules are implicated in many diseases including cancer and heart disease. However, what is less widely known is that free radicals, when in equilibrium in the body, are important in many natural processes including killing of disease-causing cancer cells and viruses.

4. The complement system involves a series of more than thirty proteins that have complementary functions with both innate and acquired immunity. The complement proteins act over a wide range of protective defenses including management of inflammation, the ability to directly kill invading microorganisms, the ability to neutralize viruses, and other immune functions. Deficiency of complement factors can lead to systemic lupus erythematosus (SLE), an autoimmune disease affecting the connective tissue and kidneys; angioedema, an allergic reaction involving tissue swelling; and recurring infections.

5. Antibodies belong to a class of proteins called globulins, named so because of their round structure, and are known collectively as immunoglobulins. Antibodies are formed in the body as part of an immune response. A similar term, antigen (see note 2, chapter 3), also begins with the prefix "anti-," meaning against. An antigen is any initiating substance, usually foreign to the body, which is recognized by and activates the adaptive immune system. When the antigen is eliminated or neutralized, the immune response is switched off. Antibodies are immune substances produced in the body by B lymphocytes that bind with antigens marking the foreign substance (the antigen) for destruction by phagocytosis.

6. Immunoglobulins have several common structural characteristics that enable them to recognize and bind to a specific antibody in a lock-and-key fashion. They also share common biological activity including the neutralization of toxins, immobilization of microorganisms, neutralization of viruses, clustering of similar microorganisms to make them more readily phagocytized, and the activation of complement to facilitate the destruction of microorganisms

7. HIV appears to infect CD4+ cells, and as the disease progresses, the number of CD4+ cells declines, sometimes to zero. (The normal range is between 500–1,600 cells per cubic millimeter.) Once below 400 cells/mm³, the immune system's ability to fight infection is severely impaired and opportunistic bacterial and fungal infections are common.

8. Interleukin-2 (IL-2), in a synthetic version of the naturally occurring cytokine, has been approved by the FDA as an immunomodulating drug (Proleukin) for the treatment of cancer. IL-2 stimulates the immune system and increases the CD4+ cells. It is given intravenously or twice daily

as a subcutaneous injection in cycles of five days every eight weeks. Though not approved as a treatment for HIV, it is used for this condition. Side effects can be severe and include flu-like symptoms, reduced number of neutrophils, aggravation of psoriasis and diabetes, and hypothyroidism.

In the beginning of treatment with IL-2, the viral load can increase up to six times pre-treatment levels. Concurrent antiviral treatment appears to help keep the viral load in check, and there appears to be no negative interactions between IL-2 and antiviral drugs. However, this IL-2 is an experimental drug and should be used only under the supervision of a physician experienced in its properties and clinical use.

9. Antioxidants are substances naturally formed in the body like glutathione, provided in the diet like carotenes, or supplemented by vitamins and minerals like vitamin C. They reduce the negative effects caused by the burning of oxygen for metabolism and other cellular processes by countering the effects of the free radicals released by these processes.

Chapter 4

1. Hormone or endocrine disrupters are manmade chemicals in the environment and pharmaceutical drugs that alter human and animal reproduction and health. Some of these hormonal disrupting substances include DDT, PCB, and DES (diethylstilboestrol). They have estrogenic effects in both males and females, and can lead to prostate cancer in men, infertility and possible cancers in women, and abnormal brain development in infants.

2. Using the waterfall analogy, treatment should aim at understanding the flow of the river rather than focusing on attempting to control the waterfall. Natural medicines are more effective at the source where the drops begin.

3. Mammals dominated the Earth after the extinction of the dinosaurs (Jurassic and Cretaceous eras). The first mammals appeared in the late Triassic era, about 200 million years ago. The Cenozoic era (65 million years ago to the present) is known as the Age of Mammals, which is distinguished by the rise of the incredible biodiversity we have on the planet today.

4. Homeopathic medications are measured by dilution increments of 10, 100, or 1000. For example, a remedy that is diluted 10 times is composed of 1 part medicinal substance to 9 parts of dilutant, usually alcohol. The nomenclature for homeopathics is in decimals (indicated by X or D), centesimals (C or CC), and by thousands (M).

Chapter 5

1. We live in what has been called the information age, where the amount of information doubles every few years. However, information is not the same as knowledge or understanding or wisdom. Knowledge comes from processing information combined with experience and teaching. It is not merely the accumulation of more and more information. Yes, we live in an information age, but of information at the expense of true knowledge. What is necessary in medicine is more wisdom and perhaps less information.

2. The scientific method is described in different ways by different authors. However, the basic agreement is that it is a system or process of deduction by which scientists, those who apply the scientific method, endeavor to construct a representation of the world that is as reliable, consistent, and objective as possible.

It has four steps: observation and description of phenomena, formulation of a hypothesis, use of the hypothesis to predict an outcome, and the performance of experiments to prove or disprove the hypothesis. If the experiment holds up the hypothesis, it becomes regarded as a theory or even as an ultimate law of nature. However, the experiment must hold up to certain standards that are designed to eliminate error that may result in false theories. To accomplish this, the scientific method attempts to minimize the researchers bias or influence on the experiment.

According to Western ideas, the scientific method is the best way ever discovered to sort truth from rumor and fact from anecdotal evidence or hearsay. There are also many criticisms of the scientific method. One of the most interesting of them is that science itself has never been studied scientifically. Some critics are concerned that science has become a dogmatic belief system and is less and less concerned with truth and more and more taken with its results. They also say that one of its most obvious failings is that it allows for only things that it has analyzed by its own methodology and does not take into consideration the importance of careful and honest observation.

The social sciences, like anthropology, have long been called pseudo-sciences for this very reason. This distinction is extremely important in the new medicine, where not all theories or practices are tested or proven scientifically, and, though may be very useful for the treatment of patients, are not accepted. Ironically, many surgical procedures have also not been proven scientifically, but are nevertheless accepted in common practice. This is a double standard that places the concept of fairness in science at risk.

3. Though there has been an explosion of interest in Chinese ideas including acupuncture, herbal medicine, kung fu, chi gong, tai chi, and even feng shui over the last decade, it is amazing how under-informed and often how misinformed Westerners remain about Chinese culture and philosophy. One of the most common misconceptions is to compare Chinese thought to Western religions.

To the Chinese, only Buddhism comes close to a religion, but even that does not fit neatly into the Western definition of religion and is more of a metaphysical psychology; the means to end suffering, rather than a religion. According to noted Chinese writer Fung Yu-Lan, Confucianism, which underscores all activity, daily life, and thought not only in China but in Japan, Korea, Taiwan, and Hong Kong, is a clearly a philosophical system and is, "no more a religion than Platonism or Aristotelianism."

The other main belief system in China, Taoism, is considered by the Chinese to be neither a religion or a philosophy, but "the way," a method or practice of "self-cultivation," or a way of becoming more in harmony with nature and more at peace with one's self. This makes writing about Chinese ideas very difficult indeed.

However, it is my purpose in this book to present only some of the basic theories as they relate to health and disease, and sickness in particular, and ask the inquisitive reader to pursue more in-depth discussions on Confucianism such as the works by Chen, or in other areas of Chinese thought or medical philosophy.

Chapter 6

1. My Chinese tai chi and qi gong (pronounced "chee gong"), and Indian yoga masters are living proof of their philosophies. Rarely ill and very active even into their eighties and nineties, these extraordinary individuals taught me much of what I know and practice in my own life. My health is excellent and my physical examinations and laboratory studies confirm excellent biochemical, hormonal, and nutritional balance. I attribute this good health largely to the teachings of these men.

2. The acid/alkaline balance is an important issue in dietary planning and in recovering from illness, especially from infection and in wound healing. When the body becomes too acidic, you are more prone to common respiratory tract infections such as colds, flu, bronchitis, and sinusitis, because bacteria and viruses that cause these illnesses thrive in acidic environments. The pH of the blood falls in a very narrow range, between 7.35 and 7.45 (the higher the pH, the more alkaline). Some people can handle more protein since they are naturally high-alkaline producers. However, people with severe chronic illness and osteoporosis, along with the elderly can lose their ability to regulate pH and should be careful with eating too much protein.

3. In my recommended diets, protein is fairly high. Adequate levels of amino acids, the building blocks of protein foods, are required for muscle and the production of many substances in the body such as neurotransmitters and immunoglobulins. While living with the Siberian Eskimo people of St. Lawrence Island, I ate a diet composed of 80 to 90 percent meat and fat, and it was one of the healthiest times of my life. There was no heart disease or cancer or diabetes among them.

However, proteins create acid in the body, and to buffer the effect of acid, the body pulls calcium (an alkaline mineral) from the bone, which can lead to osteoporosis. It is generally considered that a diet that takes more than 30 percent of its calories from protein is too acidic. If no sugar (which is highly acidic) is used and the diet is high in alkaline vegetables, and other acidic foods are eliminated (like processed cheeses and meats, fatty and fried foods) more protein can be eaten than previously thought.

It is generally thought that the body can comfortably process 40 to 60 grams of protein per day without becoming too acidic. I generally recommend an average of 65 to 85 grams of protein is per day and often advise pushing the protein even higher for certain periods of time.

4. Glycemic index is a term used to rank foods on how they affect blood sugar (glucose) levels, measured by how much your glucose rises two to three hours after eating. High glycemic-index foods are mainly carbohydrates, those foods that raise glucose the most. High-glycemic index foods include rice, potatoes, corn syrup, baked goods made from refined white flour, and fruits.

Chapter 7

1. Through oxidation, vitamins are expended in metabolic processes, and because they are not completely destroyed, they can be regenerated by chemical reactions requiring antioxidants. Both vitamins C and E have the ability to assist in regenerating oxidized nutrients.

Chapter 8

1. Soy can cause gastrointestinal allergies when eaten in large amounts, especially when using soymilk as dairy substitute. In Asia, soy is rarely used as a drink but is prepared by a variety of traditional fermentation processes to produce soy products that have less allergenicity. Other common allergic foods include cow's milk and dairy products, and wheat and wheat products.

Immune response to chronic viral diseases causes abnormally high levels of immune chemicals that contribute to inflammation with the resulting symptoms of fatigue and pain. As allergic responses appear to aggravate the immune response to viral illness, avoiding the common allergic foods helps to reduce inflammation. Soy is considerably less allergenic than dairy and wheat, but many Westerners are sensitive to soy. However, when eaten in the traditional Asian way (small amounts in fermented forms), soy is better tolerated and there are fewer allergic reactions.

2. The German-born physician, Benedict Lust, M.D., D.O., N.D., (1872–1945) is considered the father of American naturopathic medicine, which was founded in 1987. The term "nature cure" is the more common term used to describe the style of treatment and was synonymous with both medically trained and lay professionals who practiced a form of healing using only natural and safe medicines and therapies. Later, naturopathy was routed out of orthodox American medicine, as was homeopathy, and its practitioners and followers were no longer medical doctors but lay healers like John R. Christopher of Utah.

By the 1970s, naturopathy as a medical profession was nearly dead. However, with the renewed interest in natural healing and the pioneering work of modern naturopathic physicians like John Bastyr, N.D., D.C., naturopathic medicine is now growing rapidly. In this book, I use the terms "nature cure" and "nature cure doctors" to refer to those naturopaths practicing before the current era of modern naturopathic medicine.

Chapter 9

1. Hydrolysis is a chemical reaction involving water, resulting in one or more new substances, and dehalogenation is a chemical process that breaks down and removes halogen toxins (those containing chlorine, bromine, iodine, and fluorine). Halogenated compounds are used in water treatment, swimming pool chemicals, textile production, and to produce pesticides.

2. Dosages of probiotics like acidophilus are listed in billions of live organisms, or colony-forming units per gram. The recommended daily dosage for general health supplementation is 3–5 billion units. For treatment of chronic disease and during detoxification regimes, higher dosages are required.

Chapter 10

1. Throughout steps 1–10, I repeatedly point to the importance of sleep in the restoration of health and immunity. In the typical American lifestyle, which is essentially very unhealthy, the constant activity of work, recreation, getting from one place to the other, and passive activities that drain energy, like overuse of the computer and television, rob our systems of sufficient rest and disrupt the normal sleep cycle. A number of scientific studies confirm these observations.

Chapter 11

1. I studied Chinese medicine, acupuncture, and tai chi under Dr. York Why Loo from 1980 to 1983 in East San Diego and Los Angeles Chinatown, and maintained a friendship with him until his death in 1989. Dr. Loo was originally from Canton, China. He earned his M.D. in Shanghai, and later retrained in traditional Chinese medicine during the Cultural Revolution. He is well respected in the Chinese community and a recognized master of five forms of tai chi. It was an honor to have known him.

Chapter 12

1. The German Commission E was established in 1978 by the former West German government to evaluate and regulate the use of herbal medications in Germany. It is composed of scientists, physicians, pharmacists, and toxicologists. To date, more than three hundred herbs have been evaluated. The collected monographs are published as *The Complete German Commission E Monographs: Therapeutic Guide to Herbal Medicines* by Siegrid Klein and Chance Riggins.

Chapter 14

1. Dr. Thierry Hertoghe comes from a long line of endocrinologists. His great-grandfather was one of the first medical doctors in the world to use thyroid hormone to treat hypothyroidism. He is considered the world's leading authority on natural hormone balancing to treat illnesses and for aging.

2. Laboratory values for IGF-1 are from Laboratory Corporation of America.

Chapter 15

1. Although viruses are parasitic, they are also symbiotic. From the evolutionary perspective, viruses developed alongside, or even before plant and animal life; influencing immunity and participated in creating both health and disease. Over time, the human immune system is capable of achieving balance within a natural environment that is free from outside influences and within set boundaries.

Modern life, with air travel and global migration, has disrupted this balance. We are on the verge of an immune crisis of unprecedented proportions. Our immune systems must attempt to catch up, if they can, with chemical toxins, novel microorganisms, and stress. What once were symbiotic organisms may now become lethal infections.

Bibliography

Abbas, Abul K., Andrew H. Lichtman, and Jordan S. Pober. 2000. *Cellular and Molecular Immunology*. New York: W.B. Saunders Company.

Abe, Y., et al. 1994. Effectiveness of interferon, glycyrrhizin combination therapy in patients with chronic hepatitis C. *Nippon Rinsho* 52.

Aderem, Alan, and R. J. Ulevitch. 2000. Toll-like receptors in the induction of the innate immune response. *Nature* 406 Aug.

Agency for Health Care Policy and Research. 1999. Diagnosis and treatment of acute bacterial rhinosinusitis. Rockville, M.D.: Agency for Health Care Policy and Research.

Akbar, N., et al. 1998. Effectiveness of the analogue of natural schizandrin C (HpPro) in the treatment of liver disease: An experience in Indonesian patients. *Journal of Chinese Medicine* 111.

Alexander, M., H. Newmark, and R. G. Miller. 1985. Oral beta-carotene can increase the number of OKT4+ cells in human blood. *Immunology Letters* 9.

Algert, S. J., et al. 1987. Assessment of dietary intake and arginine in patients with herpes simplex. *Journal of the American Dietetic Association* 87.

Ali, Majid. 1995. *The Canary and Chronic Fatigue*. Denville, N.J.: Life Span Press.

Altman, Nathaniel. 1995. *Oxygen Healing Therapies for Optimal Health and Vitality*. Rochester, Vermont: Healing Arts Press.

Appleton, William S. 2000. *Prozac and the New Antidepressants*. New York: Penguin Putnam Inc..

Arem, R. 1999. *The Thyroid Solution*. New York: Ballantine.

Artursson, P., et al. 1987. Macrophage stimulation with some structurally related polysaccharides. *Scandinavian Journal of Immunology* 25, no. 3.

Asai, K. 1980. *Miracle Cure, Organic Germanium*. Tokyo: Japan Publications.

Askari, Fred. 1999. *Hepatitis C, The Silent Epidemic*. New York: Plenum Publishers.

Astin, J. A., et al. 2000. The efficacy of "distant healing": A systematic review of randomized trials. *Annals of Internal Medicine* 132, no. 11.

Backhyun, D., et al. 2000. High-performance liquid chromatographic analysis of saponin compounds in Bupleurum falcatum. *Journal of Chromatographic Science* 38, no. 6.

Barnum, Alex. 1993. Promising results on HIV immunity. *San Francisco Chronicle*, December 11.

Barrett, Bruce. 2000. Echinacea for upper respiratory tract infection: An assessment of randomized trials. *Healthnotes* 7, no. 3.

Batey, R. G., et al. 1998. Preliminary report of a randomized, double-blind placebo-controlled trial of a Chinese herbal medicine preparation CH-100 in the treatment of chronic hepatitis C. *Journal of Gastroenterology and Hepatology* 13.

Baur, A., et al. 1991. Alpha-lipoic acid is an effective inhibitor of human immuno-deficiency virus (HIV-1). *Klinicshe Wochenschrift* 69.

Bauer, R., et al. 1989. Influence of Echinacea extracts on phagocytotic activity. *Zeitscrift fur Phytotherapie* 10.

Baxter, Susan. 1999. *Immune Power: How to Use Your Immune System to Fight Disease—From Cancer to AIDS*. New York: Avery.

Bear, Jaya. 2000. *Amazon Magic, The Life Story of Ayahuasquero and Shaman Don Augustin Rivas Vasquez*. Taos, New Mexico: Colibri Publishing.

Beard, J. 1911. *The Enzyme Treatment of Cancer and Its Scientific Basis*. London: Chatto and Windus.

Bellini, R., et al. 1997. *Aedes albopictus* (Diptera: Culicidae) is incompetent as a vector of hepatitis C virus. *AMPIS* 105, no. 4.

Benjamini, Eli, et al. 2000. *Immunology, A Short Course.* New York: John Wiley & Sons, Inc.

Bennett, Peter, and Stephen Barrie. 1999. *7-Day Detox Miracle.* Rocklin, Calif.: Prima Publishing.

Bensky, Dan, and Randall Barolet. 1990. *Chinese Herbal Medicine, Formulas and Strategies.* Seattle: Eastland Press.

Benson, Herbert. 1975. *The Relaxation Response.* New York: Avon Books.

Berg, O., et al. 1986. Occurrence of asymptomatic sinusitis in common cold and other acute ENT infections. *Rhinology* 24.

Berkow, Robert, ed. 1982. *The Merck Manual of Diagnosis and Therapy.* Rahway, N.J.: Merck & Co.

Bermejo, B. P., et al. 1998. In vivo and in vitro anti-inflammatory activity of saikosaponins. *Life Science* 63, no. 13.

Beveridge, W. 1977. *Influenza. The Last Great Plague.* London: Heinemann.

Birdsall, T. C. 1996. Zinc picolinate: Absorption and supplementation. *Alternative Medicine Review* 1, no. 1.

Birdsall, T. C., and G. S. Kelly. 1997. Berberine: Therapeutic potential of an alkaloid found in several medicinal plants. *Alternative Medicine Review* 2, no. 2.

Birkel, D. A., and L. Edgren. 2000. Hatha Yoga: Improved vital capacity of college students. *Alternative Therapies* 6, no. 6.

Bjorkman, D. J. 1998. The effect of aspirin and nonsteroidal anti-inflammatory drugs on prostaglandins. *The American Journal of Medicine* 105, Jul 27.

Blackburn, George L. 2001. Pasteur's quadrant and malnutrition. *Nature* 409, January.

Bland, Jeffrey, ed. 1998. *Nutritional Management of Inflammatory Disorders.* Gig Harbor, Wash.: Institute for Functional Medicine.

Bland, Jeffrey S. 1997. *The 20-Day Rejuvenation Diet Program.* New Canaan, Connecticut: Keats Publishing.

————. 1999. New functional medicine paradigm: Health problems associated with dysfunctional intercellular communication. *International Journal of Integrated Medicine* 1, no. 4.

————. 2000. *Nutritional Management of the Underlying Causes of Chronic Disease.* Gig Harbor, Wash.: Institute for Functional Medicine.

Blau, S. P., and E. F. Shimberg. 1997. *How to Get Out of the Hospital Alive.* New York: Macmillan.

Bock, K., and N. Sabin. 1997. *The Road to Immunity, How To Survive and Thrive in a Toxic World*. New York: Pocket Books.

Bock, Steven J. 2000. Transfer factor and its clinical implications. *International Journal of Integrated Medicine* 2, no. 4.

Boericke, Oscar E. 1982. *Pocket Manual of Homeopathic Materia Medica*. New Delhi: D. Jain Publishers.

Bohm, David. 1980. *Wholeness and the Implicate Order*. London: Routledge and Kegan Paul.

Boik, John. 2001. *Natural Compounds in Cancer Therapy*. Princeton, Minn.: Oregon Medical Press.

Bone, Kerry. 1997. Echinacea: What makes it work? *Alternative Medicine Review* 2, no. 2.

———. 1997. Echinacea: When should it be used? *Alternative Medicine Review* 2, no. 6.

Borek, Carmia. 1997. Antioxidants and Cancer. *Science & Medicine*, Nov/Dec.

Bounnous, G., and P. Gold. 1991. The biological activity of undernatured dietary whey proteins: Role of glutathione. *Clinical Investigations in Medicine* 14, no. 4.

Bradford, Robert W. 2001. Personal communication with author, 12 April.

Breitkreutz, R., et al. 2000. Massive loss of sulfur in HIV infection. *AIDS Research and Human Retroviruses* 16, no. 3.

Brochers, A. T., et al. 2000. Shosaiko-to and other Kampo (Japanese herbal) medicines: a review of their immunomodulatory activities. *Journal of Ethnopharmacology* 73, no. 1–2.

Browder, W., et al. 1984. Modification of postoperative *C. albicans* sepsis by glucan immunostimulation. *International Journal of Immunopharmacology* 6.

Brown, Donald. 1999. St. John's wort—Drug interaction, safety, and active constituent update. *Healthnotes* 6, no. 4.

Brown, Phyllida. 2001. Cinderella goes to the ball. *Nature* 410, April 26.

Buhner, Stephen Harrod. 1999. *Herbal Antibiotics*. Pownal, Vermont: Storey Books.

Cabot, Sandra. 1999. *The Healthy Liver and Bowel Book*. Cobbitty, Australia: Dr. Sandra Cabot.

Caceres, D. D., et al. 1999 Use of visual analogue scale measurements (VAS) to assess the effectiveness of the standardized *Andrographis paniculata* extract SHA-10 in reducing the symptoms of common cold. A randomized double blind - placebo study. *Phytomedicine* 6, no. 4.

Calabrese, C., et al. 2000. A phase I trial of andrographolide in HIV positive patients and normal volunteers. *Phytotherapy Research* 14, no. 5.

Calixto, J. B., et al. 1998. A review of the plants of the genus *Phyllanthus:* Their chemistry, pharmacology, and therapeutic potential. *Medicinal Research Reviews* 18, no. 4.

Carlson, T. J. S., and S. R. King. 2000. Sangre de drago (*Croton lechleri* Muell.-Arg.)—A phytomedicine for the treatment of diarrhea. *Healthnotes* 7, no. 4.

Carr, Andrew, and D. A. Cooper. 2000. Adverse effects of antiretroviral therapy. *Lancet* 356.

Carrigan, D. R., et al. 1996. A variant human herpesvirus six as a cofactor with pathogenesis of AIDS. *Journal of Acquired Immune Deficiency Syndromes and Human Retrovirology* 13.

Castner, J. L., et al. 1998. *A Field Guide to Medicinal Plants of the Upper Amazon.* Gainesville, Florida: Feline Press.

Cathcart, R. 1981. Vitamin C, titrating to bowel tolerance, anascorbemia, and acute induced scurvy. *Medical Hypothesis* 7.

Centers for Disease Control. 2000. Prevention and control of influenza. *Morbidity and Mortality Weekly,* Atlanta, Georgia.

Cerwenka, A., and L. L. Lanier. 2001. Natural killer cells, viruses, and cancer. *Nature Reviews Immunology* 1.

Cho, J. Y., et al. 1998. Inhibitory effect of lignans from the rhizomes of *Coptis japonica* var. *dissecta* on tumor necrosis factor-alpha production in lipopolysaccharide-stimulated RAW264.7 cells. *Archives of Pharmacal Research* 21, no. 1.

———, et al. 2000. In vitro anti-inflammatory effects of neoligran woorenosides from the rhizomes of Coptis japonica. *Journal of Natural Products* 63, no. 9.

———, et al. 2001. In vitro inhibitory effect of protopanaxadiol ginsenosides on tumor necrosis factor (TNF)-alpha production and its modulation by known TNF-alpha antagonist. *Planta Medica* 67, no. 3.

Cho, Q. L., et al. 1989. Isolation of cDNA clone derived from a bloodborne non-A, non-B viral hepatitis genome. *Science* Apr 21.

Chopra, Deepak. 1989. *Quantum Healing, Exploring the Frontiers of Mind/Body Medicine.* New York: Bantam.

Choudary, Bikram. 2000. *Bikram's Beginning Yoga Class*. New York: JP Tarcher.

Civitelli, R., et al. 1992. Dietary L-lysine and calcium metabolism in humans. *Nutrition* 8.

Clarke, N. M., and J. T. May. 2000. Effect of antimicrobial factors in human milk on rhinoviruses and milk-borne cytomegalovirus in vitro. *Journal of Medical Microbiology* 49, no. 8.

Cohen, Misha, and Robert G. Gish. 2000. *The Hepatitis C Help Book*. New York: St. Martin's Press.

Cohen, S., et al. 1997. Social ties and susceptibility to the common cold. *Journal of the American Medical Association* 277.

Collier, Leslie, and John Oxford. 2000. *Human Virology*. Oxford: Oxford University Press.

Commentary. 2000. The Durban Declaration. *Nature* 406, July 6.

Cousin, Norman. 1991. *Anatomy of an Illness as Perceived by the Patient: Reflections on Healing and Regeneration*. New York: Bantam Doubleday.

Cowden, W. L., et al. 2001. *Longevity*. Tiburon, Calif.: Alternative Medicine.Com Books.

Cowley, Geoffrey. 2001. Can he find a cure? *Time*, June 11.

———, et al. 1990. Chronic Fatigue Syndrome: A modern medical mystery. *Newsweek*, November 12.

Crawford, Dorothy H. 2000. *The Invisible Enemy, A Natural History of Viruses*. London: Oxford University Press.

D'Adamo, Peter. 1996. *Eat Right For Your Type*. New York: Putnam.

———. 1996. Larch arabinogalactan. *Journal of Naturopathic Medicine* 6.

De Smet, P. A. G. M., et al, eds. 1993. *Adverse Effects of Herbal Drugs*. Berlin: Springer-Verlag.

Deguchi, K., et al. 2001. Postmenopausal changes in production of type 1 and type 2 cytokines and the effects of hormone replacement therapy. *Menopause* 8, no. 4.

DeSimone, C., et al. 1992. Effect of *Bifidobacterium bifidum* and *Lactobacillus acidophilus* on gut mucosa and peripheral blood lymphocytes. *Immunopharmacology and Immunotoxicology* 14, nos. 1&2.

Desiraju, G. R. 2001. Chemistry beyond the molecule. *Nature* 412, July 26.

Dharmananda, Sabhuti. 2000. *Ho-shou-wu, What's in an Herb Name*. Portland, Oregon: Institute for Traditional Medicine.

———. 2000. *Update on Hepatitis C Treatments.* Portland, OR: Institute for Traditional Medicine.

Di Bisceglie, A. M., and B. R. Bacon. 1999. The unmet challenges of hepatitis C. *Scientific America*, October.

Diamond, Jared. 1997. *Guns, Germs, and Steel.* New York: W.W. Norton & Co.

Diluzio, N. R. 1983. Immunopharmacology of glucan: A broad-spectrum enhancer of host defense mechanisms. *Trends in Pharmacology* 4.

Dorsey, L. 1997. The return of prayer. *Alternative Therapies* 3, no. 6

Droge, W., et al. 1991. Modulation of lymphocyte functions and immune responses by cysteine and cysteine derivatives. *American Journal of Medicine* 91, suppl. 3C.

———, et al. 1994. Functions of glutathione and glutathione disulfide in immunology and immunopathology. *FASEB J* 8.

Duesberg, Peter H. 1996. *Inventing the AIDS Virus.* Washington, D.C.: Regnery.

Eby, G. A., et al. 1984. Reduction in duration of common colds by zinc gluconate lozenges in a double-blind study. *Antimicrobial Agents and Chemotherapy* 25.

Edmund, M. B., et al. 2000. Nosocomial bloodstream infections in United States hospitals: A three-year analysis. *Clinical Infectious Disease* 2.

Eisenberg, D. M. 1993. Unconventional medicine in the United States: Prevalence, cost, and patterns of use. *New England Journal of Medicine* 328, no. 4.

Elias, Jason, and Katherine Ketcham. 1998. *Chinese Medicine for Maximum Immunity.* New York: Three Rivers Press.

Epstein, S. E., et al. 1999. Infection and atherosclerosis: Emerging mechanistic paradigms. *Circulation* 100, no. 4.

Erdelmeier, C. A., et al. 1996. Antiviral and antiphlogistic activities of *Hammelis virginiana* bark. *Planta Medica* 62, no. 3.

Ernst, E., et al. 1998. Adverse effects profile of the herbal antidepressant St. John's wort (*Hypericum perforatum* L.). *European Journal of Clinical Pharmacology* 54.

Everson, C. A. 1993. Sustained sleep deprivation impairs host defense. *American Journal of Physiology* 265.

Everson, C. A. and L. A. Toth. 2000. Systemic bacteria invasion induced by sleep deprivation. *American Journal of Physiology* 278, no. R905–R916.

Ewald, Paul W. 2000. *Plague Time: How Stealth Infections Cause Cancers, Heart Disease, and Other Deadly Ailments.* New York: The Free Press.

Fetrow, Charles W., and Juan R. Avila. 1999. *Professional's Handbook of Complementary & Alternative Medicines.* Springhouse, Penn.: Springhouse.

Fine, A. M. 2000. Oligomeric proanthocyanidin complexes: History, structure, and phytopharmaceutical applications. *Alternative Medicine Review* 5, no. 2.

Flaws, Bob. 2001. *Minor Bupleurum: My Favorite Formula.* Boulder, Colo.: Blue Poppy Press. [Internet: www.bluepoppy.com/press/download/articles/xiaochai.html]

Fletcher, D. J. 2000. Educating the immune. *Alternative Medicine,* May.

Flint, S. J., et al. 2000. *Principles of Virology, Molecular Biology, Pathogenesis, and Control.* Washington, D.C.: ASM Press.

Flodin, N. W. 1997. The metabolic roles, pharmacology, and toxicology of lysine. *Journal of the American College of Nutrition* 16.

Folkers, K., et al. 1982. Increase in levels of IgG in serum of patients treated with coenzyme Q10. *Research Communications in Chemical Pathology and Pharmacology* 38.

Fuchs, J., et al. 1993. Studies on lipoate effects on blood redux state in human immunodeficiency virus infected patients. *Arzneim-Forsch Drugs Research* 43.

Fujisawa, Y., et al. 2000. Glycyrrhizin inhibits the lytic pathway of complement: Possible mechanisms to its anti-inflammatory effect on liver cells in viral hepatitis. *Microbiology and Immunology* 44, no. 9.

Fukuda, K., et al. 1999. Inhibition of activator protein 1 activity by berberine in human hepatoma cells. *Planta Medica* 65, no. 4.

Gaby, Alan R. 1996. The role of coenzyme Q10 in clinical medicine: Part I. *Alternative Medicine Review* 1, no. 1.

Galland, L. 1997. *Power Healing: Use the New Integrated Medicine to Heal Yourself.* New York: Random House.

Gallo, M., et al. 2000. Pregnancy outcome following gestational exposure to echinacea. *Archives of Internal Medicine* 160.

Garaci, D., et al. 2000. Thymosin alpha 1 in the treatment of cancer: From basic research to clinical application. *International Journal of Immunopharmacology* 22, no. 12.

Gillis, J. C., et al. 1994. Idebenone, a review of its pharmacodynamic and pharmacokinetic properties, and therapeutic use in age-related cognitive disorders. *Drugs* 5, no. 2.

Giovannucci, E., et al. 1995. Intake of carotenoids and retinol in relation to risk of prostate cancer. *Journal of the National Cancer Institute* 87.

Goldstein, Jay A. 1996. *Betrayal by the Brain*. Binghamton, N.Y.: The Haworth Medical Press.

Goroll, A. H., et al., eds. 1981. *Primary Care Medicine*. Philadelphia: J. B. Lippincott Co..

Grachev, M. A., et al. 1989. Distemper virus in Baikal seals. *Nature* 338.

Greaves, Mel. 2000. *Cancer, The Evolutionary Legacy*. Oxford: Oxford University Press.

Greenwell, Ivy. 2001. DHEA reduces inflammation, enhances immunity, protects arteries and the brain. *Life Extension*, Aug.

Griffin, James E., and Sergio R. Ojeda. 1996. *Textbook of Endocrine Physiology*. London: Oxford University Press.

Groopman, Jerome. 1998. The shadow epidemic. *The New Yorker* May 11.

Hall, T., et al. 2001. Ginseng evaluation program, part one: Standardization phase. *HerbalGram*, no. 52.

Haltia, M. 2000. Human prion diseases. *Annals of Medicine* 32, no. 7.

Hargrove, M. E., J. Wang, and C. C. Ting. 1993. Regulation by glutathione of the activation and differentiation of IL-4-dependent activated killer cells. *Cellular Immunology* 149, no. 2.

Harper, D. R. 1998. *Molecular Virology*. Oxford: BIOS Scientific Publishers.

Hasselberger, Francis X. 1978. *Uses of Enzymes and Immobilized Enzymes*. Chicago: Nelson-Hall.

Hauer, J., and F. A. Anderer. 1993. Mechanism of stimulation of human natural killer cytotoxidity by arabinogalactan from *Larix occidentalis*. *Cancer Immunology and Immunotherapy* 36.

Hemila, H. 1995. Does vitamin C alleviate the symptoms of the common cold?—A review of current evidence. *Scandinavian Journal of Infectious Disease* 26.

Hendler, Sheldon S. 1985. *The Complete Guide to Anti-Aging Nutrients*. New York: Simon & Schuster.

Hening, Robin Marantz. 1994. *A Dancing Matrix, How Science Confronts Emerging Viruses*. New York: Vintage.

Hennecke-von Zepelin, H. H., et al. 1999. Efficacy and safety of a fixed combination phytomedicine in the treatment of the common cold (acute viral respiratory infection): Results of a randomized, double-blind, placebo-controlled, multicenter study. *Current Medical Research Opinion* 15.

Hennen, William. 2000. *Enhanced Transfer Factor.* Pleasant Grove, Utah: Woodland Publishing.

Hertoghe, Thierry. 2000. *Hormone Replacement Therapies,* Las Vegas, Nevada: December.

Herzberger, G., and M. Weiser. 1997. Homeopathic treatment of infections of various origins: A prospective study. *Biomedical Therapy* XV, no. 4.

Heuser, Gunnar, and Aristo Vojdani. 1997. Enhancement of natural killer cell activity and T and B cell function by buffered vitamin C in patients exposed to toxic chemicals: The role of protein kinase-C. *Immunopharmacology and Immunotoxicology* 19, no. 3.

Hobson, Allan J. 1994. *The Chemistry of Conscious States: How the Brain Changes Its Mind.* New York: Little, Brown.

Hooper, Edward. 1999. *The River, A Journey to the Source of HIV and AIDS.* New York: Little, Brown.

Horowitz, Leonard G. 1996. *Emerging Viruses: AIDS and Ebola, Nature, Accident, or Intentional.* Sandpoint, Idaho: Tetrahedron.

Howd, Aime. 2000. When vaccines do harm to kids. *Insight,* Feb.

Hoyle, Fred. 1983. *The Intelligent Universe.* London: Michael Joseph Limited.

Hsu, Hong-yen, and William G. Preacher, eds. 1981. *Shang Han Lun.* Los Angeles: Oriental Healing Arts Institute.

Hsu, Hong-yen, William G. Preacher, and Su-yen Wang. 1985. *The Theory of Feverish Diseases and Its Clinical Applications.* Long Beach, Calif.: Oriental Healing Arts Institute.

Husted, C., et al. 1999. Improving quality of life for people with chronic conditions: The example of t'ai shi and multiple sclerosis. *Alternative Therapies* 5, no. 5.

Hyland, Michael E. 2002. The intelligent body. *New Scientist,* May 26.

Institute of Life Sciences. 1999. Eurocell therapy: Chronic hepatitis C treatment. Seoul: Chungbuk National University.

Irwin, Donna L, ed. 1999. *Detoxification: A Clinical Monograph.* Gig Harbor, Wash.: Institute for Functional Medicine.

Irwin, M., et al. 1996. Partial night sleep deprivation reduces natural killer and cellular immune responses in humans. *Journal of the Federation of American Societies for Experimental Biology* 10, no. 5.

Jager, H. 1990. Hydrolytic enzymes in the treatment of HIV infections. *Allgemeinmedizin* 19.

Jamieson, James. 1998. What do we really know about risks and benefits of growth hormone and IFG-1? Injections, secretagogues, and testing. *Townsend Letter for Doctors and Patients*, Dec.

Janeway, C. A., et al. 1999. *Immunobiology: The Immune System in Health and Disease*. New York: Garland Press.

Jeffcoate, William J. 1999. Chronic fatigue syndrome and functional hypoadrenia—fight vainly the old ennui. *The Lancet* 353, no. 9151.

Jefferies, W. 1996. *Safe Uses of Cortisol*. 2nd ed. Springfield, Ill: C.C. Thomas.

Jeffery, D. R., et al. 1993. Transverse myelitis: Retrospective analysis of 33 cases, with differentiation of cases associated with multiple sclerosis and parainfectious events. *Archives of Neurology* 50.

Jensen, Bernard. 1978–1982. Personal communications with author. Escondido, Calif.

———. 1986. *Vibrant Health from Your Kitchen*. Escondido, Calif.: Bernard Jensen.

Joint United Nations Program on HIV/AIDS. 2000. Report on the Global HIV/AIDS Epidemic. Geneva: UNAIDS.

Julius, M., et al. 1994. Glutathione and morbidity in a community-based sample of elderly. *Journal of Clinical Epidemiology* 47.

Kahlon, J. B., et al. 1991. In vitro evaluation of the synergistic antiviral effects of acemannan in combination with azidothymidine and acyclovir. *Molecular Biotherapy* 3.

Kaiser, L., et al. 2000. Impact of zanamivir on antibiotic use for respiratory events following acute influenza in adolescents and adults. *Archives of Internal Medicine* 160.

Kastrup, Erwin K., ed. 1999. *Drug Facts and Comparisons*. St. Louis: Facts and Comparisons.

Kato, M., et al. 1994. Characterization of the immunoregulatory action of saikosaponin-d. *Cellular Immunology* 159, no. 1.

Katske, F., et al. 2001. Treatment of interstitial cystitis with a quercetin supplement. *Techniques in Urology* 7, no. 1.

Keeling, M. J., and C. A. Gilligan. 2000. Metapopulation dynamics of bubonic plague. *Nature* 407, Oct 19.

Kelley, Gregory S. 1999. Larch arabinogalactan: Clinical relevance of a novel immune-enhancing polysaccharide. *Alternative Medicine Review* 4, no. 2.

Kemeny, Margaret. 2000. The immune system: Immunity, disease and wellness. Paper presented at the CorTex, San Diego.

Kidd, Parris. 1997. Glutathione: Systemic protectant against oxidative and free radical damage. *Alternative Medicine Review* 2, no. 3.

———. 2000. The use of mushroom glucans and proteoglycans in cancer treatment. *Alternative Medicine Review* 5, no. 1.

Kim, Y. S., et al. 2000. Antiherpetic activities of acidic protein bound polysaccharide isolated form *Ganoderma lucidum* alone and in combination with interferons. *Journal of Ethnopharmcology* 72, no. 3.

Kiremidjian-Schumacher, L., and G. Stotsky. 1994. Supplementation with selenium and human immune cell functions; II. Effect on cytotoxic lymphocytes and natural killer cells. *Biological Trace Element Research* 41.

Klatz, Ronald. 1997. *Grow Young with HGH*. New York: HarperCollins.

Klenner, Frederick R. 1971. Observations on the dose and administration of ascorbic acid when employed beyond the range of a vitamin in human pathology. *Journal of Applied Nutrition* 23, nos. 3&4.

Klimas, N. G., et al. 1990. Immunological abnormalities in chronic fatigue syndrome. *Journal of Clinical Microbiology* 28, no. 6.

Kling, J. 2001. CD4+ T cell mechanism allows HIV-1 persistence. *The Scientist* 15, no. 10.

Kluger, M. J., et al. 1997. The adaptive value of fever. In *Fever, Basic Mechanisms and Management*. New York: Lippincott-Raven Press.

Kohut, M. L., et al. 2001. Prolonged exercise suppresses antigen-specific cytokine response to upper respiratory infection. *Journal of Applied Physiology* 90, no. 2.

Kolata, Gina. 2001. Kill all the bacteria! *The New York Times* Jan 7.

Koo, Linda Chih-ling. 1982. *Nourishment of Life, Health in Chinese Society*. Hong Kong: The Commercial Press.

Krause, Richard M., ed. 1998. *Emerging Infections*. San Diego: Academic Press.

Krieger, D. 1979. *The Therapeutic Touch*. Englewood Cliffs, N.J.: Prentice Hall.

Kucera, C. S., et al. 1965. Antiviral activities of extracts of the lemon balm plant. *Annals of the N.Y. Academy of Science* 130, no. 1.

Kueritzkes, Daniel R. 2000. Clinical Implications of Antiretroviral Resistance. *Medscape* vol 13. [www.medscape.com/Medscape/HIV/ClinicalMgmt/CM.v13/public/index-CM.v13.html].

Kugler, Hans J. 2001. Re-establishing Homeostasis in Brain Tissue Affected by Environmental Toxins. *American Academy of Anti-aging Medicine,* vol. 2. [www.gvi.com/gviweb/iaam/kuglervol2.html].

Kuo, Y. C., et al. 1996. Cordyceps sinensis as an immunomodulatory agent. *American Journal of Chinese Medicine* 24, no. 2.

Kurashige, S., et al. 1999. Effects of *astragali radix* extract on carcinogenesis, cytokine production, and cytotoxicity in mice treated with a carcinogen, N-butyl-N′-butanolnitrosoamine. *Cancer Investigation* 17, no. 1.

Kushi, L. H., et al. 1995. Health implications of Mediterranean diet in light of contemporary knowledge: Meat, wine, fats, and oils. *American Journal of Clinical Nutrition* 6, suppl.

Ladley, M. D. 1998. The role of growth hormone secretagogues in anti-aging therapy. Paper presented at the European International Conference on Quality of Life and Longevity Medicine, in Brussels, Belgium Sept 28–30.

Lamson, D. W., and M. S. Brignall. 2000. Antioxidants and cancer III: Quercetin. *Alternative Medicine Review* 5, no. 3.

Landis, Gary. 2001. Dinosaurs ran out of O_2. *New Scientist* 140.

Lappé, Marc. 1997. *The Tao of Immunology*. New York: Plenum Press.

Lark, Susan M., and James A. Richards. 2000. *The Chemistry of Success, Secrets of Peak Performance*. San Francisco: Bay Books.

Lau, G. K. 2000. Use of immunomodulatory therapy (other than interferon) for the treatment of chronic hepatitis B virus infection. *Journal of Gastroenterology and Hepatology* 15, Suppl.

Le Fanu, James. 1999. *The Rise and Fall of Modern Medicine*. New York: Carroll & Graft Publishers.

Lederle, F. A. 1991. Oral cobalamin for pernicious anemia: Medicine's best kept secret. *JAMA* 265.

Lee, Lita, and Lisa Turner. 1998. *The Enzyme Cure*. Tiburon, Calif.: Future Medicine Publishing.

Lentsch, A. B., and P. A. Ward. 1999. Understanding the pathogenesis of inflammation using rodent models: Identification of a transcription factor (NF Kappa B) necessary for development of inflammatory injury. *ILAR/National Resource Council, Institute of Laboratory Animal Resources Journal* 40, no. 4.

Levine, M., et al. 1996. Vitamin C pharmacokinetics in healthy volunteers: Evidence for a recommended dietary allowance. *Proceeds of the National Academy of Science U.S.A.* 93.

Lewis, R. 2000. Helper T cells "condition" antigen-presenting cells to activate killer T cells. *The Scientist* 14, no. 13, Jun 26.

Life Extension Foundation. 2000. *The Physician's Guide to Life Extension Drugs*. Hollywood, Florida: Life Extension Foundation.

Lininger, Schuyler W., ed. 1999. *The Natural Pharmacy*. Roseville, Calif.: Prima Publishing.

Linus Pauling Institute. 2000. The new recommendations for dietary antioxidants, a response and position statement by the Linus Pauling Institute. Corvallis, Oregon: Linus Pauling Institute.

Liu, J. P., et al. 2001. Chinese medicinal herbs for chronic hepatitis B. *The Cochrane Library* 1.

Liu, K. C., et al. 1999. Antiviral tannins from two *Phyllanthus* species. *Planta Medica* 65, no. 1.

Lloyd, G. E. R. 1959. *Hippocratic Writings*. New York: Penguin.

Lopez, D. A., et al. 1994. *Enzymes, the Fountain of Life*. Munchen, Germany: The Neville Press.

Machnicki, M. 1990. Biological properties of lactotransferrin. *Folia Biologica* 37.

Maciocia, Giovanni. 1989. *The Foundations of Chinese Medicine*. London: Churchill Livingston.

———. 1991. Myalgic encephalomyelitis, post-viral syndrome, chronic Epstein-Barr virus disease. *Journal of Chinese Medicine* 35, no. Jan.

Mackay, Charles R. 2001. Chemokines: Immunology's high impact factors. *Nature Immunology* 2.

Maestroni, G. J., et al. 1986. Role of the pineal gland in immunity. Circadian synthesis and release of melatonin modulates the antibody response and antagonizes the immunosuppressive effect of corticosterone. *Journal of Neuroimmunology* 13, no. 1.

Mann, D. L. 1999. Inflammatory mediators in heart failure: Homogeneity through heterogeneity. *Lancet* 354.

Martens, P., and E. Hall. 2000. Malaria on the move, human population movement and malaria transmission. *Emerging Infectious Diseases* 6, no. 2.

Martin, J. W. 2000. Stealth virus research. Rosemead, Calif.: Center for Complex Infectious Disease [www.ccid.org/stealth/svresearch.html].

Martin, M. J., et al. 1994. Cytomegalovirus-related sequence in an atypical cytopathic virus repeatedly isolated from a patient with chronic fatigue syndrome. *American Journal of Pathology* 145.

Matzinger, Polly. 2001. The real function of the immune system. Detroit, Michigan: Wayne State University [cmmg.biosci.wayne.edu/asg/polly.html].

McCutcheon, A. R., et al. 1995. Antiviral screening of British Columbian medicinal plants. *Journal of Ethnopharmacology* 49, no. 2.

McKenzie, R., et al. 1998. Low-dose hydrocortisone for treatment of chronic fatigue syndrome. *JAMA* 280.

Medawar, P. B., and J. S. Medawar. 1983. *Aristotle to Zeos, A Philosophical Dictionary of Biology*. Cambridge: Harvard University Press.

Mendal, M. A., et al. 1996. C-reactive protein and its relation to cardiovascular risk factors: A population-based cross sectional study. *British Medical Journal* 312, no. 7038.

Miller, A. L. 1996. Antioxidant flavonoids: Structure, function, and clinical usage. *Alternative Medicine Review* 1, no. 2.

Milliman, W. B., et al. 2000. Hepatitis C: A retrospective study, literature review, and naturopathic protocol. *Alternative Medicine Review* 5, no. 4.

Ming, Ou, ed. 1988. *Chinese-English Dictionary of Traditional Chinese Medicine*. Hong Kong: Joint Publishing Co.

———. 1989. *Chinese-English Manual of Commonly-Used Prescriptions in TCM*. Hong Kong: Joint Publishing.

Miric, D., et al. 1997. Triggers of acute myocardial infarction regarding its site. *International Journal of Cardiology* 60, no. 1.

Morse, Stephen S., ed. 1993. *Emerging Viruses*. New York: Oxford University Press.

Murphy, F. A., et al. 1995. Virus taxonomy: Classification and nomenclature of viruses. Sixth report of the International Committee on Taxonomy of Viruses. *Archives of Virology*.

Murphy, G. M. Jr., et al. 2001. Rate of cognitive decline in AD is accelerated by the interleukin-1alpha -889 *1 allele. *Neurology* 56, no. 11.

Murray, M. T. 1996. Clinical applications of vitamin A and carotenes. *America Journal of Natural Medicine* 3, no. 5.

Murray, Michael. *The Healing Power of Herbs*. Rocklin, Calif.: Prima Publishing, 1992.

———. 1996. A comprehensive review of vitamin C. *American Journal of Natural Medicine* 3, no. 6.

——— 1996. *Encyclopedia of Nutritional Supplements*. Rocklin, Calif.: Prima Publishing.

———. 1998. Lipoic acid—A "new breed" of antioxidant. *Natural Medicine Journal* 1, no. 3.

Mushahwar, I. K., et al. 1999. Molecular and biophysical characterization of TT virus: Evidence of a new virus family infecting humans. *Proceedings of the National Academy of Sciences* 96, March 16.

Myss, Caroline. 1996. *Anatomy of the Spirit*. New York: Harmony Books.

Nagler-Anderson, C. 2001. Man the barrier! Strategic defenses in the intestinal mucosa. *Nature Reviews Immunology* 1.

Nakaishi, H., et al. 2000. Effects of black currant anthocyanoside intake on dark adaptation and VDT work-induced transient refractive alteration in healthy humans. *Alternative Medicine Review* 5, no. 6.

Nakajima, H., et al. 1998. Herpes simplex virus myelitis: Clinical manifestations and diagnosis by the polymerase chain reaction method. *European Neurology* 39, no. 3.

Narby, Jeremy. 1998. *The Cosmic Serpent; DNA and the Origins of Knowledge*. New York: Tarcher/Putnam.

Nesse, Randolph M., and George C. Williams. 1994. *Why We Get Sick; The New Science of Darwinian Medicine*. New York: Vintage.

Neushul, Michael. 1990. Antiviral carbohydrates from marine red algae. *Hydrobiologia* 204/205.

Ng, T. B., and H. Wang. 2001. Panaxagin, a new protein from Chinese ginseng possesses anti-fungal, anti-viral, translation-inhibiting and ribonuclease activity. *Life Sciences* 68, no. 7.

Nichols, Trent W. 1997. Alpha-lipoic acid: Biological effects and clinical implications. *Alternative Medicine Review* 2, no. 3.

Novello, A., et al. 2000. West Nile virus activity, New York and New Jersey, 2000. *Morbidity and Mortality Weekly Report* 49, no. 28.

Ogayar, A., and M. Sanchez-Perez. 1998. Prions: An evolutionary perspective. *International Microbiology* 1, no. 3.

Okuda, T. 1995. Tannins, a new family of bio-active organic compounds (questions and answers). *Yakugaku Zasshi* 115, no. 2.

Oldstone, Michael B. A. 1998. *Viruses, Plagues, and History*. Oxford: Oxford University Press.

Olson, M., et al. 1997. Stress-induced immune suppression and therapeutic touch. *Alternative Therapies* 3, no. 2.

Palmblad, J., et al. 1979. Lymphocyte and granulocyte reactions during sleep deprivation. *Psychosomatic Medicine* 41.

Papadopulos-Eleopulos, E., et al. 1995. AIDS in Africa: Distinguishing fact and fiction. *World Journal of Microbiology & Biotechnology* 11.

————, et al. 1992. Oxidative stress, HIV and AIDS. *Research in Immunology* 143.

Park, K. G. M. 1993. The immunological and metabolic effects of L-arginine in human cancer. *The Proceeds of the Nutrition Society* 52.

Passwater, Richard A. 1995. *Lipoic Acid: The Metabolic Antioxidant*. New Canaan, Connecticut: Keats Publishing

Patrick, Lyn. 1999. Hepatitis C: Epidemiology and review of complementary/alternative medicine treatments. *Alternative Medicine Review* 4, no. 4.

———. 1999. Nutrients and HIV: Part 1—Beta carotene and selenium. *Alternative Medicine Review* 4, no. 6.

———. 2000. Nutrients and HIV: Part 2—Vitamins A and E, zinc, B-vitamins, and magnesium. *Alternative Medicine Review* 5, no. 1.

Peat, Ray. 2000. Growth hormone: Hormone of stress, aging, and death? *Ray Peat's Newsletter*, April.

Pelton, Ross, et al. 2000. *Drug-Induced Nutrient Depletion Handbook*. Hudson, Ohio: Lexi-Comp.

Petersen, E. W., et al. 2001. Effect of vitamin supplementation on cytokine response and on muscle damage after strenuous exercise. *American Journal of Physiology* 280, no. 6.

Pierpaoli, W., and W. Regelson. 1995. *The Melatonin Miracle*. New York: Simon & Schuster.

Pinkham, Mark Amaru. 1997. *The Return of the Serpents of Wisdom*. Kempton, Illinois: Adventures Unlimited Press.

Piraino, F., and C. R. Brandt. 1999. Isolation and partial characterization of an antiviral, RC-183, from the edible mushroom *Rozites caperata*. *Antiviral Research* 43.

Pitcher, C. J., et al. 1999. HIV-1-specific CD4(+) T cells are detectable in most individuals with active HIV-1 infection, but decline with prolonged viral suppression. *Nature Medicine* 5, May.

Pizza, G., et al. 1977. Effect of in vitro produced transfer factor on the immune response of cancer patients. *European Journal of Cancer* 13, no. 9.

———, et al. 1996. A preliminary report on the use of transfer factor for treating stage D3 hormone-unresponsive metastatic prostate cancer. *Biotherapy* 9, no. 1–3.

———, et al. 1996. Orally administered HSV-specific transfer factor prevents genital and labial herpes relapses. *Biotherapy* 9, no. 1–3.

Plotkin, Mark J. 1993. *Tales of a Shaman's Apprentice, An Ethnobotanist Searches for New Medicines in the Amazon Rain Forest*. New York: Viking.

————. 2000. *Medicine Quest*. New York: Viking.

Podda, M., et al. 1994. Alpha-lipoic acid supplementation prevents symptoms of vitamin E deficiency. *Biochemical and Biophysical Research Communications* 204.

Podmore, I. D., et al. 1998. Vitamin C exhibits pro-oxidant properties. *Nature*, no. 392.

Pray, Leslie. 2001. The mystery TT virus—What is it? *The Scientist* 15, no. 15.

Quig, David W. 2000. Molecules that detoxify. Paper presented at the 15th Annual American Association of Naturopathic Practitioners (AANP) Conference, Seattle.

Quillin, Patrick. 1994. *Beating Cancer with Nutrition*. Tulsa: Nutrition Times Press.

Rabin, Bruce S. 1999. *Stress, Immune Function, and Health*. New York: Wiley-Liss.

Rainsford, K. D. 1999. Profile and mechanisms of gastrointestinal and other side effects of nonsteroidal anti-inflammatory drugs. *American Journal of Medicine* 107(6A), no. 27S-36S.

RavenWind, Josie. 2001. João de Deus, the Miracle Man of Brazil. *Shaman's Drum* 58.

Reckeweg, Hans-Heinrich. 1980. *Homotoxicology*. Albuquerque, N.M.: Menaco Publishing.

Regelson, William, and Carol Colman. 1996. *The Super-Hormone Promise*. New York: Simon & Schuster.

Regush, Nicholas. 2000. *The Virus Within; A Coming Epidemic*. New York: Dutton.

Reichart, R. 1997. Phytotherapy alternatives for chronic active hepatitis. *Quarterly Review of Natural Medicine*, Summer.

Reiter, R. J., et al. 2000. Melatonin and its relation to the immune system and inflammation. *Annals of the New York Academy of Science*, no. 917.

Reiter, Russell J., and Jo Robinson. 1995. *Your Body's Natural Wonder Drug, Melatonin*. New York: Bantam.

Reuters. 2000. Hepatitis C virus can infect mosquito cells. *Reuters Medical News*, July.

Roitt, Ivan, et al. 1998. *Immunology*. London: Mosby.

Rosch, Eleanor. 2000. Zen and the brain: Towards an understanding of meditation and consciousness. *IONS Noetic Science Review* 54, Dec.

Rossi, M., et al. 2001. Molecular structure and activity toward DNA of baicalein, a flavone constituent of the Asian herbal medicine sho-saiko-to. *Journal of Natural Products* 64, no. 1.

Rountree, Robert, and Carol Colman. 2000. *Immunotics, A Revolutionary Way to Fight Infection, Beat Chronic Illness, and Stay Well.* New York: Putnam.

Samad, T. A., et al. 2001. Interleukin-1B—Mediated induction of Cox-2 in the CNS contributes to inflammatory pain hypersensitivity. *Nature* 410, March 22.

Sandoval, M., et al. 2000. Cat's claw inhibits TNF-alpha production and scavenges free radicals: Role in cytoprotection. *Free Radical Biology and Medicine* 29, no. 1.

Scaglione, F., et al. 1990. Immunomodulatory effects of two extracts of *Panax ginseng* C.A. Meyer. *Drugs under Experimental Clinical Research* 16, no. 10.

————, et al. 1996. Efficacy and safety of the standardized ginseng extract G115 for potentiating vaccination against the influenza syndrome and protection against the common cold. *Drugs under Experimental Clinical Research* 22, no. 2.

Schiermeier, Quirin. 2000. Testing times for BSE. *Nature* 409, Feb. 8.

Schoenherr, W. E., and K. S. Jewell. 1997. Nutritional modification of inflammatory disease. *Seminars in Veterinary Medicine and Surgery* 12, no. 3.

Scott, G. R. 1985. Rinderpest in the 1980s. *Progress in Veterinary Microbiology and Immunology* 1.

Sears, Barry. 1995. *The Zone*. New York: HarperCollins.

Seddon, J. M., et al. 1994. Dietary carotenoids, vitamins A, C, and E, and advanced age-related macular degeneration. *JAMA* 272.

Selye, H. 1956. *The Stress of Life*. New York: McGraw-Hill.

Serkedjieva, J., and S. Ivancheva. 1999. Antiherpes virus activity of extracts from the medicinal plant *Germanium sanguineum L. Journal of Ethnopharmacology* 64, no. 1.

Shabert, Judy, and Nancy Enrlich. 1994. *The Ultimate Nutrient Glutamine*. Garden Park, N.Y.: Avery Publishing Group.

Shames, R. L., and K. H. Shames. 2001. *Thyroid Power: 10 Steps to Total Health*. New York: HarperResource.

Shamgar, B. E., et al. 2000. Suppression of NK cell activity and of resistance to metastasis by stress: a role for adrenal catecholamines and β-adrenoceptors. *Neuroimmunomodulation* 8, no. 3.

Shealy, C. Norman. 1999. *Sacred Healing: The Curing Power of Energy and Spirituality*. Boston: Element Books.

Sheets, M. S., et al. 1991. Studies of the effect of acemannan on tertrovirus infections: Clinical stabilization of feline leukemia virus-infected cats. *Molecular Biotherapy* 3, no. 1.

Sherman, K. E., et al. 1998. Combination therapy with thymosin alpha and interferon for the treatment of chronic hepatitis C infections: A randomized, placebo-controlled double-blind trial. *Hepatology* 27, no. 4.

Shortridge, K. F. 1995. The next pandemic influenza virus? *Lancet* 346.

Simmons, Peter. 2001. The origin and evolution of hepatitis viruses in humans. *Journal of General Virology* 82.

Simon, P. W. 1997. Plant pigments for color and nutrition. *Horticulture Science* 32, no. 1.

Sinatra, Stephen T. 1998. *The Coenzyme Q10 Phenomenon*. Chicago, Illinois: Keats

Sinclair, Steven. 1998. Chinese herbs: A clinical review of astragalus, ligusticum, and schizandrae. *Alternative Medicine Review* 3, no. 5.

Singer, J., et al. 1993. Abstract PO-B28-2153. Paper presented at the IX International Conference on AIDS June 6–11 in Berlin, Germany.

Skotnicki, A. B. 1997. Thymus extract for cancer? A criteria-based, systematic review. *European Journal of Cancer* 33.

Song, C, and B. E. Leonard. 2000. *Fundamentals of Psychoneuroimmunology*. New York: John Wiley & Sons.

Sperry, R. 1986. The new mentalist paradigm and ultimate concern. *Perspectives in Biology and Medicine* 29, no. 3.

Spielman, Andrew, and Michael D'Antonio. 2001. *Mosquito; A Natural History of Our Most Persistent and Deadly Foe*. New York: Hyperion.

Sprietsma, J. E. 1999. Cysteine, glutathione (GSH) and zinc and copper ions together are effective, natural, intracellular inhibitors of (AIDS) viruses. *Medical Hypotheses* 52, no. 6.

Sta, F., et al. 1997. Changes in natural killer cell subpopulations in lead workers. *International Archives of Occupational and Environmental Health* 69.

Stamets, Paul. 2001. New anti-viral compounds from mushrooms. *HerbalGram* 51.

Stauder, G., and S. Kabil. 1997. Oral enzyme therapy in hepatitis C patients. *International Journal Immunotherapy* XIII.

Stites, Daniel P., et al. 1997. *Medical Immunology*. Stamford, Connecticut: Appleton & Lange.

Stoff, Jesse A., and Charles R. Pellegrino. 1988. *Chronic Fatigue Syndrome; The Hidden Epidemic*. New York: Random House.

Stolberg, Sheryl Gay. 2001 AIDS at 20: Faces of an epidemic. *The New York Times,* June 3.

Stover, C. K., et al. 2000. A small-molecule nitroimidazopyran drug candidate for the treatment of tuberculosis. *Nature* 405, June 22.

Streeten, D. H. 1999. What test for hypothalamic-pituitary-adrenocortical insufficiency? *Lancet* 354, no. SI5–SI10.

Suhadolnik, R. J., et al. 1997. Biochemical evidence for a novel low molecular weight 2-5A-dependent RNase L in chronic fatigue syndrome. *Journal of Interferon and Cytokine Research* 17, no. 7.

Svoboda, Robert. 1988. *Prakruti; Your Ayurvedic Constitution.* Albuquerque, N.M.: Geocom.

Swain, Mark G. 1998. *Fatigue As a Symptom of Liver Disease.* The Hepatitis Information Network www.hepnet.com/hepc/uldh98/swain.html.

Tandon, A., et al. 2001. Treatment of subacute hepatitis with lamivudine and intravenous glycyrrhizin: A pilot study. *Hepatology Research* 20, no. 1.

Thorley-Lawson, D. A. 2001. Epstein-Barr virus: Exploiting the immune system. *Nature Reviews Immunology* 1.

Treitinger, A., et al. 2000. Decreased antioxidant defense in individuals infected by the human immunodeficiency virus. *European Journal of Clinical Investigations* 30, no. 5.

Trevathan, Wenda R., et al., eds. 1999. *Evolutionary Medicine.* Oxford: Oxford University Press.

Tsung, Pi-Kwang. 1989. *Immune System and Chinese Herbs.* Irvine, Calif.: Institute of Chinese Herbs.

Tyler, Allen N. 1997. Influenza A virus: A possible precipitating factor in fibromyalgia. *Alternative Medicine Review* 2, no. 2.

Ubillas, R., et al. 1994. SP-303, an antiviral oligomeric proanthocyanidin from the latex of *Croton lechleri* (Sangre de Drago). *Phytomedicine* 1.

Unschuld, Paul U. 1985. *Medicine in China: A History of Ideas.* Berkeley: University of California Press.

Valerio, L. G. Jr., et al. 2001. Induction of human NAD(P)H: Quinone oxidoreductase (NQO1) expression by the flavol quercetin. *Toxicology Letters* 119, no. 1.

Van Benschoten, M. M. 2001. Clinical pharmacology of Chinese herbal medicine. *Oriental Medicine,* Summer.

Vance, R. E., et al. 1998. Mouse CD94/NKG2A is a natural killer cell receptor for the non-classical MCH class I molecule Qa1b. *Journal of Experimental Medicine* 188.

Van Damme, E. J., et al. 1997. Isolation and molecular cloning of a novel type 2 ribosome-inactivating protein with an inactive B chain from elderberry *(Sambucus nigra)* bark. *The Journal of Biological Chemistry* 272, no. 13.

Van Loon, I. M. 1997. The Golden Root: Clinical applications of *Scutellaria baicalensis* GEORGI flavonoids as modulators of the inflammatory response. *Alternative Medicine Review* 2, no. 6.

Vanderhaeghe, Lorna R., and Patrick J. D. Bouic. 1999. *The Immune System Cure*. New York: Kensington Books.

Vasilenko, A. M., and S. V. Svec. 1997. Wobenzyme in complex therapy of chronic liver diseases. Paper presented at the Second National Congress of Rheumatologists in the Ukraine, Kiev.

Vaughn, Susan. 2000. Search for cure fuels scientist's drive. *The Los Angeles Times* Dec 31.

Veith, Ilza. 1949. *The Yellow Emperor's Classic of Internal Medicine*. Berkeley: The University of California Press.

Vettori, G., et al. 1987. Prevention of recurrent respiratory infections in adults. *Minerva Medicine* 78.

Viebahn-Haensler, Renate. 1999. *The Use of Ozone in Medicine*. Heidelberg: ODREI-Publishers.

Villoldo, Alberto. 2001. *Shaman, Healer, Sage*. New York: Harmony Books.

Vogel, Verlag A. 1952. *The Nature Doctor*. Teufen, Switzerland: Druckerei und Verlagsanstalt Konstanz.

Wagner, H. 1998. *Immunomodulating Agents from Plants*. Basel: Birkhauser.

Watanabe, Myrna. 2001. No vaccine, no cure. *The Scientist* 15, no. 13.

Watson, Ronald R. 1998. *Nutrients and Foods in AIDS*. Boca Raton, Florida: CRC Press.

Weil, Andrew. 1995. *Spontaneous Healing*. New York: Alfred A. Knopf.

Weinberg, J. B., et al. 1995. Inhibition of productive human immuno-deficiency virus-1 infection by cobalamins. *Blood* 86.

Weiss, Robert A. 2001. Polio vaccines exonerated. *Nature* 410, April 26.

Wemmer, U. 1998. Reducing costs through the use of antihomotoxic medications in treating the common cold. *Biomedical Therapy* XVI, no. 1.

Wigmore, Ann. 1985. *The Wheatgrass Book*. New York: Avery.

Williams, James E. 1992. Liver and gallbladder damp heat syndrome: A case of benign nonspecific liver dysfunction with abnormal enzyme profile. *American Journal of Acupuncture* 20, no. 3.

————. 1998. Case studies on the treatment of chronic hepatitis C virus: An integrated approach using traditional Chinese medicine and acupuncture. *American Journal of Acupuncture* 26, no. 4.

Wiseman, Nigel, and Andrew Ellis. 1985. *Fundamentals of Chinese Medicine*. Cambridge: Paradigm Publications.

Witschi, A., et al. 1995. The systemic availability of oral glutathione. *European Journal of Clinical Pharmacology* 43.

Woerdenbag, H. J., et al. 1992. *Eupatorium perfoliatum* L.—Boneset. *Phytotherapy* 13.

Wohlbling, R. H., and K. Leonhardt. 1994. Local therapy of herpes simplex with dried extract of *Melissa officinalis*. *Phytomedicine* 1, no. 1.

Wolf, Fred Alan. 1986. *The Body Quantum: The New Physics of Body, Mind, and Health*. New York: MacMillan.

Womble, D., and J. H. Helderman. 1992. The impact of acemannan on the generation and function of cytotoxic T-lymphocytes. *Immunopharmacology and Immunotoxicology* 14, no. 1–2.

Xie, Zhufan, ed. 1984. *Dictionary of Traditional Chinese Medicine*. Hong Kong: The Commercial Press.

Xing, N., et al. 2001. Quercetin inhibits the expression and function of the androgen receptor in LNCaP prostate cancer cells. *Carcinogenesis* 22, no. 3.

Xu, H., and S. Lee. 2001. Activity of plant flavonoids against antibiotic-resistant bacteria. *Phytotherapy Research* 15, no. 1.

Xu, R. H., et al. 1992. Effects of *Cordyceps sinensis* on natural killer activity and colony formation of B16 melanoma. *Chinese Medicine Journal* 105, no. 2.

Yaguar, M., et al. 2001. Does the control of alanine aminotransferase levels lead to a regression of liver fibrosis in chronic hepatitis C patients? *Hepatology Research* 19, no. 2.

Yamashiki, M., et al. 1997. Effects of the Japanese herbal medicine "sho-saiko-to" (TJ-9) on in vitro interleukin-10 production by peripheral blood mononuclear cells in patients with chronic hepatitis C. *Hepatology* 25.

Yarnell, E. 2001. Proposed biomolecular theory of fasting during fevers due to infection. *Alternative Medicine Review* 6, no. 5.

Yeung, Him-che. 1983. *Handbook of Chinese Herbs and Formulas, Vol. I*. Los Angeles: Him-che Yeung.

Yoshiaki, Abe, et al. 1999. Curcumin inhibition of inflammatory cytokine production by human peripheral blood monocytes and alveolar macrophages. *Pharmacological Research* 39, no. 1.

Yoshida, T., et al. 1996. New hydrolyzable tannins, shephagenins A and B, from *Shepherdia argentea* as HIV-1 reverse transcriptase inhibitors. *Chemical and Pharmaceutical Bulletin* 44, no. 8.

Zakay-Rones, Z., et al. 1995. Inhibition of several strains of influenza virus in vitro and reduction of symptoms by an elderberry extract *(Sambucus nigra L.)* during an outbreak of influenza B Panama. *Journal of Alternative and Complementary Medicine* 1, no. 4.

Zhang, L., and I. R. Tizard. 1996. Activation of a mouse macrophage cell line by acemannan: The major carbohydrate fraction from aloe vera gel. *Immunopharmacology* 35, no. 2.

Zhang, Min Shi. 1990. An experimental study on 472 herbs relating antiviral actions on herpes simplex virus. *Journal of Integrated Chinese and Western Medicine* 10, no. 1.

Zhang, Qing Cai. 2000. *Healing Hepatitis C with Modern Chinese Medicine*. New York: Sino-Med Institute.

———. 2001. Hepatitis C and modern Chinese medicine. HepaPro Corp. (continuing education course and personal communication). Los Angeles, 14 Jan.

Zhao, B. L., et al. 1990. Scavenging effect of schizandrins on active oxygen radicals. *Cell Biology International Reports* 14, no. 2.

Zheng, M., and Y. Zheng. 1992. Experimental studies on the inhibition effects of 1000 Chinese medicinal herbs on the surface antigen of hepatitis B virus. *Journal of Traditional Chinese Medicine* 12, no. 3.

Zhu, Chun-han. 1989. *Clinical Handbook of Chinese Prepared Medicines*. Brookline, Mass.: Paradigm Publications.

Zimecki, M., et al. 1991. Immunostimulatory activity of lactotransferrin and maturation of CD-4 and CD-8 murine thymocytes. *Immunology Letters* 30.

Index

About the Author

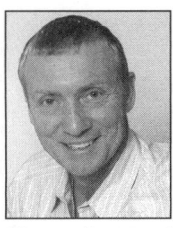 J. E. Williams, O.M.D. is a doctor of Oriental medicine with certifications in acupuncture, Chinese herbology, and naturopathic medicine, and is a Fellow of the American Association of Integrative Medicine. He practices in Southern California with an emphasis on anti-aging medicine, natural hormone balancing therapies, and immunity enhancement. Dr. Williams is widely published in medical journals and is a board member of numerous medical and nutritional organizations. He is a frequent speaker on natural therapies and integrated medicine, including continuing medical education seminars, grand rounds to medical groups and hospitals; and radio and television programs. He has traveled extensively to study ethnobotany and indigenous healing practices. For more information on viral immunity, visit www.viralimmunity.net.

Hampton Roads Publishing Company

... for the evolving human spirit

Hampton Roads Publishing Company
publishes books on a variety of subjects,
including metaphysics, health, integrative medicine,
visionary fiction, and other related topics.

For a copy of our latest catalog, call toll-free
800-766-8009, or send your name and address to:

Hampton Roads Publishing Company, Inc.
1125 Stoney Ridge Road
Charlottesville, VA 22902

e-mail: hrpc@hrpub.com
www.hrpub.com

Reader's Digest
WEBSTER'S

CANADIAN
DICTIONARY
AND THESAURUS

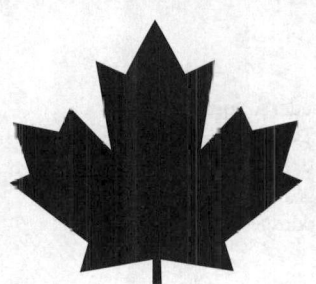

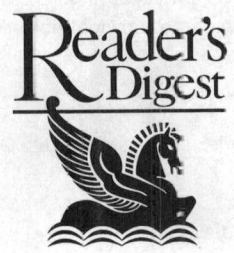

Reader's
Digest

Linguistics consultant: Prof. PKS Pandey
Canadian English pronunciation: Simon Grant
Canadian entries: Fraser Sutherland

CyberMedia
Project manager: Taru Agarwal
Team leader: Vatsala Arora
Linguistics experts: Arti Kumari, Bidisha Som, Manidipa Bhattacharyya,
  Shantanu Ghosh, Sidhartha Basu
QA: Shreya Barbara
Typesetters: Subhendu Das, Rajesh Ruhella

Geddes & Grosset
Project director: Ron Grosset
Production manager: Craig Brown
Production editor: Eleanor Cowan
Designer: Mark Mechan

Published 2005 for Reader's Digest
by Geddes & Grosset, David Dale House,
New Lanark, ML11 9DJ, Scotland

ISBN 0-88850-775-5

Typeset using Linotype Frutiger, and Bitstream Fritz Quadrata and Dutch 766 by
CyberMedia, India

Printed and bound in Poland, OZGraf S.A.

Contents

Elements of the Dictionary and Thesaurus

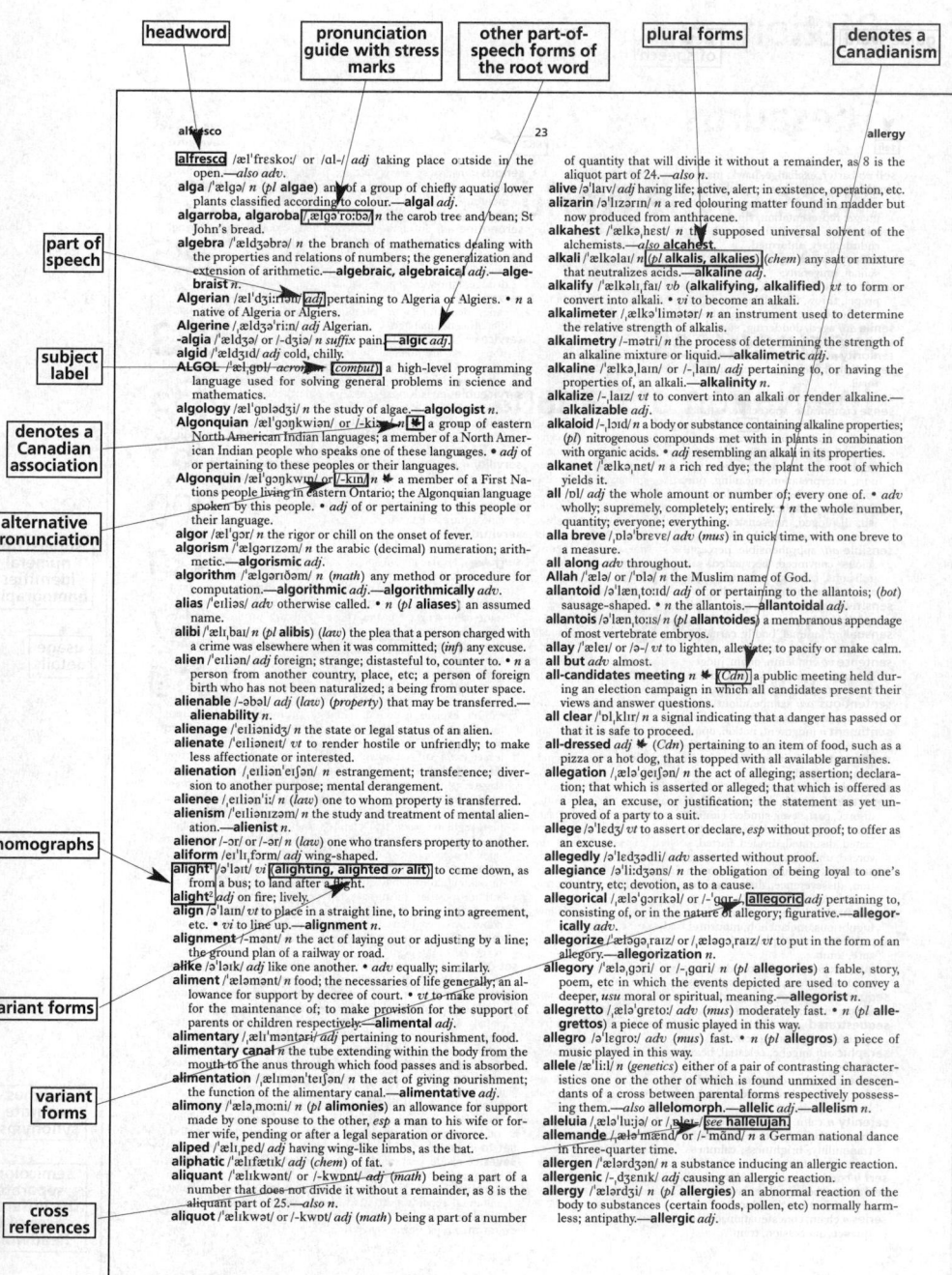

headword

pronunciation guide with stress marks

other part-of-speech forms of the root word

plural forms

denotes a Canadianism

part of speech

subject label

denotes a Canadian association

alternative pronunciation

homographs

variant forms

variant forms

cross references

alfresco /æl'freskoʊ/ or /ɑl-/ *adj* taking place outside in the open.—*also adv.*

alga /'ælgə/ *n* (*pl* **algae**) any of a group of chiefly aquatic lower plants classified according to colour.—**algal** *adj*.

algarroba, algaroba /ˌælgə'roːbə/ *n* the carob tree and bean; St John's bread.

algebra /'ældʒəbrə/ *n* the branch of mathematics dealing with the properties and relations of numbers; the generalization and extension of arithmetic.—**algebraic, algebraical** *adj*.—**algebraist** *n*.

Algerian /æl'dʒɪːriən/ *adj* pertaining to Algeria or Algiers. • *n* a native of Algeria or Algiers.

Algerine /ˌældʒə'riːn/ *adj* Algerian.

-algia /'ældʒə/ or /-dʒiə/ *n suffix* pain.—**algic** *adj*.

algid /'ældʒɪd/ *adj* cold, chilly.

ALGOL /'ælˌɡɒl/ *acronym* (*comput*) a high-level programming language used for solving general problems in science and mathematics.

algology /æl'ɡɒlədʒi/ *n* the study of algae.—**algologist** *n*.

Algonquian /æl'ɡɒŋkwiən/ or /-kiɑn/ *n* a group of eastern North American Indian languages; a member of a North American Indian people who speaks one of these languages. • *adj* of or pertaining to these peoples or their languages.

Algonquin /æl'ɡɒŋkwɪn/ or /-kɪn/ *n* a member of a First Nations people living in eastern Ontario; the Algonquian language spoken by this people. • *adj* of or pertaining to this people or their language.

algor /'ælˌɡər/ *n* the rigor or chill on the onset of fever.

algorism /'ælɡərɪzəm/ *n* the arabic (decimal) numeration; arithmetic.—**algorismic** *adj*.

algorithm /'ælɡərɪðəm/ *n* (*math*) any method or procedure for computation.—**algorithmic** *adj*.—**algorithmically** *adv*.

alias /'eɪliəs/ *adv* otherwise called. • *n* (*pl* **aliases**) an assumed name.

alibi /'æləˌbaɪ/ *n* (*pl* **alibis**) (*law*) the plea that a person charged with a crime was elsewhere when it was committed; (*inf*) any excuse.

alien /'eɪliən/ *adj* foreign; strange; distasteful to, counter to. • *n* a person from another country, etc; a person of foreign birth who has not been naturalized; a being from outer space.

alienable /-əbəl/ *adj* (*law*) (*property*) that may be transferred.—**alienability** *n*.

alienage /'eɪliənɪdʒ/ *n* the state or legal status of an alien.

alienate /'eɪliəneɪt/ *vt* to render hostile or unfriendly; to make less affectionate or interested.

alienation /ˌeɪliən'eɪʃən/ *n* estrangement; transference; diversion to another purpose; mental derangement.

alienee /ˌeɪliən'iː/ *n* (*law*) one to whom property is transferred.

alienism /'eɪliənɪzəm/ *n* the study and treatment of mental alienation.—**alienist** *n*.

alienor /'eɪliənər/ or /-ər/ *n* (*law*) one who transfers property to another.

aliform /'eɪlɪˌfɔrm/ *adj* wing-shaped.

alight /ə'laɪt/ *vi* (**alighting, alighted** *or* **alit**) to come down, as from a bus; to land after a flight.

alight *adj* on fire; lively.

align /ə'laɪn/ *vt* to place in a straight line, to bring into agreement, etc. • *vi* to line up.—**alignment** *n*.

alignment /-mənt/ *n* the act of laying out or adjusting by a line; the ground plan of a railway or road.

alike /ə'laɪk/ *adj* like one another. • *adv* equally; similarly.

aliment /'æləmənt/ *n* food; the necessaries of life generally; an allowance for support by decree of court. • *vt* to make provision for the maintenance of; to make provision for the support of parents or children respectively.—**alimental** *adj*.

alimentary /ˌælɪ'məntəri/ *adj* pertaining to nourishment, food.

alimentary canal *n* the tube extending within the body from the mouth to the anus through which food passes and is absorbed.

alimentation /ˌælɪmən'teɪʃən/ *n* the act of giving nourishment; the function of the alimentary canal.—**alimentative** *adj*.

alimony /'æləˌmoʊni/ *n* (*pl* **alimonies**) an allowance for support made by one spouse to the other, *esp* a man to his wife or former wife, pending or after a legal separation or divorce.

aliped /'æliˌped/ *adj* having wing-like limbs, as the bat.

aliphatic /ˌæli'fætɪk/ *adj* (*chem*) of fat.

aliquant /'ælikwənt/ or /-kwɒnt/ *adj* (*math*) being a part of a number that does not divide it without a remainder, as 8 is the aliquant part of 25.—*also n*.

aliquot /'ælikwət/ or /-kwɒt/ *adj* (*math*) being a part of a number

of quantity that will divide it without a remainder, as 8 is the aliquot part of 24.—*also n*.

alive /ə'laɪv/ *adj* having life; active, alert; in existence, operation, etc.

alizarin /ə'lɪzərɪn/ *n* a red colouring matter found in madder but now produced from anthracene.

alkahest /'ælkəˌhest/ *n* the supposed universal solvent of the alchemists.—*also* **alcahest**.

alkali /'ælkəˌlaɪ/ *n* (*pl* **alkalis, alkalies**) (*chem*) any salt or mixture that neutralizes acids.—**alkaline** *adj*.

alkalify /'ælkəliˌfaɪ/ *vb* (**alkalifying, alkalified**) *vt* to form or convert into alkali. • *vi* to become an alkali.

alkalimeter /ˌælkə'lɪmətər/ *n* an instrument used to determine the relative strength of alkalis.

alkalimetry /-'trɪ/ *n* the process of determining the strength of an alkaline mixture or liquid.—**alkalimetric** *adj*.

alkaline /'ælkəˌlaɪn/ or /-ˌlaɪn/ *adj* pertaining to, or having the properties of, an alkali.—**alkalinity** *n*.

alkalize /-ˌlaɪz/ *vt* to convert into an alkali or render alkaline.—**alkalizable** *adj*.

alkaloid /-ˌlɔɪd/ *n* a body or substance having alkaline properties; (*pl*) nitrogenous compounds met with in plants in combination with organic acids. • *adj* resembling an alkali in its properties.

alkanet /'ælkəˌnet/ *n* a rich red dye; the plant the root of which yields it.

all /ɔl/ *adj* the whole amount or number of; every one of. • *adv* wholly; supremely, completely; entirely. • *n* the whole number, quantity; everyone; everything.

alla breve /ˌplɑ'breɪveɪ/ *adv* (*mus*) in quick time, with one breve to a measure.

all along *adv* throughout.

Allah /'ælə/ or /'ɑlə/ *n* the Muslim name of God.

allantoid /ə'læntɔɪd/ *adj* of or pertaining to the allantois; (*bot*) sausage-shaped. • *n* the allantois.—**allantoidal** *adj*.

allantois /ə'læntoʊɪs/ *n* (*pl* **allantoides**) a membranous appendage of most vertebrate embryos.

allay /ə'leɪ/ or /ə-/ *vt* to lighten, alleviate; to pacify or make calm.

all but *adv* almost.

all-candidates meeting *n* (*Cdn*) a public meeting held during an election campaign in which all candidates present their views and answer questions.

all clear /ˌɔlˈklɪr/ *n* a signal indicating that a danger has passed or that it is safe to proceed.

all-dressed *adj* (*Cdn*) pertaining to an item of food, such as a pizza or a hot dog, that is topped with all available garnishes.

allegation /ˌælə'ɡeɪʃən/ *n* the act of alleging; assertion; declaration; that which is asserted or alleged; that which is offered as a plea, an excuse, or justification; the statement as yet unproved of a party to a suit.

allege /ə'ledʒ/ *vt* to assert or declare, *esp* without proof; to offer as an excuse.

allegedly /ə'ledʒədli/ *adv* asserted without proof.

allegiance /ə'liːdʒəns/ *n* the obligation of being loyal to one's country, etc; devotion, as to a cause.

allegorical /ˌælə'ɡɒrɪkəl/ or /-'ɡɔr-/ *adj* pertaining to, consisting of, or in the nature of allegory; figurative.—**allegorically** *adv*.

allegorize /'æləɡəˌraɪz/ or /ˌæləɡə'raɪz/ *vt* to put in the form of an allegory.—**allegorization** *n*.

allegory /'æləˌɡɒri/ or /-ˌɡɑri/ *n* (*pl* **allegories**) a fable, story, poem, etc in which the events depicted are used to convey a deeper, *usu* moral or spiritual, meaning.—**allegorist** *n*.

allegretto /ˌælə'ɡretoʊ/ *adv* (*mus*) moderately fast. • *n* (*pl* **allegrettos**) a piece of music played in this way.

allegro /ə'leɡroʊ/ *adv* (*mus*) fast. • *n* (*pl* **allegros**) a piece of music played in this way.

allele /æ'liːl/ *n* (*genetics*) either of a pair of contrasting characteristics one or the other of which is found unmixed in descendants of a cross between parental forms respectively possessing them.—*also* **allelomorph**.—**allelic** *adj*.—**allelism** *n*.

alleluia /ˌælə'luːjə/ or *also see* **hallelujah**.

allemande /ˌælə'mænd/ or /-'mɑnd/ *n* a German national dance in three-quarter time.

allergen /'ælərdʒən/ *n* a substance inducing an allergic reaction.

allergenic /-ˌdʒenɪk/ *adj* causing an allergic reaction.

allergy /'ælərdʒi/ *n* (*pl* **allergies**) an abnormal reaction of the body to substances (certain foods, pollen, etc) normally harmless; antipathy.—**allergic** *adj*.

Elements of the Dictionary and Thesaurus

guide word

new part of speech

page number

sell *vb* barter, exchange, hawk, market, peddle, trade, vend.
semblance *n* likeness, resemblance, similarity; air, appearance, aspect, bearing, exterior, figure, form, mien, seeming, show; image, representation, similitude.
seminal *adj* important, original; germinal, radical, rudimental, rudimentary, unformed.
seminary *n* academy, college, gymnasium, high school, institute, school, university.
send *vb* cast, drive, emit, fling, hurl, impel, lance, launch project, propel, throw, toss; delegate, depute, dispatch; forward, transmit; bestow, confer, give, grant.
senile *adj* aged, doddering, superannuated; doting, imbecile.
senior *adj* elder, older; higher.
seniority *n* eldership, precedence, priority, superiority.
sensation *n* feeling, sense perception; excitement, impression, thrill.
sensational *adj* exciting, melodramatic, startling, thrilling.
sense *vb* appraise, appreciate, estimate, notice, observe, perceive, suspect, understand. • *n* brains, intellect, intelligence, mind, reason, understanding; appreciation, apprehension, discernment, feeling, perception, recognition, tact; connotation, idea, implication, judgment, notion, opinion, sentiment, view; import, interpretation, meaning, purport, significance; sagacity, soundness, substance, wisdom.
senseless *adj* apathetic, inert, insensate, unfeeling; absurd, foolish, ill-judged, nonsensical, silly, unmeaning, unreasonable, unwise; doltish, foolish, simple, stupid, witless, weak-minded.
sensible *adj* apprehensible, perceptible; aware, cognizant, conscious, convinced, persuaded, satisfied; discreet, intelligent, judicious, rational, reasonable, sagacious, sage, sober, sound, wise; observant, understanding; impressionable, sensitive.
sensitive *adj* perceptive, sentient; affected, impressible impressionable, responsive, susceptible; delicate tender, touchy.
sensual *adj* animal, bodily, carnal, voluptuous; gross, lascivious, lewd, licentious, unchaste.
sentence *vb* condemn, doom, judge. • *n* decision, determination, judgment, opinion, verdict; doctrine, dogma, opinion, tenet; condemnation, conviction, doom; period, proposition.
sententious *adj* compendious, compact, concise, didactic, laconic, pithy, pointed, succinct, terse.
sentiment *n* judgment, notion, opinion; maxim, saying; emotion, tenderness; disposition, feeling, thought.
sentimental *adj* impressable, impressionable, over-emotional, romantic, tender.
sentinel *n* guard, guardsman, patrol, picket, sentry, watchman.
separate *vb* detach, disconnect, disjoin, dissever, divide, divorce, part, sever, sunder; eliminate, remove, withdraw; cleave, open. • *adj* detached, disconnected, disjoined, disjointed, dissociated, disunited, divided, parted, severed; discrete, distinct, divorced, unconnected; alone, segregated, withdrawn.
separation *n* disjunction, disjuncture, dissociation; disconnection, disseverance, disseveration, disunion; division divorce; analysis, decomposition
sepulchral *adj* deep, dismal, funereal, gloomy, grave, hollow, lugubrious, melancholy, mournful, sad, sombre, woeful.
sepulchre *n* burial place, charnel house, grave, ossuary, sepulture, tomb.
sequel *n* close, conclusion, denouement, end, termination; consequence, event, issue, result, upshot.
sequence *n* following, graduation, progression, succession; arrangement, series, train.
sequestrated *adj* hidden, private, retired secluded, unfrequented, withdrawn; seized.
seraphic *adj* angelic, celestial, heavenly, sublime; holy, pure, refined.
serene *adj* calm, collected, placid, peaceful, quiet, tranquil, sedate, undisturbed, unperturbed, unruffled bright, calm, clear, fair, unclouded.
serenity *n* calm, calmness, collectedness, composure, coolness, imperturbability, peace, peacefulness, quiescence, sedateness, tranquillity; brightness calmness, clearness, fairness, peace, quietness, stillness.
serf *n* bondman, servant, slave, thrall, villein.
serfdom *n* bondage, enslavement, enthralment, servitude, slavery, subjection, thraldom.
series *n* chain, concatenation, course, line, order, progression, sequence, succession, train.

serious *adj* earnest, grave, demure, pious, resolute, sedate, sober, solemn, staid, thoughtful; dangerous, great, important, momentous, weighty.
sermon *n* discourse, exhortation, homily lecture.
serpentine *adj* anfractuous, convoluted, crooked, meandering, sinuous, spiral, tortuous, twisted, undulating, winding.
servant *n* attendant, dependant, factotum, helper, henchman, retainer, servitor, subaltern, underling; domestic, drudge, flunky, lackey, menial, scullion, slave.
serve *vb* aid, assist, attend, help, minister oblige, succour; advance, benefit, forward, promote; content, satisfy, supply; handle, officiate, manage, manipulate, work.
service *vb* check, maintain, overhaul, repair • *n* labour, ministration, work; attendance, business, duty, employ, employment, office; advantage, benefit, good, gain, profit; avail, purpose, use, utility; ceremony, function, observance, rite, worship.
serviceable *adj* advantageous, available, beneficial, convenient, functional, handy, helpful, operative, profitable, useful.
servile *adj* dependent, menial; abject, base, beggarly, cringing, fawning, groveling, low, mean, obsequious, slavish, sneaking, sycophantic, truckling.
servility *n* bondage, dependence, slavery; abjection, abjectness, baseness, fawning, meanness, obsequiousness, slavishness, sycophancy.
servitor *n* attendant, dependant, footman, lackey, retainer, servant, squire valet, waiter.
servitude *n* bondage, enslavement, enthralment, serfdom, service, slavery, thraldom.
set¹ *vb* lay, locate, mount, place, put, stand, station; appoint, determine, establish, fix, settle; risk, stake, wager, adapt, adjust, regulate; adorn, stud, variegate, arrange, dispose, pose, post; appoint, assign, predetermine, prescribe, estimate, prize, rate, value; embarrass, perplex, pose; contrive, produce, decline, sink; congeal, concern, consolidate, harden, solidify; flow, incline, run, tend; *(with **about**)* begin, commence; *(with **apart**)* appropriate, consecrate, dedicate, devote, reserve, set aside; *(with **aside**)* abrogate, annul, omit, reject; reserve, set apart; *(with **before**)* display, exhibit, *(with **down**)* chronicle, jot down, record, register, state, write down; *(with **forth**)* display, exhibit, explain, expound, manifest, promulgate, publish, put forward, represent, show; *(with **forward**)* advance, further, promote; *(with **free**)* acquit, clear, emancipate, liberate, release; *(with **off**)* adorn, decorate, embellish; define, portion off; *(with **on**)* actuate, encourage, impel, influence, incite, instigate, prompt, spur, urge; attack, assault, set upon; *(with **out**)* display, issue, publish, proclaim, prove, recommend, show; *(with **right**)* correct, put in order; *(with **to rights**)* adjust, regulate; *(with **up**)* elevate, erect, exalt, raise; establish, found, instate; *(with **upon**)* assail, assault, attack, fly at, rush upon. • *adj* appointed, established, formal, ordained, prescribed, regular, settled determined, fixed, firm, obstinate, positive, stiff, unyielding; immovable, predetermined; located, placed, put. • *n* attitude, position, posture; scene, scenery, setting.
set² *n* assortment, collection, suit; class, circle, clique, cluster, company, coterie, division, gang, group, knot, party, school, sect.
setback *n* blow, hitch, hold-up, rebuff, defeat, disappointment, reverse.
set-off *n* adornment, decoration, embellishment, ornament; counterbalance, counterclaim, equivalent.
settle *vb* adjust, arrange, compose, regulate; account, balance, close up, conclude, discharge, liquidate, pay, pay up, reckon, satisfy, square; allay, calm, compose, pacify, quiet, repose, rest, still, tranquillize; confirm, decide, determine, make clear; establish, fix, seat; fall, gravitate, sink, subside; abide, colonize, domicile, dwell, establish, inhabit, people, place, plant, reside; *(with **on**)* determine on, fix on, fix upon; establish. • *n* bench, seat, stool.
settled *adj* established, fixed, stable; decided, deep-rooted, steady, unchanging; adjusted, arranged; methodical, orderly, quiet; common, customary, everyday, ordinary, usual, wonted.
set-to *n* combat, conflict, contest, fight.
sever *vb* divide, part, rend, separate, sunder; detach, disconnect, disjoin, disunite.
several *adj* individual, single, particular; distinct, exclusive, independent, separate; different, divers, diverse, manifold, many, sundry, various.
severance *n* partition, separation.

superscript numeral identifies homographs

usage details

commas separate synonyms

semicolons separate the different senses of the headword

How to Use This Book

Canadian Entries

All words that have a Canadian connection are indicated by the symbol ❧.

e.g.:

salal /sə'læl/ *n* ❧ a shrub of western North America with pink or white flowers and edible purple-black berries.
mainstreet /'meɪnstriːt/ *v* ❧ (*Cdn*) to campaign in an election on the main streets of towns and cities.—**mainstreeter** *n*.—**mainstreeting** *n*.

Words which are specific Candianisms, or terms that were coined in Canada are indicated by the label (*Cdn*).

Alphabetical Order

Strict alphabetical order is followed. All compound words and hyphenated words are alphabetized as if they are one word.

Headwords that contain contractions, such as St, are alphabetized as would the whole word; thus St is alphabetized just as Saint would be.

e.g.:

Saint Bernard *n* a breed of large dog with a reddish brown coat, often used as a rescue dog.
sainted /'seɪntəd/ *adj* canonized; holy; dead; much admired.
St Jean Baptist Day *n* ❧ (*Cdn*) in Quebec, common and formerly official name of a public holiday celebrated on June 24.

Abbreviations and acronyms are alphabetized as if the abbreviation is a whole word.

Capitalized headwords come before lower case headwords.

Numerals take precedence over letters.

Variations

Variant spellings appear in bold type and in brackets next to the headword.

Other terms, of a different part of speech, that are related to the headword are given at the end of an entry in bold preceded by a dash.

Inflected forms of verbs and plural forms of nouns appear in bold and in brackets following the headword.

e.g.:

eat /iːt/ *vt* (**eating, ate,** *pp* **eaten**) to take into the mouth, chew and swallow as food; to have a meal; to consume, to destroy bit by bit; (*also with* **into**) to corrode; (*inf*) to bother, cause anxiety to; (*with* **up**) to consume completely; (*inf*) to listen or absorb avidly; (*inf*) to preoccupy. • *vi* (*with* **out**) to eat away from home, *esp* in a restaurant. • *n* (*pl: inf*) food.—**eater** *n*.

Parts of Speech

Parts of speech are indicated in italic by the abbreviations shown on page 8, and the bold headword .

Other parts of speech after the main headword are indicated by a full point (.) and •.

e.g.:

bang /bæŋ/ *n* a hard blow; a sudden loud sound. • *vt* to hit or knock with a loud noise; (*door*) to slam. • *vi* to make a loud noise; to hit noisily or sharply. • *adv* with a bang, abruptly; successfully; (*inf*) precisely.

Senses and Definitions

Within entries synonyms are separated by commas (,). Different senses are separated by semicolons (;). Parts of speech are separated by full points (.).

Homographs

Words of different origins but with the same spelling are give separate, numbered entries.

e.g.:

bank[1] /bæŋk/ *n* a mound or pile; the sloping side of a river; elevated ground in a lake or the sea; a row or series of objects, as of dials, switches. • *vti* to form into a mound; to cover (a fire) with fuel so that it burns more slowly; (*aircraft*) to curve or tilt sideways.
bank[2] *n* an institution that offers various financial services, such as the safekeeping, lending and exchanging of money; the money held by the banker or dealer in a card game; any supply or store for the future, such as a *blood bank*. • *vti* (*cheques, cash, etc*) to deposit in a bank; to work as a banker.

Abbreviations and Acronyms

Headwords which are abbreviations or acronyms appear with the label *abbr* and are followed by an equals sign (=). Where doubt arises over how the abbreviation might be pronounced – for example if it could be pronounced as an acronym would, as a word – pronunciation is given.

e.g.:

HC *abbr* = Holy Communion; House of Commons.
HCF *abbr* = highest common factor.
HIV /'eɪtʃ'aɪ'viː/ *abbr* = human immunodeficiency virus, the virus that causes Aids.

Pronunciation

Pronunciation is given using the International Phonetic Alphabet (IPA) between oblique strokes (//) and is Canadian.

Where native pronunciation differs from foreign pronunciation of some foreign words this pronunciation is also given and labelled.

e.g.:

hors d'oeuvre /ˌɔr'dərv/, *Fr.* /ɑr'dœvr/ *n* (*pl* **hors d'oeuvre, hors d'oeuvres**) an appetizer served at the beginning of a meal.

Where variations occur, for example on the end syllable of a word, this is indicated by a hyphen followed by the variation.

e.g.:

horse /hɔrs/ *n* a four-legged, solid-hoofed herbivorous mammal with a flowing mane and a tail, domesticated for carrying loads or riders, etc; cavalry; a vaulting horse; a frame with legs to support something.
horseflesh /-fleʃ/ *n* horses; the flesh of a horse, *esp* for eating.
horsehair /-her/ *n* hair from the mane or the tail of a horse, used for padding, etc.

Pronunciation is not given for compound word headwords if the words appear elsewhere in the dictionary.

Primary and secondary stress marks precede the relevant symbols, *see* Key to Phonetics section on page 7.

Register

Level of registers are indicated by the following labels: formal, informal, slang, derogatory ,dialect, offensive. *See* Abbreviations.

Key to Phonetic Symbols

Vowels

1. iː   as in **see** /siː/
2. i   as in **cosy** /koːzi/
3. ɪ   as in **pit** /pɪt/
4. ɛ   as in **ten** /tɛn/
5. æ   as in **absence** /æbsəns/
6. ɑ   as in **arm** /ɑrm/
7. ɒ   as in **hot** /hɒt/
8. ɔ   as in **abort** /əˈbɔrt/
9. oː   as in **roam** /roːm/
10. ʊ   as in **put** /pʊt/
11. uː as in **root** /ruːt/
12. ə   as in **ago** /əˈgoː/
13. ɐ   as in **cup** /kɐp/
14. eɪ as in **page** /peɪdʒ/
15. əɪ as in **light** /ləɪt/
16. aɪ as in **my** /maɪ/
17. aʊ as in **now** /naʊ/
18. ɐʊ as in **house** /hɐʊs/
19. ɔɪ as in **oil** /ɔɪl/

Consonants

1. p   as in **pet** /pɛt/
2. b   as in **black** /blæk/
3. t   as in **teak** /tiːk/
4. d   as in **den** /dɛn/
5. k   as in **cat** /kæt/
6. g   as in **got** /gɒt/
7. tʃ   as in **chin** /tʃɪn/
8. dʒ   as in **juice** /dʒuːs/
9. f   as in **foil** /fɔɪl/
10. v   as in **voice** /vɔɪs/
11. θ   as in **thick** /θɪk/
12. ð   as in **them** /ðɛm/
13. s   as in **so** /soː/
14. z   as in **zoo** /zuː/
15. ʃ   as in **she** /ʃiː/
16. ʒ   as in **vision** /ˈvɪʒən/
17. h   as in **how** /haʊ/
18. m   as in **man** /mæn/
19. n   as in **no** /noː/
20. ŋ   as in **ring** /rɪŋ/
21. l   as in **lip** /lɪp/
22. r   as in **red** /rɛd/
23. j   as in **yes** /jɛs/
24. w   as in **wet** /wɛt/

Foreign Sounds

1. ʏ as in French *couture* /kʊˈtʏr/. Pronounce /i/ with the lips rounded as for English /uː/.
2. ø as in French *berceuse* /ˌbɛrˈsøz/. Pronounce /ø/ as the initial sound /e/ in /eɪ/ with the lips rounded as in English /uː/.
3. œ as in French *chef-d'oeuvre* /ʃɛˈdœvr/. Pronounce /eɪ/ with the lips rounded, like /oː/.
4. a as in French *cabochon* /kaboʃõː/. Pronounce /ɛ/ with the tongue between the positions of English /æ/ and /ɑ/.
5. ɑ as in French *agent provocateur* /aˈʒãːprovokaˌtœr/. It is pronounced with the tongue a little forward, with lips rounded as in /ɔ/.
6. x as in Gaelic *loch* /lɒx/. Pronounce /k/ without closing the air passage completely, so that the air comes out with friction.
7. ʀ as in French *rouge* /ʀuːʒ/. It resembles the German *ach* but is produced further back in the throat.
8. ɾ as in Spanish *banderilla* /ˌbandeˈriːljɑ/. Pronounce ɾ by trilling the tip of the tongue.

/ː/ denotes a long vowel as in **peak** /piːk/
/˜/ denotes a vowel is nasalized as in French **bon** /bõː/
/ˈ/ denotes a primary stress preceding the relevant syllable as in **about** /əˈbɐut/
/ˌ/ denotes secondary stress preceding the relevant syllable as in **abattoir** /ˌæbəˈtwar/
(ə) The "ə" in parenthesis denotes optional pronunciation as is heard in some varieties of Canadian English.
/-/ Hyphens preceding and/or following parts of a repeated transcription indicate that only the transcribed part changes.

Abbreviations Used in This Book

abbr	abbreviation		*n*	noun
adj	adjective		*naut*	nautical
adv	adverb		*neut*	neuter
anat	anatomy		*news*	news media
approx	approximately		*nf*	noun feminine
arch	archaic		*npl*	noun plural
archit	architecture		*n sing*	noun singular
astrol	astrology		NT	New Testament
astron	astronomy		*obs*	obsolete
Austral	Australia, Australasia		*orig*	original, originally, origin
aux	auxiliary		OT	Old Testament
biol	biology		*p*	participle
bot	botany		*pers*	person, personal
Brit	Britain, British		*philos*	philosophy
c	circa, about		*photog*	photography
cap	capital		*pl*	plural
Cdn	Canadian		*poet*	poetical
cent	century		*poss*	possessive
chem	chemical, chemistry		*pp*	past participle
compar	comparative		*prep*	preposition
comput	computing		*pres t*	present tense
conj	conjunction		*print*	printing
demons	demonstrative		*pron*	pronoun
derog	derogatory, derogatorily		*pr p*	present participle
dimin	diminutive		*psychol*	psychology
econ	economics		*pt*	past tense
eg	*exempli gratis*, for example		RC	Roman Catholic
elect	electricity		*reflex*	reflexive
esp	especially		*Scot*	Scotland
fig	figuratively		*sing*	singular
geog	geography		*sl*	slang
geol	geology		*superl*	superlative
geom	geometry		*theat*	theatre
gram	grammar		*TV*	television
her	heraldry		*TM*	trademark
hist	history		*UK*	United Kingdom
ie	*id est*, that is		*US*	United States
imper	imperative		*USA*	United States of America
incl	including		*usu*	usually
inf	informal		*var*	variant
interj	interjection		*vb*	verb
math	mathematics		*vb aux*	auxiliary verb
mech	mechanics		*vi*	intransitive verb
med	medicine		*vt*	transitive verb
mil	military		*vti*	transitive or intransitive verb
mus	music		*vulg*	vulgar, vulgarly
myth	mythology		*zool*	zoology

DICTIONARY

A

A /eɪ/ *abbr* = ampere(s).

Å *abbr* = ångström(s).

a /ə/ or /eɪ/ *adj* the indefinite article; one; any; per

A¹ *adj* (*inf*) in perfect condition; physically fit; excellent.

AA *abbr* = Alcoholics Anonymous; anti-aircraft; Automobile Association.

AAA *abbr* = Automobile Association of America; Amateur Athletics Association.

aardvark /'ɑrdvɑrk/ *n* a nocturnal African mammal with a long snout that feeds on termites.

aardwolf /'ɑrdwulf/ *n* (*pl* **aardwolves** /'ɑrd,wulvz/) the earth wolf, a South African carnivore like a hyena.

AB *abbr* ✤ = Alberta.

ab- /əb/ or /æb/ *prefix* away, from, apart.

ab /æb/ *prep* from, as in *ab initio*.

abaca /'æbəkə/ *n* Manila hemp.

aback /ə'bæk/ *adv* **taken aback** startled.

abacus /'æbəkəs/ *n* (*pl* **abaci, abacuses**) a frame with sliding beads for doing arithmetic.

Abaddon /ə'bædən/ *n* a destroying angel, the devil; hell

abaft /ə'bæft/ *adv, prep* (*naut*) behind.

abalone /'æbə'loːni/ *n* an edible mollusc having an ear-shaped shell lined with mother-of-pearl.

abandon /ə'bændən/ *vt* to leave behind; to desert; to yield completely to an emotion or urge. • *n* freedom from inhibitions.—**abandonment** *n*.

abandoned /ə'bændənd/ *adj* (*behaviour*) showing abandon, unrestrained.—**abandonedly** *adv*.

abase /ə'beɪs/ *vt* to degrade, humiliate.—**abasement** /ə'beɪsmənt/ *n*.

abash /ə'bæʃ/ *vt* to cause a feeling of shame, embarrassment or confusion.—**abashment** /-mənt/ *n*.

abashed /ə'bæʃt/ *adj* ashamed, embarrassed.

abate /ə'beɪt/ *vti* to make or become less; (*law*) to end.—**abatement** *n*.

abatis /'æbətɪs/ *n* (*pl* **abatis, abatises** /'æbətiːz/) a defence work of fallen trees with the branches towards the enemy.

abattoir /'æbə,twɑr/ *n* a slaughterhouse.

abbacy /'æbəsi/ *n* (*pl* **abbacies** /'æbəsiːs/) the office or rights of an abbot.

abbatial /ə'beɪʃəl/ *adj* of an abbey or abbot.

abbé /æ'beɪ/ *n* a French ecclesiastic.

abbess /'æbes/ *n* the woman who heads a convent of nuns.

abbey /'æbi/ *n* a building occupied by monks or nuns; a church built as part of such a building; the community of monks or nuns.

abbot /'æbət/ *n* the head of an abbey of monks.

abbreviate /ə'briːvɪ,eɪt/ *vt* to make shorter, *esp* to shorten (a word) by omitting letters.

abbreviation /ə,briːvi'eɪʃən/ *n* the process of abbreviating; a shortened form of a word.

ABC¹ /,eɪbiː'siː/ *n* the alphabet; the basic facts of a subject.

ABC² *abbr* = American Broadcasting Corporation; Australian Broadcasting Corporation.

abdicate /'æbdɪ,keɪt/ *vti* to renounce an official position or responsibility, etc.—**abdication** *n*.

abdomen /'æbdəmən/ *n* the region of the body below the chest containing the digestive organs; the belly; (*insects, etc*) the section of the body behind the thorax.—**abdominal** /æb,dɒmənl/ *adj*.—**abdominally** *adv*.

abducent /æb'duːsənt/ or /əb-/, /-'djuːs/ *adj* (*anat*) (*limb, etc*) drawn from its natural position.

abduct /əb'dʌkt/ *vt* to carry off (a person) by force; (*anat*) to draw (a limb, etc) from its natural position—**abduction** *n*.—**abductor** *n*.

abeam /ə'biːm/ *adv* (*naut*) at right angles to a ship's length, abreast.

abecedarian /eɪbiːsiː'dɛrɪən/ *adj* of the ABC, elementary; arranged alphabetically. • *n* one learning the ABC, a beginner, a learner.

abed /ə'bed/ *adv* in bed.

abelmosk /'eɪblmɒsk/ *n* an Asian herb of the mallow family yielding musk.

aberrant /ə'berənt/ *adj* deviating from that regarded as normal or right.—**aberrance, aberrancy** /æ'berənsi/ *n*.

aberration /,æbə'reɪʃən/ *n* a deviation from the normal; a mental or moral lapse.

abet /ə'bet/ *vt* (**abetting, abetted**) to encourage or assist, *esp* to do wrong.—**abetment** *n*.—**abetter**, (*esp law*) **abettor** *n*.

abeyance /ə'beɪəns/ *n* (*usu* preceded by **in**) (*law, etc*) suspended temporarily.

abhor /əb'hɔr/ *vt* (**abhorring, abhorred**) to detest, despise.

abhorrence /əb'hɒrəns/ *n* detestation.

abhorrent /əb'hɒrənt/ *adj* detestable.

abide /ə'baɪd/ *vt* (**abiding, abode** or **abided**) to endure; to put up with.

abiding /ə'baɪdɪŋ/ *adj* permanent.—**abidingly** *adv*.

abigail /'æbɪgeɪl/ *n* a lady's maid.

ability /ə'bɪlɪti/ *n* (*pl* **abilities**) the state of being able being able; power to do; talent; skill.

ab initio /,æbi'nɪʃɪoʊ/ (*Latin*) from the beginning.

abiogenesis /,eɪbaɪoʊ'dʒenəsɪs/ *n* spontaneous generation.—**abiogenetic** *adj*.

abject /'æbdʒekt/ *adj* wretched; dejected.—**abjection** *n*.—**abjectly** *adv*.

abjure /əb'dʒʊr/ *vt* to renounce.—**abjuration** *n*.—**abjurer** *n*

ablactation /,æblæk'teɪʃən/ *n* the act of weaning a child from the breast.

ablate /æb'leɪt/ *vb* (**ablating, ablated**) *vb* to remove surgically; (*astrophysics*) to melt or vaporize when entering the earth's atmosphere; (*geol*) to erode, to waste or wear away.—**ablation** *n*.

ablative /'æblətɪv/ *adj* (*gram*) expressing source, instrumentality, etc; (*astrophysics*) ablating. • *n* one of the cases of Latin nouns, expressing chiefly separation and instrumentality and sometimes place.

ablative absolute *n* a particular construction in Latin of a noun and a participle in the ablative case, agreeing in gender and number, and forming a clause by themselves, but unconnected gramatically with the rest of the sentence.

ablaut /'æblaʊt/ *n* (*linguistics*) a vowel permutation, the change of a root vowel in the derivation of a word, as *do, did* or *sing, sang, sung, song.*

ablaze /ə'bleɪz/ *adj* burning, on fire.

-able /əbəl/ *adj suffix* capable of, as in suitable.

able 'eɪbəl/ *adj* having the competence or means (to do); talented; skilled.—**ably** *adv*.

able-bodied /'eɪbəl,bɒdɪd/ *adj* fit, strong.

able-bodied seaman *n* a trained seaman in the (merchant) navy.—*also* able seaman.

abloom /ə'bluːm/ *adv* in bloom, blooming.

ablution /ə'bluːʃən/ *n* (*usu pl*) a washing or cleansing of the body by water; the ritual cleansing of vessels or hands.—**ablutionary** *adj*.

ably /'eɪbli/ *adv* in an able manner.

ABM /,eɪbiː'em/ *abbr* = antiballistic missile.

abnegate /'æbnəgeɪt/ *vt* to deny oneself (a right, etc); to renounce.—**abnegation** *n*.

abnormal /æb'nɔrml/ *adj* unusual, not average or typical; irregular.—**abnormality** *n*.—**abnormally** *adv*.

abnormality /,æbnɔr'mælɪti/ *n* (*pl* **abnormalities**) deformity; irregularity; difference or departure from a regular type or rule.

aboard /ə'bɔrd/ *adv* on or in an aircraft, ship, train, etc.—*also prep*.

abode¹ /ə'boʊd/ *n* a home, residence.

abode² *see* abide.

abolish /ə'bɒlɪʃ/ *vt* to bring to an end, do away with.—**abolisher** *n*.—**abolishment** *n*.

abolition /,æbə'lɪʃən/ *n* the act of abolishing; (*with cap*) in UK, the ending of the slave trade (1807) or slavery (1833), in US, the emancipation of the slaves (1863).

abolitionist /,æbə'lɪʃənɪst/ *n* one who is in favour of the repeal or abolition of some existing law or custom; (*often with cap*) one in favour of abolition.

abomasum /ˌæbəˈmeɪsəm/ *n* (*pl* **abomasa**) the fourth stomach of a ruminant animal.—**abomasal** *adj*.

A-bomb /ˈeɪbɒm/ *n* atomic bomb.

abominable /əˈbɒmɪnəbl/ *adj* despicable, detestable; (*inf*) very unpleasant.—**abominably** *adv*.

abominable snowman *n* a huge creature of legend resembling a man or an animal, said to be found in the Himalayas.—*also* **yeti**.

abominate /əˈbɒmɪˌneɪt/ *vt* to abhor; to regard with feelings of disgust or hatred.—**abominator** *n*.

abomination /əˌbɒmɪˈneɪʃən/ *n* detestation; a loathsome person or thing.

aboriginal /ˌæbəˈrɪdʒənəl/ *adj* existing in a place from the earliest times; of aborigines. • *n* the species of animals or plants presumed to have originated within a given area.

aborigine /ˌæbəˈrɪdʒɪni/ *n* any of the first known inhabitants of a region; (*with cap*) one of the original inhabitants of Australia before the arrival of European settlers.

abort /əˈbɔːt/ *vti* to undergo or cause an abortion; to terminate or cause to terminate prematurely. • *n* the premature termination of a rocket flight, etc.

abortion /əˈbɔːʃən/ *n* the premature expulsion of a foetus, *esp* if induced on purpose.

abortionist /əˈbɔːʃənɪst/ *n* a person who performs abortions, *esp* illegally.

abortive /əˈbɔːtɪv/ *adj* failing in intended purpose; fruitless; causing abortion.—**abortively** *adv*.

aboulia /əˈbuːlɪə/ or /-ˈbjuː-/ *see* **abulia**.

abound /əˈbaʊnd/ *vi* to be in abundance; to have in great quantities.

about /əˈbaʊt/ *prep* on all sides of; near to; with; on the point of; concerning. • *adv* all around; near; to face the opposite direction.

about-turn, about-face *n* a complete reversal in direction or opinion, etc. • *vi* to make an about-turn.

above /əˈbʌv/ *prep* over, on top of; better or more than; beyond the reach of; too complex to understand. • *adv* in or to a higher place; in addition; (*text*) mentioned earlier.

aboveboard /əˈbʌvˌbɔːd/ *adj, adv* without trickery; in open sight.

abracadabra /ˌæbrəkəˈdæbrə/ *n* a cabbalistic word used as a charm, a spell; gibberish.

abradant /æˈbreɪdənt/ *adj* having the property of rubbing away. • *n* a substance employed for abrading or scouring.

abrade /əˈbreɪd/ *vt* to wear or rub away; to remove as by friction or abrasion; to corrode, as by acids.—**abrader** *n*.

abranchiate /eɪˈbræŋkiːɪt/ or /-kɪeɪt/, **abranchial** *adj* (*zool*) devoid of gills. • *n* an animal without gills.

abrasion /əˈbreɪʒən/ *n* the act or process of rubbing away by friction, etc; a scraped area, *esp* on the body.

abrasive /əˈbreɪsɪv/ *adj* causing abrasion; harsh, irritating. • *n* a substance or tool used for grinding or polishing, etc.—**abrasively** *adv*.

abreact /ˌæbrɪˈækt/ *vt* (*psychoanal*) to remove (a complex) by acting it out or talking it out.—**abreaction** *n*.—**abreactive** *adj*.

abreast /əˈbrest/ *adv* side by side and facing the same way; informed (of); aware.

abridge /əˈbrɪdʒ/ *vt* to shorten by using fewer words but keeping the substance.

abridgment, abridgement /əˈbrɪdʒmənt/ *n* the state of being contracted or curtailed; a shortened version of a text; an epitome.

abroach /əˈbroːtʃ/ *adj, adv* letting out; broached, pierced so as to let the liquor run.

abroad /əˈbrɔːd/ *adv* in or to a foreign country; over a wide area; out in the open; in circulation, current.

abrogate /ˈæbrəˌɡeɪt/ *vt* to repeal, cancel.—**abrogator** *n*.

abrogation /ˌæbrəˈɡeɪʃən/ *n* the act of abrogating; the repeal or annulling of a law.

abrupt /əˈbrʌpt/ *adj* sudden; unexpected; curt.—**abruptly** *adv*.—**abruptness** *n*.

abruption /æbˈrʌpʃən/ or /əb-/ *n* a separation with violence; a sudden or abrupt termination.

abscess /ˈæbses/ *n* an inflamed area of the body containing pus.

abscissa /əbˈsɪsə/ *n* (*pl* **abscissas, abscissae**) (*geom*) one of the two coordinates fixing the position of a point.

abscission /əbˈsɪʒən/ *n* the act of severance; (*bot*) the shedding of parts; the breaking off in a sentence, leaving the rest to be implied.

abscond /əbˈskɒnd/ *vi* to hide, run away, *esp* to avoid punishment for a wrongdoing.

abseil /ˈæbseɪl/ or /-zaɪl/ *vi* to descend a rock face by means of a double rope attached to a higher point.—**abseiling** *n*.

absence /ˈæbsəns/ *n* the state of not being present; the time of this; a lack; inattention.

absent[1] /ˈæbsənt/ *adj* not present; not existing; inattentive.—**absently** *adv*.

absent[2] /æbˈsent/ *vt* to keep (oneself) away.

absentee /ˌæbsənˈtiː/ *n* a person who is absent, as from work or school.

absenteeism /ˌæbsənˈtiːɪzəm/ *n* persistent absence from work, school, etc.

absently /ˈæbsəntli/ *adv* in an abstracted manner.

absent-minded /ˌæbsəntˈmaɪndəd/ *adj* inattentive; forgetful.

absinthe, absinth /ˈæbsɪnθ/ *n* a potent, green, brandy-based liqueur flavoured with wormwood.

absit omen /ˌæbsɪtˈoːmen/ *interj* (*Latin*) may the foreboding caused by some unlucky word or event not come to pass.

absolute /ˈæbsəˌluːt/ or /ˌæbsəˈluːt/ *adj* unrestricted, unconditional; complete; positive; perfect; pure; not relative; (*monarch, ruler, etc*) authoritarian, despotic; (*inf*) utter, out-and-out.

absolutely /ˈæbsəˌluːtli/ or /ˌæbsəˈluːtli/ *adv* completely; unconditionally; (*inf*) I completely agree, certainly.

absolution /ˌæbsəˈluːʃən/ *n* forgiveness; remission of sin or its penalty.

absolutism /ˈæbsəluːˌtɪzəm/ *n* the state of being absolute; the principle or system of absolute government.—**absolutist** *n, adj*.

absolve /əbˈzɒlv/ or /-ˈsɒlv/ *vt* to clear from guilt or blame; to give religious absolution to; to free from a duty, obligation, etc.

absolver /əbˈzɒlvər/ or /-ˈsɒl-/ *n* one who absolves, or pronounces absolution.

absorb /əbˈzɔːb/ *vt* to take in; to soak up; to incorporate; to pay for (costs, etc); to take in (a shock) without recoil; to occupy one's attention or interest completely.—**absorber** *n*.—**absorptive** *adj*.

absorbable /əbˈzɔːbeɪbəl/ *adj* capable of being absorbed.—**absorbability** *n*.

absorbefacient /əbˈzɔːbɪˌfeɪsɪənt/ or /-sənt/ *adj* inducing or causing absorption. • *n* something that causes absorption.

absorbent /əbˈzɔːbənt/ *adj* capable of absorbing moisture, etc.—**absorbency** *n*.

absorbent cotton *n* raw cotton that has been bleached and sterilized for use as a dressing, etc.—*also* **cotton wool**.

absorbing /əbˈzɔːbɪŋ/ *adj* engrossing.—**absorbingly** *adv*.

absorption /əbˈzɔːpʃən/ *n* the process or act of absorbing; the state of being absorbed; entire preoccupation of the mind.—**absorptive** *adj*.

absorption lines *npl* dark lines in the spectrum produced by the absorption of cool vapours through which the light has passed.

absorptivity /əbˈzɔːpˌtɪvɪti/ *n* the power of absorption; (*physics*) the rate of absorption of radiation by a material.

abstain /əbˈsteɪn/ *vi* to keep oneself from some indulgence, *esp* from drinking alcohol; to refrain from using one's vote.

abstainer /-ər/ *n* one who abstains, especially from intoxicants.

abstemious /æbˈstiːmɪəs/ *adj* sparing in consuming food or alcohol.—**abstemiously** *adv*.—**abstemiousness** *n*.

abstention /əbˈstenʃən/ *n* the act of holding off or abstaining; the withholding of a vote.—**abstentious** *adj*.—**abstentionist** *n*.

abstergent /æbˈstɜːdʒənt/ *adj* possessing cleansing or purging properties. • *n* that which cleanses or purges; a detergent.

abstinence /ˈæbstɪnəns/ *n* an abstaining or refraining, *esp* from food or alcohol.

abstinent /ˈæbstɪnənt/ *adj* refraining from over-indulgence, *esp* with regard to food and drink. • *n* an abstainer.—**abstinently** *adv*.

abstract /ˈæbstrækt/ *adj* having no material existence; theoretical; (*art*) non-representational. • *n* (*writing, speech*) a summary or condensed version. • *vt* to remove or extract; to separate; to summarize.

abstract noun /-naʊn/ *n* the name of a state or quality considered apart from the object to which it belongs.

abstracted /əbˈstræktəd/ *adj* not paying attention.—**abstractedly** *adv*.—**abstractedness** *n*.

abstraction /əbˈstrækʃən/ *n* preoccupation, inattention; an abstract concept.—**abstractive** *adj*.

abstractionism /əbˈstrækʃəˌnɪzəm/ *n* the theory and art of the abstract, *esp* non-representational painting.—**abstractionist** *adj, n*.

abstruse /əbˈstruːs/ *adj* obscure; hidden; difficult to comprehend; profound.—**abstrusely** *adv*.—**abstruseness** *n*.

absurd /əb'sɜrd/ or /-'zɜrd/ adj against reason or common sense; ridiculous.—**absurdly** adv.

absurdity /əb'sɜrditi/ or /-'zɜrd-/ n (pl **absurdities**) the state of being absurd; that which is absurd.

abulia n /ə'bu:liə/ n (psychol) loss of willpower.—also **aboulia**.—**abulic** adj.

abundance /ə'bʌndəns/ n a plentiful supply; a considerable amount.

abundant /ə'bʌndənt/ adj plentiful; rich (in).—**abundantly** adv.

abuse /ə'bju:z/ vt to make wrong use of; to mistreat; to insult, attack verbally. • n misuse; mistreatment; insulting language; immoderate or illegal use of drugs or other stimulants.—**abuser** n.

abusive /ə'bju:sɪv/ adj insulting.—**abusively** adv.—**abusiveness** n.

abut /ə'bʌt/ vi (**abutting, abutted**) to adjoin, border or lean (on, against).

abutment /-mənt/, **abuttal** /-əl/ n that which borders upon something else; the solid structure that supports the extremity of a bridge or arch.

abutter /ə'bʌtər/ n (law) the owner of an adjoining property.

abuzz /ə'bʌz/ adv filled with buzzing sounds; active, alive.

abysm /ə'bɪzm/ n (arch) an abyss, a gulf.

abysmal /ə'bɪzməl/ adj extremely bad, deplorable.—**abysmally** adv.

abyss /ə'bɪs/ n a bottomless depth; anything too deep to measure; hell.

abyssal /ə'bɪsəl/ adj pertaining to oceanic depths.

AC, ac abbr = alternating current.

Ac (chem symbol) actinium.

a/c abbr = account; account current.

ac- /ək/ prefix the form of ad- before c, k, g.

acacia /ə'keɪʃə/ n a genus of shrubby or arboreous leguminous plants of warmer regions with white or yellow flowers, several species of which yield gum.

academic /ˌækə'demɪk/ adj pertaining to a school, college or university; scholarly; purely theoretical in nature. • n a member of a college or university; a scholarly person.

academically /ˈækədemɪkəli/ adv theoretically, unpractically.

academician /ˌækədə'mɪʃən/ or /əˌkædə'mɪʃən/ n a member of an Academy.

academy /ə'kædəmi/ n (pl **academies**) a school for specialized training; (Scot) a secondary school; (with cap) a society of scholars, writers, scientists, etc.

Acadian /ə'keɪdiən/ n ✤ one of the settlers in the former French colony of Acadia, or a descendant in the Maritime Provinces of Canada, southeast Quebec, or eastern Maine. • adj of Acadia, a region of Canada, Nova-Scotian.

acanthine /ə'kænθɪn/ or /-ˌθaɪn/, /ˌθi:n/ adj pertaining to or resembling the plant acanthus. • n ornamentation in the shape of the acanthus leaf.

acanthus /ə'kænθəs/ n (pl **acanthuses, acanthi**) a genus of herbaceous plants with sharp-toothed leaves; (archit) ornamentation adopted in the capitals of the Corinthian and Composite orders, and resembling the foliage of the acanthus.

a cappella /ˌɑ:kə'pelə/ or /ˌækə-/ adv (mus) after the style of church or chapel music, without accompaniment.

acarid /'ækərɪd/ n a tick or mite of the Acarina order of insects, etc, in which the divisions of head, thorax and abdomen are not apparent.—also adj.

acarpellous, acarpelous /eɪ'kɑ:rpələs/ adj (bot) without carpels.

acarpous /eɪ'kɑ:rpəs/ adj (bot) not producing fruit; sterile or barren.

acatalectic /eɪˌkætə'lektɪk/ adj (verse) with a complete number of syllables, not catalectic. —also n.

acaudal /eɪ'kɔ:dəl/, **acaudate** /eɪ'kɔ:deɪt/ adj (zool) without a tail.

acaulescent /eɪˌkɔ:'lesənt/ adj (bot) stemless or with a very short stem.—**acaulescence** n.

acc. abbr = according; account; accusative.

Accadian /ə'keɪdiən/ see Akkadian.

ACCC abbr ✤ = Association of Canadian Community Colleges.

accede /æk'si:d/ vi to take office; to agree or assent to (a suggestion).

accelerando /əkˌselə'rændo:/ or /əˌtʃel-/ adv, adj (mus) with gradual increase of speed. • n (pl **accelerandos**) a piece of music played in this way.

accelerate /ək'seləˌreɪt/ vti to move faster; to happen or cause to happen more quickly; to increase the velocity of (a vehicle, etc).—**accelerative, acceleratory** adj.

acceleration /əkˌselə'reɪʃən/ n the act of accelerating or condition of being accelerated; the rate of increase in speed or change in velocity; the power of accelerating.

accelerator /ək'seləˌreɪtər/ n a device for increasing speed; a throttle; (physics) an apparatus that imparts high velocities to elementary particles.

accent /'æksənt/ n emphasis on a syllable or word; a mark used to indicate this; any way of speaking characteristic of a region, class, or an individual; the emphasis placed on something; rhythmic stress in music or verse. • vt to express the accent, or denote the vocal division of a word by stress or modulation of the voice; to pronounce; to mark or accent a word in writing by use of a sign; to dwell upon or emphasize, as a passage of music.

accentuate /ək'sentʃuˌeɪt/ vt to emphasize.

accentuation /ækˌsentʃu'eɪʃən/ n the act of accentuating by stress or accent; speaking or writing with emphasis or distinction.

accept /ək'sept/ vt to receive, esp willingly; to approve; to agree to; to believe in; to agree to pay.

acceptable /ək'septəbəl/ or adj satisfactory; welcome; tolerable.—**acceptability** n.—**acceptably** adv.

acceptance /ək'septəns/ n the act of accepting; the act of being accepted or received with approbation; agreement; the subscription to a bill of exchange; the bill accepted or the sum contained in it.

acceptation /ˌæksep'teɪʃən/ n the act of accepting or state of being accepted or acceptable; the meaning or sense of a word or statement in which it is to be understood.

accepter, acceptor /ək'septər/ n one who accepts; the person who accepts a bill of exchange.

access /'ækses/ n approach, or means of approach; the right to enter, use, etc. • vt (comput) to retrieve (information) from a storage device; to gain access to.

accessible /ək'sesəbəl/ adj able to be reached; open (to).—**accessibility** n.—**accessibly** adv.

accession /ək'seʃən/ n the act of reaching or assuming a rank or position.—**accessiona** adj.

accessory /ək'sesəri/ adj additional; extra. • n (pl **accessories**) a supplementary part or item, esp of clothing; a person who aids another in a crime.—**accessorial** adj.

acciaccatura /ə'tʃækə'tuːrə/ n (pl **acciaccaturas, acciaccature**) a half-note or grace note below the principal note, struck at the same time as the principal note and immediately released while the latter is held.

accidence /'æksɪdəns/ n (linguistics) the part of grammar that deals with the inflections of words, which are accidents, not essentials; a book containing the rudiments of grammar; the rudiments themselves.

accident /'æksɪdənt/ n an unexpected event; a mishap or misfortune, esp one resulting in death or injury; chance.

accidental /ˌæksɪ'dentəl/ adj occurring or done by accident; non-essential; (mus) a sign prefixed to a note indicating a departure from the key signature —**accidentally** adv.

accidie /'æksɪdi/ n sloth, torpor, apathy.

accipiter /ək'sɪpɪtər/ n a generic name for birds of prey, as the common hawk.

accipitrine /-aɪn/ adj hawk-like, rapacious.

acclaim /ə'kleɪm/ vt to praise publicly (the merits of a person or thing); to welcome enthusiastically. ✤ (Cdn) elect without opposition. • vi to shout approval. • n a shout of welcome or approval.

acclamation /ˌæklə'meɪʃən/ n a shout of applause or other demonstration of hearty approval, loud united assent; an outburst of joy or praise; the adoption of a resolution viva voce; a mode of papal election. ✤ (Cdn) the act or fact of being elected without opposition.—**acclamatory** adj.

acclimatize /ə'klaɪməˌtaɪz/ vt to adapt to a new climate or environment. • vi to become acclimatized.—**acclimatization** n.

acclivity /ə'klɪvɪti/ n (pl **acclivities**) an ascent or upward slope of the earth; the talus of a rampart.—**acclivitous** adj.

accolade /'ækəˌleɪd/ n praise; approval; an award; a ceremonial touch on the shoulder with a sword to confer knighthood.

accommodate /ə'kɒməˌdeɪt/ vt to provide lodging for; to oblige; supply; to adapt, harmonize.

accommodating /-ɪŋ/ adj obliging, willing to help.—**accommodatingly** adv.

accommodation /əˌkɒmə'deɪʃən/ n lodgings; the process of adapting; willingness to help.

accommodation bill n a bill or note endorsed by one or more parties to enable the drawer to raise money upon it.

accommodation ladder *n* a ladder or stairway suspended at the gangway of a ship.

accommodative /əˈkɒməˌdeɪtɪv/ *adj* disposed or tending to accommodate.

accompaniment /əˈkʌmpənɪmənt/ *n* an instrumental part supporting a solo instrument, a voice, or a choir; something that accompanies.

accompanist, accompanyist /əˈkʌmpənɪst/ *n* one who plays a musical accompaniment.

accompany /əˈkʌmpəni/ *vt* (**accompanying, accompanied**) (*person*) to go with; (*something*) to supplement.

accomplice /əˈkɒmplɪs/ *n* a partner, *esp* in committing a crime.

accomplish /əˈkɒmplɪʃ/ *vt* to succeed in carrying out; to fulfil.

accomplished /-plɪʃd/ *adj* done; completed; skilled, expert; polished.

accomplishment /-plɪʃmənt/ *n* a skill or talent; the act of accomplishing; something accomplished.

accord /əˈkɔːd/ *vi* to agree; to harmonize (with). • *vt* to grant. • *n* consent; harmony.

accordance /əˈkɔːdəns/ *n* agreement; conformity.

accordant /əˈkɔːdənt/ *adj* corresponding; of the same mind.

according /əˈkɔːdɪŋ/ *prep* as stated by or in; (*with* **to**) in conformity with; (*with* **as**) depending on whether. • *adj* agreeing, harmonious.

accordingly /-li/ *adv* consequently; therefore; suitably.

accordion /əˈkɔːdiən/ *n* a portable keyboard instrument with manually operated folding bellows that force air through metal reeds.—**accordionist** *n*.

accost /əˈkɒst/ *vt* to approach and speak to, often to accuse of crime or to solicit sexually.

account /əˈkaʊnt/ *n* a description; an explanatory statement; a business record or statement; a credit arrangement with a bank, department store, etc; importance, consequence. • *vt* to think of or consider. • *vi* to give a financial reckoning (to); (*with* **for**) to give reasons (for); (*with* **for**) to kill, dispose of.

accountable /əˈkaʊntəbəl/ *adj* liable; responsible; explainable.—**accountability** *n*.—**accountably** *adv*.

accountancy /əˈkaʊntənsi/ *n* the profession or practice of an accountant.

accountant /əˈkaʊntənt/ *n* one whose profession is auditing business accounts.

account book *n* a book for the entering of accounts, or in which particulars of sales, purchases, etc, are kept.

accounting /əˈkaʊntɪŋ/ *n* the maintaining or auditing of detailed business accounts; accountancy.

accoutre, accouter /əˈkuːtər/ *vt* to dress; to equip; to array in military dress; to furnish with accoutrements.—**accoutrement, accouterment** *n*.

accoutrements, accouterments /əˈkuːtərmənts/ or /-ˈkuːtrə-/ *npl* equipage; dress; military equipment.

accredit /əˈkrɛdɪt/ *vt* to give credit or authority to; to have confidence in; to authorize; to stamp with authority; to believe and accept as true.—**accreditation** /-teɪʃən/ *n*.

accredited /-əd/ *adj* authorized officially; accepted as valid; certified as being of a prescribed quality.

accrescent /əˈkrɛsənt/ *adj* (*bot*) increasing; growing.

accrete /əˈkriːt/ *vi* to adhere, to grow together; to be added. • *vt* to cause to grow or unite. • *adj* (*bot*) grown into one.

accretion /əˈkriːʃən/ *n* an increase by natural growth; the addition of external parts; the growing together of parts or members naturally separate.—**accretive, accretionary** *adj*.

accrue /əˈkruː/ *vi* (**accruing, accrued**) to come as a natural increase or addition; (*money, etc*) to accumulate or be added periodically.—**accrual, accrument** *n*.

accumbent /əˈkʌmbənt/ *adj* (*bot*) reclining or recumbent; (*hist*) of the Roman style of reclining on a couch at meals.—**accumbency** *n*.

accumulate /əˈkjuːmjʊˌleɪt/ *vti* to collect together in increasing quantities, to amass.

accumulation /əˌkjuːmjʊˈleɪʃən/ *n* the act of accumulating or amassing; the addition of interest to principal; the mass accumulated.

accumulative /əˈkjuːmjʊlətɪv/ *adj* cumulative; acquisitive.

accumulator /əˈkjuːmjʊˌleɪtər/ *n* a rechargeable battery; (*horseracing*) a bet that accumulates in value over successive races; (*comput*) a storage register.

accuracy /ˈækjʊrəsi/ *n* (*pl* **accuracies**) the quality of being accurate; exactness or correctness.

accurate /ˈækjərət/ *adj* conforming with the truth or an accepted standard; done with care, exact.—**accurately** *adv*.

accursed, accurst /əˈkɜːsəd/ or /əˈkɜːst/ *adj* under or subject to a curse; ill-fated, doomed to destruction; detestable; execrable.

accusation /ˌækjuːˈzeɪʃən/ *n* the act of accusing or being accused; an allegation; the charge of guilt brought against a person.

accusative /əˈkjuːzətɪv/ *n* (*gram*) the case expressing the direct object of a word.

accusatorial /əˌkjuːzəˈtɔːriəl/, **accusatory** /əˈkjuːzəˌtɔːri/ *adj* accusing, or containing an accusation; (*of legal procedure*) in which prosecutor and judge are not the same (opposite to inquisitorial).

accuse /əˈkjuːz/ *vt* to charge with a crime, fault, etc; to blame.—**accuser** *n*.—**accusingly** *adv*.

accused /əˈkjuːzd/ *n* (*law*) (*with* **the**) the defendant in court facing a criminal charge.

accuser /-zər/ *n* one who accuses; one who formally charges an offence against another.

accustom /əˈkʌstəm/ *vt* to make used (to) by habit, use, or custom.

accustomed /əˈkʌstəmd/ *adj* usual, customary; used to.

ace /eɪs/ *n* the one spot in dice, playing cards, dominoes, etc; a point won by a single stroke, as in tennis; an expert. • *adj* (*inf*) excellent.

-acea /ˈeɪʃə/ *n suffix* forming the plural names for orders of animals, *eg* Crustacea, Crustaceae.

-aceae /ˈeɪsiiː/ *n suffix* forming plural names for families of plants, *eg* Rosaceae.

acedia /əˈsiːdiə/ *n* an abnormal condition of the mind, characterized by lassitude, listlessness, and general indifference.

acentric /eɪˈsɛntrɪk/ *adj* away from the centre; having no centre.

acephalous /əˈsɛfələs/ *adj* headless; without a leader; an ovary of a plant that has its style springing from the base instead of the apex.

acerbic /əˈsɜːbɪk/ *adj* bitter and harsh to the taste; astringent.

acerbity /əˈsɜːbɪti/ *n* (*pl* **acerbities**) sharpness of speech or manner; (of taste) bitterness.

acerose /ˈæsərˌoːz/ *adj* (*bot*) like a needle, very narrow, rigid, and tapering to a point.

acervate /əsərˌvɪt/ or /-ˌveɪt/ *adj* growing in closely compacted clusters.

acet-, aceto- /əˈsiːt/ or /ˈsɛt/, /ˈæsɛt/ *prefix* vinegar.

acetabulum /ˌæsəˈtæbjʊləm/ *n* (*pl* **acetabula, acetabulums**) the cavity of the hip bone into which the femur fits; one of the cup-like suckers on the arms of the cuttlefish; the posterior sucker of the leech; the saucer-shaped fructification of certain lichens; the receptacle of various fungi; a cup to hold vinegar.

acetanilide /ˌæsəˈtænɪlaɪd/, **acetanilid** /-ˌlɪd/ *n* a pungent white powder, formed by the action of acetyl choride on aniline, used in medicine as an antipyretic.

acetate /ˈæsəˌteɪt/ *n* a salt or ester of acetic acid; a fabric made from cellulose acetate.

acetic /əˈsiːtɪk/ *adj* of acetic acid or vinegar.

acetic acid *n* a clear liquid with a strong acid taste and sharp smell, present in a dilute form in vinegar.

acetify /əˈsɛtəˌfaɪ/ or /-ˈsiːt-/ *vt* (**acetifying, acetifed**) to turn into vinegar.—**acetification** *n*.—**acetifier** *n*.

acetometer /ˈæsɪˌtɒmətər/ *n* an instrument for gauging the strength or purity of vinegar or acetic acid.

acetone /ˈæsəˌtoːn/ *n* a clear flammable liquid used as a solvent.

acetous /ˈæsətəs/, **acetose** /-ˌtoːs/ *adj* of the nature of vinegar; sour; causing acetification.

acetylene /əsɛtɪˈliːn/ *n* a gas that burns with a hot flame, used for welding, etc.

Achates /əˈkɒtiːz/ *n* a faithful friend, from Aeneas's friend in Virgil's *Aeneid*.

ache /eɪk/ *n* a dull, continuous pain. • *vi* to suffer a dull, continuous mental or physical pain; (*inf*) to yearn.—**achy** *adj*.

achieve /əˈtʃiːv/ *vt* to perform successfully, accomplish; to gain, win. —**achievable** *adj*.—**achiever** *n*.

achievement /əˈtʃiːvmənt/ *n* a thing achieved, *esp* by great effort, courage, determination, etc; accomplishment; (*her*) an escutcheon in memory of a distinguished feat.

Achilles' heel *n* a person's vulnerable or weak point.

Achilles' tendon *n* a tendon attaching the heel to the calf muscles.

achlamydeous /ˌækləˈmɪdiəs/ *adj* having neither calyx nor corolla.

achromatic /ˌækrəˈmætɪk/ *adj* colourless; transmitting light without decomposing it.—**achromatically** *adv*.—**achromaticity, achromatism** *n*.

achromatize /əˈkroːməˌtaɪz/ vt to deprive of the power of transmitting colour; to render achromatic.—**achromatization** n.

acicula /əˌsɪkjuːlə/ n (pl **aciculae**) a spine or prickle.

acicular /əˌsɪkjulər/ adj needle-shaped.

aciculate /əˌsɪkjuˌlɪt/ or /-ˌleɪt/, **aciculated** /-ɪd/ adj in the shape of a needle; acicular.

acid /ˈæsɪd/ adj sharp, tart, sour; bitter. • n a sour substance; (chem) a corrosive substance that turns litmus red; (sl) LSD.—**acidly** adv.

acid house /-ˌhʊs/ n a party where people dance to House music; the style of popular music played.

acidic /əˈsɪdɪk/ adj containing a large proportion of the acid element; opposed to basic.

acidifier /ɒˈsɪdɪˌfaɪər/ or /-faɪr/ n a substance having the property of imparting an acid quality.

acidify /əˈsɪdɪˌfaɪ/ vti (**acidifying, acidified**) to make or become acid.—**acidification** n.

acidimeter /ˌæsəˈdɪmətər/ n an instrument for measuring the strength of acids.—**acidimetric** /ˈæˌsɪdɪˌmetrɪk/ adj.—**acidimetrically** /-ˌkəli/ adv.—**acidimetry** n.

acidity /əˈsɪdɪti/ n (pl **acidities**) the quality or condition of being acid.

acidosis /ˌæsɪˈdoːsɪs/ n an acid condition of the blood.—**acidotic** adj.

acid rain /-ˌreɪn/ n rain made acidic by air pollution from power stations, etc.

acid test /-ˌtest/ n a crucial or conclusive test.

acidulate /əˈsɪdjuˌleɪt/ vt to render slightly acid. • adj acidulous.—**acidulation** n.

acidulous /əˈsɪdjuləs/, **acidulent** /æˈsɪdjulənt/ adj somewhat acid; tart; peevish.

acierate /æˈsiːəˌreɪt/ vt (**acierating** /-ɪŋ/, **acierated** /-ɪd/) to change into steel.—**acieration** n.

acinaciform /æˌsəˈnæsəˌfɔrm/ adj (bot) resembling a scimitar in shape, as an acinaciform leaf or pod.

aciniform /əˈsɪnəˌfɔrm/ adj grape-like; clustered like grapes.

-acious /ˈeɪʃəs/ adj suffix forming adjectives meaning full of, inclined to, as mendacious.

-acity /ˈæsɪti/ n suffix forming corresponding nouns of quality, as mendacity.

acknowledge /əkˈnɒlɪdʒ/ vt to admit that something is true and valid; to show that one has noticed or recognized.

acknowledgment, acknowledgement /-mənt/ n the act of acknowledging; the admission or recognition of a truth; confession; the expression of appreciation of a favour or benefit conferred; a printed recognition by an author of others' works used or referred to; a receipt.

aclinic line /əˈklɪnɪk/ n the imaginary point near the equator where the magnetic needle has no dip, the magnetic equator.

acme /ˈækmi/ n the peak or highest point; the height of perfection.

acne /ˈækni/ n inflammation of the skin glands producing pimples.

acolyte /ˈækəˌlaɪt/ n an assistant or follower, esp of a priest.

aconite /ˈækəˌnaɪt/, **aconitum** /-nɪtəm/ n the plant wolf's-bane or monk's-hood; the drug prepared from the plant.—**aconitic** adj.

acorn /ˈeɪˈkɔrn/ n the nut of the oak tree.

acotyledon /ˌeɪˌkɒtˈliːdn/ n (bot) a plant with seeds (spores) that have no cotyledons (seed lobes).—**acotyledonous** adj.

acoustic /əˈkuːstɪk/, **acoustical** /-kəl/ adj of the sense of hearing or sound; of acoustics; (mus) not amplified, eg a guitar.—**acoustically** adv.

acoustician /ˌækuːsˈtiːʃən/ n one skilled in the study of acoustics.

acoustics /əˈkuːstɪks/ npl (room, concert hall, etc) properties governing how clearly sounds can be heard in it; (in sing) the physics of sound.—**acoustician** n.

acquaint /əˈkweɪnt/ vt to make (oneself) familiar (with); to inform; (with **with**) to introduce (to).

acquaintance /əˈkweɪntəns/ n a person whom one knows only slightly.

acquainted /əˈkweɪntəd/ adj having personal knowledge; (with **of, with**) familiar, known.

acquiesce /ˌæˈkwiˌes/ vi (with **in**) to comply with readily, or put up no opposition to.

acquiescence /ˌæˈkwiˌesəns/ n compliance; assent.—**acquiescent** adj.

acquire /əˈkwaɪr/ vt to gain by one's own efforts; to obtain.—**acquirable** adj.

acquirement /ˌæˈkwaɪrˌmənt/ n the act of acquiring; that which is acquired; mental attainment.

acquisition /ˌækwɪˈzɪʃən/ or /ˈækwəˌzɪʃən/ n the act of gaining, acquiring; someone or something that is acquired, often of special worth or talent.

acquisitive /əˈkwɪzətɪv/ adj eager or greedy for possessions.—**acquisitively** adv.—**acquisitiveness** n.

acquit /əˈkwɪt/ vt (**acquitting, acquitted**) to free from an obligation; to behave or conduct (oneself); to declare innocent.

acquittal /əˈkwɪtl/ n the act of releasing or acquitting, the state of being acquitted; a judicial discharge from accusation; the performance (of duty).

acquittance /əˈkwɪtəns/ n a discharge or release from debt or other liability; a receipt barring a further demand.

acre /ˈeɪkər/ n land measuring 4840 square yards.

acreage /ˈeɪkərɪdʒ/ n area measured in acres.

acrid /ˈækrɪd/ adj sharp and bitter of taste or smell; caustic, critical in attitude or speech.—**acridity** n.—**acridly** adv.

acrimony /ˈækrɪˌmoːni/ n pl **acrimonies** bitterness of manner or language.—**acrimonious** adj.—**acrimoniously** adv.

acro- /ˈækroː/ or /ˈækrə/ prefix topmost, extreme.

acrobat /ˈækrəˌbæt/ n a skilful performer of spectacular gymnastic feats.—**acrobatic** adj.—**acrobatically** adv.

acrobatics /ˌækrəˈbætɪks/ npl acrobatic feats.

acrocarpous /ˌækrəˈkɑrpəs/ adj (bot) having (like the mosses) the fruit at the end of the primary axis.

acrogen /ˈækrəˌdʒən/ n (bot) a nonflowering plant increasing by growth from the top, as ferns and mosses.—**acrogenic, acrogenous** adj.

acrolith /ˈækrəˌlɪθ/ n a sculptured figure, with head and extremities of stone and the rest of wood.

acromegaly /ˌækrəˈmegə i/ n a hormonal disease resulting in overdeveopment of the extremities.—**acromegalic** adj.

acronycal, acronical /əˈkrɒnəˌkəl/ adj (astron) (stars) rising at sunset and setting at sunrise.

acronym /ˈækrənɪm/ n a word formed from the initial letters of other words (as laser).

acrophobia /ˌækrəˈfoːbiə/ n dread of heights.—**acrophobe** n.—**acrophobic** adj, n.

acropolis /əˈkrɒpələs/ n the highest part or citadel of a Grecian city, the citadel itself.

acrospire /ˈækrəspɔɪr/ n (bot) the sprout of a seed.

across /əˈkrɒs/ prep from one side to the other of; on or at an angle; on the other side of. • adv crosswise; from one side to the other.

across-the-board /-ðəˌbɔrd/ adj (wage increase, cut, etc) applying equally to all; (horseracing) winning a bet if the horse comes first, second or third.

acrostic /əˈkrɒstɪk/ n a poem or word puzzle in which certain letters of each line spell a complete word, etc.—**acrostically** adv.

acrylic /əˈkrɪlɪk/ adj of or derived from acrylic acid. • n an acrylic fibre or resin.

act /ækt/ vi to perform or behave in a certain manner; to perform a specific function; to have an effect; to perform on the stage; (with **up**) (inf) to misbehave; to malfunction. • vt to portray by actions, esp on the stage; to pretend, simulate; to take the part of, as a character in a play. • n something done, a deed; an exploit; a law; a main division of a play or opera; the short repertoire of a comic, etc; something done merely for effect or show.

act of God n a direct and unforeseeable act of nature that could not reasonably have been guarded against.

acting /-ɪŋ/ n the art of an actor. • adj holding an office or position temporarily.

actin a /ækˈtɪniə/ n (pl **actiniae, actinias**) any of a genus of sea anemones that resemble flowers when the tentacles of the mouth are spread out.

actin form /ækˈtɪnɪˌfɔrm/, **actinoid** /ækˈtɪnɔɪd/ adj having the form of rays; star-shaped.

actinism /ækˈtɪnɪzm/ n the property of light by which chemical changes are caused, as in photography.—**actinic** adj.—**actinically** adv.

actinium /ækˈtɪniəm/ n a radioactive element occurring as a decay product of uranium.

actinozoan /ˌækˌtɪnoːˈzoːən/ see **anthozoan**.

action /ˈækʃən/ n the process of doing something; an operation; a movement of the body gesture; a land or sea battle; a lawsuit; the unfolding of events in a play, novel, etc; (inf) (with **the**) the centre of (social) activity.

actionable /-əbəl/ adj providing grounds for legal action.—**actionably** adv.

action painting *n* expressionist art produced by daubing, dribbling, splashing, throwing, etc, paint on to the canvas.

activate /'æktɪˌveɪt/ *vt* to make active; to set in motion; to make radioactive.—**activation** *n*.—**activator** *n*.

active /æk'tɪv/ *adj* lively, physically mobile; engaged in practical activities; energetic, busy; (*volcano*) liable to erupt; capable of producing an effect; radioactive; (*armed forces*) in full-time service. • *n* (*gram*) the verb form having as its subject the doer of the action.—**actively** *adv*.—**activeness** *n*.

active service, active duty *n* full-time service in a military force, *esp* during a war.

activist /'æktɪvɪst/ *n* an advocate of direct or militant action, *esp* in politics.—**activism** *n*.

activity /æk'tɪvɪti/ *n* (*pl* **activities**) the state of being active; energetic, lively action; specific occupations (*indoor activities*).

actor /'æktər/ *n* a person who acts in a play, film, etc.—**actress** *nf*.

ACTRA /'æktrə/ *abbr* ❧ = Alliance of Canadian Cinema, Television and Radio Artists.

actual /æk'tʃuwəl/ *adj* real; existing in fact or reality.

actuality /ˌækˌtʃuˈwæliti/ or /-ˌʃu-/ *n* (*pl* **actualities**) the state of being real or actual; that which is in full existence; reality

actualize /ˈæktʃuwəˌlaɪz/ or /-ˈʃuːə-/ *vt* to realize in action; to describe realistically; to make actual.—**actualization** *n*.

actually /'æktʃuəli/ or /'ækfəli/ *adv* as an existing fact, really; strange though it seems.

actuary /'æktʃuˌɛri/ *n* (*pl* **actuaries** /-riz/) a person who calculates insurance risks, premiums, etc.—**actuarial** *adj*.

actuate /'æktʃuˌeɪt/ *vt* to move or incite to action; to put in motion; to impel, influence.—**actuation** *n*.—**actuator** *n*.

acuity /ə'kjuːəti/ *n* sharpness of thought or vision.

aculeate /ə'kjuːliət/ *adj* pointed; (*zool*) equipped with a sting; (*bot*) having aculei or sharp prickles.

aculeus /ə'kjuːliːəs/ *n* (*pl* **aculei**) a prickle.

acumen /ə'kjuːmən/ or /'ækjəmən/ *n* sharpness of mind, perception.

acuminate /ə'kjuːmɪnət/ *adj* ending in a sharp point. • *vt* /-ˌneɪt/ (**acuminating, acuminated**) to sharpen.—**acumination** *n*.

acupuncture /'ækjuːˌpʌŋktʃər/ *n* the insertion of the tips of fine needles into the skin at certain points to treat various common ailments.—**acupuncturist** *n*.

acute /ə'kjuːt/ *adj* perceptive; sharp-witted; (*hearing*) sensitive; (*pain*) severe; very serious; (*angles*) less than 90 degrees; (*disease*) severe but not long lasting.—**acutely** *adv*.—**acuteness** *n*.

acute accent *n* a mark (ˊ) over a vowel in certain languages to indicate emphasis or special quality.

-acy /əsi/ *n suffix* forming nouns of state or quality, *eg* piracy.

ad- /əd/ or /æd/ *prefix* to, as in *adhere*.

ad[1] /æd/ *abbr* = advertisement.

ad[2] *prep* to, as in *ad absurdum*.

AD, A.D. /ˌeɪˈdiː/ *abbr* = *anno domini* (in the year of Our Lord) in dates of the Christian era, indicating the number of years since the birth of Christ.

ad absurdum /æd ˌæbˈzɜːrdəm/ or /-sɜːr-/ (*Latin*) to absurdity.

adactylous /eɪˈdæktələs/ *adj* without toes or fingers.

adage /'ædɪdʒ/ *n* a proverb, old saying.

adagio /ə'dɑːʒioʊ/ or /-dʒioʊ/ *adv* (*mus*) slowly, gracefully. • *n* (*pl* **adagios**) a slow movement.

adamant /'ædəmənt/ *adj* inflexible, unyielding. • *n* adamantine, an extremely hard substance.

adamantine /ˌædəˈmæntaɪn/ *adj* made of adamantine; impenetrable, very hard. • *n* an extremely hard substance; the diamond (—*also* **adamant**).

Adamite /'ædəmˌaɪt/ *n* a child of Adam; a member of a sect who went naked; a nudist.—**Adamitic** *adj*.

Adam's apple /'ædəmzˌæpəl/ *n* the hard projection of cartilage in the front of the neck.

Adam's needle /-niːdəl/ *n* a popular name of the yucca.

adapt /ə'dæpt/ *vti* to make or become fit; to adjust to a new purpose or circumstances.—**adaptability** *n*.—**adaptable** *adj*.—**adapter** *n*.

adaptation /ˌædæpˈteɪʃən/ *n* the process or condition of being adapted; something produced by modification; a version of a literary composition rewritten for a different medium.

adaptor /ə'dæptər/ *n* a device that allows an item of equipment to be put to new use; a device for connecting parts of differing size and shape; an electrical plug using one socket for different appliances.

adaxial /æd'æksiəl/ *adj* towards the axis.

ADC /ˌeɪdiːˈsiː/ *abbr* = aide-de-camp.

add /æd/ *vt* to combine (two or more things together); to combine numbers or amounts in a total; to remark or write further. • *vi* to perform or come together by addition.

addax /'ædæks/ *n* (*pl* **addaxes, addax**) a large North African antelope with twisted horns.

addendum /ə'dɛndəm/ *n* (*pl* **addenda**) a thing to be added; supplementary text appended to a book, etc.

adder /'ædər/ *n* the venomous viper.

adder's-tongue /'ædɔrzˌtɛŋ/ *n* a kind of fern whose spike resembles the tongue of a snake.

addict /'ædɪkt/ *n* a person who is dependent upon a drug. • *vt* to devote or give oneself up to; to practise sedulously (*usu* pejorative).—**addiction** *n*.—**addictive** *adj*.

addition /ə'dɪkʃən/ *n* the act or result of adding; something to be added; an extra part.

additional /ə'dɪʃənəl/ *adj* added, extra; supplementary.—**additionally** *adv*.

additive /'ædɪtɪv/ *adj* produced by addition. • *n* a substance added (to food, etc) to improve texture, flavour, etc.

addle /'ædəl/ *vb* (**addling, addled**) *vt* to make corrupt, putrid or confused. • *vi* to become addled. • *adj* rotten.

addle-headed, addle-pated *adj* stupid, weak-brained; muddled.

address /ə'drɛs/ *vt* to write directions for delivery on (a letter, etc); to speak or direct directly to; to direct one's skills or attention (to); (*golf*) to adjust one's stance and aim before hitting the ball; • *n* a place where a person or business resides, the details of this on a letter for delivery; a speech, *esp* a formal one; (*comput*) a specific memory location where information is stored.—**addressable** *adj*.

addressee /ˌædrɛˈsiː/ *n* a person or company to whom a letter is addressed.

Addressograph /ə'drɛsəˌɡræf/ *n* (*trademark*) an addressing machine.

adduce /ə'djuːs/ *vt* to offer as an example or evidence.

adducent /æ'duːsənt/ or /ə-/, /-'djuːs-/ *adj* bringing forward or together.

adducible, adduceable /ə'djuːsəbəl/ *adj* capable of being adduced.

adduct /ə'dʌkt/ *vt* to pull towards; (*of muscles*) to draw to a common centre.—**adduction** *n*.—**adductive** *adj*.

adductor muscle /ə'dʌktər/ *n* a muscle that draws certain parts to a common centre.

ademption /ə'dɛmpʃən/ *n* (*law*) the revocation of a grant; the lapse of a legacy.

aden- /'ædən/, **adeno-** /'ædnoː/ *prefix* gland.

adenitis /ˌædnˈaɪtɪs/ *n* inflammation of a gland.

adenoids /'ædəˌnɔɪdz/ *npl* enlarged masses of tissue in the throat behind the nose.—**adenoidal** *adj*.

adenoma /ˌædˈnoːmə/ *n* (*pl* **adenomas, adenomata**) a glandlike benign tumour.

adept /'ædɛpt/ or /ə'dɛpt/ *adj* highly proficient. • *n* a highly skilled person.—**adeptly** *adv*.—**adeptness** *n*.

adequacy /'ædəkwəsi/ *n* adequateness; sufficiency for a particular purpose.

adequate /'ædəkwət/ *adj* sufficient for requirements; barely acceptable.—**adequately** *adv*.—**adequateness** *n*.

à deux /æ'dɔː/ *Fr* /ɑdø/ for two; intimate.

adhere /əd'hɪːr/ *vi* to stick, as by gluing or suction; to give allegiance or support (to); to follow.

adherence /əd'hɪːrəns/ *n* the act or state of adhering; unwavering attachment.

adherent /əd'hɪːrənt/ *adj* sticking, attached. • *n* a supporter of a political party, idea, etc.

adhesion /əd'hiːʒən/ *n* the action or condition of adhering; the attachment of normally separate tissues in the body.

adhesive /əd'hiːsɪv/ or /-zɪv/ *adj* sticky; causing adherence. • *n* a substance used to stick, such as glue, paste, etc.—**adhesiveness** *n*.

ad hoc /æd'hɒk/ *adj* for a particular purpose.

ad hominem /æd'hɒmɪˌnɛm/ (*Latin*) to the man, personal.

adiabatic /ˌeɪdiəˈbætɪk/ or /ˌeɪdaɪə-/ *adj* (*physics*) not gaining or losing heat.—**adiabatically** *adv*.

adiaphorous /ˌædiːˈæfərəs/ or /ˌædaɪˈæ-/ *adj* (*theol*) tolerant in nonessential points of religion; morally indifferent; (*med*) neither helping nor harming.

adieu /ə'djuː/ *n* (*pl* **adieux, adieus**) farewell, goodbye; good wishes at parting.

ad infinitum /ˌædˌɪnfɪˈnaɪtəm/ *adv* without end, forever.

ad interim /ˌædˈɪntərɪm/ *adv* (*Latin*) for the meantime.

adipocere /ˈædɪpəˌsiːr/ *n* a fatty substance resulting from decomposition of animal bodies in moist places.—**adipocerous** *adj*.

adipose /ˈædɪˌpoːs/ or /-poːz/ *adj* of, like or containing animal fat; fatty.—**adiposity** *n*.

adit /ˈædɪt/ *n* an entrance or passage; an entrance to a mine more or less horizontal.

adjacent /əˈdʒeɪsənt/ *adj* nearby; adjoining, contiguous.—**adjacency** *n*.

adjective /ˈædʒəktɪv/ *n* a word used to add a characteristic to a noun or pronoun.—**adjectival** *adj*.—**adjectivally** *adv*.

adjoin /əˈdʒɔɪn/ *vt* to unite or join. • *vi* to lie next to.

adjoining /-ɪŋ/ *adj* beside, in contact with.

adjourn /əˈdʒɜrn/ *vt* to suspend (a meeting) temporarily. • *vi* (*inf*) to retire (to another room, etc).—**adjournment** *n*.

adjournment /-mənt/ *n* the act of adjourning; the postponement of a meeting.

adjudge /əˈdʒedʒ/ *vt* (**adjudging, adjudged**) to decide or award judicially; to sentence; to determine in a controversy, to adjudicate.—**adjudgment, adjudgement** *n*.

adjudicate /əˈdʒuːdɪˌkeɪt/ *vt* (*law*) to hear and decide (a case). • *vi* to serve as a judge (in or on).—**adjudicator** *n*.

adjudication /əˌdʒuːdɪˈkeɪʃən/ *n* the act of determining judicially; a judicial sentence; a court's decision.

adjunct /ˈædʒɐŋkt/ *n* something joined or added but inessential.—**adjunctive** *adj*.

adjuration /ˌædʒəˈreɪʃən/ *n* the solemn charging on oath; the oath used.

adjure /əˈdʒɜr/ or /əˈdʒʊr/ *vt* to command on oath under pain of a penalty; to charge solemnly, request earnestly.

adjust /əˈdʒɐst/ *vt* to arrange in a more proper or satisfactory manner; to regulate or modify by minor changes; to decide the amount to be paid in settling (an insurance claim). • *vi* to adapt oneself.—**adjustable** *adj*.—**adjuster** *n*.

adjustment /-mənt/ *n* the act of adjusting; arrangement.

adjutancy /ˈædʒətənsi/ *n* (*pl* **adjutancies**) the office of an adjutant.

adjutant /ˈædʒətənt/ *n* a military staff officer who assists the commanding officer.

adjutant general *n* (*pl* **adjutants general**) the chief staff officer of an army, through whom all orders, etc, are received and issued by the general commanding.

adjuvant /ˈædʒəvənt/ *adj* assisting, helpful. • *n* a helper, an auxiliary.

ad-lib /ˌædˈlɪb/ *vti* (**ad-libbing, ad-libbed**) (*speech, etc*) to improvise. • *n* an ad-libbed remark. • *adv* spontaneously, freely.—**ad-libber** *n*.

adman /ˈædmæn/ *n* (*pl* **admen**) (*inf*) a person who works in the advertising business.

admass /ˈædmæs/ or /-mɒs/ *n* the public targeted by or influenced by advertising.

admeasure /ədˈmeʒər/ *vt* (**admeasuring, admeasured**) to measure dimensions; to apportion.

admeasurement /-mənt/ *n* a measurement by a rule; adjustment of proportions; dimensions.

admin /ˌədˈmɪn/ *n* (*inf*) administration.

administer /ədˈmɪnɪstər/ *vt* to manage, direct; to give out as a punishment; to dispense (medicine, punishment, etc); to tender (an oath, etc).

administrate /ədˈmɪnɪˌstreɪt/ *vti* to manage or control the affairs of a business, institution, etc.

administration /ədˌmɪnɪˈstreɪʃən/ *n* management; the people who administer an organization; the government; (*with cap*) the executive officials of a government, their policies, and term of office.

administrative /ədˈmɪnɪˌstreɪtɪv/ *adj* of management; executive.—**administratively** *adv*.

administrator /ədˈmɪnɪˌstreɪtər/ *n* a person who manages or supervises; (*law*) one appointed to settle an estate.

admirable /ˈædmərəbəl/ *adj* deserving of admiration or approval.—**admirably** *adv*.

admiral /ˈædmərəl/ *n* the commanding officer of a fleet; a naval officer of the highest rank.

admiralty /-ti/ *n* (*pl* **admiralties**) the department of a government having authority over naval affairs; the building in which naval affairs are transacted; the office of an admiral.

admiration /ˌædmɪˈreɪʃən/ *n* a feeling of pleasurable and often surprised respect or approval; an admired person or thing.

admire /ədˈmaɪr/ *vt* to regard with honour, approval and pleasure; to express admiration for.—**admirer** *n*.—**admiring** *adj*.—**admiringly** *adv*.

admissible /ədˈmɪsɪbəl/ *adj* that may be admitted or allowed.—**admissibility, admissibleness** *n*.

admission /ədˈmɪʃən/ *n* an entrance fee; a conceding, confessing, etc; a thing conceded, confessed, etc.—**admissive** *adj*.

admit /ədˈmɪt/ *vb* (**admitting, admitted**) *vt* to allow to enter or join to concede or acknowledge as true. • *vi* to give access; (*with* **of**) to allow or permit.

admittance /ədˈmɪtəns/ *n* the act of admitting; the right to enter.

admittedly /ədˈmɪtədli/ *adv* acknowledged as fact, willingly conceded.

admix /ædˈmɪks/ *vt* to mix with something else; to add as an extra ingredient.

admixture /-tʃər/ *n* a mixture, a compound of substances mixed together.

admonish /ədˈmɒnɪʃ/ *vt* to remind or advise earnestly; to reprove gently.

admonition /ˌædməˈnɪʃən/ *n* a friendly reproof or warning.—**admonitory** *adj*.

adnate /ˈædˌneɪt/ *adj* (*bot*) with organic cohesion of unlike parts.

ad nauseam /ˌædˈnɒziˌæm/ or /-ziˌæm/ *adv* to a sickening degree.

ado /əˈduː/ *n* fuss, excitement, *esp* over trivial matters.

adobe /əˈdoːbi/ *n* a brick made of sun-dried clay; clay for making adobe bricks; a building using such bricks.

adolescence /ˌædəˈlesəns/ *n* the period of life between puberty and maturity; youth.

adolescent /ˌædəˈlesənt/ *adj* pertaining to the stage between childhood and maturity; (*inf*) immature. • *n* an adolescent person.

adopt /əˈdɒpt/ *vt* to take legally into one's family and raise as one's child; to select and pursue, *eg* a course of action; to take as one's own.—**adoption** *n*.

adoptive /əˈdɒptɪv/ *adj* made or related by adoption.

adorable /əˈdɔrəbəl/ *adj* worthy of being adored; extremely charming.—**adorably** *adv*.

adoration /ˌædəˈreɪʃən/ *n* worship, homage; profound regard.

adore /əˈdɔr/ *vt* to worship; to love deeply.—**adoringly** *adv*.

adorn /əˈdɔrn/ *vt* to decorate; to make more pleasant or attractive.—**adornment** *n*.

ad rem /ˌædˈrem/ *adj, adv* to the point or purpose.

adrenal /əˈdriːnəl/ *adj* of or near the kidney. • *n* an adrenal gland.

adrenal gland *n* one of two glands situated above the kidneys that secretes adrenaline.

adrenaline /əˈdrenəlɪn/ *n* a hormone that stimulates the heart rate, blood pressure, etc in response to stress and that is secreted by the adrenal glands or manufactured synthetically.

adrift /əˈdrɪft/ *adj, adv* afloat without mooring, drifting; loose; purposeless.

adroit /əˈdrɔɪt/ *adj* skilful and clever, sharp-witted.—**adroitly** *adv*.—**adroitness** *n*.

adscititious /ˌædsɪˈtɪʃəs/ *adj* taken in addition; added from without; additional, supplementary.

adsorb /ədˈsɔrb/ *vt* to accumulate on a surface, to collect by adsorption.—**adsorbable** *adj*.

adsorbent /-ənt/ *n* an adsorbing substance.

adsorption /ædˈsɔrpʃən/ *n* the action of a solid in condensing and holding a gas around it.

ADT /ˌeɪdiːˈtiː/ *abbr* ✦ = Atlantic Daylight Time.

adulate /ˈædʒuˌleɪt/ *vt* to flatter excessively or basely.—**adulator** *n*.—**adulatory** *adj*.

adulation /ˌædʒuˈleɪʃən/ *n* excessive flattery.—**adulatory** *adj*.

adult /əˈdɐlt/ or /ˈædɐlt/ *adj* fully grown; mature; suitable only for adults, as in pornography, etc. • *n* a mature person, etc.—**adulthood** *n*.

adulterant /əˈdɐltərənt/ *adj* adulterating. • *n* the person or thing that adulterates.

adulterate /əˈdɐltəˌreɪt/ *vt* to make impure or inferior, etc by adding an improper substance.—**adulteration** *n*.—**adulterator** *n*.

adulterer /əˈdɐltərər/ *n* a person who commits adultery.—**adulteress** *nf*.

adulterine /əˈdɐltəˌraɪn/ *adj* resulting from adulterous intercourse; fake, spurious; illegal.

adulterous /əˈdɐltərəs/ *adj* guilty of adultery.

adultery /əˈdɐltəri/ *n* (*pl* **adulteries**) sexual intercourse between a married person and someone other than their legal partner.

adumbral /'ædəmˌbrəl/ *adj* overshadowing; shady.

adumbrate /'ædəmˌbreɪt/ *vt* to foreshadow; to overshadow; to give a faint semblance of.—**adumbration** *n*.—**adumbrative** *adj*.

ad valorem /ˌædvə'lɔːrem/ *adj, adv* according to value; (*customs, duties*) levied on the value of goods as sworn to by the owner.

advance /əd'væns/ *vt* to bring or move forward; to promote; to raise the rate of; (*money*) to lend. • *vi* to go forward; to make progress; to rise in rank, price, etc. • *n* progress; improvement; a rise in value; payment beforehand; (*pl*) friendly approaches, *esp* to please. • *adj* in front; beforehand.

advanced /əd'væːnst/ *adj* in front; old; superior in development or progress.

advanced green *n* ♣ (*Cdn*) a flashing green traffic light that comes on before a steady green light, showing that oncoming traffic is halted.

advance poll *n* ♣ (*Cdn*) a poll for voters prior to the official election day.

advancement /əd'væːnsmənt/ or /-vɒns-/ *n* promotion to a higher rank; progress in development.

advantage /əd'væːntɪdʒ/ *n* superiority of position or condition; a gain or benefit; (*tennis*) the first point won after deuce. • *vt* to produce a benefit or favour to.

advantageous /ˌædvən'teɪdʒəs/ *adj* producing advantage, beneficial.—**advantageously** *adv*.

advent /'ædvent/ *n* an arrival or coming; (*with cap*) (*Christianity*) the coming of Christ; the four-week period before Christmas.

Adventist /ˌæd'ventɪst/ *n* a person who believes in Christ's second coming to set up a kingdom on earth.—**Adventism** *n*.

adventitious /ˌædven'tɪʃəs/ *adj* happening by chance; casual; fortuitous; accidental; produced out of normal and regular order; growing in an abnormal position.—**adventitiously** *adv*.—**adventitiousness** *n*.

Advent Sunday *n* the Sunday nearest (before or after) to St Andrew's Day (30 November).

adventure /əd'ventʃər/ *n* a strange or exciting undertaking; an unusual, stirring, often romantic, experience.

adventure playground *n* a children's playground equipped with materials and objects for building, climbing, hiding in, etc.

adventurer /-ər/ *n* a person who seeks adventure; someone who seeks money or power by unscrupulous means.—**adventuress** *nf*.

adventurous /-əs/ *adj* inclined to incur risk; full of risk; rash; enterprising; daring.—**adventurously** *adv*.

adverb /'ædvɜrb/ *n* a word that modifies a verb, adjective, another adverb, phrase, clause or sentence and indicates how, why, where, etc.—**adverbial** *adj*.—**adverbially** *adv*.

adversary /'ædvərˌseri/ *n* (*pl* **adversaries**) an enemy or opponent.

adversative /əd'vɜrsətɪv/ *adj* (*words*) denoting opposition or contrariety; expressing opposition.

adverse /əd'vɜrs/ or /'æd-/ *adj* hostile; contrary or opposite; unfavourable.—**adversely** *adv*.

adversity /əd'vɜrsɪti/ *n* (*pl* **adversities**) trouble, misery, misfortune.

advert[1] /əd'vɜrt/ *vt* to refer (to); to turn attention (to).

advert[2] /'ædvərt/ *n* (*inf*) an advertisement.

advertence /æd'vɜrtəns/, **advertency** /-si/ *n* attention; heedfulness.—**advertent** *adj*.

advertently /æd'vɜrtəntli/ *adv* in an intentional manner.

advertise, advertize /'ædvərˌtaɪz/ *vt* to call public attention to, *esp* in order to sell something, by buying space or time in the media, etc. • *vi* to call public attention to things for sale; to ask (for) by public notice.—**advertiser, advertizer** *n*.

advertisement, advertizement /ˌəd'vɜrtɪzmənt/ or /'ædvərˌtaɪzmənt/ *n* advertising; a public notice, *usu* paid for by the provider of a good or service.

advertising, advertizing /'ædvərˌtaɪzɪŋ/ *n* the promotion of goods or services by public notices; advertisements; the business of producing adverts.

advice /əd'vaɪz/ *n* recommendation with regard to a course of action; formal notice or communication.

advisable /əd'vaɪzəbəl/ *adj* prudent, expedient.—**advisability** *n*.

advise /əd'vaɪz/ *vt* to give advice to; to caution; to recommend; to inform. • *vi* to give advice.—**adviser, advisor** *n*.

advised /əd'vaɪzd/ *adj* acting with caution; deliberate; judicious.—**advisedly** *adv*.

advisory /əd'vaɪzəri/ *adj* having or exercising the power to advise; containing or giving advice.

advocaat /ˌædvə'kɒt/ *n* a sweet egg-based liqueur.

advocacy /'ædvəkəsi/ *n* (*pl* **advocacies**) the function of an radynamic *adj*.

advocate /'ædvəkət/ or /ˌæd'vəkeɪt/ *n* a person who argues or defends the cause of another, *esp* in a court of law; a supporter. • *vt* to plead in favour of, to recommend.

adynamia /ˌædaɪ'neɪmiə/ or /ˌædɪ'neɪ-/ *n* want of vital power, prostration, weakness.—**adynamic** *adj*.

adze, adz /ædz/ *n* a type of axe with a blade at right angles to the handle for cutting and shaping wood.

aedile, /'iːdaɪl/ *n* a Roman magistrate who exercised supervision over the temples, public and private buildings, the markets, public games, sanitation, etc, hence a municipal officer.—*also* **edile**.

aegis /'iːdʒɪs/ *n* protection, sponsorship.—*also* **egis**.

Aeolian /eɪ'oːliən/ *adj* pertaining to Aeolis in Asia Minor or to the Aeolic race; of Aeolus, the Greek god of winds.

aeolian harp *n* a stringed instrument, the wires of which are set in motion and sounded by the wind.

Aeolic /iː'ɒlɪk/ *adj* of Aeolis. • *n* the Aeolic dialect of ancient Greece.

aeon /'iːən/ or /'iːˌɒn/ *n* a period of immense duration; an age.—*also* **eon**.

aeonian /iː'oːniən/ *adj* everlasting.—*also* **eonian**.

aerate /'ereɪt/ *vt* to supply (blood) with oxygen by respiration; to supply or impregnate with air; to combine or charge a liquid with gas.—**aeration** *n*.

aerator /-ər/ *n* an apparatus for making aerated waters.

aerial /'eriəl/ *adj* belonging to or existing in the air; of aircraft or flying. • *n* a radio or TV antenna.

aerialist /'eriəlɪst/ *n* a trapeze or high-wire artist.

aerie /'eri/ or /'iːri/ *see* **eyrie**.

aeriform /'erəform/ *adj* having the form of air; gaseous; like air; unsubstantial.

aerify /'erəfaɪ/ *vt* (**aerifying, aerified**) to combine with air.—**aerification** *n*.

aero- /'eroː/ *prefix* aviation; air vessel.

aerobatics /ˌerə'bætɪks/ *npl* stunts performed while flying an aircraft.

aerobe /'eroːb/, **aerobium** /er'oːbiəm/ *n* (*pl* **aerobes, aerobia**) a microbe that cannot live without air.

aerobic /e'roːbɪk/ *adj* (*exercise*) that conditions the heart and lungs by increasing the efficient intake of oxygen by the body.

aerobics /-s/ *npl* aerobic exercises.

aerodrome /'erəˌdroːm/ *n* an airfield.

aerodynamics /ˌeroːdaɪ'næmɪks/ *n* the study of the forces exerted by air or other gases in motion, *esp* around solid bodies such as aircraft.—**aerodynamic** *adj*.—**aerodynamically** *adv*.

aerofoil /'erəˌfɔɪl/ *n* a wing, the lifting surface of an aeroplane.

aerogram, aerogramme /'erəˌgræm/ *n* a radio telegraphic message.

aerolite /'erəˌlaɪt/ *n* a stone falling from the air, a meteorite.

aerology /e'rɒlədʒi/ *n* the science that deals with the air and the atmosphere.—**aerologic, aerological** *adj*.—**aerologist** *n*.

aerometer /e'rɒmətər/ *n* an instrument for weighing the air.—**aerometric** *adj*.

aerometry /er'ɒmətri/ *n* the branch of physics concerned with air, pneumatics.

aeronaut /'erəˌnɒt/ *n* an aviator; the pilot or navigator of an aircraft.

aeronautical /ˌerə'nɒtɪkəl/, **aeronautic** /ˌerə'nɒtɪk/ *adj* of or pertaining to aeronautics or an aeronaut.—**aeronautically** *adv*.

aeronautics /-ɪks/ *n* the science dealing with the operation of aircraft; the art or science of flight.

aeroplane /'erəˌpleɪn/ *n* a power-driven aircraft.—*also* **airplane**.

aerosol /'erəˌsɒl/ *n* a suspension of fine solid or liquid particles in gas, *esp* as held in a container under pressure, with a device for releasing it in a fine spray.

aerospace /'eroːˌspeɪs/ *n* the earth's atmosphere and the space beyond. • *adj* technology for flight in aerospace.

aerostat /'erəstæt/ *n* a balloonist, a balloonist.

aerostatics /-tɪks/ *n* (*used as sing*) the science that studies the equilibrium of bodies sustained in air; the science of air navigation.—**aerostatic, aerostatical** *adj*.

aerostation /ˌerəstɪʃən/ *n* ballooning.

aeruginous /i'ruːdʒɪnəs/ *adj* of or like verdigris or copper rust.

aery /'eɪəri/ or /'iri/, /'eri/, /'iri/ *see* **eyrie**.

Aesculapian /ˌiːskuː'leɪpiən/ or /'ɛ-/ *adj* of or pertaining to Aesculapius, the Roman god of medicine, or to medicine.

aesthete /'ɛsθiːt/ *n* a person who is or pretends to be highly sensitive to art and beauty.—*also* **esthete**.

aesthetic /ɛsˈθɛtɪk/, **aesthetical** /ɛsˈθɛtɪkəl/ *adj* of or pertaining to aesthetics; concerned with beauty rather than practicality.—*also* **esthetic, esthetical.—aesthetically, esthetically** *adv*.

aestheticism /ɛsˈθɛtɪˌsɪzm/ *n* the cult of the beautiful, esp a fantastic art movement at the end of the 19th century.—*also* **estheticism.**

aesthetics /ɛsˈθɛtɪks/ *n* the philosophy of art and beauty.—*also* **esthetics.**

aestival /ˈɛstɪvəl/ *adj* of or occurring in summer.—*also* **estival.**

aestivation /ˌɛstɪˈveɪʃən/ or /ˌiːs-/ *n* (*bot*) the arrangement of petals in a flower bud; (*zool*) the spending of the dry season in a dormant state.—*also* **estivation.**

aet., aetat. *abbr* = *aetatis*, of, at, the age of.

aetiology /ˌiːtɪˈɒlədʒi/, **aetiological** /-kəl/, **aetiologist** /-ɪst/ *see* **etiology.**

af- /əf/ *prefix* the form of *ad-* before *f*.

AF *abbr* ✦ = Air Force.

afar /əˈfɑr/ *adv* at, to, or from a great distance.

affable /ˈæfəbəl/ *adj* friendly; approachable.—**affability** *n*.—**affably** *adv*.

affair /əˈfɛr/ *n* a thing done or to be done; (*pl*) public or private business; (*inf*) an event; a temporary romantic or sexual relationship.

affaire (de coeur) /æˈfɛr/ *n* a love affair.

affect[1] /əˈfɛkt/ *vt* to have an effect on; to produce a change in; to act in a way that alters or affects the feelings of.

affect[2] *vt* to pretend or feign (an emotion); to incline to or show a preference for.

affect[3] /ˈæfɛkt/ *n* an emotion, feeling or desire associated with a certain stimulus.

affectation /ˌæfɛkˈteɪʃən/ *n* a striving after or an attempt to assume what is not natural or real; pretence.

affected /əˈfɛktəd/ *adj* (*manner, etc*) assumed artificially.—**affectedly** *adv*.—**affectedness** *n*.

affecting /əˈfɛktɪŋ/ *adj* having power to excite the emotions; moving; pathetic.—**affectingly** *adv*.

affection /əˈfɛkʃən/ *n* tender feeling; liking.—**affectional** *adj*.

affectionate /əˈfɛkʃənət/ *adj* showing affection, loving.—**affectionately** *adv*.

affective /əˈfɛktɪv/ *adj* arousing the emotions, emotional.—**affectivity, affectiveness** *n*.

afferent /ˈæfərənt/ *adj* conveying inwards or to a part.

affettuoso /əˌfɛtuˈoːsoː/ *adv* (*mus*) with feeling, tender, pathetic.

affiance /æˈfiːɒns/ or /əˈfaɪəns/ *vt* to promise in marriage, betroth. • *n* faith, trust; a marriage contract.

affiche /əˈfiːʃ/ *n* a paper affixed to a wall, a poster.

affidavit /ˌæfɪˈdeɪvɪt/ *n* a statement written on oath.

affiliate /əˈfɪliˌeɪt/ *vt* to connect as a subordinate member or branch; to associate (oneself with). • *vi* to join. • *n* an affiliated person, club, etc.—**affiliation** *n*.

affinity /əˈfɪnɪti/ *n* (*pl* **affinities**) attraction, liking; a close relationship, *esp* by marriage; similarity, likeness; (*chem*) a tendency in certain substances to combine.

affirm /əˈfɜrm/ *vt* to assert confidently or positively; to confirm or ratify; (*law*) to make an affirmation.

affirmation /ˌæfərˈmeɪʃən/ *n* affirming; an assertion; a solemn declaration made by those declining to swear an oath, *eg* on religious grounds.

affirmative /əˈfɜrmətɪv/ *adj* confirming; indicating agreement. • *n* a positive word or statement, *eg* yes.—**affirmatively** *adv*.

affix /əˈfɪks/ *vt* to fasten; to add, *esp* in writing; to attach.

afflatus /əˈfleɪtəs/ *n* a breath or blast of wind; poetic or divine inspiration; creative power.

afflict /əˈflɪkt/ *vt* to cause persistent pain or suffering to; to trouble greatly.—**afflictive** *adj*.

affliction /əˈflɪkʃən/ *n* persistent pain, suffering; a cause of this.

affluence /ˈæfluəns/ *n* an abundant supply, as of thoughts, words, riches; wealth.

affluent /-ənt/ *adj* rich, well provided for.—**affluently** *adv*.

affluenza /ˈæfluˈwɒnzə/ *n* a psychological disease resulting from an excess of affluence.

afflux /ˈæflʌks/ *n* a flowing towards; an increase; an influx.

afford /əˈfɔrd/ *vt* to be in a position to do or bear without much inconvenience; to have enough time, money, or resources for; to supply, produce.

afforest /əˈfɒrəst/ or /-fɑr-/, /æ-/ *vt* to plant trees to cover with forest.—**afforestation** *n*.

affranchise /əˈfræntʃaɪz/ *v* to free from an obligation or slavery; to enfranchise.—**affranchisement** *n*.

affray /əˈfreɪ/ *n* a noisy fight.

affreightment /əˈfreɪtmənt/ *n* the hire of a ship for the transportation of goods or freight.

affright /əˈfraɪt/ *vt* (*arch*) to frighten, to terrify; to alarm; to confuse.

affront /əˈfrʌnt/ *vi* to insult or offend openly or deliberately. • *n* such an insult or offence

affusion /əˈfjuːʒən/ *n* the act of pouring upon, *esp* in baptism.

Afghan /ˈæfgæn/ *adj* pertaining to Afghanistan. • *n* a native of Afghanistan.—*also* **Afghani.**

aficionado /ˌæfɪʃəˈnɑːdoː/ or /əˌfɪsjəˈnɑːdoː/ *n* (*pl* **aficionados**) a devotee of a particular sport, activity, etc.

afield /əˈfiːld/ *adv* far away from home; to or at a distance; astray.

afire /əˈfaɪr/ *adj, adv* on fire.

aflame /əˈfleɪm/ *adj, adv* flaming, ablaze, in a glow.

afloat /əˈfloːt/ *adj* floating; at sea, on board a ship; debt-free; flooded.—*also adv*.

AFN /ˈeɪˈɛfˈɛn/ *abbr* ✦ (*Cda*) = Assembly of First Nations.

afoot /əˈfʊt/ *adj, adv* on foot; astir; on the move; in operation.

afore /əˈfɔr/ *adv, prep* in front, before; previously.

aforementioned /əˈfɔrˌmɛnʃənd/ *adj* mentioned previously.

aforesaid /-ˌsɛd/ *adj* referred to previously.

aforethought /-ˌθɔt/ *adj* premeditated.

a fortiori /ˌeɪfɔrtiˈɔri/ (*Latin*) with stronger reason, more conclusively.

afraid /əˈfreɪd/ *adj* full of fear or apprehension; regretful.

afreet /ˈæfriːt/ *n* (*Arabian myth*) an evil demon.

afresh /əˈfrɛʃ/ *adv* anew, starting again.

African /ˈæfrɪkən/ *adj* pertaining to Africa. • *n* a native of Africa.

African-Canadian *n* ✦ a Black Canadian. • *adj* pertaining to Black Canadians, or their culture, history, etc.

African violet *n* any of various African plants popular as houseplants, with purple, pink or white flowers and velvet-textured leaves.

Afrikaans /ˌæfrɪˈkɒns/ *n* a language derived from Dutch used in South Africa.

Afrikander, Africander /ˌæfrɪˈkɒndər/ *n* (any of) a breed of southern African beef cattle.

Afrikaner /ˌæfrɪˈkɒnər/ *n* a South African native white, *esp* of Dutch descent.

Afro /ˈæfroː/ *n* (*pl* **Afros**) a bushy hairstyle.

Afro- /ˈæfroː/ *prefix* Africa or African.

Afro-American /ˌæfroːəˈmɛrɪkən/ *n* a Black American. • *adj* of or relating to Black Americans, or their culture, history, etc.

afrormosia /ˌæfrɔrˈmoːzɪə/ *n* a hard wood similar to teak, used in furniture.

aft /æft/ *adv* at, near, or towards the stern of a ship or rear of an aircraft.

after /ˈæftər/ *prep* behind in place or order; following in time, later than; in pursuit of; in imitation of; in view of, in spite of; according to; about, concerning; subsequently. • *adv* later; behind. • *conj* at a time later than. • *adj* later, subsequent; nearer the stern of a ship or aircraft.

afterbirth /-ˌbɜrθ/ *n* the placenta expelled from the womb after giving birth.

afterbrain /-ˌbreɪn/ *n* that portion of the brain behind the hindbrain, the medulla oblongata.

afterburner /-ˌbɜrnər/ *n* a device in a jet engine used to provide extra thrust by igniting additional fuel.

aftercare /-ˌkɛr/ *n* care following hospital treatment, etc.

afterdamp /-ˌdæmp/ *n* the carbonic acid found in coal mines after an explosion of fire damp; choke damp.

aftereffect /-əˈfɛkt/ *n* an effect that occurs some time after its cause.

afterglow /-ˌgloː/ *n* the glow in the sky after sunset.

afterimage /-ˌɪmɪdʒ/ *n* the image that remains momentarily after the eye has been withdrawn from a bright object.

afterlife /-ˌlaɪf/ *n* life after death.

aftermath /-ˌmæθ/ *n* the result, *esp* an unpleasant one.

aftermost /-ˌmoːst/ *adj* hindmost; farthest aft, nearest to the stern.

afternoon /-ˌnuːn/ *n* the time between noon and sunset or evening.—*also adj*.

afternote /-ˌnoːt/ *n* the second or unaccented note, which takes its time from the first or accented note.

afterpains /-ˌpeɪnz/ *npl* pains after childbirth.

aftershave /-ˌʃeɪv/ *n* lotion for use after shaving.

aftertaste /-ˌteɪst/ *n* the taste that remains after eating or drinking.

afterthought /-ˌθɒt/ *n* a thought or reflection occurring later.

afterwards /-wərdz/, **afterward** /-ˌwərd/ *adv* at a later time.

afterwit /-ˌwɪt/ *n* wisdom that comes too late.

Ag (*chem symbol*) silver.

ag- /əg/ *prefix* the form of *ad-* before *g*.

aga /ˈægə/ *n* in Turkey, a commander or chief officer; a title of respect.—*also* **agha**.

again /əˈgeɪn/ or /əˈgen/ *adv* once more; besides; on the other hand.

against /əˈgenst/ or /əˈgenst/ *prep* in opposition to; unfavourable to; in contrast to; in preparation for; in contact with; as a charge on.

agalloch /əˈgæləʃ/ *n* a fragrant resinous heartwood.—*also* **eaglewood**.

agama /əˈgeɪmə/ *n* a short-tongued lizard found in India and Africa.

agami /əˈgæmi/ *n* a South American bird allied to the cranes; a trumpeter bird.

agamic /əˈgæmɪk/ *adj* (*biol*) produced without sexual action, asexual.—**agamically** *adj*.

agamogenesis /ˌægəˌmoːˈdʒenəsɪs/ *n* (*biol*) asexual reproduction.—**agamogenetic** *adj*.—**agamogenetically** *adv*.

agapanthus /ˌægəˈpænθəs/ *n* an ornamental plant with bright blue flowers.

agape /əˈgeɪp/ *adj* open-mouthed.

Agape /ˈægəˌpeɪ/ *n* the love feast of the early Christians at communion time.

agar /ˈeɪgɑr/ *n* a preparation of seaweed used for jelly, glue and bacteria culture.

agaric /ˈægərɪk/ *n* a mushroom or other fungus of the genus *Agaricus*.

agate /ˈægət/ *n* stone with striped or clouded colouring used as a gemstone.

agave /əˈgeɪvi/ *n* a genus of plants of which the chief species is the century plant.

age /eɪdʒ/ *n* the period of time during which someone or something has lived or existed; a stage of life; later years of life; a historical period; a division of geological time; (*inf: often pl*) a long time. • *vti* (**ageing** *or* **aging, aged**) to grow or make old, ripe, mature, etc.

aged /eɪdʒd/ *adj* very old; of a specified age. • *n* (*with* **the**) the elderly.

ageism /ˈeɪdʒɪzəm/ *n* discrimination on grounds of age.—*also* **agism**.—**ageist, agist** *adj*.

ageless /ˈeɪdʒləs/ *adj* timeless; appearing never to grow old.

age-long /-lɒŋ/ *see* **age-old**.

agency /ˈeɪdʒənsi/ *n* (*pl* **agencies**) action; power; means; a firm, etc empowered to act for another; an administrative government division.

agenda /əˈdʒendə/, **agendum** /-dəm/ *n* (*pl* **agendas, agendums**) a list of items or matters of business that need to be attended to.

agenesis /eɪˈdʒenəsɪs/ *n* imperfect development of the body.—**agenetic** *adj*.

agent /ˈeɪdʒənt/ *n* a person or thing that acts or has an influence; a substance or organism that is active; one empowered to act for another; a government representative; a spy.

agent general *n* ✿ the official representative of a Canadian province or Australian state in a foreign country or region.

agent provocateur *Fr.* /aˈʒɑːprɒvəkaˌtœr/ *n* (*pl* **agents provocateurs**) a person hired to tempt or provoke suspected persons into illegal acts so to incriminate themselves.

age-old /ˈeɪdʒˌoːld/ *adj* ancient.—*also* **age-long**.

agglomerate /əˈglɒməˌreɪt/ *vti* to gather into a heap; to accumulate; to collect into a mass. • *n* a heap or mass; a rock consisting of volcanic fragments.—**agglomeration** *n*.—**agglomerative** *adj*.

agglutinate /əˈgluːtɪˌneɪt/ *vti* to stick or fuse together; to form words into compounds. • *adj* glued together.—**agglutination** *n*.—**agglutinative** *adj*.

agglutination /-ˈneɪʃən/ *n* the act or condition of being united or joined together; the formation of words by combination, not inflexion.

aggrandize /əˈgrændaɪz/ *vt* to increase the power, rank, wealth, or reputation of.—**aggrandizement** *n*.

aggravate /ˈægrəˌveɪt/ *vt* to make worse; (*inf*) to annoy, irritate.—**aggravation** *n*.

aggravated /-ɪd/ *adj* (*law*) denoting a grave form of a specified offence.

aggravating /-ɪŋ/ *adj* making worse or more heinous; (*inf*) annoying, irritating.

aggregate /ˈægrəˌgeɪt/ *vt*, /ˈægrəgət/ *adj* formed of parts combined into a mass or whole; taking all units as a whole. • *n* a collection or sum of individual parts; sand, stones, etc mixed with cement to form concrete. • *vt* to collect or form into a mass or whole; to amount to (a total).—**aggregation** *n*.

aggression /əˈgreʃən/ *n* an unprovoked attack; a hostile action or behaviour.

aggressive /əˈgresɪv/ *adj* boldly hostile; quarrelsome; self-assertive, enterprising.—**aggressively** *adv*.—**aggressiveness** *n*.

aggressor /əˈgresər/ *n* a person or country that attacks first.

aggrieve /əˈgriːv/ *vt* to pain; to injure; to have a grievance; to bear heavily upon; to oppress.—**aggrieved** *adj*.—**aggrievedly** *adv*.

aggro *n* /ˈægroː/ (*sl*) aggression.

agha /ˈægə/ *see* **aga**.

aghast /əˈgæst/ *adj* utterly horrified.

agile /ˈædʒaɪl/ or /ˈædʒəl/ *adj* quick and nimble in movement; mentally acute.—**agility** /əˈdʒɪləti/ *n*.

agio /ˈædʒioː/ *n* (*pl* **agios**) the premium on changing paper money into cash or for exchanging one currency for another.—**agiotage** *n*.

agism /ˈeɪdʒɪzəm/ *see* **ageism**.

agitate /ˈædʒɪˌteɪt/ *vt* to shake, move; to disturb or excite the emotions of. • *vi* to stir up public interest for a cause, etc.—**agitation** *n*.—**agitator** *n*.

agitato /ˌædʒɪˈtɒtoː/ *adj, adv* (*mus*) in a hurried or agitated manner.

agitator /ˈædʒɪˌteɪtər/ *n* one who starts or keeps up a political or other agitation; an implement for stirring.

aglet /ˈæglət/ *n* a tag (of a shoelace, etc); a spangle, a metallic ornament; a catkin.—*also* **aiglet**.

aglow /əˈgloː/ *adj* radiant with warmth or excitement.

AGM /ˈeɪˈdʒiːˈem/ *abbr* = Annual General Meeting.

agnail /ˈægneɪl/ *n* a sore under or near the nail, a hangnail.

agnate /ˈægneɪt/ *adj* related by the father's side or with the same male ancestor. • *n* a relative by the father's side.—**agnatic** *adj*.

agnomen /ægˈnoːmən/ *n* (*pl* **agnomina**) the fourth name of a person in ancient Rome; an additional name or epithet, as *Milton, the poet*.—**agnominal** *adj*.

agnostic /ægˈnɒstɪk/ *n* one who believes that knowledge of God is impossible. • *adj* pertaining to the agnostics or their teachings; expressing ignorance.—**agnostically** *adv*.—**agnosticism** *n*.

Agnus Dei /ˌægnusˈdeiiː/ or /ˌænjus-/ *n* a figure of a lamb bearing a banner or cross, symbolic of Christ and associated emblematically with St John the Baptist; the lamb and flag; a medal of wax or precious metal stamped with the figure of the Agnus Dei and blessed by the pope for distribution on Low Sunday.

ago /əˈgoː/ *adv* in the past. • *adj* gone by; past.

agog /əˈgɒg/ *adj, adv* in agitation or expectation; eager, on the lookout.

agonic /əˈgɒnɪk/ or /-eɪ-/ *adj* making no angle.

agonistic /ˌægəˈnɪstɪk/ *adj* of athletic contests; athletic; polemic; melodramatic; strained; unnatural.

agonize /ˈægəˌnaɪz/ *vti* to suffer or cause to suffer agony; to strive.—**agonizingly** *adv*.

agony /ˈægəni/ *n* (*pl* **agonies**) extreme mental or physical suffering.

agony aunt *n* a person who replies to readers' problem letters in an agony column.

agony column *n* the column of a newspaper devoted to advertisements relating to lost friends, etc; a column in a magazine containing readers' letters with helpful replies to problems.

agoraphobia /ˌægərəˈfoːbiə/ *n* abnormal fear of crossing open places.—**agoraphobic** *adj, n*.

agouti /əˈguːti/ *n* (*pl* **agoutis, agouties**) a rodent similar to the guinea pig found in the West Indies and South America.

AGR *abbr* = advanced gas-cooled reactor.

agraphia /eɪˈgræfiə/ *n* the inability to write due to mental illness.

agrarian /əˈgreɪriən/ *adj* of or relating to fields, or their cultivation; of or relating to farmers or agricultural life. • *n* an advocate of redistribution of property in land.

agrarianism /-ˌɪzəm/ *n* the principle of a uniform division of land; agitation with respect to land tenure.

agree /ə'griː/ *vb* (**agreeing, agreed**) *vi* to be of similar opinion; to consent or assent (to); to come to an understanding about; to be consistent; to suit a person's digestion; (*gram*) to be consistent in gender, number, case, or person. • *vt* to concede, grant; to bring into harmony; to reach terms on.

agreeable /-əbəl/ *adj* likeable, pleasing; willing to agree.—**agreeableness** *n*.—**agreeably** *adv*.

agreement /-mənt/ *n* harmony in thought or opinion, correspondence; an agreed settlement between two people, etc.

ag rep /'æg,rep/ *n* ✲ (*Cdn*) (*inf*) agricultural representative, an employee of a government agriculture department who advises farmers.

agrestic /ə'grestik/ *adj* rustic; uncouth.

agriculture /'ægri,kʌltʃər/ *n* the science or practice of producing crops and raising livestock; farming.—**agricultural** *adj*.—**agriculturally** *adv*.—**agriculturist, agriculturalist** *n*.

agrimony /'ægri,moːni/ *n* (*pl* **agrimonies**) a yellow-flowered plant.

agronomics /,ægrə'nɒmiks/ *n* (*used as sing*) the part of economics concerned with the management and distribution of farming lands.—**agronomic, agronomical** *adj*.

agronomy /ə'grɒnəmi/ *n* the science of land cultivation and management, husbandry.—**agronomist** *n*.

agrostology /,ægrəs'tɒlədʒi/ *n* the branch of botany that treats of the grasses.

aground /ə'graund/ *adj, adv* on or onto the shore.

aguardiente /,əgwar'djentei/ *n* an inferior Spanish brandy.

ague /'eigjuː/ *n* malaria, an intermittent fever; the cold fit of the intermittent fever.—**aguish** *adj*.

ah /ɒ/ *interj* an exclamation of sudden emotion.

AH *abbr* = *anno Hegirae* (in the year of the Hegira) used in dates of the Muslim era.

aha /ɒ'hɒ/ or /ə'hɒ/ *interj* an exclamation of satisfaction, triumph or mockery.

ahead /ə'hed/ *adj* in or to the front; forward; onward; in advance; winning or profiting.—*also adv*.

ahem /ə'həm/ or /ə'hem/ *interj* an exclamation to call attention.

ahoy /ə'hɔi/ *interj* a term used in hailing a vessel.

A.I. *abbr* = artificial insemination; artificial intelligence.

ai /'ɒi/ *n* (*pl* **ais**) a South American three-toed sloth.

aid /eid/ *vti* to help, give assistance to. • *n* anything that helps; a specific means of assistance, *eg* money, equipment; a helper.

AID *abbr* = Agency for International Development; artificial insemination (by) donor.

aide /eid/ *n* an aide-de-camp; assistant.

aide-de-camp /,eiddə'kɒ/ *n* (*pl* **aides-de-camp**) a military officer serving as an assistant to a senior officer.

aide-mémoire /,eidme'mwar/, *Fr.* /edmei'mwaʀ/ *n* (*pl* **aides-mémoire**) a summarized document; a memorandum, etc, as an aid to the memory.

AIDS, Aids /eidz/ *n* (*acronym for* acquired immune deficiency syndrome) a condition caused by a virus, in which the body loses its immunity to infection.

AIDS-related complex /'eidzri,leitid-/ *n* a condition in which mild symptoms of AIDS (e.g. fever, weight loss) precede development of the full-blown disease.

aiglet *see* **aglet**.

aigrette, aigret /ei'gret/ or /'eigret/ *n* a small white heron; a plume arranged in imitation of the feathers of the heron, worn on helmets and as a hat decoration.

aiguille /ei'gwiːl/ *n* a sharp peak of rock.

aiguillette /,eigwi'let/ *n* an ornamental tag or lace worn on uniforms and liveries.

AIH *abbr* = artificial insemination (by) husband.

ail /eil/ *vt* to give or cause pain. • *vi* to feel pain; to be afflicted with pain.

aileron /'eilə,rɒn/ *n* a hinged section on the wing of an aircraft used for lateral control.

ailing /'eiliŋ/ *adj* unwell.

ailment /-mənt/ *n* a slight illness.

ailurophobia /ei,lurə'fɔːbiə/ or /ai-/ *n* cat fear; a morbid dread of cats and a consciousness of their presence even when they are not in sight.—**ailurophobe** *n*.

aim /eim/ *vti* to point or direct towards a target so as to hit; to direct (one's efforts); to intend. • *n* the act of aiming; purpose, intention.

aimless /'eimləs/ *adj* without purpose or object.—**aimlessly** *adv*.—**aimlessness** *n*.

ain't /eint/ *inf* = am not, is not, are not, has not, have not.

air /eər/ *n* the mixture of invisible gases surrounding the earth; the earth's atmosphere; empty, open space; a light breeze; aircraft, aviation; outward appearance, demeanour; a pervading influence; (*mus*) a melody; (*pl*) an affected manner. • *vt* to expose to the air for drying, etc; to expose to public notice; (*clothes*) to place in a warm place to finish drying.

airbag /'eərbæg/ *n* a safety device in a motor vehicle that automatically inflates to protect the occupants in the event of an accident.

air base *n* a base for military aircraft.

air bath *n* a lengthened exposure of the body to the action of the air and sun; an arrangement for drying articles by exposing them to air of any regulated temperature.

air bed *n* an inflatable mattress *usu* of plastic or rubber.

airborne /-bɔrn/ *adj* carried by or through the air; aloft or flying.

air box *n* a tube for conveying fresh air to a mine; a flue supplying air to a furnace; a chamber behind the fire box of a furnace to assist combustion by supply of air.

air brake *n* a brake operated by compressed air.

air brick *n* a brick with holes in the sides through which air for ventilation can pass.

airbrush /'eərbrʌʃ/ *n* a device for spraying paint by compressed air.

airbus *n* a jet aircraft designed for short-distance intercity flights.

Air Command *n* ✲ the Canadian air force.

air conditioning *n* regulation of air humidity and temperature in buildings, etc.

air-cooled /'eərkuːld/ *adj* cooled by having air passed over, into, or through.

air course *n* a ventilating passage in a mine.

air cover *n* protection for ground forces given by fighter aircraft; the aircraft giving this protection.

aircraft /'eərkræft/ *n* (*pl* **aircraft**) any machine for travelling through air.

aircraft carrier *n* a warship with a large flat deck, for the carrying, taking off and land of aircraft.

aircrew /'eərkruː/ *n* the crew of an aircraft.

air cushion *n* an inflatable cushion *usu* of plastic or rubber.

air drop /'eərdrɒp/ *n* a dropping by parachute of troops and supplies.

Airedale /'eərdeil/ *n* a large rough-coated terrier.

airfield /'eərfiːld/ *n* a field where aircraft can take off and land.

air force *n* the aviation branch of a country's armed forces.

air gas *n* an illuminating gas made from air charged with the vapour of petroleum, naphtha, etc.

airgun /'eərgʌn/ *n* a gun that fires pellets by compressed air.

airhead /-hed/ *n* (*sl*) a stupid person.

air hostess *n* a stewardess on a passenger aircraft.

airing /'eəriŋ/ *n* exposure to the open air for drying or freshening; exercise in the open air; exposure to public view.

airless /'eərləs/ *adj* stuffy; sultry.—**airlessness** *n*.

air letter *n* a sheet of light writing paper that is folded and sealed for sending by airmail.

airlift /-lift/ *n* the transport of cargo, troops, passengers, etc by air, *esp* in an emergency.—*also vt*.

airline /-lain/ *n* a system or company for transportation by aircraft; a beeline.

airliner /-,lainər/ *n* a large passenger aeroplane.

airlock /-lɒk/ *n* a blockage in a pipe caused by an air bubble; an airtight compartment giving access to a pressurized chamber.

airmail /-meil/ *n* mail transported by aircraft.

airman /-mən/ *n* (*pl* **airmen**) a male civilian or military pilot, etc.—**airwoman** *nf* (*pl* **airwomen**).

airmiss /-mis/ *n* the near collision of aircraft in flight.

airplane /-plein/ *see* **aeroplane**.

air plant *n* a plant that derives its nourishment from the air, an epiphyte.

airplay /-plei/ *n* the playing of a recording over radio or TV.

air pocket *n* a patch of rarefied air causing aircraft to drop abruptly.

airport /-pɔrt/ *n* a place where aircraft can land and take off, with facilities for repair, etc.

air pump *n* a machine for exhausting the air from a receiver; the pump used to exhaust the water and gases from the condenser of a steam engine.

air raid *n* an attack by military aircraft on a surface target.

airs /eərz/ *npl* affected behaviour for the purpose of impressing others.

airship /'eərʃip/ *n* a self-propelled steerable aircraft that is lighter than air.

airsick /-sɪk/ *adj* nauseated due to the motion of an aircraft.

airspace /-speɪs/ *n* the space above a nation over which it maintains jurisdiction.

airspeed /-spi:d/ *n* the speed of an aircraft relative to the outside air.

airstrip /-strɪp/ *n* an area of land cleared for aircraft to land on; a runway.

airtight /-taɪt/ *adj* too tight for air or gas to enter or escape; (*alibi, etc*) invulnerable.

airtime /-taɪm/ *n* (*radio, TV*) the time alotted to a programme, item, commercial, etc; the time at which the broadcast begins.

air-to-air /ˈɛrtuːˈɛr/ *adj* (*weaponry, communications, etc*) activated between aircraft in flight.

air valve *n* a valve regulating the supply of air to a boiler or pipe.

air vesicle *n* a dilatation of the trachea of certain insects enabling them to ascend or descend by its inflation or expiration; a vesicle filled with air in certain fishes, connected with the swim bladder.

airway /ˈɛrweɪ/ *n* an aircraft route; a ventilation passage, as in a mine; a passage for air into the lungs; (*med*) a device to maintain the airway of an unconscious person.

airworthy /-ˌwɜrði/ *adj* safe to fly.—**airworthiness** *n*.

airy /ˈɛri/ *adj* (**airier, airiest**) open to the air; breezy; light as air; graceful; lighthearted; flippant.—**airily** *adv*.—**airiness** *n*.

aisle /aɪl/ *n* a passageway, as between rows of seats; a side part of a church.

ait /eɪt/ *n* a small island in a river or lake.—*also* **eyot**.

aitch /eɪtʃ/ *n* the letter H.

aitchbone /ˈeɪtʃbo:n/ *n* the rump bone; the cut of meat lying over it.

ajar /əˈdʒar/ *adv* partly open, as a door.

AK *abbr* = Alaska.

aka, a.k.a. *or* **AKA** /ˌeɪˌkeɪˈeɪ/ *abbr* = also known as.

akimbo /əˈkɪmbo:/ *adv* having the hands on the hips and the elbows bent outwards.

akin /əˈkɪn/ *adj* related; essentially similar, compatible.

Akkadian /əˈkeɪdiən/ *n* an ancient Babylonian language preserved in cuneiform inscriptions. • *adj* of Akkad or Accad, the Babylonian city.—*also* **Accadian**.

al- /æl/ *or* /əl/ *prefix* the form of *ad-* before *l*.

-al /əl/ *adj suffix* of, of the nature of, as in *mortal, colossal*. • *n suffix esp* of verbal action, as in *approval*.

AL *abbr* = Alabama.

Al (*chem symbol*) = aluminium.

Ala. *abbr* = Alabama.

à la /ˈɑː lə/ *or* /ˈblə/ *prep* in the style of.

alabaster /ˈæləˌbæstər/ *or* /ˌæləˈbæstər/ *n* a type of soft, chalky stone used in ornaments.—**alabastrine** *adj*.

à la carte /ˌæləˈkɑrt/ *or* /ˌblɑ-/ *adj* (*menu*) with dishes listed and priced as separate items.

alack /əˈlæk/ *interj* an exclamation of blame, sorrow, or surprise.

alacrity /əˈlækrɪti/ *n* promptness, eager readiness.—**alacritous** *adj*.

alameda /ˌæləˈmiːdə/ *n* a public promenade planted with trees.

à la mode /ˌæləˈmoːd/ *or* /ˌblə-/ *adv* in the fashion. • *adj* fashionable.

alamode *n* a thin, light, glossy black silk.

alar /ˈeɪlər/ *adj* of wings; winged; winglike; wing-shaped.—*also* **alary**.

alarm /əˈlɑrm/ *n* a signal warning of danger; an automatic device to arouse from sleep or to attract attention; the fear arising from the apprehension of danger. • *vt* to give warning of danger; to fill with apprehension or fear.

alarm clock *n* a clock with an apparatus that can be set to ring loudly at a particular time.

alarming /-ɪŋ/ *adj* frightening, disconcerting.—**alarmingly** *adv*.

alarmist /-ɪst/ *n* one who keeps prophesying danger, a panic-monger.—**alarmism** *n*.

alarum /əˈlarəm/ *n* (*arch*) an alarm.

alary /ˈeɪləri/ *or* /ˈæləri/ *see* **alar**.

alas /əˈlæs/ *interj* expressive of misery, unhappiness, grief, etc.

alate /ˈeɪˌleɪt/ *adj* having wings or winglike side appendages.

alb /ælb/ *n* a white priestly vestment reaching to the feet, worn at the celebration of the Eucharist in the RC Church and in some Anglican churches.

albacore /ˈælbəˌkoːr/ *n* a large species of mackerel or tunny found in the Atlantic and Pacific Oceans.

albata an alloy imitating silver; German silver.

albatross /ˈælbəˌtrɒs/ *n* any of various large web-footed seabirds; a heavy burden, as of debt, guilt, etc; (*golf*) a score of three under par.

albeit /ɒlˈbiːɪt/ *conj* although, even though, notwithstanding.

Albertan /ælˈbɜrtən/ *n* ✽ a person who lives in, or is from, Alberta. • *adj* of or pertaining to Alberta.

albescent /ælˈbɛsənt/ *adj* shading into white; whitish; becoming white.—**albescence** *n*.

albino /ælˈbaɪno:/ *n* (*pl* **albinos**) a person lacking normal coloration, so that they have white skin and pink eyes; an animal or plant with abnormal pigmentation.

Albion /ˈælbiən/ *n* (*arch*) Britain.

album /ˈælbəm/ *n* a book with blank pages for the insertion of photographs, autographs, etc; a long-playing record, cassette, or CD.

albumen /ælˈbjuːmɪn/ *n* the white of an egg.

albumenize /-ˌaɪz/ *vt* to coat (paper) with an albuminous solution.

albuminoid /-ˌnɔɪd/ *adj* like albumen. • *n* a class of organic compounds that form the chief part of the organs and tissues of animals and plants; proteids.

albuminous /ælˈbjuːmɪnəs/ *adj* like, or containing, albumin.

albuminuria /ælˌbjuːmɪˈniəriə/ *or* /-ˈnjʊr-/ *n* the presence of albumin in the kidneys and the urine.

alburnum /ælˈbɜrnəm/ *n* the white and softer part of wood between the bark and the heartwood; sapwood.

alcahest *see* **alkahest**.

Alcaic /ælˈkeɪɪk/ *n* a kind of lyric verse form consisting of four lines of four feet devised by the 7th-century BC Greek poet Alcaeus.—*also adj*.

alcaide /ælˈkaɪd/ *or* /-ˈkeɪd/ *n* the commander of a castle in Spain; the warder of a Spanish jail.

alcalde /ɒlˈkɒldi/, **alcade** *n* a magistrate or justice in Spain or Portugal.

alcazar /ˈælkəˌzar/ *or* /ælˈkæzər/ *n* a Spanish or Moorish palace or castle.

alchemist /ˈælkəmɪst/ *n* one who studies or practises alchemy.

alchemize /-maɪz/ *vt* to transmute.

alchemy /ˈælkəmi/ *n* (*pl* **alchemies**) chemistry as practised during medieval times, with the aim of transmuting base metals into gold.—**alchemic, alchemical** *adj*.—**alchemist** *n*.

alcohol /ˈælkəhɒl/ *n* a liquid, generated by distillation and fermentation, that forms the intoxicating agent in wine, beer and spirits; a liquid containing alcohol; a chemical compound of this nature.

alcoholic /ˌælkəˈhɒlɪk/ *adj* of or containing alcohol; caused by alcohol. • *n* a person suffering from alcoholism.

alcoholism /ˈælkəˌhɒlɪzəm/ *n* a disease caused by excessive consumption of alcohol.

alcoholize /-aɪz/ *vt* to subject to the influence of alcohol; to rectify (spirits of wine).—**alcoholization** *n*.

alcoholometer /-ˌhɒlmətər/ *n* an instrument for determining the strength of spirits.

alcool /ˈælkuːl/ *n* ✽ (*Cdn*) in Quebec, unflavoured alcohol sold as a beverage.

Alcoran /ˌælkoːˈrɒn/ *or* /-ˈræn/ *n* the Koran, the Muslim bible.

alcove /ˈælˌkoːv/ *n* a recess off a larger room.

aldehyde /ˈældəˌhaɪd/ *n* a volatile fluid with a suffocating smell, obtained from alcohol.

al dente /ælˈdɛnteɪ/ *or* /æl-/ *adj* cooked but still firm to the teeth.

alder /ˈɒldər/ *n* a genus of plants growing in moist land and related to the birch.

alderman /ˈɒldərmən/ *n* (*pl* **aldermen**) in US, a member of certain municipal councils; (*formerly*) in England and Wales, a senior councillor.—**aldermanic** *adj*.

ale /eɪl/ *n* beer.

aleatory /ˈeɪliəˌtɔri/ *adj* depending on dice or chance.

alee /əˈliː/ *adj, adv* (*naut*) on the lee, to leeward.

alegar /ˈæləgər/ *or* /ˈɑl-/ *n* vinegar made from ale.

alehouse /ˈeɪlˌhɐʊs/ *n* a place where ale is sold.

alembic /əˈlɛmbɪk/ *n* an apparatus formerly used in distilling.

Alençon /əˈlɛnˌsɒn/ *or* /-sən/, *Fr.* /alɑ̃ˈsɔ̃ː/ *n* a fine lace made at Alençon in France.

alert /əˈlɜrt/ *adj* watchful; active, brisk. • *n* a danger signal. • *vt* to warn of impending danger, put in a state of readiness.—**alertly** *adv*.—**alertness** *n*.

alexandrine /ˌaləgzændrɪn/ *or* /-ˌdriːn/ *n* a heroic verse of six iambic feet, or twelve syllables.—*also adj*.

alexia /əˈlɛksiə/ *n* the inability to read, due to mental illness.

alexin /əˈlɛksɪn/ *n* a disease-resisting protein in blood serum.

alfalfa /ˈælfælfə/ *n* a deep-rooted leguminous plant grown widely for hay and forage.—*also* **lucerne**.

alfresco /æl'freskoː/ or /ɑl-/ adj taking place outside in the open.—also adv.

alga /'ælgə/ n (pl **algae**) any of a group of chiefly aquatic lower plants classified according to colour.—**algal** adj.

algarroba, algaroba /ˌælgə'roːbə/ n. the carob tree and bean; St John's bread.

algebra /'ældʒəbrə/ n the branch of mathematics dealing with the properties and relations of numbers; the generalization and extension of arithmetic.—**algebraic, algebraical** adj.—**algebraist** n.

Algerian /æl'dʒiːrɪən/ adj pertaining to Algeria or Algiers. • n a native of Algeria or Algiers.

Algerine /ˌældʒə'riːn/ adj Algerian.

-algia /'ældʒə/ or /-dʒɪə/ n suffix pain.—**algic** adj.

algid /'ældʒɪd/ adj cold, chilly.

ALGOL /'ælˌɡɒl/ acronym (comput) a high-level programming language used for solving general problems in science and mathematics.

algology /æl'ɡɒlədʒi/ n the study of algae.—**algologist** n.

Algonquian /æl'ɡɒŋkwɪən/ or /-kɪən/ n ✤ a group of eastern North American Indian languages: a member of a North American Indian people who speaks one of these languages. • adj of or pertaining to these peoples or their languages.

Algonquin /æl'ɡɒŋkwɪn/ or /-kɪn/ n ✤ a member of a First Nations people living in eastern Ontario; the Algonquian language spoken by this people. • adj of or pertaining to this people or their language.

algor /'ælɡɔr/ n the rigor or chill on the onset of fever.

algorism /'ælɡərɪzəm/ n the arabic (decimal) numeration; arithmetic.—**algorismic** adj.

algorithm /'ælɡərɪðəm/ n (math) any method or procedure for computation.—**algorithmic** adj.—**algorithmically** adv.

alias /'eɪlɪəs/ adv otherwise called. • n (pl **aliases**) an assumed name.

alibi /'ælɪˌbaɪ/ n (pl **alibis**) (law) the plea that a person charged with a crime was elsewhere when it was committed; (inf) any excuse.

alien /'eɪlɪən/ adj foreign; strange; distasteful to, counter to. • n a person from another country, place, etc; a person of foreign birth who has not been naturalized; a being from outer space.

alienable /-əbəl/ adj (law) (property) that may be transferred.—**alienability** n.

alienage /'eɪlɪənɪdʒ/ n the state or legal status of an alien.

alienate /'eɪlɪəneɪt/ vt to render hostile or unfriendly; to make less affectionate or interested.

alienation /ˌeɪlɪən'eɪʃən/ n estrangement; transference; diversion to another purpose; mental derangement.

alienee /ˌeɪlɪən'iː/ n (law) one to whom property is transferred.

alienism /'eɪlɪənɪzəm/ n the study and treatment of mental alienation.—**alienist** n.

alienor /-ɔr/ or /-ər/ n (law) one who transfers property to another.

aliform /'eɪlɪˌfɔrm/ adj wing-shaped.

alight[1] /ə'laɪt/ vi (**alighting, alighted** or **alit**) to come down, as from a bus; to land after a flight.

alight[2] adj on fire; lively.

align /ə'laɪn/ vt to place in a straight line, to bring into agreement, etc. • vi to line up.—**alignment** n.

alignment /-mənt/ n the act of laying out or adjusting by a line; the ground plan of a railway or road.

alike /ə'laɪk/ adj like one another. • adv equally; similarly.

aliment /'æləmənt/ n food; the necessaries of life generally; an allowance for support by decree of court. • vt to make provision for the maintenance of; to make provision for the support of parents or children respectively.—**alimental** adj.

alimentary /ˌælɪ'məntəri/ adj pertaining to nourishment, food.

alimentary canal n the tube extending within the body from the mouth to the anus through which food passes and is absorbed.

alimentation /ˌælɪmən'teɪʃən/ n the act of giving nourishment; the function of the alimentary canal.—**alimentative** adj.

alimony /'æləˌmoːni/ n (pl **alimonies**) an allowance for support made by one spouse to the other, esp a man to his wife or former wife, pending or after a legal separation or divorce.

aliped /'ælɪˌped/ adj having wing-like limbs, as the bat.

aliphatic /'ælɪfætɪk/ adj (chem) of fat.

aliquant /'ælɪkwənt/ or /-kwɒnt/ adj (math) being a part of a number that does not divide it without a remainder, as 8 is the aliquant part of 25.—also n.

aliquot /'ælɪkwət/ or /-kwɒt/ adj (math) being a part of a number

of quantity that will divide it without a remainder, as 8 is the aliquot part of 24.—also n.

alive /ə'laɪv/ adj having life; active, alert; in existence, operation, etc.

alizarin /ə'lɪzərɪn/ n a red colouring matter found in madder but now produced from anthracene.

alkahest /'ælkəˌhest/ n the supposed universal solvent of the alchemists.—also **alcahest**.

alkali /'ælkəlaɪ/ n (pl **alkalis, alkalies**) (chem) any salt or mixture that neutralizes acids.—**alkaline** adj.

alkalify /'ælkəlɪˌfaɪ/ vb (**alkalifying, alkalified**) vt to form or convert into alkali. • vi to become an alkali.

alkalimeter /ˌælkə'lɪmətər/ n an instrument used to determine the relative strength of alkalis.

alkalimetry /-mətri/ n the process of determining the strength of an alkaline mixture or liquid.—**alkalimetric** adj.

alkaline /'ælkəˌlaɪn/ or /-ˌlaɪn/ adj pertaining to, or having the properties of, an alkali.—**alkalinity** n.

alkalize /-ˌlaɪz/ vt to convert into an alkali or render alkaline.—**alkalizable** adj.

alkaloid /-ˌlɔɪd/ n a body or substance containing alkaline properties; (pl) nitrogenous compounds met with in plants in combination with organic acids. • adj resembling an alkali in its properties.

alkanet /'ælkəˌnet/ n a rich red dye; the plant the root of which yields it.

all /ɒl/ adj the whole amount or number of; every one of. • adv wholly; supremely, completely, entirely. • n the whole number, quantity; everyone; everything.

alla breve /ˌɒlə'breːveɪ/ adv (mus) in quick time, with one breve to a measure.

Allah /'ælə/ or /'ɒlə/ n the Muslim name of God.

all along adv throughout.

allantoid /ə'læn,tɔɪd/ adj of or pertaining to the allantois; (bot) sausage-shaped. • n the allantois.—**allantoidal** adj.

allantois /ə'læn,tɔɪs/ n (pl **allantoides**) a membranous appendage of most vertebrate embryos.

allay /ə'leɪ/ or /ə-/ vt to lighten, alleviate; to pacify or make calm.

all but adv almost.

all-candidates meeting n ✤ (Cdn) a public meeting held during an election campaign in which all candidates present their views and answer questions.

all clear /'ɒlˌklɪr/ n a signal indicating that a danger has passed or that it is safe to proceed.

all-dressed adj ✤ (Cdn) pertaining to an item of food, such as a pizza or a hot dog, that is topped with all available garnishes.

allegation /ˌælə'ɡeɪʃən/ n the act of alleging; assertion; declaration; that which is asserted or alleged; that which is offered as a plea, an excuse, or justification; the statement as yet unproved of a party to a suit.

allege /ə'ledʒ/ vt to assert or declare, esp without proof; to offer as an excuse.

allegedly /ə'ledʒədli/ adv asserted without proof.

allegiance /ə'liːdʒəns/ n the obligation of being loyal to one's country, etc; devotion, as to a cause.

allegorical /ˌælə'ɡɒrɪkəl/ or /-'ɡɑr-/, **allegoric** adj pertaining to, consisting of, or in the nature of allegory; figurative.—**allegorically** adv.

allegorize /'æləɡəˌraɪz/ or /ˌæləɡə'raɪz/ vt to put in the form of an allegory.—**allegorization** n.

allegory /'æləˌɡɒri/ or /-ˌɡɑri/ n (pl **allegories**) a fable, story, poem, etc in which the events depicted are used to convey a deeper, usu moral or spiritual, meaning.—**allegorist** n.

allegretto /ˌælə'ɡreto/ adv (mus) moderately fast. • n (pl **allegrettos**) a piece of music played in this way.

allegro /ə'leɡro/ adv (mus) fast. • n (pl **allegros**) a piece of music played in this way.

allele /ə'liːl/ n (genetics) either of a pair of contrasting characteristics one or the other of which is found unmixed in descendants of a cross between parental forms respectively possessing them.—also **allelomorph**.—**allelic** adj.—**allelism** n.

alleluia /ˌælə'luːjə/ or /ˌple-/ see **hallelujah**.

allemande /ˌælə'mænd/ or /-'mɑnd/ n a German national dance in three-quarter time.

allergen /'ælərdʒən/ n a substance inducing an allergic reaction.

allergenic /-ˌdʒenɪk/ adj causing an allergic reaction.

allergy /'ælərdʒi/ n (pl **allergies**) an abnormal reaction of the body to substances (certain foods, pollen, etc) normally harmless: antipathy.—**allergic** adj.

allerion /ə'lɛriən/ n (her) an eagle displayed without feet or beak.

alleviate /ə'li:vieit/ vt to lessen or relieve (pain, worry, etc).—**alleviation** n.—**alleviator** n.

alleviative /ə'li:vi,eitiv/ adj tending to alleviate. • n that which alleviates.

alley /'æli/ n a narrow street between or behind buildings; a bowling lane.

all fours adv on hands and knees.

All-hallowe'en /,ɒl'hælo:,wi:n/ n Hallowe'en.

All-hallows /,ɒl'hælo:z/ npl All Saints' Day, celebrated on 1 November, in honour of all the saints.

alliaceous /,æli'eiʃəs/ adj of the nature or property of garlic or the onion.

alliance /ə'laiəns/ n a union by marriage or treaty for a common purpose; an agreement for this; the countries, groups, etc in such an association.

allied /æ'laid/ or /'æ'laid/ see **ally**.

alligator /'æli,geitər/ n a large reptile similar to the crocodile but having a short, blunt snout.

alligator pear n the avocado.

all in adj (price, etc) all-inclusive.

all-in adj (inf) exhausted.

all-inclusive /,ɒlin'klu:ziv/ adj including everything.

alliteration /ə,litə'reiʃən/ n the repetition of the same sound at the beginning of two or more words in a phrase, etc.—**alliterative** adj.

allocate /'ælə,keit/ vt to distribute or apportion in shares; to set apart for a specific purpose.

allocation /,ælə'keiʃən/ n the act of alloting, allocating, or assigning; an allotment or assignment; an allowance made on an account.

allocution /,æləkju:ʃən/ n a formal address, esp as one delivered by the Pope to his clergy or to the Church generally.

allodial /æ'lo:diəl/ adj freehold; not feudal. • n land thus held.

allodium /-əm/, **allod** n (pl **allodia, allods**) freehold estate; land that is the absolute property of the owner.

allogamy /ə'lɒgəmi/ n (biol) cross-fertilization.—**allogamous** adj.

allograph /'ælə,græf/ n a signature by one person on behalf of another, opposite of autograph.—**allographic** adj.

allomorphism /,ælə'mɔrfizəm/ n (chem) the property in certain substances of assuming a different form while remaining the same in constitution.

all one adj, n in effect the same.

allopath /'æləpæθ/, **allopathist** /ə'lɒpəθist/ n one who favours or practises allopathy.

allopathy /ə'lɒpəθi/ n the orthodox medical practice of treating disease by inducing an action opposite to the disease it is sought to cure, opposite of homoeopathy.—**allopathic** adj.—**allopathically** adv.

allophone /'ælə,fo:n/ n a phonetic term describing any of various possible contextual or environmental variants of the same phoneme; ✦ (Cdn) in Quebec, an immigrant to Canada whose first language is neither English nor French. • ✦ adj having a first language as an immigrant other than English or French.—**allophonic** adj.

allot /ə'lɒt/ vt (**allotting, allotted**) to distribute, allocate.

allotment /-mənt/ n allotting; a share allotted; a small area of land rented for cultivation.

allotropy /ə'lɒtrəpi/, **allotropism** n the capability shown by certain chemical elements to assume different forms, each characterized by peculiar qualities, as the occurrence of carbon in the form of the diamond, charcoal and plumbago respectively.—**allotropic** adj.—**allotropically** adv.

allottee /ə,lɒt'i:/ n one to whom an allotment or share is granted or assigned; a plot-holder.

all out /'ɔl'aut/ adv with maximum capacity.

all-out adj using maximum effort.

all-over /'ɔl'o:vər/ adj covering the whole surface.

allow /ə'lau/ vt to permit; to acknowledge, admit as true; (money) to give, grant as an allowance at regular intervals; to estimate as an addition or deduction. • vi to admit the possibility (of).

allowable /ə'lauəbəl/ adj permissible.—**allowably** adv.

allowance /ə'lauəns/ n an amount or sum allowed or given at regular times; a discount; a portion of income not subject to income tax; permission; admission, concession.

alloy /æ'lɔi/ n a solid substance comprising a mixture of two or more metals; something that degrades the substance to which it is added. • vt to make into an alloy; to degrade or spoil by mixing with an inferior substance.

all-purpose /'ɔl,pərpəs/ adj suitable for many uses.

all right adv good enough, acceptable; without doubt. • adj satisfactory; safe, well; agreeable. • interj (used to express consent).—also **alright**.

all-round /'ɔl,raund/ adj efficient in all respects, esp sport.

All Saints' Day n (Christian Church) 1 November, a festival in honour of all the saints.

All Souls' Day /-so:lz-/ n (RC Church) the day, celebrated 2 November, in honour of the departed.

allspice /'ɒl,spais/ n an aromatic spice made from the berry of a West Indian tree.

all-star /'ɒl,star/ adj made up entirely of outstanding performers.

all there adj (sl) not mentally wanting.

all-time /'ɒl,taim/ adj unsurpassed until now.

all told adv with all counted; all in all.

allude /ə'lu:d/ vi to refer indirectly to.

allure /ə'lur/ vt to entice, charm. • n fascination; charm.—**allurement** n.

alluring /-iŋ/ adj attractive.

allusion /ə'lu:ʒən/ n alluding; an implied or indirect reference.—**allusive** adj.

allusive /ə'lu:siv/ adj having reference to something not definitely expressed.—**allusively** adv.—**allusiveness** n.

alluvion /ə'lu:viən/ n the wash of the sea or river against a shore; land added to a shore or riverbank by the action of the water; an overflow.

alluvium /ə'lu:viəm/ n (pl **alluviums, alluvia**) earth, sand, gravel, etc deposited by moving water.—**alluvial** adj.

ally /æ'lai/ vti (**allying, allied**) to join or unite for a specific purpose; to relate by similarity of structure, etc. • n (pl **allies**) a country or person joined with another for a common purpose.

Almagest /'ælmə,dʒest/ n the great astronomical treatise of Ptolemy of the 2nd century ad; (without cap) other similar treatises.

alma mater /'ælmə'mɒtər/ or /'ɒl-/, /-'meit-/ n one's school, college, or university.

almanac /'ælmə,næk/ or /'ɒl-/ n a calendar with astronomical data, weather forecasts, etc.

almanack /'ælmə,næk/ or /'ɒl-/ n (arch) an almanac.

almandine /'ælmən,di:n/ or /-dain/ n a violet-red variety of garnet, tinged sometimes with blue or yellow.

almighty /ɒl'maiti/ adj all-powerful. • n (with cap) God, the all-powerful.—**almightly** adv.—**almightiness** n.

almond /'ɒmənd/ or /'ɒl-/ n the edible kernel of the fruit of a tree of the rose family; the tree bearing this fruit. • adj (eyes, etc) oval and pointed at one or both ends.

almoner /'ɒlmənər/ n (formerly) one who dispenses or distributes alms or charity; an alms purse; a pouch or purse which in early times was suspended from the girdle.

almost /'ɒlmo:st/ adv all but, very nearly but not quite all.

alms /ɒmz/ npl money, food, etc given to the poor.

almshouse /-hɒuz/ n a house endowed by private or public charity and appropriated to the use of the poor.

aloe /'æ,lo:/ n (pl **aloes**) a succulent plant with tall spikes of flowers.

aloes /'æ,lo:z/ n (used as sing) the bitter juice of the aloe plant used in medicine.

aloft /ə'lɒft/ adv in the air, flying; high up.

alone /ə'lo:n/ adj isolated; without anyone or anything else; unassisted; unique. • adv exclusively.

along /ə'lɒŋ/ adv onward, forward; over the length of; in company and together with; in addition. • prep in the direction of the length of; in accordance with.

alongside /-said/ prep close beside. • adv at the side.

aloof /ə'lu:f/ adv at a distance; apart. • adj cool and reserved.—**aloofness** n.

alopecia /,ælə'peiʃə/ n baldness; loss of hair through skin disease.

aloud /ə'laud/ adv with a normal voice; loudly; spoken.

alow /ə'lo:/ adv (naut) to or in a lower part; below.

alp /ælp/ n a mountain peak.

alpaca /æl'pækə/ n a Peruvian llama with long fine wool; a fabric made of this wool.

alpenglow /'ælpən,glo:/ n a peculiar purple glow on the snow on the Alps seen just before sunrise and after sunset.

alpenhorn /-,hɔrn/ n a long and nearly straight horn used by the mountaineers of the Alps.

alpenstock /-,stɒk/ n a stout staff with an iron spike, used by mountain climbers.

alpha /'ælfə/ n the first letter of the Greek alphabet.

alphabet /'ælfə,bɛt/ *n* the characters used in a language arranged in conventional order.

alphabetical /,ælfə,betikəl/, **alphabetic** *adj* pertaining to an alphabet; in the order of the alphabet.—**alphabetically** *adv*.

alphabetize /'ælfəbə,taiz/ *vt* to arrange in alphabetical order.—**alphabetization** *n*.

alphanumeric /,ælfənu:'mɛrik/ or /-nju:-/, **alphameric** /,ælfə'mɛrik/ *adj* containing letters of the alphabet and numerals.—**alphanumerically, alphamerically** *adv*.

alpha particle *n* a particle of helium given off by radium.

alpha ray *n* radiation of alpha particles.

alpine /æl'pain/ *adj* (*with cap*) of the Alps; of high mountains. • *n* a mountain plant, *esp* a small herb.

alpinist /'ælpinist/ *n* a mountaineer who climbs in the Alps or in areas of similar mountains.—**alpinism** *n*.

Alps /ælps/ *npl* a high mountain range in south central Europe.

already /ɔl'redi/ *adv* by or before the time specified; before the time expected.

alright /ɔl'rait/ *adv* a frequent spelling of all right

Alsatian /æl,seiʃən/ *n* a German shepherd; a native of Alsace.

also /'ɔlsoː/ *adv* in addition, besides.

also-ran /-,ræn/ *n* a defeated contestant in a race, an election, etc.

alt /ælt/ *n* (*mus*) the high notes above the treble staff.

Alta. *abbr* ✠ = Alberta.

Altaic /æl'teiik/ *adj* pertaining to the Altaic mountain regions, partly bounding Russia and China. • *n* the language of the region.

altar /'ɒltər/ *n* a table, etc for sacred purposes in a place of worship.

altarage *n* the offerings placed upon the altar to be devoted to the church, or appropriated by the priest as stipend.

altar cloth /-,klɔθ/ *n* a general term for the coverings of the altar.

altar ledge /-,lɛdz/ *n* a step or ledge behind the altar of a church, slightly raised above it for holding lights, flowers, and other symbolical ornaments; a retable.

altarpiece /-,piːs/ *n* a painting, decorative screen or other work of art, placed over or behind an altar.

altarscreen /-,skriːn/ *n* a screen or partition separating the altar from the choir; a reredos.

altar slab /-,slæb/ *n* the top of an altar; the consecrated part of an altar (the mensa).

altarwise /-,waiz/ *adv* placed in the usual position of an altar, with the ends towards the north and south, and the front to the west.

altazimuth /,æl'tæzəməθ/ *n* an instrument for determining the altitudes and azimuths of the stars and planets.

alter /'ɒltər/ *vti* to make or become different in a small way; to change.—**alterable** *adj*.—**alterability** *n*.

alteration /,ɒltər'eiʃən/ *n* the act of altering or changing; the change or modification effected.

alterative /'ɒltə,reitiv/ or /-tərətiv/ *adj* producing change; having the power to alter. • *n* a medicine that restores the healthy functions of the body.

altercate /'ɒltər,keit/ *vi* to contend in words; to wrangle; to dispute with anger or heat.

altercation /,ɒltər'keiʃən/ *n* an angry or heated quarrel.

alter ego /'ɒltər,iːgoː/ or /'æl-/ *n* one's other self; a constant companion.

alternant /'ɒltərnənt/ *adj* alternating composed of alternate layers.

alternate[1] /'ɒltərneit/ *vt* to do or use by turns. • *vi* to act, happen, etc by turns; to take turns regularly.—**alternation** *n*.

alternate[2] *adj* occurring or following in turns.—**alternately** *adv*.

alternate angles *npl* the internal angles made by two lines with a third on opposite sides of it.

alternating current *n* an electric current that reverses its direction at regular intervals.

alternation /,ɒltər'neiʃən/ *n* the act of alternating, or state of being alternate; reciprocal succession; antiphonal singing or reading.

alternative /,ɒltər'neitiv/ *adj* presenting a choice between two things. • *n* either of two possibilities.—**alternatively** *adv*.

alternative comedy *n* a form of comedy that avoids conventional humour (e.g. racist and sexist jokes), characterized by aggressively delivered and blackly humourous stand-up routines that *usu* challenge political and social orthodoxy.

alternative medicine *n* any technique of medical treatment without use of drugs, *eg* osteopathy, acupuncture, dieting.

alternator /'ɒltər'neitər/ or /,æl-/ *n* an electric generator that produces alternating current.

althaea, althea /æl'θiːə/ *n* a genus of plants including the marshmallow and the hollyhock.

althorn /'ælt,hɔrn/ *n* a musical instrument of the saxhorn class, frequently used in military bands.

although /ɒl'ðoː/ or /ɒl'θoː, *conj* though; in spite of that.

altimeter /æl't:mitər/ *n* an instrument for measuring altitude.

altimetry /-tri/ *n* the art of measuring altitudes by the use of the altimeter.—**altimetrical** *adj*.

altissimo /æl'tisimoː/ or /ɒl-/ *adj* (*mus*) of the part or notes situated above F in alt.

altitude /'ælti,tuːd/ or /-,tjuːd/ *n* height, *esp* above sea level.—**altitudinal** *adj*.

alto /'æltoː/ or /'ɒltoː/ *n* (*pl* **altos**) the range of the highest male voice; a singer with this range; a contralto. • *adj* high.

alto clef /-klɛf/ *n* the C clef placed on the third line of the staff.

altogether /,ɒltə'gɛðər/ or /'ɒltəgɛðər/ *adv* in all; on the whole; completely.

alto-relievo, alto-rilievo /,æltoːrə'liːvoː/ *n* (*pl* **alto-relievos, alto-rilievos**) high relief; figures or other objects that stand out boldly from the background, and having more than half their thickness projecting.

altruism /'ɒl,truːizəm/ or /'æl-/ *n* unselfish concern for or dedication to the interests or welfare of others.—**altruist** *n*.—**altruistic** *adj*.—**altruistically** *adv*.

aludel /'ælju:,cɛl/ *n* one of the pear-shaped glass or earthenware pots, open at both ends, used in sublimation.

alum /ə'lɛm/ *n* a double sulphate formed of aluminium and some other element, usually an alkali metal.

alumina /ə'luːminə/ *n* the single oxide of aluminium, the most abundant of the earths; a notable constituent of common clay, alumina is largely used in dyeing and calico printing as a mordant.

aluminiferous /ə,luːmi'nifərəs/ *adj* containing or yielding alum, alumina, or aluminium.

aluminium, aluminum /ə'luːminəm/ *n* a silvery-white malleable metallic element notable for its lightness.

aluminous /ə'luːminəs/ *adj* of, containing or resembling alum or alumina.

alumna /ə'lʌmnə/ *n* (*pl* **alumnae**) a female graduate or pupil of a university or college.

alumnus /ə'lʌmnəs/ *n* (*pl* **alumni**) a former pupil or student.—**alumna** *nf* (*pl* **alumnae**).

alum root /'æləm,ruːt/ *n* a popular name given to certain astringent roots of saxifrages.

alum schist /-'ʃist/ *n* a thin-bedded fissile rock from which alum is procured.

alunite /'æljə,nait/ or /-jə-,/ *n* subsulphate of alumina and potash.

alveolar /æl'vioːlər/ *adj* of tooth sockets.

alveolate /æl'vioːleit/ *adj* with deep pits or cells resembling the honeycomb.—**alveolation** *n*.

alveolus /æl'vioːləs/ *n* (*pl* **a veoli**) a small pit, cell, cavity, or socket; the socket in which a tooth is fixed; the cell of a honeycomb.

alvine /æl'vain/ *adj* pertaining or belonging to the intestines or belly.

always /'ɒlweiz/ *adv* at all times; in all cases; repeatedly; forever.

Alzheimer's disease /'ɒltə,haimərz/ or /'ɒls-/, /'ælts-/, /'æls-/ *n* a degenerative disorder of the brain resulting in progressive senility.

A/M *abbr* ✠ (*Cdn*) = Air Marshall.

am /æm/ *see* **be**.

a.m. /'ei'em/ *abbr* = *ante meridiem*, before noon.

amadou /'æmə,duː/ *n* a styptic and a tinder prepared by steeping the solid portions of a fungus affecting trees in a solution of saltpetre; German tinder.

amah /'ɒmə/ *n* an East Indian nurse or female servant.

amalgam /ə'mælgəm/ *n* an alloy of mercury and another metal; a mixture.

amalgamate /ə'mælgə,meit/ *vt* to combine, unite.

amalgamation /ə,mælgə'meiʃən/ *n* the act or process of compounding mercury with another metal; the separation of precious metals from the mother rock by means of quicksilver; the blending or mixing of different elements or things; the union or consolidation of two or more companies or businesses into one concern, a merger.

amanuensis /ə,mænju:u'ɛnsis/ *n* (*pl* **amanuenses**) one who is employed to write at the dictation or direction of another; a secretary.

amaranth /'æmə,rænθ/ *n* an imaginary flower said by poets to be unfading; a plant of the genus *Amarantus*; a colour mixture in which magenta is the chief ingredient; red colouring added to some foods.

amaranthine /'æmə,rænθaɪn/ *adj* pertaining to the amaranth; never-fading, like amaranth; purplish.

amaryllis /,æmə'rɪlɪs/ *n* a genus of bulbous flowering plants to which the belladonna lily and narcissus belong.

amass /ə'mæs/ *vt* to bring together in a large quantity; to accumulate.—**amasser** *n*.—**amassment** *n*.

amateur /'æmətʃər/ or /-tər/ *n* one who engages in a particular activity as a hobby, and not as a profession. • *adj* of or done by amateurs.—**amateurism** *n*.

amateurish /'æmətʃərɪʃ/ or /,æmə'tʃərɪʃ/, /-'tərɪʃ/ *adj* lacking expertise.—**amateurishly** *adv*.—**amateurishness** *n*.

amatol /'æmə,tɒl/ or /-,tɔl/, /-,tɔːl/ *n* a high explosive.

amatory /'æmə,tɔri/, **amatorial** /-əl/ *adj* relating to or expressive of love.

amaurosis /,æmɔ'roːsɪs/ *n* loss or decay of sight due to partial, periodic, or complete paralysis of the optic nerve.—**amaurotic** *adj*.

amaut /ə'maut/ *n* ♣ among the Inuit, a fur-lined pouch in back of a woman's parka, used to carry an infant.

amaze /ə'meɪz/ *vt* to fill with wonder, astonish.—**amazing** *adj*.—**amazingly** *adv*.

amazement /ə'meɪzmənt/ *n* the state of being amazed; astonishment; perplexity arising from sudden surprise.

Amazon /'æmə,zɒn/ *n* (*Greek myth*) a race of women warriors; a tall strong athletic woman.—**Amazonian** *adj*.

amazon ant *n* a species of ant found in Europe and America, which seizies the neuters of other species in the pupa stage and brings them up with their own larvae.

amazonite /'æməzənaɪt/ *n* the amazon stone gemstone.

amazon stone *n* a beautiful green feldspar found near the Amazon.

ambary, ambari /æm'bɑri/ *n* (*pl* **ambaries, ambaris**) a plant of Asia that produces a jute-like fibre; the fibre.

ambassador /æm'bæsədər/ *n* the highest-ranking diplomatic representative from one country to another; an authorized messenger.—**ambassadorial** *adj*.—**ambassadress** *nf*.

ambassador extraordinary *n* an ambassador sent on a special mission.

ambassador plenipotentiary *n* an ambassador sent with full powers to make a treaty.

amber /'æmbər/ *n* a hard yellowish fossil resin, used for jewellery and ornaments, etc; the colour of amber; a yellow traffic light used to signal "caution".

ambergris /-grɪs/ or /-,grɪs/ *n* a waxy substance found in tropical seas, which is secreted by sperm whales and is used in perfumery as a fixative.

amberoid, ambroid /-ɔɪd/ *n* pressed amber; synthetic amber.

amber tree *n* the common name for various species of African evergreen shrubs with fragrant leaves.

ambidextrous /,æmbi'dekstrəs/ *adj* able to use the left and the right hand equally well.—**ambidexterity** *n*.

ambience, ambiance /'æmbiəns/ or /'æmbiãs/, *Fr*. /ãbi'ãs/ *n* surrounding influence, atmosphere.

ambient /'æmbiənt/ *adj* surrounding.

ambiguity /,æmbə'gjuːɪti/ *n* (*pl* **ambiguities** /-ɪz/) double or dubious significance; vagueness.

ambiguous /æm'bɪgjuːəs/ *adj* capable of two or more interpretations; indistinct, vague.—**ambiguously** *adv*.—**ambiguousness** *n*.

ambit /'æmbɪt/ *n* a circuit or compass; the line or sum of the lines by which a figure is bounded; the perimeter; sphere of action.

ambition /æm'bɪʃən/ *n* desire for power, wealth and success; an object of ambition.

ambitious /-ʃəs/ *adj* having or governed by ambition; resulting from or showing ambition; requiring considerable effort or ability.—**ambitiously** *adv*.

ambivalent /æm'bɪvələnt/ *adj* having mixed feelings toward the same object.—**ambivalence** *n*.

amble /'æmbəl/ *vi* to walk in a leisurely way. • *n* an easy pace. —**ambler** *n*.

amblyopia /,æmbi'oːpiə/ *n* dimness of vision; amaurosis.—**amblyopic** *adj*.

ambo /'æmbo:/ *n* (*pl* **ambos, ambones**) a pulpit; a reading desk.

amboyna, amboina /æm'bɔɪnə/ *n* a beautifully mottled and curled variegated wood used in cabinet work.

ambrosia /æm'broːʒə/ *n* (*Classical myth*) the food of the gods; anything exquisitely pleasing to taste or smell; a genus of weeds allied to wormwood.—**ambrosial, ambrosian** *adj*.

ambrotype /'æmbro:,taɪp/ *n* (*photog*) a process by which the light parts of a photograph are produced in silver, the dark parts showing as a background through the clear glass.

ambry /'æmbri/ *n* (*pl* **ambries** /-iːz/) a recess in a church wall for sacred vessels; a repository for arms; a cupboard for money tools, etc.

ambsace /'eɪmz,eɪts/ or /'æmz-/ *n* two ones, the lowest throw at dice; bad luck.

ambulacrum /,æmbju'leɪkrəm/ *n* (*pl* **ambulacra**) a perforation in the shell of echinoderms through which the tube feet are protruded.—**ambulacral** *adj*.

ambulance /'æmbjuləns/ *n* a special vehicle for transporting the sick or injured.

ambulance chaser /-,tʃeɪzər/ *n* one who attempts to profit from disaster.

ambulant /'æmbjulənt/ *adj* (*patient*) able to walk, not bed-ridden; moving from place to place.

ambulate /'æmbju,leɪt/ *vi* to walk about; to move about; to wander.—**ambulation** *n*.

ambulatory /-lə,tɔri/ *adj* of or pertaining to walking; movable; temporary; capable of walking. • *n* (*pl* **ambulatories**) a place for walking in; a covered way.

ambuscade /,æmbəs'keɪd/ *n* a strategic disposition of troops in ambush.

ambush /'æmbuʃ/ *n* the concealment of soldiers, etc to make a surprise attack; the bushes or other cover in which they are hidden. • *vti* to lie in wait; to attack from an ambush.

ambush marketing *n* the practice of taking advantage of another's official event to advertise one's own products.—*also* **ambushing**.

ameba /ə'miːbə/ *see* **amoeba**.

ameer /ə'mɪr/ *see* **amir**.

ameliorate /ə'miːliə,reɪt/ *vti* to make or become better.—**ameliorative** *adj*.—**ameliorator** *n*.

amelioration /-iə,reɪʃən/ *n* the making or growing better; improvement.

amen /ɑ'mɛn/ or /'eɪ-/ *interj* may it be so!

amenable /ə'menəbəl/ *adj* easily influenced or led, tractable; answerable to legal authority.—**amenability** *n*.—**amenably** *adv*.

amend /ə'mend/ *vt* to remove errors, *esp* in a text; to modify, improve; to alter in minor details.—**amendable** *adj*.—**amender** *n*.

amendatory /ə'mendə,tɔri/ *adj* tending to amend; corrective.

amende honorable /ə,mãdɒnɔ'ræblə/ *n* (*pl* **amendes honorables**) a public apology and reparation; a punishment formerly inflicted in France on traitors and the sacrilegious.

amendment /ə'mendmənt/ *n* the act of amending, correction; an alteration to a document, etc.

amends /ə'mendz/ *npl* (*used as sing*) compensation or recompense for some loss, harm, etc.

amenity /ə'meniti/ or /ə'miːnɪti/ *n* (*pl* **amenities**) pleasantness, as regards situation, convenience, or service.

amenorrhoea, amenorrhea /eɪ,menə'riːə/ *n* abnormal absence of menstruation.

ament /ə'ment/, **amentum** /-əm/ *n* (*pl* **aments, amenta**) a catkin, as of the willow.

amentia /ə'menʃə/ *n* want of reason; mental deficiency.

amerce /ə'mɜrs/ *vt* to punish by an arbitrary fine.—**amerceable** *adj*.—**amercement** *n*.

Amerenglish /'æmər,ɪŋlɪʃ/ or /,æmər'ɪŋlɪʃ/ *n* the English language as spoken in the United States.

American /ə'merɪkən/ *adj* belonging to or characteristic of America. • *n* an inhabitant of the US.

Americanism /ə'merɪkə,nɪzəm/ *n* a form of expression peculiar to the US; a custom peculiar to the US; attachment to the US.

Americanize /ə'merɪkə,naɪz/ *vt* to render American; to assimilate to the political and social institutions of the US.—**Americanization** *n*.

americium /,æmə'rɪʃəm/ or /-'rɪs-/ *n* a white radioactive metallic element derived from plutonium.

Amerindian /,æmə'rɪndiən/, **Amerind** /,æmə'rɪnd/ *n* an American Indian.—**Amerindic** *adj*.

ametabolic /eɪ,metə'bɒlɪk/ *adj* (*certain insects*) not undergoing metamorphosis.

amethyst /'æməθɪst/ *n* a gemstone consisting of bluish-violet quartz; the colour of an amethyst.—**amethystine** *adj*.

amiable /'eɪmɪəbəl/ *adj* friendly in manner, congenial.—**amiability** *n*.—**amiably** *adv*.

amianthus /ˌæmi'ænθəs/ *n* earth or mountain flax, a fibrous variety of asbestos.—**amianthine, amianthoid, amianthoidal** *adj*.

amicable /'æmɪkəbəl/ *adj* friendly; peaceable.—**amicability, amicableness** *n*.—**amicably** *adv*.

amice /'æmɪs/ *n* a square of white linen formerly worn on the head but now worn about the neck and shoulders by celebrant priests while saying Mass; a pilgrim's cloak.

amicus curiae /ə'mɪkus'kjuːrɪˌaɪ/ or /ə'miːkəs'kjuːrɪˌaɪ/ *n* (*pl* **amici curiae**) (*law*) a friend of the court; a disinterested adviser.

amid /ə'mɪd/, **amidst** /əmɪdst/ *prep* in or to the middle of; during.

amide /'æmaɪd/ or /'eɪm-/ *n* any of several compounds produced by the replacement of a hydrogen atom of ammonia by an acid radical or metal atom.

amidships /ə'mɪdʃɪps/ *adv* in the middle of a ship.

amine /æ'miːn/ or /ə-/ *n* any of several organic compounds formed by replacing hydrogen atoms of ammonia by one or more univalent hydrocarbon radicals.

amino acid *n* any of a group of organic acids that occur in proteins.

amir /ə'mɪr/ *n* (*formerly*) the Muslim ruler of Afghanistan.—*also* **ameer**.

amiss /ə'mɪs/ *adj* wrong, improper. • *adv* in an incorrect manner.

amity /'æmɪti/ *n* (*pl* **amities**) friendship.

ammeter /'æmiːtər/ *n* an instrument for measuring electric current in amperes.

ammo /'æmoʊ/ *n* (*sl*) ammunition.

ammonal /ə'moʊnəl/ *n* a highly explosive compound.

ammonia /ə'moʊniə/ or /-'moʊniə/ *n* a pungent colourless gas composed of nitrogen and hydrogen.

ammoniac[1] /ə'moʊniˌæk/ *n* a gum resin.—*also* **gum ammoniac**.

ammoniac[2], **ammoniacal** /ˌæmə'naɪəkəl/ *adj* of, pertaining to, like or containing ammonia.

ammonite /'æmoʊˌnaɪt/ *n* a fossil shell, twisted like a ram's horn; snakestone.—**ammonitic** *adj*.

ammonium /æ'moʊniəm/ *n* the hypothetical base of ammonia.

ammunition /ˌæmju'nɪʃən/ *n* bullets, shells, rockets, etc; any means of attack or defence; facts and reasoning used to prove a point in an argument.

amnesia /æm'niːʃə/ *n* a partial or total loss of memory.—**amnesiac, amnesic** *n, adj*.

amnesty /'æmnəsti/ *n* (*pl* **amnesties**) a general pardon, *esp* of political prisoners; a pardon granted for a limited time. • *vt* (**amnestying, amnestied**) to pardon (an offence).

amniocentesis /ˌæmnɪoʊˌsen'tiːsɪs/ *n* the extraction by hollow needle of a sample of amniotic fluid from the womb to test for foetal abnormalities.

amnion /'æmnɪən/ *n* (*pl* **amnions, amnia**) the thin innermost membrane surrounding the foetus in the womb of mammals, birds, and reptiles.—**amniotic** *adj*.

amoeba /ə'miːbə/ *n* (*pl* **amoebae** /ə,miːbaɪ/, **amoebas** /ə'miːbʊz/) a unicellular microorganism found in water, damp soil and the digestive tracts of animals.—*also* **ameba**.—**amoebic, amebic** *adj*.

amoebaean, amoebean /'æmiːbɪən/ *adj* (*verse form*) alternately answering.

amok /ə'mɛk/ *adj, adv* **run amok** to run about armed, in a state of frenzy, attacking all that come in the way; indiscriminate slaughter; headstrong violence.—*also* **amuck**.

among /ə'mʌŋ/, **amongst** /ə'mʌŋst/ *prep* in the number of, surrounded by; in the group or class of; within a group, between; by the joint efforts of.

amontillado /ə,mɒntɪ'lɑːdoʊ/, *Sp.* /ə'mɒntɪ'jɒdoː/ *n* (*pl* **amontillados**) a dry kind of light-coloured sherry.

amoral /eɪ'mɒrəl/ or /-'mɒrəl/ *adj* neither moral nor immoral; without moral sense.—**amorality** *n*.—**amorally** *adv*.

amoretto /ˌæmə'retoː/, **amorino** /ˌamə'riːnoː/ *n* (*pl* **amoretti, amorini**) (*art*) a figure of cupid and representations of children.—*also* **putto**.

amorist /'æmərɪst/ *n* an amateur in love, a philanderer.

amoroso /ˌæmə'roːsoː/ *adj* (*mus*) in a tender, amatory style.

amorous /'æmərəs/ *adj* displaying or feeling love or desire.—**amorously** *adv*.—**amorousness** *n*.

amor patriae /æ,mʊr'pætrɪˌɒi/ *n* love of one's country.

amorphous /ə'mɔrfəs/ *adj* lacking a specific shape, shapeless; unrecognizable, indefinable.—**amorphism** *n*.

amortization /ˌæmɔrtɪ'zeɪʃən/ *n* the extinction of a debt by means of a sinking fund; the act of alienating lands to a corporation in mortmain.—**amortizement** *n*.

amortize /'æmərtaɪz/ or /ə'mɔr-/ *vt* to put money aside at intervals for gradual payment of (a debt, etc).—**amortization** *n*.

amount /ə'maʊnt/ *vi* to be equivalent (to) in total, quantity or significance. • *n* the total sum; the whole value or effect; a quantity.

amour /æ'mʊr/ *n* a love affair; an intrigue.

amour propre /æ,muː-'prɒpr/ *n* self-love, vanity; self-respect.

amp /æmp/ *n* an ampere; (*inf*) an amplifier.

ampelopsis /ˌæmpɪ'lɒpsɪs/ *n* kinds of vine creeper, incl the Virginia creeper.

amperage /'æmpərɪdʒ/ or ˌæm'pɪr-/ *n* the strength of an electric current measured in amperes.

ampere /'æmpər/ *n* the standard SI unit by which an electric current is measured.

ampersand /'æmpərˌænd/ *n* the sign (&) meaning "and".

amphetamine /æm'fɛtəˌmiːn/ or /-mɪn/ *n* a drug used *esp* as a stimulant and to suppress appetite.

amphi- /'æmfi/ *prefix* of both kinds; on both sides; around.

amphibian /æm'fɪbiən/ *n* an animal living on land but breeding in water; an aircraft that can take off and land on water or land; a vehicle that can travel on land and through water.

amphibious /æm'fɪb əs/ *adj* living on both land and in water; (*mil*) involving both sea and land forces.

amphibology /ˌæm,fɪ'bɒlədʒi/, **amphiboly** /-li/ *n* (*pl* **amphibologies, amphibolies**) an ambiguous phrase, as a sentence that may be construed in two distinct ways, as "The duke yet lives that Henry shall depose"; a quibble.

amphibrach /'æmfəˌbræk/ *n* (*verse*) a foot of three syllables, the middle long, the first and last short.—**amphibrachic** *adj*.

amphimacer /æm'fɪməsər/ *n* (*verse*) a foot of three syllables, the middle short, the first and last long.

amphimixis /ˌæmfɪ'mɪksɪs/ *n* (*pl* **amphimixes**) a mingling of male and female gametes in sexual reproduction.

amphioxus /ˌæmfɪ'ɒksəs/ *n* (*pl* **amphioxi, amphioxuses**) the name of the lancelet, a fish with a body tapering at both ends, the lowest in organization of the vertebrates.

amphipod /'æmfəˌpɒd/ *n* any of the *Amphipoda* order of crustaceans having feet for both walking and swimming, including the sandhoppers and sand fleas.

amphiprostyle /ˌæm'fə'prɒstaɪl/ or /æmfɪ'prəˌstaɪl/ *adj* (*archit*) with a portico at both ends. • *n* a building of this kind, *esp* a temple.—**amphiprostylar** *adj*.

amphisbaena /ˌæmfəs'biːnə/ *n* (*pl* **amphisbaenae, amphisbaenas**) a fabled serpent with a head at each end; a kind of lizard or worm.—**amphisbaenic** *adj*.

amphitheatre, amphitheater /ˌæmfɪ'θiːətər/ *n* an oval or circular building with rising rows of seats around an open arena.

amphora /'æmfərə/ *n* (*pl* **amphorae, amphoras**) a two-handled vessel of oblong shape, used by the ancients for holding wine, etc; a Greek and Roman liquid measure, the former 9 gallons, the latter 6 gallons.

ample /'æmpəl/ *adj* large in size, scope, etc; plentiful.—**amply** *adv*.

amplification /ˌæmplɪfə'keɪʃən/ *n* the act of amplifying or expanding; enlargement.

amplifier /'æmpləˌfaɪr/ *n* a device that increases electric voltage, current, or power, or the loudness of sound.

amplify /'æmpləˌfaɪ/ *vt* (**amplifying, amplified**) to expand more fully, add details to; (*electrical signals, etc*) to strengthen.

amplitude /'æmpləˌtuːd/ or /-ˌtjuːd/ *n* largeness of extent, scope; abundance; the maximum deviation of an oscillation from the mean or zero.

amplitude modulation *n* (the transmitting of information by) the modulation of the amplitude of a radio carrier wave in accordance with the amplitude of the signal carried.

ampoule, ampul, ampule /'æmˌpʊl/ or /-ˌpʌl-/ *n* a small sealed glass vessel containing liquid, *esp* for injection.

ampulla /æm'pʊlə/ *n* (*pl* **ampullae**) an ancient vessel which contained urguents for the bath; a drinking vessel; a vessel for consecrated oil or chrism used in church rites and at the coronation of sovereigns.—**ampullar, ampullary** *adj*.

amputate /'æmpjuˌteɪt/ *vt* to cut off, *esp* by surgery.—**amputation** *n*.

amuck /ə'mʌk/ *see* **amok**.

amulet /'æmjʊlət/ *n* something worn as a charm against evil.

amuse /ə'mju:z/ *vt* to entertain or divert in a pleasant manner; to cause to laugh or smile.—**amusing** *adj.*

amusement /-mənt/ *n* that which amuses; the state of being amused; an entertainment; a pastime.

amusement arcade *n* an indoor or roofed area with mechanical games for entertainment.

amusement park *n* an outdoor area with fairground entertainments.

amygdalate /ə'mɪgdəleɪt/ *adj* of or belonging to the almond.

amygdalin /ə'mɪgdə,lɪn/ *n* a white crystalline substance obtained from the kernels of almonds.

amygdaloid /ə'mɪgdə,lɔɪd/ *adj* almond shaped. • *n* an igneous rock containing almond-shaped nodules of some mineral.

amyl /'eɪmaɪl/ or /'æmɪl/ *n* (*formerly*) the alcohol radical of many chemical compounds.

amylaceous /,æmɪ'leɪʃəs/ *adj* of starch, starchy.

amylase /'æmɪ,leɪz/ *n* an enzyme that breaks down starch and glycogen.

amylene /'æmɪ,li:n/ *n* a hydrocarbon obtained by the removal of water from amyl alcohol.

amyl nitrite *n* a drug inhaled to relieve spasms.

amyloid /'æmɪ,lɔɪd/ *n* a starchy food.

amylopsin /,æmɪ'lɒpsɪn/ *n* a pancreatic ferment converting starch into sugar.

an- /ən/ or /æn/ *prefix* the form of *ad-* before *n*.

-an /ən/, **-ain** /eɪn/, **-ane** /æn/ *adj suffix* of, of the nature of, as in *suburban, certain, humane*.

an /æn/ *adj* the indefinite article ("a"), used before words beginning with the sound of a vowel except "u".

ana- /'ænə/ *prefix* up, anew, again.

-ana /'ænə/, **-iana** *n suffix* sayings of, publications about, as *Shakespeariana*, etc.

Anabaptist /,ænə'bæptɪst/ *n* one who believes in the rebaptizing of adults on their profession of faith; one who holds the invalidity of infant baptism; (*pl*) the sect of Baptists.—**Anabaptism** *n*.

anabas /'ænəbəs/ *n* a genus of Indian fishes allied to the perch, remarkable for their power of living a long time out of water and of travelling on land.

anabasis /ə'næbəsɪs/ *n* (*pl* **anabases**) the name given to Xenophon's account of the expedition of Cyrus the Younger (401BC); an inland military expedition.

anabatic /,ænə'bætɪk/ *adj* (*of wind*) caused by upward current of air.

anabiosis /,ænə'bɪo:sɪs/ *n* a coming to life again, resuscitation.

anableps /'ænəbleps/ *n* (*pl* **anableps**) a genus of the perch family found in Guiana, remarkable for the structure of its eye.

anabolic steroid /,ænə'bɒlɪk'stɪrɔɪd/ or /'sterɔɪd/ *n* any of various synthetic steroid hormones that promote rapid muscle growth.

anabolism /ə'næbə,lɪzəm/ *n* constructive metabolism, in which simple molecules synthesize into more complex ones.—**anabolic**.

anabranch /'ænə,brɑ:ntʃ/ *n* a stream that leaves a river and rejoins it lower down.

anachronism /ə'nækrə,nɪzəm/ *n* a person, custom, or idea regarded as out of date or out of its period.—**anachronistic** *adj.*—**anachronistically** *adv.*

anacoluthia /,ænəkə'lu:θɪə/ *n* want of grammatical sequence, *esp* in a sentence.—**anacoluthic** *adj.*

anacoluthon /,ænəkə'lu:θɒn/ *n* (*pl* **anacolutha**) a sentence in which one part belongs to a different construction from the other.

anaconda /,ænə'kɒndə/ *n* a large South American semiaquatic snake that kills its prey by constriction.

Anacreontic /ə,nækri'ɒntɪk/ *adj* after the manner of Anacreon, the Greek poet (6th century BC); amatory, erotic. • *n* a poem in praise of love and wine.

anacrusis /,ænə'kru:sɪs/ *n* (*pl* **anacruses**) (*linguistics*) an unstressed syllable at the beginning of a verse.—**anacrustic** *adj.*

anadiplosis /,ænədɪ'plo:sɪs/ *n* (*rhetoric*) the repetition of the last word of a line or clause at the beginning of the next.

anadromous /ə'nædrəməs/ *adj* (*fish*) ascending from the sea to freshwater rivers to deposit spawn, as the salmon, etc.

anaemia /ə'ni:mɪə/ *n* a condition in which the blood is low in red cells or in haemoglobin, resulting in paleness, weakness, etc.—*also* **anemia**.

anaemic /ə'ni:mɪk/ *adj* suffering from anaemia; weak; pale; listless.—*also* **anemic**.

anaerobe /'ænə,ro:b/ or /ə,nɛro:b/, **anaerobium** /-bɪəm/ *n* (*pl* **anaerobes, anaerobia**) a microbe that can live without air.

anaerobiosis /,ænəro:bi'o:sɪs/ *n* life devoid of oxygen.—**anaerobic** *adj.*—**anaerobically** *adv.*

anaesthesia /,ænəs'θi:zɪə/ or /-ʒə/ *n* a partial or total loss of the sense of pain, touch, etc.—*also* **anesthesia**.

anaesthetic /,ænəs'θetɪk/ *n* a drug, gas, etc used to produce anaesthesia, as before surgery. • *adj* of or producing anaesthesia. —*also* **anesthetic**.

anaesthetist /ə'nesθətɪst/ or /ə'ni:-/ *n* a person trained to give anaesthetics.—*also* **anesthetist**.

anaesthetize /ə'nesθə,taɪz/ or /ə'ni:-/ *vt* to administer an anaesthetic.—*also* **anesthetize**.—**anaesthetization, anesthetization** *n*.

anaglyph /'ænəglɪf/ *n* an ornament or work of art carved in low relief, as distinguished from intaglio.—**anaglyphic, anaglyphical, anaglyptic, anaglyptical** *adj.*

anagnorisis /ə'nægnɔrɪsɪs/ *n* (*pl* **anagnorises**) the denouement in a drama.

anagoge, anagogy /,ænə'go:dʒi/ *n* an allegorical or mystical interpretation, a hidden sense.—**anagogic, anagogical** *adj.*—**anagogically** *adv.*

anagram /'ænə,græm/ *n* a word or sentence formed by rearranging another word or sentence.—**anagrammatic, anagrammatical** *adj.*—**anagrammatically** *adv.*

anagrammatize /,ænə'græmə,taɪz/ *vt* to make into an anagram. • *vi* to construct anagrams.—**anagrammatism** *n*.—**anagrammatist** *n*.

anal /'eɪnəl/ *adj* of or situated near the anus.

analects /'ænəlekts/, **anelecta** /,ænə'lektə/ *npl* literary passages or extracts selected from published works by different authors.—**analectic** *adj.*

analeptic /,ænə'leptɪk/ *adj* restorative. • *n* a restorative drug.

analgesia /,ænəl'dʒi:zɪə/ or /-sɪə/ *n* insensibility to pain without loss of consciousness.

analgesic /,ænəl'dʒi:zɪk/ or /-sɪk/ *adj* relieving pain. • *n* a pain-relieving drug.

analogism /ə'nælə,lɒdʒɪzəm/ *n* a reasoning from the cause to the effect; study and examination of matters and things by reference to their analogies.—**analogist** *n*.

analogize /ə'nælə,dʒaɪz/ *vt* to reason or expound by reference to analogy, to draw comparisons. • *vi* to treat or investigate by use of analogy.

analogous /ə'næləgəs/ *adj* corresponding in certain respects (to).—**analogously** *adv.*

analogue, analog /'ænə,lɒg/ *n* a word or thing analogous to something else.

analogy /ə'nælədʒi/ *n* (*pl* **analogies**) a similarity or correspondence in certain respects between two things.—**analogical, analogic** *adj.*

analysable, analyzable *adj* capable of being resolved by, or that may be subjected to, analysis.

analysand /ə'nælɪ,sænd/ *n* anyone undergoing psychoanalysis.

analyse, analyze /'ænə,laɪz/ *vt* to separate (something) into its constituent parts to investigate its structure and function, etc; to examine in detail; to psychoanalyse.

analysis /ə'næləsɪs/ *n* (*pl* **analyses** /-ɪsi:s/) the process of analysing; a statement of the results of this; psychoanalysis.

analyst /'ænəlɪst/ *n* a person who analyses; a psychoanalyst.

analytic /,ænə'lɪtɪk/, **analytical** /-kl/ *adj* pertaining to analysis.—**analytically** *adv.*

anamnesis /,ænəm'ni:sɪs/ *n* (*pl* **anamneses** /-si:z/) recollection; a patient's case history.—**anamnestic** *adj.*—**anamnestically** *adv.*

anamorphosis /,ænə'mɔrfəsɪs/ *n* (*pl* **anamorphoses** /-si:z/) the irregular and distorted representation of an object as viewed directly, but which is corrected and reduced to its proper proportion when regarded from a different point of view, or reflected by a curved mirror; the abnormal or monstrous development of a portion of a plant or flower; a gradual progression from one type to another.

ananas /ə'nænəs/ *n* a genus of tropical plants to which the pineapple belongs.

anandrous /ə'nændrəs/ *adj* without stamens.

ananthous /ə'nænθəs/ *adj* without flowers.

anapaest, anapest /'ænə,pest/ *n* a foot comprising two short syllables and one long syllable.—**anapaestic, anapestic** *adj.*

anaphora /ə'næfərə/ n (*rhetoric*) the repetition at the beginning of the succeeding clauses of sentences of the word or words used in beginning the first; that part of the Eucharistic service which starts with the Sursum Corda; the oblique ascension of a star.—**anaphoric** adj.—**anaphorically** adv.

anaphrodisia /æn,æfrə'dɪːziə/ n impotence of the sexual organs; absence of venereal desire.

anaphrodisiac /æn,æfrə'dɪːzi,æk/ adj tending to diminish sexual desire. • n a remedy that produces such an effect.

anaphylaxis /,ænəfɪ'læksɪs/ n excessive sensitivity to a substance or germ due to prior inoculation with it; an allergy.—**anaphylactic** adj.—**anaphylactically** adv.

anaplasty /,ænə'plæsti/ n the repairing of wounds by the transplantation of adjacent healthy tissue, plastic surgery.—**anaplastic** adj.

anarchism /'ænər,kɪzəm/ n lawlessness; confusion; anarchy; the doctrines of the anarchists.

anarchist /'ænərkɪst/ n a person who believes that all government is unnecessary and should be abolished.—**anarchistic** adj.

anarchy /'ænərki/ n the absence of government; political confusion; disorder, lawlessness.—**anarchic, anarchical** adj.

anarthrous /æn'ɑrθrəs/ adj without the article; destitute of joints; without articulated limbs.

anasarca /ænə'sɑrkə/ (*med*) dropsy.—**anasarcous** adj.

anastigmat /æ'næstɪg,mæt/ n a lens corrected of astigmatism.—**anastigmatic** adj.

anastomosis /ə,næstə'moːsɪs/ n (*pl* **anastomoses**) a cross-connection of arteries, rivers, etc.—**anastomotic** adj.

anastrophe /ə'næstrəfi/ n (*rhetoric*) an inversion of the sequence of words in a sentence, as "echoed the hills", for "the hills echoed".

anathema /ə'næθəmə/ n (*pl* **anathemas**) anything greatly detested; an ecclesiastical curse or denunciation accompanied by excommunication.

anathematize /ə'næθəmə,taɪz/ vt to pronounce a decree of excommunication against. • vi to curse.—**anathematization** n.

anatomist /ə'nætəmɪst/ n one possessing a knowledge of anatomy by dissection.

anatomize /ə'nætə,maɪz/ vt to dissect; to study the structure of; to analyse.—**anatomization** n.

anatomy /ə'nætəmi/ n (*pl* **anatomies**) the science of the physical structure of plants and animals; the structure of an organism.—**anatomical** adj.—**anatomically** adv.

anbury /'ænbəri/ n (*pl* **anburies**) a soft wart or tumour on horses and cattle; a disease in turnips.

ANC /'eɪ'en'siː/ abbr = African National Congress.

-ance /əns/ n suffix denoting quality or action, as in *arrogance, penance*.

ancestor /'æn,sestər/ or /-səs-/ n one from whom a person is descended, a forefather; an early animal or plant from which existing types are descended; something regarded as a forerunner.—**ancestress** nf.

ancestral /æn'sestrəl/ adj belonging to, or connected with, one's ancestors; derived from one's progenitors; lineal.

ancestry /'ænsestri/ n (*pl* **ancestries**) ancestors collectively; lineage.

anchor /'æŋkər/ n a heavy metal implement that lodges at the bottom of the sea or a river to hold a ship in position; something that gives support or stability. • vt to fix by an anchor; to secure firmly.

anchorage /'æŋkərɪdʒ/ n a safe anchoring place for ships; the charge for anchoring.

anchor ice n ✦ (*Cdn*) ice formed at the bottom of a body of water.

anchorite /'æŋkəraɪt/ n one who voluntarily secludes him or herself from society and lives a solitary life devoted to religious or philosophic meditation; a recluse; a hermit.—**anchoress** nf.

anchorman /'æŋkər,mæn/ n (*pl* **anchormen**) (*sport*) the last man in a team to compete and whose contribution is vital; the compere of a television broadcast.

anchor stock n the crossbar at the top of the shank, at right angles to the arms.

anchor watch n the watch on board ship when at anchor; the seamen on this watch.

anchovy /'æn,tʃoːvi/ or /'æntʃəvi/, /æn'tʃoːvi/ n (*pl* **anchovies, anchovy**) a small Mediterranean fish resembling a herring with a very salty taste.

anchovy pear n a West Indian fruit like the mango, used as a pickle.

anchylose /'æŋkə,loːs/ or /-,loːz/ see **ankylose**.

anchylosis /-,loːsɪs/ see **ankylosis**.

ancien régime /ɑ̃,sjæ̃reɪ'ʒiːm/, Fr. /ɑ̃sjæ̃reɪ'ʒiːm/ n (*pl* **anciens régimes**) the old order, *esp* that ruling France before the Revolution.

ancient /'eɪnʃənt/ adj very old; dating from the distant past; of the period and civilizations predating the fall of the Roman Empire; old-fashioned. • n a person who lived in the ancient period; (*pl*) the members of the classical civilizations of antiquity, *esp* of Greece and Rome.

Ancient of Days n (*Bible*) God, as described in the Book of Daniel.

ancillary /æn'sɪləri/ adj subordinate (to); auxiliary; supplementary. • n (*pl* **ancillaries**) a subordinate or auxiliary person or thing.

ancipital /æn'sɪpɪtəl/, **ancipitous** /-ɪtəʃ/ adj (*biol*) two-edged and sharp.

ancon, ancone /'æŋkən/ n (*pl* **ancones** /æn'kouniːz/ or /æŋ-/) (*archit*) a bracket or projection for the support of a cornice; the elbow.—**anconal, anconeal** adj.

and /ænd/ or /ənd/ conj in addition to; together with; plus; increasingly; as a consequence, afterwards; expressing contrast.

andalusite /,ændə'luːsaɪt/ n a silicate of alumina.

andante /æn'ɑnteɪ/ or /-dænteɪ/ adj (*mus*) moderately slow; naturally and easily. • n a movement written and to be played in andante time.

andantino /,æn,dɒn'tiːnoː/ or /,ændæn-/ adj rather slower than andante. • n (*pl* **andantinos**) a movement slower than an andante.

andesite /'ændɪ,zaɪt/ n a silicate of alumina, soda, and lime.

andiron /'ænd,aɪrn/ npl metal standards used for open fires to support the logs; fire dogs.

androgen /'ændrədʒən/ n a male sex hormone.—**androgenic** adj.

androgenous /æn'drɒdʒɛnəs/ adj (*biol*) having only male offspring.

androgynous /æn'drɒdʒɪnəs/ adj combining both sexes or bearing both male and female organs; hermaphroditical.—**androgyne** n.—**androgyny** n.

android /'ændrɔɪd/ n (*science fiction*) a robot in human form.—*also* adj.

androsphinx /'ændrə,sfɪks/ n (*pl* **androsphinxes, androsphinges**) a sphinx with the body of a lion and the head of a man.

anecdotal /'ænək,doːtəl/ adj relating to anecdotes; (*evidence, etc*) obtained from experience, not scientific.

anecdote /'ænək,doːt/ or /-ek-/ n a short entertaining account about an amusing or interesting event or person.

anemia /ə'niːmiə/ see **anaemia**.

anemic /ə'niːmɪk/ see **anaemic**.

anemograph /ə'nemə,græf/ n an instrument for registering the force or direction of the wind.

anemography /ə'nemə,grɒfi/ n the scientific description of winds, and the measurement and registration of their force and direction.—**anemographic** adj.—**anemographically** adv.

anemology /,ænə'mɒlədʒ/ n the science and literature of the winds.

anemometer /,ænə'mɒmətər/ n an instrument for measuring the force or speed of the wind.

anemone /ə'nemənɪ/ n a plant of the buttercup family.

anemophilus /,ænə'mɒfɪ,əs/ adj (flowers etc) fertilized by pollen carried by the wind, wind-pollinated.—**anemophily** n.

anemoscope /ə'nemə,skoːp/ n an apparatus for exhibiting the direction of the wind.

anent /ə'nent/ prep, adv (*Scot*) with regard or respect to; concerning.

aneroid /'ænə,rɔɪd/ adj having no liquid, as quicksilver. • n a barometer shaped like a watch, the action depending on the varying pressure of the atmosphere on the top of an elastic metal box.

aneroid barometer n a barometer that measures air pressure by its effect on the flexible lid of a box containing a partial vacuum.

anesthesia /,ænəs'θiːʒə/ or /-ziə/, see **anaesthesia**.

anesthetic /,ænəs'θetɪk/ see **anaesthetic**.

anesthetist /ə'nesθətɪst/ or /ə,niː-/ see **anaesthetist**.

anesthetize /ə'nesθə,taɪz/ or /ə,niː-/ see **anaesthetize**.

aneurysm, aneurism /'ænju,rɪzəm/ n the permanent abnormal swelling of an artery.

anew /ə'nuː/ or /-'njuː/ adv afresh; again, once more; in a new way or form.

anfractuous /æn'fræktʃuːəs/ adj winding, intricate.—**anfractuosity** n (*pl* **anfractuosities**).

angakok /'æŋɡəkɔːk/ *n* ❧ an Inuit shaman or healer.

angary /'æŋɡəri/ *n* a belligerent's right to seize and use neutral property, for which it pays indemnity.

angel /'eɪndʒəl/ *n* a messenger of God; an image of a human figure with wings and a halo; a very beautiful or kind person; (*inf*) one who gives financial backing to an enterprise.

angel cake *n* a small round cake with a round fruit on the top.

Angeleno /ˌændʒə'liːnoː/ or *n* (*pl* **Angelenos**) (*inf*) an inhabitant of the city of Los Angeles.

angelfish /'eɪndʒəlˌfɪʃ/ *n* (*pl* **angelfish, angelfishes**) a species of shark with large pectoral fins, which give to it a winged appearance.

angelic /'ændʒelɪk/, **angelical** /-əl/ *adj* belonging to or resembling an angel in nature or function.—**angelically** *adv*.

angelica /-ɪkə/ *n* the candied stalks of a fragrant plant used *esp* in cake decoration.

Angelus /'ændʒələs/ *n* (*RC Church*) a devotional exercise commemorating the Incarnation, during which the Ave Maria is twice repeated, said morning, noon, and night; the bell that is rung to announce the time of such devotions.

anger /'æŋɡər/ *n* strong displeasure, often because of opposition, a hurt, etc. • *vti* to make or become angry.

angina /æn'dʒaɪnə/ *n* sharp stabbing pains in the chest, *usu* caused by angina pectoris.

angina pectoris /'pektərɪs/ *n* a heart disease causing a spasmodic gripping pain in the chest.

angiology /ˌændʒi'ɒlədʒi/ *n* the branch of anatomy that deals with the blood vessels and lymphatics.

angioma /ændʒi'oːmə/ *n* (*pl* **angiomas, angiomata**) a tumour caused by the enlargement of a blood vessel.—**angiomatous** *adj*.

angiosperm /'ændʒiəˌspɜːrm/ *n* (*bot*) a plant having its seeds protected by a covering.—**angiospermous** *adj*.

angle[1] /'æŋɡəl/ *n* a corner; the point from which two lines or planes extend or diverge; a specific viewpoint; an individual method or approach (*eg* to a problem). • *vt* to bend at an angle; to move or place at an angle; to present information, news, etc from a particular point of view.

angle[2] *vi* to fish with a hook and line; to use hints or artifice to get something.—**angler** *n*.

angler /'æŋɡlər/ *n* one who fishes with rod and line; the name of a fish with filamentary appendage that attracts smaller fish on which it feeds.

Anglican /'æŋɡlɪkən/ *adj* belonging to or of the Church of England and other churches in communion with it. • *n* a member of the Anglican Church; a ritualist.

Anglicanism /-ɪzəm/ *n* the principles and ritual of the Anglican Church.

Anglicism /'æŋɡlɪˌsɪzəm/ *n* a form of speech, an English idiom; a principle or mannerism peculiar to England.

anglicize /'æŋɡlɪˌsaɪz/ *vt* to make or to render into English; to accord with English manners and customs.—**anglicization** *n*.

angling /'æŋɡlɪŋ/ *n* the art or act of fishing with rod and line.

Anglo- /'æŋɡloː/ or *prefix* English, British.

Anglo /æŋɡloː/ *n* ❧ (*Cdn*) (*inf*) a person who speaks English as a first language, especially in Quebec.

Anglo-American /'æŋɡloːə'merɪkən/ *adj* pertaining to England and the United States conjointly, as to commerce or population. • *n* an American citizen of English descent.

Anglo-Canadian *adj* pertaining to England and Canada, as to commerce or population. • *n* ❧ a Canadian citizen whose first language is English.

Anglo-Catholic /'kəθɒlɪk/ *adj* Catholic according to the teachings and ritual of the English Church; in the strictest Catholic sense; high church. • *n* a member of the English Church, popularly a ritualist or high churchman, who repudiates the term "Protestant".

Anglo-Catholicism /kə'θɒlɪsɪzəm/ *n* the principles and ritual of the Anglican Church interpreted in their strictest Catholic sense.

Anglo-French /'frentʃ/ *adj* English and French. • *n* the old French language introduced into England by the Normans.

Anglo-Indian /'ɪndiən/ *adj* pertaining to England and India conjointly. • *n* one of English descent born or residing in India.

Anglo-Irish /'aɪrɪʃ/ *adj* pertaining to England and Ireland, or to the English settled in Ireland and their descendants; having the father or mother of English or Irish race. • *npl* English born or resident in Ireland.

Anglomania /-'meɪniə/ *n* a predilection carried to excess for everything that is English, in the sense of being peculiar to England.

Anglo-Norman /-'nɔːrmən/ *adj* common to England and Normandy. • *n* one of the Norman settlers in England after the Conquest (AD 1066).

Anglophile /'æŋɡloːˌfaɪl/ *n* a person who loves England or anything English.—*also* **Anglophil**.

Anglophobe /'æŋɡləˌfoːb/ *n* one who hates or fears England and the English.

Anglophobia /ˌæŋɡlə'foːbiə/ *n* an intense aversion or fear of everything English.—**Anglophobe** *n*.

anglophone /'æŋɡləˌfoːn/ *adj* ❧ (*Cdn*) English-speaking. • *n* a person whose first language is English.

Anglo-Saxon /'æŋɡloː'sæksən/ *adj* pertaining to the Saxon settlers in England prior to the Conquest, or to their language. • *n* one of the Saxon settlers in England as distinguished from those on the Continent; Old English, the language of the settlers; (*pl*) the English race.

angora /æn'ɡɔːrə/ *n* a long-haired variety of cat, rabbit or goat; fabric made from the hair of angora goats or rabbits.

angostura bark /ˌæŋɡə'stʊrə/ *n* a bitter aromatic bark used for medicinal purposes.

angostura bitters *npl* a bitter flavouring made from the bark of a South American tree.

angry /'æŋɡri/ *adj* (**angrier, angriest**) full of anger; inflamed. —**angrily** *adv*.

angst /æŋst/ a feeling of anxiety, fear or remorse.

angstrom, ångström /'æŋstrəm/ or /'ɒŋ-/ *n* one hundred millionth of a centimetre, a unit used in measuring the length of light waves.

anguilliform /æn'ɡwɪləˌfɔːrm/ *adj* shaped like an eel or a serpent.

anguine /'æŋɡwɪn/ *adj* snakelike.

anguish /'æŋɡwɪʃ/ *n* agonizing physical or mental distress.

angular /'æŋɡjulər/ *adj* having one or more angles; forming an angle; measured by an angle; stiff and clumsy in manner, thin and bony.

angularity /ˌæŋɡju'lærɪti/ *n* (*pl* **angularities**) the quality of being angular in any sense.

angulate /'æŋɡjulɪt/ *adj* constructed of angles; having the form of an angle.

angulation /ˌæŋɡju'leɪʃən/ *n* the exact measurement of angles; an angular shape.

anhydride /æn'haɪdraɪd/ *n* an oxygen compound formed by substituting an acid radicle for the whole of the hydrogen in one or two molecules of water.

anhydrite /æn'haɪdraɪt/ *n* anhydrous sulphate of lime.

anhydrous /æn'haɪdrəs/ *adj* without water, applied to minerals in which the water of crystallization is not present.

ani /'æni/ *n* (*pl* **anis** /'æniːz/) a tropical American bird of the cuckoo family.

aniconic /ˌæni'kɒnɪk/ or /-kɒn-/ *adj* (*idols*) not of human or animal form.

anil /'ænɪl/ *n* the indigo plant; a dye yielded by it.

anile /'ænaɪl/ *adj* resembling an old woman; aged.—**anility** *n*.

aniline /'ænɪˌlɪn/ or /-ˌliːn/, /-ˌlaɪn/ *n* a base used in the formation of many rich dyes obtained from coal tar but more extensively from benzole. • *adj* of or pertaining to aniline.

animadversion /ˌænɪmæd'vɜːrʒən/ *n* the act of observing; capacity for perception; censure; criticism; stricture.

animadvert /ˌænɪmæd'vɜːrt/ *vi* to give the mind to; to pass comment or stricture upon, to criticize.

animal /'ænɪməl/ *n* any living organism except a plant or bacterium, typically able to move about; a lower animal as distinguished from man, *esp* mammals; a brutish or bestial person. • *adj* of or like an animal; bestial; sensual.

animalcule /ˌænɪ'mælkjuːl/, **animalculum** *n* (*pl* **animalcules, animalcula**) one of a class of minute or microscopic organisms abounding in water and infusions.—**animalcular** *adj*.

animalism /'ænɪməˌlɪzəm/ *n* the state of being animal, or actuated by animal instincts or appetites; the theory that regards humankind as merely animal; sensuality.—**animalist** *n*.—**animalistic** *adj*.

animality /ˌænɪ'mælɪti/ *n* the state or quality of being an animal, or possessing animal characteristics, animal nature.

animalize /'ænɪməˌlaɪz/ *vt* to make animal; to impart animal life, form, and attributes; to sensualize or bestialize; to convert into animal substance by assimilation.—**animalization** *n*.

animal kingdom *n* beings endowed with animal life and regarded collectively, one of the three great divisions of nature.

animal liberation *n* freeing animals from captivity and exploitation (*eg* in laboratories) by humans, action *esp* associated with organizations such as the Animal Liberation Front.

animal magnetism *n* another name for mesmerism; attractiveness, *esp* to the opposite sex.

animal rights *n* a movement that seeks to extend certain rights, such as freedom from captivity and exploitation by humans, to animals.

animal spirits *npl* vivacity; liveliness of disposition.

animal worship *n* the worship of animals as symbols of deities, as among the ancient Egyptians, Hindus, etc.

animate /'ænɪmət/ *adj*, /'ænɪˌmeɪt/ *vt* to give life to; to liven up; to inspire, encourage. • *adj* alive; lively.

animated /'ænɪˌmeɪtəd/ *adj* lively, full of spirit.

animated cartoon *n* a film made by photographing a series of drawings, giving the illusion of movement.

animation /ˌænɪˈmeɪʃən/ *n* liveliness; movement; the skill of making animated films.

animato /æˈniːmɒˌtoː/ *adv, adj (mus)* with vigour.

animator, animater /'ænɪmeɪtər/ *n* an artist who draws and produces animated cartoons.

animé /'ænɪˌmeɪ/ *n* an amber-coloured resin, resembling copal, obtained from a tropical American tree and used in varnish.

animism /'ænɪˌmɪzəm/ *n* in primitive religion, the belief that natural effects are due to spirits and that inanimate objects have spirits; the belief in a human apparitional soul, having the form and appearance of the body, existing after death as semi-human.—**animist** *n.*—**animistic** *adj.*

animosity /ˌænəˈmɒsɪti/ *n (pl* **animosities**) strong dislike; hostility.

animus /'ænɪməs/ *n* an actuating spirit; a bitter or hostile feeling (against); hostility.—*also adj.*

anion /'ænˌaɪən/ *n* the element in a body decomposed by voltaic action, which is evolved at the positive pole or anode.—**anionic** *adj.*

anise /'ænɪs/ *n* the common name for a plant (indigenous in Egypt) yielding the seeds used in aniseed.

aniseed /'ænɪˌsiːd/ *n* the seed of the anise plant, used as a flavouring.

anisette /ˌænɪˈsɛt/ *n* a liqueur prepared from aniseed.

ankh /æŋk/ *n* an Egyptian cross with a loop or handle at the top, the symbol of life.—*also* **crux ansata.**

ankle /'æŋkəl/ *n* the joint between the foot and leg, the part of the leg between the ankle and calf.

anklet /'æŋklət/ *n* an ornamental chain worn round the ankle.

ankylose /'æŋkɪˌloːz/ *vt* to consolidate or join by bony growth; to stiffen as a joint. • *vi* to grow together; to become stiff.—*also* **anchylose.**

ankylosis /ˌæŋkɪˈloːsɪs/ *n (zool)* the joining or consolidation of parts formerly or normally separate or movable by means of bony growth; *(med)* the stiffening of a joint by fibrous bands or union of bones.—*also* **anchylosis.**—**ankylotic, anchylotic** *adj.*

anna /'ænə/ *n* an Indian coin, one sixteenth of a rupee.

annals /'ænəlz/ *npl* a written account of events year by year; historical records; periodical reports or records of a society.—**annalist** *n.*—**annalistic** *adj.*

annates /əˈneɪts/ *npl (RC Church)* the sum paid to the pope by an abbot or bishop on his appointment to a benefice or see and consisting of the first year's revenue of the living, now chiefly supplied by Peter's Pence.

anneal /əˈniːl/ *vt* to fix by heat; to temper and render malleable; to bake or fuse.—**annealer** *n.*

annelid /'ænəlɪd/ *n* any of a class of invertebrates which includes the worms, whose bodies are composed of numerous segments or ring-like divisions.—**annelidan** *adj.*

annex /'ænɛks/ *vt* to attach, *esp* to something larger; to incorporate into a state the territory of (another state).

annexation /ˌænɛkˈseɪʃən/ *n* the act of annexing; that which is annexed.—**annexational** *adj.*—**annexationism** *n.*—**annexationist** *n.*

annexe /'ænɛks/ *n* an extension to a main building; something added, a supplement.

annihilate /əˈnaɪəˌleɪt/ *vt* to destroy completely; *(inf)* to defeat convincingly, as in an argument.—**annihilable** *adj.*—**annihilative** *adj.*—**annihilator** *n.*

annihilation /əˌnaɪəˈleɪʃən/ *n* the act of annihilating; nonexistence.

anniversary /ˌænɪˈvɜːrsəri/ *n (pl* **anniversaries**) the yearly return of the date of some event; a celebration of this.—*also adj.*

Anno Domini /ˌænoːˈdɒmɪˌni/ or /-ˌnaɪ/ *adv (abbr* AD) in the year of our Lord, dating from the birth of Christ. • *n (inf)* advancing age.

annotate /'ænoːˌteɪt/ or /-nə-/ *vti* to provide with explanatory notes.—**annotative** *adj.*—**annotator** *n.*

annotation /ˌænoːˈteɪʃən/ or /-nə-/ *n* the act of noting or commenting upon; a note, remark, or criticism made in a book.

announce /əˈnaʊns/ *vt* to bring to public attention; to give news of the arrival of; to be an announcer for. • *vi* to serve as an announcer.

announcement /-mənt/ *n* the act of announcing; that which is announced; a proclamation.

announcer /-ər/ *n* a person who reads the news, etc on the radio or TV.

annoy /əˈnɔɪ/ *vt* to vex, tease, irritate, as by a repeated action.—**annoyingly** *adv.*

annoyance /əˈnɔɪəns/ *n* the act of annoying or causing vexation; the state of being annoyed; the thing or act that annoys.

annual /'ænjʊəl/ *adj* of or measured by a year; yearly; coming every year; living only one year or season. • *n* a plant that lives only one year; a periodical published once a year.—**annually** *adv.*

annuitant /əˈnjuːɪtənt/ *n* one who is in receipt of, or is entitled to receive, an annuity.

annuity /əˈnjuːəti/ or /əˈnjuː-/ *n (pl* **annuities**) an investment yielding fixed payments, *esp* yearly; such a payment.

annul /əˈnʌl/ *vt (* **annulling, annulled**) to do away with; to deprive of legal force, nullify.

annular /'ænjʊlər/ or /-jə-/ *adj* ring-like; in the form of a ring or annulus. • *n* the ring of light surrounding the moon's body in an annular eclipse of the sun.

annulate /'ænjʊlət/ *adj* ringed; having ring-like bands or circles.

annulation /ˌænjʊˈleɪʃən/ *n* a ring-like formation.

annulet /'ænjuːlət/ *n* a small ring; *(archit)* a small fillet encircling a column.

annulment /əˈnʌlmənt/ *n* the act of reducing to nothing; abolition; invalidation.

annulose /'ænjʊloːs/ *adj* composed of a succession of rings; segmented.

annunciate /əˈnʌnsɪˌeɪt/ *vt* to make known officially or publicly; to announce, proclaim.—**annunciation** *n.*—**annunciative, annunciatory** *adj.*

annunciation /əˌnʌnsɪˈeɪʃən/ *n (Bible)* the intimation of the Incarnation made by the angel Gabriel to the Virgin Mary (Luke 1:28-33); the Church festival (Lady Day, 25 Mar) commemorating this.

annunciator /əˈnʌnsɪˌeɪtər/ *n* a signalling apparatus; an indicator connected with bells and telephones, to show where attendance is required.

anode /'ænoːd/ *n* the positive electrode by which electrons enter an electric circuit.

anodyne /'ænəˌdaɪn/ *n* a drug that relieves pain; anything that relieves pain or soothes.

anoestrus /æˈniːstrəs/ *n* the period of sexual inactivity in mammals between periods of estrus.—*also* **anestrus.**—**anoestrous, anestrous** *adj.*

anoint /əˈnɔɪnt/ *vt* to rub with oil; to apply oil in a sacred ritual as a sign of consecration.—**anointment** *n.*

anomalistic year /əˌnɒməˈlɪstɪk/ *n* the time occupied by the earth in passing through its orbit (365 days, 6 hours, 13 minutes, 48 seconds), from perihelion to perihelion.

anomalous /əˈnɒmələs/ *adj* deviating from the common order, abnormal.

anomaly /əˈnɒməli/ *n (pl* **anomalies**) abnormality; anything inconsistent or odd.—**anomalistic** *adj.*—**anomalistically** *adv.*

anon /əˈnɒn/ *adv* soon; at another time; *(arch)* anonymous.

anonym /'ænənɪm/ *n* an unnamed person; an assumed name.

anonymous /əˈnɒnɪməs/ *adj* having or providing no name; written or provided by an unnamed person; lacking individuality.—**anonymity** *n.*—**anonymously** *adv.*

anopheles /əˈnɒfəˌliːz/ *n (pl* **anopheles**) any of a genus of mosquitoes, which transmits the microbe of malaria.

anorak /'ænəˌræk/ *n* a waterproof jacket with a hood.

anorexia /ˌænəˈrɛksiə/ *n* loss of appetite.—**anorexic** *adj.*

anorexia nervosa /nərˈvoːsə/ *n* the psychological condition causing fear of becoming overweight and reluctance to eat even to the point of starvation and death.

anosmia /ænˈɒzmiə/ *n* the inability to smell.—**anosmatic, anosmic** *adj.*

another /ə'nʌðər/ adj a different or distinct (thing or person); an additional one of the same kind; some other.—also pron.

ansate /'ænˌseɪt/ adj with a handle, as a vase.

Anschluss /'ænʃlʊs/ n the union of Nazi Germany with Austria in 1938; the annexation of one territory by another for the benefit of the more powerful.

anserine /'ænsəˌraɪn/ or /-rɪn-/, **anserous** /'ænsəˌrəs/ adj of, relating to or resembling a goose; stupid as a goose.

answer /'ænsər/ n a spoken or written reply or response; the solution to a problem; a reaction, response. • vt to speak or write in reply; to satisfy or correspond to (eg a specific need); to justify, offer a refutation of. • vi to reply; to act in response (to); to be responsible (for); to conform (to).

answerable /'ænsərəbəl/ adj capable of being refuted; (with for or to) responsible, accountable.—**answerability** n.—**answerableness** n.

answering machine n an apparatus that records incoming telephone calls.

-ant /-ənt/ adj suffix as in repentant. • n suffix denoting agent, as in celebrant.

ant /ænt/ n any of a family of small, generally wingless insects of many species, all of which form and live in highly organized groups.

anta /'æntə/ n (pl **antae**) (archit) a square pilaster at either corner of a building, or at either side of a door.

antacid /ænt'æsɪd/ n a substance that counters excessive acidity.

antagonism /æn'tægəˌnɪzəm/ n antipathy, hostility; an opposing force, principle, etc.

antagonist /æn'tægənɪst/ n an adversary; an opponent.

antagonistic /ænˌtægə'nɪstɪk/ adj acting in opposition; opposed.—**antagonistically** adv.

antagonize /æn'tægəˌnaɪz/ vt to arouse opposition in.—**antagonization** n.

antalkali /ænt'ælkəlaɪ/ n (pl **antalkalis, antalkalies**) a substance that counteracts the presence of alkali in the system; an acid.—**antalkaline** adj, n.

Antarctic /ænt'ɑrktɪk/ or /-'ɑrtɪk/ adj of the South Pole or its surroundings. • n the Antarctic regions; the Antarctic Ocean.

ant bear n the aardvark.

ant bird n one of an extensive group of South American birds.

ant cow n an aphid or similar insect collected by ants for the sweet secretion in its body.

ante /'æntɪ/ n a player's stake in poker; (inf) money contributed as a share in a joint project.

ante- prefix in front of; earlier than.

anteater /'æntˌiːtər/ n an ant-eating animal, as the pangolin.

antecede /ˌæntɪ'siːd/ n to precede or go before in time or space.

antecedence /-'siːdəns/ n precedence; going before; priority.

antecedent /-'siːdənt/ adj prior in time, previous. • n a preceding event or happening; (pl) ancestry; (pl) the previous events of a person's life.

antechamber /'æntɪˌtʃeɪmbər/ n an anteroom.

antedate /ˌæntɪ'deɪt/ vt to carry back to an earlier period; to anticipate. • n a date esp on a document earlier than the actual date.

antediluvian /ˌæntɪdɪ'luːvɪən/ adj of or pertaining to the world before the Flood; belonging to very ancient times; antiquated; primitive. • n one who lived before the Flood; an old-fashioned person.

antelope /'æntəˌloʊp/ n (pl **antelopes, antelope**) any of the family of fast-running and graceful deer-like animals of Africa and Asia.

ante meridiem /ˌæntɪmə'rɪdɪəm/ n (abbr a.m.) the period between midnight and noon.—**antemeridian** adj.

antenatal /ˌæntɪ'neɪtəl/ adj occurring or present before birth.

antenna /æn'tenə/ n (pl **antennae**) either of a pair of feelers on the head of an insect, crab, etc; (pl **antennas**) a metal device for transmitting and receiving radio waves.

antennule /æn'tenuːl/ n a little antenna.

antependium /ˌæntɪ'pendɪəm/ n (pl **antependia**) a covering for the front of an altar.

antepenult /-pə'nʌlt/ n the last but two, usu of syllables.

antepenultimate /-pɪ'nʌltəmət/ adj pertaining to the last but two. • n that which is last but two, antepenult.

anterior /æn'tiːrɪər/ adj at or towards the front; earlier; previous.

anteroom /'æntɪˌruːm/ n an outer room leading into a larger or main room.

anthelion /æn'θiːlɪən/ n (pl **anthelia**) (meteorol) a luminous halo, opposite the sun, formed around the shadow of the head of the observer, as projected on a cloud or fog bank.

anthem /'ænθəm/ n a religious choral song; a song of praise or devotion, as to a nation.

anther /'ænθər/ n the part of a flower's stamen containing pollen.—**antheral** adj.

anthill /'ænthɪl/ n a mound thrown up by ants or termites in digging their nests.

anthologize /æn'θɒləˌdʒaɪz/ vt to compile or include in an anthology.

anthology /æn'θɒlədʒi/ n (pl **anthologies**) a collection of poetry or prose.—**anthological** adj.—**anthologist** n.

anthozoan /ˌænθə'zoʊən/ n any of a class of radiated soft marine zoophytes, which includes the sea anemones, corals, etc.—also **actinozoan**.

anthracene /'ænθrəˌsiːn/ n a complex hydrocarbon obtained from coal tar, the source of a red dye.

anthracite /'ænθrəˌsaɪt/ n a hard coal that gives off a lot of heat and little smoke.—**anthracitic** adj.

anthrax /'ænθræks/ n (pl **anthraces**) a contagious bacterial disease of cattle and sheep, etc that can be transmitted to people.

anthropo- /'ænθrəpo:/ or /-pə/ prefix man.

anthropocentric /ˌænθrəpo:'sentrɪk/ or /ˌænθrɒpo:-/ adj centring in man.—**anthropocentrism** n.

anthropoid /'ænθrəˌpɔɪd/ adj resembling man. • n one of the higher apes resembling man.—**anthropoidal** adj.

anthropology /ˌænθrə'pɒlədʒi/ n the scientific study of human beings, their origins, distribution, physical attributes and culture.—**anthropological** adj.—**anthropologist** n.

anthropometry /-'pɒmɪtri/ n the measurement of the human body; the branch of anthropology relating to such measurement of persons at various ages and in different tribes, races, occupations, etc.—**anthropometric, anthropometrical** adj.—**anthropometrist** n.

anthropomorphism /-pə'mɔrfɪzəm/ n the ascription of human behaviour to other animals or to things.—**anthropomorphic** adj.—**anthropomorphist** n.

anthropomorphize /-pə'mɔrfaɪz/ vt to invest with human qualities.

anthropomorphous /-pə'mɔrfəs/ adj in the form of a human being.

anthropophagi /-'pɒfədʒi/ npl (sing **anthropophagus**) cannibals, men-eaters.

anti- /'ænti/ or /'æntaɪ/ prefix opposed to; against.

anti-aircraft /ˌænti'erkræft/ adj for use against aircraft.

antiar /'æntiˌɑr/ n the upas tree of Java; a poison obtained from one species of it.

antibiotic /ˌæntibaɪ'ɒtik/ n any of various chemical, fungal or synthetic substances used against bacterial or fungal infections.

antibody /'æntiˌbɒdi/ n (pl **antibodies**) a protein produced by an organism in response to the action of a foreign body, such as the toxin of a parasite, that neutralizes its effects.

antic /'æntik/ n a ludicrous action intended to amuse.

Antichrist /'æntiˌkraɪst/ n (Bible) an opponent of Christ, esp the great personal opponent expected to appear before the end of the world (1 John 2:22).

Antichristian /'æntiˌkrɪstʃən/ or /'æntiˌkrɪstʃən/ n one who is an opponent of the Christian religion. • adj pertaining to Antichrist; opposed to the Christian religion.

anticipant /æn'tɪsɪpənt/ adj operating beforehand. • n one who looks forward.

anticipate /æn'tɪsɪˌpeɪt/ vt to give prior thought and attention to; to use, spend, act on in advance; to foresee and take action to thwart another; to expect. • vi to speak, act, before the appropriate time.

anticipation /ænˌtɪsɪ'peɪʃən/ n the act of taking beforehand; expectation; hope; preconception.

anticlerical /ˌænti'klerɪkəl/ adj opposed to the power of the clergy or church, esp in secular affairs. • n a person opposed to the power of the church.—**anticlericalism** n.

anticlimax /ˌænti'klaɪmæks/ or /'æntaɪ-/ n a sudden drop from the important to the trivial; an ending to a story or series of events that disappoints one's expectations.—**anticlimactic** adj.—**anticlimactically** adv.

anticlinal /ˌænti'klaɪnl/ adj (strata) inclining or folding with the convex side upwards; inclined in opposite directions.

anticlockwise /ˌænti'klɒkwaɪz/ see **counterclockwise**.

anticoagulant /ˌæntɪkoʊˈægjʊlənt/ n a substance that inhibits blood clotting.

anticyclone /ˌæntɪˈsaɪkloːn/ n a body of air rotating about an area of high atmospheric pressure.—**anticyclonic** adj.

antidepressant /ˌæntɪdəˈpresənt/ n any of various drugs used to alleviate mental depression.—also adj.

antidote /ˈæntɪˌdoːt/ n a remedy that counteracts a poison; something that counteracts harmful effects.

antifebrile /ˌæntaɪˈfiːbrəl/ or /-ˈfebrəl/, /ˌæntiː-/, /-tɪ-/ adj capable of allaying fever. • n a medicine for allaying fever.

antifreeze /ˈæntɪˌfriːz/ n a substance used, as in a car radiator, to prevent freezing up.

antigen /ˈæntɪdʒən/ or /-ˌdʒən/ n a substance introduced into the blood to stimulate production of antibodies.—**antigenic** adj.—**antigenically** adv.

antihero /ˈæntɪˌhiːroː/ n (pl **antiheroes**) a leading character in a book, film, etc who lacks the conventional heroic attributes.

antihistamine /ˌæntɪˈhɪstəmiːn/ or /-mɪn/ n any of a group of drugs that inhibit the action of histamines, used in treating allergic conditions.

antilog /ˈæntɪˌlɒg/ n an antilogarithm.

antilogarithm /ˌæntɪˈlɒgəˌrɪðəm/ n a number which a logarithm represents.—**antilogarithmic** adj.

antilogy /ænˈtɪlədʒi/ n (pl **antilogies**) a contradiction.

antimacassar /ˌæntɪməˈkæsər/ n an ornamental covering for chairbacks, etc, to prevent their being soiled (formerly by macassar oil, once used as a pomade).

antimasque /ˈæntɪˌmæsk/ n a droll or grotesque interlude between parts of a more serious nature in a masque.

antimatter /ˈæntɪˌmætər/ n matter composed of antiparticles.

antimere /ˈæntɪˌmɪr/ n (biol) one of two or more corresponding parts or organs on opposite sides of animals.—**antimeric** adj.—**antimerism** n.

antimonic /ˌæntɪˈmoːnɪk/, **antimonous** /ˈæntɪˈmoːnəs/ adj relating to, composed of, or obtained from antimony.

antimony /ˈæntɪˌmoːni/ n (pl **antimonies**) a brittle metallic element used in making alloys.—**antimonial** adj, n.

antinomy /ænˈtɪnəmi/ n (pl **antinomies**) contradiction in law or authorities or conclusions; the opposition of one law or part of a law to another.—**antinomic** adj.—**antinomically** adv.

antiparallel /ˌæntɪˈpærəˌlɛl/ or /ˌæntɪ-/, /-tɪ-/ adj running parallel, but in an opposite direction. • n one of two or more lines making equal angles with two other lines, but in contrary order.

antiparticle /ˈæntɪˌpɑrtɪkəl/ n an elementary particle with the same mass as its corresponding particle but having an equal and opposite electric charge, resulting in mutual destruction when brought into contact.

antipathetic /ˌæntɪpəˈθetɪk/, **antipathetical** /ˌæntɪpəˈθetɪkəl/ adj possessing or causing a natural antipathy or aversion (to).—**antipathetically** adv.

antipathy /ænˈtɪpəθi/ n (pl **antipathies**) a fixed dislike; aversion; an object of this.

antiperiodic /ˌæntɪˌpɪriˈɒdɪk/ adj preventive of a return in periodic or intermittent disease. • n a medicine for periodic diseases.

antipersonnel /ˌæntɪˌpərsəˈnɛl/ adj (weapon) used to destroy people rather than objects.

antiperspirant /ˌæntɪˈpərspɪrənt/ n a substance used to stem excessive perspiration.

antiphlogistic /ˌæntɪfləˈdʒɪstɪk/ adj efficacious in counteracting fever or inflammation. • n any remedy that checks inflammatory symptoms.

antiphon /ˈæntɪˌfɒn/ n a verse or sentence sung by one choir in response to another, as in church services; an anthem.

antiphonal /ænˈtɪfənəl/ adj characterized by responsive singing; sung alternately. • n a collection of antiphons.—**antiphonally** adv.

antiphonary /ænˈtɪfəˌneri/ n (pl **antiphonaries**) a book of responses used in church services; an antiphonal. • adj antiphonal or responsive.

antiphony /ænˈtɪfəni/ n (pl **antiphonies**) the alternate or responsive rendering of psalms or chants by a dual choir; a musical setting of sacred verses arranged for alternate singing.

antiphrasis /ænˈtɪfrəsɪs/ n (rhetoric) the use of words in a sense opposite to the true one.

antipodes /ænˈtɪpəˌdiːz/ npl the regions on the earth's surface opposite each other; (with cap preceded by **the**) Australia and New Zealand.—**antipodean** adj.

antipope /ˈæntɪˌpoːp/ n one who usurps or is elected to the papal office in opposition to a pope canonically elected; a rival pope.

antipyretic /ˌæntɪpaɪˈretɪk/ adj preventive of, or remedial to fever. • n a fever-allaying drug.—**antipyresis** n.

antipyrine /-ˈpaɪˌriːn/ or /-ˈpaɪrɪn/ n a drug obtained from coal tar and used to relieve neuralgia, etc, and to reduce heat in fevers.

antiquarian /ˌæntɪˈkweriən/ adj connected with the study of antiquities. • n an antiquary.

antiquary /ˈæntɪˌkweri/ n (pl **antiquaries**) a person who studies or collects antiquities.

antiquated /ˈæntɪˌkweitəd/ adj old-fashioned; obsolete.

antique /ænˈtiːk/ adj from the distant past; old-fashioned. • n a relic of the distant past; a piece of furniture, pottery, etc dating from an earlier historical period and sought after by collectors.

antiquity /ænˈtɪkwɪti/ n (pl **antiquities**) the far distant past, esp before the Middle Ages; (pl) relics dating from the far distant past.

antirrhinum /ˌæntɪˈraɪnəm/ n snapdragon.

antisabbatarian /ˌæntɪˌsæbəˈteriən/ adj opposed to the observance of the Sabbath.—also n.

antiscorbutic /ˌæntɪskərˈbjuːtɪk/ n a remedy against scurvy.—also adj.

anti-Semite /ˌæntɪˈsemaɪt/ n one who is hostile toward or discriminates against Jews as a religious or racial group.—**anti-Semitic** adj.—**anti-Semitism** n.

antiseptic /ˌæntɪˈseptɪk/ n a substance that destroys or prevents the growth of disease-producing microorganisms. • adj destroying harmful organisms; very clean; (inf) unexciting.—**antiseptically** adv.

antiserum /ˈæntɪˌsiːrəm/ n (pl **antiserums, antisera**) blood serum containing antibodies.

antisocial /ˌæntɪˈsoːʃəl/ adj avoiding the company of other people, unsocial; contrary to the interests of society in general.

antispasmodic /-spæzˈmɒdɪk/ adj counteractive to or curative of spasms. • n a medicine having such an effect.

antistatic /-ˈstætɪk/ adj (material, agent) counteracting the effects of static electricity.

antistrophe /ænˈtɪstrəfi/ n a stanza or movement of a Greek chorus alternating with the strophe, sung in moving to the right.—**antistrophic** adj.

antithesis /ænˈtɪθəsɪs/ n (pl **antitheses**) a contrast or opposition, as of ideas; the exact opposite.—**antithetical, antithetic** adj.

antitoxin /ˌæntɪˈtɒksɪn/ n a substance that acts against a specific toxin in the body; a serum containing an antitoxin, injected into a person to prevent disease.—**antitoxic** adj.

antitrade /ˈæntɪˈtreid/ or /ˌæntɪ-/ n a tropical wind blowing steadily in an opposite direction to the trade wind.

antitrust /ˌæntɪˈtrʌst/ adj (laws, regulations) restricting or opposing the activities of cartels and monopolies.

antitype /ˈæntɪˌtaɪp/ n that which a type or symbol stands for; that which preceded the type and of which the type is the representation.

antivenin /ˌæntɪˈvenɪn/ n an antidote to snake poison.

antivivisectionist /-ˌvɪvɪˈsekʃəˌnɪst/ n a person who opposes scientific experimentation on live animals.

antler /ˈæntlər/ n the branched horn of a deer or related animal.—**antlered** adj.

antlion n a neuropterous insect whose larva constructs a pitfall for ants and other insects.

antonomasia /ˌæntənoˈmeɪʒə/ n (rhetoric) the use of an attribute or epithet, or style of dignity or office, in place of the proper noun, eg "the Stagirite" for Aristotle, or the reverse, of a proper noun for a common noun, eg "some mute inglorious Milton"—**antonomastic** adj.—**antonomastically** adv.

antonym /ˈæntənɪm/ n a word that has the opposite meaning to another.

antrum /ˈæntrəm/ n (pl **antra**) (anat) a cavity, esp in the upper jawbone.

anurous /ænˈjuːrəs/ adj (zool) tailless.

anus /ˈeɪnəs/ n the excretory orifice of the alimentary canal.

anvil /ˈænvɪl/ n the heavy iron block on which metal objects are shaped with a hammer.

anxiety /æŋˈzaɪəti/ n (pl **anxieties**) the condition of being anxious; eagerness, concern; a cause of worry.

anxious /ˈæŋkʃəs/ adj worried; uneasy; eagerly wishing; causing anxiety.—**anxiously** adv.—**anxiousness** n.

any /ˈeni/ adj one out of many, some; every.

anybody /-ˌbɛdi/ or /-ˌbɒdi/ *pron* any person; an important person.

anyhow /-ˌhau/ *adv* in any way whatever; in any case.

any more, anymore /-ˈmɔr/ *adv* now; nowadays.

anyone /-ˌwʌn/ *pron* any person; anybody.

anything /-θɪŋ/ *pron* any object, event, fact, etc. • *n* a thing, no matter what kind.

anyway /-ˌwɛɪ/ *adv* in any manner; at any rate; haphazardly.

anywhere /-ˌwɛr/ *adv* in, at, or to any place.

Anzac /ˈænˌzæk/ *abbr* = Australian and New Zealand Army Corps. • *n* a member of this corps.—*also adj.*

aorist /ˈeɪərɪst/ *n* (*gram*) an indeterminate past tense of the verb expressing completed action. • *adj* indefinite; pertaining to the aorist tense.—**aoristic** *adj.*—**aoristically** *adv.*

aorta /eɪˈɔrtə/ *n* (*pl* **aortas, aortae**) the main artery that carries blood from the heart to be distributed through the body.—**aortic, aortal** *adj.*

aoudad /ˈɒuˌdæd/ or /ˈauˌdæd/ *n* a wild sheep-like animal of North Africa, somewhat resembling the chamois.

ap- /æp/ *prefix* the form of *ad-* before *p.*

apace /əˈpeɪs/ *adv* at a swift pace.

apache /əˈpæʃ/ *Fr.* /aˈpaʃ/ *n* a Parisian street ruffian, a hooligan.

Apache /əˈpætʃi/ *n* (*pl* **Apaches, Apache**) a tribe of North American Indians.

apagoge /æpəˈgoːgi/ or /-ˈgɔːg/ *n* (*logic*) the establishing of a proposition by demonstrating the untenability of its opposite.—**apagogic, apagogical** *adj.*—**apagogically** *adv.*

apanage /ˈæpənɪdʒ/ *see* **appanage**.

apart /əˈpɑrt/ *adv* at a distance, separately, aside; into two or more pieces.

apartheid /əˈpɑrtaɪt/ or /-teɪt/, /-taɪd/ *n* a policy of racial segregation implemented in South Africa.

apartment /əˈpɑrtmənt/ *n* a room or rooms in a building; a flat.

apathetic /ˌæpəˈθɛtɪk/ *adj* devoid of or insensible to feeling or emotion.—**apathetically** *adv.*

apathy /ˈæpəθi/ *n* lack of feeling; lack of concern, indifference.—**apathetic** *adj.*—**apathetically** *adv.*

apatite /ˈæpəˌtaɪt/ *n* a crystalline phosphate of lime.

ape /eɪp/ *n* a chimpanzee, gorilla, orangutan, or gibbon; any monkey; a mimic. • *vt* to imitate.

apeak /əˈpiːk/ *adv* (*naut*) nearly vertical in position.

apeman /ˈeɪpˌmæn/ *n* (*pl* **apemen**) an extinct creature supposedly intermediate in development between apes and man.

aperçu /ˌæpərˈsuː/, *Fr.* /aperˈsuː/ *n* a first view; a rapid survey; a brief outline.

aperient /əˈpɪriənt/ *adj* gently laxative; opening the bowels. • *n* a mild laxative medicine.

aperiodic /ˌeɪpɪriˈɒdɪk/ *adj* without periodicity.—**aperiodically** *adv.*—**aperiodicity** *n.*

aperitif, apéritif /əˌpɛriˈtiːf/, *Fr.* /aperiːˈtiːf/ *n* an alcoholic drink taken before a meal as an appetizer.

aperture /ˈæpərˌtʃər/ *n* an opening; a hole; a slit; in optical instruments, the (diameter of the) opening allowing or controlling the amount of light or radiation to enter.

apery /ˈeɪpəri/ *n* (*pl* **aperies**) mimicry.

apetalous /eɪˈpɛtələs/ *adj* without petals or corolla.—**apetaly** *n.*

apex /ˈeɪpɛks/ *n* (*pl* **apexes, apices**) the highest point, the tip; the culminating point; the vertex of a triangle.

aphaeresis /əˈfɪrəsɪs/ or /-ˈfɛ-/ *n* (*pl* **aphaereses**) (*linguistics*) the removal of a letter or syllable from the beginning of a word.—*also* **apheresis**.

aphagia /əˈfeɪdʒə/ *n* the inability to swallow.

aphasia /əˈfeɪʒə/ or /-ziə/ *n* loss of the power of speech or the appropriate use of words due to disease or injury of the brain.—**aphasic** *adj.*

aphelion /æpˈhiːliən/ or /əˈfiːliən/ *n* (*pl* **aphelia**) that point in the orbit of a planet or a comet which is farthest from the sun.

apheliotropic /əˌfiːliəˈtrɒpɪk/ *adj* (*bot*) turning from the sun.

apheresis /əˈfɛrəsɪs/ or /əˈfɪrəsɪs/ *see* **aphaeresis**.

aphesis /ˈæfɪsɪs/ *n* (*linguistics*) the gradual loss of an unaccented vowel at the beginning of a word, as in "squire" for "esquire".—**aphetic** *adj.*—**aphetically** *adv.*

aphid /ˈeɪfɪd/ or /ˈæfɪd/ *n* any of various small insects, such as the greenfly, that suck the juice of plants.

aphis /ˈeɪfɪs/ or /ˈæfɪs/ *n* (*pl* **aphides**) an aphid.

aphonia /əˈfoːnɪə/, **aphony** /-i/ *n* dumbness, loss of voice.—**aphonic** *adj.*

aphorism /ˈæfəˌrɪzəm/ *n* a brief, wise saying; an adage.—**aphoristic** *adj.*

aphrodisiac /ˌæfroˈdiːziæk/ or /ˌæfrəˈdɪziˌæk/ *adj* arousing sexually. • *n* a food, drug, etc that excites sexual desire.

aphtha /ˈæfθə/ or /ˈæp-/ *n* (*pl* **aphthae**) the small round white ulcers infesting the interior of the mouth; thrush.

aphyllous /əˈfɪləs/ *adj* (*bot*) without leaves.—**aphylly** *n.*

apian /ˈeɪpiən/ *adj* of, pertaining to, or like bees.

apiarian /ˌeɪpiˈɛriən/ *adj* of or relating to beekeeping.

apiarist /ˈeɪpiərɪst/ *n* a beekeeper.

apiary /ˈeɪpiˌɛri/ *n* (*pl* **apiaries**) a place with hives where bees are kept.

apical /ˈæpɪkəl/ or /ˈeɪpɪ-/ *adj* of, pertaining to, belonging to, or at the apex.—**apically** *adv.*

apices /ˈæpəˌsiːz/, /ˈeɪpə-/ *see* **apex**.

apiculate /əˈpɪkjʊlɪt/ or /-ˌleɪt/ *adj* terminated abruptly by a point, as leaves.

apiculture /ˈeɪpɪˌkʌltʃər/ *n* beekeeping.—**apicultural** *adj.*—**apiculturist** *n.*

apiece /əˈpiːs/ *adv* to, by, or for each one.

apish /ˈeɪpɪʃ/ *adj* like an ape in manners; foolish; imitative.—**apishness** *n.*

apivorous /eɪˈpɪvərəs/ *adj* feeding on bees.

aplacental /ˌeɪpləˈsɛntəl/ *adj* without a placenta.

aplanatic /ˌæpləˈnætɪk/ *adj* (*physics*) free from, or correcting, spherical or chromatic aberration.—**aplanatically** *adv.*

aplastic /əˈplæstɪk/ *adj* without plasticity; not easily moulded.

aplomb /əˈplɒm/ *n* poise; self-possession.

apnea, apnoea /æpˈniːə/ *n* partial suspension of breathing; suffocation.—**apnoeic** *adj.*

apo- /ˈæpə/ or /ˈæpoː/ *prefix* off, from, away; un-; quite.

apocalypse /əˈpɒkəlɪps/ *n* a cataclysmic event, the end of the world; revelation, *esp* that of St John; (*with cap*) the last book of the New Testament.—**apocalyptic** *adj.*—**apocalyptically** *adv.*

apocarpous /ˌæpəˈkɑrpəs/ *adj* (*bot*) having the carpels of the ovary separate or distinct.

apochromat /ˈæpəkrəˌmæt/ or /ˌæpə-/ *n* a highly achromatic lens.—**apochromatic** *adj.*

apocopate /əˈpɒkəˌpeɪt/ *vt* to cut off or drop the last letter or syllable of a word.—**apocopation** *n.*

apocope /əˈpɒkəpi/ *n* (*linguistics*) the cutting off or deletion of the last letter or syllable of a word.

Apocrypha /əˈpɒkrɪfə/ *npl* (*used as sing*) books of the Old Testament, *eg* Ecclesiasticus, accepted as an authentic part of the Holy Scriptures by the RC Church but not by Protestants.

apocryphal /əˈpɒkrɪfəl/ *adj* doubtful; untrue; invented; (*with cap*) of the Apocrypha.—**apocryphally** *adv.*

apodal /ˈæpədəl/ *adj* without feet.

apodeictic, apodictic /ˌæpəˈdɪktɪk/ *adj* clearly established, unquestionable true.—**apodeictically, apodictically** *adv.*

apodosis /əˈpɒdəsɪs/ *n* (*pl* **apodoses**) (*gram*) the latter portion, or consequent clause, of a conditional sentence.

apogamy /əˈpɒgəmi/ *n* the absence of sexual reproduction; asexual reproduction.—**apogamic** *adj.*—**apogamous** *adj.*

apogee /ˈæpəˌdʒiː/ *n* the point in the orbit of the moon or any planet where it is most distant from the earth; the highest point.

apolitical /ˌeɪpəˈlɪtɪkəl/ *adj* uninterested or uninvolved in politics.

Apollo /əˈpɒloː/ *n* (Greek, Roman myth) a sun god and god of music; (*pl* **Apollos**) a young handsome man.

apologetic /əˌpɒləˈdʒɛtɪk/ *adj* expressing an apology; contrite; presented in defence.—**apologetically** *adv.*

apologetics /-ɪks/ *n* (*used as sing*) the defence and vindication of the principles and laws of Christian belief.

apologia /ˌæpəˈloːdʒiə/ *n* a written defence of one's principles or conduct.

apologist /əˈpɒlədʒɪst/ *n* a person who makes an apology; a defender of a cause.

apologize /əˈpɒləˌdʒaɪz/ *vi* to make an apology.

apologue /ˈæpəˌlɒg/ *n* a moral fable; a fiction or allegory embodying a moral application, as *Aesop's Fables*.

apology /əˈpɒlədʒi/ *n* (*pl* **apologies**) an expression of regret for wrongdoing; a defence or justification of one's beliefs, etc; (*with* **for**) a poor substitute.

apophthegm /ˈæpəˌθɛm/ or /ˈæpəfˌθɛm/ *n* a pithy saying embodying a wholesome truth or precept, a maxim.—*also* **apothegm**.

apophyge /əˈpɒfə̩dʒiː/ n (archit) the small hollow curve of a column where it springs from the base or top of the shaft.

apoplectic /ˌæpəˈplɛktɪk/ adj of, causing, or exhibiting symptoms of apoplexy; (inf) furious.

apoplexy /ˈæpə̩plɛksi/ n a sudden loss of consciousness and subsequent partial paralysis, usu caused by a broken or blocked artery in the brain.

aport /əˈpɔːt/ adv (naut) on or towards the port or left side of a ship.

aposiopesis /ˌæpə̩saɪəˈpiːsɪs/ n (pl **aposiopeses**) (rhetoric) a sudden breaking off in speech for effect, eg "Bertrand is —what I dare not name".—**aposiopetic** adj.

apostasy /əˈpɒstəsi/ n (pl **apostasies**) abandonment of one's religion, principles or political party.

apostate /-teɪt/ n a person who commits apostasy.

apostatize /-tə̩taɪz/ vi to abandon one's faith, church or party; to change one's religion for another.

a posteriori /ˌeɪpɒ̩stiːriˈɔːraɪ/ adj (logic) inductively, from effect to cause, founded on observation of facts, effects or consequences.

apostil /əˈpɒstɪl/ n a marginal note.

apostle /əˈpɒsəl/ n the first or principal supporter of a new belief or cause; (with cap) one of the twelve disciples of Christ.

apostle spoon n a spoon having a figure of one of the Apostles at the top of the handle.

Apostles' Creed n the shortest of the three creeds, so named as containing a summary of apostolic doctrine.

apostolate /əˈpɒstələt/ n the dignity or office of an apostle, now restricted to that of the pope.

apostolic /ˌæpəˈstɒlɪk/ adj of or relating to the Apostles or their teachings; of or relating to the pope as successor to the Apostle St Peter.

Apostolic Church, Apostolic See n the Christian church as founded and governed by the Apostles on their doctrine and order. The name originally applied to the Churches of Rome, Antioch, Ephesus, Alexandria and Jerusalem.

Apostolic succession n the regular and uninterrupted transmission of ministerial authority by bishops from the Apostles.

apostrophe[1] /əˈpɒstrəfi/ n a mark (') showing the omission of letters or figures, also a sign of the possessive case or the plural of letters and figures; a breaking off in speech to appeal to someone dead or absent.—**apostrophic** adj.

apostrophe[2] n (rhetoric) a digression made in a speech or address, esp one directed at a person.

apostrophize /-̩faɪz/ vt to address by apostrophe; to omit a letter or letters; to mark an omission by the sign ('). • vi to make an apostrophe or short digressive address in speaking.

apothecaries' weight n a system of weights used for dispensing drugs, comprising the pound (12 oz), the ounce (8 drachms), the drachm (3 scruples), the scruple (20 grains), and the grain.

apothecary /əˈpɒθə̩kɛri/ n (pl **apothecaries**) (arch) one who prepares and dispenses medicines and drugs, a pharmacist.

apothecium /ˌæpəˈθiːsiəm/ n (pl **apothecia**) the shield-like receptacle of lichens.—**apothecial** adj.

apothegm /ˈæpə̩θɛm/ see **apophthegm**.

apotheosis /ə̩pɒθiˈoːsɪs/ n (pl **apotheoses**) deification; glorification of a person or thing; the supreme or ideal example.

apotheosize /əˈpɒθiə̩saɪz/ vt to exalt to the rank of a god; to deify.

appal, appall /əˈpɔːl/ vt (**appals** or **appalls**, **appalling**, **appalled**) to fill with terror or dismay.

appalling /-ɪŋ/ adj shocking, horrifying.—**appallingly** adv.

appanage /ˈæpənɪdʒ/ n provision for the younger sons of kings, etc; a perquisite; a dependency; an attribute.—also **apanage**.

apparatus /ˌæpəˈrætəs/ or /-ˈreɪt-/ n (pl **apparatus, apparatuses**) the equipment used for a specific task; any complex machine, device, or system.

apparel /əˈpɛrəl/ or /-pær-/ n clothing, dress. • vt (**apparelling, apparelled** or **appareling, appareled**) to dress; to clothe.

apparent /əˈpɛrənt/ or /-pær-/ adj easily seen, evident; seeming, but not real.—**apparently** adv.

apparition /ˌæpəˈrɪʃən/ n an appearance or manifestation, esp something unexpected or unusual; a ghost.

appassionato /ə̩pɒsiəˈnɒtoː/, It. /a̩pasjaˈnaːtə/ adj, adv (mus) with passion.

appeal /əˈpiːl/ vi to take a case to a higher court; to make an earnest request; to refer to a witness or superior authority for vindication, confirmation, etc; to arouse pleasure or sympathy. • n the referral of a lawsuit to a higher court for rehearing; an earnest call for help; attraction, the power of arousing sympathy;

a request for public donations to a charitable cause.—**appealable** adj.—**appealer** n—**appealing** adj.

appear /əˈpiːr/ vi to become or be visible; to arrive, come in person; to be published; to present oneself formally (before a court, etc); to seem, give an impression of being.

appearance /-əns/ n the act or occasion of appearing; that which appears; external aspect of a thing or person; outward show, semblance.

appease /əˈpiːz/ vt to pacify to allay; to conciliate by making concessions.—**appeasement** n.

appellant /əˈpɛlənt/ n a person who makes an appeal to a higher court.

appellate /-lət/ adj pertaining to appeals; dealing with appeals. • n the person appealed against or called upon to appear.

appellation /ˌæpəˈleɪʃən/ n the name, title or designation by which a person or thing is called or known; the act of appealing.

appellative /əˈpɛlətɪv/ n (gram) a common, as distinguished from a proper, name; the designation of a class. • adj serving to distinguish, as a name or denomination of a group or class; common, as a noun.

appellee /ˌæpəˈliː/ or /ə̩pɛl-/ n the person appealed against; the defendant in an appeal.

append /əˈpɛnd/ vt to attach; to add, esp to the end as a supplement, etc.

appendage /əˈpɛndɪdʒ/ n something appended; an external organ or part, as a tail.

appendant /əˈpɛndənt/ adj attached or annexed; attached in a subordinate capacity to another. • n that which is appended or added.

appendicectomy, appendectomy /ˌæpɛnˈdɛktəmi/ n (pl **appendicectomies, appendectomies**) surgical removal of the appendix that grows from the intestine.

appendicitis /ə̩pɛndiˈsaɪtɪs/ n inflammation of the appendix that grows from the intestine.

appendicle /əˈpɛndɪkəl/ n a small appendage.

appendix /əˈpɛndɪks/ n (pl **appendixes, appendices**) a section of supplementary information at the back of a book, etc; a small tube of tissue that forms an outgrowth of the intestine.—also **vermiform appendix**.

apperception /ˌæpərˈsɛpʃən/ n (psychol) perception with consciousness of self.—**apperceptive** adj.

appertain /ˌæpərˈteɪn/ vi to belong or pertain to, as by relation or custom.

appetence /ˈæpətəns/, **appetency** /ˈæpətənsi/ n (pl **appetences, appetencies**) desire, craving; affinity.

appetite /ˈæpə̩taɪt/ n sensation of bodily desire, esp for food; (with **for**) a strong desire or liking, a craving.

appetizer /-̩taɪzər/ n a food or drink that stimulates the appetite; something that whets one's interest.

appetizing /-̩taɪzɪŋ/ adj stimulating the appetite.—**appetizingly** adv.

applaud /əˈplɔːd/ vt to show approval, esp by clapping the hands; to praise.

applause /əˈplɔːz/ n approval expressed by clapping; acclamation.

apple /ˈæpəl/ n a round, firm, fleshy, edible fruit.

apple brandy n a liqueur distilled from cider.

applecart n upset the **applecart** to spoil one's plans.

applejack /ˈæpə̩ldʒæk/ n apple brandy.

apple-pie bed n a bed made with the sheets folded so that one's legs cannot get down.

apple-pie order n perfect order.

apple sauce /ˈæpə̩lsɒs/ n a sauce of stewed apples usu served with pork; (sl) nonsense, flattery.

appliance /əˈplaɪəns/ n a device or machine, esp for household use.

applicable /əˈplɪkəbəl/ adj that may be applied; appropriate, relevant (to).—**applicability** n.

applicant /ˈæplɪkənt/ n a person who applies, esp for a job.

application /ˌæplɪˈkeɪʃən/ n the act of applying; the use to which something is put; a petition, request; concentration, diligent effort; relevance or practical value.

applicative /ˈæplɪ̩keɪtɪv/ adj capable of being applied.

applicator /ˈæplɪ̩keɪtər/ n a device for applying something.

applicatory /ˈæplɪkə̩tɔri/ adj fit to be applied.

applied /əˈplaɪd/ adj practical.

appliqué /ˌæpliˈkeɪ/ n ornamental fabricwork applied to another fabric. • vt (**appliquéing, appliquéed**) to decorate with appliqué.

apply /ə'plaɪ/ *vb* (**applying, applied**) *vt* to bring to bear; to put to practical use; to spread, lay on; to devote (oneself) with close attention. • *vi* to make a formal, *esp* written, request; to be relevant.

appoggiatura /əˌpɒdʒə'tʊrə/ *n* (*pl* **appoggiaturas, appoggiature**) (*mus*) a grace note immediately preceding a principal note with which it is connected, and taking its time from the latter.

appoint /ə'pɔɪnt/ *vt* to fix or decide officially; to select for a job; to prescribe.

appointed /ə'pɔɪntəd/ *adj* equipped; furnished.

appointee /əˌpɔɪn'tiː/ or /ˌæpɔɪn'tiː/ *n* a person appointed.

appointment /ə'pɔɪntmənt/ *n* an appointing; a job or position for which someone has been selected; an arrangement to meet.

apportion /ə'pɔrʃən/ *vt* to divide into shares; allot.—**apportionable** *adj.*—**apportioner** *n.*—**apportionment** *n.*

appose /ə'pɔːz/ *vt* to apply; to place opposite or in juxtaposition.

apposite /'æpəzɪt/ *adj* (*remarks*) especially pertinent, appropriate.—**appositely** *adv.*

apposition /ˌæpə'zɪʃən/ *n* the act of adding; addition by application, or placing together; (*gram*) the placing of a second noun in the same case in juxtaposition to the first, which it characterizes or explains, as St Mark, the Evangelist.—**appositional** *adj.*

appraisal /ə'preɪzəl/, **appraisement** /ə'preɪzmənt/ *n* the act of appraising or valuing, *esp* the putting of a price upon with a view to sale; a valuation.

appraise /ə'preɪz/ *vt* to estimate the value or quality of.—**appraiser** *n.*

appreciable /ə'priːʃəbəl/ *adj* capable of being perceived or measured; fairly large.—**appreciably** *adv.*

appreciate /ə'priːʃɪˌeɪt/ *vt* to value highly; to recognize gratefully; to understand, be aware of; to increase the value of. • *vi* to rise in value.

appreciation /əˌpriːʃɪ'eɪʃən/ *n* gratitude, approval; sensitivity to aesthetic values; an assessment or critical evaluation of a person or thing; a favourable review; an increase in value.—**appreciative** *adj.*

apprehend /ˌæprɪ'hend/ *vt* to arrest, capture; to understand, to perceive.

apprehension /ˌæprɪ'henʃən/ *n* anxiety; the act of arresting; understanding; an idea.

apprehensive /ˌæprɪ'hensɪv/ *adj* uneasy; anxious.—**apprehensively** *adv.*

apprentice /ə'prentɪs/ *n* one being taught a trade or craft; a novice. • *vt* to take on as an apprentice.—**apprenticeship** *n.*

apprise, apprize /ə'praɪz/ *vt* to give notice to; to inform.

approach /ə'prəʊtʃ/ *vi* to draw nearer. • *vt* to make a proposal to; to set about dealing with; to come near to. • *n* the act of approaching; a means of entering or leaving; a move to establish relations; the final descent of an aircraft.

approachable /ə'prəʊtʃəbəl/ *adj* within approaching distance; easy to approach; inviting friendship.—**approachability** *n.*—**approachably** *adv.*

approbation /ˌæprə'beɪʃən/ *n* formal approval; sanction.

appropriate /ə'prəʊprɪət/ *adj* fitting, suitable. • *vt* to take for one's own use, *esp* illegally; (*money, etc*) to set aside for a specific purpose.—**appropriately** *adv.*—**appropriateness** *n.*

appropriation /əˌprəʊprɪ'eɪʃən/ *n* the act of setting apart or reserving for one's own use; a sum of money set aside for a particular purpose.

approval /ə'pruːvəl/ *n* the act of approving; favourable opinion; official permission.

approve /ə'pruːv/ *vt* to express a good opinion of; to authorize. • *vi* (*with* **of**) to consider to be favourable or satisfactory.

approx. *abbr* = approximate(ly).

approximate /ə'prɒksɪmət/ *adj* almost exact or correct. • *vt* to come near to; to be almost the same as. • *vi* to come close.—**approximately** *adv.*

approximation /əˌprɒksɪ'meɪʃən/ *n* a close estimate; a near likeness.

appulse /ə'pɒlz/ *n* a coming towards; (astron) the near approach of a planet to a conjunction with the sun or any fixed star.—**appulsive** *adj.*

appurtenance /ə'pɜːtɪnəns/ *n* that which belongs or relates to something else; an adjunct or appendage; that which belongs it, is accessory to; an estate or property.—**appurtenant** *adj, n.*

Apr. *abbr* = April.

APR. *abbr* = annual percentage rate.

après-ski /ˌæpreɪ'skiː/, *Fr.* /a'prɛ-/ *n* social activity after skiing.—*also adj.*

apricot /'æprɪˌkɒt/ or /'eɪprɪ-/ *n* a small, oval, orange-pink fruit resembling the plum and peach.

April /'eɪprəl/ *n* the fourth month of the year, having 30 days.

April Fool *n* the victim of a trick played on 1 April, **April Fool's Day.**

a priori /ˌeɪpraɪ'ɔraɪ/ (*Latin*) deductively, from cause to effect.

apron /'eɪprən/ *n* a garment worn to protect clothing; anything resembling the shape of an apron used for protection; the paved surface on an airfield where aircraft are parked, etc.

apropos /ˌæprə'pɔː/ or /'æprəˌpɔː/ *adv* at the right time; opportunely; appropriately. • *adj* appropriate. • *prep* (*with* **of**) regarding, in reference to.

apse /æps/ *n* a domed or vaulted recess, *esp* in a church.

apsis /'æpsɪs/ *n* (*pl* **apsides** /'æpsəˌdiːz/) (*astron*) one of two points in the orbit of a planet situated at the furthest or the least distance from the central body or sun; the imaginary line connecting these points.—**apsidal** *adj.*

apt /æpt/ *adj* ready or likely (to); suitable, relevant; able to learn easily.—**aptness** *n.*

apteral /'æptərəl/ *adj* (*archit*) without side columns.

apterous /'æptərəs/ *adj* without wings.

apterygial /ˌæptə'rɪdʒɪəl/ *adj* lacking wings or fins.

apteryx /'æptərɪks/ *n* the kiwi, a New Zealand bird with rudimentary wings and no tail.

aptitude /'æptɪˌtuːd/ or /-ˌtjuːd/ *n* suitability; natural talent, *esp* for learning.

apyretic /ˌæpaɪ'retɪk/ *adj* without fever, or with intermission of fever.

aq *abbr* = aqua.

aqua *n* /'ækwə/ or /-ɒ-/ (*pl* **aquae** /'eɪkwiː/, **aquas** /'ækwəz/) water as used in pharmacy.

aquaculture /-ˌkʌltʃər/ or /ɒkwə-/ *n* the cultivation and breeding of fish and other marine organisms.—*also* **aquiculture.**—**aquacultural** *adj.*—**aquaculturist** *n.*

aqua fortis *n* /-'fɔrtɪs/ or /ˌɒkwə/ impure nitric acid.

aqualung /'ækwəˌlʌŋ/ *n* portable diving gear comprising air cylinders connected to a face mask.

aquamarine /ˌækwəmə'riːn/ *n* a variety of bluish-green beryl used as a gemstone; its colour.

aquaplane /'ækwəˌpleɪn/ *n* a plank towed at high speed. • *vi* to ride on one.

aqua regia /ˌækwə'riːdʒɪə/ *n* a mixture of nitric and hydrochloric acids, capable of dissolving gold.

aquarelle /ˌækwə'rel/ or /ˌækwə'rel/ *n* a style of painting in Chinese ink and thin watercolours; a painting so executed.—**aquarellist** *n.*

aquarium /ə'kweərɪəm/ *n* (*pl* **aquariums, aquaria**) a tank, pond, etc for keeping aquatic animals or plants; a building where collections of aquatic animals are exhibited.

Aquarius /ə'kweərɪəs/ *n* (*astrol*) the eleventh sign of the zodiac, the water-carrier, operative 20 January–18 February.—**Aquarian** *adj, n.*

aquatic /ə'kwætɪk/ or /ə'kwɒtɪk/ *adj* of or taking place in water; living or growing in water.

aquatics /ə'kwætɪks/ or /ə'kwɒtɪks/ *npl* water sports.

aquatint /'ækwətɪnt/ *n* a style of etching resembling a watercolour drawing in Indian ink or in sepia; an engraving produced by this process. • *vt* to etch or engrave in aquatint.

aqua vitae /ˌækwə'viːtaɪ/ *n* unrectified alcohol; brandy and other ardent spirits.

aqueduct /'ækwəˌdekt/ *n* a large pipe or conduit for carrying water; an elevated structure supporting this.

aqueous /'eɪkwɪəs/ *adj* of, like, or formed by water.

aqueous humour *n* a limpid fluid of the eye, filling the space between the crystalline lens and the cornea.

aquiculture /'ækwɪˌkʌltʃər/ or /'ɒk-/ *n* hydroponics; another name for aquaculture.—**aquicultural** *adj.*—**aquiculturist** *n.*

aquilegia /ˌækwə'liːdʒə/ *n* columbine.

aquiline /'ækwɪˌlaɪn/ *adj* of or like an eagle; (*nose*) hooked, like an eagle's beak.

ar- /ər/ *prefix* the form of *ad-* before *r*.

-ar /ər/ *adj suffix* of, belonging to, as in *angular, popular.*

AR *abbr* = Arkansas.

Ar (*chem symbol*) argon.

Arab /'ærəb/ or /'ɛrəb/ *n* a native of Arabia; one of the Arabic races spread over the African and Syrian deserts. • *adj* pertaining to Arabia or the Arabs.

arabesque /ˌærə'bɛsk/ or /ɛrə-/ *n* a decorative design incorporating organic motifs, such as leaves and flowers in an intricate pattern; (*ballet*) a posture in which the dancer balances on one leg with one arm extending forwards and the other arm and leg extending backwards.

Arabian /ə'reɪbɪən/ *adj* of Arabia, Arab. • *n* an Arab.

Arabian camel *n* a camel with a single hump.

Arabic /'ærəbɪk/ or /'ɛrə-/ *n* the Arabian language. • *adj* of or pertaining to the Arabic language and the countries in which it is spoken.

Arabic numeral *n* one of the numbers 0, 1, 2, 3, 4, 5, etc.

arable /'ærəbəl/ or /'ɛr-/ *adj* (*land*) suitable for ploughing or planting crops.—*also n.*

arachnid /ə'ræknɪd/ *n* any of a class of animals including spiders, scorpions, mites and ticks.—**arachnidan** *adj, n.*

arachnoid /-ˌnɔɪd/ *adj* pertaining to spiders; resembling the web of a spider. • *n* the enveloping membrane of the brain and spinal cord, between the dura mater and the pia mater.

aragonite /ə'rægəˌnaɪt/ or /'ærəgə-/ *n* a variety of carbonate of lime.

arak /ə'ræk/ *see* **arrack**.

Aramaic /ˌærə'meɪɪk/ or /ˌɛrə-/ *n* the language of Palestine at the time of Christ.

araneid /ə'reɪnɪˌɪd/ *n* a member of the Arachnida order, the spider family.

araucaria /ˌærɔ'kɛrɪə/ *n* one of a genus of coniferous trees, found principally in South America and Australia, which includes the monkey puzzle.

arbalest /'ɑrbəˌlɛst/ *n* a crossbow with a drawing mechanism.

arbiter /'ɑrbɪtər/ *n* a person having absolute power of decision or absolute control.

arbitrage /'ɑrbɪtrɒdʒ/ or /-trɑdʒ/ *n* the rapid purchase and resale of stocks to maximize price discrepancy, often using confidential knowledge.—*also* **index arbitrage**.

arbitrament /'ɑrbɪtrəmənt/ *n* an arbiter's judgment; an authoritative decision.

arbitrary /'ɑrbəˌtrɛri/ *adj* not bound by rules despotic, absolute; capricious, unreasonable.—**arbitrarily** *adv.*—**arbitrariness** *n.*

arbitrate /'ɑrbɪˌtreɪt/ *vi* to act as an arbitrator. • *vt* to submit to an arbiter; to act as an arbiter upon.

arbitration /ˌɑrbɪ'treɪʃən/ *n* the settlement of disputes by arbitrating.

arbitrator /ˌɑrbɪ'treɪtər/ *n* a person chosen to settle a dispute between contending parties.

arbor[1] /'ɑrbər/ *see* **arbour**.

arbor[2] *n* the main support of a machine; an axis, a spindle.

Arbor Day *n* a day legally set apart in certain states of the US for planting trees.

arboraceous /ˌɑrbə'reɪʃəs/ *adj* pertaining to, or of the nature of, a tree or trees; living on or among trees.

arboreal /ɑr'bɔrɪəl/ *adj* of or living in trees.

arboreous /ær'bɔrɪəs/ *adj* wooded.

arborescent /ˌɑrˌbə'rɛsənt/ *adj* growing or formed like a tree.—**arborescence** *n.*

arboretum /ˌɑrbə'riːtəm/ *n* (*pl* **arbereta, arboretums**) a botanical tree garden where rare trees are cultivated and exhibited.

arboriculture /'ɑrbɒrɪˌkʌltʃər/ *n* the cultivation of trees and shrubs, forestry.

arborization, arborisation /ˌɑrbɒrɪ'zeɪʃən/ *n* a tree-like appearance.

arbor vitae /ˌɑrbər'viːtaɪ/ *n* an evergreen tree extensively cultivated in gardens, etc.

arbour /'ɑrbər/ *n* a place shaded by trees, foliage, etc; a bower.—*also* **arbor.**

arbutus /ɑr'bjuːtəs/ *n* (*pl* **arbutuses**) one of a genus of tree-like evergreen shrubs to which the strawberry tree belongs.

arc /ɑrk/ *n* a portion of the circumference of a circle or other curve; a luminous discharge of electricity across a gap between two electrodes or terminals. • *vi* to form an electric arc.

ARC *abbr* = AIDS-related complex.

ARC /ˌeɪ'ɑr'siː/ *acronym for* AIDS-related condition.

arcade /ɑr'keɪd/ *n* a series of arches supported on columns; an arched passageway; a covered walk or area lined with shops.

Arcadia /ɑr'keɪdɪə/, **Arcady** /ɑr'keɪdi/ *n* (*poet*) ideal countryside.

Arcadian /ɑr'keɪdɪən/ *adj* of or pertaining to Arcadia, a department of Greece, or its inhabitants; rurally simple. • *n* an inhabitant of Arcadia.

arcane /ɑr'keɪn/ *adj* secret or esoteric.

arcanum /ɑr'keɪnəm/ *n* (*pl* **arcana**) a secret, a mystery; a valuable elixir.

arch[1] /ɑrtʃ/ *n* a curved structure spanning an opening; the curved underside of the foot. • *vti* to span or cover with an arch; to curve, bend into an arch.

arch[2] *adj* (*criminal, etc*) principal, expert; clever, sly; mischievous.—**archly** *adv.*—**archness** *n.*

Archaean /ɑr'kiːən/ *adj* of the earliest geological period or strata.—*also* **Archean.**

archaeology /ˌɑrkɪ'lɒdʒi/ *n* the study of past human societies through their extant remains.—*also* **archeology.**—**archaeological, archeological** *adj.*—**archaeologist, archeologist** *n.*

archaeopteryx /ˌɑrkɪ'ɒptərɪks/ *n* oldest fossil bird.

archaic /ɑr'keɪɪk/ *adj* belonging to ancient times; (*language*) no longer in common use.

archaism /'ɑrkeɪɪzəm/ or /-kiːɪzəm/ *n* an archaic word or phrase.—**archaistic** *adj.*

archaize /'ɑrkeɪɪz/ *vti* to affect the archaic; to make archaic.—**archaizer** *n.*

archangel /'ɑrkeɪndʒəl/ *n* a principal angel.—**archangelic** *adj.*

archb shop /'ɑrtʃ'bɪʃəp/ *n* a bishop of the highest rank.

archb shopric /-rɪk/ *n* the jurisdiction, office or see of an archbishop.

archdeacon /-'diːkən/ *n* a clergyman ranking next under a bishop.

archdeaconry /-'diːkənri/ *n* (*pl* **archdeaconries**) the office, rank, jurisdiction, or residence of an archdeacon.

archdiocese /-'daɪəsəsz/ or /-'daɪəsɪs/, /-'daɪəsiːz/ *n* the diocese of an archbishop.—**archdiocesan** *adj.*

archducal /-'duːkəl/ or /-'djuːkəl/ *adj* of or pertaining to an archduchess, an archduchy or an archduke.

archduchess /-'dʌtʃəs/ *n* a daughter of the emperor of Austria; the wife or widow of an archduke.

archduchy /-'dʌtʃi/ *n* (*pl* **archduchies**) the territory or rank of an archduke or an archduchess.

archduke /-'duːk/ or /-'djuːk/ *n* a prince of the imperial house of Austria.

Archean *see* **Archaean.**

archegonium /ˌɑrkə'goːnɪəm/ *n* (*pl* **archegonia**) (*bot*) the pistillidium or female organ of the higher cryptogams (ferns, etc).

archenemy /ˌɑrtʃ'ɛnəmi/ *n* (*pl* **archenemies**) a principal enemy; Satan.

archeology *see* **archaeology.**

archer /'ɑrtʃər/ *n* a person who shoots with a bow and arrow.

archerfish /'ɑrtʃərˌfɪʃ/ *n* (*pl* **archerfish, archerfishes**) a scaly-finned fish of the Java seas, which catches insects by darting drops of water upon them.

archery /'ɑrtʃəri/ *n* the art or sport of shooting arrows from a bow.

archetype /'ɑrkɪˌtaɪp/ *n* the original pattern or model; a prototype.—**archetypal, archetypical** *adj.*

archfiend /'ɑrtʃˌfiːnd/ *n* a chief fiend; Satan.

archidiaconal /ˌɑrkɪdaɪ'ækənəl/ *adj* of or pertaining to an archdeacon or to his office.

archidiaconate /ˌɑrkɪdaɪ'ækəneɪt/ *n* the office of an archdeacon.

archiepiscopal /ˌɑrkɪə'pɪskəpəl/ *adj* of or pertaining to an archbishop or to his office.

archiepiscopate /ˌɑrkɪə'pɪskəpət/ or /-ˌpeɪt/, /-si/, **archiepiscopacy** /-si/ *n* the rule or dignity of an archbishop.

archil /'ɑrkɪl/ *see* **orchil.**

archimagus, archimage /'ɑrkɪˌmeɪdʒ/ *n* the high priest of the Persian magi or fire-worshippers; a chief magician.

archimandrite /ˌɑrkɪ'mændˌraɪt/ *n* (*Greek Orthodox Church*) the abbot of a monastery, or an abbot-general having the charge and superintendence of several monasteries.

Archimedean screw *n* an instrument for raising water, consisting of a flexible tube wound spirally around or within a cylinder in the form of a screw. When placed in an inclined position, with the lower end immersed in water, by the revolution of the screw the water is raised to the upper end.

archipelago /ˌɑrkɪ'pɛləˌgo/ *n* (*pl* **archipelagoes, archipelagos**) a sea filled with small islands; a group of small islands.—**archipelagic, archipelagian** *adj.*

architect /'ɑrkɪˌtɛkt/ *n* a person who designs buildings and supervises their erection; someone who plans something.

architectonic /ˌɑrkɪtekˈtɒnɪk/ *adj* pertaining to design or construction; skilled in architecture; expert in constructing; of the systematizing of knowledge.—**architectonically** *adv*.

architectonics /-nɪks/ *n* (*used as sing*) the science of architecture; structure.

architecture /ˈɑrkɪˌtektʃər/ *n* the art, profession, or science of designing and constructing buildings; the style of a building or buildings; the design and organization of a computer's parts.—**architectural** *adj*.—**architecturally** *adv*.

architrave /ˌɑrkɪˈtreɪv/ *n* an epistyle, the lowest division of an entablature, the part resting immediately on a column; the parts round a door or window.

archives /ˈɑrkaɪvs/ *npl* the location in which public records are kept; the public records themselves.—**archival** *adj*.

archivist /ˈɑrkɪvɪzst/ *n* a keeper of public records.

archivolt /ˈɑrkɪvɒlt/ *n* the undercurve of an arch or the moulding on it.

archpriest /ˈɑrtʃˈpriːst/ *n* a chief priest; a rural dean.

archway /ˈɑrtʃˌweɪ/ *n* an arched or vaulted passage, *esp* that leading into a castle.

arc light *n* light produced by a current of electricity passing between two carbon points placed a short distance from each other.

Arctic, arctic /ˈɑrktɪk/ or /ˈɑrtɪk/ *adj* of, near, or relating to the North Pole or its surroundings; (*inf*) very cold, icy. • *n* (*usu cap with* **the**) the area north of the Arctic Circle; (*without cap*) an arctic boot.

arctic boot *n* ✤ (*Cdn*) a heavy, felt-lined, rubber-soled boot worn in cold weather.

Arctic char *n* ✤ a freshwater fish of northern North America, similar to salmon.

Arctic Circle *n* an imaginary circle around the Arctic regions parallel to the equator.

Arctic cotton *n* ✤ a northern sedge whose flower heads have long white cottony hairs.

Arctic fox *n* a small species of fox, whose fine fur is used for muffs, trimmings, etc.

Arctic hare *n* ✤ a large hare of northern Canada and Greenland, whose coat is brown in summer and white in winter.

Arctic Ocean *n* the ocean that washes the northern coasts of Europe, Asia and North America.

Arctic poppy *n* ✤ a northern plant with four-petalled golden flowers.

arcuate /ˈɑrkjuːət/ or /-ˌeɪt/ *adj* bent or curved in the form of a bow.

arcuation /ˌɑrkjuːˈweɪʃən/ *n* the act of bending; the state of being bent or curved; a method of propagating trees by bending branches to the ground and covering portions of them with earth.

arc welding *n* welding using an electric arc.

ardent /ˈɑrdənt/ *adj* passionate; zealous.—**ardency** *n*.—**ardently** *adv*.

ardent spirits *npl* alocholic beverages, as brandy, whisky, etc.

ardour, ardor /ˈɑrdər/ *n* warmth of feeling; extreme intensity.

arduous /ˈɑrdʒuːəs/ *adj* difficult, laborious; steep, difficult to climb. —**arduously** *adv*.—**arduousness** *n*.

are[1] /ɑr/, /ɛr/ *see* **be**.

are[2] *n* a metric unit of measure equal to 100 square metres.

area /ˈɛriə/ *n* an expanse of land; a total outside surface, measured in square units; a specific part of a house, district, etc; scope or extent.

areca /ˈærəkə/ or /əˈriːkə/ *n* a genus of lofty palms, including the tree from which the betelnut and the astringent juice Catechu are obtained.

arena /əˈriːnə/ *n* an area within a sports stadium, etc where events take place; a place or sphere of contest or activity.

arenaceous /ˌæriˈneɪʃəs/ or /-ˌɛri-/ *adj* sandy; abounding in, or having the properties of, sand.

aren't /ˈɑrnt/ = are not.

areola /əˈriːələ/ *n* (*pl* **areolae, areolas**) a very small area; an interstice in tissue; the coloured circle or halo surrounding the nipple of the breast.—**areolar, areolate** *adj*.—**areolation** *n*.

arête /æˈret/ *n* the sharp ridge or spur of a mountain.

argali /ˈɑrgəli/ *n* (*pl* **argalis, argali**) a large wild Asiatic sheep, remarkable for its huge curved horns.

argent /ˈɑrdʒənt/ *n* (*her*) silver, represented in a drawing or engraving of a coat of arms by a plain white surface, symbolic of purity, beauty, etc. • *adj* made of or resembling silver; silvery white; bright like silver.

argentiferous /ˌɑrdʒənˈtɪfərəs/ *adj* producing or containing silver.

argentine /ˈɑrdʒənˌtaɪn/ or /-ˌtiːn/ *adj* pertaining to or resembling silver; silvery. • *n* a silvery-white slaty variety of calcite; white metal coated with silver, imitation silver.

argil /ˈɑrdʒil/ *n* clay, *esp* potter's clay or earth.

argillaceous /ˌɑrdʒəˈleɪʃəs/ *adj* of or containing clay, clayey.

argilliferous /ˌɑrdʒələˈfərəs/ *adj* producing or containing clay.

argillite /ˈɑrdʒɪˌlɔɪt/ *n* clay-slate.—**argillitic** *adj*.

argol /ˈɑrgɒl/ *n* a deposit of crude tartar on the sides of wine vessels; crude tartar from which cream of tartar is prepared.

argon /ˈɑrgɒn/ *n* an inert gaseous element.

argosy /ˈɑrgəsi/ *n* (*pl* **argosies**) a large, richly laden merchant ship.

argot /ˈɑrgo/ or /ˈɑrgət/ *n* the special vocabulary of any set of persons, as of lawyers, criminals, etc.—**argotic** *adj*.

arguable /ˈɑrgjuːəbl/ *adj* debatable; able to be asserted; plausible.—**arguably** *adv*.

argue /ˈɑrgjuː/ *vb* (**arguing, argued**) *vt* to try to prove by reasoning; to debate, dispute; to persuade (into, out of). • *vi* to offer reasons for or against something; to disagree, exchange angry words.—**arguer** *n*.

argufy /ˈɑrgjəfaɪ/ *vi* (**argufying, argufied**) (*sl*) to argue tediously, to wrangle.

argument /ˈɑrgjumənt/ or /-gjə- / *n* a disagreement; a debate, discussion; a reason offered in debate; an abstract, summary.

argumentation /ˌɑrgjumenˈteɪʃən/ *n* systematic reasoning; argument, discussion.

argumentative /ˌɑrgjuˈmentətɪv/ *adj* prone to arguing.—**argumentatively** *adv*.—**argumentativeness** *n*.

argy-bargy /ˈɑrgiˈbɑrgi/ *n* (*pl* **argy-bargies**) *n* a tedious discussion. • *vi* to argue at length.

aria /ˈɑriə/ *n* a song for one voice accompanied by instruments, *eg* in opera.

Arian /ˈɛriən/ or /ˈæ-/ *adj* pertaining to the doctrines of the Arian sect, which held that Christ is not divine.—**Arianism** *n*.

arid /ˈærəd/ or /ˈærɪd/ *adj* very dry, parched; uninteresting; dull.—**aridity** *n*.—**aridly** *adv*.

Aries /ˈɛriːz/ or /ˈær-/, /-ˈiːz/ *n* (*astrol*) the first sign of the zodiac, the Ram, operative 21 March–21 April.—**Arian** *adj, n*.

arietta /ˌɑriˈetə/ or /ˌæri-/, /ˌɛri-/ *n* a short aria, song or air.

aright /əˈraɪt/ *adv* correctly.

aril /ˈærərl/ *n* (*bot*) an accessory covering or appendage of certain seeds.

arioso /ˌɑriˈoːˌsoː/ *adj, adv* (*mus*) like an air; in a smooth melodious style.

arise /əˈraɪz/ *vi* (**arising, arose**, *pp* **arisen**) to get up, as from bed; to rise, ascend; to come into being, to result (from).

arista /əˈrɪstə/ *n* (*pl* **aristae** /əˈrɪsti/) the awn or beard of grasses; a bristle.

aristate /əˈrɪsteɪt/ *adj* bearded; having a beard or bristle, as certain grasses.

aristocracy /ˌæriˈstɒkrəsi/ or /ˈɛri-/ *n* (*pl* **aristocracies** /-siːz/) (a country with) a government dominated by a privileged minority class; the privileged class in a society, the nobility; those people considered the best in their particular sphere.

aristocrat /ˈærəstəˌkræt/ or /əˈrɪstəˌkræt/ *n* a member of the aristocracy; a supporter of aristocratic government; a person with the manners or taste of a privileged class.

aristocratic /ˌærəstəˈkrætɪk/ or /əˌrɪstəˈkrætɪk/ *adj* relating to or characteristic of the aristocracy; elegant, stylish in dress and manners.—**aristocratically** *adv*.

Aristotelian /ˌærɪstəˈtiliən/ or /əˌrɪstə-/ *adj* pertaining to, or characteristic of, Aristotle (384—322 bc) or his philosophy.

arithmetic /əˈrɪθˌmɒtiːk/ or /əˈrɪ-/ *n* (*math*) computation (addition, subtraction, etc) using real numbers; calculation.—**arithmetic, arithmetical** *adj*.—**arithmetically** *adv*.

arithmetician /-ˈtɪʃən/ *n* one skilled in the science of numbers.

Ariz. *abbr* = Arizona.

ark /ɑrk/ *n* (*Bible*) the boat in which Noah and his family and two of every kind of creature survived the Flood; a place of safety; an enclosure in a synagogue for the scrolls of the Torah.

Ark. *abbr* = Arkansas.

ark of the covenant *n* (*Bible*) the chest containing the two stone tablets inscribed with the Ten Commandments.

arm /ɑrm/ *n* the upper limb from the shoulder to the wrist; something shaped like an arm, as a support on a chair; a sleeve; power, authority; an administrative division of a large organization.

arm[2] *n* (*usu pl*) a weapon; a branch of the military service; (*pl*) heraldic bearings. • *vt* to provide with weapons, etc; to provide with something that protects or strengthens, etc; to set a fuse ready to explode. • *vi* to prepare for war or any struggle.

armada /ɑrˈmɒdə/ *n* a fleet of warships or aircraft.

armadillo /ˌɑrməˈdɪloː/ *n* (*pl* **armadillos** /-z/) a small animal from South America with a body covering of small bony plates.

Armageddon /ˌɑrməˈgedən/ *n* (*Bible*) the site of the last decisive battle between good and evil; any great decisive battle.

armament /ˈɑrməmənt/ *n* (*often pl*) all the military forces and equipment of a nation; all the military equipment of a warship, etc; the process of arming or being armed for war.

armature /ˈɑrmətʃər/ *n* a piece of iron connecting the poles of a magnet or electromagnet to preserve and increase the magnetic force; the revolving part of a dynamo; arms, armour, that which serves as a means of defence; iron bars or framework used to strengthen a building; a framework supporting clay, etc, in sculpture or modelling.

armchair /ˈɑrmtʃer/ *n* a chair with side rests for the arms. • *adj* lacking practical experience.

armed forces *npl* the military forces of a nation.—*also* **armed services.**

armful /ˈɑrmful/ *n* as much as the arms can hold.

armhole /ˈɑrmhoːl/ *n* an opening for the arm in an item of clothing.

armiger /ˈɑrmidʒər/ *n* one entitled to use heraldic bearings, an esquire.—**armigerous** *adj.*

armillary /ˈɑrmiləri/ *adj* of or resembling a bracelet; consisting of circles or rings.

armillary sphere *n* a skeleton celestial globe showing the relative positions of the stars, etc.

Arminianism /ɑrˈmɪniəˌnɪzəm/ *n* a Christian Protestant doctrine that denies Calvin's doctrine of predestination.—**Arminian** *adj, n.*

armistice /ˈɑrməstəs/ or /ˈɑrmɪtɪs/ *n* a truce, preliminary to a peace treaty.

armlet /ˈɑrmlət/ *n* an ornamental or protective band worn around the arm; a badge worn on the arm; a small arm of the sea.

armorial /ɑrˈmɔriəl/ *adj* pertaining to armour or the arms or escutcheon of a family. • *n* a book or dictionary of heraldic devices and the names of persons entitled to use them.

armour, armor /ˈɑrmər/ *n* any defensive or protective covering.

armoured, armored /ˈɑrmərd/ *adj* covered or protected with armour; equipped with tanks and armour vehicles.

armourer, armorer /ˈɑrmərər/ *n* the custodian of the arms of a battleship, etc; (formerly) a maker of arms or armour; one who had charge of the armour of another.

armour plate, armor plate *n* a plate of iron or steel affixed to a ship or tank as part of a casing for protection against shellfire.

armoury, armory /ˈɑrməri/ *n* (*pl* **armouries**, **armories**) an arsenal; a place where armour or ammunition is stored; (*Cdn*) a place where militia units train and have their headquarters.

armpit /ˈɑrmˌpɪt/ *n* the hollow underneath the arm at the shoulder.

arms /ɑrmz/ *see* **arm**[2].

army /ˈɑrmi/ *n* (*pl* **armies** /ˈɑrmiːz/) a large organized body of soldiers for waging war, *esp* on land; any large number of persons, animals, etc.

army worm *n* the larva of a moth that devastates grain and other crops, *esp* destructive in North America; the larva of a European small two-winged fly.

arnica /ˈɑrnɪkə/ *n* a genus of perennial herbs, *esp* mountain tobacco, whose roots and flowers are used to make a tincture for treating bruises.

aroma /əˈroːmə/ *n* a pleasant smell; a fragrance.

aromatherapy /əˌroːməˈθerəpi/ *n* the massage of fragrant oils into the skin to relieve tension and promote wellbeing.

aromatic /ˌerəˈmætɪk/ *adj* giving out an aroma, fragrant, spicy; odoriferous. • *n* a plant, herb or drug yielding a fragrant smell.—**aromatically** *adv.*

aromatize /əˈroːməˌtaɪz/ *vt* to render fragrant, to perfume, to scent.—**aromatization** *n.*

arose *see* **arise.**

around /əˈraʊnd/ *prep* on all sides of; on the border of; in various places in or on; approximately, about. • *adv* in a circle; in every direction; in circumference; to the opposite direction.

arousal /əˈraʊzəl/ *n* the act of awakening or stimulating; the state of being awakened or stimulated.

arouse /əˈraʊz/ *vt* to wake from sleep; to stir, as to action; to evoke.

arpeggio /ɑrˈpedʒioː/ *n* (*pl* **arpeggios** /-z/) (*mus*) the playing of notes of a chord in rapid succession, instead of simultaneously; a passage or chord so played.

arpent /ˈɑrpənt/ or /ˈɑrpɒ̃/ *n* (*Cdn*) (*hist*) a unit of land area of about one acre, *esp* in French Canada.

arquebus /ˈɑrkwəbəs/ *n* an old-fashioned handgun fired from a forked rest.—*also* **harcuebus.**

arrack /ˈærək/ *n* an alcoholic spirit distilled in some Asian countries from rice, molasses, the juice of the date palm, etc.—*also* **arak.**

arraign /əˈreɪn/ *vt* to put on trial; to indict, accuse; to censure publicly; to impeach.—**arraigner** *n.*—**arraignment** *n.*

arrange /əˈreɪndʒ/ *vt* to put in a sequence or row; to settle, make preparations for; (*mus*) to prepare a composition for different instruments other than those intended. • *vi* to come to an agreement; to make plans.—**arranger** *n.*

arrangement /əˈreɪndʒmənt/ *n* the act of putting in proper form or order; that which is ordered or disposed; the method or style of disposition; a preparatory measure; preparation; settlement; classification; adjustment; adaptation; (*pl*) plans.

arrant /ˈerənt/ *adj* notorious; unmitigated; downright, thorough; shameless.

arras /ˈærəs/ or /ˈerəs/ *n* a tapestry; hangings made of a rich figured fabric.

array /əˈreɪ/ *n* an orderly grouping, *esp* of troops; an impressive display; fine clothes; (*comput*) an ordered data structure that allows information to be easily indexed. • *vt* to set in order, to arrange; to dress, decorate.—**arrayal** *n.*

arrears /əˈrɪrz/ *npl* overdue debts; work, etc still to be completed.

arrest /əˈrest/ *vt* to stop; to capture, apprehend *esp* by legal authority; to check the development of a disease; to catch and hold the attention of. • *n* a stoppage; seizure by legal authority.

arrestee /əˈresti/ *n* one who has been arrested.

arrester /əˈrestər/ *n* one who or that which stops or seizes, or causes to be detained.

arresting /əˈrestɪŋ/ *adj* striking or attracting to the mind or eye; impressive.—**arrestingly** *adv.*

arrière-pensée *Fr.* /ˈærjer pɑ̃ˈseɪ/ *n* (*pl* **arrière-pensées**) a mental reservation.

arris /ˈærɪs/ or /ˈerɪs/ *n* (*pl* **arris**, **arrises**) (*archit*) the line or sharp edge in which two curved or straight surfaces, forming an exterior angle, meet each other.

arrival /əˈraɪvəl/ *n* arriving; a person or thing that has arrived.

arrive /əˈraɪv/ *vi* to reach any destination; to come; (*with* **at**) to reach agreement, a decision; to achieve success, celebrity.

arriviste /ˌæriːˈviːst/ *n* an ambitious person, a self-seeker.

arrogance /ˈærəgəns/ or /ˈer-/ *n* an exaggerated assumption of importance.

arrogant /ˈærəgənt/ or /ˈæ-/ *adj* overbearing; aggressively self-important.—**arrogantly** *adv.*

arrogate /ˈærəgeɪt/ *vt* to assume or lay claim to unduly or presumptuously.—**arrogation** *n.*—**arrogative** *adj.*—**arrogator** *n.*

arrondissement /æˌrɔ̃diːsˈmɑ̃/ *n* a subdivision of a French department; a municipal subdivision of Paris, etc.

arrow /ˈæroː/ or /ɛ-/ *n* a straight, pointed weapon, made to be shot from a bow; a sign used to indicate direction or location.

arrowhead /-ˌhed/ *n* the head or barb of an arrow; an aquatic plant so named from the shape of its leaves.

arrowroot /-ˌruːt/ or /-ˌrʊt/ *n* a starch obtained from the rootstocks of several species of West Indian plants.

arrowwood /-ˌwʊd/ *n* a wood once used for arrows by American Indians.

arroyo /əˈrɔɪoː/ *n* a watercourse or rivulet; the dry bed of a small stream.

arse /ɑrs/ *n* (*vulg*) the buttocks.

arsenal /ˈɑrsənəl/ *n* a workshop or store for weapons and ammunition.

arsenate /ˈɑrsəˌneɪt/ or /-ˌnɪt/ *n* a salt formed by combination of arsenic acid with any base.

arsenic /ˈɑrsəˌnɪk/ *n* a soft grey metallic element, highly poisonous.

arsenical /ɑrˈsenɪkəl/ *adj* pertaining to or containing arsenic.

arsenious, arsenous /ɑrˈsiːniəs/ *adj* pertaining to or containing arsenic.

arsenite /ˈɑrsəˌnaɪt/ *n* a salt of arsenious acid.

arsis /ˈɑrsɪs/ *n* (*poet*) the part of a metrical foot where the accent is placed.

arson /'ɑrsən/ *n* the crime of using fire to destroy property deliberately.—**arsonist** *n*.

art[1] /ɑrt/ *n* human creativity; skill acquired by study and experience; any craft and its principles; the making of things that have form and beauty; any branch of this, as painting, sculpture, etc; drawings, paintings, statues, etc; (*pl*) the creative and nonscientific branches of knowledge, *esp* as studied academically.

art[2] (*arch*) the second person singular indicative mood and present tense of the verb to be.

art deco /-'dɛko/ *n* a style of design and architecture popular in the 1920s and 1930s and characterized by bold geometrical lines.

artefact /'ɑrtə,fækt/ *see* **artifact**.

artel /ɑr'tɛl/ *n* a workers' guild in the former USSR.

artemisia /ɑrtə'miːʒə/ or /-'miːʃə/, *n* a large genus of plants to which the common wormwood belongs, yielding a volatile oil (the chief ingredient of absinthe).

arterial /ɑr'tiːriəl/ *adj* pertaining to an artery or the arteries; contained in an artery; (*blood*) oxygenated, of a lighter red colour than venous blood; (*road*) major, with many branches.

arterialize /-,aiz/ *vt* to convert as venous blood into arterial blood by exposure to oxygen in the lungs.—**arterialization** *n*.

arteriosclerosis /ɑr,tiːriːo:sklə'ro:səs/ *n* (*med*) hardening of the walls of the arteries due to the action of fatty deposits, which impairs blood circulation.—**arteriosclerotic** *adj*.

artery /'ɑrtəri/ *n* (*pl* **arteries**) a tubular vessel that conveys blood from the heart; any main channel of transport or communication.

artesian well /ɑr'tiʒən/ *n* a well in which water rises to the surface by internal pressure.

artful /'ɑrtfʊl/ *adj* skilful at attaining one's ends; clever, crafty.—**artfully** *adv*.—**artfulness** *n*.

arthritis /ɑr'θraitis/ *n* painful inflammation of a joint.—**arthritic** *adj*.

arthropod /'ɑrθrə,pɒd/ *n* a member of the largest group of invertebrate animals with jointed legs, such as the butterfly, spider, crab, centipede.

artichoke /'ɑrti,tʃo:k/ *n* a thistle-like plant with a scaly flower head, parts of which are eaten as a vegetable.

article /'ɑrtəkəl/ *n* a separate item or clause in a written document; an individual item on a particular subject in a newspaper, magazine, etc; a particular or separate item; (*gram*) a word placed before a noun to identify it as definite or indefinite. • *vt* ✦ (*Cdn*) serve a period of apprenticeship as a law student.

articled /-d/ *adj* apprenticed to, as an articled clerk to a solicitor.

articular /ɑr'tikjuːlər/ or /-jə-/ *adj* of a joint or structural components in a joint.

articulate /ɑr'tikjuːlət/ *adj* capable of distinct, intelligible speech, or expressing one's thoughts clearly; jointed. • *vti* to speak or express clearly; to unite or become united (as) by a joint.—**articulatedly** *adv*.—**articulateness** *n*.

articulated lorry, articulated truck *n* a large vehicle composed of a tractor and one or more trailers connected by flexible joints for greater manoeuvrability.—*also* **trailer truck**.

articulation /ɑr,tikjuː'leiʃən/ *n* the act of jointing; the act of speaking distinctly; a distinct utterance; the state of being articulated; a joint or juncture between bones; the point of separation of organs or parts of a plant; a node or joint of the stem, or the space between two nodes.—**articulatory** *adj*.

articulator /ɑr'tikjuː,leitər/ or /-jə-/ *n* one who pronounces distinctly; any organ of the mouth, etc, that moves to produce speech sounds.

artifact /'ɑrtə,fækt/ *n* a product of human craftsmanship, *esp* a simple tool or ornament.—*also* **artefact**.

artifice /'ɑrtə,fis/ *n* a clever contrivance or stratagem; a trick, trickery.

artificer /ɑr'tifəsər/ or /'ɑrtəfə-/ *n* a skilled or artistic worker; a maker or constructor; an inventor.

artificial /,ɑrtə'fiʃəl/ *adj* lacking natural qualities; man-made.—**artificiality** *n*.—**artificially** *adv*.

artificial insemination *n* injection of semen into the womb by artificial means so that conception takes place without sexual intercourse.

artificial intelligence *n* (*comput*) the ability to imitate intelligent human behaviour.

artificial respiration *n* the forcing of air into and out of the lungs of somebody whose breathing has stopped.

artillery /ɑr'tiləri/ *n* (*pl* **artilleries**) large, heavy guns; the branch of the army that uses these.

artisan /'ɑrti,zæn/ or /-,sæn/ *n* a skilled workman.

artist /'ɑrtist/ *n* one who practises fine art, *esp* painting; one who does anything very well.—**artistic** *adj*.

artiste /ɑr'tiːst/ *n* a professional, *usu* musical or theatrical, entertainer.

artistic /ɑr'tistik/ *adj* pertaining to art or to artists; characterized by aesthetic feeling or conformity to the principles of a school of art or design.—**artistically** *adv*.

artistry /'ɑrtistri/ *n* artistic quality, ability, work, etc.

artless /'ɑrtləs/ *adj* simple, natural; without art or skill.—**artlessly** *adv*.—**artlessness** *n*.

art nouveau /,ɑrt'nuːvo:/ or /,ɑr-/ *n* a style of art and decoration that developed in the late 19th century, characterized by flowing curves and designs in imitation of nature.

arty /'ɑrti/ *adj* (**artier, artiest**) (*inf*) having a pretentious or affected interest in art.

arty-crafty, artsy-craftsy *adj* (*inf*) relating to arts and crafts, *esp* when affecting a simple, traditional style.

arum /'ɛrəm/ *n* a genus of plants with small flowers within a hood-shaped leaf.

arundinaceous /ə,rɛndi'neiʃəs/ *adj* pertaining to or resembling a reed or cane.

-ary /'ɛri/ or /əri/ *adj suffix, n suffix* connected with, as *dictionary*.

Aryan /'ɛriən/ *n* a member of the Indo-European race; according to Nazi belief, a Caucasian, *esp* of the Nordic type, with no Jewish blood. • *adj* pertaining to the Aryans, or to their language.

As (*chem symbol*) arsenic.

as[1] /æz/ *adv* equally; for instance; when related in a certain way. • *conj* in the same way that; while; when; because. • *prep* in the role or function of.

as[2] /æs/ *n* (*pl* **asses**) a Roman weight equivalent to the libra or pound; a Roman copper coin.

ASA /'ei'es'ei/ *abbr* = ✦ (*Cdn*) Acetylsalicylic acid; (*Brit*) Amateur Swimming Association; (*US*) American Standards Association.

asafoetida, asafetida /,æsə'fetədə/ or /-'fiːtədə/ *n* a foul-smelling gum resin obtained from the roots of several large umbelliferous plants and used in medicine.

ASAP, a.s.a.p. /'ei'sæp/ or /'æsæp/ *abbr* = as soon as possible.

asbestos, asbestus /æs'bestəs/ or /æz-/ *n* a fine fibrous mineral used for making incombustible and chemical-resistant materials.

asbestosis /,æsbes'to:sis/ or /,æz-/ *n* (*med*) a disease of the lungs caused by the inhalation of asbestos fibres.

ascend /ə'send/ *vti* to go up; to succeed to (a throne).

ascendancy, ascendency /ə'sendənsi/ *n* governing or dominating influence; power; sway.

ascendant, ascendent /-dənt/ *adj* rising upwards; dominant.

ascender /ə'sendər/ *n* one who ascends; the top part of letters such as b, d, h.

ascension /ə'senʃən/ *n* the act of ascending or rising.—**ascensional** *adj*.

Ascension *n* the ascent of Christ into heaven after the Resurrection.

Ascension Day *n* a movable feast commemorating the Ascension, celebrated on the Thursday next but one before Whit Sunday.—*also* **Holy Thursday**.

ascent /ə'sent/ *n* an ascending; an upward slope; the means of, the way of ascending.

ascertain /,æsər'tein/ *vt* to acquire definite knowledge of, to discover positively.—**ascertainable** *adj*.

ascetic /ə'setik/ *adj* self-denying, austere. • *n* a person who practises rigorous self-denial as a religious discipline; any severely abstemious person.—**ascetically** *adv*.—**asceticism** *n*.

ascidian /ə'sidiən/ *n* a type of mollusc with a leathery tunic resembling a double-necked bottle, a sea squirt.—*also adj*.

ascidium /-əm/ *n* (*pl* **ascidia**) (*bot*) a pitcher-shaped or flask-shaped organ peculiar to certain plants, as the pitcher plants.

ASCII /'æski/ *acronym* (*comput*) = *American Standard Code for Information Interchange*, a standard code of 128 alphanumeric characters for storing and exchanging information.

ascomycete /,æsko'mai,sit/ or /-,mai'siːt/ *n* one of a family of the fungi, including most of the lichens, which form free spores within elongated spore cases.—**ascomyetous** *adj*.

ascorbic acid /ə'skɔrbik/ *n* vitamin C, found *esp* in citrus fruit and fresh green vegetables.

ascribe /ə'skraib/ *vt* to attribute, impute or refer; to assign.—**ascribable** *adj*.—**ascription, adscription** *n*.

ascus /ˈæskəs/ n (pl **asci**) the spore case of lichens and fungi.

asdic /ˈæzdɪk/ n an apparatus for locating submarines; an echo sounder; sonar.

asepsis /eɪˈsepsɪs/ or /ə-/ n an absence of disease or putrefaction; a surgical method aiming at this —**aseptic** adj.

asexual /eɪˈsekʃuːəl/ adj lacking sex or sexual organs; (*reproduction*) produced without the union of male and female germ cells.—**asexuality** n.—**asexually** adv.

ash[1] /æʃ/ n a tree with silver-grey bark; the wood of this tree.

ash[2] n powdery residue of anything burnt; fine, volcanic lava.

ashamed /əˈʃeɪmd/ adj feeling shame or guilt.—**ashamedly** adv.

ash can /ˈæʃˌkæn/ n a container for household refuse, a garbage can.

ashen /ˈæʃən/ adj like ashes, esp in colour; pale.

Ashkenazi /ˌæʃkəˈnɒzi/ n (pl **Ashkenazim**) a Jew from Germany or eastern Europe.

ashlar, ashler /ˈæʃlər/ n a squared stone used in building; masonry of this; thin slabs of building stone squared for facing walls.

ashlaring /-ɪŋ/ n a wall faced with ashlar; a low wall of a garret, built close to where the rafters reach the floor

ashore /əˈʃɔːr/ adv to or on the shore; to or on land.—*also* adj.

ashram /ˈæʃrəm/ n a Hindu religious retreat.

ashtray /ˈæʃtreɪ/ n a small receptacle for tobacco ash and cigarette stubs.

Ash Wednesday n the first day of Lent; a special day set apart for fasting.

ashy /ˈæʃi/ adj (**ashier, ashiest**) of ashes; ash-coloured, pale.

Asian /ˈeɪʒən/ adj of or relating to the continent of Asia, its inhabitants or languages.—*also* n.

Asiatic cholera n a virulent form of cholera.

aside /əˈsaɪd/ adv on or to the side; in reserve; away from; notwithstanding. • n words uttered and intended as inaudible, esp as spoken by an actor to the audience and supposedly unheard by the other actors on the stage.

asinine /ˈæsəˌnaɪn/ adj silly, stupid.—**asininity** n.

ask /æsk/ or /ɒsk/ vt to put a question to, inquire of; to make a request of or for; to invite; to demand, expect. • vi to inquire about.—**asker** n.

askance, askant /əˈskæns/ or /əˈskænt/ adv with a sideways glance; with distrust.

askew /əˈskjuː/ adv to one side; awry.—*also* adj.

aslant /əˈslænt/ adv not at right angles; obliquely. • prep slantingly across, athwart.

asleep /əˈsliːp/ adj sleeping; inactive; numb. • adv into a sleeping condition.

asocial /eɪˈsoʊʃəl/ adj not capable of or avoiding social contact; antisocial.

asp /æsp/ n a small poisonous snake.

asparagus /əˈspærəgəs/ or /-ˈspær-/ n a plant cultivated for its edible young shoots.

aspartame /ˈæspərˌteɪm/ n an artificial sweetener derived from an amino acid.

aspect /ˈæsˌpekt/ n the look of a person or thing to the eye; a particular feature of a problem, situation, etc; the direction something faces; view; (*astrol*) the position of the planets with respect to one another, regarded as having an influence on human affairs.

aspen /ˈæspən/ n a species of poplar with leaves that have tremble in the slightest breeze. • n (*arch*) quivering.

aspergillus /ˌæspərˈdʒɪləs/ n (pl **aspergilli**) a genus of microscopic fungi, to which several of the moulds belong.

asperity /əˈsperəti/ n (pl **asperities**) hardship, severity; sharpness of temper.

asperse /əˈspɜːrs/ vt to slander; (*rare*) to besprinkle, to bespatter.—**asperser** n.—**aspersive** adj.

aspersions /əˈspɜːrʒənz/ or /-ʃənz/ n pl slander; an attack on a person's reputation.

aspersorium /ˌæspərˈsɔːriəm/ n (pl **aspersoria, aspersoriums**) a vessel containing holy water for sprinkling; a brush or metallic instrument used for sprinkling the water.

asphalt /ˈæsˌfɒlt/ or /ˈæʃ-/ n a hard, black bituminous substance, used for paving roads, etc. • vt to surface with asphalt.—**asphaltic** adj.

asphodel /ˈæsfəˌdel/ n one of several plants of the lily family; (*poet*) the daffodil; (*poet*) an immortal, unfading flower that bloomed in the meadows of Elysium (possibly the narcissus).

asphyxia /æsˈfɪksiə/ n unconsciousness due to lack of oxygen or excess of carbon dioxide in the blood.

asphyxiate /-siˌeɪt/ vt to suffocate.—**asphyxiation** n.—**asphyxiator** n.

aspic /ˈæsˌpɪk/ n a savoury jelly used to coat fish, game, etc.

aspidistra /ˌæspɪˈdɪstrə/ n an Asian plant with broad leaves, grown as a house plant

aspirant /ˈæspɪrənt/ or /əˈspaɪrənt/ n someone who aspires to something.

aspirate[1] /ˈæspərət/ n the sound of h.

aspirate[2] /ˈæspəˌreɪt/ vt to pronounce with an h; to suck out using an aspirator.

aspiration /ˌæspɪˈreɪʃən/ n strong desire; ambition; the act of aspirating; the act of breathing; the withdrawal of air or fluid from a body cavity—**aspiratory** adj.

aspirator /ˈæspɪˌreɪtər/ n a device used to suck (air, fluid, etc) from a (body) cavity.

aspire /əˈspaɪr/ vi to des re eagerly; to aim at high things.—**aspirer** n.—**aspiring** adj.

aspirin /ˈæspɪˌrɪn/ or /-ˌrɪn/ n (pl **aspirin, aspirins**) acetylsalicylic acid, a pain-relieving drug.

asquint /əˈskwɪnt/ adv, adj with a squint, to or out of the corner of the eye; obliquely.

ass /æs/ n a donkey; a silly, stupid person; (sl) the arse, the buttocks.

assagai /ˈæsəˌgaɪ/ see **assegai**.

assai /æˈsaɪ/ adv (mus) very, more, extremely.

assail /əˈseɪl/ vt to attack violently either physically or verbally. —**assailable** adj.—**assailer** n.—**assailment** n.

assailant /-ənt/ n an attacker.

assassin /əˈsæsɪn/ n a murderer, esp one hired to kill a leading political figure, etc.

assassinate /-ˌeɪt/ vt to kill a political figure, etc; to harm (a person's reputation, etc).—**assassination** n.

assault /əˈsɒlt/ n a violent attack; (*law*) an unlawful threat or attempt to harm another physically. • vti to make an assault (on); to rape.—**assaulter** n.

assault course n an obstacle course used for military training.

assay /əˈseɪ/ or /ˈæseɪ/ n, vb the analysis of the quantity of metal in an ore or alloy, esp the standard purity of gold or silver; a test. • vt (**assaying, assayed**) to subject to analysis; to determine the quantity or proportion of one or more of the constituents of a metal.—**assayable** adj.—**assayer** n.

assegai, assagai /ˈæsəˌgaɪ/ n (pl **assegais, assagais**) (*S Africa*) a light hardwood javelin or spear for casting or stabbing.

assemblage /əˈsemblɪdʒ/ n a gathering of persons or things; (*art*) a form of collage.

assemble /-bəl/ vti to bring together; to collect; to fit together the parts of; (*comput*) to translate using an assembler.

assembler /-blər/ n (*comput*) a program that converts low-level mnemonic symbols into machine code.

assembly /-bli/ n (pl **assemblies**) assembling or being assembled; a gathering of persons, esp for a particular purpose; the fitting together of parts to make a whole machine, etc.

assembly line n a series of machines, equipment and workers through which a product passes in successive stages to be assembled.

assemblyman /əˈsemblimən/ n (pl **assemblymen**) a member of a legislative assembly.—**assemblywoman** nf (pl **assemblywomen**)

assent /əˈsent/ vi to express agreement to something. • n consent or agreement.—**assentor, assenter** n.

assentation /ˌæsenˈteɪʃən/ n compliance with the opinion of another, in flattery or obsequiousness.

assert /əˈsɜːrt/ vt to declare, affirm as true; to maintain or enforce (eg rights).—**assertible** adj.

assertion /əˈsɜːrʃən/ n an asserting; a statement that something is a fact, usu without evidence.

assertive /əˈsɜːrtɪv/ adj self-assured, positive, confident; dogmatic.—**assertively** adv.—**assertiveness** n.

assess /əˈses/ vt to establish the amount of, as a tax; to impose a tax or fine; to value, for the purpose of taxation; to estimate the worth, importance, etc of.—**assessable** adj.

assessment /-mən-/ n the act of assessing or determining an amount to be paid; an official valuation of property, or income, for the purpose of taxation; the specific sum levied as tax, or assessed for damages.

assessor /-ər/ *n* a person appointed to assess property or persons for taxation; an expert appointed to assist a judge or magistrate as an adviser on special points of law.—**assessorial** *adj.*

asset /'æset/ *n* anything owned that has value; a desirable thing; (*pl*) all the property, accounts receivable, etc of a person or business; (*pl*) (*law*) property usable to pay debts.

asset-stripping *n* the practice of buying a company in order to sell off its assets at a profit.—**asset-stripper** *n.*

asseverate /ə'sevə‚reɪt/ *vt* to declare solemnly; to affirm or aver positively.—**asseveration** *n.*

asshole /'æs‚hoːl/ *n* (*sl*) a stupid person; (*vulg*) the anus.

assibilate /ə'sɪbə‚leɪt/ *vt* (*phonetics*) to pronounce with a hissing sound; to alter to a sibilant.—**assibilation** *n.*

assiduity /‚æsɪ'dʒuːɪtɪ/ or /-'djuːɪtɪ/ *n* (*pl* **assiduities**) close application, steady attention; diligence; (*usu pl*) constant attentions.

assiduous /ə'sɪdʒʊəs/ or /-djʊəs/ *adj* persistent or persevering; diligent.—**assiduously** *adv.*—**assiduousness** *n.*

assign /ə'saɪn/ *vt* to allot; to appoint to a post or duty; to ascribe; (*law*) to transfer (a right, property, etc).—**assignable** *adj.* —**assigner** *n.*

assignat /'æsɪg‚næt/ *n* a money or currency bond secured on state lands, issued by the French Revolutionary Government (1789–96).

assignation /‚æsɪg'neɪʃən/ *n* the act of assigning; a meeting, *esp* one made secretly by lovers.

assignee /‚æsaɪ'niː/ *n* (*law*) one to whom an assignment of anything is made, either in trust or for his or her own use and enjoyment.

assignment /ə'saɪnmənt/ *n* the act of assigning; something assigned to a person, such as a share, task, etc.

assignor /-ər/ *n* (*law*) one who assigns or transfers an interest.

assimilate /ə'sɪmə‚leɪt/ *vt* to absorb; to digest; to take in and understand fully; to be ascribed; to be like.—**assimilable** *adj.* —**assimilation** *n.*

assimilative /ə'sɪmə‚leɪtɪv/, **assimilatory** /-‚tɔrɪ/ *adj* having the power of assimilating, or causing assimilation, tending to produce assimilation.

assist /ə'sɪst/ *vti* to support or aid.—**assister** *n.*

assistance /ə'sɪstəns/ *n* help; furtherance; aid; succour; support.

assistant /-tənt/ *n* one who or that which assists; a helper; an auxiliary; a subordinate. • *adj* helping; lending aid; auxiliary.

assize /ə'saɪz/ *n* (*pl* **assizes**) a court or session of justice for the trial by jury of civil or criminal cases; (*usu pl*) (*formerly*) the sessions held periodically in each county of England by judges of the Supreme Court; (*usu pl*) the time or place of holding the assize.

associable /ə'soːʃɪəbəl/ or /-ʃəbəl/ *adj* capable of being joined or associated; liable to be affected by sympathy with kindred parts or organs.

associate /ə'soːʃi‚eɪt/ or /-si-/ *vt* ; /ə'soːʃət/ or /-'siət/ *n, adj* to join as a friend, business partner or supporter; to bring together; to unite; to connect in the mind. • *vi* to combine or unite with others; to come together as friends, business partners or supporters. • *adj* allied or connected; having secondary status or privileges. • *n* a companion, business partner, supporter, etc; something closely connected with another; a person admitted to an association as a subordinate member.

association /ə'soːsi'eɪʃən/ *n* an organization of people joined together for a common aim; the act of associating or being associated; a connection in the mind, memory, etc.

association football *n* football played with a round ball that is not handled, soccer.

associationism *n* (*psychol*) the mental connection existing between an object and the ideas related to it.

associative /ə'soːʃi‚eɪtɪv/ *adj* tending to or characterized by association; (*math*) having elements whose result is the same despite the grouping.

assonance /'æsənəns/ *n* a correspondence in sound between words or syllables.—**assonant** *adj, n.*—**assonantal** *adj.*

assort /ə'sɔrt/ *vt* to arrange in groups according to kind. • *vi* to agree in kind.—**assortative, assortive** *adj.*—**assorter** *n.*

assorted /-ɪd/ *adj* distributed according to sorts; miscellaneous.

assortment /-mənt/ *n* a collection of people or things of different sorts.

asst *abbr* = assistant.

assuage /ə'sweɪdʒ/ *vt* to soften the intensity of; to soothe.—**assuager** *n.*—**assuagement** *n.*—**assuasive** *adj.*

assume /ə'suːm/ or /-'sjuːm/ *vt* to take on, to undertake; to usurp; to take as certain or true; to pretend to possess.—**assumable** *adj.*—**assumer** *n.*

assuming /ə'suːmɪŋ/ or /-juː-/ *adj* presumptuous.

assumption /ə'sʌmpʃən/ *n* something taken for granted; the taking on of a position, *esp* of power; (*with cap*) the ascent of the Virgin Mary into heaven; (*RC Church*) the Christian feast in remembrance of this, celebrated 15 August.—**assumptive** *adj.*

assurance /ə'ʃʊrəns/ *n* a promise, guarantee; a form of life insurance; a feeling of certainty, self-confidence.

assure /ə'ʃʊr/ or /ə‚ʃər/ *vt* to make safe or certain; to give confidence to; to state positively; to guarantee, ensure.—**assurable** *adj.*—**assurer** *n.*

assured /ə'ʃʊrd/ or /ə‚ʃərd/ *adj* certain; convinced; self-confident.—**assuredness** *n.*

assuredly /ə'ʃʊrədlɪ/ or /ə‚ʃərədlɪ/ *adv* certainly.

assurgent /ə'sərdʒənt/ *adj* ascending, rising; (*bot*) rising in a curve.

Assyrian /ə'sɪrɪən/ *adj* pertaining to Assyria, an ancient kingdom of Mesopotamia, or to its inhabitants or language. • *n* the language spoken in Assyria; an inhabitant of Assyria.

Assyriology /ə'sɪrɪˌɒlədʒɪ/ *n* the science or study of the extinct language and the antiquities of Assyria.—**Assyriologist** *n.*

astatic /eɪ'stætɪk/ or /ə-/ *adj* having a tendency not to stand still; unstable.—**astatically** *adv.*—**astaticism** *n.*

astatine /'æstə‚tiːn/ *n* a radioactive element.

aster /'æstər/ *n* a kind of plant with round composite flowers; a Michaelmas daisy.

-aster /'æstər/ *n suffix* petty imitation, as in *poetaster.*

asteriated /æs'tɪrɪ‚eɪtɪd/ *adj* (*crystal, etc*) radiated; having the form of a star.

asterisk /'æstərɪsk/ *n* a sign (*) used in writing or printing to mark omission of words, a footnote or other reference, etc. • *vt* to mark with an asterisk.

asterism /'æstə‚rɪzəm/ *n* a group or cluster of stars; three asterisks placed in the form of a triangle (***) or (***) to direct attention to a particular passage; the star-like appearance in certain crystals.

astern /ə'stərn/ *adv* behind a ship or aircraft; at or towards the rear of a ship, etc; backward.

asternal /eɪ'stərnəl/ *adj* (*anat*) (*ribs*) not joined to the sternum or breastbone.

asteroid /'æstərɔɪd/ *n* any of the small planets between Mars and Jupiter. • *adj* star-like; star-shaped.—*also* **asteroidal.**

asthenia /æs'θiːnɪə/ *n* debility, weakness.—**asthenic** *adj.*

asthma /'æzmə/ *n* a chronic respiratory condition causing difficulty with breathing.—**asthmatic** *adj.*—**asthmatically** *adv.*

asthmatic /æz'mætɪk/ *adj* of or suffering from or good for asthma. • *n* an asthmatic person.—**asthmatically** *adv.*

astigmatism /ə'stɪgmə‚tɪzəm/ *n* a defective condition of the eye or lens causing poor focusing.—**astigmatic** *adj.*—**astigmatically** *adv.*

astir /ə'stər/ *adv* moving or bustling about; out of bed.

astomatous /eɪ'stɒmətəs/ *adj* (*biol*) lacking a mouth; without breathing pores.

astonish /ə'stɒnɪʃ/ *vt* to fill with sudden or great surprise.—**astonishing** *adj.*—**astonishment** *n.*

astound /ə'staʊnd/ *vt* to astonish greatly.—**astounding** *adj.* —**astoundingly** *adv.*

astraddle /ə'strædəl/ *adv* astride, straddling.

astragal /'æstrəgəl/ *n* (*archit*) a small moulding or bead of semicircular form; a ring of moulding round the top or bottom of a column.

astragalus /ə'strægələs/ *n* (*pl* **astragali**) the ball of the ankle joint; the lower bone into which the tibia articulates.

Astrakhan /'æstrə‚kæn/ *n* the dark curly fleece of lambs from Astrakhan in Russia; a cloth with a curled pile made from or imitating this.

astral /'æstrəl/ *adj* of or from the stars.

astray /ə'streɪ/ *adv* off the right path; into error.

astride /ə'straɪd/ *adv* with a leg on either side. • *prep* extending across.

astringent /ə'strɪndʒənt/ *adj* that contracts body tissues; stopping blood flow, styptic; harsh; biting. • *n* an astringent substance.—**astringency** *n.*

astro- /'æstro‚/ *prefix* (*astrophysics*) of a star or stars.

astrodome /'æstrə‚doːm/ *n* a large sports stadium covered with a domed translucent roof.

astrolabe /ˈæstrəˌleɪb/ or /-trə-/ *n* an instrument formerly used for taking altitudes of the sun and stars.

astrology /əˈstrɒlədʒi/ *n* the study of planetary positions and motions to determine their supposed influence on human affairs.—**astrologer, astrologist** *n*.—**astrological** *adj*.—**astrologically** *adv*.

astrometry /əˈstrɒmətri/ *n* the art by which the apparent relative magnitude of the stars is determined.—**astrometric, astrometrical** *adj*.

astronaut /ˈæstrəˌnɒt/ *n* one trained to make flights in outer space.

astronautics /ˌæstrəˈnɒtiks/ *npl* (*used as sing*) the scientific study of space flight and technology.

astronomical, astronomic /ˌæstrəˈnɒmɪkəl/ *adj* enormously large; of or relating to astronomy—**astronomically** *adv*.

astronomical clock *n* a clock that keeps sidereal time.

astronomical year *n* a year the length of which is determined by astronomical observations.

astronomy /əˈstrɒnəmi/ *n* the scientific investigation of the stars and other planets.—**astronomer** *n*.

astrophotography /ˌæstrəʊfəˈtɒɡrəfi/ *n* photography of the heavenly bodies.—**astrophotographic** *adj*.

astrophysics /ˌæstrəʊˈfɪzɪks/ *n* (*used as sing*) the branch of astronomy that deals with the physical and chemical constitution of the stars.—**astrophysical** *adj*.—**astrophysicist** *n*.

astute /əˈstjuːt/ or /-ˈstjuːt-/ *adj* clever, perceptive; crafty, shrewd.—**astutely** *adv*.—**astuteness** *n*.

asunder /əˈsʌndər/ *adv* apart in direction or position; into pieces.

asylum /əˈsaɪləm/ *n* a place of safety, a refuge; (*formerly*) an institution for the blind, the mentally ill, etc.

asymmetric /ˌeɪsəˈmetrɪk/, **asymmetrical** /ˌeɪsəˈmetrɪkəl/ *adj* lacking symmetry.—**asymmetrically** *adv*.

asymmetry /eɪˈsɪmətri/ or /æˈsɪm-/ *n* a lack of symmetry or proportion between the parts of a thing.

asymptote /ˈæsɪmpˌtoʊt/ or /ˈæsɪmˌtoʊt/ *n* (*geom*) the line that continually approaches nearer to a given curve without ever meeting it.—**asymptotic, asymptotical** *adj*.

asyndeton /əˈsɪndətən/ *n* (*pl* **asyndetons, asyndeta**) (*gram*) a figure of speech in which conjunctions are omitted, as "I came, I saw, I conquered"; such a figure.

At (*chem symbol*) astatine.

at- /æt/ *prefix* the form of *ad-* before *t*.

at /æt/ *prep* on; in; near; by; used to indicate location or position.

at. no. *abbr* = atomic number.

ataraxia /ˌætəˈræksiə/, **ataraxy** /ˈætəˌræksi/ *n* impassivity; peace of mind.

atavism /ˈætəˌvɪzəm/ *n* the appearance in plants or animals of characteristics typical in more remote ancestors; reversion to a more primitive type.—**atavistic** *adj*.—**atavistically** *adv*.

ataxia /əˈtæksiə/ *n* irregularities in the functions of the body, *esp* muscular coordination, or in the course of a disease.—**ataxic, atactic** *adj*.

ate /ɒɪt/ *see* eat.

-ate /eɪt/ or /ət/ *adj suffix* having or furnished with, as *foliate*. • *n* *suffix* forming the equivalent of *pp*, as in *associate*.

atelier /ætəlˈjeɪ/ *n* a workshop; the studio of a painter or sculptor.

a tempo, a tempo primo /æˈtempoʊ/ *n* (*mus*) a direction to a musician to restore the original time after acceleration or retardation.

a tempo giusto *n* (*mus*) a direction to a performer to sing or play in strict time.

Athanasian Creed /ˌæθəˈneɪʃən/ *n* one of the three creeds thus named as containing an exposition of the doctrines of the Trinty and incarnation of Christ, which Athanasius, bishop of Alexandria (c.296–373), defended.

Athapaskan /ˌæθəˈpæskən/ *n* ♣ a large group of First Nations languages in northwest Canada: a member of a First Nations people who speaks one of these languages. • *adj* of or pertaining to these peoples or their languages. — *also* **Athabaskan**.

atheism /ˈeɪθiˌɪzəm/ *n* belief in the nonexistence of God.—**atheist** *n*.—**atheistic, atheistical** *adj*.

atheling /ˈæθəlɪŋ/ *n* an Anglo-Saxon title of honour conferred on royal children and young nobles.

athenaeum, atheneum /ˌæθəˈniːəm/ or /-ˈneɪəm/ *n* a public institution, club or building devoted to the purposes or study of literature, science and art; a literary club; (*with cap*) the temple of Athena in ancient Athens, where scholars met.

Athenian /əˈθiːniən/ *adj* pertaining to Athens, the capital of Greece. • *n* a native or citizen of Athens.

athermanous /eɪˈθɜːrmənəs/ *adj* resisting the passage of heat; nonconducting.—**athermany** *n*.

atherosclerosis /ˌæθəroʊskləˈroʊsɪs/ *n* (*pl* **atheroscleroses**) a degenerative disease of the arteries characterized by deposition of fatty material on the inner arterial walls.—**atherosclerotic** *adj*.

athirst /əˈθɜːrst/ *adj* thirsty; eager (for).

athlete /ˈæθliːt/ *n* a person trained in games or exercises requiring skill, speed, strength, stamina, etc.

athlete's foot *n* a fungal infection of the feet.

athletic /æθˈletɪk/ *adj* of athletes or athletics; active, vigorous.—**athletically** *adv*.—**athleticism** *n*.

athletics /æθˈletɪks/ *n* (*used as sing or pl*) running, jumping, throwing sports, games, etc.

athwart /əˈθwɔːrt/ *prep* across, from side to side. • *adv* crosswise; obliquely; across the course or direction of a ship; adversely (to).

atigi /ˈætəɡi/ or /əˈtiːɡi/ *n* ♣ a type of Inuit parka.

atilt /əˈtɪlt/ *adv* in the position or with the action of a person making a thrust; tilted.

-ation /ˈeɪʃən/ *n suffix* denoting action or its result, as in *flirtation, vacation*.

atlantes /ətˈlæntiːz/ *see* **atlas²**.

Atlantic /ətˈlæntɪk/ *adj* of, near or relating to the Atlantic Ocean.

Atlantic Canadian *n* ♣ a person who lives in or is from New Brunswick, Nova Scotia, Prince Edward Island, or Newfoundland. • *adj* of or pertaining to such a person.

Atlantic salmon *n* ♣ a salmon of the coastal North Atlantic Ocean and its tributaries.

atlas¹ /ˈætləs/ *n* a book containing maps, charts and tables.

atlas² *n* (*pl* **atlantes**) (*a-chit*) a figure or half-figure of a man, used in place of a column or pilaster to support an entablature.—*also* **telamon**.

ATM /ˌeɪtiːˈem/ *abbr* = automated teller machine.

atmo- /ætmoʊ/ or /ætmə/ *prefix* vapour, air, atmosphere.

atmometer /ætˈmɒmətər/ *n* an instrument for measuring the rate and amount of evaporation from a moist surface.—**atmometry** *n*.

atmosphere /ˈætməsˌfɪr/ *n* the gaseous mixture that surrounds the earth or the other stars and planets; a unit of pressure equal to the pressure of the atmosphere at sea level; any dominant or surrounding influence; special mood or aura.—**atmospheric, atmospherical** *adj*.

atmospherics /ˌætməsˈfɪrɪks/ or /ˈfɛrɪks/ *n pl* interference in radio reception, etc caused by atmospheric disturbances.

atoll /ˈætɒl/ *n* a coral reef enclosing a central lagoon.

atom /ˈætəm/ *n* the smallest particle of a chemical element; a tiny particle, bit.

atomic /əˈtɒmɪk/ *adj* pertaining to or consisting of atoms; extremely minute.—**atomically** *adv*.

atomic bomb *n* a bomb whose explosive power derives from the atomic energy released during nuclear fission or fusion.—*also* **A-bomb**.

atomic energy *n* the energy derived from nuclear fission.

atomicity /ˌætəˈmɪsɪti/ *n* the number of atoms in a molecule of an element; equivalence; the combining capacity of an element, valency.

atomic theory *n* the theory that elemental bodies consist of ultimate atoms of definite weight, and that atoms of different elements unite chemically with each other in fixed proportions.

atomic weight *n* the weight of the atom of any element as compared with another taken as a standard, *usu* hydrogen, taken as 1.

atomism /ˈætəˌmɪzəm/ *n* the doctrine of atoms, atomic theory.—**atomist** *n*.—**atomistic, atomistical** *adj*.

atomize /ˌætəˈmaɪz/ *vt* to reduce to a fine spray or minute particles.—**atomization** *n*.

atomizer /ˈætəˌmaɪ zər/ *n* a device for atomizing liquids, *usu* perfumes or cleaning agents.

atonal /eɪˈtoʊnəl/ *adj* (*mus*) avoiding traditional tonality; not written in any established key.—**atonality** *n*.—**atonally** *adv*.

atone /əˈtoʊn/ *vi* to give satisfaction or make amends (for).—**atonable, atoneable** *adj*.—**atoner** *n*.

atonement /əˈtoʊnmənt/ *n* satisfaction, reparation; (*Christianity*: *with cap*) the reconciliation of humankind with God through Christ's self-sacrifice.

atonic /əˈtɒnɪk/ *adj* (*word, etc*) unaccented; lacking tone, or vital energy. • *n* an unaccented word or syllable; a medicine to allay excitement.—**atonicity** *n*.

atony /'ætəni/ *n* lack of tone; debility; weakness of any organ.

atop /ə'tɒp/ *adv* on or at the top.

atrip /ə'trɪp/ *adv* (*naut*) (*anchor*) just clear of the ground.

atrium /'eɪtrɪəm/ *n* (*pl* **atria** /'eɪtrɪə/, **atriums** /'eɪtrɪəms/) an auricle of the heart; the unroofed courtyard of a Roman house; an entrance hall that rises up several storeys, often with a glass roof.

atrocious /ə'trəʊʃəs/ *adj* extremely brutal or wicked; (*inf*) very bad, of poor quality.—**atrociously** *adv*.

atrocity /ə'trɒsɪti/ *n* (*pl* **atrocities**) a cruel act; something ruthless, wicked, repellent.

atrophy /'ætrəfi/ *n* (*pl* **atrophies**) a wasting away or failure to grow of a bodily organ. • *vti* (**atrophying, atrophied**) to cause or undergo atrophy.

atropine, atropin /'ætrə,piːn/ or /'ætrə,pɪn/ *n* a crystalline alkaloid of a very poisonous nature extracted from the deadly nightshade (belladonna), having the singular property of producing dilatation of the pupil of the eye.

attacca /ə'tækə/ *n* (*mus*) a direction to a performer at the end of a movement to follow on with the next without pause.

attach /ə'tætʃ/ *vt* to fix or fasten to something; to appoint to a specific group; to ascribe, attribute. • *vi* to become attached; to adhere.—**attachable** *adj*.—**attacher** *n*.

attaché /ætæ'ʃeɪ/ or /,ætə'ʃeɪ/ *n* a technical expert on a diplomatic staff.

attaché case *n* a flat case for carrying documents, etc.

attached /ə'tætʃt/ *adj* fixed; feeling affection for.

attachment /ə'tætʃmənt/ *n* a fastening; affection, devotion; something attached; a device or part fixed to a machine, implement, etc; the act of attaching or being attached.

attack /ə'tæk/ *vt* to set upon violently; to assault in speech or writing; to invade, as of a disease. • *vi* to make an assault. • *n* an assault; a fit of illness; severe criticism; an enthusiastic beginning of a performance, task, undertaking, etc.—**attacker** *n*.

attain /ə'teɪn/ *vt* to succeed in getting or arriving at; to achieve. • *vi* to come to or arrive at by growth or effort.—**attainable** *adj*.—**attainability** *n*.

attainder /ə'teɪndər/ *n* loss of estate and civil rights following conviction for high treason.

attainment /ə'teɪnmənt/ *n* something attained; an accomplishment.

attaint /ə'teɪnt/ *vt* to subject to attainder; to infect; to stain, to disgrace.

attar /'ætər/ *n* a fragrant essential oil extracted from rose petals and used in making perfume.

attempt /ə'tempt/ *vt* to try to accomplish, get, etc. • *n* an endeavour or effort to accomplish; an attack, assault.—**attemptable** *adj*.—**attempter** *n*.

attend /ə'tend/ *vt* to take care of; to go with, accompany; to be present at. • *vi* to apply oneself (to); to deal with, give attention to.—**attender** *n*.

attendance /ə'tendəns/ *n* attending; the number of people present; the number of times a person attends.

attendant /ə'tendənt/ *n* a person who serves or accompanies another; someone employed to assist or guide. • *adj* accompanying, following as a result; being in attendance.

attention /ə'tenʃən/ *n* the application of the mind to a particular purpose, aim, etc; awareness, notice; care, consideration; (*usu. pl*) an act of civility or courtesy; (*usu. pl*) indications of admiration or love; (*mil*) a soldier's formal erect posture.

attentive /ə'tentɪv/ *adj* observant, diligent; courteous.—**attentively** *adv*.—**attentiveness** *n*.

attenuate /ətenju,eɪt/ *vt* to make thin; to weaken; to reduce the force or severity of. • *vi* to become thin; to weaken.—**attenuation** *n*.

attest /ə'test/ *vt* to state as true; to certify, as by oath; to give proof of. • *vi* to testify, bear witness (to).—**attestable** *adj*.—**attestation** *n*.—**attester, attestor** *n*.

attestation /,æte'steɪʃən/ *n* the act of attesting; testimony or evidence given on oath or by official declaration; swearing in.

attic /'ætɪk/ *n* the room or space just under the roof; a garret.

Attic *adj* pertaining to Attica in Greece; classical; elegant. • *n* a dialect of ancient Athens.

Attic order *n* a square column of any of the five Greek orders of architecture.

atticism /'ætə,sɪzəm/ *n* an elegant expression; (*with cap*) a peculiarity of style or idiom characterizing the Attic rendering of the Greek language.

Attic salt, Attic wit *n* delicate wit.

attire /ə'taɪr/ *vt* to clothe; to dress up. • *n* dress, clothing.

attitude /'ætɪ,tuːd/ or /'ætɪ,tjuːd/ *n* posture, position of the body; a manner of thought or feeling; behaviour; the position of an aircraft or spacecraft in relation to certain reference points.—**attitudinal** *adj*.

attitudinize /,ætɪ'tuːdɪ,naɪz/ or /,ætɪ'tjuː-/ *vi* to assume affected postures, to pose for effect.—**attitudinizer** *n*.

attorn /ə'tərn/ *vti* to transfer; to make legal acknowledgment of a new landlord.—**attornment** *n*.

attorney /ə'tərni/ *n* (*pl* **attorneys**) one legally authorized to act for another; a lawyer.

attorney general *n* (*pl* **attorneys general, attorneys generals**) the chief law officer of of a state or nation acting as its legal representative and advising the chief executive on legal matters.

attract /ə'trækt/ *vt* to pull towards oneself; to get the admiration, attention, etc of. • *vi* to be attractive.—**attractable** *adj*.—**attractor** *n*.

attraction /ə'trækʃən/ *n* the act of attraction; the power of attracting, *esp* charm; (*physics*) the mutual action by which bodies tend to be drawn together.

attractive /ə'træktɪv/ *adj* pleasing in appearance, etc; arousing interest; able to draw or pull.—**attractively** *adv*.—**attractiveness** *n*.

attribute /ə'trɪbjuːt/ *vt* to regard as belonging to; to ascribe, impute (to). • *n* a quality, a characteristic of.—**attributable** *adj*.

attribution /,ætrɪ'bjuːʃən/ *n* the act of attributing, *esp* a work of art, etc to a particular creator; a designation; a function.—**attributional** *adj*.

attributive /ə'trɪbjutɪv/ *adj* expressing an attribute; (*gram*) qualifying. • *n* a word joined to and describing a noun; an adjective or adjective phrase.—**attributively** *adv*.

attributive *adj* pertaining to, of the nature of, or expressing, an attribute; (*gram*) qualifying. • *n* a word denoting an attribute; a word joined to and describing a noun; an adjective or adjectival phrase.

attrition /ə'trɪʃən/ *n* a grinding down by or as by friction; a relentless wearing down and weakening; natural wastage or reduction of a workforce by not employing replacements for those who resign or leave.—**attritional** *adj*.—**attritive** *adj*.

attune /ə'tjuːn/ or /ə'tuːn/ *vt* to bring (a person or thing) into harmony with; to adapt.

at. wt. *abbr* = atomic weight.

atypical /eɪ'tɪpɪkəl/ *adj* not according to type; without definite typical character.—**atypically** *adv*.

Au (*chem symbol*) gold.

aubade /oː'bɒd/ *n* a musical announcement of dawn; a sunrise song.

auberge *Fr.* /oː'bɛRʒ/ *n* an inn.

aubergine /'oːbər,ʒiːn/ *n* a plant producing a smooth, dark-purple fruit; this fruit used as a vegetable.—*also* **eggplant**.

aubrietia, aubretia /ɒ'briːʃə/ *n* a small purple-flowered perennial plant.

auburn /'ɒbərn/ *adj* reddish brown.

au contraire *Fr.* /oː kɔ̃:'tRɛR/ *adv* on the contrary.

au courant *Fr.* /oːkuː'Rɑ̃/ *adj* well-informed, *esp* in current affairs.

auction /'ɒkʃən/ *n* a public sale of items to the highest bidder. • *vt* to sell by or at an auction.

auction bridge *n* a form of bridge in which the players contract to take a certain number of tricks, with extra tricks counting towards game.

auctioneer /,ɒkʃə'niːr/ *n* one who conducts an auction.

audacious /ɒ'deɪʃəs/ *adj* daring, adventurous; bold; rash; insolent.—**audaciously** *adv*.—**audaciousness** *n*.

audacity /ɒ'dæsɪti/ *n* (*pl* **audacities**) boldness; daring; spirit; presumptuousness; impudence; effrontery.

audible /'ɒdɪbəl/ *adj* heard or able to be heard.—**audibility** *n*.—**audibly** *adv*.

audience /'ɒdɪəns/ *n* a gathering of listeners or spectators; the people addressed by a book, play, film, etc; a formal interview or meeting, *esp* one in which one's views are heard.

audile /'ɒdaɪl/ *adj* received through hearing.

audio /'ɒdɪoː/ *n* sound; the reproduction, transmission or reception of sound.

audio frequency *n* a frequency audible to the human ear.

audiometer /,ɒdɪ'ɒmɪtər/ *n* an instrument for gauging the power of hearing.—**audiometric** *adj*.—**audiometrically** *adv*.—**audiometry** *n*.

audiotypist /ˌɒdiəˈtaɪpɪst/ *n* a typist who works from a recording.

audiovisual /-ˈvɪʒʊəl/ *adj* using both sound and vision, as in teaching aids.

audit /ˈɒdɪt/ *n* the inspection and verification of business accounts by a qualified accountant • *vt* to make such an inspection.

audition /ɒˈdɪʃən/ *n* a trial to test a performer. • *vti* to test or be tested by audition.

auditor /ˈɒdɪtər/ *n* a person qualified to audit business accounts.—**auditorial** *adj*.

auditorium /ˌɒdɪˈtɔriəm/ *n* (*pl* **auditoriums** /ˌɒdɪˈtɔriəms/, **auditoria**) the part of a building allotted to the audience; a building or hall for speeches, concerts, etc.

auditory /ˈɒdɪˌtɔri/ *adj* of or relating to the sense of hearing.

au fait /oːˈfeɪ/ *adj* fully informed about; competent.

au fond *Fr.* /oːˈfõ/ fundamentally.

auf Wiedersehen *Ger.* /aʊfˈviːdərˌzeɪən/ *interj, n* till we meet again.

Aug. *abbr* = August.

auger /ˈɒgər/ *n* a tool for boring holes, a large gimlet.

aught /ɒt/ *n* anything; any part. • *adv* (*arch*) in any degree, in any way; at all.—*also* **ought**.

augite /ˈɒdʒaɪt/ or /ˈɒg-/ *n* a variety of pyroxene of a black or dark green colour.—**augitic** *adj*.

augment /ɒgˈment/ *vti* to increase.—**augmentable** *adj*.—**augmenter, augmentor** *n*.

augmentation /ˌɒgmenˈteɪʃən/ *n* enlargement, addition, increase; (*mus*) the increase in time value of the notes of a theme; (*her*) an additional charge to a coat of arms bestowed as a mark of honour.

augmentative /ɒgˈmentətɪv/ *adj* having the quality or power of augmenting; (*gram*) increasing in force the idea of a word. • *n* a word or affix that expresses with greater force the idea conveyed by the term from which it is derived, opposite of diminutive.

au gratin /ˌoːˈgræˈtæ̃/ *adj* topped with breadcrumbs or breadcrumbs and cheese, and cooked until crisp.

augur /ˈɒgər/ *vti* to prophesy; to be an omen (of).—**augural** *adj*.

augury /ˈɒgjəri/ *n* (*pl* **auguries**) the art or practice of foretelling events by reference to natural signs or omens; an omen; prediction; presage.

August /ˈɒgəst/ *n* the eighth month of the year, having 31 days.

august /ɒˈgʌst/ *adj* imposing; majestic.

Augustan /ˈɒgəstən/ *adj* of or pertaining to Augustus Caesar, emperor of Rome, or his reign, during which Roman literature gained its highest point; of or pertaining to the period of the highest stage of literary excellence in other countries.

auk /ɒk/ *n* a northern sea bird with short wings used as paddles.

au lait /oːˈleɪ/ *adj* with milk.

auld lang syne /ˌoːld læŋˈsaɪn/ or /ˌɒld læŋˈsaɪn/ *n* days of old; long ago.

au naturel /ˌoːnætʃəˈrel/ *adj, adv* in the natural state; cooked plainly; raw; nude.

aunt /ɒnt/ or /ænt/ *n* a father's or mother's sister an uncle's wife.

auntie, aunty /ˈænti/ or /ˈɒnti/ *n* (*pl* **aunties** /ˈæntiːz/) (*inf*) aunt.

au pair /oːˈpeːr/ *n* a person, *esp* a girl, from abroad who performs domestic chores, child-minding, etc in return for board and lodging.

aura /ˈɔrə/ *n* (*pl* **auras, aurae**) a particular quality or atmosphere surrounding a person or thing.

aural /ˈɔrəl/ *adj* of the ear or the sense of hearing.—**aurally** *adv*.

aural *adj* of the air or an aura.

au revoir /oːrəˈvwɑr/ *n* goodbye for the present

aureate /ˈɔriət/ *adj* golden; gilded golden yellow.

aureole /ˈɔriˌoːl/, **aureola** /ˈɔriˌoːlə/ *n* (*art*) a halo, radiance, or luminous cloud encircling the figures of Christ, the virgin and the saints in sacred pictures; anything resembling an aureole.

auric /oːˈriːk/ *adj* of or pertaining to gold.

auricle /ˈɔrɪkəl/ *n* the external part of the ear; either of the two upper chambers of the heart.

auricula /ɔrˈɪkjʊlə/ *n* (*pl* **auriculas, auriculae**) a species of primrose with leaves the shape of a bear's ear.

auricular /ɔrˈɪkjʊlər/ *adj* of or received by the ear; shaped like an ear; spoken privately; relating to the auricles of the heart.

auriculate /ɔrˈɪkjʊlət/ *adj* ear-shaped; having ears or ear-like appendages.

auriferous /ɔrˈɪfərəs/ *adj* gold-bearing; yielding or containing gold.

aurochs /ˈɔrɒks/ *n* (*pl* **aurochs**) an extinct wild ox of North Africa, Europe and Asia.

aurora /əˈrɔrə/ *n* (*pl* **auroras** /əˈrɔrəs/, **aurorae** /əˈrɔri/) either of the luminous bands seen in the night sky in the polar regions.—*also* **northern lights**.

aurora australis /-ɒˈstreɪlɪs/ *n* the aurora seen at the South Pole.

aurora borealis /-ˌbɔriˈælɪs/ *n* the aurora seen at the North Pole.

aurora trout *n* ✴ a brightly spotted brook trout of northern Ontario.

aurous /ˈɔrəs/ *adj* of or bearing gold.

auscultate /ˈɒskəlˌteɪt/ *v* to examine by auscultation.—**auscultator** *n*.—**auscultatory** *adj*.

auscultation /ˌɒskəlˈteɪʃən/ *n* a listening to the sounds of the heart, lungs, etc in the chest for medical diagnosis.

auspex /ˈɒsˌpeks/ *n* (*pl* **auspices** /ˈɒspɪsɪz/) one who divined by observation of birds in ancient Rome.

auspice /ˈɒspɪs/ *n* (*pl* **auspices** /ˈɒspɪsɪz/) an omen; (*pl*) sponsorship; patronage.

auspicious /ɒˈspɪʃəs/ *adj* showing promise, favourable.—**auspiciously** *adv*.

Aussie /ˈɒzi/ or /ˈɒsi/ *n* (*s.*) an Australian.

austere /ɒˈstiːr/ *adj* stern, forbidding in attitude or appearance; abstemious; severely simple, plain.—**austerely** *adv*.—**austereness** *n*.

austerity /ɒˈsteriti/ *n* (*pl* **austerities** /ˈɒspəsəs/)being austere; economic privation.

austral /ˈɒstrəl/ *adj* southern; (*with cap*) Australian.

Australasian /ˌɒstrəˈleɪʒən/ *adj* of or pertaining to Australasia (Australia, New Zealand and adjacent islands). • *n* a native or inhabitant of Australasia.

Australian /ɒˈstreɪliən/ *adj* of or pertaining to Australia. • *n* a native or inhabitant of Australia.

Australoid /ˈɒstrəlɔɪd/ *adj* of the variety of human population that includes the Australian aborigines. • *n* an Australoid person.

autarchy /ˈɒtɑrki/ *n* (*pl* **autarchies** /ˈɒtɑrkiːz/) absolute or autocratic rule or sovereignty; a country governed in such a way; autarky.—**autarchic, autarchical** *adj*.

autarky /ˈɒtɑrki/ *n* (*pl* **autarkies** /ˈɒtɑrkiːz/) self-sufficiency, *esp* in the economic sphere; the policy of encouraging economic self-sufficiency.—**autarkic, autarkical** *adj*.

authentic /ɒˈθentik/ *adj* genuine, conforming to truth or reality; trustworthy, reliable.—**authentically** *adv*.—**authenticity** *n*.

authenticate /ɒˈθentɪˌkeɪt/ *vt* to demonstrate the authenticity of; to make valid; to verify.—**authentication** *n*.—**authenticator** *n*.

author /ˈɒθər/ *n* a person who brings something into existence; the writer of a book, article, etc. • *vt* to be the author of.—**authoress** *nf*.—**authorial** *adj*.

authoritarian /əˌθɒrɪˈteriən/ or /-θɒr-/, /ɒ-/ *adj* favouring strict obedience; dictatorial. • *n* a person advocating authoritarian principles.—**authoritarianism** *n*.

authoritative /əˈθɒrɪˌteɪtɪv/ or /-θɒr-/, /ɒ-/ *adj* commanding or possessing authority; accepted as true; official.—**authoritatively** *adv*.

authority /əˈθɒrɪti/ or /-θɒr/, /ɒ-/ *n* (*pl* **authorities** /əˈθɒrətiːz/) the power or right to command; (*pl*) officials with this power; influence resulting from knowledge, prestige, etc; a person, writing, etc cited to support an opinion; an expert.

authorize /ˈɒθəˌraɪz/ *vt* to give authority to, to empower; to give official approval to, sanction.—**authorization** *n*.

Authorized Version /ˈɒθəˌraɪzd vərzən/ *n* the version of the Bible published by the sanction of James I of England in 1611 and appointed to be read in churches.—*also* **King James Bible, King James Version**.

authorship /ˈɒθərʃɪp/ *n* the writing profession; origin (of book).

autism /ˈɒtɪzəm/ *n* (*psychiatry*) a mental state, *usu* of children, marked by disregard of external reality.—**autistic** *adj*.

auto /ˈɒtoː/ *n* (*pl* **autos** /ˈɒtoːz/) (*inf*) an automobile.

auto- /ˈɒtoː/ or /ˈɒtoː/ *prefix* self; by oneself or itself.

autobahn /ˈɒtoːˌbɒn/ *n* a German, Austrian or Swiss motorway.

autobiography /ˌɒtoːbaɪˈɒgrəfi/ *n* (*pl* **autobiographies** /ˌɒtoːbaɪˈɒgrəfiːz/) the biography of a person written by himself or herself.—**autobiographer** *n*.—**autobiographical** *adj*.

autocephalous /ˌɒtoːˈsefələs/ *adj* having its own head; independent.

autochondriac /ˌɒtoːˈkɒndriˌæk/ *n* a person who is preoccupied with his or her car.

autochthon /ɒˈtɒkθən/ *n* (*pl* **autochthons, autochthones**) an earliest known inhabitant, an aboriginal.

autochthonous /-nəs/, **autochthonal** /-nəl/ *adj* pertaining to primitive inhabitants; indigenous, native to the soil.—**autochthonism, autochthony** *n*.

autoclave /ˈɒtəˌkleɪv/ *n* a strong container used for chemical reactions at high temperatures and pressures; a device for sterilizing implements using steam at high pressure.

autocracy /ɒˈtɒkrəsi/ *n* (*pl* **autocracies**) government by one person with absolute power.

autocrat /ˈɒtəˌkræt/ *n* an absolute ruler; any domineering person.—**autocratic** *adj*.—**autocratically** *adv*.

autocross /ˈɒtəˌkrɒs/ *n* cross-country motor racing.

Autocue /ˈɒtəˌkjuː/ *n* (*trademark*) a prompting device used in TV, etc, which provides speakers with a script that remains invisible to the audience.—*also* **Teleprompter**.

auto-da-fé /ˌɒtəʊdæˈfeɪ/ or /ˌɒtəzˈ/, *Fr.* /ˈautodəˈfe/ *n* (*pl* **autos-da-fé**) a public judgment by the Spanish Inquisition upon prisoners tried for heresy and other offences against the religious or civil law; the subsequent execution of such sentences by burning.

autoeroticism /ˌɒtəːəˈrɒtɪˌsɪzm/, **autoerotism** /-ˈerəˌtɪzəm/ *n* self-produced sexual emotion.—**autoerotic** *adj*.

autogamy /ɒˈtɒgəmi/ *n* self-fertilization.—**autogamous** *adj*.

autogenesis /ˌɒtəˈdʒɛnəsɪs/, **autogeny** /ɒtəˈdʒɛni/ *n* spontaneous generation.—**autogenetic** *adj*.

autogenous /ɒˈtɒdʒənəs/ *adj* self-generated; produced independently.

autogiro, autogyro /ˌɒtəˈdʒaɪrəʊ/ *n* (*pl* **autogyros, autogiros**) an aircraft like a helicopter but with unpowered rotor blades.

autograph /ˈɒtəˌɡrɑːf/ *n* a pers on's signature. • *vt* to write one's signature in or on.—**autographic** *adj*.—**autographically** *adv*.

autography /ɒˈtɒɡrəfi/ *n* one's own handwriting; a lithographic process by which copies of writings or drawings are reproduced in facsimile.

autolysis /ɒˈtɒlɪsɪs/ *n* the destruction of cells of a body by the action of its own serum.—**autolytic** *adj*.

automaker /ˈɒtəˌmeɪkər/ *n* a manufacturer of automobiles.

automat /ˈɒtəˌmæt/ *n* in US, a restaurant equipped with slot machines for dispensing food and drink; a vending machine.

automate /ˈɒtəˌmeɪt/ *vt* to control by automation; to convert to automatic operation.

automated telling machine *n* a device that provides cash and other banking services automatically when activated by a plastic card issued to customers; a cash dispenser.—*also* **autoteller**.

automatic /ˌɒtəˈmætɪk/ *adj* involuntary or reflexive; self-regulating; acting by itself. • *n* an automatic pistol or rifle.—**automatically** *adv*.

automatic pilot *n* a device that can maintain an aircraft or ship on a previously set course.—*also* **autopilot**.

automatic transmission *n* a system in a motor vehicle for changing gears automatically.

automation /ˌɒtəˈmeɪʃən/ *n* the use of automatic methods, machinery, etc in industry.

automatism /ɒˈtɒməˌtɪzəm/ *n* automatic action; involuntary action; mechanical routine; the doctrine that assigns all animal functions to the active operation of physical laws.—**automatist** *n*.

automaton /əˈtɒməˌtɒn/ *n* (*pl* **automatons, automata**) any automatic device, *esp* a robot; a human being who acts like a robot.

automatous /əˈtɒmətəs/ *adj* spontaneous; of the nature of an automaton.

automobile /ˈɒtəməˌbiːl/ *n* a *usu* four-wheeled vehicle powered by an internal combustion engine.—*also* **motor car**.

automotive /ˌɒtəˈmoʊtɪv/ *adj* relating to motor vehicles.

autonomy /ɒˈtɒnəmi/ *n* (*pl* **autonomies**) freedom of self-determination; independence, self-government.—**autonomous** *adj*.

Auto Pact /ˈɒtəˌpækt/ *n* ✲ (*Cdn*) (*inf*) an agreement between Canada and the US that removed tariffs from the sale of motor vehicles and parts between the two countries.

autopilot /ˈɒtəˌpaɪlət/ *n* automatic pilot.

autoplasty /-ˌplæsti/ *n* the process of repairing lesions by application of tissue removed from another part of the same body.—**autoplastic** *adj*.

autopsy /ˈɒˌtɒpsi/ *n* (*pl* **autopsies**) a post-mortem examination to determine the cause of death.

autoroute /ˈɒtəˌruːt/ *n* a French motorway.

autostrada /ˈɒtəˌstrædə/ *n* an Italian motorway.

autosuggestion /ˌɒtəsəˈdʒɛstʃən/ or /-səɡˈdʒɛst/ *n* (*psychoanal*) self-applied suggestion.—**autosuggestive** *adj*.

autoteller *see* **automated telling machine**.

autotoxin /ˌɒtəˈtɒksɪn/ *n* a poisonous substance produced by changes within an organism.—**autotoxic** *adj*.

autumn /ˈɒtəm/ *n* the season between summer and winter.—*also* fall.

autumnal /ɒˈtʌmnəl/ *adj* belonging or peculiar to autumn or fall; produced or gathered in autumn; pertaining to the period of life when middle age is past. • *n* a plant that flowers in autumn.

aux. /ɒks/ *abbr* = auxiliary.

auxiliary /ɒɡˈzɪljəri/ or /-ˈzɪləri/ *adj* providing help, subsidiary; supplementary. • *n* (*pl* **auxiliaries**) a helper; (*gram*) a verb that helps form tenses, moods, voices, etc of other verbs, as *have, be, may, shall*, etc.

AV /ˈeɪˈviː/ *abbr* = ad valorem; audiovisual; Authorized Version.

avadavat /ˌævədəˈvæt/ *n* a small Asian finch-like bird, kept as a caged bird for its song.

avail /əˈveɪl/ *vti* to be of use or advantage to. • *n* benefit, use or help.

available /əˈveɪləbəl/ *adj* ready for use; obtainable, accessible.—**availability** *n*.—**availably** *adv*.

avalanche /ˈævəˌlæntʃ/ *n* a mass of snow, ice, and rock tumbling down a mountainside; a sudden overwhelming accumulation or influx.

avalanche lily *n* ✲ a plant of the lily family with a large yellow flower found near the snow line on mountains.

avant-garde /ˌævɒntˈɡɑːd/, *Fr.* /avɑ̃ˈɡard/ *n* (*arts*) those ideas and practices regarded as in advance of those generally accepted. • *adj* pertaining to such ideas and practices and their creators.—**avant-gardism** *n*.

avarice /ˈævərɪs/ *n* greed for wealth.—**avaricious** *adj*.—**avariciously** *adv*.

avast /əˈvæst/ *interj* (*naut*) stop! cease! hold!

avatar /ˈævəˌtɑr/ *n* (*Hinduism*) the descent to earth of a deity in an incarnate form; manifestation or embodiment; transference of personality.

avdp. *abbr* = avoirdupois.

ave /ˈɑːveɪ/ *interj* hail; farewell. • *n* an Ave Maria; a salutation.

Ave, ave *abbr* = avenue.

Ave Maria /ˈɑːveɪməˈriːə/ *n* (*RC Church*) Hail Mary.

avenge /əˈvɛndʒ/ *vt* to get revenge for.—**avenger** *n*.

avens /ˈævənz/ *n* (*pl* **avens**) the popular name of plants to which the herb bennet belongs.

aventurine /əˈvɛntʃəˌriːn/ *n* a brown, gold-spangled kind of Venetian glass; a variety of micaceous quartz or feldspar.

avenue /ˈævəˌnjuː/ *n* a street, drive, etc, *esp* when broad; means of access; the way to an objective.

aver /əˈvɜr/ *vt* (**averring, averred**) to state as true; to assert.—**averment** *n*.

average /ˈævərɪdʒ/ *n* the result of dividing the sum of two or more quantities by the number of quantities; the usual kind, amount, quality, etc. • *vt* to calculate the average of; to achieve an average number of.

averse /əˈvɜrs/ *adj* unwilling; opposed (to).

aversion /əˈvɜrʒən/ or /-ʃən/ *n* antipathy; hatred; something arousing hatred or repugnance.

avert /əˈvɜrt/ *vt* to turn away or aside from; to prevent, avoid.—**avertible, avertable** *adj*.

avian /ˈeɪvɪən/ *adj* of or pertaining to birds.

aviary /ˈeɪviˌeri/ *n* (*pl* **aviaries**) a building or large cage for keeping birds.

aviate /ˈeɪviət/ *vi* to pilot or travel in an aircraft.

aviation /ˌeɪviˈeɪʃən/ *n* the art or science of flying aircraft.

aviator /ˈeɪviˌeɪtər/ *n* a pilot, *esp* in the early history of flying.

aviculture /ˈeɪviˌkʌltʃər/ *n* the breeding and rearing of birds.—**aviculturist** *n*.

avid /ˈævɪd/ *adj* eager, greedy.—**avidly** *adv*.

avidity /əˈvɪdɪti/ *n* greediness; eagerness; strong appetite.

avifauna *n* /ˈeɪviˌfɒnə/ (*pl* **avifaunae**) the birds of a region regarded collectively.—**avifaunal** *adj*.

avionics /ˌeɪviˈɒnɪks/ *n* (*used as sing*) the application of electronics in aviation.—**avionic** *adj*.

avocado /ˌævəˈkɒdəʊ/ *n* (*pl* **avocados**) a thick-skinned, pear-shaped fruit with yellow buttery flesh.

avocet /ˈævəˌsɛt/ *n* one of several species of wading birds, characterized by very long legs and an extremely slender curved bill.

avoid /ə'vɔɪd/ *vt* to keep clear of, shun; to refrain from.—**avoider** *n.*

avoidable *adj* able to be avoided.

avoidance /ə'vɔɪdəns/ *n* the act of annulling or making void; the act of shunning; the state of being vacant.

avoirdupois /ˌævədə'pɔɪz/ *n* the system of weights based on the pound of 16 ounces; (*inf*) excess weight.

avow /ə'vaʊ/ *vt* to declare confidently; to acknowledge.—**avowed** *adj.*—**avowedly** *adv.*—**avower** *n.*

avowal /ə'vaʊəl/ *n* an open declaration; a frank acknowledgment; a confession.

avulsion /ə'vʌlʃən/ *n* a separation by violence; the sudden removal of land, without change of ownership, caused by a flood, etc.

avuncular /ə'vʌŋkjʊlər/ *adj* like an uncle.

await /ə'weɪt/ *vti* to wait for; to be in store for.

awake /ə'weɪk/ *vb* (**awaking, awoke** *or* **awaked,** *pp* **awoken** *or* **awaked**) *vi* to wake; to become aware. • *vt* to rouse from sleep; to rouse from inaction. • *adj* roused from sleep, not asleep; active; aware.

awaken /ə'weɪkən/ *vti* to awake.

awakening /-ɪŋ/ *n* the act of rousing from sleep; a revival of religion, or activity of a particular religious sect. • *adj* rousing; exciting; alarming.

award /ə'wɔːd/ *vt* to give, as by a legal decision; to give (a prize, etc); to grant. • *n* a decision, as by a judge; a prize.

aware /ə'wɛr/ *adj* realizing, having knowledge; conscious; fully conversant with and sympathetic towards (*ecologically aware*).—**awareness** *n.*

awash /ə'wɒʃ/ *adj* filled or overflowing with water.

away /ə'weɪ/ *adv* from a place; in another place or direction; off, aside; far. • *adj* absent; at a distance.

awe /ɔː/ *n* a mixed feeling of fear, wonder and dread. • *vt* to fill with awe.

aweather /ə'wɛðər/ *adv* (*naut*) on the weather side, or towards the wind. • *n* opposed to the alee.

aweigh /ə'weɪ/ *adj, adv* (*naut*) (*anchor*) atrip, just drawn out of the ground and hanging perpendicularly.

awesome /'ɔːsəm/ *adj* inspiring awe; (*inf*) marvellous, terrific.

awestricken /'ɔːstrɪkən/, **awestruck** /'ɔːstrʌk/ *adj* struck with awe.

awful /'ɔːfəl/ *adj* very bad; unpleasant. • *adv* (*inf*) very.—**awfulness** *n.*

awfulize *vt* to envisage a situation as being worse than it is.—*also* **catastrophize.**

awfully /'ɔːfəli/ *or* /'ɔːfli/ *adv* in an awful manner; excessively; (*inf*) very.

awhile /ə'waɪl/ *adv* for a short time.

awkward /'ɔːkwəd/ *adj* lacking dexterity, clumsy; graceless; embarrassing; embarrassed; inconvenient; deliberately obstructive or difficult to deal with.—**awkwardly** *adv.*—**awkwardness** *n.*

awl /ɔːl/ *n* a small pointed tool for boring or piercing, used by shoemakers, etc.

awn /ɔːn/ *n* the beard or bristle-like appendage of the outer glume of wheat, barley, and numerous grasses.

awning /'ɔːnɪŋ/ *n* a structure, as of canvas, extended above or in front of a window, door, etc to provide shelter against the sun or rain.

awoke /ə'wəʊk/ *see* **awake.**

AWOL /'eɪwɒl/ *abbr* = absent without leave.

awry /ə'raɪ/ *adv* twisted to one side. • *adj* contrary to expectations, wrong.

axe, ax /æks/ *n* (*pl* **axes**) a tool with a long handle and bladed head for chopping wood. etc. • *vt* to trim, split, etc with an axe.

axial /'æksɪəl/ *adj* of, forming or round an axis.—**axially** *adv.*

axil /'æksɪl/ *n* (*bot*) the angle formed by the upper side of an organ or branch with the stem or trunk to which it is attached.

axile /'æksɪl/ *or* /-saɪl/ *adj* (*bot*) of, lying or situated in, or attached to, an axis.

axilla /æk'sɪlə/ *n* (*pl* **axillae, axillas**) the armpit, or cavity in the junction of the arm and shoulder; the axil of a leaf.

axillary /æk'sɪləri/ *adj* of or pertaining to the armpit; (*bot*) pertaining to, springing from, or situated in, the axil. • *n* (*pl* **axillaries**) a feather from the axilla of a bird.

axiom /'æksɪəm/ *n* a widely held or accepted truth or principle.

axiomatic /ˌæksɪə'mætɪk/ *adj* pertaining to, or of the nature of, an axiom.—**axiomatically** *adv.*

axis[1] /'æksɪs/ *n* (*pl* **axes**) a real or imaginary straight line about which a body rotates; the centre line of a symmetrical figure; a reference line of a coordinate system; (*with cap*) a partnership, alliance, *esp* of Germany and Italy, 1936 to the end of World War II.—**axial** *adj.*

axis[2] *n* (*pl* **axises**) a small deer of India and Asia with slender antlers.

axle /'æksəl/ *n* a rod on or with which a wheel turns; a bar connecting two opposite wheels, as of a car.

axletree /-ˌtriː/ *n* a bar connecting the opposite wheels of a carriage, on the rounded ends of which the wheels revolve.

axolotl /'æksə,lɒtəl/ *n* a Mexican amphibian like the salamander, having gills.

ay[1], **aye**[1] /eɪ/ *or* /aɪ/ *adv* (*arch*) for ever, always; continually.

ay[2], **aye**[2] /aɪ/ *adv, interj* yes; even so; indeed. • *n* (*pl* **ayes**) an affirmative answer or vote in a parliamentary division; the members so voting.

ayah /'aɪjə/ *n* a native Indian nurse or lady's maid.

Ayatollah /ˌaɪjə'tɒlə/ *n* a Shiite Muslim leader; a title of respect.

aye-aye /'aɪaɪ/ *n* a small nocturnal quadruped, native to Madagascar and allied to the emurs.

AZ *abbr* = Arizona.

azalea /ə'zeɪlɪə/ *n* a flowering shrub-like plant.

azan /ɑ'zɑːn/ *n* the call to public prayers in Islamic countries.

azedarach /ə'zedəræk/ *n* an Asian tree, the bark or root of which was formerly used as a drug.

Azilian /ə'zɪlɪən/ *adj* of a Mesolithic geological stage characterized by bone harpoon heads and painted stone pebbles.

azimuth /'æzɪməθ/ *n* (*astron*) a vertical arc from the zenith to the horizon; the angular distance of this from the meridian.—**azimuthal** *adj.*

azoic /ə'zoɪk/ *or* /-eɪ-/ *adj* without life; (*geol*) without fossils, older than the lowermost series of rocks containing traces of organic life.

azote /ə'zoʊt/ *or* /æ-/ *n* an old name for nitrogen.

AZT /'eɪ'zed'tiː/ *abbr* = azidothymidine, a drug that has been effective in alleviating symptoms in some AIDS sufferers.

Aztec /'æztek/ *adj* pertaining to the Aztec race that ruled Mexico before the Spanish conquest. • *n* a member of the Aztec race.

azure /'æʒər/ *or* /-zjər/ *adj* sky-blue.

azurite /'æʒə,raɪt/ *n* blue carbonate of copper; blue malachite or chessylite; lazulite.

azygous /'eɪzaɪgəs/ *adj* (*anat*) single, as a muscle or vein; not one of a pair.

B

B *abbr* = boron.

b *abbr* = born; billion.

BA /'biː'eɪ/ *abbr* = Bachelor of Arts; British Airways; British Academy.

Ba *abbr* = barium.

baa /bɒ/ *n* the bleat of a sheep. • *vi* to bleat as a sheep.

baba /'bɒbə/ *n* a small sponge cake soaked in (*usu* rum) flavoured syrup.

Babbitt metal /'bæbɪt/ *n* an anti-friction alloy of copper, tin and zinc, used in crank and axle bearings, etc.

Babbittry /'bæbɪtri/ *n* (*derog*) businessman's or middle-class person's standards or blinkered outlook.—**Babbitt** *n*.

babble /'bæbəl/ *vi* to make sounds like a baby; to talk incoherently, endlessly or senselessly; to give away secrets; to murmur, as a brook. • *n* incoherent talk; chatter; a murmuring sound.—**babbler** *n*.

babe /beɪb/ *n* a baby; a naive person; (*sl*) a girl or young woman.

Babel /'beɪbəl/ or /'bæbəl/ *n* (*Bible*) the tower in Shinar (Genesis 11); a lofty structure; a confused and meaningless sound of voices; a scene of confusion and noise.

babirusa, babiruossa, babirussa /bɒbəˌruːsə/ *n* the wild hog of Eastern Asia.

baboon /bæ'buːn/ or /bə-/ *n* a large, short-tailed monkey.

babul /bə'buːl/ *n* the rind of the East Indian acacia.

baby /'beɪbi/ *n* (*pl* **babies**) a newborn child or infant; a very young animal; (*sl*) a girl or young woman; a personal project. • *vt* (**babying, babied**) to pamper.—*also adj.*—**babyish** *adj*.

baby beef *n* ✸ (*Cdn*) meat from young beef cattle, older than those producing veal.

baby bonus *n* ✸ (*Cdn*) a government allowance paid to families.

baby boom *n* a sharp rise in the birth rate.

baby-boomer *n* a person born in the period immediately after World War II when the birthrate increased sharply (*baby boom*).

baby break *n* a period, often five years, when a parent raises children before returning to work.

baby burst *n* a sudden fall in birth rate.

baby carriage *n* a perambulator.

baby grand *n* a small grand piano.

Babylonian /ˌbæbə'loːnɪən/ *adj* of or pertaining to the ancient kingdom of Babylonia; magnificent; luxurious. • *n* an inhabitant of Babylonia; its language.

baby-sit /'beɪbiˌsɪt/ *vti* (**baby-sitting, baby-sat**) to look after a baby or child while the parents are out.—**baby-sitter** *n*.

baby snatcher *n* (*inf*) one who marries or has a liaison with a much younger person; a person who steals a baby.

baby wipe *n* a disposable paper towel, ready moistened.

baccalaureate /ˌbækə'lɔːrɪət/ *n* the university degree awarded to a Bachelor of Arts etc; a commencement address.

baccarat /'bækəˌrɒ/ or /ˌbækə'rɒ/, /bɒ-/ *n* a card game where players bet against the banker.

baccate /'bækeɪt/ *adj* having many berries; berry-shaped.

bacchanal /ˌbækə'nɒl/ or /ˌbɒk-/ *n* a priest of Bacchus, the god of wine; a drunken reveler; a drunken feast.—**bacchanalian** *adj*.

bacchanalia /ˌbækə'neɪlɪə/ or /ˌbɒk-/ *npl* drunken revels.

bacchant /'bækənt/ *n* (*pl* **bacchants, bacchantes**) a priest or votary of Bacchus; a drunkard.—**bacchante** *nf* (*pl* **bacchantes**).

Bacchic /'bækɪk/ or /'bɒkɪk/ *adj* pertaining to Bacchus or the feasts in his honour; riotous, or mad with drink.

bacciferous /bæk'sɪfərəs/ *adj* bearing or producing berries.

bacciform /'bæksəˌfɔːm/ *adj* berry-shaped.

baccivorous /bæk'sɪvərəs/ *adj* eating or subsisting on berries.

bachelor /'bætʃələr/ or /'bætʃlər/ *n* an unmarried man; a person who holds a degree from a college or university.—**bachelorhood** *n*.

bachelor apartment *n* ✸ (*Cdn*) an apartment that has one large room serving as a bedroom and living room, together with a kitchenette and bathroom.

bachelor's buttons *npl* the popular name for a double-flowered buttercup with blossoms resembling buttons.

bacillary /bə'sɪləri/ or /'bæsəˌlɛri/, **bacillar** *adj* of, like, caused by, or consisting of bacilli; rod-shaped.

bacilliform /bə'sɪləˌfɔːm/ *adj* rod-shaped, like a bacillus.

bacillus /bə'sɪləs/ *n* (*pl* **bacilli** /bəsɪl'aɪ/) any of a genus of rod-shaped bacteria; (*loosely*) bacteria in general.

back[1] /bæk/ *n* the rear surface of the human body from neck to hip; the corresponding part in animals; a part that supports or fits or makes firm the back of anything; the part farthest from the front; (*sport*) a player or position behind the front line. • *adj* at the rear; (*streets, etc*) remote or inferior; (*pay, etc*) of or for the past; backward. • *adv* at or towards the rear; to or towards a former condition, time, etc; in return or requital; in reserve or concealment. • *vti* to move or go backwards; to support; to bet on; to provide or be a back for; to supply a musical backing for a singer; (*with* **down**) to withdraw from a position or claim; (*with* **off**) to move back (or away, etc); (*with* **out**) to withdraw from an enterprise; to evade keeping a promise, etc; (*with* **up**) to support; to move backwards; to accumulate because of restricted movement; (*comput*) to make a copy (of a data file, etc) for safekeeping.

back[2] *n* a large shallow cistern or vat used by brewers, etc, for liquids.

backache /'bækeɪk/ *n* an ache or pain in the back.

back bacon *n* round, lean bacon cut from a pork loin.

back bay *n* ✸ (*Cdn*) a shallow bay of a lake.

backbencher /-bentʃər/ *n* in UK, Australia, etc, a member of parliament who does not hold office.

backbite /-baɪt/ *vt* (**backbiting, backbit**, *pp* **backbitten** or **backbit**) to talk spitefully or ill of behind a person's back.—**backbiter** *n*.—**backbiting** *n*.

backboard /'bækbɔːd/ *n* a board at the back of a cart; a board worn at the back to support the back; a thin wooden backing used for picture frames, mirrors, etc.

backbone /-boːn/ *n* the spinal column; main support; strength, courage.

backbreaking /-breɪkɪŋ/ *adj* arduous; physically exhausting.

back channel *n* a person who acts as a secret intermediary, *esp* in diplomacy; ✸ (*Cdn*) a backwater or side channel of a river.

backchat /-tʃæt/ *n* (*inf*) cheeky repartee.

backcomb /-koːm/ *vt* (*hair*) to comb towards the roots to give body.

back concession *n* ✸ (*Cdn*) a land concession distant from heavily populated areas.

backdate /-deɪt/ *vt* to declare valid from some previous date.

backdoor /-dɔːr/ *adj* indirect, concealed, devious.

backdown /-daʊn/ *n* the act of backing down; the withdrawal of a claim, etc.

backdrop /-drɒp/ *n* a curtain, often scenic, at the back of a stage; background.

back end /-ɛnd/ *n* (*dial*) autumn.

backer /-ər/ *n* a patron; one who bets on a contestant.

backfire /-faɪr/ *vi* (*cars*) to ignite prematurely causing a loud bang from the exhaust; to have the opposite effect from that intended, *usu* with unfortunate consequences.—*also n*.

back forty *n* ✸ (*Cdn*) (*inf*) the area at the rear of a rural property.

backgammon /'bækˌgæmən/ or /bæk'gæmən/ *n* a board game played by two people with pieces moved according to throws of the dice.

background /-graʊnd/ *n* the distant part of a scene or picture; an inconspicuous position; social class, education, experience; circumstances leading up to an event.

backhand /-hænd/ *n* (*tennis, etc*) a stroke played with the hand turned outwards.

backhanded /'bækˌhændəd/ or /bæk'hændəd/ *adj* backhand; (*compliment*) indirect, ambiguous.—*also adv*.—**backhandedly** *adv*.

backhander /-ˌhændər/ *n* a backhanded stroke; (*inf*) a backhanded remark; (*sl*) a bribe.

backing /-ɪŋ/ *n* support; supporters; a lining to support or strengthen the back of something; musical accompaniment to a (*esp* pop) singer.

backlash /-læʃ/ *n* a violent and adverse reaction; a recoil in machinery.

backlist /-lɪst/ *n* books published in past years that are still in print.

backlog /-lɒg/ *n* an accumulation of work, etc still to be done.

back number *n* a former issue (of a magazine, etc); an out-of-date person.

backpack /-pæk/ *n* a rucksack; an equipment pack carried on the back of an astronaut, etc. • *vi* to travel, hike, etc wearing a backpack.

back pay /-peɪ/ *n* an increase in wages or salary paid retrospectively.

back-pedal /-ˌpedəl/ *vi* (**back-pedalling, back-pedalled** *or* **back-pedaling, back-pedaled**) to work the pedals of a bicycle backwards; to modify or withdraw one's original argument or action.

back-seat driver /ˈsiːt/ *n* a passenger in a car who irritates the driver with persistent unwanted advice.

backside /ˈbæksaɪd/ *n* (*inf*) buttocks.

backslide /-slaɪd/ *vi* (**backsliding, backslid, *pp* backslid** *or* **backslidden**) to return to one's (bad) old ways.—**backslider** *n*.

backspace /-speɪs/ *vi* to move a typewriter carriage or cursor of a word processor back one space.

backspin /-spɪn/ *n* (*sport*) a backward spin in a ball to slow it down.

backsplit /ˈbæksplɪt/ *n* ✤ (*Cdn*) a house with floors raised half a storey at the rear.

backstage /ˈbæksteɪdʒ/ *or* /bækˈsteɪdʒ/ *adv* behind the stage of a theatre in areas hidden from the audience; (*inf*) away from public view.—*also adj*.

backstairs /-ˈsterz/ *npl* stairs in the back part of a house; stairs for private use. • *adj* indirect; underhand; secret; intriguing.

backstay /-steɪ/ *n* (*naut*) a long rope extending from the masthead to the side of a ship, supporting the mast.

backstitch /-stɪtʃ/ *n* an overlapping stitch. • *vt* to sew with this stitch.

backstroke /-strəʊk/ *n* (*swimming*) a stroke using backward circular sweeps of the arms whilst lying face upwards.

backsword /-sɔːd/ *n* a sword with one sharp edge, a broadsword; a stick with a basket handle used in the game of singlestick.

back-to-back *adj* facing in opposite directions, often with the backs touching.

backtrack /ˈbɒktræk/ *vi* to return along the same path; to reverse or recant one's opinion, action, etc.

backup /-ʌp/ *n* an alternate or auxiliary; support, reinforcement; (*comput*) a copy of a data file, etc.

backward /-wərd/ *adj* turned toward the rear or opposite way; shy; slow or retarded. • *adv* backwards.—**backwardness** *n*.

backwards /-ˌwərdz/ *adv* towards the back; with the back foremost; in a way opposite the usual; into a less good or favourable state or condition; into the past.

backwash /-wɒʃ/ *n* water receding from the action of an oar, propeller, etc; the consequences of an event.

backwater /-wɒtər/ *n* a pool of still water fed by a river; a remote, backward place.

backwoods /-wʊdz/ *npl* uncleared forest land; an isolated, thinly populated area.—**backwoodsman** *n* (*pl* **backwoodsmen**).

backyard /-ˈjɑːd/ *n* a yard at the back of a house.

baclava /ˌbʌkləˈvɒ/ *see* **baklava**.

bacon /ˈbeɪkən/ *n* salted and smoked meat from the back or sides of a pig; **to bring home the bacon** to succeed; to help materially; **to save one's bacon** to have a narrow escape.

bacteria /bækˈtɪːrɪə/ *npl* (*sing* **bacterium**) microscopic unicellular organisms *usu* causing disease.—**bacterial** *adj*.

bactericide /bækˈtɪrɪˌsaɪd/ *n* a substance that destroys bacteria.—**bactericidal** *adj*.

bacteriology /bækˌtɪriˈɒlədʒi/ *n* the scientific study of bacteria.—**bacteriological** *adj*.—**bacteriologist** *n*.

bacteriolysis /bækˌtiːriˈɒlɪsɪs/ *n* destruction of bacteria by a serum.—**bacteriolytic** *adj*.

bacterium /bækˈtɪːrɪəm/ *see* **bacteria**.

Bactrian camel *n* a camel with two humps.

bad[1] /bæd/ *adj* (**worse, worst**) not good; not as it should be; inadequate or unfit; rotten or spoiled; incorrect or faulty; wicked; immoral; mischievous; harmful; ill; sorry, distressed.—**badness** *n*.

bad[2] *see* **bid**.

bad blood *n* enmity, hostility.

bad debt *n* a debt that is not recoverable.

baddie, baddy /ˈbædi/ *n* (*pl* **baddies**) (*inf*) a villain.

badderlocks /ˈbædərˌlɒks/ *n* a large dark-green edible seaweed.

bade /beɪd/ *see* **bid**.

badge /bædʒ/ *n* an emblem, symbol or distinguishing mark.

badger /ˈbædʒər/ *n* a hibernating, burrowing black and white mammal related to the weasel. • *vt* to pester or annoy persistently.

badinage /ˈbædɪˌnɒʒ/ *n* light or playful raillery or banter.

badlands /ˈbædlændz/ *npl* ✤ barren, dry, heavily eroded areas of land in northwestern North America.

badly /ˈbædli/ *adv* (**worse, worst**) poorly; inadequately; unsuccessfully; severely; (*inf*) very much.

badminton /ˈbædmɪntən/ *n* a court game for two or four players played with light rackets and a shuttlecock volleyed over a net.

badmouth *vt* (*sl*) to speak ill of; to slander.

baffle /ˈbæfəl/ *vt* to bewilder or perplex; to frustrate; to make ineffectual. • *n* a plate or device used to restrict the flow of sound, light or fluid.—**bafflement** *n*.—**baffling** *adj*.

bag /bæg/ *n* a *usu* flexible container of paper, plastic, etc that can be closed at the top; a satchel, suitcase, etc; a handbag; a purse; game taken in hunting; a bag-like shape or part; (*derog*) an old, unpleasant or ugly woman; (*inf: in pl*) plenty (of). • *vti* (**bagging, bagged**) to place in a bag; to kill in hunting; (*inf*) to get; to make a claim on; to hang loosely.

bagasse /bəˈgæs/ *n* sugar-cane refuse after crushing, used as a fuel.

bagatelle /ˌbægəˈtel/ *n* something of little value; a piece of light music *usu* for piano; a board game in which balls struck with a cue or by a spring are aimed at holes or pinned spaces.

bagel /ˈbeɪgəl/ *n* a ring-shaped bread roll, hard and glazed on the outside, soft in the centre.

bagful /ˈbægfʊl/ *n* (*pl* **bagfuls**) as much as will fill one bag.

baggage /ˈbægɪdʒ/ *n* suitcases; luggage; **bag and baggage** with one's entire possessions; entirely.

baggataway /bəˈgætəwe/ *n* ✤ an early form of lacrosse played by Indian peoples in eastern North America.

bagging /ˈbægɪŋ/ *n* the act of putting into bags; a coarse cloth or other material used for bags; filtration through canvas bags.

baggy /ˈbægi/ *adj* (**baggier, baggiest**) hanging loosely in folds.—**baggily** *adv*.—**bagginess** *n*.

bag lady *n* (*pl* **bag ladies**) a homeless woman who wanders the streets carrying her possessions in shopping bags or carrier bags.

bagman /ˈbægmæn/ *n* (*pl* **bagmen**) (*formerly*) a travelling salesman who carried his wares in saddlebags; a person who collects or distributes illegally obtained money for another; ✤ (*Cdn*) (*inf*) a person who raises funds for a political candidate or party.

bagnio /ˈbænjəʊ/ *n* (*pl* **bagnios**) a brothel; a bath house; an oriental prison.

bagpipe /ˈbægpaɪp/ *n* (*often pl*) a musical instrument consisting of an air-filled bag fitted with pipes.

bail[1] /beɪl/ *n* money lodged as security that a prisoner, if released, will return to court to stand trial; such a release; the person pledging such money. • *vt* to free a person by providing bail; (*with* **out**) to help out of financial or other difficulty; (*government, bank, etc*) to assist a floundering business.—**bailable** *adj*.

bail[2] *vti* (*usu with* **out**) to scoop out (water) from (a boat).

bail[3] *n* (*cricket*) either of two wooden crosspieces that rest on the three stumps; a bar separating horses in an open stable; a metal bar that holds the paper against the roller of a typewriter.

bailee /beˈliː/ *n* (*law*) the person to whom goods are delivered in trust.

bailey /ˈbeɪli/ *n* the outer wall of a castle; a castle yard.

Bailey bridge /ˈbeɪli/ *n* a prefabricated bridge of steel easily and quickly assembled for temporary use.

bailie /ˈbeɪli/ *n* (*Scot*) a municipal officer corresponding to an alderman.

bailiff /ˈbeɪlɪf/ *n* in UK, the agent of a landlord or landowner; a sheriff's officer who serves writs and summonses; a minor official in some US courts, *usu* a messenger or usher; ✤ (*Cdn*) a person who repossesses property for private clients.

bailiwick /ˈbeɪlɪwɪk/ *n* the district within which a bailiff has jurisdiction; a person's special sphere of knowledge or activity or jurisdiction.

bailment /ˈbeɪlmənt/ *n* (*law*) a delivery of goods in trust to another; the action of becoming surety for one in custody.

bailor /ˈbeɪlər/ *n* (*law*) one who delivers goods in trust.

bail-out *n* assistance by a bank, government, etc, to help (a company) in financial trouble.

bailsman /ˈbeɪlzmən/ *n* (*pl* **bailsmen**) one who gives bail for another.

bain-marie /ˌbæmæˈriː/ *n* (*pl* **bains-marie**) a vessel that holds hot water for cooking or warming food.

bairn /bɛrn/ n (Scot) a child.

bait /beɪt/ n food attached to a hook to entice fish or make them bite; any lure or enticement. • vt to put food on a hook to lure; to set dogs upon (a badger, etc); to persecute, worry or tease, esp by verbal attacks; to lure, to tempt; to entice.

baize /beɪz/ n a coarse, green woollen fabric used to cover snooker tables.

bake /beɪk/ vt (pottery) to dry and harden by heating in the sun or by fire; (food) to cook by dry heat in an oven. • vi to do a baker's work; to dry and harden in heat; (inf) to be very hot. • n all the food baked at one time or baking; a party or picnic featuring one baked item, eg a clambake.

bakeapple /'beɪk,æpəl/ n ✤ (Cdn) cloudberry.

baked beans npl cooked haricot beans canned in tomato sauce.

bakehouse /'beɪkhʊs/ n a bakery.

Bakelite /'beɪkə,laɪt/ n (trademark) a hard synthetic resin used for dishes, etc.

baker /'beɪkər/ n a person who bakes and sells bread, cakes, etc.

baker's dozen n thirteen.

bakery /'beɪkəri/ n (pl **bakeries**) a room or building for baking; a shop that sells bread, cakes, etc; baked goods.

baking powder n a leavening agent containing sodium bicarbonate and an acid-forming substance.

baking soda n sodium bicarbonate.

baklava /,bæklə'vɒ/ or /'bækləvə/ n a cake made with thin, flaky pastry, honey and nuts.—also **baclava**.

baksheesh /'bækʃiːʃ/ n a present of money as a bribe or tip to expedite service.

balaclava (helmet) /,bælə'klɒvə/ n a woollen hood that covers the ears and neck.

balalaika /,bælə'laɪkə/ n a Russian, three-stringed guitar with a triangular body.

balance /'bæləns/ n a device for weighing, consisting of two dishes or pans hanging from a pivoted horizontal beam; equilibrium; mental stability; the power to influence or control; a remainder.—**in the balance** a state of uncertainty.—**on balance** having considered all aspects or factors. • vt to weigh; to compare; to equalize the debit and credit sides of an account. • vi to be equal in power or weight, etc; to have the debits and credits equal.—**balanceable** adj.—**balancer** n.

balance of payments n the difference between a country's total receipts from abroad and total payments abroad over a given period.

balancer /'bælənsər/ n one who or that which keeps anything in equilibrium; an acrobat; (pl) halter.

balance sheet n a statement of assets and liabilities.

balance wheel n a wheel that regulates the speed of a clock or watch.

balas /'bæləs/ n a variety of spinel ruby of a pale rose-red colour.

balata /'bælətə/ n dried gum from a South American tree, used as a substitute for guttapercha.

balcony /'bælkəni/ n (pl **balconies**) a projecting platform from an upper storey enclosed by a railing; an upper floor of seats in a theatre, etc, often projecting over the main floor.—**balconied** adj.

bald /bɒld/ adj lacking a natural or usual covering, as of hair, vegetation, or nap; (tyre) having little or no tread; (truth) plain or blunt; bare, unadorned.—**baldly** adv.—**baldness** n.

baldachin /'bɒldəkɪn/ n a canopy, esp over a throne or altar; a rich brocade fabric used for this.

balderdash /'bɒldər,dæʃ/ n nonsense.

balding /'bɒldɪŋ/ adj becoming bald.

baldric /'bɒldrɪk/ n a broad belt, often richly ornamented, worn round the waist, or over one shoulder and across the breast.

bale[1] /beɪl/ n a large bundle of goods, as raw cotton, compressed and bound. • vt (hay etc) to make into bales. • vi (with **out**) to parachute from an aircraft, usu in an emergency.

bale[2] n a great evil; woe.

baleen /bə'liːn/ n whalebone.

baleful /'beɪlfʊl/ adj evil; harmful; deadly; ominous.—**balefully** adv.—**balefulness** n.

balk see **baulk**.

ball[1] /bɒl/ n a spherical or nearly spherical body or mass; a round object for use in tennis, football, etc; a throw or pitch of a ball; a missile for a cannon, rifle, etc; any rounded part or protuberance of the body; (pl: sl) testicles; nonsense. • interj (pl) (sl) nonsense! • vti to form into a ball; (vulg sl) to have sexual intercourse with.

ball[2] n a formal social dance; (inf) a good time.—**ballroom** n.—**ballroom dancing** n.

ballad /'bæləd/ n a narrative song or poem; a slow, sentimental, esp pop, song.—**balladeer** n.—**balladry** n.

ballade /bæ'lɒd/ n a poem of (usu) three eight-line stanzas and an envoy, all with the same rhymes and refrain.

balladmonger /'bæləd,mʌŋgər/ n a dealer in ballads; an inferior poet, a poetaster.

ballast /'bæləst/ n heavy material carried in a ship or vehicle to stabilize it when it is not carrying cargo; crushed rock or gravel, etc used in railway tracks.

ball bearing n a device for lessening friction by having a rotating part resting on small steel balls; one of these balls.

ball boy n (tennis) a boy who retrieves balls that go out of play.—**ball girl** nf.

ballcock n a device that uses a floating ball to regulate the flow of water in a cistern, tank, etc.

ballerina /,bælə'riːnə/ n a female ballet dancer.

ballet /'bæleɪ/ or /bæ'leɪ/ n a theatrical representation of a story, set to music and performed by dancers; the troupe of dancers.

balletomane /bə'lɛtoː,meɪn/ n an enthusiastic lover of ballet.—**balletomania** n.

ball hockey n ✤ (Cdn) a game with the rules of ice hockey, but played in a gymnasium or arena and using a hard plastic ball instead of a puck.

ballicater /bælɪ'kætər/ n ✤ (Cdn) in Newfoundland, ice formed along a shoreline from waves and freezing spray.

ballistic /bə'lɪstɪk/ adj relating to the flight of projectiles.

ballistic missile n a missile whose trajectory is initially guided then ballistic.

ballistics /bə'lɪstɪks/ n (used as sing) the scientific study of projectiles and firearms.

ballonet /,bælə'net/ n a small balloon; a subdivision of a balloon's or an airship's gasbag for controlling descent.

balloon /bə'luːn/ n a large airtight envelope that rises up when filled with hot air or light gases, often fitted with a basket or gondola for carrying passengers; a small inflatable rubber pouch used as a toy or for decoration; a balloon-shaped line enclosing speech or thoughts in a strip cartoon. • vti to inflate; to swell, expand; to travel in a balloon.—**balloonist** n.

balloon jib, balloon sail n (naut) a light triangular sail used by yachts in a slight breeze.

ballooning n the art or practice of managing balloons or making balloon ascents.

ballot /'bælət/ n a paper used in voting; the process of voting; the number of votes cast; the candidates offering themselves for election. • vi (**balloting, balloted**) to vote.—**balloter** n.

ballot box n a secure container for ballot papers.

ballpoint pen n a pen with a tiny ball, which rotates against an inking cartridge, as its writing tip.

ball valve n a valve that is opened or shut by the rising or falling of a ball.

ballyhoo /'bælɪ,hu:/ or /bælɪ'hu:/ n vulgar, noisy publicity or advertisement.

ballyrag /'bælɪ,ræg/ vb (**ballyragging, ballyragged**) vt to hustle, to jeer at. • vi to indulge in horseplay.—also **bullyrag**.

balm /bɒm/ n a fragrant ointment used in healing and soothing; anything comforting and soothing.

balm of Gilead n any of various fragrant resins, as that of the evergreen terebinth tree of Arabia or the balsam fir; a North American poplar with broad heart-shaped leaves.

balmoral /bæl'mɒrəl/ n a laced boot; a Scottish bonnet of wool; a petticoat.

balmy /'bɒmi/ adj (**balmier, balmiest**) having a pleasant fragrance; soothing; (weather) mild, warm.

balneology /,bælni'ɒlədʒi/ n the science of therapeutic baths and their effect.—**balneological** adj.—**balneologist** n.

baloney /bə'loːni/ n (inf) foolish talk; nonsense.—also **boloney**.

balsa /'bɒlsə/ n lightweight wood from a tropical American tree.

balsam /'bɒlsəm/ n a fragrant, resinous substance; the tree yielding it.—**balsamic** adj.

balsam fir n a North American evergreen pine with flat needles and yielding balsam.

balsamiferous /,bɒlsə,mɪfərəs/ adj producing or yielding balsam.

Baltimore oriole n an American bird nearly related to the starlings with bright orange and black plumage.

baluster /'bæləstər/ n any of the small posts of a railing, as on a staircase.—**balustered** adj.

balustrade /'bælə,streɪd/ *n* an ornamental row of balusters joined by a rail.

bambino /bæm'biːnoː/ *n* (*pl* **bambinos, bambini**) a child or baby; (*RC Church*) a figure of the infant Christ wrapped in swaddling clothes, exhibited in churches from Christmas to Epiphany.

bamboo /bæm'buː/ *n* (*pl* **bamboos**) any of various, often tropical, woody grasses, used for furniture.

bamboo shoots *npl* the edible shoots of certain bamboos.

bamboozle /bæm'buːzəl/ *vt* (*inf*) to deceive; to mystify.—**bamboozlement** *n*.—**bamboozler** *n*.

ban¹ /bæn/ *n* a condemnation, an official prohibition. • *vt* (**banning, banned**) to prohibit, *esp* officially; to forbid.

ban² *n* (*feudal*) a public proclamation or summons to arms.

banal /bə'næl/ *adj* trite, commonplace.—**banally** *adj*.

banality /bə'nælɪti/ *n* (*pl* **banalities**) anything trite or trivial; a commonplace remark, etc.

banana /bə'nænə/ *n* a herbaceous plant bearing its fruit in compact, hanging bunches.

banana belt *n* ♣ (*Cdn*) (*inf*) a region with a relatively warm climate, such as southwestern Ontario or British Columbia.

banana republic *n* (*derog*) a small country, *esp* in Central America, that is dominated by foreign interests.

banana skin *n* (*inf*) an unforeseen occurrence that causes embarrassment.

banana split *n* ice cream served on a lengthwise sliced banana and topped with syrup, nuts, cream, etc.

banausic /bə'nɒsɪk/ *adj* merely mechanical; mean, illiberal.

band¹ /bænd/ *n* a strip of material used for binding; a stripe; (*radio*) a range of wavelengths.

band² *n* a group of people with a common purpose; a group of musicians playing together, an orchestra; ♣ (*Cdn*) a First Nations community recognized as an administrative unit by the federal government. • *vti* to associate together for a particular purpose.

bandage /'bændɪdʒ/ *n* a strip of cloth for binding wounds and fractures. • *vt* to bind a wound.

bandanna, bandana /bæn'dænə/ *n* a large coloured handkerchief.

B and B, B & B *abbr* = bed and breakfast; ♣ (*Cdn*) bilingualism and biculturalism.

bandbox *n* a light box of pasteboard, etc, for holding collars or hats.

bandeau /'bændoː/ or /-'doː/ *n* (*pl* **bandeaux**) a band for the hair; a fitting band inside a hat.

banderilla /ˌbændə'riːjə/ or /-'riːljə/ *n* a barbed dart, used by a banderillero in bullfights to exasperate the bull.

banderillero *n* (*pl* **banderilleros**) a bullfighter's assistant.

banderole, banderol /'bændə,roːl/ *n* a long narrow flag with a cleft end; a streamer; a small flag carried at the head of a lance or mast; a scroll or band with an inscription.—*also* **bannerol**.

bandicoot /'bændɪ,kuːt/ *n* a large rat, native to India and Sri Lanka, very destructive to rice fields and gardens; the name given to rat-like marsupials of several species found in Australia and Tasmania.

bandit /'bændɪt/ *n* (*pl* **bandits, banditti**) a robber.—**banditry** *n*.

bandmaster /'bænd,mæstər/ *n* the conductor of a musical, *esp* brass, band

bandoleer, bandolier /ˌbændə'liːr/ *n* a belt worn over the chest with pockets for holding ammunition.

bandore, bandora /bæn'dɑr/ or /'tændər/ *n* an ancient stringed instrument resembling a zither.—*also* **pandora, pandore**.

band saw *n* a motorized, toothed steel belt used for sawing.

bandsman /'bændzmən/ *n* (*pl* **bandsmen**) a player in a musical, *esp* brass, band.

bandstand /'bænd,stænd/ *n* a platform for a musical band.

bandwagon /'bænd,wægən/ *n* a wagon for carrying a band in a parade; a movement, idea, etc that is (thought to be) heading for success.

bandwidth /'bændwɪdθ/ *n* the range of frequencies within a given waveband for radio or other types of transmission.

bandy¹ /'bændi/ *vt* (**bandying, bandied**) to pass to and fro; (*often with* about) (*rumours, etc*) to spread freely; to exchange words, *esp* angrily.

bandy² *adj* (**bandier, bandiest**) having legs curved outwards at the knee.

bandy-legged /-legɪd/ or /-legd/ *adj* bandy.

bane /beɪn/ *n* a person causing distress or misery; something bringing destruction or death; a poison.—**baneful** *adj*.

baneberry /'beɪn,beri/ or /-bəri/ *n* (*pl* **baneberries**) a plant of the buttercup family bearing white or red poisonous berries; its berry.—*also* **herb Christopher, cohosh**.

bang¹ /bæŋ/ *n* a hard blow; a sudden loud sound. • *vt* to hit or knock with a loud noise; (*door*) to slam. • *vi* to make a loud noise; to hit noisily or sharply. • *adv* with a bang, abruptly; successfully; (*inf*) precisely.

bang² *n* (*pl*) hair cut straight across the forehead to form a fringe; false hair so worn. • *vt* to cut the hair across the forehead to form a fringe.

bang³ *see* **bhang**.

bangbelly /'bæŋbeli/ *n* ♣ (*Cdn*) in Newfoundland, a baked or fried dumpling-like pudding, cake, or pancake.

banger /'bæŋgər/ *n* an exploding firework; (*sl*) a sausage; (*sl*) an old car.

bangle /'bæŋgəl/ *n* a bracelet worn on the arm or ankle.

banian /'bænjən/ *see* **banyan**.

banish /'bænɪʃ/ *vt* to exile from a place; to drive away; to get rid of.—**banishment** *n*.

banister /'bænɪstər/ *n* the railing or supporting balusters in a staircase.—*also* **bannister**.

banjo /'bændʒoː/ *n* (*pl* **banjos, banjoes**) a stringed musical instrument with a drum-like body and a long fretted neck.—**banjoist** *n*.

bank¹ /bæŋk/ *n* a mound or pile; the sloping side of a river; elevated ground in a lake or the sea; a row or series of objects, as of dials, switches. • *vti* to form into a mound; to cover (a fire) with fuel so that it burns more slowly; (*aircraft*) to curve or tilt sideways.

bank² *n* an institution that offers various financial services, such as the safekeeping, lending and exchanging of money; the money held by the banker or dealer in a card game; any supply or store for the future, such as a *blood bank*. • *vti* (*cheques, cash etc*) to deposit in a bank; to work as a banker.

bank account *n* money deposited in a bank and credited to the depositor.

bank bill *n* a note or a bill of exchange of a bank payable on demand or at a future specified time.

bankbook *n* a book in which a record is kept of deposits and withdrawals of money into a personal account.

bank discount *n* a deduction made according to the current rate of interest.

banker /-ər/ *n* a person who runs a bank; the keeper of the bank at a gaming table.

banker's card *see* **cheque card**.

bank holiday *n* (*Brit*) in UK, a weekday when banks are officially closed; a day observed as a public holiday.

banking /-kɪŋ/ *n* the activity or occupation of running a bank. • *adj* of or concerning a bank.

banknote *n* a promissory note issued by a bank, which serves as money.

bank rate *n* the rate at which a central bank will discount bills; ♣ (*Cdn*) the minimum interest rate set by the central bank on short-term loans to other banks.

bankrupt /'bæŋkrʌpt/ *n* a person, etc legally declared unable to pay his debts; one who becomes insolvent. • *adj* judged to be insolvent; financially ruined; devoid of resources, ideas, etc. • *vt* to make bankrupt.—**bankruptcy** *n*.

banksia /'bæŋksiə/ *n* any of an Australian genus of flowering shrubs with evergreen leaves.

banner /'bænər/ *n* a flag or ensign; a headline running across a newspaper page; a strip of cloth bearing a slogan or emblem carried between poles in a parade.

banneret /'bænərət/ or /-'ret/ *n* (*hist*) an order of knighthood conferred on the field of battle for distinguished service or a deed of valour; the person on whom the degree was conferred and who ranked between a baron and a knight.

bannerette /'bænə,ret/ *n* a little banner or flag.

bannerol /'bænə,roːl/ *see* **banderole**.

bannister /'bænɪstər/ *see* **banister**.

bannock /'bænək/ *n* (*Scot*) a thick flat cake made of oatmeal or barley and baked on a griddle; ♣ (*Cdn*) a bread made of flour, water, and fat, cooked over an outdoor fire.

banns /bænz/ *npl* public declaration of intention, *esp* in church, to marry.

banquet /'bæŋkwət/ *n* a feast; an elaborate and sometimes formal dinner in honour of a person or occasion. • *vt* (**banqueting, banqueted**) to hold a banquet.—**banqueter** *n*.

banquette /bæŋ'kɛt/ *n* a cushioned bench; a step along the inside of a parapet on which soldiers stood to fire upon the enemy; the footway of a bridge when raised above the carriageway.

banshee /'bænʃiː/ *n* (*folklore*) a female fairy whose wail portends a death in the family.

bantam /'bæntəm/ *n* a dwarf breed of domestic fowl; a small, aggressive person; (*boxing*) a bantamweight; ✹ (*Cdn*) a level of amateur sports competition for children aged 13 to 15.

bantamweight /-ˌweɪt/ *n* a boxing weight (112–118 lbs; 51–53.5 kg) between featherweight and flyweight.

banter /'bæntər/ *vt* to tease good-humouredly.—**banterer** *n*.

Bantu /'bæntuː/ *n* (*pl* **Bantu, Bantus**) one of a group of Southern African peoples or their language.

banyan /'bænjən/ *n* an Indian fig tree with vast, rooting branches.—*also* **banian.**

banzai /'bɒn'zaɪ/ or /bæn'zaɪ/ *interj* a Japanese greeting or salute.

baobab /'beɪoːˌbæb/ *n* an African tree with an enormously thick trunk.

bap /bæp/ *n* a large soft bread roll.

baptism /'bæptɪzəm/ *n* the sprinkling of water on the forehead, or complete immersion in water, as a rite of admitting a person to a Christian church; any initiating experience.—**baptismal** *adj.*—**baptismally** *adv.*

Baptist /'bæptɪst/ *n* a member of a Protestant Christian denomination holding that the true church is of believers only, who are all equal, that the only authority is the Bible, and that adult baptism by immersion is necessary.

baptistry /'bæptɪstri/, **baptistery** /'bæptɪstəri/ *n* (*pl* **baptistries, baptisteries**) the part of a church where baptism takes place.

baptize /'bæptaɪz/ or /bæp'taɪz/ *vt* to christen, to name.—**baptizer** *n*.

bar[1] /bɑr/ *n* a straight length of wood or metal; a counter where alcoholic drinks or other refreshments are served; a place with such a counter; an oblong piece, as of soap; anything that obstructs or hinders; a band or strip; a strip or bank of sand or mud near and in line with the shore or across a river or harbour; (*mil*) a badge signifying a second award; (*with cap*) barristers or lawyers collectively; the legal profession; (*mus*) a vertical line dividing a staff into measures; (*mus*) a measure. • *vt* (**barring, barred**) to secure or fasten as with a bar; to exclude or prevent; to oppose. • *prep* except for.

bar[2] *n* a unit of atmospheric pressure.

barachois /bɑrəˌʃwɒ/ ✹ (*Cdn*) in Atlantic Canada, a shallow coastal lagoon or pond created by the formation of a sand bar.

barathea /ˌbɑrə'θiə/ *n* a type of fine woollen material.

barb /bɑrb/ *n* the sharp backward point of a fish-hook, etc; one of the sharp parts combined to form barbed wire; a pointed or critical remark; a beard-like growth. • *vt* to provide with a barb.—**barbed** *adj.*

barbarian /bɑr'beriən/ *n* an uncivilized, primitive person; a cruel vicious person.—*also adj.*

barbaric /bɑr'berik/ or /bɑr'bærɪk/ *adj* of or suitable for barbarians.—**barbarically** *adv.*

barbarism /'bɑrbərɪzəm/ *n* a barbarous act; the state of being a barbarian; an expression or word that is tasteless or not standard; an object or act that offends.

barbarity /bɑr'berəti/ or /-'bærɪti/ *n* (*pl* **barbarities**) savage cruelty; a vicious act.

barbarize /'bɑrbəˌraɪz/ *vti* to make or become barbarous.

barbarous /'bɑrbərəs/ *adj* uncivilized, cruel, coarse.—**barbarously** *adv.*

Barbary ape *n* a tailless macaque monkey of North Africa and Gibraltar.

barbate /'bɑrbeɪt/ *adj* tufted, bearded.

barbecue /'bɑrbəˌkjuː/ *n* a metal frame for grilling food over an open fire; an open-air party where barbecued food is served. • *vt* (**barbecuing, barbecued**) to cook on a barbecue.

barbed wire /bɑrbd/ *n* wire with barbs at close intervals.—*also* **barbwire.**

barbel /'bɑrbəl/ *n* a freshwater fish with beard-like filaments at its mouth; such a filament.—**barbelled** *adj.*

barbell /'bɑrˌbɛl/ *n* a metal rod with weights at each end, used in weightlifting.

barber /'bɑrbər/ *n* a person who cuts hair and shaves beards.

barberry /'bɑrˌberi/ or /-bəri/ *n* (*pl* **barberries**) a thorny shrub with yellow flowers; its red berry.

barbershop /'bɑrbərˌʃɒp/ *n* the business premises of a barber.

barbet /'bɑrbət/ *n* a tropical bird with tufts of feathers at the base of the bill.

barbette /bɑr'bɛt/ *n* a raised platform for guns to fire over a parapet; a type of armoured turret in a warship.

barbican /'bɑrbɪkən/ *n* a defensive tower over the gate or drawbridge of a castle or fortification.

barbitone /'bɑrbɪtoːn/, **barbital** /'bɑrbɪˌtɒl/ *n* a habit-forming, toxic, hypnotic and sedative drug.

barbiturate /bɑr'bɪtʃʊrət/ or /-ˌreɪt/ *n* a sedative drug.

barbotte /'bɑrbət/ *n* ✹ (*Cdn*) a large catfish.

barbule /'bɑrbjuːl/ *n* a minute barb; a filament fringing the barb of a feather.

barbwire /'bɑrbˌwaɪər/ *see* **barbed wire.**

barcarole, barcarolle /'bɑrkəˌroːl/ *n* a Venetian gondolier's song; an instrumental piece resembling this.

bar code /'bɑrkoːd/ or /ˌbɑr'koːd/ *n* a striped pattern on a package, book cover, etc, containing information about the price that can be read by a computer for stock control, etc.

bard /bɑrd/ *n* a poet.—**bardic** *adj.*

bare /bɛr/ *adj* without covering; unclothed, naked; simple, unadorned; mere; without furnishings. • *vt* to uncover; to reveal.—**bareness** *n*.

bareback /'bɛrˌbæk/ *adj* on a horse with no saddle.—*also adv.*

barefaced /'bɛrfeɪst/ *adj* with the face shaven or uncovered; shameless.—**barefacedly** *adv.*

barefoot /'bɛrfʊt/, **barefooted** /-ɪd/ *adj* with the feet bare.—*also adv.*

barège, barege /bə'reɪʒ/ *n* a thin gauze-like fabric, *usu* of silk and worsted.

barehanded /'bɛrˌhændɪd/ *adj* without using weapons.

barely /'bɛrli/ *adv* openly; merely, scarcely.

bargain /'bɑrɡən/ *n* an agreement laying down the conditions of a transaction; something sold at a price favourable to the buyer; **into the bargain** as well; in addition. • *vt* to make a bargain, to haggle; (*with* **for**) to expect or hope for.

barge /bɑrdʒ/ *n* a flat-bottomed vessel, used to transport freight along rivers and canals; a large boat for excursions or pleasure trips. • *vi* to lurch clumsily; (*with* **in**) to interrupt (a conversation) rudely; (*with* **into**) to enter abruptly.

bargeboard /-bɔrd/ *n* a board placed at a gable to conceal the roof timbers.

barge couple *n* one of two beams bounding a gable, mortised and tenoned together and used for strengthening a building.

barge course *n* the tiling that projects beyond the principal rafters in a building; a wall coping constructed of bricks set on edge.

bargee /bɑr'dʒiː/ *n* the owner of or one employed on a barge; a bargeman.

barilla /bə'rɪlə/ *n* an alkali made from kinds of marine plant or seaweed.

barite /'bɛraɪt/ *see* **barytes.**

baritone /'bɛrɪˌtoːn/ or /'bæri-/ *n* the adult male voice ranging between bass and tenor; a singer with such a voice.—*also adj.*

barium /'bɛriəm/ or /'bæ-/ *n* (*chem*) a white metallic element.

barium sulphate /-ˌsɔlfeɪt/ *n* a white insoluble fine heavy powder which is opaque to X-rays, swallowed by a patient before X-ray of the alimentary canal.

bark[1] /bɑrk/ *n* the harsh or abrupt cry of a dog, wolf, etc; a similar sound, such as one made by a person. • *vi* to make a loud cry like a dog; to speak or shout sharply or angrily.

bark[2] *n* the outside covering of a tree trunk. • *vt* to remove the bark from; to scrape; to skin (the knees, etc).

bark[3] *see* **barque.**

barkentine /'bɑrkənˌtiːn/ *see* **barquentine.**

barker /'bɑrkər/ *n* one who or that which barks; a person who shouts his wares, etc, *usu* at a fairground.

barking /'bɑrkɪŋ/ *n* the process of stripping bark from trees; the process of tanning leather or dyeing with bark.

barley /'bɑrli/ *n* a grain used in making beer and whisky, and for food.

barleycorn /'bɑrliˌkɔrn/ *n* a grain of barley; (*formerly*) a measure of length, one-third of an inch (0.85 cm).

barley sugar /'bɑrliˌʃʊɡər/ *n* a transparent amber-coloured sweet.

barm /bɑrm/ *n* the froth on fermenting liquor used as leaven in breadmaking, yeast.

barmaid /'bɑrmeɪd/ *n* a female serving alcohol in a bar.

barman /'bɑrmən/ *n* (*pl* **barmen**) a man serving alcohol in a bar.

Barmecide /'bɑrmə,saɪd/, **Barmedcidal** *adj* like the Barmecide's feast in *The Arabian Nights*; imaginarily satisfying; unreal, illusory.

bar mitzvah /bɑr'mɪtzvə/ *n* (*Judaism*) the ceremony marking the thirteenth birthday of a boy, who then assumes full religious obligations; the boy himself.

barn /'bɑrn/ *n* a farm building used for storing grain, hay, etc, and sheltering animals.

barnacle /'bɑrnəkəl/ *n* a marine crustacean that attaches itself to rocks and ship bottoms.

barnacle goose *n* a wild European grey-winged goose that breeds in the Arctic.

Barnardo boy *n* ✹ (*Cdn*) (*hist*) one of the orphaned or homeless boys who were sent from Britain to Canada to serve as farm or domestic workers.

barn dance *n* a social dance featuring several dance forms (as square dancing).

barn owl *n* any of a genus of owl with brownish plumage above and white plumage below.

barn raising *n* ✹ a gathering of people who put up the framework of a neighbour's barn, often followed by a party.

barnstorm /'bɑrnstɔrm/ *vi* to tour (rural areas) as an actor, or making speeches in a political campaign, or demonstrating flying stunts.—**barnstormer** *n*.

barograph /'bærə,grɑf/ *n* a self-recording aneroid barometer.—**barographic** *adj*.

barogram /'bærə,græm/ *n* the record traced by a barograph.

barometer /bə'rɒmɪtər/ *n* an instrument for measuring atmospheric pressure and imminent changes in the weather; anything that marks change.—**barometric** *adj*.—**barometrically** *adv*.

baron /'bærən/ or /'bɛrən/ *n* a member of a rank of nobility, the lowest in the British peerage; a powerful businessman.—**baroness** *nf*.

baronage /'bærənɪdʒ/ or /'bɛr-/ *n* the whole body of barons; the dignity or rank of a baron.

baronet /'bærənət/ or /,berə'nɛt/, /bær-/ *n* the lowest hereditary title of honour in Britain.

baronetage /-ɪdʒ/ *n* the collective body of baronets; the dignity or rank of a baronet.

baronetcy /-si/ *n* (*pl* **baronetcies**) the dignity or rank of a baronet.

baronial /bə'roːnɪəl/ *adj* pertaining to or suitable for a baron.

barony /'bærəni/ *n* (*pl* **baronies**) the rank or lands of a baron; (*Scot*) a large manor; (*Ir*) a division of a county

baroque /bə'roːk/ *adj* extravagantly ornamented, *esp* in architecture and decorative art.

baroscope /'bærəskoːp/ *n* an instrument for indicating variations in the pressure of the atmosphere without actual measurement of its weight.—**baroscopic** *adj*.

barouche /bə'ruːʃ/ *n* a 19th-century roomy four-wheeled carriage for four with a folding top.

barque /bɑrk/ *n* (*poet*) a ship; a three-masted vessel with the foremast and main mast square-rigged and the mizzen fore-and-aft.—*also* **bark**.

barquentine, barquantine /'bɑrkən,tiːn/ *n* a three-masted vessel with the foremast square-rigged and the main mast and mizzen-mast fore-and-aft or schooner-rigged.—*also* **barkentine**.

barrack /'bærək/ or /'bɛr-/ *vti* to shout or protest at.—**barracker** *n*.

barracks /'bærəks/ or /'bɛr-/ *n* (*used as sing*) a building for housing soldiers.

barracuda /,berə'kuːdə/ or /'bær-/ *n* (*pl* **barracuda, barracudas**) a fierce fish with edible flesh.

barrage /bə'rɒʒ/ *n* a man-made dam across a river; heavy artillery fire; (*of protests, questions, etc*) continuous and heavy delivery.

barrage balloon /bə'rɒʒbə,luːn/ *n* a large balloon anchored to the ground and trailing cables or nets, used as a defence against low-flying enemy aircraft.

barranca /bə'rænkə/, **barranco** /-koː/ *n* (*pl* **barrancas, barrancos**) a deep mountain gully or ravine.

barratry /'bærətri/ *n* the defrauding or injury of a ship's owner, freighter or insurer by the master or crew; the practice of inciting and encouraging lawsuits or litigation.—**barrator** *n*.—**barratrous** *adj*.

barre /bɑr/ *n* a horizontal rail used for ballet practice.

barred *see* **bar**[1].

barrel /'bærəl/ or /'bɛr-/, /'bɑrəl/ *n* a cylindrical container, *usu* wooden, with bulging sides held together with hoops; the amount held by a barrel; a tubular structure, as in a gun. • *vt* (**barrelling, barrelled** *or* **barreling, barreled**) to put into barrels.

barrel-jumping *n* ✹ (*Cdn*) a sport in which a skater jumps over a line of barrels lying on their sides.

barrel organ *n* a mechanical piano or organ played by a revolving cylinder with pins that operate the keys or valves to produce sound.

barren /'bærən/ or /'bɛr-/ *adj* infertile; incapable of producing offspring; unable to bear crops; unprofitable; (*with* **of**) lacking in.

barrens /'bɛrənz/ *npl* ✹ (*Cdn*) an expanse of flat land that may support shrubs and bushes but not trees, especially (*cap*) a large treeless, sparsely populated area in northern Canada.

barricade /,bærɪ'keɪd/ or /,beri-/ *n* a barrier or blockade used in defence to block a street an obstruction. • *vt* to block with a barricade.

barrier /'bærɪər/ or /'bɛr-/ *n* anything that bars passage, prevents access, controls crowds, etc, such as a fence; obstruction; hindrance.

barrier reef *n* an exposed coral reef separated from the shore by a navigable channel.

barring /'bɑrɪŋ/ *prep* excepting; leaving out of account.

barrister /'bærɪstər/ or /'bɛr-/ *n* a qualified lawyer who has been called to the bar in England; ✹ (*Cdn*) a lawyer who pleads cases in a court of law. The term is used mainly by the Canadian legal profession as all Canadian lawyers are both barristers and solicitors.

barrister and solicitor *n* ✹ (*Cdn*) a lawyer.

barrow[1] /'bæroː/ or /'bɛr-/ *n* a wheelbarrow or hand-cart used for carrying loads.

barrow[2] *n* a prehistoric burial mound.

Barsac /'bɑrsæk/ *n* a French white wine.

bar sinister *n* (*her*) in error for **bend sinister**, the badge of illegitimacy.

Bart *abbr* = baronet.

barter /'bɑrtər/ *vt* to trade commodities or services without exchanging money. • *vi* to haggle or bargain. • *n* trade by the exchanging of commodities.—**barterer** *n*.

bartizan /'bɑrtɪzən/ or /,bɑrtɪ'zæn/ *n* an overhanging turret at the top of a tower or wall.

barytes /bə'raɪtiːz/ *n* a white crystalline mineral of great weight, consisting mainly of barium sulphate.—*also* **barite, heavy spar**.

baryon /'bærɪ,ɒn/ *n* an elementary particle (nucleon or hyperon) with a mass greater than or equal to that of the proton.

basal /'beɪsəl/ *adj* pertaining to, at or forming the base; fundamental. • *n* a basal part.—**basally** *adv*.

basalt /'bæsɒlt/ *n* hard, compact, dark-coloured igneous rock.—**basaltic** *adj*.

bascule /'bæskjuːl/ *n* a mechanical arrangement on the seesaw principle by which the lowering of one end raises the other; a kind of drawbridge so operated.

base[1] /beɪs/ *n* the bottom part of anything; the support or foundation; the fundamental principle; the centre of operations (*eg* military); (*baseball*) one of the four corners of the diamond. • *vt* to use as a basis; to found (on); (*with* **at, in**) to place, to station.—**basal** *adj*.

base[2] *adj* low in morality or honour; worthless; menial.—**basely** *adv*.—**baseness** *n*.

baseball /'beɪsbɒl/ *n* the US national game, involving two teams that score runs by hitting a ball and running round four bases arranged in a diamond shape on the playing area.

baseborn /'beɪsbɔrn/ *adj* (*arch*) of low or mean birth; illegitimate; mean.

baseless /'beɪsləs/ *adj* without a base; unfounded.

baseline /'beɪslaɪn/ *n* the line at each end of a games court marking the limit of play; (*baseball*) the line between any two consecutive bases; a measured line in a survey area from which triangulations are calculated.

baseman /-mən/ *n* (*pl* **basemen**) (*baseball*) a fielder placed at the first, second, and third bases respectively.

basement /'beɪsmənt/ *n* the part of a building that is partly or wholly below ground level.

base metal *n* any metal other than the precious metals.

bash /bæʃ/ *vt* (*inf*) to hit hard; to dent by striking. • *n* (*inf*) a heavy blow; (*inf*) a try or attempt; (*sl*) a party.

bashful /-fʊl/ *adj* easily embarrassed, shy.—**bashfully** *adv*.—**bashfulness** *n*.

bashibazouk /,bæʃɪbə'zuːk/ *n* a volunteer or irregular in the Turkish army.

BASIC /'beɪsɪk/ n (*comput*) a simple programming language: *Be-ginners' All-purpose Symbolic Instruction Code*.

basic /'beɪsɪk/ adj fundamental; simple. • n (*often pl*) a basic principle, factor, etc; the rudiments.—**basically** adv.

basicity /beɪ'sɪsɪtɪ/ n the state of being a base; (*chem*) the power of an acid to unite with one or more atoms of a base.

basic slag n the phosphates of lime and oxidized impurities left as a brittle powder in steelmaking and used as a fertilizer.

basidium /bə'sɪdɪəm/ n (*pl* **basidia**) the cell to which the spores of certain fungi are attached.—**basidial** adj.

basify /'beɪsɪfaɪ/ vt (**basifying, basified**) to convert into a base, make basic.

basil /'bæzəl/ n a plant with aromatic leaves used for seasoning food.

basilar /'bæsɪlər/, **basilary** adj (*anat*) pertaining to or situated at the base, *esp* of the skull.

basilica /bə'sɪlɪkə/ or /'bæzɪl-/ n a church with a broad nave, side aisles, and an apse; (*RC Church*) a church with special cere-monial rites.—**basilican** adj.

basilisk /'bæzɪlɪsk/ n a fabulous creature dealing death by its gaze, sometimes identified with the cockatrice; a lizard with an inflatable crest. • adj pertaining to the basilisk; penetrating or malignant.

basin /'beɪsən/ n a wide shallow container for liquid; its contents; any large hollow, often with water in it; a tract of land drained by a river.

basinet /'bæsɪnət/ n a light steel helmet of medieval times, often with a visor.

basis /'beɪsɪs/ n (*pl* **bases**) a base or foundation; a principal con-stituent; a fundamental principle or theory.

bask /bæsk/ vi to lie in sunshine or warmth; to enjoy someone's approval.

basket /'bæskət/ n a container made of interwoven cane, wood strips, etc; the hoop through which basketball players throw the ball to score.

basketball /-ˌbɔl/ n a game in which two teams compete to score by throwing the ball through an elevated net basket or hoop; this ball.

basket hilt n the hilt of a sword shaped like a basket.

basking shark n a large shark of northern seas, which is harm-less and has the habit of basking at the surface in the sun.

basque /bæsk/ n a woman's jacket with a short skirt.

Basque /bæsk/ or /bɒsk/ n one of a people inhabiting the western Pyrenees; their language.

bas-relief /ˌbɒrɪ'liːf/ or /ˌbæs-/ n a low relief; a form of relief in which the figures stand out very slightly from the ground.—*also* **basso-rilievo**.

bass[1] /bæs/ n (*mus*) the range of the lowest male voice; a singer or instrument with this range. • adj of, for or in the range of a bass.

bass[2] n (*pl* **bass**) any of numerous freshwater food and game fishes.

bass clef /beɪs/ n (*mus*) the character C placed at the beginning of the bass staff.

basset[1] /'bæsət/, **basset hound** n a smooth-haired hound with short legs.

basset[2] vi (**basseting, basseted**) (*geol*) to crop out at the sur-face. • n an outcrop.

basset horn n a tenor clarinet.

bassinet /ˌbæsə'net/ n a wickerwork or wooden cradle with a hood; a pram.

bassist /'beɪsɪst/ n a player of the double bass.

basso /'bæsoː/ n (*pl* **bassos, bassi**) one who sings bass.

bassoon /bə'suːn/ n an orchestral, deep-toned woodwind instru-ment.—**bassoonist** n.

basso profundo /-proːˈfundoː/ n (*pl* **basso profundos**) the low-est bass voice; a singer with such a voice.

basso-rilievo /-rɪ'ljeɪvoː/ n (*pl* **basso-rilievos**) a bas-relief.

bass viol /bæs/ n a large stringed instrument of the violin class for playing bass, the violoncello.

bast /bæst/ n the tough inner fibrous bark of various trees, espe-cially of the lime; rope or matting made from this bark.

basta /'bæstɒ/ *interj* enough!

bastard /'bæstərd/ n a person born of unmarried parents; (*offen-sive*) an unpleasant person; (*inf*) a person (can be positive or derogatory); (*inf*) a difficult task, situation, etc. • adj illegiti-mate (by birth); false; not genuine.—**bastardy** n.

bastardize /'bæstərdaɪz/ vt to declare illegitimate; to falsify or corrupt.—**bastardization** n.

baste[1] /beɪst/ vt to drip fat over (roasting meat, etc).

baste[2] vt to sew with long loose stitches as a temporary seam.

bastinado /ˌbæstɪ'neɪdoː/ n (*pl* **bastinadoes**) a caning of the soles of the feet as a form of torture. • vt. (**bastinadoing, bastinadoed**) to torture in this way.

bastion /'bæstɪən/ n a tower at the corner of a fortification; any strong defence; one who strongly upholds or supports a princi-ple, etc.—**bastioned** adj.

basuco /bʊ'zuːkoː/ n the dregs of cocaine after refining, which are packaged and sold in Colombia.

bat[1] /bæt/ n a wooden club used in cricket, baseball, etc; a bats-man; a paddle used in table tennis. • vb (**batting, batted**) vt to hit as with a bat. • vi to take one's turn at bat.

bat[2] n a nocturnal, mouse-like flying mammal with forelimbs modified to form wings.

bat[3] vt (**batting, batted**) (*one's eyelids*) to wink or flutter.

batch /bætʃ/ n the quantity of bread, etc produced at one time; one set, group, etc; an amount of work for processing by a com-puter in a single run.

bate /beɪt/ vt to lessen or reduce; to deduct.

bateau /bæ'toː/ or /'bætoː/ n (*pl* **bateaux**) a light boat used *esp* on Canadian rivers.

bath /bæθ/ n water for washing the body; a bathing; a bathtub; (*pl*) a building with baths for public use; a municipal swim-ming pool. • vti to give a bath to; to bathe.

bath chair n a wheeled chair for invalids.

bathe /beɪð/ vt to dampen with any liquid. • vi to have a bath; to go swimming; to become immersed.—**bather** n.

bathometer /bə'θɒmətər/ n an apparatus for measuring depths.

bathos /'beɪθɒs/ n anticlimax; descent from the elevated to the ordinary in speech or writing.

bathrobe /'bæθˌroːb/ n a loose-fitting garment of absorbent fab-ric for use after bathing or as a dressing gown.

bathroom /-ruːm/ n a room with a bath or shower and usually a lavatory and washbasin.—*also* **lavatory**.

bathtub /-tʌb/ n a *usu* fixed tub for bathing.

bathymetry /bæ'θɪmɪtrɪ/ n the art or science of sounding or of measuring sea depths.—**bathymetric** adj.—**bathymetri-cally** adv.

bathyscaphe /'bæθɪˌskæf/ n a submersible vessel for deep-sea observation and exploration.

bathysphere /-ˌsfɪːr/ n a hollow steel sphere for descending to great depths in the sea.

batik /bə'tiːk/ n a method of printing coloured designs on fabric; fabric produced by this method.

batiste /bæ'tiːst/ or /bə-/ n a kind of cambric; a fabric like cambric.

batman /'bætmən/ n (*pl* **batmen**) (*mil*) in UK, an officer's servant.

baton /bə'tɒn/ n a staff serving as a symbol of office; a thin stick used by the conductor of an orchestra to beat time; a hollow cylinder carried by each member of a relay team in succession; a policeman's truncheon.

batrachian /bə'treɪkɪən/ n one of the amphibians, which includes frogs and toads. • adj of or pertaining to frogs or toads.

batsman /'bætsmən/ n (*pl* **batsmen**) (*cricket, baseball*) the player whose turn it is to bat.

battalion /bə'tælɪən/ n an army unit consisting of three or more companies; a large group.

batten[1] /'bætən/ n a strip of wood or metal; a strip of wood put over a seam between boards. • vt to fasten or supply with battens.

batten[2] vt to make fat by rich living; to fertilize or enrich. • vi to grow or become fat; to thrive at the expense of others.

batter /'bætər/ vt to beat with repeated blows; to wear out with heavy use; to criticize strongly and at length. • vi to strike heav-ily and repeatedly. • n a mixture of flour, egg, and milk or water used in cooking.—**batterer** n.

battering ram /'bætərɪŋˌræm/ n (*hist*) a military machine for breaching the walls of besieged places, consisting of a large beam with an iron head resembling the head of a ram.

battery /'bætərɪ/ n (*pl* **batteries**) a set of heavy guns; a small unit of artillery; an electric cell that supplies current; an unlawful beating; an arrangement of hens' cages designed to increase egg laying.

battle /'bætəl/ n a combat or fight between two opposing individ-uals or armies; a contest; any struggle towards a goal. • vti to fight; to struggle.—**battler** n.

battle-axe, battle-ax /-ˌæks/ n (*pl* **battle-axes**) an old-fash-ioned two-headed axe; (*inf*) a domineering woman.

battle cruiser *n* a heavy-gunned ship with higher speed and lighter armour than a battleship.

battle cry *n* a war cry; a slogan used to rally supporters of a political campaign, etc.

battledore /'bætəl,dor/ *n* a wooden bat used in washing, baking, etc; a bat used in **battledore and shuttlecock**, a forerunner of badminton.

battlefield /'bætəl,fi:ld/ *n* the land on which a battle is fought.

battlement /-mənt/ *n* a parapet or wall with indentations, from which to shoot.

battle royal *n* (*pl* **battles royal**) a fight with many combatants; a general engagement; a melee.

battleship /-ʃɪp/ *n* a large, heavily armoured warship.

battue /bæ'tu:/ or /-'tju:/ *n* (*hunting*) the driving up of game by beaters towards the guns; wholesale slaughter.

batty /'bæti/ *adj* (**battier, battiest**) (*inf*) crazy; eccentric.—**battiness** *n*.

bauble /'bɔbəl/ *n* a showy toy; a shining ball hung on a Christmas tree as a decoration; a worthless trifle or ornament.

baud /bɔd/ *n* (*comput*) a unit used in measuring the speed of electronic data transmissions.

baulk /bɔk/ *vt* to obstruct or foil. • *vi* to stop and refuse to move and act.—*also* **balk**.

bauxite /'bɔksaɪt/ *n* aluminium ore.

bawd /bɔd/ *n* a woman who runs a brothel; a prostitute.

bawdy /'bɔdi/ *adj* (**bawdier, bawdiest**) humorously indecent; obscene, lewd.—**bawdily** *adv*.—**bawdiness** *n*.

bawl /bɔl/ *vti* to shout; to weep loudly. • *n* a loud shout; a noisy weeping.—**bawler** *n*.—**bawling** *n*.

bay[1] /beɪ/ *n* a type of laurel tree.

bay[2] *n* a wide inlet of a sea or lake; an inward bend of a shore.

bay[3] *n* an alcove or recess in a wall; a compartment used for a special purpose.

bay[4] *vti* to bark (at). • *n* the cry of a hound or a pursuing pack.— **at bay** the position of one forced to turn and fight.

bay[5] *adj* reddish brown. • *n* a horse of this colour.

bayberry /'beɪ,beri/ *n* (*pl* **bayberries**) any of various shrubs, *esp* the wax myrtle of North America; the grey waxy berry of the wax myrtle; a West Indian tree with fragrant leaves used in bay rum.

bay boat *n* ✹ in Newfoundland, a ship that carries passengers, mail and supplies to coastal communities.

bay leaf *n* the leaf of the laurel dried and used as a flavouring for food.

bayman /'beɪmən/ *n* ✹ (*Cdn*) a person who lives beside or near a bay.

bayonet /,beɪə'net/ *n* a blade for stabbing attached to the muzzle of a rifle. • *vt* (**bayoneting, bayoneted** or **bayonetting, bayonetted**) to kill or stab with a bayonet.

bayou /'baɪu:/ *n* in the southern US, the marshy inlet or outlet of a lake or river.

bay rum *n* a perfumed cosmetic obtained from the leaves of the bayberry.

bay window *n* a window projecting from the outside wall of a house.

bazaar /bə'zar/ *n* a marketplace; a street full of small shops; a benefit sale for a church, etc.

bazooka /bə'zu:kə/ *n* a portable anti-tank weapon that fires rockets from a long tube.

BBC *abbr* = British Broadcasting Corporation.

BC *abbr* = Before Christ; ✹ British Columbia.

BD *abbr* = Bachelor of Divinity.

bdellium /'dɛliəm/ *n* a fragrant gum used medicinally and as a perfume; the African and Asian tree yielding it.

be- /bi/ *prefix* all over, thoroughly, as in *bespatter*; to make, as in *bedim*; to call, as in *bedevil*; to form a transitive verb from an intrasitive, as in *bewail*.

Be (*chem symbol*) beryllium.

be /bi:/ *vi* (*pr t* **am, are, is**, *pt* **was, were**, *pp* **been**) to exist; to live; to take place.

beach /bi:tʃ/ *n* a flat, sandy shore of the sea. • *vi* to bring (a boat) up on the beach from the sea.

beachcomber /-,komər/ *n* a person who hangs about the shore on the lookout for wreckage or plunder; a long curling wave rolling in from the ocean.—**beachcombing** *n*.

beachhead /-hɛd/ *n* an area of seashore captured from the enemy by an advance force in preparation for a full-scale landing of troops and equipment.

beach music *n* a style of pop music originating on the coast of South Carolina, based on soul music and rhythm and blues.

beacon /'bi:kən/ *n* a light, *esp* on a high place, tower, etc, for warning or guiding. • *vi* to guide, to act as a beacon.

bead /bi:d/ *n* a small ball pierced for stringing; (*pl*) a string of beads (*pl*) a rosary; a bubble or droplet of liquid; the sight of a rifle.—**beaded** *adj*.

beading /-ɪŋ/ *n* moulding or edging in the form of a series of beads a wooden strip, rounded on one side, used for trimming.—*also* **beadwork**.

beadle /'bi:dəl/ *n* an officer of a parish or church; a mace-bearer; (*formerly*) an officer in a law court.

beady /'bi:di/ *adj* (**beadier, beadiest**) (*eyes*) small, round and bright, sometimes calculating or unfriendly.—**beadily** *adv*.— **bead ness** *n*.

beagle /'bi:gəl/ *n* a small hound with short legs and drooping ears.

beak /bi:k/ *n* a bird's bill; any projecting part; the nose.—**beaked** *adj*.

beaker /'bi:kər/ *n* a large drinking cup, or the amount it holds; a cylindrical vessel with a pouring lip used by chemists and pharmacists.

beam /bi:m/ *n* a long straight piece of timber or metal; the crossbar of a balance; a ship's breadth at its widest point; a slender shaft of light, etc; a radiant look, smile, etc; a steady radio or radar signal for guiding aircraft or ships. • *vt* (*light, etc*) to send out; to smile with great pleasure.

beamy /-i/ *adj* (**beamier, beamiest**) emitting rays of light; resembling a beam in size and weight; (*ship*) broad; (*inf*) having broad hips.

bean /bi:n/ *n* a plant bearing kidney-shaped seeds; a seed or pod of such a plant; any bean-like seed.

bean bag /-bæg/ *n* a small cloth bag filled with dried beans and used in games; a larger cloth bag filled with plastic granules and used for sitting on.

bean curd *n* soft cheese made from soya milk.—*also* **tofu**.

beanfeast *n* (*inf*) an annual dinner given by an employer for his employees; (*inf*) any festive meal.

bean sprout *n* the shoot of the mung bean used in Chinese cooking.

bear[1] /bɛr/ *vb* (**bearing, bore**, *pp* **borne**) *vt* to carry; to endure; to support, to sustain; to conduct (oneself); to produce or bring forth; (*with* **out**) to show to be true, confirm. • *vi* to be productive; (*with* **down**) to press or weigh down; to overwhelm; (*with* **on** *or* **upon**) to have reference to, be relevant to; (*with* **out**) to confirm the truth of; (*with* **up**) to endure with courage; (*with* **with**) to listen to patiently.

bear[2] *n* (*pl* **bears, bear**) a large mammal with coarse black, brown or white fur, short legs, strong claws and feeding mainly on fruit and insects; a gruff or ill-mannered person; a teddy bear a speculator who sells stock in anticipation of a fall in price so that he may buy them back at a lower price.

bearable /-əbəl/ *adj* endurable.—**bearably** *adv*.

bear baiting /-,beɪtɪŋ/ *n* the former sport of setting dogs to attack captive bears.

beard /bi:rd/ *n* hair covering a man's chin; similar bristles on an animal or plant. • *vt* to defy, oppose openly.—**bearded** *adj*.

beardless /'bi:rdləs/ *adj* without a beard; youthful.

bearer /'bɛrər/ *n* a person who bears or presents; a person who carries something (a coffin, etc).

bear garden *n* (*formerly*) a place where bears were kept for sport; any scene or place of tumult or disorder.

bear hug /'bɛr,həg/ *n* (*wrestling*) a hold in which the opponent's arms and chest are pinned in a tight embrace; any tight embrace.

bearing /'bɛrɪŋ/ *n* demeanour; conduct; a compass direction; (*with* **on, upon**) relevance; a machine part on which another part slides, revolves, etc; (*usu pl*) one's position, orientation.

bearing rein *n* a short fixed rein for holding up the head of a horse.—*also* **checkrein**.

bearish /'bɛrɪʃ/ *adj* resembling a bear in qualities; rude, surly.— **bearishly** *adv*.—**bearishness** *n*.

bear's breech /'bɛrz,britʃ/ *n* one of two tall plants of the acanthus genus with purple-tinged white flowers.

bearpaw /'bɛrpɔ/ *n* ✹ (*Can*) an almost circular type of snowshoe.

bear's ear /-,ɪr/ *see* **auricula**.

bearskin /'bɛrskɪn/ *n* the skin of a bear used as a garment, rug, etc; a tall furry cap worn by a guardsman in the British army.

beast /bi:st/ *n* a large, wild, four-footed animal; a brutal, vicious person; (*inf*) something difficult, an annoyance.

beastings /'biːstɪŋz/ *see* **beestings**.

beastly /'biːstli/ *adj* (**beastlier, beastliest**) (*inf*) disagreeable. • *adv* (*inf*) very (*beastly cold*).

beat /biːt/ *vb* (**beating, beaten,** *pp* **beat**) *vt* to strike, dash or pound repeatedly; to flog; to overcome or counteract; to win against, to arrive first; to find too difficult for; (*mus*) to mark (time) with a baton, etc; (*eggs, etc*) to mix by stirring vigorously; (*esp wings*) to move up and down; (*a path, way, etc*) to form by repeated trampling; (*sl*) to baffle; (*with* **up**) (*inf*) to cause grievous bodily harm to by severe and repeated blows and kicks. • *vi* to hit, pound, etc repeatedly; to throb; (*naut*) to sail against the wind. • *n* a recurrent stroke, pulsation, as in a heartbeat or clock ticking; rhythm in music or poetry; the area patrolled by a police officer.—**beatable** *adj*.

beaten /'biːtən/ *adj* defeated; (*metal*) shaped or formed by pounding; (*a path*) formed by constant trampling.

beater /'biːtər/ *n* an implement for beating, such as an attachment for an electric food mixer; one who rouses game birds from cover.

beatific /ˌbiːə'tɪfɪk/ *adj* showing great happiness; making blessed.—**beatifically** *adv*.

beatify /bi'ætɪˌfaɪ/ *vt* (**beatifying, beatified**) (*RC Church*) to declare that one who has died is among the blessed in heaven; to make blissfully happy.—**beatification** *n*.

beating /'biːtɪŋ/ *n* the act of striking or thrashing; throbbing or pulsation; a defeat.

beatitude /bi'ætɪˌtuːd/ *or* /-ˌtjuːd/ *n* blessedness; heavenly happiness; (*with cap*) (*Bible*) one of Christ's eight sayings in the Sermon on the Mount (Matthew 5).

beau *Fr.* /boʊ/ *n* (*pl* **beaus, beaux**) a woman's suitor or sweetheart.

Beaufort scale *Fr.* /'boʊfərt/ *n* an international system of indicating wind strength, from 0 (calm) to 12 (hurricane).

beau geste *Fr.* /boʊ'ʒɛst/ *n* (*pl* **beaux gestes**) a fine gesture; a gesture that appears noble but is meaningless.

beau ideal *Fr.* /ˌboʊiːdeɪ'æl/ *n* (*pl* **beaux ideals**) ideal excellence, a standard of perfection.

beaujolais *Fr.* /'boʊʒəˌleɪ/ *n* (*often with cap*) a popular fruity red or white wine from Burgundy in France.

beau monde *Fr.* /boʊ'mɒnd/ *n* the fashionable world.

beaut /bjuːt/ *adj* (*sl*) good. • *n* (*sl*) beauty.

beauteous /'bjuːtiəs/ *adj* (*poet*) beautiful.

beautician /bjuː'tɪʃən/ *n* one who works in a beauty salon offering cosmetic treatments.

beautiful /'bjuːtɪˌfʊl/ *adj* having beauty; very enjoyable.—**beautifully** *adv*.

beautify /'bjuːtɪˌfaɪ/ *vti* (**beautifying, beautified**) to make or become beautiful.—**beautification** *n*.

beauty /'bjuːti/ *n* (*pl* **beauties**) the combination of qualities in a person or object that cause delight or pleasure; a very attractive woman or girl; good looks; a very fine specimen.

beauty salon, beauty parlour, beauty shop *n* an establishment that offers cosmetic beauty treatments.

beauty sleep *n* sleep taken before midnight, supposed to be more restorative than that taken later.

beauty spot *n* a scenic location; a small birthmark or artificial patch on the cheek, regarded as a mark of beauty.

beaver[1] /'biːvər/ *n* a large semi-aquatic dam-building rodent; its fur; a hat made from beaver fur. • *vi* (*often with* **away**) to work hard (at).

beaver[2] *n* the lower or moveable part of a helmet's face guard.

beaver dam *n* ✿ a dam of mud and sticks built by beavers across a narrow body of water.

beaver fever *n* ✿ (*Cdn*) an intestinal infection leading to diarrhea, often caused by drinking water contaminated by wildlife feces.

bebop /'biːbɒp/ *see* **bop**.

becalm /bi'kɑːm/ *vt* to make calm; to make (a ship) motionless from lack of wind.—**becalmed** *adj*.

became /bi'keɪm/ *or* /bɪ-/ *see* **become**.

because /bi'kɒz/ *or* /-'kʌz/ *conj* since; for the reason that.

because of *prep* by reason of.

beccafico /ˌbɛkə'fiːkoʊ/ *n* (*pl* **beccaficos**) a small bird of the warbler family, eaten as a delicacy in Italy.

béchamel sauce /ˌbeɪʃə'mɛl/ *n* a thick, rich white sauce.

bêche-de-mer /ˌbɛʃdə'mɛr/ *n* (*pl* **bêches-de-mer**) the trepang, a sea slug dried and eaten as a food in China; a form of pidgin English used in the islands of the Pacific.—*also* **beach-la-mar**.

beck[1] /bɛk/ *n* a wave or nod with the finger or head.

beck[2] *n* a brook, a mountain stream.

becket /'bɛkət/ *n* (*naut*) a rope loop, a hook, or a bracket for securing sails, tackle, etc.

beckon /'bɛkən/ *vti* to summon by a gesture.—**beckoner** *n*.—**beckoning** *adj*.

becloud /bi'klaʊd/ *or* /bɪ-/ *vt* to obscure by clouds, to dim.

become /bi'kʌm/ *vb* (**becoming, became,** *pp* **become**) *vi* to come or grow to be. • *vt* to be suitable for.

becoming /-ɪŋ/ *adj* appropriate; seemly; suitable to the wearer.—**becomingly** *adv*.

becquerel /'bɛkəˌrɛl/ *n* the SI unit of radiation activity.

bed /bɛd/ *n* a piece of furniture for sleeping on; the mattress and covers for this; a plot of soil where plants are raised; the bottom of a river, lake, etc; any flat surface used as a foundation; a stratum. • *vt* (**bedding, bedded**) to put to bed; to embed; to plant in a bed of earth; to arrange in layers.

BEd *abbr* = Bachelor of Education.

bed and breakfast /bɛd ənd 'brɛkfəst/ *n* overnight accommodation and breakfast the following morning, as offered in hotels and guesthouses, etc.—**bed-and-breakfast** *adj*.

bedaub /bi'dɒb/ *vt* to smear all over.

bedbug /'bɛdˌbʌg/ *n* a bloodsucking wingless insect that infests dirty bedding.

bedchamber /-ˌtʃeɪmbər/ *n* a bedroom.

bedclothes /-kloʊðz/ *npl* sheets, blankets, etc for a bed.

bedding /-ɪŋ/ *n* bedclothes; litter (straw, etc) for animals; a bottom layer, foundation.

bedding plant *n* a young plant suitable for a garden bed.

bedeck /bi'dɛk/ *vt* to cover with finery, to adorn.

bedevil /bi'dɛvəl/ *vt* (**bedevilling, bedevilled** *or* **bedeviling, bedevilled**) to plague or bewilder.—**bedevilment** *n*.

bedew /bi'duː/ *or* /-'djuː/ *vt* to moisten, to sprinkle.

bedfellow /'bɛdˌfɛloʊ/ *n* a sharer of a bed; an associate, ally, etc, *esp* a temporary one.

bedim /bi'dɪm/ *vt* (**bedimming, bedimmed**) to make dim.

bedizen /bi'daɪzən/ *or* /-'dɪzən/ *vt* to adorn or dress gaudily.—**bedizenment** *n*.

bedlam /'bɛdləm/ *n* (*arch*) a madhouse; uproar.

Bedouin /'beduːɪn/ *n* (*pl* **Bedouins, Bedouin**) an Arab desert nomad; a gypsy.

bedpan /'bɛdpæn/ *n* a vessel used as a lavatory by a bedridden person; a warming pan.

bedplate /-pleɪt/ *n* the base plate or frame or platform on which a machine is fixed.

bedraggle /bi'drægəl/ *or* /bɪ-/ *vt* to make untidy or dirty by dragging in the wet or dirt.—**bedraggled** *adj*.

bedridden /'bɛdˌrɪdən/ *adj* confined to bed through illness.

bedrock /-rɒk/ *n* solid rock underlying soil, etc; the base or bottom; fundamentals.

bedroom /-ruːm/ *n* a room for sleeping in. • *adj* suggestive of sexual relations; (*area, suburb, etc*) inhabited by commuters.

bedside /-saɪd/ *n* the space beside a bed. • *adj* situated or conducted at the bedside; suitable for someone bedridden.

bedsitter, bedsit, bedsitting room *n* a single room with sleeping and cooking facilities.

bedsore /-sɔr/ *n* an ulcerous sore caused by pressure, common in bedridden persons.

bedspread /-sprɛd/ *n* a covering for a bed, *usu* decorative.

bedstead /-stɛd/ *n* a frame for the spring and mattress of a bed.

bedstraw /-strɔ/ *n* a plant of the madder family used formerly as straw for stuffing beds.

bee[1] /biː/ *n* a social, stinging four-winged insect that is often kept in hives to make honey; any of numerous insects that also feed on pollen and nectar and are related to wasps.

bee[2] /biː/ *n* a social meeting for work on behalf of a neighbour or a charitable object.

bee[3] /biː/ *n* (*naut*) strips of wood bolted each side of a bowsprit, through which the fore topmast stays are reeved.

beebread /-ˌbrɛd/ *n* a brown bitter substance consisting of the pollen of flowers collected and stored by bees as food for larvae.

beech /biːtʃ/ *n* a tree with smooth silvery-grey bark; its wood.

beechmast /'biːtʃmæst/ *n* beechnuts collectively.

beechnut /-nʌt/ *n* the triangular nut of the beech, which yields an oil.

bee-eater *n* any of the numerous species of bee-eating birds.

beef /biːf/ *n* (*pl* **beefs**) the meat of a full-grown cow, steer, etc; (*inf*) muscular strength; (*inf*) a complaint, grudge; (*pl* **beeves**) cows, ox, steers, etc bred for their meat. • *vt* (*with* **up**) to add weight, strength or power to.

beefburger *n* a flat grilled or fried cake of minced beef.
beefcake /-keɪk/ *n* (*sl*) muscular men displayed provocatively, *esp* in photographs.
beefeater /-ˌiːtər/ *n* an eater of beef; (*inf*) in UK, a yeoman of the royal guard, attending the sovereign on state occasions.
beef tea *n* stewed beef juice.
beefy /ˈbiːfi/ *adj* (**beefier, beefiest**) brawny, muscular.
beehive /ˈbiːhaɪv/ *n* a container for keeping honeybees; a scene of crowded activity.
beekeeper /-ˌkiːpər/ *n* one who keeps bees for producing honey.—**beekeeping** *n*.
beeline /-laɪn/ *n* the straight course pursued by a bee returning laden to the hive; a direct line or course.
Beelzebub /biˈelzəˌbʌb/ *n* the devil, Satan; a fallen angel, next in power to Satan.
bee moth *n* a moth that lays its eggs in beehives, and whose larvae feed upon the wax.
been /biːn/ *see* **be**.
beep /biːp/ *n* the brief, high-pitched sound of a horn or electronic signal. • *vti* to make or cause to make this sound.
beer /biːr/ *n* an alcoholic drink made from malt, sugar, hops and water fermented with yeast.
beer parlour *n* ✲ (*Cdn*) a room in a hotel or tavern where beer is sold and consumed.
beery /ˈbiːri/ *adj* (**beerier, beeriest**) smelling or tasting of beer.
beestings /ˈbiːstɪŋz/ *npl* the first milk given by a cow after calving.—*also* **biestings, beastings**.
beeswax /ˈbiːzwæks/ *n* wax secreted by bees, refined and used for polishing.
beeswing /-wɪŋ/ *n* a gauze-like crust that occurs in port and some other wines, indicative of age.
beet /biːt/ *n* a red, edible root used as a vegetable, in salads, etc; a source of sugar.
beetle[1] /ˈbiːtəl/ *n* any of an order of insects having hard wing covers.
beetle[2] *n* a heavy wooden mallet for driving wedges, etc; a club for beating linen, etc, in washing. • *vt* to use a beetle on; to beat with a heavy wooden mallet.
beetle[3] *vi* to be prominent; to jut out, overhang, as a cliff.—**beetling** *adj*.
beetroot /ˈbiːtruːt/ *n* (*pl* **beetroot**) the fleshy root of beet used as a vegetable, in salads, etc.—*also* **red beet**.
beeves /biːvz/ *see* **beef**.
beezer /ˈbiːzər/ *n* (*sl*) a fellow; (*sl*) a nose.
befall /biˈfɔl/ *vti* (**befalling, befell,** *pp* **befallen**) to happen or occur to.
befit /biˈfit/ *vt* (**befitting, befitted**) to be suitable or appropriate for; to be right for.—**befitting** *y adv*.
befog /biˈfɒg/ *vt* (**befogging, befogged**) to involve in a fog, to confuse.
befool /biˈfuːl/ *vt* to make a fool of.
before /biˈfɔr/ *prep* ahead of; in front of; in the presence of; preceding in space or time; in preference to; rather than. • *adv* beforehand; previously; until now. • *conj* earlier than the time that; rather than.
beforehand /-hænd/ *adv* ahead of time; in anticipation.
befoul /biˈfaʊl/ *vt* to make foul, to soil.—**befouler** *n*.—**befoulment** *n*.
befriend /biˈfrend/ *vt* to be a friend to, to favour.
befuddle /biˈfʌdəl/ *vt* to confuse, stupefy, often with drink.
beg /beg/ *vti* (**begging, begged**) to ask for money or food; to ask earnestly; to implore.
began /biˈgæn/ *see* **begin**.
beget /biˈget/ *vt* (**begetting, begot** *or* **begat,** *pp* **begotten** *or* **begot**) to become the father of; to cause.—**begetter** *n*.
beggar /ˈbegər/ *n* a person who begs or who lives by begging; a pauper; (*inf*) a person. • *vt* to reduce to poverty; (*description*) to render inadequate.
beggarly /-li/ *adj* like, or in the condition of, a beggar; poor; mean, contemptible.—**beggarliness** *n*.
beggary /ˈbegəri/ *n* the state of a beggar; extreme poverty; beggars collectively.
begin /biˈgɪn/ *vti* (**beginning, began,** *pp* **begun**) to start doing, acting, etc; to originate.
beginner /biˈgɪnər/ *or* /bi-/ *n* one who has just started to learn or do something; a novice.
beginning /-ɪŋ/ *n* source or origin; commencement.

begird /biˈgɜrd/ *or* /bi-/ *vt* (**begirding, begirded** *or* **begirt**) to gird round, to encompass, surround.
begone biˈgɒn/ *interj* go away! be off!
begonia /bəˈgoːnjə/ *or* /-niə/ *n* a tropical plant cultivated for its showy petalless flowers and ornamental lopsided leaves.
begorra /bəˈgɔrə/ *interj* by God.
begot /biˈgɒt/, **begotten** /-ˈkɒtən/ *see* **beget**.
begrime /biˈgraɪm/ *vt* to make grimy, to soil deeply.
begrudge /biˈgrʌdʒ/ *vt* to grudge; to envy.—**begrudgingly** *adv*.
beguile /biˈgaɪl/ *vt* (**beguiling, beguiled**) to cheat or deceive; to charm; to fascinate.—**beguilement** *n*.—**beguiler** *n*.—**beguilingly** *adv*.
beguine /biˈgiːn/ *n* a West Indian dance in bolero rhythm; the music for this.
begum /ˈbeɪgəm/ *n* a Muslim queen or lady of high rank.
begun /biˈgʌn/ *see* **begin**.
behalf /biˈhæf/ *n* **in** *or* **on behalf of** in the interest of; for.
behave /biˈheɪv/ *vti* to act in a specified way; to conduct (oneself) properly.
behaviour, behavior /biˈheɪvjər/ *n* way of behaving; conduct or action.—**behavioural, behavioral** *adj*.
behaviourism, behaviorism /-ˌɪzəm/ *n* the doctrine that human action is governed by external stimuli.—**behaviourist, behaviorist** *adj, n*.—**behaviouristic, behavioristic** *adj*.
behead /biˈhed/ *vt* to cut the head off.
beheld /biˈheld/ *see* **behold**.
behemoth /bəˈhiːmoθ/ *or* /ˈbiːəˌmoθ/ *n* (*Bible*) an enormous animal described in Job, possibly the hippopotamus.
behest /biˈhest/ *n* a command; a precept.
behind /biˈhaɪnd/ *prep* at the rear of; concealed by; later than; supporting. • *adv* in the rear; slow; late.
behindhand /-hænd/ *adj, adv* late, in arrears.
behold /biˈhoːld/ *vb* (**beholding, beheld**) *vt* to look at; to observe • *vi* to see.—**beholder** *n*.
beholden /-ən/ *adj* indebted to; bound under an obligation.
behoof /biˈhuːf/ *or* /bi-/ *n* advantage; interest; profit; use; behalf.
behove, behoove /biˈhuːv/ *vt* to be necessary or fit for, to be incumbent.
beige /beɪʒ/ *n* a very light brown.
being /ˈbiːɪŋ/ *n* life; existence; a person or thing that exists; nature or substance.
bejewel /biˈdʒuːəl/ *vt* (**bejewelling, bejewelled** *or* **bejeweling, bejeweled**) to ornament or furnish with jewels.
bel /bel/ *n* a unit equal to 10 decibels.
belabour, belabor /biˈleɪbər/ *vt* to beat soundly, to thump; to criticize severely.
belated /biˈleɪtəd/ *adj* coming late.—**belatedly** *adv*.
belay /biˈleɪ/ *vti* (**belaying, belayed**) to secure (a rope) by winding it round a spike, piton; to secure by a rope.
belch /beltʃ/ *vti* to expel gas from the stomach by the mouth; to eject violently from inside.—*also n*.
beleaguer /bəˈliːgər/ *vt* to besiege, to blockade; to harass.
belemnite /ˈbeləmˌnaɪt/ *n* a pointed fossil internal bone or shell of an extinct family of cuttlefish.
bel esprit /ˌbeleˈspriː/ *n* (*pl* **beaux esprits**) a person of wit or genius.
belfry /ˈbelfri/ *n* (*pl* **belfries**) the upper part of a tower, in which bells are hung.
Belgian /ˈbeldʒən/ *adj* of or pertaining to Belgium or its inhabitants. • *n* a native or inhabitant of Belgium.
Belial /ˈbiːliəl/ *n* a demon or devil; a fallen angel.
belie /bəˈlaɪ/ *vt* (**belying, belied**) to show to be a lie; to misrepresent; to fail to live up to (a hope, promise).—**belier** *n*.
belief /bəˈliːf/ *n* a principle or idea considered to be true; religious faith.
believe /bəˈliːv/ *vt* to accept as true; to think; to be convinced of. • *vi* to have religious faith.—**believable** *adj*.—**believer** *n*.
believing /-ɪŋ/ *adj* trustful.
belittle /biˈlɪtəl/ *vt* (*a person*) to make feel small; to disparage.—**belittlement** *n*.—**belittler** *n*.—**belittlingly** *adv*.
bell[1] /bel/ *n* a hollow metal object which rings when struck; anything bell-shaped; the sound made by a bell.
bell[2] *n* the cry of a stag in rut. • *vi* to make this cry.
belladonna /ˌbeləˈdɒnə/ *n* the deadly nightshade plant, whose flowers, leaves and stalk are poisonous.
bellbird /ˈbelbərd/ *n* an American bird whose note resembles a bell; an Australian bird with a similar call.

bell buoy *n* a buoy with a warning bell activated by wave movement.

belle /bɛl/ *n* a pretty woman or girl.

belles-lettres /bɛl'lɛtr/ *n* (*used as sing*) artistic literature, including poetry, essays, etc.—**belletrist** *n*.—**belletristic** *adj*.

bellfounder *n* a person who casts bells.—**bellfoundry** *n*.

bellhop, bellboy /'bɛlhɒp/ *n* one who carries luggage, runs errands, etc in a hotel or club.

bellicose /'bɛlɪˌkoːs/ *adj* war-like; ready to fight.—**bellicosity** *n*.

belligerent /bə'lɪdʒərənt/ *adj* at war; of war; war-like; ready to fight or quarrel.—**belligerence** *n*.—**belligerently** *adv*.

bell jar *n* a protective glass cover in the shape of a bell.

bellman /'bɛlmən/ *n* (*pl* **bellmen**) one who uses a bell for public announcement, a town crier.

bell metal *n* an alloy of copper and tin, used for the manufacture of bells.

bellow /'bɛloː/ *vi* to roar; to make an outcry. • *vt* to utter loudly. • *n* the roar of a bull; any deep roar.

bellows /'bɛloːz/ *n* (*used as pl or sing*) a device for creating and directing a stream of air by compression of its collapsible sides.

bellpull *n* a rope or handle for a bell.

bell punch *n* a punch with a signal bell used for punching tickets and checking the number of fares issued.

bellpush *n* a button that operates a bell.

bellwether /'bɛlˌwɛðər/ *n* the leading sheep of a flock with a bell round its neck.

belly /'bɛli/ *n* (*pl* **bellies**) the lower part of the body between the chest and the thighs; the abdomen; the stomach; the underside of an animal's body; the deep interior, as of a ship. • *vti* (**bellying, bellied**) to swell out; to bulge.

bellyache /-ˌeɪk/ *n* (*inf*) a pain in the stomach. • *vi* (*sl*) to complain constantly.

bellyband /-ˌbænd/ *n* a band that encircles the belly of a horse, a saddle girth.

bellybutton /-ˌbʌtən/ *n* (*inf*) the navel.

belly dance *n* a solo dance performed by a woman with sinuous, provocative movements of the belly and hips.—**belly dancer** *n*.

belly-flop /-flɒp/ *vt* (**belly-flopping, belly-flopped**) to dive in such a way that the body lands almost flat against the water.—**belly flop** *n*.

bellyful /-ˌful/ *n* (*sl*) as much as one can tolerate of something.

belong /bɪ'lɒŋ/ *vi* to have a proper place; to be related (to): (*with* **to**) to be a member; to be owned; (*inf*) to fit in socially.

belongings /-ɪŋz/ *npl* personal effects, possessions.

beloved /bə'lʌvəd/ or /-lʌvd/ *adj* dearly loved. • *n* one who is dearly loved.

below /bə'loː/ *prep* lower than; unworthy of. • *adv* in or to a lower place; south of; beneath; later (in a book, etc).

belt /bɛlt/ *n* a band of leather, etc worn around the waist; any similar encircling thing; a belt as an award for skill, *eg* in boxing, judo; a continuous moving strap passing over pulleys and so driving machinery; a distinctive region or strip; (*sl*) a hard blow. • *vt* to surround, attach with a belt; to thrash with a belt; (*sl*) to deliver a hard blow; (*sl*) to hurry; (*with* **out**) (*sl*) to sing or play loudly; (*with* **up**) (*inf*) to wear a seat belt; (*sl:often imper*) to be quiet.

Beltane /'bɛlteɪn/ *n* a Celtic festival formerly observed in Scotland on old May Day and in Ireland on June 21 by the kindling of huge bonfires.

beluga /bə'luːgə/ *n* a large sturgeon; its caviar; a white whale.

belvedere /'bɛlvəˌdiːr/ *n* a raised turret or summerhouse for viewing scenery.

bema /'biːmə/ *n* the inner part of the chancel in a Greek church; a speaker's platform; a platform in a synagogue from which services are led.

bemire /bə'maɪr/ *vt* to soil with mire; to be stuck in mud.

bemoan /bɪ'moːn/ *vti* to lament.

bemuse /bə'mjuːz/ *vt* to muddle; to preoccupy.—**bemused** *adj*.—**bemusement** *n*.

ben /bɛn/ *n* (*Scot*) a mountain.

bench /bɛntʃ/ *n* a long hard seat for two or more persons; a long table for working at; the place where judges sit in a court of law; the status of a judge; judges collectively; (*sport*) the place where reserves, etc, sit during play.

bencher /'bɛntʃər/ *n* one who sits on a bench; in UK, a senior member of an Inn of Court, one of a group that has the government of the society.

bench mark *n* a surveyor's mark for making measurements; something that serves as a standard.

bench warrant *n* a warrant issued by a court or judge for someone's arrest.

bend /bɛnd/ *vb* (**bending, bent**) *vt* to form a curve; to make crooked; to turn, *esp* from a straight line; to adapt to one's purpose, distort. • *vi* to turn, *esp* from a straight line; to yield from pressure to form a curve; (*with* **over** *or* **down**) to curve the body; to give in. • *n* a curve, turn; a bent part; (*pl: used as sing or pl*) decompression sickness in divers.—**bendable** *adj*.

bender /'bɛndər/ *n* one who or that which bends; (*sl*) a bout of drinking.

bend sinister *n* (*her*) a bar or band drawn from the upper corner of the shield at the left (sinister) to the opposite base at the right (dexter), a sign of illegitimacy.

beneath /bə'niːθ/ *prep* underneath; below; unworthy. • *adv* in a lower place; underneath.—*also adj*.

benedict /'bɛnəˌdɪkt/ *n* a newly married man, *esp* if previously a confirmed bachelor.

benedicite *n* a blessing, a grace; (*with cap*) a Christian hymn or canticle sung at morning prayer when the Te Deum is not used.

Benedictine /ˌbɛnə'dɪktiːn/ *adj* of or relating to the order of St Benedict. • *n* a monk of the Benedictine order; a kind of liqueur made from herbs and spices.

benediction /ˌbɛnə'dɪkʃən/ *n* a blessing; an invocation of a blessing, *esp* at the end of a church service.—**benedictory** *adj*.

Benedictus /ˌbɛnə'dɪktʊs/ *n* the Song of Zacharias (Luke 1) used as a canticle after the second lesson at morning prayer when the Jubilate is not sung.

benefaction /ˌbɛnə'fækʃən/ *n* the act of doing good; the money or help given.

benefactor /'bɛnəˌfæktər/ *n* a patron.—**benefactress** *nf*.

benefice /'bɛnəfɪs/ *n* a church office yielding an income to a clergyman.

beneficence /bə'nɛfəsəns/ *n* active kindness, the act of doing good; a benefaction.

beneficent /-sənt/ *adj* generous; conferring blessings.—**beneficence** *n*.—**beneficently** *adv*.

beneficial /ˌbɛnə'fɪʃəl/ *adj* advantageous.—**beneficially** *adv*.

beneficiary /ˌbɛnə'fɪʃɪeri/ *n* (*pl* **beneficiaries**) a person who receives or will receive benefit, as from a will, etc.

benefit /'bɛnəfɪt/ *n* advantage; anything contributing to improvement; (*often pl*) allowances paid by a government, insurance company, etc; a public performance, bazaar, etc, the proceeds of which are to help some person or cause. • *vb* (**benefiting, benefited**) *vt* to help. • *vi* to receive advantage.

benefit of clergy *n* a sanctioning by the church; (*hist*) exemption from trial by a secular court.

benefit society, benefit association *n* an association for mutual insurance against sickness, etc.

benevolence /bə'nɛvələns/ *n* inclination to do good; kindness; generosity; (*formerly*) a royal tax levied under the guise of a gratuity to the sovereign.—**benevolent** *adj*.—**benevolently** *adv*.

Bengali /bɛn'gɒli/ or /-gæli/ *n* a native or inhabitant of the Bengal province of India; the language spoken in Bengal. • *adj* of or pertaining to Bengal, its inhabitants or language.

Bengal light /'bɛŋgɒl/ *n* a firework used also for signals, giving a steady bright blue light.

benighted /bə'naɪtəd/ or /bɪ-/ *adj* overtaken by night; in moral darkness or ignorance.

benign /bə'naɪn/ *adj* favourable; kindly; gentle or mild; (*med*) not malignant.—**benignly** *adv*.

benignant /bə'nɪgnənt/ *adj* kind; benign.—**benignancy** *n*.

benignity /-nɪti/ *n* (*pl* **benignities**) kindliness.

benison /'bɛnɪzən/ *n* (*arch*) a benediction or blessing.

benne /'bɛni/ *n* the sesame, an Asian annual cultivated for its seeds, which yield a valuable oil.

Bennett buggy ✽ (*Cdn*) (*hist*) a motor vehicle hitched to horses or oxen, used during the economic depression of the 1930s by drivers who could not afford gasoline.

bent[1] /bɛnt/ *see* **bend**.

bent[2] *n* aptitude; inclination of the mind. • *adj* curved or crooked; (*with* **on**) strongly determined; (*sl*) dishonest.

bent[3] *n* a kind of coarse stiff grass; a withered grass stalk; a heath.

benthos /'benθɒs/ *n* the flora and fauna at the bottom of the sea; the sea bottom itself.—**benthic, benthonic** *adj*.

bentwood /'bentwʊd/ *adj* (*furniture*) made of wood that is bent and shaped by heat.

benumb /bɪ'nʌm/ *vt* to make numb.—**benumbed** *adj*.

benzene /'benziːn/ *n* a mixture of hydrocarbons from petroleum used as a solvent, in the manufacture of plastics, and as motor fuel.

benzine /'benziːn/, **benzol** /ben'zɒl/ *n* a volatile mixture of lighter hydrocarbons from petroleum, used as a solvent and as motor fuel.

benzoin /'benzoʊɪn/ *n* a resin of the benjamin tree of Sumtra, used chiefly in cosmetics, perfumes and incense.—**benzoic** *adj*.

Beothuk /bɪ'ɒθʊk/ *n* ❦ a member of an extinct Indian people of Newfoundland; the language of this people. • *adj* of or pertaining to this people or their language.

bequeath /bɪ'kwiːθ/ or /-'kwiːð/ *vt* (*property, etc*) to leave by will; to pass on to posterity.—**bequeathal** *n*.—**bequeather** *n*.

bequest /bɪ'kwest/ *n* act of bequeathing; something that is bequeathed, a legacy.

berate /bɪ'reɪt/ *vt* to scold severely.

berberine /'bɜrbərˌin/ *n* an alkaloid used in dyeing and medicine, and obtained as a bitter yellow substance from the barberry and other plants.

berceuse *Fr.* /bɛr'sœz/ *n* (*pl* **berceuses**) a cradle song; a tender or soothing musical composition.

bereave /bɪ'riːv/ *vt* to deprive (of) a loved one through death.—**bereaved** *adj*.—**bereavement** *n*.

bereft /bɪ'reft/ *adj* deprived; bereaved.

beret /bə'reɪ/ or /be-/ *n* a flat, round, brimless, soft cap.

berg /bɜrg/ *n* an iceberg.

bergamot /'bɜrgəˌmɒt/ *n* a variety of lemon, the rind of which yields a valuable oil used in perfumery; the oil of the bergamot; a variety of pear; a variety of mint; a coarse kind of tapestry.

bergschrund /'bɜrkʃrʊnt/ *n* a crevasse between a glacier and the side of its valley.

beriberi /ˌberi'beri/ *n* a disease of the nervous system, due to lack of vitamin B.

berkelium /bɜr'kiːliəm/ or /'bɜrkliːəm/ *n* a radioactive metallic element derived from americium.

berlin /bɜr'lɪn/ *n* a fine dyed knitting wool; an 18th-century four-wheeled carriage with a hood behind.

berm, berme /bɜrm/, *Fr.* /bɛrmə/ *n* a ledge between a ditch and rampart; a narrow shelf along a slope; a shoulder of a road.

Bermuda grass /bɜr'mjuːdə/ *n* a valuable variety of pasture grass.

Bermuda shorts *npl* close-fitting knee-length shorts.

Bermuda-rigged *adj* (*naut*) rigged with a high tapering mainsail.

berry /'beri/ *n* (*pl* **berries**) any small, juicy, stoneless fruit (*eg* blackberry, holly berry). • *vti* (**berrying, berried**) to bear, produce or gather berries.

berry ground *n* ❦ in Newfoundland, a high, treeless area where wild berries can be picked.

berserk /bə'zɜrk/ or /bər-/ *adj* frenzied; destructively violent.—*also adv*.

berth /bɜrθ/ *n* a place in a dock for a ship at mooring; a built-in bed, as in a ship or train; (*inf*) a job. • *vt* to put into or furnish with a berth; to moor a ship. • *vi* to occupy a berth.

bertha /'bɜrθə/ *n* a wide lace collar.

Bertillon system /'bɜrtəˌlɒn/, *Fr.* /bɛrtijõ/ *n* a method of identifying criminals by body measurements.

beryl /'berɪl/ *n* a (*usu* green) precious stone.

beryllium /bə'rɪliəm/ *n* a hard lightweight silvery-white metallic element used in making alloys.

beseech /bɪ'siːtʃ/ *vt* (**beseeching, beseeched** *or* **besought**) to implore, to entreat; to beg earnestly for.

beset /bɪ'set/ *vt* (**besetting, beset**) to surround or hem in; to attack from all sides; to harass.

besetting /-ɪŋ/ *adj* constantly harassing.

beside /bɪ'saɪd/ *prep* at, by the side of, next to; in comparison with; in addition to; aside from; **beside oneself** extremely agitated.

besides /-z/ *prep* other than; in addition; over and above. • *adv* in addition; also; except for that mentioned; moreover.

besiege /bɪ'siːdʒ/ *vt* to hem in with armed forces to close in on; to overwhelm, harass, etc.

besmear /bɪ'smɪr/ *vt* to smear with sticky stuff; to soil.

besmirch /bɪ'smɜrtʃ/ *vt* to sully; to make dirty, to soil.

besom /'biːzəm/ *n* a broom made of twigs; (*Scot*) a naughty or silly woman.

besotted /bɪ'sɒtəd/ *adj* muddled with drunkenness or infatuation; dull, stupid.—**besottedly** *adv*.

besought /bɪ'sɒt/ *see* **beseech**.

bespangle /bɪ'spæŋɡəl/ *vt* to adorn with spangles; to dot or sprinkle with something that glitters.

bespatter /bɪ'spætər/ *vt* to soil by spattering; to spot with mud; to asperse with calumny.

bespeak /bɪ'spiːk/ *vt* (**bespeaking, bespoke,** *pp* **bespoken** *or* **bespoke**) to speak for beforehand; to order or arrange in advance; to indicate, as by signs or marks.

bespoke /bɪ'spoʊk/ *adj* (*clothes*) custom-made; (*tailor*) making such clothes.

besprent /bɪ'sprent/ *adj* (*poet*) sprinkled; scattered.

besprinkle /bɪ'spriŋkəl/ *vt* to sprinkle over (with).

best /best/ *adj* (*superl* of **good**) most excellent; most suitable, desirable, etc; largest; above all others. • *n* one's utmost effort; the highest state of excellence. • *adv* (*superl* of **well**) in or to the highest degree. • *vt* to defeat, outdo.

bestial /'biːstiəl/ or /'bes-/ *adj* brutal; savage.—**bestially** *adv*.

bestiality /ˌbiːsti'æliti/ or /best-/ *n* (*pl* **bestialities**) brutal or brutish behaviour; a brutal or savage action or practice; sexual intercourse by a person with an animal.

bestialize /'biːstiəlˌaɪz/ or /best-/ *vt* to make like a beast; to degrade to the level of a brute.

bestiary /'biːstiˌeri/ or /best-/ *n* (*pl* **bestiaries**) a medieval treatise on beasts.

bestir /bɪ'stɜr/ *vt* (**bestirring, bestirred**) to put into brisk or vigorous action; to rouse, exert (oneself).

best man *n* the principal attendant of the bridegroom at a wedding.

bestow /bɪ'stoʊ/ *vt* to present as a gift or honour.—**bestowal** *n*.—**bestower** *n*.

bestrew /bɪ'struː/ *vt* (**bestrewing, bestrewed,** *pp* **bestrewed** *or* **bestrewn**) to strew or scatter over; to lie scattered over.

bestride /bɪ'straɪd/ *vt* (**bestriding, bestrode,** *pp* **bestridden**) to stand, sit on or mount with the legs astride.

best seller /ˌbest'selər/ *n* a book or other commodity that sells in vast numbers; the author of such a book.—**best-selling** *adj*.

bet /bet/ *n* a wager or stake; the thing or sum staked; a person or thing likely to bring about a desired result; (*inf*) belief, opinion. • *vti* (**betting, bet** *or* **betted**) to declare as in a bet; to stake (money, etc) in a bet (with someone).

beta /'beɪtə/ *n* the second letter of the Greek alphabet; (*astron*) the second star in a constellation; (*chem*) the second of two or more isomerous modifications of the same compound; (*biol*) the second subspecies or permanent variety of a species.

beta blocker *n* a drug that subdues cardiac activity, used in the treatment of high blood pressure.

betake /bɪ'teɪk/ *vt* (**betaking, betook,** *pp* **betaken**) to have recourse (to), to resort; to take oneself (to), to go.

beta particle *n* an electron or positron ejected from the nucleus of an atom during radioactive disintegration.

beta ray *n* a stream of penetrating rays emitted by radioactive substances.

beta wave *n* an electrical rhythm of the brain associated with normal waking consciousness.

betel /'biːtəl/ *n* an Asian pepper, the leaves of which are mixed with betel nuts and chewed as a stimulant or narcotic.

bête noir /ˌbeɪt'nwɑr/, *Fr.* /bɛt'nwɑr/ *n* (*pl* **bêtes noires**) pet hate.

betel nut *n* the seed of the betel palm.

betel palm *n* a palm tree of tropical Asia with feathery leaves and scarlet or orange fruit.

bethel /'beθəl/ *n* a hallowed spot; a seamen's church; in UK, a nonconformist chapel.

betide /bɪ'taɪd/ *vt* to happen to, to befall. • *vi* to come to pass.

betimes /bɪ'taɪmz/ *adv* (*arch*) in good time; before it is too late; early, soon.

bêtise /beɪ'tiːz/ *n* folly; an ill-chosen remark.

betoken /bɪ'toʊkən/ *vt* to signify, to indicate by signs; to augur, to foreshadow.

betony /'betəni/ *n* (*pl* **betonies**) a purple-flowered woodland plant formerly used in medicine and as a dye.

betook *see* **betake**.

betray /bɪ'treɪ/ or /bɪ-/ *vt* to aid an enemy; to expose treacherously; to be a traitor to; to reveal unknowingly.—**betrayal** *n*.—**betrayer** *n*.

betroth /bɪ'troʊð/ *vt* to promise in marriage.

betrothal /-əl/ *n* the state of being engaged to marry; a mutual promise for future marriage made between a man and a woman.

betrothed /bɪ'troːð̩d/ or /-ðəd/ *adj* affianced, engaged to be married. • *n* a fiancé or fiancée.

better[1] /'bɛtər/ *adj* (*compar of* **good**) more excellent; more suitable; improved in health; larger. • *adv* (*compar of* **well**) in a more excellent manner; in a higher degree; more. • *n* a person superior in position, etc; a more excellent thing, condition, etc. • *vt* to outdo; to surpass.

better[2] *n* someone who bets.

betterment /-mənt/ *n* an improvement.

between /bɪ'twiːn/ *prep* the space, time, etc separating (two things); (*bond, etc*) connecting from one or the other.

betweentimes /-ˌtaɪmz/, **betweenwhiles** /-hwaɪlz/ *adv* at or during intervals.

betwixt /bɪ'twɪkst/ *prep* between; in the space that separates.

bevel /'bɛvəl/ *n* an angle other than a right angle; the inclination that one surface makes with another when not at right angles; a tool for setting of angles. • *vb* (**bevelling, bevelled** *or* **beveling, beveled**) *vt* to cut on the slant. • *vi* to slant or incline.

bevel gear *n* a gear in which the axis or shaft of the driving wheel forms an angle with the shaft of the wheel driven.

beverage /'bɛvərɪdʒ/ *n* a drink, *esp* one other than water.

beverage room *n* ✦ (*Cdn*) a bar or other establishment where alcoholic drinks are sold and consumed.

bevy /'bɛvi/ *n* (*pl* **bevies**) a flock of quails; a large group (*esp* of girls).

bewail /bɪ'weɪl/ *vt* to mourn or weep aloud for, to lament. • *vi* to express grief.—**bewailer** *n*.—**bewailing** *n*.

beware /bɪ'wɛr/ *vti* to be wary or careful (of).

bewilder /bɪ'wɪldər/ *vt* to perplex; to confuse hopelessly.—**bewilderingly** *adv*.—**bewilderment** *n*.

bewitch /bɪ'wɪtʃ/ *vt* to cast a spell over; to fascinate or enchant.

bewitching /-ɪŋ/ *adj* fascinating, enchanting, captivating, alluring.—**bewitchingly** *adv*.

bey /beɪ/ *n* a Turkish title of respect; a title similar to Mr; (*formerly*) a governor of a province or district in the Turkish dominions.

beyond /bɪ'jɒnd/ *prep* further on than; past; later than; outside the reach of (*beyond help*). • *adv* further away. • *n* (*with* **the**) life after death.

bezant /'bɛzənt/ or /bɪ'zænt/ *n* a gold coin of Byzantium or Constantinople, issued in the Middle Ages and current in Europe until the fall of the Eastern Empire, 1472; (*her*) a small circle of gold representing the coin.

bezel /'bɛzəl/ *n* the sloping edge of a chisel; the rim that holds a gem in its setting; the groove in which the glass of a watch is fitted.

bezique /bə'ziːk/ *n* a game of cards for two, three, and four persons using two decks of cards with sixes and cards below omitted.

bezoar /'biːˌzɔr/ or /'biːzoˌɑr/ *n* a calcareous concretion found in the intestines of certain animals.

BGen *abbr* = ✦ (*Cdn*) Brigadier General.

bhang /bæŋ/ *n* the dried leaves of Indian hemp, chewed or smoked as an intoxicant or narcotic, hashish.—*also* **bang**.

bhp *abbr* = brake horsepower.

Bi (*chem symbol*) bismuth.

bi- /baɪ/ *prefix* having two; doubly; happening twice during; every two; using two or both; joining or involving two; having twice the amount of acid or base.

BIA *abbr* ✦ (*Cdn*) = Business Improvement Association.

bi and bi *abbr* ✦ (*Cdn*) = bilingualism and biculturalism.

biannual /baɪ'ænjuəl/ *adj* occurring twice a year.—**biannually** *adv*.

bias /'baɪəs/ *n* a slanting or diagonal line, cut or sewn across the grain in cloth; a weight inside a bowl in a game of bowls slanting its course when rolled; partiality; prejudice. • *vt* (**biasing, biased** *or* **biassing, biassed**) to prejudice.

biathlon /baɪ'æθlɒn/ *n* (*sport*) an athletic event combining cross-country skiing and rifle shooting.

biauriculate /ˌbaɪə'rɪkjuːlɪt/, **biauricular** /-lər/ *adj* having two auricles, as the heart of the higher vertebrates; (*bot*) having two ear-like projections at the base, as a leaf.

biaxial /baɪ'æksɪəl/ *adj* having two (optic) axes.—**biaxially** *adv*.

bib[1] /bɪb/ *n* a cloth or plastic cover tied around a baby or child to prevent food spillage on clothes; the upper part of dungarees or an apron.

bib[2] *vi* (**bibbing, bibbed**) (*arch*) to drink, to tipple.

bib[3] *n* a kind of fish, whiting pout.

bibelot /'bɪbˌloː/ *n* a trinket, a knickknack.

Bible /'baɪbəl/ *n* the sacred book of the Christian Church; the Old and New Testaments; (*without cap*) an authoritative book on a particular subject.

biblical /'bɪblɪkəl/ *adj* of or referring to the Bible.—**biblically** *adv*.

Biblicist /bɪblɪsɪst/ *n* a biblical scholar; a fundamentalist.—**Biblicism** *n*.

biblio- /'bɪblioː/ or /-ə/ *prefix* book or books.

bibliography /ˌbɪbli'ɒɡrəfi/ *n* (*pl* **bibliographies**) a list of writings on a given subject or by a given author; the study of the history of books and book production. —**bibliographer** *n*.—**bibliographic** *adj*.—**bibliographical** *adj*.

bibliolatry /ˌbɪbli'ɒlətri/ *n* book worship; excessive reverence for the letter of the Bible.—**bibliolater** *n*.—**bibliolatrous** *adj*.

bibliomania /ˌbɪblio'meɪnɪə/ *n* a mania for acquiring rare and curious books.—**bibliomaniac** *adj, n*.

bibliophile, bibliophil /'bɪbliːˌfaɪl/ *n* a book lover.—**bibliophilistic** *adj*.—**bibliophism** *n*.

bibliopole /'bɪblioːˌpoːl/, **bibliopolist** /-ɪst/ *n* a bookseller, *esp* one who deals in rare works.—**bibliopolic** *adj*.—**bibliopoly** *n*.

bibliotheca /ˌbɪblio'θiːkə/ *n* (*pl* **bibliothecas, bibliothecae**) a library; a list of books.

bibulous /'bɪbjuːləs/ *adj* readily absorbing or imbibing fluids; spongy; addicted to drink.—**bibulously** *adv*.—**bibulousness** *n*.

bicameral /baɪ'kæmərəl/ *adj* (*legislature*) having two chambers.

bicarbonate /baɪ'kɑrbəneɪt/ or /-nət/ *n* sodium bicarbonate.

bicentenary /ˌbaɪsən'tenəri/ or /-'tiːnəri/ *adj* occurring every two hundred years. • *n* (*pl* **bicentenaries**) a two hundredth anniversary or its celebration.

bicentennial /ˌbaɪsen'tenɪəl/ *adj* lasting or occurring every two hundred years. • *n* a bicentenary, the two hundredth anniversary of an event, or its celebration.

bicephalous /baɪ'sefələs/, **bicephalic** /ˌbaɪsə'fælɪk/ *adj* (*biol*) two-headed.

biceps *n* /'baɪˌseps/ (*pl* **biceps, bicepses**) the muscle with two points of origin, *esp* the large muscle in the upper arm.

bichloride /baɪ'kloːraɪd/ *n* (*chem*) a compound of two or more atoms of chlorine combined with a base; dichloride.

bicipital /baɪ'sɪpətl/ *adj* (*anat*) having two heads, as a biceps muscle; dividing into two parts at either extremity.

bicker /'bɪkər/ *vi* to squabble, quarrel.—*also* **n.**—**bickerer** *n*.

bicoastal /baɪ'koːstəl/ *adj* pertaining to both the west and east coasts of the United States.

biconcave /baɪ'kɒŋkeɪv/ or /baɪ'kɒnkeɪv/ *adj* hollow on both sides.—**biconcavity** *n*.

biconvex /baɪ'kɒnveks/ *adj* rounded on both sides.

bicultural /baɪ'kʌltʃərəl/ *adj* ✦ with or involving two cultures, *esp*, in Canada, French and English.—**biculturalism** *n*.

bicorn /'baɪˌkɔrn/, **bicornuate** *adj* having two horns.

bicuspid /baɪ'kʌspɪd/ *adj* having two points or prominences.—*also* **bicuspidate**. • *n* one of the two double-pointed teeth forming the first pair of molars on either side of the jaw, above and below.

bicycle /'baɪˌsɪkəl/ *n* a vehicle consisting of a metal frame on two wheels, driven by pedals and having handlebars and a seat. • *vti* to ride or travel on a bicycle.—**bicyclist, bicycler** *n*.

bid[1] /bɪd/ *n* an offer of an amount one will pay or accept; (*cards*) a statement of the number of tricks that a player intends to win. • *vi* (**bidding, bid**) to make a bid.—**bidder** *n*.

bid[2] *vt* (**bidding, bade** *or* **bid**, *pp* **bidden** *or* **bid**) to command or ask; to summon; (*farewell, etc*) to express.

biddable /'bɪdəbəl/ *adj* docile, obedient; worth bidding on.—**biddability** *n*.—**biddably** *adv*.

bidding /-ɪŋ/ *n* an order; command; an invitation; the act of offering a price at auction.

biddy[1] /'bɪdi/ *n* (*pl* **biddies**) (*inf*) a woman, *esp* an old or meddlesome one.

biddy[2] *n* (*pl* **biddies**) (*dial*) a fowl or chicken.

bide /baɪd/ *vb* (**biding, bided** *or* **bode**) *vi* to wait; to dwell. • *vt* to endure, suffer; to wait for.

bidentate /baɪ'denˌteɪt/ *adj* having two teeth, or two tooth-like processes.

bidet /biː'deɪ/ *n* a low, bowl-shaped bathroom fixture with running water for bathing the crotch and anus.

biennial /baɪ'enɪəl/ *adj* lasting two years; occurring every two years. • *n* a plant that lasts for two years.—**biennially** *adv*.

bier /biːr/ *n* a portable framework on which a coffin is put.

biestings /'biːstɪŋz/ *see* **beestings**.

bifacial /baɪˈfeɪʃəl/ *adj* having two faces or fronts; (*leaves*) having upper and lower surfaces that are dissimilar; having opposite surfaces alike.

bifarious /baɪˈferɪəs/ *adj* (*bot*) two-fold; two-rowed; pointing in two ways.

biff /bɪf/ *n* (*sl*) a blow. • *vt* to hit, strike.

bifid /ˈbaɪˌfɪd/ *adj* divided by a deep cleft, partially divided into two.—**bifidity** *n*.—**bifidly** *adv*.

bifilar /baɪˈfɪlər/ *adj* two-threaded; fitted with two threads.—**bifilarly** *adv*.

bifocal /baɪˈfoʊkəl/ *adj* (*spectacles*) having two different focuses.

bifocals /ˈbaɪˌfoʊkəlz/ *npl* spectacles with bifocal lenses for near and distant vision.

bifoliate /baɪˈfoʊlɪeɪt/ *adj* (*bot*) having two leaves.

bifurcate /ˈbaɪfərˌkeɪt/ or /baɪˈfərkeɪt/, /-kət/ *vti* to divide into two branches.—**bifurcation** *n*.

big /bɪg/ *adj* (**bigger, biggest**) large; of great size; important; influential; grown-up; pregnant; generous; boastful.—**bigness** *n*.

bigamist /ˈbɪgəmɪst/ *n* a person guilty of bigamy.

bigamy /ˈbɪgəmi/ *n* (*pl* **bigamies**) the act of marrying a second time when one is already legally married.—**bigamous** *adj*.—**bigamously** *adv*.

big bang theory /ˈbɪgˈbæŋ/ *n* (*astron*) the theory that the universe originated in a cataclysmic explosion and is still expanding.

big brother *n* an older brother; a person who fills that protective role; (*with caps*) a ruthless and sinister dictator, corporation, etc that wields absolute power.

big business *n* large corporations and enterprises collectively, *esp* when regarded as exploitative.

big cat *see* cat.

big deal *n* an important achievement. • *interj* (*sl*) an expression of scorn or contempt.

big dipper *n* a roller coaster; (*with caps*) the seven main stars in the constellation Ursa Major.

big dry *n* a period of drought longer than normal.

Bigfoot /ˈbɪgfʊt/ *n* ♣ Sasquatch.

big game *n* large animals or fish hunted for sport; an important, *usu* risky objective.

biggin[1] /ˈbɪgɪn/ *n* a close-fitting child's hood or cap.

biggin[2] *n* a small building; a cottage.

bighead /ˈbɪgˌhɛd/ *n* (*inf*) a boastful or conceited person.—**bigheaded** *adj*.

bighorn /ˈbɪgˌhɔrn/ *n* (*pl* **bighorns, bighorn**) the wild sheep of the Rocky Mountains.

bighouse /ˈbɪgˌhaʊs/ *n* ♣ a communal dwelling used by some Indian peoples of the Pacific Northwest coast of North America; *sl* a prison.

bight /baɪt/ *n* a loop or bend of a rope, in distinction from the ends; a bend in a coastline forming an open bay; a small bay between two headlands.

bigmouth /ˈbɪgˌmaʊθ/ *n* (*inf*) a loud-mouthed, bragging or indiscreet person.

big name *n* a famous person, *esp* in entertainment.

bigot /ˈbɪgət/ *n* an intolerant person who blindly supports a particular political view or religion.—**bigoted** *adj*.

bigotry /ˈbɪgətri/ *n* (*pl* **bigotries**) the state or condition of a narrow-minded, intolerant person; blind and obstinate attachment to a particular creed, party or opinion; intolerance; fanaticism.

big screen *n* (*inf*) the cinema (industry).

big shot *n* (*inf*) an important person.

big stick *n* the threat of force.

big time /ˈbɪgˌtaɪm/ *n* the top level in any profession.

big top *n* a large circus tent.

bigwig /ˈbɪgwɪg/ *n* (*inf*) an important person.

bijou /ˈbiːʒuː/ or /biˈʒuː/ *n* (*pl* **bijoux**) a jewel; any small and elegantly finished article. • *adj* (*often derog*) small and elegant.

bijouterie /biːˈʒuːtəri/ *n* bijoux collectively, jewellery.

bijugate /ˈbaɪdʒuːˌgeɪt/, **bijugous** /-dʒuːgəs/ *adj* (*bot*) having two pairs of leaflets; having two heads in profile, one of which overlaps the other.

bike /baɪk/ *n* (*inf*) a bicycle; a motorcycle.

bikini /bɪˈkiːni/ *n* (*pl* **bikinis**) a scanty two-piece swimsuit for women.

bilabiate /baɪˈleɪbɪeɪt/ *adj* (*bot*) having two lips, as a flower.

bilateral /baɪˈlætərəl/ *adj* having two sides; affecting two parties reciprocally.—**bilaterally** *adv*.

bilberry /ˈbɪlbɛri/ *n* (*pl* **bilberries**) an edible dark-blue berry.

bilbo /ˈbɪlˌboː/ *n* (*pl* **bilboes**) a rapier or sword; (*pl*) a long bar of iron with sliding shackles for the feet and a lock at the end, formerly used as fetters.

bile /baɪl/ *n* a gall, a thick bitter fluid secreted by the liver; bad temper.

bilge /bɪldʒ/ *n* the lowest part of a ship's hull; filth that collects there.

bilge keel *n* a piece of timber secured edgeways under the bottom of a vessel to prevent heavy rolling.

bilge water *n* foul water in a ship's bilge.

bilharzia /bɪlˈhɑrtsɪə/ *n* a tropical disease caused by a parasitic worm.

biliary /ˈbɪlɪˌɛri/ or /ˈbɪljəri/ *adj* of or pertaining to the bile; conveying bile.

bilingual /baɪˈlɪŋgwəl/ or /-gjuːəl/ *adj* written in two languages; able to speak two languages.—**bilingualism** *n*.—**bilingually** *adv*.

bilious /ˈbɪljəs/ or /ˈbɪlɪəs/ *adj* suffering from or caused by disorder of the bile; peevish.—**biliously** *adv*.—**biliousness** *n*.

bilirubin /ˌbɪlɪˈruːbɪn/ *n* an orange or yellow pigment in the bile.

biliverdin /ˌbɪlɪˈvərdɪn/ *n* a green pigment in the bile, the oxidized form of bilirubin.

bilk /bɪlk/ *vt* to deceive or defraud, as by evading a payment; to leave in the lurch; (*cribbage*) to spoil the score of an opponent. • *n* a swindler; the act of spoiling the score of an opponent at cribbage.—**bilker** *n*.

bill of exchange *n* a written order to pay a certain sum of money to the person named.

bill of fare *n* a menu.

bill of health *n* a ship's certificate of health; a report on a situation or condition, *usu* favourable.

bill of lading *n* a receipt issued to a shipper by a carrier, listing the goods received for shipment.

bill of rights *n* a charter or summary of basic human rights.

bill of sale *n* a written statement transferring ownership by sale.

bill[1] /bɪl/ *n* a bird's beak.

bill[2] *n* a statement for goods supplied or services rendered, the money due for this; a list as a menu or theatre programme; a poster or handbill; a draft of a proposed law, to be discussed by a legislature; a bill of exchange; a piece of paper money; (*law*) a written declaration of charges and complaints filed. • *vt* to make out a bill of (items); to present a statement of charges to; to advertise by bills; (*a performer*) to book.

billabong /ˈbɪləˌbɒŋ/ *n* an Australian word for a pond or a stagnant pool connected to a river.

billboard /ˈbɪlˌbɔrd/ *n* a large panel designed to carry outdoor advertising; a hoarding.

billet[1] /ˈbɪlət/ *n* a written order to provide lodging for military personnel; the lodging; a position or job. • *vt* (**billeting, billeted**) to assign to lodging by billet.

billet[2] *n* a small stick or log of wood, as for fuel; (*archit*) a moulding ornament, resembling a billet of wood.

billet-doux /ˌbɪleɪˈduː/ or /ˌbɪli-/ *n* (*pl* **billets-doux**) a love letter.

bill fold /ˈbɪlˌfoʊld/ *n* a notecase or wallet.

billhook /ˈbɪlˌhʊk/ *n* a small curved cutting tool with a hooked point.

billiards /ˈbɪljərdz/ *n* a game in which hard balls are driven by a cue on a felt-covered table with raised, cushioned edges.

billing /ˈbɪlɪŋ/ *n* the order in which actors' names are listed.

billingsgate /ˈbɪlɪŋzˌgeɪt/ *n* coarse or profane language; virulent abuse.

billion /ˈbɪljən/ *n* (*pl* **billions, billion**) a thousand millions, the numeral 1 followed by 9 zeros; in UK, a million million, a trillion.—**billionaire** *n*.—**billionth** *adj, n*.

billon /ˈbɪljən/ *n* an alloy of gold and silver, with a large proportion of copper or other base metal, used in coinage of low value.

billow /ˈbɪloʊ/ *n* a large wave; any large swelling mass or surge, as of smoke. • *vi* to surge or swell in a billow.—**billowy** *adj*.

billposter /ˈbɪlˌpoʊstər/ *n* a person who pastes up bills.

billsticker /ˈbɪlˌstɪkər/ *n* a billposter.

billy /ˈbɪli/, **billycan** /-ˌkæn/ *n* (*pl* **billies, billycans**) (*Austral*) a can used as a kettle by campers.

billy-goat *n* a male goat.

bilobate /baɪˈloʊˌbeɪt/, **bilobed** /ˈbaɪloʊbd/ *adj* divided into two lobes or segments, with two lobes.

bilocular /baɪˈlɒkjuːlər/, **biloculate** /ˌbaɪlɒkjuːˈleɪt/ *adj* divided into, or containing, two cells.

biltong /'bɪltɒŋ/ n (S Africa) strips of meat, salted and dried in the sun.

bimanous /baɪ'meɪnəs/ adj (zool) having two hands.

bimbo /'bɪmbɔː/ n (pl **bimbos, bimboes**) (sl) an attractive, but brainless, young woman, often one who has an affair with a prominent person.

bimetallic /ˌbaɪmə'tælɪk/ adj of or containing two metals; of or based on bimetallism.

bimetallism /baɪ'metəlɪzəm/ n a monetary system using both gold and silver as a standard currency at a fixed relative value.— **bimetallist** n.

bimonthly /baɪ'mʌnθlɪ/ adj every two months; loosely twice a month.

bin /bɪn/ n a box or enclosed space for storing grain, coal, etc; a dustbin. • vt (**binning, binned**) to put or store in a bin; (inf) to discard, throw away.

binary /'baɪnərɪ/ or /-ɛrɪ/ adj made up of two parts; double; denoting or of a number system in which the base is two, each number being expressed by using only two digits, specifically 0 and 1.

binary star n a double star or sun whose members revolve round their common centre of gravity.

binate /'baɪ,neɪt/ adj (bot) occurring or growing in pairs.— **binately** adv.

binaural /baɪ'nɔrəl/ adj of or used with both ears; (sound) transmitted from two sources.— **binaurally** adv.

bind /baɪnd/ vb (**binding, bound**) vt to tie together, as with rope; to hold or restrain; to encircle with a belt, etc; to fasten together the pages of (a book) and protect with a cover; to obligate by duty, love, etc; (with **over**) to compel, as by oath or legal restraint; (often with **up**) to bandage. • vi to become tight or stiff; to stick together; to be obligatory; (sl) to complain. • n anything that binds; (inf) a difficult situation.

binder /'baɪndər/ n a folder for keeping loose papers together; a bookbinder; something used to bind; a sheaf-binding machine.

bindery /'baɪndərɪ/ n (pl **binderies**) a bookbinder's workshop.

binding /'baɪndɪŋ/ n the covering of a book holding the pages together.

bindweed /'baɪnd,wiːd/ n a common name for twining plants belonging to the genus Convolvulus.

bine /baɪn/ n the slender stem of a twining plant, esp hop; one of these plants.

binge /bɪndʒ/ n (inf) a heavy drinking session; immoderate indulgence in anything.

bingo /'bɪngɔː/ n a game of chance in which players cover numbers on their cards according to the number called aloud. • interj, n a cry of delight, surprise or success.

binnacle /'bɪnəkəl/ n a turret-shaped box containing a ship's compass.

binocular /baɪ'nɒkjʊlər/ or /bɪ-/ adj for or using both eyes.

binoculars /bɪ'nɒkjʊlərz/ npl a viewing device for use with both eyes, consisting of two small telescope lenses joined together.

binomial /baɪ'nɔːmɪəl/ n (math) an expression or quantity consisting of two terms connected by the sign plus (+) or minus (-). • adj consisting of two terms; pertaining to binomials; (biol) using two names, esp of classification by genus and species.— **binomially** adv.

binomial theorem n the general algebraic formula, discovered by Newton, by which any power of a binomial quantity may be found with performing the progressive multiplication.

binturong /'bɪntuːrɒŋ/ or /'bɪntjuːˌrɒn/ n a prehensile-tailed civet of India.

binucleate /baɪ'nuːkliˌeɪt/, **binucleated, binuclear** adj having two nuclei.

bio- /'baɪɔː/ prefix life.

biochemistry /-'kemɪstrɪ/ n the chemistry of living organisms.— **biochemical** adj.— **biochemist** n.

biodegradable /-dɪ'greɪdəbəl/ adj readily decomposed by bacterial action.

bioengineering /-ˌendʒɪ'niːrɪŋ/ n the application of engineering principles in the biological and medical sciences.— **bioengineer** n.

biofeedback /-'fiːd,bæk/ n the practice of monitoring and recording involuntary mental and physiological processes (eg brainwaves) in order to attempt to bring them under conscious control.

biogenesis /ˌbaɪɔː'dʒenəsɪs/ n the theory that only living matter can produce living matter; the science of life development.— **biogenetic** adj.— **biogenetically** adv.

biography /baɪ'ɒgrəfɪ/ n (pl **biographies**) an account of a person's life written by another; biographical writings in general.— **biographer** n.— **biographical** adj.

biology /baɪ'ɒlədʒɪ/ n the study of living organisms.— **biological** adj.— **biologically** adv.— **biologist** n.

biometry /baɪ'ɒmətrɪ/, **biometrics** n (used as sing) the statistics of biology or probable duration of life.— **biometric, biometrical** adj.— **biometrically** adv.— **biometrician** n.

bionics /baɪ'ɒnɪks/ n the study of electronically operated mechanical systems that function like living organisms.— **bionic** adj.

bionomics /ˌbaɪɔː'nɒmɪks/ n (used as sing) ecology.— **bionomic, bionomical** adj.— **bionomist** n.

biophysics /baɪ'ɒ:fɪzɪks/ n the application of physics to biology.— **biophysical** adj.— **biophysicist** n.

bioplasm /'baɪɔːplæzəm/ n living germinal matter, living protoplasm.— **bioplasmic** adj.

biopsy /'baɪ,ɒpsɪ/ n (n **biopsies**) the removal of parts of living tissue for medical diagnosis.

biorhythm /'baɪɔːˌrɪðəm/ n a cyclical pattern in physiological activity said to determine a person's intellectual, emotional and physical moods and behaviour.— **biorhythmic** adj.

biosphere /'baɪɔˌsfiːr/ n the regions of the earth's surface and atmosphere inhabited by living things.

biosynthesis /ˌbaɪɔː'sɪnθəsɪs/ n (pl **biosyntheses**) the formation of chemical compounds by living organisms.— **biosynthetic** adj.— **biosynthetically** adv.

biotechnology /ˌbaɪɔːtek'nɒlədʒɪ/ n the commercial and industrial application of biological processes, such as the use of microorganisms to dye cloth.

biotic /baɪ'ɒtɪk/ adj of life or specific life conditions.

biotin /'baɪətɪn/ n a factor of the vitamin B group found in liver and egg yolk.

biparous /'bɪpərəs/ adj producing two at once in time or place; (zool) producing two at a birth; (bot) having two branches.

bipartisan /baɪ'pɑrtɪzən/ adj of, representing or supported by two political parties.— **bipartisanship** n.

bipartite /baɪ'pɑrˌtaɪt/ adj having two parts; involving two.— **bipartition** n.

biped /'baɪˌped/ n an animal having two feet.— also adj.— **bipedal** adj.

bipinnate /baɪ'pɪnˌeɪt/ adj (bot) having lobes that are lobed themselves.— **bipinnately** adv.

biplane /'baɪˌpleɪn/ n an aeroplane with two sets of wings.

bipod /'baɪˌpɒd/ n a stand with two legs for supporting a weapon, etc.

bipolar /baɪ'poːlər/ adj having two poles or opposite extremities; of or affecting both the earth's poles; having or expressing two directly opposite ideas or qualities.— **bipolarity** n.

biquadratic /ˌbaɪkwɒd'rætɪk/ adj (math) pertaining to the fourth power. • n the fourth power, arising from the multiplication of a square number or quantity by itself.

birch /bɑrtʃ/ n a tree with a smooth white bark and hard wood; a bundle of birch twigs used for thrashing. • vt to flog.— **birchen** adj.

bird /bɜrd/ n any class of warm-blooded, egg-laying vertebrates with a feathered body, scaly legs, and forelimbs modified to form wings; (sl) a woman; (sl) time in prison; **for the birds** useless, worthless, unimportant; **get** or **give the bird** (inf) to boo an entertainer off the stage.

birdbrain /'bɜrd,breɪn/ n (inf) a stupid or frivolous person.— **bird-brained** adj.

bird course n ✦ (Cdn) (sl) a school or university course requiring little effort.

bird of passage n a migratory bird; a transient person.

bird of prey n a meat-eating bird (as a hawk, owl, falcon, etc) that hunts other animals for food.

birdie /'bɜrdɪ/ n (inf) a small bird; (golf) a score of one stroke under par for a hole.

birdlime /'bɜrd,laɪm/ n a viscous substance used for snaring small birds; a thing that snares. • vt to smear or trap with birdlime.

birdseed /'bɜrd,siːd/ n a mixture of seeds for feeding wild or caged birds.

bird's-eye /'bɜrdz,aɪ/ adj seen from above; dappled to resemble the eye of a bird. • n any of several plants with flowers resembling a bird's eye.

bird watcher *n* one who makes a study of birds in the wild.—**bird watching** *n*.

bireme /'baɪriːm/ *n* an ancient galley with two tiers of oars.

biretta /bɪ'retə/ *n* a square cap with three corners worn by Roman Catholic clergy.

Biro /'baɪroʊ/ *n* (*trademark*) (*pl* **Biros**) a ball-point pen.

birr /bər/ *vi* to make a whirring sound, like that of a spinning wheel. • *n* a whirring sound.

birth /bərθ/ *n* the act of being born; childbirth; the origin of something; lineage, ancestry.

birth control *n* the use of contraceptive drugs or devices to limit reproduction.

birth rate /-reɪt/ *n* the number of births per thousand of population per year.

birthday /'bərθdeɪ/ *n* the day of birth; the anniversary of the day of birth.

birthmark /'bərθmɑːrk/ *n* a patch or blemish on the body dating from birth.

birthright /-raɪt/ *n* privileges or property that a person is believed entitled to by birth.

birthstone /-stoːn/ *n* a gem symbolizing the month of one's birth.

bis /biːs/ *or* /bɪs/ *adv* twice; (*mus*) for a second time; encore.

biscuit /'bɪskət/ *n* ♣ (*Cdn*) a small baked cake made with shortening and leavened with baking powder or soda; (*Brit*) a small, flat, dry, sweet or plain cake baked from dough.—*also* **cookie**. • *adj* pale brown in colour.

bise /biːz/ *n* a piercing dry northeast wind prevalent in Switzerland.

bisect /baɪ'sekt/ *vt* to split into two equal parts; (*geom*) to divide into two equal parts.—**bisection** *n*.

bisector /-ər/ *n* a line bisecting.

bisexual /baɪ'sekʃʊəl/ *adj* sexually attracted to both sexes having the characteristics of both sexes. • *n* a person sexually attracted to both sexes.—**bisexualism, bisexuality** *n*.

bishop /'bɪʃəp/ *n* a high-ranking clergyman governing a diocese or church district; a chessman that can move in a diagonal direction.

bishopric /'bɪʃəprɪk/ *n* the office, dignity or jurisdiction of a bishop; a diocese.

bismuth /'bɪzməθ/ *n* one of the elements, a light reddish-coloured metal of brittle texture.—**bismuthal, bismuthic** *adj*.

bison /'baɪsən/ *or* /'baɪzən/ *n* (*pl* **bison**) a wild ox of Europe and America.—*also* **buffalo**.

bisque[1] /bɪsk/ *n* a thick cream soup made from shellfish.

bisque[2] *n* an unglazed white porcelain, used for statuettes, etc, biscuit porcelain.

bisque[3] *n* (*croquet, tennis, golf*) a stroke allowed to an inferior player or side.

bissextile /bɪs'sekstɪl/ *or* /-taɪl/, /-təl/ *n* a leap year. • *adj* pertaining to a leap year.

bister /'bɪstər/ *see* **bistre**.

bistort /'bɪstɔːrt/ *n* a herb with twisted roots, snakeweed.

bistoury /'bɪstuːri/ *n* (*pl* **bistouries** /-iːz/) a surgeon's knife, a scalpel.

bistre /'bɪstər/ *n* a warm brown pigment made from wood soot. • *adj* of this colour.—*also* **bister**.

bistro /'biːstroː/ *or* /'bɪstroː/ *n* (*pl* **bistros**) a small restaurant.

bisulcate /baɪ'sʌlkeɪt/ *adj* having two furrows or grooves; cloven-footed.

bisulphate, bisulfate /baɪ'sʌlfeɪt/ *n* a salt of sulphuric acid in which half of its hydrogen is replaced by a positive element.

bisulphite, bisulfite /baɪ'sʌlfaɪt/ *n* a salt of sulphurous acid, half the hydrogen of which is replaced by the base.

bit part *n* a small acting role in a play, film, etc.

bit[1] /bɪt/ *n* a small amount or piece; in US, a small coin worth one eighth of a dollar; a small part in a play, film, etc, a bit part.—**a bit** slightly, rather.

bit[2] *n* a metal mouthpiece in a bridle used for controlling a horse; a cutting or boring attachment for use in a brace, drill, etc. • *vt* (**bitting, bitted**) to put a bridle upon; to put the bit in the mouth of.

bit[3] *n* (*comput*) a unit of information in binary notation equivalent to either of two digits, 0 or 1.

bit[4] *see* **bite**.

bitch /bɪtʃ/ *n* a female dog or wolf; (*sl*) a spiteful woman; (*inf*) an unpleasant or difficult situation. • *vi* (*inf*) to grumble; to act spitefully; (*with* **up**) to make a mess of, to ruin.

bite /baɪt/ *vb* (**biting, bit**, *pp* **bitten**) *vt* to grip or tear with the teeth; to sting or puncture, as an insect; to cause to smart; to take the bait. • *vi* to press or snap the teeth (into, at, etc); (*with*

back) to stop oneself from saying something offensive, embarrassing, etc. • *n* the act of biting with the teeth; a sting or puncture by an insect.

biting /'baɪtɪŋ/ *adj* severe; critical, sarcastic.—**bitingly** *adv*.—**bitingness** *n*.

bitt /bɪt/ *n* (*usu pl*) (*naut*) a post of wood or iron to which cables are made fast. • *vt* to put round the bitts.

bitter /'bɪtər/ *adj* having an acrid or sharp taste; sorrowful; harsh; resentful; cynical; (*weather*) extremely cold.—**bitterly** *adj*.—**bitterness** *n*.

bitter end *n* final extremity.

bittern[1] /'bɪtərn/ *n* a wading bird of the heron family, with a booming cry.

bittern[2] *n* the liquid that remains after cystallization of common salt from sea water or the brine of salt springs.

bitters /'bɪtərz/ *npl* liquor in which herbs or roots are steeped.

bittersweet /'bɪtər,swiːt/ *n* the woody nightshade, the roots and leaves of which when chewed produce first a bitter then a sweet taste; a variety of apple. • *adj* simultaneously sweet and bitter; pleasantly sad.

bitty /'bɪti/ *adj* (**bittier, bittiest**) small, tiny; made up of scraps of something.

bitumen /bɪ'tjuːmən/ *or* /-tuː-/ *n* any of several substances obtained as residue in the distillation of coal tar, petroleum, etc, or occurring naturally as asphalt.—**bituminous** *adj*.

bituminize /bɪtjuːmə,naɪz/ *or* /-tuː-/ *vt* to make into or mix with bitumen.—**bituminization** *n*.

bivalent /baɪ'veɪlənt/ *adj* (*chem*) having a valency of two; (*genetics*) having two homologous chromosomes; (*logic*) having two truth values. • *n* an element, one of the atoms of which can replace two atoms of hydrogen; (*genetics*) a pair of homologous chromosomes.—**bivalency** *n*.

bivalve /'baɪ,vælv/ *n* any mollusc having two valves or shells hinged together, as a clam.—**bivalvular** *adj*.

bivouac /'bɪvə,wæk/ *n* a temporary camp, *esp* one without tents or other cover. • *vi* (**bivouacking, bivouacked**) to spend the night in a bivouac.

biweekly /baɪ'wiːkli/ *adj* every two weeks; twice a week. • *n* (*pl* **biweeklies**) a periodical published every two weeks.

bizarre bɪ'zɑːr/ *adj* odd, unusual.

Bk (*chem symbol*) berkelium.

blab /blæb/ *vti* (**blabbing, blabbed**) to reveal (a secret); to gossip. • *n* a gossip.—**blabber** *n*.

black /blæk/ *adj* of the darkest colour, like coal or soot; having dark-coloured skin and hair; without light; wicked; sad, dismal; sad sullen; angry; (*coffee, etc*) without milk. • *n* black colour; (*often with* **cap**) of the black-skinned population, *usu* of African origin; Australian Aborigine; black clothes, *esp* when worn in mourning; (*chess, draughts*) black pieces.—**in the black** without debts, in credit. • *vt* to make black; to blacken; (*shoes*) to polish with blacking; to boycott; (*with* **out**) (*lights*) to extinguish, obliterate; (*broadcast*) to prevent transmission. • *vi* (*with* **out**) to lose consciousness or vision.—**blackly** *adv*.—**blackness** *n*.

black-and-blue *adj* livid with bruises.

black and white *n* writing, print; a line drawing; a photograph not in colour. • *adj* black-and-white.

black-and-white *adj* (*film, photography*) in black and white, not colour; (*ideas, etc*) highly simplistic.

black art *n* black magic, witchcraft.

blackball /-,bɔl/ *vt* to ostracize.

black belt *n* a black belt awarded to an expert of the highest skill in judo or karate; a person who holds a black belt.

blackberry /'blæk,beri/ *or* /-bəri/ *n* (*pl* **blackberries**) a woody bush with thorny stems and berry-like fruit; its black or purple edible fruit (—*also* **bramble**). • *vt* to gather blackberries.

blackbird /-,bərd/ *n* any of various birds, the male of which is almost all black.

black blizzard *n* ♣ (*Cdn*) a dust storm of soil blown by high winds.

blackboard /-,bɔrd/ *n* a black or dark green board written on with chalk.

black book *n* a record of offenders; **in someone's black books** in disfavour; **little black book** (*sl*) an address book with names and telephone numbers of women.

black box *n* a flight recorder on an aircraft.

black bread *n* rye bread.

black bryony *n* a European climbing plant with small green flowers and poisonous red berries.

blackcap /ˈblækˌkæp/ n the popular name of several black-crested birds.

blackcock /-ˌkɒk/ n the male of the European black grouse or black game.

black comedy n a comedy with a tragic theme.

Black Death n the name given to the bubonic plague that ravaged Europe and Asia in the 14th century.

black duck n ✻ a wild duck of North America, mainly dark brown with a purple patch on its wings.

black economy n undeclared economic activity.

blacken /ˈblækən/ vt to make black; to defame.

black eye n (inf) discoloration around the eye caused by a blow; (sl) shame.

blackfish /-ˌfɪʃ/ n (pl **blackfish**, **blackfishes**) a female salmon immediately after spawning; a common name for several species of British and American fish.

black flag n the flag of a pirate with a skull and crossbones emblazoned upon it.

Blackfoot /ˈblækfʊt/ n ✻ (pl same or **Blackfeet**) a member of a First Nations or Native American people in western Canada and Montana. • adj of or pertaining to these peoples or their languages.

blackfly n (pl **blackflies**) any of various dark insects, esp a North American fly that sucks the blood of mammals.

black frost n a severe frost without a rime that damages vegetation.

blackguard /ˈblægərd/ or /-ˌɑrd/ n a villain, scoundrel.—**blackguardism** n.—**blackguardly** adj.

blackhead /ˈblækˌhed/ n a small spot or pimple clogging a pore in the skin.

black hole /ˈblækˌhoːl/ n a hypothetical, invisible region in space.

black ice /ˈblækˌaɪs/ n a thin transparent coating of ice on roads or other surfaces.

blacking /ˈblækɪŋ/ n black shoe polish.

blackish /ˈblækɪʃ/ adj rather black.—**blackishly** adv.—**blackishness** n.

blackjack (oak) n a dark shrubby oak of North America.

blackjack[1] /ˈblækˌdʒæk/ n a gambling game with cards in which players try to obtain points better than the banker's but not more than 21.—also **pontoon**, **twenty-one**, **vingt-et-un**.

blackjack[2] n a large leather vessel or drinking cup; a short leather club with a flexible handle. • vt to hit with a blackjack.

black lead n plumbago, graphite.

blackleg /-ˌleg/ n a person who takes a striker's place, a scab; a person who endeavours to obtain money by cheating at races or cards, a rook; a disease affecting sheep and cattle. • vti (**blacklegging**, **blacklegged**) to act or injure, as a blackleg.

black letter n the old English or Gothic type used in early manuscripts and the first printed books. • adj written or printed in black letter.

blacklist /-lɪst/ n a list of those censored, refused employment, regarded as suspicious politically or generally not to be trusted. • vt to put on such a list.

black magic n sorcery, witchcraft.

blackmail /ˈblækˌmeɪl/ vt to extort money by threatening to disclose discreditable facts. • n the crime of blackmailing.—**blackmailer** n.

Black Maria n a prison van, a patrol wagon.

black market n the illegal buying and selling of goods, esp banned goods, eg drugs, or when rationing is in force.—**black marketeer, black marketer** n.

black mass n a travesty of the Mass used by Satanists.

blackout /ˈblækˌaʊt/ n the darkness when all lights are switched off; temporary loss of consciousness or electricity; a breakdown of communications between a spacecraft and ground control; a closing down of radio or TV broadcasting due to strike action or government ban.

black power n a movement of black people whose goal is political, social and economic equality with whites.

black pudding n a dark sausage with a large proportion of blood.

black robe n ✻ (Cdn) (hist) a Roman Catholic priest, esp a Jesuit, who was a missionary among Indian peoples.

Black Rod n in UK, the usher belonging to the order of the Garter and the House of Lords, so called from the black rod of the office.

black sheep n a person regarded as disreputable or a disgrace by their family.

Blackshirt n a fascist, esp a member of Mussolini's Italian Fascist party.

blacksmith /ˈblækˌsmɪθ/ n a metal worker, esp one who shoes horses.

black spot n an area where traffic accidents frequently happen; a difficult or dangerous place; a disease affecting leaves, esp of roses.

blackthorn /-ˌθɔrn/ n the sloe; a walking stick cut from the stem of the sloe.

black widow n a poisonous spider found in America, the female of which devours its mate.

bladder /ˈblædər/ n a sac that fills with fluid, esp one that holds urine flowing from the kidneys; any inflatable bag.

bladderwort /-ˌwɜrt/ n any of a genus of water plants, some of which trap insects.

bladderwrack /-ˌræk/ n a type of seaweed with trailing fronds containing small air bladders.

blade /bleɪd/ n the cutting edge of a tool or knife; the broad, flat surface of a leaf; a straight, narrow leaf of grass; the flat part of an oar or paddle; the runner of an ice skate.—**bladed** adj.

blah[1] /blɒ/ n (sl) nonsense, exaggeration; a blunder.

blah[2] adj (sl) boring; mediocre.

blain /bleɪn/ n an inflamed sore, a blister.

blame /bleɪm/ vt to hold responsible for; to accuse. • n responsibility for an error; reproof.—**blamable, blameable** adj.

blameful /ˈbleɪmfʊl/ adj meriting blame; guilty.—**blamefully** adv.—**blamefulness** n.

blameless /-ləs/ adj innocent; free from blame.—**blamelessly** adv.—**blamelessness** n.

blameworthy /-ˌwɜrði/ adj deserving blame.—**blameworthiness** n.

blanch /blɑːntʃ/ vt to whiten or bleach; to make pale; (vegetables, almonds, etc) to scald. • vi to turn pale.

blancmange /bləˈmɒndʒ/ n a dessert made from gelatinous or starchy ingredients (as cornflour) and milk.

bland /blænd/ adj mild; gentle; insipid.—**blandly** adv.—**blandness** n.

blandish /ˈblændɪʃ/ vti to flatter in order to coax; to cajole.

blandishment /-mənt/ n (usu pl) a winning expression or action, an artful caress, cajolery.

blank (cartridge) n a powder-filled cartridge without a bullet.

blank /blæŋk/ adj (paper) bearing no writing or marks; vacant; (mind) empty of thought; (look) without expression; (denial, refusal) utter, complete; (cheque) signed but with no amount written in. • n an empty space, esp one to be filled out on a printed form; an empty place or time.—**blankly** adv.—**blankness** n.

blank cheque, blank check n a signed cheque with the amount left blank to be filled by the payee; complete freedom of action.

blank verse n unrhymed verse.

blanket /ˈblæŋkət/ n a large, soft piece of cloth used for warmth, esp as a bed cover; (of snow, smoke) a cover or layer. • adj applying to a wide variety of cases or situations. • vt to cover.

blanket coat n ✻ a coat made from a blanket, esp a Hudson's Bay blanket.

blare /blɛr/ vti to sound harshly or loudly. • n a loud, harsh sound.

blarney /ˈblɑrni/ n wheedling talk, flattery. • vt (**blarneying, blarneyed**) to influence or talk over by soft wheedling speeches; to humbug with flattery.

Blarney Stone n a stone in the wall of Blarney Castle, Cork, kissing which a person is said to become an adept in flattery.

blasé /blɒˈzeɪ/ or /ˈblɒzeɪ/ adj bored, indifferent; sated with pleasure.

blaspheme /blæsˈfiːm/ or /ˈblæsfiːm/ vt to speak irreverently of (God, a divine being or sacred things). • vi to utter blasphemy.—**blasphemer** n.

blasphemous /ˈblæsfəməs/ adj impious, grossly insulting (to God, etc).

blasphemy /ˈblæsfəmi/ n (pl **blasphemies**) impious speaking; speaking irreverently of God, a divine being or sacred things.

blast /blɑːst/ n a sharp gust of air; the sound of a horn; an explosion; an outburst of criticism. • vt to wither; to blow up, explode; to criticize sharply. • vi to make a loud, harsh sound; to set off explosives, etc; (with **off**) to be launched.

blasted /ˈblɑːstəd/ adj withered; (inf) damned.

blastema /blæsˈtiːmə/ n (pl **blastemas, blastemata**) (biol) the point of growth of an organ as yet unformed, from which it is developed.—**blastemal, blastemic, blastematic** adj.

blast furnace n a smelting furnace using compressed air.

blasto- /'blæsto:/ or /-tə/ *prefix* bud; germination.

blastoderm /-ˌdərm/ *n* a layer of embryonic cells in an egg from which an organism is formed.—**blastodermic** *adj*.

blastoff /'blæst͜ˌof/ *n* the launch of a space vehicle or rocket; the time when this takes place.

blastogenesis /ˌblæsto:'ʒenəsis/ *n* reproduction by budding.—**blastogenic, blastogenetic** *adj*.

blatant /'bleitənt/ *adj* noisy; glaringly conspicuous.—**blatancy** *n*.—**blatantly** *adv*.

blather /'blæðər/ *see* **blether**.

blatherskite /-ˌskait/ *n* a blethering or blustering person.

blaze[1] /bleiz/ *n* an intensive fire; a bright light; splendour; an outburst (of emotion). • *vi* to burn brightly; to shine with a brilliant light; to be excited, as with anger.

blaze[2] *n* a white mark on the face of a horse or other quadruped; a white mark cut on a tree to serve as a guide. • *vt* to mark, as trees, by removing a portion of the bark; to indicate, as a path or boundary, by blazing trees; **blaze a trail** to act as a pioneer.

blaze[3] *vt* to proclaim, to publish widely.

blazer /'bleizər/ *n* a lightweight jacket, often in a bright colour representing membership of a sports club, school, etc.

blazon /'bleizən/ *vt* to proclaim publicly; to adorn; to describe (heraldic or armorial bearings) in technical terms. • *n* the terminology of coats of arms.—**blazoner** *n*.—**blazonment** *n*.

blazonry /-ri/ *n* (*pl* **blazonries**) a heraldic device; the art of describing and explaining coats of arms; decoration, as with heraldic devices; a bright display.

bldg. *abbr* = building.

bleach /bli:tʃ/ *vti* to make or become white or colourless. • *n* a substance for bleaching.—**bleachable** *adj*.—**bleacher** *n*.

bleachers /-ərz/ *npl* the unroofed seats at a baseball field or sports ground.

bleaching powder *n* a white powder, chloride of lime, used for bleaching.

bleak[1] /bli:k/ *adj* cold; exposed; bare; harsh; gloomy; not hopeful.—**bleakly** *adv*.—**bleakness** *n*.

bleak[2] *n* (*pl* **bleak, bleaks**) a small European river fish with brilliant silvery scales.

blear /blir/ *adj* (*eyes*) sore or dim with inflammation. • *vt* to make (eyes) sore or watery; to dim or blur.

bleary /'bli:ri/ *adj* (**blearier, bleariest**) (*eyesight*) dim with water or tears; obscure, indistinct.—**blearily** *adv*.—**bleariness** *n*.

bleary-eyed /-ˌaid/ *adj* with eyes dulled by tears or tiredness; dull.

bleat /bli:t/ *vi* to cry as a sheep, goat or calf; to complain. • *n* a bleating cry or sound.—**bleater** *n*.—**bleatingly** *adv*

bleb /bleb/ *n* a small blister; a bubble in water or glass.

bleed /bli:d/ *vb* (**bleeding, bled**) *vi* to lose blood; to ooze sap, colour or dye; to die for a country or an ideal; to sympathize (often ironically). • *vt* to remove blood or sap from; (*inf*) to extort money or goods from.

bleeder /'bli:dər/ *n* one who bleeds, *esp* blood from another; (*inf*) a person with haemophilia; (*sl*) an annoying person.

bleep /bli:p/ *vi* to emit a high-pitched sound or signal (*eg* a car alarm). • *n* a small portable electronic radio receiver that emits a bleep to convey a message.—*also* **bleeper**.

blemish /'blemiʃ/ *n* a flaw or defect, as a spot. • *vt* to mar; to spoil.

blench /blentʃ/ *vi* to flinch; to blanch.

blend /blend/ *vt* (*varieties of tea, etc*) to mix or mingle; to mix so that the components cannot be distinguished. • *vi* to mix, merge; to shade gradually into each other, as colours; to harmonize. • *n* a mixture.

blende /blend/ *n* any of various minerals composed mainly of metallic sulphides; a yellow to brownish-black zinc ore, sphalerite.

blender /'blendər/ *n* something or someone that blends; an electrical device for preparing food.—*also* **liquidizer**.

blenny /'bleni/ *n* (*pl* **blennies, blenny**) a small elongated spiny-finned sea fish.

blepharitis /ˌblefə'raitis/ *n* inflammation of the eyelids.—**blepharitic** *adj*.

blesbok /'blesˌbok/ *n* (*pl* **blesboks, blesbok**) a South African white-faced antelope.

bless /bles/ *vt* (**blessing, blessed** *or* **blest**) to consecrate; to praise; to call upon God's protection; to grant happiness; to make the sign of the cross over.

blessed /'blesəd/ *or* /blest/ *adj* holy, sacred; fortunate; blissful; beatified.—**blessedly** *adv*.—**blessedness** *n*.

blessing /'blesiŋ/ *n* a prayer or wish for success or happiness; a cause of happiness; good wishes or approval; a grace said before or after eating.

blest /blest/ *see* **bless**.

blet /blet/ *n* a decayed spot in fruit.

blether /'bleðər/ *vi* (*inf*) to talk foolishly. • *n* (*inf*) foolish talk; one who talks it.—*also* **blather**.

blew /blu/ *see* **blow**[2].

blight /blait/ *n* any insect, disease, etc that destroys plants; anything that prevents growth or destroys; somone or something that spoils. • *vt* to destroy; to frustrate.

blimp /blimp/ *n* a small, nonrigid airship; any airship; a soundproof cover for a camera.

blind /blaind/ *adj* sightless; unable to discern or understand; not directed by reason; (*exit*) hidden, concealed; closed at one end. • *n* something that deceives; a shade for a window; (*sl*) a drinking bout. • *vti* to make sightless, to deprive of insight; to dazzle (with facts, a bright light, etc); to deceive.—**blindly** *adv*.—**blindness** *n*.

blind alley *n* a street closed at one end; an occupation or inquiry that leads to nothing.

blind date *n* a date between two individuals who have never met before; either individual on a blind date.

blinder /-ər/ *n* a horse's blinkers.

blindfish /-ˌfiʃ/ *n* (*pl* **blindfish, blindfishes**) a diminutive fish of a pale colour and with rudimentary eyes, which inhabits underground waters.

blindfold /-ˌfo:ld/ *n* a cloth or bandage used to cover the eyes. • *adj* having the eyes covered, so as not to see; reckless. • *vt* to cover the eyes with a strip of cloth, etc; to hamper sight or understanding; to mislead.

blind man's buff *n* a game in which a blindfold person tries to catch and identify others.

blind spot *n* a point on the retina of the eye that is insensitive to light; a place where vision is obscured; a subject on which someone is ignorant.

blindstorey, blindstory /'blaindˌstori/ *n* (*pl* **blindstoreys, blindstories**) (*archit*) the storey below the clerestory, admitting no light.

blindworm /-ˌwərm/ *n* the slowworm, a small, slender limbless lizard with very small eyes.

blini, blinis /'blini/ *npl* (*sing* **blin**) buckwheat pancakes.

blink /bliŋk/ *vi* to open and close the eyes rapidly; (*light*) to flash on and off; (*with* at) to ignore. • *vt* (*with* at) to be amazed or surprised. • *n* a glance, a glimpse; a momentary flash.

blinker /-ər/ *n* one who blinks; that which obscures the sight or mental perception; (*pl*) a screen for a horse's eye, to prevent it from seeing sideways; (*sl*) the eyes.

blip /blip/ *n* a trace on a radar screen; a recurring sound; a temporary setback. • *vi* (**blipping, blipped**) to make a blip.

bliss /blis/ *n* supreme happiness; spiritual joy.—**blissful** *adj*.—**blissfully** *adv*.

blister /'blistər/ *n* a raised patch on the skin, containing water, as caused by burning or rubbing; a raised bubble on any other surface. • *vti* to cause or form blisters; to lash with words.

blistering /'blistəriŋ/ *adj* (*criticism*) scornful, cruel.

BLit, BLitt *abbr* = Bachelor of Literature.

blithe /blaiθ/ *or* /blaið/ *adj* happy, cheerful, gay.—**blithely** *adv*.—**blitheness** *n*.

blithering /'bliðəriŋ/ *adj* (*inf*) stupid, idiotic.

blithesome /'blaiðsəm/ *or* /blaiθ-/ *adj* blithe, merry.—**blithesomely** *adv*.—**blithesomeness** *n*.

blitz /blits/ *n* heavy aerial bombing; any sudden destructive attack; a determined effort. • *vt* to subject to a blitz.

Blitzkrieg /'blitsˌkri:g/ *n* warfare in which blitz is employed; any swift combined action.

blizzard /'blizərd/ *n* a severe storm of wind and snow.

bloat /blo:t/ *vti* to swell as with water or air; to puff up, as with pride; to cure or dry (fish) in smoke.—**bloated** *adj*.

bloater /'blo:tər/ *n* a herring or mackerel smoked and partially dried, but not split open.

blob /blob/ *n* a drop of liquid; a round spot (of colour, etc).

bloc /blok/ *n* a group of parties, nations, etc united to achieve a common purpose.

block /blok/ *n* a solid piece of stone or wood, etc; a piece of wood used as a base (for chopping, etc); a group or row of buildings; a number of things as a unit; the main body of a petrol engine;

a building divided into offices; an obstruction; a child's building brick; (*sl*) the head. • *vt* to impede or obstruct; to shape; (*often with* **out**) to sketch roughly. • *vi* to obstruct an opponent in sports.—**blocker** *n*.

blockade /blɒˈkeɪd/ *n* (*mil*) the obstruction of an enemy seaport by warships; any strategic barrier. • *vt* to obstruct in this way.— **blockader** *n*.

blockage /ˈblɒkɪdʒ/ *n* an obstruction.

blockbuster /ˈblɒkˌbʌstər/ *n* (*sl*) a very heavy bomb of great penetrative power; a conspicuously powerful or effective person or thing; one who engages in blockbusting.

blockbusting /-ˌbʌstɪŋ/ *n* the practice of persuading house owners to sell their houses quickly by convincing them that property values will drop.

blockhead /ˈblɒkˌhed/ *n* a dolt, a stupid person.

block heater *n* ❧ an electric heater that is connected to the engine block of a motor vehicle and allows easier starting in cold weather.

blockhouse /ˈblɒkˌhaʊs/ *n* a small fort, *usu* of timber; a log house; a concrete fortification with loopholes for observation or firing from.

block letter *n* a handwritten capital letter similar to a printed letter.

block vote *n* at a conference, a total vote represented by one delegate.

bloke /bloʊk/ *n* (*inf*) a man.

blond, blonde /blɒnd/ *adj* having light-coloured hair and skin; light-coloured. • *n* a blond person.—**blondness, blondeness** *n*.

blonde lace *n* a silk lace.

blood /blʌd/ *n* the red fluid that circulates in the arteries and veins of animals; the sap of a plant; the essence of life; kinship; descent; hatred; anger; bloodshed; guilt of murder.

blood-and-thunder *adj* melodramatic. • *n* a sensational story or play.

blood bank *n* a place where blood is taken from blood donors and stored.

blood bath *n* a massacre.

blood brother *n* one of two men or boys pledged to treat the other as a brother, as confirmed by the ceremonial mingling of blood.

blood cell *n* a red or white cell present in the blood.

blood count *n* the determination of the numbers of red and white corpuscles in a sample of blood.

bloodcurdling /ˈblʌdˌkɜːrdlɪŋ/ *adj* exciting terror, horrifying, chilling.

blood donor *n* a person who donates his or her blood for transfusion.

blood donor clinic *n* ❧ (*Cdn*) a temporary location where people can donate blood.

blooded /ˈblʌdɪd/ *adj* having a specific kind of blood (*hot-blooded*); of fine breed; initiated.

blood group *n* any of the classes of human blood.—*also* **blood type**.

blood heat *n* the normal heat of the human blood in health (37°C, 98.4°F).

bloodhound /ˈblʌdˌhaʊnd/ *n* a large breed of hound used for tracking; a detective.

bloodless /ˈblʌdlɪs/ *adj* without blood or slaughter; unfeeling.— **bloodlessly** *adv.*—**bloodlessness** *n*.

bloodletting /ˈblʌdˌletɪŋ/ *n* phlebotomy; bloodshed, *eg* a massacre.

blood money *n* money obtained at the cost of another's life; the reward paid for the discovery or capture of a murderer; compensation paid to the next of kin of a person slain by another.

blood poisoning *n* septicaemia.

blood pressure *n* the pressure of the blood in the arterial system.

blood pudding *n* blood sausage.

blood-red /blʌdˈred/ *adj* red as blood.

blood relation, blood relative *n* a person related by descent, not marriage.

bloodroot /ˈblʌdruːt/ *n* ❧ a woodland plant of eastern North America with white flowers and a red root.

blood sausage *n* a dark sausage with a large proportion of blood.

bloodshed /ˈblʌdˌʃed/ *n* killing.

bloodshot /ˈblʌdˌʃɒt/ *adj* (*eye*) suffused with blood, red and inflamed.

blood sport *n* any sport in which an animal is hunted and killed.

bloodstain /ˈblʌdˌsteɪn/ *n* a stain made by blood.

bloodstained /ˈblʌdˌsteɪnd/ *adj* stained with blood; responsible for killing.

bloodstock /ˈblʌdˌstɒk/ *n* thoroughbred horses collectively.

bloodstone /ˈblʌdˌstoʊn/ *n* a dark green quartz flecked with red jasper; heliotrope.

bloodstream /ˈblʌdˌstriːm/ *n* the flow of blood through the blood vessels in the human body.

bloodsucker /ˈblʌdˌsʌkər/ *n* an animal that sucks blood, a leech; a person who sponges or preys on another, an extortionist.— **bloodsucking** *adj, n*.

blood test *n* an examination of a blood specimen to ascertain blood group, alcohol intake, etc.

bloodthirsty /ˈblʌdˌθɜːrsti/ *adj* (**bloodthirstier, bloodthirstiest**) eager for blood, cruel, warlike.—**bloodthirstiness** *n*.

blood type *see* **blood group**.

blood vessel *n* in the body, a vein, artery, or capillary.

bloody /ˈblʌdi/ *adj* (**bloodier, bloodiest**) stained with or covered in blood; bloodthirsty; cruel, murderous; (*sl*) as an intensifier (*a bloody good hiding*). • *vt* (**bloodying, bloodied**) to cover with blood.—**bloodily** *adv.*—**bloodiness** *n*.

Bloody Caesar *n* ❧ (*Cdn*) a drink made with vodka and a mixture of tomato and clam juice.

Bloody Mary *n* (*pl* **Bloody Marys**) a drink made with vodka and tomato juice.

bloody-minded /ˈblʌdiˌmaɪndəd/ *adj* (*inf*) deliberately obstructive.—**bloody-mindedness** *n*.

bloom[1] /bluːm/ *n* a flower or blossom; the period of being in flower; a period of most health, vigour, etc; a youthful, healthy glow; the powdery coating on some fruit and leaves. • *vi* to blossom; to be in one's prime; to glow with health etc.

bloom[2] *n* a rough mass of incandescent iron for hammering or rolling into bars. • *vt* to make (iron) into bloom.

bloomer /ˈbluːmər/, **blooper** /ˈbluːpər/ *n* (*inf*) a stupid mistake.

bloomers /ˈbluːmərz/ *npl* (*inf*) baggy knickers.

blooming /ˈbluːmɪŋ/ *adj* blossoming, flowering; flourishing; (*sl*) confounded, bloody.—**bloomingly** *adv*.

blossom /ˈblɒsəm/ *n* a flower, *esp* one that produces edible fruit; a state or time of flowering. • *vi* to flower; to begin to develop.—**blossomy** *adj*.

blot /blɒt/ *n* a spot or stain, *esp* of ink; something that diminishes or spoils the beauty of; a blemish in reputation. • *vt* (**blotting, blotted**) to spot or stain; to obscure; to disgrace; to absorb with blotting paper.

blotch /blɒtʃ/ *n* a spot or discoloration on the skin; any large blot or stain. • *vt* to cover with blotches.—**blotched** *adj.*— **blotchily** *adv.*—**blotchy** *adj*.

blotter /ˈblɒtər/ *n* a piece of blotting paper.

blotting paper *n* absorbent paper used to dry freshly written ink.

blotto /ˈblɒtoʊ/ *adj* (*sl*) very drunk.

blouse /blaʊz/ or /bluːs/ *n* a shirt-like garment worn by women.

blow[1] /bloʊ/ *n* a hard hit, as with the fist; a sudden attack; a sudden misfortune; a setback.

blow[2] *vb* (**blowing, blew**, *pp* **blown**) *vi* to cause a current of air; to be moved or carried (by air, the wind, etc); (*mus*) to make a sound by forcing in air with the mouth; (*often with* **out**) to burst suddenly; to breathe hard; (*with* **out**) to become extinguished by a gust of air; (*gas or oil well*) to erupt out of control; (*with* **over**) to pass without consequence. • *vt* to move along with a current of air; to make a sound by blowing; to inflate with air (*a fuse, etc*) to melt; (*inf*) to spend (money) freely; (*sl*) to leave; (*sl*) to divulge a secret; (*sl*) to bungle; (*often with* **up**) to burst by an explosion; (*with* **out**) to extinguish by a gust; (*storm*) to dissipate (itself) by blowing; (*with* **over**) to pass over or pass by; (*with* **up**) to enlarge a photograph; (*with* **up**) (*inf*) to lose one's temper.

blow[3] *vi* (**blowing, blew**, *pp* **blown**) to blossom, to flower. • *n* a mass of blossom; the state or condition of flowering.

blow-by-blow /ˈbloʊbaɪˌbloʊ/ *adj* told or shown in great detail.

blow-dry /ˈbloʊˌdraɪ/ *vi* (**blow-drying, blow-dried**) to style recently washed hair with a hand-held drier.

blower /ˈbloʊər/ *n* one who blows; a braggart; a device for producing a stream of gas or air.

blowfly /ˈbloʊˌflaɪ/ *n* (*pl* **blowflies**) a fly that lays its eggs in rotting meat.

blowhole /ˈbloʊˌhoʊl/ *n* a nostril of a whale; a vent for the escape of gas, air, etc; a hole in ice used for breathing by whales, seals, etc; a hole of gas in metal capturing during the solidifying process.

blowlamp /ˈbloʊlæmp/, **blowtorch** /-ˌtɔːrtʃ/ *n* a gas-powered torch that produces a hot flame for welding, etc.

blown /bloːn/ *adj* swollen or bloated.

blowout /bloːˌaʊt/ *n* (*inf*) a festive social event; a bursting of a container (as a tyre) by pressure on a weak spot; an uncontrolled eruption of a gas or oil well.

blowpipe /bloːˌpaɪp/ *n* a tube through which a current of air or gas is driven upon a flame to concentrate its heat on a substance, *eg* glass, to fuse it; a long tube of cane or reed used to discharge arrows by the force of the breath.

blowup /bloːˌʌp/ *n* an explosion; an enlarged photograph; (*sl*) an angry outburst.

blowy /ˈbloːi/ *adj* (**blowier, blowiest**) breezy, windy.

blowzy, blowsy /ˈbloːzi/ *adj* (**blowzier, blowziest** *or* **blowsier, blowsiest**) (*esp a woman*) fat and ruddy, slatternly.—**blowzily, blowsily** *adv*.—**blowziness, blowsiness** *n*.

blubber[1] /ˈblʌbər/ *vi* to weep loudly.

blubber[2] *n* whale fat; excessive fat on the body.

bludgeon /ˈblʌdʒən/ *n* a short, heavy stick used for striking. • *vti* to strike with a bludgeon; to bully or coerce.

blue /bluː/ *adj* (**bluer, bluest**) of the colour of the clear sky; depressed; (*film*) indecent, obscene. • *n* the colour of the spectrum lying between green and violet; (*with* **the**) the sky, the sea; (*pl: with* **the**) (*inf*) a depressed feeling; (*pl: with* **the**) a style of vocal and instrumental jazz; a representative in a sport of a university, *esp* Oxford or Cambridge; the badge worn or honour bestowed; in UK, a member or adherent of the Tory party. • *vt* (**blueing** *or* **bluing, blued**) to make or dye blue; to dip in blue liquid; (*sl*) to squander.

blue baby *n* one born with a heart condition causing a blueness of the skin.

bluebell /ˈbluːˌbel/ *n* any of several plants with a one-sided cluster of blue bell-shaped flowers.

bluebird /ˈbluːˌbərd/ *n* any of various small songbirds prevalent in North America.

blue blood *n* royal or aristocratic descent.

bluebonnet /ˈbluːˌbɒnɪt/ *n* a Scottish cap of blue cloth; a name given to the Scottish troops before the Union, 1707; a Scotsman.

blue book *n* a governmental official report, etc, bound in blue paper covers; a directory of socially prominent persons; a booklet in which students answer examination questions.

bluebottle /ˈbluːˌbɒtəl/ *n* a large fly; (*inf*) a policeman.

blue box *n* 🍁 (*Cdn*) a blue container for discarded household items that are picked up for recycling.

blue cheese *n* cheese with veins of blue mould.

blue chip *adj* (*stocks, shares*) providing a reliable return.

blue-collar /ˌbluːˈkɒlər/ *adj* of or pertaining to manual workers.

blue devils *npl* low spirits; mental depression; delirium tremens.

bluegrass /ˈbluːˌɡræs/ *n* any of several rich pasture grasses with bluish green blades, *esp* in Kentucky; improvisatory country music played on unamplified instruments.

blue gum *n* a lofty eucalyptus tree of Australia, valuable for its timber and essential oil.

blueing /ˈbluːɪŋ/ *n* the process of imparting a blue tint; the indigo, etc, used by washerwomen.—*also* **bluing**.

bluejacket /ˈbluːˌdʒækət/ *n* a seaman in the British or US navy.

blue jay *n* 🍁 a crested jay of eastern and central North America with a large tail and blue, black and white plumage.

blue line *n* 🍁 in ice hockey, one of two lines on the ice surface between the centre and the goals.

blue mould *n* a minute fungus that attacks bread and other foodstuffs.

Bluenose /ˈbluːnoːz/ *n* a puritanical person.

Bluenoser /ˈbluːnoːzər/ *n* 🍁 (*Cdn*) (*inf*) a Nova Scotian.

blue peter *n* a small blue flag with a white square in the centre, hoisted when a ship is about to sail.

blueprint /ˈbluːˌprɪnt/ *n* a blue photographic print of plans; a detailed scheme, template of work to be done; basis or prototype for future development.

blue ribbon *n* in UK, the broad ribbon of a dark blue colour worn by members of the order of the Garter; a prized distinction; a mark of success; a thin blue strip worn as a badge of teetotalism.

blue rinse *n* a rinse giving a blue tint to grey hair.

blue-rinse *adj* (*inf*) describing mature, assured, social women and their background.

blues /bluːz/ *npl* (*used as sing or pl*) depression, melancholy; a type of melancholy folk music originating among Black Americans.

bluestocking /-ˌstɒkɪŋ/ *n* a woman of literary tastes or occupation.

bluestone /-ˌstoːn/ *n* a grey sandstone used for building, etc; copper sulphate in crystalline form.

blue whale *n* a rorqual, the largest mammal known.

bluey /ˈbluːi/ *n* (*Austral*) a bushman's bundle.

bluff[1] /blʌf/ *adj* rough in manner; abrupt, outspoken; ascending steeply with a flat front. • *n* a broad, steep bank or cliff.—**bluffness** *n*.

bluff[2] *vti* to mislead or frighten by a false, bold front. • *n* deliberate deception.—**bluffer** *n*.

bluff[3] *n* 🍁 a steep cliff or bank; 🍁 (*Cdn*) in western Canada, a grove or clump of leafy trees.

bluing /ˈbluːɪŋ/ *see* **blueing**.

blunder /ˈblʌndər/ *vi* to make a foolish mistake; to move about clumsily. • *n* a foolish mistake.—**blunderer** *n*.—**blundering** *adj*.—**blunderingly** *adv*.

blunderbuss /-ˌbʌs/ *n* (*hist*) a short gun or firearm with a wide bore, firing many balls; a clumsy person.

blunge /blʌndʒ/ *vt* (*pottery*) to mix clay with water.

blunt /blʌnt/ *adj* not having a sharp edge or point; rude, outspoken, unsubtle. • *vti* to make or become dull.—**bluntly** *adv*.—**bluntness** *n*.

blur /blər/ *n* a stain, smear; an ill-defined impression. • *vti* (**blurring, blurred**) to smear; to make or become indistinct in shape, etc; to dim.—**blurred** *adj*.—**blurredly** *adv*.—**blurry** *adj*.

blurb /blərb/ *n* a promotional description, as on a book cover; an exaggerated advertisement.

blurt /blərt/ *vt* (*with* **out**) to utter impulsively.

blush /blʌʃ/ *n* a red flush of the face caused by embarrassment or guilt; any rosy colour. • *vi* (*with* **for, at**) to show embarrassment, modesty, joy, etc involuntarily, by blushing; to become rosy.

blusher /ˈblʌʃər/ *n* a cosmetic that gives colour to the cheeks.

blush wine *n* rose wine, a blend of red and white wines.

bluster /ˈblʌstər/ *vi* to make a noise like the wind; to bully. • *n* a blast, as of the wind; bullying or boastful talk, often to hide shame or embarrassment.—**blusterer** *n*.—**blustery** *adj*.—**blusteringly, blusterously** *adv*.

Blvd *abbr* = Boulevard.

B-movie *n* (*cinema*) a film made as a supporting feature, *esp* in the 1940s and 1950s.

BMus *abbr* = Bachelor of Music.

bn *abbr* = battalion; billion.

BNA *abbr* = (*hist*) British North America.

BO *abbr* = (*inf*) body odour.

boa /ˈboːa/ *n* any of various large South American snakes that crush their prey; a long fluffy scarf of feathers.

boa constrictor *n* the largest boa, remarkable for its length and power of destroying its prey by constriction.

boar /bɔr/ *n* a male pig, a wild hog.

board[1] /bɔrd/ *n* meals, *esp* when provided regularly for pay; a long, flat piece of sawed wood, etc; a flat piece of wood, etc for some special purpose; pasteboard; a council; a group of people who supervise a company; the side of a ship (*overboard*); 🍁 (*pl*) a low solid barrier surrounding the ice surface of an indoor skating or hockey rink. • *vt* to provide with meals and lodging at fixed terms; to come onto the deck of (a ship); to get on (a train, bus, etc). • *vi* to provide with meals, or room and meals, regularly for pay; (*with* **up**) to cover with boards; **to take on board** to appoint to a position; to adopt new ideas.

boarder /ˈbɔrdər/ *n* one who is provided with board.

board game *n* a game as chess, chequers, etc, played by moving pieces on a marked board.

boarding /ˈbɔrdɪŋ/ *n* light timber collectively; a covering of planks; the act of supplying, or state of being supplied with, food and lodging for a stipulated sum; the act of entering a ship or aircraft; 🍁 in ice hockey, the infraction of bodychecking an opponent into the boards with excessive force.

boarding house *n* a house for boarders.

boarding school *n* a school where the students are boarded.

boardroom /ˈbɔrdˌruːm/ *n* a room where meetings of a company's board are held.

board rule *n* a figured scale for finding the number of square feet in a board without calculation.

boardwalk /ˈbɔrdˌwɒk/ *n* a footway of boards, *esp* by the sea.

boarish /ˈbɔrɪʃ/ *adj* coarse; brutal; cruel.

boart *see* **bort**.

boast[1] /boːst/ *vi* to brag. • *vt* to speak proudly of; to possess with pride. • *n* boastful talk.—**boaster** *n*.—**boastingly** *adv*.

boast[2] *vt* to dress stone with a broad chisel and mallet; to dress a block in outline for a statue, etc, prior to more detailed or delicate work.

boastful /'boːstfʊl/ *adj* given to boasting.—**boastfully** *adv*.—**boastfulness** *n*.

boat /boːt/ *n* a small, open, waterborne craft; (*inf*) a ship. • *vi* to travel in a boat, *esp* for pleasure.

boatbill(ed heron) /-ˌbɪld'herən/ *n* a South American wading bird with a boat-shaped bill.

boater /-ər/ *n* a stiff flat straw hat.

boathook /-ˌhʊk/ *n* a hooked pole for drawing a boat to land, fending off, etc.

boathouse /-ˌhɑʊs/ *n* a shed for boats.

boating /-ɪŋ/ *n* rowing, sailing, etc, for pleasure.

boatman /-mən/ *n* (*pl* **boatmen**) a person who works on, deals in, or operates boats.

boat people *npl* refugees fleeing by boat.

boatswain /'boːsən/ *n* a ship's officer in charge of hull maintenance and related work.—*also* **bosun**.

boat train *n* a train for steamer or ferry passengers.

bob /bɒb/ *vb* (**bobbing, bobbed**) *vi* to move abruptly up and down, often in water; to nod the head; to curtsey. • *vt* (*hair*) to cut short. • *n* a jerking motion up and down; the weight on a pendulum, plumb line, etc; a woman's or girl's short haircut.

bobbery *n* (*pl* **bobberies**) a rumpus, a row, a noisy disturbance; a pack of hunting dogs.

bobbin /'bɒbɪn/ *n* a reel or spool on which yarn or thread is wound.

bobbinet /'bɒbɪˌnɛt/ *n* a machine-made cotton netting or lace in imitation of pillow lace.

bobble /'bɒbəl/ *n* a small woolly ball used for ornament or trimming; a bobbing movement; (*inf*) a mistake; a fumble. *vti* to bob up and down; to make a mistake; to fumble with (a ball).

bobby /'bɒbi/ *n* (*pl* **bobbies**) (*sl*) a policeman.

bobby pin *n* a clip for holding hair in position; a hairgrip.

Bobcat /'bɒbˌkæt/ *n* (*pl* **bobcats, bobcat**) a medium-sized feline of eastern North America with a black-spotted reddish-brown coat and a short tail.

bobolink /'bɒbəˌlɪŋk/ *n* an American migratory songbird.—*also* **reedbird, ricebird**.

Bobsled /'bɒbˌslɛd/, **bobsleigh** /'bɒbˌsleɪ/ *n* a long racing sled. • *vi* (**bobsledding, bobsledded**) to ride or race on a bobsled.

bobstay /'bɒbˌsteɪ/ *n* (*naut*) a rope holding the bowsprit down to the stem.

bobtail /'bɒbˌteɪl/ *n* a short tail or a tail cut short; an animal with a docked tail; the rabble (*rag-tag and bobtail*). • *adj* with a docked tail.—**bobtailed** *adj*.

Boche /bɒʃ/ *n* (*pl* **Boche**) (*sl*) a German, *esp* a soldier.

bock /bɒk/ *n* a variety of lager beer of double strength; a glass of beer.

bode /boːd/ *vt* to be an omen of.

bodega /boː'deɪɡə/ *n* a wine vault, cellar or shop where wine is sold from the cask; a store specializing in Hispanic groceries.

bodice /'bɒdɪs/ *n* the upper part of a woman's dress.

bodiless /'bɒdiːləs/ *adj* without a body, incorporeal.—**bodilessness** *n*.

bodily /'bɒdɪli/ *adj* physical; relating to the body. • *adv* in the flesh; as a whole; altogether.

bodkin /'bɒdkɪn/ *n* a large blunt needle, a tool for piercing holes; a pin for fastening hair; a small dagger.

body /'bɒdi/ *n* (*pl* **bodies**) the whole physical substance of a person, animal, or plant; the trunk of a person or animal; a corpse; the principal part of anything; a distinct mass; substance or consistency, as of liquid; a richness of flavour; a person; a distinct group of people. • *vt* (**bodying, bodied**) to give shape to.

body bag *n* a large plastic sack, *usu* zipped, to carry a corpse from the scene of a disaster.

bodybuilding /-ˌbɪldɪŋ/ *n* strengthening and enlarging the muscles through exercise and diet for competitive display.— **bodybuilder** *n*.

bodyguard /-ˌɡɑrd/ *n* a person or persons assigned to guard someone.

body language *n* gestures, unconscious bodily movements, etc, that function as a means of communication.

body politic *n* the collective body of people living under an organized political government.

body-snatcher *n* (*formerly*) one who stole corpses from graves for dissection by anatomists.

body stocking *n* a woman's tight-fitting garment that covers the torso and sometimes the legs.

body warmer *n* a sleeveless, quilted outer garment.

bodywork /'bɒdiˌwɜrk/ *n* the outer shell of a motor vehicle.

Boeotian /bi'oːʃən/ *adj* pertaining to Boeotia in central Greece, noted for its moist and heavy atmosphere; dull, stupid. • *n* an inhabitant of Boeotia; a dull, stupid person.

Boer /bɔr/ or /'boːr/, /bʊr/ *n* a Dutch-descended South African.— *also adj*.

boffin /'bɒfɪn/ *n* (*inf*) a military research scientist.

boffo /'bɒfoː/ *adj* (*sl*) wonderful, amazing.

bog /bɒɡ/ or /bɔɡ/ *n* wet, spongy ground; quagmire. • *vb* (**bogging, bogged**) *vt* to sink or submerge in a bog or quagmire. • *vi* to sink or stick in a bog.—**boggy** *adj*.

bogan /'boːɡən/ *n* ✤ (*Cdn*) a stagnant backwater of a lake or river.

bogey[1] /'boːɡi/ *n* (*pl* **bogeys**) (*golf*) one stroke more than par on a hole.

bogey[2] *n* (*pl* **bogeys**) a goblin; a cause of worry.—*also* **bogy** (*pl* **bogies**).

bogeyman /'boːɡiˌmæn/ *n* (*pl* **bogeymen**) an imaginary monster commonly used to frighten children.

boggle /'bɒɡəl/ *vi* to be surprised; to hesitate (at). • *vt* to confuse (the imagination, mind, etc).

bogie /'boːɡi/ *n* an assembly of four or six wheels on a rail carriage.

bogle /'boːɡəl/ *n* a goblin, a spectre; a scarecrow.

bogus /'boːɡəs/ *adj* counterfeit, spurious.

bogy /'boːɡi/ or /'bʊɡi/ *see* **bogey**[2].

bohea *n* a black China tea of the lowest quality.

Bohemian /boː'hiːmiən/ *adj* of or pertaining to Bohemia in Czechoslovakia; unconventional. • *n* an inhabitant of Bohemia; a person who disregards social conventions or evinces a wild or roving disposition; a gipsy.

Bohemianism /-ˌɪzəm/ *n* the life or habits of a person, *usu* artistic or literary, who by natural inclination leads a free and easy unconventional existence.

boil[1] /bɔɪl/ *vi* to change rapidly from a liquid to a vapour by heating; to bubble when boiling; to cook in boiling liquid; to be aroused with anger; (*with* **down**) to reduce by boiling; to condense; (*with* **over**) to overflow when boiling; to burst out in anger. • *vt* to heat to boiling point; to cook in boiling water.—**boilable** *adj*.

boil[2] *n* an inflamed, pus-filled, painful swelling on the skin.

boiler /'bɔɪlər/ *n* a container in which to boil things; a storage tank in which water is heated and steam generated; a device for providing central heating and hot water.

boilersuit /-suːt/ *n* coveralls.

boiling point *n* the temperature at which a liquid boils; the point at which a person loses his temper; the point of crisis.

boisterous /'bɔɪstərəs/ *adj* wild, noisy; stormy; loud and exuberant.—**boisterously** *adv*.

bola, bolas /'boːlə/ *n* a South American hunting implement consisting of two or more balls of iron or stone attached to the ends of a leather cord, used to entangle the legs of an animal.

bold /boːld/ *adj* daring or courageous; fearless; impudent; striking to the eye. • *n* boldface type.—**boldly** *adv*.—**boldness** *n*.

boldface type /-ˌfeɪs/ *n* type characters with thickened, heavy strokes.

bole[1] /boːl/ *n* the trunk or stem of a tree.

bole[2] *n* friable clay or clayey shale, *usu* coloured by oxide of iron.

bolection /boː'lɛkʃən/ *n* (*archit*) a raised moulding on a panel.

bolero /boː'lɛroː/ *n* (*pl* **boleros**) a lively Spanish dance; the music accompanying such a dance; a short jacket-shaped bodice.

boletus /boː'liːtəs/ *n* (*pl* **boletuses, boleti**) any of a large genus of thick-stemmed fungi containing edible or poisonous species.

bolide /'boːˌlaɪd/ or /-ˌlɪd/ *n* a large meteor that explodes on coming into contact with air, a fire ball.

boll /boːl/ *n* the pod of a plant, *esp* of cotton or flax.

boll weevil *n* an American weevil that infests cotton bolls.

bollard /'bɒlərd/ *n* a strong post on a wharf around which mooring lines are secured; one of a line of posts closing off a street to traffic; an illuminated marker on a traffic island.

bolometer /boː'lɒmətər/ *n* an instrument for measuring radiation.—**bolometric** *adj*.—**bolometrically** *adv*.

boloney /bə'loːni/ *see* **baloney**.

Bolshevik /'bɒlʃəˌvɪk/ or /'bɒl-/ *n* (*pl* **Bolsheviks, Bolsheviki**) a Russian communist; a revolutionary; an opponent of an existing social order.

Bolshevism /-ˌvɪzm/ *n* the doctrines and practices of the Bolsheviks; the communist form of government adopted in Russia in March 1917.—**Bolshevist** *adj, n.*

bolshie, bolshy /'bɒlʃi/ *adj* (*sl*) left-wing; rebellious. • *n* (*pl* **bolshies**) (*often with cap*) a Bolshevik; a revolutionary.

bolster /'bɒlstər/ *n* a long narrow pillow; any bolster-like object or support. • *vt* (*often with* **up**) to support or strengthen.—**bolsterer** *n.*—**bolsteringly** *adv.*

bolt[1] /boʊlt/ *n* a bar used to lock a door, etc; an arrow for a crossbow; a flash of lightning; a threaded metal rod used with a nut to hold parts together; a roll (of cloth, paper etc); a sudden dash. • *vt* to lock with a bolt; to eat hastily; to say suddenly; to blurt (out); to abandon (a party, group, etc). • *vi* (*horse*) to rush away suddenly • *adv* erectly upright.—**bolter** *n*

bolt[2] *vt* to sift or separate coarser from finer particles; to examine with care, to investigate; to separate.—*also* **boult.**—**bolter** *n.*

bolthole /-ˌhoʊl/ *n* an escape route; a safe and secret hiding place; a person's private refuge.

boltrope /-ˌroʊp/ *n* (*naut*) a rope to which the edges of sails are sewn.

bolus /'boʊləs/ *n* (*pl* **boluses**) a medicine in the form of a soft rounded mass, larger than an ordinary pill, to be swallowed at once; anything disagreeable, which must be accepted.

bomb /bɒm/ *n* a projectile containing explosives incendiary material, or chemicals used for destruction; (*with* **the**) the hydrogen or atomic bomb; (*sl*) a lot of money. • *vt* to attack with bombs. • *vi* to fail, to flop.

bomb site /bɒmsaɪt/ *n* an area devastated by bombing; a vacant area cleared after a bombing raid.

bombard /bɒm'bɑrd/ *vt* to attack with bombs or artillery; to attack verbally.—**bombardment** *n.*

bombardier /ˌbɒmbər'dɪr/ *n* the crew member who releases the bombs in a bomber; in Britain and Canada a noncommissioned artillery officer.

bombardier beetle *n* any of various coleopterous insects that, when irritated, expel a fluid from the abdomen with a slight report.

bombast /'bɒmˌbæst/ *n* pretentious or boastful language.—**bombastic** *adj.*—**bombastically** *adv.*

bombazine /ˌbɒmbə'ziːn/ or /'bɒmbəˌziːn/ *n* a twilled fabric of which the warp is silk and the weft worsted.

bombe /bɒm/, *Fr.* /bõb/ *n* a frozen dessert moulded into a round shape.

bomber /'bɒmər/ *n* a person who bombs; an aeroplane that carries bombs.

bomber jacket *n* a waist-length bloused jacket with a zip.

bombshell /'bɒmˌʃel/ *n* a shocking surprise.

bombsight /'bɒmsaɪt/ *n* a manual or electronic device for aiming bombs.

bombycid /'bɒmbəˌsɪd/ *n* any of a family of moths, including the silkworm moth.

bona fide /'boʊnəˌfaɪd/ or /'boʊnə-/, /ˌboʊnə'faɪdi/ *adj* in good faith; genuine or real.

bona fides /'boʊnə'faɪˌdiz/ or /-ˌfaɪdz/ *n* good faith; honourable dealing.

bonanza /bə'nænzə/ *n* a rich vein of ore; any source of wealth; unexpected good fortune or luck.

bonbon /'bɒnˌbɒn/ *n* a small piece of candy, a sweet.

bond /bɒnd/ *n* anything that binds, fastens, or unites; (*pl*) shackles; an obligation imposed by a contract, promise, etc; the status of goods in a warehouse until taxes are paid; an interest-bearing certificate issued by the government or business, redeemable on a specified date; surety against theft, absconding, etc. • *vt* to join, bind, or otherwise unite; to provide a bond for; to place or hold (goods) in bond; to put together bricks or stones so that they overlap to give strength. • *vi* to hold together by means of a bond.—**bondable** *adj.*—**bonder** *n.*

bondage /'bɒndɪdʒ/ *n* slavery, captivity.

bondstone /'bɒndˌstoʊn/ *n* a long stone running through a wall and so binding it.

bone /boʊn/ *n* the hard material making up the skeleton; any constituent part of the skeleton; (*pl*) the skeleton: the essentials or basics of anything. • *vti* to remove the bones from, as meat; (*with* **up**) (*inf*) to study hard.—**boneless** *adj*

bone black *n* a black pigment made partly from charcoal obtained by roasting animal bones.

bone china *n* china made from clay mixed with bone ash.

bone-dry /'boʊn'draɪ/ *adj* completely dry.

bonehead /'boʊnˌhed/ *n* (*sl*) a fool.

bone meal *n* fertilizer or feed made of crushed or ground bone.

bone of contention *n* a source of strife.

bonesetter *n* one who treats fractures or dislocated limbs without medical qualification to do so.

bonfire /'bɒnˌfaɪr/ *n* an outdoor fire.

bongo[1] /'bɒŋgoʊ/ *n* (*pl* **bongos**) either of a pair of small drums of different pitch struck with the fingers.

bongo[2] *n* (*pl* **bongo, bongos**) a large striped African antelope.

bonhomie /ˌbɒnɒ'mi/, *Fr.* /bɔnɔ'mi/ *n* good-heartedness; a frank good-natured manner.—**bonhomous** *adj.*

bonito /bɒ'nitoʊ/ or /bə-/ *n* (*pl* **bonitos, bonito**) one of several species of warm-sea game fishes allied to the tuna.

bon mot /bɒn'moʊ/, *Fr.* /bɔn'mo/ *n* (*pl* **bons mots**) a witty saying, a fitting remark.

bonne *Fr.* /bɒn/ *n* a French nursemaid.

bonnet /'bɒnət/ *n* a hat with a chin ribbon, worn by women and children; a case or covering, *usu* of sheet metal, placed over a motor.—*also* **hood.**

bonny, bonnie /'bɒni/ *adj* (**bonnier, bonniest**) healthy, attractive looking.

bonsai /'bɒnˌsaɪ/ or /bɒn'saɪ/ *n* (*pl* **bonsai**) a miniature tree or shrub that has been dwarfed by selective pruning; the art of cultivating bonsai.

bonspiel /'bɒnˌspiːl/ or /-ˌspəl/ *n* (*Scot*) a curling match between players of different clubs.

bontebok /'bɒntəˌbɒk/ *n* (*pl* **bonteboks, bontebok**) a pied antelope of South Africa.

bon ton /bɒn'toːn/ *n* the style of persons in high life; good breeding; fashionable society; height of fashion.

bonus /'boʊnəs/ *n* (*pl* **bonuses**) an amount paid over the sum due as interest, dividend, or wages.

bon vivant /bõviː'vã/ *n* (*pl* **bons vivants**) a gourmet.

bon voyage /ˌbɒnvɔɪ'ɒdʒ/, *Fr.* /bõvwɒ'jɒʒ/ or /-vɔɪ'jɒʒ/ *n, interj* an expression used to wish travellers a pleasant trip.

bony /'boʊni/ *adj* (**bonier, boniest**) of or resembling bones; having large or prominent bones; full of bones.

bonze /bɒnz/ *n* a Buddhist monk.

boo /buː/ *interj* an expression of disapproval. • *n* (*pl* **boos**) hooting. • *vb* (**booing, booed**) *vi* to low like an ox; to groan. • *vt* to hoot at.

boob /buːb/ *n* a stupid awkward person; a blunder.

booby /'buːbi/ *n* (*pl* **boobies**) a foolish person; the loser in a game.

booby prize *n* a prize of little value for the lowest score.

booby trap *n* a trap for playing a practical joke on someone; a camouflaged explosive device triggered by an unsuspecting victim.

boodle /'buːdəl/ *n* money paid for votes or undue political influence; graft; lot, caboodle.

boogie /'buɡi/ or /'buːɡi/ *vi* (**boogieing, boogied**) to dance to pop music or jazz. • *n* fast, rhythmic music for dancing.

boogie-woogie /ˌbuɡi'wuːɡi/ or /ˌbuːɡi'wuːɡi/ *n* a style of jazz piano.

boohoo /ˌbuː'huː/ *vi* (**boohooing, boohooed**) to weep noisily or to pretend to do so. • *n* (*pl* **boohoos**) the sound of noisy weeping.

book /bʊk/ *n* a bound set of printed or blank pages; a literary composition of fact or fiction; the script or libretto of a play or musical; (*pl*) written records of transactions or accounts; a book or record of bets. • *vt* to make a reservation in advance; to note a person's name and address for an alleged offence. • *vi* to make a reservation.

bookcase /-ˌkeɪs/ *n* a piece of furniture with shelves for books.

book club *n* an organization that sells books to its members at cheaper prices, *usu* by mail order.

book end /-ˌend/ *npl* a prop at the end of a row of books to keep them upright.

bookie /-i/ *n* (*inf*) a bookmaker.

bookish /-ɪʃ/ *adj* fond of reading.—**bookishness** *n.***book learning** *n* theoretical, not practical, knowledge.—**book-learned** *adj.*

bookkeeping /-ˌkiːpɪŋ/ *n* the systematic recording of business accounts.—**bookkeeper** *n.*

booklet /-lɪt/ *n* a small book, *usu* with a paper cover; a pamphlet.

bookmaker /-ˌmeɪkər/ *n* a person who takes bets on horse races, etc and pays out winnings; a manufacturer or publisher of books.

bookman /-mən/ *n* (*pl* **bookmen**) a literary man, a scholar; one who works in publishing.

bookmark(er) /-ˌmarkər/ *n* a thing to mark a place in a book.

bookplate /-ˌpleɪt/ *n* a label in a book with the owner's name on it.

bookseller /-ˌselər/ *n* a person who sells books.

bookstall /-stɔl/ *n* a stall for the sale of books, magazines, etc.

bookworm /-ˌwɜrm/ *n* an insect that feeds on books; a person who reads a lot.

Boolean algebra *n* (*math*) a system of symbolic logic used in the manipulation of sets and other mathematical entities, and in computing science.

boom[1] /buːm/ *n* ✽ a raft of limber or logs fastened together for transportation across a body of water.

boom[2] *n* a spar on which a sail is stretched; a barrier across a harbour; a long pole carrying a microphone.

boom[3] *vi* to make a deep, hollow sound. • *n* a resonant sound, as of the sea.

boom[4] *vi* to flourish or prosper suddenly. • *n* a period of vigorous growth (*eg* in business, sales, prices).

boomer /ˈbuːmər/ *n* the male of the great kangaroo; one who starts or promotes a boom; (*sl*) a migratory worker.

boomerang /ˈbuːməˌræŋ/ *n* a curved stick that, when thrown, returns to the thrower; an action that unexpectedly rebounds and harms the agent.—*also vi.*

booming ground *n* ✽ (*Cdn*) a section of a body of water where logs are collected into booms.

boom town /ˈbuːmˌtaʊn/ *n* a town that suddenly grows and increases in economic prosperity.

boon[1] /buːn/ *n* something useful or helpful; a blessing; a favour.

boon[2] *adj* bountiful; convivial, jolly; specially friendly (*boon companion*).

boondocks /ˈbuːnˌdɒks/ *npl* (*sl*) a wild, inhospitable area; a dull, provincial region.—**boondock** *adj.*

boondoggle /ˈbuːnˌdɒgəl/ *n* ✽ (*Cdn*) (*inf*) work of little value done merely to appear busy or to provide an income for employees, *esp* a project funded by a government. • *vi* do such work.

boor /ˈbʊr/ *n* an ill-mannered or coarse person.—**boorish** *adj.*—**boorishly** *adv.*—**boorishness** *n.*

boost /buːst/ *vt* (*sales, etc*) to increase; to encourage, to improve; to push; to help by advertising or promoting. • *n* a push.

booster /-ər/ *n* a thing or person that increases the effectiveness of another mechanism; the first stage of a rocket, which usually breaks away after launching; a substance that increases the effectiveness of medication.

boosterism /-ˌɪzəm/ *n* the practice of boosting an image or product commercially.

booster shot, booster injection *n* a supplementary dose of medicine, *esp* a vaccine.

boot[1] /buːt/ *n* a strong covering for the foot and lower part of the leg; (*sl: with* **the**) dismissal from employment; the rear compartment of a car used for holding luggage, etc.—*also* **trunk**. • *vt* to kick; to get rid of by force; (*comput*) to bring a program from a disc into the memory.

boot[2] *n* (*arch*) advantage, use; **to boot** as well. • *vi* (*arch*) to avail.

bootblack /ˈbuːtˌblæk/ *n* one who shines shoes.

booted *adj* wearing boots.

bootee /buːˈtiː/ *n* a knitted or soft shoe for a baby.

booth /buːθ/ *n* a stall for selling goods; a small enclosure for voting; a public telephone enclosure.

bootjack /ˈbuːtˌdʒæk/ *n* an appliance for drawing off boots.

bootleg /-ˌleg/ *vt* (**bootlegging, bootlegged**) to smuggle illicit alcohol; to deal in illegally made records and tapes of live music, etc.—**bootlegger** *n.*

bootless /-ləs/ *adj* useless, unavailing.—**bootlessly** *adv.*—**bootlessness** *n.*

bootlicker /-ˌlɪkər/ *n* a person who ingratiates himself or herself to gain favour, a toady.

boots /buːts/ *n* (*pl* **boots**) in UK, the servant in an hotel who cleans the boots of the guests.

boots and saddles *n* a cavalry signal to mount.

booty /ˈbuːti/ *n* (*pl* **booties**) spoils obtained as plunder.

booze /buːz/ *vi* (*inf*) to drink alcohol excessively. • *n* alcohol.—**boozer** *n.*

boozy /ˈbuːzi/ *adj* (**boozier, booziest** (*sl*) addicted to drink; drunk.—**boozily** *adv.*

bop /bɒp/ *n* a style of 1940s jazz music.—*also* **bebop**.

bora /ˈboːrə/ *or* /ˈbɔrə/ *n* a fierce dry northeast wind that blows on the coasts of the Adriatic Sea.

boracic /bəˈræsɪk/ *see* **boric**.

boracic acid *see* **boric acid**.

borage /ˈbɒrədʒ/ *n* a blue-flowered herb used in salads, etc.

borax /ˈbɔræks/ *n* a mineral composed of the sodium salt compounded of boracic acid chiefly from the dried beds of certain lakes, used in the manufacture of glass, enamel, antiseptics, soaps, etc; (*sl*) shoddy merchandise.

Bordeaux /bɔrˈdoː/ *n* any of several red, white or rosé wines from around Bordeaux in France.

bordello /bɔrˈdeloː/ *n* (*pl* **bordellos**) a brothel.

border /ˈbɔrdər/ *n* the edge, rim, or margin; a dividing line between two countries; a narrow strip along an edge. • *vi* (*with* **on, upon**) to be adjacent; to approach, to verge on. • *vt* to form a border.

bordereau *Fr.* /bɔrdəˈroː/ *n* (*pl* **bordereaux**) a memorandum of contents, a docket.

borderer /ˈbɔrdərər/ *n* a dweller on a frontier.

borderland /ˈbɔrdərˌlænd/ *n* land forming a border or frontier; an uncertain or debatable district; an intermediate state.

borderline /ˈbɔrdərˌlaɪn/ *n* a boundary. • *adj* on a boundary; doubtful, indefinite.

bordure /ˈbɔrdjʊr/ *n* (*her*) a border round a shield.

bore[1] /bɔr/ *to* drill so as to form a hole; to weary, by being dull or uninteresting. • *n* a hole made by drilling; the diameter of a gun barrel; a dull or uninteresting person.

bore[2] *see* **bear**[1].

bore[3] *n* a tidal wave that breaks in the estuaries of some rivers and, impeded by a narrowing channel, rises in a ridge and courses along with great force and noise.

boreal /ˈbɔriəl/ *adj* of or pertaining to the north, or to the north wind; situated on the northern side; of a northern character.

Boreas /-əs/ *n* the north wind personified.

boredom /ˈbɔrdəm/ *n* tedium.

boric /ˈbɔrɪk/ *adj* of or yielding boron.—*also* **boracic**.

boric acid *n* a white solid acid used in manufacturing a mild antiseptic.

boring /ˈbɔrɪŋ/ *adj* dull, tedious; making holes.

born /bɔrn/ *pp* of **bear**[1]. • *adj* by birth, natural.

born-again /ˈbɔrnəˌgen/ *adj* having undergone a revival of personal faith or conviction.

borne /bɔrn/ *see* **bear**[1].

bornite /ˈbɔrˌnaɪt/ *n* a valuable ore of copper.

boron /ˈbɔrˌɒn/ *n* a nonmetallic element found in borax.

borough /ˈbərəʊ/ *n* a self-governing, incorporated town; an administrative area of a city, as in London or New York.

borough English *n* (*formerly*) a custom existing in some parts of England by which an estate descended to the youngest son instead of the eldest, or, if there were no son, to the youngest brother.

borrow /ˈbɒrəʊ/ *vt* to obtain (an item) with the intention of returning it; (*an idea*) to adopt as one's own; (*loan, money*) to obtain from a financial institution at definite rates of interest.—**borrower** *n.*

borscht /bɔrʃt/, **borsch** *Russ.* /bɔrʃtʃ/ *n* a type of soup (orig from Russia) made with beetroot.

borstal system /ˈbɔrstəlˌsɪstəm/ *n* (*often cap*) (*formerly*) a reformatory system by which the sentence depended on the prisoner's conduct; now called a youth custody centre.

bort /bɔrt/, **bortz** *n* an imperfect or inferior diamond used for polishing other stones; a fragment of diamond made in the cutting.—*also* **boart**.

borzoi /ˈbɔrˌzɔɪ/ *n* (*pl* **borzois**) a tall hound with a long, silky coat and a long head, a Russian wolfhound.

boscage, boskage /ˈbɒskɪdʒ/ *n* ground covered with trees and shrubs; woods; thickets; a wooded landscape.

bosh /bɒʃ/ *n* (*inf*) nonsense.—*also interj*.

bosk /bɒsk/ *n* a small wood, a thicket.

bosky /ˈbɒski/ *adj* (**boskier, boskiest**) wooded, bushy.—**boskiness** *n.*

bosom /ˈbʊzəm/ *n* the breast of a human being, *esp* a woman; the part of a dress that covers it; the seat of the emotions. • *adj* (*friend*) very dear, intimate.

boss[1] /bɒs/ *n* (*inf*) the manager or foreman; a powerful local politician. • *vt* to domineer; to be in control.

boss[2] *n* a protuberant part; a stud or knob, an ornamental projection of a ceiling. • *vt* to ornament with studs or knobs.

bossa nova /ˌbɒsə'nəʊvə/ *n* a dance from Brazil similar to the samba; the music for this.

bossy /'bɒsi/ *adj* (**bossier, bossiest**) (*inf*) domineering, fond of giving orders.—**bossily** *adv*.—**bossiness** *n*.

Boston bluefish *n* ✤ (*Cdn*) pollack.

bosun /'bəʊsən/ *see* **boatswain**.

bot /bɒt/ *n* the larva of the botfly, which infests horses, cattle, sheep, etc; (*pl*) the disease that it causes.—*also* **bott**

botanical /bə'tænɪkəl/, **botanic** *adj* pertaining to plants and botany.—**botanically** *adv*.

botanize /'bɒtəˌnaɪz/ *vi* to study plants, *esp* on a field trip.—**botanizer** *n*.

botany /'bɒtəni/ *n* (*pl* **botanies**) the study of plants.—**botanist** *n*.

botch /bɒtʃ/ *n* a poorly done piece of work. • *vt* to mend or patch clumsily; to put together without sufficient care.—**botcher** *n*.

botchy /'bɒtʃi/ *adj* (**botchier, botchiest**) clumsily made or done; marked with botches.—**botchily** *adv*.—**botchiness** *n*.

botfly /'bɒtˌflaɪ/ *n* (*pl* **botflies**) any of many winged insects with larvae parasitic on humans and livestock.

both /bəʊθ/ *adj, pron* the two together; the one and the other. • *conj* together equally.—*also* **aav**.

bother /'bɒðər/ *vt* to perplex or annoy; to take the time or trouble. • *n* worry; trouble; someone who causes problems, etc.

botheration /ˌbɒðəreɪ'ʃən/ *n* bother.—*also* **interj**.

bothersome /'bɒðərsəm/ *adj* causing bother.

bothy /'bɒθi/ *n* (*pl* **bothies**) (*Scot*) a small cottage or hut, *esp* a hut or barrack serving as farm servants' quarters; a shelter for climbers on mountains.

bo tree /'bəʊˌtriː/ *n* the peepul, the sacred tree of the Buddhists.

botryoidal /ˌbɒtri'ɔɪdəl/ *adj* resembling a bunch of grapes.—**botryoidally** *adv*.

bott /bɒt/ *see* **bot**.

bottle green *adj* dark green.

bottle[1] /'bɒtəl/ *n* a glass or plastic container for holding liquids; its contents; (*sl*) courage, nerve. • *vt* to put in bottles; to confine as if in a bottle.

bottle[2] *n* (*dial*) a quantity of hay or grass bundled up.

bottleneck /-ˌnek/ *n* a narrow stretch of a road where traffic is held up; a congestion in any stage of a process.

bottlenose /-ˌnəʊz/ *n* a dolphin with a sharp protruding beak; a moderately large toothed whale with a prominent beak.

bottom /'bɒtəm/ *n* the lowest or deepest part of anything; the base or foundation; the lowest position (*eg* in a class); the buttocks; (*naut*) the part of a ship's hull below water; the seabed. • *vt* to be based or founded on; to bring to the bottom, to get to the bottom of. • *vi* to become based; to reach the bottom; (*with* **out**) to flatten off after dropping sharply.

bottomlands /-ˌlændz/ *npl* rich flat low-lying land along watercourses in the western states of the US.

bottomless /-ləs/ *adj* very deep; without limit.

bottom line *n* the crux; the line at the bottom of a financial report that shows the net profit or loss; the final result.—**bottom-line** *adj*.

bottomry /'bɒtəmri/ *n* (*pl* **bottomries**) the borrowing of money by the owner on the security of his or her ship. • *vt* to pledge (a ship) thus.

botulism /'bɒtʃʊˌlɪzəm/ *n* a type of severe food poisoning.

bouclé, boucle /buː'kleɪ/ *n* a type of looped yarn or fabric.

boudoir /buː'dwɑr/ *n* a woman's bedroom.

bouffant /buː'fɒnt/ *adj* puffed out; (*of hair*) backcombed.

bougainvillea, bougainvillaea /ˌbuːgən'vɪliə/ *n* a tropical plant with large rosy or purple bracts.

bough /baʊ/ *n* a branch of a tree.

bought /bɒt/ *see* **buy**.

bougie /'buːˌdʒi/ or /-ˌʒi/ *n* a wax candle; (*med*) a slender flexible tube for inserting into the gullet, etc; a catheter.

bouillabaisse /ˌbuːjə'beɪs/ *n* a French fish stew.

bouillon /'buːˌjɒ/ or /-ˌljɒn/, /'buːˌljən/, *Fr.* /buː'jɔ̃/ *n* a clear seasoned stock or broth.

boulder /'bəʊldər/ *n* a large stone or mass of rock rounded by the action of erosion.

boule[1] /'buːl/ *n* an imitation gemstone.

boule[2] /'buːli/ *n* in ancient Athens, a higher popular assembly; (*with cap*) the lower house of the modern Greek legislative assembly.

boule[3] /buːl/ *see* **boulle**.

boules *n* (*used as sing*) a French game similar to bowls played with small, hard balls.

boulevard /'buːləˌvɑrd/ *n* a broad, often tree-lined road; ✤ (*Cdn*) a strip of grass between a sidewalk and a roadway; a median in the centre of a road that separates opposite directions of traffic.

boulevardier *Fr.* /buːlvɑr'djeɪ/ *n* a frequenter of a boulevard, *esp* a Parisian; a man about town.

bouleversement *Fr.* /buːˌvɛrs'mɑ̃/ *n* an overturning, overthrow.

boulle /buːl/ *n* decorative inlaying for cabinetwork, consisting of brass or other metal, tortoiseshell, etc, worked into scrolls or other patterns; the articles so ornamented.—*also* **boule, buhl.**

boult *see* **bolt**[2].

bounce /baʊns/ *vi* to rebound; to jump up suddenly; (*sl: cheque*) to be returned because of lack of funds; (*with* **back**) to recover easily, *eg* from misfortune or ill health. • *vt* to cause a ball to bounce; (*sl*) to put (a person) out by force; (*sl*) to fire from a job. • *n* a leap or springiness; capacity for bouncing; sprightliness; boastfulness, arrogance.

bouncer /'baʊnsər/ *n* (*sl*) a man hired to remove disorderly people from nightclubs, etc.

bouncing /'baʊnsɪŋ/ *adj* big, healthy, etc.

bouncy /'baʊnsi/ *adj* able to spring or bound; elastic; vigorous, lively.—**bouncily** *adv*.—**bounciness** *n*.

bound[1] /baʊnd/ *see* **bind**

bound[2] *n* (*usu pl*) the limit or boundary. • *vt* to limit, confine or surround; to name the boundaries of.

bound[3] *n* a jump or leap. • *vi* to jump or leap.

bound[4] *adj* (*with* **for**) intending to go to, on the way to.

boundary /'baʊndri/ or /-dəri/ *n* (*pl* **boundaries**) the border of an area; the limit; (*cricket*) the limit line of a field; a stroke that goes beyond the boundary line.

bounden /'baʊndən/ *adj* (*duty*) obligatory.

bounden duty *n* a moral obligation.

bounder /'baʊndər/ *n* one who or that which bounds; (*inf*) an insolent, ill-bred man, who makes himself disagreeable to those whom he meets.

boundless /'baʊndləs/ *adj* unlimited, vast.—**boundlessly** *adv*.—**boundlessness** *n*.

bounteous /'baʊntiəs/ *adj* giving freely, bountiful, generous; plentiful.—**bounteously** *adv*.—**bounteousness** *n*.

bountiful /'baʊntɪˌfʊl/ *adj* generous in giving.—**bountifully** *adv*.—**bountifulness** *n*.

bounty /'baʊnti/ *n* (*pl* **bounties**) generosity in giving; the gifts given; a reward or premium.

bouquet /buː'keɪ/ or /bɒ:-/ *n* a bunch of flowers; the perfume given off by wine.

bouquet garni /buː'keɪgɑr'niː/ *n* (*pl* **bouquets garnis**) herbs tied in a small bundle used for flavouring stews, soups, sauces, etc.

bourbon /'bɜrbən/ or /'bʊrbə̃/ *n* a whiskey distilled in the US from corn mash.

bourdon /'bʊrdən/ *n* the bass drone of the bagpipe; a bass stop of an organ.

bourgeois /bʊr'ʒwɒ/ *n* (*pl* **bourgeois**) a member of the bourgeoisie or middle class, a conventional and unimaginative individual. • *adj* smug, respectable, conventional; mediocre.

bourgeoisie /ˌbʊrʒwɒ'ziː/ *n* the class between the lower and upper classes, mostly composed of professional and business people.—*also* **middle class.**

bourn, bourne[1] /bɔrn/ or /bʊrn/ *n* a small stream, a rivulet.

bourn, bourne[2] *n* (*arch*) a boundary; a destination, goal; a realm.

bourrée /buː'reɪ/ *n* (*mus*) a composition of a lively character, similar to the gavotte; the music for this.

bourse /bʊrs/ *n* a stock exchange for the transaction of business; (*with cap*) the stock exchange of Paris.

bouse /baʊs/ or /baʊz/ *vi* (*naut*) to pull or haul hard.—*also* **bowse.**

boustrophedon /ˌbuːstrə'fiːdən/, /ˌbuː-/ *n* an ancient mode of writing lines alternately from left to right and from right to left.—**boustrophedonic** *adj*.

bout /baʊt/ *n* a spell, a turn, a period spent in some activity; a contest or struggle, *esp* boxing or wrestling; a time of illness.

boutique /buː'tiːk/ *n* a small shop, usually selling fashionable clothing and accessories.

boutonniere, boutonnière /ˌbuːtəˈniːr/ *n* a buttonhole; a spray of flowers worn in it.

bouzouki /buːˈzuːki/ *n* (*pl* **bouzoukis**) a Greek stringed instrument similar to the mandolin.

bovine /ˈboʊˌvaɪn/ *adj* relating to cattle; dull; sluggish. • *n* an ox, cow etc.

bow[1] /baʊ/ *vi* to bend the knee or to lean the head (and chest) forward as a form of greeting or respect or shame; (*with* **before**) to accept, to submit; (*with* **out**) to withdraw or retire gracefully. • *vt* to bend downwards; to weigh down; to usher in or out with a bow. • *n* a lowering of the head (and chest) in greeting.

bow[2] /boʊ/ *n* a weapon for shooting arrows; an implement for playing the strings of a violin; a decorative knot of ribbon, etc. • *vti* to bend, curve.

bow[3] /baʊ/ *n* the forward part of a ship.—**bow compass** /boʊ/ *n* (*geom*) a compass with jointed legs.

bowdlerize /ˈbaʊdlərˌaɪz/ *vt* to expurgate, to remove indelicate words from.—**bowdlerism** *n*.—**bowdlerization** *n*.

bowel /ˈbaʊəl/ *n* the intestine; (*pl*) entrails; (*pl*) the deep and remote part of anything.

bower[1] /ˈbaʊər/ *n* an arbour, a shady recess; (*poet*) dwelling.

bower *n* (*naut*) an anchor carried at the bow of a ship.

bower[3] *n* (*cards*) one of the two highest cards in some card games, or the second and third highest (when the joker is used).

bowerbird /-ˌbərd/ *n* one of various Australian birds belonging to the starling family.

bowhead /ˈboʊˌhɛd/ *n* an Arctic whale with a large mouth; Greenland whale.

bowie knife /ˈboʊiˌnaɪf/ or /ˈboʊ-/ *n* a long hunting knife, a sheath knife.

bowing /ˈboʊɪŋ/ *n* a playing upon an instrument of the violin class with a bow; the particular style of execution.

bowl[1] /boʊl/ *n* a wooden ball having a bias used in bowling; (*pl*) a game played on a smooth lawn with bowls. • *vti* to play the game of bowls; (*cricket*) to send a ball to a batsman; to dismiss (a batsman) by hitting the wicket with a bowled ball; (*with* **over**) to knock over; (*inf*) to astonish.

bowl[2] *n* a deep, rounded dish; the rounded end of a pipe; a sports stadium.

bow-legged /ˈboʊˌlɛɡəd/ *adj* having legs that curve outwards between the thigh and the ankle; bandy.

bowler[1] /ˈboʊlər/ *n* a person who plays bowls; (*cricket*) the player who delivers the ball.

bowler[2] *n* a stiff felt hat.—*also* **derby**.

bowline /ˈboʊlən/ *n* (*naut*) a knot used in making a fixed end loop; (*naut*) a rope from the weather side of a square sail to the bow to keep the ship near the wind.

bowling /ˈboʊlɪŋ/ *n* a game in which a heavy wooden ball is bowled along a bowling alley at ten wooden skittles; the game of bowls.

bowling alley *n* a long narrow wooden lane, *usu* one of several in a building designed for them.

bowling green *n* a smooth lawn for bowls.

bowman[1] /ˈboʊmən/ *n* (*pl* **bowmen**) an archer.

bowman[2] /ˈbaʊmən/ *n* (*pl* **bowmen**) (*naut*) the oarsman nearest the bow.

bowsaw *n* a saw with a blade under tension for cutting curves.

bowse *see* **bouse**.

bowsprit /ˈboʊˌsprɪt/ or *n* a large boom or spar running out from the stem of a (sailing) ship to carry its sails forward.

bowstring /ˈboʊˌstrɪŋ/ *n* the string of a bow.

bow tie /ˈboʊˌtaɪ/ *n* a necktie tied in the shape of a bow.

bow window /boʊˈwɪndoʊ/ *n* a curved bay window.

bow-wow /ˈbaʊwaʊ/ or /-ˈwaʊ/ *n* a dog's bark; a child's name for a dog. • *vi* to bark like a dog.

bowyer /ˈboʊjər/ *n* a maker or seller of archery bows.

box[1] /bɒks/ *n* a container or receptacle for holding anything; (*theatre*) a compartment with seats; (*inf*) a television set. • *vt* to put into a box; to enclose; (*with* **in**) to restrict.

box[2] *vt* to hit using the hands or fists. • *vi* to fight with the fists. • *n* a blow on the head or ear with the fist.

box[3] *n* an evergreen shrub or small tree yielding a hard close-grained wood; the wood. • *adj* of box or boxwood.

boxcar /-ˌkɑr/ *n* an enclosed freight car.

boxer /ˈbɒksər/ *n* a person who engages in boxing; a breed of dog with smooth hair and a stumpy tail.

boxer shorts *npl* loose underpants that resemble the pants worn by boxers.

box girder *n* a girder constructed from rectangular metal plates.

boxing /ˈbɒksɪŋ/ *n* the skill or sport of fighting with the fists.

Boxing Day the weekday following December 25, Christmas, when traditionally presents are given to tradesmen, employees, etc.

box lacrosse *n* ✤ (*Cdn*) a form of lacrosse played indoors. — *also* (*inf*) **boxla**.

box office *n* a theatre ticket office; the popularity of a play, film, actor.—**box-office** *adj*.

box pleat *n* a double pleat in cloth made by two facing folds.

boxwood /ˈbɒksˌwʊd/ *n* the hard wood of the box tree; the tree itself.

boy /bɔɪ/ *n* a male child; a son; a lad; a youth. • *interj* an exclamation of surprise or joy.

boyar /boʊˈjɑr/ *n* (*formerly*) a Russian landed proprietor of an old aristocratic order abolished by Peter I.

boycott /ˈbɔɪˌkɒt/ *vt* to refuse to deal with or trade with in order to punish or coerce.—*also n*.

boyfriend /ˈbɔɪˌfrɛnd/ *n* a male friend with whom a person is romantically or sexually involved.

boyhood /-ˌhʊd/ *n* the time, or state, of being a boy.

boyish /-ɪʃ/ *adj* like a boy; puerile; with the appeal of a boy.—**boyishly** *adv*.—**boyishness** *n*.

Boy Scout *n* a scout; (*without cap*) (*inf*) a man with a strong sense of duty.

boysenberry /ˈbɔɪzənˌbɛri/ or /ˈbɔɪsən-/ *n* (*pl* **boysenberries**) (the fruit of) a hybrid shrub developed by crossing the loganberry and various blackberries and raspberries.

BP, B/P *abbr* = blood pressure.

BQ *abbr* ✤ (*Cdn*) = Bloc Québécois.

Bq (*symbol*) bequerel.

Br *abbr* = British; (*chem symbol*) bromine; brother.

br'er /brər/ *n* (*dial*) brother.

bra /brɒ/ *n* a brassiere.

brace /breɪs/ *n* a prop; a support to stiffen a framework; a hand tool for drilling; (*pl* **brace**) a pair, *esp* of game; (*pl*) straps for holding up trousers; a dental appliance for straightening the teeth. • *vt* to steady.

brace and bit *n* a revolving tool for boring.

bracelet /ˈbreɪslət/ *n* an ornamental chain or band for the wrist; (*pl: sl*) handcuffs.

bracer[1] /ˈbreɪsər/ *n* something that braces; a pick-me-up.

bracer[2] *n* a wrist guard in archery.

brachial /ˈbrækiəl/ *adj* of, pertaining to, or like the arm.

brachiate /ˈbrækiət/ or /ˈbreɪ-/, /-eɪt/ *adj* having arms; (*bot*) having branches in pairs, nearly horizontal and each pair at right angles to the next.—**brachiation**.

brachiopod /ˈbrækioˌpɒd/ or /ˈbreɪ-/ *n* an animal like a mollusc with two spirally coiled armlike appendages, one on each side of the mouth.

brachy- /ˈbræki/ *prefix* short.

brachycephalic /ˌbrækisəˈfælɪk/, **brachycephalous** /ˌbrækisəˈfələs/ *adj* (*anat*) having the skull short in proportion to its breadth, short-headed.—**brachycephaly** *n*.

brachylogy /brəˈkɪlədʒi/ *n* (*pl* **brachylogies**) conciseness; a condensed expression.—**brachylogous** *adj*.

brachypterous /brəˈkɪptərəs/ *adj* (*insects*) short-winged.

brachyuran /ˌbrækijuərən/ *adj* of or belonging to a group of ten-footed crustaceans, including the crabs, marked by an undeveloped abdomen.—*also* **brachyurous**. • *n* a member of this group.

bracing /ˈbreɪsɪŋ/ *adj* refreshing, invigorating.—**bracingly** *adv*.

bracken /ˈbrækən/ *n* a large, coarse fern; a wide area of these growing on hills or moorland.

bracket /ˈbrækət/ *n* a projecting metal support for a shelf; a group or category of people classified according to income; (*pl*) a pair of characters (), [], {}, used in printing or writing as parentheses. • *vt* to support with brackets; to enclose by brackets; (*people*) to group together.

brackish /ˈbrækɪʃ/ *adj* somewhat salty; nauseating.—**brackishness** *n*.

bract /brækt/ *n* a modified leaf growing from a flower stem or enveloping a head of flowers.—**bracteal** *adj*.

bracteate /ˈbræktieɪt/ *adj* (*plant*) furnished with bracts. • *n* a plate or dish made of a thin beaten precious metal and decorated.

brad /bræd/ *n* a slender flat nail with a projection on one side.

bradawl /-ˌɒl/ *n* a small boring tool for making holes for brads.

brady- /'breɪdɪ/ *prefix* slow.

brae /breɪ/ *n* (*Scot*) a hillside; sloping ground.

brag /bræg/ *vti* (**bragging, bragged**) to boast. • *n* a boast or boastful talk.—**bragger** *n*.

braggadocio /ˌbrægə'doːtʃioː/ or /-doːʃoː/ *n* (*pl* **braggadocios**) bragging talk, empty boasting; a boaster, braggart.

braggart /'brægərt/ *n* a loud arrogant boaster.

Brahma[1] /'brɑːmə/ *n* (*Hinduism*) a supreme god; divine essence.

Brahma[2] *n* a useful variety of large domestic fowl with feathered legs.

Brahman[1] /'brɑːmən/ *n* (*pl* **Brahmans**) (*Hinduism*) a member of the highest caste, formerly consisting only of priests; Brahma.—**Brahmanic, Brahmanical** *adj*.

Brahman[2] *n* (*pl* **Brahmans, Brahman**) a breed of Indian cattle with a large hump used in crossbreeding beef cattle.

Brahmani /'brɑːmənɪ/ *n* (*pl* **Brahmanis**) a female Brahman.

Brahmanism /'brɑːmənˌɪzəm/ *n* the religion or doctrines of the Brahmans.—**Brahmanist** *n*.

Brahmin /'brɑːmɪn/ *n* a Brahman; a member of an upper-class New England family.

braid /breɪd/ *vt* to interweave three or more strands (of hair, straw, etc); to make by such interweaving. • *n* a narrow band made by such interweaving for decorating clothing; a plait.—**braider** *n*.

brail /breɪl/ *n* (*naut*) one of certain ropes used to gather up the foot and leeches of a sail prior to furling. • *vt* (*usu with* **up**) to haul in by the brails.

Braille /breɪl/ *n* printing for the blind, using a system of raised dots that can be understood by touch.—*also adj*.

brain /breɪn/ *n* nervous tissue contained in the skull of vertebrates that controls the nervous system; intellectual ability; (*inf*) a person of great intelligence; (*often pl*) the chief planner of an organization or enterprise. • *vt* to shatter the skull of; (*sl*) to hit on the head.

brainchild /-ˌtʃaɪld/ *n* (*pl* **brainchildren**) the result of creative thought; a clever and original idea or plan.

brain death *n* the irreversible cessation of brain activity, but not of the heartbeat, widely accepted as a criterion of death.

brain drain *n* the loss of highly skilled scientists, technicians, academics, etc through emigration.

brainless /-ləs/ *adj* (*inf*) stupid.—**brainlessness** *n*.

brainpan /-ˌpæn/ *n* the cranium.

brainstorm /-ˌstorm/ *n* a violent mental disturbance; a brain wave.

brainteaser /-ˌtiːzər/ *n* a mathematical puzzle; a difficult problem.

brainwash /-wɒʃ/ *vt* to change a person's ideas or beliefs by physical or mental conditioning, *usu* over a long period.—**brainwasher** *n*.—**brainwashing** *n*.

brain wave *n* an electrical impulse in the brain; (*inf*) a bright idea.

brainy /'breɪnɪ/ *adj* (**brainier, brainiest**) (*inf*) having a good mind; intelligent.—**braininess** *n*.

braise /breɪz/ *vt* (*meat, vegetables, etc*) to sauté lightly and cook slowly in liquid with the lid on.

brake[1] /breɪk/ *n* a device for slowing or stopping the motion of a wheel by friction. • *vt* to retard or stop by a brake. • *vi* to apply the brake on a vehicle; to become checked by a brake.

brake[2] *n* bracken.

brake[3] *n* a place overgrown with brushwood, etc; a thicket.

brake horsepower *n* the rate of work of an engine measured in terms of its resistance to a brake.

brakeman /'breɪkmən/ *n* (*pl* **brakemen**) a person in charge of a brake; a guard on a train; the person at the back of a bobsled team.

brake shoe *n* that part of a brake which presses against the wheel.

bramble /'bræmbəl/ *n* a prickly shrub or vine, *esp* of blackberries and raspberries.—**brambly** *adj*

brambling /'bræmblɪŋ/ *n* a migratory European finch with bright plumage.

bran /bræn/ *n* the husks of grain separated by sieving from the flour; a food containing these.

branch /brɑːntʃ/ *n* an offshoot extending from the trunk or bough of a tree or from the parent stem of a shrub; a separately located subsidiary or office of an enterprise or business; a part of something larger, *eg* a road or railway. • *vi* to possess branches; to divide into branches; to come out (from a main part) as a branch; (*with* **out**) to extend or enlarge one's interests, activities, etc.

branchia /'bræŋkɪə/ *n* (*pl* **branchiae**) a respiratory organ of fishes and some amphibians, a gill.—**branchial** *adj*.

branchiate /'bræŋkɪeɪt/ *adj* having permanent gills.

branchio- /'bræŋkɪoː/ *prefix* gills.

branchiopod /-ˌpɒd/ *n* one of a group of crustaceans, including the water flea, the gills of which are situated on the feet.

branch plant *n* ✻ (*Cdn*) a factory or business owned by a company based in another country.

brand /brænd/ *n* an identifying mark on cattle, imprinted with hot iron; a burning piece of wood; a mark of disgrace; a trademark; a particular make (of goods). • *vt* to burn a mark with a hot iron; to fix in the memory; to denounce.

brandish /'brændɪʃ/ *vt* (*a weapon, etc*) to wave or flourish in a threatening manner.—**brandisher** *n*.

brandling /'brændlɪŋ/ *n* a small brownish-red earthworm used as bait by freshwater anglers.

brand name *n* the name by which a certain commodity is known.—**brand-name** *adj*.

brand-new /'brænd'njuː/ *adj* entirely new and unused.

brandy /'brændɪ/ *n* (*pl* **brandies**) an alcoholic liquor made from distilled wine or fermented fruit juice.

brant /brænt/ *n* the brent goose, the smallest species of the wild goose.

brash[1] /bræʃ/ *adj* bold; loud-mouthed; reckless.—**brashly** *adv*.—**brashness** *n*.

brash[2] *n* broken, loose and angular fragments of rock underlying alluvial deposits; small broken pieces of ice; hedge clippings.

brash[3] *n* acid eructation; a fit of sickness; a rash; a burst of rain.

brasilin /'bræzəˌlɪn/ or /brə'zɪlɪn/ *see* **brazilin**.

brass /brɑːs/ *n* an alloy of copper and zinc; (*inf*) impudence; nerve; cheek; money; (*often pl*) the brass instruments of an orchestra or band; (*sl*) officers or officials of high rank.

brassard, brassart /'bræsˌɑːd/ *n* armour for the upper arm; an armlet for the upper arm.

brass band *n* a band that uses brass and percussion instruments.

brasserie /ˌbræsə'riː/ *n* a bar and restaurant.

brassica /'bræsɪkə/ *n* any of a group of plants that includes cabbages, turnips and mustards.—**brassicaceous** *adj*.

brassie /'bræsɪ/ *n* (*golf*) a wooden club orig with a brass sole, now No 2 wood.

brassiere /brə'zɪːr/ *n* a woman's undergarment for protecting and supporting the breasts, a bra.

brass tacks *npl* (*inf*) basic facts.

brassy /'brɑːsɪ/ *adj* (**brassier, brassiest**) like brass; brazen; cheeky.—**brassily** *adv*.—**brassiness** *n*.

brat /bræt/ *n* an ill-mannered, annoying child.

bratpack /-pæk/ *n* a group of precociously young actors, writers, etc.

brattice /'brætɪs/ *n* (*mining*) a wooden partition or separating wall in a level or shaft to form an air passage. • *vt* to divide by a brattice.

bratwurst /'brætwərst/ *n* a type of seasoned German sausage made from pork.

bravado /brə'vɑːdoː/ *n* (*pl* **bravadoes, bravados**) pretended confidence; swaggering.

brave /breɪv/ *adj* showing courage; not timid or cowardly; fearless; handsome; of excellent appearance. • *vt* to confront boldly; to defy. • *n* a North American Indian warrior.—**bravely** *adv*.

bravery /'breɪvərɪ/ *n* (*pl* **braveries**) the quality of being brave; courage, fearlessness; finery, magnificence.

bravo /'brɑːvoː/ *interj* well done! • *n* (*pl* **bravoes, bravos**) a cry or shout of "bravo!"

bravura /brə'vjʊərə/ *n* bold daring; dash; (*mus*) a passage requiring spirit and technical brilliance.

brawl /brɔːl/ *n* a loud quarrel; a noisy fight. • *vi* to quarrel loudly.—**brawler** *n*.

brawn /brɔːn/ *n* strong, well-developed muscles; physical strength; pickled pork.

brawny /-nɪ/ *adj* (**brawnier, brawniest**) muscular, tough.—**brawnily** *adv*.—**brawniness** *n*.

bray /breɪ/ *n* the sound of a donkey; any harsh sound. • *vi* (**braying, brayed**) to make similar sounds.—**brayer** *n*.

bray[2] *vt* (**braying, brayed**) to pound or beat fine or small.

brayer /-ər/ *n* (*print*) a hand roller used to rub down and temper ink.

braze[1] /breɪz/ *vt* to solder with an alloy of brass and zinc.—**brazer** *n*.

braze[2] /breɪz/ *vt* to cover or ornament with brass; to colour like brass.

brazen /ˈbreɪzən/ *adj* made of brass; shameless. • *vt* (*usu with* **out**) to face a situation boldly and shamelessly.—**brazenness** *n*.

brazier[1] /ˈbreɪzɪər/ or /-ʒər/ *n* a metal container for hot coals.

brazier[2] *n* a worker in brass.

brazil /brəˈzɪl/ *n* brazilwood; a dye of various tints of *esp* red and orange obtained from brazilin.

brazilin /ˈbrzəˌlɪn/ or /brəˈzɪlɪn/ *n* the colouring substance extracted from brazilwood.—*also* **brasilin**.

brazil nut *n* a large three-cornered nut, the seed of a tall tree of Brazil.

brazilwood /brəˈzɪlwʊd/ *n* a very heavy wood of a red colour from various species of Central and South American trees.

breach /briːtʃ/ *n* a break or rupture; violation of a contract, promise, etc; a break in friendship. • *vt* to make an opening in.

breach of promise *n* the breaking of a promise to marry.

breach of the peace *n* a public disturbance.

bread /bred/ *n* a dough, made from flour, yeast and milk, that is baked; nourishment; (*sl*) money; **bread and butter** (*inf*) one's livelihood. • *vt* to coat meat, fish, etc with breadcrumbs before cooking.

bread-and-butter /-ən'bʌtər/ *adj* (*job*) providing a basic income; (*issues, etc*) fundamental, basic; (*letter*) thanking for hospitality.

breadbasket /-ˌbæskət/ *n* a basket for holding bread; (*sl*) the stomach; a source of food.

breadboard /-ˌbɔrd/ *n* a wooden board for cutting bread on; board used for constructing experimental electric circuits.

breaded /-əd/ *adj* coated with breadcrumbs.

breadfruit /-fruːt/ *n* (*pl* **breadfruits, breadfruit**) the fruit of a tree growing in the Pacific islands, which, when roasted, is eaten as bread.

breadline /-laɪn/ *n* a queue for bread ration; **on the breadline** poverty-stricken, only just able to subsist.

breadth /bredθ/ *n* measurement from side to side, width; extent; liberality (*eg* of interests).

breadthways /-ˌweɪz/, **breadthwise** /-ˌwaɪz/ *adv* from side to side.

breadwinner /ˈbredˌwɪnər/ *n* the principal wage-earner of a family.

break /breɪk/ *vb* (**breaking, broke,** *pp* **broken**) *vt* to smash or shatter; to tame; (*rules*) to violate; to discontinue; to cause to give up a habit; (*fall*) to lessen the severity of; to ruin financially; (*news*) to impart; to decipher or solve; (*with* **down**) to crush or destroy; to analyse; (*with* **in**) to intervene; to train. • *vi* to fall apart; (*voice*) to assume a lower tone at puberty; to cut off relations with; to suffer a collapse, as of spirit; (*news*) to become public in a sudden and sensational manner; (*with* **down**) to fail completely; to succumb emotionally; (*with* **even**) to suffer neither profit nor loss (after taking certain action); (*with* **in**) to force a way in; (*with* **out**) to appear, begin; to erupt; to throw off restraint, escape; (*with* **up**) to disperse; to separate; to collapse. • *n* a breaking; an interruption; a gap; a sudden change, as in weather; a rest or a short holiday; an escape; (*snooker, billiards*) a continuous run of points; (*sl*) a fortunate opportunity.

breakable /ˈbreɪkəbəl/ *adj* able to be broken. • *n* a fragile object.

breakage /breɪkədʒ/ *n* the action of breaking; something broken.

breakaway /ˈbreɪkəweɪ/ *n* secession, disassociation.

break dancing /breɪkdænsɪŋ/ *n* dancing that involves acrobatic movements.

breakdown /ˈbreɪkdaʊn/ *n* a mechanical failure; failure of health; nervous collapse; an analysis.

breakdown truck *n* a vehicle for towing away smashed or damaged cars, etc.

breaker[1] /ˈbreɪkər/ *n* a large wave that crashes onto the shore, reef, etc.

breaker[2] *n* (*naut*) a small cask for holding water.

breakeven /ˌbreɪkˈiːvən/ *n* the point at which costs are covered but no profit is made.

breakfast /ˈbrekfəst/ *n* the first meal of the morning; the food consumed. • *vi* to have breakfast.

break-in /ˈbreɪkˌɪn/ *n* the unlawful entering of premises, *esp* by thieves.

breakneck /ˈbreɪknɛk/ *adj* dangerously steep or fast.

break of day *n* dawn.

break-out /ˈbreɪkˌaʊt/ *n* an escape, *esp* from prison.

breakthrough /ˈbreɪkˌθruː/ *n* the action of breaking through an obstruction; an important advance or discovery.

break-up /ˈbreɪkʌp/ *n* separation; collapse; dispersal; ✸ (*Cdn*) the thawing of ice in spring in a frozen river or lake.—*also* **spring break-up.**

breakwater /ˈbreɪkˌwɔtər/ *n* a barrier that protects a harbour or area of coast against the force of the waves.

bream[1] /briːm/ *n* (*pl* **bream**) a freshwater fish.

bream[2] *vt* (*naut*) to clear (a ship's bottom) of shells, seaweed, etc, by heating and scraping.

breast /brest/ *n* the chest; one of the two mammary glands; the seat of the emotions. • *vt* to oppose, confront; to arrive at the top of; to confess (*make a clean breast of*).

breastbone /ˈbrestboːn/ *n* (*anat*) the flat narrow bone in the centre of the chest that connects the ribs, the sternum.

breast-feed /ˈbrestfiːd/ *vt* (**breast-feeding, breast-fed**) to allow a baby to suck milk from the breast.

breastplate /ˈbrestpleɪt/ *n* armour covering the front of the body; a part of the vestment of a Jewish high priest.

breaststroke /ˈbrestˌstroːk/ *n* a swimming stroke in which both arms are brought out sideways from the chest.

breastwork /brestˌwɜrk/ *n* a hastily constructed work thrown up breast-high for defence; the parapet of a building.

breath /breθ/ *n* the inhalation and exhalation of air in breathing; the air taken into the lungs; life; a slight breeze; (*scandal*) a hint.

Breathalyzer, Breathalyser /breθəlaɪzər/ *n* (*trademark*) a device for measuring the amount of alcohol in a person's breath.

breathe /briːð/ *vi* to inhale and exhale, to respire air; to take a rest or pause; to exist or live; to speak or sing softly; to whisper. • *vt* to emit or exhale; to whisper or speak softly.

breather /ˈbriːðər/ *n* a pause during exercise to recover one's breath.

breathing /ˈbriːðɪŋ/ *n* respiration; air in gentle motion; a gentle influence; a pause; (*phonetics*) an accent (') whether an initial vowel is aspirated or not.

breathing space *n* a pause in which to recover, get organized or get going.

breathless /ˈbreθləs/ *adj* out of breath; panting; gasping; unable to breathe easily because of emotion.—**breathlessly** *adv*.—**breathlessness** *n*.

breathtaking /ˈbreθˌteɪkɪŋ/ *adj* very exciting.

breathy /ˈbrɛθi/ *adj* (**breathier, breathiest**) (*voice*) not clear sounding.—**breathily** *adv*.—**breathiness** *n*.

breccia /ˈbretʃiə/ *n* a rock of angular fragments cemented by lime, etc.—**brecciated** *adj*.

bred *see* **breed.**

bree /briː/ *n* (*Scot*) broth; juice or liquor in which something has been steeped or boiled.

breech /briːtʃ/ *n* the back part of a gun barrel.

breech delivery, breech birth *n* the birth of a baby buttocks or feet first.

breeches /-əz/ *npl* trousers extending just below the knee.

breeches buoy *n* a lifebuoy on a hawser to take people off a wreck.

breeching /-ɪŋ/ *n* the harness that passes round a horse's hindquarters; a strong rope to check the recoil of a gun.

breechloader /-loːdər/ *n* a gun loaded at the breach.—**breechloading** *adj*.

breed /briːd/ *vb* (**breeding, bred**) *vt* to engender; to bring forth; (*dogs*) to raise; to give rise to. • *vi* to produce young; to be generated. • *n* offspring; lineage or race; species (of animal).—**breeder** *n*.

breeder reactor *n* a nuclear reactor that produces more fissile material than it consumes.

breeding /ˈbriːdɪŋ/ *n* the bearing of offspring; one's education and training; refined behaviour.

breeze[1] /briːz/ *n* a light gentle wind; something easy to do. • *vi* (*inf*) to move quickly or casually.

breeze[2] *n* sifted ashes and cinders used in burning bricks; house sweepings, refuse.

breeze block *n* a lightweight building brick composed mainly of the ashes of coal and coke.

breezy /ˈbriːzi/ *adj* (**breezier, breeziest**) windy; nonchalant; light-hearted, cheerful.—**breezily** *adv*.—**breeziness** *n*.

brent (goose) /brent/ *n* the smallest species of the wild goose.—*also* **brant.**

brethren /ˈbreðrən/ *see* **brother.**

Breton /ˈbretən/ *adj* of or relating to Brittany, its people or language. • *n* an inhabitant of Brittany; the Celtic language of Brittany.

breve /briːv/ *n* a mark (^) used to indicate a short vowel; (*mus*) the longest note now used, equal to two whole notes (two semi-breves or four minims).

brevet /brə'vet/ *n* (*mil*) a commission to an officer in the army conferring a higher rank but without increase of pay; a warrant; a licence. • *adj* conferred by brevet; nominal, honorary. • *vt* (**brevetting, brevetted** *or* **breveting, breveted**) to confer brevet rank on.—**brevetcy** *n*.

brevi- /'brevɪ/ *prefix* short.

breviary /'briːvɪərɪ/ or /'briːˌvɪərɪ/, /'brev-/ *n* (*pl* **breviaries**) (*RC Church*) a book containing the daily offices and prayers.

brevirostrate /'brevɪˈrɒsˌtreɪt/ *adj* (*birds*) short-billed.

brevity /'brevɪtɪ/ *n* (*pl* **brevities**) briefness; conciseness.

brew /bruː/ *vt* to make (beer, ale, etc) from malt and hops by boiling and fermenting; to infuse (tea, etc); to plot, scheme. • *vi* to be in the process of being brewed; to be about to happen. • *n* a brewed drink.

brewage /-ədʒ/ *n* something made by brewing; the brewing process.

brewer /'bruːər/ *n* a person who brews, *usu* beer.

brewery /'bruːərɪ/ *n* (*pl* **breweries**) a place where beer, etc is brewed.

briar /'braɪər/ *see* **brier**.

bribe /braɪb/ *n* money or gifts offered illegally to gain favour or influence; the gift to achieve this. • *vt* to offer or give a bribe to.—**bribable** *adj*.—**briber** *n*.

bribery /-ərɪ/ *n* (*pl* **briberies**) the giving or taking of bribes.

bric-a-brac /'brɪkəˌbræk/ *n* curios, ornamental or rare odds and ends.

brick /brɪk/ *n* a baked clay block for building; a similar shaped block of other material. • *vt* to lay or wall up with brick.

brickbat /-bæt/ *n* a piece of brick, *esp* one used as a weapon; an unfavourable remark.

bricklayer /'brɪkleɪər/ *n* a person who lays bricks.

brick red *n* a greyish red colour.—**brick-red** *adj*.

brickwork /'brɪkwɜːk/ *n* a structure formed of bricks.

bridal /'braɪdəl/ *adj* relating to a bride or a wedding.

bride /braɪd/ *n* a woman about to be married or recently married.

bridegroom /'braɪdgruːm/ or /-grʊm/ *n* a man about to be married or recently married.

bridesmaid /'braɪdzmeɪd/ *n* a young girl or woman attending the bride during a wedding.

bridge¹ /brɪdʒ/ *n* a structure built to convey people or traffic over a river, road, railway line, etc; the platform on a ship where the captain gives directions; the hard ridge of bone in the nose; an arch to raise the strings of a guitar, etc; a mounting for false teeth. • *vt* to be or act as a bridge; to be a connecting link between.—**bridgeable** *adj*.

bridge² *n* a card game for two teams of two players based on whist.

bridgeboard /'brɪdʒbɔːd/ *n* a notched board into which the ends of the steps of wooden stairs are fastened.

bridge financing *n* ✲ (*Cdn*) bridge loan.

bridgehead /-hed/ *n* a defensive work covering the end of a bridge nearest the enemy; a foothold in enemy territory.

bridge loan *n* a temporary loan made to cover a short period before more permanent financing is arranged.

bridgework /-wɜːk/ *n* a false tooth or teeth secured to the natural teeth.

bridging /-ɪŋ/ *n* a piece of wood between two beams to keep them apart.

bridging loan *n* a loan, *usu* short-term, advanced to cover the gap between the settlement of two transactions, *esp* between buying a new house and selling the old one.

bridle /'braɪdəl/ *n* the headgear of a horse, controlling its movements; a restraint or check; (*naut*) a mooring cable. • *vt* to put a bridle on (a horse); to restrain or check. • *vi* to draw one's head back as an expression of anger, scorn, etc.—**bridler** *n*.

bridle path *n* a trail suitable for horse riding.

bridoon /brɪ'duːn/ *n* the light snaffle and rein of a military bridle.

brie /briː/ *n* creamy white soft cheese.

brief /briːf/ *n* a summary of a client's case for the instruction of a barrister in a trial at law; an outline of an argument, *esp* that setting out the main contentions; (*pl*) men's or women's close-fitting underpants or knickers. • *vt* to provide with a precise summary of the facts. • *adj* short, concise.—**briefly** *adv*.—**briefness** *n*.

briefcase /'briːfkeɪs/ *n* a flat case for carrying documents, etc.

brier /'braɪər/ *n* a plant with a thorny or prickly woody stem; a mass of these; a tobacco pipe made from the root of the brier.—*also* **briar**.—**briery, briary** *adj*.

brig /brɪg/ *n* a two-masted square-rigged vessel; a naval prison, *esp* on a ship.

brigade /brɪ'geɪd/ *n* an army unit, smaller than a division, commanded by a brigadier; a group of people organized to perform a particular function.

brigadier /brɪgə'dɪə/ *n* an officer commanding a brigade and ranking next below a major general.

brigand /'brɪgənd/ *n* a bandit, *usu* one of a roving gang.

brigantine /'brɪgənˌtiːn/ *n* a small two-masted vessel, square-rigged on the foremast only and with raking masts.

bright /braɪt/ *adj* clear, shining; brilliant in colour or sound; favourable or hopeful; intelligent, illustrious.—**brightly** *adv*—**brightness** *n*.

Bright's disease *n* a kidney disease characterized by the presence of albumin in the urine.

brighten /'braɪtən/ *vti* to make or become brighter.—**brightener** *n*.

brill /brɪl/ *n* (*pl* **brill, brills**) a European flatfish resembling the turbot.

brilliance /'brɪljəns/ *n* intense radiance, lustre, splendour.

brilliancy /-sɪ/ *n* the quality of being brilliant; shining quality, lustrousness, shining brightness.

brilliant /'brɪljənt/ *adj* sparkling, bright; splendid; very intelligent.—**brilliantly** *adv*.

brilliantine /'brɪljənˌtiːn/ *n* a cosmetic oil giving a gloss to the hair; a shiny fabric of cotton and mohair.

brim /brɪm/ *n* the rim of a hollow vessel; the outer edge of a hat. • *vi* (**brimming, brimmed**) to fill or be filled to the brim; (*with* **over**) to overflow.

brimful /'brɪmˌfʊl/ *adj* completely full; overflowing.

brimstone /'brɪmstəʊn/ *n* sulphur; a yellow butterfly.

brin /brɪn/ *n* ✲ (*Cdn*) in Newfoundland, a burlap bag.

brindled /'brɪndəld/ *adj* streaked brown or grey, or with flecks of a darker colour.

brine /braɪn/ *n* salt water; the sea.

bring /brɪŋ/ *vt* (**bringing, brought**) to fetch, carry or convey "here" or to the place where the speaker will be; to cause to happen (*eg* rain, relief), to result in; to lead to an action or belief; to sell for; (*with* **about**) to induce, to effect; (*with* **down**) to cause to fall by or as if by shooting; (*with* **forth**) to give birth to; (*with* **forward**) to present something for consideration; to transfer a total figure from the bottom of a page to the top of the next page; (*with* **in**) to yield a profit or return; to return a verdict in court; to introduce (a legislative bill); to earn (an income); (*with* **off**) to achieve a success, often against odds; accomplish; (*with* **out**) to cause to appear; to produce (a play) or publish (a book); to demonstrate clearly, expose to view; to help someone with encouragement; (*with* **over**) to convince a person to change their loyalties; (*with* **round**) to convince a person to change their opinion; to get someone to agree or give support; to restore a person to consciousness, revive; (*with* **up**) to educate, rear a child; to raise (a matter) for discussion; to vomit.—**bringer** *n*.

brink /brɪŋk/ *n* the verge of a steep place; the edge of the sea; the point of onset; the threshold of danger.

brinkmanship /'brɪŋkmənˌʃɪp/, **brinksmanship** *n* the pursuing of a policy, *esp* in international relations, that brings serious risk of danger in order to gain advantage.

briny /'braɪnɪ/ *adj* (**brinier, briniest**) salty. • *n* the sea.—**brininess** *n*.

brio /'briːəʊ/ *n* vivacity.

brioche /'briːɒʃ/ or /bri'ɒːʃ/ *n* a small, slightly sweet, bread roll.

briony /'braɪənɪ/ *see* **bryony**.

briquette, briquet /brɪ'ket/ *n* a compacted brick *usu* of fine compressed material, *esp* charcoal.

brisk /brɪsk/ *adj* alert; vigorous; sharp in tone.—**briskly** *adv*—**briskness** *n*.

brisket /'brɪskət/ *n* meat from the breast of an animal.

brisling /'brɪzlɪŋ/ or /'brɪs-/ *n* a small fish like a sardine.

bristle /'brɪsəl/ *n* a short, coarse hair. • *vi* to stand up, as bristles; to have the bristles standing up; to show anger or indignation; to be thickly covered (with).

bristly /'brɪslɪ/ *adj* (**bristlier, bristliest**) covered with bristles; rough.—**bristliness** *n*.

Bristol board *n* a thick smooth white pasteboard.

brit /brɪt/ *n* the young of the herring and sprat; small animals upon which whales feed.

Brit /brɪt/ *n* (*inf*) a British person.

Brit. *abbr* = Britain; British.

Britannia /brɪˈtænjə/ *n* Britain or its former empire personified.

Britannia metal *n* a white metal alloy of tin, copper, antimony and bismuth, resembling pewter.

Britannic /brɪˈtænɪk/ *adj* of Britain; British.

Briticism /ˈbrɪtəˌsɪzəm/ *n* a word, phrase, etc, peculiar to or characteristic of British English.

British /ˈbrɪtɪʃ/ *adj* of or pertaining to Great Britain or its inhabitants; pertaining to the ancient Britons. • *n* the people of Britain; the language of the ancient Britons.

British Columbian *n* ✤ a person who lives in or is from British Columbia. • *adj* of British Columbia.

Britisher /-ər/ *n* a British subject.

Britishism /-ˌʃɪzəm/ *n* a Briticism.

Briton /brɪtən/ *n* a native of Great Britain, *esp* before the Anglo-Saxon conquest.

brittle /brɪtəl/ *adj* easily cracked or broken; fragile; sharp-tempered.—**brittleness** *n*.

britzka /ˈbrɪtskə/, **britzska** /ˈbrɪtʃkɒ/ *n* an open carriage with a hooded top and space for reclining.

bro /broː/ *n* (*inf*) mate, buddy.

broach /broːtʃ/ *vt* (*a topic*) to introduce for discussion; to pierce (a container) and draw out liquid.

broad /brɒd/ *adj* of large extent from side to side; wide; spacious; giving an overall view or idea; (*humour*) coarse; strongly marked in dialect or pronunciation. • *n* (*sl*) a woman.—**broadly** *adv*.—**broadness** *n*.

broad arrow *n* an arrow with a broad barbed head; a UK government mark to distinguish its property.

broad bean *n* a plant widely grown for its large flat edible seed.

Broad Church *n* a section or party intermediate between the High and the Low Church of England; any group that opposes rigid dogma.—**Broad-Church** *adj*.

broad seal *n* the official seal of a nation.

broadcast /-kæst/ *n* a programme on radio or television. • *vti* (**broadcasting, broadcast**) to transmit on radio or television; to make known widely; to scatter seed.—**broadcaster** *n*.

broadcloth /-klɒθ/ *n* a fine woollen cloth with a smooth finished surface.

broaden /ˈbrɒdən/ *vti* to grow or make broad; to widen.

broadloom /ˈbrɒdluːm/ *adj* (*carpets*) woven on a wide loom.

broad-minded /brɒdˈmaɪndɪd/ *adj* tolerant; liberal in outlook.—**broad-mindedly** *adv*.—**broad-mindedness** *n*.

broadsheet /ˈbrɒdʃiːt/ *n* a large sheet of paper printed on one side only; a large format newspaper, approx 15 by 24 inches (38 by 61cms).

broadside /ˈbrɒdsaɪd/ *n* the entire side of a ship above the waterline; a simultaneous volley from one side of a warship; a sheet printed on one side containing information of a popular nature or an attack on some public person; any verbal or written attack.

broad-spectrum /-ˈspɛktrəm/ *adj* efficacious against a wide range (of diseases, microorganisms).

broadsword /ˈbrɒdsɔːrd/ *n* a cutting sword with a broad straight blade.

Brobdingnagian /brɒbdɪŋˈnægiən/ *adj* resembling one of the giant inhabitants of the land of Brobdingnag in Swift's *Gulliver's Travels*; gigantic.

brocade /broˈkeɪd/ *n* a heavy fabric woven with raised patterns, orig in gold and silver. • *vt* to work with a raised pattern.

brocatelle, brocatel /ˌbrɒkəˈtɛl/ *n* a figured brocade of silky texture; a variegated marble from Italy and Spain.

broccoli /ˈbrɒkəli/ *n* (*pl* **broccoli**) a kind of cauliflower with loose heads of tiny green buds.

broch /brɒk/ or *Scot.* /brɒx/ *n* (*Scot*) a dry-built circular tower of the Iron Age.

brochette /brɒˈʃɛt/ or /brəˈʃɛt/ *n* (food cooked on) a skewer or small spit.

brochure /ˈbroˈʃʊr/ or /-ˈʃər/, /ˈbroːʃər/ *n* an advertising booklet.

brock /brɒk/ *n* (*dial*) a badger.

brogan /ˈbroːgən/ *n* a sturdy ankle-high work shoe.

brogue /broːg/ *n* a sturdy shoe; a dialectical accent, *esp* Irish.

broil[1] /brɔɪl/ *vti* to cook by exposure to direct heat; to grill.

broil[2] *n* a noisy quarrel, a tumult. • *vi* to be heated with passion.

broiler /brɔɪlər/ *n* a pan, grill, etc for broiling; a bird fit for broiling.

broke /broːk/ *pt* of **break**. • *adj* (*inf*) hard up, having no money.

broken /ˈbroːkən/ *pp* of **break**. • *adj* splintered, fractured; violated; ruined; tamed; disconnected, interrupted; overwhelmed by sorrow or ill fortune; (*speech*) imperfect.—**brokenly** *adv*.—**brokenness** *n*.

broken-down /-daʊn/ *adj* extremely infirm; worn out.

brokenhearted *adj* grief-stricken; very sad.

broken-winded *adj* (*horse*) having the heaves.

broker /ˈbroːkər/ *n* an agent who negotiates contracts of purchase and sale (as of commodities or securities); a power broker; a stockbroker.

brokerage /ˈbroːkərɪdʒ/ *n* a broker's business; the commission charged by a broker.

bromate /ˈbroːmeɪt/ *n* a salt of bromic acid.

brome (grass) /broːm/ *n* any of a genus of oat-like grasses with drooping clusters of spikelets.

bromic acid *n* a compound of bromine and oxygen.

bromide /ˈbroːmaɪd/ *n* a compound of bromine; a sedative; (*sl*) a bore; a trite remark.

bromine /ˈbroːmiːn/ *n* an evil-smelling nonmetallic element related to chlorine and iodine.—**bromic** *adj*.

bronchi /ˈbrɒŋkaɪ/ *see* **bronchus**.

bronchia /ˈbrɒŋkɪə/ *npl* (*sing* **bronchium**) the bronchial tubes.

bronchial /-əl/ *adj* of or pertaining to the bronchial tubes.

bronchial tube *n* either of the two main branches of the windpipe.

bronchitis /brɒŋˈkaɪtɪs/ *n* inflammation of the lining of the bronchial tubes.—**bronchitic** *adj*.

bronchopneumonia /ˌbrɒŋkonəˈmoːnjə/ or /-nuːˈmoː/, /njuːˈmoː/ *n* diffuse inflammation of the lungs and bronchi.

bronchus /ˈbrɒŋkəs/ *n* (*pl* **bronchi**) one of the two principal branches of the windpipe or trachea.

bronco /ˈbrɒŋkoː/ *n* (*pl* **broncos**) a wild or half-tamed horse of North America.

broncobuster /-ˌbʌstər/ *n* a cowboy who breaks in broncos.—**broncobusting** *n*.

brontosaur, brontosaurus /ˌbrɒntəˈsɔːrəs/ *n* (*pl* **brontosauruses**) a large plant-eating dinosaur.—**brontosaurian** *adj*.

Bronx cheer *n* (*inf*) a rude sound made with the lips; a raspberry.

bronze /brɒnz/ *n* a copper and tin alloy, sometimes other elements; any object cast in bronze; a reddish-brown colour. • *adj* made of, or like, or of the colour of bronze; (*skin*) tanned.—**bronzy** *adj*.

Bronze Age *n* the age succeeding the Stone Age, the ornaments and weapons of that period being made of bronze.

brooch /broːtʃ/ *n* an ornament held by a pin or a clasp.

brood /bruːd/ *vi* to incubate or hatch (eggs); to ponder over or worry about. • *n* a group having a common nature or origin, *esp* the children in a family; the number produced in one hatch.

broody /ˈbruːdi/ *adj* (**broodier, broodiest**) contemplative, moody; (*inf*) wanting to have a baby.—**broodily** *adv*.—**broodiness** *n*.

brook[1] /brʊk/ *n* a freshwater stream.

brook[2] *vt* to tolerate.—**brookable** *adj*.

brooklet /-lət/ *n* a small brook.

broom[1] /bruːm/ *n* a bundle of fibres or twigs attached to a long handle for sweeping.

broom[2] *n* a shrub bearing large yellow flowers.

broomball /ˈbruːmbɒl/ *n* ✤ a game similar to ice hockey in which players run rather than skate and use brooms or broom handles to propel a large ball.

broomstick /ˈbruːmstɪk/ or /ˈbrʊm-/ *n* the handle of a broom.

Bros *abbr* = Brothers.

brose /broːz/ *n* (*Scot*) a kind of porridge made by pouring boiling water or milk on meat liquor on oatmeal.

broth /brɒθ/ *n* a thin or thick soup made by boiling meat, etc in water.

brothel /ˈbrɒθəl/ *n* a house where prostitutes work.

brother /ˈbrɛðər/ *n* a male sibling; a friend who is like a brother; a fellow member of a group, profession or association; a lay member of a men's religious order; (*pl* **brethren**) used chiefly in formal address or in referring to the members of a society or sect.

Brother Jonathan *n* (*hist*) a humorous personification of the US.

brotherhood /-hʊd/ *n* the state or quality of being a brother, brotherliness; a fraternity, an association.

brother-in-law /-ɪnlɒ/ *n* (*pl* **brothers-in-law**) the brother of a husband or wife; the husband of a sister.

brotherly /-li/ *adj* like a brother; kind; affectionate.—**brotherliness** *n*.

brougham /ˈbruːəm/ or /bruːm/, /ˈbroːəm/ *n* a light closed four-wheeled carriage for one or two horses.

brought /brɒt/ *see* **bring**.

brouhaha /ˈbruːhɒhɒ/ *n* a fuss; uproar.

brow /braʊ/ *n* the forehead; the eyebrows; the top of a cliff; the jutting top of a hill.

browbeat /ˈbraʊbiːt/ *vt* (**browbeating, browbeat,** *pp* **browbeaten**) to intimidate with threats, to bully.

brown /braʊn/ *adj* having the colour of chocolate, a mixture of red, black and yellow; tanned. • *n* a brown colour. • *vi* to make or become brown, *esp* by cooking.—**brownish** *adj.*—**brownness** *n*.

brown bear *n* a large wild bear of a brownish colour that lives in forests in temperate areas of Asia, North America and Europe.

brown bread *n* bread made from wholemeal flour.

brown coal *n* lignite.

brown cow *n* ♣ (*Cdn*) a drink made from a mixture of coffee liqueur and milk or cream.

brownie /ˈbraʊni/ *n* a square of flat, rich chocolate cake; a friendly helpful elf; (*with cap*) ♣ a member of the junior branch of the Girl Scout or Guide movement.

Brownie point *n* a credit gained by having scored some success.

brown rice *n* unpolished rice.

brown study *n* a reverie.

brown sugar *n* sugar that is unrefined or partially refined.

browned-off *adj* (*sl*) fed up, depressed.

Brownian movement *n* a rapid whirling movement frequently seen in microscopic particles suspended in water or other liquids.

Browning /ˈbraʊnɪŋ/ *n* an automatic or semi-automatic gas-operated rifle; an automatic machine gun.

brownshirt /-ʃɜːt/ *n* (*often cap*) a member of the Nazi Party; a storm trooper.

brownstone /ˈbraʊnstoːn/ *n* a kind of sandstone; a house built of this.

browse /braʊz/ *vti* to nibble, to graze; to examine (a book) at one's leisure or casually.—**browser** *n*.

brucellosis /ˌbruːsəˈloːsɪs/ *n* an infectious disease of livestock, *esp* cattle, which can be passed to human beings.

bruin /ˈbruːɪn/ *n* the brown bear personified.

bruise /bruːz/ *vt* to injure and discolour (body tissue, surface of fruit) without breaking the skin; to break down (as leaves and berries) by pounding; to inflict psychological pain on. • *vi* to inflict a bruise; to undergo bruising. • *n* contusion of the skin; a similar injury to plant tissue; an injury, *esp* to the feelings.

bruiser /ˈbruːzər/ *n* a tough, pugnacious man; a boxer.

bruit /bruːt/ *n* a report; a rumour; fame. • *vt* to report; to noise abroad.

brumal /ˈbruːməl/ *adj* of or like winter, wintry.

brume /bruːm/ *n* fog, mist; a thick vapour.—**brumous** *adj*.

brunch /brʌntʃ/ *n* breakfast and lunch combined.

brunette, brunet /bruːˈnet/ *adj* having dark-brown or black hair, often with dark eyes. • *n* a brunette person.

brunt /brʌnt/ *n* the main force or shock of a blow; the hardest part.

brush[1] /brʌʃ/ *n* a device made of bristles set in a handle, used for grooming the hair, painting or sweeping; a short unfriendly meeting or exchange of words; a fox's bushy tail; a light stroke or graze, made in passing. • *vt* to groom or sweep with a brush; to remove with a brush; (*with* **aside**) to ignore, to regard as little account; (*with* **up**) to refresh one's memory of or skill in a subject; to wash and tidy oneself. • *vi* to touch lightly or graze; (*with* **up**) to smarten one's appearance.—**brusher** *n*.

brush[2] *n* brushwood.

brush-off /-ɒf/ *n* a curt dismissal.

brush-up /-ʌp/ *n* a smartening of one's appearance; refreshment of memory or skill.

brushwood /ˈbrʌʃwʊd/ *n* rough, close bushes; a thicket, a coppice; small wood or twigs suitable for the fire.

brushwork /ˈbrʌʃwɜːk/ *n* a particular or characteristic style of painting.

brusque /bresk/ or /brʌsk/, /bruːsk/ *adj* blunt and curt in manner.—**brusquely** *adv.*—**brusqueness** *n*.

Brussels carpet *n* a strong kind of woollen carpet.

Brussels lace *n* a fine, expensive lace with a floral pattern made orig in Brussels.

Brussels sprout *n* a plant of the cabbage family with a small edible green head.

brut /bruːt/ *adj* (*wines*) dry, unsweetened.

brutal /ˈbruːtəl/ *adj* inhuman; savage, violent; severe.—**brutally** *adv*.

brutality /bruːˈtælɪti/ *n* (*pl* **brutalities**) the quality of being brutal; pitiless cruelty; a brutal act.

brutalize /ˈbruːtəˌlaɪz/ *vt* to treat brutally; to degrade.—**brutalization** *n*.

brute /bruːt/ *n* any animal except man; a brutal person; (*inf*) an unpleasant or difficult person or thing. • *adj* (*force*) sheer, physical.

brutish /ˈbruːtɪʃ/ *adj* brutal; stupid; savage, violent; coarse.—**brutishly** *adv.*—**brutishness** *n*.

bryology /braɪˈɒlədʒi/ *n* the scientific study of mosses.—**bryological** *adj.*—**bryologist** *n*.

bryony /ˈbraɪəni/ *n* (*pl* **bryonies**) any of several climbing plants of Europe and North Africa; black bryony; white bryony.—*also* **briony**.

bryozoan /ˌbraɪəˈzoːən/ *n* any small animal belonging to the class Polyzoa, forming moss-like colonies by budding.

BSc /ˌbiːesˈsiː/ *abbr* = Bachelor of Science.

Bt. *abbr* = Baronet.

bub /bʌb/ *n* (*inf*) a boy; brother.

bubble /ˈbʌbəl/ *n* a film of liquid forming a ball around air or gas; a tiny ball of gas or air in a liquid or solid; a transparent dome; a scheme that collapses. • *vi* to boil; to rise in bubbles; to make a gurgling sound.

bubble and squeak *n* meat and vegetables fried together.

bubble bath *n* perfumed crystals or liquid added to a bath to soften the water and produce foam; a bath to which this has been added.

bubble gum *n* chewing gum that can be blown into large bubbles.

bubbly /ˈbʌbli/ *adj* (**bubblier, bubbliest**) having bubbles, effervescent; cheerful, high-spirited. • *n* (*inf*) champagne.

bubo /ˈbjuːboː/ or /ˈbuː-/ *n* (*pl* **buboes**) an inflamed swelling in the groin or armpit.—**bubonic** *adj*.

bubonic plague *n* a highly infectious often fatal disease contracted from fleas from infected rats.

bubonocele /bjuːˈbɒnəsiːl/ *n* a rupture or hernia in the groin.

bucca /ˈbʌkəl/ *adj* pertaining to the cheek or the mouth.

buccaneer /ˌbʌkəˈnɪər/ *n* a sea robber, a pirate. • *vi* to be a pirate.

buccinator /ˈbʌksɪneɪtər/ *n* a flat muscle of the cheek, also called the trumpeter's muscle from its use in blowing wind instruments.

Buchmanism *see* **Oxford Group**.

buck[1] /bʌk/ *n* the male of animals such as the deer, hare, rabbit, antelope; (*inf*) a dashing young man; (*sl*) a dollar. • *vti* (*horse*) to rear upwards quickly; (*inf*) to resist; (*with* **up**) (*inf*) to make or become cheerful; to hurry up.

buckaroo /ˌbʌkəˈruː/ or /ˌbʌkəˈruː/ *n* (*pl* **buckaroos**) a cowboy.

buckbean /ˈbʌkbiːn/ *n* a water plant with pinkish flowers.

buckboard /ˈbʌkbɔːd/ *n* a light four-wheeled carriage with a flexible board bearing the seats.

bucket /ˈbʌkɪt/ *n* a container with a handle for carrying liquid or substances in small pieces; (*comput*) a direct-access storage area from which data can be retrieved; (*inf*) a wastepaper bin. • *vi* to drive fast or recklessly; to pour with rain.

bucket seat *n* a single, contoured seat with an adjustable back as in a car, etc.

bucket shop *n* (*sl*) a dishonest brokerage firm; a business that sells cheap airline tickets.

buckeye /ˈbʌkaɪ/ *n* a North American tree with white or reddish flowers growing in clusters, the American horse chestnut; its nut: a native of Ohio.

buckjumper *n* a vicious untrained horse that endeavours to throw its rider by arching its back and drawing its feet together.

buckle /ˈbʌkəl/ *n* a fastening or clasp for a strap or band; a bend or bulge. • *vti* to fasten with a buckle; to bend under pressure, etc; (*with* **down**) (*inf*) to apply oneself diligently.

buckler /ˈbʌklər/ *n* a small shield; protection. • *vt* to defend.

bucko /ˈbʌkoː/ *n* (*pl* **buckoes**) (*naut: sl*) a swaggering bully; (*Irish*) a young man.

buckpasser /ˈbʌkˌpæsər/ *n* (*inf*) one who regularly shifts the blame or responsibility to someone else.

buckram /'bɛkrəm/ n a coarse linen or cotton cloth stiffened with dressing. • adj made of, or resembling, buckram; stiff, precise. • vt (**buckraming, buckramed**) to stiffen with or bind in buckram.

buckshee /'bɛkˌʃi/ n (sl) an extra allowance, a windfall. • adj, adv free, for nothing.

buckshot /'bɛkʃɒt/ n shot of a large size for shooting game.

buckskin /'bɛkskɪn/ n a soft leather of deerskin, etc; (pl) breeches or shoes made of this; (hist) a native American. • adj made of buckskin.

buckthorn /-θɔrn/ n any of several shurbs or trees with small greenish flowers, black berries and thorny branches.

bucktooth /-ˌtuːθ/ n (pl **buckteeth**) a projecting front tooth.

buckwheat /-wiːt/ n a plant cultivated for its triangular seeds, which are ground into meal and used as a cereal.

bucolic /bjuːˈkɒlɪk/ adj pastoral; rustic. • n a pastoral poem; a rustic.—**bucolically** adv.

bud¹ /bʌd/ n an embryo shoot, flower, or flower cluster of a plant; an early stage of development. • vi (**budding, budded**) to produce buds; to begin to develop.

bud² n (inf) buddy.

Buddha /'buːdə/ or /'bʊdə/ n one who has arrived at the state of perfect enlightenment; an image of Siddharta Gautama, founder of Buddhism.

Buddhism /'buːdɪzəm/ or /'bʊd-/ n a system of ethics and philosophy based on teachings of Buddha.

Buddhist /-dɪst/ n a follower of Buddhism.

budding /'bʌdɪŋ/ n being in an early stage of development; promising or showing promise.

buddle /'bʌdəl/ n an inclined trough in which ore is separated from earth by the action of running water. • vt to wash ore in a buddle.

buddleia /'bʌdliə/ n a shrub with lilac or yellow flowers.

buddy /'bʌdi/ n (pl **buddies**) (inf) a friend; a term of informal address; one who helps and supports another, esp an AIDS sufferer. • vi (**buddying, buddied**) to help as a buddy.

budge¹ /bʌdʒ/ vti to shift or move.

budge² n lambskin dressed with the wool outwards.

budgerigar /'bʌdʒərɪˌɡɑr/ n a small Australian parrot bred as a cage bird in many varieties of different colours.

budget /'bʌdʒət/ n an estimate of income and expenditure within specified limits of a country, a business, etc; the total amount of money for a given purpose; a stock or supply; **on a budget** restricting one's expenditure. • vb (**budgeting, budgeted**) vi to make a budget. • vt to put on a budget; to plan; (with **for**) to allow for or save money for a purpose or aim.—**budgetary** adj.

budgie /'bʌdʒi/ n (inf) a budgerigar.

buff /bʌf/ n a heavy, soft, brownish-yellow leather; a dull brownish yellow; (inf) a devotee, fan; (inf) a person's bare skin. • adj made of buff; of a buff colour. • vt to clean or shine, orig with leather or a leather-covered wheel.

buffalo /'bʌfəloʊ/ n (pl **buffalo, buffaloes** or **buffalos**) a wild ox; a bison.

buffer¹ /'bʌfər/ n anything that lessens shock, as of collision; something that serves as a protective barrier; a temporary storage area in a computer.

buffer² n (sl) a good-tempered somewhat foolish person; an elderly man.

buffer zone, buffer state n an area intended to separate; a neutral area.

buffet car n a railway coach where light refreshments are served.

buffet¹ /'bʌfət/ n a blow with the hand or fist. • vb (**buffeting, buffeted**) vt to hit with the hand or fist; to batter (as of the wind). • vi to make one's way esp under difficult conditions.—**buffeter** n.

buffet² /bəˈfeɪ/ or /bʊˈfeɪ/, /bʊˈfeɪ/ n a counter where refreshments are served; a meal at which guests serve themselves food.

buffeting n repeated battering.

buffo /'bʊfoʊ/ n (pl **buffi, buffos**) a comic actor, esp in an opera. • adj comic; burlesque.

buffoon /bəˈfuːn/ n a clown, a jester; a silly person.

buffoonery n ridiculous behaviour.

bug¹ /bʌɡ/ n a continuing source of irritation.

bug² n an insect with sucking mouth parts; any insect; (inf) a germ or virus; (sl) a defect, as in a machine; (sl) a hidden microphone; an obsession, an enthusiasm. • vt (**bugging, bugged**) (sl) to plant a hidden microphone; (sl) to annoy, anger, etc.

bugbear /'bʌɡbɛr/ n an object that causes great fear and anxiety.

buggy /'bʌɡi/ n (pl **buggies**) a light four-wheeled, one-horse carriage with one seat; a small pushchair for a baby; a small vehicle.

bughouse /bʌɡˌhaʊs/ n (sl) a mental home. • adj crazy.

bugle¹ /'bjuːɡəl/ n a valveless brass instrument like a small trumpet, used esp for military calls. • vti to signal by blowing a bugle.—**bugler** n.

bugle² n an elongated glass bead, usu black.

bugle³ n bugleweed.

bugleweed /-wiːd/ n a plant of Europe and Asia with spikes or clusters of small blue or white flowers.

bugloss /'bjuːˌɡlɒs/ n any of various plants with hairy leaves and stems.

buhl /buːl/ see **boulle**.

build /bɪld/ vb (**building, built**) vt to make or construct, to establish, base; (with **up**) to create or develop gradually. • vi to put up buildings; (with **up**) to grow or intensify; (health, reputation) to develop. • n the way a thing is built or shaped; the shape of a person; the physical appearance or weight or size of a person.—**builder** n.

building /-ɪŋ/ adj the skill or occupation of constructing houses, boats, etc; something built with walls and a roof.

building society n a company that pays interest on deposits and issues loans to enable people to buy their own houses.—also **savings and loan association**.

built-in /ˌbɪltˈɪn/ adj incorporated as an integral part of a main structure; inherent.

built-up /ˈbɪltʌp/ adj made higher, stronger, etc with added parts; having many buildings on it, eg built-up area.

bulb /bʌlb/ n the underground bud of plants such as the onion and daffodil; a glass bulb in an electric light; a rounded shape.—**bulbous** adj.

bulbiferous /bʌlˈbɪfərəs/ adj (plants) producing bulbs.

bulbil /'bʌlˌbɪl/ n (bot) a small bulb formed at the side of an old one; a small solid or scaly bud, which detaches itself from the stem, becoming an independent plant.

bulbul /'bʊlbʊl/ n an Eastern songbird; (poet) the Persian nightingale.

bulge /bʌldʒ/ n a swelling; a rounded projected part; a significant rise in numbers (of population). • vti to swell or bend outward.—**bulgy** adj.

bulimia /buːˈliːmiə/ n insatiable hunger, voracity.

bulimia nervosa /- nərˈvoʊsə/ n an illness characterized by bouts of compulsive eating followed by self-induced vomiting.

bulk /bʌlk/ n magnitude; great mass; volume; the main part; **in bulk** in large quantities. • adj total, aggregate; (goods) not packaged.

bulk buying n the large-scale buying of one commodity usu at a cost reduction; the purchase by one country of the total output of a product of another country.

bulk carrier n a ship carrying as cargo one unpackaged commodity.

bulkhead /bʌlkˈhɛd/ n a wall-like partition in the interior of a ship, aircraft or vehicle.

bulky /bʌlki/ adj (**bulkier, bulkiest**) large and unwieldy.—**bulkily** adv.—**bulkiness** adj.

bull¹ /bʊl/ n an adult male bovine animal; a male whale or elephant; a speculator who buys in anticipation of reselling at a profit; the bull's-eye; (sl) nonsense; bullshit. • adj male; rising in price.

bull² n an official edict issued by the pope, with the papal seal on it.

bull³ n a ludicrous inconsistency in language.—also **Irish bull**.

bulla /'bʊlə/ n (pl **bullae**) a lead seal on a papal document; a blister.—**bullous** adj.

bullace /'bʊləs/ n a wild European species of plum cultivated as the damson.

bullate /'bʊlət/ or /-eɪt/, /bʌl-/ adj blistered; puffy.

bulldog /ˌbʊldɛɡ/ n a variety of dog of strong muscular build, remarkable for its courage and ferocity, formerly used for baiting bulls; a short-barrelled pistol with a large calibre. • adj characterized by the courage of a bulldog; tenacious.

bulldog clip n a spring clip with a powerful grip.

bulldoze /'bʊldoʊz/ vt to demolish with a bulldozer; (inf) to force.

bulldozer /bʊlˌdoʊzər/ n an excavator with caterpillar tracks for moving earth.

bullet /'bʊlət/ n a small metal missile fired from a gun or rifle.

bulletin /'bʊlətɪn/ n an announcement; a short statement of news or of a patient's progress.

bulletin board *n* a board on which notices are posted.

bulletproof /'bulətpru:f/ *adj* providing protection against bullets.

bullfight /'bul,faɪt/ *n* a combat between armed men and a bull or bulls.

bullfighting /-ɪŋ/ *n* the sport of goading and then killing bulls, popular in Spain, etc.—**bullfighter** *n*.

bullfinch /-,fɪntʃ/ *n* a common brightly coloured European songbird.

bullfrog /-,frɒg/ *n* a large North American frog found in marshy places, remarkable for its loud bellowing croak.

bullheaded /-,hedəd/ *adj* stubborn; stupid.—**bullheadedly** *adv*.—**bullheadedness** *n*.

bullion /'buljən/ *n* gold or silver in mass before coinage.

bull-necked /-,nekt/ *adj* having a short thick neck.

bullock /'bulək/ *n* a gelded bull; steer.

bullring /-rɪŋ/ *n* an arena for bullfighting.

bull's-eye /'bulz,aɪ/ *n* (*darts, archery*) the centre of a target; something resembling this; a direct hit; a large round peppermint boiled sweet.

bullwhip /-wɪp/ *n* a whip with a long lash for driving cattle. • *vt* (**bullwhipping, bullwhipped**) to whip with this.

bullshit /'bul,ʃɪt/ *n* (*vulg sl*) nonsense; exaggeration, pretentious talk. • *vti* (**bullshitting, bullshitted**) (*vulg sl*) to claim knowledge that is lacking; to talk boastfully.—**bullshitter** *n*.

bull terrier *n* a dog bred by a cross between the bulldog and the terrier.

bully (beef) *n* canned corned beef.

bully /'buli/ *n* (*pl* **bullies**) a person, adult or child, who hurts or intimidates others weaker than himself or herself. • *vb* (**bullying, bullied**) *vt* to intimidate, oppress or hurt. • *vi* (*with* **off**) (*hockey*) to cross sticks in a bully-off to start a match. • *adj* (*inf*) very good, as in *bully for you*.

bully boy *n* a hoodlum, a ruffian, *usu* one hired to beat up someone.

bullyrag /-,ræg/ *see* **ballyrag**.

bulrush /'bulrʌʃ/ *n* a tall marsh plant.

bulwark /'bulwərk/ *or* /-work/ *n* a defensive wall or rampart; (*naut*) a fence-like structure projecting above the deck of a ship; an object or person acting as a means of defence.

bum /bʌm/ *n* (*inf*) a tramp; an idle person; (*inf*) a devotee, as of skiing or tennis; (*sl*) buttocks or anus. • *adj* broken; useless. • *vti* (**bumming, bummed**) to beg, to sponge; to live as a vagabond; (*with* **around**) to be idle, to loaf about.

bumble /'bʌmbəl/ *vi* to do or say something clumsily or in a confused way; to stumble.—**bumbler** *n*.

bumblebee /-,bi:/ *n* a large, furry bee.

bumbleberry pie *n* (*Cdn*) a pie with a filling of mixed berries.

bumboat /'bʌm,boːt/ *n* a boat used for conveying provisions, fruit, etc, for sale to vessels lying off shore.

bummer /'bʌmər/ *n* a worthless person who sponges on others; a low politician; an unpleasant experience, *esp* due to drug taking.

bump /bʌmp/ *vi* to knock with a jolt. • *vt* to hurt by striking or knocking; (*inf*) to refuse a booked passenger a seat on a flight because of overbooking by the airline; (*with* **into**) to collide with; (*inf*) to meet by chance; (*with* **off**) (*sl*) to kill, murder; (*with* **up**) (*inf*) to increase prices, size or bulk. • *n* a jolt; a knock the noise made by a bump or a collision; a swelling or lump; one of the bulges on the head supposedly indicating a special faculty.

bumper /'bʌmpər/ *n* a shock-absorbing bar fixed to the front and rear of a motor vehicle; a brimming glass for a toast. • *adj* exceptionally large.

bumpkin /'bʌmpkɪn/ *n* an awkward or simple country person.

bumptious /'bʌmpʃəs/ *adj* offensively conceited or self-assertive.—**bumptiously** *adv*.—**bumptiousness** *n*.

bumpy /'bʌmpi/ *adj* (**bumpier, bumpiest**) having many bumps; rough; jolting, jerky.—**bumpily** *adv*.—**bumpiness** *n*.

bum steer *n* (*sl*) false or deceptive information or advice.

bun /bʌn/ *n* a roll made of bread dough and currants, spices and sugar; a bun-shaped coil of hair at the nape of the neck.

bunch /bʌntʃ/ *n* a cluster; a number of things growing or fastened together; (*inf*) a group of people. • *vi* to group together. • *vt* to make into a bunch.—**bunchy** *adj*.—**bunchiness** *n*.

buncombe /'bʌŋkəm/ *see* **bunkum**.

bund¹, Bund /bund/ *or* /bunt/ *n* (*pl* **bunds, Bünde**) a league, a confederacy.

bund² /bund/ *n* an embankment to protect land against inundation.

bundle /'bʌndəl/ *n* a number of things fastened together; a fastened package; (*sl*) a large sum of money. • *vt* to put together in bundles; to push hurriedly into.—**bundler** *n*.

bung /bʌŋ/ *n* a cork or rubber stopper. • *vt* to close up with or as with a bung; (*sl*) to throw, toss.

bungalow /'bʌngə,ləʊ/ *n* a one-storey house.

bungle /'bʌŋgəl/ *n* a mistake or blunder; something carried out clumsily. • *vt* to spoil something through incompetence or clumsiness.—**bungler** *a*.—**bungling** *adj, n*.

bunion /'bʌnjən/ *n* a lump on the side of the first joint of the big toe.

bunk /bʌŋk/ *n* a narrow, shelf-like bed; a bunk bed.

bunk² *n* (*sl*) a hurried departure.

bunk³ *n* (*sl*) buncombe.

bunk bed *n* one of two or three single beds arranged one above the other in a compact unit.

bunker /'bʌŋkər/ *n* a large storage container, *esp* for coal; a sand pit forming an obstacle on a golf course; an underground shelter.

bunkhouse /'bʌŋkhaʊs/ *n* a building where workers are housed temporarily, *esp* one for loggers or miners.

bunkum /'bʌŋkəm/ *n* idle or showy speech; nonsense.—*also* **buncombe**.

bunny /'bʌni/ *n* (*pl* **bunnies**) a pet name for a rabbit; a nightclub waitress dressed to resemble a rabbit.

Bunsen burner /'bʌnsən'bɜːnər/ *n* a burner that mixes gas and air to produce a smokeless flame of great heat.

bunt¹ /bʌnt/ *vti* (*animal*) to butt; (*baseball*) to tap (the ball) within the infield. • *n* this stroke.

bunt² *n* a species of fungus that produces the smut disease in wheat.

bunt³ *n* the bulge of a sail, net, etc.

bunting¹ /-ɪŋ/ *n* a cotton fabric used for making flags; a line of pennants and decorative flags.

bunting² *n* a bird allied to the finches and sparrows.

buntline /'bʌntlaɪn/ *n* (*naut*) one of the ropes attached to the foot rope of a square sail to draw the sail up to the yard.

buoy /bɔɪ/ *or* /'bu:i/ *n* a bright, anchored, marine float used for mooring and for making obstacles. • *vt* to keep afloat; (*usu with* **up**) to hearten or raise the spirits of; to mark with buoys.

buoyancy /'bɔɪənsi/ *n* ability to float or rise; cheerfulness; resilience.

buoyant /'bɔɪənt/ *adj* able to float; light, elastic; not easily depressed, cheerful.—**buoyantly** *adv*.

bur /bɜːr/ *n* a prickly seed-case of a plant; a person hard to shake off; a rough edge left after drilling or cutting; a burr. • *vt* (**burring, burred**) to pick burs off.

burble /'bɜːbəl/ *vi* to make a gurgling sound; to speak incoherently, *esp* from excitement.—**burbler** *n*.

burbot /'bɜːbət/ *n* (*pl* **burbot, burbots**) a freshwater fish like the eel.

burden /'bɜːdən/ *n* a load; something worrisome that is difficult to bear; responsibility. • *vt* to weigh down, to oppress.

burden² *n* the chorus or refrain of a song; a topic dwelt on in speech or writing.

burdensome /-səm/ *adj* onerous; oppressive; heavy.—**burdensomely** *adv*.

burdock /'bɜːdɒk/ *n* a large wayside weed with prickly flowers and rough broad leaves.

bureau /'bjʊrəʊ/ *n* (*pl* **bureaus, bureaux**) a writing desk; a chest of drawers; a branch of a newspaper, magazine or wire service in an important news centre; a government department.

bureaucracy /'bjʊrɒkrəs/ *n* (*pl* **bureaucracies**) a system of government where the administration is organized in a hierarchy; the government collectively; excessive paperwork and red tape.

bureaucrat /'bjʊrə,kræt/ *or* /-roː-/, /-kræt/ *n* an official in a bureaucracy, *esp* one who adheres inflexibly to this system.—**bureaucratic** *adj*.—**bureaucratically** *adv*.

burette, buret /bjuː'ret/ *n* a graduated glass tube, *usu* with a tap, for measuring the volume of liquids.

burg /bɜːg/ *n* a town; (*formerly*) a fortified town.

burgee /bɜː'dʒiː/ *n* a swallow-tailed flag or pennant flown on the mast of a yacht to show membership of a club or of a merchant vessel to show ownership.

burgeon /'bɜːdʒən/ *vt* to start to increase rapidly; (*plant*) to bloom copiously.

burger /'bɜːgər/ *n* (*inf*) hamburger.

burgess /'bɜːdʒəs/ *n* in UK, a citizen or freeman of a borough; (*formerly*) a member of parliament for a borough or university; in US, a representative sent by a town to the colonial legislative body of Virginia or Maryland.

Burgh /'bʌrə/ *n* (*Scot*) a borough.—**burghal** *adj*.

burgher /'bərgər/ *n* a citizen or freeman of a burgh or borough; a prosperous person of the middle classes.

burglar /'bərglər/ *n* a person who trespasses in a building with the intention of committing a crime, such as theft.

burglary /-ləri/ *n* (*pl* **burglaries**) the act or crime of breaking into a house or any building with intent to commit a felony, *esp* theft.

burgle /'bərgəl/, **burglarize** /'bərglə̩raɪz/ *vti* to commit burglary (in or on).

burgomaster /'bərgo̩ˌmæstər/ *n* the chief magistrate of a municipal town in Holland, Belgium or Germany.

burgonet /'bərgə̩net/ *n* a kind of steel cap or helmet of the 16th century.

Burgundy /'bərgəndi/ *n* (*pl* **Burgundies**) a dryish wine, red or white, made in the Burgundy region of eastern France; a similar wine produced elsewhere; a dark purplish red colour.

burial /'beriəl/ *n* the act of burying; interment of a dead body.

burial ground *n* a graveyard.

burin /'bjʊrɪn/ *n* a chisel used for engraving metal, wood or marble; (*archaeol*) a primitive tool with a chisel-shaped head.

burke /bərk/ *vt* to murder by suffocation; to dispose of quietly; to hush up.

burl /bərl/ *n* a small knot or lump in thread or cloth; a knot in wood; a wood veneer with knots in it. • *vt* to pick knots, etc, from, as in finishing cloth.

burlap /'bərlæp/ *n* a coarse fabric made of jute, hemp, etc, used for bagging or in upholstery.

burlesque /bərlesk/ *n* a caricature; a literary or dramatic satire. • *vti* (**burlesquing, burlesqued**) to make fun of, to caricature. • *adj* of or like burlesque; mockingly imitative.

burly /'bərli/ *adj* (**burlier, burliest**) heavily built; sturdy.—**burliness** *n*.

burn[1] /bərn/ *vb* (**burning, burned** or **burnt**) *vt* to destroy by fire; to injure by heat. • *vi* to be on fire; to feel hot; to feel passion; (*inf*) to suffer from sunburn; (*with* **off**) to clear ground by burning all vegetation; to get rid of (surplus gas, energy) by burning or using up; (*with* **out**) (*fire*) to go out; (*person*) to lose efficiency through exhaustion, excess or overwork. • *n* a scorch mark or injury caused by burning.

burn[2] *n* (*Scot*) a small stream, a brook.

burner *n* the part of a lamp or stove that produces a flame.

burnet /bər'net/ *n* a brown-flowered plant of the rose family.

burning /'bərnɪŋ/ *adj* intense, passionate; urgent.—**burningly** *adj*.

burning glass *n* a double convex lens used to focus the sun's rays on combustible substances to ignite them.

burnish /'bərnɪʃ/ *vt* to make shiny by rubbing; to polish. • *n* lustre; polish.—**burnishable** *adj*.—**burnisher** *n*.

burnous, burnoose /bər'nu:s/ or /'bərnu:s/ *n* a long, hooded cloak worn by Arabs.

burnt /bərnt/ see **burn**.

burnt offering *n* something offered and burnt upon an altar as a sacrifice or an atonement for sin.

burnt sienna *n* an orange-reddish pigment used in painting.

burp /bərp/ *vi* to belch. • *vt* to pat a baby on the back to cause it to belch. • *n* a belch.

burr[1] /bər/ see **bur**.

burr[2] *n* a whirring sound; a gruff pronunciation of the letter *r*. • *vti* to pronounce with a burr.

burrito /bə'ri:to:/ *n* a tortilla baked with a savoury filling.

burro /'bəro:/ *n* (*pl* **burros**) a donkey.

burrow /'bəro:/ *n* an underground hide or tunnel dug by a rabbit, badger or fox, etc for shelter. • *vi* to dig a burrow; to live in a burrow; to hide (oneself); to grope into the depths of one's pockets.—**burrower** *n*.

burry /'bəri/ *adj* (**burrier, burriest**) full of burs; rough; prickly.

bursa /'bərsə/ *n* (*pl* **bursae, bursas**) (*anat*) a sac or sac-like cavity, *esp* between joints, full of a fluid that lessens friction.—**bursal** *adj*.

bursar /'bərsər/ *n* a treasurer; a person in charge of the finances of a college or university; a student holding a bursary.—**bursarial** *adj*.

bursary /-ri/ *n* (*pl* **bursaries**) a scholarship awarded to a student.—**bursarial** *adj*.

burst /bərst/ *vb* (**bursting, burst**) *vt* to break open; to cause to explode. • *vi* to emerge suddenly; to explode; to break into pieces; to give vent to. • *n* an explosion; a burst; a volley of shots; a sudden increase of activity; a spurt.—**burster** *n*.

burton /'bərtən/ *n* (*naut*) a tackle formed of two or more blocks or pulleys; **go for a burton** to die; to be no longer useful.

bury /'beri/ *vt* (**burying, buried**) (*bone, corpse*) to place in the ground; to inter; to conceal, to cover; to blot out of the mind; **bury the hatchet** to make peace; to be reconciled.

bus /bʌs/ *n* (*pl* **buses, busses**) a motor coach for public transport. • *vti* (**busing, bused** or **bussing, bussed**) to transport or travel by bus; to take by bus children from one area to another, *esp* to balance racial numbers.

busby /'bʌzbi/ *n* (*pl* **busbies**) a tall, fur hat, *esp* one worn by a guardsman.

bush[1] /bʊʃ/ *n* a low shrub with many branches; a cluster of shrubs forming a hedge; woodland; (*with* **the**) uncultivated land, *esp* in Africa, Australia, New Zealand, Canada; a thick growth, *eg* of hair; a fox's tail or brush.

bush[2] *n* a metal lining of a hole in which an axle turns to reduce wear by friction.—*also* **bushing**. • *vt* to furnish with a bush.

bushbaby /-beɪbi/ *n* (*pl* **bushbabies**) a small tree-dwelling nocturnal lemur from Africa.

bush camp *n* ✹ (*Cdn*) the headquarters or living quarters of a mining or logging company in the bush.

bushed /bʊʃt/ *adj* (*inf*) tired, exhausted; (*Austral*) lost in the bush; ✹ (*Cdn*) driven insane because of isolation in the wilderness.

bushel[1] /'bʊʃl/ *n* a dry measure containing eight gallons (UK) or 64 pints (US); a vessel of such a capacity; a large quantity.

bushel[2] *vt* (**bushelling, bushelled** or **busheling, busheled**) to patch or repair, *esp* clothes.—**busheller, busheler** *n*.

bush fever *n* ✹ (*Cdn*) a mental disorder resulting from isolation in the wilderness.

bushfire /ˌbʊʃ'faɪr/ *n* a fire, often widespread, in bush or scrubland.

bushing /'bʊʃɪŋ/ see **bush**[2].

bush lot *n* ✹ (*Cdn*) a woodlot.

bushman /'bʊʃmən/ *n* (*pl* **bushmen**) a woodsman; (*Austral*) a settler in the bush or newly opened country; (*with cap*) one of a tribe of South African aboriginals near the Cape of Good Hope.

bushmaster /-ˌmæstər/ *n* a large deadly South American snake with brown and grey markings.

bush pilot *n* ✹ (*Cdn*) a pilot who flies small aircraft into isolated or wilderness areas.

bush plane *n* ✹ (*Cdn*) a small plane used for flying into isolated or wilderness areas, *usu* equipped with floats or skis.

bushranger /-ˌreɪndʒər/ *n* a frontiersman; (*Austral: formerly*) a criminal who escaped and lived a lawless life in the bush.

bush road *n* ✹ (*Cdn*) a road cut through bush.

bush telegraph *n* a means of communicating news by drumbeat across a large area; (*inf*) a means of spreading gossip.

bushwhack /'bʊʃˌwæk/ *vi* to work one's way through the bush; to ambush.

bushwhacker /-ər/ *n* a backwoodsman; a guerrilla fighter; an implement for cutting brushwood.

bushworker /'bʊʃwərkər/ *n* ✹ (*Cdn*) a logger.

bushy /'bʊʃi/ *adj* (**bushier, bushiest**) covered with bushes; (*hair*) thick.—**bushiness** *n*.

business /'bɪznəs/ *n* trade or commerce; occupation or profession; a firm; a factory; one's concern or responsibility; a matter; the agenda of a business meeting.

businesslike /-ˌlaɪk/ *adj* efficient, methodical, practical.

businessman /-mæn/ *n* (**businessmen**) a person who works for an industrial or commercial company, *esp* as an executive.—**businesswoman** *nf* (*pl* **businesswomen**).

busing see **bussing**.

busker /'bʌskər/ *n* a street entertainer.—**busking** *n*.

buskin /'bʌskɪn/ *n* a half boot or high shoe; a high boot once worn by tragic actors to increase their height; a tragic drama.

busman's holiday *n* a holiday spent doing what one usually does at work.

buss /bʌs/ *n* a smacking kiss. • *vt* to kiss.

bussing /-ɪŋ/ *n* the transport of children to a school in another district to achieve racially balanced classes.—*also* **busing**.

bust[1] /bʌst/ *n* the chest or breast of a human being, *esp* a woman; a sculpture of the head and chest.

bust[2] /bʌst/ *vti* (**busting, busted** or **bust**) (*inf*) to burst or break; to make or become bankrupt or demoted; to hit; to arrest. • *n* (*inf*) a failure; financial collapse; a punch; a spree; an arrest.

bustard /'bʌstərd/ *n* any of a genus of large swift-running birds of Europe and Africa.

buster /'bʌstər/ n a person or thing that busts; something very large; a frolic; a violent wind; (with cap) (inf) boy, man, a form of address.

bustle[1] /'bʌsəl/ vi to move or act noisily, energetically or fussily. • n noisy activity, stir, commotion.—**bustler** n.—**bustling** adj.

bustle[2] n a pad placed beneath the skirt of a dress to cause it to puff up at the back.

bust-up /'bʌstəp/ n (inf) a fight or quarrel; a noisy brawl; the permanent ending of a relationship.

busy /'bɪzi/ adj (**busier, busiest**) occupied; active; crowded; full; industrious; (painting) having too much detail; (room, telephone) engaged, in use. • vt (**busying, busied**) to occupy; to make or keep busy (esp oneself).—**busily** adv.—**busyness** n.

busybody /'bɪzi,bɒdi/ n (pl **busybodies**) a meddlesome person.

but /bʌt/ prep save; except. • conj in contrast; on the contrary, other than. • adv only; merely; just. • n an objection.

butane /'bjuːteɪn/ or /bju:'teɪn/ n an inflammable gas used as a fuel.

butch /bʊtʃ/ adj (sl) tough; aggressively male; (often of a woman) male-looking.

butcher /'bʊtʃər/ n a person who slaughters meat; a retailer of meat; a ruthless murderer. • vt to slaughter; to murder ruthlessly; to make a mess of or spoil.

butcher's-broom n a low-growing evergreen shrub with rigid branched stems and spiny leaves.

butcherbird /-,bərd/ n any of a genus of shrikes that suspend their slaughtered prey from thorns.

butchery /'bʊtʃəri/ n (pl **butcheries**) the preparation of meat for sale; slaughter.

butler /'bʌtlər/ n a manservant, usu the head servant of a household, etc.

butt[1] /bʌt/ vti to strike or toss with the head or horns, as a bull, etc; (with in) to interfere, to enter into unasked. • n a push with the head or horns.—**butter** n.

butt[2] n a large cask for wine or beer.

butt[3] n a mound of earth behind targets; a person who is the target of ridicule or jokes; (pl) the target range.

butt[4] n the thick or blunt end; the stump; (sl) a cigarette; fag end; (sl) the buttocks. • vti to join end to end.

butte /bjuːt/ n an abrupt isolated hill or ridge.

butter /'bʌtər/ n a solidified fat made from cream by churning. • vt to spread butter on; (with up) (inf) to flatter.

butter bean n a variety of lima bean cultivated for its large flat pale edible seeds.

buttercup /-,kʌp/ n any of various plants with ye low, glossy, cup-shaped flowers.

butterfingers /-,fɪŋgərz/ n (used as sing) a person who lets (a ball, etc) slip through his or her fingers.—**butterfingered** adj.

butterfly /-,flaɪ/ n (pl **butterflies**) an insect with a slender body and four usu brightly coloured wings; a swimming stroke.

buttermilk /-,mɪlk/ n the sour liquid that remains after separation from the cream in buttermaking.

butternut /-,nʌt/ n a North American tree of the walnut family; its large oily nut; its hard wood; the colour of the butternut, a brownish grey, the colour of the Confederate uniform in the American Civil War; one who wore the uniform of the Confederate army.

butterscotch /-,skɒtʃ/ n a sauce made of melted butter and brown sugar; a kind of hard toffee made from this; its flavour; a brownish-yellow colour.

butter tart n ✽ (Cdn) a small tart with a filling of butter, eggs, brown sugar, and raisins.

butterwort /-,wərt/ n a violet-flowered bog plant with leaves that secrete a viscid fluid to entrap small insects.

buttery[1] /'bʌtəri/ adj like or tasting of butter; insincere.

buttery[2] n (pl **butteries**) a storeroom for wine or food.

buttock /'bʌtək/ n either half of the human rump.

button /'bʌtən/ n a disc or knob of metal, plastic, etc used as a fastening; a badge; a small button-like sweet; an electric bell push; a knob at the point of a fencing foil. • vti to fasten with a button or buttons.

buttonhole /-,hoʊl/ n the slit through which a button is passed; a single flower in the buttonhole. • vt to make buttonholes; to sew with a special buttonhole stitch; (person) to keep in conversation.

buttonhook /-,hʊk/ n a tool for fastening buttons on shoes or gloves.

buttress /'bʌtrəs/ n a projecting structure for strengthening a wall. • vt to support or prop.

butyraceous /,bjuːtə'reɪʃəs/ adj like butter in consistency, appearance or properties.

butyrate /'bjuːtə,reɪt/ n a salt of butyric acid.

butyric acid /'bjuːtərɪk/ n a colourless liquid obtained from butter, also present in cod-liver oil and sweat glands.

buxom /'bʌksəm/ adj plump and healthy; (woman) big-bosomed.—**buxomness** n.

buy /baɪ/ vt (**buying, bought**) to purchase (for money); to bribe or corrupt; to acquire in exchange for something; (inf) to believe; (with off) to pay someone to ensure that some undesired action is not taken; (with out) to purchase a controlling interest in or share of; to secure the release of (e.g. a person from the army) by payment; (with up) to purchase the total supply of something; to acquire a controlling interest in. • n a purchase.

buyer /baɪr/ n a person who buys; a customer; an employee who buys on behalf of his or her employer, esp a company or store.

buyer's market n a market in which, because the supply exceeds the demand, the buyers control the price.

buzz /bʌz/ vi to hum like an insect; to gossip; to hover (about). • vt spread gossip secretly; (inf) to telephone. • vi (with off) to go away. • n the humming of bees or flies; a rumour; (sl) a telephone call; (sl) a thrill, a kick.

buzzard /'bʌzərd/ n a large bird of prey of the hawk family.

buzzer /'bʌzər/ n a device producing a buzzing sound.

buzz saw n a circular saw.

buzzword /'bʌz,wərd/ n (inf) a vogue or jargon word; a word or phrase that was once a technical or specialist term and which has suddenly become popular, often used mainly for effect.—also **fuzzword**.

bwana /'bwɒnɑ/ n (E Africa) an employer, a boss; (with cap) a form of address.

by /preɪ/ beside; next to; via; through the means of; not later than. • adv near to; past; in reserve, aside.

by-, bye- /baɪ/ prefix subordinate, side, secret.

by and by adv presently, before long; later; eventually; in the future.—**by-and-by** n.

by and large adv on the whole.

by-blow /'baɪ,bloʊ/ n a side blow; a bastard.

bye /baɪ/ n something subordinate or incidental; an odd man in a knockout competition; (cricket) a run scored without the ball being hit by the batsman; (golf) holes left after a match is decided; (lacrosse) a goal.

bye-bye[1] /'baɪ,baɪ/ or /,baɪ'baɪ/ interj (inf) goodbye.

bye-bye[2] n sleep; bed.

by-election, bye-election /'baɪɪ,lɛkʃən/ n an election held other than at a general election.

bygone /'baɪ'gɒn/ adj past. • n (pl) past offences or quarrels.

bylaw, bye-law /'baɪ,lɔː/ n a rule or law made by a local authority or a company.

by-line /'baɪlaɪn/ n a line under a newspaper article naming its author.

bypass /-,pæs/ n a main road built to avoid a town; a channel redirecting the flow of something around a blockage; (med) an operation to redirect the flow of blood into the heart. • vt (**bypassing, bypassed**) to go around; to avoid, to act by ignoring the usual channels.

bypath /-,pæθ/ n a secluded path.

byplay /-,pleɪ/ n action or dumb show aside from the main action.

byproduct, by-product /-,prɒdəkt/ n something useful produced in the process of making something else.

byre /baɪr/ n a shed for cows.

byroad /'baɪ,roʊd/ n an unfrequented or side road.

byssus /'bɪsəs/ n (pl **byssuses, byssi**) a tuft of long soft silky filaments by which certain molluscs attach themselves to rocks; a fine linen used by the ancient Egyptians for wrapping mummies.

bystander /'baɪ,stændər/ n a chance onlooker.

byte /baɪt/ n (comput) a set of eight bits treated as a unit.

by the by, by the bye adv incidentally.

by the way adv incidentally.

byway /'baɪweɪ/ n a side road; a specialist or abstruse interest or area of study.

byword /'baɪ,wərd/ n a well-known saying; a perfect example; an object of derision.

Byzantine /'bɪzən,tiːn/ or /-,taɪn/ adj of or pertaining to Byzantium, the ancient capital of the Eastern Roman Empire; (archit) in the style of the Eastern Empire. • n an inhabitant of Byzantium.

C

C *abbr* = Celsius, centigrade; (*math*) third known quantity; (*roman numerals*) 100; (*chem symbol*) = carbon.

c. *abbr* = carat; cent(s); century.

c. *abbr* = circa, about.

© (*symbol*) = copyright.

CA *abbr* = California; Chartered Accountant.

Ca (*chem symbol*) = calcium.

CAA *abbr* = ✢ Canadian Automobile Association; (*Brit*) Civil Aviation Authority.

cab /kæb/ *n* a taxicab; the place where the driver sits in a truck, crane, etc.

cabal /kə'bæl/ *n* a conspiracy, a secret plot; a small group of people united in perpetrating this; a clique. • *vi* (**caballing, caballed**) to form a cabal, to plot.

cabala, cabbala /kə'bɒlə/ or /'kæbələ/ *n* a mystic interpretation of Scripture by Jewish rabbis; occult lore.—*also* **kabala, kabbala.—cabalism, cabbalism** *n.—***cabalist, cabbalist** *n.—***cabalistic, cabbalistic** *adj.*

caballero /ˌkæbə'ljɛroː/ *n* (*pl* **caballeros**) a Spanish knight or gentleman; a horseman; a Spanish dance.

cabaret /'kæbəˌreɪ/ *n* entertainment given in a restaurant or nightclub.

cabbage /'kæbədʒ/ *n* a garden plant with thick leaves formed *usu* into a compact head, used as a vegetable.

cabbage rose *n* a large full rose.

cabby, cabbie /'kæbi/ *n* (*pl* **cabbies**) (*inf*) a person who drives a cab for hire.

caber /'keɪbər/ *n* a rough pole, *usu* cut from a tree, tossed as a trial of strength at Highland games.

cabin /'kæbɪn/ *n* a small house, a hut; a room in a ship; the area where passengers sit in an aircraft.

cabin cruiser *n* a powerful motorboat with living accommodation.

cabinet /'kæbɪnət/ *n* a case or cupboard with drawers or shelves; a case containing a TV, radio, etc; (*often with cap*) a body of official advisers to a government; the senior ministers of a government.

cabinetmaker /-ˌmeɪkər/ *n* a person who makes fine furniture.

cable /'keɪbəl/ *n* a strong thick rope often of wire strands; an anchor chain; an insulated cord that carries electric current; a cablegram; a bundle of insulated wires for carrying cablegrams, TV signals, etc; (*naut*) a cable length. • *vti* to send a message by cablegram.

cable car /-ˌkɑr/ *n* a car drawn by a moving cable, as up a steep incline.

cablegram /-ˌgræm/ *n* a message transmitted by telephone line, submarine cable, satellite, a cable.

cable-laid /-ˌleɪd/ *adj* (*rope*) composed of three triple strands.

cable length *n* (*naut*) (*UK*) a unit of length, about 100 fathoms, 608 feet or one tenth of a nautical mile, (*US*) 120 fathoms, 720 feet.

cable stitch *n* a pattern of knitting stitches resembling a cable.

cable television *n* TV transmission to subscribers by cable.

cabman /'kæbmən/ *n* (*pl* **cabmen**) the driver of a cab.

cabochon /'kæbəˌʃɒn/, *Fr.* /kabɔ'ʃɔ̃ː/ *n* a precious stone polished but not faceted.

caboodle /kə'buːdəl/ *n* (*sl*) a lot, a set (*the whole caboodle*).

caboose /kə'buːs/ *n* the guard's car at the rear of a freight train; a kitchen on a ship's deck; ✢ (*Cdn*) a portable wooden cabin, *esp* one on runners that are pulled over snow.

cabriolet /ˌkæbrioː'leɪ/ *n* a covered carriage with two or four wheels drawn by one horse; a car body with a folding hood and fixed sides.

cacao /kæ'kæoː/ or /-'keɪoː/ *n* a tropical tree; its seed, from which cocoa and chocolate are obtained.

cachalot /'kæʃəˌlɒt/ or /-ˌlɒt/ *n* the sperm whale.

cache /kæʃ/ *n* a secret hiding place; a store of weapons or treasure; a store of food left for use by travellers, etc. • *vt* to place in a cache.

cache (memory) *n* a small high-speed memory for easy access and frequent reference to computer data.

cachepot /'kæʃˌpoː/ or /-ˌpɒt/ *n* an ornamental pot to hold a flowerpot.

cachet /kæ'ʃeɪ/ or /'kæʃeɪ/ *n* a mark of authenticity; any distinguishing mark; prestige.

cachexia /kə'kɛksɪə/, **cachexy** /-ksi/ *n* (*med*) a bad state of general health, weakness.—**cachectic** *adj.*

cachinnate /'kækəˌneɪt/ *vi* to laugh loudly and unrestrainedly.—**cachinnation** *n.*

cachou[1] /'kæʃuː/ *see* **catechu**.

cachou[2] *n* a lozenge for sweetening the breath.

cachucha /kə'tʃuːtʃə/ *n* a quick Spanish dance; the music for it.

cacique /kə'siːk/ *n* a West Indian or American Indian chief; a political boss.

cackle /'kækəl/ *n* the clucking sound of a hen; shrill or silly talk or laughter. • *vi* to utter with a cackle.

caco- /'kækoː/ *prefix* bad.

cacodemon, cacodaemon /ˌkækə'diːmən/ *n* an evil spirit.

cacodyl /'kækəˌdɪl/ or /-daɪl/ *n* an evil-smelling compound of arsenic and methyl.

cacoethes /ˌkækoː'iːθiːz/ *n* a bad habit or propensity of the body or mind; an uncontrollable urge.—**cacoethic** *adj.*

cacography /kə'kɒɡrəfi/ *n* bad handwriting or spelling, the opposite of calligraphy and orthography.—**cacographic** *adj.*

cacophonous /kə'kɒfənəs/ *adj* harsh, ill-sounding, discordant.

cacophony /kə'kɒfəni/ *n* (*pl* **cacophonies**) an ugly sound, a discord.

cactus /'kæktəs/ *n* (*pl* **cactuses, cacti**) a plant with a thick fleshy stem that stores water and is often studded with prickles.

cad /kæd/ *n* (*inf*) a man who behaves in an ungentlemanly or dishonourable way.—**caddish** *adj.—***caddishly** *adv.—***caddishness** *n.*

cadastre, cadaster /kə'dæstər/ *n* a register of the real estate of a district or county as a basis for taxation.—**cadastral** *adj.*

cadaver /kə'dævər/ *n* a dead body.—**cadaveric** *adj.*

cadaverous /-əs/ *adj* gaunt, haggard; pallid, livid.—**cadaverousness** *n.*

caddie, caddy /'kædi/ *n* (*pl* **caddies**) a person who carries a golfer's clubs.—*vi* (**caddying, caddied**) to perform as a caddie.

caddis /'kædɪs/ *n* the larva of the mayfly used as bait.

caddy /'kædi/ *n* (*pl* **caddies**) a small box or tin for storing tea.

cade /keɪd/ *n* a lamb, etc, bred by hand.

cadence /'keɪdəns/ *n* a falling of the voice; the intonation of the voice; rhythm; measured movements as in marching.

cadent /kə'dent/ *adj* rhythmic; falling.

cadenza /kə'dɛnzə/ *n* (*mus*) an ornamental flourish at the close of a movement.

cadet /kə'det/ *n* a student at an armed forces academy, police college, etc; a school pupil in a school army training corps.

cadge /kædʒ/ *vti* to beg or obtain by begging.—**cadger** *n.*

cadi /'kɒdi/ or /'keɪ-/ *n* a minor Mohammedan judge.

cadmium /'kædmɪəm/ *n* a whitish metallic element.

cadre /'kædrə/ or /'kɒ-/, /-dreɪ/ *n* a permanent nucleus or framework of a political or military unit.

caduceus /kə'duːsɪəs/ or /-'djuː-/, /-ʃɪəs/, /-ʃəs/ *n* (*pl* **caducei**) the winged wand of Hermes (Mercury) entwined with two serpents, the emblem of the medical profession; an ancient herald's wand.

caducity /-sɪti/ or /-'djuː-/ *n* the quality or condition of being caducous; senility.

caducous /-kəs/ *adj* (*biol*) (*parts of a plant*) falling off quickly or before maturity; fleeting; perishable.

caecum /'siːkəm/ *n* (*pl* **caeca**) the pouch at the beginning of the large intestine containing the vermiform appendix.—*also* **cecum.—caecal** *adj.*

Caesar /'siːzər/ *n* the title of Roman emperors, *esp* Julius Caesar (*c.* 100–44 bc); (*without cap*) any ruler.

Caesarean section, Cesarean section /sə'zɛrɪən'sɛkʃən/ *n* the removal of a child from the womb by a surgical operation involving the cutting of the abdominal wall.

caesium /'siːzɪəm/ *n* a rare silvery alkaline metal.—*also* **cesium.**

caesura /sɪ'zjuːrə/ or /-'dʒuːrə/ *n* (*pl* **caesuras, caesurae**) a natural pause in the rhythm of a verse line.—**caesural** *adj*.

CAF *abbr* ♣ = Canadian Armed Forces.

cafe, café /'kæfeɪ/ *n* a small restaurant, a coffee bar, a nightclub, etc.

café au lait /-oː'leɪ/ *n* coffee with milk; a light brown colour.

café noir /-'nwɑr/, *Fr.* /kafeɪ'nwɑr/ *n* coffee without milk.

cafeteria /kæfə'tiːriə/ *n* a self-service restaurant.

cafetière /kæfiti'er/ *n* a *usu* glass coffee pot with a plunger to press down coffee grounds.

caffeine /'kæfiːn/ or /kæf'iːn/ *n* a stimulant present in coffee and tea.—**caffeinic** *adj*.

caftan /'kæftæn/ *n* a long-sleeved, full-length, voluminous garment originating in the Middle East.—*also* **kaftan**.

cage /keɪdʒ/ *n* a box or enclosure with bars for confining an animal, bird, prisoner, etc; a car for raising or lowering miners. • *vt* to shut in a cage, to confine.

cagey, cagy /'keɪdʒi/ *adj* (**cagier, cagiest**) (*inf*) wary, secretive, not frank.—**cagily** *adv*.—**caginess** *n*.

cahier /kɒ'jeɪ/ *n* sheets of paper put loosely together, a notebook.

cahoots /kə'huːts/ *npl* partnership; **in cahoots** in league or partnership.

CAI *abbr* = Computer-Aided Instruction.

caiman /'keɪmən/ *n* (*pl* **caimans**) an alligator of South and Central America.—*also* **cayman**.

caique, caïque /kaɪ'iːk/ *n* a skiff or light rowing boat used on the Bosphorus in Turkey.

cairn /kern/ *n* a stone mound placed as a monument or marker.

cairngorm /'kerngorm/ *n* (a gemstone of) a yellow or brown variety of quartz or rock crystal.

caisse populaire /kes popjuːleər/ *a* ♣ (*Cdn*) a credit union in Québec and other French-speaking parts of Canada.

caisson /'keɪsɒn/ *n* a watertight chamber used for carrying out underwater repairs or construction work; an apparatus for floating or lifting a vessel.

caitiff /'keɪtɪf/ *n* (*arch*) a coward; a rascal. • *adj* (*arch*) base, despicable, cowardly.

cajole /kə'dʒoːl/ *vti* to persuade or soothe by flattery or deceit.—**cajoler** *n*.—**cajolingly** *adv*.

cajolery, cajolement *n* (*pl* **cajoleries, cajolements**) the action or practice of cajoling; persuasion by false arts.

Cajun /'keɪdʒən/ *n* ♣ an inhabitant of Louisiana descended from 18th-century French-Canadians who were expelled by the British; the dialect spoken by Cajuns.

cake /keɪk/ *n* a mixture of flour, eggs, sugar, etc baked in small, flat shapes or a loaf; a small block of compacted or congealed matter. • *vti* to encrust; to form into a cake or hard mass.

cakewalk /'keɪkˌwɒk/ *n* an elaborate step dance; a task accomplished without difficulty.

Cal *abbr* = California; Calorie.

cal *abbr* = calendar; calibre; calorie.

Calabar bean /'kæləˌbɑr/ *n* a West African plant; its poisonous bean.

calabash /'kæləˌbæʃ/ *n* the fruit of the calabash tree of tropical America, used when dried as a vessel for liquids, etc.

calaboose /'kæləˌbuːs/ *n* (*inf*) a jail.

calamanco /kæləˈmæŋkoː/ *n* (*pl* **calamancoes, calamancos**) a glossy woollen fabric, brocaded or checkered.

calamander /'kæləˌmændər/ *n* a fine variety of Indian ebony of a very hard texture.

calamari /kæləˈmɑri/ *n* squid eaten as a food.

calamary /'kæləˌmeri/ *n* (*pl* **calamaries**) squid.

calamine /'kæləˌmaɪn/ *n* a zinc oxide powder used in skin lotions, etc for its soothing effect.

calamint /'kæləˌmɪnt/ *n* an aromatic herb of the mint family.

calamite /'kæləˌmaɪt/ *n* a fossil plant resembling a horsetail.

calamitous /kə'læmɪtəs/ *adj* producing or resulting from calamity; disastrous.—**calamitously** *adv*.—**calamitousness** *n*.

calamity /kæ'lɒmɪti/ *n* (*pl* **calamities**) a disastrous event, a great misfortune; adversity.

calamus /'kæləməs/ *n* (*pl* **calami**) any of a genus of palms producing the rattan canes; the sweet flag.

calando /kə'lændoː/ *adv* (*mus*) gradually; slower and softer.

calash /kə'læʃ/ *n* a light carriage with low wheels and a folding removable top; (*Canada*) a two-wheeled single-seater carriage; a hood formerly worn by women.—*also* **caleche**.

calcar /'kælˌkɑr/ *n* (*pl* **calcaria**) a tube or spur at the base of a petal or sepal; a furnace used in glass-making

calcareous /'kælkeriəs/ *adj* of the nature of, or containing, lime.—**calcareousness** *n*.

calceiform /'kælsɪˌfɔrm/ or /kæl'siː-/, **calceolate** /-ələt/ *adj* (*bot*) slipper-shaped.

calceolaria /kælsiəˈleriə/ *n* any of a genus of South American ornamental plants with slipper-shaped flowers.

calcic /'kælsɪk/ *adj* of or containing calcium.

calciferous /kæl'sɪfərəs/ *adj* containing or yielding carbonate of lime

calcify /'kælsəfaɪ/ *vb* (**calcifying, calcified**) *vt* to convert into lime • *vi* to harden by conversion into lime.

calcimine /-ˌmaɪn/ *n* a white or tinted wash for walls or ceilings.—*also* **kalsomine**.

calcination /kælsəˈneɪʃən/ *n* the act or process of reducing to powder by heat.

calcine /'kælˌsaɪn/ or /-sɪn/ *vt* to reduce a substance to chalky powder by the action of heat; to burn to ashes. • *vi* to undergo calcination.

calcite /'kælˌsaɪt/ *n* crystallized carbonate of lime.—**calcitic** *adj*.

calcium /'kælsiəm/ *n* the chemical element prevalent in bones and teeth.

calcium carbide *n* a fusion of coal or coke with lime in an electrical furnace, which, with water, produces acetylene gas.

calcium carbonate *n* a compound occurring naturally in limestone, chalk, and in bones and shells.

calcsinter /'kælkˌsɪntər/ *n* a crystalline deposit from lime springs.

calcspar /-ˌspɑr/ *n* calcite, a crystalline carbonate of lime.

calculate /'kælkjuˌleɪt/ *vti* to reckon or compute by mathematics; to suppose or believe; to plan.—**calculable** *adj*.

calculated /-ˌleɪtəd/ *adj* adapted or suited (to); deliberate, cold-blooded, premeditated.—**calculatedly** *adv*.

calculating /-ˌleɪtɪŋ/ *adj* shrewd, scheming.—**calculatingly** *adv*.

calculation /-ˌleɪʃən/ *n* the act of calculating; the result obtained from this; an estimate.—**calculational** *adj*.

calculator /-ˌleɪtər/ *n* a device, *esp* a small, electronic, hand-held one, for doing mathematical calculations rapidly; one who calculates.

calculous /-ləs/ *adj* stony; gritty.

calculus /-ləs/ *n* (*pl* **calculi, calculuses**) an abnormal, stony mass in the body; (*math*) a mode of calculation using symbols.

caldera /kæl'derə/ or /kɒl-/ *n* a deep caldron-like cavity on the summits of extinct volcanoes.

caldron /'kɒldrən/ *see* **cauldron**.

caleche /kə'leʃ/ *see* **calash**.

calèche /kə'leʃ/ *n* (*Cdn*) a two-wheeled, one-horse carriage, often used to carry tourists.

Caledonian /kælə'doːniən/ *adj* pertaining to Caledonia, the ancient name of Scotland; Scottish. • *n* a native of Scotland.

calefacient /kælə'feɪsiənt/ or /-ʃiənt/, /-ʃənt/ *adj* producing or exciting heat. • *n* a heat-producing substance.—**calefaction** *n*.

calendar /'kæləndər/ *n* a system of determining the length and divisions of a year; a chart or table of months, days and seasons; a list of particular, scheduled events.

calendar month *n* a solar month reckoned according to the calendar, as distinguished from the lunar month.

calender /'kæləndər/ *n* a press with rollers for finishing the surface of cloth, paper, etc. • *vt* to press in a calender.—**calenderer** *n*.

calender [2] *n* a mendicant dervish.

calends /'kæləndz/ *npl* in the Roman calendar, the first day of each month.—*also* **kalends**.

calendula /kə'lendjulə/ *n* any of a genus of plants, including the marigold, from which a medical tincture is obtained.

calenture /'kæləntʃər/ *n* a tropical fever with delirium.

calf [1] /kɑf/ *n* (*pl* **calves**) the young of a cow, seal, elephant, whale, etc; the leather skin of a calf.

calf [2] *n* (*pl* **calves**) the fleshy back part of the leg below the knee.

calf love *n* puppy love; an immature infatuation.

calfskin /'kæfskɪn/ *n* the skin of a calf made into leather.

Calgarian /kæl'geriən/ *n* ♣ a person who lives in or is from Calgary, Alberta.

Calgary redeye *n* ♣ (*Cdn*) a drink made from beer and tomato juice.—*also* **redeye**.

calibrate /'kæləˌbreɪt/ *vt* to measure the calibre of a gun; to adjust or mark units of measurement on a measuring scale or gauge.—**calibration** *n*.—**calibrator** *n*.

calibre, caliber /'kæləbər/ *n* the internal diameter of a gun barrel or tube; capacity, standing, moral weight.

calico /'kælə,koː/ n (pl **calicoes, calicos**) a kind of cotton cloth. • adj made of this.

calif /'keɪlɪf/ or /'kæ-/ see **caliph**.

Calif. abbr = California.

califate /'kælɪfət/ or /-,feɪt/ see **caliphate**.

californium /,kælə'fɔːniəm/ n an artificial radioactive metallic element.

calipash /'kæləpæʃ/ or /kælə'pæʃ/ n the part of a turtle belonging to the upper shell, enclosing a dull greenish gelatinous edible substance.

calipee /'kæləpi/ or /kælə'piː/ n the part of a turtle belonging to the lower shell, enclosing a light yellow gelatinous edible substance.

caliper /'kæləpər/ see **calliper**.

caliph /'keɪlɪf/ or /'kæ-/ n the former title assumed by the successors of Mohammed as rulers; title of a Turkish sultan.—also **calif**.

caliphate /'kælɪfət/ or /-,feɪt/ n the office, dignity or government of a caliph.—also **califate**.

calisthenics /,kælɪs'θenɪks/ npl light gymnastic exercises.—also—**callisthenics**.—**calisthenic, callisthenic** adj.

calix /'keɪlɪks/ or /'kæl-/ n (pl **calices**) a chalice; a cup-like cavity or organ.

calk[1] /kɒk/ see **caulk**.

calk[2] n the part of a horseshoe that projects downwards to prevent slipping; a semicircular piece of iron nailed to the heel of a boot.

call /kɒl/ vi to shout or cry out; to pay a short visit; to telephone; (with **in**) to pay a brief or informal visit; (with **on**) to pay a visit; to ask, to appeal to. • vt to summon; to name; to describe as specified; to awaken; to give orders for; (with **down**) to invoke; (with **in**) to summon for advice or help; to bring out of circulation; to demand payment of (a loan); (with **off**) to cancel; (an animal) to call away in order to stop, divert; (with **out**) to cry aloud; to order (workers) to come out on strike; to challenge to a duel; to summon (troops) to action; (with **up**) to telephone; to summon to military action, as in time of war; to recall. • n a summons; the note of a bird; a vocation, esp religious; occasion; a need; a demand; a short visit; the use of a telephone; a cry, a shout.

calla (lily) /'kælə/ n an ornamental plant of the arum family with a large white spathe that enfolds a yellow spadix.

callant /kælənt/, **callan** /-ən/ n (Scot) a lad, a youth.

call box n a telephone booth; a roadside box containing a telephone for making emergency calls.

callboy /'kɒl,bɔɪ/ n a prompter's attendant who tells actors when to go on.

caller[1] /-ər/ n one who calls, esp by telephone; one who pays a brief visit.

caller[2] adj (Scot) (food) cool, fresh; in season; (fish) recently caught.

call girl /-,gɜːl/ n (inf) a prostitute who makes appointments by telephone.

callibogus /kælə'boːgəs/ n ✿ (Cdn) a drink made from spruce beer, rum and molasses.

calligraphy /kə'lɪgrəfi/ n handwriting; beautiful writing.—**calligrapher, calligraphist** n.—**calligraphic** adj.—**calligraphically** adv.

calling /'kɒlɪŋ/ n the act of summoning; a summons or invitation; a vocation, trade or profession; the state of being divinely called.

calliope /kə'laɪəpi/ n a steam organ; (with cap) the muse of epic poetry.

calliper /'kælɪpər/ n a metal framework for supporting a crippled or weak leg; paper thickness measured in microns; (pl) a two-legged measuring instrument. • vt to measure with or use callipers.—also **caliper**.

callisthenics /,kælɪs'θenɪks/ see **calisthenics**.

call loan n a loan subject to recall without notice.

callosity /kə'lɒsɪti/ n (pl **callosities**) the state or quality of being hardened; a callus.

callous /'kæləs/ adj (skin) hardened; (person) unfeeling.—**calloused** adj.—**callously** adv.—**callousness** n.

callow /'kæloː/ adj inexperienced, undeveloped.—**callowness** n.

call sign n a signal identifying a particular radio transmitter.

call-up /'kɒl,ʌp/ n a summons to military service.

callus /'kæləs/ n (pl **calluses**) a hardened, thickened place on the skin.

calm /kɒm/ or /kɒlm/ adj windless; still, unruffled; quiet, peaceful. • n the state of being calm; stillness; tranquillity. • vti to become or make calm.—**calmly** adv.—**calmness** n.

calmative /'kɒmətɪv/ or /'kælm-/ adj (med) sedating. • n a sedative.

calomel /'kælə,mel/ n a preparation of mercury used as a purgative.

caloric /kə'lɒrɪk/ adj of or pertaining to heat or calories.—**calorically** adv.

calorie /'kæləri/ n a unit of quantity of heat also called a kilocalorie; a measure of food energy.—also **calory**.

calorific /kə'lɒrɪfɪk/ adj heat-producing; (inf) causing fat.—**calorifically** adv.

calorimeter /,kælə'rɪmətər/ n an instrument for measuring quantities of heat.—**calorimetric, calorimetrical** adj.—**calorimetry** n.

calory /'kæləri/ see **calorie**.

calotte /kə'lɒt/ n a small plain skullcap of satin, etc, worn by priests.

calotype /'kælətɔɪp/ n a photographic process in which the image is received on paper prepared with iodide of silver.

caloyer /'kæləjər/ n a Greek monk of the order of St Basil.

calpac, calpack /'kæl,pæk/ n a tall brimless sheepskin cap worn by Turks and Armenians.—also **kalpak**.

caltrop, caltrap, calthrop /'kæltrəp/ any of various plants with prickly fruit; an iron instrument with four spikes, placed in ditches, etc, to hinder the advance of troops.

calumet /'kælju,met/ n the tobacco pipe of the North American Indians, smoked as a symbol of peace or to ratify treaties.

calumniate /kə'lʌmni,eɪt/ vt to accuse falsely and maliciously. • vi to utter calumnies.—**calumniation** n.—**calumniator** n.

calumny /'kæləmni/ n (pl **calumnies**) a slander; a lie, a false accusation.—**calumnious** adj.—**calumniously** adv.

calvados /'kælvə,dɒs/ n apple brandy distilled in Normandy in France.

calvary /'kælvəri/ n (pl **calvaries**) a place or representation of the crucifixion of Christ; an experience of intense mental suffering; (with cap) the place where Christ was crucified.

calve /kæv/ vti to give birth to a calf; (glacier, iceberg) to break up and release ice.

calves /kævz/ see **calf**.

Calvinism /'kælvɪn,ɪzəm/ n the doctrines of John Calvin (1509–64) the French theologian and reformer, esp those relating to predestination and election.—**Calvinist** n.—**Calvinistic** adj.

calvities /'kælvɪʃɪ,iːz/ n (med) baldness.

calx /kælks/ n (pl **calxes, calces**) the powder left when a metal or mineral has been subjected to great heat.

calycine /'keɪlə,saɪn/, **calycinal** /-əl/ adj having a calyx; of or on the calyx.

calycle /'kælɪkəl/, **calyculus** /-'kjuːləs/ n (pl **calycles, calyculi**) a whorl of small bracts forming a secondary calyx below the true one.

calypso /kə'lɪpsoː/ n (pl **calypsos**) a West Indian folk song that comments on current events or personalities.

calyptra /kə'lɪptrə/ n (bot) the hood-like covering of the spore case of mosses.—**calyptrate** adj.

calyx /'keɪlɪks/ or /'kæliks/ n (pl **calyxes, calyces**) the outer series of leaves that form the cup from which the petals of a flower spring.

cam /kæm/ n a device to change rotary to reciprocating motion.

camas /'kæməs/ n ✿ North American plant of the lily plants with edible bulbs, once consumed by some First Nations or Native American peoples.

camaraderie /,kɒmə'rɒdəri/ or /,kæmə'rædəri/, /,kæmə'rɒdəri/ n friendship, comradeship.

camarilla /,kæmə'rɪlə/, Sp. /,kɑmɑ'riːljɑ/ n a political clique, a cabal.

camber /'kæmbər/ n a slight upward curve in the surface of a road, etc. • vti to curve upwards slightly.—**cambered** adj.

cambist /'kæmbɪst/ n an expert in exchanges; a dealer in bills of exchange.

cambium /'kæmbiəm/ n (pl **cambiums, cambia**) the formative layer of cellular tissue that lies between the young wood and the bark of exogenous trees.—**cambial** adj.

Cambrian /'kæmbriən/ adj of Wales; (geol) of the earliest Palaeozoic period, before the Silurian. • n the strata underlying the Silurian rocks, now classed with them.

cambric /'kæmbrɪk/ or /'kæm-/ n a fine white linen or cotton cloth.

camcorder n a portable video recorder with built-in sound recording facilities.

came /keɪm/ see **come**.

camel /'kæməl/ n a large four-footed, long-necked animal with a humped back; a fawny-beige colour.—also adj.

cameleer /'kæmə,li:r/ n a camel driver.

camellia /kə'mi:liə/ n an oriental evergreen shrub with showy blooms.—also **japonica**.

camelopard /'kæmələ,pard/ or /kə'mɛl'-/ n the giraffe.

camel's hair, camelhair n the hair of a camel; cloth from this; its fawn-tan colour; the hair from a squirrel's tail used as a paintbrush.—**camel's-hair, camelhair** adj.

Camembert /'kæməmbər/ n a soft white cheese originating in Normandy.

cameo /'kæmio:/ n (pl **cameos**) an onyx or other gem carved in relief, often showing a head in profile; an outstanding bit role, esp in a motion picture; a short piece of fine writing.

camera /'kæmrə/ or /-ərə/ n the apparatus used for taking still photographs or television or motion pictures; a judge's private chamber; **in camera** in private, esp of a legal hearing exluding the public; **off camera** outside the area being filmed; **on camera** being filmed, before the camera.

cameraman /-,mæn/ n (pl **cameramen**) a film or television camera operator.

camera obscura /-ɒb'skju:rə/ n a darkened chamber or box in which, by means of lenses, external objects are exhibited on paper, glass, etc.

camera-ready /-,rɛdi/ adj (printing) ready for photographic platemaking.

camera-shy /-,ʃaɪ/ adj unwilling to, or against, being filmed or photographed.

camion /'kæmiən/, Fr. /ka'mjõ:/ n a heavy truck, a wagon.

camise /kə'mi:s/ n a light loose robe, a chemise.

camisole /'kæmɪ,so:l/ n a woman or girl's loose sleeveless underbodice.

camlet /'kæmlət/ n a kind of light cloth.

camomile /'kæmə,maɪl/ see **chamomile**.

Camorra /kə'mɒrə/ n a secret terrorist organization in southern Italy; a lawless clique.

camouflage /'kæmə,flɒʒ/ n a method (esp using colouring) of disguise or concealment used to deceive an enemy; a means of putting people off the scent. • vt to conceal by camouflage.

camp[1] /kæmp/ n the ground on which tents or temporary accommodation is erected; the occupants of this, such as holidaymakers or troops; the supporters of a particular cause. • vi to lodge in a camp; to pitch tents.—**camping** n.

camp[2] adj (sl) theatrical, exaggerated; effeminate; homosexual. • vi (with **up**) to make or give an exaggerated display of camp characteristics.

campaign /kæm'peɪn/ n a series of military operations; a series of operations with a particular objective, such as election of a candidate or promotion of a product; organized course of action. • vi to take part in or conduct a campaign.—**campaigner** n.

campanile /,kæmpə'ni:leɪ/ n a bell tower detached from the body of a church.

campanology /,kæmpə'nɒlədʒi/ n the art of bell ringing.—**campanologist** n.

campanula /kæm'pænjʊlə/ n a plant with bell-shaped flowers.

campanulate /kæm'pænjʊlət/ adj (flower) bell-shaped.

camper /'kæmpər/ n one who lives in a tent; a person on a camping holiday; a vehicle equipped with all domestic facilities.

campfire /'kæmp,faɪr/ n an outdoor fire at a camp; a social gathering around such a fire.

camp follower n a civilian, esp a prostitute, who provides unofficial services to military personnel; a person who is sympathetic to the aims of a particular group but is not a member

camphene /'kæmfi:n/ or /kæm'fi:n/ n rectified oil of turpentine.

camphor /'kæmfər/ n a solid white transparent essential oil with a pungent taste and smell used to repel insects, as a stimulant in medicine, etc.—**camphoric** adj.

camphorate /'kæmfə,reɪt/ vt to saturate or treat with camphor.

camphor tree n a species of laurel that yields camphor.

campion /'kæmpiən/ n any of various wild plants of the pink family, the commonest having red or white flowers.

camp meeting n an outdoor religious meeting.

campsite /'kæmp,saɪt/ n a camping ground, often with facilities for holiday-makers.

campstool /-,stu:l/ n a folding stool or seat.

campus /'kæmpəs/ n (pl **campuses**) the grounds, and sometimes buildings, of a college or university.

camshaft /'kæm,ʃæft/ n the rotating shaft to which cams are fitted to lift valves in engines.

Can abor ✲ = Canada; Canadian.

can[1] /kæn/ vt (pt **could**) to be able to; to have the right to; to be allowed to.

can[2] n a container, usu metal, with a separate cover in which petrol, film, etc is stored; a tin in which meat, fruit, drinks, etc are hermetically sealed; the contents of a can; (sl) jail; (sl) a lavatory; **in the can** (film) shot and edited and ready for showing; (inf) accomplished, agreed, tied up. • vti (**canning, canned**) to preserve (foods) in a can.—**canner** n.

Canada balsam /'kænədə,bɒlsəm/ n a resin obtained from a species of fir.

Canada Day /-deɪ/ n ✲ a national Canadian holiday, July 1, commemorating its dominion status (established 1867).

Canada goose /-,gu:s/ n ✲ a large grey goose with a black head and neck and a white throat patch.

Canada jay n ✲ grey jay.

Canada lily n ✲ a lily of eastern North America with large yellow, orange or spotted flowers.

Canada mayflower n ✲ a woodland lily of eastern North America with white flowers and red berries.

Canadarm /,kænə'darm/ n ✲ (Trademark) a mechanical arm on a spacecraft, used to release, retrieve and repair satellites and other equipment.

Canadian /kə'neɪdiən/ adj ✲ of or pertaining to Canada. • n a native of Canada.

Canadian football n ✲ a form of football resembling American football but with a wider field, three downs and 12 players.

Canadianism /kə'neɪdiə,nɪzəm/ n ✲ a form of expression peculiar to Canada; a custom peculiar to Canada.

Canadianize /kə'neɪdiə,naɪz/ vt ✲ to render Canadian; to assimilate to the political and social institutions of Canada. — **Canadianization** n.

Canadian whisky n ✲ whisky distilled from rye and other grains.

Canadien, Canadienne /kə'neɪdjen/ n ✲ a French Canadian.

canaille /kə'neɪl/, Fr. /ka'naj/ n a rabble, the lowest orders.

canal /kə'næl/ n an artificial waterway cut across land; a duct in the body. • vt (**canalling, canalled** or **canaling, canaled**) to provide with canals.

canalize, canalise /'kænə,laɪz/ vt to provide with a canal or channel. • vi to flow in or into a channel; to establish new channels or outlets.—**canalization, canalisation** n.

Can-Am /'kæn,æm/ adj ✲ pertaining to an event, esp in sports, with Canadian and US participants. • n an event with Canadian and US participants.

canapé /'kænə,peɪ/ n a small piece of pastry, bread or toast with a savoury spread or topping.

canard /kə'nɑrd/ n a false report, an absurd story, a baseless rumour.

canary /kə'neri/ n (pl **canaries**) a small finch, usu greenish to yellow in colour, kept as a songbird.

canasta /kə'næstə/ n a card game played with two packs of cards, for two to six players.

cancan /'kænkæn/ n an energetic dance performed by women, involving high kicks and the lifting of frothy petticoats.

cancel /'kænsəl/ vt (**cancelling, cancelled** or **canceling, canceled**) to cross out; to obliterate; to annul, suppress; (reservation etc) to call off; to countermand; (with **out**) to make up for.—**canceller, canceler** n.

cancellation, cancelation /kænsə'leɪʃən/ n the act of cancelling; annulment; something that has been cancelled; the mark made by cancelling.

cancellous /'kænsələs/, cancellate /-lət/, cancellated /-tɪd/ adj (med) marked with cross lines or ridges.

cancer /'kænsər/ n the abnormal and uncontrollable growth of the cells of living organisms, esp a malignant tumour; an undesirable or dangerous expansion of something.—**cancerous** adj.

Cancer /'kænsər/ n (astron) the Crab, a northern constellation; (astrol) the 4th sign of the zodiac, operative 21 June–21 July.—**Cancerian** adj.

cancroid /'kæŋ,krɔɪd/ or /'kæn-/ adj resembling a cancer; like a crab.

candela /,kæn'di:lə/ or /-'delə/ n a unit of luminous intensity.

candelabrum /,kændə'læbrəm/ n (pl **candelabra**) a branched and ornamented candlestick or lampstand.

candescent /kæn'desən/ adj glowing; white-hot.—**candescence** n

candid /'kændɪd/ adj frank, outspoken; unprejudiced; (photograph) informal.—**candidly** adv.—**candidness** n.

candidate /ˈkændɪdeɪt/ or /-ˌdət/ *n* a person who has nomination for an office or qualification for membership or award; a student taking an examination.—**candidacy** *n*.—**candidature** *n*.

candid camera *n* a small camera for photographing people unexpectedly or unknowingly.

candied /ˈkændiːd/ *adj* preserved in or encrusted with sugar.

candle /ˈkændəl/ *n* a stick of wax with a wick that burns to give light. • *vt* to check the freshness of eggs by examining in front of a light.

candle ice /ˈkændəlˈʌɪs/ *n* ✦ ice that has deteriorated into candle-like icicles.

candlelight /-ˌlʌɪt/ *n* the light produced by a candle or candles.

Candlemas (Day) *n* the Feast of the Purification of the Virgin Mary (2 February).

candlepower /-ˌpaʊr/ *n* a unit of measurement of the intensity of a light source, measured in candelas.

candlestick /-stɪk/ *n* a holder for one or more candles.

candlewick /-wɪk/ *n* a cotton fabric with raised pattern of tufted yarn.—*also adj.*

candour, candor /ˈkændər/ *n* sincerity, openness, frankness.

CANDU /ˈkændjuː/ *n* ✦ (*Cdn*) a nuclear reactor that uses fuel bundles and a system that moderates heat with heavy water.

candy /ˈkændi/ *n* (*pl* **candies**) a solid confection of sugar or syrup with flavouring, fruit, nuts, etc, a sweet. • *vb* (**candying, candied**) *vt* to preserve by coating with candy; to encrust with crystals. • *vi* to become candied.

candyfloss /-ˌflɒs/ *n* a confection of spun sugar.—*also* **cotton candy**.

candy-striped *adj* (*cloth*) with narrow stripes of colour on a white background.

candytuft /-ˌtʌft/ *n* a plant with pink, white or purple tufted flowers.

cane /keɪn/ *n* the slender, jointed stem of certain plants, as bamboo; a plant with such a stem, as sugar cane; (*usu with* **the**) a stick of this used for corporal punishment; strips of this used in furniture making etc or for supporting plants; a walking stick. • *vt* to thrash with a cane; to weave cane into; (*inf*) to beat, eg in a game.

canebrake /ˈkeɪnbreɪk/ *n* a thicket of canes.

canella /kəˈnelə/ *n* an aromatic and tonic bark of a West Indian tree.

canescent /kəˈnesənt/ *adj* (*biol*) growing white, hoary.

cane sugar *n* sugar made from sugar cane.

cangue /kæŋ/ *n* (*formerly*) a square wooden collar worn as a punishment by criminals in China.

canine /ˈkeɪnaɪn/ *adj* of or like a dog; of the family of animals that includes wolves, dogs and foxes; pertaining to a canine tooth. • *n* a dog or other member of the same family of animals; in humans, a pointed tooth next to the incisors.

canister /ˈkænɪstər/ *n* a small box or container *usu* of metal for storing tea, flour, etc; a tube containing tear gas which explodes and releases its contents on impact.

canker /ˈkæŋkər/ *n* an erosive or spreading sore; a foot disease in horses; an ear disease in cats and dogs; a fungal disease of trees; a corrupting influence.—**cankerous** *adj*.

cankerworm /-wɔrm/ *n* a caterpillar destructive to trees or plants.

CanLit ✦ (*Cdn*) (*inf*) *abbr* = Canadian literature.

canna /ˈkænə/ *n* a showy American tropical plant.

cannabin /ˈkænəˌbɪn/ *n* a narcotic resin extracted from hemp.

cannabis /ˈkænəbɪs/ *n* a narcotic drug obtained from the hemp plant; the hemp plant.—*also* **hashish, marijuana**.—**cannabic** *adj.*

canned /kænd/ *adj* stored in sealed tins; recorded for reproduction; (*sl*) drunk.

canned hunt *n* (*sl*) an organized big-game hunt carried out within an area from which the quarry cannot escape.

cannel (coal) /ˈkænəl/ *n* a hard bituminous coal burning with a clear bright flame.

cannelloni /ˌkænəˈloʊni/ *npl* stuffed pasta tubes.

cannelure /ˈkænəljʊr/ or /-lʊr/ *n* a groove or fluting.

cannery /ˈkænəri/ *n* (*pl* **canneries**) a building, etc, where foods are canned.

cannibal /ˈkænəbəl/ *n* a person who eats human flesh; an animal that feeds on its own species. • *adj* relating to or indulging in this practice.—**cannibalism** *n*.—**cannibalistic** *adj*.

cannibalize /-ˌlaɪz/ *vti* to strip (old equipment) of parts for use in other units.—**cannibalization** *n*.

cannikin /ˈkænɪkɪn/ *n* a small can.

cannon /ˈkænən/ *n* (*pl* **cannon**) a large mounted piece of artillery; an automatic gun on an aircraft; (*pl* **cannons**) (*billiards*) a

carom. • *vi* to collide with great force (with into); to rebound; (*billiards*) to make a carom.

cannonade /ˌkænənˈeɪd/ *n* a heavy, continuous artillery attack. • *vti* to attack with cannon.

cannonball /ˈkænənˌbɒl/ *n* the heavy, round shot fired from a cannon; (*tennis*) a low, fast service stroke. • *vi* to move along at great speed.

cannoneer /ˌkænəˈnɪr/ *n* an artilleryman.

cannon fodder *n* soldiers regarded as expendable in war.

cannonry /ˈkænənri/ *n* (*pl* **cannonries**) artillery.

cannot /kæˈnɒt/ or /kə-/, /ˈkænɒt/ = can not.

cannula /ˈkænjʊlə/ *n* (*pl* **cannulas, cannulae**) (*med*) a small tube for inspecting or withdrawing fluids.

canny /ˈkæni/ *adj* (**cannier, canniest**) knowing, shrewd; cautious, careful; thrifty.—**cannily** *adv*.—**canniness** *n*.

canoe /kəˈnuː/ *n* a narrow, light boat propelled by paddles.—*also vi* (**canoeing, canoed**).—**canoeist** *n*.

canola /kəˈnoʊlə/ *n* ✦ (*Cdn*) the seeds of a variety of the rape plant, used to make cooking oil.

canon /ˈkænən/ *n* a decree of the Church; a general rule or standard, criterion; a list of the books of the Bible accepted as genuine; the works of any author recognized as genuine; a list of canonized saints; a member of a cathedral chapter; a part of the mass containing words of consecration; (*mus*) a round.

canoness /ˈkænənəs/ *n* (*RC Church*) one of a number of women living under canon law but not compelled to take religious vows.

canonical /kəˈnɒnɪkəl/ *adj* pertaining to a rule or canon; according to or established by ecclesiastical laws; belonging to the canon of scripture. • *n* (*pl*) the official dress of the clergy.—**canonically** *adv*.

canonical hour *n* (*RC Church*) one of the hours appointed by ecclesiastical law for daily prayer: matins with lauds, prime, sext, nones, vespers, and compline.

canonist /ˈkænənɪst/ *n* an expert in canon law.—**canonistic** *adj*.

canonize /ˈkænəˌnaɪz/ *vt* (*RC Church*) to officially declare (a person) a saint.—**canonization** *n*.

canon law *n* rules or laws relating to faith, morals and discipline that regulate church government, as laid down by popes and councils.

canonry /ˈkænənri/ *n* (*pl* **canonries**) the office of a cathedral canon.

canoodle /kəˈnuːdəl/ *vti* (*sl*) to cuddle, to fondle.

canopy /ˈkænəpi/ *n* (*pl* **canopies**) a tent-like covering over a bed, throne, etc; any roof-like structure or projection; the transparent cover of an aeroplane's cockpit; the tops of trees in a forest; the sky regarded as a covering. • *vt* (**canopying, canopied**) to cover with or as with a canopy.

cans /kænz/ *npl* (*sl*) headphones.

cant¹ /kænt/ *n* insincere or hypocritical speech; language specific to a group (eg thieves, lawyers); cliched talk, meaningless jargon. • *vi* to talk in or use cant.

cant² *n* an inclination or tilt; a slanting surface, bevel. • *vti* to slant, to tilt; to overturn by a sudden movement.

can't /kænt/ = can not.

cantabile /kænˈtæbiˌleɪ/ *adv* (*mus*) in a lyrical flowing style.

Cantabrigian /ˌkæntəˈbrɪdʒɪən/ *n* a student or graduate of Cambridge University; an inhabitant of Cambridge.—*also adj.*

cantaloupe, cantaloup /ˈkæntəloʊp/ *n* a variety of melon with orange flesh.

cantankerous /kænˈtæŋkərəs/ *adj* ill-natured, bad-tempered, quarrelsome.—**cantankerously** *adv*.—**cantankerousness** *n*.

cantata /kænˈtɑːtə/ or /tɒtə-/ *n* (*mus*) a composition for voices of a story or religious text.

cantatrice *Fr.* /kɑ̃taˈtriːs/, *It.* /ˌkantaˈtriːtʃe/ *n* a female singer, *esp* one who sings in operas.

canteen /kænˈtiːn/ *n* a restaurant attached to factory, school, etc, catering for large numbers of people; a flask for carrying water; (a box containing) a set of cutlery.

canter /ˈkæntər/ *n* a horse's three-beat gait resembling a slow, smooth gallop.—*also vti*.

Canterbury bell /ˈkæntərbəri/ *n* a large variety of campanula with handsome bell-shaped blossoms.

cantharides /kænˈθærɪˌdiːz/ *npl* (*sing* **cantharis**) (*med*) a diuretic preparation made from dried Spanish flies, formerly considered an aphrodisiac.—*also* **Spanish fly**.

canthus /ˈkænθəs/ *n* (*pl* **canthi**) the angle made by the meeting of the eyelids.

canticle /'kæntɪkəl/ *n* a song taken from the Bible (eg the Magnificat).

cantilever /'kæntɪˌliːvər/ *n* a projecting beam that supports a balcony, etc.

cantilever bridge *n* a bridge supported by cantilevers springing from piers.

cantle /'kæntəl/ *n* a corner; a piece; the rising rear part of a saddle.

canto /'kæntoː/ *n* (*pl* **cantos**) a division of a long poem.

canton /'kæntɒn/ *n* a political and administrative division of Switzerland.—**cantonal** *adj*.

Cantonese /ˌkæntəˈniːz/ *n* (*pl* **Cantonese**) a Chinese language deriving from Canton; an inhabitant or native of Canton.—*also adj*.

cantonment /kænˈtɒnmənt/ *n* a part of a town or village allotted to a body of troops; in India, a permanent military station.

cantor /'kæntər/ or /-tɔr/ *n* a singer of liturgical solos in a synagogue; the leader of singing in a church choir.

cantorial /-'toːriəl/ *adj* of or pertaining to a precentor's or the north side of the choir of a church.

cantrip /'kæntrɪp/ *n* a prank, a piece of mischief; a magic spell.

Canuck /kəˈnʊk/ *n* ✹ (*Cdn*) (*inf*) a Canadian.—*also adj*.

canvas /'kænvəs/ *n* a strong coarse cloth of hemp or flax, used for tents, sails, etc, and for painting on; a ship's sails collectively; a tent or tents; an oil painting on canvas.

canvasback /-ˌbæk/ *n* (*pl* **canvasbacks, canvasback**) a North American duck esteemed for the delicacy of its flesh.

canvass /'kænvəs/ *vti* to go through (places) or among (people) asking for votes, opinions, orders, etc.—*also n*.—**canvasser** *n*.

canyon /'kænjən/ *n* a long, narrow valley between high cliffs.

canzone *It*. /kanˈtsoːne/, **canzona** /-ˌnɒ/ *n* (*pl* **canzoni, canzone**) a song or air resembling the madrigal; an instrumental piece in the style of a madrigal.

canzonet, canzonette /ˌkænzəˈnet/ *n* a short light song.

caoutchouc /kauˈtʃʊk/ *n* rubber.—*also adj*.

cap /kæp/ *n* any close-fitting headgear, visored or brimless; the special headgear of a profession, club, etc; the top of a mushroom or toadstool; a cap-like thing, as an artificial covering for a tooth; a top, a cover; a percussion cap in a toy gun; a type of contraceptive device; (*sport*) the head gear presented to a player chosen for a team. • *vt* (**capping, capped**) to put a cap on; to cover (the end of); to award a degree at a university; to seal (an oil or gas well); to equal, outdo or top; to limit the level of a tax increase, etc; (*sport*) to choose a player for a team.

capability /ˌkeɪpəˈbɪləti/ *n* (*pl* **capabilities**) the quality of being capable; an undeveloped faculty.

capable /'keɪpəbəl/ *adj* able or skilled to do; competent, efficient; susceptible (of); adapted to.—**capably** *adv*.

capacious /kəˈpeɪʃəs/ *adj* able to hold a great deal; roomy.—**capaciousness** *n*.

capacitance /kəˈpæsɪtəns/ *n* (a measure of) the ability of a system to store an electric charge.

capacitate /-ˌteɪt/ *vt* to make capable; to enable; to qualify.—**capacitation** *n*.

capacitor /-tər/ *n* a device for storing electric charge.

capacity /kəˈpæsɪti/ *n* (*pl* **capacities**) the power of holding or grasping; cubic content; mental ability or power; character; the position held; legal competence; the greatest possible output or content.

cap-a-pie /ˌkæpəˈpiː/ *adv* from head to foot.

caparison /kəˈpærɪsən/ *n* an ornamental covering for a horse; rich clothing. • *vt* to cover (a horse) with rich clothing; to adorn with rich dress.

cape[1] /keɪp/ *n* a headland or promontory running into the sea.

cape[2] *n* a sleeveless garment fastened at the neck and hanging over the shoulders and back.

Cape Bretoner /ˌkeɪpˈbretnər/ *n* ✹ (*Cdn*) a person who lives in or is from the island of Cape Breton, Nova Scotia.

capelin, caplin /'kæplɪn/ or /'keɪp-/ *n* a small sea fish of the smelt family, largely used as bait for cod

caper[1] /'keɪpər/ *vi* to skip about playfully, to frolic. • *n* a playful leap or skip; (*sl*) an escapade; (*sl*) a criminal activity.

caper[2] *n* a low, prickly Mediterranean shrub; its pickled flower buds, used in cooking (eg caper sauce).

capercaillie /kæpərˈkeɪli/, **capercailzie** /-lzi/ *n* the largest Old World grouse.

capetian /kəˈpiːʃən/ *adj* of or pertaining to the dynasty founded by Hugh Capet, who ascended the French throne in 1987.

Capias /'kæpiəs/ or /'keɪp-/ *n* (*law*) a writ for arrest.

capillarity /ˌkæpɪˈlɛrɪti/ *n* (*pl* **capillarities**) the power possessed by porous bodies of drawing up a fluid; surface tension.

capillary /'kæpɪˌlɛri/ *adj* of or as fine as a hair; (*tube, pipe*) of a hair-like calibre; (*anat*) of the capillaries. • *n* (*pl* **capillaries**) one of the very fine blood vessels connecting arteries and veins.

capital /'kæpɪtəl/ *adj* of or pertaining to the head; (*offence*) punishable by death; serious; chief, principal; leading, first-class; of, or being the seat of government; of capital or wealth; relating to a large letter, upper-case; (*inf*) excellent. • *n* a city that is the seat of government of a country; a large letter; accumulated wealth used to produce more; stock or money for carrying on a business; a city, town, etc pre-eminent in some special activity.—**capitally** *adv*.

capital[1] *n* the head or top part of a column or pillar.

capital gain *n* the profit made on the sale of an asset.

capital goods *npl* goods (eg machinery) used to produce other goods.

capital sm /'kæpɪtəˌlɪzəm/ *n* the system of individual ownership of wealth; the dominance of such a system.

capital st /-lɪst/ *n* a person who has money invested in business for profit; a supporter of capitalism. • *adj* of or favouring capitalism.—**capitalistic** *adj*.

capital ze /-ˌlaɪz/ *vti* (*with* **on**) to use (something) to one's advantage; to convert into money or capital; to provide with capital; to write in or print in capital letters.—**capitalization** *n*.

capital y /-liː/ *adv* in a capital manner; excellently.

capital punishment *n* the death penalty for a crime.

capitate /'kæpɪteɪt/ *adj* (*bot*) shaped like a head; head-like.

capitation /ˌkæpɪˈteɪʃən/ *n* a direct, uniform tax imposed on each person, a tax per head.

capitol /'kæpɪtəl/ *n* (*with* **the**) the building where the US Congress meets; the temple of Jupiter on the Capitoline in Rome.

capitular /kəˈpɪtʃjʊlər/ *adj* of or pertaining to a chapter. • *n* a member of a cathedral chapter.

capitulary *n* (*pl* **capitularies**) a statue passed in a chapter, as of knights or canons; (*pl*) the body of statues of a chapter or of an ecclesiastical council.

capitulate /kəˈpɪtʃjʊleɪt/ *vi* to surrender on terms; to give in.—**capitulation** *n*.—**capitulator** *n*.—**capitulatory** *adj*.

capo /'keɪpoː/ *n* (*pl* **capos**) a device attached across the fingerboard of a guitar to raise the pitch of the strings.

capon /'keɪpɒn/ *n* a castrated cockerel fattened for eating.

caponize /-pənaɪz/ *vt* to make a cock a capon by castration.

caporal /'kæpərəl/ or /'kæpɔˌræl/ *n* a French tobacco.

capote /kəˈpoːt/ *n* a long coarse cloak; a long mantle for women; ✹ (*Cdn*) (*hist*) a long coat with a hood, tied with a colourful sash

cappuccino /ˌkæpəˈtʃiːnoː/ *n* (*pl* **cappuccinos**) frothy, milky coffee *usu* served sprinkled with chocolate powder.

capreolate /'kæpriˌoːlət/ *adj* (*bot*) furnished with tendrils.

capriccio /kəˈpriːtʃioː/ *n* (*pl* **capriccios, capricci**) a light musical composition in a fantastic, whimsical style.

capriccioso /kəˌpriːtʃiˈoːsoː/ *adv* (*mus*) in a free, fantastic style.

caprice /kəˈpriːs/ *n* a passing fancy; an impulsive change in behaviour, opinion, etc; a whim.

capricious /kəˈpriːʃəs/ or /-prɪ-/ *adj* unstable, inconstant; unreliable.—**capriciously** *adv*.—**capriciousness** *n*.

Capricorn /'kæprɪˌkɔrn/ *n* (*astron*) the Goat, a southern constellation; (*astrol*) the tenth sign of the zodiac, operative 21 December–19 January.—**Capricornean** *adj*.

caprification /ˌkæprɪfɪˈkeɪʃən/ *n* a process of accelerating the ripening of the fig by puncturing it.

caprine /'kæpraɪn/ *adj* of, pertaining to, or like a goat.

capriole /'kæpriˌoːl/ *n* a leap of a horse made without advancing; a caper. • *vi* to execute a capriole, to kick up the heels.

capsaicin /kæpˈseɪəsɪn/ *n* an alkaloid extracted from several species of capsicum.

capsicum /'kæpsɪkəm/ *n* a tropical plant with bell-shaped fruits containing hot or mild seeds; the fruit of this plant used as a vegetable.—*also* **red** or **green pepper**.

capsize /'kæpsaɪz/ or /kæpˈsaɪz/ *vti* to upset or overturn.

capstan /'kæpstən/ *n* an upright drum around which cables are wound to haul them in the spindle in a tape recorder that winds the tape past the head.

capsulate, capsulated /'kæpsəˌleɪt/ *adj* furnished with or enclosed in a capsule.—**capsulation** *n*.

capsule /'kæpsəl/ or /-sjəl/ *n* a small gelatin case enclosing a drug to be swallowed; a metal or plastic container; (*bot*) a seed case; the orbiting and recoverable part of a spacecraft.—**capsular** *adj*.

capsulize /-aɪz/ *vt* to present (information) in a concise or condensed form.—**capsulization** *n*.

captain /'kæptən/ *n* a chief, leader; the master of a ship; the pilot of an aircraft; a rank of army, naval and marine officer; the leader of a team, as in sports; a leading employer in industry; a policeman responsible for a precinct. • *vt* to be captain of.—**captaincy** *n*.

captaincy, captainship *n* (*pl* **captaincies, captainships**) the rank, post, or commission of a captain.

caption /'kæpʃən/ *n* a heading in a newspaper, to a chapter, etc; a legend or title describing an illustration; a subtitle. • *vti* to provide with a caption.

captious /-ʃəs/ *adj* ready to find fault or take offence; carping, quibbling.—**captiously** *adv*.

captivate /'kæptɪˌveɪt/ *vt* to fascinate; to charm.—**captivating** *adj*.—**captivation** *n*.—**captivator** *n*.

captive /'kæptɪv/ *n* one kept confined; a prisoner; a person obsessed by an emotion. • *adj* taken or kept prisoner; unable to avoid being addressed (*a captive audience*); unable to refuse (a product) through a lack of choice (*a captive market*); captivated.

captivity /kæp'tɪvɪti/ *n* (*pl* **captivities**) the state of being a captive; a period of imprisonment.

captor /'kæptər/ *n* a person or animal who takes a prisoner.

capture /-tʃər/ *vt* to take prisoner; (*fortress, etc*) to seize; to catch; to gain or obtain by skill, attraction, etc, to win. • *n* the act of taking a prisoner or seizing by force; anything or anyone so taken.

capuche /kə'puːtʃ/ or /-puːʃ/ *n* a monk's hood or cowl; the hood of a cloak.

capuchin /'kæpjuːtʃɪn/ or /-puː-/, /-ʃɪn/ *n* a monkey with hair resembling a cowl; a pigeon with cowl-like feathers; a woman's cloak and hood; (*with cap*) a Franciscan monk of the mendicant order.

capybara /ˌkæpə'bɑrə/ *n* a large South American rodent that lives mostly in water.

car /kɑr/ *n* a self-propelled motor vehicle, an automobile, a motorcar; the passenger compartment of a train, airship, lift, cable railway, etc; a railway carriage.

carabineer, carabinier /ˌkærəbə'nɪr/ *see* **carbineer**.

carabiner /ˌkærə'binər/ or /'kærə-/ *n* (*climbing*) a type of shackle with a snap link, used to secure a rope.

caracal /'kerəˌkæl/ or /'kærə-/ *n* a kind of lynx; its fur.

caracole, caracol /'kerəˌkoːl/ or /'kærə-/ *vi* (*horse*) to make a half turn to the right or left. • *n* a half turn, right or left; a spiral staircase.

carafe /kə'ræf/ *n* an open-topped bottle for serving water or wine at table.

carageen /'kærəˌgin/ *see* **carrageen**.

caramel /'kerəməl/ or /'kɑrməl/ *n* burnt sugar, used in cooking to colour or flavour; a type of sweet tasting of this.

caramelize /'kerəməˌlaɪz/ or /'kærə-/, /'kɑrmə-/ *vti* to turn or be turned into caramel.

carapace /'kerəˌpeɪs/ or /'kærə-/ *n* the upper shell of the tortoise, turtle, crab, etc.

carat /'kerət/ or /'kæ-/ *n* a measure of weight for precious stones; a measure of the purity of gold.—*also* **karat**.

caravan /'kerəˌvæn/ or /'kærə-/ *n* a large enclosed vehicle that is equipped to be lived in and may be towed by a car.—*also* **trailer**; a band of merchants travelling together for safety. • *vi* (**caravanning, caravanned**) to travel with a caravan, *esp* on holiday.

caravanserai /ˌkerə'vænsəraɪ/, **caravansary** /-səri/ *n* (*pl* **caravanserais, caravansaries**) in the East, a large inn surrounding a spacious courtyard, where caravans rest at night.

caravel, caravelle /'kɑrəˌvɛl/ *n* an ancient small light fast Spanish ship with broad bows, a narrow high poop, four masts and lateen sails.—*also* **carvel**.

caraway /'kɑrəˌweɪ/ *n* a biennial plant with pungent aromatic seeds used as a flavouring.

carbide /'kɑrˌbaɪd/ *n* a compound of carbon with another element, *esp* calcium carbide.

carbine /'kɑrbaɪn/ *n* a light, semiautomatic or automatic rifle.

carbineer /'kɑrbəniːr/ *n* a mounted soldier armed with a carbine.—*also* **carabineer, carabinier**.

carbo-, carb- /'kɑrbo/ *prefix* carbon.

carbohydrate /ˌkɑrboː'haɪdreɪt/ *n* a compound of carbon, hydrogen and oxygen, *esp* in sugars and starches as components of food. • *npl* starchy foods.

carbolic acid /kɑr'bɒlɪk/ *n* phenol.

carbolize /'kɑrbəˌlaɪz/ *vt* to sterilize with carbolic acid.

carbon /'kɑrbən/ *n* a nonmetallic element, a constituent of all organic matter; a duplicate made with carbon paper.

carbon-12 *n* an isotope of carbon, used as the standard for atomic weight.

carbon-14 *n* a radioisotope used in medicine as a tracer and in carbon dating.

carbonaceous /ˌkɑrbə'neɪʃəs/ *adj* pertaining to, composed of or resembling carbon.

carbonado /ˌkɑrbə'neɪdoː/ or /-nɑ-/ *n* (*pl* **carbonadoes, carbonados**) a piece of meat cut crossways for grilling.

carbonate /'kɑrbəneɪt/ *n* a salt of carbonic acid. • *vt* to treat with carbon dioxide, as in making soft, fizzy drinks.—**carbonated** *adj*.

carbon copy *n* a copy of typed or written material made by using carbon paper; (*inf*) an exact copy of something or someone.

carbon dating *n* a scientific method of dating material by measuring the amount of carbon-14 it contains.

carbon dioxide *n* a gas formed by combustion and breathing and absorbed by plants.

carbonic /'kɑrbɒnɪk/ *adj* of or obtained from carbon.

carbonic acid *n* a weakly acidic solution of carbon dioxide in water.

carboniferous /ˌkɑrbə'nɪfərəs/ *adj* coal-bearing, yielding carbon; (*with cap*) of or relating to strata of the Palaeozoic Age from which coal is derived.

carbonize /'kɑrbəˌnaɪz/ *vt* to convert into carbon or a carbon residue.—**carbonization** *n*.

carbon monoxide *n* a colourless, odourless, highly poisonous gas.

carbon paper *n* a sheet of paper covered with a dark, waxy pigment inserted between sheets of paper for making copies of writing or typing.

carborundum /ˌkɑrbə'rʌndəm/ *n* (*trademark*) a compound of carbon and silicon used for polishing and grinding.

carboy /'kɑrbɔɪ/ *n* a, *usu* cushioned, container of glass, plastic or metal for the safe transportation of liquids.

carbuncle /'kɑrˌbʌŋkəl/ *n* a red, knob-shaped gemstone, *esp* a garnet; a large inflamed boil; a pimple.—**carbuncular** *adj*.

carburet /'kɑrbəˌreɪt/ or /-rɛt/, /-bə-/ *vt* (**carburetting, carburetted** *or* **carbureting, carbureted**) to combine with carbon.

carburetor, carburettor /'kɑrbəˌreɪtə/ *n* a device in an internal-combustion engine for making an explosive mixture of air and fuel vapour.

carburize /'kɑrbəˌraɪz/ or /-bə-/ *vt* to combine with carbon.—**carburization** *n*.

carcanet /'kɑrkəˌnɛt/ *n* (*arch*) a collar of jewels.

carcass /'kɑrkəs/ *n* the dead body of an animal; a framework, skeleton or shell; (*derog*) the body of a living person.

carcinogen /kɑr'sɪnədʒən/ *n* a substance that produces cancer.—**carcinogenic** *adj*.

carcinoma /ˌkɑrsɪ'noːmə/ *n* (*pl* **carcinomas, carcinomata**) a tumour caused by a cancer.

card[1] /kɑrd/ *n* a small piece of cardboard; a piece of this with a figure or picture for playing games or fortune-telling; a piece of this filed in a card index; a membership card; a piece of card with a person or firm's name, address or with an invitation, greeting, message, etc; (*inf*) an entertaining or eccentric person; a small piece of plastic identifying a person for banking purposes, eg a cheque card, credit card; (*pl*) card games; (*pl*) card playing; (*pl*) employees insurance and tax documents held by the employer.

card[2] *n* a toothed instrument for combing cotton, wool or flax fibres off. • *vt* (*wool, etc*) to comb.

cardamom, cardamum, cardamon /'kɑrdəməm/ *n* a tropical Asian plant the seed pods of which are used as a spice.

cardboard /'kɑrdbɔrd/ *n* thick stiff paper, often with a clay coating, for boxes, cartons, etc. • *adj* made of this; lacking substance; makeshift.

card-carrying *adj* being an official member of a political party, organization, etc.

card catalogue *n* a catalogue, each item of which is entered on a separate card.

card file *n* a filing system in which each item is entered separately on a single card.

cardi- /'kɑrdi/ or /-dɪ/, /-də/ *prefix* heart.

cardiac /'kɑrdiˌæk/ *adj* relating to the heart. • *n* a person suffering a disorder of the heart; a drug to stimulate the heart.

cardiac arrest *n* heart failure.

cardialgia /ˌkardiˈældʒiə/ or /-dʒə/ n heartburn.—**cardialgic** adj.

cardigan /ˈkardɪgən/ n a knitted sweater fastening up the front.

cardinal /ˈkardɪnəl/ adj of chief importance, fundamental; of a bright red. • n an official appointed by the Pope to his councils; bright red.—**cardinally** adv.

cardinalate /-leɪt/, **cardinalship** /-ʃp/ n the office, rank, or dignity of a cardinal; the body of cardinals.

cardinal numbers npl numbers that express how many (1, 2, 3, 4 etc).

cardinal points npl the four chief points of the compass: north, south, east, west.

cardinal virtues npl justice, prudence, temperance, and fortitude.

cardio- /ˈkardiˌoː/ prefix heart.

cardiogram /ˈkardioˌgræm/ n an electrocardiogram.

cardiograph /-ˌgræf/ n a device for recording heart movements; an electrocardiograph.

cardiology /ˌkardiˈɒladʒi/ n the branch of medicine concerned with the heart and its diseases.—**cardiological** adj.—**cardiologist** n.

cardiopulmonary /ˌkardioːˈpelmoˌneri/ or /-pol/ adj of or concerned with or affect the heart and lungs.

cardiovascular /-ˈvæskjʊlər/ adj of or pertaining to the heart and the blood vessels.

carditis /karˈdaɪtɪs/ n inflammation of the muscular tissue of the heart.

cardoon /karˈduːn/ n a plant related to and resembling the artichoke and used as a vegetable in Spain and France.

cards /kards/ see **card**[1].

cardsharp(er) /kardˈʃarp(ər)/ n a person who cheats at cards.

care /ker/ n anxiety; concern; serious attention, heed; consideration; charge, protection; the cause or object of concern or anxiety. • vt to feel concern; to agree, like, or be willing (to do something); **care of** at the address of, c/o; **in, into care** (person) taken charge of by a local authority by court order. • vi (usu with **for** or **about**) to feel affection or regard; to have a desire (for); to provide for, have in one's charge.

careen /kəˈriːn/ vt to bring (a ship) over on one side for calking, cleansing, or repairing. • vi to incline to one side, as a ship under press of sail.

career /kəˈriːr/ n progress through life; a profession, occupation, esp with prospects for promotion. • vi to rush rapidly or wildly.

careerist /-ɪst/ n a person who is ambitious to advance in a chosen profession.

career woman n a woman primarily interested in her job and in furthering her career.

carefree /ˈkerˈfriː/ adj without cares, lively, light-hearted.

careful /ˈkerfʊl/ adj painstaking; cautious; thoughtful.—**carefully** adv.—**carefulness** n.

careless /ˈkerləs/ adj not careful; unconcerned, insensitive; carefree.—**carelessly** adv.—**carelessness** n.

carer /ˈkerər/ n one who takes on (professionally) the care of a dependent person.

caress /kəˈres/ n any act or expression of affection; an embrace. • vt to touch or stroke lovingly.—**caresser** n.—**caressingly** adv.

caret /ˈkærət/ n a mark (^) showing where something omitted in text is to be inserted.

caretaker /ˈkerˌteɪkər/ n a person put in charge of a place or thing; (government) one temporarily in control.

careworn /ˈkerwornˌ/ adj showing signs of stress, worry.

cargo /ˈkargoː/ n (pl **cargoes, cargos**) the load carried by a ship, truck, aircraft, etc; freight.

Carib /ˈkerɪb/ n (pl **Caribs, Carib**) a member of an Indian people of the Lesser Antilles and neighbouring parts of the South American coast, or of their descendants; their language. • adj of or pertaining to the Carib people or language.

Caribbean /ˌkerəˈbiən/ or /kəˈrɪbiən/ adj of or pertaining to the Caribbean Sea and its islands. • n the Caribbean Sea.

caribou /ˈkærɪˌbuː/ or /ˈkærə-/ n (pl **caribou, caribous**) a large North American reindeer; ✦ (Cdn) a drink made from red wine and diluted alcohol.

caricature /ˈkærɪkətʃər/ n a likeness made ludicrous by exaggeration or distortion of characteristic features. • vt to make a caricature of, to parody.—**caricaturist** n.

caries /ˈkeˌriːz/ n (pl **caries**) decay of bones or teeth.

carillon /ˈkærələn/ or /-ɒn/ n a chime of bells diatonically tuned and played by hand or machinery; a simple air adapted for playing on a set of bells.

carina /kəˈriːnə/ n (pl **carinae, carinas**) a keel; the two lower petals of a papilionaceous flower (as the furze) partially joined; the keel of the breastbone of birds.

carinate /ˈkærɪˌneɪt/, **carinated** /-ɪd/ adj shaped like a keel.

caring /ˈkerɪŋ/ adj compassionate; of or dealing with people's welfare, usu professionally.

carious /ˈkeriəs/ adj affected with caries; decayed.

carjacking /ˈkarˌdʒækɪŋ/ n the violent hijacking and theft of a car, possibly involving the abduction or kidnapping of the driver or passenger.

carling /ˈkarlɪŋ/ n a ship's timber running fore and aft from one transverse deck beam to another, serving as a foundation for the planks of the deck.

Carlovingian /ˌkarləvɪnjiən/ see **Carolingian**.

carmagnole /ˈkarmənˌjoːl/ n a popular song and dance of the time of the French Revolution; a costume adapted by the revolutionists; a bombastic report from the French armies during the Revolution.

Carmelite /ˈkarməˌlaɪt/ n a member of a mendicant order founded on Mount Carmel in the 12th century, a white friar; a variety of pear; a kind of fine woollen cloth. • adj of or belonging to the order of Carmelites.

carminative /karˈmɪnətɪv/ or /ˈkar-/ n a medicine that expels wind and relieves colic and flatulence. • adj expelling wind.

carmine /ˈkarmaɪn/ n a rich crimson pigment; the essential colouring principle of cochineal.

carnage /ˈkarnɪdʒ/ n great slaughter.

carnal /ˈkarnəl/ adj of the flesh; sexual; sensual; worldly.—**carnality** n.—**carnally** adv.

carnal knowledge n sexual intercourse.

carnation /karˈneɪʃən/ n a garden flower, the clove pink.

carnelian /karˈniːljən/ see **cornelian**.

carnet /ˈkarneɪ/ n a customs permit or licence, esp for a vehicle; a book of tickets, etc.

carnival /ˈkarnəvəl/ n public festivities and revelry; a travelling fair with sideshows, etc.

carnivore /ˈkarnəˌvor/ n a flesh-eating mammal.

carnivorous /karˈnɪvərəs/ adj (animals) feeding on flesh; (plants) able to trap and digest insects.

carob /ˈkerəb/ or /ˈkær-/ n an edible, sugary pod of a Mediterranean tree.

carol /ˈkerəl/ or /ˈkæ-/ n a joyful song or hymn; a Christmas hymn. • vi (**carolling, carolled** or **caroling, caroled**) to sing carols; to sing with happiness.

Caroline /ˈkerəlaɪn/ or /ˈkerə/, **Carolean** /-liːən/ adj belonging to the period of Charles I or Charles II.

Carolingian /ˈkerəˈlɪndʒiən/ or /ˈkærə-/ adj of or pertaining to the medieval Frankish dynasty that once ruled France. • n a member of this dynasty.—also **Carlovingian**.

Carolinian /ˌkerəˈlɪniən/ or /ˈkærə-/ adj of or pertaining to either North or South Carolina

carom /ˈkerəm/ or /ˈkærəm/ n (billiards) a shot in which the cue ball hits two others successively. • vi to make a carom.—also **cannon**.

carotic (artery) /kəˈrɒtɪd/ n one of the two principal arteries, one on either side of the neck, which convey blood from the aorta to the head.—**carotidal** adj.

carousal /kəˈrəzəl/ or /ˈkærə-/ n a feast or festival; a noisy drinking bout or revel.

carouse /kəˈrauz/ vi to drink and have fun.—**carousal** n.—**carouser** n.

carousel /ˈkærəˌsel/ or /ˌkærəˈsel/ n a merry-go-round; a revolving circular platform, as in an airport luggage conveyor.

carp[1] /karp/ vi to find fault, esp continually.

carp[2] n (pl **carp, carps**) a brown and yellow freshwater fish.

carpal /ˈkarpəl/ adj pertaining to the carpus or wrist.

car park n a parking lot.

carpe diem /ˌkarpeɪˈdiːem/ (Latin) seize the day; take advantage of a present opportunity.

carpel /ˈkarpəl/ n a simple pistil, or one of the parts of a compound pistil or ovary of a flower.—**carpellary** adj.

carpellate /-ˌleɪt/ adj having a carpel.

carpenter /ˈkarpəntər/ n a person skilled in woodwork, esp in house building.—**carpentry** n.

carpenter bee n a bee that makes nests in wood.

carpentry /ˈkarpəntri/ n the art of cutting, framing, and joining timber; work done by a carpenter.

carpet /'kɑrpət/ *n* a woven fabric for covering floors; any thick covering. • *vt* to cover with carpet; (*inf*) to issue a reprimand, to have on the carpet to rebuke.

carpetbag /-ˌbæg/ *n* a carrying bag formerly made of carpeting.

carpetbagger /-ˌbægər/ *n* an outsider, *esp* a nonresident who meddles in politics.

carpeting /-ɪŋ/ *n* cloth for carpets; carpets in general.

carpet sweeper *n* a mechanical device for removing dirt, etc, from a carpet.

carphone *n* a cellular telephone fitted in and operated from a car.

carpology /kɑr'pɒlədʒi/ *n* the branch of botany that treats of the structure of fruits in general.—**carpological** *adj*.—**carpologist** *n*.

carpophore /'kɑrpəfɔr/ *n* (*bot*) a slender prolongation of the axis that bears the carpels.

carport /'kɑrpɔrt/ *n* an open-sided shelter for a car extending from the side of a house.

carpus /'kɑrpəs/ *n* (*pl* **carpi**) the bones between the forearm and the hand, forming the wrist in man and the corresponding bones in other animals.

carrack /'kerək/ or /'kæ-/ *n* a large round-built vessel formerly used by the Portuguese and Spaniards in the East Indian and American trade.

carrageen, carragheen /'kerəˌgiːn/ or /'kærə-/ *n* a seaweed very common on the rocks of the Irish coast that, when dried and bleached, is known as Irish moss and is used for blancmanges, soup, etc.—*also* **carageen**.

carrel /'kerəl/ or /'kærəl/ *n* a small study room or cubicle, *esp* in a library.

carriage /'kerɪdʒ/ or /'kærədʒ/ *n* the act of carrying, transport; the cost of this; deportment, bearing; behaviour; a rail coach or compartment; a wheeled coach drawn by horses; a frame with wheels to carry a gun; the moving part of a typewriter.

carriage dog *n* the spotted Dalmatian.

carrick bend /'kerɪk/ or /'kæ-/ *n* (*naut*) a particular kind of knot for splicing two hawsers together.

carrick bitt *n* (*naut*) one of the bitts supporting the windlass.

carrier /'keriər/ or /'kær-/ *n* one who carries or transports goods, *esp* for hire; a device for carrying; a person or animal transmitting an infectious disease without being affected by it; an aircraft carrier; a plastic or paper bag with handles for holding things; a portable seat for a baby, a carrycot.

carrier pigeon *n* a homing pigeon used to carry messages.

carrier wave *n* an electromagnetic wave that can be modulated in frequency, amplitude, etc, to transmit (radio, TV, etc) signals.

carrion /'keriən/ or /'kær-/ *n* the dead putrefying flesh of an animal.

carrion crow *n* the common crow of Europe.

Carronade /ˌkerə'neɪd/ *n* a short cannon of large bore for close range, formerly used in the navy.

carron oil *n* a mixture of linseed oil and lime water used as a liniment for burns.

carrot /'kerət/ or /'kæ-/ *n* a plant grown for its edible, fleshy orange root; an inducement, often illusory.

carroty /'kerəti/ *adj* orange-red in colour.

carry /'keri/ or /'kæ-/ *vb* (**carrying, carried**) *vt* to convey or transport; to support or bear; to involve, have as a result; to hold (oneself); to extend or prolong; to gain by force; to win over; to stock; to be pregnant; (*with* **away**) to delight; to arouse to extreme enthusiasm; to remove violently; (*with* **forward**) (*book-keeping*) to transfer (a total) to the next column, page, etc; (*with* **off**) to cause to die; to remove by force, capture; (*situation*) to handle successfully; (*with* **out**) to perform (a task, etc); to accomplish; (*with* **over**) to carry forward; (*with* **through**) to complete. • *vi* (*with* **away**) to be filled with joy or emotion; (*with* **on**) to persevere; to conduct a business, etc; (*inf*) to have an affair; (*inf*) to cause a fuss; (*with* **through**) to enable to survive; to persist.

carryall /'kerɪɒl/ or /'kæri-/ *n* an overnight or holdall bag.

carrycot /'kerikɒt/ or /'kæri-/ *n* a baby carrier, a portable cot.

carrying place *n* ✤ (*Cdn*) a portage.

carry-out /-ɐʊt/ *n* food or drink sold by a restaurant but consumed elsewhere.—*also adj*.

carsick /'kɑrsɪk/ *adj* ill or queasy from the motion of a moving vehicle.—**carsickness** *n*.

cart /kɑrt/ *n* a two-wheeled vehicle drawn by horses; any small vehicle for carrying loads. • *vt* to carry in a cart; (*inf*) to transport with effort.

cartage /'kɑrtɪdʒ/ *n* conveyance in a cart; the charge made for this.

carte blanche /'kɑrt'blɑnʃ/, *Fr.* /kɑrt'blɑ̃ʃ/ *n* (*pl* **cartes blanches**) full authority to act as one thinks best.

cartel /kɑr'tel/ *n* an association of business firms to coordinate production, prices, etc to avoid competition and maximize profits; a union of political parties to achieve common aims.

Cartesian /kɑr'tiːʒən/ or /-iːziən/ *adj* pertaining to the French philosopher René Descartes (1596–1650) or his philosophy. • *n* a follower of Descartes or his philosophy.

Carthaginian /ˌkɑrθə'dʒɪniən/ *adj* pertaining to ancient Carthage, a city of North Africa.

Carthusian /kɑr'θjuːziən/ or /-'θuːʒən/ *n* one of an order of monks founded (1086) by St Bruno in the Grande Chartreuse, France.

cartilage /'kɑrtəlɪdʒ/ *n* tough, elastic tissue attached to the bones of animals; gristle.—**cartilaginous** *adj*.

cartload /'kɑrtloːd/ *n* the amount a cart will hold.

cartogram /'kɑrtəˌgræm/ *n* a map showing statistical information in diagrammatic form.

cartography /kɑr'tɒgrəfi/ *n* the drawing and publishing of maps.—**cartographer** *n*.—**cartographic, cartographical** *adj*.

carton /'kɑrtən/ *n* a cardboard box or container.

cartoon /kɑr'tuːn/ *n* a humorous picture dealing with current events; a comic strip; an animated cartoon; a full-size preparatory sketch for reproduction on a fresco, etc.—**cartoonist** *n*.

cartouche, cartouch /kɑr'tuːʃ/ *n* a cartridge; a canvas cartridge case; an ornament in the form of an unrolled scroll; on Egyptian monuments, etc, an oval figure containing the name or title of a sovereign or deity.

cartridge /'kɑrtrɪdʒ/ *n* the case that contains the explosive charge and bullet in a gun or rifle; a sealed case of film for a camera; the device containing the stylus on the end of the pick-up arm of a record player.

cartridge belt *n* a belt with loops for holding spare cartridges.

cartridge clip *n* a detachable container for cartridges in an automatic firearm.

cartulary /'kɑrtʃəˌleri/ *n* (*pl* **cartularies**) a collection or register of charters.—*also* **chartulary**.

cartwheel /'kɑrtwiːl/ *n* an acrobatic handspring in which the body revolves with the weight on each hand in turn and the legs spread like the spokes of a wheel.

caruncle /'kærˌəŋkəl/ or /kə'rʌŋkəl/ *n* a small fleshy excrescence on a bird's head, as the comb or wattle of a fowl; an appendage surrounding the hilum of a seed.—**caruncular, caruncutate** *adj*.

carve /kɑrv/ *vt* to shape by cutting; to adorn with designs; to cut up (meat, etc); (*with* **up**) to cut into pieces or shares; (*sl*) to share out illegal proceeds; to slash someone with a knife or razor.

carvel /'kɑrvəl/ *see* **caravel**.

carvel-built /-ˌbɪlt/ *adj* (*vessel*) with the outer boards or plates meeting flush, not overlapping.

carving /-ɪŋ/ *n* a figure or design carved from wood, stone, etc; the act of carving.

caryatid /ˌkæˌriætɪd/ *n* (*pl* **caryatids, caryatides**) a figure of a woman in long robes supporting an entablature.—**caryatic, caryatidic, caryatidal, caryatidean** *adj*.

caryophyllaceous /ˌkæriə'fɪleɪʃəs/ *adj* (*flowers*) belonging to the pink family.

caryopsis /ˌkær'ɪɒpsɪs/ *n* (*pl* **caryopses, caryopsides**) a small dry fruit with the thin pericarp adherent to the seed, as in wheat, etc.

CAS *abbr* ✤ (*Cdn*) = Children's Aid Society.

casaba /kə'sɒbə/ *n* a variety of winter melon with a yellow rind and sweet flesh.—*also* **cassaba**.

Casanova /ˌkæsə'noːvə/ or /ˌkæsə-/ *n* a man of amorous reputation.

cascade /kæs'keɪd/ *n* a small, steep waterfall; a shower, as of sparks, etc. • *vti* to fall in a cascade.

cascara /kæs'kɑrə/ *n* Californian bark used as an aperient; a bark canoe.

cascarilla /ˌkæskə'rɪlə/ *n* the bark of a West Indian shrub, possessing aromatic and bitter properties; the shrub itself, from which is obtained a white bitter crystalline substance, cascarillin.

case¹ /keɪs/ *n* a covering; a suitcase; its contents; the binding covering a book.

case² *n* an instance; a state of affairs; a condition, circumstance; a lawsuit; an argument for one side; (*sl*) a character; a person of a specific type; (*med*) a patient under treatment; (*gram*) the relationship between nouns, pronouns and adjectives in a sentence; **in case** in order to prevent, lest.

case-harden /'keɪsˌhɑːrdən/ vt to make the surface (of iron or steel) harder than the interior.

case-hardened /-dənd/ adj with a hard surface; made callous.

case history n a record of a person's medical background, etc.

casein /'keɪsiːn/ or /'keɪsiːɪn/ n a protein in the curd matter of milk.

case knife n a sheath knife.

case law n law as settled by precedent.

casemate /'keɪsmeɪt/ n a bomb-proof vault or battery in a fortification; an armoured enclosure for a gun in a warship; a hollow moulding.

casement /'keɪsmənt/ n a window or its frame with a side hinge for opening.

caseous /'keɪsiəs/ adj like cheese, cheesy.

casern, caserne /kə'zərn/ n a lodging or barrack for soldiers in a garrison town.

case study n an analysis arrived at from studying more than one case history.

casework /'keɪsˌwɜːrk/ n social work based on the close monitoring of individuals or families.—**caseworker** n.

cash[1] /kæʃ/ n money in coins or notes; immediate payment, as opposed to that by cheque or on credit; ✦ (Cdn) a cash register. • vt to give or get cash for; (with in) to exchange something for money; (inf) to gain an advantage or seize an opportunity to profit from; (sl) to die. • vi (with in) to exploit for profit; to take advantage of.—**cashable** adj.

cash[2] n (pl **cash**) the name of various Eastern coins of low value.

cash and carry n, adj (a policy of) selling for cash without delivery of goods.

cash-book n a book in which a register is kept of money received or paid out.

cash crop n a crop grown for market not for consumption.

cashew /'kæʃuː/ or /kæ'ʃuː/ n the small, edible nut of a tropical tree.

cash flow n money which is paid into and out of a business during its operations.

cashier[1] /kæ'ʃiːr/ n a person in charge of the paying and receiving of money in a bank, shop, etc.

cashier[2] vt to dismiss (an officer) from military service; to discharge.

cashmere /'kæʃˌmiːr/ n a fine wool from Kashmir goats; a material made from this.

cash on delivery n delivery to be paid for to a postman or carrier.

cash register n an automatic or electronic machine that shows and records the amount placed in it.

casimere see **cassimere**.

casing /'keɪsɪŋ/ n any protective or outer covering; the material for this.

casino /kə'siːnoː/ n (pl **casinos**) a room or building where gambling takes place.

cask /kæsk/ n a barrel of any size, esp one for liquids; its contents.

casket /'kæskɪt/ n a small box or chest for jewels, etc; a coffin.

casque /kæsk/ n (poet) a helmet.

cassaba /kə'sɒbə/ see **casaba**.

cassava /kə'sɒvə/ n a plant of tropical America and Africa cultivated for its tuberous roots, which yield a nutritious starch from which cassava bread and tapioca are made.

casse-croûte /kæs'kruːt/ n ✦ (Cdn) in Quebec, a small place of business that sells snacks.

casserole /'kæsəˌroːl/ n a covered dish for cooking and serving; the food so cooked and served. • vt to cook in a casserole.

cassette /kə'set/ n a case containing magnetic tape or film for loading into a tape recorder or camera.

cassia /'kæsiə/ or /'kæʃə/ n one of several tropical leguminous plants, the leaves of several species of which constitute the drug senna.

cassimere /'kæsəˌmiːr/ n a thin twilled woollen cloth used for men's garments.—also **casimere**.

cassiterite /kə'sɪtəˌraɪt/ n a native tin dioxide; the principal ore of tin.

cassock /'kæsək/ n a long close-fitting black garment worn by certain clergy and by choristers.

cassowary /'kæsəˌweri/ n (pl **cassowaries**) a large running bird resembling the ostrich, inhabiting Australia and New Guinea.

cast /kæst/ vb (**casting, cast**) vt to throw or fling to throw off or shed; to record; to direct; to shape in a mould; to calculate; to select actors, etc for a play; to throw a fishing line into the water. • vi to throw, hurl; (with **off**) to untie a ship from its moorings; (knitting) to loop off stitches from a needle without letting them unravel; (with **on**) to loop the first row of stitches onto a needle. • n act of casting; a throw; a plaster form for immobilizing an injured limb; a mould for casting; type or quantity; a tinge of colour; the actors assigned roles in a play; the set of actors; a slight squint in the eye.

castanets /ˌkæstə'nets/ npl hollow shell-shaped pieces of wood held between the fingers and rattled together, esp to accompany Spanish dancing.

castaway /'kæstəweɪ/ adj shipwrecked; discarded. • n a shipwrecked person.

cast down adj depressed.

caste /kæst/ n any of the Hindu hereditary social classes; an exclusive social group.

castellan /'kæstələn/ n the governor of a castle.

castellated /-leɪtəd/ adj having turrets and battlements, as a castle.

caster /'kæstər/ see **castor**.

castigate /'kæstɪˌgeɪt/ vt to chastise; to punish; to correct.—**castigation** n.

casting vote /'kæstɪŋ/ n the deciding vote used by the chairman of a meeting when the votes on each side are equal.

cast iron /'kæst'aɪrən/ n an iron-carbon alloy melted and run into moulds.

cast-iron adj made of cast iron; untiring; rigid, unadaptable.

castle /'kæsəl/ n a fortified building; a chess piece.—also **rook**.

castoff /'kæstɒf/ n a rejected item; a rough estimate of the number of pages of a finished book, etc.

cast-off adj laid aside or rejected.—**castoff** n.

castor /'kæstər/ n a small container with a perforated top for sprinkling salt, sugar, etc; a small swivelled wheel on a table leg, etc.—also **caster**.

castor oil /'kæstər/ n a vegetable oil used as a cathartic and lubricant.

castrate /'kæstreɪt/ vt to remove the testicles of, to geld.—**castration** n.—**castrator** n.

castrato /kæs'trɒtoː/ n (pl **castrati, castratos**) a male castrated in childhood to prevent a change of voice at the age of puberty; an artificial male soprano.

casual /'kæʒʊəl/ or /'kæʒjʊəl/ adj accidental, chance; unplanned; occasional; careless, offhand; unmethodical; informal. • n someone who works occasionally. (pl) informal or leisure clothing, shoes.—**casually** adv.—**casualness** n.

casualty /'kæʒʊəlti/ n (pl **casualties**) a person injured or killed in a war or in an accident; something damaged or destroyed.

casuarina /ˌkæsjuˈriːnə/ n a tree of Australia and southeast Asia having jointed branches.

casuist /'kæʒuːɪst/ or /'kæʒuːɪst/ n one who studies or resolves cases of conscience; one skilled in casuistry.—**casuistic, casuistical** adj.—**casuistically** adv.

casuistry /'kæʒuːɪstri/ n (pl **casuistries**) the study or application of rules of right and wrong; sophistical or equivocal reasoning, esp on moral matters.

casus belli /'kæsəs'beli/ or /ˌkeɪsəs-/ n (pl **casus belli**) an act or occurrence justifying war.

CAT /kæt/ (acronym) n computerized axial tomography.—also **computer-aided** or **computer-assisted tomography**; the production of detailed three-dimensional images from scans of cross-sections of internal organs (**CAT scans**) using a computer-controlled X-ray machine (**CAT scanner**).

cat /kæt/ n a small, domesticated feline mammal kept as a pet; a wild animal related to this; lions, tigers, etc.—also **big cat**; (inf) a spiteful woman; (sl) a man.

cata- /'kætə/ prefix down; wrongly; thoroughly.

catabolism /kə'tæbəˌlɪzəm/ n a downward series of changes by which complex bodies are broken down into simpler forms.—**catabolic** adj.—**catabolically** adv.

catabolize /-aɪz/ vti to subject to or undergo catabolism.

catachresis /ˌkætə'kriːsɪs/ n (pl **catachreses**) misapplication of words; formation of words on a false analogy.—**catachrestic** adj.—**catachrestically** adv.

cataclysm /'kætəˌklɪzəm/ n a violent disturbance or disaster.—**cataclysmic** adj.

catacomb /'kætəˌkoːm/ n (usu pl) an underground burial place.

catadromous /kə'tædrəməs/ adj going down to the sea to spawn.

catafalque /'kætəˌfɒlk/ n a temporary structure erected, usu in a church, to support the coffin on the occasion of a lying in state.

Catalan /ˈkætəˌlæn/ *adj* of or pertaining to Catalonia, a province of Spain, or to its inhabitants or language. • *n* an inhabitant of Catalonia; the language of Catalonia.

catalectic /ˌkætəˌlɛktɪk/ *adj* (*poetry*) lacking a syllable in the last foot.

catalepsy /ˈkætəˌlɛpsi/ *n* (*pl* catalepsies) a state of temporary rigidity and unconsciousness.—**cataleptic** *adj*.

catalogue, catalog /ˈkætəˌlɒg/ *n* a list of books, names, etc in systematic order. • *vti* to list, to make a catalogue of.—**cataloger, cataloguer** *n*.

catalogue raisonné /ˈkætəˌlɒgˈreɪzɒˌneɪ/, *Fr.* /kataˈlɔgʀɛzɔˈneɪ/ *n* a catalogue of books, paintings, etc, classed according to their subjects.

catalpa /kəˈtælpə/ *n* an American tree with trumpet-shaped flowers.

catalyse /ˈkætəˌlaɪz/ *vt* to accelerate or retard (a chemical reaction) by catalysis.—**catalyser** *n*.

catalysis /kəˈtælɪsɪs/ *n* (*pl* catalyses) the acceleration or retardation of a chemical reaction by the action of a catalyst.—**catalytic** *adj*.

catalyst /ˈkætəlɪst/ *n* a substance which accelerates or retards a chemical reaction without itself undergoing any permanent chemical change; a person or thing which produces change.

catalytic converter *n* a filter device in vehicles to reduce pollution from exhaust produced by combustion, eg carbon monoxide, nitrogen oxide, etc.

catamaran /ˌkætəməˈræn/ *n* a (sailing) boat with twin hulls; a raft of logs.

catamenia /ˌkætəˈmiːniə/ *n* menstruation.—**catamenial** *adj*.

catamite /ˈkætəmaɪt/ *n* a boy kept by a sodomite.

catamount /ˈkætəmaunt/, **catamountain** /-eɪn/ *n* the wild cat; the puma, cougar, or mountain lion.

cataplasm /ˌkætəˌplæzəm/ *n* a poultice.

cataplexy /ˈkætəˌplɛksi/ *n* (*pl* cataplexies) a sudden shock to the nerves causing paralysis.

catapult /ˈkætəpʊlt/ or /-pɛlt/ *n* a slingshot; a device for launching aircraft from the deck of an aircraft carrier. • *vt* to shoot forwards as from a catapult.

cataract /ˈkætəˌrækt/ *n* a waterfall, *esp* a large sheet one; a disease of the eye causing dimming of the lens and loss of vision.

catarrh /kəˈtɑr/ *n* inflammation of a mucous membrane, *esp* in the nose and throat, causing a flow of mucus.—**catarrhal** *adj*.

catarrhine /ˈkætəˌraɪn/ *adj* of or pertaining to a group of monkeys and apes of the Old World, which have the nostrils close together and pointing downwards.

catastrophe /kəˈtæstrefi/ *n* a great disaster.—**catastrophic** *adj*.—**catastrophically** *adv*.

catastrophize /-aɪz/ *vt* to envisage a situation as being worse than it is.—*also* **awfulize**.

catatonia /ˌkætəˈtɒniə/ *n* a form of schizophrenia in which a trance-like state is punctuated by periods of hyperactivity.—**catatonic** *adj*.

Catawba /kəˈtɒbə/ *n* (*pl* Catawba, Catawbas) a member of a North American Indian people formerly of North and South Carolina; a light red variety of American grape; a light wine made from this grape.

catbird /ˈkætbərd/ *n* a kind of American thrush.

catboat /-boːt/ *n* a small boat with one sail on a single mast near the bows.

cat burglar *n* a burglar who enters by climbing.

catcall /-ˌkɒl/ *n* a shrill whistle or cry used to express disapproval. • *vt* to express disapproval by a catcall.

catch /kætʃ/ *vb* (**catching, caught**) *vt* to take hold of, to grasp; to capture; to ensnare or trap; to be on time for; to detect; to apprehend; to become infected with (a disease); to attract (the eye); (*inf*) to see, hear, etc; to grasp (a meaning); (*with* **out**) (*inf*) to detect (a person) in a mistake; (*cricket*) to catch a ball hit by a batsman before it touches the ground, making him "out". • *vi* to become entangled; to begin to burn; (*with* **on**) (*inf*) to become popular; to understand; (*with* **up**) to reach or come level with (eg a person ahead); to make up for lost time, deal with a backlog. • *n* the act of catching; the amount or number caught; a device for fastening; someone worth catching; a hidden difficulty.

catch-all /ˈkætʃˌɒl/ *adj*, *n* (something) intended to cover all eventualities.

catcher /-ər/ *n* (*baseball*) the player who stands behind the batter to catch the ball.

catching /-ɪŋ/ *adj* infectious; attractive.

catchment /-mənt/ *n* the collecting or the drainage of water.

catchment area *n* the area from which a body of water is fed, eg a river or reservoir; a geographic area served by a particular institution.

catchpenny /-ˌpeni/ *n* (*pl* catchpennies) an article of little value got up attractively to effect a quick sale.

catch phrase /-freɪz/ *n* a well-known phrase or slogan, *esp* one associated with a particular group or person.

catchpole /-ˌpoːl/ *n* a sheriff's officer; a constable in medieval England.

catch-22 /-twɛntiˈtuː/ *n* a predicament from which a victim is powerless to escape due to conditions beyond his or her control.

catchup /-əp/ *see* **ketchup**.

catchweight /-ˌweɪt/ *n* a weight left to the choice of an owner of a horse. • *adv* without being handicapped.

catchword /-wərd/ *n* a guide word; a word or expression, briefly popular, representative of a person or point of view; a cue in the theatre.

catchy /ˈkætʃi/ *adj* (**catchier, catchiest**) easily remembered, as a tune.—**catchiness** *n*.

catechetic /ˌkætəˈkɛtɪk/, **catechetical** /-əl/ *adj* instructing orally; proceeding by question and answer; of catechism.—**catechetically** *adv*.

catechin /ˈkætətʃɪn/ or /-kɪn/ *n* a tannic acid extracted from catechu.

catechism /ˈkætəˌkɪzəm/ *n* a simple summary of the principles of religion in question and answer form, used for instruction; continuous questioning.—**catechismal** *adj*.

catechize /ˈkætəˌkaɪz/ *vt* to instruct by question and answer.—**catechization** *n*.—**catechist, catechizer** *n*.

catechu /ˈkætətʃuː/ *n* a brown astringent substance obtained from tropical plants and used in the arts and as a medicine.—*also* **cachou, cutch**.

catechumen /ˌkætəˈkjuːmən/ *n* one who is under religious instruction prior to receiving baptism; a beginner in the first principles of knowledge.

categorical /ˌkætəˈgɒrɪkəl/ or /-gɒr-/ *adj* unconditional, absolute; positive, explicit.—**categorically** *adv*.

categorical imperative *n* (*philos*) in Kantian ethics, the absolute and unconditional command of moral law.

categorize /ˈkætəgəˌraɪz/ *vt* to place in a category.—**categorization** *n*.

category /ˈkætəgəri/ *n* (*pl* categories) a class or division of things.

catena /kəˈtiːnə/ *n* (*pl* catenae, catenas) a series of notions; things connected with each other like the links of a chain; a systematic arrangement of selections from authors to illustrate a doctrine.

catenary /ˈkætəˌneri/ *n* (*pl* catenaries) a curve formed by a hanging chain. • *adj* of or resembling a chain.—*also* **catenarian**.

catenate /ˈkætəneɪt/ *vt* (*biol*) to link together.—**catenation** *n*.

catenulate /kəˈtenjuːleɪt/ *adj* (*bot*) consisting of little links.

cater /ˈkeɪtər/ *vi* (*with* **for** *or* **to**) to provide with what is needed or desired, *esp* food and service, as for parties.—**caterer** *n*.

cateran /ˈkætərən/ *n* a kern; a Highland or Irish irregular soldier; a Highland freebooter.

caterpillar /ˈkætərˌpɪlər/ *n* the worm-like larvae of a butterfly or moth; the ribbed band in place of wheels on a heavy vehicle; a vehicle (eg tank, tractor) equipped with such tracks.

caterwaul /-ˌwɒl/ *vi* to make a howling noise like a cat. • *n* a cry.

catfish /ˈkætfɪʃ/ *n* (*pl* catfish, catfishes) a large, *usu* freshwater, fish with whisker-like feelers around the mouth.

catgut /ˈkætgʌt/ *n* a strong cord made from animal intestines, used for the strings of musical instruments, sports rackets, and surgical ligatures.

catharsis /kəˈθɑrsɪs/ *n* (*pl* catharses) emotional relief given by art, *esp* tragedy; (*med*) purgation; (*psychoanal*) relief obtained by the uncovering of buried repressions, etc.

cathartic /-tɪk/ *adj* bringing about catharsis; purgative. • *n* a purgative medicine.—**cathartically** *adv*.

cathead /ˈkæthɛd/ *n* a beam projecting from a ship's bows to which the anchor is secured.

cathedra /ˈkæθiːdrə/ or /kəˈθiːdrə/ *n* (*pl* cathedrae) a bishop's throne in the cathedral of his diocese; an official or professional chair.

cathedral /kəˈθiːdrəl/ *n* the chief church of a diocese. • *adj* having or belonging to a cathedral.

Catherine wheel /ˈkæθərɪn/ *n* a rotating firework.—*also* **pinwheel**.

catheter /'kæθətər/ *n* a flexible tube inserted into the bladder for drawing off urine.

catheterize /-ˌraɪz/ *vt* to insert a catheter into.—**catheterization** *n*.

cathode /'kæθoːd/ *n* (*elect*) the negative terminal, the electrode by which current leaves.—**cathodal** *adj*.—**cathodic, cathodical** *adj*.

cathode rays /-reɪz/ *n* (one of the electrons in) a stream of electrons emitted by a cathode in a vacuum tube.

cathode-ray tube *n* a vacuum tube in which electron beams are directed onto a fluorescent screen to produce luminous images, as used in television sets.

Catholic /'kæθlɪk/ or /-əl-/ *n* a member of the Roman Catholic Church. • *adj* relating to the Roman Catholic Church; embracing the whole body of Christians.—**Catholicism** *n*.

catholic /'kæθlɪk/ or /-əl-/ *adj* universal, all-embracing; broad-minded, liberal; general, not exclusive.

Catholic Epistles *npl* the Epistles of the Apostles addressed to believers generally, ie James 1 and 2, Peter 1, 2 and 3, John, and Jude.

Catholicism /kəˈθɒlɪˌsɪzəm/ *n* the belief of, or adherence to, the Catholic Church or faith, *esp* to that of the Roman Catholic Church.

catholicity /ˌkæθəˈlɪsɪti/ *n* the quality of being catholic; universality, comprehensiveness; accordance with Catholic, *esp* Roman Catholic, church doctrine.

catholicize /kəˈθɒlɪˌsaɪz/ *vt* to convert to the Roman Catholic Church.—**catholicization** *n*.

catholicon /-ɪˌkɒn/ or /-ɪkən/ *n* a universal remedy a panacea.

cathouse /'kætˌhʊs/ *n* a brothel.

cation /'kætˌaɪən/ or /-aɪɒn/ *n* a positively charged ion.—**cationic** *adj*.

catkin /'kætkɪn/ *n* a hanging spike of small flowers, eg on birch, willow and hazel trees.

cat-like /-ˌlaɪk/ *adj* like a cat; stealthy noiseless.

catmint /-ˌmɪnt/, **catnip** /-ˌnɪp/ *n* a strongly-scented plant attractive to cats.

catnap /-ˌnæp/ *n* a short, light or intermittent sleep, a snooze, a doze.—*also vi* (**catnapping, catnapped**).

cat-o'-nine-tails /ˌkætəˈnaɪnˌteɪlz/ *n* (*pl* **cat-o'-nine-tails**) a whip with nine lashes of knotted cord, formerly used as a punishment in the army and navy.

catoptric /kəˈtɒpˌtrɪk/, **catoptrical** /-əl/ *adj* of or pertaining to mirrors or reflected light.

Cat scan, Cat scanner *see* **CAT**.

cat's cradle *n* a game of making designs with string looped over the fingers.

cat's-eye /'kætsˌaɪ/ *n* a hard semi-transparent variety of quartz.

cat's-paw /'kætsˌpɒ/ *n* a person used as a tool by another, a dupe; (*naut*) a light breeze that slightly ripples the surface of the water.

catsup /'kætsəp/ *see* **ketchup**.

cattery /'kætəri/ *n* (*pl* **catteries**) a place for boarding or breeding cats.

cattle /'kætəl/ *npl* domesticated bovine mammals such as bulls and cows.

cattle-grid /-grɪd/ *n* a metal grid over a ditch allowing the passage of people and vehicles, but not cattle, sheep, etc.

cattleman /-mən/ or /-ˌmæn/ *n* (*pl* **cattlemen**) one who tends or drives cattle; a breeder of cattle.

cattle prod /-prɒd/ *n* an electrified prod for driving cattle.

catty[1] /'kæti/ *adj* (**cattier, cattiest**) (*inf*) spiteful, mean.—**cattily** *adv*.—**cattiness** *n*.

catty[2] *n* (*pl* **catties**) an East Indian weight equal to one and a third pounds; a name applied to a Chinese kin or pound; a Siamese coin.

catwalk /'kætˌwɒk/ *n* a narrow, raised pathway on a stage, bridge, etc; fashion modelling (*with* **the**).

Caucasian /kɒˈkeɪʒən/ *adj* of the light-skinned racial group of humankind; of or relating to the Caucasus Mountains. • *n* a Caucasian person.—**Caucasoid** *adj*.

Caucasus /'kɒkəsəs/ *n* a mountain range in the southwest USSR (*with* **the**).—*also* **Caucasus Mountains**.

caucus /'kɒkəs/ *n* (*pl* **caucuses**) a private meeting of leaders of a political party or faction, *usu* to plan strategy.

caudal /'kɒdəl/ *adj* of or pertaining to a tail.—**caudally** *adv*.

caudate /'kɒdeɪt/, **caudated** /-ɪd/ *adj* having a tail; having a tail-like appendage.

caudex /'kɒdɛks/ *n* (*pl* **caudices, caudexes**) the main trunk or axis of a plant.

caudle /'kɒdəl/ *n* a warm drink made of wine or ale, spiced or sugared, and mixed with bread, eggs, etc.

caught /kɒt/ *see* **catch**.

caul /kɒl/ *n* the membrane covering a foetus; part of this covering the head of some infants at birth.

cauldron /'kɒldrən/ *n* a large kettle or boiling pot; a state of violent agitation.—*also* **caldron**.

caulescent /kɒˈlesənt/ *adj* having a true stem or stalk.

caulicle /'kɒlɪkəl/ *n* a small or rudimentary stem.

cauliflower /'kɒlɪflaʊr/ *n* a kind of cabbage with an edible white flower-head used as a vegetable.

cauliflower ear *n* a thickening condition of the ear, common to boxers, caused by repeated blows.

cauline /'kɒˌlaɪn/ *adj* of, on or belonging to a stem.

caulk /kɒk/ *vt* to make (a boat) watertight by stopping up the seams with pitch.—*also* **calk.**—**caulker, calker** *n*.

causal /'kɒzəl/ *adj* forming or being a cause; involving, expressing or implying a cause.—**causally** *adv*.

causality /kɒˈzælɪti/ *n* (*pl* **causalities**) the relationship between cause and effect.

causation /-ˈzeɪʃən/ *n* causality; the act of causing something to happen.—**causational** *adj*.

causative /'kɒzəˌtɪv/ *adj* that causes; effective as a cause; expressing causation.

cause /kɒz/ *n* that which produces an effect; reason, motive, purpose, justification; a principle for which people strive; a lawsuit. • *vt* to bring about, to effect; to make (to do something).—**causer** *n*.

cause célèbre /'kɒzsəˈleb/ or /ˌkoːz-/, /seɪ-/, /-ˈlebrə/, *Fr.* /koːzeɪˈleˌbʀ/ *n* (*pl* **causes célèbres**) a famous lawsuit, trial or celebrated issue.

causeless /'kɒzləs/ *adj* without cause; groundless.

causerie /ˌkoːzəˈriː/ *n* a discursive conversational article; an informal chat.

causeway /'kɒzˌweɪ/ *n* a raised road across wet ground or water.

caustic /'kɒstɪk/ *adj* burning tissue, etc by chemical action; corrosive; sarcastic, cutting. • *n* a caustic substance.—**caustically** *adv*.—**causticness, causticity** *n*.

caustic potash *n* potassium hydroxide, a white substance acting as a powerful bleach, much used in medicine and manufacturing.

caustic soda *n* sodium hydroxide, a white solid substance, largely used in soap making.

cauterize /'kɒtərˌaɪz/ *vt* to burn with a caustic substance or a hot iron so as to destroy dead tissue, stop bleeding, etc; to deaden.—**cauterization** *n*.

cautery /'kɒtəri/ *n* (*pl* **cauteries**) a burning or searing; an instrument or drug used for such a purpose.

caution /'kɒʃən/ *n* care for safety, prudence; a warning, *esp* a formal one, to a suspect or accused person. • *vt* to warn (against); to admonish.

cautionary /-ˌɛri/ *adj* of a warning nature.

cautious /'kɒʃəs/ *adj* careful, circumspect.—**cautiously** *adv*.—**cautiousness** *n*.

cavalcade /ˌkævəlˈkeɪd/ *n* a procession of riders on horseback; a dramatic sequence or procession.

cavalier /ˌkævəˈliːr/ *adj* free and easy, careless; offhand, brusque. • *n* a horseman; a lady's escort; (*with cap*) a royalist in the English Civil War.—**cavalierly** *adv*.

cavalry /'kævəlri/ *n* (*pl* **cavalries**) combat troops originally mounted on horseback.

cavatina /ˌkævəˈtiːnə/ *n* (*pl* **cavatine**) a short simple melody.

cave /keɪv/ *n* a hollow place inside the earth open to the surface. • *vti* (*with* **in**) to collapse or make collapse; (*inf*) to yield, submit.—**cave-in** *n*.

caveat /'keɪvɪˌæt/ *n* (*law*) a process to suspend proceedings; a warning.

caveat emptor /-ˈemptɔr/ (*Latin*) let the buyer beware.

cavefish *n* (*pl* **cavefish, cavefishes**) a fish belonging to the family Amblyopsidae, species of which inhabit cave streams of the US.

caveman /'keɪvˌmæn/ *n* (*pl* **cavemen**) a prehistoric cave dweller; (*inf*) a person who acts in a primitive or crude manner.

cavern /'kævərn/ *n* a large cave.—**cavernous** *adj*.

cavetto /kəˈvetoː/ *n* (*pl* **cavetti**) (*archit*) a round concave moulding.

caviar, caviare /'kævɪˌɑr/ *n* salted roe of the sturgeon or other large fish.

cavil /'kævəl/ *vi* (**cavilling, cavilled** *or* **caviling, caviled**) to make trifling objections, to find fault. • *n* a trifling objection.—**caviller** *n*.

caving /'keɪvɪŋ/ *n* the sport of exploring caves.—**caver** *n*.

cavity /'kævɪti/ *n* (*pl* **cavities**) a hole; a hollow place, *esp* in a tooth.

cavort /kə'vɔrt/ *vi* to frolic, prance.

cavy /'keɪvi/ *n* (*pl* **cavies**) one of several kinds of small rodent including the guinea pig.

caw /kɒ/ *n* the cry of the crow, rook, or raven. • *vi* to utter this cry.

CAW *abbr* ✤ = Canadian Auto Workers.

cay /keɪ/ *n* a small low island.

cayenne /kaɪ'ɛn/, **cayenne pepper** *n* a hot red pepper made from capsicum.

cayman /'keɪmən/ *see* **caiman**.

Cayuse /kaɪ'uːs/ or /keɪ-/ *n* (*pl* **Cayuse, Cayuses**) a member of an American Indian tribe of Oregon and Washington; their language.

CB *abbr* = Citizens' Band; ✤ Cape Breton (Island).

CBC *abbr* ✤ = Canadian Broadcasting Corporation.

CC *abbr* ✤ = Companion of the Order of Canada.

CD *abbr* = compact disc; corps diplomatique.

Cd (*chem symbol*) = cadmium.

cd *abbr* = candela.

CDIC *abbr* ✤ = Canada Deposit Insurance Corporation.

Cdn. *abbr* ✤ = Canadian.

CD-ROM /'siː'diː'rɒm/ *abbr* = compact disc read only memory: a CD used for distributing text and images in electronic publishing, for computer software, and for permanent storage of computer data.

CDV *abbr* = CD-video; compact video disc.

Ce (*chem symbol*) = cerium.

cease /siːs/ *vti* to stop, to come to an end; to discontinue.

ceasefire /'siːsfaɪr/ *n* a period of truce in a war, uprising, etc.

ceaseless /-ləs/ *adj* without ceasing; incessant.—**ceaselessly** *adv*.

cecum /'siːkəm/ *see* **caecum**.

cedar /'siːdər/ *n* a large coniferous evergreen tree; its wood.—**cedarwood** *n*.

cede /siːd/ *vt* to yield to another, give up, *esp* by treaty; to assign or transfer the title of.—**ceder** *n*.

cedilla /sə'dɪlə/ *n* a character written under a c in certain languages (ç) to indicate that it is pronounced as an (s) not (k).

CEGEP /ˌseɪ'dʒɛp/ *abbr* ✤ = in Quebec, a college that prepares students for university and offers training in professions and trades.

ceil /siːl/ *vt* to overlay or cover the inner surface of a roof; to furnish with a ceiling.

ceiling /'siːlɪŋ/ *n* the inner roof of a room; the lining of this; any upper limit; the highest altitude a particular aircraft can fly.

celadon /'sɛləˌdɒn/ *n* a soft pale sea-green colour; porcelain or fine earthenware of such a colour. • *adj* having the colour of celadon.

celandine /'sɛlənˌdaɪn/ *n* one of several kinds of wild plant with star-shaped yellow flowers.

celebrant /'sɛləbrənt/ *n* one who celebrates, *esp* the principal officiating priest in offering mass or celebrating the Eucharist.

celebrate /'sɛləˌbreɪt/ *vt* to make famous; to praise, extol; to perform with proper rites; to mark with ceremony; to keep (festival).—**celebrant** *n*.

celebrated /-d/ *adj* famous.

celebration /-'breɪʃən/ *n* the act of celebrating; an observance or ceremony to celebrate anything.

celebrity /sə'lɛbrəti/ *n* (*pl* **celebrities**) fame; a famous or well-known person.

celeriac /sə'lɛriˌæk/ *n* a variety of celery with a turnip-like root.

celerity /sə'lɛrɪti/ *n* quickness, dispatch.

celery /'sɛləri/ *n* (*pl* **celeries**) a vegetable with long juicy edible stalks.

celesta, celeste /sə'lɛstə/ *n* a kind of glockenspiel with a keyboard.

celestial /sə'lɛstəl/ *adj* in or of the sky; heavenly; divine.—**celestially** *adv*.

celestite /'sɛləsˌtaɪt/ *n* native strontium sulphate.

celiac /'siːliˌæk/ *see* **coeliac**.

celibacy /'sɛlɪbəsi/ *n* (*pl* **celibacies**) the unmarried state; complete sexual abstinence.

celibate /'sɛlɪbət/ *n* a person who remains unmarried, *esp* one who has taken religious vows; a person who abstains from sexual intercourse.—*also adj*.

cell /sɛl/ *n* a small room for one in a prison or monastery; a small cavity as in a honeycomb; a device that converts chemical energy into electricity; a microscopic unit of living matter; a small group of people bound by common aims within an organization or political party.—**cellular** *adj*.

cellar /'sɛlər/ *n* a basement; a stock of wines.

cellarage /'sɛlərədʒ/ *n* cellars collectively; the space occupied by cellars; a charge for storage in cellars.

cellarer /-ər/ *n* an official in a monastery who superintends the cellar and distribution of provisions; an official of the chapter who has charge of the temporals.

cellarete, cellaret /ˌsɛlə'rɛt/ *n* a case for holding bottles of wine or liquor.

cellnet *n* a portable radio telephone used in cellular radio.

cello /'tʃɛloː/ *n* (*pl* **cellos**) the violoncello, a large four-stringed bass instrument of the violin family, held between the knees.—**cellist** *n*.

cellophane /'sɛləˌfeɪn/ *n* a thin transparent paper made from cellulose, used for wrapping.

cellphone /'sɛlfoːn/ *n* (*trademark*) a cellular telephone, a portable mobile telephone operated by cellular radio.

cellular /'sɛljuːlər/ *adj* of, resembling or containing cells; (*textiles*) of an open texture.

cellular radio *n* a computer-controlled radio communications system for Cellphones, etc, using a network of transmitters serving small zones called cells, as users move between cells the transmitters/receivers are transferred automatically.

cellule /'sɛljuːl/ *n* a small cell or cavity.

cellulite /'sɛljuːˌlaɪt/ *n* a form of fat on the hips, thighs and buttocks that causes puckering of the skin surface.

celluloid /'sɛljuːˌlɔɪd/ *n* a type of plastic made from cellulose nitrate and camphor; a plastic coating on film; cinema film.

cellulose /'sɛljuːˌloːs/ or /-loːz/ *n* a starch-like carbohydrate forming the cell walls of plants, used in making paper, textiles, film, etc.

cellulose acetate *n* a compound used in the manufacture of artificial textiles, film, and varnishes.

celsius /'sɛlsiəs/ *adj* pertaining to a thermometer scale with a freezing point of 0 degrees and a boiling point of 100 degrees.

Celt /kɛlt/ or /sɛlt/ *n* a member of an ancient people who inhabited pre-Roman Britain, Gaul and Spain.

celt /sɛlt/ *n* a prehistoric edged instrument or weapon of stone or bronze, resembling a chisel or blade of an axe, found in ancient tumuli.

Celtic /'kɛltɪk/ or /'sɛltɪk/ *adj* of or relating to the Celts; the language of the Celts, including Scots or Irish Gaelic, Manx, Welsh, Cornish and Breton.

Celticist, Celtist *n* a student of Celtic antiquities, languages, etc.

cement /sə'mɛnt/ *n* a powdered substance of lime and clay, mixed with water, etc to make mortar or concrete, which hardens upon drying; any hard-drying substance. • *vt* to bind or glue together with or as if with cement; to cover with cement.—**cementer** *n*.

cementation /ˌsimɛn'teɪʃən/ or /ˌsɛmən-/ *n* the act of cementing; a process for converting iron into steel, glass into porcelain, etc.

cemetery /'sɛməˌtɛri/ or /-tri/ *n* (*pl* **cemeteries**) a place for the burial of the dead.

cenobite /'sɛnəˌbaɪt/ or /'sinə-/ *see* **coenobite**.

cenotaph /'sɛnəˌtæf/ *n* a monument to a person who is buried elsewhere.—**cenotaphic** *adj*.

Cenozoic /ˌsinə'zoːɪk/ or /ˌsɛnə-/ *adj* of the third geological period, Tertiary.

cense /sɛns/ *vt* to perfume with incense.

censer /'sɛnsər/ *n* a covered cup-shaped vessel pierced with holes in which incense is burned.

censor /'sɛnsər/ *n* an official with the power to examine literature, films, mail, etc and remove or prohibit anything considered obscene, objectionable, etc. • *vt* to act as a censor.—**censorable** *adj*.—**censorial** *adj*.—**censorship** *n*.

censorious /sɛn'sɔriəs/ *adj* expressing censure; fault-finding.—**censoriously** *adv*.—**censoriousness** *n*.

censure /'sɛnʃər/ *n* an expression of disapproval or blame. • *vt* to condemn as wrong; to reprimand.—**censurable** *adj*.

census /'sɛnsəs/ *n* (*pl* **censuses**) an official count of the population, including details of age, sex, occupation, etc; any official count.

cent /sɛnt/ *n* a hundredth of a dollar; (*inf*) a negligible amount of money.

centaur /'sɛnˌtɔr/ *n* a fabulous monster, half man, half horse; an expert horseman; (*astron*) a southern constellation.

centaury /'sɛnˌtɔri/ *n* (*pl* **centauries**) a medicinal herb.

centavo /sɛn'tævoː/ *n* (*pl* **centavos**) the hundredth part of a dollar or peso in use in the South American republics.

centenarian /ˌsɛntə'nɛriːən/ *n* one who is one hundred years old or more.—*also adj*.

centenary /ˌsentɪˈnəri/ or /senˈtenəri/ *n* (*pl* **centenaries**) a hundredth anniversary or its celebration. • *adj* of a hundred years.

centennial /senˈteniəl/ or /-jəl/ *adj* happening every hundred years. • *n* a centenary.

center /ˈsentər/ *see* **centre**.

centerboard /-ˌbɔrd/ *see* **centreboard**.

centerfold /-ˌfoːld/ *see* **centrefold**.

centerpiece /ˈsentərˌpiːs/ *see* **centrepiece**.

centesimal /senˈtesiməl/ *adj* counting or counted by hundredths. • *n* a hundredth part.

centi- /ˈsenti/ *prefix* one hundredth.

centiare, centare /senˈtɛr/ *n* a square metre, equal to the hundredth part of an are.

centigrade /ˈsentɪˌɡreɪd/ *adj* Celsius.

centigram, centigramme /-ˌɡræm/ *n* one hundredth of a gram.

centilitre, centiliter /ˌliːtər/ *n* one hundredth of a litre.

centime *Fr.* /ˈsɑ̃ːtiːm/ *n* a small french coin, the hundredth part of a franc.

centimetre, centimeter /ˈsentiˌmiːtər/ *n* one hundredth of a metre.

centimetre-gram-second /-ˈɡræmˈsækənd/ *n* a unit system in which the centimetre, the gram and the mean solar second are taken respectively as the units of length, mass, and time (*usu abbr* **cgs units**).

centipede /ˈsentiˌpiːd/ *n* a crawling creature with a long body divided into numerous segments each with a pair of legs.

centner /ˈsentnər/ *n* a weight divisible first into a hundred parts and then into smaller parts; in many European countries the commercial name for a hundredweight.

cento /ˈsentoː/ *n* (*pl* **centos**) a literary or musical composition formed by selections from various authors or composers and arranged in a new order.

central /ˈsentrəl/ *adj* in, at, from or forming the centre; main, principal; important.—**centrally** *adv.*—**centrality** *n.*

central bank *n* a national bank that handles government transactions as opposed to private business.

central heating *n* a system of heating by pipes from a central boiler or other heat source.

centralism /-ˌlɪzəm/ *n* the policy or process of bringing under central control.—**centralist** *adj, n.*

centralize /ˈsentrəˌlaɪz/ *vt* to draw to the centre; to place under the control of a central authority, *esp* government.—**centralization** *n.*

central nervous system *n* in vertebrates, the brain and spinal cord which coordinates an animal's activity.

central processing unit *n* (*comput*) the part of a computer that performs logical and arithmetical operations on data in accordance with program instructions.

centre /ˈsentər/ *n* the approximate middle point or part of anything, a pivot; interior; point of concentration; a place where a particular activity goes on (*shopping centre*); source; political moderation; (*sport*) a player at the centre of the field, etc., a centre-forward. • *adj* of or at the centre. • *vt* (**centring, centred**) to place in the centre; to concentrate; to be fixed; (*football, hockey*) to kick or hit the ball into the centre of the pitch.—*also* **center**.

centre bit *n* a carpenter's tool turning upon a centre, for boring holes.

centreboard *n* a keel so constructed that it may be raised within the hull of a vessel or lowered, extensively used by racing craft; a yacht with this.—*also* **centerboard**.

centrefold *n* a colour illustration spread across the two facing pages in the middle of a newspaper or magazine.—*also* **centerfold**.

centre ice *n* ✸ the central area of a rink on which ice hockey is played or the exact spot in the centre where the puck is dropped during faceoffs at the start of each period and after a goal is scored.

centre of gravity *n* that point of a body through which the resultant of all the forces acting upon it in consequence of the earth's attraction will pass.

centrepiece /ˈsentərˌpiːs/ *n* a central ornament or decoration.—*also* **centerpiece**.

centric, centrical /ˈsentrɪk/ *adj* placed in the centre; central.—**centricity** *n.*

centrifugal /ˈsentrɪˈfjuːɡəl/ or /-ˈtrɪfˌəɡəl/ *adj* moving away from the centre of rotation.—**centrifugally** *adv.*

centrifugal force *n* an imaginary force which acts outwards on a rotating body or one moving along a curved path.

centrifuge /ˈsentrɪˌfjuːdʒ/ *n* a device used to separate milk, blood, etc, by rotating at very high speed.—**centrifugation** *n.*

centripetal /senˈtrɪpətəl/ *adj* tending to move towards the centre.—**centripetally** *adv.*

centrist /ˈsentrɪst/ *n* a person of moderate political opinions, etc.—**centrism** *n.*

centrobaric /ˌsentroˈbærɪk/ *adj* relating to the centre of gravity or to the method of its determination.

centroid /ˈsentroɪd/ *n* the centre of mass or gravity of a body.

centurion /senˈtʃuriən/ or /-ˈtʃər-/ *n* an officer commanding a hundred Roman soldiers.

century /ˈsentʃəri/ *n* (*pl* **centuries**) a period of a hundred years; a set of a hundred; (*cricket*) 100 runs made by a batsman in a single innings; a company of a Roman legion.

century home *n* ✸ (*Cdn*) a house that is about a hundred years old.

century plant *n* a name of the American aloe, from the supposition that it flowered once only in a hundred years.

cep /sep/ *n* an edible woodland fungus with a shiny brown cap and a white underside.

cephalagia /səˈfæləˌdʒiə/ *n* a headache.

cephalic /səˈfælɪk/ *adj* of the head.

cephalic index *n* the relation of the length of the head to its breadth.

cephalization /ˌsefəlɪˈzeɪʃən/ *n* the tendency in animal development to localize important parts or organs in or near the head.

cephalopod /ˈsefələˌpɒd/ *n* a marine mollusc, such as an octopus, characterized by a well-developed head and eyes and a ring of sucker-bearing tentacles.—**cephalopodan** *n, adj.*

cephalothorax /ˌsefəloˈθɔrˌæks/ *n* (*pl* **cephalothoraxes, cephalothoraces**) the anterior part of the body in the higher crustaceans, spiders, etc.

ceraceous /səˈreɪʃəs/ *adj* resembling wax.

ceramic /səˈræmɪk/ *adj* of earthenware, porcelain, or brick. • *n* something made of ceramic; (*pl*) the art of pottery.

ceramics *n sing* work executed wholly or partly in clay and baked; the art of pottery.—**ceramist, ceramicist** *n.*

cerastes /səˈræstiːz/ *n* (*pl* **cerastes**) the horned viper.

cerate /ˈsɪrˌeɪt/ or /ˈsɪrɪt/ *n* a thick ointment of wax, etc.

ceratodus /ˌsɪˈrætədəs/ or /ˌserəˈtoːdəs/ *n* (*pl* **ceratoduses**) a genus of Australian fishes containing the barramunda, or native salmon.

cere[1] /sɪr/ *n* a wax-like membrane at the base of the bill of many birds, as the parrot.

cere[2] *vt* to cover or close with cerecloth.

cereal /ˈsɪriəl/ *n* a grass grown for its edible grain, eg wheat, rice; the grain of such grasses; a breakfast food made from such grains. • *adj* of corn or edible grain.

cerebellum /ˌserəˈbeləm/ *n* (*pl* **cerebellums, cerebella**) a part of the brain below and behind the cerebrum which coordinates voluntary movements.—**cerebellar** *adj.*

cerebral /ˈserəbrəl/ or /səˈriːbrəl/ *adj* of or relating to the cerebrum; intellectual.—**cerebrally** *adv.*

cerebral hemisphere *n* one of the two lateral halves of the cerebrum.

cerebral palsy *n* a disability caused by brain damage before, during or immediately after birth resulting in poor muscle coordination.

cerebrate /ˈserəˌbreɪt/ *vi* to use the brain; to think.

cerebration /ˌserəˈbreɪʃən/ *n* the conscious or unconscious action of the brain; thought or thinking.

cerebrospinal /ˌsəˈriːbroːˈspaɪnəl/ *adj* of the brain and spinal cord.

cerebrum /ˈserəbrəm/ or /səˈriːbrəm/ *n* (*pl* **cerebrums, cerebra**) the front part of the brain of vertebrates; the dominant part of the brain in man, associated with intellectual function; the brain as a whole.

cerecloth /ˈsɪrklɒθ/ *n* a cloth saturated with wax or some gummy substance, used for wrapping embalmed bodies in.

cerement /ˈsɪrmənt/ *n* a grave cloth or shroud; (*pl*) grave clothes.

ceremonial /ˌserəˈmoːniəl/ *adj* of or with ceremony; formal. • *n* a set of rules for ceremonies.—**ceremonially** *adv.*

ceremonialism /-niəˌlɪzəm/ *n* adherence to, or fondness for, ceremonial observance; ritualism.—**ceremonialist** *n.*

ceremonious /-niəs/ *adj* observant of ceremony; marked by formality; overpolite.—**ceremoniously** *adv.*

ceremony /ˈserəˌmoːni/ *n* (*pl* **ceremonies**) a sacred rite; formal observance or procedure; behaviour that follows rigid etiquette.

cerise /səˈriːz/ or /-ˈriːs/ *n* a light and clear red.—*also adj.*

cerium /ˈsɪriəm/ *n* a grey metallic element used in various metallurgical and nuclear applications.

cero- /'sɪroː/ or /'seroː/, /-ə/ prefix wax.

cert abbr = certified; certificate; (sl) certainty.

certain /'sərtən/ adj sure, positive; unerring, reliable; sure to happen, inevitable; definite, fixed; some; one; unnamed, unspecified.

certainly /-tɪnli/ or /-tənli/ adv without doubt; yes.

certainty /-tənti/ n (pl **certainties**) something undoubted, inevitable; the condition of being certain.

certificate /sər'tɪfɪkɪt/ n a document formally attesting a fact; a testimonial of qualifications or character.—**certificated** adj.

certified public accountant n an accountant who has qualified by passing official examinations; a chartered accountant.

certify /'sərtɪfaɪ/ vt (**certifying, certified**) to declare in writing or attest formally; to endorse with authority.—**certification** n.

certiorari /ˌsərʃioː'rarɪ/ n a writ issuing from a superior court calling for the records of an inferior court, or to remove a case from a court below.

certitude /'sərtəˌtjuːd/ or /-ˌtjuːd/ n freedom from doubt.

cerulean /sə'ruːlɪən/ adj deep blue.

cerumen /sə'ruːmən/ n wax of the ear.—**ceruminous** adj.

ceruse /'sɪruːs/ or /sɪ'ruːs/ n white lead used as a pigment and from which a cosmetic is prepared.

cervical /'sərvɪkəl/ adj of the neck of the womb.

cervical smear n (med) a sample of cells taken from the cervix for detection of cancer; the taking of the sample.

cervine /'sərvaɪn/ adj of or pertaining to the deer family; of a tawny or fawn colour.

cervix /'sərvɪks/ n (pl **cervixes, cervices**) the neck of the womb.

cesium /'siziəm/ see **caesium**.

cespitose /'sespɪˌtoːs/ adj (bot) growing in tufts.

cess[1] /ses/ vt to impose a tax; to assess. • n a rate or tax, esp the land tax.

cess[2] n (Irish) luck or fortune.

cessation /se'seɪʃən/ n a stoppage; a pause.

cession /'seʃən/ n a giving up, a surrender; something ceded.

cessionary /'seʃəˌneri/ n (pl **cessionaries**) (law) a giving or yielding up.

cesspool /'sespuːl/, **cesspit** /-pɪt/ n a covered cistern for collecting liquid waste or sewage; (fig) a place of sin and depravity.

cestoid /'sestɔɪd/ adj of or pertaining to the Cestoda, an order of parasitic flat worms to which the tapeworms belong. • n a flat intestinal worm.

cetacean /sə'teɪʃən/ n a member of an order of aquatic, usu marine, mammals that includes whales, dolphins and porpoises. • adj belonging to this order.—also **cetaceous**.

ceteris paribus /'setərɪs'pærɪˌbus/ (Latin) other things being equal.

CF abbr ♣ = Canadian Forces.

Cf (chem symbol) californium.

cf. abbr = compare (Latin confer).

CFB abbr ♣ = Canadian Forces Base.

CFC abbr = chlorofluorocarbon.

CGA abbr ♣ = Certified General Account.

CGM abbr = Computer Graphics Metafile, a file format for graphics which uses mainly vector notation.

cgs abbr = centimetre-gram-second.

ch. abbr = chapter; church; (chess) check.

cha-cha(-cha) /'tʃɒtʃɒ/ n a ballroom dance orig from Latin America; the music for this.

chablis /ʃæ'bliː/ or /ʃə-/, /'ʃæbli/ n (often with cap) a dry white wine from Chablis, France.

chacma n a South African baboon.

chaconne /ʃə'kɒn/, Fr. /ʃɑ'kɔn/ n an old Spanish dance; the music for such a dance.

chad /tʃæd/ n (comput) the little scraps of paper or cardboard left by the punching of holes in computer cards or paper tape.

chafe /tʃeɪf/ vti to restore warmth by rubbing; to make or become sore by rubbing; to irritate; to feel irritation, to fret.

chafer /'tʃeɪfər/ n any of various large beetles.

chaff[1] /tʃæf/ n husks of grain separated from the seed by threshing or winnowing; cut hay or straw; worthless stuff.

chaff[2] vt to banter; to make a game of. • vi to use bantering language. • n good-natured teasing, banter.

chaffer /'tʃæfər/ vt to bargain, haggle. • n the act of bargaining.

chaffinch /'tʃæfɪntʃ/ n a European songbird.

chaffy /'tʃæfi/ adj resembling, or full of, chaff; anything light or worthless.

chafing dish /'tʃeɪfɪŋ/ n a vessel for heating or cooking food on a table; a small portable grate for coals.

chagrin /ʃə'grɪn/, Brit. /'ʃægrɪn/ n annoyance; vexation; disappointment.

chain /tʃeɪn/ n a series of connected links or rings; a continuous series; a series of related events; a bond; a group of shops, hotels, etc owned by the same company; a unit of length equal to 66 feet; a range of mountains; a group of islands; (pl) anything that restricts or binds; fetters. • vt to fasten with a chain or chains.

chain gang n a group of prisoners chained together.

chain mail n flexible armour formed of metal links interwoven.

chain reaction n a process in which a chemical, atomic or other reaction stimulates further reactions, eg combustion or nuclear fission; a series of events, each of which stimulates the next.

chain saw n a power-driven saw with teeth linked as in a chain.

chain-smoke /'tʃeɪnˌsmoːk/ vti to smoke (cigarettes) one after the other.—**chain-smoker** n.

chain stitch n an embroidery stitch that resembles the links of a chain.

chain store n one of a series of retail stores owned by one company.

chair /tʃer/ n a separate seat for one, with a back and legs; a seat of authority; a chairman; a professorship; the electric chair. • vt to preside as chairman of.

chair lift /-ˌlɪft/ n a series of seats suspended from a cable for carrying sightseers or skiers uphill.

chairman /-mən/ n (pl **chairmen**) a person who presides at a meeting; the president of a board or committee.—**chairwoman** nf (pl **chairwomen**).—also **chairperson**.

chaise /ʃeɪz/ n a light two-wheeled carriage; any carriage.

chaise longue /ˌʃeɪz'lɒŋ/ or /-'lɑundʒ/ n (pl **chaise longues, chaises longues**) a couch-like chair with a long seat.

chalcedony /kæl'sedəni/ n (pl **chalcedonies**) a form of quartz used as a gemstone.

chalco- /'kælkoː/ or /-kə/ prefix copper.

chalcopyrite /ˌkælkə'paɪraɪt/ n a copper ore.

Chaldean, Chaldaean /kæl'diːən/ adj pertaining to Chaldea, or ancient Babylon, or its language. • n the language of ancient Babylon.

chalet /ʃæl'eɪ/ n a Swiss hut; any similar building used in a holiday camp, as a ski lodge, etc.

chalice /'tʃælɪs/ n a large cup with a base; a communion cup.

chalk /tʃɒk/ n calcium carbonate, a soft white limestone; such a stone or a substitute used for drawing or writing. • vt to write, mark or draw with chalk; (with **up**) (inf) to score, get, achieve; to charge or credit.

chalky /'tʃɒki/ adj (**chalkier, chalkiest**) containing or resembling chalk.—**chalkiness** n.

challenge /'tʃæləndʒ/ vt to summon to a fight or contest; to call in question; to object to; to hail and interrogate; to demand proof of identity. • n the act of challenging; a summons to a contest; a calling in question; a problem that stimulates effort.—**challenger** n.—**challenging** adj.

challis /'ʃæli/ or /ʃæ'liː/ n a light all-wool fabric.

chalybeate /kə'lɪbɪət/ or /-'lɪbɪeɪt/ adj (water) impregnated with iron.

chamber /'tʃeɪmbər/ n a room, esp a bedroom; a deliberative body or a division of a legislature; a room where such a body meets; a compartment; a cavity in the body of an organism; part of a gun cylinder holding the cartridge; (pl) a judge's office.

chamberlain /'tʃeɪmbərlɪn/ n an official in charge of the household of a monarch or nobleman; a steward, treasurer or factor of a municipal corporation.

chambermaid /'tʃeɪmbərˌmeɪd/ n a woman employed to clean bedrooms in a hotel, etc.

chamber music n music for performance by a small group, as a string quartet.

chamber of commerce n (often cap) an organization of representatives from local businesses formed to promote and protect their interests.

chamber pot n a vessel for urine.

chameleon /kə'miːlɪən/ n a lizard capable of changing colour to match its surroundings; a person of variable moods or behaviour; an adaptable person.—**chameleonic** adj.

chamfer /'tʃæmfər/ n a flat surface made in wood or metal by paring off an angle, a bevel. • vt to groove, channel or flute.—**chamferer** n.

chamois /'ʃæmwɒ/ n (pl **chamois**) a small antelope found in Europe and Asia; a piece of chamois leather.

chamois leather, chammy (leather) *n* a soft, pliable leather formerly made from chamois skin, and now obtained from sheep, goats and deer; a piece of this for polishing.—*also* **shammy (leather)**.

chamomile /'kæmə,maıl/ or /-,miːl/ *n* an aromatic plant with daisy-like flowers used medicinally for its soothing property and as a hair lightener, and in making camomile tea.—*also* **camomile**.

champ[1] /tʃæmp/ *vti* to munch noisily, chomp; **champ at the bit** to be impatient.

champ[2] *n* (*inf*) a champion.

champagne /ʃæm'peɪn/ *n* a sparkling white wine; a pale straw colour.

champaign /ʃæm'peɪn/ *n* flat open country, a level expanse. • *adj* level, open.

champerty /'tʃæmpərtı/ *n* (*pl* **champerties**) (*law*) the maintenance of a party in a suit on condition that, if successful, the property is shared; the offence of aiding another's lawsuit in order to share in gains from it.—**champertous** *adj*.

champignon /ʃæm'pɪnjən, *Fr.* /ʃɑ̃pi'njoʊn/ *n* an edible mushroom that grows in circular clusters.

champion /'tʃæmpɪən/ *n* a person who fights for another; one who upholds a cause; a competitor successful against all others. • *adj* first-class; (*inf*) excellent. • *vt* to defend; to uphold the cause of.

championship /-ʃɪp/ *n* the act of championing; the process of determining a champion; a contest held to find a champion.

champlevé /ʃɑ̃lə'veɪ/ *n* enamel bearing indentations filled with colour.—*also adj*.

chance /tʃæns/ *n* a course of events; fortune; an accident, an unexpected event; opportunity; possibility; probability; risk. • *vti* to risk; to happen; to come upon unexpectedly. • *adj* accidental, not planned.

chancel /'tʃænsəl/ *n* the part of a church around the altar, for the clergy and the choir.

chancellery, chancellory /'tʃænsələrɪ/ or /-slərɪ/ *n* (*pl* **chancelleries, chancellories**) a chancellor's department or office; an office attached to an embassy.

chancellor /'tʃænsələr/ *n* a high government official, as, in certain countries, a prime minister; in some universities, the president or other executive officer.—**chancellorship** *n*.

chance-medley /'tʃæns,medlɪ/ *n* (*law*) justifiable homicide in self-defence; inadvertency.

chancery /'tʃænsərɪ/ *n* (*pl* **chanceries**) originally in England, next to Parliament the highest court of justice, since 1873 a division of the High Court of Justice; the office for public records; in US a court of equity.

chancre /'ʃæŋkər/ *n* a syphilitic ulcer.—**chancrous** *adj*.

chancy /'tʃænsɪ/ *adj* (**chancier, chanciest**) (*inf*) risky, uncertain.—**chancily** *adv*.

chandelier /,ʃændə'lɪːr/ *n* an ornamental hanging frame with branches for holding lights.

chandler /'tʃændlər/ *n* a dealer or merchant, *esp* in candles, oil, soap, etc.

chandlery /-rɪ/ *n* (*pl* **chandleries**) a chandler's shop or stock.

change /tʃeɪndʒ/ *vt* to make different, to alter; to transform; to exchange; to put fresh clothes on. • *vi* to become different, to undergo alteration; to put on fresh clothes; to continue one's journey by leaving one station, etc, or mode of transport and going to and using another. • *n* alteration, modification; substitution; variety; a fresh set, *esp* clothes; money in small units; the balance of money returned when given in a larger denomination as payment.—**changer** *n*.

changeable /'tʃeɪndʒəbəl/ *adj* able to be changed; altering rapidly between different conditions; inconstant.—**changeability** *n*.—**changeably** *adv*.

changeful /'tʃeɪndʒfəl/ *adj* often changing.

changeless /-ləs/ *adj* constant, immutable.—**changelessly** *adv*.—**changelessness** *n*.

changeling /-lɪŋ/ *n* a child secretly left in place of another.

change of life *n* (*inf*) the menopause.

changeover /-oʊ,vər/ *n* a complete change of system, method, state, attitude, etc.

channel[1] /'tʃænəl/ *n* the bed or the deeper part of a river, harbour, etc; a body of water joining two larger ones; a navigable passage; a means of passing or conveying or communicating; a band of radio frequencies reserved for a particular purpose, eg television station; a path for an electrical signal; a groove or line along which

liquids, etc may flow. • *vt* (**channelling, channelled** *or* **channeling, channeled**) to form a channel in; to groove; to direct.

channel[2] *n* a projection from a ship's side to spread the shrouds and keep them clear of the bulwarks.

chanson /ʃɑ̃sɔ̃/ *n* (*pl* **chansons**) a song.

chant /tʃænt/ *vti* to sing; to recite in a singing manner; to sing or shout (a slogan) rhythmically. • *n* sacred music to which prose is sung; sing-song intonation; a monotonous song; a rhythmic slogan, *esp* as sung or shouted by sports fans, etc.

chanter /'tʃæntər/ *n* a person who chants; the tenor or treble pipe of a bagpipe on which the melody is played.

chanterelle /,tʃæntə'rɛl/ *n* an edible yellow mushroom.

chantey /'ʃæntɪ/, **chanty** /'tʃɒntɪ/ *n* (*pl* **chanteys, chanties**) a shanty.

chanticleer /'tʃæntɪ'klɪːr/ *or* /,tʃɒn-/, /,ʃæn-/, /,ʃɒn-/ *n* a rooster.

chantry /'tʃæntrɪ/ *n* (*pl* **chantries**) a chapel endowed for the saying or singing mass daily for the soul of the founder; such an endowment.

chaology /'keɪɒlədʒɪ/ *n* the study of chaos theory.—**chaologist** *n*.

chaos /'keɪɒs/ *n* utter confusion, muddle.

chaos theory *n* (*physics*) the theory that the behaviour of dynamic systems is haphazard rather than mathematical.

chaotic /keɪ'ɒtɪk/ *adj* completely without order or arrangement.—**chaotically** *adv*.

chap[1] /ʃæp/ *vti* (**chapping, chapped**) (*skin*) to make or become split or rough in cold weather. • *n* a chapped place in the skin.

chap[2] *n* (*inf*) a man.

chap[3] /ʃɒp/ or /tʃæp/ *n* (*usu pl*) one of the jaws or its fleshy covering; the mouth of a channel.

chaparejos /,tʃæpə'reɪɒs/ or /,ʃæp-/ *npl* a cowboy's leather leg coverings.—*also* **chaps**.

chaparral /,ʃæpə'ræl/ or /,tʃæp-/ *n* a dense thicket.

chapati, chapatti /tʃə'pɒtɪ/ or /-'pæti/ *n* (*pl* **chapattis, chapatis** in Indian cookery, flat unleavened bread.

chapbook /'tʃæpbʊk/ *n* a small book of ballads, romances, etc, formerly hawked by a chapman.

chape /tʃeɪp/ *n* the metal tip of a scabbard; the part attaching a scabbard to a belt.

chapeau /ʃæ'poʊ/ *n* (*pl* **chapeaux, chapeaus**) a hat or head covering.

chapel /'tʃæpəl/ *n* a building for Christian worship, not as large as a church; an association or trade union of printers in a printing office.

chaperon, chaperone /'ʃæpə,roʊn/ *n* a woman who accompanies a girl at social occasions for propriety. • *vt* to attend as a chaperon.—**chaperonage** *n*.

chapfallen /'tʃæp,fɔlən/ *adj* with the jaw hanging down, dejected, dispirited.—*also* **chopfallen**.

chapiter /'tʃæpɪtər/ *n* (*archit*) the upper part or capital of a column.

chaplain /'tʃæplən/ *n* a clergyman serving in a religious capacity with the armed forces, or in a prison, hospital, etc.—**chaplaincy** *n*.

chaplet /'tʃæplət/ *n* a wreath or garland encircling the head; a rosary; a round moulding carved into beads, olives, etc.—**chapleted** *adj*.

chapman /'tʃæpmən/ *n* (*pl* **chapmen**) formerly a merchant or trader; a hawker.

chaps /tʃæps/ or /ʃæps/ *npl* chaparejos.

chapter /'tʃæptər/ *n* a main division of a book; the body or meeting of canons of a cathedral or members of a monastic order; a sequence of events; an organized branch of a society or association.

chapterhouse *n* a room for the meetings of a cathedral chapter.

char[1] /tʃɑr/ *n* a charwoman. • *vti* (**charring, charred**) to work as a charwoman.

char[2] *vb* (**charring, charred**) *vt* to burn to charcoal or carbon. • *vi* to scorch.

char[3] *n* (*pl* **char, chars**) a red-bellied fish allied to the salmon.—*also* **charr**.

character /'kærəktər/ *n* the combination of qualities that distinguishes an individual person, group or thing; moral strength; reputation; disposition; a person of marked individuality; an eccentric; (*inf*) a person; a person in a play or novel; a guise, role; a letter or mark in writing, printing, etc.

characterful /-fʊl/ *adj* full of character, unusual.

characteristic /,kærəktə'rıstık/ *adj* marking or constituting the particular nature of (a person or thing). • *n* a characteristic or distinguishing feature.—**characteristically** *adv*.

characterize /'kærıktə,raız/ *vt* to describe in terms of particular qualities; to designate; to be characteristic of, mark.—**characterization** *n*.

characterless /-ləs/ *adj* ordinary, undistinguished.

charade /ʃəˈreɪd/ *n* a travesty; an absurd pretence; (*usu pl*) a game of guessing a word from the acted representation of its syllables and the whole.

charcoal /ˈtʃɑrkoːl/ *n* the black carbon matter obtained by partially burning wood and used as fuel, as a filter or for drawing.

chard /tʃɑrd/ *n* a type of beet with edible leaves and stalks.

charge /tʃɑrdʒ/ *vt* to ask as the price; to record as a debt; to load, to fill, saturate; to lay a task or trust on; to burden; to accuse; to attack at a run; to build up an electric charge (in). • *n* a price charged for goods or service; a build-up of electricity; the amount which a receptacle can hold at one time; the explosive required to fire a weapon; trust, custody; a thing or person entrusted; a task, duty; accusation; an attack.

chargeable /ˈtʃɑrdʒəbəl/ *adj* liable to be charged.—**chargeability** *n.*

charge account *n* an account with a store, etc, to which the cost of goods are charged for later payment.

charge card *n* a type of credit card issued by a chain store or other organization.

chargé d'affaires /ˌʃɑrʒeɪdæˈfer/ *n* (*pl* **chargés d'affaires**) an ambassador's deputy; a minor diplomat.

charger /ˈtʃɑrdʒər/ *n* a cavalry horse; a device for charging a battery.

charily /ˈtʃerəli/ *adv* reluctantly; cautiously.

chariness /-inəs/ *n* a being chary.

chariot /ˈtʃæriət/ *n* a two-wheeled vehicle driven by two or more horses in ancient warfare, races, etc.—**charioteer** *n.*

charisma, charism /kəˈrɪzmə/ *n* (*pl* **charismata, charisms**) personal quality enabling a person to influence or inspire others; a God-given power or gift.—**charismatic** *adj.*

charitable /ˈtʃærɪtəbəl/ or /ˈtʃerɪ-/ *adj* of or for charity; generous to the needy, benevolent; lenient in judging others, kindly.—**charitableness** *n.*—**charitably** *adv.*

charity /ˈtʃærɪti/ or /ˈtʃerɪ-/ *n* (*pl* **charities**) leniency or tolerance towards others; generosity in giving to the needy; a benevolent fund or institution.

charivari /ˌʃɑrɪˈvɑri/ *n* a mock serenade of discordant music; hurly-burly.—*also* **shivaree**.

charlatan /ˈʃɑrlətən/ *n* a person who pretends to be what he or she is not; one who professes knowledge dishonestly, *esp* of medicine.—**charlatanism, charlatanry** *n.*

Charleston /ˈtʃɑrlstən/ *n* a lively dance with sidekicks from the knee.

charlock /ˈtʃɑrlɒk/ *n* wild mustard.

charlotte /ˈtʃɑrlət/ *n* a pudding of stewed fruit covered with breadcrumbs.

charlotte russe /ˈruːs/ *n* whipped cream custard enclosed in a sponge cake.

charm /tʃɑrm/ *n* an alluring quality, fascination; a magic verse or formula; something thought to possess occult power; an object bringing luck; a trinket on a bracelet. • *vt* to delight, captivate; to influence as by magic.—**charmer** *n.*

charming /ˈtʃɑrmɪŋ/ *adj* delightful, attractive.—**charmingly** *adv.*

charnel house /ˈtʃɑrnəlˌhɛʊs/ *n* a vault containing corpses or bones.

charpoy /ˈtʃɑrpɔɪ/ *n* a light portable Indian bedstead.

charqui /ˈtʃɑrki/ *n* beef cut into strips and sun-dried.

charr /tʃɑr/ *see* **char³**.

chart /tʃɑrt/ *n* a map, *esp* for use in navigation; an information sheet with tables, graphs, etc; a weather map; a table, graph, etc; (*pl with* **the**) a list of the most popular music recordings. • *vt* to make a chart of; to plan (a course of action).

charter /ˈtʃɑrtər/ *n* a document granting rights, privileges, ownership of land, etc; the hire of transportation. • *vt* to grant by charter; to hire.

Charter /ˈtʃɑrtər/ *n* ✹ (*Cdn*) the Charter of Rights and Freedoms, part of the constitution of Canada.

chartered accountant *n* an accountant who has qualified by passing the official examinations; a certified public accountant.

Chartism /ˈtʃɑrtɪzəm/ *n* a democratic reforming movement in England for the extension of political power to the working class, embodied in the People's Charter of 1838.—**Chartist** *adj, n.*

Chartreuse /ʃɑrˈtrəz/, *Fr.* /ʃɑrˈtrøz/ *n* (*trademark*) a yellowish green liqueur; (*without cap*) its colour.

chartulary /ˈkɑrtʃəˌleri/ *see* **cartulary**.

charwoman /ˈtʃɑrˌwʊmən/ *n* (*pl* **charwomen**) a woman employed to clean a house.

chary /ˈtʃeri/ *adj* (**charier, chariest**) cautious; sparing; (*with* **of**) unwilling to risk.

chase¹ /tʃeɪs/ *vt* to pursue; to run after; to drive (away); to hunt; (*inf: usu with* **up**) to pursue in a determined manner. • *n* pursuit; a hunt; a quarry hunted; a steeplechase.

chase² *Fr.* /tʃæs/ *n* a frame for securing a page of type; a groove; that part of a cannon in front of the trunnions.

chase³ *vt* to work or emboss precious metals; to cut a screw.

chaser /ˈtʃeɪsər/ *n* a horse used in steeplechasing; a person that chases; (*inf*) a drink taken after another, as in beer after a whisky.

chasm /ˈkæzəm/ *n* a deep cleft, an abyss, a gaping hole; a wide difference in opinions, etc.—**chasmal, chasmic** *adj.*

chassé /ˈʃæseɪ/ *n* a rapid gliding step in dancing. • *vi* to perform a chassé.

chasseur /ʃæˈsɜr/ *n* a French light-armed foot or cavalry soldier; a domestic dressed in military or hunting costume.

chassis /ˈtʃæsi/ or /ˈʃæsi/ *n* (*pl* **chassis**) the frame, wheels, engine of a car, aeroplane or other vehicle.

chaste /tʃeɪst/ *adj* pure, abstaining from unlawful sexual intercourse; virgin; modest; restrained, unadorned.—**chastely** *adv.*—**chasteness** *n.*

chasten /ˈtʃeɪsən/ *vt* to correct by suffering, discipline; to restrain.—**chastener** *n.*

chastise /tʃæsˈtaɪz/ or /ˈtʃæstaɪz/ *vt* to punish; to beat; to scold.—**chastisement** *n.*

chastity /ˈtʃæstɪti/ *n* sexual abstinence; virginity; purity.

chasuble /ˈtʃæzubəl/ or /ˈtʃæzju-/, /-su-/ *n* a rich sleeveless vestment worn over the alb by a priest celebrating mass.

chat /tʃæt/ *vti* (**chatting, chatted**) to talk in an easy or familiar way; (*with* **up**) (*inf*) to talk in a flirtatious way with another person. • *n* informal conversation.

chateau, château /ʃæˈtoː/ or /ˈʃætoː/ *n* (*pl* **chateaus, châteaux**) a castle or large country estate in France; ✹ (*Cdn*) (*hist*) in French Canada, the residence of a seigneur or governor. • ✹ *adj* (*Cdn*) (*cap*) in the architectural style of such a residence.

chatelaine /ˈʃætəˌleɪn/ *n* the lady of a country house; a bunch of chains to which are attached keys, etc, worn at the waist by ladies.

chatoyant /ʃəˈtɔɪənt/ *adj* changing in colour or lustre.—**chatoyancy** *n.*

chatroom /ˈtʃætˌtrum/ *n* (*comput*) on the Internet, a function on a website that allows several Internet users to type messages to each other in real time, simultaneously.

chat show *n* a television or radio programme with informal interviews and conversation.

chattel /ˈtʃætəl/ *n* (*usu pl*) goods, possessions; (*law*) personal property except freehold.

chatter /ˈtʃætər/ *vi* to talk aimlessly and rapidly; (*animal, etc*) to utter rapid cries; (*teeth*) to rattle together due to cold or fear. • *n* idle rapid talk; the sound of chattering.— **chatterer** *n.*

chatterbox /-ˌbɒks/ *n* an incessant talker.

chatty /ˈtʃæti/ *adj* (**chattier, chattiest**) talkative, full of gossip.—**chattily** *adv.*—**chattiness** *n.*

chauffeur /ˈʃoːfər/ or /ʃoːˈfər/ *n* a person who drives a car for someone else. • *vt* to drive as a chauffeur.—**chauffeuse** *nf.*

chautauqua /ʃəˈtɒkwə/ or /tʃə-/ *n* ✹ (*hist*) a public cultural entertainment in North America that included music, lectures and theatre.

chauvinism /ˈʃoːvəˌnɪzəm/ *n* aggressive patriotism; excessive devotion to a belief, cause, etc, *esp* a man's belief in the superiority of men over women.—**chauvinist** *n.*—**chauvinistic** *adj.*

chaw /tʃɒ/ *vt* (*dial*) to chew, to munch, *esp* tobacco. • *n* a plug of tobacco.

cheap /tʃiːp/ *adj* low-priced, inexpensive; good value; of little worth, inferior; vulgar.—**cheaply** *adv.*—**cheapness** *n.*

cheapen /ˈtʃiːpən/ *vti* to make or become cheap; to lower the value, worth or reputation of.

cheap-jack /ˈtʃiːpdʒæk/ *n* (*inf*) a person who sells cheap or worthless goods. • *adj* worthless, inferior.

cheapskate /-skeɪt/ *n* (*inf*) a mean or dishonourable person.

cheat /tʃiːt/ *vti* to defraud, to swindle; to deceive; to play unfairly. • *n* a fraud, deception; a person who cheats.—**cheater** *n.*

check /tʃek/ *vti* to bring or come to a stand; to restrain or impede; to admonish, reprove; to test the accuracy of, verify; (*with* **in**) to sign or register arrival at a hotel, work, an airport, etc; (*with* **out**) to settle the bill and leave a hotel; to investigate. • *n* repulse; stoppage; a pattern of squares; a control to test accuracy; a tick against listed items; a bill in a restaurant; a cheque; (chess) a threatening of the king; a money order to a bank.—also **check**.

checkbook /'tʃɛk,bʊk/ see **chequebook**.

check digit n (comput) a digit added to data digits to test accuracy and check for corruption.

checker[1] /'tʃɛkər/ see **chequer**.

checker[2] n a cashier in a supermarket.

checkerboard /-,bɔrd/ n a draughtboard.

checkered /'tʃɛkərd/ see **chequered**.

check list /'tʃɛklɪst/ n a list of items used for reference or verification.

checkmate /-meɪt/ n (chess) the winning position when the king is threatened and unable to move; utter defeat. • vt (chess) to place in checkmate; to defeat, foil.

checking account n a bank account, usu with no interest, from which money is withdrawn by cheques or cash cards; a current account.

checkout /-aʊt/ n a place where traffic may be halted for inspection; the place in a store where goods are paid for.

checkpoint /-pɔɪnt/ n a place where visitors' passports or other official documents may be examined.

checkrein /-,reɪn/ see **bearing rein**

checkroom /-ruːm/ n a temporary repository for luggage, coats, etc.

checkup /-,ʌp/ n a thorough examination; a medical examination, usu repeated at intervals.

Cheddar /'tʃɛdər/ n a type of hard, white or yellow cheese originally made in Cheddar, England.

cheechako /tʃiː'tʃæko:/ n ✻ a newcomer or neophyte, esp in the Canadian North and Alaska.

cheek /tʃiːk/ n the side of the face below the eye; (sl) buttock; impudence; ✻ (Cdn) the edible cheek of a fish, esp cod.

cheeky /'tʃiːki/ adj (**cheekier, cheekiest**) disrespectful, impudent.—**cheekily** adv.—**cheekiness** n.

cheep /tʃiːp/ n the frail squeak of a young bird. • vi to make such a sound.

cheer /tʃiːr/ n a shout of applause or welcome; a frame of mind, spirits; happiness. • vt to gladden; to encourage; to applaud.

cheerful /'tʃɪrfʊl/ adj in good spirits; happy.—**cheerfully** adv.—**cheerfulness** n.

cheerleader /-,lidər/ n a person who leads organized cheering, esp at a sports event.

cheerless /-ləs/ adj dismal, depressing.

cheers /tʃɪrz/ interj (inf) an expression used in offering a toast, as a form of farewell or thanks.

cheery /'tʃɪri/ adj (**cheerier, cheeriest**) lively, genial, merry.—**cheerily** adv.—**cheeriness** n.

cheese /tʃiːz/ n the curds of milk pressed into a firm or hard mass; a boss or important person (big cheese).

cheeseburger /'tʃiːz,bərgər/ n a hamburger with melted cheese on top.

cheesecake /-keɪk/ n a cake made with cottage or cream cheese; (sl) attractive women or men displayed as sex objects in photographs, etc.

cheesecloth /-klɒθ/ n a thin cotton fabric.

cheeseparing /-'pɛrɪŋ/ adj niggardly, mean.

cheesy /-i/ adj (**cheesier, cheesiest**) like cheese.—**cheesiness** n.

cheetah /'tʃiːtə/ n a large spotted cat, similar to a leopard.

chef /ʃɛf/ n a professional cook.

chef-d'oeuvre /ʃeɪ'də:vr/, Fr. /ʃe'dœ,vr/ n (pl **chefs-d'oeuvre**) a masterpiece.

cheiro-, chiro- /'kaɪrou/ or /-rə/ prefix hand.

chela /'kiːlə/ n (**chelae**) a claw-like pincer of the crab, etc.—**cheliferous** adj.

chelonian /kə'loːniən/ n any of the order of reptiles, including turtles and tortoises.—also adj.

chemical /'kɛmɪkəl/ n a substance used in, or arising from, a chemical process. • adj of, used in, or produced by chemistry.—**chemically** adv.

chemical engineering n the branch of engineering dealing with the design, construction, and manufacture of plant used in industrial chemical processes.

chemical warfare n warfare in which poison gases and other chemicals are used.

chemin de fer /ʃə,mædə'fer/ n a gambling game, a kind of baccarat.

chemise /ʃə'miːz/ n a woman's undergarment; a loose-fitting dress.

chemisette /ʃɛmi'zɛt/ n a short bodice worn over the breast; lace, etc, filling the neck opening of a dress.

chemist /'kɛmɪst/ n a pharmacy; a manufacturer of medicinal drugs; a person skilled in chemistry.

chemistry /'kɛməstri/ n (pl **chemistries**) the science of the properties of substances and their combinations and reactions; chemical structure.

chemotherapy /,kiːmo:'θɛrəpi/ n the treatment of disease, esp cancer, by drugs and other chemical agents.

chenille /ʃə'niːl/ n silk or worsted cord.

cheque /tʃɛk/ see **check**.

chequebook n a book containing blank cheques to be drawn on a bank.—also **checkbook**.

chequer /'tʃɛkər/ n a pattern of squares.—also **checker**; a flat counter used in the game of checkers.—also **draughtsman**; (pl) a game for two players who each move twelve round flat pieces over a checkerboard.—also **draughts**.

chequered adj marked with a variegated pattern; having a career marked by fluctuating fortunes.—also **checkered**.

cherish /'tʃɛrɪʃ/ vt to tend lovingly, foster; to keep in mind as a hope, ambition, etc.—**cherisher** n.

cheroot /ʃə'ruːt/ n a cigar cut square at each end.

cherry /'tʃɛri/ n (pl **cherries**) a small red, pitted fruit; the tree bearing it; a bright red colour.

cherry picker n a crane, usu on a truck, with a long elbow-jointed arm carrying a platform that can be raised and lowered.

chersonese /'kərsə,niːs/ n (poet) a peninsula.

chert /ʃərt/ n an impure flint-like quartz or hornstone.—**cherty** adj.

cherub /'tʃɛrəb/ n (pl **cherubim**) an angel of the second order; a winged child or child's head; (pl **cherubs**) an angelic, sweet child.—**cherubic** adj.

chervil /'tʃərvɪl/ n an aromatic herb used for flavouring.

Cheshire cheese /'tʃɛʃiːr/ or /-ər/ n a mild flavoured cheese, originally made in Cheshire England.

chess[1] /tʃɛs/ n a game played by two people with 32 pieces on a chessboard.

chess[2] n one of the flooring planks of a pontoon bridge.

chessboard /'tʃɛsbɔrd/ n a board chequered with 64 squares in two alternate colours, used for playing chess or draughts.

chessman /-mæn/ n (pl **chessmen**) any of the 16 pieces used by each player in chess.

chest /tʃɛst/ n a large strong box; the part of the body enclosed by the ribs, the thorax.

chesterfield /'tʃɛstər,fiːld/ n a large, stuffed couch with straight ends; a man's overcoat.

chestnut /'tʃɛsnət/ n a tree or shrub of the beech family; the edible nut of a chestnut; the wood of the chestnut; a horse with chestnut colouring; (inf) an old joke. • adj of the colour of a chestnut, a deep reddish brown.

chest of drawers n a piece of furniture containing several drawers.

chesty /'tʃɛsti/ adj (**chestier, chestiest**) (inf) prone to chest infections; having a large chest or bosom.—**chestily** adv.—**chestiness** n.

cheval-de-frise /ʃə,vældə'friːz/ n (pl **chevaux-de-frise**) a fence constructed of a bar armed with long spikes.

cheval glass /ʃə'væl/ n a full-length mirror which can swivel in its frame.

chevalier /,ʃəvə'liːr/ or /ʃə'væljeɪ/ n a knight; a horseman; a member or knight of an honourable order; the lowest title or rank of the old French nobility; a gallant.

chevet /ʃə'veɪ/ n an apse; a group of apses.

cheviot /'tʃɛviət/ or /'tʃ-/ n a rough cloth made from the wool of sheep bred on the Cheviot Hills along the border between England and Scotland.

chevron /'ʃɛvrən/ or /-rɒn/ n the V-shaped bar on the sleeve of a uniform, showing rank.

chevrotain /'ʃɛvrə,teɪn/ or /-tɪn/ n a small musk deer.

chew /tʃuː/ vt to grind between the teeth, to masticate; (with over) to ponder, think over; (with up) to spoil by chewing. • n the act of chewing; something to chew, as a sweet or tobacco.—**chewable** adj.—**chewer** n.

chewing gum n a flavoured gum made from chicle, for chewing.

chewed-up (sl) made nervous or worried.

chewy /'tʃuːi/ adj (**chewier, chewiest**) needing to be chewed.

chez /ʃeɪ/ prep at the home of.

chi /kaɪ/ n the 22nd letter of the Greek alphabet.

Chianti /ki'ænti/ n a dry red or white wine from Italy.

chiaroscuro /kɪˌɑrəˈsjuːroː/ or /-ˈskjɜroː/ n (pl **chiaroscuros**) the effects of light and shade; the treatment of this in painting, drawing, or engraving; the use of contrast and relief in literature. • adj pertaining to such treatment.—**chiaroscurism** n.—**chiaroscurist** n.

chiasma, chiasm /kaɪˈæzmə/ n (pl **chiasmas, chiasmata, chiasms**) the central body of nervous matter formed by the junction and the crossing of the fibres of the optic nerves. —**chiasmal** adj.—**chiasmic** adj.

chiasmus /kaɪˈæzməs/ n (pl **chiasmi**) a figure of speech by which the order of words in the first of two parallel clauses is reversed in the second, eg "to stop too fearful and too faint to go".—**chiastic** adj.

chibouk, chibouque /tʃɪˈbuːk/ n a long Turkish tobacco pipe.

chic /ʃiːk/ n elegance, style. • adj stylish.

chicane /ʃɪˈkeɪn/ n a hand at bridge without trumps; a barrier or obstacle on a motor-racing course; chicanery.

chicanery /ʃɪˈkeɪnəri/ n (pl **chicaneries**) underhand dealing, trickery; verbal subterfuge.

Chicano /tʃɪˈkɒnoː/ or /-ˈkænoː/ n (pl **Chicanos**) a Mexican-American.—also adj.

chick /tʃɪk/ n a young bird; (sl) a young attractive woman or girl.

chickadee /ˈtʃɪkəˌdiː/ n the American blackcap titmouse.

chickaree /ˈtʃɪkəˌriː/ n the American red squirrel.

chicken /ˈtʃɪkən/ n a young, domestic fowl; its flesh. • adj cowardly, timorous. • vi (with **out**) (inf) to suffer a failure of nerve or courage.

chicken feed n poultry food; (inf) a trifling amount of money.

chicken-hearted /-ˌhɑrtɪd/, **chicken-livered** adj cowardly.

chickenpox /-ˌpɒks/ n a contagious viral disease that causes a rash of red spots on the skin.

chicken wire n light wire netting with a hexagonal mesh.

chickpea /ˈtʃɪkˌpiː/ n (the seed eaten as a vegetable of) an Asian leguminous plant.

chickweed /-wiːd/ n a small white-flowered plant of the pink family.

chicle /ˈtʃɪkəl/ or /-liː/ n the milky gum of a tropical American tree used to make chewing gum.

chicory /ˈtʃɪkəri/ n (pl **chicories**) a salad plant; its dried, ground, roasted root used to flavour coffee or as a coffee substitute.

chide /tʃaɪd/ vt (**chiding, chided** or **chid**; pp **chided, chid** or **chidden**) to rebuke, scold.—**chider** n.—**chidingly** adv.

chief /tʃiːf/ adj principal, most important. • n a leader; the head of a tribe or clan.

chiefly /ˈtʃiːfli/ adv especially; mainly; for the most part.

chieftain /ˈtʃiːftən/ n the head of a Scottish clan; a chief.

chiffchaff /ˈtʃɪftʃæf/ n a European warbler.

chiffon /ˈʃəˈfɒn/ n a thin gauzy material. • adj made of chiffon; (pie filling, etc) having a light fluffy texture.

chiffonier, chiffonnier /ˌʃɪfəˈniːr/ n a high chest of drawers; a wide, low cupboard.

chignon /ˈʃiːnjɔ̃/ n a mass of hair worn in a roll at the back of the head, a bun.

chigoe /ˈtʃɪgoː/ n a species of West Indian and South American flea that burrows beneath the skin of the feet, causing irritation and ulcers.—also **jigger**.

chihuahua /tʃəˈwɒwɒ/ n a tiny dog with erect ears, originally from Mexico.

chilblain /ˈtʃɪlbleɪn/ n an inflamed swelling on the hands, toes, etc, due to cold.

child /tʃaɪld/ n (pl **children**) a young human being; a son or daughter; offspring; an innocent or immature person.

child abuse n physical, mental or sexual maltreatment of a child by parents or any other adult.

childbearing /ˈtʃaɪldˌbɛrɪŋ/ n pregnancy and childbirth.—also adj.

childbirth /-ˌbɜrθ/ n the process of giving birth to children.

child care /-ˌkɛr/ n care by an authority of homeless children or those from a disturbed home background.

childe /tʃaɪld/ n a term formerly applied to the scions of knightly houses before their admission into knighthood; a youth of noble birth.

childhood /ˈtʃaɪldhʊd/ n the period between birth and puberty in humans.

childish /ˈtʃaɪldɪʃ/ adj of, like or suited to a child; foolish.—**childishly.**—**childishness** n.

child labour n illegal employment of children below a certain age.

childless adj having no children.

child-like /ˈtʃaɪldlaɪk/ adj like a child; innocent, simple, candid.

children /ˈtʃɪldrən/ see **child**.

child's play n an easy task.

chili /ˈtʃɪli/ n (pl **chilies**) the hot-tasting pod of some of the capsicums, dried and used as flavouring.

chiliad /ˈkɪliˌæd/ n a thousand; a thousand years.—**chiliadal, chiliadic** adj.

chiliasm /ˈkɪliˌæzəm/ n the doctrine of the milennium.—**chiliast** n.—**chiliastic** adj.

chili con carne /ˈtʃɪlikɒnˈkɑrni/ n a spicy stew of minced beef, beans, onions and tomatoes flavoured with chilli powder or chillies.

chill /tʃɪl/ n a sensation of coldness; an illness caused by exposure to cold and marked by shivering; anything that dampens or depresses. • adj shivering with cold; feeling cold; unemotional, formal. • vti to make or become cold; to harden by cooling; to depress.

chillum /ˈtʃɪləm/ n the bowl of a hookah; a hookah; smoking.

chilly /ˈtʃɪli/ adj (**chillier, chilliest**) cold; unfriendly.—**chilliness** n.

chilopod /ˈkaɪloˌpɒd/ or /-lə-/ n any of an order of the class Myriopoda, containing the centipedes.

chime[1] /tʃaɪm/ n the harmonious sound of a bell; accord; harmony; (pl) a set of bells or metal tubes, etc tuned in a scale; their ringing. • vi to ring (a bell); (with **in**) (inf) to join in in agreement; to interrupt a conversation; (with **with**) to agree. • vt to indicate the hour by chiming, as a clock.

chime[2], **chimb** n the rim formed by the ends of the staves of a cask.

chimera, chimaera /kaɪˈmiːrə/ or /kɪ-/ n (Greek myth) a fire-breathing monster with body parts from various different animals; a fantastic hybrid; an impossible fancy.

chimere /tʃɪˈmɪr/ or /ʃɪ-/ n a loose silk robe worn by an Anglican bishop, either sleeveless or with lawn sleeves.

chimeric /kaɪˈmɛrɪkəl/ or /kɪ-/, **chimerical** /-kəl/ adj merely imaginary; fantastic, visionary; unreal.—**chimerically** adv.

chimney /ˈtʃɪmni/ n (pl **chimneys**) a passage for smoke, hot air or fumes, a funnel; a chimney stack; the vent of a volcano; a vertical crevice in rock large enough to enter and climb.

chimneypiece n a mantelpiece.

chimneypot n a pipe extending a chimney at the top.

chimney stack n the chimney above roof level.

chimney sweep n a person who removes soot from chimneys.

chimo /ˈtʃimoː/ interj ✦ (Cdn) used to give a friendly greeting, esp in the Canadian North.

chimp /tʃɪmp/ n (inf) chimpanzee.

chimpanzee /ˌtʃɪmpænˈziː/ n an African anthropoid ape.

chin /tʃɪn/ n the part of the face below the mouth.

china /ˈtʃaɪnə/ n fine porcelain; articles made from this.

china clay n kaolin.

Chinatown /ˈtʃaɪnəˌtaʊn/ n the Chinese quarter of any city.

chinch /tʃɪntʃ/ n a tropical American insect destructive to corn crops; a bedbug.

chinchilla /tʃɪnˈtʃɪlə/ n a small South American rodent with soft grey fur; a breed of domestic cat; a breed of rabbit.

chine /tʃaɪn/ n the backbone or spine of an animal; a piece of the backbone of an animal with adjacent parts cut for cooking; a ridge; a rocky ravine or large fissure in a cliff.

Chinese /tʃaɪˈniːz/ adj of or pertaining to China. • n (pl **Chinese**) an inhabitant of China.

Chinese chequers n a board game played with marbles.

Chinese gooseberry see **kiwi fruit**.

Chinese lantern n a collapsible paper lantern.

Chinese puzzle n an intricate puzzle based on fitting boxes within boxes; any very difficult puzzle or complex problem.

Chinese restaurant syndrome n an ailment characterized by chest pain, dizziness, flushing, allegedly caused by consuming in quantity monosodium glutamate found in Chinese food.

Chinese white n a white pigment; white zinc oxide.

chink[1] /tʃɪŋk/ n a narrow opening; a crack or slit.

chink[2] n the sound of coins clinking together.

chino /ˈtʃiːnoː/ n (pl **chinos**) a strong, hardwearing twilled cotton; (pl) trousers made of this fabric.

chinoiserie /ʃɪnˌwɒzəˈriː/ n (an object or objects in) a style of decoration copying Chinese motifs.

Chinook /ʃəˈnuːk/ n a jargon of native and foreign words used on the northwest Pacific coast by Indians and whites.

chinook n a warm dry southwesterly wind of the eastern slopes of the Rocky Mountains; a warm moist wind blowing onto the northwest coast of America.

Chinook jargon *n* ✷ (*hist*) a pidgin language made up of English, French and Indian languages, used by traders on the Pacific Northwest coast of North America.

chinquapin /'tʃɪŋkəpɪn/ *n* the dwarf chestnut of the US; its nut.

chintz /tʃɪnts/ *n* a glazed cotton cloth printed with coloured designs.

chintzy /'tʃɪnsi/ *adj* (**chintzier, chintziest**) of or describing furniture, decor, etc covered in chintz; cheap; tasteless in a flowery way.

chinwag /'tʃɪnwæg/ *vi* (**chinwagging, chinwagged** (*sl*) to talk, to gossip. • *n* (*sl*) a chatty conversation, a gossip.

chip /tʃɪp/ *vt* (**chipping, chipped**) to knock small pieces off; to shape or make by chipping. • *n* a small piece cut or broken off; a mark left by chipping; a thin strip of fried potato, french fry; a potato chip; a counter used in games; a tiny piece of semiconducting material, such as silicon, printed with a microcircuit and used as part of an integrated circuit.

chipboard /'tʃɪpbɔrd/ *n* a thin stiff material made from compressed wood shavings and other waste pieces combined with resin.

Chipewyan /tʃɪpə'waɪən/ *n* ✷ a member of a First Nations people in the northern Canadian Prairies and subarctic Northwest Territories; the Athapaskan language of this people. • *adj* of or pertaining to this people or their language.

chipmunk /'tʃɪpmʌŋk/ *n* a small, striped, squirrel-like animal of North America.

Chippendale /'tʃɪpən,deɪl/ *adj* of the light style of furniture introduced in the middle of the 13th century by the furniture maker and designer, Thomas Chippendale (1718–79)

chipper /'tʃɪpər/ *adj* active; lively, cheerful.

chip shot *n* a short, lofted approach shot in golf.

chip wagon *n* ✷ (*Cdn*) a mobile vehicle that sells French fries and other snacks.

chiro-, cheiro- /'kaɪroʊ/ *prefix* hand

chirography /kaɪ'rɒgrəfi/ *n* the art of writing, calligraphy; judgment of character by the handwriting.—**chirographer** *n.*—**chirographic, chirographical** *adj*.

chiromancy /'kaɪroʊ,mænsi/ *n* palmistry.—**chiromancer** *n*.

chiropody /kɪ'rɒpədi/ or /ʃɪ-/ *n* the care and treatment of the feet.—**chiropodist** *n*.

chiropractic /,kaɪroʊ'præktɪk/ *n* the manipulation of joints, *esp* of the spine, to alleviate nerve pressure as a method of curing disease.—**chiropractor** *n*.

chirp /tʃɜrp/ *n* the sharp, shrill note of some bird or a grasshopper. • *vi* to make this sound.—**chirper** *n*.

chirpy /'tʃɜrpi/ *adj* (**chirpier, chirpiest**) lively, cheerful.—**chirpily** *adv.*—**chirpiness** *n*.

chirr /tʃɜr/ *n* the shrill rasping sound of a grasshopper. • *vi* to make this sound.—*also* **churr**.

chirrup /'tʃɜrəp/ *vi* (*birds*) to twitter; to make a clicking sound to a horse. • *n* chirruping sound.—**chirruper** *n.*—**chirrupy** *adj*.

chisel /'tʃɪzəl/ *n* a tool with a square cutting end. • *vt* (**chiselling, chiselled** *or* **chiseling, chiseled**) to cut or carve with a chisel; (*sl*) to defraud.—**chiseller** *n*.

chit[1] /tʃɪt/ *n* a voucher or a sum owed for drink, food, etc; a note; a requisition.

chit[2] *n* a child; (*derog*) an impudent girl.

chitchat /'tʃɪttʃæt/ *n* gossip, trivial talk.

chitin /'kaɪtɪn/ *n* the white horny substance that forms the outer covering of many invertebrate animals.—**chitinoid** *adj.*—**chitinous** *adj*.

chiton /'kaɪtən/ *n* in ancient Greece, a knee-length tunic; a full-length woman's dress; a genus of molluscs.

chitterlings /'tʃɪtər,lɪŋz/, **chitlins** /'tʃɪtlɪnz/, **chitlings** /'tʃɪtlɪŋz/ *npl* the small edible entrails of pigs.

chivalrous /'ʃɪvəlrəs/ *adj* relating to chivalry; war-like; high-spirited; brave, gallant; generous to the weak.—**chivalrously** *adv*.

chivalry /'ʃɪvəlri/ *n* (*pl* **chivalries**) the medieval system of knighthood; knightly qualities, bravery, courtesy, respect for women.—**chivalric** *adj.*—**chivalrous** *adj.*—**chivalrously** *adv*.

chive /tʃaɪv/, **chives** /tʃaɪvz/ *n* a plant whose onion-flavoured leaves are used in cooking and salads.

chivvy, chivy /'tʃɪvi/ *vt* (**chivvying, chivvied** *or* **chivying, chivied**) to annoy, harass, nag.

chloral (hydrate) /'klɔrəl/ *n* a bitter white crystalline compound used as a sedative or anaesthetic.

chlorate /'klɔreɪt/ *n* a salt of chloric acid.

chlor-, chloro- /'klɔro/ *prefix* green.

chloric /'klɔrɪk/ *adj* pertaining to or containing chlorine.

chloric acid *n* an acid containing hydrogen, oxygen, and chlorine.

chloride /'klɔraɪd/ *n* any compound containing chlorine.—**chloridic** *adj*.

chloride of lime *n* a compound of chlorine with lime used in bleaching.

chlorinate /'klɔrə,neɪt/ *vt* to treat or combine with chlorine; to disinfect with chlorine.—**chlorination** *n*.

chlorine /'klɔriːn/ or /'klɔr-/ *n* a nonmetallic element, a yellowish-green poisonous gas used in bleaches, disinfectants, and in industry.

chloro-, chlor- /'klɔro/ *prefix* green.

chlorofluorocarbon /,klɔroʊ'fluːroʊ,kɑrbən/ *n* any of various compounds containing carbon, chlorine, fluorine and hydrogen, used in refrigerants, aerosol propellants, etc, and thought to be harmful to the earth's atmosphere.

chloroform /'klɔrə,fɔrm/ *n* a colourless volatile liquid formerly used as an anaesthetic.

chlorophyll, chlorophyl /'klɔrəfɪl/ *n* the green photosynthetic colouring matter in plants.

chlorosis /klə'roʊsɪs/ or /klɔr-/ *n* a disease affecting young women, characterized by anaemia.—**chlorotic** *adj*.

chock /tʃɒk/ *n* a block of wood or other material used as a wedge. • *vt* to secure with a chock.

chock-a-block /'tʃɒkə,blɒk/ *adj* completely full.—*also* **chock-full**.

chocolate /'tʃɒklət/ or /'tʃɜkələt/ *n* a powder or edible solid made of the roasted, pounded cacao bean; a drink made by dissolving this powder in boiling water or milk; a sweet with a centre and chocolate coating. • *adj* flavoured or coated with chocolate; dark reddish brown.—**chocolaty** *adj*.

chocolate-box *adj* sweetly pretty; oversentimental.

choice /tʃɔɪs/ *n* act of choosing; the power to choose; selection; alternative; a thing chosen; preference; the best part. • *adj* of picked quality, specially good.—**choicely** *adv.*—**choiceness** *n*.

choir /kwaɪr/ *n* an organized group of singers, *esp* of a church; the part of a church before the altar used by them.

choirboy /'kwaɪr,bɔɪ/ *n* one of the young trebles in a choir.

choirmaster /-,mæstər/ *n* one who trains and conducts the singers in a choir.

choke /tʃoʊk/ *vti* to stop the breath of, stifle; to throttle; to suffocate; to block (up); to check, *esp* emotion, to choke back or up. • *n* a fit of choking; a choking sound; a valve that controls the flow of air in a carburettor.

chokebore /'tʃoʊk,bɔr/ *n* a shotgun with a bore narrowing towards the muzzle.

chokedamp /-,dæmp/ *n* carbonic acid gas generated in mines.

choker /-ər/ *n* a necklace worn tight round the neck; a high collar.

chole- /'kɒlər/ *n* bile; irascibility, anger.

cholera /'kɒlərə/ *n* a severe, infectious intestinal disease.

choleric /'kɒlərɪk/ *adj* irascible; tending to anger; angry.

cholesterol /kə'lɛstə,rɒl/ **cholesterin** *n* a substance found in animal tissues, blood and animal fats, thought to be a cause of hardening of the arteries.

chomp /tʃɒmp/ *vt* to chew noisily and with relish, champ.

chondr-, chondri-, chondro- /'kɒndro/ *prefix* cartilage.

chondrify /-faɪ/ *vti* (**chondrifying, chondrified**) to change into cartilage.—**chondrification** *n*.

choose /tʃuːz/ *vb* (**choosing, chose**, *pp* **chosen**) *vt* to select (one thing) rather than another. • *vi* to decide, to think fit.—**chooser** *n*.

choosy /'tʃuːzi/ *adj* (**choosier, choosiest**) (*inf*) cautious, fussy, particular.—**choosily** *adv.*—**choosiness** *n*.

chop /tʃɒp/ *vt* (**chopping, chopped**) to cut by striking; to cut into pieces. • *n* a cut of meat and bone from the rib, loin, or shoulder; a downward blow or motion; **get the chop** (*sl*) to be dismissed from one's employment; to be killed.

chop *n* a mark or brand denoting quality.

chopfallen /'tʃɒp,fɔlən/ *see* **chapfallen**.

chopper /'tʃɒpər/ *n* a tool for chopping; a cleaver; a small hand axe; (*sl*) a helicopter.

choppy /-i/ *adj* (**choppier, choppiest**) (*sea*) running in rough, irregular waves; jerky.—**choppily** *adv.*—**choppiness** *n*.

chops /tʃɒps/ *npl* the jaws or cheeks.

chopsticks /'tʃɒpstɪks/ *n* a pair of wooden or plastic sticks used in Asian countries to eat with.

chop suey /tʃɒp'suːi/ *n* a Chinese-American dish consisting of stir-fried vegetables and meat or seafood served with rice.

choral[1] /'kɔrəl/ *adj* relating to, sung by, or written for, a choir or chorus.—**chorally** *adv*.

choral², **chorale** /kər'æl/ n a slow hymn or psalm sung to a traditional or composed melody, esp by a choir.

chord¹ /kɔrd/ n (mus) three or more notes played simultaneously.—**chordal** adj.

chord² n a straight line joining the ends of an arc; a feeling of sympathy, recognition or remembering (strike a chord).

chore /tʃɔr/ n a piece of housework; a regular or tedious task.

chorea /kə'riə/ n a neurological disorder characterized by jerky involuntary movements, esp of the arms, legs and face.—**choreal, choreic** adj.

choreograph /'kɔriə,græf/ vt to devise the steps for a ballet, dance, etc.

choreography /'kɔri'ɒgrəfi/ n the art of devising ballets or dances.—**choreographer** n.—**choreographic** adj.—**choreographically** adv.

choric /'kɔrik/ adj of or for a Greek chorus.

chorion /'kɔriən/ n the exterior membrane of a seed or foetus.—**chorionic, chorial** adj.

chorister /'kɔristər/ n a member of a choir.

chorizo /tʃə'ri:zo:/ n (pl chorizos) a spicy pork sausage.

chorography /ko:'rɒgrəfi/ or /kə-/ n the geographical description of a region.—**chorographer** n.—**chorographic, chorographical** adj.

choroid /'kɔrɔid/ n the vascular membrane of the retina.

chorology /ko:'rɒlədʒi/ n the study of the geographical distribution of plants and animals.

chortle /'tʃɔrtəl/ vi to chuckle exultantly.—also n.

chorus /'kɔrəs/ n (pl choruses) a group of singers and dancers in the background to a play, musical, etc; a group of singers, a choir; music sung by a chorus; a refrain; an utterance by many at once. • vt (chorusing, chorused) to sing, speak or shout in chorus.

chorus girl n one who sings and dances in the chorus of a musical.—**chorus boy** nm.

chose /tʃoːz/, **chosen** /'tʃoːzən/ see choose.

chough /tʃʌf/ n a red-legged crow.

chow /tʃaʊ/ n a breed of thick-coated dog, originally from China.—also chow chow; (sl) food.

chowder /'tʃaʊdər/ n a thick clam and potato soup.

chow mein /,tʃaʊ'meɪn/ n a Chinese-American dish of fried, crispy noodles with meat and vegetables.

chrestomathy /krɛs'tɒməθi/ n (pl chrestomathies) a collection of extracts for learning a foreign language; a phrasebook; an anthology.

chrism /'krɪzəm/ n consecrated oil.—**chrismal** adj.

chrisom /'krɪzəm/ n an infant's baptismal robe.

Christ /kraɪst/ n Jesus of Nazareth, regarded by Christians as the Messiah.

christen /'krɪsən/ vt to enter the Christian Church by baptism; to give a name to; (inf) to use for the first time.—**christener** n.—**christening** n.

Christendom /'krɪsəndəm/ n all Christians, or Christian countries regarded as a whole.

Christian /'krɪstʃən/ n a person who believes in Christianity. • adj relating to, believing in, or based on the doctrines of Christianity; kind, gentle, humane.

Christian Era n the present era reckoned from the birth of Christ.

Christianity /,krɪstʃi'ænəti/ or /-ti'æn-/ n the religion based on the teachings of Christ.

Christianize /'krɪstʃə,naɪz/ vt to convert to Christianity.—**Christianization** n.—**Christianizer** n.

Christianly adj like or befitting a Christian.

Christian name n a name given when one is christened; (loosely) any forename.

Christian Science n a system of religion founded by Mary Baker Eddy, 1866, in which sin and disease are regarded as mental errors to be overcome by faith.—**Christian Scientist** n.

Christlike /'kraɪst,laɪk/ adj resembling Christ.

Christmas /'krɪsməs/ n (pl Christmases) an annual festival (25 December) in memory of the birth of Christ.

Christmas card n a greeting card, usu decorative, sent at Christmas.

Christmas Eve n the day and esp the night before Christmas Day.

Christmas rose n the black hellebore.

Christmastide n Christmas Eve (24 December) to Epiphany (6 January).

Christmas tree n an evergreen tree decorated at Christmas; an imitation tree.

Christology /krɪs'tɒlədʒi/ n the branch of theology that studies Christ's nature.—**Christological** adj.—**Christologist** n.

chrom-, chromo- /krɔːm/ prefix colour.

chromate /'krɔː,meɪt/ n a salt or ester of chromic acid.

chromatic /krɔː'mætɪk/ adj of or in colour; (mus) using tones outside the key in which the passage is written.—**chromatically** adv.—**chromaticism** n.

chromatics n sing the science of colour.

chromatic scale n a twelve-note musical scale that proceeds by semitones.

chromatin /'krɔːmətɪn/ n a protoplasmic substance in a cell nucleus forming chromosomes.—**chromatinic** adj.

chromatography /,krɔːmə'tɒgrəfi/ n the separation of the components of a substance by passing it over or through a substance that absorbs selectively.—**chromatograph** n.—**chromatographer** n.—**chromatographic** adj.—**chromatographically** adv.

chrome /krɔːm/ n chromium; a chromium pigment; something plated with an alloy of chromium.

-chrome /krɔːm/ adj suffix coloured. • n suffix colour, pigment.

chrome green n a green pigment made from a compound of chromium.

chrome red n a red pigment made from a compound of chromium.

chrome yellow n a yellow pigment made from a compound of chromium.

chromic /'krɔːmɪk/ adj of chromium.

chromium /'krɔːmiːəm/ n a hard metallic element used in making steel alloys and electroplating to give a tough surface.

chromo-, chrom- /'krɔːmoː/ prefix colour.

chromogen /'krɔːmədʒən/ n the colouring matter of plants.—**chromogenic** adj.

chromolithography /,krɔːmoːlɪ'θɒgrəfi/ n the art of printing in colours from stone.—**chromolithograph** n.—**chromolithographer** n.—**chromolithographic** adj.

chromosome /'krɔːmə,soːm/ n any of the microscopic rod-shaped bodies bearing genes.

chromosphere /-,sfiːr/ n the rose-coloured outer gaseous envelope of the sun above the photosphere.—**chromospheric** adj.

chron- /krɒn/, **chrono-** /-ə/ prefix time.

chronic /'krɒnɪk/ adj (disease) long-lasting; regular; habitual.—**chronically** adv.—**chronicity** n.

chronicle /'krɒnɪkəl/ n a record of events in chronological order; an account; a history. • vt to record in a chronicle.—**chronicler** n.

chronogram /'krɒnə,græm/ n an inscription which includes in it the date of some event.—**chronogrammatic, chronogrammatical** adj.

chronograph /'krɒnə,græf/ or /'krɔːnə-/ n an instrument for recording minute intervals of time; a stopwatch.—**chronographer** n.—**chronographic** adj.

chronologic /'krɒnə,lɒdʒɪk/, **chronological** /,krɒnə'lɒdʒɪkəl/ adj arranged in order of occurrence.—**chronologically** adv.

chronology /'krɒnə,lədʒi/ n (pl chronologies) the determination of the order of events, eg in history; the arrangement of events in order of occurrence; a table of events listed in order of occurrence.—**chronologist** n.

chronometer /-,nɒmətər/ n a very accurate instrument for measuring time exactly.

chronometry /-,nɒmətri/ n the scientific measurement of time.—**chronometric, chronometrical** adj.—**chronometrically** adv.

chronoscope /'krɒnə,skoːp/ n an instrument for measuring by electricity the velocity of a projectile.—**chronoscopic** adj.

chrys- /kraɪs/, **chryso-** /-ə/ prefix gold.

chrysalis /'krɪsəlɪs/ n (pl chrysalises, chrysalides) the pupa of a moth or butterfly, enclosed in a cocoon.

chrysanthemum /krɪ'sænθəməm/ n a plant with a brightly coloured flower head.

chryselephantine /,krɪsɛlə'fæntaɪn/ adj composed (or overlaid) partly with gold and partly with ivory.

chrysoberyl /'krɪsə,bɛrəl/ n a yellowish-green gem.

chrysolite /'krɪsə,laɪt/ n a green-coloured and sometimes transparent gem.—**chrysolitic** adj.

chrysoprase /-,preɪz/ n a variety of chalcedony of an apple-green colour.

chthonian /'kθoːniən/ or /'θɒ:-/ **chthonic** /'kθɒnɪk/ or /'θɒnɪk/ adj (Greek gods) of the underworld, as opposed to Olympian.

chub /tʃʌb/ n (pl **chub, chubs**) a small freshwater fish of the carp family.

chubby /'tʃʌbi/ adj (**chubbier, chubbiest**) plump.—**chubbiness** n.

chuck[1] /tʃʌk/ vt to throw, to toss; (inf) to stop, to give up. • n (usu with **the**) a giving up; dismissal.

chuck[2] n a device on a lathe, etc, that holds the work or drill; a cut of beef from the neck to the ribs.

chuck[3] vt to make a noise like a hen calling to her chickens. • n a hen's call.

chuck[4] n (dial) darling.

chuck[5] n ✳ on the Pacific Northwest coast of North America, a large body of water.

chuckle /'tʃʌkəl/ vt to laugh softly; to gloat. • n a quiet laugh.—**chuckler** n.

chuck wagon n a provision cart.

chuff[1] /tʃʌf/ n a surly fellow, a boor.

chuff[2] vi to make a puffing sound, as a steam engine. • n such a sound.

chug /tʃʌg/ n the explosive sound of a car exhaust, etc. • vi (**chugging, chugged**) to make such a sound.

chukker /'tʃʌkər/, **chukka** /'tʃʌkə/ n each period of play in a game of polo.

chum[1] /tʃʌm/ n (inf) a close friend, esp of the same sex. • vi (**chumming, chummed**) to be friendly (with); to room together.

chum[2] n ✳ a Salmon of the Pacific Northwest coast of North America.

chummy /'tʃʌmi/ adj (**chummier, chummiest**) friendly, close to.—**chummily** adv.—**chumminess** n.

chump /tʃʌmp/ n (inf) a stupid person; a fool.

chunk /tʃʌŋk/ n a short, thick piece or lump, as wood, bread, etc.—**chunky** adj.

chunky /'tʃʌŋki/ adj (**chunkier, chunkiest**) short and thick; (clothing) of heavy material.—**chunkily** adv.—**chunkiness** n.

Chunnel /'tʃʌnəl/ n (inf) the Channel Tunnel linking England and France.

church /tʃɜrtʃ/ n a building for public worship, esp Christian worship; the clerical profession; a religious service; (with cap) all Christians; (with **the**) a particular Christian denomination.

churchgoer /-ˌgoʊər/ n one who goes to church regularly.—**churchgoing** adj, n.

churchman /-mən/ n (pl **churchmen**) a member of the Church; a clergyman.—**churchwoman** n (pl **churchwomen**).

churchwarden /-'wɔrdən/ n in the Anglican church, an elected lay representative who administers the secular matters of a parish church.

churchyard /-jɑrd/ n the yard around a church often used as a burial ground.

churl /tʃɜrl/ n formerly one of the lowest orders of freemen; a peasant; a surly ill-bred person.

churlish /'tʃɜrlɪʃ/ adj surly, ill-mannered.—**churlishly** adv.—**churlishness** n.

churn /tʃɜrn/ n a large metal container for milk; a device that can be vigorously turned to make milk or cream into butter. • vt to agitate in a churn; to make (butter) this way; to stir violently; (with **out**) (inf) to produce quickly or one after the other or without much effort.

churr /tʃɜr/ see **chirr**.

chute /ʃuːt/ n an inclined trough or a passage for sending down water, logs, rubbish, etc; a fall of water, a rapid; an inclined slide for children; a slide into a swimming pool.

chutney /'tʃʌtni/ n a relish of fruits, spices, and herbs.

chutzpah, chutzpa /'hʊtzpə/ or /-ʔets-/, /xuːts-/, /-pɒ/ n shameless audacity, presumption, or gall.

chyle /kaɪl/ n a milk-like fluid separated from digested matter in the stomach, absorbed by the lacteal vessels and assimilated into the blood.—**chylaceous, chylous** adj.

chyme /kaɪm/ n the pulpy mass of digested food prior to the separation of the chyle.

CI abbr ✳ (Cdn) = Collegiate Institute.

Ci (symbol) curie.

CIA /ˌsiːaɪ'eɪ/ abbr = Central Intelligence Agency.

ciao It. /tʃaʊ/ interj used to express greeting or farewell.

ciborium /sə'bɔriəm/ n (pl **ciboria**) a covered chalice for holding the sacrament; a canopy over an altar.

cicada /sɪ'keɪdə/ or /-'kɑdə/, **cicala** /-lə/ n (pl **cicadas, cicadae** or **cicalas, cicale**) a large fly-like insect with transparent wings, the male producing a loud chirp or drone.

cicatrix /ˈsɪkətrɪks/ n (pl **cicatrices**) the scar remaining after a wound has healed; a sca-like mark.—**cicatricial** adj.—**cicatricose** adj.

cicatrize /'sɪkəˌtraɪz/ vt to heal a wound by inducing the skin to form a cicatrix; to mark with scars.—**cicatrization** n.—**cicatrizer** n.

cicely /'sɪsəli/ n (pl **cicelies**) a species of umbelliferous plants allied to chervil.

cicerone /'sɪsəˌroːni/ n (pl **cicerones, ciceroni**) a guide who explains the antiquities and chief features of a place.

CID /ˌsiːaɪ'diː/ abbr = Criminal Investigation Department.

-cide /saɪd/ n suffix killing, or killer of, as in regicide.

cider /ˈsaɪdər/ n fermented apple juice as a drink.

cigar /sɪ'gɑr/ n a compact roll of tobacco leaf for smoking.

cigarette /ˌsɪgə'ret/ or /'sɪgəret/ n shredded tobacco rolled in fine paper for smoking.

cilia /'sɪliə/ npl (sing **cilium**) the hair of the eyelids; long minute hair-like appendages on the margins of vegetable bodies; the minute vibrating filaments lining or covering certain organs.—**ciliated** adj.

cilice /'sɪlɪs/ n haircloth.

Cimmerian /sɪ'mɪriən/ adj intensely dark; gloomy; pertaining to the Cimmerii, a legendary people mentioned by Homer as living in perpetual darkness.

C in C abbr = Commander in Chief.

cinch /sɪntʃ/ n (sl) a firm hold, an easy job; a saddle band or girth.

cinchona /sɪŋ'koːnə/ n a South American tree that yields quinine and other drugs.

cinchonism /'sɪŋkəˌnɪzəm/ n a medical condition characterized by buzzing in the ears, deafness, etc, caused by the excessive use of quinine.

cincture /'sɪŋktʃər/ n a belt or girdle worn round the waist; a raised or carved ring at the bottom and top of a pillar.

cinder /'sɪndər/ n a tiny piece of partly burned wood, etc; (pl) ashes from wood or coal.—**cindery** adj.

cine- /'sɪneɪ/ or /'sɪni/ prefix motion picture or cinema, as in cinecamera, cinefilm.

cineast, cineaste /'sɪneɪ,æst/ or /'sɪni-/, Fr. /siːnɒ'æst/ n a film enthusiast.

cinema /'sɪnəmə/ n a place where motion pictures are shown; film as an industry or art form.—**cinematic** adj.—**cinematically** adv.

cinematography /ˌsɪnəmə'tɒgrəfi/ n the art or science of motion-picture photography.—**cinematographic** adj.—**cinematographer** n.

cinéma vérité /ˌsɪneɪ,məveri'teɪ/ n cinema photography of real-life scenes and situations, etc, to create realism.

cineraria /ˌsɪnə'rɛəriə/ n a genus of garden plants of the aster family with bright flowers.

cinerarium /-iəm/ n (pl **cineraria**) a place for keeping a person's ashes after cremation.

cinerary /ˌsɪnə'rɛəri/ adj of, pertaining to, or containing, ashes.

cinereous /sɪ'nɪəriəs/ adj ash-grey.

cingulum /'sɪŋgjʊləm/ n (pl **cingula**) belt.

cinnabar /'sɪnəˌbɑr/ n red sulphide of mercury. • adj vermilion.

cinnamon /'sɪnəmən/ n a tree of the laurel family; its aromatic edible bark; a spice made from this; a yellowish-brown colour. • adj yellowish brown.—**cinnamonic, cinamic** adj.

cinnamon stone n a variety of the garnet.

cinque /sɪŋk/ n a five at dice or cards.

cinquecento /ˌtʃɪŋkwɪ'tʃento/ n the 16th century and Italian fine art of that period. • adj designed or executed in such Italian style.

cinquefoil /'sɪŋkfɔɪl/ n a plant with leaves divided into five lobes; (archit) ornamentation resembling five leaves.

cipaille /si'paɪ/ n ✳ (Cdn) a pie made up of alternating layers of meat and vegetables.

cipher /'saɪfər/ n the numeral 0, zero; any single Arabic numeral; a thing or person of no importance, a nonentity; a method of secret writing. • vt to convert (a message) into cipher.—also **cypher**.

circa /'sɜrkə/ prep about.

circadian /sər'keɪdiən/ adj of or pertaining to biological processes that occur in 24-hour cycles.

circinate /'sɜrsɪˌneɪt/ adj (leaf) rolled up with the tip inwards.

circle /'sɜrkəl/ n a perfectly round plane figure; the line enclosing it; anything (built) in the form of a circle; the curved seating area above the stalls in a theatre; a group, set or class (of people); extent, scope, as of influence. • vti to encompass; to move in a circle; to revolve (round); to draw a circle round.—**circler** n.

circlet /'sərklət/ *n* a small circle; a circular band or hoop.

circuit /'sərkɪt/ *n* a distance round; a route or course; an area so enclosed; the path of an electric current; a visit to a particular area by a judge to hold courts; the area itself; a chain or association, eg of cinemas controlled by one management; sporting events attended regularly by the same competitors and at the same venues; a motor-racing track.—**circuital** *adj*.

circuit breaker *n* a switch that interrupts an electric circuit under certain abnormal conditions.

circuitous /sər'kjuːɪtəs/ *adj* roundabout, indirect.—**circuitously** *adv*.

circuitry /'sərkətri/ *n* (*pl* **circuitries**) the plan of an electric circuit; the components of a circuit.

circular /'sərkjulər/ *adj* shaped like a circle, round; (*argument*) using as evidence the conclusion which it is seeking to prove; moving round a circle. • *n* an advertisement, etc addressed to a number of people.—**circularity, circularness** *n*.

circularize /-julə,raɪz/ *vt* to make circular; to send circulars to; to canvass.—**circularization** *n*.—**circularizer** *n*.

circular saw *n* a power-driven saw with a circular blade.

circulate /'sərkju,leɪt/ *vti* to pass from hand to hand or place to place; to spread or be spread about; to move round, finishing at the starting point.—**circulative** *adj*.—**circulator** *n*.—**circulatory** *adj*.

circulating decimal *n* the recurring decimal.

circulating library *n* a lending library.

circulation /,sərkju'leɪʃən/ *n* the act of circulating; a movement to and fro; the regular cycle of blood flow in the body; the number of copies sold of a newspaper, etc; currency.

circum- /'sərkəm/ or /sər'kəm/ *prefix* round, about.

circumambient /,sərkəm'æmbiənt/ *adj* enclosing, or being surrounded, on all sides.—**cicumambience, cicumabiency** *n*.

circumcise /'sərkəm,saɪz/ *vt* to cut off the foreskin of a male in a religious rite or for medical reasons; to cut off the clitoris and/or labia minora of a female for socio-cultural reasons.—*see* **clitoridectomy**.

circumcision /'sərkəm,sɪʒən/ *n* the act of circumcising; spiritual purification.

circumference /sər'kəmfərəns/ *n* the line bounding a circle, a ball, etc; the length of this line.—**circumferential** *adj*.

circumflex /'sərkəm,fleks/ *n* an accent (^) placed over a vowel to indicate contraction, length, etc.—**circumflexion** *n*.

circumfuse /,sərkəm'fjuːz/ *vt* to pour or spread around; to bathe (with).—**circumfusion** *n*.

circumlocution /-lə'kjuːʃən/ *n* the use of more words than are necessary; a roundabout or evasive expression.—**circumlocutory** *adj*.

circumnavigate /-'nævɪ,geɪt/ *vt* to sail or fly completely round (the world).—**circumnavigable** *adj*.—**circumnavigation** *n*.—**circumnavigator** *n*.

circumnutate /-nju:'teɪt/ *vi* (*bot*) to turn successively to all points of the compass.—**circumnutation** *n*.

circumpolar /-'poːlər/ *adj* near the north or south pole; (*astron*) always above the horizon.

circumscribe /'sərkəm,skraɪb/ *vt* to draw a line around; to enclose; to limit or restrict.—**circumscription** *n*.

circumspect /-,spekt/ *adj* prudent, cautious; careful; discreet.—**circumspection** *n*.—**circumspective** *adj*.

circumstance /-,stæns/ *n* an occurrence, an incident; a detail; ceremony; (*pl*) a state of affairs; condition in life.

circumstantial /,sərkəm'stænʃəl/ *adj* detailed; incidental; (*law*) strongly inferred from direct evidence.—**circumstantially** *adv*.

circumstantiality /-,stænʃi'ælɪti/ *n* (*pl* **circumstantialities**) the state of being circumstantial; fullness of detail.

circumstantiate /-'stænʃi,eɪt/ *vt* to describe or verify in detail.—**circumstantiation** *n*.

circumvallate /-'væl,eɪt/ *vt* to surround with a rampart.—**circumvallation** *n*.

circumvent /,sərkəm'vent/ *vt* to evade, bypass; to outwit.—**circumventer, circumventor** *n*.—**circumvention** *n*.

circumvolution /-və'luːʃən/ *n* the act of rolling round; the state of being rolled round; a coil.—**circumvolutory** *adj*.

circus /'sərkəs/ *n* (*pl* **circuses**) a large arena for the exhibition of games, feats of horsemanship, etc; a travelling show of acrobats, clowns, etc; a company of people travelling round giving displays; houses built in a circle; an open space in a town where streets meet; (*inf*) noise, disturbance; loud, extravagant behaviour.

cirque /sərk/ *n* a natural amphitheatre or ring.

cirrhosis /sɪ'roːsɪs/ *n* a hardened condition of the tissues of an organ, *esp* the liver.—**cirrhosed** *adj*.—**cirrhotic** *adj*.

cirriped /'sɪrɪ,ped/, **cirripede** /'sɪrɪ,piːd/ *adj* having feet resembling cirri; pertaining to the Cirripedia, a subclass of parasitic crustaceans, as the barnacles and acorn shells.

cirrocumulus /,sɪro'kjuːmjuləs/ *n* (*pl* **cirrocumuli**) a cloud broken up into small fleecy masses.

cirrostratus /-'strætəs/ *n* (*pl* **cirrostrati**) a horizontal or slightly inclined light fleecy cloud.

cirrouse, cirrous /'sɪrəs/ *adj* terminating in a curl, tuft, or tendril.

cirrus /'sɪrəs/ *n* (*pl* **cirri**) thin, wispy clouds.

CIS /'siː'aɪ'es/ *abbr* = Commonwealth of Independent States: a federation of former Soviet republics, such as Russia, Ukraine, who wish to retain voluntary links with one another.

cis- /sɪs/ *prefix* on this side of.

cisalpine /sɪs'æl,paɪn/ *adj* this side of the Alps with regard to Rome, south of the Alps.

cisco /'sɪskoː/ *n* (*pl* **ciscoes, ciscos**) the Canadian lake herring; ♣ (*Cdn*) a North American freshwater whitefish.

cismontane /sɪs'mɒn,teɪn/ *adj* on this (northern) side of the Alps.

cist /sɪst/ or /kɪst/ *n* a prehistoric stone tomb consisting of two rows of stone and covered with a flat stone slab; a box or chest.

Cistercian /sɪs'tərʃən/ *n* one of a Benedictine order of monks, founded 1098 at Citeaux, France. • *adj* pertaining to the Cistercians.

cistern /'sɪstərn/ *n* a tank or reservoir for storing water, *esp* in a toilet.

citadel /'sɪtədel/ or /-dəl/ *n* a fortress in or near a city.

citation /saɪ'teɪʃən/ *n* a quotation; a source or authority cited; a commendation, *esp* for bravery; (*law*) a summons to appear.

cite /saɪt/ *vt* to summon officially to appear in court; to quote; to give as an example or authority.—**citable, citeable** *adj*.

cithara /'sɪθərə/ *n* an ancient lyre.—*also* **kithara**.

citify /'sɪtɪ,faɪ/ *vt* (**citifying, citifed**) to assume city ways, habits, dress.

citizen *n* a member of a city, state or nation.—**citizenship** *n*.

Citizenship Court *n* ♣ (*Cdn*) a federal court that awards Canadian citizenship.

citizenry /'sɪtɪzənri/ *n* (*pl* **citizenries**) citizens collectively.

citizen's band *n* a shortwave band reserved for private radio communication.

citrate /'sɪtreɪt/ *n* a salt or ester of citric acid.

citric /'sɪtrɪk/ *adj* of or obtained from citrus fruits or citric acid.

citric acid *n* a sour acid found in fruits and used as a flavouring.

citrine /-trɪn/ or /-,triːn/ *adj* lemon-coloured.

citron /-trən/ *n* a large fruit-like a lemon; the tree bearing it; a yellow-green colour.

citronella /,sɪtrə'nelə/ *n* a fragrant Asian grass which yields an aromatic oil used in soap, perfumes, and in insect repellents.

citrus /'sɪtrəs/ *n* (*pl* **citruses**) a genus of trees including the lemon, orange, etc; the fruit of these trees. • *adj* of or relating to citrus trees or shrubs or their fruit.

cittern /'sɪtərn/ *n* a medieval stringed instrument.

city /'sɪti/ *n* (*pl* **cities**) an important or cathedral town; a town created a city by charter; the people of a city; business circles, *esp* financial services.—*also* **adj**.

city editor *n* the editor in charge of local news.

city fathers *npl* the people who take part in running a city.

city hall *n* the townhall; the government of a city or its officers; (*inf*) bureaucracy.

city slicker *n* (*inf*) one who adopts city ways; a suave, unreliable person.

city-state /-,steɪt/ *n* (*hist*) a sovereign state comprising a city and its surrounding territory.

civet /'sɪvət/ *n* a cat-like animal of central Africa and South Asia; the pungent substance secreted by this animal used in perfumery.

civic /'sɪvɪk/ *adj* of a city, citizen or citizenship. • *npl* the principles of good citizenship; the study of citizenship.—**civically** *adv*.

civic holiday *n* ♣ (*Cdn*) a public holiday held in most Canadian provinces, *usu* on the first Monday in August.

civil /'sɪvəl/ *adj* of citizens or the state; not military or ecclesiastical; polite, obliging; (*law*) relating to crimes other than criminal ones or to private rights.—**civilly** *adv*.

civil defence *n* the organization of civilians against enemy attack.

civil disobedience *n* refusal to pay taxes, etc, as part of a political campaign; nonviolent protest to achieve an end.

civil engineer *n* an engineer who designs and constructs roads, bridges, etc.

civilian /sɪ'vɪljən/ n a person who is not a member of the armed forces.

civility /sɪ'vɪlɪti/ n (pl **civilities**) good manners, politeness.

civil rights npl the personal rights of a citizen.

civil service n those employed in the service of a state apart from the military.—**civil servant** n.

civil war n a war between citizens of the same state or country.

civilization /ˌsɪvɪlaɪ'zeɪʃən/ n the state of being civilized; the process of civilizing; an advanced stage of social culture; moral and cultural refinement.

civilize /'sɪvɪˌlaɪz/ vt to bring out from barbarism to educate in arts and refinements.—**civilizer** n.

civilized /'sɪvɪˌlaɪzd/ adj no longer in a savage or uncultured state.

civvy /'sɪvɪ/ adj (sl) civilian. • n (pl **civvies**) (sl) civilian clothes.

Cl (chem symbol) = chlorine.

cl abbr = centilitre(s).

clack /klæk/ vt to make a sudden, sharp sound; to chatter rapidly and continuously. • n a sudden, sharp sound as of wood striking wood.

clad[1] /klæd/ see **clothe**.

clad[2] vt (**cladding, clad**) to bond one material to another for protection (iron cladding).—**cladding** n.

claim /kleɪm/ vt to demand as a right; to call for to require; to profess (to have); to assert; to declare to be true. • n the act of claiming; a title, right to something; a thing claimed, esp a piece of land for mining.—**claimable** adj.—**claimer** n.

claimant /-mənt/ n a person who makes a claim.

clairvoyance /kler'vɔɪəns/ n the power of seeing things not present to the senses, second sight.

clairvoyant /kler'vɔɪənt/ n a person with the gift of clairvoyance. • adj possessing clairvoyance; having remarkable insight.

clam /klæm/ n edible marine bivalve mollusc. • vb (**clamming, clammed**) vt to gather clams. • vi (with **up**) (inf) to remain silent, refuse to talk.

clamant /'kleɪmənt/ adj insistent, crying; clamorous.

clambake /'klæmbeɪk/ n clams baked with seaweed; a picnic at which baked clams form the chief dish.

clamber /'klæmbər/ or /'klæmər/ vi to climb with difficulty, using the hands as well as the feet. • n a climb performed in this way.—**clamberer** n.

clammy /'klæmɪ/ adj (**clammier, clammiest**) damp and sticky.—**clammily** adv.—**clamminess** n.

clamour, clamor /'klæmər/ n a loud confused noise; an uproar; an insistent demand. • vi to demand loudly; to make an uproar.—**clamorous** adj.

clamp /klæmp/ n a device for gripping objects tightly together. • vt to grip with a clamp; to attach firmly. • vi (with **down**) to put a stop to forcefully. • vt to attach a wheelclamp to a wheel to immobilize an illegally parked car.

clan /klæn/ n a group of people with a common ancestor, under a single chief; people with the same surname; a party or clique.

clandestine /klæn'destɪn/ or /-taɪn/ adj done secretly; surreptitious; sly.—**clandestinely** adv.

clang /klæŋ/ n a loud metallic sound. • vti to make or cause to make a clang.

clangour, clangor /'klæŋər/ n a sharp clang; repeated clanging.—**clangourous, clangorous** adj.—**clangourously, clangorously** adv.

clank /klæŋk/ n a short, harsh metallic sound. • vt to make or cause to make a clank.

clannish /'klænɪʃ/ adj closely united and excluding others.—**clannishly** adv.

clansman /'klænzmən/ n (pl **clansmen**) a member of a clan.—**clanswoman** nf (pl **clanswomen**).

clap /klæp/ vti (**clapping, clapped**) to strike (the hands) together sharply; to applaud in this way; to slap (wings) loudly; to put or place suddenly or vigorously. • n the sound of hands clapping; a sudden sharp noise; a sudden sharp slap.

clapboard /'klæpbɔrd/ or /'klæbɔrd/ n a narrow thin board used for building by overlapping each piece.

clapper /'klæpər/ n the tongue of a bell.

claptrap /'klæptræp/ n flashy display, empty words.

claque /klæk/ n an organized body of people paid to applaud or express disapproval at theatres; interested admirers.

clarence /'klærəns/ or /'klerəns/ n a closed four-wheeled carriage with a curved front.

claret /'klærət/ or /'kle-/ n a dry red wine of Bordeaux in France; its purple-red colour.

claret cup n a summer drink composed of iced claret, lemon, brandy, etc.

clarify /'klærɪˌfaɪ/ or /'kle-/ vti (**clarifying, clarified**) to make or become clear or intelligible; to free or become free from impurities.—**clarification** n.—**clarifier** n.

clarinet /ˌklærɪ'net/ or /ˌkle-/ n an orchestral woodwind instrument.—**clarinettist** n.

clarion /'klæriən/ or /'kle-/ n a shrill trumpet formerly used in war; a rousing sound. • adj ringing.

clarity /'klærɪtɪ/ or /'kle-/ n clearness.

clarkia /'klarkiə/ n a bright-flowered garden plant.

clary /'kleri/ n (pl **claries**) meadow and wild sage.

clash /klæʃ/ n a loud noise of striking weapons, cymbals, etc; a contradiction, disagreement; a collision. • vti to make or cause to make a clash by striking together; to conflict; to collide; to be at variance (with); (colours) to be unsuitable or not pleasing when put together.—**clasher** n.

clasp /klæsp/ n a hold, an embrace; a catch or buckle. • vt to grasp firmly, to embrace; to fasten with a clasp.—**clasper** n.

clasp knife n a knife with a blade or blades that shut into the handle.

class /klæs/ n a division, a group; a kind; a set of students who are taught together; a grade of merit or quality; standing in society, rank; (inf) high quality, excellence; style. • vt to put into a class.

class-conscious adj aware of and taking part in the conflict between labouring and other classes.—**class-consciousness** n.

classic /'klæsɪk/ adj of the highest class or rank, esp in literature; of the best Greek and Roman writers; of music conforming to certain standards of form, complexity, etc; traditional; authoritative. • n a work of literature, art, cinema, etc of the highest excellence; a definitive work of art.

classical /'klæsɪkəl/ adj influenced by, of or relating to ancient Roman and Greek art, literature and culture; traditional; serious refined.—**classicality** n.—**classically** adv.

classical college n ✷ (Cdn) (hist) in Quebec, a private school that offered an eight-year program leading to a university undergraduate degree.

classicism /'klæsɪˌsɪzəm/, **classicalism** /'klæsɪkəˌlɪzəm/ n the use of ancient Roman and Greek style.

classicist /'klæsɪˌsɪst/, **classicalist** /'klæsɪkəˌlɪst/ n a scholar of the classics.—**classicistic** adj.

classics /'klæsɪks/ n (with **the**) the study of ancient Greek and Roman literature; any literature considered to be a model of its type.

classification /ˌklæsɪfɪ'keɪʃən/ n the organization of knowledge into categories; a category or a division of a category into which knowledge or information has been put.—**classificational** adj.—**classificatory** adj.

classified /'klæsɪˌfaɪd/ adj arranged by a system of classification; (information) secret and restricted to a select few; (advertisements) grouped according to type.

classify /'klæsɪˌfaɪ/ vt (**classifying, classified**) to arrange in classes, to categorize; to restrict for security reasons.—**classifiable** adj.—**classifier** n.

classless /'klæsləs/ adj not divided into classes; not belonging to a particular class.—**classlessness** n.

classmate /-meɪt/ n a member of the same class in a school, college, etc.

classroom /-ruːm/ n a room where pupils or students are taught.

classy /'klæsɪ/ adj (**classier, classiest**) (sl) stylish; elegant.—**classily** adv.—**classiness** n.

clastic /'klæstɪk/ adj (geol) composed of fragments.

clatter /'klætər/ n a rattling noise; noisy talk. • vti to make or cause a clatter.—**clattery** adj.

clause /klɔz/ n a single article or stipulation in a treaty, law, contract, etc; (gram) a short sentence; a division of a sentence.—**clausal** adj.

claustral /'klɔstrəl/ adj of or pertaining to a cloister, cloistral.

claustrophobia /ˌklɔstrə'fəʊbiə/ n a morbid fear of confined spaces.—**claustrophobe** n.—**claustrophobic** adj.—**claustrophobically** adv.

clavate /'kleɪveɪt/, **claviform** /-fɔrm/ adj club-shaped.

clavichord /'klævɪˌkɔrd/ n a medieval keyboard instrument, the predecessor of the piano.—**clavichordist** n.

clavicle /'klævkəl/ *n* one of the two bones that connect the shoulder blades with the breast bone, the collarbone.—**clavicular** *adj*.

clavier /'klævɪər/ *n* a musical instrument with a keyboard; the keyboard.

claw /klɒ/ *n* the sharp hooked nail of an animal or bird; the pointed end or pincer of a crab, etc; a claw-like thing. • *vti* to seize or tear with claws or nails; to clutch or scratch (at); (*with* **back**) to recover (something) with difficulty; to get back money by taxing; to take back part of what was handed out, *esp* by taxation.—**clawer** *n*.

claw hammer *n* a hammer with a claw for drawing out nails.

clay /kleɪ/ *n* a sticky ductile earthy material.—**clayey** *adj*.

claymore /'kleɪmɔr/ *n* a large two-edged sword formerly used in Scotland.

clay pigeon *n* a brittle clay disc or other object propelled into the air as a shooting target; someone in a vulnerable position.

CLC /'si:'ɛl'si:/ *abbr* ♣ = Canadian Labour Congress.

clean /kliːn/ *adj* free from dirt or impurities; unsoiled; morally or ceremonially pure; complete, decisive; free of errors; free of suggestive language; not carrying firearms or drugs. • *adv* entirely; outright; neatly. • *vti* to remove dirt from; (*with* **out**) to remove dirt out of; (*sl*) to take away everything from someone, *esp* money; (*with* **up**) to leave clean; (*sl*) to get rid of corrupt people, a system, etc; to gain a large profit.—**cleanable** *adj*.—**cleanness** *n*.

clean-cut /'kliːn,kʌt/ *adj* sharply defined, clear-cut; well-shaped.

cleaner /-ər/ *n* a substance or device used for cleaning; a person employed to clean; (*pl*) a dry cleaner.

clean-limbed *adj* having well-proportioned or shapely limbs.

cleanly /-li/ *adj* (**cleanlier, cleanliest**) clean in habits or person; pure; neat. • *adv* in a clean manner.—**cleanliness** *n*.

cleanse /klɛnz/ *vt* to make clean or pure.—**cleansable** *adj*.

cleanser /-ər/ *n* something that cleanses, *esp* a detergent, face cream, etc.

clear /kliːr/ *adj* bright, not dim; transparent; without blemish; easily seen or heard; unimpeded, open; free from clouds; quit (of); plain, distinct, obvious; keen, discerning; positive, sure; without debt. • *adv* plainly; completely; apart from. • *vti* to make or become clear; to rid (of), remove; to free from suspicion, vindicate; to disentangle; to pass by or over without touching; to make as a profit; (*with* **off**) (*inf*) to depart; (*with* **up**) to explain; to tidy up; (*weather*) to become fair.—**clearness** *n*.

clearance /'kliːrəns/ *n* the act of clearing; permission, authority to proceed; the space between two objects in motion.

clear-cut /'kliːr,kʌt/ *adj* having a sharp, clearly defined outline, as if chiselled; straightforward and open.

clear-headed /-,hɛdɪd/ *adj* showing sense, alertness, judgment.—**clear-headedly** *adv*.—**clear-headedness** *n*.

clearing /-ɪŋ/ *n* a tract of land cleared of trees, etc for cultivation.

clearing bank *n* a bank that uses a clearing house to exchange cheques and credits with other banks.

clearing house /-,həʊs/ *n* an office where cheques are sorted and exchanged by the clearing banks; a central agency for the collection, classification and distribution of information.

clearly /-li/ *adv* in a clear manner; evidently.

clear-sighted /-,sɔɪtɪd/ *adj* discerning, objective.

clearstory /-,stɔːri/ *see* **clerestory**.

cleat /kliːt/ *n* a wedge; a strip of wood nailed crossways to a footing, etc; a projection for making ropes fast to.

cleavage /'kliːvɪdʒ/ *n* the way a thing splits; divergence; the hollow between the breasts.

cleave[1] /kliːv/ *vti* (**cleaving, cleft, cleaved** *or* **clove,** *pp* **cleft, cleaved** *or* **cloven**) to divide by a blow; split; to sever.—**cleavable** *adj*.

cleave[2] *vi* (**cleaved, clave**) to be faithful to; to stick.

cleaver /'kliːvər/ *n* a butcher's heavy chopper.

cleavers /'kliːvərz/ *n* goose-grass.

cleek /kliːk/ *n* an iron-headed golf club with a narrow straight face; (*Scot*) a large hook or crook.

clef /klɛf/ *n* a sign on a music stave that indicates the pitch of the notes.

cleft /klɛft/ *n* a fissure or crack.

cleft palate *n* a congenital fissure of the hard palate in the roof of the mouth.

cleistogamy /klɔɪ'stɒɡæmi/ *n* (*bot*) self-fertilization without opening of the flower.—**cleistogamous, cleistogamic** *adj*.

clematis /'klɛmətɪs/ *or* /klə'mætɪs/ *n* a climbing plant with large colourful flowers.

clemency /'klɛmənsi/ *n* (*pl* **clemencies**) mercy, leniency; mildness, *esp* of weather.

clement /'klɛmənt/ *adj* merciful, gentle; (*weather*) mild.

clench /klɛntʃ/ *vt* (*teeth, fist*) to close tightly; to grasp. • *n* a firm grip.

clerestory /'kliːr,stɔri/ *or* /-stɔri/ *n* (*pl* **clerestories**) the upper story, with windows, of the nave of a church.—*also* **clearstory.**—**clerestoried, clearstoried** *adj*.

clergy /'klɜrdʒi/ *n* (*pl* **clergies**) ministers of the Christian church collectively.

clergyman /-,mən/ *n* (*pl* **clergymen**) a member of the clergy.

cleric /'klɛrɪk/ *n* a member of the clergy.

clerical /'klɛrɪkəl/ *adj* of or relating to the clergy or a clergyman; of or relating to a clerk or a clerk's work.—**clerically** *adv*.

clerical collar *n* a narrow stiff white collar buttoned at the back and worn by the clergy.—*also* **dog collar.**

clericalism /-,lɪzəm/ *n* clerical influence, *esp* of an undue kind.

clerihew /'klɛrɪ,hju:/ *n* a short nonsensical or satirical poem, *usu* in four lines of varying length, eg Sir Christopher Wren / Said, "I'm going to dine with some men. / If anyone calls, / Say I'm designing St Paul's."

clerk /klɑrk/ *n* an office worker who types, keeps files, etc; a layman with minor duties in a church; a public official who keeps the records of a court, town, etc.—**clerkdom** *n*.—**clerkship** *n*.

clerkly /-li/ *adj* (**clerklier, clerkliest**) pertaining to a clerk, or to penmanship. • *adv* in a scholarly manner.

clever /'klɛvər/ *adj* able; intelligent; ingenious; skilful, adroit.—**cleverly** *adv*.—**cleverness** *n*.

clew /klu:/ *n* a ball of thread; the corner of a sail to which a sheet is attached. • *vt* to truss up (sails) to the yard of a ship.

cliché /kli:'ʃeɪ/ *or* /'kli:-/ *n* a hackneyed phrase; something that has become commonplace.—**cliché'd, clichéd** *adj*.

click /klɪk/ *n* a slight, sharp sound. • *vi* to make such a sound; (*inf*) to establish immediate friendly relations with; to succeed; (*inf*) to become plain or evident; to fall into place.—**clicker** *n*.

client /'klaɪənt/ *n* a person who employs another professionally; a customer.—**cliental** *adj*.

clientele /,klaɪən'tɛl/ *or* /,kli:ɒn'tɛl/ *n* clients, customers.

cliff /klɪf/ *n* a high steep rock face.

cliffhanger /-,hæŋər/ *n* the perilous situation at the climax of each episode of a serialized film or book; any dramatic or suspenseful situation.—**cliffhanging** *adj*.

climacteric /klaɪ'mæktərɪk/ *or* /,klaɪmæk'tɛrɪk/ *n* a critical period, a turning point, *esp* in the life of an individual; the male menopause. • *adj* forming a crisis.—*also* **climacterical.**

climate /'klaɪmət/ *n* the weather characteristics of an area; the prevailing attitude, feeling, atmosphere.—**climatic, climatical, climatal** *adj*.

climatology /,klaɪmə'tɒlədʒi/ *n* the science of climates.—**climatologic, climatological** *adj*.—**climatologist** *n*.

climax /'klaɪmæks/ *n* the highest point; a culmination; sexual orgasm; the highlight or most interesting part of a story, drama or music. • *vti* to reach, or bring to a climax.—**climactic, climactical** *adj*.

climb /klaɪm/ *vti* to mount with an effort; to ascend; to rise; (*plants*) to grow upwards by clinging onto walls, fences or other plants; (*with* **down**) to descend from a higher level; to retreat from a position previously held, eg in a debate or argument; to yield. • *n* an ascent.

climber /'klaɪmər/ *n* a mountaineer or rock climber; a climbing plant; a socially ambitious person.

clime /klaɪm/ *n* (*poet*) a country, region, or tract.

clinch /klɪntʃ/ *vt* (*argument, etc*) to confirm or drive home. • *vi* (*boxing*) to grip the opponent with the arms to hinder his punching. • *n* the act of clinching; (*inf*) an embrace.

clincher /'klɪntʃər/ *n* a decisive point in an argument.

cling /klɪŋ/ *vi* (**clinging, clung**) to adhere, to be attached (to); to keep hold by embracing or entwining.—**clinger** *n*.

clingstone /'klɪŋstoːn/ *n* a fruit, eg the peach, with pulp adhering to the stone.—*also* **adj**.

clinic /'klɪnɪk/ *n* a place where outpatients are given medical care or advice; a place where medical specialists practise as a group; a private or specialized hospital; the teaching of medicine by treating patients in the presence of students.

clinical /'klɪnɪkəl/ *adj* of or relating to a clinic; based on medical observation; plain, simple; detached, cool, objective.—**clinically** *adv*.

clink[1] /klɪŋk/ n a slight metallic ringing sound. • vti to make or cause to make such a sound.

clink[2] n (sl) prison.

clinker /'klɪŋkər/ n very hard-burnt brick; a mass of partly vitrified brick; slag; a fine specimen.

clinker-built /-ˌbɪlt/ adj built so that the planks of a boat overlap each other like weather-boarding.

clinkstone /-ˌstoːn/ n an igneous rock that emits a clinking sound when struck.

clinometer /klaɪˈnɒmɪtər/ n an instrument for measuring the angles of slopes or the dip of rock strata; a kind of plumb level.—**clinometric, clinometrical** adj.—**clinometry** n.

clinquant /'klɪŋkənt/ adj glittering. • n tinsel.

clip[1] /klɪp/ vt (**clipping, clipped**) to cut or trim with scissors or shears; to punch a small hole in, esp a ticket; (words) to shorten or slur; (inf) to hit sharply. • n the piece clipped off; a yield of wool from sheep; an extract from a film; (inf) a smart blow; speed.

clip[2] vt (**clipping, clipped**) to hold firmly; to secure with a clip. • n any device that grips, clasps or hooks; a magazine for a gun; a piece of jewellery held in place by a clip.

clipboard /'klɪpbɔrd/ n a writing board with a spring clip for holding paper.

clip joint /-ˌdʒɔɪnt/ n (sl) a place, such as nightclub or restaurant, that overcharges or defrauds its customers.

clipper /'klɪpər/ n a fast sailing ship.

clippers /-s/ n a hand tool, sometimes electric, for cutting hair; nail clippers.

clipping /'klɪpɪŋ/ n an item cut from a publication, film, etc, a cutting.

clique /kliːk/ n a small exclusive group, a set.—**cliquey, cliquish** adj.

clitoridectomy /ˌklɪtərɪˈdɛktəmi/ n (pl **clitoridectomies**) the excision of the clitoris, performed for cultural reasons, and often referred to as female circumcision or female genital mutilation.

clitoris /'klɪtərɪs/ n a small sensitive erectile organ of the vulva.—**clitoral** adj.

cloaca /kloːˈeɪkə/ n (pl **cloacae**) a sewer; the cavity receiving the alimentary canal and urinary duct in birds, reptiles, many fishes, and the lower mammals.—**cloacal** adj.

cloak /kloːk/ n a loose sleeveless outer garment; a covering; something that conceals, a pretext. • vt to cover as with a cloak; to conceal.

cloak-and-dagger /'kloːkənˈdæɡər/ adj involving intrigue or espionage; undercover.

cloakroom /'kloːkruːm/ n a room where overcoats, luggage, etc, may be left.

clobber /'klɒbər/ vt (sl) to hit hard and repeatedly; to defeat; to criticize severely.

cloche /kloːʃ/ or /klɒʃ/ n a bell-shaped glass or plastic cover for food or outdoor plants; a woman's bell-shaped hat.

clock[1] /klɒk/ n a device for measuring time; any timing device with a dial and displayed figures; a dandelion head after flowering. • vt to time (a race, etc) using a stopwatch or other device; (inf) to register a certain speed; (sl) to hit; (with **off, out**) to stop work, esp by registering the time of one's departure on a card; (with **on, in**) to start work, esp by registering the time of one's arrival on a card.

clock[2] n a woven or embroidered ornament on a sock or stocking.

clockwise /'klɒkwaɪz/ adv moving in the direction of a clock's hands.—also adj.

clockwork /-wɜrk/ n the mechanism of a clock or any similar mechanism with springs and gears. • adj mechanically regular.

clod /klɒd/ n a lump of earth or clay; a stupid person.

cloddish /'klɒdɪʃ/ adj stupid; phlegmatic.

clodhopper /'klɒdˌhɒpər/ n (inf) a clumsy person; (usu pl) a large heavy shoe.

clog /klɒɡ/ n a wooden-soled shoe. • vt (**clogging, clogged**) to cause a blockage in; to impede, obstruct.

cloggy /'klɒɡi/ adj (**cloggier, cloggiest**) lumpy, clogging; adhesive, sticky.—**clogginess** n.

cloisonné /ˌklwɒzɒˈneɪ/, Fr. /klwazɔˈneɪ/ n enamel decoration with the colours of the pattern set in spaces partitioned off by wires. • adj inlaid with partitions; decorated in outline with bands of metal.

cloister /'klɔɪstər/ n a roofed pillared walk, usu with one side open, in a convent, college, etc; a religious retreat. • vt to confine or keep apart as if in a convent.

cloistered /'klɔɪstərd/ adj solitary, secluded.

cloistral /'klɔɪstrəl/ adj pertaining to or confined in a cloister; secluded; claustral.

clone /kloːn/ n a group of organisms or cells derived asexually from a single ancestor; an individual grown from a single cell of its parent and genetically identical to it; (inf) a person or thing that resembles another. • vt to propagate a clone from; to make a copy of.—**clonal** adj.

clonus /'kloːnəs/ n (pl **clonuses**) (med) a series of convulsive spasms.—**clonic** adj.—**clonicity** n.

close[1] /kloːz/ adj near; reticent, secret; nearly alike; nearly even or equal; dense, compact; cut short; sultry, airless; narrow; careful; restricted. • adv closely; near by. • n a courtyard; the entrance to a courtyard; the precincts of a cathedral.—**closely** adv.—**closeness** n.

close[2] vt to make closed; to stop up (an opening); to draw together; to conclude; to shut; (with **down**) to wind up, eg a business. • vi to come together; to complete; to finish. • n a completion, end.

close call n a close shave, a narrow escape.

close(d) corporation n a corporation in which vacancies are filled up by its members

closed /kloːzd/ adj shut up, with no opening; restricted; not open to question or debate; not open to the public, exclusive.

closed book n something too difficult to understand; something put aside for ever.

closed circuit n the transmission of TV signals by cable to receivers connected in a particular circuit.

closed shop n a firm employing only members of a trade union.

close-fisted /'kloːzˌfɪstɪd/ adj mean with money.

close-hauled /-ˌhɔld/ adj with sails trimmed to keep as near to the wind as possible.

close(d) season n certain months in the year in which it is illegal to kill certain game, protected wild birds, fish, etc.

close shave, close thing n a close call, a narrow escape.

closet /'klɒzət/ n a small room or a cupboard for clothes, supplies, etc; a small private room. • vt to enclose in a private room for a confidential talk.

close-up /'kloːzˌʌp/ n a film or television shot taken from very close range; a close examination.

closure /'kloːʒər/ n closing; the condition of being closed; something that closes; (parliament, etc) a decision to end further debate and move to an immediate vote.

clot /klɒt/ n a thickened mass, esp of blood; (sl) an idiot. • vti (**clotting, clotted**) to form into clots, to curdle, coagulate.

cloth /klɒθ/ n (pl **cloths**) woven, knitted or pressed fabric from which garments, etc are made; a piece of this; a tablecloth; clerical dress; (with **the**) the clergy.

cloth binding n a book binding of linen over cardboard.

clothe /kloːð/ vt (**clothing, clothed** or **clad**) to cover with garments; to dress; to surround, endow (with).

clothes /kloːz/ or /kloːðz/ npl garments, apparel.

clotheshorse /-ˌhɔrs/ n a wooden or metal frame for drying linen, etc; a dressy person.

clothesline /-laɪn/ n a rope on which washing is hung to dry.

clothespin /-pɪn/ n a plastic, wooden or metal clip for attaching washing to a line.

clothier /'kloːðiːər/ n one who manufactures or sells cloth and clothes.

clothing /'kloːðɪŋ/ n clothes.

cloud /klaʊd/ n a visible mass of water vapour floating in the sky; a mass of smoke, etc; a threatening thing, a gloomy look; a multitude; **on cloud nine** (inf) blissfully happy; **under a cloud** suspected of wrongdoing, disgraced. • vt to darken or obscure; to confuse; to depress.—**cloudless** adj.

cloudberry /'klaʊdˌbɛri/ n ✿ a low-growing North American plant of the raspberry family with amber-coloured fruit.

cloudburst /-bɜrst/ n a sudden rainstorm.

cloud chamber n (physics) a chamber filled with vapour used for detecting the tracks of high-energy particles.

cloud-cuckoo-land /klaʊdˈkʊkuːˌlænd/ n a realm of fantasy, imagination and impossible dreams.

cloudlet /'klaʊdlɪt/ n a small cloud.

cloudy /'klaʊdi/ adj (**cloudier, cloudiest**) of or full of clouds; not clear; gloomy.—**cloudily** adv.—**cloudiness** n.

clout /klaʊt/ n a blow; (sl) power, influence.

clove[1] /kloːv/ see **cleave**.

clove² *n* a segment of a bulb, as garlic.

clove³ *n* the dried flower bud of a tropical tree, used as a spice.

clove hitch *n* a knot used to secure a rope around a spar or pole.

cloven /'klo:vən/ *adj* divided; split.—*see also* **cleave**.

cloven hoof *n* the split hoof of oxen, sheep, etc; the mark of the Devil; an evil influence.

clove pink *n* the carnation.

clover /'klo:vər/ *n* a low-growing plant with three leaves used as fodder; a trefoil; **in clover** (*inf*) luxury.

cloverleaf /'klo:vər,li:f/ *n* connecting roads built in the shape of a clover leaf.

clown /klaʊn/ *n* a person who entertains with jokes, antics, etc, *esp* in a circus; a clumsy or boorish person. • *vi* to act the clown, behave comically or clumsily.—**clownish** *adj*.

cloy /klɔɪ/ *vt* to sicken with too much sweetness or pleasure.—**cloyingly** *adv*.

club /klʌb/ *n* a heavy stick used as a weapon; a stick with a head for playing golf, etc; an association of people for athletic, social, or common purposes; its premises; a suit of playing cards with black clover-like markings. • *vb* (**clubbing, clubbed**) *vt* to beat with or use as a club. • *vi* to form into a club for a common purpose.

clubbable, clubable /'klʌbəbəl/ *adj* suitable for a club, sociable.

clubfoot /'klʌb,fut/ *n* a congenital malformation of the foot.

clubhaul /-,hɔl/ *vt* (*naut*) to tack by dropping the lee anchor as soon as the wind is out of the sails, bringing the ship's head to the wind.

clubhouse /-haʊs/ *n* premises used by a club.

club moss /-mɒs/ *n* the lycopodium.

club sandwich *n* a three-layered sandwich.

cluck /klʌk/ *n* the call of a hen. • *vi* to make such a noise.

clue /klu:/ *n* a guide to the solution of a mystery or problem. • *vt* (**cluing, clued**) (*with* **in, up**) to provide with helpful information.

clueless /'klu:ləs/ *adj* (*inf*) stupid, incompetent.

clumber /'klʌmbər/ *n* a breed of spaniel, a field spaniel.

clump /klʌmp/ *n* a cluster of trees; a cluster of bacteria; a lump; (*of hair*) a handful; the sound of heavy footsteps.

clumsy /'klʌmzi/ *adj* (**clumsier, clumsiest**) unwieldy; awkward; lacking tact, skill or grace.—**clumsily** *adv*.—**clumsiness** *n*.

clung /klʌŋ/ *see* **cling**.

clunk /klʌŋk/ *n* a dull metallic sound. • *vi* to make this sound.

clupeid /'klu:pi,ɪd/ *n* one of the genus of fishes to which the herring belongs.—*also adj*.

cluster /'klʌstər/ *n* a bunch, *esp* of things growing or tied together; a swarm; a group. • *vti* to form or arrange in a cluster.—**clustery** *adj*.

clutch¹ /klʌtʃ/ *vt* to seize, to grasp tightly; to snatch at. • *n* a tight grip; a device for throwing parts of a machine into or out of action; the pedal operating this device; (*pl*) power.

clutch² *n* a nest of eggs; a brood of chicks.

clutter /'klʌtər/ *n* a disordered mess; confusion. • *vti* to litter; to put into disorder.

Clydesdale /'klaɪdzdeɪl/ *n* a heavy breed of carthorse.

clypeal, clypeate /'klɪpi,eɪt/ *adj* shield-shaped.

clypeus /'klɪpiəs/ *n* (*pl* **clypei**) a shield-like part of an insect's head.

clyster /'klɪstər/ *n* a liquid injected into the lower intestines by a syringe, an enema.

CM *abbr* ✤ = Member of the Order of Canada.

Cm (*chem symbol*) curium.

cm *abbr* = centimetre.

CMA *abbr* ✤ = Canadian Medical Association; Canadian Management Accountant.

CMHC *abbr* ✤ = Canada Mortgage and Houshing Corporation.

CN *abbr* ✤ = Canada National (Railways).

CNIB *abbr* ✤ = Canada National Institute for the Blind.

CNN /'si:,ɛnen/ *abbr* = Cable News Network.

CO *abbr* = Colorado; Commanding Officer.

Co (*chem symbol*) = cobalt.

Co. *abbr* = Company; County.

co- /ko:/ *prefix* together with, jointly.

c/o *abbr* = care of.

coach /ko:tʃ/ *n* a long-distance bus; a railway carriage; a large, covered four-wheeled horse-drawn carriage; a sports instructor; a tutor in a specialized subject. • *vti* to teach or train.

coach dog *n* a Dalmatian dog.

coachman /'ko:tʃmən/ *n* (*pl* **coachmen**) the driver of a horse carriage.

coaction /ko:'ækʃən/ or /'ko:,ækʃən/ *n* compulsion; an acting together.—**coactive** *adj*.—**coactivity** *n*.

coadjutor /ko:'ædjutər/ *n* a helper; an assistant to a bishop.—**coadjutrix** *nf*.

coadunate /-nɪt/ or /-,neɪt/ *adj* (*bot*) united, growing together.—**coadunation** *n*.—**coadunative** *adj*.

coagulant /ko:'ægjulənt/ *n* a substance that causes coagulation.

coagulate /-,leɪt/ *vti* to change from a liquid to partially solid state, to clot, curdle.—**coagulation** *n*.—**coagulative** *adj*.—**coagulator** *n*.

coagulum /-ləm/ *n* (*pl* **coagula**) a clot (of blood); a curdled mass.

coal /ko:l/ *n* a black mineral used for fuel; a piece of this; an ember.

coalesce /,ko:ə'les/ *vi* to come together and form one, to merge.—**coalescence** *n*.—**coalescent** *adj*.

coalfield /'ko:lfi:ld/ *n* a region yielding coal.

coalfish /-fɪʃ/ *n* (*pl* **coalfish, coalfishes**) the pollock.

coal gas *n* gas obtained from coal and formerly used for lighting and heating.

coalition /,ko:ə'lɪʃən/ *n* a temporary union of parties or states.—**coalitional** *adj*.—**coalitionist, coalitioner** *n*.

Coal Measure *n* that part of the Carboniferous series in which coal is found.

coal oil /'ko:l,ɔɪl/ *n* petroleum; kerosene.

coal tar /-,tɑr/ *n* a thick opaque liquid distilled from bituminous coal and from which many rich dye colours are obtained.

coaming /'ko:mɪŋ/ *n* the raised wood or iron border round the outside of a ship's hatch.

coaptation /,ko:æp'teɪʃən/ *n* the adjustment or adaptation of parts to one another.

coarse /kɔrs/ *adj* rough; large in texture; rude, crude; inferior.—**coarsely** *adv*.—**coarseness** *n*.

coarse-grained /'kɔrs,greɪnd/ *adj* having a coarse grain; ill-tempered; gross.

coarsen /'kɔrsən/ *vti* to make or become coarse.

coast /ko:st/ *n* an area of land bordering the sea; the seashore. • *vi* to sail along a coast; to travel down a slope without power; to proceed with ease.—**coastal** *adj*.

coaster /'ko:stər/ *n* a ship engaged in coastal trade; a tray for a decanter; a small mat for drinks; a roller coaster.

coastguard *n* an organization which monitors the coastline and provides help for ships in difficulties, prevents smuggling, etc.

coastline /'ko:stlaɪn/ *n* the outline of the shore.

coast-to-coast-to-coast *adj, adv* ✤ (*Cdn*) between the coasts of the Atlantic, Pacific and Arctic oceans.

coat /ko:t/ *n* a sleeved outer garment; the natural covering of an animal; a layer. • *vt* to cover with a layer or coating.

coat hanger *n* a piece of wood, wire or plastic curved to fit the shoulders for hanging a garment from a hook.

coati /ko:'ɒti/, **coatimundi** /,ko:tə'mʌndi/ *n* a raccoon-like South American animal.

coating /'ko:tɪŋ/ *n* a surface coat or layer; material for coats.

coat of arms *n* the heraldic bearings of a family, city, institution, etc.

coat of mail *n* chain mail.

coax /ko:ks/ *vt* to persuade gently; to obtain by coaxing; to make something work by patient effort.—**coaxer** *n*.—**coaxingly** *adv*.

coaxial /ko:'æksiəl/ *adj* having a common axis.

coaxial cable *n* a transmission cable having a double conductor separated by insulating material, as for a television.

cob¹ /kɒb/ *n* a sturdy riding horse; a corn cob; a round lump of coal; a male swan.

cob² *n* a composition of clay and straw used for building.

cobalt /'ko:bɒlt/ *n* a metallic element; a deep blue pigment made from it.

cobalt-60 *n* a radioisotope used in radiotherapy.

cobalt-blue *n* a greenish-blue pigment derived from cobalt.

cobalt bomb *n* a radioisotope (cobalt-60) used in radiotherapy; a nuclear weapon made from a hydrogen bomb encased in cobalt.

cobber /'kɒbər/ *n* (*Austral*) (*sl*) a chum, a pal.

cobble¹ /'kɒbəl/ *n* a cobblestone, a rounded stone used for paving. • *vt* to pave with cobblestones.

cobble² *vt* to repair, to make (shoes); to put together roughly or hastily.

cobbler¹ /'kɒblər/ *n* a person who mends shoes; a clumsy workman.

cobbler² *n* an iced drink of wine or spirits, fruit and sugar; fruit covered with a rich crust as a pudding.

cobelligerent /,ko:bə'lɪdʒərənt/ *n* a power cooperating with another in carrying on a war.

cobnut /ˈkɒbnʌt/ n a large hazelnut

Cobol /ˈkɒbɒl/ n (comput) a high-level programming language for general business use (Common Business Oriented Language).

cobra /ˈkɒbrə/ n a venomous hooded snake of Africa and India.

cobweb /ˈkɒbwɛb/ n a spider's web; a flimsy thing; an entanglement.—**cobwebbed** adj.—**cobwebby** adj.

coca /ˈkoːkə/ n either of two South American shrubs; their leaves, chewed as a stimulant.

Coca-Cola n (trademark) a brown-coloured carbonated soft drink flavoured with coca leaves, etc.

cocaine, cocain /koˈkeɪn/ n an intoxicating addictive drug obtained from coca leaves, used in anaesthesia.

cocainism /koˈkeɪˌnɪzəm/ n a morbid state resulting from excess of cocaine.

cocainize /koˈkeɪnˌaɪz/ vt to subject to, or render insensible by, cocaine; to treat with cocaine.—**cocainization** n.

cocci /ˈkɒki/ see **coccus**.

coccus /ˈkɒkəs/ n (pl **cocci**) a spherical bacterium one of the separable carpels of a dry fruit.—**coccal, coccoid** adj.

coccyx /ˈkɒksɪks/ n (pl **coccyges**) a small triangular bone at the base of the spine.—**coccygeal** adj.

cochineal /ˈkɒtʃəˌniːl/ or /-ˈniːl/ n a scarlet dye obtained from dried insects.

cochlea /ˈkɒklɪə/ n (pl **cochleae**) the spiral-shaped cavity of the inner ear.

cochleate /lɪˌeɪt/ or /-ɪt/, **cochleated** /-əd/ adj shell-shaped, screw-like.

cock[1] /kɒk/ n the adult male of the domestic fowl; the male of other birds; a tap or valve; the hammer of a gun; a cocked position. • vt to set erect, to stick up; to set at an angle; to bring the hammer (of a gun) to firing position; (with **up**) to make a complete mess of.—**cockup** n.

cock[2] n a small pile of hay.

cockade /kɒˈkeɪd/ n a rosette worn on the hat as a badge.

cock-a-hoop /ˌkɒkəˈhuːp/ adj elated, exultant.

Cockaigne /kɒkˈeɪn/ n an imaginary land of plenty.—also **Cockayne**.

cock-a-leekie /ˌkɒkəˈliːki/ n soup made of chicken boiled with leeks, etc.

cockalorum /ˌkɒkəˈlɔːrəm/ n a young cock; a perky or self-important person.

cock-and-bull story /ˈkɒkənˌbʊl/ n an incredible story.

cockatoo /ˌkɒkəˈtuː/ n (pl **cockatoos**) a large crested parrot.

cockatrice /ˈkɒkətrɪs/ or /-ˌtriːs/ n a fabulous serpent possessing the power of killing by a glance of its eye, a basilisk.

Cockayne see **Cockaigne**.

cockchafer /ˈkɒkˌtʃeɪfər/ n a large winged beetle.

cockcrow /ˈkɒkˌkroː/ n the time of dawn, early morning.

cocked hat n a hat with turned-up brims pointed in front and behind; **to knock into a cocked hat** to beat easily.

cockerel /ˈkɒkərəl/ n a young cock, rooster.

cocker spaniel /ˈkɒkər/ n a small breed of spaniel.

cockeyed /ˈkɒkaɪd/ adj (inf) having a squint; slanting; daft, absurd.

cockfight /ˈkɒkˌfaɪt/ n an organized fight between gamecocks.

cockhorse /ˈkɒkˌhɔːs/ n a rocking horse.

cockle[1] /ˈkɒkəl/ n an edible shellfish with a rounded shell.

cockle[2] vti to curl up, to pucker. • n a wrinkle, a bulge.

cockle[3] n a purple-flowered weed, the plant corncockle or darnel.

cockleshell /ˈkɒkəlˌʃel/ n the shell of a cockle; a frail boat.

cockloft /ˈkɒkˌlɒft/ n a small upper loft; a garret.

cockney /ˈkɒkni/ n (pl **cockneys**) a person born in the East End of London; the dialect of this area.

cockpit /ˈkɒkpɪt/ n the compartment of a small aircraft for the pilot and crew, the flight deck; an arena for cock fighting; the driver's seat in a racing car.

cockroach /ˈkɒkroːtʃ/ n a nocturnal beetle-like insect.

cockscomb /ˈkɒkskoːm/ n a cock's crest; a jester's cap resembling a cock's comb; a decorative plant with red or yellow flowers; a vain young fop.—also **coxcomb**.

cockshy /ˈkɒkʃaɪ/ n (pl **cockshies**) a thing set up to be thrown at; a throw at a cockshy.

cocksure /ˈkɒkʃʊr/ or /-ˌʃər/ adj quite certain; over-confident.

cocktail /ˈkɒkteɪl/ n an alcoholic drink containing a mixture of spirits or other liqueurs; an appetizer, usu containing shellfish, served as the first course of a meal.

cocky /ˈkɒki/ adj (**cockier, cockiest**) cheeky; conceited; arrogant.—**cockily** adv.—**cockiness** n.

coco /ˈkoːkoː/ n (pl **cocos**) the coconut palm.

cocoa /ˈkoːkoː/ n a powder of ground cacao seeds; a drink made from this.

cocoa bean n the seed of the cacao plant.

cocoa butter n a waxy substance derived from cocoa beans and used in perfumery, confectionery, etc.

coconut /ˈkoːkəˌnʌt/ n the fruit of the coconut palm.

coconut matting n rough matting made from the fibrous outer husks of coconuts.

coconut palm n a tall palm tree that is grown widely in the tropics for its fruit, the coconut.

coconut shy n a fairground stall where coconuts are set up as targets.

cocoon /kəˈkuːn/ n a silky case spun by some insect larvae for protection in the chrysalis stage; a cosy covering. • vt to wrap in or as in a cocoon; to protect oneself by cutting oneself off from one's surroundings.

cocotte[1] /kəˈkɒt/ n a small fireproof dish for cooking and individual serving of food.

cocotte[2] n a promiscuous woman.

COD abbr = cash on delivery; collect on delivery.

cod /kɒd/ n (pl **cod, cods**) a large edible fish of the North Atlantic.

coda /ˈkoːdə/ n (mus) a passage at the end of a composition or section to give a greater sense of finality; a supplementary section at the end of a novel.

coddle /ˈkɒdəl/ vt to treat as an invalid, to pamper; to cook (eggs) in lightly boiling water.—**coddler** n.

code /koːd/ n a system of letters, numbers or symbols used to transmit secret messages, or to simplify communication; a systematic body of laws; a set of rules or conventions; (comput) a set of program instructions. • vt to put into code.

codeine /ˈkoːdiːn/ n an analgesic substance.

codeword, codename n a word used in planning and when referring to a secret operation.

codex /ˈkoːdeks/ n (pl **codices**) a volume of ancient manuscripts.

codger /ˈkɒdʒər/ n (sl) a buffer, an old man.

codicil /ˈkoːdəsɪl/ or /ˈkɒd-/ n an addition to a will modifying, adjusting, or supplementing its contents.—**codicillary** adj.

codify /ˈkoːdəˌfaɪ/ or /ˈkɒd-/ vt (**codifying, codified**) to collect or arrange (laws, rules, regulations, etc) into a system.—**codifier** n.—**codification** n.

codlin /ˈkɒdlɪn/ n a kind of stewing apple.

codling n a young cod.

cod-liver oil /ˈkɒd ˌlɪvər/ n oil derived from the livers of cod and related fish which is rich in vitamins A and D.

codpiece /ˈkɒdpiːs/ n a baggy appendage once worn in front of men's breeches.

codswallop /ˈkɒdzˌwɒləp/ n (sl) nonsense.

cod tongue /ˈkɒd ˌtʌŋ/ n • (Cdn) the tongue of a codfish, fried in pork fat.

co-ed /ˈkoːed/ or /koːˈed/ adj (inf) coeducational. • n (inf) a girl attending a coeducational school or college.

coeducation /ˌkoːedʒʊˈkeɪʃən/ n the teaching of students of both sexes in the same institution.—**coeducational** adj.—**coeducationally** adv.

coefficient /ˌkoːɪˈfɪʃənt/ n (math) a numerical or constant factor in an algebraic term.

coelacanth /ˈsiːləˌkænθ/ n a type of primitive fish that is extinct except for one species.

coelenterate /siːˈlentəˌreɪt/ n any of a group of aquatic creatures with a bulbous or tube-shaped body and a mouth surrounded by tentacles, such as sea anemones, jellyfish and corals.—also adj.

coeliac /ˈsiːlɪæk/ adj of or pertaining to the abdomen. • n a person with celiac disease.—also **celiac**.

coeliac disease n a chronic digestive disease of young children, causing malnutrition and diarrhoea.

coenobite /ˈsenoˌbaɪt/ or /ˈsiːno-/ n one of a religious order living in a convent or in community.—also **cenobite**.

coequal /koːˈiːkwəl/ adj having complete equality.—**coequality** n.—**coequally** adv.

coerce /koːˈɜːs/ vt to compel; to force by threats.—**coercible** adj.—**coercion** n.

coercion /koːˈɜːʃən/ n the act of coercing; forcible compulsion; government by force.—**coercionary** adj.—**coercionist** n.

coercive /koːˈɜːsɪv/ adj having the power to force; compelling.—**coerciveness** n.

coessential /ˌkoːɪˈsenʃəl/ adj of the same substance.—**coessentiality, coessentialness** n.

coeternal /ˌkoʊˈiːtərnəl/ *adj* equally eternal.—**coeternally** *adv*.

coeval /koʊˈiːvəl/ *adj* contemporaneous. • *n* a person of the same age, a contemporary.—**coevality** *n*.—**coeally** *adv*.

coexist /ˌkoʊəgˈzɪst/ *vi* to exist together at the same time; to live in peace together.—**coexistence** *n*.—**coexistent** *adj*.

coextensive /ˌkoʊəkˈstɛnsɪv/ *adj* extending over the same space or time; equally extensive.

C of E *abbr* = Church of England.

coffee /ˈkɒfi/ *n* a drink made from the seeds of the coffee tree; the seeds, or the shrub; a light-brown colour.

coffee bean *n* the seed of the coffee plant.

coffee house /-ˌhaʊs/, **coffee bar** /-ˌbɑr/, **coffee shop** /-ˌʃɒp/ *n* a refreshment house where coffee is served.

coffee mill /-ˌmɪl/ *n* a machine for grinding coffee beans.

coffeepot /-ˌpɒt/ *n* a pot for making coffee in.

coffee table /-ˌteɪbəl/ *n* a low table for holding drinks, books, etc.

coffee table book *n* a large book for display, not reading.

coffer /ˈkɒfər/ *n* a strong chest for holding money or valuables.

cofferdam /ˈkɒfərˌdæm/ *n* a watertight structure enclosing a submerged area which can be pumped dry to allow construction or essential repair work.

coffin /ˈkɒfɪn/ *n* a box for a dead body to be buried or cremated in.

coffin bone *n* a bone inside a horse's hoof.

coffle /ˈkɒfəl/ *n* a gang of slaves, animals, etc chained together.

cog[1] /kɒg/ *n* a tooth-like projection on the rim of a wheel.

cog[2] *vti* (**cogging, cogged**) to load dice in order to cheat. • *n* a trick.

cogent /ˈkoʊdʒənt/ *adj* persuasive, convincing.—**cogently** *adv*.—**cogency** *n*.

cogitate /ˈkɒdʒəˌteɪt/ *vi* to think deeply, to ponder.—**cogitation** *n*.—**cogitator** *n*.

cognac /ˈkɒnjæk/ *n* a superior grape brandy distilled in France.

cognate /ˈkɒgneɪt/ *adj* having a common source or origin; kindred, related.—**cognation** *n*.

cognition /kɒgˈnɪʃən/ *n* the mental act of perceiving; knowledge.—**cognitive** *adj*.

cognizable /ˈkɒgnɪzəbəl/ or /ˌkɒgˈnaɪzəbəl/, /ˈkɒn-/ *adj* knowable; (*law*) within the cognizance of a court.

cognizance /ˈkɒgnɪzəns/ or /ˈkɒn-/ *n* judicial knowledge or notice; extent of knowledge; awareness, perception; (*her*) a distinctive crest or badge.

cognizant /ˈkɒgnɪzənt/ or /ˈkɒn-/ *adj* aware, informed (of).

cognize /ˈkɒgˌnaɪz/ or /kɒgˈnaɪz/ *vt* to have cognition of.

cognomen /kɒgˈnoʊmɛn/ *n* (*pl* **cognomens, cognomina**) a surname; a nickname.

cognoscente /ˌkɒgnəˈʃɛnti/ or /-ˈsɛnti/ *n* (*pl* **cognoscenti**) (*usu pl*) a connoisseur.

cogwheel /ˈkɒgwiːl/ *n* a wheel with a toothed rim for gearing.

cohabit /koʊˈhæbɪt/ *vi* to live together as husband or wife.—**cohabitant, cohabiter** *n*.—**cohabitation** *n*.

cohere /koʊˈhɪr/ *vi* to stick together; to remain united; to be consistent.

coherent /koʊˈhɪrənt/ *adj* cohering; capable of intelligible speech; consistent.—**coherently** *adv*.—**coherence** *n*.

cohesion /koʊˈhiːʒən/ *n* the act of cohering or sticking together; the force that causes this; interdependence.—**cohesive** *adj*.

cohort /ˈkoʊhɔrt/ *n* a tenth part of a Roman legion; any group of persons banded together; a follower, a comrade.

coif /kɔɪf/ *n* a close-fitting cap.

coiffeur /kwɒˈfər/ *n* a hairdresser.—**coiffeuse** *nf*.

coiffure /kwɒˈfjʊr/ *n* a hairstyle.

coil[1] /kɔɪl/ *vti* to wind in rings or folds; to twist into a circular or spiral shape. • *n* a coiled length of rope; a single ring of this; (*elect*) a spiral wire for the passage of current; an intrauterine contraceptive device.—**coiler** *n*.

coil[2] *n* (*arch*) tumult, disturbance.

coin /kɔɪn/ *n* a piece of legally stamped metal used as money. • *vt* to invent (a word, phrase); to make into money, to mint; to make a lot of money quickly.

coinage /ˈkɔɪnɪdʒ/ *n* the act of coining; the issue of coins, currency; a coined word.

coincide /ˌkoʊɪnˈsaɪd/ *vi* to occupy the same portion of space; to happen at the same time; to agree exactly, to correspond.

coincidence /koʊˈɪnsɪdəns/ *n* the act of coinciding; the occurrence of an event at the same time as another without apparent connection.

coincident /-dənt/ *adj* coinciding.

coincidental /koʊˌɪnsɪˈdɛntəl/ *adj* happening by coincidence.—**coincidentally** *adv*.

coin-op /ˈkɔɪnɒp/ *n* a self-service launderette, etc where the machines are operated by coins.

Cointreau /ˈkwɒntroʊ/ (*trademark*) *n* a clear liqueur with orange flavouring.

coir /kɔɪər/ *n* the prepared fibre of the husks of coconuts.

coitus /ˈkɔɪtəs/ or /ˈkoʊɪt-/, **coition** /ˈkɔɪʃən/ *n* sexual intercourse.—**coital** *adj*.

coitus interruptus /ˈkɔɪtəsˌɪntəˈrʌptəs/ *n* the interruption of coitus by withdrawal of the penis before ejaculation.

Coke /ˈkoʊk/ *n* (*trademark*) short for Coca-Cola.

coke[1] /koʊk/ *n* coal from which gas has been expelled. • *vt* to convert (coal) into coke.

coke[2] *n* (*sl*) cocaine.

col /kɒl/ *n* a pass between mountain peaks; an atmospheric depression between two anticyclones.

col- *prefix* the form of *com-* before *l*.

Col. *abbr* = Colonel.

cola[1] /ˈkoʊlə/ *see* **colon**[1].

cola[2] *n* a carbonated drink flavoured with extracts from the kola nut and coca leaves.—*also* **kola**.

colander /ˈkɒləndər/ or /ˈkʌl-/ *n* a bowl with holes in the bottom for straining cooked vegetables, pasta, etc.

cola nut *see* **kola nut**.

colcannon /kɒlˈkænən/ *n* an Irish dish of boiled cabbage and potatoes mashed together and seasoned with salt, pepper, etc.

colchicum /ˈkɒltʃɪkəm/ or /ˈkɒlkɪ-/ *n* meadow saffron; a narcotic made from its seeds.

colcothar /ˈkɒlkoʊˌθər/ *n* red peroxide of iron used as a pigment.

cold /koʊld/ *adj* lacking heat or warmth; lacking emotion, passion or courage; unfriendly; dead; (*scent*) faint; (*sl*) unconscious. • *adv* (*inf*) without prior knowledge or preparation; completely. • *n* absence of heat; the sensation caused by this; cold weather; a virus infection of the respiratory tract.—**coldish** *adj*.—**coldly** *adv*.—**coldness** *n*.

cold-blooded /ˈkoʊldˌblʌdɪd/ *adj* having a body temperature that varies with the surrounding air or water, as reptiles and fish; without feeling; callous; ruthless; in cold blood.—**cold-bloodedness** *n*.

cold chisel *n* a tempered chisel for cutting cold iron.

cold cream *n* a creamy preparation for cleansing and softening the skin.

cold feet *n* (*inf*) fear.

cold frame *n* an unheated plant frame with a glass top for protecting seedlings, etc.

cold front *n* the forward edge of a cold air mass approaching a warmer mass.

cold-shoulder *vt* (*inf*) to treat with indifference or hostility.—**cold shoulder** *n*.

cold sore *n* one or more blisters appearing near the mouth, caused by the virus herpes simplex.

cold storage *n* storage in refrigerated areas; (*with* **in**) (*inf*) abeyance, being set aside for future use.

cold sweat *n* a cooling and moistening of the skin usually associated with fear or shock.

cold turkey *n* (*sl*) sudden withdrawal of narcotic drugs from an addict as a cure; the symptoms (*eg* nausea, vomiting, cramps) resulting from this withdrawal.

cold war *n* enmity between two nations characterized by military tension and political hostility.

cole /koʊl/ *n* cabbage plants in general.

coleopteran /ˌkoʊliˈɒptəˌrən/ or /ˌkoʊli-/ *n* (*pl* **coleopterans, coleoptera**) any of the beetles, an order of insects having the outer pair of wings formed into hard sheaves for the inner pair.—**coleopterous** *adj*.

coleslaw /ˈkoʊlˌslɔ/ *n* raw shredded cabbage, carrots, onions in a dressing, used as a salad.

coleus /ˈkoʊliəs/ *n* (*pl* **coleuses**) a plant cultivated for its variegated foliage.

colic /ˈkɒlɪk/ *n* acute spasmodic pain in the abdomen.—**colicky** *adj*.

coliseum /ˌkɒləˈsiːəm/ *n* a large building, such as a stadium, used for sports events and other public entertainments; (*with cap*) the Colosseum.

colitis /kəˈlaɪtɪs/ *n* inflammation of the colon.—**colitic** *adj*.

collaborate /kəˈlæbəˌreɪt/ *vi* to work jointly or together, *esp* on a literary project; to side with the invaders of one's country.—**collaboration** *n*.—**collaborator** *n*.—**collaborative** *adj*.

collage /kə'lɒʒ/ *n* art made up from scraps of paper, material and other odds and ends pasted onto a hard surface.

collagen /'kɒlədʒən/ *n* a protein present in connective tissue and bones which yields gelatin when boiled.

collapse /kə'læps/ *vi* to fall down; to come to ruin, to fail; to break down physically or mentally. • *n* the act of collapsing; a breakdown, prostration.

collapsible, collapsable /-ɪbəl/ *adj* designed to fold compactly.—**collapsibility** *n*.

collar /'kɒlər/ *n* the band of a garment round the neck; a decoration round the neck, a choker; a band of leather or chain put round an animal's neck. • *vt* to put a collar on; (*inf*) to seize; to arrest.

collarbone /-,bo:n/ *n* one of the two bones that connect the shoulder blades with the breast bone, the clavicle.

collate /'kɒleɪt/ or /'kɒ-/, /kə'leɪt/ *vt* to examine and compare (manuscripts, etc); to put (pages) together in sequence; (*bishop*) to appoint to a benefice.—**collation** *n*—**collator** *n*.

collateral /kə'lætərəl/ *n* security pledged for the repayment of a loan. • *adj* side by side; accompanying but secondary; descended from the same ancestor but not directly.—**collaterally** *cdv*.

collation /ko:'leɪʃən/ or /'kɒ-/, /kə-/ *n* the act of collating, a comparison; a light meal; the presentation to a benefice by a bishop, who is the patron.

colleague /'kɒli:g/ *n* an associate in the same profession or office; a fellow worker.

collect[1] /kə'lɛkt/ *vti* to bring together, gather or assemble; to regain command of (oneself); to concentrate (thoughts, etc); to ask for or receive money or payment. • *adj* (*telephone call*) paid for by the person called.

collect[2] /'kɒlɛkt/ *n* a short comprehensive prayer for a particular occasion.

collectible, collectable /kə'lɛktəbəl/ *adj* (*antiques, etc*) of interest to a collector. • *n* an object worth collecting.

collectanea *npl* passages selected from various authors; a miscellany.

collected /kə'lɛktəd/ *adj* self-possessed, cool.—**collectedly** *adv*.

collection /kə'lɛkʃən/ *n* act of collecting; an accumulation; money collected at a meeting, etc; a group of things collected for beauty, interest, rarity or value; the periodic showing of a designer's fashions; a regular gathering of post from a postbox.

collective /kə'lɛktɪv/ *adj* viewed as a whole, taken as one; combined, common; (*gram*) used in the singular to express a multitude. • *n* a collective enterprise, as a farm.—**collectively** *adv*.

collective bargaining *n* negotiations on working conditions between representatives of employees and management.

collective farm *n* a farm or number of smallholdings run on a cooperative basis, usually under state supervision.

collective noun *n* a singular noun covering a number of person or things (eg *family*, *flock*).

collectivism /kə'lɛktə,vɪzəm/ *n* the political or economic theory of collective ownership of the means of production and distribution by the state or people.—**collectivist** *n* —**collectivistic** *adj*.

collectivize /kə'lɛktə,vaɪz/ *vt* to bring into public ownership in accordance with the principle of collectivism.—**collectivization** *n*.

collector /kə'lɛktər/ *n* a person who collects things, eg stamps, butterflies, as a hobby or so as to inspect them, as tickets.

colleen /kɒ'li:n/ *n* (*Irish*) a girl.

college /'kɒlədʒ/ *n* an institution of higher learning; a school offering specialized knowledge; the buildings housing a college; an organized body of professionals.

collegian /kə'li:dʒən/ *n* a student or recent graduate of a college.

collegial /kə'li:dʒi:ıt/, **collegial** *adj* of or belonging to a college; containing, connected with or having the status of a college.

collegiate institute *n* ✸ (*Cdn*) a secondary school that chiefly prepares students for university.

collet /'kɒlət/ *n* the part of a ring in which the stone is set.

collide /kə'laɪd/ *vi* to come into violent contact (with); to dash together; to conflict; to disagree.

collie /'kɒli/ or /'ko:li/ *n* a breed of dog with a pointed muzzle and long hair, used as a sheepdog.

colligate /'kɒlə,geɪt/ *vt* to bind together; to bring (isolated facts) under a general principle.—**colligation** *n*.—**colligative** *adj*.

collimate /'kɒlə,meɪt/ *vt* to bring into the same line; to make parallel.—**collimation** *n*.

collinear /kə'lɪniər/ or /ko:-/ *adj* in the same straight line.—**collinearity** *n*.

collision /kə'lɪʒən/ *n* state of colliding together; a violent impact of moving bodies, a crash; a clash of interests, etc.

collision course *n* one that, if continued on, will end in disaster.

collocate /'kɒlə,keɪt/ *vt* to place together; to arrange.

collocation /,kɒlə'keɪʃən/ *n* a placing in a particular order; an arrangement, relative situation.

collodion /kə'lo:diən/ *n* a preparation of soluble pyroxylin with ether, used in photography.

colloid /'kɒlɔɪd/ *adj* like glue or jelly; (*chem*) of a gummy noncrystalline kind. • *n* a viscid inorganic transparent substance.—**colloidal** *adj*.—**colloidality** *n*.

collop /'kɒləp/ *n* a slice of meat.

colloquial /kə'lo:kwiəl/ *adj* used in familiar but not formal talk, not literary.—**colloquially** *adv*.

colloquialism /-,lɪzəm/ *n* a colloquial word or phrase.

colloquium /kə'lo:kwiəm/ *n* (*pl* **colloquiums, colloquia**) a conference, seminar.

colloquy /'kɒləkwi/ *n* (*pl* **colloquies**) a conversation; a written dialogue.

collotype /'kɒlə,taɪp/ *n* a gelatine photographic plate used for printing from in ink.—**collotypic** *adj*.

collude /kə'lu:d/ *vi* to act together; to conspire, *esp* to defraud.

collusion /kə'lu:ʒən/ *n* the act of colluding; an agreement to commit fraud or deception.—**collusive** *adj*.

collyrium /kə'lɪriəm/ *n* (*pl* **collyria, collyriums**) an eye salve.

collywobbles /'kɒli,wɒbəlz/ *npl* (*si*) abdominal pain or discomfort; nervousness.

colobus /'kɒləbəs/ *n* any of a genus of long-tailed African monkeys with shortened or absent thumbs.

colocynth /'kɒləsɪnθ/ *n* a kind of cucumber; the pulp it yields dried and powdered and used as a purgative.

cologne /kə'lo:n/ *n* eau-de-Cologne, a scented liquid.

colon[1] /'ko:lən/ *n* (*pl* **colons, cola**) the part of the large intestine from the caecum to the rectum.—**colonic** *adj*.

colon[2] *n* (*pl* **colons**) a punctuation mark (:) between the semicolon and the full stop, *usu* written before an explanation or a list.

colonel /'kɜrnəl/ *n* a commissioned officer junior to a brigadier but senior to a lieutenant colonel.—**colonelcy, colonelship** *n*.

colonial /kə'lo:niəl/ *adj* of or pertaining to a colony or colonies; (*with cap*) pertaining to the thirteen British colonies that became the US. • *n* a person who takes part in founding a colony, a settler.—**colonially** *adv*.

colonialism /-,lɪzəm/ *n* the policy of acquiring and governing colonies.—**colonialist** *adj, n*.

colonist /'kɒlənɪst/ *n* a person who settles in a colony.

colonize /-,naɪz/ *vt* to establish a colony in; to settle in a colony.—**colonization** *n*.—**colonizer** *n*.

colonnade /-'neɪd/ *n* a range of columns placed at regular intervals; a similar row, as of trees.

colony /'kɒləni/ *n* (*pl* **colonies**) an area of land acquired and settled by a distant state and subject to its control; a community of settlers; a group of people of the same nationality or interests living in a particular area; a collection of organisms in close association.

colophon /'kɒlə,fɒn/ or /-fən/ *n* a publisher's imprint or decorative device on a book; (*formerly*) an inscription at the end of a book giving the printer's or writer's name.

color /'kʌlər/ *see* **colour**.

colorable /'kʌlərəbəl/ *see* **colourable**.

colored /'kʌlərd/ *see* **coloured**.

colorfast /'kʌlər,fæst/ *see* **colourfast**.

colorful /-,fʊl/ *see* **colourful**.

coloring /-ɪŋ/ *see* **colouring**.

colorist /-ɪst/ *see* **colourist**.

colorize /-,aɪz/ *see* **colourize**.

colorless /-ləs/ *see* **colourless**.

Colorado beetle /,kɒlə'rædo:/ or /,kɒlə'rædo:/ *n* a yellowish beetle with ten longitudinal black stripes on its back, destructive to potatoes.

colorant /'kʌlərənt/ *n* a colouring matter.

coloration /,kʌlə'reɪʃən/ *n* colouring.

coloratura, colorature /,kɒlərə'tʊrə/ or /-'tjʊrə/, /kɒl-/ *adj* (*mus*) highly ornamented or florid. • *n* a vocal passage sung in this way.

colorific /,kʌlə'rɪfɪk/ *adj* producing colour.

colorimeter /,kʌlə'rɪmətər/ *n* an instrument for measuring the intensity of colour, strength of dyes, etc.—**colorimetric, colorimetrical** *adj*.—**colorimetry** *n*.

Colosseum /ˌkɒləˈsiːəm/ n a large amphitheatre in Rome built in the 1st century.

colossal /kəˈlɒsəl/ adj gigantic, immense; (inf) amazing, wonderful.—**colossally** adv.

colossus /kəˈlɒsəs/ n (pl **colossi, colossuses**) a gigantic statue; something immense.

colostomy /kəˈlɒstəmi/ n (pl **colostomies**) a surgical opening into the bowl forming an artificial anus.

colostrum /kəˈlɒstrəm/ n the first milk secreted after parturition; biestings.—**colostral** adj.

colotomy /kəˈlɒtəmi/ n (pl **colotomies**) an incision in the colon.

colour /ˈkʌlər/ n the eye's perception of wavelengths of light with different colours corresponding to different wavelengths; the attribute of objects to appear different according to their differing ability to absorb, emit, or reflect light of different wavelengths; colour of the face or skin; pigment; dye; paint; (literature) use of imagery, vividness; (mus) depth of sound; (pl) a flag; a symbol of a club, team, etc. • vt to give colour to, paint; to misrepresent; to influence. • vi to emit colour; (face) to redden in anger or embarrassment; to blush; to change colour, to ripen.—also **color**.

colourable /ˈkʌlərəbəl/ adj capable of being coloured; specious, plausible.—also **colorable**.

colour bar n discrimination based on race, esp by White races against other races.

colour-blind adj unable to distinguish colours, esp red and green.—**colour blindness** n.

colour code n a system of identifying by colours, eg of electrical wires.

coloured /ˈkʌlərd/ adj possessing colour; biased, not objective; of a darker skinned race. • n a person of a darker skinned race.—also **colored**.

colourfast /ˈkʌlərˌfæst/ adj of a material made with non-running or non-fading colours after washing.—also **colorfast**.

colour filter n (photog) a thin plate or layer for adjusting depth and brightness of required colours.

colourful /-ˌfʊl/ adj full of colour; vivid.—also **colorful**.—**colourfully** adv.

colouring /-ɪŋ/ n appearance in term of colour; disposition or use of colour; a substance for giving colour.—also **coloring**.

colourist /-ɪst/ n an artist whose works are characterized by beauty of colour.—also **colorist**.—**colouristic** adj.

colourize /-ˌaɪz/ vt to add colour to a black-and-white film using a special device.—also **colorize**.

colourless adj lacking colour; dull, uninteresting, characterless.—also **colorless**.—**colourlessly** adv.—**colourlessness** n.

colporteur /ˈkɛlˌpɔrtər/ n a person who hawks books, esp bibles.

colt /koːlt/ n a young male horse; a young, inexperienced person; an inexperienced player of a sport.

colter /ˈkoːltər/ see **coulter**.

coltish /-ɪʃ/ adj like a colt; frisky; inexperienced.

coltsfoot /ˈkoːltsfʊt/ n (pl **coltsfoots**) a yellow-flowered weed.

colubrine /ˈkɒljuˌbraɪn/ adj of, like or pertaining to snakes.

columbarium /kɒləmˈbɛriəm/ n (pl **columbaria**) a dovecote; a place with niches for cinerary urns.

Columbian /kəˈlɛmbiən/ adj pertaining to the US.

Columbine /ˈkɒləmˌbaɪn/ n a female character or dancer in a pantomime, sweetheart of Harlequin.

columbine[1] /ˈkɒləmˌbaɪn/ adj pertaining to or like a dove or pigeon.

columbine[2] n a garden plant, aquilegia.

columbium /kəˈlɛmbiəm/ n a metallic element now called niobium.

Columbus Day /kəˈlɛmbəs/ n a legal holiday in most US states, 12 October, commemorating Columbus' landing in the Americas, 1492.

columella /ˌkɒljuːˈmɛlə/ or /-jə-/ n (pl **columellae**) (biol) a central axis or column.—**columellar** adj.

column /ˈkɒləm/ n a round pillar for supporting or decorating a building; something shaped like this; a vertical division of a page; a narrow-fronted deep formation of troops; a long line of people; a feature article appearing regularly in a newspaper, etc.—**columnar** adj.—**columned, columnated** adj.

columnist /-nɪst/ or /-mɪst/ n a journalist who contributes a regular newspaper or magazine column.

colza /ˈkɒlzə/ n rape seed.

colza oil n an oil made from rape seed.

coma[1] /ˈkoːmə/ n (pl **comas**) deep prolonged unconsciousness.

coma[2] n (pl **comae**) (astron) the nebulous hair-like envelope around the nucleus of a comet; (bot) the silky hairs at the end of a seed; the branches forming the leafy head of a tree.—**comal** adj.

comate /ˈkoːˌmeɪt/ adj (bot) hairy.

comatose /ˈkoːməˌtoːs/ adj in a coma; lethargic, sleepy.

comb /koːm/ n a toothed instrument for separating hair, wool, etc; a part of a machine like this; the crest of a cock; a honeycomb. • vt to arrange (hair) or dress (wool) with a comb; to seek for thoroughly.

combat /ˈkɒmbæt/ vti to strive against, oppose; to do battle. • n a contest; a fight; struggle.—**combatable** adj.—**combater** n.

combatant /kɒmˈbætənt/ or /kəm-/, /ˈkɒmbætənt/, /ˈkɛm-/ adj fighting. • n a person engaged in a fight or contest.

combative /ˌkɒmˈbætɪv/ or /ˌkəm-/ adj aggressive, keen to fight.

comber /ˈkoːmər/ n a wool-combing machine; a long curling wave, a breaker.

combination /ˌkɒmbɪˈneɪʃən/ n the act of combining; a union of separate parts; persons allied for a purpose; a sequence of numbers which opens a combination lock; a motorcycle and sidecar.

combination lock /-lɒk/ n a lock which can only be opened by moving a set of dials to show a specific sequence of numbers.

combinations npl an all-in-one undergarment also covering the arms and legs.

combine /kəmˈbaɪn/ vti to join together; to unite intimately; to possess together; to cooperate; (chem) to form a compound with. • n an association formed for commercial or political purposes; a machine for harvesting and threshing grain.—**combinable** adj.—**combiner** n.

combo /ˈkɒmboː/ n (pl **combos**) a small jazz band; (inf) any small group.

combust /kəmˈbʌst/ vt to burn.

combustible /kəmˈbʌstəbəl/ adj capable of burning; easily set alight; excitable. • n a combustible thing.—**combustibility, combustibleness** n.

combustion /kəmˈbʌstʃən/ n the process of burning; the process in which substances react with oxygen in air to produce heat.

combustion chamber n the space in the cylinder of an engine in which the gas compressed by the piston is exploded.

come /kʌm/ vi (**coming, came**, pp **come**) to approach; to arrive; to reach; to happen (to); to originate; to turn out (to be); to occur in a certain order; to be derived or descended; to be caused; to result; to be available; (sl) to experience a sexual orgasm; (with **about**) to happen; (naut) to change to a new tack; (with **across**) to meet with unexpectedly; to communicate the intended information or impression; to provide what is expected; (sl) to pay up; (with **along**) to make progress; (with **at**) to find out; to attack; (with **away**) to get detached; to leave with; (with **between**) to cause the estrangement of (two people); (with **by**) to obtain, esp by chance; to pass; (with **down**) to descend; to fall; to suffer an illness; to leave university; (with **down on**) to reprimand; (with **forward**) to offer oneself for some duty, volunteer; (with **from**) (inf) to have an awareness of the circumstances causing one's attitudes or actions; to understand what someone means; (with **in**) to enter, arrive; (race) to finish in a certain position; to perform a certain function; to become popular or fashionable; (money) to be received as income; to turn out to be; (with **into**) to enter; to receive as an inheritance; (with **of**) to result from; (with **off**) to become detached; to fall from; to emerge from or finish something in a specified way; to succeed; to be reduced in price, etc; (inf) to happen; (inf) to have the intended effect; (with **on**) to advance, make progress; (electricity, etc) to begin functioning; to enter on to the stage or set; (with **out**) to become public or be published; to go on strike; to declare oneself in public; to present oneself openly as homosexual; to transpire; to make one's debut; (with **over**) to change sides; to communicate effectively; to make an impression; (inf) to become affected with a certain feeling; (with **round, around**) to recover one's normal state; to look in as a visitor; to regain consciousness; to change one's opinion, accede to something; (with **to**) to regain consciousness, revive; (total) to amount to; (with **through**) to overcome; to survive; (with **under**) to be subjected to; to be classed among; (with **up**) to approach; to grow; to come to a higher place or rank; (sun) to rise; to occur; to arise for discussion, etc; (with **upon**) to discover or meet unexpectedly; (with **up with**) to overtake; to put forward for discussion.

comeback /ˈkʌmbæk/ n (inf) a return to a career or to popularity; (inf) a witty answer.

comedian /kə'mi:diən/ *n* an actor of comic parts; an entertainer who tells jokes; a person who behaves in a humorous manner.

comedienne /kə,mi:di'ɛn/ *nf* a female comedian.

comedown /'kʌmdaun/ *n* a downfall; a disappointment.

comedy /'kɒmədi/ *n* (*pl* **comedies**) an amusing play or film; drama consisting of amusing plays; an amusing occurrence; humour.—**comedic** *adj*.

comehither /'kʌm,hiðər/ *adj* (*sl*) flirtatious; charmingly seductive.

comely /'kʌmli/ or /kɒmli/ *adj* (**comelier, comeliest**) pleasing to the eye, good-looking.—**comeliness** *n*.

come-on /'kʌm,ɒn/ *n* (*inf*) an enticement, lure.

comer /'kʌmər/ *n* (*inf*) a person or thing showing promise of success.

comestible /kə'mɛstibəl/ *n* (*usu pl*) anything to eat.

comet /'kɒmət/ *n* a celestial body that travels round the sun, with a visible nucleus and a luminous tail.—**cometary, cometic** *adj*.

comeuppance /kʌm'ʌpəns/ *n* (*inf*) a deserved retribution.

comfit /'kʌmfit/ *n* a candy; a sugared almond.

comfort /'kʌmfərt/ *vti* to bring consolation to; to soothe; to cheer. • *n* consolation; relief; bodily ease; (*pl*) things between necessities and luxuries.—**comforting** *adj*.

comfortable /'kʌmftərbəl/ or /-fərtəbəl/, /-frtəbəl/ *adj* promoting comfort; at ease; adequate; (*inf*) financially well off.—**comfortably** *adv*.

comforter /'kʌmfərtər/ *n* one who comforts; a woollen scarf; a baby's dummy teat; a quilted bedcover.

comfort station *n* (*inf*) a public lavatory.

comfrey /'kʌmfri/ *n* a tall bell-flowered hairy plant.

comfy /'kʌmfi/ *adj* (**comfier, comfiest**) (*inf*) comfortable.

comic /'kɒmɪk/ *adj* of comedy; causing amusement. • *n* a comedian; an entertaining person; a paper or book with strip cartoons.

comical /'kɒmɪkəl/ *adj* funny, laughable; droll, ludicrous.—**comically** *adv*.

comic book /'kɒmɪk,buk/ *n* a book or magazine containing stories told in strip cartoons.

comic opera *n* a musical play with a comic theme.

comic relief *n* a humorous scene or character in a tragedy that alleviates tension.

comic strip *n* a series of drawings that depict a story in stages.

coming /'kʌmɪŋ/ *adj* approaching next; of future importance or promise.

comitia /kɒ'mɪʃiə/ or /-'mɪʃə/ *n* (*pl* **comitia**) one of the three Roman public assemblies for passing laws, declaring war, etc.

comity /'kɒmɪti/ *n* (*pl* **comities**) civility, politeness; acts of international courtesy.

comma /'kɒmə/ *n* a punctuation mark (,) that indicates a slight pause or break in a sentence or separates items in a list.

command /kə'mænd/ *vti* to order; to bid; to control; to have at disposal; to evoke, compel; to possess knowledge or understanding of; to look down over; to be in authority (over), to govern. • *n* an order; control; knowledge; disposal; position of authority; something or someone commanded; an instruction to a computer; ✚ (*cap*) (*Cdn*) one of the three main branches of the Canadian armed forces.

commandant /,kɒmən'dænt/ or /-'dɒnt/, /'kɒm-/ *n* an officer in command of troops or a military establishment, *esp* a fortress.

commandeer /,kɒmən'di:r/ *vt* to seize for military purposes; to appropriate for one's own use.

commander /kə'mændər/ *n* a person who commands, a leader; a naval officer ranking next below a captain.—**commandership** *n*.

commander in chief *n* the commander of a state's entire forces.

commanding /-ɪŋ/ *adj* in command; dominating; impressive.

commandment /kə'mændmənt/ *n* a command; a divine law, *esp* one of the Ten Commandments in the Bible.

command module *n* the operational part of a spacecraft.

commando /kə'mændoʊ/ *n* (*pl* **commandos, commandoes**) a member of an elite military force trained to raid enemy territory.

comme il faut /,kɒmi:l'fo:/, *Fr.* /kɒmi:l'fo:/ as it should be; correct; well bred.

commemorate /kə'mɛmə,reɪt/ *vt* to keep in the memory by ceremony or writing; to be a memorial of.—**commemoration** *n*.—**commemorative, commemoratory** *adj*.—**commemorator** *n*.

commence /kə'mɛns/ *vti* to begin

commencement /-mənt/ *n* a start; a ceremony of conferring degrees; the day of this.

commend /kə'mɛnd/ *vt* to speak favourably of, to praise; to recommend; to entrust.—**commendable** *adj*.—**commendably** *adv*.—**commendatory** *adj*.

commendation /,kɒmən'deɪʃən/ *n* the act of commending, praise; an award.

commensal /kə'mɛnsəl/ *adj* (*biol*) living together, but not at the expense of another; (*person, organization*) living and feeding with another. • *n* one of two commensal plants or animals; a dinner companion.—**commensalism, commensality** *n*.

commensurable /kə'mɛnʃərəbəl/ or /-sjərəbəl/ *adj* measurable by the same standard; divisible without a remainder by the same quantity; proportionate (to).—**commensurability** *n*.

commensurate /kə'mɛnsəret/ or /-fərət/, /-sjərət/ *adj* having the same extent or measure proportionate.—**commensuration** *n*.

comment /'kɒmənt/ *n* a remark, observation, criticism; an explanatory note; talk, gossip. • *vi* to make a comment (upon); to annotate.—**commenter** *n*.

commentary /'kɒmən,teri/ *n* (*pl* **commentaries**) a series of explanatory notes or remarks; a verbal description on TV or radio of an event as it happens, *esp* sport.—*also* **running commentary.**—**commentarial** *adj*.

commentate /'kɒmən,teit/ *vt* to act as a commentator.

commentator /'kɒmən,teitər/ *n* one who reports and analyses events, trends, etc, as on television.

commerce /'kɒmərs/ *n* trade in goods and services on a large scale between nations or individuals.

commercial /kə'mərʃəl/ *adj* of or engaged in commerce; sponsored by an advertiser; intended to make a profit. • *n* a broadcast advertisement.—**commerciality** *n*.—**commercially** *adv*.

commercial art *n* art designed for use in all aspects of advertising and packaging.—**commercial artist** *n*.

commercialism /kə'mərʃə,lizəm/ *n* commercial methods or principle.—**commercialist** *n*.—**commercialistic** *adj*.

commercialize /-,laiz/ *vt* to put on a business basis; to exploit for profit.—**commercialization** *n*.

commercial traveller *n* a sales representative or travelling salesman.

commie /'kɒmi/ *n* (*pl* **commies**) (*derog*) a communist.

commination /,kɒmɪ'neiʃən/ *n* a threatening of divine punishment and vengeance, denunciation, cursing.—**comminatory** *adj*.

commingle /kə'mɪŋɡəl/ *vti* to mix together, to mingle.

comminute /'kɒmɪ,njuːt/ *vt* to reduce to minute particles or powder.—**comminution** *n*.

commiserate /kə'mɪzə,reit/ *vti* to sympathize (with); to feel pity for.—**commiseration** *n*.—**commiserator** *n*.

commissar /'kɒmɪ,sɑr/ *n* (*formerly*) a head of a government department in the USSR.

commissariat /,kɒmɪ'sɛriət/ *n* a supply of provisions; the department in charge of this, as for an army.

commissary /'kɒmɪsɛri/ or /kə'mɪs-/ *n* (*pl* **commissaries**) a store, as in an army camp, where food and supplies are sold; a restaurant in a film studio, factory, etc.—**commissarial** *adj*.

commission /kə'mɪʃən/ *n* authority to act; a document bestowing this; appointment as a military officer of the rank of lieutenant or above; a body of people appointed (by government) for specified duties; a task or duty or business committed to someone; a special order for something, *esp* a picture or other art object; a percentage on sales paid to a salesman or agent; brokerage. • *vt* to empower or appoint by commission; to employ the service of; to authorize.—**commissional, commissionary** *adj*.

commissioner /kə'mɪʃənər/ *n* a person empowered by a commission; various types of civil servant; a member of a commission.

commissure /'kɒmɪ,sjuːr/ *n* (*anat*) a line of junction, a seam; the point of union between two bodies.—**commissural** *adj*.

commit /kə'mɪt/ *vti* (**committing, committed**) to entrust; to consign (to prison); to do, to perpetrate a crime, etc; to pledge, to involve.—**committer** *n*.

commitment /-mənt/ *n* the act of committing; an engagement that restricts freedom; an obligation; an order for imprisonment or confinement in a mental institution.—*also* **committal.**

committed /-əd/ *adj* dedicated; pledged by a commitment.

committee /kə'mɪti/ *n* a body of people appointed from a larger body to consider or manage some matter.

commode /kə,moːd/ *n* a chamber pot enclosed in a stool; a chest of drawers.

commodious /kə'moːdiəs/ *adj* roomy; (*arch*) useful.

commodity /kə'mɒdəti/ *n* (*pl* **commodities**) an article of trade; a useful thing; (*pl*) goods.

commodore /ˈkɒməˌdɔr/ *n* a naval officer ranking below a rear admiral and above a captain; the senior commander of a fleet; the president of a yacht club.

common /ˈkɒmən/ *adj* belonging equally to more than one; public; usual, ordinary; widespread; familiar; frequent; easily obtained, not rare; low, vulgar; (*noun*) applying to any of a class. • *n* a tract of open public land; (*pl*) the common people; the House of Commons.—**commonality** *n*.—**commonly** *adv*.—**commonness** *n*.

commonage /ˈkɒmənədʒ/ *n* the right of pasturing on common land.

commonalty /ˈkɒmənəlti/, **commonality** /ˌkɒməˈnælɪti/ *n* (*pl* **commonalties, commonalities**) the common people.

common chord *n* a note accompanied by its third and fifth.

common denominator *n* a common multiple of the denominators of two or more fractions; a characteristic in common.

commoner /ˈkɒmənər/ *n* an ordinary person, not a member of the nobility.

common law *n* the body of law developed in England based on custom and judicial precedents, as distinct from statute law. • *adj* denoting a marriage recognized in law not by an official ceremony, but after a man and woman have cohabited for a number of years.

common market *n* a grouping of nations formed to facilitate trade by removing tariff barriers; (*with caps*) the European Union.

common measure *n* a number that will divide two or more numbers without a remainder.

commonplace /ˈkɒmənˌpleɪs/ *adj* ordinary, unremarkable. • *n* a platitude; an ordinary thing.

Commons /ˈkɒmənz/ *n* (*with* **the**) the House of Commons, the lower House of the British Parliament.

common sense *n* ordinary, practical good sense.—**common-sense** *adj*.

common time *n* (*mus*) two or four beats in a bar.

commonweal /ˈkɒmənˌwiːl/ *n* the public good.

commonwealth /-ˌwelθ/ *n* a political community; a sovereign state, republic; a federation of states; (*with cap*) an association of sovereign states and dependencies ruled or formerly ruled by Britain.

commotion /kəˈmoːʃən/ *n* a violent disturbance; agitation; upheaval.—**commotional** *adj*.

communal /kəˈmjuːnəl/ or /ˈkɒm-/ *adj* of a commune or community; shared in common.—**communality** *n*.—**communally** *adv*.

communalism /-ˌlɪzəm/ *n* a political system based on local self-government.—**communalist** *n*.—**communalistic** *adj*.

communalize /-ˌlaɪz/ *vt* to make over to a community.—**communalization** *n*.

communard /ˈkɒmjʊˌnɑrd/ *n* one who advocates government by communes.

commune[1] /ˈkɒmjuːn/ *n* a group of people living together and sharing possessions; the smallest administrative division in several European countries.

commune[2] /kəˈmjuːn/ *vi* to converse intimately; to communicate spiritually.

communicable /kəˈmjuːnɪkəbəl/ *adj* able to be communicated; (*disease*) easily passed on.—**communicability, communicableness** *n*.

communicant /kəˈmjuːnɪkənt/ *n* a person who receives Holy Communion.

communicate /kəˈmjuːnəˌkeɪt/ *vti* to impart, to share; to succeed in conveying information; to pass on; to transmit, *esp* a disease; to be connected.—**communicator** *n*.—**communicatory** *adj*.

communication /kəˌmjuːnəˈkeɪʃən/ *n* the act of communicating; information; a connecting passage or channel; (*pl*) connections of transport; (*pl*) means of imparting information, as in newspapers, radio, television.

communications satellite *n* an artificial satellite orbiting the earth used to relay telephone, radio and TV signals.

communicative /kəˈmjuːnɪkətɪv/ or /-ˌkeɪtɪv/ *adj* inclined to talk and give information.

communion /kəˈmjuːniən/ *n* common possession, sharing; fellowship; an emotional bond with; union in a religious body; (*with cap*) Holy Communion, the Christian sacrament of the Eucharist when bread and wine are consecrated and consumed.—**communional** *adj*.

communiqué /kəˌmjuːnəˈkeɪ/ or /kəˈmjuːnəˌkeɪ/ *n* an official communication, *esp* to the press or public.

communism /ˈkɒmjʊˌnɪzəm/ *n* a social system under which private property is abolished and the means of production are owned by the people; (*with cap*) a political movement seeking the overthrow of capitalism based on the writings of Karl Marx; the system as instituted in the former USSR and elsewhere.—**communistic** *adj*.

communist /-nɪst/ *n* a supporter of communism; (*with cap*) a member of a Communist party.

community /kəˈmjuːnɪti/ *n* (*pl* **communities**) an organized political or social body; a body of people in the same locality; the general public, society; any group having work, interests, etc in common; joint ownership; common character; a group of plants and animals of a region, dependent on each other for life and survival.

community centre *n* a place providing social and recreational facilities for a local community.

community hall *n* ✹ (*Cdn*) a hall in a community that is used for local events such as dances and suppers.

commutative /kəˈmjuːtətɪv/ *n* relating to or involving substitution; (*math*) having a result that is independent of the order in which the elements are combined; (*addition, etc*) showing this property.

commutator /ˈkɒmjuːˌteɪtər/ *n* a device for reversing the direction of electric current.

commute /kəˈmjuːt/ *vti* to travel a distance daily from home to work; to exchange (for); to change (to); to reduce (a punishment) to one less severe.—**commutable** *adj*.—**commutation** *n*.

commuter /-ər/ *n* a person who commutes to and from work.

commutershed *n* ✹ the area from which it is possible to commute to a large city.

comose /ˈkoːmoːs/ *adj* hairy; tufted.

compact[1] /ˈkɒmpækt/ *n* an agreement; a contract, a treaty.

compact[2] *adj* closely packed; condensed; terse; firm; taking up space neatly. • *vt* to press or pack closely; to compose (of). • *n* a small cosmetic case, *usu* containing face powder and a mirror.—**compacter** *n*.—**compactly** *adv*.—**compactness** *n*.

compact disc /ˈkɒmpækt/ *n* a small mirrored disc containing music (or audio-visual material) encoded digitally in metallic pits which are read optically by a laser beam.

compact video disc *n* a laser disc, similar to an audio compact disc, which plays sound and pictures.

companion[1] /kəmˈpænjən/ *n* an associate in an activity; a partner; a friend; one of a pair of matched things; a low-ranking member of an order of knighthood.—**companionship** *n*.

companion[2] *n* a wooden shelter over a companionway.

companionable /-əbəl/ *adj* friendly, sociable.—**companionability** *n*.—**companionably** *adv*.

companionway /-ˌweɪ/ *n* a ladder or staircase on a ship.

company /ˈkɒmpəni/ *n* (*pl* **companies**) any assembly of people; an association of people for carrying on a business, etc; a society; a military unit; the crew of a ship; companionship, fellowship; a guest, visitor(s).

comparable /ˈkɒmpərəbəl/ or /kəmˈpɛrəbəl/ *adj* able or suitable to be compared (*with* **with**); similar.—**comparably** *adv*.—**comparability** *n*.

comparative /kəmˈpɛrətɪv/ or /-ˈpærətɪv/ *adj* estimated by comparison; relative, not absolute; (*gram*) expressing more.—**comparatively** *adv*.

compare /kəmˈpɛr/ *vt* to make one thing the measure of another; to observe similarity between, to liken; to bear comparison; (*gram*) to give comparative and superlative forms of (an adjective). • *vi* to make comparisons; to be equal or alike.—**comparer** *n*.

comparison /kəmˈpærɪsən/ *n* the act of comparing; an illustration; a likeness; (*gram*) the use of *more* or *er* with an adjective.

compartment /kəmˈpɑrtmənt/ *n* a space partitioned off; a division of a railway carriage; a separate section or category.—**compartmental** *adj*.—**compartmented** *adj*.

compartmentalize /ˌkɒmpɑrtˈmɛntəˌlaɪz/ *vt* to divide into categories, *esp* excessively.—**compartmentalization** *n*.

compass /ˈkʌmpəs/ *n* a circuit, circumference; an extent, area; the range of a voice; an instrument with a magnetic needle indicating north, south, east, west; (*often pl*) a two-legged instrument for drawing circles, etc.—**compassable** *adj*.

compassion /kəmˈpæʃən/ *n* sorrow for another's sufferings; pity.

compassionate /-ət/ *adj* showing compassion; merciful.—**compassionately** *adv*.

compass points *n* north, south, east, west, etc.

compatible /kəmˈpætəbəl/ *adj* agreeing or fitting in (with); of like mind; consistent; (*body organ*) able to be transplanted successfully.—**compatibly** *adv*.—**compatibility** *n*.

compatriot /kəm'peɪtrɪət/ n a fellow countryman.—also adj.—**compatriotic** adj.

compeer /'kɒmpiːr/ or /-'piːr/ n an equal; a companion.

compel /kəm'pel/ vt (**compelling, compelled**) to force, constrain; to oblige; to obtain by force.—**compeller** n.

compelling /-ɪŋ/ adj evoking powerful feelings, eg interest, admiration.

compendious /kəm'pendɪəs/ adj containing much in a small space, succinct.

compendium /kəm'pendɪəm/ n (pl **compendiums, compendia**) an abridgement; a summary; a collection: an assortment of things in one box.

compensate /'kɒmpənˌseɪt/ vti to counterbalance; to make up for; to recompense.—**compensator** n.—**compensatory, compensative** adj.

compensation /ˌkɒmpən'seɪʃən/ n the act of compensating; a sum given to compensate, esp for loss or injury; an exaggerated display of ability in one area as a cover-up for a lack in another.

compete /kəm'piːt/ vi to strive; to contend; to take part in a competition, esp sporting.

competence /'kɒmpətəns/ n the quality of being capable; sufficiency; capacity; an adequate income to live on.

competency /-si/ n (pl **competencies**) competence; (law) the capacity to testify in court.

competent /-tənt/ adj fit, capable; adequate; with enough skill for; legally qualified.—**competently** adv.

competition /ˌkɒmpə'tɪʃən/ n act of competing; rivalry; a contest in skill or knowledge; a match.

competitive /kəm'petɪtɪv/ adj of, or involving, competition; of sufficient value in terms of price or quality to ensure success against rivals.—**competitively** adv.—**competitiveness** n.

competitor /kəm'petɪtər/ n a person who competes; an opponent; a rival.

compile /kəm'paɪl/ vt to collect or make up from various sources; to amass; to gather data, etc for a book; (comput) to translate high-level program instructions into machine code using a compiler.—**compilation** n.

compiler /-'paɪlər/ n a person who compiles a book, etc; (comput) a program that translates high-level program instructions into machine code.

complacence /kəm'pleɪsəns/ **complacency** /-ˌsiː/ n (pl **complacencies, complacences**) self-satisfaction; gratification.

complacent /kəm'pleɪsənt/ adj self-satisfied.—**complacently** adv.—**complacency, complacence** n.

complain /kəm'pleɪn/ vi to find fault, to grumble; to be ill; (poet) to express grief, to make a mourning sound.—**complainer** n.

complainant /kəm'pleɪnənt/ n (law) a plaintiff.

complaint /kəm'pleɪnt/ n a statement of some grievance; a cause of distress or dissatisfaction; an illness.

complaisant /kəm'pleɪzənt/ adj disposed to please, obliging; compliant.—**complaisance** n.

complement /'kɒmpləmənt/ n something making up a whole; a full allowance (of equipment or number); the entire crew of a ship, including officers. • vt to make complete.

complementary /ˌkɒmplɪ'mentəri/ adj completing; together forming a balanced whole.

complete /kəm'pliːt/ adj entire; free from deficiency; finished; thorough. • vt to make complete; to finish.—**completeness** n.—**completer** n.—**completive** adj.

completely /-li/ adv entirely, utterly.

completion /kəm'pliːʃən/ n the act of completing; accomplishment; fulfilment.

complex /'kɒmpleks/ adj having more than one part; intricate, not simple; difficult. • n a complex whole; a collection of interconnected parts, buildings or units; a group of mostly unconscious impulses, etc strongly influencing behaviour; (inf) an undue preoccupation; a phobia.—**complexity** n (pl **complexities**).

complex fraction n (math) a fraction with fractions for the numerator or denominator or both.

complexion /kəm'plekʃən/ n a colour, texture and look of the skin; aspect, character.

complexity /kəm'pleksəti/ n (pl **complexities**) the state of being complex, complexness.

complex number n (math) a number having both real and imaginary parts.

complex sentence n a sentence with one principal clause and one or more subordinate clauses.

compliance, compliancy /kəm'plaɪəns/ n the act of complying with another's wishes; acquiescence.

compliant /-ənt/ adj yielding, submissive.—**compliantly** adv.

complicate /'kɒmpləˌkeɪt/ vt to make intricate or involved; to mix up.

complicated /-əd/ adj intricately involved; difficult to understand.

complication /ˌkɒmpli'keɪʃən/ n a complex or intricate situation; a circumstance that makes (a situation) more complex; (med) a condition or disease following an original illness.

complicity /kəm'plisiti/ n (pl **complicites**) partnership in wrongdoing.

compliment /'kɒmpləmənt/ n a polite expression of praise, a flattering tribute; (pl) a formal greeting or expression of regard. • vt to pay a compliment to, to flatter; to congratulate (on).

complimentary /ˌkɒmplə'mentəri/ adj conveying or expressing a compliment; given free of charge.

complin, compline /'kɒmplɪn/ or /-plaɪn/ n (RC Church) the last service of the day following vespers.

comply /kəm'plaɪ/ vi (**complying, complied**) to act in accordance (with); to yield, to agree.—**complier** n.

compo /'kɒmpoː/ n (pl **compos**) a mixture of plaster, stucco, etc; (sl) compensation.

component /kəm'poːnənt/ adj going to the making of a whole, constituent. • n a component part.—**componential** adj.

comport /kəm'pɔːrt/ vti to conduct (oneself); to be compatible, to accord (with).—**comportment** n.

compose /kəm'poːz/ vt to make up, to form; to construct in one's mind, to write; to arrange, to put in order; to settle, to adjust; to tranquillize; (print) to set up type. • vi to create musical works, etc.

composed /-'poːzd/ adj calm, self-controlled.—**composedly** adv.

composer /-'poːzər/ n a person who composes, esp music.

composite /'kɒmpəzɪt/ adj made up of distinct parts or elements; (archit) blending Ionic and Corinthian orders; (bot) having many flowers in the guise of one, as the daisy. • n a composite thing or flower.

composition /ˌkɒmpə'zɪʃən/ n the act or process of composing; a work of literature or music, a painting; a short written essay; the general make-up of something; a chemical compound.—**compositional** adj.

compositor /kəm'pɒzɪtər/ n a person who puts together, or sets up, type for printing.

compos mentis /ˌkɒmpəs'mentis/ adj of sound mind, sane.

compost /'kɒmpoːst/ n a mixture of decomposed organic matter for fertilizing soil.

composure /kəm'poːʒər/ n the state of being composed, calmness.

compote /'kɒmpoːt/ or /-pɒt/ n fruit preserved in syrup.

compound[1] /'kɒmpaʊnd/ n a substance or thing made up of a number of parts or ingredients, a mixture; a compound word made up of two or more words. • vt to combine (parts, elements, ingredients) into a whole, to mix; to intensify by adding new elements; to settle (debt) by partial payment. • vi to become joined in a compound; to come to terms of agreement. • adj compounded or made up of several parts: not simple.—**compounder** n.

compound[2] n an enclosure in which a building stands.

compound eye n the eye in insects consisting of numerous separate visual units.

compound fracture n a fracture in which the shattered bone protrudes through the skin.

compound interest n interest paid on the principal sum of capital and the interest that it has accrued.

compound sentence n a sentence with more than one principal clause.

comprador /ˌkɒmprə'dɔːr/ n a native agent for a foreign company in China or Japan.

comprehend /ˌkɒmpri'hend/ vt to grasp with the mind, to understand; to include, to embrace.—**comprehendible** adj.—**comprehension** n.

comprehensible /-'hensɪəl/ adj capable of being understood.—**comprehensibly** adv.—**comprehensibility** n.

comprehensive /-'hensɪv/ adj wide in scope or content, including a great deal; (car insurance policy) covering most risks including third party, fire, theft. • n a comprehensive school.—**comprehensively** adv.—**comprehensiveness** n.

compress /kəm'pres/ *vt* to press or squeeze together; to bring into a smaller bulk; to condense. • *n* a soft pad for compressing an artery, etc; a wet or dry bandage or pad for relieving inflammation or discomfort.—**compressed** *adj.*—**compressible** *adj.*—**compressive** *adj.*

compression /kəm'preʃən/ *n* the act of compressing; the increase in pressure in an engine to compress the gases so that they explode.—**compressional** *adj.*

compressor /-'presər/ *n* a machine for compressing air or other gases.

comprise /kəm'praɪz/ *vt* to consist of, to include.—**comprisable** *adj.*—**comprisal** *n*.

compromise /'kɒmprə,maɪz/ *n* a settlement of a dispute by mutual concession; a middle course or view between two opposed ones. • *vti* to adjust by compromise; to lay open to suspicion, disrepute, etc.—**compromiser** *n*.

compromised /'kɒmprəmaɪzd/ *adj* (*reputation*) open to disrepute, tarnished.

comptroller /kən'troːlər/ or /kɒmp-/ *n* the form of controller used in some titles.

compulsion /kəm'pʊlʃən/ *n* the act of compelling; something that compels; an irresistible urge.

compulsive /-sɪv/ *adj* compelling; acting as if compelled.—**compulsively** *adv*.

compulsory /-səri/ *adj* enforced, obligatory, required by law, etc; involving compulsion; essential.—**compulsorily** *adv*.

compunction /kəm'pʌŋksən/ *n* pricking of the conscience; remorse; scruple.—**compunctious** *adj*.

computation /,kɒmpju:'teɪʃən/ *n* the act or process of computing; a reckoning, an estimate.—**computational** *adj*.

compute /kəm'pju:t/ *vt* to determine mathematically; to calculate by means of a computer. • *vi* to reckon; to use a computer.—**computability** *n*.—**computable** *adj*.—**computation** *n*.

computer /kəm'pju:tər/ *n* an electronic device that processes data in accordance with programmed instructions.

computer-aided tomography, computer-asisted tomography *see* **CAT**.

computer game *n* a game on cassette or disk to play on a home computer by means of operating the keys according to the images appearing on the screen.

computer graphics *n* the production and manipulation of pictorial images on a computer screen.

computerize /kəm'pju:tə,raɪz/ *vt* to equip with computers; to control or perform (a process) using computers; to store or process data using a computer.—**computerization** *n*.

computerized axial tomography *see* **CAT**.

computer language *n* a code used to provide instructions and data to a computer.

computer literate *adj* capable of or proficient in using computers.

computer virus *n* a program introduced into a computer system with the intention of sabotaging or destroying data.

comrade /'kɒmræd/ *n* a companion; a fellow member of a Communist party.—**comradely** *adv*.—**comradeship** *n*.

comsat /'kɒm,sæt/ *n* communications satellite.

con[1] /kɒn/ *vt* (**conning, conned**) (*inf*) to swindle, trick. • *n* (*inf*) a confidence trick.

con[2] *n* against, as in **pro and con**.

con[3] *prep* with.

con[4] *vt* (**conning, conned**) to direct the course of (a ship).

con[5] *vt* (**conning, conned**) to study; to learn by heart.

con[6] *n* (*sl*) a convict.

con- /kɒn/ or /kɒn/ *prefix* com-.

con amore *It.* /,kɒnæ'mɔreɪ/ *adj, adv* (*mus*) with love.

conation /koː'neɪʃən/ *n* (*psychol*) the faculty of voluntary agency, including volition and desire.

conative /'kɒnətɪv/ or /'kɒːn-/ *adj* (*verb*) expressing endeavour or effort; pertaining to the faculty of conation.

con brio *It.* /kɒn'briː/ *adj, adv* (*mus*) with spirit.

Conc. *abbr* ✦ (*Cdn*) = concession.

concatenate /kən'kætɪ,neɪt/ *vt* to link together. • *adj* linked.

concatenation /-'neɪʃən/ *n* a string of connected ideas or events.

concave /'kɒnkeɪv/ or /kɒn'keɪv/ *adj* curving inwards, hollow. • *n* a concave line or surface.—**concavity** *n* (*pl* **concavities**).

concavo-concave /kɒn'keɪvoːkɒn'keɪv/ *adj* hollow on both surfaces, as a lens.

concavo-convex /-kɒn'veks/ *adj* concave on one side, convex on the other.

conceal /kən'si:l/ *vt* to hide, to keep from sight; to keep secret.—**concealment** *n*.

concede /ken'si:d/ *vt* to grant; to admit to be true, to allow; to agree to be certain in outcome.—**conceder** *n*.

conceit /kən'si:t/ *n* an over-high opinion of oneself; vanity; a far-fetched comparison, a quaint fancy.

conceited /-əd/ *adj* full of conceit, vain.—**conceitedly** *adv*.

conceivable /kən'si:vəbəl/ *adj* capable of being imagined or believed; possible.—**conceivably** *adv*.

conceive /kən'si:v/ *vti* to become pregnant (with); to form in the mind; to think out, to imagine; to understand; to express.

concenter /kən'sentər/ *see* **concentre**.

concentrate /'kɒnsən,treɪt/ *vt* to bring or converge together to one point; to direct to a single object or purpose; to collect one's thoughts or efforts; (*chem*) to increase the strength of by diminishing bulk, to condense. • *n* a concentrated product, *esp* a food reduced in bulk by eliminating fluid; a foodstuff relatively high in nutrients.—**concentrator** *n*.

concentration /,kɒnsən'treɪʃən/ *n* the act or process of concentrating; the direction of attention to a single object; a drawing together of forces; the simultaneous firing of many weapons.—**concentrative** *adj*.

concentration camp *n* a camp where persons (as prisoners of war, political prisoners, and refugees) are detained or confined.

concentre /kən'sentər/ *vti* to bring or come to a common centre.—*also* **concenter**.

concentric /kən'sentrɪk/, **concentrical** /-əl/ *adj* having a common centre.—**concentrically** *adv*.—**concentricity** *n*.

concept /'kɒnsept/ *n* a general idea, *esp* an abstract one.

conceptacle /kən'septəkəl/ *n* (*bot*) that which holds anything; a follicle.

conception /kən'sepʃən/ *n* the act of conceiving; the fertilizing of an ovum by a sperm; a thing conceived; an idea, a notion.—**conceptional** *adj*.

conceptual /kən'septʃuəl/ *adj* of mental conception or concepts.

conceptualism /-,lɪzəm/ *n* (*philos*) the theory that universal truths exist in the mind apart from any concrete embodiment.—**conceptualist** *n*.—**conceptualistic** *adj*.

conceptualize /-,laɪz/ *vt* to form a concept of in the mind based on evidence, experience, etc.—**conceptualization** *n*.

concern /kən'sɜrn/ *vt* to relate or apply to; to fill with anxiety; to interest (oneself) in; to take part, to be mixed up (in). • *n* a thing that concerns one; anxiety, misgiving; interest in or regard for a person or thing; a business or firm.

concerned /kən'sɜrnd/ *adj* troubled, worried; interested.—**concernedly** *adv*.

concerning /-ɪŋ/ *prep* about; regarding.

concert /'kɒnsərt/ *n* a musical entertainment; harmony; agreement or union; **in concert** working together; (*musicians*) playing together.

concerted /kən'sɜrtəd/ *adj* planned or arranged by mutual agreement; combined; (*mus*) arranged in separate parts for musicians or singers.

concertina /,kɒnsər'ti:nə/ *n* a hexagonal musical instrument, similar to an accordion, which produces sound by squeezing bellows which pass air over metal reeds.

concertino /,kɒntʃər'ti:no:/ *n* (*pl* **concertini**) a short concerto.

concerto /kən'tʃɜrto:/ *n* (*pl* **concertos, concerti**) a musical composition for a solo instrument and orchestra.

concert pitch *n* a pitch slightly above normal; a state of exceptional efficiency.

concession /kə'nseʃən/ *n* the act of conceding; something conceded; a grant of rights, land, etc by a government, corporation, or individual; the sole right to sell a product within an area; a reduction in price (of admission, travel, etc) for certain people; ✦ (*Cdn*) a tract of surveyed farmland that is subdivided into individual lots.—**concessionary** *adj*.—**concessible** *adj*.

concessionaire, concessioner /kən,seʃə'nɛr/ *n* a person holding a concession.

concessive /kən'sesɪv/ *adj* of or expressing concession.

conch /kɒntʃ/ or /kɒŋk/ *n* (*pl* **conchs, conches**) a tropical marine spiral shell, sometimes used as a trumpet.

concha /'kɒŋkə/ *n* (*pl* **conchae**) the external ear or its cavity; (*archit*) the dome of a semicircular apse.—**conchal** *adj*.

conchiferous /kɒŋ'kɪfərəs/ *adj* producing shells.

conchology /-'kɒlədʒi/ *n* the branch of zoology that studies molluscs and their shells.—**conchological** *adj*.—**conchologist** *n*.

concierge /ˌkɔsi'erʒ/ or /kɒn-/ *n* a resident doorkeeper or janitor, *esp* in France.

conciliar /kən'sıliər/ *adj* of or pertaining to ecclesiastical councils.

conciliate /kən'sılieıt/ *vt* to win over from hostility; to make friendly; to appease; to reconcile.—**conciliation** *n*.—**conciliator** *n*.—**conciliatory** *adj*.

concinnity /kən'sınəti/ *n* (*pl* **concinnities**) neatness, elegance, *esp* in speech or writing.—**concinnous** *adj*.

concise /kən'sɔıs/ *adj* brief, condensed, terse.—**concisely** *adv*.—**conciseness** *n*.

concision /kən'sıʒən/ *n* conciseness; (*arch*) mutilation.

conclave /'kɒnkleıv/ *n* a private or secret meeting; a meeting of cardinals in seclusion to choose a pope; the meeting place.—**conclavist** *n*.

conclude /kən'kluːd/ *vti* to bring or come to an end, to finish; to effect, to settle; to infer; to resolve.

conclusion /kən'kluːʒən/ *n* concluding; the end or close; an inference; a final opinion; (*logic*) a proposition deduced from premises.

conclusive /-sıv/ *adj* decisive; convincing, removing all doubt.—**conclusively** *adv*.

concoct /kən'kɒkt/ *vt* to make by combining ingredients; to devise, to plan; to invent (a story).—**concocter, concoctor** *n*.—**concoctive** *adj*.

concoction /-'kɒkʃən/ *n* the act of concocting; something concocted; a mixture; a lie.

concomitance /kən'kɒmıtəns/ *n* the state of being concomitant; coexistence.

concomitant /-'kɒmıtənt/ *n* an accompanying thing or circumstance.—*also adj*.

concord /'kɒnkɔrd/ or /'kɒŋ-/ *n* agreement, harmony; a treaty; grammatical agreement.—**concordant** *adj*.

concordance /kən'kɔrdəns/ or /kəŋ-/ *n* agreement; an alphabetical index of words in a book or in the works of an author with their contexts.

concordant /-kɔrdənt/ *adj* agreeing, harmonious.

concordat /kən'kɔrdæt/ *n* a compact or agreement, *esp* between church and state.

concourse /'kɒnkɔrs/ or /'kɒŋ-/ *n* a crowd; a gathering of people or things, eg events; an open space or hall where crowds gather, eg a railway or airport terminal.

concrescence /kən'kresəns/ *n* (*biol*) a growing together, coalescence.—**concrescent** *adj*.

concrete /'kɒnkriːt/ or /'kɒŋ-/ *adj* having a material existence; (*gram*) denoting a thing, not a quality, not abstract; actual, specific (*a concrete example*); made of concrete. • *n* anything concrete; a mixture of sand, cement, etc with water, used in building. • *vti* to form into a mass, to solidify; to build or cover with concrete.

concretion /kən'kriːʃən/ *n* a solidified mass; a stone-like mass found in some parts of the body, calculus.—**concretionary** *adj*.

concubinage /kɒn'kjuːbınədʒ/ or /kɒŋ-/ *n* the act of living with a woman without being legally married.

concubine /'kɒŋkjuˌbaın/ or /'kɒn-/ *n* a secondary wife (in polygamous societies); (*formerly*) a mistress of a king or nobleman.—**concubinage** *n*.

concupiscence /kən'kjuːpısəns/ *n* sexual desire, lust.—**concupiscent** *adj*.

concur /kən'kər/ or /kəŋ-/ *vi* (**concurring, concurred**) to happen together, to coincide; to cooperate; to be of the same opinion, to agree.—**concurrence** *n*.

concurrence /-əns/ *n* the act of concurring; agreement; consent.

concurrent /-ənt/ *adj* existing, acting or occurring at the same time; coinciding.—**concurrently** *adv*.

concuss /kən'kʌs/ *vt* to shake violently, to agitate; to cause concussion of the brain.

concussion /kən'kʌʃən/ *n* the violent shock of an impact or explosion; loss of consciousness caused by a violent blow to the head.—**concussive** *adj*.

condemn /kən'dem/ *vt* to express strong disapproval of; to find guilty; to blame or censure; to declare unfit for use; to force into unwillingly.—**condemnable** *adj*.—**condemnation** *n*.—**condemnatory** *adj*.—**condemner** *n*.

condense /kən'dens/ *vt* to reduce to a smaller compass, to compress; to change from a gas into a liquid; to concentrate; to express in fewer words. • *vi* to become condensed.—**condensable, condensible** *adj*.—**condenser** *n*.—**condensation** *n*.

condensed milk *n* milk that has been sweetened and reduced by evaporation.

condenser /kən'densər/ *n* an apparatus for reducing gases or vapour to a liquid or solid form; a device for storing electricity; a lens for concentrating light.

condescend /ˌkɒndə'send/ *vi* to waive one's superiority; to deign, to stoop; to act patronizingly.—**condescension** *n*.

condescending /-ıŋ/ *adj* kindly in a lordly fashion to inferiors; patronizing.

condescension /-'senʃən/ *n* a condescending act or manner.

condign /kən'daın/ *adj* deserved, merited; suitable.

condiment /'kɒndəmənt/ *n* a seasoning or relish.

condition /kən'dıʃən/ *n* the state or nature of things; anything required for the performance, completion or existence of something else; physical state of health; an abnormality, illness; a prerequisite; (*pl*) attendant circumstances. • *vt* to be essential to the happening or existence of; to stipulate; to agree upon; to make fit; to make accustomed (to); to bring about a required effect by subjecting to certain stimuli.

conditional /-əl/ *adj* depending on conditions; not absolute; (*gram*) expressing condition. • *n* a conditional clause or conjunction.—**conditionality** *n*.—**conditionally** *adv*.

conditioner /-ər/ *n* a person or thing that conditions; a creamy substance for bringing the hair into a glossy condition.

conditioning /-ıŋ/ *n* a bringing into a required state or state of fitness for an objective.

condo /'kɒndoː/ *n* (*pl* **condos, condoes**) (*inf*) a condominium.

condole /kən'doːl/ *vt* (*with* **with**) to express sympathy for another.—**condolatory** *adj*.—**condoler** *n*.

condolence /kən'doːləns/ **condolement** /-mənt/ *n* sympathy.

con dolore *It. adv* (*mus*) mournfully.

condom /'kɒndəm/ *n* a sheath for the penis, used as a contraceptive and to prevent infection.

condominium /ˌkɒndə'mınıəm/ *n* (*pl* **condominiums**) a block of apartments, each apartment being individually owned; joint rule; a country ruled by more than one other country.

condone /kən'doːn/ *vt* to overlook, to treat as nonexistent; to pardon an offence.—**condonation** *n*.—**condoner** *n*.

condor /'kɒndɔr/ *n* a large South American vulture.

condottiere /ˌkɒndɒt'jeri/ *n* (*pl* **condottieri**) a military adventurer, a captain of mercenaries.

conduce /kən'duːs/ or /-duːs/ *vi* to tend to bring about, to contribute (to)—**conducer** *n*.

conducive /-'duːsıv/ or /-djuːsıv/ *adj* leading to or helping to cause or produce a result.

conduct /'kɒndʌkt/ *vti* to lead; to guide; to convey; to direct (an orchestra); to carry on or manage (a business); to transmit (electricity, heat); to behave (oneself). • *n* management, direction; behaviour.—**conductible** *adj*.—**conductibility** *n*.

conductance /kən'dʌktəns/ *n* the ability of a specified system to conduct electricity.

conduction /kən'dʌkʃən/ *n* the conducting or transmission of heat or electricity through a medium; the transmission of nerve impulses.

conductive /-tıv/ *adj* having the power to transmit heat or electricity.—**conductivity** *n* (*pl* **conductivities**).

conductor /kən'dʌktər/ *n* a person who conducts an orchestra; one in charge of passengers on a train, or who collects fares on a bus; a substance that conducts heat or electricity.—**conductress** *nf*.

conduit /'kɒnduıt/ or /-djuıt/ *n* a channel or pipe that carries water, etc.

conduplicate /kɒn'duːplıkıt/ or /-'djuː-/ *adj* (*bot*) folded lengthwise along the middle.—**conduplication** *n*.

condyle /'kɒndıl/ or /-daıl/ *n* the rounded head at the end of a bone fitting into another bone.—**condylar** *adj*.

condyloid /-də,lɔıd/ *adj* shaped like, resembling or connected with a condyle.

cone /koːn/ *n* a solid pointed figure with a circular or elliptical base; any cone-shaped object (*an ice-cream cone*); a warning bollard on roads, etc; the scaly fruit of the pine, fir, etc.

coney /'koːni/ *see* **cony**.

confab /'kɒnfæb/ *n* (*inf*) an informal talk, chat.

confabulate /kən'fæbjuˌleıt/ *vi* to talk familiarly together.—**confabulation** *n*.—**confabulator** *n*.—**confabulatory** *adj*.

confection /kən'fekʃən/ *n* candy, ice cream, preserves, etc; anything overfussy, fanciful or ornate.

confectionary /-ˌɛri/ *n* (*pl* **confectionaries**) a place where confectionery is made or sold. • *adj* of or pertaining to confectionery.

confectioner /-ər/ *n* a person who makes or sells confectionery.

confectionery /-ˌɛri/ *n* (*pl* **confectioneries**) candies.

confederacy /kən'fɛdərəsi/ *n* (*pl* **confederacies**) a union of states, an alliance; a combination of persons for illegal purposes; (*with cap*) the Confederate States of America.

confederate /kən'fɛdərət/ *adj* banded together by treaty, united in confederation. • *vti* to bring or come into alliance or confederacy. • *n* a member of a confederacy; a partner in design, an accomplice; an ally.

Confederate States *npl* in US history, the eleven Southern States that seceded from the Union in 1861, leading to the Civil War in which they were defeated in 1865.

confederation /kənˌfɛdə'reɪʃən/ *n* the act or state of confederating; an alliance of individuals, organizations, states or cantons (as in Switzerland); (*with cap*) ✤ the political union of most British colonies in North America in 1867 to form the Dominion of Canada, subsequently expanded to include the present provinces and territories.—**confederationism** *n*.—**confederationist** *n*.

confer /kən'fər/ *vt* (**conferring, conferred**) to grant or bestow; to compare views or take counsel; to consult.—**conferment, conferral** *n*.—**conferrable** *adj*.—**conferrer** *n*.

conferee, conferree /ˌkɑnfə'ri:/ *n* one on whom something is conferred; a member of a conference.

conference /'kɑnfərəns/ *n* a meeting for discussion or consultation.—**conferential** *adj*.

conferva /kən'fərvə/ *n* (*pl* **confervae, confervas**) a genus containing green freshwater algae.—**conferval** *adj*.—**confervoid** *adj*.

confess /kən'fɛs/ *vt* to acknowledge or admit; to disclose (sins) to a confessor; (*priest*) to hear confession of. • *vi* to make or hear a confession.

confessedly /-ədli/ *adv* avowedly.

confession /kən'fɛʃən/ *n* admission or acknowledgement of a fault or sin, *esp* to a confessor; a thing confessed; a statement of one's religious beliefs, creed.—**confessionary** *adj*.

confessional /-əl/ *n* an enclosure in a church where a priest hears confessions.

confessor /-sər/ *n* a priest who hears confessions and grants absolution; one who confesses.

confetti /kən'fɛti/ *npl* small bits of coloured paper thrown at weddings.

confidant /ˌkɑnfi'dɑnt/ or /'kɑnfiˌdɑnt/, /-dænt/ *n* a person trusted with one's secrets.—**confidante** *nf*.

confide /kən'faɪd/ *vti* to put confidence (in); to entrust; to impart a confidence or secret.—**confider** *n*.

confidence /'kɑnfidəns/ *n* firm trust, faith; belief in one's own abilities; boldness; something revealed confidentially.

confidence trick *n* the persuading of a victim to hand over valuables as proof of confidence.

confident /'kɑnfidənt/ *adj* full of confidence; positive, assured.—**confidently** *adv*.

confidential /ˌkɑnfi'dɛnʃəl/ *adj* spoken or written in confidence, secret; entrusted with secrets.—**confidentiality, confidentialness** *n*.—**confidentially** *adv*.

confiding /kən'faɪdɪŋ/ *adj* unsuspicious.—**confidingly** *adv*.

configuration /kənˌfɪgjʊ'reɪʃən/ or /-gə'reɪʃən/ *n* arrangement of parts; external shape, general outline; aspect; (*astrol*) the relative position of the planets; the make-up of a computer system.—**configurational, configurative** *adj*.

confine /'kɑnfaɪn/ *n*; /kən'faɪn/ *vt* to restrict, to keep within limits; to keep shut up, as in prison, a sickbed, etc; to imprison. • *n* (*pl*) borderland, edge, limit.—**confinable, confineable** *adj*.

confined /-nd/ *adj* narrow, enclosed, of limited space.

confinement /kən'faɪnmənt/ *n* a being confined; the period of childbirth.

confirm /kən'fərm/ *vt* to make stronger; to establish firmly; to make valid, to ratify; to corroborate; to administer rite of confirmation to.

confirmation /ˌkɑnfər'meɪʃən/ *n* the act of confirming; convincing proof; the rite by which people are admitted to full communion in Christian churches.

confirmatory /kən'fərməˌtɔri/, **confirmative** /-meɪtɪv/ *adj* giving extra proof; corroborative.

confirmed /kən'fərmd/ *adj* habitual; settled in belief, mode of life, etc; having undergone the rite of confirmation.

confiscate /'kɑnfiˌskeɪt/ *vt* to appropriate to the state as a penalty; to seize by authority.—**confiscable** *adj*.—**confiscation** *n*.—**confiscator** *n*.—**confiscatory** *adj*.

conflagration /ˌkɑnflə'greɪʃən/ *n* a massively destructive fire.—**conflagrative** *adj*.

conflation /kən'fleɪʃən/ *n* a fusing together; a combining of two variant readings of a text into one.—**conflate** *vt*.

conflict /'kɑnflɪkt/ *n* a fight; a contest; strife, quarrel; emotional disturbance. • *vi* to be at variance; to clash (with); to struggle.—**confliction** *n*.—**conflictive, conflictory** *adj*.

conflicting /-ɪŋ/ *adj* contradictory.

confluence /'kɑnfluəns/, **conflux** /'kɑnˌflʌks/ *n* the point where two rivers meet; a coming together.

confluent /-ənt/ *adj* flowing or running together. • *n* a tributary river or stream.

confocal /kɑn'foːkəl/ *adj* having a common focus.

conform /kən'fɔrm/ *vi* to comply, to be obedient (to); to act in accordance with. • *vt* to adapt; to make like.—**conformer** *n*.

conformable /-əbəl/ *adj* compliant; corresponding, adapted (to); in parallel order.—**conformability, conformableness** *n*.—**conformably** *adv*.

conformation /ˌkɑnfɔr'meɪʃən/ *n* arrangement of parts, structure; adaptation.

conformist /kən'fɔrmɪst/ *n* one who conforms to established rules, standards, etc; compliance with the rites and doctrines of an established church. —**conformism** *n*.

conformity /kən'fɔrmɪti/, **conformance** /-məns/ *n* (*pl* **conformities, conformances**) correspondence; agreement; conventional behaviour; compliance.

confound /kən'faʊnd/ *vt* to mix up, to obscure; to perplex, to astound; to overthrow; to mistake one thing for another.—**confounder** *n*.

confounded /-ɪd/ *adj* astonished; confused; annoying; (*inf*) damned.—**confoundedly** *adv*.

confraternity /ˌkɑnfrə'tərnəti/ *n* (*pl* **confraternities**) a brotherhood or society of men associated for a common purpose.—**confraternal** *adj*.

confrère /'kɑnˌfrɛr/ *n* an associate, a colleague.

confront /kən'frʌnt/ *vt* to stand in front of, to face; to bring face to face (with); to encounter; to oppose.—**confronter** *n*.

confrontation /ˌkɑnfrʌn'teɪʃən/ *n* the coming face to face with; hostility without actual warfare, *esp* between nations.

Confucian /kən'fju:ʃən/ *adj* pertaining to Confucius, the Chinese philosopher. • *n* a follower of the teachings of Confucius.

confuse /kən'fju:z/ *vt* to throw into disorder; to mix up; to mistake one thing for another; to perplex, to disconcert; to embarrass; to make unclear.—**confusable** *adj*.—**confusing** *adj*.—**confusingly** *adv*.

confused /-d/ *adj* perplexed; disordered; mentally unbalanced.—**confusedly** *adv*.

confusion /kən'fju:ʒən/ *n* the act or state of being confused; disorder; embarrassment, discomfiture; lack of clarity.

confute /kən'fju:t/ *vt* (*argument, etc*) to prove wrong; to convict of error; to overcome in argument.—**confutation** *n*.—**confutative** *adj*.—**confuter** *n*.

conga /'kɑŋgə/ *n* a Cuban dance in which the dancers move along in a long line; music for this. • *vi* (**congaing, congaed**) to do this dance.

congé /'kɒ̃ʒeɪ/ *n* dismissal; (*arch*) a formal bow, *esp* at parting.

congeal /kən'dʒi:l/ *vti* to change from a liquid to a solid by cooling, to jell.—**congealment** *n*.

congelation /ˌkɑndʒə'leɪʃən/ *n* the act of congealing; a congealed state or substance.

congener /'kɑndʒənər/ *n* a person or thing of the same kind as another.

congeneric /ˌkɑndʒə'nɛrɪk/ *adj* of the same genus or origin.

congenial /kən'dʒi:niəl/ *adj* of a similar disposition or with similar tastes, kindred; suited, agreeable (to).—**congenially** *adv*.—**congeniality, congenialness** *n*.

congenital /kən'dʒɛnɪtəl/ *adj* existing or dating since birth, as in certain defects.—**congenitally** *adv*.

conger eel /'kɑŋgər/ *n* a large marine eel.

congeries /'kɑndʒəˌri:z/ or /kɑn'dʒi:ri:z / *n* (*used as sing or pl*) a gathered mass, a heap; a conglomeration.

congest /kən'dʒɛst/ vt to overcrowd. • vi (med) to affect with congestion.—**congested** adj.—**congestible** adj.

congestion /kən'dʒɛstʃən/ n an overcrowding; (med) an excessive accumulation of blood in any organ; an accumulation of traffic causing obstruction.—**congestive** adj.

conglobate /kən'gloːbeɪt/ or /'kɒngloːˌbeɪt/ vti to form into a mass.—**conglobation** n.

conglomerate /kən'glɒməˌrət/ adj stuck together in a mass. • vt to gather into a ball. • n a coarse-grained rock of embedded pebbles; a large corporation consisting of companies with varied and often unrelated interests.—**conglomeratic, conglomeritic** adj.

conglomeration /kənˌglɒmə'reɪʃən/ n the act of conglomerating; a mass stuck together; a miscellaneous collection.

conglutinate /kən'gluːtɪnˌeɪt/ vt to glue together. • adj glued together; united by an adhesive substance.—**conglutination** n.—**conglutinative** adj.

congou /'kɒnguː/ n a kind of black Chinese tea.

congratulate /kən'grætʃəˌleɪt/ or /-'grædʒ-/ vt to express sympathetic pleasure at success or good fortune of, to compliment; to feel satisfied or pleased with oneself.—**congratulation** n.—**congratulator** n.—**congratulatory** adj.

congratulations /kənˌgrætʃə'leɪʃəns/ npl an expression of joy or pleasure.

congregate /'kɒngrəˌgeɪt/ vti to flock together, to assemble; to gather into a crowd or mass.—**congregator** n.

congregation /ˌkɒngrə'geɪʃən/ n a gathering, an assembly; a body of people assembled for worship.

congregational /-əl/ adj of a congregation; (with cap) of or pertaining to Congregationalism.

Congregationalism /-ˌlɪzəm/ n a form of church government in which each congregation has management of its own affairs.—**Congregationalist** adj, n.

congress /'kɒngrɛs/ n an association or society; an assembly or conference, esp for discussion and action on some question; (with cap) the legislature of the US, comprising the Senate and the House of Representatives.

congressional /kən'grɛʃənəl/ adj of, or relating to, a congress.—**congressionalist** n.

Congressman /'kɒngrɛsmən/ n (pl **Congressmen**) a member of Congress.—**Congresswoman** nf (pl **Congresswomen**).

congruent /-wənt/ or /-ənt/ adj in agreement; harmonious; (geom) having identical shape and size so that all parts correspond.—**congruence, congruency** n.

congruous /'kɒngruəs/ adj accordant; fit.—**congruity** r.

conic /'kɒnɪk/, **conical** /-əl/ adj of a cone; cone-shaped.

conics /-ɪks/ n (used as sing) the branch of geometry that deals with conic sections.

conic section n a curve formed from a cone—an ellipse, a parabola, or a hyperbola.

conidium /kə'nɪdɪəm/ (pl **conidia**) a reproductive cell formed of certain fungi.—**conidial** adj.

conifer /'kɒnɪfə/ or /'kɒː-/ n any evergreen trees and shrubs with true cones (as pines) and others (as yews).—**coniferous** adj.

coniferous /'kənɪfərəs/ adj bearing fruit cones.

conine, conin /'kɒnɪˌɪn/ or /'kɒːnɪn/ n a very poisonous alkaloid existing in the hemlock.

conium /'kɒːnɪəm/ or /kɒː'naɪəm/ n a genus of biennial poisonous plants including the hemlock.

conjectural /kən'dʒɛktʃərəl/ adj depending on conjecture, doubtful.—**conjecturally** adv.

conjecture /kən'dʒɛktʃər/ n a guess, guesswork. • vt to make a conjecture, to guess, surmise.—**conjecturer** n.—**conjecturable** adj.—**conjectural** adj.

conjoin /kən'dʒɔɪn/ vt to join together; to connect or associate. • vi to be joined.—**conjoinedly** adv.—**conjoiner** n.

conjoint /kən'dʒɔɪnt/ adj united, combined; cooperating.—**conjointly** adv.

conjugal /'kɒndʒʊgəl/ adj of or relating to marriage.—**conjugality** n.—**conjugally** adv.

conjugate /'kɒndʒʊˌgeɪt/ vt to give the parts of (a verb); to unite.—**conjugable** adj.—**conjugation** n.—**conjugator** n.—**conjugative** adj.

conjugation /ˌkɒndʒʊ'geɪʃən/ n the act of conjugating; a group of verbs with the same inflections; the union of cells in reproduction.—**conjugational** adj.

conjunct /kən'dʒʌŋkt/ adj, n joined together; associated.

conjunction /kən'dʒʌŋkʃən/ n (gram) a word connecting words, clauses or sentences; a union; a simultaneous occurrence of events; the apparent proximity of two or more planets.—**conjunctional** adj.

conjunctiva /ˌkɒndʒʌŋk'tɪvə/ or /kɒn'dʒʌŋktɪvə/ n (pl **conjunctivas, conjunctivae**) the mucous membrane that lines the inner surface of the eyelids and the exposed area of the eyeball.—**conjunctival** adj.

conjunctive /kən'dʒʌŋktɪv/ adj serving to unite; closely connected; (gram) of or pertaining to conjunctions. • n a conjunction.—**conjunctively** adv.

conjunctivitis /kənˌdʒʌŋkɪ'vaɪtɪs/ n inflammation of the conjunctiva.

conjuncture /kən'dʒʌŋktʃər/ n a combination of many circumstances or causes; a critical time.—**conjunctural** adj.

conjuration /ˌkɒndʒʊ'reɪʃən/ n the act of conjuring or invoking; an incantation; an enchantment; a solemn entreaty.

conjure /'kɒndʒər/ or /'kʌr-/ vti to practise magical tricks; to call up (spirits) by invocation.

conjurer, conjuror /'kɒndʒərər/ or /'kʌn-/ n one who conjures or is skilled in sleight of hand.

conk /kɒŋk/ n (sl) the nose or head. • n a blow to the nose or head. • vt to hit, esp on the head. • vi (with out) (sl) (machine) to break down entirely; to collapse suddenly from exhaustion.

conker /'kɒŋkər/ n (inf) the horse chestnut; (pl) a children's game using conkers on a string.

con man n (inf) a swindler, one who defrauds by means of a confidence trick.

con moto /kɒn'moːtoː/, It. /kɒn'mɔtə/ adj (mus) spirited.

connate /kɒ'neɪt/ adj inborn, congenital; (leaves) united at the base.

connatural /kən'nætʃərəl/ adj congenital; having the same nature.

connect /kə'nɛkt/ vti to fasten together, to join; to relate together, to link up; (trains, buses, etc) to be timed to arrive as another leaves so that passengers can continue their journey; to establish a link by telephone; (sl) to punch or kick; to uncover (a source of drugs).—**connectible, connectable** adj.—**connector, connecter** n.

connection /kə'nɛkʃən/ n the act of connecting; the state of being connected; a thing that connects; a relationship, bond; a train, bus, etc timed to connect with another; an opportunity to transfer between trains, buses, etc; context; a link between components in an electric circuit; a relative; (sl) a supply or the supplier of illicit drugs; (pl) clients, customers.—**connectional** adj.

connective /kə'nɛktɪv/ adj serving to connect.—**connectively** adv.

connectivity /kə'nɛktɪvɪti/ n the ability of computers of different kinds to communicate.

conning tower n the armoured pilot house of a submarine.

conniption /kə'nɪpʃən/ n (sl) a fit of hysteria or rage.

connivance /kə'naɪvəns/ n the act of conniving; pretence of ignorance; passive cooperation in a crime or fault; collusion.

connive /kə'naɪv/ vi to permit tacitly; to wink (at); to plot.—**conniver** n.

connivent /-ənt/ adj converging.

connoisseur /ˌkɒnə'sər/ or /-'sʊr/ n a trained discriminating judge, esp of the fine arts.

connotation /ˌkɒnə'teɪʃər/ n a consequential meaning, an implication.—**connotative, connotive** adj.

connote /kə'noːt/ vt to imply; to indicate; to mean.

connubial /kə'nuːbɪəl/ or /-njuː-/ adv of or relating to marriage.—**connubiality** n—**connubially** adv.

conoid /'koːnɔɪd/ n (geom) a solid formed by revolution of a conic section about its axis. • adj somewhat conical.—also **conoidal**.

conquer /'kɒŋkər/ vt to gain victory (over), to defeat; to acquire by conquest; to overcome, to master. • vi to be victor.—**conqueror** n.

conquest /'kɒŋˌkwɛst/ or /'kɒŋ-/ n conquering; the winning of a person's affection; a person or thing conquered.

conquistador /kɒn'kwɪstəˌdɔr/ n (pl **conquistadors, conquistadores**) a member of the Spanish forces that conquered Mexico and Peru in the 16th century.

Cons. abbr = Conservative.

consanguineous /ˌkɒnsæŋ'gwɪnɪəs/ or /-sæn-/, **consanguine** /-'sæŋgwɪn/ adj related by blood or birth.—**consanguinity** n.

conscience /'kɒnʃəns/ n the knowledge of right and wrong that affects a person's action and behaviour; the sense of guilt or virtue induced by actions, behaviour, etc; an inmost thought; conscientiousness.

conscience clause n a clause in an act giving relief to persons having religious scruples to some requirement in it.

conscience investment n the investment in companies whose activities do not offend the investor's moral principles.—*also* **ethical investment**.

conscience money n money paid, *usu* anonymously, to atone for some dishonest act or illegal monetary gain.

conscience-stricken adj feeling extreme guilt or remorse.

conscientious /ˌkɒnʃi'enʃəs/ adj following the dictates of the conscience; scrupulous; careful, thorough.—**conscientiously** adv.—**conscientiousness** n.

conscientious objector n a person who refuses to serve in the military forces on moral or religious grounds.

conscionable /'kɒnʃənəbəl/ adj governed by conscience, just.—**conscionably** adv.

conscious /'kɒnʃəs/ adj aware (of); awake to one's surroundings; *(action)* realized by the person who does it, deliberate.—**consciously** adv.

consciousness /-nəs/ n the state of being conscious; perception; the whole body of a person's thoughts and feelings.

conscript /'kɒnˌskrɪpt/ for n, adj, for vb enrolled into service by compulsion; drafted. • n a conscripted person (as a military recruit). • /kən'skrɪpt/ vt to enlist compulsorily.

conscription /kən'skrɪpʃən/ n compulsory military or naval service; the persons enrolled.—**conscriptional** adj.

consecrate /'kɒnsəˌkreɪt/ vt to set apart as sacred, to sanctify; to devote (to).—**consecration** n.—**consecrator** n.—**consecratory, consecrative** adj.

consecration /ˌkɒnsə'kreɪʃən/ n the act of consecrating; a setting apart or devoting to a sacred use or office; *(with cap)* *(RC Church)* the part of Mass when the bread and wine are blessed.

consecution /ˌkɒnsə'kjuːʃən/ n a following on; a logical sequence.

consecutive /kən'sekjʊtɪv/ adj following in regular order without a break; successive; *(gram)* expressing consequence.—**consecutively** adv.

consensual /kən'senʃʊəl/ adj caused by sympathetic action.

consensus /kən'sensəs/ n an opinion held by all or most; general agreement, *esp* in opinion.

consent /kən'sent/ vi to agree (to); to comply; to acquiesce. • n agreement, permission; concurrence.—**consenter** n.

consequence /'kɒnsəkwəns/ n a result, an outcome; importance; *(pl)* an unpleasant result of an action; a game in which each player writes part of a story without knowing what has gone before.

consequent /-kwənt/ adj occurring as a result.

consequential /ˌkɒnsə'kwenʃəl/ adj pompous, self-important; resultant.—**consequentiality, consequentialness** n.—**consequentially** adv.

consequently /-ˌkwentli/ adv as a result, therefore.

conservancy /kən'sɜːrvənsi/ n *(pl* **conservancies**) in UK, an authority controlling a river or port; conservation.

conservation /ˌkɒnsər'veɪʃən/ n the act of conserving; preservation of the environment and natural resources.—**conservational** adj.—**conservationist** n.

conservation of energy n the fact that the amount of energy in a closed system remains the same although its form changes.

conservatism /kən'sɜːrvəˌtɪzəm/ n opposition to change; a political ideology favouring preservation and defence of tradition.

conservative /-tɪv/ adj traditional, conventional; cautious; moderate. • n a conservative person; *(with cap)* a member of the Conservative Party in Britain and other countries.—**conservatively** adv.

conservatoire /kən'sɜːrvəˌtwɑr/ n an institution for instruction in music.

conservator /kən'sɜːrvəˌtər/ or /'kɒnsərˌveɪtər/ n a custodian, a keeper; a preserver; a member of a conservancy.

conservatory /kən'sɜːrvəˌtɔri/ or /-triː/ n *(pl* **conservatories**) a greenhouse attached to a house; a conservatoire.

conserve /kən'sɜːrv/ vt to keep from loss or injury; to preserve (a foodstuff) with sugar. • n a type of jam using whole fruit.—**conservable** adj.—**conserver** n.

consider /kən'sɪdər/ vti to reflect (upon), to contemplate; to examine, to weigh the merits of; to take into account; to regard as; to be of the opinion; to act with respect; to allow for.—**considerer** n.

considerable /kən'sɪdərəbəl/ adj a fairly large amount; worthy of respect.—**considerably** adv.

considerate /kən'sɪdərət/ adj careful of the feelings of others.—**considerately** adv.

consideration /kənˌsɪdə'reɪʃən/ n the act of considering; deliberation; a point of importance; an inducement; thoughtfulness; deference; a payent.

considered /kən'sɪdərd/ adj well thought out.

considering /kən'sɪdərɪŋ/ prep in view of. • adv all in all. • conj seeing that.

consign /kə'saɪn/ vt to hand over, to commit; to send goods addressed (to).—**consignable** adj.—**consignation** n.

consignee /ˌkɒn'saɪniː/ or /kənˌsaɪ'niː/ n the person to whom goods are consigned.

consignment /kən'saɪnmənt/ n consigning; goods, etc consigned.

consignor /ˌkɒn'saɪnər/ or /kən'saɪnˌɔr/, /-ər/ n the person by whom goods are consigned.

consist /kən'sɪst/ vi to be made up (of); to be comprised (of).

consistency /kən'sɪstənsi/ n *(pl* **consistencies**) degree of density, *esp* of thick liquids; the state of being consistent.

consistent /kən'sɪstənt/ adj compatible, not contradictory; uniform in thought or action.—**consistently** adv.

consistory /kən'sɪstəri/ n a solemn assembly or the place where it meets; the ecclesiastical court of the pope and cardinals, of an Anglican bishop, or of Presbyterian presbyters.—**consistorial, consistorian** adj.

consolation /ˌkɒnsə'leɪʃən/ n someone or something that offers comfort in distress.—**consolatory** adj.

consolation prize n a prize for the runner up or loser in a competition.

console¹ /kən'soːl/ vt to bring consolation to, to cheer in distress.—**consolable** adj.—**consoler** n.

console² /'kɒnsoːl/ n a desk containing the controls of an electronic system; the part of an organ containing the pedals, stops, etc; an ornamental bracket supporting a shelf or table.

consolidate /kə'sɒlɪˌdeɪt/ vti to solidify; to establish firmly, to strengthen; to combine into a single whole.—**consolidator** n.

consolidated school n ✻ *(Cdn)* a school that replaces several existing schools in an area.

consolidation /kənˌsɒlɪ'deɪʃən/ n the act of consolidating; solidification.

consols /'kɒnˌsɒlz/ or /kən'sɒlz/ npl British government securities consolidated into a single stock.

consommé /'kɒnsəˌmeɪ/ or /ˌkɒnsə'meɪ/ n a clear soup made from meat stock.

consonance /'kɒnsənəns/, **consonancy** /-i/ n *(pl* **consonance, consonancies**) agreement of sounds; harmony; concord.

consonant /-nənt/ n a letter of the alphabet that is not a vowel; the sound representing such a letter. • adj consistent, in keeping (with).—**consonantal** adj.

consort /'kɒnˌsɔrt/ n, a husband or wife, *esp* of a reigning queen or king; a ship sailing with another. • vti to associate, to keep company with (often dubious companions).—**consorter** n.

consortium /kən'sɔrtiəm/ or /-'sɔrʃəm/ n *(pl* **consortia**) an international banking or financial combination.—**consortial** adj.

conspectus /kən'spektəs/ n a general sketch or digest of some subject, a synopsis.

conspicuous /kən'spɪkjʊəs/ adj easily seen, prominent; outstanding, eminent.—**conspicuousness** n.—**conspicuously** adv.

conspiracy /kən'spɪrəsi/ n *(pl* **conspiracies**) a secret plan for an illegal act; the act of conspiring.

conspirator /kən'spɪrətər/ n one who conspires.—**conspiratorial, conspiratory** adj.—**conspiratorially** adv.

conspire /kən'spaɪr/ vti to combine secretly for an evil purpose; to plot, to devise.

con spirito *It.* /kɒn'spɪrɪtoː/ adj, adv *(mus)* with spirit.

constable /'kɒnstəbəl/ n in UK, a policeman or policewoman of the lowest rank; a governor of a royal castle.

constabulary /kən'stæbjuːˌleri/ n *(pl* **constabularies**) in UK, a police force.—*also adj*.

constancy /'kɒnstənsi/ n being constant; steadfastness; fidelity.

constant /'kɒnstənt/ adj fixed; unchangeable; unchanging; faithful; firm and steadfast; continual. • n *(math, physics)* a quantity that does not vary.

constantly /-li/ adv continually, continuously, often.

constellate /'kɒnstəˌleɪt/ vti to form into a constellation.

constellation /ˌkɒnstəˈleɪʃən/ n a group of fixed stars; an assembly of the famous.—**constellatory** adj.

consternate /ˈkɒnstər.neɪt/ vt to dismay.

consternation /ˌkɒnstərˈneɪʃən/ n surprise and alarm; shock; dismay.

constipate /ˈkɒnstɪˌpeɪt/ vt to cause constipation in.—**constipated** adj.

constipation /ˈkɒnstɪˈpeɪʃən/ n infrequent and difficult movement of the bowels.

constituency /kənˈstɪtʃʊənsi/ n (pl **constituencies**) a body of electors; the voters in a particular district or area.

constituent /kənˈstɪtʃʊənt/ adj forming part of a whole, component; having the power to revise the constitution. • n a component part; a member of an elective body; a voter in a district.

constitute /ˈkɒnstɪˌtuːt/ or /-ˌtjuːt/ vt to set up by authority, to establish; to frame, to form; to appoint; to compose, to make up.—**constituter, constitutor** n.

constitution /ˌkɒnstɪˈtuːʃən/ or /-ˌtjuːʃən/ n fundamental physical condition; disposition; temperament; structure, composition; the system of basic laws and principles of a government, society, etc; a document stating these specifically.

constitutional /-əl/ adj of or pertaining to a constitution authorized or limited by a constitution, legal; inherent, natural. • a walk for the sake of one's health.—**constitutionally** adv.—**constitutionality** n.

constitutionalism /-nəˌlɪzəm/ n constitutional government; adherence to constitutional principles.—**constitutionalist** n.

constitutive /ˈkɒnstɪˌtuːtɪv/ or /-ˌtjuːtɪv/ adj having the power to enact, constituent; elemental; essential; productive.

constrain /kənˈstreɪn/ vt to compel, to force; to hinder by force; to confine, to imprison.—**constrainer** n.

constrained /kənstreɪnd/ adj enforced; embarrassed, inhibited; showing constraint.

constraint /kənˈstreɪnt/ n compulsion; forcible confinement; repression of feeling; embarrassment; a condition that restricts freedom.

constrict /kənˈstrɪkt/ vt to draw together, to squeeze, to compress.

constricted /-ɪd/ adj narrowed, cramped.

constriction /-ʃən/ n compression; tightness.—**constrictive** adj.

constrictor /-ər/ n a constrictive muscle; a snake that crushes its prey.

construct /kənˈstrʌkt/ n & vt to make, to build, to fit together; to compose. • n a structure; an interpretation; an arrangement, esp of words in a sentence.—**constructible** adj.—**constructor, constructer** n.

construction /kənˈstrʌkʃən/ n a constructing; anything constructed; a structure, building; interpretation, meaning; (gram) two or more words grouped together to form a phrase, clause or sentence.—**constructional** adj.

construction holiday n ❀ (Cdn) in Quebec, a compulsory holiday for all construction workers during the last two weeks of July, often taken by other workers.

constructive /kənˈstrʌktɪv/ adj helping to improve, promoting development.—**constructively** adv.

constructivism /-ˌɪzəm/ n nonrepresentational art, esp sculpture based on movement and using machine-made materials.

construe /kənˈstruː/ vti (**construing, construed**) to translate word for word; to analyse grammatically; to take in a particular sense, to interpret.—**construer** n.

consubstantiation /ˌkɒnsəbˌstænʃɪˈeɪʃən/ n the doctrine that the body and blood of Christ are in a mysterious manner substantially present in the Eucharistic elements after Consecration.

consuetude /ˈkɒnswɪˌtuːd/ n an established custom.—**consuetudinary** adj.

consul /ˈkɒnsəl/ n a government official appointed to live in a foreign city to attend to the interests of his country's citizens and business there.—**consular** adj.

consulate /-ət/ or /-ˌsjəl-/ n the official residence of a consul; the office of a Roman consul.

consult /kənˈsʌlt/ vti to seek advice from, esp a doctor or lawyer; to seek information from, eg a work of reference; to deliberate, to confer.—**consulter, consultor** n.

consultant /kənˈsʌltənt/ n a specialist who gives professional or technical advice; a senior physician or surgeon in a hospital; a person who consults another.—**consultancy** n (pl **consultancies**).

consultation /ˌkɒnsəlˈteɪʃən/ n the act of consulting; a conference, esp with a professional adviser.—**consultative, consultatory, consultive** adj.

consultative /kənˈsʌltətɪv/ or /-ˌteɪtɪv/, **consultatory** /-ˌtɔri/ adj advisory; deliberative.

consumable /kənˈsuːməbəl/ adj able to be consumed. • n (usu pl) something bought to be used.

consume /kənˈsuːm/ or /-ˈsjuːm/ vti to destroy; to use up; to eat or drink up; to waste away; to utilize economic goods.

consumer /kənˈsuːmər/ or /-ˈsjuː-/ n a person who uses goods and services, the end user.

consumer goods npl commodities for domestic consumption which are not used for the production of other goods and services.

consumerism /-ˌɪzəm/ n protection of the interests of consumers; encouragement to buy consumer goods.

consumer price index n an index of the prices of the food, clothing and housing necessary for life.

consummate[1] /ˈkɒnsəˌmeɪt/ or /-sjə-/ adj, vt to bring to perfection, to be the crown of; (marriage) to complete by sexual intercourse.—**consummation** n.—**consummative, consummatory** adj.—**consummator** n.

consummate[2] adj complete, perfect, highly skilled.

consumption /kənˈsʌmpʃən/ n the act of consuming; the state of being consumed or used up; (econ) expenditure on goods and services by consumers; tuberculosis.

consumptive /kənˈsʌmptɪv/ adj tending to consume; affected with consumption. • n a person with tuberculosis.

contact /ˈkɒnˌtækt/ n touch, touching; connection; an acquaintance, esp one willing to provide help or introductions in business, etc; a connection allowing the passage of electricity; (med) a person who has been in contact with a contagious disease. • vti to establish contact with.—**contactual** adj.

contact lens n a thin correctional lens placed over the cornea of the eye.

contagion /kənˈteɪdʒən/ n the communicating of a disease by contact; a disease spread in this way; a corrupting influence.

contagious /-dʒəs/ adj (disease) spread by contact; capable of spreading disease by contact; (influence) catching, infectious.—**contagiousness** n.

contain /kənˈteɪn/ vt to hold, to enclose; to comprise, to include; to hold back or restrain within fixed limits.

container /kənˈteɪnə/ n a receptacle, etc designed to contain goods or substances; a standardized receptacle used to transport commodities.

containerize /-ˌaɪz/ vt to put or convey (cargo) in large standardized containers.

containment /kənˈteɪnmənt/ n the prevention of the expansion of a hostile power; the prevention of the release of dangerous quantities of radioactive material from a nuclear reactor.

containment building n a building enclosing a nuclear reactor to limit the spread of radiation, esp in the event of an accident.

contaminate /kənˈtæmɪneɪt/ vt to render impure by touch or mixing, to pollute, esp by radioactive contact.—**contaminant** n.—**contaminator** n.

contamination /kəntæmɪˈneɪʃən/ n the act of contaminating; the state of being contaminated; a thing that contaminates.

conte /kɔ̃t/ n a short story.

contemn /kənˈtem/ vt to despise; to disregard scornfully.—**contemner, contemnor** n.—**contemnible** adj.

contemplate /ˈkɒntəmˌpleɪt/ vti to look at steadily; to reflect upon, to meditate; to have in view to intend.—**contemplator** n.

contemplation /ˌkɒntəmˈpleɪʃən/ n the act of contemplating; pious meditation; intention.

contemplative /kənˈtempləˌtɪv/ adj thoughtful, meditative, of or given to contemplation; dedicated to religious contemplation.—**contemplatively** adv.—**contemplativeness** n.

contemporaneous /kənˌtempəˈreɪniəs/ adj existing or occurring at the same time; of the same period.—**contemporaneously** adv.—**contemporaneity** n.

contemporary /kənˈtempəˌreri/ adj living or happening at the same time; of about the same age; present day; of or following present-day trends in style, art, fashion, etc. • n (pl **contemporaries**) a person living at the same time; a person of the same age.—**contemporarily** adv.

contempt /kənˈtempt/ n the feeling one has towards someone or something considered low, worthless etc; the condition of being despised; disregard.

contemptible /-ɪbəl/ adj deserving contempt.—**contemptibly** adv.—**contemptibility** n.

contemptuous /kən'temptʃʊəs/ adj showing or feeling contempt; disdainful.—**contemptuously** adv.—**contemptuousness** n.

contend /kən'tend/ vti to take part in a contest, to strive (for); to quarrel; to maintain (that), to assert or argue strongly for.—**contender** n.

content¹ /'kɒntent/ n (usu pl) what is in a container; (usu pl) what is in a book; substance or meaning.

content² /kən'tent/ adj satisfied (with), not desiring more; willing (to); happy; pleased. • n quiet satisfaction. • vt to make content; to satisfy.—**contentment** n.

contented /kən'tentəd/ adj content; gratified, satisfied.—**contentedly** adv.

contention /kən'tenʃən/ n contending, struggling, arguing; a point in dispute; an assertion in an argument.—**contentional** adj.

contentious /kən'tenʃəs/ adj tending to argue; likely to cause dispute, controversial.—**contentiously** adv.

conterminous /kɒn'tɜːmɪnəs/ adj having a common boundary (with), contiguous.—also **coterminous**.

contest /kɒn'test/ vti, n to call in question, to dispute; to fight to gain, to compete for; to strive. • n a struggle, an encounter; a competition; a debate; a dispute.—**contestable** adj.—**contestation** n.—**contester** n.

contestant /kən'testənt/ n a competitor in a contest; a person who contests.

context /'kɒntekst/ n the parts of a written work or speech that precede and follow a word or passage, contributing to its full meaning; associated surroundings, setting.—**contextual** adj.—**contextually** adv.

contextualize /kən'tekstʃʊəˌlaɪz/ vt to place in or treat as part of a context.

contexture /kən'tekstʃər/ n a structure; a fabric; a style of composition.—**contextural** adj.

contiguous /kən'tɪgjʊəs/ adj touching, adjoining; near; adjacent.—**contiguity** n.

continent¹ /'kɒntɪnənt/ n one of the six or seven main divisions of the earth's land; (with cap) the mainland of Europe, excluding the British Isles; a large extent of land.

continent² adj able to control urination and defecation; practising self-restraint; chaste.—**continence, continency** n.

continental /ˌkɒntɪ'nentəl/ adj of a continent; (with cap) of or relating to Europe, excluding the British Isles; of or relating to the former thirteen British colonies later forming the USA. • n an inhabitant of the Continent.—**continentalism** n.—**continentalist** n.—**continentally** adv.

continental breakfast n a light morning meal of coffee and rolls.

continental drift n (geol) the (theoretical) gradual process of separation of the continents from their original solid land mass.

continental shelf n the sea bed, under relatively shallow seas, bordering a continent.

contingency /kən'tɪndʒənsi/ n (pl contingencies) a possibility of a future event or condition; something dependent on a future event.

contingent /kən'tɪndʒənt/ adj possible, that may happen; chance; dependent (on); incidental (to). • n a possibility; a quota of troops.—**contingently** adv.

continual /kən'tɪnjʊəl/ adj frequently repeated, going on all the time.—**continuality** n.—**continually** adv.

continuance /kən'tɪnjʊəns/ n uninterrupted succession; duration.

continuant /kə'tɪnjʊənt/ n a consonant whose sound can be prolonged, as f, v.

continuation /kənˌtɪnjʊ'eɪʃən/ n a continuing; prolongation; resumption; a thing that continues something else, a sequel, a further instalment.

continue /kən'tɪnjuː/ vt to go on (with); to prolong; to extend; to resume, to carry further. • vi to remain, to stay; to last; to preserve.—**continuable** adj.—**continuer** n.—**continuingly** adv.

continuity /ˌkɒntə'njuːɪti/ or /-'njuː-/ n (pl continuities) continuousness; uninterrupted succession; the complete script or scenario in a film or broadcast.

continuous /kən'tɪnjʊəs/ adj continuing; occurring without interruption.—**continuously** adv.—**continuousness** n.

continuum /kən'tɪnuːəm/ n (pl continua, continuums) a continuous and homogeneous whole.

contort /kən'tɔːt/ vti to twist out of a normal shape, to pull awry.—**contorted** adj.—**contortion** n.—**contortional** adj.

contortionist /kən'tɔːʃənɪst/ n a person who can twist his or her body into unusual postures, esp as entertainment.—**contortionistic** adj.

contour /'kɒnˌtʊr/ n the outline of a figure, land, etc; the line representing this outline; a contour line. • adj made according to a shape or form (contour chair).

contour line n a line on a map that passes through all points at the same altitude.

contra /'kɒntrə/ n a thing that may be argued against.

contra- /'kɒntrə/ prefix against.

contraband /'kɒntrəˌbænd/ n smuggled goods; smuggling. • adj illegal to import or export.—**contrabandist** n.

contraband of war n certain commodities used in warfare; the traffic in them with belligerent states; goods supplied to one belligerent and seizable by another.

contrabass /'kɒntrəˌbeɪs/ n an instrument sounding an octave lower than another instrument of the same class; the largest instrument of the violin class, the double bass.—**contrabassist** n.

contrabassoon /ˌkɒntrəbə'suːn/ n the largest instrument of the oboe class.—**contrabassoonist** n.

contraception /ˌkɒntrə'sepʃən/ n the deliberate prevention of conception, birth control.

contraceptive /ˌkɒntrə'septɪv/ n a contraceptive drug or device.—also adj.

contract /'kɒntrækt/ vt, n to draw closer together; to confine; to undertake by contract; (debt) to incur; (disease) to become infected by; (word) to shorten by omitting letters. • vi to shrink; to become smaller or narrower; to make a contract; (with out) to decide not to take part in or join, eg a pension scheme. • n a bargain; an agreement to supply goods or perform work at a stated price; a written agreement enforceable by law.—**contractibility** n.—**contractible** adj.

contract bridge n a form of bridge in which the players contract to take a certain number of tricks.

contractile /kən'træktɪl/ adj able or causing to grow smaller.—**contractility** n.

contraction /kən'trækʃən/ n the act of contracting; the state of being contracted; a contracted word; a labour pain in childbirth.—**contractional** adj.—**contractive** adj.

contractor /'kɒnˌtræktər/ n a person who makes a business contract, esp a builder; something that draws together, eg a muscle.

contractual /kən'træktʃuːəl/ adj of a contract.—**contractually** adv.

contradance /'kɒntrəˌdɒns/ see **contredanse**.

contradict /ˌkɒntrə'dɪkt/ vti to assert the contrary or opposite of; to deny; to be at variance (with); to lack consistency.—**contradictable** adj.—**contradicter, contradictor** n.

contradiction /ˌkɒntrə'dɪkʃən/ n the act of contradicting; a denial.—**contradictory** adj.

contradistinction /ˌkɒntrədɪ'stɪŋkʃən/ n a distinction by opposite qualities.—**contradistinctive** adj.

contradistinguish /-dɪ'stɪŋgwɪʃ/ vt to mark the difference between two things by contrasting their opposite qualities.

contralto /kən'trɒltəʊ/ or /-'træltəʊ/ n (pl contraltos) a singing voice having a range between tenor and mezzo-soprano; a person having this voice.

contraposition /ˌkɒntrəpə'zɪʃən/ n opposition, antithesis.

contraption /kən'træpʃən/ n (inf) a device, a gadget.

contrapuntal /ˌkɒntrə'pentəl/ adj of or according to counterpoint.—**contrapuntally** adv.

contrapuntist /-ɪst/ n one skilled in the rules of counterpoint.

contrariety /ˌkɒntrə'raɪəti/ n (pl contrarieties) opposition; inconsistency, discrepancy.

contrariwise /'kɒntrəriwaɪz/ adv on the other hand; conversely.

contrary /'kɒnˌtreri/ adj opposed; opposite in nature; wayward, perverse. • n (pl contraries) the opposite. • adv in opposition to; in conflict with.—**contrarily** adv.—**contrariness** n.

contrast /kɒn'træst/ vi to show marked differences. • vt to compare so as to point out the differences. • n the exhibition of differences; difference of qualities shown by comparison; the degree of difference between colours or tones when put together.

contravene /ˌkɒntrə'viːn/ vt to infringe (a law), to transgress; to conflict with, to contradict.—**contravener** n.—**contravention** n.

contredanse /'kɒntrə,dɒns/ *n* a dance in which the partners are arranged in opposite lines; the music for this.—*also* **contradance**.

contretemps /'kɒntrə,tɑ̃/ *n* (*pl* **contretemps**) a confusing, embarrassing or awkward occurrence.

contribute /kən'trɪbjuːt/ *vti* to give to a common stock or fund; to write (an article) for a magazine or newspaper; to furnish ideas, etc.—**contributive** *adj*.

contribution /,kɒntrɪ'bjuːʃən/ *n* the act of contributing; something contributed; a literary article; a payment into a collection.

contributor /-ər/ *n* a person who contributes, *esp* the writer of an article for a newspaper, etc; a factor, a contributory cause.—**contributorial** *adj*.

contributory /kən'trɪbjutəri/ or /kən'trɪbju,tɔri/ *adj* giving, donating; partly responsible, sharing in.

con trick *n* (*inf*) confidence trick.

contrite /'kɒntraɪt/ or /kən'traɪt/ *adj* deeply repentant, feeling guilt.—**contritely** *adv*.—**contrition** *n*.

contrivance /kən'traɪvəns/ *n* something contrived, *esp* a mechanical device, invention; inventive ability; an artificial construct; a stratagem.

contrive /kən'traɪv/ *vt* to plan ingeniously; to devise, to design, to manage; to achieve, *esp* by some ploy or trick; to scheme.—**contriver** *n*.

contrived /-'traɪvd/ *adj* skilful but overdone; (*writing*) not spontaneous or natural or flowing.

control /kən'troːl/ *v, n* restraint; command, authority; a check; a means of controlling; a standard of comparison for checking an experiment; (*pl*) mechanical parts by which a car, aeroplane, etc is operated. • *vt* (**controlling, controlled**) to check; to restrain; to regulate; to govern; (*experiment*) to verify by comparison.

controllable /-əbəl/ *adj* able to be controlled.—**controllably** *adv*.

controller /kən'troːlər/ *n* a person who controls, *esp* one in charge of expenditure or finances.

control tower *n* a tower at an airport from which flight directions are given.

controversial /,kɒntrə'vərʃəl/ *adj* causing controversy, open to argument.—**controversialism** *n*.—**controversialist** *n*.—**controversially** *adv*.

controversy /'kɒntrə,vərsi/ or /kən'trɒvərsi/ *n* (*pl* **controversies**) a discussion of contrary opinions; dispute, argument.

controvert /'kɒntrə,vərt/ or /-'vərt/ *vt* to contend against; to refute; to disprove.—**controverter** *n*.—**controvertible** *adj*.

contumacious /,kɒntju:'meɪʃəs/ *adj* resisting authority, insubordinate; obstinate.

contumacy /kɒn'tjuːməsi/ or /'kɒntjuməsi/ *n* (*pl* **contumacies**) stubborn resistance to authority, *esp* contempt of court.—**contumacious** *adj*.

contumelious /,kɒntju:'miːliəs/ *adj* haughtily contemptuous or offensive; supercilious.

contumely /kɒn'tjuːmli/ or /'kɒntju:mli/ *n* (*pl* **contumelies**) haughty and contemptuous rudeness; scornful and insolent abuse; reproach, disgrace.

contuse /kən'tjuːz/ or /-,tuːz/ *vt* to wound or bruise without breaking the skin.—**contusive** *adj*.

contusion /kən'tuːʃən/ or /-tjuː-/ *n* a wound that does not break the skin, a bruise.—**contusioned** *adj*.

conundrum /kə'nʌndrəm/ *n* a riddle involving a pun; a puzzling question.

conurbation /,kɒnər'beɪʃən/ *n* a vast urban area around and including a large city.

convalesce /,kɒnvə'les/ *vi* to recover health and strength after an illness; to get better.—**convalescence** *n*.

convalescent /-'lesənt/ *adj* recovering health; aiding the recovery of full health. • *n* a patient recovering after an illness.

convection /kən'vekʃən/ *n* the transmission of heat through a liquid by currents; the process whereby warmer air rises while cooler air drops.—**convectional** *adj*.—**convective** *adj*.

convector /kən'vektər/ *n* a heater that circulates warm air.

convene /kən'viːn/ *vti* to call together for a meeting.—**convenable** *adj*.—**convener** *n*.

convenience /kən'viːniəns/ *n* what suits one; a useful appliance.

convenience food *n* food that is easily and quickly prepared.

convenience store *n* a small store open for extended hours that sells packaged, canned, or bottled foods and drinks as well as common household items.

convenient /-iənt/ *adj* handy; suitable; causing little or no trouble.—**conveniently** *adv*.

convent /'kɒnvənt/ or /-vent/ *n* a house of a religious order, *esp* an establishment of nuns.

conventicle /kən'ventɪkəl/ *n* a meeting house; a secret meeting; an assembly for worship *usu* by a schism; (*formerly*) a prohibited meeting of Nonconformists or Covenanters.

convention /kən'venʃən/ *n* a political or ecclesiastical assembly or meeting; an agreement between nations, a treaty; established usage, social custom.

conventional /-əl/ *adj* of or based on convention or social custom; not spontaneous; lacking imagination or originality; following accepted rules; (*weapons*) non-nuclear.—**conventionality** *n* (*pl* **conventionalities**).—**conventionally** *adj*.

conventionalism /-,ɪzəm/ *n* that which is received as established by usage, etc; adherence to established usage.—**conventionalist** *n*.

conventionalize /-,aɪz/ *vt* to make conventional.—**conventionalization** *n*.

conventual /kən'ventʃuəl/ *adj* belonging to a convent. • *n* a member or inmate of a convent.

converge /kən'vərdʒ/ *vti* to come or bring together.—**convergence, convergency** *n*—**convergent** *adj*.

conversable /kən'vərsəbəl/ *adj* disposed to converse, sociable.

conversant /kən'vərsənt/ *adj* well acquainted; proficient; familiar (with).—**conversance, conversancy** *n*.

conversation /,kɒnvər'seɪʃən/ *n* informal talk or exchange of ideas, opinions, etc between people.—**conversational** *adj*.—**conversationally** *adv*.

conversationalist /-ʃənəl st/, **conversationist** /-ɪst/ *n* a person who is good at conversation.

conversation piece *n* originally an 18th-century picture showing a group in an outdoor or indoor setting; something unusual or novel that provokes conversation; a play that focuses interest on dialogue as much as on action.

conversazione *It*. /,kɒnvə'so'tsjɒne/ *n* (*pl* **conversazioni, conversaziones**) a meeting for conversation, *esp* on literary or scientific topics.

converse[1] /'kɒn,vərs/ *n*; /kən'vərs/ *vi* to engage in conversation (with). • *n* familiar talk, conversation.—**converser** *n*.

converse[2] /'kɒn,vərs/ *n*; /'kɒnvərs/ *adj* opposite, contrary. • *n* something that is opposite or contrary.—**conversely** *adv*.

conversion /kən'vərʒən/ *n* change from one state, or from one religion, to another; something converted from one use to another; an alteration to a building undergoing a change in function; (*rugby*) a score after a try by kicking the ball over the crossbar.—**conversional, conversionary** *adj*.

convert /kən'vərt/ *vti* to change from one thing, condition or religion to another; to alter; to apply to a different use; (*rugby*) to make a conversion after a try. • *n* a converted person, *esp* one who has changed religion.

converter, convertor /kən'vərtər/ *n* one who converts; an iron retort used for converting pig iron into steel in the Bessemer process; a kind of electrical induction coil.

converter reactor *n* a nuclear reactor that changes fertile material to fissile material.

convertible /kən'vərtɪbəl/ *adj* able to be converted. • *n* an automobile with a folding or detachable roof.—**convertibility** *n*.

convex /kɒn'veks/ *adj* curving outward like the surface of a sphere.—**convexly** *adv*—**convexity** *n*.

convexo-concave /kɒn'veksoːkɒn'keɪv/ or /kən-/ *adj* convex on one side, concave on the other.

convexo-convex /-kɒn'veks/ *adj* curving outwards on both sides, as a lens.

convey /kən'veɪ/ *vt* to transport; to conduct; to transmit; to make known, to communicate; (*law*) to make over (property).—**conveyable** *adj*.—**conveyor, conveyer** *n*.

conveyance /kən'veɪəns/ *n* the act of conveying; a means of transporting, a vehicle; (*law*) the act of transferring property.—**conveyancer** *n*.

conveyancing /-ənsɪŋ/ *n* the business of drawing up deeds, leases, etc, and investigating titles to property.

conveyor belt *n* a continuous moving belt or linked plates for moving objects in a factory.

convict /kən'vɪkt/ *vt* to prove or pronounce guilty. • /'kɒn,vɪkt/ *n* a convicted person serving a prison sentence.

conviction /kən'vɪkʃən/ *n* act of convicting; a settled opinion; a firm belief.

convince /kən'vɪns/ vt to persuade by argument or evidence; to satisfy by proof.—**convincer** n.—**convincible** adj.

convincing /-ɪŋ/ adj compelling belief.—**convincingly** adv.

convivial /ken'vɪvɪəl/ adj sociable, jovial.—**conviviality** n.—**convivially** adv.

convocation /ˌkɒnvə'keɪʃən/ n the act of convoking an assembly, esp of bishops, clergy or heads of a university; an assembly of clergy.—**convocational** adj.—**convocator** n.

convoke /kən'vo:k/ to call or summon together; to convene.—**convoker** n.

convolute /'kɒnvə'lu:t/ vt to form into a rolled or coiled shape. • adj (bot) rolled upon itself; coiled.

convoluted /-əd/ adj twisted; coiled; complicated, difficult to understand.

convolution /ˌkɒnvə'lu:ʃən/ n a rolling together, a coiling; a fold, a twist; a complicated or confused matter.

convolve /kən'vɒlv/ vt to roll together.

convolvulus /kən'vɒlvjuləs/ n (pl **convolvuluses, convolvuli**) a twining plant with bell-shaped flowers.

convoy /'kɒnvɔɪ/ n a group of ships or vehicles travelling together for protection. • vt to travel thus.

convulse /kən'vʌls/ vt to agitate violently; to shake with irregular spasms. • vi (inf) to cause to shake with uncontrollable laughter.—**convulsive** adj.—**convulsively** adv.

convulsion /ken'vʌlʃən/ n a violent involuntary contraction of a muscle or muscles; an agitation, tumult; (pl) a violent fit of laughter.

cony, coney /'ko:ni/ n (pl **conies, coneys**) rabbit, or the skin or fur of a rabbit used in making clothes.

coo /ku:/ n the note of the pigeon; a soft murmuring sound. • vt (**cooing, cooed**) to utter the cry of a dove or pigeon; to speak softly; to act or murmur in a loving manner.

cook /kʊk/ vt to prepare (food) by heat; (inf) to fake (accounts, etc); to subject to great heat. • vi to be a cook; to undergo cooking; (with up) to plot; to make up a story. • n a person who cooks; one whose job is to cook.—**cookable** adj.

cookbook /'kʊkˌbʊk/, **cookery book** n a book of recipes and other information for preparing food.

cook-chill n (catering) a method in which meals are pre-cooked, chilled rapidly and then reheated as required.

cooker /'kʊkər/ n an electric or gas appliance for cooking.

cookery /'kʊkəri/ n the art or practice of cooking.

cookhouse /'kʊkhəʊs/ n a kitchen, esp outdoors.

cookie[1], cooky /'kʊki/ n (pl **cookies**) a small flat sweet cake; (sl) a person.

cookie[2] n (comput) a small file which is transmitted to, and stored on, the hard disk of a computer, which acts as a sort of identification.

cookout /'kʊkˌɛʊt/ n a meal cooked and eaten outdoors, a barbecue.

cool /ku:l/ adj moderately cold; calm; indifferent; unenthusiastic; cheeky. • vti to make or become cool. • n coolness; composure.—**coolly** adv.—**coolness** n.

coolant /'ku:lənt/ n a fluid or other substance for cooling machinery.

cooler /'ku:lə/ n that which cools; a vessel for cooling liquids, etc; a drink of spirits; (sl) prison.

cool-headed /'ku:lhedəd/ adj not easily excited.

coolie, cooly /'ku:li/ n (pl **coolies**) an Indian or Chinese hired labourer.

cooling tower n a tall hollow construction used in some industries, in which water is cooled and reused.

coon /ku:n/ n a raccoon; (derog) a black person.

cooncan /ku:n'kæn/ n a card game for two.

coop /ku:p/ n a small pen for poultry. • vt to confine as in a coop.

co-op /'ko:ɒp/ n a cooperative.

cooper /'ku:pər/ n one who makes and repairs barrels, etc.

cooperage /-ədʒ/ n the business or workshop of a cooper; the price for a cooper's work.

cooperate /ko:'ɒpəˌreɪt/ vi to work together, to act jointly.—**cooperation** n.—**cooperator** n.

cooperative /ko:'ɒpərtɪv/ or /-rətɪv/ adj willing to cooperate; helpful. • n an organization or enterprise owned by, and operated for the benefit of, those using its services.—**cooperatively** adv.

co-opt /ko:'ɒpt/ vt to elect or choose as a member by the agreement of the existing members.—**co-optation, co-option** n.—**co-optative, co-optive** adj.

coordinate /ko:'ɔrdɪˌneɪt/ vt to integrate (different elements, etc) into an efficient relationship; to adjust to; to function

harmoniously. • n an equal person or thing; any of a series of numbers that, in a given frame of reference, locate a point in space; (pl) separate items of clothing intended to be worn together. • adj equal in degree or status.—**coordinately** adv.—**coordinator** n.

coordination /ko:ˌɔrdɪ'neɪʃən/ n the act of coordinating; the state of being coordinated; balanced and harmonious movement of the body.

coot /ku:t/ n a European water-bird with dark plumage and a white spot on the forehead; a silly person.

cootie /'ku:ti/ n (sl) a louse.

cop[1] /kɒp/ vb (**copping, copped**) vt (sl) to arrest, catch. • vi (with out) (sl) to fail to perform, to renege. • n (sl) capture; a policeman.

cop[2] n a conical ball of thread on a spindle.

copaiba /ko:'peɪbə/ or /-'paɪ-/ n an aromatic resinous balsam from various South American and West Indian trees.

copal /'ko:pəl/ n a gum resin used in varnishes.

coparcenary /ko:'pɒrsəˌneɪri/ n joint heirship.

coparcener /-sənər/ n a coheir.

copartner /'ko:ˌpɑrtnər/ n a joint partner.—**copartnership** n.

cope[1] /'ko:p/ vi to deal successfully with; to contend on even terms (with).

cope[2] n a large semicircular ecclesiastical vestment worn by bishops and priests over the surplice; a canopy, esp of heaven.

Copernican /kə'pərnɪkən/ adj of or relating to Copernicus and his teaching that the earth and planets revolve around the sun.

copestone /'ko:pˌsto:n/ n the top stone of a structure; a crowning touch.

copier /'kɒpiər/ n a copying machine, a photocopier.

copilot /'ko:ˌpaɪlət/ n a second pilot in an aircraft.

coping /'ko:pɪŋ/ n the top masonry of a wall.

coping saw n a saw with a U-shaped frame and narrow blade used for cutting outlines in wood.

copious /'ko:piəs/ adj plentiful, abundant.—**copiously** adv.—**copiousness** n.

cop-out /'kɒpˌɛʊt/ n (sl) an evasion; a means of avoiding responsibility.

copper[1] /'kɒpər/ n a reddish ductile metallic element; a bronze coin. • adj made of, or of the colour of, copper. • vt to cover with copper.—**coppery** adj.

copper[2] n (sl) a police officer.

copper-bottomed adj to be trusted; financially sound.

copperhead /'kɒpərˌhed/ n a South American snake.

copperplate /'kɒpərˌpleɪt/ n a polished plate of copper for engraving or printing; a print from this; copybook writing.

coppersmith /'kɒpərˌsmɪθ/ n a worker in copper.

copra /'kɒprə/ n the dried kernel of the coconut after the oil has been removed.

copro- /'kɒpro:/ prefix dung.

coprolite /'kɒpro:ˌlaɪt/ n fossil dung.—**coprolitic** adj.

coprophagous /'kɒprɒfəgəs/ adj feeding on dung, as certain beetles.—**coprophagy** n.

coprophilia /ˌkɒpro:'fɪliə/ n an abnormal interest in faeces; love of obscenity.

coprophilous /-'fɪləs/ adj growing in dung.

copse /kɒps/ n a thicket of small trees and shrubs.

Copt /kɒpt/ n a native Egyptian Christian.

copter /'kɒptər/ n a helicopter.

Coptic /'kɒptɪk/ adj pertaining to the Copts, their church or their language. • n the language spoken by Copts.

copula /'kɒpjʊlə/ n (pl **copulas, copulae**) a link, a connecting part; (gram) a word that joins the subject and predicate in a sentence or proposition.—**copular** adj.

copulate /'kɒpjʊˌleɪt/ vi to have sexual intercourse.—**copulation** n.—**copulatory** adj.

copulative /-tɪv/ adj joining, uniting; (gram) serving as a copula; uniting ideas as well as words. • n a copulative conjunction.

copy /'kɒpi/ n (pl **copies**) a reproduction; a transcript; a single specimen of a book; a model to be copied; a manuscript for printing; newspaper text; text for an advertisement; subject matter for a writer. • vt (**copying, copied**) to make a copy of, to reproduce; to take as a model, to imitate.

copybook /-bʊk/ n a book of handwriting exercises.

copy-edit vt to correct and prepare text for printing.

copyhold /-ˌho:ld/ n (English law) a tenure of estate by copy of the court roll or custom of the manor.

copyholder /-ər/ *n* a tenant by copyhold; (*print*) a reader's assistant.

copyist /'kɒpiɪst/ *n* one who copies.

copyright /'kɒpi,raɪt/ *n* the exclusive legal right to the publication and sale of a literary, dramatic, musical, or artistic work in any form. • *adj* protected by copyright.

copywriter /-,raɪtər/ *n* a writer of advertising or publicity copy.— **copywriting** *n*.

coq au vin /,kɒko:'væ/ *n* a dish of chicken cooked in wine.

coquet /ko:'kɛt/ *vi* (**coquetting, coquetted**) to flirt with; to seek to attract attention or admiration; to trifle.

coquetry /'ko:kɪtri/ *n* (*pl* **coquetries**) the act of coquetting; flirtatious behaviour.

coquette /ko:'kɛt/ *n* a woman who trifles with men's affections.— **coquettish** *adj*.

coquito /ko:'ki:to:/ *n* (*pl* **coquitos**) a tall Chilean palm producing edible nuts and palm honey.

coracle /'kɒrəkəl/ or /'kɒ-/ *n* a boat with a wicker frame covered with leather.

coracoid /'kɒrə,kɔɪd/ or /'kɒ-/ *n* a hook-like process of the scapula or bladebone.

coral /'kɒrəl/ or /kɒ-/ *n* the hard skeleton secreted by certain marine polyps. • *adj* made of coral, *esp* jewellery; of the colour of coral, deepish pink.

coralline /'kɒrə,laɪn/ or /kɒ-/, **coralloid** /-lɔɪd/ or /kɒ-/ *adj* consisting of, or like, coral; of a colour like coral. • *n* a coral-like seaweed or animal.

coral reef *n* a formation or bank of coral.

coral tree *n* an American tree with blood-red flowers.

corban *n* an offering to God in fulfilment of a vow.

corbeil /'kɒrbəl/ or /-,bɛl/ *n* (*archit*) a sculptured basket of flowers, fruit, etc.

corbel /'kɒrbəl/ *n* a stone or timber projection from a wall to support something. • *vt* (**corbelling, corbelled** *or* **corbeling, corbeled**) to furnish with or support by corbel.

corbicula *n* (*pl* **corbiculae**) the receptacle for pollen in the honey bee.

cord /kɒrd/ *n* a thick string or thin rope; something that binds; a slender electric cable; a ribbed fabric, *esp* corduroy; (*pl*) corduroy trousers; any part of the body resembling string or rope (*spinal cord*).

cordage /-ɪdʒ/ *n* a quantity of cords or ropes; ropes and rigging collectively.

cordate /'kɒrdeɪt/ *adj* heart-shaped.

cordial /'kɒrdʒəl/ or /-diəl/ *adj* hearty, warm; friendly; affectionate. • *n* a fruit-flavoured drink.—**cordially** *adv*.—**cordialness** *n*.

cordiality /kɒrdiæ'lɪti/ *n* (*pl* **cordialities**) sincere sympathethic geniality; sincerity; heartiness.

cordiform /'kɒrdə,fɔrm/ *adj* heart-shaped.

cordillera /kɒr'dɪlərə/ or /-,kɒrdɪ'ljɛrə/ *n* a continuous ridge or chain of mountains, *esp* of the Andes mountains.

cordite /'kɒr,daɪt/ *n* an explosive used in bullets and shells.

cordless /'kɒrdləs/ *adj* (*electrical device*) operated by a battery.

cordon /'kɒrdən/ *n* a chain of police or soldiers preventing access to an area; a piece of ornamental cord or ribbon given as an award. • *vt* (*with* **off**) (*area*) to prevent access to.

cordon bleu *Fr.* /,kɒrdɔ̃'blu/ or /,kɒrdɔ̃-/ *n* the highest distinction in any profession; a first-class cook.—*also adj*.

cordon sanitaire /,kɒrdɒn,sani'tɛr/ *n* a barrier around an infected area; a buffer zone.

cordovan /'kɒrdəvən/ *n* a Spanish leather made of goatskin or split horsehide, tanned and dressed.—*also* **cordwain**.

cords /'kɒrdz/ *npl* (*inf*) corduroy trousers.

corduroy /'kɒrdə,rɔɪ/ or /-djʊ-/ *n* a strong cotton fabric with a velvety ribbed surface; (*pl*) trousers of this.

corduroy road *n* a roadway formed of logs laid crosswise across swampy ground, etc.

cordwain /'kɒrd,weɪn/ *see* **cordovan**.

cordwainer /-ər/ *n* (*arch*) a worker in leather; a shoemaker.

core /kɒr/ *n* the innermost part, the heart; the inner part of an apple, etc containing seeds; the region of a nuclear reactor containing the fissile material; (*comput*) a form of magnetic memory used to store one bit of information. • *vt* to remove the core from.—**corer** *n*.

coreopsis /,kɒri'ɒpsɪs/ or /,kɒri-/ *n* a kind of plant with rayed flowers and seeds with two small horns at the end.

corespondent /,kɒrɪ'spɒndənt/ *n* (*law*) a person named as having committed adultery with the husband or wife from whom a divorce is sought.—**corespondency** *n*.

corgi /'kɒrgi/ *n* (*pl* **corgis**) a Welsh breed of dog with short legs and a sturdy body.

coriaceous /,kɒri'eɪʃəs/ *adj* of leather; leathery.

coriander /'kɒri,ændər/ *n* a plant with aromatic seeds used for flavouring food.

Corinthian /kə'rɪnθiən/ *adj* of or pertaining to Corinth, a Greek city noted for its luxury and licentiousness; luxurious; conducted by amateurs; (*archit*) denoting the Corinthian order. • *n* a man about town; a gentleman yachtsman or sportsman.

Corinthian order *n* the lightest and most ornate of the classic orders of architecture, with a bell-shaped capital and ornamented with acanthus leaves.

corium /'kɒriəm/ *n* (*pl* **coria**) the innermost layer of skin of the cuticle.

cork /kɒrk/ *n* the outer bark of the cork oak used *esp* for stoppers and insulation; a stopper for a bottle, *esp* made of cork. • *adj* made of cork. • *vt* to stop up with a cork; to give a taste of cork to (*wine*).

corkage /'kɒrkɪdʒ/ *n* a charge made by a restaurant for serving wine, *esp* when brought in by the customer from outside.

corked /-d/ *adj* (*wine*) contaminated by a decayed cork.

corker /'kɒrkər/ *n* (*sl*) something conclusive or superlatively good; a flagrant lie.

corkscrew /'kɒrkskru:/ *n* a tool for drawing corks from wine bottles. • *adj* spiral-shaped, resembling a corkscrew.

corky /'kɒrki/ *adj* made of, or like, cork.

corm /kɒrm/ *n* the bulb-like underground stem of the crocus, etc; a solid bulb.—**cormous** *adj*.

cormel /'kɒrməl/ *n* a new corm developing from a mature one.

cormorant /'kɒrmərənt/ *n* a large voracious sea bird with dark plumage and webbed feet.

corn[1] /kɒrn/ *n* a grain or seed of a cereal plant; plants that yield grain; maize; (*sl*) something corny.

corn[2] *n* a small hard painful growth on the foot.

corn[3] *vt* to preserve or cure, as with salt.

corn(ed) beef *n* cooked salted beef.

corn circle *see* **crop circle**.

corncob /-'kɒb/ *n* the central part of an ear of maize to which the corn kernels are attached; a corncob pipe.

corncockle *n* a plant with purplish flowers that grows among corn.

corncrake /-,kreɪk/ *n* a bird with a harsh cry, the landrail.

corncrib /-,krɪb/ *n* a storehouse for corn.

cornea /'kɒrniə/ *n* (*pl* **corneas, corneae**) the transparent membrane in front of the eyeball.—**corneal** *adj*.

cornel /'kɒrnəl/ *n* the cornelian cherry or dogwood, yielding an acrid edible red berry.

cornelian /'kɒrnilian/ *n* a dull-red semi-transparent form of chalcedony.—*also* **carnelian**.

corneous /'kɒrniəs/ *adj* horny.

corner /'kɒrnər/ *n* the point where sides or streets meet; an angle; a secret or confined place; a difficult or dangerous situation; (*football, hockey*) a free kick from the corner of the pitch; a monopoly over the supply of a good or service giving control over the market price; one of the opposite angles in a boxing ring. • *vt* to force into a corner; to monopolize supplies of (a commodity). • *vi* to turn round a corner; to meet at a corner or angle.

cornerstone /-,stoʊn/ *n* the principal stone, *esp* one at the corner of a foundation; an indispensable part; the most important thing or person.

cornet /'kɒrnət/ *n* a tapering valved brass musical instrument; a cone-shaped wafer for ice cream.

cornetist, cornettist /kɒr'nɛtɪst/ *n* a performer on the cornet.

cornfield /-,fi:ld/ *n* a field planted with corn or other cereal plants.

cornflakes /-,fleɪks/ *npl* a breakfast cereal made from split and toasted maize.

cornflour /-,flaʊr/ *n* a type of corn or maize flour used for thickening sauces.—*also* **cornstarch**.

cornflower /-,flaʊr/ *n* a blue-flowered wild plant growing in cornfields.

cornice /'kɒrnɪs/ *n* a plaster moulding round a ceiling or on the outside of a building.

corniche /'kɒrnɪʃ/ or /kɒr'ni:ʃ/ *n* a coastal road, *esp* one along a cliff offering spectacular views.

corniculate /kɔr'nɪkjuːlɪt/ or /-ˌleɪt/ adj horned; spurred.

Corn Laws npl British laws (1436–1834) for regulating the import and export of corn, repealed 1846–9.

corn pone n a type of Indian cornbread made with milk and eggs.

cornstalk /-ˌstɒk/ n a stem of corn; (sl) a youth or girl of Australian birth.

cornstarch /-ˌstɑːtʃ/ see **cornflour**.

cornucopia /ˌkɔrnjuˈkoːpiə/ n a horn-shaped container overflowing with fruits, flowers, etc; great abundance, an inexhaustible store.

cornute /kɔr'njuːt/ or /-'nuːt/, **cornuted** /-əd/ adj (biol) horned; horn-like.

corny /'kɔrni/ adj (**cornier, corniest**) (inf) hackneyed; banal; trite; overly sentimental.—**cornily** adv.—**corniness** n.

corolla /kə'rɒlə/ or /-'roːlə/ n the inner envelope of a flower composed of two or more petals.

corollary /kə'rɒləri/ n (pl **corollaries**) an additional inference from a proposition already proved; a result.

corona /kə'roːnə/ n (pl **coronas, coronae**) a top; a crown: a luminous halo or envelope round the sun or moon; the flat projecting part of a cornice.

coronal /kə'roːnəl/ adj pertaining to the corona. • n a crown or garland.

coronary /'kɔrəˌneri/ or /'kɑrə-/ adj pertaining to the arteries supplying blood to the heart. • n (pl **coronaries**) a coronary artery; coronary thrombosis.

coronary thrombosis n blockage of one of the coronary arteries by a blood clot.

coronation /ˌkɔrə'neɪʃən/ or /ˌkɑrə-/ n the act or ceremony of crowning a sovereign.

coroner /'kɔrənər/ or /'kɑr-/ n a public official who inquires into the causes of sudden or accidental deaths.—**coronership** n.

coronet /'kɔrəˌnet/ or /'kɑr-/, /-net/ n a small crown; an ornamental headdress.

corpora /'kɔrpərə/ see **corpus**.

corporal[1] /'kɔrpərəl/ or /-prəl/ n a noncommissioned officer below the rank of sergeant.—**corporalship** n.

corporal[2] adj of or relating to the body; physical, not spiritual.—**corporality** n.—**corporally** adv.

corporal[3] n a communion cloth.

corporate /'kɔrpərət/ or /-prət/ adj legally united into a body; of or having a corporation; united.—**corporately** adv.

corporation /ˌkɔrpə'reɪʃən/ n a group of people authorized by law to act as one individual; a city or town council.—**corporative** n.

corporator /-'reɪtər/ n a member of a corporation.

corporeal /kɔr'pɔriəl/ adj having a body or substance, material.—**corporeality, corporealness** n.—**corporeally** adv.

corposant /'kɔrpəˌsænt/ or /-ˌzænt/ n a flame-like electric discharge from a ship's mast and rigging in thundery weather, St. Elmo's fire.

corps /kɔr/ n (pl **corps**) an organized subdivision of the military establishment; a group or organization with a special function (medical corps).

corps de ballet /ˌkɔrdəbæ'leɪ/ n all the dancers in a ballet company.

corps diplomatique /ˌkɔrdɪplɒmæ'tiːk/ n all the ambassadors at a particular capital, the diplomatic corps.

corpse /kɔrps/ n a dead body. • vi (theat sl) to laugh or create laughter mischievously on stage.

corpulent /'kɔrpjulənt/ adj fleshy, fat.—**corpulence, corpulency** n.

corpus /'kɔrpəs/ n (pl **corpora**) a body or collection, esp of written works; the chief part of an organ.

Corpus Christi /ˌkrɪsti/ n (RC Church) a festival in honour of the Eucharist, held on the Thursday after Trinity Sunday.

corpuscle /'kɔrpəsəl/ n a red or white blood cell.—**corpuscular** adj.

corpus delicti /-dɪ'lɪkˌtaɪ/ n (law) the essence of a crime charged.

corral /'kɔræl/ n a pen for livestock; an enclosure with wagons; a strong stockade. • vt (**corralling, corralled**) to form a corral; to put or keep in a corral.

correct /kə'rekt/ vt to set right, to remove errors from; to reprove, to punish; to counteract, to neutralize; to adjust. • adj free from error; right, true, accurate; conforming to a fixed standard; proper.—**correctable, correctible** adj.—**correctly** adv.—**correctness** n.—**corrector** n.

correction /kə'rekʃən/ n the act of correcting; punishment.—**correctional** adj.

correctitude /kə'rektɪˌtuːd/ or /-ˌtjuːd/ n correctness, esp of conduct.

corrective /kə'rektɪv/ adj serving to correct or counteract. • n that which corrects.—**correctively** adv.

correlate /ˌkɒrə'leɪt/ vti to have or to bring into mutual relation; to correspond to one another. • n either of two things so related that one implies the other.—**correlation** n.—**correlative** adj.

correlation /ˌkɒrə'leɪʃən/ or /ˌkɑ-/ n reciprocal relation; similarity or parallelism of relation or law; the interdependence of functions, organs, natural forces, or phenomena.—**correlational** adj.

correlative /kə'relətɪv/ adj having or expressing reciprocal or mutual relation. • n the antecedent to a pronoun.—**correlativeness, correlativity** n.

correspond /ˌkɒrə'spɒnd/ or /ˌkɑ-/ vi to answer, to agree; to be similar (to); to tally; to communicate by letter.

correspondence /ˌkɒrə'spɒndəns/ or /ˌkɑ-/ n communication by writing letters; the letters themselves; agreement.

correspondence school n an institution offering tuition (**correspondence courses**) by post.

correspondent /ˌkɒrə'spɒndənt/ n a person who writes letters; a journalist who gathers news for newspapers, radio or television from a foreign country. • adj similar, analogous.

corridor /'kɒrɪdɔr/ or /'kɑr-/, /-dər/ n a long passage into which compartments in a train or rooms in a building open; a strip of land giving a country without a coastline access to the sea.

corrie /'kɒri/ or /'kɑri/ n (Scot) a round hollow on a hillside.

corrigendum /ˌkɒrɪ'dʒendəm/ or /ˌkɑr-/ n (pl **corrigenda**) an error in a book, etc, for which a correction slip is printed.

corrigible /'kɒrədʒəbəl/ or /'kɑr-/ adj capable of being amended, correct, or reformed.—**corrigibility** n.

corroborant /kə'rɒbərənt/ adj corroborating. • n a corroborating fact.

corroborate /kə'rɒbəˌreɪt/ vt to confirm; to make more certain; to verify.—**corroboration** n.—**corroborative** adj.—**corroborator** n.

corroboree /kə'rɒbəri/ n an Australian festivity and dance.

corrode /kə'roːd/ vti to eat into or wear away gradually, to rust; to disintegrate.—**corrodant, corrodent** n.—**corroder** n.—**corrodible** adj.—**corrosion** n.

corrosion /kə'roːʒən/ n the act of corroding; a corroded condition.

corrosive /kə'roːzɪv/ adj causing corrosion. • n a corrosive substance, as acid.—**corrosively** adv.—**corrosiveness** n.

corrosive sublimate n a poisonous compound of mercury.

corrugate /'kɒruˌgeɪt/ or /'kɑr-/ vt to form into parallel ridges and grooves.—**corrugated** adj.—**corrugation** n.

corrugated iron n sheet iron pressed in alternate parallel ridges and grooves and galvanized.

corrugated paper n paper used for packaging with one surface in parallel ridges.

corrupt /kə'rʌpt/ adj dishonest; taking bribes; depraved; rotten, putrid. • vti to make or become corrupt; to infect; to taint.—**corrupter, corruptor** n.—**corruptive** adj.—**corruptly** adv.—**corruptness** n.

corruptible /kə'rʌptəbəl/ adj open to corruption.—**corruptibility** n.

corruption /kə'rʌpʃən/ n the act of corrupting; the state of being corrupted; physical dissolution.—**corruptionist** n.

corsage /kɔr'sɒʒ/ n a small bunch of flowers for pinning to a dress; the part of a woman's dress covering the bust.

corsair /'kɔrsər/ or /ˌkɑr,ser/ n a pirate; a pirate ship.

corse /kɔrs/ n (poet) a corpse.

corselet, corslet /'kɔrslɪt/ or /'kɔrsə,let/ n light body armour, esp for the breast.

corset /'kɔrsət/ n a close-fitting undergarment, worn to support the torso.

corsetière /ˌkɔrsə'tɪr/ or /-'tjer/ n a woman who makes and fits corsets.—**corsetier** nm.

cortege, cortège /'kɔrˌteʒ/ n a train of attendants; a retinue; a funeral procession.

Cortes /'kɔrtez/, Sp. /'kɔrtes/ n the national and legislative assembly of Spain and (formerly) Portugal.

cortex /'kɔrˌteks/ n (pl **cortices**) an outer layer of tissue of any organ, eg the outer grey matter of the brain; the outer tissue of a plant stem; bark of a tree.—**cortical** adj.

corticate /'kɔrtəˌkɒt/ or /-ˌkeɪt/, **corticated** adj covered with bark or a bark-like substance.—**cortication** n.

cortisone /'kɔrtəˌzoːn/ n a hormone produced by the adrenal glands, the synthetic version of which is used to treat arthritis, allergies and skin disorders, etc.

corundum /kə'rʌndəm/ *n* a hard mineral of many colours used as an abrasive and as gemstones.

coruscate /'kɒrə,skeɪt/ or /'kʌr-/ *vi* to sparkle, to flash.—**coruscation** *n*.

corvée /kɔr'veɪ/ *n* the exacting of unpaid labour in the feudal system.

corves /kɔrvz/ *see* **corf**.

corvette /'kɔr,vet/ *n* a fast escort warship.

corvine /'kɔr,vaɪn/ *adj* of or pertaining to a crow or raven.

corymb /'kɒrɪmb/, or /'kʌr-/, /-ɪm/ *n* an inflorescence with the flowers all nearly at the same level and the lower stalks are the longest.—**corymbose, corybous** *adj*.

coryphaeus /,kɒrə'fiːəs/ *n* (*pl* **coryphaei**) the leader of the chorus in ancient Greek drama.

coryphée /,kɒrɪ'feɪ/ or /,kɔr-/ *n* a ballet dancer.

coryza /kə'raɪzə/ *n* a severe cold in the head with inflammation of the mucous membrane of the nose.

cos /kɒs/ *abbr* = cosine.

cosec /'kɒ,sek/ *abbr* = cosecant.

cosecant /kɒ'siːkənt/ *n* (*geom*) the secant of the complement of the given angle or arc of 90°.

coseismal /kɒ'saɪsməl/ or /-'saɪz-/, **coseismic** /-mɪk/ *adj* showing simultaneous shocks of an earthquake.

cosh /kɒʃ/ *vt* (*sl*) to bludgeon.

cosher /'kɒʃər/ *vt* to pamper, to coddle.

cosignatory /kɒ'sɪgnə,tɔːri/ *n* a person signing along with another.

cosine /kɒ'saɪn/ *n* a trigonometrical function of an angle that in a right-angled triangle is equal to the ratio of the length of the adjacent side to the hypotenuse.

cosmetic /kɒz'metɪk/ *n* a preparation for improving the beauty, *esp* of the face. • *adj* beautifying or correcting faults in the appearance.—**cosmetically** *adv*.

cosmetic bag ✳ (*Cdn*) a small, zippered, waterproof bag for holding cosmetics and related items.

cosmetic surgery *n* surgery carried out to improve the appearance.

cosmic /,kɒzmɪk/, **cosmical** /-əl/ *adj* of or pertaining to the universe and the laws that govern it; vast in extent, intensity, or comprehensiveness.—**cosmically** *adv*.

cosmo- /'kɒzmɔː/ or /-mə/ *prefix* universe.

cosmogony /kɒz'mɒgəni/ *n* (*pl* **cosmogonies**) the origin of the universe; a theory or treatise on this.—**cosmogonal** *adj*.—**cosmogonic, cosmogonical** *adj*.—**cosmogonist** *n*.

cosmography /kɒz'mɒgrəfi/ *n* the description and mapping of the universe or the earth as a whole.—**cosmographer, cosmographist** *n*.—**cosmographic, cosmographical** *adj*.

cosmology /kɒz'mɒlədʒi/ *n* the science of the nature, origins, and development of the universe.—**cosmological, cosmologic** *adj*.—**cosmologist** *n*.

cosmonaut /'kɒzmə,nɒt/ *n* a Russian astronaut.

cosmopolitan /,kɒzmə'pɒlɪtən/ *adj* of all parts of the world; free from national prejudice; at home in any part of the world. • *n* a well-travelled person; a person without national prejudices.—**cosmopolitanism** *n*.

cosmopolite /kɒz'mɒpə,laɪt/ *n* a citizen of the world, a person without patriotism; an animal or plant found worldwide.—**cosmopolitism** *n*.

cosmos /kɒz'mɒːs/ or /-məs/ *n* the universe as an ordered whole; any orderly system.

Cossack /'kɒsæk/ *n* a member of a Russian people skilled as horsemen. • *adj* pertaining to Cossacks.

cosset /'kɒset/ *vt* to make a pet of; to pamper.

cost /kɒst/ *vt* (**costing, cost**) to involve the payment, loss, or sacrifice of; to have as a price; to estimate and fix the price of. • *n* a price; an expense; expenditure of time, labour, etc; a loss, a penalty; (*pl*) the expenses of a lawsuit.

costa /'kɒstə/ *n* (*pl* **costae**) a rib.—**costal** *adj*.

costard /'kɒstərd/ *n* a large kind of English apple; (*arch*) a head.

costate /'kɒs,teɪt/ or /'kɒs-/ *adj* ribbed.

cost-effective /,kɒstə'fektɪv/ *adj* giving a satisfactory return for the amount spent on outlay.

costive /'kɒstɪv/ *adj* constipated.

costly /'kɒstli/ *adj* (**costlier, costliest**) expensive; involving great sacrifice.—**costliness** *n*.

costmary /'kɒst,meri/ *n* (*pl* **costmaries**) a perennial plant with fragrant leaves, formerly used for flavouring ale.

cost-of-living index *n* consumer price index.

costume /'kɒ,stjuːm/ or /-,tuːm/ *n* a style of dress, *esp* belonging to a particular period, fashion, etc; clothes of an unusual or historical nature, as worn by actors in a play, etc; fancy dress.

costume jewellery *n* imitation gems or cheap jewellery worn for decorative effect.

costumer /-ər/, **costumier** /-ɪər/ *n* a dealer in fancy dress for the theatre, etc.

cosy /'kɒːzi/ *adj* (**cosier, cosiest**) warm and comfortable; snug; friendly for an ulterior motive. • *n* a cover to keep a thing warm.—*also* **cozy**.—**cosily** *adv*.—**cosiness** *n*.

cot¹ /'kɒt/ *n* a child's box-like bed; a narrow collapsible bed.

cot² *abbr* = cotangent.

cotangent /'kɒː'tændʒənt/ *n* a trigonometrical function of an angle that in a right-angled triangle is equal to the ratio of the length of the adjacent side to the opposite side.

cot death *n* the sudden death of a baby during sleep from an unexplained cause.—*also* **crib death**.

cote /kɒːt/ *n* a shed or shelter for animals or birds, *esp* doves.

cotenant /kɒː'tenənt/ or /'kɒ,ten-/ *n* a joint tenant.—**cotenancy** *n*.

coterie /'kɒːtəri/ *n* a small circle of people with common interests; a social clique.

coterminous /,kɒː'tɜːmənəs/ *see* **conterminous**.

cotidal /kɒː'taɪdəl/ *adj* (*chart lines*) joining those places where high tide occurs at the same time.

cotillion /kə'tɪljən/ or /kɒ-/ *n* a brisk, lively dance for eight or more people; music for such a dance; a formal ball.

cotoneaster /kə,tɒ:ni'æstər/ *n* an ornamental shrub of the rose family with red or orange berries.

cotta /'kɒtə/ *n* (*pl* **cottae, cottas**) a short surplice.

cottage /'kɒtədʒ/ *n* a small house, *esp* in the country.

cottage cheese *n* a soft cheese made from loose milk curds.

cottage industry *n* manufacture carried out in the home, eg weaving, basketry.

cottager /-ər/ *n* a person who lives or holidays in a cottage.

cotter¹, cottar /'kɒtər/ *n* a farm labourer who has the use of a cottage for which he works in lieu of rent.

cotter² /'kɒtər/ *n* a bolt, wedge, etc used to secure parts of machinery to prevent movement.

cotter pin *n* a split pin that secures (a cotter, etc) by spreading the ends after insertion.

cotton /'kɒtən/ *n* soft white fibre of the cotton plant; fabric or thread made of this; thread. • *adj* made of cotton. • *vi* (*with* **on**) (*inf*) to realize the meaning of, to understand; to take a liking to.—**cottony** *adj*.

cotton batting, cotton batten *n* ✳ (*Cdn*) a form of cotton wool used in first aid and for crafts.

cotton candy *see* **candyfloss**.

cotton grass *n* a plant with long silky hairs.

cottontail *n* an American rabbit.

cotton wool *n* raw cotton that has been bleached and sterilized for use as a dressing, etc; absorbent cotton; a state of being protected.

cotyledon /,kɒtə'liːdən/ *n* a seed lobe or rudimentary leaf or leaves of an embryo; kinds of plant, chiefly evergreens.—**cotyledonal** *adj*.—**cotyledonary** *adj*—**cotyledonous, cotyledonoid** *adj*.

cotyloid /,kɒtə'lɔɪd/, **cotyloidal** /-əl/ *adj* cup-shaped.

couch /kʊtʃ/ *n* a piece of furniture, with a back and armrests, for seating several persons; a bed, *esp* as used by psychiatrists for patients. • *vt* to express in words in a particular way; to lie down; to deposit in a bed or layer; (*arch*) to crouch ready for springing; to depress or remove (a cataract in the eye).—**coucher** *n*.

couchant /'kʊtʃənt/ *adj* (*her*) lying down with the head up.

couch grass *n* a kind of coarse grass that spreads rapidly.

couching /'kʊtʃɪŋ/ *n* the operation of removing a cataract from the eye by depressing or removing the crystalline lens; a stye of embroidery.

couch potato *n* (*sl*) a person who would rather watch television in leisure time than participate in sports, etc.

cougar /'kuːgər/ *n* a puma.

cough /kɒf/ *vi* to expel air from the lungs with a sudden effort and noise; (*with* **up**) (*inf*) to hand over or tell unwillingly. • *n* the act of coughing; a disease causing a cough.

cough drop *n* a lozenge that when sucked relieves a cough.

cough syrup *n* a medicinal liquid to relieve coughing.

could /kʊd/ or /kəd/ *see* **can¹**.

couldn't /kʊdənt/ = could not.

coulee /'kuːli/ *n* a dry ravine with sloping sides; a flow of lava.

coulisse /ku:'li:s/ *n* a piece of grooved timber in which anything slides; one of the side scenes of a stage; (*pl*) the space between the side scenes.

couloir /ku:lwαr/ *n* a steeply ascending gorge in a mountainside.

coulomb /'ku:lɒm/ *n* an SI unit of electric charge; the quantity of electricity conveyed by a current of one ampere in one second.

coulter /'ko:ltər/ *n* a vertical blade at the front of a ploughshare.— *also* **colter**.

coumarin /'ku:mərɪn/ *n* an aromatic crystalline substance obtained from the tonka bean and used in perfumes and medicines.—**coumaric** adj.

council /'kaʊnsəl/ *n* an elected or appointed legislative or advisory body; a central body uniting a group of organizations; an executive body whose members are equal in power and authority.— **councillor, councilor** n.—**councillorship, councilorship** n.

councillor, councilor /-ər/ *n* a member of a council.—**councillorship, councilorship** n.

councilman /-mən/ *n* (*pl* **councilmen**) a member of a council, a councillor.

counsel /'kaʊnsəl/ *n* advice; consultation, deliberate purpose or design; a person who gives counsel, a lawyer or a group of lawyers; a consultant. • *vb* (**counselling** *or* **counseling, counselled** *or* **counseled**) *vt* to advise; to recommend. • *vi* to give or take advice.

counselling, counseling /-ɪŋ/ *n* professional guidance for an individual or a couple from a qualified person.

counsellor, counselor /-ər/ *n* one who gives advice, *esp* legal advice, an adviser a lawyer.

count[1] /kaʊnt/ *n* a European noble.

count[2] *vt* to number, to add up; to reckon; to consider to be; to call aloud (beats or time units); to include or exclude by counting; (*with* **against**) to have an adverse effect. • *vi* to name numbers or add up items in order; to mark time; to be of importance or value; to rely (upon); (*with* **on**) to rely on; (*with* **out**) (*inf*) to exclude, leave out; to pronounce after a count a floored boxer to be the loser. • *n* an act of numbering or reckoning; the total counted; a separate and distinct charge in an indictment; rhythm.

countdown /'kaʊntdaʊn/ *n* the descending count backwards to zero, eg to the moment a rocket lifts off.

countenance /'kaʊntənəns/ *n* the whole form of the face; appearance; support. • *vt* to favour, give approval to.

counter[1] /'kaʊntər/ *n* one who or that which counts; a disc used for scoring, a token; a table in a bank or shop across which money or goods are passed.

counter[2] *adv* contrary; adverse; in an opposite direction; in the wrong way. • *adj* opposed; opposite. • *n* a return blow or parry; an answering move. • *vti* to oppose; to retort; to give a return blow; to retaliate.

counter- /'kaʊntər/ *prefix* rival; opposed; reversed; matched.

counteract /ˌkaʊntər'ækt/ *vt* to act in opposition to so as to defeat or hinder; to neutralize.—**counteraction** n.—**counteractive** adj.

counterattack /'kaʊntərəˌtæk/ *or n* an attack in response to an attack. • *vt* to make a counterattack.

counterattraction /'kaʊntərəˌtrækʃən/ *n* a rival attraction; attraction in an opposite direction.

counterbalance /'kaʊntərˌbæləns/ *n* a weight balancing another. • *vt* to act as a counterbalance; to act against with equal power.

counterchange /ˌkaʊntər'tʃeɪndʒ/ *vti* to interchange; to chequer.

countercharge /'kaʊntərˌtʃɑrdʒ/ *n* an opposing charge, *esp* by an accused person against his or her accuser. • *vt* to charge in opposition to another.

countercheck /-ˌtʃɛk/ *n* a check on a check; an opposing check; (*arch*) a retort.

counterclaim /'kaʊntərˌkleɪm/ *n* an opposing claim, *esp* by a defendant in a lawsuit.—**counterclaimant** n.

counterclockwise /ˌkaʊntər'klɒkˌwaɪz/ *adj* moving in a direction contrary to the hands of a clock as viewed from the front.— *also adv*.—*also* **anticlockwise**.

counterespionage /ˌkaʊntər'espiəˌnɒʒ/ *n* spying on or exposing enemy spies.

counterfeit /'kaʊntərˌfɪt/ *vt* to imitate; to forge; to feign, simulate. • *adj* made in imitation, forged; feigned, sham. • *n* an imitation, a forgery.—**counterfeiter** n.

counterfoil /-ˌfɔɪl/ *n* a detachable section of a cheque or ticket, kept as a receipt or record; a stub.

counterintelligence /ˌkaʊntərɪn'telɪdʒəns/ *n* activities intended to frustrate enemy espionage and intelligence-gathering operations.

counterirritant /ˌkaʊntər'ɪrɪtənt/ *n* an application or action irritating the body surface to relieve internal inflammation.— **counterirritation** n.

countermand /-'mænd/ *vt* to revoke or annul, as an order or command; to cancel the orders of another. • *n* a command cancelling another.

countermarch /'kaʊntərˌmɑrtʃ/ *vti* to march in the reverse direction. • *n* such a march.

countermeasure /-ˌmeʒər/ *n* an action taken to neutralize or retaliate against some threat or danger, etc.

countermine /-ˌmaɪn/ *n* a mine made to intercept that of an enemy. • *vi* to make a countermine; to counterplot.

counteroffensive /-əˌfensɪv/ *n* a counterattack, *esp* by defenders of a position.

counterpane /-ˌpeɪn/ *n* a bedspread.

counterpart /-ˌpɑrt/ *n* a thing exactly like another, a duplicate; a corresponding or complementary part or thing.

counterplot /-ˌplɒt/ *n* a plot to defeat another plot. • *vi* (**counterplotting, counterplotted**) to plot in retaliation.

counterpoint /-ˌpɔɪnt/ *n* (*mus*) a melody added as an accompaniment to another. • *vt* to set in contrast.

counterpoise /-ˌpɔɪz/ *n* a weight, force or influence that balances another; equilibrium. • *vt* to counterbalance.

counterproductive /-prəˌdʌktəv/ *adj* producing a contrary effect on productivity or usefulness; hindering the desired end.

Counter-Reformation /ˌkaʊntərˌrefər'meɪʃən/ *n* the reforming movement in the Roman Catholic Church following the Protestant Reformation.

counter-revolution /-ˌrevə'lu:ʃən/ *n* a revolution undoing the work of a previous one.—**counter-revolutionary** adj, n.

countersign /'kaʊntərˌsaɪn/ *vt* to authenticate a document by an additional signature. • *n* an additional signature to a document to attest it; a word to be given in answer to a sentry's challenge; an additional mark.—**countersignature** n.

countersink /-ˌsɪŋk/ *vt* (**countersinking, countersunk**) to enlarge the upper part of a hole so that the screw head will sit flush with, or below, the surface; to drive (a screw) into such a hole. • *n* a tool for countersinking.

countertenor /-ˌtenər/ *n* a high tenor voice with an alto range; a person who sings countertenor.

counterterrorism /ˌkaʊntər'terərɪzəm/ *n* terrorist act(s) perpetrated in revenge for former terrorist act(s).

countervail /ˌkaʊntər'veɪl/ *or* /'kaʊntər-/ *vt* to counterbalance, compensate for.

counterweight /'kaʊntərˌweɪt/ *n* a counterbalancing weight or power.

countess /'kaʊntəs/ *n* a woman with the rank of count or earl; the wife or widow of a count.

counting house *n* a book-keeping office or department.

countless /'kaʊntləs/ *adj* innumerable.

countrified, countryfied /'kʌntrɪˌfaɪd/ *adj* in the manner of the country; rural.

country /'kʌntri/ *n* (*pl* **countries**) a region or district; the territory of a nation; a state; the land of one's birth or residence; rural parts; country-and-western. • *adj* rural.

country-and-western *n* a style of white folk music of the southeastern US.—*also* **country music**.

country club *n* a social and sporting facility in a rural setting.

country dance *n* a dance with the couples face to face in two lines.

country house *n* a gentleman's country residence.

countryman /-mən/ *n* (*pl* **countrymen**) a person who lives in the country; a person from the same country as another.— **countrywoman** nf (*pl* **countrywomen**).

countryside /-ˌsaɪd/ *n* a rural district.

county /'kaʊnti/ *n* (*pl* **counties**) in US, an administrative subdivision of a state; in UK, an administrative subdivision for local government.—*also adj*.

county palatine *n* a county having royal powers in the administration of justice.

county town, county seat *n* the capital of a county.

coup /ku:/ *n* a sudden telling blow; a masterstroke; a coup d'état.

coup de grâce /ˌku:də'grɒs/ *n* (*pl* **coups de grâce**) a finishing or fatal blow.

coup d'état /ˌkuːdeɪˈtɒ/ *n* (*pl* **coups d'état**) a sudden and unexpected bold stroke of policy; the sudden overthrow of a government.

coup de théâtre /kuːdəterˈætrə/, *Fr.* /ˌkuːttɛɪˈɑːtʀ/ *n* (*pl* **coups de théâtre**) a sudden dramatic or sensational action.

coupé /kuːp/, *Fr.* /kuːˈpeɪ/ *n* a closed, four-seater, two-door automobile with a sloping back.

couple /ˈkʌpəl/ *n* two of the same kind connected together; a pair; a husband and wife; a pair of equal and parallel forces. • *vt* to link or join together. • *vi* to copulate.

couplet /ˈkʌplət/ *n* two consecutive lines of verse that rhyme with each other.

coupling /ˈkʌplɪŋ/ *n* a device for joining parts of a machine or two railway carriages.

coupon /ˈkuːpɒn/ or /ˈkjuː-/ *n* a detachable certificate on a bond, presented for payment of interest; a certificate entitling one to a discount, gift, etc.

courage /ˈkʌrɪdʒ/ *n* bravery; fortitude; spirit.—**courageous** *adj*.—**courageously** *adv*.—**courageousness** *n*.

coureur de bois *Fr.* /kuːrœrdəˈbwɑ/ (*pl* **coureurs de bois**) *n* ✹ (*Cdn*) (*hist*) a French or Metis fur trader.

courgette /kurˈʒet/ *n* a zucchini.

courier /ˈkuriːər/ *n* a messenger, *esp* diplomatic; a tourist guide; a carrier of illegal goods between countries.

course /kɔːrs/ *n* a race; a path or track; a career; a direction or line of motion; a regular sequence; the portion of a meal served at one time; conduct; behaviour; the direction a ship is steered; a continuous level range of brick or masonry of the same height; the chase of a hare by greyhounds a length of time; an area set aside for a sport or a race; a series of studies; any of the studies. • *vt* to hunt. • *vi* to move swiftly along an indicated path; to chase with greyhounds.

courser /ˈkɔːrsər/ *n* one who courses; a dog trained for coursing; (*poet*) a swift and spirited horse.

coursing /ˈkɔːrsɪŋ/ *n* the sport of pursuing game with hunting dogs.

court /kɔːrt/ *n* an uncovered space surrounded by buildings or walls; a short street; a playing space, as for tennis, etc; a royal palace; the retinue of a sovereign; (*law*) a hall of justice; the judges, etc engaged there; address; civility; flattery. • *vt* to seek the friendship of; to woo; to flatter; to solicit; to risk. • *vi* to carry on a courtship.

courteous /ˈkɔːrtiːəs/ *adj* polite; obliging.—**courteously** *adv*.—**courteousness** *n*.

courtesan /ˌkɔːrtɪˈzæn/ or /ˈkɔːrt-/ *n* (*formerly*) a prostitute, or mistress of a courtier.

courtesy /ˈkɔːrtɪsi/ *n* (*pl* **courtesies**) politeness and kindness; civility; a courteous manner or action.

courthouse /ˈkɔːrtˌhaus/ *n* a public building that houses law courts.

courtier /ˈkɔːrtiːər/ *n* one in attendance at a royal court.

courtly /ˈkɔːrtli/ *adj* (**courtlier, courtliest**) well-mannered, polite; of a court.—**courtliness** *n*.

court martial /ˈkɔːrtˌmɑːrʃəl/ *n* (*pl* **courts martial, court martials**) a court of justice composed of naval or military officers for the trial of disciplinary offences.

court-martial *vt* (**court-martialling, court-martialled** *or* **court-martialing, court-martialed**) to try by court martial.

court plaster *n* a superior kind of sticking plaster, originally used by ladies at court for ornamental patches on the face.

courtship /-ˌʃɪp/ *n* the act of wooing.

courtyard /-ˌjɑːrd/ *n* an enclosed space adjoining or in a large building.

couscous /ˈkuːskuːs/ *n* a North African dish of cracked wheat steamed and served with a meat and vegetable stew.

cousin /ˈkʌzən/ *n* the son or daughter of an uncle or aunt.—**cousinly** *adj*.—**cousinship** *n*.

couture /kuːˈtʃuːr/ or /-ˈtur/, /-ˈtjuːr/, *Fr.* /kuˈtyʀ/ *n* the design and manufacture of expensive fashion clothes.

couturier /kuːˈturiˌeɪ/, *Fr.* /kutyˌʀjeɪ/ *n* a designer of expensive fashion clothes.—**couturière** *nf*.

couvade /kuːˈvɒd/ *n* a primitive custom by which when a child is born the father takes to his bed, where he receives the attentions *usu* given to the mother.

cove /koːv/ *n* a small sheltered bay or inlet in a body of water; a curved moulding at the juncture of a wall and ceiling.—*also* **coving**.

coven /ˈkʌvən/ *n* an assembly of witches.

covenant /ˈkʌvənənt/ *n* a written agreement; a solemn agreement of fellowship and faith between members of a church; an agreement to pay annually a sum to a charity. • *vt* to promise by a covenant. • *vi* to enter into a formal agreement.—**covenantal** *adj*.—**covenanted** *adj*.

covenantee /ˌkʌvənənˈtiː/ *n* one in whose favour a covenant is made.

covenantor /ˈkʌvənəntər/ *n* one who enters into a covenant.

cover /ˈkʌvər/ *vt* to overspread the top of anything with something else; to hide; to save from punishment; to shelter; to clothe; to understudy; to insure against damage, loss, etc; to report for a newspaper; to include; to make a journey over; (*male animal*) to copulate. • *vi* to spread over, as a liquid does; to provide an excuse or alibi (for); to work, eg as a salesman, in a certain area; to have within firing range. • *n* that which is laid on something else; a bedcover; a shelter; a covert; an understudy; something used to hide one's real actions, etc; insurance against loss or damage; a place laid at a table for a meal.—**coverer** *n*.

coverage /ˈkʌvərɪdʒ/ *n* the amount, extent, etc covered by something; the amount of reporting of an event for newspaper, television, etc.

coverall /-ˌɔːl/ *n* (*usu pl*) a one-piece garment that completely covers and protects one's clothing.

cover charge *n* a charge made by a restaurant over and above the cost of the food and service.

cover girl *n* an attractive girl whose picture is used on magazine covers.

covering /ˈkʌvərɪŋ/ *n* that which covers or protects; dress.

covering letter *n* a letter containing an explanation of an accompanying item.

coverlet /ˈkʌvərlət/ *n* a bedspread.

coversine /ˈkoːvərs/ *n* the versed sine of the complement of an angle or arc.

covert /ˈkoːvərt/ or /koːˈvərt/, /kʌ-/ *adj* covered; secret, concealed. • *n* a place that protects or shelters; a thicket; shelter for game.—**covertly** *adv*.

coverture /ˈkoːvərtʃər/ *n* a cover; shelter; (*law*) the status of a married woman.

cover-up /ˈkʌvərˌʌp/ *n* something used to hide one's real activities, etc; a concerted effort to keep an act or situation from being made public.

covet /ˈkʌvət/ *vt* to desire earnestly; to lust after; to long to possess (what belongs to another).—**coveter** *n*.—**covetous** *adj*.—**covetousness** *n*.

covetous /ˈkʌvətəs/ *adj* avaricious, grasping, acquisitive.—**covetousness** *n*.

covey /ˈkʌvi/ *n* a hatch or brood of birds, *esp* partridges.

coving /ˈkoːvɪŋ/ *n* a curved moulding at the juncture of a wall and ceiling.—*also* **cove**.

cow[1] /kaʊ/ *n* the mature female of domestic cattle; the mature female of various other animals, as the whale, elephant, etc; (*sl*) a disagreeable woman.

cow[2] *vt* to take the spirit out of, to intimidate.

coward /ˈkaʊərd/ *n* a person lacking courage; one who is afraid.

cowardice /ˈkaʊərdɪs/ *n* lack of courage.

cowardly /ˈkaʊərdli/ *adj* of, or like, a coward.—**cowardliness** *n*.

cowbane /ˈkaʊˌbeɪn/ *n* water hemlock.

cowbird /-ˌbɜːrd/ *n* an American blackbird so called from its accompanying cattle.

cowboy /-ˌbɔɪ/ *n* a person who tends cattle or horses.—*also* **cowhand**; (*inf*) one who is engaged in dubious business activities.

cowcatcher /-ˌkætʃər/ *n* a wedge-shaped iron frame on the front of a locomotive to push aside obstacles.

cower /ˈkaʊər/ *vi* to crouch or sink down through fear, etc; to tremble.

cowfish /ˈkaʊfɪʃ/ *n* (*pl* **cowfish, cowfishes**) a name given to various fishes and other marine animals, as the dolphin.

cowgirl /-ˌgɜːrl/ *n* a woman who works as a cowhand.

cowherd /-ˌhɜːrd/ *n* a person employed to tend cattle.

cowhide /-ˌhaɪd/ *n* the tanned and dressed skins of cows; a stout flexible whip made of rawhide.

cowl /kaʊl/ *n* a hood; the hooded habit of a monk; the draped neckline of a woman's dress or sweater; a chimney corner.

cowlick /ˈkaʊˌlɪk/ *n* a tuft of hair turned up or brushed over the forehead.

cowling /ˈkaʊlɪŋ/ *n* the metal covering of an aeroplane engine.

coworker /'koːwərkər/ *n* a fellow worker.

cowpat /'kauˌpæt/ *n* a piece of cow dung.

cow pony /-ˌpoːni/ *n* a mustang used by cowboys.

cowpox /-ˌpɒks/ *n* a disease of cows that produces vesicles from which the vaccine for inoculation against smallpox is obtained.

cowpuncher /-ˌpəntʃər/, **cowpoke** /-ˌpoːk/ *n* a cowboy.

cowry, cowrie /'kauri/ *n* (*pl* **cowries**) a marine mollusc with a glossy, brightly speckled shell.

cowslip /'kauˌslip/ *n* a common wild plant with small fragrant yellow flowers.

cox /kɒks/ *n* a coxswain. • *vt* to act as a coxswain.

coxa /'kɒksə/ *n* (*pl* **coxae**) the hip joint.—**coxal** *adj*.

coxalgia /kɒksˈældʒiə/ or /-dʒə/ *n* a pain in, or disease of, the hip joint.—**coxalgic** *adj*.

coxcomb /'kɒkskoːm/ *n* a cockscomb; a vain conceited person, a fop.

coxcombry /'kɒkskəmri/ *n* (*pl* **coxcombries**) affected airs, foppishness.

coxswain /'kɒksən/ or /-swein/ *n* a person who steers a boat, *esp* a lifeboat or racing boat.—*also* **cockswain**.

coy /kɔɪ/ *adj* playfully or provocatively demure; bashful.—**coyly** *adv*.—**coyness** *n*.

coyote /kaɪˈoːti/ or /'kaɪoːt/ *n* (*pl* **coyotes, coyote**) a small prairie wolf of North America.

coypu /'kɔɪpuː/ *n* (*pl* **coypus, coypu**) an aquatic beaver-like animal, originally from South America.

coz /kʌz/ *n* (*arch*) cousin.

cozen /'kʌzən/ *vt* to cheat, to beguile; to act deceitfully.—**cozenage** *n*.—**cozener** *n*.

cozy /'koːzi/ *see* **cosy**.

cp. *abbr* = compare.

CP *abbr* = Communist Party.

CP *abbr* ✺ = Canadian Pacific; Canadian Press.

Cpl *abbr* = Corporal.

CPP *abbr* ✺ = Canada Pension Plan.

CPS *abbr* ✺ = Canadian Parks Service.

CPU *abbr* = central processing unit.

Cr (*chem symbol*) chromium.

cr. *abbr* = credit; creditor.

crab /kræb/ *n* any of numerous chiefly marine broadly built crustaceans. • *vi* (**crabbing, crabbed**) to fish for crabs; to complain.

crab-apple *n* a wild apple.

crabbed /kræbd/ *adj* bad-tempered, morose; (*writing*) cramped; hard to decipher.

crabby /'kræbi/ *adj* bad-tempered.—**crabbily** *adv*.—**crabbiness** *n*.

crab louse *n* a species of body louse.

crabstick /'kræbstik/ *n* a cudgel; a surly person.

crack /kræk/ *vt* to burst, break or sever; to utter a sharp, abrupt cry; to injure; to damage mentally; to open a bottle; (*sl*) to make (a joke); (*inf*) to break open (a safe); to decipher (a code). • *vi* to make a sharp explosive sound; (*inf*) to lose control under pressure; to shift erratically in vocal tone; (*with* **up**) (*inf*) to be unable to cope; (*sl*) to take the drug crack. • *n* a chink or fissure; a narrow fracture; a sharp sound; a sharp resonant blow; an altered tone of voice; a chat, gossip; a wisecrack; (*inf*) an attempt; an expert; (*sl*) the drug cocaine packaged in the form of pellets.

crackbrained /'kræk,breind/ *adj* crazy.

crackdown /-ˌdaun/ *n* repressive action to quell disorder, etc.

cracked /krækt/ *adj* split, broken; blemished; insane; legally imperfect.

cracker /'krækər/ *n* a firework that explodes with a loud crack; a paper tube that when pulled explodes harmlessly and releases a paper hat and plastic toy; a thin, crisp biscuit; (*sl*) a person or thing of great ability or excellence.

crackerjack /'krækərˌdʒæk/ *n* (*sl*) a fine specimen.

crackers /'krækərz/ *adj* (*sl*) crazy.

crackhead /'krækhɛd/ *n* (*sl*) a person who is addicted to the drug crack.

crack house /-ˌhɛus/ *n* (*sl*) a place where the drug crack is made available by dealers.

cracking /-ɪŋ/ *adj* (*inf*) fast-moving; excellent. • *n* the act of hacking into computer games; **to get cracking** to start to do something with vim and vigour.

crackle /'krækəl/ *vi* to make a slight, sharp explosive noise. • *vt* to cover with a delicate network of minute cracks. • *n* a noise of frequent and slight cracks and reports; a surface glaze on glass or porcelain.—**crackly** *adj*.

crackling /'kræklɪŋ/ *n* (*usu pl*) the browned crisp rind of roast pork.

cracknel /'kræknəl/ *n* a thick puffy dry fancy biscuit.

crackpot /'krækpɒt/ *n* (*inf*) an eccentric, a crazy person. • *adj* (*inf*) crazy, unpractical.

cracksman /'kræksmən/ *n* (*pl* **cracksmen**) a burglar.

-cracy /krəsi/ *n suffix* government by, as in *democracy*.

cradle /'kreidəl/ *n* a baby's crib or a small bed, often on rockers; infancy; birthplace or origin; a case for a broken limb; a framework of timbers, *esp* for supporting a boat; the rest for a telephone handset. • *vt* to rock or place in a cradle; to nurse or train in infancy.

cradlesong /-ˌsɒŋ/ *n* a lullaby.

cradling /'kreidlɪŋ/ *n* the open timbers or ribs of a vaulted ceiling.

craft /kræft/ *n* manual skill; a skilled trade; the members of a skilled trade; cunning; (*pl* **craft**) a boat, ship, or aircraft.

craftsman /'kræftsmən/ *n* (*pl* **craftsmen**) a person skilled in a particular craft.—**craftsmanship** *n*.—**craftswoman** *nf* (*pl* **craftswomen**).

crafty /'kræfti/ *adj* (**craftier, craftiest**) cunning, wily.—**craftily** *adv*.—**craftiness** *n*.

crag /kræg/ *n* a rough steep rock or cliff.

craggy /'krægi/, **cragged** /-d/ *adj* (**craggier, craggiest**) full of crags; rugged.—**cragginess** *n*.

crake /kreik/ *n* the corncrake.

cram /kræm/ *vb* (**cramming crammed**) *vt* to pack tightly, to stuff; to fill to overflowing; (*inf*) to prepare quickly for an examination. • *vi* to eat greedily.

crambo /'kræmbo:/ *n* (*pl* **cramboes**) a game in which rhymes have to be found for a given word.

cramp /kræmp/ *n* a spasmodic muscular contraction of the limbs; (*pl*) abdominal spasms and pain; a clamp. • *vt* to affect with muscular spasms; to confine narrowly; to hamper; to secure with a cramp. • *vi* to suffer from cramps.

cramped /kræmpd/ *adj* restricted, narrow; (*handwriting*) small and irregular.

crampon /'kræmpɒn/, **crampoon** /'kræmpu:n/ *n* a metal frame with spikes attached to boots for walking or climbing on ice.

cranberry /'kræn,bɛri/ or /-bəri/ *n* (*pl* **cranberries**) a small red sour berry; the shrub it grows on.

crane /krein/ *n* a large wading bird with very long legs and neck, and a long straight bill; a machine for raising, shifting, and lowering heavy weights. • *vti* to stretch out (the neck).

crane fly *n* the daddy-longlegs.

cranesbill *n* a kind of wild geranium.

craniology /ˌkreini'ɒlədʒi/ *n* the scientific study of skulls and their characteristics.—**craniological** *adj*.—**craniologist** *n*.

craniometer /-'ɒmətər/ *n* an instrument for measuring the skull.

craniometry /-'ɒmətri/ *n* the measurement and study of skulls.—**craniometric, craniometrical** *adj*.

craniotomy /-'ɒtəmi/ *n* (*pl* **craniotomies**) the operation of crushing the head of a dead fetus for facilitating delivery; the operation of opening the skull for neurosurgery.

cranium /'kreiniəm/ *n* (*pl* **craniums, crania**) the skull, *esp* the part enclosing the brain.—**cranial** *adj*.

crank /kræŋk/ *n* a right-angled arm attached to a shaft for turning it; (*inf*) an eccentric person, *usu* one with strange or unorthodox opinions; an irritable or rude person. • *vt* to provide with a crank; to turn or wind; (*with* **up**) (*engine*) to start with a crank handle; (*inf*) to speed up; (*sl*) to inject a narcotic drug.

crankcase /'kræŋkkeis/ *n* the housing for a crankshaft in an internal combustion engine, etc.

crankpin /'kræŋk,pin/ *n* a cylindrical pin parallel with the shaft axis of a crank upon which the connecting rod acts to turn the crank.

crankshaft /'kræŋkʃæft/ *n* a shaft with one or more cranks for transmitting motion.

cranky /'kræŋki/ *adj* (**crankier, crankiest**) (*inf*) eccentric; shaky; cross.—**crankily** *adv*.—**crankiness** *n*.

cranny /'kræni/ *n* (*pl* **crannies**) a fissure, crack, crevice.

crap /kræp/ *n* (*sl*) nonsense; (*vulg*) faeces. • *vi* (**crapping, crapped**) (*vulg*) to defecate.—**crappy** *adj*.

crape /kreip/ *n* crepe; a black gauze-like crimped silk material used for mourning.

craps /kræps/ *n* (*sing or pl*) a gambling game played with two dice.

crapshooter /'kræpʃu:tər/ *n* a player of craps.

crapulence /'kræpju:ləns/ *n* sickness from drinking to excess.—**crapulent, crapulous** *adj*.

craquelure /'krækə,luːr/ n a network of tiny cracks found on old paintings caused by cracking of the varnish.

crash /kræʃ/ n a loud, sudden confused noise; a violent fall or impact; a sudden failure, as of a business or a computer; a collapse, as of the financial market. • adj done with great speed, suddenness or effort. • vti to clash together with violence; to make a loud clattering noise; (aircraft) to land with a crash; to involve a car in a collision with one or more other vehicles or with a hard object; to collapse, to ruin; (inf) to intrude into (a party); (with out) vi (sl) to fall asleep; to pass out; to stay the night somewhere other than home.

crash dive n an emergency dive by a submarine.

crash helmet n a cushioned helmet worn by airmen, motorcyclists, etc for protection.

crash-land /'kræʃ,lænd/ vti (aircraft) to make an emergency landing without lowering the undercarriage, or to be landed in this way.—**crash-landing** n.

crass /kræs/ adj gross; dense; very stupid.—**crassly** adv.—**crassness, crassitude** n.

-crat /kræt/ n suffix a supporter or member of a particular form of government or class.

cratch /krætʃ/ n a rack for fodder.

crate /kreɪt/ n an open box of wooden slats, for shipping (sl) an old vehicle or aircraft. • vt to pack in a crate.

crater /'kreɪtər/ n the mouth of a volcano; a cavity caused by the landing of a meteorite, the explosion of a bomb, shell, etc; an ancient Greek goblet.—**craterous** adj.

cravat /krə'væt/ n a neckcloth.

crave /kreɪv/ vt to have a strong desire (for); to ask humbly, to beg.—**craving** n.

craven /'kreɪvən/ adj spiritless, cowardly. • n a coward.

craw /krɔː/ n a bird's crop.

crawfish /'krɔːfɪʃ/ n (pl crawfish) a crayfish; the spiny lobster.

crawl /krɔːl/ vi to move along the ground on hands and knees; to move slowly and with difficulty; to creep; (inf) to seek favour by servile behaviour; to swarm (with). • n the act of crawling; a slow motion; a racing stroke in swimming.—**crawler** n.

crayfish /'kreɪfɪʃ/ n (pl crayfish) any of numerous freshwater crustaceans; the spiny lobster.

crayon /'kreɪɒn/ or /-ən/ n a stick or pencil of coloured chalk; a drawing done with crayons. • vt to draw with a crayon.—**crayonist** n.

craze /kreɪz/ n a passing infatuation; excessive enthusiasm; a crack in pottery glaze. • vt to produce cracks; to render insane.—**crazed** adj.

crazy /'kreɪzi/ adj (**crazier, craziest**) (inf) mad, insane; foolish; ridiculous; unsound; madly in love with; (paving) composed of irregular pieces.—**crazily** adv.—**craziness** n.

crazy paving n ✤ a form of paving in which stones of different shapes and sizes are pieced together.

creak /kriːk/ vi to make a shrill grating sound. • n such a sound.

creaky /'kriːki/ adj (**creakier, creakiest**) apt to creak.—**creakiness** n.

cream /kriːm/ n the rich, fatty part of milk; the choicest part of anything; a yellowish white colour; a type of face or skin preparation; any preparation of the consistency of cream (eg shoe cream). • vt to add or apply cream to; to beat into a soft, smooth consistency; to skim cream from; to remove the best part of. • vi to form cream or scum; to break into a creamy froth.

cream cheese n soft cheese made from soured milk or cream.

creamer /'kriːmər/ n a machine or dish for separating cream from milk; a jug for cream or milk; a powder used as a substitute for cream in drinks.

creamery /'kriːməri/ n (pl creameries) a place where dairy products are made or sold.

cream of tartar n purified tartar or argol, potassium bitartrate.

creamy adj (**creamier, creamiest**) like cream.—**creaminess** n.

crease /kriːs/ n a line made by folding; a wrinkle; (cricket) a line made by a batsman or bowler marking the limits of their position. • vti to make or form creases; to become creased; (sl) to find something very funny; ✤ a marked area in front of the goal in ice hockey or lacrosse.

create /kri'eɪt/ vt to cause to come into existence to form out of nothing. • vi to make something new, to originate; (sl) to make a fuss.

creatine, creatin /'kriə,tiːn/ n a white crystalline substance in muscular tissue.

creation /kri'eɪʃən/ n the act of creating; the thing created; the whole world or universe; a production of the human mind; (with cap) the universe as created by God.—**creational** adj.

creationism /-,nizəm/ n the belief in special creation, not evolution; the belief that God creates a soul for every human being at birth.—**creationist** adj, n.

creative /kri'eɪtɪv/ adj of creation; having the power to create; imaginative, original, constructive.—**creatively** adv.—**creativeness** n.—**creativity** n.

creator /kri'eɪtər/ n one who creates, esp God.

creature /'kriːtʃər/ n a living being; a created thing; one dependent on the influence of another.—**creatural, creaturely** adj.

crèche /kreʃ/ or /kreɪʃ/ n a day nursery for very young children.

credence /'kriːdəns/ n belief or trust, esp in the reports or testimony of another.

credentials /krə'denʃəls/ npl documents proving the identity, honesty or authority of a person.

credibility gap n a gap between what is claimed in official statements and the true facts of a situation.

credible /'kredibəl/ adj believable; trustworthy.—**credibility, credibleness** n.—**credibly** adv.

credit /'kredɪt/ n belief; trust; honour; good reputation; approval; trust in a person's ability to pay; time allowed for payment; a sum at a person's disposal in a bank; the entry in an account of a sum received; the size of the account on which this is entered; (educ) a distinction awarded for good marks in an examination; (pl) a list of those responsible for a film, television programme, etc. • vt to believe; to trust; to have confidence in; to attribute to; to enter on the credit side of an account.

creditable /'kredɪtəbəl/ adj worthy of praise.—**creditableness, creditability** n.—**creditably** adv.

credit card n a card issued by a bank, department store, etc authorizing the purchase of goods and services on credit.

creditor /'kredɪtər/ n a person to whom money is owed.

credit rating n an appraisal of a person's or a business's creditworthiness.

credits npl a list of those involved in the production of a film or television show.

creditworthy /'kredɪt,wɜːði/ adj worthy of being given credit as judged by the capacity to earn, repay debts promptly, etc.—**creditworthiness** n.

credo /'kriːdoʊ/ or /'kreɪ-/ n (pl credos) a creed.

credulous /'kredjʊləs/ adj over-ready to believe; easily imposed on.—**credulously** adv.—**credulity** n.

Cree /kriː/ n ✤ a member of a First Nations people living in Canada east of the Rocky Mountains; the Algonquian language of this people. • adj of or pertaining to this people or their language.

creed /kriːd/ n a system of religious belief or faith; a summary of Christian doctrine; any set of principles or beliefs.—**creedal, credal** adj.

creek /kriːk/ n a natural stream of water smaller than a river.

creel /kriːl/ n a wicker fishing basket; a wickerwork cage.

creep /kriːp/ vi (**creeping, crept**) to move slowly along the ground, as a worm or reptile; (plant) to grow along the ground or up a wall; to move stealthily or slowly; to fawn; to cringe; (flesh) to feel as if things were creeping over it. • n (inf) a dislikable or servile person; (pl: inf) shrinking horror.

creeper /'kriːpər/ n a creeping or climbing plant.

creepy /'kriːpi/ adj (**creepier, creepiest**) making one's flesh crawl; causing fear or disgust.—**creepily** adv.—**creepiness** n.

creepy-crawly /'kriːpi,krɔːli/ n (pl creepy-crawlies) (inf) a small crawling insect.

cremate /'kriːmeɪt/ or /krɪ'meɪt/, /krə-/ vt to burn (a corpse) to ashes.—**cremation** n.—**cremationism** n.—**cremationist** n.

crematorium /'kriːmə,tɔːriəm/ n (pl crematoriums, crematoria) a place where bodies are cremated.

crematory /'kriːmə,tɔːri/ adj pertaining to cremation. • n (pl crematories) a place for burning the dead, a crematorium.

crème, creme /kriːm/, Fr. /krɛm/ n cream.

crème de la crème /,kreɪm dəlɑ'krɛm/ n the cream of the cream, the very best.

crème de menthe /,krɛmdə'mɒnθ/ or /-'mɛnθ/, /-'mɪnt/ n a green-coloured peppermint liqueur.

crenate /'kriːneɪt/, **crenated** adj (leaves) scalloped.—**crenation, crenature** n.

crenellated, crenelated /'krenə,leɪtɪd/ adj having battlements.—**crenellation, crenelation** n.

crenulate, crenulated /'krɛnju:ˌleɪt/ *adj* (*leaves*) finely notched, indented.—**crenulation** *n*.

Creole /'kri:o:l/ *n* a descendant of European settlers in the West Indies or South America; a white descendant of French settlers in the southern US; a person of mixed European and Negro ancestry; the language of any of these groups.

creole /'kri:o:l/ *n* a language combining two or more original languages, one of which is European.

creosol /'kri:ə,so:l/ *n* an oily liquid resembling phenol, a constituent of creosote.

creosote /'kri:ə,so:t/ *n* an oily substance derived from tar used as a wood preservative. • *vt* to treat with creosote.—**creosotic** *adj*.

crepe /kreɪp/, **crêpe** /krɛp/ *n* a thin, crinkled cloth of silk, rayon, wool, etc.—*also* **crape** ; thin paper like crepe; a thin pancake.

crepe de Chine /ˌkreɪpdə'ʃiːn/ *n* a silk crepe.

crepe paper, crêpe paper *n* a thin soft coloured paper that resembles crepe.

crepe rubber *n* a type of ribbed rubber used for the soles of shoes.

crêpe suzette /ˌkreɪsuː'zɛt/, *Fr.* /krɛɪp'syzɛt/ *n* (*pl* **crêpes suzettes**) a thin orange-flavoured pancake with a hot liqueur sauce.

crepitate /'krɛpɪˌteɪt/ *vi* to make a slight, sharp crackling noise.—**crepitation** *n*.

crept /krɛpt/ *see* **creep**.

crepuscular /krə'pʌskjuːlər/ *adj* pertaining to or resembling twilight; active at twilight, as certain animals.

crescendo /krə'ʃɛndo:/ *adv* (*mus*) gradually increasing in loudness or intensity; moving to a climax. • *n* (*pl* **crescendos, crescendi**) a crescendo passage or effect.

crescent /'krɛsənt/ *n* the figure of the moon in its first or last quarter; a narrow, tapering curve; a curving street. • *adj* crescent-shaped; (*arch*) increasing.—**crescentic** *adj*.

cresol /'kri:ˌsɒl/ *n* a phenol obtained from coal and wood tar.

cress /krɛs/ *n* any of various plants with pungent leaves, used in salads.

cresset /'krɛsɪt/ *n* a light set on a beacon; an open frame of iron containing fire, used as a torch.

crest /krɛst/ *n* a plume of feathers on the head of a bird; the ridge of a wave; the summit of a hill; a distinctive device above the shield on a coat of arms. • *vti* to mount to the top of; to take the form of a crest; to provide or adorn with a crest, to crown.—**crested** *adj*.

crestfallen /'krɛstˌfɔlən/ *adj* dejected.

cresting /'krɛstɪŋ/ *n* an ornamental finish, *esp* along a rooftop; ornamentation on top of furniture, a mirror, etc.

Cretaceous /krɪ'teɪʃəs/ *n* a geological group between the Jurassic and Tertiary formations. • *adj* of the last Mesozoic era.

cretaceous /krɪ'teɪʃəs/ *adj* composed of or like chalk; chalky.

Cretan /'kri:tən/ *adj* of or pertaining to Crete or its inhabitants.

cretin /'krɛtɪn/ *n* a person suffering from mental and physical retardation due to a thyroid disorder; (*inf*) an idiot.—**cretinism** *n*.—**cretinoid, cretinous** *adj*.

cretonne /kri:'tɒn/ *n* an unglazed cotton fabric printed with coloured patterns on one side.

cretons /kri:tɒns/ *npl* ♣ (*Cdn*) in Quebec, a spread of shredded pork and onions cooked in pork fat and served cold.

crevasse /krə'væs/ *n* a deep cleft in a glacier; a deep crack.

crevice /'krɛvɪs/ *n* a crack, a fissure.

crew /kru:/ *n* the people operating a ship or aircraft; a group of people working together. • *vi* to act as a member of the crew of a ship, etc.

crewcut *n* a very short hairstyle for men.

crewel /'kru:əl/ *n* a fine twisted or worsted yarn used in embroidery.—**crewelist** *n*.

crew neck *n* a plain closely-fitting neckline in sweaters.

crib /krɪb/ *n* a rack for fodder, a manger; a child's cot with high sides; a model of the manger scene representing the birth of Jesus; (*inf*) something copied from someone else; (*inf*) a literal translation of foreign texts used (*usu* illicitly) by students in examinations, etc. • *vti* (**cribbing, cribbed**) (*inf*) to copy illegally, plagiarize.

cribbage /'krɪbˌɪdʒ/ *n* a card game for two to four players.

crib death *see* **cot death**.

cribellum /krɪ'bɛləm/ *n* (*pl* **cribella**) a spinning organ in front of the spinnerets of certain spiders.

cribriform /'krɪbrɪˌfɔrm/ *adj* with small holes like a sieve.

crick /krɪk/ *n* a painful stiffness of the muscles of the neck. • *vt* to produce a crick in.

cricket[1] /'krɪkɪt/ *n* a leaping grasshopper-like insect.

cricket[2] *n* a game played with wickets, bats, and a ball, by eleven players on each side.—**cricketer** *n*.

cried /kraɪd/ *see* **cry**.

crier /'kraɪər/ *n* one who cries; an officer who makes public proclamations.

crime /kraɪm/ *n* a violation of the law; an offence against morality or the public welfare; wrong-doing; (*inf*) a shame, disappointment.

criminal /'krɪmɪnəl/ *adj* of the nature of, or guilty of, a crime. • *n* a person who has committed a crime.—**criminality** *adv*.—**criminally** *adv*.

Criminal Code *n* ♣ a Canadian federal statute containing most laws concerning crimes and the legal procedures dealing with them.

criminal conversation *n* (*formerly*) a legal action for damages for illegal sexual intercourse; adultery.

criminology /ˌkrɪmə'nɒlədzi/ *n* the scientific study of crime.—**criminological, criminologic** *adj*.—**criminologist** *n*.

crimp[1] /krɪmp/ *vt* to press into small folds; to frill; to corrugate; (*hair*) to curl.—**crimper** *n*.

crimp[2] *n* a person luring or pressganging sailors aboard a vessel. • *vt* to decoy thus.

crimson /'krɪmzən/ *n* a deep-red colour inclining to purple. • *adj* crimson-coloured. • *vti* to dye with crimson; to blush.

cringe /krɪndʒ/ *vi* to shrink in fear or embarrassment; to cower; to behave with servility; to fawn.

cringle /'krɪŋgəl/ *n* a loop of rope containing a metal ring for another rope to pass through.

crinite /'kraɪˌnəɪt/ *adj* hairy.

crinkle /'krɪŋkəl/ *vt* to wrinkle; to corrugate; to crimp; to rustle. • *vi* to curl; to be corrugated or crimped. • *n* a wrinkle.—**crinkly** *adj*.

crinoid /'krɪˌnɔɪd/ *adj* lily-shaped. • *n* a stone lily, a kind of sea urchin.

crinoline /'krɪnəˌlɪn/ *n* a hooped skirt made to project all round; a stiff fabric for stiffening a garment.

crinum /'krɪnəm/ *n* any of several handsome tropical plants.

cripple /'krɪpəl/ *vt* to deprive of the use of a limb; to disable. • *n* a lame or otherwise disabled person. • *adj* lame.

crippling /'krɪplɪŋ/ *adj* harmful; unbearable.

crisis /'kraɪsɪs/ *n* (*pl* **crises**) a turning point; a critical point in a disease; an emergency; a time of serious difficulties or danger.

crisp /krɪsp/ *adj* dry and brittle; bracing; brisk; sharp and incisive; decided; very clean and tidy. • *n* a potato snack; in US, a potato chip. • *vt* to make crisp.—**crisply** *adv*.—**crispness** *n*.

crispate /'krɪspeɪt/, **crispated** *adj* curled; (*bot*) with a wavy margin.—**crispation** *n*.

crispy /'krɪspi/ *adj* (**crispier, crispiest**) crisp.—**crispily** *adv*.—**crispiness** *n*.

crisscross /'krɪsˌkrɒs/ *vti* to intersect; to mark with cross lines. • *n* an intersecting; a mark of a cross; a game of noughts and crosses. • *adj* crossing; in cross lines. • *adv* crosswise.

cristate /'krɪsteɪt/, **cristated** /-ɪd/ *adj* crested; tufted.

criterion /kraɪ'tɪrɪən/ *n* (*pl* **criteria**) a standard, law or rule by which a correct judgment can be made.

critic /'krɪtɪk/ *n* a person skilled in judging the merits of literary or artistic works; one who passes judgment; a fault-finder; ♣ (*Cdn*) a member of an opposition party in a legislature who is responsible for review and criticism of a specific government ministry.

critical /'krɪtɪkəl/ *adj* skilled in criticism; censorious; relating to the turning point of a disease; crucial.—**critically** *adv*.

criticism /'krɪtɪsɪzəm/ *n* being critical; an adverse comment; a review or analysis of a book, play, work of art, etc by a critic.

criticize /'krɪtɪˌsaɪz/ *vt* to pass judgment on; to find fault with; to examine critically.—**criticizer** *n*.

critique /ˌkrɪ'ti:k/ *n* a critical article or review.

critter /'krɪtər/ *n* (*dial*) a creature.

croak /kro:k/ *n* a deep hoarse discordant cry. • *vti* to utter a croak; (*inf*) to die, to kill.—**croakily** *adv*.—**croakiness** *n*.—**croaky** *adj*.

Croatian, Croat /kro:æt/ *adj* of or pertaining to Croatia, its people or language. • *n* an inhabitant of Croatia; the language of Croatia, a dialect of Serbo-Croatian.

crochet /kro:'ʃeɪ/ or /'kro:-/ *n* a kind of knitting done with a hooked needle. • *vti* (**crocheting, crocheted**) to do this; to make crochet articles.—**crocheter** *n*.

crocidolite /ˌkro'sɪdəˌlaɪt/ n blue asbestos.

crock[1] /krɒk/ n an earthenware pot.

crock[2] n a broken-down horse; (sl) a worn-out or unfit person. • vti to become or make unfit.

crock[3] n soot on a kettle, etc. • vt to blacken with soot.

crockery /'krɒkəri/ n china dishes, earthenware vessels, etc.

crocket /'krɒkət/ n a small curved ornament on the angles of spires, canopies, etc.

crocodile /'krɒkəˌdaɪl/ n a large amphibious reptile, similar to an alligator; its skin, used to make handbags, shoes, etc; a line of schoolchildren walking in pairs.

crocodile tears npl insincere grief.

crocodilian /ˌkrɒkə'dɪliən/ adj pertaining to crocodiles. • n any of the order of reptiles that includes alligators and crocodiles.

crocus /'krɒkəs/ n (pl **crocuses**) a bulbous plant with yellow, purple, or white flowers.

croft /krɒft/ n a small plot of land with a rented farmhouse, esp in Scotland.—**crofter** n.

croissant /krə'sõ/, Fr. /kʀwa'sõ/ n a rich bread roll.

crokinole /'krɒkəˌnoːl/ n ✽ (Cdn) a game in which wooden discs are flicked toward a central hole in a circular board.

Cro-Magnon man /kroːˈmægnən/ or /-ˈmægnən/ n a race of man living in late Palaeolithic times.

cromlech /'krɒmˌlek/ n a prehistoric monument of rough stones in a circle and usu surrounding a lofty pillar of stone.

crone /kroːn/ n a withered old woman.

crony /'kroːni/ n (pl **cronies**) an intimate friend.

crook /kruk/ n a shepherd's hooked staff; a bend, a curve; a swindler, a dishonest person. • adj (sl) unwell. • vti to bend or to be bent into the shape of a hook.

crooked /'krukəd/ adj bent, twisted; dishonest.—**crookedly** adv.—**crookedness** n.

croon /kruːn/ vi to hum in a low gentle voice. • vt to sing songs in a soft gentle manner.—**crooner** n.

crop /krɒp/ n a year's or a season's produce of any cultivated plant; harvest; any collection of things appearing at the same time; a pouch in a bird's gullet; a hunting whip; hair cut close or short. • vti (**cropping, cropped**) to clip short; to bite off or eat down (grass); (land) to yield; to sow, to plant; (geol) to come to the surface; to sprout; (with up) (inf) to occur or appear by chance or unexpectedly.

crop circle n a circular patch of corn in a cornfield that has been flattened by an as yet unexplained whirling movement.

crop-eared /-ˌɪrd/ adj with clipped ears; short-haired.

cropper /-ər/ n a thing that crops; a cloth-facing machine; a pouter pigeon; (sl) a heavy fall.

croquet /kro'keɪ/ or /'krɒkeɪ/ n a game played with mallets, balls and hoops. • vt (**croqueting, croqueted**) to drive away an opponent's ball by striking one's own placed in contact with it.

croquette /kro'ket/ n a ball of minced meat, fish or potato seasoned and fried brown.

crosier /'kroːʒər/ or /-ziər/ n the pastoral staff of a bishop.—also **crozier**.

cross /krɒs/ n a figure formed by two intersecting lines; a wooden structure, consisting of two beams placed across each other, used in ancient times for crucifixion; the emblem of the Christian faith; a symbol or mark (X); a focal point in a town; a burden, or affliction; a device resembling a cross; a cross-shaped medal; a hybrid. • vti to pass across; to intersect; to meet and pass; to place crosswise; to mark with a cross; to make the sign of the cross over; to thwart, to oppose; to modify (a breed) by intermixture (with). • adj transverse; reaching from side to side; intersecting; out of temper, peevish.—**crosser** n.—**crossly** adv.—**crossness** n.

crossbar /-bar/ n a horizontal bar, as that across goal posts or a bicycle frame.

crossbill /-bɪl/ n a bird whose mandibles cross when the bill is closed.

crossbow /-boː/ n a bow set crosswise on the stock from which bolts are shot along a groove.

crossbreed /-briːd/ vt (**crossbreeding, crossbred**) to breed animals by mating different varieties. • n an animal produced in this way.

crosscheck /-tʃek/ vt to verify by checking different opinions or sources.

cross-country /krɒs'kʌntri/ adj across fields; denoting cross-country racing or skiing.—also n

crosscurrent /'krɒsˌkʌrənt/ n a current that flows across another in water or air; ideas running counter to those generally held.

crosse /krɒs/ n a long-handled racket in which the ball is caught and carried in lacrosse.

cross-examine /ˌkrɒsɪg'zæmɪn/ vt to question closely; (law) to question (a witness) who has already been questioned by counsel on the other side.—**cross-examiner** n.—**cross-examination** n.

cross-eyed /'krɒsˌaɪd/ adj squinting.—**cross-eye** n.

cross-fertilization /krɒsˌfɜːtɪlaɪˈzeɪʃən/ n fertilization of the ovules of a flower by the pollen of another.

cross-fertilize /krɒs'fɜːtɪˌlaɪz/ vt to fertilize (a plant) with pollen from another.

crossfire /'krɒsˌfaɪr/ n converging gunfire from two or more positions; animated debate or argument.

cross-grained /greɪnd/ adj contrary or awkward; with an irregular grain or fibre.

crosshatch /-hætʃ/ vt to shade with crossed lines.

crossing /-ɪŋ/ n an intersection of roads or railway lines; a place for crossing a street; the crossbreeding of animals and plants.

cross-legged /-legɪd/ or /-legd/ adj seated with one leg crossed over the other.

crosspatch /-pætʃ/ n (inf) a bad-tempered person.

crosspiece /-piːs/ n a transverse piece.

cross-platform adj (comput) applies to the use of software and files on computer with a different hardware system.

cross-purpose /-pɜːpəs/ n a contrary purpose; **be at cross-purposes** to talk without either party realizing that the other is talking about a different thing.

cross-question /krɒs'kwestʃən/ vt to question to elicit details or test the accuracy of an account already given.—**cross-questioning** n.

cross-refer /ˌkrɒsri'fɜr/ vt to mark (text, a book, etc) in such a way as to direct the reader to another page, etc with more information.

cross-reference /'krɒsˌrefərəns/ n a note directing the reader to a different section of a book or document.

crossroad /-roːd/ n a road crossing another; (pl) where two roads cross; (fig) the time when a decisive action has to be made.

cross section /-ˌsekʃən/ n a cutting at right angles to length; the surface then shown; a random selection of the public.—**cross-sectional** adj.

cross-stitch /-stɪtʃ/ n a stitch formed of two stitches of the same length, one crossing the other.

crosstalk /-stɒk/ n interference in lines of communication, esp telephone lines; a quick-witted flow of conversation; repartee.

crosstie /-taɪ/ n a railway sleeper.

crosstree /-triː/ n (naut) one of several pieces of timber across the head of a lower mast to support the mast above.

crosswalk /-wɒk/ n a street crossing for pedestrians.

crosswind /-wɪnd/ n a side or unfavourable wind.

crosswise /-waɪz/, **crossways** /-weɪz/ adv in the manner of a cross.

crossword (puzzle) /-wɜːd/ n a puzzle in which interlocking words be inserted vertically and horizontally in a squared diagram are indicated by clues.

crotch /krɒtʃ/ n the region of the body where the legs fork, the genital area; any forked region.

crotchet /'krɒtʃət/ n (mus) a note equal to the duration of a half-minim.—also **quarter note**.

crotchety /'krɒtʃəti/ adj peevish, ill-tempered.—**crotchetiness** n.

crouch /kreutʃ/ vi to squat or lie close to the ground; to cringe, to fawn.

croup[1] /kruːp/ n inflammation of the windpipe causing coughing and breathing problems, esp in children.—**croupous, croupy** adj

croup[2], **croupe** n the rump or buttocks of certain animals; the place behind the saddle of a horse.

croupier /'kruːpiər/ or /-piˌeɪ/ n a person who presides at a gaming table and collects or pays out the money won or lost.

crouton /'kruːˌtɒn/ n a small piece of fried or toasted bread sprinkled onto soups.

crow /kroː/ n any of various usu large, glossy, black birds; a cawing cry; the shrill sound of a cock. • vi (**crowing, crowed** or **crew**) to make a sound like a cock; to boast in triumph; to utter a cry of pleasure.—**crower** n.

crowbar /-bar/ n an iron bar for use as a lever.

crowberry /'kro:bɛri/ *n* an evergreen shrub with black berries; the edible berry of this shrub.

crowd /kraʊd/ *n* a number of people or things collected closely together; a dense multitude, a throng; (*inf*) a set; a clique. • *vti* to press closely together; to fill to excess; to push, to thrust; to importune.—**crowded** *adj*.

crowfoot /'kro:fʊt/ *n* (*pl* **crowfoots**) any of several kinds of buttercup with yellow or white flowers and leaves like a crow's foot.

crown /kraʊn/ *n* a wreath worn on the head; the head covering of a monarch; regal power; the sovereign; the top of the head; the top of a tree; a summit; a reward; the part of a tooth above the gum. • *vt* to invest with a crown; to adorn or dignify; to complete; to reward; to put an artificial crown on a tooth; (*sl*) to strike on the head; ✲ (*cap*) the sovereign, considered as the head of state.

Crown attorney *n* ✲ (*Cdn*) a lawyer who prosecutes crimes on behalf of the Crown. —*also* **Crown counsel, Crown prosecutor**.

crown colony *n* a British colony subject to the control of the home government.

Crown corporation *n* ✲ (*Cdn*) a corporation owned by a federal or provincial government.

Crown counsel *n* ✲ Crown attorney.

crown glass *n* a fine, thick kind of glass.

crown land *n* ✲ in the UK and Canada, land or real property belonging to the sovereign.

crown prince *n* the heir apparent to a throne.

crown princess *n* the heiress apparent to a throne; the wife of a crown prince.

Crown prosecutor *n* ✲ Crown attorney.

crown saw *n* a kind of circular saw.

crownwork *n* the covering or replacement of the crown of a tooth; the making of crowns; a fortified outwork.

crow's-foot /'kro:z,fʊt/ *n* (*pl* **crow's-feet**) a wrinkle at the corner of the eye; an arrangement of cords to suspend an awning; a decorative embroidery stitch.

crow's-nest /-,nɛst/ *n* a lookout or watchtower on the main topmast of a sailing vessel.

crozier *see* **crosier**.

CRT /ˌsiːˌɑrˈtiː/ *abbr* = cathode-ray tube.

CRTC *abbr* ✲ = Canadian Radio-television and Telecommunications Commission.

cruces /'kruːsiːz/ *see* **crux**.

crucial /'kruːʃəl/ *adj* decisive; severe; critical.—**crucially** *adv*.

cruciate /'kruːʃət/ *adj* (*bot*) cross-shaped.

crucible /'kruːsəbəl/ *n* a heat-resistant container for melting ores, etc.

crucifer /'kruːsəfər/ *n* any of many plants with four petals arranged like a cross, as the mustard, etc; the bearer of a large cross in a religious procession.

crucifier /'kruːsəfaɪr/ *n* one who crucifies.

crucifix /'kruːsəfɪks/ *n* a cross with the sculptured figure of Christ.

crucifixion /ˌkruːsəˈfɪkʃən/ *n* a form of execution by being nailed or bound to a cross by the hands and feet; (*with cap*) the death of Christ in this manner.

cruciform /'kruːsəˌfɔrm/ *adj* cross-shaped.

crucify /'kruːsəˌfaɪ/ *vt* (**crucifying, crucified**) to put to death on a cross; to cause extreme pain to; to defeat utterly in an argument; to ridicule mercilessly.

crud /krʌd/ *n* (*sl*) a deposit of encrusted filth; nuclear waste; a contemptible person.

crude /kruːd/ *adj* in a natural state; unripe; raw; immature; harsh in colour; unfinished, rough; lacking polish; blunt; vulgar. • *n* crude oil.—**crudely** *adv*.—**crudeness** *n*.

crude oil *n* unrefined petroleum.

crudités /ˌkruːdɪˈteɪ/ or /-diː-/, *Fr.* /kʀydiˈteɪ/ *npl* coarsely chopped raw vegetables eaten with a dip.

crudity /'kruːdɪti/ *n* (*pl* **crudities**) crudeness; a crude act or expression.

cruel /'kruːəl/ *adj* (**crueller, cruellest**) disposed to give pain to others; merciless; hard-hearted; fierce; painful; unrelenting.—**cruelly** *adv*.—**cruelty** *n*.

cruelty /-ti/ *n* (*pl* **cruelties**) inhumanity; savageness; a cruel act.

cruet /'kruːət/ *n* a small glass bottle for vinegar and oil, used at the table; a set of containers holding salt, pepper, vinegar.

cruise /kruːz/ *vi* to sail to and fro; to wander about; to move at the most efficient speed for sustained travel. • *vt* to cruise over or about. • *n* a voyage from place to place for military purposes or in a liner for pleasure.

cruise missile *n* a subsonic low-flying guided missile.

cruiser /-ər/ *n* fast warship smaller than a battleship; a pleasure yacht or motorboat.

crumb /krʌm/ *n* a fragment of bread; the soft part of bread; a little piece of anything; (*sl*) a despicable person. • *vi* to cover food with breadcrumbs before cooking.

crumble /'krʌmbəl/ *vt* to break into crumbs; to cause to fall into pieces. • *vi* to disappear gradually, to disintegrate.—**crumbly** *adj*.

crumby /'krʌmi/ *adj* (**crumbier, crumbiest**) in crumbs; soft.—**crumbiness** *n*.

crummy /'krʌmi/ *adj* (**crummier, crummiest**) (*sl*) dirty, squalid, worthless; slightly ill.—**crumminess** *n*.

crump /krʌmp/ *n* a bursting shell; the crunching or exploding sound of this. • *vi* to explode. • *vt* to shell; to hit (a ball) hard.

crumpet /'krʌmpɪt/ *n* a soft cake with holes on one side, often eaten toasted; (*sl*) a sexually attractive woman.

crumple /'krʌmpəl/ *vti* to twist or crush into wrinkles; to crease; to collapse. • *n* a wrinkle or crease made by crumpling.—**crumply** *adj*.

crunch /krʌntʃ/ *vti* to crush with the teeth; to tread underfoot with force and noise; to make a sound like this; to chew audibly. • *n* the sound or act of crunching; (*with* **the**) (*inf*) the crucial moment, the time of vital decision.

crunchy /'krʌntʃi/ *adj* (**crunchier, crunchiest**) crisp; able to be crunched.—**crunchily** *adv*.—**crunchiness** *n*.

crupper /'krʌpər/ *n* a looped leather band attached to the back of a saddle and passing under the horse's tail; the hindquarters of a horse.

crural /'krʊrəl/ *adj* of the leg or thigh; leg-shaped.

crus /krʌs/ or /kruːs/ *n* (*pl* **crura**) the leg proper; a part resembling a leg.

crusade /kruːˈseɪd/ *n* a medieval Christian military expedition to recover the Holy Land; a vigorous concerted action for the defence of a cause or the advancement of an idea. • *vi* to engage in a crusade.—**crusader** *n*.

cruse /kruːz/ *n* a small earthenware pot or dish for holding liquids.

crush /krʌʃ/ *vt* to press between two opposite bodies; to squeeze; to break by pressure; to bruise; to ruin; to quell, to defeat; to mortify. • *vi* to be pressed out of shape or into a smaller compass. • *n* a violent compression or collision; a dense crowd; (*inf*) a large party; a drink made from crushed fruit; (*sl*) an infatuation.—**crushable** *adj*.—**crusher** *n*.

crust /krʌst/ *n* any hard external coating or rind; the exterior solid part of the earth's surface; a shell or hard covering; (*sl*) a means of livelihood. • *vti* to cover or become covered with a crust.—**crusty** *adj* (**crustier, crustiest**).—**crustily** *adv*.—**crustiness** *n*.

crustacean /krʌsˈteɪʃən/ *n* any aquatic animal with a hard shell, including crabs, lobsters, shrimps, and barnacles.—*also adj*.—**crustaceous** *adj*.

crutch /krʌtʃ/ *n* a staff with a crosswise head to support the weight of a lame person; something that supports; a prop; the crotch.

crux /krʌks/ *n* (*pl* **cruxes, cruces**) a difficult problem; the essential or deciding point.

cry /kraɪ/ *vb* (**crying, cried**) *vi* to call aloud; to proclaim; to exclaim vehemently; to implore; to shed tears; (*with* **off**) (*inf*) to cancel (an agreement, arrangement, etc), to renege; (*with* **out**) to shout due to fear or pain. • *vt* to utter loudly and publicly; (*with* **out for**) to be in dire need of. • *n* (*pl* **cries**) an inarticulate sound; an exclamation of wonder or triumph; an outcry; clamour; an urgent appeal; a spell of weeping; a battle cry; a catchword; the particular sound made by an animal or bird.

crybaby /-,beɪbi/ *n* (*pl* **crybabies**) a child who weeps easily; a person who cries or complains often.

cryo- /kraɪo:/ or /-ə/ *prefix* frost; freezing.

cryoextraction /ˌkraɪo:kˈstrækʃən/ *n* the extraction of juice from grapes that have been frozen before pressing to obtain a higher level of sugar and fruitier taste.

cryogen /'kraɪo:dʒən/ *n* a substance for producing freezing temperatures.

cryogenics /ˌkraɪo:ˈdʒɛnɪks/ *n sing* the science of very low temperatures and their effects.

cryolite /'kraɪo:ˌlaɪt/ *n* a mineral from which aluminium is produced.

cryometer /kraɪˈɒmətər/ *n* an instrument for measuring very low temperatures.—**cryometry** *n*.

cryonic suspension /kraɪˈɒnɪk/ *n* the process of freezing a corpse in the hope that it may be restored to life in the future.

cryonics /kraɪˈɒnɪks/ *n* (*sing*) the use of extreme cold to preserve living tissue (eg organs) for future use.

cryosurgery /ˌkraɪoˈsɜrdʒəri/ *n* surgery involving freezing to destroy or remove diseased tissue.

crypt /krɪpt/ *n* an underground chamber or vault, *esp* under a church, used as a chapel or for burial.

crypt- /krɪpt/, **crypto-** /ˈkrɪpto/ *prefix* hidden.

cryptaesthesia, cryptesthesia /ˌkrɪptəsˈθiːsiə/ *n* clairvoyance; extrasensory perception.

cryptic /ˈkrɪptɪk/, **cryptical** /-əl/ *adj* hidden, secret; mysterious.

cryptogam /ˈkrɪptəˌgæm/ *n* a plant without stamens or pistil, a non-flowering plant, as mosses, ferns, etc.—**cryptogamic, cryptogamous** *adj*.

cryptogram /-ˌgræm/ *n* a coded message, cipher.

cryptograph /-ˌgræf/ *n* a piece of writing in cipher.

cryptography /krɪpˈtɒgrəfi/ *n* the art of code writing and breaking.—**cryptographer** *n*.—**cryptographic** *adj*.

cryptozoology /ˌkrɪptəzuˈɒlədʒi/ *n* the study of creatures whose existence has yet to be proved, eg the yeti, the Loch Ness monster.

crystal /ˈkrɪstəl/ *n* a solid piece, eg of quartz, geometrically shaped owing to regular arrangement of its atoms; very clear, brilliant glass; articles of such glass, as goblets; (*sl*) the drug methamphetamine packaged and sold as a stimulant in powdered form.—*also* **crystal meth**. • *adj* made of crystal.—**crystalline** *adj*.

crystal gazing *n* fortune telling by peering into a ball of crystal.

crystalline /ˈkrɪstəˌlaɪn/ or /-ˌiːn/ *adj* pertaining to or having the form of a crystal; clear; transparent.—**crystallinity** *n*.

crystalline lens *n* a transparent biconvex solid body enclosed in a capsule between the vitreous and acqueous humours of the eye.

crystallize /ˈkrɪstəˌlaɪz/ *vti* to form crystals; to give definite form; to express clearly the theme and content of an argument, proposition, etc.—**crystallization** *n*.

crystallography /ˌkrɪstəˈlɒgrəfi/ *n* the science of the forms and structure of crystals.—**crystallographer** *n*.—**crystallographic** *adj*.

crystalloid /ˈkrɪstəˌlɔɪd/ *adj* resembling a crystal; of a crystalline structure, opposite to colloid. • *n* a crystalloid substance; one of certain bodies that in solution diffuse readily through animal membranes.

Cs (*chem symbol*) = caesium.

c/s *abbr* = cycles per second.

CSB *abbr* ✳ = Canada Savings Bond.

CSC *abbr* ✳ = Correctional Services of Canada.

CS gas *n* an irritant gas used in quelling riots and disturbances.

CST *abbr* = Central Standard Time.

Cst. *abbr* ✳ (*Cdn*) = Constable.

CT *abbr* = Connecticut.

ct *abbr* = carat; cent; court.

CTC *abbr* ✳ = Canadian Transport Commission.

ctenidium /təˈniːdiəm/ *n pl* **ctenidia**) one of the respiratory organs of molluscs.

ctenoid /ˈtiːnɔɪd/ *adj* having a comb-like margin.

CTV *abbr* ✳ = Canadian Television Network.

Cu (*chem symbol*) = copper.

cu. *abbr* = cubic.

cub /kʌb/ *n* a young carnivorous mammal; a young, inexperienced person; (*with cap*) a Cub Scout. • *vi* (**cubbing, cubbed**) to bring forth cubs.

cubage /ˈkjuːˌbædʒ/, **cubature** /-ˌbætʃər/ *n* the act of determining the contents of a solid; the contents so measured.

cubbyhole /ˈkʌbiˌhoʊl/ *n* a small or snug place; a pigeonhole.

cube /kjuːb/ *n* a solid body with six equal square sides or faces; a cube-shaped block; the product of a number multiplied by itself twice. • *vt* to raise (number) to the third power, or cube; to cut into cube-shaped pieces.

cubeb /ˈkjuːbɛb/ *n* a species of pepper of Asia; its small spicy berry dried and used as a stimulant.

cube root *n* the number that gives the stated number when cubed.

cube van *n* ✳ (*Cdn*) a truck with a cube-like storage compartment at the rear.

cubic /ˈkjuːbɪk/ *adj* having the form or properties of a cube; three-dimensional.

cubical /-əl/ *adj* of or pertaining to volume; cube-shaped.

cubicle /-əl/ *n* a small separate sleeping compartment in a dormitory, etc.

cubiculum /kjuːˈbɪkjuːləm/ *n* (*pl* **cubicula**) a burial chamber in a catacomb.

cubism /ˈkjuːˌbɪzəm/ *n* a style of painting in which objects are depicted as fragmented and reorganized geometrical forms.—**cubist** *n*.—**cubistic** *adj*.—**cubistically** *adv*.

cubit /ˈkjuːbɪt/ *n* an ancient measure of about 18 inches; the forearm from the elbow to the wrist.

cubital /-əl/ *adj* of the forearm.

cuboid /ˈkjuːbɔɪd/ *adj* like a cube. • *n* a regular solid contained by parallelograms.

Cub Scout *n* a junior branch of the Scout Association.

cuckold /ˈkʌkoʊld/ *n* a man whose wife has committed adultery.—**cuckoldry** *n*.

cuckoo /ˈkuːkuː/ or /ˈkʊkuː/ *n* a bird with a dark plumage, a curved bill and a characteristic call that lays its eggs in the nests of other birds. • *adj* (*inf*) crazy, silly.

cuckoo clock *n* a clock that strikes the hours with a cuckoo call.

cuckoopint /-ˌpɪnt/ *n* a European plant with large leaves, purple flowers and bearing red berries.

cuckoo spit *n* a white froth exuded by froghopper larvae on the leaves of plants.

cucullate /kjuːˈkɛlˌeɪt/ or /-ˌ-/, /ˈkjuːkəˌleɪt/, /-lɪt/, **cucullated** /-təd/ *adj* hooded; hood-shaped

cucumber /ˈkjuːˌkʌmbər/ *n* a long juicy fruit used in salads and as a pickle; the creeping plant that bears it.

cucurbit /kjuːˈkɜrbɪt/ *n* any of an order of succulent, climbing, tendril-bearing plants with a fleshy fruit, including cucumbers, pumpkins, melons, etc.

cud /kʌd/ *n* the food that a ruminating animal brings back into the mouth to chew again; **chew the cud** to consider and mull over.

cudbear /ˈkʌdˌbɛr/ *n* a purple dye made from lichens.

cuddle /ˈkʌdəl/ *vt* to embrace or hug closely. • *vt* to nestle together. • *n* a close embrace.

cuddlesome /-səm/ *adj* tempting to cuddle.

cuddly /ˈkʌdli/ *adj* (**cuddlier, cuddliest**) given to cuddling; tempting to cuddle.

cuddy /ˈkʌdi/ *n* (**cuddies**) (*naut*) the cabin of a half-decked boat; a small cabin, a galley.

cudgel /ˈkʌdʒəl/ *n* a short thick stick for beating. • *vt* (**cudgelling, cudgelled** *or* **cudgeling, cudgeled**) to beat with a cudgel.—**cudgeller, cudgeler** *n*.

cudweed /ˈkʌdwiːd/ *n* a plant with a fine down, belonging to the aster-family.

cue[1] /kjuː/ *n* the last word of a speech in a play, serving as a signal for the next actor to enter or begin to speak; any signal to do something; a hint. • *vt* (**cueing** *or* **cuing, cued**) to give a cue to.

cue[2] *n* a tapering rod used in snooker, billiards, and pool to strike the cue ball.

cue ball *n* (*snooker, etc*) the ball that a player strikes in order to hit other balls.

cuff[1] /kʌf/ *n* a blow with the fist or the open hand. • *vt* to strike such a blow.

cuff[2] *n* the end of a sleeve; a covering round the wrist; the turn-up on a trouser leg.

cufflink /ˈkʌflɪŋk/ *n* a decorative clip for fastening the edges of a shirt cuff.

cuirass /kwɪˈræs/ *n* defensive armour for the breast and back, a breastplate.

cuirassier /ˌkwɪrəˈsɪr/ *n* a cavalry soldier armed with a cuirass.

cuisine /kwɪˈziːn/ *n* a style of cooking or preparing food; the food prepared.

cuisse /kwɪs/ *n* defensive armour for the thighs.

culch /kʌltʃ/ *n* materials forming a spawning bed for oysters; oyster spawn.

cul-de-sac /ˈkʌldəˌsæk/ or /ˈkʊl-/ *n* (*pl* **culs-de-sac, cul-de-sacs**) a street blocked off at one end; a blind alley; a position, job leading nowhere.

-cule /kjuːl/ *n suffix* forming diminutives, as *animalcule*.

culinary /ˈkʌlɪˌnɛri/ or /ˈkjuː-/, /ˈkʌl-/ *adj* of or relating to cooking.

cull /kʌl/ *vt* to select; to pick out, gather. • *n* the selection of certain animals with the intention of killing them.—**culler** *n*.

cullet /ˈkʌlət/ *n* broken or refuse glass for recycling.

culm[1] /kʌlm/ *n* the stem of grasses.

culm[2] *n* inferior anthracite coal.

culminate /'kʌlmɪˌneɪt/ *vti* to reach the highest point of altitude, rank, power, etc; (*astron*) to reach the meridian; to bring to a head or the highest point.—**culminant** *adj.*—**culmination** *n.*

culottes /kuːˈlɒts/ or /'kuː-/ *npl* a women's flared trousers that resemble a skirt.

culpable /'kʌlpəbəl/ *adj* deserving censure; criminal; blameworthy.—**culpably** *adv.*—**culpability** *n.*

culprit /'kʌlprɪt/ *n* a person accused, or found guilty, of an offence.

cult /kʌlt/ *n* a system of worship; devoted attachment to a person, principle, etc; a religion regarded as unorthodox or spurious; its body of adherents; a current fashion.—**cultic** *adj.*—**cultism** *n.*—**cultist** *n.*

cultivate /'kʌltɪˌveɪt/ *vt* to till and plant; to improve by care, labour, or study; to seek the society of; to civilize or refine.—**cultivated** *adj.*

cultivation /'kʌltəˈveɪʃən/ *n* the act of cultivating; the state of being cultivated; tillage; culture.

cultivator /'kʌltɪˌveɪtər/ *n* a machine for breaking up soil for cultivation; someone who cultivates.

Cultrate /'kʌlˌtreɪt/, **cultrated** /-ɪd/ *adj* (*bot*) shaped like a pruning knife; pointed and sharp-edged.

cultural /'kʌltʃərəl/ *adj* pertaining to culture.—**culturally** *adv.*

cultural sovereignty *n* ✤ (*Cdn*) the authority of a country to maintain its own culture, rather than another, more dominant one.

culture /'kʌltʃər/ *n* appreciation and understanding of the arts; the skills, arts, etc of a given people in a given period; the entire range of customs, beliefs, social forms, and material traits of a religious, social, or racial group; the scientific cultivation of plants to improve them and find new species; improvement of the mind, manner, etc; a growth of bacteria, etc in a prepared substance. • *vt* to cultivate bacteria for study or use.

cultured /'kʌltʃərd/ *adj* educated to appreciate the arts; having good taste; artificially grown, as cultured pearls.

cultured pearl *n* a pearl induced to grow artificially by the injection of a foreign body into the closed shell.

culture shock *n* loss of bearings and distress caused by an uprooting from a familiar environment or culture.

culverin /'kʌlvərɪn/ *n* a 16th-century long cannon with serpent-shaped handles.

culvert /'kʌlvərt/ *n* a drain or conduit under a road.

cum /kʌm/ *prep* with.

cumarin *see* **coumarin**.

cumber /'kʌmbər/ *vt* to hamper, to burden. • *n* a hindrance.

cumbersome /-səm/ *adj* inconveniently heavy or large, unwieldy.

cumin, cummin /'kʌmɪn/ or /kjuː-/ *n* a plant cultivated for its seeds which are used as a spice.

cummerbund /'kʌmərˌbʌnd/ *n* a sash worn as a waistband, *esp* with a man's tuxedo.

cumshaw /'kʌmˌʃɔ/ *n* in China, a present or bonus.

cumulate /'kjuːmjʊˌleɪt/ *vt* to accumulate; to combine into one; to build up by adding new material.—**cumulation** *n.*

cumulative /'kjuːmjʊlətɪv/ *adj* augmenting or giving force; growing by successive additions; gathering strength as it grows.—**cumulatively** *adv.*

cumulative voting *n* a system of voting in which each voter has as many votes as there are candidates, and may give all to one candidate.

cumulus /'kjuːmjʊləs/ *n* (*pl* **cumuli**) a cloud form having a flat base and rounded outlines.

cuneate /'kjuːniət/ *adj* wedge-shaped.

cuneiform /kjuːˈneɪəˌfɔrm/ or /-ˈniːə-/, /'kjuːnɪ-/ *adj* wedge-shaped.—*also* **cuneal**. • *n* the wedge-shaped characters of ancient Assyrian and Persian writing.

cunnilingus /ˌkʌnɪˈlɪŋɡəs/ *n* sexual stimulation of the female genitals by the tongue.

cunning /'kʌnɪŋ/ *adj* ingenious; sly; designing; subtle. • *n* slyness, craftiness.

cup /kʌp/ *n* a small, bowl-shaped container for liquids, *usu* with a handle; the amount held in a cup; a drink made from a mixture of drinks with one main ingredient (eg *claret cup*); one of two shaped supporting parts of a brassiere; an ornamental cup used as a trophy. • *vt* (**cupping, cupped**) to take or put as in a cup; to curve (the hands) into the shape of a cup.

cupbearer /'kʌpˌbɛrər/ *n* one who serves wine at a banquet, *esp* an officer of a royal household.

cupboard /'kʌbərd/ *n* a closet or cabinet with shelves for cups, plates, utensils, food etc.

cupel /'kjuːpəl/ *n* a small flat vessel used to assay precious metals. • *vt* (**cupelling, cupelled** *or* **cupeling, cupeled**) to refine precious metals from lead in a cupel.

cupful /'kʌpˌfʊl/ *n* (*pl* **cupfuls**) as much as a cup will contain.

Cupid /'kjuːpɪd/ *n* the god of love in Roman mythology.

cupidity /kjuːˈpɪdɪti/ *n* greed of gain; covetousness.

cupola /'kjuːpələ/ *n* a dome, *esp* of a pointed or bulbous shape; a furnace for melting metals.—**cupolated** *adj.*

cupreous /'kjuːpriəs/ or /'kuː-/ *adj* of or like copper; coppery.

cupric /'kjuːprɪk/ or /'kuː-/, **cuprous** /-prəs/ *adj* containing copper.

cupriferous /kjuːˈprɪfərəs/ or /kuː-/ *adj* yielding copper.

cuprite /'kjuːpreɪt/ *n* red oxide of copper.

cupule /'kjuːpjuːl/ *n* (*biol*) a cup-shaped part, as of the acorn.

CUPW *abbr* ✤ = Canadian Union of Postal Workers.

cur /kər/ *n* a mongrel dog; a despicable person.

curable /'kjərəbəl/ or /'kjur-/ *adj* able to be cured, remediable.—**curability** *n.*—**curably** *adv.*

curaçao /ˌkjʊrəˈsoː/ or /ˌkjərəˈsoː/ *n* an orange-flavoured liqueur.

curacy /'kjərəʃi/ or /'kjurə-/ *n* (*pl* **curacies**) the office or district of a curate.

curare, curari /kjʊˈrɑri/ or /kʊ-/ *n* a substance extracted from vines and used by South American Indians to poison arrows.

curarine /-rɪn/ *n* an alkaloid extract of curare used as a muscle relaxant.

curarize /-raɪz/ *vt* to poison with curare.—**curarization** *n.*

curassow /'kjərəˌsoː/ or /'kjurə-/ *n* a large turkey-like bird of South America.

curate /'kjʊrət/ or /'kjərət/ *n* an assistant of a vicar or rector.

curative /'kjʊrətɪv/ or /'kjərə-/ *adj* tending to cure. • *n* a curative agent or drug.

curator /'kjəreɪtər/ or /'kjʊ-/, /kjʊˈreɪtər/ *n* a superintendent of a museum, art gallery, etc.—**curatorial** *adj.*

curb /kərb/ *vt* to restrain; to check; to keep in subjection. • *n* that which checks, restrains, or subdues; a line of raised stone forming the edge of a pavement.—*also* **kerb**.

curbing /-ɪŋ/ *n* curbstones collectively; material for curbstones.—*also* **kerbing**.

curb roof *n* a roof with a double slope, the lower being steeper.

curbstone /'kərbstoːn/ *n* the stone edge of a path.—*also* **kerbstone**.

curcuma /'kərkjuːmə/ *n* one of several kinds of plant including turmeric.

curd /kərd/ *n* the coagulated part of soured milk, used to make cheese.—**curdy** *adj.*—**curdiness** *n.*

curdle /'kərdəl/ *vti* to turn into curds; to coagulate; (*with* **the blood**) to cause terror.—**curdler** *n.*

cure /kjər/ or /'kjʊr/ *n* the act or art of healing; a remedy; restoration to health. • *vt* to heal; to rid of; to preserve meat or fish by drying, salting, etc.

curé /kjuˈreɪ/, *Fr.* /kYˈReɪ/ *n* a French parish priest.

curettage /kjuˈretɪdʒ/ or /-rɪˈtɒdʒ/ *n* surgical scraping to remove growths or dead tissue, etc.

curette, curet /kjuˈret/ *n* a surgical instrument for scraping a body cavity. •*vt* (**curetting, curetted**) to scrape with this.

curfew /'kərfjuː/ *n* a signal, as a bell, at a fixed evening hour as a sign that everyone must be indoors; the signal or hour.

curia /'kjʊriə/ or /'kjə-/ *n* (*pl* **curiae**) the papal court; a senate house of ancient Rome; one of the divisions of the Roman people; a medieval court of justice.

curie /'kjʊri/ or /kjʊˈriː/ *n* a unit of radioactivity.

curio /'kjʊrioː/ *n* (*pl* **curios**) an item valued as rare or unusual.

curiosity /ˌkjʊriˈɒsɪti/ *n* (*pl* **curiosities**) the quality of being curious; inquisitiveness; a strange, rare or interesting object.

curious /'kjʊriəs/ *adj* anxious to know; prying, inquisitive; strange, remarkable, odd.—**curiously** *adv.*—**curiousness** *n.*

curium /'kjʊriəm/ *n* an artificially made radioactive metallic element derived from plutonium.

curl /kərl/ *vti* to form into a curved shape, to coil; to twist into ringlets; to proceed in a curve, to bend; to play at curling; (*with* **up**) to rest with the body in a curved shape and the legs drawn up; to relax in a comfortable place; (*inf*) to give up; to be embarrassed and sickened by. • *n* a ringlet of hair; a spiral form, a twist; a bend or undulation.

curler /'kərlər/ *n* a small pin or roller used for curling the hair; a person who plays curling.

curlew /'kərluː/ *n* a bird with a long curved bill and long legs.

curlicue /'kərliˌkjuː/ *n* an exaggerated ornamental curl.

curling /'kərlıŋ/ n a Scottish game in which two teams slide large smooth stones on ice into a target circle.

curling stone n a heavy round flat stone with a handle used in curling.

curling tongs n a pair of tongs heated to curl hair.

curly /'kərli/ adj (**curlier, curliest**) full of curls.—**curliness** n.

curmudgeon /kər'mʌdʒən/ n an ill-natured churlish person; a miser.—**curmudgeonly** adj.

currant /'kərənt/ n a small variety of dried grape; a shrub that yields a red or black fruit.

currency /'kərənsi/ n (pl **currencies**) the time during which a thing is current; the state of being in use; the money current in a country.

current /'kərənt/ adj generally accepted; happening now; presently in circulation. • n a body of water or air in motion, a flow; the transmission of electricity through a conductor; a general tendency.

current account n a bank account, usu with no interest, from which money is withdrawn by cheques or cash cards; a checking account.

currently /-li/ adv at the present time.

curricle /'kərikəl/ n a two-wheeled open carriage drawn by two horses abreast.

curriculum /kə'rıkjʊləm/ n (pl **curricula, curriculums**) a prescribed course of study.—**curricular** adj.

curriculum vitae /-'viːtaɪ/ n (pl **curricula vitae**) a brief survey of one's career.

currier /'kəriər/ n a leather dresser.—**curriery** n.

currish /'kərıʃ/ adj snappy; quarrelsome; rude.

curry[1] /'kəri/ n (pl **curries**) a spicy dish with a hot sauce; curry seasoning. • vt (pl **currying, curried**) to flavour with curry.

curry[2] vt (**currying, curried**) to rub down and groom (a horse); to dress leather after tanning; to beat; (with **favour**) to use flattery to ingratiate.

currycomb /'kəri,koːm/ n a metal comb for grooming horses.

curse /kərs/ n a calling down of destruction or evil; a profane oath; a swear word; a violent exclamation of anger; a scourge. • vti to invoke a curse on; to swear, to blaspheme; to afflict, to torment.

cursed /'kərsəd/ or /kərst/ adj damnable.

cursive /'kərsıv/ adj running; flowing. • n a script with the letters joined, as in handwriting.

cursor /'kərsər/ n a flashing indicator on a computer screen indicating position; the transparent slide on a slide rule.

cursorial /kər'soriəl/ adj (bird) with limbs adapted for running or walking.

cursory /'kərsəri/ adj hasty, passing; superficial, careless.—**cursorily** adv.

curt /kərt/ adj short; abrupt; concise; rudely brief.—**curtly** adv.—**curtness** n.

curtail /kər'teɪl/ vt to cut short; to reduce; to deprive of part (of).—**curtailment** n.

curtain /'kərtən/ n a cloth hung as a screen at a window, etc; the movable screen separating the stage from the auditorium; (pl: sl) the end, death. • vt to enclose in, or as with, curtains.

curtain call n (theat) a call from the audience for performers to appear at the end to receive applause.

curtain lecture n a private reprimand from a wife to her husband.

curtain-raiser n a short play preceding the main one; an introductory item.

curtilage /'kərtəlıdʒ/ n (law) a yard, garden or enclosure of a house, included in the same fence.

curtsy, curtsey /'kərtsi/ n (pl **curtsies, curtseys**) a formal gesture of greeting or respect, involving bending the knees, made by women. • vi (**curtsying, curtsied** or **curtseying, curtseyed**) to make a curtsy.

curvaceous /kər'veɪʃəs/ adj (inf) having an attractive body with shapely curves.

curvature /'kərvətʃər/ n a bending; a curved form.

curve /kərv/ n a bending without angles; a bent form or thing; (geom) a line of which no part is straight. • vti to form into a curve, to bend.—**curvy** adj (**curvier, curviest**).

curvet /kər'vet/ n a particular leap of a horse; a frisk or bound. •vi (**curvetting, curvetted** or **curveting, curveted**) to leap as a horse; to frisk or bound.

Curvilinear /,kərvi'lıniər/, **curvilineal** /-əl/ adj consisting of or bounded by curved lines.—**curvilinearity** n.

cusec /'kjuːsek/ n a unit of flow of one cubic foot of water per second.

cushion /'kʊʃən/ n a case stuffed with soft material for resting on; the elastic border around a snooker table; the air mass supporting a hovercraft. • vt to furnish with cushions; to protect by padding; to give protection against difficulties, etc; to soften the effect of.—**cushiony** adj.

cushy /'kʊʃi/ adj (**cushier, cushiest**) (inf) easy, comfortable.

cusp /kʌsp/ n an apex or point; the point at each end of a crescent moon; (astrol) the transitional point of a house; (archit) the pointed intersection between two arcs; a cone-shaped point on a tooth; a fold or flap of a heart valve.

cuspid /'kʌspɪd/ n a canine tooth.

cuspidate /'kʌspɪ,deɪt/ or /-dɪt/, **cuspidal** /-pɪ,dəl/ adj of, like or having a cusp; (leaves, etc) ending in a point.

cuspidor /'kʌspɪ,dor/ n a spittoon.

cuss /kʌs/ n (sl) an annoying person; a curse. • vt (sl) to curse.

cussed /'kʌsɪd/ adj (sl) cursed; stubborn, perverse.

cussedness /-nəs/ n (sl) contrariness.

custard /'kʌstərd/ n a sauce mixture of milk, eggs and sugar.

custard apple /'kʌstərd'æpəl/ n a West Indian tree; its dark fruit with a soft edible pulp.

custodian /kə'stoːdiən/ n one who has the care of anything; a keeper; a caretaker.

custody /'kʌstədi/ n (pl **custodies**) guardianship; imprisonment; security.—**custodial** adj.

custom /'kʌstəm/ n a regular practice; usage; traditions of a people or a society; frequent repetition of the same act; business patronage; (pl) duties on imports.

customary /-əri/ adj habitual; conventional; common.—**customarily** adv.

custom-built /-'bɪlt/ adj made to a customer's specifications.

customer /-mər/ n a person who buys from a shop or business, esp regularly; (inf) a person.

custom house /'kʌstəm,haʊs/ n an office or building where duties are paid on exported or imported goods and vessels are entered and cleared.

cut /kʌt/ vb (**cutting, cut**) vt to cleave or separate with a sharp instrument; to make an incision in; to wound with a sharp instrument; to divide; to trim; to intersect; to abridge; to diminish; to pass deliberately without recognition; to wound the feelings deeply; to reduce or curtail; to grow a new tooth through the gum; to divide (a pack of cards) at random; to switch off (a light, an engine); (inf) to stay away from class, school, etc; (with **back**) to prune vegetation; to economize; (with **down**) to fell a tree; to reduce expenditure, consumption, etc; to make a smaller garment from an old one; to kill; (with **off**) to take away by cutting or slicing; to stop abruptly, esp a telephone conversation; to sever relations; to be so placed as to foil something, eg an escape; (with **out**) to delete; to cut into shapes; (inf) to force out a rival; to give up an indulgence or habit; (with **up**) to cut into pieces; to wound with a knife; (inf) to affect deeply. • vi to make an incision; to perform the work of an edged instrument; to grow through the gums; (cinema) to change to another scene, to stop photographing; (with **in**) to butt in; to interpose oneself; to interrupt with comments; to drive between two vehicles, leaving insufficient space; (with **out**) (engine) to stop working. • n an incision or wound made by a sharp instrument; a gash; a sharp stroke; a sarcastic remark; a passage or channel cut out; a slice; a block on which an engraving is cut; the fashion or shape of a garment; the deliberate ignoring of an acquaintance; the division of a pack of cards; a diminution in price below another merchant; (sl) a share, as of profits. • adj divided or separated; gashed; having the surface ornamented or fashioned; not wrought or hand-made; reduced in price.

cutaneous /kju:'teɪniəs/ adj pertaining to the skin.

cutaway /'kʌtə,weɪ/ n a drawing (of a machine) with part of the exterior covering cut away to show the internal mechanism; (film) a scene shot separately from but relevant to the main action.

cutback /'kʌtbæk/ n a reduction, esp in expenditure; a flashback.

cutch /kʌtʃ/ see catechu.

cute /kjuːt/ adj (inf) acute, shrewd; pretty or attractive, esp in a dainty way.—**cutely** adv.—**cuteness** n.

cut glass n flint glass cut into facets or figures.

cuticle /'kjuːtıkəl/ n the skin at the base of the fingernail or toe nail; epidermis.—**cuticular** adj.

cutie /'kjuːti/ n (sl) a bright smart girl.

cutis /'kju:tɪs/ *n* (*pl* **cutes, cutises**) the vascular layer of the skin, below the epidermis.

cutlass /'kʌtləs/ *n* a sailor's short heavy sword.

cutler /'kʌtlər/ *n* a maker of or dealer in knives.

cutlery /'kʌtləri/ *n* knives, forks, etc for eating and serving food.

cutlet /'kʌtlət/ *n* a neck chop of lamb, etc; a small slice cut off from the ribs or leg; minced meat in the form of a cutlet.

cutoff /'kʌt,ɔf/ *n* a short or straight road; a new shorter channel cut by a river across a bend; a device for stopping steam from entering a cylinder.

cutout /-,aʊt/ *n* a switch to cut off an electric light from a circuit.

cutpurse /-pərs/ *n* a pickpocket.

cutter /'kʌtər/ *n* someone or something that cuts; a small, swift sailing vessel; a light boat carried by larger ships.

cutthroat /'kʌtθro:t/ *n* a murderer. • *adj* merciless; (*razor*) having a long blade in a handle.

cutthroat trout /-trʌʊt/ *n* ☙ a North American trout with a red or orange marking under its jaw.

cutting /'kʌtɪŋ/ *n* a piece cut off or from; an incision; a newspaper clipping; a slip from a plant for propagation; a passage or channel cut out; the process of editing a film or recording; a recording. • *adj* (*wind*) sharp, biting; (*remarks*) hurtful.

cuttlebone /'kʌtəlbo:n/ *n* the internal bone of the cuttlefish, used for polishing, etc.

cuttlefish /-fɪʃ/ *n* (*pl* **cuttlefish, cuttlefishes**) a marine creature with a flattened body that squirts ink when threatened.

cutwater /'kʌt,wɔtər/ *n* the fore part of a ship's prow.

cutwork /-,wərk/ *n* appliqué work.

CV *abbr* = curriculum vitae.

CWB *abbr* ☙ = Canadian Wheat Board.

cwt. *abbr* = hundredweight.

cyan /'saɪæn/ *n* a blue colour, one of the primary colours.

cyanamide, cyanamid /saɪ'ænə,maɪd/ *n* a chemical compound of calcium carbide and nitrogen, used as a fertilizer.

cyanate /'saɪ,neɪt/ *n* a compound of cyanic acid with a base.

cyanic acid /saɪ'ænɪk/ *n* a strong acid composed of cyanogen and oxygen.

cyanide /'saɪ,naɪd/ *n* a poison.

cyanogen /saɪ'ænədʒən/ *n* a colourless poisonous gas burning with a purple flame and with the odour of peach blossom.

cyanosis /,saɪə'no:sɪs/ *n* a condition of the body in which its surface becomes blue due to insufficient aeration of the blood.— **cyanotic** *adj*.

cyanotype /,saɪno:'təɪp/ *n* a photographic process in which the picture is taken in Prussian blue; a blueprint.

cyber café /,saɪbər'kæfeɪ/ *n* a café for use by the customers to enable them to browse the Internet.

cybernetics /-'nɛtɪks/ *n* (*sing*) the study of communication and control functions in living organisms, and in mechanical and electronic systems.—**cybernetic** *adj*.

cyberphobia /-'fo:bɪə/ *n* a morbid fear or intense dislike of computers.—**cyberphobic** *adj*.

cyberspace /-'speɪs/ *n* all of the data stored on a large computer or network through which a virtual reality user can move.

cyclamen /'sɪkləmən/ *n* a plant of the primrose family, with pink, purple or white flowers.

cycle /'saɪkəl/ *n* a recurring series of events or phenomena; the period of this; a body of epics or romances with a common theme; a group of songs; a bicycle, motorcycle, or tricycle. • *vi* to go in cycles; to ride a bicycle or tricycle.

cyclic /'saɪklɪk/ or /'sɪk-/, **cyclical** /'saɪklɪkəl/ or /'sɪk-/ *adj* moving or recurring in cycles.—**cyclically** *adv*.

cyclist /'saɪklɪst/ *n* a person who rides a bicycle.

cycloid /'saɪklɔɪd/ *n* a curve traced by a point on a circle as it rolls along a straight line.—**cycloidal** *adj*.

cyclometer /saɪ'klɒmɪtər/ *n* an instrument for registering the revolutions of a wheel.—**cyclometry** *n*.

cyclone /'saɪklo:n/ *n* a violent circular storm; an atmospheric movement in which the wind blows spirally round towards a centre of low barometric pressure.—**cyclonic** *adj*.

Cyclopean /,saɪklə'pi:ən/ or /-'klo:pɪən/ *adj* pertaining to the Cyclops, the legendary one-eyed giant; one-eyed; huge and rough; vast, massive; (*archit*) built of huge stones without mortar.

cyclopedia, cyclopaedia /,saɪklə'pi:dɪə/ *n* an encyclopedia.— **cyclopedic, cyclopaedic** *adj*.

cyclorama /,saɪklo:'ræmə/ *n* a series of moving pictures extended circularly so as to appear in natural perspective to the viewer standing in the centre.—**cycloramic** *adj*.

cyclotron /'saɪklə,trɒn/ *n* an apparatus for accelerating charged particles in a magnetic field.

cygnet /'sɪgnət/ *n* a young swan.

cylinder /'sɪlɪndər/ *n* a hollow figure or object with parallel sides and circular ends; an object shaped like a cylinder; any machine part of this shape; the piston chamber in an engine.— **cylindrical** *adj*.—**cylindrically** *adv*.

cylindroid /'sɪlɪn,drɔɪd/ *adj* like a cylinder. • *n* a solid body resembling a cylinder but with the ends elliptical.

cyma /'saɪmə/ *n* (*pl* **cymae, cymas**) (*archit*) ogee moulding of a cornice.

cymbal /'sɪmbəl/ *n* (*mus*) one of a pair of two brass plates struck together to produce a ringing or clashing sound.—**cymbalist** *n*.

cyme /saɪm/ *n* a flower cluster in which the main stem ends in a flower, while from each side of the main stem secondary stems branch off to end a flower, and tertiary stems from those, etc.— **cymose** *adj*.

Cymric /'kɪmrɪk/ *adj* pertaining to the Cymry, or the Welsh. • *n* the Welsh language.

cynic /'sɪnɪk/ *n* a morose, surly, or sarcastic person; a sceptic about people, motives and actions; one of a sect of ancient Greek philosophers.—**cynicism** *n*.

cynical /'sɪnɪkəl/ *adj* sceptical of or sneering at goodness; shameless in admitting unworthy motives.—**cynically** *adv*.

cynosure /'sɪnə,ʃʊr/ or /'saɪnə-/ *n* a centre of attraction or admiration.

cypher /'saɪfər/ *see* **cipher**.

cypress /'saɪprəs/ *n* an evergreen tree with hard wood.

Cyprian /'sɪprɪən/ *adj* of Cyprus; of Aphrodite, the Greek goddess of love; wanton, lascivious. • *n* a native of Cyprus; a prostitute.

cyprinid /'sɪprɪ,nɪd/ *n* any of a family of freshwater fishes, including the carp.

cyprinoid /'sɪprɪ,nɔɪd/ *adj* of or resembling a cyprinid; carp-like.

Cypriot /'sɪprɪət/ *adj* pertaining to Cyprus, or to its inhabitants. • *n* a native of Cyprus.

Cyrillic /sɪ'rɪlɪk/ *adj* of or pertaining to St Cyril, or to the Slavonic alphabet. • *n* the alphabet of the Slavonic languages.

cyst /sɪst/ *n* a closed sac developing abnormally in the structure of plants or animals.—**cystic** *adj*.

cystic fibrosis /'sɪstɪk/ *n* a congenital disorder in young children characterized by chronic respiratory and digestive problems.

cystitis /sɪ'staɪtɪs/ *n* inflammation of the urinary bladder.

cystocele /'sɪsto:,si:l/ *n* a hernia caused by protrusion of the bladder.

cystoid /'sɪs,tɔɪd/ *adj* cyst-like. • *n* a growth resembling a cyst.

cystolith /'sɪsto:,lɪθ/ or /-tə-/ *n* a stone in the bladder.

cystoscope /'sɪstə,sko:p/ *n* an instrument for examining the urinary bladder.—**cystoscopic** *adj*.—**cystoscopy** *n*.

cystotomy /sɪs'tɒtəmi/ *n* (*pl* **cystotomies**) the opening of the human bladder for the removal of a stone, etc.

cyt-, cyto- /'saɪto:/ or /-ə/ *prefix* cell.

cytogenesis, cytogeny *n* cell formation in plants and animals.

cytology /saɪ'tɒlədʒi/ *n* the scientific study of cells; cell structure.—**cytological** *adj*.—**cytologist** *n*.

cytoplasm /'saɪto:,plæzəm/ *n* the substance of a cell as opposed to its nucleus.—**cytoplasmic** *adj*.

cytoscreening *n* the examination of smear tests for indications of cervical cancer.

czar /zar/ *see* **tsar**.

czardas /'tʃardæʃ/ *n* a Hungarian national dance with varying tempos; the music for it.

czarevitch /'zarəvɪtʃ/ *see* **tsarevitch**.

czarina, czaritsa /zar'i:nə/ *see* **tsarina, tsaritsa**.

Czech /tʃɛk/ *n* a native, or the language, of the Czech Republic.

D

D (*symbol*) (*mus*) the second note of the C major scale; (*chem*) deuterium ; five hundred.

d. *abbr* = penny or pennies (*UK currency before 1971*).

DA *abbr* = District Attorney.

dab[1] /dæb/ *vt* (**dabbing, dabbed**) to touch lightly with something moist or soft. • *n* a quick light tap; a small lump of anything moist or soft.—**dabber** *n*.

dab[1] *n* a species of European flounder.

dab[3] *n* (*inf*) a dab hand.

dabble /'dæbəl/ *vi* to move hands, feet, etc gently in water or another liquid; (*usu with* **at, in, with**) to do anything in a superficial or dilettante way. • *vt* to splash.—**dabbler** *n*.

dabchick /'dæb,tʃɪk/ *n* a water bird, the little grebe.

dab hand *n* (*inf*) an adept person, an expert.

da capo /dæ'kæpo:/ *adj, adv* (*mus*) from the beginning.

dace /deɪs/ *n* (*pl* **dace**) a small freshwater fish of the carp family.

dacha /'dætʃə/ *n* in Russia, a house in the country used as a holiday and summer residence.

dachshund /'dækshənt/ or /dɒk-/ *n* a breed of short-legged, long-bodied hound.

dacoit /də'kɔɪt/ *n* one of a group of robbers in India and Burma, who plunder in bands.—*also* **dakoit**.

dactyl /'dæktɪl/ *n* a poetic foot of three syllables, one long and two short.—**dactylic** *adj, n*.

dactylogram /dæk'tɪlə,græm/ *n* a fingerprint.

dactylography /,dæktə'lɒgrəfi/ *n* the science of fingerprints.—**dactylographer** *n*.—**dactylographic** *adj*.

dactylology /-'lɒlədʒi/ *n* the art of communicating ideas with the fingers; sign language.

dad /dæd/ *n* (*inf*) father.

Dada /'dɒdɒ/ *n* a school of art and literature that aims at suppressing all relations between thought and expression.—**Dadaism** *n*.— **Dadaist** *n*—**Dadaistic** *adj*.

daddy /'dædi/ *n* (*pl* **daddies**) (*inf*) father.

daddy longlegs /-'lɒŋ,legz/ *n* (*inf*) any of various spiders or insects with long, slender legs, *esp* a crane fly.

dado /'deɪdo:/ *n* (*pl* **dadoes**) the lower part of a room wall when separately panelled or decorated.

daff /dæf/ *vi* (*Scot*) to sport, to play.

daffodil /'dæfədɪl/ *n* a yellow spring flower, a narcissus; its pale yellow colour.

daft /dæft/ *adj* (*inf*) silly, weak-minded; giddy; mad.—**daftly** *adv*.—**daftness** *n*.

dagger /'dægər/ *n* a short weapon for stabbing; a reference mark used in printing (†).—*also* **obelisk**.

dago /'deɪgo:/ *n* (*pl* **dagos, dagoes**) (*offensive*) a foreigner, *esp* from Spain or Portugal.

daguerreotype /də'gero:,taɪp/ *n* an early photographic process using a copper plate; a picture taken by this process.—**daguerreotypy** *n*.

dahlia /'deɪliə/ *n* a half-hardy tuberous perennial of the aster family grown for its colourful blooms.

daily /'deɪli/ *adj, adv* (happening) every day; constantly, progressively. • *n* (*pl* **dailies**) a newspaper published every weekday; (*inf*) a charwoman.

dainty /'deɪnti/ *adj* (**daintier, daintiest**) delicate; choice; nice, fastidious. • *n* (*pl* **dainties**) a titbit, a delicacy.—**daintily** *adv*.—**daintiness** *n*.

daiquiri /'dækəri/ *n* (*pl* **daiquiris**) a cocktail of rum, sugar and lime juice.

dairy /'deəri/ *n* (*pl* **dairies**) a building or room where milk is stored and dairy products made; a shop selling these; a company supplying them.

dairy cattle *npl* cows reared for milk production.

dairying /-ɪŋ/ *n* the business or occupation of a dairy farmer.

dairyman /-mən/ *n* (*pl* **dairymen**) a person who works in a dairy or deals in dairy products.

dairy products *npl* milk and products made from it, *eg* butter, cheese, yogurt.

dais /'daɪəs/ or /'deɪs/ *n* a low platform at one end of a hall or room.

daisy /'deɪzi/ *n* (*pl* **daisies**) any of various plants with a yellow centre and white petals.

daisywheel /'deɪzi,wi:l/ *n* (*comput*) a flat, wheel-shaped, printing device with characters at the ends of spokes.

dal /dɒl/ *n* a split-grain pulse commonly used in Indian cooking.—*also* **dhal**.

Dalai Lama /,dɒlaɪ'lɒmə/ *n* the chief lama of Tibet.

dale /deɪl/ *n* a valley.

dalliance /'dæliəns/ *n* idle or frivolous time-wasting; trifling; flirtation.

Dall sheep, Dall's sheep /dɒl/ *n* ♣ a wild, thin-horned sheep of the mountainous parts of northwest Canada and Alaska.

dally /'dæli/ *vi* (**dallying, dallied**) to lose time by idleness or trifling; to play or trifle (with); to flirt.—**dallier** *n*.

dallymoney *n* (*sl*) alimony paid by one partner in a former sexual relationship to the other.

Dalmatian /dæl'meɪʃən/ *n* a large short-haired dog with black spot-like markings on a white body.

dalmatic /dæl'mætɪk/ *n* a loose vestment with open sides worn *esp* by a bishop.

dam[1] /dæm/ *n* an artificial embankment to retain water; water so contained. • *vt* (**damming, dammed**) to retain (water) with such a barrier; to stem, obstruct, restrict.

dam[2] *n* the mother of a four-footed animal.

damage /'dæmədʒ/ *n* injury, harm; loss; (*inf*) price, cost; (*pl*) (*law*) payment in compensation for loss or injury. • *vt* to do harm to, to injure.—**damageable** *adj*.—**damager** *n*.—**damaging** *adj*.

damask /'dæməsk/ *n* a reversible, figured, woven fabric, *esp* linen or silk. • *adj* made of this; having a pinkish colour like a damask rose.

damask rose *n* a rose with greyish-pink blooms and a sweet fragrance used in perfume making.

dame /deɪm/ *n* the comic, female role in a pantomime *usu* played by a man; (*sl*) a woman; (*with cap*) the title of a woman who has been awarded an order of chivalry equivalent to the title of a Knight; the wife of a knight or baronet.

dammar, damar /'dæmər/ *n* a resin used for varnish.

damn /dæm/ *vt* to condemn, censure; to ruin; to curse; to consign to eternal punishment. • *vti* to prove guilty. • *interj* (*sl*) expressing irritation or annoyance. • *n* (*sl*) something having no value. • *adj, adv* damned.

damnable /'dæmnəbəl/ *adj* deserving damnation; despicable; hateful; offensive; wicked; (*inf*) annoying.—**damnably** *adv*.

damnation /dæm'neɪʃən/ *n* the state of being condemned to hell; the act of damning. • *interj* expressing annoyance, irritation, etc.

damnatory /'dæmnətori/ *adj* assigning to, or containing a threat of, damnation.

damned /dæmd/ *adj* (*inf*) damnable; extremely.—*also adv*.

damnify /'dæmni,faɪ/ *vt* **damnifying, damnified**) (*law*) to cause loss or damage to.

damp /dæmp/ *n* humidity, moisture; in mines, poisonous or foul gas. • *adj* slightly wet, moist. • *vt* to moisten; (*with* **down**) to stifle, reduce.—**damply** *adv*.—**dampness** *n*.

dampen /'dæmpən/ *vti* to make or become damp. • *vt* to stifle.—**dampener** *n*.

damper /-ər/ *n* a depressive influence; a metal plate in a flue for controlling combustion; (*mus*) a device for stopping vibration in stringed instruments; (*Austral*) unleavened bread.

damsel /'dæmzəl/ *n* (*formerly*) a girl.

damselfly /'dæmzəl,flaɪ/ *n* (*pl* **damselflies**) an insect resembling the dragonfly but having wings that fold when at rest.

damson /'dæmzən/ *n* a small, dark-purple variety of plum; the colour of this; the tree on which this fruit grows.

dance /dæns/ *vti* to move rhythmically, *esp* to music; to skip or leap lightly; to execute (steps); to cause to dance or to move up and down. • *n* a piece of dancing; a dance performance of an artistic nature; a party with music for dancing; music for accompanying dancing.—**dancer** *n*.—**dancing** *adj, n*.

D and C *n* (*med*) dilation (of the cervix) and curettage (of the womb).

dandelion /'dændɪˌlaɪən/ *n* a common wild plant with ragged leaves, a yellow flower and a fluffy seed head.

dander[1] /'dændər/ *n* scurf from various animals, *eg* cats, dogs, that may be allergenic; temper; fighting spirit.

dander[2] *vi* (*Scot*) to saunter. • *n* a sauntering stroll.

Dandie Dinmont /'dændɪˌdɪnˌmɒnt/ or /-mənt/ *n* a breed of terrier.

Dandify /'dændəˌfaɪ/ *vt* to give the character or style of a dandy to; to make trim or smart like a dandy.—**dandification** *n*.

dandle /'dændəl/ *vt* to play with (a baby) on the knee, to fondle.—**dandler** *n*.

dandruff /'dændrəf/ *n* scales of skin on the scalp, under the hair, scurf.—**dandruffy** *adj*.

dandy /'dændɪ/ *n* (*pl* **dandies**) a man who likes to dress too fashionably. • *adj* (**dandier, dandiest**) (*inf*) excellent, fine.—**dandyish** *adj*.—**dandyism** *n*.

dandy-brush *n* a stiff brush for grooming horses.

Dane /deɪn/ *n* a native or citizen of Denmark.

Danegeld /'deɪngeld/ *n* an annual tax imposed in England in the reign of Ethelred II to maintain forces against the Danes.

Danelaw, Danelagh /'deɪnlɒ/ *n* the code of laws established by the Danes on their settlement in England; that part of the country where these laws were in force.

dang /dæŋ/ *adj, adv, interj, n* a euphemistic form of **damn**.

danger /'deɪndʒər/ *n* exposure to injury or risk; a source of harm or risk.

dangerous /'deɪndʒərəs/ *adj* involving danger; unsafe; perilous.—**dangerously** *adv*.—**dangerousness** *n*.

dangle /'dæŋgəl/ *vi* to hang and swing loosely. • *vt* to carry something so that it hangs loosely; to display temptingly.—**dangler** *n*.

Danish /'deɪnɪʃ/ *adj* of the people or language of Denmark. • *n* the language of Denmark.

Danish pastry *n* a sweet pastry topped with fruity icing and nuts.

dank /dæŋk/ *adj* disagreeably damp.—**dankly** *adv*.—**dankness** *n*.

danseur /dɒ̃'sɜr/ *n* a professional dancer, a ballet dancer.—**danseuse** *nf*.

dap /dæp/ *vb* (**dapping, dapped**) *vi* to drop bait gently into water. • *vt* to dip lightly; to bounce (a ball). • *n* a bounce.

daphne /'dæfnɪ/ *n* a genus of small evergreen shrubs with fragrant flowers, allied to the laurel.

dapper /'dæpər/ *adj* nimble; neat in appearance, spruce.

dapple /'dæpəl/ *vti* to mark with or show patches of a different colour; to variegate. • *adj* marked in such a way. • *n* something so marked.

dapple-grey /-'greɪ/ *adj* mottled with darker grey. • *n* a horse of this colour.

Dardanian /dɑr'deɪnɪən/, **Dardan** /dɑrdən/ *adj* pertaining to Dardania, an ancient city of Troy, in Asia Minor, or its people. • *n* a Trojan.

dare /der/ *vti* (**daring, dared** *or* **durst**) to be bold enough; to venture, to risk; to defy, to challenge. • *n* a challenge.—**darer** *n*.

daredevil /'derˌdevəl/ *n* a rash, reckless person. • *adj* daring, bold; courageous.—**daredevilry, daredeviltry** *n*.

daring /'derɪŋ/ *adj* fearless; courageous; unconventional. • *n* adventurous courage.—**daringly** *adv*.

dark /dɑrk/ *adj* having little or no light; of a shade of colour closer to black than white; (*person*) having brown or black skin or hair; gloomy; (*inf*) secret, unknown; mysterious. • *n* a dark state or colour; ignorance; secrecy.—**darkly** *adv*.—**darkness** *n*.

darken /'dɑrkən/ *vti* to make or become dark or darker.—**darkener** *n*.

dark horse *n* a competitor about whom little is known; a person of reserved character; a surprise political candidate.

darkish /'dɑrkɪʃ/ *adj* quite dark.

darkroom /'dɑrkruːm/ *n* a room for processing photographs in darkness or safe light.

darksome /-səm/ *adj* gloomy.

darling /'dɑrlɪŋ/ *n* a dearly loved person; a favourite. • *adj* lovable; much admired.

darn[1] /dɑrn/ *vt* to mend a hole in fabric or a garment with stitches. • *n* an area that has been darned.—**darner** *n*.

darn[2] *interj* a form of **damn** as a mild oath.—*also adj*.

darnel /'dɑrnəl/ *n* a kind of rye grass.

darning /'dɑrnɪŋ/ *n* a patch made by darning; material, garments, etc to be darned.

dart /dɑrt/ *n* a small pointed missile; a sudden movement; a fold sewn into a garment for shaping it; (*pl*) an indoor game in which darts are thrown at a target. • *vti* to move rapidly; to send out rapidly.

dartboard /'dɑrtbɔrd/ *n* a circular cork or wooden target used in the game of darts.

darter /'dɑrtər/ *n* one of several kinds of bird or fish.

Darwinian /dɑr'wɪnɪən/ *adj* pertaining to Charles Darwin, the naturalist (1809–82) or Darwinism. • *n* an evolutionist.

Darwinism /'dɑrwɪˌnɪzəm/ *n* the theory of natural selection advocated by Darwin.—**Darwinist** *n*.

dash /dæʃ/ *vti* to fling violently; to rush quickly; (*hopes*) to shatter; (*one's spirits, etc*) to depress, confound; to write quickly. • *n* a short race; a rush; a small amount of something added to food; a tinge; a punctuation mark (—); a dashboard; vigour, verve; display.

dashboard /'dæʃbɔrd/ *n* an instrument panel in a car.

dasher /'dæʃər/ *n* one who or that which dashes; a dashing person; the part of a churn that agitates cream; ♣ one of the boards surrounding a hockey rink.

dashing /'dæʃɪŋ/ *adj* debonair; spirited, stylish, dapper.—**dashingly** *adv*.

dastard /'dæstərd/ *n* a malicious coward.

dastardly /'dæstərdlɪ/ *adj* mean, cowardly; base.—**dastardliness** *n*.

dasyure /'dæsiʊr/ *n* a small carnivorous Australian marsupial.

DAT *abbr* = digital audio tape.

data /'dætə/ or /'deɪtə/ *npl* (*sing* **datum**) (*often used as sing*) facts, statistics, or information either historical or derived by calculation or experimentation.

data bank, database /'dætəˌbeɪs/ or /'deɪtə-/ *n* a large store of information for analysis, *esp* one held in a computer.

data capture *n* the process of translating information into computer-readable form.

data processing *n* the analysis of information stored in a computer for various uses, *eg* stock control, statistical research, mathematical modelling, etc.

data warehouse *n* a system which collects data from a wide range of sources, and is processed as a management tool regarding trends, marketing etc.

date[1] /deɪt/ *n* a day or time of occurrence; a statement of this in a letter, etc; a period to which something belongs; a duration; an appointment, *esp* with a member of the opposite sex. • *vt* to affix a date to; to note the date of; to reckon the time of; (*inf*) to make a date with; (*inf*) to see frequently a member of the opposite sex. • *vi* to reckon from a point in time; to show signs of belonging to a particular period.—**datable, dateable** *adj*.—**dater** *n*.

date[2] *n* the sweet fruit of the date palm, a palm tree of tropical regions.

dated /'deɪtəd/ *adj* old-fashioned; out of style; bearing a date.—**datedness** *n*.

dateless /'deɪtləs/ *adj* without a date; timeless; classic.

dateline /-laɪn/ *n* a line on a newspaper story giving the date and place of writing. • *vt* to provide with a dateline.

date line *n* the line running north to south along the 180-degree meridian, east of which is one day earlier than west of it.—*also* **International Date Line**.

dative /'deɪtɪv/ *adj* (*gram*) denoting an indirect object. • *n* the dative case.—**datival** *adj*.—**datively** *adv*.

datum /'dætəm/ or /'deɪtəm/ *n* (*pl* **data**) a single unit of information; a thing given or taken for granted; something known or assumed as fact and made the basis of reasoning or calculation; an assumption or premise from which inferences are drawn; (*pl* **datums**) (*geol*) a level, line or point used as a reference in surveying.

datura /də'tjʊrə/ *n* any of several kinds of strongly scented narcotic plant.

daub /dɒb/ *vt* to smear or overlay (with clay, etc); to paint incompetently. • *n* a smear; a poor painting.—**dauber** *n*.

daughter /'dɒtər/ *n* a female child or descendant; a female member of a family, race, etc; a woman in relation to her native country or place; (*physics*) a nucleus, particle, etc, produced from another by radioactive decay; (*biol*) a cell produced by the division of another.

daughter-in-law /-ɪnˌlɔ/ *n* (*pl* **daughters-in-law**) the wife of one's son.

daughterly /-lɪ/ *adj* of or befitting a daughter.—**daughterliness** *n*.

daunt /dɒnt/ *vt* to intimidate; to discourage.—**daunter** *n*.—**dauntingly** *adv*.

dauntless /'dɔntləs/ adj incapable of being discouraged; intrepid, fearless.—**dauntlessly** adv.—**dauntlessness** n.

dauphin /'dɔfɪn/ or /do:fæ̃/ n the title of the eldest son of the king of France, 1349–1830.

dauphine, dauphiness /'do:fi,neɪ/ n the wife of the dauphin.

davenport /'dævən,pɔrt/ n a large sofa, often able to be converted into a bed; a small ornamental writing desk.

davit /'dævət/ or /'deɪvət/ n a small crane with tackle for raising or lowering a lifeboat, etc over a ship's side.

Davy Jones /,deɪvɪ'dʒoːnz/ n the spirit of the sea.

Davy Jones's locker n the seabed, the deep, esp as the grave of those who die at sea.

daw /dɔ/ n a bird of the crow family; a jackdaw.

dawdle /'dɔdəl/ vi to move slowly and waste time, to loiter.—**dawdler** n.

dawn /dɔn/ vi (day) to begin to grow light; to begin to appear. • n daybreak; a first sign.

day /deɪ/ n the time when the sun is above the horizon; the twenty-four hours from midnight to midnight; daylight; a particular period of success or influence; (usu pl) a period, an epoch.

daybook /'deɪbuk/ n a diary; an account book for recording the day's transactions.

daybreak /'deɪbreɪk/ n the first appearance of daylight, dawn.

daydream /'deɪdriːm/ n a reverie. • vi to have one's mind on other things; to fantasize.—**daydreamer** n.

daylight /'deɪlaɪt/ n the light of the sun; dawn; publicity; a visible gap; the dawning of sudden realization or understanding.

day release n ✸ (Cdn) a release of a jailed prisoner during the day or for a short period of time in order to hold a job or to attend school.

days /deɪz/ adv during the day regularly.

daytime /'deɪtaɪm/ n the time of daylight.

day-to-day /'deɪtə'deɪ/ adj daily; routine.

daze /deɪz/ vt to stun, to bewilder. • n confusion, bewilderment.—**dazedly** adv.—**dazedness** n.

dazzle /'dæzəl/ vt to confuse the sight of or be partially blinded by strong light; to overwhelm with brilliance. • n the act of dazzling; a thing that dazzles; an overpoweringly strong light; bewilderment.—**dazzlement** n.—**dazzler** n.—**dazzlingly** adv.

dB, db abbr = decibels.

DBS abbr = direct broadcasting by satellite.

DC abbr = District of Columbia.

dc, DC abbr = direct current.

DD abbr = Doctor of Divinity.

D-day /'diːdeɪ/ n the date (June 6, 1944) of the Allied cross-channel invasion of France during World War II; any date set aside for an important event.

DDT abbr = dichlorodiphenyltrichloroethane, a chemical used as an insecticide.

de prep from, concerning; of.

de- /dɪ/ or /diː/ prefix down; off; completely; un-.

de-accessioning /,diːæk'seʃənɪŋ/ n the disposal, usu by selling, of an artefact or painting in a public collection.

deacon /'diːkən/ n (Anglican, RC churches) an ordained member of the clergy ranking below a priest; (Presbyterian churches) a lay church officer who assists the minister.—**deaconship** n.

deaconess /,diːkə'nes/ or /'diːkənəs/ n a churchwoman appointed to do work in a parish; a member of an institution or order trained to carry on systematic charitable work; in a convent, the nun who attends to the altar.

deactivate /diː'æktɪ,veɪt/ vt (bomb) to make inactive or harmless.—**deactivation** n.—**deactivator** n.

dead /ded/ adj without life; inanimate, inert; no longer used; lacking vegetation; emotionally or spiritually insensitive; without motion; (fire, etc) extinguished; (limb, etc) numb; (colour, sound etc) dull; (a ball) out of play; complete, exact; unerring. • adv in a dead manner; completely; utterly. • n a dead person; the quietest time.—**deadness** n.

deadbeat /'dedbiːt/ n (inf) a lazy or socially inept person; a vagrant.

dead duck n (sl) a person or thing destined to fail.

deadhead /'dedhed/ n ✸ a sunken or submerged log, esp one that is a hazard to water traffic.

deaden /'dedən/ vt to render numb or insensible; to deprive of vitality; to muffle.—**deadener** n.—**deadeningly** adv.

dead end n a cul-de-sac; a hopeless situation.

dead-end /'ded,end/ adj (job) holding no chance of advancement; having no hope of success in the future (dead-end kids).

deadening /'dedənɪŋ/ n material for soundproofing a room.

deadeye /'dedaɪ/ n an expert marksman; (naut) a round, laterally flattened wooden block pierced with three holes through which the lanyards are passed, used for extending the shrouds.

deadfall /'dedfɔl/ n a trap with a falling weight, which can kill or disable; a tangled mass of fallen trees.

deadhead /'dedhed/ n a person who has a free pass on trains or to places of amusement, etc; a transport vehicle travelling empty; ✸ a sunken or submerged log. • vt to remove dead flower heads from (a plant); to provide free admission to. • vi to travel or gain admission without payment; to drive an empty transport vehicle.

dead heat n a race in which two or more finish equal, a tie.

dead letter n a law or rule that is no longer enforced; a letter that cannot be delivered and is returned to the sender.

deadlight /'dedlaɪt/ n (naut) a storm shutter for a cabin window; a skylight not made to open.

deadline /'dedlaɪn/ n the time by which something must be done.

deadlock /'dedlɒk/ n a clash of interests making progress impossible; a standstill.—also vt.

deadly /'dedli/ adj (**deadlier, deadliest**) fatal; implacable; (inf) tedious. • adv death-like; intensely.—**deadliness** n.

deadly nightshade n a poisonous plant with purple flowers and black berries.—also **belladonna**.

deadpan /'dedpæn/ adj (inf) deliberately expressionless or emotionless.—also adv.

dead reckoning n the taking of a ship's position by log and compass, not astronomical observations.

dead set adv with determination.

dead weight n a very heavy load; an oppressive burden.

dead wood /'dedwud/ n (inf) a useless person or thing.

deaf /def/ adj unable to hear; hearing badly; not wishing to hear.—**deafly** adv.—**deafness** n.

deafen /'defən/ vt to deprive of hearing.—**deafeningly** adv.

deaf-mute n a deaf and dumb person.

deal¹ /diːl/ vb (**dealing, dealt**) vt (a blow) to deliver, inflict; (cards etc) to distribute; (with **with**) to do business with; (problem, task) to solve. • vi to do business (with); to trade (in). • n a portion, quantity; (inf) a large amount; a dealing of cards; a business transaction.

deal² n fir or pine wood.—also adj.

dealer /'diːlər/ n a trader; a person who deals cards; (sl) a seller of illegal drugs.

dealings /'diːlɪŋs/ npl personal or business transactions.

dealt /delt/ see **deal**

dean /diːn/ n the head of a cathedral chapter; a college fellow in charge of discipline; the head of a university or college faculty.—**deanship** n.

deanery /'diːnəri/ n (pl **deaneries**) the office or residence of a dean.

dear /dɪr/ adj loved, precious; charming; expensive; a form of address in letters. • n a person who is loved. • adv at a high price.—**dearness** n.

dearie, deary /'dɪri/ n (pl **dearies**) (inf) a darling, a dear.

dearly /'dɪrli/ adv with great affection; at a high price or rate.

dearth /dərθ/ n scarcity, lack.

death /deθ/ n the end of life, dying; the state of being dead; the destruction of something.

deathbed /'deθbed/ n the bed in which a person dies or is about to die.

death blow /-,blou/ n a blow causing death.

death duty n a tax paid on an inheritance after a death.—also **death tax**.

deathless /-lɪs/ adj immortal.—**deathlessly** adv.—**deathlessness** n.

deathly /'deθli/ adj like death, pale, still; deadly. • adv in a manner causing or tending to death; to a degree resembling death; (inf) extremely (deathly quiet).—**deathliness** n.

death mask n a plaster cast of a face taken immediately after death.

death rate n the yearly proportion of deaths to population.—also **mortality rate**.

death rattle n a deep gurgling noise sometimes made by a dying person.

death row n the section of a prison housing inmates sentenced to death.

death's head /'dɛθs,hɛd/ *n* a skull or representation of a skull, emblematic of death.

death's-head moth *n* a large moth with skull-like markings.

death tax *see* **death duty**.

deathtrap *n* an unsafe place, thing or structure.

death warrant *n* official authorization for the execution of a person condemned to death; anything that guarantees the destruction of hope or expectation.

deathwatch beetle *n* a small beetle that makes a ticking sound, superstitiously supposed to forebode death.

deathwatch /'dɛθ,wɒtʃ/ *n* a vigil beside a dying person; a guard over a criminal prior to execution.

death wish *n* a *usu* unconscious wish for one's own death or that of another.

deb /dɛb/ *n* (*inf*) a debutante.

debacle /deɪ'bɒkəl/ or /-'bækəl/, /də-/ *n* a sudden disastrous break-up or collapse; a break-up of river ice.

debar /di:'bɑr/ *vt* (**debarring, debarred**) to exclude, to bar.—**debarment** *n*.

debark /di:'bɑrk/ or /dɪ-/ *vti* to land from a ship, to disembark.—**debarkation** *n*.

debase /dɪ'beɪs/ *vt* to lower in character or value; (*coinage*) to degrade.—**debasement** *n*.—**debaser** *n*.

debatable /dɪ'beɪtəbəl/ *adj* open to question, disputed.—**debatably** *adv*.

debate /də'beɪt/ *n* a formal argument; a discussion, *esp* in parliament. • *vt* to consider, contest. • *vi* to discuss thoroughly; to join in debate.—**debater** *n*.

debauch /də'bɒtʃ/ *vti* to corrupt, dissipate; to lead astray, to seduce.—**debaucher** *n*.

debauchee /,dɛbɔ'tʃi:/ or /-'ʃi:/ *n* a dissolute person, a libertine.

debauchery /də'bɒtʃəri/ *n* (*pl* **debaucheries**) depraved over-indulgence; corruption; profligacy.

debenture /də'bɛntʃər/ *n* a bond with guaranteed interest and forming a first charge on assets; a certificate acknowledging a debt; a certificate entitling a refund of customs duty.

debilitate /də'bɪlɪ,teɪt/ *vt* to weaken, to enervate.—**debilitation** *n*.—**debilitative** *adj*.

debility /də'bɪlɪti/ *n* (*pl* **debilities**) weakness, infirmity.

debit /'dɛbɪt/ *n* the entry of a sum owed, opposite to the credit; the left side of a ledger used for this. • *vt* to charge to the debit side of a ledger.

debonair, debonnaire /,dɛbə'nɛr/ *adj* having a carefree manner; courteous, gracious, charming.—**debonairly** *adv*.

debouch /də'bəʊtʃ/ or /-'bu:ʃ/ *vi* to march or to flow out from a narrow space to open ground.—**debouchment** *n*.

debrief /di:'bri:f/ *vt* (*diplomat, etc*) to make a report following a mission; to obtain such information.—**debriefing** *n*.

debris /də'bri:/ or /de-/ *n* (*pl* **debris**) broken and scattered remains, wreckage.

debt /dɛt/ *n* a sum owed; a state of owing; an obligation.

debtor /'dɛtər/ *n* a person, company, etc who owes money to another.

debug /di:'bʌg/ *vt* (**debugging, debugged**) (*inf*) (*room, etc*) to clear of hidden microphones; (*machine, program, plan, etc*) to locate and remove errors from; to remove insects from.

debunk /di:'bʌŋk/ *vt* (*inf*) (*claim, theory*) to expose as false.—**debunker** *n*.

debut /deɪ'bju:/ or /'deɪ-/ *n* a first appearance as a public performer or in society. • *vi* to make one's debut.

debutant /'dɛbju:,tɒnt/ or /'deɪ-/ *n* one making a debut, *esp* a sportsman.

debutante /'dɛbju:,tɒnt/ or /'deɪ-/ *n* a young woman making her first appearance in upper-class society; a young woman regarded as wealthy, aristocratic and indolent.

Dec. *abbr* = December.

decade /'dɛkeɪd/ or /de'keɪd/ *n* a period of ten years; a group of ten.—**decadal** *adj*.

decadence /'dɛkədəns/, **decadency** /-si/ *n* a state of deterioration in standards, *esp* of morality.

decadent /'-dənt/ *adj* deteriorating; self-indulgent.—**decadently** *adv*.

decaffeinated /di:'kæfɪ,neɪtəd/ *adj* (*coffee, tea, carbonated drinks, etc*) with caffeine reduced or removed.

decagon /'dɛkə,gɒn/ *n* a ten-sided plane figure.—**decagonal** *adj*.

decahedron /,dɛkə'hi:drən/ *n* a solid with ten faces.—**decahedral** *adj*.

decalcify /di:'kælsɪ,faɪ/ *vt* (**decalcifying, decalcified**) to deprive (bone etc) of its lime.

decalitre, decaliter /'dɛkə,li:tər/ *n* a unit of ten litres.

Decalogue /'dɛkə,lɒg/ *n* the Ten Commandments.

decametre, decameter /'dɛkə,mi:tər/ *n* a unit of ten metres.

decamp /dɪ'kæmp/ *vi* to leave suddenly or secretly.—**decampment** *n*.

decanal /'dɪkeɪnəl/ or /'dɛkə-/ *adj* of a dean or his office; of the south side of the choir of a church, etc.

decant /dɪ'kænt/ *vt* (*wine, etc*) to pour from one vessel to another, leaving sediment behind.—**decantation** *n*.

decanter /dɪ'kæntər/ *n* an ornamental bottle (*usu* glass) for holding wines, etc.

decapitate /dɪ'kæpɪ,teɪt/ *vt* to behead.—**decapitation** *n*.—**decapitator** *n*.

decapod /'dɛkə,pɒd/ *adj* having ten feet or ten arms. • *n* a ten-footed crustacean, or ten-armed cephalopod.—**decapodal, decapodan, decapodous** *adj*.

decarbonate /di:'kɑrbə,neɪt/ *vt* to deprive of carbon dioxide.—**decarbonation** *n*.

decarbonize /-,naɪz/ *vt* take carbon or carbon deposit from.—**decarbonization** *n*.

decare /dɪ'kɛr/ *n* a measure of 1,000 square metres.

decasyllable /'dɛkə,sɪləbəl/ *n* a ten-syllabled line or word.—**decasyllabic** *adj, n*.

decathlon /də'kæθlɒn/ *n* a track-and-field contest consisting of ten events.—**decathlete** *n*.

decay /dɪ'keɪ/ *vti* to rot, to decompose; to deteriorate, to wither. • *n* the act or state of decaying; a decline, collapse.

decease /dɪ'si:s/ *n* death. • *vi* to die.

deceased /dɪ'si:st/ *adj* dead. • *n* the dead person.

deceit /dɪ'si:t/ *n* the act of deceiving; cunning; treachery; fraud.

deceitful /-fʊl/ *adj* treacherous; insincere; misleading.—**deceitfully** *adv*.—**deceitfulness** *n*.

deceive /dɪ'si:v/ *vt* to cheat; to mislead; to delude; to impose upon.—**deceivable** *adj*.—**deceiver** *n*.—**deceivingly** *adv*.

decelerate /di:'sɛlə,reɪt/ *vt, vi* to reduce speed.—**deceleration** *n*.—**decelerator** *n*.

December /dɪ'sɛmbər/ *n* the twelfth and last month of the year with 31 days.

Decembrist /-brɪst/ *n* one of the conspirators who took part in the insurrection against Tsar Nicholas I of Russia, on his accession, December 1825.

decency /'di:sənsi/ *n* (*pl* **decencies**) being decent; conforming to accepted standards of proper behaviour.

decennial /dɪ'sɛniəl/ *adj* lasting for, or occurring, every ten years.—**decennially** *adv*.

decennium /-iəm/ *n* (*pl* **decenniums, decennia**) a ten-year period, a decade.

decent /'di:sənt/ *adj* respectable, proper; moderate; not obscene; (*inf*) quite good; (*inf*) kind, generous.—**decently** *adv*.

decentralize /di:'sɛntrə,laɪz/ *vt* (*government, organization*) to divide among local centres.—**decentralist** *adj, n*.—**decentralization** *n*.

deception /də'sɛpʃən/ or /di:-/ *n* the act of deceiving or the state of being deceived; illusion; fraud.

deceptive /də'sɛptɪv/ or /di:-/ *adj* apt to mislead; ambiguous; unreliable.—**deceptively** *adv*.—**deceptiveness** *n*.

deci- /'dɛsɪ/ *prefix* one tenth.

decibel /'dɛsɪbəl/, /-,bɛl/ *n* a unit for measuring sound level.

decide /dɪ'saɪd/ *vti* to determine, to settle; to give a judgment on; to resolve.—**decidable** *adj*.

decided /-ɪd/ *adj* unhesitating; clearly marked.

decidedly /-ɪdli/ *adv* definitely, certainly.

decider /-ər/ *n* a deciding round, a final heat.

deciduous /dɪ'sɪdʒʊəs/ or /-djʊəs/ *adj* (*trees, shrubs*) shedding all leaves annually, at the end of the growing season.—**deciduousness** *n*.

decilitre, deciliter /'dɛsɪ,li:tər/ *n* a unit equal to one-tenth of a litre.

decillion /dɪ'sɪljən/ *n* in UK, the tenth power of a million, a unit followed by 60 zeros; in US, the eleventh power of a thousand, a unit followed by 33 zeros.—**decillionth** *adj*.

decimal /'dɛsɪməl/ *adj* of tenths, of numbers written to the base 10. • *n* a tenth part; a decimal fraction.—**decimally** *adv*.

decimal classification *see* **Dewey Decimal System**.

decimal currency *n* currency in which units are divisible by ten.

decimal fraction *n* a fraction whose denominator is ten or a power of ten, indicated by figures after a decimal point.

decimalize /-ˌlaɪz/ *vt* to express as a decimal or to convert to a decimal system.—**decimalization** *n*.

decimal point *n* a dot written before the numerator in a decimal fraction (*eg* $0.5 = \frac{1}{2}$).

decimal system *n* a system of weights and measures in which units are related in multiples or submultiples of ten.

decimate /ˈdɛsɪˌmeɪt/ *vt* to kill every tenth person; to reduce by one tenth; to kill a great number.—**decimation** *n*.—**decimator** *n*.

decimetre, decimeter /ˈdɛsɪˌmiːtər/ *n* a measure of length, one tenth of a metre.

decipher /dɪˈsaɪfər/ *vt* to decode; to make out (indistinct writing, meaning, etc).—**decipherable** *adj*.—**decipherer** *n*—**decipherment** *n*.

decision /dɪˈsɪʒən/ *n* a settlement; a ruling; a judgment; determination, firmness; (*boxing*) a win on points.—**decisional** *adj*.

decisive /-ˈsaɪsɪv/ *adj* determining the issue, positive; conclusive, final.—**decisively** *adv*.—**decisiveness** *n*.

deck /dɛk/ *n* the floor on a ship, aircraft, bus or bridge; a pack of playing cards; the turntable of a record-player; the playing mechanism of a tape recorder; (*sl*) the ground, the floor. • *vt* to cover; to adorn.

deck chair *n* a folding chair made of canvas suspended in a frame.

deck hand /ˈdɛkˌhænd/ *n* a seaman who performs manual tasks.

deckle edge *n* the ragged edge, as on handmade paper.—**deckle-edged** *adj*.

deckle /ˈdɛkəl/ *n* a gauge on a papermaking machine for determining the width.

declaim /dɪˈkleɪm/ *vti* to state dramatically; to recite.—**declaimer** *n*.

declamation /ˌdɛkləˈmeɪʃən/ *n* the art of declaiming according to rhetorical rules; impassioned oratory; distinct and correct enunciation of words in vocal music.

declamatory /dɪˈklæməˌtɔːri/ *adj* pertaining to, or characterized by, declamation; noisy in style; appealing to the passions.—**declamatorily** *adv*.

declaration /ˌdɛkləˈreɪʃən/ *n* the act of declaring or proclaiming; that which is declared; an assertion; publication; a statement reduced to writing.

declarative /dɪˈklɛrətɪv/ or /dɪ-/ *adj* making a declaration.—**declaratively** *adv*.

declaratory /-əˌtɔːri/ *adj* declarative; explanatory, affirmative.—**declaratorily** *adv*.

declare /dɪˈklɛr/ *vt* to affirm, to proclaim; to admit possession of (dutiable goods). • *vi* (*law*) to make a statement; (*with against, for*) to announce one's support.—**declarable** *n*.

déclassé /ˌdeɪˈklæseɪ/ *adj* fallen in the social scale.

declassify /diːˈklæsɪˌfaɪ/ *vt* (**declassifying, declassified**) to remove a document, etc from the list of official secrets.—**declassification** *n*.

declension /dɪˈklɛnʃən/ *n* (*gram*) variation in the form of a noun and its modifiers to show case and number; a complete set of such variations of a noun, etc.—**declensional** *adj*.

declination /ˌdɛklɪˈneɪʃən/ *n* a downward bend; (*astron*) the angular distance of a star and the celestial equator; (*compass*) the angle between true north and the magnetic north.—**declinational** *adj*.

decline /dɪˈklaɪn/ *vi* to refuse; to move down; to deteriorate, fall away; to fail; to diminish; to draw to an end; to deviate. • *vt* to reject, to refuse; (*gram*) to give the cases of a declension. • *n* a diminution; a downward slope; a gradual loss of physical and mental faculties.—**declinable** *adj*.—**decliner** *n*.

declivity /dɪˈklɪvɪti/ *n* (*pl* **declivities**) a downward slope.—**declivitous** *adj*.

decoct /dɪˈkɒkt/ *vt* to boil anything to extract its essence.

decoction /dɪˈkɒkʃən/ *n* an extract obtained by boiling or digesting in hot water; the act of decocting.

decode /diːˈkoʊd/ *vt* to translate a code into plain language.

decoder /-ər/ *n* one who decodes; (*comput*) a device for converting data from one form to another, *eg* binary to decimal.

decollate /dɪˈkɒlˌeɪt/ *vt* to separate (collated papers); (*arch*) to behead.—**decollator** *n*.

decollation /ˌdiːkɒˈleɪʃən/ *n* the act of decollating; (*art*) a representation of a beheading, *esp* of St John the Baptist.

décolletage /ˌdeɪkɒlˈtɒʒ/ *n* a low-cut dress or neckline.

décolleté /deɪˈkɒlteɪ/ *adj* having a low neckline.

decolonize /diːˈkɒləˌnaɪz/ *vt* to allow a colony to become independent.

decolorize /diːˈkʌləˌraɪz/ *vt* to remove colour from, to bleach.—**decoloration** *n*.—**deco orization** *n*.

decompose /ˌdiːkəmˈpoʊz/ *vti* to separate or break up into constituent parts, *esp* as part of a chemical process; to resolve into its elements. • *vi* to decay.—**decomposable** *adj*.—**decomposition** *n*.

decompress /ˌdiːkəmˈprɛs/ *vt* to decrease the pressure on, *esp* gradually; to return (a diver, etc) to a condition of normal atmospheric pressure.—**decompression** *n*.—**decompressive** *adj*.—**decompressor** *n*.

decompression sickness *n* a condition affecting divers, astronauts, etc, resulting from too rapid a return from high pressure to atmosphere and characterized by cramps and paralysis.

decongestant /ˌdiːkənˈdʒɛstənt/ *n* a medical preparation that relieves congestion, *eg* catarrh.

deconsecrate /diːˈkɒnsɪˌkreɪt/ *vt* to transfer (a church) from ecclesiastical use.—**deconsecration** *n*.

decontaminate /-ˈtæməˌneɪt/ *vt* to free from (radioactive, etc) contamination.—**decontamination** *n*.—**decontaminator** *n*.

decontrol /ˌdiːkənˈtroʊl/ *vt* (**decontrolling, decontrolled**) to release from control, *esp* government control.

décor, decor /ˈdeɪkɔːr/ or /dəˈkɔːr/ *n* general decorative effect, *eg* of a room; scenery and stage design.

decorate /ˈdɛkəˌreɪt/ *vt* to ornament; to paint or wallpaper; to honour with a badge or medal.

decoration /ˌdɛkəˈreɪʃən/ *n* decorating; an ornament; a badge or an honour.

decorative /ˈdɛkrətɪv/ *adj* ornamental, pretty to look at.—**decoratively** *adv*.—**decorativeness** *n*.

decorator /ˈdɛkəˌreɪtər/ *n* a person who decorates, *esp* houses.

decorous /ˈdɛkərəs/ *adj* proper, decent; showing propriety and dignity.—**decorously** *adv*.—**decorousness** *n*.

decorticate /diːˈkɔːrtɪˌkeɪt/ *vt* to remove the bark, rind, or husk from; to remove the cortex of an organ by surgery. • *vi* to peel or come off, as bark, skin.—**decortication** *n*.—**decorticator** *n*.

decorum /dɪˈkɔːrəm/ *n* what is correct in outward appearance, propriety of conduct, decency.

decoy /ˈdiːkɔɪ/ *vt* to lure into a trap. • *n* anything intended to lure into a snare.—**decoyer** *n*.

decrease /ˈdiːkris/ *n*, /dɪˈkriːs/ *vti* to make or become less. • *n* a decreasing; the amount of diminution.—**decreasingly** *adv*.

decree /dɪˈkriː/ *n* an order, edict or law; a judicial decision. • *vt* (**decreeing, decreed**) to decide by sentence in law; to appoint.—**decreeable** *adj*.—**decreer** *n*.

decrement /ˈdɛkrɪmənt/ *n* a decrease; the amount of this; (*math*) a negative increment of a variable.—**decremental** *adj*.

decrepit /dɪˈkrɛpɪt/ *adj* worn out by the infirmities of old age; in the last stage of decay.—**decrepitly** *adv*.

decrepitate /dɪˈkrɛpɪˌteɪt/ *vti* to heat (a salt, mineral) until it crackles; to crackle under extreme heat.—**decrepitation** *n*.

decrepitude /-ˌtuːd/ or /ˌtjuːd/ *n* the state or condition of being decrepit; feebleness and decay, *esp* that due to old age.

decrescendo /ˌdiːkrɛˈʃɛndoʊ/ or /ˌdeɪkrɪ-/ *n* (*pl* **decrescendos**) (*mus*) a sign (>) that the volume of sound is to be gradually reduced; a gradual decrease in force of tone or a passage where this occurs. • *adj* gradually diminishing in loudness.—*also* **diminuendo**.

decrescent /dɪˈkrɛsənt/ *adj* growing less; (*moon*) waning.—**decrescence** *n*.

decretal /dɪˈkriːtəl/ *n* (*RC Church*) a papal decree; a book of edicts. • *adj* of a decree or decretal.

decry /dɪˈkraɪ/ *vt* (**decrying, decried**) to disparage, to censure as worthless.—**decrial** *n*.—**decrier** *n*.

dectet /dɛkˈtɛt/ *n* a group of eight musicians or voices.

decumbent /dɪˈkʌmbənt/ *adj* lying down, prostrate, reclining; (*bot*) resting on the ground, trailing.—**decumbence, decumbency** *n*.

decuple /ˈdɛkjuːpəl/ *adj* tenfold. • *n* a number repeated ten times. • *vt* to increase tenfold.

decurion /diːˈkjuːriən/ *n* a Roman officer commanding ten men.

decurrent /dɪˈkʌrənt/ *adj* (*plant*) running or extending downward.

decussate /dɪˈkʌsɪt/ *adj*, /ˌdiːˈkʌseɪt/ *vti* to intersect in the form of an X. • *adj* X-shaped; (*leaves*) in pairs, at right angles to those above and below.—**decussation** *n*.

dedicate /ˈdɛdɪˌkeɪt/ vt to consecrate (to some sacred purpose); to devote wholly or chiefly; to inscribe (to someone).—**dedicatee** n.—**dedicator** n.—**dedicatory, dedicative** adj.

dedicated /ˈdɛdɪˌkeɪtəd/ adj devoted to a particular cause, profession, etc; single-minded; assigned to a particular function.

dedication /ˌdɛdɪˈkeɪʃən/ n the act of dedicating; a dedicatory inscription in a book, etc; devotion to a cause, ideal, etc.

deduce /dɪˈduːs/ or /-ˈdjuːs/ vt to derive (knowledge, a conclusion) from reasoning; infer.—**deducible** adj.

deduct /dɪˈdʌkt/ vt to take (from); to subtract.

deductible /-ɪbəl/ adj capable of being deducted; allowable as a deduction against income tax.—**deductibility** n.

deduction /dɪˈdʌkʃən/ n deducting; the amount deducted; deducing; a conclusion that something is true because it necessarily follows from a set of general premises known to be valid.—**deductive** adj.—**deductively** adv.

deed /diːd/ n an act; an exploit; a legal document recording a transaction.

deem /diːm/ vti to judge; to think, to believe.

deep /diːp/ adj extending or placed far down or far from the outside; fully involved; engrossed; profound, intense; heartfelt; penetrating; difficult to understand; secret; cunning; sunk low; low in pitch; (colour) of high saturation and low brilliance. • adv in a deep manner; far in, into. • n that which is deep; the sea.—**deeply** adv.—**deepness** n.

deepen /ˈdiːpən/ vt to make deeper in any sense; to increase. • vi to become deeper.—**deepener** n.

deepfreeze /ˈdiːpˌfriːz/ n a refrigerator in which food is frozen and stored.

deep-freeze vt (**deep-freezing, deep-froze** or **deep-freezed**, pp **deep-frozen, deep-freezed**) to freeze (food) so that it keeps for a long period of time; to store in a freezer. • n a freezer.

deep-fry vt (**deep-frying, deep-fried**) to fry food in deep fat in order to cook or brown it without turning.—**deep-fryer** n.

deep-laid adj (plans, etc) secret and elaborate.

deep-rooted adj (feelings, opinions, etc) firmly established; ingrained; deep-seated.

deep-seated adj having its seat far beneath the surface; deep-rooted.

Deep South n the southeastern states of the USA.

deep space n the region of outer space beyond our solar system.

deer /diːr/ n (pl **deer, deers**) a four-footed animal with antlers, esp on the males, including stag, reindeer, etc.

deerhound /ˈdiːrhaʊnd/ n a large rough-haired greyhound.—also **Scottish deerhound**.

deerstalker /-ˌstɔːkər/ n a person who hunts deer; a soft hat peaked at the front and back.

de-escalate /diːˈɛskəˌleɪt/ vti to reduce the intensity of.—**de-escalation** n.

deface /dɪˈfeɪs/ vt to disfigure; to obliterate.—**defaceable** adj.—**defacement** n.—**defacer** n.

de facto /diːˈfæktoː/ or /deɪ-/ adv in fact; in reality.—also adj.

defalcate /diːˈfælkeɪt/ or /-ˈfɔl-/, /dɪ-/ vi to embezzle money held in trust.—**defalcation** n.—**defalcator** n.

defamation /ˌdɛfəˈmeɪʃən/ or /ˌdiːf-/ n the act of injuring someone's good name or reputation without justification, either orally or in writing; the condition of being defamed.

defamatory /dɪˈfæmətəri/ adj containing that which is injurious to the character or reputation of someone.—**defamatorily** adv.

defame /dɪˈfeɪm/ vt to destroy the good reputation of; to speak evil of.—**defamer** n.

default /dɪˈfɔlt/ or /dɪˈ-/ n neglect to do what duty or law requires; failure to fulfil a financial obligation; (comput) a basic setting or instruction to which a program reverts. • vi to fail in one's duty (as honouring a financial obligation, appearing in court).

defaulter /-ər/ n one who defaults; one who fails to appear in court when required, or to make a proper account of money or property entrusted to his charge; on the Stock Exchange, one who fails to meet his engagements.

defeasance /dɪˈfiːzəns/ n (law) annulment; a condition annexed to a deed, which being performed renders the deed void.

defeasible /dɪˈfiːzɪbəl/ adj able to be annulled.—**defeasibility** n.

defeat /dɪˈfiːt/ or /dɪ-/ vt to frustrate; to win a victory over; to baffle. • n a frustration of plans; overthrow, as of an army in battle; loss of a game, race, etc.—**defeater** n.

defeatism /-ɪzəm/ n disposition to accept defeat.—**defeatist** n, adj.

defecate /ˈdɛfəˌkeɪt/ vi to empty the bowels. • vt (chem) to free from impurities, to refine.—**defecation** n.—**defecator** n.

defect /dɪˈfɛkt/ vi, /ˈdiːfɛkt/ n a deficiency; a blemish, fault. • vi to desert one's country or a cause, transferring one's allegiance (to another).—**defector** n.

defection /dɪˈfɛkʃən/ n desertion of duty or allegiance.

defective /-tɪv/ adj having a defect; faulty; incomplete. • n a person defective in physical or mental powers.—**defectively** adv.—**defectiveness** n.

defence, defense /dəˈfɛns/ n resistance or protection against attack; a means of resisting an attack; protection; vindication; (law) a defendant's plea; the defending party in legal proceedings; (sport) defending (the goal, etc) against the attacks of the opposing side; the defending players in a team.—**defenceless, defenseless** adj.—**defencelessness, defenselessness** n.

defend /dəˈfɛnd/ or /dɪ-/ vt to guard or protect; to maintain against attack; (law) to resist, as a claim; to contest (a suit).—**defendable** adj.—**defender** n.

defendant /dəˈfɛndənt/ or /dɪ-/ n a person accused or sued in a lawsuit.

defensible /dəˈfɛnsɪbəl/ or /dɪ-/ adj able to be defended or justified.—**defensibly** adv.—**defensibility** n.

defensive /dəˈfɛnsɪv/ or /dɪ-/ adj serving to defend; in a state or posture of defence.—**defensively** adv.—**defensiveness** n.

defer[1] /dəˈfər/ vt (**deferring, deferred**) to put off to another time; to delay.—**deferrable, deferable** adj.—**deferrer** n.

defer[2] vi (**deferring, deferred**) to yield to another person's wishes, judgment or authority.

deference /ˈdɛfərəns/ n a deferring or yielding in judgment or opinion; polite respect.

deferent /ˈdɛfərənt/ adj deferential (anat) conveying (a fluid, etc) away.

deferential /ˌdɛfəˈrɛnʃəl/ adj expressing deference or respect.—**deferentially** adv.

deferment /dɪˈfərmənt/ or /dɪ-/ n a delay; postponement.

deferral /dəˈfərəl/ n a deferment.

deferred /dɪˈfərd/ or /dɪ-/ adj postponed; (stock, shares) having its dividend payable after other shares.

defiance /dəˈfaɪəns/ n the act of defying; wilful disobedience; a challenge.

defiant /-ənt/ adj characterized by defiance; challenging.—**defiantly** adv.

deficiency /dəˈfɪʃənsi/ or /dɪ-/ n (pl **deficiencies**) being deficient; lack, shortage; deficit.

deficient /dəˈfɪʃənt/ or /dɪ-/ adj insufficient, lacking.—**deficiently** adv.

deficit /ˈdɛfɪsɪt/ n the amount by which an amount falls short of what is required; excess of expenditure over income, or liabilities over assets.

defilade /ˌdɛfɪˈleɪd/ vt to raise (a rampart) to protect defensive lines from guns placed in a high position. • n protection provided in this way.

defile[1] /dəˈfaɪl/ or /diː-/ vt to pollute or corrupt.—**defilement** n.—**defiler** n.

defile[2] n a long, narrow pass or way, through which troops can pass only in single file. • vt to march in single file.

define /dəˈfaɪn/ vt to fix the bounds or limits of; to mark the limits or outline of clearly; to describe accurately; to fix the meaning of.—**definable** adj.—**definer** n.

definite /ˈdɛfɪnɪt/ adj defined; having distinct limits; fixed; exact; clear.—**definiteness** n.

definitely /-li/ adv certainly; distinctly. • interj used to agree emphatically.

definition /ˌdɛfɪˈnɪʃən/ n a description of a thing by its properties; an explanation of the exact meaning of a word, term, or phrase; sharpness of outline.—**definitional** adj.

definitive /-tɪv/ adj defining or limiting; decisive, final.—**definitively** adv.—**definitiveness** n.

definitude /dɪˈfɪnəˌtʊd/ or /-ˌtjuːd/ n the quality of being definite; definiteness, precision.

deflagrate /ˈdɛfləˌgreɪt/ or /ˈdiː-/ vt to set fire to. • vi to cause to burn with sudden and sparkling combustion.—**deflagration** n.

deflate /dəˈfleɪt/ or /dɪ-/ vt to release gas or air from; to reduce in size or importance; to reduce the money supply, restrict credit, etc to reduce inflation in the economy.—**deflator** n.

deflation /dəˈfleɪʃən/ or /di-/ *n* deflating; a reduction in the supply of money, causing a fall in prices.—**deflationary** *adj.*—**deflationist** *adj, n*.

deflect /dəˈflekt/ or /di-/ *vti* to turn or cause to turn aside from a line or proper course.—**deflective** *adj.*—**deflector** *n*.

deflection /dɪˈflekʃən/ or /di-/ *n* the action of deflecting or the state of being deflected from a straight line or regular path; deviation; the turning of a magnetic needle away from its zero; the amount of this.

defloration /ˌdiːflɔrˈeɪʃən/ *n* a deflowering.

deflower /diːˈflaʊr/ *vt* to deprive of virginity; to corrupt the beauty, innocence of.—**deflowerer** *n*.

defoliant /diːˈfoːliənt/ *n* a chemical that kills foliage.

defoliate /-ˌeɪt/ *vt* to strip (a plant or tree) of its leaves.—**defoliation** *n*.—**defoliator** *n*.

deforce /diːˈfɔrs/ *vt* (*law*) to keep (property) out of the legal owner's possession by force; (*Scots law*) to resist (an officer of law in execution of his duty).—**deforcement** *n*.

deforest /diːˈfɔrəst/ or /-fɔrəst/ *vt* to clear of trees.—**deforestation** *n*.—**deforester** *n*.

deform /dəˈfɔrm/ or /di-/ *vt* to spoil the natural form of; to put out of shape.—**deformer** *n*.

deformation /ˌdefɔrˈmeɪʃən/ or /ˌdiː-/ *n* the act of deforming; a change for the worse; a perverted form of word.

deformed /dəˈfɔrmd/ or /di-/ *adj* misshapen; warped.

deformity /dɪˈfɔrmɪti/ *n* (*pl* **deformities**) the condition of being deformed; a deformed part of the body; a defect.

defraud /dɪˈfrɒd/ *vt* to remove (money, rights, etc) from a person by cheating or deceiving.—**defraudation** *n*.—**defrauder** *n*.

defray /dɪˈfreɪ/ *vt* to provide money (to pay expenses, etc).—**defrayable** *adj.*—**defrayal** *n*.—**defrayer** *n*.

defrock /diːˈfrɒk/ *vt* to expel from the priesthood, to unfrock.

defrost /diːˈfrɒst/ *vt* to unfreeze; to free from frost or ice. • *vi* to become unfrozen.

deft /deft/ *adj* skilful, adept; nimble.—**deftly** *adv.*—**deftness** *n*.

defunct /dɪˈfʌŋkt/ *adj* no longer being in existence or function or in use.—**defunctive** *adj*.

defuse /diːˈfjuːz/ *vt* to disarm an explosive (bomb or mine) by removing its fuse; to decrease tension in a (crisis) situation.

defy /dɪˈfaɪ/ *vt* (**defying, defied**) to resist openly and without fear; to challenge (a person) to attempt something considered dangerous or impossible; to resist attempts at, to elude.—**defier** *n*.

dégagé /deɪˈgæʒeɪ/ *adj* unconstrained, at ease.

degauss /diːˈgaʊs/ *vt* to neutralize or remove a magnetic field.—**degausser** *n*.

degeneracy /dɪˈdʒenərəsiː/ *n* (*pl* **degeneracies**) the condition or quality of being degenerate; an instance of degeneracy; something that is degenerate.

degenerate /-eɪt/ *vi*, /dɪˈdʒenərət/ *adj* having declined in physical or moral qualities; sexually deviant. • *vi* to become or grow worse. • *n* a degenerate person.—**degenerately** *adv*.

degeneration /dɪˌdʒenəˈreɪʃən/ *n* the act, state, or process of growing worse; degeneracy; decline; the morbid impairment of any structural tissue or organ.

degenerative /-tɪv/ *adj* of the nature of, or tending to, degenerate.—**degeneratively** *adv*.

deglutinate /diːˈgluːtɪnˌeɪt/ *vt* to extract gluten from; to unglue.—**deglutination** *n*.

deglutition /ˌdiːgluːˈtɪʃən/ *n* the power to swallow, a swallowing.

degradable /diːˈgreɪdəbəl/ or /dɪ-/ *adj* capable of being broken down by biological or chemical action.

degradation /ˌdegrəˈdeɪʃən/ *n* a degrading or being degraded in quality, rank or status; a degraded state; (*geol*) a lowering of land by erosion; (*RC Church*) the unfrocking of a priest.

degrade /dɪˈgreɪd/ *vt* to reduce in rank or status; to disgrace; to decompose; to be lowered by erosion.—**degrader** *n*.

degrading /-ɪŋ/ *adj* humiliating; (*geol*) eroding.—**degradingly** *adv*.

degree /dəˈgriː/ *n* a step in an ascending or descending series; a stage in intensity; the relative quantity in intensity; a unit of measurement in a scale; an academic title awarded as of right or as an honour.

degression /dɪˈgreʃən/ *n* a going down; a decrease, *esp* in taxation rate.—**degressive** *adj*.

dehisce /diːˈhɪs/ *vi* (*fruits, seed pods, etc*) to burst open.

dehiscent /-ənt/ *adj* (*fruits*) opening to release seeds.—**dehiscence** *n*.

dehorn /diːˈhɔrn/ *vt* to cut back, or deprive of, horns.—**dehorner** *n*.

dehumanize /diːˈhjuːmənaɪz/ *vt* to remove human qualities from; to deprive of personality or emotion, to render mechanical.—**dehumanization** *n*.

dehydrate /diːˈhaɪdreɪt/ *vt* to remove water from. • *vi* to lose water, *esp* from the bodily tissues.—**dehydration** *n*.—**dehydrator** *n*.

dehypnotize /diːˈhɪpnəˌtaɪz/ *vt* to rouse from a hypnotic state.

de-ice /diːˈaɪs/ *vt* to prevent the formation of or to remove ice from a surface.—**de-icer** *n*.

deicide /ˈdiːəˌsaɪd/ *n* the killing of a god; the killer of a god.—**deicidal** *adj*.

deictic /ˈdaɪktɪk/ *adj* (*gram*) demonstrative; (*logic*) proving directly.—**deictically** *adv*.

deific /diːˈɪfɪk/ *adj* making, or tending to make, divine.

deify /ˈdiːəˌfaɪ/ *vt* (**deifying, deified**) to make into a god; to worship as a god, glorify.—**deification** *n*.—**deifier** *n*.

deign /deɪn/ *vi* to condescend; to think it worthy to do (something).

deil /diːl/ *n* (*Scot*) the devil.

deism /ˈdiːˌɪzəm/ *n* belief in the existence of God, but not religious revelation.—**deist** *n*.—**deistic, deistical** *adj*.

deity /ˈdiːɪti/ or /ˈdeɪ-/ *n* (*pl* **deities**) a god or goddess; the rank or essence of a god; (*with cap*) God.

déjà vu /ˌdeɪʒɑˈvuː/ or /-ʒɑ-/ *n* the illusion that you have already experienced the present situation.

deject /dəˈdʒekt/ *vt* to have a depressing effect on.

dejecta /dɪˈdʒektə/ *npl* excrement, droppings.

dejected /dɪˈdʒektɪd/ or /dɪ-/ *adj* morose, depressed.—**dejectedly** *adv.*—**dejectedness** *n*.

dejection /dəˈdʒekʃən/ *n* depression; lowness of spirits.

de jure /dɪˈdʒʊriː/ or /deɪˈjʊreɪ/ *adv* according to the law, by right.

deke /diːk/ *n* a fake shot or movement in ice hockey, *esp* to draw an opponent out of position. • *vti* to deceive an opponent with a fake shot or movement.

delaine /dɪˈkleɪn/ *n* a light fabric of wool and cotton.

delate /dəˈleɪt/ *vt* (*formerly*) to inform against (a person); to report (an offence).—**delation** *n*.—**delator** *n*.

delay /dəˈleɪ/ *vt* to postpone to detain, obstruct. • *vi* to linger. • *n* a delaying or being delayed; the time period during which something is delayed.—**delayer** *n*.

delayed penalty *n* a penalty in ice hockey that has been signalled by the referee but for which play has not yet been stopped.

dele /ˈdiːli/ *vt* (**deleing, de ed**) (*print*) to take out a letter, etc, in proofreading. • *n* a mark that a letter, etc, is to be deleted.

delectable /dəˈlektəbəl/ *adj* delightful, delicious.—**delectability** *n.*—**delectably** *adv*.

delectation /ˌdiːlekˈteɪʃən/ *n* delight, enjoyment.

delegate /ˈdeləgeɪt/ *vt* to appoint as a representative; to give powers or responsibilities to (an agent or assembly). • *n* a deputy or an elected representative.—**delegable** *adj*.

delegation /ˌdeləˈgeɪʃən/ *n* the act of delegating; a group of people empowered to represent others.

delete /dəˈliːt/ *vt* to strike out (something written or printed); to erase.

deleterious /ˌdeləˈtɪriːəs/ *adj* harmful or destructive.

deletion /dəˈliːʃən/ *n* the act of deleting; a word, passage, etc, deleted from a text; the absence of a normal part of a chromosome.

delft, delftware /ˈdelftweɪr/ *n* a type of blue-glazed earthenware, originally from Delft in Holland.

deli /ˈdeli/ *n* (*pl* **delis**) (*inf*) a delicatessen.

deliberate /dəˈlɪbərət/ *vt* to consider carefully. • *vi* to discuss or debate thoroughly; to consider. • *adj* well thought out; intentional; cautious.—**deliberately** *adv.*—**deliberateness** *n.*—**deliberator** *n*.

deliberation /ˌdəlɪbəˈreɪʃən/ *n* careful consideration; thorough discussion; caution.

deliberative /dəˈlɪbəˌrətɪv/ *adj* of or appointed for deliberation; as a result of deliberation.—**deliberatively** *adv*.

delicacy /ˈdeləkəsi/ *n* (*pl* **delicacies**) delicateness; sensibility; a luxurious food.

delicate /ˈdeləkət/ *adj* fine in texture; fragile, not robust; requiring tactful handling; of exquisite workmanship; requiring skill in techniques.—**delicately** *adv.*—**delicateness** *n*.

delicatessen /ˌdeləkəˈtesən/ *n* a store selling prepared foods, *esp* imported delicacies.

delicious /dəˈlɪʃəs/ *adj* having a pleasurable effect on the senses, *esp* taste; delightful.—**deliciously** *adv*.—**deliciousness** *n*.

delict /dəˈlɪkt/ or /ˈdiː-/ *n* a legal offence.

delight /dəˈlaɪt/ *vt* to please greatly. • *vi* to have or take great pleasure (in). • *n* great pleasure; something that causes this.—**delighter** *n*.

delighted /-ɪd/ *adj* very pleased; filled with delight.—**delightedly** *adv*.—**delightedness** *n*.

delightful /-fʊl/ *adj* giving great pleasure.—**delightfully** *adv*.—**delightfulness** *n*.

delimit /diːˈlɪmɪt/ **delimitate** *vt* to fix or mark the boundaries of.—**delimitation** *n*.—**delimitative** *adj*.

delineate /dəˈlɪniˌeɪt/ *vt* to describe in great detail; to represent by drawing.—**delineation** *n*.—**delineative** *adj*.

delineator /-ər/ *n* one who delineates; an adjustable tailor's pattern.

delinquency /dəˈlɪŋkwənsi/ *n* (*pl* **delinquencies**) neglect of or failure in duty; a misdeed; a fault; antisocial or illegal behaviour, *esp* by young people.—*also* **juvenile delinquency**.

delinquent /-kwənt/ *adj* negligent; guilty of an offence. • *n* a person guilty of a misdeed, *esp* a young person who breaks the law.

deliquesce /ˌdɛləˈkwɛs/ *vi* to melt and become liquid by absorbing moisture from the atmosphere.—**deliquescence** *n*.—**deliquescent** *adj*.

delirious /dəˈlɪːriəs/ *adj* mentally confused, light-headed; wildly excited.—**deliriously** *adv*.—**deliriousness** *n*.

delirium /dəˈlɪːriəm/ *n* (*pl* **deliriums, deliria**) a state of mental disorder, *esp* caused by a feverish illness; wild enthusiasm.

delirium tremens /ˈtrɛmɛnz/ *n* a disorder of the brain, causing delusions and violent trembling, as the result of excessive drinking.

deliver /dəˈlɪvər/ *vt* (*goods, letters, etc*) to transport to a destination; to distribute regularly; to liberate, to rescue; to give birth; to assist at a birth; (*blow*) to launch; (*baseball*) to pitch; (*speech*) to utter.—**deliverable** *adj*.—**deliverer** *n*.

deliverance /dəˈlɪvərəns/ *n* the act of rescuing or liberating.

delivery /dəˈlɪvəri/ *n* (*pl* **deliveries**) the act of delivering; anything delivered or communicated; the manner of delivering (a speech, etc); the manner of bowling in cricket, etc; the act of giving birth.

dell /dɛl/ *n* a small hollow, *usu* with trees.

delocalize /diːˈloʊkəˌlaɪz/ *vt* to deprive of local character; to remove from a locality.—**delocalization** *n*.

delouse /diːˈlaʊs/ *vt* to rid the lice from.

Delphic /ˈdɛlfɪk/, **Delphian** /-fiən/ *adj* relating to the ancient Greek city or its famous oracle which imparted enigmatic prophecies; obscure or ambiguous in meaning.

delphinium /dɛlˈfɪniəm/ *n* a garden plant with spikes of, *usu* blue, flowers.

delta /ˈdɛltə/ *n* the fourth letter of the Greek alphabet; an alluvial deposit at the mouth of a river.—**deltaic** *adj*.

delta wing *n* a triangular-shaped aircraft wing.

deltoid /ˈdɛltɔɪd/ *adj* of the shape of the letter delta; triangular. • *n* (*anat*) a muscle that lifts the upper arm.

delude /dəˈluːd/ *vt* to mislead, to deceive.—**deluder** *n*.

deluge /ˈdɛljuːʒ/ or /-juːdʒ/ *n* a flood; anything happening in a heavy rush. • *vt* to inundate.

delusion /dəˈluːʒən/ *n* a false belief; a persistent false belief that is a symptom of mental illness.—**delusional** *adj*.

delusive /dəˈluːsɪv/ *adj* deluding or tending to delude; deceptive; false.—**delusively** *adv*.

delusory /dəˈluːsəri/ *adj* delusive.

deluxe /dəˈlʌks/ *adj* luxurious, of superior quality.

delve /dɛlv/ *vti* to search deeply; to dig.—**delver** *n*.

demagnetize /diːˈmæɡnəˌtaɪz/ *vt* to remove the magnetic properties of.—**demagnetization** *n*.—**demagnetizer** *n*.

demagogic /ˌdɛməˈɡɒdʒɪk/ or /-ˈɡɒɡɪk/, /-ˈɡoʊdʒɪk/, **demagogical** *adj* of, pertaining to, or characteristic of a demagogue.—**demagogically** *adv*.

demagogue, demagog /ˈdɛməˌɡɒɡ/ *n* a political orator who derives power from appealing to popular prejudices.

demagoguery /-ˈɡɒɡəri/ *n* demagogy; the rhetoric of a demagogue.

demagogy /-ˈɡɒɡi/ or /-ˈɡɒɡi/ *n* the principles or practice of a demagogue; rule by a demagogue.

demand /dəˈmænd/ *vt* to ask for in an authoritative manner. • *n* a request or claim made with authority for what is due; an urgent claim; desire for goods and services shown by consumers.—**demandable** *adj*.—**demander** *n*.

demandant /-dənt/ *n* a plaintiff.

demanding /-ɪŋ/ *adj* constantly making demands; requiring great skill, concentration or effort.—**demandingly** *adv*.

demantoid /dəˈmæntɔɪd/ *n* an emerald green garnet used as a gem.

demarcate /ˈdiːmɑːˌkeɪt/ *vt* to delimit; to define or mark the bounds of.—**demarcator** *n*.

demarcation, demarkation /ˌdiːmɑːˈkeɪʃən/ *n* the act of marking off a boundary or setting a limit to; a limit; the strict separation of the type of work done by members of different trade unions.

démarche /deɪˈmɑːʃ/ *n* a diplomatic announcement of policy or plan.

demark /diːˈmɑːk/ *vt* to demarcate.

dematerialize /ˌdiːməˈtɪːriəˌlaɪz/ *vti* to deprive of or give up material form.—**dematerialization** *n*.

deme /diːm/ *n* a territorial subdivision or township of ancient Greece; (*biol*) a group within a species with similar cell structure, etc.

demean /dəˈmiːn/ *vt* to lower in dignity.—**demeaning** *adj*.

demeanour, demeanor /dəˈmiːnər/ *n* behaviour; bearing.

dement /dəˈmɛnt/ *vt* to make insane, to drive mad.

demented /-əd/ *adj* crazy, insane.—**dementedly** *adv*.

dementia /dɪˈmɛnʃə/ or /-ʃiə/ *n* the failure or loss of mental powers.

demerge /diːˈmɜːdʒ/ *vt* to separate a previously merged business corporation into several companies.—**demerger** *n*.

demerit /diːˈmɛrɪt/ *n* a fault, a defect; a mark recording poor work by a student, etc.

demersal /dəˈmɜːsəl/ *adj* (*zool*) found in deep water or on the sea bottom.

demesne /dəˈmiːn/ or /-ˈmeɪn/ *n* (*law*) one's own land; (*hist*) a landed estate attached to a manor; a domain.

demi- /ˈdɛmi/ *prefix* half.

demigod /ˈdɛmiˌɡɒd/ *n* a being that is part mortal part god; a god-like individual.—**demigoddess** *nf*.

demijohn /-ˌdʒɒn/ *n* a large bottle, often in a wicker case.

demilitarize /diːˈmɪlətəˌraɪz/ *vt* to remove armed forces, weapons systems, etc from.—**demilitarization** *n*.

demimondaine /ˈdɛmimɒnˌdeɪn/ or /-mɔ̃ˌdeɪn/ *n* a member of the demimonde, a courtesan.

demimonde /ˈdɛmiˌmɒnd/ or /-ˈmɔ̃d/ *n* a class of women not recognized by society, *esp* in 19th-century France, because of promiscuity; any socially disreputable group.

demise /dəˈmaɪz/ *n* (*formal*) death; termination, end. • *vt* to give or grant by will. • *vi* to pass by bequest or inheritance.—**demisable** *adj*.

demisemiquaver /ˌdɛmiˈsɛmiˌkweɪvər/ *n* (*mus*) a note with a time value of half a semiquaver.—*also* **thirty-second note**.

demitasse /ˈdɛmiˌtæs/ *n* a small cup (of black coffee).

demiurge /ˈdɛmiˌɜːdʒ/ *n* in Platonic philosophy, the creator of the world; in Gnostic philosophy, an agent of the Supreme Being in the creation of man and the material universe; in ancient Greece, the chief magistrate of some states.—**demiurgic** *adj*.

demo /ˈdɛmoʊ/ *n* (*pl* **demos**) (*inf*) a demonstration.

demob /diːˈmɒb/ *vt* (**demobbing, demobbed**) (*inf*) to demobilize. • *n* (*inf*) demobilization.

demobilize /diːˈmoʊbəˌlaɪz/ *vt* to discharge from the armed forces.—**demobilization** *n*.

democracy /dəˈmɒkrəsi/ *n* (*pl* **democracies**) a form of government by the people through elected representatives; a country governed by its people; political, social or legal equality.

democrat /ˈdɛməˌkræt/ *n* a person who believes in or promotes democracy; (*with cap*) a member of the Democratic Party in the US.

democratic /ˌdɛməˈkrætɪk/ *adj* of, relating to, or supporting the principles of democracy; favouring or upholding equal rights; (*with cap*) of or pertaining to the Democratic Party in the US.—**democratically** *adv*.

democratize /dəˈmɒkrəˌtaɪz/ *vt* to make democratic. • *vi* to become democratic.—**democratization** *n*.

démodé /deɪmoʊˈdeɪ/ *adj* out of fashion.

demodulate /diːˈmɒdjʊˌleɪt/ *vt* to extract a modulating (radio, video, etc) wave or signal from a modulated carrier wave.—**demodulator** *n*.—**demodulation** *n*.

demography /dəˈmɒɡrəfi/ *n* the study of population statistics concerning birth, marriage, death and disease.—**demographer, demographist** *n*.—**demographic** *adj*.—**demographically** *adv*.

demoiselle /ˌdɛmwæˈzɛl/ *n* a damsel; a small crane of North Africa, southeast Europe and central Asia.

demolish /dəˈmɒlɪʃ/ vt (a building) to pull down or knock down; (an argument) to defeat; (inf) to eat up.—**demolisher** n.—**demolishment** n.

demolition /ˌdeməˈlɪʃən/ n a demolishing or being demolished, esp by explosives.—**demolitionist** adj, n.

demon /ˈdiːmən/ n an evil spirit; a cruel person; someone who is very skilled, energetic, hard-working, etc.—**demonic** adj.—**demonically** adv.

demonetize /diːˈmɒnɪˌtaɪz/ vt to withdraw (coin) from circulation; to abandon (gold etc) as a currency.—**demonetization** n.

demoniac, demoniacal /dəˈmoʊnɪˌæk/ or /ˈdiːməˌnaɪæk/ adj of or like a demon; possessed by evil; frenzied, energetic. • n a person possessed by a demon.—**demoniacally** adv.

demonism /ˈdiːməˌnɪzəm/ n belief in demons; the nature of a demon.—**demonist** n.

demonize /-aɪz/ vt to make into or represent as a demon.

demonolater /-əletər/ n a demon worshipper.—**demonolatry** n.

demonology /-ˈnɒlədʒi/ n the study of demons and superstitions about them.—**demonologist** n.

demonstrable /dəˈmɒnstrəbəl/ adj able to be demonstrated or proved.—**demonstrability** n.—**demonstrably** adv.

demonstrate /ˈdemənˌstreɪt/ vt to indicate or represent clearly; to provide certain evidence of, prove; to show how something (a machine, etc) works. • vi to show one's support for a cause, etc by public parades and protests; to act as a demonstrator of machinery, etc.—**demonstrational** adj.

demonstration /ˌdemənˈstreɪʃən/ n proof by evidence; a display or exhibition; a display of feeling; a public manifestation of opinion, as by a mass meeting, march, etc; a display of armed force.

demonstrative /dəˈmɒnstrətɪv/ adj displaying one's feelings openly and unreservedly; indicative; conclusive; (gram) describing an adjective or pronoun indicating the person or thing referred to.—**demonstratively** adv.—**demonstrativeness** n.

demonstrator /ˈdemənˌstreɪtər/ n a person who shows consumer goods to the public; one who or that which shows how a machine, etc works; a person who takes part in a public protest.

demoralize /dɪˈmɒrəˌlaɪz/ vt to lower the morale of, discourage.—**demoralization** n.—**demoralizer** n.

demos /ˈdiːˌmɒs/ n in ancient Greece, the common people of a state; the population personified.

demote /diːˈmoʊt/ or /də-/ vt to reduce in rank or position.—**demotion** n.

demotic /dəˈmɒtɪk/ adj pertaining to the people; in the simplified style of ancient Egyptian writing.

demulcent /dəˈmʌlsənt/ adj softening; soothing. • n a medicine that allays irritation.

demur /dəˈmər/ vi (**demurring, demurred**) to raise objections.—**demurral** n.

demure /dəˈmjʊr/ adj modest, reserved; affectedly quiet and proper; coy.—**demurely** adv.—**demureness** n.

demurrage /dəˈmɜrɪdʒ/ n a charge for keeping a ship, truck, etc beyond the time agreed for unloading.

demurrer /dəˈmɜrər/ n (law) a plea that an opponent's facts are irrelevant; exception taken.

demy /dɪˈmaɪ/ n (pl **demies**) a size of paper for printing (22½ x 17½ ins) or writing (20 x 15½ ins).

demystify /diːˈmɪstəˌfaɪ/ vt (**demystifying, demystified**) to remove the mystery from; clarify.—**demystification** n.

den /den/ n a cave or lair of a wild beast; a place where people gather for illegal activities; a room in a house for relaxation or study.

denarius /dəˈneriəs/ n (pl **denarii**) in ancient Rome, a silver coin; a gold coin worth 25 silver denarii.

denary /ˈdiːnəri/ adj of ten; decimal.

denationalize /diːˈnæʃənəˌlaɪz/ vt to transfer (industry, etc) from state control to private ownership.—**denationalization** n.

denaturalize /diːˈnætʃərəˌlaɪz/ vt to make unnatural; to deprive of acquired citizenship.—**denaturalization** n.

denature /diːˈneɪtʃər/ vt to modify the nature of; to change the properties of (a protein) by the action of an acid or heat; to render (alcohol) unfit for consumption.—**denaturant** n.—**denaturation** n.

dendriform /ˈdendrɪˌfɔrm/ or /-drə-/ adj branching, like a tree.

dendrite /ˈdendraɪt/ n a stone or mineral with tree-like markings; a fine branch of one of the nerve cells that conduct impulses.—**dendritic** adj.

dendrochronology /ˌdendroʊkrəˈnɒlədʒi/ n the dating of past events by studying the annual growth rings in trees.—**dendrochronological** adj.

dendroid /ˈdendrɔɪd/ adj resembling a tree in appearance.

dendrology /denˈdrɒlədʒi/ n the scientific study of trees.—**dendrologic, dendrological** adj.—**dendrologist** n.

dene /diːn/ n a low sandy tract near sea, a dune.

Dene /deneɪ/ n ✿ (Cdn) n a member of a First Nations people in the Canadian north. • adj of or pertaining to this people.

denegation /ˌdenəˈɡeɪʃən/ n a denial.

dengue /ˈdeŋɡɪ/ n a tropical disease transmitted by the mosquito, causing fever and pain in the joints.

deniable /dɪˈnaɪəbəl/ adj able to be denied; questionable.—**deniably** adv.

denial /dɪˈnaɪəl/ n the act of denying; a refusal of a request, etc; a refusal or reluctance to admit the truth of something.

denier[1] /ˈdenjər/ n a unit of weight used to measure the fineness of silk, nylon or rayon fibre, esp as used in women's tights, etc.

denier[2] /dɪˈnaɪr/ one who denies.

denigrate /ˈdenɪˌɡreɪt/ vt to disparage the character of; to belittle.—**denigration** n.—**denigrator** n.

denim /ˈdenəm/ n a hard-wearing cotton cloth, esp used for jeans; (pl) denim trousers or jeans.

denizen /ˈdenɪzən/ n an inhabitant, resident; an animal or plant established in a region where it is not native.

denominate /dəˈnɒmɪˌneɪt/ vt to give a name to; to designate.

denomination /dəˌnɒmɪˈneɪʃən/ n a name or title; a religious group comprising many local churches, larger than a sect; one of a series of related units, esp monetary.

denominational /dɪˌnɒmɪˈneɪʃənəl/ adj of, belonging to or controlled by a religious denomination.—**denominationally** adv.

denominationalism /-ɪzəm/ n denominational spirit, policy or principles; adherence to these.—**denominationalist**.

denominative /diːˈnɒmɪnətɪv/ adj giving a name; (gram) formed from a substantive or adjectival stem; connotative. • n a verb formed from a substantive or adjectival stem.

denominator /dɪˈnɒmɪˌneɪtər/ n the part of a fractional expression written below the fraction line.

denotation /ˌdiːnoʊˈteɪʃən/ n the action of denoting; expression by marks, signs or symbols; a sign, indication; a mark by which a thing is made known; designation, meaning.

denotative /ˌdiːnoʊˈteɪtɪv/ adj having the power to denote or point out; significant.—**denotatively** adv.

denote /diːˈnoʊt/ vt to indicate, be the sign of; to mean.—**denotement** n.

denouement, dénouement /ˌdeɪnuːˈmɑ̃/ n the resolution of a plot or story; the solution, the outcome.

denounce /dɪˈnaʊns/ vt to condemn or censure publicly; to inform against; to declare formally the ending of (treaties, etc).—**denouncement** n.—**denouncer** n.

dense /dens/ adj difficult to see through; massed closely together; dull-witted, stupid.—**densely** adv.—**denseness** n.

density /ˈdensɪti/ n (pl **densities**) the degree of denseness or concentration; stupidity; the ratio of mass to volume.

dent /dent/ n a depression made by pressure or a blow. • vti to make a dent or become dented.

dental /ˈdentəl/ adj of or for the teeth.—**dentally** adv.

dental floss n waxed thread for cleaning between the teeth.

dental hygienist n a professionally trained and qualified person who checks and cleans teeth.—also **hygienist**.

dentate /ˈdenteɪt/ adj toothed, notched.

denticle /ˈdentɪkəl/ n a small tooth or tooth-like projection.

denticulate /denˈtɪkjʊlət/ or /-ˌleɪt/ adj (leaf) having small teeth.

dentiform /ˈdentəˌfɔrm/ adj tooth-shaped.

dentifrice /ˈdentəfrɪs/ n toothpowder or toothpaste.

dentil /ˈdentɪl/ n (arch) a small, square, projecting block on a moulding.

dentin, dentine /ˈdentiːn/ n the hard, bone-like substance forming the main part of teeth.

dentist /ˈdentɪst/ n a person qualified to treat tooth decay, gum disease, etc.

dentistry /-ɪstri/ n the area of medicine dealing with the care of teeth and the treatment of diseases of the teeth and gums; the practice of this as a profession.

dentition /denˈtɪʃən/ n the process or period of cutting the teeth; the arrangement of the teeth.

dentoid /ˈdenˌtɔɪd/ adj tooth-shaped.

denture /'dɛntʃər/ n (usu pl) a set of artificial teeth.

denude /dɪ'nuːd/ or /-'njuːd/ vt to make naked; to deprive, strip.—**denudation** n.—**denuder** n.

denunciate /dɪ'nʌnsɪˌeɪt/ vt (rare) to denounce.—**denunciator** n.

denunciation /dɪˌnʌnsɪ'eɪʃən/ n the act of denouncing; a threat.—**denunciator** n.—**denunciatory** adj.

deny /dɪ'naɪ/ or /də-/ vt (**denying, denied**) to declare to be untrue; to repudiate; to refuse to acknowledge; to refuse to assent to a request, etc.

deodand /'diːoʊˌdænd/ n (law) (hist) a chattel that, having caused death, was forfeited to the crown.

deodar /'diːəˌdɑr/ n a tall Himalayan cedar tree yielding a valuable timber.

deodorant /diː'oːdərənt/ n a substance that removes or masks unpleasant odours.

deodorize /diː'oːdəˌraɪz/ vt to remove the odour or smell from.—**deodorization** n.—**deodorizer** n.

deoxidize /diː'ɒksəˌdaɪz/ vt to deprive of oxygen.

dépanneur /'depənər/ n ♣ (Cdn) in Quebec, a small store with extended hours that sells food and other items.

depart /də'pɑrt/ vi to go away, leave; to deviate (from).

departed /-əd/ adj (time, etc) long past; (person) recently dead.

department /də'pɑrtmənt/ n a unit of specialized functions into which an organization or business is divided; a province; a realm of activity.

departmental /ˌdiːpɑrt'mɛntəl/ adj of, having, or organized into departments.—**departmentally** adv.

departmentalism /-ɪzəm/ n departmental structure, esp a bureaucratic one.

departmentalize /-aɪz/ vt to split into departments; to subdivide.—**departmentalization** n.

department store n a large store divided into various departments selling different types of goods.

departure /də'pɑrtʃər/ n a departing; a deviating from normal practice; a new venture, course of action, etc.

depend /də'pɛnd/ or /dɪ-/ vi to be determined by or connected with anything; to rely (on), put trust (in); to be reliant on for support, esp financially.

dependable /-əbəl/ adj able to be relied on.—**dependably** adv.—**dependability** n.

dependant, dependent /-dənt/ or /di-/ n a person who is dependent on another, esp financially.

dependence, dependance /-dəns/ n the state of being dependent; reliance, trust; a physical or mental reliance on a drug, person, etc.

dependency /-si/ n (pl **dependencies**) dependence; a territory controlled by another country.

dependent, dependant adj relying on another person, thing, etc for support, money, etc; contingent; subordinate.

depersonalize /diː'pɜrsənəˌlaɪz/ vt to eliminate the individual character from a person, organization, etc; to make impersonal.—**depersonalization** n.

depict /də'pɪkt/ or /di-/ vt to represent pictorially; to describe.—**depicter, depictor** n.—**depiction** n.

depilate /'dɛpɪˌleɪt/ vt to remove hair from.—**depilation** n.—**depilator** n.

depilatory /də'pɪləˌtori/ n (pl **depilatories**) a substance for removing superfluous hair. • adj removing hair.

deplane /diː'pleɪn/ vti to alight or unload from an aircraft.

deplete /di'pliːt/ vt to use up a large quantity of.—**depletion** n.—**depletive** adj.

deplorable /diː'plɔrəbəl/ adj shocking; extremely bad.—**deplorably** adv.

deplore /diː'plɔr/ vt to regret deeply; to complain of; to deprecate.—**deplorer** n.—**deploringly** adv.

deploy /diː'plɔɪ/ vt (military forces) to distribute and position strategically. • vi to adopt strategic positions within an area.—**deployment** n.

deplume /diː'pluːm/ vt to strip of feathers, to pluck; to strip of position, honour, etc.—**deplumation** n.

depolarize /diː'poːləˌraɪz/ vt to deprive of or counteract the polarity of.—**depolarization** n.

depone /diː'poːn/ vti (Scot) to testify upon oath, to depose.

deponent /diː'poːnənt/ adj (gram) (verb) passive in form but active in meaning. • n (gram) a deponent verb; (law) one who makes a deposition.

depopulate /diː'pɒpjuˌleɪt/ vt to reduce the population of.—**depopulation** n.—**depopulator** n.

deport /diː'pɔrt/ vt to expel (an undesirable person) from a country; to behave (in a certain manner).—**deportable** adj.

deportation /ˌdiːpɔr'teɪʃən/ n forcible removal from a country, esp of an undesirable person.

deportee /ˌdiːpɔr'tiː/ n a deported person.

deportment /diː'pɔrtmənt/ n manners; bearing; behaviour.

depose /diː'poːz/ vt to remove from power; to testify, esp in court.—**deposable** adj.—**deposer** n.

deposit /diː'pɒzət/ or /də-/ vt to place or lay down; to pay money into a bank or other institution for safekeeping, to earn interest, etc; to pay as a first instalment; to let fall, leave. • n something deposited for safekeeping; money put in a bank; money given in part payment or security; material left in a layer, eg sediment.

depositary /diː'pɒzɪteri/ n (pl **depositaries**) the person to whom something is entrusted; a depository.

deposition /ˌdepə'zɪʃən/ or /ˌdiːp-/ n the act of depositing or deposing; a being removed from office or power; a sworn testimony, esp in writing.

depositor /diː'pɒzɪtər/ n a person who deposits money in a bank, etc.

depository /-ˌtori/ n (pl **depositories**) a place where anything is deposited; a depositary.

depot /'depo/ or /'diːpo/ n a warehouse, storehouse; a place for storing military supplies; a military training centre; a bus or railway station.

deprave /di'preɪv/ vt to pervert; to corrupt morally.—**depravation** n.—**depraver** n.

depraved /-'preɪvd/ adj morally debased; corrupt; made bad or worse.—**depravedly** adv.

depravity /di'præviti/ n (pl **depravities**) moral corruption; extreme wickedness.

deprecate /'dɛprɪˌkeɪt/ vt to criticize, esp mildly or politely; to belittle.—**deprecation** n.—**deprecative** adj.—**deprecator** n.

deprecative /'dɛprɪkətɪv/ adj deprecatory.

deprecatory /-'kətəri/ adj apologetic; disapproving, belittling.

depreciate /dɪ'priːʃiˌeɪt/ vti to make or become lower in value.—**depreciator** n.—**depreciatory, depreciative** adj.

depreciation /dɪˌpriːʃi'eɪʃən/ or /-si'eɪʃən/ n a fall in value, esp of an asset through wear and tear; an allowance for this deducted from gross profit; disparagement.

depredate /'dɛprəˌdeɪt/ vt to pillage; to rob; to lay waste; to prey upon.—**depredator** n.

depredation /ˌdɛprə'deɪʃən/ n plundering; pillage.

depress /diː'prɛs/ vt to push down; to sadden, dispirit; to lessen the activity of.—**depressing** adj.—**depressingly** adv.

depressant /-ənt/ adj causing depression. • n a substance that reduces the activity of the nervous system; a drug that acts as a depressant.

depressed /diː'prɛst/ or /dɪ-/ adj cast down in spirits; lowered in position; flattened from above, or vertically.

depression /diː'prɛʃən/ n excessive gloom and despondency; an abnormal state of physiological inactivity; a phase of the business cycle characterized by stagnation, widespread unemployment, etc; a falling in or sinking; a lowering of atmospheric pressure, often signalling rain.

depressive /-sɪv/ adj depressing; tending to suffer from mental depression.—**depressively** adv.

depressor /-sər/ n one who or that which depresses; a muscle that draws down an organ or part.

deprive /diː'praɪv/ or /də-/ vt to take a thing away from; to prevent from using or enjoying.—**deprivation** n.

deprived /-'praɪvd/ adj lacking the essentials of life, such as adequate food, shelter, education, etc.

dept. abbr = department.

depth /dɛpθ/ n deepness; the distance downwards or inwards; the intensity of emotion or feeling; the profundity of thought; intensity of colour; the mid point of the night or winter; the lowness of sound or pitch; the quality of being deep.

depth charge n a bomb designed to explode under water, used against submarines.

depurate /'dɛpjuˌreɪt/ vti to free or become free from impurities.—**depuration** n.—**depurative** adj.—**depurator** n.

deputation /ˌdɛpju'teɪʃən/ n a person or group appointed to represent others.

depute /dɪ'pjuːt/ vt to appoint as one's representative; to delegate.

deputize /'dɛpjuˌtaɪz/ vi to act as deputy.—**deputization** n.

deputy /'depjuti/ *n* (*pl* **deputies**) a delegate, representative, or substitute.

deputy minister *n* ✤ (*Cdn*) a civil servant who acts as a deputy to the head of a government department or ministry.

deracinate /diː'ræsɪ.neɪt/ *vt* to tear up by the roots.—**deracination** *n*.

derail /diː'reɪl/ *vti* (*train*) to cause to leave the rails.—**derailment** *n*.

derailleur /diː'reɪlər/ *n* a system of gearing on a bicycle.

derange /diː'reɪndʒ/ *vt* to throw into confusion; to disturb; to make insane.—**deranged** *adj*.—**derangement** *n*.

derby /'dɑːbi/ *n* (*pl* **derbies**) a bowler hat.

deregulate /diː'regjʊ.leɪt/ *vt* to remove (*eg* government) regulations or controls from (an industry, etc).—**deregulation** *n*.

derelict /'derə.lɪkt/ *adj* abandoned, deserted and left to decay; negligent. • *n* a person abandoned by society; a wrecked ship or vehicle.

dereliction /.derɪ'lɪkʃən/ *n* neglect (of duty); abandonment.

deride /də'raɪd/ *vt* to scorn, mock.

de rigueur /dərɪ'gɜːr/ *adj* required by fashion or etiquette.

derisible /dɪ'rɪzɪbəl/ *adj* open to derision.

derision /də'rɪʒən/ *n* ridicule.

derisive /də'raɪsɪv/ *adj* full of derision; mocking, scornful.—**derisively** *adv*.—**derisiveness** *n*.

derisory /-səri/ *adj* showing or deserving of derision.

derivation /.derɪ'veɪʃən/ *n* the tracing of a word to its root; origin; descent.—**derivational** *adj*.

derivative /də'rɪvətɪv/ *adj* derived from something else; not original. • *n* something that is derived; a word formed by derivation; (*math*) the rate of change of one quantity with respect to another.—**derivatively** *adv*.

derive /də'raɪv/ *vt* to take or receive from a source; to infer, deduce (from). • *vi* to issue as a derivative (from).—**derivable** *adj*.—**deriver** *n*.

dermal /'dɜːməl/ *adj* of the skin; consisting of skin.

dermatitis /.dɜːmə'taɪtɪs/ *n* inflammation of the skin.

dermatology /.dɜːmə'tɒlədʒi/ *n* the science of the skin and its diseases.—**dermatologic, dermatological** *adj*.—**dermatologist** *n*.

dermic /'dɜːmɪk/ *adj* dermal.

dermis /'dɜːmɪs/ *n* the fine skin below the epidermis containing blood vessels.

derogate /'derə.geɪt/ *vti* to detract (from); to lose face; to degenerate; to take a part (from).—**derogation** *n*.

derogatory /də'rɒgətəri/ *adj* disparaging; deliberately offensive.—**derogatorily** *adv*.

derrick /'derɪk/ *n* any crane-like apparatus; a tower over an oil well, etc, holding the drilling machinery.

derring-do /.derɪŋ'duː/ *n* bravery, reckless valour.

derringer /'derɪndʒər/ *n* a pocket pistol with a short barrel of very large calibre.

dervish /'dɜːvɪʃ/ *n* a member of a Muslim religious order vowing chastity and poverty, noted for frenzied, whirling dancing.

desalinate /diː'sælɪ.neɪt/ *vt* to remove the salt from (seawater, etc).—**desalination** *n*.—**desalinator** *n*.

descant /'des.kænt/ *n* a musical accompaniment sung or played in counterpoint to the main melody.—*also vi*.

descend /də'send/ *vi* to come or climb down; to pass from a higher to a lower place or condition; (*with* **on, upon**) to make a sudden attack upon, or visit unexpectedly; to sink in morals or dignity; to be derived. • *vt* to go, pass, or extend down.

descendant /də'sendənt/ *n* a person who is descended from an ancestor; something derived from an earlier form.

descendent *adj* descending; sinking.

descendible /-əbəl/ *adj* (*law*) that may be inherited; transmissible.

descent /də'sent/ *n* a descending; a downward motion or step; a way down; a slope; a raid or invasion; lineage, ancestry.

describe /də'skraɪb/ *vt* to give a verbal account of; to trace out.—**describable** *adj*.—**describer** *n*.

description /də'skrɪpʃən/ *n* a verbal or pictorial account; a sort, a kind.

descriptive /də'skrɪptɪv/ *adj* tending to or serving to describe.—**descriptively** *adv*.—**descriptiveness** *n*.

descry /də'skraɪ/ *vt* (**descrying, descried**) to catch sight of.

desecrate /'desə.kreɪt/ *vt* to violate a sacred place by destructive or blasphemous behaviour.—**desecration** *n*.—**desecrator, desecrater** *n*.

desegregate /diː'segrə.geɪt/ *vt* to abolish (racial or sexual) segregation in.—**desegregation** *n*.

desert /də'zɜːt/ *n* (*often pl*) a deserved reward or punishment.

desert *vt* to leave, abandon, with no intention of returning; to abscond from the armed forces without permission.—**deserter** *n*.—**desertion** *n*.

desert /'dezət/ *n* a dry, barren region, able to support little or no life; a place lacking in some essential quality.

desertification /də.zɜːtɪfɪ'keɪʃən/ *n* the transformation of fertile land into arid waste or desert through soil erosion, overcultivation, etc.

desertion /dɪ'zɜːʃən/ *n* deserting; being forsaken.

deserve /də'zɜːv/ *vt* to merit or be suitable for (some reward, punishment, etc).

deserved /-vəd/ *adj* justly earned, merited.—**deservedly** *adv*.—**deservedness** *n*.

deserving /-ɪŋ/ *adj* worthy of support, *esp* financially.

deshabille /.dezæ'biːeɪ/ or /.deɪzæ'biːl/ *see* **dishabille**.

desiccate /'desɪ.keɪt/ *vti* to dry or become dried up; to preserve (food) by drying.—**desiccation** *n*.—**desiccative** *adj*.

desiccator /-ər/ *n* an apparatus for drying foods and other substances.

desiderate /də'zɪdər.eɪt/ *vt* to feel the lack of, to desire earnestly.—**desideration** *n*.—**desiderative** *adj*.

desideratum /də.zɪdə'rætəm/ or /-.sɪd-/ *n* (*pl* **desiderata**) anything desired; a want or desire generally felt and recognized.

design /də'zaɪn/ *vt* to plan to create; to devise; to make working drawings for; to intend. • *n* a working drawing; a mental plan or scheme; the particular form or disposition of something; a decorative pattern; purpose; (*pl*) dishonest intent.

designate /'dezɪg.neɪt/ *vt* to indicate, specify; to name; to appoint to or nominate for a position, office. • *adj* (*after noun*) appointed to office but not yet installed.—**designator** *n*.

designation /.dezɪg'neɪʃən/ *n* the act of designating; nomination; a distinguishing name or title.

designedly /də'zaɪnədli/ *adv* intentionally.

designer /də'zaɪnər/ *n* a person who designs things; a person who is renowned for creating high-class fashion clothes. • *adj* (*inf*) trendy, of the latest, *esp* expensive, fashion.

designer drug *n* a synthetic narcotic or hallucinogenic substance which mimics the chemical structure and effects of banned drugs but is not yet covered by anti-drug laws.

designing /-ɪŋ/ *adj* crafty, scheming. • *n* the art or practice of making designs.

desirable /də'zaɪrəbəl/ *adj* arousing (sexual) desire; advisable or beneficial; worth doing.—**desirability** *n*.—**desirably** *adv*.

desire /də'zaɪr/ *vt* to long or wish for; to request, ask for. • *n* a longing for something regarded as pleasurable or satisfying; a request; something desired; sexual craving.

desirous /-əs/ *adj* desiring; craving.

desist /də'sɪst/ *vi* to stop (doing something).—**desistance** *n*.

desk /desk/ *n* a piece of furniture with a writing surface and *usu* drawers; a counter behind which a cashier, etc sits; the section of a newspaper responsible for a particular topic.

desktop *n* the surface of a desk; (*comput*) the backdrop on a computer screen on which icons and windows appear.

desktop publishing *n* the use of a computer with sophisticated page-layout programs and a laser printer to produce professional-looking printed matter.

desman /'desmən/ *n* (*pl* **desmans**) a small amphibious animal similar to a mole.

desmoid /-.mɔɪd/ *adj* having the characteristics of, or resembling, a ligament; (*tumour*) fibrous.

desolate /'desələt/ *adj* solitary, lonely; devoid of inhabitants; laid waste; forlorn, disconsolate; overwhelmed with grief. • *vt* to depopulate; to devastate, lay waste; to make barren or unfit for habitation; to leave alone, forsake, abandon; to overwhelm with grief.—**desolately** *adv*.—**desolateness** *n*.—**desolator, desolater** *n*.

desolated /'desə.leɪtəd/ *adj* wretched, lonely, miserable.

desolation /.desə'leɪʃən/ *n* destruction, ruin; a barren state; loneliness; wretchedness.

despair /də'sper/ *vi* to have no hope. • *n* utter loss of hope; something that causes despair.

despatch /də'spætʃ/ *see* **dispatch**.

desperado /.despə'rɑːdoʊ/ *n* (*pl* **desperadoes, desperados**) a violent criminal.

desperate /'despərət/ *adj* (almost) hopeless; reckless through lack of hope; urgently requiring (money, etc); (*remedy*) extreme, dangerous.—**desperately** *adv*.—**desperateness** *n*.

desperation /ˌdɛspəˈreɪʃən/ *n* loss of hope; recklessness from despair.

despicable /dəˈspɪkəbəl/ or /ˈdɛspɪk-/ *adj* contemptible, worthless.—**despicableness** *n*.—**despicably** *adv*.

despise /dəˈspaɪz/ *vt* to regard with contempt or scorn; to consider as worthless, inferior.

despite /dəˈspaɪt/ *prep* in spite of.

despoil /dəˈspɔɪl/ *vt* to plunder, rob.—**despoiler** *n*.—**despoilment** *n*.

despoliation /dəˌspoːliˈeɪʃən/ *n* despoilment; pillage.

despond /dəˈspɒnd/ *vi* to lose hope, to be dejected. • *n* despondency.

despondency /-dɛnsi/, **despondence** /-ɒns/ *n* a being despondent; depression or dejection of spirits through loss of resolution or hope.

despondent /dəˈspɒndənt/ *adj* dejected, depressed.—**despondently** *adv*.

despot /ˈdɛspɒt/ *n* a ruler possessing absolute power; a tyrant.

despotic /-ˈspɒtɪk/, **despotical** /-kəl/ *adj* of, pertaining to, or of the nature of a despot or of despotism; arbitrary, tyrannical.—**despotically** *adv*.

despotism /-zəm/ *n* absolute power, tyranny; a state governed by a despot.

desquamate /ˈdɛskwəˌmeɪt/ *vti* to peel or scale off.—**desquamation** *n*.

dessert /dəˈzɜrt/ *n* the sweet course at the end of a meal.

dessertspoon /-ˌspuːn/ *n* a spoon in between a teaspoon and a tablespoon in size, used for eating desserts.

destination /ˌdɛstɪˈneɪʃən/ *n* the place to which a person or thing is going.

destine /ˈdɛstɪn/ *vt* to set aside for some specific purpose; to predetermine; intend.

destiny /ˈdɛstɪni/ *n* (*pl* **destinies**) the power supposedly determining the course of events; the future to which any person or thing is destined; a predetermined course of events.

destitute /ˈdɛstɪˌtuːt/ or /-ˈtjuːt/ *adj* (*with* **of**) lacking some quality; lacking the basic necessities of life, very poor.

destitution /ˌdɛstɪˈtuːʃən/ or /-ˈtjuːʃən/ *n* extreme poverty.

destream /diːˈstriːm/ *vt* ✸ (*Cdn*) to teach students in an undivided group, rather than according to categories based on their academic abilities.—**destreaming** *n*.

destroy /dəˈstrɔɪ/ *vt* to demolish, ruin, to put an end to; to kill.

destroyer /-ər/ *n* one who or that which destroys; a fast small warship.

destruct /dəˈstrʌkt/ *vt* to destroy deliberately (a missile, etc). • *n* the act of destructing (a missile, etc).

destructible /-ɪbəl/ *adj* subject to destruction; able to be destroyed.—**destructibility** *n*.

destruction /dəˈstrʌkʃən/ *n* the act or process of destroying or being destroyed; ruin.

destructionist /-ɪst/ *n* an anarchist.

destructive /-tɪv/ *adj* causing destruction; (*with* **of** *or* **to**) ruinous; (*criticism*) intended to discredit, negative.—**destructively** *adv*.—**destructivity** *n*.

destructor /-ər/ *n* a furnace for burning up rubbish, etc; an explosive device for blowing up a malfunctioning rocket, etc.

desuetude /dəˈsuːɪˌtuːd/ or /-ˈtjuːd/ *n* disuse, discontinuance.

desultory /ˈdɛsəlˌtɔri/ *adj* going aimlessly from one activity or subject to another, not methodical.—**desultorily** *adv*.—**desultoriness** *n*.

detach /dəˈtætʃ/ *vt* to release; to separate from a larger group; (*mil*) to send off on special assignment.

detachable /-əbəl/ *adj* able to be detached.—**detachability** *n*.—**detachably** *adv*.

detached /dəˈtætʃd/ *adj* separate; free from bias or emotion; (*house*) not joined to another; aloof.

detachment /-mənt/ *n* indifference; freedom from emotional involvement or bias; the act of detaching; a thing detached; a body of troops detached from the main body and sent on special service; ✸ (*Cdn*) the office or headquarters of a police force in a district.

detail /dəˈteɪl/ or /ˈdiːteɪl/ *vt* to describe fully; (*mil*) to set apart for a particular duty. • *n* an item; a particular or minute account; (*art*) treatment of smaller parts; a reproduction of a smaller part of a picture, statue, etc; a small detachment for special service.

detailed /ˈdiːteɪld/ or /diːˈteɪld/, /dəˈteɪld/ *adj* giving full details; thorough.

detain /dɪˈteɪn/ *vt* to place in custody or confinement; to delay.—**detainment** *n*.

detainee /ˌdiːteɪˈniː/ or /dəˈteɪˌniː/ *n* a person who is held in custody.

detainer /-ər/ *n* the (wrongful) detaining of person or goods; a writ for holding on another charge a person already arrested.

detect /dəˈtɛkt/ *vt* to discover the existence or presence of; to notice.

detectable /-əbəl/ *adj* able to be detected.—**detectability** *n*.

detection /dəˈtɛkʃən/ *n* a discovery or a being discovered; the job or process of detecting.

detective /dəˈtɛktɪv/ *n* a person or a police officer employed to find evidence of crimes.

detector /-ər/ *n* a device for detecting the presence of something.

detent /ˈdəˌtɛnt/ *n* a catch for locking machinery or regulating the striking of a clock.

détente, detente /deɪˈtɑ̃t/ *n* relaxation of tension between countries.

detention /dəˈtɛnʃən/ *n* the act of detaining or withholding; a being detained; confinement; the act of being kept in (school after hours) as a punishment.

deter /dəˌtər/ *vt* (**deterring, deterred**) to discourage or prevent (from acting).—**determent** *n*.

deterge /dəˈtɜrdʒ/ or /dɪ-/ *vt* to cleanse, as a wound.

detergent /dəˈtɜrdʒənt/ *n* a cleaning agent, *esp* one made from a chemical compound rather than fats, as soap. • *adj* having cleaning power.

deteriorate /dɪˈtiːriəˌreɪt/ *vt* to make or become worse.—**deterioration** *n*.—**deteriorative** *adj*.

determinable /diːˈtɜrmɪnəbəl/ or /dɪ-/ *adj* capable of being definitely ascertained; defined with clearness; terminable.—**determinability** *n*.—**determinably** *adv*.

determinant /dəˈtɜrmɪnənt/ *adj* determining. • *n* something that determines, a decisive factor; (*math*) an algebraic term expressing the sum of certain products arranged in a square or matrix.

determinate /dəˈtɜrmɪnət/ *adj* definitely bounded in time, space, position, etc; fixed; clearly defined; distinct; resolute, decisive; (*bot*) having the terminal flower bud opening first, followed by those on lateral branches.—**determinately** *adv*.—**determinateness** *n*.

determination /dəˌtɜrmɪˈneɪʃən/ *n* the act or process of making a decision; a decision resolving a dispute; firm intention; resoluteness.

determinative /dəˈtɜrmɪnətɪv/ *adj* determining, limiting, or defining; tending to define the genus or species. • *n* that which serves to determine the quality or character of something else; a demonstrative pronoun; an ideograph.—**determinatively** *adv*.

determine /dəˈtɜrmɪn/ *vt* to fix or settle officially; to find out; to regulate; to impel. • *vi* to come to a decision.

determined /-mɪnd/ *adj* full of determination, resolute.—**determinedly** *adv*.—**determinedness** *n*.

determiner /-mɪnər/ *n* one who or that which determines; (*gram*) a word that limits the meaning of a noun, *esp* an article or possessive pronoun.

determinism /-ɪzəm/ *n* the theory that all events, including human actions, are determined by preceding causes, thereby precluding free will.—**determinist** *n*.—**deterministic** *adj*.—**deterministically** *adv*.

deterrent /-ənt/ *n* something that deters; a nuclear weapon that deters attack through fear of retaliation. • *adj* deterring.—**deterrence** *n*.

detest /dɪˈtɛst/ *vt* to dislike intensely.—**detester** *n*.

detestable /-əbəl/ *adj* intensely disliked, abhorrent.—**detestably** *adv*.

detestation /ˌdiːtɛˈsteɪʃən/ *n* extreme dislike; a detestable person or thing.

dethrone /diːˈθroːn/ *vt* to remove from a throne, to depose.—**dethronement** *n*.—**dethroner** *n*.

detinue /ˈdɛtɪˌnjuː/ or /-ˌnuː/ *n* (*law*) a writ for recovery of property wrongfully detained.

detonate /ˈdɛtəˌneɪt/ *vti* to explode or cause to explode rapidly and violently.

detonation /-ˈneɪʃən/ *n* a sudden explosion with a loud report.

detonator /ˈdɛtəˌneɪtər/ *n* a device that sets off an explosion.

detour /ˈdiːtʊər/ *n* a deviation from an intended course, *esp* one serving as an alternative to a more direct route. • *vti* to make or send by a detour.

detoxification centre *n* an institution that treats alcoholism or drug addiction.

detoxify /diːˈtɒksɪˌfaɪ/ *vt* (**detoxifying, detoxified**) to extract poison or toxins from.—**detoxification** *n*.

detract /diˈtrækt/ *vt* to take away. • *vi* to take away (from).—**detractor** *n*.

detraction /diˈtrækʃən/ *n* defamation; slander; depreciation.—**detractive** *adj*.—**detractively** *adv*

detrain /diˈtrein/ *vt, vi* to set down or alight from a train.—**detrainment** *n*.

detriment /ˈdetrimənt/ *n* (a cause of) damage or injury.

detrimental /ˌdetriˈmentəl/ *adj* harmful.—**detrimentally** *adv*.

detrition /diˈtriʃən/ *n* a wearing down by rubbing or friction.

detritus /dəˈtraitəs/ *n* debris; loose matter, *esp* formed by rubbing away or erosion of a larger mass (*eg* a rock).—**detrital** *adj*.

de trop /dəˈtro:/ *adj* too much; out of place; (*person*) not wanted.

detumescence /ˌdi:tuːˈmesəns/ or /ˌ-tjuː-/ *n* the diminution of a swelling, *esp* of an erect penis.—**detumescent** *adj*.

deuce[1] /djuːs/ or /djuːs/ *n* a playing card or dice with two spots; (*tennis*) the score of forty-all.

deuce[2] *interj* (*inf*) the devil!—an exclamation of surprise or annoyance.

deuced /ˈdjuːsd/ or /ˈduːst/ *adj* (*inf*) confounded.

deus ex machina /ˌdeiuseksˈmækmə/ or /ˌdiːəs-/ *n* divine intervention; an artificial solution of difficulties, *esp* in a play.

deuter(o)- /ˈduːtəro:/ or /ˌdju:-/ *prefix* second.

deuteragonist /ˌduːtəˈrægənist/ or /ˌdju:-/ *n* (*Greek drama*) the second principal actor.

deuterium /duːˈtiːriəm/ or /djuː-/ *n* heavy hydrogen, used as a moderator in nuclear reactors to slow the rate of fission.

deuterocanonical /ˌduːtəroːkæˈnɒnikəl/ or /ˌdjuː-/ *adj* of or belonging to a second canon or to the Apocrypha.

deuterogamy /ˌduːtərˈɒgəmi/ or /ˌdjuːt-/ *n* a second marriage.

deuteron /ˈduːtəˌrɒn/ or /ˈdjuː-/ *n* the nucleus of a heavy hydrogen atom.

deutoplasm /-ˌplæzəm/ *n* the albuminous part of the yolk that provides food for the embryo in an egg.—**deutoplasmic** *adj*.

Deutschmark, Deutsche Mark /ˈdoitʃmɑːk/ *n* the monetary unit of Germany.

deutzia /ˈdjuːtsiə/ or /ˈdoit-/ *n* a small shrub of the saxifrage family with clusters of white flowers.

deva /ˈdeivə/ *n* (*Hinduism*) a god.

devaluate /diːˈvæljuːeit/ *vt* to devalue.

devalue /diːˈvæljuː/ *vt* (**devaluing, devalued**) to reduce the exchange value of (a currency).—**devaluation** *n*.

devastate /ˈdevəˌsteit/ *vt* to lay waste; to destroy; to overwhelm.—**devastatingly** *adv*.—**devastation** *n*.—**devastator** *n*.

develop /dəˈveləp/ *vt* to evolve; to bring to maturity; to show the symptoms of (*eg* a habit, a disease); to treat a photographic film or plate to reveal an image; to improve the value of. • *vi* to grow (into); to become apparent.

developer /-ər/ *n* a person who develops; a person or organization that develops property; a reagent for developing photographs.

developing country *n* a poor country that is attempting to improve its social conditions and encourage industrial growth.

development /-mənt/ *n* the process of growing or developing; a new situation that emerges; a piece of land or property that has been developed.—**developmental** *adj*.

deviant /ˈdiːviənt/ *adj* that which deviates from an accepted norm. • *n* a person whose behaviour deviates from the accepted standards of society.—**deviance, deviancy** *n*.

deviate /ˈdiːviˌeit/ *vi* to diverge from a course, topic, principle, etc.—**deviator** *n*.

deviation /ˌdiːviˈeiʃən/ *n* a deviating from normal behaviour, official ideology, etc; deflection of a compass needle by magnetic disturbance; (*statistics*) difference from a mean.

device /diˈvais/ *n* a machine, implement, etc for a particular purpose; an invention; a scheme, a plot.

devil /ˈdevəl/ *n* (*with cap*) in Christian and Jewish theology, the supreme spirit of evil, Satan; any evil spirit; an extremely wicked person; (*inf*) a reckless, high-spirited person; (*inf*) someone or something difficult to deal with; (*inf*) a person. • *vb* (**devilling, devilled** *or* **deviling, deviled**) *vt* to cook food with a hot seasoning. • *vi* to act as a drudge to someone; to do research for an author or barrister.

devilfish /-fiʃ/ *n* (**devilfish, devilfishes**) the manta, a very large ray; a large species of octopus.

devilish /-iʃ/ *adj* fiendish; mischievous. • *adv* (*inf*) very.—**devilishly** *adv*.—**devilishness** *n*.

devil-may-care /ˌdevəlmeiˈkeər/ *adj* audacious, contemptuous of authority.

devilment /-mənt/ *n* mischievous behaviour.

devilry /ˈdevəlri/ (*pl* **dev lries**) wickedness; malicious mischief.

devil's advocate *n* a person who advocates an opposing cause, *esp* for the sake of argument.

devious /ˈdiːviəs/ *adj* indirect; not straightforward; underhand, deceitful.—**deviously** *adv*.—**deviousness** *n*.

devisable /-əbəl/ *adj* capable of being imagined; (*law*) (*real estate*) capable of being bequeathed.—**devisability** *n*.

devise /dəˈvaiz/ *vt* to invert, contrive; to plan; (*law*) to leave (real estate) by will. • *n* (*law*) a bequest (of real estate); property so bequeathed.—**deviser** *n*.

devisee /ˌdevəˈziː/ or /ˌdiˈvaizi/ *n* (*law*) a person to whom (real estate) has been bequeathed.

devisor /-ər/ *n* (*law*) a person who bequeathes, *esp* real estate.

devitalize /diːˈvaitəˌlaiz/ *vt* to deprive of vitality or vigour.—**devitalization** *n*.

devitrify /diːˈvitrəˌfai/ *vt* (**devitrifying, devitrified**) to deprive of glassy quality, to make opaque.—**devitrification** *n*.

devoid /dəˈvoid/ *adj* (*with* **of**) lacking; free from.

devoirs /dəˈvwɑːz/ *npl* civilities; one's best.

devolution /ˌdevəˈluːʃən/ or /ˌdiː-/ *n* a transfer of authority, *esp* from a central government to regional governments; a passing on from one person to another.

devolve /dəˈvɒlv/ *vi* to hand on or be handed on to a successor or deputy.—**devolvement** *n*.

devote /dəˈvoːt/ *vt* to give or use for a particular activity or purpose.

devoted /-əd/ *adj* zealous; loyal; loving.—**devotedly** *adv*.—**devotedness** *n*.

devotee /ˌdevəˈtiː/ or /ˌdiː-/ *n* (*with* **of** *or* **to**) a person who is enthusiastically or fanatically devoted to something; a religious zealot.

devotion /dəˈvoːʃən/ *n* given to religious worship; piety; strong affection or attachment (to); ardour; (*pl*) prayers.

devotional /-əl/ *adj* of devotions; devout. • *n* a brief religious service.

devour /dəˈvaur/ *vt* to eat up greedily; to consume; to absorb eagerly by the senses or mind.

devout /dəˈvaut/ *adj* very religious, pious; sincere, dedicated.—**devoutly** *adv*.—**devoutness** *n*.

dew /duː/ or /djuː/ *n* air moisture, deposited on a cool surface, *esp* at night.

dew point *n* the air temperature at which dew forms.

dewberry /ˈduːberi/ or /ˈdjuː-/ *n* (*pl* **dewberries**) a kind of trailing blackberry plant; its dark blue fruit.

dewclaw /ˈduːklɔː/ or /ˈdjuː-/ *n* a rudimentary toe above a dog's paw or above the hoof of a deer, etc.

Dewey Decimal System /ˈduːi/ or /ˈdjuː-/ *n* a method of classifying library books into ten main subject areas.—*also* **decimal classification**.

dewlap /-læp/ *n* a flap of skin hanging under the throat of some animals, *eg* cows; loose skin on the throat of an elderly person.

dewy /ˈduːi/ or /ˈdjuː-/ *adj* (**dewier, dewiest**) wet with dew.—**dewily** *adv*.—**dewiness** *n*.

dewy-eyed /-ˌaid/ *adj* sentimental, naive.

dexter /ˈdekstər/ *adj* right; (*her*) to the viewer's left and the wearer's right.

dexterity /deksˈterəti/ *n* manual skill, adroitness.

dexterous /ˈdekstrəs/ *adj* possessing manual skill; quick, mentally or physically; adroit; clever.—**dexterously** *adv*.—**dexterousness** *n*.

dextral /ˈdekstrəl/ *adj* on the right-hand side; right-handed; (*shell*) with whorls going to the right.—**dextrality** *n*.—**dextrally** *adv*.

dextrin, dextrine /ˈdekstrin/ *n* a white gummy substance found in plant sap, etc, and used as gum and a thickening agent.

dextrorotation /dekstroːroːˈteiʃən/ *n* right-handed or clockwise rotation.—**dextrorotary, dextrorotatory** *adj*.

dextrorse /ˈdekstrɔːs/ *adj* (*bot*) twining spirally from left to right.—**dextrorsely** *adv*.

dextrose /ˈdekstroːs/ *n* a form of glucose found in fruit, honey and animal tissues.

dextrous /ˈdekstrəs/ *adj* dexterous.

DFC *abbr* = Distinguished Flying Cross.

DFO *abbr* ✷ (*Cdn*) = Department of Fisheries and Oceans.

dhak /dæk/ *n* an Indian tree with brilliant red flowers.

dhal /dɒl/ *see* dal.

dharma /ˈdɑːrmə/ *n* (*Hinduism, Buddhism*) the law requiring virtue and righteousness; its practice in daily life.

dhobi /'dəʊbi/ *n* (*pl* **dhobis**) in India, a laundryman.

dhole /dəʊl/ *n* (*pl* **dholes, dhole**) an Asian wild dog that hunts in packs.

dhoti /'dəʊti/ *n* (*pl* **dhotis**) a loincloth worn by men in India.

dhow /daʊ/ *n* an Arab coastal vessel with a triangular sail.

DHS *abbr* ✦ (*Cdn*) = District High School.

di- /daɪ/ *prefix* two; twice; double.

diabase /'daɪəbeɪs/ *n* dolerite, a dark coloured igneous rock.

diabetes /ˌdaɪə'biːtiːz/ *n* a medical disorder marked by the persistent and excessive discharge of urine.

diabetes mellitus /-mə'lɪtəs/ *n* a breakdown in the body's ability to absorb carbohydrates caused by a deficiency of insulin, which results in abnormally high levels of sugar in the blood and urine.

diabetic /ˌdaɪə'betɪk/ *adj* of or suffering from diabetes. • *n* a person with diabetes.

diablerie /diː'æbləri/ or /daɪ-/ *n* a devil's work, sorcery; devil-lore; mischief.

diabolic /ˌdaɪə'bɒlɪk/ *adj* devilish; cruel, wicked.—**diabolically** *adv.*—**diabolicalness** *n.*

diabolical /ˌdaɪə'bɒlɪkəl/ *adj* diabolic; (*inf*) extremely bad or annoying.

diabolism /daɪ'æbəˌlɪzəm/ *n* devil worship; witchcraft.—**diabolist** *n.*

diabolize /-ˌlaɪz/ *vt* to make into or represent as a devil.

diaconal /daɪ'ækənəl/ or /diː-/ *adj* of or pertaining to a deacon.

diaconate /daɪ'ækəˌneɪt/ or /diː/, /-nət/ *n* the office or dignity of a deacon; deacons collectively.

diacritic /ˌdaɪə'krɪtɪk/ *adj* diacritical. • *n* a diacritical mark.

diacritical /ˌdaɪə'krɪtɪkəl/ *adj* distinguishing, distinctive, *esp* of accents, etc attached to letters to indicate pronunciation.—**diacritically** *adv.*

diacritical mark *n* a mark, such as an accent, used above or below a letter to indicate differences in sound.

diactinic /ˌdaɪæk'tɪnɪk/ *adj* transparent to actinic rays.—**diactinism** *n.*

diadelphous /ˌdaɪə'delfəs/ *adj* (*flowers*) with stamens in two bundles.

diadem /ˌdaɪə'dem/ *n* a crown or jewelled headband worn by royalty.

diaeresis /daɪ'ərəsɪs/ *see* **dieresis**.

diagnose /ˌdaɪəg'nəʊs/ or /-'nəʊz/, /'daɪəgnəʊs/, /-ˌnəʊz/ *vt* to ascertain by diagnosis.—**diagnosable, diagnoseable** *adj.*

diagnosis /ˌdaɪəg'nəʊsɪs/ *n* (*pl* **diagnoses**) the identification of a disease from its symptoms; the analysis of the nature or cause of a problem.—**diagnostician** *n.*

diagnostic /ˌdaɪəg'nɒstɪk/ *adj* of or aiding diagnosis; characteristic. • *n* a symptom distinguishing a disease; a characteristic; (*pl: used as sing*) the art of diagnosing.—**diagnostically** *adv.*

diagonal /daɪ'ægənəl/ *adj* slanting from one corner to an opposite corner of a polygon. • *n* a straight line connecting opposite corners.—**diagonally** *adv.*

diagram /'daɪəˌgræm/ *n* a figure or plan drawn in outline to illustrate the form or workings of something. • *vt* (**diagramming, diagrammed** *or* **diagraming, diagramed**) to demonstrate in diagram form.

diagrammatic, diagrammatical *adj* having the form or nature of a diagram; of or pertaining to diagrams.—**diagrammatically** *adv.*

diagraph /'daɪəˌgræf/ *n* an instrument for enlarging maps, etc mechanically.

dial /'daɪəl/ *n* the face of a watch or clock; a graduated disk with a pointer used in various instruments; the control on a radio or television set indicating wavelength or station; the numbered disk on a telephone used to enter digits to connect calls; an instrument for telling the time by the sun's shadow. • *vt* (**dialling, dialled** *or* **dialing, dialed**) to measure or indicate by a dial; to make a telephone connection by using a dial or numbered keypad.

dialect /'daɪəˌlekt/ *n* the form of language spoken in a particular region or social class.—**dialectal** *adj.*—**dialectally** *adv.*

dialectic /'daɪəˌlektɪk/ *n* the pursuit of truths in philosophy through logical debate.—**dialectical** *adj.*—**dialectically** *adv.*

dialectology /-ˌtɒlədʒi/ *n* the study of dialects.—**dialectological** *adj.*—**dialectologist** *n.*

dialogue, dialog /'daɪəˌlɒg/ *n* a conversation, *esp* in a play or novel; an exchange of opinions, negotiation.

dial tone *n* a sound heard over the telephone indicating that the line is clear.

dialyse, dialyze /'daɪəˌlaɪz/ *vt* to separate crystalline from colloid parts of a mixture by filtration.—**dialysation, dialyzation** *n.*

dialyser, dialyzer /-ˌlaɪzer/ *n* a machine for dialysing, *esp* one that act as a kidney.

dialysis /daɪ'æləsɪs/ *n* (*pl* **dialyses**) the removal of impurities from the blood by filtering it through a membrane.—**dialytic** *adj.*—**dialytically** *adv.*

diamagnetic /ˌdaɪəmæg'netɪk/ *adj* cross-magnetic, tending to point east and west.—**diamagnetically** *adv.*

diamagnetism /-'mægnəˌtɪzəm/ *n* the property of certain bodies when under the influence of magnetism and freely suspended of taking a position at right angles to the magnetic meridian.

diamanté /ˌdiːə'mɒnteɪ/ *adj* glittering with rhinestones, sequins or imitation jewels. • *n* a material ornamented in this way.

diameter /daɪ'æmətər/ *n* a straight line bisecting a circle; the length of this line.

diametric /ˌdaɪə'metrɪk/, **diametrical** /-əl/ *adj* of or along a diameter; completely opposed.—**diametrically** *adv.*

diamond /'daɪmənd/ or /'daɪə-/ *n* a valuable gem, a crystallized form of pure carbon; (*baseball*) the playing field, *esp* the infield; a suit of playing cards denoted by a red lozenge. • *adj* composed of, or set with diamonds; shaped like a diamond; denoting the 60th (or 75th) anniversary of an event.

diamondback /-ˌbæk/ *n* a large rattlesnack with diamond-shaped markings.

dianthus /daɪ'ænθəs/ *n* (*pl* **dianthuses**) any of a large genus of ornamental plants, including carnations and pinks.

diapason /ˌdaɪə'peɪzən/ or /-sən/ *n* the entire compass of a voice or instrument; a recognized musical standard of pitch; the foundation stops of an organ.

diaper /'daɪpər/ *n* a nappy.

diaphanous /daɪ'æfənəs/ *adj* (*fabrics*) delicate, transparent.—**diaphanously** *adv.*—**diaphanousness** *n.*

diaphoretic /ˌdaɪəfə'retɪk/ *adj* causing profuse perspiration. • *n* a diaphoretic drug.

diaphragm /'daɪəˌfræm/ *n* the midriff, a muscular structure separating the chest from the abdomen; any thin dividing membrane; a device for regulating the aperture of a camera lens; a contraceptive cap covering the cervix; a thin vibrating disk used in a telephone receiver, microphone, etc.—**diaphragmatic** *adj.*—**diaphragmatically** *adv.*

diarchy /'daɪərki/ *n* (*pl* **diarchies**) government by two independent authorities.—*also* **dyarchy**.

diarist /'daɪərɪst/ *n* one who keeps a diary; the author of a diary.

diarrhoea, diarrhea /ˌdaɪə'riːə/ *n* excessive looseness of the bowels.—**diarrhoeal, diarrheal, diarrhoeic, diarrheic** *adj.*

diary /'daɪəri/ *n* (*pl* **diaries**) a daily record of personal thoughts, events, or business appointments; a book for keeping a daily record.

Diaspora /daɪ'æspərə/ *n* the dispersion of the Jews after the Babylonian captivity; the Jewish communities outside Israel; (*without cap*) the dispersion of any peoples outside their native area.

diastase /'daɪəˌsteɪz/ *n* any enzyme that converts starch into sugar.—**diastatic, diastasic** *adj.*

diastole /daɪ'æstəliː/ *n* the dilation of the chambers of the heart during which they fill with blood.—**diastolic** *adj.*

diatessaron /ˌdaɪə'tesəˌrɒn/ *n* the combination of the four Gospels into a single narrative.

diathermancy /ˌdaɪə'θɜrmənsi/ *n* the property of transmitting radiant heat.—**diathermanous** *adj.*

diathermic /-mɪk/ *adj* having diathermancy; allowing heat rays to pass freely.

diathermy /'daɪəˌθɜrmi/ *n* the use of electric current to warm or destroy body tissues as part of medical treatment.

diathesis /daɪ'æθəsɪs/ *n* (*pl* **diatheses**) a constitutional tendency, *esp* to disease; a predisposing factor.

diatom /'daɪəˌtɒm/ *n* a microscopic alga found in fresh and seawater and in soil.—**diatomaceous** *adj.*

diatomite /daɪ'ætəˌmɔɪt/ *n* soft earth formed from the shells of diatoms and used as a filter, etc.

diatonic /ˌdaɪə'tɒnɪk/ *adj* (*mus*) using only the major and minor scales, as opposed to the chromatic scale.—**diatonically** *adv.*—**diatonicism** *n.*

diatribe /'daɪəˌtraɪb/ *n* a lengthy and abusive verbal attack.

dib /dɪb/ *vti* (**dibbing, dibbed**) to dibble; (*fishing*) to drop bait gently into water; to dip lightly.

dibasic /daɪ'beɪsɪk/ adj containing two atoms of hydrogen replaceable by a basic radical.—**dibasicity** n.

dibber /'dɪbər/ n a dibble.

dibble /-əl/ n a pointed tool used to make holes in the ground for seedlings. • vt to make a hole in the ground with a dibber.

dicast /'daɪ,kæst/ n in ancient Athens, a juryman.

dice /daɪs/ n (the pl of die² but used as sing) a small cube with numbered sides used in games of chance. • vt to gamble using dice; to cut (food) into small cubes.

dicentra /daɪ'sentrə/ n a member of a genus of perennial plants with heart-shaped flowers.

dicephalous /daɪ'sefələs/ adj two-headed.

dicey /'daɪsi/ adj (**dicier, diciest**) (inf) risky.

dichloride /daɪ'klɔɪraɪd/ see **bichloride**.

dichogamous /ˌdaɪkɒ'gæməs/, **dichogamic** /-mɪk/ adj (bot) with stamens and pistils maturing at different times, preventing self-fertilization.—**dichogamy** n.

dichotomy /daɪ'kɒtəmi/ n (pl **dichotomies**) a division into two parts.—**dichotomous, dichotomic** adj.

dichroic /daɪ'kroʊɪk/, **dichroitic** /ˌdaɪkroʊ'ɪtɪk/ adj (crystal) showing two colours; dichromatic.

dichroism /'daɪkroʊɪzəm/ n the property by which a crystallized body exhibits different colours according to the direction of light transmitted through it.

dichromatic /ˌdaɪkroʊ'mætɪk/ adj two-coloured.—also **dichroic**; being able to see only two of the three primary colours, colourblind; (biol) having one of two varieties of seasonal coloration.—**dichromatism** n.

dichromic /daɪ'kroʊmɪk/ adj seeing only two of the three primary colours, dichromatic.

dick /dɪk/ n (sl) a detective; (sl) a person.

dickens /'dɪkɪnz/ interj (inf) the devil.

dicker /'dɪkər/ vi to barter or trade on a small scale; to haggle.• n a barter; a deal; haggling.

dicky, dickey[1] /'dɪki/ n (pl **dickies, dickeys**) a false shirt-front; a seat at the back of a sports car.

dicky, dickey[2] adj (**dickier, dickiest**) (sl) shaky, unsound.

dicrotic /daɪ'krɒtɪk/ adj having a double or secondary pulse beat.—**dicrotism** n.

dicta /'dɪktə/ see **dictum**.

Dictaphone /'dɪktə,foʊn/ n (trademark) a machine that records dictation and later reproduces it for typing.

dictate /'dɪkteɪt/ or /dɪk'teɪt/ vt to say or read for another person to write or for a machine to record; to pronounce, order with authority. • vi to give dictation; to give orders (to). • n an order, rule, or command; (usu pl) an impulse, ruling principle.

dictation /dɪk'teɪʃən/ n the act of dictating words to be written down by another; the thing dictated; an authoritative utterance.

dictator /dɪk'teɪtər/ n a ruler with absolute authority, usu acquired by force.

dictatorial /dɪktə'tɔɪriəl/ adj like a dictator; tyrannical; domineering.—**dictatorially** adv.

dictatorship /dɪk'teɪtərʃɪp/ n the office or government of a dictator; a country governed by a dictator; absolute power.

diction /'dɪkʃən/ n a way of speaking, enunciation; a person's choice of words.

dictionary /'dɪkʃəˌneri/ n (pl **dictionaries**) a reference book containing the words of a language or branch of knowledge alphabetically arranged, with their meanings, pronunciation, origin, etc.

Dictograph /'dɪktə,græf/ n (trademark) a sound recording instrument used for recording or monitoring telephone conversations.

dictum /'dɪktəm/ n (pl **dictums, dicta**) an authoritative pronouncement.

did /dɪd/ see **do**.

Didache /'dɪdə,kiː/ n the title of a 2nd-century AD treatise on Christian doctrine and order, discovered 1883.

didactic /daɪ'dæktɪk/ or /də-/ adj intended to teach; instructive; in a lecturing manner.—**didactically** adv.—**didacticism** n.

didactics /-tɪks/ n (used as sing) the art of teaching.

diddle /'dɪdəl/ vi (sl) to cheat.—**diddler** n.

didn't /'dɪdənt/ = did not.

didymium /dɪ'dɪmiəm/ n a mixture of rare earths, formerly thought to be an element, used for colouring glass.

didymous /'dɪdəməs/ adj (biol) growing in pairs; paired or double.

die[1] /daɪ/ vb (**dying, died**) vi to cease existence; to become dead; to stop functioning; to feel a deep longing; (with out) to become extinct. • vi to experience a particular form of death.

die[2] n a dice.

die[3] n (pl **dies**) an engraved stamp for pressing coins; a casting mould; a tool used in cutting the threads of screws or bolts, etc.

diecious /daɪ'iːʃəs/ see **dioecious**.

diehard /'daɪhɑrd/ n a person who prolongs futile resistance, usu an extreme conservative.

dielectric /ˌdaɪə'lektrɪk/ adj nonconducting. • n any medium, as glass, that transmits electric force by induction.

dieresis /daɪ'erəsɪs/ n (pl **diereses**) a sign (¨) placed over the second of two separate vowels to show that each has a separate sound in pronunciation, as Zoë; a division in a line of verse.—also **diaeresis**.—**dieretic, diaeretic** adj.

diesel /'diːzəl/ n a vehicle driven by a diesel engine.

diesel engine n an internal combustion engine in which ignition is produced by the heat of highly compressed air alone.

diesel oil n a form of petroleum for diesel engines, ignited by the heat of compression.

diesis /'daɪəsɪs/ (pl **dieses**) n the double dagger used in printing (‡); (mus) the difference between a greater and lesser semitone.

diet[1] /'daɪət/ n food selected to adjust weight, to control illness, etc; the food and drink usually consumed by a person or animal. • vt to put on a diet. • vi to eat according to a special diet.—**dieter** n.

diet[2] n a legislative assembly in some countries.

dietary /'daɪəˌteri/ adj pertaining to a diet.

dietetic /ˌdaɪə'tetɪk/, **dietetical** /-əl/ adj regulating food or diet.—**dietetically** adv.

dietetics /-ɪks/ n (used as sing) the scientific study of diet and nutrition.

differ /'dɪfər/ vi to be unlike, distinct (from); to disagree.

difference /'dɪfrəns/ n the act or state of being unlike; disparity; a distinguishing feature; the amount or manner of being different; the result of the subtraction of one quantity from another; a disagreement or argument.

different /-ənt/ adj distinct, separate; unlike, not the same; unusual.—**differently** adv.

differentia /ˌdɪfər'enʃiə/ n (pl **differentiae**) (logic) what distinguishes a thing from others, esp one subclass from another of the same class.

differential /-ʃəl/ adj of or showing a difference; (math) relating to increments in given functions. • n something that marks the difference between comparable things; the difference in wage rates for different types of labour, esp within an industry.—**differentially** adv.

differential calculus n the branch of calculus dealing with the rate of change of given functions with respect to their variables.

differential gear n a type of gear that allows powered wheels in a motor vehicle to turn at different speeds (eg when cornering).

differentiate /ˌdɪfə'renʃiˌeɪt/ vt to make different; to become specialized; to note differences; (math) to calculate the derivative of.

differentiation /-ənʃi'eɪʃən/ n the act of differentiating; (biol) specialization; (math) the calculation of a differential.

difficult /'dɪfɪkəlt/ adj hard to understand; hard to make, do, or carry out; not easy to please.

difficulty /-,kəlti/ n (pl **difficulties**) the state of being difficult; a problem, etc that is hard to deal with; an obstacle; a troublesome situation; a disagreement.

diffidence /'dɪfɪdəns/ n lack of confidence in one's own ability; shyness, modesty.

diffident /-dənt/ adj shy, lacking self-confidence, not assertive.—**diffidently** adv.

diffract /dɪ'frækt/ vti to cause, or cause to undergo, diffraction.—**diffractive** adj.

diffraction /-ʃən/ n the breaking up of a ray of light into coloured bands of the spectrum, or into a series of light and dark bands.

diffuse /dɪ'fjuːz/ vt to spread widely in all directions. • vti (gases, fluids, small particles) to intermingle. • adj spread widely, not concentrated; wordy, not concise.—**diffusely** adv.

diffusion /-ən/ n the act of diffusing; a spreading abroad; the passing by osmosis through animal membranes.

diffusive /-sɪv/ adj extending; spreading widely.—**diffusively** adv.—**diffusiveness** n.

dig /dɪg/ vt (**digging, dug**) to use a tool or hands, claws, etc in making a hole in the ground; to unearth by digging; to excavate; to investigate; to thrust (into); to nudge; (sl) to understand, approve. • n (sl) a thrust; an archaeological excavation; a cutting remark.

digamist /'dɪɡəmɪst/ *n* one who marries for a second time.—**digamous** *adj*.—**digamy** *n*.

digamma /daɪ'ɡæmə/ *n* a letter of the ancient Greek alphabet, in sound approaching that of V or W.

digastric /daɪ'ɡæstrɪk/ *adj* (*muscle*) with two swollen ends. • *n* a neck muscle that helps lower the jaw.

digenesis /daɪ'dʒenəsɪs/ *n* (*biol*) an alternating process of reproduction, sexual in one generation, asexual in the following.—**digenetic** *adj*.

digest[1] /daɪ'dʒest/ or /də-/ *vt* to convert (food) into assimilable form; to reduce (facts, laws, etc) to convenient form by classifying or summarizing; to form a clear view of (a situation) by reflection. • *vi* to become digested.

digest[2] *n* an abridgment of any written matter; a periodical synopsis of published or broadcast material.

digester /-tər/ *n* one who makes a digest; a thing that digests; an apparatus for extracting the essence of a substance by heat.

digestible /-təbəl/ *adj* capable of being digested.—**digestibility, digestibly** *adv*.

digestion /-ʃən/ *n* the act or process of digesting.—**digestional** *adj*.

digestive /-tɪv/ *adj* pertaining to, performing, or aiding, digestion. • *n* a thing that aids digestion; a sweet wholemeal biscuit.

digger /'dɪɡər/ *n* an implement or machine for digging; (*inf*) an Australian or New Zealander (used as a form of address).

digispeak /,dɪdʒɪ'piːk/ *n* (*comput*) the use of acronyms in online communication in which frequently-used terms or phrases are abbreviated.

digit /'dɪdʒɪt/ *n* any of the basic counting units of a number system, including zero; a human finger or toe.

digital /'dɪdʒətəl/ *adj* of, having or using digits; using numbers rather than a dial to display measurements; of or pertaining to a digital computer or digital recording.—**digitally** *adv*.

digital audio tape *n* a magnetic tape capable of being used in digital recording, giving high-quality audio reproduction.

digital clock *n* a clock that displays the time in figures.

digital computer *n* a computer that processes information in the form of characters and digits in electronic binary code.

digitalin /,dɪdʒɪ'tælɪn/ *n* a poison extracted from foxglove leaves.

digitalis /-lɪs/ *n* a drug derived from foxglove leaves, used as a heart stimulant.

digital recording *n* the conversion of sound into discrete electronic pulses (representing binary digits) for recording.

digital watch *n* a watch that displays the time in figures.

digitate /'dɪdʒɪ,teɪt/, **digitated** /-ɪd/ *adj* having separate fingers or toes.—**digitation** *n*.

digitigrade /'dɪdʒɪtɪ,ɡreɪd/ *adj* (cats, dogs, etc) walking on the toes. • *n* an animal that walks in this way.

digitize /'dɪdʒɪ,taɪz/ *vt* (*data, images*) to translate into digital form for input into a computer.—**digitization** *n*.

diglot /'daɪ,ɡlɒt/ *adj* bilingual. • *n* a book with the text in two languages.

dignified /,dɪɡnə'faɪd/ *adj* possessing dignity; noble; serious.—**dignifiedly** *adv*.

dignify /,dɪɡnə'faɪ/ *vt* (**dignifying, dignified**) to confer dignity; to exalt; to add the appearance of distinction (to something).

dignitary /'dɪɡnə,teri/ *n* (*pl* **dignitaries**) a person in a high position or rank.

dignity /'dɪɡnɪti/ *n* (*pl* **dignities**) noble, serious, formal in manner and appearance; sense of self-respect, worthiness; a high rank, *eg* in the government.

digraph /'daɪɡræf/ *n* a combination of two sounds or characters to represent one simple sound, as *ph* in *phone*.—**digraphic** *adj*.—**digraphically** *adv*.

digress /daɪ'ɡres/ *vi* to stray from the main subject in speaking or writing.—**digression** *n*.

digressive /-ɪv/ *adj* tending to digress; deviating from the subject.—**digressively** *adv*.—**digressiveness** *n*.

dihedral /daɪ'hiːdrəl/ *adj* (*angle*) having two intersecting plane faces or sides. • *n* a dihedral angle; the angle between aircraft wings for improving stability.

dik-dik /'dɪkdɪk/ *n* a small East African antelope.

dike[1] /daɪk/ *see* **dyke**[2].

dike[2] *n* an embankment to prevent flooding or form a barrier to the sea; a ditch; a causeway.—*also* **dyke**.

dilapidate /dɪ'læpɪ,deɪt/ *vt* to bring into partial ruin by neglect or misuse. • *vi* to become dilapidated.

dilapidated /-əd/ *adj* in a state of disrepair; shabby.

dilapidation /dɪ,læpɪ'deɪʃən/ *n* a state of damage or disrepair.

dilatation /,daɪlə'teɪʃən/ *n* a dilating, *esp* as part of a medical procedure; an abnormal enlargement of an organ, etc.—**dilatational** *adj*.

dilatation and curettage *n* a surgical procedure for opening the cervix and scraping the uterus.

dilate /'daɪ,leɪt/ *vti* to make wider or larger; to increase the width of; to expand, amplify, enlarge; to extend in time, protract, prolong, lengthen. • *vi* to become wider or larger; to spread out, widen, enlarge, expand; to discourse or write at large; to enlarge.—**dilatable** *adj*.—**dilatabilty** *n*.

dilation /daɪ'leɪʃən/ *n* the action or process of dilating; something dilated.

dilator /daɪ'leɪtər/ *n* that which dilates; a surgical instrument for opening or expanding an orifice; a muscle that dilates the parts on which it acts.

dilatory /'dɪlə,tori/ *adj* tardy; causing or meant to cause delay.—**dilatorily** *adv*.—**dilatoriness** *n*.

dilemma /dɪ'lemə/ *n* a situation where each of two alternative courses is undesirable; any difficult problem or choice.—**dilemmatic** *adj*.

dilettante /,dɪlə'tɒnt/ or /'dɪlə-/, /-,tænti/ *n* (*pl* **dilettantes, dilettanti**) a person who dabbles in a subject for amusement only.

diligence[1] /'dɪlɪdʒəns/ *n* careful attention; assiduity; industry.

diligence[2] /'dɪlɪdʒəns/, *Fr* /diːliː'ʒɑ̃s/ *n* (*formerly*) a French stagecoach.

diligent /'dɪlɪdʒənt/ *adj* industrious; done with proper care and effort.—**diligently** *adv*.

dill /dɪl/ *n* a yellow-flowered herb whose leaves and seeds are used for flavouring and in medicines.

dillydally /'dɪli,dæli/ *vi* (**dillydallying, dillydallied**) (*inf*) to dawdle, loiter.

dilute /daɪ'luːt/ or /dɪ-/ *vt* to thin down, *esp* by mixing with water; to weaken the strength of. • *adj* diluted.—**diluter, dilutor** *n*.—**diluteness** *n*.

dilution /-'luːʃən/ *n* the act of diluting; a weak liquid.

diluvial /daɪ'luːvɪəl/ or /də-/, **diluvian** /-ən/ *adj* pertaining to, produced by, or resulting from, a deluge or flood, *esp* the Flood of the Bible.

diluvium /-vɪəm/ (*pl* **diluviums, diluvia**) *n* (*formerly*) geological deposits caused by water action, drift.

dim /dɪm/ *adj* (**dimmer, dimmest**) faintly lit; not seen, heard, understood, etc clearly; gloomy; unfavourable; (*inf*) stupid. • *vti* (**dimming, dimmed**) to make or cause to become dark.—**dimly** *adv*.—**dimness** *n*.

dime /daɪm/ *n* a US or Canadian coin worth ten cents.

dimension /də'menʃən/ or /daɪ-/ *n* any linear measurement of width, length, or thickness; extent; size.

dimensional /-əl/ *adj* of or pertaining to dimension or magnitude; (*geom*) of or pertaining to (a specified number of) dimensions.—**dimensionality** *n*.—**dimensionally** *adv*.

dimerous /'daɪmərəs/ *adj* (*flowers*) having two members in each whorl; (*insects*) having a foot composed of two parts.

dimeter /'dɪmɪtər/ *n* (a line of) verse of two measures, a measure being one or two feet, according to the metre.

diminish /dɪ'mɪnɪʃ/ *vti* to make or become smaller in size, amount, or importance.—**diminishable** *adj*.—**diminishment** *n*.

diminuendo /də,mɪnju'endoː/ *see* **decrescendo**.

diminution /,dɪmɪ'njuːʃən/ or /-njuː-/ *n* act or process of being made smaller.

diminutive /dɪ'mɪnjutɪv/ or /-njə-/ *adj* very small. • *n* a word formed by a suffix to mean small (*eg duckling*) or to convey affection (*eg Freddie*).

dimity /dɪ'məti/ (*pl* **dimities**) *n* a light, strong striped or figured cotton cloth used for curtains, etc.

dimmer /'dɪmər/ *n* a switch for reducing the brightness of an electric light.

dimorphism /daɪ'mɔrfɪzəm/ *n* the quality of assuming, crystallizing or existing in two forms.—**dimorphic, dimorphous** *adj*.

dimple /'dɪmpəl/ *n* a small hollow, *usu* on the cheek or chin. • *vti* to make or become dimpled; to reveal dimples.—**dimply** *adj*.

dimwit /'dɪmwɪt/ *n* (*inf*) an idiotic person, a fool.—**dimwitted** *adj*.—**dimwittedly** *adv*.—**dimwittedness** *n*.

din /dɪn/ *n* a loud persistent noise. • *vt* (**dinning, dinned**) to make a din; (*with* **into**) to instil by continual repetition.

dinar /'dɪnɑr/ n the monetary unit of Yugoslavia and various North African countries.

dine /daɪn/ vi to eat dinner. • vt to entertain to dinner.

diner /'daɪnər/ n a person who dines; a dining car on a train; a small, cheap eating place.

dinette /daɪ'nɛt/ n a small area in a house for eating in.

ding /dɪŋ/ vi to sound, as a bell, with a continuous monotonous tone. • vt to impress by noisy repetition. • n the ringing sound of a bell.

ding-dong /'dɪŋ,dɒŋ/ n the sound of a metallic body produced by blows, as a bell; (inf) a violent argument. • adj characterized by a rapid succession of blows; (insults, etc) vigorously maintained. • vi to ring as or like a bell. • vt to assail with constant repetition; to repeat with mechanical regularity.

dinghy /'dɪŋɪ/ or /'dɪŋgɪ/ n (pl dinghies) a small open boat propelled by oars or sails; a small inflatable boat.

dingle /'dɪŋgəl/ n a small wooded hollow.

dingo /'dɪŋgoʊ/ n (pl dingoes) an Australian wild dog.

dingy /'dɪndʒɪ/ adj (dingier, dingiest) dirty-looking, shabby.—**dingily** adv.—**dinginess** n.

dining car n a restaurant car on a train.

dining room n a room used for eating meals.

dinkum /'dɪŋkəm/ adj genuine, honest.

dinky /'dɪŋkɪ/ adj (dinkier, dinkiest) (inf) small; of no consequence, unimportant; (Scot) neat and attractive, smart.

dinner /'dɪnər/ n the principal meal of the day; a formal meal in honour of a person or occasion.

dinner jacket n a tuxedo.

dinosaur /'daɪnə,sɔr/ n any of an order of extinct reptiles, typically enormous in size; (inf) a person or thing regarded as outdated.

dinothere /'daɪnə,θiːr/ n a huge, extinct animal like an elephant.

dint /dɪnt/ n (arch) a mark left by a blow, a dent; **by dint of** by force of. • vt make a dint in.

diocesan /daɪ'ɒsɪsən/ or /-zən/ adj of or pertaining to a diocese; the bishop of a diocese.

diocese /'daɪəsiːs/ n the district over which a bishop has authority.

diode /'daɪ,oʊd/ n a semiconductor device for converting alternating to direct current; a basic thermionic valve with two electrodes.

dioecious /daɪ'iːʃəs/ adj (bot, zool) having male and female organs respectively in separate individuals.—also **diecious**.

dioptase /daɪ'ɒp,teɪs/ n a vitreous emerald green ore of copper.

dioptre, diopter /daɪ'ɒptər/ n a unit for measuring the refractive power of a lens.

dioptric /daɪ'ɒptrɪk/, **dioptrical** /-əl/ adj assisting vision by means of the refraction of light in viewing distant objects.

dioptrics /daɪ'ɒp,trɪks/ n (used as sing) the area of optics dealing with the refraction of light.

diorama /,daɪə'rɑmə/ n a miniature three-dimensional scene, esp in a museum; any small-scale model with figures; a device for producing changing effects using special lighting on a translucent picture.—**dioramic** adj.

diorite /'daɪə,raɪt/ n a granite-like rock consisting of felspar and hornblende.

dioxide /daɪ'ɒks,aɪd/ n an oxide with two molecules of oxygen to one molecule of the other constituents.

dip /dɪp/ vt (dipping, dipped) to put (something) under the surface (as of a liquid) and lift quickly out again; to immerse (as a sheep in an antiseptic solution). • vi to go into water and come out quickly; to suddenly drop down or sink out of sight; to read superficially; to slope downwards. • n a dipping of any kind; a sudden drop; a mixture in which to dip something.

dip., Dip. abbr = diploma.

diphtheria /dɪf'θɪrɪə/ or /dɪp-/ n an acute infectious disease causing inflammation of the throat and breathing difficulties.—**diphtherial** adj.

diphtheritic /,dɪfθə'rɪtɪk/, **diphtheric** /-'θɛrɪk/ adj of or like diphtheria; affected by diphtheria.

diphthong /'dɪfθɒŋ/ or /'dɪp-/ n the union of two vowel sounds pronounced in one syllable; a ligature.—**diphthongal** adj.

diphyllous /daɪ'fɪləs/ adj (bot) having two leaves.

diploblastic /,dɪplə'blæstɪk/ adj (zool) with two germ layers.

diplodocus /dɪ'plɒdəkəs/ or /-'loːdə-/ (pl diplocouses) n an extinct reptile with a very long tail and neck and a small head.

diploe /'dɪploʊ,iː/ n the soft spongy tissue between the two layers of the skull.—**diploic** adj.

diploma /dɪ'ploʊmə/ n (pl diplomas) a certificate given by a college or university to its graduating students; the course of study leading to a diploma; (pl often diplomata) an official document, a charter.

diplomacy /dɪ'ploʊməsɪ/ n (pl diplomacies) the management of relations between nations; skill in handling affairs without arousing hostility.

diplomat /'dɪplə,mæt/ n a person employed or skilled in diplomacy.

diplomatic /,dɪplə'mætɪk/, **diplomatical** /-kə/ adj of diplomacy; employing tact and conciliation; tactful.—**diplomatically** adv.

diplomatic corps n all the ambassadors at a particular capital, the corps diplomatique.

diplomatic immunity n the exemption from local laws and taxes accorded to foreign diplomats in the country where they are stationed.

diplomatist n a diplomat.

dipole /'daɪ,poʊl/ n two equal and opposite electric charges or magnetic poles a small distance apart; a molecule in which the centres of negative and positive charge do not coincide; a directional aerial consisting of two metal rods.—**dipolar** adj.

dipper /'dɪpər/ n a ladle; any of various diving birds; ✦ (Cdn) a small lidless saucepan.

dippy /'dɪpɪ/ n (dippier, dippiest) (sl) eccentric; crazy.

dipso /'dɪpsoʊ/ n (pl dipsos) (inf) a dipsomaniac.

dipsomania /,dɪpsə'meɪnɪə/ n a compulsive craving for alcohol.

dipsomaniac /-'meɪnɪ,æk/ n a person with an uncontrollable craving for alcohol. • adj of or having dipsomania.—**dipsomaniacal** adj.

dipstick /'dɪpstɪk/ n a rod with graduated markings to measure fluid level.

dipteral /'dɪptərəl/ adj (archit) having a double row of columns, as a temple, etc.

dipteran /'dɪptərən/ n any of a large order of insects including flies, mosquitoes, midges, having one pair of true wings and piercing or sucking mouthparts.

dipterous /'dɪptərəs/ adj (insects) two-winged; (seeds) with appendages resembling wings.

diptych /'dɪptɪk/ n a pair of paintings or carvings on two panels hinged together.

dire /daɪr/ adj dreadful; ominous; desperately urgent.—**direly** adv.—**direness** n.

direct /dɪ'rɛkt/ or /daɪ-/ adj straight; in an unbroken line, with nothing in between; frank; truthful. • vt to manage, to control; to tell or show the way; to point to, to aim at; (a letter or parcel) to address; to carry out the organizing and supervision of; to train and lead performances; to command. • vi to determine a course; to act as a director.—**directness** n.

direct current n an electric current that flows in one direction only.

direct debit n ✦ (Cdn and Brit) a pre-arranged regular debit of a bank account, usu to make a recurring payment.

direct deposit n (US) the transfer of money, electronically, from one bank account to another.

direction /dɪ'rɛkʃən/ or /daɪ-/ n management, control; order, command; a knowing or telling what to do, where to go, etc; any way in which one may face or point; (pl) instructions.

directional /-ʃənəl/ adj relating to direction in space; (aerial) transmitting in one direction only.—**directionality** n.—**directionally** adv.

direction finder n a device used to locate the direction of incoming radio signals, used in navigation.

directive /dɪ'rɛktɪv/ or /daɪ-/ adj directing; authoritatively guiding or ruling. • n an order, instruction.

directly /dɪ'rɛktlɪ/ or /daɪ-/ adv in a direct manner; immediately; in a short while.

Directoire /,dɪrɛk'twɑr/ adj of or imitating the low-necked high-waisted dress or curving informal furniture of the Directoire period in France (1795–99).

director /dɪ'rɛktər/ or /daɪ-/ n person who directs, esp the production of a show for stage or screen; one of the persons directing the affairs of a company or an institution.—**directorial** adj.— **directorship** n.

directorate /-ət/ n a board of directors; the position of a director.—also **directorship**.

directory /-tərɪ/ or /daɪ-/ n (pl directories) an alphabetical or classified list, as of telephone numbers, members of an organization, charities, etc.

direct tax n a tax paid by the actual person or organization on which it is levied.

direful /'daɪr,fʊl/ adj dreadful, dire.—**direfully** adv.

dirge /'dərdʒ/ *n* a song or hymn played or sung at a funeral; a slow, mournful piece of music.

dirigible /'dɪrɪdʒəbəl/ or /dɪ'rɪdʒ-/ *adj* able to be steered. • *n* an airship.

dirk /dərk/ *n* a small dagger, *esp* as formerly worn by Scottish Highlanders.

dirndl /'dərndəl/ *n* a woman's full skirt with a tight waistband.

dirt /dərt/ *n* filth; loose earth; obscenity; scandal. • *adj* made of dirt.

dirt-cheap /-,tʃi:p/ *adj* (*inf*) very cheap.

dirty /'dərti/ *adj* (**dirtier, dirtiest**) filthy; unclean; dishonest; mean; (*weather*) stormy; obscene. • *vti* (**dirtying, dirtied**) to make or become dirty.—**dirtily** *adv.*—**dirtiness** *n*.

Dirty Thirties *n* ✤ (*Cdn*) (*inf*) the economic depression of the 1930s.

dis- /dɪs/ *prefix* not, the reverse of; away from, apart; deprive of.

disability /,dɪsə'bɪləti/ or /'dɪs-/ *n* (*pl* **disabilities**) a lack of physical, mental or social fitness; something that disables, a handicap.

disable /dɪs'eɪbəl/ *vt* to make useless; to cripple; (*law*) to disqualify.—**disablement** *n*.

disabled /dɪs'eɪbəld/ *adj* having a physical handicap.

disabuse /,dɪsə'bju:z/ *vt* to free from a mistaken impression.

disaccord /,dɪsə'kɔrd/ *vi* to disagree, to be at variance. • *n* disagreement, incongruity.

disadvantage /,dɪsəd'væntɪdʒ/ *n* an unfavourable condition or situation; loss, damage. • *vt* to put at a disadvantage.

disadvantaged /-tɪdʒd/ *adj* deprived or discriminated against in social and economic terms.

disadvantageous /,dɪs,ædvən'teɪdʒəs/ *adj* causing disadvantage; unfavourable.—**disadvantageously** *adv*.

disaffected /,dɪsə'fektɪd/ *adj* discontented, no longer loyal.—**disaffectedly** *adv.*—**disaffection** *n*.

disaffirm /,dɪsə'fɪrm/ *vt* (*law*) to set aside, to reverse.—**disaffirmation** *n*.

disafforest /,dɪsə'fɔrəst/ or /'dɪse,fɔr-/ *vt* to change from the legal state of forest to that of ordinary land; to remove forest from.—**disafforestation** *n*.

disagree /,dɪsə'gri:/ *vi* (**disagreeing, disagreed**) to differ in opinion; to quarrel; (*with* **with**) to have a bad effect on.—**disagreement** *n*.

disagreeable /-əbəl/ *adj* nasty, bad tempered.—**disagreeableness** *n.*—**disagreeably** *adv*.

disagreement /-mənt/ *n* refusal to agree; a difference; a quarrel or dispute.

disallow /,dɪsə'laʊ/ *vt* to refuse to allow or to accept the truth or value of.—**disallowance** *n*.

disannul /,dɪsə'nʌl/ *vt* (**disannulling, disannulled**) to annul completely; to make void.

disappear /,dɪsə'pɪːr/ *vi* to pass from sight completely; to fade into nothing.—**disappearance** *n*.

disappoint /,dɪsə'pɔɪnt/ *vt* to fail to fulfil the hopes of (a person).—**disappointed** *adj.*—**disappointing** *adj.*—**disappointingly** *adv*.

disappointment /-mənt/ *n* the frustration of one's hopes; annoyance due to failure; a person or thing that disappoints.

disapprobation /,dɪs,æprə'beɪʃən/ *n* disapproval, condemnation.

disapproval /,dɪsə'pru:vəl/ *n* the action or fact of disapproving; condemnation of what is wrong.

disapprove /,dɪsə'pru:v/ *vti* to express or have an unfavourable opinion (of).—**disapprovingly** *adv*.

disarm /dɪs'ɑrm/ *vt* to deprive of weapons or means of defence; to defuse (a bomb); to conciliate. • *vi* to abolish or reduce national armaments.

disarmament /-'ɑrməmənt/ *n* the reduction or abolition of a country's armed forces and weaponry.

disarming /-'ɑrmɪŋ/ *adj* allaying opposition, conciliating; ingratiating, endearing.—**disarmingly** *adv*.

disarrange /,dɪsə'reɪndʒ/ *vt* to make untidy; to disorganize.—**disarrangement** *n*.

disarray /,dɪsə'reɪ/ *n* disorder, confusion; undress. • *vt* to put into disorder.

disarticulate /,dɪsɑr'tɪkjʊ,leɪt/ *vt* to separate, to take to pieces.—**disarticulation** *n.*—**disarticulator** *n*.

disaster /dɪ'zæstər/ *n* a devastating and sudden misfortune; utter failure.—**disastrous** *adj.*—**disastrously** *adv*.

disavow /,dɪsə'vaʊ/ *vt* to deny, disclaim; to repudiate.—**disavowal** *n.*—**disavower** *n*.

disband /dɪs'bænd/ *vt* to disperse; to break up and separate.—**disbandment** *n*.

disbar /dɪs'bɑr/ *vt* (**disbarring, disbarred**) to deprive (a barrister) of the right to practice.—**disbarment** *n*.

disbelief /,dɪsbə'li:f/ *n* a disbelieving; mental rejection of a statement or assertion; positive unbelief.

disbelieve /-'li:v/ *vt* to believe to be a lie. *vi* to have no faith (in).—**disbeliever** *n*.

disburden /dɪs'bərdən/ *vt* to throw off a burden; to relieve of anything annoying or oppressive. • *vi* to ease one's mind.—**disburdenment** *n*.

disburse /dɪs'bərs/ *vt* to pay out.—**disburser** *n*.

disbursement /-mənt/ *n* a paying out (of money); expenditure.

discalced /dɪs'kælst/ *adj* (*friars, etc*) barefoot, wearing sandals.

discard /dɪs'kɑrd/ *vti* to cast off, get rid of; (*cards*) to throw away a card from one's hand. • *n* something discarded; (*cards*) a discarded card.

disc brake, disk brake *n* a brake in which two flat discs press against a central plate on the wheel hub.

discern /dɪ'sərn/ *vt* to perceive; to see clearly.—**discernible** *adj.*—**discernibly** *adv*.

discerning /-ɪŋ/ *adj* discriminating; perceptive.—**discerningly** *adv.*—**discernment** *n*.

discharge /dɪs'tʃɑrdʒ/ *vt* to unload; to send out, emit; to release, acquit; to dismiss from employment; to shoot a gun; to fulfil, as duties. • *vi* to unload; (*gun*) to be fired; (*fluid*) to pour out. • *n* the act or process of discharging; something that is discharged; an authorization for release, acquittal, dismissal, etc.

disciple /dɪ'saɪpəl/ *n* a person who believes in and helps to spread another's teachings, a follower; (*with cap*) one of the twelve apostles of Christ.—**discipleship** *n*.

disciplinarian /,dɪsɪplɪ'nɛriən/ *n* a person who insists on strict discipline.

disciplinary /'dɪsɪplɪ,nɛri/ *adj* of or for discipline.

discipline /'dɪsɪplɪn/ *n* a field of learning; training and conditioning to produce obedience and self-control; punishment; the maintenance of order and obedience as a result of punishment; a system of rules of behaviour. • *vt* to punish to enforce discipline; to train by instruction; to bring under control.—**disciplinable** *adj.*—**disciplinal** *adj*.

disc jockey *n* (*inf*) a person who announces records on a programme of broadcast music, or in discotheques.

disclaim /dɪs'kleɪm/ *vi* to deny connection with; to renounce all legal claim to.

disclaimer /-ər/ *n* a denial of legal responsibility; a written statement embodying this.

disclose /dɪs'kloːz/ *vt* to bring into the open, to reveal.—**disclosure** *n*.

disclosure /-'kloːʒər/ *n* the act of revealing anything secret; discovery; an uncovering.

disco /'dɪskoː/ *n* (*pl* **discos**) (*inf*) a discotheque.

discography /,dɪs'kɒɡrəfi/ *n* (*pl* **discographies**) a classified list or survey of gramophone records or CDs.—**discographer** *n*.

discoid /'dɪskɔɪd/ *adj* round and flat like a disc.—*also* **discoidal**. • *n* anything with the shape of a disc.

discolour, discolor /dɪs'kələr/ *vti* to ruin the colour of; to fade, stain.—**discolouration** *n*.

discomfit /dɪs'kəmfɪt/ *vt* to defeat; to rout; to frustrate; to thwart; to disconcert.

discomfiture /-fɪtʃər/ *n* defeat; disappointment; confusion.

discomfort /dɪs'kəmfərt/ or /'dɪs-/ *n* uneasiness; something causing this. • *vt* to make uncomfortable; to make apprehensive or uneasy.

discommode /,dɪskə'moːd/ *vt* to put to inconvenience.

discompose /,dɪskəm'poːz/ *vt* to disturb the calmness of; to ruffle.—**discomposure** *n*.

disconcert /,dɪskən'sərt/ *vt* to confuse; to upset; to embarrass.—**disconcerting** *adj.*—**disconcertingly** *adv*.

disconnect /,dɪskə'nekt/ *vt* to separate or break the connection of.—**disconnection** *n*.

disconnected /-əd/ *adj* not connected, detached; disjointed; incoherent.—**disconnectedly** *adv.*—**disconnectedness** *n*.

disconsolate /dɪs'kɒnsələt/ *adj* miserable; dejected.—**disconsolately** *adv.*—**disconsolation** *n*.

discontent /,dɪskən'tent/ *n* lack of contentment, dissatisfaction.—*also* **discontentment**. • *adj* not content; dissatisfied; discontented. • *vt* to deprive of contentment; to dissatisfy.

discontented /-əd/ *adj* feeling discontent; unhappy, unsatisfied.—**discontentedly** *adv*.

discontinuance /ˌdɪskən'tɪnjuːəns/ *n* a discontinuing or breaking off; interruption; (*law*) the termination of a suit by the plaintiff.

discontinuation /-'tɪnjuː'eɪʃən/ *n* a discontinuing; discontinuance; a breach or interruption of continuity.

discontinue /-tɪnjuː/ *vti* to stop or come to a stop; to give up, *esp* the production of something; (*law*) to terminate (a suit).

discontinuity /ˌdɪskɒntɪ'njuːiti/ *n* (*pl* **discontinuities**) a being discontinuous; lack or failure of continuity or sequence; a break or gap in a structure; (*geol*) a point at which the character of the earth alters abruptly; (*math*) a function that is discontinuous.

discontinuous /ˌdɪskən'tɪnjuːəs/ *adj* not continuous, incoherent, intermittent; (*math*) of a function that varies discontinuously and whose differential coefficient may therefore become infinite.—**discontinuously** *adv*.

discord /'dɪskɔrd/ *n* lack of agreement, strife; (*mus*) a lack of harmony; harsh clashing sounds.

discordant /-dənt/ *adj* at variance; inharmonious, jarring; incongruous.—**discordance, discordancy** *n*.—**discordantly** *adv*.

discotheque, discothèque /'dɪskə tek/ *n* an occasion when people gather to dance to recorded pop music; a club or party, etc where this takes place; equipment for playing such music.

discount /'dɪskaunt/ *n* a reduction in the amount or cost; the percentage charged for doing this. • *vt* to deduct from the amount, cost; to allow for exaggeration; to disregard; to make less effective by anticipation. • *vi* to make and give discounts.—**discountable** *adj*.—**discounter** *n*.

discountenance /dɪs'kauntənəns/ *vt* to refuse moral support to; to discourage, frown upon.

discourage /dɪs'kɒrɪdʒ/ *vt* to deprive of the will or courage (to do something); to try to prevent; to hinder.—**discouragingly** *adv*.

discouragement /-mənt/ *n* the action or fact of discouraging; the state or feeling of being discouraged; something that discourages; a disheartening or deterring influence.

discourse /'dɪskɔrs/ *n* a formal speech or writing; conversation. • *vi* to talk or write about.

discourteous /dɪs'kɔrtiəs/ *adj* lacking in courtesy, rude.—**discourteously** *adv*.—**discourteousness** *n*.

discourtesy /dɪs'kɔrtəsi/ *n* (*pl* **discourtesies**) lack of courtesy or consideration; rudeness; an inconsiderate or rude act

discover /dɪs'kʌvər/ *vt* to see, find or learn of for the first time.—**discoverable** *adj*.—**discoverer** *n*.

discovert /dɪs'kʌvərt/ *adj* (*law*) (*single woman, divorcée, widow*) without a husband.—**discoverture** *n*.

discovery /dɪs'kʌvəri/ *n* (*pl* **discoveries**) the act of discovering or state of being discovered; something discovered; (*law*) a process obliging on the parties to an action to disclose relevant facts or documents.

discredit /dɪs'kredɪt/ *n* damage to a reputation; doubt; disgrace; lack of credibility. • *vt* to damage the reputation of; to cast doubt on the authority or credibility of.

discreditable /dɪs'kredɪtəbəl/ *adj* bringing discredit or disgrace.—**discreditably** *adv*.

discreet /dɪs'kriːt/ *adj* wisely cautious, prudent; unobtrusive.—**discreetly** *adv*.—**discreetness** *n*.

discrepancy /dɪs'krepənsi/ *n* (*pl* **discrepancies**) difference; a disagreement, as between figures in a total.

discrepant /-pənt/ *adj* inconsistent; not tallying.—**discrepantly** *adv*.

discrete /dɪs'kriːt/ *adj* individually distinct; discontinuous.—**discretely** *adv*.—**discreteness** *n*.

discretion /dɪs'kreʃən/ *n* the freedom to judge or to choose; prudence; wise judgment; skill.

discretionary /-ˌeri/ *adj* left to or done at one's own discretion.

discriminate /dɪ'skrɪmɪˌneɪt/ *vi* to be discerning in matters of taste or judgment; to make a distinction; to treat differently, *esp* unfavourably due to prejudice.

discriminating /-ˌneɪtɪŋ/ *adj* judicious; discerning; discriminatory.—**discriminatingly** *adv*.

discrimination /dɪˌskrɪmɪ'neɪʃən/ *n* prejudicial treatment of a person, minority group, etc, based on sex, religion, race, etc; penetration, discernment.

discriminative /dɪs'krɪmɪˌnətɪv/ *adj* serving to discriminate or distinguish; discerning; discriminatory.—**discriminatively** *adv*.

discriminator /dɪsˌkrɪmɪ'reɪtər/ *n* one who or that which discriminates; (*electronics*) a circuit that converts a property of a signal into an amplitude variation.

discriminatory /-nə'tɔri/ *adj* discriminating; showing prejudice or favouritism; biased.—**discriminatorily** *adv*.

discursive /dɪ'skɜrsɪv/ *adj* wandering from one subject to another; digressive.—**discursively** *adv*.—**discursiveness** *n*.

discus /'dɪskəs/ *n* (*pl* **discuses, disci**) a heavy disk with a thickened middle, thrown by athletes.

discuss /dɪs'kʌs/ *vt* to talk over; to investigate by reasoning or argument.—**discussible, discussable** *adj*.

discussion /-ʃən/ *n* an argument; a debate; the airing of a question.

disdain /dɪs'deɪn/ *vt* to scorn, treat with contempt. • *n* scorn; a feeling of contemptuous superiority.—**disdainful** *adj*.—**disdainfully** *adv*.

disdainful /dɪs'deɪnful/ *adj* showing or feeling disdain; contemptuous; haughty.—**disdainfully** *adv*.—**disdainfulness** *n*.

disease /dɪ'ziːz/ *n* an unhealthy condition in an organism caused by infection, poisoning, etc; sickness; a harmful condition or situation.—**diseased** *adj*.

disembark /dɪs'ɪmbɑrk/ *vti* to land from a ship, debark.—**disembarkation** *n*.

disembarrass /ˌdɪsɪm'bærəs/ *vt* to free from embarrassment; to relieve (of); to disentangle.—**disembarrassment** *n*.

disembody /ˌdɪsɪm'bɒdi/ *vt* (**disembodying, disembodied**) to free (a soul, spirit, etc) from the body.—**disembodiment** *n*.

disembogue /ˌdɪsɪm'boːg/ *vti* (**disemboguing, disembogued**) (*river etc*) to discharge, pour forth (its water).

disembowel /ˌdɪsɪm'bauəl/ *vt* (**disembowelling, disembowelled** *or* **disemboweling, disemboweled**) to remove the entrails of; to remove the substance of.—**disembowelment** *n*.

disenchant /ˌdɪsɪn'tʃænt/ *vt* to disillusion.—**disenchantment** *n*.

disencumber /ˌdɪsɪn'kʌmbər/ *vt* to free from burden or hindrance.

disendow /ˌdɪsɪn'dau/ *vt* to deprive (a church) of endowments.—**disendowment** *n*.

disenfranchise /ˌdɪsɪn'fræntʃaɪz/ *see* **disfranchise**.

disengage /ˌdɪsɪn'geɪdʒ/ *vti* to separate or free from engagement or obligation; to detach. to release.—**disengaged** *adj*.—**disengagement** *n*.

disentail /ˌdɪsɪn'teɪl/ *vt* to release from entail.—*also n*.

disentangle /ˌdɪsɪn'tæŋgəl/ *vt* to untangle; to free from complications.—**disentanglement** *n*.

disenthrall, disenthral /ˌdɪsɪn'θrɒl/ *vt* (**disenthralling, disenthralled**) to free from bondage, to emancipate.

disestablish /ˌdɪsɪ'stæblɪʃ/ *vt* to displace from a settled position; to sever (church) from connection with the state.—**disestablishment** *n*.

disesteem /ˌdɪsɪ'stiːm/ *vt* to regard with disfavour, to dislike. • *n* lack of favour or regard.

diseur *Fr.* /diː'zɜr/ *n* a reciter of monologues for entertainment.—**diseuse** *nf*.

disfavour, disfavor /dɪs'feɪvər/ *n* dislike; disapproval. • *vt* to treat with disfavour.

disfeature /dɪs'fiːtʃər/ *vt* to disfigure.

disfigure /dɪs'fɪgər/ *vt* to spoil the beauty or appearance of.—**disfigurer** *n*.

disfigurement /-mənt/, **disfiguration** /-ˌeɪʃən/ *n* the act of disfiguring; a disfigured state; a thing that disfigures; a blemish, a defect.

disfranchise /dɪs'fræntʃaɪz/ *vt* to deprive of the right to vote.—*also* **disenfranchise**.—**disfranchisement, disenfranchisement** *n*.

disgorge /dɪs'gɔrdʒ/ *vt* to emit violently from the throat, to vomit; to empty; to surrender (*eg* stolen property).—**disgorgement** *n*.

disgrace /dɪs'greɪs/ *n* a loss of trust, favour, or honour; something that disgraces. • *vt* to bring disgrace or shame upon.—**disgracer** *n*.

disgraceful /-ful/ *adj* causing or deserving disgrace, shameful.—**disgracefully** *adv*.—**disgracefulness** *n*.

disgruntled /dɪs'grʌntəld/ *adj* dissatisfied, resentful.—**disgruntlement** *n*.

disguise /dɪs'gaɪz/ *vt* to hide what one is by appearing as something else; to hide what (a thing) really is. • *n* the use of a changed appearance to conceal identity; a false appearance.—**disguisedly** *adv*.—**disguiser** *n*.

disgust /dɪs'gʌst/ *n* sickening dislike; repugnance; aversion. • *vt* to cause disgust in.—**disgustedly** *adv*.

dish *n* /dɪʃ/ any of various shallow concave vessels to serve food in; the amount of food served in a dish; the food served; a shallow concave object, as a dish aerial; (*inf*) an attractive person. • *vt* (*with* **out**) (*inf*) to distribute freely; (*with* **up**) to serve food at mealtimes; (*inf*) to present (*eg* facts).

dishabille *Fr.* /ˌdɪsæˈbiːl/ *n* a partly clad state, undress.—*also* **deshabille**.

dish aerial, dish antenna *n* a microwave antenna used in radar, telescopes, telecommunications, etc having a concave reflector.

disharmonize /dɪsˈhɑːrməˌnaɪz/ *vt* to put out of harmony; to set at variance.

disharmony /dɪsˈhɑːrməni/ *n* (*pl* **disharmonies**) a lack of harmony between sounds; discord; a discordant situation, etc.—**disharmonious** *adj*.

dishcloth /ˈdɪʃklɒθ/ *n* a cloth for washing dishes.

dishearten /dɪsˈhɑːrtən/ *vt* to discourage.—**dishearteningly** *adv*.—**disheartenment** *n*.

dishevelled, disheveled /dɪˈʃevəld/ *adj* rumpled, untidy.—**dishevelment** *n*.

dishonest /dɪsˈɒnəst/ *adj* not honest.—**dishonestly** *adv*.—**dishonesty** *n*.

dishonour, dishonor /dɪsˈɒnər/ *n* loss of honour; disgrace, shame. • *vt* to bring shame on, to disgrace; to refuse to pay, as a cheque.

dishonourable, dishonorable /-əbəl/ *adj* lacking honour, disgraceful.—**dishonourably, dishonorably** *adv*.

dishtowel /ˈdɪʃˌtaʊəl/ *n* a towel for drying dishes.

dishwasher /-ˌwɒʃər/ *n* an appliance for washing dishes; a person employed to wash dishes.

dishwater /-ˌwɒtər/ *n* water used for washing dishes; something that looks like or tastes like this.

dishy /ˈdɪʃi/ *adj* (**dishier, dishiest**) (*inf*) physically attractive, good-looking.

disillusion /ˌdɪsɪˈluːʒən/ *vt* to free from (mistaken) ideals or illusions. • *n* the state of being disillusioned.—**disillusionment** *n*.

disincentive /ˌdɪsɪnˈsentɪv/ *n* a discouragement to action or effort.

disinclination /ˌdɪsˌɪnkləˈneɪʃən/ *n* reluctance, unwillingness.

disinclined /ˌdɪsɪnˈklaɪnd/ *adj* unwilling.

disinfect /ˌdɪsɪnˈfekt/ *vt* to destroy germs.—**disinfection** *n*.

disinfectant /ˌdɪsɪnˈfektənt/ *n* any chemical agent that inhibits the growth of or destroys germs.

disinformation /ˌdɪsˌɪnfərˈmeɪʃən/ *n* false information given out by intelligence agencies to mislead foreign spies.

disingenuous /ˌdɪsɪnˈdʒenjuːəs/ *adj* insincere, not candid or straightforward.—**disingenuously** *adv*.—**disingenuousness** *n*.

disinherit /ˌdɪsɪnˈherɪt/ *vt* to deprive of the right to an inheritance.—**disinheritance** *n*.

disintegrate /dɪsˈɪntəˌɡreɪt/ *vti* to break or cause to break into separate pieces.—**disintegration** *n*.—**disintegrator** *n*.

disinter /dɪsˈɪntər/ *vt* (**disinterring, disinterred**) to take out of a grave; to bring out from obscurity, to unearth.—**disinterment** *n*.

disinterest /dɪsˈɪntərest/ *n* lack of partiality or bias. • *vt* to cease to concern (oneself).

disinterested /dɪsˈɪntrestəd/ *adj* impartial; objective.—**disinterestedly** *adv*.—**disinterestedness** *n*.

disjoin /ˈdɪsˌdʒɔɪn/ *or* /-ˈdʒɔɪn/ *vt* to separate. • *vi* to become detached.

disjoint /dɪsˈdʒɔɪnt/ *vt* to dislocate; to take to pieces. • *adj* (*math*) having no elements in common; (*obs*) disjointed.

disjointed /-ˌdʒɔɪntəd/ *adj* incoherent, muddled, *esp* of speech or writing.—**disjointedly** *adv*.—**disjointedness** *n*.

disjunction /dɪsˈdʒʌŋkʃən/ *n* severance, disconnection.—*also* **disjuncture**; (*logic*) a compound proposition presenting alternative terms only one of which is true.

disjunctive /dɪsˈdʒʌŋktɪv/ *adj* disjoining; alternative; (*gram*) marking an adverse or oppositional sense; syntactically independent; (*logic*) presenting alternative terms.—**disjunctively** *adv*.

disk[1] /dɪsk/ *n* a disc; a cylindrical pad of cartilage between the vertebrae; a gramophone record.

disk[2] *n* any flat, thin circular body; something resembling this, as the sun; (*comput*) a storage device in a computer, either floppy or hard.

disk brake *see* **disc brake**.

disk drive *n* (*comput*) a mechanism that allows a computer to read data from, and write data to, a disk.

dislike /dɪsˈlaɪk/ *vt* to consider unpleasant. • *n* aversion, distaste.—**dislikable, dislikeable** *adj*.

dislocate /ˈdɪsloʊˌkeɪt/ *vt* to put (a joint) out of place, to displace; to upset the working of.

dislocation /ˌdɪsloʊˈkeɪʃən/ *n* the act of dislocating; a joint put out of its socket; an imperfection in a crystalline structure; (*geol*) a displacement of stratified rocks, a fault.

dislodge /dɪsˈlɒdʒ/ *vt* to force or move out of a hiding place, established position, etc.—**dislodgment, dislodgement** *n*.

disloyal /dɪsˈlɔɪəl/ *adj* unfaithful; false to allegiance, disaffected.—**disloyally** *adv*.

disloyalty /-ti/ (*pl* **disloyalties**) *n* the state of being unfaithful; a disloyal act.

dismal /ˈdɪsməl/ *adj* gloomy, miserable, sad; (*inf*) feeble, worthless. —**dismally** *adv*.

dismantle /dɪsˈmæntəl/ *vt* to pull down; to take apart.—**dismantlement** *n*.

dismast /dɪsˈmæst/ *vt* to deprive (a ship) of a mast or masts.

dismay /dɪsˈmeɪ/ *n* apprehension, discouragement. • *vt* to fill with dismay.

dismember /dɪsˈmembər/ *vt* to cut or tear off the limbs from; to cut or divide into pieces.—**dismemberment** *n*.

dismiss /dɪsˈmɪs/ *vt* to send away; to remove from an office or employment; to stop thinking about; (*law*) to reject a further hearing (in court); (*cricket*) to bowl a batsman or side out.—**dismissible** *adj*.

dismissal /-əl/ *n* the act of dismissing; a removal from office, etc.

dismissive /-ˈmɪsɪv/ *adj* rejecting; offhand.—**dismissively** *adv*.

dismount /dɪsˈmaʊnt/ *vti* to alight from a horse or bicycle; to remove from a mount or setting.

disobedience /ˌdɪsoʊˈbiːdiəns/ *or* /-əˈbiː-/ *n* the withholding of obedience; a refusal to obey; violation of a command by omitting to conform to it, or of a prohibition by acting in defiance of it; an instance of this.

disobedient /-ənt/ *adj* failing or refusing to obey.—**disobediently** *adv*.

disobey /ˌdɪsoʊˈbeɪ/ *or* /-əˈbeɪ/ *vt* (**disobeying, disobeyed**) to refuse to follow orders.

disoblige /ˌdɪsoʊˈblaɪdʒ/ *vt* to ignore the wishes of; to inconvenience.—**disobligingly** *adv*.

disorder /dɪsˈɔːrdər/ *n* lack of order; untidiness; a riot; an illness or interruption of the normal functioning of the body or mind. • *vt* to throw into confusion; to upset.

disorderly /-li/ *adj* untidy; unruly, riotous.—**disorderliness** *n*.

disorganize /dɪsˈɔːrɡəˌnaɪz/ *vt* to confuse or disrupt an orderly arrangement.—**disorganization** *n*.

disorient /dɪsˈɔːriənt/, **disorientate** /-ɪd/ *vt* to cause the loss of sense of time, place or identity; to confuse.—**disorientation** *n*.

disown /dɪsˈoʊn/ *vt* to refuse to acknowledge as one's own.

disparage /dɪsˈpærɪdʒ/ *vt* to belittle.—**disparagingly** *adv*.—**disparagement** *n*.

disparate /ˈdɪspərət/ *adj* unequal, completely different.—**disparately** *adv*.—**disparateness** *n*.

disparity /dɪsˈperəti/ *n* (*pl* **disparities**) essential difference; inequality.

dispassionate /dɪsˈpæʃənət/ *adj* unemotional; impartial.—**dispassionately** *adv*.—**dispassionateness** *n*.

dispatch /dɪsˈpætʃ/ *vt* to send off somewhere; to perform speedily; to kill. • *n* a sending off (of a letter, a messenger etc); promptness; haste; a written message, *esp* of news.—*also* **despatch**.—**dispatcher** *n*.

dispel /dɪˈspel/ *vt* (**dispelling, dispelled**) to drive away and scatter.

dispensable /dɪˈspensəbəl/ *adj* able to be done without; unimportant.—**dispensability** *n*.

dispensary /dɪˈspensəri/ *n* (*pl* **dispensaries**) a place in a hospital, a chemist shop, etc where medicines are made up and dispensed; a place where medical treatment is available.

dispensation /ˌdɪspenˈseɪʃən/ *or* /-pən-/ *n* the act of distributing or dealing out; exemption from a rule, penalty, etc.

dispense /dɪˈspens/ *vt* to deal out, distribute; to prepare and distribute medicines; to administer.

dispenser /dɪˈspensər/ *n* a person who dispenses medicines; a machine, etc, that dispenses measured quanitites or units of something.

dispermous /daɪˈspɜːrməs/ *adj* (*bot*) two-seeded.

dispersal /dɪˈspɜːrsəl/ *n* the act of dispersing; dispersion.

disperse /dɪ'spɜrs/ vt to scatter in different directions; to cause to evaporate; to spread (knowledge); to separate (light, etc) into different wavelengths. • vi to separate, become dispersed.—**dispersedly** adv.

dispersion /dɪ'spɜrʒən/ n a dispersing, or state of being dispersed; (physics) the separation of light into colours by diffraction or refraction; (statistics) the scattering of data about a mean.

dispersive /dɪ'spɜrsɪv/ adj tending to disperse; producing dispersion.—**dispersively** adv.

dispirit /dɪ'spɪrɪt/ vt to depress the spirits of; to dishearten; to render cheerless.

dispirited /-əd/ adj depressed, discouraged.—**dispiritedly** adv.

displace /dɪs'pleɪs/ vt to take the place of, to oust; to remove from a position of authority.

displaced person n a person who has become a refugee from their own country, eg due to war or famine.

displacement /-mənt/ n the act of displacing; substitution; apparent change of position; the weight of water displaced by a solid body immersed in it.

display /dɪs'pleɪ/ vt to show, expose to view; to exhibit ostentatiously. • n a displaying; an eye-catching arrangement; exhibition; a computer monitor for presenting visual information.

displease /dɪs'pliːz/ vt to cause offence or annoyance to.

displeasure /-'pleʒər/ n a feeling of being displeased; dissatisfaction.

disport /dɪ'spɔrt/ vt to amuse or divert (oneself). • vi to display gaily.

disposable /dɪ'spozəbəl/ adj designed to be discarded after use; available for use. • n something disposable, eg a baby's nappy.

disposal /dɪ'spozəl/ n a disposing of something; order, arrangement.

dispose /dɪ'spoz/ vt to place in order, arrange; to influence. • vi to deal with or settle; to give, sell or transfer to another; to throw away.

disposed /dɪ'spozd/ adj inclined (towards something).

disposition /ˌdɪspə'zɪʃən/ n a natural way of behaving towards others; tendency; arrangement.—**dispositional** adj.

dispossess /ˌdɪspə'zes/ vt to deprive, rid (of); to eject.—**dispossession** n.—**dispossessor** n.

dispraise /dɪs'preɪz/ vt to disparage; to censure. • n depreciation; a reproach.—**dispraisingly** adv.

disproof /dɪs'pruːf/ n a disproving or refuting; evidence that refutes.

disproportion /ˌdɪsprə'pɔrʃən/ n a lack of symmetry, a being out of proportion. • vt to render or make out of due proportion.—**disproportional** adj.—**disproportionally** adv.

disproportionate /ˌdɪsprə'pɔrʃənət/ adj out of proportion.—**disproportionately** adv.

disprove /dɪs'pruːv/ vt to prove (a claim, etc) to be incorrect.—**disprovable** adj.

disputable /dɪs'pjuːtəbəl/ or /'dɪspjətəbəl/ adj likely to cause dispute, arguable.—**disputability** n.—**disputably** adv.

disputant /'dɪspjuːtənt/ n a person involved in a dispute.

disputation /ˌdɪspjuː'teɪʃən/ n an argument; an exercise in debate.

disputatious /ˌdɪspjuː'teɪʃəs/ adj fond of argument, contentious.—**disputatiously** adv.—**disputatiousness** n.

dispute /dɪs'pjuːt/ vt to make the subject of an argument or debate; to query the validity of. • vi to argue. • n an argument; a quarrel.

disqualify /dɪs'kwɒlɪˌfaɪ/ vt (**disqualifying, disqualified**) to make ineligible because of a violation of rules; to make unfit or unsuitable, to disable.—**disqualifier** n.—**disqualification** n.

disquiet /dɪs'kwaɪət/ vt to trouble, disturb; to make uneasy or restless. • n disturbance; uneasiness, anxiety, worry; restlessness. • adj restless; uneasy; disturbed.—**disquieting** adj.

disquietude /dɪs'kwaɪəˌtuːd/ or /-ˌtjuːd/ n restlessness; disturbance; a feeling, occasion or cause of disquiet.

disquisition /ˌdɪskwɪ'zɪʃən/ n a careful examination of a subject.

disregard /ˌdɪsrɪ'gɑrd/ vt to pay no attention to; to consider as of little or no importance. • n lack of attention, neglect.

disrelish /dɪs'relɪʃ/ vt to dislike.—also n.

disrepair /ˌdɪsrɪ'per/ or /-ri-/ n a worn-out condition through neglect of repair.

disreputable /dɪs're'pjuːtəbəl/ adj of bad reputation; not respectable; discreditable.—**disreputably** adv.

disrepute /ˌdɪsrɪ'pjuːt/ or /'dɪsrɪˌpjuːt/ n disgrace, discredit.

disrespect /ˌdɪsrə'spekt/ n lack of respect, rudeness.—**disrespectful** adj.—**disrespectfully** adv.

disrobe /dɪs'roːb/ vti to undress; to uncover.

disrupt /dɪs'rʌpt/ vti to break up; to create disorder or confusion; to interrupt.—**disruption** n.

disruptive /dɪs'rʌptɪv/ adj causing disruption.—**disruptively** adv.

dissatisfaction /ˌdɪsætɪs'fækʃən/ n disapproval; discontent; something that dissatisfies.

dissatisfactory /-'fæktəri/ adj unsatisfactory.

dissatisfy /dɪ'sætɪsˌfaɪ/ vt (**dissatisfying, dissatisfied**) to fail to please, to make discontented.

dissect /'daɪsekt/ vt to cut apart (a plant, an animal, etc) for scientific examination; to analyse and interpret in fine detail.—**dissection** n.—**dissector** n.

disseise, disseize /dɪs'siːz/ vt to deprive of possession; to dispossess unlawfully.—**disseisor, disseizor** n.

disseisin, disseizin /-zɪn/ n the act of unlawfully dispossessing a person or an estate.

dissemble /dɪ'sembəl/ vti to pretend or to conceal (eg true feelings) by pretence.—**dissemblance** n.—**dissembler** n.

disseminate /dɪ'semɪˌneɪt/ vt to spread or scatter (ideas, information, etc) widely.—**dissemination** n.—**disseminator** n.

dissension /dɪ'senʃən/ n disagreement, esp when resulting in conflict.

dissent /dɪ'sent/ vi to hold a different opinion; to withhold assent. • n a difference of opinion.—**dissenter** n.

dissentient /dɪ'senʃənt/ adj disagreeing with the majority. • n a person who dissents.

dissepiment /dɪ'sepɪmənt/ n (biol) a calcareous or membraneous partition, a septum.

dissertate /ˌdɪsər'teɪt/ vi to hold forth, to discourse.—**dissertator** n.

dissertation /-ʃən/ n a written thesis, esp as required for a university degree, etc.

disservice /dɪs'ərvɪs/ n an ill turn, a harmful action.

dissever /-vər/ vti to cut apart, to disunite.—**disseverance, disseverment** n.

dissident /'dɪsɪdənt/ adj disagreeing. • n a person who disagrees strongly with government policies, esp one who suffers harassment or imprisonment as a result.—**dissidence** n.

dissimilar /dɪ'sɪmɪlər/ adj unlike, different.—**dissimilarly** adv.

dissimilarity /'dɪsɪmɪ'lerɪti/ n (pl **dissimilarities**) lack of similarity; a difference, distinction.

dissimulate /dɪ'sɪmjuˌleɪt/ vt to dissemble.—**dissimulation** n.—**dissimulator** n.

dissipate /'dɪsɪˌpeɪt/ vt to scatter, dispel; to waste, squander (money, etc). • vi to separate and vanish.—**dissipater, dissipator** n.

dissipated /-əd/ adj dissolute, indulging in excessive pleasure; scattered, wasted.—**dissipatedly** adv.—**dissipatedness** n.

dissipation /'dɪsɪˌpeɪʃən/ n dispersion; wastefulness; frivolous or dissolute living.

dissociate /dɪ'soːsiˌeɪt/ or -ʃiˌeɪt/ vti to separate or cause to separate the association of (people, things, etc) in consciousness; to repudiate a connection with.—**dissociation** n.

dissociation /dɪ'soːsiˌeɪʃən/ or /-ʃiˌeɪʃən/ n a dissociating or being dissociated; (chem) decomposition of a molecule into single atoms, etc; (psychol) the separation of an attitude, belief, etc, from the rest of the personality.

dissoluble /dɪ'sɒljubəl/ adj soluble.—**dissolubility** n.

dissolute /dɪsə'luːt/ adj lacking moral discipline, debauched.—**dissolutely** adv.—**dissoluteness** n.

dissolution /dɪsə'luːʃən/ n separation into component parts; the dissolving of a meeting or assembly (eg parliament); the termination of a business or personal relationship; death; the process of dissolving.

dissolve /dɪ'sɒlv/ vt to cause to pass into solution; to disperse (a legislative assembly); to melt; (partnership, marriage) to break up legally, annul. • vi to become liquid; to fade away; to be overcome by emotion.—**dissolvable** adj.—**dissolver** n.

dissolvent /-vənt/ adj able to dissolve. • n a substance that dissolves.

dissonance /'dɪsənəns/ n a harsh or inharmonious sound; discord; lack of agreement; (mus) an incomplete or unfulfilled chord requiring resolution into harmony.

dissonant /-nənt/ adj inharmonious; discordant; disagreeing; (mus) producing dissonance.—**dissonantly** adv.

dissuade /dɪ'sweɪd/ vt to prevent or discourage by persuasion.—**dissuasion** n.—**dissuasive** adj.

dissyllable /daɪ'sɪləbəl/ or /'daɪ-/ n a word of two syllables.—also **disyllable.**—**dissyllabic, disyllabic** adj.

dissymmetry /dɪˈsɪmɪtri/ *n* (*pl* **dissymmetries**) an absence or lack of symmetry; symmetry in opposite directions, like right and left hands.—**dissymmetrical, dissymmetric** *adj*.

distaff /ˈdɪstæf/ *n* the stick on which wool for flax is wound for spinning; (*arch*) a woman, women.

distaff line *n* the female line of a family.

distal /ˈdɪstəl/ *adj* (*anat*) relatively distant from the centre of the body or point of attachment.—**distally** *adv*.

distance /-təns/ *n* the amount of space between two points or things; a distant place or point; remoteness, coldness of manner. • *vt* to place at a distance, physically or emotionally; to out-distance in a race, etc.

distant /-ənt/ *adj* separated by a specific distance; far-off in space, time, place, relation, etc; not friendly, aloof.—**distantly** *adv*.

distaste /dɪsˈteɪst/ *n* aversion; dislike.

distasteful /-fʊl/ *adj* unpleasant, offensive.—**distastefully** *adv*.—**distastefulness** *n*.

distemper /dɪsˈtempər/ *n* an infectious and often fatal disease of dogs and other animals; a type of paint made by mixing colour with egg or glue instead of oil; a painting made with this.

distend /dɪsˈtend/ *vti* to swell or cause to swell, *esp* from internal pressure.

distensible /dɪsˈtensəbəl/ *adj* able to be distended.

distension, distention /-ʃən/ *n* a distending or being distended; a swelling.

distich /ˈdɪstɪk/ *n* (*pl* **distichs**) (*poetry*) a couplet.

distichous /-əs/ *adj* (*bot*) arranged in two rows on opposite sides of an axis.—**distichously** *adv*.

distil, distill /ˈdɪstɪl/ *vti* (**distils** *or* **distills, distilling, distilled**) to treat by, or cause to undergo, distillation; to purify; to extract the essence of; to let or cause to fall in drops.

distillate /ˈdɪstɪlət/ *or* /-leɪt/, /-ˈstɪl-/ *n* a product of distillation.

distillation /ˌdɪstɪˈleɪʃən/ *n* the conversion of a liquid into vapour by heat and then cooling the vapour so it condenses again, separating out the liquid's constituents or purifying it in the process; a distillate.—**distillatory** *adj*.

distiller /dɪˈstɪlər/ *n* an individual or organization that distils, *eg* a brewery.

distillery /-əri/ *n* (*pl* **distilleries**) a place where distilling, *esp* of alcoholic spirits, is carried on.

distinct /dɪˈstɪŋkt/ *adj* different, separate (from); easy to perceive by the mind or senses.—**distinctly** *adv*.—**distinctness** *n*.

distinction /dɪˈstɪŋkʃən/ *n* discrimination, separation; a difference seen or made; a distinguishing mark or characteristic; excellence, superiority; a mark of honour.

distinctive /dɪˈstɪŋktɪv/ *adj* clearly marking a person or thing as different from another; characteristic.—**distinctively** *adv*.—**distinctiveness** *n*.

distingué *Fr.* /diːstæ̃ˈgeɪ/ *adj* of superior manner, distinguished, striking.

distinguish /dɪˈstɪŋgwɪʃ/ *vt* to see or recognize as different; to mark as different, characterize; to see or hear clearly; to confer distinction on; to make eminent or known. • *vi* to perceive a difference.—**distinguishable** *adj*.

distinguished /dɪˈstɪŋgwɪʃt/ *adj* eminent, famous; dignified in appearance or manners.

Distinguished Flying Cross *n* a US military decoration for gallantry or heroism in flying operations.

distort /dɪˈstɔrt/ *vt* to pull or twist out of shape; to alter the true meaning of, misrepresent.

distortion /-ʃən/ *n* a distorting or being distorted; a distorted feature; (*optics*) a faulty image; (*electronics*) an unwanted change in a signal, etc.—**distortional** *adj*.

distract /dɪˈstrækt/ *vt* to draw (*eg* the mind or attention) to something else; to confuse.—**distractingly** *adv*.

distracted /-əd/ *adj* bewildered, confused.—**distractedly** *adv*.

distraction /-ʃən/ *n* something that distracts the attention; an amusement; perplexity; extreme agitation.—**distractive** *adj*.—**distractively** *adv*.

distrain /dɪˈstreɪn/ *vt* to seize and hold goods or chattels as security for payment of a debt.—**distrainer, distrainor** *n*.—**distrainment** *n*.

distrainee /-ˈniː/ *n* a person who is distrained upon.

distraint /dɪˈstreɪnt/ *n* the act of distraining for debt; seizure.

distrait /dɪˈstreɪt/ *adj* absent-minded, preoccupied.

distraught /dɪˈstrɔt/ *adj* extremely distressed.

distress /dɪˈstres/ *n* physical or emotional suffering, as from pain, illness, lack of money, etc; a state of danger, desperation. • *vt* to cause distress to.—**distressingly** *adv*.

distressful /-fʊl/ *adj* suffering or causing distress.—**distressfully** *adv*.—**distressfulness** *n*.

distributary /dɪˈstrɪbjuˌteri/ *n* (*pl* **distributaries**) a river branch that does not return to the main stream.

distribute /dɪˈstrɪbjuːt/ *or* /ˈdɪ-/ *vt* to divide and share out; to spread, disperse throughout an area.—**distributable** *adj*.

distribution /-ʃən/ *n* a distributing or a being distributed; allotment; a thing distributed; diffusion; the geographical range or occurence of an organism; classification; (*law*) the apportioning of an estate among the heirs; (*commerce*) the marketing of goods to customers, their handling and transport; (*statistics*) the way numbers denoting characteristics in a statistical population are distributed.—**distributional** *adj*.

distributor /-tər/ *n* an agent who sells goods, *esp* wholesale; a device for distributing current to the spark plugs in an engine.

district /ˈdɪstrɪkt/ *n* a territorial division defined for administrative purposes; a region or area with a distinguishing character.

district attorney *n* in US a lawyer who is the state's prosecutor in a judicial district.

district municipality *n* ✤ (*Cdn*) in British Columbia, an administrative unit for a thinly-populated area.

District of Columbia *n* a federal area whose boundary is that of Washington, the capital.

distrust /dɪsˈtrʌst/ *n* suspicion, lack of trust. • *vt* to withhold trust or confidence from; to suspect.—**distrustful** *adj*.—**distrustfully** *adv*.—**distrustfulness** *n*.

disturb /dɪˈstɜrb/ *vt* to interrupt; to cause to move from the normal position or arrangement; to destroy the quiet or composure of.

disturbance /-əns/ *n* a disturbing or being disturbed; an interruption; an outbreak of disorder and confusion.

disturbed /dɪˈstɜrbd/ *adj* showing symptoms of emotional illness.

disulphate, disulfate /daɪˈsʌlfeɪt/ *n* a sulphate containing one atom of hydrogen, replaceable by a basic element.

disulphide, disulfide /-faɪd/ *n* a sulphide in which two atoms of sulphur are contained.

disunite /dɪʃˈjuːnaɪt/ *vt* to divide, disrupt. • *vi* to separate.

disuse /dɪsˈjuːz/ *n* the state of being neglected or unused.—**disused** *adj*.

disyllable /daɪˈsɪləbəl/ *see* **dissyllable**.

ditch /dɪtʃ/ *n* any long narrow trench dug in the ground. • *vt* to make a ditch in; (*sl*) to drive (a car) into a ditch; (*sl*) to make a forced landing of (an aircraft); (*sl*) to get rid of.

dither /ˈdɪðər/ *vi* to hesitate, vacillate. • *n* a state of confusion; uncertainty.—**ditherer** *n*.

dithyramb /ˈdɪðɪˌræm/ *or* /-ˈræmb/ *n* a hymn sung in honour of Dionysus, the Greek god of wine; an impassioned speech or writing.—**dithyrambic** *adj, n*.—**dithyrambically** *adv*.

dittany /ˈdɪtəni/ (*pl* **dittanies**) *n* an aromatic pink-flowered plant of the mint family formerly believed to have magical properties.

ditto /ˈdɪto/ *n* (*pl* **dittos**) the same again, as above—used in written lists and tables to avoid repetition. • *vt* (**dittoing, dittoed**) to repeat.

ditto marks *npl* two small marks (') placed under an item repeated.

ditty /ˈdɪti/ *n* (*pl* **ditties**) a simple song.

diuretic /ˌdaɪjʊˈretɪk/ *n* a substance or drug that acts to increase the discharge of urine.—*also adj*.

diurnal /daɪˈɜrnəl/ *adj* occurring daily; of the daytime; having a daily cycle.—**diurnally** *adv*.

diva /ˈdiːvə/ *n* (*pl* **divas, dive**) an accomplished female opera singer; a prima donna.

divalent /daɪˈveɪlənt/ *adj* (*chem*) having a valence of two.

divan /dɪˈvæn/ *n* a long couch without back or sides; a bed of similar design.

dive /daɪv/ *vi* (**diving, dived** *or* **dove, dived**) to plunge head-first into water; (*aircraft*) to descend or fall steeply; (*diver, submarine*) to submerge; to plunge (*eg* the hand) suddenly into anything; to dash headlong, lunge. • *n* a headlong plunge; a submerging of a submarine, etc; a sharp descent; a steep decline; (*sl*) a disreputable public place.

dive bomber *n* an aircraft designed to release its bombs during a steep dive for superior accuracy.—**dive-bomb** *vt*.

diver /-ər/ *n* a person who dives; a person who works or explores underwater from a diving bell or in a diving suit; any of various aquatic birds.

diverge /daɪˈvɜːdʒ/ *vi* to branch off in different directions from a common point; to differ in character, form, etc; to deviate from a path or course.—**divergence** *n*.—**divergent** *adj*.

divers /ˈdaɪvərz/ *adj* (*arch*) various; sundry.

diverse /ˈdaɪvərs/ *adj* different; assorted, various.—**diversely** *adv*.—**diverseness** *n*.

diversify /daɪˈvɜːsɪˌfaɪ/ *vb* (**diversifying, diversified**) *vt* to vary; to invest in a broad range of securities to lessen risk of loss. • *vi* to engage in a variety of commercial operations to reduce risk.—**diversification** *n*.

diversion /daɪˈvɜːʒən/ or /dɪ-/ *n* turning aside from a course; a recreation, amusement; a drawing of attention away from the principal activity; a detour when a road is temporarily closed to traffic.—**diversionary** *adj*.

diversity /ˈdaɪvɜːsɪti/ or /dɪ-/ *n* (*pl* **diversities**) the condition or quality of being diverse; unlikeness; a difference, distinction; variety.

divert /daɪˈvɜːt/ *vt* to turn aside from one course onto another; to entertain, amuse.

diverticulitis /ˌdaɪvərˌtɪkjuˈlaɪtɪs/ *n* inflammation of a diverticulum.

diverticulum /ˌdaɪvərtɪˈkjuləm/ *n* (*pl* **diverticula**) a pocket or side branch off a passage or cavity in the body, esp the intestine.

divertimento /dɪˌvɜːtɪˈmentoː/ or /dɪˌvɜːr-/ *n* (*pl* **divertimenti, divertimentos**) a light, pleasant vocal or instrumental composition.

divertissement /diːˈvɜːtɪsmənt/, *Fr.* /diːvɛrtiːsˈmɑ̃/ *n* an amusement; a recreation, a light entertainment, a ballet, etc, as an interlude between the acts of a play; an entr'acte; (*mus*) a divertimento.

divest /daɪˈvest/ *vt* to strip of clothing, equipment etc; to deprive of rights, property, power, etc.—**d vestiture, divestment** *n*.

divide /dɪˈvaɪd/ *vt* to break up into parts; to distribute, share out; to sort into categories; to cause to separate from something else; to separate into opposing sides; (*parliament*) to vote or cause to vote by division; (*math*) to ascertain how many times one quantity contains another. • *vi* to become separated; to diverge; to vote by separating into two sides. • *n* a watershed; a split.—**dividable** *adj*.

divided highway *see* **dual carriageway**.

dividend /ˈdɪvɪˌdend/ *n* a number which is to be divided; the money earned by a company and divided among the shareholders; a bonus derived from some action.

divider /dɪˈvaɪdər/ *n* something that divides; a screen, furniture or plants, etc used to divide up a room; (*pl*) measuring-compasses.

divi-divi /ˈdɪvɪˌdɪvɪ/ (*pl* **divi-divis**) *n* a South American tropical plant; its astringent husks used for dyeing and tanning.

divination /ˌdɪvɪˈneɪʃən/ *n* the art of foretelling the future or discovering hidden knowledge by supernatural means; intuitive perception.—**divinatory** *adj*.

divine /dɪˈvaɪn/ *adj* of, from, or like God or a god; (*inf*) excellent. • *n* a clergyman; a theologian. • *vt* to foretell the future by supernatural means; to discover intuitively; to dowse. • *vi* to practise divination.—**divinely** *adv*.—**diviner** *n*.

diving bell *n* an open-bottomed chamber for working under water, supplied with compressed air.

diving board *n* a platform or springboard for diving from.

diving suit *n* a watertight suit with a helmet and air supply, used by divers.

divining rod *n* a forked twig used for dowsing.

divinity /dɪˈvɪnɪti/ *n* (*pl* **divinities**) any god; theology; the quality of being God or a god.

divisible /dɪˈvɪsɪbəl/ *adj* able to be divided.—**divisibility** *n*.

division /dɪˈvɪʒən/ *n* a dividing or being divided; a partition, a barrier; a portion or section; a military unit; separation; (*Parliament*) a separation into two opposing sides to vote; a disagreement; (*math*) the process of dividing one number by another.—**divisional** *adj*.

divisive /dɪˈvaɪsɪv/ or /dɪˈvaɪsɪv/, /-zɪv/ *adj* creating disagreement or disunity.—**divisively** *adv*.—**divisiveness** *n*.

divisor /dɪˈvaɪzər/ *n* a number that is to be divided into another number (the dividend).

divorce /dɪˈvɔːs/ *n* the legal dissolution of marriage; separation. • *vt* to terminate a marriage by divorce; to separate.

divorcé, divorcee /ˌdɪvɔːˈsiː/ *n* a divorced person.—**divorcée** *nf*.

divorcement /dɪˈvɔːsmənt/ *n* the act or process of divorcing.

divot /ˈdɪvət/ *n* a lump of turf dug from the ground while making a golf swing, etc.

divulge /daɪˈvʌldʒ/ or /dɪ/ *vt* to tell or reveal.—**divulgence** *n*.

divvy /ˈdɪvi/ *n* (*pl* **divvies**) in the UK, a dividend; in the US, a portion. • *vt* (**divvying, divvied**) (*usu with* **up**) to share out.

Dixie /ˈdɪksi/ *n* the southern States of the US.

Dixieland /-ˌlænd/ *n* Dixie; a New Orleans jazz style.

dizzy /ˈdɪzi/ *adj* (**dizzier, dizziest**) confused; causing giddiness or confusion; (*sl*) silly; foolish. • *vt* to make dizzy; to confuse.—**dizzily** *adv*.—**dizziness** *n*.

DJ *abbr* = disc jockey; dinner jacket.

dl *abbr* = decilitre.

DM *abbr* = Deutschmark; ✤ (*Cdn*) Deputy Minister.

dm *abbr* = decimetre.

DMus *abbr* = Doctor of Music.

DMZ *abbr* = demilitarized zone.

DNA *abbr* = deoxyribonucleic acid, the main component of chromosomes that stores genetic information.

DND *abbr* ✤ (*Cdn*) = Department of National Defence.

do /duː/ *vt* (*pres t* **does, doing, did,** *pp* **done**) to perform; to work; to end, to complete; to make; to provide; to arrange; to tidy; to perform; to cover a distance; to visit; (*sl*) to serve time in prison; (*sl*) to cheat, to rob; (*sl*) to assault; (*with* **in**) (*inf*) to kill; to tire out. • *vi* to act or behave; to be satisfactory; to manage. • *n* (*pl* **dos, do's**) (*inf*) a party; (*inf*) a hoax. *Do* has special uses where it has no definite meaning, as in asking questions (*Do you like milk?*), emphasizing a verb (*I do want to go*), and standing for a verb already used (*My dog goes where I do*).

DOA *abbr* = dead on arrival.

Doberman (pinscher) /ˈdoːbərmən(ˈpɪnʃər)/ *n* a breed of dog with a smooth glossy black-and-tan coat and docked tail.

doc /dɒk/ *n* (*inf*) doctor.

docent /ˈdoːsənt/ *n* a person licensed to teach in a university, but of lower grade and authority than a professor.

docile /ˈdɒsaɪl/ or /ˈdoː-/ *adj* easily led; submissive.—**docilely** *adv*.—**docility** *n*.

dock[1] /dɒk/ *vt* (*an animal's tail*) to cut short; (*wages, etc*) to deduct a portion of.

dock[2] *n* a wharf; an artificial enclosed area of water for ships to be loaded, repaired, etc; (*pl*) a dockyard. • *vt* to come or bring into dock; to join (spacecraft) together in space.

dock[3] *n* an enclosed area in a court of law reserved for the accused.

dockage /ˈdɒkɪdʒ/ *n* the provision of accommodation for the docking of vessels; money paid for the use of a dock.

docker /-ər/ *n* a labourer who works at the docks.—*also* **longshoreman** *n*.

docket /ˈdɒkət/ *n* a label or document recording the contents of a package, delivery instructions, payment advice, or details of payment of customs dues; in US, a list of lawsuits to be tried by a court. • *vt* (*goods*) to put a docket on; (*lawsuit*) to enter on a docket.

dockyard /-jɑːd/ *n* an area with docks and facilities for repairing and refitting ships.

doctor /ˈdɒktər/ *n* a person qualified to treat diseases or physical disorders; the highest academic degree; the holder of such a degree. • *vt* to treat medically; (*machinery, etc*) to patch up; to tamper with, falsify; (*inf*) to castrate or spay.—**doctoral** *adj*.

doctorate /-tərət/ *n* the highest degree in any discipline given by a university, conferring the title of doctor.

doctrinaire /ˌdɒktrɪˈnɛr/ *adj* obsessed by theory rather than by experience. • *n* a person so obsessed.—**doctrinairism** *n*.

doctrine /-trɪn/ *n* a principle of belief.—**doctrinal** *adj*.—**doctrinally** *adv*.

document /ˈdɒkjumənt/ *n* a paper containing information or proof of anything. • *vt* to provide or prove with documents.—**documental** *adj*.—**documentation** *n*.

documentary /-ˈmentəri/ *adj* consisting of documents; presenting a factual account of an event or activity. • *n* (*pl* **documentaries**) a nonfiction film.

dodder /ˈdɒdər/ *vi* to tremble or shake through old age or weakness; to walk slowly and shakily.—**dodderer** *n*.—**doddery** *adj*.

dodecagon /doːˈdekəgon/ *n* a geometric figure with twelve angles and sides.

dodecahedron /ˌdoːdəkəˈhiːdrən/ *n* a solid figure with twelve faces.—**dodecahedral** *adj*.

dodge /dɒdʒ/ *vi* to move quickly in an irregular course. • *vt* to evade (a duty) by cunning; to avoid by a sudden movement or shift of position; to trick. • *n* a sudden movement; (*inf*) a clever trick.—**dodger** *n*.

dodgy /'dɒdʒi/ *adj* (**dodgier, dodgiest**) (*inf*) cunning; risky.

dodo /'dəʊdəʊ/ *n* (*pl* **dodos, dodoes**) a large, clumsy bird, now extinct.

doe /dəʊ/ *n* (*pl* **does, doe**) a female deer, rabbit, or hare.

DOE *abbr* ✝ (*Cdn*) = Department of the Environment.

doer /'duːər/ *n* a person who acts, as opposed to thinking or talking; an active energetic person.

does /dʌs/ *see* **do**.

doeskin /'dəʊskɪn/ *n* the skin of a doe; a fine woollen cloth with a smooth finish.

doesn't /'dʌzənt/ = does not.

doff /dɒf/ *vt* to take off (*esp* one's hat) in greeting or as a sign of respect.

dog /dɒg/ *n* a canine mammal of numerous breeds, commonly kept as a domestic pet; the male of the wolf or fox; a despicable person; a device for gripping things. • *vt* (**dogging, dogged**) to pursue relentlessly.—**dog-like** *adj*.

dogan /'dəʊgən/ *n* ✝ (*Cdn*) (*hist sl*) a Roman Catholic, especially one who is Irish.

dogcart *n* a light, two-wheeled carriage with cross seats back to back.

dog collar *n* a collar for a dog; (*inf*) a clerical collar.

dog days *npl* the warmest days of the year.

doge /dəʊdʒ/ *n* (*formerly*) the chief magistrate in republican Venice and Genoa.

dog-eared *adj* worn, shabby; (*book*) having the corners of the pages turned down.—**dog-ear** *vt*.

dogfight /'dɒgfaɪt/ *n* (*loosely*) a fiercely disputed contest; combat between two fighter planes, *esp* at close quarters.

dogfish /-fɪʃ/ *n* (*pl* **dogfish, dogfishes**) any of various small shark-like fish.

dogged /'dɒgəd/ *adj* tenacious.—**doggedly** *adv*.—**doggedness** *n*.

doggerel /'dɒgərəl/ *n* trivial or worthless verse.

doggish *adj* like a dog, surly; (*sl*) showily stylish.—**doggishly** *adv*.—**doggishness** *n*.

doggo /'dɒgəʊ/ *adv* (*sl*) silent and still; **lie doggo** to lie low, stay hidden.

doggone /'dɒgɒn/ *interj* (*sl*) darn, damn. • *adj* (*sl*) cursed, confounded. • *vt* (*sl*) to damn.

doggy /'dɒgi/ *adj* (**doggier, doggiest**) of or like a dog; fond of dogs; (*sl*) showily stylish. • *n* (*pl* **doggies**) a pet name for a dog; a little dog.—*also* **doggie**.

doghouse /'dɒghaʊs/ *n* a dog kennel; **in the doghouse** (*inf*) in disgrace.

dogleg /-leg/ *n* something having a sharp angle or a sharp bend, as a road or fairway on a golf course. • *adj* crooked like a dog's hind leg.—*also* **doglegged**.

dogma /'dɒgmə/ *n* (*pl* **dogmas, dogmata**) a belief taught or held as true, *esp* by a church; a doctrine; a belief.

dogmatic /dɒg'mætɪk/, **dogmatical** /-əl/ *adj* pertaining to a dogma; forcibly asserted as if true; overbearing.—**dogmatically** *adv*.

dogmatics /-ɪks/ *n* (*used as sing*) the study of religious dogmas; doctrinal theology.

dogmatize /-ˌtaɪz/ *vt* to assert in a dogmatic manner.—**dogmatism** *n*.—**dogmatist** *n*.

do-gooder /duː'gʊdər/ *n* a well-meaning person, *esp* if naive or ineffectual.—**do-gooding** *n*.

dog paddle *n* an elementary form of swimming in which the arms and legs paddle rapidly in the water.—**dog-paddle** *vi*.

dog rose *n* a prickly wild rose.

dogsbody /'dɒgzˌbɒdi/ *n* (*pl* **dogsbodies**) (*inf*) a drudge.

dogtooth /-ˌtuːθ/ (*pl* **dogteeth**) *n* a canine tooth; (*archit*) a small conical ornament resembling a petal in Early English architecture.

dogtrot /'dɒgtrɒt/ *n* a gentle trot; a covered passageway.

dogwatch /-wɒtʃ/ *n* (*naut*) one of two watches on board ship of two hours each, between 4 and 8 pm.

dogwood /-wʊd/ *n* any of several shrubs with clusters of small flowers.

doily /'dɔɪli/ *n* (*pl* **doilies**) a small ornamented mat, laid under food on dishes, *eg* cakes.—*also* **doyley**.

doing /'duːɪŋ/ *n* an action or its result; (*pl*) things done; actions.

doit /dɔɪt/ *n* a small old Dutch copper coin; a thing of little value.

do-it-yourself /'duːɪtjʊər'sɛlf/ *n* domestic repairs, woodwork, etc undertaken as a hobby or to save money.—*also adj*.—**do-it-yourselfer** *n*.

dolabriform /dɒ'læbrɪˌfɔrm/, **dolabrirate** *adj* (*bot*) hatchet-shaped.

Dolby /'dɒlbi/ *n* (*trademark*) an electronic noise-reduction system used in sound-recording and playback systems.

dolce /'dɒltʃeɪ/ /-reɪf/ *adj* soft. • *adv* (*mus*) gently.

doldrums /'dɒldrəmz/ or /'dɒl-/ *npl* inactivity; depression; boredom; the regions of the ocean about the equator where there is little wind.

dole /dəʊl/ *n* (*inf*) money received from the state while unemployed; a small portion. • *vt* to give (out) in small portions.

doleful /'dəʊlfʊl/ *adj* sad, gloomy.—**dolefully** *adv*.—**dolefulness** *n*.

dolerite /'dɒləˌraɪt/ *n* a dark-coloured basic igneous rock composed of augite, felspar and iron; basaltic greenstone.

dolichocephalic /ˌdɒlɪˌkɒsɪ'fælɪk/ *adj* with a skull long in proportion to its breadth, long-headed.—**dolichocephaly** *n*.

doll /dɒl/ *n* a toy in the form of a human figure; a ventriloquist's dummy; (*sl*) a woman

dollar /'dɒlər/ *n* the unit of money in the US, Canada, Australia and many other countries.

dollop /'dɒləp/ *n* (*inf*) a soft mass or lump; a portion, serving.

dolly /'dɒli/ *n* (*pl* **dollies**) (*inf*) a child's word for a doll; a wheeled platform for a camera. • *vi* (**dollying, dollied**) to manouevre a camera dolly.

Dolly Varden /ˌdɒli'vɑrdən/ *n* ✝ a brightly spotted trout of western North America; a large hat lop-sided hat worn by women; a sponge cake made with spices and dried fruit.

dolman /'dɒlmən/ *n* (*pl* **dolmans**) a loose robe; a short cloak.

dolman sleeve *n* a full, wide sleeve narrowing to a wristband.

dolmen /'dɒlmən/ *n* a prehistoric structure of two or more erect stones supporting a horizontal slab.

dolomite /'dɒləˌmaɪt/ *n* a white mineral obtained from sedimentary rock; a sedimentary rock similar to limestone.—**dolomitic** *adj*.

doloroso /ˌdɒlə'rɔːsɔː/, *Fr.* /ˌdɒlə'rɔsə/ *adv* (*mus*) sadly.

dolorous /'dɒlərəs/ *adj* mournful, doleful.—**dolorously** *adv*.—**dolorousness** *n*.

dolour, dolor /'dɒlər/ *n* grief, sorrow, distress.

dolphin /'dɒlfɪn/ *n* a marine mammal with a beak-like snout, larger than a porpoise but smaller than a whale.

dolphinarium /ˌdɒlfɪ'neriəm/ *n* (*pl* **dolphinariums, dolphinaria**) a large pool or aquarium for keeping and displaying dolphins.

dolt /dəʊlt/ *n* a dull or stupid person.—**doltish** *adj*.—**doltishly** *adv*.—**doltishness** *n*.

Dom /dɒm/ *n* (*RC Church*) the title of certain dignitaries; a former Portuguese title of rank, as Don.

domain /də'meɪn/ *n* an area under the control of a ruler or government; a field of thought, activity, etc.

domain name *n* (*comput*) an Internet site, service or computer main representing a business or an organization.

dome /dəʊm/ *n* a large, rounded roof; something high and rounded.—*also vt*.

domed /'dəʊmd/ *adj* having, or shaped like, a dome.

dome fastener *n* ✝ a small fastener for articles of clothing or other items that has a rounded portion that snaps into a socket.

domesday /'duːmzdeɪ/ *n* the day of God's Last Judgment of mankind.—*also* **doomsday**.

Domesday Book *n* the record of William I's survey of England in 1086.

domestic /də'mɛstɪk/ *adj* belonging to the home or family; not foreign; (*animals*) tame. • *n* a servant in the home. —**domestically** *adv*.

domestic science *n* the study of household skills; home economics.

domesticate /də'mɛstɪˌkeɪt/ *vt* to tame; to make home-loving and fond of household duties.—**domestication** *n*.

domesticity /ˌdɒmə'stɪsɪti/ or /dɒm-/ *n* (*pl* **domesticities**) home life; being domestic.

domicile /'dɒməˌsaɪl/ or /-sɪl/ *n* a house; a person's place of residence. • *vt* to establish, to settle permanently.—**domiciliary** *adj*.

domiciliate /ˌdɒmə'sɪliˌeɪt/ or /ˌdɒːmə-/ *vt* to domicile.—**domiciliation** *n*.

dominant /'dɒmənənt/ *adj* commanding, prevailing over others; overlooking from a superior height. • *n* (*mus*) the fifth note of a diatonic scale.—**dominance** *n*.—**dominantly** *n*.

dominate /'dɒmə,neɪt/ *vt* to control or rule by strength; to hold a commanding position over; to overlook from a superior height.—**domination** *n*.—**dominator** *n*.

domineer /,dɒmə'nɪːr/ *vti* to act in an arrogant or tyrannical manner.—**domineeringly** *adv*.

dominical /də'mɪnɪkəl/ *adj* pertaining to Christ as Lord, or to Sunday.

dominie /'dɒmɪnɪ/ *n* (*Scot*) a schoolteacher; (*inf*) a clergyman.

dominion /də'mɪnjən/ *n* a territory with one ruler or government; the power to rule; authority.

Dominion Day *n* ♣ former name for Canada Day.

domino /'dɒmə,noː/ *n* (*pl* **dominoes, dominos**) a flat oblong tile marked with up to six dots; (*pl*) a popular game *usu* using a set of 28 dominoes; a loose cloak, *usu* worn with an eye mask, at masquerades.

Don /dɒn/ *n* a Spanish title for a gentleman or nobleman.—**Doña** *nf*.

don[1] *vt* (**donning, donned**) to put on; to invest with; to assume.

don[2] *n* a head, fellow or tutor at Oxford or Cambridge universities; (*loosely*) any university teacher; a Mafia leader.

donate /'dɒneɪt/ or /dɒ'neɪt/ *vt* to give as a gift or donation, *esp* to a charity.—**donator** *n*.

donation /dɒ'neɪʃən/ *n* a donating; a contribution or gift, *esp* to a charity.

donative /'dɒnətɪv/ *n* a gift; largess, a donation. • *adj* given by donation.

done[1] /dʌn/ *see* **do**.

done[2] *adj* completed; cooked sufficiently; socially acceptable; (*with* **for**) (*sl*) doomed; dead; exhausted; discarded.

donee /dɒ'niː/ *n* a person to whom a gift is made.

donjon /'dʌndʒən/ or /'dɒn-/ *n* the central tower of a castle, a keep.

donkey /'dɒŋkɪ/ *n* (*pl* **donkeys**) a small animal resembling a horse.

donkey engine *n* a portable auxiliary engine.

donkey jacket *n* a thick waterproof jacket, *esp* worn by labourers.

donkey's years *npl* (*inf*) a very long time.

donkey-work /'dɒŋkɪ,wɜːk/ *n* the groundwork; drudgery.

Donna /'dɒnə/ *n* a term of respect to a lady in Italy.

donnish /'dɒnɪʃ/ *adj* (*inf*) resembling a university don.—**donnishly** *adv*.—**donnishness** *n*.

donor /'dɒːnər/ *n* a person who donates something, a donator; a person who gives their blood, organs, etc for medical use.

don't /dɒnt/ = do not.

donut /'dɒː,nʌt/ *n* (*sl*) a doughnut.

doodad /'duː,dæd/ *n* (*inf*) a small item whose name is lost or forgotten.

doodle /'duː,dəl/ *vi* to scribble aimlessly. • *vt* to draw (something) absentmindedly. • *n* a meaningless drawing or scribble.—**doodler** *n*.

doom[1] /duːm/ *n* a grim destiny; ruin. • *vt* condemn to failure, destruction, etc.

doom[2] *see* **doum**.

doomsday /'duːmzdeɪ/ *n* the day of God's Last Judgment of mankind.—*also* **domesday**.

door /dɔːr/ *n* a movable barrier to close an opening in a wall; a doorway; a means of entry or approach.

doorjamb /'dɔː,dʒæm/ *n* one of the two vertical sides of a door frame; a doorpost.

doorkeeper /-kiːpər/ *n* a person guarding a door.

doorman /-mæn/ or /-mən/ *n* (*pl* **doormen**) a uniformed attendant stationed at the entrance to large hotels, offices, etc.

doormat /-mæt/ *n* a mat placed at the entrance to a doorway for wiping one's feet; (*inf*) a submissive or easily bullied person.

doornail /-neɪl/ *n* (*formerly*) a large nail with which doors were studded; **dead as a doornail** most certainly dead.

doorplate /-pleɪt/ *n* a plate with the name of the occupant of a building.

doorpost /-pɔːst/ *n* the straight vertical side-post of a door, jamb.

doorstop /-stɒp/ *n* a device for preventing a door from moving or fixed to the bottom of a door to prevent it hitting a wall when opening, etc.

doorway /-weɪ/ *n* an opening in a wall, etc filled by a door.

dope /dɒːp/ *n* a thick pasty substance used for lubrication; (*inf*) any illegal drug, such as cannabis or narcotics; (*sl*) a stupid person; (*sl*) information. • *vt* to treat with dope. • *vi* to take addictive drugs.

dopey, dopy /'dɒːpɪ/ *adj* (**dopier, dopiest**) (*sl*) stupid; (*inf*) half asleep.—**dopiness** *n*.

doppelgänger, doppelganger /'dɒpəl,ɡeŋər/ *n* a ghostly double of a living person.

doré /dɒ'reɪ/ *n* ♣ (*Cdn*) a walleye (fish).

Dorian /'dɔːrɪən/ *adj* of or relating to an early Greek race that overthrew the Mycenaean civilization. • *n* a member of that race.

Doric /'dɒrɪk/ *adj* of the Dorians or their dialect; of or belonging to the oldest and simplest style of Greek architecture. • *n* the dialect of the Dorians; any broad dialect.

dormant /'dɔːmənt/ *adj* sleeping; quiet, as if asleep; inactive.—**dormancy** *n*.

dormer /'dɔːmər/ *n* an upright window that projects from a sloping roof.

dormitory /'dɔːmɪtɔrɪ/ *n* (*pl* **dormitories**) a large room with many beds, as in a boarding school.

dormouse /'dɔːmaʊs/ *n* (*pl* **dormice**) a small mouse-like creature that hibernates in winter.

dorp /dɔːp/ *n* (*S Africa*) a small town.

dorsal /'dɔːsəl/ *adj* of, on, or near the back.—**dorsally** *adv*.

Dorset /'dɔːsət/ *n* ♣ a member of an extinct Indian people living in the Eastern Arctic prior to their being displaced by the Inuit.

dorsiventral /,dɔːsɪ'ventrə/ *adj* (*leaves*) having a differentiated back and front.

dory[1] /'dɔːrɪ/ *n* (*pl* **dories**) a light flat-bottomed boat with a sharp bow and high sides.

dory[2] *n* (*pl* **dories**) an edible yellow seafish.—*also* **John Dory**.

dosage /'dɒːsɪdʒ/ *n* the administration of a medicine in doses; the size of a dose; the operation of dosing.

dose /dɒːs/ *n* the amount of medicine, radiation, etc administered at one time; a part of an experience; (*sl*) a venereal disease. • *vt* to administer a dose (of medicine) to.

doss /dɒs/ *vi* (*sl*) to sleep, *esp* in a dosshouse.

dossal, dossel /'dɒsəl/ *n* a hanging of silk or damask at the back and sides of an altar.

dosshouse /'dɒs,haʊs/ *n* (*sl*) a cheap lodging house.

dossier /'dɒsɪ,eɪ/ *n* a collection of documents about a subject or person, a file.

DOT *abbr* ♣ = Department of Transport; Department of Transportation.

dot /dɒt/ *n* a small round speck, a point; the short signal in Morse code. • *vt* (**dotting, dotted**) to mark with a dot; to scatter (about).—**dotter** *n*.

dotage /'dɒːtɪdʒ/ *n* weakness and infirmity caused by old age.

dotard /'dɒːtəd/ *n* a person in their dotage.

dote /dɒːt/ *vi* (*with* **on** *or* **upon**) to show excessive affection.—**doter** *n*.

dot matrix printer /dɒt'meɪtrɪks/ *n* (*comput*) a printer in which each printed character is formed by pins selected from a rectangular array.

dotted /'dɒtɪd/ *see* **dot**.

dotterel, dottrel /'dɒtərəl/ *n* a small plover of Europe and Asia, now rare; a similar Australian bird.

dottle /'dɒtəl/ *n* a remnant of tobacco left in a smoked pipe.

dotty /'dɒtɪ/ *adj* (**dottier, dottiest**) (*inf*) eccentric, slightly mad.—**dottily** *adv*.—**dottiness** *n*.

double /'dʌbəl/ *adj* twice as large, as strong, etc; designed or intended for two; made of two similar parts; having two meanings, characters, etc; (*flowers*) having more than one circle of petals. • *adv* twice; in twos. • *n* a number or amount that is twice as much; a person or thing identical to another; (*film*) a person closely resembling an actor and who takes their place to perform stunts, etc; (*pl*) a game between two pairs of players. • *vti* to make or become twice as much or as many; to fold, to bend; to bend sharply backwards; to sail around; to have an additional purpose.—**doubly** *adv*.

double agent *n* a spy secretly acting for two governments at the same time.

double-barrelled, double-barreled /-'bærəld/ *adj* (*gun*) having two barrels; (*surname*) having two parts; (*question*) serving a double purpose.

double bass /-beɪs/ *n* the largest instrument of the violin family.—**double bassist** *n*.

double boiler *n* two saucepans fitting into each other so that the contents of the upper are cooked while boiling in the lower.

double-breasted /-'brestɪd/ *adj* (*suit*) having one half of the front overlap the other.

double cream *n* cream with a high fat content.

double-cross /-,krɒs/ *vt* to betray an associate, to cheat. • **double cross** *n*.—**double-crosser** *n*.

double-dealing /'dʌbəl.diːlɪŋ/ n treachery, deceit.—**double-dealer** n.

double-edged /-.ɛdʒd/ adj acting in two ways; (remarks) having two possible meanings (eg well-meaning or malicious).

double entendre /.dʌbəlɒn'tɒndrə/ n a word or phrase with two meanings, one of which is usu indecent.

double entry n (bookkeeping) a system where each transaction is entered as a debit in one account and a credit in another.—**double-entry** adj.

double-faced /'dʌbəl.feɪst/ adj having two faces; hypocritical.

double-jointed /-.dʒɔɪntɪd/ adj having joints which allow the limbs, figures, etc an unusual degree of flexibility.

double-park /-.pɑːrk/ vt to park alongside a car which is already parked beside the kerb.

double-quick /-'kwɪk/ adj, adv very quick. • vti to march quickly.

double standard n a principle that is applied more strictly to one person or group than to another.

doublet /'dʌblət/ n (formerly) a man's close-fitting jacket; one of a pair of similar things.

doublethink /'dʌbəlθɪŋk/ n a belief in two conflicting ideas, principles, etc.

doubleton /-tən/ n two cards only of a suit (in a player's hand).

doubloon /dʌ'bluːn/ n an old Spanish gold coin.

doubt /dʌut/ vi to be uncertain or undecided. • vt to hold in doubt; to distrust; to be suspicious of. • n uncertainty; (often pl) lack of confidence in something, distrust.—**doubter** n.

doubtful /'dʌutful/ adj feeling doubt; uncertain; suspicious.—**doubtfully** adv.—**doubtfulness** adv.

doubtless /-ləs/ adv no doubt; probably. • adj assured; certain.—**doubtlessly** adv.—**doubtlessness** n.

douce /duːs/ adj (Scot) sober; sedate; prudent; modest.

douceur Fr. /duː'sœr/ n a gift for services rendered, or to secure favour; a bribe.

douche /duːʃ/ n a jet of water directed on or into a part of the body; a device for applying this. • vt to cleanse or treat with a douche.

dough /doː/ n a mixture of flour and water, milk, etc used to make bread, pastry, or cake; (inf) money.

doughboy /-bɔɪ/ n a boiled dumpling; (sl) a soldier.

doughnut /-nʌt/ n a small, fried, usu ring-shaped, cake.—also **donut**.

doughty /'dʌuti/ adj (**doughtier**, **doughtiest**) valiant; strong.—**doughtily** adv.—**doughtiness** n.

doughy /'doːi/ (**doughier**, **doughiest**) adj soft, like dough.—**doughiness** n.

doum, doom /duːm/ or /dʌum/ n an Egyptian palm tree.

dour /dʊr/ or /dʌur/ adj stern; sullen; grim.—**dourly** adv.—**dourness** n.

douse /dʌus/ vt to plunge into or soak with water; to put out, extinguish.

dove[1] /dʌv/ see **dive**.

dove[2] n a small bird of the pigeon family; (politics, diplomacy) an advocate of peace or a peaceful policy.

dovecote, dovecot /'dʌvkɔːt/ n a shelter and breeding place for domesticated pigeons.

dovetail /-teɪl/ n a wedge-shaped joint used in woodwork. • vt to fit or combine together.

dowager /'dʌuədʒər/ n a widow possessing property or title from her husband; (inf) a dignified elderly woman.

dowdy /'dʌudi/ adj (**dowdier**, **dowdiest**) poorly dressed, not stylish.—**dowdily** adv.—**dowdiness** n.

dowel /'dʌuəl/ n a headless wooden or metal pin used for fastening wood or stone. • vt (**doweling**, **doweled** or **dowelling**, **dowelled**) to fasten with dowels.

dower /'dʌuər/ n a widow's share of her husband's estate.

down[1] adv towards or in a lower physical position; to a lying or sitting position; toward or to the ground, floor, or bottom; to a source or hiding place; to or in a lower status or in a worse condition; from an earlier time; in cash; to or in a state of less activity; ♣ in Canadian and US football, one of a series of attempts by the team on offence to advance the ball ten yards. • adj occupying a low position, esp lying on the ground; depressed, dejected. • prep in a descending direction in, on, along, or through. • n a low period (as in activity, emotional life, or fortunes); (inf) a dislike, prejudice. • vti to go or cause to go or come down; to defeat; to swallow.

down[2] /dʌun/ n soft fluffy feathers or fine hairs.

down[3] /dʌun/ n (usu pl) a tract of bare hilly land used for pasturing sheep; banks or rounded hillocks of sand.

downbeat /'dʌunbiːt/ adj (mus) the first beat in the bar, the downward gesture of a conductor's baton; (inf) dismal; relaxed.

downcast /-kæst/ adj dejected; (eyes) directed downwards.

downer /-ər/ n (sl) a depressant drug, esp a barbiturate; a depressing experience or situation.

downfall /-fɒl/ n a sudden fall (from power, etc); a sudden or heavy fall of rain or snow.

downgrade /-greɪd/ n a descending slope. • vt to reduce or lower in rank or position; to disparage.

download /-loːd/ vt copy or transfers software or data from one storage device or computer to another; ♣ (Cdn) shift responsibilities or costs from one level of government to a lower one. • n a transfer of software or data.

down payment n a deposit.

downpour /-pɔr/ n a heavy fall of rain.

downright /-rɔɪt/ adj frank; absolute. • adv thoroughly.

downscale, down-market /-skeɪl/ or /-mɑrkɪt/ adj (goods, services) of inferior quality.

downside /-saɪd/ n the less appealing or advantageous aspect of something.

downsize /-saɪz/ vt to produce a smaller version of (eg a car); to reduce the numbers in a workforce by means of redundancy.

Down's syndrome n a chromosomal abnormality resulting in a flat face, slanting eyes and mental retardation.

downstage /dʌun'steɪdʒ/ or /'dʌun-/ adv to the front of the stage.

downstairs /-'stɑrz/ adv to or on a lower floor. • adj on the ground floor or a lower floor. • n (used as sing or pl) the lower part of a house, the ground floor.

down-to-earth /-tə'ərθ/ adj practical, sensible.

downtown /dʌun'tʌun/ n the main business district of a town or city.—also adj.

downtrodden /-.trɒdən/ adj oppressed, trampled underfoot.

downturn /-tərn/ n a decline in (economic) activity or prosperity.

down under n (inf) Australia or New Zealand.

downward /-wərd/ adj moving from a higher to a lower level, position or condition. • adv towards a lower place, position, etc; from an earlier time to a later.—also **downwards**.

downwind /-wɪnd/ adv in the direction the wind is blowing.—also adj.

downy /'dʌuni/ adj (**downier**, **downiest**) like, covered with, or made of, down.

dowry /'dʌuəri/ n (pl **dowries**) the money or possessions that a woman brings to her husband at marriage.

dowse /dʌuz/ vi to search for water, treasure, etc with a divining rod.—**dowser** n.

doxology /dɒk'sɒlədʒi/ n (pl **doxologies**) a hymn of praise to God.

doxy /'dɒksi/ n (pl **doxies**) (arch) a sweetheart, a prostitute.

doyen /'dɔɪən/ or /-'ɛn/, /'dwɒjã/ n a senior member of a group; an expert in a field; the oldest example of a category.—**doyenne** nf.

doyley /'dɔɪli/ see **doily**.

doze /doːz/ vi to sleep lightly. • n a light sleep, a nap.—**dozer** n.

dozen /'dʌzən/ n a group of twelve.—**dozenth** adj.

dozy /'doːzi/ adj (**dozier**, **doziest**) drowsy; (inf) stupid.—**dozily** adv.—**doziness** n.

DPhil, D.Phil abbr = Doctor of Philosophy.

Dr abbr = Doctor; debtor.

drab /dræb/ adj (**drabber**, **drabbest**) dull, uninteresting; of a dull brown colour. • n a dull yellowy brown colour; cloth of this colour.—**drably** adv.—**drabness** n.

drabble /'dræbəl/ vt to make wet or dirty by dragging through mud or water.

dracaena /drə'siːnə/ n any of a genus of tropical liliaceous palm-like plants.

drachm /dræm/ n in UK, a unit of capacity (¹/₈th fluid ounce); in US, a dram; a drachma.

drachma /'drækmə/ n (pl **drachmas, drachmae**) the monetary unit of Greece.

draconian /drə'koːnɪən/ or /dreɪ-/ adj (laws, etc) very cruel, severe; (with cap) of the 7th-century Athenian statesman Draco or his extremely harsh laws.

draft /dræft/ n a rough plan, preliminary sketch; an order for the payment of money by a bank; a smaller group selected from a larger for a specific task; conscription. • vt to draw a rough sketch or outline of; to select for a special purpose; to conscript.—also **draught**.

draftboard, draftsboard see **draughtboard**.

draftee /dræf'ti/ n a conscript.

draftsman /'drɑːftsmən/ see **draughtsman**.

drafty /'drɑːfti/ see **draughty**.

drag /dræg/ vb (**dragging, dragged**) vt to pull along by force; to draw slowly and heavily; to search (in water) with a dragnet or hook. • vi to trail on the ground; to move slowly and heavily; (sl) to draw on a cigarette. • n something used for dragging, a dragnet, a heavy harrow; something that retards progress; a braking device; (sl) something boring or tedious; (sl) women's clothes worn by a man; (sl) a draw at a cigarette.

dragée /'dræʒeɪ/ n a coated nut or ball of sugar; a silver coated ball used as a cake decoration; a pill coated with sugar.

draggle /'drægəl/ vt to wet or soil by dragging in the mud or along the ground. • vi to become dirty or wet by dragging.

dragnet /'drægnet/ n a net for scouring a riverbed, pond, etc to search for anything; a coordinated hunt for an escaped criminal, etc.

dragon /'drægən/ n a mythical winged reptile; an authoritarian or grim person, esp a woman.

dragonfly /-ˌflaɪ/ n (pl **dragonflies**) an insect with a long slender abdomen, large eyes and iridescent wings.

dragoon /drə'guːn/ n a soldier on horseback, a cavalryman. • vt to force into submission by bullying commands.

drail /dreɪl/ n a weighted fishhook for dragging through water.

drain /dreɪn/ vt to draw off liquid gradually; to make dry by removing liquid gradually; to exhaust physically or mentally; to drink the entire contents of a glass. • vi to flow away gradually; to become dry as liquid trickles away. • n a sewer, pipe, etc by which water is drained away; something that causes exhaustion or depletion.—**drainer** n.

drainage /'dreɪnɪdʒ/ n a draining; a system of drains; something drained off.

draining board, drainboard /-bɔːd/ n a sloping, usu grooved, surface beside a sink for draining washed dishes.

drainpipe /-paɪp/ n a pipe that carries waste liquid, sewage, etc out of a building.

drake /dreɪk/ n a male duck.

dram /dræm/ n a small drink of spirits; a small amount; a unit of capacity (⅛th fluid ounce); a unit of weight (avoirdupois 27.243 grains or 0.00265 ounce/apothecaries' weight 3 scruples or 60 grains).

drama /'drɑːmə/ or /'dræmə/ n a play for the stage, radio or television; dramatic literature as a genre; a dramatic situation or a set of events.

dramatic /drə'mætɪk/ adj of or resembling drama; exciting, vivid.—**dramatically** adv.

dramatics /drə'mætɪks/ n (used as sing or pl) the producing or performing of plays; (used as sing) exaggerated behaviour, histrionics.

dramatis personae /ˌdræmətɪspər'soʊnaɪ/ or /-miː/ n the characters in a play.

dramatist /'dræmətɪst/ n a person who writes plays.

dramatization /ˌdræmətɪ'zeɪʃən/ n the action or process of dramatizing; an event or novel, etc, adapted to the form of a play.

dramatize /'dræməˌtaɪz/ vt to write or adapt in the form of a play; to express in an exaggerated or dramatic form.—**dramatizer** n.

dramaturge, dramaturg /-ˌtɜːdʒ/ n a playwright; a literary adviser; an expert in dramaturgy.

dramaturgy /-ˌtɜːdʒi/ n the art of dramatic composition; representation and stage effect.—**dramaturgic, dramaturgical** adj.

drank /dræŋk/ see **drink**.

drape /dreɪp/ vt to cover or hang with cloth; to arrange in loose folds; to place loosely or untidily. • n a hanging cloth or curtain; (pl) curtains.

draper /'dreɪpər/ n a seller of cloth.

drapery /'dreɪpəri/ n (pl **draperies**) fabrics or curtains, esp as arranged in loose folds; the trade of a draper.

drastic /'dræstɪk/ adj acting with force and violence.—**drastically** adv.

drat /dræt/ interj (sl) a euphemism for damn.

dratted /'drætəd/ adj (sl) confounded; annoying.

draught /drɑːft/ n a current of air, esp in an enclosed space; the pulling of a load using an animal, etc; something drawn; a dose of medicine or liquid; an act of swallowing; the depth of water required to float a ship; beer, wine, etc stored in bulk in casks; a flat counter used in the game of draughts; (pl) (used as sing) a game for two players using 24 round pieces on a draughtboard.

draughtboard n a square board identical to a chessboard used for playing draughts.—also **draftboard, draftsboard**.

draughtsman /'drɑːftsmən/ n (pl **draughtsmen**) a person who makes detailed drawings or plans.—also **draftsman**.—**draughtsmanship, draftsmanship** n.

draughtsman[2] n (pl **draughtsmen**) a flat counter used in the game of draughts.—also **checker, draftsman**.

draughty /'drɑːfti/ adj (**draughtier, draughtiest**) letting in or exposed to drafts of air.—also **drafty**.—**draughtiness, draftiness** n.

Dravidian /drə'vɪdiːən/ adj pertaining to an ancient race and their languages, spoken in southern India and Sri Lanka. • n a member of this race; a family of languages spoken by the Dravidians.

draw /drɔː/ vti (**drawing, drew,** pp **drawn**) to haul, to drag; to cause to go in a certain direction; to pull out; to attract; to delineate, to sketch; to receive (as a salary); to bend (a bow) by pulling back the string; to leave (a contest) undecided; to write up, to draft (a will); to produce or allow a current of air; to draw lots; to get information from; (ship) to require a certain depth to float; (with **on**) to approach; to use (a resource); to withdraw (money) from (an account, etc); to put on (clothes); (with **out**) to extract; to prolong, extend; to cause (someone) to speak freely; to take (money) from an account; (with **up**) to bring or come to a standstill; to draft (a document); to straighten oneself; to form soldiers into an array. • n the act of drawing; (inf) an event that attracts customers, people; the drawing of lots; a drawn game.

drawback /'drɔːbæk/ n a hindrance, handicap.

drawbridge /-brɪdʒ/ n a bridge (eg over a moat) designed to be drawn up.

drawee /ˌdrɔː'iː/ n one on whom an order, bill of exchange, or a draft is drawn.

drawer /'drɔːər/ or /drɔːr/ n a person who draws; a person who draws a cheque; a sliding box-like compartment (as in a table, chest, or desk); (pl) knickers, underpants.

drawing /'drɔːɪŋ/ n a figure, plan, or sketch drawn by using lines.

drawing pin n a thumbtack.

drawing room n a room where visitors are entertained, a living room.

drawl /drɔːl/ vt to speak slowly and with elongated vowel sounds. • n a drawling speech.—**crawler** n.—**drawlingly** adv.

drawn[1] /drɔːn/ see **draw**.

drawn[2] adj looking strained because of tiredness or worry.

drawstring /'drɔːstrɪŋ/ n a string or tape threaded through fabric which when pulled gathers it up or closes an opening (eg in a purse).

dray /dreɪ/ n a low, stoutly built cart used for heavy loads.

dread /dred/ n great fear or apprehension. • vt to fear greatly.

dreadful /'dredfʊl/ adj full of dread; causing dread; extreme (dreadful tiredness); (sl) bad, disagreeable.—**dreadfully** adv.—**dreadfulness** n.

dreadlocks /-lɒks/ npl hair worn in long matted strands by male Rastafarians.

dreadnought, dreadnaught /-nɔːt/ n a battleship with main armament entirely of big guns; a heavy cloth; an overcoat of this cloth.

dream /driːm/ n a stream of thoughts and images experienced during sleep; a day-dreaming state, a reverie; an ambition; an ideal. • vb (**dreaming, dreamt** or **dreamed**) vi to have a dream during sleep; to fantasize. • vt to dream of; to imagine as a reality; (with **up**) to devise, invent.—**dreamer** n.

dreamy /'driːmi/ adj (**dreamier, dreamiest**) given to dreaming, unpractical; (inf) attractive, wonderful.—**dreamily** adv.—**dreaminess** n.

dreary /-ri/ adj (**drearier, dreariest**) dull; cheerless.—**drearily** adv.—**dreariness** n.

dredge[1] /dredʒ/ n a device for scooping up material from the bottom of a river, harbour, etc. • vt to widen, deepen, or clean with a dredge; to scoop up with a dredge; (with **up**) (inf) to discover, reveal, esp through effort.

dredge[2] vt to coat (food) by sprinkling.

dredger[1] /'dredʒər/ n a vessel fitted with dredging equipment.

dredger[2] n a container with a perforated lid for sprinkling.

dreggy /'dregi/ adj (**dreggier, dreggiest**) full of dregs; like dregs.

dregs /dregz/ npl solid impurities that settle on the bottom of a liquid; residue; (inf) a worthless person or thing.

drench /drentʃ/ vt to soak, saturate.

dress /drɛs/ *n* clothing; a one-piece garment worn by women and girls comprising a top and skirt; a style or manner of clothing. • *vt* to put on or provide with clothing; to decorate; (*wound*) to wash and bandage; (*animal*) to groom; to arrange the hair; to prepare food (*eg* poultry, fish) for eating by cleaning, gutting, etc; (*with* **up**) to attire in best clothes; to improve the appearance of. • *vi* to put on clothes; to put on formal wear for an occasion; (*with* **up**) to put on fancy dress, etc.

dressage /drə'sɒʒ/ *n* the training of a horse in deportment and obedience.

dress circle *n* the first tier of seats in a theatre above the stalls.

dresser /'drɛsər/ *n* a person who assists an actor to dress; a type of kitchen sideboard.

dressing /-ɪŋ/ *n* a sauce or stuffing for food; manure spread over the soil; dress or clothes; the bandage, ointment, etc applied to a wound.

dressing-down /'drɛsɪŋ'daʊn/ *n* a severe scolding.

dressing gown *n* a loose garment worn when one is partially clothed.

dressmaker /'drɛs,meɪkər/ *n* a person who makes clothes.—**dressmaking** *n*.

dress rehearsal *n* rehearsal in full costume.

dressy /'drɛsi/ *adj* (**dressier, dressiest**) stylish; elaborate; showy.—**dressily** *adv*.—**dressiness** *n*.

drew /'druː/ *see* **draw**.

dribble /'drɪbəl/ *vi* to flow in a thin stream or small drips; to let saliva trickle from the mouth. • *vt* (*soccer, basketball, hockey*) to move (the ball) along little by little with the foot, hand, stick, etc. • *n* the act of dribbling; a thin stream of liquid.—**dribbler** *n*.

driblet /'drɪblət/ *n* a small amount; a drop, trickle.

dried /draɪd/ *see* **dry**.

drier /'draɪər/ *see* **dry, dryer**.

drift /drɪft/ *n* a heap of snow, sand, etc deposited by the wind; natural course, tendency; the general meaning or intention (of what is said); the extent of deviation (of an aircraft, etc) from a course; an aimless course; the action or motion of drifting. • *vt* to cause to drift. • *vi* to be driven or carried along by water or air currents; to move along aimlessly; to be piled into heaps by the wind.

driftage /'drɪftədʒ/ *n* matter that drifts ashore; deviation from a course caused by air or sea currents.

drifter /-ər/ *n* a person who wanders aimlessly.

driftwood /'drɪftwʊd/ *n* wood cast ashore by tides.

drill¹ /drɪl/ *n* an implement with a pointed end that bores holes; the training of soldiers, etc; repetitious exercises or training as a teaching method; (*inf*) correct procedure or routine. • *vt* to make a hole with a drill; to instruct or be instructed by drilling.

drill² *n* a machine for planting seeds in rows; a furrow in which seeds are planted; a row of seeds planted in this way.—*also vt*.

drilling platform *n* the fixed or mobile structure supporting the equipment and accommodation facilities, etc for drilling an offshore oil well.

drilling rig *n* the machinery required to drill an oil well.

drily /'draɪli/ *see* **dry**.

drink /drɪŋk/ *vb* (**drinking, drank**, *pp* **drunk**) *vt* to swallow (a liquid); to take in, absorb; to join in a toast. • *vi* to consume alcoholic liquor, *esp* to excess. • *n* liquid to be drunk; alcoholic liquor; (*sl*) the sea.—**drinker** *n*.

drip /drɪp/ *vti* (**dripping, dripped**) to fall or let fall in drops. • *n* a liquid that falls in drops; the sound of falling drops; (*med*) a device for administering a fluid slowly and continuously into a vein; (*inf*) a weak or ineffectual person.—**dripper** *n*.

drip-dry /'drɪp,draɪ/ *adj* (*clothing*) drying easily and needing relatively little ironing.—*also vti*.

dripping /'drɪpɪŋ/ *n* fat that drips from meat during roasting.

drive /draɪv/ *vb* (**driving, drove**, *pp* **driven**) *vt* to urge, push or force onward; to direct the movement or course of; to convey in a vehicle; to carry through strongly; to impress forcefully; to propel (a ball) with a hard blow. • *vi* to be forced along; to be conveyed in a vehicle; to work, to strive (at). • *n* a trip in a vehicle; a stroke to drive a ball (in golf, etc); a driveway; a military attack; an intensive campaign; dynamic ability; the transmission of power to machinery.

drive-in /'draɪv,ɪn/ *n* a cinema, restaurant, etc, where customers are served in their cars.—*also adj*.

drivel /'drɪvəl/ *n* nonsense. • *vi* (**drivelling, drivelled** *or* **driveling, driveled**) to talk nonsense.—**driveller, driveler** *n*.

driven /-ən/ *see* **drive**.

driver /'draɪvər/ *n* one who or that which drives; a chauffeur; (*golf*) a wooden club used from the tee.

drive shed *n* ✴ (*Cdn*) a large shed for storing vehicles or farm machinery.

driveway /-,weɪ/ *n* a road for vehicles, often on private property.

drizzle /'drɪzəl/ *n* fine light rain.—*also vi*.—**drizzly** *adj*.

drogue /droːg/ *n* a sea anchor; a small parachute that slows down or stabilizes something (as a jet aircraft); a funnel-shaped device that enables an aeroplane to be refuelled from a tanker plane while in flight; a buoy at the end of a harpoon line; a windsock.

droit /drɔɪt/ *Fr*. /drwa/ *n* equity; a right of ownership, *esp* in land; custom; duty.

droke /droːk/ *n* ✴ (*Cdn*) in the Atlantic Provinces, a grove of trees; a steep-sided valley.

droll /droːl/ *adj* oddly amusing; whimsical.—**drollness** *n*.—**drolly** *adv*.

drollery /'droːləri/ *n* (*pl* **drolleries**) the quality of being droll; buffoonery; a droll act.

dromedary /'drɒmə,deri/ *n* (*pl* **dromedaries**) a one-humped camel.

drone /droːn/ *n* a male honey-bee; a lazy person; a deep humming sound; a monotonous speaker or speech; an aircraft piloted by remote control. • *vi* to make a monotonous humming sound; to speak in a monotonous manner.

drool /druːl/ *vi* to slaver, dribble; to show excessive enthusiasm for.

droop /druːp/ *vi* to bend or hang down; to become weak or faint. • *n* the act or an instance of drooping.

droopy /'druːpi/ *adj* (**droopier, droopiest**) drooping; tending to droop; (*sl*) tired, depressed.—**droopily** *adv*.—**droopiness** *n*.

drop /drɒp/ *n* a small amount of liquid in a roundish shape; something shaped like this, as a sweet; a tiny quantity; a sudden fall; the distance down; (*pl*) liquid medicine, etc dispensed in small drops. • *vb* (**dropping, dropped**) *vi* to fall in drops; to fall suddenly; to go lower, to sink; to come (in); (*with* **in**) to visit (with) informally; (*with* **out**) to abandon or reject (a course, society, etc). • *vt* to let fall, to cause to fall; to lower or cause to descend; to set down from a vehicle; to mention casually; to cause (the voice) to be less loud; to give up (as an idea).—**dropper** *n*.

drop-dead *adv* slang reference to a very attractive individual; drop-dead gorgeous.

drop kick *n* a kick made by dropping the ball onto the ground and kicking as it bounces.—**drop-kick** *vt*.

droplet /'drɒplət/ *n* a tiny drop (as of liquid).

dropout /-aʊt/ *n* a student who abandons a course of study; a person who rejects normal society.

droppings /-ɪŋz/ *npl* animal dung.

dropsy /-si/ *n* an unnatural accumulation of serious fluid in any cavity of the body or its tissues.—**dropsical** *adj*.

droshky, drosky /'drɒʃki/ *n* (*pl* **droshkies, droskies**) a light four-wheeled open Russian carriage.

dross /drɒs/ *n* a surface scum on molten metal; rubbish, waste matter.

drought /draʊt/ *n* a long period of dry weather.—**droughty** *adj*.

drove¹ /droːv/ *see* **drive**.

drove² *n* a group of animals driven in a herd or flock, etc; a large moving crowd of people.

drover /'droːvər/ *n* a person whose occupation is to drive cattle.

drown /draʊn/ *vti* to die or kill by suffocation in water or other liquid. • *vt* to flood; to drench; to become deeply immersed in some activity; to blot out (a sound) with a louder noise; to remove (sorrow, etc) with drink.

drowse /draʊz/ *vi* to be nearly asleep.

drowsy /'draʊzi/ *adj* (**drowsier, drowsiest**) sleepy; soporific; lethargic; inactive.—**drowsily** *adv*.—**drowsiness** *n*.

drub /drʌb/ *vt* (**drubbing, drubbed**) to thrash; to defeat convincingly.

drudge /drʌdʒ/ *vi* to do boring or very menial work. • *n* a person who drudges, *esp* a servant.—**drudger** *n*.—**drudgingly** *adv*.

drudgery /'drʌdʒəri/ *n* (*pl* **drudgeries**) dull, boring work.

drug /drʌg/ *n* any substance used in medicine; a narcotic. • *vt* (**drugging, drugged**) to administer drugs to; to stupefy.

drugget /'drʌgɪt/ *n* a coarse woollen or cotton fabric; a rug made of this.

druggist /'drʌgɪst/ *n* a pharmacist.

drugstore /-stɔr/ *n* a retail store selling medicines and other miscellaneous articles such as cosmetics, film, etc.

druid /'dru:ɪd/ *n* (*often with cap*) a priest of the ancient inhabitants (probably Celtic) of Britain, Gaul and Germany; a member of a modern society reviving druidism.—**druidic, druidical** *adj.*

druidism /'dru:ɪˌdɪzəm/ *n* the beliefs, manners, rites and customs of the druids.

drum /drʌm/ *n* a round percussion instrument, played by striking a membrane stretched across a hollow cylindrical frame; the sound of a drum; anything shaped like a drum, as a container for liquids. • *vb* (**drumming, drummed**) *vi* to play a drum; to beat or tap rhythmically. • *vt* (*with* **in**) to instil (knowledge) into a person by constant repetition; (*with* **up**) to summon as by drum; to create (business, etc) by concerted effort; to originate.

drumhead /'drʌmhed/ *n* the membrane stretched across the end of a drum.

drummer /'drʌmər/ *n* a person who plays a drum; (*inf*) a travelling salesman.

drumstick /-stɪk/ *n* a stick for beating a drum; the lower part of a cooked leg of poultry.

drunk[1] /drʌŋk/ *see* **drink**.

drunk[2] *adj* intoxicated with alcohol. • *n* a drunk person.

drunkard /'drʌŋkərd/ *n* an habitual drunk.

drunken /-kən/ *adj* intoxicated; caused by excessive drinking.—**drunkenly** *adv.*—**drunkenness** *n.*

drupe /dru:p/ *n* a fleshy fruit with a stone, as a plum.—**drupaceous** *adj.*

drupelet /-lət/ *n* a small drupe in a compound fruit, *eg.* raspberry.

druse /dru:z/ *n* a crust of crystals; a rock cavity lined with this.

Druse, Druze *n* a member of a fanatical politico-religious sect in Syria and Lebanon.

dry /draɪ/ *adj* (**drier, driest**) free from water or liquid; thirsty; marked by a matter-of-fact, ironic or terse manner of expression; uninteresting, wearisome; (*bread*) eaten without butter, etc; (*wine*) not sweet; not selling alcohol. • *vti* (**drying, dried**) to make or become dry; (*with* **out**) to be treated for alcoholism or drug addiction.—**drily, dryly** *adv.*—**dryness** *n.*

dryad /'draɪˌæd/ or /-əd/ *n* (*pl* **dryads, dryades**) (*Greek myth*) a wood nymph.

dry-clean /'draɪˌkli:n/ *vt* to clean with solvents as opposed to water.—**dry-cleaner** *n.*—**dry-cleaning** *n.*

dry dock *n* a dock that can be drained of water to make ship repairs easier.

dryer /'draɪr/ *n* a device for drying, as a tumble-drier; a clothes horse.—*also* **drier.**

dry ice *n* solid carbon dioxide.

dry rot *n* decay of timber caused by a fungus; any form of moral decay or corruption.

dry run *n* (*inf*) a rehearsal.

dry-salt /'draɪˌsɒlt/ *vt* to cure (meat, etc) by salting and drying.

drysalter /-sɒltər/ *n* (*formerly*) a dealer in dyes, oils, etc.—**drysaltery** *n.*

DSC *abbr* = Distinguished Service Cross.

DSM *abbr* = Distinguished Service Medal.

DSO *abbr* = Distinguished Service Order.

dt, DT *abbr* = delirium tremens.

DTP *abbr* = desktop publishing.

dual /'dju:əl/ or /'dju:-/ *adj* double; consisting of two.

dual carriageway *n* a road with traffic travelling in opposite directions separated by a central reservation.—*also* **divided highway.**

dualism /-ˌlɪzəm/ *n* a twofold division; (*philos*) the doctrine that the universe is based on two principles, *eg* good and evil, mind and matter.—**dualist** *n.*—**dualistic** *adj.*—**dualistically** *adv.*

duality /-ˌlɪti/ *n* (*pl* **dualities**) the condition or quality of being two or in two parts, dualism; dichotomy.

dub[1] /dʌb/ *vt* (**dubbing, dubbed**) to confer knighthood on; to nickname.

dub[2] *vt* (**dubbing, dubbed**) to replace the soundtrack of (a film), *eg* with one in a different language; to add sound effects or music to (a film, broadcast, etc); to transfer (a recording) to a new tape.

dubbin, dubbing /'dʌbɪn/ or /'dʌbɪŋ/ *n* a grease for softening and waterproofing leather.

dubiety /dju:'baɪəti/ or /dju:-/ *n* (*pl* **dubieties**) doubtfulness, uncertainty; a matter of doubt.

dubious /'dju:bɪəs/ or /'dju:-/ *adj* doubtful (about, of); uncertain as to the result; untrustworthy.—**dubiously** *adv.*—**dubiousness** *n.*

ducal /'dju:kəl/ or /'dju:-/ *adj* of or pertaining to a duke, a dukedom or a duchy.—**ducally** *adv.*

ducat /'dʌkət/ *n* a gold or silver coin formerly in use in Europe; (*pl*) (*sl*) money.

duce /'du:tʃeɪ/ *n* a chief, a leader; (*with cap*) the title used by the Italian Fascist dictator, Benito Mussolini (1922–43).

duchess /'dʌtʃəs/ *n* the wife or widow of a duke; a woman having the same rank as a duke in her own right.

duchy /'dʌtʃi/ *n* (*pl* **duchies**) the territory of a duke, a dukedom.

duck[1] /dʌk/ *vt* to dip briefly in water; to lower the head suddenly, *esp* to avoid some object; to avoid, dodge. • *vi* to dip or dive; to move the head or body suddenly; to evade a duty, etc. • *n* a ducking movement.

duck[2] *n* (*pl* **ducks, duck**) a water bird related to geese and swans; the female of this bird; its flesh used as food.

duck[3] *n* a plain cotton cloth; (*pl*) trousers or light clothes made from this and worn in hot climates.

duckbill, duck-billed platypus /'dʌkbɪl/ *n* an Australian egg-laying furred mammal with webbed feet and a broad bill.—*also* **platypus.**

duckboard /-bɔrd/ *n* a path of wooden slats laid over muddy or wet ground.

duckish /'dʌkɪʃ/ *n* (*Cdn*) in Newfoundland, twilight or the time between sunset and darkness.

duckling /-lɪŋ/ *n* a young duck.

duckweed /-wi:d/ *n* a common floating freshwater plant.

ducky, duckie /'dʌki/ *adj* (**duckier, duckiest**) (*inf*) fine; satisfactory; cute. • *n* (*pl* **duckies**) (*inf*) a term of endearment, darling.

duct /dʌkt/ *n* a channel or pipe for fluids, electric cable, etc; a tube in the body for fluids to pass through.

ductile /'dʌktaɪl/ *adj* malleable; yielding.

dud /dʌd/ *adj* (*sl*) worthless. • *n* (*sl*) anything worthless; an ineffectual person.

dude /du:d/ *n* a dandy; a city person on holiday in a ranch.

dudeen /du:'di:n/ or /θu:-/ *n* a short clay tobacco pipe.

dudgeon /'dʌdʒən/ *n* resentment, indignation; (*arch*) the hilt of a dagger.

due /dju:/ or /dju:/ *adj* owed as a debt; immediately payable; fitting, appropriate; appointed or expected to do or arrive. • *adv* directly, exactly. • *n* something due or owed; (*pl*) fees.

duel /'dju:əl/ or /'dju:-/ *n* combat with weapons between two persons over a matter of honour, etc; conflict of any kind between two people, sides, ideas, etc. • *vi* (**duelling, duelled** *or* **dueling, dueled**) to fight in a duel.—**duellist, duelist** *n.*

duello /du:'eloʊ/ or /dju:-/ *n* (*pl* **duellos**) the duelists' code.

duenna /du:'enə/ or /dju:-/ *n* an older woman acting as a chaperone of young women in Spanish or Portuguese families.

duet /dju:'et/ or /dju:-/ *n* a musical composition for two performers.—**duettist** *n.*

duffel, duffle /'dʌfəl/ *n* a coarse, heavy woollen cloth.

duffel bag, duffle bag *n* a large cylindrical drawstring bag for personal belongings.

duffel coat, duffle coat *n* a heavy, hooded overcoat, fastened with toggles.

duffer /'dʌfər/ *n* an incompetent person, *esp* an elderly one.

dug /dʌg/ *see* **dig**.

dugong /'du:gɒŋ/ *n* an aquatic herbivorous mammal resembling the seal and walrus; the sea cow.

dugout /'dʌgaʊt/ *n* a boat made from the hollowed out tree trunk; a rough underground shelter.

duiker /'daɪkər/ *n* (*pl* **duikers, duiker**) a small South African antelope.

duke /du:k/ or /dju:k/ *n* the highest order of British nobility; the title of a ruler of a European duchy.

dukedom /'du:kdəm/ or /dju:k-/ *n* a duchy; the rank, position or title of a duke.

dulcet /'dʌlsət/ *adj* sweet-sounding, melodious.—**dulcetly** *adv.*

dulcimer /'dʌlsɪmər/ *n* a musical instrument with wire strings that are struck with a hammer; a folk-music instrument with *usu* three strings that are played by plucking.—*also* **dulcimore.**

dulia /du:'laɪə/ or /dju:-/ *n* the veneration paid to saints and angels as the servants of God.

dull /dʌl/ *adj* not sharp or pointed; not bright or clear; stupid; boring; not active. • *vti* to make or become dull.—**dully** *adv.*—**dullness** *n.*

dullard /'dʌlərd/ *n* a slow-witted person.

dulse /dʌls/ *n* a red edible seaweed found on rocks.

duly /'duːli/ or /'djuː-/ adv properly; suitably.

dumb /dʌm/ adj not able to speak; silent; (inf) stupid.—**dumbly** adv.—**dumbness** n.

dumbbell n /'dʌmˌbel/ one of a pair of heavy weights used for muscular exercise; (sl) a fool.

dumbfound, dumfound /'dʌmfaʊnd/ or /dʌm'faʊnd/ vti to astonish, surprise.

dumbwaiter /'dʌmˌweɪtər/ n a stand with revolving shelves for holding food; a revolving tray for holding food; a small elevator or lift for carrying food, etc, between floors.

dum-dum /'dʌmdʌm/ n (sl) a foolish person.

dumdum (bullet) n a soft-nosed, expanding bullet.

dumdum n (sl) a stupid person; a dummy.

dummy /'dʌmi/ n (pl **dummies**) a figure of a person used to display clothes; (sl) a soother or pacifier for a baby; a stupid person; an imitation; (bridge) the exposed cards of the dealer's partner.

dump /dʌmp/ vt to drop or put down carelessly in a heap; to deposit as rubbish; to abandon or get rid of; to sell goods abroad at a price lower than the market price abroad; (with **on**) (sl) to censure strongly the words or actions of others. • n a place for refuse; a temporary store; (inf) a dirty, dilapidated place; (pl) (inf) despondency, low spirits.—**dumper** n.

dumpling /'dʌmplɪŋ/ n a rounded piece of dough cooked by boiling or steaming; a short, fat person.

dumpster /'dʌmpstər/ n a large garbage can.

dumpy /'dʌmpi/ adj (**dumpier, dumpiest**) short and thick.—**dumpily** adv.—**dumpiness** n.

dun[1] /dʌn/ adj (**dunner, dunnest**) greyish-brown.—**dunness** n.

dun[2] vt (**dunning, dunned**) to press persistently for payment of a debt.

dunce /dʌns/ n a person who is stupid or slow to learn.

dunderhead /'dʌndərˌhed/ n a stupid person, a dunce.—**dunderheaded** adj.

dune /duːn/ or /djuːn/ n a hill of sand piled up by the wind.

dung /dʌŋ/ n excrement; manure; filth. • vt to spread with manure.—**dungy** adj.

dungaree /ˌdʌŋgə'riː/ n a coarse cotton cloth; (pl) overalls or trousers made from this.

dungeon /'dʌndʒən/ n an underground cell for prisoners.

dunghill /'dʌŋhɪl/ n a heap of dung.

dunk /dʌŋk/ vti to dip (cake, etc) into liquid, eg coffee.

dunlin /'dʌnlɪn/ n a small red-backed sandpiper of northern regions.

dunnage /'dʌnɪdʒ/ n loose wood, etc, used to pack cargo or keep it out of bilge water in a ship's hold; baggage.

dunnite /'dʌnaɪt/ n a powerful explosive used esp in shells.

duo /'duːoʊ/ or /'djuːoʊ/ n (pl **duos, dui**) a pair of performers; (inf) two persons connected in some way.

duodecimal /ˌdjuːoʊ'desɪməl/ adj of twelve; proceeding by twelves. • n a twelfth; a system of computing by twelves.

duodecimo /-ˌmoʊ/ n (pl **duodecimos**) a book of sheets folded into twelve leaves; this book size.—also **twelvemo**.

duodenary /-'denəri/ adj duodecimal.

duodenum /ˌduːoʊ'diːnəm/ or /ˌdjuː-/, /duː'ɒdənəm/ n (pl **duodena, duodenums**) the first part of the small intestine.—**duodenal** adj.

duologue /'duːəˌlɒg/ or /'djuː-/ n a play with two actors; a conversation between two people.

Duo-Tang /'duːoʊˌtæŋ/ or /'djuː/ n ✹ (Cdn) (trademark) a folder of light cardboard that has three flexible metal fasteners to be inserted through the holes of looseleaf paper.

dup vt (**dupping, dupped**) (arch) to open.

dupe /duːp/ or /djuːp/ n a person who is cheated. • vt to deceive; to trick.—**dupable** adj.—**duper** n.—**dupery** n.

duple /'duːpəl/ or /'djuː-/ adj double; (mus) of two beats to the bar.

duplex /'duːˌpleks/ or /'djuː-/ adj having two parts, double. • n a flat or apartment on two floors.—**duplexity** n.

duplicate /'duːplɪkət/ or /'djuː-/ adj in pairs, double; identical; copied exactly from an original. • n one of a pair of identical things; a copy. • vt to make double; to make an exact copy of; to repeat.—**duplicable** adj.

duplication /ˌduːplɪ'keɪʃən/ or /ˌdjuː-/ n the act of duplicating; a copy; multiplication by two.—**duplicative** adj.

duplicator /'duːplɪˌkeɪtər/ or /'djuː-/ n a machine for making copies, esp of a document.

duplicity /duː'plɪsɪti/ or /djuː-/ n (pl **duplicities**) treachery; deception.—**duplicitous** adj.

durable /'dʊrəbəl/ or /'djʊ-/ adj enduring, resisting wear, etc.—**durability** n.—**durably** adv.

duralumin /duː'ræljuːmɪn/ or /djuː-/ n a strong alloy of aluminium with copper, magnesium, manganese and silicon.

dura mater /ˌdʊrə'meɪtər/ or /ˌdjʊr-/ n the tough outer membrane that envelops the brain and spinal cord.

duramen /duː'reɪmən/ or /djuː-/ n the inner heartwood of a tree.

durance /'dʊrəns/ or /'djʊr-/ n imprisonment.

duration /dʊ'reɪʃən/ or /djʊ-/ n the time in which an event continues.

durbar /'dərbar/ n (formerly) a state levee or reception in India and Africa.

duress /dʊ'res/ or /djʊ'-/, /'dʊ-/, /'djʊ-/ n compulsion by use of force or threat; unlawful constraint; imprisonment.

durian, durion /'dʊriən/ n an oval fruit with a foul smell and a pleasant taste; the Asian tree that bears it.

during /'djʊrɪŋ/ prep throughout the duration of; at a point in the course of.

durmast /'dərmæst/ n a dark European oak yielding a tough wood.

durst /dərst/ see **dare**.

dusk /dʌsk/ n (the darker part of) twilight.

dusky /'dʌski/ adj (**duskier, duskiest**) having a dark colour.—**duskily** adv.—**duskiness** n.

dust /dʌst/ n fine particles of solid matter. • vt to free from dust; to sprinkle with flour, sugar, etc.

dustbin /'dʌstbɪn/ or /'dʌsbɪn/ n a container for household refuse.—also **garbage can, trash can**.

dust bowl n a drought area subject to dust storms.

dust cover n a dust jacket.

duster (coat), dustcoat n a coat for keeping off dust, worn esp by early motorists.

duster /'dʌstər/ n a cloth for dusting; a device for dusting; a duster coat; a light housecoat.

dustman /'dʌstmən/ or /'dʌsmən/ n (pl **dustmen**) a garbageman.

dust jacket n a paper cover for a book.

dust wrapper n a dust jacket.

dusty /'dʌsti/ adj (**dustier, dustiest**) covered with dust.—**dustily** adv.—**dustiness** n.

Dutch /dʌtʃ/ adj pertaining to Holland, its people, or language. • n the Dutch language.

Dutch courage n courage obtained from alcohol; alcoholic drink.

Dutch elm disease n a fungal disease which withers the foliage of elm trees and eventually kills them.

Dutch oven n a metal box for cooking before an open fire.

Dutch treat n a meal, etc, where each pays for himself or herself.

Dutch uncle n a person with stern kindness.

duteous /'duːtiːəs/ or /'djuːt-/ adj (poet) dutiful.—**duteously** adv.—**duteousness** n.

dutiable /'duːtiːəbəl/ or /'djuːt-/ adj (goods, etc) subject to duty.—**dutiability** n.

dutiful /'duːtɪfʊl/ or /'djuːt-/ adj performing one's duty; obedient.—**dutifully** adv.—**dutifulness** n.

duty /'duːti/ or /'djuːti/ n (pl **duties**) an obligation that must be performed for moral or legal reasons; respect for one's elders or superiors; actions and responsibilities arising from one's business, occupation, etc; a tax on goods or imports, etc.

duty-free /-'friː/ adj free from tax or duty.

duumvir /duː'ʌmvər/ or /'duːəm-/ /djuː-/ n (pl **duumvirs, duumviri**) in ancient Rome, either of two officers of high rank acting together in one capacity or public function; either member of a duumvirate.

duumvirate /duː'ʌmvɪrət/ or /djuː-/ n a governing body of two; two such people.

duvet /duː'veɪ/ n a thick, soft quilt used instead of bedclothes.—also **continental quilt**.

DVD /'diː'viː'diː/ abbr = digital video disc.

dwarf /dwɔrf/ n (pl **dwarfs, dwarves**) a person, animal or plant of abnormally small size. • vt to stunt; to cause to appear small.

dwarfish /'dwɔrfɪʃ/ adj like a dwarf; very small.—**dwarfishness** n.

dweeb /dwiːb/ n (sl) a bore or person perhaps considered unfashionable, a dull person.—adj **dweeby, dweebish**.

dwell /dwel/ vi (**dwelling, dwelt** or **dwelled**) to live (in a place); (with **on**) to focus the attention on; to think, talk, or write at length about.—**dweller** n.

dwelling /'dwelɪŋ/ n the house, etc where one lives, habitation.

dwindle /'dwɪndəl/ vi to shrink, diminish; to become feeble.

Dy (chem symbol) dysprosium.

dyad /'daɪæd/ *n* a pair; (*chem*) a bivalent atom, element, or radical.—**dyadic** *adj*.

dyarchy /'daɪˌɑrki/ *see* **diarchy**.

dye /daɪ/ *vt* (**dyeing, dyed**) to give a new colour to. • *n* a colouring substance, *esp* in solution; a colour or tint produced by dyeing.—**dyer** *n*.

dyeing /'daɪɪŋ/ *n* the process or work of giving colour to fabrics using dyes.

dyed-in-the-wool /ˌdaɪdɪnðə'wʊl/ *adj* uncompromising in attitude or opinion.

dyestuff /'daɪˌstʌf/ *n* material yielding a dye.

dying[1] /'daɪɪŋ/ *see* **die**[1].

dying[2] *adj* passing away from life; decaying physically; drawing to a close; expiring. • *n* death.

dyke[1] /daɪk/ *see* **dike**[2].

dyke[2] *n* (*derog*) a lesbian.

dynamic /daɪ'næmɪk/ *adj* relating to force that produces motion; (*person*) forceful, energetic.—**dynamically** *adv*.

dynamics /-s/ *n* (*used as sing*) the branch of science that deals with forces and their effect on the motion of bodies.

dynamism /'daɪnəˌmɪzəm/ *n* dynamic influence or power; (*philos*) the theory that the universe is constituted of forces.—**dynamist** *n*.—**dynamistic** *adj*.

dynamite /'daɪnəˌmaɪt/ *n* a powerful explosive; a potentially dangerous situation; (*inf*) an energetic person or thing. • *vt* to blow up with dynamite.—**dynamiter** *n*.

dynamo /'daɪnəˌmoː/ *n* (*pl* **dynamos**) a device that generates electric current.

dynamoelectric /ˌdaɪnəˌmoːɪ'lektrɪk/, **dynamoelectrical** /-moː'ɪlektrɪkəl/ *adj* of or denoting the production of electricity from mechanical energy or of mechanical energy from electricity.

dynamometer /ˌdaɪnə'mɒmɪtər/ *n* an instrument for measuring energy expended.

dynast /'daɪˌnæst/ *n* a ruler, *usu* a hereditary one.

dynasty /'daɪnəsti/ *n* (*pl* **dynasties**) a line of hereditary rulers or leaders of any powerful family or similar group.—**dynastic** *adj*.—**dynastically** *adv*.

dyne /daɪn/ *n* a unit of force, causing in one gram an acceleration per second of one centimetre per second; the unit of force in the cgs system.

dys- /dɪs/ *prefix* bad, unfavourable.

dysentery /'dɪsənˌteri/ or /-tri/ *n* painful inflammation of the large intestine with associated diarrhoea.—**dysenteric** *adj*.

dysergy /dɪsˈɜːrdʒi/ *n* (*business*) the possibility that the merger of two companies will produce a combined operation of less productivity and efficiency, the opposite of synergy.

dysfunction /dɪs'fʌŋkʃən/ *n* a failure in normal functioning.—**dysfunctional** *adj*.

dysgenic /dɪs'dʒenɪk/ *adj* having a bad effect on the hereditary qualities of a race.

dysgenics /dɪs'dʒenɪks/ *n* used as sing) the study of the causes of reduction in quality of a race.

dyslexia /dɪs'leksiə/ *n* impaired ability in reading or spelling.—**dyslexic** *adj*, *n*.

dysmenorrhoea, dysmenorrhea /ˌdɪsmenə'riːə/ *n* painful menstruation.—**dysmenorrhoeal, dysmenorrheal** *adj*.

dyspepsia /dɪs'pepsiə/ *n* indigestion, *esp* chronic.

dyspeptic /dɪs'peptɪk/ *adj* of or afflicted with indigestion. • *n* a dyspeptic sufferer.

dysphagia /dɪs'feɪdʒə/ or /-dʒiə/ *n* difficulty in swallowing.—**dysphagic** *adj*.

dysphasia /ˌdɪs'feɪʒə/ or /-ziə/ *n* a deficiency in the use or understanding of language.—**dysphasic** *adj*.

dysphoria /dɪs'fɔriə/ *n* morbid restlessness, fidgets.—**dysphoric** *adj*.

dyspnoea, dyspnea /dɪsp'niːə/ *n* shortness of breath, difficulty in breathing.—**dyspnoeal, dyspneal, dyspneic, dyspnoeic** *adj*.

dysprosium /dɪs'proːziəm/ *n* a soft metallic element used in lasers and magnetic alloys.

dystrophy /'dɪstrəfi/ *n* various hereditary disorders causing progressive weakening of the muscles (*muscular dystrophy*).—**dystrophic** *adj*.

dysuria /dɪs'jʊriə/ *n* difficulty in passing urine.—**dysuric** *adj*.

E

E. *abbr* = east; eastern.

E- /i:/ *prefix* used to indicate a standard system (for packaging, weight, content, etc) within the European Community.

each /i:tʃ/ *adj* every one of two or more.

eager /'i:gər/ *adj* enthusiastically desirous (of); keen (for); marked by impatient desire or interest.—**eagerly** *adv.*—**eagerness** *n*.

eager beaver *n* (*inf*) an exceptionally diligent person.

eagle /'i:gəl/ *n* a bird of prey with keen eyes and powerful wings; (*golf*) a score of two strokes under par.

eagle-eyed /-ˌaɪd/ *adj* having very sharp eyesight.

eagle owl *n* a type of large owl, also known as the great horned owl.

eaglet /'i:glət/ *n* a young eagle.

ear[1] /i:r/ *n* (the external part of) the organ of hearing; the sense or act of hearing; attention; something shaped like an ear.

ear[2] *n* the part of a cereal plant (*eg* corn, maize) that contains the seeds.

earache /'i:rˌeɪk/ *n* a pain in the ear.

eardrum /-ˌdrʌm/ *n* the membrane within the ear that vibrates in response to sound waves.

eared /'i:rd/ *adj* having ears.

earing /'i:rɪŋ/ *n* (*naut*) a rope attaching the upper corner of a sail to a yard or stanchion.

earl /ərl/ *n* a member of the British nobility ranking between a marquis and a viscount.—**countess** *nf*.

earldom /ərldəm/ *n* the position or estate of an earl.

early /'ərli/ *adj* (**earlier, earliest**) before the expected or normal time; of or occurring in the first part of a period or series; of or occurring in the distant past or near future.—*also adv.*—**earliness** *n*.

earmark /'i:rmɑːrk/ *vt* to set aside for a specific use; to put an identification mark on. • *n* a distinguishing mark.

earn /ərn/ *vt* to gain (money, etc) by work or service; to acquire; to deserve; to earn interest (on money invested, etc).

earnest /'ərnɪst/ *adj* sincere in attitude or intention.—**earnestly** *adv.*—**earnestness** *n*.

earnings /'ərnɪŋz/ *npl* wages or profits; something earned.

earphone /'i:rˌfoːn/ *n* a device held to or worn over the ear, through which sound is transmitted; a headphone.

earpiece /'i:rpiːs/ *n* a telephone earphone.

earplug /-plʌg/ *n* a piece of wadding or wax inserted in the ear to prevent noise or water penetration.

earring /'i:rɪŋ/ *n* an ornament worn on the ear lobe.

earshot /'i:rʃɒt/ *n* hearing distance.

ear-splitting /-ˌsplɪtɪŋ/ *adj* very loud.

earth /ərθ/ *n* the world that we inhabit; solid ground, as opposed to sea; soil; the burrow of a badger, fox, etc; a connection between an electric device or circuit with the earth; (*inf*) a large amount of money. • *vt* to cover with or bury in the earth; to connect an electrical circuit or device to earth.

earthborn /'ərθbɔrn/ *adj* mortal.

earthbound /-ˌbaʊnd/ *adj* confined to the earth; heading towards the earth.

earthen /'ərθən/ *adj* composed of earth; made of baked clay.

earthenware /-ˌwɛr/ *n* pottery, etc made from baked clay.

earthly /-li/ *adj* (**earthlier, earthliest**) of the earth; material, worldly.—**earthliness** *n*.

earthquake /-ˌkweɪk/ *n* a violent tremor of the earth's crust.

earth science *n* any of the sciences (*eg* geology) concerned with the nature and composition of the earth.

earthward /-wərd/, **earthwards** *adv* towards the earth.

earthwork /-ˌwərk/ *n* an excavation of earth; a fortification.

earthworm /-ˌwərm/ *n* any of various common worms that live in the soil.

earthy /'ərθi/ *adj* (**earthier, earthiest**) of or resembling earth; crude.—**earthiness** *n*.

earwax /'i:rˌwæks/ *n* cerumen, the brown wax found in the ear.

earwig /'i:rwɪg/ *n* a small insect with a pincer-like appendage at the end of its body.

ease /i:z/ *n* freedom from pain, discomfort or disturbance; rest from effort or work; effortlessness; lack of inhibition or restraint, naturalness. • *vt* to relieve from pain, trouble, or anxiety; to relax, make less tight, release; to move carefully and gradually. • *vi* (*often with* **off**) to become less active, intense, or severe.

easeful /-fəl/ *adj* restful.

easel /'i:zəl/ *n* a supporting frame, *esp* one used by artists to support their canvases while painting.

easement /'izmənt/ *n* relief; something that gives ease or relief; (*law*) right of way over someone else's land.

easily /'i:zɪli/ *adv* with ease; by far; probably.

east /'i:st/ *n* the direction of the sunrise; the compass point opposite west; (*with cap preceded by* **the**) the area of the world east of Europe. • *adj, adv* in, towards, or from the east.

Easter /'i:stər/ *n* the Christian festival observed on a Sunday in March or April in commemoration of the resurrection of Christ.

easterly /'i:stərli/ *adj* situated towards or belonging to the east, coming from the east. • *n* (*pl* **easterlies**) a wind from the east.

eastern /'i:stərn/ *adj* of or in the east.

Eastern Canadian *n* ✤ a person who lives in or is from Ontario, Quebec, or one of the provinces east of them. • *adj* of or pertaining to such a person.

easterner /'i:stərnər/ *n* someone from the east.

easternmost /-ˌmoːst/ *adj* farthest to the east.

easting /'i:stɪŋ/ *n* the distance travelled by a vessel eastwards from a given meridian.

eastward /'i:stwərd/ *adj* towards the east.—**eastwards** *adv*.

easy /'i:zi/ *adj* (**easier, easiest**) free from pain, trouble, anxiety; not difficult or requiring much effort; (*manner*) relaxed; lenient; compliant; unhurried; (*inf*) open to all alternatives. • *adv* with ease.—**easiness** *n*.

easy chair *n* a comfortable chair.

easygoing /-ˌgoːɪŋ/ *adj* placid, tolerant, relaxed.

eat /i:t/ *vt* (**eating, ate,** *pp* **eaten**) to take into the mouth, chew and swallow as food; to have a meal; to consume, to destroy bit by bit; (*also with* **into**) to corrode; (*inf*) to bother, cause anxiety to; (*with* **up**) to consume completely; (*inf*) to listen or absorb avidly; (*inf*) to preoccupy. • *vi* (*with* **out**) to eat away from home, *esp* in a restaurant. • *n* (*pl: inf*) food.—**eater** *n*.

eatable /'i:təbəl/ *adj* suitable for eating; fit to be eaten. • *n* (*pl*) food.

eating disorder *n* a psychological disorder identified by unusual or abnormal eating patterns.

eau de Cologne /ˌoːdəkəˈloːn/ *n* (*pl* **eaux de Cologne**) a perfume originally from Cologne.

eau de vie /oːdəˈviː/ *n* brandy.

eaves /i:vz/ *npl* the overhanging edge of a roof.

eavesdrop /'i:vzdrɒp/ *vi* (**eavesdropping, eavesdropped**) to listen secretly to a private conversation.—**eavesdropper** *n*.

ebb /ɛb/ *n* the flow of the tide out to sea; a decline. • *vi* (*tide water*) to flow back; to become lower, to decline.

ebon /'ɛbən/ *n* (*poet*) ebony.

ebonite /'ɛbəˌnaɪt/ *n* a hard black rubber substance.

ebonize /'ɛbənaɪz/ *vt* to make black by staining like ebony.

ebony /'ɛbəni/ *n* (*pl* **ebonies**) a hard heavy wood. • *adj* black as ebony.

ebracteate /iːˈbræktɪət/ *adj* without bracts.

ebullient /ɪˈbʌlɪənt/ or /-bʊl-/ *adj* exuberant, enthusiastic, boiling.—**ebullience, ebulliency** *n*.—**ebulliently** *adv*.

ebullition /ˌɛbəˈlɪʃən/ or /ˌɛbjuː-/ *n* boiling; an outburst (of passion, feeling, etc).

EC *abbr* = European Community; East Central.

eccentric /ɪkˈsɛntrɪk/ or /ɛk-/ *adj* deviating from a usual or accepted pattern; unconventional in manner or appearance, odd; (*circles*) not concentric; off centre; not precisely circular. • *n* an eccentric person.—**eccentrically** *adv*.

eccentricity /-trɪsɪti/ *n* (*pl* **eccentricities**) strangeness of behaviour; an eccentric or unusual habit.

ecclesiastic[1] /ɪˌkliːziˈæstɪk/ *n* a member of the clergy.

ecclesiastic[2], **ecclesiastical** /-əl/ *adj* of or relating to the Christian Church or clergy.—**ecclesiastically** *adv*.

ecclesiasticism /-tɪˌsɪzəm/ *n* excessive attachment to the forms, usages, organization and privileges of the Christian Church.

ecclesiology /ɪˌkliːzɪˈɒlədʒi/ or /ɪ-/ *n* the study of the Christian Church and its development; the study of church architecture and decoration.—**ecclesiological** *adj*.—**ecclesiologist** *n*.

ecdysis /ˈɛkdaɪsɪs/ (*pl* **ecdyses**) *n* sloughing of skin, moulting.

ECG /ˈiːsiːˈdʒiː/ *abbr* = electrocardiogram.

echelon /ˈɛʃəˌlɒn/ or /ˈeɪʃəˌlɔ̃/ *n* a stepped formation of troops, ships, or aircraft; a level (of authority) in a hierarchy.

echidna /ɪˈkɪdnə/ *n* (*pl* **echidnas, echidnae**) an Australian nocturnal, toothless, spiny, egg-laying animal.

echinoderm /ɪˈkaɪnəˌdɜːm/ *n* one of a class of animals which includes starfish and sea urchins.

echinus /ˈɪkaɪnəs/ *n* (*pl* **echini**) a sea urchin.

echo /ˈɛkoː/ *n* (*pl* **echoes**) a repetition of sound caused by the reflection of sound waves; imitation; the reflection of a radar signal by an object. • *vb* (**echoing, echoed**) *vi* to resound; to produce an echo. • *vt* to repeat; to imitate; to send back (a sound) by an echo.

echo chamber *n* a room with walls that reflect sound, used for making acoustic measurements and creating special sound effects.

echoic /ɛˈkoːɪk/ *adj* like an echo; imitative.

echolocation /ˈɛkoːloːˌkeɪʃən/ *n* finding unseen objects by means of reflected sound waves.

echo sounder *n* an instrument for determining the depth beneath a ship using sound waves.—**echo sounding** *n*.

éclair /eɪˈklɛr/ or /ɪ-/ *n* a small oblong shell of choux pastry covered with chocolate and filled with cream.

eclampsia /ɛkˈlæmpsiə/ *n* (*med*) a serious condition occurring in the last three months of pregnancy, caused by toxins in the blood and causing convulsions.

éclat /eɪˈklɑː/ *n* success; applause; striking effect; social distinction.

eclectic /ɪkˈlɛktɪk/ *adj* selecting from or using various styles, ideas, methods, etc; composed of elements from a variety of sources. • *n* a person who adopts an eclectic method—**eclectically** *adv*.—**eclecticism** *n*.

eclipse /ɪˈklɪps/ *n* the obscuring of the light of the sun or moon by the intervention of the other; a decline into obscurity, as from overshadowing by others. • *vt* to cause an eclipse of; to overshadow, darken; to surpass.—**eclipser** *n*.

ecliptic /ɪˈklɪptɪk/ *n* the apparent path of the sun's motion relative to the stars.—**ecliptically** *adv*.

eclogue /ˈɛkˌlɒg/ *n* a short, *esp* pastoral poem.

eco- /ˈiːkoː/ *prefix* ecology; ecological.

ecology /ɪˈkɒlədʒi/ *n* (the study of) the relationships between living things and their environments.—**ecological** *adj*.—**ecologist** *n*.

e-commerce /ɪˈkɒmɜːs/ *n* electronic commerce; undertaking business transactions online.

econometrics /ɪˌkɒnəˈmetrɪks/ *n sing* the application of mathematical and statistical methods in economics.

economic /ˌɛkəˈnɒmɪk/ or /ˌiːk-/ *adj* pertaining to economics or the economy; (*business, etc*) capable of producing a profit.

economical /-əl/ *adj* thrifty.—**economically** *adv*.

economics /ˌiːkəˈnɒmɪks/ *n sing* the social science concerned with the production, consumption and distribution of goods and services; (*pl*) financial aspects.

economist /ɪˈkɒnəmɪst/ *n* an expert in economics.

economize /ɪˈkɒnəˌmaɪz/ *vti* to spend money carefully; to save; to use prudently.—**economization** *n*.

economy /ɪˈkɒnəmi/ *n* (*pl* **economies**) careful use of money and resources to minimize waste; an instance of this; the management of the finances and resources, etc of a business, industry or organization; the economic system of a country.

ecosphere /ˈiːkoːˌsfɪr/ *n* the parts of the universe where life can exist.

ecosystem /-ˌsɪstəm/ *n* (*ecology*) a system comprising a community of living organisms and its surroundings.

ecru /ˈeɪkruː/ *n* beige.

ecstasy /ˈɛkstəsi/ *n* (*pl* **ecstasies**) intense joy; (*sl: often with cap*) the synthetic amphetamine-based drug MDMA, which reduces social and sexual inhibitions.—**ecstatic** *adj*.—**ecstatically** *adv*.

ECT /ˈiːsiːˈtiː/ *abbr* = electroconvulsive therapy.

ecto-, ect- /ˈɛktoː/ *prefix* outside.

ectoderm /ˈɛktoːˌdɜːm/ *n* the outer layer of an embryo or skin.

ectomorph /-ˌmɔːf/ *n* a person with a lightly built physique.—**ectomorphic** *adj*.—**ectomorphy** *n*.

-ectomy /ˈɛktəmi/ *suffix* denoting surgical removal of a part.

ectopic /ɛkˈtɒpɪk/ *adj* (*anat*) in an abnormal position; (*fertilized egg*) developing abnormally outside the uterus.

ectoplasm /ˈɛktoːˌplæzəm/ *n* the outer layer of the cytoplasm of a cell; a substance supposedly exuded from the body of spiritualist mediums during trances.—**ectoplasmic** *adj*.

ectype /ˈɛkˌtaɪp/ *n* a reproduction or imitation of an original design.

ECU *abbr* = European Currency Unit; *see* **euro**.

ecumenical /ˌɛkjuːˈmɛnɪkəl/ or /ˌiːk-/ *adj* of the whole Christian Church; seeking Christian unity worldwide.—**ecumenicalism, ecumenicism** *n*.—**ecumenically** *adv*.

eczema /ˈɛksɪmə/ or /ɛkˈziːmə/ *n* inflammation of the skin causing itching and the formation of scaly red patches.—**eczematous** *adj*.

edacious /iˈdeɪʃəs/ *adj* gluttonous, greedy.—**edacity** *n*.

Edam /ˈiːdæm/ *n* a mild-flavoured round Dutch cheese, *usu* with a red waxy rind.

EDC *abbr* ✦ (*Cdn*) = Export Development Corporation.

eddy /ˈɛdi/ *n* (*pl* **eddies**) a swiftly revolving current of air, water, fog, etc. • *vi* (**eddying, eddied**) to move round and round.

edelweiss /ˈeɪdəlˌvaɪs/ *n* a small white-flowered alpine herb.

edema /ɪˈdiːmə/ *see* **oedema**.

Eden /ˈiːdən/ *n* (*Bible*) the garden where Adam and Eve lived after the creation; a paradise.

edentate /iˈdɛnˌteɪt/ or /ɪ-/ *adj* (*zool*) toothless.

edge /ɛdʒ/ *n* the border, brink, verge, margin; the sharp cutting side of a blade; sharpness, keenness; force, effectiveness. • *vt* to supply an edge or border to; to move gradually.—**edger** *n*.

edgeways /ˈɛdʒˌweɪz/, **edgewise** /-ˌwaɪz/ *adv* with the edge forwards; sideways.

edging /ˈɛdʒɪŋ/ *n* any border for decoration or strengthening.

edgy /ˈɛdʒi/ *adj* (**edgier, edgiest**) irritable.—**edgily** *adv*.—**edginess** *n*.

edible /ˈɛdɪbəl/ *adj* fit or safe to eat.—**edibility, edibleness** *n*.

edict /ˈiːˌdɪkt/ *n* a decree; a proclamation.—**edictal** *adj*.

edifice /ˈɛdɪfɪs/ *n* a substantial building; any large or complex organization or institution.—**edificial** *adj*.

edify /ˈɛdɪˌfaɪ/ *vt* (**edifying, edified**) to improve the moral character or mind of (a person).—**edification** *n*.—**edifier** *n*.—**edifyingly** *adv*.

edile /ˈiːdaɪl/ *see* **aedile**.

edit /ˈɛdɪt/ *vt* to prepare (text) for publication by checking facts, grammar, style, etc; to be in charge of a publication; (*cinema*) to prepare a final version of a film by selection and arrangement of photographed sequences.

edition /ɪˈdɪʃən/ *n* a whole number of copies of a book, etc printed at a time; the form of a particular publication.

editio princeps /ɪˌdɪʃioːˈprɪnseps/ (*pl* **editiones principes**) *n* the first printed edition of a book.

editor /ˈɛdɪtər/ *n* a person in charge of a newspaper or other publication; a person who edits written material for publication; one who prepares the final version of a film; a person in overall charge of the form and content of a radio or television programme.—**editorship** *n*.

editorial /ˌɛdɪˈtɔːriəl/ *adj* of or produced by an editor. • *n* an article expressing the opinions of the editor or publishers of a newspaper or magazine.—**editorialist** *n*.—**editorially** *adv*.

EDP *abbr* = Electronic Data Processing.

educable, educatable /ˈɛdʒʊkəbəl/ or /-dʒʊ-/ *adj* able to be educated.

educate /ˈɛdʒʊˌkeɪt/ or /-dʒʊ-/ *vt* to train the mind, to teach; to provide schooling for.—**educator** *n*.

education /ˌɛdʒʊˈkeɪʃən/ or /-dʒʊ-/ *n* the process of learning and training; instruction as imparted in schools, colleges and universities; a course or type of instruction; the theory and practice of teaching.—**educational** *adj*.—**educationally** *adv*.

educationalist /-əlɪst/, **educationist** /-ɪst/ *n* an expert in education.

educative /ˈɛdʒʊˌkətɪv/ or /-dʒʊ-/ *adj* educating.

educe /ɛˈdjuːs/ *vt* to elicit (information, etc); to infer.—**educible** *adj*.

edulcorate /əˈdʌlkəˌreɪt/ *vt* to free from acids and other impurities by washing.—**edulcoration** *n*.

edutainment /ˌɛdʒʊˈteɪnmənt/ or /-dʒʊ-/ *n* programmes or classes aimed at combining information with material of an entertaining nature.

EEC /ˈiːˈiːˈsiː/ *abbr* = European Economic Community (now European Union).

EEG /ˈiːˈiːˈdʒiː/ *abbr* = electroencephalogram.

eel /iːl/ *n* a snake-like fish.

eelpout /-ˌpaʊt/ *n* a type of freshwater fish, found in Europe, North America and Asia; another name for the burbot.

e'en /iːn/ *n* (*poet*) evening.

e'er /er/ *adv* (*poet*) ever.

eerie /ˈiːri/ *adj* (**eerier, eeriest**) causing fear; weird.—**eerily** *adv.*—**eeriness** *n.*

efface /ɪˈfeɪs/ *vt* to rub out, obliterate; to make (oneself) humble or inconspicuous.—**effaceable** *adj.*—**effacement** *n.*—**effacer** *n.*

effect /ɪˈfekt/ *n* the result of a cause or action by some agent; the power to produce some result; the fundamental meaning; an impression on the senses; an operative condition; (*pl*) personal belongings; (*pl: theatre, cinema*) sounds, lighting, etc to accompany a production. • *vt* to bring about, accomplish.—**effecter** *n.*—**effectible** *adj.*

effective /-tɪv/ *adj* producing a specified effect; forceful, striking in impression; actual, real; operative.—**effectively** *adv.*—**effectiveness** *n.*

effectual /ɪˈfektʃuːəl/ *adj* able to produce the desired effect.—**effectuality, effectualness** *n.*—**effectually** *adv.*

effectuate /-ˌeɪt/ *vt* to make happen.—**effectuation** *n.*

effeminate /ɪˈfemənət/ *adj* (*man*) displaying what are regarded as feminine qualities.—**effeminacy, effeminateness** *n.*

effendi /eˈfendi/ (*pl* **effendis**) *n* a Turkish title of respect, equivalent to sir or Mr.

efferent /ˈefərənt/ *adj* (*anat*) conveying or discharging outwards.

effervesce /ˌefərˈves/ *vt* (*liquid*) to froth and hiss as bubbles of gas escape; to be exhilarated.—**effervescence** *n.*—**effervescent** *adj.*—**effervescible** *adj.*

effete /ɪˈfiːt/ *adj* decadent, weak.—**effeteness** *n.*

efficacious /ˌefɪˈkeɪʃəs/ *adj* achieving the desired result.—**efficacy, efficaciousness** *n.*

efficiency unit *n* ♣ (*Cdn*) a hotel room or temporarily let small apartment that has some cooking and washing facilities.

efficient /ɪˈfɪʃənt/ or /ɪ-/ *adj* achieving results without waste of time or effort; competent.—**efficiently** *adv.*—**efficiency** *n* (*pl* **efficiencies**).

effigy /ˈefɪdʒi/ *n* (*pl* **effigies**) a sculpture or portrait; a crude figure of a person, *esp* for exposure to public contempt and ridicule.

effloresce /ˌeflɔːˈres/ *vi* to blossom; (*chem*) to turn to powder when exposed to air, to crystallize; to become encrusted with crystals as a result of loss of water.—**efflorescence** *n.*—**efflorescent** *adj.*

effluence /ˈefluːəns/, **efflux** /ˈefˌlʌks/ *n* something that flows out.

effluent /ˈefluːənt/ *adj* flowing out. • *n* that which flows out, *esp* sewage.

effluvium /ɪˈfluːviəm/ *n* (*pl* **effluvia, effluviums**) an offensive vapour or smell.—**effluvial** *adj.*

effort /ˈefərt/ *n* exertion; an attempt, try; a product of great exertion.—**effortful** *adj.*

effortless /-ləs/ *adj* done with little effort, or seemingly so.—**effortlessly** *adv.*—**effortlessness** *n.*

effrontery /ɪˈfrʌntəri/ *n* (*pl* **effronteries**) impudent boldness, insolence.

effulgent /ɪˈfeldʒənt/ *adj* radiant, brilliant.—**effulgence** *n.*

effuse /ɪˈfjuːz/ *vt* (*liquid, words*) to flow or pour out.

effusion /ɪˈfjuːʒən/ *n* a pouring out; an unrestrained outpouring, as of emotion; something poured out.

effusive /ɪˈfjuːsɪv/ *adj* gushing, emotionally unrestrained; demonstrative.—**effusiveness** *n.*

eft /eft/ *n* a newt.

e.g., eg, eg. *abbr* = for example (*Latin exempli gratia*).

egad /iːˈɡæd/ *interj* (*arch*) an exclamation of surprise, pleasure or admiration.

egalitarian /ɪˌɡælɪˈteriən/ *adj* upholding the principle of equal rights for all.—*also n.*—**egalitarianism** *n.*

egest /ɪˈdʒest/ *vt* to excrete.—**egestion** *n.*

egesta /ɪˈdʒestə/ *npl* excrement.

egg[1] /eɡ/ *n* the oval hard-shelled reproductive cell laid by birds, reptiles and fish; the egg of the domestic poultry used as food; ovum.—**eggy** *adj.*

egg[2] *vt* (*with* **on**) to incite (someone to do something).

egger /ˈeɡər/ *n* a type of large moth.

egghead /ˈeɡˌhed/ *n* (*inf*) an intellectual.

eggnog /ˈeɡnɒɡ/ *n* a drink made from egg, beaten up with hot milk, sugar and brandy.

eggplant /-plænt/ *see* **aubergine.**

eggshell /ˈeɡʃel/ *n* the hard outer covering of an egg. • *adj* fragile; (*paint*) having a slight sheen.

egis /ˈiːdʒɪs/ *see* **aegis.**

eglantine /ˈeɡlənˌtaɪn/ *n* the sweetbrier; the wild rose.

ego /ˈiːɡoː/ *n* (*pl* **egos**) the self; self-image, conceit.

egocentric /ˌiːɡoːˈsentrɪk/ *adj* self-centred.—**egocentricity** *n.*

egoism /ˈiːɡoːˌɪzəm/ *n* self-concern; self-centredness.—**egoist** *n.*—**egoistic, egoistical** *adj.*—**egoistically** *adv.*

egotism /-tɪzəm/ *n* excessive reference to oneself; conceit.—**egotist** *n.*—**egotistic, egotistical** *adj.*—**egotistically** *adv.*

ego trip *n* (*inf*) an activity undertaken to boost one's own self-esteem or importance in the eyes of others.—**ego-trip** *vi.*

egregious /ɪˈɡriːdʒəs/ *adj* outstandingly bad.—**egregiousness** *n.*

egress /ˈiːˌɡres/ *n* the way out, exit.

egression /ɪˈɡreʃən/ *n* the act of going out or emerging; egress.

egret /ˈiːɡret/ *n* a type of heron.

Egyptology /ˌiːdʒɪpˈtɒlədʒi/ *n* the study of Egyptian antiquities and hieroglyphics.—**Egyptologist** *n.*

eh /eɪ/ *interj* an exclamation of inquiry or surprise.

eider /ˈaɪdər/ *n* a large marine duck, the down of which has commercial value as a filling for quilts etc.

eiderdown /-ˌdaʊn/ *n* the down of the eider duck used for stuffing quilts, etc; a thick quilt with a soft filling.

eidolon /aɪˈdoːlɒn/ *n* (*pl* **eidolons, eidola**) *n* an apparition or phantom.

eight /eɪt/ *n, adj* one more than seven; the symbol for this (8, VIII, viii); (the crew of) an eight-oared rowing boat.

eighteen /eɪˈtiːn/ *n, adj* one more than seventeen; the symbol for this (18, XVIII, xviii).—**eighteenth** *adj.*

eighteenmo /eɪˈtiːnmoː/ *n* (*pl* **eighteenmos**) *n* a book whose sheets are folded into eighteen leaves.

eightfold /ˈeɪtfoːld/ *adj, adv* consisting of eight units; being eight times as great or many.

eighth /eɪtθ/ *adj, n* one after seventh; one of eight equal parts.

eighty /ˈeɪti/ *n* (*pl* **eighties**) eight times ten; the symbol for this (80, LXXX, lxxx); (*pl*) the numbers from 80 to 89.—**eightieth** *adj, n.*

einsteinium /aɪnˈstaɪniəm/ *n* an artificial radioactive element.

eisteddfod /aɪsˈteðˌvɒd/ or /-fəd/ *n* (*pl* **eisteddfods, eisteddfodau**) a Welsh competitive festival of the arts, *esp* singing.—**eisteddfodic** *adj.*

either /ˈaɪðər/ or /ˈiːðər/ *adj, n* the one or the other of two; each of two. • *conj* correlative to *or.*

ejaculate /ɪˈdʒækjuˌleɪt/ *vti* to emit a fluid (as semen); to exclaim.—**ejaculation** *n.*—**ejaculator** *n.*—**ejaculatory** *adj.*

eject /ɪˈdʒekt/ *vt* to turn out, to expel by force. • *vi* to escape from an aircraft or spacecraft using an ejector seat.—**ejection** *n.*—**ejector** *n.*

ejecta /ɪˈdʒektə/ *npl* matter discharged by an erupting volcano.

ejector seat *n* an escape seat, *esp* in combat aircraft, that can be ejected with its occupant in an emergency by means of explosive bolts.

e-journal /ˌiːˈdʒərnəl/ *n* an online publication that can be accessed on the Web, commonly used in the academic world.

eke /iːk/ *vt* (*with* **out**) to supplement; to use (a supply) frugally; to make (a living) with difficulty.

elaborate /ɪˈlæbəˌreɪt/ *vt*, /ɪˈlæbərət/ *adj* highly detailed; planned with care and exactness. • *vt* to work out or explain in detail.—**elaborateness** *n.*—**elaboration** *n.*—**elaborative** *adj.*—**elaborator** *n.*

élan /eɪˈlɑ̃/ *n* verve, spirit.

eland /ˈiːlənd/ *n* an African antelope with spirally twisted horns.

elapse /ɪˈlæps/ *vi* (*time*) to pass by.

elasmobranch /ɪˈlæzməˌbræŋk/ *n* (*pl* **elasmobranchs**) a member of a class of fish that includes sharks and skates.

elastic /ɪˈlæstɪk/ or /ɪ-/ *adj* returning to the original size and shape if stretched or squeezed; springy; adaptable. • *n* fabric, tape, etc incorporating elastic thread.—**elastically** *adv.*—**elasticity** *n.*

elasticated /-keɪtəd/ *adj* made elastic by the use of elastic thread.

elate /ɪˈleɪt/ or /ɪ-/ *vt* to fill with happiness or pride.—**elated** *adj.*—**elatedness** *n.*—**elation** *n.*

elbow /ˈelboː/ *n* the joint between the forearm and upper arm; the part of a piece of clothing covering this; any sharp turn or bend, as in a pipe. • *vt* to shove away rudely with the elbow; to jostle.

elbow grease *n* (*inf*) effort, hard work.

elbowroom /ˈelboːˌruːm/ *n* space to move, scope.

elder[1] /'ɛldər/ n a tree or shrub with flat clusters of white or pink flowers.

elder[2] n an older person; an office bearer in certain churches.—**eldership** n.

elderberry /-ˌberi/ n (pl **elderberries**) (the fruit of) an elder.

elderly /-li/ adj quite old.—**elderliness** n.

eldest /'ɛldəst/ n oldest, first born.

El Dorado, eldorado /ˌɛldə'rædo:/ n an imaginary land of vast wealth.

eldritch, eldrich /'ɛldrɪtʃ/ adj (Scot) weird; hideous.

elecampane /ˌɛləkæm'peɪn/ n a plant of the aster family, from the roots of which a tonic medicine is made.

elect /ɪ'lɛkt/ or /i-/ vti to choose by voting; to make a selection (of); to make a decision on. • adj chosen for an office but not installed.

election /ɪ'lɛkʃən/ or /i-/ n the public choice of a person for office, esp a politician.

electioneer /ɪ,lɛkʃə'ni:r/ or /i-/ vi to work on behalf of a candidate for election.—**electioneering** n.

elective /ɪ'lɛktɪv/ or /i-/ adj pertaining to, dependant on, or exerting the power of, choice.—**electivity, electiveness** n.

elector /ɪ'lɛktər/ or /i-/ n a person who has a vote at an election.—**electorship** n.

electoral /ɪ'lɛktərəl/ or /i-/, /-'tɔrəl/ adj of elections or electors.

electoral officer n ♣ (Cdn) a public official who oversees the running of an election.

electorate /ɪ'lɛktərɪt/ or /i-/ n the whole body of qualified electors.

electric /ɪ'lɛktrɪk/ or /i-/ adj of, producing or worked by electricity; exciting, thrilling. • npl electric fittings.

electrical /-kəl/ adj of or relating to electricity.—**electrically** adv.

electric chair n a chair used in executing condemned criminals by electrocution.

electric eel n an eel-like fish capable of giving an electric shock.

electric eye n a photoelectric cell.

electric guitar n a guitar that is electronically amplified.

electrician /ˌi:lɛk'trɪʃən/ or /ˌɛl-/, /ˌɪlɛk-/ n a person who installs and repairs electrical devices.

electricity /ˌi:lɛk'trɪsɪti/ or /ˌɛl-/, /ˌɪlɛk-/ n a form of energy comprising certain charged particles, such as electrons and protons; an electric current.

electrify /ɪ'lɛktrəˌfaɪ/ or /i-/ vt (**electrifying, electrified**) to charge with electricity; to modify or equip for the use of electric power; to astonish or excite.—**electrifiable** adj.—**electrification** n.—**electrifier** n.

electro-, electr- /ɪ'lɛktro:/ or /i-/ prefix of or by electricity.

electrocardiogram /-'kardiəˌgræm/ or /i-/ n the tracing made by an electrocardiograph.

electrocardiograph /-'kardiəˌgræf/ n a device for recording the electrical activity of the heart.—**electrocardiographic, electrocardiographical** adj.—**electrocardiography** n.

electrochemistry /-'kɛmɪstri/ or /i-/ n the area of chemistry dealing with chemical changes caused by electricity.—**electrochemical** adj.—**electrochemist** n.

electroconvulsive therapy /-kən'vʌlsɪv/ n treatment of certain types of mental illness by passing an electric current through the brain.

electrocute /ɪ'lɛktrəˌkju:t/ or /i-/ vt to kill or execute by electricity.—**electrocution** n.

electrode /ɪ'lɛkˌtro:d/ or /i-/ n a conductor through which an electric current enters or leaves an electrolyte, gas discharge tube or thermionic valve.

electrodynamics /-daɪ'næmɪks/ n sing the area of physics dealing with electric currents.—**electrodynamic, electrodynamical** adj.

electroencephalogram /-ɛn'sɛfələˌgræm/ n the tracing produced by an electroencephalograph.

electroencephalograph /-ˌgræf/ n a device for recording the electrical activity of the brain.—**electro-encephalographic** adj.—**electroencephalographically** adv.—**electroencephalography** n.

electrokinetics /ɪ,lɛktro:kɪ'nɛtɪks/ or /i-/, /-trə-/ n sing the area of physics dealing with electricity in motion.—**electrokinetic** adj.

electrolysis /ˌɪlɛk'trɒləsɪs/ or /ˌi:-/, /ˌɛl-/ n the passage of an electric current through an electrolyte to effect chemical change; the destruction of living tissue, esp hair roots, by the use of an electric current

electrolyte /ɪ'lɛktrəˌlaɪt/ or /i-/ n a solution that conducts electricity.

electrolyze /-ˌlaɪz/ vt to cause to undergo electrolysis.—**electrolyzation** n.—**electrolyzer** n.

electromagnet /ɪ,lɛktro:'mægnət/ or /i-/ n a metal core rendered magnetic by the passage of an electric current through a surrounding coil.

electromagnetic /-tɪk/ adj pertaining to, or produced by, electromagnetism.—**electromagnetically** adv.

electromagnetism /-tɪ,zəm/ n magnetism produced by an electric current; the area of science dealing with the relations between electricity and magnetism.

electrometallurgy /-'mɛtə,lərdʒi/ n metallurgy using a slow electric current to precipitate certain metals from their solutions, or to separate metals from their ores.—**electrometallurgical** adj.—**electrometallurgist** n.

electrometer /ˌɪlɛk'trɒmətər/ or /i-/ n an instrument for measuring electricity.—**electrometric, electrometrical** adj.—**electrometry** n.

electromotive /ɪ,lɛktrə'mo:tɪv/ or /i-/ adj producing an electric current.

electromotive force n a source of energy producing an electric current; the amount of energy drawn from such a source per unit current of electricity passing through it, measured in volts.

electron /ɪ'lɛktrɒn/ or /i-/ a a negatively charged elementary particle that forms the part of the atom outside the nucleus.

electronegative /ɪ,lɛktro:'nɛgətɪv/ or /i-/ adj with a negative electrical charge.

electronic /ˌɪlɛk'trɒnɪk/ or /i-/, /ˌi-/, /ˌɛl-/ adj of or worked by streams of electrons flowing through semiconductor devices, vacuum or gas; of or concerned with electrons or electronics.—**electronically** adv.

electronic mail n messages, etc, sent and received via computer terminals, email, e-mail.

electronic publishing n the use of the Internet to publish and distribute material, whether text, databases or other types of information.

electronics /-ɪks/ n sing the study, development and application of electronic devices; (pl) electronic circuits.

electron microscope n a powerful microscope that uses a stream of electrons instead of light to produce magnified images.

electronvolt n a unit of energy equivalent to the energy gained by an electron that has been accelerated through a potential difference of one volt.

electrophorus /ˌɪlɛk'trɒfərəs/ or /ˌi:-/ n (pl **electrophori**) an instrument for generating static electricity by induction.

electroplate /ɪ'lɛktrəˌpleɪt/ or /i-/, /-'tro:-/ vt to plate or cover with metal (eg silver) by electrolysis. • n electroplated objects.—**electroplater** n.

electropositive /ɪ,lɛktro:'pɒzɪtɪv/ or /i-/ adj with a positive electrical charge.

electroscope /ɪ'lɛktrə,sko:p/ or /i-/ n an instrument for showing the presence or quality of electricity.—**electroscopic** adj.

electrostatics /-'stætɪks/ or /-tro:-/ n sing the branch of physics concerned with static electric charges.—**electrostatic** adj.—**electrostatically** adv.

electrotherapeutics /-'θɛrəpju:tɪks/ n sing the area of medicine dealing with the use of electrotherapy.

electrotherapy /-'θɛrəpi/ n the treatment of disease using electricity.—**electrotherapist** n.

electrotype /ɪ'lɛktrə,taɪp/ or /i-/ n (print) a facsimile made by covering a mould or plate of the original with a coating of copper or nickel. • vt to make a copy in this way.—**electrotyper** n.

electrum /ɪ'lɛktrəm/ or /-/ n an alloy of gold and silver.

electuary /ɪ'lɛktʃuːeri/ or /i-/ n (pl **electuaries**) a medicinal drug mixed with honey or syrup.

eleemosynary /ˌɛlə'mɒsəneri/ or /ɛliə-/, /-'mɒz-/ adj dependent on charity. (money) given as charity.

elegant /'ɛləgənt/ adj graceful; refined; dignified and tasteful in manner and appearance.—**elegance, elegancy** n.—**elegantly** adv.

elegiac /ɛ'lədʒaɪˌək/ adj characteristic of elegy; mournful.

elegize /'ɛlə,dʒaɪz/ vt to write an elegy about.—**elegist** n.

elegy /'ɛlədʒi/ n (pl **elegies**) a slow mournful song or poem.

element /'ɛləmənt/ n a constituent part; any of the 105 known substances composed of atoms with the same number of protons in their nuclei; a favourable environment for a plant or animal; a wire that produces heat in an electric cooker, kettle, etc;

any of the four substances (earth, air, fire, water) that in ancient and medieval thought were believed to constitute the universe; (*pl*) atmospheric conditions (wind, rain, etc); (*pl*) the basic principles, rudiments.

elemental /ɛləˈmɛntəl/ *adj* of elements or primitive natural forces.—**elementally** *adv*.

elementary /ˌɛləˈmɛntəri/ or /-tri/ *adj* concerned with the basic principles of a subject.—**elementariness** *n*.

elementary particle *n* any of the subatomic particles, such as electrons, protons and neutrons, not made up of other particles.

elemi /ˈɛləmi/ *n* (*pl* **elemis**) a resin used in medicines and varnishes.

elenchus /ɪˈlɛŋkəs/ *n* (*pl* **elenchi**) (*logic*) refutation of an argument.—**elenctic** *adj*.

elephant /ˈɛləfənt/ *n* (*pl* **elephants, elephant**) a large heavy mammal with a long trunk, thick skin, and ivory tusks.—**elephantoid** *adj*.

elephantiasis /ˌɛləfənˈtaɪəsɪs/ *n* (*pl* **elephantiases**) a disease in which the limbs or scrotum become enormously enlarged.—**elephantiasic** *adj*.

elephantine /ˈɛləfænˌtaɪn/ or /-ˌtiːn/, /ˌɛləˈfænˌtaɪn/, /-ˌtiːn/ *adj* of or like elephants; very big or clumsy.

elevate /ˈɛləveɪt/ *vt* to lift up; to raise in rank; to improve in intellectual or moral stature.

elevated /-ˌveɪtəd/ *adj* raised; (*fig*) inflated; (*inf*) tipsy.

elevation /ˌɛləˈveɪʃən/ *n* a raised place; the height above the earth's surface or above sea level; the angle to which a gun is aimed above the horizon; a drawing that shows the front, rear, or side view of something.

elevator /ˈɛləˌveɪtər/ *n* a cage or platform for moving something from one level to another; a moveable surface on the tailplane of an aircraft to produce motion up and down; a lift; a building for storing grain.

eleven /ɪˈlɛvən/ *adj, n* one more than ten; the symbol for this (11, XI, xi); (*soccer, etc*) a team of eleven players.—**eleventh** *adj, n*.

elf /ɛlf/ *n* (*pl* **elves**) a mischievous fairy.—**elfin** *adj*.—**elfish, elvish** *adj*.

elflock /ˈɛlfˌlɒk/ *n* an intricately twisted lock of hair.

elicit /ɪˈlɪsɪt/ or /i-/ *vt* to draw out (information, etc).—**elicitable** *adj*.—**elicitation** *n*.—**elicitor** *n*.

elide /ɪˈlaɪd/ or /i-/ *vt* (*linguistics*) to cut off a syllable or vowel.

eligible /ˈɛlɪdʒəbəl/ *adj* suitable to be chosen, legally qualified; desirable, *esp* as a marriage partner.—**eligibility** *n*.—**eligibly** *adv*.

eliminate /ɪˈlɪməˌneɪt/ or /i-/ *vt* to expel, get rid of; to eradicate completely; (*sl*) to kill; to exclude (*eg* a competitor) from a competition, *usu* by defeat.—**eliminable** *adj*.—**elimination** *n*.—**eliminative, eliminatory** *adj*.—**eliminator** *n*.

elision /ɪˈlɪʒən/ or /i-/ *n* (*linguistics*) the cutting off of a syllable or vowel.

elite, élite /ɪˈliːt/ or /eɪ-/ *n* a superior group; (*typewriting*) a letter size having twelve characters to the inch.

elitism /-ˌɪzəm/ *n* leadership or rule by an elite; advocacy of such a system.—**elitist** *n*.

elixir /ɪˈlɪksər/ or /i-/ *n* (*alchemy*) a substance thought to have the power of transmuting base metals into gold, or of conferring everlasting life; any medicine claimed as a cure-all; a sweet syrup containing a medicine.

Elizabethan /ɪˌlɪzəˈbiːθən/ or /i-/ *adj* pertaining to Queen Elizabeth I of England and her reign (1558–1603), *esp* its architecture and literature; pertaining to Queen Elizabeth II of Great Britain and her reign (1952–). • *n* a person alive in the reign of Elizabeth I.

elk /ɛlk/ *n* (*pl* **elks, elk**) the largest existing deer of Europe and Asia.

ell /ɛl/ *n* an old measure of length used for cloth, based on the length of a man's arm, approximately equal to 45 inches (1.15 metres).

ellipse /ɪˈlɪps/ or /i-/ *n* (*geom*) a closed plane figure formed by the plane section of a right-angled cone; a flattened circle.

ellipsis /ɪˈlɪpsɪs/ or /i-/ *n* (*pl* **ellipses**) the omission of words needed to complete the grammatical construction of a sentence; the mark (...) used to indicate such omission.

ellipsoid /ɪˈlɪpˌsɔɪd/ or /i-/ *n* (*geom*) an elliptical spheroid; an oval.—**ellipsoidal** *adj*.

elliptic /ɪˈlɪptɪk/ or /i-/, **elliptical** /-əl/ *adj* of or like an ellipse; having a part understood.—**elliptically** *adv*.

ellipticity /ˌɪlɪpˈtɪsəti/ *n* (*geom*) the extent of deviation of an oval from a circle or sphere.

elm /ɛlm/ *n* a tall deciduous shade tree with spreading branches and broad top; its hard heavy wood.

elocution /ˌɛləˈkjuːʃən/ *n* skill in public speaking.—**elocutionary** *adj*.—**elocutionist** *n*.

elongate /iːˈlɒŋˌgeɪt/ or /ˈiːlɒŋˌgeɪt/ *vti* to make or become longer.—**elongation** *n*.

elope /ɪˈloʊp/ or /i-/ *vi* to run away secretly with a lover, *esp* to get married.—**elopement** *n*.—**eloper** *n*.

eloquence /ˈɛləkwəns/ *n* skill in the use of words; speaking with fluency, power or persuasiveness.

eloquent /ˈɛləkwənt/ *adj* (*speaking, writing, etc*) fluent and powerful.

else /ɛls/ *adv* besides; otherwise.

elsewhere /ˈɛlsˌwɛr/ *adv* in another place.

elucidate /ɪˈluːsɪˌdeɪt/ or /i-/ *vt* to make clear, to explain.—**elucidation** *n*.—**elucidative, elucidatory** *adj*.—**elucidator** *n*.

elude /ɪˈluːd/ or /i-/ *vt* to avoid stealthily; to escape the understanding or memory of a person.—**eluder** *n*.—**elusion** *n*.

elusive /ɪˈluːsɪv/ or /i-/ *adj* escaping; baffling; solitary, difficult to contact.—**elusiveness** *n*.

elver /ˈɛlvər/ *n* a young eel.

elves, elvish /ˈɛlvɪʃ/ *see* **elf**.

Elysian /ɪˈlɪziən/ or /ɪˈlɪʒ-/, /ɪˈliː-/ *adj* of or resembling Elysium; paradisiacal, blissful.

Elysium /ɪˈlɪziəm/ or /ɪˈlɪʒ-/, /ɪˈliː-/ *n* the ancient Greek paradise; a condition of perfect happiness.

elytron /ˈɛləˌtrɒn/, **elytrum** /-trəm/ *n* (*pl* **elytra**) one of the hard wing cases of a beetle.—**elytroid, elytrous** *adj*.

em /ɛm/ *n* (*print*) a measure of width, equal to one sixth of an inch (approx 4 mm).

emaciate /ɪˈmeɪsɪˌeɪt/ or /i-/ *vti* to make or become very thin and weak.—**emaciated** *adj*.—**emaciation** *n*.

email, e-mail /ˌiːˈmeɪl/ *n* short for electronic mail.

emanate /ˈɛməˌneɪt/ *vi* to issue from a source.—**emanative** *adj*.—**emanator** *n*.—**emanatory** *adj*.

emanation /ˌɛməˈneɪʃən/ *n* something coming from or caused by something else.—**emanational** *adj*.

emancipate /ɪˈmænsəˌpeɪt/ or /i-/ *vt* to liberate, *esp* from bondage or slavery.—**emancipative** *adj*.—**emancipator** *n*.—**emancipatory** *adj*.

emancipation /ɪˌmænsəˈpeɪʃən/ or /i-/ *n* the act of freeing; freedom, liberation.—**emancipationist** *n*.

emarginate /iˈmɑːrdʒənɪt/ or /-ˌneɪt/, /ɪ-/, **emarginated** *adj* (*leaf*) notched at the edges or tip.—**emargination** *n*.

emasculate /ɪˈmæskjʊˌleɪt/ or /i-/ *vt* to castrate; to deprive of vigour, strength, etc.—**emasculation** *n*.—**emasculative, emasculatory** *adj*.—**emasculator** *n*.

embalm /ɛmˈbɒm/ or /ɪm-/ *vt* to preserve (a dead body) with drugs, chemicals, etc.—**embalmer** *n*.—**embalmment** *n*.

embank /ɛmˈbæŋk/ or /ɪm-/ *vt* to enclose or protect with an embankment.

embankment /-mənt/ *n* an earth or stone mound made to hold back water or to carry a roadway.

embargo /ɛmˈbɑːrgoʊ/ or /ɪm-/ *n* (*pl* **embargoes**) an order of a government forbidding ships to enter or leave its ports; any ban or restriction on commerce by law; a prohibition, ban. • *vt* (**embargoing, embargoed**) to lay an embargo on; to requisition.

embark /ɛmˈbɑːrk/ or /ɪm-/ *vti* to put or go on board a ship or aircraft to begin a journey; to make a start in any activity or enterprise.—**embarkation** *n*.—**embarkment** *n*.

embarrass /ɛmˈbɛrəs/ or /ɪm-/ *vt* to make (a person) feel confused, uncomfortable or disconcerted.—**embarrassing** *adj*.—**embarrassment** *n*.

embassy /ˈɛmbəsi/ *n* (*pl* **embassies**) a person or group sent to a foreign government as ambassadors; the official residence of an ambassador.

embattle /ɛmˈbætl/ or /ɪm-/ *vt* to arrange troops for battle; to prepare for battle.—**embattled** *adj*.

embay /ɛmˈbeɪ/ or /ɪm-/ *vt* to bring or drive a ship into a bay.

embed /ɛmˈbɛd/ or /ɪm-/ *vt* (**embedding, embedded**) to fix firmly in surrounding matter.—**embedment** *n*.

embellish /ɛmˈbɛlɪʃ/ or /ɪm-/ *vt* to decorate, to adorn.—**embellisher** *n*.—**embellishment** *n*.

ember /ˈɛmbər/ *n* a piece of glowing coal or wood in a fire; (*pl*) the smouldering remains of a fire.

embezzle /ɛmˈbɛzəl/ or /ɪm-/ *vt* to steal (money, securities, etc entrusted to one's care).—**embezzlement** *n*.—**embezzler** *n*.

embitter /ɛm'bɪtər/ or /ɪm-/ vt to cause to feel bitter.—**embitterment** n.

emblazon /ɛm'bleɪzən/ or /ɪm-/ vt to make bright with colour; to ornament with heraldic devices.—**emblazonment** n.

emblazonry /-ri/ n heraldic decoration, blazonry.

emblem /'ɛmbləm/ n a symbol; a figure adopted and used as an identifying mark.

emblematic /ˌɛmblə'mætɪk/, **emblematical** /-əl/ adj of emblems; symbolic.—**emblematically** adv.

emblements /'ɛmbləmənts/ npl (law) the annual crops produced by the labour of the cultivator; the profit from these crops.

embody /ɛm'bɒdi/ or /ɪm-/ vt (**embodying, embodied**) to express in definite form; to incorporate or include in a single book, law, system, etc.—**embodiment** n.

embolden /ɛm'bo:ldən/ or /ɪm-/ vt to inspire with courage; to make bold.

embolism /'ɛmbəˌlɪzəm/ n the obstruction of a blood vessel by a blood clot, air bubble, etc.—**embolismic** adj.

embolus /'ɛmbələs/ n (pl **emboli**) material obstructing a blood vessel, eg a blood clot or air bubble.

embonpoint /ˌɑ̃bɔ̃'pwɑ̃/ n plumpness.

emboss /ɛm'bɒs/ or /ɪm-/ vt to ornament with a raised design.—**embosser** n.—**embossment** n.

embouchure /'ɒmbuˌʃʊr/ n the mouth of a river; (mus) the mouthpiece of a wind instrument; the correct positioning of the mouth when playing a wind instrument.

embowel /ɛm'baʊəl/ or /ɪm-/ vt (**embowelling, embowelled** or **emboweling, emboweled**) (arch) to remove the intestines from, disembowel; to embed, to bury.

embower /ɛm'baʊər/ or /ɪm-/ vt (arch) to cover with, or as with, a bower.

embrace /ɛm'breɪs/ or /ɪm-/ vt to take and hold tightly in the arms as a sign of affection; to accept eagerly (eg an opportunity); to adopt (eg a religious faith); to include. • n the act of embracing, a hug.—**embraceable** adj.—**embracement** n.

embracer /-ər/ n one who embraces; (law) one who attempts to influence a jury corruptly.

embracery /ɛm'breɪsəri/ n (law) the act of attempting to corrupt or influence a jury.

embranchment /ɛm'bræntʃmənt/ n the act of branching out.

embrasure /ɛm'breɪʒər/ or /ɪm-/ n an opening in a wall or parapet from which to fire guns; a window or door having its sides slanted on the inside.

embrocate /'ɛmbroˌkeɪt/ vt to rub a diseased or injured part of the body with a lotion.

embrocation /ˌɛmbro'keɪʃən/ n a liniment for applying to, or rubbing, an injured part of the body.

embroider /ɛm'brɔɪdər/ or /ɪm-/ vt to ornament with decorative stitches; to embellish (eg a story).—**embroiderer** n

embroidery /-dri/ n (pl **embroideries**) decorative needlework; elaboration or exaggeration (of a story, etc).

embroil /ɛm'brɔɪl/ or /ɪm-/ vt to involve (a person) in a conflict, argument, or problem.—**embroiler** n.—**embroilment** n.

embryo /'ɛmˌbrio:/ n (pl **embryos**) an animal during the period of its growth from a fertilized egg up to the third month; a human product of conception up to about the second month of growth; a thing in a rudimentary state.—**embryoid** adj.

embryology /ˌɛmbri'ɒlədʒi/ n the scientific study of embryos.—**embryological, embryologic** adj.—**embryologist** n.

embryonic /ˌɛmbri'ɒnɪk/, **embryonal** /-'ɒnəl/ adj immature, existing at an early stage.—**embryonically** adv.

emend /i'mɛnd/ or /ɪ-/ vt to correct mistakes in written material.—**emendable** adj.—**emendation** n.

emerald /'ɛmərəld/ n a rich green gemstone; its colour.

emerge /i'mɜrdʒ/ or /ɪ-/ vi to appear up out of, to come into view; to be revealed as the result of investigation; n ✱ (Cdn) (inf) a section of a hospital that handles emergencies.—**emergence** n.—**emergent** adj.

emergency /i'mɜrdʒənsi/ or /ɪ-/ n (pl **emergencies**) an unforeseen situation demanding immediate action; a serious medical condition requiring instant treatment.

emergicentre /ɪˌmɜrdʒi'sɛntər/ n walk-in facility for minor ailments and injuries often located in shopping malls or along highways.

emeritus /i'mɛrɪtəs/ adj retired but still holding one's title or rank.—also n.

emersed /i'mɜrst/ adj (bot) rising out of water.

emersion /i'mɜrʃən/ n the act of emerging.

emery /'ɛmɔri/ n a hard granular mineral used for grinding and polishing; a hard abrasive powder.

emery board n a nailfile made from cardboard covered with powdered emery.

emery paper n a stiff paper covered with powdered emery.

emetic /i'mɛtɪk/ n a medicine that induces vomiting.—also adj.—**emetically** adv.

emf, EMF abbr = electromotive force.

emigrant /'ɛmɪgrənt/ n a person who emigrates.

emigrate /'ɛmɪˌgreɪt/ vi to leave one's country for residence in another.—**emigration** n.

émigré /'ɛmɪˌgreɪ/ n an emigrant, usually someone forced to emigrate.

eminence /'ɛmɪnəns/, **eminency** /-i/ n (pl **eminences, eminencies**) high rank or position; a person of high rank or attainments; (with cap) the title for a cardinal of the RC Church; a raised piece of ground, a high place.

eminent /'ɛmɪnənt/ adj famous; conspicuous; distinguished.—**eminently** adv.

emir /ɛ'mɪr/ n a ruler in parts of Africa and Asia.

emirate /'ɛmərət/ or /-ˌreɪt/ n the territory governed by an emir.

emissary /'ɛmɪˌsɛri/ n (pl **emissaries**) a person sent on a mission on behalf of another, esp a government.

emit /i'mɪt/ or /i-/ vt (**emitting, emitted**) to send out (light, heat, etc); to put into circulation; to express, to utter.—**emission** n.—**emissive** adj.—**emitter** n.

Emmenthal(er), Emmental /'ɛmənˌtɒl/ n a hard Swiss cheese with lots of holes.

emmet /'ɛmɪt/ n (dial) an ant.

emollient /i'mɒliənt/ or /i-/ adj softening and soothing, esp the skin. • n a preparation used for skin care.—**emollience** n.

emolument /i'mɒljumənt/ or /ɛ-/ n a fee received, salary.

emote /i'mo:t/ or /i-/ vi to display emotion theatrically.

emoticon n (comput) an icon representing emotion made up of standard keyboard characters.

emotion /i'mo:ʃən/ or /i-/ n a strong feeling of any kind.

emotional /-əl/ adj of emotion; inclined to express excessive emotion.—**emotionality** n.—**emotionally** adv.—**emotionalism** n.

emotive /i'mo:tɪv/ adj characterized by or arousing emotion.—**emotiveness, emotivity** n.

empale /ɛm'peɪl/ see **impale**.

empanel /ɛm'pænəl/ or /m-/ vt (**empanelling, empanelled** or **empaneling, empaneled**) (law) to enrol (for a jury); to enter on a jury list.—also **impanel**.

empathize /'ɛmpəˌθaɪz/ vi to treat with or feel empathy.

empathy /'ɛmpəθi/ n the capacity for participating in and understanding the feelings or ideas of another.—**empathic, empathetic** adj.

emperor /'ɛmpərər/ n the sovereign ruler over an empire.—**emperorship** n.

emperor penguin n an Antarctic penguin, the largest species known.

empery /'ɛmpəri/ n (pl **emperies**) (arch) power, dominion.

emphasis /'ɛmfəsɪs/ n (pl **emphases**) particular stress or prominence given to something; force or vigour of expression; clarity of form or outline.

emphasize /'ɛmfəˌsaɪz/ vt to place stress on.

emphatic /ɛm'fætɪk/ or /ɪm-/ adj spoken, done or marked with emphasis; forceful, decisive.—**emphatically** adv.—**emphaticalness** n.

emphysema /ˌɛmfɪ'ziːmə/ or /-'siː-/ n a medical condition marked by the distension of the air sacs in the lungs, causing breathlessness.—**emphysematous** adj.

empire /'ɛmpaɪr/ n a large state or group of states under a single sovereign, usu an emperor; nations governed by a single sovereign state; a large and complex business organization.

empiric /ɛm'pɪrɪk/ or /ɪm-/ adj empirical. • n an empirical worker; a quack.

empirical /-əl/ adj based on observation, experiment or experience only, not theoretical.—**empirically** adv.—**empiricalness** n.

empiricism /ɛm'pɪrɪˌsɪzəm/ or /ɪm-/ n (philos) the theory that experience is the only source of knowledge; the use of empirical methods.—**empiricist** n.

emplacement /ɛm'pleɪsmənt/ or /ɪm-/ n a position prepared for a gun or artillery.

emplane /ɛm'pleɪn/ vti to put on board a plane; to board a plane.

employ /ɛmˈplɔɪ/ or /ɪm-/ vt to give work and pay to; to make use of.—**employable** adj.

employee /-i/ n a person who is hired by another person for wages.

employer /-ər/ n a person, business, etc that employs people.

employment /-mənt/ n an employing; a being employed; occupation or profession.

empoison /ɛmˈpɔɪzən/ vt to taint, corrupt.

emporium /ɛmˈpɔːrɪəm/ or /ɪm-/ n (pl **emporiums, emporia**) a large shop carrying many different items.

empower /ɛmˈpaʊər/ or /ɪm-/ vt to give official authority to.—**empowerment** n.

empress /ˈɛmprəs/ n the female ruler of an empire; the wife or widow of an emperor.

empty /ˈɛmptɪ/ or /ˈɛmti/ adj (**emptier, emptiest**) containing nothing; not occupied; lacking reality, substance, or value; hungry. • vb (**emptying, emptied**) vt to make empty; to transfer or discharge (the contents of something) by emptying. • vi to become empty; to discharge contents. • n (pl **empties**) empty containers or bottles.—**emptily** adv.—**emptiness** n.

empty-handed /-ˌhændəd/ adj with nothing in one's hands; without gain.

empty-headed /-ˌhɛdəd/ adj scatterbrained.

empyema /ˌɛmpaɪˈiːmə/ or /ˌɛmpi-/ n (pl **empyemata**) a collection of pus, esp in the chest.—**empyemic** adj.

empyrean /ɛmˈpaɪˈriːən/ or /ˌɛmpɪ-/, /ˌɛmpiːˈriən/ n (arch) the highest heaven. • adj pertaining to the highest heaven; celestial.

EMS abbr = European Monetary System.

EMU abbr = European Monetary Union.

emu /ˈiːmjuː/ n a fast-running Australian bird, related to the ostrich.

emulate /ˈɛmjʊˌleɪt/ vt to try to equal or do better than; to imitate; to rival or compete.—**emulation** n.—**emulative** adj.—**emulator** n.

emulous /ˈɛmjʊləs/ adj wanting to excel; competitive.

emulsify /ɪˈmʌlsəˌfaɪ/ vti (**emulsifying, emulsified**) to make or become an emulsion.—**emulsification** n.—**emusifier** n.

emulsion /ɪˌmʌlʃən/ n a mixture of mutually insoluble liquids in which one is dispersed in droplets throughout the other; a light-sensitive substance on photographic paper or film.—**emulsive** adj.

emunctory /ɪˈmʌŋktərɪ/ n (pl **emunctories**) (anat) an excretory duct or canal. • adj excretory.

en /ɛn/ or /ɪn/ n (print) a measure of width, equal to half an em.

enable /ɪˈneɪbəl/ or /ɛ-/ vt to give the authority or means to do something; to make easy or possible.—**enabler** n.

enact /ɪˈnækt/ or /ɛ-/ vt to make into law; to act (a play, etc).—**enactive** adj.—**enactment** n.—**enactor** n.—**enactory** adj.

enamel /ɪˈnæməl/ n a glass-like substance used to coat the surface of metal or pottery; the hard outer layer of a tooth; a usu glossy paint that forms a hard coat. • vt (**enamelling, enamelled** or **enameling, enameled**) to cover or decorate with enamel.—**enameller, enameler, enamellist, enamelist** n.—**enamelwork** n.

enamour, enamor /ɪˈnæmər/ or /ɛ-/ vt to inspire with love.—**enamoured, enamored** adj.

enarthrosis /ˌɛnɑrˈθrəʊsɪs/ n (pl **enarthroses**) (anat) a ball-and-socket joint.

en bloc /ɑ̃ˈblɒk/ adv in a mass.

encage /ɛnˈkeɪdʒ/ vt to shut up in, or as in, a cage.

encamp /ɛnˈkæmp/ vt to place or stay in a camp.—**encampment** n.

encapsulate /ɛnˈkæpsʊˌleɪt/ vt to enclose or be enclosed in, as a capsule; to summarize.—**encapsulation** n.

encase /ɛnˈkeɪs/ vt to enclose (as if) in a case.—**encasement** n.

encaustic /ɛnˈkɒstɪk/ adj (ceramics) with colours burned in. • n the art of painting in melted wax; a piece of work done by this method.

enceinte /ɛnˈsænt/, Fr. /ɑ̃ˈsæ̃t/ adj pregnant.

encephalic /ˌɛnsəˈfælɪk/ or /ˌɛnk-/ adj of the brain.

encephalitis /ɛnˌsefəˈlaɪtɪs/ or /ˌɛnkɛf-/ n inflammation of the brain.—**encephalitic** adj.

encephalogram /ɛnˈsefələˌgræm/ or /ɛnˈkɛf-/ n an electroencephalogram.—**encephalograph** n.

enchain /ɛnˈtʃeɪn/ vt to hold fast with, or as with, a chain.—**enchainment** n.

enchant /ɛnˈtʃænt/ vt to bewitch, to delight.—**enchanter** n.—**enchantment** n.—**enchantress** nf.

enchase /ɛnˈtʃeɪs/ vt to engrave, to emboss.

encircle /ɛnˈsɜrkəl/ vt to surround; to move or pass completely round.—**encirclement** n.

enclasp /ɪnˈklæsp/ or /ɛn-/ vt to clasp.

enclave /ˈɒnkleɪv/ or /ˈɛn-/ n an area of a country's territory entirely surrounded by foreign territory.

enclitic /ɛnˈklɪtɪk/ adj (linguistics) attached to the preceding word and treated as a suffix, eg "thee" in "prithee". • n an enclitic word.—**enclitically** adv.

enclose /ɪnˈkloːz/ or /ɛn-/ vt to shut up or in; to put in a wrapper or parcel, usu together with a letter.—**enclosable** adj.—**encloser** n.

enclosure /ɪnˈkloːʒər/ or /ˈɛn-/ n an enclosing; an enclosed area; something enclosed with a letter, in a parcel, etc.

encomiast /ɛnˈkoːmiˌæst/ n a composer of an encomium.—**encomiastic** adj.

encomium /ɛnˈkoːmiəm/ n (pl **encomiums, encomia**) a usu formal expression of high praise in speech or writing.

encompass /ɛnˈkʌmpəs/ or /ɪn-/ vt to encircle or enclose; to include.—**encompassment** n.

encore /ˈɒŋkɔr/ or /ˈɒn-/ interj once more! • n a call for the repetition of a performance.—also vt.

encounter /ɛnˈkaʊntər/ vt to meet, esp unexpectedly; to fight, engage in battle with; to be faced with (problems, etc). • n a meeting; a conflict, battle.

encourage /ɪnˈkʌrədʒ/ or /ɛn-/ vt to inspire with confidence or hope; to urge, incite; to promote the development of.—**encouragement** n.—**encourager** n.—**encouragingly** adv.

encroach /ɪnˈkroːtʃ/ or /ɛn-/ vi to infringe another's territory, rights, etc; to advance beyond an established limit.—**encroacher** n.—**encroachingly** adv.—**encroachment** n.

encrust /ɛnˈkrʌst/ vt to cover with a hard crust; to form a crust on the surface of; to decorate a surface with jewels.—**encrustation** n.

encumber /ɛnˈkʌmbər/ or /ɪn-/ vt to weigh down; to hinder the function or activity of.—**encumberingly** adv.

encumbrance /ɛnˈkʌmbrəns/ or /ɪn-/ n something that is a hindrance or burden.

encumbrancer /-ər/ n a person who has a legal claim on an estate.

encyclical /ɛnˈsɪklɪkəl/ adj circulated widely.—also **encyclic**. • n a letter addressed by the pope to all Roman Catholic bishops.

encyclopedia, encyclopaedia /ɛnˌsʌɪkləˈpiːdɪə/ or /ɪn-/, /ən-/ n a book or series of books containing information on all branches of knowledge, or treating comprehensively a particular branch of knowledge, usu in alphabetical order.

encyclopedic, encyclopaedic /-ˈpiːdɪk/ adj comprehensive.—**encyclopedically, encyclopaedically** adv.

encyclopedist, encyclopaedist /-ɪst/ n a compiler of an encyclopedia.

encyst /ɪnˈsɪst/ or /ɛn-/, /ən-/ vti (biol) to enclose, or become enclosed in, a cyst or vesicle.—**encystment** n.

end /ɛnd/ n the last part; the place where a thing stops; purpose; result, outcome. • vt to bring to an end; to destroy. • vi to come to an end; to result (in). • adj final; ultimate.

end-, endo- /ɛndoː/ or /-də/ prefix within.

endanger /ɪnˈdeɪndʒər/ or /ɛn-/, /ən-/ vt to put in danger.—**endangerment** n.

endear /ɪnˈdiːr/ or /ɛn-/, /ən-/ vt to make loved or more loved.—**endearing** adj.—**endearingly** adv.

endearment /-mənt/ n something that endears; a word or words of affection.

endeavour, endeavor /ɪnˈdɛvər/ or /ɛn-/, /ən-/ vi to try or attempt (to). • n an attempt.

endemic /ɛnˈdɛmɪk/ adj (disease) locally prevalent; (plant) peculiar to a locality. • n an endemic disease; an endemic plant.—**endemicity** n.—**endemically** adv.

ending /-ɪŋ/ n reaching or coming to an end; the final part.

endive /ˈɛndaɪv/ n an annual or biennial herb widely cultivated as a salad plant; a variety of chicory used in salads.

endless /ˈɛndləs/ adj unending; uninterrupted; extremely numerous.—**endlessly** adv.—**endlessness** n.

endo-, end- /ˈɛndoː/ prefix within.

endocarditis /ˌɛndoːkɑrˈdəʊtɪs/ n inflammation of the endocardium.—**endocarditic** adj.

endocardium /ˌɛndoːˈkɑrdɪəm/ n (pl **endocardia**) the membrane lining the heart cavities.

endocarp /ˈɛndoːˌkɑrp/ n the inner coat or shell of a fruit.—**endocarpal, endocarpic** adj.

endocrine /'endo:ˌkraɪn/ or /-ˌkrɪn/ adj secreting internally, specifically producing secretions that are distributed in the body by the bloodstream.—*also* **endocrinal.** • = an endocrine gland.

endocrine gland n a gland that secretes hormones directly into the bloodstream, *eg* the pituitary and thyroid.

endocrinology /ˌendo:krɪ'nɒlədʒɪ/ n the scientific study of endocrine glands and hormones.—**endocrinologic, endocrinological** adj.—**endocrinologist** n.

endoderm /'endo:ˌdərm/ n the inner layer of embryonic cells in an egg from which an organism is formed.—*also* **entoblast, entoderm.**—**endodermal, endodermic, entodermal, entodermic** adj.

endogamy /en'dɒgəmɪ/ n the practice of marrying only within the same tribe.—**endogamous** adj.

endogenous /en'dɒdʒɪnəs/ adj growing from or on the inside.—**endogeny** n.

endomorph /'endo:ˌmorf/ n a mineral enclosed within another mineral; a person with a heavily built physique.—**endomorphic** adj.—**endomorphy** n.

endomorphism /-'morfɪzəm/ n (*gecl*) metamorphosis of molten rock within older rock.

endoparasite /ˌendo:'pærəˌsaɪt/ n an internal parasite.—**endoparasitic** adj.

endoplasm /'endo:ˌplæzəm/ n (*biol*) the inner layer of protoplasm.

endorsation /ɪnˌdɔr'seɪʃən/ n ✦ (*Cdn*) endorsement.

endorse /ɪn'dɔrs/ or /en-/, /ən-/ vt to write one's name, comment, etc on the back of to approve; to record an offence on a driving licence; to support.—**endorsable** adj.—**endorsee** n.—**endorsement** n.—**endorser** n.

endoscope /'endo:ˌskoːp/ n a medical instrument for examining the interior of the body.—**endoscopic** adj.—**endoscopist** n.—**endoscopy** n.

endosmosis /ˌendɒs'moːsɪs/ n (*biol*) osmosis inwards through the porous membrane of a cell, etc, by a surrounding liquid.

endosperm /'endo:ˌspərm/ n the albumen of a seed.—**endospermic** adj.

endothelium /ˌendo:'θiːlɪəm/ n (*pl* **endothelia**) (*anat*) a tissue which lines blood vessels.

endow /ɪn'dau/ or /en-/, /ən-/ vt to give money or property to provide an income for; to provide with a special power or attribute.—**endower** n.

endowment /-mənt/ n an endowing: an income, etc settled on an individual or organization; a natural quality or gift.

endpaper /'endˌpeɪpər/ n either of two folded sheets of paper pasted against the inside covers of a book and attached to the first and last pages.

end product n the final result of a manufacturing or other process.

endue /ɪn'djuː/ or /en-/, /ən-/ vt (**enduing, endued**) to provide with a quality or power.—*also* **indue.**

endurance /ɪn'dʊrəns/ or /en-/, /ən-/ n the ability to withstand pain, hardship, strain, etc.

endure /ɪn'djʊr/ or /en-/, /ən-/, /-'djər/, /-dər/ vt to undergo, tolerate (hardship, etc) *esp* with patience. • vi to continue in existence, to last out.—**endurable** adj.—**endurability** n.—**endurably** adv.

enduring /-ɪŋ/ adj lasting, permanent.—**enduringly** adv.

endways /'endˌweɪz/ adv on end, with the end foremost.

enema /'enɪmə/ n (*pl* **enemas, enemata**) the injection of a liquid into the rectum to void the bowels; the liquid injected.

enemy /'enəmɪ/ n (*pl* **enemies**) a person who hates or dislikes and wishes to harm another; a military opponent; something harmful or deadly.

energetic /ˌenər'dʒetɪk/ adj lively, active; done with energy.—**energetically** adv.

energetics /-ɪks/ n sing the science of energy.

energize /'enərdʒaɪz/ vt to fill with energy; to invigorate; to apply an electric current to.—**energizer** n.

energy /'enərdʒɪ/ n (*pl* **energies**) capacity of acting or being active; vigour, power; (*physics*) capacity to do work.

enervate /'enərˌveɪt/ vt to lessen the strength or vigour of; to enfeeble in mind and body.—**enervation** n.—**enervative** adj.—**enervator** n.

enface /en'feɪs/ or /ɪn-/ vt to write or stamp on the face of a document.

enfant terrible /ˌɑ̃fɑ̃te'riːbl/ n (*pl* **enfants terribles**) a person who makes awkward remarks.

enfeeble /ɪn'fiːbəl/ or /en-/, /ən-/ vt to make feeble.—**enfeeblement** n.—**enfeebler** n.

enfeoff /en'fef/ or /-'fiːf/ vt (*law*) to give a freehold property to; to convey.—**enfeoffment** n.

enfilade /ˌenfɪ'leɪd/ n gunfire directed (at troops, etc) in a line from end to end.—*also* vt.

enfold /ɪn'foːld/ or /en-/, /ən-/ vt to wrap up; to hug in the arms.—**enfolder** n.—**enfoldment** n.

enforce /en'fɔrs/ or /ɪn-/, /ən-/ vt to compel obedience by threat; to execute with vigour.—**enforceable** adj.—**enforcement** n.—**enforcer** n.

enfranchise /en'fræntʃaɪz/ or /ɪn-/ vt to admit to citizenship; to grant the vote to.—**enfranchisement** n.—**enfranchiser** n.

engage /ɪn'geɪdʒ/ or /en-/, /ən-/ vt to pledge as security; to promise to marry; to keep busy; to hire; to attract and hold, *esp* attention or sympathy; to cause to participate; to bring or enter into conflict; to begin or take part in a venture; to connect or interlock, to mesh.—**engager** n.

engaged /ɪn geɪdʒd/ or /en-/, /ən-/ adj entered into a promise to marry; reserved, occupied or busy.

engagement /ɪn'geɪdʒmənt/ or /en-/, /ən-/ n the act or state of being engaged; a pledge: an appointment agreed with another person; employment; a battle.

engaging /-ɪŋ/ adj pleasing, attractive.—**engagingly** adv.—**engagingness** n.

engender /ɪn'dʒendər/ or /en-/, /ən-/ vt to bring into existence.—**engenderment** n.

engine /'endʒɪn/ n a machine by which physical power is applied to produce a physical effect; a locomotive; (*formerly*) a mechanical device, such as a large catapult, used in war.

engineer /ˌendʒɪ'nɪr/ n a person trained in engineering; a person who operates an engine, etc; a member of a military group devoted to engineering work; a designer or builder of engines. • vt to contrive, plan, *esp* deviously.

engineering /-ɪŋ/ n the art or practice of constructing and using machinery; the art and science by which natural forces and materials are utilized in structures or machines.

English /'ɪŋglɪʃ/ adj of, relating to, or characteristic of England, the English people, or the English language. • n the language of the English people, the US and many areas formerly under British control; English language and literature as a subject of study.

engorge /ɪn'gɔrdʒ/ or /en-/, /ən-/ vt to congest with blood; to consume (food) greedily.—**engorgement** n.

engrained /ɪn'greɪnd/ or /en-/, /ən-/ *see* **ingrained.**

engrave /ɪn'greɪv/ or /en-/, /ən-/ vt to produce by cutting or carving a surface; to cut to produce a representation that may be printed from; to lodge deeply (in the mind, etc).—**engraver** n.

engraving /-ɪŋ/ n a print made from an engraved surface.

engross /ɪn'groːs/ or /en-/, /ən-/ vt to occupy (the attention) fully; to copy in large handwriting; to prepare the final text of.—**engrossing** adj.—**engrossment** n.

engulf /ɪn'gʌlf/ or /en-/, /ər-/ vt to flow over and enclose; to overwhelm.—**engulfment** n.

enhance /ɪn'hæns/ or /en-/, /ən-/ vt to increase in value, importance, attractiveness, etc; to heighten.—**enhancement** n.—**enhancer** n.

enigma /ɪ'nɪgmə/ or /ɛ-/, /ə-/ n someone or something that is puzzling or mysterious.—**enigmatic, enigmatical** adj.—**enigmatically** adv.

enjoin /ɪn'dʒɔɪn/ or /en-/, /ən-/ vt to command, order someone with authority; to forbid to prohibit.—**enjoiner** n.—**enjoinment** n.

enjoy /ɪn'dʒɔɪ/ or /en-/, /ən-/ vt to get pleasure from, take joy in; to use or have the advantage of; to experience.—**enjoyment** n.

enjoyable /-əbəl/ adj giving enjoyment.—**enjoyably** adv.

enkindle /ɪn'kɪndəl/ or /en-/, /ən-/ vt to set on fire; (*fig*) to inflame.

enlace /ɪn'leɪs/ or /en-/, /ər-/ vt to entwine; to enfold.—**enlacement** n.

enlarge /ɪn'lɑrdʒ/ or /en-/, /ən-/ vti to make or grow larger; to reproduce (a photograph) in a larger form; to speak or write at length (on).

enlargement /-mənt/ n an act, instance, or state of enlarging; a photograph, etc that has been enlarged.

enlarger /-ər/ n a device for making photographic enlargements.

enlighten /ɪn'laɪtən/ or /en-/, /ən-/ vt to instruct; to inform.—**enlightening** adj.—**enlightenment** n.

enlightened /-'laɪtənd/ adj well-informed, tolerant, unprejudiced.

enlist /ɪnˈlɪst/ or /ɛn-/, /ən-/ vt to engage for service in the armed forces; to secure the aid or support of. • vi to register oneself for the armed services.—**enlistee** n.—**enlistment** n.

enliven /ɪnˈlaɪvən/ or /ɛn-/, /ən-/ vt to make more lively or cheerful.—**enlivening** adj.—**enlivenment** n.

en masse /ãˈmæs/ adv all together; in a large group.

enmesh /ɪnˈmɛʃ/ or /ɛn-/, /ən-/ vt to catch in a net; to entangle.—also **inmesh, immesh**.

enmity /ˈɛnmɪti/ n (pl **enmities**) hostility, esp mutual hatred.

ennage /ɛˈneɪdʒ/ n (print) the number of ens in a text.

ennea- /ˈɛnɪə/ prefix nine.

ennead /ˈɛnɪˌæd/ n a set of nine.—**enneadic** adj.

enneagon /ˈɛnɪəˌgɒn/ n a plane figure with nine sides and nine angles.

ennoble /ɪˈnoːbəl/ or /ɛn-/, /ən-/ vt to make noble, dignify; to raise (a person) to a rank of nobility.—**ennoblement** n.—**ennobler** n.

ennui /ˈɒnwiː/ n boredom, apathy.

enology /ɪˈnɒlədʒi/ see **oenology**.

enormity /ɪˈnɔːrmɪti/ n (pl **enormities**) great wickedness; a serious crime; huge size, magnitude.

enormous /ɪˈnɔːrməs/ adj extremely large.—**enormously** adv.

enough /ɪˈnʌf/ or /iː-/, /ɛ-/, /ə-/ adj adequate, sufficient. • adv so as to be sufficient; very; quite. • n a sufficiency. • interj stop!

enounce /ɪˈnaʊns/ vt to proclaim, to enunciate.

en passant /ˌãpæˈsã/ adv in passing.

enquire, enquirer see **inquire**.

enquiry see **inquiry**.

enrage /ɪnˈreɪdʒ/ or /ɛn-/, /ən-/ vt to fill with anger.—**enraged** adj.—**enragement** n.

enrapture /ɪnˈræptʃər/ or /ɛn-/, /ən-/ vt to fill with pleasure or delight.

enrich /ɪnˈrɪtʃ/ or /ɛn-/, /ən-/ vt to make rich or richer; to ornament; to improve in quality by adding to.—**enricher** n.—**enrichment** n.

enrol, enroll /ɪnˈroːl/ or /ɛn-/, /ən-/ vti (**enrols** or **enrolls, enrolling, enrolled**) to enter or register on a roll or list; to become a member of a society, club, etc; to admit as a member.—**enrollee** n.—**enroller** n.—**enrolment, enrollment** n.

en route /ãˈruːt/ adv along or on the way.

ensanguine /ɛnˈsæŋgwɪn/ vt to smear or cover with blood.

ensconce /ɪnˈskɒns/ or /ɛn-/, /ən-/ vt to establish in a safe, secure or comfortable place.

ensemble /ɒnˈsɒmbəl/ n something regarded as a whole; the general effect; the performance of the full number of musicians, dancers, etc; a complete harmonious costume.

enshrine /ɪnˈʃraɪn/ or /ɛn-/, /ən-/ vt to enclose (as if) in a shrine; to cherish as sacred.—also **inshrine**.—**enshrinement** n.

enshroud /ɪnˈʃraʊd/ or /ɛn-/, /ən-/ vt to cover with, or as with, a shroud.

ensiform /ˈɛnsɪˌfɔːrm/ adj sword-shaped.

ensign /ˈɛnsaɪn/ or /-sən/ n a flag; the lowest commissioned officer in the US Navy.

ensilage /ˈɛnsɪlɪdʒ/ or /ˈɪn-/ n storage in a pit or silo; silage.

ensile /ɪnˈsaɪl/ or /ɛn-/ vt to store in a silo.—**ensilability** n.

enslave /ɪnˈsleɪv/ or /ɛn-/ vt to make into a slave; to subjugate.—**enslavement** n.—**enslaver** n.

ensnare /ɪnˈsnɛr/ or /ɛn-/, /ən-/ vt to trap in, or as in, a snare.—**ensnarement** n.

ensue /ɪnˈsuː/ or /ɪnˈsjuː/, /ɛn-/, /ən-/ vi (**ensuing, ensued**) to occur as a consequence or in time.—**ensuing** adj.

en suite /ãˈswiːt/ adv, adj in a single unit.

ensure /ɪnˈʃʊr/ or /ɛn-/, /ən-/ vt to make certain, sure, or safe.—**ensurer** n.

enswathe /ɪnˈswɒθ/, or /ɛn-/, /ən-/ vt to wrap, swathe.

ENT /ˈiːˈɛnˈtiː/ abbr = ear, nose, and throat.

entablature /ɪnˈtæblətʃər/ or /ɛn-/ n the part of a building resting on top of columns.

entablement /ɪnˈteɪbəlmənt/ or /ɛn-/ n a platform for a statue, above the dado and base.

entail /ɪnˈteɪl/ or /ɛn-/, /ən-/ vt to involve, necessitate as a result; to restrict the inheritance of property to a designated line of heirs. • n the act of entailing or the estate entailed.—**entailer** n.—**entailment** n.

entangle /ɪnˈtæŋgəl/ or /ɛn-/, /ən-/ vt to tangle, complicate; to involve in a tangle or complications.—**entanglement** n.—**entangler** n.

entelechy /ɛnˈtɛləki/ or /ɪn-/ n (pl **entelechies**) (philos) actuality.

entente (cordiale) Fr. /ãˌtãtkɔːrdiˈæl/ n a friendly understanding or relationship between two or more countries.

enter /ˈɛntər/ vi to go or come in or into; to come on stage; to begin, start; (with **for**) to register as an entrant. • vt to come or go into; to pierce, penetrate; (an organization) to join; to insert; (proposal, etc) to submit; to record (an item) in a diary, etc.—**enterable** adj.—**enterer** n.

enteric /ɛnˈtɛrɪk/, **enteral** /-rəl/ adj intestinal.—**enterally** adv.

enteritis /ɛntəˈraɪtɪs/ n inflammation of the intestines, usu causing diarrhoea.

enteron /ˌɛntəˈrɒn/ (pl **entera**) the alimentary canal.

enterotomy /ˌɛntəˈrɒtəmi/ n (pl **enterotomies**) dissection of, or an incision into, the bowels.

enterprise /ˈɛntərˌpraɪz/ n a difficult or challenging undertaking; a business project; readiness to engage in new ventures.—**enterpriser** n.

enterprising /-ɪŋ/ adj adventurous, energetic and progressive.—**enterprisingly** adv.

entertain /ˌɛntərˈteɪn/ vt to show hospitality to; to amuse, please (a person or audience); to have in mind; to consider.

entertainer /-ər/ n a person who entertains in public, esp professionally.

entertaining /-ɪŋ/ adj amusing; diverting.—**entertainingly** adv.

entertainment /-mənt/ n entertaining; amusement; an act or show intended to amuse and interest an audience, etc.

enthral, enthrall /ɪnˈθrɒl/ or /ɛn-/, /ən-/ vt (**enthrals** or **enthralls, enthralling, enthralled**) to captivate.—**enthralment, enthrallment** n.

enthrone /ɪnˈθroːn/ or /ɛn-/, /ən-/ vt to install ceremonially, as a monarch or bishop.—**enthronement** n.

enthuse /ɪnˈθuːz/ or /-ˈθjuːz/, /ɛn-/, /ən-/ vti to fill with or express enthusiasm.

enthusiasm /ɪnθuːziˌæzəm/ or /-ˈθjuːz-/, /ɛn-/, /ən-/ n intense interest or liking; something that arouses keen interest.

enthusiast /ɪnθuːziˌæst/ or /-ˈθjuːz-/, /ɛn-/, /ən-/, /-ɪəst/ n a person filled with enthusiasm for something.

enthusiastic /-ɪk/ adj filled with enthusiasm.—**enthusiastically** adv.

enthymeme /ˈɛnθɪˌmiːm/ n (logic) a syllogism in which one premise is suppressed.

entice /ɪnˈtaɪs/ or /ɛn-/, /ən-/ vt to attract by offering some pleasure or reward.—**enticement** n.—**enticer** n.—**enticing** adj.

entire /ɪnˈtaɪr/ or /ɛn-/, /ən-/ adj whole; complete.—**entireness** n.

entirely /-li/ adv fully; completely.

entirety /-əti/ or /-ti/ n (pl **entireties**) completeness; the total.

entitle /ɪnˈtaɪtəl/ or /ɛn-/, /ən-/ vt to give a title to; to give a right (to).—**entitlement** n.

entity /ˈɛntɪti/ n (pl **entities**) existence, being; something that has a separate existence.

entoblast /ɛntoˈblæst/, **entoderm** /-dɛrm/ see **endoderm**.

entomb /ɪntuːm/ or /ɛn-/, /ən-/ vt to place in, or as in, a tomb.—**entombment** n.

entomic /ɛnˈtɒmɪk/ adj of insects.

entomo-, entom- /ˈɛntəmoː/ prefix insect.

entomology /ˌɛntəˈmɒlədʒi/ n the branch of zoology that deals with insects.—**entomological, entomologic** adj.—**entomologist** n.

entomophagous /ˌɛntəˈmɒfəgəs/ adj insect-eating.

entomophilous /-fələs/ adj fertilized by insects.

entopic /ɛnˈtɒpɪk/ adj (anat) in a normal position.

entourage /ˌɒntʊˈrɒʒ/ n a retinue, group of attendants.

entozoic /ˌɛntəˈzoɪk/ adj living within an animal.

entozoan /ˌɛntəˈzoːən/ n (pl **entozoa**) a parasite which lives inside an animal.

entr'acte /ˈɒntrækt/ n a light entertainment, a ballet, etc, as an interlude between the acts of a play or opera.

entrails /ˈɛntreɪlz/ npl the insides of the body, the intestines.

entrain /ɪnˈtreɪn/ or /ɛn-/, /ən-/ vti to put or get onto a train.

entrance¹ /ˈɛntrəns/ n the act of entering; the power or authority to enter; a means of entering; an admission fee.

entrance² /ɪnˈtræns/ vt to put into a trance; to fill with great delight.—**entrancement** n.—**entrancing** adj.

entrant /ˈɛntrənt/ n a person who enters (eg a competition, profession).

entrap /ɪntræp/ or /ɛn-/, /ən-/ vt (**entrapping, entrapped**) to catch, as if in a trap; to lure into a compromising or incriminatory situation.—**entrapment** n.—**entrapper** n.

entreat /ɪn'triːt/ or /ɛn-/, /ən-/ vt to request earnestly; to implore, beg.—**entreaty** n (pl **entreaties**).

entrecôte /'ɒntrəˌkoːt/ n a boned cut of beef from between the ribs.

entrée, entree /'ɒntreɪ/ or /'ɑ̃treɪ/ n a dish served before the main meal; in US, the principal dish of a meal; the right or power of admission.

entremets Fr. /ˌɒntrə'meɪ/ n (pl **entremets**) a dessert.

entrench /ɪn'trɛntʃ/ or /ɛn-/, /ən-/ vt to dig a trench as a defensive perimeter; to establish (oneself) in a strong defensive position.—**entrencher** n.—**entrenchment** n.

entrepôt /'ɒntrəˌpoː/ n an intermediate centre of trade and transhipment.

entrepreneur /ˌɒntrəprə'nər/ n a person who takes the commercial risk of starting up and running a business enterprise.—**entrepreneurial** adj.—**entrepreneurship** n.

entresol /'ɒntrəˌsɒl/ n a floor between the ground and first floor, a mezzanine.

entropy /'ɛntrəpi/ n (pl **entropies**) a measure of the unavailable energy in a closed thermodynamic system; disorder, disorganization.

entrust /ɪn'trʌst/ or /ɛn-/, /ən-/ vt (usu with **with**) to confer as a responsibility, duty, etc; (usu with **to**) to place something in another's care.—**entrustment** n.

entry /'ɛntri/ n (pl **entries**) the act of entering a place of entrance; an item recorded in a diary, journal, etc; a person or thing taking part in a contest.

entwine /ɪn'twaɪn/ or /ɛn-/, /ən-/ vt to twine together or around.—**entwinement** n.

enucleate /ɪ'njuːkliˌeɪt/ or /ɪ'nuːk-/ vt to remove the nucleus from.

E number n a series of numbers with the prefix **E** used to identify food additives within the European Union.

enumerate /ɪ'njuːməˌreɪt/ or /ɪ'nuː-/ vt to count; to list.—**enumeration** n.—**enumerator** n.

enunciate /ɪ'nʌnsiˌeɪt/ vt to state definitely; to pronounce clearly.—**enunciation** n.—**enunciator** n.—**enunciative** adj.

enure /ɪ'njʊr/ see **inure**.

enuresis /ˌɛnjʊ'riːsɪs/ n urinary incontinence; bedwetting.—**enuretic** adj.

envelop /ɪn'vɛləp/ vt to enclose completely (as it) with a covering.—**envelopment** n.

envelope /'ɛnvəˌloːp/ or /'ɒn-/ n something used to wrap or cover, esp a gummed paper container for a letter; the bag containing the gas in a balloon or airship.

envenom /ɪn'vɛnəm/ or /ɛn-/, /ən-/ vt to put poison into; (fig) to embitter.

enviable /'ɛnviəbəl/ adj causing envy; fortunate.—**enviably** adv.

envious /'ɛnviəs/ adj filled with envy.—**enviously** adv.

environ /ɪn'vaɪrən/ or /ɛn-/, /ən-/ vt to surround or enclose.

environment /-mənt/ n external conditions and surroundings, esp those that affect the quality of life of plants, animals and human beings.—**environmental** adj.—**environmentally** adv.

environmentalist /-ˌmɛntəlɪst/ n a person who is concerned with improving the quality of the environment.—**environmentalism** n.

environs /ɪn'vaɪrənz/ or /'ɛnvɪrənz/ npl the surrounding area or outskirts of a district or town.

envisage /ɪn'vɪzədʒ/ or /ɛn-/, /ən-/ vt to have a mental picture of.—**envisagement** n.

envoy /'ɒnvɔɪ/ or /'ɛn-/ n a diplomatic agent; a representative.

envy /'ɛnvi/ n (pl **envies**) resentment or discontent at another's achievements, possessions, etc; an object of envy. • vt (**envying, envied**) to feel envy of.—**envier** n.

enwrap /ɪn'ræp/ or /ɛn-/, /ən-/ vt to wrap up.

enzootic /ˌɛnzoʊ'ɒtɪk/ adj (disease) affecting animals in a particular district.

enzyme /'ɛnzaɪm/ n a complex protein, produced by living cells, that induces or speeds chemical reactions in plants and animals.

eon /'iːɒn/ see **aeon**.

eonian /'iːɒniən/ see **aeonian**.

eonism n (psychiatry) a tendency in a male to adopt female clothing and mannerisms, transvestitism.

eosin, eosine /'iːoːsɪn/ n a pink coal tar dye.—**eosinic** adj.

EP abbr = Extended Play (gramophone record).

epact /'iːpækt/ n (astron) the difference between the solar and the lunar month, about eleven days in the year.

eparch /'ɛpɑrk/ n (Greek Orthodox Church) a metropolitan or other bishop; a governor of an eparchy.

eparchy /'ɛpɑrki/, **eparchate** /-keɪt/ n (pl **eparchies, eparchates**) a Greek province; the diocese of an eparch.—**eparchial** adj.

epaulette, epaulet /ˌɛpɔ'lɛt/ or /'ɛpəˌlɛt/ n a piece of ornamental fabric or metal worn on the shoulder, esp on a uniform.

épée /ɛɪ'peɪ/ n a sword used in fencing.—**épéeist** n.

epenthesis /ɛ'pɛnθɪsɪs/ or /ɪ-/ n (pl **epentheses**) n (linguistics) the insertion of a letter or syllable in the middle of a word.

epergne /ɪ'pərn/ n a branched centrepiece or ornamental stand for a dinner table.

epexegesis /ɛˌpɛksi'dʒiːsɪs/ n (pl **epexegeses**) (linguistics) the use of additional words to clarify a meaning.—**epexegetic, epexegetical** adj.

ephah /'iːfə/ n a Hebrew dry measure, equal to about one bushel (33 litres).

ephebe /'ɛfiːb/ n a young citizen (aged 18 to 20) of ancient Greece.

ephedrine /'ɛfədrɪn/ n an alkaloid used to treat asthma and hay fever.

ephemeral /ɪ'fɛmərəl/ or /ɪ'fiːm-/ adj existing only for a very short time. • n an ephemeral thing or organism.—**ephemerality, ephemeralness** n.

ephemeris /ɪ'fɛmərɪs/ or /ɪ'fiːm-/ n (pl **ephemerides**) an astronomical almanac showing the daily positions of the sun, moon and planets.

ephod /'iːfɒd/ or /'ɛfɒd/ n a vestment worn by a Jewish priest.

ephor /'ɛfɔr/ n (pl **ephors, ephori**) a magistrate in ancient Greece.

epi-, ep- /'ɛpi/ prefix upon, at, in addition.

epiblast /'ɛpiˌblæst/ n the outer layer of the embryonic cells in an egg from which an organism is formed.—**epiblastic** adj.

epic /'ɛpɪk/ n a long poem narrating the deeds of a hero; any literary work, film, etc in the same style. • adj relating to or resembling an epic.

epicarp /'ɛpɪkɑrp/ n the outer skin of a fruit.

epicene /'ɛpɪˌsiːn/ adj having characteristics of both sexes; lacking characteristics of either sex, sexless.

epicentre, epicenter /'ɛpɪˌsɛntər/ n the area of the earth's surface directly above the focus of an earthquake.—**epicentral** adj.

epicure /'ɛpɪˌkjʊr/ n a person who has cultivated a refined taste in food, wine, literature, etc.—**epicurism, epicureanism** n.

epicurean /ˌɛpɪkjʊ'riːən/ adj given to sensuous enjoyment.

epicycle /'ɛpɪˌsaɪkəl/ n (geom) a small circle, the centre of which is situated on the circumference of a larger circle.—**epicyclic** adj.

epicycloid /ˌɛpɪ'saɪklɔɪd/ n (geom) a curve described by a point in the circumference of one circle which rolls round the circumference of another circle.

epidemic /ˌɛpɪ'dɛmɪk/ adj, n (a disease) attacking many people at the same time in a community or region.—**epidemical** adj.

epidemiology /ˌɛpɪdiː'ɒlədʒi/ n the area of medicine dealing with epidemic diseases.—**epidemiological** adj.—**epidemiologist** n.

epidermis /ˌɛpɪ'dərmɪs/ n an outer layer, esp of skin.—**epidermal, epidermic, epidermoid** adj.

epidiascope /ˌɛpɪ'daɪˌskoːp/ n a projector for magnifying opaque as well as transparent pictures.

epidural /ˌɛpɪ'dərəl/ or /-'dʊrəl/, /-'dj-/ n a spinal anaesthetic used for the relief of pain during childbirth.

epigastrium /ˌɛpɪ'gæstriəm/ n (pl **epigastria**) the upper part of the abdomen.

epigenesis /ˌɛpɪdʒə'nɛsɪs/ n the theory that an organism is created by the division or segmentation of a fertilized egg cell; a form of geological metamorphism of rock brought about by outside forces; the depositing of ore in already formed rock.—**epigenesist, epigenist** n.—**epigenetic** adj.—**epigenetically** adv.

epiglottis /ˌɛpɪ'glɒtɪs/ n (**epiglottises, epiglottides**) a thin flap of cartilaginous tissue over the entrance to the larynx.—**epiglottal, epiglottic** adj.

epigram /'ɛpɪˌgræm/ n a short witty poem or saying.—**epigrammatic** adj.—**epigrammatically** adv.

epigrammatize /-'græməˌtaɪz/ vti to compose an epigram (about).—**epigrammatist** n.

epigraph /'ɛpɪˌgræf/ n a quotation at the beginning of a book or chapter; an inscription on a building or monument.—**epigraphic, epigraphical** adj.

epigraphy /ɛ'pɪgrəfi/ n the study of inscriptions.—**epigraphist, epigrapher** n.

epilepsy /'ɛpɪˌlɛpsi/ n a disorder of the nervous system marked typically by convulsive attacks and loss of consciousness.

epileptic /ˌɛpɪˈlɛptɪk/ adj of or affected with epilepsy. • n a person affected with epilepsy.—**epileptically** adv.

epilogue /ˈɛpəˌlɒg/ n the concluding section of a book or other literary work; a short speech addressed by an actor to the audience at the end of a play.—**epilogist** n.

epiphany /ɛˈpɪfəni/ or /ɪ-/ n (pl **epiphanies**) a moment of sudden revelation or insight; (with cap) a festival of the Christian Church in commemoration of the coming of the Magi to Christ.

epiphenomenon /ˌɛpɪfɪˈnɒmɪnən/ n (pl **epiphenomena**) a by-product; (med) an attendant symptom.

epiphyte /ˈɛpɪˌfaɪt/ n (bot) a plant which grows on another plant but is not fed by it.—**epiphytic** adj.

episcopacy /ɪˈpɪskəpəsi/ n (pl **episcopacies**) the system of church government by bishops.

episcopal /ɪˈpɪskəpəl/ adj of bishops; governed by bishops.—**episcopally** adv.

episcopalian /ɪˌpɪskəˈpeɪliən/ adj pertaining to episcopacy. • n a member or supporter of an episcopal church.—**episcopalianism** n.

episcopate /ɪˈpɪskəpət/ n the office of a bishop.

episiotomy /ɛˌpizɪˈɒtəmi/ or /ɛˌpɪz-/ n (pl **episiotomies**) a cut made in the perineum during childbirth to prevent tearing.

episode /ˈɛpɪˌsoːd/ n a piece of action in a dramatic or literary work; an incident in a sequence of events.

episodic /-ɪk/, **episodical** /-ɪkəl/ adj happening at irregular intervals; digressive.—**episodically** adv.

epispastic /ˌɛpɪˈspæstɪk/ adj producing a blister.

epistaxis /ˌɛpɪˈstæksɪs/ n (med) nosebleed.

epistemology /ɪˌpɪstɪˈmɒlədʒi/ n the science of the processes and grounds of knowledge.

epistle /ɪˈpɪsəl/ n (formal) a letter; (with cap) a letter written by one of Christ's Apostles to various churches and individuals.

epistler /-ər/ n someone who reads the Epistle in the communion service; one who writes an epistle.

epistolary /ɪˈpɪstəˌlɛri/ adj pertaining to, contained in, or conducted by letters.

epistrophe /ɪˈpɪstrəfi/ n (rhetoric) the practice of ending several successive clauses or sentences with the same word.

epistyle /ˈɛpɪˌstaɪl/ n an architrave.

epitaph /ˈɛpɪˌtæf/ n an inscription in memory of a dead person, usu on a tombstone.—**epitaphic** adj.—**epitaphist** n.

epithalamium /ˌɛpɪθəˈleɪmiəm/ n (pl **epithalamia**) a nuptial song or poem.—**epithalamic** adj.

epithelioma /ˌɛpɪθiːliˈoʊmə/ n (pl **epitheliomas**, **epitheliomata**) a cancer of the epithelium.—**epitheliomatous** adj.

epithelium /ˌɛpɪˈθiːliəm/ n (pl **epithelia**) any of the cells that line the surface of the membranes of the body.—**epithelial** adj.

epithet /ˈɛpɪˌθɛt/ n a descriptive word or phrase added to or substituted for a person's name (Vlad the Impaler).—**epithetic**, **epithetical** adj.

epitome /ɪˈpɪtəmi/ n a typical example; a paradigm; personification; a condensed account of a written work.—**epitomic**, **epitomical** adj.—**epitomist** n.

epitomize /ɪˈpɪtəˌmaɪz/ vt to be or make an epitome of.—**epitomization** n.—**epitomizer** n.

epoch /ˈɛpɒk/ or /ˈiːpɒk/, /ˈɛpək/ n a date in time used as a point of reference; an age in history associated with certain characteristics; a unit of geological time.—**epochal** adj.

epode /ˈɛpˌoːd/ n a kind of lyric poem; the last part of a lyric ode.

eponym /ˈɛpəˌnɪm/ n a person after whom something is named; a name so derived.—**eponymous, eponymic** adj.—**eponymy** n.

epopee /ˈɛpəˌpiː/ or /ˌɛpəˈpiː/ n an epic poem; epic poetry.

EPOS /ˈiːpɒs/ abbr = Electronic Point Of Sale.

epos /ˈɛpˌɒs/ n early unwritten epic poetry; an epic poem; the subject of an epic poem.

epoxy /ɪˈpɒksi/ adj (chem) of or containing an oxygen atom and two other groups, usually carbon, which are themselves linked with other groups.

epoxy resin n a strong synthetic resin containing epoxy groups, used in laminates and adhesives.

epsilon /ˈɛpsɪˌlɒn/ n the 5th letter of the Greek alphabet.

equable /ˈɛkwəbəl/ adj level, uniform; (climate) free from extremes of hot and cold; even-tempered.—**equability**, **equableness** n.—**equably** adv.

equal /ˈiːkwəl/ adj the same in amount, size, number, or value; impartial, regarding or affecting all objects in the same way; capable of meeting a task or situation. • n a person that is equal.

• vt (**equalling, equalled** or **equaling, equaled**) to be equal to, esp to be identical in value; to make or do something equal to.—**equally** adv.

equality /iːˈkwɒlɪti/ n (pl **equalities**) being equal.

equalization payment n ♣ (Cdn) a transfer of funds from the federal government to a poorer province to ensure that all provinces have about the same level of public services and taxation.

equalize /ˈiːkwəˌlaɪz/ vti to make or become equal; (games) to even the score.—**equalization** n.—**equalizer** n.

equanimity /ˌɛkwəˈnɪmɪti/ n (pl **equanimities**) evenness of temper; composure.—**equanimous** adj.

equate /iˈkweɪt/ vt to make, treat, or regard as comparable. • vi to correspond as equal.

equation /iˈkweɪʒən/ n an act of equalling; the state of being equal; a usu formal statement of equivalence (as in logical and mathematical expressions) with the relations denoted by the sign (=); an expression representing a chemical reaction by means of chemical symbols.—**equational** adj.

equator /iˈkweɪtər/ n an imaginary circle passing round the globe, equidistant from the North and South poles.—**equatorial** n.

equerry /ˈɛkwəri/ or /iˈkwɛri/ n (pl **equerries**) an officer in the British royal household.

equestrian /iˈkwɛstriən/ adj pertaining to horses and riding; on horseback. • n a skilled rider.—**equestrienne** nf.—**equestrianism** n.

equi- /ˈɛkwɪ/ or /ˈiːkwɪ/ prefix equal.

equiangular /ˌɛkwɪˈæŋgjuːlər/ or /ˈiːkwɪ-/ adj having equal angles.

equidistant /ˌɛkwɪˈdɪstənt/ or /ˈiːkwɪ-/ adj at equal distances.—**equidistance** n.

equilateral /ˌɛkwɪˈlætərəl/ or /ˈiːkwɪ-/ adj having all sides equal.

equilibrate /ˈiːkwɪˌbreɪt/ or /ˈɛkwɪˈlaɪbreɪt/ vti to balance.—**equilibration** n.—**equilibrator** n.

equilibrist /ɪˈkwɪləbrɪst/ n a tightrope walker; an acrobat.—**equilibristic** adj.

equilibrium /ˌiːkwɪˈlɪbriəm/ or /ˈɛkwɪ-/ n (pl **equilibriums**, **equilibria**) a state of balance of weight, power, force, etc.

equine /ˈɛkwaɪn/ or /ˈiːk-/ adj of or resembling a horse.

equinox /ˈɛkwɪˌnɒks/ or /ˈiːk-/ n the two times of the year when night and day are equal in length (around 21 March and 23 September).—**equinoctial** adj.

equip /ɪˈkwɪp/ vt (**equipping, equipped**) to provide with all the necessary tools or supplies.—**equipper** n.

equipage /ˈɛkwɪpɪdʒ/ n a carriage with horses and liveried attendants.

equipment /ɪˈkwɪpmənt/ n the tools, supplies and other items needed for a particular task, expedition, etc.

equipoise /ˈɛkwɪˌpɔɪz/ or /ˈiːkwɪ-/ n balance, equilibrium.

equipollent /ˌikwɪˈpɒlənt/ adj equal in power.—**equipollence** n.

equiponderant /ˌikwɪˈpɒndərənt/ vti to make or be equal in weight.—**equiponderant** adj.

equisetum /ˌɛkwɪˈsitəm/ n (pl **equisetums, equiseta**) a plant of the group that includes horsetails.

equitable /ˈɛkwɪtəbəl/ adj just and fair; (law) pertaining to equity as opposed to common or statute law.—**equitableness** n.—**equitably** adv.

equitation /ˌɛkwɪˈteɪʃən/ n horsemanship.

equity /ˈɛkwɪti/ n (pl **equities**) fairness; (law) a legal system based on natural justice developed into a body of rules supplementing the common law; (pl) ordinary shares in a company.

equivalence /iˈkwɪvələns/ or /ɪ-/, **equivalency** /-i/ n (pl **equivalences, equivalencies**) equality of value or power; (chem) the property of having equal valency.

equivalent /ɪˈkwɪvələnt/ adj equal in amount, force, meaning, etc; virtually identical, esp in effect or function. • n an equivalent thing.

equivocal /ɪˈkwɪvəkəl/ adj ambiguous; uncertain; questionable; arousing suspicion.—**equivocality, equivocacy** n.—**equivocally** adv.

equivocate /ɪˈkwɪvəˌkeɪt/ vi to use ambiguous language, esp in order to confuse or deceive.—**equivocation** n.—**equivocator** n.—**equivocatory** adj.

equivoque, equivoke /ˈɛkwɪˌvoːk/ or /iˈkwɪ-/ n a pun; an ambiguous expression.

Er (chem symbol) erbium.

era /ˈɛrə/ or /ˈiːrə/ n an historical period typified by some special feature; a chronological order or system of notation reckoned from a given date as a basis.

eradiate /ɪˈreɪdɪˌeɪt/ *vti* to emit rays, to radiate.—**eradiation** *n*.

eradicate /ɪˈrædɪˌkeɪt/ *vt* to obliterate.—**eradicable** *adj*.—**eradication** *n*.—**eradicator** *n*.

erase /ɪˈreɪs/ *vt* to rub out, obliterate; to remove a recording from magnetic tape; to remove data from a computer memory or storage medium.—**erasable** *adj*.—**erasion** *n*.

eraser /-ər/ *n* a piece of rubber, etc for rubbing out marks or writing.

erasure /ɪˈreɪʃər/ *n* an erasing; something rubbed out.

erbium /ˈɜːbɪəm/ *n* a soft metallic element of the rare earth group.

ere /ɛr/ *prep, conj* (*poet*) before.

erect /ɪˈrekt/ *adj* upright; not leaning or lying down; (*sexual organs*) rigid and swollen with blood from sexual stimulation. • *vt* to construct, set up.—**erectable** *adj*.—**erecter, erector** *n*.—**erectness** *n*.

erectile /ɪˈrektaɪl/ *adj* (*penis, clitoris, etc*) able to become enlarged and rigid through sexual stimulation.—**erectility** *n*.

erection /ɪˈrekʃən/ *n* construction; something erected, as a building; swelling, *esp* of the penis, due to sexual excitement.

erector /ɪˈrektər/ *n* a person who, or a thing that, erects; a muscle that erects.

eremite /ˈɛrɪˌmaɪt/ *n* a hermit.—**eremitic, eremitica** *adj*.—**eremitism** *n*.

erethism /ˈɛrɪˌθɪzəm/ *n* (*med*) an abnormal degree of excitement in an organ or tissue of the body.

erg /ɜːɡ/ *n* the unit for measuring work or energy.

ergo /ˈɜːɡoʊ/ or /ˈɜːr-/ *adv* therefore.

ergometer /ɜːrˈɡɒmɪtər/ *n* an instrument for measuring work performed or force produced.

ergonomics /ˌɜːɡəˈnɒmɪks/ *n sing* the study of the interaction between people and their working environment with the aim of improving efficiency.—**ergonomic** *adj*.—**ergonomically** *adv*.—**ergonomist** *n*.

ergot /ˈɜːɡət/ *n* a disease of rye and other cereals caused by a fungus; this fungus; a medicine derived from an ergot fungus.

ergotism /ˈɜːɡətˌɪzəm/ *n* a toxic condition in humans caused by ergot fungus or chronic excessive use of an ergot drug.

erica /ˈɛrɪkə/ *n* a genus of flowering plants, including the heaths.

ericaceous /ˌɛrɪˈkeɪʃəs/ *adj* of the heath family.

eristic /ɛrˈɪstɪk/, **eristical** /-əl/ *adj* (*logic*) seeking to win an argument rather than find the truth.

ermine /ˈɜːmɪn/ *n* (*pl* **ermines, ermine**) the weasel in its winter coat; the white fur of the winter coat; a rank or office whose official robe is edged with ermine.

Ermite /ɜːrˈmaɪt/ *n* ♣ a creamy blue-veined cheese made in Quebec.

erne, ern /ɜːrn/ *n* the sea eagle.

erode /ɪˈroʊd/ *vt* to eat or wear away gradually.

erogenous /ɪˈrɒdʒɪnəs/ *adj* sexually arousing; sensitive to sexual stimulation.

erosion /ɪˈroʊʒən/ *n* the act of eroding; gradual destruction or eating away; an eroded part.—**erosive, erosional** *adj*.

erotic /ɪˈrɒtɪk/, **erotical** /-əl/ *adj* of sexual love; sexually stimulating.—**erotically** *adv*.

erotica /ɪˈrɒtɪkə/ *n* sexually explicit literature or art.

eroticism /ɪˈrɒtɪˌsɪzəm/, **erotism** /-tɪzəm/ *n* erotic nature; sexually arousing themes in literature and art; sexual desire.

erotomania /ɪˌroʊtəˈmeɪnɪə/ *n* excessive sexual desire.—**erotomaniac** *n*.

err /ɜːr/ or /ɛr/ *vi* to be or do wrong.

errand /ˈɛrənd/ *n* a short journey to perform some task, *usu* on behalf of another; the purpose of this journey.

errant /ˈɛrənt/ *adj* going astray, *esp* doing wrong; moving aimlessly.

errantry /ˈɛrəntri/ *n* (*pl* **errantries**) the state or conduct of a knight errant.

erratic /ɪˈrætɪk/ *adj* capricious; irregular; eccentric, odd.—**erratically** *adv*.

erratum /ɛˈrætəm/ *n* (*pl* **errata**) a written or printed error; a page bearing a list of corrigenda.—*also* **corrigendum**.

erroneous /ɪˈroʊnɪəs/ *adj* incorrect; mistaken.—**erroneously** *adv*.

error /ˈɛrər/ *n* a mistake, an inaccuracy; a mistaken belief or action; (*statistics*) the difference between an approximation of a value and the actual value, *usu* expressed as a percentage.

ersatz /ˈɛrˌzæts/ or /ˈɜːrˌzæts/ *adj* made in imitation; synthetic.

Erse /ɜːrs/ *n* Scottish Gaelic; Irish Gaelic.—*also adj*.

erstwhile /ˈɜːrstˌwaɪl/ *adv* formerly. • *adj* former.

eructation /ˌiːrʌkˈteɪʃən/ *n* the act of belching.

erudite /ˈɛruːˌdaɪt/ or /ˈɛrjə-/ *adj* scholarly, having great knowledge.—**eruditely** *adv*.—**erudition** *n*.

erupt /ɪˈrʌpt/ *vi* to burst forth; to break out into a rash; (*volcano*) to explode, ejecting ash and lava into the air.—**eruptible** *adj*.

eruption /ɪˈrʌpʃən/ *n* the ejection of lava from a volcano; an outbreak; a rash, pimples.—**eruptional** *adj*.—**eruptive** *adj*.

eryngo, eringo /ɪˈrɪŋɡoʊ/ or /ɪ-/ *n* (*pl* **eryngoes, eryngos, eringoes, eringos**) one of a genus of plants including the sea holly.

erysipelas /ˌɛrɪˈsɪpɪləs/ *n* an acute bacterial disease, characterized by a fever and skin inflammation.—**erysipelatous** *adj*.

erythema /ˌɛrɪˈθiːmə/ *n* (*med*) a superficial patchy redness of the skin.—**erythematic, erythematous, erythemic** *adj*.

erythrocyte /ɪˈrɪθroʊˌsaɪt/ *n* a red blood corpuscle.—**erythrocytic** *adj*.

Es (*chem symbol*) einsteinium.

escalade /ˌɛskəˈleɪd/ *n* the act of scaling the walls of a fortified place by ladders.

escalate /ˈɛskəˌleɪt/ *vi* to increase rapidly in magnitude or intensity.—**escalation** *n*.

escalator /ˈɛskəˌleɪtər/ *n* a motorized set of stairs arranged to ascend or descend continuously.

escallop /eˈskæləp/ *n* a scallop.

escalope /ˈɛskəˌlɒp/ *n* a thin cut of meat, *esp* veal.

escapade /ˈɛskəˌpeɪd/ *n* a wild or mischievous adventure.

escape /ɪˈskeɪp/ *vt* to free oneself from confinement, etc; to avoid, remain unnoticed; to be forgotten. • *vi* to achieve freedom; (*gas, liquid*) to leak. • *n* an act or instance of escaping; a means of escape; a leakage of liquid or gas; a temporary respite from reality.—**escapable** *adj*.—**escaper** *n*.

escapee /ɪˈskeɪpi/ or /ɪskeɪˈpi/ *n* a person who has escaped, *esp* a prisoner.

escapement /ɪˈskeɪpmənt/ *n* a device in a watch or clock by which the motions of the pendulum or balance are regulated.

escape velocity *n* the minimum velocity required for a rocket, etc to escape the gravitational pull of the earth or other celestial body.

escapism /ɪˈskeɪpɪzəm/ *n* the tendency to avoid or retreat from reality into fantasy.—**escapist** *n, adj*.

escapologist /ˌɛskeɪˈpɒlədʒɪst/ *n* a performer who escapes from handcuffs, locked boxes, etc.—**escapology** *n*.

escargot /ˌɛskɑrˈɡoʊ/ or /esˈkɑrɡoʊ/ *n* a snail prepared as food.

escarp /ɪˈskɑrp/ *n* a steep bank in front of a rampart.

escarpment /-mənt/ *n* a steep side of a ridge or plateau.

eschatology /ˌɛskəˈtɒlədʒi/ *n* (*pl* **eschatologies**) the study of death, judgment, heaven and hell, and how humanity relates to them.

escheat /ɪsˈtʃiːt/ *n* (*law*) (*formerly*) the lapsing of property to the state in the absence of an heir or by forfeiture; property that passes to the state in this way. • *vt* to confiscate property by escheat. • *vi* to revert to the state by escheat.

eschew /esˈtʃuː/ *vt* to avoid as habit, *esp* on moral grounds.—**eschewal** *n*.—**eschewer** *n*.

escort /ˈɛskɔrt/ *n* a person, group, ship, aircraft, etc accompanying a person or thing to give protection, guidance, or as a matter of courtesy; a person who accompanies another on a social occasion. • *vt* to attend as escort.

escritoire /ˌɛskrɪˈtwɒr/ *n* a writing desk.

escrow /ˈɛskroʊ/ *n* (*law*) a contract kept by a third party until the fulfilment of a condition.

escudo /esˈkuːdoʊ/, *Sp.* /esˈkuːðo/, *Port.* /ɪʃˈkuːdu/ *n* (*pl* **escudos**) formerly the monetary unit of Portugal, now the euro.

esculent /ˈɛskjulənt/ *adj* edible.

escutcheon /ɪˈskʌtʃən/ *n* a shield bearing a coat of arms.

esker, eskar /ˈɛskər/ *n* (*geol*) a ridge of gravel, glacially deposited.

Eskimo /ˈɛskɪˌmoʊ/ *n* (*pl* **Eskimos, Eskimo**) the Inuit people; a group of peoples of eastern Siberia; a member of these peoples; their language.—*also adj*.

Eskimo dog *n* a powerful type of dog with a thick coat bred to pull sledges.

esophagus /iˈsɒfəɡəs/ *see* **oesophagus**.

esoteric /ˌɛsoʊˈtɛrɪk/ *adj* intended for or understood by a select few; secret; private.—**esoterically** *adv*.—**esotericism** *n*.

ESP /ˌiːɛsˈpi/ *abbr* = extrasensory perception.

esp. *abbr* = especially.

espadrille /ˈɛspəˌdrɪl/ *n* a flat shoe *usu* having a fabric upper and rope soles.

espalier /ɛˈspæljər/ *n* a plant (as a fruit tree) trained to grow flat against a support; the trellis on which such plants are trained.

esparto /ɛˈspɑrtoː/ *n* (*pl* **espartos**) either of two Spanish and Algerian grasses used *esp* in paper-making.

especial /ɪˈspɛʃəl/ *adj* notably special, unusual; particular to one person or thing.—**especially** *adv*.

Esperanto /ˌɛspəˈræntoː/ *n* an artificial international language.

espionage /ˈɛspiəˌnɒʒ/ *n* spying or the use of spies to obtain information.

esplanade /ˌɛspləˈneɪd/ or /-ˈnɒd/, /ˈɛsp-/ *n* a level open space for walking or driving, *esp* along a shore.

espouse /ɪˈspaʊz/ *vt* to adopt or support a cause.—**espousal** /ɛˈspaʊzəl/ *n*.—**espouser** *n*.

espresso /ɛˈspresoː/ *n* (*pl* **espressos**) coffee brewed by forcing steam through finely ground darkly roasted coffee beans; an apparatus for making espresso.

esprit /ɛˈspriː/ or /ˈɛspriː/ *n* wit; liveliness.

esprit de corps /-dəˈkɔr/ *n* a sense of loyalty and attachment to a group to which one belongs.

espy /ɛˈspaɪ/ or /ɪ-/ *vt* (**espying, espied**) to catch sight of.—**espial** *n*.—**espier** *n*.

Esq *abbr* = esquire.

esquire /ɪˈskwaɪr/ or /ɛˈskwaɪr/ *n* a general courtesy title used instead of Mr in addressing letters.

essay /ˈɛseɪ/ *n* a short prose work *usu* dealing with a subject from a limited or personal point of view; an attempt. • *vt* (**essaying, essayed**) to try, to attempt.

essayist /ˈɛseɪɪst/ *n* an essay writer.

essence /ˈɛsəns/ *n* that which makes a thing what it is; a substance distilled or extracted from another substance and having the special qualities of the original substance; a perfume.

essential /ɪˈsɛnʃəl/ or /iː-/ *adj* of or containing the essence of something; indispensable, of the greatest importance. • *n* (*often pl*) indispensable elements or qualities.—**essentiality, essentialness** *n*.—**essentially** *adv*.

essential oil *n* any of various plant oils used in perfumery.

establish /ɪˈstæblɪʃ/ *vt* to set up (*eg* a business) permanently; to settle (a person) in a place or position; to get generally accepted; to place beyond dispute, prove as a fact.—**establisher** *n*.

established *adj* (*church, religion*) officially recognized as the national church or religion of a country.

establishment /-mənt/ *n* the act of establishing; a commercial organization or other large institution; the staff and resources of an organization; a household; (*with cap*) those people in institutions such as the government, civil service and commerce who use their power to preserve the social, economic and political status quo.

establishmentarian /ɪˌstæblɪʃmənˈtɛriən/ *adj, n* of an established church; supporting the established church system. • *n* a person who advocates official recognition of a church or religion.—**establishmentarianism** *n*.

estaminet *Fr.* /ɛsˈtæmiˈneɪ/ *n* a café.

estancia /ɛsˈtɒnsiːə/ *n* a cattle ranch in Latin America.

estate /əˈsteɪt/ *n* landed property; a large area of residential or industrial development; a person's total possessions, *esp* at their death; a social or political class.

estate agent *see* **realtor**.

estate car *n* a car with extra carrying space reached through a rear door.—*also* **station wagon**.

esteem /ɪˈstiːm/ *vt* to value or regard highly; to consider or think. • *n* high regard, a favourable opinion.

ester /ˈɛstər/ *n* (*chem*) a compound of acid and alcohol.

esthete /ˈɛsˌθiːt/ or, **esthetics** /ɛsˈθɛtɪks/ *see* **aesthete, aesthetics**.

estheticism /ɛsˈθɛtɪˌsɪzəm/ *see* **aestheticism**.

estimable /ˈɛstɪməbəl/ *adj* worthy of esteem; calculable.

estimate /ˈɛstəmət/ *vt* to judge the value, amount, significance of; to calculate approximately. • *n* an approximate calculation; a judgment or opinion; a preliminary calculation of the cost of a particular job.—**estimative** *adj*.

estimation /ˌɛstəˈmeɪʃən/ *n* estimating; an opinion, judgment; esteem.

estimator /ˈɛstəˌmeɪtər/ *n* someone or something that estimates.

estival /ˈɛstəvəl/ or /ɛsˈtaɪvəl/ *see* **aestival**.

estivation /ˌɛstəˈveɪʃən/ *see* **aestivation**.

estop /ɛˈstɒp/ *vt* (**estopping, estopped**) (*law*) to prohibit by estoppel.

estoppel /ɛˈstɒpəl/ *n* (*law*) a legal impediment arising as a result of one's previous action.

estrange /ɪˈstreɪndʒ/ *vt* to alienate the affections or confidence of.—**estranged** *adj*.—**estrangement** *n*.

estrogen /ˈɛstrədʒən/ *see* **oestrogen**.

estrus /ˈɛstrəs/, *Brit.* /ˈiːstrəs/ *see* **oestrus**.

estuarine /ˈɛstʃuːəraɪn/ *adj* pertaining to, or formed in, an estuary.

estuary /ˈɛstʃuːˌɛri/ *n* (*pl* **estuaries**) an arm of the sea at the mouth of a river.

esurient /ɪˈsʊriənt/ *adj* voracious, greedy.—**esurience** *n*.

ETA *abbr* = Estimated Time of Arrival.

eta /ˈeɪtə/ or /ˈiːtə/ *n* the 7th letter of the Greek alphabet.

étagère /ˌeɪtæˈjər/ *n* an ornamental stand.

et al *abbr* = *et alii*, and others.

etc, etc. *abbr* = et cetera.

et cetera, etcetera /ɛtˈsɛtərə/ or /-ˈsɛtrə/ *n* and so forth.

etceteras /ɛtˈsɛtərəz/ or /-ˈsɛtrəz/ *npl* the usual extra things or persons.

etch /ɛtʃ/ *vti* to make lines on (metal, glass) *usu* by the action of acid; to produce (as a design) by etching; to delineate clearly.—**etcher** *n*.

etching /ˈɛtʃɪŋ/ *n* the art or process of producing designs on and printing from etched plates; an impression made from an etched plate.

ETD *abbr* = Estimated Time of Departure.

eternal /ɪˈtɜːrnəl/ or /iː-/ *adj* continuing forever without beginning or end, everlasting; unchangeable; (*inf*) seemingly endless.—**eternality, eternalness** *n*.—**eternally** *adv*.

eternalize /-aɪz/ *vt* to make eternal.—**eternalization** *n*.

eternity /ɪˈtɜːrnɪti/ or /iː-/ *n* (*pl* **eternities**) infinite time; the timelessness thought to constitute life after death; (*inf*) a very long time.

etesian /ɪˈtiːʒən/ *adj* (*winds*) blowing from the northwest in the Mediterranean for about forty days each summer.

ethane /ˈɛθeɪn/ or /ˈiːθ-/ *n* a colourless gaseous hydrocarbon found in natural gas and used *esp* as fuel.

ethene /ˈɛθiːn/ *see* **ethylene**.

ether /ˈiːθər/ *n* (*chem*) a light flammable liquid used as an anaesthetic or solvent; the upper regions of space, the invisible elastic substance formerly believed to be distributed evenly through all space.—**etheric** *adj*.

ethereal /ɪˈθɪəriəl/ *adj* delicate; spiritual; celestial.—**ethereality, etherealness** *n*.—**ethereally** *adv*.

etherealize /-ˌaɪz/ *vt* to make ethereal; to regard as ethereal.—**etherealization** *n*.

etherize /ˈiːθəraɪz/ *vt* (*patient*) to anaesthetize, using ether.—**etherization** *n*.

ethic /ˈɛθɪk/ *n* a moral principle or set of principles. • *adj* ethical.

ethical /ˈɛθɪkəl/ *adj* of or pertaining to ethics; conforming to the principles of proper conduct, as established by society, a profession, etc; (*med*) legally available only on prescription.—**ethically** *adv*.—**ethicalness, ethicality** *n*.

ethical investment *n* the investment in companies whose activities do not offend the investor's moral principles.—*also* **conscience investment**.

ethics /ˈɛθɪks/ *n sing* the philosophical analysis of human morality and conduct; system of conduct or behaviour, moral principles.—**ethicist** *n*.

Ethiopian /ˌiːθiˈoːpiən/ *adj* of or pertaining to Ethiopia, its languages or people.—*also n*.

ethmoid /ˈɛθmɔɪd/ *adj* (*anat*) denoting a light, spongy bone that forms the roof of the nose.—*also* **ethmoidal**. • *n* the ethmoid bone.

ethnic, ethnical /ˈɛθnɪk/ *adj* of races or large groups of people classed according to common traits and customs.—**ethnically** *adv*.

ethnic cleansing *n* the planned expulsion, extermination or removal of people from a religious or ethnic minority within an area, region or country.

ethno- /ˈɛθnoː/ *prefix* indicating race; people; culture.

ethnography /ɛθˈnɒɡrəfi/ *n* the area of anthropology dealing with the scientific description of human races.—**ethnographer** *n*.—**ethnographic, ethnographical** *adj*.

ethnology /ɛθˈnɒlədʒi/ *n* the scientific study of the origins and culture, etc of different races and peoples.—**ethnologic, ethnological** *adj*.—**ethnologist** *n*.

ethology /iːˈθɒlədʒi/ *n* the scientific study of animal behaviour.—**ethologic, ethological** *adj*.—**ethologist** *n*.

ethos /'iˌθɒs/ *n* the distinguishing character, sentiment, moral nature, or guiding beliefs of a person, group, or institution.

ethyl /'eθɪl/ *n* the radical from which common alcohol and ether are derived.

ethylene /'εθəˌliːn/ *n* a colourless sweet-smelling gaseous hydrocarbon obtained from petroleum and used to manufacture chemicals including polythene.—*also* **ethene**.

etiolate /'iːtɪəˌleɪt/ *vti* (*green plants*) to bleach by depriving of light; to make or become pale and sickly.—**etiolation** *n*.

etiology /ˌiːtɪ'ɒlədʒi/ *n* (*pl* **etiologies**) the study of causation, *esp* causes of diseases.—*also* **aetiology**.—**etiological** *adj*.—**etiologist** *n*.

etiquette /'etɪkət/ or /-ket/ *n* the form of conduct or behaviour prescribed by custom or authority to be observed in social, official or professional life.

Etruscan /ɪ'trʌskən/ *n* an inhabitant of ancient Etruria (now Tuscany); the language of ancient Etruscans.—*also adj*.

étude /'eɪ'tuːd/ or /-'tjuːd/, /'eɪ-/ (*mus*) a short study or exercise for a solo instrument.

étui /'εˌtwiː/ *n* (*pl* **étuis**) a pocket case for sewing implements and other small articles.

etymology /ˌetɪ'mɒlədʒi/ *n* (*pl* **etymologies**) the study of the source and meaning of words; an account of the source and history of a word.—**etymological, etymologic** *adj*.—**etymologist** *n*.

etymon /'etɪˌmɒn/ *n* (*pl* **etymons, etyma**) the root of a word, or its original meaning.

EU *abbr* = European Union.

Eu (*chem symbol*) europium.

eucalyptol /ˌjuːkə'lɪptɒl/ or /-toːl/ *n* a liquid contained in eucalyptus oil.

eucalyptus, eucalypt /ˌjuːkə'lɪptəs/ *n* (*pl* **eucalyptuses, eucalypti** *or* **eucalypts**) any of a genus of mostly Australian evergreen trees cultivated for their resin, oil, and wood; a type of oil obtained from its leaves.

Eucharist /'juːkərɪst/ *n* the Christian sacrament of communion in which bread and wine are consecrated; the consecrated elements in communion.—**Eucharistic, Eucharistical** *adj*.

euchre /'juːkər/ *n* a card game for two, three or four players.

Euclidean /juː'klɪdɪən/ *adj* pertaining to or accordant with the geometrical principles of Euclid, the Greek mathematician (*fl* 3rd century BC).

eudemonism, eudaemonism /juː'diːmənˌɪzəm/ *n* the ethical doctrine that regards happiness as the chief end in moral conduct.

eudiometer /ˌjuːdɪ'ɒmətər/ *n* an instrument for measuring the amount of oxygen in the air.

eugenics /juː'dʒenɪks/ *n sing* the science of improving the human race by selective breeding.—**eugenic** *adj*—**eugenically** *adv*.—**eugenicist** *n*.

euhemerism /juː'hiːmərˌɪzəm/ or /-'hemər-/ *n* the theory that the classical deities are deified heroes and that the myths connected with them are based on real history.—**euhemerist** *n*.—**euhemeristic** *adj*.—**euhemeristically** *adv*.

eulogize /'juːləˌdʒaɪz/ *vt* to extol in speech or writing.—**eulogist, eulogizer** *n*.—**eulogistic, eulogistical** *adj*.—**eulogistically** *adv*.

eulogy /'juːlədʒi/ *n* (*pl* **eulogies**) a speech or piece of writing in praise or celebration of someone or something.

eunuch /'juːnək/ *n* a castrated man.

euonymus /juː'ɒnɪməs/ *n* a genus of small trees, containing the spindle tree.

euphemism /'juːfəˌmɪzəm/ *n* a mild or inoffensive word substituted for a more unpleasant or offensive term; the use of such inoffensive words.—**euphemistic** *adj*.—**euphemistically** *adv*.

euphonic /juː'fɒnɪk/, **euphonical** /-əl/ *adj* sounding pleasant to the ear.—**euphonically** *adv*.

euphonium /juː'fəʊnɪəm/ *n* a brass musical instrument with its oval bell pointed backwards.

euphony /'juːfəni/ *n* (*pl* **euphonies**) a pleasing sound, *esp* words.—**euphonious** *adj*.

euphorbia /juː'fɔːbɪə/ *n* a member of the large genus of plants of the spurge family.

euphoria /juː'fɔːrɪə/ *n* a feeling of elation.—**euphoric** *adj*.—**euphorically** *adv*.

euphuism /'juːfjuːˌɪzəm/ *n* an affected style of prose using elaborate antithesis, alliteration, and conceits; the pedantic or affected use of words or language.—**euphuist** *n*.—**euphuistic, euphuistical** *adj*.

Eurasian /jʊr'eɪʒən/ or /jə-/ *adj* of Europe and Asia (Eurasia) taken as one continent; of mixed European and Asian descent.—*also n*.

eureka /jʊ'riːkə/ or /jə-/ *interj* used to express triumph on a discovery.

eurhythmics /jʊ'rɪðmɪks/ *see* **eurythmics**.

euro /'jʊrəʊ/ or /'jər/ *n* the name for the European unit of currency.

Euro- /'jʊrəʊ/ or /'jər-/ *prefix* Europe; European.

Euro-Canadian *n* a Canadian of European origin or descent. • *adj* pertaining to Canadians of European origin or descent.

Eurocrat /'jʊrəʊˌkræt/ or /'jər-/ *n* a member of the administration of the European Community.

Europe /'jʊrəp/ or /'jər-/ *n* a continent extending from Asia in the east to the Atlantic Ocean in the west.

European /ˌjʊrə'pɪən/ or /'jər-/ *adj* relating to or native to Europe. • *n* a native or inhabitant of Europe; a person of European descent.

European Economic Community *or* **European Community** *n* the official name of the European Common Market, whose members aim to eliminate all obstacles to the free movement of goods, services, capital and labour between the member countries and to set up common external commercial, agricultural, and transport policies.

europium /jʊ'rəʊpɪəm/ *n* a soft metallic element of the rare earth group.

eurythmics /juː'rɪðmɪks/ *npl* the art of representing musical harmony by physical gestures.—*also* **eurhythmics**.

Eustachian tube /juː'steɪʃən/ or /-ʃɪən/ *n* a tube that leads from the middle ear to the pharynx.

euthanasia /ˌjuːθə'neɪʒə/ *n* the act or practice of killing painlessly, *esp* to relieve incurable suffering.

eV *abbr* = electronvolt.

evacuate /ɪ'vækjuˌeɪt/ or /i-/ *vti* to move (people, etc) from an area of danger to one of safety; to leave or make empty; to discharge wastes from the body.—**evacuation** *n*.—**evacuative** *adj*.—**evacuator** *n*.

evacuee /ɪˌvækjuː'iː/ or /ɪ-/ *n* an evacuated person.

evade /ɪ'veɪd/ or /i-/ *vt* to manage to avoid, *esp* by dexterity or slyness.—**evadable** *adj*.—**evader** *n*.

evaluate /ɪ'væljuˌeɪt/ or /i-/ *vt* to determine the value of; to assess.—**evaluation** *n*.—**evaluator** *n*.

evanescent /ˌevə'nesənt/ *adj* fading away, vanishing; ephemeral.—**evanescence** *n*.

evangel /ɪ'vændʒəl/ or /i-/ *n* the Christian gospel.

evangelical /ˌiːvæn'dʒelɪkəl/ or /ˌevən-/ *adj* of or agreeing with Christian teachings, *esp* as presented in the four Gospels; pertaining to various Christian sects that believe in salvation through personal conversion and faith in Christ.—**evangelicalism** *n*.

evangelism /ɪ'vændʒəˌlɪzəm/ or /i-/ *n* preaching the Christian gospel; missionary zeal.

evangelist /-lɪst/ *n* a person who preaches the gospel; one of the writers of the four Gospels.—**evangelistic** *adj*.—**evangelistically** *adv*.

evangelize /ɪ'vændʒəˌlaɪz/ or /i-/ *vt* to preach or spread the gospel; to seek converts to a particular cause.—**evangelization** *n*.—**evangelizer** *n*.

evaporate /ɪ'væpəˌreɪt/ or /i-/ *vti* to change into a vapour; to remove water from; to give off moisture; to vanish; to disappear.—**evaporable** *adj*.—**evaporation** *n*.—**evaporative** *adj*.—**evaporator** *n*.

evaporated milk *n* tinned unsweetened milk thickened by evaporation.

evasion /ɪ'veɪʒən/ or /i-/ *n* the act of evading; a means of evading, *esp* an equivocal reply or excuse.—**evasive** *adj*.—**evasively** *adv*.—**evasiveness** *n*.

eve /iːv/ *n* the evening or the whole day, before a festival; the period immediately before an event; (*formerly*) evening.

evection /ɪ'vekʃən/ or /i-/ *n* (*astron*) a periodical irregularity of the moon's motion.

even /'iːvən/ *adj* level, flat; smooth; regular, equal; balanced; exact; divisible by two. • *vti* to make or become even; (*with* **up**) to balance (debts, etc). • *adv* exactly; precisely; fully; quite; at the very time; used as an intensive to emphasize the identity of something (*he looked content, even happy*), to indicate something unexpected (*she refused even to look at him*), or to stress the comparative degree (*she did even better*).—**evenly** *adv*.—**evenness** *n*.

even-handed /-ˌhændəd/ *adj* impartial, fair.—**even-handedness** *n*.

evening /'iːvnɪŋ/ *n* the latter part of the day and early part of the night.

evening primrose *n* a plant with yellow flowers that open in the evening.

evens /'iːvənz/ *npl* (*bet*) winning the same as the stake if successful; offered at such odds, as a horse.—*also* **even money**.

evensong /'iːvənˌsɒŋ/ *n* vespers; evening prayers.

event /ɪ'vent/ or /i-/ *n* something that happens; a social occasion; contingency; a contest in a sports programme.

even-tempered /ˌiːvən'tempərd/ *adj* calm.

eventful /ɪ'ventfəl/ or /i-/ *adj* full of incidents; momentous.

eventide /'iːvənˌtaɪd/ *n* (*formerly*) evening.

eventual /ɪ'ventʃʊəl/ *adj* happening at some future unspecified time; ultimate.—**eventually** *adv*.

eventuality /ɪˌventʃʊælɪti/ *n* (*pl* **eventualities**) a possible occurrence.

eventuate /ɪ'ventʃʊˌeɪt/ *vi* to result.—**eventuation** *n*.

ever /'ɛvər/ *adv* always, at all times; at any time; in any case.

evergreen /'ɛvərˌgriːn/ *adj* (*plants, trees*) having foliage that remains green all year.—*also* **n**.

everlasting /ˌɛvər'læstɪŋ/ *adj* enduring forever; (*plants*) having flowers that may be dried without loss of form or colour.—**everlastingly** *adv*.

evermore /ˌɛvər'mɔr/ *adv* forever.

evert /ɪ'vɜrt/ *vt* to turn inside out.—**eversible** *adj*.—**eversion** *n*.

every /'ɛvri/ *adj* being one of the total.

everybody /'ɛvriˌbɒdi/ or /-ˌbɛdi/, **everyone** /-ˌwʌn/ *pron* every person.

everyday /-ˌdeɪ/ or /-'deɪ/ *adj* happening daily; commonplace; worn or used on ordinary days.

everything /-θɪŋ/ *pron* all things, all; something of the utmost importance.

everywhere /-ˌwɛr/ *adv* in every place.

evict /ɪ'vɪkt/ *vt* to expel from land or from a building by legal process; to expel.—**eviction** *n*.—**evictor** *n*.

evidence /'ɛvɪdəns/ *n* an outward sign; proof, testimony, *esp* matter submitted in court to determine the truth of alleged facts. • *vt* to demonstrate clearly; to give proof or evidence for.

evident /'ɛvɪdənt/ *adj* easy to see or understand.—**evidently** *adv*.

evidential /ˌɛvɪ'denʃəl/ *adj* relating to, providing, or based on evidence.—**evidentially** *adv*.

evil /'iːvəl/ or /-ɪl/ *adj* wicked; causing or threatening distress or harm. • *n* a sin; a source of harm or distress.—**evilly** *adv*.—**evilness** *n*.

evildoer /-ˌduːər/ *n* a wicked person.—**evildoing** *n*.

evil eye *n* a stare superstitiously believed to inflict harm; the power to cause harm in this manner.

evince /ɪ'vɪns/ *vt* to indicate that one has (*eg* a quality); to demonstrate.—**evincible** *adj*.—**evincive** *adj*.

eviscerate /ɪ'vɪsəˌreɪt/ *vt* to take out the intestines of, disembowel.—**evisceration** *n*.—**eviscerator** *n*.

evocative /ɪ'vɒkətɪv/ or /-ɪ-/ *adj* serving to evoke.—**evocatively** *n*.

evoke /ɪ'voːk/ or /ɪ-/ *vt* to call forth or up.—**evocable** *adj*.—**evocation** *n*.—**evoker** *n*.

evolution /ˌɛvə'luːʃən/ or /ˌiːvə-/, /-'ljuːʃən/ *n* a process of change in a particular direction; the process by which something attains its distinctive characteristics; a theory that existing types of plants and animals have developed from earlier forms.—**evolutionary, evolutional** *adj*.

evolutionist /-ɪst/ *adj* pertaining to evolution. • *n* someone who believes in the theory of evolution.

evolve /iː'vɒlv/ or /ɪ-/ *vi* to develop by or as if by evolution.—**evolvable** *adj*.—**evolvement** *n*.

ewe /juː/ *n* a female sheep.

ewer /'juːər/ *n* a large pitcher or jug with a wide spout.

ex[1] /ɛks/ *n* (*inf*) a former husband, wife, etc.

ex[2] *prep* out of, from.

ex- *prefix* out, forth; quite, entirely; formerly.

exacerbate /ɛk'sæsərˌbeɪt/ or /ɪg-/ *vt* to make more violent, bitter, or severe.—**exacerbatingly** *adv*.—**exacerbation** *n*.

exact /ɪg'zækt/ *adj* without error, absolutely accurate; detailed. • *vt* to compel by force, to extort; to require.—**exactable** *adj*.—**exactness** *n*.—**exactor, exacter** *n*.

exacting /ɪg'zæktɪŋ/ *adj* greatly demanding; requiring close attention and precision.—**exactingness** *n*.

exaction /ɪg'zækʃən/ *n* the extortion of money, etc; an outrageous demand; something exacted.

exactitude /ɪg'zæktɪˌtuːd/ or /-ˌtjuːd/ *n* (the state of) being exact.

exactly /ɪg'zæktli/ *adv* in an exact manner; precisely. • *interj* quite so!

exactor /ɪg'zæktər/ *n* ♣ (*Cdn*) a bet on the first-and second-place finishers in a horse race, specifying their order of finishing.

exaggerate /ɪg'zædʒəˌreɪt/ *vt* to enlarge (a statement, etc) beyond what is really so or believable.—**exaggeration** *n*.—**exaggerative** *adj*.—**exaggerator** *n*.

exalt /ɪg'zɒlt/ *vt* to raise up, *esp* in rank, power, or dignity.—**exalted** *adj*.—**exalter** *n*.

exaltation /ˌɛgzɒl'teɪʃən/ *n* elevation; rapture; a flock of larks.

exam /ɪg'zæm/ *n* (*inf*) an examination.

examination /ɪgˌzæmɪ'neɪʃən/ *n* an examining, close scrutiny; a set of written or oral questions designed as a test of knowledge; the formal questioning of a witness on oath.—**examinational** *adj*.

examination for discovery *n* ♣ (*Cdn*) a meeting before the start of a trial in civil law to disclose what evidence will be presented.

examine /ɪg'zæmɪn/ *vt* to look at closely and carefully, to investigate; to test, *esp* by questioning.—**examinable** *adj*.—**examiner** *n*.

examinee /ɪgˌzæmɪ'niː/ *n* a person who is being tested in an examination.

example /ɪg'zæmpəl/ *n* a representative sample; a model to be followed or avoided; a problem to be solved in order to show the application of some rule; a warning to others.

exanimate /ɛks'ænɪmət/ *adj* dead, defunct, lifeless.—**exanimation** *n*.

exarch /'ɛksark/ *n* a bishop of the Eastern Orthodox Church; the governor of a province under the Byzantine Empire.

exarchate, exarchy /ɛk'sarkɪt/ or /-ˌkeɪt/, /'ɛksˌar-/ *n* the area of jurisdiction of an exarch.

exasperate /ɪg'zæspəˌreɪt/ *vt* to annoy intensely.—**exasperatedly** *adv*.—**exasperating** *adj*.—**exasperation** *n*.

Excalibur /ɛks'kælɪbər/ *n* in legend, King Arthur's sword.

ex cathedra /ˌɛkskə'θiːdrə/ *adj* with authority.

excavate /'ɛkskəˌveɪt/ *vt* to form a hole or tunnel by digging; to unearth; to expose to view (historical remains, etc) by digging away a covering.—**excavation** *n*.—**excavator** *n*.

exceed /ɛk'siːd/ or /ɪk-/ *vt* to be greater than or superior to; to go beyond the limit of.—**exceedable** *adj*.—**exceeder** *n*.

exceedingly /-ɪŋli/ *adv* very, extremely.

excel /ɛk'sɛl/ or /ɪk-/ *vb* (**excelling, excelled**) *vt* to outdo, to be superior to. • *vi* (*with* **in, at**) to do better than others.

excellence /'ɛksələns/ *n* that in which one excels; superior merit or quality; (*with cap*) a title of honour given to certain high officials.—*also* **Excellency**.

excellent /'ɛksələnt/ *adj* very good, outstanding.—**excellently** *adv*.

excelsior /ɛk'sɛlsiˌɔr/ or /ɪk-/ *interj* higher. • *n* soft wood shavings for stuffing.

except /ɛk'sept/ or /ɪk-/ *vt* to exclude, to leave out. • *prep* not including; other than.—**exceptable** *adj*.

excepting /-'septɪŋ/ *prep* except, not including.

exception /ɛk'sepʃən/ or /ɪk-/ *n* the act of excepting; something excepted; an objection.

exceptionable /-əbəl/ *adj* open to objection.—**exceptionably** *adv*.

exceptional /ɛk'sepʃənəl/ or /ɪk-/ *adj* unusual, forming an exception; superior.—**exceptionally** *adv*.

excerpt /'ɛksɜrpt/ or /'ɛgz-/ *n* an extract from a book, film, etc. • *vt* to select or quote (a passage from a book).—**exerptible** *adj*.—**excerption** *n*.

excess /'ɛksɛs/ or /ɪk'-/ *n, adj* the exceeding of proper established limits; the amount by which one thing or quantity exceeds another; (*pl*) overindulgence in eating or drinking; unacceptable conduct.

excessive /ɛk'sɛsəv/ *adj* greater than what is acceptable, too much.—**excessively** *adv*.—**excessiveness** *n*.

exchange /ɛks'tʃeɪndʒ/ *vt* to give and take (one thing in return for another); to give to and receive from another person. • *n* the exchanging of one thing for another; the thing exchanged; the conversion of money in one currency into a sum of equivalent value in another currency; the system of settling commercial debts between foreign governments, *eg* by bills of exchange; a place where things and services are exchanged, *esp* a marketplace for securities; a centre or device in which telephone lines are interconnected.—**exchangeable** *adj.*—**exchangeability** *n.*—**exchanger** *n.*

exchange rate *n* the rate at which one foreign currency may be exchanged for another.

exchequer /ɛks'tʃɛkər/ *n* (*with cap*) the British governmental department in charge of finances; (*inf*) persona finances.

excise[1] /'ɛksaɪz/ *n* a tax on the manufacture, sale, or use of certain articles within a country.—**excisable** *adj.*

excise[2] /ɛk'saɪz/ *vt* to remove by cutting out.—**excision** *n.*

exciseman /'ɛksaɪzˌmæn/ *n* (*pl* **excisemen**) (*formerly*) an officer employed to collect and enforce excise.

excitable /ɛk'saɪtəbəl/ *adj* easily excited.—**excitability, excitableness** *n.*

excitant /'ɛksɪtənt/ or /ɪk'saɪtənt/ *n* a stimulant. • *adj* stimulating.

excitation /ˌɛksaɪ'teɪʃən/ or /-sɪ-/ *n* the act of exciting; the state of excitement.—**excitative, excitatory** *adj.*

excite /ɛk'saɪt/ or /ɪk-/ *vt* to arouse the feelings of, *esp* to generate feelings of pleasurable anticipation; to cause to experience strong emotion; to stir up, agitate; to rouse to activity; to stimulate a physiological response, *eg* in a bodily organ.

excited /-əd/ *adj* experiencing or expressing excitement.—**excitedly** *adv.*—**excitedness** *n.*

excitement /ɛk'saɪtmənt/ or /ɪk-/ *n* a feeling of strong, *esp* pleasurable, emotion; something that excites.

exciting /ɪk'saɪtɪŋ/ *adj* causing excitement; stimulating.—**excitingly** *adv.*

exclaim /ɪk'skleɪm/ *vti* to shout out or utter suddenly and with strong emotion.—**exclaimer** *n.*

exclamation /ˌɛksklə'meɪʃən/ *n* a sudden crying out; a word or utterance exclaimed.—**exclamational** *adj.*

exclamation point, exclamation mark *n* the punctuation mark (!) placed after an exclamation.

exclamatory /ɪk'sklæməˌtɔri/ *adj* of or expressing exclamation.—**exclamatorily** *adv.*

exclave /'ɛkskleɪv/ *n* a small part of a country lying within the territory of another country.

exclude /ɛk'sklu:d/ *vt* to shut out, to keep out; to reject or omit; to eject.—**excluder** *n.*—**exclusion** *n.*

exclusive /ɛk'sklu:sɪv/ or /ɪks-/ *adj* excluding all else; reserved for particular persons; snobbishly aloof; fashionable, high-class, expensive; unobtainable or unpublished elsewhere; sole, undivided.—**exclusively** *adv.*—**exclusiveness** *n.*—**exclusivity** *n.*

excogitate /ɛks'kɒdʒɪˌteɪt/ *vt* to devise, to invent; to discover by thinking.—**excogitation** *n.*—**excogitative** *adj.*

excommunicate /ˌɛkskə'mju:nɪˌkeɪt/ *vt* to bar from association with a church; to exclude from fellowship.—**excommunication** *n.*—**excommunicative** *adj.*—**excommunicator** *n.*

excoriate /ɛks'kɔriˌeɪt/ *vt* to strip of the skin; to flay.—**excoriation** *n.*

excrement /'ɛkskrəmənt/ *n* waste matter discharged from the bowels.—**excremental, excrementitious** *adj.*

excrescence /ɛk'skrɛsəns/ *n* an outgrowth, *esp* abnormal, from a plant or animal; a disfigurement.

excrescent /ɛk'skrɛsənt/ *adj* pertaining to excrescence; superfluous.

excreta /ɛk'skri:tə/ or /ɪk-/ *npl* waste matter discharged from the body, faeces, urine.

excrete /ɪk'skri:t/ *vt* to eliminate or discharge wastes from the body.—**excreter** *n.*—**excretion** *n.*—**excretive, excretory** *adj.*

excruciate /ɪk'skru:ʃiˌeɪt/ *vt* to inflict severe pain upon; to torture.—**excruciation** *n.*

excruciating /-ˌeɪtɪŋ/ *adj* intensely painful or distressful; (*inf*) very bad.—**excruciatingly** *adv.*

exculpate /'ɛkskəlˌpeɪt/ *vt* to free (a person) from alleged fault or guilt.—**exculpable** *adj.*—**exculpation** *n.*

exculpatory /-'kəlpəˌtɔri/ *adj* tending or serving to exculpate.

excurrent /ɛks'kərənt/ *adj* (*bot*) (*leaf*) having a midrib running beyond the edge; (*tree*) having a projecting stem; (*zool*) having a duct, etc, whose contents flow out.

excursion /ɪk'skərʃən/ *n* a pleasure trip; a short journey.

excursionist /-ɪst/ *n* someone going on an excursion.

excursive /ɛks'kərsɪv/ *adj* digressing, rambling.—**excursively** *adv.*

excursus /ɛk'skərsəs/ or /ɪk-/ *n* (*pl* **excursuses, excursus**) a dissertation added as a supplement to a work, giving additional information on certain points; a digression from the main subject of a work.

excusable /ɪk'skju:zəbəl/ *adj* able to be excused.—**excusably** *adv.*

excuse /ɪk'skju:z/ *vt* to pardon; to forgive; to give a reason or apology for; to be a reason or explanation of; to let off. • *n* an apology, a plea in extenuation.

ex-directory /ˌɛksdaɪ'rɛktəri/ *adj* (*telephone number*) not listed in the telephone directory by request.

execrable /'ɛksɪkrəbəl/ *adj* appalling.—**execrableness** *n.*

execrate /'ɛksɪˌkreɪt/ *vt* to denounce as evil; to abhor.—**execration** *n.*—**execrative, execratory** *adj.*

executant /ɪg'zɛkjutənt/ *n* a person who executes or performs, *esp* an artist, musician, etc.

execute /'ɛksɪˌkju:t/ *vt* to carry out, put into effect; to perform; to produce (*eg* a work of art); to make legally valid; to put to death by law.—**executable** *adj.*—**executer** *n.*

execution /ˌɛksɪ'kju:ʃən/ *n* the act or process of executing; the carrying out or suffering of a death sentence; the style or technique of performing, *eg* music.

executioner /-ər/ *n* a person who executes a death sentence upon a condemned prisoner.

executive /ɪg'zɛkjutɪv/ *n* a person or group concerned with administration or management of a business or organization; the branch of government with the power to put laws, etc into effect. • *adj* having the power to execute decisions, laws, decrees, etc.

executor /-ər/ *n* a person appointed by a testator to see the terms of a will implemented.—**executorial** *adj.*—**executorship** *n.*

executory /ɪg'zɛkjuˌtɔri/ *adj* (*law*) pertaining to the execution of laws; to be carried out at a future date.

executrix /ɪg'zɛkjutrɪks/ *n* (*pl* **executrices, executrixes**) a female executor.

exegesis /ˌɛksɪ'dʒɪsɪs/ *n* (*p*° **exegeses**) an explanation or interpretation of a text or passage, *esp* of the Bible.

exegetic, exegetical /ˌɛksə'dʒɛtɪk/ *adj* expository; interpretative.

exegetics /ˌɛksə'dʒɛtɪks/ *n sing* the study of exegesis.

exemplar /ɪg'zɛmplər/ or /-ˌplɑr/ *n* a model; a typical instance or example.

exemplary /ɪg'zɛmpləri/ *adj* deserving imitation; serving as a warning.—**exemplarily** *adv.*—**exemplariness** *n.*

exemplify /ɪg'zɛmplɪˌfaɪ/ *vt* (**exemplifying, exemplified**) to illustrate by example; to be an instance or example of.—**exemplification** *n.*—**exemplifier** *n.*

exempt /ɪg'zɛmpt/ *adj* not liable, free from the obligations required of others. • *vt* to grant immunity (from).—**exemptible** *adj.*—**exemption** *n.*

exercise /'ɛksərˌsaɪz/ *n* the use or application of a power or right; regular physical or mental exertion for health, amusement or acquisition of some skill; something performed to develop or test a specific ability or skill; (*often pl*) manoeuvres carried out for military training and discipline. • *vt* to use, exert, employ; to engage in regular physical activity to strengthen the body, etc; to train (troops) by means of drills and manoeuvres; to engage the attention of; to perplex.—**exercisable** *adj.*

exergue /ɛg'zərg/ or /'ɛk-/ *n* the space below the principal design on a coin or medal for the insertion of a date, etc.—**exergual** *adj.*

exert /ɪg'zərt/ *vt* to bring (*eg* strength, influence) into use.

exertion /ɪg'zərʃən/ *n* an exerting; a strenuous effort.—**exertive** *adj.*

exeunt /'ɛksɪˌənt/ (*Latin*) they go off, a stage direction.

exfoliate /ɛks'fo:liˌeɪt/ *vi* to flake off; (*tree*) to shed bark.—**exfoliation** *n.*

ex gratia /ɛks'greɪʃə/ *adj* given as a favour or where no legal obligation exists.

exhalant /ɛks'heɪlənt/ or /ɪgz-/ *adj* exhaling. • *n* a duct, organ, etc used for exhaling.

exhale /ɛks'heɪl/ or /ɪgz-/ *vt* to breathe out.—**exhalation** *n.*

exhaust /ɛg'zɒst/ or /ɪg-/ *vt* to use up completely; to make empty; to use up, tire out; (*subject*) to deal with or develop completely. • *n* the escape of waste gas or steam from an engine; the device through which these escape.—**exhausted** *adj.*—**exhauster** *n.*—**exhaustible** *adj.*—**exhausting** *adj.*

exhaustion /ɛg'zɒstʃən/ or /ɪg-/ *n* the act of exhausting or being exhausted; extreme weariness.

exhaustive /ɛg'zɒstɪv/ or /ɪg-/ *adj* comprehensive, thorough.—**exhaustively** *adv.*

exhibit /ɛg'zɪbɪt/ or /ɪg-/ *vt* to display, *esp* in public; to present to a court in legal form. • *n* an act or instance of exhibiting, something exhibited; something produced and identified in court for use as evidence.—**exhibitor** *n.*—**exhibitory** *adj.*

exhibition /ˌɛgsɪ'bɪʃən/ *n* a showing, a display; a public show; an allowance made to a student; ❧ (*Cdn*) a large fair that includes agricultural exhibits and craft displays.

exhibitioner /-ər/ *n* a student who holds an exhibition.

exhibitionism /-ˌnɪzəm/ *n* an excessive tendency to show off one's abilities; a compulsion to expose oneself indecently in public.—**exhibitionist** *n*.—**exhibitionistic** *adj*.

exhilarant /ɛg'zɪlərənt/ or /ɪg-/ *adj* exhilarating. • *n* something that exhilarates.

exhilarate /ɛg'zɪləˌreɪt/ or /ɪg-/ *vt* to make very happy; to invigorate.—**exhilarating** *adj*.—**exhilaration** *n*.—**exhilarator** *n*.

exhort /ɛg'zɔrt/ or /ɪg-/ *vt* to urge or advise strongly.—**exhortation** *n*.—**exhortative, exhortatory** *adj*.—**exhorter** *n*.

exhume /ɛks'u:m/ or /ɪgz-/, /ɛgz-/, /-hju:m/ *vt* to dig up (a dead person) for detailed examination.—**exhumation** *n*.—**exhumer** *n*.

exigency, exigence /'ɛksɪdʒənsi/ or /ɛg'zɪdʒən-/, /ɪg-/ *n* (*pl* **exigencies, exigences**) a pressing need; emergency.

exigent /'ɛksɪdʒənt/ or /ɛgz-/ *adj* urgent; exacting.—**exigently** *adv*.

exigible /'ɛksɪdʒəbəl/ *adj* (*debt etc*) liable to be exacted.

exiguous—**exiguity** /ɛg'zɪgjʊəs/ or /ɪg-/ *adj* very small in amount, measure.—**exiguity, exiguousness** *n*.

exile /'ɛksaɪl/ or /'ɛgzaɪl/ *n* prolonged absence from one's own country, either through choice or as a punishment; an exiled person. • *vt* to banish, to expel from one's native land.—**exilic, exilian** *adj*.

exist /ɛg'zɪst/ or /ɪg-/ *vi* to have being; to just manage a living; to occur in a specific place under specific conditions.

existence /ɛg'zɪstəns/ or /ɪg-/ *n* the state or fact of existing; continuance of life; lifestyle; everything that exists.

existent /ɛg'zɪstənt/ or /ɪg-/ *adj* real, actual; existing; current.

existential /ˌɛgzɪ'stɛnʃəl/ or /ˌɛksɪs-/ *adj* of or pertaining to existence; existentialist.

existentialism /-ˌlɪzəm/ *n* (*philos*) a movement stressing personal freedom and responsibility in relation to existence.—**existentialist** *n, adj*.

exit /'ɛksɪt/ or /'ɛgzɪt/ *n* a way out of an enclosed space; death; a departure from a stage. • *vi* to leave, withdraw; to go offstage.

ex libris /ɛks'li:brɪːs/ *adj* from the library of. • *n* (*pl* **ex libris**) a book plate.

exocrine /'ɛksoˌkraɪn/ *adj* secreting though a duct; of or relating to exocrine glands or their secretions.

exocrine gland *n* a gland that releases secretions through a duct, *eg* a sweat gland.

exoderm *see* **ectoderm**.

exodus /'ɛksədəs/ *n* the departure of many people; (*with cap*) the departure of the Israelites from Egypt led by Moses; (*Bible*) the second book of the Old Testament.

ex officio /ˌɛksə'fɪʃɪo/ or /-'fɪs-/ *adv, adj* by virtue of an official position.

exogamy /ɛk'sɒgəmi/ *n* the practice of marrying only outside one's own tribe.—**exogamous** *adj*.

exogenous /ɛk'sɒdʒənəs/ *adj* (*biol*) produced by external growth; a used or influenced by external factors.—**exogenously** *adv*.

exonerate /ɪg'zɒnəˌreɪt/ *vt* to absolve from blame; to relieve from a responsibility, obligation.—**exoneration** *n*.—**exonerative** *adj*.—**exonerator** *n*.

exophthalmos, exophthalmus /ˌɛksɒf'θælməs/ *n* protrusion of the eyeball.—**exophthalmic** *adj*.

exorbitant /ɪg'zɔrbɪtənt/ *adj* (*prices, demands, etc*) unreasonable, excessive.—**exorbitance** *n*.

exorcise, exorcize /'ɛksɔrˌsaɪz/ or /-ər-/ *vt* to expel an evil spirit (from a person or place) by ritual and prayer.—**exorciser, exorcizer** *n*.—**exorcism** *n*.—**exorcist** *n*.

exordium /ɛk'sɔrdiəm/ *n* (*pl* **exordiums, exordia**) the opening part of a speech or composition.—**exordial** *adj*.

exoteric /ɛkso'tɛrɪk/ *adj* accessible to ordinary people; external.—**exoterically** *adv*.—**exotericism** *n*.

exotic /ɛg'zɒtɪk/ or /ɪg-/ *adj* foreign; strange; excitingly different or unusual.—**exotically** *adv*.—**exoticism** *n*.—**exoticness** *n*.

exotica /-ɪkə/ *npl* exotic items, *esp* as a collection.

expand /ɛk'spænd/ or /ɪk-/ *vt* to increase in size, bulk, extent, importance; to describe in fuller detail. • *vi* to become larger; to become more genial and responsive.—**expandable, expandible** *adj*.—**expander** *n*.

expanse /ɛk'spæns/ or /ɪk-/ *n* a wide area of land, etc; the extent of a spread-out area.

expansible /ɛk'spænsəbəl/ or /ɪk-/ *adj* capable of expansion, or of being expanded.—**expansibility** *n*.

expansile /-saɪl/ *adj* capable of expansion, or of causing expansion.

expansion /-ʃən/ *n* the act of expanding or being expanded; something expanded; the amount by which something expands; the fuller development of a theme, etc.—**expansionary** *adj*.

expansive /-sɪv/ *adj* able to or having the capacity to expand or cause expansion; comprehensive; (*person*) genial, communicative.—**expansively** *adv*.—**expansiveness** *n*.

ex parte /ɛks'parti/ *adj* (*law*) on behalf of one side only; partisan.

expatiate /ɛk'speɪʃiˌeɪt/ or /ɪk-/ *vi* to speak or write at length; to enlarge.—**expatiation** *n*.—**expatiator** *n*.

expatriate /ɛks'peɪtriət/ or /-'pætriət/ *adj* living in another country; self-exiled or banished. • *n* an expatriate person. • *vti* to exile (oneself) or banish (another person). —**expatriation** *n*.

expect /ɛk'spɛkt/ or /ɪk-/ *vt* to anticipate; to regard as likely to arrive or happen; to consider necessary, reasonable or due; to think, suppose.

expectant /ɛk'spɛktənt/ or /ɪk-/ *adj* expecting, hopeful; filled with anticipation; pregnant.—**expectantly** *adv*.—**expectancy, expectance** *n*.

expectation /ˌɛkspɛk'teɪʃən/ *n* the act or state of expecting; something that is expected to happen; (*pl*) prospects for the future, *esp* of inheritance.—**expectative** *adj*.

expectorant /ɛk'spɛktərənt/ *n* a medicine that promotes expectoration.

expectorate /ɛk'spɛktəˌreɪt/ *vti* to bring up (mucus) from the respiratory tract by coughing; to spit.—**expectoration** *n*.—**expectorator** *n*.

expedience, expediency /ɛk'spi:diənsi/ or /ɪk-/ *n* (*pl* **expediencies, expediences**) fitness, suitability; an inclination towards expedient methods.—**expediential** *adj*.

expedient /ɛk'spi:diənt/ or /ɪk-/ *adj* suitable or desirable under the circumstances. • *n* a means to an end; a means devised or used for want of something better.—**expediently** *adv*.

expedite /'ɛkspəˌdɔɪt/ *vt* to carry out promptly; to facilitate.—**expediter, expeditor** *n*.

expedition /ˌɛkspə'dɪʃən/ *n* a journey to achieve some purpose, as exploration, etc; the party making this journey; speedy efficiency, promptness.

expeditionary /ˌɛkspə'dɪʃəˌnɛri/ *adj* of or constituting an expedition.

expeditious /ˌɛkspə'dɪʃəs/ *adj* speedy; efficient.—**expeditiously** *adv*.

expel /ɛk'spɛl/ or /ɪk-/ *vt* (**expelling, expelled**) to drive out, to eject; to banish.—**expellable** *adj*.—**expellee** *n*.—**expeller** *n*.

expend /ɛk'spɛnd/ or /ɪk-/ *vt* to spend (money, time, energy, etc); to use up, consume.—**expender** *n*.

expendable /ɛk'spɛndəbəl/ or /ɪk-/ *adj* able to be consumed, not worth keeping; available for sacrifice to achieve some objective.—**expendability** *n*.

expenditure /ɛk'spɛndɪtʃər/ or /ɪk-/ *n* the act or process of expending money, etc; the amount expended.

expense /ɛk'spɛns/ or /ɪk-/ *n* a payment of money for something, expenditure; a cause of expenditure; (*pl*) money spent on some activity (*eg* travelling on business); reimbursement for this.

expense account *n* an account of expenses to be reimbursed to an employee.

expensive /ɛk'spɛnsɪv/ or /ɪk-/ *adj* causing or involving great expense; costly.—**expensively** *adv*.—**expensiveness** *n*.

experience /ɛk'spi:riəns/ or /ɪk-/ *n* observation or practice resulting in or tending towards knowledge; knowledge gained by seeing and doing; a state of being affected from without (as by events); an affecting event. • *vt* to have experience of.

experienced /-ənst/ *adj* wise or skilled through experience.

experiential /ɛkˌspi:ri'ɛnʃəl/ or /ɪk-/ *adj* of or based on experience.

experiment /ɛk'spɛrɪmənt/ or /ɪk-/, /-ˌmɛnt/ *n* any test or trial to find out something; a controlled procedure carried out to discover, test, or demonstrate something. • *vi* to carry out experiments.—**experimentation** *n*.—**experimenter** *n*.

experimental /ɛkˌspɛri'mɛntəl/ or /ɪk-/ *adj* of, derived from, or proceeding by experiment; empirical; provisional.—**experimentalism** *n*.—**experimentally** *adv*.

expert /'ɛkspərt/ *adj* thoroughly skilled; knowledgeable through training and experience. • *n* a person with special skills or training in any art or science.—**expertly** *adv*.—**expertness** *n*.

expertise /ˌɛkspər'tiːz/ *n* expert knowledge or skill.

expiate /'ɛkspɪˌeɪt/ *vt* to pay the penalty for; to make amends for.—**expiation** *n*.—**expiator** *n*.—**expiatory** *adj*.

expire /ɛk'spaɪr/ or /ɪk-/ *vti* to come to an end; to lapse or become void; to breathe out; to die.—**expiration** *n*.—**expirer** *n*.

expiry /ɛk'spaɪəri/ or /ɪk-/ *n* (*pl* **expiries**) the ending of a period of validity, *eg* of a passport.

explain /ɛk'spleɪn/ or /ɪk-/ *vt* to make plain or clear; to give a reason for, account for.—**explainable** *adj*.—**explainer** *n*.

explanation /ˌɛksplə'neɪʃən/ *n* an act or process of explaining; something that explains, *esp* a statement.

explanative, explanatory /ɛk'splænəˌtori/ or /ɪk-/ *adj* serving as an explanation.—**explanatorily** *adv*.

expletive /'ɛksplətɪv/ or /ɪk'spliːtəv/ *n* a violent exclamation or swearword.

explicable /'ɛksplɪkəbəl/ or /ɪk'splɪkəbəl/ *adj* able to be explained.

explicate /'ɛksplɪˌkeɪt/ *vt* to analyse the implications of; to explain in great detail.—**explication** *n*.—**explicative, explicatory** *adj*.—**explicator** *n*.

explicit /ɛk'splɪsɪt/ or /ɪk-/ *adj* clearly stated, not merely implied; outspoken, frank; graphically detailed.—**explicitly** *adv*.—**explicitness** *n*.

explode /ɛk'sploːd/ or /ɪk-/ *vti* to burst or cause to blow up with a loud noise, as in the detonation of a bomb; (*emotions*) to burst out; (*population*) to increase rapidly; to expose (a theory, etc) as false.—**exploder** *n*.

exploit /'ɛksplɔɪt/ or /ɪk-/ *n* a bold achievement. • *vt* to utilize, develop (raw materials, etc); to take unfair advantage of, *esp* for financial gain.—**exploitable** *adj*.—**exploitation** *n*.—**exploitative** *adj*.

exploratory, explorative /ɛk'splorəˌtori/ or /ɪk-/ *adj* for the purpose of exploring or investigating.

explore /ɛk'splor/ or /ɪk-/ *vti* to examine or inquire into; to travel through (a country) for the purpose of (geographical) discovery; to examine minutely.—**exploration** *n*.—**explorer** *n*.

explosion /ɛk'sploːʒən/ or /ɪk-/ *n* an act or instance of exploding; a sudden loud noise caused by this; an outburst of emotion; a rapid increase or expansion.

explosive /ɛk'sploːsɪv/ or /ɪk-/ *adj* liable to or able to explode; liable or threatening to burst out with violence and noise. • *n* an explosive substance.—**explosively** *adv*.

exponent /ɛk'spoːnənt/ or /ɪk-/ *n* a person who explains or interprets something; a person who champions, advocates, or exemplifies; (*math*) an index of the power to which an expression is raised.

exponential /ˌɛkspo'nɛnʃəl/ or /-tʃəl/ *adj* of, relating to or having an exponent; (*math*) having a variable in an exponent; able to be expressed by an exponential function. • *n* an exponential function.—**exponentially** *adv*.

exponential function *n* a mathematical function in which the constant quantity of the expression is raised to the power of a variable quantity, i.e. the exponent.

export /'ɛksˌport/ *vt* to send out (goods) of one country for sale in another. • *n* the act of exporting; the article exported.—**exportable** *adj*.—**exportation** *n*.—**exporter** *n*.

exposé /ˌɛkspo'zeɪ/ *n* a revelation of crime, dishonesty, etc.

expose /ɛk'spoːz/ or /ɪk-/ *vt* to deprive of protection or shelter; to subject to an influence (as light, weather); to display, reveal; to uncover or disclose.—**exposable** *adj*.—**exposal** *n*.—**exposer** *n*.

exposed /ɪk'spoːzd/ or /ɛk-/ *adj* open to view; not shielded or protected.—**exposedness** *n*.

exposition /ˌɛkspo'zɪʃən/ *n* a public show or exhibition; a detailed explanation; a speech or writing explaining a process, thing, or idea.—**expositional** *adj*.

expositive, expository /ɛk'spozɪˌtori/ or /ɪk-/ *adj* of, pertaining to or conveying exposition; explanatory.—**expositively, expositorily** *adv*.

ex post facto /ˌɛkspo'st'fækto/ *adj* (*law*) enacted retrospectively. • *adv* after the fact.

expostulate /ɛk'spostʃəˌleɪt/ or /ɪk-/ *vi* to argue with, *esp* to dissuade.—**expostulation** *n*.—**expostulator** *n*.—**expostulatory, expostulative** *adj*.

exposure /ɛk'spoːʒər/ or /ɪk-/ *n* an exposing or state of being exposed; time during which light reaches and acts on a photographic film, paper or plate; publicity.

expound /ɛk'spaʊnd/ or /ɪk-/ *vt* to explain or set forth in detail.—**expounder** *n*.

express /ɛk'sprɛs/ or /ɪk-/ *vt* to represent in words; to make known one's thoughts, feelings, etc; to represent by signs, symbols, etc; to squeeze out. • *adj* firmly stated, explicit; (*train, bus, etc*) travelling at high speed with few or no stops. • *adv* at high speed, by express service. • *n* an express train, coach, etc; a system or company for sending freight, etc at rates higher than standard.—**expresser** *n*.—**expressible** *adj*.

expression /ɛk'sprɛʃən/ or /ɪk-/ *n* an act of expressing, *esp* by words; a word or phrase; a look; intonation; a manner of showing feeling in communicating or performing (*eg* music); (*math*) a collection of symbols serving to express something.—**expressional** *adj*.—**expressionless** *adj*.

expressionism /-ˌnɪzəm/ *n* a style of art, literature, music, etc that seeks to depict the subjective emotions aroused in the artist by objects and events, not objective reality.—**expressionist** *n*.—**expressionistic** *adj*.

expressive /ɛk'sprɛsɪv/ or /ɪk-/ *adj* serving to express; full of expression.—**expressively** *adv*.—**expressiveness** *n*.

expressly /ɛk'sprɛsli/ or /ɪk-/ *adv* explicitly; for a specific purpose.

expressway /ɛk'sprɛsweɪ/ or /ɪk-/ *n* a motorway.

expropriate /ɛks'proːpriˌeɪt/ *vt* to remove (property) from its owner; to dispossess.—**expropriable** *adj*.—**expropriation** *n*.—**expropriator** *n*.

expulsion /ɛk'spʌlʃən/ or /ɪk-/ *n* the act of expelling or being expelled.—**expulsive** *adj*.

expunge /ɛk'spʌndʒ/ or /ɪk-/ *vt* to obliterate, to erase.—**expunction** *n*.—**expunger** *n*.

expurgate /'ɛkspərˌgeɪt/ *vt* to cut from a book, play, etc any parts supposed to be offensive or erroneous.—**expurgation** *n*.—**expurgator** *n*.—**expurgatory, expurgatorial** *adj*.

exquisite /'ɛkskwɪzɪt/ or /ɛk'skwɪzɪt/ *adj* very beautiful, refined; sensitive, showing discrimination; acutely felt, as pain or pleasure.—**exquisitely** *adv*.

exsanguinate /ɛk'sæŋwɪˌneɪt/ *vt* to drain of blood.—**exsanguination** *n*.

exsanguine /ɛk'sæŋwɪn/ *adj* bloodless.

exscind /ɛk'sɪnd/ *vt* to cut off; to cut out, excise.

exsert /ɛk'sərt/ or /ɪk-/ *vt* to thrust outwards.—**exsertile** *adj*.—**exsertion** *n*.

exsiccate /'ɛksɪˌkeɪt/ *vt* to dry up.—**exsiccation** *n*.

extant /'ɛkstənt/ or /ɛk'stænt/, /ɪk-/ *adj* still existing.

extemporaneous /ɛkˌstɛmpə'reɪniəs/ or /ɪkˌstɛm-/, **extemporary** /ɛk'stɛmpəˌreri/ or /ɪk-/ *adj* spoken, acted, etc without preparation.—**extemporaneously, extemporarily** *adv*.

extempore /ɛk'stɛmpəri/ or /ɪk-/ *adv, adj* without preparation, impromptu.

extemporize /-ˌraɪz/ *vi* to do something extemporaneously.—**extemporization** *n*.

extend /ɛk'stɛnd/ or /ɪk-/ *vt* to stretch or spread out; to stretch fully; to prolong in time; to cause to reach in distance, etc; to enlarge, increase the scope of; to hold out (*eg* the hand); to accord, grant; to give, offer, (*eg* sympathy). • *vi* to prolong in distance or time; to reach in scope.

extended family /ɛk'stɛndəd/ *n* a family with three or more generations of blood relations living as a unit.

extendible, extendable /-ˌcəbəl/ *adj* able to be extended.—**extendibility, extendability** *n*.

extensible /ɛk'stɛnsɪbəl/ or /ɪk-/, **extensile** *adj* extendible.—**extensibility, extensibleness** *n*.

extension /-ʃən/ *n* the act of extending or state of being extended; extent, scope; an added part, *eg* to a building; an extra period; a programme of extramural teaching provided by a college, etc; an additional telephone connected to the principal line.

extensive /ɛk'stɛnsɪv/ or /ɪk-/ *adj* large; having a wide scope or extent.—**extensively** *adv*.—**extensiveness** *n*.

extensometer /ˌɛkstɛn'somɪtər/ *n* a type of micrometer for measuring the expansion of a body.

extensor /ɛk'stɛnsər/ or /ɪk-/ *n* a muscle that extends or straightens a limb.

extent /ɛk'stɛnt/ or /ɪk-/ *n* the distance over which a thing is extended; the range or scope of something; the limit to which something extends.

extenuate /ɛk'stɛnjʊˌeɪt/ or /ɪk-/ vt to make (guilt, a fault, or offence) seem less.—**extenuating** adj.—**extenuator** n.—**extenuatory** adj.

extenuation /ɛkˌstɛnjʊ'eɪʃən/ or /ɪk-/ n an extenuating or being extenuated, partial justification; something that extenuates, an excuse.

exterior /ɛk'stiːrɪər/ or /ɪk-/ adj of, on, or coming from the outside; external; (paint, etc) suitable for use on the outside. • n the external part or surface; outward manner or appearance.

exteriorize /ɛk'stiːrɪəraɪz/ or /ɪk-/ vt to externalize; (med) to move (an organ, etc) out of the body, usu to facilitate surgery.

exterminate /ɛk'stɜːrmɪˌneɪt/ or /ɪk-/ vt to destroy completely.—**exterminable** adj.—**extermination** n.—**exterminatory** adj.

exterminator /ɛk'stɜːrmɪˌneɪtər/ or /ɪk-/ n one who or that which exterminates; a person who is employed to destroy pests, etc.

extern, externe /'ɛkstɜːrn/ n a non-resident doctor.

external /ɛk'stɜːrnəl/ or /ɪk-/ adj outwardly perceivable; of, relating to, or located on the outside or outer part. • n an external feature.—**externally** adv.

externality /ˌɛkstɜːr'næliti/ or /ɪk-/ n (pl externalities) a being external or externalized; something external; (philos) a being external to the perceiving mind.

externalize /ɛk'stɜːrnəˌlaɪz/ or /ɪk-/ vt to make external; to attribute an external existence to; to express (feelings, etc) esp in words; (psychol) to project (opinions, feelings) onto others or one's surroundings.—**externalization** n.

exterritorial /ˌɛkstɛrɪ'tɔːrɪəl/ adj extraterritorial.—**exterritoriality** n.

extinct /ɛk'stɪŋkt/ or /ɪk-/ adj (animals) not alive, no longer existing; (fire) not burning, out; (volcano) no longer active.—**extinction** n.

extine n (bot) the outer coat of the pollen grain.

extinguish /ɪk'stɪŋgwɪʃ/ vt to put out (a fire, light, etc); to bring to an end.—**extinguishable** adj.—**extinguishment** n.

extinguisher /-ər/ n a device for putting out a fire.

extirpate /'ɛkstər̩peɪt/ vt to destroy totally, as by uprooting.—**extirpation** n.—**extirpative** adj.—**extirpator** n.

extol, extoll /ɪk'stoːl/ vt (extols or extolls, extolling, extolled) to praise highly.—**extoller** n.—**extollment, extolment** n.

extort /ɪk'stɔːrt/ vt to obtain (money, promises, etc) by force or improper pressure.—**extorter** n.—**extortive** adj.

extortion /ɛk'stɔːrʃən/ or /ɪk-/ n the act or practice of extorting; the criminal instance of this; oppressive or unjust exaction.—**extortionary** adj.—**extortioner, extortionist** n.

extortionate /-ʃənət/ adj exorbitant; excessively high in price.—**extortionately** adv.

extra /'ɛkstrə/ adj additional. • adv unusually; in addition. • n something extra or additional, esp a charge; a special edition of a newspaper; a person who plays a non-speaking role in a film.

extra- /'ɛkstrə/ prefix outside, beyond.

extra-billing /'ɛkstrəˌbɪlɪŋ/ n ✲ (Cdn) the charging of fees by a doctor to a patient in excess of what a public health insurance pays.

extract /ɪk'strækt/ vt to take or pull out by force; to withdraw by chemical or physical means; to abstract, excerpt. • n the essence of a substance obtained by extraction; a passage taken from a book, play, film, etc.—**extractable, extractible** adj.—**extractability, extractibility** n.

extraction /ɪk'strækʃən/ n the act of extracting; lineage; something extracted.

extractive /ɪk'stræktɪv/ adj tending or serving to extract.

extractor /ɛk'stræktər/ n one who extracts; a thing that extracts, esp a device for removing teeth or delivering a baby; a device for extracting stale air or fumes from a room.—also **extractor fan**.

extracurricular /ˌɛkstrəkə'rɪkjʊlər/ adj not part of the regular school timetable; beyond one's normal duties or activities.

extradite /'ɛkstrəˌdɔɪt/ vt to surrender (an alleged criminal) to the country where the offence was committed.—**extraditable** adj.—**extradition** n.

extrados /ɛk'streɪdɒs/ n (pl extrados, extradoses) (archit) the upper or outer curve of an arch.

extragalactic /ˌɛkstrəgə'læktɪk/ adj outside the Galaxy.

extrajudicial /-dʒuː'dɪʃəl/ adj out of the ordinary course of legal proceedings.

extramarital /-'mɛrɪtəl/ adj occurring outside marriage, esp sexual relationships.

extramundane /-'mʊndeɪn/ adj beyond the material world.

extramural /-'mjʊrəl/ adj (course, studies) outside the usual courses run by a university, etc; outside a city's walls or boundaries.—**extramurally** adv.

extraneous /ɪk'streɪnɪəs/ adj coming from outside; not essential.—**extraneously** adv.

extraordinary /ɛk'strɔːrdɪneri/ or /ˌɛkstrə'ɔːrdɪneri/ adj not usual or regular; remarkable, exceptional.—**extraordinarily** adv.—**extraordinariness** n.

extrapolate /ɛk'stræpəˌleɪt/ vti to infer (unknown data) from known data.—**extrapolation** n.—**extrapolator** n.

extrasensory perception /ˌɛkstrə'sɛnsəri/ n the claimed ability to obtain information by means other than the ordinary physical senses.

extraterritorial /-ˌtɛrɪ'tɔːrɪəl/ adj outside territorial boundaries; (embassy etc) outside the jurisdiction of the country in which it is.—also **exterritorial**.

extraterritoriality /-ˌtɛrɪˌtɔːrɪə'lɪti/ n exemption granted to foreign diplomats from the legal jurisdiction of the country to which they are posted; a country's jurisdiction over its nationals abroad.

extravagant /ɪk'strævəgənt/ adj lavish in spending; (prices) excessively high; wasteful; (behaviour, praise, etc) lacking in restraint, flamboyant, profuse.—**extravagantly** adv.—**extravagance** n.

extravaganza /ɪkˌstrævə'gænzə/ n an elaborate musical production; a spectacular show, play, film, etc.

extravagate /ɛk'strævəˌgeɪt/ vi (arch) to wander; to be extravagant.—**extravagation** n.

extravasate /ɛk'strævəˌseɪt/ vt (anat) to force blood, etc out of its proper vessel; to exude. • vi to flow out.—**extravasation** n.

extraversion /ˌɛkstrə'vɜːrʒən/ see extroversion.

extravert /-ˌvɜːrt/ see extrovert.

extreme /ɪk'striːm/ adj of the highest degree or intensity; excessive, immoderate, unwarranted; very severe, stringent; outermost. • n the highest or furthest limit or degree; (often pl) either of the two points marking the ends of a scale or range.—**extremely** adv.—**extremeness** n.

extremist /ɪk'striːmɪst/ n a person of extreme views, esp political.—**extremism** n.

extremity /ɪk'strɛmɪti/ n (pl extremities) the utmost point or degree; the most remote part; the utmost violence, vigour, or necessity; the end; (pl) the hands or feet.

extricable /'ɛkstrɪkəbəl/ adj able to be extricated.

extricate /-ˌkeɪt/ vt to release from difficulties; to disentangle.—**extrication** n.

extrinsic /ɛk'strɪnsɪk/ adj external; not inherent or essential.—**extrinsically** adv.

extrorse /ɛk'strɔːrs/ adj (bot) turned outwards.

extroversion /ˌɛkstrə'vɜːrʒən/ n the state of having thoughts and activities directed towards things other than oneself.—also **extraversion**.

extrovert /'ɛkstrəˌvɜːrt/ n a person more interested in the external world than his own thoughts and feelings.—also **extravert**.—**extroverted, extraverted** adj.

extrude /ɪk'struːd/ vt to force or push out; to mould (metal or plastic) by forcing through a shaped die.—**extrusion** n.—**extrusive** adj.

exuberant /ɪg'zuːbərənt/ or /-'zjuː-/ adj lively, effusive, high-spirited; profuse.—**exuberance** n.—**exuberantly** adv.

exuberate /-ˌreɪt/ vi to be exuberant; (arch) to abound.

exudate /'ɛgzjʊˌdeɪt/ n exuded matter, eg sweat.

exudation /-'deɪʃən/ n an exuding or being exuded; exuded matter, eg sweat.—**exudative** adj.

exude /ɪg'zjuːd/ or /-'zuːd/ vt to cause or allow to ooze through pores or incisions, as sweat, pus; to display (confidence, emotion) freely.

exult /ɪg'zʌlt/ vi to rejoice greatly.—**exultation** n.

exultant /ɪg'zʌltənt/ adj exulting, joyful; triumphant.—**exultantly** adv.

exuviae /ɪg'zuːvi/ or /-iː/ npl the cast-off skins, shells, etc, of animals.—**exuvial** adj.

exuviate /-vɪˌeɪt/ vt (skin) to shed, slough.—**exuviation** n.

eyas /'aɪəs/ n a young hawk.

eye /aɪ/ n the organ of sight; the iris; the faculty of seeing; the external part of the eye; something resembling an eye, as the hole in a needle, the leaf-bud on a potato, etc. • vt (**eyeing** or **eying, eyed**) to look at; to observe closely.

eyeball /'aɪbɒl/ *n* the ball of the eye. • *vt* (*sl*) to stare at.

eyebright /-braɪt/ *n* a plant with small white and purplish flowers, formerly used as a lotion to treat disorders of the eye.

eyebrow /-braʊ/ *n* the hairy ridge above the eye.

eye-catching /-kætʃɪŋ/ *adj* attractive or striking in appearance.—**eye-catcher** *n*.

eyeful /-fʊl/ *adj* (*inf*) a close look, gaze; an attractive vision, *esp* a woman.

eyeglass /-glæs/ *n* a lens for correcting defective vision, a monocle.

eyeglasses *npl* spectacles.

eyelash /-læʃ/ *n* the fringe of fine hairs along the edge of each eyelid.

eyeless /-ləs/ *adj* without eyes; blind

eyelet /-lət/ *n* a small hole for a rope or cord to pass through, as in sails, garments, etc.

eyelid /-lɪd/ *n* the lid of skin and muscle that moves to cover the eye.

eye-liner /-ˌlaɪnər/ *n* a cosmetic used to apply a line round the eye.

eye-opener /-ˌoːpənər/ *n* something that comes as a shock or surprise.

eyephone /-foːn/ *n* a device in the style of a headset which provides the user with stereoscopic images and stereo sound used in virtual reality simulation.

eyepiece /-piːs/ *n* the lens or lenses at the end nearest the eye of an optical instrument, *eg* a telescope.

eyeprint /-prɪnt/ *n* the pattern of veins in the retina, which is unique to an individual and used as a means of identification.

eye-shadow /-ʃædoː/ *n* a coloured powder applied to accentuate or decorate the eyelids.

eyeshot /-ʃɒt/ *n* seeing distance.

eyesight /-saɪt/ *n* the faculty of seeing.

eyesore /-soːr/ *n* anything offensive to the sight.

eyespot /-spɒt/ *n* a rudimentary visual organ; (*on butterflies, etc*) a marking resembling an eye.

eyetooth /-tuːθ/ *n* (*pl* **eyeteeth**) a canine tooth in the upper jaw.

eyewash /-wɒʃ/ *n* (*inf*) nonsense, drivel.

eye-witness /-ˌwɪtnəs/ *n* a person who sees an event, such as an accident or a crime, and can describe what happened.

eyrie /'ɛri/ or /'iːri/ *n* the nest of an eagle or other bird of prey; any high inaccessible place or position.—*also* **aerie**.

F

F *abbr* = Fahrenheit; (*chem symbol*) fluorine.

f, F /ɛf/ *n* the 6th letter of the English alphabet.

fa /fɑ/ *n* (*music*) the fourth note in the sol-fa musical notation.—*also* **fah.**

fabaceous /ˈfæbeɪʃən/ *adj* (*bot*) bean-like.

Fabian /ˈfeɪbiən/ *adj* pertaining to the tactics of the Roman general, Fabius Maximus; cautiously persistent; watchful. • *n* a member of the Fabian Society.

Fabian Society *n* a society seeking socialism by moral persuasion.

fable /ˈfeɪbəl/ *n* a story, often with animal characters, intended to convey a moral; a lie, fabrication; a story involving mythical, legendary or supernatural characters or events.

fabled /ˈfeɪbəld/ *adj* related in fables; fictitious.

fabric /ˈfæbrɪk/ *n* cloth made by knitting, weaving, etc; framework, structure.

fabricate /ˈfæbrɪˌkeɪt/ *vt* to construct, manufacture; to concoct (*eg* a lie); to forge.—**fabrication** *n.*—**fabricator** *n.*

fabulist /ˈfæbjʊlɪst/ *n* a writer of fables; a liar.

fabulous /ˈfæbjʊləs/ *adj* told in fables; incredible, astonishing; (*inf*) very good.—**fabulously** *adv.*

façade, facade /fəˈsɒd/ *n* the main front or face of a building; an outward appearance, *esp* concealing something hidden.

face /feɪs/ *n* the front part of the head containing the eyes, nose, mouth, chin, etc; facial expression; the front or outer surface of anything; external show or appearance; dignity, self respect; impudence, effrontery; a coal face. • *vt* to be confronted by (a problem, etc); to deal with (an opponent, problem, etc) resolutely; to be opposite to; to turn (a playing card) face upwards; to cover with a new surface. • *vi* to turn the face in a certain direction; to be situated in or have a specific direction.

face card *n* the king, queen or jack in a pack of cards.

faceless /-ləs/ *adj* lacking a face; anonymous.

face-lift /-lɪft/ *n* plastic surgery to smooth and firm the face; an improvement or renovation, *esp* to the outside of a building.

faceoff /ˈfeɪsɒf/ *n* ♣ the act of starting or restarting play in hockey or lacrosse by dropping or placing the puck or ball between two opposing players' sticks; a direct confrontation.

facer /-ər/ *n* someone who, or something which, faces; (*inf*) an unexpected setback.

face-saving *adj* allowing the preservation of dignity and prevention of humiliation.

facet /ˈfæsət/ *n* a small plane surface (as on a cut gem); an aspect of character, a problem, issue, etc.

facetiae /fəˈsiːʃɪˌiː/ *npl* witty sayings; books characterized by coarse wit.

face-time *n* (*sl*) a spell of duty, *esp* by US Secret Service agents guarding the President or others.

facetious /fəˈsiːʃəs/ *adj* joking, *esp* in an inappropriate manner.—**facetiously** *adv.*—**facetiousness** *n.*

face value *n* the value indicated on the face of (*eg* a coin or share certificate); apparent worth or significance.

facia /ˈfeɪʃə/ or /ˈfæʃə/, /-iə/ *see* **fascia.**

facial /ˈfeɪʃəl/ *adj* of or pertaining to the face. • *n* a beauty treatment for the face.—**facially** *adv.*

facies /ˈfeɪʃiːz/ *n* (*pl* **facies**) the general appearance of a person or a group of plants, animals or rocks; the face.

facile /ˈfæsaɪl/ or /ˈfæsɪl/ *adj* easy to do; superficial.

facilitate /fəˈsɪlɪˌteɪt/ *vt* to make easier; to help forward.—**facilitator** *n.*—**facilitation** *n.*

facility /fəˈsɪlɪti/ *n* (*pl* **facilities**) the quality of being easily done; aptitude, dexterity; something, *eg* a service or equipment, that makes it easy to do something.

facing /ˈfeɪsɪŋ/ *n* a lining at the edge of a garment; a covering on a surface for decoration or protection.

facsimile /fækˈsɪmɪli/ *n* an exact copy of a book, document, etc; a method of transmitting printed matter (text and graphics) through the telephone system.—*also* **fax.**

fact /fækt/ *n* a thing known to have happened or to exist; reality; a piece of verifiable information; (*law*) an event, occurrence, etc as distinguished from its legal consequences.

faction¹ /ˈfækʃən/ *n* a small group of people in an organization working together in a common cause against the main body; dissension within a group or organization.—**factional** *adj.*—**factionally** *adv.*—**factious** *adj.*

faction² *n* a book, film, etc based on facts but presented as a blend of fact and fiction.

factitious /fækˈtɪʃəs/ *adj* contrived, artificial.—**factitiously** *adv.*

factitive /ˈfæktɪtɪv/ *adj* (*gram*) causative.

factor /ˈfæktər/ *n* any circumstance that contributes towards a result; (*math*) any of two or more numbers that, when multiplied together, form a product; a person who acts for another; ♣ a company that buys invoices at a discount and then collects payments on them; ♣ (*Cdn*) (*hist*) a person in charge of a fur-trading post.

factor8 /-eɪt/ *n* a blood-clotting agent used in the treatment of haemophilia.

factorage /ˈfæktərɪdʒ/ *n* a factor's commission.

factorial /fækˈtɔːriəl/ *n* (*math*) an integer multiplied by all lower integers, *eg* $4 \times 3 \times 2 \times 1$.

factorize /ˈfæktəˌraɪz/ *vt* to reduce to factors.—**factorization** *n.*

factory /ˈfæktəri/ *n* (*pl* **factories**) a building or buildings where things are manufactured; ♣ (*Cdn*) (*hist*) a large fur-trading post.

factory farm *n* a farm, which rears livestock intensively ,using modern manufacturing processes.—**factory farming** *n.*

factory ship *n* a ship that processes the catch of a fishing fleet.

factotum /fækˈtoːtəm/ *n* a person employed to do all kinds of work.

facts of life *npl* knowledge of human sexual reproduction.

factual /ˈfæktʃʊəl/ *adj* based on, or containing, facts; actual.—**factually** *adv.*

facula /ˈfækjʊlə/ *n* (*pl* **faculae**) a bright spot or streak on the surface of the sun.

facultative /ˈfækəltətɪv/ *adj* enabling; optional; contingent.

faculty /ˈfækəlti/ *n* (*pl* **faculties**) any natural power of a living organism; special aptitude; a teaching department of a college or university, or the staff of such a department.

fad /fæd/ *n* a personal habit or idiosyncrasy; a craze.—**faddish, faddy** *adj.*—**faddism** *n.*—**faddist** *n.*

fade /feɪd/ *vi* to lose vigour or brightness of colour gradually; to vanish gradually. • *vt* to cause (an image or a sound) to increase or decrease in brightness or intensity gradually.—*also n.*

fadeless /-ləs/ *adj* unfading.

fading /-ɪŋ/ *n* decay; loss of colour; (*radio*) a deterioration in quality of reception.

faeces /ˈfiːsiːz/ *npl* excrement.—*also* **feces.**—**faecal, fecal** *adj.*

faerie, faery /ˈfeɪəri/ *n* (*pl* **faeries**) (*arch*) the fairy world; enchantment.

Faeroese /ˌferoˈiːz/ *n* (*pl* **Faeroese**) an inhabitant of the Faeroes in the North Atlantic; the language of the Faeroes.—*also adj.*—*also* **Faroese.**

fag /fæg/ *vti* (**fagging, fagged**) to become or cause to be tired by hard work. • *n* (*formerly*) a British public schoolboy who performs chores for senior pupils; (*inf*) drudgery; (*sl*) a cigarette.

fag-end *n* the useless remains of anything; (*sl*) a cigarette-end.

faggot, fagot /ˈfægət/ *n* a bundle of sticks for fuel; (*sl*) a nasty old woman.

faggoting, fagoting /-ɪŋ/ *n* a method of decorating textile fabrics.

fah /fɑ/ *see* **fa.**

Fahrenheit /ˈfærənˌhaɪt/ *adj* of, using, or being a temperature scale with the freezing point of water marked at 32° and the boiling point at 212°.

faïence, faience /ˈfaɪɑːs/, *Fr.* /fajˈɑːs/ *n* a type of decorated earthenware.

fail /feɪl/ *vi* to weaken, to fade or die away; to stop operating; to fall short; to be insufficient; to be negligent in duty, expectation, etc; (*exam, etc*) to be unsuccessful; to become bankrupt. • *vt* to disappoint the expectations or hopes of; to be unsuccessful in an exam, etc; to leave, to abandon; to grade (a candidate) as not passing a test, etc. • *n* failure in an examination.

failing /-ɪŋ/ *n* a fault, weakness. • *prep* in default or absence of.

faille /faɪl/ or /feɪl/ *n* a soft silk, used for dresses and hat trimmings.

fail-safe *adj* designed to operate safely even if a fault develops; foolproof.

failure /ˈfeɪljər/ *n* failing, non-performance, lack of success; the ceasing of normal operation of something; a deficiency; bankruptcy; an unsuccessful person or thing.

fain /feɪn/ *adv* (*arch*) willingly; gladly. • *adj* willing; glad.

fainéant, faineant /ˈfeɪˌneɪɑ̃/, *Fr.* /fɛneɪˈɑ̃/ *adj* indolent.

faint /feɪnt/ *adj* dim, indistinct; weak, feeble; timid; on the verge of losing consciousness. • *vi* to lose consciousness temporarily from a decrease in the supply of blood to the brain, as from shock. • *n* an act or condition of fainting.—**faintly** *adv*.—**faintness** *n*.

faint-hearted *adj* lacking courage and resolution.

fainting /-ɪŋ/ *n* a sudden and temporary loss of consciousness.

fair[1] /feər/ *adj* pleasing to the eye; clean, unblemished; (*hair*) light-coloured; (*weather*) clear and sunny; (*handwriting*) easy to read; just and honest; according to the rules; moderately large; average. • *adv* in a fair manner; squarely.—**fairness** *n*.

fair[2] /feər/ *n* a gathering for the sale of goods, *esp* for charity; a competitive exhibition of farm, household, or manufactured goods; a fun-fair.

fair game *n* a legitimate target for attack or ridicule.

fairground /ˈfeərɡraʊnd/ *n* an open area where fairs are held.

fairing /ˈfeərɪŋ/ *n* a structure attached to the exterior of an aircraft, ship, motor vehicle, etc to reduce drag.

fairly /ˈfeərli/ *adv* in a fair manner; justly; moderately.

fair play *n* justice, honesty; impartiality.

fairway /ˈfeərweɪ/ *n* a navigable channel; the mowed part of a golf course between the tee and the green.

fair-weather *adj* (*friend*) unreliable in troubled times.

fairy /ˈfeəri/ *n* (*pl* **fairies**) an imaginary supernatural being, *usu* in human form.

fairyland /ˈfeəriˌlænd/ *n* the country of fairies; a beautiful, enchanting place.

fairy ring *n* a dark or bare ring in grass caused by fungi.

fairy story, fairy tale *n* a story about fairies; an incredible story; a fabrication.

fait accompli /ˌfeɪtəˈkɒmpliː/ or /-əˈkɔ̃pli/, *Fr.* /fɛtakɔ̃ˈpliː/ *n* (*pl* **faits accomplis**) something already done; an irreversible act.

faith /feɪθ/ *n* trust or confidence in a person or thing; a strong conviction, *esp* a belief in a religion; any system of religious belief; fidelity to one's promises, sincerity.

faithful /ˈfeɪθful/ *adj* loyal; true; true to the original, accurate.—**faithfully** *adv*.—**faithfulness** *n*.

faithless /-ləs/ *adj* treacherous, disloyal; untrustworthy.—**faithlessly** *adv*.—**faithlessness** *n*.

fake /feɪk/ *vt* to make (an object) appear more real or valuable in order to deceive; to pretend, simulate. • *n* a faked article, a forgery; an impostor. • *adj* counterfeit, not genuine.—**faker** *n*.

fakir /ˈfeɪkiːr/ or /fəˈkiːr/ *n* a Muslim or Hindu religious mendicant or ascetic.

Falangist /fəˈlændʒɪst/ *n* a supporter of the Spanish Falange, a fascist party founded in 1933.

falbala /fɒlˈbɒlə/ or /fælˈbælə/ *n* a flounce on a dress.

falcate /ˈfælkeɪt/, **falciform** /ˈfælsɪˌfɔrm/ *adj* sickle-shaped.

falchion /ˈfɒltʃən/ *n* a broad, curved sword.

falcon /ˈfɒlkən/ or /ˈfæl-/ *n* a type of hawk trained for use in falconry.

falconer /-ər/ *n* a person who hunts with, or who breeds and trains hawks for hunting.—**falconry** *n*.

falconet /-ət/ *n* a small falcon.

falderal /ˈfɒldəˌrɒl/ *n* a trifling ornament.

faldstool /ˈfɒldstuːl/ *n* an armless chair, used by a bishop.

fall /fɒl/ *vi* (**falling, fell**, *pp* **fallen**) to descend by force of gravity; to come as if by falling; to collapse; to drop to the ground; to become lower, weaker, less; to lose power, status, etc; to lose office; to slope in a downward direction; to be wounded or killed in a battle; to pass into a certain state; to become pregnant; to take place, happen; to be directed by chance; to come by inheritance; (*with* **about**) to laugh uncontrollably; (*with* **back**) to retreat; (*with* **behind**) to fail to keep up with; to become in arrears with; (*with* **for**) to fall in love with; to be fooled by (a lie, trick, etc); (*with* **out**) to quarrel; to leave one's place in a military formation;

(*with* **through**) to fail to happen. • *n* act or instance of falling; something which falls; the amount by which something falls; a decline in status, position; overthrow; a downward slope; a decrease in size, quantity, value; (*US*) autumn; (*wrestling*) a scoring move by pinning both shoulders of an opponent to the floor at once.

fallacious /fəˈleɪʃəs/ *adj* misleading.—**fallaciously** *adv*.—**fallaciousness** *n*.

fallacy /ˈfæləsi/ *n* (*pl* **fallacies**) a false idea; a mistake in reasoning.

fallal /fəˈlɒl/ *n* a piece of finery, an ornament.

fallen /ˈfɒlən/ *adj* sunk to a lower state or condition; overthrown.

fall guy *n* (*inf*) a person who is easily cheated; a scapegoat.

fallible /ˈfælɪbəl/ *adj* liable to make mistakes.—**fallibly** *adv*.—**fallibility** *n*.

Fallopian tube /fəˈloːpiən/ *n* either of the two tubes through which the egg cells pass from the ovary to the uterus.

fall-out /ˈfɒlaʊt/ *n* a deposit of radioactive dust from a nuclear explosion; a by-product.

fallow[1] /ˈfæloː/ *adj* (*land*) ploughed and left unplanted for a season or more.

fallow[2] *adj* yellowish-brown.

fallow deer *n* a small European deer with a brownish-yellow coat which becomes spotted with white in summer.

false /dɒls/ *adj* wrong, incorrect; deceitful; artificial; disloyal, treacherous; misleading, fallacious.—**falsely** *adv*.—**falseness** *n*.

falsehood /ˈfɒlshud/ *n* being untrue; the act of deceiving; a lie.

falsetto /ˈfælseto/ *n* (*pl* **falsettos**) an artificial tone higher in key than the natural compass of the voice.

falsify /ˈfælsɪˌfaɪ/ *vt* (**falsifying, falsified**) to misrepresent; to alter (a document, etc) fraudulently; to prove false.—**falsification** *n*.

falsity /ˈfælsɪti/ *n* (*pl* **falsities**) the quality of being false; an error, a lie.

falter /ˈfæltər/ *vi* to move or walk unsteadily, to stumble; to hesitate or stammer in speech; to be weak or unsure, to waver.—**falteringly** *adv*.

fame /feɪm/ *n* the state of being well known; good reputation.—**famed** *adj*.

Fameuse /fəˈmuːz/ *n* ✹ (*Cda*) snow apple.

familiar /fəˈmɪljər/ *adj* well-acquainted; friendly; common; well-known; too informal, presumptuous. • *n* a spirit or demon supposed to aid a witch, etc; an intimate.—**familiarly** *adv*.—**familiarity** *n*.

familiarize /-ˌraɪz/ *vt* to make well known or acquainted; to make (something) well known.—**familiarization** *n*.

family /ˈfæmɪli/ or /ˈfæmli/ *n* (*pl* **families**) parents and their children; a person's children; a set of relatives; the descendants of a common ancestor; any group of persons or things related in some way; a group of related plants or animals; a unit of a crime syndicate (as the Mafia).

family allowance *n* ✹ (*Cda*) formerly, a monthly payment by the federal government to mothers who had children who were under 18 years of age; (*Brit*) formerly, the name for child benefit.

family circle *n* close relatives.

family name *n* a surname.

family planning *n* birth control.

family tree *n* a genealogical diagram.

famine /ˈfæmɪn/ *n* an acute scarcity of food in a particular area; an extreme scarcity of anything.

famish /ˈfæmɪʃ/ *vti* to make or be very hungry.

famous /ˈfeɪməs/ *adj* renowned; (*inf*) excellent.—**famously** *adv*.

famulus /ˈfæmjʊləs/ *n* (*pl* **famuli**) a magician's assistant.

fan[1] /fæn/ *n* a handheld or mechanical device used to set up a current of air. • *vt* (**fanning, fanned**) to cool, as with a fan; to ventilate; to stir up, to excite; to spread out like a fan.

fan[2] *n* an enthusiastic follower of some sport, hobby, person, etc.

fanatic /fəˈnætɪk/ *n* a person who is excessively enthusiastic about something.—**fanatical** *adj*.—**fanatically** *adv*.

fanaticism /fəˈnætɪˌsɪzəm/ *n* excessive enthusiasm.

fanaticize /ˈfænətɪˌsaɪz/ *vti* to make or become fanatical.

fan belt *n* the belt that drives the cooling fan in a car engine.

fancied /ˈfænsɪd/ *adj* imaginary.

fancier /ˈfænsɪər/ *n* a person with a special interest in something, *esp* plant or animal breeding.

fanciful /ˈfænsɪful/ *adj* not factual, imaginary; indulging in fancy; elaborate or intricate in design.—**fancifully** *adv*.

fan club *n* an organized group of followers of a celebrity.

fancy /'fænsi/ n (pl **fancies**) imagination; a mental image; a whim; fondness. • adj (**fancier, fanciest**) not based on fact, imaginary; elegant or ornamental. • vt (**fancying, fancied**) to imagine; to have a fancy or liking for; (inf) to be sexually attracted to.

fancy dress n a costume worn at masquerades or parties, usu representing an animal, historical character, etc.

fancy-free adj uncommitted, carefree.

fancy man n (sl) a woman's lover; a pimp.

fancy woman n (sl) a mistress, prostitute.

fancywork n ornamental needlework.

fandango /fæn'dæŋgoː/ n (pl **fandangos**) a Spanish dance, music for this dance, tomfoolery.

fanfare /'fænfɛr/ n a flourish of trumpets.

fang /fæŋ/ n a long sharp tooth, as in a canine; the long hollow tooth through which venomous snakes inject poison.

fan hitch n ♣ (Cdn) in the North, a method of harnessing a dog sled in which the lead dog is on a long trace, with the other dogs arranged in a fan-shaped pattern.

fanlight /'fænlɑɪt/ n a semicircular window with radiating bars like the ribs of a fan.

fanny /'fæni/ n (pl **fannies**) (US sl) the buttocks.

fantail /'fænteɪl/ n a pigeon with a tail that opens out like a fan.

fantan /'fæntæn/ n a Chinese gambling game in which players make guesses about hidden counters.

fantasia /fæn'teɪʒə/ or /-ziə/ n an improvised musical or prose composition.

fantasize /'fæntəˌsɑɪz/ vt to imagine in an extravagant way. • vi to daydream.

fantast /'fæntæst/ n a visionary or dreamer.

fantastic /fæn'tæstɪk/ adj unrealistic, fanciful; unbelievable; imaginative; (inf) wonderful.—**fantastically** adv.

fantasy /'fæntəsi/ n (pl **fantasies**) imagination; a product of the imagination, esp an extravagant or bizarre notion or creation; an imaginative poem, play or novel.

fanzine /'fænziːn/ n a magazine produced by and for the fans of a celebrity, football club, etc.

FAO abbr = Food and Agricultural Organization.

far /fɑr/ adj (**farther, farthest** or **further, furthest**) remote in space or time; long; (political views, etc) extreme. • adv very distant in space, time, or degree; to or from a distance in time or position, very much.—**farness** n.

farad /'fɛrəd/ n a unit of electrical capacitance.

faradic /fə'rædɪk/ adj pertaining to the phenomenon of induced electricity or to faradization.

faradize /'fɛrəˌdɑɪz/ vt to treat by use of a faradic current.—**faradization** n.—**faradizer** n.

farandole /ˌfɛrən'dɒl/ n a lively dance, originating in Provence.

faraway /'fɑrəwei/ adj distant, remote; dreamy.

farce /fɑrs/ n a style of light comedy; a drama using such comedy; a ludicrous situation.—**farcical** adj.—**farcically** adv.

farceur /'fɑrsər/, **farceuse** /-juːz/ n a writer of or actor in a farce; a wit.

farcy /'fɑrsi/ n (pl **farcies**) a disease of horses, closely allied to glanders.

fardel /'fɑrdəl/ n (arch) a bundle or burden.

fare /fɛr/ n money paid for transportation; a passenger in public transport; food. • vi to be in a specified condition.

Far East n the countries of East and Southeast Asia including China, Japan, North and South Korea, Indochina, eastern Siberia and adjacent islands.

farewell /fɛr'wɛl/ interj goodbye.—also n.

far-fetched adj unlikely.

far-flung adj spread over a wide area; remote.

farina /fə'riːnə/ n flour or meal obtained by grinding the seeds of cereals and leguminous plants; starch.

farinaceous /ˌfɛrɪ'neɪʃəs/ adj consisting of, or made from, farina; mealy.

farinose /'fɛrɪˌnoːz/ adj producing farina; resembling farina.

farm /fɑrm/ n an area of land (with buildings) on which crops and animals are raised. • vt to grow crops or breed livestock; to cultivate, as land; to breed fish commercially; (with **out**) to put out (work, etc) to be done by others, to subcontract.

farmer /-ər/ n a person who manages or operates a farm.

farmer's sausage n ♣ (Cdn) a sausage of seasoned, coarsely grown raw pork, bound in a casing but not in links.

farm hand /-hænd/ n a worker on a farm.

farmhouse /-hʊʊs/ n a house on a farm.

farming /-ɪŋ/ adj pertaining to, or engaged in, agriculture. • n the business or practice of agriculture.

farmstead /-stɛd/ n a farm with the buildings belonging to it.

farmyard /-jɑrd/ n a yard close to or surrounded by farm buildings.

faro /'fɑroː/ n a gambling card game.

farouche /fə'ruːʃ/ adj sullen; unsociable.

far-out adj (sl) weird, bizarre; fantastic, wonderful. • interj used to express delight.

farrago /fə'rɒgoː/ n (pl **farragoes**) a confused collection.—**farraginous** adj.

far-reaching adj having serious or widespread consequences.

farrier /'fɛriər/ n a person who shoes horses.

farrow /'fɛroː/ n a litter of pigs. • vti to give birth to (pigs).

far-seeing adj having foresight.

fart /fɑrt/ vi (vulg) to expel wind from the anus.—also n.

farther /'fɑrðər/ adj at or to a greater distance. • adv to a greater degree.

farthest /-ðɪst/ adj at or to the greatest distance. • adv to the greatest degree.

farthing /'fɑrðɪŋ/ n a former British monetary unit.

farthingale /'fɑrðɪŋˌgeɪl/ n a hooped support worn beneath a skirt to expand it at the hip line.

fasces /'fæsiːz/ npl a bundle of rods with an axe used in ancient Rome as a symbol of authority.

fascia /'feɪʃə/ or /'fæʃə/, /-iə/ n (pl **fasciae**) the instrument panel of a motor vehicle, the dashboard; the flat surface above a shop front, with the owner's name, etc.—also **facia**.

fascicle /'fæsɪkəl/ n one part of a book published by instalments.—also **fascicule**; a small collection, group or bundle; (bot) a cluster of leaves, roots, etc.

fascicular /fæ'sɪkjʊlər/, **fasciculate** /-lət/ adj (bot) arranged in fascicles.

fascicule /'fæsɪkjʊl/ n a fascicle.

fasciculus /'fæsɪkjʊləs/ n (pl **fasciculi**) (anat) a bundle of nerve fibres; a fascicle.

fascinate /'fæsɪˌneɪt/ vt to hold the attention of, to attract irresistibly.—**fascination** n.

fascinating /-ɪŋ/ adj having great interest or charm.

fascine /fæ'siːn/ or /fə-/ n a long bundle of sticks bound together, used for fortifying ditches, building earthworks, etc.

Fascism /'fæʃɪzəm/ n a system of government characterized by dictatorship, belligerent nationalism, racism, and militarism.—**Fascist** n, adj.

fash /fæʃ/ vti (Scot) to bother, worry. • n worry; trouble.

fashion /'fæʃən/ n the current style of dress, conduct, speech, etc; the manner or form of appearance or action. • vt to make in a particular form; to suit or adapt.—**fashioner** n.

fashionable /-əbəl/ adj conforming to the current fashion; attracting or frequented by people of fashion.—**fashionably** adv.

fast[1] /fæst/ adj swift, quick; (clock) ahead of time; firmly attached, fixed; (colour, dye) non-fading; wild, promiscuous. • adv firmly, thoroughly, rapidly, quickly.

fast[2] vi to go without all or certain foods. • n a period of fasting.

fastback /'fæstbæk/ n a car with a roof that slopes to the back.

fast breeder reactor n a nuclear reactor that produces more fissile material than it uses.

fasten /'fæsən/ vti to secure firmly; to attach; to fix or direct (the eyes, attention) steadily.

fastener /-ər/, **fastening** /-ɪŋ/ n a clip, catch, etc for fastening.

fast food n food, such as hamburgers, kebabs, pizzas, etc prepared and served quickly.

fast-forward vt to move (video or music tape, etc) on at high speed.

fastidious /'fæstɪdiəs/ adj hard to please; daintily refined; oversensitive.—**fastidiously** adv.—**fastidiousness** n.

fastigiate /fæ'stɪdʒɪət/ or /-ieɪt/ adj (biol) narrowing at the apex.

fastness /'fæstnəs/ n swiftness; colourfast quality; a stronghold.

fast track n a hectic and competitive lifestyle or career.—**fast-track** adj.

fat /fæt/ adj (**fatter, fattest**) plump; thick; fertile; profitable. • n an oily or greasy material found in animal tissue and plant seeds; the richest or best part of anything; a superfluous part.—**fatness** n.

fatal /'feɪt(ə)l/ adj causing death; disastrous (to); fateful.—**fatally** adv.

fatalism /'feɪtəˌlɪzəm/ n belief that all events are predetermined by fate and therefore inevitable; acceptance of this doctrine.—**fatalist** n.—**fatalistic** adj.

fatality /fə'tælɪti/ *n* (*pl* **fatalities**) a death caused by a disaster or accident; a person killed in such a way; a fatal power or influence.

fat cat *n* (*sl*) a rich person.

fate /feɪt/ *n* the ultimate power that predetermines events, destiny; the ultimate end, outcome; misfortune, doom, death.

fated /'feɪtəd/ *adj* doomed; destined by fate.

fateful /-ful/ *adj* having important, *usu* unpleasant, consequences.—**fatefully** *adv*.

Fates /feɪts/ *npl* (*Greek myth*) the three goddesses of destiny, Atropos, Clotho and Lachesis.

fathead /'fæthed/ *n* (*inf*) an idiot.

father /'fɒðər/ *n* a male parent; an ancestor; a founder or originator; (*with cap*) God; a title of respect applied to monks priests, etc. • *vt* to be the father of; to found, originate.—**fatherhood** *n*.

father-in-law *n* (*pl* **fathers-in-law**) the father of one's husband or wife.

fatherland /-,lænd/ *n* one's native country.

fatherless *adj* without a living father.

fatherly /-li/ *adj* pertaining to a father; kind, affectionate, as a father. • *adv* like a father.

fathom /'fæðəm/ *n* a nautical measure of 6 feet (1.83 m). • *vt* to measure the depth of; to understand.

fatidic /'feɪtɪdɪk/, **fatidical** *adj* having the gift of prophecy.

fatigue /fə'tiːg/ *n* tiredness from physical or mental effort; the tendency of a material to break under repeated stress; any of the menial or manual tasks performed by military personnel; (*pl*) the clothing worn on fatigue or in the field. • *vti* (**fatiguing, fatigued**) to make or become tired.

fatling /'fætlɪŋ/ *n* a young animal fattened for slaughter.

fatten /'fætən/ *vt* to make fat or fleshy; to make abundant.—**fattening** *adj*.

fat transfer *n* a cosmetic surgery procedure to take fat from parts of the body, *eg* hips, and insert it in the face to reduce wrinkling.

fatty /'fæti/ *adj* (**fattier, fattiest**) resembling or containing fat. • *n* (*pl* **fatties**) (*inf*) a fat person.

fatty acid *n* any of various organic carboxylic acids (*eg* palmitic, stearic and oleic) present in fats and oils.

fatuous /'fætʃuəs/ *adj* foolish, idiotic.—**fatuously** *adv*.—**fatuousness** *n*.—**fatuity** *n*.

fatwa, fatwah /'fætwə/ *n* a decision by a mufti or Muslim judge.

faubourg /'fəːbʊr/ or /-bərg/, *Fr*. /foː'bʊr/ *n* a suburb, *esp* of Paris in France.

faucal /'fɔːsəl/ *adj* (*anat*) of the fauces; (*sound*) deeply guttural.

fauces /'fɔːsiːz/ *n* (*pl* **fauces**) (*anat*) the upper part of the throat.

faucet /'fɔːsət/ *n* a fixture for draining off liquid (as from a pipe or cask); a device controlling the flow of liquid through a pipe or from a container.—*also* **tap**.

faugh /fɔː/ (*conventionalized pronunciation; sound produced by expulsion of air, often with vibration of lips*) *interj* an expression of disgust or abhorrence.

fault /fɒlt/ *n* a failing, defect; a minor offence; (*tennis, etc*) an incorrect serve or other error; a fracture in the earth's crust causing displacement of strata. • *vt* to find fault with, blame. • *vi* to commit a fault.

fault-finding *adj* censorious, critical.—**fault-finder** *n*.

faultless /-ləs/ *adj* without fault; perfect; blameless.—**faultlessly** *adv*.—**faultlessness** *n*.

faulty /-ti/ *adj* (**faultier, faultiest**) imperfect; defective; wrong.—**faultily** *adv*.—**faultiness** *n*.

faun /fɒn/ *n* (*Roman myth*) a woodland deity, half man, half beast.

fauna /'fɒnə/ *n* (*pl* **faunas, faunae**) the animals of a region, period, or specific environment.

faute de mieux *Fr*. /,foːtdə'mjuː/ in the absence of anything better.

fauteuil /foː'tɜːl/, *Fr*. /foː'tœj/ *n* an armchair; a stall in a theatre.

faux pas /fo'pɒ/ *n* (*pl* **faux pas**) an embarrassing social blunder.

faveolate /fə'viːə,leɪt/ *adj* honeycombed.

favonian /fə'vonɪən/ *adj* of or pertaining to the west wind; (*poet*) favourable.

favour, favor /'feɪvər/ *n* goodwill; approval; a kind or helpful act; partiality; a small gift given out at a party; (*usu pl*) a privilege granted or conceded, *esp* sexual. • *vt* to regard or treat with favour; to show support for; to oblige (with); to afford advantage to, facilitate.

favourable, favorable /'feɪvərəbəl/ or /'feɪvrə-/ *adj* expressing approval; pleasing; propitious; conducive (to).—**favourably, favorably** *adv*.

favourite, favorite /'feɪvərɪt/ or /'feɪvr-/ *n* a favoured person or thing; a competitor expected to win. • *adj* most preferred.

favouritism, favoritism /'feɪvərɪ,tɪzəm/ or /'feɪvr-/ *n* the showing of unfair favour.

fawn[1] /fɒn/ *n* a young deer; a yellowish-brown colour. • *adj* fawn-coloured.

fawn[2] *vi* (*dogs, etc*) to crouch, etc in a show of affection; to flatter in an obsequious manner.—**fawner** *n*.—**fawning** *n*.

fax /fæks/ *n* a document sent by facsimile transmission; a device for sending faxes. • *vt* to send (a document) by facsimile transmission.

fay /feɪ/ *n* a fairy.

faze /feɪz/ *vt* (*inf*) to disturb; to discompose, to disconcert; to daunt.

FBI /'ɛf'biː'aɪ/ *abbr* = Federal Bureau of Investigation.

FC *abbr* (Brit) = Football Club.

FD *abbr* ✠ (*Cdn*) = Forest District.

Fe (*chem symbol*) iron.

fealty /'fiːəlti/ *n* (*pl* **fealties**) (*feudal society*) the loyalty due from a vassal to his feudal lord.

fear /fiːr/ *n* an unpleasant emotion excited by danger, pain, etc; a cause of fear; anxiety; deep reverence. • *vt* to feel fear, be afraid of; to be apprehensive, anxious; to be sorry. • *vi* to be afraid or apprehensive.—**fearless** *adj*.—**fearlessly** *adv*.—**fearlessness** *n*.

fearful /-ful/ *adj* causing intense fear; timorous; apprehensive (of); (*inf*) very great, very bad.—**fearfully** *adv*.

fearless /-ləs/ *adj* brave, intrepid.—**fearlessly** *adv*.—**fearlessness** *n*.

fearnought, fearnaught /'fiːrnɒt/ *n* a strong woollen cloth.

fearsome /'fiːrsəm/ *adj* causing fear, frightful.

feasible /'fiːzəbəl/ *adj* able to be done or implemented, possible.—**feasibly** *adv*.—**feasibility** *n*.

feast /fiːst/ *n* an elaborate meal prepared for some special occasion; something that gives abundant pleasure; a periodic religious celebration. • *vi* to have or take part in a feast. • *vt* to entertain with a feast.—**feaster** *n*.

feat /fiːt/ *n* an action of remarkable strength, skill, or courage.

feather /'feðər/ *n* any of the light outgrowths that form the covering of a bird, consisting of a hollow central shaft with a vane of fine barbs on each side; a plume; something resembling a feather; the water thrown up by the turn of the blade of an oar. • *vt* to ornament with feathers; to turn (an oar or propeller blade) so that the edge is foremost.—**feathering** *n*.—**feathery** *adj*.

feather bed *n* a mattress stuffed with feathers.

featherbrain /-breɪn/, **featherhead** /-hed/ *n* (*inf*) a silly, forgetful person.

featherbrained /-breɪnd/ *adj* frivolous, giddy.

featheredge /-edʒ/ *n* a thin piece of board with one wedge-shaped side.

featherstitch /-stɪt/ *n* a zigzag stitch with a featherlike appearance.

featherweight /-,weɪt/ *n* a lightweight thing or person; an insignificant thing or person; a boxer weighing from 118–126 lbs (53.5–57 kg); a wrestler weighing from 127–137 lbs (58–62 kg).

feathery /'feðəri/ *adj* like or covered with feathers.—**featheriness** *n*.

feature /'fiːtʃər/ *n* any of the parts of the face; a characteristic trait of something; a special attraction or distinctive quality of something; a prominent newspaper article, etc; the main film in a cinema programme. • *vti* to make or be a feature of (something).

featureless /-ləs/ *adj* lacking prominent or distinctive features.

Feb. *abbr* = February.

febrifuge /'febrə,fjudʒ/ *n* a drug that reduces fever.—**febrifugal** *adj*.

febrile /'fiːbraɪl/ or /'feb-/ *adj* of fever; feverish.

February /'februəri/ or /'febjuəri/, /-uːəri/ *n* (*pl* **Februaries**) the second month of the year, having 28 days (or 29 days in leap years).

feces /'fiːsiːz/ *see* **faeces**.

feckless /'fekləs/ *adj* incompetent, untrustworthy.—**fecklessly** *adv*.—**fecklessness** *n*.

feculent /'fekjulənt/ *adj* muddy, turbid; full of dregs or sediment.—**feculence** *adj*.

fecund /'fiːkənd/ or /'fek-/ *adj* fertile, prolific.—**fecundity** *n*.

fecundate /-,deɪt/ *vt* to impregnate.—**fecundation** *n*.

fed /fed/ *see* **feed**.

fedayee /,fedaː'jiː/ *n* (*pl* **fedayeen**) an Arab commando or guerrilla.

federal /ˈfedərəl/ or /ˈfedr-/ *adj* designating, or of a union of states, etc, in which each member surrenders some of its power to a central authority; of a central government of this type.—**federalism** *n*.—**federalist** *n*.—**federally** *adv*.

federalize /-ˌlaɪz/ *vt* to unite (states, etc) in a federal union; to put under federal authority.—**federalization** *n*.

federate /ˈfedəˌreɪt/ *vti* to unite in a federation. • *adj* united in a league; on a federal basis.—**federative** *adj*.

federation /ˌfedəˈreɪʃən/ *n* a union of states, groups, etc, in which each subordinates its power to a central authority; a federated organization.

fedora /fəˈdɔːrə/ *n* a soft felt hat with a curled brim and a crown creased lengthways.

fee /fiː/ *n* the price paid for the advice or service of a professional; a charge for some privilege, as membership of a club; (*law*) an inheritance in land.

feeble /ˈfiːbəl/ *adj* weak, ineffective.—**feebly** *adv*.—**feebleness** *n*.

feeble-minded /-ˌmaɪndəd/ *adj* mentally defective; of low intelligence.

feed /fiːd/ *vb* (**feeding, fed**) *vt* to give food to; to give as food to; to supply with necessary material; to gratify. • *vi* to consume food. • *n* food for animals; material fed into a machine; the part of a machine supplying this material.

feedback /ˈfiːdbæk/ *n* a return to the input of part of the output of a system; information about a product, service, etc returned to the supplier for purposes of evaluation.

feeder /ˈfiːdər/ *n* a person or thing that feeds; a baby's feeding-bottle; a device for supplying material to a machine; a subsidiary road, railway, etc acting as a link with the central transport network.

feel /fiːl/ *vb* (**feeling, felt**) *vt* to perceive or explore by the touch; to find one's way by cautious trial; to be conscious of, experience; to have a vague or instinctual impression of; to believe, consider. • *vi* to be able to experience the sensation of touch; to be affected by; to convey a certain sensation when touched. • *n* the sense of touch; feeling; a quality as revealed by touch.

feeler /ˈfiːlər/ *n* a tactile organ (as a tentacle or antenna) of an animal; a tentative approach or suggestion to test another person's reactions.

feel-good *adj* that which generates the feeling of well-being; feel-good factor.

feeling /-ɪŋ/ *n* the sense of touch; mental or physical awareness; a physical or mental impression; a state of mind; sympathy; emotional sensitivity; a belief or opinion arising from emotion; (*pl*) emotions, sensibilities.

feet /fiːt/ *see* **foot**.

feign /feɪn/ *vt* to invent; to pretend.

feint /feɪnt/ *n* a pretended attack, intended to take the opponent off his guard, as in boxing.—*also vi*.

feldspar /ˈfeldspɑːr/ *n* any member of the group of hard rock-forming minerals.—*also* **felspar**.—**feldspathic, felspathic** *adj*.

felicitate /fəˈlɪsɪˌteɪt/ *vt* to congratulate.—**felicitation** *n*.

felicitous /fəˈlɪsɪtəs/ *adj* (*words, etc*) apt, well-chosen; agreeable in manner; happy.—**felicitously** *adv*.

felicity /fəˈlɪsɪti/ *n* (*pl* **felicities**) happiness; apt and pleasing style in writing, speech, etc.

feline /ˈfiːlaɪn/ *adj* of cats; cat-like.—**felinity** *n*.

fell¹ /fel/ *see* **fall**.

fell² *vt* to cut, beat, or knock down; to kill, to sew (a seam) by folding one raw edge under the other.

fell³ *n* a skin, hide, pelt.

fell⁴ *adj* (*poet*) cruel, fierce, bloody, deadly.

fellah /ˈfelə/ *n* (*pl* **fellahs, fellahin, fellaheen**) an Arab peasant.

fellatio /fəˈleɪʃɪo/ *n* sexual stimulation of the penis with the mouth.

felloe /ˈfeloː/, **felly** /ˈfeli/ *n* (*pl* **felloes, fellies**) one of the curved pieces of wood which form the outer section of a wheel; the outer section of a wheel, the circumference.

fellow /ˈfeloː/ *n* an associate; a comrade; an equal in power, rank, or position; the other of a pair, a mate; a member of the governing body in some colleges and universities; a member of a learned society; (*inf*) a man or boy. • *adj* belonging to the same group or class.

fellowship /ˈfeloːʃɪp/ *n* companionship; a mutual sharing; a group of people with the same interests; the position held by a college fellow.

felo de se /ˈfeloːdəˌseɪ/ *n* (*pl* **felones de se, felos de se**) the act of suicide; a person who commits suicide.

felon /ˈfelən/ *n* a person guilty of a felony.

felonious /fəˈloːnɪəs/ *adj* done with the intention of committing a crime; criminal; malignant.—**feloniously** *adv*.—**feloniousness** *n*.

felony /ˈfeləni/ *n* (*pl* **felonies**) (*formerly*) a grave crime.

felspar /ˈfelspɑːr/ *see* **feldspar**.

felt¹ /felt/ *see* **feel**.

felt² *n* a fabric made from woollen fibres, often mixed with fur or hair, pressed together. • *vti* to make into or become like felt.

felting /-ɪŋ/ *n* the material from which felt is made; the process of manufacturing felt.

felucca /fɪˈlʌkə/ *n* a small boat with oars and lateen sails, used in the Mediterranean.

female /ˈfiːmeɪl/ *adj* of the sex that produces young; of a woman or women; (*pipe, plug, etc*) designed with a hollow part for receiving an inserted piece. • *n* a female animal or plant.

feminine /ˈfemɪnɪn/ *adj* of, resembling, or appropriate to women; (*gram*) of that gender to which words denoting females belong.—**femininity** *n*.

feminism /ˈfemɪˌnɪzəm/ *n* the movement to win political, economic and social equality for women.—**feminist** *adj, n*.

feminize /ˈfemɪˌnaɪz/ *vti* to make or become feminine.—**feminization** *n*.

femme de chambre *Fr.* /famdəˈʃɑːbr/ *n* (*pl* **femmes de chambre**) a chambermaid.

femme fatale /ˌfæmfæˈtæl/, *Fr.* /famfəˈtal/ *n* (*pl* **femmes fatales**) a dangerously seductive woman.

femur /ˈfiːmər/ *n* (*pl* **femurs, femora**) the thighbone.—**femoral** *adj*.

fen /fen/ *n* an area of low-lying marshy or flooded land.

fence /fens/ *n* a barrier put round land to mark a boundary, or prevent animals, etc from escaping; a receiver of stolen goods. • *vt* to surround with a fence; to keep (out) as by a fence. • *vi* to practise fencing; to make evasive answers; to act as a fence for stolen goods.—**fencer** *n*.

fencing /ˈfensɪŋ/ *n* fences; material for making fences; the art of fighting with foils or other types of sword.

fend /fend/ *vi* (*with* **for**) to provide a livelihood for.

fender /ˈfendər/ *n* anything that protects or fends off something else, as old tyres along the side of a vessel, or the part of a car body over the wheel.

fenestrated /ˈfenəstreɪtəd/ or /fəˈnes-/, **fenestrate** /ˈfenəstreɪt/ or /fəˈnes-/ *adj* having windows.

fenestration /ˌfenəˈstreɪʃən/ *n* the design and arrangement of windows in a building.

feng shui /ˈfeŋʃuːi/ *n* a form of geomancy with its base in Chinese mythology concerning the positioning of buildings and household items and their relationship to their surroundings as they affect people.

fennec /ˈfenɪk/ *n* a type of small fox, found in Africa.

fennel /ˈfenəl/ *n* a European herb of the carrot family grown for its foliage and aromatic seeds; a herb grown for its edible bulbous stem tasting of aniseed.

fennelflower *n* one of a variety of Mediterranean plants, with white, blue or yellow flowers.—*also* **love-in-a-mist**.

fenny /ˈfeni/ *adj* marshy.

fenugreek /ˈfenjuːˌgriːk/ *n* a Mediterranean plant with white flowers and pungent seeds.

feoff /fiːf/ or /fef/ *see* **fief**.

feral /ˈfiːrəl/ or /ˈferəl/, **ferine** /ˈfiːraɪn/ or /ˈferaɪn/ *adj* wild, untamed; like a wild beast.

fer-de-lance /ˌferdəˈlɒns/ *n* a yellowish, highly poisonous snake of tropical America.

feretory /ˈferəˌtɔːri/ *n* (*pl* **feretories**) a shrine for the relics of a saint; a chapel for keeping this.

ferial /ˈferɪəl/ *adj* (*RC: Church*) (*a day*) ordinary, not a festival or a fast.

ferment /ˈfɜːment/ *n* an agent causing fermentation, as yeast; excitement, agitation. • *vti* to (cause to) undergo fermentation; to (cause to) be excited or agitated.—**fermentable** *adj*.—**fermenter** *n*.

fermentation /ˌfɜːmenˈteɪʃən/ *n* the breakdown of complex molecules in organic components caused by the influence of yeast or other substances.

fermentative /ˌfɜːmenˈteɪtɪv/ *adj* of or pertaining to fermentation; capable of or causing fermentation.

fermion /ˈfɜːmɪˌɒn/ *n* a type of subatomic particle.

fermium /ˈfəːmiəm/ n an artificially-produced radioactive metallic element.

fern /fəːn/ n any of a large class of nonflowering plants having roots, stems, and fronds, and reproducing by spores.—**ferny** adj.

fernery /ˈfəːnəri/ n (pl **ferneries**) a place for growing ferns.

ferny /ˈfəːni/ adj (**fernier, ferniest**) full of ferns; of or characteristic of ferns.

ferocious /fəˈrəʊʃəs/ adj savage, fierce.—**ferociously** adv.—**ferocity, ferociousness** n.

ferrate /ˈfɛreɪt/ n a salt of ferric acid.

ferret /ˈfɛrɪt/ n a variety of the polecat, used in unearthing rabbits. • vt to drive out of a hiding-place; (with **out**) to reveal by persistent investigation. • vi to hunt with ferrets.—**ferreter** n.—**ferrety** adj.

ferriage /ˈfɛriɪdʒ/ n the act of conveying by ferry; the fare paid for this.

ferric /ˈfɛrɪk/ adj of or containing iron.

ferriferous /fɛˈrɪfərəs/ adj yielding iron.

Ferris wheel /ˈfɛrɪs/ n a large upright revolving wheel with suspended seats, popular in amusement parks.

ferroconcrete /ˌfɛroˈkɒŋkriːt/ n reinforced concrete.

ferrocyanic acid /ˌfɛroˈsaɪænɪk-/ n an acid formed by the union of iron and cyanogen.

ferromagnetism /ˌfɛroˈmægnəˌtɪzəm/ n magnetism possessed by iron, and some other metals, which is retained even after the removal of the magnetizing field.—**ferromagnetic** adj.

ferromanganese /ˌfɛroˈmæŋgəˌniːz/ or /-niːs/ n an alloy of iron and manganese.

ferrotype /ˈfɛroˌtaɪp/ n a photograph taken on a sensitized iron plate.

ferrous /ˈfɛrəs/ adj containing iron.

ferruginous /fəˈruːdʒɪnəs/ adj containing, or impregnated with, iron; rust-coloured, reddish brown.

ferrule /ˈfɛruːl/ n a metal ring or cap on a cane, umbrella, etc, to keep it from splitting.—also **ferule**.

ferry /ˈfɛri/ vt (**ferrying, ferried**) to convey (passengers, etc) over a stretch of water; to transport from one place to another, esp along a regular route. • n (pl **ferries**) a boat used for ferrying; a ferrying service; the location of a ferry.—**ferryman** n (pl **ferrymen**).

fertile /ˈfəːtaɪl/ or /-təl/ adj able to bear offspring; (land) easily supporting plants and vegetation; (animals) capable of breeding; (eggs) able to grow and develop; prolific; (mind, brain) inventive.—**fertility, fertileness** n.

fertility /ˈfəːtɪlɪti/ n the state or quality of being fertile.

fertilize /ˈfəːtɪˌlaɪz/ vt to make (soil) fertile by adding nutrients; to impregnate; to pollinate.—**fertilization** n.

fertilizer /ˈfəːtɪˌlaɪzər/ n natural organic or artificial substances used to enrich the soil.

ferula /ˈfɛrʊlə/ n (pl **ferulas, ferulae**) a genus of plants of the parsley family, from one of which asafoetida is produced.

ferule /ˈfɛruːl/ see **ferrule**.

fervency /ˈfəːvənsi/ n earnestness; ardour.

fervent /ˈfəːvənt/, **fervid** /ˈfəːvɪd/ adj passionate; zealous.—**fervently, fervidly** adv.—**fervency** n.

fervour, fervor /ˈfəːvər/ n intensity of feeling; zeal; warmth.

fescue /ˈfɛskjuː/ n a kind of grass, often grown for pasture and fodder.

fesse /fɛs/ n (her) a broad horizontal band across the middle of a shield.

festal /ˈfɛstəl/ adj of a feast or holiday; festive.—**festally** adv.

fester /ˈfɛstər/ vti to become or cause to become infected; to suppurate; to rankle.

festival /ˈfɛstɪvəl/ n a time of celebration; performances of music, plays, etc given periodically.

festive /ˈfɛstɪv/ adj merry, joyous.—**festively** adv.—**festiveness** n.

festivity /ˈfɛstɪvɪti/ n (pl **festivities**) a festive celebration.

festoon /fɛˈstuːn/ n a decorative garland of flowers, etc hung between two points. • vt to adorn as with festoons.—**festoonery** n.

feta /ˈfɛtə/ n a type of white goat's milk cheese, esp popular in Greece.

fetal /ˈfiːtəl/ adj pertaining to the fetus.—also **foetal**.

fetch[1] /fɛtʃ/ vt to go for and bring back; to cause to come; (goods) to sell for (a certain price); (inf) to deal (a blow, slap, etc); (with **up**) to come to stand, arrive at; **fetch and carry** to run errands for another.—**fetcher** n.

fetch[2] n an apparition of a living person, a wraith; a person's double.

fetching /ˈfɛtʃɪŋ/ adj attractive.—**fetchingly** adv.

fête, fete /feɪt/ n a festival; a usu outdoor sale, bazaar or entertainment in aid of charity. • vt to honour or entertain (as if) with a fête.

Fête nationale /fet ˌnasjɔˈnæl/ n ✺ (Cdn) in Quebec, official name of St Jean Baptiste Day.

fetial /ˈfiːʃəl/ n (pl **fetiales**) a priestly herald in ancient Rome who performed rites accompanying a declaration of war or peace.

feticide /ˈfiːtɪˌsaɪd/ n the destruction of a fetus in the womb.—also **foeticide**.

fetid /ˈfɛtɪd/ or /ˈfiːtɪd/ adj stinking.—also **foetid**.

fetish, fetich /ˈfɛtɪʃ/ n an object believed by primitive peoples to have magical properties; any object or activity regarded with excessive devotion.

fetishism, fetichism /ˈfɛtɪˌʃɪzəm/ n the transfer of sexual desire to an inanimate object, or to some part of the body other than the sexual organs; worship of, or belief in, fetishes—**fetishist, fetichist** n.

fetlock /ˈfɛtlɒk/, **fetterlock** /-ər-/ n the joint on a horse's leg behind and above the hoof.

fetter /ˈfɛtər/ n (usu pl) a shackle for the feet; anything that restrains. • vt to put into fetters; to impede, restrain.—**fetterer** n.

fettle /ˈfɛtəl/ n good condition or repair.

fettucine, fettuccine, fettucini /fɛtʊˈtʃiːni/ n a kind of pasta cut in strips.

fetus /ˈfiːtəs/ n (pl **fetuses** the unborn young of an animal, esp in its later stages; in humans, the offspring in the womb from the fourth month until birth—also **foetus** (pl **foetuses**).—**fetal, foetal** adj.

feud /fjuːd/ n a state of hostilities, esp between individuals, families, or clans; a dispute.—also vi.

feudal /ˈfjuːdəl/ adj pertaining to feudalism; (inf) old-fashioned, redundant.

feudalism /-ˌlɪzəm/ n the economic and social system in medieval Europe, in which land, worked by serfs, was held by vassals in exchange for military and other services to overlords.—**feudalist** n.—**feudalistic** adj.

feudality /-lɪti/ n (pl **feudalities**) the state of being feudal; a feudal estate.

feudalize /-ˌlaɪz/ vt to make feudal.—**feudalization** n.

feudatory /ˈfjuːdəˌtɔri/ adj pertaining to, or held by, feudal tenure.

feudist /ˈfjuːdɪst/ n someone taking part in a feud or argument.

feuilleton /ˌfəjəˈtɒ̃/, Fr. /fœjtɔ̃/ n in France, etc, the section of a newspaper containing reviews, fiction, etc; an article in this; serialization in a newspaper.—**feuilletonist** n—**feuilletonistic** adj.

fever /ˈfiːvər/ n an abnormally increased body temperature; any disease marked by a high fever; a state of restless excitement.—**fevered** adj.

feverfew /ˈfiːvərˌfjuː/ n a perennial European herb, formerly used to reduce fevers.

feverish /ˈfiːvərɪʃ/, **feverous** /ˈfiːvərəs/ adj having a fever; indicating a fever; restlessly excited.—**feverishly** adv.—**feverishness** n.

few /fjuː/ adj, n a small number, not many.—**fewness** n.

fey /feɪ/ adj strange and unusual.—**feyness** n.

fez /fɛz/ n (pl **fezzes**) a red brimless high cap, usu with black tassel, worn esp by men in eastern Mediterranean countries.

ff abbr = and the following pages; (mus) fortissimo—very loud.

fiacre /fiˈækr/ n a type of horse-drawn carriage.

fiancé /ˌfiɒnˈseɪ/ or /ˌfiˈɒnseɪ/, /-ɔ̃-/ n a person engaged to be married.—**fiancée** nf.

fiasco /fiˈæskoʊ/ n (pl **fiascos, fiascoes**) a complete and humiliating failure.

fiat /ˈfiˌæt/ or /faɪˈæt/ n an order by authority; a decree.

fib /fɪb/ n a lie about something unimportant. • vi (**fibbing, fibbed**) to tell a gib.—**fibber** n.

fibre, fiber /ˈfaɪbər/ n a natural or synthetic thread, eg from cotton or nylon, which is soun into yarn; a material composed of such yarn; texture; strength of character; a fibrous substance, roughage.—**fibred, fibered** adj.

fibreglass, fiberglass /-glæs/ n glass in fibrous form, often bonded with plastic, used in making various products.

fibre optics, fiber optics /-ˌɒptɪks/ n sing the transmission of information in the form of light signals along thin transparent fibres of glass.—**fibre-optic, fiber-optic** adj.

fibril /'faɪbrɪl/, **fibrilla** /-lə/ *n* (*pl* **fibrils, fibrillae**) a small fibre.— **fibrilar, fibrillar, fibrillose** *adj*.

fibrillation /ˌfaɪbrɪ'leɪʃən/ *n* the rapid and irregular twitching of muscle fibres, *esp* in the heart.

fibrin /'faɪbrɪn/ *n* a white protein in the blood, which causes coagulation.

fibrinous /'faɪbrɪnəs/ *adj* composed of, or resembling, fibrin.

fibroid /'faɪbrɔɪd/ *adj* (*anat*) containing or resembling fibre. • *n* a benign tumour in the uterus.

fibroin /ˌfaɪ'brɔːɪn/ *n* a protein that is the main constituent of silk and cobwebs.

fibroma /ˌfaɪ'broːmə/ *n* (*pl* **fibromata, fibromas**) a benign fibrous tumour.

fibrosis /ˌfaɪ'broːsɪs/ *n* the abnormal growth of fibrous tissue in an organ or part of the body.

fibrositis /ˌfaɪbrə'saɪtɪs/ *n* inflammation of fibrous tissues, *esp* muscles.

fibrous /'faɪbrəs/ *adj* composed of fibres.—**fibrousness** *n*.

fibula /'fɪbjulə/ *n* (*pl* **fibulae, fibulas**) the outer of the two bones of the lower leg.—**fibular** *adj*.

fiche /fiːʃ/ *n* (*pl* **fiche**) a microfiche.

fichu /'fɪʃuː/ or /fiːʃuː/ *n* a woman's light three-cornered scarf worn over the neck and shoulders.

fickle /'fɪkəl/ *adj* inconstant; capricious.—**fickleness** *n*.

fictile /'fɪktaɪl/ *adj* moulded from clay; able to be moulded from clay.

fiction /'fɪkʃən/ *n* an invented story; any literary work with imaginary characters and events, as a novel, play, etc; such works collectively.—**fictional** *adj*.—**fictionally** *adv*.

fictitious /'fɪktɪʃəs/ *adj* imaginary, not real; feigned.—**fictiously** *adv*.

fictive /'fɪktɪv/ *adj* pertaining to fiction; creating or created by the imagination.—**fictively** *adv*.

fid /'fɪd/ *n* (*naut*) an iron or wooden bar used to support a topmast; a pin used to open the strands of a rope.

fid. *abbr* = fidelity.

fiddle /'fɪdəl/ *n* (*inf*) a violin; (*sl*) a swindle. • *vt* (*inf*) to play on a violin; (*sl*) to swindle; to falsify. • *vi* to handle restlessly, to fidget.—**fiddler** *n*.

fiddle-de-dee /ˌfɪdəldi'diː/ *interj* an expression of incredulity or impatience.

fiddle-faddle /'fɪdəlˌfædəl/ *n* nonsense; trifles. • *vi* to fuss over unimportant matters.

fiddlehead /'fɪdəlˌhed/ *n* an ornament at the prow of a ship.

fiddler /'fɪdlər/ *n* one who fiddles; (*inf*) a violinist.

fiddlestick[1] /'fɪdəlstɪks/ *n* a bow for playing the violin.

fiddlesticks[2] *interj* nonsense!

fiddling /'fɪdlɪŋ/ *adj* trifling, petty.

fidelity /fɪ'delɪti/ *n* (*pl* **fidelities**) faithfulness, loyalty; truthfulness; accuracy in reproducing sound.

fidget /'fɪdʒɪt/ *vi* to (cause to) move restlessly. • *n* nervous restlessness; a fussy person.—**fidgetingly** *adv*.—**fidgety** *adj*.

fiducial /'fɪduːʃəl/ or /fɪ'djuː-/ *adj* (*physics*) taken as a standard of reference; based on trust or faith.—**fiducially** *adv*.

fiduciary /fɪ'duːʃəri/ or /fɪ'djuː-/ *adj* of, held or given in trust; (*paper currency*) depending on public confidence for value. • *n* a trustee.

fie /faɪ/ *interj* for shame; an expression of disgust or dismay.

fief /fiːf/ *n* (*feudalism*) heritable land held by a vassal; an area in which one has control or influence.—*also* **feoff**.

field[1] /fiːld/ *n* an area of land cleared of trees and buildings, used for pasture or crops; an area rich in a natural product (*eg* gold, coal); a battlefield; a sports ground; an area affected by electrical, magnetic or gravitational influence, etc; the area visible through an optical lens; a division of activity, knowledge, etc; all competitors in a contest; (*comput*) a section of a record in a database. • *vt* (*cricket, baseball, etc*) to catch or stop and return the ball as a fielder; to put (*eg.* a team) into the field to play; (*inf*) to handle (*eg* questions) successfully.

field[2] *see* **fjeld**.

field day *n* a day of sports and athletic competition; (*inf*) any day of unusual happenings or success.

fielder /'fiːldər/ *n* (*cricket, baseball, etc*) a person who is not in the batting side, a person who fields.—*also* **fieldsman** (*pl* **fieldsmen**).

field event *n* (*usu pl*) an athletic competition involving jumping or throwing, as opposed to running.

fieldfare *n* a European thrush, which migrates to Britain for winter.

field glasses *npl* small, portable binoculars for use outdoors.

field hockey *n* an outdoor game played by two teams of 11 players with a ball and clubs curved at one end.—*also* **hockey**.

fieldmouse *n* a small, noctural mouse that lives in woods and fields.

fieldwork *n* research done outside the laboratory or place of work by scientists, archaeologists, social workers, etc.—**fieldworker** *n*.

fiend /fiːnd/ *n* an evil spirit; an inhumanly wicked person; (*inf*) an avid fan.—**fiendish** *adj*.—**fiendishly** *adv*.

fierce /fiːrs/ *adj* ferociously hostile; angry, violent; intense; strong, extreme.—**fiercely** *adv*.—**fierceness** *n*.

fiery /'fiːri/ *adj* (**fierier, fieriest**) like or consisting of fire; the colour of fire; intensely hot; spicy; passionate, ardent; impetuous; irascible.—**fierily** *adv*.—**fieriness** *n*.

fiesta /fi'estə/ *n* a religious celebration, a festival, *esp* in Spain and Latin America.

fife /faɪf/ *n* a type of small flute with a shrill sound used *esp* in military music to accompany drums.—**fifer** *n*.

fife rail /'faɪfreɪl/ *n* (*naut*) a rail round the mast holding belaying pins.

fifteen /fɪf'tiːn/ or /'fɪf-/ *adj, n* one more than fourteen; the symbol for this (15, XV, xv); the first point scored by a side in a game of tennis; a rugby football team.—**fifteenth** *adj, n*.

fifth /fɪfθ/ *adj, n* last of five; (being) one of five equal parts; (*mus*) an interval of three tones and a semitone; a gear in a motor vehicle used when driving at speed.—**fifthly** *adv*.

fifth column *n* a subversive organization within a country, which is ready to give help to an enemy.—**fifth columnist** *n*.

fifty /'fɪfti/ *adj, n* (*pl* **fifties**) five times ten; the symbol for this (50, L, l).—**fiftieth** *adj*.

fifty-fifty /'fɪftɪ'fɪfti/ *adj, adv* (*inf*) evenly, equally; (*chance*) an equal possibility of winning.

fig /fɪg/ *n* a tree yielding a soft, pear-shaped fruit; a thing of little or no importance.

fig. *abbr* = figure; figuratively.

fight /faɪt/ *vb* (**fighting, fought**) *vi* to engage in battle in war or in single combat; to strive, struggle (for). • *vt* to engage in or carry on a conflict with; to achieve (one's way) by fighting; to strive to overcome; (*with* **off**) to repel; to ward off or repress through effort. • *n* fighting; a struggle or conflict of any kind; a boxing match.—**fighting** *n*.

fighter /'faɪtər/ *n* a person who fights; a person who does not yield easily; an aircraft designed to destroy enemy aircraft.

fighting chance *n* a small chance of success given supreme effort.

figment /'fɪgmənt/ *n* something imagined or invented.

figurant /'fɪgjurənt/ *n* a ballet dancer who performs as one of a group.—**figurante** *nf*.

figuration /ˌfɪgju'reɪʃən/ *n* the giving of form; representation; a figure, a shape; (*mus*) the use of florid counterpoint.

figurative /'fɪgjurətɪv/ or /-gər-/ *adj* metaphorical, not literal; using or full of figures of speech; emblematic; pictorial.—**figuratively** *adv*.

figure /'fɪgjuər/ or /'fɪgər/ *n* a character representing a number; a number; value or price; bodily shape or form; a graphic representation of a thing, person or animal; a design; a geometrical form; a statue; appearance; a personage; (*dancing, skating*) a set of steps or movements; (*pl*) arithmetic. • *vt* to represent in a diagram or outline; to imagine; (*inf*) to consider; (*inf*) to believe; (*with* out) (*inf*) to solve. • *vi* to take a part (in), be conspicuous (in); to calculate.—**figurer** *n*.

figured /-ərd/ *adj* depicted as a figure; adorned with figures.

figurehead /'fɪgjurˌhed/ or /'fɪgər-/ *n* a carved figure on the bow of a ship; a nominal head or leader.

figure of speech *n* an expression not intended to be taken literally, as a metaphor or simile.

figure skating *n* ice skating in which prescribed figures are outlined.

figurine /ˌfɪgju'riːn/ or /'fɪg-/ *n* a statuette.

filagree /'fɪləˌgriː/ *see* **filigree**.

filament /'fɪləmənt/ *n* a slender thread or strand; a fibre; the fine wire in an electric light bulb that is made incandescent by current; (*bot*) the anther-bearing stalk of a stamen.—**filamentary, filamentous** *adj*.

filar /'faɪlər/ *adj* of or pertaining to thread; (*microscope, etc*) having fine threads in the eyepiece for measuring tiny distances.

filature /'fɪlətʃər/ *n* the reeling of silk from cocoons; a place where this is done.

filbert /'fɪlbərt/ n the edible nut of the cultivated hazel.

filch /fɪltʃ/ vt to steal (something of little value), to pilfer.—**filcher** n.

file[1] /faɪl/ n a container for keeping papers, etc, in order; an orderly arrangement of papers; a line of persons or things; (comput) a collection of related data under a specific name. • vt to dispatch or register; to put on public record. • vi to move in a line; to apply.—**filer** n.

file[2] n a tool, usu steel, with a rough surface for smoothing or grinding. • vt to cut or smooth with, or as with, a file; to polish, improve.—**filer** n.

filefish /'faɪl,fɪʃ/ n (pl **filefish, filefishes**) a tropical fish, of the family of triggerfish, with a narrow body and rough skin.

filester see **fillister**.

filet / fi'leɪ/ or /'fɪlət/ n a net with a square mesh.

filial /'fɪlɪəl/ adj of, or expected from, a son or daughter.—**filially** adv.—**filialness** n.

filiation /,fɪlɪ'eɪʃən/ n the relation of child to father; lineage, line of descent; the formation of branches of a society, etc; a branch so formed.

filibeg /'fɪlɪ,beg/ n a kilt.—also **philabeg**.

filibuster /'fɪlɪ,bʌstər/ n a member of a legislature who obstructs a bill by making long speeches. • vti to obstruct (a bill) by such methods.—**filibusterer** n.

filiform /'fɪlɪ,fɔrm/ adj threadlike.

filigree /'fɪlɪ,griː/ n a kind of lace-like ornamental work in precious metal. • vt (**filigreeing, filigreed**) to decorate with filigree.—also **filagree**.

filing /'faɪlɪŋ/ n a particle rubbed off with a file.

Filipino /,fɪlɪ'piːnoː/ n (pl **Filipinos**) a native or inhabitant of the Philippines.—also adj.

fill /fɪl/ vt to put as much as possible into; to occupy wholly; to put a person into (a position or job, etc); (US) to supply the things called for (in an order, etc); to close or plug (holes, etc); (with **in**) to complete (a form, design, etc) by writing or drawing; (inf) to provide with the latest news or facts; (with **out**) to make fuller or heavier; to fill in (a form, etc). • vi to become full; (with **in**) to act as a substitute for; (with **out**) to become fuller or heavier. • n enough to make full or to satisfy; anything that fills.

filler /'fɪlər/ n one who or that which fills; a substance used to plug a hole or increase the bulk of something.

fillet /'fɪlət/ or /fɪ'leɪ/ n a thin boneless strip of meat or fish; a ribbon, etc worn as a headband; (archit) a narrow band used between mouldings. • vt to bone and slice (fish or meat).

filling /'fɪlɪŋ/ n a substance used to fill a tooth cavity; the contents of a sandwich, pie, etc. • adj (meal, etc) substantial.

filling station n a place where petrol is sold to motorists, a service station.

fillip /'fɪlɪp/ n a blow with the nail of the finger; a stimulus.

fillister, filister /'fɪlɪstər/ n a plane used to cut grooves, rabbets, etc.—also **filester**.

filly /'fɪlɪ/ n (pl **fillies**) a young female horse, usu less than four years.

film /fɪlm/ n a fine, thin skin, coating, etc; a flexible cellulose material covered with a light-sensitive substance used in photography; a haze or blur; a motion picture. • vti to cover or be covered as with a film; to photograph or make a film (of).—**filmic** adj.

film card see **microfiche**.

film star n a leading cinema actor or actress.

filmy /'fɪlmɪ/ adj (**filmier, filmiest**) gauzy, transparent; blurred, hazy.—**filmily** adv.—**filminess** n.

filose /'faɪloːs/ adj threadlike.

filter /'fɪltər/ n a device or substance straining out solid particles, impurities, etc, from a liquid or gas; a device for removing or minimizing electrical oscillations, or sound or light waves, of certain frequencies; a traffic signal at certain road junctions that allows vehicles to turn left or right while the main lights are red. • vti to pass through or as through a filter; to remove with a filter.—**filterable, filtrable** adj.

filter tip n the porous tip of a cigarette designed to reduce the intake of tar during smoking.—**filter-tipped** adj.

filth /fɪlθ/ n dirt; obscenity.

filthy /'fɪlθɪ/ adj (**filthier, filthiest**) dirty, disgusting; obscene; (inf) extremely unpleasant.—**filthily** adv.—**filthiness** n.

filtrate /'fɪltreɪt/ vt to filter. • n a liquid that has been filtered.—**filtration** n.

fimbriate /'fɪmbrɪ,eɪt/ **fimbriated** /-ɪd/ adj (bot) fringed.

fin /fɪn/ n an organ by which a fish, etc steers itself and swims; a rubber flipper used for underwater swimming; any fin-shaped object used as a stabilizer, as on an aircraft or rocket. • vb (**finning, finned**) vi (fish, whale, etc) to agitate the fins. • vt to furnish with fins.

finable, fineable /'faɪn,æbəl/ adj liable to a fine.

finagle /fɪ'neɪgəl/ vt (inf) to obtain or achieve through cunning or deceit; to use trickery or deceit on someone.

final /'faɪnəl/ adj of or coming at the end; conclusive. • n (often pl) the last of a series of contests; a final examination.—**finally** adv.

finale /fɪ'nælɪ/ n the concluding part of any public performance; the last section in a musical composition.

finalist /'faɪnəlɪst/ n a contestant in a final.

finality /faɪ'nælɪtɪ/ or /fə-/ n (pl **finalities**) the state or quality of being final; completeness, conclusiveness.

finalize /'faɪnə,laɪz/ vt to make complete, to bring to an end.—**finalization** n.

finally /'faɪnəlɪ/ or /'faɪnlɪ/ adv at last; lastly; completely.

finance /'faɪ,næns/ or /fɪ'næns/ n the management of money; (pl) money resources. • vt to supply or raise money for.

financial /faɪ'nænʃəl/ or /fɪ-/ adj of finance.—**financially** adv.

financier /faɪnən'sɪr/ or /fɪ-/ n a person skilled in finance.

finback /'fɪnbæk/ n a whale with a prominent dorsal fin; the rorqual.

finch /fɪntʃ/ n any of numerous songbirds of the Fringillidae family.

find /faɪnd/ vb (**finding, found**) vt to discover by chance; to come upon by searching; to perceive; to recover (something lost); to reach, attain; to decide and declare to be; (with **out**) to discover; to solve; to detect in an offence. • vi to reach a decision (as by a jury). • n a discovery, something found.—**findable** adj.

finder /'faɪndər/ n one who or that which finds; a discoverer; a device for sighting the field of view of a camera, telescope, etc.

fin de siècle /,fæ̃də'sjɛkl/ adj of or typical of the end of a century, esp the 19th century. • n the end of a century.

finding /'faɪndɪŋ/ n a discovery; the conclusion reached by a judicial enquiry.

fine[1] /faɪn/ adj very good; with no impurities, refined; (weather) clear and bright; not heavy or coarse; very thin or small; sharp; subtle; elegant. • adv in a fine manner; (inf) very well.—**finely** adv.—**fineness** n.

fine[2] n a sum of money imposed as a punishment. • vt to punish by a fine.—**finable, fineable** adj.

fine arts npl painting, sculpture, engraving, etc valued for their aesthetic qualities.

fine-draw /-drɔː/ vt (**fine-drawing, fine-drew, pp fine-drawn**) to sew up (a darn) so neatly that the join cannot be noticed; to draw out (wire) to an extreme fineness.—**fine-drawn** adj.

finely /'faɪnlɪ/ adv in a fine manner; discriminatingly; subtly; in tiny pieces.

fineness /'faɪnnɪs/ n the state or quality of being fine; the quantity of pure metal contained in an alloy.

finery /'faɪnərɪ/ n (pl **fineries**) elaborate clothes, jewellery, etc.

finespun /'faɪn,spʌn/ adj delicate, fine; over-subtle.

finesse /fɪ'nɛs/ n delicacy or subtlety of performance; skilfulness, diplomacy in handling a situation; (bridge) an attempt to take a trick with a card lower than a higher card held by an opponent. • vt to achieve by finesse; to play (a card) as a finesse.

fine-tooth(ed) comb /'faɪn'tuːθt/ n a comb with closely set fine teeth for trapping nits, etc.

fine-tune /-'tuːn/ or /-'tjuːn/ vt to make fine adjustments to something in order to improve its effectiveness.

finger /'fɪŋgər/ n one of the digits of the hand, usu excluding the thumb; anything shaped like a finger; (inf) the breadth of a finger. • vt to touch with fingers; (mus) to use the fingers in a certain way when playing; to mark this way on music; (sl) to inform against.—**fingerer** n.

fingerboard /-,bɔrd/ n the part of a violin, guitar, etc against which the strings are pressed by the fingers.

finger bowl n a small bowl containing water for rinsing the fingers at the table.

fingered /'fɪŋgərd/ adj marked by handling; having a finger or fingers; (mus) marked to show how the fingers are used.

fingering /'fɪŋgərɪŋ/ n the manner of using the fingers in playing a musical instrument; the indication of this in a musical score.

fingering[2] n a fine knitting yarn.

fingerling /'fɪŋgərlɪŋ/ n a young fish, esp a trout.

fingernail /-,neɪl/ n the nail on a finger.

fingerpost n a direction post in the shape of a pointing finger.

fingerprint /-ˌprɪnt/ *n* the impression of the ridges on a fingertip, *esp* as used for purposes of identification.—*also vt*.

fingerstall /-ˌstɔl/ *n* a protective covering for a finger.

finial /ˈfɪnɪəl/ *n* (*archit*) a pointed ornament at the top of a spire, gable, etc.—**finialed** *adj*.

finical /ˈfɪnɪkəl/ *adj* fastidious, over-particular, fussy; affectedly fine.—**finicality** *n*.—**finically** *adv*.

finicky /ˈfɪnɪki/ **finicking** *adj* too particular, fussy.

fining /ˈfaɪnɪŋ/ *n* the act or process of clarifying or refining; a liquid used to clarify wine, beer, etc.

finis /ˈfiːniː/ or /ˈfɪnɪs/ *n* the end, used at the conclusion of books, films, etc.

finish /ˈfɪnɪʃ/ *vt* to bring to an end, to come to the end of; to consume entirely; to perfect; to give a desired surface effect to. • *vi* to come to an end. • *n* the last part, the end; anything used to finish a surface; the finished effect; means or manner of completing or perfecting; polished manners, speech, etc.—**finisher** *n*.

finishing school *n* a private school for girls which teaches social etiquette.

finite /ˈfaɪnaɪt/ *adj* having definable limits; (*verb form*) having a distinct grammatical person and number.—**finitely** *adv*—**finiteness** *n*.

Finn /fɪn/ *n* a native of Finland.

finnan haddock, Finnan haddie /ˌfɪnən ˈhædi/ *n* a kind of smoked haddock, named after *Findon*, a Scottish fishing village.

finned /fɪnd/ *adj* having a fin or fins.

Finnish /ˈfɪnɪʃ/ *adj* of or relating to Finland or its language. • *n* the language of Finland.

finny /ˈfɪni/ *adj* (**finnier, finniest**) pertaining to, or abounding in, fish; having a fin or fins.

fino /ˈfiːnoː/ *n* (*pl* **finos**) a dry sherry.

Fiord /fjɔːd/ *n see* **fjord**.

fir /fɜr/ *n* a kind of evergreen, cone-bearing tree; its timber.

fire /ˈfaɪr/ *n* the flame, heat and light of combustion; something burning; burning fuel in a grate to heat a room; an electric or gas fire; a destructive burning; a strong feeling; a discharge of firearms. • *vti* to ignite; to supply with fuel; to bake (bricks, etc) in a kiln; to excite or become excited; to shoot (a gun, etc); to hurl or direct with force; to dismiss from a position.—**fireable** *adj*.—**firer** *n*.

fire alarm *n* a device that uses a bell, hooter, etc to warn of a fire.

firearm /ˈfaɪrˌɑrm/ *n* a handgun.

fireball /-ˌbɔl/ *n* a ball of fire; a meteor; the hot gas cloud created by a nuclear explosion.

firebox /-ˌbɒks/ *n* the furnace in a steam locomotive.

firebrand /-ˌbrænd/ *n* a piece of burning wood; a person who starts trouble.

firebreak /ˈfaɪrbreɪk/ *n* a strip of land cleared of vegetation to halt the spread of a fire.

firebrick /-brɪk/ *n* a brick made of fireclay to withstand the action of fire.

fire brigade *n* an organized body specially trained and equipped for fighting fires.

firebug /-ˌbʌg/ *n* (*inf*) an arsonist.

fireclay /-ˌkleɪ/ *n* a fire-resisting clay.

firecracker /-ˌkrækər/ *n* a small explosive firework.

firedamp /-ˌdæmp/ *n* a combustible mine gas, chiefly methane.

firedog /-ˌdɒg/ *n* a metal standard used for open fires to support the logs; andirons.

fire-eater /-ˌitər/ *n* a performer who pretends to eat fire; a quarrelsome person.—**fire-eating** *adj, n*.

fire engine *n* a vehicle equipped for fire-fighting.

fire escape *n* a means of exit from a building, *esp* a stairway, for use in case of fire.

fire extinguisher *n* a container with a spray nozzle, holding water or chemicals for putting out a fire

firefighter /-ˌfaɪtər/ *n* a person who fights fires, *esp* a member of a fire department; fireman.

firefly /-ˌflaɪ/ *n* (*pl* **fireflies**) a winged nocturnal beetle whose abdomen glows with a soft intermittent light.

fireguard /-ˌgɑrd/ *n* a protective grating placed in front of a fire.

fire hall *n* ✤ (*Cdn*) a fire station.

fire insurance *n* insurance against loss by fire.

fire irons *npl* tools for tending a domestic fire, *esp* a poker, tongs, and shovel.

firelighter /-ˌlaɪtər/ *n* a prepared block of ignitable material used for lighting a fire.

firelock /-ˌlɒk/ *n* a flintlock.

fireman /-mən/ *n* (*pl* **firemen**) a member of a fire brigade; fire-fighter; a person employed to tend furnaces.

fireplace /ˈfaɪrˌpleɪs/ *n* a place for a fire, *esp* a recess in a wall; the area surrounding this.

fireplug /-ˌplʌg/ *n* a connection in a water main for a hose; a hydrant.

fire power /-ˈpauər/ *n* the amount of fire that a military unit can deliver on a target.

fireproof /-ˌpruːf/ *adj* not easily destroyed by fire. • *vt* to make fireproof.

fire raiser *n* an arsonist.—**fire raising** *n*.

firescreen /-skriːn/ *n* a movable ornamental screen for keeping the heat of a fire off the face; a screen for decorating an empty fireplace.

fireship /-ʃɪp/ *n* a ship filled with explosives to set an enemy's ships on fire.

fireside /-ˌsaɪd/ *n* the area in a room nearest the fireplace; home.

fire station *n* a building where firemen and fire-fighting equipment are based.—*also* **firehouse, station house**.

firetrap /-ˌtræp/ *n* a building easily set on fire or hard to get out of if on fire.

firewarden /-wɔrdən/ *n* an officer responsible for protecting forests against fire.

firewater /-wɒtər/ *n* (*inf*) strong alcoholic drink.

firewood /-ˌwʊd/ *n* wood for fuel.

firework /-ˌwɜrk/ *n* a device packed with explosive and combustible material used to produce noisy and colourful displays; (*pl*) such a display; (*pl*) a fit of temper, an outburst of emotions.

firing /ˈfaɪrɪŋ/ *n* baking in intense heat, *esp* of clay; fuel; the act of discharging a firearm; the act of adding fuel to a fire.

firing line *n* the front line of a military position; the forefront of any activity.

firing squad *n* a detachment with the task of firing a salute at a military funeral or carrying out an execution.

firkin /ˈfɜrkɪn/ *n* a small wooden barrel containing butter, etc; (*Brit*) a measure of one quarter of a barrel (41 litres/9 gallons).

firm¹ /fɜrm/ *adj* securely fixed; solid, compact; steady; resolute; definite. • *vti* to make or become firm.—**firmly** *adv*.—**firmness** *n*.

firm² *n* a business partnership; a commercial company.

firmament /ˈfɜrməmənt/ *n* the sky, viewed poetically as a solid arch or vault.—**firmamental** *adj*.

first /fɜrst/ *adj* before all others in a series; 1st; earliest; foremost, as in rank, quality, etc. • *adv* before anyone or anything else; for the first time; sooner. • *n* any person or thing that is first; the beginning; the winning place, as in a race; low gear; the highest award in a university degree.

first aid /-ˈeɪd/ *n* emergency treatment for an injury, etc, before regular medical aid is available.

first-born /ˈfɜrstˌbɔrn/ or /-ˈbɔrn/ *adj* eldest. • *n* the eldest child in a family.

first-class /-ˈklæs/ *adj* of the highest quality, as in accommodation, travel. • *n* the best accommodation on a plane, train, etc; the highest class in an examination, etc.

first-degree burn /ˈfɜrstdɪˈgri/ *n* (*med*) a mild burn causing a painful reddening of the skin but no blistering or charring.

first fruits *npl* fruit which is the first to ripen; the earliest returns or results from an enterprise.

firsthand /ˈfɜrstˈhænd/ *adj* obtained directly from a source.

First Lady *n* the wife of the US president.

firstling /ˈfɜrstlɪŋ/ *n* the first offspring.

firstly /ˈfɜrstli/ *adv* in the first place.

First Ministers *npl* ✤ (*Cdn*) the Prime Minister and the premiers of the provinces.

First Nations *npl* ✤ (*Cdn*) Indian peoples or their communities, not including the Inuit or Metis peoples. • *adj* of or pertaining to such a people or community.

first night *n* the opening performance of a play.

First Peoples *npl* ✤ the aboriginal peoples of a country, in Canada including First Nations, Inuit, and Metis peoples.

first person *n* (*gram*) pronouns and verbs referring to the person speaking.

first-rate /ˈfɜrstˈreɪt/ *adj, adv* of the best quality; (*inf*) excellent.

firth /fɜrθ/ *n* an arm of the sea, *esp* a river mouth.—*also* **frith**.

fiscal /ˈfɪskəl/ *adj* of or relating to public revenue; financial. • *n* a prosecuting official in some countries.

fish /fɪʃ/ *n* (*pl* **fish, fishes**) any of a large group of cold-blooded animals living in water, having backbones, gills for breathing and fins; the flesh of fish used as food. • *vi* to catch or try to catch fish; (*with* **for**) to try to obtain by roundabout methods. • *vt* (*often with* **out**) to grope for, find, and bring to view.—**fishable** *adj*.

fish² *n* a rigid strip of wood or metal used to strengthen a mast, joint, etc. • *vt* to strengthen or join with a fish.

fish and brewis *n* ✤ (*Cdn*) a dish of salt cod and hardtack soaked in water and then cooked with fried salt pork.

fish-eye lens /'fiʃ,aɪ/ *n* a wide-angled lens with a curved protruding front.

fisher /'fiʃər/ *n* a person who fishes; (*zool*) another name for the pekan, a marten found in North America.

fisherman /'fiʃərmən/ *n* (*pl* **fishermen**) a person who fishes for sport or for a living; a ship used in fishing.

fishery /'fiʃəri/ *n* (*pl* **fisheries**) the fishing industry; an area where fish are caught.

fishfinger *n* a small oblong piece of fish covered in breadcrumbs.—*also* **fish stick**.

fish flake *n* ✤ (*Cdn*) a large rack on which to dry fish.

fishing /'fiʃɪŋ/ *n* the art, sport or business of catching fish.

fishing rod *n* a wooden, metal or fibreglass rod used with a line to catch fish.

fishing stage *n* ✤ (*Cdn*) a shed used for preparing freshly caught fish before they are dried.

fish meal *n* granules of dried fish used as fertilizer and food for livestock.

fishmonger /'fiʃ,mɒŋgər/ or /-mɐŋ-/ *n* a shop that sells fish.

fishnet /'fiʃnet/ *n* a coarse open-mesh fabric.—*also adj*.

fishplate /'fiʃ,pleɪt/ *n* an iron plate, one of a pair used to join railway rails.

fishpond /'fiʃ,pɒnd/ *n* a pond in which fish are kept.

fish stick *see* **fishfinger**.

fishway /'fiʃwaɪ/ *n* ✤ (*Cdn*) a lock built to assist fish in passing a waterfall or other obstacle on their way upstream to spawn.

fishwife /'fiʃwaɪf/ *n* (*pl* **fishwives**) a woman who guts or sells fish; a coarse, scolding woman.

fishy /'fiʃi/ *adj* (**fishier, fishiest**) like a fish in odour, taste, etc; (*inf*) creating doubt or suspicion.—**fishily** *adv*.—**fishiness** *n*.

fissile /'fisaɪl/ *adj* capable of undergoing nuclear fission; easily split.—**fissility** *n*.

fission /'fiʃən/ *n* a split or cleavage; the reproductive division of biological cells; the splitting of the atomic nucleus resulting in the release of energy, nuclear fission.—**fissionable** *adj*.

fissiparous /fi'sɪpərəs/ *adj* multiplying or propagating by fission.

fissiped /'fisi,ped/, **fissipedal** *adj* (*zool*) having the toes separated, *eg* dogs, cats, etc.

fissirostral /'fisi'rɒstrəl/ *adj* (*birds*) with a deeply cleft beak, *eg* swallows.

fissure /'fiʃər/ *n* a narrow opening or cleft. • *vti* to split.

fist /fist/ *n* the hand when tightly closed or clenched.

fistic /'fistɪk/ *adj* (*joc*) of or pertaining to boxing.

fisticuffs /'fisti,kʌfs/ *npl* a fight with the fists.

fistula /'fistjʊlə/ *n* (*pl* **fistulas, fistulae**) an abnormal passage, as from an abscess to the skin.

fistulous /-ləs/ *adj* resembling a fistula; hollow, like a pipe.

fit¹ /fit/ *adj* (**fitter, fittest**) suited to some purpose, function, etc; proper, right; healthy; (*sl*) inclined, ready. • *n* the manner of fitting. • *vb* (**fitting, fitted**) *vt* to be suitable to; to be the proper size, shape, etc, for; to adjust so as to fit; (*with* **out**) to equip, to outfit. • *vi* to be suitable or proper; to have the proper size or shape.—**fittable** *adj*.—**fitly** *adv*.—**fitness** *n*.

fit² *n* any sudden, uncontrollable attack, as of coughing; an outburst, as of anger; a short period of impulsive activity; a seizure involving convulsions or loss of consciousness.

fitch /fitʃ/ *n* the polecat; the hair of a polecat; a brush made of this.

fitful /'fitful/ *adj* marked by intermittent activity; spasmodic.—**fitfully** *adv*.—**fitfulness** *n*.

fitment /'fitmənt/ *n* a piece of equipment, *esp* fixed furniture.

fitter /'fitər/ *n* a person who specializes in fitting clothes; a person skilled in the assembly and operation of a particular piece of machinery.

fitting /'fitɪŋ/ *adj* appropriate; suitable, right. • *n* an act of one that fits, *esp* a trying on of altered clothes; a small often standardized electrical part.—**fittingly** *adv*.—**fittingness** *n*.

five /faɪv/ *adj, n* one more than four; the symbol for this (5, V, v).

fivefold /'faɪvfəʊld/ *adj, adv* having five units or members; being five times as great or as many.

fiver /'faɪvər/ *n* (*inf*) in UK, a £5 note; in US, a $5 bill.

fives /faɪvz/ *n sing* a ball game similar to squash, played in a walled court.

fix /fiks/ *vt* to fasten firmly; to set firmly in the mind; to direct (one's eyes) steadily at something; to make rigid; to make permanent; to establish (a date, etc) definitely; to set in order; to repair; to prepare (food or meals); (*inf*) to influence the result or action of (a race, jury, etc) by bribery; (*inf*) to punish. • *vi* to become fixed; (*inf*) to prepare or intend. • *n* the position of a ship, etc, determined from the bearings of two known positions; (*inf*) a predicament; (*inf*) a situation that has been fixed; (*inf*) something whose supply becomes continually necessary or greatly desired, as a drug, entertainment, activity, etc.—**fixable** *adj*.

fixated /fik'seɪtɪd/ *adj* having a fixation.

fixation /fik'seɪʃən/ *n* a fixing; (*psychol*) an unhealthy obsession, *esp* one leading to arrested emotional development.

fixative /'fiksətɪv/ *n* a substance used to fix things in position; a substance that prevents (colours, perfumes, etc) fading or evaporating.

fixed /fikst/ *adj* firm; not moving; lasting; intent.—**fixedly** *adv*.—**fixedness** *n*.

fixer /'fiksər/ *n* a chemical that fixes photographs, making the image permanent; (*sl*) a person who fixes something, *esp* by illegal means.

fixings /'fiksɪŋz/ *npl* trimmings.

fixity /'fiksɪti/ *n* (*pl* **fixities**) the state of being fixed; stability; permanence.

fixture /'fikstʃər/ *n* what is fixed to anything, as to land or to a house; a fixed article of furniture; a firmly established person or thing; a fixed or appointed time or event.

fizz /fiz/ *vi* to make a hissing or sputtering sound. • *n* this sound; any effervescent drink.—**fizzy** *adj*.—**fizziness** *n*.

fizzle /'fizəl/ *vi* to make a weak fizzing sound; (*with* **out**) (*inf*) to end feebly, die out, *esp* after a promising start.

fjeld /fjeld/ or /fjel/ *n* in Scandinavia, a high, barren plateau.—*also* **field**.

fjord /fi'ɔrd/ or /fjɔrd/ or /fiːɔrd/ *n* a long, narrow inlet of the sea between high cliffs, *esp* in Norway.—*also* **fiord**.

F/L *abbr* ✤ (*Cdn*) = Flight Lieutenant.

fl. *abbr* = fluid; floor; *floruit* (flourished).

flab /flæb/ *n* (*inf*) fat.

flabbergast /'flæbər,gæst/ *vt* (*inf*) to astonish, startle.

flabby /'flæbi/ *adj* (**flabbier, flabbiest**) fat and soft; weak and ineffective.—**flabbily** *adv*.—**flabbiness** *n*.

flabellate /fləˈbelˌeɪt/ or '-ɪt/, **flabelliform** /-ɪˌform/ *adj* (*bot*) fan-shaped.

flabellum /fləˈbeləm/ *n* (*pl* **flabella**) (*RC*) a large fan.

flaccid /'flæsɪd/ or /'flæks d/ *adj* not firm or stiff; limp, weak.—**flaccidity** *n*.

flack /flæk/ *see* **flak**.

flacon /'flækən/, *Fr* /flaˈkɔ̃/ *n* a small bottle or flask.

flag¹ /flæg/ *vi* (**flagging, flagged**) to grow limp; to become weak, listless.

flag² *n* a piece of cloth, *usu* with a design, used to show nationality, party, a particular branch of the armed forces, etc, or as a signal. • *vt* (**flagging, flagged**) to decorate with flags; to signal to (as if) with a flag; (*usu with* **down**) to signal to stop.

flag³ *n* a hard, flat stone used for paving, a flagstone. • *vt* (**flagging, flagged**) to pave with flagstones.

flag⁴ *n* a plant with a sword-shaped leaf, the iris; a long thin plant blade.

flag day *n* a day on which charitable donations are solicited in exchange for small flags; (*with caps*) in US, 14 June, the anniversary of the adoption of the stars and stripes, 1777.

flagellant /'flædʒələnt/ or /flə'dʒelənt/ *n* a person who scourges himself or herself or others as a sign of religious penance or for sexual gratification.—**flagellantism** *n*.

flagellate /'flædʒə,leɪt/ *vt* to scourge, to whip.—**flagellation** *n*.—**flagellator** *n*..

flagelliform /flə'dʒelɪˌform/ *adj* long, tapering and flexible; shaped like the thong of a whip.

flagellum /flə'dʒeləm/ *n* (*pl* **flagella, flagellums**) (*biol, zool*) a whiplike appendage; (*bot*) a runner.

flageolet¹ /,flædʒə'let/ or 'flædʒ-/ or /,flædʒə'leɪ/ *n* a small flute resembling the treble recorder.

flageolet² *n* a type of edible bean.

flagging /'flægɪŋ/ *n* a pavement of flagstones.

flagitious /fləˈdʒɪʃəs/ *adj* atrocious, abominably wicked.—**flagitiously** *adv*.—**flagitiousness** *n*.

flag of convenience *n* a flag of a country flown by a ship registered there by the owners to benefit from less rigorous taxes or safety regulations.

flagon /ˈflægən/ *n* a pottery or metal container for liquids with a handle and spout and often a lid.

flagrant /ˈfleɪgrənt/ *adj* conspicuous, notorious.—**flagrancy, flagrance** *n*.—**flagrantly** *adv*.

flagrante delicto /fləˈgræntidiˈlɪkˌtoː/ *adv* in the very act, red-handed.

flagrante delicto *see* **in flagrante delicto**.

flagship /ˈflægʃɪp/ *n* the ship that carries the admiral and his flag; the most important vessel of a shipping line; the chief or leading item of a group or collection.

flagstaff /ˈflægstæf/, **flagpole** /ˈflægpoːl/ *n* a pole on which a flag is displayed.

flagstone /ˈflægstoːn/ *n* hard, evenly stratified rock easily split into slabs for paving.

flag-waver /ˈflægˌweɪvər/ *n* an excessively patriotic person, a jingoist.

flail /fleɪl/ *n* a tool for threshing by hand. • *vt* to beat with a flail. • *vi* (*usu with* **about**) to wave (the arms, etc) wildly.

flair /fler/ *n* natural ability, aptitude; discernment; (*inf*) stylishness, sophistication.

flak /flæk/ *n* shells fired by anti-aircraft guns; criticism, opposition.—*also* **flack**.

flake /fleɪk/ *n* a small piece of snow; a small thin layer chipped from a larger mass of something. • *vt* to form into flakes. • *vi* (*with* **out**) (*inf*) to collapse or fall asleep from exhaustion.—**flaker** *n*.

flaky /ˈfleɪki/ *adj* (**flakier, flakiest**) of or resembling flakes; liable to flake; (*sl*) nervous; (*sl*) odd, eccentric.—**flakily** *adv*.—**flakiness** *n*.

flam /flæm/ *vt* (**flamming, flammed**) (*dial*) to deceive.

flambé, flambée /ˈflɒmbeɪ/ *or* /flɒmˈbeɪ/, /flæm-/ *adj* (*food*) covered with flaming brandy or other spirit.—*also vt*.

flambeau /ˈflæmboː/ *n* (*pl* **flambeaux, flambeaus**) a lighted, flaming torch; a large ornamental candlestick.

flamboyant /flæmˈbɔɪənt/ *adj* brilliantly coloured; ornate; strikingly elaborate; dashing, exuberant.—**flamboyance, flamboyancy** *n*.—**flamboyantly** *adv*.

flame /fleɪm/ *n* the burning gas of a fire, appearing as a tongue of light; the state of burning with a blaze; a thing like a flame; an intense emotion; (*inf*) a sweetheart. • *vi* to burst into flame; to become bright red with emotion.

flamen /ˈfleɪmən/ *n* (*pl* **flamens, flamines**) in ancient Rome, a priest devoted to the service of a special deity.

flamenco /fləˈmeŋkoː/ *n* (*pl* **flamencos**) a type of vigorous Spanish dance and music of gipsy origin.

flame-thrower /-ˌθroːər/ *n* a weapon that shoots a jet of flaming liquid.

flaming /ˈfleɪmɪŋ/ *adj* emitting flames; very hot; gaudy; exaggerated; intense.—**flamingly** *adv*.

flamingo /fləˈmɪŋˌgoː/ *n* (*pl* **flamingos, flamingoes**) any of several wading birds with rosy-pink plumage and long legs and neck.

flammable /ˈflæməbəl/ *adj* easily set on fire.—**flammability** *n*.

flamy /-i/ *adj* (**flamier, flamiest**) resembling flame; flame-coloured.

flan /flæn/ *n* an open case of pastry or sponge cake with a sweet or savoury filling.

flânerie *Fr.* /flɑnˈʀi/ *or* /flɑnə-/ *n* idleness.

flâneur *Fr.* /flɑˈnœr/ *n* an idle person, a lounger.

flange /flændʒ/ *n* a raised edge, as on a wheel rim to keep it on a rail; a projecting rib. • *vt* to provide with a flange.—**flanged** *adj*.

flank /flæŋk/ *n* the fleshy part of the side from the ribs to the hip; the side of anything; the right or left side of a formation of troops. • *vt* to attack the flank of; to skirt the side of; to be situated at the side of.

flanker /ˈflæŋkər/ *n* (*mil*) a soldier or fortification used to protect a flank.

flannel /ˈflænəl/ *n* a soft light cotton or woollen cloth; a small cloth for washing the face and hands; (*sl*) nonsense, equivocation; (*pl*) trousers of such cloth. • *vt* (**flannelling, flannelled** *or* **flanneling, flanneled**) to wash with a flannel; (*inf*) to flatter.—**flannelly** *adj*.

flannelette /ˌflænəˈlɛt/ *n* a soft cotton fabric.

flap /flæp/ *vi* (**flapping, flapped**) to move up and down, as wings; to sway loosely and noisily, as curtains in the wind, etc; to move or hang like a flap; (*inf*) to get into a panic or fluster. • *n* the motion or noise of a flap; anything broad and flexible, either hinged or hanging loose; a light blow with a flat object; (*inf*) agitation, panic.

flapdoodle /ˈflæpˌduːdəl/ *n* (*inf*) nonsense.

flapjack /ˈflæpdʒæk/ *n* a kind of pancake; a cake made with oats and syrup.

flapper /ˈflæpər/ *n* someone who, or something which, flaps; (*inf*) a fashionable young woman of the 1920s.

flare /fler/ *vi* to burn with a sudden, bright, unsteady flame; to burst into emotion, *esp* anger; to widen out gradually. • *n* an unsteady flame; a sudden flash; a bright light used as a signal or illumination; a widened part or shape.

flare-up /-ˌʌp/ *n* a sudden burst of fire; (*inf*) a sudden burst of emotion.

flash /flæʃ/ *n* a sudden, brief light; a brief moment; a sudden brief display; (*TV, radio*) a sudden brief news item about an important event; (*photog*) a device for producing a brief intense light; a sudden onrush of water; **flash in the pan** a misfire; a showy start not followed up. • *vi* to send out a sudden, brief light; to sparkle; to come or pass suddenly; (*sl*) to expose the genitals indecently. • *vt* to cause to flash; to send (news, etc) swiftly; (*inf*) to show off. • *adj* (*inf*) flashy.—**flasher** *n*.

flashback /ˈflæʃbæk/ *n* an interruption in the continuity of a story, etc, by telling or showing an earlier episode.

flashboard /-ˌbɔrd/ *n* a board placed on a dam to increase its height and hence the depth of the water contained.

flashbulb /-ˌbʌlb/ *n* a small bulb giving an intense light used in photography.

flash flood *n* a sudden brief flood caused by a heavy rainfall.

flash gun *n* (*photog*) a device for holding and operating a flashbulb.

flashing /ˈflæʃɪŋ/ *n* a piece of lead or other metal, used to keep a roof watertight.

flashlight /ˈflæʃlɔɪt/ *n* an electric torch; a flash of electric light used to take photographs in dark conditions.

flashpoint /ˈflæʃpɔɪnt/ *n* the lowest temperature at which vapour, as from oil, will ignite with a flash; the point where a situation will erupt into violence.

flashy /ˈflæʃi/ *adj* (**flashier, flashiest**) pretentious; showy, gaudy.—**flashily** *adv*.—**flashiness** *n*.

flask /flæsk/ *n* a slim-necked bottle; a vacuum flask.

flasket /ˈflæskɪt/ *n* a small flask; a long, shallow basket.

flat /flæt/ *adj* (**flatter, flattest**) having a smooth level surface; lying spread out; broad, even, and thin; not fluctuating; (*tyre*) deflated; dull, tedious; (*drink*) not fizzy; (*battery*) drained of electric current. • *adv* in a flat manner or position; exactly; (*mus*) below true pitch. • *n* anything flat, *esp* a surface, part, or expanse; a flat tyre; a set of rooms on one floor of a building .—*also* **apartment**.—**flatly** *adv*.—**flatness** *n*.

flatcar /-ˌkɑr/ *n* an open, sideless rail truck.

flatfish /-ˌfɪʃ/ *n* (*pl* **flatfish, flatfishes**) any of an order of marine fishes that as adults have both eyes on one side.

flatfoot /-ˌfʊt/ *n* (*pl* **flatfeet, flatfoots**) a condition in which the arch of the instep is flattened; (*sl*) a policeman.

flat-footed /-ˌfʊtɪd/ *adj* having flatfoot; (*inf*) awkward; (*inf*) unprepared; (*inf*) determined, blunt.—**flat-footedly** *adv*.—**flat-footedness** *n*.

flatiron /ˈflætˌaɪrn/ *n* an iron used for clothes, linen, etc, heated by being placed upon a hot stove, etc.

flat spin *n* a spin or manoeuvre in which an aircraft is more horizontal than vertical; (*inf*) a confused or agitated state.

flatten /ˈflætən/ *vti* to make or become flat.—**flattener** *n*.

flatter /ˈflætər/ *vt* to praise excessively or insincerely, *esp* out of self-interest or to win favour; to display to advantage; to represent as more attractive, etc than reality; to gratify the vanity of; to encourage falsely.—**flatterer** *n*.—**flattering** *adj*.—**flatteringly** *adv*.

flattery /ˈflætəri/ *n* (*pl* **flatteries**) compliments; insincere praise.

flattie /ˈflæti/ *n* (*inf*) a woman's shoe with a flat heel.

flatting /-ɪŋ/ *n* (*metallurgy*) the process of rolling metal into flat sheets.

flatulence, flatulency /ˈflætjʊləns/ *n* wind in the stomach; windiness, verbosity; pomposity.

flatulent /ˈflætjʊlənt/ *adj* causing or affected with intestinal gas; pretentious, vain.—**flatulently** *adv*.

flatways, flatwise /-ˌwaɪz/ *adv* flat side downwards.

flatworm /-ˌwɜːm/ *n* any of various parasitic worms having a flattened body.

flaunt /flɒnt/ *vi* to move or behave ostentatiously (*flag*) to wave in the wind. • *vt* to display.—**flaunter** *n*.—**flauntingly** *adv*.

flaunty /ˈflɒnti/ *adj* (**flauntier, flauntiest**) inclined to flaunting.

flautist /ˈflɔːtɪst/ or /ˈflaʊ-/ *n* a flute player.—*also* **flutist**.

flavescent /fləˈvesənt/ *adj* turning yellow; yellowish.

flavin, flavine /ˈfleɪvɪn/ *n* a yellow dye and antiseptic.

flavorous /ˈfleɪvərəs/ *adj* tasty.

flavour, flavor /ˈfleɪvər/ *n* the taste of something in the mouth; a characteristic quality. • *vt* to give flavour to.—**flavourer, flavorer** *n*.—**flavoursome, flavorsome** *adj*.

flavouring, flavoring /-ɪŋ/ *n* any substance used to give flavour to food.

flaw /flɔ/ *n* a defect; a crack. • *vti* to make or become flawed.

flaw[2] *n* a gust of wind, a squall.

flawless *adj* perfect.—**flawlessly** *adv*.—**flawlessness** *n*.

flax /flæks/ *n* a blue-flowered plant cultivated for its fibre and seed; the fibre of this plant.

flaxen /ˈflæksən/, **flaxy** /-si/ *adj* made of flax; pale yellow.

flaxseed /ˈflækssiːd/ *n* the seed of the flax plant, from which linseed oil is obtained.

flay /fleɪ/ *vt* to strip off the skin; to berate, criticize severely.—**flayer** *n*.

flea /fliː/ *n* a small wingless jumping bloodsucking insect.

fleabane /-beɪn/ *n* a plant of the aster family.

fleabite /-ˌbaɪt/ *n* the bite of a flea; a minor inconvenience.

fleabitten /-ˌbɪtn/ *adj* marked with fleabites; (*inf*) shabby, wretched; (*horses*) flecked with red spots on a light ground.

fleam /fliːm/ *n* a lancet used for bleeding cattle.

flea market *n* an open-air street market, *usu* selling second-hand articles.

fleapit /ˈfliːpɪt/ *n* (*inf*) a shabby cinema or theatre.

flèche /fleʃ/ or /fleɪʃ/ *n* (*archit*) a slender spire, *esp* at the intersection of the nave and transept.

fleck /flek/ *n* a spot or speckle of colour; a tiny particle. • *vt* to mark with flecks.

flection /ˈflekʃən/ *see* **flexion**.

fled /fled/ *see* **flee**.

fledge /fledʒ/ *vt* (*birds*) to rear until ready to fly; to cover or provide with feathers, *esp* an arrow.

fledgling, fledgeling /ˈfledʒlɪŋ/ *n* a young bird just fledged; an inexperienced person, a trainee.

flee /fliː/ *vti* (**fleeing, fled**) to run away from danger, etc; to pass away quickly, to disappear.—**fleer** *n*.

fleece /fliːs/ *n* the woollen coat of sheep or similar animal. • *vt* to remove wool from; to defraud.

fleecy /ˈfliːsi/ *adj* (**fleecier, fleeciest**) like a fleece, woolly.—**fleecily** *adv*.—**fleeciness** *n*.

fleer /ˈfliːr/ *n* a derisive look, sneer. • *vti* to sneer (at), to mock.

fleet[1] /fliːt/ *n* a number of warships under one command; (*often with cap*) a country's navy; any group of cars, ships, buses, etc, under one control.

fleet[2] *adj* swift moving; nimble.—**fleetly** *adv*.—**fleetness** *n*.

fleeting /ˈfliːtɪŋ/ *adj* brief, transient.—**fleetingly** *adv*.

Fleming /ˈflemɪŋ/ *n* a native or inhabitant of Flanders.

Flemish /ˈflemɪʃ/ *adj* of the people of Flanders, or their language.

flense /flens/, **flench** /flentʃ/ *vt* (*whale, seal*) to strip blubber from.

flesh /fleʃ/ *n* the soft substance of the body, *esp* the muscular tissue; the pulpy part of fruits and vegetables; meat; the body as distinct from the soul; all mankind; a yellowish-pink colour. • *vt* (*usu with* **out**) to give substance to.

fleshings /ˈfleʃɪŋz/ *npl* flesh-coloured tights.

fleshly /ˈfleʃli/ *adj* (**fleshlier, flesh iest**) having to do with the body and its desires, material, sensual.—**fleshliness** *n*

flesh wound *n* a superficial wound.

fleshy /ˈfleʃi/ *adj* (**fleshier, fleshiest**) of or resembling flesh; plump; succulent; sensual.—**fleshiness** *n*.

fleur-de-lis /ˌflɜːdəˈliː/, **fleur-de-lys** /-ˈliːs/ *n* (*pl* **fleurs-de-lis, fleurs-de-lys**) a heraldic lily, the emblem of France.

fleury /ˈflɔːri/ *adj* (*her*) decorated with a fleur-de-lis.—*also* **flory**.

flew /fluː/ *see* **fly**.

flews /fluːz/ *npl* the pendulous lips of a bloodhound, etc.

flex /fleks/ *vti* to bend (a limb or joint, etc); to contract (a muscle). • *n* an insulated cable used to connect electric appliances to the mains.—*also* **cord**.

flexible /ˈfleksɪbəl/ *adj* easily bent, pliable; adaptable, versatile; docile.—**flexibility** *n*.—**flexibly** *adv*.

flexile /ˈfleksɪl/ *adj* supple; docile; flexible.—**flexility** *n*.

flexion /ˈflekʃən/ *n* the act or process of bending; a curve; (*gram*) an inflection.—*also* **flection**.

flexitime, flextime /ˈfleksˌtaɪm/ *n* the staggering of working hours to enable each employee to work the full quota of time but at periods most convenient for the individual.

flexor /ˈfleksər/ *n* a muscle that acts to bend a joint or limb.

flexuous, flexose /ˈfleksjuəs/ *adj* winding, sinuous; unsteady.—**flexuosity** *n*.

flexure /ˈflekʃər/ *n* the act of bending; the state of being bent; (*math*) the curving of a line or surface.—**flexural** *adj*.

flibbertigibbet /ˈflɪbərtiˌdʒɪbət/ *n* an impish, flighty or gossipy person.

flick /flɪk/ *n* a light stroke or blow; (*inf*) a cinema film. • *vt* to strike or propel with a flick; a flicking movement.

flicker /ˈflɪkər/ *vi* to burn unsteadily, as a flame; to move quickly to and fro. • *n* a flickering moment of light or flame; a flickering movement.—**flickeringly** *adv*.—**flickery** *adj*.

flick knife /-ˌnaɪf/ *n* a knife with a retractable blade released by pressing a button.

flier /ˈflaɪər/ *see* **flyer**.

flies *see* **fly**.

flight[1] /flaɪt/ *n* the act, manner, or power of flying; distance flown; a group of creatures or things flying together; an aircraft scheduled to fly a certain trip; a trip by aircraft; a set of stairs, as between landings; a mental act of soaring beyond the ordinary; a set of feathers on a dart or arrow.

flight[2] *n* an act or instance of fleeing.

flight-deck *n* the cockpit of an aircraft.

flightless /ˈflaɪtləs/ *adj* (*birds, insects*) incapable of flying.

flight recorder *n* a device that records information about the flight performance of an aircraft.

flighty /ˈflaɪti/ *adj* (**flightier, flightiest**) irresponsible, capricious, frivolous.—**flightily** *adv*.—**flightiness** *n*.

flimflam /ˈflɪmflæm/ *vt* (**flimflamming, flimflammed**) to deceive. • *n* nonsense; a trick.

flimsy /ˈflɪmzi/ *adj* (**flimsier, flimsiest**) weak, insubstantial; light and thin; (*excuse etc*) unconvincing. • *n* (*pl* **flimsies**) thin paper; copy written on this.—**flimsily** *adv*.—**flimsiness** *n*

flinch /flɪntʃ/ *vi* to draw back, as from pain or fear; to wince.—**flincher** *n*.—**flinchingly** *adv*.

flinders /ˈflɪndərz/ *npl* fragments.

fling /flɪŋ/ *vb* (**flinging, flung**) *vt* to cast, throw aside, *esp* with force; to put or send suddenly or without warning. • *vi* to kick out violently; to move or rush quickly or impetuously. • *n* the act of flinging; a lively dance; a period of pleasurable indulgence.—**flinger** *n*.

flint /flɪnt/ *n* a very hard rock that produces sparks when struck with steel; an alloy used for producing a spark in lighters.

flint glass *n* a lustrous kind of glass; lead glass.

flintlock /ˈflɪntlɒk/ *n* a type of old-fashioned gun fired by sparks from a flint.

flinty /ˈflɪnti/ *adj* (**flintier, flintiest**) like flint, hard; cruel.—**flintily** *adv*.—**flintiness** *n*.

flip[1] /flɪp/ *n* a drink made from any alcoholic beverage sweetened and mixed with beaten egg.

flip[2] *vb* (**flipping, flipped**) *vt* to toss with a quick jerk, to flick; to snap (a coin) in the air with the thumb; to turn or turn over. • *vi* to move jerkily; (*inf*) to burst into anger.

flip-flop /ˈflɪpflɒp/ *n* a backward handspring; an electronic circuit that can assume either of two states when activated; a rubber-soled sandal with a strap that fits between the toes.—*also* **thong**.

flippant /ˈflɪpənt/ *adj* impertinent; frivolous.—**flippancy** *n*.—**flippantly** *adv*.

flipper /ˈflɪpər/ *n* a limb adapted for swimming; a flat rubber shoe expanded into a paddle, used in underwater swimming.

flipper pie *n* ✤ (*Cdn*) a pie with a filling of seal flippers and vegetables.

flip side *n* the reverse side of a gramophone record; the less attractive or well-known aspect of a person or thing.

flirt /flɜːt/ *vi* to make insincere amorous approaches; to trifle or toy (*eg* with an idea). • *n* a person who toys amorously with the opposite sex.—**flirtation** *n*.—**flirter** *n*.—**flirtingly** *adv*.

flirtatious /flərˈteɪʃəs/ *adj* fond of flirting, coquettish.—**flirtatiously** *adv*.

flit /flɪt/ *vi* (**flitting, flitted**) to move lightly and rapidly; to vacate (a premises) stealthily. • the act of flitting, a removal.

flitch /flɪtʃ/ *n* a side of bacon, salted and cured; a plank cut from a tree.

flitter /ˈflɪtər/ *vi* to flit about; to flicker, flutter.

flivver /ˈflɪvər/ *n* (*sl*) an old or cheap car.

float /floːt/ *vi* to rest on the surface of or be suspended in a liquid; to move lightly; to wander aimlessly. • *vt* to cause to float; to put into circulation; to start up a business, *esp* by offering shares for sale. • *n* anything that floats; a cork or other device used on a fishing line to signal that the bait has been taken; a low flat vehicle decorated for exhibit in a parade; a small sum of money available for cash expenditures.—**floatable** *adj*.

floatage /ˈfloːtɪdʒ/ *see* **flotage**.

floatation /floːˈteɪʃən/ *see* **flotation**.

floater /ˈfloːtər/ *n* something that floats; a person lacking strong political convictions; (*inf*) a blunder.

floating /ˈfloːtɪŋ/ *adj* swimming, or buoyed up, on the surface of a liquid; (*anat*) displaced; (*vote, etc*) not settled; (*capital*) in circulation, available for use.

floccose /ˈflɒkˌoːs/ *adj* tufted.

floccule /ˈflɒkjuːl/ *n* a mass of fleecy material; a small tuft or flake.

flocculent /ˈflɒkjʊlənt/ *adj* woolly or flaky.—**flocculence, flocculency** *n*.

flocculus /ˈflɒkjʊləs/ *n* (*pl* **flocculi**) a tufted mass; (*astron*) a mass of gas appearing as a mark on the sun.—*also* **plage**.

floccus /ˈflɒkəs/ *n* (*pl* **flocci**) down, such as that found on young birds; a tuft of hair.

flock[1] /flɒk/ *n* a group of certain animals as birds, sheep, etc, living and feeding together; a group of people or things. • *vi* to assemble or travel in a flock or crowd.

flock[2] *n* a tuft of wool or cotton fibre; woollen or cotton waste used for stuffing furniture.—**flocky** *adj*.

floe /floː/ *n* a sheet of floating ice.

flog /flɒg/ *vt* (**flogging, flogged**) to beat harshly with a rod, stick or whip; (*sl*) to sell.—**flogger** *n*.—**flogging** *n*.

flong /flɒŋ/ *n* (*printing*) paper used for stereotyping.

flood /flʌd/ *n* an overflowing of water on an area normally dry; the rising of the tide; a great outpouring, as of words. • *vt* to cover or fill, as with a flood; to put too much water, fuel, etc on or in. • *vi* to gush out in a flood; to become flooded.—**floodable** *adj*.—**flooder** *n*.

floodgate /ˈflʌdɡeɪt/ *n* a gate for controlling the flow of water, a sluice.

floodlight /-ˌlaɪt/ *n* a strong beam of light used to illuminate a stage, sports field, stadium, building exterior, etc. • *vt* (**floodlighting, floodlit**) to illuminate with floodlights.

flood tide *n* the rising or inflowing tide.

floor /flɔr/ *n* the inside bottom surface of a room, flooring; the bottom surface of anything, as the ocean; a storey in a building; the area in a legislative assembly where the members sit and debate; the lower limit, the base. • *vt* to provide with a floor; to knock down (a person) in a fight; (*inf*) to defeat; (*inf*) to shock, to confuse.

floorage /ˈflɔrɪdʒ/ *n* the area of a floor.

floorboard /ˈflɔrbɔrd/ *n* one of the boards making up a floor.

flooring /-ɪŋ/ *n* material for making or covering a floor; a floor.

floor plan *n* a scale drawing of the layout of a floor of a building.

floor show *n* entertainment with singers and dancers, etc in a nightclub.

floozy, floozie, floosie /ˈfluːzi/ *n* (*pl* **floozies, floosies**) (*sl*) a disreputable woman.

flop /flɒp/ *vi* (**flopping, flopped**) to sway or bounce loosely; to move in a heavy, clumsy or relaxed manner; (*inf*) to fail. • *n* a flopping movement; a collapse; (*inf*) a complete failure.

floppy /ˈflɒpi/ *adj* (**floppier, floppiest**) limp, hanging loosely. • *n* (*pl* **floppies**) a floppy disk.—**floppily** *adv*.—**floppiness** *n*.

floppy disk *n* (*comput*) a flexible magnetic disk in a protective casing used for data storage and retrieval.

flora /ˈflɔrə/ *n* (*pl* **floras, florae**) the plants of a region or a period.

floral /ˈflɔrəl/ or /ˈflɒ-/ *adj* pertaining to flowers.—**florally** *adv*.

Florentine /ˈflɒrənˌtiːn/ or /-taɪn/ *n* a native or inhabitant of Florence.—*also adj*.

florescence /flɔˈresəns/ or /flɑ-/ *n* the process, state or time of flowering.

floret /ˈflɔrit/ *n* one of the small flowers forming the head of a plant.

floriated, floreated /ˈflɔriˌeɪtəd/ *adj* ornamented with floral decorations; flowery.

floribunda /ˌflɑrɪˈbʌndə/ or /ˌflɔr-/ *n* any of several varieties of hybrid roses with large clusters of flowers.

floriculture /ˈflɑrɪˌkʌltʃər/ or /ˈflɔr-/ *n* the cultivation of flowers.—**floricultural** *adj*.—**floriculturist** *n*

florid /ˈflɔrɪd/ or /ˈflɑ-/ *adj* flowery; elaborate; (*complexion*) ruddy.—**floridity** *n*.—**floridly** *adv*.

florist /ˈflɔrɪst/ *n* a person who sells or grows flowers and ornamental plants.

flory /ˈflɔri/ *see* **fleury**.

floss /flɒs/ *n* a mass of short silky fibres, as from the rough outside of the silkworm's cocoon; fine silk used in embroidery; dental floss.

flossy /-i/ *adj* (**flossier, flossiest**) like floss, silky, downy; (*sl*) flashy.

flotage /ˈfloːtɪdʒ/ *n* flotation; a craft afloat; flotsam.—*also* **floatage**.

flotation /floːˈteɪʃən/ *n* the act or process of floating; the launching of a business venture.—*also* **floatation**.

flotilla /fləˈtɪlə/ *n* a small fleet of ships.

flotsam /ˈflɒtsəm/ *n* wreckage or debris found floating in the sea.

flounce[1] /flaʊns/ *vi* to move in an emphatic or impatient manner. • *n* the act of flouncing, a plunge.

flounce[2] *n* a frill of material sewn to the skirt of a dress. • *vt* to add flounces to.

flouncing /-ɪŋ/ *n* a material used for making flounces.

flounder[1] /ˈflaʊndər/ *vi* to move awkwardly and with difficulty; to be clumsy in thinking or speaking.

flounder[2] *n* (*pl* **flounder, flounders**) a small flatfish used as food.

flour /flaʊr/ *n* the finely ground powder of wheat or other grain. • *vt* to sprinkle with flour.—**floury** *adj*.

flourish /ˈflɔrɪʃ/ or /ˈflɛrɪʃ/ *vi* (*plants*) to grow luxuriantly; to thrive, prosper; to live and work at a specified time. • *vt* to brandish dramatically. • *n* embellishment; a curve made by a bold stroke of the pen; a sweeping gesture; a musical fanfare.—**flourisher** *n*.

flout /flaʊt/ *vt* to treat with contempt, to disobey openly. • *n* an insult.—**flouter** *n*.—**floutingly** *adv*.

flow /floː/ *vi* (*liquids*) to move (as if) in a stream; (*tide*) to rise; to glide smoothly; (*conversation, etc*) to continue effortlessly; to be characterized by smooth and easy movement; to hang free or loosely; to be plentiful. • *n* a flowing; the rate of flow; anything that flows; the rising of the tide.

flow chart /-ˌtʃɑrt/ *n* a diagram representing the sequence of and relationships between different steps or procedures in a complex process, *eg* manufacturing.

flower /ˈflaʊr/ *n* the seed-producing structure of a flowering plant, blossom; a plant cultivated for its blossoms; the best or finest part. • *vt* to cause to bear flowers. • *vi* to produce blossoms; to reach the best stage.

floweret /ˈflaʊrət/ or /ˈflaʊrˈɛt/ *n* a little flower.

flowerpot /-ˌpɒt/ *n* a pot used to contain a growing plant.

flowery /ˈflaʊri/ *adj* full of or decorated with flowers; (*language*) full of elaborate expressions.—**floweriness** *n*.

flown /floːn/ *see* **fly**.

fl. oz. *abbr* = fluid ounce.

flu /fluː/ *n* (*inf*) influenza.

fluctuate /ˈflɛktʃuːˌeɪt/ *vi* (*prices, etc*) to be continually varying in an irregular way.—**fluctuation** *n*.

flue[1] /fluː/ *n* a shaft for the passage of smoke, hot air, etc, as in a chimney.

flue[2] *n* soft downy matter; fluff.

flue[3] *n* a type of fishing net.

fluent /ˈfluːənt/ *adj* able to write and speak a foreign language with ease; articulate, speaking and writing easily and smoothly; graceful.—**fluency** *n*.—**fluently** *adv*.

fluff /flʌf/ *n* soft, light down; a loose, soft mass, as of hair; (*inf*) a mistake, bungle. • *vt* to pat or shake until fluffy; (*inf*) to forget, to bungle.

fluffy /ˈflʌfi/ *adj* (**fluffier, fluffiest**) like fluff; soft and downy; feathery.—**fluffily** *adv*.—**fluffiness** *n*.

fluid /ˈfluːɪd/ *n* a substance able to flow freely, as a liquid or gas does. • *adj* able to flow freely; able to change rapidly or easily.—**fluidal** *adj*.—**fluidity** *n*.—**fluidly** *adv*.

fluid ounce *n* a US unit of capacity equal to one sixteenth of a US pint; a UK unit of capacity equal to one twentieth of an imperial pint

fluke[1] /fluːk/ *n* a flatfish; a flattened parasitic worm.

fluke[2] *n* the part of an anchor that fastens in the sea bed, river bottom, etc; the barbed end of a harpoon; one of the lobes of a whale's tail.

fluke[3] *n* a stroke of luck. • *vti* to make or score by a fluke.

fluky, flukey /ˈfluːki/ *adj* (**flukier, flukiest**) obtained by luck; uncertain.—**flukiness** *n*.

flume /fluːm/ *n* a channel for water; a ravine with a stream; a chute with a flow of water into a swimming pool. • *vt* to transport or divert by a flume.

flummery /ˈflʌməri/ *n* (*pl* **flummeries**) (*inf*) an empty compliment; a pudding, a kind of custard or blancmange.

flummox /ˈflʌməks/ *vt* (*inf*) to bewilder, perplex.

flung /flʌŋ/ *see* **fling**.

flunk /flʌŋk/ *vti* (*sl*) to fail, as in school work; to shirk.

flunky, flunkey /ˈflʌŋki/ *n* (*pl* **flunkies, flunkeys**) a servile person, toady; a person who does menial work; a liveried servant.

fluor /ˈfluːɔr/ *see* **fluorspar**.

fluoresce /fləˈres/ *vi* to display fluorescence.

fluorescence /fləˈresəns/ *n* the property of producing light when acted upon by radiant energy; light so produced.—**fluorescent** *adj*.

fluorescent lamp /fləˈresənt/ *n* a glass tube coated with a fluorescent substance that emits light when acted upon by ultraviolet radiation.

fluoridate /ˈflɔːrɪˌdeɪt/ *vt* to add fluoride to drinking water to reduce tooth decay.—**fluoridation** *n*.

fluoride /ˈflɔːraɪd/ *n* any of various compounds of fluorine.

fluorinate /ˈflɔːrɪˌneɪt/ *vt* to treat or mix with fluorine.—**fluorination** *n*.

fluorine, fluorin /ˈflɔːriːn/ *n* a chemical element, a pale greenish-yellow corrosive gas.

fluoroscope /ˈflɔːrəˌskoːp/ *n* an instrument with a fluorescent screen, used for studying X-ray images.—**fluoroscopy** *n*.

fluorspar /ˈfluːɔrspɑr/ *n* a transparent, or semi-transparent, material, composed of calcium fluoride.—*also* **fluor**.

flurry /ˈflɔːri/ *n* (*pl* **flurries**) a sudden gust of wind, rain, or snow; a sudden commotion. • *vti* (**flurrying, flurried**) to (cause to) become flustered.

flush[1] /flʌʃ/ *n* a rapid flow, as of water; sudden, vigorous growth; a sudden excitement; a blush; a sudden feeling of heat, as in a fever. • *vi* to flow rapidly; to blush or glow; to be washed out by a sudden flow of water. • *vt* to wash out with a sudden flow of water; to cause to blush; to excite. • *adj* level, or in one plane with another surface; (*inf*) abundant, well-supplied, *esp* with money.—**flusher** *n*.

flush[2] *vt* to make game birds fly away suddenly.—**flusher** *n*.

flush[3] *n* (*poker, etc*) a hand of cards all of the same suit.

fluster /ˈflʌstər/ *vti* to make or become confused. • *n* agitation or confusion.

flute /fluːt/ *n* an orchestral woodwind instrument in the form of a straight pipe (with finger holes and keys) held horizontally and played through a hole located near one end; a decorative groove. • *vi* to play or make sounds like a flute; to cut grooves in.—**fluty** *adj*.

fluter /ˈfluːtər/ *n* a person who makes flutes; a tool used in making flutes; a flute player.

fluting /ˈfluːtɪŋ/ *n* decorative channels or grooves in pillars, etc; pleats like this in a skirt, etc.

flutist /ˈfluːtɪst/ *n* a flute player, flautist.

flutter /ˈflʌtər/ *vi* (*birds*) to flap the wings; to wave about rapidly; (*heart*) to beat irregularly or spasmodically. • *vt* to cause to flutter. • *n* rapid, irregular motion; nervous excitement; commotion, confusion; (*inf*) a small bet.—**flutterer** *n*.—**fluttery** *adj*.

fluty /ˈfluːti/ *adj* (**flutier, flutiest**) soft and clear like the sound of a flute.—**flutily** *adv*.—**flutiness** *n*.

fluvial /ˈfluːviəl/, **fluviatile** /ˈfluːviəˌtaɪl/ *adj* of or found in streams and rivers.

flux /flʌks/ *n* a continual flowing or changing; a substance used to help metals fuse together, as in soldering.

fluxion /ˈflʌkʃən/ *n* a flowing; an excessive flow; (*math*) differential calculus.—**fluxional, fluxionary** *adj*.

fly[1] /flaɪ/ *n* (*pl* **flies**) a two-winged insect; a natural or imitation fly attached to a fish-hook as bait.

fly[2] *vb* (**flying, flew,** *pp* **flown**) *vi* to move through the air, *esp* on wings; to travel in an aircraft; to control an aircraft; to take flight, flee; to pass quickly; (*inf*) to depart quickly. • *vt* to cause to fly, as a kite; to escape, flee from; to transport by aircraft. • *n* a flap that conceals buttons, a zip, etc on trousers; material forming the outer roof of a tent; a device for regulating machinery, a flywheel.—**flyable** *adj*.

fly[3] *adj* (*inf*) sly, astute.

flyaway /ˈflaɪəweɪ/ *adj* (*hair etc*) loose; (*person*) flighty.

flyblow /ˈflaɪˌbloː/ *n* the egg or larva of a fly. • *vt* (**flyblowing, flyblew,** *pp* **flyblown**) to contaminate (meat, etc) by laying eggs (*esp* of a blowfly) in it.

flyby /ˈflaɪˌbaɪ/ *n* (*pl* **flybys**) a flight past a target, *esp* by a spacecraft past a celestial body to collect scientific data.

fly-by-night /-naɪt/ *adj* (*inf*) unreliable, untrustworthy; transitory. • *n* an untrustworthy person, *esp* one who evades responsibilities or debts by flight.

flycatcher /ˈflaɪˌkætʃər/ *n* a bird that catches insects on the wing.

flyer /flaɪr/ *n* something that flies or moves very fast; a pilot.—*also* **flier**.

fly fishing /ˈflaɪˌfɪʃɪŋ/ *n* fishing using artificial flies as lures.—**fly-fish** *vi*.

flying /ˈflaɪɪŋ/ *adj* capable of flight; fleeing; fast-moving. • *n* the act of flying an aircraft, etc.

flying boat *n* a sea plane in which the boat forms the fuselage and float.

flying buttress *n* a buttress connected to a wall by an arch, serving to resist outward pressure.

flying colours *npl* great success; triumph.

flying doctor *n* a doctor who visits patients (*eg* in isolated communities) by aircraft.

flying fish /ˈflaɪɪŋˈfɪʃ/ *n* any of numerous fishes of warm seas with winglike fins used in gliding through the air.

flying fox *n* a large fruit bat of Africa and Asia.

flying saucer *n* an unidentified flying disc-shaped object, purportedly from outer space.

flying squad *n* a small detachment of police officers mobilized for swift action.

flying squirrel *n* a nocturnal squirrel with folds of skin joining its legs, enabling it to glide.

flying start *n* a start in a race when the competitor is already moving when passing the starting line; a promising start in anything.

flyleaf /ˈflaɪliːf/ *n* (*pl* **flyleaves**) the blank leaf at the beginning or end of a book.

flyover /ˈflaɪˌoːvər/ *n* a bridge that carries a road or railway over another; a fly-past.

flypaper /ˈflaɪˌpeɪpər/ *n* paper with a sticky poisonous coating that is hung up to trap and kill flies.

fly-past /ˈflaɪpæst/ *n* a processional flight of aircraft.

flyte /flaɪt/ *see* **flite**.

flytrap /ˈflaɪtræp/ *n* any of various insect-eating plants; a device for catching flies.

flyweight /ˈflaɪweɪt/ *n* a boxer weighing not more than 112 pounds (51 kg).

flywheel /ˈflaɪwiːl/ *n* a heavy wheel which stores energy by inertia, used to regulate machinery.

FM *abbr* = Field Marshal; frequency modulation.

Fm (*chem symbol*) fermium.

f-number /ˈef ˌnʌmbər/ *n* (*photog*) a number used to calculate the ratio of light passing through a lens.

FO *abbr* (*Brit*) = Foreign Office.

foal /foːl/ *n* the young of the horse or a related animal. • *vti* to give birth to a foal.

foam /foːm/ *n* froth or fine bubbles on the surface of liquid; something like foam, as frothy saliva; a rigid or springy cellular mass made from liquid rubber, plastic, etc. • *vi* to cause or emit foam.

foamy /-i/ *adj* (**foamier, foamiest**) of, like, or covered with foam.—**foamily** *adv*.—**foaminess** *n*.

f.o.b. *abbr* = free on board.

fob[1] /fɒb/ *n* the chain or ribbon for attaching a watch to a waistcoat; any object attached to a watch chain; a small pocket in a waistcoat for a watch.

fob[2] *vt* (**fobbing, fobbed**) (*with* **off**) to cheat; to put off; to palm off (upon).

focal /ˈfoːkəl/ *adj* of or pertaining to a focus.—**focally** *adv*.

focalize /ˈfoːkəˌlaɪz/ *vti* to (cause to) focus.—**focalization** *n*.

focal length *n* the distance between the focal point and optical centre of a lens or mirror.

fo'c's'le, fo'c'sle /ˈfoːksəl/ *see* **forecastle**.

focus /ˈfoːkəs/ *n* (*pl* **focuses, foci**) a point where rays of light, heat, etc meet after being bent by a lens, curved mirror, etc; correct adjustment of the eye or lens to form a clear image; a centre of activity or interest. • *vt* (**focusing, focused** *or* **focussing, focussed**) to adjust the focus of; to bring into focus; to concentrate.—**focusable** *adj.*—**focuser** *n*.

fodder /ˈfɒdər/ *n* dried food for cattle, horses, etc.

FOE *abbr* = Friends of the Earth.

foe /foː/ *n* an enemy, an adversary.

foehn /feɪn/ *Gr.* /fœn/ *see* **föhn**.

foeman *n* (*arch*) an adversary in war.

foetal /ˈfiːtəl/ *see* **fetal**.

foeticide /ˈfoːtɪˌsaɪd/ *see* **feticide**.

foetid /ˈfetɪd/ *or* /ˈfiːt-/ *see* **fetid**.

foetus /ˈfiːtəs/ *see* **fetus**.

fog[1] /fɒg/ *n* (a state of poor visibility caused by) a large mass of water vapour condensed to fine particles just above the earth's surface; a state of mental confusion; (*photog*) cloudiness on a developed photograph. • *vti* (**fogging, fogged**) to make or become foggy.

fog[2] *n* a second growth of grass in autumn; winter pasture; (*Scot*) moss.

fogbound /ˈfɒgbaʊnd/ *n* unable to function due to fog.

fogey, fogy /ˈfoːgi/ *n* (*pl* **fogeys, fogies**) a person of old-fashioned or eccentric habits.—**fogeyish, fogyish** *adj*.

foggy /ˈfɒgi/ *adj* (**foggier, foggiest**) thick with fog; mentally confused; indistinct, opaque.—**foggily** *adv.*—**fogginess** *n*.

foghorn /ˈfɒghɔːn/ *n* a horn (in a ship, etc) sounded in a fog as a warning.

fogy *see* **fogey**.

föhn /fən/ *n* a warm, dry, Alpine wind.—*also* **foehn**.

foible /ˈfɔɪbəl/ *n* a slight weakness or failing; an idiosyncrasy; the weakest part of the blade of a sword.

foil[1] /fɔɪl/ *vt* to defeat; to frustrate; to trample a trail to spoil scent. • *n* (*arch*) the trail of hunted game.—**foilable** *adj*.

foil[2] *n* a very thin sheet of metal; a backing for a mirror or gem; anything that sets off or enhances another by contrast; (*archit*) a small arc or space in the tracery of a window. • *vt* to cover, back or adorn with foil; to set off.

foil[3] *n* a long, thin blunted sword used for fencing.

foison /ˈfɔɪzən/ *n* (*arch*) an abundance.

foist /fɔɪst/ *vt* (*with* **in** *or* **into**) to introduce stealthily or without permission; (*with* **off** *or* **on**) to pass off as genuine.

folacin /ˈfɒləsɪn/ *or* /ˈfoːl-/ *see* **folic acid**.

fold[1] /foːld/ *vt* to cover by bending or doubling over so that one part covers another; to wrap up, envelop; to interlace (one's arms); to clasp (one's hands); to embrace; to incorporate (an ingredient) into a food mixture by gentle overturnings. • *vi* to become folded; to fail completely; to collapse, *esp* to go out of business. • *n* something folded, as a piece of cloth; a crease or hollow made by folding.—**foldable** *adj*.

fold[2] *n* a pen for sheep; a group of people or institutions having a common belief, activity, etc. • *vt* to pen in a fold.

-fold *suffix* times repeated, *eg* tenfold.

foldaway /ˈfoːldəˌweɪ/ *adj* (*bed, etc*) collapsible.

folder /ˈfoːldər/ *n* a folded cover or large envelope for holding loose papers.

folderol /ˈfɒldəˌrɒl/ *see* **falderal**.

folding /-ɪŋ/ *n* the act or process of folding. • *adj* which folds or can be folded.

foliaceous /ˌfoːliˈeɪʃəs/ *adj* resembling or having leaves; (*rock*) having thin layers.

foliage /ˈfoːliədʒ/ *n* leaves, as of a plant or tree.

foliar /ˈfoːliər/ *adj* of or pertaining to leaves.

foliate /ˈfoːliət/ *adj* resembling or having leaves. • *vti* to beat (metal) into foil; to divide into thin layers; to produce leaves; (*archit*) to decorate with foils; to number the leaves of (a book).

foliation /ˌfoːliˈeɪʃən/ *n* (*bot*) the act of producing leaves or the state of having leaves; the act or process of beating a metal into thin plates.

folic acid /ˈfɒlɪk/ *or* /ˈfoːlɪk/ *n* a B-complex vitamin used in treating anaemia.—*also* **folacin**.

folio /ˈfoːlioː/ *n* (*pl* **folios**) a large sheet of paper folded once to make two leaves of a book; a book of sheets in this size, the largest commonly used; the number of a page in a book. • *vt* (**folioing, folioed**) to number the pages of.

foliose /ˈfoːliˌoːs/ *adj* (*bot*) having many leaves; of or resembling leaves.

folk /foːk/ *n* (*pl* **folk, folks**) a people of a country or tribe; people in general, *esp* those of a particular area; relatives; folk music. • *adj* of or originating among the ordinary people.—**folkish** *adj*.

folk etymology *n* the perversion of a word in an attempt to explain it, as "sparrow grass" for "asparagus."

folklore /ˈfoːklɔːr/ *n* the traditional beliefs, customs, legends, etc of a people; the study of these.—**folkloric, folkloristic** *adj.*—**folklorist** *n*.

folk music *n* traditional music.

folk song *n* a traditional song.

folksy /ˈfoːksi/ *adj* (**folksier, folksiest**) (*inf*) simple, plain; friendly.—**folksiness** *n*.

folktale *n* an anonymous, timeless, and placeless tale circulated orally among a people.

follicle /ˈfɒlɪkəl/ *n* any small sac, cavity, or gland.—**follicular, folliculate, folliculated** *adj*.

follow /ˈfɒloː/ *vt* to go or come after; to pursue; to go along (a path, road, etc); to copy; to obey; to adopt, as an opinion; to watch fixedly; to focus the mind on; to understand the meaning of; to monitor the progress of; to come or occur after in time; to result from; (*with* **through**) to pursue (an aim) to a conclusion; (*with* **up**) to pursue a question, inquiry, etc, that has been started. • *vi* to go or come after another; to result; (*with* **on**) (*cricket*) to take a second innings immediately after a first; (*with* **suit**) to play a card of the same suit; to do the same thing; (*with* **through**) (*sport*) to continue a stroke or motion of a bat, club, etc after the ball has been struck; (*with* **up**) to pursue steadily; to supplement.—**followable** *adj*.

follower /-wər/ *n* a disciple or adherent; a person who imitates another.

following /-wɪŋ/ *n* a body of adherents or believers. • *adj* next after; now to be stated.

follow-on /-ˌɒn/ *n* (*cricket*) an immediate return to bat by a side which has scored a certain number of runs fewer than its opponents in the first innings.

follow-through /-ˌθruː/ *n* (*golf, tennis, etc*) the continuation of a swing after hitting the ball.

follow-up /-ˌʌp/ *n* the continuing after a beginning; a steady pursuit.

folly /ˈfɒli/ *n* (*pl* **follies**) a lack of sense; a foolish act or idea; an extravagant and fanciful building which serves no practical purpose.

foment /foːˈmɛnt/ *vt* to stir up (trouble); to bathe with warm water or lotions.—**fomenter** *n*.

fomentation /ˌfoːmɛnˈteɪʃən/ *n* the act of formenting; instigation; the application of a warm lotion to ease pain or swelling.

fond /fɒnd/ *adj* loving, affectionate; doting, indulgent; (*arch*) overcredulous, simple; (*with* **of**) having a liking for.—**fondly** *adv.*— **fondness** *n*.

fondant /ˈfɒndənt/ *n* a soft sugar mixture for sweets and icings; a sweet made from this.

fondle /ˈfɒndəl/ *vt* to caress.—**fondler** *n.*—**fondlingly** *adv*.

fondue /fɒnˈduː/ *n* melted cheese used as a dip with small pieces of bread.

font[1] /fɒnt/ *n* a receptacle for baptismal water; a receptacle for holy water.—**fontal** *adj*.

font[2] *see* **fount**[1].

fontanameter /fɒnˈtænəˌmətər/ *n* a device for measuring the pressure within the skull of a foetus in the womb.

fontanelle, fontanel /ˌfɒntəˈnɛl/ *n* one of the open spaces in between the bones of an infant's skull.

food /fuːd/ *n* any substance, *esp* a solid, taken in by a plant or animal to enable it to live and grow; anything that nourishes.

foodie /ˈfuːdi/ *n* (*sl*) a person whose main focus is food whether reading about it, preparing it or eating it.

food poisoning *n* an acute illness caused by harmful bacteria or toxins in food.

food processor *n* an electric appliance used to perform various functions when preparing food, as chopping, mixing and grating.

foodstuff /ˈfuːdstʌf/ *n* a substance used as food.

fool /fuːl/ *n* a person lacking wisdom or common sense; (*Middle Ages*) a jester; a dupe; a cold dessert made from whipped cream mixed with fruit purée. • *vt* to deceive, make a fool of. • *vi* to act jokingly; to spend time idly; to tease or meddle with.

foolery /'fu:ləri/ *n* (*pl* **fooleries**) foolish behaviour, buffoonery.

foolhardy /'fu:l,hɑrdi/ *adj* (**foolhardier, foolhardiest**) foolishly bold; rash.—**foolhardiness** *n.*

foolish /'fu:lɪʃ/ *adj* unwise; ridiculous; ill-judged.—**foolishly** *adv.*—**foolishness** *n.*

foolproof /'fu:lpru:f/ *adj* proof against failure; easy to understand; easy to use.

foolscap /'fulskæp/ or /'fu:l-/ *n* a large size of writing paper.

fool's errand *n* a pointless undertaking.

fool's paradise *n* illusory happiness.

foot /fut/ *n* (*pl* **feet**) the end part of the leg, on which one stands; anything a resembling foot, as the lower part of a chair, table, etc; the lower part or edge of something, bottom; a measure of length equal to 12 inches (30.48 cm); the part of a garment that covers the foot; an attachment on a sewing machine that grips the fabric; a group of syllables serving as a unit of metre in verse. • *vi* to dance. • *vt* to walk, dance over or on; to pay the entire cost of (a bill).

footage /'futədʒ/ *n* measurement in feet, *esp* film exposed.

foot-and-mouth disease /'fu:tn'mauθ/ *n* a contagious disease of cattle.

football /'futbɒl/ *n* a field game played with an inflated leather ball by two teams; the ball used.—**footballer** *n.*

footboard /'futbord/ *n* a treadle on a machine; a step on a carriage.

footbridge /'futbrɪdʒ/ *n* a narrow bridge for pedestrians.

footer /'futər/ *n* (*sl*) football.

footfall /'futfɔl/ *n* the sound of a footstep.

foot-fault *n* (*tennis*) overstepping the base line when serving. • *vi* to commit a foot-fault.

footgear /'futgi:r/ *n* shoes and socks, etc.

foothill /'futhɪl/ *n* a hill at the foot of higher hills.

foothold /'futho:ld/ *n* a ledge, etc for placing the foot when climbing, etc; a place from which further progress may be made.

footie /'fu:ti/*see* **footy**.

footing /'futɪŋ/ *n* the basis upon which something rests; status, relationship; a foothold; (*archit*) a projecting course at the base of a wall.

footle /'futəl/ *vi* to potter.

footlights /'futlaɪts/ *npl* a row of lights in front of a stage floor.

footling /'fu:tlɪŋ/ *adj* trifling.

footloose /'futlu:s/ *adj* free, untramelled.

footman /'futmən/ *n* (*pl* **footmen**) a liveried servant or attendant.

footmark /'futmɑrk/ *n* a footprint.

footnote /'futno:t/ *n* a note or comment at the foot of a page.

footpad /'futpæd/ *n* (*arch*) a highwayman on foot.

footpath /'futpæθ/ *n* a narrow path for pedestrians.

foot-pound /'fu:t,paund/ *n* a unit of energy, equal to the work required to raise a one pound weight through one foot; equivalent to 0.042 joule.

footprint /'futprɪnt/ *n* the impression left by a foot.

foot-rot *n* an inflammation of the feet of sheep and cattle; a plant disease affecting stalks and trunks; (*sl*) athlete's foot.

foots /'futs/ *npl* the sediment of oil or sugar.

footsie /'futsi/ *n* (*inf*) amorous touching together of feet; (*inf*) clandestine dealings.

footslog /'futslɒg/ *vt* (**footslogging, footslogged**) (*inf*) to march.

footsore /'futsor/ *adj* having painful feet from excessive walking.

footstalk /'futstɔk/ *n* (*bot*) the supporting stem of a plant or flower; (*zool*) the attachment of a barnacle.

footstall /'futstɔl/ *n* a woman's stirrup (used on a sidesaddle).

footstool /'futstu:l/ *n* a stool for the feet of a seated person.

footwear /'futwer/ *n* shoes and socks, etc.

footwork /'futwork/ *n* skilful use of the feet in boxing, football, dancing, etc.

footy /'fu:ti/ or /'futi/ *n* (*sl*) football.—*also* **footie**.

foozle /'fu:zəl/ *n* (*golf*) a bungled shot. • *vi* to bungle (a shot).

fop /fɒp/ *n* someone obsessed with fashion and appearance.

foppery /'fɒpəri/ *n* (*pl* **fopperies**) the appearance, manner or dress of a fop.

foppish /'fɒpɪʃ/ *adj* affected in dress and manners.—**foppishly** *adv.*—**foppishness** *n.*

for /fər/ or /fɔr/ *prep* because of, as a result of; as the price of, or recompense of; in order to be, to serve as; appropriate to, or adapted to; in quest of; in the direction of; on behalf of; in place

of; in favour of; with respect to; notwithstanding, in spite of; to the extent of; throughout the space of; during. • *conj* because.

for- *prefix* expressing prohibition or neglect; bad effect; intensity.

forage /'fɒrədʒ/ or /'far-/ *n* food for domestic animals, *esp* when taken by browsing or grazing; a search for provisions. • *vi* to search for food.—**forager** *n.*

foramen /fɒ'reɪmen/ *n* (*pl* **foraminia, foramens**) a short passage or opening, *esp* in a bone.

foraminifer /,fɒrə'mɪnɪfər/ *n* a member of a group of protozoa having a shell with very minute apertures, through which parts of its body pass.

forasmuch as /,fɒrəz'mʌtʃ/ *conj* seeing that, since.

foray /'fɒreɪ/ *n* a sudden raid. • *vti* to plunder.—**forayer** *n.*

forbad, forbade /fɔr'bæd/ or /for-/ *see* **forbid**.

forbear /fɔr'bɛr/ *vb* (**forbearing, forbore,** *pp* **forborne**) *vi* to endure, to avoid. • *vt* to hold oneself back from.—**forbearer** *n.*—**forbearingly** *adv.*

forbearance /fɔr'bɛrəns/ *n* patience; self-control.

forbid /fɔr'bɪd/ *vt* (**forbidding, forbad** or **forbade,** *pp* **forbidden** or **forbid**) to command (a person) not to do something; to render impossible, prevent.—**forbiddance** *n.*—**forbidder** *n.*

forbidding /-ɪŋ/ *adj* unfriendly, solemn, strict.—**forbiddingly** *adv.*

forbore /fɔr'bor/, **forborne** /-'born/ *see* **forbear**.

force /fors/ *n* strength, power, effort; (*physics*) (the intensity of) an influence that causes movement of a body or other effects; a body of soldiers, police, etc prepared for action; effectiveness; violence, compulsion; legal or logical validity. • *vt* to compel or oblige by physical effort, superior strength, etc; to achieve by force; to press or drive against resistance; to produce with effort; to break open, penetrate; to impose, inflict; to cause (plants, animals) to grow at a greater rate than normal.—**forceable** *adj.*—**forcer** *n.*

forced /forst/ *adj* compulsory; strained.—**forcedly** *adv.*—**forcedness** *n.*

force-feed *vt* (**force-feeding, force-fed**) to compel a person to swallow food.

forceful /'forsful/ *adj* powerful, effective.—**forcefully** *adv.*—**forcefulness** *n.*

force majeure /,fors mæ'ʒɜr/ *n* compelling force, unavoidable circumstances.

forcemeat /'forsmi:t/ *n* finely chopped meat, seasoned and used as a stuffing.

force pump *n* a pump that forces water beyond the range of atmospheric pressure.

forceps /'forseps/ *n* (*pl* **forceps, forcipes**) an instrument for grasping and holding firmly, or exerting traction upon objects, *esp* by jewellers and surgeons.

forcible /'forsəbəl/ *adj* powerful; done by force.—**forcibleness** *n.*—**forcibly** *adv.*

ford /ford/ *n* a shallow crossing place in a river, stream, etc. • *vt* to wade across.—**fordable** *adj.*

fore /for/ *adj* in front. • *n* the front. • *adv* in, at or towards the front. • *interj* (*golf*) a warning cry to anybody who may be hit by the ball.

fore- *prefix* in front; beforehand.

fore-and-aft /'forən'æft/ *adj* (*naut*) (situated) at both bow and stern.

forearm[1] /'forɑrm/ *n* the arm between the elbow and the wrist.

forearm[2] /fo'ɑrm/ *vt* to arm in advance.

forebear /'forber/ *n* (*usu pl*) an ancestor.

forebode /for'bo:d/ *vt* to be a sign or warning (of trouble, etc) in advance; to have a premonition of (an event).—**foreboder** *n.*

foreboding /for'bo:dɪŋ/ *n* a feeling that evil is going to happen, a presentiment.

forecast /'forkæst/ *vt* (**forecasting, forecast** or **forecasted**) to predict (an event, the weather, etc) through rational analysis; to serve as a forecast of. • *n* a prediction, *esp* of weather; foresight.—**forecaster** *n.*

forecastle /'fo:ksəl/ *n* the forward part of a ship containing the crew's quarters.—*also* **fo'c's'le, fo'c'sle.**

foreclose /for'klo:z/ *vt* to remove the right of redeeming (a mortgage); to bar, exclude; to hinder.—**foreclosable** *adj.*—**foreclosure** *n.*

forecourt /'forkort/ *n* an enclosed space in front of a building, as in a filling station.

forefather /'for,foðər/ *n* (*usu pl*) an ancestor.

forefinger /'fɔr,fɪŋgər/ *n* the finger next to the thumb.
forefoot /'fɔrfut/ *n* (*pl* **forefeet**) a front foot of an animal; (*naut*) the foremost piece of the keel.
forefront /'fɔrfrʌnt/ *n* the very front, vanguard.
foregather /fɔr'gæðər/ *see* **forgather**.
forego[1] /fɔr'goː/ *see* **forgo**.
forego[2] *vt* (**foregoing, forewent**, *pp* **foregone**) to precede.—**foregoer** *n*.
foregoing /fɔr'goːɪŋ/ or /'fɔr-/ *adj* going before, preceding.
foregone conclusion /fɔr'gɒn-/ or /'fɔr,gɒn-/ *n* an inevitable result, easily predictable.
foreground /'fɔrgraʊnd/ *n* the part of a picture or view nearest the spectator's vision.
forehand /'fɔrhænd/ *n* (*tennis, etc*) a stroke made with the hand facing forwards; the part of a horse in front of the rider. • *adj* (*tennis stroke*) made with the palm leading.
forehanded /-əd/ *adj* thrifty; well-off.—**forehandedness** *n*.
forehead /'fɔrhɛd/ *n* the part of the face above the eyes.
foreign /'fɒrən/ or /fɒrən/ *adj* of, in, or belonging to another country; involving other countries; alien in character; introduced from outside.
foreigner /-ər/ *n* a person from another country; a stranger.
foreignism /'fɒrɪn,ɪzəm/ or /'far-/ *n* a foreign mannerism, custom or saying, or an imitation of any of these.
foreign office *n* the government department which handles foreign affairs.—*also* **state department**.
forejudge /fɔr'dʒʌdʒ/ *vti* to judge before hearing evidence.
foreknow /fɔr'noː/ *vt* (**foreknowing, foreknew**, *pl* **foreknown**) to know beforehand.—**foreknowledge** *n*.
foreland /'fɔrlænd/ *n* a promontory, a headland.
foreleg /'fɔrlɛg/ *n* a front leg of an animal.
forelock /'fɔrlɒk/ *n* the lock of hair growing above the forehead.
foreman /'fɔrmən/ *n* (*pl* **foremen**) a person who supervises workers in a factory, etc; the spokesperson of a jury.—**forewoman** *nf* (*pl* **forewomen**).
foremast /'fɔrmæst/ or /-məst/ *n* the mast nearest the bow of a sailing vessel.
foremost /'fɔrmoːst/ *adj* first in importance; most advanced in rank or position. • *adv* in the first place.
forenoon /'fɔrnuːn/ *n* time before midday; morning.
forensic /fə'rɛnsɪk/ *adj* of, belonging to or used in courts of law.—**forensicality** *n*.—**forensically** *adv*.
forensic medicine *n* the application of medical expertise to legal and criminal investigations.
foreordain /ˌfɔrɔr'deɪn/ *vt* to arrange in advance; to predestine.—**foreordainment, foreordination** *n*.
forepeak /'fɔrpiːk/ *n* (*naut*) the end of a ship's hold in the angle of the bow.
foreplay /'fɔrpleɪ/ *n* mutual sexual stimulation before intercourse.
forerun /fɔr'rʌn/ *vt* (**forerunning, foreran**, *pp* **forerun**) to precede, to foreshadow.
forerunner /'fɔr,rʌnər/ *n* a person or thing that comes in advance of another; a portent.
foresail /'fɔrseɪl/ or /-səl/ *n* (*naut*) the largest sail on the foremast of a sailing vessel.
foresee /fɔr'siː/ *vt* (**foreseeing, foresaw**, *pp* **foreseen**) to be aware of beforehand.—**foreseeable** *adj*.—**foreseer** *n*.
foreshadow /fɔr'ʃædoː/ *vt* to represent or indicate beforehand.—**foreshadower** *n*.
foresheet /'fɔrʃiːt/ *n* a rope for controlling a foresail; (*pl*) the inner part of a boat's bows.
foreshore /'fɔrʃɔr/ *n* a strip of land next to the shore; the shore between the high and low water marks.
foreshorten /fɔr'ʃɔrtən/ *vt* in drawing, etc, to shorten some lines of (an object) to give the illusion of proper relative size.
foresight /'fɔrsaɪt/ *n* foreseeing; the power to foresee; prudent provision for the future.—**foresighted** *adj*.—**foresightedness** *n*.
foreskin /'fɔrskɪn/ *n* the loose skin that covers the end of the penis.
forest /'fɒrəst/ or /'farəst/ *n* a thick growth of trees, etc covering a large tract of land; something resembling a forest. • *vt* to plant with trees; to make into forest.—**forestal, forestial** *adj*.
forestall /fɔr'stɒl/ *vt* to prevent by taking action beforehand; to anticipate.—**forestaller** *n*.—**forestalment, forestallment** *n*.
forestation /fɒrə'steɪʃən/ or /farə-/ *n* the planting of trees over a large area.

forestay /'fɔrsteɪ/ *n* (*naut*) a strong rope reaching from the top of the foremast to the bow of a vessel.
forester /'fɒrəstər/ or /'farə-/ *n* a person trained in forestry.
forestry /'fɒrəstri/ or /'farə-/ *n* the science of planting and cultivating forests.
foretaste /'fɔrteɪst/ *n* partial experience in advance; anticipation. • *vt* to taste before possession; to have a foretaste of.
foretell /fɔr'tɛl/ *vt* (**foretelling, foretold**) to forecast, to predict.—**foreteller** *n*.
forethought /'fɔrθɒt/ *n* thought for the future; provident care.—**forethoughtful** *adj*.
foretime /'fɔr,taɪm/ *n* the past, old times.
foretoken /'fɔr,toːkən/ *vt* to portend, foreshadow. • *n* an omen.
foretop /'fɔrtɒp/ or /-təp/ *n* (*naut*) a platform at the head of the foremast.
fore-topgallant mast /'fɔr,tɒp,gæl,ənt,mæst/ or /-tə,gæl-/, /-məst/ *n* the mast above the fore-topmast, carrying the fore-topgallant sail.
fore-topmast /fɔr'tɒpmæst/ or /-məst/ *n* (*naut*) the mast immediately above the foremast, carrying the fore-topsail.
for ever, forever /fər'ɛvər/ or /fɔr'ɛvər/ *adv* for all future time; continually.
for evermore, forevermore /fər,ɛvər'mɔr/ or /fɔr-/ *adv* for ever.
forewarn /fɔr'wɔrn/ *vt* to warn beforehand.—**forewarner** *n*.—**forewarningly** *adv*.
forewent /-'wɛnt/ *see* **forego**[2].
forewind /'fɔrwɪnd/ *n* (*naut*) a favourable wind.
forewoman /'fɔr,wʊmən/ *n* (*pl* **forewomen**) a person who supervises workers in a factory, etc; the spokesperson of a jury.
foreword /'fɔrwərd/ *n* an introduction to a book to explain its purpose, often by someone other than the author.
forfeit /'fɔrfət/ *n* something confiscated or given up as a penalty for a fault; (*pl*) a game in which a player redeems a forfeit by performing a ludicrous task. • *vt* to lose or be penalized by forfeiture.—**forfeiter** *n*.—**forfeiture** *n*.
forfend /fɔr'fɛnd/ *vt* to protect; (*arch*) to avert, ward off.
forficate /'fɔrfɪkət/ or /-,keɪt/ *adj* (*zool*) scissor-shaped, forked.
forgather /fɔr'gæðər/ *vi* to assemble, meet.—*also* **foregather**.
forgave /fɔr'geɪv/ or /fɔr-/ *see* **forgive**.
forge[1] /fɔrdʒ/ *n* (a workshop with) a furnace in which metals are heated and shaped. • *vt* to shape (metal) by heating and hammering; to counterfeit (*eg* a signature). • *vi* to commit forgery.—**forgeable** *adj*.—**forger** *n*.
forge[2] *vt* to move steadily forward with effort.
forgery /'fɔrdʒəri/ *n* (*pl* **forgeries**) fraudulently copying; a forged copy; a spurious thing.
forget /fər'gɛt/ *vti* (**forgetting, forgot**, *pp* **forgotten**) to be unable to remember; to overlook or neglect; **forget oneself** to lose self-control; to act unbecomingly.—**forgettable** *adj*.—**forgetter** *n*.
forgetful /fər'gɛtful/ *adj* apt to forget, inattentive.—**forgetfully** *adv*.—**forgetfulness** *n*.
forget-me-not /fər'gɛtmi,nɒt/ *n* a plant with bright-blue or white flowers.
forgive /fər'gɪv/ *vt* (**forgiving, forgave**, *pp* **forgiven**) to cease to feel resentment against (a person); to pardon. • *vi* to be merciful or forgiving.—**forgivable** *adj*.—**forgiveness** *n*.—**forgiver** *n*.
forgiving /-ɪŋ/ *adj* willing to forgive; merciful, kind.—**forgivingly** *adv*.
forgo /fɔr'goː/ *vt* (**forgoing, forwent**, *pp* **forgone**) to give up, abstain from.—*also* **forego**.—**forgoer** *n*.
forgot /fər'gɒt/, **forgotten** *see* **forget**.
fork /fɔrk/ *n* a small, *usu* metal, instrument with two or more thin prongs set in a handle, used in eating and cooking; a pronged agricultural or gardening tool for digging, etc; anything that divides into prongs or branches; one of the branches into which a road or river divides; the point of separation. • *vi* to divide into branches; to follow a branch of a fork in a road, etc. • *vt* to form as a fork; to dig, lift, etc with a fork; (*with* **out**) (*sl*) to pay or hand over (money, goods, etc).
forked /fɔrkt/ *adj* shaped like a fork; branching, opening into two or more parts; zigzag, *eg* lightning.
fork-lift truck /'fɔrk,lɪft/ *n* a vehicle with power-operated prongs for raising and lowering loads.
forlorn /fɔr'lɔrn/ *adj* alone; wretched.—**forlornly** *adv*.
forlorn hope *n* a faint hope; a desperate enterprise.

form /fɔrm/ *n* general structure; the figure of a person or animal; a mould; a particular mode, kind, type, etc; arrangement; a way of doing something requiring skill; a conventional procedure; a printed document with blanks to be filled in; a class in school; condition of mind or body; a chart giving information about racehorses; changed appearance of a word to show inflection; (*sl*) a criminal record. • *vt* to shape; to train; to develop (habits); to constitute. • *vi* to be formed.—**formable** *adj*.

form² *see* **forme**.

formal /'fɔrməl/ *adj* in conformity with established rules or habits; regular; relating to the outward appearance only; ceremonial; punctilious; stiff.—**formally** *adv*.

formaldehyde /fɔr'mældə,haid/ or /fər-/ *n* a colourless pungent gas used in solution as a disinfectant and preservative.

formalin /'fɔrməlin/ *n* an aqueous solution of formaldehyde used as an antiseptic or preservative.—*also* **formol**.

formalism /'fɔrmə,lizəm/ *n* strict observance of outward form or conventional usage.—**formalist** *n*.—**formalist c** *adj*.

formality /fɔr'mæliti/ *n* (*pl* **formalities**) strict observance of established rules or customs; an act or procedure required by law or convention.

formalize /'fɔrmə,laiz/ *vt* to make formal; to clothe with legal formality.—**formalization** *n*.

format /'fɔrmæt/ *n* the size, form, shape in which books, etc are issued; the general style or presentation of something *eg* a television programme; (*comput*) the arrangement of data on magnetic disk, etc for access and storage. • *vt* (**formatting, formatted**) to arrange in a particular form, *esp* for a computer.

formate /'fɔrmeit/ *n* a salt of formic acid.

formation /fɔr'meiʃən/ *n* form of making or producing; that which is formed; structure; regular array or prearranged order; (*geol*) a group of strata with common characteristics.—**formational** *adj*.

formative /'fɔrmətiv/ *adj* pertaining to formation and development; shaping; (*gram*) used in forming words.—**formatively** *adv*.—**formativeness** *n*.

forme /fɔrm/ *n* a frame with type assembled in it for printing.—*also* **form**.

former /'fɔrmər/ *adj* of or occurring in a previous time; the first mentioned (of two).—**formerly** *adv*.

formerly /'fɔrmərli/ *adv* previously; heretofore.

formic /'fɔrmik/ *adj* of or pertaining to ants or formic acid.

Formica /fɔr'maikə/ *n* (*trademark*) a heat-resistant laminated sheeting.

formic acid /'fɔrmik/ *n* a colourless pungent liquid found *esp* in ants and many plants.

Formicary /'fɔrmi,keri/, **formicarium** *n* (*pl* **formicaries, formicaria**) an anthill.

formication /,fɔrmi'keiʃən/ *n* an irritation of the skin, resembling the sensation made by insects crawling over it.

formidable /fɔr'midəbəl/ or /'fɔrmid-/ *adj* causing fear or awe; difficult to defeat or overcome; difficult to handle.—**formidability** *n*.—**formidably** *adv*.

formless /'fɔrmləs/ *adj* without distinct form, shapeless.—**formlessness** *n*.

formol *see* **formalin**.

formula /'fɔrmjulə/ *n* (*pl* **formulas, formulae**) a set of symbols expressing the composition of a substance; a general expression in algebraic form for solving a problem; a prescribed form; a formal statement of doctrines; a list of ingredients, as for a prescription or recipe; a fixed method according to which something is to be done; a prescribed recipe for baby food.—**formulaic** *adj*.

formularize /'fɔrmju:lər,aiz/ or /-mjə-/ *vt* to formulate.—**formularization** *n*.—**formularizer** *n*.

formulary /'fɔrmju,leri/ *n* (*pl* **formularies**) a book of prescribed forms, or of prayers, ritual, etc; (*med*) a book giving details of the formulas and preparation of pharmaceutical products. • *adj* of formulas or ritual.

formulate /'fɔrmju,leit/ *vt* to express in a formula; to devise.—**formulation** *n*.—**formulator** *n*.

formulism /'fɔrmju,lizəm/ *n* adherence to formulas.—**formulist** *adj*, *n*.

fornicate¹ /'fɔrni,keit/ *vi* to have sexual intercourse without being married.—**fornication** *n*.—**fornicator** *n*.

fornicate², **fornicated** *adj* (*archit*) vaulted, arched.

fornix /'fɔr,niks/ *n* (*pl* **fornices**) (*anat*) an arch-shaped part.

forsake /fɔr'seik/ *vt* (**forsaking, forsook, *pp* forsaken**) to desert; to give up, renounce.—**forsaker** *n*.

forsooth /fɔr'su:θ/ *adv* (*arch*) in truth.

forswear /fɔr'swer/ *vt* (**forswearing, forswore, *pp* forsworn**) *vt* to reject, renounce; to deny; to perjure (oneself).

forsythia /fɔr'siθiə/ *n* a widely cultivated, yellow-flowered shrub.

fort /fɔrt/ *n* a fortified place for military defence.

forte¹ /'fɔrtei/ *n* something at which a person excels.

forte² *adv* (*mus*) loudly.

forte-piano /,fɔrtəpi'æno/ or /-'pjæno:/ *adj*, *adv* (*music*) loud, then soft.

forth /fɔrθ/ *adv* forwards; onwards; out; into view; **and so forth** and the like.

forthcoming /fɔrθ'kʌmiŋ/ or /'fɔrθ-/ *adj* about to appear; readily available; responsive.—**forthcomingness** *n*.

forthright /'fɔrθrait/ or /fɔrθ'rait/ *adv* frank, direct, outspoken; decisive.—**forthrightly** *adv*.—**forthrightness** *n*.

forthwith /fɔrθ'wiθ/ or /-'wið/ *adv* immediately, without delay.

fortification /,fɔrtəfi'keiʃən/ *n* the act or process of fortifying; a wall, barricade, etc built to defend a position.

fortify /'fɔrtə,fai/ *vt* (**fortifying, fortified**) to strengthen physically, emotionally, etc; to strengthen against attack, as with forts; to support; (*wine, etc*) to add alcohol to; (*milk*) to add vitamins to.—**fortifiable** *adj*.—**fortifier** *n*.

fortissimo /fɔr'tisə,mo:/ *adv* (*mus*) very loud. • *n* (*pl* **fortissimos, fortissimi**) (*mus*) a passage played very loudly.

fortitude /'fɔrti,tu:d/ or /-,tju:d/ *n* courage in adversity; patient endurance, firmness.—**fortitudinous** *adj*.

fortnight /'fɔrtnait/ *n* a period of two weeks or fourteen consecutive days.

fortnightly /'fɔrt,naitli/ *adj*, *adv* once a fortnight.

Fortran /'fɔrtræn/ *n* (*comput*) a high-level programming language used for scientific and mathematical problem-solving.

fortress /'fɔrtrəs/ *n* a strong fort or fortified town.

fortuitous /fɔr'tu:itəs/ or /-'tju:-/ *adj* happening by chance.—**fortuitously** *adv*.—**fortuitousness** *n*.

fortuity /fɔr'tu:iti/ or /-'tju:-/ *n* (*pl* **fortuities**) fortuitousness; accident, chance.

fortunate /'fɔrtʃənət/ *adj* having or occurring by good luck.—**fortunately** *adv*.

fortune /'fɔrtʃən/ *n* the supposed arbitrary power that determines events; luck; destiny; prosperity, success; vast wealth.

fortune hunter *n* someone who seeks to become rich, *esp* by marrying for money.

fortune-teller /'fɔrtʃən,telər/ *n* a person who claims to foretell a person's future.—**fortune-telling** *n*.

forty /'fɔrti/ *n* (*pl* **forties**) four times ten, the symbol for this (40, XL, xl).—*also adj*.—**fortieth** *adj*.

forty-five /,fɔrti'faiv/ *n* a gramophone record played at 45 revolutions per minute; (*with cap*) the Jacobite rebellion of 1745.

forty-niner /,fɔrti'nainər/ *n* a pioneer who went to California in 1849 to look for gold.

forty-ouncer (*Cdn*) ✦ (*inf*) a forty-ounce bottle of alcoholic liquor.

forty-ninth parallel *n* ✦ (*Cdn*) the parallel of 49° north of the equator, *esp* as forming the border between Canada and the US.

forty winks *n* (*sing or pl*) a nap.

forum /'fɔrəm/ *n* (*pl* **forums, fora**) an assembly or meeting to discuss topics of public concern; a medium for public debate, as a magazine; the marketplace and centre of public affairs in ancient Rome.

forward /'fɔrwərd/ *adj* at, toward, or of the front; advanced; onward; prompt; bold; presumptuous; of or for the future. • *vt* to promote; to send on. • *n* (*sport*) an attacking player in various games. • *adv* toward the front; ahead.—**forwardness** *n*.

forwardly /-li/ *adv* pertly; promptly; forwards.

forwards /-s/ *adv* towards the front, in an onward direction.

forwent /fɔr'went/ *see* **forgo**.

forzando /fɔr'tsando:/ *adv* (*music*) with sudden emphasis.

fossa /'fɔsə/ *n* (*pl* **fossae**) (*anat*) a groove, pit or cavity.

Fosse, foss /fɔs/ *n* a ditch or moat, *esp* in a fortification.

fossick /'fɔsik/ *vt* to search for by picking over, to rummage.—**fossicker** *n*.

fossil /'fɔsil/ *n* the petrified remains of an animal or vegetable preserved in rock; (*inf*) a thing or person regarded as outmoded or redundant. • *adj* of or like a fossil; dug from the earth.

fossiliferous /,fɔsi'lifərəs/ *adj* containing fossils.

fossilize /-aɪz/ *vti* to change or become changed into a fossil.—**fossilization** *n.*

fossorial /fɒˈsɔːrɪəl/ *adj* (*zool*) used for digging.

foster /ˈfɒstər/ *vt* to encourage; to bring up (a child that is not one's own). • *adj* affording, giving, sharing or receiving parental care although not related.—**fosterer** *n.*

fosterage /ˈfɒstərɪdʒ/ *n* the act of fostering.

fosterling /ˈfɒstərlɪŋ/ *n* a foster child.

foudroyant /fuːˈdrɔɪənt/, Fr /fuːdRwaˈjɑ̃/ *adj* sudden and overwhelming; dazzling, like lightning.

fought /fɔːt/ *see* **fight**.

foul /faʊl/ *adj* stinking, loathsome; extremely dirty; indecent; wicked; (*language*) obscene; (*weather*) stormy; (*sports*) against the rules. • *adv* unfairly. • *vt* to make filthy; to dishonour; to obstruct; to entangle (a rope, etc); to make a foul against, as in a game; (*with* **up**) to contaminate; to ruin, bungle; to cause to become blocked or entangled. • *vi* to be or become fouled; (*with* **up**) to become blocked or entangled. • *n* (*sports*) a hit, blow, move, etc that is foul.—**foully** *adv.*—**foulness** *n.*

foulard /fuːˈlɑːrd/ *n* a light silk, or silk-cotton, fabric; a scarf made of this fabric.

foul-mouthed /ˈfaʊlˈmaʊθd/ or /-maʊθt/ *adj* using abusive or obscene language.

foul play *n* fouls in sport; violent crime, murder.

found[1] /faʊnd/ *see* **find**.

found[2] *vt* to bring into being; to establish (as an institution) often with provision for future maintenance.

found[3] *vt* to melt and pour (metal) into a mould to produce castings.

foundation /faʊnˈdeɪʃən/ *n* an endowment for an institution; such an institution; the base of a house, wall, etc; a first layer of cosmetic applied to the skin; an underlying principle, etc; a supporting undergarment, as a corset.—**foundational** *adj.*—**foundationary** *adj.*

founder[1] /ˈfaʊndər/ *n* one who founds an institution, a benefactor.

founder[2] *n* a person who casts metal.

founder[3] *vi* (*ship*) to fill with water and sink; to collapse; to fail.

found-in *n* ✤ (*Cdn*) a person arrested for being discovered in a place where illegal activities go on.

founding people *n* ✤ (*Cdn*) the French or English, considered as one of the two peoples that founded the nation-state of Canada.

foundling /ˈfaʊndlɪŋ/ *n* a deserted child whose parents are unknown.

foundry /ˈfaʊndri/ *n* (*pl* **foundries**) a workshop or factory where metal castings are produced.

fount[1] /faʊnt/ *n* a set of printing type or characters of one style and size.—*also* **font**.

fount[2] *n* a source.

fountain /ˈfaʊntən/ *n* a natural spring of water; a source; an artificial jet or flow of water; the basin where this flows; a reservoir, as for ink. • *vti* to (cause to) flow or spurt like a fountain.

fountainhead *n* a spring from which a stream flows; a first source.

fountain pen *n* a pen with an internal reservoir or cartridge of ink which supplies the nib.

four /fɔːr/ *n* one more than three; the symbol for this (4, IV, iv); the fourth in a series or set; something having four units as members (as a four-cylinder engine); a four-oared boat or its crew.—*also adj.*

fourchette /fʊrˈʃet/ *n* (*anat*) a fold of skin situated at the rear of the vulva.

four flush /ˈfɔːrˌflʌʃ/ *n* a poker hand with four cards of one suit.

four-flusher /-ər/ *n* a bluffer.

fourfold /ˈfɔːrfoːld/ *adj* having four units or members; being four times as great or as many.—*also adv.*

fourhanded /ˈfɔːrˌhændɪd/ *adj* for four players; (*mus*) for two players.

four-letter word *n* any of various words regarded as offensive or obscene typically containing four letters.

four-poster /ˈfɔːrˈpoːstər/ *n* a bed with four posts and a canopy.

fourscore /fɔːrˈskɔːr/ *n* eighty.

foursome /ˈfɔːrsəm/ *n* a group or set of four; (*golf*) a game between two pairs in which each pair has one ball.

Foursquare /ˈfɔːrˈskwer/ *adj* square; firm. • *adv* squarely; firmly.

four-stroke /ˈfɔːrˈstroːk/ *adj* (*internal-combustion engine*) having a piston that operates a cycle of four strokes for every explosion.

fourteen /fɔːrˈtiːn/ *n, adj* four and ten; the symbol for this (14, XIV, xiv).—**fourteenth** *adj.*

fourth /fɔːrθ/ *adj* next after third. • *n* one of four equal parts of something.—**fourthly** *adv.*

fourth dimension *n* time as added to the three spatial dimensions (length, breadth, depth).

fourth estate *n* journalists or the press in general.

Fourth of July *n* Independence Day of USA.

fowl /faʊl/ *n* any of the domestic birds used as food, as the chicken, duck, etc; the flesh of these birds. • *vi* to hunt or snare wildfowl.—**fowler** *n.*—**fowling** *n.*

fox /fɒks/ *n* (*pl* **foxes, fox**) any of various small, alert wild mammals of the dog family; the fur of the fox; a sly, crafty person. • *vt* to deceive by cunning. • *vi* (*inf*) to bemuse, puzzle.

foxglove /ˈfɒksglʌv/ *n* a tall plant with spikes of purple or white flowers.

foxhole /ˈfɒkshoːl/ *n* a pit dug in the ground as a protection against enemy fire.

foxhound /ˈfɒkshaʊnd/ *n* any of various large swift powerful hounds of great endurance used in hunting foxes.

foxtail /ˈfɒksteɪl/ *n* a type of grass found in Europe, Asia and South America.

fox-terrier *n* any of a breed of small lively terriers formerly used to dig out foxes.

foxtrot /ˈfɒkstrɒt/ *n* a dance for couples in 4/4 time. • *vi* (**foxtrotting, foxtrotted**) to dance the foxtrot.

foxy /ˈfɒksi/ *adj* (**foxier, foxiest**) reddish-brown; crafty; resembling a fox; physically attractive.—**foxily** *adv.*—**foxiness** *n.*

foyer /ˈfɔɪeɪ/ *n* an anteroom; an entrance hallway, as in a hotel or theatre.

FP *abbr* = (*US*) fireplug; former pupil.

Fr (*chem symbol*) francium.

fr *abbr* = franc.

Fra /frɑ/ *n* (*title*) a friar.

fracas /ˈfrækəs/ or /ˈfrækɒ/, /ˈfreɪkəs/ *n* (*pl* **fracas, fracases**) uproar; a noisy quarrel.

fraction /ˈfrækʃən/ *n* a small part, amount, etc; (*math*) a quantity less than a whole, expressed as a decimal or with a numerator and denominator.—**fractionary** *adj.*—**fractionally** *adv.*

fractional /ˈfrækʃənəl/ *adj* of or pertaining to fractions; inconsiderable, very small.

fractional distillation *n* the process used for separating a mixture of liquids into component parts by distillation.

fractionate /ˈfrækʃəˌneɪt/ *vt* to separate (elements of a mixture) by distillation.—**fractionation** *n.*

fractionize /-aɪz/ *vt* to divide into fractions.—**fractionization** *n.*

fractious /ˈfrækʃəs/ *adj* quarrelsome; peevish.—**fractiously** *adv.*—**fractiousness** *n.*

fracture /ˈfræktʃər/ *n* the breaking of any hard material, *esp* a bone. • *vti* to break; to cause to suffer a fracture.—**fracturable** *adj.*—**fractural** *adj.*

fragile /ˈfrædʒaɪl/ or /-dʒəl/ *adj* easily broken; frail; delicate.—**fragilely** *adv.*—**fragility, fragileness** *n.*

fragment /ˈfrægmənt/ *n* a piece broken off or detached; an incomplete portion. • *vti* to break or cause to break into fragments.—**fragmentation** *n.*

fragmentary /ˈfrægmənˌteri/ *adj* consisting of fragments; incomplete.—**fragmentarily** *adv.*—**fragmentariness** *n.*

fragrance /ˈfreɪgrəns/, **fragrancy** /-si/ *n* (*pl* **fragrances, fragrancies**) a pleasant scent, a perfume.

fragrant /ˈfreɪgrənt/ *adj* sweet-scented.—**fragrantly** *adv.*

frail[1] /freɪl/ *adj* physically or morally weak; fragile.—**frailly** *adv.*—**frailness** *n.*

frail[2] *n* a rush basket; the quantity of fruit held in a frail.

frailty /ˈfreɪlti/ *n* (*pl* **frailties**) physical or moral weakness; infirmity; a failing.

fraise /freɪz/ *n* a palisade of pointed sticks, used in a rampart; a type of neck ruff; a tool used to enlarge a drill hole.

framboesia, frambesia /fræmˈbiːzɪə/ *n* an infectious tropical disease, causing red skin eruptions and joint pain.—*also* **yaws**.

frame /freɪm/ *vt* to form according to a pattern; to construct; to put into words; to enclose (a picture) in a border; (*sl*) to falsify evidence against (an innocent person). • *n* something composed of parts fitted together and united; the physical make-up of an animal, *esp* a human body; the framework of a house; the structural case enclosing a window, door, etc; an ornamental border, as around a picture; (*snooker*) a triangular mould for setting up balls before play; (*snooker*) a single game.—**framable, frameable** *adj.*—**framer** *n.*

frame of reference *n* an arbitrary system of axes for describing the position or motion of something or from which physical laws are derived; a set or system (as of facts and ideas) serving to orient; a viewpoint, a theory.

frame-up /-ˌʌp/ *n* (*sl*) a conspiracy to have someone falsely accused of a crime.

framework /-ˌwɜːk/ *n* a structural frame; a basic structure (as of ideas); frame of reference.

franc /fræŋk/ *n* a unit of money in Switzerland and formerly of Belgium and France (now the euro).

franchise /ˈfræntʃaɪz/ *n* the right to vote in public elections; authorization to sell the goods of a manufacturer in a particular area. • *vt* to grant a franchise.—**franchisement** *n*.

Franciscan /frænˈsɪskən/ *n* a member of the Order of Friars Minor founded by St Francis of Assisi in 1209.

francium /ˈfrænsiəm/ *n* a radioactive metallic element.

francize /ˈfrænsaɪz/ *vt* ✸ (*Cdn*) to cause a person or group to adopt French as the official and working language of business, employment, and education.—**francization** *n*.

Franco- /ˈfræŋko/ *prefix* France; French.

Franco-Canadian *n* ✸ (*Cdn*) a French Canadian. • *adj* French-Canadian; pertaining to France and Canada.

francolin /ˈfræŋkolɪn/ *n* a kind of partridge, found in Africa and Asia.

Francophile /ˈfræŋkoˌfaɪl/ *n* a lover of France or its customs, etc.

francophone /ˈfræŋkoˌfoʊn/ *adj esp* ✸ (*Cdn*) French-speaking. • *n* a person whose first language is French.

frangible /ˈfrændʒɪbəl/ *adj* fragile, easily broken.—**frangibility** *n*.

frangipane /ˈfrændʒɪˌpeɪn/ *n* a paste or cake made with almonds and cream.

frangipani /ˌfrændʒɪˈpæni/ *n* (*pl* **frangipanis, frangipani**) a tropical American shrub, the flowers of which are used to make a perfume.

Frank /fræŋk/ *n* a member of a West Germanic people who conquered Gaul in the 4th century AD.—**Frankish** *adj*.

frank *adj* free and direct in expressing oneself; honest, open. • *vt* to mark letters, etc with a mark denoting free postage. • *n* a mark indicating free postage.—**frankly** *adv*.—**frankness** *n*.

Frankenstein /ˈfræŋkənˌstaɪn/ *n* a work that ruins its originator.

frankfurter /ˈfræŋkˌfɜːtər/ *n* a type of smoked sausage.

frankincense /ˈfræŋkɪnˌsens/ *n* a fragrant gum resin.

franklin /ˈfræŋklɪn/ *n* a middle-class landowner in 14th and 15th century England.

frantic /ˈfræntɪk/ *adj* violently agitated; furious, wild.—**frantically, franticly** *adv*.

frap /fræp/ *vt* (**frapping, frapped**) (*naut*) to bind tightly.

frappé /ˈfræpeɪ/ *adj* iced; chilled.

frater[1] /ˈfreɪtər/ *n* a friar.

frater[2] *n* (*arch*) a refectory.

fraternal /frəˈtɜːnəl/ *adj* of or belonging to a brother or fraternity; friendly, brotherly.—**fraternalism** *n*.—**fraternally** *adv*.

fraternity /frəˈtɜːnɪti/ *n* (*pl* **fraternities**) brotherly feeling; a society of people with common interests.

fraternize /ˈfrætərnaɪz/ *vt* to associate in a friendly manner.—**fraternization** *n*.

fratricide /ˈfætrɪˌsaɪd/ *n* the murder of a brother; a person guilty of this.—**fratricidal** *adj*.

Frau /frau/ *n* (*pl* **Frauen, Fraus**) (a title of) a married German woman.

fraud /frɔd/ *n* deliberate deceit; an act of deception; (*inf*) a deceitful person; an impostor.

fraudulent /ˈfrɔdjulənt/ *adj* deceiving or intending to deceive; obtained by deceit.—**fraudulence, fraudulency** *n*.—**fraudulently** *adv*.

fraught /frɔt/ *adj* filled or loaded (with); (*inf*) anxious; difficult.

Fräulein /ˈfrɔɪlaɪn/ *n* (*pl* **Fräulein, Fräuleins**) (a title of) an unmarried German woman.

fraxinella /ˌfræksɪˈnelə/ *n* a white-flowered Eurasian plant.

fray[1] /freɪ/ *n* a fight, a brawl.

fray[2] *vti* (*fabric, etc*) to (cause to) wear away into threads, *esp* at the edge of; (*nerves, temper*) to make or become irritated or strained.

frazil /ˈfræzəl/ *n* the ice that forms in a stream.

frazzle /ˈfræzəl/ *vt* to exhaust; to fray, tatter. • *n* (*inf*) a state of exhaustion.

freak[1] /friːk/ *n* an unusual happening; any abnormal animal, person, or plant; (*inf*) a person who dresses or acts in a notably

unconventional manner; an ardent enthusiast. • *vi* (*with* **out**) (*inf*) to hallucinate under the influence of drugs; to experience intense emotional excitement.—**freakish** *adj*.

freak[2] *vt* to variegate; to spot or streak.

freakish /ˈfriːkɪʃ/ *adj* very unusual; changing suddenly.—**freakishly** *adv*.—**freakishness** *n*.

freckle /ˈfrekəl/ *n* a small brownish spot on the skin. • *vti* to make or become spotted with freckles.—**freckled, freckly** *adj*.

free /friː/ *adj* (**freer, freest**) not under the control or power of another; having social and political liberty; independent; able to move in any direction; not burdened by obligations; not confined to the usual rules; not exact; generous; frank; with no cost or charge; exempt from taxes, duties, etc; clear of obstruction; not fastened. • *adv* without cost; in a free manner. • *vt* (**freeing, freed**) to set free; to clear of obstruction, etc.—**freely** *adv*.

freebie /ˈfriːbi/ *n* (*sl*) something provided free of charge.

freeboard /ˈfriːbɔːd/ *n* the part of the side of a ship between the upper side of the deck and the water-line.

freebooter /ˈfriːˌbuːtər/ *n* a pirate; a plunderer.

freeborn /ˈfriːbɔːn/ *adj* born of free parents, as opposed to in slavery.

freedman /ˈfriːdmən/ *n* (*pl* **freedmen**) an emancipated slave.

freedom fighter /ˈfriːdəm/ *n* a person violently resisting an oppressive political regime.

freedom /ˈfriːdəm/ *n* being free; exemption from obligation; unrestricted use; a right or privilege.

free enterprise *n* the freedom of business from government intervention or control.

free fall *n* the descent of a body under the force of gravity alone, as a parachutist before the parachute opens.

free fight *n* an indiscriminate contest, a melée.

free-for-all /ˈfriːfərˌɔl/ *n* (*inf*) a disorganized fight or brawl involving as many participants as are willing.

free hand /ˈfriːˌhænd/ *n* freedom to act as desired.

freehand *adj* (*drawing, etc*) drawn by the hand without the aid of instruments.

freehanded /-ˈhænˌdɪd/ *adj* generous; liberal.—**freehandedly** *adv*.—**freehandedness** *n*.

freehold /ˈfriːˌhoʊld/ *n* tenure without rent; absolute ownership; an estate so held.—**freeholder** *n*.

free house *n* in the UK, a public house which is allowed to sell drinks from more than one brewer.

free kick *n* (*soccer, rugby*) a place kick awarded because of a foul or infringement by an opponent.

freelance /ˈfriːlæns/ *n* a person who pursues a profession without long-term commitment to any employer.—*also* **freelancer**. • *vt* to work as a freelance.

free-living /ˈfriːlɪvɪŋ/ *n* (*organisms*) not parasitic.—**free-liver** *n*.

freeload /ˈfriːlowd/ *vi* to impose upon another's hospitality.—**freeloader** *n*.

free love *n* sexual intercourse without the restraints of marriage.

freeman /ˈfriːmən/ *n* (*pl* **freemen**) someone who is not a slave; someone with civic rights.

freemartin /ˈfriːˌmɑːtən/ *n* a sexually imperfect and sterile cow calf, born as the twin of a bull calf.

Freemason /ˈfriːˌmeɪsən/ *n* a member of the secretive fraternity (Free and Accepted Masons) dedicated to mutual aid.

freemasonry /ˈfriːˌmeɪsənri/ *n* mutual help between persons of similar interests.

free port *n* a port where goods are received and shipped free of customs duty.

free-range /ˈfriːˌreɪndʒ/ *adj* (*hens*) allowed to roam freely, not confined in a battery; (*eggs*) produced by hens raised in this way.

freesheet *n* a newspaper distributed free of charge.

freesia /ˈfriːʒə/ *or* /ˈfriːziə/ *n* a sweet-scented African plant of the iris family.

freespoken /ˈfriːˈspoʊkən/ *adj* outspoken, blunt.—**freespokenness** *n*.

freestanding /ˈfriːˌstændɪŋ/ *adj* (*furniture*) standing on its own; not attached.

freestone /ˈfriːstoʊn/ *n* a type of limestone or sandstone that is suitable for working.

freestyle /ˈfriːstaɪl/ *n* a swimming competition in which the competitor chooses the stroke.

freethinker /ˌfriːˈθɪŋkər/ *n* a person who rejects authority in religion, etc; a sceptic.

free trade *n* trade based on the unrestricted international exchange of goods with tariffs used only as a source of revenue.—**free-trader** *n*.

free verse *n* verse without a fixed metrical pattern.

freeway /ˈfriːweɪ/ *n* in North America, a fast road, a motorway.

freewheel /friːˈwiːl/ *n* a device for temporarily disconnecting and setting free the back wheel of a bicycle from the driving gear. • *vi* to ride a bicycle with the gear disconnected; to drive a car with the gear in neutral.—**freewheeler** *n*.

free will /ˈfriːˈwɪl/ *n* voluntary choice or decision; freedom of human beings to make choices that are not determined by prior causes or by divine intervention.

freeze /friːz/ *vb* (**freezing, froze,** *pp* **frozen**) *vi* to be formed into, or become covered by ice; to become very cold; to be damaged or killed by cold; to become motionless; to be made speechless by strong emotion; to become formal and unfriendly. • *vt* to harden into ice; to convert from a liquid to a solid with cold; to make extremely cold; to act towards in a stiff and formal way; to act on *usu* destructively by frost; to anaesthetize by cold; to fix (prices, etc) at a given level by authority; to make (funds, etc) unavailable to the owners by authority.—**freezable** *adj*.

freeze-dry /ˈfriːzˌdraɪ/ *vt* (**freeze-drying, freeze-dried**) to preserve (food) by rapid freezing and then drying in a vacuum.

freeze-frame *n* a frame of a motion picture or television film that is repeated to give the illusion of a static picture.

freezer /ˈfriːzər/ *n* a compartment or container that freezes and preserves food for long periods.

freezing /-ɪŋ/ *adj* very cold.

freezing point *n* the temperature at which a liquid solidifies.

freeze-up /ˈfriːzˌʌp/ *n esp* ♣ (*Cdn*) the freezing of a body of water, *esp* in the autumn.

freight /freɪt/ *n* the transport of goods by water, land, or air; the cost for this; the goods transported. • *vt* to load with freight; to send by freight.

freightage /ˈfreɪtɪdʒ/ *n* the conveyance of cargo; the cargo conveyed; a charge made for transporting cargo.

freight car *n* a rail truck for carrying freight.

freighter /ˈfreɪtər/ *n* one who freights; a ship or aircraft carrying freight.

French /frentʃ/ *adj* of France, its people, culture, etc. • *n* the language of France.

French bread *n* bread in a long, slender loaf.

French Canada *n* ♣ Quebec and other parts of Canada where mainly French is spoken.

French Canadian *n* ♣ a Canadian whose first language is French. • *adj* **French-Canadian** pertaining to French-speaking Canadians.

French chalk *n* a soapstone used as a dry lubricant and to mark cloth, etc.

French doors *see* **French windows**.

French dressing *n* a salad dressing made from vinegar, oil and seasonings.

French French (*Cdn*) ♣ (*inf*) French as spoken in France, as distinguished from that spoken in French Canada.

French fries, french fries *npl* thin strips of potato fried in oil, etc, chips.

French horn *n* an orchestral brass instrument with a narrow conical tube wound twice in a circle, a funnel shaped mouthpiece, and a flaring bell.

Frenchify /ˈfrentʃɪˌfaɪ/ *vti* (**Frenchifies, Frenchifying, Frenchified**) (*inf*) to make or become French.

French immersion *n* ♣ (*Cdn*) an educational program in which English-speaking students are taught entirely in French.

French leave *n* leave taken without permission; a hasty or secret departure.

French letter *n* a condom.

French polish *n* a shellac varnish for furniture.

French roof *n* a mansard roof.

French toast *n* toast with one side buttered and the other toasted; bread soaked in milk and batter and fried lightly.

French windows *npl* a pair of casement windows extending to the floor that are placed in an outside wall and open on to a patio, garden, etc.—*also* **French doors**.

frenetic /frəˈnetɪk/ *adj* frantic, frenzied.—**frenetically** *adv*.

frenzy /ˈfrenzi/ *n* (*pl* **frenzies**) wild excitement; violent mental derangement. • *vt* (**frenzying, frenzied**) to infuriate, to madden.—**frenzied** *adj*.—**frenziedly** *adv*.

frequency /ˈfriːkwənsi/ *n* (*pl* **frequencies**) repeated occurrence; the number of occurrences, cycles, etc in a given period.

frequency modulation *n* the transmission of signals by radio waves whose frequency varies according to the amplitude of the signal.

frequent /ˈfriːkwənt/ *adj* coming or happening often. • *vi* to visit often; to resort to.—**frequenter** *n*.—**frequently** *adv*.

frequentative /frɪˈkwentətɪv/ *adj* (*gram*) expressing repetition and intensity (of a verb). • *n* a frequentative verb.

fresco /ˈfreskəʊ/ *n* (*pl* **frescos, frescoes**) a picture painted on walls covered with damp freshly laid plaster. • *vt* (**frescoing, frescoed**) to paint in fresco.

fresh /freʃ/ *adj* recently made, grown, etc; not salted, pickled, etc; not spoiled; lively, not tired; not worn, soiled, faded, etc; new, recent; inexperienced; cool and refreshing; (*wind*) brisk; (*water*) not salt; (*inf*) presumptuous, impertinent. • *adv* newly.—**freshly** *adv*.—**freshness** *n*.

freshen /ˈfreʃən/ *vi* to make or become fresh.—**freshener** *n*.

fresher /ˈfreʃər/ *n* (*pl* **freshers**) a freshman.

freshet /ˈfreʃət/ *n* a flood caused by melting snow or heavy rain; a stream of fresh water.

freshman /ˈfreʃmən/ *n* (*pl* **freshmen**) a first year student at university, college or high school.

freshwater /ˈfreʃˌwɒtər/ *adj* of a river; not sea-going.

fret[1] /fret/ *vti* (**fretting, fretted**) to make or become worried or anxious; to wear away or roughen by rubbing.

fret[2] *n* a running design of interlacing small bars. • *vt* (**fretting, fretted**) to furnish with frets.

fret[3] *n* any of a series of metal ridges along the finger-board of a guitar, banjo, etc used as a guide for depressing the strings.

fretful /ˈfretfʊl/ *adj* troubled; peevish; irritable; impatient.—**fretfully** *adv*.—**fretfulness** *n*.

fretsaw /ˈfretsɔː/ *n* a narrow saw held under tension in a frame used for cutting intricate designs in wood or metal.

fretwork /ˈfretwɜːk/ *n* decorative carving consisting of frets.

Freudian /ˈfrɔɪdiən/ *adj* of or pertaining to the psychoanalytic theories of Sigmund Freud. • *n* a psychoanalyst who follows the theories of Freud.—**Freudianism** *n*.

Freudian slip *n* a slip of the tongue said to betray an unconscious feeling.

Fri. *abbr* = Friday.

friable /ˈfraɪəbəl/ *adj* easily crumbled.—**friability** *n*.

friar /ˈfraɪr/ *n* a member of certain Roman Catholic religious orders.

friarbird /-ˌbɜːd/ *n* an Australasian songbird with a tongue specially adapted to extract nectar.

friary /ˈfraɪri/ *n* (*pl* **friaries**) a monastery of friars.

fribble /ˈfrɪbəl/ *vt* to fritter away. • *n* a trifler.—**fribbler** *n*.

fricandeau, fricando /ˌfrɪkənˈdəʊ/ or /ˈfrɪkənˌdəʊ/ *n* (*pl* **fricandeaus, fricandeaux, fricandoes**) a dish made from spiced, stewed veal.

fricassee /ˈfrɪkəˌsiː/ or /-ˈsiː/ *n* a dish made of stewed poultry, rabbit, etc in a white sauce. • *vt* (**fricasseeing, fricasseed**) to cook in this way.

fricative /ˈfrɪkeɪtɪv/ *n* (*phonetics*) a sound, *eg* "f" produced by the friction of breath in a narrow opening. • *adj* pertaining to a fricative.

friction /ˈfrɪkʃən/ *n* a rubbing of one object against another; conflict between differing opinions, ideas, etc; the resistance to motion of things that touch.—**frictional** *adj*.

friction clutch *n* a clutch that transmits motion by friction.

Friday /ˈfraɪdeɪ/ or /-di/ *n* the sixth day of the week.

fridge /frɪdʒ/ *n* (*inf*) a refrigerator.

fried /fraɪd/ *see* **fry**[1].

friend /frend/ *n* a person whom one knows well and is fond of; an ally, supporter, or sympathizer. • *vt* (*arch*) to befriend.—**friendless** *adj*.—**friendship** *n*.

friendly /ˈfrendli/ *adj* (**friendlier, friendliest**) like a friend; kindly; favourable. • *n* a sporting game played for fun, not in competition.—**friendlily** *adv*.—**friendliness** *n*.

friendly society *n* an association for mutual insurance against sickness, etc.

friendship /ˈfrendʃɪp/ *n* the state of being friends; intimacy united with affection or esteem; mutual attachment; goodwill.

frier /ˈfraɪər/ *see* **fry**[1].

frieze[1] /friːz/ *n* a decorative band along the top of the wall of a room; (*archit*) the part of an entablature between the architrave and cornice, often filled with sculpture.

frieze[2] *n* a coarse woollen cloth with a rough shaggy nap on one side.

frigate /ˈfrɪgət/ *n* a warship smaller than a destroyer used for escort, anti-submarine, and patrol duties.

frigate bird *n* a swift-flying tropical sea bird.

fright /fraɪt/ *n* sudden fear; a shock; (*inf*) something unsightly or ridiculous in appearance.

frighten /ˈfraɪtən/ *vt* to terrify, to scare; to force by frightening.—**frightener** *n*.—**frighteningly** *adv*.

frightful /ˈfraɪtful/ *adj* terrible, shocking; (*inf*) extreme, very bad.—**frightfully** *adv*.—**frightfulness** *n*.

frigid /ˈfrɪdʒɪd/ *adj* extremely cold; not warm or friendly; unresponsive sexually.—**frigidity** *n*.—**frigidly** *adv*.

Frigid Zone *n* either of the areas within the Arctic or Antarctic circles.

frigorific /ˌfrɪgəˈrɪfɪk/ *adj* (*arch*) causing cold.

frijol /ˈfriːˌhoːl/ or /friːˈhoːl/ *n* (*pl* **frijoles**) a type of bean, widely cultivated for eating in Mexico.

frill /frɪl/ *n* a piece of pleated or gathered fabric used for edging; something superfluous, an affectation. • *vt* to decorate with a frill or frills.—**frilled** *adj*.—**frilly** *adj*.

fringe /frɪndʒ/ *n* a decorative border of hanging threads; hair hanging over the forehead; an outer edge; a marginal or minor part. • *vt* to be or make a fringe for. • *adj* at the outer edge; additional; minor; unconventional.

fringe benefit *n* a benefit given by an employer to supplement an employee's wages; any additional advantage.

frippery /ˈfrɪpəri/ *n* (*pl* **fripperies**) cheap, gaudy clothes or ornaments; trivia.

Frisbee /ˈfrɪzbi/ *n* (*trademark*) a plastic disc that is spun through the air for recreation or sport.

frisette /frɪˈset/ *n* a curly fringe, *esp* of false hair.—*also* **frizette**.

frisk /frɪsk/ *vi* to leap playfully. • *vt* (*inf*) to search (a person) by feeling for concealed weapons, etc. • *n* a gambol, dance, or frolic.—**frisker** *n*.

frisky /ˈfrɪski/ *adj* (**friskier**, **friskiest**) lively, playful.—**friskily** *adv*.—**friskiness** *n*.

frisson /ˈfriːsɒn/ or /-sɔ̃/ *n* an emotional thrill, a shiver of excitement.

frit, fritt /frɪt/ *n* the mixture of sand and fluxes from which glass is made. • *vt* (**fritting, fritted**) to make into frit.

frith /frɪθ/ *see* **firth**.

frit fly *n* a small fly destructive to grain.

fritillary /frɪˈtɪləri/ or /ˈfrɪtɪˌleri/ *n* (*pl* **fritillaries**) a flowering plant of the lily kind, the petals of which are variegated with purple, dice-shaped marks; a butterfly with brownish wings spotted with black or silver.

fritt *see* **frit**.

fritter[1] /ˈfrɪtər/ *n* a slice of fruit or meat fried in batter.

fritter[2] *vt* (*with* **away**) to waste; to break into tiny pieces.—**fritterer** *n*.

frivol /ˈfrɪvəl/ *vb* (**frivolling, frivolled** or **frivoling, frivoled**) *vi* to behave in a frivolous way; to trifle. • *vt* to squander.

frivolity /frɪˈvɒlɪti/ *n* (*pl* **frivolities**) a trifling act, thought, or action.

frivolous /ˈfrɪvələs/ *adj* irresponsible; trifling; silly.—**frivolously** *adv*.—**frivolousness** *n*.

frizette /frɪˈzet/ *n see* **frisette**.

frizz /frɪz/ *vti* (*hair*) to (cause to) form into small tight curls. • *n* hair that is frizzed.—**frizzer** *n*.

frizzle[1] /ˈfrɪzəl/ *vt* to frizz. • *n* a small tight curl.—**frizzler** *n*.

frizzle[2] *vti* to sizzle, as in frying; to scorch by frying.

frizzy /ˈfrɪzi/, **frizzly** /ˈfrɪzli/ *adj* (**frizzier, frizz est** or **frizzlier, frizzliest**) (*hair*) in tight wiry curls.—**frizziness, frizzliness** *n*.

fro /froː/ *adv* away from; backward; **to and fro** back and forward.

frock /frɒk/ *n* a dress; a smock; a loose wide-sleeved gown worn by a monk. • *vt* to put on a frock; to invest with the office of priest.

frock coat *n* a double-breasted skirted coat for men.

frog[1] /frɒg/ *n* a small tailless web-footed jumping amphibian.

frog[2] *n* a decorative loop used to fasten clothing; an attachment on a belt for carrying a sword.—**frogged** *adj*.

frog[3] *n* a section of rail where two lines cross.

frog[4] *n* a tender horny substance growing in the middle of the sole of a horse's foot.

frogfish /ˈfrɒgfɪʃ/ *n* (*pl* **frogfish, frogfishes**) a variety of angler fish.

froggy /ˈfrɒgi/ *adj* (**froggier, froggiest**) resembling or containing a frog or frogs.

froghopper /ˈfrɒgˌhɒpər/ *n* a small jumping insect whose larvae secrete a spittle-like protective covering.

frogman /ˈfrɒgmən/ *n* (*pl* **frogmen**) a person who wears rubber suit, flippers, oxygen supply, etc and is trained in working underwater.

frogmarch /ˈfrɒgmɑːtʃ/ *vt* to carry an unwilling person by the legs and arms face down; to move (a person) by force.—*also n*.

frolic /ˈfrɒlɪk/ *n* a lively party or game; merriment, fun. • *vi* (**frolicking, frolicked**) to play happily.—**frolicker** *n*.

frolicsome /ˈfrɒlɪksəm/, **frolicky** *adj* fond of frolicking; playful.

from /frəm/ or /frɒm/ *prep* beginning at, starting with; out of; originating with; out of the possibility or use of.

fromage frais /frɒmɒʒ ˈfreɪ/ *n* a smooth white curd cheese eaten plain or with added fruit as a dessert.

fromenty /ˈfrɒmənti/ *see* **frumenty**.

frond /frɒnd/ *n* a large leaf with many divisions, *esp* of a palm or fern.

frondescence /frɒnˈdesərs/ *n* (*bot*) the act of producing leaves; foliage.—**frondescent** *adj*.

frons /frɒnz/ *n* (*pl* **frontes**) a plate found on the head of an insect.

front /frʌnt/ *n* outward behaviour; (*inf*) an appearance of social standing; etc; the part facing forward; the first part; a forward or leading position; the promenade of a seaside resort; the advanced battle area in warfare; a person or group used to hide another's activity; an advancing mass of cold or warm air. • *adj* at, to, in, on, or of the front. • *vti* to face; to stand or be situated opposite to or over against; to serve as a front (for); to have the front turned in a particular direction.

frontage /ˈfrʌntɪdʒ/ *n* the front part of a building or plot of land; the width or extent of the front of a shop, building, piece of land, etc.

frontal /ˈfrʌntəl/ *adj* of or belonging to the front; of or pertaining to the forehead. • *n* a decorative covering for the front of an altar; a small pediment over a window or door.—**frontally** *adv*.

front bench *n* in the British House of Commons, either of the two rows of benches occupied by the leading figures (**front benchers**) in the Government or Opposition.

front door *n* a main entrance to a building.

frontier /frʌnˈtɪr/ or /frɒn-/, /ˈfrʌn-/, /frɒn-/ *n* the border between two countries; the limit of existing knowledge of a subject.

frontispiece /ˈfrʌntɪsˌpiːs/ *n* an illustration opposite the title page of a book; (*archit*) the main face of a building.

frontlet /ˈfrʌntlət/ *n* a band worn on the forehead; an animal's forehead.

frontrunner /ˈfrʌntˌrʌnər/ *n* the favourite to win a race, election, etc.

frontward /ˈfrʌntwərd/ **frontwards** *adj, adv* towards the front.

frost /frɒst/ *n* temperature at or below freezing point; a coating of powdery ice particles; coldness of manner. • *vt* to cover (as if) with frost or frosting; to give a frost-like opaque surface to (glass).

frostbite /ˈfrɒstbaɪt/ *n* injury to a part of the body by exposure to cold.—**frostbitten** *adj*

frosting /ˈfrɒstɪŋ/ *n* icing for a cake.

frosty /ˈfrɒsti/ *adj* (**frostier, frostiest**) cold with frost; cold or reserved in manner, chilly, distant.—**frostily** *adv*.—**frostiness** *n*.

froth /frɒθ/ *n* foam; foaming saliva; frivolity. • *vi* to emit or gather foam.

frothy /-i/ *adj* (**frothier, frothiest**) full of or composed of froth; frivolous; insubstantial.—**frothily** *adv*.—**frothiness** *n*.

froufrou /ˈfruːfruː/ *n* the rustling sound made by the material, *esp* silk, of a dress etc, when in motion.

froward /ˈfrɒwərd/ *adj* (*arch*) obstinate; wayward.

frown /fraʊn/ *vi* to contract the brow as in anger or thought; (*with* **upon**) to regard with displeasure or disapproval. • *n* a wrinkled brow; a stern look.—**frowner** *n*.—**frowningly** *adv*.

frowst /fraʊst/ *n* (*inf*) a close, stuffy atmosphere.

frowsty /-i/ *adj* stuffy; musty.

frowzy, frowsy /ˈfraʊzi/ *adj* (**frowzier, frowziest** or **frowsier, frowsiest**) dirty and untidy; unkempt.

froze /froːz/ *see* **freeze**.

frozen[1] /ˈfroːzən/ *see* **freeze**.

frozen[2] *adj* formed into or covered by ice; damaged or killed by cold; (*food, etc*) preserved by freezing; motionless; made speechless by strong emotion; formal and unfriendly; extremely cold; (prices, wages, etc) fixed at a given level; (funds, etc) unrealizable.

FRS *abbr* = Fellow of the Royal Society.

fructiferous /frɛk'tɪfərəs/ *adj* (*plant etc*) bearing fruit.

fructify /'frɛktɪˌfaɪ/ *vb* (**fructifies, fructifying, fructified**) *vt* to make fruitful, fertilize. • *vi* to bear fruit; to become fruitful.—**fructification** *n*.

fructose /'frʌktiːs/ or /-oːz-/, /'frɛk-/ *n* a type of sugar found in ripe fruit and honey.

fructuous /'frɛktjʊəs/ *adj* fruitful.

frugal /'fruːɡəl/ *adj* economical, thrifty; inexpensive, meagre.—**frugality** *n*.—**frugally** *adv*.

frugivorous /fruː'dʒɪvərəs/ *adj* fruit-eating.

fruit /fruːt/ *n* the seed-bearing part of any plant; the fleshy part of this used as food; the result or product of any action. • *vti* to bear or cause to bear fruit.

fruitage /'fruːtɪdʒ/ *n* the process of bearing fruit; a collective term for all fruits.

fruiter /'fruːtər/ *n* a fruit grower; a fruit tree.

fruiterer /'fruːtərər/ *n* a dealer in fruit.

fruitful /'fruːtfʊl/ *adj* producing lots of fruit; productive.—**fruitfully** *adv*.—**fruitfulness** *n*.

fruition /fruː'ɪʃən/ *n* a coming to fulfilment, realization.

fruitless /'fruːtləs/ *adj* unproductive; pointless; useless.—**fruitlessly** *adv*.—**fruitlessness** *n*.

fruit machine *n* a coin-operated gambling machine, using symbols of fruit to indicate a winning combination.

fruit salad *n* a dish of various fruits sliced and mixed.

fruity /'fruːti/ *adj* (**fruitier, fruitiest**) like, or tasting like, fruit; (*inf*) (*voice*) mellow; (*inf*) salacious.—**fruitiness** *n*.

frumenty /'fruːmənti/ *n* a sort of porridge, made from hulled wheat and boiled milk.—*also* **fromenty, furmenty**.

frump /frʌmp/ *n* a drab and dowdy woman.—**frumpish, frumpy** *adj*.

frustrate /'frʌstreɪt/ *vt* to prevent from achieving a goal or gratifying a desire; to discourage, irritate, tire; to disappoint.—**frustrater** *n*.—**frustratingly** *adv*.—**frustration** *n*.

frustule /'frʌstjuːl/ *n* the shell of a diatom.

frustum /'frʌstəm/ *n* (*pl* **frustums, frusta**) (*geom*) the part of a cone, pyramid, etc, left after the top is cut off.

frutescent /fruː'tɛsənt/ *adj* pertaining to, having the form of, or resembling a shrub.

fruticose /'fruːtɪˌkoːs/ or /-ˌkoːz/ *adj* resembling a shrub.

fry[1] /fraɪ/ *vti* (**frying, fried**) to cook over direct heat in hot fat. • *n* (*pl* **fries**) a dish of things fried.

fry[2] *n* (*pl* **fries**) recently hatched fishes; the young of a frog, etc.

fryer /'fraɪr/ *n* a person who fries; a pan, etc, for frying in; a piece of meat for frying.—*also* **frier**.

f-stop *n* any of the standard settings of the aperture in a camera lens.

ft. *abbr* = foot or feet.

FTA *abbr* = Free Trade Agreement.

FTP /ˌɛftiːpiː/ *abbr* = File Transfer Protocol, a protocol used for moving files over a network such as the Internet.

fuchsia /'fjuːʃə/ *n* any of a genus of decorative shrubs with purplish-red flowers.

fuchsine, fuchsin /'fuːksɪn/ *n* a crystalline substance, made into a dark red dye.

fucus /'fjuːkəs/ *n* (*pl* **fuci, fucuses**) a kind of large brown flat seaweed.—**fucoid, fucoidal** *adj*.

fuddle /'fʌdəl/ *vt* to make drunk; to make confused.

fuddy-duddy /'fʌdɪˌdʌdi/ *n* (*pl* **fuddy-duddies**) a person with old-fashioned or staid views.

fudge[1] /fʌdʒ/ *n* a soft sweet made of butter, milk, sugar, flavouring, etc; (*print*) a piece of late matter inserted in the stop-press column of a newspaper; a made-up story. • *vi* to refuse to commit oneself; to cheat; to contrive by imperfect or improvised means. • *vt* to fake; to fail to come to grips with; to make or do anything in a bungling, careless manner.

fudge[2] *n* nonsense. • *interj* expressing annoyance or disbelief.

fuehrer *see* **führer**.

fuel /'fjuːəl/ *n* material burned to supply heat and power, or as a source of nuclear energy; anything that serves to intensify strong feelings. • *vti* (**fuelling, fuelled** *or* **fueling, fueled**) to supply with or obtain fuel.—**fueller, fueler** *n*.

fug /fʌg/ *n* (*inf*) a hot, stale atmosphere.

fugacious /fjuː'ɡeɪʃəs/ *adj* fleeting; elusive; volatile; (*bot*) (*petals, etc*) falling off very early.—**fugaciously** *adv*.—**fugaciousness** *n*.

fugacity /-'ɡæsɪti/ *n* fugaciousness; the property of a gas to escape or expand.

fugitive /'fjuːdʒɪtɪv/ *n* a person who flees from danger, pursuit, or duty. • *adj* fleeing, as from danger or justice; fleeting, transient; not permanent.—**fugitively** *adv*.

fugleman /'fjuːɡəlmən/ *n* (*pl* **fuglemen**) (*formerly*) a soldier who stands in front of others to demonstrate drill; a ringleader.

fugue /fjuːɡ/ *n* a polyphonic musical composition with its theme taken up successively by different voices.—**fugal** *adj*.—**fugally** *adv*.

fuguist /'fjuːɡɪst/ *n* a composer of fugues.

führer /'fjʊrər/ *n* (*German*) a leader, *esp* a dictator; (*with cap*) the title of Adolf Hitler (1889-1945), leader of the German Nazi party.

-ful /fʊl/ *adj suffix* full of, *eg* doleful. • *n suffix* the amount needed to fill, *eg* cupful.

fulcrum /'fʊlkrəm/ or /'fɛl-/ *n* (*pl* **fulcrums, fulcra**) the fixed point on which a lever turns; a critical factor determining an outcome.

fulfil, fulfill /fʊl'fɪl/ *vt* (**fulfils** *or* **fulfills, fulfilling, fulfilled**) to carry out (a promise, etc); to achieve the completion of; to satisfy; to bring to an end, complete.—**fulfiller** *n*.—**fulfilment, fulfillment** *n*.

fulgent /'fɛldʒənt/ *adj* (*poet*) shining, radiant.—**fulgency** *n*.—**fulgently** *adv*.

fulgurate /ˌfɛlɡju'reɪt/ *vi* to flash (like lightning).—**fulgurant** *adj*.

fulgurite /'fɛlɡjʊˌraɪt/ *n* rock or sand that has been vitrified by lightning.

fuliginous /fjuː'lɪdʒɪnəs/ *adj* sooty, smoky.—**fuliginously** *adv*.

full[1] /fʊl/ *adj* having or holding all that can be contained; having eaten all one wants; having a great number (of); complete; having reached to greatest size, extent, etc. • *n* the greatest amount, extent etc. • *adv* completely, directly, exactly.

full[2] *vt* to clean and thicken (cloth) by beating.

fullback *n* (*football, rugby, hockey, etc*) one of the defensive players at the back; the position held by this player.

full-blooded *adj* vigorous, hearty.—**full-bloodedly** *adv*.

full-blown *adj* in full bloom; matured, fully developed.

full-bodied *adj* (*flavour*) characterized by richness and fullness.

full dress *n* dress worn for formal or ceremonial occasions.—**full-dress** *adj*.

fuller[1] /'fʊlər/ *n* someone who fulls cloth.

fuller[2] *n* a tool used for grooving and shaping iron; a groove made by this.

fuller's earth *n* a type of clay used for fulling.

full face *adj, adv* seen from in front.

full-frontal *adj* (*inf*) (*nude person or photograph*) with the genitals clearly visible; unrestrained.—**full frontal** *n*.

full house *n* (*poker*) a hand with three cards of the same value and a pair.—*also* **full hand**; (*theatre, etc*) a performance for which all seats are sold; (*bingo*) a complete set of winning numbers.

full moon *n* the moon at its phase when the whole disc is illuminated; the period of this.

fullness /'fʊlnəs/ *n* the state of being full; **fullness of time** the proper or destined time.—*also* **fulness**.

full-scale *adj* actual size.

full-stop *n* the punctuation mark (.) at the end of a sentence.—*also* **period**.

full time *n* the finish of a match.

full-time *adj* working or lasting the whole time.—**full-timer** *n*.

fully /'fʊli/ *adv* thoroughly, completely; at least.

fully-fledged *adj* (*bird*) mature; having full status.—*also* **full-fledged**.

fulmar /'fʊlmər/ *n* an Arctic sea bird.

fulminant /'fɛlmɪnənt/ or /'fʊl-/ *adj* fulminating; sudden; (*pain*) sharp, piercing.

fulminate /'fɛlmɪˌneɪt/ or /'fʊl-/ *vi* to issue protests with violence or threats; to inveigh (against). • *vt* to utter or exclaim, as a denunciation. • *n* an explosive compound of fulminic acid.—**fulmination** *n*.—**fulminator** *n*.—**fulminatory** *adj*.

fulminic acid /fɛl'mɪnɪk/ or /fʊl-/ *n* an unstable acid composed of cyanogen and oxygen.

fulness *see* **fullness**.

fulsome /'fʊlsəm/ *adj* excessively praising, obsequious.—**fulsomely** *adv*.—**fulsomeness** *n*.

fulvous /'fɛlvəs/ *adj* tawny.

fumarole /'fju:mə,roːl/ n a small hole in a volcano from which gases issue.

fumatorium n (pl **fumatoriums, fumatoria**) an airtight room where insects, plants, etc, are fumigated.

fumble /'fembəl/ vi to grope about. • vt to handle clumsily; to say or act awkwardly; to fail to catch (a ball) cleanly. • n an awkward attempt.—**fumbler** n.—**fumblingly** adv.

fume /fju:m/ n (usu pl) smoke, gas or vapour, esp if offensive or suffocating. • vi to give off fumes; to express anger. • vt to subject to fumes.—**fumer** n.—**fumingly** adv.

fumigate /'fju:mɪ,geɪt/ vt to disinfect or exterminate (pests, etc) using fumes.—**fumigation** n.—**fumigator** n.

fumitory /'fju:mɪtəri/ n (pl **fumitories**) a plant, found mainly in Europe, the leaves of which were formerly used as a treatment for skin diseases.

fun /fʌn/ n (what provides) amusement and enjoyment. • vi (**funning, funned**) to joke.

funambulist /fju:'næmbjʊlɪst/ n a tightrope walker.

function /'fʌŋkʃən/ n the activity characteristic of a person or thing; the specific purpose of a certain person or thing; an official ceremony or social entertainment; (math) a quantity whose value depends on the varying value of another. • vi to perform a function; to act, operate.

functional /-əl/ adj of a function or functions; practical, not ornamental; (disease) affecting the functions only, not organic.—**functionally** adv.

functionalism /-ə,lɪzəm/ n the theory and practice of design for practical application.—**functionalist** adj, n.

functionary /-ɛri/ n (pl **functionaries**) a person in an official capacity.

fund /fʌnd/ n a supply that can be drawn upon; a sum of money set aside for a purpose; (pl) ready money. • vt to provide funds for; to convert a (debt) into stock; to place in a fund.

fundament /fʌndəmənt/ n foundation, basis; (euphemism) the buttocks; the anus.

fundamental /,fʌndə'mentəl/ adj basic; essential. • n that which serves as a groundwork; an essential.—**fundamentality, fundamentalness** n.—**fundamentally** adv.

fundamentalism /-,lɪzəm/ n belief in the literal truth of the Bible, Koran etc.—**fundamentalist** adj, n.—**fundamentalistic** adj.

fundus /'fʌndəs/ n (pl **fundi**) (anat) the base or deepest part of an organ.

funeral /'fju:nərəl/ n the ceremony associated with the burial or cremation of the dead; a procession accompanying a coffin to a burial.

funeral director n a person who manages funerals.

funereal /fju:'niːriəl/ adj suiting a funeral, dismal, mournful.—**funereally** adv.

fungal /'fʌŋɡəl/ adj of or pertaining to a fungus; caused by a fungus.

fungible /'fʌndʒəbəl/ adj (law) replaceable by another, similar specimen. • n a fungible thing, eg a coin.

fungicide /'fʌŋɡɪ,saɪd/ n a substance that destroys fungi.—**fungicidal** adj.

fungiform /'fʌndʒə,fɔrm/ adj resembling a mushroom.

fungoid /'fʌŋɡɔɪd/ adj resembling a fungus.

fungous /'fʌŋɡəs/ adj of, pertaining to or like fungi; fungal; developing suddenly.

fungus /'fʌŋɡəs/ n (pl **fungi, funguses**) any of a major group of lower plants, as mildews, mushrooms, yeasts, etc, that lack chlorophyll and reproduce by spores.—**fungic** adj.

funicular /fə'nɪkjʊlər/ adj of rope or its tension. • n a cable railway ascending a mountain.

funiculus /fju:'nɪkjuːləs/ n (pl **funiculi**) (anat) a small cord, ligature or fibre.

funk /fʌŋk/ n (inf) panic, fear; a coward; funky music. • vti (inf) to show fear; to shirk.—**funker** n.

funky[1] /'fʌŋki/ adj (**funkier, funkiest**) panicky; fearful.

funky[2] adj (**funkier, funkiest**) (inf) (pop, jazz music, etc) soulful, bluesy; fashionable.—**funkiness** n.

funnel /'fʌnəl/ n an implement, usually a cone with a wide top and tapering to a narrow tube, for pouring fluids, powders, into bottles, etc; a metal chimney for the escape of smoke, steam, etc. • vti (**funnelling, funnelled** or **funneling, funneled**) to pour or cause to pour through a funnel.

funny /'fʌni/ adj (**funnier, funniest**) causing laughter; puzzling, odd; (inf) unwell, queasy. • n (pl **funnies**) a joke; (pl) comic strips, esp in a newspaper.—**funnily** adv.—**funniness** n.

funny bone n the part of the elbow where a sensitive nerve rests close to the bone, producing a tingling sensation if struck.

fur /fər/ n the short, soft, fine hair on the bodies of certain animals; their skins with the fur attached; a garment made of fur; a fabric made in imitation of fur; a fur-like coating, as on the tongue. • vti (**furring, furred**) to cover or become covered with fur.

furbelow /'fərbə,loː/ n a flounce or other trimming on clothing.

furbish /'fərbɪʃ/ vt to polish, to burnish; to renovate.—**furbisher** n.

furcate /'fər,keɪt/ vi to fork, divide. • adj forked, branching.—**furcation** n.

furfur /'fərfər/ n (pl **furfures**) scurf, dandruff.

furfuraceous /,fərfə'reɪʃəs/ adj resembling bran; resembling dandruff.

Furies /'fjʊriːz/ see **fury**.

furioso /'fjʊrɪoːsoː/ adv (mus) wildly.

furious /'fjʊriəs/ or /'fjʊr-/ adj full of anger; intense; violent, impetuous.—**furiously** adv.—**furiousness** n.

furl /fɜːl/ vt to roll up (a sail, flag, etc) tightly and make secure; to fold up, close.—**furlable** adj.—**furler** n.

furlong /'fərlɒŋ/ n 220 yards, one-eighth of a mile (201 metres).

furlough /'fərloː/ n leave of absence from duty, esp for military personnel. • vt to grant a furlough to.

furmenty /'fərmənti/ see **frumenty**.

furnace /'fərnəs/ n an enclosed chamber in which heat is produced to burn refuse, smelt ore, etc.

furnish /'fərnɪʃ/ vt to provide (a room, etc) with furniture; to equip with what is necessary; to supply.—**furnisher** n.

furnishings /-ɪŋz/ npl furniture, carpets, etc.

furniture /'fərnɪtʃər/ n the things in a room, etc that equip it for living, as chairs, beds, etc; equipment.

furore, furor /'fjʊrɔr/ or /'fjər-, /-ər/ n fury, indignation; widespread enthusiasm.

furrier /'fəriər/ n a dealer in furs.

furriery /-i/ n (pl **furrieries**) the fur trade; a collective name for furs.

furrow /'fərə/ n the groove in the earth made by a plough; a groove or track resembling this; a wrinkle. • vti to make furrows in; to wrinkle.—**furrower** n.—**furrowy** adj.

furry /'fəri/ adj (**furrier, furriest**) like, made of, or covered with, fur.—**furrily** adv.—**furriness** n.

further /'fərðər/ adv at or to a greater distance or degree; in addition. • adj more distant, remote; additional. • vt to help forward, promote.—**furtherer** n.

furtherance /'fərðərəns/ n a helping forward.

furthermore /,fərðər'mor/ adv moreover, besides.

furthermost /-'moːst/ adj most remote.

furthest /'fərðəst/ adj at or to the greatest distance.

furtive /'fərtɪv/ adj stealthy, sly.—**furtively** adv.—**furtiveness** n.

furuncle /'fjʊrʌŋkəl/ n (med) a boil.—**furuncular** adj.

fury /'fjəri/ or /'fjʊri/ n (pl **furies**) intense rage; a frenzy; a violently angry person; (with cap) (Greek, Roman myth) one of the three winged goddesses of vengeance with serpents for hair, Alecto, Megaera, and Tisiphone.

furze /fərz/ n gorse.

fuscous /'fʌskəs/ adj dark-coloured, esp brownish-black.

fuse /fju:z/ vti to join or become joined by melting; to (cause to) melt by the application of heat; to equip a plug, circuit, etc with a fuse; to (cause to) fail by blowing a fuse. • n a tube or wick filled with combustible material for setting off an explosive charge; a piece of thin wire that melts and breaks when an electric current exceeds a certain level.—also **fuze**.

fusee /fju:'zi:/ n a large-headed match; a conical spindle in a clock, around which the chain is wound.—also **fuzee**.

fuselage /'fju:zə,lɒʒ/ or /'fju:s-/, /-lɒdʒ/, /-lɪdʒ/ n the body of an aircraft.

fusel oil /'fju:zəl/ or /-səl/ n a poisonous liquid mixture of various alcohols, formed as a byproduct of distillation.

fusible /'fju:zəbəl/ adj able to be fused; (metal, alloy) having a melting point below 148.9 °C (300 °F) and used in fuses, etc.—**fusibility** n.—**fusibly** adv.

fusiform /'fju:zə,fɔrm/ adj spindle-shaped.

fusil /'fju:zəl/ or /-sɪl/ n a light flintlock musket.

fusilier, fusileer /,fju:zə'li:r/ n (formerly) a British soldier armed with a flintlock musket; a soldier in certain infantry regiments.

fusillade /ˌfjuːzəˈleɪd/ or /-ˌlɒd/, /-sə-/ *n* a firing of shots in continuous or rapid succession; an outburst, as of criticism. • *vt* to attack or shoot down by fusillade.

fusion /ˈfjuːʒən/ *n* the act of melting, blending or fusing; a product of fusion; union, partnership; nuclear fusion.

fuss /fʊs/ *n* excited activity, bustle; a nervous state; (*inf*) a quarrel; (*inf*) a showy display of approval. • *vi* to worry over trifles; to whine, as a baby.—**fusser** *n*.

fussy /ˈfʊsi/ *adj* (**fussier, fussiest**) worrying over details; hard to please; fastidious; over-elaborate.—**fussily** *adv*.—**fussiness** *n*.

fustian /ˈfʊstiən/ or /-tʃən/ *n* a kind of coarse twilled cotton cloth, *eg* corduroy; ranting language, bombast. • *adj* made of fustian; turgid.

fustic /ˈfʊstɪk/ *n* a large tropical American tree; its wood; the yellow obtained from it.

fusty /ˈfʊsti/ *adj* (**fustier, fustiest**) smelling of mould or damp; outmoded in ideas or opinions.—**fustily** *adv*.—**fustiness** *n*.

futhark, futharc, futhork, futhorc /ˈfuːθɔːrk/ *n* a phonetic alphabet made up of runes.

futile /ˈfjuːtaɪl/ or /-təl/ *adj* useless; ineffective.—**futilely** *adv*.—**futility** *n*.

futon /ˈfuːtɒn/ *n* a light cotton mattress.

futtock /ˈfʊtək/ *n* (*naut*) one of the upright curved ribs of a ship, springing from the keel.

future /ˈfjuːtʃər/ *adj* that is to be; of or referring to time yet to come. • *n* the time to come; future events; likelihood of eventual success; (*gram*) the future tense; (*pl*) commodities purchased at a prescribed price for delivery at some future date.

futurism /ˈfjuːtʃəˌrɪzəm/ *n* a movement in art, music, and literature begun in Italy about 1909 marked by an effort to give formal expression to the energy of mechanical processes; a point of view that finds meaning or fulfillment in the future.—**futurist** *adj, n*.

futuristic /ˌfjuːtʃəˈrɪstɪk/ *adj* forward-looking in design, appearance, intention, etc.—**futuristically** *adv*.

futurity /fjuːˈtʃərɪti/ or /-ˈtʃʊr/ *n* (*pl* **futurities**) time or events yet to come.

futurology /ˌfjuːtʃəˈrɒlədʒi/ *n* the forecasting of future trends in human affairs.—**futurologist** *n*.

fuze /fjuːz/ *see* **fuse**.

fuzee /fjuːˈzi/ or /ˈfjuːˌzi/ *see* **fusee**.

fuzz /fʊz/ *n* fine light particles of fibre (as of down or fluff); a blurred effect; fluff; (*sl*) police. • *vi* to fly off in minute particles; to become blurred.

fuzzword /ˈfʊzwərd/ *see* **buzzword**.

fuzzy /ˈfʊzi/ *adj* (**fuzzier, fuzziest**) like fuzz; fluffy; blurred.—**fuzzily** *adv*.—**fuzziness** *n*.

-fy /faɪ/ *vb suffix* to make, *eg solidify*.

G

G /dʒiː/ (*symbol*) (*mus*) the 5th note of the scale of C; gravitational constant; (*physcs*) conductance; giga; (*sl*) grand ($1000 or £1000).

g *abbr* = gallons(s); gram(s); gravity; acceleration due to gravity.

Ga (*chem symbol*) gallium.

GA, Ga. (*US*) *abbr* = Georgia.

gab /gæb/ *vi* (**gabbing, gabbed**) (*inf*) to talk in a rapid or thoughtless manner, chatter. • *n* (*inf*) idle talk.—**gabber** *n*.

gabardine /'gæbərˌdiːn/ or /-'diːn/ *n* a firm cloth of wool, rayon, or cotton; gaberdine.

gabble /'gæbəl/ *vti* to talk or utter rapidly or incoherently; to utter inarticulate or animal sounds.—**gabbler** *n*.

gabbro /'gæbroː/ *n* (*pl* **gabbros**) a dark igneous rock like granite.—**gabbroic** *adj*.

gabby /'gæbi/ *adj* (**gabbier, gabbiest**) (*inf*) talkative.

gabelle /gə'bɛl/ *n* (*formerly*) a tax on salt in France.

gaberdine /'gæbərˌdiːn/ or /-'diːn/ *n* (*formerly*) a long, loose upper garment worn by pilgrims, Jews etc; a raincoat; gaberdine.

gabion /'geɪbiən/ *n* (*formerly*) a large cylindrical basket filled with earth or stones, used in military defence; a similar metal container used in engineering and underwater construction.

gable /'geɪbəl/ *n* the triangular upper part of a wall enclosed by the sloping ends of a pitched roof.—**gabled** *adj*.

gablet /'geɪblət/ *n* a small ornamental gable used for the summit of niches etc.

gad /gæd/ *vi* (**gadding, gadded**) (*usu with* **about**) to wander restlessly or idly in search of pleasure.—**gadder** *n*.

gadabout /'gædəˌbaʊt/ *n* (*inf*) a person that wanders restlessly in search of pleasure or amusement.

gadfly /'gædflaɪ/ *n* (*pl* **gadflies**) any of various flies that bite or annoy livestock; an irritating person.

gadget /'gædʒɪt/ *n* a small, often ingenious, mechanical or electronic tool or device.—**gadgety** *adj*.

gadgetry /'gædʒɪtri/ *n* gadgets; the use of gadgets.

gadoid /'geɪdɔɪd/ *adj, n* (a fish) of the cod family.

gadolinite /'gædəlɪˌnaɪt/ *n* a silicate of yttrium.

gadolinium /ˌgædə'lɪniəm/ *n* a magnetic metallic element of the rare earth group.—**gadolinic** *adj*.

gadroon /gə'druːn/ *n* an ornamental edge of inverted fluting; a decorative border, *esp* on silver.

gadwall /'gædwɒl/ *n* (*pl* **gadwalls, gadwall**) a large freshwater duck, prized as game.

Gael /geɪl/ *n* a person who speaks Gaelic, *esp* a Scottish Highlander or Irishman.

Gaelic /'geɪlɪk/ *n* the Celtic language of Ireland, the Scottish Highlands, and the Isle of Man.—*also adj*.

gaff /gæf/ *n* a pole with a sharp hook for landing large fish; (*naut*) a high boom or yard for hoisting a sail aft of a mast; (*Brit sl*) one's home. • *vt* to land (a fish) with a gaff.

gaffe /gæf/ *n* a social blunder.

gaffer /'gæfər/ *n* an old man, often a countryman; an overseer or foreman; the senior electrician of a film crew.

gaff-topsail /'gæf'tɒpˌseɪl/ *n* (*naut*) a light sail set above a gaff.

gag /gæg/ *n* something put over or into the mouth to prevent talking; any restraint of free speech; a joke. • *vb* (**gagging, gagged**) *vt* to cause to retch; to keep from speaking, as by stopping the mouth of. • *vi* to retch; to tell jokes.

gaga /'gɒgɒ/ *adj* (*inf*) senile; slightly crazy.

gage /geɪdʒ/ *see* **gauge**.

gaggle /'gægəl/ *n* a flock of geese when not in flight; (*inf*) a disorderly collection of people.

gahnite /'gɒnˌaɪt/ *n* a greenish and dark-brown mineral.

gaiety /'geɪəti/ *n* (*pl* **gaieties**) happiness, liveliness; colourful appearance.

gaige /geɪdʒ/ *n* the Chinese word for "radical reform" or peristroika.

gaily /'geɪli/ *adv* in a cheerful manner; with bright colours.

gain /geɪn/ *vt* to obtain, earn, *esp* by effort; to win in a contest; to attract; to get as an addition (*esp* profit or advantage); to make an increase in; to reach. • *vi* to make progress; to increase in weight. • *n* an increase *esp* in profit or advantage; an acquisition.

gainful /'geɪnfʊl/ *adj* profitable.—**gainfully** *adv*.—**gainfulness** *n*.

gainsay /geɪn'seɪ/ or /'geɪnseɪ/ *vt* (**gainsaying, gainsaid**) (*formal*) to dispute; to deny.—**gainsayer** *n*.

gait /geɪt/ *n* a manner of walking or running; the sequence of footsteps made by a moving horse.

gaiter /'geɪtər/ *n* a cloth or leather covering for the lower leg.

gal[1] /gæl/ *n* (*sl*) a girl.

gal[2], **gall.** *abbr* = gallon.

gala /'gɑːlə/ or /'geɪlə/ *n* a celebration, festival.

galactic /gə'læktɪk/ *adj* of a galaxy; huge.

galago /gə'leɪgoː/ *n* (*pl* **galagos**) an African genus of lemurs; a bushbaby.

galantine /'gælənˌtiːn/ *n* a dish composed of chicken, veal or other white meat, boned, seasoned, tied up, boiled, shaped and served cold in its own je ly.

galatea /ˌgælə'tiːə/ *n* a cotton fabric, often with blue and white stripes.

Galatians /gə'leɪʃənz/ *n sing* (*New Testament*) the epistles of St Paul addressed to the Galatians.

galavant /'gæləˌvænt/ *see* **gallivant**.

galaxy /'gæləksi/ *n* (*pl* **galaxies**) any of the systems of stars in the universe; any splendid assemblage; (*with cap*) the galaxy containing the Earth's solar system; the Milky Way.

galbanum /'gælbənəm/ *n* an odorous and bitter gum resin used in medicine.

gale /geɪl/ *n* a strong wind, specifically one between 32 to 63 mph; an outburst.

galea /'geɪliə/ *n* (*pl* **galeae**) (*bot, zool*) a helmet-like structure.—**galeate, galeated** *adj*.

galena /gə'liːnə/ *n* a sulphide of lead.

Galenic /gə'lɛnɪk/ *adj* of Galen (*c.*AD130*c.*200), the Greek physician and philosopher, or his works.

Galilean[1] /ˌgælə'liːən/ *adj* of Galilee or its inhabitants • *n* a native of Galilee; (*often pl*) a Christian; (*with* **the**) Jesus Christ.

Galilean[2] /ˌgælə'liːən/ *adj* of or pertaining to Galileo (1564-1642), the Italian astronomer and mathematician.

galilee /ˈgæləˌliː/ *n* a small chapel or porch at the western entrance to a church.

galingale, galangal /'gælɪŋˌgeɪl/ *n* a kind of sedge; the aromatic root of an Asian plant.

galiot, galliot /'gæliət/ *n* a heavily built two-masted Dutch trading vessel; (*formerly*) a small light galley used in the Mediterranean.

galipot /'gælɪˌpɒt/ *n* a white resinous juice that exudes from pine trees.

galivant /'gælɪˌvænt/ *see* **gallivant**.

gall[1] /gɒl/ *n* bile; bitter feeling; (*inf*) impudence.

gall[2] *n* a diseased growth on plant tissue produced by fungi, insect parasites, or bacteria.

gall[3] *n* a skin sore caused by rubbing. • *vt* to chafe or hurt by rubbing; to irritate.

gallant /'gælənt/ *adj* dignified, stately; brave; noble; (*man*) polite and chivalrous to women.—**gallantly** *adv*.—**gallantness** *n*.—**gallantry** *n* (*pl* **gallantries**).

gallantry /'gæləntri/ *n* (*pl* **gallantries**) (an act of) bravery, dashing courage; courtliness, a polite act.

gall bladder /'gɒl,blædər/ *n* a membranous sac attached to the liver in which bile is stored.

galleass /'gæliˌæs/ *n* a large low-built three-masted vessel propelled by sails and oars, and carrying twenty or more guns.

galleon /'gæliən/ *n* a large sailing ship of the 15th–18th centuries.

gallery /'gæləri/ *n* (*pl* **galleries**) a covered passage for walking; a long narrow outside balcony; a balcony running along the inside wall of a building; (the occupants of) an upper area of seating in a theatre; a long narrow room used for a special purpose, *eg* shooting practice; a room or building designed for the exhibition of works of art; the spectators at a golf tournament, tennis match, etc.—**galleried** *adj*.

galley /ˈgæli/ *n* a long, *usu* low, ship of ancient or medieval times, propelled by oars; the kitchen of a ship, aircraft; (*print*) a shallow tray for holding type; proofs printed from such type.—*also* **galley proof**.

galliard /ˈgæliˌard/ *n* a lively dance in triple time.

Gallic /ˈgælɪk/ *adj* of or pertaining to France; of ancient Gaul or its people.

gallic /ˈgælɪk/ *adj* of or made of gallnuts; (*chem*) of or containing gallium in the trivalent state.

Gallican /ˈgælɪkən/ *adj* of the Roman Catholic Church in France.

Gallicanism /-ˌnɪzəm/ *n* the doctrine of the national party in the French Roman Catholic Church, tending to restrict papal control, opposed to Ultramontanism.

Gallice /ˈgælɪs/ *adv* in French.

Gallicism /ˈgælɪˌsɪzəm/ *n* a French expression or idiom.

Gallicize, Gallicise /ˈgælɪˌsaɪz/ *vt* to make French in manners, idiom etc.

galligaskins /ˌgælɪˈgæskɪnz/ *npl* trousers, leggings worn in the 16th and 17th centuries.

gallimaufry /ˌgælɪˈmɒfri/ *n* (*pl* **gallimaufries**) a medley, a hotch-potch.

gallinaceous /ˌgælɪˈneɪʃəs/ *adj* of or relating to a group of heavy-bodied largely land-loving birds including pheasants and domestic fowl.

galling /ˈgælɪŋ/ *adj* irritating, exasperating.

gallipot /ˈgælɪˌpɒt/ *n* a small glazed pot, *esp* for medicine.

gallium /ˈgæliəm/ *n* a metallic element that is liquid at room temperature and is used in thermometers, semiconductor devices, etc.

gallivant /ˈgælɪˌvænt/ *vi* (*inf*) to go about in search of amusement.—*also* **galivant, galavant**.

galliwasp /ˈgælɪˌwɒsp/ *n* a West Indian lizard.

gallnut /ˈgɒlˌnʌt/ *n* a round excrescence produced on the oak by the puncturing of the leaf buds by an insect, the gall beetle.

gallon /ˈgælən/ *n* a unit of liquid measure comprising 4 quarts or 3.78 litres (in UK, 4.54 litres); (*pl*) (*inf*) a large amount.

galloon /gəˈluːn/ *n* a narrow braid or trimming of silk, gold lace, embroidery etc.

gallop /ˈgæləp/ *n* the fastest gait of a horse, etc; a succession of leaping strides; a fast pace. • *vti* to go or cause to go at a gallop; to move swiftly.—**galloper** *n*.

gallowglass /ˈgæloˌglæs/ *n* a heavily armed footsoldier; a chief's retainer in Ireland in the 13th-16th centuries.

gallows /ˈgæloˌz/ *n* (*pl* **gallowses, gallows**) a wooden frame used for hanging criminals.

gallstone /ˈgɒlstoˌn/ *n* a small solid mass in the gall bladder.

Gallup poll /ˈgæləp/ *n* a sampling of public opinion, *esp* to help forecast an election.

galop /ˈgæləp/ *n* a dance.

galore /gəˈlɔr/ *adv* in great quantity; in plentiful supply.

galosh /gəˈlɒʃ/ *n* a waterproof overshoe.

galumph /gəˈlʌmf/ *vi* (*inf*) to prance triumphantly, or clumsily.

galvanic /gælˈvænɪk/ *adj* producing electricity by chemical action; stimulating (people) into action.—**galvanically** *adv*.

galvanism /ˈgælvəˌnɪzəm/ *n* (*arch*) electricity produced by the chemical action of certain bodies or an acid on a metal; the medical use of this.

galvanize /ˈgælvəˌnaɪz/ *vt* to apply an electric current to; to startle; to excite; to plate (metal) with zinc.—**galvanization** *n*.—**galvanizer** *n*.

galvanometer /ˌgælvəˈnɒmətər/ *n* an instrument for detecting or measuring small electric currents.—**galvanometric, galvanometrical** *adj*.—**galvanometry** *n*.

galvanoscope /-skɒp/ *n* an instrument for measuring the direction and presence of electricity by movements of a magnetic needle.

gam[1] /gæm/ *n* a school of whales; a visit by one captain of a whaler to another; • *vb* (**gams, gammed, gamming**) *vt* to call upon the captain of a whaler. • *vi* (*whales*) to gather together in schools.

gam[2] *n* (*sl*) a well-shaped leg.

gambado /gæmˈbɒdoː/ (*pl* **gambados, gambadoes**) *n* a kind of leather legging used by horsemen; a flourish or curvet.

gambier, gambir /ˈgæmbiər/ or /ˈgæmbiːr/ *n* a vegetable extract used medicinally as an astringent, and also for tanning and dyeing.

gambit /ˈgæmbɪt/ *n* (*chess*) an opening in which a piece is sacrificed to gain an advantage; any action to gain an advantage.

gamble /ˈgæmbəl/ *vi* to play games of chance for money; to take a risk for some advantage. • *vt* to risk in gambling, to bet. • *n* a risky venture; a bet.—**gambler** *n*.—**gambling** *n*.

gamboge /gæmˈboːdʒ/ or /-ˈbuːʒ/ *n* a yellow gum resin from SE Asia, used as a pigment and as a purgative.—*also* **cambogia**; a bright yellow colour.

gambol /ˈgæmbəl/ *vi* (**gambolling, gambolled** *or* **gamboling, gamboled**) to jump and skip about in play; to frisk. • *n* a caper, a playful leap.

gambrel /ˈgæmbrəl/ *n* the hock of a horse; a bent stick of wood or metal resembling a horse's leg, used by butchers; a gambrel roof.

gambrel roof *n* a curved roof with a small gable at each end; a roof with a double slope on each side so that each side is shaped like a horse's leg.

game[1] /geɪm/ *n* any form of play, amusement; activity or sport involving competition; a scheme, a plan; wild birds or animals hunted for sport or food, the flesh of such animals. • *vi* to play for a stake. • *adj* (*inf*) brave, resolute; (*inf*) willing.—**gamely** *adv*.—**gameness** *n*.

game[2] *adj* (*limbs*) injured, crippled, lame.

game-breaking *adj* ♣ a play in sports that turns a close game suddenly and decisively in favour of one team.

gamecock /ˈgeɪmkɒk/ *n* (*formerly*) a cock bred and trained for fighting.

gamekeeper /ˈgeɪmˌkiːpər/ *n* a person who breeds and takes care of game birds and animals, as on an estate.—**gamekeeping** *n*.

game misconduct *n* ♣ a penalty in ice hockey that expels a player for the remainder of the game.

game point *n* (*tennis*) the situation when the next point scored wins the game for one side or player.

gamesmanship /ˈgeɪmzmənʃɪp/ *n* (*inf*) the art of winning games by questionable acts just short of cheating.

gamesome /ˈgeɪmsəm/ *adj* sportive.

gamester /ˈgeɪmstər/ *n* a gambler.

gamete /ˈgæmiːt/ or /gəˈmiːt/ *n* a reproductive cell that unites with another to form the cell that develops into a new individual.—**gametal, gametic** *adj*.

gamic /ˈgæmɪk/ *adj* (*zool*) having a sexual character.

gamin /ˈgæmɪn/ *n* a mischievous urchin.

gamine /ˈgæmiːn/ or /gæˈmiːn/ *n* a boyish girl or woman with impish appeal.

gaming /ˈgeɪmɪŋ/ *n* the act of playing games for stakes; gambling.—*also adj*.

gamma /ˈgæmə/ *n* the third letter of the Greek alphabet.

gamma radiation, gamma rays *n* shortwave electromagnetic radiation from a radioactive substance.

gammer /ˈgæmər/ *n* (*rare*) (*usu humorous*) an old woman.

gammon /ˈgæmən/ *n* cured or smoked ham; meat from the hindquarters of a side of bacon.

gamogenesis /ˌgæmoːˈdʒenəsɪs/ *n* (*bot*) sexual reproduction.

gamopetalous /-ˈpetələs/ *adj* with petals united at the base.

gamophyllous /-ˈfɪləs/ *adj* (*flowers*) with leaves cohering at the edges.

gamosepalous /-ˈsepələs/ *adj* (*flowers*) with sepals united at the edges to form a calyx.

gamut /ˈgæmət/ *n* a complete range or series; (*mus*) the whole range of notes of a voice or instrument.

gamy, gamey /ˈgeɪmi/ *adj* (**gamier, gamiest**) having the strong smell or flavour of cooked game; (*inf*) spirited, lively.—**gaminess** *n*.

-gamy /gəmi/ *n suffix* marriage; sexual union.

gander /ˈgændər/ *n* an adult goose; (*inf*) a quick look.

gang /gæŋ/ *n* a group of persons, *esp* labourers, working together; a group of persons acting or associating together, *esp* for illegal purposes. • *vti* to form into or act as a gang.—**ganged** *adj*.

gangland /-lænd/ *n* the criminal fraternity.

gangling /-glɪŋ/, **gangly** /ˈgæŋgli/ *adj* tall, thin and awkward in appearance and movement.

ganglion /-gliən/ *n* (*pl* **ganglia, ganglions**) a mass of nerve cells from which nerve impulses are transmitted.—**ganglionic** *adj*.

gangplank /-plæŋk/ *n* a moveable ramp by which to board or leave a ship.

gangrene /-griːn/ *n* death of body tissue when the blood supply is obstructed.—**gangrenous** *adj*.

gangsta /-stə/ *n* a variant of rap music with its source the US West Coast with lyrics focused on gang culture; ~ **rapper** a performer of this style of music. • *adj* belonging to gangsta music.

gangster /'gæŋstər/ *n* a member of a criminal gang.

gangue, gang /gæŋ/ *n* the earth or matrix in which ore is found

gangway /'gæŋweɪ/ *n* a passageway, *esp* an opening in a ship's side for loading, etc; a gangplank.

ganister, gannister /'gænɪstər/ *n* a kind of siliceous clay rock or hard sandstone; a refractory material used for lining furnaces.

ganja /'gændʒə/ or /'gɒn-/ *n* marijuana.

gannet /'gænət/ *n* any of various large voracious fish-eating sea birds.

ganoid /'gænɔɪd/ *adj* (*fish*) having enamelled bony scales, like the sturgeon. • *n* a ganoid fish.

gantlet /'gɒntlɪt/ or /'gɒnt-/, /'gænt-, *see* **gauntlet**.

gantry /'gæntri/ *n* (*pl* **gantries**) a metal framework, often on wheels, for a travelling crane; a wheeled framework with a crane, platforms, etc for servicing a rocket to be launched.

gaol /dʒeɪl/, **gaolbird, gaoler** *see* **jail, jailbird, jailer**.

gap /gæp/ *n* a break or opening in something, as a wall or fence; an interruption in continuity, an interval; a mountain pass; a divergence, disparity. • *vt* (**gapping, gapped**) to make a gap in.—**gappy** *adj*.

gape /geɪp/ *vi* to open the mouth wide; to stare in astonishment, *esp* with the mouth open; to open widely. • *n* the act of gaping; a wide opening.—**gaping** *adj*.—**gapingly** *adv*.

gaper /'geɪpər/ *n* a person who gapes; one of various types of shellfish that have a space between the valves.

gap year *n* a break of one year between school and college or university planned for the student to access work or experience seen as valuable in terms of personal development.

gar /gɑr/ *n* (*pl* **gar, gars**) a garfish.

garage /gə'rɒʒ/ or /-'rɒdʒ/, /-'rædʒ/, /-'ræʒ/ *n* an enclosed shelter for motor vehicles; a place where motor vehicles are repaired and serviced, and fuel sold. • *vt* to put or keep in a garage.

garage sale *n* a sale of unwanted household goods, held in a garage or other part of the house.

garb /gɑrb/ *n* clothing, style of dress. • *vt* to clothe.

garbage /'gɑrbɪdʒ/ *n* food waste; unwanted or useless material; rubbish; (*comput*) useless data.

garbageman /-,mæn/ *n* (*pl* **garbagemen**) a person employed to remove garbage.

garbage mitt *n* ✽ a heavy mitt worn by a garbage collector.

garble /'gɑrbəl/ *vt* to distort (a message, story, etc) so as to mislead.—**garbler** *n*.

garboard (strake) /'gɑrbɔrd/ *n* (*naut*) the plank or plate on a ship's bottom next to the keel.

garbology /gɑr'bɒlədʒi/ *n* the study of the disposal of waste material.—**garbologist** *n*.

garburator /'gɑrbə,reɪtər/ *n* ✽ (*Cdn*) a garbage disposal unit for a household.

garçon /gɑr'sɔ̃/ *n* a waiter.

garden /'gɑrdən/ *n* an area of ground for growing herbs, fruits, flowers, or vegetables; a yard; a fertile, well-cultivated region; a public park or recreation area, *usu* laid-out with plants and trees. • *vi* to make, or work in, a garden.—**gardener** *n*.—**gardening** *n*.

gardenia /gɑr'diːniə/ *n* a tree or shrub with beautiful fragrant white or yellow flowers.

garfish /'gɑrfɪʃ/ *n* (*pl* **garfish, garfishes**) a long, slender freshwater fish with a spearlike snout and a thick-scaled body.

gargantuan /gɑr'gæntʃʊən/ *adj* colossal, prodigious.

garget /'gɑrgət/ *n* a disease in cattle

gargle /'gɑrgəl/ *vti* to rinse the throat by breathing air from the lungs through liquid held in the mouth. • *n* a liquid for this purpose; the sound made by gargling.—**gargler** *n*.

gargoyle /'gɑrgɔɪl/ *n* a grotesquely carved face or figure, *usu* acting as a spout to drain water from a gutter; a person with an ugly face.—**gargoyled** *adj*.

garibaldi /,gerɪ'bɒldi/ or /,gær-/ *n* a type of loose blouse, *orig* red.

garish /'gerɪʃ/ or /'gæ-/ *adj* crudely bright, gaudy.—**garishly** *adv*.—**garishness** *n*.

garland /'gɑrlənd/ *n* a wreath of flowers or leaves worn or hung as decoration. • *vt* to decorate with a garland.

garlic /'gɑrlɪk/ *n* a bulbous herb cultivated for its compound bulbs used in cookery; its bulb.—**garlicky** *adj*.

garment /'gɑrmənt/ *n* an item of clothing.

garner /'gɑrnər/ *vt* to gather, store.

garnet /'gɑrnət/ *n* a semiprecious stone, red, yellow or green in colour.

garnish /'gɑrnɪʃ/ *vt* to decorate; to decorate (food) with something that adds colour or flavour. • *n* something used to garnish food.—**garnisher** *n*.—**garniture** *n*.

garnishee /,gɑrnɪ'ʃiː/ *vt* (**garnisheeing, garnisheed**) (*law*) to warn by garnishment. • *n* (*law*) the person into whose hands the property of another is attached pending the satisfaction of the claims of a third party.

garnishment /'gɑrnɪʃmənt/ *n* embellishment; (*law*) notice to holder of another's attached property not to give it to him but to account for it in court; a summons; (*arch*) notice to third party to appear in suit.

garniture /'gɑrnɪtʃər/ *n* embellishment, trimmings (*esp* on a dish of food).

garpike /'gɑrpaɪk/ *n* the garfish.

garret /'gerət/ or /'gær-/ *n* an attic.

garrison /'gerɪsən/ or /'gær-/ *n* troops stationed at a fort; a fortified place with troops. • *vt* to station (troops) in (a fortified place) for its defence.

garrote, garrote, garotte /gə'rɒt/ *n* a method of execution by strangling with an iron collar; the iron collar used. • *vt* to execute by garrotte; to half-throttle and rob.—**garrotter, garroter, garotter** *n*.

garrulous /'gerʊləs/ or /'gær-/ *adj* excessively talkative.—**garrulously** *adv*.—**garrulousness, garrulity** *n*.

garter /'gɑrtər/ *n* an elasticated band used to support a stocking or sock.

garth /gɑrθ/ *n* a courtyard surrounded by a cloister; (*arch*) a yard, garden or paddock.

gas /gæs/ *n* (*pl* **gases, gasses**) an air-like substance with the capacity to expand indefinitely and not liquefy or solidify at ordinary temperatures; any mixture of flammable gases used for lighting or heating; any gas used as an anaesthetic; any poisonous substance dispersed in the air, as in war; (*inf*) empty talk; gasoline. • *vt* (**gases** *or* **gasses, gassing, gassed**) to poison or disable with gas; (*inf*) to talk idly and at length.

gasbag /'gæsbæg/ *n* (*inf*) an idle talker.

gas bar *n* ✽ (*Cdn*) a gas station that consists of pumps and a kiosk only.

gas chamber *n* an airtight room where animals or people are killed by poisonous gas.

gasconade /,gæskə'neɪd/ *n* (*rare*) boastful or blustering talk. • *vi* to bluster, to boast.

gaseous /'gæsiəs/ or /'gæʃəs/ *adj* having the form of or being gas; of or being related to gases; lacking substance or solidity.—**gaseousness** *n*.

gash /gæʃ/ *n* a long, deep, open cut. • *vt* to cut deep.

gasholder *n* a circular hollow tank, open at the bottom and closed at the top, for storing gas prior to distribution.

gasify /'gæsɪ,faɪ/ *vti* (**gasifying, gasified**) to turn into gas.—**gasification** *n*.

gasket /'gæskət/ *n* a piece or ring of rubber, metal, etc sandwiched between metal surfaces to act as a seal.

gaslight /'gæslaɪt/ *n* a type of lamp using a jet of gas to provide illumination.

gasman /-,mæn/ *n* (*pl* **gasmen**) an employee of a gas company who reads meters, etc.

gasolier, gaselier /,gæsə'lɪr/ *n* a branched hanging support for gas lights.

gasoline, gasolene /'gæsə,liːn/ *n* (*US*) a liquid fuel or solvent distilled from petroleum.—*also* **petrol**.—**gasolinic** *adj*.

gasometer /gæ'sɒmɪtər/ *n* an instrument for measuring gas; a gasholder.

gasometry /gæ'sɒmɪtri/ *n* the science or process of measuring gas.

gasp /gæsp/ *vi* to draw in the breath suddenly and audibly, as from shock; to struggle to catch the breath. • *vt* to utter breathlessly. • *n* the act of gasping.—**gaspingly** *adv*.

gaspereau /'gæspərəʊ/ *n* ✽ a fish that is a member of the herring family, found mainly off the Atlantic coast of North America.

gassy /'gæsi/ *adj* (**gassier, gassiest**) impregnated with or like a gas; given to pretentious talk; inflated.

gastr-, gastro- /'gæstrəʊ/ *prefix* stomach.

gastric /'gæstrɪk/ *adj* of, in, or near the stomach.

gastric juice *n* digestive fluid secreted by glands in the stomach lining.

gastric ulcer *n* an ulcer of the lining of the stomach.

gastritis /gæ'straɪtɪs/ *n* inflammation of the stomach.—**gastritic** *adj*.

gastroenteric /ˌgæstroːɛnˈterɪk/ *adj* of or pertaining to the stomach or intestinal tract.

gastroenteritis /-ɛntəˈrɔɪtɪs/ *n* inflammation of the mucous membrane of the stomach and intestines.—**gastroenteritic** *adj.*

gastrointestinal /-ɪnˈtɛstɪnəl/ or /-ɪntɛsˈtaɪnəl/ *adj* of or pertaining to the stomach or intestines.

gastrology /gæsˈtrɒlədzi/, **gastroenterology** /-ɛntəˈrɒlədʒi/ *n* the study of diseases of the stomach and intestinal tract.

gastronome /ˈgæstrəˌnoːm/, **gastronomer** /-ər/, **gastronomist** /-ɪst/ *n* a connoisseur of food.

gastronomy /gæˈstrɒnəmi/ *n* the art and science of good eating.—**gastronomic, gastronomical** *adj.*—**gastronomically** *adj.*

gastropod /ˈgæstrəˌpɒd/ *n* any of a large class of molluscs (as snails) with a flattened foot for moving and *usu* with stalk-like sense organs.—**gastropodan** *adj, n.*—**gastropodous** *adj.*

gastrula /ˈgæstrʊlə/ *n* (*pl* **gastrulas, gastrulae**) the fertilized ovum at a certain period in its development.

gasworks /ˈgæswɜːks/ *n sing* a place where gas is manufactured.

gate /geɪt/ *n* a movable structure controlling passage through an opening in a fence or wall; a gateway; a movable barrier; a structure controlling the flow of water, as in a canal; a device (as in a computer) that outputs a signal when specified input conditions are met; the total amount or number of paid admissions to a football match, etc. • *vt* to supply with a gate; to keep within the gates (of a university) as a punishment; ✹ (*Cdn*) keep an inmate in prison for the full length of a sentence, by re-arresting the inmate upon release after he or she has served less than the full term.

gâteau, gateau /ˈgæˈtoː/ *n* (*pl* **gâteaux, gateaux**) a large cream cake.

gate-crasher /ˈgeɪtˌkræʃər/ *n* a person who attends a party, etc without being invited.—**gatecrash** *vi.*

gatefold /ˈgeɪtfoːld/ *n* an oversize page in a book or magazine that is folded in.

gatehouse /-hʊs/ *n* a house built over or beside a gate.

gatekeeper /-ˌkiːpər/ *n* a person who controls entrance to a gate.

gate-leg(ged) table /ˈgeɪtlɛg/ *n* a table with drop leaves supported by movable legs.

gatepost /ˈgeɪtpoːst/ *n* a post on which a gate is hung, or to which it is attached when closed.

gateway /ˈgeɪtweɪ/ *n* an opening for a gate; a means of entrance or exit.

gather /ˈgæðər/ *vt* to bring together in one place or group; to get gradually; to collect (as taxes); to harvest; to draw (parts) together; to pucker fabric by pulling a thread or stitching; to understand, infer. • *vi* to come together in a body; to cluster around a focus of attention; (*sore*) to swell and fill with pus.—**gatherable** *adj.*—**gatherer** *n.*

gathering /-ɪŋ/ *n* the act of gathering or assembling together; an assembly; folds made in a garment by gathering.

Gatling gun /ˈgætlɪŋ/ *n* a machine gun with clustered barrels, which are discharged in succession by turning a handle.

GATT /gæt/ *abbr* = General Agreement on Tariffs and Trade.

gauche /goːʃ/ *adj* socially inept; graceless, tactless.—**gauchely** *adv.*—**gaucheness** *n.*

gaucherie /ˌgoːʃəˈriː/ or /ˈgoːʃəˌriː/ *n* awkwardness, tactlessness; a tactless or awkward act.

gaucho /ˈgaʊtʃoː/ *n* (*pl* **gauchos**) a cowboy of the pampas of South America.

gaud /gɒd/ *n* a piece of finery, a trinket or ornament.

gaudery /ˈgɒdi/ *n* (*pl* **gauderies**) cheap, showy finery.

gaudy /ˈgɒdi/ *adj* (**gaudier, gaudiest**) excessively ornamented; tastelessly bright.—**gaudily** *adv.*—**gaudiness** *n.*

gauffer /ˈgɒfər/ or /ˈgɒf-/ *see* **goffer**.

gauge /geɪdʒ/ *n* measurement according to some standard or system; any device for measuring; the distance between rails of a railway; the size of the bore of a shotgun; the thickness of sheet metal, wire, etc. • *vt* to measure the size, amount, etc of.—*also* **gage.**—**gaugeable, gagable** *adj.*—**gauger, gager** *n.*

Gaul /gɒl/ *n* an ancient region of Western Europe corresponding roughly to modern France and Belgium; a native of Gaul.

Gaullism /ˈgoːlɪzəm/ *n* the policies pertaining to General de Gaulle, first president of the Fifth Republic in France (1959–69); the political movement based on de Gaulle's policies and principles.—**Gaullist** *n, adj.*

gaunt /gɒnt/ *adj* excessively thin as from hunger or age; looking grim or forbidding.—**gauntness** *n.*

gauntlet[1] /ˈgɒntlət/ *n* a knight's armoured glove; a long glove, often with a flaring cuff.—*also* **gantlet** *n.*

gauntlet[2] *n* (*formerly*) a type of military punishment in which a victim was forced to run between two lines of men who struck him as he passed.

gaur /ˈgaʊər/ *n* a large fierce, dark-coloured ox found in SE Asia and India.

gauss /gaʊs/ *n* (*pl* **gauss, gausses**) the unit of measurement for magnetic flux density.

gauze /gɒz/ *n* any very thin, loosely woven fabric, as of cotton or silk; a firm woven material of metal or plastic filaments; a surgical dressing.

gauzy /ˈgɒzi/ *adj* (**gauzier, gauziest**) like gauze, thin, transparent.—**gauzily** *adv.*—**gauziness** *n.*

gave /geɪv/ *see* **give**.

gavel /ˈgævəl/ *n* a hammer used by a chairman, auctioneer, judge, etc to command proceedings.

gavial /ˈgeɪvɪəl/ *n* an Indian crocodile with a long narrow snout.

gavotte /gəˈvɒt/ *n* a lively dance of French peasant origin.

gawk /gɒk/ *vi* to stare at stupidly.

gawky /ˈgɒki/ *adj* (**gawkier, gawkiest**) clumsy, awkward, ungainly.—**gawkily** *adv.*—**gawkiness** *n.*

gay /geɪ/ *adj* joyous and lively; colourful; homosexual. • *n* a homosexual.—**gayness** *n.*

gaze /geɪz/ *vi* to look steadily. • *n* a steady look.—**gazer** *n.*

gazebo /gəˈziːboː/ *n* (*pl* **gazebos, gazeboes**) a summerhouse or belvedere, elevated to command a wide view.

gazelle /gəˈzɛl/ *n* (*pl* **gazelles, gazelle**) any of numerous small swift Asian or African antelopes.

gazette /gəˈzɛt/ *n* a newspaper, now mainly in newspaper titles; an official publication listing government appointments, legal notices, etc.

gazetteer /ˌgæzəˈtiːr/ *n* an index of geographical place names.

gazpacho /gəˈspætʃoː/ *n* a Spanish soup of tomatoes and other vegetables, served cold.

GB *abbr* = Great Britain.

Gd (*chem symbol*) gadolinium.

GDP /ˈdʒiːˌdiːˌpiː/ *abbr* = Gross Domestic Product.

Ge /geɪ/ (*chem symbol*) germanium.

gear /giːr/ *n* clothing; equipment, *esp* for some task or activity; a toothed wheel designed to mesh with another; (*often pl*) a system of such gears meshed together to transmit motion; a specific adjustment of such a system; a part of a mechanism with a specific function. • *vt* to connect by or furnish with gears; to adapt (one thing) to conform with another.

gearbox /ˈgiːrbɒks/ *n* a metal case enclosing a system of gears.

gearing /ˈgiːrɪŋ/ *n* a particular arrangement of gears.

gearshift /ˈgiːrʃɪft/ *n* a lever used to engage or change gear, *esp* in a motor vehicle.

gearwheel /-wiːl/ *n* a cogwheel.

gecko /ˈgɛkoː/ *n* (*pl* **geckos, geckoes**) a small lizard of warm regions that feeds on insects.

gee /dʒiː/ *vi* (**geeing geed**) (*often with* **up**) to make a horse go faster. • *interj* a mild oath.

geese /giːs/ *see* **goose**.

geezer /ˈgiːzər/ *n* (*sl*) an old man.

Geiger counter /ˈgaɪgər/ *n* an electronic device for detecting and measuring radioactive emissions.

geisha /ˈgeɪʃə/ *n* (*pl* **geisha, geishas**) a Japanese girl trained as an entertainer to serve as a hired companion to men.

gel /dʒɛl/ *n* a jelly-like substance, as that applied to style and sculpt hair before drying it. • *vti* (**gelling, gelled**) to become or cause to become a gel.—*also* **jell**.

gelatin, gelatine /ˈdʒɛlətɪn/ *n* a tasteless, odourless substance extracted by boiling bones, hoofs, etc and used in food, photographic film, medicines, etc.

gelatinize /dʒɪˈlætɪˌnaɪz/ *vt* to make or become gelatinous; to coat with gelatin.—**gelatinization** *n.*—**gelatinizer** *n.*

gelatinous /dʒəˈlætɪnəs/ *adj* of or like gelatin; jelly-like in consistency.

gelation /dʒəˈleɪʃən/ *n* solidification (of liquids) by cold.

geld /gɛld/ *vt* (**gelding, gelded** *or* **gelt**) to castrate, *esp* a horse.

gelding /ˈgɛldɪŋ/ *n* a castrated horse.

gelid /ˈdʒɛlɪd/ *adj* intensely cold; icy.—**gelidity** *n.*

gelignite /ˈdʒɛlɪgˌnəɪt/ *n* an explosive consisting of nitroglycerin absorbed in a base of wood pulp mixed with sodium or potassium nitrate.

gem /dʒɛm/ *n* a precious stone, *esp* when cut and polished for use as a jewel; a person or thing regarded as extremely valuable or beloved. • *vt* (**gemming, gemmed**) to decorate or set with gems.

Geminate /'dʒɛmɪnət/, **geminated** /-ɪd/ *adj* growing or occurring in pairs.

gemination /-'neɪʃən/ *n* duplication; (*rhetoric*) the repetition of a word, etc, for effect.

Gemini /'dʒɛmɪˌnaɪ/ or /-ˌniː/ *n* the third sign of the zodiac, represented by the twins Castor and Pollux, operative 21 May–20 June.—**Geminian** *adj*.

gemma /'dʒɛmə/ *n* (*pl* **gemmae**) a growth on an animal or plant budding off as a separate individual.

gemmate /'dʒɛmˌeɪt/ *vi* to have buds; to propagate by gemmae.—**gemmation** *n*.—**gemmiparous** *adj*.

gemmule /'dʒɛmjuːl/ *n* a small bud or gemma; an ovule; a cell produced by certain moulds.

gemot, gemote /gə'moːt/ *n* an assembly or local court in pre-Norman England.

gemsbok /'gɛmzbɒk/ *n* (*pl* **gemsbok, gemsboks**) a large, straight-horned South African antelope with a broad black stripe along its length.

gemstone /'dʒɛmstoːn/ *n* a mineral or substance used as a gem.

gendarme /'ʒɒndɑrm/ *n* an armed policeman in France and Belgium.

gendarmerie, gendarmery /ʒɒn'dɑrməri/ *n* a force of gendarmes.

gender /'dʒɛndər/ *n* the classification by which words are grouped as feminine, masculine, or neuter; (*inf*) the sex of a person.

gene /dʒiːn/ *n* any of the complex chemical units in the caromosomes by which hereditary characteristics are transmitted.

genealogy /ˌdʒiːni'ɒlədʒi/ or /-ælədʒi/ *n* (*pl* **genealogies**) a recorded history of one's ancestry; the study of family descent; lineage.—**genealogical** *adj*.—**genealogist** *n*.

genera /'dʒɛnərə/ *see* **genus**.

generable /-əbəl/ *adj* capable of being generated.

general /'dʒɛnərəl/ *adj* not local, special, or specialized; cf or for a whole genus, relating to or covering all instances or individuals of a class or group; widespread, common to many; not specific or precise; holding superior rank, chief. • *n* something that involves or is applicable to the whole; a commissioned officer above a lieutenant general; a leader, commander; the title of the head of some religious orders.—**generalness** *n*.

general anaesthetic *n* an anaesthetic effecting the whole body and producing unconsciousness.

general delivery *n* the department of a post office that will hold mail until it is called for.—*also* **poste restante**.

general election *n* a national election to choose representatives in every constituency.

generalissimo /ˌdʒɛnərə'liːsimoː/ *n* (*pl* **generalissimos**) a military commander of combined air, naval and ground forces.

generality /ˌdʒɛnə'ræliti/ *n* (*pl* **generalities**) the quality or state of being general; a vague or inadequate statement.

generalization /ˌdʒɛnərəlaɪ'zeɪʃən/ or /-li-/ *n* general inference; induction; a general notion formed by attributing the characteristic(s) of a particular part or member (of a class, community etc) to the whole.

generalize /'dʒɛnərəˌlaɪz/ *vti* to form general conclusions from specific instances; to talk (about something) in general terms.—**generalization** *n*.—**generalizer** *n*.

generally /'dʒɛnərəli/ *adv* widely; popularly; usually; not specifically.

general practitioner *n* a non-specialist doctor who treats all types of illnesses in the community.

general-purpose /'dʒɛnərəl'pərpəs/ *adj* having all kinds of uses.

generalship /'dʒɛnərəlˌʃɪp/ *n* the office of general; military skill; management skill.

general staff *n* officers who advice and assist a military commander.

general strike *n* a strike of all workers in a city, region or country.

generate /'dʒɛnəˌreɪt/ *vt* to bring into existence; to produce.

generation /ˌdʒɛnə'reɪʃən/ *n* the act or process of generating; a single succession in natural descent; people of the same period; production, as of electric current.

generation gap *n* the difference in attitudes and understanding between one generation and another.

generative /'dʒɛnərətɪv/ *adj* pertaining to generation; having the power to generate.

generator /'dʒɛnəˌreɪtər/ *n* one who or that which generates; a machine that changes mechanical energy to electrical energy.

generic /dʒə'nɛrɪk/ *adj* of a whole class, kind, or group.—**generically** *adv*.

generosity /-'rɒsiti/ *n* (*pl* **generosities**) the quality of being generous; liberality; munificence; a generous act.

generous /'dʒɛnərəs/ *adj* magnanimous; of a noble nature; willing to give or share; large ample.—**generously** *adv*.—**generousness** *n*.

genesis /'dʒɛnəsis/ *n* (*pl* **geneses**) the beginning, origin; (*with cap*) the first book of the Old Testament.

genet /'dʒɛnɪt/ *n* an animal of southern Europe, western Asia and Africa, related to the civet and valued for its fur; any fur made in imitation of genet.

genetic /dʒə'nɛtɪk/, **genetical** /-əl/ *adj* of or relating to the origin, development or causes of something; of or relating to genes or genetics.—**genetically** *adv*.

genetic code *n* the order of genetic information in a cell, which determines hereditary characteristics.

genetic engineering *n* the modification of genetic information in the cell of a plant or animal to improve yield, performance, etc.

genetic fingerprinting *n* the analysis of bodily tissue or fluids to identify the unique genetic character of an individual, as used in criminal investigations the determination of paternity, etc.

genetics /dʒə'nɛtiks/ *n sing* the branch of biology dealing with heredity and variation in plants and animals.—**geneticist** *n*.

genial /'dʒiːnɪəl/ *adj* kindly, sympathetic and cheerful in manner; mild, pleasantly warm.—**geniality, genialness** *n*.—**genially** *adv*.

genial [2] *adj* of the chin.

geniculate /dʒə'nɪkjuːlɪt/ or /-ˌleɪt/, **geniculated** /-td/ *adj* having knee-like joints; bent at a sharp angle.

genie /'dʒiːni/ *n* (*pl* **genies, genii**) (*fairy tales*) a spirit with supernatural powers which can fulfil your wishes.—*also* **jinni**.

genital /'dʒɛnɪtəl/ *adj* of reproduction or the sexual organs.

genitals, genitalia /ˌdʒɛnɪ'teɪliə/ *npl* the (external) sexual organs.—**genitalic** *adj*.

genitive /'dʒɛnɪtɪv/ *adj* (*gram*) of or belonging to the case of nouns, pronouns and adjectives expressing ownership or relation. • *n* the genitive case.—**genitival** *adj*.

genius /'dʒiːnjəs/ *n* (*pl* **geniuses**) a person possessing extraordinary intellectual power; (*with* **for**) natural ability, strong inclination.

genocide /'dʒɛnəˌsaɪd/ *n* the systematic killing of a whole race of people.—**genocidal** *adj*.

genre /'ʒɑrə/ or /'ʒɒnrə/ *n* a distinctive type or category, *esp* of literary composition; a style of painting in which everyday objects are treated realistically.

gens /dʒɛnz/ *n* (*pl* **gentes**) in ancient Rome, a clan or house; one of a number of related families claiming a common ancestor or having a name or religious rites etc in common.

gent /dʒɛnt/ *n* (*inf*) a gentleman.

genteel /dʒɛn'tiːl/ *adj* polite or well-bred; affectedly refined.—**genteelly** *adv*.—**genteelness** *n*.

gentes *see* **gens**.

gentian /'dʒɛnʃən/ or /-ʃiən/ *n* an alpine plant, *usu* with blue flowers.

gentian violet *n* a crystalline substance used as an antiseptic.

gentile /'dʒɛntaɪl/ *n* a person who is not a Jew.—*also adj*.

gentility /dʒɛn'tɪliti/ *n* (*pl* **gentilities**) refinement, good manners.

gentle /'dʒɛntəl/ *adj* belonging to a family of high social station; refined, courteous; generous; kind; kindly; patient; not harsh or rough.—**gentleness** *n*.—**gently** *adv*.

gentleman /-mən/ *n* (*pl* **gentlemen**) a man of good family and social standing; a courteous, gracious and honourable man; a polite term of address.—**gentlemanly** *adj*.

gentleman-at-arms /-æt'ɑrmz/ *n* (*pl* **gentlemen-at-arms**) one of the bodyguard of the UK sovereign on state occasions.

gentlewoman /-ˌwumən/ *n* (*pl* **gentlewomen**) a woman of noble or gentle birth; a lady.

gentrify /'dʒɛntrɪfaɪ/ *vt* (**gentrifying, gentrified**) to convert a working-class house or district to more expensive middle-class tastes.—**gentrification** *n*.

gentry /'dʒɛntri/ *n* people of high social standing; (*formerly*) landed proprietors not belonging to the nobility.

genuflect /'dʒɛnjuˌflɛkt/ *vi* to act in a servile way; to bend the knee in worship or respect.—**genuflection** *n*.—**genuflector** *n*.

genuine /'dʒɛnjʊn/ or /-aɪn/ *adj* not fake or artificial, real; sincere.—**genuinely** *adv.*—**genuineness** *n*.

genus /'dʒiːnəs/ or /'dʒɛnəs/ *n* (*pl* **genera**) (*biol*) a taxonomic division of plants and animals below a family and above a species; a class of objects divided into several subordinate species.

geo- /'dʒiːoː/ *prefix* earth.

geocentric /,dʒiːoː'sɛntrɪk/ *adj* viewed as from the centre of the earth; having the earth as a centre.—**geocentrically** *adj*.

geod *abbr* = geodesic; geodesy; geodetic.

geode /'dʒiːoːd/ *n* a cavity lined with crystals, *usu* within a rock.

geodesic /,dʒiːoː'diːsɪk/ or /-'dɛsɪk/ *adj* geodetic.—*also* **geodesical**. • *n* (*math*) the shortest distance between two points on a curved surface, determined by triangulation.

geodesic dome *n* a lightweight domed structure made of interlocking polygons.

geodesy /dʒiːɒdɪsi/ *n* the mathematical determination of the exact positions of geographical points and the shape and size of the earth.—**geodesic** *adj.*—**geodic** *adj*.

geodetic /dʒiːoː'dɛtɪk/, **geodetical** /-əl/ *adj* of, pertaining to, determined by, or carried out by geodesy.

geography /,dʒiː'ɒɡræfi/ *n* (*pl* **geographies**) the science of the physical nature of the earth, such as land and sea masses, climate, vegetation, etc, and their interaction with the human population; the physical features of a region.—**geographer** *n.*—**geographical, geographic** *adj.*—**geographically** *adv*.

geologize /dʒiː'ɒlə,dʒaɪz/ *vti* to study geology or the geology of.

geology /dʒiː'ɒlədʒi/ *n* the science relating to the history and structure of the earth's crust, its rocks and fossils.—**geological, geologic** *adj.*—**geologically** *adv.*—**geologist, geologer** *n*.

geomancy /'dʒiːoː,mænsi/ *n* divination by figures or lines.—**geomancer** *n.*—**geomantic** *adj*.

geometer /dʒiː'ɒmɪtər/, **geometrician** /-mətvɪsɪən/ *n* one who studies or is skilled in geometry.

geometric /,dʒiːə'mɛtrɪk/, **geometrical** /-əl/ *adj* pertaining to, or done by, geometry; (*design, etc*) consisting of simple geometric shapes.—**geometrically** *adv*.

geometric progression *n* a sequence in which the terms differ by a constant ratio (e.g. 1, 2, 4, 8, 16...).

geometrize /dʒiː'ɒmə,traɪz/ *vti* to work or make by geometrical methods; to study geometry.

geometry /dʒiː'ɒmətri/ *n* the branch of mathematics dealing with the properties, measurement, and relationships of points, lines, planes, and solids.—**geometric, geometrical** *adj.*—**geometrically** *adv*.

geophagy /dʒiː'ɒfədʒi/, **geophagia, geophagism** *n* the practice of eating certain kinds of clay, earth or chalk.—**geophagist** *n.*—**geophagous** *adj*.

geophysics /,dʒiːoː'fɪzɪks/ *n sing* the physics of the earth.—**geophysical.**—*adj.*—**geophysicist** *n*.

geopolitics /,dʒiːoː'pɒlɪtɪks/ *n sing* the study of the relationship between the geographical situation of a nation and its politics; the study of the effect of a nation's geography on its politics, *esp* in relation to that nation's relationship with other nations.

geoponic /,dʒiːoː'pɒnɪk/ *adj* agricultural.

geoponics /-s/ *n sing* the scientific study of agriculture.

georgette /dʒɔr'dʒɛt/ *n* a thin silk fabric.

Georgian /'dʒɔrdʒən/ *adj* of the times or reigns of the four Georges (1714–1830) or of George V (1910–36) who ruled Britain; pertaining to Georgia in the US; pertaining to Georgia in the Caucasus. • *n* a person from Georgia; a person who lived in Georgian times; one who lives as if he or she belonged to Georgian times.

Georgic /'dʒɔrdʒɪk/, **georgical** /-əl/ *adj* of or pertaining to husbandry; rural. • *n* a poem on agriculture; (*with cap: pl*) a poem on agriculture by Virgil.

geothermal /,dʒiːoː'θɜrməl/, **geothermic** /-mɪk/ *adj* of, relating to, or using the heat of the earth's interior.

geotropism /dʒiː'ɒtrə,pɪzəm/ *n* (*bot*) a tendency in the roots of certain plants to turn in the direction of the earth.—**geotropic** *adj.*—**geotropically** *adv*.

geranium /dʒə'reɪniəm/ *n* a garden plant with red, pink or white flowers.

gerbil, gerbille /'dʒɜrbɪl/ *n* a type of burrowing desert rodent of Asia and Africa.—*also* **jerbil**.

gerent /'dʒɪrənt/ *n* (*rare*) a ruler, a manager.

gerfalcon /'dʒɜr,fɔlkən/ or /-,fɔkən/, /-,fæl-/ *see* **gyrfalcon**.

geriatric /,dʒɛri'ætrɪk/ *adj* relating to geriatrics or old people; (*inf*) old, decrepit. • an aged person.

geriatrics /-s/ *n sing* a branch of medicine dealing with the diseases and care of old people.—**geriatrician, geriatrist** *n*.

germ /dʒɜrm/ *n* a simple form of living matter capable of growth and development into an organism; any microscopic, disease-causing organism; an origin or foundation capable of growing and developing.

German /'dʒɜrmən/ *adj* of or relating to Germany, its people or their language. • *n* a native of Germany.

german *adj* of the same stock or parentage; germane.

germander /dʒɜr'mændər/ *n* a plant of the mint family.

germane /dʒɜr'meɪn/ *adj* relevant.—**germanely** *adv.*—**germaneness** *n*.

Germanic /dʒɜr'mænɪk/ *adj* of Germans or Germany or of a German-speaking nation. • *n* the family of languages derived from Indo-European that comprises the English, Dutch, German, Scandinavian and Gothic languages.

Germanism /'dʒɜrmən,ɪzəm/ *n* a German idiom, custom, or characteristic.

germanium /dʒɜr'meɪniəm/ *n* a rare metallic element used in transistors.

Germanize /'dʒɜrmə,naɪz/ *vti* to make or become German in language, custom, manners etc.—**Germanization** *n*.

German measles *n sing* a mild contagious disease similar to measles.—*also* **rubella**.

Germanophile /dʒɜr'mænə,faɪl/ *n* a lover of Germany or its customs, etc.

Germanophobe /-,foːb/ *n* a person who has an irrational fear of Germany.—**Germanophobia** *n*.

German shepherd *n* any of a breed of large smooth-haired dogs often used by the police and for guarding property.—*also* **Alsatian**.

German silver *n* an alloy of nickel, copper and zinc.—*also* **nickel silver**.

germ cell *n* a reproductive cell.

germicide /'dʒɜrmɪ,saɪd/ *n* a substance used to destroy germs.—**germicidal** *adj*.

germinal /'dʒɜrmɪnəl/ *adj* incipient; of or pertaining to a germ or germs or seed buds; in the French revolutionary calendar, the seventh month (March 22-April 20).

germinate /'dʒɜrmɪ,neɪt/ *vti* to start developing; to sprout, as from a seed.—**germinable, germinative** *adj.*—**germination germinator** *n*.

germ warfare *n* the use of disease-causing bacteria against enemy forces.

gerontocracy /,dʒɛrɒn'tɒkrəsi/ *n* (*pl* **gerontocracies**) government by old men.—**gerontocratic** *adj*.

gerontology /,dʒɛrən'tɒlədʒi/ *n* the study of aging and its effects and problems.—**gerontological** *adj.*—**gerontologist** *n*.

gerrymander /,dʒɛri'mændər/ *vt* to rearrange the boundaries of (voting districts) to favour a particular party or candidate.

gerund /'dʒɛrənd/ *n* the participle of a verb used as a noun.—**gerundial** *adj*.

gerundive /dʒɛ'rɛndɪv/ *adj* of or like a gerund. • *n* a passive verbal adjective.

gesso /'dʒɛsoː/ *n* (*pl* **gessoes**) a prepared ground of plaster for painting on; plaster of Paris.

gestalt /gə'ʃtɒlt/ *n* (*pl* **gestalts, gestalten**) an integral pattern or system of phenomena forming a functional unit in which the whole is more than the sum of its parts.

Gestapo /gə'stɒpoː/ *n* the secret police of Nazi Germany.

gestate /'dʒɛsteɪt/ *vt* to carry (young) in the womb during pregnancy; to develop (a plan, etc) gradually in the mind.—**gestational, gestative** *adj.*—**gestatory** *adj*.

gestation /dʒɛ'steɪʃən/ *n* the act or period of carrying young in the womb; pregnancy.

gesticulate /dʒɛ'stɪkjʊ,leɪt/ *vi* to make expressive gestures, *esp* when speaking.—**gesticulation** *n.*—**gesticulative** *adj.*—**gesticulator** *n*.

gesture /'dʒɛstʃər/ *n* movement of part of the body to express or emphasize ideas, emotions, etc. • *vi* to make a gesture.—**gestural** *adj.*—**gesturer** *n*.

get /gɛt/ *vb* (**getting, got**, *pp* **got, gotten**) *vt* to obtain, gain, win; to receive; to acquire; to go and bring; to catch; to persuade; to cause to be; to prepare; (*inf*) (*with vb aux* **have** *or* **has**) to be obliged to; to possess; (*inf*) to strike, kill, baffle; defeat, etc; (*inf*) to understand; (*with* **across**) to cause to be understood; (*with* **in**) to bring in; (*crops, etc*) to gather; to insert; (*with* **off**) to acquit, to secure favourable treatment of; (*letters*) to post (*with* **out**) to cause to leave or escape; to cause to become known or published; (*with* **out of**) to avoid doing; (*with* **over**) to communicate effectively. • *vi* to come; to go; to arrive; to come to be; to manage or contrive; (*with* **about, around**) to be up and on one's feet, *esp* after being unwell; to be socially active; (*news, gossip*) to become circulated; (*with*) **across**) to be understood; (*with* **at**) to reach; (*inf*) to mean, imply; to irritate, pester relentlessly; (*inf*) to criticize; (*inf*) to corrupt, bribe, influence illegally; (*with* **away**) to escape; (*with* **by**) (*inf*) to manage, to survive; (*with* **in**) (*vehicle, etc*) to enter; to arrive; (*university, college, etc*) to be offered a place; (*with* **off**) to come off, down, or out of; to be acquitted; to escape the consequences of; to begin, depart; (*with* **on**) to go on or into; to put on; to proceed; to grow older; to become late; to manage; to succeed; (*with* **on with**) to establish a friendly relationship; (*with* **out**) to go out or away; to leave or escape; to take out; to become known or published; (*with* **over**) to overcome; to recover from; to forget; (*with* **round, around**) to evade, circumvent; to coax, cajole; (*with* **through**) to use up, spend, consume; to finish; to manage to survive; (*examination, test*) to succeed or pass; to contact by telephone; (*with* **up**) to rise to one's feet; to get out of bed; (*inf*) to organize; (*inf*) to dress in a certain style; (*inf*) to be involved in (mischief, etc).—**getable, gettable** *adj*.

get-at-able /gɛt'ætəbəl/ *adj* accessible.

getaway /'gɛtəweɪ/ *n* the act of escaping; a start in a race, etc.

get-together /'gɛtəˌgɛðər/ *n* (*inf*) an informal social gathering or meeting.

get-up /'gɛtʌp/ *n* (*inf*) dress, costume.

get-up-and-go /-ən'goʊ/ *n* (*inf*) energy, enthusiasm.

getter /'gɛtər/ *n* one who gets or acquires.

geum /'dʒiːəm/ *n* a genus of the rose family, with yellow, orange, red or white flowers.

gewgaw /'guːgɔː/ or /'gjuː-/ *n* a showy ornament; a trinket.

geyser /'gaɪzər/ *n* a natural spring from which columns of boiling water and steam gush into the air at intervals; a water heater.

GG = *abbr* Governor General; ✿ (*Cda*) Governor General's Award.

gharry, gharri /'gæri/ *n* (*pl* **gharries**) a cart or carriage in India that is available for hire.

ghastly /'gæstli/ *adj* (**ghastlier, ghastliest**) terrifying, horrible; (*inf*) intensely disagreeable; pale, unwell looking.—**ghastliness** *n*.

ghat, ghaut /gɒt/ *n* in India, a mountain pass or a chain of mountains; a landing-place with steps; a flight of steps to a river or a temple.

ghazi /'gɒzi/ *n* (*pl* **ghazies**) a Muslim slayer of infidels; a Turkish title bestowed on distinguished commanders; a warrior champion.

ghee /giː/ *n* clarified butter.

gherkin /'gɜrkɪn/ *n* a small cucumber used for pickling.

ghetto /'gɛtoʊ/ *n* (*pl* **ghettos, ghettoes**) a section of a city in which members of a minority group live, *esp* because of social, legal or economic pressure.

ghetto blaster *n* (*inf*) a large portable stereo cassette player and radio with built-in speakers.

ghillie /'gɪli/ *n* (*pl* **ghillies**) a gillie.

ghost /goʊst/ *n* the supposed disembodied spirit of a dead person, appearing as a shadowy apparition; a faint trace or suggestion; a false image in a photographic negative. • *vt* to ghostwrite.

ghostly /'goʊstli/ *adj* (**ghostlier, ghostliest**) of or like a ghost.—**ghostliness** *n*.

ghost town *n* a town abandoned by most or all of its inhabitants.

ghostwrite /'goʊstˌraɪt/ *vt* (**ghostwriting, ghostwrote**, *pp* **ghostwritten**) to write books, speeches, articles, etc for another who professes to be the author.—**ghostwriter** *n*.

ghoul /guːl/ *n* (*Muslim folklore*) an evil spirit that robs graves and feeds on the dead; a person with macabre tastes or interests.—**ghoulish** *adj*.—**ghoulishly** *adv*.

GHQ *abbr* = General Headquarters.

GI /dʒiː'aɪ/ *n* (*pl* **GI's, GIs**) (*inf*) a private soldier in the US Army.

giant /'dʒaɪənt/ *n* a huge legendary being of great strength; a person or thing of great size, strength, intellect, etc. • *adj* incredibly large.—**giantess** *nf*.

giant panda *n* a large black and white bear-like herbivore.—*also* **panda**.

giaour /'dʒaʊr/ *n* (*derog*) a Muslim term for an unbeliever, *esp* a Christian.

gibber /'dʒɪbər/ *vi* to utter meaningless or inarticulate sounds.

gibberish /-ɪʃ/ *n* unintelligible talk, nonsense.

gibbet /'dʒɪbət/ *n* a gallows; a structure from which bodies of executed criminals were hung and exposed to public scorn.

gibbon /'gɪbən/ *n* a small tailless ape of southeastern Asia and the East Indies.

gibbous /'gɪbəs/ *adj* protuberant; humped; irregularly rounded; (*moon*) between full and half.

gibe *n* a taunt, sneer. • *vti* to jeer, scoff (at).—*also* **jibe**.—**giber, jiber** *n*.—**gibingly, jibingly** *adv*.

giblets /'dʒɪbləts/ *npl* the edible internal organs of a bird.

gid *n* a disease in sheep, marked by staggering.

giddy /'gɪdi/ *adj* (**giddier, giddiest**) frivolous, flighty; having a feeling of whirling around as if about to lose balance and fall; causing giddiness. • *vti* (**giddying, giddied**) to make giddy, to become giddy.—**giddily** *adv*.—**giddiness** *n*.

gie /giː/ *vt* (*Scot*) to give.

GIFT /gɪft/ *abbr* = Gamete Intra-Fallopian Transfer; a technique that helps infertile couples to have children.

gift *n* something given; the act of giving; a natural ability. • *vt* to present with or as a gift.—**giftedness** *n*.

gifted /'gɪftəd/ *adj* having great natural ability.

gig¹ /gɪg/ *n* a light two-wheeled horse-drawn carriage; a long, light boat.

gig² *n* (*inf*) a single booking for a jazz or pop band, etc; a single night's performance. • *vi* (**gigging, gigged**) to perform a gig.

giga- /'gɪgə/ or /'dʒɪgə/, /'gɛɪgə/ *prefix* one billion (10⁹); (*comput*) 2³⁰.

gigantesque /dʒaɪˌgæn'tɛsk/ *adj* as if by or for a giant.

gigantic /dʒaɪ'gæntɪk/ *adj* exceedingly large.—**gigantically** *adv*.—**giganticness** *n*.

giggle /'gɪgəl/ *vi* to laugh in a nervous or silly manner. • *n* a laugh in this manner; (*inf*) a prank, a joke.—**giggler** *n*.—**giggly** *adj*.

gigolo /'dʒɪgə loʊ/ or /'ʒɪg-/ *n* (*pl* **gigolos**) a man paid to be a woman's escort.

gigot /ʒiː'goʊ/ or /'dʒɪgət/ *n* a leg of mutton.

gigue /ʒiːg/ *n* a lively tune; a dance similar to a jig.

gild¹ /gɪld/ *see* **guild**.

gild² *vt* (**gilding, gilded** *or* **gilt**) to coat with gold leaf; to give a deceptively attractive appearance to.—**gilder** *n*

gilder /'gɪldər/ *see* **guilder**.

gilding /-ɪŋ/ *n* the art or process of overlaying or covering with gold leaf; gold leaf applied to a surface; a superficial covering.

gill¹ /gɪl/ *n* an organ, *esp* in fish, for breathing in water.

gill² /dʒɪl/ *n* in US, a liquid measure equal to 4 fluid ounces (0.25 pint or 23.6 millimetres; in UK, 5 fluid ounces (0.25 pint) or 28.4 millimetres.

gillie, gilly /'gɪli/ *n* (*pl* **gil ies**) (*Scot*) a Highland attendant, *esp* one who accompanies a shooting or fishing party.—*also* **ghillie**.

gills /gɪls/ *npl* the wattle below the beak of a bird, as in certain domestic fowl; one of the radiating plates under the cap of a mushroom; a person's cheeks or jowls.

gillyflower /'dʒɪliˌflaʊr/ *n* one of various scented plants of the mustard family, *eg* wallflower, stock, etc.

gilt¹ /gɪlt/ *see* **gild**.

gilt² *n* gilding; a substance used for this.

gilt-edged /'gɪltˌɛdʒd/ *adj* (*securities*) considered a secure investment.

gimbal /'dʒɪmbəl/ or /'gɪmbəl/ *n* (*usu pl*) one of two rings moving within each other at right angles, used to suspend a ship's compass, etc.

gimcrack /'dʒɪmkræk/ *adj* showy, cheap and useless.

gimlet /'gɪmlət/ *n* a small tool with a screw point for boring holes.

gimmick /'gɪmɪk/ *n* a trick or device for attracting notice, advertising or promoting a person, product or service.—**gimmickry** *n*.—**gimmicky** *adj*.

gimp /gɪmp/ *n* an interlaced silk twist or trimming interwoven with wire or cord, used for furniture, dresses etc.—*also* **guimpe**.

gin¹ /dʒɪn/ *n* an alcoholic spirit distilled from grain and flavoured with juniper berries.

gin² *n* a trap for catching small animals; a type of crane; a machine for separating the seeds from raw cotton. • *vt* (**ginning, ginned**) to trap with a gin; to separate seeds from cotton.

ginger /'dʒɪndʒər/ *n* a tropical plant with fleshy roots used as a flavouring; the spice prepared by drying and grinding; (*inf*) vigour; a reddish-brown.—**gingery** *adj*.

ginger ale, ginger beer *n* a carbonated soft drink flavoured with ginger.

gingerbread /'dʒɪndʒər,brɛd/ *n* a cake flavoured with ginger.

gingerly /'dʒɪndʒərli/ *adv* with care or caution. • *adj* cautious.—**gingerliness** *n*.

ginger snap /'dʒɪndʒər,snæp/ *n* a ginger-flavoured biscuit.

gingham /'ɡɪŋəm/ *n* a cotton fabric with stripes or checks.

gingival /dʒɪn'dʒaɪvəl/ *adj* of the gums.

gingivitis /,dʒɪndʒɪ'vəɪtɪs/ *n* inflammation of the gums.

ginglymus /'dʒɪndʒli,məs/ *n* (*pl* **ginglymi**) (*anat*) a joint like a hinge.

gink /ɡɪŋk/ *n* (*sl*) a boy or man, *esp* an eccentric one.

ginkgo /'ɡɪŋkɡoː/ *n* (*pl* **ginkgoes**) a Japanese tree with hand-some fan-shaped foliage; the maidenhair tree.

ginseng /'dʒɪnsɛŋ/ *n* a plant found in China and North America; its root, said to have an invigorating effect on the mind and body.

gip /dʒɪp/ *see* **gyp**.

Gipsy /'dʒɪpsi/ *see* **Gypsy**.

giraffe /dʒɪ'ræf/ *n* (*pl* **giraffes**, **giraffe**) a large cud-chewing mammal of Africa, with very long legs and neck.

girandole /'dʒɪrən,doːl/, **girandola** *n* a branched chandelier; a revolving firework or water jet; a pendant or earring with small stones around a larger one; one of several mines connected in a group.

girasol /'dʒɪrə,sɒl/, **girosol**, **girasole** /-,soːl/ *n* a variety of opal; the fire opal.

gird /ɡərd/ *vt* (**girding**, **girded** *or* **girt**) to encircle or fasten with a belt; to surround; to prepare (oneself) for action.

girder /'ɡərdər/ *n* a large steel beam for supporting joists, the framework of a building, etc.

girdle /'ɡərdəl/ *n* a belt for the waist.

girl /ɡərl/ *n* a female child; a young woman; (*inf*) a woman of any age.—**girlhood** *n*.—**girlish** *adj*.

girlfriend /'ɡərlfrɛnd/ *n* a female friend, *esp* with whom one is ro-mantically involved.

Girl Guide *n* a member of the Girl Guides, a scouting organiza-tion founded in Britain in 1910.

girlie /'ɡərli/ *n* a little girl; a young woman; (*inf*) a woman.

girlie magazine *n* a magazine that contains photographs of nude or semi-nude females.

girlish /'ɡərlɪʃ/ *adj* of or like a girl.—**girlishly** *adv*.—**girlishness** *n*.

Girl Scout *n* a member of the Girl Scouts, a youth organization founded in the US in 1912.

giro /'dʒaɪroː/ *n* (*pl* **giros**) a credit-transfer system between finan-cial organizations; a payment so made.

Girondist /ʒɪ'rɒndɪst/ *n* a member of the Gironde, the moderate Republican party during the Revolution in France (179193).

girt[1] /ɡərt/ *see* **gird**.

girt[2] *adj* (*naut*) moored so taut by two cables as not to swing to the wind or tide.

girth /ɡərθ/ *n* the thickness round something; a band put around the belly of a horse, etc to hold a saddle or pack.

gist /dʒɪst/ *n* the principal point or essence of anything.

gîte /ʒiːt/ *n* self-catering holiday accommodation in France.

give /ɡɪv/ *vb* (**giving**, **gave**, *pp* **given**) *vt* to hand over as a pres-ent; to deliver; to hand over in or for payment; to pass (regards etc) along; to act as host or sponsor of; to supply; to yield; (*advice*) to offer; (*punishment, etc*) to inflict; to sacrifice; to perform; (*with* **away**) to make a gift of; to give (the bride) to the bridegroom; to sell cheaply; to reveal, betray; (*with* **in**) to deliver, hand in (a document, etc); (*with* **off**) to emit (fumes, etc); (*with* **out**) to discharge; to make public, to announce; to emit; to distribute; (*with* **over**) to devote time to a specific activity; to cease (an activity); to transfer to another; to set aside for a particular purpose; (*with* **up**) to hand over; to stop, renounce; to cease; to resign (a position); to stop trying; to de-spair of; to surrender; to devote oneself completely (to). • *vi* to bend, move, etc from force or pressure; (*inf*) to be happening; (*with* **in**) to concede, admit defeat; (*with* **out**) to become used up or exhausted; to fail; (*with* **over**) (*inf*) to stop (an activity). • *n* capacity or tendency to yield to force or strain; the quality or state of being springy; (*with* **in**) to submit; (*with* **out**) to become worn out; (*with* **up**) to accept defeat or failure to do something, to surrender.—**givable**, **giveable** *adj*.

give-and-take /'ɡɪvən'teɪk/ *n* mutual concessions; free-flowing exchange of ideas and conversation.

giveaway /'ɡɪvəweɪ/ *n* (*inf*) an unintentional revelation; a free gift to encourage sales; a freesheet.

given[1] /'ɡɪvən/ *see* **give**.

given[2] *adj* accustomed (to) by habit, etc; specified; assumed; granted.

giver /'ɡɪvər/ *n* a person who gives.

gizzard /'ɡɪzərd/ *n* the second stomach of a bird, used for grinding food.

glabrous /'ɡleɪbrəs/ *adj* without hair, smooth-skinned.

glacé /'ɡlæseɪ/ *or* /ɡlæ'seɪ/ *adj* candied, covered in icing, as fruit. • *vt* (**glacéing**, **glacéed**) to cover with icing; to candy.

glacial /'ɡleɪʃəl/ *or* /-sɪəl/ *adj* extremely cold; of or relating to gla-ciers or a glacial epoch.—**glacially** *adv*.

glaciate /'ɡleɪsɪ,eɪt/ *vti* to subject to glacial action; to cover or become covered with glaciers.—**glaciation** *n*.

glacier /'ɡleɪʃər/ *or* /-ʃɪər/, /-sɪər/ *n* a large mass of snow and ice moving slowly down a mountain.

glacis /'ɡlæsi/ *or* /-sɪs/, /'ɡleɪ-/ *n* (*pl* **glacis**) a sloping bank of earth in front of a fortification for its defence; a slope (on a tank) to throw off hostile shot.

glad /ɡlæd/ *adj* (**gladder**, **gladdest**) happy; causing joy; very willing; bright.—**gladly** *adv*.—**gladness** *n*.

gladden /'ɡlædən/ *vti* to make or become glad.—**gladdener** *n*.

glade /ɡleɪd/ *n* an open space in a wood or forest.

gladiate /'ɡlædi,eɪt/ *adj* sword-shaped.

gladiator /'ɡlædi,eɪtər/ *n* (*ancient Rome*) a person trained to fight with men or beasts in a public arena.—**gladiatorial** *adj*.

gladiolus /,ɡlædi'oːləs/ *n* (*pl* **gladiolus**, **gladioli**) any of a genus of the iris family with sword-like leaves and tall spikes of funnel-shaped flowers.

gladsome /'ɡlædsəm/ *adj* joyous.

glair /ɡlɛr/ *n* white of egg; size made from this; a sticky sub-stance; any sticky or glairy matter. • *vt* to smear with glair.—**glaireous** *adj*.

glairy /'ɡlɛri/ *adj* (**glairier**, **glairiest**) like or smeared with glair.—**glairiness** *n*.

glamorize, **glamourize** /'ɡlæmə,raɪz/ *vt* to make glamorous.—**glamorization**, **glamourization** *n*.—**glamorizer**, **glamour-izer** *n*.

glamour, **glamor** /'ɡlæmər/ *n* charm, allure; attractiveness, beauty.—**glamorous**, **glamourous** *adj*.—**glamorousness**, **glamourousness** *n*.

glance /ɡlæns/ *vi* to strike obliquely and go off at an angle; to flash; to look quickly. • *n* a glancing off; a flash; a quick look.—**glancingly** *adv*.

gland /ɡlænd/ *n* an organ that separates substances from the blood and synthesizes them for further use in, or for elimina-tion from, the body.

glanders /'ɡlændərz/ *n* (*sing or pl*) a contagious bacterial disease *esp* of horses, often fatal.—**glandered** *adj*.—**glanderous** *adj*.

glandular /'ɡlændjulər/ *adj* of, having or resembling glands; (*plants*) covered with hair tipped with glands.

glare /ɡlɛr/ *n* a harsh, uncomfortably bright light, *esp* painfully bright sunlight; an angry or fierce stare. • *vi* to shine with a steady, dazzling light; to stare fiercely.

glaring /'ɡlɛrɪŋ/ *adj* dazzling; obvious, conspicuous.—**glaringly** *adv*.—**glaringness** *n*.

glasnost /'ɡlæznɒst/ *or* /'ɡlæs-/ *n* the Russian word for "openness," applied to the policy, initiated by President Gorbachev of the former USSR, of greater frankness and openness in Soviet affairs.—**glasnostian** *adj*.

glass /ɡlæs/ *n* a hard brittle substance, *usu* transparent; glassware; a glass article, as a drinking vessel; (*pl*) spectacles or binoculars; the amount held by a drinking glass. • *adj* of or made of glass. • *vt* to equip, enclose, or cover with glass.

glass-blowing *n* the art, skill or process of blowing air into molten glass and shaping it.—**glass-blower** *n*.

glassware /'ɡlæswer/ *n* objects made of glass, *esp* drinking vessels.

glasswort /'ɡlæswərt/ *n* a fleshy plant of marshy areas, from which soda was formerly obtained for use in making glass.

glassy /'ɡlæsi/ *adj* (**glassier**, **glassiest**) resembling glass; smooth; expressionless, lifeless.—**glassily** *adv*.—**glassiness** *n*.

glaucoma /ɡlɒ'koːmə/ *n* a disease of the eye caused by pressure.—**glaucomatous** *adj*.

glaucous /'ɡlɒkəs/ *adj* sea-green; covered with bloom of a blueish-white colour, green with a bluish-grey tinge.

glaze /ɡleɪz/ *vt* to provide (windows etc) with glass; to give a hard glossy finish to (pottery, etc); to cover (foods, etc) with a glossy surface. • *vi* to become glassy or glossy. • *n* a glassy finish or coating.—**glazer** *n*.

glazier /'gleɪzɪər/ or /-ʒər/ n a person who fits glass in windows.—**glaziery** n.

glazing /'gleɪzɪŋ/ n a glaze; the operation of setting glass or applying a glaze; windowpanes; glass; semi-transparent colours passed thinly over other colours to tone down their effect.

gleam /gliːm/ n a subdued or moderate beam of light; a brief show of some quality or emotion, esp hope. • vi to emit or reflect a beam of light.—**gleamingly** adv.

glean /gliːn/ vti to collect (grain left by reapers); to gather (facts, etc) gradually.—**gleanable** adj.—**gleaner** n.

gleaning /'gliːnɪŋ/ n the act of collecting after reapers; (often pl) that which is collected laboriously from various sources.

glee /gliː/ n joy and gaiety; delight; (mus) a song in parts for three or more male voices.—**gleeful** adj.—**gleefully** adv.—**gleefulness** n.

gleeful /'gliːfʊl/ adj merry, joyous; triumphant.—**gleefully** adv.—**gleefulness** n.

gleet /gliːt/ n a thin mucous discharge, esp from the urethra, resulting from gonorrhoeal disease.

glen /glɛn/ n a narrow valley.

glengarry /glɛn'gærɪ/ n (pl glengarries) (often cap) a boat-shaped cap originating in Scotland.

glib /glɪb/ adj (glibber, glibbest) speaking or spoken smoothly, to the point of insincerity; lacking depth and substance.—**glibly** adv.—**glibness** n.

glib ice n ✶ (Cdn) extremely slippery ice on a roadway.

glide /glaɪd/ vti to move smoothly and effortlessly; to descend in an aircraft or glider with little or no engine power. • n a gliding movement.—**glidingly** adv.

glider /'glaɪdər/ n an engineless aircraft carried along by air currents.

gliding /-ɪŋ/ n the sport of flying gliders.

glim /glɪm/ n (sl) a light, a candle.

glimmer /'glɪmər/ vi to give a faint, flickering light; to appear faintly. • n a faint gleam; a glimpse, an inkling.

glimmering /-ɪŋ/ n a faint gleam; a glimpse, an inkling.

glimpse /glɪmps/ n a brief, momentary view. • vt to catch a glimpse of.—**glimpser** n.

glint /glɪnt/ n a brief flash of light; a brief indication. • vti to (cause to) gleam brightly.

glioma /glaɪ'oːmə/ n (pl gliomata, gliomas) a tumour of rapid growth on the brain, spinal cord, or auditory nerve.

glissade /glɪ'sɒd/ or /-'seɪd/ vi to slide down a snow-covered slope without the aid of skis. • n a sliding ballet step.—**glissader** n.

glissando /glɪ'sændoʊ/ or /-'sɒndoʊ/ n (pl glissandi, glissandos) (mus) a run by sliding the fingers over the keys of a piano; a quick slur on a violin.

glisten /'glɪsən/ vi to shine, as light reflected from a wet surface.—**glisteningly** adv.

glister /'glɪstər/ vi (poet) to sparkle, to glitter.—also n.

glitch /glɪtʃ/ n a malfunction in a, usu electronic, system.

glitter /'glɪtər/ vi to sparkle; (usu with with) to be brilliantly attractive. • n a sparkle; showiness, glamour; tiny pieces of sparkling material used for decoration.—**glittering** adj.—**glittery** adj.

glitz /glɪts/ n (sl) gaudiness; ostentatious glamour.—**glitzy** adj (glitzier, glitziest).

gloaming /'gloːmɪŋ/ n twilight.

gloat /gloːt/ vi to gaze or contemplate with wicked or malicious satisfaction.—**gloatingly** adv.

global /'gloːbəl/ adj worldwide; comprehensive.—**globally** adv.

global village n the world considered as a single community because of instantaneous communications.

global warming n the process caused by a blanket of 'greenhouse gases' building up around the earth trapping heat from the sun. Carbon dioxide, released by burning fossil fuels is one of the main causes.—see **greenhouse effect**.

globate /'gloː,beɪt/, **globated** /-ɪd/ adj globe-shaped.

globe /gloːb/ n anything spherical or almost spherical; the earth, or a model of the earth.

globeflower /'gloːb,flaʊr/ n a plant with round yellow flowers.

globetrotter /'gloːb,trɒtər/ n a person who travels widely.—**globetrotting** n, adj.

globin /'gloːbɪn/ n a constituent of red blood corpuscles.

globoid /'gloːbɔɪd/ adj nearly globular. • n a globoid figure.

globose /'gloː,boːs/, **globous** /-bəs/ adj globe-like, spherical.

globosity /-'bɒsɪtɪ/, **globoseness** n.

globular /'glɒbjʊlər/ adj spherical.

globule /'glɒbjuːl/ n a small spherical particle; a drop, pellet; a blood corpuscle.

globulin /'glɒbjʊlɪn/ n an albuminous protein forming one of the constituents of blood, muscle, and the cellular tissue of plants.

glockenspiel /'glɒkən,spiːl/ or /-,ʃpiːl/ n an orchestral percussion instrument with tuned metal bars, played with hammers.

glomerate /'glɒmərɪt/ adj gathered into a roundish head or mass; compactly clustered.

glomerule /glə'merjʊl/ n a clustered flowerhead.

gloom /gluːm/ n near darkness; deep sadness. • vti to look sullen or dejected; to make or become cloudy or murky.

gloomy /'gluːmɪ/ adj (gloomier, gloomiest) almost dark, obscure; depressed, dejected.—**gloomily** adv.—**gloominess** n.

gloria /'glɔːrɪə/ n a halo or aureole; a light fabric of silk, etc; (with cap) a prayer of praise, esp the Gloria in excelsis and Gloria patri a musical setting of these.

glorify /'glɔːrɪ,faɪ/ vt (glorifying, glorified) to worship; to praise, to honour; to cause to appear more worthy, important, or splendid than in reality.—**glorifiable** adj.—**glorification** n.—**glorifier** n.

glorious /'glɔːrɪəs/ adj having or deserving glory; conferring glory or renown; beautiful; delightful.—**gloriously** adv.—**gloriousness** n.

glory /'glɔːrɪ/ n (pl glories) great honour or fame, or its source; adoration; great splendour or beauty; heavenly bliss. • vi (glorying, gloried) (with in) to exult, rejoice proudly.

gloss¹ /glɒs/ n the lustre of a polished surface; a superficially attractive appearance. • vt to give a shiny surface to; (with over) to hide (an error, etc) or make seem right or inconsequential.—**glosser** n.

gloss² n an explanation of an unusual word (in the margin or between the lines of a text); a misleading explanation; a glossary. • vt to provide with glosses; to give a misleading sense of.—**glosser** n.

glossa /'glɒsə/ n (pl glossae, glossas) the tongue, esp of insects.—**glossal** adj.

glossary /'glɒsərɪ/ n (pl glossaries) a list of specialized or technical words and their definitions.—**glossarial** adj.—**glossarist** n.

glossitis /glɒ'saɪtɪs/ n inflammation of the tongue.

glossography /glɒ'sɒgrəfɪ/ n the making of glossaries or glosses.—**glossographer** n.

glossy /'glɒsɪ/ adj (glossier, glossiest) having a shiny or highly polished surface; superficial; (magazines) lavishly produced. • n (pl glossies) a magazine with many colour pictures, printed on coated paper, esp a fashion magazine.—**glossily** adv.—**glossiness** n.

glottal /'glɒtəl/ adj of, pertaining to, or produced by the glottis.

glottis /'glɒtɪs/ n (glottises, glottides) the opening between the vocal cords in the larynx.—**glottidean** adj.

glove /glʌv/ n a covering for the hand; a baseball player's mitt; a boxing glove. • vt to cover (as if) with a glove.

glover /'glʌvər/ n a maker or seller of gloves.

glow /gloʊ/ vi to shine (as if) with an intense heat; to emit a steady light without flames; to be full of life and enthusiasm; to flush or redden with emotion. • n a light emitted due to intense heat; a steady, even light without flames; a reddening of the complexion; warmth of emotion or feeling.

glower /'glaʊər/ vi to scowl; to stare sullenly or angrily. • n a scowl, a glare.—**gloweringly** adv.

glow-worm n a beetle that emits light from the abdomen.

gloxinia /glɒk'sɪnɪə/ n a tropical plant with showy bell-shaped flowers, cultivated as a houseplant.

glucose /'gluːkoːs/ or /-oːz/ n a crystalline sugar occurring naturally in fruits, honey, etc.

glue /gluː/ n a sticky, viscous substance used as an adhesive. • vt (gluing, glued) to join with glue.—**gluer** n.

gluey /'gluːɪ/ adj (gluier, glueist) like glue, sticky.

glum /glʌm/ adj (glummer, glummest) sullen; gloomy.—**glumly** adv.—**glumness** n.

glumaceous /gluː'meɪʃəs/ adj bearing or resembling glumes.

glume /gluːm/ n the husk of corn or grasses.

glut /glʌt/ vt (glutting, glutted) to over-supply (the market). • n a surfeit, an excess of supply.

gluteal /'gluːtɪəl/ adj pertaining to the buttocks.

gluten /'gluːtən/ n a sticky elastic protein substance, esp of wheat flour, that gives cohesiveness to dough.—**glutenous** adj.

gluteus /'gluːtɪəs/ n (pl glutei) any of the three muscles that form the buttocks.

glutinous /'glu:tɪnəs/ *adj* resembling glue, sticky.—**glutinousness, glutinosity** *n*.

glutton /'glʌtən/ *n* a person who eats and drinks to excess; a person who has a tremendous capacity for something (*eg* for work); a wolverine.—**gluttonous** *adj*.

gluttony /'glʌtəni/ *n* the act or habit of eating and drinking to excess.

glyceride /'glɪsəˌraɪd/ *n* an ester of glycerol.

glycerin, glycerine /'glɪsəˌrɪn/ *n* the popular and commercial name for glycerol.

glycerol /'glɪsəˌrɒl/ *n* a colourless, syrupy liquid made from fats and oils, used in making skin lotions, explosives, etc.—**glyceric** *adj*.

glycogen /'glaɪkədʒən/ *n* a white insoluble starch-like substance obtained from the livers of animals and humans.

glycol /'glaɪkɒl/ *n* a viscid liquid intermediate between glycerine and alcohol; antifreeze.

glycosuria /ˌglaɪkə'sjʊərɪə/ *n* a disease marked by excess sugar in the urine.—**glycosuric** *adj*.

glyph /glɪf/ *n* (*arch*) a perpendicular fluting.—**glyphic** *adj*.

glyptic /'glɪptɪk/ *adj* pertaining to engraving on gems; figured. • *n* the art of engraving designs on precious stones, ivory, etc.

glyptography /glɪp'tɒgrəfi/ *n* the art of cutting designs or engraving on a gem.

gm *abbr* = gram(s).

Gm *abbr* = genetically modified.

G-man *n* (*pl* **G-men**) (*inf*) an agent of the FBI.

GMT /ˌdʒiːɛm'tiː/ *abbr* = Greenwich Mean Time.

gnarl /nɑrl/ *n* a knot on the trunk or branch of a tree.

gnarled /nɑrld/ *adj* (*tree trunks*) full of knots; (*hands*) rough, knobbly; crabby in disposition.

gnash /næʃ/ *vti* to grind (the teeth) in anger or pain. • *n* a grinding of the teeth.—**gnashingly** *adv*.

gnat /næt/ *n* any of various small, two-winged insects that bite or sting.

gnathic /'næθɪk/, **gnathial**, /'næθɪəl/ *adj* of or pertaining to jaws.

gnaw /nɒ/ *vti* (**gnawing, gnawed**, *pp* **gnawed** *or* **gnawn**) to bite away bit by bit; to torment, as by constant pain.—**gnawable** *adj*.—**gnawer** *n*.

gneiss /nəɪs/ *n* a granite-like rock formed by layers of quartz, mica, etc.—**gneissic, gneissoid, gneissose** *adj*.

gnocchi /'njɒki/ *npl* small dumplings made from flour, semolina or potatoes.

gnome /nɒːm/ *n* (*folklore*) a dwarf who dwells in the earth and guards its treasure; a small statue of a gnome used as a garden decoration; a small and ugly person; (*sl*) an international banker or financier.—**gnomish** *adj*.

gnomic /'nɒːmɪk/ *adj* dealing in or containing pithy or sententious sayings; didactic.—**gnomically** *adv*.

gnomon /'nɒːmɒn/ *n* the indicator on a sundial that casts a shadow to indicate the time of day.—**gnomonic** *adj*.—**gnomonically** *adv*.

gnosis /'nɒːsɪs/ *n* (*pl* **gnoses**) higher knowledge, mysticism or insight.

gnostic /'nɒstɪk/ *adj* of, pertaining to, or having knowledge; (*with cap*) pertaining to the Gnostics or Gnosticism.—*also* **gnostical**. • *n* (*with cap*) a member of an early Christian sect seeking salvation by knowledge, not faith.

Gnosticism /'nɒstɪˌsɪzəm/ *n* the doctrine of the Gnostics.

GNP /'dʒiːɛnˌpiː/ *abbr* = Gross National Product.

gnu /nuː/ *or* /njuː/ *n* (*pl* **gnus, gnu**) either of two large African antelopes with an ox-like head.—*also* **wildebeest**.

GNWT *abbr* ✤ = Government of the Northwest Territories.

go[1] /gɒː/ *vb* (**going, went**, *pp* **gone**) *vi* to move on a course; to proceed; to work properly; to act, sound, as specified; to result; to become; to be accepted or valid; to leave, to depart; to die; to be allotted or sold; to be able to pass (through); to fit (into); to be capable of being divided (into); to belong; (*with* **about**) to handle (a task, etc) efficiently; to undertake (duties, etc); (*sailing*) to change tack; (*with* **into**) to enter; to become a member of; to examine or investigate; to discuss; (*with* **off**) to explode; to depart; (*food, etc*) to become stale or rotten; to fall asleep; to proceed, occur in a certain manner; to take place as planned; to stop liking (something or someone); (*with* **on**) to continue; to happen; to talk effusively; to nag; to enter on stage; (*with* **out**) to depart; (*light, fire, etc*) to become extinguished; to cease to be fashionable; to socialize; (*radio or TV show*) to be broadcast; to spend time with, *esp* a person of the opposite sex; (*with* **over**) to change one's loyalties (to); to be received or regarded in a certain

way; to examine and repair (something); (*with* **round**) to circulate; to be sufficient for everyone; (*with* **slow**) to work at a slow rate as part of an industrial dispute; (*with* **through**) to continue to the end (with); to be approved; to use up completely; to experience (an illness, etc); to search thoroughly; (*with* **together**) to match, to be mutually suited; (*inf*) to associate frequently, *esp* as lovers; (*with* **up**) in the UK, to enter or return to college or university; (*with* **with**) to match; to accompany; to associate frequently, *esp* as lovers; (*with* **without**) to be deprived of or endure the lack of (something). • *vt* to travel along; (*inf*) to put up with. • *n* (*pl* **goes**) a success; (*inf*) a try; (*inf*) energy.

go[2] *n* a Japanese board game.

goa /gɒːə/ *n* an Asian gazelle, the male of which has horns that curve backwards.

goad /gɒːd/ *n* a sharp-pointed stick for driving cattle, etc; any stimulus to action. • *vt* to drive (as if) with a goad; to irritate, nag persistently.

go-ahead *n* (*inf*) permission to proceed. • *adj* (*inf*) enterprising, ambitious.

goal /gɒːl/ *n* the place at which a race, trip, etc is ended; an objective; the place over or into which the ball or puck must go to score in some games; the score made; the position of goalkeeper.

goalie /'gɒːli/ *n* (*inf*) a goalkeeper.

goalkeeper /'gɒːlˌkiːpər/ *n* a player who defends the goal.—**goalkeeping** *n*.

goat /gɒːt/ *n* a mammal related to the sheep that has backward curving horns, a short tail, and *usu* straight hair; a lecherous man.

goatee /gɒː'tiː/ *n* a small pointed beard.

goatherd /'gɒːthərd/ *n* a person who looks after goats.

goatish /-ɪʃ/ *adj* pertaining to or like a goat; (*arch*) lustful; ranksmelling.—**goatishly** *adv*.—**goatishness** *n*.

goatsbeard, goat's-beard *n* a European grass-like plant with yellow flowers; an American plant with compound leaves and small white flowers.

goatskin /'gɒːtskɪn/ *n* the skin of a goat; a bottle or garment made of this.

goatsucker /'gɒːtˌsʌkər/ *n* a nocturnal bird with dull mottled plumage.—*also* **nightjar**.

gob[1] /gɒb/ *n* (*sl*) the mouth.

gob[2] *n* a lump or clot of something; (*inf*) spittle. • *vi* (**gobbing, gobbed**) (*inf*) to spit.

gobbet /'gɒbət/ *n* a lump of something.

gobble /'gɒbəl/ *vt* to eat greedily; (*often with* **up**) to take, accept or read eagerly. • *vi* to make a throaty gurgling noise, as a male turkey.

gobbledygook, gobbledegook /'gɒbəldiˌguk/ *or* /-ˌguːk/ *n* (*sl*) nonsense, pretentious jargon.

gobbler /'gɒblər/ *n* (*inf*) a turkey cock.

go-between *n* a messenger, an intermediary.

goblet /'gɒblət/ *n* a large drinking vessel with a base and stem but without a handle.

goblin /'gɒblɪn/ *n* an evil or mischievous elf.

goby /'gɒːbi/ *n* (*pl* **goby, gobies**) a sea fish with a large head and a long thin body.

go-cart *n* a small cart for children to play in or pull; a stroller; a handcart.

god /gɒd/ *n* any of various beings conceived of as supernatural and immortal, *esp* a male deity; an idol; a person or thing deified; (*with cap*) in monotheistic religions, the creator and ruler of the universe.

godchild /'gɒdtʃaɪld/ *n* (*pl* **godchildren**) the child a godparent sponsors.

goddaughter /'gɒdˌdɔːtər/ *n* a female godchild.

goddess /'gɒdəs/ *n* a female deity; a woman of superior charms or excellence.

godfather /'gɒdˌfɒðər/ *n* a male godparent; the head of a Mafia crime family or other criminal organization.

god-fearing *adj* religious.

godforsaken /'gɒdfərˌseɪkən/ *or* /ˌgɒdfər'seɪkən/ *adj* desolate, wretched.

godhead /'gɒdhɛd/ *n* the divine nature, deity; God.

godhood /'gɒdhʊd/ *n* the quality or condition of being a god; divinity.

godless /'gɒdləs/ *adj* irreligious; wicked.—**godlessly** *adv*.—**godlessness** *n*.

godlike /'gɒdlaɪk/ *adj* like a god, divine.

godly /'gɒdli/ *adj* (**godlier, godliest**) religious; holy; devout; devoted to God.—**godliness** *n*.

godmother /'gɒd‚mʌðər/ *n* a female godparent.

godown /gəʊ'daʊn/ *n* in India and China, a warehouse or storeroom.

godparent /'gɒd‚peərənt/ *n* a person who sponsors a child, as at baptism or confirmation, taking responsibility for its faith.

godsend /'gɒdsend/ *n* anything that comes unexpectedly and when needed or desired.

godson /'gɒdsʌn/ *n* a male godchild.

Godspeed /'gɒdspi:d/ *n* success, good luck.

godwit /'gɒdwɪt/ *n* any of a genus of wading birds with a long bill, related to the snipes but resembling curlews.

goer /'gəʊər/ *n* a regular attender; something, as a car, that goes fast; an enthusiastic person.

gofer /'gəʊfər/ *n* (*inf*) a person who runs errands, as in an office.

goffer /'gəʊfər/ or /'gɒ-/ *vt* to make wavy or frilly with a hot iron, to crimp.—*also* **gauffer**.

go-getter *n* (*inf*) an ambitious person.

goggle /'gɒgəl/ *vi* to stare with bulging eyes. • *npl* large spectacles, sometimes fitting snugly against the face, to protect the eyes.

goggle-eyed *adj* with wide staring eyes.

go-go dancer *n* a scantily-clad dancer employed in a disco or nightclub.

going /'gəʊɪŋ/ *n* an act or instance of going, a departure; the state of the ground, *eg* for walking, horse-racing; rate of progress. • *adj* that goes; commonly accepted; thriving; existing.

going-over *n* (*pl* **goings-over**) (*inf*) a thorough inspection; (*sl*) a beating.

goings-on /‚gəʊɪnz'ɒn/ *npl* events or actions, *esp* when disapproved of.

goiter, goitre /'gɔɪtər/ *n* an abnormal enlargement of the thyroid gland.—**goitrous** *adj*.

gold /gəʊld/ *n* a malleable yellow metallic element used *esp* for coins and jewellery; a precious metal; money, wealth; a yellow colour. • *adj* of, or like, gold.

goldbeater's skin *n* a membrane prepared from the large intestine of an ox used to separate layers of gold in goldbeating.

goldbeating *n* the process of beating gold until it is very thin.—**goldbeater** *n*.

gold card *n* a credit card that entitles the cardholder to extra benefits.

gold-digger *n* a person who mines gold; (*inf*) a woman who uses feminine charms to extract money or gifts from men.—**gold-digging** *adj*.

golden /'gəʊldən/ *adj* made of or relating to gold; bright yellow; priceless; flourishing.—**goldenly** *adv*.—**goldenness** *n*.

golden age *n* the fabled early age of innocence and perfect human happiness; the flowering of a nation's civilization or art.

golden calf *n* (*Bible*) a golden calf made by Aaron and worshipped by the Israelites; wealth worshipped as a god.

golden eagle *n* a large eagle of the Northern hemisphere.

golden fleece *n* (*Greek myth*) the ram's fleece in search of which Jason sailed with the Argonauts; an order of knighthood in Austria and Spain.

golden handcuffs *npl* financial incentives to induce an employee to remain in a particular job for an agreed period.

golden handshake *n* (*inf*) financial compensation awarded an employee for loss of employment.

golden mean *n* neither too much nor too little; moderation.

goldenrod /'gəʊldənrɒd/ *n* a tall plant of the aster family with yellow flowers.

golden rule *n* a guiding principle.

goldeye /'gəʊldaɪ/ *n* ✦ a silvery freshwater of central North America, often smoked for food.—*also* **Winnipeg goldeye**.

goldfield /'gəʊldfi:ld/ *n* a district containing gold deposits and diggings.

gold-filled *adj* coated with gold.

goldfinch /'gəʊldfɪntʃ/ *n* a common European finch with yellow and black wings.

goldfish /'gəʊldfɪʃ/ *n* (*pl* **goldfish**, **goldfishes**) a small gold-coloured fish of the carp family, kept in ponds and aquariums.

goldilocks /'gəʊldɪlɒks/ *n* any of various plants with yellow flowers, *eg* the buttercup; (*with cap*) a name for someone, *usu* female, with golden hair.

gold leaf *n* gold beaten into very thin sheets, used for gilding.

gold mine *n* a mine where gold is extracted; (*inf*) a source of wealth.

gold plate *n* vessels of gold; a thin covering of gold.—**gold-plated** *adj*.

gold rush *n* a rush to a new gold field, as to the Yukon in 1897.

goldsmith /'gəʊldsmɪθ/ *n* a worker in gold; a dealer in gold plate.

gold standard *n* a monetary standard in which the basic currency unit equals a specified quantity of gold.

golf /gɒlf/ *n* an outdoor game in which the player attempts to hit a small ball with clubs around a turfed course into a succession of holes in the smallest number of strokes.—**golfer** *n*.

golf ball *n* a hard dimpled ball used in golf; the spherical printing head in some typewriters.

golf club *n* a club with a wooden or metal head used in golf; a golf association or its premises.

golf course, golf links *n* a tract of land laid out for playing golf.

golliard /'gɒlɪərd/ *n* a medieval wandering jester or scholar.

golliwog, golliwogg /'gɒlɪwɒg/ *n* a cloth doll with a black face.

golly[1] /'gɒlɪ/ *n* (*inf*) a golliwog.

golly[2] *interj* expressing surprise.

gonad /'gəʊnæd/ *n* a primary sex gland that produces reproductive cells, such as an ovary or testis.—**gonadal, gonadic** *adj*.

gondola /'gɒndələ/ *n* a long, narrow black boat used on the canals of Venice; a cabin suspended under an airship or balloon; an enclosed car suspended from a cable used to transport passengers, *esp* skiers up a mountain; a display structure in a supermarket, etc.

gondolier /‚gɒndə'lɪːr/ *n* a person who propels a gondola with a pole.

gone[1] /gɒn/ *see* **go**[1].

gone[2] *adj* departed; dead; lost; (*inf*) in an excited state; (*inf*) pregnant for a specified period.

goner /ˈ/ (*sl*) a person or thing that is ruined, dead, or about to die.

gonfalon /'gɒnfələn/ *n* a banner, *usu* with streamers, hung from a crossbar, used in ecclesiastical processions; a military flag or standard with a pointed edge.

gong /gɒn/ *n* a disk-shaped percussion instrument struck with a *usu* padded hammer; (*sl*) a medal. • *vi* to sound a gong.

Gongorism /'gɒngə‚rɪzəm/ *n* (a passage of) a florid pedantic Spanish literary style resembling euphuism.

goniometer /‚gəʊnɪ'ɒmɪtər/ *n* an instrument for measuring solid angles; an instrument used to determine the location of a distant radio station.—**goniometry** *n*.

gonorrhoea, gonorrhea /‚gɒnə'rɪə/ *n* a venereal disease causing a discharge of mucous and pus from the genitals.—**gonorrhoeal, gonorrheal, gonorrhoeic, gonorrheic** *adj*.

goo /gu:/ *n* (*sl*) sticky matter; sickly sentimentality.

good /gʊd/ *adj* (**better, best**) having the right or proper qualities; beneficial; valid; healthy or sound; virtuous, honourable; enjoyable, pleasant, etc; skilled; considerable. • *n* something good; benefit; something that has economic utility; (*with* **the**) good persons; (*pl*) personal property; commodities; (*pl*) the desired or required articles. • *adv* (*inf*) well; fully.—**goodish** *adj*.

goodbye /gʊd'baɪ/ *interj* a concluding remark at parting; farewell.—*also n*.

good-for-nothing *adj* useless, worthless. • a worthless person.

Good Friday *n* the Friday before Easter, commemorating the Crucifixion of Christ.

good-humoured *adj* genial, cheerful.—**good-humouredly** *adv*.—**good-humouredness** *n*.

good-looking *adj* handsome.

goodly /'gʊdlɪ/ *adj* (**goodlier, goodliest**) considerable; ample.—**goodliness** *n*.

goodman /'gʊdmən/ *n* (*pl* **goodmen**) (*formerly*) the master of a house, a husband; a man not born into the aristocracy.

good-natured *adj* amiable, easy-going.—**good-naturedly** *adv*.—**good-naturedness** *n*.

goodness /'gʊdnəs/ *n* the state of being good; the good element in something; kindness; virtue. • *interj* an exclamation of surprise.

Good Samaritan *n* a person who helps those in distress (after the compassionate figure mentioned in the Bible.—Luke 10:33).

goods and services tax *n* ✦ a federal value-added tax.

good-tempered *adj* having a pleasant and kindly nature.

good turn *n* a favour; an act of kindness.

goodwill /gʊd'wɪl/ or /'gʊdwɪl/ *n* benevolence; willingness; the established custom and reputation of a business.

goodwoman *n* (*pl* **goodwomen**) (*formerly*) the mistress of a house, a wife; a woman not born into the aristocracy.

goody /'gʊdɪ/ *n* (*pl* **goodies**) something pleasant or sweet; a goody-goody. • *interj* an expression (*usu* used by a child) signifying pleasure.

goody-goody /'gʊdɪ‚gʊdɪ/ *adj* insufferably virtuous. • *n* (*pl* **goody-goodies**) a goody-goody person.

gooey /'gu:i/ *adj* (**gooier, gooiest**) (*inf*) soft and sticky; sweet; sentimental.

goof /gu:f/ *n* (*sl*) a stupid person; a blunder. • *vi* (*sl*) to bungle.

goofy /'gu:fi/ *adj* (**goofier, goofiest**) (*sl*) silly, stupid.—**goofily** *adv*.—**goofiness** *n*.

goon /gu:n/ *n* (*sl*) a thug; a stupid person.

goop /gu:p/ *n* (*sl*) any sticky, semi-liquid substance; (*sl*) a rude person.

goosander /gu:'sændər/ *n* a web-footed migratory waterfowl.

goose[1] /gu:s/ *n* (*pl* **geese**) a large, long-necked, web-footed bird related to swans and ducks; its flesh as food; a female goose as distinguished from a gander; (*inf*) a foolish person.

goose[2] *vt* (*sl*) to poke (a person) between the buttocks.

gooseberry /'gu:z,beri/ or /-bəri/, /'gu:z-/ *n* (*pl* **gooseberries**) the acid berry of a shrub related to the currant and used *esp* in jams and pies.

goose bumps, goose pimples, goose flesh /'gu:sbʌmps/ *n* a roughening of the skin caused *usu* by cold or fear.

goosegrass *n* a species of creeping plant on which geese feed.

gooseneck /'gu:snek/ *n* (*naut*) a bent iron fitted to the extremity of a boom or yard.

goose step *n* a stiff-legged marching step used by some armies when passing in review.

goose-step *vi* (**goose-stepping, goose-stepped**) to march in a stiff-legged manner using the goose step.

gopher /'go:fər/ *n* a North American burrowing, rat-like rodent; a ground squirrel; a burrowing tortoise.

gopherwood *n* the wood Noah's Ark is reputed to have been made from, possibly cypress; the yellowwood.

gore[1] /gor/ *n* (clotted) blood from a wound.

gore[2] *n* a tapering section of material used to shape a garment, sail, etc.

gore[3] *vt* to pierce or wound as with a tusk or horns.

gorge /gordʒ/ *n* a ravine. • *vt* to swallow greedily; to glut. • *vi* to feed gluttonously.—**gorgeable** *adj*.—**gorger** *n*.

gorgeous /'gordʒəs/ *adj* strikingly attractive; brilliantly coloured; (*inf*) magnificent.—**gorgeously** *adv*.—**gorgeousness** *n*.

Gorgon /'gorgən/ *n* (*Greek myth*) one of three female monsters with live snakes for hair whose looks turned the beholder to stone; (*without cap*) any ugly or formidable woman.

gorgonian /gor'go:niən/ *n* any of a genus of flexible branching coral.

Gorgonzola /,gorgən'zo:lə/ *n* a semi-hard blue-veined cheese with a rich flavour, originating in Italy.

gorilla /gə'rilə/ *n* an anthropoid ape of western equatorial Africa related to the chimpanzee but much larger.

gormand /gurmənd/ *see* **gourmand**.

gormandize /'gur,mondaiz/ *vti* to eat like a glutton.—**gormandizer** *n*.

gorse /gors/ *n* a spiny yellow-flowered European shrub.

gory /'gori/ *adj* (**gorier, goriest**) bloodthirsty; causing bloodshed; covered in blood.—**gorily** *adv*.—**goriness** *n*.

gosh /gɒʃ/ *interj* an exclamation of surprise.

goshawk /'gɒshɒk/ *n* any of several long-tailed hawks with short rounded wings.

gosling /'gɒzlɪŋ/ *n* a young goose.

go-slow *n* a deliberate slowing of the work rate by employees as a form of industrial action.

gospel /'gɒspəl/ *n* the life and teachings of Christ contained in the first four books of the New Testament; (*with cap*) one of these four books; anything proclaimed or accepted as the absolute truth.

gospeller, gospeler /'gɒspələr/ *n* the reader of the gospel in a communion service; an evangelist.

gossamer /'gɒsəmər/ *n* very fine cobwebs; any very light and flimsy material. • *adj* light as gossamer.

gossip /'gɒsɪp/ *n* one who chatters idly about others; such talk. • *vi* to take part in or spread gossip.—**gossiper** *n*.—**gossipingly** *adv*.—**gossipy** *adj*.

gossipmonger /'gɒsɪp,mʌŋgər/ or /-mɒngər/ *n* a gossip.

got *see* **get**.

gotchie /gɒtʃi:/ *n* (*Cdn*) ✤ (*sl*) boys' or men's underwear.

Goth /gɒθ/ *n* any member of a Germanic people that conquered most of the Roman Empire in the 3rd–5th centuries AD.

Gothic /'gɒθɪk/ *adj* of a style of architecture with pointed arches, steep roofs, elaborate stonework, etc. • *n* German black letter type; a bold type style without serifs.—**Gothically** *adv*.

gotten *see* **get**.

gouache /gu:'ɒʃ/ or /gwɒʃ/ *n* a method of painting with opaque watercolours.

Gouda /'gu:də/ *n* a type of large flat round Dutch cheese.

gouge /gaudʒ/ *n* a chisel with a concave blade used for cutting grooves. • *vt* to scoop or force out (as if) with a gouge.

gouger /-ər/ *n* one who or that which gouges; a swindler.

goujons /'gu:ʒɒs/ *npl* narrow fried strips of fish or chicken in breadcrumbs.

goulash /'gu:læʃ/ *n* a rich stew made with beef or veal seasoned with paprika.

gourami /'gu:rəmi/ or /-'rɒmi/ *n* (*pl* **gourami, gouramis**) an oriental fish cultivated for food.

gourd /gurd/ *n* any trailing or climbing plant of a family that includes the squash, melon, pumpkin, etc; the fruit of one species or its dried, hollowed-out shell, used as a cup, bowl, etc or ornament.

gourmand /gur'mɒnd/ *n* a person who likes good food and drink, often to excess.—*also* **gormand**.—**gourmandism** *n*.

gourmandise, gormandise /'gurmən,daiz/ *n* the (sometimes excessive) love of good food.

gourmet /gur'mei/ or /'gur-/, /'gor-/ *n* a person who likes and is an excellent judge of fine food and drink.

gout /gaut/ *n* a disease causing painful inflammation of the joints; *esp* of the great toe.—**gouty** *adj*.—**goutiness** *n*.

Gov., gov *abbr* = government; governor.

govern /'gʌvərn/ *vti* to exercise authority over; to rule, to control; to influence the action of; to determine.—**governable** *adj*.—**governability, governableness** *n*.

governance /'gʌvərnəns/ *n* the action, function, or power of government.

Governor General *n* ✤ (*pl* **Governors-General**) the representative of the Crown as head of state in a country in the Commonwealth of Nations.

governess /'gʌvərnəs/ *n* a woman employed in a private home to teach and train the children.

government /'gʌvərnmənt/ or /'gʌvərmənt/ *n* the exercise of authority over a state, organization, etc; a system of ruling, political administration, etc; those who direct the affairs of a state, etc.—**governmental** *adj*.

Government House *n* ✤ an official residence of the Crown's representative, *esp* a Lieutenant-Governor.

governor /'gʌvərnər/ or /'gʌvənər/ *n* a person appointed to govern a province, etc; the elected head of any state of the US; the director or head of a governing body of an organization or institution; (*sl*) an employer; a mechanical device for automatically controlling the speed of an engine.—**governorship** *n*.

Gov. Gen. *abbr* ✤ = Governor General.

Govt, govt *abbr* = government.

gowan /'gauən/ *n* (*Scot*) the daisy.

gown /gaun/ *n* a loose outer garment, specifically a woman's formal dress, a nightgown, a long, flowing robe worn by clergymen, judges, university teachers, etc; a type of overall worn in the operating room. • *vt* to dress in a gown, to supply with a gown.

goy /gɔi/ *n* (*pl* **goyim, goys**) (*sl*) Jewish for Gentile.

GP *abbr* = general practitioner.

GPO *abbr* = general post office.

Gr. *abbr* = Grecian; Greece; Greek.

grab /græb/ *vt* (**grabbing, grabbed**) to take or grasp suddenly; to obtain unscrupulously; (*inf*) to catch the interest or attention of. • *n* a sudden clutch or attempt to grasp; a mechanical device for grasping and lifting objects.—**grabber** *n*.

grabble /'græbəl/ *vi* to feel about, to grope.—**grabbler** *n*.

grace /greis/ *n* beauty or charm of form, movement, or expression; good will; favour; a delay granted for payment of an obligation; a short prayer of thanks for a meal. • *vt* to decorate; to dignify.

graceful /-fʊl/ *adj* having beauty of form, movement, or expression.—**gracefully** *adv*.—**gracefulness** *n*.

graceless /-ləs/ *adj* unattractive; lacking sense of what is proper; clumsy.—**gracelessly** *adv*.—**gracelessness** *n*.

grace note *n* (*mus*) an ornamental note.

Graces *npl* (*Greek myth*) the three sister goddesses who are the givers of charm and beauty.

gracile /'græsail/ or /-sil/ *adj* slender.—**gracility** *n*.

gracious /'greiʃəs/ *adj* having or showing kindness, courtesy, etc; compassionate; polite to supposed inferiors; marked by luxury, ease, etc; *interj* an expression of surprise.—**graciously** *adv*.—**graciousness** *n*.

grackle /ˈgrækəl/ n an Asian bird like a starling; an American bird with shiny black plumage; the crow blackbird.

grad /græd/ n (sl) a graduate.

gradate /ˈgreɪdeɪt/ vti to change or cause to change gradually from one stage, degree, colour, etc to another; to arrange by grade or degree.

gradation /greɪˈdeɪʃən/ or /grə-/ n a series of systematic steps in rank, degree, intensity, etc; arranging in such stages; a single stage in a gradual progression; progressive change.—**gradational** adj.

grade /greɪd/ n a stage or step in a progression; a degree in a scale of quality, rank, etc; a group of people of the same rank, merit, etc; the degree of slope; a sloping part; a mark or rating in an examination, etc. • vt to arrange in grades; to give a grade to; to make level or evenly sloping.

grade crossing n a place where a road and rail line or two rail lines cross at the same level, a level crossing.

gradient /ˈgreɪdɪənt/ n a sloping road or railway; the degree of slope in a road, railway, etc.

gradin, gradine /ˈgreɪdiːn/ n one of a tier of seats; a ledge at the back of an altar.

gradual /ˈgrædʒʊəl/ adj taking place by degrees.—**gradually** adv.—**gradualness** n.

graduate /ˈgrædʒʊət/ n a person who has completed a course of study at a school, college, or university; a receptacle marked with figures for measuring contents. • adj holding an academic degree or diploma; of or relating to studies beyond the first or bachelor's degree.—**graduator** n.

graduation /grædʒʊˈeɪʃən/ n graduating or being graduated; the ceremony at which degrees are conferred by a college or university; an arranging or marking in grades or stages.

Graeco- see **Greco-**.

graffiti /grəˈfiːti/ npl (sing **graffito**) inscriptions or drawings, often indecent, on a wall or other public surface.

graft /grɑːft/ n a shoot or bud of one plant inserted into another, where it grows permanently; the transplanting of skin, bone, etc; the getting of money or advantage dishonestly.—**grafter** n.—**grafting** n.

grail /greɪl/ n in medieval legend, the dish or chalice that was used by Christ at the Last Supper, and the object of many knights' quests.—also **Holy Grail**.

grain /greɪn/ n the seed of any cereal plant, as wheat, corn, etc; cereal plants; a tiny, solid particle, as of salt or sand; a unit of weight, 0.0648 gram; the arrangement of fibres, layers, etc of wood, leather, etc; the markings or texture due to this; natural disposition. • vt to form into grains; to paint in imitation of the grain of wood, etc. • vi to become granular.—**grainer** n.

grainy /ˈgreɪni/ adj (**grainier, grainiest**) resembling grains in form or texture.—**graininess** n.

gram[1] /græm/ n the basic unit of weight in the metric system, equal to one thousandth of a kilogram (one twenty-eighth of an ounce).

gram[2] n any of various leguminous plants grown for their edible seeds.

gram. abbr = grammar; grammatical.

grama (grass) /ˈgrɑːmə/ n a low pasture grass of western and southwestern USA and South America.

gramarye, gramary /ˈgræməri/ n (arch) magic, necromancy.

gramercy /ˈgræmɔːrsi/ interj (arch) an expression of great thanks; expressing great surprise.

gramineous /grəˈmɪniəs/ adj of or like grass; grassy.

graminivorous /ˌgræmɪˈnɪvərəs/ adj feeding on grasses.

grammar /ˈgræmər/ n the study of the forms of words and their arrangement in sentences; a system of rules for speaking and writing a language; a grammar textbook; the use of language in speech or writing judged with regard to correctness of spelling, syntax, etc.

grammarian /grəˈmeɪriən/ n one who studies grammar; the author of a grammar.

grammatical /grəˈmætɪkəl/ adj conforming to the rules of grammar.—**grammatically** adv.

gramophone /ˈgræməˌfoːn/ n a record player, esp an old mechanical model with an acoustic horn.—also **phonograph**.

grampus /ˈgræmpəs/ n (pl **grampuses**) a marine mammal, as the blackfish or killer whale.

granadilla /ˌgrænəˈdɪlə/ n a passion-fruit.

granary /ˈgrænəri/ or /ˈgreɪn-/ n (pl **granaries**) a building for storing grain.

grand /grænd/ adj higher in rank than others; most important; imposing in size, beauty, extent, etc; distinguished; illustrious;

comprehensive; (inf) very good; delightful. • n a grand piano; (inf) a thousand pounds or dollars.—**grandly** adv.—**grandness** n.

grand-aunt n a father's or mother's aunt.—also **great-aunt**.

grandchild /ˈgræntʃaɪld/ n (pl **grandchildren**) the child of a person's son or daughter.

granddad /ˈgrændæd/ n (inf) grandfather; an old man.

granddaughter /ˈgrænˌdɔːtər/ n the daughter of a person's son or daughter.

grand duke n the ruler of a state or principality.

grandee /grænˈdiː/ n a high-ranking person.

grandeur /ˈgrændər/ or /-djər/, /-dʒər/ n splendour; magnificence; nobility; dignity.

grandfather /ˈgrænˌfɔːðər/ or /ˈgrænd-/ n the father of a person's father or mother.

grandfather clock n a large clock with a pendulum in a tall, upright case.

grandiloquent /ˌgrænˈdɪləkwənt/ adj using pompous words.—**grandiloquence** n.

grandiose /ˈgrændiˌoːs/ or /ˈgræn-/ adj having grandeur; imposing; pompous and showy—**grandiosely** adv.—**grandiosity** n.

grand jury n a jury in the US that examines evidence in a case to determine whether an indictment should be made.

grandma /ˈgrændmə/ or /ˈgrænmə/, /-mɒ/, **grandmama** n (inf) grandmother.

grand mal /grɑːˈmæl/ n severe epilepsy.

grand master /grændˈmæstər/ n an expert player (as of chess) who has scored consistently well in international competition.

grandmother /ˈgrænˌmʌðər/ or /ˈgrænd-/ n the mother of a person's father or mother.

grandnephew /ˈgrændˌnɛfjuː/ or /ˈgræn-/ n a nephew's or niece's son.—also **great-nephew**.

grandniece /ˈgrændniːs/ or /ˈgræn-/ n a nephew's or niece's daughter.—also **great-niece**.

grand opera n opera in which the whole text is set to music.

grandpa /ˈgrændpə/ or /ˈgræn-/, /-pɒ/, **grandpapa** n (inf) grandfather.

grandparent /ˈgrænˌpɛrənt/ or /ˈgrænd-/ n a grandfather or grandmother.

grand piano n a large piano with a horizontal harp-shaped case.

Grand Prix /grɑːˈpriː/ n (pl **Grand Prix**) any of a series of formula motor races held in different countries throughout the season; an important contest in other sports, including horse racing, tennis, and athletics.

grand slam n (tennis, golf) a winning of all the major international championships in a season; (bridge) a bidding for and winning all the tricks in a deal; (baseball) a home run hit when there is a runner on each base.

grandson /ˈgrænsən/ or /ˈgrænd-/ n the son of a person's son or daughter.

grandstand /ˈgrændstænd/ or /ˈgræn-/ n the main structure for seating spectators at a sporting event.

grand tour n (formerly) a trip round Europe taken by the sons of wealthy Englishmen to complete their education; (inf) a sightseeing or educational tour.

grand-uncle n a father's or mother's uncle.—also **great-uncle**.

grange /greɪndʒ/ n a country house with outbuildings etc; a local lodge of a powerful agricultural association; (with the) this association; (formerly) an outlying farm building where a monastery or local lord stored crops or tithes; (arch) a granary.

grangerize /ˈgrændʒəˌraɪz/ vt interleave (a book) with illustrations taken from other books; to remove illustrations, etc, from books for this purpose.—**grangerism** n.—**grangerization** n.

granite /ˈgrænɪt/ n a hard, igneous rock consisting chiefly of feldspar and quartz; unyielding firmness of endurance.—**granitic, granitoid** adj.

granivorous /grəˈnɪvərəs/ adj grain-eating; living on seeds.—**granivore** n.

granny, grannie /ˈgræni/ n (pl **grannies**) (inf) a grandmother; (inf) an old woman.

granny knot n a wrongly tied reef knot, which is insecure.

grant /grɑːnt/ vt to consent to; to give or transfer by legal procedure; to admit as true • n the act of granting; something granted, esp a gift for a particular purpose; a transfer of property by deed; the instrument by which such a transfer is made.

grantee /grænˈtiː/ n the person to whom property is transferred by deed, etc.

granter /ˈgræntər/ n one who grants.

grantor /ˈgrænˈtɔr/ *n* one who transfers property by deed, etc.

granular /ˈgrænjʊlər/ *adj* consisting of granules; having a grainy texture.—**granularity** *n*.

granulate /ˈgrænjʊˌleɪt/ *vt* to form or crystallize into grains or granules. • *vi* to collect into grains or granules; to become roughened and grainy in surface texture.—**granulation** *n*.—**granulative** *adj*.—**granulator, granulater** *n*.

granule /ˈgrænjuːl/ *n* a small grain or particle.

grape /greɪp/ *n* a small round, juicy berry, growing in clusters on a vine; a dark purplish red.—**grapey, grapy** *adj*.

grape fern *n* a fern with cresent-shaped fronds, moonwort.

grapefruit /ˈgreɪpfruːt/ *n* (*pl* **grapefruit, grapefruits**) a large, round, sour citrus fruit with a yellow rind.

grape hyacinth *n* any of various small plants of the lily family bearing tight clusters of blue grape-like flowers.

grapeshot /ˈgreɪpʃɒt/ *n* cannon shot packed in layers, scattering when fired.

grapevine /-vaɪn/ *n* a type of woody vine on which grapes grow; an informal means of communicating news or gossip.

graph /græf/ *n* a diagram representing the successive changes in the value of a variable quantity or quantities. • *vt* to illustrate by graphs.

-graph *n suffix* a writing or recording device; something written, drawn or recorded.

-grapher /-ər/ *n suffix* denoting a person with specified skills; denoting a person who writes or draws in a certain way.

graphic /ˈgræfɪk/, **graphical** /ˈgræfɪkəl/ *adj* described in realistic detail; pertaining to a graph, lettering, drawing, painting, etc.—**graphically** *adv*.—**graphicalness, graphicness** *n*.

graphic arts *npl* the fine and applied arts involving design, illustration and printing.

graphics /ˈgræfɪks/ *n sing or pl* the use of drawings and lettering; the drawings, illustrations, etc used in a newspaper, magazine, television programme, etc; information displayed in the form of diagrams, illustrations and animation on a computer monitor.

graphite /ˈgræfaɪt/ *n* a soft, black form of carbon used in pencils, for lubricants, etc.—**graphitic** *adj*.

graphology /grəˈfɒlədʒi/ *n* the study of handwriting, *esp* as a clue to character.—**graphological** *adj*.—**graphologist** *n*.

graph paper *n* ruled paper for drawing graphs and diagrams.

-graphy /grəfi/ *n suffix* denoting a form of writing, representation or description.

grapnel /ˈgræpnəl/ *n* a small anchor with multiple claws.

grapple /ˈgræpəl/ *vt* to seize or grip firmly. • *vi* to struggle hand-to-hand with; to deal or contend with. • *n* a grapnel; an act of grappling, a wrestle; a grip.—**grappler** *n*.

grappling iron, grappling hook *n* an iron bar with claws at one end for anchoring a boat, securing a ship alongside or raising sunken objects.

grasp /græsp/ *vt* to grip, as with the hand; to seize; to understand. • *vi* to try to clutch, seize; (*with* **at**) to take eagerly. • *n* a firm grip; power of seizing and holding; comprehension.—**graspable** *adj*.—**grasper** *n*.

grasping /ˈgræspɪŋ/ *adj* greedy, avaricious.—**graspingly** *adv*.—**graspingness** *n*.

grass /græs/ *n* any of a large family of plants with jointed stems and long narrow leaves including cereals, bamboo, etc; such plants grown as lawn; pasture; (*sl*) marijuana; (*sl*) an informer. • *vi* to cover with grass; (*sl*) to inform, betray.

grass hockey *n* ✦ (*Cdn*) field hockey.

grasshopper /ˈgræsˌhɒpər/ *n* any of a group of plant-eating, winged insects with powerful hind legs for jumping.

grassland /ˈgræslænd/ *n* land reserved for pasture; land, such as prairie, where grass dominates.

grass roots /ˈgræsruːts/ *npl* (*inf*) the common people, the ordinary members of a political or other organization; the basic level, the essentials.

grass snake *n* a small nonpoisonous European snake with a greenish body and yellow markings.

grass widow, grass widower *n* (*inf*) a person whose spouse is frequently absent.

grassy /ˈgræsi/ *adj* (**grassier, grassiest**) abounding in, covered with, or like, grass.—**grassiness** *n*.

grate[1] /greɪt/ *n* a frame of metal bars for holding fuel in a fireplace; a fireplace; a grating.

grate[2] *vt* to grind into particles by scraping; to rub against (an object) or grind (the teeth) together with a harsh sound; to irritate. • *vi* to rub or rasp noisily; to cause irritation.

grateful /ˈgreɪtfʊl/ *adj* appreciative; welcome.—**gratefully** *adv*.—**gratefulness** *n*.

grater /ˈgreɪtər/ *n* a metal implement with a jagged surface for grating food.

gratification /ˌgrætɪfɪˈkeɪʃən/ *n* the act of gratifying; satisfaction; pleasure; (*arch*) a reward or recompense.

gratify /ˈgrætɪˌfaɪ/ *vt* (**gratifying, gratified**) to please; to indulge.—**gratification** *n*.—**gratifier** *n*.—**gratifyingly** *adv*.

grating[1] /ˈgreɪtɪŋ/ *n* a open framework or lattice of bars placed across an opening.

grating[2] *adj* harsh; irritating.—**gratingly** *adv*.

gratis /ˈgrætɪs/ or /ˈgreɪ-/ *adj, adv* free of charge.

gratitude /ˈgrætɪˌtuːd/ or /-ˌtjuːd/ *n* a being thankful for favours received.

gratuitous /grəˈtuːətəs/ or /-ˈtjuːətəs/ *adj* given free of charge; done without cause, unwarranted.—**gratuitously** *adv*.—**gratuitousness** *n*.

gratuity /grəˈtuːɪti/ or /-ˈtjuːɪti/ *n* (*pl* **gratuities**) money given for a service, a tip.

grav /græv/ *n* a unit of acceleration equal to standard free fall (1 grav = 9.8 metres (32 feet) per second).

gravamen /grəˈveɪmən/ *n* (*pl* **gravamens, gravamina**) the principal part of a legal complaint or accusation.

grave[1] /greɪv/ *n* a hole dug in the ground for burying the dead; any place of burial, a tomb.

grave[2] *adj* serious, important; harmful; solemn, sombre; (*sound*) low in pitch. • *n* an accent (ˋ) over a vowel.—**gravely** *adv*.—**graveness** *n*.

gravel /ˈgrævəl/ *n* coarse sand with small rounded stones. • *vt* (**gravelling, gravelled** *or* **graveling, graveled**) to cover or spread with gravel.—**gravelish** *adj*.

gravelly /ˈgrævəli/ *adj* like gravel; (*voice*) deep and rough-sounding.

graven /ˈgreɪvən/ *adj* engraved; fixed indelibly.

graven image *n* an idol.

graver /ˈgreɪvər/ *n* an engraving tool.

gravestone /ˈgreɪvstoːn/ *n* a stone marking a grave, *usu* inscribed with the name and details of the deceased.

graveyard /ˈgreɪvjɑrd/ *n* a burial-ground, cemetery.

gravid /ˈgrævɪd/ *adj* pregnant.—**gravidity, gravidness** *n*.—**gravidly** *adv*.

gravimeter /grəˈvɪmɪtər/ *n* an instrument for measuring the specific gravity of liquid or solid bodies; an instrument for measuring gravity at particular geographical locations.—**gravimetry** *n*.

gravimetric /ˌgrævɪˈmɛtrɪk/, **gravimetrical** /-kəl/ *adj* of or relating to measurement by weight; determined by weight.—**gravimetrically** *adv*.

gravitate /ˈgrævəˌteɪt/ *vi* to move or tend to move under the force of gravitation.—**gravitater** *n*.

gravitation /ˌgrævəˈteɪʃən/ *n* a natural force of attraction that tends to draw bodies together.—**gravitational** *adj*.—**gravitationally** *adv*.

gravitative /-tɪv/ *adj* pertaining to or determined by gravitation; likely to gravitate, causing something to gravitate.

gravity /ˈgrævɪti/ *n* (*pl* **gravities**) importance, *esp* seriousness; weight; the attraction of bodies toward the centre of the earth, the moon, or a planet.

gravy /ˈgreɪvi/ *n* (*pl* **gravies**) the juice given off by meat in cooking; the sauce made from this juice; (*sl*) money easily obtained.

gravy boat *n* a small boat-shaped dish for holding and serving gravy or sauces.

gravy train *n* (*sl*) a source of easy money.

gray /greɪ/ *see* **grey**.

graybeard *see* **greybeard**.

graylag (goose) /ˈgreɪˌlæg/ *n* the common wild goose of Europe and Asia.

grayling /ˈgreɪlɪŋ/ *n* (*pl* **grayling, graylings**) a freshwater fish.

gray matter *see* **grey matter**.

gray squirrel *see* **grey squirrel**

graywacke *see* **greywacke**.

graze[1] /greɪz/ *vi* to feed on growing grass or pasture. • *vt* to put (animals) to feed on growing grass or pasture.—**grazer** *n*.

graze[2] *vt* to touch lightly in passing; to scrape, scratch. • *n* an abrasion, *esp* on the skin, caused by scraping on a surface.—**grazingly** *adv*.

grazier /ˈgreɪziər/ *n* a person who grazes cattle and prepares them for the market.

grazing /-ɪŋ/ *n* pasture; the crops, plants, etc, growing on this for animals to feed from.

grease /griːs/ *n* melted animal fat; any thick, oily substance or lubricant. • *vt* to smear or lubricate with grease.

greasepaint /'griːspeɪnt/ *n* make-up used by actors.

greaser /'griːsər/ *n* (*sl*) a mechanic; a motorcyclist, often a member of a gang; a member of the engine room crew on a commercial ship; (*derog*) an unpleasant, fawning person.

greasy /'griːsi/ *adj* (**greasier, greasiest**) covered with grease; full of grease; slippery; oily in manner.—**greasily** *adv*.—**greasiness** *n*.

great /greɪt/ *adj* of much more than ordinary size, extent, etc; much above the average; intense; eminent; most important; more distant in a family relationship by one generation; (*often with* at) (*inf*) skilful; (*inf*) excellent; fine. • *n* (*inf*) a distinguished person.—**greatly** *adv*.—**greatness** *n*.

great-aunt *n* a parent's aunt.—*also* **grand-aunt**.

greatcoat /'greɪtkoːt/ *n* a large heavy coat.

Great Dane *n* a breed of very large smooth-haired dogs.

great divide *n* a watershed between major drainage systems; a significant point of division, *esp* death.

great-nephew *n* a nephew's or niece's son.—*also* **grandnephew**.

great-niece *n* a nephew's or niece's daughter.—*also* **grandniece**.

great-uncle *n* a parent's uncle.—*also* **grand-uncle**.

great tit *n* a common yellow, black and white Eurasian tit.

Great War *n* the First World War 1914–18.

Great White North *n* ♣ (*Cdn*) (*inf*) Canada.

greave /griːv/ *n* armour for the lower leg.

greaves /-z/ *npl* the sediment of melted tallow; (*often* -ing) armour to protect the legs from the ankle to the knee.

grebe /griːb/ *n* any of a family of swimming and diving birds.

Grecian /'griːʃən/ *adj* pertaining to Greece; in the Greek style; Greek. • *n* a native or inhabitant of Greece; a Greek scholar.

Grecism *n* a Greek idiom, phrase, spirit or style; a reverent imitation of these, *eg* in architecture or literature.

Grecize *vti* to give a Greek form to; to imitate Greek.

Greco- /'griːko/ *or* /'greko/ *prefix* Greek.

Greco-Roman *adj* of or relating to the ancient Greek and Romans.

greed /griːd/ *n* excessive desire, *esp* for food or wealth.

greedy /'griːdi/ *adj* (**greedier, greediest**) wanting more than one needs or deserves; having too strong a desire for food and drink.—**greedily** *adv*.—**greediness** *n*.

Greek /griːk/ *adj* of Greece, its people, or its language. • *n* a native of Greece; the language used by Greeks; (*inf*) something unintelligible.

Greek cross *n* a cross with four equal arms.

Greek fire *n* (*ancient history*) a weapon used in sea battles consisting of an unidentified substance that ignited on contact with water.

green /griːn/ *adj* of the colour green; covered with plants or foliage; having a sickly appearance; unripe; inexperienced, naive; not fully processed or treated; concerned with the conservation of natural resources; (*inf*) jealous. • *n* a colour between blue and yellow in the spectrum; the colour of growing grass; something of a green colour; (*pl*) green leafy vegetables, as spinach, etc; (*often with cap*) a person concerned with the future of the earth's environment; a grassy plot, *esp* the end of a golf fairway.—**greenish** *adj*.—**greenly** *adv*.—**greenness** *n*.—**greeny** *adj*.

greenback /'griːnbæk/ *n* a legal-tender note of US currency.

green bean *n* any of various beans with narrow edible pods.

green belt /'griːnbelt/ *n* a belt of parkland, farms, etc surrounding a community, designed to prevent urban sprawl.

Green Chamber *n* ♣ (*Cdn*) the Canadian Senate.

greenery /'griːnəri/ *n* (*pl* **greeneries**) green vegetation.

green-eyed /-aɪd/ *adj* jealous.

green-eyed monster *n* jealousy.

greenfinch /'griːnfɪntʃ/ *n* a European and Asian bird with yellow and green plumage.

green fingers *n* gardening expertise. Us and Canadian equivalent—**green thumb**.

greenfly /'griːnflaɪ/ *n* (*pl* **greenflies**) an insect pest that infests garden plants and crops.

greengage /'griːngeɪdʒ/ *n* a small greenish sweet variety of plum.

greenheart /'griːnhɑrt/ *n* a tropical American tree that yields a dark durable timber; the timber.

greenhorn /'griːnhɔrn/ *n* an inexperienced person; a person easily duped.

greenhouse /'griːnhaus/ *n* a heated building, mainly of glass, for growing plants.

greenhouse effect *n* action of radiant heat from the sun passing through the glass of greenhouses etc., warming the contents inside, where such heat is thus trapped; application of the same effect to a planet's atmosphere.—*see* **global warming**.

greening /'griːnɪŋ/ *n* a type of cooking apple that is green when ripe.

greening[2] *n* growing awareness of the environment.

green light *n* permission to proceed with a plan, etc.

green pepper *n* the unripe fruit of the sweet pepper eaten raw or cooked.

greenroom *n* the actors' rest room in a theatre, the room where they can receive visitors.

greensand /'griːnsænd/ *n* a green sandstone.

greenshank *n* a large European wading bird with greenish legs and feet.

greenstone /-stoːn/ *n* New Zealand jade; any green igneous rock that contains chlorite or epidote.

green thumb *see* **green fingers**.

greensward /-swɔrd/ *n* (*arch*) (a stretch of) turf.

green tea *n* a drink made from dried unfermented tea leaves.

Greenwich Mean Time *n* the time of the meridian of Greenwich, England, used as the basis of worldwide standard time.

greenwood /'griːnwʊd/ *n* leafy woodland.

greet /griːt/ *vt* to address with friendliness; to meet (a person, event, etc) in a specified way; to present itself to.—**greeter** *n*.

greeting /-ɪŋ/ *n* the act of welcoming with words or gestures; an expression of good wishes; (*pl*) a message of regards.

gregarious /grɪ'geriəs/ *adj* (*animals*) living in flocks and herds; (*people*) sociable, fond of company.—**gregariously** *adv*.—**gregariousness** *n*.

Gregorian /grə'gɔriən/ *adj* pertaining to or established by Gregory, the name of various popes.

Gregorian calendar *n* the reformed calendar introduced in 1582 by Pope Gregory XIII and currently in use.

gremlin /'gremlɪn/ *n* an imaginary creature blamed for disruption of any procedure or of malfunction of equipment, *esp* in an aircraft.

grenade /grə'neɪd/ *n* a small bomb thrown manually or projected (as by a rifle or special launcher).

grenadier[1] /ˌgrenə'diːr/ *n* a soldier of the British Grenadier Guards, the first regiment of the household infantry; (*formerly*) a foot soldier who threw grenades; (*formerly*) a company made up of the tallest and strongest soldiers in the regiment.

grenadier[2] *n* a sea fish with a large head and a long, narrow tail.

grenadine[1] /'grenəˌdiːn/ *n* a gauze-like dress fabric.

grenadine[2] *n* a syrup made from pomegranates; a red-orange colour.

gressorial /gre'sɔriəl/ *adj* adapted for walking; (*birds*) having three toes of the feet forward, two of them connected, and one behind.

grew /gruː/ *see* **grow**.

grey /greɪ/ *n* any of a series of neutral colours ranging between black and white; something (as an animal, garment, cloth, or spot) of a grey colour. • *adj* grey in colour; having grey-coloured hair; darkish; dreary; vague, indeterminate.—*also* **gray**.—**greyish** *adj*.—**greyness** *n*.

greybeard /'greɪbɪrd/ *n* an old man, *esp* one considered to be wise; an earthenware jug.—*also* **graybeard**.

grey economy *n* the term used to describe unofficial trading which is not accounted for in a country's official economic statistics.

greyhound /'greɪhaund/ *n* any of a breed of tall and slender dogs noted for its great speed and keen sight.

grey jay *n* ♣ (*Cdn*) a North American jay with grey, black and white plumage.—*also* **Canada jay**.

grey matter *n* grey-coloured nerve tissue of the brain and spinal cord; (*inf*) brains, intelligence.

grey squirrel *n* a common squirrel with grey fur orig from North America.

greywacke /'greɪˌwækə/ *or* /-wækə/ *n* a hard conglomerate rock of pebbles and sand.—*also* **graywracke**.

grid /grɪd/ *n* a gridiron, a grating; an electrode for controlling the flow of electrons in an electron tube; a network of squares on a map used for easy reference; a national network of transmission lines, pipes, etc for electricity, water, gas, etc.

griddle /'grɪdəl/ *n* a flat metal surface for cooking.

griddlecake *n* a pancake.

gridiron /'grɪdaɪrn/ *n* a framework of iron bars for cooking; anything resembling this, as a field used for American football.

gridlock /ˈgrɪdlɒk/ *n* a traffic jam that halts all traffic at a street crossing; the breakdown of an organization or a system.

grid road *n* ✦ (*Cdn*) a road that follows the surveyed divisions of an area or community.

grief /griːf/ *n* extreme sorrow caused as by a loss; deep distress. **grief-stricken** *adj* full of sorrow.

grievance /ˈgriːvəns/ *n* a circumstance thought to be unjust and cause for complaint.

grieve /griːv/ *vti* to feel or cause to feel grief.—**griever** *n*.— **grieving** *adj, n*.

grievous /ˈgriːvəs/ *adj* causing or characterized by grief; deplorable; severe.—**grievously** *adv*.—**grievousness** *n*.

griffin /ˈgrɪfɪn/, **griffon**[1] /ˈgrɪfən/ *n* a mythical animal with the body and tail of a lion and an eagle's beak and wings.—*also* **gryphon**.

griffon[2] /ˈgrɪfən/ *n* a small dog with a wire-haired coat; a large hawk with a pale body and black wings, found in Africa, Asia and warm parts of Europe.

grig /grɪg/ *n* an extravagantly vivacious person; the sandeel; a young eel; a hen with short legs; heather.

grill /grɪl/ *vt* to broil by direct heat using a grill or gridiron; (*inf*) to question relentlessly. • *n* a device on a cooker that radiates heat downward for broiling or grilling; a gridiron; broiled or grilled food; a grille; a grillroom.—**griller** *n*.

grillage /ˈgrɪlɪdʒ/ *n* an arrangement of planks and crossbeams forming a foundation in loose or marshy soil.

grille, grill /grɪl/ *n* an open grating forming a screen.

grillroom *n* a restaurant that specializes in grilled food.

grilse /grɪls/ *n* (*pl* **grilses, grilse**) a young salmon returning from the sea to spawn for the first time.

grim /grɪm/ *adj* (**grimmer, grimmest**) hard and unyielding, stern; appearing harsh, forbidding; repellent, ghastly in character.—**grimly** *adv*.—**grimness** *n*.

grimace /ˈgrɪməs/ *n* a contortion of the face expressing pain, anguish, humour, etc. • *vi* to contort the face in pain, etc.—**grimacer** *n*.—**grimacingly** *adv*.

grimalkin /grɪˈmælkɪn/ or /-ˈmɒlkɪn/ *n* an old she-cat; a spiteful, bad-tempered old woman.

grime /graɪm/ *n* soot or dirt, rubbed into a surface, as the skin. • *vt* to dirty, soil with grime.

grimy /ˈgraɪmɪ/ *adj* (**grimier, grimiest**) dirty, soiled.—**griminess** *n*.

grin /grɪn/ *vi* (**grinning, grinned**) to smile broadly as in amusement; to show the teeth in pain, scorn, etc. • *n* a broad smile.— **grinner** *n*.

grind /graɪnd/ *vb* (**grinding, ground**) *vt* to reduce to powder or fragments by crushing; to wear down, sharpen, or smooth by friction; to rub (the teeth) harshly together; to oppress, tyrannize; to move or operate by a crank. • *vi* to be crushed, smoothed, or sharpened by grinding; to jar or grate; to work monotonously; to rotate the hips in an erotic manner. • *n* the act or sound of grinding; hard monotonous work.

grinder /ˈgraɪndər/ *n* someone or something that grinds; a molar tooth.

grindstone /ˈgraɪndstoːn/ *n* a circular revolving stone for grinding or sharpening tools.

gringo /ˈgrɪŋgoː/ *n* (*pl* **gringos**) (*offensive*) among Hispanics, a foreigner, *esp* North Americans.

grip /grɪp/ *n* a secure grasp; the manner of holding a bat, club, racket, etc; the power of grasping firmly; mental grasp; mastery; a handle; a small travelling bag. • *vt* (**gripping, gripped**) to take firmly and hold fast.

gripe /graɪp/ *vt* to cause sharp pain in the bowels of; (*sl*) to annoy. • *vi* (*sl*) to complain.—**griper** *n*.—**gripingly** *adv*.

grippe /grɪp/ *n* (*formerly*) influenza.

gripper /-ər/ *n* one who or that which grips; a mechanical device for seizing and holding.

grisaille /grɪˈzeɪl/ or /-ˈzaɪl/ *n* a method of painting in grey tints so as to represent a solid body in relief; a decorative painting in grey monochrome, *esp* on glass.

griseous /ˈgrɪʃəs/ *adj* bluish-grey.

grisette *n* a lively young French working girl, *esp* a flirtatious one; an edible toadstool.

griskin *n* the lean part of a loin of pork.

grisly /ˈgrɪzlɪ/ *adj* (**grislier, grisliest**) terrifying; ghastly; arousing horror.—**grisliness** *n*.

grison *n* a carnivorous mammal of Central and South America, which resembles a weasel.

grist /grɪst/ *n* grain that is to be or has been ground; matter forming the basis of a story or analysis.

gristle /ˈgrɪsəl/ *n* cartilage, *esp* in meat.—**gristly** *adj*.—**gristliness** *n*.

grit[1] /grɪt/ *n* rough particles, as of sand; firmness of spirit; stubborn courage. • *vt* (**gritting, gritted**) to clench or grind together (*eg* the teeth); to spread grit on (*eg* an icy road).

Grit[2] /grɪt/ *n* ✦ (*Cdn*) (*inf*) a member or supporter of the Liberal Party of Canada.

grits /grɪts/ *npl* oats, hulled and coarsely ground; coarsely ground maize, boiled in water or milk as a food.—*also* **hominy grits**.

gritty /-tɪ/ *adj* (**grittier, grittiest**) composed of, containing, or resembling, grit; courageous.—**grittily** *adv*.—**grittiness** *n*.

grivet /ˈgrɪvət/ *n* a green and white Ethiopian monkey with a long tail.

grizzle /ˈgrɪzəl/ *vt* (*inf*) to fret; to complain. • *vti* to (cause to) become grey. • *n* a grey colour; hair that is, or is becoming, grey; a wig of grey hair.—**grizzled** *adj*.

grizzled /ˈgrɪzəld/ *adj* streaked with grey; grey-haired.

grizzly /ˈgrɪzlɪ/ *adj* (**grizzlier, grizzliest**) greyish; grizzled. • *n* (*pl* **grizzlies**) the grizzly bear.

grizzly bear *n* a large powerful bear of North America.

groan /groːn/ *vi* to utter a deep moan; to make a harsh sound (as of creaking) under sudden or prolonged strain. • *n* a deep moan; a creaking sound.—**groaner** *n*.—**groaningly** *adv*.

groat /groːt/ *n* (*formerly*) a British silver coin worth fourpence; a trifling sum.

groats /groːts/ *npl* hulled grain broken into fragments, *esp* oats.

grocer /ˈgroːsər/ or /-ʃər/ *n* a dealer in food and household supplies.

grocery /ˈgroːsərɪ/ or /-ʃərɪ/, /-ʃrɪ/ *n* (*pl* **groceries**) a grocer's shop; (*pl*) goods, *esp* from a grocer.

grog /grɒg/ *n* rum diluted with water, often spiced and served hot.

groggy /ˈgrɒgɪ/ *adj* (**groggier, groggiest**) (*inf*) weak and unsteady, *usu* through illness, exhaustion or alcohol.—**groggily** *adv*.—**grogginess** *n*.

grogram /ˈgrɒgrəm/ *n* a coarse cloth of silk or silk and mohair or wool.

groin /grɔɪn/ *n* the fold marking the junction of the lower abdomen and the thighs; the location of the genitals.

grommet /ˈgrɒmət/ *n* a plastic or rubber ring used to protect wire, a cable, etc passing through a hole; a ring formed of a strand of rope laid round, used in pipe joints or sails.—*also* **grummet**; (*formerly*) a cannon-wad made of rope, and rammed between the powder and the ball.

gromwell /ˈgrɒmˌwel/ or /-wəl/ *n* a herb of the borage family.

groom /gruːm/ *n* a person employed to care for horses; a bridegroom. • *vt* to clean and care for (animals); to make neat and tidy; to train (a person) for a particular purpose.—**groomer** *n*.—**grooming** *n*.

groomsman /ˈgruːmzmən/ *n* (*pl* **groomsmen**) one who attends a bridegroom; a best man.

groove /gruːv/ *n* a long, narrow channel; a spiral track in a gramophone record for the stylus; a settled routine. • *vt* to make a groove in.

groovy /ˈgruːvɪ/ *adj* (**groovier, grooviest**) (*sl*) excellent.

grope /groːp/ *vi* to search about blindly as in the dark; to search uncertainly for a solution to a problem. • *vt* to find by feeling; (*sl*) to fondle sexually. • *n* the act of groping.—**groper** *n*.—**gropingly** *adv*.

grosbeak /ˈgroːsbiːk/ *n* any finch-like bird of Europe or America with a large stout conical bill.

groschen /ˈgroːʃən/ *n* (*pl* **groschen**) a 10-pfennig coin used in Germany; a silver coin formerly current in Germany; in Austria, a coin with a value of one hundredth of a schilling.

grosgrain /ˈgroːgreɪn/ *n* a stout double-corded silk; a fabric or ribbon of this.

gros point /ˈgroːpɔɪnt/ *n* a large needlepoint stitch covering two vertical and two horizontal threads; a piece of needlework done in this.

gross /groːs/ *adj* fat and coarse-looking; flagrant, dense, thick; lacking in refinement; earthy; obscene; total, with no deductions. • *n* (*pl* **grosses**) an overall total; (*pl* **gross**) twelve dozen. • *vt* to earn as total revenue.—**grossly** *adv*.—**grossness** *n*.

gross domestic product *n* the total value of goods and services produced by a country in one year.

gross national product *n* the gross domestic product plus income earned from abroad.

grot[1] /grɒt/ *n* (*poet*) a grotto.

grot^2 *n* (*Brit sl*) unpleasant mess.—**grotty** *adj* (**grottier, grottiest**) nasty, unattractive; in bad condition; unsatisfactory.

grotesque /grəʊ'tesk/ *adj* distorted or fantastic in appearance, shape, etc; ridiculous; absurdly incongruous. • *n* a grotesque person or thing; a decorative device combining distorted plant, animal and human forms.—**grotesquely** *adv*.—**grotesqueness** *n*.

grotesquery, grotesquerie /-'teskəri/ *n* (*pl* **grotesqueries**) something that is fantastic or distorted in shape, etc.

grotto /'grɒtəʊ/ *n* (*pl* **grottoes, grottos**) a cave, *esp* one with attractive features.

grotty /'grɒti/ *see* **grot**.

grouch /graʊtʃ/ *vi* (*inf*) to grumble or complain. • *n* (*inf*) a grumble; a person who grumbles.—**groucher** *n*.

grouchy /'graʊtʃi/ *adj* (**grouchier, grouchiest**) bad-tempered.—**grouchily** *adv*.—**grouchiness** *n*.

ground /graʊnd/ *n* the solid surface of the earth; soil; the background, as in design; the connection of an electrical conductor with the earth; (*pl*) a basis for belief, action, or argument; the area about and relating to a building; a tract of land; sediment. • *vti* to set on the ground; to run aground or cause to run aground; to base, found, or establish; to instruct in the first principles of; to prevent (aircraft) from flying.

ground control *n* the communications and tracking equipment and staff that monitor aircraft and spacecraft in flight and during takeoff and landing.

ground cover *n* low-growing shrubs, plants and other foliage on the ground.

ground floor *n* the floor of a building on a level with the ground.

ground hog /'graʊndhɒg/ *n* a woodchuck.

grounding /-ɪŋ/ *n* basic general knowledge of a subject.

ground ivy *n* a trailing Eurasian plant with bluish-purple flowers.

groundless /-ləs/ *adj* without reason.—**groundlessly** *adv*.

groundnut /-nʌt/ *n* a climbing plant of North America with an underground nut; a peanut.

ground rule *n* a fundamental rule or principle.

groundsel /'graʊnsəl/ *n* a weed of the aster family with yellow flowers.

groundsheet /'graʊndʃiːt/ *n* a waterproof sheet placed on the ground in, or as part of, a tent.

groundsman /'graʊndzmən/ *n* (*pl* **groundsmen**) a man who looks after a cricket pitch, football pitch, park, etc.

groundswell /'graʊndswel/ *n* a large rolling wave; a wave of popular feeling.

groundwork /'graʊndwɜːk/ *n* foundation, basis.

group /gruːp/ *n* a number of persons or things considered as a collective unit; a small musical band of players or singers; a number of companies under single ownership; two or more figures forming one artistic design. • *vti* to form into a group or groups.

grouper /'gruːpər/ *n* (*pl* **grouper, groupers**) an edible sea fish.

groupie /'gruːpi/ *n* a devoted fan.

group therapy *n* (*psychol*) the simultaneous treatment of patients with similar problems through mutual discussion and exchange of experiences.

grouse^1 /graʊs/ *n* (*pl* **grouse, grouses**) a game bird; its flesh as food.

grouse^2 *vi* (*inf*) to complain.—**grouser** *n*.

grout /graʊt/ *n* a thin mortar used as between tiles. • *vt* to fill with grout.—**grouter** *n*.

grove /grəʊv/ *n* a small wood, generally without undergrowth.

grovel /'grɒvəl/ *vi* (**grovelling, grovelled** *or* **groveling, groveled**) to lie and crawl in a prostrate position as a sign of respect, fear or humility.—**groveller, groveler** *n*.—**grovellingly, grovelingly** *adv*.

grow /grəʊ/ *vb* (**growing, grew, pp grown**) *vi* to come into being; to be produced naturally; to develop, as a living thing; to increase in size, quantity, etc; (*with* **on**) to become more accustomed or acceptable to; (*with* **up**) to mature; to arise, develop. • *vt* to cause or let grow; to raise, to cultivate.—**growable** *adj*.—**grower** *n*.

growing pains *npl* muscular discomfort sometimes experienced by growing children; difficulties experienced in the early stages of a project.

growl /graʊl/ *vi* to make a rumbling, menacing sound such as an angry dog makes. • *vt* to express in a growling manner. • *n* a growling noise; a grumble.—**growler** *n*.

growler /'graʊlər/ *n* one who growls; (*arch*) a four-wheeled cab; a small iceberg; a beer jug or beer can.

grown-up *n* a fully grown person, an adult. • *adj* mature, adult; fit for an adult.

growth /grəʊθ/ *n* the act or process of growing; progressive increase, development; something that grows or has grown; an abnormal formation of tissue, as a tumour.

groyne /grɔɪn/ *n* a timber structure to stop the shifting of sand on a beach.

grub /grʌb/ *vb* (**grubbing, grubbed**) *vi* to dig in the ground; to work hard. • *vt* to clear (ground) of roots; to uproot. • *n* the worm-like larva of a beetle; (*sl*) food.

grubber /'grʌbər/ *n* one who or that which grubs; a grub hoe.

grubby /'grʌbi/ *adj* (**grubbier, grubbiest**) dirty.—**grubbily** *adv*.—**grubbiness** *n*.

grudge /grʌdʒ/ *n* a deep feeling of resentment or ill will. • *vt* to be reluctant to give or admit something.—**grudger** *n*.—**grudging** *adj*.—**grudgingly** *adv*.

gruel /'gruːəl/ *n* a thin porridge cooked in water or milk.

grueling, gruelling /'gruːəlɪŋ/ *adj* severely testing, exhausting.

gruesome /'gruːsəm/ *adj* causing horror or loathing.

gruff /grʌf/ *adj* rough or surly; hoarse.—**gruffly** *adv*.—**gruffness** *n*.

grugru /'gruːgruː/ *n* the larva of a South American weevil, cooked for food as a delicacy; the palm tree on which this lives.

grumble /'grʌmbəl/ *vti* to mutter in discontent; to make a rumbling sound. • *n* a complaint; a grumbling sound.—**grumbler** *n*.—**grumblingly** *adv*.

grump /grʌmp/ *n* (*inf*) a bad-tempered person.

grumpy /'grʌmpi/ *adj* (**grumpier, grumpiest**) bad-tempered, peevish.—**grumpily** *adv*.—**grumpiness** *n*.

grunt /grʌnt/ *vi* to make a gruff guttural sound like a pig; to say or speak in such a manner. • *n* a low gruff sound; (*sl*) a US infantry man.

grunter /'grʌntər/ *n* one who or that which grunts; an edible marine American fish; a pig.

Gruyère /'gruːjer/ *n* a hard, pale yellow Swiss cheese *usu* with holes.

gryphon *see* **griffin**.

GSC *abbr* ✠ = Geological Survey of Canada.

GST *abbr* ✠ (*Cdn*) = Goods and Services Tax.

G-string /'dʒiːstrɪŋ/ *n* a string on an instrument tuned to the note G; a string or strip worn round the waist and between the legs.

G-suit /'dʒiːsuːt/ *n* a (gravity) suit designed to counteract the physiological effects of acceleration on airmen and astronauts.

GT /'dʒiːti/ *abbr* = *gran turismo*, a sporty touring car.

GTA *abbr* ✠ = Greater Toronto Area.

guaco /'gwɒkəʊ/ *n* (*pl* **guacos**) a tropical American plant, used as an antidote to snakebites.

guaiacum /'gwaɪəkəm/ *n* any of various tropical and West Indian shrubs or trees; the wood from these; a gum obtained from them, used medicinally and in the manufacture of varnishes.

guan /gwɒn/ *n* an American bird similar to a turkey.

guanaco /gwə'nɒkəʊ/ *n* (*pl* **guanacos, guanaco**) the wild llama of South America.

guanine /'gwɒniːn/ *n* a nitrogenous base component of the nucleic acids, DNA and RNA, also found in guano.

guano /'gwɒːnəʊ/ *n* (*pl* **guanos**) dung of sea birds used as manure; a similar artificially produced fertilizer.

guarantee /ˌgærən'tiː/ *or* /ˌgærən-/ *n* a pledge or security for another's debt or obligation; a pledge to replace something if it is substandard, etc; an assurance that something will be done as specified; something offered as a pledge or security; a guarantor. • *vt* (**guaranteeing, guaranteed**) to give a guarantee for; to promise.

guaranteed investment certificate *n* ✠ (*Cdn*) a certificate issued by a financial institution that guarantees a fixed interest rate on a sum of money for a fixed term.

guarantor /'gærənˌtɔːr/ *or* /ˌgærən'tɔːr/, /'gæ-/ *n* a person who gives a guaranty or guarantee.

guaranty /'gærənti/ *or* /ˌgærən-/ *n* (*pl* **guaranties**) (*law*) a guarantee.

guard /gɑːd/ *vt* to watch over and protect; to defend; to keep from escape or trouble; to restrain. • *vi* to keep watch (against); to act as a guard. • *n* defence; protection; a posture of readiness for defence; any device to protect against injury or loss; a person or group that guards; (*boxing, fencing, cricket*) a defensive attitude; a railway official in charge of a train; (*with cap: pl*) a regiment of British or European household troops.—**guardable** *adj*.—**guarder** *n*.

guarded /'gɑːdəd/ *adj* discreet; cautious.—**guardedly** *adv*.—**guardedness** *n*.

guardhouse /'gɑrdhɐʊs/ *n* a building used by a military guard when not walking a post; a military jail for temporary confinement.

guardian /'gɑrdɪən/ *n* a custodian; a person legally in charge of a minor or someone incapable of taking care of their own affairs.—**guardianship** *n*.

guardrail /'gɑrdreɪl/ *n* a railing, *eg* at the side of a road, to prevent falling; a short metal rod placed inside the rails to keep a train's wheels on the track.

guardsman /'gɑrdzmən/ *n* (*pl* **guardsmen**) an officer or soldier of the British Guards; an officer or solider of the US National Guard.

guard's van *n* the railway carriage where the guard travels, *usu* at the back of a train.—*also* **caboose**.

guava /'gwɒvə/ *n* a tropical American shrubby tree widely cultivated for its sweet acid yellow fruit.

gubernatorial /ˌguːbərnəˈtɔriəl/ *adj* pertaining to a governor or to his office.

gudgeon /'gʌdʒən/ *n* a small edible freshwater fish; a fish used as bait in fishing; a person who is easily imposed upon; an iron pin or shaft on which a wheel revolves; (*naut*) one of the sockets into which a rudder is fixed.

guelder-rose /'gɛldər/ *n* a cultivated variety of cranberry bush with large heads of sterile flowers.

Guelph, Guelf /gwɛlf/ *n* a member of a powerful Italian political party in the Middle Ages, which supported the pope and sought the independence of Italy; a member of a secret society in 19th-century Italy, supporting Italian independence.

guerdon /'gɜrdən/ *n* (*poet*) reward. • *vt* to reward, to recompense.

guernsey /'gɜrnzi/ *n* a particular breed of dairy cattle originally from the island of Guernsey; a close-fitting knitted woollen jersey; (*Austral*) a woollen top worn by a football player.

guerrilla, guerilla /gəˈrɪlə/ *n* a member of a small force of irregular soldiers, making surprise raids.—*also adj*.

guess /gɛs/ *vt* to form an opinion of or state with little or no factual knowledge; to judge correctly by doing this; to think or suppose. • *n* an estimate based on guessing.—**guessable** *adj*.—**guesser** *n*.

guesstimate /'gɛstɪmət/ *n* (*inf*) an estimate based mainly on guesswork.

guesswork /'gɛswɜrk/ *n* the process or result of guessing.

guest /gɛst/ *n* a person entertained at the home, club, etc of another; any paying customer of a hotel, restaurant, etc; a performer appearing by special invitation.

guesthouse *n* a private home or boarding-house offering accommodation.

guestroom *n* a room kept for guests.

guffaw /gʌˈfɔ/ *n* a crude noisy laugh. • *vi* to laugh boisterously.

guidance /'gaɪdəns/ *n* leadership; advice or counsel.

guide /gaɪd/ *vt* to point out the way for; to lead; to direct the course of; to control. • *n* a person who leads or directs others; a person who exhibits and explains points of interest; something that provides a person with guiding information; a device for controlling the motion of something; a book of basic instruction; a Girl Guide.—**guidable** *adj*.—**guider** *n*.—**guiding** *adj*, *n*.

guidebook /'gaɪdbʊk/ *n* a book containing directions and information for tourists.

guided missile *n* a military missile whose course is controlled by radar or internal instruments, etc.

guideline /'gaɪdlaɪn/ *n* a principle or instruction which determines conduct or policy.

guidepost /'gaɪdpoʊst/ *n* a direction post; a guiding principle.

guidon /'gaɪdən/ *n* a forked or pointed military flag, used *esp* by troops of light cavalry.

guild /gɪld/ *n* a club, society; an association of people with common interests formed for mutual aid and protection, as craftsmen in the Middle Ages.—*also* **gild**.

guilder /'gɪldər/ *n* a coin of the Netherlands, or of Netherlands Antilles and Surinam; a gold or silver coin formerly in circulation in Germany, Austria and the Netherlands.—*also* **gilder, gulden**.

guildhall /gɪldˈhɒl/ or /'gɪld-/ *n* the meeting place of a guild or corporation.

guile /gaɪl/ *n* craftiness, deceit.—**guileful** *adj*.—**guilefully** *adv*.—**guilefulness** *n*.

guileless /-ləs/ *adj* without guile; ingenuous.—**guilelessly** *adv*.—**guilelessness** *n*.

guillemot /'gɪlɪˌmɒt/ *n* a small sea bird of the auk family.

guilloche /gɪˈlɒʃ/ *n* (*archit*) an ornament resembling braided ribbons.

guillotine /'gɪləˌtiːn/ or /'giːə-/ *n* an instrument for beheading by a heavy blade descending between grooved posts; a device or machine for cutting paper; a rule for limiting time for discussion in a legislature. • *vt* to execute (someone) by guillotine.—**guillotiner** *n*.

guilt /gɪlt/ *n* the fact of having done a wrong or committed an offence; a feeling of self-reproach from believing one has done a wrong.

guiltless /-ləs/ *adj* innocent.

guilty /'gɪlti/ *adj* (**guiltier, guiltiest**) having guilt; feeling or showing guilt.—**guiltily** *adv*.—**guiltiness** *n*.

guimpe /gæmp/ or /gɪmp/ *n* a short blouse worn under a pinafore dress; a piece of cloth used to disguise a low-cut neckline; the starched cloth that covers the shoulders and front of a nun's habit; gimp.

guinea /'gɪni/ *n* a former English gold coin equal to 21 shillings (£1.05).

guinea fowl *n* a domestic African bird of the pheasant family.

guinea pig *n* a rodent-like animal commonly kept as a pet, and often used in scientific experiments; a person or thing subject to an experiment.

guipure (lace) /giːˈpyuːr/ *n* a coarse lace in which the pattern is supported by bars connecting the motifs rather than founded on a net base; a kind of gimp.

guise /gaɪz/ *n* an external appearance, aspect; an assumed appearance or pretence.

guitar /gɪˈtɑr/ *n* a stringed musical instrument with a long, fretted neck, and a flat body, which is plucked with a plectrum or the fingers.—**guitarist** *n*.

gular /'gjuːlər/ *adj* of, in or pertaining to the gullet or throat.

gulch /gʌltʃ/ *n* a deep, narrow ravine.

gulden /'gʊldən/ *see* **guilder**.

gules /gjuːlz/ *n* (*her*) the colour red, also indicated by vertical parallel lines.

gulf /gʌlf/ *n* a large area of ocean reaching into land; a wide, deep chasm; a vast separation.

Gulf Stream *n* a warm ocean current flowing from the Gulf of Mexico northward towards Europe.

gulfweed /'gʌlfwiːd/ *n* brown seaweed with air bladders which floats in dense masses in warm Atlantic waters.—*also* **sargasso, sargasso weed**.

gull /gʌl/ *n* any of numerous long-winged web-footed sea birds.

gullet /'gʌlət/ *n* the esophagus; the throat.

gullible /'gʌləbəl/ *adj* easily deceived.—**gullibility** *n*.—**gullibly** *adv*.

gully /'gʌli/ *n* (*pl* **gullies**) a narrow trench cut by running water after rain; (*cricket*) a fielding position between the slips and point. • *vt* (**gullying, gullied**) to make gullies in.

gulp /gʌlp/ *vt* to swallow hastily or greedily; to choke back as if swallowing. • *n* a gulping or swallowing; a mouthful.—**gulper** *n*.—**gulpingly** *adv*.

gum[1] /gʌm/ *n* the firm tissue that surrounds the teeth.

gum[2] /gʌm/ *n* a sticky substance found in certain trees and plants; an adhesive; chewing gum. • *vb* (**gumming, gummed**) *vt* to coat or unite with gum. • *vi* to become sticky or clogged; (*with* **up**) (*inf*) to mess up, prevent from working properly.

gum ammoniac *n* a gum resin.—*also* **ammoniac**.

gum arabic *n* the gum obtained from certain species of acacia trees and used in the manufacture of adhesives and in pharmacy.

gumbo /'gʌmboʊ/ *n* (*pl* **gumbos**) a rich soup thickened with okra.

gumboil /'gʌmbɔɪl/ *n* an abscess in the gum.

gumboot /'gʌmbuːt/ *n* a rubber, waterproof boot, a wellington.

gumma /'gʌmə/ *n* (*pl* **gummas, gummata**) a syphilitic tumour.—**gummatous** *adj*.

gummy /'gʌmi/ *adj* (**gummier, gummiest**) sticky; revealing the gums, toothless.—**gummily** *adv*.—**gumminess** *n*.

gumption /'gʌmpʃən/ *n* (*inf*) shrewd practical common sense; initiative.

gum resin *n* a mixture of gum and resin exuded from certain plants and trees.

gumtree *n* a eucalyptus, or one of various other trees that yield gum.

gun /gʌn/ *n* a weapon with a metal tube from which a projectile is discharged by an explosive; the shooting of a gun as a signal or salute; anything like a gun. • *vb* (**gunning, gunned**) *vi* to shoot or hunt with a gun; (*with* **for**) to search out in order to hurt or kill. • *vt* (*inf*) to shoot (a person); (*sl*) to advance the throttle of an engine.

gunboat /'gʌnboʊt/ *n* a small armed ship.

gunboat diplomacy *n* the threat of force used to back diplomatic activity.

guncotton *n* a highly explosive substance formed by the action of nitric and sulphuric acid upon cotton, or some other vegetable fibre.

gun dog *n* a dog trained to flush out or retrieve game shot by hunters.

gunfire /'gʌn,faɪr/ *n* repeated and consecutive gunshots the use of guns, etc, rather than other military options.

gunk /gʌŋk/ *n* (*inf*) dirty, greasy, matter; gunge.

gunman /'gʌnmən/ *n* (*pl* **gunmen**) an armed gangster a hired killer.

gunmetal /'gʌnmetəl/ *n* bronze with a dark tarnish; its dark-grey colour.

gunnel /'gʌnəl/ *see* **gunwale**.

gunner /'gʌnər/ *n* a soldier, etc who helps fire artillery a naval warrant officer in charge of a ship's guns.

gunnery /'gʌnəri/ *n* the science of the design and operation of large guns.

gunny /'gʌni/ *n* (*pl* **gunnies**) a strong coarse fabric made from jute used for sacking.

gunpoint /'gʌnpɔɪnt/ *n* the muzzle of a gun; the threat of being shot.

gunpowder /'gʌn,paʊdər/ *n* an explosive powder used in guns, for blasting, etc.

gunrunning /'gʌn,rʌnɪŋ/ *n* the smuggling of firearms into a country.—**gunrunner** *n*.

gunshot /'gʌnʃɒt/ *n* the range of a gun; the instance of shooting a gun or the shot fired from it.

gun-shy *adj* afraid of a loud noise; markedly distrustful.

gunslinger /'gʌn,slɪŋər/ *n* (*sl*) a gunman or gunfighter.

gunstock /'gʌnstɒk/ *n* the wooden or metal mounting of a gun barrel.

gunwale /'gʌnəl/ *n* the upper edge of a ship's or boat's side.—*also* **gunnel**.

guppy /'gʌpi/ *n* (*pl* **guppies**) a small vividly-coloured fish of South America and the West Indies popular for aquariums.

gurgitation /,gɜːdʒə'teɪʃən/ *n* a whirling motion, a surging.

gurgle /'gɜːgəl/ *vi* (*liquid*) to make a low bubbling sound; to utter with this sound. • *n* a bubbling sound.—**gurglingly** *adv*.

gurnard /'gɜːnərd/ *n* (*pl* **gurnard, gurnards**) a spiny sea fish with an armoured head.

guru /'guːruː/ or /'guruː/ *n* (*pl* **gurus**) a Hindu or Sikh spiritual teacher; an influential leader or teacher, *esp* of a religious cult.

gush /gʌʃ/ *vi* to issue plentifully; to have a sudden flow; to talk or write effusively. • *vt* to cause to gush. • *n* a sudden outpouring.—**gushingly** *adv*.

gusher /'gʌʃər/ *n* an effusive person; an oil well from which oil spouts forth.

gushy /'gʌʃi/ *adj* (**gushier, gushiest**) expressing excessive admiration.—**gushily** *adv*.—**gushiness** *n*.

gusset /'gʌsət/ *n* a small triangular piece of cloth inserted in a garment to strengthen or enlarge a part.

gust /gʌst/ *n* a sudden brief rush of wind; a sudden outburst. • *vi* to blow in gusts.

gustation /gʌ'steɪʃən/ *n* the act of tasting; the ability to taste; taste.—**gustatory** *adj*.

gusto /'gʌstoː/ *n* great enjoyment, zest.

gusty /'gʌsti/ *adj* (**gustier, gustiest**) windy; irritable.—**gustily** *adv*.—**gustiness** *n*.

gut /gʌt/ *n* (*often pl*) the bowels or the stomach; the intestine; tough cord made from animal intestines; (*pl*) (*sl*) daring; courage. • *vt* (**gutting, gutted**) to remove the intestines from; to destroy the interior of.

gutless /-ləs/ *adj* (*inf*) cowardly, lacking determination.—**gutlessness** *n*.

gutsy /'gʌtsi/ *adj* (**gutsier, gutsiest**) (*sl*) brave, courageous; passionate; greedy.

gutta /,gʌtə/ *n* (*pl* **guttae**) (*archit*) a small loop-like ornament, *esp* in a Doric entablature; (*med*) (*formerly*) a drop.

gutta-percha /,gʌtəpɜːtʃə/ *n* the flexible hardened juice of a tropical tree; one of several trees yielding this.

guttate /'gʌteɪt/ **guttated** *adj* (*plants*) spotted; drop-like.

gutter /'gʌtər/ *n* a channel for carrying off water, *esp* at a roadside or under the eaves of a roof; a channel or groove to direct something (as of a bowling alley); the lowest condition of human life. • *adj* marked by extreme vulgarity or indecency. • *vt* to provide with a gutter. • *vi* to flow in rivulets; (*candle*) to melt unevenly; (*candle flame*) to flutter.—**guttering** *n*.

guttering /'gʌtərɪŋ/ *n* the system of gutters, pipes, etc, on exterior walls for carrying off rain water; material for making gutters.

guttersnipe /'gʌtər,snaɪp/ *n* a dirty child who plays in the streets, *esp* slum areas.

guttural /'gʌtərəl/ *adj* formed or pronounced in the throat; harsh-sounding.—**gutturally** *adv*.—**gutturalness, gutturality, gutturalism** *n*.

gutturalize /-,laɪz/ *vt* to form (a sound) in the throat; to speak in a harsh manner.—**gutturalization** *n*.

guy /gaɪ/ *n* a rope, chain, etc, for fixing or steadying anything. • *vt* to fix or steady with a guy.

guy² *n* (*Brit*) an effigy of Guy Fawkes made from old clothes stuffed with newspapers, etc burnt on the anniversary of the Gunpowder Plot (5 November); (*inf*) a man or boy; (*pl*) (*inf*) men or women; a shabby person. • *vt* to tease.

guzzle /'gʌzəl/ *vti* to gulp down food or drink greedily.—**guzzler** *n*.

gybe /dʒaɪb/ *vti* (*sail, boom*) to swing over from one side to the other; (*yacht*) to alter course in this way.—*also* **jibe**.

gym /dʒɪm/ *n* (*inf*) a gymnasium.

gymkhana /dʒɪm'kɑːnə/ *n* a meeting featuring sports contests or athletic skills, *esp* horse-riding.

gymnasium /dʒɪm'neɪziəm/ *n* (*pl* **gymnasiums, gymnasia**) a room or building equipped for physical training and sports.

gymnast /'dʒɪmnæst/ or /-nəst/ *n* a person skilled in gymnastics.

gymnastic /dʒɪm'næstɪk, *adj* pertaining to gymnastics.—**gymnastically** *adv*.

gymnastics /-'næstɪks/ *n sing* training in exercises devised to strengthen the body; (*pl*) gymnastic exercises; (*pl*) feats of dexterity or agility.

gymnosophist /dʒɪm'nɒsəfɪst/ *n* one of a class of ancient Hindu philosophers who lived bare-footed and lightly clothed or naked.

gymnosperm /'dʒɪmnoː,spɜːm/ *n* a plant whose seeds are not enclosed in a covering; a conifer or a conifer-like plant.—**gymnospermous** *adj*.

gynaecocracy, gynecocracy /,gaɪnə'kɒkrəsi/ *n* (*pl* **gynaecocracies, gynecocracies**) female rule or supremacy.—**gynaecocratic, gynecocratic** *adj*.

gynaecology, gynecology /,gaɪnə'kɒlədʒi/ *n* the branch of medicine that deals with the diseases and disorders of the female reproductive system.—**gynaecological, gynecological, gynaecologic, gynecologic** *adj*.—**gynaecologist, gynecologist** *n*.

gynarchy *n* (*pl* **gynarchies**) gynaecocracy.

gynoecium /gaɪ'niːsiəm/ or /dʒ-/ *n* (*pl* **gynoecia**) (*bot*) the female organs of a flower.

gynopathy /gaɪnɒ'pæθi/ *n* the condition of feeling threatened by women.—**gynopathic** *adj*.

gynophore *n* the long stalk on which the pistil is situated, as in the passion flower.—**gynophoric** *adj*.

gyp /dʒɪp/ *vt* (**gypping, gypped**) (*sl*) to cheat (someone). • *n* a swindle; a swindler; a college servant at Cambridge University; (*sl*) acute pain.—*also* **gip**.

gypsum /'dʒɪpsəm/ *n* a chalk-like mineral used to make plaster of Paris and fertilizer.—**gypseous, gypsiferous** *adj*.

Gypsy /'dʒɪpsi/ *n* (*pl* **Gypsies**) a member of a travelling people, orig from India, now spread throughout Europe and North America; (*without cap*) a person who looks or lives like a Gypsy.—*also* **Gipsy** (*pl* **Gipsies**).

gyral /'dʒaɪrəl/ *adj* rotatory whirling; pertaining to a gyrus.

gyrate /'dʒaɪreɪt/ *vi* to revolve; to whirl or spiral.—**gyration** *n*.—**gyratory** *adj*.

gyre /'dʒaɪr/ *vt* (*poet*) to gyrate. • (*poet*) a gyration.

gyrfalcon /'dʒɜːr,fɔːlkən/ *n* a large northern falcon, often used for hunting.—*also* **gerfalcon**.

gyro /'dʒaɪroː/ *n* (*pl* **gyros**) (*inf*) a gyroscope; a gyrocompass.

gyrocompass /'dʒaɪroː,kʌmpəs/ *n* a compass mounted on a gyroscope to keep it stable.

gyroscope /'dʒaɪroː,skoːp/ *n* a wheel mounted in a ring so that its axis is free to turn in any direction, so that when spinning rapidly it keeps its original plane of rotation.—**gyroscopic** *adj*.

gyrose /'dʒaɪroːs/ *adj* (*bot*) turned round like a crook.

gyrostabilizer /'dʒaɪroː,steɪbɪ,laɪzər/ *n* a device of two or more gyroscopes to prevent rolling of a ship or aircraft.

gyrostat /'dʒaɪroː,stæt/ *n* a gyrostabilizer.

gyrus /'dʒaɪrəs/ *n* (*pl* **gyri**) a convolution (of the brain).

gyve /dʒaɪv/ *vt* to fetter. • *n* (*usu pl*) shackles.

H

H /eɪtʃ/ (chem symbol) hydrogen.

ha /hɒ/ *interj* used to express surprise, triumph, etc.—*also* **hah**.

ha. *abbr* = hectare(s).

Habakkuk /ˈhæbəkək/ or /həˈbæk-/ *n* (*Bible*) one of the minor Old Testament book of prophets.

habeas corpus /ˌheɪbiəsˈkɔrpəs/ *n* a writ requiring that a prisoner be brought before a court, *esp* to ascertain the legality of his or her detention.

haberdasher /ˈhæbərˌdæʃər/ *n* a dealer in sewing accessories; a dealer in men's clothing.—**haberdashery** *n*.

habergeon /ˈhæbərdʒən/ *n* a sleeveless coat of chain mail covering the neck and breast.

habile /ˈhæbɪl/ *adj* skillful.

habiliment /həˈbɪlɪmənt/ *n* (*often pl*) clothing, attire.

habilitate /həˈbɪlɪˌteɪt/ *vi* to qualify for a post. • *vt* to provide working capital for a mine.—**habilitation** *n*.—**habilitator** *n*.

habit /ˈhæbɪt/ *n* a distinctive costume, as of a nun, etc; a thing done often and hence easily; a usual way of doing things; an addiction, *esp* to narcotics. • *vt* to clothe.

habitable /-əbəl/ *adj* capable of being lived in.—**habitability** *n*.—**habitably** *adv*.

habitant /ˌhæbiːˈtã/ ✽ (*Cdn*) (*hist*) a French settler in rural Quebec.

habitat /ˈhæbɪˌtæt/ *n* the normal environment of an animal or plant.

habitation /ˌhæbɪˈteɪʃən/ *n* the act of inhabiting; a dwelling or residence.—**habitational** *adj*.

habited /ˈhæbɪtəd/ *adj* wearing a habit or a dress.

habit-forming /-ˌfɔrmɪŋ/ *adj* addictive.

habitual /həˈbɪtʃʊəl/ *adj* having the nature of a habit; regular.—**habitually** *adv*.—**habitualness** *n*.

habituate /həˈbɪtʃuˌeɪt/ *vt* to accustom.—**habituation** *n*.

habitude /ˌhæbɪˈtjud/ or /-ˈtuːd/ *n* a custom or tendency; familiarity.—**habitudinal** *adj*.

habitué /həˈbɪtʃuˌeɪ/ *n* a frequent visitor to a place.

hacienda /ˌhæsiˈɛndə/ *n* (in Spanish-speaking countries) a large estate or ranch; the main house on such an estate.

hack¹ /hæk/ *vt* to cut or chop (at) violently; to clear (vegetation) by chopping; (*comput*) to gain illegal access to confidential data. • *n* a gash or notch; a harsh, dry cough.

hack² *n* a riding horse for hire; an old worn-out horse; a mediocre or unexceptional writer; a coach for hire; (*inf*) a taxicab. • *vti* to ride a horse cross-country. • *adj* banal, hackneyed.

hackbut /ˈhækˌbʌt/ *n* a type of arquebus.—*also* **hagbut**.

hacker /ˈhækər/ *n* a person who hacks; (*inf*) (*comput*) a person who uses computers as a hobby, *esp* one who uses a personal computer to gain illegal access to the computer systems of government departments or large corporations.

hacking /ˈhækɪŋ/ *adj* (*cough*) short, dry, spasmodic.

hackles /ˈhækəlz/ *npl* the hairs on the back of a dog, cat, etc, which stick out when the animal is angry or afraid.

hackney /ˈhækni/ *n* a horse for driving or riding; any of an English breed of high-stepping horses; a carriage or vehicle for hire.

hackneyed /ˈhækniːd/ *adj* made trite or banal through overuse.

hacksaw /ˈhæksɒ/ *n* a fine-toothed saw for cutting metal.

had /hæd/ *see* **have**.

haddock /ˈhædək/ *n* (*pl* **haddocks, haddock**) an important Atlantic food fish related to the cod.

Hades /ˈheɪdiːz/ *n* (*Greek myth*) the home of the dead; (*inf*) hell.—**Hadean** *adj*.

Hadith /ˈhædɪθ/ or /hæˈdiːθ/ *n* (*pl* **Hadith, Hadiths**) the traditions surrounding Muhammed and his sayings; an appendix to the Koran.

hadj /hædʒ/ *n* (*pl* **hadjes**) a pilgrimage to Mecca, required of all Muslims.—*also* **hajj** (*pl* **hajjes**).

hadji /ˈhædʒi/ *n* (*pl* **hadjis**) a Muslim who has made the pilgrimage to Mecca.—*also* **haji, hajji** (*pl* **hajjis, hajis**).

hadn't /ˈhædənt/ = had not.

haema-, haemo- /ˈhɛmɒ/ or /-mə/, /hɛmˈoː/, /-ə/ *prefix* blood.

haemal /-məl/ *adj* of or relating to the blood, blood vessels or the part of the body that contains the heart.

haematic /hiːˈmætɪk/ *adj* of, containing, acting on, or relating to blood. • *n* a drug that increases the level of haemoglobin in blood.

haematite /ˈhɛmətaɪt/ *n* native ferric oxide, an important iron ore.

haematoid /ˈhiːmətɔɪd/ *adj* relating to blood; blood-like.

haemoptysis /ˈhiːmoːtaɪsɪs/ or /ˈhiːmə-/ *n* the spitting or coughing up of blood or mucus containing blood.

hafiz /ˈhɒfɪz/ *n* a Muslim who knows the Koran by heart; a title of respect; the guardian of the Mosque.

hafnium /ˈhæfniəm/ *n* a silvery metallic element found in zirconium.

haft /hæft/ *n* the handle of a weapon or tool.

hag /hæg/ *n* an ugly or unpleasant old woman; a witch.—**haggish** *adj*.—**haggishness** *n*.

Haggadah /həˈgædə/ or /hægæˈdæ/ *n* (*pl* **Haggadoth**) (*Judaisim*) a parable or illustration of a commentary on Scripture; a book containing the order for the traditional Passover feast; a narrative of the flight from Egypt that is the main part of the Passover feast.

haggard /ˈhægərd/ *n adj* having an exhausted, untidy look.—**haggardly** *adv*.—**haggardness** *n*.

haggis /ˈhægɪs/ *n* (*pl* **haggises, haggis**) a traditional Scottish dish made of minced offal with suet, onions, oatmeal, seasonings, etc.

haggle /ˈhægəl/ *vi* to bargain; barter; to dispute over terms; to cavil. • *n* the act of haggling.—**haggler** *n*.

hagiography /ˌhægiˈɒgrəfi/ *n* (*pl* **hagiographies**) the history or legends of the saints; an uncritical biography.—**hagiographer, hagiographist** *n*.—**hagriographic, hagiographical** *adj*.

hah *see* **ha**.

ha-ha¹ /hɒˈhɒ/ *interj* an exclamation of mockery; an outburst of laughter.—*also* **haw-haw**.

ha-ha² *n* a fence sunk in the ground as a boundary of a park or garden.

Haida /ˈhaɪdə/ *n* ✽ a member of a First Nations people on the Pacific Northwest coast of Canada; the language of this people. • *adj* of or pertaining to this people or their language.

haiku /ˈhaɪkuː/ *n* (*pl* **haiku**) a Japanese verse form of three lines.

hail¹ /heɪl/ *vt* to greet; to summon by shouting or signalling, as a taxi; to welcome with approval, to acclaim. • *vi* (*with* **from**) to come from. • *interj* an exclamation of tribute, greeting, etc. • *n* a shout to gain attention; a distance within which one can be heard calling.—**hailer** *n*.

hail² *n* frozen raindrops; something, as abuse, bullets, etc, sent forcefully in rapid succession. • *vti* to pour down like hail.

Hail Mary *n* (*RC Church*) a prayer to the Virgin Mary beginning with these words.

hailstone /ˈheɪlstoːn/ *n* a pellet of hail.

hailstorm /-stɔrm/ *n* a sudden storm of hail.

hair /hɛr/ *n* a threadlike growth from the skin of mammals; a mass of hairs, *esp* on the human head; a threadlike growth on a plant.

haircut /ˈhɛrkʌt/ *n* a shortening and styling of hair by cutting it; the style of cutting.

hairdo /-duː/ *n* (*pl* **hairdos**) a particular style of hair after cutting, etc.

hairdresser /-ˌdrɛsər/ *n* a person who cuts, styles, colours, etc, hair.—**hairdressing** *n*.

hairgrip /-grɪp/ *n* a clip for holding hair in position; a bobby pin.

hairless /-ləs/ *adj* without hair; having little hair.

hairline /-laɪn/ *n* a very thin line; the outline of the hair on the head.

hairnet /-nɛt/ *n* a net used to keep the hair in place.

hairpiece /-piːs/ *n* a wig or toupee; an additional piece of hair attached to a person's real hair.

hairpin /-pɪn/ *n* U-shaped pin used to hold hair in place.

hairpin bend *n* a sharply curving bend in a road, etc.

hair-raising /-ˌreɪzɪŋ/ *adj* terrifying, shocking.

hair's-breadth *n* a very small space or amount.

hairsplitting /-splɪtɪŋ/ *adj* making petty distinctions; quibbling. • *n* the act of making petty distinctions.—**hairsplitter** *n*.

hairspring /-sprɪŋ/ n a slender, hair-like coil spring, as in a watch.

hairstyle /-staɪl/ n the way in which hair is arranged.—**hairstylist** n.

hairweaving /-wiːvɪŋ/ n the technique of attaching strands of false hair to the follicles of the head.

hairy /ˈhɛrɪ/ adj (**hairier, hairiest**) covered with hair; (inf) difficult, dangerous.—**hairiness** n.

haji, hajji see **hadji**.

hajj see **hadj**.

hake /heɪk/ n (pl **hake, hakes**) a marine food fish related to the cod.

hakim /ˈhɒkɪm/ n a judge, administrator or governor of an Islamic country; a Muslim physician.

Halakah, Halacha /həˈlɒxə/ n (pl **Halakoth, Halachoth**) (Judaism) traditional law containing minor precepts in addition to the Mosaic law; legal literature in general.

halal /hæˈlæl/ n meat from animals butchered according to Muslim law. • adj of or pertaining to such meat.—also **hallal**.

halation /həˈleɪʃən/ n (photog, TV) a halo-like appearance round an object, caused by light reflection.

halberd, halbert /ˈhælbərd/ n a medieval weapon consisting of a long staff to which an axe with a spear-like point was affixed.

halberdier /ˌhælbərˈdiːr/ n a soldier armed with a halberd.

halcyon /ˈhælsɪən/ adj calm, gentle, peaceful. • n a fabled bird (probably the kingfisher) that nested at sea and calmed it.

hale /heɪl/ adj healthy and strong.

half /hæf/ n (pl **halves**) either of two equal parts of something; (inf) a half-price ticket for a bus, etc; (inf) half a pint. • adj being a half; incomplete; partial. • adv to the extent of a half; (inf) partly.

half-and-half n something half one thing and half another, esp a mixture of mild and bitter beer. • adj partly one thing and partly another. • adv in two equal parts.

halfback /ˈhæfbæk/ n (football, hockey) a player occupying a position between the forwards and the fullbacks; a player in this position in other sports.

half-baked adj (inf) poorly planned or thought-out; (inf) stupid.

half-brother n a brother through one parent only.

half-caste n a person whose parents are of different races.

half cock n the middle position of a gun's hammer; **at half cock** not prepared.—**half-cocked** adj.

half-hearted /hæfˈhɑrtəd/ adj with little interest, enthusiasm, etc.—**half-heartedly** adv.—**half-heartedness** n.

half-hour n 30 minutes; the point 30 minutes after the beginning of an hour.

half-life n the time taken for half the atoms in a radioactive substance to decay.

half-mast n the position to which a flag is lowered as a sign of mourning.

half-measure n (often pl) an inadequate action; a compromise.

half-moon n the moon at its phase when half the disc is illuminated; something shaped like this. • adj in the shape of a half-moon.

half-nelson n a wrestling hold, pinning the arm of an opponent behind the back from behind.

half note n (mus) a note with the time value of half of a semibreve.—also **minim**.

halfpenny /ˈheɪpənɪ/ or /ˈheɪpnɪ/ (pl **halfpence**) n a bronze coin worth two farthings in pre-decimal British currency.

half-sister n a sister through one parent only.

half title n a short title on the page before the title page of a book, a bastard title.

half-term n a short holiday in the middle of a school term.

half-time /hæfˈtaɪm/ n (sport) an interval between two halves of a game.

halftone /ˈhæfˈtoːn/ n an illustration printed from a relief plate, showing light and shadow by means of minute dots.

half-track n a (military) vehicle with wheels in front but driven by caterpillar tracks at the rear.

half-truth n a statement that is only partly true.

half volley n (tennis, etc) the striking of the ball the instant it bounces.

halfway /ˈhæfweɪ/ or /hæfˈweɪ/ adj midway between two points, etc.

halfwit /ˈhæfwɪt/ n a stupid or silly person; a mentally retarded person.—**halfwitted** adj.—**halfwittedly** adv.—**halfwittedness** n.

halibut /ˈhælɪbət/ n (pl **halibut, halibuts**) a large marine flatfish used as food.

halide /ˈhælaɪd/ or /ˈheɪl-/ n a compound containing halogen; a haloid.

Haligonian /ˌhælɪˈɡoːnɪən/ n ✤ a person who lives in or is from Halifax, Nova Scotia.

halitosis /ˌhælɪˈtoːsɪs/ n bad-smelling breath.

hall /hɒl/ n a public building with offices, etc; a large room for exhibits, gatherings, etc; the main house on a landed estate; a college building, esp a dining room; a vestibule at the entrance of a building; a hallway.

hallal see **halal**.

Hallel /hæˈleɪl/ or /ˈhælɛl/ n (Judaism) Psalms 113-118 chanted as part of morning services during Passover and other festivals.

hallelujah, halleluiah /ˌhæləˈluːjə/ or /ˌhɒleɪ-/ interj an exclamation of praise to God. • n a praising of God; a musical composition having this as its theme.—also **alleluia**.

halliard see **halyard**.

hallmark /ˈhɒlmɑrk/ n a mark used on gold, silver or platinum articles to signify a standard of purity, weight, date of manufacture; a mark or symbol of high quality; a characteristic feature. • vt to stamp with a hallmark.

hallo see **hello**.

hallow /ˈhæloː/ vt to make or regard as holy.—**hallowed** adj.—**hallowedness** n.—**hallower** n.

Hallowe'en, Halloween /ˌhæləˈwiːn/ or /ˌhɒlə-/ n the eve of All Saints' Day, October 31.

Hallowmas /ˈhæloːməs/ or /-ˌmæs/ n (formerly) All Saints' Day, November 1.

Hallstatt, Hallstadt /ˈhɒlʃˌæt/ adj of or denoting the final period of the Bronze Age and the first period of the Iron Age (9th – 4th centuries BC).

hallucinate /həˈluːsəˌneɪt/ vti to have or cause to have hallucinations.—**hallucinator** n.

hallucination /həˌluːsəˈneɪʃən/ n the apparent perception of sights, sounds, etc, that are not actually present; something perceived in this manner.—**hallucinational, hallucinative** adj.—**hallucinatory** adj.

hallucinogen /həˈluːsənədʒən/ n a drug that produces hallucinations.—**hallucinogenic** adj.

hallux /ˈhæləks/ n (pl **halluces**) the big toe; the first digit on the back foot of an amphibian, bird, mammal, or reptile.

halm see **haulm**.

halo /ˈheɪloː/ n (pl **haloes, halos**) a circle of light, as around the sun; a symbolic ring of light around the head of a saint in pictures; the aura of glory surrounding an idealized person or thing. • vt (**haloing, haloed**) to surround with a halo.

halogen /ˈhælədʒən/ or /ˈheɪ-/ n any of the five chemical elements fluorine, chlorine, bromine, iodine and astatine.—**halogenous** adj.

halt[1] /hɒlt/ n a temporary interruption or cessation of progress; a minor station on a rail line. • vti to stop or come to a stop.

halt[2] vi to falter; to hesitate.—**halting** adj.

halter /ˈhɒltər/ n a rope or strap for tying or leading an animal; a style of women's dress top tied behind the neck and waist leaving the back and arms bare. • vt to put a halter on (a horse, etc).

halve /hæv/ vt to divide equally into two; to reduce by half; (golf) to play one hole in the same number of strokes as one's opponent.

halves /hævz/ see **half**.

halyard /ˈhæljərd/ n a line for hoisting or lowering a sail, yard, or flag.—also **halliard**.

ham /hæm/ n the upper part of a pig's hind leg, salted, smoked, etc; the meat from this area; (inf) the back of the upper thigh; (inf) an actor who overacts; (inf) a licensed amateur radio operator. • vti (**hamming, hammed**) to speak or move in an exaggerated manner, to overact.

hamadryad /ˌhæməˈdraɪæd/ n (pl **hamadryads, hamadryades**) (Greek myth) a wood nymph; a giant cobra, the king cobra.

hamadryas /ˌhæməˈdraɪəs/ n a North African baboon, the male of which has a heavy mane of silvery hair.

hamal /həˈmɒl/ or /-ˈmɒl/ n a porter in several Muslim countries.—also **hammal, hammaul**.

Hamburg /ˈhæmbərɡ/ n a rich, black grape; a breed of black domestic fowl.

hamburger /ˈhæmˌbərɡər/ n ground beef; a cooked patty of such meat, often in a bread roll with pickle, etc.

hame[1] /heɪm/ n either of two curved bars for the traces on the collar of a draught horse.

hame[2] n (Scot) home.

ham-handed /hæm'hændəd/, **ham-fisted** /hæm'fıstəd/ *adj* (*inf*) clumsy.

Hamite /'hæmaıt/ *n* a descendant of Ham, son of Noah; a member of the Hamitic race.

Hamitic /hə'mıtık/ *adj* relating to Ham, the races descended from him, or the languages they speak. • *n* any of a group of languages spoken in North Africa.

hamlet /'hæmlət/ *n* a very small village.

hammal, hammaul *see* **hamal**.

hammer /'hæmər/ *n* a tool for pounding, driving nails, etc, having a heavy head and a handle; a thing like this in shape or use, as the part of the gun that strikes the firing pin; a bone of the middle ear; a heavy metal ball attached to a wire thrown in athletic contests; **hammer and tongs** with great force. • *vti* to strike repeatedly, as with a hammer; to drive, force, or shape, as with hammer blows; (*inf*) to defeat utterly.—**hammerer** *n*.

hammerhead /'hæmər,hed/ *n* a shark with a mallet-shaped head.

hammock /'hæmək/ *n* a length of strong cloth or netting suspended by the ends and used as a bed.

hammy /'hæmi/ *adj* (**hammier, hammiest**) (*inf*) overacting; exaggerated.

hamper[1] /'hæmpər/ *vt* to hinder; to interfere with; to encumber.—**hamperer** *n*.

hamper[2] *n* a large, *usu* covered, basket for storing or transporting food and crockery, etc.

hamster /'hæmstər/ *n* a small short-tailed rodent with cheek pouches.

hamstring /'hæmstrıŋ/ *n* any of the tendons at the back of the thigh that flex and rotate the leg. • *vt* (**hamstringing, hamstrung**) to cripple by severing the hamstring of; to render useless, to thwart.

hamulus /'hæmjuləs/ *n* (*pl* **hamuli**) a small hook-like projection at the end of the bones or between the fore and hind wings of a bee or bee-like insect.—**hamular** *adj*.

hand /hænd/ *n* the part of the arm below the wrist, used for grasping; a side or direction; possession or care; control; an active part; a promise to marry; skill; one having a special skill; handwriting; applause; help; a hired worker; a source; one of a ship's crew; anything like a hand, as a pointer on a clock; the breadth of a hand, four inches when measuring the height of a horse; the cards held by a player at one time; a round of card play ; (*inf*) applause. • *adj* of, for, or controlled by the hand. • *vt* to give as with the hand; to help or conduct with the hand. • *vi* (*with* **on**) to pass to the next.

handbag /'hændbæg/ *n* a woman's small bag for carrying personal items.—*also* **bag, pocket book, purse**.

handbill /'hændbıl/ *n* a small printed notice to be passed out by hand.

handbook /'hændbuk/ *n* a book containing useful instructions.

handcart /'hændkart/ *n* a small cart pulled or pushed by hand.

handcuff /'hændkəf/ *n* (*usu pl*) either of a pair of connected steel rings for shackling the wrists of a prisoner. • *vt* to manacle.

handed /'hændəd/ *adj* having or involving (a specified kind or number of) hands.

handfast /'hændfæst/ *vt* (*formerly*) to pledge or betroth; to grip with the hand. • *n* a contract of betrothal.

handful /'hændful/ *n* as much as will fill the hand; a few; (*inf*) a person who is difficult to handle or control.

handicap /'hændı,kæp/ *n* a mental or physical impairment; a contest in which difficulties are imposed on, or advantages given to, contestants to equalize their chances; such a difficulty or advantage; any hindrance. • *vt* (**handicapping, handicapped**) to give a handicap to; to hinder.—**handicapper** *n*.

handicapped /-kæpt/ *adj* mentally or physically disabled.

handicraft /'hændı,kræft/ *n* a skill involving the hands, such as basketwork, pottery, etc; an item of pottery, etc made by hand.

handiwork /'hændıwərk/ *n* handmade work; something done by a person or thing.

handkerchief /'hæŋkərtʃıf/ or /-,tʃiːf/ *n* a small cloth for blowing the nose, etc.

handle /'hændəl/ *vt* to touch, hold, or move with the hand; to manage or operate with the hands; to manage, deal with; to buy and sell (goods). • *vi* to react in a specified way. • *n* a part of anything designed to be held or grasped by the hand.—**handleable** *adj*.—**handling** *n*.

handlebar /'hændəl,bar/ *n* (*often pl*) the curved metal bar with a grip at each end used to steer a bicycle, etc; a bushy moustache with curved ends.

handler /'hændlər/ *n* a person who trains or controls animals, such as a police dog.

handless /'hændləs/ *adj* awkward, clumsy.

handmade /-meıd/ *adj* made by hand, carefully crafted.

handmaid(en) /'hændmeıd/ or /-,meıdən/ *n* a female servant.

hand-out /'hændaut/ *n* an item of food, clothing, etc, given free to the needy; a statement given to the press to replace or supplement an oral presentation.

hand-picked *adj* carefully selected.

handrail /'hændreıl/ *n* a narrow rail for gripping as a support.

hands-on *adj* involving active participation and operating experience.

handsaw /'hænd,sɒ/ *n* any saw that is used in one hand only.

handsel /'hænsəl/ *n* (*formerly*) a good-luck gift on beginning something; a housewarming present; a New Year gift. • *vt* to give a handsel to; to inaugurate; to be first to use something.

handset /'hændset/ *n* a telephone earpiece and mouthpiece as a single unit.

handshake /'hændʃeık/ *n* a grasping and shaking of a person's hand as a greeting or when concluding an agreement.

handsome /'hænsəm/ *adj* good-looking; dignified; generous; ample.—**handsomely** *adv*.—**handsomeness** *n*.

handspike /'hændspaık/ *n* an iron-shod bar or pipe used as a lever.

handspring /'hændsprıŋ/ *n* (*gymnastics*) a leaping forwards or backwards from a standing position into a handstand then back onto the feet.

handstand /'hændstænd/ *n* the act of supporting the body on the hands with the feet in the air.

hand-to-hand *adj* (*fighting*) at close quarters.

hand-to-mouth *adj* having barely enough food or money to survive.—*also adv*.

handwriting /'hænd,raıtıŋ/ *n* writing done by hand; a style of such writing.—**handwritten** *adj*.

handy /'hændi/ *adj* (**handier, handiest**) convenient, near; easy to use; skilled with the hands.—**handily** *adv*.—**handiness** *n*.

handyman /'hændi,mæn/ *n* (*pl* **handymen**) a person who does odd jobs.

hang /hæŋ/ *vb* (**hanging, hung**) *vt* to support from above, *esp* by a rope, chain, etc, to suspend; (*door, etc*) to attach by hinges to allow to swing freely; to decorate with pictures, or other suspended objects; (*wallpaper*) to stick to a wall; to exhibit (works of art); to prevent (a jury) from coming to a decision; (*pt, pp* **hanged**) to put to execute or kill by suspending by the neck. • *vi* to be suspended, so as to dangle loosely; (*clothing, etc*) to fall or flow in a certain direction; to lean, incline, or protrude; to depend; to remain in the air; to be in suspense; to fall or droop; (*pt, pp* **hanged**) to die by hanging; (*with* **about, around**) to loiter; (*with* **back**) to hesitate, be reluctant; (*with* **out**) to meet regularly at a particular place. • *n* the way in which anything hangs; (*sl*) a damn.

hangar /'hæŋər/ *n* a large shelter where aircraft are built, stored or repaired.—*also vt*.

hangbird /'hæŋbərd/ *n* the Baltimore oriole; any North American bird that builds a hanging nest.

hangdog /'hæŋdɒg/ *adj* abject or ashamed in appearance or manner.

hanger /'hæŋər/ *n* a device on which something is hung; one who hangs things.

hanger-on *n* (*pl* **hangers-on**) a sycophantic follower.

hang-glider /'hæŋ,glaıdər/ *n* an unpowered aircraft consisting of a metal frame over which a lightweight material is stretched, with a harness for the pilot suspended below.—**hang gliding** *n*.

hanging /'hæŋıŋ/ *n* the act of executing a person by suspending them by the neck; something hung, as a picture; (*pl*) decorative draperies hung on walls. • *adj* suspended in the air; undecided; overhanging; situated on a steep slope.

hangman /'hæŋmæn/ or /-mən/ *n* (*pl* **hangmen**) a person who executes prisoners by hanging them.

hangnail /'hæŋneıl/ *n* a thin strip of torn skin at the root of a fingernail.

hangout /'hæŋaut/ *n* a favourite meeting place.

hangover /'hæŋ,oːvər/ *n* the unpleasant after-effects of excessive consumption of alcohol; something surviving from an earlier time.

hang-up /'hæŋʌp/ *n* an emotional preoccupation with something.

hank /hæŋk/ *n* a coiled or looped bundle of wool, rope, etc.

hanker /'hæŋkər/ *vi* (*with* **after, for**) to desire longingly.—**hankerer** *n*.—**hankering** *n*.

hanky, hankie /'hæŋki/ *n* (*pl* **hankies**) (*inf*) a handkerchief.

hanky-panky /'hæŋki'pæŋki/ *n* (*inf*) foolish behaviour; dishonesty; illicit sexual relations.

Hansard /'hænsərd/ *n* the official, printed verbatim reports of British parliamentary proceedings.

hanse /'hænsə/ *n* a medieval guild of merchants; a fee paid by new members of such a guild; (*with cap*) a town of the Hanseatic League; the Hanseatic League.—**hanseatic** *adj*.

Hanseatic League /,hænsi'ætik/ *n* a confederacy of merchants or commercial towns in northern Germany and elsewhere, which lasted from the 14th–19th centuries.

hansom (cab) /'hænsəm/ *n* a light two-wheeled covered horse-drawn carriage, with the driver's seat raised behind.

hap /hæp/ *vb* (**happing, happed**) *vi* (*arch*) to happen or befall. • *vt* to cover up; to wrap up warmly. • *n* (*arch*) chance; luck; a fortunate accident; a covering of any kind.

haphazard /hæp'hæzərd/ *adj* not planned; random. • *adv* by chance.—**haphazardly** *adv*.—**haphazardness** *n*.

hapless /'hæpləs/ *adj* unfortunate, unlucky.—**haplessness** *n*.

haploid /'hæplɔid/ *adj* (*cell nucleus, organism*) possessing only half the normal number of chromosomes. • *n* a single set of unpaired chromosomes.

haply /'hæpli/ *adv* (*formerly*) by chance.

happen /'hæpən/ *vi* to take place; to be, occur, or come by chance.

happening /-ɪŋ/ *n* an occurrence; an improvization.

happy /'hæpi/ *adj* (**happier, happiest**) fortunate; having, expressing, or enjoying pleasure or contentment; pleased; appropriate, felicitous.—**happily** *adv*.—**happiness** *n*.

happy-go-lucky *adj* irresponsible; carefree.

happy hour *n* a particular time of day when a bar, hotel, etc, sells drinks at reduced prices

happy medium *n* a middle course between extremes.

hapteron /'hæptərən/ *n* (*pl* **haptera**) the tissue in seaweed and related plants that enables them to attach themselves to a host object.

haptic /'hæptik/ *adj* of or relating to the sense of touch.

harakiri /'hærə,kiri/ *n* ritual suicide by disembowelment.—*also* **harikari**.

harangue /'hæræŋ/ *n* a tirade; a lengthy, forceful speech. • *vti* to make a harangue, to address vehemently.—**haranguer** *n*.

harass /hə'ræs/ or /'hərəs/, /'hærəs/ *vt* to annoy, to irritate; to trouble (an enemy) by constant raids and attacks.—**harasser** *n*.—**harassment** *n*.

harbinger /'harbindʒər/ *n* a person or thing that announces or presages the arrival of another, a forerunner.

harbour, harbor /'harbər/ *n* a protected inlet for anchoring ships; any place of refuge. • *vt* to shelter or house; (*grudge, etc*) to keep in the mind secretly. • *vi* to take shelter.—**harbourer, harborer** *n*.

harbourage, harborage /'harbərədʒ/ *n* a port or anchorage for ships.

hard /hard/ *adj* firm, solid, not easily cut or punctured; difficult to comprehend; difficult to accomplish; difficult to bear, painful; severe, unfeeling, ungenerous; indisputable, intractable; (*drugs*) addictive and damaging to health; (*weather*) severe; (*currency*) stable in value; (*news*) definite, not speculative; (*drink*) very alcoholic; (*water*) having a high mineral content that prevents lathering with soap; (*colour, sound*) harsh. • *adv* with great effort or intensity; earnestly, with concentration; so as to cause hardness; with difficulty; with bitterness or grief; close, near by.—**hardness** *n*.

hardback /'hardbæk/ *n* a book bound with a stiff cover.—*also adj*.

hard-bitten /'hard,bitən/ *adj* (*inf*) tough, seasoned.

hardboard /'hard,bord/ *n* a stiff board made of compressed wood chips.

hard-boiled *adj* (*eggs*) boiled until solid; (*inf*) unfeeling.

hard cash *n* payment in coins and notes as opposed to cheque, credit card, etc.

hard copy *n* output (as from microfilm or a computer) on paper.

hard core *n* the stubborn inner group in an organization that is resistant to change; the heavy foundation material for a road.

hard-core *adj* of a hard core; utterly entrenched; (*pornography*) showing sexual acts in explicit detail.

hard disk *n* (*comput*) a rigid magnetic disk in a sealed unit capable of much greater storage capacity than a floppy disk.

harden /'hardən/ *vti* to make or become hard.—**hardener** *n*.

hard-headed /'hard,hedəd/ *adj* shrewd and unsentimental; practical.—**hard-headedly** *adv*.—**hard-headedness** *n*.

hardhearted /'hard,hartəd/ *adj* unfeeling; cruel.—**hardheartedly** *adv*.—**hardheartedness** *n*.

hard-hitting *adj* forcefully effective.

hard line *n* an aggressive unyielding policy.—**hard-line** *adj*.—**hardliner** *n*.

hardly /'hardli/ *adv* scarcely; barely; with difficulty; not to be expected.

hardpan /'hardpæn/ *n* a hard, impervious layer of clay below the soil; a solid foundation.

hardrock mining /'hard-rok/ *n* ♣ mining performed underground in large formations of igneous or metamorphic rock.

hard sell *n* an aggressive selling technique.

hardship /'hardʃip/ *n* something that causes suffering or privation.

hard shoulder *n* in UK, a raised strip of land alongside a motorway for vehicles to make emergency stops.

hardtack /'hardtæk/ *n* a hard, saltless biscuit formerly eaten by seamen.

hard-up *adj* (*inf*) short of money.

hardware /'hardwer/ *n* articles made of metal as tools, nails, etc; (*comput*) the mechanical and electronic components that make up a computer system.

hardwood /'hardwud/ *n* the close-grained wood of deciduous trees.

hardy /'hardi/ *adj* (**hard er, hardiest**) bold, resolute; robust; vigorous; able to withstand exposure to physical or emotional hardship.—**hardily** *adv*.—**hardiness** *n*.

hare /her/ *n* (*pl* **hare, hares**) any of various timid, swift, long-eared mammals, resembling but larger than the rabbit.

harebell /'herbel/ *n* the bluebell; the wild hyacinth.

harebrained /'herbreind/ *adj* flighty; foolish.

harelip /'herlip/ *n* a congenital deformity of the upper lip in the form of a vertical fissure.—**harelipped** *adj*.

harem /'herəm/ *n* the *usu* secluded part of a Muslim household where the women live; the women in a harem.

haricot /'heri,ko/ *n* a type of French bean with an edible light-coloured seed.

harikari *see* harakiri.

hark /hark/ *vi* to listen; (*with* **back**) to retrace a course; to revert (to).

harken /'harkən/ *see* **hearken**.

harlequin /'harləkwin/ *n* the performer in a pantomime who wears parti-coloured garments and carries a wand. • *adj* fantastic or full of trickery; colourful.

harlequinade /,harləkwi'neid/ *n* a play or the part of a pantomime in which Harlequin plays a leading role; buffoonery.

harlot /'harlət/ *n* (*formerly*) a prostitute.—**harlotry** *n*.

harm /harm/ *n* hurt; damage; injury. • *vt* to inflict hurt, damage, or injury upon.—**harmer** *n*.

harmattan /har'mætən/ *n* a hot dust-laden wind that blows from the interior to the west coast of Africa.

harmful /'harmful/ *adj* hurtful.—**harmfully** *adv*.—**harmfulness** *n*.

harmless /'harmləs/ *adj* not likely to cause harm.—**harmlessly** *adv*.—**harmlessness** *n*.

harmonic /har'monik/ *adj* (*mus*) of or in harmony. • *n* an overtone; (*pl*) the science of musical sounds.—**harmonically** *adv*.

harmonica /har'monikə/ *n* a small wind instrument that produces tones when air is blown or sucked across a series of metal reeds; a mouth-organ.

harmonious /har'moniəs/ *adj* fitting together in an orderly and pleasing manner; agreeing in ideas, interests, etc; melodious.—**harmoniously** *adv*.

harmonium /har'moniəm/ *n* a keyboard musical instrument whose tones are produced by thin metal reeds operated by foot bellows.

harmonize /'harmə naiz/ *vi* to be in harmony; to sing in harmony. • *vt* to make harmonious.—**harmonization** *n*.

harmonized sales tax *n* ♣ (*Cdn*) a tax on goods and services, combining the federal goods and services tax and the provincial sales tax.

harmony /'harməni/ *n* (*pl* **harmonies**) a pleasing agreement of parts in colour, size, etc; agreement in action, ideas, etc; the pleasing combination of musical tones in a chord; a collation of parallel narratives, *esp* of the Gospels, with a commentary.

harness /'harnəs/ *n* the leather straps and metal pieces by which a horse is fastened to a vehicle, plough, etc; any similar fastening or attachment, *eg* for a parachute, hang-glider. • *vt* to put a harness on; to control so as to use the power of.—**harnesser** *n*.

harp /hɑrp/ *n* a stringed musical instrument played by plucking. • *vi* (*with* **on** *or* **upon**) to talk persistently (on some subject).—**harpist, harper** *n*.

harpoon /hɑrˈpuːn/ *n* a barbed spear with an attached line, for spearing whales, etc. • *vt* to strike with a harpoon.—**harpooner** *n*.

harpsichord /ˈhɑrpsɪˌkɔrd/ *n* a musical instrument resembling a grand piano whose strings are plucked by a mechanism rather than struck.—**harpsichordist** *n*.

harpy /ˈhɑrpi/ *n* (*pl* **harpies**) a grasping, vicious person.

harquebus *see* **arquebus**.

harridan /ˈherɪdən/ *n* a disreputable, shrewish old woman.

harrier /ˈhæriər/ *n* a small breed of hound used for hunting hares; a cross-country runner.

harrow /ˈhero:/ *n* a heavy frame with spikes, spring teeth, or disks for breaking up and levelling ploughed ground. • *vt* to draw a harrow over (land); to cause mental distress to.—**harrower** *n*.—**harrowing** *adj, n*.—**harrowment** *n*.

harry /ˈheri/ *vt* (**harrying, harried**) to torment or harass.

harsh /hɑrʃ/ *adj* unpleasantly rough; jarring on the senses or feelings; rigorous; cruel.—**harshly** *adv*.—**harshness** *n*.

hart /hɑrt/ *n* (*pl* **hart, harts**) a male deer, especially the red deer, aged five years or more.

hartal /ˈhɑrtəl/ *n* (*Hinduism*) the closing of shops as a sign of mourning or as a political gesture.

hartebeest, hartbeest /ˈhɑrtəˌbiːst/ *n* the South African antelope.

hartshorn /ˈhɑrtʃɔrn/ *n* the antler of a hart; sal volatile.

harum-scarum /ˌherəmˈskɛrəm/ *adj* (*inf*) rash, reckless. • *n* a giddy rash person.

haruspex /həˈruːspɛks/ *n* (*pl* **haruspices**) in ancient Rome, a soothsayer who foretold events by inspecting the entrails of sacrificial animals.

harvest /ˈhɑrvəst/ *n* (the season of) gathering in the ripened crops; the yield of a particular crop; the reward or product of any exertion or action. • *vti* to gather in (a crop). • *vt* to win by achievement.—**harvester** *n*.—**harvesting** *n*.

harvester /-ər/ *n* a person who harvests; a harvesting machine *esp* a combine harvester.

harvest excursion *n* ✤ (*Cdn*) (*hist*) an organized, low-priced train excursion for workers travelling to western Canada to harvest grain crops.

harvest moon *n* the full moon nearest the time of the September equinox.

has /hæz/ *see* **have**.

has-been *n* (*inf*) a person or thing that has lost its former popularity or celebrity status.

hash[1] /hæʃ/ *n* a chopped mixture of reheated cooked meat and vegetables. • *vt* to chop up (meat or vegetables) for hash; to mix or mess up.

hash[2] *n* (*inf*) hashish.

hashish /ˈhæʃiːʃ/ *or* /ˈhæ-/ *n* resin derived from the leaves and shoots of the hemp plant, smoked or chewed as an intoxicant.

hasn't /ˈhæzənt/ = has not.

hasp /hæsp/ *n* a hinged fastening for a door, etc, *esp* a metal piece fitted over a staple and fastened as by a bolt or padlock.

hassock /ˈhæsək/ *n* a firm cushion used as a footstool or seat.

hast /hæst/ (*arch*) *the second person sing of* **have**, used with **thou**.

hastate /ˈhæsteɪt/ *adj* spear-shaped (of a leaf).

haste /heɪst/ *n* quickness of motion; urgency. • *vi* (*poet*) to hasten.

hasten /ˈheɪsən/ *vt* to accelerate; to cause to hurry. • *vi* to move or act with speed.—**hastener** *n*.

hasty /ˈheɪsti/ *adj* (**hastier, hastiest**) done in a hurry; rash, precipitate.—**hastily** *adv*.—**hastiness** *n*.

hat /hæt/ *n* a covering for the head. • *vt* (**hatting, hatted**) to cover with a hat.

hatband /ˈhætbænd/ *n* a band or ribbon around the base of a hat; a black cloth band worn as a token of mourning.

hatbox /ˈhætbɒks/ *n* a box or case for a hat or hats.

hatch[1] /hætʃ/ *n* a small door or opening (as on an aircraft or spaceship); an opening in the deck of a ship or in the floor or roof of a building; a lid for such an opening; a hatchway.

hatch[2] *vt* to produce (young) from the egg, *esp* by incubating; to devise (*eg* a plot). • *vi* to emerge from the egg; to incubate.—**hatchable** *adj*.—**hatcher** *n*.

hatch[3] *vt* (*drawing, engraving*) to shade using closely spaced parallel lines or incisions.—**hatching** *n*.

hatchback /ˈhætʃbæk/ *n* a sloping rear end on a car with a door; a car of this design.

hatchery /ˈhætʃəri/ *n* (*pl* **hatcheries**) a place for hatching eggs, *esp* of fish.

hatchet /ˈhætʃət/ *n* a small axe with a short handle.

hatchet job *n* (*inf*) devastating or malicious verbal or written criticism.

hatchet man *n* a person hired to perform unpleasant tasks; a critic specializing in invective.

hatchment /ˈhætʃmənt/ *n* (*her*) a diamond-shaped tablet bearing a dead person's armorial bearings, placed on a house or tomb.

hatchway /ˈhætʃweɪ/ *n* an opening in a ship's deck or in a floor or roof; a passage giving access to an enclosed space (as a cellar).

hate /heɪt/ *vt* to feel intense dislike for. • *vi* to feel hatred; to wish to avoid. • *n* a strong feeling of dislike or contempt; the person or thing hated.—**hater** *n*.

hateful /ˈheɪtful/ *adj* deserving or arousing hate.—**hatefully** *adv*.—**hatefulness** *n*.

hath /hæθ/ (*arch*) *the third person sing of* **have**.

hatred /ˈheɪtrəd/ *n* intense dislike or enmity.

hatter /ˈhætər/ *n* a person who makes or sells hats.

hat trick *n* (*cricket*) the taking of three wickets with three successive bowls; the scoring of three successive goals, points, etc in any game.

hauberk /ˈhɒbərk/ *n* a coat of armour, often sleeveless, formed of chain mail, which reached below the knees.

haugh /hɒ/ *n* (*Scot*) a small, low-lying riverside meadow.

haughty /ˈhɒti/ *adj* (**haughtier, haughtiest**) having or expressing arrogance.—**haughtily** *adv*.—**haughtiness** *n*.

haul /hɒl/ *vti* to move by pulling; to transport by truck, etc. • *n* the act of hauling; the amount gained, caught, etc, at one time; the distance over which something is transported.

haulage /ˈhɒlɪdʒ/ *n* the transport of commodities; the charge for this.

hauler /-ər/ *n* a person or business that transports goods by road.

haulm /hɒm/ *n* the stalk of potatoes, peas, etc, *esp* after the crop has been gathered.—*also* **halm**.

haunch /hɒntʃ/ *n* the part of the body around the hips; the leg and loin of a deer, sheep, etc.—**haunched** *adj*.

haunt /hɒnt/ *vt* to visit often or continually; to recur repeatedly to. • *vi* to linger; to appear habitually as a ghost. • *n* a place often visited.—**haunter** *n*.

haunted /ˈhɒntəd/ *adj* supposedly visited by ghosts; obsessed; anxious, worried.

haunting /ˈhɒntɪŋ/ *adj* constantly recurring in the mind; unforgettable.—**hauntingly** *adv*.

Hausa /ˈhausə/ *or* /-zə/ *n* a member of the negroid people of West Africa living chiefly in Nigeria; the language of these people.

haustellum /hɒˈstɛləm/ *n* (*pl* **haustella**) the tip of the proboscis of the housefly or similar insects used for sucking foods.

hautbois, hautboy /ˈhoːbɔɪ/ *n* (*pl* **hautbois, hautboy**) (*arch*) the oboe.

haute couture /ˌoːtkuːˈtʃʊr/ *or* /-ˈtuːr/, /hoːt-/ *n* high fashion.

haute cuisine /ˌoːtkwiˈziːn/ *n* high-class cooking.

hauteur /oːˈtər/ *n* arrogance, haughtiness.

Havana (cigar) *n* a cigar rolled from Cuban tobacco.

have /hæv/ *vt* (**has, having**, *pp* **had**) to have in one's possession; to possess as an attribute; to hold in the mind; to experience; to give birth to; to allow, or tolerate; to arrange or hold; to engage in; to cause, compel, or require to be; to to be obliged; (*sl*) to have sexual intercourse with; to be pregnant with; (*inf*) to hold at a disadvantage; (*inf*) to deceive; to accept or receive; to consume food, drink, etc; to show some quality; to perplex.

haven /ˈheɪvən/ *n* a place where ships can safely anchor; a refuge.

have-not province *n* ✤ (*Cdn*) province that receives equalization payments from the federal government because it does not have sufficient tax revenue.

haven't /ˈhævənt/ = have not.

have province *n* ✤ (*Cdn*) a province that has enough tax revenue that it is ineligible to receive equalization payments from the federal government.

haver /ˈheɪvər/ *vi* (*Scot*) to talk foolishly or in consequently; to dither. • *n* (*pl*) nonsense.

haversack /ˈhævərˌsæk/ *n* a canvas bag similar to a knapsack but worn over one shoulder.

havoc /ˈhævək/ *n* widespread destruction or disorder. • *vt* (**havocking, havocked**) to lay waste.

haw /hɒ/ *n* (the berry of) the hawthorn.

Hawaiian /hə'waɪən/ *adj* pertaining to Hawaii, its inhabitants or its language. • *n* an inhabitant of Hawaii; a Polynesian language spoken in Hawaii.

hawfinch /'hɔfɪntʃ/ *n* a rare European finch with a stout bill, brown plumage and black-and-white wings.

haw-haw *see* **ha-ha**[1].

hawk[1] /hɔk/ *n* any of numerous birds of prey; a person who advocates aggressive or intimidatory action. • *vti* to hunt with a hawk; to strike like a hawk.—**hawkish** *adj*.—**hawkishly** *adv*.

hawk[2] *vti* to clear the throat (of) audibly. • *n* the sound of this.

hawk[3] *vt* to offer goods for sale, as in the street; to spread gossip. • *vi* to peddle.

hawker /'hɔkər/ *n* a person who goes about offering goods for sale; a person who hunts with a trained hawk.

hawk-eyed *adj* keen-sighted; vigilant.

hawkweed /'hɔkwiːd/ *n* a yellow-flowered plant of the aster family.

hawse /hɔz/ *n* (*naut*) the part of a ship's bows where the hawseholes are situated; the distance from the bow of an anchored ship to the anchor. • *vi* (*naut*) to pitch violently when at anchor.

hawsehole /'hɔzhoːl/ *n* (*naut*) one of the two holes in the upper part of a ship's bows through which the anchor cables pass when the vessel is moored.

hawser /'hɔzər/ *n* (*naut*) a heavy rope for towing, mooring, etc.

hawthorn /'hɔθɔrn/ *n* any of a genus of spring-flowering spiny shrubs or trees with white or pink flowers and red fruit.

hay /heɪ/ *n* grass cut and dried for fodder.

haybox /'heɪbɒks/ *n* an airtight box packed with hay or any other natural insulating material used to keep partially cooked food warm and allow to cook by retained heat.

haycock /-kɒk/ *n* a conical pile of hay left in the fields to dry out.

hay fever *n* an allergic reaction to pollen, causing irritation of the nose and eyes.

haymaker /-meɪkər/ *n* one who lifts and spreads hay; either of two machines used in haymaking; a wild punch.

haystack /-stæk/, **hayrick** /-rɪk/ *n* a pile of stacked hay ready for storing.

haywire /-waɪr/ *adj* (*inf*) out of order; disorganized.

hazard /'hæzərd/ *n* a risk; a danger; an obstacle on a golf course. • *vt* to risk; to venture.—**hazardable** *adj*.

hazardous /-əs/ *adj* dangerous; risky.—**hazardously** *adv*.—**hazardousness** *n*.

haze /heɪz/ *n* a thin vapour of fog, smoke, etc. in the air; slight vagueness of mind. • *vti* to make or become hazy.

hazel /'heɪzəl/ *n* a tree with edible nuts; a light-brown colour. • *adj* light-brown.

hazelnut /-ˌnʌt/ *n* the edible nut of the hazel.

hazy /'heɪzi/ *adj* (**hazier, haziest**) misty; vague.—**hazily** *adv*.—**haziness** *n*.

HBC /'eɪtʃ'biː'siː/ *abbr* ♣ = Hudson's Bay Company.

H-bomb *n* a hydrogen bomb.

HC *abbr* = Holy Communion; House of Commons.

HCF *abbr* = highest common factor.

HDTV *abbr* = high-definition television.

HE *abbr* = high explosive; His Eminence; His (or Her) Excellency.

He (*chem symbol*) helium.

he /hiː/ *pron* the male person or animal named before; a person (male or female). • *n* a male person or animal.

head /hed/ *n* the part of an animal or human body containing the brain, eyes, ears, nose and mouth; the top part of anything; the foremost part; the chief person; (*pl*) a unit of counting; the striking part of a tool; mind; understanding; the topic of a chapter, etc; crisis, conclusion; pressure of water, steam, etc; the source of a river, etc; froth, as on beer. • *adj* at the head, top or front; coming from in front; chief, leading. • *vt* to command; to lead; to cause to go in a specified direction; to set out; to travel (in a particular direction); to strike (a football) with the head.—**headless** *adj*.

headache /'hedeɪk/ *n* a continuous pain in the head; (*inf*) a cause of worry or trouble.—**headachy** *adj*.

headband /-bænd/ *n* a ribbon or band worn around the head; a narrow strip of cloth stitched to the top of the spine of a book for protection or decoration.

headboard /-bɔrd/ *n* a board that forms the head of a bed, etc.

headdress /-dres/ *n* a decorative covering for the head.

headed /-əd/ *adj* having (a specified kind of) head; having a heading.

header /-ər/ *n* a dive with the head first; (*soccer*) the action of striking the ball with the head.

headfirst /hed'fərst/ *adj* with the head in front; recklessly.—*also adv*.

headgear /'hedgiːr/ *n* a covering for the head, a hat, cap, etc.

head-hunt /-hʌnt/ *vt* to cut off and preserve the heads of enemies as trophies; a person who recruits executive personnel.—**head-hunter** *n*.—**head-hunting** *n*.

heading /-ɪŋ/ *n* something forming the head, top, or front; the title, topic, etc of a chapter, etc; the direction in which a vehicle is moving.

headland /-lænd/ *n* a promontory; unploughed land at the ends of a furrow.

headless /-ləs/ *adj* being without a head; leaderless.

headlamp /-læmp/, **head light** /-laɪt/ *n* a light at the front of a vehicle.

headline /-laɪn/ *n* printed lines at the top of a newspaper article giving the topic; a brief news summary. • *vt* to give featured billing or publicity to.

headlong /-lɒŋ/ *adj, adv* with the head first; with uncontrolled speed or force; rashly.

headman /-mən/ *n* (*pl* **headmen**) the chieftain or leader of a tribe; a foreman or overseer.

headmaster /-ˌmæstər/, **headmistress** /-ˌmɪstrəs/ *n* the principal of a school.—**headmastership, headmistress-ship** *n*.

headmost /-moʊst/ *adj* foremost.

head-on *adj, adv* with the head or front foremost; without compromise.

head over heels *adv* as if somersaulting; completely, utterly, deeply.

headphone /-foʊn/ *n* one of two radio receivers held to the head by a band.

headquarters /-ˌkwɔrtərz/ *n* the centre of operations of one in command. as in an army; the main office in any organization.

headrest /-rest/ *n* a support for the head.

headroom /-ruːm/ *n* space overhead, as in a doorway or tunnel.

heads-up *adj* self-assured and excellent.

headset /-set/ *n* a set of headphones, *usu* with a microphone.

headshrinker /-ˌʃrɪŋkər/ *n* (*sl*) a psychiatrist.

headstall /-stɔl/ *n* the part of a bridle that fits round a horse's head.

head start *n* an early start. any other competitive advantage.

headstone /-stoʊn/ *n* a marker placed at the head of a grave.

headstrong /-strɒŋ/ *adj* determined to do as one pleases; obstinate.

head waiter *n* the head of the dining-room staff in a restaurant.

headwaters /-ˌwɔtərz/ *npl* the small streams that are the source of a river.

headway /-weɪ/ *n* forward motion; progress.

headwind /-wɪnd/ *n* a wind blowing against the direction of a ship or aircraft.

headword /-wərd/ *n* a term placed at the beginning (as of an entry in a dictionary).

headwork /-wərk/ *n* mental work; the decoration on the keystone of an arch.

heady /'hedi/ *adj* (**headier, headiest**) (*alcoholic drinks*) intoxicating; invigorating; exciting; impetuous.—**headily** *adv*.—**headiness** *n*.

heal /hiːl/ *vti* to make or become healthy; to cure; (*wound, etc*) to repair by natural processes.—**healable** *adj*.—**healer** *n*.—**healingly** *adv*.

health /helθ/ *n* physical and mental well-being; freedom from disease, etc; the condition of body or mind; a wish for one's health and happiness, as in a toast.

health card *n* ♣ (*Cdn*) a card identifying a person as eligible to receive medical services paid by a public insurance plan.

health farm *n* a residential establishment for improving health through a strict regime of diet and exercise.

health foods *npl* foods that are organically grown, unprocessed and additive-free.

healthful /-ful/ *adj* healthy.—**healthfully** *adv*.—**healthfulness** *n*.

health maintenance organization *n* a health care organization which meets medical needs in return for a fee.

healthy /'helθi/ *adj* (**healthier, healthiest**) having or producing good health; beneficial; sound.—**healthily** *adv*.—**healthiness** *n*.

heap /hiːp/ *n* a mass or pile of jumbled things; (*pl*) (*inf*) a large amount. • *vt* to throw in a heap; to pile high; to fill (a plate, etc) full or to overflowing.—**heaper** *n*.

hear /hiːr/ *vb* (**hearing, heard**) *vt* to perceive by the ear; to listen to; to conduct a hearing of (a law case, etc); to be informed of; to learn. • *vi* to be able to hear sounds; (*with* **of** *or* **about**) to be told.—**hearable** *adj*.—**hearer** *n*.

hearing /'hiːrɪŋ/ *n* the sense by which sound is perceived by the ear; an opportunity to be heard; the distance over which something can be heard, earshot.

hearing aid *n* a small electronic amplifier worn behind the ear to improve hearing.

hearken /'harkən/ *vi* to listen to.—*also* **harken.**—**hearkener** *n*.

hearsay /'hiːrseɪ/ *n* rumour, gossip.

hearse /hərs/ *n* a vehicle for transporting a coffin to a funeral.

heart /hart/ *n* the hollow, muscular organ that circulates the blood; the central, vital, or main part; the human heart as the centre of emotions, *esp* sympathy, courage, etc; a conventional design representing a heart; one of a suit of playing cards marked with such a symbol in red.

heartache /'harteɪk/ *n* sorrow or grief.

heart attack *n* a sudden instance of abnormal heart functioning, *esp* coronary thrombosis.

heartbeat /'hartbiːt/ *n* the rhythmic contraction and dilation of the heart.

heartbreak /'hartbreɪk/ *n* overwhelming sorrow or grief.—**heartbreaker** *n*.

heartbreaking /-ɪŋ/ *adj* causing heartbreak; pitiful.—**heartbreakingly** *adv*.

heartbroken /'hart,broːkən/ *adj* overcome by sorrow or grief.—**heartbrokenly** *adv*.—**heartbrokenness** *n*.

heartburn /'hartbərn/ *n* a burning sensation in the lower chest.

hearten /'hartən/ *vt* to encourage; to cheer up.—**hearteningly** *adv*.

heart failure *n* the inability of the heart to supply enough blood to the body; a cessation of heart activity leading to death.

heartfelt /'hartfɛlt/ *adj* deeply felt; sincere.

hearth /harθ/ *n* the floor of a fireplace and surrounding area; this as symbolic of house and home.

hearthstone /'harθstoːn/ *n* a stone forming a hearth; soft stone used to whiten hearths, floors, steps, etc.

heartily /'hartɪli/ *adv* in a vigorous or enthusiastic way; sincerely.

heartland /'hartlænd/ *n* the central or most vital part of an area, region, etc.

heartless /-ləs/ *adj* lacking compassion; unfeeling.—**heartlessly** *adv*.—**heartlessness** *n*.

heart-rending *adj* causing much mental anguish.

heartsease /-siːz/ *n* the wild pansy.

heartsick /-sɪk/ *adj* extremely unhappy, despondent.—**heartsickness** *n*.

heartstrings /-strɪŋz/ *npl* deepest feelings.

heart-throb /-θrɒb/ *n* (*inf*) the object of a person's infatuation; a heartbeat.

heart-to-heart *n* an intimate conversation. • *adj* intimate; candid.

heartwood /-wʊd/ *n* the central older wood of a tree, *usu* harder and darker than the outer rings.—*also* **duramen**.

hearty /'harti/ *adj* (**heartier, heartiest**) warm and friendly; (*laughter, etc*) unrestrained; strong and healthy; nourishing and plentiful.—**heartiness** *n*.

heat /hiːt/ *n* energy produced by molecular agitation; the quality of being hot; the perception of hotness; hot weather or climate; strong feeling, *esp* ardour, anger, etc; a single bout, round, or trial in sports; the period of sexual excitement and readiness for mating in female animals; (*sl*) coercion. • *vti* to make or become warm or hot; to make or become excited.

heated /'hiːtəd/ *adj* made hot; excited, impassioned.—**heatedly** *adv*.—**heatedness** *n*.

heater /-ər/ *n* a device that provides heat; (*sl*) a pistol.

heath /hiːθ/ *n* an area of uncultivated land with scrubby vegetation; any of various shrubby plants that thrive on sandy soil, *eg* heather.

heathen /'hiːðən/ *n* (*pl* **heathens, heathen**) anyone not acknowledging the God of Christian, Jew, or Muslim belief; a person regarded as irreligious, uncivilized, etc. • *adj* of or denoting a heathen; irreligious; pagan.—**heathendom** *n*.

heathenish /-ɪʃ/ *adj* relating to or resembling a heathen or heathenish culture; rude, ignorant or uncultured.—**heathenishly** *adv*.—**heathenishness** *n*.

heathenism /-,nɪzəm/ *n* ignorance of God; paganism; idolatry.

heather /'hiːðər/ *n* a common evergreen shrub of northern and alpine regions with small sessile leaves and tiny *usu* purplish pink flowers.—**heathery** *adj*.

heating /'hiːtɪŋ/ *n* a system of providing heat, as central heating; the warmth provided.

heat wave *n* a prolonged period of unusually hot weather.

heave /hiːv/ *vb* (**heaving, heaved**) *vt* to lift or move, *esp* with great effort; to utter (a sigh, etc) with effort; (*inf*) to throw. • *vi* to rise and fall rhythmically; to vomit; to pant; to gasp; to haul; (**heaving, hove**) (*with* **to**) (*ship*) to come to a stop. • *n* the act or effort of heaving.—**heaver** *n*.

heaven /'hɛvən/ *n* (*usu pl*) the visible sky; (*sometimes cap*) the dwelling place of God and his angels where the blessed go after death; any place or state of great happiness; (*pl*) *interj* an exclamation of surprise.

heavenly /-li/ *adj* of or relating to heaven or heavens; divine; (*inf*) excellent, delightful.—**heavenliness** *n*.

heavy /'hɛvi/ *adj* (**heavier, heaviest**) hard to lift or carry; of more than the usual, expected, or defined weight; to an unusual extent; hard to do; stodgy, hard to digest; cloudy; (*industry*) using massive machinery to produce basic materials, as chemicals and steel; (*ground*) difficult to make fast progress on; clumsy; dull, serious. • *n* (*pl* **heavies**) (*theatre*) a villain; (*sl*) a person hired to threaten violence, a thug.—**heavily** *adv*.—**heaviness** *n*.

heavy duty *adj* made to withstand heavy strain or rough usage.

heavy-handed *adj* clumsy; tactless; oppressive.—**heavy-handedly** *adv*.—**heavy-handedness** *n*.

heavy metal *n* a type of rock music characterized by a heavy beat and reliance on loudly amplified instruments.

heavy spar *see* **barium sulphate**.

heavy water *n* deuterium oxide, water in which the normal hydrogen content has been replaced by deuterium.

heavyweight /'hɛvi,weɪt/ *n* a professional boxer weighing more than 175 pounds (79 kg) or wrestler weighing over 209 pounds (95 kg); (*inf*) a very influential or important individual.

hebdomad /hɛb'dɒməd/ *n* (*formerly*) seven; a group of seven; a week.

hebdomadal /-əl/ *adj* weekly.—**hebdomadally** *adv*.

Hebe /'hiːbi/ *n* (*Greek myth*) the goddess of youth.

hebetate /'hɛbəteɪt/ *vti* to make or become dull. • *adj* (*plant*) having a blunt or soft point.—**hebetation** *n*.

hebetude /'hɛbətjuːd/ *n* mental dullness or lethargy.—**hebetudinous** *adj*.

Hebraic /hɪ'breɪk/, **Hebraical** /-əl/ *adj* of or pertaining to the Hebrews, Jewish language or literature.—**Hebraically** *adv*.

Hebraism /hɪ'breɪzəm/ *n* a linguistic usage, custom or idiom borrowed from and characteristic of the Hebrew language, or to the Jewish people or culture.

Hebraist /hɪ'breɪɪst/ *n* one who studies or is learned in the Hebrew language and culture.—**Hebraistic, Hebraistical** *adj*.—**Hebraistically** *adv*.

Hebrew /hɪ'bruː/ *n* a member of an ancient Semitic people; an Israelite; a Jew; the ancient Semitic language of the Hebrews; its modern form. • *adj* pertaining to the Hebrew people; Jewish.

Hecate /'hɛkəti/ *n* (*Greek myth*) a goddess of the underworld.

hecatomb /'hɛkə,tuːm/ in ancient Greece, the ritual sacrifice of 100 oxen; any large sacrifice or slaughter.

heck /hɛk/ *interj* an expression of surprise or grief.

heckle /'hɛkəl/ *vti* to harass (a speaker) with questions or taunts.—**heckler** *n*.

hect- /hɛkt/, **hecto-** /hɛktoː/ *prefix* hundred.

hectare /'hɛktər/ *n* a metric measure of area, equivalent to 10,000 square metres (2.47 acres).

hectic /'hɛktɪk/ *adj* involving intense excitement or activity.—**hectically** *adv*.

hectogram /'hɛktə,græm/ *n* a metric unit of mass equivalent to 100 grams (3.527 ounces).

hectograph /-,græf/ *n* a process for copying a manuscript by transferring it onto a layer of gelatin coated with glycerin; the machine that uses this process. • *vt* to copy in this way.—**hectographic** *adj*.—**hectographically** *adv*.

hector /'hɛktər/ *vt* to bully; to annoy. • *n* a bully.

he'd = /'hiːɪd/ he had, he would.

hedge /hɛdʒ/ *n* a fence consisting of a dense line of bushes or small trees; a barrier or means of protection against something, *esp* financial loss; an evasive or noncommittal answer or statement. • *vt* to surround or enclose with a hedge; to place secondary bets as a precaution. • *vi* to avoid giving a direct answer in an argument or debate.—**hedger** *n*.—**hedgy** *adj*.

hedgehog /'hɛdʒhɒg/ *n* a small insectivorous mammal with sharp spines on the back.

hedgerow /'hɛdʒ,roː/ *n* a line of shrubs or trees separating or enclosing fields.

hedonism /'hedə,nızəm/ *n* the doctrine that personal pleasure is the chief good.—**hedonistic** *adj.*—**hedonist** *n.*

heebie-jeebies /,hi:bi'dʒi:biz/ *npl* (*sl*) nervousness, jitters.

heed /hi:d/ *vt* to pay close attention (to). • *n* careful attention.—**heeder** *n.*

heedful /'hi:dful/ *adj* paying attention; mindful.—**heedfully** *adv.*—**heedfulness** *n.*

heedless /-ləs/ *adj* inattentive; thoughtless.—**heedlessly** *adv.*—**heedlessness** *n.*

heehaw /'hi:hɔ/ *n* (an imitation of) the bray of a donkey, a crude laugh. • *vi* to bray like a donkey.

heel /hi:l/ *n* the back part of the foot, under the ankle; the part covering or supporting the heel in stockings, socks etc, or shoes; a solid attachment forming the back of the sole of a shoe; (*inf*) a despicable person. • *vt* to furnish with a heel; to follow closely; (*inf*) to provide with money, etc. • *vi* to follow along at the heels of someone.—**heelless** *adj.*

heel² /vti/ to tilt or become tilted to one side, as a ship.

heelball /'hi:lbɒl/ *n* a black, waxy substance used to blacken the heels and soles of shoes; a waxy substance used in brass rubbing.

heeler /'hi:lər/ *n* a person who works for a local political organization, *esp* a ward heeler; (*Austral*) a dog that herds cattle by snapping at their heels.

heeltap /'hi:ltæp/ *n* a small layer of leather in the heel of a shoe; the dregs of an alcoholic drink left at the bottom of a glass.

heft /heft/ *vt* to asses the weight of an object by holding it in the hand; to lift; to become used to. • *n* weight; the main part.

hefty /'hefti/ *adj* (**heftier, heftiest**) (*inf*) heavy; large and strong; big.—**heftily** *adv.*—**heftiness** *n.*

Hegelian /he'geiliən/ *adj* relating to or pertaining to the German philosopher Georg Hegel (1770-1831) or his theories.—**Hegelianism** *n.*

hegemony /hə'dʒemoni/ *n* (*pl* **hegemonies**) leadership, domination, *esp* of one nation over others.—**hegemonic** *adj.*

Hegira /'hedʒırə/ or /hı'gi:rə/ *n* the flight of Mohammed from Mecca in AD 622, marking the start of the Muslim era.—*also* **Hejira**.

heifer /'hefər/ *n* a young cow that has not calved.

height /hait/ *n* the topmost point; the highest limit; the distance from the bottom to the top; altitude; a relatively great distance above a given level; an eminence; a hill.

heighten /'haitən/ *vti* to make or come higher or more intense.—**heightener** *n.*

heinous /'hainəs/ *adj* outrageously evil; wicked.—**heinously** *adj.*—**heinousness** *n.*

heir /-er/ *n* a person who inherits or is entitled to inherit another's property, title, etc.—**heirless** *adj.*

heirdom /-'erdəm/ *n* succession by right of blood inheritance.

heiress /-'erəs/ *n* a woman or girl who is an heir, *esp* to great wealth.

heirloom /-'erlu:m/ *n* any possession handed down from generation to generation.

heist /haist/ *n* (*sl*) a robbery. • *vt* (*sl*) to steal.—**heister** *n.*

Hejira /'hedʒırə/ or /hı'gi:rə/ *see* **Hegira**.

held /held/ *see* **hold¹**.

heliacal /hı'laiəkəl/ *adj* emerging from or passing into the light of the sun.

helianthus /,hi:lı'ænθəs/ *n* any of a genus of plants with large yellow flowers, including the sunflower and Jerusalem artichoke.

helical /'helikəl/ *adj* like a helix, spiral.—**helically** *adv.*

helicoid /'helikɔid/ *adj* resembling a flattened spiral. • *n.* a spirally curved geometrical figure.

helicopter /'heli,kɒptər/ *n* a kind of aircraft lifted and moved, or kept hovering, by large rotary blades mounted horizontally.

heliculture /'heli,kʌltʃər/ *n* the rearing of snails for food

helio- /'hi:lio/ *prefix* sun.

heliocentric /,hi:lio'sentrik/ *adj* having the sun as the centre; measured or viewed from the sun's centre.—**heliocentrically** *adv.*—**heliocentricity, heliocentricism** *n.*

heliochrome /-'kro:m/ *n* a photograph in natural colours.

heliograph /-'græf/ *n* a signalling device using the sun's rays reflected by a mirror.—**heliographer** *n.*—**heliographic** *adj.*—**heliography** *n.*

heliogravure /-grə'vjuːr/ *n* photogravure, the process of photoengraving or etching.

heliolatry /-'lætri/ *n* sun worship.

heliometer /,hi:lı'ɒmətər/ *n* a refracting telescope used to measure small angular distances between celestial bodies.

heli-skiing *n* the use of helicopters to take skiers to high, uncrowded off-piste slopes

heliostat /'hi:lia,stæt/ *n* an instrument that sends signals by reflecting the light of the sun in a constant direction.

heliotrope /-,tro:p/ *n* a genus of plants whose flowers follow the course of the sun; a green-hued variety of chalcedony with small red spots; a bloodstone; the bluish-pink colour of the flower heliotrope; an instrument used in geodetic surveying.—**heliotropic** *adj*

heliotropism /,hi:li'ɒtrə,p zəm/ *n* the movement of flowers or leaves towards the sun.—**heliotropic** *adj.*

heliport /'heli,pɔrt/, **helipad** /-,pæd/ *n* a landing and takeoff place for a helicopter.

helium /'hi:liəm/ *n* a light nonflammable gaseous element.

helix /'hi:liks/ *n* (*pl* **helices, helixes**) a spiral line, as a line coiled round; (*zool*) a snail or its shell; (*anat*) the folded rim of the external ear ; (*archit*) a small volute on a capital.

hell /hel/ *n* (*Christianity*) the place of punishment of the wicked after death; the home of devils and demons; any place or state of supreme misery or discomfort; (*inf*) a cause of this. • *interj* (*inf*) an exclamation of anger, surprise, etc.

he'll /'hi:l/ = he will.

hellbent /'hel,bent/ *adj* (*inf*) rashly determined.

hellebore /'heli,bor/ *n* any of a genus of mostly poisonous plants, including the Christmas rose.

Hellene /'helən/, **Hellenian** /'heli:n/ *n* a Greek.

Hellenic /'helənik/ or /-'li:nik/ *adj* of or relating to classical Greece and the Greeks; relating to classical and modern Greeks and their language. • *n* a branch of the Indo-European family of languages made up of Greek and its dialects.

Hellenism /-,nizəm/ *n* the national character of the Greeks; the ideals and principles of classical Greece; the love of Greek culture and art.

Hellenist /-,nist/ *n* a non-Greek, especially a Jew, who spoke Greek in classical times; a student of Greek culture and language.

Hellenistic /-,nistik/ *adj* relating to or characteristic of classical Greece; relating to Greeks or to Hellenism.

Hellenize /-,naiz/ *vt* to adopt classical Greek culture or customs; to use or study the Greek language.—**Hellenization** *n.*—**Hellenizer** *n.*

hellish /'heliʃ/ *adj* of, pertaining to, or resembling hell; very wicked; (*inf*) very unpleasant.—**hellishly** *adv.*—**hellishness** *n.*

hello /hə'loʊ/ *interj* an expression of greeting. • *n* (*pl* **hellos**) the act of saying "hello."—*also* **hallo, hullo** (*pl* **hallos, hullos**).

helm¹ /helm/ *n* (*naut*) the tiller or wheel used to steer a ship; any position of control or direction, authority. • *vt* to steer; to control.

helm² /helm/ *n* (*arch*) a helmet. • *vt* to provide or cover with a helmet.

helmet /'helmət/ *n* protective headgear worn by soldiers, policemen, divers, etc.—**helmeted** *adj.*

helminth /'helminθ/ *n* a worm, *esp* an intestinal one, a fluke.

helminthic /hel'minθik/ *adj* pertaining to worms. • *n* a drug used to treat intestinal worms.

helminthoid /hel'minθɔid/ *adj* worm-shaped.

helminthology /,helminθ'ɒladʒi/ *n* the study of parasitic worms.

helmsman /'helmsmən/ *n* (*pl* **helmsmen**) a person who steers.—**helmswoman** *nf* (*pl* **helmswomen**).

helot /'helət/ *n* a serf or slave; (*with cap*) in ancient Sparta, a state-owned slave.

helotry /'helətri/ *n* slavery or serfdom; the class of slaves or serfs.

help /help/ *vt* to make things better or easier for; to aid; to assist; to remedy; to keep from; to serve or wait on. • *vi* to give aid; to be useful.—*interj* used to ask for assistance. • *n* the action of helping; aid; assistance; a remedy; a person that helps, *esp* a hired person.—**helper** *n.*

helpful /'helpful/ *adj* giving help; useful.—**helpfully** *adv.*—**helpfulness** *n.*

helping /-iŋ/ *n* a single portion of food.

helpless /-ləs/ *adj* unable to manage alone, dependent on others; weak and defenceless.—**helplessly** *adv.*—**helplessness** *n.*

helpmate /-meit/, **helpmeet** /-mi:t/ *n* a helpful companion, *esp* a wife or husband.

help-wanted index *n* ✸ (*Cdn*) a seasonally-adjusted measure of employment, based on jobs that are advertised.

helter-skelter /,heltər'skeltər/ *adv* in confused haste. • *adj* disorderly. • *n* a tall spiral slide *usu* found in an amusement park.

helve /helv/ *n* the handle of a tool.

Helvetia /hɛl'viːʃə/ or /-ʃiə/ n the Latin name for Switzerland.

Helvetian /hɛl'viːʃən/ adj of or relating to Helvetia; Swiss. • n a native or citizen of Switzerland.

hem /hɛm/ n the edge of a garment, etc, turned back and stitched or fixed. • vt (**hemming, hemmed**) to finish (a garment) with a hem; (with **in**) to enclose, confine.—**hemmer** n.

he-man n (pl **he-men**) (inf) an excessively masculine or strongly built male.

hematite /'hiːmə,taɪt/ n native ferric oxide, an important iron ore.—also **haematite**.

hematology /,hiːmə'tɒlədʒi/ n the branch of medicine dealing with blood and its diseases.—**hematologic, hematological** adj.—**hematologist** n.

hemi- /'hɛmi/ prefix half; partial.

hemicycle /'hɛmi,saɪkəl/ n a half-circle, semicircle.—**hemicyclic** adj.

hemidemisemiquaver /-dɛmi,sɛmikweɪvər/ n (mus) a sixty-fourth note.

hemihedral /hɛmi'hɛdrəl/ adj (crystal) having only half the normal number of faces.

hemiplegia /-'pliːdʒiə/ n paralysis of one side.—**hemiplegic** adj, n.

hemisphere /-'sfiːr/ n half of a sphere or globe; any of the halves (northern, southern, eastern, or western) of the earth.—**hemispheric, hemispherical** adj.—**hemispherically** adv.

hemistitch /'hɛmistɪk/ n half of a line of verse.

hemline /'hɛmlaɪn/ n the bottom edge of a skirt or dress.

hemlock /'hɛmlɒk/ n a poisonous plant with small white flowers; a poison made from this plant.

hemmer /'hɛmər/ n one who stitches hems; a machine for hemming.

hemoglobin /,hiːmə'gloːbɪn/ n the oxygen-carrying red colouring matter of the red blood corpuscles.

hemophilia /-'fiːliə/ n a hereditary condition in which the blood fails to clot normally.—**hemophiliac, hemophile** n.—**hemophilic** adj.

hemorrhage /'hɛmərɪdʒ/ n the escape of blood from a blood vessel; heavy bleeding. • vi to bleed heavily.—**hemorrhagic** adj.

hemorrhoids /'hɛmə,rɔɪd/ npl swollen or bleeding veins around the anus.—also **piles**.—**hemorrhoidal** adj.

hemp /'hɛmp/ n a widely cultivated Asian herb of the mulberry family; its fibre, used to make rope, sailcloth, etc; a narcotic drug obtained from different varieties of this plant.—also **cannabis, marijuana**.—**hempen** adj.

hemstitch /'hɛmstɪtʃ/ n an ornamental stitch.—**hemstitcher** n.

hen /hɛn/ n the female of many birds, esp the chicken.

henbane /'hɛnbeɪn/ n a poisonous, sticky, hairy plant of the nightshade family.

hence /hɛns/ adv from here; from this time; from this reason.

henceforth /hɛns'fɔrθ/, **henceforward** /-'fɔrwərd/ adv from now on.

henchman /'hɛntʃmən/ n (pl **henchmen**) a trusted helper or follower.

hendecagon /hɛn'dɛkə,gɒn/ n an eleven-sided plane figure.—**hendecagonal** adj.

hendecasyllable /-'sɪləbəl/ n a verse of eleven syllables.—**hendecasyllabic** adj.

hendiadys /hɛn'daɪədɪs/ n the use of two connected words to express one idea, as "with might and main."

henna /'hɛnə/ n a tropical plant; a reddish-brown dye extracted from its leaves used to tint the hair or skin. • vt to dye with henna.

hennery /'hɛnəri/ n (pl **henneries**) a poultry farm.

henotheism /'hɛnə,θiːɪzəm/ n the worship of one god while recognizing the existence of others.—**henotheist** n, adj.—**henotheistic** adj.

henpeck /'hɛnpɛk/ vt to nag and domineer over (one's husband).—**henpecked** adj.

henry /'hɛnri/ n (pl **henries, henrys**) a unit of electrical inductance.

hent /hɛnt/ vt (arch) to seize; to grasp. • n (arch) a clutching; intention; anything that has been gasped by the mind.

hepat- /'hɛpæt/, **hepato-** /'hɛpæto/ prefix liver.

hepatic /hɪ'pætɪk/ adj of, like, or pertaining to the liver. • n a drug for treating the liver.

hepatitis /,hɛpə'taɪtɪs/ n inflammation of the liver.

heptad /'hɛptæd/ n a group of seven; the number seven; an atom or element with the valency of seven.

heptagon /'hɛptəgɒn/ n a polygon of seven angles and seven sides.—**heptagonal** adj.

heptahedron /,hɛptə'hiːdrən/ n (pl **heptahedrons, heptahedra**) a solid figure with seven plane faces.—**heptahedral** adj.

heptameter /hɛp'tɒmətər/ n a verse line of seven metrical feet.

heptarchy /hɛp'tɑrki/ n (pl **heptarchies**) government by seven rulers; a state divided into seven regions each with its own ruler; the seven kingdoms of Anglo-Saxon England.

Heptateuch /'hɛptə,tjuːk/ n (Bible) the first seven books of the Old Testament.

her /hər/ pron the objective and possessive case of the personal pronoun **she**. • adj of or belonging to a female.

herald /'hɛrəld/ n a person who conveys news or messages; a forerunner, harbinger; (Middle Ages) an official at a tournament. • vt to usher in; to proclaim.

heraldic /-ɪk/ adj of a herald or heraldry.—**heraldically** adv.

heraldry /-ri/ n (pl **heraldries**) the study of genealogies and coats of arms; ceremony; pomp.—**heraldist** n.

herb /hɜrb/ or /'ɜrb/ n any seed plant whose stem withers away annually; any plant used as a medicine, seasoning, etc.

herbaceous /hɜr'beɪʃəs/ or /'ɜrb-/ adj of or like herbs; green and leafy.

herbage /'hɜrbɪdʒ/ or /'ɜrb-/ n pasturage; the succulent parts of herbs.

herbal /'hɜrbəl/ or /'ɜrb-/ adj of herbs. • n a book listing and describing plants with medicinal properties.

herbalist /-ɪst/ n a person who practises healing by using herbs; a person who grows or deals in herbs.

herbarium /hɜr'bɛriəm/ or /'ɜrb-/ n (pl **herbariums, herbaria**) a (place or container for a) systematic collection of dried plants.—**herbarial** adj.

herb Christopher see **baneberry**.

herbicide /'hɜrbi,saɪd/ or /'ɜrb-/ n a substance for destroying plants.—**herbicidal** adj.

herbivore /'hɜrbi,vɔːr/ or /'ɜrb-/ n a plant-eating animal.

herbivorous /-əs/ adj herb-eating; (animals) plant-eating.—**herbivorousness** n.

herby /'hɜrbi/ or /'ɜrb-/ adj (**herbier, herbiest**) herb-like; rich in herbs.

herculean /,hɜrkjuˈliən/ or /-kjuː-/ adj of extraordinary strength, size, or difficulty; (with cap) of or like the Roman god Hercules.

herd /hɜrd/ n a large number of animals, esp cattle, living and feeding together. • vi to assemble or move animals together. • vt to gather together and move as if a herd; to tend, as a herdsman.—**herder** n.

herdsman /'hɜrdsmən/ n (pl **herdsmen**) a person who tends a herd of animals.

here /hiːr/ adv at or in this place; to or into this place; now; on earth.

hereabout /,hiːrə'baʊt/, **hereabouts** /-ə'baʊts/ adv in this area.

hereafter /hiːr'æftər/ adv after this, in some future time or state. • n (with **the**) the future, life after death.

hereat /-'æt/ adv (arch) because of this.

hereby /-baɪ/ adv by this means.

hereditable /hɪ'rɛdɪtəbəl/ adj that may be inherited, heritable.—**hereditability** n.—**hereditably** adv.

hereditament /'hɛrɪdɪtəmənt/ or /hɪ'rɛdɪ-/ n (law) property capable of being inherited.

hereditary /hɪ'rɛdɪtəri/ adj descending by inheritance; transmitted to offspring.—**hereditarily** adv.—**hereditariness** n.

heredity /hɪ'rɛdɪti/ n (pl **heredities**) the transmission of genetic material that determines physical and mental characteristics from one generation to another.

herein /hiːr'ɪn/ adv (formal) in this place, document, etc.

hereinafter /,hiːrɪn'æftər/ adv (formerly) afterwards of this.

hereof /hiːr'ɒf/ adv of this.

heresiarch /he'riːzi,ɑrk/ n the leader or fonder of a heretical movement or sect.

heresy /'hɛrəsi/ n (pl **heresies**) a religious belief regarded as contrary to the orthodox doctrine of a church; any belief or opinion contrary to established or accepted theory.

heretic /'hɛrətɪk/ n a dissenter from an established belief or doctrine.—**heretical** adj.—**heretically** adv.

hereto /hiːr'tuː/ adv (formal) to this matter, document, etc.

heretofore /,hiːrtuˈfɔr/ adv (formal) until now.

hereunder /hiːr'ʌndər/ adv (formal) below.

hereupon /,hiːrə'pɒn/ adv (formal) on this matter, issue, etc; immediately after this.

herewith /hiːr'wɪð/ or /-'wɪθ/ adv (formal) with this.

heriot /'herɪət/ n a tribute, usu cattle paid to a feudal lord on the death of a tenant by his heir.

heritable /'herɪtəbəl/ adj able to be inherited, hereditable.—**heritably** adv.

heritage /'herɪtɪdʒ/ n something inherited at birth; anything deriving from the past or tradition; historical sites, traditions, practices, etc regarded as the valuable inheritance of contemporary society; ✤ designated as worthy of preservation because of historic, architectural, or environmental value.

heritor /'herɪtər/ n (law) one who inherits; a proprietor.

hermaphrodite /hər'mæfrə,daɪt/ n an animal or organism with both male and female reproductive organs; a plant with stamens and pistils in the same floral envelope.—**hermaphroditic** adj.—**hermaphroditically** adv.

hermaphrodite brig n a brig square-rigged forward and schooner-rigged aft.

hermaphroditism /-dɪ,tɪzəm/, **hermaphrodism** ,-dɪzəm/ n the state of being an hermaphrodite.

hermeneutics /,hərmɪ'nuːtɪks/ or /-'njuː-/ n sing the science of interpretation, esp of the Bible.—**hermeneutic, hermeneutical** adj.—**hermeneutically** adv.

hermetic /hər'metɪk/, **hermetical** /-əl/ adj perfectly closed and airtight; of alchemy, magical.—**hermetically** adv.

hermit /'hɜrmɪt/ n a person who lives in complete solitude, esp for religious reasons; a recluse.—**hermitic, hermitical** adj.—**hermitically** adv.

hermitage /'hɜrmɪtɪdʒ/ n the dwelling place of a hermit; a secluded retreat.

hern /hɜrn/ n (arch) the heron.

hernia /'hɜrniə/ n (pl **hernias, herniae**) the protrusion of an organ, esp part of the intestine, through an opening in the wall of the cavity in which it sits; a rupture.—**hernial** adj.—**herniated** adj.

hero /hi'roː/ n (pl **heroes**) a person of exceptional bravery; a person admired for superior qualities and achievements; the central male character in a novel, play, etc

heroic /'hi'rɔɪk/ adj of, worthy of, or like a hero; having the qualities of a hero; daring, risky; (poetry) of or about heroes and their deeds, epic; (language) grand, high-flown. • n heroic verse; (pl) melodramatic talk or behaviour.—**heroically** adv.

heroic age n the age in which the legendary heroes of a nation, esp ancient Greece and Rome, are fabled to have lived in.

heroic couplet n a rhyming couplet in iambic pentameter, used in English heroic verse.

heroic verse n a verse form used in epic poetry, ie the hexameter in Greek and Latin poetry, the iambic pentameter in English, and the Alexandrine in French.

heroin /'herʊɪn/ n a powerfully addictive drug derived from morphine.

heroine /'herʊɪn/ n a woman with the attributes of a hero; the leading female character in a novel, film or play.

heroism /'herʊ,ɪzəm/ n the qualities or conduct of a hero; bravery.

heron /'herən/ n a long wading bird with long legs and neck.

heronry /'herənri/ n (pl **heronries**) a heron rookery; a breeding place for herons.

herpes /'hɜrpiːz/ n any of several virus diseases marked by small blisters on the skin or mucous membranes.—**herpetic** adj.

herpetology /,hɜrpɪ'tɒlədʒi/ n the study of snakes and amphibians.—**herpetologist** n.

Herr /her/, Ger. /her/ n (pl **Herren**) a title, the German equivalent of Mister or Sir.

herring /'herɪŋ/ n (pl **herrings, herring**) a small food fish of commercial importance.

herringbone /'herɪŋ,boːn/ n a kind of cross-stitch; a zigzag pattern used in brickwork; (skiing) a method of walking uphill with the skis pointing outwards. • vt to work in cross-stitch; to decorate with a herringbone pattern. • vi to ascend a ski slope in herringbone fashion.

herring choker n ✤ (Cdn) (sl) a New Brunswicker.

hers /hɜrz/ pron something or someone belonging to her.

herself /hər'self/ pron the reflexive form of **she** or **her**.

hertz /hɜrts/ n (pl **hertz**) the unit of frequency equal to one cycle per second.

he's /'hiːz/ = he is; he has.

Hesiodic /'hiːsɪədɪk/ adj pertaining to or in the style of Hesiod, a Greek didactic poet of the 8th century BC.

hesitancy /'hezɪtənsi/ n (pl **hesitancies**) an act of hesitating; the state of being hesitant; indecision.

hesitant /'hezɪtənt/ adj hesitating; indecisive; reluctant; shy.—**hesitantly** adv.

hesitate /,hezɪ'teɪt/ vi to be slow in acting due to uncertainty or indecision; to be reluctant (to); to falter or stammer when speaking.—**hesitater** n.—**hesitatingly** adv.

hesitation /,hezɪ'teɪʃən/ n the act of hesitating; a pause in speech.

Hesperian /'hespiːrɪən/ adj of or relating to the Hesperides; western. • n a native or inhabitant of a western land.

Hesperides /'hesperədiːz/ n (Greek myth) (pl) the nymphs who guarded the golden apples given by Gaia to Hera on her marriage to Zeus; (sing) the garden containing the golden apples.

Hesperus /'hesperəs/ n the evening star, esp Venus.

Hessian /'heʃən/ adj pertaining to the German state of Hesse. • n a native or inhabitant of Hesse; a mercenary soldier.

hessian /'heʃən/ n a coarse cloth made of jute.

hest /'hest/ n (arch) a behest; a command.

hetaera, hetaira /hɪ'tiːrə/ n (pl **hetaerae, hetaeras, hetairai**) a female prostitute or courtesan, esp in ancient Greece.—**hetaeric, hetairic** adj.

heter- /'hetər/, **hetero-** /'hetəroː/ prefix another; abnormal; different, other, unequal.

heterocercal /,hetəroː'siːrəl/ adj (fish) having the upper lobe of the tail longer than the lower lobe.

heterochromatic /-krə'mætɪk/ adj of different colours.

heteroclite /-'klaɪt/ n an irregularly inflected or unusual word; an unusual person or thing. • adj irregular; deviating from the ordinary.—also **heteroclitic**.

heterodox /'hetəroː,dɒks/ adj contrary to established beliefs or opinions; unorthodox; heretical.

heterodoxy /-,dɒksi/ n (pl **heterodoxies**) the state of being heterodox; an unorthodox doctrine or opinion; heresy.

heterodyne /-daɪn/ vt to impose (a radio frequency wave) on a transmitting wave to produce pulsations of audible frequency. • adj having or produced by combining waves of different lengths.

heterogamous /,hetə'rɒgəməs/ adj (bot) bearing two kinds of flowers that differ sexually.

heterogeneous /,hetəroː'dʒiːnəs/ adj opposite or dissimilar in character, quality structure, etc; not homogeneous; disparate.—**heterogeneity** n.—**heterogeneously** adv.

heterogenesis /,hetəroː'dʒenəsɪs/ n the production by certain organisms of offspring differing in structure and habit from the parent, but reverting in subsequent generations to the original type.—**heterogenetic** adj.

heterogenous /,hetə'rɒdʒənəs/ adj (biol) originating outside the body; foreign.—**heterogeny** n.

heterologous /,hetə'rɒləgəs/ adj (biol) abnormal in type or structure; derived from a different species; consisting of the same elements in varying proportions.—**heterology** n.

heteromorphism /,hetəroː'mɔrfɪzəm/ n (biol) deviation from the natural form or structure.—**heteromorphic** adj.

heteronomous /,hetə'rɒnəməs/ adj differing from the normal type; subject to external law, rule or authority.—**heteronomously** adv.

heteronym /'hetərə,nɪm/ n a word spelled in the same way as another or others but having a different meaning, as brake (in a vehicle) and brake (fern).—**heteronymous** adj.

heterophyllous /,hetəroː'fɪləs/ adj (plants) having leaves of different forms on the same stem.—**heterophylly** n.

heterosexual /,hetəroː'sekʃʊəl/ adj sexually attracted to the opposite sex. • n a heterosexual person.—**heterosexuality** n.—**heterosexually** adv.

hetman /'hetmən/ n (pl **hetmen**) (formerly) a Cossack prince or general.

het-up /het'ʌp/ adj (inf) agitated, annoyed.

heulandite /'hjuːlən,daɪt/ n a vitreous transparent brittle mineral.

heuristic /hjʊ'rɪstɪk/ adj assisting or leading to discovery or invention.—**heuristically** adv.

hew /hjuː/ vb (**hewing, hewed**, pp **hewed, hewn**) vt to strike or cut with blows using an axe, etc; to shape with such blows. • vi to conform (to a rule, principle, etc).—**hewer** n.

hex /heks/ vt to bewitch; to bring bad luck. • n a magic spell; a curse; a witch.

hex- /heks/, **hexa-** /heksə/ prefix six.

hexachord /'heksə,kɔrd/ n (mus) a diatonic series of six notes with a semitone between third and fourth.

hexad /'hɛksæd/ *n* a group or series of six; the number or sum of six; a chemical element, atom, or radical that can be combined with, or replaced by, six atoms of hydrogen.—**hexadic** *adj*.

hexagon /'hɛksəgɒn/ *n* a polygon having six sides and six angles.—**hexagonal** *adj*.—**hexagonally** *adv*.

hexagram /hɛksə,græm/ *n* a plane figure having six angles and six sides; a six-pointed star formed by two intersecting triangles; a group of six lines which may be combined into 64 different patterns in I Ching.

hexahedron /,hɛksə'hi:drɒn/ *n* a solid bounded by six plane faces.—**hexahedral** *adj*.

hexameter /hɛk'sæmɪtər/ *n* a line of Greek or Latin verse consisting of six feet the last usually being a spondee; a verse line consisting of six metric feet.—**hexametric, hexametrical** *adj*.

hexapod /'hɛksə,pɒd/ *n* any of a large class of anthropods; an animal with six legs; an insect. • *adj* having six legs.—*also* **hexapodous**.

Hexateuch /'hɛksə,tu:k/ or /-,tju:k/ *n* (*Bible*) the first six books of the Old Testament.

hey /heɪ/ *interj* an expression of joy, surprise or to call attention.

heyday /'heɪdeɪ/ *n* a period of greatest success, happiness, etc.

HF *abbr* = high frequency.

Hf (*chem symbol*) = hafnium.

Hfx. *abbr* ✹ = Halifax (Nova Scotia).

Hg (*chem symbol*) = mercury.

HGV *abbr* = heavy goods vehicle.

hi /haɪ/ *interj* an exclamation of greeting.

hiatus /haɪ'eɪtəs/ *n* (*pl* **hiatuses, hiatus**) a break in continuity; a lacuna; (*med*) an aperture; (*phonetics*) the concurrence of two vowels in two successive syllables.—**hiatal** *adj*.

hibernaculum /haɪbər'nækju:ləm/ *n* (*pl* **hibernacula**) the winter quarters of a hibernating animal; the bud-scales of a winter bud.

hibernal *adj* /'haɪbərnəl/ of or happening in winter; wintry.

hibernate /'haɪbərneɪt/ *vi* to spend the winter in a dormant condition like deep sleep; to be inactive.—**hibernation** *n*.—**hibernator** *n*.

Hibernian /haɪ'bərnɪən/ *adj* relating to Ireland. • *n* a native or inhabitant of Ireland.

hibiscus /hɪ'bɪskəs/ or /haɪ-/ *n* any plant of a tropical or subtropical genus of plants with large showy flowers.

hiccup, hiccough /'hɪkəp/ *n* a sudden involuntary spasm of the diaphragm followed by inhalation and closure of the glottis producing a characteristic sound; (*inf*) a minor setback. • *vt* (**hiccuping, hiccuped** *or* **hiccupping, hiccupped**) to have hiccups.

hic jacet /hɪk'dʒeɪsɛt/ or /hɪk'dʒækɛt/ *n* (*Latin* here lies) an inscription on tombstones.

hick /hɪk/ *n* (*inf*) an unsophisticated person, *esp* from a rural area.

hickory /'hɪkərɪ/ *n* (*pl* **hickories**) a North American tree of the walnut family; its wood; its smooth-shelled edible nut.

hid /hɪd/ *see* **hide**[1].

hidalgo /hɪ'dælgɒ:/ *n* (*pl* **hidalgoes**) a low-ranking Spanish nobleman.

hidden /'hɪdən/ *adj* concealed or obscured.

hide[1] /haɪd/ *vb* (**hiding, hid**, *pp* **hidden, hid**) *vt* to conceal, put out of sight; to keep secret; to screen or obscure from view. • *vi* to conceal oneself. • *n* a camouflaged place of concealment used by hunters, bird-watchers, etc.—**hider** *n*.

hide[2] *n* the raw or dressed skin of an animal; (*inf*) the human skin.

hide[3] *n* an ancient English measure of land.

hide-and-seek *n* a children's game in which one player must find the others, who have hidden themselves.

hidebound /'haɪdbaʊnd/ *adj* obstinately conservative and narrow-minded; (*animals*) having a tight or contracted hide that impedes movement; (*trees*) having a tight bark that restricts growth.

hideous /'hɪdɪəs/ *adj* visually repulsive; horrifying.—**hideously** *adv*.—**hideousness** *n*.

hiding[1] /'haɪdɪŋ/ *n* (*inf*) a thrashing, a beating.

hiding[2] *n* concealment.

hiding place *n* a place of concealment.

hidrosis /hɪdroːsɪs/ or /haɪ-/ *n* perspiration; any skin disease affecting the sweat glands.

hidrotic /hɪdro:tɪk/ or /haɪ-/ *adj* of or promoting perspiration. • *n* a drug that stimulates sweating.

hie /haɪ/ *vti* (**hieing** *or* **hying, hied**) (*poet*) to speed; to hasten.

hier- /haɪr/, **hiero-** /haɪrɒ/ *prefix* sacred.

hierarch /'haɪər,ɑrk/ *n* the chief ruler of an ecclesiastical body; a person at a high level of hierarchy.

hierarchism /haɪər'ɑrkɪzəm/ *n* hierarchical principles; government by a hierarchy.—**hierarchist** *n*.

hierarchy /haɪər'ɑrkɪ/ *n* (*pl* **hierarchies**) a group of persons or things arranged in order of rank, grade, etc.—**hierarchical, hierarchic** *adj*.—**hierarchically** *adv*.

hieratic /haɪər'ætɪk/ *adj* of or relating to priests; sacred; consecrated; of or relating to a cursive form of hieroglyphics used by priests in ancient Egypt. • *n* the Egyptian hieratic script.—**hieratically** *adv*.

hierocracy /haɪər'ɒkrəsɪ/ *n* (*pl* **hierocrocies**) government by priests or ecclesiastics.

hieroglyph /'haɪr,əglɪf/ *n* a character used in a system of hieroglyphic writing.

hieroglyphic /haɪr'əglɪfɪk/ *n* a sacred character or symbol; (*pl*) the picture writings of the ancient Egyptians and others. • *adj* pertaining to hieroglyphs; emblematic.—**hieroglyphically** *adv*.

hierology /,haɪ'rɒlədʒɪ/ *n* (*pl* **hierologies**) the sacred literature of people; a biography of a saint.

hierophant /'haɪrə,fænt/ *n* in ancient Greece, a priest who initiated novices into the sacred mysteries; a person who explains arcane mysteries.

hifalutin /,haɪfə'lu:tin/ *see* **highfalutin**.

hi-fi *n* /'haɪfaɪ/ (*inf*) high fidelity; equipment for reproducing high quality musical sound.

higgle /'hɪgəl/ *vi* to dispute over trifling matters; to haggle.

higgledy-piggledy /,hɪgəldɪ'pɪgəldɪ/ *adj, adv* (*inf*) in confusion; jumbled up.

high /haɪ/ *adj* lofty, tall; extending upward a (specified) distance; situated at or done from a height; above others in rank, position, etc; greater in size, amount, cost, etc than usual; raised or acute in pitch; (*meat*) slightly bad; (*inf*) intoxicated; (*inf*) under the influence of drugs. • *adv* in or to a high degree, rank, etc. • *n* a high level, place, etc; an area of high barometric pressure; (*inf*) a euphoric condition induced by alcohol or drugs.

high and dry *adj* helpless; stranded; (*ship*) out of the water.

high and mighty *adj* (*inf*) arrogant.

High Arctic *n* ✹ (*Cdn*) the part of the Arctic within the Arctic Circle.—*also* **High North**.

highball /'haɪbɒl/ *n* a cool drink with spirits, soda, etc, served in a tall glass.

highborn *adj* of noble birth.

highboy /-bɔɪ/ *n* (*US*) a chest of drawers on legs; a tallboy.

highbrow /-braʊ/ *n* (*inf*) an intellectual. • *adj* (*inf*) interested in things requiring learning.

High Church *n* the part of the Anglican Church that attaches great importance to the authority of the Church, its sacraments and priesthood.—**High-Church** *adj*.

high-class *adj* of good quality; of or appropriate to the upper social classes.

High Commission *n* ✹ a diplomatic mission representing one member country in the Commonwealth of Nations in another.—**High Commissioner** *n*

higher /haɪər/ *adj* more high. • *adv* in or to a higher position.

higher education *n* education at college or university level.

higher-up *n* (*inf*) a person of higher rank.

high explosive *n* a very powerful chemical explosive, such as gelignite.

highfalutin /,haɪfə'lu:tin/, **highfaluting** /-tɪŋ/ *adj* (*inf*) pretentious; pompous.—*also* **hifalutin**.

high fidelity *n* the high quality reproduction of sound.

high-five *n* an action or gesture as a greeting, acclamation or celebration where two people slap their open right hands together at head height or above.

high-flown *adj* extravagantly ambitious; bombastic.

high-flyer, high-flier *n* an ambitious person; a person of great ability in any profession.—**high-flying** *adj*.

high frequency *n* any radio frequency between 3 and 30 megahertz.

high-handed *adj* overbearing, arbitrary.—**high-handedly** *adv*.—**high-handedness** *n*.

high-hat *vti* (**high-hatting, high-hatted**) to affect superiority; to treat patronizingly. • *n* a person who behaves in this way.

highjack, highjacker *see* **hijack**.

high jinks *npl* (*inf*) mischievous sport or tricks.

high jump *n* an athletic event in which a competitor jumps over a high bar; (*inf*) (*with* **the**) a severe reprimand.

highland /ˈhaɪlənd/ *adj* of or in mountains. • *n* a region with many hills or mountains; (*pl*) mountainous country; (*with cap*) the mountainous region occupying most of northern Scotland.

highlander *n* a person who lives in a highland area; (*with cap*) an inhabitant of the Scottish Highlands.

Highland fling *n* a lively Scottish dance by one person.

highlife /ˈhaɪlaɪf/ *n* (*W Africa*) a style of jazz music combining American and African elements.

high life *n* fashionable society; its manner of living.—**high-life** *adj*.

highlight /ˈhaɪlaɪt/ *n* the lightest area of a painting, etc; the most interesting or important feature; (*pl*) a lightening of areas of the hair using a bleaching agent. • *vt* to bring to special attention; to give highlights to.

highly /ˈhaɪlɪ/ *adv* highly, very much; favourably; at a high level, wage, rank, etc.

highly strung *adj* nervous and tense; excitable; high-strung.

High Mass *n* (*RC Church*) a ceremonial mass, usu at the high altar, at which a deacon or subdeacon assist the celebrant.

high-minded /haɪˈmaɪndəd/ *adj* having high ideals, etc.—**high-mindedness** *n*.

highness /ˈhaɪnəs/ *n* the state or quality of being high; (*with cap and poss pron*) a title used in speaking to or of royalty.

High North *n* ✤ High Arctic.

high-pitched *adj* (*sound*) shrill; (*roof*) steep.

high-powered, high-power *adj* (*lens, etc*) producing great magnification; energetic; powerful; highly competent.

high priest *n* a chief priest, *esp* the principal priest of the Jewish hierarchy; an unofficial leader of fashion, etc.

high-rise *adj* (*building*) having multiple storeys. • *n* a building of this kind.

highroad *n* a chief road, a highway; an easy course or method.

high roller *n* a gambler; an extravagant person; a leader of fashion.—**high rolling** *adj*, *n*.

high school *n* a secondary school.

high seas *npl* open ocean waters outside the territorial limits of any nation.

high season *n* the busiest time of the year for a holiday resort, etc.

high-sounding *adj* imposing, pompous.

high-spirited *adj* courageous; lively.—**high-spiritedness** *n*.

high-strung *adj* strung to a high pitch; extremely sensitive; highly strung.

hightail /ˈhaɪteɪl/ *vi* to leave in a great rush.

high tide *n* the tide at its highest level; the time of this; an acme.

high time *adv* (*inf*) fully time. • *n* an especially good or enjoyable time.

high treason *n* treason against the ruler or state.

high-up *n* (*inf*) a person of high status or position.

high water *n* high tide.—**highwater** *adj*.

highwater mark *n* the highest point reached by a high tide; any maximum.

highway /ˈhaɪweɪ/ *n* a public road; a main thoroughfare.

highwayman /ˈhaɪweɪmən/ *n* (*pl* **highwaymen**) one who robs travellers on a highway.

high wire *n* a high tightrope.

hijack /ˈhaɪdʒæk/ *vt* to steal (goods in transit) by force; to force (an aircraft) to make an unscheduled flight. • *n* an act of hijacking.—*also* **highjack**.—**hijacker, highjacker** *n*.

hike /haɪk/ *vi* to take a long walk. • *vt* (*inf*) to pull up, to increase. • *n* a long walk; a tramp.—**hiker** *n*.

hilarious /hɪˈleərɪəs/ *adj* highly amusing.—**hilariously** *adv*.—**hilariousness** *n*.—**hilarity** *n*.

hilarity /hɪˈlerɪtɪ/ *n* mirth; merriment; cheerfulness.

hill /hɪl/ *n* a natural rise of land lower than a mountain; a heap or mound; an slope in a road, etc. *vt* to bank up; to draw earth around (plants) in mounds; ✤ (*Cdn*) (*cap*) Parliament Hill.

hillbilly /ˈhɪlbɪlɪ/ *n* (*pl* **hillbillies**) (*inf*) a person from the mountainous areas of southeastern US; country music.—*also adj*.

hillock /ˈhɪlək/ *n* a small hill.—**hillocked, hillocky** *adj*.

hilly /ˈhɪlɪ/ *adj* (**hillier, hilliest**) abounding with or characterized by hills; rugged.—**hilliness** *n*.

hilt /hɪlt/ *n* the handle of a sword, dagger, tool, etc.

hilum /ˈhaɪləm/ *n* (*pl* **hila**) a scar on the surface of a seed indicating where it was attached to the seed grain; the nucleus of a starch grain.

him /hɪm/ *pron* the objective case of **he**.

himation /hɪˈmæʃən/ *n* (*pl* **himatia**) in ancient Greece, a square-shaped cloak draped around the body.

himself /hɪmˈself/ *pron the reflexive* (he killed himself) *or emphatic* (he himself was lucky) *form of* **he, him**.

Himyaritic /ˈhɪmjəˌraɪt/ *n* an extinct language of the Semitic family of the Afro-Asian family; an Arabian dialect. • *adj* of or relating to the Hymarite people of Arabia or their language.

hind[1] /haɪnd/ *adj* (**hinder, hindmost** *or* **hindermost**) situated at the back; rear.

hind[2] *n* (*pl* **hinds, hind**) a female deer.

hinder /ˈhɪndər/ *vt* to obstruct, delay or impede. • *vi* to impose instructions or impediments. • *adj* belonging to or constituting the back or rear of anything.—**hinderer** *n*.

Hindi /ˈhɪndi/ *n* the official language of India; a group of dialects of northern India.

hindmost /ˈhaɪndməʊst/, **hindermost** /ˈhɪndərməʊst/ *adj* farthest behind.

hindquarters /ˈhaɪndˌkwɔːtərz/ *npl* the hind legs and accompanying parts of a quadruped.

hindrance /ˈhɪndrəns/ *n* the act of hindering; an obstacle, impediment.

hindsight /ˈhaɪndsaɪt/ *n* understanding an event after it has occurred.

Hindu /ˈhɪnduː/ *n* (*pl* **Hindus**) any of several peoples of India; a follower of Hinduism.

Hinduism /ˈhɪnduːˌɪzəm/ *n* the dominant religion of India, characterized by an emphasis on religious law, a caste system and belief in reincarnation.

hinge /hɪndʒ/ *n* a joint or flexible part on which a door, lid, etc turns; a natural joint, as of a clam; a small piece of gummed paper for sticking stamps in an album. • *vti* to attach or hang by a hinge; to depend.

hinny /ˈhɪni/ *n* (*pl* **hinnies**) the sterile offspring of a male horse and a female donkey or ass. • *vi* to neigh.

hint /hɪnt/ *n* an indirect or subtle suggestion; a slight mention; a little piece of practical or helpful advice. • *vt* to suggest or indicate indirectly. • *vi* to give a hint.—**hinter** *n*.

hinterland /ˈhɪntərˌlænd/ *n* the land behind that bordering a coast or river; a remote area.

hip[1] /hɪp/ *n* either side of the body below the waist and above the thigh.

hip[2] *n* the fruit of the wild rose.

hip[3] *interj* used as part of a cheer (*hip, hip, hurrah*).

hip[4] *adj* (*sl*) stylish, up-to-date.

hippie, hippy /ˈhɪpi/ *n* (*pl* **hippies**) (*sl*) a person who adopts an alternative lifestyle, *eg* involving mysticism, psychedelic drugs, or communal living, to express alienation from conventional society.

hippo /ˈhɪpəʊ/ *n* (*pl* **hippos**) (*inf*) a hippopotamus.

hippocras /ˈhɪpəˌkræs/ *n* an old English cordial of spiced wine.

Hippocratic oath /ˈhɪpəˌkrætɪk/ *n* an oath taken by a doctor to observe the code of medical ethics derived from Hippocrates, a Greek physician of the 5th century BC.

hippodrome /ˈhɪpəˌdrəʊm/ *n* a dance hall, music hall, etc; in ancient Greece, a stadium for horse and chariot races.

hippogriff /ˈhɪpəˌɡrɪf/ *n* (*Greek myth*) a monster with a griffin's head, wings and claws, and the body of a horse.

hippopotamus /ˈhɪpəˌpɒtəməs/ *n* (*pl* **hippopotamuses, hippopotami**) a large African water-loving mammal with thick dark skin, short legs, and a very large head and muzzle.

hircine /ˈhɜːsaɪn/ *or* /-sɪn/ *adj* of or resembling a goat; smelling like a goat.

hire /haɪr/ *vt* to pay for the services of (a person) or the use of (a thing). • *n* the payment for the temporary use of anything; the fact or state of being hired.—**hirable, hireable** *adj*.—**hirer** *n*.

hireling /ˈhaɪrlɪŋ/ *n* a person who works only for money, *esp* for doing something unpleasant.

hire-purchase *n* a system by which a person takes possession of an article after paying a deposit and then becomes the owner only after payment of a series of instalments is completed.

hirsute /hɜːˈsuːt/ *or* /ˈhɜːsuːt/, /-sjuːt/ *adj* covered in hair; of or pertaining to hair.—**hirsuteness** *n*.

his /hɪz/ *poss pron* of or belonging to *him*.—*also adj*.

Hispanic /hɪˈspænɪk/ *adj* of or derived from Spain, Spanish or Spanish-speaking countries. • *n* a person of Hispanic descent, *esp* in the US.

Hispanicism /hɪˈspænɪˌsɪzəm/ *n* a word or expression borrowed from Spanish.

hispid /ˈhɪspɪd/ *adj* bristly; covered with stiff hairs.—**hispidity** *n*.

hiss /hɪs/ *vi* to make a sound resembling a prolonged *s*; to show disapproval by hissing. • *vt* to say or indicate by hissing. • *n* the act or sound of hissing.—**hisser** *n*.

hist. *abbr* = history; historian; historical.

hist- /ˈhɪst/, **histo-** /ˈhɪstoː/ *prefix* tissue.

histamine /ˈhɪstəmɪn/ or /ˈhɪstəmiːn/ *n* a substance released by the tissues in allergic reactions, acting as an irritant.—**histaminic** *adj*.

histogenesis /ˌhɪstəˈdʒenəsɪs/ *n* the formation of organic tissue.—**histogenetic** *adj*.—**histogenetically** *adv*.

histogram /ˌhɪstəˈɡræm/ *n* a statistical diagram representing frequency distribution in terms of columns.

histology /hɪsˈtɒlədʒi/ *n* the study of the microscopic structure of animal and plant tissues.—**histologic, histological** *adj*.—**histologically** *adv*.—**histologist** *n*.

historian /hɪˈstɔːriən/ *n* a person who writes or studies history.

historic /hɪˈstɒrɪk/ *adj* (potentially) important or famous in history.

historical /hɪˈstɒrɪkəl/ *adj* belonging to or involving history or historical methods; concerning actual events as opposed to myth or legend; based on history.—**historically** *adv*.—**historicalness** *n*.

historicity /hɪˈstɒrɪsɪti/ *n* historical authenticity; genuineness.

historiography /hɪˌstɔːriˈɒɡrəfi/ *n* the principles of historical writing, *esp* that based on the use of primary sources and techniques of research; the study of methods of historical research and writing.—**historiographic, historiographical** *adj*.—**historiographically** *adv*.

historiographer /hɪˌstɔːriˈɒɡrəfər/ *n* a writer of history, *esp* an official historian.

history /ˈhɪstəri/ or /ˈhɪstri/ *n* (*pl* **histories**) a record or account of past events; the study and analysis of past events; past events in total; the past events or experiences of a specific person or thing; an unusual or significant past.

histrionic /ˌhɪstrɪˈɒnɪk/, **histrionical** /-əl/ *adj* of actors or the theatre; melodramatic.—**histrionically** *adv*.

histrionics /ˌhɪstrɪˈɒnɪks/ *n* (*used as sing or pl*) the art of theatrical representation; melodramatic behaviour or tantrums to attract attention.

hit /hɪt/ *vti* (**hitting, hit**) to come against (something) with force; to give a blow (to), to strike; to strike with a missile; to affect strongly; to arrive at; (*with* **on**) to discover by accident or unexpectedly. • *n* a blow that strikes its mark; a collision; a successful and popular song, book, etc; (*inf*) an underworld killing; (*sl*) a dose of a drug.

hit-and-run *n* a motor vehicle accident in which the driver leaves the scene without stopping or informing the authorities.

hitch /hɪtʃ/ *vt* to move, pull, etc with jerks; to fasten with a hook, knot, etc; to obtain a ride by hitchhiking. • *vi* to hitchhike. • *n* a tug; a hindrance, obstruction; a kind of knot used for temporary fastening; (*inf*) a ride obtained from hitchhiking.—**hitcher** *n*.

hitchhike /ˈhɪtʃhaɪk/ *vt* to travel by asking for free lifts from motorists along the way.—**hitchhiker** *n*.

hither /ˈhɪðər/ *adv* (*formal*) to or towards this place.

hitherto /ˈhɪðərtuː/ *adv* (*formal*) until this time.

hit list *n* (*sl*) a list of people to be eliminated, etc.

hit man *n* a hired assassin.

Hittite /ˈhɪtˌaɪt/ *n* a member of an ancient people of Asia Minor; the language of these people. • *adj* of or pertaining to the Hittite people or their language or inscriptions.

HIV /ˈeɪtʃˈaɪˈviː/ *abbr* = human immunodeficiency virus, the virus that causes Aids.

hive /haɪv/ *n* a shelter for a colony of bees; a beehive; the bees of a hive; a crowd of busy people; a place of great activity. • *vt* to gather (bees) into a hive. • *vi* to enter a hive; (*with* **off**) to separate from a group.

hives /haɪvz/ *n* (*used as sing or pl*) a rash on the skin often caused by an allergy; nettle rash.

hiya /ˈhaɪjə/ *interj* an exclamation of greeting.

HM *abbr* = Her (or His) Majesty ('s).

HMCS /ˈeɪtʃˈemˈsiːˈes/ *abbr* ✠ = Her Majesty's Canadian Ship.

HMS /ˈeɪtʃˈemˈes/ *abbr* = Her (or His) Majesty's Ship.

Ho (*chem symbol*) = holmium.

ho /hoː/ *interj* an exclamation used to attract attention.

hoard /hɔːd/ *n* an accumulation of food, money, etc, stored away for future use. • *vti* to accumulate and store away.—**hoarder** *n*.

hoarding /ˈhɔːdɪŋ/ *n* a temporary screen of boards erected around a construction site; a billboard.

hoarfrost /ˈhɔːˈfrɒst/ *n* a covering of minute ice crystals.—*also* **white frost.**

hoarse /hɔːs/ *adj* (*voice*) rough, as from a cold; (*person*) having a hoarse voice.—**hoarsely** *adv*.—**hoarseness** *n*.

hoary /ˈhɔːri/ *adj* (**hoarier, hoariest**) white or grey with age; having whitish or greyish hairs; (*joke, etc*) ancient, hackneyed.—**hoarily** *adv*.

hoax /hoːks/ *n* a deception; a practical joke. • *vt* to deceive by a hoax.—**hoaxer** *n*.

hob /hɒb/ *n* a ledge near a fireplace for keeping kettles, etc hot; a flat surface on a cooker incorporating hot plates or burners.

hobble /ˈhɒbəl/ *vi* to walk unsteadily, to limp. • *vt* to fasten the legs of (horses, etc) loosely together to prevent straying. • *n* a limp; a rope, etc, used to hobble a horse.—**hobbler** *n*.

hobbledehoy /ˈhɒbəldɪˌhɔɪ/ *n* (*arch*) (*pl* **hobbledehoys**) an inexperienced and awkward young person.

hobby /ˈhɒbi/ *n* (*pl* **hobbies**) a spare-time activity carried out for personal amusement; (*arch*) a hobbyhorse.—**hobbyist** *n*.

hobbyhorse *n* a child's toy comprising a stick with a horse's head; a rocking horse; a favourite topic for discussion.

hobgoblin /ˈhɒbˌɡɒblɪn/ *n* a mischievous goblin.

hobnail /ˈhɒbnɪl/ *n* a short nail with a wide head, used on the soles of heavy shoes.—**hobnailed** *adj*.

hobnob /ˈhɒbnɒb/ *vi* (**hobnobbing, hobnobbed**) to spend time with in a friendly manner.

hobo /ˈhoːboː/ *n* (*pl* **hoboes, hobos**) a migrant labourer; a tramp.—**hoboism** *n*.

hock[1] /hɒk/ *vt* (*sl*) to give something in security for a loan.—**hocker** *n*.

hock[2] *n* the joint bending backward on the hind leg of a horse, etc.

hock[3] *n* a variety of German white wine.

hockey /ˈhɒki/ *n* an outdoor game played by two teams of 11 players with a ball and clubs curved at one end.—*also* **field hockey**; ice hockey.

hockshop /ˈhɒkˌʃɒp/ *n* (*inf*) a pawnshop.

hocus /ˈhoːkəs/ *vt* (**hocusses, hocussing, hocussed** or **hocuses, hocusing, hocused**) to cheat or trick; to dupe; to doctor alcohol in order to stupefy a person so as to cheat him or her; to stupefy with a drug. • *n* a trick; drugged alcohol.

hocus-pocus /ˌhoːkəsˈpoːkəs/ *n* meaningless words used by a conjurer; sleight of hand; deception. • *vti* (**hocus-pocuses, hocus-pocusing, hocus-pocused** or **hocus-pocusses, hocus-pocussing, hocus-pocussed**) to play tricks (on).

hod /hɒd/ *n* a trough on a pole for carrying bricks or mortar on the shoulder; a coal scuttle.

hodgepodge /ˈhɒdʒpɒdʒ/ *n* a jumble.

hoe /hoː/ *n* a long-handled tool for weeding, loosening the earth, etc. • *vti* (**hoeing, hoed**) to dig, weed, till, etc, with a hoe.

hog /hɒɡ/ *n* a domesticated male pig raised for its meat; (*inf*) a selfish, greedy, or filthy person. • *vt* (**hogging, hogged**) to take more than one's due; to hoard greedily.

hogfish /-fɪ/ *n* (*pl* **hogfish, hogfishes**) a fish with a bristled head of warm Atlantic waters; the wrasse.

Hogmanay /ˌhɒɡməˈneɪ/ *n* (*Scot*) New Year's Eve.

hogshead /ˈhɒɡzhed/ *n* a large cask or barrel; one of several measures of liquid capacity, *esp* one of 63 gallons (238.5 litres).

Hogtown /ˈhɒɡtaʊn/ *n* ✠ (*Cdn*) (*sl*) Toronto, Canada.

hogwash /ˈhɒɡwɒʃ/ *n* swill fed to pigs; rubbishy or nonsensensical writing or speech.

hoi polloi /ˌhɔɪpəˈlɔɪ/ *n* (*often derog*) the common people; the masses.

hoist /hɔɪst/ *vt* to raise aloft, *esp* with a pulley, crane, etc. • *n* a hoisting; an apparatus for lifting to a higher flower; a lift, elevator.—**hoister** *n*.

hoity-toity /ˌhɔɪtiˈtɔɪti/ *adj* arrogant or haughty. • *interj* an exclamation of surprise.

hokey-pokey /ˌhoːkiˈpoːki/ *n* hocus-pocus; a cheap ice cream sold in slabs.

hol- /hɒl/, **holo-** /ˈhɒloː/ *prefix* whole.

hold[1] /hoːld/ *vb* (**holding, held**) *vt* to take and keep in one's possession; to grasp; to maintain in a certain position or condition; to retain; to contain; to own, to occupy; to support, sustain; to remain firm; to carry on, as a meeting; to regard; to believe, to consider; to bear or carry oneself; (*with* **back**) to withhold; to restrain; (*with* **down**) to restrain; (*inf*) to manage to retain one's job, etc; (*with* **forth**) to offer (*eg* an inducement); (*with* **off**) to keep apart; (*with* **up**) to delay; to hinder; to commit an armed robbery. • *vi* to go on being firm, loyal, etc; to remain unbroken or unyielding; to be true or valid; to continue; (*with* **back**) to refrain; (*with* **forth**) to speak at length; (*with* **off**) to wait, to refrain; (*with* **on**) to maintain a grip on; to persist; (*inf*) to keep a telephone line open. • *n* the act or manner of holding; grip; a dominating force on a person.—**holdable** *adj*.—**holder** *n*.

hold[2] *n* the storage space in a ship or aircraft used for cargo.

holdall /ˈhoːldɒl/ *n* a portable container for miscellaneous articles.—*also* **carryall**.

holder /ˈhoːldər/ *n* one who holds; a device for holding things; a person who has control of something; one who is in possession of a financial document.

holdfast /ˈhoːldfæst/ *n* a hook or clamp; the act of gripping strongly; the organ by which seaweed and related plants attach themselves to a host object.

holding /ˈhoːldɪŋ/ *n* (*often pl*) legally held property, *esp* land, stocks, and bonds; ✹ the action of illegally blocking or obstructing an opponent in a sports contest.

hold-up /ˈhoːldʌp/ *n* a delay; an armed robbery.

hole /hoːl/ *n* a hollow place; a cavity; a pit; an animal's burrow; an aperture; a perforation; a small, squalid, dingy place; (*inf*) a difficult situation; (*golf*) a small cavity into which the ball is hit; the tee, the fairway, etc leading to this. • *vti* to make a hole in (something); to drive into a hole; (*with* **up**) to hibernate; (*inf*) to hide oneself.

holey /ˈhoːli/ *adj* full of holes.

holiday /ˈhɒlɪˌdeɪ/ *n* a period away from work, school, etc for travel, rest or recreation; a day of freedom from work, etc, *esp* one set aside by law. • *vi* to spend a holiday.—*also* **vacation**.

holiday-maker /ˈhɒlədeɪˌmeɪkər/ *n* a vacationer.

holily /ˈhoːlɪli/ *adv* in a holy manner.

holiness /ˈhoːlɪnəs/ *n* sanctity; (*with cap and poss pron*) the title of the Pope.

holism /ˈhoːlɪzəm/ *n* (*philos*) the creation by creative evolution of wholes that are greater than the sum of the parts; (*med*) consideration of the whole body in the treatment of disease.—**holistic** *adj*.—**holistically** *adv*.

holland /ˈhɒlənd/ *n* an unbleached linen either glazed or unglazed used for furnishing.

hollandaise sauce /ˈhɒlənˌdeɪz/ *n* a rich sauce of egg yolks, lemon juice, butter, etc.

Hollands /ˈhɒləndz/ *n* a kind of Dutch gin sold in stone bottles.

hollow /ˈhɒloː/ *adj* having a cavity within or below; recessed, concave; empty or worthless. • *n* a hole, cavity; a depression, a valley.• *vti* to make or become hollow.—**ho lowly** *adv*.—**hollowness** *n*.

hollow-eyed *adj* with the eyes deep-set or sunken from tiredness, etc.

holly /ˈhɒli/ *n* (*pl* **hollies**) an evergreen shrub with prickly leaves and red berries.

hollyhock /ˈhɒliˌhɒk/ *n* a tall-stemmed plant with spikes of large flowers.

holmium /ˈhoːlmiəm/ *n* a malleable white metallic element.

holoblastic /ˌhɒloˈblæstɪk/ or /ˌhoːloː-/ *adj* wholly germinal.

holocaust /ˈhɒləˌkɒst/ *n* a great destruction of life, *esp* by fire; (*with cap and* **the**) the mass extermination of European Jews by the Nazis 1939–45.—**holocaustal, holocaustic** *adj*.

hologram /ˈhɒləˌgræm/ *n* an image made without the use of a lens on photographic film by means of interference between two parts of a laser beam, the result appearing as a meaningless pattern until suitably illuminated, when it shows as a three-dimensional image.

holograph /-ˌgræf/ *n* a document wholly in the handwriting of the author.

holography /həˈlɒgrəfi/ *n* the technique of making or using holograms.—**holographic** *adj*.—**holographically** *adv*.

holohedral /ˌhɒləˈhiːdrəl/ *adj* showing all the planes necessary for the perfect symmetry of the crystal system.

holophrastic /-ˈfræstɪk/ *adj* (*linguistics*) describing the stage in language development where most utterances are single words; having the force of a whole phrase; polysynthetic.

holothurian /-ˈθuːriən/ *n* any echinoderm of the class that contains the sea cumcumber. • *adj* of, related or belonging to the holothurians.

holpen /ˈhoːlpən/ or /ˈhoː-/ *vb* (*arch*) a past participle of *help*.

holster /ˈhoːlstər/ *n* a leather case attached to a belt for a pistol.—**holstered** *adj*.

holt /hoːlt/ *n* an otter's den; the burrowed lair of any animal; (*poet*) a wood; a wooded hill.

holus-bolus /ˈhoːləsˌboːləs/ *adv* (*inf*) at a gulp, all at once.

holy /ˈhoːli/ *adj* (**holier, holiest**) dedicated to religious use; without sin; deserving reverence. • *n* (*pl* **holies**) a holy place, innermost shrine.

Holy Communion *n* the celebration of the Eucharist.

Holy Ghost *n* (*Christianity*) the third person of the Trinity.

Holy Grail *n* in medieval legend, the dish or chalice that was used by Christ at the Last Supper, and the object of many knights' quests.

holy jumpin' *interj* ✹ (*Cdn*) (*sl*) used to express astonishment or disbelief.

Holy Land *n* Palestine.

Holy Spirit *n* the Holy Spirit.

holystone /ˈhoːliˌstoːn/ *n* sandstone used by sailors to scour ships' decks. • *vt* to scrub a ship's deck with holystone.

Holy Thursday *see* **Ascens on Day**.

Holy Week *n* the week before Easter Sunday.

hom- /ˈhoːm/, **homo-** /ˈhoːmoː/ *prefix* same; like.

homage /ˈhɒmɪdʒ/ or /ˈɒm/ *n* a public demonstration of respect or honour towards someone or something.

hombre /ˈɒmbreɪ/ or /ˈhɒm-/ *n* (*sl*) a man.

homburg /ˈhɒmbərg/ *n* a man's soft felt hat with a narrow curled brim and a lengthwise dent in the crown.

home /hoːm/ *n* the place where one lives; the city, etc where one was born or reared; a place thought of as home; a household and its affairs; an institution for the aged, orphans, etc. • *adj* of one's home or country; domestic. • *adv* at, to, or in the direction of home; to the point aimed at. • *vi* (*birds*) to return home; to be guided onto a target; to head for a destination; to send or go home.

home child ✹ (*Cdn*) (*hist*) one of the orphaned or homeless children who were sent from Britain to Canada to serve as farm or domestic workers.

home economics *n* (*sing or pl*) the art and science of household management, nutrition, etc.

home-grown /hoːmˈgroːn/ *adj* grown or produced at home or nearby; characteristic of a particular locale.

home ice *n* ✹ the rink or arena where a hockey team or curling rink normally plays when not playing away from home.

homeland /ˈhoːmlænd/ *n* the country where a person was born.

homely /ˈhoːmli/ *adj* (**homelier, homeliest**) simple, everyday; crude; not good-looking.—**homeliness** *n*.

home-made /ˈhoːmmeɪd/ *adj* made, or as if made, at home.

homeopathy, homoeopathy /ˌhoːmiˈɒpəθi/ *n* the system of treating disease by small quantities of drugs that cause symptoms similar to those of the disease.—**homeopath, homeopathist** *n*.—**homeopathic** *adj*.—**homeopathically** *adv*.

homer /ˈhoːmər/ *n* (*baseball*) a home run; a homing pigeon; (*inf*) work done on an informal basis, without declaring the earnings.

Homeric /hoːˈmerɪk/ or /hə-/ *adj* pertaining to the poet Homer, or his works; heroic.—**Homerically** *adv*.

home run *n* (*baseball*) a hit that allows the batter to touch all bases and score a run.

homesick /ˈhoːmsɪk/ *adj* longing for home.—**homesickness** *n*.

homespun /-spʌn/ *adj* cloth made of yarn spun at home; coarse cloth like this.

homestead /-sted/ *n* a farmhouse with land and buildings.—**homesteader** *n*

home stretch, home straight *n* the part of a race track between the last turn and the finish line; the final part.

home truth *n* an unpleasant fact that a person has to face about himself or herself.

homeward /ˈhoːmwərd/ *adj* going towards home. • *adv* homewards.

homewards /-wərdz/ *adv* towards home.

homework /-wərk/ *n* work, *esp* piecework, done at home; schoolwork to be done outside the classroom; preliminary study for a project.

homey /ˈhoːmi/ *adj*, **homeyness** *n see* **homy**.

homicidal /hɒmɪˈsaɪdəl/ *adj* characterized by homicide; likely to commit suicide.

homicide /ˈhɒmɪˌsaɪd/ *n* the killing of a person by another; a person who kills another.—**homicidal** *adj*.—**homicidally** *adv*.

homiletic /ˌhɒmɪˈletɪk/, **homiletical** /-əl/ *adj* of or relating to a homily or sermon; of or relating to homiletics.—**homiletically** *adv*.

homiletics /ˈletɪks/ *n sing* the art of writing or preaching sermons.

homily /ˈhɒmɪli/ *n* (*pl* **homilies**) a sermon; moralizing talk or writing.—**homilist** *n*.

homing /ˈhoːmɪŋ/ *adj* (*pigeon*) trained to fly home after being transported long distances; (*missile, etc*) designed to guide itself onto a target.

hominid /ˈhɒmɪnɪd/ *adj* of or relating to the zoological species that includes present-day man and his ancestors. • *n* a member of this species.

hominoid /ˈhɒmɪ̩nɔɪd/ *adj* resembling man; of or belonging to primates.

hominy (grits) /ˈhɒmɪni/ *n* ground maize boiled in water to make a thin porridge.

homo[1] /ˈhoːmoː/ *n* any member of the genus *Homo* that includes modern man.

homo[2] *n* (*pl* **homos**) (*inf*) a male homosexual.

homocentric /̩hoːmoːˈsentrɪk/ or /̩hɒmoː-/ *adj* concentric; having the same centre.

homogeneous /̩hɒməˈdʒiːnɪəs/ or /̩hoːmə-/ *adj* composed of parts that are of identical or a similar kind or nature; of uniform structure.—**homogeneity, homogeneousness** *n*.

homogenize /həˈmɒdʒə̩naɪz/ *vt* to break up the fat particles (in milk or cream) so they do not separate; to make or become homogeneous.—**homogenization** *n*.—**homogenizer** *n*.

homograph /ˈhɒmə̩græf/ *n* a word spelled the same as another word but with a different meaning and derived from a different root.

homologous /həˈmɒləgəs/ *adj* corresponding in relative position, structure, and descent.

homologue, homolog /ˈhɒmə̩lɒg/ *n* something that exhibits homology.

homology /həˈmɒlədʒi/ *n* (*pl* **homologies**) a similarity often attributed to a common origin; affinity of structure.—**homological** *adj*.—**homologically** *adv*.

homonym /ˈhɒmənɪm/ *n* a word with the same spelling or pronunciation as another, but a different meaning.—**homonymic** *adj*.—**homonymy** *n*.

Homoousian /̩hoːmoːˈuːsɪən/ *n* a Christian who believes that Jesus is of the same essence as God.

homophobia /̩hoːməˈfoːbɪə/ *n* fear and hatred of homosexuals; persecution of homosexuals.—**homophobe** *n*.—**homophobic** *adj*.

homophone /ˈhɒmə̩foːn/ *n* a letter or group of letters having the same sound as another letter or group of letters; one of a group of words with identical pronunciations but with different meanings or spellings or both.—**homophony** *n*.

homophonous /həˈmɒfənəs/ *adj* alike in sound but different in meaning; relating to or denoting a homophone.

homoplastic /̩hɒməˈplæstɪk/ *adj* similar in structure; derived from a donating individual of a tissue graft of the same species as the recipient.

Homo sapiens /̩hoːmoːˈseɪpɪənz/ *n* the species designating mankind.

homosexual /̩hoːmoːˈsekʃʊəl/ *adj* sexually attracted towards a person of the same sex. • *n* a homosexual person.—**homosexuality** *n*.—**homosexually** *adv*.

homunculus /həˈmʌŋkjʊləs/ *n* (*pl* **homunculi**) a dwarf; a miniature man.

homy /ˈhoːmi/ *adj* (**homier, homiest**) cosy, home-like.—*also* **homey**.—**hominess, homeyness** *n*.

Hon. *abbr* = Honourable.

hon *abbr* = honorary; honourable.

hone /hoːn/ *n* a stone for sharpening cutting tools. • *vt* to sharpen (as if) on a hone.

honest /ˈɒnəst/ *adj* truthful; trustworthy; sincere or genuine; gained by fair means; frank, open.—**honestness** *n*.

honestly /ˈɒnəstli/ *adv* in an honest manner; really.

honesty /ˈɒnəsti/ *n* (*pl* **honesties**) the quality of being honest; a European plant with purple flowers that forms transparent seed pods.

honey /ˈhʌni/ *n* (*pl* **honeys**) a sweet sticky yellowish substance that bees make as food from the nectar of flowers; sweetness; its colour; (*inf*) darling. • *adj* of, resembling honey; much loved.

honeybee /ˈhʌni̩biː/ *n* the common bee of the genus that produces honey.

honey bucket *n* ✲ (*sl*) a container for human waste, *esp* in an outdoor toilet.

honeycomb /-̩koːm/ *n* the structure of six-sided wax cells made by bees to hold their honey, eggs, etc; anything arranged like this. • *vt* to fill with holes like a honeycomb.

honeydew /-̩djuː/ *n* a sugary deposit on leaves secreted by aphids; a variety of melon with yellowish skin and pale green flesh.—**honeydewed** *adj*.

honeyed, honied /ˈhʌniːd/ *adj* flattering; of, containing, or resembling honey.—**honeyedly, honiedly** *adv*.

honeymoon /ˈhʌni̩muːn/ *n* the vacation spent together by a newly married couple.—*also vi*.—**honeymooner** *n*.

honeysuckle /-̩sʌkəl/ *n* a climbing shrub with small fragrant flowers.

hong /hɒŋ/ *n* (*formerly*) in China, a factory or warehouse, or a commercial establishment owned by a foreigner.

honk /hɒŋk/ *n* (a sound resembling) the call of the wild goose; the sound made by an old-fashioned motor horn. • *vti* to cry like a goose; to sound (a motor horn); (*sl*) to be sick.

honky-tonk /ˈhɒŋkɪ̩tɒŋk/ *n* a style of ragtime piano playing.

honorarium /ˈɒnə̩rɛrɪəm/ *n* (*pl* **honorariums, honoraria**) a voluntary payment for professional services for which no fees are nominally due.

honorary /ˈɒnəreri/ *adj* given as an honour; (*office*) voluntary, unpaid.

honorific /ˈɒnərɪfɪk/ *adj* conferring honour.—**honorifically** *adv*.

honour, honor /ˈɒnər/ *n* high regard or respect; glory; fame; good reputation; integrity; chastity; high rank; distinction; (*with cap*) the title of certain officials, as judges; cards of the highest value in certain card games. • *vt* to respect greatly; to do or give something in honour of; to accept and pay (a cheque when due, etc).—**honourer, honorer** *n*.

honourable, honorable /ˈɒnə̩rəbəl/ *adj* worthy of being honoured; honest; upright; bringing honour; (*with cap*) a title of respect for certain officials, as Members of Parliament, when addressing each other.—**honourably, honorably** *adv*.

hooch /huːtʃ/ *n* (*US sl*) alcoholic liquor, *esp* when illicitly distilled or obtained.

hood[1] /hʊd/ *n* a loose covering to protect the head and back of the neck; any hood-like thing as the (folding) top of a car, etc; (*US*) the hinged metal covering over an automobile engine—*see* **bonnet**.

hood[2] *n* (*inf*) a hoodlum.

hoodlum /ˈhʊdləm/ *n* a gangster; a young hooligan.—**hoodlumism** *n*.

hoodoo /ˈhuːduː/ *n* (*pl* **hoodoos**) voodoo; a person or thing thought to bring bad luck. • *vt* (**hoodooing, hoodooed**) to bring ill luck to.—**hoodooism** *n*.

hoodwink /ˈhʊdwɪŋk/ *vt* to mislead by trickery.—**hoodwinker** *n*.

hooey /ˈhuːi/ *n* nonsense; humbug. • *interj* conveying disbelief.

hoof /huːf/ *n* (*pl* **hoofs, hooves**) the horny covering on the ends of the feet of certain animals, as horses, cows, etc.

hook /hʊk/ *n* a piece of bent or curved metal to catch or hold anything; a fishhook; something shaped like a hook; a strike, blow, etc, in which a curving motion is involved. • *vt* to seize, fasten, hold, as with a hook; (*rugby*) to pass the ball backwards from a scrum.

hookah /ˈhʊkə/ *n* an oriental tobacco-pipe with a long tube connected to a container of water, which cools the smoke as it is drawn through.

hooked /hʊkd/ *adj* shaped like a hook; (*sl*) addicted.—**hookedness** *n*.

hooker /ˈhʊkər/ *n* (*sl*) a prostitute; (*rugby football*) a player in the scrum whose task is to hook the ball.

hooking /ˈhʊkɪŋ/ *n* ✲ an illegal check in ice hockey in which a player hooks an opponent with a stick, *usu* from behind.

hookworm [1] /ˈhʊkwɜrm/ *n* a parasitic worm with hooked mouthparts that can bore through the skin and cause disease.

hooky /ˈhʊki/ *n* truancy from school.

hooligan /ˈhuːlɪgən/ *n* a lawless young person.—**hooliganism** *n*.

hoop /huːp/ *n* a circular band of metal or wood; an iron band for holding together the staves of barrels; anything like this, as a child's toy or ring in a hoop skirt. • *vt* to bind (as if) with hoops.—**hooped** *adj*.

hooper /ˈhuːpər/ *n* a cooper; the wild swan.

hoopla /ˈhuːplə/ *n* (*inf*) noise; bustle; (*inf*) misleading publicity.

hoopoe /ˈhuːpuː/ *n* a bird with a fanlike crest and pinky brown plumage.

hooray, hoorah /huˈreɪ/ *see* **hurrah**.

hoosegow /'huːsgaʊ/ *n* (*sl*) jail.

Hoosier /huːʒər/ *n* the nickname used for a native or resident of Indiana.

hoot /huːt/ *n* the sound that an owl makes; a similar sound, as made by a train whistle; a shout of scorn; (*inf*) laughter; (*inf*) an amusing person or thing. • *vi* to utter a hoot; to blow a whistle, etc. • *vt* to express (scorn) of (someone) by hooting.—**hooter** *n*.

hooves /huːvz/ *see* **hoof**.

hop[1] /hɒp/ *vi* (**hopping, hopped**) to jump up on one leg; to leap with all feet at once, as a frog, etc; (*inf*) to make a quick trip. • *n* a hopping movement; (*inf*) an informal dance; a trip, *esp* in an aircraft.

hop[2] *n* a climbing plant with small cone-shaped flowers; (*pl*) the dried ripe cones, used for flavouring beer.

hope /hoːp/ *n* a feeling that what is wanted will happen; the object of this; a person or thing on which one may base some hope. • *vt* to want and expect. • *vi* to have hope (for).—**hoper** *n*.

hopeful /'hoːpfʊl/ *adj* filled with hope; inspiring hope or promise of success. • *n* a person who hopes to or looks likely to be a success.—**hopefulness** *n*.

hopefully /-li/ *adv* in a hopeful manner; it is hoped.

hopeless /'hoːpləs/ *adj* without hope; offering no grounds for hope or promise of success; impossible to solve; (*inf*) incompetent.—**hopelessly** *adv*.—**hopelessness** *n*.

hoplite /'hɒplaɪt/ *n* in ancient Greece, a heavily armed foot soldier.

hopper /'hɒpər/ *n* a hopping insect; a funnel-shaped container with an opening at the bottom from which its contents can be discharged into a receptacle.

hopscotch /'hɒpskɒtʃ/ *n* a children's game in which the players hop through a sequence of squares drawn on the ground.

horary /'hɒrəri/ *adj* of or pertaining to or lasting an hour; noting the hours; hourly.

Horatian /hə'reɪʃən/ *adj* of or pertaining to the Roman poet Horace (658 BC) or his works.

horde /hɔːd/ *n* a crowd or throng; a swarm.

horizon /hə'raɪzən/ *n* the apparent line along which the earth and sky meet; the limit of a person's knowledge, interest, etc.

horizontal /hɒrə'zɒntəl/ *adj* level; parallel to the plane of the horizon.—**horizontally** *adv*.—**horizontalness** *n*.

hormone /'hɔːmoːn/ *n* a product of living cells formed in one part of the organism and carried to another part, where it takes effect; a synthetic compound having the same purpose.—**hormonal** *adj*.

horn /hɔːn/ *n* a bony outgrowth on the head of certain animals; the hard substance of which this is made; any projection like a horn; a wind instrument, *esp* the French horn or trumpet; a device to sound a warning. • *vt* to wound with a horn; (*with* in) to intrude.

hornbeam /'hɔːnbiːm/ *n* a tree of the birch family.

hornbill /-bɪl/ *n* a tropical bird with a horny protuberance on its large beak.

hornblende /-blend/ *n* a dark mineral of silica with magnesium, lime or iron.

hornbook /-bʊk/ *n* a framed child's primer made of a thin slab of wood or paper on which numbers, the alphabet and the Lord's Prayer were printed and protected with a covering of transparent horn; any elementary primer.

horned /hɔːnd/ *adj* having horns.

hornet /'hɔːnət/ *n* a large wasp with a severe sting.

hornpipe /'hɔːnpaɪp/ *n* a lively dance, formerly associated with British sailors; the music for such a dance; an obsolete wind instrument.

hornswoggle /-ˌswɒgəl/ *vt* to deceive; to swindle.

horny /'hɔːni/ *adj* (**hornier, horniest**) like horn; hard; callous; (*sl*) sexually aroused.—**hornily** *adv*.—**horniness** *n*.

horologe /'hɒrəˌlɒdʒ/ or /-ˌloːdʒ/ *n* any instrument that tells the time; a timepiece.

horology /hə'rɒlədʒi/ *n* the science of measuring time; the art of making clocks, watches, etc.—**horologic, horological** *adj*.—**horologist, horologer** *n*.

horoscope /'hɒrəˌskoːp/ *n* a chart of the zodiacal signs and positions of planets, etc, by which astrologers profess to predict future events, *esp* in the life of an individual.

horrendous /hə'rendəs/ *adj* horrific; (*inf*) disagreeable.—**horrendously** *adv*.

horrible /'hɒrəbəl/ *adj* arousing horror; (*inf*) very bad, unpleasant, etc.—**horribleness** *n*.—**horribly** *adv*.

horrid /'hɒrɪd/ *adj* terrible; horrible.—**horridly** *adv*.—**horridness** *n*.

horrific /hə'rɪfɪk/ *adj* arousing horror; horrible.—**horrifically** *adv*.

horrify /'hɒrəˌfaɪ/ *vt* (**horrifying, horrified**) to fill with horror; to shock.—**horrification** *n*.—**horrifyingly** *adv*.

horripilation /hɒrɪpə'leɪʃən/ *n* gooseflesh; the bristling of the skin caused by chill or fright.

horror /'hɒrər/ *n* the strong feeling caused by something frightful or shocking; strong dislike; a person or thing inspiring horror. • *adj* (*film, story, etc*) designed to frighten.

hors de combat *Fr.* /ɔːdəkõ'ba/ *adj* excluded from competition; unrivalled; unequalled; disabled.

hors d'oeuvre /ˌɔːr'dɜːv/, *Fr.* /ɔːr'dœvr/ *n* (*pl* **hors d'oeuvre, hors d'oeuvres**) an appetizer served at the beginning of a meal.

horse /hɔːs/ *n* a four-legged, solid-hoofed herbivorous mammal with a flowing mane and a tail, domesticated for carrying loads or riders, etc; cavalry; a vaulting horse; a frame with legs to support something.

horsebox /'hɔːsbɒks/ *n* a trailer used for transporting a horse.

horse brass *n* a decorative brass ornament attached to a horse's harness.

horse chestnut *n* a large tree with large palmate leaves and erect clusters of flowers.

horseflesh /-fleʃ/ *n* horses; the flesh of a horse, *esp* for eating.

horsehair /-hər/ *n* hair from the mane or the tail of a horse, used for padding, etc.

horse latitude *n* either of two oceanic regions between 30 degrees north and 30 degrees south latitude, marked by calms.

horse laugh *n* a boisterous, *usu* derisive laugh.

horseleech /-liːtʃ/ *n* a large carnivorous leech; an insatiable person.

horseman /-mən/ *n* (*pl* **horsemen**) a person skilled in the riding or care of horses; ✹ (*Cdn*) (*inf*) a member of the Royal Canadian Mounted Police.—**horsemanship** *n*.

horseplay /-pleɪ/ *n* rough, boisterous fun.

horsepower /-ˌpaʊər/ *n* (*pl* **horsepower**) a unit for measuring the power of engines, etc, equal to 746 watts or 33,000 footpounds per minute.

horseradish /-ˌrædɪʃ/ *n* a tall herb of the mustard family; a sauce or relish made with its pungent root.

horse sense *n* common sense.

horseshoe /-ʃuː/ *n* a flat U-shaped, protective metal plate nailed to a horse's hoof; anything shaped like this.

horsetail /-teɪl/ *n* a plant with jointed stems and whorls of small dark toothlike leaves; the tail of a horse, *esp* when used as a symbol of rank or as a standard.

horse-trade /-treɪd/ *n* a negotiation marked by shrewd bargaining and mutual concessions.—*also vi*.

horsewhip /-wɪp/ *n* a whip with a long thong used on horses. • *vt* (**horsewhipping, horsewhipped**) to flog with a horsewhip.

horsewoman /-ˌwʊmən/ *n* (*pl* **horsewomen**) a woman skilled at riding.

horsy, horsey /'hɔːsi/ *adj* (**horsier, horsiest**) of or resembling a horse; preoccupied with horses, horse racing, etc.—**horsily** *adv*.—**horsiness** *n*.

hortatory /'hɔːtətəri/, **hortative** /'hɔːtətɪv/ *adj* exhorting; encouraging.—**hortatorily** *adv*.

horticulture /'hɔːtɪˌkʌltʃər/ *n* the art or science of growing flowers, fruits, and vegetables.—**horticultural** *adj*.—**horticulturally** *adv*.—**horticulturist** *n*.

hosanna, hosannah /hoː'zænə/ *interj* an exclamation of praise to God. • *n* the cry of hosanna; a shout of praise.

hose[1] /hoːz/ *n* a flexible tube used to convey fluids. • *vt* to spray with a hose.

hose[2] *n* (*pl* **hose, hosen**) stockings, socks, tights collectively.

Hosea /hoː'zeɪə/ *n* (*Bible*) an Old Testament book containing the oracles of Hosea, a Hebrew prophet of the 8th century BC.

hoser /'hoːzər/ *n* ✹ (*Cdn*) (*sl*) an ignorant and boorish man, fond of drinking beer.

hosier /'hoːziər/ or /'hoːʒər/ *n* a person who sells stockings, socks, etc.

hospice /'hɒspɪs/ *n* a home for the care of the terminally ill; a place of rest and shelter for travellers.

hospitable /hɒ'spɪtəbəl/ or /'hɒsp-/ *adj* offering a generous welcome to guests or strangers; sociable.—**hospitableness** *n*.—**hospitably** *adv*.

hospital /'hɒspɪtəl/ *n* an institution where the sick or injured are given medical treatment.

hospitality /ˌhɒspɪ'tælɪti/ *n* (*pl* **hospitalities**) the act, practice, or quality of being hospitable.

hospitalize /'hɒspɪtə,laɪz/ *vt* to place in a hospital.—**hospitalization** *n*.

hospitaler, hospitaller /'hɒspɪtələr/ *n* (*often cap*) a member of a medieval charitable religious order, *esp* one who worked in a hospital.

host[1] /'hoːst/ *n* a person who receives or entertains a stranger or guest at his house; an animal or plant on or in which another lives; a compere on a television or radio programme. • *vti* to act as a host (to a party, television programme, etc).

host[2] *n* a very large number of people or things.

host[3] *n* the wafer of bread used in the Eucharist or Holy Communion.

hostage /'hɒstɪdʒ/ *n* a person given or kept as security until certain conditions are met.

hostel /'hɒstəl/ *n* a lodging place for the homeless, travellers, or other groups.—**hosteler, hosteller** *n*.—**hosteling, hostelling** *n*.

hostelry /'hɒstəlri/ *n* (*pl* **hostelries**) (*formerly*) an inn.

hostess /'hoːstəs/ *n* a woman acting as a host; a woman who entertains guests at a nightclub, etc.

hostile /'hɒstaɪl/ or /'hɒstəl/ *adj* of or being an enemy; unfriendly.—**hostilely** *adv*.

hostility /hɒ'stɪlɪti/ *n* (*pl* **hostilities**) enmity, antagonism; (*pl*) deliberate acts of warfare.

hostler /'hɒslər/ or /'ɒslər/ *see* **ostler**.

hot /hɒt/ *adj* (**hotter, hottest**) of high temperature; very warm; giving or feeling heat; causing a burning sensation on the tongue; full of intense feeling; following closely; electrically charged; (*inf*) recent, new; (*inf*) radioactive; (*inf*) stolen. • *adv* in a hot manner.—**hotly** *adv*.—**hotness** *n*.

hot air *n* (*sl*) empty talk.

hotbed /'hɒtbɛd/ *n* a bed of heated earth enclosed by low walls and covered by glass for forcing plants; ideal conditions for the growth of something, *esp* evil.

hot-blooded *adj* easily excited.—**hot-bloodedness** *n*.

hotchpotch /'hɒtʃpɒtʃ/ *n* a thick meat and vegetable stew; a hodgepodge.

hot dog *n* a sausage, *esp* a frankfurter, served in a long soft roll.

hotel /ho:'tɛl/ *n* a commercial establishment providing lodging and meals for travellers, etc.

hotelier /ho:'tɛliər/ *n* the owner or manager of a hotel.

hotfoot /'hɒtfʊt/ *adv* with all speed; quickly.

hothead /'hɒthɛd/ *n* an impetuous person.—**hot-headed** *adj*.—**hot-headedly** *adv*.—**hot-headedness** *n*.

hothouse /'hɒthʊs/ *n* a heated greenhouse for raising plants; an environment that encourages rapid growth.

hot line /'hɒtlaɪn/ *n* a direct telephone link between heads of government for emergency use.

hotplate *n* a heated surface for cooking or keeping food warm ; a small portable heating device.

hotpot /'hɒtpɒt/ *n* a dish of meat cooked with potatoes in a tight-lidded pot.

hot seat *n* (*inf*) a dangerous position; (*sl*) the electric chair.

Hottentot /'hɒtən,tɒt/ *n* (*pl* **Hottentots, Hottentot**) a member of a people of the Cape of Good Hope region of South Africa, with pale brown skin; any of the languages spoken by these people.

hot water *n* (*inf*) trouble.

houmous, houmus /'hʊməs/ *see* **hummus**.

hound /haʊnd/ *n* a dog used in hunting; a contemptible person. • *vt* to hunt or chase as with hounds; to urge on by harassment.—**hounder** *n*.

hour /aʊr/ *n* a period of 60 minutes, a 24th part of a day; the time for a specific activity; the time; a special point in time; the distance covered in an hour; (*pl*) the customary period for work, etc.

hourglass /'aʊrglæs/ *n* an instrument for measuring time by trickling sand in a specified period.

houri /'hʊri/ *n* (*pl* **houris**) a beautiful woman of the Muslim paradise; a voluptuous young woman.

hourly /'aʊrli/ *adj* occurring every hour; done during an hour; frequent. • *adv* at every hour; frequently.

house /haʊs/ *n* a building to live in, *esp* by one person or family; a household; a family or dynasty including relatives, ancestors and descendants; the audience in a theatre; a business firm; a legislative assembly; house music. • *vt* to provide accommodation or storage for; to cover, encase.

house arrest *n* detention in one's own house, as opposed to prison.

houseboat /'haʊsbo:t/ *n* a boat furnished and used as a home.

housebound /'haʊsbaʊnd/ *adj* confined to the house through illness, injury, etc.

housebreaker /'haʊs,breɪkər/ *n* a burglar; a person employed to demolish buildings.—**housebreaking** *n*.

house-broken /'haʊs,bro:kən/ *adj* (*dogs, cats, etc*) trained not to mess in the house; (*inf*) well-mannered.

housefly /'haʊsflaɪ/ *n* (*pl* **houseflies**) a common fly found in houses, which is attracted by food and can spread disease.

household /'haʊsho:ld/ *n* all those people living together in the same house. • *adj* pertaining to running a house and family; domestic; familiar.

householder /'haʊs,ho:ldər/ *n* the person who owns or rents a house.

housekeeper /'haʊs,ki:pər/ *n* a person who runs a home, *esp* one hired to do so.

housekeeping /'haʊs,ki:pɪŋ/ *n* the daily running of a household; (*inf*) money used for domestic expenses; routine maintenance of equipment, records, etc in an organization.

housel /'haʊzəl/ *n* (*formerly*) the Eucharist.

house league *n* ✦ (*Cdn*) a sports league whose teams are formed from members of the same school or organization.

houseleek /'haʊsliːk/ *n* a plant with a rosette of succulent leaves and pink flowers that grows on walls.

housemaid /'haʊsmeɪd/ *n* a female servant employed to do housework.

houseman /'haʊsmən/ *n* (*pl* **housemen**) an intern.

housemaster /'haʊs,mæstər/ *n* a male teacher at a boarding school responsible for the pupils in his house.

house martin *n* a type of swallow with a forked tail.

house music *n* a pop music style, using electronic bass and synthesizers, a fast hypnotic beat and sporadic vocals, that originated in Chicago.

house party *n* a party, *usu* in a large house, where the guests stay over for several days; the guests themselves.

house plant /'haʊsplænt/ *n* an indoor plant.

houseproud /'haʊs,praʊd/ *adj* concerned with tidiness and cleanliness, often to excess.

house warming /'haʊs,wɔrmɪŋ/ *n* a party given to celebrate moving into a new house.

housewife /'haʊswaɪf/ *n* (*pl* **housewives**) the woman who keeps house.—**housewifely** *adj*.—**housewifeliness** *n*.—**housewifery** *n*.

housework /'haʊswərk/ *n* the cooking, cleaning, etc, involved in running a home.—**houseworker** *n*.

housing /'haʊzɪŋ/ *n* houses collectively; the provision of accommodation; a casing enclosing a piece of machinery, etc; a slot or groove in a piece of wood, etc, to receive an insertion.

hove /ho:v/ *see* **heave**.

hovel /'hævəl/ or /'hɒv-/ *n* a small miserable dwelling. • *vt* (**hoveling, hoveled** or **hovelling, hovelled**) to shelter in a hovel.

hover /'hʌvər/ *vi* (*bird, etc*) to hang in the air stationary; to hang about, to linger.—**hoverer** *n*.—**hoveringly** *adv*.

hovercraft /'hʌvər,kræft/ *n* a land or water vehicle that travels supported on a cushion of air.

how /haʊ/ *adv* in what way or manner; by what means; to what extent; in what condition.

howbeit /haʊ'bi:ɪt/ *conj* (*arch*) though; although.

howdah /'haʊdə/ *n* a seat fixed on the back of an elephant or camel.

how do you do *interj* a formal greeting, *esp* when meeting for the first time.

how-do-you-do, how-d'ye-do *n* (*inf*) a difficult situation, mess.

howdy /'haʊdi/ *n* (*inf*) how do you do; hello.

however /haʊ'ɛvər/ *adv* in whatever way or degree; still; nevertheless.

howitzer /'haʊɪtsər/ *n* a short cannon that fires shells at a steep trajectory.

howl /haʊl/ *vi* to utter the long, wailing cry of wolves, dogs, etc; to utter a similar cry of anger, pain, etc; to shout or laugh in pain, amusement, etc. • *vt* to utter with a howl; to drive by howling. • *n* the wailing cry of a wolf, dog, etc; any similar sound.

howler /'haʊlər/ *n* (*inf*) a stupid mistake.

howsoever /,haʊso:'ɛvər/ *conj* still; nevertheless. • *adv* by whatever means; in whatever manner.

hoy /hɔɪ/ *n* a coastal vessel; a freight barge. • *interj* a cry used to call attention.

hoya /'hɔɪə/ n a plant with pink, yellow or white flowers.

hoyden /'hɔɪdən/ n a tomboy; a wild girl.—**hoydenish** adj.

HP abbr = hire purchase; horsepower; high pressure; Houses of Parliament.

HQ abbr = headquarters.

hr abbr = hour.

HRH abbr = His or Her Royal Highness.

HST /'eɪtʃ'es'ti:/ abbr ✽ (Cdn) = Harmonized sales tax.

HT abbr = high tension.

HTML /'eɪtʃti:emel/ abbr = HyperText Markup Language, the basic language in which pages on the Internet are written.

HTTP /'eɪtʃti:ti:pi:/ abbr = HyperText Transport Protocol, the structure used to connect the many servers on the Web.

hub /hʌb/ n the centre part of a wheel; a centre of activity.

hubba-hubba /'hʌbə,hʌbə/ interj an exclamation of delight.

hubble-bubble /'hʌbəl,bʌbəl/ n a bubbling noise; confused talk; a hookah.

hubbub /'hʌbʌb/ n a confused noise of many voices; an uproar.

hubby /'hʌbi/ n (pl **hubbies**) (inf) a husband.

hubcap /'hʌbkæp/ n a metal cap that fits over the hub of a car wheel.

hubris /'hju:brɪs/ n arrogance, presumption.—**hubristic** adj.

huckaback /'hʌkə,bæk/ n an absorbent linen or cotton fabric used for towels, etc.

huckleberry /'hʌkəlberi/ n (pl **huckleberries**) a North American shrub with dark-blue berries; the fruit of this plant.

huckster /'hʌkstər/ n a person using aggressive or questionable methods of selling.—**hucksterism** n.

huddle /'hʌdəl/ vti to crowd together in a confined space; to curl (oneself) up. • n a confused crowd or heap.—**huddler** n.

Hudibrastic /,hju:dɪ'bræstɪk/ adj mock-heroic, in the style of Hudibras, a poem by Samuel Butler (161280).

Hudson's Bay blanket n ✽ (Cdn) a woollen blanket with a creamy white background and a pattern of white coloured stripes.

hue /hju:/ n colour; a particular shade or tint of a colour.

hued /hju:d/ adj having a colour or hue as specified.

huff /hʌf/ n a state of smouldering resentment. • vi to blow; to puff.

huffish /'hʌfɪʃ/ adj prone to fits of anger or petulance.

huffy /'hʌfi/ adj (**huffier, huffiest**) disgruntled, moody.—**huffily** adv.—**huffiness** n.

hug /hʌg/ vb (**hugging, hugged**) vt to hold or squeeze tightly with the arms; to cling to; to keep close to. • vi to embrace one another. • n a strong embrace.—**huggable** adj.—**hugger** n.

huge /hju:dʒ/ or /ju:dʒ/ adj very large, enormous.—**hugely** adv.—**hugeness** n.

huggermugger /'hʌgər,mʌgər/ n secrecy, concealment; confusion. • adj secret, clandestine; confused, jumbled. • adv in confusion. • vt to conceal, to hush up. • vi to muddle.

hula /'hu:lə/, **hula-hula** n a Polynesian dance performed by men or women; the music for this.

hulk /hʌlk/ n the body of a ship, esp if old and dismantled; a large, clumsy person or thing.

hulking /'hʌlkɪŋ/, **hulky** /-i/ adj unwieldy, bulky.

hull /hʌl/ n the outer covering of a fruit or seed; the framework of a ship. • vt to remove the hulls of; to pierce the hull of (a ship, etc).—**huller** n.—**hull-less** adj.

hullabaloo, hullaballoo /,heləbə'lu:/ n (pl **hullabaloos, hullaballoos**) a loud commotion, uproar.

hullo /ha'lo:/ see **hello**.

hum /hʌm/ vb (**humming, hummed**) vi to make a low continuous vibrating sound; to hesitate in speaking and utter an inarticulate sound; (inf) to be lively, busy; (sl) to stink. • vt to sing with closed lips. • n a humming sound; a murmur; (sl) a stink.

human /'hju:mən/ or /'ju:-/ adj of or relating to human beings; having the qualities of humans as opposed to animals; kind, considerate. • n a human being.—**humanness** n.

human being n a member of the races of Homo sapiens; a man, woman or child.

humane /hju:'meɪn/ or /ju:-/ adj kind, compassionate, merciful.—**humanely** adv.—**humaneness** n.

human immunodeficiency virus n either of two strains of a virus, also know as HIV, that inhibits the body from developing resistance to diseases and can lead to the development of AIDS.

human interest adj (newspaper story, etc) appealing to the emotions.

humanism /'hju:mə,nɪzəm/ or /'ju:-/ n belief in the promotion of human interests, intellect and welfare.

humanist /'hju:mənɪst/ or /'ju:-/ n one versed in the knowledge of human nature; a student of the humanities.—**humanistic** adj.

humanitarian /hju:mænɪ'tɛriən/ or /ju:-/ adj concerned with promoting human welfare. • n a humanitarian person.—**humanitarianism** n.—**humanitarianist** n.

humanity /hju:'mænɪti/ or /ju:-/ n (pl **humanities**) the human race; the state or quality of being human or humane; philanthropy; kindness; (pl) the study of literature and the arts, as opposed to the sciences.

humanize /'hju:mə,naɪz/ or /'ju:-/ vti to make or become human.—**humanization** n.—**humanizer** n.

humankind /'hju:mən,kaɪnd/ or /'ju:-/ n the human species; humanity.

humanly /'hju:mənli/ or /ju:-/ adv in a way characteristic of humans; within the limits of human capabilities.

humanoid /'hju:mənɔɪd/ or /'ju:-/ adj resembling a human being in appearance or character. • n a humanoid thing.

humble /'hʌmbəl/ adj having a low estimation of one's abilities; modest, unpretentious; servile. • vt to lower in condition or rank; to humiliate.—**humbleness** n.—**humbly** adv.

humblebee /'hʌmbəl,bi:/ n the bumblebee.

humble pie n apology, usu under pressure.

humbug /'hʌmbʌg/ n fraud, sham, hoax; an insincere person; a peppermint-flavoured sweet. • vt (**humbugging, humbugged**) to cheat or impose upon; to hoax.—**humbugger** n.—**humbuggery** n.

humdinger /'hʌm,dɪŋər/ n (inf) a remarkable person or thing.

humdrum /'hʌmdrʌm/ adj dull, ordinary, boring.—**humdrumness** n.

humerus /'hju:mərəs/ n (pl **humeri**) the bone extending from the shoulder to the elbow in humans.—**humeral** adj.

humid /'hju:mɪd/ adj (air) moist, damp.—**humidly** adv.—**humidness** n.

humidex /'hju:mɪdeks/ n ✽ (Cdn) a measure of the amount of discomfort caused by a combination of heat and humidity in the air.

humidifier /hju:'mɪdɪ,faɪr/ n a device employed to increase the amount of water vapour in a room.

humidifier fever n a collection of symptoms, thought to be caused by micro-organisms found in humidifiers and including lethargy, headache and eye irritation, that affect those who work in totally air-conditioned buildings.—also **sick building syndrome**.

humidify /hju:'mɪdɪ,faɪ/ vt (**humidifying, humidified**) to make humid.—**humidification** n.—**humidifier** n.

humidity /hju:'mɪdɪti/ n (a measure of the amount of) dampness in the air.

humidor /'hju:mɪ,dɔr/ n a humid cabinet or room where cigars are kept moist.

humiliate /hju:'mɪli,eɪt/ vt to cause to feel humble; to lower the pride or dignity of.—**humiliatingly** adv.—**humiliator** n.—**humiliatory** adj.

humiliation /,hju:mɪli'eɪʃən/ n the act of humiliation; the state of being humiliated; mortification; abasement.

humility /hju:'mɪlɪti/ n (pl **humilities**) the state of being humble; modesty.

hummingbird /'hʌmɪŋ,bərd/ n a tiny brightly coloured tropical bird with wings that vibrate rapidly, making a humming sound.

hummock /'hʌmək/ n a hillock.—**hummocky** adj.

hummus /'hʌməs/ n a dip or appetizer of puréed chick peas, sesame seeds and garlic.—also **houmous, houmus**.

humoresque /,hju:mə'resk/ n a light musical piece.

humorist /'hju:mərɪst/ or /ju:-/ n a person who writes or speaks in a humorous manner.—**humoristic** adj.

humorous /'hju:mərəs/ or /ju:-/ adj funny, amusing; causing laughter.—**humorously** adv.—**humorousness** n.

humour, humor /'hju:mər/ or /'ju:mər/ n the ability to appreciate or express what is funny, amusing, etc; the expression of this; temperament, disposition; state of mind; (formerly) any of the four fluids of the body (blood, phlegm, yellow and black bile) that were thought to determine temperament. • vt to indulge; to gratify by conforming to the wishes of.—**humourful, humorful** adj.

humourless, humorless /-ləs/ adj done or said without humour; lacking a sense of humour.—**humourlessness, humorlessness** n.

humourology, humorology /hju:mə'rɒlədʒi/ n the study of humour.

hump /hʌmp/ *n* a rounded protuberance; a fleshy lump on the back of an animal (as a camel or whale); a deformity causing curvature of the spine. • *vt* to hunch; to arch.

humpback /'hʌmpbæk/ *n* a hunchback.—**humpbacked** *adj*.

humph /hʌmf/ *interj* expressing annoyance.

humus /'hju:məs/ *n* dark brown or black organic matter in the soil formed from partially decomposed leaves, plants, etc.

Hun /hʌn/ *n* one of the ancient Tartar races that overran Europe in the 4th and 5th centuries; a vandal; (*Hist derog*) a German.

hunch /hʌntʃ/ *n* a hump; (*inf*) an intuitive feeling. • *vt* to arch into a hump. • *vi* to move forward jerkily.

hunchback /'hʌntʃbæk/ *n* a person with curvature of the spine.

hunchbacked /-bækt/ *adj* having an abnormal convex curvature of the thoracic spine.

hundred /'hʌndrəd/ *adj, n* (*pl* **hundreds, hundred**) ten times ten; the symbol for this (100, C, c); the hundredth in a series or set.

hundredfold /-ˌfo:ld/ *adj, adv* one hundred times as great or many.

hundredth /'hʌndrədθ/ *adj* the last of a hundred.

hundredweight /'hʌndrədˌweɪt/ *n* (*pl* **hundredweight, hundredweights**) a unit of weight, equal to 110 pounds in US and 112 pounds in the UK.

hung /hʌŋ/ *see* **hang**.

Hungarian /hʌŋ'gerɪən/ *adj* pertaining to Hungary, its inhabitants, or language. • *n* an inhabitant of Hungary; the language spoken in Hungary.

hunger /'hʌŋgər/ *n* (a feeling of weakness or emptiness from) a need for food; a strong desire. • *vi* to feel hunger; to have a strong desire (for).

hunger strike *n* refusal to take food as a protest.

hung-over /hʌŋ'o:vər/ *adj* (*sl*) suffering from a hangover.

hungry /'hʌŋgrɪ/ *adj* (**hungrier, hungriest**) desiring food; craving for something; greedy.—**hungrily** *adv*.—**hungriness** *n*.

hunk /hʌŋk/ *n* (*inf*) a large piece, lump, etc; (*sl*) a sexually attractive man.—**hunky** *adj*.

hunker /'hʌŋkər/ *vi* to squat, crouch down. • *npl* the haunches or buttocks.

hunkydory /ˌhʌŋki'dorɪ/ *adj* first-rate.

hunt /hʌnt/ *vti* to seek out to kill or capture (game) for food or sport; to search (for); to chase. • *n* a chase; a search; a party organized for hunting.

hunter /'hʌntər/ *n* a person who hunts; a horse used in hunting.—**huntress** *nf*.

hunting /'hʌntɪŋ/ *n* the art or practice of one who hunts; a pursuit; a search.

huntsman /'hʌntsmən/ *n* (*pl* **huntsmen**) a person who manages a hunt and looks after the hounds.

hurdle /'hərdəl/ *n* a portable frame of bars for temporary fences or for jumping over by horses or runners; an obstacle. (*pl*) a race over hurdles.—**hurdler** *n*.

hurdy-gurdy /'hərdɪˌgərdi/ *n* (*pl* **hurdy-gurdies**) a mechanical instrument such as a barrel organ.

hurl /hərl/ *vt* to throw violently; to utter vehemently. • *n* a violent throw; a ride in a car.—**hurler** *n*.

hurling /'hərlɪŋ/, **hurley** /'hərli/ *n* an Irish form of field hockey.

hurly-burly /'hərliˌbərli/ *n* (*pl* **hurly-burlies**) uproar; confusion.

hurrah /hə'ro/ *interj* an exclamation of approval or joy.—*also* **hooray, hoorah**.

hurricane /'hʌriˌkein/ *n* a violent tropical cyclone with winds of at least 74 miles (119 kilometres) per hour.

hurried /'həri:d/ *adj* performed with great haste.—**hurriedly** *adv*.—**hurriedness** *n*.

hurry /'həri/ *n* (*pl* **hurries**) rush; urgency; eagerness to do, go, etc. • *vb* (**hurrying, hurried**) *vt* to cause to move or happen more quickly. • *vi* to move or act with haste.—**hurryingly** *adv*.

hurt /hərt/ *vb* (**hurting, hurt**) *vt* to cause physical pain to; to injure, damage; to offend. • *vi* to feel pain; to cause pain.—**hurter** *n*.

hurtful /'hərtful/ *adj* causing hurt, mischievous.—**hurtfully** *adv*.—**hurtfulness** *n*.

hurtle /'hərtəl/ *vti* to move or throw with great speed and force.

husband /'hʌzbənd/ *n* a man to whom a woman is married. • *vt* to conserve; to manage economically.—**husbander** *n*.

husbandman /-mən/ *n* (*pl* **husbandmen**) a farmer.

husbandry /'hʌzbəndri/ *n* management of resources; farming.

hush /hʌʃ/ *vti* to make or become silent. • *n* a silence or calm.

hush-hush /hʌʃ'hʌʃ/ *adj* (*inf*) secret.

hush money *n* (*sl*) money paid to a person to keep a discreditable fact secret.

husk /hʌsk/ *n* the dry covering of certain fruits and seeds; any dry, rough, or useless covering. • *vt* to strip the husk from.—**husker** *n*.

husky[1] /'hʌski/ *adj* (**huskier, huskiest**) (*voice*) hoarse; rough-sounding; hefty, strong.—**huskily** *adv*.—**huskiness** *n*.

husky[2] *n* (*pl* **huskies**) an Arctic sled dog.

hussar /hʊ'zɑr/ *n* a member of any of various European light cavalry regiments, *usu* with an elegant dress uniform.

hussy /'hʌsi/ *n* (*pl* **hussies**) a cheeky woman; a promiscuous woman.

hustings /'hʌstɪŋz/ *n* (*pl or sing*) the process of, or a place for, political campaigning.

hustle /'hʌsəl/ *vt* to jostle or push roughly or hurriedly; to force hurriedly; (*sl*) to obtain by rough or illegal means. • *vi* to move hurriedly. • *n* an instance of hustling.—**hustler** *n*.

hut /hʌt/ *n* a very plain or crude little house or cabin.

hutch /hʌtʃ/ *n* a pen or coop for small animals; a hut.

huzzah /'hʌzə/ *interj* (*formerly*) hurrah.

hyacinth /'haɪəsɪnθ/ *n* a plant of the lily family with spikes of bell-shaped flowers; the orange gemstone jacinth; a light violet to moderate purple.—**hyacinthine** *adj*.

Hyades /'haɪəˌdi:z/ *n* (*Greek myth*) five nymphs, the daughters of Atlas, the five stars in the constellation Taurus.

hyaline /'haɪəlɪn/ or /-ˌlaɪn/, /-ˌli:n/ *adj* glassy; transparent.

hybrid /'haɪbrɪd/ *n* the offspring of two plants or animals of different species; a mongrel. • *adj* crossbred.—**hybridism** *n*.—**hybridity** *n*.

hybridize /'haɪbrɪˌdaɪz/ *vti* to produce hybrids; to interbreed.—**hybridizable** *adj*.—**hybridization** *n*.—**hybridizer** *n*.

hydatid /'haɪdətɪd/ *n* a watery cyst in animal tissue; a large bladder containing the larvae of the tapeworm.—*also adj*.

hydr- /haɪdr/, **hydro-** /haɪdro/ *prefix* water, fluids.

hydra /'haɪdrə/ *n* (*pl* **hydras, hydrae**) (*usu with cap*) a legendary many-headed water serpent; any of numerous freshwater polyps having a mouth surrounded by tentacles.

hydrangea /haɪ'dreɪndʒə/ or /-dʒiə/ *n* a shrub with large heads of white, pink, or blue flowers.

hydrant /'haɪdrənt/ *n* a large pipe with a valve for drawing water from a water main; a fireplug.

hydrate /'haɪdreɪt/ *n* a chemical compound of water with some other substance. • *vt* to (cause to) combine with or absorb water.—**hydration** *n*.—**hydrator** *n*.

hydraulic /haɪ'drɒlɪk/ *adj* operated by water or other liquid, *esp* by moving through pipes under pressure; of hydraulics.—**hydraulically** *adv*.

hydraulics /haɪ'drɒlɪks/ *n sing* the science dealing with the mechanical properties of liquids, as water, and their application in engineering.

hydric /'haɪdrɪk/ *adj* of or containing hydrogen; of or containing water.

hydride /'haɪdraɪd/ *n* any compound of hydrogen and another element.

hydriodic /ˌhaɪdrɪ'ɒdɪk/ or /-draɪ-/ *adj* composed of hydrogen and iodine.

hydro[1] /'haɪdro:/ *n* (*pl* **hydros**) a hotel or resort offering hydropathic treatment.

hydro[2] *n* ✻ (*Cdn*) electricity, especially hydroelectricity.

hydrocarbon /ˌhaɪdro:'kɑrbən/ *n* any organic compound containing only hydrogen and carbon.

hydrocele /'haɪdrəˌsi:l/ *n* an accumulation of fluid in a body cavity, *esp* in the scrotum.

hydrocephalus /ˌhaɪdrə'sefələs/, **hydrocephaly** /-i/ *n* an accumulation of fluid in the brain.—**hydrocephalic** *adj*.

hydrochloric acid *n* a strong, highly corrosive acid that is a solution of the gas hydrogen chloride in water.

hydrochloric /ˌhaɪdrə'klorɪk/ *adj* composed of hydrogen and chlorine.

hydrocyanic /ˌhaɪdrəsaɪ'ænɪk/ *adj* composed of hydrogen and cyanic.

hydrodynamics /ˌhaɪdro:daɪ'næmɪks/ *n sing* the science of the mechanical properties of fluids.—**hydrodynamic** *adj*.—**hydrodynamically** *adv*.

hydroelectricity /ˌhaɪdro:ɪlɛk'trɪsɪti/ *n* electricity generated by water power.—**hydroelectric** *adj*.

hydrofluoric /ˌhaɪdrɔ:ˈflʊrɪk/ *adj* composed of hydrogen and fluorine.

hydrofoil /ˈhaɪdrəˌfɔɪl/ *n* a vessel equipped with vanes that lift the hull out of the water to allow fast cruising speeds.

hydrogen /ˈhaɪdrədʒən/ *n* a flammable, colourless, odourless, tasteless, gaseous chemical element, the lightest substance known.

hydrogenate /haɪˈdrɒdʒɪˌneɪt/ or /ˈhaɪdrədʒəˌneɪt/ *vt* to combine with or treat with hydrogen.—**hydrogenation** *n*.—**hydrogenator** *n*.

hydrogen bomb *n* a powerful bomb that produces explosive energy through the fusion of hydrogen nuclei.

hydrography /haɪˈdrɒɡrəfi/ *n* the study, surveying and mapping of the oceans, seas, lakes, and rivers as on a chart.—**hydrographer** *n*.—**hydrographic, hydrographical** *adj*.

hydrokinetics /ˌhaɪdrɔ:kɪˈnetɪks/ *n sing* the branch of physics concerned with the study of fluids in motion.

hydrology /haɪˈdrɒlədʒi/ *n* the science of the properties of water and its distribution on the earth and in the atmosphere.—**hydrologic, hydrological** *adj*.—**hydrologist** *n*.

hydrolysis /haɪˈdrɒlɪsɪs/ *n* the chemical breakdown of organic compounds by interaction with water.

hydrolyze /ˈhaɪdrəˌlaɪz/ *vti* to decompose by hydrolysis.—**hydrolyzation** *n*.—**hydrolyzer** *n*.

hydromechanics /ˌhaɪdrɔ:mɪˈkænɪks/ *n sing* the science of the use of fluids as motive-power also called hydrodynamics.

hydromel /ˈhaɪdrəˌmel/ *n* a mixture of honey and water that is fermented to make mead.

hydrometer /haɪˈdrɒmɪtər/ *n* a device for measuring the densities of liquids.—**hydrometric, hydrometrical** *adj*.—**hydrometry** *n*.

hydropathy /haɪˈdrɒpəθi/ *n* the use of water to treat diseases.—**hydropathic, hydropathical** *adj*.—**hydropathist, hydropath** *n*.

hydrophane /ˈhaɪdrəˌfeɪn/ *n* a partially opaque, white type of opal that becomes translucent in water.

hydrophobia /ˌhaɪdrəˈfoːbiə/ *n* a morbid fear of water; rabies.—**hydrophobic** *adj*.

hydrophone /ˈhaɪdrəˌfoːn/ *n* an instrument that detects sound through water.

hydrophyte /ˈhaɪdrəˌfaɪt/ *n* a plant that will grow only in water or sodden soil.—**hydrophitic** *adj*.

hydroplane /ˈhaɪdrəˌpleɪn/ *n* a light motor boat that skims through the water at high speed with its hull raised out of the water; a fin that directs the vertical movement of a submarine; an attachment to an aircraft that enables it to glide along the surface of water. • *vi* (of a boat) to rise out of the water in the manner of a hydroplane.

hydroponics /ˌhaɪdrəˈpɒnɪks/ *n sing* the growing of plants in chemical nutrients without soil.—**hydroponically** *adv*.

hydroscope /ˈhaɪdrəˌskoːp/ *n* any instrument that makes observations of underwater objects.

hydrosphere /ˈhaɪdrəˌsfiːr/ *n* the moisture-bearing envelope that surrounds the earth.

hydrostatics /ˌhaɪdrəˈstætɪks/ *n sing* the branch of physics concerned with the study of fluids at rest.—**hydrostatic** *adj*.

hydrotherapy /ˌhaɪdrəˈθerəpi/ *n* (*pl* **hydrotherapies**) the treatment of certain diseases and physical conditions by the external application of water.—**hydrotherapist** *n*.

hydrous /ˈhaɪdrəs/ *adj* containing water.

hyena /haɪˈiːnə/ *n* a nocturnal, carnivorous, scavenging mammal like a wolf.—*also* **hyaena**.

Hygeia /haɪˈdʒiːə/ *n* (*Greek myth*) the goddess of health.

hygiene /ˈhaɪdʒiːn/ *n* the principles and practice of health and cleanliness.—**hygienic** *adj*.—**hygienically** *adv*.

hygienist /haɪˈdʒenɪst/ or /haɪˈdʒiːnɪst/ *n* a person skilled in the practice of hygiene.

hygrometer /haɪˈɡrɒmɪtər/ *n* an instrument for measuring the humidity of the atmosphere.—**hygrometric** *adj*.—**hygrometrically** *adv*.—**hygrometry** *n*.

hygroscope /ˈhaɪɡrəˌskoːp/ *n* an instrument that shows changes in the humidity of the atmosphere.

hygroscopic /ˌhaɪɡrəˈskɒpɪk/ *adj* readily absorbing and retaining moisture from the air.—**hygroscopically** *adv*.

hylozoism /ˌhaɪləˈzoːɪzəm/ *n* (*philos*) the doctrine that life is a property of matter; materialism.—**hylozoic** *adj*.—**hylozoist** *n*.

Hymen /ˈhaɪmen/ *n* (*Greek myth*) the god of marriage.

hymen *n* the mucous membrane partly closing the vaginal orifice.—**hymenal** *adj*.

hymeneal /ˌhaɪmɪˈniːəl/ *adj* of marriage, nuptial.

hymenopteran /ˌhaɪməˈnɒptərən/ *n* (*pl* **hymenopterans, hymenopterana**) any of a large order of insects that have two pairs of membranous wings —**hymenopterous** *adj*.

hymn /hɪm/ *n* a song of praise to God or other object of worship.

hymnal /ˈhɪmnəl/ *n* a hymn book.

hymn book *n* a book of hymns.

hymnology /hɪmˈnɒlədʒi/ *n* the study of the composition of hymns.—**hymnologist** *n*

hyoid /ˈhaɪɔɪd/ *adj* U-shaped; of or relating to the hyoid bone at the base of the tongue.

hyoscine /ˈhaɪəˌsiːn/ *see* **scopolamine**.

hyp- /hɪp/ or /haɪp/ **hypo-** *prefix* below; slightly.

hype¹ /haɪp/ *n* (*sl*) a hypodermic needle. • *vi* (*sl*) to inject a narcotic drug with a needle.

hype² *n* (*sl*) deception; aggressive or extravagant publicity. • *vt* to publicize or promote a product, etc in this manner.

hyped-up *adj* aggressively publicized; (*sl*) stimulated as if by injection of a drug.

hyper- /ˈhaɪpər/ *prefix* above; too; exceeding.

hyperactive /ˌhaɪpərˈæktɪv/ *adj* abnormally active.—**hyperactivity** *n*.

hyperesthesia, hyperaesthesia /ˌhaɪpərəsˈθiːziə/ *n* increased sensitivity of any of the sense organs.—**hyperaesthetic** *adj*.

hyperbola /haɪˈpɜːbələ/ *n* (*pl* **hyperbolas, hyperbolae**) (*geom*) a curve formed by a plane intersecting a cone at a greater angle to its base than its side.

hyperbole /haɪˈpɜːbəli/ *n* a figure of speech using absurd exaggeration.

hyperbolic /ˌhaɪpərˈbɒlɪk/, **hyperbolical** /-əl/ *adj* pertaining to or containing hyperbole, exaggerated; pertaining to or of the nature of a hyperbola.

hyperborean /ˌhaɪpərbɔ:ˈriːən/ *adj* of or relating to the extreme north. • *n* an inhabitant of the extreme north; (*Greek myth*) (*with cap*) one of the people who lived in the sunny land beyond the north wind.

hypercritical /ˌhaɪpərˈkrɪtɪkəl/ *adj* excessively critical.—**hypercritically** *adv*.—**hypercriticism** *n*.

hypermetric /ˌhaɪpərˈmetrɪk/ *adj* beyond the normal metre of a line; having one syllable too many.

hypersensitive /ˌhaɪpərˈsensɪtɪv/ *adj* extremely vulnerable; abnormally sensitive to a drug, pollen, etc.—**hypersensitivity** *n*.

hypersonic /ˌhaɪpərˈsɒnɪk/ *adj* travelling at speeds at least five times faster than sound; of sound frequencies above 1,000 megahertz.—**hypersonics** *n*.

hypertension /ˌhaɪpərˈtenʃən/ *n* abnormally high blood pressure.—**hypertensive** *adj*

hypertext /ˈhaɪpərtekst/ *n* computer software/hardware that allows the user to pick up on one word in a document as a route to another area of the document or a different document.

hyperthyroidism /ˌhaɪpərˈθaɪrɔɪˌdɪzəm/ *n* the overproduction of the thyroid hormone by the thyroid gland.—**hyperthyroid** *adj*.

hypertrophy /haɪˈpɜːtrəfi/ *n* (*pl* **hypertrophies**) abnormal enlargement of an organ or part.—**hypertrophic** *adj*.

hypervitaminosis /ˌhaɪpərˌvaɪtəmɪˈnoːsɪs/ *n* the pathological condition that results from the excessive intake of vitamins.

hyphen /ˈhaɪfən/ *n* a punctuation mark (-) used to join two syllables or words, or to divide words into parts. • *vt* to hyphenate.

hyphenate /ˈhaɪfəˌneɪt/ *vt* to join by a hyphen.—**hyphenation** *n*.

hypnosis /hɪpˈnoːsɪs/ *n* (*pl* **hypnoses**) a relaxed state resembling sleep in which the mind responds to external suggestion.

hypnotherapy /ˌhɪpnoːˈθerəpi/ *n* the use of hypnosis in treatment of emotional and psychological disorders.

hypnotic /hɪpˈnɒtɪk/ *adj* of or producing hypnosis; (*person*) susceptible to hypnosis. • *n* a drug causing sleep; a person susceptible to hypnosis.—**hypnotically** *adv*.

hypnotism /ˈhɪpnəˌtɪzəm/ *n* the act of inducing hypnosis; the study and use of hypnosis.—**hypnotist** *n*.

hypnotize /ˈhɪpnəˌtaɪz/ *vt* to put in a state of hypnosis; to fascinate.—**hypnotizer** *n*.

hypo- /ˈhaɪpoː/ *prefix* below; slightly.

hypocaust /ˈhaɪpəˌkɒst/ *n* the hot-air chamber under a Roman bath.

hypochondria /ˌhaɪpəˈkɒndriə/ *n* chronic anxiety about health, often with imaginary illnesses.

hypochondriac /ˌhəɪpə'kɒndriˌæk/ *n* a person suffering from hypochondria. • *adj* pertaining to or affected with hypochrondria.—**hypochondriacally** *adv*.

hypocorism /ˌhəɪpəkə'rɪzəm/ *n* a diminutive pet name; a euphemism.—**hypocoristic, hypocoristical** *adj*.

hypocrisy /hɪ'pɒkrəsi/ *n* (*pl* **hypocrisies**) a falsely pretending to possess virtues, beliefs, etc; an example of this.—**hypocritical** *adj*.—**hypocritically** *adv*.

hypocrite /'hɪpəkrɪt/ *n* a person who pretends to be what he or she is not.

hypocycloid /ˌhəɪpə'səɪklɔɪd/ *n* (*geom*) a curve traced by the point on the circumference of a circle, which rolls on to the inside of another circle.

hypodermic /ˌhəɪpə'dərmɪk/ *adj* injected under the skin. • *n* a hypodermic needle, syringe or injection.

hypodermic syringe *n* a syringe with a hollow (hypodermic) needle through which blood samples can be drawn.

hypogastrium /ˌhəɪpə'gæstriəm/ *n* (*pl* **hypogastria**) the middle part of the lower region of the abdomen.

hypogeal /ˌhəɪpə'dʒiːəl/, **hypogean** /-ən/, **hypogeous** /-əs/ *adj* (*bot*) underground; occuring or living underground.

hypogene /'həɪpəˌdʒiːn/ *adj* (*rocks*) formed under the surface of the ground.

hypostasis /həɪ'pɒstəsɪs/ *n* (*pl* **hypostates**) the essential personality of a substance; (*Christianity*) any of the three persons of the Godhead which together make up the Holy Trinity; (*med*) an excess of blood in the organs as the result of poor circulation.—**hypostatic** *adj*.

hypostatize /həɪ'pɒstətaɪz/ *vt* to regard as real; to embody or personify.—**hypostatization** *n*.

hypostyle /'həɪpəˌstaɪl/ *n* a roof supported by columns; a covered colonnade; a pillared hall or court.

hypotenuse /həɪ'pɒtəˌnuːs/ or /-ˌnjuːz/, /-ˌnuːz/ *n* the side opposite to the right angle in a right-angled triangle.

hypothecate /həɪ'pɒθɪˌkeɪt/ or /hɪ-/ *vt* to pledge (a property) without delivery of title or possession.—**hypothecation** *n*.—**hypothecator** *n*.

hypothermia /ˌhəɪpəʊ'θɜːmiə/ *n* an abnormally low body temperature.

hypothesis /həɪ'pɒθɪsɪs/ *n* (*pl* **hypotheses**) something assumed for the purpose of argument; a theory to explain some fact that may or may not prove to be true; supposition; conjecture.

hypothesize /həɪ'pɒθɪˌsaɪz/ *vti* to form or assume as a hypothesis.

hypothetical /ˌhəɪpə'θetɪkəl/ *adj* based on hypothesis, conjectural.—**hypothetically** *adv*.

hypothyroidism /ˌhəɪpəʊ'θaɪrɔɪˌdɪzəm/ *n* deficient activity of the thyroid glands.

hypsometry /hɪp'sɒmətri/ *n* the science of measuring altitude.—**hypsometric** *adj*

hyrax /'haɪræks/ *n* (*pl* **hyraxes, hyraces**) a small African hamster-like mammal related to the elephant.

hyson /'haɪsən/ *n* Chinese green tea.

hyssop /'hɪsəp/ *n* an aromatic plant with blue flowers formerly used in medicine.

hysterectomy /ˌhɪstə'rektəmi/ *n* (*pl* **hysterectomies**) surgical removal of the womb.

hysteresis /ˌhɪstə'riːsɪs/ *n*. (*pl* **hystereses**) magnetic inertia.—**hysteretic** *adj*.

hysteria /hɪ'steriə/ or /-'stiːriə/ *n* a mental disorder marked by excitability, anxiety, imaginary organic disorders, etc; frenzied emotion or excitement.

hysteric /hɪ'sterɪk/ *n* a hysterical person; (*pl*) fits of hysteria; (*inf*) uncontrollable laughter.

hysterical /hɪ'sterɪkəl/ *adj* caused by hysteria; suffering from hysteria; (*inf*) extremely funny.—**hysterically** *adv*.

hysterotomy /ˌhɪstər'ɒtəmi/ *n* (*pl* **hysterotomies**) a surgical incision into the womb.

Hz *abbr* = hertz.

I

I[1] /aɪ/ *pron* the person who is speaking or writing, used in referring to himself or herself.

I[2] (*chem symbol*) iodine.

I. *abbr* = island(s); isle(s).

IAEA *abbr* = International Atomic Energy Authority.

iamb /ˈaɪæmb/, **iambus** /aɪˈæmbəs/ *n* (*pl* **iambi, iambs, iambuses**) a metrical foot consisting of two syllables, the first short or unstressed and the second long or stressed.—**iambic** *adj*.

-iana, -ana *n suffix* sayings of, publications about, as *Shakespeariana*, etc.

-iatric, -iatrical *adj* pertaining to doctors and medicine.

Iberian /aɪˈbɪːriən/ *adj* pertaining to Spain and Portugal; pertaining to Iberia, the ancient name of the southwest European peninsula now comprising Spain and Portugal.

ibex /ˈaɪbɛks/ *n* (*pl* **ibexes, ibices, ibex**) any of various wild mountain goats with large horns.

ibid *abbr* = *ibidem*, in, in the same book, page, etc.

ibis /ˈaɪbɪs/ *n* (*pl* **ibises, ibis**) a wading bird with a curved bill.

Ibo /ˈiːboː/ *n* (*pl* **Ibo, Ibos**) a member of a Black people of southern Nigeria; their language.

ICBM *abbr* = intercontinental ballistic missile.

ice /aɪs/ *n* water frozen solid; a sheet of this; a portion of ice cream or water ice. • *vti* (*often with* **up** *or* **over**) to freeze; to cool with ice; to cover with icing.

ice age *n* a period when much of the earth's surface was covered in glaciers; (*with caps*) the Pleistocene glacial epoch.

iceberg /ˈaɪsbɜːrg/ *n* a great mass of mostly submerged ice floating in the sea.

iceblink /ˈaɪsblɪŋk/ *n* a streak of whiteness on the horizon caused by the reflection of light from masses of ice in the distance.

icebound /ˈaɪsbaʊnd/ *adj* (*ship, etc*) surrounded, and immobilized, by ice.

icebox /ˈaɪsbɒks/ *n* a compartment in a refrigerator for making ice.

icebreaker, iceboat /ˈaɪsboːt/ *n* a powerful and reinforced vessel for breaking a channel through ice.

ice bridge *n* ✺ (*Cdn*) a formation of ice across a body of water strong enough to support motor or other traffic.

icecap *n* a mass of slowly spreading glacial ice.

ice cream *adj* a sweet frozen food, made from flavoured milk or cream.

ice dance *n* a type of ballroom dancing by skaters on ice.

icefall /ˈaɪsfɔl/ *n* a steep part of a glacier, resembling a frozen waterfall.

ice field /ˈaɪsfiːld/ *n* an extensive field of floating ice.

ice fishing *n* ✺ the activity of fishing through holes cut in the ice of a lake or river.

ice floe *n* a sheet of floating ice.

ice hockey *n* an indoor or outdoor hockey game played on ice by two teams of six skaters with curved sticks and a flat disk called a puck.

ice hole *n* ✺ (*Cdn*) a hole cut in ice so that people may fish.

Icelander /ˈaɪslændər/ *n* a native or inhabitant of Iceland.

Icelandic /aɪsˈlændɪk/ *adj* of or pertaining to Iceland or its language, literature and people. • *n* the language of Iceland.

ice pack *n* a field of broken and drifting ice, consisting of great masses packed together; a cloth or small bag filled with crushed ice for soothing sores and swellings on the body.

ice pick *n* a pointed awl with a handle for chipping or breaking up ice.

ice plant *n* a type of plant with leaves that glisten as if covered with ice.

ice road *n* ✺ (*Cdn*) a road built across a frozen body of water.

ice skate *n* a boot with a steel blade fixed to the sole for skating on ice.—*also vi.*—**ice skater** *n*.

ichneumon /ɪkˈnjuːmən/ *n* a North African mongoose.

ichneumon fly *n* an insect that lays its eggs in the bodies of other insects.

ichnite /ˈɪknaɪt/, **ichnolite** /-nolaɪt/ *n* a fossil footprint.

ichor /ˈaɪkɔr/ *n* (*Greek myth*) the ethereal fluid believed to run, instead of blood, in the veins of the classical gods.—**ichorous** *adj*.

ichtny- /ˈɪkθɪniː/, **ichthyo-** /ˈɪkθɪoː/ *prefix* fish.

ichthyic /ˈɪkθɪk/ *adj* pertaining to fishes.

ichthyoid /ˈɪkθɔɪd/, **ichthyidal** /-əl/ *adj* resembling a fish.

ichthyology /ˌɪkθɪˈɒlədʒi/ *n* the study of fish.—**ichthyologic, ichthyological** *adj*.—**ichthyologist** *n*.

ichthyophagous /ˌɪkθɪˈɒfəgəs/ *adj* fish-eating.—**ichthyophagy** *n*.

ichthyornis /ˌɪkθɪˈɔrnɪs/ *n* an extinct species of toothed fish-eating bird.

ichthyosaur /ˈɪkθɪəsɔr/ **ichthyosaurus** /-rəs/ *n* (*pl* **ichthyosaurs, ichthosauri**) a gigantic, extinct, marine reptile.

ichthyosis /ɪkθɪˈoːsɪs/ *n* a disease in which the skin becomes dry and scaly.

icicle /ˈaɪsɪkəl/ *n* a hanging tapering length of ice formed when dripping water freezes.—**icicled** *adj*.

icily /ˈaɪsɪli/ *adv* in an icy manner, coldly.

iciness /-nəs/ *n* the state of being icy, coldness.

icing /ˈaɪsɪŋ/ *n* a semi-solid sugary mixture used to cover cakes, etc.—*also* **frosting**.

icon /ˈaɪkɒn/ *n* an image; (*Eastern Church*) a sacred image, *usu* on a wooden panel; a symbol on a computer screen that represents something or some process or function in the computer.—*also* **ikon**.—**iconic, iconical** *adj*.

iconoclast /aɪˈkɒnəˌklæst/ *n* a person who attacks revered or traditional beliefs, opinions etc.—**iconoclasm** *n*.—**iconoclastic** *adj*.—**iconoclastically** *adv*.

iconography /ˌaɪkəˈnɒgrəfi/ *n* (*pl* **iconographies**) the art of representation by means of images (statues), pictures, or engravings; the study of this art.—**iconographer** *n*.—**iconographic, iconographical** *adj*.

iconolatry /ˌaɪkəˈnɒlətri/ *n* the worship of images.

iconology /ˌaɪkəˈnɒlədʒi/ *n* the study of icons.

icosahedron /ˌaɪkəsəˈhiːdrən/ *n* (*pl* **icosahedrons, icosahedra**) (*geom*) a solid bounded by 20 plane faces.

icterus /ˈɪktərəs/ *n* jaundice.—**icteric** *adj*.

ictus /ˈɪktəs/ *n* (*pl* **ictuses, ctus**) a stress in verse.

icy /ˈaɪsi/ *adj* (**icier, iciest**) full of, made of, or covered with ice; slippery or very cold; cold in manner.

ID *abbr* = identification.

ID card *n* an identity card.

I'd /aɪd/ = I had; I should; I would.

id /ɪd/ *n* (*psychoanal*) the primitive psychological instincts in the unconscious which are the source of psychic activity.

ide /aɪd/ *n* a small European fish.

idea /aɪˈdiːə/ *n* a mental impression of anything; a vague impression, notion; an opinion or belief; a scheme; a supposition; a person's conception of something; a significance or purpose.

ideal /aɪˈdiːəl/ *or* /-diːl/ *adj* existing in the mind or as an idea; satisfying an ideal, perfect. • *n* the most perfect conception of anything; a person or thing regarded as perfect; a standard for attainment or imitation; an aim or principle.—**ideally** *adv*.—**idealness** *n*.

idealism /aɪˈdiəˌlɪzəm/ *n* the pursuit of high ideals; the conception or representation of things in their ideal form as against their reality.—**idealist** *n*.—**idealistic** *adj*.—**idealistically** *adv*.

ideality /ˌaɪdiˈælɪti/ *n* (*pl* **idealities**) the quality of being ideal; the faculty to form ideals.

idealize /aɪˈdiəˌlaɪz/ *vt* to consider or represent as ideal.—**idealization** *n*.—**idealizer** *n*.

ideate /ˈaɪdiˌeɪt/ *vti* to imagine.

idée fixe /ˌiːdeɪˈfiːks/ *n* (*pl* **idées fixes**) a fixed idea; an obsession.

identical /aɪˈdɛntɪkəl/ *adj* exactly the same; having the same origin.—**identically** *adv*.—**identicalness** *n*.

identifiable /aɪˈdɛntɪˌfaɪəbəl/ *adj* able to be identified.—**identifiableness** *n*.

identification /aɪˌdɛntɪfɪˈkeɪʃən/ *n* the act of identifying; the state of being identified; that which identifies.

identify /aɪˈdɛntɪˌfaɪ/ *vt* (**identifying, identified**) to consider to be the same, equate; to establish the identity of; to associate closely; to regard (oneself) as similar to another.—**identifier** *n*.

identity /aɪˈdɛntɪti/ *n* (*pl* **identities**) the state of being exactly alike; the distinguishing characteristics of a person, personality; the state of being the same as a specified person or thing.

identity card *n* a card carrying personal details, a photograph, etc of an individual as carried by staff of an organization, journalists, etc.

ideogram, ideograph /ˈɪdɪəˌɡræm/ or /ˈɪdɪəˌɡræf/ *n* a symbol, as in Chinese writing, used instead of a word to represent an idea or thing; a graphic sign.

ideography /ˌɪdɪˈɒɡræfi/ *n* the direct representation of ideas by symbols.—**ideographic, ideographical** *adj*.

ideologist /ˌaɪdɪˈɒlədʒɪst/, **ideologue** /ˈaɪdɪəˌlɒɡ/ or /ˈɪd-/, /-ˈdiː-/ *n* one occupied with ideals or ideals; a theorist.

ideology /ˌaɪdɪˈɒlədʒi/ or /ˌɪd-/ *n* (*pl* **ideologies**) the doctrines, beliefs or opinions of an individual, social class, political party, etc.—**ideological, ideologic** *adj*.

ides /aɪdz/ *n* the 15th day of March, May, July, or October and the 13th day of any other month in the ancient Roman calender.

idiocy /ˈɪdɪəsi/ *n* (*pl* **idiocies**) mental deficiency; stupidity, imbecility; something stupid or foolish.

idiom /ˈɪdɪəm/ *n* an accepted phrase or expression with a different meaning from the literal; the usual way in which the words of a language are used to express thought; the dialect of a people, region, etc; the characteristic style of a school of art, literature, etc.—**idiomatic, idiomatical** *adj*.—**idiomatically** *adv*.

idiopathy /ˌɪdɪˈɒpəθi/ *n* a disease whose cause is unknown.—**idiopathic** *adj*.

idiosyncrasy /ˌɪdɪəˈsɪŋkrəsi/ *n* (*pl* **idiosyncrasies**) a type of behaviour or characteristic peculiar to a person or group; a quirk, eccentricity.—**idiosyncratic** *adj*.—**idiosyncratically** *adv*.

idiot /ˈɪdɪət/ *n* a severely mentally retarded adult; (*inf*) a foolish or stupid person.

idiot board *n* an autocue.

idiotic /-ˈɒtɪk/ *adj* stupid; senseless.—**idiotically** *adv*.

idiot strings *npl* ✤ (*Cdn*) strings attached to children's winter gloves or mittens to prevent them from being lost.

idle /ˈaɪdəl/ *adj* not employed, unoccupied; not in use; averse to work; useless; worthless. • *vt* to waste or spend (time) in idleness. • *vi* to move slowly or aimlessly; (*engine*) to operate without transmitting power.—**idleness** *n*.—**idler** *n*.—**idly** *adv*.

idler /ˈaɪdlər/ *n* someone who idles; a lazy person.

idol /ˈaɪdəl/ *n* an image or object worshipped as a god; a person who is intensely loved, admired or honoured.

idolatry /aɪˈdɒlətri/ *n* the worship of idols; excessive admiration or devotion.—**idolatrous** *adj*.—**idolater** *n*.

idolize /ˈaɪdəˌlaɪz/ *vt* to make an idol of, for worship; to love to excess.—**idolization** *n*.—**idolizer** *n*.

idyll, idyl /ˈɪdɪl/ *n* a short simple poem, *usu* evoking the romance and beauty of rural life; a romantic or picturesque event or scene; a romantic or pastoral musical composition.—**idyllist** *n*.

idyllic /ɪˈdɪlɪk/ *adj* pertaining to or of the nature of an idyll, pastoral; romantic, picturesque.—**idyllically** *adv*.

i.e. *abbr* = *id est*, that is.

if /ɪf/ *conj* on condition that; in the event that; supposing that; even though; whenever; whether.

iffy /ˈɪfi/ *adj* (*inf*) uncertain, unreliable.

igloo /ˈɪɡluː/ *n* (*pl* **igloos**) an Eskimo house built of blocks of snow and ice.

igneous /ˈɪɡnɪəs/ *adj* of fire; (*rocks*) produced by volcanic action or intense heat beneath the earth's surface.

ignite /ɪɡˈnaɪt/ *vti* to set fire to; to catch fire; to burn or cause to burn.—**ignitable** *adj*.

ignition /ɪɡˈnɪʃən/ *n* an act or instance of igniting; the starting of an internal combustion engine; the mechanism that ignites an internal combustion engine.

ignoble /ɪɡˈnoːbəl/ *adj* dishonourable, despicable; base, of low birth.—**ignobly** *adv*.

ignominious /ˌɪɡnəˈmɪnɪəs/ *adj* bringing disgrace or shame; humiliating, degrading.—**ignominiously** *adv*.

ignominy /ˈɪɡnɒmɪni/ or /-məni/ *n* (*pl* **ignominies**) disgrace, dishonour; a cause of ignominy, a disgraceful act.

ignoramus /ˌɪɡnəˈreɪməs/ or /-ˈræməs/ *n* (*pl* **ignoramuses**) an ignorant person.

ignorance /ˈɪɡnərəns/ *n* the state of being ignorant; a lack of knowledge.

ignorant /ˈɪɡnərənt/ *adj* lacking knowledge; uninformed, uneducated; resulting from or showing lack of knowledge.—**ignorance** *n*.—**ignorantly** *adv*.

ignore /ɪɡˈnɔr/ *vt* to disregard; to deliberately refuse to notice someone.—**ignorable** *adj*.—**ignorer** *n*.

iguana /ɪɡˈwɒnə/ *n* any of a family of large lizards of tropical America.—**iguanian** *adj*, *n*.

iguanodon /ɪˈɡwɒnəˌdɒn/ *n* a gigantic, extinct, herbivorous lizard.

ihram /ɪˈræm/ or /-ˈrɒm/ *n* the distinctive white robes worn by Muslims on pilgrimage to Mecca.

ikebana /ˌɪkəˈbænə/ *n* the Japanese art of flower arranging.

ikon *see* **icon**.

ileac /ˈɪliːækl/, **ileal** /-æl/ *adj* (*anat*) pertaining to the ileum.

ileum /ˈɪlɪəm/ *n* (*anat*) the lower part of the small intestine.

ilk /ɪlk/ *n* a type or sort.

ill /ɪl/ *adj* (**worse, worst**) not in good health; harmful; bad; hostile; faulty; unfavourable. • *adv* badly, wrongly; hardly, with difficulty. • *n* trouble; harm; evil.

ill. *abbr* = illustrated; illustration.

I'll /aɪl/ = I shall; I will.

ill-advised *adj* unwise.

ill at ease *adj* uneasy, embarrassed.

ill-bred *adj* bad-mannered.—**ill-breeding** *n*.

ill-considered *adj* lacking consideration; not thought out properly.

ill-disposed *adj* unfavourably inclined (towards).

illegal /ɪˈliːɡəl/ *adj* against the law.—**illegally** *adv*.—**illegality** *n*.

illegible /ɪˈledʒɪbəl/ *adj* impossible to read.—**illegibility, illegibleness** *n*.—**illegibly** *adv*.

illegitimate /ˌɪləˈdʒɪtəmət/ *adj* born of parents not married to each other; contrary to law, rules, or logic.—**illegitimacy, illegitimateness** *n*.—**illegitimately** *adv*.

ill-fated *adj* unlucky.

ill-favoured, ill-favored *adj* unattractive; unpleasant.

ill-founded *adj* not based on reliable facts; unsubstantiated.

ill-gotten *adj* illegally or dishonestly acquired.

ill-humoured, ill-humored *adj* bad tempered; sullen.—**ill-humour, ill humor** *n*.

illiberal /ɪˈlɪbərəl/ *adj* narrow-minded; mean.—**illiberality, illiberalness** *n*.—**illiberally** *adv*.

illicit /ɪˈlɪsɪt/ *adj* improper; unlawful.—**illicitly** *adv*.

illimitable /ɪˈlɪmɪtəbəl/ *adj* limitless, infinite.—**illimitability** *n*.

illiterate /ɪˈlɪtərət/ *adj* uneducated, *esp* not knowing how to read or write. • *n* an illiterate person.—**illiteracy** *n*.—**illiterately** *adv*.

ill-mannered *adj* rude.

ill-natured *adj* spiteful.

illness /ˈɪlnəs/ *n* a state of ill-health; sickness.

illogical /ɪˈlɒdʒɪkəl/ *adj* not logical or reasonable.—**illogicality, illogicalness** *n*.—**illogically** *adv*.

ill-starred *adj* unlucky.

ill-timed *adj* occurring or done at an unsuitable time.

ill-treat *vt* to treat unkindly, unfairly, etc.—**ill-treatment** *n*.

illume /ɪˈluːm/ *vt* (*poet*) to light up, illuminate.

illuminant /ɪˈluːmɪnənt/ *n* a substance or device that illuminates.

illuminate /ɪˈluːmɪˌneɪt/ *vt* to give light to; to light up; to make clear; to inform; to decorate as with gold or lights.—**illumination** *n*.—**illuminative** *adj*.—**illuminator** *n*.

illuminati /ɪˌluːmɪˈnæti/ or /-ˈnɒti/ *npl* (*sing* **illuminato**) a name given to persons professing special spiritual or intellectual enlightenment.

illumination /ɪˌluːmɪˈneɪʃən/ *n* a supply of light; the act of illuminating; the state of being illuminated; (*Brit, esp pl*) decorative coloured lights used in public places.

illumine /ɪˈluːmɪn/ *vt* (*poet*) to illuminate.

illuminism /-ɪzəm/ *n* the belief in and profession of special spiritual and intellectual enlightenment.

ill-usage *n* ill-use, abuse.

ill-use *vt* to treat badly, etc. • *n* abuse.

illusion /ɪˈluːʒən/ *n* a false idea or conception; an unreal or misleading image or appearance.—**illusional, illusionary** *adj*.

illusionism /-ˌnɪzəm/ *n* (*philos*) a disbelief in objective existence.

illusionist /ɪˈluːʒənɪst/ *n* a magician or conjuror.—**illusionism** *n*.

illusory /ɪˈluːsəri/ or /-zəri/, **illusive** /ɪˈluːsɪv/ *adj* deceptive; based on illusion.—**illusorily** *adv*.—**illusoriness** *n*.

illustrate /ˈɪləˌstreɪt/ *vt* to explain, as by examples; to provide (books, etc) with explanatory pictures, charts, etc; to serve as an example.—**illustratable** *adj*.—**illustrative** *adj*.—**illustrator** *n*.

illustration 257 immure

illustration /ˌɪləˈstreɪʃən/ n the act of illustrating; the state of being illustrated; an example that explains or corroborates; a picture or diagram in a book, etc.—**illustrational** adj.

illustrious /ɪˈlʌstriəs/ adj distinguished, famous.—**illustriousness** n.

ill-will n antagonism, hostility.

I'm /aɪm/ = I am.

image /ˈɪmɪdʒ/ n a representation of a person or thing; the visual impression of something in a lens, mirror, etc; a copy; a likeness; a mental picture; the concept of a person, product, etc held by the public at large. • vt to make a representation of; to reflect; to imagine.

imagery /ˈɪmɪdʒri/ n (pl **imageries**) the work of the imagination; mental pictures; figures of speech; images in general or collectively.

imaginable /ɪˈmædʒɪnəbl/ adj able to be imagined.—**imaginably** adv.

imaginal /ɪˈmædʒɪnəl/ adj pertaining to an image; pertaining to an imago.

imaginary /ɪˈmædʒɪneri/ adj existing only in the imagination.—**imaginarily** adv.

imagination /ɪˌmædʒɪˈneɪʃən/ n the image-forming power of the mind, or the power of the mind that modifies the conceptions, esp the higher form of this power exercised in art and poetry; creative ability; resourcefulness in overcoming practical difficulties, etc.

imaginative /ɪˈmædʒɪnətɪv/ adj having or showing imagination; produced by imagination.—**imaginatively** adv.

imagine /ɪˈmædʒɪn/ vt to form a mental image of; to believe falsely; (inf) to suppose; to guess. • vi to employ the imagination.—**imaginer** n.

imagist /-ɪst/ n a member of a group of poets, active between 1912 and 1917, who sought clarity of expression through use of precise images.

imago /ɪˈmeɪgo/ n (pl **imagoes, imagines**) an insect in its fully developed state; an idealized mental image of oneself or another.

imam /ɪˈmæm/ or /-mɒm/ n a leader of prayer in a mosque; a title given to various Muslim religious leaders.

imamate /ɪˈmæmeɪt/ n a region controlled by an imam; the rank or term of office of an imam.

imaret /ˌɪməˈret/ n a hostel in Turkey giving accommodation to pilgrims or travellers.

IMAX /ˈaɪmæks/ n ✹ (Cdn) (trademark) a form of cinematography in which extra-large film is shot and then projected on a giant screen.

imbalance /ɪmˈbæləns/ n a lack of balance, as in proportion, emphasis, etc.

imbecile /ˈɪmbəsəl/ or /-sɪl/, /-saɪl/ n an adult with a mental age of a three- to eight-year-old child; an idiotic person. • adj stupid or foolish.

imbecility /-sɪlɪti/ n (pl **imbecilities**) mental or physical weakness.

imbed vt (**imbedding, imbedded**) to embed.

imbibe /ɪmˈbaɪb/ vti to drink, esp alcoholic liquor; to absorb mentally.—**imbiber** n.

imbibition /ˌɪmbɪˈbɪʃən/ n (chem) the process of a gel or solid absorbing a liquid; (photog) the process, used in colour printing, of using gelatine to absorb dyes.

imbricate /ˈɪmbrɪkeɪt/, **imbricated** /-əd/ adj (tiles, leaves) overlapping.—**imbrication** n.

imbroglio /ɪmˈbroːliːo/ n (pl **imbroglios**) a complicated, confusing situation; a confused misunderstanding.

imbrue /ɪmˈbruː/ vt (**imbruing, imbrued**) to wet or moisten; to soak; to drench, esp in blood.—also **embrue**.

IMF abbr = International Monetary Fund.

imitable /ˈɪmɪtəbl/ adj able to be imitated.—**imitability, imitableness** n.

imitate /ˈɪmɪteɪt/ vt to try to follow as a pattern or model; to mimic humorously, impersonate; to copy, reproduce.—**imitator** n.

imitation /ˌɪmɪˈteɪʃən/ n an act or instance of imitating; a copy; an act of mimicking or impersonation.—**imitational** adj.

imitative /ˈɪmɪteɪtɪv/ adj imitating or inclined to imitate; characterized by imitation; copying an original, esp something superior.

immaculate /ɪˈmækjulət/ adj spotless; flawless; pure, morally unblemished.—**immaculacy, immaculateness** n.—**immaculately** adv.

Immaculate Conception n (RC Church) the doctrine that the Virgin Mary was conceived without original sin.

immanent /ˈɪmənənt/ adj (qualities) inherent; (God) pervading the universe.—**immanence, immanency** n.

immaterial /ˌɪməˈtiːriəl/ adj spiritual as opposed to physical; unimportant.—**immateriality, immaterialness** n.

immaterialism /ˌɪməˈtiːriəˌlɪzəm/ n (philos) the doctrine that matter has no existence independent of the mind.—**immaterialist** n.

immaterialize /-ˌlaɪz/ vt to make immaterial.

immature /ˌɪməˈtʃur/ or /-ˈtʃər/ adj not mature.—**immaturity, immatureness** n.

immeasurable /ɪˈmeʒərəbl/ adj not able to be measured; immense, limitless.—**immeasurably** adv.

immediate /ɪˈmiːdiət/ adj acting or occurring without delay; next nearest, without intervening agency; next in relationship; in close proximity, near to; directly concerning or touching a person or thing.—**immediacy, immediateness** n.

immediately /-li/ adv without delay; directly; near, close by. • conj as soon as.

immemorial /ˌɪməˈmoːriəl/ adj existing in the distant past, beyond the reach of memory.—**immemorially** adv.

immense /ɪˈmens/ adj very large in size or extent; limitless; (inf) excellent.—**immensely** adv.

immensity /-sɪti/ n (pl **immensities**) the character of being immense; immeasurableness; infinite space; vastness in extent or bulk.

immeasurable /ɪˈmenʃərəbl/ adj immeasurable.

immerse /ɪˈmers/ vt to plunge into a liquid; to absorb or engross; to baptize by total submergence.—**immersible** adj.

immersion /ɪˈmerʒən/ n the act of immersing; the state of being immersed; baptism by dipping the whole person into water.

immesh /ɪˈmeʃ/ see **enmesh**.

immethodical /ˌɪməˈθɒdɪkəl/ adj without method or order.

immigrant /ˈɪmɪgrənt/ n a person who immigrates; a person recently settled in a country but not born there.

immigrate /ˈɪmɪˌgreɪt/ vi to come into a new country, esp to settle permanently.—**immigration** n.—**immigrator** n.—**immigratory** adj.

imminent /ˈɪmɪnənt/ adj about to happen; impending.—**imminence** n.—**imminently** adv.

immiscible /ɪˈmɪsɪbəl/ adj incapable of being mixed.—**immiscibility** n.

immobile /ɪˈmoːbaɪl/ or /-bəl/ adj not able to be moved; motionless.—**immobility** n.

immobilize /ɪˈmoːbəˌlaɪz/ vt to make immobile.—**immobilization** n.

immoderate /ɪˈmɒdərət/ adj excessive, unrestrained.—**immoderately** adv.—**immoderation, immoderateness** n.

immodest /ɪˈmɒdəst/ adj lacking in modesty or decency.—**immodestly** adv.—**immodesty** n.

immolate /ˈɪməˌleɪt/ vt to kill as a sacrifice.—**immolation** n.—**immolator** n.

immoral /ɪˈmɒrəl/ adj against accepted standards of proper behaviour; sexually degenerate; corrupt; wicked.—**immorally** adv.

immorality /ˌɪməˈrælɪti/ n (pl **immoralities**) the quality of being immoral; an immoral act or practice.

immortal /ɪˈmɔːrtəl/ adj living for ever; enduring; having lasting fame. • n an immortal being or person; (pl) the gods of classical mythology.—**immortality** n.—**immortally** adv.

immortalize /-ˌlaɪz/ vt to render immortal; to bestow lasting fame upon.—**immortalization** n.

immortelle /ˌɪmɔːrˈtel/ n a type of flower that retains its colour when dried.

immovable /ɪˈmuːvəbl/ adj firmly fixed; impassive, unyielding; (property) land, buildings, etc.—**immovability, immovableness** n.—**immovably** adv.

immune /ɪˈmjuːn/ adj not susceptible to a specified disease through inoculation or natural resistance; conferring immunity; exempt from a certain obligation, tax, duty, etc.

immunity /ɪˈmjuːnɪti/ n (pl **immunities**) the state of being immune.

immunize /ˈɪmjuˌnaɪz/ vt to make immune, esp against infection.—**immunization** n.

immuno- /ˈɪmjuːno/ or /ɪˈmjuːno/ prefix immunity.

immunology /ˈɪmjuːnɒlədʒi/ n the branch of medical science dealing with immunity to disease.—**immunologic, immunological** adj.—**immunologist** n.

immure /ɪˈmjʊr/ vt to enclose within walls; to shut up (in prison), confine.

immutable /ɪˈmjuːtəbəl/ *adj* not capable of change; unalterable.—**immutability, immutableness** *n*.—**immutably** *adv*.

imp /ɪmp/ *n* a mischievous child; a little devil.

impact /ˈɪmpækt/ *n* violent contact; a shocking effect; the force of a body colliding with another. • *vt* to force tightly together. • *vi* to hit with force.—**impaction** *n*.

impacted /ɪmˈpæktəd/ *adj* (*tooth*) unable to emerge through the gum because of an obstruction, *esp* proximity to another tooth.

impair /ɪmˈpɛr/ *vt* to make worse, less, etc.—**impairer** *n*.—**impairment** *n*.

impaired /ɪmˈpɛrd/ *adj* ✻ (*Cdn*) affected by alcohol or narcotics so as to prevent the safe driving of a motor vehicle.

impala /ɪmˈpælə/ *n* (*pl* **impalas, impala**) a type of African antelope.

impale /ɪmˈpeɪl/ *vt* to fix on, or pierce through, with something pointed.—**impalement** *n*.—**impaler** *n*.

impalpable /ɪmˈpælpəbəl/ *adj* not able to be sensed by touch; difficult to apprehend or grasp with the mind.—**impalpability** *n*.—**impalpably** *adv*.

impanel *see* **empanel**.

imparity /ɪmˈpærɪti/ *n* (*pl* **imparities**) inequality; disproportion; disparity.

impart /ɪmˈpɑrt/ *vt* to give, convey; to reveal, disclose.—**imparter** *n*.

impartial /ɪmˈpɑrʃəl/ *adj* not favouring one side more than another, unbiased.—**impartiality, impartialness** *n*.—**impartially** *adv*.

impartible /ɪmˈpɑrtəbəl/ *adj* (*law*) which cannot be partitioned.

impassable /ɪmˈpæsəbəl/ *adj* (*roads, etc*) incapable of being travelled through or over.—**impassability, impassableness** *n*.—**impassably** *adv*.

impasse /ˈɪmpæs/ *n* a situation from which there is no escape; a deadlock.

impassioned /ɪmˈpæʃənd/ *adj* passionate; ardent.—**impassionedly** *adv*.

impassive /ɪmˈpæsɪv/ *adj* not feeling or showing emotion; imperturbable.—**impassively** *adv*.—**impassiveness, impassivity** *n*.

impaste /ɪmˈpeɪst/ *vt* (*art*) to paint (onto canvas) in thick layers.—**impastation** *n*.

impasto /ɪmˈpæstoː/ *n* (*art*) the effect produced by applying thick layers of paint to a canvas; the technique of applying paint in thick layers.

impatiens /ɪmˈpeɪʃəns/ or /-ənz/ *n* (*pl* **impatiens**) one of a genus of plants of this name, including balsam and touch-me-not.

impatient /ɪmˈpeɪʃənt/ *adj* lacking patience; intolerant of delay, etc; restless.—**impatience** *n*.—**impatiently** *adv*.

impeach /ɪmˈpiːtʃ/ *vt* to question a person's honesty; to try (a public official) on a charge of wrongdoing.—**impeachable** *adj*.—**impeacher** *n*.—**impeachment** *n*.

impearl /ɪmˈpɜrl/ *vt* (*arch*) to adorn with pearls; to make like pearls.

impeccable /ɪmˈpɛkəbəl/ *adj* without defect or error; faultless.—**impeccability** *n*.—**impeccably** *adv*.

impecunious /ˌɪmpɪˈkjuːniəs/ *adj* having little or no money.—**impecuniousness, impecuniosity** *n*.

impedance /ɪmˈpiːdəns/ *n* the total resistance in an electric circuit to the flow of alternating current.

impede /ɪmˈpiːd/ *vt* to obstruct or hinder the progress of.—**impeder** *n*.—**impedingly** *adv*.

impediment /ɪmˈpɛdəmənt/ *n* something that impedes; an obstruction; a physical defect, as a stammer that prevents fluency of speech.—**impedimental** *adj*.

impedimenta /ɪmˌpɛdəˈmɛntə/ *npl* heavy items of baggage, *esp* military equipment.

impel /ɪmˈpɛl/ *vt* (**impelling, impelled**) to urge or force into doing something; to propel.—**impeller** *n*.

impend /ɪmˈpɛnd/ *vi* to be imminent; to threaten.—**impending** *adj*.

impenetrable /ɪmˈpɛnətrəbəl/ *adj* unable to be pierced or penetrated; incomprehensible; unable to be seen through.—**impenetrability** *n*.—**impenetrably** *adv*.

impenitent /ɪmˈpɛnɪtənt/ *adj* not sorry or feeling guilty; unrepentant.—**impenitence, impenitency** *n*.

imperative /ɪmˈpɛrətɪv/ *adj* urgent, pressing; authoritative; obligatory; designating or of the mood of a verb that expresses a command, entreaty, etc. • *n* a command; (*gram*) the imperative mood of a verb.

imperator /ˌɪmpəˈrætər/ or /-tər/, /-ˈreɪ-/ *n* (*ancient Rome*) a commander-in-chief; a title given to a victorious general; a title given to the head of state.

imperceptible /ˌɪmpərˈsɛptəbəl/ *adj* not able to be detected by the mind or senses; slight, minute, gradual.—**imperceptibility** *n*.—**imperceptibly** *adv*.

impercipient /ˌɪmpərˈsɪpiənt/ *adj* lacking perception.

imperfect /ɪmˈpɜrfɪkt/ *adj* havingfaults,flaws,mistakes, etc; defective; incomplete; (*gram*) designating a verb tense that indicates a past action or state as incomplete or continuous. • (*gram*) an imperfect tense.

imperfection /ˌɪmpərˈfɛkʃən/ *n* the state or quality of being imperfect; a defect, fault.

imperforate /ɪmˈpɜrfərət/ *adj* not perforated; (*anat*) without the normal opening.

imperial /ɪmˈpiːriəl/ *adj* of an empire, emperor, or empress; majestic; of great size or superior quality; of the British non-metric system of weights and measures.—**imperially** *adv*.

imperialism /ɪmˈpiːriəˌlɪzəm/ *n* the policy of forming and maintaining an empire, as by subjugating territories, establishing colonies, etc.—**imperialist** *n*.—**imperialistic** *adj*.—**imperialistically** *adv*.

imperil /ɪmˈpɛrɪl/ *vt* (**imperiling, imperiled** *or* **imperilling, imperilled**) to put in peril, to endanger.

imperious /ɪmˈpiːriəs/ *adj* tyrannical; arrogant.—**imperiously** *adv*.

imperishable /ɪmˈpɛrɪʃəbəl/ *adj* indestructible, not subject to decay; permanently enduring.—**imperishability** *n*.

imperium /ɪmˈpiːriəm/ *n* (*pl* **imperia**) supreme power; an empire.

impermanent /ɪmˈpɜrmənənt/ *adj* not permanent.—**impermanence, impermanency** *n*.

impermeable /ɪmˈpɜrmiəbəl/ *adj* not allowing fluids to pass through; impervious.—**impermeability** *n*.

impermissible /ˌɪmpərˈmɪsəbəl/ *adj* not permissible.

impersonal /ɪmˈpɜrsənəl/ *adj* not referring to any particular person; cold, unfeeling; not existing as a person; (*verb*) occurring only in the third person singular, *usu* with "it" as subject.—**impersonality** *n*.—**impersonally** *adv*.

impersonate /ɪmˈpɜrsəˌneɪt/ *vt* to assume the role of another person as entertainment or for fraud.—**impersonation** *n*.—**impersonator** *n*.

impertinent /ɪmˈpɜrtɪnənt/ *adj* impudent; insolent; irrelevant.—**impertinence** *n*.—**impertinently** *adv*.

imperturbable /ˌɪmpərˈtɜrbəbəl/ *adj* not easily disturbed; calm; impassive.—**imperturbability** *n*.—**imperturbably** *adv*.—**imperturbation** *n*.

impervious /ɪmˈpɜrviəs/ *adj* incapable of being penetrated, as by water; not readily receptive (to) or affected (by).

impetigo /ˌɪmpəˈtaɪɡoː/ *n* (*pl* **impetigos**) a contagious bacterial skin disease.—**impetiginous** *adj*.

impetrate /ˈɪmpəˌtreɪt/ *vt* to obtain by supplication, *esp* by prayer.—**impetration** *n*.

impetuous /ɪmˈpɛtʃʊəs/ *adj* acting or done suddenly with impulsive energy.—**impetuosity** *n*.—**impetuously** *adv*.

impetus /ˈɪmpɪtəs/ *n* (*pl* **impetuses**) the force with which a body moves against resistance; driving force or motive.

impiety /ɪmˈpaɪəti/ *n* (*pl* **impieties**) want of piety; ungodliness; an act of irreverence or wickedness.

impinge /ɪmˈpɪndʒ/ *vi* (*with* **on, upon**) to have an impact; to encroach.—**impingement** *n*.—**impinger** *n*.

impious /ˈɪmpiəs/ *adj* showing lack of reverence; wicked.—**impiously** *adv*.

impish /ˈɪmpɪʃ/ *adj* of or like an imp.—**impishly** *adv*.—**impishness** *n*.

implacable /ɪmˈplækəbəl/ *adj* not able to be appeased or pacified; inflexible, inexorable.—**implacability** *n*.—**implacably** *adv*.

implant /ɪmˈplænt/ *vt* to plant firmly; to fix (ideas, etc) firmly in the mind. • *n* something implanted in tissue surgically.—**implantation** *n*.—**implanter** *n*.

implausible /ɪmˈplɔzəbəl/ *adj* not plausible.—**implausibility** *n*.—**implausibly** *adv*.

implead /ɪmˈpliːd/ *vt* to sue, prosecute.

implement /ˈɪmpləmənt/ *n* something used in a given activity. • *vt* to carry out, put into effect.—**implemental** *adj*.—**implementation** *n*.—**implementer, implementor** *n*.

implicate /ˈɪmplɪˌkeɪt/ *vt* to show to have a part, *esp* in a crime; to imply.—**implicative** *adj*.

implication /ˌɪmplɪˈkeɪʃən/ *n* an implicating or being implicated; that which is implied; an inference not expressed but understood; deduction.

implicit /ɪm'plɪsɪt/ *adj* implied rather than stated explicitly; unquestioning, absolute.—**implicitly** *adv.*—**implicitness, implicity** *n.*

implode /ɪm'pləʊd/ *vi* to collapse inwards.

implore /ɪm'plɔːr/ *vt* to request earnestly; to plead, entreat.—**imploration** *n.*—**implorer** *n.*—**imploringly** *adv.*

imply /ɪm'plaɪ/ *vt* (**implying, implied**) to hint, suggest indirectly; to indicate or involve as a consequence.

impolite /ɪmpə'laɪt/ *adj* not polite, rude.—**impolitely** *adv.*—**impoliteness** *n.*

impolitic /ɪm'pɒlɪtɪk/ *adj* contrary to good policy; unwise; injudicious; indiscreet.—**impoliticly** *adv.*

imponderable /ɪm'pɒndərəbəl/ *adj* not able to be weighed or measured. • *n* something difficult to measure or assess.—**imponderability** *n.*—**imponderably** *adv.*

import /ɪm'pɔːt/ or /'ɪmpɔːt/ *vt* to bring (goods) in from a foreign country for sale or use; to mean; to signify. • *vi* to be of importance, to matter. • *n* something imported; meaning; importance.—**importable** *adj.*—**importer** *n.*

importance /ɪm'pɔːtəns/ *n* the quality of being important; a high place in public estimation; high self-esteem.

important /ɪm'pɔːtənt/ *adj* having great significance or consequence; (*person*) having power, authority, etc.—**importantly** *adv.*

importation /-'teɪʃən/ *n* the act or business of importing; imported goods.

importunate /ɪm'pɔːtʃənət/ *adj* persistent in asking or demanding.

importune /ɪm'pɔːtjuːn/ or /-'tjuːn/ *vt* to ask urgently and repeatedly.—**importuner** *n.*—**importuning** *n.*

importunity /ˌɪmpɔː'tjuːnɪti/ or /-'tjuː-/ *n* (*pl* **importunities**) persistent solicitation or demand; incessant insistence; urgency.

impose /ɪm'pəʊz/ *vt* to put (a burden, tax, punishment) on or upon; to force (oneself) on others; to lay pages of type or film and secure them. • *vi* (*with* **on** *or* **upon**) to take advantage of; to cheat or defraud.—**imposable** *adj.*—**imposer** *n.*

imposing /-ɪŋ/ *adj* impressive because of size, appearance, dignity, etc.—**imposingly** *adv.*

imposition /ˌɪmpə'zɪʃən/ *n* the act of imposing; something imposed, as a tax; an unfair burden; (*print*) the arrangement of pages of type or film in the correct order.

impossibility /ɪmˌpɒsə'bɪlɪti/ *n* (*pl* **impossibilites**) the character of being impossible; that which cannot be, or be supposed to be, done.

impossible /ɪm'pɒsəbəl/ *adj* not capable of existing, being done, or happening; (*inf*) unendurable, outrageous.—**impossibly** *adv.*

impost /'ɪmpəʊst/ *n* a tax or duty, *esp* imposed by customs.

impostor, imposter /ɪm'pɒstər/ *n* a person who acts fraudulently by impersonating another.

imposture /ɪm'pɒstʃər/ *n* a fraud, deception.

impotent /'ɪmpətənt/ *adj* lacking in necessary strength, powerless; (*man*) unable to engage in sexual intercourse.—**impotence, impotency** *n.*—**impotently** *adv.*

impound /ɪm'paʊnd/ *vt* to take legal possession of; to shut up (an animal) in a pound.—**impoundage, impoundment** *n.*—**impounder** *n.*

impoverish /ɪm'pɒvərɪʃ/ *vt* to make poor; to deprive of strength.—**impoverishment** *n.*

impracticable /ɪm'præktɪkəbəl/ *adj* not able to be carried out, not feasible.—**impracticability** *n.*—**impracticably** *adv.*

impractical /ɪm'præktɪkəl/ *adj* not practical; not competent in practical skills.—**impracticality** *n.*—**impractically** *adv.*

imprecate /'ɪmprəˌkeɪt/ *vti* to invoke evil (on); to curse or utter curses.—**imprecatory** *adv.*

imprecation /ˌɪmprə'keɪʃən/ *n* a curse.

imprecise /ˌɪmprə'saɪs/ *adj* not precise; ill-defined.—**imprecisely** *adv.*—**imprecision** *n.*

impregnable /ɪm'preɡnəbəl/, **impregnatable** *adj* secure against attack, unyielding.—**impregnability** *n.*—**impregnably** *adv.*

impregnate /ɪm'preɡˌneɪt/ *vt* to cause to become pregnant, to fertilize; to saturate, soak (with); to imbue, pervade.—**impregnation** *n.*—**impregnator** *n.*

impresario /ˌɪmprə'sɑːriəʊ/ or /-'seəriəʊ/ *n* (*pl* **impresarios**) the manager of an opera, a concert series, etc.

impress[1] /ɪm'pres/ *vt* to make a strong, *usu* favourable, impression on; to fix deeply in the mind; to stamp with a mark; to imprint. • *n* an imprint.—**impresser** *n.*—**impressible** *adj.*

impress[2] *vt* to coerce into military service.—**impressment** *n.*

impression /ɪm'preʃən/ *n* the effect produced in the mind by an experience; a mark produced by imprinting; a vague idea, notion; the act of impressing or being impressed; a notable or strong influence on the mind or senses; the number of copies of a book printed at one go.—*also* **printing**; an impersonation or act of mimicry.—**impressional** *adj.*

impressionable ɪm'preʃənəbəl/ or /-'preʃnəbəl/ *n* easily impressed or influenced.—**impressionability** *n.*—**impressionably** *adv.*

impressionism /ɪm'preʃəˌnɪzəm/ *n* painting, writing, etc in which objects are painted or described so as to reproduce only their general effect or impression without selection or elaboration of details.—**impressionist** *n.*—**impressionistic** *adj.*

impressive /ɪm'presɪv/ *adj* tending to impress the mind or emotions; arousing wonder or admiration.—**impressiveness** *n.*

impressment /-mənt/ *n* the act of seizing (things) for public use or conscripting (people) into public service.

imprest /'ɪmprest/ *n* a sum of money advanced.

imprimatur /ˌɪmprɪ'mætər/ or /-'meɪtər/, /-tʊr/ *n* permission or licence to publish a book, etc; an authoritative mark of approval; sanction.

imprint /ɪm'prɪnt/ *vt* to stamp or impress a mark on, etc; to fix firmly in the mind. • *n* a mark made by imprinting; a lasting effect; a note in a book giving the facts of publication.—**imprinter** *n.*

imprison /ɪm'prɪzən/ *vt* to put in a prison; to confine, as in a prison.—**imprisoner** *n.*—**imprisonment** *n.*

improbable /ɪm'prɒbəbəl/ *adj* unlikely to be true or to happen.—**improbability** *n.*—**improbably** *adv.*

improbity /ɪm'prəʊbɪti/ *n* (*pl* **improbities**) wickedness, dishonesty.

impromptu /ɪm'prɒmptuː/ or /-'tjuː/ *adj, adv* unrehearsed, unprepared. • *n* something impromptu, as a speech.

improper /ɪm'prɒpər/ *adj* lacking propriety, indecent; incorrect; not suitable or appropriate.—**improperly** *adv.*

improper fraction *n* a fraction in which the numerator is greater than or equal to the denominator, as $^4/_3$.

impropriety /ˌɪmprə'praɪəti/ *n* (*pl* **improprieties**) the quality of being improper; indecency; an improper act, etc.

improve /ɪm'pruːv/ *vt* to make or become better.—**improvable** *adj.*—**improver** *n.*—**improvingly** *adj.*

improvement /ɪm'pruːvmənt/ *n* the act of improving or being improved; an alteration that improves or adds to the value of something.

improvident /ɪm'prɒvɪdənt/ *adj* lacking foresight or thrift; wanting care to provide for the future; careless.—**improvidence** *n.*

improvisation /ˌɪmprəvaɪ'zeɪʃən/ *n* the act of improvising; the act of composing poetry, music, etc, extemporaneously; an impromptu.—**improvisational** *adj.*

improvise /'ɪmprəˌvaɪz/ *vti* to compose, perform, recite, etc without preparation; to make or do with whatever is at hand.—**improviser** *n.*

imprudent /ɪm'pruːdənt/ *adj* rash, lacking discretion; unwise.—**imprudence** *n.*—**imprudently** *adv.*

impudent /'ɪmpjʊdənt/ *adj* disrespectfully bold; impertinent.—**impudence** *n.*—**impudently** *adv.*

impugn /ɪm'pjuːn/ *vt* to oppose or challenge as false; to discredit.—**impugnation, impugnent** *n.*—**impugner** *n.*

impuissant *Fr.* /ɛpɥi'sɑ̃/ *adj* powerless, weak.—**impuissance** *n.*

impulse /'ɪmpʌls/ *n* a sudden push or thrust; a stimulus transmitted through a nerve or a muscle; a sudden instinctive urge to act.

impulsion /ɪm'pʌlʃən/ *n* the act of impelling; the state of being impelled; impetus; an irrational urge, compulsion.

impulsive /ɪm'pʌlsɪv/ *adj* tending to act on impulse; forceful, impelling; acting momentarily.—**impulsively** *adv.*—**impulsiveness** *n.*

impunity /ɪm'pjuːnɪti/ *n* (*pl* **impunities**) exemption or freedom from punishment or harm.

impure /ɪm'pjʊr/ or /-pjɔː/ *adj* unclean; adulterated.

impurity /ɪm'pjʊrɪti/ or /-pjɔː-/ *n* (*pl* **impurities**) a being impure; an impure substance or constituent.

impute /ɪm'pjuːt/ *vt* to attribute (*esp* a fault or misbehaviour) to another.—**imputable** *adj.*—**imputation** *n.*—**imputative** *adj.*—**imputer** *n.*

In (*chem symbol*) indium

in *abbr* = inch(es).

in /ɪn/ *prep* inside; within; at; as contained by; during; at the end of; not beyond; affected by; being a member of; wearing; using; because of; into. • *adv* to or at a certain place; so as to be contained by a certain space, condition, etc; (*games*) batting, in play. • *adj* that is in power; inner; inside; gathered, counted, etc; (*inf*) currently smart, fashionable, etc.

inability /ˌɪnəˈbɪlɪti/ *n* (*pl* **inabilities**) lack of ability.

in absentia /ˌɪnæbˈsenʃə/ or /-ˈʃiə/, /-tiə/ *adv* in the absence of.

inaccessible /ˌɪnækˈsesɪbəl/ *adj* not accessible, unapproachable.—**inaccessibility** *n*.—**inaccessibly** *adv*.

inaccurate /ɪnˈækjʊrət/ *adj* not accurate, imprecise.—**inaccuracy** *n*.—**inaccurately** *adv*.

inaction /ɪnˈækʃən/ *n* idleness, inertia.

inactive /ɪnˈæktɪv/ *adj* not active.—**inactively** *adv*.—**inactivity** *n*.

inadequate /ɪnˈædəkwət/ *adj* not adequate; not capable.—**inadequacy** *n*.—**inadequately** *adv*.

inadmissible /ˌɪnədˈmɪsəbəl/ *adj* not admissible, *esp* as evidence.—**inadmissibility** *n*.—**inadmissibly** *adv*.

inadvertent /ˌɪnədˈvɜrtənt/ *adj* not attentive or observant, careless; due to oversight.—**inadvertence, inadvertency** *n*.—**inadvertently** *adv*.

inadvisable /ˌɪnədˈvaɪzəbəl/ *adj* not advisable; inexpedient.—**inadvisability** *n*.—**inadvisably** *adv*.

inalienable /ɪnˈɛliənəbəl/ *adj* that cannot or should not be surrendered or transferred to another.—**inalienability** *n*.—**inalienably** *adv*.

inalterable /ɪnˈɒltərəbəl/ *adj* unalterable.—**inalterability** *n*.

inamorata /ɪnˌæməˈrætə/ *n* (*pl* **inamoratas**) a woman with whom one is in love; a sweetheart.

inamorato /ɪnˌæməˈrætoː/ *n* (*pl* **inamoratos**) a man who is in love, a lover.

inane /ɪˈneɪn/ *adj* lacking sense, silly.—**inanely** *adv*.

inanimate /ɪnˈænəmət/ *adj* not animate; showing no signs of life; dull.—**inanimately** *adv*.—**inanimateness, inanimation** *n*.

inanition /ˌɪnəˈnɪʃən/ *n* emptiness; exhaustion from lack of nourishment.

inanity /ɪnˈænɪti/ *n* (*pl* **inanities**) (*arch*) emptiness; silliness; frivolity; a silly action or remark.

inapplicable /ˌɪnəˈplɪkəbəl/ or /ɪnˈæplɪk-/ *adj* not applicable.—**inapplicability** *n*.

inapposite /ɪnˈæpəzɪt/ *adj* not apposite, unsuitable.—**inappositely** *adv*.

inappreciable /ˌɪnəˈpriːʃəbəl/ *adj* not to be appreciated or estimated; of no consequence.

inappreciative /ˌɪnəˈpriːʃətɪv/ *adj* unappreciative.

inapproachable /ˌɪnəˈproːtʃəbəl/ *adj* not approachable, inaccessible.

inappropriate /ˌɪnəˈproːpriət/ *adj* unsuitable.—**inappropriately** *adv*.—**inappropriateness** *n*.

inapt /ɪnˈæpt/ *adj* inappropriate; unfit, unskilful.—**inaptitude** *n*.

inarticulate /ˌɪnɑrˈtɪkjʊlət/ *adj* not expressed in words; incapable of being expressed in words; incapable of coherent or effective expression of ideas, feelings, etc.—**inarticulately** *adv*.

inartistic /ˌɪnɑrˈtɪstɪk/ *adj* not artistic; not appreciative of art.—**inartistically** *adv*.

inasmuch /ˌɪnəzˈmʌtʃ/ *adv* in like degree; (*with* **as**) seeing that; because.

inattentive /ˌɪnəˈtentɪv/ *adj* not attending; neglectful.—**inattention** *n*.

inaudible /ɪnˈɒdəbəl/ *adj* unable to be heard.—**inaudibility** *n*.—**inaudibly** *adv*.

inaugural /ɪˈnɒɡjʊrəl/ or /-ɡər-/ *n* of or pertaining to an inauguration; a speech made at an inauguration.

inaugurate /ɪˈnɒɡjʊˌreɪt/ or /-ɡər-/ *vt* to admit ceremonially into office; to open (a building, etc) formally to the public; to cause to begin, initiate.—**inauguration** *n*.—**inaugurator** *n*.

inauspicious /ˌɪnɒˈspɪʃəs/ *adj* ill-starred; unlucky; unfavourable; unfortunate.

inboard /ˈɪnbɔrd/ *adv, adj* towards the centre or within an aircraft, ship, etc.

inborn /ˈɪnbɔrn/ *adj* present from birth; hereditary.

inbred /ɪnˈbred/ or /ˈɪn-/ *adj* innate; produced by inbreeding.

inbreed /ɪnˈbriːd/ *vti* (**inbreeding, inbred**) to breed by continual mating of individuals of the same or closely related stocks.

in-built /ˈɪnbɪlt/ *adj* built in.

Inc. *abbr* = Incorporated.

incalculable /ɪnˈkælkjʊləbəl/ *adj* beyond calculation; unpredictable.—**incalculability** *n*.—**incalculably** *adv*.

incalescent /ˌɪnkəˈlesənt/ *adj* (*chem*) increasing in heat.—**incalescence** *n*.

in camera /ɪnˈkæmərə/ *adv* in private; in a judge's chamber as opposed to open court.

incandesce /ˌɪnkænˈdes/ *vi* to glow with heat.

incandescent /ˌɪnkænˈdesənt/ *adj* glowing or luminous with intense heat.—**incandescence** *n*.

incantation /ˌɪnkænˈteɪʃən/ *n* words chanted in magic spells or rites.—**incantational, incantatory** *adj*.

incapable /ɪnˈkeɪpəbəl/ *adj* lacking capability; not able or fit to perform an activity.—**incapability** *n*.—**incapably** *adv*.

incapacitate /ˌɪnkəˈpæsɪˌteɪt/ *vt* to weaken, to disable; to make ineligible.—**incapacitation** *n*.

incapacity /ˌɪnkəˈpæsɪti/ *n* (*pl* **incapacities**) lack of power or strength, inability; ineligibility.

incarcerate /ɪnˈkɑrsəˌreɪt/ *vt* to put in prison, to confine.—**incarceration** *n*.—**incarcerator** *n*.

incarnate /ɪnˈkɑrnət/ *adj* endowed with a human body; personified. • *vt* to give bodily form to; to be the type or embodiment of.—**incarnation** *n*.

incautious /ɪnˈkɒʃəs/ *adj* not cautious, reckless.—**incautiously** *adv*.—**incautiousness, incaution** *n*.

incendiarism /ɪnˈsendiəˌrɪzəm/ *n* the act of burning illegally; arson.

incendiary /ɪnˈsendieri/ *adj* pertaining to arson; (*bomb*) designed to start fires; tending to stir up or inflame. • *n* (*pl* **incendiaries**) a person that sets fire to a building, etc maliciously, an arsonist; an incendiary substance (as in a bomb); a person who stirs up violence, etc.

incense¹ /ɪnˈsens/ *vt* to make extremely angry.

incense² *n* a substance that gives off a fragrant odour when burned; the fumes so produced; any pleasant odour.

incentive /ɪnˈsentɪv/ *n* a stimulus; a motive. • *adj* serving as a stimulus to action.

incept /ɪnˈsept/ *vt* (*biol*) to ingest.

inception /ɪnˈsepʃən/ *n* the beginning of something.

inceptive /ɪnˈseptɪv/ *adj* noting a beginning, initial.

incertitude /ɪnˈsɜrtɪˌtuːd/ or /-ˌtjuːd/ *n* doubt, uncertainty.

incessant /ɪnˈsesənt/ *adj* never ceasing; continual, constant.—**incessancy** *n*.—**incessantly** *adv*.

incest /ˈɪnsest/ *n* sexual intercourse between persons too closely related to marry legally.

incestuous /ɪnˈsestʃʊəs/ *adj* involving incest; guilty of incest.

inch /ɪntʃ/ *n* a measure of length equal to $1/_{12}$ foot (2.54 cm); a very small distance or amount. • *vti* to move very slowly, or by degrees.

inchmeal /ˈɪntʃˌmiːl/ *adv* inch by inch, gradually.

inchoate /ɪnˈkoːət/ or /-eɪt/, /ˈɪn-/ *adj* just begun; at a very early stage.—**inchoation** *n*.—**inchoative** *adj*.

incidence /ˈɪnsɪdəns/ *n* the degree or range of occurrence or effect.

incident /ˈɪnsɪdənt/ *adj* likely to happen as a result; falling upon or affecting. • *n* something that happens; an event, *esp* a minor one; a minor conflict.

incidental /ˌɪnsɪˈdentəl/ *adj* happening in connection with something more important; happening by chance. • *npl* miscellaneous items, minor expenses.

incidental music *n* background music for a film, play, etc.

incidentally /ˌɪnsɪˈdentəli/ *adv* in passing, as an aside.

incinerate /ɪnˈsɪnəˌreɪt/ *vt* to reduce to ashes.—**incineration** *n*.

incinerator /-ər/ *n* a furnace for burning rubbish.

incipient /ɪnˈsɪpiənt/ *adj* beginning to be or appear; initial.—**incipience, incipiency** *n*.

incise /ɪnˈsaɪz/ *vt* to cut or carve into a surface; to engrave.—**incised** *adj*.

incision /ɪnˈsɪʒən/ *n* incising; a cut made into something, *esp* by a surgeon into a body.

incisive /ɪnˈsaɪsɪv/ *adj* keen, penetrating; decisive; biting.—**incisively** *adv*.—**incisiveness** *n*.

incisor /ɪnˈsaɪzər/ *n* any of the front cutting teeth at the front of the mouth.

incite /ɪnˈsaɪt/ *vt* to urge to action; to rouse.—**incitement** *n*.—**inciter** *n*.—**incitingly** *adv*.

incivility /ˌɪnsɪˈvɪlɪti/ *n* (*pl* **incivilities**) lack of civility or courtesy; impoliteness.

incl. *abbr* = including; inclusive.

inclement /ɪnˈklemənt/ *adj* (*weather*) rough, stormy; lacking mercy; harsh.—**inclemency** *n*.

inclination /ˌɪnklɪˈneɪʃən/ *n* a propensity or disposition, *esp* a liking; a deviation from the horizontal or vertical; a slope; inclining or being inclined; a bending movement, a bow.—**inclinational** *adj*.

incline /ɪn'klaɪn/ *vi* to lean, to slope; to be disposed towards an opinion or action. • *vt* to cause to bend (the head or body) forwards; to cause to deviate, *esp* from the horizontal or vertical. • *n* a slope.—**inclinable** *adj.*—**incliner** *n.*

inclinometer /ˌɪnklɪ'nɒmətər/ *n* an instrument used to measure the angle made by an aircraft with the horizontal.

include /ɪn'kluːd/ *vt* to enclose, contain; to comprise as part or a larger group, amount, etc.—**includable, includible** *adj.*—**inclusion** *n.*

inclusive /ɪn'kluːsɪv/ *adj* comprehensive; including the limits specified.—**inclusively** *adv.*

incognito /ˌɪnkɒg'niːtoː/ *adj, adv* under an assumed name or identity. • *n* (*pl* **incognitos**) a person appearing or living incognito; the name assumed by such a person.—**incognita** *nf* (*pl* **incognitas**).

incognizant /ɪn'kɒgnɪzənt/ *adj* (*usu with* **of**) unaware.—**incognizance** *n.*

incoherent /ˌɪnko'hiːrənt/ *adj* lacking organization or clarity; inarticulate in speech or thought.—**incoherence, incoherency** *n.*—**incoherently** *adv.*

incombustible /ˌɪnkəm'bʌstɪbəl/ *adj* not able to be burned or ignited. • *n* an incombustible substance.—**incombustibility** *n.*—**incombustibly** *adv.*

income /'ɪnkʌm/ or /'ɪnkəm/ *n* the money etc received for labour or services, or from property, investments, etc.

incomer /'ɪnˌkʌmər/ *n* one who comes in; one who succeeds, as a tenant.

income tax *n* a tax levied on the net income of a person or business.

incoming /'ɪnˌkʌmɪn/ *adj* coming; accruing. • *n* the act of coming in; that which comes in; income.

incommensurable /ˌɪnkə'menʃərəbəl/ *adj* not able to be measured or judged comparatively.—**incommensurability** *n.*—**incommensurably** *adv.*

incommensurate /ˌɪnkə'menʃərət/ *adj* not commensurate; disproportionate; inadequate; incommensurable.

incommode /ˌɪnkə'moːd/ *vt* to give inconvenience or trouble to; to disturb.—**incommodious** *adj.*

incommunicable /ˌɪnkə'mjuːnɪkəbəl/ *adj* not capable of being communicated.—**incommunicability** *n.*—**incommunicably** *adv.*

incommunicado /ˌɪnkəmjuːnɪ'kædoː/ *adj* not allowed to communicate with others.

incommunicative /ˌɪnkə'mjuːnɪkətɪv/ *adj* not disposed to give information, reserved.

incommutable /ˌɪnkə'mjuːtəbəl/ *adj* which cannot be exchanged or commuted.

incomparable /ɪn'kɒmpərəbəl/ or /-prəbəl/ *adj* beyond comparison, matchless; not amenable to comparison.—**incomparability** *n.*—**incomparably** *adv.*

incompatible /ˌɪnkəm'pætɪbəl/ *adj* not able to exist together in harmony; antagonistic; inconsistent.—**incompatibility** *n.*—**incompatibly** *adv.*

incompetent /ɪn'kɒmpətənt/ *adj* lacking the necessary ability, skill, etc. • *n* an incompetent person.—**incompetence, incompetency** *n.*—**incompetently** *adv.*

incomplete /ˌɪnkəm'pliːt/ *adj* unfinished; lacking a part or parts.—**incompletely** *adv.*—**incompleteness, incompletion** *n.*

incomprehensible /ɪnˌkɒmprə'hensɪbəl/ *adj* not to be understood or grasped by the mind; inconceivable.—**incomprehensibility** *n.*—**incomprehensibly** *adv.*

incomprehension /ɪnˌkɒmprə'henʃən/ *n* failure to understand.

incompressible /ˌɪnkəm'presɪbəl/ *adj* incapable of being reduced in volume by pressure; resisting pressure.—**incompressibility** *n.*—**incompressibly** *adv.*

incomputable /ˌɪnkəm'pjuːtəbəl/ *adj* incalculable, which cannot be reckoned.

inconceivable /ˌɪnkən'siːvəbəl/ *adj* impossible to comprehend; (*inf*) unbelievable.—**inconceivably** *adv.*

inconclusive /ˌɪnkən'kluːsɪv/ *adj* leading to no definite result; ineffective; inefficient.—**inconclusively** *adv.*—**inconclusiveness** *n.*

incondensable, incondensible /ˌɪnkən'densəbəl/ *adj* which cannot be condensed or compressed.

inconformity /ˌɪnkən'fɔːmətɪ/ *n* lack of conformity.

incongruity /ɪnkɒŋ'gruːɪtɪ/ *n* (*pl* **incongruities**) unsuitableness of one thing to another, inconsistency; absurdity.

incongruous /ɪn'kɒŋgruəs/ *adj* lacking harmony or agreement of parts; unsuitable; inappropriate.—**incongruously** *adv.*—**incongruousness, incongruence** *n.*

inconsequential /ɪnˌkɒnsə'kwenʃəl/, **inconsequent** /ɪn'kɒnsəkwənt/ *adj* not following logically; irrelevant.—**inconsequence** *n.*—**inconsequentiality** *n.*—**inconsequentially, inconsequently** *adv.*

inconsiderable /ˌɪnkən'sɪdərəbəl/ *adj* trivial.—**inconsiderably** *adv.*

inconsiderate /ˌɪnkən'sɪdərət/ *adj* uncaring about others; thoughtless.—**inconsiderately** *adv.*—**inconsideration** *n.*

inconsistency /ˌɪnkən'sɪstənsɪ/ *n* (*pl* **inconsistencies**) the quality of being inconsistent; incongruity.—**inconsistently** *adv.*

inconsistent /ˌɪnkən'sɪstənt/ *adj* not compatible with other facts; contradictory; irregular, fickle.

inconsolable /ˌɪnkən'soːləbəl/ *adj* not able to be comforted.—**inconsolability** *n.*—**inconsolably** *adv.*

inconsonant /ɪn'kɒnsənənt/ *adj* not in harmony or agreement.—**inconsonance** *n.*

inconspicuous /ˌɪnkən'spɪkjuəs/ *adj* not conspicuous.—**inconspicuously** *adv.*—**inconspicuousness** *n.*

inconstant /ɪn'kɒnstənt/ *adj* subject to change; unstable; variable; fickle; capricious.—**inconstancy** *n.*

inconsumable /ˌɪnkən'suːməbəl/ or /-'sjuː-/ *adj* which cannot be consumed or used up.

incontestable /ˌɪnkən'testəbəl/ *adj* not admitting of question or doubt; incontrovertible.—**incontestability** *n.*—**incontestably** *adv.*

incontinent /ɪn'kɒntɪnən/ *adj* unable to control the excretion of bodily wastes; lacking self-restraint.—**incontinence** *n.*

incontrovertible /ˌɪnkɒntrə'vɜːtɪbəl/ *adj* not admitting of controversy; indisputable.—**incontrovertibility** *n.*—**incontrovertibly** *adv.*

inconvenience /ˌɪnkən'viːnɪəns/ *n* want of convenience; unfitness; that which incommodes; disadvantage. • *vt* to put to inconvenience; to annoy.—**inconvenient** *adj.*

inconvertible /ˌɪnkən'vɜːtɪbəl/ *adj* incapable of being converted into or exchanged for something else.—**inconvertibility** *n.*—**inconvertibly** *adv.*

inconvincible /ˌɪnkən'vɪnsəbəl/ *adj* unable or unwilling to be convinced.

incoordination /ˌɪnkoːˌɔːdɪ'neɪʃən/ *n* lack of coordination.

incorporate /ɪn'kɔːpəˌreɪt/ *vt* to combine; to include; to embody; to merge; to form into a corporation. • *vi* to unite into one group or substance; to form a corporation. • *adj* united; formed into a corporation.—**incorporation** *n.*—**incorporative** *adj.*—**incorporator** *n.*

incorporeal /ˌɪnkɔː'pɔːrɪəl/ *adj* not corporeal, without substance; spiritual; (*law*) intangible, and existing only in contemplation of the law.—**incorporeally** *adv.*—**incorporeity, incorporeality** *n.*

incorrect /ˌɪnkə'rekt/ *adj* faulty; inaccurate; improper.—**incorrectly** *adv.*—**incorrectness** *n.*

incorrigible /ɪn'kɒrɪdʒɪbəl/ *adj* not able to be corrected, reformed or altered.—**incorrigibility** *n.*—**incorrigibly** *adv.*

incorrupt /ˌɪnkə'rʌpt/, **incorrupted** /-ɪd/ *adj* free from physical or moral taint; unimpaired; upright, *esp* above the influence of corruption or bribery; honest.

incorruptible /ˌɪnkə'rʌptɪbəl/ *adj* incapable of physical corruption, decay or dissolution; incapable of being bribed; not liable to moral perversion or contamination.—**incorruptibility** *n.*—**incorruptibly** *adv.*

increase /ɪn'kriːs/ *vti* to make or become greater in size, quality, amount, etc. • *n* increasing or becoming increased; the result or amount by which something increases.—**increasable** *adj.*—**increaser** *n.*—**increasingly** *adv.*

incredible /ɪn'kredɪbəl/ *adj* unbelievable; (*inf*) wonderful.—**incredibility** *n.*—**incredibly** *adv.*

incredulity /ˌɪnkrə'djuːlɪtɪ/ *n* scepticism; disbelief.

incredulous /ɪn'kredjuləs/ *adj* not able or willing to accept as true; unbelieving.—**incredulously** *adv.*—**incredulousness** *n.*

increment /'ɪnkrəmənt/ *n* (the amount of) an increase; an addition.—**incremental** *adj.*

increscent /ɪn'kresənt/ *adj* (*moon*) waxing, growing.

incriminate /ɪn'krɪmɪˌneɪt/ *vt* to involve in or indicate as involved in a crime or fault.—**incrimination** *n.*—**incriminator** *n.*—**incriminatory** *adj.*

incubate /ˈɪŋkjʊbeɪt/ *vti* to sit on and hatch (eggs); to keep (eggs, embryos, etc) in a favourable environment for hatching or developing; to develop, as by planning.—**incubation** *n.*—**incubative, incubatory** *adj.*

incubator /ˈɪŋkjʊˌbeɪtər/ *n* an apparatus in which eggs are hatched by artificial heat; an apparatus for nurturing premature babies until they can survive unaided.

incubus /ˈɪŋkjʊbəs/ *n* (*pl* **incubi, incubuses**) an evil spirit believed in folklore to have intercourse with women as they sleep; something oppressive or disturbing, as a nightmare.

inculcate /ˈɪnkəlˌkeɪt/ *vt* to teach by frequent repetition or urging.—**inculcation** *n.*—**inculcator** *n.*

inculpate /ɪnˈkʌlpeɪt/ or /ˈɪn-/ *vt* to blame, censure; to incriminate.—**inculpation** *n.*—**inculpative, inculpatory** *adj.*

incumbency /ɪnˈkʌmbənsi/ *n* (*pl* **incumbencies**) a duty or obligation; a term of office.

incumbent /ɪnˈkʌmbənt/ *adj* resting (on or upon) one as a duty or obligation; currently in office. • *n* the holder of an office, etc.

incunabulum /ˌɪnkjuˈnæbjʊləm/ *n* (*pl* **incunabula**) any book printed before 1500; the early stages of anything.—**incunabular** *adj.*

incur /ɪnˈkər/ *vt* (**incurring, incurred**) to bring upon oneself (something undesirable).—**incurrable** *adj.*

incurable /ɪnˈkjʊrəbəl/ *adj* incapable of being cured; beyond the power of skill or medicine; lacking remedy; incorrigible. • *n* a person diseased beyond cure.—**incurability** *n.*—**incurably** *adv.*

incurious /ɪnˈkjʊriəs/ *adj* indifferent, heedless.—**incuriosity** *n.*

incursion /ɪnˈkərʒən/ *n* an invasion or raid into another's territory, etc.—**incursive** *adj.*

incurvate /ɪnˈkərvɪt/ or /-ˌveɪt/, /ˈɪnkər-/ *vti* to curve inwards. • *adj* curved or bent inwards.—**incurvation** *n.*

incus /ˈɪnkəs/ *n* (*pl* **incudes**) a bone found in the middle ear.

incuse /ɪŋˈkjuːz/ *n* a design stamped onto a coin.

indebted /ɪnˈdetəd/ *adj* in debt; obliged; owing gratitude.—**indebtedness** *n.*

indecency /ɪnˈdisənsi/ *n* (*pl* **indecencies**) lack of decency, modesty, or good manners; something indecent, vulgar, or obscene.

indecent /ɪnˈdiːsənt/ *adj* offending against accepted standards of decent behaviour.—**indecently** *adv.*

indecent assault *n* a sexual assault not involving rape.

indecent exposure *n* the offence of deliberately exposing one's genitals in public.

indeciduous /ˌɪndɪˈsɪdʒuːəs/ *adj* (*bot*) not deciduous; evergreen.

indecipherable /ˌɪndəˈsaɪfərəbəl/ *adj* which cannot be deciphered; illegible.

indecision /ˌɪndɪˈsɪʒən/ *n* not able to make a decision; hesitation.

indecisive /ˌɪndɪˈsaɪsɪv/ *adj* inconclusive; irresolute.—**indecisively** *adv.*—**indecisiveness** *n.*

indeclinable /ˌɪndɪˈklaɪnəbəl/ *adj* (*gram*) which cannot be declined, having no inflected forms.

indecorous /ɪnˈdekərəs/ *adj* violating decorum, or any accepted rule of conduct.—**indecorum** *n.*

indeed /ɪnˈdiːd/ *adv* truly, certainly. • *interj* expressing irony, surprise, disbelief, etc.

indefatigable /ˌɪndɪˈfætɪgəbəl/ *adj* tireless.—**indefatigability** *n.*—**indefatigably** *adv.*

indefeasible /ˌɪndɪˈfiːzəbəl/ *adj* not to be defeated or made void, as a title.—**indefeasibility** *n.*—**indefeasibly** *adv.*

indefensible /ˌɪndɪˈfensəbəl/ *adj* unable to be defended or justified.—**indefensibility** *n.*—**indefensibly** *adv.*

indefinable /ˌɪndɪˈfaɪnəbəl/ *adj* that cannot be defined.—**indefinably** *adv.*

indefinite /ɪnˈdefənɪt/ *adj* not certain, undecided; imprecise, vague; having no fixed limits.—**indefinitely** *adv.*—**indefiniteness** *n.*

indefinite article *n* the word "a" or "an."

indehiscent /ˌɪndɪˈhɪsənt/ *adj* (*bot*) not opening when mature.—**indehiscence** *n.*

indelible /ɪnˈdeləbəl/ *adj* not able to be removed or erased; (*pen, ink, etc*) making an indelible mark.—**indelibility** *adv.*—**indelibly** *adv.*

indelicacy /ɪnˈdelɪkəsi/ *n* (*pl* **indelicacies**) lack of delicacy; something offensive to modesty or refined taste.

indelicate /ɪnˈdelɪkət/ *adj* improper; rough, crude; tactless.—**indelicately** *adv.*

indemnify /ɪnˈdemnəˌfaɪ/ *vt* (**indemnifying, indemnified**) to insure against loss, damage, etc; to repay (for damage, loss, etc).—**indemnification** *n.*—**indemnifier** *n.*

indemnity /ɪnˈdemnɪti/ *n* (*pl* **indemnities**) compensation for damage or loss; insurance against future loss or injury.

indemonstrable /ˌɪndɪˈmɒnstrəbəl/ or /ɪnˈdɛmən-/ *adj* which cannot be demonstrated or proved.

indent /ɪnˈdent/ *vt* to make notches in; to begin (a line of text) farther in from the margin than the rest. • *vi* to form an indentation. • *n* a dent or notch.—**indentor** *n.*

indentation /ˌɪndenˈteɪʃən/ *n* a being indented; a notch, cut, inlet, etc; a dent; a spacing in from the margin—*also* **indention, indent.**

indenture /ɪnˈdentʃər/ *n* a written agreement, a contract binding one person to work for another. • *vt* to bind by indentures.

indépendantiste /æˌdeɪpãndãˈtiːst/ *n* ✹ (*Cdn*) a person who supports the political independence of Quebec. • of or pertaining to the movement for the political independence of Quebec.

independence /ˌɪndɪˈpendəns/ *n* the state of being independent.

Independence Day *n* the anniversary of the adoption of the American Declaration of Independence on 4 July 1776.

independency /ˌɪndɪˈpendənsi/ *n* (*pl* **independencies**) a self-governing political unit.

independent /ˌɪndɪˈpendənt/ *adj* freedom from the influence or control of others; self-governing; self-determined; not adhering to any political party; not connected with others; not depending on another for financial support. • *n* a person who is independent in thinking, action etc.—**independently** *adv.*

in-depth /ˈɪnˌdepθ/ *adj* detailed, thorough.

indescribable /ˌɪndɪˈskraɪbəbəl/ *adj* unable to be described; too beautiful, horrible, intense, etc for words.—**indescribability** *n.*—**indescribably** *adv.*

indestructible /ˌɪndɪˈstrʌktəbəl/ *adj* not able to be destroyed.—**indestructibility** *n.*—**indestructibly** *adv.*

indeterminable /ˌɪndɪˈtərmɪnəbəl/ *adj* which cannot be ascertained, settled or classified.

indeterminate /ˌɪndɪˈtərmɪnət/ *adj* vague, uncertain; not defined or fixed in value.—**indeterminancy, indetermination** *adv.*—**indeterminately** *adv.*

indeterminism /ˌɪndɪˈtərmɪˌnɪzəm/ *n* (*philos*) the doctrine that the will has a certain freedom, independent of motives.

index /ˈɪndeks/ *n* (*pl* **indexes, indices**) an alphabetical list of names, subjects, items, etc mentioned in a printed book, *usu* listed alphabetically at the end of the text; a figure showing ratio or relative change, as of prices or wages; any indication or sign; a pointer or dial on an instrument; the exponent of a number. • *vt* to make an index of or for.—**indexer** *n.*

index arbitrage *see* **arbitrage.**

index finger *n* the forefinger.

Indiaman /ˈɪndiəmən/ *n* (*pl* **Indiamen**) (*formerly*) a commercial sailing vessel involved in trade with India.

Indian /ˈɪndiən/ *n* a native of India; an American Indian, the original inhabitants of the continent of America; the language of the people of India; a member of the aboriginal peoples of North and South America; ✹ (*Cdn*) one of three categories of aboriginal people (Indians, Inuit and Metis); ✹ (*Cdn*) a status Indian. • *adj* of or pertaining to a native of India; of or pertaining to the aboriginal peoples of North and South America.

Indian agent *n* ✹ (*Cdn*) a federal government official who administers programs on a First Nations reserve or in a region.

Indian corn *n* maize.

Indian file *n* single file.

Indian ink *n* a solid black pigment; a black ink made from this.—*also* **India ink.**

Indian paintbrush *n* ✹ a North American plant with flowers hidden by brightly coloured bracts.

Indian pear *n* ✹ a North American shrub with white flowers; the edible fruit of this shrub.

Indian summer *n* a period of unusually warm weather in the autumn.

indiarubber *n* an elastic gummy substance obtained from the milky juice of several tropical trees and used for rubbing out pencil marks.

Indic /ˈɪndɪk/ *adj* a term sometimes applied to the Indo-European languages of India, *eg* Sanskrit, Hindi, Bengali, etc.

indicant /ˈɪndɪkənt/ *n* something which indicates.

indicate /'ɪndɪˌkeɪt/ *vt* to point out; to show or demonstrate; to be a sign or symptom of; to state briefly, suggest.—**ind catable** *adj.*—**indication** *n.*—**indicatory** *adj.*

indicative /ɪn'dɪkətɪv/ *adj* serving as a sign (of); (*gram*) denoting the mood of the verb that affirms or denies.

indicator /'ɪndɪˌkeɪtər/ *n* a thing that indicates or points; a measuring device with a pointer, etc; an instrument showing the operating condition of a piece of machinery, etc; a device giving updated information, such as a departure board in a railway station or airport; a flashing light used to warn of a change in direction of a vehicle.

indices /'ɪndɪˌsez/ *see* **index**.

indicia /ɪn'dɪʃɪə/ *npl* (*sing* **indicium**) distinguishing markings.

indict /ɪn'daɪt/ *vt* to charge with a crime; to accuse.

indictable /ɪn'daɪtəbəl/ *adj* subject to being indicted; making one liable to indictment.

indictment /ɪn'daɪtmənt/ *n* a formal written statement framed by a prosecuting authority charging a person of a crime.

indifferent /ɪn'dɪfrənt/ or /-fərənt/ *adj* showing no concern; uninterested; unimportant; impartial; average; mediocre.—**indifference** *n.*—**indifferently** *adv.*

indifferentism /ɪn'dɪfrənˌtɪzəm/ *n* systematic indifference, *esp* with regard to religion.—**indifferentist** *n.*

indigen, indigene /'ɪndɪdʒiːn/ *n* a native (person, animal, etc).

indigenous /ɪn'dɪdʒənəs/ *adj* existing naturally in a particular country, region, or environment; native.

indigent /'ɪndɪdʒənt/ *adj* poor, needy.—**indigence** *n.*

indigestible /ˌɪndɪ'dʒestəbəl/ *adj* difficult or impossible to digest.—**indigestibility** *n.*

indigestion /ˌɪndɪ'dʒestʃən/ *n* a pain caused by difficulty in digesting food.

indigestive /ˌɪndɪ'dʒestɪv/ *adj* pertaining to, or having, indigestion.

indign /ɪn'daɪn/ *adj* (*arch*) unworthy; disgraceful.

indignant /ɪn'dɪgnənt/ *adj* expressing anger, *esp* at mean or unjust action.—**indignantly** *adv.*

indignation /ˌɪndɪg'neɪʃən/ *n* anger at something regarded as unfair, wicked, etc.

indignity /ɪn'dɪgnɪti/ *n* (*pl* **indignities**) humiliation; treatment making one feel degraded, undignified.

indigo /'ɪndɪˌgoʊ/ *n* (*pl* **indigos, indigoes**) a deep blue dye or colour.

indirect /ˌɪndɪ'rekt/ or /-daɪ-/ *adj* not straight; roundabout; secondary; dishonest.—**indirectly** *adv.*—**indirectness** *n.*

indirect evidence *n* circumstantial or inferential evidence.

indirection /ˌɪndə'rekʃən/ or /-daɪ-/ *n* indirect means or procedure; lack of direction; deceit.

indirect object *n* (*gram*) a person or thing affected by a verb but less directly than the object.

indirect speech *n* reported speech.

indirect tax *n* a tax levied on goods and services (which increases prices) rather than directly on individuals or companies.

indiscernible /ˌɪndɪ'sɜrnəbəl/ *adj* not discernible.—**indiscernibly** *adv.*

indiscipline /ɪn'dɪsɪplɪn/ *n* lack of discipline.

indiscreet /ˌɪndɪ'skriːt/ *adj* not discreet; tactless.—**indiscreetly** *adv.*

indiscrete /ˌɪndɪ'skriːt/ *adj* not separated into distinct parts.

indiscretion /ˌɪndɪ'skreʃən/ *n* an indiscreet act; rashness.—**indiscretionary** *adj.*

indiscriminate /ˌɪndɪ'skrɪmɪnət/ *adj* not making a careful choice; confused; random; making no distinctions.—**indiscriminately** *adv.*—**indiscrimination** *n.*—**indiscriminative** *adj.*

indispensable /ˌɪndɪ'spensəbəl/ *adj* absolutely essential.—**indispensability** *n.*—**indispensably** *adv.*

indispose /ˌɪndɪ'spoʊz/ *vt* to make unfit or unwell; to disincline.

indisposed /ˌɪndɪ'spoʊzd/ *adj* ill or sick; reluctant; disinclined.

indisposition /ˌɪndɪspə'zɪʃən/ *n* disinclination; a slight illness.

indisputable /ˌɪndɪ'spjuːtəbəl/ *adj* unquestionable; certain.—**indisputability** *n.*—**indisputably** *adv.*

indissoluble /ˌɪndɪ'sɒljʊbəl/ *adj* permanent; not able to be dissolved or destroyed.—**indissolubility** *n.*—**indissolubly** *adv.*

indistinct /ˌɪndɪ'stɪŋkt/ *adj* not clearly marked; dim; not distinct.—**indistinctly** *adv.*—**indistinctness** *n.*

indistinctive /ˌɪndɪ'stɪŋktɪv/ *adj* not capable of making distinctions; lacking distinctive characteristics.—**indistinctiveness** *n.*

indistinguishable /ˌɪndɪ'stɪŋgwɪʃəbəl/ *adj* not distinguishable; lacking identifying characteristics.—**indistinguishability** *n.*—**indistinguishably** *adv.*

indite /ɪn'daɪt/ *vt* (*arch*) to write.

indium /'ɪndɪəm/ *n* a soft metallic element used in alloys and electronic circuitry.

individual /ˌɪndɪ'vɪdʒuəl/ *adj* existing as a separate thing or being; of, by, for, or relating to a single person or thing. • *n* a single thing or being; a person.

individualist /-ɪst/ *n* a person who thinks or behaves with marked independence.—**individualism** *n.*—**individualistic** *adj.*—**individualistically** *adv.*

individuality /ˌɪndɪvɪdʒʊ'ælɪti/ *n* (*pl* **individualities**) the condition of being individual; separate or distinct existence; distinctive character.

individualize /ˌɪndɪ'vɪdʒʊəˌlaɪz/ *vt* to mark as distinct, particularize; to distinguish individually.—**individualization** *n.*

individually /ˌɪndɪ'vɪdʒʊəli/ *adv* in a distinctive manner; one by one; separately; personally.

individuate /ˌɪndɪ'vɪdʒʊˌeɪt/ *vt* to individualize.—**individuation** *n.*

indivisible /ˌɪndɪ'vɪzɪbəl/ *adj* not divisible.—**indivisibility** *n.*—**indivisibly** *adv.*

Indo-Canadian /ˌɪndoʊkə'neɪdɪən/ *n* ♣ a Canadian born on the Indian subcontinent, *esp* India. • *adj* pertaining to such Canadians.

indocile /ɪn'dɒsaɪl/ or /-doʊ-/ *adj* unteachable; intractable.—**indocility** *n.*

indoctrinate /ɪn'dɒktrɪˌneɪt/ *vt* to systematically instruct in doctrines, ideas, beliefs, etc.—**indoctrination** *n.*—**indoctrinator** *n.*

Indo-European /ˌɪndoʊjʊrə'pɪən/ or /-jər-/ *adj* of a family of languages (including English) spoken in most of Europe and Asia as far east as northern India. —*also n.*

indolent /'ɪndələnt/ *adj* idle; lazy.—**indolence** *n.*—**indolently** *adv.*

indomitable /ɪn'dɒmɪtəbəl/ *adj* not easily discouraged or defeated.—**indomitability** *n.*—**indomitably** *adv.*

indoor /'ɪndɔr/ *adj* done, used, or situated within a building.

indoors /ɪn'dɔrz/ *adv* in or into a building.

indorse /ɪn'dɔrs/ *see* **endorse**.

indraft /'ɪndræft/ *n* an inlet or inward current.

indubitable /ɪn'duːbɪtəbəl/ or /-'djuː-/ *adj* not capable of being doubted.—**indubitability** *n.*—**indubitably** *adv.*

induce /ɪn'duːs/ or /-'djuːs/ *vt* to persuade; to bring on; to draw (a conclusion) from particular facts; to bring about (an electric or magnetic effect) in a body by placing it within a field of force.—**inducer** *n.*—**inducible** *adj.*

inducement /-mənt/ *n* something that induces; a stimulus; a motive.

induct /ɪn'dʌkt/ *vt* to place formally in an office, a society, etc; to enrol (*esp* a draftee) in the armed forces.

inductance /-əns/ *n* the property of an electric circuit by which an electromotive force is produced by a variation in the current in the same or a neighbouring circuit; the measure of inductance in an electric circuit.

inductile /ɪn'dʌktɪl/ *adj* not ductile, not pliant.

induction /ɪn'dʌkʃən/ *n* the act or an instance of inducting, *eg* into office; reasoning from particular premises to general conclusions; the inducing of an electric or magnetic effect by a field of force.—**inductional** *adj.*

inductive /ɪn'dʌktɪv/ *adj* proceeding by or producing induction; operating by induction; susceptible to being acted on by induction.

inductor /ɪn'dʌktər/ *n* one who inducts; (*elect*) that part of an apparatus that acts inductively.

indue /ɪn'duː/ or /-'djuː/ *see* **endue**.

indulge /ɪn'dʌldʒ/ *vt* to satisfy (a desire); to gratify the wishes of; to humour. • *vi* to give way to one's desire.—**indulger** *n.*

indulgence /-əns/ *n* indulging or being indulged; a thing indulged in; a favour or privilege; (*RC Church*) a remission of punishment still due for a sin after the guilt has been forgiven.

indulgent /ɪn'dʌldʒənt/ *adj* indulging or characterized by indulgence; lenient.—**indulgently** *adv.*

induline, indulin /'ɪnduˌliːn/ or /-lɪn/, /-djuː-/ *n* a dark blue dye.

indult /'ɪnˌdʌlt/ *n* (*RC Church*) a licence from the Pope authorizing something not sanctioned by Church law.

induplicate /-əns/ /ɪn'duːplɪkɪt/ or /-'djuː-/, **induplicated** /-ɪd/ *adj* (*bot*) bent inwards.

indurate /'ɪndjʊˌreɪt/ *vt* to make hard or callous. • *vi* to grow hard or callous.—**induration** *n.*—**indurative** *adj.*

indusium /ɪnˈduːzɪəm/ or /-ˈdjuː-/ n (pl **indusia**) (bot) the covering of the growing spores in many ferns.—**indusial** adj.

industrial /ɪnˈdʌstrɪəl/ adj relating to or engaged in industry; used in industry; having many highly developed industries.—**industrially** adv.

industrialism /ɪnˈdʌstrɪəˌlɪzəm/ n social and economic organization characterized by large industries, machine production, urban workers, etc.

industrialist /ɪnˈdʌstrɪəlɪst/ n a person who owns or manages an industrial enterprise.

industrialize /ɪnˈdʌstrɪəˌlaɪz/ vti to make or become industrial.—**industrialization** n.

industrial league n ✦ (Cdn) a sports league, esp for ice hockey, whose teams are sponsored by businesses.

industrial relations n the relations between employees and employers.

industrious /ɪnˈdʌstrɪəs/ adj hard-working.—**industriously** adv.—**industriousness** n.

industry /ˈɪndəstri/ n (pl **industries**) organized production or manufacture of goods; manufacturing enterprises collectively; a branch of commercial enterprise producing a particular product; any large-scale business activity; the owners and managers of industry; diligence.

indwelling /ɪnˈdwelɪŋ/ vti (**indwelling, indwelt**) to dwell (in).

inebriate /ɪˈniːbrɪˌeɪt/ vt to intoxicate, esp with alcoholic drink. • n a drunkard. • adj inebriated.—**inebriation** n.

inebriated /-ɪd/ adj drunken.

inedible /ɪnˈedɪbəl/ adj not fit to be eaten.—**inedibility** n.

inedited /ɪnˈedɪtɪd/ adj unpublished; not edited.

ineducable /ɪnˈedʒʊkəbəl/ or /-djʊ-/ adj impossible to educate, esp due to mental deficiency.

ineffable /ɪnˈefəbəl/ adj too intense or great to be spoken; unutterable; too sacred to be spoken.—**ineffability** n.—**ineffably** adv.

ineffaceable /ˌɪnɪˈfeɪsəbəl/ adj which cannot be effaced.—**ineffaceability** n.

ineffective /ˌɪnɪˈfektɪv/ adj not effective.—**ineffectively** adv.—**ineffectiveness** n.

ineffectual /ˌɪnɪˈfektʃʊəl/ adj not effectual; futile.—**ineffectuality** n.—**ineffectually** adv.

inefficacious /ˌɪnefɪˈkeɪʃəs/ adj not having the power to produce a desired effect.—**inefficacy** n.

inefficiency /ˌɪnɪˈfɪʃənsi/ n (pl **inefficiences**) the quality or condition of being inefficient; an instance of inefficiency or incompetence.

inefficient /ˌɪnɪˈfɪʃənt/ adj not efficient.—**inefficiently** adv.

inelastic /ˌɪnɪˈlæstɪk/ adj not elastic; inflexible, unyielding.—**inelastically** adv.—**inelasticity** n.

inelegant /ɪnˈeləgənt/ adj ungraceful; lacking refinement or polish.—**inelegance** n.

ineligible /ɪnˈelɪdʒəbəl/ adj not eligible.—**ineligibility** n.

ineluctable /ˌɪnɪˈlektəbəl/ adj not possible to escape from or avoid.—**ineluctably** adv.

inept /ɪnˈept/ or /ɪˈnept/ adj unsuitable; unfit; foolish; awkward; clumsy.—**ineptitude** n.—**ineptly** adv.

inequality /ˌɪnɪˈkwɒlɪti/ n (pl **inequalities**) lack of equality in size, status, etc; unevenness.

inequitable /ɪnˈekwɪtəbəl/ adj unjust, unfair.—**inequitably** adv.

inequity /ɪnˈekwɪti/ n (pl **inequities**) lack of equity; injustice.

ineradicable /ˌɪnɪˈrædɪkəbəl/ adj which cannot be eradicated.

inert /ɪˈnɜːt/ adj without power to move or to resist; inactive; dull; slow; with few or no active properties.—**inertly** adv.—**inertness** n.

inertia /ɪˈnɜːʃə/ n (physics) the tendency of matter to remain at rest (or continue in a fixed direction) unless acted on by an outside force; disinclination to act.

inertial /ɪnˈɜːʃɪəl/ adj of, or pertaining to, inertia.

inescapable /ˌɪnɪˈskeɪpəbəl/ adj which cannot be escaped, inevitable.

inessential /ˌɪnɪˈsenʃəl/ adj not essential.

inestimable /ɪnˈestɪməbəl/ adj not to be estimated; beyond measure or price; incalculable; invaluable.—**inestimably** adv.

inevitable /ɪnˈevɪtəbəl/ adj sure to happen; unavoidable. • n something that is inevitable.—**inevitability** n.—**inevitably** adv.

inexact /ˌɪnɪgˈzækt/ adj not strictly true or correct.—**inexactitude** n.—**inexactly** adv.

inexcusable /ˌɪnɪkˈskjuːzəbəl/ adj without excuse; unpardonable.—**inexcusably** adv.

inexhaustible /ˌɪnɪgˈzɔːstɪbəl/ adj not to be exhausted or spent; unfailing; unwearied.—**inexhaustibility** n.—**inexhaustibly** adv.

inexorable /ɪnˈeksərəbəl/ adj unable to be persuaded by persuasion or entreaty, relentless.—**inexorability** n.—**inexorably** adv.

inexpedient /ˌɪnɪkˈspiːdɪənt/ adj unsuitable to circumstances; inadvisable.—**inexpedience, inexpediency** n.

inexpensive /ˌɪnɪkˈspensɪv/ adj cheap.—**inexpensively** adv.

inexperience /ˌɪnɪkˈspiːrɪəns/ n want of experience or of the knowledge that comes by experience.

inexperienced /-d/ adj lacking experience; unpractised; unskilled; unversed.

inexpert /ɪnˈekspɜːt/ adj unskilled; lacking the knowledge or dexterity derived from practice.

inexpiable /ɪnˈekspiəbəl/ adj which cannot be expiated.

inexplicable /ˌɪnɪkˈsplɪkəbəl/ or /ɪnˈeks-/ adj not to be explained, made plain, or intelligible; not to be interpreted or accounted for.—**inexplicability** n.—**inexplicably** adv.

inexplicit /ˌɪnɪkˈsplɪsɪt/ adj not clear.

inexpressible /ˌɪnɪkˈspresɪbəl/ adj incapable of being expressed, uttered, or described.—**inexpressibly** adv.

inexpressive /ˌɪnɪkˈspresɪv/ adj lacking expression or distinct significance.

inextensible /ˌɪnekˈstensəbəl/ or /-ɪk-/ adj which cannot be extended.—**inextensibility** n.

inextinguishable /ˌɪnɪkˈstɪŋgwɪʃəbəl/ adj which cannot be extinguished, unquenchable.

in extremis /ˌɪnekˈstreɪmɪs/ or /-triːmɪs/, /-tremɪs/ adv close to death; in a very difficult situation.

inextricable /ɪnˈekstrɪkəbəl/ or /ˌɪnɪkˈstrɪk-/ adj that cannot be disentangled, solved, or escaped from.—**inextricably** adv.

infallible /ɪnˈfælɪbəl/ adj incapable of being wrong; dependable; reliable.—**infallibility** n.—**infallibly** adv.

infamous /ˈɪnfəməs/ adj having a bad reputation; notorious; causing a bad reputation; scandalous.

infamy /ˈɪnfəmi/ n (pl **infamies**) ill fame; public disgrace; ignominy.

infancy /ˈɪnfənsi/ n (pl **infancies**) early childhood; the beginning or early existence of anything.

infant /ˈɪnfənt/ n a very young child; a baby.

infanta /ɪnˈfæntə/ n a title for a Spanish princess, not the heir apparent.

infante /ɪnˈfænti/ n a title for a Spanish prince, not the heir apparent.

infanticide /ɪnˈfæntɪˌsaɪd/ n the killing of an infant; a person who does this.—**infanticidal** adj.

infantile /ˈɪnfənˌtaɪl/ adj of infants; like an infant, babyish.

infantile paralysis n poliomyletis.

infantry /ˈɪnfəntri/ n (pl **infantries**) soldiers trained to fight on foot.

infatuate /ɪnˈfætʃuːˌeɪt/ or /-tjuː-/ vt to inspire with intense, foolish, or short-lived passion.—**infatuated** adj.—**infatuatedly** adv.

infatuation /-ˈeɪʃən/ n an extravagant passion.

infect /ɪnˈfekt/ vt to contaminate with disease-causing microorganisms; to taint; to affect, esp so as to harm.—**infective** adj.

infection /ɪnˈfekʃən/ n an infecting or being infected; an infectious disease; a diseased condition.

infectious /ɪnˈfekʃəs/ adj (disease) able to be transmitted; causing or transmitted by infection; tending to spread to others.—**infectiousness** n.

infectious hepatitis n an infectious disease which causes inflammation of the liver.

infectious mononucleosis n an infectious disease characterized by inflammation of the lymph glands.—also **glandular fever**.

infelicitous /ˌɪnfəˈlɪsɪtəs/ adj unfortunate; unhappy; inappropriate; ill-timed.

infelicity /ˌɪnfɪˈlɪsɪti/ n (pl **infelicities**) misfortune; unhappiness; inapproriateness; an infelicitous act or expression.

infer /ɪnˈfɜː/ vt (**inferring, inferred**) to conclude by reasoning from facts or premises; to accept as a fact or consequence.—**inferable** adj.—**inferrer** n.

inference /ˈɪnfərəns/ n an inferring; something inferred or deduced; a reasoning from premises to a conclusion.—**inferential** adj.

inferior /ɪnˈfiːriər/ adj lower in position, rank, degree, or quality. • n an inferior person.—**inferiority** n.

inferiority complex n (psychol) an acute sense of inferiority expressed by a lack of confidence or in exaggerated aggression.

infernal /ɪnˈfɜːnəl/ adj of hell; hellish; fiendish; (inf) irritating, detestable.—**infernally** adv.

inferno /ɪnˈfɜːnoː/ n (pl **infernos**) hell; intense heat; a devastating fire.

infertile /ɪnˈfɜːtaɪl/ adj not fertile.—**infertility** n.

infest /ɪnˈfest/ vt to overrun in large numbers, usu so as to be harmful; to be parasitic in or on.—**infestation** n.—**infester** n.

infidel /ˈɪnfɪdəl/ n a person who does not believe in a certain religion; a person who has no religion.

infidelity /ˌɪnfɪˈdeliti/ n (pl **infidelities**) unfaithfulness, esp in marriage.

infield /ˈɪnfiːld/ n (cricket) the area of the ground near the wicket; (baseball) the area of the field enclosed by the baselines.

infielder /ˈɪnfiːldər/ n (baseball, cricket) a player in an infield position.

infighting /ˈɪnˌfaɪtɪŋ/ n (boxing) exchanging punches at close quarters; intense competition within an organization.—**infighter** n.

infiltrate /ˈɪnfɪlˌtreɪt/ vti to filter or pass gradually through or into; to permeate; to penetrate (enemy lines, etc) gradually or stealthily, eg as spies.—**infiltration** n.—**infiltrator** n.

infinite /ˈɪnfɪnɪt/ adj endless, limitless; very great; vast.—**infinitely** adv.

infinitesimal /ˌɪnfɪnɪˈtesɪməl/ adj immeasurably small.—**infinitesimally** adv.

infinitive /ɪnˈfɪnɪtɪv/ n (gram) the form of a verb without reference to person, number or tense.—**infinitival** adj.

infinitude /ɪnˈfɪnɪˌtuːd/ or /-tjuːd/ n the condition or quality of being infinite; infinity.

infinity /ɪnˈfɪnɪti/ n (pl **infinities**) the condition or quality of being infinite; an unlimited number, quantity, or time period.

infirm /ɪnˈfɜːm/ adj physically weak, esp from old age or illness; irresolute.

infirmary /ɪnˈfɜːməri/ n (pl **infirmaries**) a hospital or place for the treatment of the sick.

infirmity /ɪnˈfɜːməti/ n (pl **infirmities**) being infirm; a physical weakness.

infix /ˈɪnfɪks/ vt to fix or insert in.

in flagrante delicto /ˌɪn fləˌgrænti dɪˈlɪktoː/ adv in the very act of commiting the crime, red-handed.—also **flagrante delicto**.

inflame /ɪnˈfleɪm/ vti to arouse, excite, etc, or to become aroused, excited, etc; to undergo or cause to undergo inflammation.—**inflamingly** adv.

inflammable /ɪnˈflæməbəl/ adj able to catch fire, flammable; easily excited.—**inflammability** n.

inflammation /ˌɪnfləˈmeɪʃən/ n an inflaming or being inflamed; redness, pain, heat, and swelling in the body, due to injury or disease.

inflammatory /ɪnˈflæmətəri/ or /-tri/ adj rousing excitement, anger, etc; of or caused by inflammation.—**inflammatorily** adv.

inflatable /ɪnˈfleɪtəbəl/ adj able to be inflated.

inflate /ɪnˈfleɪt/ vti to fill or become filled with air or gas; to puff up with pride; to increase beyond what is normal, esp the supply of money or credit.—**inflatedly** adv.—**inflater, inflator** n.

inflation /ɪnˈfleɪʃən/ n an inflating or being inflated; an increase in the currency in circulation or a marked expansion of credit, resulting in a fall in currency value and a sharp rise in prices.

inflationary /-ˌneri/ adj pertaining to or causing inflation.

inflationist /-ist/ n, adj (someone) in favour of a policy of an increased issue of money and availability of credit, with inflation as a consequence.

inflect /ɪnˈflekt/ vt to change the form (of a word) by inflection; to vary the tone of (the voice).—**inflective** adj.—**inflector** n.

inflection /ɪnˈflekʃən/ n a bend; the change in the form of a word to indicate number, case, tense, etc; a change in the tone of the voice.—**inflectional** adj.

inflexible /ɪnˈfleksɪbəl/ adj not flexible; stiff, rigid; fixed; unyielding.—**inflexibility** n.—**inflexibly** adv.

inflict /ɪnˈflɪkt/ vt to impose (pain, a penalty, etc) on a person or thing.—**inflicter, inflictor** n.—**infliction** n.

inflorescence /ˌɪnfləˈresəns/ n the producing of blossoms; the arrangement of flowers on a stem; a flower cluster; flowers collectively.—**inflorescent** adj.

inflow /ˈɪnfloː/ n something which flows in.

influence /ˈɪnfluːəns/ n the power to affect others; the power to produce effects by having wealth, position, ability, etc; a person with influence. • vt to have influence on.—**influenceable** adj.

influent /ˈɪnfluːənt/ adj flowing in.

influential /ˌɪnfluːˈenʃəl/ adj having or exerting great influence.—**influentially** adv.

influenza /ˌɪnfluːˈenzə/ n a contagious feverish virus disease marked by muscular pain and inflammation of the respiratory system.—**influenzal** adj.

influx /ˈɪnflʌks/ n a sudden inflow of people or things to a place.

info /ˈɪnfoː/ n (sl) information.

inform /ɪnˈfɔːm/ vt to provide knowledge of something to. • vi to give information to the police, etc, esp in accusing another.

informal /ɪnˈfɔːməl/ adj not formal; not according to fixed rules or ceremony, etc; casual.—**informally** adv.

informality /-ˈmæliti/ n (pl **informalities**) the lack of regular, customary, or legal form; an informal act.

informant /ɪnˈfɔːmənt/ n a person who gives information.

information /ˌɪnfərˈmeɪʃən/ n something told or facts learned; news; knowledge; data stored in or retrieved from a computer.—**informational** adj.

information technology n (the study of) the collection, retrieval, use, storage and communication of information using computers and microelectronic systems.

information theory n mathematical and statistical analysis of information communication systems.

informative /ɪnˈfɔːmətɪv/, **informatory** /-təri/ adj conveying information, instructive.—**informatively** adv.

informer /ɪnˈfɔːmər/ n a person who informs on another, esp to the police for a reward.

infra- /ˈɪnfrə/ prefix below; within; beneath; after.

infraction /ɪnˈfrækʃən/ n a violation of a law, pact, etc.

infra dig /ˌɪnfrə ˈdɪg/ adj (inf) beneath one's dignity.

infrangible /ɪnˈfrændʒɪbəl/ adj unbreakable; inviolable.—**infrangibility** n.

infrared /ˌɪnfrəˈred/ n (radiation) having a wavelength longer than light but shorter than radio waves; of, pertaining to, or using such radiation.

infrasonic /ˌɪnfrəˈsɒnɪk/ adj (soundwaves) having a frequency below the audible range.—**infrasound** n.

infrastructure /ˈɪnfrəˌstrʌktʃər/ n the basic structure of any system or organization; the basic installations, such as roads, railways, factories, etc that determine the economic power of a country.

infrequent /ɪnˈfriːkwənt/ adj seldom occurring; rare.—**infrequence, infrequency** n.—**infrequently** adv.

infringe /ɪnˈfrɪndʒ/ vt to break or violate, esp an agreement or a law.—**infringement** n.

infundibular /ˌɪnfenˈdɪbjʊlər/, **infundibulate** /-leɪt/ adj funnel-shaped.

infuriate /ɪnˈfjʊriˌeɪt/ vt to enrage; to make furious.—**infuriating** adj.—**infuriatingly** adv.

infuse /ɪnˈfjuːz/ vt to instil or impart (qualities, etc); to inspire; to steep (tea leaves, etc) to extract the essence.—**infuser** n.

infusible[1] /ɪnˈfjuːzɪbəl/ adj incapable of being fused or melted.—**infusibility** n.

infusible[2] adj capable of being infused.—**infusibility** n.

infusion /ɪnˈfjuːʒən/ n the act of infusing; something obtained by infusing.

infusorial earth /ˌɪnfjuːˈsɔːriəl/ n a silicious deposit composed chiefly of the shells of microscopic vegetable organisms called diatoms, used as a polishing powder and in the manufacture of dynamite.

ingenious /ɪnˈdʒiːniəs/ adj clever, resourceful, etc; made or done in an original or clever way.—**ingeniously** adv.—**ingeniousness** n.

ingénue /ˌæʒəˈnjuː/ or /-nuː/ n a naive young woman.

ingenuity /ˌɪndʒɪˈnjuːɪti/ n (pl **ingenuities**) skill in contriving or inventing; resourcefulness.

ingenuous /ɪnˈdʒenjuəs/ adj naive, innocent; candid.—**ingenuously** adv.—**ingenuousness** n.

ingest /ɪnˈdʒest/ vt to take (as food) into the body.—**ingestion** n.—**ingestive** adj.

ingle /ˈɪŋgəl/ n (arch) a fireplace.

inglenook /ˈɪŋgəlˌnʊk/ n (a seat in) a recess by a large open fireplace.

inglorious /ɪnˈglɔːriəs/ adj disgraceful, shameful; obscure.

ingot /'ɪngət/ *n* a brick-shaped mass of cast metal, *esp* gold or silver.

ingrain /'ɪngreɪn/ *vt* to make a deep impression upon; (*arch*) to dye.—*also* **engrain**.

ingrained /ɪn'greɪnd/ or /'ɪn-/ *adj* (*habits, feelings, etc*) firmly established; (*dirt*) deeply embedded.—*also* **engrained**.

ingrate /'ɪngreɪt/ *adj* (*arch*) ungrateful. • *n* an ungrateful person.

ingratiate /ɪn'greɪʃɪˌeɪt/ *vt* to bring oneself into another's favour.—**ingratiating, ingratiatory** *adj*.—**ingratiation** *n*.

ingratitude /ɪn'grætɪˌtuːd/ or /-ˌtjuːd/ *n* absence of gratitude; insensibility to kindness.

ingredient /ɪn'griːdɪənt/ *n* something included in a mixture; a component.

ingress /'ɪngres/ *n* entrance.

in-group /'ɪngruːp/ *n* a group favouring its own members at the expense of members of other groups.

ingrowing /'ɪnˌgroʊɪn/ *adj* (*toe nail, etc*) growing abnormally into the flesh.

ingrowth /'ɪnˌgroʊθ/ *n* the process of growing inwards; something which grows inwards.

inguinal /'ɪngwɪnəl/ *adj* of the groin or its vicinity.

ingurgitate /ɪn'gərdʒɪˌteɪt/ *vt* to swallow greedily.—**ingurgitation** *n*.

inhabit /ɪn'hæbɪt/ *vt* to live in; to occupy; to reside.

inhabitable /ɪn'hæbɪtəbəl/ *adj* fit for habitation.—**inhabitability** *n*.—**inhabitation** *n*.

inhabitant /-tənt/ *n* a person or animal inhabiting a specified place.—**inhabitancy, inhabitance** *n*.

inhalant /ɪn'heɪlənt/ *n* a medicine, etc that is inhaled.

inhalation /-hə'leɪʃən/ *n* the act of inhaling.

inhale /ɪn'heɪl/ *vti* to breathe in.

inhaler /ɪn'heɪlər/ *n* a device that dispenses medicines in a fine spray for inhalation.

inharmonic /ˌɪnhɑr'mɒnɪk/, **inharmonious** /ˌɪnhɑr'moʊnɪəs/ *adj* lacking harmony; discordant.

inhere /ɪn'hiːr/ *vi* to be inherent.

inherent /ɪn'hɛrənt/ or /ɪn'hiːr-/ *adj* existing as an inseparable part of something.—**inherence, inherency** *n*.—**inherently** *adv*.

inherit /ɪn'hɛrɪt/ *vt* to receive (property, a title, etc) under a will or by right of legal succession; to possess by genetic transmission. • *vi* to receive by inheritance; to succeed as heir.—**inheritor** *n*.

inheritable /-əbəl/ *adj* capable of being inherited.

inheritance /-əns/ *n* the action of inheriting; something inherited.

inhibit /ɪn'hɪbɪt/ *vt* to restrain; to prohibit.—**inhibitor, inhibiter** *n*.

inhibition /ˌɪnhɪ'bɪʃən/ *n* an inhibiting or being inhibited; a mental process that restrains or represses an action, emotion, or thought.

inhospitable /ˌɪnhɒ'spɪtəbəl/ or /ɪn'hɒsp-/ *adj* not hospitable; affording no shelter; barren; cheerless.—**inhospitably** *adv*.—**inhospitality** *n*.

in-house /'ɪnhɐʊs/ or /-'hɐʊs/ *adj* within an organization.

inhuman /ɪn'hjuːmən/ or /ɪn'juːmən/ *adj* lacking in the human qualities of kindness, pity, etc; cruel, brutal, unfeeling; not human.

inhumane /ˌɪnhjuː'meɪn/ *adj* not humane; inhuman.

inhumanity /ˌɪnhjuː'mænɪti/ *n* (*pl* **inhumanites**) the quality of being inhuman; cruelty.

inhume /ɪn'hjuːm/ *vt* to bury, inter.—**inhumation** *n*.—**injumer** *n*.

inimical /ɪ'nɪmɪkəl/ *adj* hostile; adverse, unfavourable.—**inimically** *adv*.

inimitable /ɪ'nɪmɪtəbəl/ *adj* impossible to imitate; matchless.—**inimitably** *adv*.

iniquitous /ɪ'nɪkwɪtəs/ *adj* marked by iniquity.

iniquity /ɪ'nɪkwɪti/ *n* (*pl* **iniquities**) wickedness; great injustice.

initial /ɪ'nɪʃəl/ *adj* of or at the beginning. • *n* the first letter of each word in a name; a large letter at the beginning of a chapter, etc. • *vt* (**initialing, initialed** *or* **initialling, initialled**) to sign with initials.—**initialer, initialler** *n*.—**initially** *adv*.

initialize /ɪ'nɪʃəˌlaɪz/ *vt* (*comput*) to format (a disk) to suit a particular processor.—**initialization** *n*.

initiate /ɪ'nɪʃɪˌeɪt/ *vt* to bring (something) into practice or use; to teach the fundamentals of a subject to; to admit as a member into a club, etc, *esp* with a secret ceremony. • *n* an initiated person.—**initiator** *n*.—**initiatory** *adj*.

initiation /-'eɪʃən/ *n* the act of initiating; a formal, often secret, ceremony of admission.

initiative /ɪ'nɪʃətɪv/ or /ɪ'nɪʃɪətɪv/ *n* the action of taking the first step; ability to originate new ideas or methods.

inject /ɪn'dʒɛkt/ *vt* to force (a fluid) into a vein, tissue, etc, *esp* with a syringe; to introduce (a remark, quality, etc) to interject.—**injectable** *adj*.

injection /ɪn'dʒɛkʃən/ *n* an injecting; a substance that is injected.—**injective** *adj*.

injector /-ər/ *n* someone who, or something which, injects; a device for injecting fuel into an internal combustion engine; a device for filling the boiler of a steam engine with water.

injudicious /ˌɪndʒuː'dɪʃəs/ *adj* not judicious; indiscreet; unwise.

injunction /ɪn'dʒʌŋkʃən/ *n* a command; an order; a court order prohibiting or ordering a given action.—**injunctive** *adj*.

injure /'ɪndʒər/ *vt* to harm physically or mentally; to hurt, do wrong to.—**injurer** *n*.

injurious /ɪn'dʒʊrɪəs/ *adj* causing injury.

injury /'ɪndʒəri/ *n* (*pl* **injuries**) physical damage; harm.

injury time *n* (*sport*) time added to compensate for stoppages through injuries to players.

injustice /ɪn'dʒʌstɪs/ *n* the state or practice of being unfair; an unjust act.

ink /ɪŋk/ *n* a coloured liquid used for writing, printing, etc; the dark protective secretion of an octopus, etc. • *vt* to cover, mark, or colour with ink.

inkhorn /'ɪŋkhɔrn/ *n* (*formerly*) a container for ink.

inkling /'ɪŋklɪŋ/ *n* a hint; a vague notion.

inkstand /'ɪŋkstænd/ *n* a stand for an ink bottle.

inkwell /'ɪŋkˌwɛl/ *n* a container for ink.

inky /'ɪŋki/ *adj* (**inkier, inkiest**) like very dark ink in colour; black; covered with ink.—**inkiness** *n*.

inlaid /'ɪnleɪd/ *see* **inlay**.

inland /'ɪnlænd/ or /-lənd/ *adj* of or in the interior of a country. • *n* an inland region. • *adv* into or toward this region.—**inlander** *n*.

in-law *n* a relative by marriage.

inlay /'ɪnleɪ/ or /ɪn'leɪ/ *vt* (**inlaying, inlaid**) to decorate a surface by inserting pieces of metal, wood, etc. • *n* inlaid work; material inlaid.—**inlaid** *adj*.

inlet /'ɪnlɛt/ or /-lət/ *n* a narrow strip of water extending into a body of land; an opening; a passage, pipe, etc for liquid to enter a machine, etc. • *vt* (**inletting, inletted**) to inlay; to insert.

in loco parentis /ɪn ˌloːkoː pə'rɛntɪs/ (*Latin*) in the place of a parent.

inmate /'ɪnmeɪt/ *n* a person confined with others in a prison or institution.

in memoriam /ɪn mə'mɔriəm/ (*Latin*) in memory of.

inmost /'ɪnmoːst/ *adj* farthest within; most secret.

inn /ɪn/ *n* a small hotel; a restaurant or tavern, *esp* in the countryside.

innards /'ɪnərdz/ *npl* (*inf*) the stomach and intestines, internal organs.

innate /ɪ'neɪt/ or /'ɪ-/ *adj* existing from birth; inherent; instinctive.—**innately** *adv*.

inner /'ɪnər/ *adj* further within; inside, internal; private, exclusive. • *n* (*archery*) the innermost ring on a target.

inner city *n* the central area of a city, *esp* as affected by overcrowding and poverty.

innermost /'ɪnərˌmoːst/ *adj* furthest within.

inner tube *n* the separate inflatable tube within a pneumatic tire.

innervation /ˌɪnər'veɪʃən/ *n* the arrangement of nerve filaments in the body; special activity or stimulus in any part of the nervous system.

inning /'ɪnɪŋ/ *n* (*baseball*) a team's turn at bat.

innings /-z/ *n* (*pl* **innings**) (*cricket*) a turn at bat for a batsman or side; the number of runs scored at this time; an opportunity to demonstrate one's abilities.

innkeeper /'ɪnˌkiːpər/ *n* a person who owns or manages an inn.

innocence /'ɪnəsəns/ *n* the condition or quality of being innocent.

innocent /'ɪnəsənt/ *adj* not guilty of a particular crime; free from sin; blameless; harmless; inoffensive; simple, credulous, naive. • *n* an innocent person, as a child.—**innocence** *n*.—**innocently** *adv*.

innocuous /ɪ'nɒkjʊəs/ *adj* harmless.—**innocuously** *adv*.—**innocuousness** *n*.

innominate /ɪ'nɒmɪnət/ *adj* without a name.

innovate /'ɪnəˌveɪt/ *vi* to introduce new methods, ideas, etc; to make changes.—**innovation** *n*.—**innovative, innovatory** *adv*.

innovator /-ər/ *n* one who introduces, or seeks to introduce, new things.

innoxious /ɪˈnɒkʃəs/ *adj* harmless.

Innu /ˈɪnuː/ *n* ❀ a member of a First Nations people of Labrador and northern Quebec; the language of this people. • *adj* of or pertaining to this people or their language.

innuendo /ˌɪnjʊˈendoʊ/ *n* (*pl* **innuendos, innuendoes**) a hint or sly remark, *usu* derogatory; an insinuation.

Innuit /ˈɪnjuːɪt/ or /ˈɪnuɪt/ *see* **Inuit**.

innumerable /ɪˈnuːmərəbəl/ or /-ˈnjuː-/, **innumerous** /-əs/ *adj* too many to be counted; very numerous.—**innumerability** *n*.—**innumerably** *adv*.

innumerate /ɪˈnuːmərət/ or /-ˈnjuː-/ *adj* lacking knowledge or understanding of mathematics and science; not numerate.—*also n*.

inobservance /ˌɪnəbˈzɜrvəns/ *n* inattention; failure to observe (law, etc).—**inobservant** *adj*.

inoculate /ɪˈnɒkjʊˌleɪt/ *vt* to inject a serum or a vaccine into, *esp* in order to create immunity; to protect as if by inoculation.—**inoculation** *n*.—**inoculative** *adj*.

inodorous /ɪnˈoʊdərəs/ *adj* without odour.

inoffensive /ˌɪnəˈfensɪv/ *adj* harmless, not offensive.

inofficious /ˌɪnəˈfɪʃəs/ *adj* contrary to moral duty.

inoperable /ɪnˈɒprəbəl/ or /-ˈɒpərəbəl/ *adj* not suitable for surgery.—**inoperability** *n*.

inoperative /ɪnˈɒprətɪv/ or /-ˈɒpərətɪv/ *adj* not working; producing no effect.

inopportune /ɪnˈɒpərˌtuːn/ or /-ˌtjuːn/ *adj* unseasonable; untimely.—**inopportuneness, inopportunity** *n*.

inordinate /ɪnˈɔːrdɪnət/ *adj* excessive.—**inordinately** *adv*.

inorganic /ˌɪnɔːrˈgænɪk/ *adj* not having the structure or characteristics of living organisms; denoting a chemical compound not containing carbon.—**inorganically** *adv*.

inorganic chemistry *n* the chemistry of all substances except those containing carbon.

inosculate /ɪnˈɒskjʊˌleɪt/ *vti* (*anat, of blood vessels, fibres, etc*) to join closely, be closely joined.—**inosculation** *n*.

inpatient /ˈɪnˌpeɪʃənt/ *n* a patient being treated while remaining in hospital.

in perpetuum /ˌɪn pərˈpetuːʊm/ *adv* perpetually, forever.

in posse /ɪn ˈpɒsi/ *adj, adv* having a possible but not an actual existence, potential.

input /ˈɪnpʊt/ *n* what is put in, as power into a machine, data into a computer, etc. • *vt* (**inputting, input** *or* **inputted**) to put in; to enter (data) into a computer.

inquest /ˈɪnkwest/ *n* a judicial inquiry held by a coroner, *esp* into a case of violent or unexplained death; (*inf*) any detailed inquiry or investigation.

inquietude /ɪnˈkwaɪəˌtuːd/ or /-ˌtjuːd/ *n* unease, disquiet.

inquiline /ˈɪnkwɪˌlaɪn/ *n* (*zool*) an animal which lives in the abode of another but does not harm it, *eg* a hermit crab.—**inquilinous** *adj*.

inquire /ɪnˈkwaɪr/ *vi* to request information about; (*usu with* **into**) to investigate. • *vt* to ask about.—*also* **enquire**.—**inquirer, enquirer** *n*.

inquiry /ɪnˈkwaɪri/ *n* (*pl* **inquiries**) the act of inquiring; a search by questioning; an investigation; a question; research.—*also* **enquiry**.

inquisition /ˌɪnkwəˈzɪʃən/ *n* a detailed examination or investigation; (*with cap and* **the**) (*RC Church*) formerly the tribunal for suppressing heresy.—**inquisitional** *adj*.

inquisitive /ɪnˈkwɪzɪtɪv/ *adj* eager for knowledge; unnecessarily curious; prying.—**inquisitively** *adv*.—**inquisitiveness** *n*.

inquisitor /ɪnˈkwɪzɪtər/ *n* a person who questions searchingly or forcefully; (*often cap*) a member of the Inquisition.

inquisitorial /ɪnˈkwɪzɪˈtɔːriəl/ *adj* of or resembling an inquisitor; prying.—**inquisitorially** *adv*.

in re /ɪn ˈriː/ or /-ˈreɪ/ *prep* in the matter of.

inroad /ˈɪnroʊd/ *n* a raid into enemy territory; an encroachment or advance.

inrush /ˈɪnrʌʃ/ *n* a sudden inward flow or influx.

insalivate /ɪnˈsæləˌveɪt/ *vt* to mix (food) with saliva while chewing.—**insalivation** *n*.

insalubrious /ˌɪnsəˈluːbriəs/ *adj* (*climate, place*) unhealthy.—**insalubrity** *n*.

insane /ɪnˈseɪn/ *adj* not sane, mentally ill; of or for insane people; very foolish.—**insanely** *adv*.

insanitary /ɪnˈsænɪteri/ *adj* unclean, likely to cause infection or ill-health.—**insanitariness, insanitation** *n*.

insanity /ɪnˈsænɪti/ *n* (*pl* **insanities**) derangement of the mind or intellect; lunacy; madness.

insatiable /ɪnˈseɪʃəbəl/ *adj* not easily satisfied; greedy.—**insatiability** *n*.—**insatiably** *adv*.

insatiate /ɪnˈseɪʃiət/ *adj* insatiable.

inscribe /ɪnˈskraɪb/ *vt* to mark or engrave (words, etc) on (a surface); to add (a person's name) to a list; to dedicate (a book) to someone; to autograph; to fix in the mind.—**inscribable** *adj*.

inscription /ɪnˈskrɪpʃən/ *n* an inscribing; words, etc inscribed on a tomb, coin, stone, etc.—**inscriptional** *adj*.

inscrutable /ɪnˈskruːtəbəl/ *adj* hard to understand, incomprehensible; enigmatic.—**inscrutability** *n*.—**inscrutably** *adv*.

insect /ˈɪnsekt/ *n* any of a class of small arthropods with three pairs of legs, a head, thorax, and abdomen and two or four wings.

insectary /ɪnˈsektəri/ or /ˈɪnˌsek-/, /ˈɪnsekˌteri/ *n* (*pl* **insectaries**) a place for keeping insects.

insecticide /ɪnˈsektəˌsaɪd/ *n* a substance for killing insects.—**insecticidal** *adj*.

insectivore /ɪnˈsektɪˌvɔr/ *n* an order of mammals that are small, nocturnal, and feed on insects or other invertebrates; any insect-eating plant or animal.—**insectivorous** *adj*.

insecure /ˌɪnsɪˈkjʊr/ *adj* not safe; feeling anxiety; not dependable.—**insecurely** *adv*.

insecurity /-ˈkjʊrɪti/ *n* (*pl* **insecurities**) the condition of being insecure; lack of confidence or sureness; instability; something insecure.

inseminate /ɪnˈsemɪˌneɪt/ *vt* to fertilize; to impregnate.—**insemination** *n*.—**inseminator** *n*.

insensate /ɪnˈsenseɪt/ *adj* not feeling sensation; stupid; without regard or feeling; cold.

insensible /ɪnˈsensəbəl/ *adj* unconscious; unaware; indifferent; imperceptible.—**insensibility** *n*.—**insensibly** *adv*.

insensitive /ɪnˈsensɪtɪv/ *adj* not sensitive, unfeeling.

insentient /ɪnˈsenʃənt/ *adj* inert; inanimate.

inseparable /ɪnˈseprəbəl/ or /-ˈsepərəbəl/ *adj* not able to be separated; closely attached, as romantically.—**inseparability** *n*.—**inseparably** *adv*.

insert /ɪnˈsɜrt/ *vt* to put or fit (something) into something else. • *n* something inserted.—**insertion** *n*.

insertion /ɪnˈsɜrʃən/ *n* the act of inserting; something which is inserted.

in-service /ˈɪnˌsɜrvɪs/ *adj* (*training*) given during employment.

inessorial /ˌɪnseˈsɔriəl/ *adj* (*ornithology*) adapted for perching.

inset /ˈɪnset/ *n* something inserted within something larger; an insert. • *vt* (**insetting, inset**) to set in, insert.—**insetter** *n*.

inshore /ˈɪnʃɔr/ *adj, adv* near or towards the shore.

inshrine *see* **enshrine**.

inside /ɪnˈsaɪd/ or /ˈɪn-/ *n* the inner side, surface, or part; (*pl: inf*) the internal organs, stomach, bowels. • *adj* internal; known only to insiders; secret. • *adv* on or in the inside; within; indoors; (*sl*) in prison. • *prep* in or within.

inside job *n* (*inf*) a crime committed with the help of someone connected with the victim or premises involved.

inside out *adj* reversed; with the inner surface facing the outside.

insider /ɪnˈsaɪdər/ *n* a person within a place or group; a person with access to confidential information.

insidious /ɪnˈsɪdiəs/ *adj* marked by slyness or treachery; more dangerous than seems evident.—**insidiously** *adv*.—**insidiousness** *n*.

insight /ˈɪnsaɪt/ *n* the ability to see and understand clearly the inner nature of things, *esp* by intuition; an instance of such understanding.—**insightful** *adj*.

insignia /ɪnˈsɪɡniə/ *n* (*pl* **insignias, insignia**) a mark or badge of authority; a distinguishing characteristic.

insignificant /ˌɪnsɪɡˈnɪfɪkənt/ *adj* having little or no importance; trivial; worthless; small, inadequate.—**insignificance, insignificancy** *n*.—**insignificantly** *adv*.

insincere /ˌɪnsɪnˈsɪr/ *adj* not sincere; hypocritical.—**insincerely** *adv*.—**insincerity** *n*.

insinuate /ɪnˈsɪnjʊˌeɪt/ *vt* to introduce or work in slowly, indirectly, etc; to hint.—**insinuator** *n*.

insinuation /-ˈeɪʃən/ *n* the act of insinuating; an indirect or sly hint.

insipid /ɪnˈsɪpɪd/ *adj* lacking any distinctive flavour; uninteresting, dull.—**insipidity, insipidness** *n*.—**insipidly** *adv*.

insist /ɪnˈsɪst/ *vi* (*often with* **on** *or* **upon**) to take and maintain a stand. • *vt* to demand strongly; to declare firmly.—**insister** *n*.

insistent /ɪnˈsɪstənt/ *adj* insisting or demanding.—**insistence, insistency** *n*.—**insistently** *adv*.

in situ /ɪn ˈsɪtjuː/ or /-sɪtuː/ or /ˈsiː-/ *adj* in the original or natural place or position.

insobriety /ˌɪnsəˈbraɪətɪ/ *n* drunkenness.

in so far, insofar /ˌɪnsoˈfɑːr/ *adv* to such a degree or extent.

insole /ˈɪnsoːl/ *n* the inner sole of a shoe, etc; a thickness of material used as a inner sole.

insolent /ˈɪnsələnt/ *adj* disrespectful; impudent, arrogant; rude.—**insolence** *n*.—**insolently** *adv*.

insoluble /ɪnˈsɒljʊbəl/ *adj* incapable of being dissolved; impossible to solve or explain.—**insolubility** *n*.—**insolubly** *adv*.

insolvent /ɪnˈsɒlvənt/ *adj* unable to pay one's debts; bankrupt.—**insolvency** *n*.

insomnia /ɪnˈsɒmnɪə/ *n* abnormal inability to sleep.

insomniac /-ɪˌæk/ *n* a person who suffers from insomnia.

insomuch /ˌɪnsoˈmʌtʃ/ *adv* (*with* **as** *or* **that**) to such an extent; (*with* **as**) inasmuch.

insouciant /ɪnˈsuːsɪənt/ *adj* calm and unconcerned, carefree.—**insouciance** *n*.

inspect /ɪnˈspɛkt/ *vt* to look at carefully; to examine or review officially.—**inspection** *n*.—**inspectional** *adj*.—**inspective** *adj*.

inspector /-ər/ *n* an official who inspects in order to ensure compliance with regulations, etc; a police officer ranking below a superintendent.—**inspectorate** *n*.—**inspectoral, inspectorial** *adj*.—**inspectorship** *n*.

inspectorate /-rət/ *n* the office, district or rank of an inspector; a body of inspectors.

inspiration /ˌɪnspɪˈreɪʃən/ *n* an inspiring; any stimulus to creative thought; an inspired idea, action, etc.—**inspirational** *adj*.

inspiratory /ɪnˈspɪrətəri/ *adj* pertaining to inhalation.

inspire /ɪnˈspaɪr/ *vt* to stimulate, as to some creative effort; to motivate by divine influence; to arouse (a thought or feeling) in (someone); to cause.—**inspiring** *adj*.—**inspiringly** *adv*.

inspirit /ɪnˈspɪrɪt/ *vt* to put life into, invigorate; to animate, cheer.

inst. *abbr* = instant (this month).

instability /ˌɪnstəˈbɪlɪtɪ/ *n* (*pl* **instabilities**) lack of stability; inconstancy.

install, instal /ɪnˈstɔːl/ *vt* (**installs** *or* **instals, installing, installed**) to formally place in an office, rank, etc; to establish in a place; to settle in a position or state.—**installer** *n*.

installation /ˌɪnstəˈleɪʃən/ *n* the act of installing or being installed; machinery, equipment, etc that has been installed.

installment, instalment /ɪnˈstɔːlmənt/ *n* a sum of money to be paid at regular specified times; any of several parts, as of a magazine story or television serial.

instance /ˈɪnstəns/ *n* an example; a step in proceeding; an occasion. • *vt* to give as an example.

instant /ˈɪnstənt/ *adj* immediate; (*food*) concentrated or precooked for quick preparation. • *n* a moment; a particular moment.

instantaneous /ˌɪnstənˈteɪnɪəs/ *adj* happening or done very quickly.—**instantaneously** *adv*.—**instantaneousness, instantaneity** *n*.

instanter /ɪnˈstæntər/ *adv* (*law*) immediately.

instantly /ˈɪnstəntlɪ/ *adv* immediately.

instate /ɪnˈsteɪt/ *vt* to install in an office or rank.

instead /ɪnˈstɛd/ *adv* in place of the one mentioned.

instep /ˈɪnstɛp/ *n* the upper part of the arch of the foot, between the ankle and the toes.

instigate /ˈɪnstɪˌɡeɪt/ *vt* to urge on, goad; to initiate.—**instigation** *n*.—**instigator** *n*.

instill, instil /ɪnˈstɪl/ *vt* (**instills** *or* **instils, instilling, instilled**) to put (an idea, etc) in or into (the mind) gradually.—**instillation** *n*.—**instiller** *n*.

instinct /ˈɪnstɪŋkt/ *n* the inborn tendency to behave in a way characteristic of a species; a natural or acquired tendency; a knack.

instinctive /ɪnˈstɪŋktɪv/, **instinctual** /-tʊəl/ *adj* of, relating to, or prompted by instinct.—**instinctively, instinctually** *adv*.

institute /ˈɪnstɪˌtuːt/ or /-ˌtjuːt/ *vt* to organize, establish; to start, initiate. • *n* an organization for the promotion of science, art, etc; a school, college, or department of a university specializing in some field.—**instructor, instituter** *n*.

institution /ˌɪnstɪˈtuːʃən/ or /-ˈtjuː-/ *n* an established law, custom, etc; an organization having a social, educational, or religious purpose; the building housing it; (*inf*) a long-established person or thing.

institutional /-əl/ *adj* of or resembling an institution; dull, routine.

institutionalize /ˌɪnstɪˈtuːʃənəˌlaɪz/ or /-ˈtjuː-/ *vt* to make or become an institution; to place in an institution; to make a person dependent on an institutional routine and unable to cope on their own.—**institutionalization** *n*.

instruct /ɪnˈstrʌkt/ *vt* to provide with information; to teach; to give instructions to; to authorize.—**instructible** *adj*.—**instructor** *n*.—**instructress** *nf*.

instruction /ɪnˈstrʌkʃən/ *n* an order, direction; the act or process of teaching or training; knowledge imparted; (*comput*) a command in a program to perform a particular operation; (*pl*) orders, directions; detailed guidance.—**instructional** *adj*.

instructive /ɪnˈstrʌktɪv/ *adj* issuing or containing instructions; giving information, educational.—**instructively** *adv*.

instructor /-ər/ *n* someone who instructs; a teacher.

instrument /ˈɪnstrəmənt/ *n* a thing by means of which something is done; a tool or implement; any of various devices for indicating, measuring, controlling, etc; any of various devices producing musical sound; a formal document. • *vt* to orchestrate.

instrument panel *n* a panel in a vehicle or machine in which instruments monitoring speed, engine status, etc are mounted.

instrumental /ˌɪnstrəˈmɛntəl/ *adj* serving as a means of doing something; helpful; of, performed on, or written for a musical instrument or instruments.—**instrumentality** *n*.—**instrumentally** *adv*.

instrumentalist /-ˈmɛntəlɪst/ *n* a person who plays a musical instrument.

instrumentation /ˌɪnstrəmɛnˈteɪʃən/ *n* the arrangement of a musical composition for different instruments; the use or provision of tools or instruments.

insubordinate /ˌɪnsəˈbɔːdɪnət/ *adj* not submitting to authority; rebellious.—**insubordination** *n*.

insubstantial /ˌɪnsəbˈstænʃəl/ *adj* unreal, imaginary; weak or flimsy.—**insubstantiality** *n*.—**insubstantially** *adv*.

insufferable /ɪnˈsʌfərəbəl/ *adj* intolerable; unbearable.—**insufferably** *adv*.

insufficient /ˌɪnsəˈfɪʃənt/ *adj* not sufficient.—**insufficiency, insufficience** *n*.—**insufficiently** *adv*.

insufflate /ˈɪnsəˌfleɪt/ *vt* to blow (air, powder) into or onto.—**insufflation** *n*.—**insufflator** *n*.

insular /ˈɪnsʊlər/ or /ˈɪnsjʊ-/ *adj* of or like an island or islanders; narrow-minded; illiberal.—**insularity, insularism** *n*.

insulate /ˈɪnsəˌleɪt/ or /ˈɪnsjə-/ *vt* to set apart; to isolate; to cover with a nonconducting material in order to prevent the escape of electricity, heat, sound, etc.—**insulation** *n*.—**insulator** *n*.

insulation /ˌɪnsəˈleɪʃən/ or /-sjə-/ *n* the act of insulating; the material used for insulating.

insulator /ˈɪnsəˌleɪtər/ or /ˈɪnsjə-/ *n* something which insulates; a non-conductor of electricity, heat or sound.

insulin /ˈɪnsəlɪn/ or /ˈɪnsjə-/ *n* a hormone that controls absorption of sugar by the body, secreted by islets of tissue in the pancreas.

insult /ɪnˈsʌlt/ *vt* to treat with indignity or contempt; to offend. • *n* an insulting remark or act.—**insulter** *n*.

insuperable /ɪnˈsuːpərəbəl/ or /ɪnˈsjuː-/, /-prəbəl/ *adj* unable to be overcome.—**insuperability** *n*.—**insuperably** *adv*.

insupportable /ˌɪnsəˈpɔːtəbəl/ *adj* unbearable, intolerable.

insurable /ɪnˈʃʊərəbəl/ *adj* able to be insured.

insurable earnings *npl* ✦ (*Cdn*) income on which unemployment premiums are paid.

insurance /ɪnˈʃʊərəns/ or /-ˈʃərəns/ *n* insuring or being insured; a contract purchased to guarantee compensation for a specified loss by fire, death, etc; the amount for which something is insured; the business of insuring against loss.

insure /ɪnˈʃʊr/ or /-ˈʃər/ *vt* to take out or issue insurance on; to ensure. • *vi* to contract to give or take insurance.

insurer /ɪnˈʃʊrər/ or /-ˈʃərər/ *n* someone who insures, an underwriter; a company which sells insurance.

insurgent /ɪnˈsɔːdʒənt/ *adj* rebellious, rising in revolt. • *n* a person who fights against established authority, a rebel.—**insurgence** *n*.—**insurgency** *n*.

insurmountable /ˌɪnsərˈmaʊntəbəl/ *adj* which cannot be overcome, insuperable.

insurrection /ˌɪnsəˈrɛkʃən/ *adj* a rising or revolt against established authority.—**insurrectional** *adj*.—**insurrectionary** *n*, *adj*.—**insurrectionism** *n*.—**insurrectionist** *n*.

intact /ɪnˈtækt/ *adj* unimpaired; whole.

intaglio /ɪnˈtælioː/ n (pl **intaglios**) a design carved or engraved below the surface; a printing technique using engraved surfaces.—**intagliated** adj.

intake /ˈɪnteɪk/ n the place in a pipe etc where a liquid or gas is taken in; a thing or quantity taken in, as students, etc; the process of taking in.

intangible /ɪnˈtændʒəbəl/ adj that cannot be touched, incorporeal; representing value but without material being, as good will; indefinable. • n something that is intangible.—**intangibility** n.—**intangibly** adv.

integer /ˈɪntɪdʒər/ n any member of the set consisting of the positive and negative whole numbers and zero, such as -5, 0, 5.

integral /ˈɪntəɡrəl/ or /ɪnˈteɡrəl/ adj necessary for completeness; whole or complete; made up of parts forming a whole. • n the result of a mathematical integration.—**integrally** adv

integral calculus n (maths) the determination of definite and indefinite integrals and their use in the solution of differential equations.

integrant /ˈɪntəɡrənt/ adj component, making part of a whole.

integrate /ˈɪntəˌɡreɪt/ vti to make whole or become complete; to bring (parts) together into a whole to remove barriers imposing segregation upon (racial groups); to abolish segregation; (math) to find the integral of.—**integration** n.—**integrative** adj.

integrated circuit n a small electronic circuit assembled from microcomponents mounted on chips of semiconducting material.

integrator /ˈɪntəˌɡreɪtər/ n someone who, or something which, integrates.

integrity /ɪnˈteɡriti/ n honesty, sincerity; completeness, wholeness; an unimpaired condition.

integument /ɪnˈteɡjʊmənt/ n a natural covering as skin, a rind, a husk, etc.—**integumental, integumentary** adj.

intellect /ˈɪntəˌlekt/ n the ability to reason or understand; high intelligence; a very intelligent person.—**intellective** adj.

intellection /ˌɪntəˈlekʃən/ n thought.

intellectual /ˌɪntəˈlektʃʊəl/ adj of, involving, or appealing to the intellect; requiring intelligence. • n an intellectual person.—**intellectuality** n.—**intellectually** adv.

intellectualism /ˌɪntəˈlektʃʊəˌlɪzəm/ n the use of the intellect; (philos) the theory that all knowledge is derived from the intellect; (derog) excessive emphasis on the value of the intellect.—**intellectualist** n.

intellectualize /ɪntəˈlektʃʊəˌlaɪz/ vt to make intellectual; to use the intellect on. • vi to become intellectual; to use the intellect.—**intellectualization** n.

intelligence /ɪnˈtelɪdʒəns/ n the ability to learn or understand; the ability to cope with a new situation; news or information; those engaged in gathering secret, esp military, information.

intelligence quotient n a measure of a person's intelligence, calculated by dividing mental age by actual age and multiplying by 100.

intelligent /ɪnˈtelɪdʒənt/ adj having or showing intelligence; clever, wise, etc.—**intelligently** adv.

intelligentsia /ɪnˌtelɪˈdʒentsiə/ n intellectuals collectively.

intelligible /ɪnˈtelɪdʒəbəl/ adj able to be understood; clear.—**intelligibility** n.—**intelligibly** adv.

intemperate /ɪnˈtempərət/ or /-prət/ adj indulging excessively in alcoholic drink; unrestrained; (climate) extreme.—**intemperance** n.—**intemperately** adv.

intend /ɪnˈtend/ vt to mean, to signify; to propose, have in mind as an aim or purpose.—**intender** n.

intendancy /-dənsi/ n (pl **intendancies**) the rank or office of an intendant.

intendant /-dənt/ n a superintendent or manager (esp under a monarch in France, Spain and Portugal).

intended /-dɪd/ adj planned. • n (inf) a fiancé or fiancée.

intendment /-mənt/ n the true meaning of something, as fixed by law.

intense /ɪnˈtens/ adj very strong, concentrated; passionate, emotional.—**intensely** adv.

intensify /ɪnˈtensəˌfaɪ/ vti (**intensifying, intensified**) to make or become more intense.—**intensification** n.

intensity /ɪnˈtensiti/ n (pl **intensities**) the state or quality of being intense; density, as of a negative plate; the force or energy of any physical agent.

intensive /ɪnˈtensɪv/ adj of or characterized by intensity; thorough; denoting careful attention given to patients right after surgery, etc.—**intensively** adv.

intensive care n 24-hour monitoring and treatment of acutely ill patients in hospital; the specialized unit administering this.

intent /ɪnˈtent/ adj firmly directed; having one's attention or purpose firmly fixed. • n intention; something intended; purpose or meaning.—**intently** adv.—**intentness** n.

intention /ɪnˈtenʃən/ n a determination to act in a specified way; anything intended.

intentional /ɪnˈtenʃənəl/ adj done purposely.—**intentionality** n.—**intentionally** adv.

inter /ɪnˈtər/ vt (**interring, interred**) to bury.

inter- /ˈɪntər/ prefix between, among.

interact /ˌɪntərˈækt/ vi to act upon each other.—**interaction** n.—**interactional** adj.

interactive /ˌɪntərˈæktɪv/ adj interacting; allowing two-way communication between a device, such as a computer or compact video disc, and its user.—**interactivity** n.

inter alia /ˌɪntər ˈeɪliə/ or /ˈæliə/ adv among other things.

interbreed /ˌɪntərˈbriːd/ vti (**interbreeding, interbred**) to breed within the same breed or family; to breed by crossing one species with another.

intercalary /ɪnˈtərkələri/ or /-ˈkæləri/ adj inserted into the calendar to harmonize it with the solar year, eg February 29 as inserted in the leap year.

intercalate /ɪnˈtərkəˌleɪt/ vt to insert (an intercalary day) into the calendar.—**intercalation** n.

intercede /ˌɪntərˈsiːd/ vi to intervene on another's behalf; to mediate.—**interceder** n.

intercellular /ˌɪntərˈseljulər/ adj lying between cells.

intercept /ˌɪntərˈsept/ vt to stop or catch in its course. • n a point of intersection of two geometric figures; interception by an interceptor.—**interception** n.—**interceptive** adj.

interceptor interceptor /ˌɪntərˈseptər/, n a high-speed fighter aircraft used to intercept and destroy enemy aircraft.

intercession /ˌɪntərˈseʃən/ n the act of interceding, esp by prayer; mediation.—**intercessional, intercessory** adj.—**intercessor** n.—**intercessorial** adj.

interchange /ˌɪntərˈtʃeɪndʒ/ vt to give and receive one thing for another; to exchange, to put (each of two things) in the place of the other; to alternate. • n an interchanging; a junction on a motorway designed to prevent traffic intersecting.—**interchangeable** /-əbəl/ adj able to be interchanged.—**interchangeability** n.—**interchangeably** adv.

intercollegiate /ˌɪntərkəˈliːdʒət/ adj between or among colleges or universities.

intercolumniation /-kəˌlʌmniˈeɪʃən/ n the distance between pillars; the spacing between pillars.—**intercolumniar** adj.

intercom /ˈɪntərˌkɒm/ n (inf) a system of intercommunicating, as in an aircraft.

intercommunicate /ˌɪntərkəˈmjuːnɪˌkeɪt/ vi to have mutual communication; to have passage to each other.—**intercommunicable** adj.—**intercommunication** n.

interconnect /ˌɪntərkəˈnekt/ vti to connect by reciprocal links.—**interconnection** n.

intercontinental /ˌɪntərˌkɒntɪˈnentəl/ adj between continents.

intercostal /ˌɪntərˈkɒstəl/ adj (anat) lying between the ribs.

intercourse /ˈɪntərˌkɔrs/ n a connection by dealings or communication between individuals or groups; sexual intercourse, copulation.

intercross /ˌɪntərˈkrɒs/ vti to crossbreed.

intercurrent /ˌɪntərˈkʌrənt/ adj occurring at the same time; (disease) occurring during the course of another.—**intercurrence** n.

interdependence /ˌɪntərdiˈpendəns/ or /-dɪ-/, **interdependency** n dependence on each other.—**interdependent** adj.

interdict /ˈɪntərdɪkt/ vt to prohibit (an action); to restrain from doing or using something. • n an official prohibition.—**interdiction** n.—**interdictory** adj.

interdisciplinary /ˌɪntərˈdɪsəplɪnˌeri/ adj involving two or more different branches of knowledge.

interest /ˈɪntrəst/ or /-tərəst/ n a feeling of curiosity about something; the power of causing this feeling; a share in, or a right to, something; anything in which one has a share; benefit; money paid for the use of money; the rate of such payment. • vt to excite the attention of; to cause to have a share in; to concern oneself with.

interested /-ɪd/ or /-təˌrestəd/ adj having or expressing an interest; affected by personal interest, not impartial.—**interestedly** adv.

interesting /ˈɪntrəstɪŋ/ or /ˈɪntəˌrestɪŋ/ n engaging the attention.

interface /'ɪntərˌfeɪs/ *n* a surface that forms the common boundary between two things; an electrical connection between one device and another, *esp* a computer. • *vt* (*elect*) to modify the input and output configurations of (devices) so that they may connect and communicate with each other; to connect using an interface; to be interactive (with).—**interfacial** *adj*.—**interfacially** *adv*.

interfacing /'ɪntərˌfeɪsɪŋ/ *n* a layer of fabric between the neck, etc of a garment and its facing to give body.

interfere /ˌɪntər'fiːr/ *vi* to clash; to come between; to intervene; to meddle; to obstruct.—**interfering** *adj*.

interference /ˌɪntər'fiːrəns/ *n* an interfering; (*radio, TV*) the interruption of reception by atmospherics or by unwanted signals.

interferometer /ˌɪntərfə'rɒmɪtər/ *n* (*physics*) an instrument used to measure the length of light waves by interference phenomena.

interferon /ˌɪntər'fiəˌrɒn/ *n* a protein, produced by cells in response to a virus, which then prevents the virus from growing.

interfuse /ˌɪntər'fjuːz/ *vti* to mix, blend.—**interfusion** *n*.

intergalactic /ˌɪntərgə'læktɪk/ *adj* occurring or existing between galaxies.

interglacial /ˌɪntər'gleɪʃəl/ or /-siəl/ *adj* occurring between two glacial periods.

intergrade /'ɪntərˌgreɪd/ *vi* (*usu biol*) to change form gradually.—**intergradation** *n*.

interim /'ɪntərɪm/ *n* an intervening period of time. • *adj* provisional, temporary. • *adv* meanwhile.

interior /ɪn'tiːriːər/ *adj* situated within; inner; inland; private. • *n* the interior part, as of a room, country, etc.

interior angle *n* the angle between two adjacent sides of a polygon.

interior design *n* the art or business of an interior designer— *also* **interior decoration**.

interior designer *n* a person whose profession is the planning of the decor and furnishings of the interiors of houses, offices, etc.—*also* **interior decorator**.

interj. *abbr* = interjection.

interject /ˌɪntər'dʒekt/ *vt* to throw in between; to interrupt with.—**interjector** *n*.—**interjectory** *adj*.

interjection /ˌɪntər'dʒekʃən/ *n* an interjecting; an interruption; an exclamation.—**interjectional** *adj*.—**interjectionally** *adv*.

interlace /ˌɪntər'leɪs/ *vti* to combine (as if) by lacing or weaving together.—**interlacement** *n*.

interlard /ˌɪntər'lɑrd/ *vt* to insert something foreign into.

interleaf /'ɪntərˌliːf/ *n* (*pl* **interleaves**) an additional, blank leaf inserted into a book.

interleave /ˌɪntər'liːv/ *vti* to insert an extra page (*usu* blank) in a book.

interline /ˌɪntər'laɪn/ *vt* to write between lines.—**interlinear** *adj*.—**interlineation** *n*.

interlining /'ɪntərˌlaɪnɪŋ/ *n* an extra lining between the lining and the outer fabric of a garment, etc; the material for this.

interlink /ˌɪntər'lɪŋk/ *vt* to link together.

interlock /ˌɪntər'lɒk/ *vti* to lock or become locked together; to join with one another.

interlocution /ˌɪntərlə'kjuːʃən/ *n* dialogue, discussion.

interlocutor /ˌɪntər'lɒkjutər/ *n* a person who takes part in a conversation.—**interlocutress, interlocutrix** *nf*.

interlocutory /ˌɪntər'lɒkjutəri/ *adj* conversational; (*law*) pronounced during legal proceedings.

interlope /'ɪntərˌloːp/ *vi* to intrude in a matter in which one has no real concern.

interloper /-ər/ *n* a person who meddles; an intruder.

interlude /'ɪntərˌluːd/ *n* anything that fills time between two events, as music between acts of a play.

interlunar /ˌɪntər'luːnər/ *adj* coming between the old and the new moon.

intermarry /ˌɪntər'meri/ or /-mæri/ *vi* (**intermarrying, intermarried**) (*different races, religions, etc*) to become connected by marriage; to marry within one's close family.—**intermarriage** *n*.

intermediary /ˌɪntər'miːdiːeri/ *n* (*pl* **intermediaries**) a mediator. • *adj* acting as a mediator; intermediate.

intermediate /ˌɪntər'miːdiət/ *adj* in the middle; in between.

interment /ɪn'tərmənt/ *n* burial.

intermezzo /ˌɪntər'metsoː/ *n* (*pl* **intermezzos, intermezzi**) a short musical composition between parts of an opera, play, etc; a movement between sections of an extended instrumental work; a similar composition intended as an independent work.

interminable /ɪn'tərmɪnəbəl/ *adj* lasting or seeming to last forever; endless.—**interminably** *adv*.

intermingle /ˌɪntər'mɪŋgəl/ *vti* to mingle or mix together.

intermission /ˌɪntər'mɪʃən/ *n* an interval of time between parts of a performance.

intermit /ˌɪntər'mɪt/ *vb* (**intermitting, intermitted**) *vt* to cause to cease for a time; to suspend. • *vi* to cease for a time; to be suspended.

intermittent /ˌɪntər'mɪtənt/ *adj* stopping and starting again at intervals; periodic.—**intermittence, intermittency** *n*.—**intermittently** *adv*.

intermix /ˌɪntər'mɪks/ *vti* to mix together.

intermixture /ˌɪntər'mɪkstʃər/ *n* the act of mixing together; a mixture.

intern[1] /'ɪntərn/ *vt* to detain and confine within an area, *esp* during wartime.—**internment** *n*.

intern[2] *n* a doctor serving in a hospital, *usu* just after graduation from medical school, a houseman.

intern[3], **interne** *n* an apprentice journalist, teacher, etc.

internal /ɪn'tərnəl/ *adj* of or on the inside; of or inside the body; intrinsic; domestic.—**internality** *n*.—**internally** *adv*.

internal combustion engine *n* an engine producing power by the explosion of a fuel-and-air mixture within the cylinders.

international /ˌɪntər'næʃənəl/ *adj* between or among nations; concerned with the relations between nations; for the use of all nations; of or for people in various nations. • *n* a sporting competition between teams from different countries; a member of an international team of players.—**internationality** *n*.—**internationally** *adv*.

International Date Line *n* the line running north to south along the 180-degree meridian, east of which is one day earlier than west of it.

internationalism /ˌɪntər'næʃənəˌlɪzəm/ *n* an attitude, belief, or policy favouring the promotion of cooperation and understanding between nations.—**internationalist** *n*.

interne /'ɪnˌtərn/ *see* **intern**[3].

internecine /ˌɪntər'nesiːn/ or /-aɪn/, /-niːs-/ *adj* extremely destructive to both sides.

internee /ˌɪntər'niː/ *n* a person who is interned.

Internet /'ɪntərnet/ *n* the worldwide system of linked computer networks.

internist /ɪn'tərnɪst/ *n* a physician who specializes in internal diseases.

internode /'ɪntərˌnoːd/ *n* (*bot*) the space on a plant stem between two nodes or leaf joints.—**internodal** *adj*.

internuncial /ˌɪntər'nʌnʃəl/ *adj* pertaining to an internuncio; (*anat*) transmitting nervous signals.

internuncio /ˌɪntər'nʌnˌʃoː/ or /-ʃiˌoː/, /-siˌoː/, /-'nʌntsiˌoː/ *n* a representative of the Pope.

interpellate /ɪn'tərpeˌleɪt/ *vt* to question (an official) about government policy or about personal conduct.—**interpellation** *n*.—**interpellator** *n*.

interpenetrate /ˌɪntər'penəˌtreɪt/ *vt* to penetrate thoroughly. • *vi* to penetrate each other.—**interpenetration** *n*.—**interpenetrative** *adj*.

interplanetary /ˌɪntər'plænəteri/ *adj* between or among planets.

interplay /'ɪntərˌpleɪ/ *n* the action of two things on each other, interaction.

interplead /ˌɪntər'pliːd/ *vi* (**interpleading, interpleaded, interplead, interpled**) (*law*) to discuss a point incidentally arising, or concerning a third party.

interpleader /-ər/ *n* (*law*) the discussion of a point incidentally arising or concerning a third party.

Interpol /'ɪntərˌpɒl/ (*acronym*) International Criminal Police Organization.

interpolate /ɪn'tərpəˌleɪt/ *vt* to change (a text) by inserting new material; to insert between or among others; (*math*) to estimate a value between two known values.—**interpolator** *n*.—**interpolation** *n*.

interpose /ˌɪntər'poːz/ *vti* to place or come between; to intervene (with); to interrupt (with).—**interposer** *n*.—**interposition** *n*.

interpret /ɪn'tərprət/ *vt* to explain; to translate; to construe; to give one's own conception of, as in a play or musical composition. • *vi* to translate between speakers of different languages.—**interpretational** *adj*.

interpretation /-'teɪʃən/ *n* an act or instance of interpreting; an explanation; a rendering (of a piece of music, theatre, etc).

interpreter /ɪnˈtɜrprətər/ n a person who translates orally for persons speaking in different languages; (*comput*) a program that translates an instruction into machine code.

interracial /ˌɪntərˈreɪʃəl/ adj between or among races.

interregnum /ˌɪntərˈrɛgnəm/ n (pl **interregnums, interregna**) the period between two reigns, governments, etc; a suspension of normal government; a pause in a continuous series.

interrelate /ˌɪntərəˈleɪt/ vti to be or place in a mutually dependant or reciprocal relationship.—**interrelation** n.—**interrelationship** n.

interrogate /ɪnˈtɛrəˌgeɪt/ vti to question, *esp* formally.—**interrogation** n.—**interrogational** adj.—**interrogator** n.

interrogative /ˌɪntəˈrɒgətɪv/ adj asking a question. • n a word used in asking a question.—**interrogatively** adv.

interrogatory /ˌɪntəˈrɒgətəri/ adj questioning. • n (pl **interrogatories**) examination by questions.—**interrogatorily** adv.

interrupt /ˌɪntəˈrʌpt/ vt to break into (a discussion, etc) or break in upon (a speaker, worker, etc); to make a break in the continuity of. • vi to interrupt an action, talk, etc.—**interrupter** n.—**interruptive** adj.

interruption /-ˈrʌpʃən/ n the act of interrupting; a hindrance; a remark interposed in a conversation, etc.

intersect /ˌɪntərˈsɛkt/ vti to cut or divide by passing through or crossing; (*lines, roads, etc*) to meet and cross each other.

intersection /ˈɪntərˌsɛkʃən/ n an intersecting; the place where two lines, roads, etc meet or cross.—**intersectional** adj.

interspace /ˈɪntərˌspeɪs/ n a space between things.

intersperse /ˌɪntərˈspɜrs/ vt to scatter or insert among other things; to diversify with other things scattered here and there.—**interspersion** n.

interstate /ˈɪntərˌsteɪt/ adj between or among different states of a federation.

interstellar /ˌɪntərˈstɛlər/ adj between or among stars.

interstice /ɪnˈtɜrstɪs/ n a crack; a crevice; a minute space.

interstitial /ˌɪntərˈstɪʃəl/ adj occurring in interstices.

intertexture /ˌɪntərˈtɛkstʃər/ n the act or product of interweaving.

intertribal /ˌɪntərˈtraɪbəl/ adj between or among tribes.

intertwine /ˌɪntərˈtwaɪn/ vti to twine or twist closely together.

interval /ˈɪntərvəl/ n a space between things; the time between events; (*mus*) the difference of pitch between two notes.

intervene /ˌɪntərˈviːn/ vi to occur or come between; to occur between two events, etc; to come in to modify, settle, or hinder some action, etc.—**intervener, intervenor** n.—**intervention** n.—**interventional** adj.

interventionist /ˌɪntərˈvɛnʃənɪst/ n a person who favours intervention. • adj of or in favour of intervention.—**interventionism** n.

interview /ˈɪntərˌvjuː/ n a meeting in which a person is asked about his or her views, etc, as by a newspaper or television reporter; a published account of this; a formal meeting at which a candidate for a job is questioned and assessed by a prospective employer. • vt to have an interview with.—**interviewer** n.

interviewee /-vjuːˈiː/ n a person who is interviewed.

interweave /ˌɪntərˈwiːv/ vti (**interweaving, interwove** or **interweaved**, pp **interwoven** or **interweaved**) to weave together, interlace; to intermingle.

interwind /ˈɪntərwɪnd/ vt (**interwinding, interwound**) to wind together.

intestate /ɪnˈtɛsteɪt/ adj having made no will. • n a person who dies intestate.—**intestacy** n.

intestine /ɪnˈtɛstaɪn/ or /-ɪn/ n the lower part of the alimentary canal between the stomach and the anus.—**intestina** adj.

intifada /ˌɪntəˈfɑːdə/ n the Arabic word for "uprising," *esp* the uprising in Israel in 1987 of Palestinian inhabitants.

intimacy /ˈɪntɪməsi/ n (pl **intimacies**) close or confidential friendship; familiarity; sexual relations.

intimate /ˈɪntɪmət/ adj most private or personal; very close or familiar, *esp* sexually; deep and thorough. • n an intimate friend. • vt to indicate; to make known; to hint or imply.—**intimately** adv.

intimation /-ˈmeɪʃən/ n the act of intimating; a notice, announcement.

intimidate /ɪnˈtɪmɪˌdeɪt/ vt to frighten; to discourage, silence, etc *esp* by threats.—**intimidation** n.—**intimidator** n.

intinction /ɪnˈtɪŋʃən/ n (*Eastern Church*) the practice of administering both parts of Holy Communion at the same time by dipping the bread into the wine.

into /ˈɪntuː/ or /ˈɪntə/ prep to the interior or inner parts of; to the middle; to a particular condition; (*inf*) deeply interested or involved in.

intolerable /ɪnˈtɒlərəbəl/ adj unbearable.—**intolerably** adv.

intolerance /ɪnˈtɒlərəns/ n lack of toleration of the opinions or practices of others; inability to bear or endure.—**intolerant** adj.

intonate /ˈɪntəˌneɪt/ vti to recite in a singing voice, chant.

intonation /ˌɪntəˈneɪʃən/ n intoning; variations in pitch of the speaking voice; an accent.—**intonational** adj.

intone /ɪnˈtoːn/ vti to speak or recite in a singing tone; to chant.—**intoner** n.

in toto /ɪn ˈtoːtoː/ adv completely; as a whole; entirely.

intoxicant /ɪnˈtɒksɪkənt/ n something that intoxicates, *esp* a drug or an alcoholic drink.—*also* adj.

intoxicate /ɪnˈtɒksɪˌkeɪt/ vt to make drunken; to elate; to poison.—**intoxicatingly** adv.

intoxication /-ˈkeɪʃən/ n drunkenness; great excitement; poisoning.

intra- /ˈɪntrə/ prefix within.

intracranial /ˌɪntrəˈkreɪniə/ adj within the skull.

intractable /ɪnˈtræktəbəl/ adj unmanageable, uncontrollable; (*problem, illness, etc*) difficult to solve, alleviate, or cure.—**intractability** n.—**intractably** adv.

intrados /ɪnˈtreɪdɒs/ n (pl **intrados, intradoses**) the inner and lower curve of an arch.

intramural /ˌɪntrəˈmjʊrəl/ adj (*education*) within an institution or organization.

intranet /ˈɪntrənɛt/ n a system that works in a similar way to the Internet, but which has limited access and may work, for example, in an office.

intransigent /ɪnˈtrænzɪdʒənt/ or /-sɪdʒənt/ adj unwilling to compromise, irreconcilable.—**intransigence** n.—**intransigently** adv.

intransitive /ɪnˈtrænzɪtɪv/ or /-sɪtɪv/ adj (*gram*) denoting a verb that does not take a direct object.—**intransitively** adv.

intrauterine /ˌɪntrəˈjuːtərɪn/ or /-ˌraɪn/ adj inside the uterus.

intrauterine device n a small loop or coil inserted into the uterus as a contraceptive.

intravenous /ˌɪntrəˈviːnəs/ adj into a vein.—**intravenously** adv.

in-tray /ˈɪntreɪ/ n a tray holding documents, etc, awaiting attention.

intrench /ɪnˈtrɛntʃ/ see **entrench**.

intrepid /ɪnˈtrɛpɪd/ adj bold fearless; brave.—**intrepidity** n.—**intrepidly** adv.

intricate /ˈɪntrɪkət/ adj difficult to understand; complex, complicated; involved, detailed.—**intricacy** n.—**intricately** adv.

intrigue /ɪnˈtriːg/ n a secret or underhand plotting; a secret or underhanded plot or scheme; a secret love affair. • vb (**intriguing, intrigued**) vi to carry on an intrigue. • vt to excite the interest or curiosity of.—**intriguer** n.

intrinsic /ɪnˈtrɪnzɪk/ adj belonging to the real nature of a person or thing; inherent.—**intrinsically** adv.

intro- /ˈɪntroː/ prefix within, into.

intro n (pl **intros**) (*inf*) introduction.

introduce /ˌɪntrəˈdjuːs/ vt to make (a person) acquainted by name (with other persons); to bring into use or establish; to present (legislation, etc) for consideration or approval; to present a radio or television programme to bring into or insert.—**introducer** n.

introduction /ˌɪntrəˈdʌkʃən/ n an introducing or being introduced; the presentation of one person to another; preliminary text in a book; a preliminary passage in a musical composition.

introductory /ˌɪntrəˈdʌktəri/ adj serving as an introduction; preliminary.—**introductorily** adv.

introit /ˈɪntrɔɪt/ n (*RC Church, Church of England*) a psalm or passage of scripture sung by the choir as the priest approaches the altar before Mass or Holy Communion.

intromission /ˌɪntrəˈmɪʃən/ a insertion; introduction.

intromit /ˌɪntrəˈmɪt/ vt to insert.—**intromittent** adj.

introspect /ˌɪntrəˈspɛkt/ vi to examine one's own thoughts and feelings.

introspection /-ˈspɛkʃən/ n examination of one's own mind and feelings, etc.—**introspectional, introspective** adj.

introversion /ˌɪntrəˈvɜrʒən/ n the act of introverting; the state of being introverted; the direction of, or tendancy to direct, one's thoughts and concerns inward.

introvert /ˈɪntrəˌvɜrt/ vt to turn or direct inward. • vi to produce introversion in. • n a person who is more interested in his or her own thoughts, feelings, etc than in external objects or events. • adj characterized by introversion.—**introversive** adj.

intrude /ɪnˈtruːd/ vti to force (oneself) upon others unasked.—**intruder** n.—**intrudingly** adv.

intrusion /ɪn'truːʒən/ *n* the act or an instance of intruding; the forcible entry of molten rock into and between existing rocks.—**intrusional** *adj*.

intrusive /ɪn'truːsɪv/ *adj* intruding; tending to intrude; (*rocks*) formed by intrusion.—**intrusively** *adv*.

intrust /ɪn'trʌst/ *see* **entrust**.

intubate /'ɪntjuˌbeɪt/ or /-tjʊ-/ *vt* (*med*) to insert a tube into (the larynx, etc).—**intubation** *n*.

intuit /ɪn'tuːɪt/ or /-tjuː-/ *vt* to know by intuition.

intuition /ˌɪntuː'tʃən/ or /-tjuː-/ *n* a perceiving of the truth of something immediately without reasoning or analysis; a hunch, an insight.—**intuitional** *adj*.—**intutionally** *adv*.

intuitive /ɪn'tuːɪtɪv/ or /-tjuː-/ *adj* perceiving or perceived by intuition.—**intuitively** *adv*.

intuitivism /-vɪzəm/ *n* the doctrine that ethical principles are matters of intuition.—**intuitivist** *n*.

intuitonism /-nˌɪzəm/, **intuitionalism** /-nəlɪm/ *n* the doctrine that the immediate perception of truth is by intuition.—**intuitionist, intuitionalist** *n*.

intumescence /ˌɪntuː'mesəns/, **intumescency** /-si/ *n* a swelling up; a tumid state.—**intumescent** *adj*.

intussusception /ˌɪntəssə'sepʃən/ *n* (*med*) the protrusion of the upper part of the intestinal canal into the lower part; (*biol*) the expansion of a cell.

intwine /ɪn'twaɪn/ *see* **entwine**.

inuit /'ɪnjuːɪt/ or /'ɪnʊɪt/ *n* (*pl* **Inuit, Inuits**) an Eskimo from Greenland or North America.—*also* **Innuit**.

Inuk /ɪ'nuːk/ *n* ❀ a member of the Inuit people.

Inukshuk /'ɪnʊkˌʃʊk/ *n* ❀ a figure of a human made from stones, used by the Inuit as a marker.

Inuktitut /ɪn'ʊktɪtʊt/ *n* ❀ the language of the Inuit.

inulin /'ɪnuːlɪn/ *n* a starchy constituent of many plants.

inunction /ɪn'ʌŋkʃən/ *n* the act of applying ointment; the act of anointing or smearing with oil.

inundate /'ɪnənˌdeɪt/ *vt* to cover as with a flood; to deluge.—**inundation** *n*.—**inundator** *n*.

inure /ɪ'njʊr/ *vt* to accustom to, *esp* to something unpleasant.—*also* **enure**.—**inurement, enurement** *n*.

inurn /ɪn'ɜrn/ *vt* to put (ashes) in an urn.

inutile /ɪn'juːˈl/ *adj* useless.

invade /ɪn'veɪd/ *vt* to enter (a country) with hostile intentions; to encroach upon; to penetrate; to crowd into as if invading.—**invader** *n*.

in vacuo /ɪn 'vækjʊoː/ *adv* in a vacuum.

invaginate /ɪn'vædʒɪˌneɪt/ *vt* (*anat*) to fold back a part of a tubular organ on itself so that it is sheathed.

invagination /-'neɪʃən/ *n* the process of invaginating; the state of being invaginated.

invalid[1] /ɪn'vælɪd/ *adj* not valid.

invalid[2] /'ɪnvəˌlɪd/ *n* a person who is ill or disabled. • *vt* to cause to become an invalid; to disable; to cause to retire from the armed forces because of ill-health or injury.

invalidate /ɪn'vælɪˌdeɪt/ *vt* to render not valid; to deprive of legal force.—**invalidation** *n*.

invalidity /ˌɪnvə'lɪdɪti/ *n* (*pl* **invalidities**) a lack of validity; a state of illness or disability.

invaluable /ɪn'væljʊbəl/ or /-juːəbəl/ *adj* too valuable to be measured in money.—**invaluably** *adv*.

Invar /'ɪnˌvɑr/ *n* (*trademark*) an alloy of nickel and steel, used in scientific instruments because of its invariability.

invariable /ɪn'veəriəbəl/ *adj* never changing; constant.—**invariability** *n*.—**invariably** *adv*.

invasion /ɪn'veɪʒən/ *n* the act of invading with military forces; an encroachment, intrusion.

invasive /ɪn'veɪsɪv/ *adj* marked by military aggression; tending to spread; tending to infringe.

invective /ɪn'vektɪv/ *n* the use of violent or abusive language or writing.

inveigh /ɪn'veɪ/ *vi* to speak violently or bitterly (against).—**inveigher** *n*.

inveigle /ɪn'veɪgəl/ or /-'viːgəl/ *vt* to entice or trick into doing something.—**inveiglement** *n*.—**inveigler** *n*.

invent /ɪn'vent/ *vt* to think up; to think out or produce (a new device, process, etc); to originate; to fabricate (a lie, etc).—**inventible, inventable** *adj*.—**inventor** *n*.

invention /ɪn'venʃən/ *n* something invented; inventiveness.—**inventional** *adj*.

inventive /ɪn'ventɪv/ *adj* pertaining to invention; skilled in inventing.—**inventiveness** *n*.

inventory /'ɪnvənˌtɒri/ *n* (*pl* **inventories**) an itemized list of goods, property, etc, as of a business; the store of such goods for such a listing; a list of the property of an individual or an estate. • *vt* (**inventorying, inventoried**) to make an inventory of; to enter in an inventory.—**inventoriable** *adj*.—**inventorial** *adj*.

inveracity /ˌɪnvə'ræsəti/ *n* (*pl* **inveracities**) untruthfulness.

inverse /'ɪnvərs/ or /-'vərs/ *adj* reversed in order or position; opposite, contrary. • *n* an inverse state or thing.—**inversely** *adv*.

inversion /ɪn'vərʒən/ *n* an inverting or being inverted; something inverted.—**inversive** *adj*.

invert /ɪn'vərt/ *vt* to turn upside down or inside out; to reverse in order, position or relationship.—**invertible** *adj*.

invertebrate /ɪn'vərtəbreɪt/ *adj* without a backbone.—*also* **invertebral**. • *n* an animal without a backbone.

inverted comma *n* a quotation mark.

invest /ɪn'vest/ *vt* to commit (money) to property, stocks and shares, etc for profit; to devote effort, time, etc on a particular activity; to install in office with ceremony; to furnish with power, authority, etc. • *vi* to invest money.

investigate /ɪn'vestɪˌgeɪt/ *vti* to search (into); to inquire, examine.—**investigative, investigatory** *adj*.

investigation /ɪnˌvestɪ'geɪʃən/ *n* the act of investigating; an inquiry; a search to uncover facts, etc.—**investigational** *adj*.

investigator /-ər/ *n* one who investigates, *esp* a private detective.

investiture /ɪn'vestɪˌtʃər/ *n* the act or right of giving legal possession; the ceremony of investing a person with an office, robes, title, etc.

investment /ɪn'vestmənt/ *n* the act of investing money productively; the amount invested; an activity in which time, effort or money has been invested.

investor /ɪn'vestər/ *n* a person who invests money.

inveterate /ɪn'vetərət/ *adj* firmly established, ingrained; habitual.—**inveteracy** *n*.—**inveterately** *adv*.

invidious /ɪn'vɪdiəs/ *adj* tending to provoke ill-will, resentment or envy; (*decisions, etc*) unfairly discriminating.—**invidiously** *adv*.—**invidiousness** *n*.

invigorate /ɪn'vɪgəˌreɪt/ *vt* to fill with vigour and energy; to refresh.—**invigorating** *adj*.—**invigoration** *n*.—**invigorative** *adj*.—**invigorator** *n*.

invincible /ɪn'vɪnsɪbəl/ *adj* unconquerable.—**invincibility** *n*.—**invincibly** *adv*.

inviolable /ɪn'vaɪələbəl/ *adj* not to be broken or harmed.—**inviolability** *n*.—**inviolably** *adv*.

inviolate /ɪn'vaɪələt/ *adj* not violated; unbroken, unharmed.—**inviolacy** *n*.

invisible /ɪn'vɪzɪbəl/ *adj* unable to be seen; hidden.—**invisibility** *n*.—**invisibly** *adv*.

invitation /ˌɪnvɪ'teɪʃən/ *n* a message used in inviting.

invite /ɪn'vaɪt/ *vt* to ask to come somewhere or do something; to ask for; to give occasion for; to tempt; to entice. • *n* (*inf*) an invitation.

inviting /ɪn'vaɪtɪŋ/ *adj* attractive, enticing.—**invitingly** *adv*.

in vitro /ɪn 'viːtroː/ *adv, adj* (*biological experiments, etc*) occurring outside the living body and in an artificial environment.

in vivo /ɪn 'viːvoː/ *adv, adj* (*biological processes, etc*) occurring inside the living body.

invocation /ˌɪnvə'keɪʃən/ *n* the act of invoking; a formula used in invoking.—**invocatory** *adj*.

invoice /'ɪnvɔɪs/ *n* a document listing goods dispatched, *usu* with particulars of their price and quantity; to demand due settlement. • *vt* to submit an invoice for or to.

invoke /ɪn'voːk/ *vt* to call on (God, etc) for help, blessing, etc; to resort to (a law, etc) as pertinent; to implore.

involucel /ɪn'vɒljuːˌsel/ *n* (*bot*) a bract around part of a flower head.

involucre /'ɪnvəˌluːkər/ *n* (*bot*) a ring of bracts around the base of a flower cluster.

involuntary /ɪn'vɒlənteri/ *adj* not done by choice; not consciously controlled.—**involuntarily** *adv*.—**involuntariness** *n*.

involute /'ɪnvəˌluːt/, **involuted** *adj* intricate; (*bot*) folded or rolled inwards (*eg* leaves, flowers); curled spirally.

involution /ˌɪnvə'luːʃən/ *n* something which is involute; the act of involving; involvement, complication; (*anat*) the return of an organ or tissue to its normal size after distension; (*math*) the process of raising an arithmetical or algebraic quantity to a given power.

involve /ɪn'vɒlv/ *vt* to affect or include; to require; to occupy, to make busy; to complicate; to implicate.—**involvement** *n*.

invulnerable /ɪn'vʌlnərəbəl/ *adj* not capable of being wounded or hurt in any way.—**invulnerability** *n*.—**invulnerable** *adj*.

inward /'ɪnwərd/ *adj* situated within or directed to the inside; relating to or in the mind or spirit. • *adv* inwards.

inwardly /'ɪnwərdli/ *adv* within; in the mind or spirit; towards the inside or centre.

inwards /'ɪnwərdz/ *adv* towards the inside or interior; in the mind or spirit.

inweave /ɪn'wiːv/ *vt* (**inweaving, inwove** *or* **inweaved**, *pp* **inwoven** *or* **inweaved**) to weave in.

inwrought /ɪn'rɒt/ *or* /'ɪnrɒt/ *adj* worked into or onto (fabric, etc); adorned with figures or patterns.

Io /'aɪoː/ (*chem symbol*) ionium.

iodic /aɪ'ɒdɪk/ *adj* pertaining to, or containing, iodine.

iodide /'aɪədaɪd/ *n* a compound of iodine.

iodine /'aɪədaɪn/ *or* /-diːn/ *n* a nonmetallic element, found in seawater and seaweed, whose compounds are used in medicine and photography.

iodism /'aɪədɪzəm/ *n* poisoning caused by overdoses of iodine.

iodize /'aɪədaɪz/ *vt* to treat or combine with iodine.

iodoform /aɪ'oːdə‚fɔrm/ *n* a compound of iodine, used as an antiseptic.

ion /'aɪɒn/ *or* /'aɪən/ *n* an electrically charged atom or group of atoms formed through the gain or loss of one or more electrons.

Ionic /aɪ'ɒnɪk/ *adj* of a Greek style of architecture that is characterized by ornamental scrolls on the tops of columns.

ionic *adj* of or occurring in the form of ions.

ionize /'aɪə‚naɪz/ *vti* to change or become changed into ions.—**ionization** *n*.

ionosphere /aɪ'ɒnə‚sfiːr/ *n* the series of ionized layers high in the stratosphere from which radio waves are reflected.—**ionospheric** *adj*.

iota /aɪ'oːtə/ *n* the ninth letter of the Greek alphabet; a very small quantity; a jot.

IOU /‚aɪoː'juː/ *n* (*pl* **IOUs**) a written note promising to pay a sum of money to the holder.

IPA *abbr* = International Phonetic Alphabet.

ipecac /'ɪpɪ‚kæk/, **ipecacuanha** /‚ɪpɪ‚kækjuː'ænə/ *n* a South American plant, the root of which is made into a medicine used as an emetic and purgative.

ipso facto /‚ɪpsoː'fæktoː/ *adv* by the fact or act itself.

IQ *abbr* = Intelligence Quotient.

Ir (*chem symbol*) iridium.

IRA *abbr* = Irish Republican Army.

Iranian /ɪ'reɪnɪən/ *or* /-'rɒnɪən/ *n* a native or inhabitant of Iran; a branch of the Indo-European group of languages including Persian; modern Persian.—*also adj*.

irascible /ɪ'ræsɪbəl/ *adj* easily angered; hot-tempered.—**irascibility** *n*.—**irascibly** *adv*.

irate /aɪ'reɪt/ *adj* enraged, furious.—**irately** *adv*.

IRB /'aɪ'ɑr'biː/ *abbr* ✤ (*Cdn*) = Immigration and Refugee Board.

IRC *abbr* = Internet Relay Chat, a type of "meeting to chat" facility on the Internet which takes place in a chatroom.

ire /aɪr/ *n* anger; wrath.

irenic /aɪ'riːnɪk/, **irenical** /-əl/ *adj* aiming at peace

iridaceous /‚ɪrɪ'deɪʃəs/ *adj* (*bot*) of, or pertaining to the iris family.

iridescent /‚ɪrɪ'desənt/ *adj* exhibiting a spectrum of shimmering colours, which change as the position is altered.—**iridescence** *n*.

iridium /ɪ'rɪdɪəm/ *n* a metallic element that is extraordinarily resistant to corrosion.

iris[1] /'aɪrɪs/ *n* (*pl* **irises, irides**) the round, pigmented membrane surrounding the pupil of the eye.

iris[2] *n* (*pl* **irises**) a perennial herbaceous plant with sword-shaped leaves and brightly coloured flowers.

Irish /'aɪrɪʃ/ *adj* of Ireland or its people. • *n* the Celtic language of Ireland.

Irish bull *see* **bull**[3].

Irish coffee *n* coffee mixed with Irish whiskey and topped with fresh cream.

Irish moss *see* **carrageen**.

Irish stew *n* a stew of mutton, onions and potatoes.

iritis /aɪ'raɪtɪs/ *n* (*med*) inflammation of the iris.

irk /ɔrk/ *vt* to annoy, irritate.

irksome /ir'kutsk/ *adj* tedious; tiresome.

iron /'aɪrn/ *n* a metallic element, the most common of all metals; a tool, etc of this metal; a heavy implement with a heated flat underface for pressing cloth; (*pl*) shackles of iron; firm strength; power; any of certain golf clubs with angled metal heads. • *adj* of iron; like iron, strong and firm. • *vti* to press with a hot iron; (*with* **out**) to correct or settle a problem through negotiation or similar means.—**ironer** *n*.

Iron Age *n* the period when most tools and weapons were made of iron, following the Bronze Age in around 1100 BC.

ironbark /'aɪrnbɑrk/ *n* a type of eucalyptus tree.

ironbound /-baʊnd/ *adj* bound with iron; unyielding.

ironclad /‚aɪrn'klæd/ *adj* covered in iron; difficult to change or break.

iron curtain *n* the name of the physical and ideological barrier which once separated the former Soviet Union and Communist Eastern Europe from the rest of Europe.

iron gray *adj* a slightly greenish dark grey.

ironic /aɪ'rɒnɪk/, **ironical** /-əl/ *adj* of or using irony.—**ironically** *adv*.

ironing /'aɪrnɪŋ/ *n* the act of ironing; items of clothing, etc, for ironing.

ironing-board *n* a narrow flat surface to iron clothes on.

iron lung *n* a large respirator that encloses all of the body but the head.

iron maiden *n* a medieval instrument of torture consisting of a hinged coffin-like box fitted with spikes which was closed around the victim.

ironmonger /'aɪrn‚mʌŋgər/ *n* a dealer in metal utensils, tools, etc; a hardware shop.—**ironmongery** *n*.

iron rations *npl* emergency food rations for military use.

ironstone /'aɪrn‚stoːn/ *n* a type of iron ore; a type of hardwearing earthenware.

ironwood /'aɪrnwʊd/ *n* a name given to the timber of certain trees, which is of exceptional hardness and durability.

ironwork /'aɪrn‚wɔrk/ *n* articles made of iron, *esp* decorative railings, etc.

ironworks /-s/ *n* (*pl or sing* a factory where iron is smelted, cast, or wrought.

irony /aɪrəni/ *or* /'aɪrni/ *n* (*pl* **ironies**) an expression in which the intended meaning of the words is the opposite of their usual sense; an event or result that is the opposite of what is expected.

Iroquoian /‚ɪrə'kwɔɪən/ *n* ✤ a speaker of one of a grouping of Indian languages in eastern North America; the language spoken by a people using one of these languages. • *adj* of or pertaining to this people or their language.

Iroquois /‚ɪrə'kwɔɪ/ *n* ✤ a member of one of several Indian peoples mainly of Ontario, Quebec, and New York State; the language of one of these peoples. • *adj* of or pertaining to these peoples or their languages.

irradiance /ɪ'reɪdɪənj/ *n* the act of emitting rays of light; lustre.

irradiant /ɪ'reɪdɪənt/ *adj* emitting rays of light; shining brightly.

irradiate /ɪ'reɪdɪ‚eɪt/ *vt* to shine upon; to light up; to enlighten; to radiate; to expose to X-rays or other radiation. • *vi* to emit rays; to shine.—**irradiative** *adj*.—**irradiator** *n*.

irradiation /ɪ‚reɪdɪ'eɪʃən/ *n* the act of irradiating; the condition of being irradiated; the apparent extension of the edges of an illuminated object seen against a dark background; the use of radiation in medicine.

irrational /ɪ'ræʃənəl/ *adj* not rational, lacking the power of reason; senseless; unreasonable; absurd.—**irrationality** *n*.—**irrationally** *adv*.

irrational number *n* a real number (*eg* π) that cannot be expressed as the result of dividing one integer by another.

irreclaimable /‚ɪrɪ'kleɪməbəl/ *adj* which cannot be reclaimed.

irreconcilable /ɪ'rekən‚saɪləbəl/ *adj* not able to be brought into agreement; incompatible.—**irreconcilability** *n*.—**irreconcilably** *adv*.

irrecoverable /‚ɪrɪ'kʌvərəbəl/ *adj* beyond recovery.—**irrecoverably** *adv*.

irrecusable /‚ɪrɪ'kjuːzəbəl/ *adj* which must be accepted.

irredeemable /‚ɪrɪ'diːməbəl/ *adj* not able to be redeemed.—**irredeemably** *adv*.

irredentist /‚ɪrɪ'dentɪst/ *n* an advocate of the return of a country of neighbouring regions claimed by another on language and other grounds.—**irredentism** *n*.

irreducible /‚ɪrɪ'duːsɪbəl/ *adj* unable to be reduced from one form, state, degree, etc to another.—**irreducibility** *n*.—**irreducibly** *adv*.

irrefragable /ɪ'refrəgəbəl/ *adj* irrefutable, unanswerable.

irrefrangible /ˌɪrɪ'frændʒɪbəl/ *adj* inviolable; (*physics*) which cannot be refracted.

irrefutable /ˌɪrɪ'fjuːtəbəl/ or /ɪ'rɛfjutəbəl/ *adj* unable to deny or disprove; indisputable.—**irrefutability** *adv.*—**irrefutably** *adv.*

irregular /ɪ'rɛgjulər/ *adj* not regular, straight or even; not conforming to the rules; imperfect; (*troops*) not part of the regular armed forces.—**irregularly** *adv.*

irregularity /-'lɛrɪti/ *n* (*pl* **irregularities**) departure from a rule, order or method; crookedness.

irrelative /ɪ'rɛlətɪv/ *adj* unconnected, unrelated.

irrelevant /ɪ'rɛləvənt/ *adj* not pertinent; not to the point.—**irrelevance, irrelevancy** *n.*—**irrelevantly** *adv.*

irreligion /ˌɪrəʊlɪdʒən/ *n* lack of religious belief; disregard for, or hostility towards, religion.

irreligious /ˌɪrɪ'lɪdʒəs/ *adj* impious, irreverent.

irremediable /ˌɪrə'miːdɪəbəl/ *adj* which cannot be remedied.

irremissible /ˌɪrə'mɪsɪbəl/ *adj* unpardonable; (*obligation*) binding.

irremovable /ˌɪrɪ'muːvəbəl/ *adj* not removable.—**irremovability** *adv.*—**irremovably** *adv.*

irreparable /ɪ'rɛpərəbəl/ *adj* that cannot be repaired, rectified or made good.—**irreparably** *adv.*

irreplaceable /ˌɪrə'pleɪsəbəl/ *adj* unable to be replaced.—**irreplaceability** *n.*

irrepressible /ˌɪrə'prɛsɪbəl/ *adj* unable to be controlled or restrained.—**irrepressibly** *adv.*

irreproachable /ˌɪrə'prəʊtʃəbəl/ *adj* blameless; faultless.—**irreproachability** *adv.*—**irreproachably** *adv.*

irresistible /ˌɪrə'zɪstɪbəl/ *adj* not able to be resisted; overpowering; fascinating; very charming, alluring.—**irresistibility** *adv.*—**irresistibly** *adv.*

irresolute /ɪ'rɛzəˌluːt/ *adj* lacking resolution, uncertain, hesitating.—**irresolutely** *adv.*—**irresoluteness, irresolution** *n.*

irresolvable /ˌɪrə'zɒlvəbəl/ *adj* which cannot be resolved or solved.

irrespective /ˌɪrə'spɛktɪv/ *adj* (*with* **of**) regardless.—**irrespectively** *adv.*

irresponsible /ˌɪrə'spɒnsɪbəl/ *adj* not showing a proper sense of the consequences of one's actions; unable to bear responsibility.—**irresponsibility** *n.*—**irresponsibly** *adv.*

irresponsive /ˌɪrə'spɒnsɪv/ *adj* not responsive.

irretentive /ˌɪrɪ'tɛntɪv/ *adj* not retentive.

irretrievable /ˌɪrə'triːvəbəl/ *adj* that cannot be recovered; irreparable.—**irretrievability** *n.*—**irretrievably** *adj.*

irreverent /ɪ'rɛvərənt/, **irreverential** /-ʃəl/ *adj* not reverent, disrespectful.—**irreverence** *n.*—**irreverently** *adv.*

irreversible /ˌɪrə'vɜːsɪbəl/ *adj* not able to be reversed; unable to be revoked or altered.—**irreversibility** *n.*—**irreversibly** *adv.*

irrevocable /ɪ'rɛvəkəbəl/ or /ˌɪrɪ'vəʊk-/ *adj* unable to be revoked, unalterable.—**irrevocability** *n.*—**irrevocably** *adv.*

irrigate /'ɪrəˌgeɪt/ *vt* to supply (land) with water as by means of artificial ditches, pipes, etc; (*med*) to wash out (a cavity, wound, etc).—**irrigable** *adj.*—**irrigation** *n.*—**irrigative** *adj.*—**irrigator** *n.*

irritable /'ɪrɪtəbəl/ *adj* easily annoyed, irritated, or provoked; (*med*) excessively sensitive to a stimulus.—**irritability** *n.*—**irritably** *adv.*

irritant /'ɪrɪtənt/ *adj* irritating; causing irritation. • *n* something that causes irritation.

irritate /'ɪrɪˌteɪt/ *vt* to provoke to anger; to annoy; to make inflamed or sore.—**irritative** *adj.*—**irritator** *n.*

irritation /-'teɪʃən/ *n* the act of irritating; the state of being irritated; someone who, or something which, irritates.

irrupt /ɪ'rʌpt/ *vi* to enter forcibly or suddenly.—**irruption** *n.*

is *see* **be.**

ISBN /'ɔɪɛsbiːɛn/ *abbr* = International Standard Book Number.

ISDN /'ɔɪɛsdiːɛn/ *abbr* = Integrated Services Digital Network. A means of transmitting data, voice and video digitally over a telecommunications line.

isinglass /'aɪzɪŋˌglæs/ *n* a gelatin prepared from fish bladders; mica, *esp* in thin sheets.

Islam /'ɪzlæm/ or /-lɒm/, /-'læm/ *n* the Muslim religion, a monotheistic religion founded by Mohammed; the Muslim world.—**Islamic** *adj.*

island /'aɪlənd/ *n* a land mass smaller than a continent and surrounded by water; anything like this in position or isolation.

islander /-ər/ *n* a native or inhabitant of an island.

isle /aɪl/ *n* an island, *esp* a small one.

islet /'aɪlət/ *n* a small island.

-ism /'ɪzəm/ *n suffix* indicating a system or doctrine, as *Protestantism*; a state or condition, as *barbarism*; action, as *criticism*; a peculiarity or idiom, as *archaism, gallicism*; a morbid condition caused by abuse of drugs, as *alcoholism.*

isn't /'ɪzənt/ = is not.

isobar /'aɪsoˌbɑr/ *n* a line on a map connecting places of equal barometric pressure.—**isobaric** *adj.*—**isobarism** *n.*

isochromatic /ˌaɪsoʊkroʊ'mætɪk/ *adj* of the same colour; (*photog*) giving equal intensity to different colours.

isochronal /aɪ'sɒkrəʊnəl/, **isochronous** /-əs/ *adj*

isoclinal /ˌaɪsoʊ'klaɪnəl/, **isoclinic** /-'klɪnɪk/ *adj* having the same dip or inclination.

isodynamic /ˌaɪsoʊdaɪ'næmɪk/ *adj* having equal force.

isogon /ˌaɪsoʊ'gɒn/ *n* (*geom*) a figure with equal angles.

isohel /'aɪsoʊˌhɛl/ *n* a line on a map, linking places with the same hours of sunshine.

isohyet /ˌaɪsoʊ'haɪɪt/ *n* a line on a map, linking places with the same rainfall.

isolate /'aɪsoʊˌleɪt/ *vt* to set apart from others; to place alone; to quarantine a person or animal with a contagious disease; to separate a constituent substance from a compound.—**isolator** *n.*

isolation /ˌaɪsoʊ'leɪʃən/ *n* the state of being isolated; the act of isolating.

isolationism /ˌaɪsoʊ'leɪʃəˌnɪzəm/ *n* a policy of refraining from involvement in international affairs.—**isolationist** *adj, n.*

isolation pay *n* ✹ (*Cdn*) a supplement to a salary given as additional compensation for someone who works in a remote area, *esp* in the North.

isomer /'aɪsəmər/ *n* any of two or more chemical compounds whose molecules contain the same atoms but in different arrangements.—**isomeric** *adj.*—**isomerism** *n.*

isometric /ˌaɪsoʊ'mɛtrɪk/, **isometrical** /-əl/ *adj* having equality of measure; relating to muscular contraction involving little shortening of the muscle; (*drawing*) projecting an image to scale in three dimensions with the axis equally inclined.—**isometrically** *adv.*

isometrics /-s/ *n* (*sing or pl*) physical exercises in which muscles are contracted against each other or in opposition to fixed objects.

isomorphism /ˌaɪsoʊ'mɔrfɪsm/ *n* (*biol*) similarity in form; (*chem*) the quality of having the same crystalline form despite being formed of different elements.—**isomorphic, isomorphous** *adj.*

isopod /'aɪsoʊˌpɒd/ *n* a type of crustacean with seven pairs of equal legs, *eg* the woodlouse.

isosceles /aɪ'sɒsɪˌliːz/ *adj* denoting a triangle with two equal sides.

isoseismic /ˌaɪsoʊ'saɪzmɪk/, **isoseismal** /-məl/ *adj* pertaining to points at which earthquake shock is of the same intensity. • *n* a line on a map, linking these points.

isotherm /'aɪsoʊˌθɜrm/ *n* a line on a map connecting points of the same temperature.—**isothermal** *adj.*

isotope /'aɪsəˌtoʊp/ *n* any of two or more forms of an element having the same atomic number but different atomic weights.—**isotopic** *adj.*—**isotopically** *adv.*

Israelite /'ɪzrɪəˌlaɪt/ or /-rəˌlaɪt/ *n* (*Bible*) a descendant of the Hebrew patriarch Jacob.

issuable /'ɪsuːəbəl/ *adj* which can be issued.

issuance /'ɪʃuːəns/ *n* the act of issuing.

issue /'ɪsuː/ *n* an outgoing; an outlet; a result; offspring; a point under dispute; a sending or giving out; all that is put forth at one time (an issue of bonds, a periodical, etc). • *vb* (**issuing, issued**) *vi* to go or flow out; to result (from) or end (in); to be published. • *vt* to let out; to discharge; to give or deal out, as supplies; to publish.

isthmian /'ɪsmɪən/ or /'ɪsθ-/ *adj* of or pertaining to an isthmus.

isthmus /'ɪsməs/ or /'ɪsθ-/ *n* (*pl* **isthmuses, isthmi**) a narrow strip of land having water at each side and connecting two larger bodies of land.—**isthmoid** *adj.*

istle /'ɪstli/ *n* a tough fibre made from a species of Mexican agave, used to make cord.—*also* **ixtle.**

it /ɪt/ *pron* the thing mentioned; the subject of an impersonal verb; a subject or object of indefinite sense in various constructions. • *n* the player, as in tag, who must catch another.

it'll /'ɪtəl/ = it will; it shall.

it's /ɪts/ = it is; it has.

Italian /ɪˈtæljən/ adj of Italy or its people. • a native of Italy; the Italian language.

Italianate /ɪˈtæljəˌneɪt/ adj Italian in style or character.

Italic /aɪˈtælɪk/ or /ɪ-/ adj (language) of ancient Italy.

italic /aɪˈtælɪk/ or /ɪ-/ adj denoting a type in which the letters slant upward to the right (this is italic type). • n (usu pl) italic type or handwriting.

italicize /ɪˈtælɪˌsaɪz/ vi to write in italics. • vt to underline a word to indicate italics.—**italicization** n.

itch /ɪtʃ/ n an irritating sensation on the surface of the skin causing a need to scratch; an insistent desire. • vi to have or feel an irritating sensation in the skin; to feel a restless desire.

itchy /ˈɪtʃi/ adj (**itchier, itchiest**) pertaining to or affected with an itch.—**itchiness** n.

item /ˈaɪtəm/ n an article; a unit; a separate thing; a bit of news or information.

itemize /ˈaɪtəˌmaɪz/ vt to specify the items of; to set down by items.—**itemization** n.

iterate /ˈɪtəˌreɪt/ vt to say or do again or repetitively.—**iteration** n.—**iterative** adj.

ithyphallic /ˌɪθɪˈfælɪk/ adj (poet) in the manner of the rites or hymns to Bacchus.

itinerancy /aɪˈtɪnərənsi/ or /ɪ-/, **itineracy** /-rəsi/ n (pl **itinerancies, itineracies**) the act of travelling from place to place, esp to carry out an official duty.

itinerant /aɪˈtɪnərənt/ adj travelling from place to place. • n a traveller.

itinerary /aɪˈtɪnərəri/ or /ɪ-/ n (pl **itineraries**) a route; a record of a journey; a detailed plan of a journey.

its /ɪts/ poss pron relating to or belonging to **it**.

itself /ɪtˈself/ pron the reflexive and emphatic form of **it**.

IUD abbr = intrauterine device.

I've /aɪv/ = I have.

IVF abbr = in vitro fertilization: a technique for helping infertile couples to have children, in which a woman's eggs are fertilized by the father's sperm in a laboratory and then re-implanted in the womb.

ivory /ˈaɪvəri/ n (pl **ivories**) the hard, creamy-white substance forming the tusks of elephants, etc; any substance like ivory; creamy white. • adj of or like ivory; creamy white.

ivory tower n a place or situation which excludes the realities of everyday life.—**ivory towered** adj.

ivy /ˈaɪvi/ n (pl **ivies**) a climbing or creeping vine with a woody stem and evergreen leaves.—**ivied** adj.

ixtle /ˈɪkstli/ or /ˈɪst-/ see **istle**.

J

J *abbr* = joule(s).

jab /dʒæb/ *vti* (**jabbing, jabbed**) to poke or thrust roughly; to punch with short, straight blows. • *n* a sudden thrust or stab; (*inf*) an injection with a hypodermic needle.

jabber /ˈdʒæbər/ *vti* to speak or say rapidly, incoherently, or foolishly. • *n* such talk.—**jabberer** *n*.

jabiru /ˈdʒæbɪˌruː/ *n* a stork-like bird of tropical America; an Australian stork.

jaborandi /ˌdʒæbəˈrændi/ *n* a tropical American plant that yields an alkaloid used to stimulate perspiration and as a diuretic.

jabot /ˈʒæboʊ/ *n* an ornamental frill worn down the front of a blouse or shirt.

jacamar /ˈdʒækəmɑr/ *n* a South American bird similar to a kingfisher.

jacana, jaçana /ˈdʒækənə/ or /-sənə/ *n* a small tropical wading bird.

jacaranda /ˌdʒækəˈrændə/ *n* a South American tree with hard, heavy wood; any one of several similar trees; the fragrant wood from such trees.

jacinth /ˈdʒæsɪnθ/ or /ˈdʒeɪ-/ *n* a reddish-orange gem, a variety of zircon.

jack /dʒæk/ *n* any of various mechanical or hydraulic devices used to lift something heavy; a playing card with a knave's picture on it, ranking below the queen; a small flag flown on a ship's bow as a signal or to show nationality; (*bowls*) a small white ball used as a target. • *vt* (*with* **in**) (*sl*) to abandon (an attempt at something); (*with* **up**) to raise (a vehicle) by means of a jack; to increase (prices, etc); (*sl*) to inject a narcotic drug.

jackal /ˈdʒækəl/ *n* (*pl* **jackals, jackal**) any of various wild dogs of Africa and Asia.

jackanapes /ˈdʒækəˌneɪps/ *n* a conceited or upstart person; a pert child; (*arch*) a monkey.

jackass /ˈdʒækæs/ *n* a male donkey; a fool.

jackboot /ˈdʒækbuːt/ *n* a leather military boot extending above the knee; authoritarian rule, oppression.

jackdaw /ˈdʒækdɔː/ *n* a black bird like the crow but smaller.

jackeroo, jackaroo /ˌdʒækəˈruː/ (*pl* **jackeroos, jackaroos**) (*Austral sl*) a young person training to be a manager on a sheep or cattle station.

jacket /ˈdʒækət/ *n* a short coat; an outer covering, as the removable paper cover of a book. • *vt* to cover with a jacket or cover.—**jacketed** *adj*.

jackfruit /ˈdʒækfruːt/ *n* an East Indian tree or its fruit, which is similar to breadfruit.

jack-in-the-box *n* a toy consisting of a box from which a figure on a spring pops out when the lid is lifted.

jackknife /ˈdʒæknaɪf/ *n* (*pl* **jackknives**) a pocket-knife; a dive in which the diver touches his feet with knees straight and then straightens out. • *vi* to dive in this way; (*articulated truck*) to lose control so that the trailer and cab swing against each other.

jack-of-all-trades *n* (*pl* **jacks-of-all-trades**) a person who does many different types of work.

jack-o'-lantern *n* a lantern made from a hollowed-out pumpkin with holes cut in it to resemble a face; a will-o'-the-wisp.

jackpot /ˈdʒækpɒt/ *n* the accumulated stakes in certain games, as poker; **hit the jackpot** (*sl*) to win; to gain an enormous amount.

jack rabbit /ˈdʒækˌræbət/ *n* a large hare with long ears, common in North America.

jacksnipe /ˈdʒæksnaɪp/ *n* (*pl* **jacksnipes, jacksnipe**) a kind of small snipe; a sandpiper.

jack-tar *n* (*inf*) a sailor.

Jacobean /ˌdʒækəˈbiːən/ *adj* pertaining to the time or reign of James I of England and VI of Scotland. • *n* a person of this period, *esp* a poet.

Jacobin /ˈdʒækəbɪn/ *n* a French Dominican friar; a member of a violent democratic faction that exercised a powerful influence in the French Revolution; an extreme revolutionary.—**Jacobinic, Jacobinical** *adj*.—**Jacobinism** *n*.

Jacobite /ˈdʒækəˌbaɪt/ *n* a supporter of James II of England and VII of Scotland after his abdication or of his descendants.—*also adj*.—**Jacobitism** *n*.

jaconet /ˈdʒækənət/ *n* a fine soft white cotton material resembling cambric.

jacquard /ˈdʒækɑrd/ *n* a loom for weaving patterns; a pattern woven on a jacquard loom.

jactitation /ˌdʒæktɪˈteɪʃən/ *n* boasting; (*med*) a restless, feverish tossing of the body in illness; (*law*) a false pretence of being married to another, or likely to harm another person.

jacuzzi /dʒəˈkuːzi/ *n* (*trademark*) a device that swirls water in a bath; a bath containing such a device.

jade /dʒeɪd/ *n* a hard, ornamental semiprecious stone; its light green colour.

jaded /ˈdʒeɪdəd/ *adj* tired, exhausted; satiated.—**jadedly** *adv*.—**jadedness** *n*.

jadeite /ˈdʒeɪdɔɪt/ *n* a form of jade found in Burma.

jag[1] /dʒæg/ *n* a sharp, tooth-like notch or projection. • *vt* (**jagging, jagged**) to cut into notches; to prick.

jag[2] *n* (*sl*) intoxication from drugs or alcohol; (*sl*) a drinking spree.

jagged /ˈdʒægəd/ *adj* having sharp notches or projecting points; notched or ragged.—**jaggedly** *adv*.—**jaggedness** *n*.

jaggery, jaggary, jagghery /ˈdʒægəri/ *n* a coarse East Indian sugar made from palm sap.

jaggy /ˈdʒægi/ *adj* (**jaggier, jaggiest**) jagged.

jaguar /ˈdʒægwɑr/ or /-juɑr/ *n* (*pl* **jaguars, jaguar**) a large American black-spotted yellow wild cat similar to the leopard.

jail /dʒeɪl/ *n* a prison; imprisonment. • *vt* to send to or confine in prison.

jailbird /ˈdʒeɪlbərd/ *n* a person who is or has been confined in jail.

jailer, jailor /ˈdʒeɪlər/ *n* a person in charge of prisoners in a jail.

Jain /dʒaɪn/ *n* an adherent of Jainism. • *adj* pertaining to the Jains or their religious system.—*also* **Jaina, Jainist**.

Jainism /-ˌnɪzəm/ *n* a Hindu religion of India similar to Buddhism.

jalap, jalop /ˈdʒæləp/ *n* the root of a Mexican plant used formerly as a purgative; the plant itself or similar plants; the resin from the plant.—**jalapic** *adj*.

jalopy /dʒəˈlɒpi/ *n* (*pl* **jalopies**) an old battered vehicle.

jalousie /ˈʒæləˌziː/ *n* a blind with slats like a Venetian blind or a louvred shutter; a louvre window.

jam[1] /dʒæm/ *n* a preserve made from fruit boiled with sugar until thickened; (*inf*) something easy or desirable.

jam[2] *vb* (**jamming, jammed**) *vt* to press or squeeze into a confined space; to crowd full with people or things; to cause (machinery) to become wedged and inoperable; to cause interference to a radio signal rendering it unintelligible. • *vi* to become stuck or blocked; (*sl*) to play in a jam session. • *n* a crowded mass or congestion in a confined space; a blockage caused by jamming; (*inf*) a difficult situation.—**jammer** *n*.

jamb /dʒæm/ *n* the straight vertical side-post of a door, fireplace, etc.

jamboree /ˌdʒæmbəˈriː/ *n* a large party or spree; a large, *usu* international, gathering of Scouts.

jam-packed *adj* filled to capacity.

jam session *n* (*sl*) an unrehearsed performance by jazz, rock or other musicians, *usu* for their own enjoyment.

Jan. *abbr* = January.

jangle /ˈdʒæŋgəl/ *vi* to make a harsh or discordant sound, as bells. • *vt* to cause to jangle; to irritate.—*also n*.

janitor /ˈdʒænɪtər/ *n* a person who looks after a building, doing routine maintenance, etc.—**janitorial** *adj*.

janizary, janissary /ˈdʒænɪˌzɛri/ *n* (*pl* **janizaries, janissaries**) (*formerly*) a foot-guard of the Turkish sultans; a Turkish infantryman.

Jansenism /ˈdʒænsəˌnɪzəm/ *n* the doctrine of sovereign and irresistible grace, promulgated in the 17th century in opposition to the Jesuits; the religion based on these doctrines.—**Jansenist** *n, adj*.—**Jansenistic** *adj*.

January /ˈdʒænjuːˌɛri/ *n* (*pl* **Januaries**) the first month of the year, having 31 days.

japan /dʒə'pæn/ *vt* (**japanning, japanned**) to cover with a hard black glossy lacquer.

Japanese /ˌdʒæpə'niːz/ *adj* of Japan, its people or language. • *n* the language of Japan; an inhabitant of Japan.

jape /dʒeɪp/ *n* a joke, jest.—**japer** *n.*—**japery** *n.*

japonica /dʒə'pɒnɪkə/ *n* any of various species of Japanese plants, Japanese quince, pear, etc; the camellia.

jar[1] /dʒɑr/ *vb* (**jarring, jarred**) *vi* to make a harsh, discordant noise; to have an irritating effect (on one); to vibrate from an impact; to clash. • *vt* to jolt. • *n* a grating sound; a vibration due to impact; a jolt.

jar[2] *n* a short cylindrical glass vessel with a wide mouth. (*inf*) a pint of beer.

jardiniere /ˌʒɑrdɪ'njer/ *n* an ornamental flower-stand of porcelain or metal; mixed diced vegetables stewed in a sauce and served around a meat dish.

jargon[1] /dʒɑrgən/ *n* the specialized or technical vocabulary of a science, profession, etc; obscure and *usu* pretentious language. • *vi* to talk in jargon.—**jargonistic** *adj.*

jargon[2], **jargoon** *n* a translucent, colourless, yellowish, or smoky kind of zircon.

jargonize /-ˌnaɪz/ *vti* to put into or talk in jargon.—**jargonization** *n.*

jarl /dʒɑrl/ *n* an Old Norse chief, a noble.

jasmine, jasmin /'dʒæzmɪn/ *n* any of a genus of climbing shrubs with fragrant white or yellow flowers.

jasper /'dʒæspər/ *n* an opaque, many-shaded variety of quartz that, when polished, is made into a variety of ornamental articles and jewellery; a style of porcelain with a dull surface of green or blue.

jaundice /'dʒɒndɪs/ *n* a condition characterized by yellowing of the skin, caused by excess of bile in the bloodstream bitterness; resentment; prejudice.

jaundiced /'dʒɒndɪst/ *adj* affected with jaundice; jealous, envious, disillusioned.

jaunt /dʒɒnt/ *n* a short journey, *usu* for pleasure • *vi* to make such a journey.

jaunty /'dʒɒnti/ *adj* (**jauntier, jauntiest**) sprightly or self-confident in manner.—**jauntily** *adv.*—**jauntiness** *n.*

Javanese /ˌdʒævə'niːz/ *n* (*pl* **Javanese**) a native or inhabitant of Java; the language of Java.—*also adj.*

javelin /'dʒævəlɪn/ *n* /-vlɪn/ *n* a light spear, *esp* one thrown some distance in a contest.

javex /'dʒæveks/ *n* ✳ (*Cdn*) (*trademark*) a chlorine bleach used for cleaning.

jaw /dʒɒ/ *n* one of the bones in which teeth are set; either of two movable parts that grasp or crush something, as in a vice; (*sl*) a friendly chat, gossip; argument. • *vi* (*sl*) to talk boringly and at length.

jawbone /'dʒɒboːn/ *n* a bone of the jaw, *esp* of the lower jaw.

jawbreaker *n* a machine for crushing rocks, etc; (*inf*) a word that is difficult to pronounce.

jay /dʒeɪ/ *n* any of several birds of the crow family with raucous voices, roving habits, and destructive behaviour to other birds.

jaycee /dʒeɪ'siː/ *n* a young member of a Junior Chamber of Commerce.

jaywalk /'dʒeɪwɒk/ *vi* to walk across a street carelessly without obeying traffic rules or signals.—**jaywalker** *n.*

jazz /dʒæz/ *n* a general term for American popular music, characterized by syncopated rhythms and embracing ragtime, blues, swing, jive, and bebop; (*sl*) pretentious or nonsensical talk or actions. • *vt* (*with* **up**) (*inf*) to play (a piece of music) in a jazz style; to enliven, add colour to.

jazzerati /ˌdʒæzə'rɒti/ *npl* famous or accomplished jazz musicians.

jazzy /'dʒæzi/ *adj* (**jazzier, jazziest**) of or like jazz; (*sl*) lively.—**jazzily** *adj.*—**jazziness** *n.*

jealous /'dʒeləs/ *adj* apprehensive of or hostile toward someone thought of as a rival; envious of, resentful; anxiously vigilant or protective.—**jealously** *adv.*—**jealousness** *n.*

jealousy /'dʒeləsi/ *n* (*pl* **jealousies**) suspicious fear or watchfulness, *esp* the fear of being supplanted by a rival.

jean /dʒiːn/ *n* a hardwearing twilled cotton cloth; (*pl*) trousers made from this or denim.

jeep /dʒiːp/ *n* a small robust vehicle with heavy duty tires and four-wheel drive for use on rough terrain, *esp* by the military.

jeer /dʒiːr/ *vt* to laugh derisively. • *vi* to scoff (at). • *n* a jeering remark.—**jeerer** *n.*—**jeeringly** *adv*

jehad *see* **jihad.**

Jehovah /dʒə'hoːvə/ *n* (*Bib'e*) Hebrew name of God in the OT.

jejune /dʒɪ'dʒuːn/ *adj* lacking significance, dull; naive; lacking in nourishment.—**jejunely** *adv.*—**jejuneness** *n.*

jell /dʒel/ *vti* to become or make into jelly; to crystallize, as a plan.—*also* **gel.**

Jell-O /'dʒeloː/ *n* (*US, proprietary*) a sweet gelatin dessert; jelly.

jelly /'dʒeli/ *n* (*pl* **jellies**) a jam made with fruit juice; a gelatinous food made from fruit syrup or meat juice; any substance like this. • *vt* (**jellying, jellied**) to turn into jelly, to congeal.—**jellied** *adj.*

jellyfish /'dʒelɪfɪʃ/ *n* (*pl* **jellyfish, jellyfishes**) a sea creature with a nearly transparent body and long tentacles.

jennet /'dʒenɪt/ *n* a small Spanish horse; a female donkey.

jenny /'dʒeni/ *n* (*pl* **jennies**) a machine for spinning; a female of some animals, a wren or donkey.

jeopardize /'dʒepərˌdaɪz/ *vt* to endanger, put at risk.

jeopardy /'dʒepərdi/ *n* (*pl* **jeopardies**) great danger or risk.

jequirity /dʒɪ'kwɪrəti/ *n* (*pl* **jequirities**) an Indian shrub with parti-coloured seeds.

jerbil /'dʒɜrbɪl/ *see* **gerbil.**

jerboa /dʒɜr'boːə/ *n* a small desert rodent with long hind legs and a long tail.

jeremiad /ˌdʒerə'maɪəd/ or /-æd/ *n* a long mournful lament or complaint.

jerk[1] /dʒɜrk/ *n* a sudden sharp pull or twist; a sudden muscular contraction or reflex; (*inf*) a stupid person. • *vti* to move with a jerk; to pull sharply; to twitch.

jerk[2] *vt* to preserve (meat) by cutting it into long strips and drying it in the sun. • *n* jerked meat (—*also* **jerky**).

jerkin /'dʒɜrkɪn/ *n* a close-fitting sleeveless jacket. **jerkiness** *n.*

jerky[1] /'dʒɜrki/ *see* **jerk**[2].

jerky[2] *adj* (**jerkier, jerkiest**) moving with jerks.—**jerkily** *adv.*—**jerkiness** *n.*

jeroboam /ˌdʒerə'boːəm/ *n* a huge bottle four times ordinary size, *esp* for champagne.

jerry-built *adj* cheaply and flimsily constructed.—**jerry-builder** *n.*—**jerry-building** *n.*

jerry can *n* a flat-sided container for liquids, *esp* fuel or water, with a capacity of about five gallons (25 litres).

jersey /'dʒɜrzi/ *n* (*pl* **jerseys**) any plain machine-knitted fabric of natural or artificial fibres a knitted sweater.

Jerusalem artichoke *n* (the edible tuber of) the North American sunflower.

jess, jesse /dʒes/ *n* a short leather strap fixed to the leg of a hawk or falcon.

jest /dʒest/ *n* a joke; a thing to be laughed at. • *vi* to jeer; to joke.

jester /'dʒestər/ *n* a person who makes jokes, *esp* an entertainer employed in a royal household in the Middle Ages.

Jesuit /'dʒezjuɪt/ or /'dʒez-/, /-juɪt/ *n* a member of the Catholic Society of Jesus, founded by Ignatius Loyola in 1534; an insidious, crafty intriguer.—**Jesuitic, Jesuitical** *adj.*

Jesuitism /-ˌtɪzəm/, **Jesuitry** /-tri/ *n* (a following of) the principles, system, or practices of the Jesuits; subtle duplicity; disingenuousness.

Jesus (Christ) /'dʒiːzəs/ *n* the Jewish religious teacher and founder of Christianity.

Jesus freak *n* (*sl*) a fervent Christian, *esp* a young member of an evangelical group.

jet[1] /dʒet/ *n* a hard black compact mineral that can be polished and is used in jewellery; a lustrous black.—**jet-black** *adj.*

jet[2] *n* a stream of liquid or gas suddenly emitted; a spout for emitting a jet; a jet-propelled aircraft. • *vti* (**jetting, jetted**) to gush out in a stream; (*inf*) to travel or convey by jet.

jet engine *n* an engine, such as a gas turbine, producing jet propulsion.

jet lag /-ˌlæg/ *n* fatigue caused by disruption of the daily bodily rhythms, associated with crossing time zones at high speed.—**jet-lagged** *adj.*

jet propulsion *n* propulsion of aircraft, boats, etc, by the discharge of gases from a rear vent.—**jet-propelled** *adj.*

jetsam /'dʒetsəm/ *n* cargo thrown overboard from a ship in distress to lighten it, *esp* such cargo when washed up on the shore.

jet set *n* the wealthy and fashionable social elite who travel widely for pleasure.—**jetsetter** *n.*

jet stream *n* the jet of exhaust gases from a jet engine; high-altitude winds.

jettison /'dʒetɪsən/ or /-zər/ *vt* to abandon, to throw overboard.

jetty /'dʒeti/ *n* (*pl* **jetties**) a wharf; a small pier.

Jew /dʒuː/ *n* a person descended, or regarded as descended, from the ancient Israelites; a person whose religion is Judaism.

jewel /'dʒuːəl/ *n* a precious stone; a gem; a piece of jewellery; someone or something highly esteemed; a small gem used as a bearing in a watch. • *vt* (**jewelling, jewelled** *or* **jeweling, jeweled**) to adorn or provide with jewels.

jeweller, jeweler /'dʒuːələr/ *n* a person who makes, repairs or deals in jewellery, watches, etc.

jewellery, jewelry /'dʒuːləri/ *or* /'dʒuːəlri /, /'dʒuːlri/ *n* jewels such as rings, brooches, etc, worn for decoration.

Jewish /'dʒuːɪʃ/ *adj* of or like Jews.

Jewry /'dʒuri/ *n* (*pl* **Jewries**) the Jewish people.

jew's harp *n* a small metal musical instrument that makes a twanging sound when held between the lips and plucked.

Jezebel /'dʒɛzə‚bɛl/ *n* a woman of abandoned or licentious demeanour.

jib[1] /dʒɪb/ *n* a triangular sail extending from the foremast in a ship. • *vti* (**jibbing, jibbed**) to pull (a sail) round to the other side; (*sail*) to swing round.—**jibber** *n*.

jib[2] *n* the projecting arm of a crane.

jib[3] *vi* to refuse to go on; to balk.

jibe /dʒaɪb/ *see* **gybe**.

jiffy, jiff /dʒɪfi/ *n* (*pl* **jiffies, jiffs**) (*inf*) a very short time.

jig /dʒɪg/ *n* a lively springing dance; the music for this; a device used to guide a tool. • *vt* (**jigging, jigged**) to dance in lively manner, as in a jig; to jerk up and down rapidly.

jigger[1] /'dʒɪgər/ *see* **chigoe**.

jigger[2] *n* any of various mechanical devices that operate with a jigging motion; a small glass for spirits; a person or thing that jigs; (*naut*) small tackle, a small sail.

jiggermast /-‚mæst/ *n* the stern mast in a two-masted sailing vessel; a small aftermost mast in a four-master.

jiggery-pokery /‚dʒɪgəri'poːkəri/ *n* (*inf*) underhand work; trickery.

jiggle /'dʒɪgəl/ *vt* to jerk; to move (something) up and down lightly. • *n* a jerky movement.

jigsaw /'dʒɪgsɒ/ *n* a saw with a narrow fine-toothed blade for cutting irregular shapes. • *vt* to cut with a jigsaw.

jigsaw (puzzle) *n* a picture mounted on wood or stiff cardboard and then cut up into irregular pieces, which are then assembled for amusement.

jihad /dʒɪ'hæd/ *n* a holy war waged by Muslims against non-believers; a crusade for or against a cause.—*also* **jehad**.

jilt /dʒɪlt/ *vt* to discard (a lover) unfeelingly, *esp* without warning.—**jilter** *n*.

jimjams /'dʒɪmdʒæmz/ *npl* (*sl*) delirium tremens; nervous jitters.

jingle /'dʒɪŋgəl/ *n* a metallic tinkling sound like a bunch of keys being shaken together; a catchy verse or song with light rhythm, simple rhymes, etc. • *vti* (to cause) to make a light tinkling sound.—**jingler** *n*.

jingly /-li/ *adj* (**jinglier, jingliest**) tinkling.

jingo /'dʒɪŋgoː/ *n* (*pl* **jingoes**) a blustering patriot, a warmonger.

jingoism /-‚ɪzəm/ *n* advocacy of an aggressive foreign policy.—**jingoist** *adj, n*.—**jingoistic** *adj*.—**jingoistically** *adv*.

jink /dʒɪŋk/ *n* a rapid swerve from side to side in order to dodge; (*pl*) high spirits. • *vti* to move nimbly; to dodge.

jinni /dʒɪ'niː/ *n* (*pl* **jinn**) (*fairy tales*) a spirit with supernatural powers that can fulfil your wishes.—*also* **genie**.

jinx /dʒɪŋks/ *n* (*inf*) someone or something thought to bring bad luck.

JIT *abbr* = just-in-time.

jitter /'dʒɪtər/ *vi* (*inf*) to feel nervous or to act nervously. • *npl* (*inf*) (*with* **the**) an uneasy nervous feeling; fidgets.

jitterbug /'dʒɪtər‚bʌg/ *n* a fast acrobatic dance for couples, *esp* popular in the 1940s. • *vi* (**jitterbugging, jitterbugged**) to dance the jitterbug.

jittery /'dʒɪtəri/ *adj* (*inf*) nervous.—**jitteriness** *n*.

jive /dʒaɪv/ *n* improvised jazz played at a fast tempo; dancing to this music; (*sl*) foolish, exaggerated, or insincere talk. • *vti* to dance the jive.

Jnr, jnr *abbr* = Junior.

job /'dʒɒb/ *n* a piece of work done for pay; a task; a duty; the thing or material being worked on; work; employment; (*sl*) a criminal enterprise; (*inf*) a difficult task. • *adj* hired or done by the job. • *vti* (**jobbing, jobbed**) to deal in (goods) as a jobber; to sublet (work, etc).

jobber /'dʒɒbər/ *n* a person who jobs; a person who buys and sells goods as a middleman; in UK, a broker.

jobbery /'dʒɒbəri/ *n* profiting personally from a public office.

jobless /'dʒɒbləs/ *adj* unemployed. • *n* unemployed people collectively.—**joblessness** *n*.

job lot *n* a miscellaneous collection of items sold as one lot; any miscellaneous collection of cheap items.

jock /dʒɒk/ *n* (*inf*) a jockey; a jockstrap; a male athlete; a disc jockey.

jockey /'dʒɒki/ *n* (*pl* **jockeys**) a person whose job is riding horses in races. • *vti* (**jockeying, jockeyed**) to act as a jockey; to manœuvre for a more advantageous position; to swindle or cheat.

jockstrap /'dʒɒkstræp/ *n* a support for the genitals worn by men participating in sport, an athletic supporter.

jocose /dʒə'koːs/ *adj* playful, humorous.—**jocosely** *adv*.—**jocoseness** *n*.

jocosity /-'kɒsɪti/ *n* (*pl* **jocosities**) a being jocose; a playful action; a humorous remark.

jocular /'dʒɒkjʊlər/ *adj* joking; full of jokes.—**jocularity** *n*.—**jocularly** *adv*.

jocund /'dʒɒkənd/ *adj* merry, cheerful; jovial.—**jocundity** *n*.—**jocundly** *adv*.

jodhpurs /'dʒɒdpəz/ *npl* riding breeches cut loose at the hips but close-fitting from knee to ankle.

joe job *n* ✦ (*Cdn*) a low-paying or monotonous job.

joey /'dʒoːi/ *n* (*pl* **joeys**) (*Austral inf*) a young kangaroo; any young animal or a small child.

jog /dʒɒg/ *vb* (**jogging, jogged**) *vt* to give a slight shake or nudge to; to rouse, as the memory. • *vi* to move up and down with an unsteady motion; to run at a relaxed trot for exercise; (*horse*) to run at a jogtrot. • *n* a slight shake or push; a nudge; a slow walk or trot.—**jogger** *n*.

joggle /'dʒɒgəl/ *vti* to move or shake slightly. • *n* a slight jolt.

jogtrot /'dʒɒgtrɒt/ *n* a slow even-paced trot. • *vi* (**jogtrotting, jogtrotted**) to move at a slow even-paced trot.

john /dʒɒn/ *n* (*sl*) a toilet; an easy prey.

John Barleycorn *n* a personification of malt liquor.

John Dory /dʒɒn'dɔri/ *n* an edible yellow seafish, the dory.

Johnny Canuck *n* ✦ (*inf*) a Canadian; Canada.

joie de vivre /'ʒwɑː'viːvrə/ *n* great enjoyment of life.

join /dʒɔɪn/ *vti* to bring and come together (with); to connect; to unite; to become a part or member of (a club, etc); to participate (in a conversation, etc); (*with* **up**) to enlist in the armed forces; to unite, connect. • *n* a joining; a place of joining.

joinder /'dʒɔɪndər/ *n* the act of joining; (*law*) the coupling of two or more causes of action into the same declaration; the coupling of two issues or two parties.

joiner /'dʒɔɪnər/ *n* a carpenter, *esp* one who finishes interior woodwork; (*inf*) a person who is involved in many clubs and activities, etc.

joinery /'dʒɔɪnəri/ *n* the trade of a joiner; the work of a joiner.

joint /dʒɔɪnt/ *n* a place where, or way in which, two things are joined; any of the parts of a jointed whole; the parts where two bones move on one another in an animal; a division of an animal carcass made by a butcher; (*sl*) a cheap bar or restaurant; (*sl*) a gambling or drinking den; (*sl*) a cannabis cigarette. • *adj* common to two or more; sharing with another. • *vt* to connect by a joint or joints; to divide (an animal carcass) into parts for cooking.

joint account *n* a bank account accessible to two or more people, for deposting or withdrawing funds.

jointer /'dʒɔɪntər/ *n* a tool for pointing; a kind of plane; someone or something that forms joints.

jointly /-li/ *adv* in common; together.

joint stock *n* capital held in common and distributed as shares among the owners.

joint-stock company *n* a company whose capital is owned jointly by stockholders who may sell their individual shares.

jointure /'dʒɔɪntʃər/ *n* landed estate or other property settled on a woman in consideration of her marriage, to be enjoyed by her after the death of her husband; the provision made to enable this; (*arch*) a joining or being joined.

joint venture *n* the sharing of expertise or commercial risk by two or more businesses, etc.•

joist /dʒɔɪst/ *n* any of the parallel beams supporting floorboards or the laths of a ceiling.

jojoba /ho:'ho:bə/ *n* a broad-leaved evergreen shrub with edible seeds yielding a valuable oil.

joke /dʒoːk/ *n* something said or done to cause laughter; a thing done or said merely in fun; a person or thing to be laughed at. • *vi* to make jokes.—**jokingly** *adv*.

joker /'dʒo:kər/ *n* a person who jokes; (*sl*) a person; an extra playing card made use of in certain games.

jokey, joky /-ki/ *adj* (**jokier, jokiest**) full, or fond, of jokes.

jollify /'dʒɒlɪˌfaɪ/ *vti* (**jollifying, jollified**) to make merry, *esp* with drink; to make jolly.—**jollification** *n*.

jollity /'dʒɒlɪti/ *n* (*pl* **jollities**) the state of being jolly.

jolly /'dʒɒli/ *adj* (**jollier, jolliest**) merry; full of fun; delightful; (*inf*) enjoyable. • *vti* (**jollying, jollied**) (*inf*) to try to make (a person) feel good; to make fun of (someone).

Jolly Jumper *n* ♣ (*Cdn*) (*trademark*) a swing that suspends a baby in a harness in a standing position, allowing the baby to freely exercise his or her legs.

Jolly Roger *n* a pirate's flag with a white skull and crossbones on a black background.

jolt /dʒo:lt/ *vt* to give a sudden shake or knock to; to move along jerkily; to surprise or shock suddenly. • *n* a sudden jar or knock; an emotional shock.—**joltingly** *adv*.—**jolty** *adj*.

jonquil /'dʒɒnkwɪl/ *n* a species of narcissus.

jooal *see* **joual**.

jorum /'dʒɔrəm/ *n* a large drinking vessel; its contents, *esp* punch.

josh /dʒɒʃ/ *vi* (*sl*) to tease gently. • *n* (*sl*) friendly teasing; a teasing joke.—**josher** *n*.—**joshingly** *adv*.

joss /dʒɒs/ *n* a Chinese god or idol.

joss stick *n* a stick of incense.

jostle /'dʒɒsəl/ *vti* to shake or knock roughly; to collide or come into contact (with); to elbow for position. • *n* a jostling; a push.

jot /dʒɒt/ *n* a very small amount. • *vt* (**jotting, jotted**) to note (down) briefly.—**jotter** *n*.

jotting /'dʒɒtɪŋ/ *n* something noted down, *esp* a memorandum.

joual[1] /ʒu:'ɒl/ *n* a French Canadian dialect also spoken in Maine that has nonstandard French grammar and pronunciation with English syntax and a substantial English vocabulary.—*also* **jooal**.

joual[2] *n* ♣ (*Cdn*) a form of urban, working-class French in Quebec that has non-standard syntax and many borrowings from English.

joule /dʒu:l/ *n* (*physics*) a unit of energy equal to work done when a force of one newton acts over a distance of one metre.

jounce /dʒauns/ *vti* to bump; to jolt (someone or something). • *n* a bump, a jolt.

journal /'dʒɜrnəl/ *n* a daily record of happenings as a diary; a newspaper or periodical; (*bookkeeping*) a book of original entry for recording transactions; that part of a shaft or axle that turns in a bearing.

journalese /ˌdʒɜrnə'li:z/ *n* a facile style of writing found in many magazines, newspapers, etc.

journalism /'dʒɜrnəˌlɪzəm/ *n* the work of gathering news for or producing a newspaper, magazine or news broadcast.

journalist /-ɪst/ *n* a person who writes for or edits a newspaper, etc; one who keeps a diary.—**journalistic** *adj*.—**journalistically** *adv*.

journalize /'dʒɜrnəˌlaɪz/ *vt* to enter in a journal; to keep a daily record.—**journalization** *n*.—**journalizer** *n*.

journey /'dʒɜrni/ *n* (*pl* **journeys**) a travelling or going from one place to another; the distance covered when travelling. • *vi* (**journeying, journeyed**) to make a journey.—**journeyer** *n*.

journeyman /'dʒɜrnɪmən/ *n* (*pl* **journeymen**) a person whose apprenticeship is completed and who is employed by another a reliable workman.

joust /dʒaust/ *n* a fight on horseback between two knights with lances. • *vi* to engage in a joust, to run at the tilt.—**jouster** *n*.

Jove /dʒo:v/ *n* the Roman god Jupiter; **by Jove** a mild oath; an exclamation of surprise.

jovial /'dʒo:viəl/ *adj* full of cheerful good humour.—**joviality** *n*.—**jovially** *adv*.

Jovian /'dʒo:viən/ *adj* (*Roman myth*) of or like Jove or Jupiter.

jowl[1] /dʒaul/ *n* the lower jaw; (*usu pl*) the cheek.

jowl[2] *n* the loose flesh around the throat; the similar flesh in an animal, as a dewlap.

jowly /'dʒauli/ *adj* (**jowlier, jowliest**) having heavy jowls.—**jowliness** *n*

joy /dʒɔɪ/ *n* intense happiness; something that causes this; its expression.

joyful /'dʒɔɪfʊl/ *adj* filled with, expressing, or causing joy, glad.—**joyfully** *adv*.—**joyfulness** *n*.

joyless /'dʒɔɪləs/ *adj* not occasioning joy, unhappy; bleak.—**joylessly** *adv*.—**joylessness** *n*.

joyous /'dʒɔɪəs/ *adj* joyful, very happy.—**joyously** *adv*.—**joyousness** *n*.

joyride /'dʒɔɪraɪd/ *n* (*inf*) a car ride, often in a stolen vehicle and at reckless speed, just for pleasure.—**joy-rider** *n*.—**joyriding** *n*.

joystick /'dʒɔɪstɪk/ *n* (*inf*) the control lever of an aircraft; (*comput*) a device for controlling cursor movement on a monitor *usu* for computer games.

JP *abbr* = Justice of the Peace.

Jr., jr *abbr* = Junior.

jt *abbr* = joint.

jubilant /'dʒu:bɪlənt/ *adj* triumphant; expressing joy; rejoicing.—**jubilance** *n*.—**jubilantly** *adv*.

Jubilate /'dʒu:bɪlæteɪ/ or /ju:bɪ-/ *n* (*Bible*) the 100th psalm, *esp* as a canticle in morning service; (*mus*) a setting of the 100th psalm.

jubilate /'dʒu:bɪˌleɪt/ *vi* to exult, to show joy.—**jubilation** *n*.

jubilee /dʒu:bɪ'li:/ or /'dʒu:-/ *n* a 50th or 25th anniversary; a time of rejoicing.

Judaic /dʒu:'deɪɪk/, **Judaical** /-kəl/ *adj* of the Jews or Judaism.—**Judaically** *adv*.

Judaism /'dʒu:deɪˌɪzəm/ *n* the religion of the Jews, based on the Old Testament and the Talmud.—**Judaist** *n*.—**Judaistic** *adj*.

Judaize /'dʒu:deɪˌaɪz/ *vi, vt* to make or become Judaistic in belief, customs, precepts, etc.—**Judaization** *n*.

Judas /'dʒu:dəs/ *n* a traitor who pretends to be a friend; (*without cap*) a peephole, as in a cell door.

judder /'dʒʌdər/ *vi* to vibrate violently. • *n* a spasmodic or rapid shaking.

Judean /dʒu:'di:ən/ *adj* of, pertaining to, or from, the ancient region of Judaea.

judge /dʒʌdʒ/ *n* a public official with authority to hear and decide cases in a court of law; a person chosen to settle a dispute or decide who wins; a person qualified to decide on the relative worth of anything. • *vti* to hear and pass judgment (on) in a court of law; to determine the winner of (a contest) or settle (a dispute); to form an opinion about; to criticize or censure; to suppose, think.—**judgeable** *adj*.—**judgingly** *adv*.

judgeship /-ʃɪp/ *n* the office of a judge; his or her jurisdiction.

judgment, judgement /'dʒʌdʒmənt/ *n* a judging; a deciding; a legal decision; an opinion; the ability to come to a wise decision; censure.

judgmental, judgemental /dʒʌdʒ'mentəl/ *adj* of or depending on judgment; tending to make moral or personal judgments.—**judgmentally, judgementally** *adv*.

Judgment Day *n* (*Christianity*) the time of God's final judgment of mankind; (*without cap*) a final judgment; a day of reckoning.

judicable /'dʒu:dɪkəbəl/ *adj* that may be judged; liable to be judged.

judicator /'dʒu:dɪˌkeɪtər/ *n* one who judges.

judicatory /'dʒu:dɪkəˌtɔri/ *n* (*pl* **judicatories**) a system of courts, a judiciary. • *adj* of or pertaining to the administration of justice.

judicature /'dʒu:dɪkətʃər/ or /-'dɪkətʃər/ *n* a court or courts of justice; the power of dispensing justice by legal trial and judgment; jurisdiction; a body of judges; a tribunal.

judicial /dʒu:'dɪʃəl/ *adj* of judges, courts, or their functions.—**judicially** *adv*.

judiciary /dʒu:'dɪʃiːri/ *adj* of judges or courts. • *n* (*pl* **judiciaries**) the part of government that administers justice; a system of courts in a country; judges collectively.

judicious /dʒu:'dɪʃəs/ *adj* possessing or characterized by sound judgment.—**judiciously** *adv*.—**judiciousness** *n*.

judo /'dʒu:do:/ *n* a Japanese system of unarmed combat, adapted as a competitive sport from jujitsu.—**judoist** *n*.

jug /dʒʌg/ *n* a vessel for holding and pouring liquids, with a handle and curved lip; a pitcher; (*sl*) prison. • *vt* (**jugging, jugged**) to stew meat (*esp* hare) in an earthenware pot; (*sl*) to put into prison.—**jugful** *n*.

jugate /dʒu:'geɪt/ *adj* coupled together; (*bot*) having leaflets in pairs.

juggernaut /'dʒʌgərˌnɒt/ *n* a terrible, irresistible force; a large heavy truck; (*with cap*) a Hindu god; his idol, dragged annually in processional car, under whose wheels devotees formerly threw themselves.

juggle /'dʒʌgəl/ *vi* to toss up balls, etc and keep them in the air. • *vt* to manipulate skilfully; to manipulate so as to deceive. • *n* the act of juggling; manipulation.—**jugglery** *n*.

juggler /'dʒʌglər/ *n* one who juggles, a conjurer; a manipulator, a cheat.

jugular /'dʒʌgjulər/ *adj* (*anat*) of the neck or throat. • *n* a jugular vein.

jugular vein *n* (*anat*) any of the large veins in the neck carrying blood from the head.

juice /dʒuːs/ *n* the liquid part of fruit, vegetables or meat; liquid secreted by a bodily organ; (*inf*) vitality; (*inf*) electric current; (*inf*) engine fuel.

juicer /dʒuːsər/ *n* a mechanical or electrical device for extracting juice from fruit and vegetables; (*sl*) a person who drinks to excess.

juicy /ˈdʒuːsi/ *adj* (**juicier, juiciest**) full of juice; (*inf*) very interesting; (*inf*) highly profitable.—**juicily** *adv.*—**juiciness** *n.*

jujitsu /dʒuːˈdʒitsuː/ *n* a traditional Japanese system of unarmed defence in which an opponent's strength is used against him.

juju /ˈdʒuːdʒuː/ *n* an object of superstitious worship in West Africa used as a fetish or charm; the magic attributed to this.—**jujuism** *n.*

jujube /ˈdʒuːdʒuːb/ *n* a gelatinous, fruit-flavoured lozenge; the fruit of any of several small trees of the buckthorn family; the trees themselves.

jukebox /ˈdʒuːkbɒks/ *n* a coin-operated automatic record or CD player.

Jul. *abbr* = July.

julep /ˈdʒuːlɛp/ *n* a tall drink of bourbon or brandy and sugar over crushed ice, garnished with mint.

Julian /ˈdʒuːliən/ *adj* of or pertaining to Julius Caesar or to the Julian calendar.

Julian calendar *n* a calendar introduced in 46BC by Julius Caesar, in which the year was made to consist of 365 days with a leap year of 366 days every fourth year.

julienne /ˌdʒuːliˈɛn/ *adj* (*vegetables*) cut into very thin strips. • *n* a clear soup containing such vegetable.

July /dʒuːˈlaɪ/ *n* (*pl* **Julies**) the seventh month of the year, having 31 days.

jumble /ˈdʒʌmbəl/ *vt* (*often with* **up**) to mix together in a disordered mass. • *n* items mixed together in a confused mass; articles for a jumble sale.—**jumbly** *adj.*

jumbo /ˈdʒʌmbəʊ/ *n* (*pl* **jumbos**) something very large of its kind. • *adj* very large.

jumbo jet *n* a very large jet airliner.

jumbuck /ˈdʒʌmbək/ *n* (*Austral*) a sheep.

jump /dʒʌmp/ *vi* to spring or leap from the ground, a height, etc; to jerk; to pass suddenly, as to a new topic; to rise suddenly, as prices; (*sl*) to be lively; (*often with* **at**) to act swiftly and eagerly; (*with* **at**) to accept or agree too eagerly; (*with* **on**) (*inf*) to reprimand or criticize harshly. • *vt* to leap or pass over (something); to leap upon; to cause (prices, etc) to rise; to fail to turn up (for trial when out on bail); (*inf*) to attack suddenly; (*inf*) to react to prematurely; (*sl*) to leave suddenly. • *n* a jumping; a distance jumped; a sudden transition; an obstacle; a nervous start.

jumper /ˈdʒʌmpər/ *n* a knitted garment for the upper body; a sleeveless dress for wearing over a blouse, etc.

jumper cable, jump lead *n* one of two cables for transferring electric charge from one battery to another, used to start a car with a flat battery by using the battery of another vehicle.

jump jet *n* (*inf*) a jet aircraft that can take off and land vertically.

jump-start *vt* to start a motor vehicle by pushing it in low gear so the engine turns over or by using jump leads; (*inf*) to set (a sluggish system, etc) in motion.

jumpsuit /ˈdʒʌmpsuːt/ *n* a one-piece garment, as worn by paratroopers.

jumpy /ˈdʒʌmpi/ *adj* (**jumpier, jumpiest**) moving in jerks, etc; apprehensive; easily startled.—**jumpily** *adv.*—**jumpiness** *n.*

Jun. *abbr* = June.

jun., Jun. *abbr* = junior.

junction /ˈdʒʌŋkʃən/ *n* a place or point where things join; a place where roads or railway lines, etc meet, link or cross each other.—**junctional** *adj.*

juncture /ˈdʒʌŋktʃər/ *n* a junction; a point of time; a crisis.

June /dʒuːn/ *n* the sixth month of the year, having 30 days.

jungle /ˈdʒʌŋgəl/ *n* an area overgrown with dense tropical trees and other vegetation, etc; any scene of wild confusion, disorder, or of ruthless competition for survival.

jungly /-li/ *adj* (**junglier, jungliest**) pertaining to or covered with jungle.

junior /ˈdʒuːnjər/ *adj* younger in age; of more recent or lower status; of juniors. • *n* a person who is younger, of lower rank, etc; a young person employed in minor capacity in an office; a student in the third year of college or school; (*US inf*) (*with cap*) the younger son, often used after the name if the same as the father's; ✦ (*Cdn*) a level of amateur competition in ice hockey for teenage players. • *adj* of or pertaining to this level.

junior miss *n* a girl in her teens; a clothes size for girls and slim women.

juniper /ˈdʒuːnɪpər/ *n* an evergreen shrub that yields purple berries.

junk[1] /dʒʌŋk/ *n* a flat-bottomed sailing vessel prevalent in the China Seas.

junk[2] *n* discarded useless objects; (*inf*) rubbish, trash; (*sl*) any narcotic drug, such as heroin. • *vt* (*inf*) to scrap. • *adj* cheap, worthless; showy but without substance.

junk bond *n* an interest-bearing certificate held without security, used in junk debt.

junk debt *n* a method of funding takeovers by lending money unsecured in return for a higher yield and other benefits.—*also* **mezzanine debt.**

Junker /ˈdʒʌŋkər/ *n* (*formerly*) a member of the Prussian aristocracy known for its political conservatism and militarism.

junker /ˈdʒʌŋkər/ *n* (*sl*) a jalopy.

junket /ˈdʒʌŋkɛt/ *n* curdled milk, sweetened and flavoured; a picnic; an excursion, *esp* one by an official at public expense. • *vi* to go on a junket.

junketeer /dʒʌŋkəˈtiːr/ *n* to make a practice of going on free trips. • *vi* someone who does this.

junk food *n* a snack or fast food with little nutritional value.

junkie, junky /ˈdʒʌŋki/ *n* (*pl* **junkies**) (*sl*) an addict of a particular activity, food, etc; a drug addict.

junk mail *n* unsolicited mail, *eg* advertising leaflets.

Juno /ˈdʒuːnoʊ/ *n* (*Roman myth*) the queen of the gods, sister and wife of Jupiter; a queenly woman.—**Junoesque** *adj.*

junta /ˈhʊntə/ *or* /ˈhɛn /, /ˈdʒʌn-/ *n* a group of people, *esp* military, who assume responsibility for the government of a country following a coup d'état or revolution.

Jupiter /ˈdʒuːpɪtər/ *n* (*Roman myth*) the king of the gods, Jove; (*astron*) the largest planet in the solar system.

jural /ˈdʒʊrəl/ *adj* of law; of moral rights and obligations.—**jurally** *adv.*

Jurassic /dʒʊˈræsɪk/ *adj* (geol) of or pertaining to the middle system of the Mesozoic Era marked by the existence of dinosaurs and the appearance of birds and mammals. • *n* the Jurassic period.

jurat /ˈdʒʊræt/ *n* (law) a record of the time, place, etc, of an affidavit.

juridical, juridic /dʒʊˈrɪdɪkəl/ *adj* of judicial proceedings or law.—**juridically** *adv.*

jurisconsult /ˌdʒʊrɪskənˈsʌlt/ *n* one learned in law, a jurist.

jurisdiction /ˌdʒʊrɪsˈdɪkʃən/ *n* the right or authority to apply the law; the exercise of such authority; the limits of territory over which such authority extends.—**jurisdictional** *adj.*—**jurisdictionally** *adv.*

jurisprudence /ˌdʒʊrɪsˈpruːdəns/ *n* the science or philosophy of law; a division of law.—**jurisprudential** *adj.*—**jurisprudentially** *adv.*

jurisprudent /ˌdʒʊrɪsˈpruːdənt/ *adj, n* (a person) skilled in law.

jurist /ˈdʒʊrɪst/ *n* an expert on law; a judge.—**juristic** *adj.*—**juristically** *adv.*

juror /ˈdʒʊrər/ *n* a member of a jury; a person who takes an oath.

jury[1] /ˈdʒʊri/ *or* /ˈdʒəri/ *n* (*pl* **juries**) a body of *usu* 12 people sworn to hear evidence and to deliver a verdict on a case; a committee or panel that decides winners in a contest.

jury[2] *adj* (*naut*) makeshift, temporary.

juryman /ˈdʒʊrimæn/ *n* (*pl* **jurymen**) a male juror.

jury-rigged *adj* (*yacht, etc*) rigged in a temporary or makeshift way.

jurywoman /ˈdʒʊriˌwʊmən/ *n* (*pl* **jurywomen**) a female juror.

jussive /ˈdʒʌsɪv/ *adj* (*gram*) imperative, expressing command. • *n* (*gram*) a jussive word, mood or form.

just /dʒʌst/ *adj* fair, impartial; deserved, merited; proper, exact; conforming strictly with the facts. • *adv* exactly; nearly; only; barely; a very short time ago; immediately; (*inf*) really; justly, equitably; by right.—**justly** *adv.*—**justness** *n.*

justice /ˈdʒʌstəs/ *n* justness, fairness; the use of authority to maintain what is just; the administration of law; a judge.

justice of the peace *n* a magistrate who summarily tries minor cases within his or her jurisdiction.

justiciable /dʒʌˈstɪʃəbəl/ *adj* subject to trial; able to be settled by law.—**justiciability** *n.*

justiciar /dʒʌˈstɪʃiːr/ *n* (*formerly*) in England, the administrator of justice, chief justice.

justiciary /dʒʌˈstɪʃieri/ *n* (*pl* **justiciaries**) an officer who administers justice; a justiciar. • *adj* of or pertaining to the administration of justice.

justifiable /ˈdʒʌstɪˌfaɪəbəl/ *adj* capable of being justified or defended.—**justifiability** *n.*—**justifiably** *adv.*

justification /ˌdʒʊstɪfɪˈkeɪʃən/ *n* the act of justifying; vindication or defence; a showing adequate reason; absolution; (*print*) the spacing out of type to the full length of a line.

justify /ˈdʒʊstɪˌfaɪ/ *vt* (**justifying, justified**) to prove or show to be just or right; to vindicate; to space out (a line of type) so that it fills the required length.

just-in-time *adj* pertaining to a method of inventory control in production industries, where components are delivered just before they are needed.

jut /dʒʊt/ *vti* (**jutting, jutted**) to project; to stick out. • *n* a part that projects.

jute /dʒuːt/ *n* the fibre of either of two tropical plants used for making sacking, etc.

juvenescent /ˌdʒuːvɪˈnəsərt/ *adj* becoming young.—**juvenescence** *n*.

juvenile /ˈdʒuːvəˌnaɪl/ *adj* young; immature; of or for young persons: ✤ (*Cdn*) of or pertaining to amateur sports competition for teenagers. • *n* a young person

juvenile delinquency *n* (*pl* **delinquencies**) antisocial or illegal behaviour by young people *usu* under 18.—**juvenile delinquent** *n*.

juvenilia /ˌdʒuːvəˈnɪliə/ or /-ˈnaɪljə/ *npl* works produced in an artist's or author's youth.

juvenility /-lɪti/ *n* (*pl* **juvenilities**) the state of being juvenile; youthfulness; a childish act.

juxtapose /ˌdʒʊkstəˈpoːz/ *vt* to place side by side, *esp* for comparison.—**juxtaposition** *n*.

K

K *abbr* = **kelvin**(s); one thousand; *(comput)* 1024 words, bits or bytes; *(chem symbol)* potassium.

kabbala, kabala /kə'bɒlə/ or /'kæbələ/ *see* **cabbala**.

kabloona /kə'blu:nə/ *n* ❧ *(pl* same or **kabloonas**) a person who is not an Inuit, *esp* a white person.

kabuki /kə'bu:ki/ *n* classical Japanese theatre.

Kabyle /kə'baɪl/ or /-'bi:l/ *n* *(pl* **Kabyles, Kabyle**) an Algerian Berber, or his dialect.

Kaddish /'kædɪʃ/ *n* *(pl* **Kaddishim**) a Jewish daily prayer, used by mourners for the year following, and on the anniversary of, someone's death.

kaftan /'kæftən/ or /-,tæn/, /kɒf'tɒn/ *see* **caftan**.

kaiak /'kaɪæk/ *see* **kayak**.

kainite /'kaɪnaɪt/ *n* a mineral fertilizer.

Kaiser /'kaɪzər/ *n* *(formerly)* the title of the emperors of Germany and Austria.

kaka /'kɒkɒ/ *n* a New Zealand parrot with a long beak.

kakapo /'kɒkə,po:/ *n* an owl-like parrot, a flightless nocturnal bird nesting in burrows in New Zealand.

kakemono /,kækə'mo:no:/ *n* a Japanese hanging picture of paper or silk, mounted on rollers.

kaki /'kɒki/ *n* *(pl* **kakis**) the Japanese persimmon.

kale, kail /keɪl/ *n* a variety of cabbage with crinkled leaves.

kaleidoscope /kə'laɪdə,sko:p/ *n* a small tube containing bits of coloured glass reflected by mirrors to form symmetrical patterns as the tube is rotated; anything that constantly changes.—**kaleidoscopic** *adj.*—**kaleidoscopically** *adv.*

kalends /'kæləndz/ *see* **calends**.

kaleyard, kailyard /'keɪl,jɑrd/ *n* *(Scot)* a kitchen garden.

Kali /'kɒli/ *n* *(Hindu myth)* the goddess of destruction.

kalif, khalif /'kɒlɪf/ or /'kælɪf/ *see* **caliph**.

kalmia /'kælmɪə/ *n* the American mountain laurel.

Kalmuck, Kalmyk /'kælmʌk/ *n* *(pl* **Kalmucks, Kalmuck, Kalmyks, Kalmyk**) *n* a member of a Mongolian Buddhist people; the variety of the Mongolian language. • *adj* of or pertaining to the Kalmuck or their language.

kalong /'kɒlɒŋ/ *n* a large Indonesian or tropical fruitbat; a flying fox.

kalpak /'kæl,pæk/ *see* **calpac**.

kalsomine /'kɒlsə,maɪn/ or /-,mɪn/ *see* **calcimine**.

Kamasutra /'kɒmə'su:trə/ *n* an ancient Hindu manual on erotic love.

kame /keɪm/ *n* *(Scot)* an elongated gravel or sand mound or hill of glacial origin; a comb.

kami /'kɒmi/ *n* *(pl* **kami**) a divinity or demigod in the Shinto religion of Japan, from whom the Japanese emperors were supposed to have been descended.

kamik /'kɒmɪk/ or /'kæm-/ *n* ❧ an Inuit boot made from caribou hide.

kamikaze /,kæmɪ'kɒzi/ *n* *(World War II)* a Japanese aircraft packed with explosives for making a suicidal crashing attack; the pilot of such an aircraft.

kamseen /kæm'si:n/, **kamsin** /'kæmsɪn/ *see* **khamsin**.

kangaroo /,kæŋgə'ru:/ *n* *(pl* **kangaroos**) an Australian marsupial with short forelegs and strong, large hind legs for jumping.

kangaroo court *n* an illegal court operated by an unauthorized body, which perverts the proper course of justice.

Kantian /'kæntɪən/ *adj* of the German philosopher Immanuel Kant (1724–1804) or his philosophy.

kaolin /'keɪəlɪn/ *n* a white clay used in porcelain, etc.

kapellmeister /kə'pɛl,maɪstər/ *n* *(pl* **kapellmeister**) the musical director of an orchestra etc, *esp* in an 18th-century aristocratic household.

kapok /'keɪpɒk/ *n* the silky fibres around the seeds of a tropical tree, used for stuffing cushions, etc.

kappa /'kæpə/ *n* the tenth letter of the Greek alphabet.

kaput /kæ'pʊt/ *adj* *(sl)* broken, ruined.

karabiner /,kærə'bi:nər/ or /'kærə-/ *n* *(mountaineering)* a spring-loaded hook for securing ropes.

karakul /'kærə,kʊl/ *n* (the black fur of) a breed of sheep from the Bukhara region of central Asia.

karaoke /,kɛri'o:ki:/ *n* a CD music system that plays recordings of popular songs with the vocal part removed to allow amateurs to sing along.

karat /'kɛrət/ *n* a measure of weight for precious stones; a measure of the purity of gold.—*also* **carat**.

karate /kə'rɒti/ *n* a Japanese system of unarmed combat using sharp blows of the feet and hands.

Karen /kə'rɛn/ *n* *(pl* **Karens, Karen**) *n* a member of a Thai people in Burma, or their language.

karma /'kɒrmə/ *n* *(Buddhism, Hinduism)* the sum of a person's actions during one of their existences, held to determine their destiny in the next; *(inf)* a certain aura that a person or place is felt to possess.—**karmic** *adj.*

karoo, karroo /kə'ru:/ *n* *(pl* **karoos, karroos**) *(S Africa)* *(sometimes with a cap)* a series of clayey tablelands, *usu* barren except in the wet season; a system of rocks in, or a period; of this period.

kart /kɑrt/ *n* a small motorized vehicle used in racing.—*also* **go-kart**.

karting /-ɪŋ/ *n* kart racing.

karyo- /'kærio:/ *prefix* = nucleus.

katydid /'keɪtɪdɪd/ *n* a large green North American insect like a grasshopper.

kauri /kau'ri/ *n* *(pl* **kauris**) a New Zealand pine with oval leaves from which a resinous gum is extracted; the wood or gum from this tree.

kava /'kɒvə/ *n* a Polynesian shrub; an intoxicating and narcotic drink made from it.

kayak /'kaɪæk/ *n* an Eskimo canoe made of skins on a wooden frame.—*also* **kaiak**.

kazoo /kə'zu:/ *n* *(pl* **kazoos**) a small tube-shaped musical instrument through which one hums to vibrate a membrane-covered hole at the end or side

KB *abbr* = kilobyte.

KBE *abbr* = Knight Commander of the Order of the British Empire.

kc *abbr* = kilocycle.

KCB *abbr* = Knight Commander of the Order of the Bath.

KE *abbr* = kinetic energy.

kebab /kə'bɒb/ or /-'bæb/ *n* small cubes of grilled meat and vegetables, *usu* served on a skewer.

keck /kɛk/ *vi* to make a sound as if about to vomit; to feel or express loathing.

keddah /'kɛdə/ *n* in India and Burma, an enclosure for catching wild elephants.

kedge /kɛdʒ/ *n* a small anchor for kedging a ship. • *vt* to move (a ship) by hauling on a cable attached to a kedge.

kedgeree /'kɛdʒəri/ or /-'ri:/ *n* a dish containing fish, rice and hard-boiled eggs.

keef /ki:f/ *see* **kif**.

keek /ki:k/ *vt* *(Scot)* to peep cheekily.

keel /ki:l/ *n* one of the main structural members of a ship extending along the bottom from stem to stern to which the frame is attached; any structure resembling this. • *vti* (to cause) to turn over.

keelhaul /'ki:lhɒl/ *vt* *(formerly)* to drag under water beneath the bottom of a ship from one side to the other; to reprimand sternly.

keelson /'ki:lsən/ *n* a beam of timber laid on the middle of the floor timbers over the keel of a vessel to strengthen it.—*also* **kelson**.

keen[1] /ki:n/ *adj* eager, enthusiastic; intellectually acute, shrewd; having a sharp point or fine edge; *(senses)* perceptive, penetrating; extremely cold and piercing; intense; *(prices)* very low so as to be competitive.—**keenly** *adv.*—**keenness** *n*.

keen[2] *n* a dirge or lament for the dead. • *vi* to lament the dead.

keep /ki:p/ *vb* *(keeping, kept)* *vt* to celebrate, observe; to fulfil; to protect, guard; to take care of; to preserve; to provide for; to make regular entries in; to maintain in a specified state; to hold for the future; to hold and not let go; (*with* **at**) to harass (a person) into continuing (some task, etc); (*with* **back**) to refuse to disclose; to restrain; (*with* **down**) to repress; to subdue; (*with* **from**) to abstain or restrain from; to preserve as a secret (from someone); (*with* **to**) to cause to adhere strictly to; (*with* **up**) to persist in; to continue; to maintain in good condition. • *vi* to stay in a specified condition; to continue, go on; to refrain or restrain oneself to stay fresh, not spoil; (*with* **at**) to persist; (*with* **away**) to prevent from approaching; (*with* **down**) to stay hidden; (*with* **on**) to talk or nag continuously; (*with* **to**) to (cause to) adhere strictly to; (*with* **up**) to maintain the same pace, level of knowledge, etc as another; to stay informed; to continue relentlessly. • *n* food and shelter; care and custody; the inner stronghold of a castle.

keeper /'ki:pər/ *n* one who guards, watches, or takes care of persons or things.

keeping /-ɪŋ/ *n* care, charge; observance; agreement, conformity.

keepsake /-seɪk/ *n* something kept in memory of the giver.

kef /kef/ *see* **kif**.

keg /keg/ *n* a small barrel.

kelp /kelp/ *n* a large brown seaweed.

kelpie /'kelpi/ *n* (*pl* **kelpies**) in Scottish folklore, a malevolent water sprite, supposed to take the form of a horse.

Keltic /'keltɪk/ *see* **Celtic**.

kelvin /'kelvɪn/ *n* a unit of temperature of the Kelvin scale

Kelvin scale *n* temperature on a scale where absolute zero (-273.15° Celsius) is taken as zero degrees.

ken /ken/ *n* understanding; view; sight. • *vt* (**kenning, kenned** *or* **kent**) to know; to recognize at sight.

kendo /'kendo:/ *n* a Japanese style of fencing with bamboo staves.

kennel /'kenəl/ *n* a small shelter for a dog, a doghouse; (*often pl*) a place where dogs are bred or kept. • *vt* (**kennelling, kennelled** *or* **kenneling, kenneled**) to keep in a kennel.

keno /ki:no/ *n* a game of chance, similar to bingo played with numbered balls and cards.

kenosis /kɪ'no:sɪs/ *n* (*theology*) the self-limitation of Christ in laying aside his divinity and becoming man.—**kerotic** *adj*.

kentledge /'kentlədʒ/ *n* (*naut*) ballast of scrap metal.

kepi /'kepi/ *or* /'keɪpi/ *n* (*pl* **kepis**) a French military peaked cap.

kept /kept/ *see* **keep**.

keratin /'kerətɪn/ *n* a tough, fibrous protein, the substance of hair, nails, feathers, etc.

keratitis /kerə'taɪtɪs/ *n* inflammation of the cornea.

keratose /'kerə,to:s/ *adj* (*sponges*) having a horn-like skeleton.

kerb /kɜrb/ *n* a line of raised stone forming the edge of a pavement; a curb.

kerbing /'kɜrbɪŋ/ *n* kerbstones collectively; material for kerbstones, curbing.

kerbstone /'kɜrbsto:n/ *n* the stone edge of a path, curbstone.

kerchief /'kɜrtʃɪf/ *or* /-tʃi:f/ *n* a piece of square cloth worn on the head.

kerf /kɜrf/ *n* a cut or slit made by a saw, etc.

kermes /'kɜrmiz/ *n* the dried bodies of female scale insects from which a dye of a deep cherry red colour is obtained; an oak tree found in Europe and Asia, on which these insects live.

kermis /'kɜrmɪs/ *n* an open-air festival or fair.

kern [1], **kerne** /kɜrn/ *n* (*formerly*) a lightly armed Irish or Scottish medieval foot-soldier; a troop of these; (*arch*) a peasant.

kern [2] *n* (*print*) the part of a type or character that overhangs the following piece of type or character.

kernel /'kɜrnəl/ *n* the inner edible part of a fruit or nut; the essential part of anything.

kerosene, kerosine /'kerə,si:n/ *n* a fuel oil distilled from petroleum, paraffin.

kersey /'kɜrzi/ *n* a coarse smooth-faced woollen cloth.

kerseymere /'kɜrzɪmɪːr/ *n* a twilled cloth of fine wool.

kestrel /'kestrəl/ *n* a type of small falcon.

ketch /ketʃ/ *n* a small two-masted sailing vessel.

ketchup /'ketʃəp/ *n* any of various thick sauces, *esp* one made from puréed tomato, for meat, fish, etc.—*also* **catchup, catsup**.

ketone /'ki:to:n/ *n* a class of chemical compounds, the simplest being acetone.

kettle /'ketəl/ *n* a container with a handle and spout for boiling water.

kettledrum /'ketəl,drəm/ *n* a musical instrument consisting of a hollow metal body with a parchment head, the tension of which controls the pitch and is adjusted by screws.

kevel /'kevəl/ *n* (*naut*) a cleat for belaying ropes.

key [1] /ki:/ *n* a device for locking and unlocking something; a thing that explains or solves, as the legend of a map, a code, etc; a controlling position, person, or thing; one of a set of parts or levers pressed in a keyboard or typewriter, etc; (*mus*) a system of related tones based on a keynote and forming a given scale; style or mood of expression; a roughened surface for improved adhesion of plaster, etc; an electric circuit breaker. • *vt* to furnish with a key; to bring into harmony. • *adj* controlling; important.

key [2] *n* a low island or reef.

keyboard /'ki:bɔrd/ *n* a set of keys in a piano, organ, microcomputer, etc.

keyhole /'ki:ho:l/ *n* an opening (in a lock) into which a key is inserted.

keyhole surgery *n* surgery performed through small incisions in the body using fibre-optic tubes both for internal examination and as conduits for tiny surgical instruments.

Keynesianism /'keɪnziə,nɪzəm/ *n* the economic theories based on the works of the English economist John Maynard Keynes (1883–1946).—**Keynesian** *adj*.

keynote /'ki:no:t/ *n* the basic note of a musical scale; the basic idea or ruling principle. • *vt* to give the keynote of; to give the keynote speech at.

keypad /'ki:pæd/ *n* a small *usu* hand-held keyboard of numbered buttons used to tap in a telephone number, operate a calculator, etc.

key signature *n* the sharps or flats at the beginning of a musical stave to indicate the key.

keystone /'ki:sto:n/ *n* the middle stone at the top of an arch, holding the stones or other pieces in place.

keystroke /'ki:stro:k/ *n* the depressing of a key on a typewriter, computer keyboard, etc.

kg /'keɪdʒi:/ *abbr* = kilogram(s).

KGB /keɪdʒi:'bi:/ *abbr* = (*formerly*) the secret police of the USSR.

khaddar, khadi /'kodi/ *n* an Indian homespun cotton cloth.

khaki /'kæki/ *or* /'koki/, /'korki/ *adj* dull yellowish-brown. • *n* (*pl* **khakis**) strong, twilled cloth of this colour; (*often pl*) a khaki uniform or trousers.

khamsin /'kæmsɪn/ *n* a hot southerly wind, *esp* in Egypt, that blows for about 50 days in spring.—**kamseen, kamsin**.

khan /kon/ *or* /kæn/ *n* the title of a ruler, prince, or governor in Asia.

khanate /'kon,eɪt/ *or* /'kæn-/ *n* the rule or jurisdiction of a khan.

khedive /kɪ'di:v/ *n* the title of the viceroy of Egypt (1867–1914).

khoraschot /'xorəʃot/ *n* the policy in the former USSR, initiated by President Gorbachev, of the decentralized economic accountability of managers in industrial production and other enterprises.

kHz *abbr* = kilohertz.

kiang /ki'æŋ/ *n* a wild ass of Tibet.

kibble /'kɪbəl/ *vt* to grind coarsely. • *n* a raiseable bucket used in wells, mines etc.

kibbutz /kɪ'buts/ *n* (*pl* **kibbutzim**) an agricultural commune in Israel.

kibbutznik /kɪ'butsnɪk/ *n* a person who lives in a kibbutz.

kibe /kaɪb/ *n* ulcerated chilblain, *esp* one on the heel.

kiblah, kibla /'kɪblɔ/ *n* the point to which Muslims turn at prayer, Mecca.

kibosh /'kaɪbɒʃ/ *n* (*sl*) nonsense.

kick /kɪk/ *vt* to strike with the foot; to drive, force, etc as by kicking; to score (a goal, etc) by kicking; (*with* **about, around**) (*inf*) to abuse physically or mentally; to discuss or analyse (a problem, etc) in a relaxed unsystematic manner; (*with* **out**) (*inf*) to eject, dismiss; (*with* **up**) (*inf*) to cause (trouble, etc). • *vi* to strike out with the foot; to recoil, as a gun; (*inf*) to complain; (*with* **about, around**) (*inf*) to wander idly; to be unused or forgotten; (*with* **off**) (*football*) to give the ball the first kick to start play; (*inf*) to start. • *n* an act or method of kicking; a sudden recoil; (*inf*) a thrill; (*inf*) an intoxicating effect.—**kicker** *n*.

kickback /'kɪkbæk/ *n* a recoil; (*inf*) a returning of part of a sum of money received in payment.

kickoff /'kɪkɒf/ *n* (*football*) a kick putting the ball into play; the beginning or start of proceedings, *eg* a discussion.

kickshaw /'kɪkʃɔ/ *n* a trifle, trinket; (*arch*) a small, light, fancy dish, a delicacy.

kickstand /'kɪkstænd/ *n* a retractable stand for parking a bicycle or motorbike.

kid /kɪd/ *n* a young goat; soft leather made from its skin; (*inf*) a child. • *vti* (**kidding, kidded**) (*inf*) to tease or fool playfully; (*goat*) to bring forth young.—**kidder** *n*.

kiddy, kiddie /'kɪdi/ *n* (*pl* **kiddies**) (*inf*) a child.

kidnap /'kɪdnæp/ *vt* (**kidnapping, kidnapped** *or* **kidnaping, kidnaped**) to seize and hold to ransom, as of a person.—**kidnapper, kidnaper** *n*.

kidney /'kɪdni/ *n* (*pl* **kidneys**) either of a pair of glandular organs excreting waste products from the blood as urine; an animal's kidney used as food.

kidney bean *n* any of various cultivated beans, *esp* a large dark red bean seed.

kidney stone *n* a hard mineral deposit in the kidney.

kidskin /'kɪdskɪn/ *n* a soft leather made from the skin of a young goat.

kief /kiːf/ *see* **kif**.

kier /kiːr/ *n* a vat in which cloth is boiled for bleaching.

kieselguhr /'kiːzəlˌgʊr/ *n* mineral remains of algae, used for filtering and insulation purposes etc.

kif /kɪf/ *n* a drowsy state of well-being produced by marijuana; marijuana itself; any drug producing a similar state.—*also* **keef, kef, kief**.

kill /kɪl/ *vt* to cause the death of; to destroy; to neutralize (a colour); to spend (time) on trivial matters; to turn off (an engine, etc); (*inf*) to cause severe discomfort or pain to. • *n* the act of killing; an animal or animals killed.—**killer** *n*.

killdeer /'kɪldiːr/ *n* ✽ a large North American plover with a mournful call.

killer whale /'kɪlər/ *n* a carnivorous black-and-white toothed whale.

killick /'kɪlɪk/, **killock** *n* (*naut*) a heavy stone used as an anchor; a small anchor.

killing /'kɪlɪŋ/ *adj* (*inf*) tiring; very amusing; causing death, deadly. • *n* the act of killing, murder; (*inf*) a sudden (financial) success.—**killingly** *adv*.

killjoy /'kɪldʒɔɪ/ *n* a person who spoils other people's enjoyment.

kiln /kɪln/ *n* a furnace or large oven for baking or drying (lime, bricks, etc).

kilo /'kiːloː/ *n* (*pl* **kilos**) kilogram; kilometre.

kilo- /'kiːloː/ *prefix* one thousand.

kilobyte /'kɪləbəɪt/ *n* 1024 bytes.

kilocalorie /'kɪləˌkæləri/ *n* a Calorie.

kilocycle /'kɪləˌsəɪkəl/ *n* a kilohertz.

kilogram /'kɪləgræm/ *n* a unit of weight and mass, equal to 1000 grams or 2.2046 pounds.

kilohertz /'kɪləˌhɜrts/ *n* one thousand cycles per second, 1000 hertz.

kilolitre, kiloliter /'kɪləˌliːtər/ *n* one thousand litres.

kilometre, kilometer /kɪ'lɒmɪtər/ *or* /'kɪləˌmiːtər/ *n* a unit of length equal to 1000 metres or 0.62 mile.—**kilometric** *adj*.

kiloton /'kɪləˌtɒn/ *n* a unit of explosive force equal to 1000 tons of TNT.

kilowatt /'kɪləˌwɒt/ *n* a unit of electrical power, equal to 1000 watts.

kilowatt-hour *n* a unit of energy equal to work done by one kilowatt in one hour.

kilt /kɪlt/ *n* a knee-length skirt made from tartan material pleated at the sides, worn as part of the Scottish Highland dress for men and women.

kilter /'kɪltər/ *n* good working order; good condition (*out of kilter*).

kimono /kɪ'moːnoː/ *or* /-nə/ *n* (*pl* **kimonos**) a loose Japanese robe.

kin /kɪn/ *n* relatives; family.—*see* **kith**.

kind[1] /kaɪnd/ *n* sort; variety; class; a natural group or division; essential character.

kind[2] *adj* sympathetic; friendly; gentle; benevolent.—**kindness** *n*.

kindergarten /'kɪndərˌgɑrtən/ *n* a class or school for very young children.

kind-hearted /'kaɪndˌhɑrtɪd/ *adj* benevolent; kind, warm.—**kind-heartedly** *adv*.

kindle /'kɪndəl/ *vt* to set on fire; to excite (feelings, interest, etc). • *vi* to catch fire; to become aroused or excited.

kindling /'kɪndlɪŋ/ *n* material, such as bits of dry wood, for starting a fire.

kindly /'kaɪndli/ *adj* (**kindlier, kindliest**) kind; gracious; agreeable; pleasant. • *adv* in a kindly manner; favourably.—**kindliness** *n*.

kindred /'kɪndrəd/ *n* a person's family or relatives; family relationship; resemblance. • *adj* related; like, similar.

kine /kaɪn/ *n* (*pl*) (*arch*) cattle.

kinematic /ˌkɪnə'mætɪk/ *or* /ˌkaɪ-/ *adj* of pure motion, without reference to force etc.

kinematics /-s/ *n sing* the science of pure motion.

kinetic /kɪ'nɛtɪk/ *or* /kaɪ-/ *adj* of or produced by movement.—**kinetically** *adv*.

kinetic art *n* sculpture, etc that moves or has moving parts.

kinetic energy *n* energy derived from motion.

kinetics /kɪ'nɛtɪks/ *or* /kaɪ-/ *n* (*used as sing*) the science of the effects of forces in producing or changing motion; the study of the mechanisms and rates of chemical reactions.

king /kɪŋ/ *n* the man who rules a country and its people; a man with the title of ruler, but with limited power to rule; man supreme in a certain sphere; something best in its class; the chief piece in chess; a playing card with a picture of a king on it, ranking above a queen; (*draughts*) a piece that has been crowned.

King Charles spaniel *n* a small breed of spaniel with black and brown markings.

kingcup /'kɪŋkʌp/ *n* the marsh marigold; any of various yellow-flowered, five-petalled plants, such as the buttercup or clematis.

kingdom /'kɪŋdəm/ *n* a country headed by a king or queen; a realm, domain; any of the three divisions of the natural world: animal: vegetable, mineral.

kingfisher /'kɪŋˌfɪʃər/ *n* a short-tailed diving bird that feeds chiefly on fish.

King James Bible, King James Version *n* the version of the Bible published by the sanction of James I of England and VI of Scotland in 1611 and appointed to be read in churches.—*also* **Authorized Version**.

kinglet /'kɪŋlət/ *n* a minor king; a small bird with a yellow crown found throughout North America.

kingly /'kɪŋli/ *adj* (**kinglier, kingliest**) of, resembling, or fit for a king.—**kingliness** *n*.

king-of-arms /'kɪŋəv'ɑrmz/ *n* (*pl* **kings-of-arms**) chief officer of the Heralds' College.

kingpin /'kɪŋpɪn/ *n* (*sl*) the chief person in a company, group, etc; the pin in a car, etc that attaches the stub axle to the axle beam and allows limited movement to the stub axle; the foremost pin in tenpin bowling; the central pin in ninepins; the crux of an argument.

kingship /'kɪŋʃɪp/ *n* the office or authority of a king; the art of ruling as king.

king-size /'kɪŋˌsaɪz/, **king-sized** *adj* larger than standard size.

kink /kɪŋk/ *n* a tight twist or curl in a piece of string, rope, hair, etc; a painful cramp in the neck, back, etc; a minor problem in some course of action; a personality quirk; (*Brit sl*) a sexual deviation; (*pl*) (*Scot*) a convulsive fit of laughter; (*US*) a bright, original idea. • *vt* to form kinks.

kinkajou /'kɪŋkəˌdʒuː/ *n* nocturnal long-tailed quadruped of Central and Southern America similar to a racoon.—*also* **honeybear**; a short-tailed primate with spiny protrusions from the neck.—*also* **potto**.

kinky /'kɪŋki/ *adj* (**kinkier, kinkiest**) full of kinks; (*inf*) eccentric; (*inf*) sexually bizarre.—**kinkiness** *n*.

kinnikinnick /ˌkɪnɪkɪ'nɪk/ *n* ✽ (*hist*) among some Indian peoples, a substitute for tobacco made from dried wild berries and leaves.

kino (gum) /'kinoː/ *n* an astringent vegetable gum of a dark red colour, used in medicine, tanning etc.

kinsfolk /'kɪnzfoːk/ *n* blood relations.

kinship /'kɪnʃɪp/ *n* blood relationship; close connection.

kinsman /'kɪnzmən/, **kinswoman** /-ˌwʊmən/ *n* (*pl* **kinsmen, kinswomen**) a relative, *esp* by blood.

kiosk /'kiːɒsk/ *n* a small open structure used for selling newspapers, confectionery, etc; a public telephone booth.

kip /kɪp/ *vi* (**kipping, kipped**) (*sl*) to sleep. • *n* (*sl*) sleep, a lodging.

kipper /'kɪpər/ *n* a kippered herring, etc. • *vt* to cure (fish) by salting and drying or smoking.

kirk /kɜrk/ *n* (*Scot*) a church.

kirsch /kiːrʃ/, **kirschwasser** /'kɪrʃˌvɒsər/ *n* a type of brandy made from cherries.

kismet /'kɪzmɛt/ *or* /'kɪs-/ *n* fate, destiny.

kiss /kɪs/ *vti* to touch with the lips as an expression of love, affection or in greeting; to touch the lips with those of another person as a sign of love or desire; to touch lightly. • *n* an act of kissing; a light, gentle touch.—**kissable** *adj*.

kissagram /'kɪsə,græm/ *n* a celebratory telegram or message delivered with a kiss.

kiss-and-tell /'kɪsən,tel/ *adj* (*inf*) pertaining to the publication of memoirs that reveal hitherto secret details.

kisser /'kɪsər/ *n* one who kisses; (*sl*) the mouth or face.

kiss of life *n* mouth-to-mouth resuscitation.

kist /kɪst/ *n* (*Scot*) a chest or box; (*arch*) a cist; (*S Africa*) a large chest or box used for storing linen, *esp* for a trousseau.

kit /kɪt/ *n* clothing and personal equipment, etc; tools and equipment for a specific purpose; a set of parts with instructions ready to be assembled. • *vt* (**kitting, kitted**) (*usu with out or up*) to provide with kit.

kitchen /'kɪtʃən/ *n* a place where food is prepared and cooked.

kitchenette /,kɪtʃɪ'net/ *n* a small kitchen.

kitchen garden *n* a garden where vegetables are grown for domestic use.

kite /kaɪt/ *n* a bird of prey with long narrow wings and a forked tail; a light frame covered with a thin covering for flying in the wind.

kith /kɪθ/ *n* friends and relations, now only in **kith and kin**.

kithara /'kɪθərə/ *see* **cithara**.

kitsch /kɪtʃ/ *n* art, literature, etc regarded as pretentious, inferior, or in poor taste.—*also adj*.—**kitschy** *adj*.

kitten /'kɪtən/ *n* a young cat; the young of other small mammals. • *vti* to give birth to kittens.

kittenish /'kɪtənɪʃ/ *adj* like a kitten, playful; (*woman*) flirtatious.

kittiwake /'kɪti,weɪk/ *n* either of two types of gull with blacktipped wings.

kittle /'kɪtəl/ *adj* (*Scot*) difficult to manage, capricious. • *vt* (*Scot*) to tickle; to cause (someone) to be puzzled or to bother someone.

kitty /'kɪti/ *n* (*pl* **kitties**) the stakes in a game of poker or other gambling game; a shared fund of money; affectionate name for a cat or kitten.

kiwi /'kiːwiː/ *n* (*pl* **kiwis**) a flightless bird of New Zealand; (*inf*) a New Zealander.

kiwi fruit *n* a fruit of an Asian vine.—*also* **Chinese gooseberry**.

KKK *abbr* = Ku Klux Klan.

kl *abbr* = kiloliter.

klaxon /'klæksən/ *n* a type of old-fashioned motor horn.

kleptomania /,klepto'meɪniə/ *n* an uncontrollable impulse to steal.—**kleptomaniac** *n*.

klipspringer /'klɪp,sprɪŋər/ *n* a small antelope of South Africa.

kloof /kluːf/ *n* a ravine, a deep narrow valley, in South Africa.

klystron /'klaɪstrɒn/ *n* an electronic device that generates and amplifies microwaves.

km *abbr* = kilometre(s).

knack /næk/ *n* an ability to do something easily; a trick; a habit.

knacker /'nækər/ *n* one who buys worn-out horses or old houses, ships, etc, for destruction.

knackwurst /'nækwɔrst/ *n* a type of spicy German sausage.

knap /næp/ (**knapping, knapped**) *vt* to break, snap or hit something.

knapsack /'næpsæk/ *n* a bag for carrying equipment or supplies on the back.

knapweed /'næpwiːd/ *n* a purple-flowered weed.

knar /nɑr/ *see* **knur**.

knave /neɪv/ *n* (*formerly*) a tricky or dishonest man; the jack in a pack of playing cards.—**knavish** *adj*—**knavishly** *adv*.

knavery /'neɪvəri/ *n* (*pl* **knaveries**) dishonesty; fraud; deceit.

knead /niːd/ *vt* to squeeze and press together (dough, clay, etc) into a uniform lump with the hands; to make (bread, etc) by kneading; to squeeze and press with the hands.—**kneader** *n*.

knee /niː/ *n* the joint between the thigh and the lower part of the human leg; anything shaped like a bent knee. • *vt* (**kneeing, kneed**) to hit or touch with the knee.

kneecap /'niːkæp/ *n* the small bone covering and protecting the front part of the knee-joint. • *vt* (**kneecapping, kneecapped**) to maim by shooting into the kneecap.

knee-deep /-'diːp/ *adj* deep enough to cover the knees; deeply involved.

knee jerk /-,jɜrk/ *n* an involuntary jerk when the tendon below the knee is tapped.

kneejerk *adj* responding automatically.

kneel /niːl/ *vi* (**kneeling, kneeled** *or* **knelt**) to go down on one's knee or knees; to remain in this position.—**kneeler** *n*.

knell /nel/ *n* the sound of a bell rung slowly and solemnly at a death or funeral; a warning of death, failure, etc. • *vi* (*bell*) to ring a knell; to summon, announce, etc (as if) by a knell.

knelt /nelt/ *see* **kneel**.

knew /nuː/ *or* /njuː/ *see* **know**.

knickerbocker /'nɪkər,bɒkər/ *n* a New Yorker; a descendant of the founders of the original city.

knickerbockers /-s/ *npl* baggy breeches fastened by a band at the knee.

knickers /'nɪkərz/ *npl* an undergarment covering the lower body and having separate leg holes, worn by women and girls.

knickknack /'nɪknæk/ *n* a small ornament or trinket.—*also* **nicknack**.

knife /naɪf/ *n* (*pl* **knives**) a flat piece of steel, etc, with a sharp edge set in a handle, used to cut or as a weapon; a sharp blade forming part of a tool or machine. • *vt* to cut or stab with a knife.

knife edge /'naɪf,edʒ/ *n* the sharp edge of a knife; anything resembling this, such as the blade of an ice skate; a sharp wedge used as a pivot for a balance; a critical or precarious situation.

knight /naɪt/ *n* (*Middle Ages*) a medieval mounted soldier; a man who for some achievement is given honorary rank entitling him to use "Sir" before his given name; a chessman shaped like a horse's head. • *vt* to make (a man) a knight.—**knightly** *adj*.—**knightliness** *n*.

knight-errant /'naɪt'erənt/ *n* (*pl* **knights-errant**) a quixotic person; (*Middle Ages*) a knight who went in quest of adventure, to show his prowess, chivalry etc.

knight-errantry /-i/ *n* the practices or customs of knights-errant; quixotic behaviour.

knighthood /'naɪt,hud/ *n* the character, rank, or dignity of a knight; the order of knights.

knit /nɪt/ *vb* (**knitting, knitted** *or* **knit**) *vt* to form (fabric or a garment) by interlooping yarn using knitting needles or a machine; to cause (*eg* broken bones) to grow together; to link or join together closely; to draw (the brows) together. • *vi* to make knitted fabric from yarn by means of needles; to grow together; to become joined or united. • *n* a knitted garment or fabric.—**knitter** *n*.

knitting /'nɪtɪŋ/ *n* work being knitted.

knitting needle *n* a long thin eyeless needle, *usu* made of plastic or steel, used in knitting.

knitwear /'nɪtweər/ *n* knitted clothing.

knives /naɪvz/ *see* **knife**.

knob /nɒb/ *n* a rounded lump or protuberance; a handle, *usu* round, of a door, drawer, etc.

knobby /'nɒbi/ *adj* (**knobbier, knobbiest**) full of knobs.

knobkerrie /'nɒb,keri/ *n* a round-headed stick used as a weapon in South Africa.

knock /nɒk/ *vi* to strike with a sharp blow; to rap on a door; to bump, collide; (*engine*) to make a thumping noise; (*with* **off**) (*inf*) to finish work; (*with* **up**) (*tennis, etc*) to practise before a match. • *vt* to strike; (*inf*) to criticize; (*with* **about, around**) to wander around aimlessly; to treat roughly; (*with* **back**) (*inf*) to drink, swallow quickly; to reject, refuse; (*with* **down**) to indicate a sale at an auction; (*with* **down** *or* **off**) to hit so as to cause to fall; (*with* **off**) (*inf*) to do or make hastily and without effort; to reduce in price; to discontinue, *esp* work; (*sl*) to kill; (*sl*) to steal; (*with* **out**) to make unconscious or exhausted; to eliminate in a knockout competition; (*inf*) to amaze; (*with* **up**) (*inf*) to make or arrange hastily; (*cricket*) to score a certain number of runs; to rouse; (*sl*) to make pregnant. • *n* a knocking, a hit, a rap.

knockabout /'nɒkə,baut/ *adj* rough, boisterous.

knockdown *adj* cheap; (*furniture*) easy to dismantle.

knocker /'nɒkər/ *n* a device hinged against a door for use in knocking; (*Brit sl: usu pl*) a woman's breasts.

knock-kneed *adj* having inward-curving legs.

knockout /'nɒkaut/ *n* a punch or blow that produces unconsciousness; a contest in which competitors are eliminated at each round; (*inf*) an attractive or extremely impressive person or thing.

knoll /nəul/ *n* a small round hill.

knot /nɒt/ *n* a lump in a thread, etc formed by a tightened loop or tangling; a fastening made by tying lengths of rope, etc; an ornamental bow; a small group, cluster; a hard mass of wood where a branch grows out from a tree, which shows as a roundish, cross-grained piece in a board; a unit of speed of one nautical mile per hour; something that ties closely, *esp* the bond of marriage. • *vti* (**knotting, knotted**) to make or form a knot (in); to entangle or become entangled.—**knotter** *n*.

knotgrass /'nɒtgræs/ *n* a weed with a jointed stem and green flowers; any of various similar plants.

knothole /'nɒthoːl/ *n* a hole in wood once filled by a knot.

knotting /'nɒtɪŋ/ *n* a kind of lace work made with knots; a sealer applied to knots before priming wood as protection from sap.

knotty /'nɒti/ *adj* (**knottier, knottiest**) full of knots; hard to solve; puzzling.—**knottiness** *n*.

know /noː/ *vt* (**knowing, knew,** *pp* **known**) to be well informed about; to be aware of; to be acquainted with; to recognize or distinguish.—**knowable** *adj*.

know-all /'noːˌɔl/ *n* a know-it-all.

know-how /-ˌhaʊ/ *n* practical skill, experience.

knowing /-ɪŋ/ *adj* having knowledge; shrewd; clever; implying a secret understanding.—**knowingly** *adv*.—**knowingness** *n*.

know-it-all /-ɪtˌɔl/ *n* a person who acts as if they know about everything.

knowledge /'nɒlɪdʒ/ *n* what one knows; the body of facts, etc accumulated over time; fact of knowing; range of information or understanding; the act of knowing.

knowledgeable /'nɒlɪdʒəbəl/ *adj* having knowledge or intelligence; well-informed.—**knowledgeably** *adv*.

known /noːn/ *see* **know**.

knuckle /'nʌkəl/ *n* a joint of the finger, *esp* at the roots of the fingers; the knee of an animal used as food. • *vi* (*with* **down**) (*inf*) to apply oneself in earnest (to some task, duty, etc); (*with* **under**) to submit, to give in.

knuckle-duster /-ˌdʌstər/ *n* a metal device that fits over the knuckles, used for inflicting severe injury by punching.

knur, knurr /nər/ *n* a knot either in a tree trunk or in wood; a hard lump.—*also* **knar**.

knurl /nərl/ *n* a small ridge, *esp* one of a series on a metal surface to prevent slippage.

KO /'keɪoː/ *abbr* = knockout.

koa /'koːə/ *n* a Hawaiian tree; the hard wood it produces used in making furniture.

koala /koːˈɑlə/ *n* an Australian tree-dwelling marsupial with thick, grey fur.

koan /'koːæn/ *n* an insoluble riddle used as a meditation exercise in Zen Buddhism.

kob /kɒb/ *n* a South African water antelope.

kobold /'koːbəld/ *n* a household goblin or elf; a spirit of mines and other underground places.

Kohinoor, Koh-i-nor /'koːɪˌnuːr/ *n* a famous, very large Indian diamond, which has belonged to the British Crown since 1849.

kohl /koːl/ *n* a fine powder, as of antimony, used for darkening the eyelids.

kohlrabi /koːlˈræbi/ *n* (*pl* **kohlrabies**) a variety of cabbage with a thick stem, used as a vegetable.

kokanee /koːˈkæni/ *n* ✤ (*Cdn*) a form of non-migratory salmon of lakes in western Canada.

kola nut /'koːlə/ *n* the seed of either of two tropical trees which has stimulant properties and is chewed or used in making sweet drinks.—*also* **cola nut**.

kolinsky /kəˈlɪnski/ *n* (*pl* **kolinskies**) an Asian mink; its fur.

kolkhoz /'kɒlkɒz/ or /kɛlkˈhɒz/ *n* a collective farm in Russia.

koodoo /'kuːduː/ *n* an African striped antelope with long spiral horns.—*also* **kudu**.

kook /kuːk/ *n* (*inf*) a person regarded as silly, eccentric, etc.

kookaburra /'kʊkəˌbərə/ *n* an Australian kingfisher with a harsh cry like loud laughter.

kooky, kookie /'kuːki/ *adj* (**kookier, kookiest**) (*inf*) crazy; eccentric.

kop /kɒp/ *n* (*S Africa*) an isolated hill.

kopeck, kopek /'koːpɛk/ *n* a Russian coin, one hundred of which comprise one ruble.

kopje /'kɒpi/ *n* (*S Africa*) a hillock or small hill.

Koran /kɔrˈæn/ or /kə-/ *n* the sacred book of the Muslims.—**Koranic** *adj*.

Korean /kəˈriːən/ *n* a native or inhabitant of Korea; the language spoken in North and South Korea. • *adj* of or pertaining to Korea, its language or people.

kosher /'koːʃər/ *adj* (*Judaism*) clean or fit to eat according to dietary laws; (*inf*) acceptable, genuine. • *n* kosher food.

koto /'koːtoː/ *n* (*pl* **kotos**) *n* a Japanese musical instrument with silk strings, similar to a zither.

kowtow /'kaʊtaʊ/ *vi* to show exaggerated respect (to) by bowing.

kph *abbr* = kilometres per hour.

Kr (*chem symbol*) krypton.

kraal /krɑl/ *n* an African village consisting of a group of huts surrounded by a pallisade; a sheepfold, or cattle pen. • to pen sheep or cattle in a kraal.

krait /kraɪt/ *n* a deadly Asian rock snake.

kraken /'krækən/ *n* a gigantic fabled sea monster supposed to live in the sea off Norway.

kremlin /'krɛmlɪn/ *n* a Russian citadel; (*with cap and* **the**) the citadel in Moscow, housing the former palace, cathedrals, and the Russian government; (*with cap*) the central government of Russia.

kriegspiel /'kriːɡspiːl/ *n* (*sometimes with cap*) (*mil*) a game with blocks or models representing the various sections of an army as if in actual warfare, used in training; a chess game for two players, each playing on their own board with their own pieces, unseen by the other, with the moves regulated by a third person also with a board unseen by either player.

krill /krɪl/ *n* (*pl* **krill**) the tiny shrimp-like plankton eaten by many whales.

kris /kriːs/ *n* a Malaysian or Indonesian knife or dagger with a wavy blade.—*also* **crease, creese**.

Krishna /'krɪʃnə/ *n* a great deity of later Hinduism.—**Krishnaism** *n*.

krona /'kroːnə/ *n* (*pl* **kronor**) the monetary unit of Sweden.

króna /'kroːnə/ *n* (*pl* **krónur**) the monetary unit of Iceland.

krone /'kroːnə/ *n* (*pl* **kroner**) the monetary unit of Denmark and Norway.

krypton /'krɪptɒn/ *n* a colourless, odourless gas used in fluorescent lights and lasers.

Kt *abbr* = Knight.

kudlik /'kuːdlɪk/ *n* ✤ an Inuit soapstone lamp in which seal oil is burned.

kudos /'kuːdoːz/ or /-doːs/, /-dɒs/ *n* (*used as sing*) (*inf*) fame, glory, prestige.

kudu /'kuːduː/ *see* **koodoo**.

Kufic /'kuːfɪk/ *see* **Cufic**.

Ku Klux Klan /ˌkuːklʌksˈklæn/ *n* an American secret society hostile to Blacks, Jews, Catholics, etc.

kulak /'kuːlæk/ *n* an independent well-to-do peasant in Russia.

kumiss /'kuːmɪs/ *n* a spirit made in central Asia from fermented mare's milk and sometimes used as a medicine.

kümmel /'kʊməl/ *n* a liqueur flavoured with caraway seeds.

kumquat /'kʌmkwɒt/ *n* a small fruit like an orange with a sweet rind.

kung fu /kʊŋˈfuː/ *n* a Chinese system of unarmed combat.

Kurd /kərd/ *n* a native of Kurdistan, an area of plateaus and mountains covering eastern Turkey, northern Iraq, western Iran, and Armenia.

Kurdish /'kərdɪʃ/ *adj* pertaining to the Kurds or to their language. • *n* the language of the Kurds.

kvass, kvas /kvæs/ *n* a Russian rye beer that has stale bread as one of its ingredients.—*also* **quass**.

kw. *abbr* = kilowatt(s).

kwashiorkor /ˌkwɒʃɪˈɔrkɔr/ *n* a disease, *esp* of children, caused by protein deficiency and characterized by a distended stomach and changes in skin pigmentation.

kwh *abbr* = kilowatt-hour(s).

kyanize /'kaɪəˌnaɪz/ *vt* to preserve wood from dry rot by injecting corrosive sublimate.—**kyanization** *n*.

kymograph /'kaɪməˌɡræf/ *n* an instrument for recording pressure, oscillations, sound waves, etc, *eg* an apparatus for determining the pressure of blood, by means of a stylus on a continually rotating drum of paper; (*phonetics*) an instrument to measure muscular strength in the tongue, lips, etc; an instrument that records the angular oscillations of an aircraft in the air.—*also* **cymograph**.

Kyrie (eleison) /'kiːriˌeɪ/ *n* a prayer, part of a mass; a musical setting of this; the response in an Anglican communion service.

L

L, l /ɛl/ *n* the 12th letter of the English alphabet; something shaped like an L.

l *abbr* = litre(s).

La (*chem symbol*) lanthanum.

la /lɑ/ *n* the name given to the sixth note of the diatonic scale in solmization.

laager /'lɒgər/ *n* (*S Africa*) a camp in a circle of wagons.—*also* **lager**.

Lab. *abbr* ✠ = Labrador.

lab /læb/ *n* (*inf*) laboratory.

labarum /'læbərəm/ *n* (*pl* **labara**) a banner used in Christian processions.

label /'leɪbəl/ *n* a slip of paper, cloth, metal, etc attached to anything to provide information about its nature, contents, ownership, etc; a term of generalized classification. • *vt* (**labelling, labelled** *or* **labeling, labeled**) to attach a label to; to designate or classify (as).—**labeller, labeler** *n*.

labellum /lə'beləm/ *n* (*pl* **labella**) the lower petal of an orchid.

labia /'leɪbiə/ *npl* (*sing* **labium**) the lips of the female genitals, comprising the outer pair (*labia majora*) and the inner pair (*labia minora*).

labial /'leɪbiəl/ *adj* of the lips or labia.

labialize /-aɪz/ *vt* (*phonetics*) to pronounce (a sound) by rounding one's lips.—**labialization** *n*.

labiate /-eɪt/ *adj, n* (*bot*) (a plant) with the corolla or calyx divided into two parts, resembling lips.

labile /'leɪbaɪl/ *or* /-bɪl/ *adj* (*chem*) unstable.

labiodental /ˌleɪbioˈdentəl/ *adj* (*phonetics*) (*sound*) formed by the lips and teeth.

labionasal /-'neɪsəl/ *adj* (*phonetics*) (*sound*) formed by the lips and nose.

labium /'leɪbiəm/ *see* **labia**.

labor *see* **labour**.

Labor Day *n* the first Monday in September in US and Canada, a legal holiday honouring labour.

laboratory /'læbrəˌtɔri/ *or* /lə'bɒrə-, lə'bɒrətri/ *n* *pl* **laboratories**) a room or building where scientific work and research is carried out.

laborious /lə'bɔriəs/ *adj* requiring much work; hard-working; laboured.—**laboriously** *adv*.—**laboriousness** *n*.

labour, labor /'leɪbər/ *n* work, physical or mental exertion; a specific task; all wage-earning workers; workers collectively; the process of childbirth. • *vi* to work; to work hard; to move with difficulty; to suffer (delusions, etc); to be in childbirth. • *vt* to develop in unnecessary detail.

Labour Day *n* ✠ a public holiday to honour workers, held in Canada and the United States on the first Monday in September, elsewhere on May.

laboured, labored /-bərd/ *adj* done with effort; strained.—**labouredly, laboredly** *adv*.

labourer, laborer /-bərər/ *n* a person who labours, *esp* a person whose work requires strength rather than skill.

labour or labor union *n* an organized association of employees of any trade or industry for the protection of their income and working conditions.

Labradorian *n* ✠ (*Cdn*) a person who lives in or is from Labrador.

Labrador retriever *n* a breed of large, smooth-coated sporting dog.

labradorite /læbrə'dɔraɪt/ *n* a type of feldspar.

labret /'læbrɪt/ *n* a shell, etc, worn as an ornament in the lip.

labrum /'leɪbrəm/ *n* (*pl* **labra** /-brə/) the liplike shield of an insect's mouth.

laburnum /lə'bɜrnəm/ *n* a small tree or shrub with hanging yellow flowers.

labyrinth /'læbərɪnθ/ *n* a structure containing winding passages through which it is hard to find one's way; a maze.—**labyrinthine** *adj*.

lac[1] /læk/ *n* a resinous substance secreted by certain insects.

lac[2] *see* **lakh**.

lace /leɪs/ *n* a cord, etc used to draw together and fasten parts of a shoe, a corset, etc; a delicate ornamental fabric of openwork design using fine cotton, silk, etc. • *vt* to fasten with a lace or laces; to intertwine, weave; to fortify (a drink, etc) with a dash of spirits.

lacerate /'læsəˌreɪt/ *vt* to tear jaggedly; to wound (feelings, etc).—**laceration** *n*.

laches /'lætʃɪz/ *or* /'leɪ-/ *n* (*law*) undue delay in claiming one's rights, etc.

lachrimatory /'lækrɪmətəri/ *n* (*pl* **lachrimatories**) a vessel used to hold tears, found in ancient Roman tombs.

lachrimal /'lækrɪməl/ *adj* of tears; relating to the glands that secrete tears.—*also* **lacrimal**.

lachrymose /'lækrɪˌmoʊs/ *adj* tending to shed tears; sad.—**lachrymosity** *n*.

laciniate /lə'sɪniət/, **laciniated** /-əd/ *adj* (*biol*) cut into narrow lobes, fringed.

lack /læk/ *n* the fact or state of not having any or not having enough; the thing that is needed. • *vti* to be deficient in or entirely without.

lackadaisical /ˌlækə'deɪzɪkəl/ *adj* showing lack of energy or interest; listless.—**lackadaisically** *adv*.

lackey /'læki/ *n* a male servant of low rank; a servile hanger-on.

lacklustre, lacklustre /'lækˌlʌstər/ *adj* lacking in brightness or vigour; dull.

laconic /lə'kɒnɪk/ *adj* using few words; concise.—**laconically** *adv*.—**laconicism** *n*.

lacquer /'lækər/ *n* a glossy varnish. • *vt* to coat with lacquer, to make glossy.

lacrimal *see* **lachrymal**.

lacrosse /lə'krɒs/ *n* a game played by two teams of 10 players with the aim of throwing a ball through the opponents' goal using a long stick topped with a netted pouch for catching and carrying the ball.

lact-, lacto- /'læktoʊ/ *prefix* milk.

lactate /læk'teɪt/ *vi* (*mammals*) to secrete milk.

lactation /-'teɪʃən/ *n* the secretion of milk.—**lactational** *adj*.

lacteal /'læktiəl/ *adj* pertaining to, or resembling, milk; (*anat*) conveying chyle.

lactescent /læk'tesənt/ *adj* milky; (*plant, insect*) yielding a milky juice.—**lactescence** *n*.

lactic /'læktɪk/ *adj* of or relating to milk; obtained from sour milk or whey; involving the production of lactic acid.

lactic acid *n* an organic acid normally present in sour milk.

lactiferous /læk'tɪfərəs/ *adj* producing milk, or a milky juice.

lacto-, lact- /'læktoʊ/ *prefix* milk.

lactometer /læk'tɒmɪtər/ *n* an instrument used for determining the quality of milk.

lactose /'læktoʊs/ *or* /-toʊz/ *n* a sugar present in milk.

lacuna /lə'kjuːnə/ *n* (*pl* **lacunas, lacunae**) a gap, *esp* a missing portion in a text.—**lacunary** *adj*.

lacustrine /lə'kʌstraɪn/ *adj* pertaining to lakes; growing by lakesides.

lacy /'leɪsi/ *adj* (**lacier, laciest**) resembling lace.—**lacily** *adv*.—**laciness** *n*.

lad /læd/ *n* a boy; a young man; a fellow, chap.

ladder /'lædər/ *n* a portable metal or wooden framework with rungs between two vertical supports for climbing up and down; something that resembles a ladder in form or use.

ladder back chair *n* a type of chair with a tall slatted back.

laddie /'lædi/ *n* a boy; a young lad.

lade /leɪd/ *vt* (**lading, laded,** *pp* **laden** *or* **laded**) (*ship*) to load (with cargo); (*with* **with**) to burden; to spoon up (liquid), *eg* with a ladle.

laden /'leɪdən/ *adj* loaded with cargo; burdened.

la-di-da, la-de-da /ˌlɑːdiˈdɑː/ *adj* (*inf*) affected; foppish. • *n* an affected or foppish person

ladies' room *n* a public lavatory for women.

lading /'leɪdɪŋ/ *n* the act of lading; that which is loaded; cargo; freight.

ladle /'leɪdəl/ *n* a long-handled, cup-like spoon for scooping liquids; a device like a ladle in shape or use. • (*with* **out**) (*inf*) to give (money, etc) generously.—**ladleful** *n*.

lady /'leɪdɪ/ *n* (*pl* **ladies**) a polite term for any woman; (*with cap*) a title of honour given to various ranks of women in the British peerage.

Lady Day *n* 25 March, the feast of the Annunciation.

ladybug /'leɪdɪ,bʌg/, **ladybird** /-,bɜrd/ *n* a small, *usu* brightly coloured beetle.

lady-in-waiting *n* (*pl* **ladies-in-waiting**) a female member of a royal household, who attends upon a queen or princess.

lady-killer *n* (*inf*) a man who is or thinks he is particularly attractive to women.

ladylike /'leɪdɪ,laɪk/ *adj* like or suitable for a lady; refined, polite.

ladylove /'leɪdɪlʌv/ *n* (*arch*) a sweetheart.

ladyship /'leɪdɪʃɪp/ *n* a title used in speaking to or of a woman with the rank of Lady.

lady-slipper *n* an orchid with flowers resembling slippers.

lady's-smock *n* a flowering plant, also known as the cuckooflower.

laevorotation *see* **levorotation**.

laevulose *see* **levulose**.

lag[1] /læg/ *vi* (**lagging, lagged**) to fall behind, hang back; to fail to keep pace in movement or development; to weaken in strength or intensity. • *n* a falling behind; a delay.

lag[2] *vt* (**lagging, lagged**) to insulate (pipes, etc) with lagging.

lag[3] *n* (*sl*) a convict; a term of imprisonment.

lagan /'lægən/ *n* goods, or wreckage, lying on the seabed.—*also* **ligan**.

lager[1] /'lɒgər/ *n* a light beer that has been aged for a certain period.

lager[2] *see* **laager**.

laggard /'lægərd/ *n* a person who lags behind; a loiterer. • *adj* backward, slow.—**laggardly** *adv*.

lagging /'lægɪŋ/ *n* insulating material used to lag pipes, boilers, etc.

lagoon /lə'guːn/ *n* a shallow lake or pond, *esp* one connected with a larger body of water; the water enclosed by a circular coral reef.

laic /'leɪɪk/, **laical** /-əl/ *adj* non-clerical, lay; secular.

laicize /'leɪɪ,saɪz/ *vt* to make non-clerical or lay; to open to lay persons.—**laicization** *n*.

laid /'leɪd/ *see* **lay**[2].

laid-back /'leɪd,bæk/ *adj* relaxed, easy-going.

laid paper *n* paper impressed with fine lines from the wires on which the pulp is laid.

lain /leɪn/ *see* **lie**[2].

lair /lɛr/ *n* the dwelling or resting place of a wild animal; (*inf*) a secluded place, a retreat.

laird /lɛrd/ *n* (*Scot*) a landowner.

laissez-faire, laisser-faire /ˌleseɪ'fɛr/ *n* the policy of non-interference with individual freedom, *esp* in economic affairs.—**laissez-faireism, laisser-faireism** *n*.

laity /'leɪtɪ/ *n* laymen, as opposed to clergymen.

lake[1] /leɪk/ *n* a large inland body of water.

lake[2] *n* a purplish-red pigment, originally made from lac.

lake boat *n* ✦ (*Cdn*) a commercial boat or ship that sails on the Great Lakes.

Lake Wobegon effect *n* a propensity to attribute quality to the average, from the novel by Garrison Keillor.

lakehead /'leɪkhɛd/ *n* ✦ (*Cdn*) the area along a lakeshore most distant from the lake's outlet.

lakh /læk/ or /lɒk/ *n* (*India*) 100,000, *esp* rupees.

lam[1] /læm/ *vt* (**lamming, lammed**) (*inf*) to beat or thrash.

lam[2] *n* a sudden flight, *esp* to evade capture by the authorities.

lama /'lɒmə/ *n* a monk or priest of Lamaism.

Lamaism /-,ɪzəm/ *n* a form of Buddhism in Tibet and Mongolia.—**lamaist** *n*.—**Lamaistic** *adj*.

lamasery /-,sɛrɪ/ *n* (*pl* **lamaseries**) a monastery of lamas.

lamb /læm/ *n* a young sheep; its flesh as food; (*inf*) an innocent or gentle person. • *vi* to give birth to a lamb; to tend (ewes) at lambing time.

lambada /ləm'bɒdə/ *n* (the music for) a lively erotic dance of Brazilian origin, in which couples dance with their stomachs touching.

lambast, lambaste /læm'beɪst/ *vt* (*inf*) to beat or censure severely.

lambda /'læmdə/ *n* the Greek letter L.

lambdoid /læm'dɔɪd/ *adj* shaped like lambda.

lambent /'læmbənt/ *adj* (*flame*) playing lightly over a surface; marked by radiance; brilliant.—**lambency** *n*.

lambert /'læmbərt/ *n* a measure of brightness, the brightness of a surface radiating one lumen per square centimetre.

lambkin /'læmkɪn/ *n* a little lamb.

lambrequin /'læmbrɪkɪn/ or /'læmbər-/ *n* a short hanging over a door, mantelpiece, etc.

lambrusco /lɒm'bruskoː/ or /læm-/, /-'bruːs-/ *n* a sparkling red Italian wine.

lambskin /'læmskɪn/ *n* the skin of a lamb with the wool on or as leather, for making clothes, etc.

lame /leɪm/ *adj* disabled or crippled, *esp* in the feet or legs; stiff and painful; weak, ineffectual. • *vt* to make lame.—**lamely** *adv*.—**lameness** *n*.

lamé /læ'meɪ/ or /'læmeɪ/ *n* a fabric interwoven with metallic threads.

lame duck *n* a weak, ineffectual person; an elected official serving between the end of his or her term and the inauguration of a successor.

lamella /lə'melə/ *n* (*pl* **lamellae, lamellas**) a thin plate, scale, or film.—**lamellar, lamellate, lamellose** *adj*.

lamelliform /lə'melɪ,fɔrm/ *adj* lamella-shaped.

lament /lə'mɛnt/ *vti* to feel or express deep sorrow (for); to mourn. • *n* a lamenting; an elegy, dirge, etc mourning some loss or death.—**lamenter** *n*.

lamentable /lə'mɛntəbəl/ or /'læmɛntəbəl/ *adj* distressing, deplorable.—**lamentably** *adv*.

lamentation /ˌlæmɛn'teɪʃən/ *n* a lamenting; a lament, expression of grief.

lamented /lə'mɛntəd/ *adj* grieved for.

lamia /'leɪmɪə/ *n* (*pl* **lamias, lamiae**) (*myth*) a monster, half snake, half woman.

lamina /'læmɪnə/ *n* (*pl* **laminae, laminas**) a thin plate, scale or layer; the expanded part of a foliage leaf.—**laminose** *adj*.

laminate /'læmɪneɪt/ *vt* to cover with one or more thin layers; to make by building up in layers. • *n* a product made by laminating. • *adj* laminated.—**laminator** *n*.

laminated /-əd/ *adj* built in thin sheets or layers; covered by a thin film of plastic, etc.

lamination /ˌlæmɪ'neɪʃən/ *n* divisibility, or division, into thin plates.

Lammas /'læməs/ *n* (*RC Church*) a feast held on August 1; (*formerly*) a harvest festival celebrated on August 1.

lammergeier, lammergeyer /'læmərgaɪər/ *n* a vulture found in southern Europe, Africa and Asia, the bearded vulture.

lamp /læmp/ *n* any device producing light, either by electricity, gas, or by burning oil, etc; a holder or base for such a device; any device for producing therapeutic rays.

lampas /'læmpəs/ *n* a disease of horses, which causes swelling in the roof of the mouth; a type of flowered silk.

lampblack /'læmpblæk/ *n* fine charcoal or soot.

lampion /'læmpiən/ *n* a small lamp.

lamplighter /'læmp,laɪtər/ *n* (*formerly*) someone who lit street lamps.

lampoon /læm'puːn/ *n* a piece of satirical writing attacking someone. • *vt* to ridicule maliciously in a lampoon.—**lampooner** *n*.—**lampoonery** *n*.

lamppost /'læmppoːst/ *n* a post supporting a street lamp.

lamprey /'læmprɪ/ *n* (*pl* **lamprey, lampreys**) an animal resembling an eel but having a jawless, round sucking mouth.

LAN /læn/ (*abbr*) local area network: a number of computers in close proximity linked together in order to transfer information and share peripherals such as printers.

lanate /'leɪneɪt/ *adj* woolly.

lance /læns/ *n* a long wooden spear with a sharp iron or steel head. • *vt* to pierce (as if) with a lance; to open a boil, etc with a lancet.

lance corporal *n* a noncommissioned officer of the lowest rank in the British army.

lanceolate /'lænsɪələt/ *adj* (*bot*) tapering to a point at either end.

lancer /'lænsər/ *n* a cavalry soldier formerly armed with a lance; (*pl*) a kind of dance, a quadrille.

lancet /'lænsət/ *n* a small, *usu* two-edged, pointed surgical knife.

lancet arch *n* a sharply pointed arch.

lanceted /-əd/ *adj* (*archit*) with one or more lancet arches or windows.

lancet window *n* a tall narrow window with a lancet arch.

lancewood /'lænswʊd/ *n* a tough, elastic wood.

land /lænd/ *n* the solid part of the earth's surface; ground, soil; a country and its people; property in land. • *vt* to set (an aircraft) down on land or water; to put on shore from a ship; to bring to a particular place; to catch (a fish); to get or secure (a job, prize, etc); to deliver (a blow). • *vi* to go ashore from a ship; to come to port; to arrive at a specified place; to come to rest.

landamman /'lændəmæn/ *n* (*Switzerland*) the chief official in some cantons.

landau /'lændau/ *n* a four-wheeled horse-drawn carriage with a roof that folds down.

landaulet, landaulette /,lændə'lət/ *n* a small landau.

land claim *n* ✤ (*Cdn*) a legal claim by a First Nations people to the use or ownership of an area of land.

landed /'lændəd/ *adj* consisting of land; owning land.

landed immigrant *n* ✤ (*Cdn*) a person granted official status as an immigrant to Canada.

landfall /-fɒl/ *n* a sighting of land, *esp* from a ship at sea; the land sighted.

landfill /-fɪl/ *n* a large pit in which refuse is buried between layers of soil.—*also adj.*

landgrave /-greɪv/ *n* (*formerly*) a title given to certain counts in Germany.

landgravine /-grə,vain/ *n* the wife of a landgrave; the title given to a woman landgrave.

landing /'lændɪŋ/ *n* the act of coming to shore or to the ground; the place where persons or goods are loaded or unloaded from a ship; a platform at the end of a flight of stairs.

landing craft *n* a small military vessel designed for landing troops and equipment ashore.

landing gear *n* the undercarriage of an aircraft.

landing stage *n* a platform for landing goods or people from a ship.

landing strip *n* an airstrip.

landlady /'lænd,leidi/ *n* (*pl* **landladies**) a woman who owns and rents property; a woman who owns and runs a boarding house, pub, etc.

landlocked /'lændlɒkt/ *adj* surrounded by land.

landlord /-lɔrd/ *n* a man who owns and rents property; a man who owns and runs a boarding house, pub, etc.

landlubber /'lænd,lʌbər/ *n* a person who has had little experience of the sea.

landmark /'lændmɑrk/ *n* any prominent feature of the landscape distinguishing a locality; an important event or turning point.

landmass /-,mæs/ *n* a large expanse of land.

land mine *n* an explosive charge shallowly buried in the ground, *usu* detonated by stepping or driving on it.

Land of the Midnight Sun *n* ✤ (*Cdn*) (*inf*) the Arctic.

landowner /-o:nər/ *n* a person who owns land.—**landowning** *adj, n.*

landscape /-skeɪp/ *n* an expanse of natural scenery seen in one view; a picture of natural, inland scenery. • *vt* to make (a plot of ground) more attractive, as by adding lawns, bushes, trees, etc.

landscape gardening *n* the decorative design and planting of gardens and grounds in imitation of natural scenery.—**landscape gardener** *n.*

landscapist /'lændskeɪpɪst/ *n* an artist who paints landscapes.

landslide /'lændslaɪd/ *n* the sliding of a mass of soil or rocks down a slope; an overwhelming victory, *esp* in an election.

landsman /'lændzməns/ *n* (*pl* **landsmen**) a person who resides and works on land, as opposed to the sea.

Landtag /'lændtæk/ *n* (*Germany, Austria*) the parliament of an individual state.

landward /'lændwərd/ *adv, adj* towards the land.—**landwards** *adv.*

lane /lein/ *n* a narrow road, path, etc; a path or strip specifically designated for ships, aircraft, cars, etc; one of the narrow strips dividing a running track, swimming pool, etc for athletes and swimmers; one of the narrow passages along which balls are bowled in a bowling alley.

laneway /'leinwei/ *n* ✤ (*Cdn*) a lane, *esp* behind a row of buildings.

langlauf /'læŋ,lʌuf/ *n* cross-country skiing.—**langläufer** *n.*

langouste *Fr.* /lã'gu:st/ or /'lɒŋgu:st/ *n* the spiny lobster.

langoustine *Fr.* /,lãgu:'sti:n/ or /'lɒŋgus,ti:n/ *n* a large prawn or small lobster.

langsyne /læŋ'zain/ *adv* (*Scot*) long ago.

language /'læŋgwɪdʒ/ *n* human speech or the written symbols for speech; any means of communicating; a special set of symbols used for programming a computer; the speech of a particular nation, etc; the particular style of verbal expression characteristic of a person, group, profession, etc.

langue d'oc *Fr.* /,lãg'dɒk/ *n* a form of medieval French spoken in the South of France.

languid ,'læŋgwid/ *adj* lacking energy or vitality; apathetic; drooping, sluggish.—**languidly** *adv.*—**languidness** *n.*

languish /'læŋgwɪʃ/ *vi* to lose strength and vitality; to pine; to suffer neglect or hardship; to assume a pleading or melancholic expression.—**languisher** *n.*—**languishment** *n.*

languor /'læŋgər/ *n* physical or mental fatigue or apathy; dreaminess; oppressive stillness.—**languorous** *adj.*

langur /lɛŋ'gu:r/ *n* a long-tailed monkey, found in South Asia.

laniard *n see* **lanyard**.

laniary /'læni'eri/ *n* (*pl* **laniaries**) a canine tooth.

laniferous /læni'fərəs/, **lanigerous** /-nidʒ-/ *adj* wool-bearing.

lank /læŋk/ *adj* tall and thin; long and limp.—**lankly** *adv.*—**lankness** *n.*

lanky /'læŋki/ *adj* (**lankier, lankiest**) lean, tall, and ungainly.—**lankily** *adv.*—**lankiness** *n.*

lanner /'lænər/ *n* a falcon found in Mediterranean countries, North Africa and South Asia; the female of this species.

lanneret /-ət/ *n* the male lanner falcon.

lanolin, lanoline /'lænəlɪn/ *n* wool grease used in cosmetics, ointments, etc.

lantern /'læntərn/ *n* a portable transparent case for holding a light; a structure with windows on top of a door or roof to provide light and ventilation; the light-chamber of a lighthouse.

lantern jaw *n* a long thin jaw.

lanthanide /'lænθə,naid/ *n* any of a series of related chemical elements with atomic numbers from 57 (lanthanum) to 71 (lutetium).

lanthanum /'lænθənəm/ *n* a metallic element.

lanyard /'lænjərd/ or /-jɑrd/ *n* a rope used for fastening things on board a ship; a cord worn round the neck to hold a knife, whistle, etc.

laodicean /,leio:di'si:ən/ *adj* indifferent, *esp* towards religion.

lap[1] /læp/ *vti* (**lapping, lapped**) to take in (liquid) with the tongue; (*waves*) to flow gently with a splashing sound.

lap[2] *n* the flat area from waist to knees formed by a person sitting; the part of the clothing covering this.

lap[3] *n* an overlapping; a part that overlaps; one complete circuit of a race track. • *vb* (**lapping, lapped**) *vt* to fold (over or on); to wrap. • *vi* to overlap; to extend over something in space or time.

laparotomy /,læpər'ɒtəmi/ *n* (*pl* **laparotomies**) (*med*) the operation of cutting the abdominal wall.

lapdog /'læpdɒg/ *n* a dog small and docile enough to be held on the lap.

lapel /lə'pɛl/ *n* a part of a suit, coat, jacket, etc folded back and continuous with the collar.—**lapelled** *adj.*

lapidary /'læpɪ,deri/ *adj* of or relating to stones; inscribed on stone; concise, like an inscription. • *n* (*pl* **lapidaries**) a cutter or engraver of gems.—**lapidarian** *adj.*

lapidate /'læpideit/ *vt* to stone (to death).—**lapidation** *n.*

lapidify *vti* (**lapidifying, lapidified**) to turn to stone.

lapis lazuli /,læpis'læzulai/ or /-li/, /-ju-/ *n* an azure, opaque, semi-precious stone.

lap of honour *n* a ceremonial circuit of the field by a winning person or team.

lappet /'læpit/ *n* a small, loose flap.

lapse /læps/ *n* a small error; a decline or drop to a lower condition, degree, or state; a moral decline; a period of time elapsed; the termination of a legal right or privilege through disuse. • *vi* to depart from the usual or accepted standard, *esp* in morals; to pass out of existence or use; to become void or discontinued; (*time*) to slip away.—**lapsable, lapsible** *adj.*—**lapser** *n.*

lapsus /-əs/ *n* (*pl* **lapsus**) a slip or error.

laptop /'læptɒp/ *n* a small portable computer that can comfortably be used on the lap.

lapwing /'læpwiŋ/ *n* a crested plover.

larboard /'lɑrbərd/ *n* (*naut*) (*formerly*) the port or left side of a ship.

larceny /'lɑrsəni/ *n* (*pl* **larcenies**) the theft of someone else's property.—**larcenist, larcener** *n.*—**larcenous** *adj.*

larch /lɑrtʃ/ *n* a cone-bearing tree of the pine family.

lard /lɑrd/ *n* melted and clarified pig fat. • *vt* to insert strips of bacon or pork fat (in meat) before cooking; to embellish.

larder /'lɑrdər/ *n* a room or cupboard where food is stored.

lares /'leri:z/ *npl* (*Roman myth*) the household gods.

large /lɑrdʒ/ *adj* great in size, amount, or number; bulky; big; spacious; bigger than others of its kind; operating on a big scale.—**largeness** *n.*

large intestine *n* the section of the digestive system comprising the caecum, colon and rectum.

largely /lɑrdʒli/ *adv* much, in great amounts; mainly, for the most part.

largen /-ən/ *vt* to make larger, to enlarge.

large-scale /-skeɪl/ *adj* drawn on a big scale to reveal much detail; extensive.

largess, largesse /lɑrˈdʒes/ or /-ˈʒes/ *n* the generous distribution of money, gifts, favours, etc; generosity.

larghetto /lɑrˈgeto:/ *adv* (*mus*) slowly. • *n* (*pl* **larghettos**) a passage of music played in this way.

largish /ˈlɑrdʒɪʃ/ *adj* quite large.

largo /ˈlɑrgo:/ *adv* (*mus*) slow and dignified. • *n* (*pl* **largos**) a passage of music played in this way.

lariat /ˈleriət/ or /ˈlæriət/ *n* a rope for tethering grazing horses; a lasso.

lark[1] /lɑrk/ *n* any of a family of songbirds.

lark[2] *n* a playful or amusing adventure; a harmless prank. • *vi* (*usu with* **about**) to have fun, frolic.—**larky** *adj*.

larkspur /ˈlɑrkspər/ *n* an annual delphinium.

larrigan /ˈlærɪgən/ *n* a knee-high leather boot worn by trappers.

larrikin /ˈlærɪkɪn/ *n* (*Austral sl*) a hooligan.

larrup /ˈlærəp/ *vt* (*dial*) to thrash, flog.

larva /ˈlɑrvə/ *n* (*pl* **larvae**) the immature form of many animals after emerging from an egg before transformation into the adult state, *eg* a caterpillar.—**larval** *adj*.

laryngeal /ləˈrɪndʒiəl/ *adj* pertaining to, or situated near, the larynx.

laryngitis /ˌlerɪnˈdʒaɪtɪs/ *n* inflammation of the larynx.—**laryngitic** *adj*.

laryngo-, laryng- /ˈlerɪŋgo:/ *prefix* larynx.

laryngology /ˌlerɪŋˈgɒlədʒi/ *n* the medical study of the larynx.—**laryngologist** *n*.

laryngoscope /ˌlerɪŋgəˈskoːp/ *n* a medical instrument for examining the larynx.—**laryngoscopy** *n*.

laryngotomy /ˌlerɪŋˈgɒtəmi/ *n* (*pl* **laryngotomies**) (*med*) the operation of cutting into the larynx.

larynx /ˈlerɪŋks/ *n* (*pl* **larynxes, larynges**) the structure at the upper end of the windpipe, containing the vocal cords.

lasagna, lasagne /ləˈzɒnjə/ *n* pasta formed in thin wide strips; a dish of lasagne baked in layers with cheese, minced meat and tomato sauce.

lascar /ˈlæskər/ *n* an East Indian sailor.—*also* **lashkar**.

lascivious /ləˈsɪviəs/ *adj* lecherous, lustful; arousing sexual desire.—**lasciviously** *adv*.—**lasciviousness** *n*.

lase /leɪz/ *vi* (*gem, gas*) able to act as a laser.

laser /ˈleɪzər/ *n* a device that produces an intense monochromatic beam of coherent light or other electromagnetic radiation.

laser printer *n* a computer printer that uses a laser beam and photoconductive drum to produce high quality text output.

lasertripsy /-ˌtrɪpsi/ *n* a medical procedure for removing kidney stones, etc, by the use of laser beams.

lash /læʃ/ *vt* to strike forcefully (as if) with a lash; to fasten or secure with a cord, etc; to attack with criticism or ridicule. • *vi* to move quickly and violently; (*rain, waves, etc*) to beat violently against; (*with* **out**) to attack suddenly either physically or verbally; (*inf*) to spend extravagantly (on). • *n* the flexible part of a whip; an eyelash; a stroke (as if) with a whip.—**lasher** *n*.

lashkar *see* **lascar**.

lass /læs/, **lassie** /ˈlæsi/ *n* a young woman or girl.

Lassa fever *n* an infectious viral disease of Africa.

lassitude /ˈlæsɪˌtuːd/ or /-ˌtjuːd/ *n* weariness.

lasso /ləˈsuː/ or /ˈlæsoː/ *n* (*pl* **lassos, lassoes**) a long rope or leather thong with a running noose for catching horses, cattle, etc. • *vt* (**lassoes** *or* **lassos, lassoing, lassoed**) to catch (as if) with a lasso.—**lassoer** *n*.

last[1] /læst/ *n* a shoemaker's model of the foot on which boots and shoes are made or repaired. • *vt* to shape with a last.

last[2] *vi* to remain in existence, use, etc; to endure. • *vt* to continue during; to be enough for.

last[3] *adj* being or coming after all the others in time or place; only remaining, the most recent; least likely; conclusive. • *adv* after all the others; most recently; finally. • *n* the one coming last.

last-ditch *adj* being a final effort to avoid disaster.

last hurrah *n* a final appearance; a swan song.

lasting /-ɪŋ/ *adj* enduring.—**lastingly** *adv*.

lastly /-li/ *adv* at the end, in the last place, finally.

last-minute *adj* at the last possible time when something can be done.

last rites *npl* the sacraments prescribed for a person near death.

last straw *n* a final addition to one's burdens that results in collapse or defeat.

last word *n* the final remark in an argument; a definitive statement; the latest fashion.

Lat. *abbr* = Latin.

lat. *abbr* = latitude.

latch /lætʃ/ *n* a fastening for a door, gate, or window, *esp* a bar, etc that fits into a notch. • *vti* to fasten with a latch.

latchet /ˈlætʃət/ *n* (*arch*) a strap or lace for fastening a shoe.

latchkey /ˈlætʃkiː/ *n* the key of an outer door.

late /leɪt/ *adj, adv* after the usual or expected time; at an advanced stage or age; near the end; far on in the day or evening; just prior to the present; deceased; not long past; until lately; out of office.—**lateness** *n*.

latecomer /ˈleɪtˌkʌmər/ *n* a person or thing that arrives late.

lateen /ləˈtiːn/ *n* a triangular sail used on boats in the Mediterranean.—**lateenrigged** *adj*.

lately /ˈleɪtli/ *adv* recently, in recent times.

latent /ˈleɪtənt/ *adj* existing but not yet visible or developed.—**latency** *n*.—**latently** *adv*.

later /ˈleɪtər/ *adv* subsequently; afterwards.—*also compar of* **late**.

lateral /ˈlætərəl/ *adj* of, at, from, towards the side.—**laterally** *adv*.

lateral thinking *n* a solving of problems by employing unorthodox thought processes.

latest /ˈleɪtest/ *adj* most recent or fashionable. • *n* (*inf: with* **the**) the most up-to-date fashion, news, etc.—*also superl of* **late**.

latex /ˈleɪteks/ *n* (*pl* **latexes, latices**) the milky juice produced by certain plants, used in the manufacture of rubber.

lath /læθ/ *n* (*pl* **laths**) a thin narrow strip of wood used in constructing a framework for plaster, etc.

lathe /leɪð/ *n* a machine that rotates wood, metal, etc for shaping.

lather /ˈlæðər/ *n* a foam made by soap or detergent mixed with water; frothy sweat; a state of excitement or agitation. • *vti* to cover with or form lather.—**lathery** *adj*.

lathi /ˈlæti/ *n* a long, heavy stick, carried by policemen in India.

Latin /ˈlætɪn/ *adj* of ancient Rome, its people, their language, etc; denoting or of the languages derived from Latin (Italian, Spanish, etc), the peoples who speak them, their countries, etc. • *n* a native or inhabitant of ancient Rome; the language of ancient Rome; a person, as a Spaniard or Italian, whose language is derived from Latin.

Latinate /ˈlætɪˌneɪt/ *adj* of, resembling or derived from Latin.

Latinist /-ˌnɪst/ *n* a Latin scholar.

Latinity /-ˌnɪti/ *n* Latin style.

Latinize /-ˌnaɪz/ *vt* to translate into Latin; to give Latin characteristics to.—**Latinization** *n*.—**Latinizer** *n*.

Latino /ləˈtiːnoː/ *n* a person of Latin American origin living in the US.

latish /ˈleɪtɪʃ/ *adj* somewhat late.

latitude /ˈlætɪˌtuːd/ or /-ˌtjuːd-/ *n* the distance from north or south of the equator, measured in degrees; a region with reference to this distance; extent; scope; freedom from restrictions on actions or opinions.—**latitudinal** *adj*.—**latitudinally** *adv*.

latitudinarian /ˌlætɪˌtuːdɪˈnerɪən/ *adj* claiming or showing freedom of thought, *esp* regarding religion. • *n* a person with such an outlook.—**latitudinarianism** *n*.

latria /ˈlætriə/ *n* (*RC Church*) supreme worship, offered to God alone.

latrine /ləˈtriːn/ *n* a lavatory, as in a military camp.

-latry /lətri/ *n suffix* worship, *esp* excessively.

latter /ˈlætər/ *adj* later; more recent; nearer the end; being the last mentioned of two.

latter-day *adj* present-day; modern.

latterly /ˈlætərli/ *adv* recently.

lattice /ˈlætɪs/ *n* a network of crossed laths or bars.—**latticed** *adj*.

laud /lɒd/ *vt* to praise; to extol.

laudable /ˈlɒdəbəl/ *adj* praiseworthy.—**laudability** *n*.—**laudably** *adv*.

laudanum /ˈlɒdənəm/ *n* (*formerly*) any of various opium preparations; a solution of opium in alcohol.

laudation /lɒˈdeɪʃən/ *n* praise.

laudatory /ˈlɒdətɔri/, **laudative** /-tɪv/ *adj* expressing praise.

laugh /læf/ *vi* to emit explosive inarticulate vocal sounds expressive of amusement, joy or derision. • *vt* to utter or express with laughter; (with **off**) to dismiss as of little importance make a joke of. • *n* the act or sound of laughing; (*inf*) an amusing person or thing.—**laugher** *n*.—**laughing** *adj*, *n*.—**laughingly** *adv*.

laughable /'læfəbəl/ *adj* causing laughter; ridiculous.—**laughably** *adv*.

laughing gas *n* nitrous oxide.

laughing stock *n* an object of ridicule.

laughter /'læftər/ *n* the act or sound of laughing.

launch[1] /lontʃ/ *vt* to throw, hurl or propel forward; to cause (a vessel) to slide into the water; (*rocket, missile*) to set off; to put into action; to put a new product onto the market. • *vi* to involve oneself enthusiastically. • *n* the act or occasion of launching.

launch[2] *n* an open, or partly enclosed, motor boat.

launch pad, launching pad *n* a platform from which a spacecraft is launched.

launder /'lɒndər/ *vti* to wash and iron clothes. • *vt* to legitimize (money) obtained from criminal activity by passing it through foreign banks, or investing in legitimate businesses, etc.—**launderer** *n*.

launderette /lɒn'drɛt/ *n* an establishment equipped with coin-operated washing machines and driers for public use.

laundress /'lɒndrɛs/ *n* a woman who earns her living by doing laundry.

Laundromat /'lɒndrəmæt/ *n* (*trademark*) a launderette.

laundry /'lɒndri/ *n* (*pl* **laundries**) a place where clothes are washed and ironed; clothes sent to be washed and ironed.

laureate /'lɒriət/ *adj* crowned with laurel leaves as a mark of honour. • *n* the recipient of an honour or distinction; a poet laureate.—**laureateship** *n*.

laurel /'lɒrəl/ *n* an evergreen shrub with large, glossy leaves; the leaves used by the ancient Greeks as a symbol of achievement.

lava /'lævə/ *n* molten rock flowing from a volcano; the solid substance formed as this cools.

lavabo /lə'veɪbɔː/ or /-'væbɔː/ *n* (*pl* **lavaboes, lavabos**) (*RC Church*) the ritual washing of the celebrant's hands at the Eucharist; a washbasin.

lavation /lə'veɪʃən/ *n* the act of washing.

lavatory /'lævətɔri/ *n* (*pl* **lavatories**) a sanitary device for the disposal or faeces and urine; a room equipped with this.—*also* **bathroom, toilet**.

lavender /'lævəndər/ *n* the fragrant flowers of a perennial shrub dried and used in sachets; a pale purple.

laver /'leɪvər/ or /'lævər/ *n* an edible seaweed.

lavish /'lævɪʃ/ *vt* to give or spend freely. • *adj* abundant, profuse; generous; extravagant.—**lavishly** *adv*.—**lavishness** *n*.

law /lɒ/ *n* all the rules of conduct in an organized community as upheld by authority; any one of such rules; obedience to such rules; the study of such rules, jurisprudence; the seeking of justice in courts under such rules; the profession of lawyers, judges, etc; (*inf*) the police; a sequence of events occurring with unvarying uniformity under the same conditions; any rule expected to be observed.

law-abiding *adj* obeying the law.

lawbreaker /'lɒ'breɪkər/ *n* a person who violates the law.—**lawbreaking** *adj*, *n*.

lawful /'lɒfʊl/ *adj* in conformity with the law; recognized by law.—**lawfully** *adv*.—**lawfulness** *n*.

lawgiver /'lɒ,gɪvər/ *n* a maker of a code of laws.

lawless /'lɒləs/ *adj* not regulated by law; not in conformity with law, illegal.—**lawlessly** *adv*.—**lawlessness** *n*.

lawmaker /'lɒmeɪkər/ *n* a maker of laws, a legislator.

lawn[1] /lɒn/ *n* a fine sheer cloth of linen or cotton.—**lawny** *adj*.

lawn[2] *n* land covered with closely cut grass, *esp* around a house.

lawn darts *n* an outdoor game of darts using a lawn as a board, at which are fired foot-long metal darts.

lawn mower *n* a hand-propelled or power-driven machine to cut lawn grass.

lawn tennis *n* tennis played on a grass court.

lawrencium /lɒ'rensiəm/ *n* a radioactive metallic element.

lawsuit /'lɒsuːt/ *n* a suit between private parties in a law court.

lawyer /'lɔɪər/ *n* a person whose profession is advising others in matters of law or representing them in a court of law.

lax /læks/ *adj* slack, loose; not tight; not strict or exact.—**laxly** *adv*.—**laxness** *n*.

laxative /'læksətɪv/ *n* a substance that promotes emptying of the bowels.—*also adj*.

laxity /'læksɪti/ *n* the state or quality of being lax, laxness.

lay[1] /leɪ/ *see* **lie**[2].

lay[2] *vt* (**laying, laid**) to put down; to allay or suppress; to place in a resting position; to place or set; to place in a correct position; to produce (an egg); to devise; to present or assert; to stake a bet; (with **down**) to put down; to surrender, relinquish; to begin to build; to establish (guidelines, rules, etc); to store, *esp* wine; to record tracks in a music studio; (with **in**) to store, to stockpile; (with **off**) to suspend from work temporarily or permanently; (with **on**) to supply, provide; to install (electricity, etc); (with **out**) to plan in detail; to arrange for display; to prepare (a corpse) for viewing; (*inf*) to spend money, *esp* lavishly; (with **up**) to store for future use; to disable or confine through illness. • *vi* (*inf*) to leave (a person or thing) alone; (with **into**) to attack physically or verbally. • *n* a way or position in which something is situated.

lay[3] *n* a simple narrative poem, *esp* as intended to be sung; a ballad.

lay[4] *adj* of or pertaining to those who are not members of the clergy; not belonging to a profession.

layabout /'leɪə,baʊt/ *n* a loafer, lazy person.

lay-by /'leɪbaɪ/ *n* (*Austral*) a deposit payment system that reserves an article for a purchaser until full settlement; (*Brit*) a pull-in place for motorists to stop at the side of a main road.—**lay by** *vt* to set aside or save for future needs.

layer /'leɪər/ *n* a single thickness, fold, etc; the runner of a plant fastened down to take root; a hen that lays. • *vti* to separate into layers; to form by superimposing layers; to (cause to) take root by propagating a plant shoot still attached to its parent.

layette /leɪ'ɛt/ *n* a complete set of clothes, equipment and accessories for a newborn baby.

lay figure *n* a jointed model of the human body used by artists for hanging drapery on; a person regarded as a puppet or nonentity.

laying /'leɪŋ/ *n* a sitting of eggs; the first coat of plaster.

layman /'leɪmən/ *n* (*pl* **laymen**) a person who is not a member of the clergy; a non-specialist, someone who does not possess professional knowledge.—**laywoman** *nf* (*pl* **laywomen**).

layoff /'leɪɒf/ *n* a period of involuntary unemployment.

layout /'leɪaʊt/ *n* the manner in which anything is laid out, *esp* arrangement of text and pictures on the pages of a newspaper or magazine, etc; the thing laid out.

layover /'leɪ,oʊvər/ *n* (*US*) a stop on a journey.

lazar /'læzər/ *n* (*arch*) a leper.

lazaret, lazarette /,læzə'rɛt/ (*also* **lazaretto** /-'rɛtoʊ/) *n* (*pl* **lazarettos, lazarets, lazarettes**) (*naut*) a part of a ship's hold; (*formerly*) a hospital for people suffering from infectious diseases.

laze /leɪz/ *vti* to idle or loaf.

lazulite /'læzəlaɪt/ *n* an azure blue mineral.

lazy /'leɪzi/ *adj* (**lazier, laziest**) disinclined to work or exertion; encouraging or causing indolence; sluggishly moving.—**lazily** *adv*.—**laziness** *n*.

lazybones /'leɪzi,boʊnz/ *n* a lazy person.

lb *abbr* = pound(s) weight.

lbw /,elbiː'dʌbəl,juː/ *abbr* = (*cricket*) leg before wicket.

LC *abbr* ✸ (*Cdn*) = Liquor Commission.

LCBO *abbr* ✸ = Liquor Control Board of Ontario.

LCD /,elsiː'diː/ *abbr* = liquid-crystal display; (*also without cap*) lowest common denominator.

LCdr *abbr* ✸ (*Cdn*) = Lieutenant Commander.

LCol *abbr* ✸ (*Cdn*) = Lieutenant Colonel.

L/Cpl *abbr* ✸ = Lance Corporal.

lea[1] /liː/ *n* (*poet*) a meadow, grassland.

lea[2] *n* a measure of yarn, varying from 80 yards (approx 73 metres) for wool to 300 yards (approx 274 metres) for linen.

leach /liːtʃ/ *vt* to wash (soil, ore, etc) with a filtering liquid; to extract (a soluble substance) from some material. • *vi* to lose soluble matter through a filtering liquid.—**leacher** *n*.

lead[1] /liːd/ *vb* (**leading, led**) *vt* to show the way, *esp* by going first; to direct or guide on a course; to direct by influence; to be head of (an expedition, orchestra, etc); to be ahead of in a contest; to live, spend (one's life); (with **on**) to lure or entice, *esp* into mischief. • *vi* to show the way, as by going first; (with **to**) to tend in a certain direction; to be or go first. • *n* the role of a leader; first place; the amount or distance ahead; anything that leads, as a clue; the leading role in a play, etc; the right of playing first in cards or the card played.

lead[2] /lɛd/ *n* a heavy, soft, bluish-grey, metallic element; a weight for sounding depths at sea, etc; bullets; a stick of graphite, used in pencils; (*print*) a thin strip of metal used to space lines of type.

• *adj* of or containing lead. • *vt* (**leading, leaded**) to cover, weight, or space out with lead.

leaden /'lɛdən/ *adj* made of lead; very heavy; dull grey; gloomy.— **leadenly** *adv*.

leader /'liːdər/ *n* the person who goes first; the principle first violin-player in an orchestra; the director of an orchestra; the inspiration or head of a movement, such as a political party; a person whose example is followed; the leading editorial in a newspaper; the leading article.

leadership /'liːdərʃɪp/ *n* the act of leading; the ability to be a leader; the leaders of an organization or movement collectively.

lead glass *n* flint glass.

lead-in /'liːdɪn/ *n* introductory material; the connection between a radio transmitter or receiver with an aerial or transmission cable.

leading[1] /'liːdɪŋ/ *adj* capable of guiding or influencing; principal; in first position.

leading[2] /'lɛdɪŋ/ *n* a covering of lead; (*print*) the body of a type, larger than the size, giving space.

leading article /'liːdɪŋ-/ *n* an article in a newspaper stating editorial opinion on a given subject; the leader.

leading light *n* the most important member of a group or organization.

leading question *n* a question worded so as to suggest the desired answer.

leadsman /'liːdsmən/ *n* (*pl* **leadsmen**) a sailor who heaves the lead.

lead time /'liːd-/ *n* the period between the design of a product and its manufacture.

leaf /liːf/ *n* (*pl* **leaves**) any of the flat, thin (*usu* green) parts growing from the stem of a plant; a sheet of paper; a very thin sheet of metal; a hinged or removable part of a table top. • *vi* to bear leaves; (*with* **through**) to turn the pages of.

leafage /'liːfɪdʒ/ *n* foliage.

leafless /-ləs/ *adj* without leaves.

leaflet /'liːflət/ *n* a small or young leaf; a sheet of printed information (often folded), *esp* advertising matter distributed free. • *vi* to distribute leaflets (to).

leaf mold *n* compost or soil composed of decaying leaves and other vegetable matter; any of various fungal diseases of plants.

leafy /'liːfi/ *adj* (**leafier, leafiest**) having many or broad leaves; resembling leaves.—**leafiness** *n*.

league[1] /liːg/ *n* an association of nations, groups, etc for promoting common interests; an association of sports clubs that organizes matches between members; any class or category. • *vti* (**leaguing, leagued**) to form into a league.

league[2] *n* (*formerly*) a varying measure of distance, averaging about three miles (5km).

leak /liːk/ *n* a crack or hole through which liquid or gas may accidentally pass; the liquid or gas passing through such an opening; confidential information made public deliberately or accidentally. • *vi* to (let) escape though an opening; to disclose information surreptitiously.—**leaker** *n*.

leakage /'liːkədʒ/ *n* the act of leaking; that which enters or escapes by leaking.

leaky /'liːki/ *adj* (**leakier, leakiest**) leaking or likely to leak.— **leakiness** *n*.

leal /liːl/ *adj* (*Scot*) loyal.

lean[1] /liːn/ *adj* thin, with little flesh or fat; spare; meagre. • *n* meat with little or no fat.—**leanness** *n*.

lean[2] *vb* (**leaning, leaned** *or* **leant**) *vi* to bend or slant from an upright position; to rest supported (on or against); to rely or depend for help (on). • *vt* to cause to lean.

leaning /'liːnɪŋ/ *n* inclination, tendency.

leant /lɛnt/ *see* **lean**[1].

lean-to /'liːnˌtuː/ *n* (*pl* **lean-tos**) a building whose rafters rest on another building.

leap /liːp/ *vb* (**leaping, leaped** *or* **leapt**) *vi* to jump; (*with* **at**) to accept something offered eagerly. • *vt* to pass over by a jump; to cause to leap. • *n* an act of leaping; bound; space passed by leaping; an abrupt transition.—**leaper** *n*.

leapfrog /'liːpˌfrɒg/ *n* a game in which one player vaults over another's bent back. • *vi* (**leapfrogging, leapfrogged**) to vault in this manner; to advance in alternate jumps.

leap year *n* a year with an extra day (29 February) occurring every fourth year.

learn /lərn/ *vti* (**learning, learned** *or* **learnt**) to gain knowledge of or skill in; to memorize; to become aware of, realize.— **learner** *n*.

learned /'lərnəd/ *adj* having learning; erudite; acquired by study, experience, etc.—**learnedly** *adv*.

learning /'lərnɪŋ/ *n* a gaining of knowledge; the acquiring of knowledge or skill through study.

lease /liːs/ *n* a contract by which an owner lets land, property, etc to another person for a specified period. • *vt* to grant by or hold under lease.—**leaseable** *adj*.—**leaser** *n*.

leaseback /'liːsbæk/ *n* the process of selling an asset, *esp* a building, and then renting it.

leasehold /'liːshoʊld/ *n* the act of holding by lease; the land, buildings, etc held by lease.—**leaseholder** *n*.

leash /liːʃ/ *n* a cord, strap, etc by which a dog or animal is held in check. • *vt* to hold or restrain on a leash.

least /liːst/ *adj* smallest in size, degree, etc; slightest. • *adv* to the smallest degree. • *n* the smallest in amount.

leastways /'liːstweɪz/ *adv* at least.

leather /'lɛðər/ *n* material made from the skin of an animal prepared by removing the hair and tanning; something made of leather. • *vt* to cover with leather; to thrash.

leatherback /'lɛðərˌbæk/ *n* the largest existing sea turtle, having a flexible shell.

Leatherette /ˌlɛðə'rɛt/ *n* (*trademark*) an imitation leather.

leatherjacket /'lɛðərdʒækɪt/ *n* a tropical fish with a leathery skin; the larva of the cranefly.

leathern /'lɛðərn/ *adj* (*arch*) made of, or resembling, leather.

leatherneck /'lɛðərnɛk/ *n* (*sl*) a member of the US Marine Corps.

leathery /'lɛðəri/ *adj* like leather; tough and flexible.

leave[1] /liːv/ *n* permission to do something; official authorization to be absent; the period covered by this.

leave[2] *vb* (**leaving, left**) *vt* to depart from; to cause or allow to remain in a specified state; to cause to remain behind; to refrain from consuming or dealing with; to have remaining at death, to bequeath; to have as a remainder; to allow to stay or or continue doing without interference; to entrust or commit to another; to abandon. • *vi* to depart; (*with* **off**) to stop, desist.—**leaver** *n*.

leaved /'liːvd/ *adj* having leaves.

leaven /'liːvən/ *n* a substance to make dough rise, *esp* yeast; something that changes or enlivens. • *vt* to raise with leaven; to modify, to enliven.—**leavening** *n*.

leaves /'liːvz/ *see* **leaf**.

leave-taking *n* a departure, farewell.

leavings /'liːvɪŋz/ *npl* leftovers; remnants; refuse.

leben /'leɪbən/ *n* a food made from soured milk, eaten in North Africa and the Levant.

Lebensraum /'leɪbənsˌraʊm/ *n* a piece of territory claimed by another country on the basis that it is needed to accommodate the country's expanding population.

lech /lɛtʃ/ *vt* (*sl*) to lust after.

lecher /'lɛtʃər/ *n* a lecherous man.

lecherous /-əs/ *adj* characterized by or encouraging lechery.

lechery /-əri/ *n* (*pl* **lecheries**) unrestrained sexuality; debauchery.

lecithin /'lɛsɪθɪn/ *n* any of a group of fatty compounds found in plant and animal tissues, used as an emulsifier and antioxidant.

lectern /'lɛktərn/ *n* a reading stand in a church; any similar reading support.

lection /'lɛkʃən/ *n* a reading from scripture for a particular day; a variant reading of a text.

lectionary /-əri/ *n* (*pl* **lectionaries**) a book listing lessons from scripture to be read at religious services on particular days.

lector /'lɛktɔr/ *n* a lecturer or reader at a university.

lecture /'lɛktʃər/ *n* an informative talk to a class, etc; a lengthy reprimand. • *vti* to give a lecture (to); to reprimand.—**lecturer** *n*.

lectureship /-ʃɪp/ *n* the position of lecturer.

LED /lɛd/ *or* /ˌeliː'diː/ *abbr* = light-emitting diode.

led /lɛd/ *see* **lead**[1].

lederhosen /'leɪdərˌhoʊzən/ *npl* leather shorts with braces worn by men in Austria and Bavaria.

ledge /lɛdʒ/ *n* a narrow horizontal surface resembling a shelf projecting from a wall, rock face, etc; an underwater ridge of rocks; a rock layer containing ore.—**ledgy** *adj*.

ledger /'lɛdʒər/ *n* a book in which a record of debits, credits, etc is kept.

ledger line *n* a short line added above or below a musical staff to extend its range.—*also* **leger line**.

lee /liː/ *n* a shelter; the side or part away from the wind.

leech /liːtʃ/ *n* a blood-sucking worm; a person who clings to or exploits another.

leek /liːk/ *n* a vegetable that resembles a greatly elongated green onion.

leer /liːr/ *n* a sly, oblique or lascivious look. • *vi* to look with a leer.—**leeringly** *adv*.

leery /'liːri/ *adj* (**leerier, leeriest**) (*with* **of**) suspicious, wary.

lees /liːz/ *npl* sediment in the bottom of a wine bottle, etc.

leeward /'liːwərd/ *adj, n* (*naut*) (in) the quarter towards which the wind blows.

leeway /'liːweɪ/ *n* the distance a ship or aircraft has strayed sideways of its course; freedom of action as regards expenditure of time, money, etc.

left[1] /lɛft/ *see* **leave**[2].

left[2] *adj* of or on the side that is towards the west when one faces north; worn on the left hand, foot, etc. • *n* the left side; (*often cap*) of or relating to the left in politics; the left hand; (*boxing*) a blow with the left hand.

left-hand *adj* of or towards the left side of a person or thing; for use by the left hand.

left-handed /lɛft'hændəd/ *adj* using the left hand in preference to the right; done or made for use with the left hand; ambiguous, backhanded. • *adv* with the left hand.—**left-handedly** *adv*.—**left-handedness** *n*.

left-hander /-'hændər/ *n* a left-handed person; a blow delivered with the left fist.

left-luggage office *n* (*Brit*) a place at an airport, railway station, etc., where luggage may be left for a small charge with an attendant for safekeeping; a checkroom in the US.

leftist /'lɛftɪst/ *adj* tending to the left in politics. • *n* a person tending towards the political left.—**leftism** *n*.

leftovers /'lɛft,oʊvərz/ *npl* unused portions of something, esp uneaten food.

leftward /'lɛftwərd/ *adj, adv* on or toward the left.—**leftwards** *adv*.

left-wing /'lɛftwɪŋ/ *adj* of or relating to the liberal faction of a political party, organization, etc.—**left-winger** *n*.

lefty /'lɛfti/ *n* (*pl* **lefties**) (*inf*) a left-winger; (*US sl*) a left-handed person.

leg /lɛg/ *n* one of the limbs on which humans and animals support themselves and walk; the part of a garment covering the leg; anything shaped or used like a leg; a branch or limb of a forked object; a section, as of a trip; any of a series of games or matches in a competition.

legacy /'lɛgəsi/ *n* (*pl* **legacies**) money, property, etc left to someone in a will; something passed on by an ancestor or remaining from the past.

legal /'liːgəl/ *adj* of or based on law; permitted by law; of or for lawyers.—**legally** *adv*.

legalese /,liːgə'liːz/ *n* legal language as used in documents.

legalism /'liːgə,lɪzəm/ *n* observance of the letter rather than the spirit of the law, red tape.—**legalist** *n*.—**legalistic** *adj*.—**legalistically** *adv*.

legality /lɪ'gæliti/ or /liː-/ *n* (*pl* **legalities**) conformity with the law.

legalize /'liːgə,laɪz/ *vt* to make lawful.—**legalization** *n*.

legal tender *n* a currency which a creditor is legally bound to accept in payment of a debt.

legate /'lɛgət/ *n* an envoy, *esp* from the Pope; an official emissary.—**legatine** *adj*.

legatee /,lɛgə'tiː/ *n* a person to whom a legacy is bequeathed.

legation /lɪ'geɪʃən/ *n* a diplomatic minister and staff; the headquarters of a diplomatic minister.—**legationary** *adj*.

legato /lə'gɑːtoʊ/ *adj, adv* (*mus*) smoothly and evenly.

leg before wicket *n* (*cricket*) the dismissal of a batsman for illegally preventing the ball from hitting the wicket by obstructing it with his or her leg.

leg bye *n* (*cricket*) a run made when the ball touches any part of the batsman except the hand.

legend /'lɛdʒənd/ *n* a story handed down from the past; a notable person or the stories of his or her exploits; an inscription on a coin, etc; a caption; an explanation of the symbols used on a map.—**legendry** *n*.

legendary /'lɛdʒənd,ɛri/ *adj* of, based on, or presented in legends; famous, notorious.

legerdemain /,lɛdʒərdə'meɪn/ *n* trickery, sleight of hand.

leger line *see* **ledger line**.

legged /'lɛgd/ *adj* having legs.

leggings /'lɛgɪŋz/ *npl* protective outer coverings for the lower legs; a leg-hugging fashion garment for women.

leggy /'lɛgi/ *adj* (**leggier, leggiest**) having long and shapely legs.—**legginess** *n*.

leghorn /'lɛghɔrn/ *n* fine plaited straw; a hat made of this; (*with cap*) a breed of domestic fowl.

legible /'lɛdʒɪbəl/ *adj* able to be read.—**legibility** *n*.—**legibly** *adv*.

legion /'liːdʒən/ *n* an infantry unit of the ancient Roman army; a large body of soldiers; a large number, a multitude.

legionary /-əri/ *adj* of a legion. • *n* (*pl* **legionaries**) a member of a legion; a soldier in a legion of the ancient Roman army.

legionnaire /,liːdʒə'nɛr/ *n* a member of certain military forces or associations.

Legionnaire's disease *n* a serious and sometimes fatal bacterial infection which causes symptoms like pneumonia (first identified after an outbreak at an American Legion convention in 1976).

legislate /'lɛdʒɪs,leɪt/ *vi* to make or pass laws. • *vt* to bring about by legislation.

legislation /,lɛdʒɪs'leɪʃən/ *n* the act or process of law-making; the laws themselves.

legislative /'lɛdʒɪsleɪtɪv/ *adj* of legislation or a legislature; having the power to make laws.

legislator /'lɛdʒɪs,leɪtər/ *n* a member of a legislative body.

legislature /'lɛdʒɪs,leɪtʃər/ *n* the body of people who have the power of making laws.

legist /'lɛdʒɪst/ *n* someone versed in the law.

legit /lɪ'dʒɪt/ *adj* (*sl*) legitimate.

legitimate /lɪ'dʒɪtəmət/ *adj* lawful; reasonable, justifiable; conforming to accepted rules, standards, etc; (*child*) born of parents married to each other.—**legitimacy** *n*.—**legitimately** *adv*.

legitimatize /lɪ'dʒɪtɪmə,taɪz/ *vt* to legitimize.

legitimist /'lɪdʒɪtɪmɪst/ *n* a supporter of a hereditary title to a monarchy.—**legitimism** *n*.

legitimize /lɪ'dʒɪtɪ,maɪz/ *vt* to make or declare legitimate.—**legitimization** *n*.

legume /'lɛgjuːm/ *n* any of a large family of plants having seeds growing in pods, including beans, peas, etc; the pod or seed of such a plant used as food.

leguminous /lɪ'gjuːmɪnəs/ *adj* (*bot*) belonging to a family of flowering and pod-bearing plants.

legwork /'lɛgwərk/ *n* (*inf*) work that involves a lot of walking.

lei / leɪi/ or /leɪ/ *n* a garland of flowers worn around the neck, given as a token of affection in Hawaii.

leister /'liːstər/ *n* a pronged spear used for catching salmon.

leisure /'liːʒər/ or /'lɛ-/ *n* ease, relaxation, *esp* freedom from employment or duties. • *adj* free and unoccupied.—**leisured** *adj*.

leisurely /-li/ *adj* relaxed, without hurry.

leitmotif, leitmotiv /'laɪtmoʊ,tiːf/ *n* a dominant theme.

lemma /'lɛmə/ *n* (*pl* **lemmas, lemmata**) (*logic*) a premise believed to be true.

lemming /'lɛmɪŋ/ *n* a small arctic rodent; one of a group wilfully heading on a course for destruction.

lemon /'lɛmən/ *n* (a tree bearing) a small yellow oval fruit with an acid pulp; pale yellow; (*sl*) a person or thing considered disappointing or useless.—**lemony** *adj*.

lemonade /,lɛmə'neɪd/ *n* a lemon-flavoured drink.

lemon grass *n* a tropical grass with lemon-scented leaves used in cooking and which yields an aromatic oil.

lemur /'liːmər/ *n* a Madagascan arboreal primate related to the monkey.

lemuroid /-ɔɪd/, **lemurine** /-,raɪn/ or /-,riːn/ *adj* pertaining to, or resembling, a lemur.

lend /lɛnd/ *vb* (**lending, lent**) *vt* to give the use of something temporarily in expectation of its return; to provide (money) at interest; to give, impart. • *vi* to make loans.—**lender** *n*.

length /lɛŋkθ/ or /lɛŋθ/ *n* the extent of something from end to end, *usu* the longest dimension; a specified distance or period of time; something of a certain length taken from a larger piece; a long expanse; (*often pl*) the degree of effort put into some action.

lengthen /'lɛŋkθən/ or /'lɛŋ-/ *vti* to make or become longer.

lengthwise /'lɛŋkθwaɪz/ or /lɛŋθ-/, **lengthways** /-weɪz/ *adv* in the direction of the length.

lengthy /'lɛŋkθi/ or /'lɛŋθi/ *adj* (**lengthier, lengthiest**) long, *esp* too long.—**lengthily** *adv*.—**lengthiness** *n*.

lenient /liːnɪənt/ *adj* not harsh or severe; merciful.—**leniency, lenience** *n*.—**leniently** *adv*.

lenitive /'lɛnɪtɪv/ *adj* easing pain.

lenity /'lɛnɪtɪ/ *n* (*pl* **lenities**) clemency, mercy; leniency.

leno /'liːnoʊ/ *n* (*pl* **lenos**) a way of weaving fabric; a fabric woven in this way.

lens /lɛnz/ *n* a curved piece of transparent glass, plastic, etc used in optical instruments to form an image; any device used to focus electromagnetic rays, sound waves, etc; a similar transparent part of the eye that focuses light rays on the retina.

Lent /lɛnt/ *n* the forty weekdays from Ash Wednesday to Easter, observed by Christians as a period of fasting and penitence.— **Lenten** *adj*.

lent /lɛnt/ *see* **lend**.

lentamente /ˌlɛntəˈmɛntɛɪ/ *adv* (*mus*) slowly.

lenticular /lɛnˈtɪkjʊlər/ *adj* doubly convex.

lentigo /'lɛntɪɡoʊ/ *n* (*pl* **lentigines**) a freckle.

lentil /'lɛntɪl/ *n* any of several leguminous plants with edible seeds; their seed used for food.

lento /'lɛntoʊ/ *adj, adv* (*mus*) slow, slowly. • *n* (*pl* **lentos**) a piece of music played in this way.

Leo /'liːoʊ/ *n* (*astrol*) the fifth sign of the zodiac, in astrology operative July 22–August 21; (*astron*) the Lion, a constellation in the northern hemisphere.

Leonid /'liːənɪd/ *n* (*pl* **Leonids, Leonides**) (*astron*) one of the meteors that fall in showers during the November of certain years, their chief point being in the constellation of Leo.

leonine /'liːənaɪn/ *adj* of or like a lion.

leopard /'lɛpərd/ *n* a large tawny feline with black spots found in Africa and Asia.—*also* **panther**.—**leopardess** *nf*.

leotard /'liːətard/ *n* a skintight one-piece garment worn by dancers and others engaged in strenuous exercise.

leper /'lɛpər/ *n* a person with leprosy.

lepidopteran /lɛpɪˈdɒtərən/ or /ˌlɛpɪdoʊˈtɛrən/ *n* (*pl* **lepidopterans, lepidoptera**) any of a large order of insects, such as moths or butterflies, that as adults have four wings covered with minute, often coloured, scales and that as larvae are caterpillars.—**lepidopterous** *adj*.

lepidopterist /lɛpɪˈdɒtɛrɪst/ *n* an expert on moths and butterflies.

lepidosiren /ˌlɛpɪdoʊˈsaɪrən/ *n* an eel-like mudfish found in South America

leporine /lɛpəˈriːn/ or /-ˈraɪn/ *adj* pertaining to hares; hare-like.

leprechaun /'lɛprəˌkɒn/ *n* (*Irish folklore*) a fairy.

leprosy /'lɛprəsɪ/ *n* a chronic infectious bacterial disease of the skin, often resulting in disfigurement.—**leprous** *adj*.

lepton /'lɛptɒn/ *n* (*phys*) any of various elementary particles, such as electrons and muons, that participate in weak interactions with other elementary particles.

lesbian /'lɛzbɪən/ *n* a female homosexual. • *adj* of or characteristic of lesbians.—**lesbianism** *n*.

lèse-majesté, lese-majesty /liːzˈmædʒəstɪ/ *n* high treason; a crime against royalty.

lesion /'liːʒən/ *n* any change in an organ or tissue caused by injury or disease; an injury.

less /'lɛs/ *adj* not so much, not so great, etc; fewer; smaller. • *adv* to a smaller extent. • *n* a smaller amount. • *prep* minus.

lessee /'lɛsiː/ *n* a person who holds property under a lease.

lessen /'lɛsən/ *vti* to make or become less.

lesser /-ər/ *adj* less in size, quality or importance.

lesson /'lɛsən/ *n* something to be learned or studied; something that has been learned or studied; a unit of learning or teaching; (*pl*) a course of instruction; a selection from the Bible, read as a part of a church service.

lessor /'lɛsɔr/ *n* a person who lets property on a lease.

lest /lɛst/ *conj* in order, or for fear, that not; that.

let[1] /'lɛt/ *n* a stoppage; (*tennis*) a minor obstruction of the ball that requires a point to be replayed.

let[2] *vb* (**letting, let**) *vt* to allow, permit; to rent; to assign (a contract); to cause to run out, as blood; as an auxiliary in giving suggestions or commands (*let us go*); (*with* **down**) to lower; to deflate; to disappoint; to untie; to lengthen; (*with* **off**) to allow to leave (a ship, etc); to cause to explode or fire; to release, excuse from (work, etc); to deal leniently with, refrain from punishing; to allow (gas, etc) to escape; (*with* **out**) to release; to reveal; to rent out; to make a garment larger; (*with* **up**) to relax; to cease. • *vi* to be rented; (*with* **on**) (*inf*) to pretend; (*inf*) to reveal (a secret, etc); to pretend. • *n* the letting of property or accommodation.

let-down /'lɛtdaʊn/ *n* a disappointment.

lethal /'liːθəl/ *adj* deadly.—**lethality** *n*.—**lethally** *adv*.

lethargy /'lɛθɑrdʒɪ/ *n* (*pl* **lethargies**) an abnormal drowsiness; sluggishness; apathy.—**lethargic** *adj*.—**lethargically** *adv*.

let's /lɛts/ = let us.

letter /'lɛtər/ *n* a symbol representing a phonetic value in a written language; a character of the alphabet; a written or printed message; (*pl*) literature; learning; knowledge; literal meaning. • *vt* to mark with letters.

letter bomb *n* an explosive device concealed in an envelope and sent through the post.

letter box *n* a slit in the doorway of a house or building through which letters are delivered; a postbox.

lettered /'lɛtərd/ *adj* literate; highly educated; marked with letters.

letterhead /'lɛtərˌhɛd/ *n* a name, address, etc printed as a heading on stationery; stationery printed with a heading.

lettering /'lɛtərɪŋ/ *n* the act or process of inscribing with letters; letters collectively; a title; an inscription.

letterpress /'lɛtərˌprɛs/ *n* a method of printing; the printed matter of a book, as opposed to the illustrations.

lettuce /'lɛtəs/ *n* a plant with succulent leaves used in salads.

letup *n* a relaxation of effort.

leukemia, leukaemia /luːˈkiːmɪə/ *n* a chronic disease characterized by an abnormal increase in the number of white blood cells in body tissues and the blood.

leukocyte /'luːkəˌsɔɪt/ *n* a white blood cell.

leukoma /luːˈkoʊmə/ *n* a white, opaque scar on the cornea of the eye.

leukorrhea *n* a mucous discharge from the vagina.

leukotomy /luːˈkɒtəmɪ/ *n* (*pl* **leukotomies**) the severing of nerve fibres in the frontal lobes of the brain formerly used to relieve certain severe mental disorders.

lev /lɛv/ *n* (*pl* **leva**) the monetary unit of Bulgaria.

levanter /lɪˈvæntər/ *n* an easterly wind in the Mediterranean.

levantine /lɪˈvæntaɪn/ or /-ˈlɛvən-/ *n* a kind of reversible silk cloth.

levator /lɪˈveɪtər/ *n* (*anat*) a muscle that serves to raise a part of the body.

levee[1] /'lɛvɪ/ *n* a reception of visitors formerly held by a sovereign or other important person on rising from bed; a reception *usu* in honour of a particular person; ✦ (*Cdn*) a public reception held on New Year's Day by the Governor General or by the Lieutenant-Governor of a province.

levee[2] *n* an embankment beside a river.

level /'lɛvəl/ *n* a horizontal line or plane; a position in a scale of values; a flat area or surface; an instrument for determining the horizontal. • *adj* horizontal; having a flat surface; at the same height, rank, position, etc; steady. • *vti* (**leveling, leveled** *or* **levelling, levelled**) to make or become level; to demolish; to raise and aim (a gun, criticism, etc).—**levelly** *adv*.

level crossing *n* (*Brit*) a place where a road crosses a railway line on the same level *esp* where gates or barriers close the road to allow trains to pass; a grade crossing in the US.

leveler, leveller /'lɛvələr/ *n* one who levels; an advocate of social equality.

level-headed /ˌlɛvəlˈhɛdəd/ *adj* having an even temper and sound judgment.—**level-headedly** *adv*.

lever /'liːvər/ *n* a bar used for prising or moving something; a means to an end; a device consisting of a bar turning about a fixed point; any device used in the same way, *eg* to operate machinery. • *vt* to raise or move (as with) a lever.

leverage /'lɛvərɪdʒ/ or /'liːvər-/ *n* the action of a lever; the mechanical advantage gained by the use of a lever; power, influence.

leveret /'lɛvərət/ *n* a hare less than a year old.

leviable /'lɛvɪəbəl/ *adj* subject to a levy; (*goods*) which may be levied upon or seized.

leviathan /ləˈvaɪəθən/ *n* something huge.

levigate /'lɛvɪˌɡeɪt/ *vt* to grind to a fine powder.

Levis /'liːˌvaɪz/ *n* (*trademark*) jeans made from (blue or black) denim.

levitate /'lɛvɪˌteɪt/ *vti* to rise or cause to rise into the air and float without support.—**levitation** *n*.

levity /'lɛvɪtɪ/ *n* (*pl* **levities**) excessive frivolity; lack of necessary seriousness.

levorotation /ˌliːvoʊroʊˈteɪʃən/ *n* left-handed or counterclockwise rotation.—*also* **laevorotation. levorotatory** *adj*.

levulose /'liːvjʊˌloʊs/ or /-ˌloʊz/ *n* a fruit found in sugar.—*also* **laevulose.**

levy /'lɛvɪ/ *vt* (**levying, levied**) to collect by force or authority, as a tax, fine, etc; an amount levied; to enrol or conscript troops;

to prepare for or wage war. • *n* (*pl* **levies**) a levying; the amount levied.—**levier** *n*.

lewd /lju:d/ *adj* indecent; lustful; obscene.—**lewdly** *adv.*—**lewdness** *n*.

lewis /'luːɪs/ *n* an appliance for lifting heavy blocks of stone.

lewisite /'luːɪˌsaɪt/ *n* a blistering liquid obtained from arsenic and acetylene, used in gas form in chemical warfare.

lexical /'lɛksɪkəl/ *adj* of or pertaining to words in a language; of a lexicon or dictionary.—**lexically** *adv.*

lexicographer /ˌlɛksɪ'kɒgrəfər/ *n* a person skilled in lexicography.

lexicography /-grəfi/ *n* the process of writing or compiling a dictionary; the principles and practices of dictionary making.—**lexicographic, lexicographical** *adj.*—**lexicographically** *adv.*

lexicology /ˌlɛksɪ'kɒlədʒi/ *n* the branch of linguistics dealing with the meaning and use of words.—**lexicological** *adj.*—**lexicologist** *n*.

lexicon /'lɛksɪkɒn/ *n* a dictionary; a special vocabulary, as of a specific language, branch of knowledge, etc.

lexis /'lɛksɪs/ *n* the total of words or vocabulary in a language.

ley /leɪ/, **ley-line** *n* a straight line joining two landmarks, supposedly of prehistoric origin.

LF *abbr* = low frequency.

LGen *abbr* ✠ (*Cdn*) = Lieutenant General.

Li (*chem symbol*) lithium.

li /liː/ *n* the Chinese equivalent of a mile, equivalent to approximately 590 yards.

liability /ˌlaɪə'bɪlɪti/ *n* (*pl* **liabilities**) a being liable; something for which one is liable; (*inf*) a handicap, disadvantage; (*pl*) debts, obligations, disadvantages.

liable /ˌlaɪəbəl/ *adj* legally bound or responsible; subject to; likely (to).

liaise /li'eɪz/ *vi* to form a connection and retain contact with.

liaison /li'eɪzɒn/ or /ˌliːeɪ'zɒn/ *n* intercommunication as between units of a military force; an illicit love affair; a thickening for sauces, soups, etc, as egg yolks or cream.

liana, liane /li'ænə/ *n* a climbing plant found in tropical forests.

liar /'laɪər/ *n* a person who tells lies.

Lias /'laɪəs/ *n* (*geol*) the lowest division of rocks of the Jurassic system.—**Liassic** *adj.*

lib /lɪb/ *n* (*inf*) liberation.

libation /lɪ'beɪʃən/ *n* the act of pouring wine or oil on the ground, as a sacrifice; the liquid so poured out; a drink.

libel /'laɪbəl/ *n* any written or printed matter tending to injure a person's reputation unjustly; (*inf*) any defamatory or damaging assertion about a person. • *vt* (**libeling, libeled** or **libelling, libelled**) to utter or publish a libel against.—**libeler, libeller** *n*.—**libelous, libellous** *adj.*

liberal /'lɪbərəl/ *adj* ample, abundant; not literal or strict; tolerant; (*education*) contributing to a general broadening of the mind, non-specialist; favouring reform or progress. • *n* a person who favours reform or progress.—**liberally** *adv.*

liberalism /'lɪbərəˌlɪzəm/ *n* liberal opinions, principles or politics.

liberality /ˌlɪbə'rælɪti/ *n* (*pl* **liberalities**) generosity; breadth of mind.

liberalize /'lɪbərəˌlaɪz/ *vti* to make or become less strict.—**liberalization** *n*.

liberate /'lɪbəˌreɪt/ *vt* to set free from foreign occupation, slavery, etc.—**liberator** *n*.

liberation /ˌlɪbə'reɪʃən/ *n* the act of liberating; the state of being liberated; the pursuit of social, political or economic equality by or on behalf of those being discriminated against.

liberation priest *n* a priest who is active in working for social and political justice.

liberation theology *n* the belief that Christianity requires commitment to social and political change, as well as faith, *esp* in South America.

libertarian /ˌlɪbər'tɛriən/ *n* a person who advocates liberty, *esp* in conduct or thought; a believer in free will.—**libertarianism** *n*.

liberticide /lɪ'bɜːrtɪsaɪd/ *n* a destroyer of liberty; the destruction of liberty.

libertine /'lɪbərˌtiːn/ or /-ˌtaɪn/ *n* a dissolute person; a freethinker. • *adj* unrestrained, morally or socially; licentious.—**libertinism, libertinage** *n*.

liberty /'lɪbərti/ *n* (*pl* **liberties**) freedom from slavery, captivity, etc; the right to do as one pleases; freedom; a particular right, freedom, etc granted by authority; an impertinent attitude; authorized leave granted to a sailor.

libidinous /lɪ'bɪdɪnəs/ *adj* lustful, lascivious.

libido /'lɪbɪˌdoː/ *n* (*pl* **libidos**) the sexual urge.—**libidinal** *adj.*

Libra /'liːbrə/ *n* (*astrol*) the 7th sign of the zodiac, operative 24 September–23 October; a constellation represented as a pair of scales.—**Libran** *n, adj.*

librarian /laɪ'brɛriən/ *n* a person in charge of a library or trained in librarianship.

librarianship, library science *n* the profession of organizing collections of books, etc for reference by others.

library /'laɪˌbreri/ *n* (*pl* **libraries**) a collection of books, tapes, records, photographs, etc for reference or borrowing; a room, building or institution containing such a collection; (*comput*) a set of, *usu* general purpose, programs or subroutines for use in programming.

librate /laɪ'breɪt/ *vi* to waver; to balance.—**libratory** *adj.*

libration /laɪ'breɪʃən/ *n* the act of oscillating; the act of balancing; an apparent irregularity in the motion of the moon or a satellite.

librettist /lɪ'brɛtɪst/ *n* a writer of a libretto.

libretto /lɪ'brɛtoː/ *n* (*pl* **libretti, librettos**) the text to which an opera, oratorio, etc is set.—**librettist** *n*.

Libyan /'lɪbiən/ *n* a native or inhabitant of Libya.—*also adj.*

lice /laɪs/ *see* **louse**.

license /'laɪsəns/ *n* a formal or legal permission to do something specified; a document granting such permission; freedom to deviate from rule, practice, etc; excessive freedom, an abuse of liberty.—*also* **licence**. • *vt* to grant a license to or for; to permit.—**licenser, licensor** *n*.

license plate *n* (*US*) a plate on the front or rear of a motor vehicle that displays its registration number.—*also* **numberplate**.

licensee /ˌlaɪsən'siː/ *n* a person who is granted a licence.

licentiate /laɪ'sɛnʃiət/ or /-ʃət/ *n* a person holding a certificate of competence in a profession; a degree between that of bachelor and doctor in some universities; one licensed to preach.—**licentiateship** *n*.

licentious /laɪ'sɛnʃəs/ *adj* morally unrestrained; lascivious.—**licentiousness** *n*.

lichee /'liːtʃi/ *see* **litchi**.

lichen /'laɪkən/ *n* any of various small plants consisting of an alga and a fungus living in symbiotic association, growing on stones, trees, etc.

lichenology /ˌlaɪkə'nɒlədʒi/ *n* the study of lichens.

lich gate /'lɪtʃgeɪt/ *n* (*Brit*) a roofed gate of a churchyard, under which a coffin can be rested.—*also* **lych gate**.

lichi /'liːtʃi/ *see* **litchi**.

licit /'lɪsɪt/ *adj* lawful.—**licitly** *adv.*

lick /lɪk/ *vt* to draw the tongue over, *esp* to taste or clean; (*flames, etc*) to flicker around or touch lightly; (*inf*) to thrash; (*inf*) to defeat. • *n* a licking with the tongue; (*inf*) a sharp blow; (*inf*) a short, rapid burst of activity.

lickerish /'lɪkərɪʃ/ *adj* lustful; greedy.

lickety-split /ˌlɪkəti'splɪt/ *adv* very fast.

licking /'lɪkɪŋ/ *n* (*inf*) a severe beating; a defeat.

lickspittle /'lɪkˌspɪtəl/ *n* a servile flatterer.

licorice /'lɪkərɪʃ/ or /-rɪs/ *n* a black extract made from the root of a European plant, used in medicine and confectionery; a licorice-flavoured sweet.—*also* **liquorice**.

lictor /'lɪktər/ *n* an official serving a magistrate in ancient Rome.

lid /lɪd/ *n* a removable cover as for a box, etc; an eyelid.—**lidded** *adj.*

lido /'liːdoː/ or /'laɪ-/ *n* (*pl* **lidos**) an open air swimming pool and recreational complex for public use.

lie[1] /laɪ/ *n* an untrue statement made with intent to deceive; something that deceives or misleads. • *vi* (**lying, lied**) to speak untruthfully with an intention to deceive; to create a false impression.

lie[2] *vi* (**lying, lay**, *pp* **lain**) to be or put oneself in a reclining or horizontal position; to rest on a support in a horizontal position; to be in a specified condition; to be situated; to exist. • *n* the way in which something is situated.

lied /liːd/ or /liːt/ *n* (*pl* **lieder**) a German song or ballad.

lie detector *n* a polygraph device used by police and security services that monitors sharp fluctuations in involuntary physiological responses as evidence of stress, guilt, etc when deliberately lying.

lief /liːf/ *adv* (*arch*) willingly.

liege /liːdʒ/ or /liːʒ/ *n* (*feudalism*) a lord or sovereign.—*also* **liege lord**; a subject or vassal.

lien /liːn/ *or* /ˈliːən/ *n* (*law*) a right to keep another's property pending payment of a debt due to the holder.

lierne /liˈərn/ *n* (*archit*) a cross-rib or branch rib in vaulting.

lieu /luː/ *or* /ljuː/ *n* place; stead (*esp in lieu of*, in place of, instead of).

lieutenant /ˈlɛftənənt/ *or* /ˈluː-/ *n* a commissioned army officer ranking below a captain; a naval officer next below a lieutenant commander; a deputy, a chief assistant to a superior.—**lieutenancy** *n*.

Lieutenant-Governor (*pl* **Lieutenant-Governors**) *n* ♣ (*Cdn*) the representative of the Crown in a province.

life /laɪf/ *n* (*pl* **lives**) that property of plants and animals (ending at death) that enables them to use food, grow, reproduce, etc; the state of having this property; living things collectively; the time a person or thing exists; one's manner of living; one's animate existence; vigour, liveliness; (*inf*) a life sentence; a biography. • *adj* of animate being; lifelong; using a living model; of or relating to or provided by life insurance.

life-belt /ˈlaɪfbɛlt/ *n* an inflatable ring to support a person in the water; a safety belt.

lifeblood /-blɛd/ *n* the blood necessary to life; a vital element.

lifeboat /-boːt/ *n* a small rescue boat carried by a ship; a specially designed and equipped rescue vessel that helps those in distress along the coastline.

life buoy /-bɔɪ/ *n* a ring-shaped buoyant device to keep a person afloat.

life cycle *n* a sequence of stages through which a living being passes during its lifetime.

lifeguard /-gɑrd/ *n* an expert swimmer employed to prevent drownings.

life jacket *n* a sleeveless jacket or vest of buoyant material to keep a person afloat.

lifeless /-ləs/ *adj* dead; unconscious; dull.—**lifelessly** *adv*.—**lifelessness** *n*.

lifelike /-laɪk/ *adj* resembling a real life person or thing.

lifeline /-laɪn/ *n* a rope for raising or lowering a diver; a rope for rescuing a person, *eg* as attached to a lifebelt; a vitally important channel of communication or transport.

lifelong /-lɒŋ/ *adj* lasting one's whole life.

life peer *n* a British peer whose title lapses with death.

life preserver *n* a club used as a weapon of self-defence; a lifebelt or life jacket.

lifer /laɪfər/ *n* (*sl*) a person sentenced to prison for life.

life raft *n* a raft kept on board ship for use in emergencies.

lifesaving /ˈlaɪfseɪvɪŋ/ *adj* something (as drugs) designed to save lives. • *n* the skill or practice of saving lives, *esp* from drowning.—**lifesaver** *n*.

life science *n* a science dealing with living organisms and life processes, such as biology, zoology, etc.

life sentence *n* imprisonment for life, or a long period, as punishment for a grave offence.

life-size, life-sized *adj* of the size of the original.

lifestyle /ˈlaɪfstaɪl/ *n* the particular attitudes, living habits, etc of a person.

lifetime /-taɪm/ *n* the length of time that a person lives or something lasts.

lift /lɪft/ *vt* to bring to a higher position, raise; to raise in rank, condition, etc; (*sl*) to steal; to revoke. • *vi* to exert oneself in raising something; to rise; to go up; (*fog, etc*) to disperse; (*with off*) (*rocket, etc*) to take off. • *n* act or fact of lifting; distance through which a thing is lifted; elevation of mood, etc; elevated position or carriage; a ride in the direction in which one is going; help of any kind; (*Brit*) a cage or platform for moving something from one level to another.—*also* **elevator**; upward air pressure maintaining an aircraft in flight.—**lifter** *n*.

liftoff /ˈlɪftɒf/ *n* the vertical thrust of a spacecraft, etc at launching; the time of this.

ligament /ˈlɪɡəmənt/ *n* a band of tissue connecting bones; a unifying bond.

ligan /ˈlaɪɡən/ *see* **lagan**.

ligate /lɪˈɡeɪt/ *vt* to tie up (with a ligature).—**ligation** *n*.

ligature /ˈlɪɡətʃər/ *n* a tying or binding together; a tie, bond, etc; two or more printed letters joined together, as æ; a thread used to suture a blood vessel, etc in surgery.

light[1] /laɪt/ *n* the agent of illumination that stimulates the sense of sight; electromagnetic radiation such as ultraviolet, infrared or X-rays; brightness, illumination; a source of light, as the sun, a lamp, etc; daylight; a thing used to ignite something; a

window; knowledge, enlightenment; aspect or appearance. • *adj* having light; bright; pale in colour. • *adv* palely. • *vt* (**lighting, lit** *or* **lighted**) to ignite; to cause to give off light; to furnish with light; to brighten, animate.

light[2] *adj* having little weight; not heavy; less than usual in weight, amount, force, etc; of little importance; easy to bear; easy to digest; happy; dizzy, giddy; not serious; moderate; moving with ease; producing small products. • *adv* lightly. • *vi* (**lighting, lit** *or* **lighted**) to come to rest after travelling through the air; to dismount, to alight; to come or happen on or upon; to strike suddenly, as a blow.—**lightly** *adv*.—**lightness** *n*.

lighten[1] /ˈlaɪtən/ *vti* to make or become light or lighter; to shine, flash.—**lightener** *n*.

lighten[2] *vti* to make or become lighter in weight; to make or become more cheerful; to mitigate.—**lightener** *n*.

lighter[1] /ˈlaɪtər/ *n* a small device that produces a naked flame to light cigarettes.

lighter[2] *n* a large barge used in loading or unloading larger ships.

lighterage /ˈlaɪtərɪdʒ/ *n* the transport of goods by lighter; the price paid for the service; lighters collectively.

light-fingered *adj* thievish.

light-headed *adj* dizzy; delirious.—**light-headedly** *adv*.

light-hearted /ˈlaɪtˌhɑrtəd/ *adj* carefree.—**light-heartedly** *adv*.

lighthouse /ˈlaɪthʊs/ *n* a tower with a bright light to guide ships.

lighting /ˈlaɪtɪŋ/ *n* the process of giving light; equipment for illuminating a stage, television set, etc; the distribution of light on an object, as in a work of art.

lightning /ˈlaɪtnɪŋ/ *n* a discharge or flash of electricity in the sky. • *adv* fast, sudden.

lightning conductor *or* **rod** *n* a metal rod placed high on a building and grounded to divert lightning from the structure.

light opera *n* an operetta.

light pen *n* a pen-shaped photoelectric device used to communicate with a computer by pointing at the monitor; a similar device used for reading bar codes.

lightship /ˈlaɪtʃɪp/ *n* a ship equipped with a warning beacon and moored at a place dangerous to navigation.

lightsome /ˈlaɪtsəm/ *adj* (*arch, poet*) carefree; graceful, nimble.

lights out *n* (a signal indicating) the time prescribed for retiring to bed, as in a military barracks.

lightweight /ˈlaɪtweɪt/ *adj* of less than average weight; trivial, unimportant. • *n* a person or thing of less than average weight; a professional boxer weighing 130-135 pounds (59-61 kg); a person of little importance or influence.

light-year *n* the distance light travels in one year.

lignaloes *see* **eaglewood**.

ligneous /ˈlɪɡnɪəs/ *adj* of or like wood.

ligniform /ˈlɪɡnɪˌfɔrm/ *adj* resembling wood.

lignify /ˈlɪɡnɪˌfaɪ/ *vti* (**lignifies, lignifying, lignified**) (*bot*) to make or become wood, or woody.—**lignification** *n*.

lignin /ˈlɪɡnɪn/ *n* a woody fibre.

lignite /ˈlɪɡnaɪt/ *n* a soft brownish-black coal with the texture of the original wood.—**lignitic** *adj*.

lignum vitae /ˌlɪɡnəmˈvaɪtɪ/ *or* /-ˈviːtaɪ/ *n* the heavy hard wood of the South American guaiacum tree.

ligroin /ˈlɪˌɡroːɪn/ *n* a solvent distilled from petroleum.

ligulate /ˈlɪɡjʊlət/ *adj* (*bot*) strap-shaped.

ligule /ˈlɪɡjuːl/ *n* (*bot*) a membranous appendage at the top of a sheathing petiole in grasses; one of the rays of a composite plant.

likable, likeable /ˈlaɪkəbəl/ *adj* attractive, pleasant, genial, etc.—**likably, likeably** *adv*.

like[1] /laɪk/ *adj* having the same characteristics; similar; equal. • *adv* (*inf*) likely. • *prep* similar to; characteristic of; in the mood for; indicative of; as for example. • *conj* (*inf*) as; as if. • *n* an equal; counterpart.

like[2] *vt* to be pleased with; to wish. • *vi* to be so inclined.

likelihood /ˈlaɪklɪhʊd/ *n* probability.

likely /ˈlaɪkli/ *adj* (**likelier, likeliest**) reasonably to be expected; suitable; showing promise of success.• *adv* probably.—**likeliness** *n*.

like-minded *adj* sharing the same tastes, ideas, etc.—**likemindedness** *n*.

liken /ˈlaɪkən/ *vt* to compare.

likeness /ˈlaɪknəs/ *n* a being like; something that is like, as a copy, portrait, etc; appearance, semblance.

likewise /ˈlaɪkwaɪz/ *adv* the same; also.

liking /ˈlaɪkɪŋ/ *n* fondness; affection; preference.

lilac /'laɪlək/ or /-lɒk/, /-læk/ n a shrub with large clusters of tiny, fragrant flowers; a pale purple. • adj lilac coloured.

Lilliputian /ˌlɪlɪ'pjuːʃən/ adj tiny; petty. • n a tiny person, a midget.

Li-Lo /'laɪlo/ n (pl **Li-Los**) (trademark) an inflatable rubber or plastic mattress.

lilt /lɪlt/ n a light rhythmic song or tune; a springy motion. • vi (music, song) to have a lilt; to move buoyantly.—**lilting** adj.

lily /'lɪlɪ/ n (pl **lilies**) a bulbous plant having typically trumpet-shaped flowers; its flower.

lily-livered adj cowardly.

lily of the valley n a small plant of the lily family with white bell-shaped flowers.

lily-white adj pure white; (inf) pure, incorruptible.

lima bean n a kind of bean that produces flat, edible pale green seeds; its edible seed.

limb /lɪm/ n a projecting appendage of an animal body, as an arm, leg, or wing; a large branch of a tree; a participating member, agent; an arm of a cross.—**limbless** adj.

limbate /'lɪmˌbeɪt/ adj (bot) with a border of a different colour.

limber[1] /'lɪmbər/ adj flexible, able to bend the body easily. • vt to make limber. • vi to become limber; (with **up**) to stretch and warm the muscles in readiness for physical exercise.

limber[2] n the detachable wheeled section of a gun carriage.

limbo[1] /'lɪmbo/ n (pl **limbos**) (Christianity) the abode after death assigned to unbaptized souls; a place for lost, unwanted, or neglected persons or things; an intermediate stage or condition between extremes.

limbo[2] n (pl **limbos**) a West Indian dance that involves bending over backwards and passing under a horizontal bar that is progressively lowered.

lime[1] /laɪm/ n a white calcium compound used for making cement and in agriculture. • vt to treat or cover with lime.

lime[2] n a small yellowish-green fruit with a juicy, sour pulp; the tree that bears it; its colour.

lime[3] n the linden tree.

limekiln /'laɪmkɪln/ n a furnace for making lime.

limelight /'laɪmlaɪt/ n intense publicity; a type of lamp, formerly used in stage lighting, in which lime was heated to produce a brilliant flame.

limen /'laɪmən/ n (pl **limens, limina**) (psychol) the point at which the effect of a stimulus is just discernible.

limerick /'lɪmərɪk/ n a type of humorous verse consisting of five lines.

limestone /'laɪmstoːn/ n a type of rock composed mainly of calcium carbonate.

limey /laɪmɪ/ n (pl **limeys**) (US sl) a British person.

limit /'lɪmɪt/ n a boundary; (pl) bounds; the greatest amount allowed; (inf) as much as one can tolerate. • vt to set a limit to; to restrict.—**limitable** adj.

limitary /'lɪmɪˌtərɪ/ adj restrictive; restricted.

limitation /ˌlɪmɪ'teɪʃən/ n the act of limiting or being limited; a hindrance to ability or achievement.

limited /'lɪmɪtəd/ adj confined within bounds; lacking imagination or originality.

limited liability n in UK, responsibility for the debts of a company only to the extent of the amount of capital stock held.

limitless /'lɪmɪtləs/ adj boundless, immense.—**limitlessly** adv.—**limitlessness** n.

limn /lɪm/ vt to paint or draw.—**limner** n.

limnology /lɪm'nɒlədʒɪ/ n the scientific study of freshwater bodies (eg. lakes and ponds) in terms of their support for plant and animal life, physical geography, chemical composition, etc.

limo /'lɪmo/ n (inf) **limousine**.

limousine /ˌlɪmə'ziːn/ or /'lɪməˌziːn/ n (sl) a large luxury car.

limp[1] /lɪmp/ vi to walk with or as with a lame leg. • n a lameness in walking.—**limper** n.—**limpingly** adv.

limp[2] adj not firm; lethargic; wilted; flexible.—**limply** adv.—**limpness** n.

limpet /'lɪmpət/ n a mollusc with a low conical shell that clings to rocks.

limpid /'lɪmpɪd/ adj perfectly clear; transparent.—**limpidity** n.

limpkin /'lɪmpkɪn/ n a kind of American wading bird.

limy /'laɪmɪ/ adj (**limier, limiest**) containing, or resembling, lime.

linage /'laɪnɪdʒ/ n the number of written or printed lines or a page.

linchpin /'lɪntʃpɪn/ n a pin passed through an axle to keep a wheel in position; a person or thing regarded as vital to an organization, project, etc.

linden /'lɪndən/ n a tree with deciduous heart-shaped leaves and small fragrant yellow flowers.

line[1] /laɪn/ vt (**lining, lined**) to put, or serve as, a lining in.

line[2] n a length of cord, rope, or wire; a cord for measuring, making level; a system of conducting fluid, electricity, etc; a thin threadlike mark; anything resembling such a mark, as a wrinkle; edge, limit, boundary; border, outline, contour; a row of persons or things, as printed letters across a page; a succession of persons, lineage; a connected series of things; the course a moving thing takes; a course of conduct, actions, etc; a whole system of transportation a person's trade or occupation; a field of experience or interest (inf) glib, persuasive talk; a verse; the forward combat position in warfare fortifications, trenches or other defences used in war; a stock of goods; a piece of information; a short letter, note; (pl) all the speeches of a character in a play; • vb (**lining, lined**) vt to mark with lines; to form a line along; to cover with lines; to arrange in a line. • vi to align.

lineage /'lɪnɪdʒ/ n direct descent from an ancestor; ancestry.

lineal /'lɪnɪəl/ adj hereditary; direct; linear.—**lineally** adv.

lineament /'lɪnɪəmənt/ n (usu pl) a facial feature.

linear /'lɪnɪər/ adj of, made of, or using a line or lines; narrow and long; in relation to length only.—**linearity** n.—**linearly** adv.

linear accelerator n a device for accelerating elementary particles in a straight line by successively activating electric fields at regular intervals along their path.

lineate /'lɪnɪˌeɪt/ adj marked with lines.

lineation /ˌlɪnɪ'eɪʃən/ n the drawing, or arrangement, of lines.

line drawing n a drawing made with solid lines.

line-engraving n an engraving with fine lines; the art of this type of engraving.

linen /'lɪnən/ n thread or cloth made of flax; household articles (sheets, cloths, etc) made of linen or cotton cloth.

line-out n (Rugby Union) the method of restarting a game after the ball has been put into touch, the forwards forming two opposing parallel lines at right angles to the touch-line and jumping for the ball that is thrown in.

line printer n a high-speed computer printer that prints each line as a single unit instead of character by character.

liner /'laɪnər/ n a large passenger ship or aircraft travelling a regular route.

linesman /'laɪnzmən/ n (pl **linesmen**) an official in certain games who assists the referee in deciding when the ball is out of play, etc.

lineup /'laɪnʌp/ n an arrangement of persons or things in a line, eg for inspection.

ling. abbr = linguistics.

ling[1] /lɪŋ/ n a type of heather.

ling[2] n (pl **ling, lings**) a sea fish of northern waters used as food.

linger /'lɪŋgər/ vi to stay a long time; to delay departure; to dawdle or loiter; to dwell on in the mind; to remain alive though on the point of death.—**lingerer** n.—**lingering** adj.—**lingeringly** adv.

lingerie /lɔ̃ʒə'reɪ/ or /lɒ̃-/, /-'riː/ n women's underwear and nightclothes.

lingo /'lɪŋgo/ n (pl **lingoes**) (inf) a dialect, jargon, etc.

lingua franca /ˌlɪŋgwə'fræŋkə/ n (pl **lingua francas, linguae francae**) a language used for communication between speakers of different languages.

lingual /'lɪŋgwəl/ adj of, or pronounced with, the tongue.—**lingually** adv.

linguiform /'lɪŋgwɪˌfɔrm/ adj tongue-shaped.

linguist /'lɪŋgwɪst/ n a person who is skilled in speaking foreign languages.

linguistic /lɪŋ'gwɪstɪk/ adj of or pertaining to language or linguistics.—**linguistically** adv.

linguistics /lɪŋ'gwɪstɪks/ n used as sing) the science of language.

lingulate /'lɪŋgjuˌleɪt/ adj tongue-shaped.

liniment /'lɪnɪmənt/ n a soothing medication, usu applied to the skin.

lining /'laɪnɪŋ/ n a material used to cover the inner surface of a garment, etc any material covering an inner surface.

link /lɪŋk/ n a single loop or ring of a chain; something resembling a loop or ring or connecting piece; a person or thing acting as a connection, as in a communication system, machine or organization. • vti to connect or become connected.

linkage /'lɪŋkɪdʒ/ n a linking; a series or system of links.

linkboy /'lɪŋkbɔɪ/ n (formerly) someone who guided others through dark streets with a torch.

linkman /'lɪŋkmən/ n (pl **linkmen**) (radio, TV) a presenter who links items, reports, etc, esp on a sports programme.

links /lɪŋks/ npl (also used as sing) flat sandy soil; a golf course, esp by the sea.

linkup n a linking together.

linn /lɪn/ n (Scot) a waterfall; the pool beneath a waterfall; a ravine.

Linnaean, Linnean /lɪ'neɪəs/ or /lɪ'niːəs/ adj pertaining to the Swedish naturalist Linnaeus or to his system of classification.

linnet /'lɪnət/ n a small brown or grey songbird.

lino /'laɪnoʊ/ n (inf) (pl **linos**) linoleum.

linocut /'laɪnoʊˌkʌt/ n a design cut in relief on a piece of linoleum; a print made from this.

linoleum /lɪ'noʊliəm/ n a floor covering of coarse fabric backing with a smooth, hard decorative coating.

Linotype /'laɪnoʊtaɪp/ n (trademark) a typesetting machine that casts lines in one piece.

linsang /'lɪnsæŋ/ n a type of civet, found in Indonesia and Borneo.

linseed /'lɪnsiːd/ n the seed of flax, from which linseed oil is made.

linseed oil n oil made from flax seeds, used in paint and varnish.

linsey-woolsey /ˌlɪnzi'wʊlzi/ n a sturdy coarse fabric of linen or cotton and wool mixed.

linstock /'lɪnstɒk/ n (formerly) a staff holding a match, used to light a cannon.

lint /lɪnt/ n scraped and softened linen used to dress wounds; fluff.

lintel /'lɪntəl/ n the horizontal crosspiece spanning a doorway or window.

lintwhite /'lɪntˌwaɪt/ n (Scot, arch) a linnet.

lion /'laɪən/ n a large, flesh-eating feline mammal with a shaggy mane in the adult male; a person of great courage or strength.—**lioness** nf.

lion-hearted adj extremely brave.

lionize /'laɪənaɪz/ vt to treat as or make famous.—**lionization** n.—**lionizer** n.

lip /lɪps/ n either of the two fleshy flaps that surround the mouth; anything like a lip, as the rim of a jug; (sl) insolent talk. • vt (**lipping, lipped**) to touch with the lips; to kiss; to utter.

lipid /'lɪpɪd/ n an organic compound in fats, which is soluble in solvents but insoluble in water.

lipo- /'lɪpoʊ:/, **lip-** /lɪp/ prefix fat, fatty.

lipoid /'lɪpɔɪd/, **lipoidal** /-əl/ adj fatty, resembling fat. • n a fat-like substance.

liposuction /'lɪpoʊsʌkʃən/ or /'ləɪ-/ n cosmetic surgery involving the removal of fat from under the skin of the thighs, stomach, etc using a suction device inserted through an incision.

lipped /lɪpt/ adj having lips or rounded edges.

lip-read vt (**lip-reading, lip-read**) to understand another's speech by watching their lip movements.

lip service n support expressed but not acted upon.

lipstick /'lɪpstɪk/ n a small stick of cosmetic for colouring the lips; the cosmetic itself.

lip-sync, lip-synch vt to move the lips in time with a prerecorded soundtrack (of dialogue or music) on film or television.

liquate /lɪ'kweɪt/ vt to melt (metals) to separate or purify them.—**liquation** n.

liquefacient /ˌlɪkwə'feɪʃənt/ adj serving to liquefy. • n something that liquefies.

liquefy /'lɪkwəfaɪ/ vti (**liquefying, liquefied**) to change to a liquid.—**liquefaction** n.—**liquefier** n.

liquescent /lɪ'kwesənt/ adj becoming liquid.

liqueur /lɪ'kjʊər/ or /-kjʊr/ n a sweet and variously flavoured alcoholic drink.

liquid /'lɪkwɪd/ n a substance that, unlike a gas, does not expand indefinitely and, unlike a solid, flows readily. • adj in liquid form; clear; limpid; flowing smoothly and musically, as verse; (assets) readily convertible into cash.—**liquidity** n.

liquidate /'lɪkwɪˌdeɪt/ vt to settle the accounts of; to close a (bankrupt) business and distribute its assets among its creditors; to convert into cash; to eliminate, kill.

liquidation /ˌlɪkwɪ'deɪʃən/ n the act of liquidating or paying off; the settlement of the affairs of a bankrupt person or business.

liquidator /'lɪkwɪˌdeɪtər/ n an official who winds up a business.

liquidize /'lɪkwɪˌdaɪz/ vt to make liquid.

liquidizer /'lɪkwɪˌdaɪzər/ n a domestic appliance for liquidizing and blending foods.

liquid paraffin n an oily distillate of petroleum used as a laxative.—also **mineral oil**.

liquor /'lɪkər/ n an alcoholic drink; any liquid, esp that in which food has been cooked.

liquor commission n ✦ (Cdn) in some provinces and territories, a government body that regulates the distribution and sales of alcoholic beverages. —also **liquor control board**.

liquorice /'lɪkərɪʃ/ or /-rɪs/ n see **licorice**.

liquor store n a place where alcohol is sold for consumption off the premises.—also **off-licence, package store**.

lira /'liːrə/ n (pl **lire, liras**) the monetary unit of Turkey and former monetary unit of Italy, replaced by the euro.

lisle /laɪl/ n a fine tightly-twisted cotton thread.

lisp /lɪsp/ vi to substitute the sounds th (as in thin) for s or th (as in then) for z; a speech defect or habit involving such pronunciation; to utter imperfectly. • vt to speak or utter with a lisp.—also n.—**lisper** n.

lissom /'lɪsəm/ adj lithe; supple; agile, etc.—**lissomeness** n.

list¹ /lɪst/ n a series of names, numbers, words, etc written or printed in order. • vt to make a list of; to enter in a directory, etc.

list² vti to tilt to one side, as a ship. • n such a tilting.

listed /'lɪstəd/ adj (company, etc) having its shares quoted on a stock exchange; (building) of architectural interest and protected from demolition or alteration without permission.

listed building n in UK, a building officially designated as of historic or architectural interest and protected from alteration or demolition.

listen /'lɪsən/ vi to try to hear; to pay attention, take heed; (with in) to intercept radio or telephone communications; to tune into a radio broadcast; to eavesdrop.

listener /'lɪsənər/ n a person who listens; a person listening to a radio broadcast.

listeriosis /lɪˌstiːri'oʊsɪs/ n chronic food poisoning caused by the bacteria Listeria.

listing /'lɪstɪŋ/ n a list, or an individual entry therein; the act of making a list; (pl) a guide giving details of events, eg music, theatre, taking place in a particular area, published in a newspaper or magazine.

listless /'lɪstləs/ adj lacking energy or enthusiasm because of illness, dejection, etc; languid.—**listlessly** adv.—**listlessness** n.

lit /lɪt/ see **light¹, light²**.

lit. abbr = literal; literary; literature; litre.

litany /'lɪtəni/ n (pl **litanies**) a type of prayer in which petitions to God are recited by a priest and elicit set responses by the congregation; any tedious or automatic recital.

litchi /'liːtʃi/ n a fruit consisting of a soft, sweet white pulp in a thin brown shell; the tree that bears this fruit.—also **lichee, lichi**.

-lite /laɪt/ n suffix stone; mineral; fossil.

liter /'liːtər/ see **litre**.

literacy /'lɪtərəsi/ n the ability to read and write.

literal /'lɪtərəl/ adj in accordance with the exact meaning of a word or text; in a basic or strict sense; prosaic, unimaginative; real.—**literalness, literality** n.—**literally** adv.

literalism /'lɪtərəˌlɪzəm/ n adherence to the literal sense of a word or saying.—**literalist** n.

literary /'lɪtərˌeri/ adj of or dealing with literature; knowing much about literature.—**literarily** adv.—**literariiness** n.

literate /'lɪtərət/ adj able to read and write; educated.—also n.

literati /ˌlɪtə'rɒti/ npl educated people.

literatim /ˌlɪtə'rætɪm/ adv letter for letter.

literature /'lɪtərətʃər/ or /'lɪtrə-/ n the writings of a period or of a country, esp those valued for their excellence; of style or form; all the books and articles on a subject; (inf) any printed matter.

-lith /lɪθ/ n suffix stone or rock.

litharge /'lɪθɑrdʒ/ n an oxide of lead.

lithe /laɪð/ adj supple, flexible.—**litheness** n.

lithesome /'laɪðsəm/ adj lithe, supple.

lithia /'lɪθiə/ n an oxide of lithium.

lithic /'lɪθɪk/ adj of or pertaining to stone.

lithium /'lɪθiəm/ n the lightest metallic element.

litho /'lɪθoʊ/ n (pl **lithos**) a lithograph; lithography.

lithograph /ˌlɪθə'græf/ n a print, etc made by lithography.—**lithographic** adj.—**lithographically** adv.

lithography /lɪ'θɒɡrəfi/ n printing from a flat stone or metal plate, parts of which have been treated to repel ink.—**lithographer** n.

lithoid /'lɪθɔɪd/, **lithoidal** /-əl/ adj stonelike.

lithology /lɪ'θɒlədʒi/ n the study of rocks and their physical characteristics.—**lithologic, lithological** adj.

lithophyte /'lɪθəˌfaɪt/ n a stony polyp; a plant which grows on a rocky surface.

lithosphere /'lɪθəˌsfiːr/ n the solid outer part of the earth.

lithotomy /lɪ'θɒtəmi/ n (pl **lithotomies**) (med) the operation of cutting into the bladder to remove a stone.—**lithotomic** adj.

lithotripter, lithotriptor /ˌlɪθə'trɪptər/ n an instrument that fragments kidney or bladder stones, etc by ultrasound without the need for invasive surgery.

lithotrity /lɪ'θɒtrəti/ n (pl **lithotrities**) (med) the operation of crushing a stone in the bladder.

litigant /'lɪtɪgənt/ n a person engaged in a lawsuit

litigate /'lɪtɪˌgeɪtʃən/ vti to bring or contest in a lawsuit.—**litigator** n.

litigation /lɪtɪ'geɪʃən/ n the act or processs of carrying on a lawsuit; a judicial contest.

litigious /lɪ'tɪdʒəs/ adj of or causing lawsuits; fond of engaging in lawsuits; contentious.—**litigiousness** n.

litmus /'lɪtməs/ n a colouring material obtained from certain lichens that turns red in acid solutions and blue in alkaline solutions.

litotes /laɪ'təʊtiːz/ n (pl **litotes**) (rhetoric) understatement for effect.

litre, liter /'liːtər/ n a measure of liquid capacity in the metric system, equivalent to 1.76 pints.—also **litre**.

Litt.D, Lit.D abbr = Doctor of Letters; Doctor of Literature.

litter /'lɪtər/ n rubbish scattered about; young animals produced at one time; straw, hay, etc used as bedding for animals; a stretcher for carrying a sick or wounded person. • vt to make untidy; to scatter about carelessly.

littérateur /ˌlɪtəræˈtər/ n a writer.

litterbug /'lɪtərˌbʌg/ n a person who drops refuse in public places.

little /'lɪtl/ adj not great or big, small in size, amount, degree, etc; short in duration; small in importance or power; narrowminded. • n small in amount, degree, etc. • adv less, least, slightly; not much; not in the least.

little people npl (folklore) supernatural beings such as fairies, elves and leprechauns.

littoral /'lɪtərəl/ adj of or along the seashore.

liturgics /lɪ'tɜːdʒɪks/ n sing the study of liturgies.

liturgist /'lɪtərdʒɪst/ n someone who studies or composes liturgies.

liturgy /'lɪtərdʒi/ n (pl **liturgies**) the prescribed form of service of a church.—**liturgical** adj.—**liturgically** adv.

livable /'lɪvəbəl/ adj worth living; suitable for living in.

live¹ /lɪv/ vi to have life; to remain alive; to endure; to pass life in a specified manner; to enjoy a full life; to reside; (with **in, out**) (employee) to reside at (or away from) one's place of work; (with **together**) (unmarried couple) to cohabit. • vt to carry out in one's life; to spend; pass; (with **down**) to survive or efface the effects of (a crime or mistake) by waiting until it is forgotten or forgiven.

live² adj having life; of the living state or living beings; of present interest; still burning; unexploded; carrying electric current; broadcast during the actual performance.

liveable /'lɪvəbəl/ see **livable**.

livelihood /'laɪvlɪˌhʊd/ n employment; a means of living.

livelong /'laɪvlɒŋ/ adj of the whole length of (the day).

lively /'laɪvli/ adj (**livelier, liveliest**) full of life; spirited; exciting; vivid; keen. • adv in a lively manner.—**liveliness** n.

liven /'laɪvən/ vti to make or become lively.—**livener** n.

liver /'lɪvər/ n the largest glandular organ in vertebrate animals, which secretes bile, etc and is important in metabolism; the liver of an animal used as food; a reddish-brown colour.

liveried /'lɪvəˌriːd/ adj wearing a livery.

liverish /'lɪvərɪʃ/ adj suffering from liver disorder; peevish.

liverwort /'lɪvərˌwɜːt/ n a cryptogamous plant, found in wet places.

liverwurst /'lɪvərˌwɜːst/ n sausage made with liver.

livery /'lɪvəri/ n (pl **liveries**) an identifying uniform, as that worn by a servant.

liveryman /'lɪvərɪmən/ n (pl **liverymen**) a keeper of a livery stable; a member of a livery company.

liveyer /'laɪvjər/ n ✤ (Cdn) (inf) a permanent resident of Newfoundland or Labrador.

lives /laɪvz/ see **life**.

livestock /'laɪvstɒks/ n (farm) animals raised for use or sale.

live wire n (inf) a lively, energetic person.

livid /'lɪvɪd/ adj (skin) discoloured, as from bruising; greyish in colour; (inf) extremely angry.—**lividly** adv.—**lividness, lividity** n.

living /'lɪvɪŋ/ adj having life; still in use; true to life, vivid; of life, for living in. • n a being alive; livelihood; manner of existence.

living room n a room in a house used for general entertainment and relaxation.

living wage n a wage sufficient to maintain a reasonable standard of comfort.

lixiviate /'lɪksɪvɪˌeɪt/ vt to wash (soil, ore, etc) with a filtering liquid; to extract (a soluble substance) from some material.—**lixiviation** n.

lizard /'lɪzərd/ n a reptile with a slender body, four legs, and a tapering tail.

llama /'læmə/ n a South American animal, related to the camel, used for carrying loads and as a source of wool.

llano /'læno/ or /'ljæ-/ n (pl **llanos**) one of the vast, level plains of South America.

LLB /'ɛl'ɛl'biː/ abbr = Bachelor of Laws.

LLD /'ɛl'ɛl'diː/ abbr = Doctor of Laws.

LLM /'ɛl'ɛl'ɛm/ abbr = Master of Laws.

lm abbr = lumen.

LNG /'ɛl'ɛn'dʒiː/ abbr = liquefied natural gas.

lo /loʊ/ interj behold!, see!

loach /loʊtʃ/ n an edible freshwater fish.

load /'loʊd/ n an amount carried at one time; something borne with difficulty; a burden; (often pl) (inf) a great amount. • vt to put into or upon; to burden; to oppress; to supply in large quantities; to alter, as by adding a weight to dice or an adulterant to alcoholic drink; to put a charge of ammunition into (a firearm); to put film into (a camera); (comput) to install a program in memory. • vi to take on a load.—**loader** n.

loaded /'loʊdəd/ adj (sl) having plenty of money; drunk; under the influence of drugs.

loadstar /'loʊdstɑr/ see **lodestar**.

loadstone /'loʊdstoʊn/ see **lodestone**.

loaf¹ /'loʊf/ n (pl **loaves**) a mass of bread of regular shape and standard weight; food shaped like this; (sl) the head.

loaf² vi to pass time in idleness.—**loafer** n.

loam /'loʊm/ n rich and fertile soil.

loamy /'loʊmi/ adj (**loamier, loamiest**) consisting of or full of loam.—**loaminess** n.

loan /'loʊn/ n the act of lending; something lent, esp money. • vti to lend.—**loanable** adj.—**loaner** n.

loath /'loʊθ/ adj unwilling.—also **loth**.—**loathly** adv.

loathe /'loʊð/ vt to dislike intensely; to detest.—**loather** n.—**loathing** n.

loathsome /'loʊðsəm/ adj giving rise to loathing; detestable.—**loathsomeness** n.

loaves /'loʊvz/ see **loaf**¹.

lob /lɒb/ vti (**lobbing, lobbed**) to toss or hit (a ball) in a high curve. • n a high-arching throw or kick.

lobar /'loʊbər/ adj of or relating to a lobe.

lobate /'loʊbeɪt/ adj having lobes; loblike.

lobby /'lɒbi/ n (pl **lobbies**) an entrance hall of a public building; a person or group that tries to influence legislators. • vti (**lobbying, lobbied**) to try to influence (legislators) to support a particular cause or take certain action.

lobbyist /-ɪst/ n someone employed to lobby.

lobe /loʊb/ n a rounded projection, as the lower end of the ear; any of the divisions of the lungs or brain.

lobelia /lə'biːliə/ n a genus of garden plants, usually with blue flowers.

loblolly /'lɒblɒli/ n (pl **loblollies**) a type of American pine tree; (naut) gruel.

lobotomy /lə'bɒtəmi/ n (pl **lobotomies**) surgical incision into the lobe of an organ; a leukotomy.

lobscouse /'lɒbskaʊs/ n a sailor's dish of meat, vegetables and ship's biscuit.

lobster /'lɒbstər/ n (pl **lobsters, lobster**) any of a family of edible sea crustaceans with four pairs of legs and a pair of large pincers.

lobster roll ✤ (Cdn) a long bread roll filled with lobster salad.

lobster supper n ✤ (Cdn) in the Maritime Provinces, a full meal featuring boiled lobsters that is sold and served to the public in a community hall.

lobule /'lɒbjuːl/ n a small lobe.—**lobular, lobulate** adj.

local /'loʊkəl/ adj of or belonging to a particular place; serving the needs of a specific district; of or for a particular part of the body. • n an inhabitant of a specific place; (inf) a pub serving a particular district.—**locally** adv.—**localness** n.

locale /loːˈkæl/ *n* a place or area, *esp* in regard to the position or scene of some event.

localism /ˈloːkəˌlɪzəm/ *n* a word, idiom or custom restricted to a particular locality; narrowness of outlook.

locality /loːˈkælɪti/ *n* (*pl* **localities**) a neighbourhood or a district; a particular scene, position, or place; the fact or condition of having a location in space and time.

localize /ˈloːkəˌlaɪz/ *vt* to limit, confine, or trace to a particular place.—**localization** *n*.

locate /loːˈkeɪt/ or /ˈloː-/ *vt* to determine or indicate the position of something; to set in or assign to a particular position.

location /loːˈkeɪʃən/ *n* a specific position or place; a locating or being located; a place outside a studio where a film is (partly) shot; (*comput*) an area in memory where a single item of data is stored.

locative /ˈlɒkətɪv/ *adj, n* (a grammatical case) indicating place.

loc. cit. *abbr* = loco citato (Latin *in the place cited*).

loch /lɒk/, *Scot.* /lɒx/ *n* (*Scot*) a lake.

loci /ˈloːkaɪ/ *see* **locus**.

lock[1] /lɒk/ *n* a fastening device on doors, etc, operated by a key or combination; part of a canal, dock, etc in which the level of the water can be changed by the operation of gates; the part of a gun by which the charge is fired; a controlling hold, as used in wrestling. • *vt* to fasten with a lock; to shut; to fit, link; to jam together so as to make immovable. • *vi* to become locked; to interlock.—**lockable** *adj*.

lock[2] *n* a curl of hair; a tuft of wool, etc.

lockage /ˈlɒkɪdʒ/ *n* a system of canal locks; the act of going through a lock; the fee paid for so doing.

locker /ˈlɒkər/ *n* a small cupboard, chest, etc that can be locked, *esp* one for storing possessions in a public place.

locker room *n* room equipped with lockers for storing possessions in a public place.

locket /ˈlɒkət/ *n* a small ornamental case, *usu* holding a lock of hair, photograph or other memento, hung from the neck.

lockjaw /ˈlɒkdʒɔː/ *n* tetanus.

lockout /ˈlɒkaʊt/ *n* the exclusion of employees from a workplace by an employer, as a means of coercion during an industrial dispute.

locksmith /ˈlɒksmɪθ/ *n* a person who makes and repairs locks and keys.

lockup /ˈlɒkʌp/ *n* a jail; a garage or storage room; ✦ (*Cdn*) a period of time in which members of the media are allowed to examine a government budget, but not report on it, while locked in a room just before the budget is released in a legislature.

loco /ˈloːkoː/ *adj* (*sl*) crazy.

locomotion /ˌloːkəˈmoːʃən/ *n* motion, or the power of moving, from one place to another.

locomotive /-ˈmoːtɪv/ *n* an electric, steam, or diesel engine on wheels, designed to move a railway train. • *adj* of locomotion.

locomotor /-ˈmoːtər/ *adj* of or pertaining to locomotion. locomotive.

locular /ˈlɒkjulər/, **loculate** /-ˌleɪt/ *adj* (*biol*) split into compartments.

loculus /ˈlɒkjuləs/, **locule** *n* (*pl* **loculi, locules**) (*biol*) a small cavity or cell.

locum /ˈloːkəm/ *n* (*inf*) a locum tenens.

locum tenens /ˈloːkəmˈtiːnənz/ *n* (*pl* **locum tenentes**) a person who stands in for a professional colleague, *esp* for a doctor, chemist or clergyman.

locus /ˈloːkəs/ *n* (*pl* **loci**) a place; (*math*) the path of a point or curve, moving according to some specific rule; the aggregate of all possible positions of a moving or generating element.

locust /ˈloːkəst/ *n* a type of large grasshopper often travelling in swarms and destroying crops; a type of hard-wooded leguminous tree.

locution /ləˈkjuːʃən/ *n* a word, phrase or expression; an act or mode of speaking.

lode /loːd/ *n* an ore deposit.

lodestar /ˈloːdstɑːr/ *n* a star, *usu* the North Star, used to guide navigation.—*also* **loadstar**.

lodestone /ˈloːdstoːn/ *n* a magnetic oxide of iron; a piece of this oxide, used as a magnet or a crude compass.—*also* **loadstone**.

lodge /lɒdʒ/ *n* a small house at the entrance to a park or stately home; a country house for seasonal leisure activities; a resort hotel or motel; the local chapter or hall of a fraternal society; a beaver's lair. • *vt* to house temporarily; to shoot, thrust, etc firmly (in); to bring before legal authorities; to confer upon. • *vi* to live in a place for a time; to live as a paying guest; to come to rest and stick firmly (in).

lodger /ˈlɒdʒər/ *n* a person who lives in a rented room in another's home.

lodging /ˈlɒdʒɪŋ/ *n* a temporary residence; (*pl*) accommodation rented in another's house.

lodgment, lodgement /ˈlɒdʒmənt/ *n* the act of lodging; the state of being lodged; an accumulation of something deposited; (*mil*) a foothold in enemy territory.

loess /ˈloːɛs/ *n* a light brown deposit of fine silt and clay found in Asia, Europe and America.—**loessial, loessal** *adj*.

loft /lɒft/ *n* a space under a roof; a storage area under the roof of a barn or stable; a gallery in a church or hall. • *vt* to send into a high curve.

lofty /ˈlɒfti/ *adj* (**loftier, loftiest**) (*objects*) of a great height, elevated; (*person*) noble, haughty, superior in manner.—**loftily** *adv*.—**loftiness** *n*.

log[1] /lɒg/ *n* a section of a felled tree; a device for ascertaining the speed of a ship; a record of speed, progress, etc, *esp* one kept on a ship's voyage or aircraft's flight. • *vb* (**logging, logged**) *vt* to record in a log; to sail or fly (a specified distance). • *vi* (*with* **on, off**) (*comput*) to establish or disestablish communication with a mainframe computer from a remote terminal in a multiuser system.—**logger** *n*.

log[2] *n* a logarithm.

loganberry /ˈloːgənˌbɛri/ *n* (*pl* **loganberries**) a hybrid developed from the blackberry and the red raspberry.

logarithm /ˈlɒgəˌrɪðəm/ *n* the exponent of the power to which a fixed number (the base) is to be raised to produce a given number, used to avoid multiplying and dividing when solving mathematical problems.—**logarithmic** *adj*.—**logarithmically** *adv*.

logbook /ˈlɒgbʊk/ *n* an official record of a ship's or aircraft's voyage or flight; an official document containing details of a vehicle's registration.

log drive *n* ✦ (*Cdn*) the transportation of logs from forests to mills by floating them down rivers.

loge /loːʒ/ *n* a box in a theatre.

loggerhead /ˈlɒgərˌhɛd/ *n* (*arch*) a blockhead; (*pl*) a dispute, confrontation (*to be at loggerheads with someone*); (*zool*) a type of turtle.

loggia /ˈloːdʒə/ or /ˈlɒ-/ *n* (*pl* **loggias, loggie**) a covered open gallery or balcony on the side of a building.

logging /ˈlɒgɪŋ/ *n* the business of cutting down timber.

logic /ˈlɒdʒɪk/ *n* correct reasoning, or the science of this; way of reasoning; what is expected by the working of cause and effect.—**logician** *n*.

logical /ˈlɒdʒɪkəl/ *adj* conforming to the rules of logic; capable of reasoning according to logic.—**logically** *adv*.—**logicality** *n*.

logician /ləˈdʒɪʃən/ *n* someone versed in logic.

logistics /ləˈdʒɪstɪks/ *n* (*used as sing*) the science of the organization, transport and supply of military forces; the planning and organization of any complex activity.—**logistic** *adj*.—**logistically** *adv*.

log jam *n* a blockage of logs floating in a watercourse; a deadlock, standstill.

logo /ˈloːgoː/ *n* (*pl* **logos**) (*inf*) a logotype.

logo- /ˈlɒgoː/ or /-ə/ *prefix* word, speech.

logogram /ˈlɒgəˌgræm/, **logograph** /-ˌgræf/ *n* a sign or letter representing a word or phrase.

logographer /ləˈgɒgrəfər/ *n* an annalist or writer of speeches in ancient Greece.

logography /ləˈgɒgrəfi/ *n* a method of printing in which a type represents a word instead of a letter.

logogriph /ˈlɒgəˌgrɪf/ *n* a word puzzle based on an anagram.

logomachy /ləˈgɒməki/ *n* (*pl* **logomachies**) a dispute over words.

loggorhea /ˌlɒgəˈriə/ *n* excessive or incoherent talkativeness.

Logos /ˈlɒgɒs/ *n* (*Christianity*) the Divine Word; the second person of the Trinity, Jesus Christ.

logotype /ˈlɒgəˌtaɪp/ *n* a printed symbol representing a corporation, product, etc; a trademark, emblem.

logrolling /ˈlɒgˌroːlɪŋ/ *n* in US, the undemocratic trading of votes between politicians to ensure the passage of legislation of mutual interest.

-logue, -log /lɒg/ *n suffix* indicating a particular type of speech or writing, as in monologue, travelogue.

logwood /ˈlɒgwʊd/ *n* a wood of a deep-red colour, used in dyeing.

-logy /lədʒi/ *n suffix* science, theory or doctrine of, *eg astrology*; type of writing or discourse, *eg phraseology*.

logy /'lo:gi/ *adj* (**logier, logiest**) dull, sluggish.

loin /lɔin/ *n* (*usu pl*) the lower part of the back between the hip-bones and the ribs; the front part of the hindquarters of an animal used for food.

loincloth /'lɔinklɒθ/ *n* a cloth worn around the loins.

loiter /'lɔitər/ *vi* to linger or stand about aimlessly.—**loiterer** *n*.

loll /lɒl/ *vi* to lean or recline in a lazy manner, to lounge; (*tongue*) to hang loosely.—**loller** *n*.

lollapalooza, lollapaloosa /lɒləpə'lu:zə/ *n* (*sl*) something or someone exceptional.

Lollard /'lɒlərd/ *n* (*hist*) a follower of the 14th-century English religious reformer, John Wycliff.

lollipop /'lɒli,pɒp/ *n* a flat boiled sweet at the end of a st ck.

lollop /'lɒləp/ *vi* to run or walk with an ungainly, bouncing rhythm.

lolly /'lɒli/ *n* (*pl* **lollies**) (*inf*) a lollipop; (*Brit sl*) money.

loment /'lo:mənt/ *n* a plant pod that breaks at maturity into single-seeded joints.

London Pride *n* a type of saxifrage plant with pink flowers.

lone /lo:n/ *adj* by oneself; isolated; without comparisons, solitary.—**loneness** *n*.

lonely /'lo:nli/ *adj* (**lonelier, loneliest**) isolated; unhappy at being alone; (*places*) remote, rarely visited.—**loneliness** *n*.

loner /'lo:nər/ *n* a person who avoids the company of others.

lonesome /'lo:nsəm/ *adj* having or causing a lonely feeling.—**lonesomely** *adv*.

long. *abbr* = longitude.

long[1] /lɒŋ/ *adj* measuring much in space or time; having a greater than usual length, quantity, etc; tedious, slow; far-reaching; well-supplied. • *adv* for a long time; from start to finish; at a remote time.

long[2] *vi* to desire earnestly, *esp* for something not likely to be attained.

longanimity /,lɒŋgə'nimiti/ *n* long-suffering, forbearance.

longboat /'lɒŋbo:t/ *n* the largest boat carried aboard a ship.

longbow /'lɒŋbo:/ *n* a large hand-drawn bow.

longcloth /-klɒθ/ *n* a fine cotton fabric.

long-distance *adj* travelling or communicating over long distances.

longe /lʌndʒ/ *see* **lunge**[2].

longeron /'lɒndʒərən/ *n* the principal longitudinal spar of an aircraft's fuselage.

longevity /lɒn'dʒɛviti/ *n* long life.

longhand /'lɒŋhænd/ *n* ordinary handwriting, as opposed to shorthand.

long-headed *adj* shrewd.

longhorn /'lɒŋhɔrn/ *n* a breed of long-horned cattle.

longhouse /'lɒŋhaus/ *n* ❦ among some North American Indian peoples, a traditional dwelling shared by several families.

longicorn /'lɒndʒikɔrn/ *n* a type of beetle with long antennae.

longing /'lɒŋiŋ/ *n* an intense desire.—**longingly** *adv*.

longitude /'lɒŋgi,tu:d/ or /'lɒndʒ-/, /-tju:d/ *n* distance east or west of the prime meridian, expressed in degrees or time.

longitudinal /'lɒŋgi,tu:dinəl/ or /'lɒndʒ-/, /-tju:d-/ *adj* of or in length; running or placed lengthways; of longitude.—**longitudinally** *adv*.

long johns *npl* (*inf*) warm underpants with long legs.

long jump *n* an athletic event consisting of a horizontal running jump.

long-lived *adj* having or tending to live a long time.

long-playing *adj* of or relating to an LP record.

long-range *adj* reaching over a long distance or period of time.

longshore /'lɒŋʃɔr/ *adj* found on, or pertaining to, the shore.

longshoreman /'lɒŋʃɔrmən/ *n* (*pl* **longshoremen**) a person who loads and unloads ships at a port.

long shot *n* a wild guess; a competitor, etc who is unlikely to win; a project that has little chance of success.

long-sighted *adj* only seeing distant objects clearly.—**long-sightedly** *adv*.

long-standing *adj* having continued for a long time.

long-suffering *adj* enduring pain, provocation, etc patiently.

long-term *adj* of or extending over a long time.

longueur /lɒŋ'gər/, *Fr.* /lo:n'gœr/ *n* a tedious period of time.

long wave *n* a radio wave of a frequency less than 300 kHz.

longways /'lɒŋweiz/, **longwise** /'lɒŋwaiz/ *adv* in the direction of the length (of something), lengthways.

long-winded /'lɒŋwaindəd/ *adj* speaking or writing at great length; tiresome.—**long-windedly** *adv*.—**long-windedness** *n*.

loo /lu:/ *n* (*pl* **loos**) (*Brit inf*) a lavatory, a toilet.

looby /'lu:bi/ *n* (*pl* **loobies**) a clumsy, stupid person.

loofah /'lu:fə/ *n* the fibrous skeleton of a type of gourd used as a sponge for scrubbing.—*also* **luffa**.

look /luk/ *vi* to try to see; to see; to search; to appear, seem; to be facing in a specified direction; (*with* **in**) to pay a brief visit; (*with* **up**) to improve in prospects. • *vt* to direct one's eyes on; to have an appearance befitting. • *n* the act of looking; a gaze, glance; appearance; aspect; (*with* **after**) to take care of; (*with* **over**) to examine; (*with* **up**) to research (for information, etc) in book; to visit.

look-alike *n* a person that looks like another.

looker /'lukər/ *n* (*inf*) an attractive woman.

looker-on *n* (*pl* **lookers-on**) a spectator.

look-in *n* a brief visit.

looking glass *n* a mirror.

lookout /'lukaut/ *n* a place for keeping watch; a person assigned to watch.

look-see *n* (*inf*) a brief inspection.

loom[1] /lu:m/ *n* a machine or frame for weaving yarn or thread. • *vt* to weave on a loom.

loom[2] *vi* to come into view indistinctly and often threateningly; to come ominously close, as an impending event.

loon[1] /lu:n/ *n* a large fish-eating diving bird.

loon[2] *n* (*sl*) a clumsy or stupid person; a crazy person.

loonie /'lu:ni/ *n* ❦ (*Cdn*) a one-dollar coin.

loony, looney /'lu:ni/ *n* (*pl* **loonies**) (*sl*) a lunatic. • *adj* (**loonier, looniest**) (*sl*) crazy, demented.—**looniness** *n*.

loop /lu:p/ *n* a figure made by a curved line crossing itself; a similar rounded shape in cord, rope, etc crossed on itself; anything forming this figure; (*comput*) a set of instructions in a program that are executed repeatedly; an intrauterine contraceptive device; a segment of film or magnetic tape. • *vt* to make a loop of; to fasten with a loop. • *vi* to form a loop or loops.

looper /'lu:pər/ *n* a caterpillar that crawls by arching itself into loops.

loophole /'lu:pho:l/ *n* a means of evading an obligation, etc; a slit in a wall for looking or shooting through.

loopy /'lu:pi/ *adj* (**loopier, loopiest**) (*inf*) slightly mad, cracked.

loose /lu:s/ *adj* free from confinement or restraint; not firmly fastened; not tight or compact; not precise; inexact; (*inf*) relaxed. • *vt* to release; to unfasten; to untie; to detach; (*bullet*) to discharge. • *vi* to become loose.—**loosely** *adv*.—**looseness** *n*.

loose cannon *n* a person who acts independently and often obstreperously.

loose-leaf *adj* having pages or sheets that can easily be replaced or removed.

loosen /'lu:zən/ *vti* to make or become loose or looser.—**loosener** *n*.

loosestrife /'lu:sstraif/ *n* a kind of plant with golden or purple flowers.

loot /lu:t/ *n* goods taken during warfare, civil unrest, etc; (*sl*) money. • *vti* to plunder, pillage.—**looter** *n*.

lop /lɒp/ *vt* (**lopping, lopped**) to sever the branches or twigs from a tree; to cut off or out as superfluous.

lope /lo:p/ *vi* to move or run with a long bounding stride.—*also n*.—**loper** *n*.

lop-eared *adj* having drooping ears.

lophobranchiate /'lɒfə,bræŋki:it/ *adj* (*fish*) with gills arranged in tufts.

lopsided /lɒp'saidəd/ *adj* having one side larger in weight, height, or size than the other; badly balanced.—**lopsidedly** *adv*.—**lopsidedness** *n*.

loquacious /lo:'kweiʃəs/ *adj* talkative.—**loquaciously** *adv*.—**loquacity** *n*.

loquat /'lo:kwɒt/ *n* an evergreen tree found in China and Japan; its edible fruit.

loquitur /'lɒkwitər/ (*theatre*) (*formerly*) he or she speaks (as a stage direction).

lord /lɔrd/ *n* a ruler, master or monarch; a male member of the nobility; (*with cap and* **the**) God; a form of address used to certain peers, bishops and judges.

lordling /'lɔrdliŋ/ *n* a young or minor lord.

lordly /-li/ *adj* (**lordlier, lordliest**) noble; haughty; arrogant.—**lordliness** *n*.

Lord Mayor *n* the mayor of the City of London and certain other UK boroughs and towns—*also* **Lord Provost** in Scotland.

lordosis /lɔr'doːsɪs/ n forward curvature of the spine.

Lord Privy Seal n a British cabinet minister without specific responsibilities.

Lord Provost see **Lord Mayor.**

Lord's Day n (with **the**) Sunday.

lordship /'lɔrdʃɪp/ n the rank or authority of a lord; rule, dominion; (with **his** or **your**) a title used in speaking of or to a lord.

Lord's Prayer n (with **the**) the prayer taught by Jesus to His disciples beginning 'Our Father'.

lords spiritual npl the bishops and archbishops who are members of the British House of Lords.

lords temporal npl the peers other than bishops and archbishops in the British House of Lords.

lore /lɔr/ n knowledge; learning, esp of a traditional nature; a particular body of tradition.

lorgnette /lɔr'njɛt/ n a long-handled opera glass; a pair of spectacles fixed to a long handle, into which they fold.

lorica /loːˈraɪkə/ n (pl **loricae**) the hard outer shell of certain animals.—**loricate, loricated** adj.

lorikeet /'lɔrɪˌkiːt/ or /'lɒrɪ-/ n a small, brightly coloured parrot.

loris /'lɔrɪs/ n (pl **loris**) a small, nocturnal, climbing primate, found in South and South-East Asia.

lorn /lɔrn/ adj (poet) forsaken; forlorn.

lorry /'lɔri/ n (pl **lorries**) (esp Brit) a large motor vehicle for transporting heavy loads.—also **truck.**

lory /'lɔri/ n (pl **lories**) a small parrot with brilliant plumage.

lose /luːz/ vb (**losing, lost**) vt to have taken from one by death, accident, removal, etc; to be unable to find; to fail to keep, as one's temper; to fail to see, hear, or understand; to fail to have, get, etc; to fail to win; to cause the loss of; to wander from (one's way, etc); to squander. • vi to suffer (a) loss.—**losable** adj.—**loser** n.

losel /'luːzəl/ n (dial) a worthless person.

loss /lɒs/ n a losing or being lost; the damage, trouble caused by losing; the person, thing, or amount lost.

loss leader n an item sold at a price below its value in order to attract customers.

lost /lɒst/ adj no longer possessed; missing; not won; destroyed or ruined; having wandered astray; wasted.

lot /lɒt/ n an object, such as a straw, slip of paper, etc drawn from others at random to reach a decision by chance; the decision thus arrived at; one's share by lot; fortune; a plot of ground; a group of persons or things; an item or set of items put up for auction; (often pl) (inf) a great amount; much; (inf) sort. • vt (**lotting, lotted**) to divide into lots.

lota, lotah /'loːtə/ n a brass or copper water pot.

loth see **loath.**

Lothario /lə'θɑrɪo/ or /-'θerɪo/ n (pl **Lotharios**) a libertine.

lotion /'loːʃən/ n a liquid for cosmetic or external medical use.

lottery /'lɒtəri/ n (pl **lotteries**) a system of raising money by selling numbered tickets that offer the chance of winning a prize; an enterprise, etc which may or may not succeed.

lotto /'lɒtoː/ n a game of chance based on the drawing of prize numbers.

lotus /'loːtəs/ n a type of waterlily; (Greek legend) a plant whose fruit induced contented forgetfulness.

lotus-eater n a person dedicated to a life of idle pleasure.

lotus position n an erect sitting position in yoga with the legs crossed close to the body.

louche /luːʃ/ adj untrustworthy, shady.

loud /laud/ adj characterized by or producing great noise; emphatic; (inf) obtrusive or flashy.—**loudly** adv.—**loudness** n.

louden /-ən/ vi to grow louder. • vt to make louder.

loudspeaker /'laudˌspiːkər/ n a device for converting electrical energy into sound.

lough /lɒx/, Ir. /lɒx/ n a lake; an arm of the sea.

louis, louis d'or /'luːi/ n (pl **louis, louis d'or**) (formerly) a French gold coin, with a value of 20 francs.

lounge /laundʒ/ vi to move, sit, lie, etc in a relaxed way; to spend time idly. • n a room with comfortable furniture for sitting, as a waiting room at an airport, etc; a comfortable sitting room in a hotel or private house.

lounger /'laundʒər/ n a comfortable couch or chair for relaxing on; a person who lounges.

lour /laur/ vi to look sullen; to become dark, gloomy, threatening.—also **lower.**—**louringly, loweringly** adv.

louse /laus/ n (pl **lice**) any of various small wingless insects that are parasitic on humans and animals; any similar but unrelated insects that are parasitic on plants; (inf) (pl **louses**) a mean, contemptible person.

lousy /'lauzi/ adj (**lousier, lousiest**) infested with lice; (sl) disgusting, of poor quality, or inferior; (sl) well supplied (with).—**lousily** adv.—**lousiness** n.

lout /laut/ n a clumsy, rude person.—**loutish** adj.

louver, louvre /'luːvər/ n one of a set of slats in a door or window set parallel and slanted to admit air but not rain.—**louvered, louvred** adj.

lovable /'lʌvəbəl/ adj easy to love or feel affection for.—**lovability** n.—**lovably** adv.

lovage /'lʌvɪdʒ/ n a European herb used as a seasoning in food.

love /lʌv/ n a strong liking for someone or something; a passionate affection for another person; the object of such affection; (tennis) a score of zero. • vti to feel love (for).

love affair n a romantic or sexual relationship between two people.

lovebird /'lʌvbərd/ n any of various small parrots.

love child n an illegitimate child.

love-in-a-mist n a flowering garden plant, fennelflower.

loveless /'lʌvləs/ adj without love; not feeling or receiving love.—**lovelessly** adv.

lovelock /'lʌvlɒk/ n a curl worn on the forehead.

lovelorn /'lʌvlɔrn/ adj pining from love.

lovely /'lʌvli/ adj (**lovelier, loveliest**) beautiful; (inf) highly enjoyable. • n (pl **lovelies**) a lovely person.—**loveliness** n.

lovemaking /'lʌvˌmeɪkɪŋ/ n sexual activity, esp intercourse, between lovers.

lover /'lʌvər/ n a person in love with another person; a person, esp a man, having an extramarital sexual relationship; (pl) a couple in love with each other; someone who loves a specific person or thing.

lovesick /'lʌvsɪk/ adj languishing through love.—**lovesickness** n.

lovey-dovey /'lʌvi dʌvi/ adj (sl) displaying affection in an excessive or exaggerated manner.

loving /'lʌvɪŋ/ adj affectionate.—**lovingly** adv.—**lovingness** n.

loving cup n a large cup with two or more handles passed round a group for all to drink from.

low[1] /loː/ n the sound a cow makes, a moo. • vi to make this sound.

low[2] adj not high or tall; below the normal level; less in size, degree, amount, etc than usual; deep in pitch; depressed in spirits; humble, of low rank; vulgar, coarse; not loud. • adv in or to a low degree, level, etc. • n a low level, degree, etc; a region of low barometric pressure.

Low Arctic n ✦ (Cdn) the Arctic south of the Arctic Circle.

lowborn /'loːbɔrn/, **lowbred** /'loːbrɛd/ adj of humble birth.

lowboy /'loːbɔɪ/ n a table with drawers.

lowbrow /'loːbrau/ n (inf) a person regarded as uncultivated and lacking in taste.—also adj.

low comedy n comedy reliant on farce or physical slapstick.

lowdown /'loːdaun/ n (sl: with **the**) the true, pertinent facts

low-down adj (inf) mean, contemptible.

lower case n small letters (not capitals) used for printing.

lower class n the class of people having the lowest status in society.

lower house, lower chamber n one of the two chambers in a bicameral legislature, such as the US House of Representatives or the British House of Commons.

lower[1] /'loːər/ adj below in place, rank, etc; less in amount, degree, etc. • vt to let or put down; to reduce in height, amount, etc; to bring down in respect, etc. • vi to become lower.—**lowerable** adj.

lower[2] /laur/ or /'loːər/ see **lour.**

lowermost adj lowest.

low frequency n a radio frequency between 300 and 30 kilohertz.

low-key, low-keyed adj of low intensity, subdued.

lowland /'loːlənd/ n low-lying land; (pl) a flat region. • adj of or pertaining to lowlands.—**lowlander** n.

low-level language n (comput) a programming language that corresponds more to machine language than human language.

lowlife n (pl **lowlifes**) (sl) a criminal.

lowly /'loːli/ adj (**lowlier, lowliest**) humble, of low status; meek.—**lowliness** n.

Low Mass n a Mass without music or elaborate ritual.

low-rise adj (building) having only one or two storeys.—also n.

low spirited adj unhappy, depressed.

low-tech adj of or involving low technology.

low technology n unsophisticated technology limited to the provision of basic human needs.

low tension *adj* using, conveying, or operating at a low voltage.

low tide *n* (the time of) the tide when it is at its lowest level; a low point.

low water *n* low tide.

lox[1] /lɒks/ *n* a type of smoked salmon.

lox[2] *n* liquid oxygen.

loyal /'lɔɪəl/ *adj* firm in allegiance to a person, cause, country, etc, faithful; demonstrating unswerving allegiance.—**loyally** *adv.*—**loyalty** *n.*

loyalist /-ɪst/ *n* a person who supports the established government, *esp* during a revolt.—**loyalism** *n.*

lozenge /'lɒzɪndʒ/ *n* a four-sided diamond-shaped figure; a cough drop, sweet, etc, originally diamond-shaped.

LP *n* a long-playing record, *usu* 12 inches (30.5 cm) in diameter and played at a speed of 33 $\frac{1}{3}$ revolutions per minute.

LPG *abbr* = liquefied petroleum gas.

Lr (*chem symbol*) lawrencium.

LSD *n* a powerful hallucinatory drug (lysergic acid diethylamide).

Lt *abbr* = lieutenant.

Ltd *abbr* = limited liability (used by private companies only).

LU (*chem symbol*) lutetium.

luau /'lu:au/ *n* a sumptuous feast in Hawaii; a warm welcome; an unexpected source of wealth; a bonanza.

lubber /'lʌbər/ *n* a clumsy person.

lubricant /'lu:brɪkənt/ *n* a substance that lubricates.

lubricate /'lu:brɪˌkeɪt/ *vt* to coat or treat (machinery, etc) with oil or grease to lessen friction; to make smooth, slippery, or greasy. • *vi* to act as a lubricant.—**lubrication** *n.*

lubricator /-ər/ *n* person who or thing that lubricates; a device used for oiling machines.

lubricity /-sɪti/ *n* slipperiness; evasiveness; lewdness.

lucarne /lu:'kɑrn/ *n* a dormer window, *esp* in a spire.

lucent /'lu:sənt/ *adj* bright, shining.—**lucency** *n.*

lucerne /lu:'sɜrn/ *see* **alfalfa**.

lucid /'lu:sɪd/ *adj* easily understood; sane.—**lucidly** *adv.*—**lucidity** *n.*

Lucifer /'lu:sɪfər/ *n* Satan.

luck /lʌk/ *n* chance; good fortune.

luckless /'lʌkləs/ *n* unfortunate, unlucky.—**luck essly** *adv.*—**lucklessness** *n.*

lucky /'lʌki/ *adj* (**luckier, luckiest**) having or bringing good luck.—**luckily** *adv.*—**luckiness** *n.*

lucrative /'lu:krətɪv/ *adj* producing wealth or profit; profitable.—**lucratively** *adv.*—**lucrativeness** *n.*

lucre /'lu:kər/ *n* (*derog*) riches, money.

lucubrate /'lu:kjuˌbreɪt/ *vi* to study, *esp* by night.— **ucubrator** *n.*

lucubration /ˌlu:kjuˈbreɪʃən/ *n* study. *esp* nocturnal; (*often pl*) a literary compositon produced as the result of protracted study.

ludicrous /'lu:dɪkrəs/ *adj* absurd, laughable.—**ludicrously** *adv.*

luff /lʌf/ *n* (*naut*) the part of ship towards the wind. • *vti* (*naut*) to turn (a ship) into the wind.

luffa *see* **loofah**.

Luftwaffe /'luft,vɒfə/ *n* the German Air Force.

lug[1] /lʌg/ *vt* (**lugging, lugged**) to pull or drag along with effort.

lug[2] *n* an ear-like projection by which a thing is held or supported.

luge /lu:ʒ/ *n* a small one-person toboggan.

luggage /'lʌgɪdʒ/ *n* the suitcases and other baggage containing the possessions of a traveller.

lugger /'lʌgər/ *n* a small vessel rigged with one or more lugsails.

lugsail /'lʌgseɪl/ or /-səl/ *n* a square sail, with no boom or lower yard, which hangs nearly at right angles to the mast.

lugubrious /lu:'gu:brɪəs/ or /lu-/ *adj* mournful, dismal.—**lugubriously** *adv.*

lugworm /'lʌgwɜrm/ *n* a marine worm used as bait.

lukewarm /'lu:kwɔrm/ *adj* barely warm, tepid; lacking enthusiasm.

lull /lʌl/ *vt* to soothe, to calm; to calm the suspicions of, *esp* by deception. • *n* a short period of calm.

lullaby /'lʌləˌbaɪ/ *n* (*pl* **lullabies**) a song to lull children to sleep.

lulu /'lu:lu:/ *n* (*inf*) a wonderful or remarkable person or thing.

lumbago /lʌm'beɪgo:/ *n* rheumatic pain in the lower back.

lumbar /'lʌmbər/ *adj* of or in the loins.

lumber[1] /'lʌmbər/ *n* timber, logs, beams, boards, etc, roughly cut and prepared for use; articles of unused household furniture that are stored away; any useless articles. • *vi* to cut down timber and saw it into lumber. • *vt* to clutter with lumber; to heap in disorder.

lumber[2] *vi* to move heavily or clumsily.—**lumberer** *n.*

lumbering[1] /'lʌmbərɪŋ/ *adj* moving clumsily and heavily.—**lumberingly** *adv.*

lumbering[2] *n* the cutting down and sawing of trees into timber as a business.

lumberjack /'lʌmbərˌdʒæk/ *n* a person employed to fell trees and transport and prepare timber.

lumbrical /'lʌmbrɪkəl/ or /-brək-/ *adj* wormlike.

lumen /'lu:mən/ *n* (*pl* **lumina, lumens**) the SI unit of light flux; (*anat*) a duct within a tubular organ.

luminary /'lu:mɪnɛri/ *n* (*pl* **luminaries**) a body that gives off light, such as the sun; a famous or notable person.

luminescent /ˌlu:mɪ'nɛsənt/ *adj* emitting light but not heat.—**luminescence** *n.*

luminosity /ˌlu:mɪ'nɒsɪti/ *n* (*pl* **luminosities**) the quality of being luminous; something luminous; (*astron*) the degree of light emitted by a star when compared with the sun.

luminous /'lu:mɪnəs/ *adj* emitting light; glowing in the dark; clear, easily understood.—**luminously** *adv.*

lump /lʌmp/ *n* a small, compact mass of something, *usu* without definite shape; an abnormal swelling; a dull or stupid person. • *adj* in a lump or lumps. • *vt* to treat or deal with in a mass. • *vi* to become lumpy.

lumper /'lʌmpər/ *n* a docker.

lumpfish /'lʌmpfɪʃ/ *n* (*pl* **lumpfish, lumpfishes**) a sea fish found in the North Atlantic, with horny spines and a sucker with which it clings to objects.

lumpish /'lʌmpɪʃ/ *adj* like a lump; heavy; dull, stupid.

lump sum *n* a sum of money (*esp* cash) paid as a whole and not in instalments.

lumpy /'lʌmpi/ *adj* (**lumpier, lumpiest**) filled or covered with lumps.—**lumpily** *adv.*— **umpiness** *n.*

lunacy /'lu:nəsi/ *n* (*pl* **lunacies**) insanity; utter folly.

lunar /'lu:nər/ *adj* of or like the moon.

lunar eclipse *n* an eclipse when the earth passes between the sun and the moon.

lunar month *n* a month measured by the complete revolution of the moon, 29.5 days.

lunar year *n* a year of twelve lunar months, 354.33 days.

lunate /'lu:neɪt/, **lunated** *adj* crescent-shaped.

lunatic /'lu:nətɪk/ *adj* insane; utterly foolish. • *n* an insane person.

lunatic fringe *n* the members of an organization regarded as being fanatical or extreme.

lunation /lu:'neɪʃən/ *n* a lunar month, the time taken for the moon to revolve once around the earth.

lunch /lʌntʃ/ *n* a light meal, *esp* between breakfast and dinner; **out to lunch** (*sl*) crazy; eccentric. • *vi* to eat lunch.—**luncher** *n.*

luncheon /'lʌntʃən/ *n* lunch, *esp* a formal lunch.

luncheon meat *n* processed meat in tins ready to eat.

lune /lu:n/ *n* (*geom*) a figure formed on a plane or sphere by two intersecting arcs of circles.

lunette /lu:'nɛt/ *n* anything shaped like a crescent; an arched opening in a vaulted roof to admit light.

lung /lʌŋ/ *n* either of the two sponge-like breathing organs in the chest of vertebrates.

lunge[1] /lʌndʒ/ *n* a sudden forceful thrust, as with a sword; a sudden plunge forward. • *vti* to move, or cause to move, with a lunge.—**lunger** *n.*

lunge[2] *n* a long halter for training a horse; the use of this in training horses. • *vt* to train with a lunge.—**longe**.

lungfish /'lʌŋfɪʃ/ *n* (*pl* **lungfish, lungfishes**) a freshwater fish with lungs as well as gills.

lungi /'lʊŋgi:/ *n* a long piece of cloth worn as a skirt or loincloth by Indian men.

lungwort /'lʌŋwɔrt/ *n* a Eurasian plant with dark-coloured leaves spotted with white.

lunisolar /ˌlu:nɪ'so:lər/ *adj* pertaining to the sun and moon; produced by the sun and moon in unison.

lunula, lunule /'lu:njolə/ *n* (*pl* **lunulae, lunules**) the white crescent-shaped part near the root of the fingernail.

lupine[1] /'lu:pɪn/ *n* a garden plant of the pea family.

lupine[2] /'lu:paɪn/ *adj* of or resembling a wolf.

lupulin /lu:'pulɪn/ or /lə-/, r-/pju:-/ *n* a powder, obtained from hops, used as a sedative.

lupus /'lu:pəs/ *n* any of several diseases marked by lesions of the skin.

lurch /lɜrtʃ/ *vi* to lean or pitch suddenly to the side. • *n* a sudden roll to one side.—**lurchingly** *adv.*

lurdan /'lərdən/ *adj* (*arch*) stupid. • *n* a stupid person.

lure /lʊr/ or /lər/ *n* something that attracts, tempts or entices; a brightly coloured fishing bait; a device used to recall a trained hawk; a decoy for wild animals. • *vt* to entice, attract, or tempt.—**luringly** *adv*.

lurid /'lʊrɪd/ or /lər-/ *adj* vivid, glaring; shocking; sensational.—**luridly** *adv*.—**luridness** *n*.

lurk /lərk/ *vi* to lie hidden in wait; to loiter furtively.—**lurker** *n*.

luscious /'lʌʃəs/ *adj* delicious; richly sweet; delighting any of the senses.—**lusciously** *adv*.—**lusciousness** *n*.

lush¹ /lʌʃ/ *adj* tender and juicy; of or showing abundant growth.—**lushly** *adv*.—**lushness** *n*.

lush² *n* (*sl*) an alcoholic.

lust /lʌst/ *n* strong sexual desire (for); an intense longing for something. • *vi* to feel lust.—**lustful** *adj*.—**lustfully** *adv*.

lustral /'lʌstrəl/ *adj* of or relating to ceremonial purification; of or relating to a lustrum.

lustrate /'lʌstreɪt/ *vt* to purify by sacrifice or ceremonial washing.—**lustration** *n*.

lustre, luster /'lʌstər/ *n* gloss; sheen; brightness; radiance; brilliant beauty or fame; glory; a chandelier with pendants of cut glass; a fabric with a lustrous surface; a substance used to give lustre to an object; a metallic glaze on pottery; the quality and intensity of light reflected from the surface of minerals.—**lusterless** *adj*.—**lustrous** *adj*.

lustreware, lusterware /'lʌstər,wɛr/ *n* earthenware decorated with luster.

lustrum /'lʌstrəm/ *n* (*pl* **lustrums, lustra**) a period of five years.

lusty /'lʌsti/ *adj* (**lustier, lustiest**) strong; vigorous; healthy.—**lustily** *adv*.—**lustiness** *n*.

lute¹ /luːt/ *n* an old, round-backed stringed musical instrument plucked with the fingers.

lute² *n* clay or cement used to make joints airtight, etc.

lutenist /'luːtənɪst/, **lutist** /'luːtɪst/ *n* a lute player.

luteous /'luːtiəs/ *adj* greenish-yellow.

lutetium /luːˈtiːʃiəm/ *n* a metallic element.

Lutheran /'luːθərən/ *adj* pertaining to Martin Luther (1483-1546), the German religious reformer, or to the Lutheran Church and its doctrines. • *n* a follower of Martin Luther; a member of the Lutheran Church.—**Lutheranism** *n*.

Lutheran Church *n* the Protestant church founded by Martin Luther in Germany in the 16th century.

lux /lʌks/ *n* (*pl* **lux**) a unit of illumination.

luxate /'lʌks,eɪt/ *vt* to put out of joint.—**luxation** *n*.

luxuriant /lʌgˈʒʊriənt/ or /lʌkˈʃʊr-/ *adj* profuse, abundant; ornate; fertile.—**luxuriance** *n*.

luxuriate /lʌgˈʒʊri,eɪt/ or /lʌkˈʃʊr-/ *vi* to enjoy immensely, to revel (in).—**luxuriation** *n*.

luxurious /lʌgˈʒʊriəs/ or /lʌkˈʃʊr-/ *adj* constituting luxury; indulging in luxury; rich, comfortable.—**luxuriously** *adv*.—**luxuriousness** *n*.

luxury /'lʌkʃəri/ or /'lʌgʒəri/ *n* (*pl* **luxuries**) indulgence and pleasure in sumptuous and expensive food, accommodation, clothes, etc; (*often pl*) something that is costly and enjoyable but not indispensable. • *adj* relating to or supplying luxury.

lx *abbr* = lux.

lycanthrope /'laɪkən,θroʊp/ *n* a werewolf; (*med*) a sufferer from lycanthropy.

lycanthropy /-i/ *n* the supposed power of changing from a human being into a werewolf; (*med*) a form of mental illness in which the sufferer believes himself or herself to be a wolf.

lycée /liːˈseɪ/ *n* (*pl* **lycées**) a state secondary school in France.

lyceum /laɪˈsiːəm/ *n* a public lecture hall.

lychee /'liːtʃi/ *see* **lichee**.

lych gate /'lɪtʃgeɪt/ *see* **lich gate**.

lychnis /'lɪknɪs/ *n* a genus of flowering plants, including the ragged robin and campion.

lycopod /'laɪkə,pɒd/ *n* a kind of moss, also known as the club moss.

lycopodium /ˌlaɪkəˈpoʊdiəm/ *n* any of a genus of perennial plants, the club mosses; an inflammable yellow powder in the spore cases of certain species, used in fireworks.

Lycra /'laɪkrə/ *n* (*trademark*) an elastic synthetic material used for tight-fitting garments, such as bicycle shorts and swimwear.

lyddite /'lɪdaɪt/ *n* a powerful explosive, composed chiefly of picric acid.

lye /laɪ/ *n* an alkaline solution.

lying /'laɪŋ/ *see* **lie¹, lie²**.

lying-in *n* (*pl* **lyings-in, lying-ins**) childbirth.

Lyme disease /laɪm/ *n* an infectious disease, carried by ticks, that produces fever, pains in the joints and a rash, and can result in paralysis or chronic fatigue, and, rarely, death.

lymph /lɪmf/ *n* a clear, yellowish body fluid, found in intercellular spaces and the lymphatic vessels.

lymphatic /lɪmˈfætɪk/ *adj* of, relating to, or containing lymph; sluggish. • *n* a vessel that contains or conveys lymph.

lymph node *n* any of numerous nodules of tissue distributed along the course of lymphatic vessels that produce lymphocytes.

lympho- /'lɪmfə-/ *prefix* lymph; lymph tissue; lymphatic system.

lymphocyte /'lɪmfə,saɪt/ *n* a white blood cell formed in the lymph nodes, which helps to protect against infection.—**lymphocytic** *adj*.

lymphoid /'lɪmfɔɪd/ *adj* relating to lymph glands; resembling lymph.

lymphoma /lɪmˈfoʊmə/ *n* (*pl* **lymphomata**) a tumour of the lymphoid tissue.

lyncean /'lɪn,siən/ *adj* pertaining to or resembling the lynx; sharp-eyed.

lynch /lɪntʃ/ *vt* to murder (an accused person) by mob action, without lawful trial, as by hanging.—**lyncher** *n*.—**lynching** *n*.

lynx /lɪŋks/ *n* (*pl* **lynxes, lynx**) a wild feline of Europe and North America with spotted fur.

lynx-eyed /-aɪd/ *adj* keen-sighted.

lyonnaise /ˌliːəˈnɒz/, *Fr.* /ljɔˈnɛz/ *adj* (*cooking*) with onions.

lyrate /'laɪrət/ **lyrated** *adj* lyre-shaped.

lyre /laɪr/ *n* an ancient musical instrument of the harp family.

lyrebird /'laɪrbərd/ *n* an Australian bird with a tail shaped like a lyre.

lyric /'lɪrɪk/ *adj* denoting or of poetry expressing the writer's emotion; of, or having a high voice with a light, flexible quality. • *n* a lyric poem; (*pl*) the words of a popular song.

lyrical /'lɪrɪkəl/ *adj* lyric; (*inf*) expressing rapture or enthusiasm.—**lyrically** *adv*.

lyricism /'lɪrɪ,sɪzəm/ *n* lyrical quality or expression.

lyricist /'lɪrɪsɪst/ *n* a person who writes lyrics, *esp* for popular songs.

lyrist /'laɪrɪst/ *n* a lyric poet; a lyre player.

lysergic acid /laɪˈsərdʒɪk/ *see* **LSD**.

lysin /'laɪsɪn/ *n* a specific antibody in blood that can destroy cells.

lysine /'laɪsiːn/ *n* an amino acid formed by the digestion of dietary protein.

-lysis /lɪsɪs/ *n suffix* disintegration; decomposition.

lysis /'laɪsɪs/ *n* (*pl* **lyses**) (*biol*) the process of destroying cells with a lysin; (*med*) the gradual abatement of an acute disease.

-lyte /'laɪt/ *n suffix* denoting a substance able to be disintegrated or decomposed.

-lytic /'lɪtɪk/ *adj suffix* indicating a disintegration or decomposition.

M

M *abbr* = mega-; medium; motorway.

M. *abbr* = Master; Monsieur

m *abbr* = metre(s); mile(s); million(s).

MA *abbr* = Master of Arts; Massachusetts.

ma /mɒ/ *n* (*inf*) mother.

ma'am /mæm/ or /məm/ *n* madam (used as a title of respect, *esp* when addressing royalty).

macabre /mə'kɒbrə/ or /-'kæbrə/, /-'kɒb/ *adj* gruesome; grim; of death.

macaco /mə'kɒkoː/ *n* (*pl* **macacos**) one of various lemurs, *esp* the ruffled lemur and the ring-tailed lemur.

macadam /mə'kædəm/ *n* a road surface composed of successive layers of small stones compacted into a solid mass.

macadamia /ˌmækə'deɪmɪə/ *n* an Australian tree bearing white flowers and an edible seed (**macadamia nut**).

macadamize /mə'kædəˌmaɪz/ *vt* to surface (a road) with macadam.—**macadamization** *n*.

macaque /mə'kæk/ *n* a short-tailed monkey of Asia and Africa.

macaroni /ˌmækə'roːni/ *n* (*pl* **macaronis, macaronies**) a pasta made chiefly of fine wheat flour and made into tubes; an 18th-century dandy who copied continental mannerisms etc.

macaronic /ˌmækə'rɒnik/ *adj* (*verse*) using words from more than one language, or a mixture of everyday words and Latin words or words with Latin endings. • *n* (*often pl*) macaronic verse.

macaroon /ˌmækə'ruːn/ *n* a small cake or biscuit made with sugar, egg whites and ground almonds or coconut.

macaw /mə'kɔː/ *n* a large parrot with brightly coloured plumage.

Maccabean /ˌmækə'biːən/ *adj* pertaining to the Maccabees, a family of Jewish patriots who led a successful revolt against the Syrians, or to its most famous member, Judas Maccabaeus.

maccaboy /'mækəˌbɔɪ/ *n* a kind of snuff, *usu* rose-scented.

mace[1] /meɪs/ *n* a staff used as a symbol of authority by certain institutions.

mace[2] *n* an aromatic spice made from the external covering of the nutmeg.

macédoine /'mæsɪˌdwɒn/, *Fr.* /masei'dwan/ *n* a dish of mixed fruits, served hot or cold; a dish of diced vegetables, *usu* in jelly or syrup; any mixture.

macerate /'mæsəˌreɪt/ *vti* to soften or become soft or separated through soaking; to make or become thin.—**maceration** *n*.—**macerator** *n*.

Mach /mɒk/ or /mæk/ *see* **Mach number**.

machete /mə'ʃeti/ or /mə'tʃeti/ *n* a large knife used for cutting, or as a weapon.

Machiavellian /ˌmækɪə'veliən/ *adj* cunning; deceitful.

machicolation /məˌtʃɪkə'leɪʃən/ *n* (*arch*) a projecting parapet, *usu* found on medieval castles, with openings for dropping stones, etc, on assailants; such an opening.—**machicolated** *adj*.

machinate /'mækɪˌneɪt/ or /'mæʃ-/ *vti* to scheme, plan, *esp* to do harm.—**machinator** *n*.

machination /ˌmæʃɪ'neɪʃən/ or /ˌmækɪ-/ *n* (*usu pl*) an artifice; an intrigue; a plot; the act of plotting or intriguing.

machine /mə'ʃiːn/ *n* a structure of fixed and moving parts, for doing useful work; an organization functioning like a machine; the controlling group in a political party; a device, as the lever, etc that transmits, or changes the application of energy. • *vt* to shape or finish by machine-operated tools. • *adj* of machines; done by machinery.

machine code, machine language *n* (*comput*) programming instructions in binary or hexadecimal code.

machine gun *n* an automatic gun, firing a rapid stream of bullets.—*also vt*.

machine-readable /mə'ʃiːn'riːdəbəl/ *adj* directly usable by a computer.

machinery /mə'ʃiːnəri/ *n* machines collectively; the parts of a machine; the framework for keeping something going.

machine tool *n* a mechanized tool for cutting or shaping metals, wood, etc.

machinist /mə'ʃiːnɪst/ *n* one who makes, repairs, or operates machinery.

machismo /mə'tʃɪzmoː/ or /-'kɪzmoː/ *n* strong or assertive masculinity; virility.—**macho** *adj*.

Mach number /mɒk/ *n* the ratio of the speed of a body in a particular medium to the speed of sound in the same medium. Mach 1 is equal to the speed of sound.

mackerel /'mækrəl/ *n* (*pl* **mackerel, mackerels**) a common oily food fish.

Mackinaw (coat) /'mækɪˌnɒ/ *n* a short, double-breasted coat made of a heavy woollen plaid material.

mackintosh /'mækɪnˌtɒʃ/ *n* a waterproof raincoat.

mackle /'mækəl/ *n* (*printing*) a blurred or imprecise impression, which produces the effect of a double printing.—*also* **macule**.

macle /'mækəl/ *n* a type of crystal in two parts, containing carbon impurities, sometimes used as a gemstone.

macramé /'mækrəˌmeɪ/ *n* (the art of) knotting or weaving coarse thread to produce ornamental work.

macro- /'mækroː/ *prefix* = long, large.

macrobiotic /ˌmækrobaɪ'ɒtik/ *adj* (*diet*) composed of an extremely restricted range of foods, *usu* vegetables and whole grains.

macrocephalic /ˌmækrosə'fælik/ *adj* having an unusually large skull.—*also* **megacephalic** *adj*.—**macrocephaly** *n*.

macrocosm /'mækroˌkɒzəm/ *n* the universe; any complex system.—**macrocosmic** *adj*.

macroeconomics /ˌmækroˌiːkə'nɒmɪks/ *n* (*used as sing*) the study of the economy in terms of total national income, production and investment.—**macroeconomic** *adj*.

macron /'mækrɒn/ *n* a mark placed over a letter to indicate a stressed or long vowel (-).

macropterous /mæ'krɒptərəs/ *adj* (*zool*) large-winged.

macroscopic /ˌmækro'skɒpɪk/ *adj* visible to the naked eye; regarded in terms of large elements.

macrospore /'mækroˌspɔr/ *see* **megaspore**.

macula /'mækjulə/ *n* (*pl* **maculae**) a spot or mark on the skin; a coloured area near the retina, where vision is *esp* sharp.—**macular** *adj*.—**maculation** *n*.

macule[1] /'mækjuːl/ *see* **mackle**.

mad /mæd/ *adj* (**madder, maddest**) insane; frantic; foolish and rash; infatuated; (*inf*) angry.

madam /'mædəm/ *n* a polite term of address to a woman; a woman in charge of a brothel; (*inf*) a precocious little girl.

madame /mə'dæm/ or /'mædəm/ *n* (*pl* **mesdames**) the title of a married French woman; used as a title equivalent to Mrs.

madcap /'mædkæp/ *adj* reckless, impulsive.—*also n*.

madden /'mædən/ *vti* to make or become insane, angry, or wildly excited.—**maddening** *adj*.—**maddeningly** *adv*.

madder[1] /'mædər/ *see* **mac**.

madder[2] *n* a plant of the genus from whose root a red dye and pigment are extracted; the red dye so obtained; a synthetic pigment used in paints and inks.

madding /'mædɪŋ/ *adj* (*arch*) raging; furious; causing (someone or something) to be raging.

made /meɪd/ *see* **make**.

Madeira /mə'diːrə/ *n* a rich strong, white wine made in the North Atlantic island of Madeira.

madeleine /'mædəˌlen/ *n* a small sponge cake with a coating of red jam covered with coconut.

mademoiselle /ˌmædmwə'zel/ *n* (*pl* **mesdemoiselles**) the title of an unmarried French girl or woman; used as a title equivalent to Miss; a French teacher or governess.

made-to-order /'meɪdtə'ɔrdər/ *adj* produced to a customer's specifications; being ideally suited for a particular purpose.

madhouse /'mædhɒus/ *n* (*inf*) as mental institution; a state of uproar or confusion.

madly /'mædli/ *adv* in an insane manner; at great speed, force; (*inf*) excessively.

madman /'mædmæn/ *n* (*pl* **madmen**) an insane person.

madness /'mædnəs/ *n* insanity; foolishness; excitability.

Madonna /mə'dɒnə/ *n* the Virgin Mary, *esp* as seen in pictures or statues.

madras /mə'drɑːs/ *n* a strong cotton or silk material, *usu* striped.

madrepore /'mædrə͵pɔr/ *n* any of several corals, often forming tropical coral reefs.—**madreporic** *adj*.

madrigal /'mædrɪgəl/ *n* a 16th-century love song or pastoral poem in the form of an unaccompanied part-song; 14th-century Italian song derived from a pastoral poem.—**madrigalist** *n*.

maduro /mə'dʊrɔː/ *adj* (*cigar*) dark and full-flavoured. • *n* (*pl* **maduros**) such a cigar.

madwoman /'mæd͵wʊmən/ *n* (*pl* **madwomen**) an insane person.

madwort /-͵wɔrt/ *n* a small herb with yellow or white flowers, formerly reputed to cure madness; a type of small, low-growing, flowering plant with hairy leaves and blue flowers.

maelstrom /'meɪlstrəm/ *n* a whirlpool; a state of turbulence or confusion.

maenad /'miːnæd/ *n* (**maenads, maenades**) (*Greek myth*) a female adherent of Dionysus; a frantic, agitated woman.—*also* **menad**.

maestoso /maɪ'stɔːzɔː/ *adj, adv* (*mus*) in a majestic manner.

maestro /'maɪstrɔː/ *n* (*pl* **maestros**) a master of an art, *esp* a musical composer, conductor, or teacher.

mae west /meɪ'wɛst/ *n* (*inf*) an inflatable life jacket.

Mafia /'mɒfiə/ or /'mæ-/ *n* a secret society composed chiefly of criminal elements, originating in Sicily.

mafioso /͵mæfi'ɔːsɔː/ or /͵mɒ-/ *n* (*pl* **mafiosos, mafiosi**) a member of the Mafia.

mag. *abbr* = magazine.

magazine /͵mægə'ziːn/ *n* a military store; a space where explosives are stored, as in a fort; a supply chamber, as in a camera, a rifle, etc; a periodical publication containing articles, fiction, photographs, etc.

magdalen, magdalene /'mægdələn/ *n* a reformed prostitute; (*rare*) an institution for housing and reforming prostitutes.

magenta /mə'dʒɛntə/ *n* a purplish-red dye; purplish red.—*also adj*.

maggot /'mægət/ *n* a wormlike larva, as of the housefly.—**maggoty** *adj*.—**maggotiness** *n*.

magi /'meɪdʒaɪ /, **magian** /'meɪdʒiən/ *see* **magus**.

magic /'mædʒɪk/ *n* the use of charms, spells, etc to supposedly influence events by supernatural means; any mysterious power; the art of producing illusions by sleight of hand, etc. • *adj* of or relating to magic; possessing supposedly supernatural powers; (*inf*) wonderful. • *vt* (**magicking, magicked**) to influence, produce or take (away) by or as if by magic.—**magical** *adj*.—**magically** *adv*.

magician /mə'dʒɪʃən/ *n* one skilled in magic; a conjurer.

magisterial /͵mædʒɪ'stiːriəl/ *adj* of, or suitable for a magistrate; authoritative.—**magisterially** *adv*.

magistracy /'mædʒɪstrəsi/ *n* (*pl* **magistracies**) the office, jurisdiction or dignity of a magistrate; magistrates collectively.

magistral /-əl/ *adj* or or pertaining to a master or teacher, magisterial; (*med*) specially prescribed; (*fortification*) in a strategic position.

magistrate /'mædʒɪstreɪt/ or /-͵strət/ *n* a public officer empowered to administer the law.—**magistrateship, magistrature** *n*.

magma /'mægmə/ *n* (*pl* **magmas, magmata**) a stratum of hot molten rock within the earth's crust, which solidifies on the surface as lava.

Magna Carta, Magna Charta /͵mægnə'kɑrtə/ *n* in England, the Great Charter, forming the basis of civil liberty, granted by King John to the barons, church and freemen in 1215.

magnanimity /͵mægnə'nɪməti/ *n* (*pl* **magnanimities**) generosity.

magnanimous /mæg'nænɪməs/ *adj* noble and generous in conduct or spirit, not petty.—**magnanimously** *adv*.

magnate /'mægneɪt/ or /-nət/ *n* a very wealthy or influential person.

magnesia /mæg'niːʒə/ or /-ʃə/, /-ʒə/ *n* a magnesium compound used as a mild laxative.

magnesium /mæg'niːziəm/ *n* a white metallic element that burns very brightly.

magnet /'mægnət/ *n* any piece of iron or steel that has the property of attracting iron; anything that attracts.

magnetic /mæg'nɛtɪk/ *adj* of magnetism or a magnet; producing or acting by magnetism; having the ability to attract or charm people.—**magnetically** *adv*.

magnetic declination *n* deviation of the magnetic needle from true north; the measure of this.

magnetic equator *n* the imaginary point near the equator where the magnetic needle has no dip, the aclinic line.

magnetic field *n* any space in which there is an appreciable magnetic force.

magnetic needle *n* a thin piece of magnetized iron, steel, etc, used in a compass and other instruments, that indicates the direction of a magnetic field.

magnetic north *n* the northerly direction of the earth's magnetic field, as pointed to by a compass needle.

magnetic pole *n* either of the two variable points in the regions of the earth's northern and southern poles to which a magnetic needle points.

magnetic resonance imaging *n* a method of viewing the body's internal organs by the use of radio waves.

magnetics /mæg'nɛtɪks/ *n sing* the science of magnetism.

magnetic tape *n* a thin plastic ribbon with a magnetized coating for recording sound, video signals, computer data, etc.

magnetism /'mægnə͵tɪzəm/ *n* the property, quality, or condition of being magnetic; the force to which this is due; personal charm.

magnetize /'mægnɪ͵taɪz/ *vt* to make magnetic; to attract strongly.—**magnetization** *n*.—**magnetizer** *n*.

magneto /mæg'niːtɔː/ *n* (*pl* **magnetos**) a small generator with permanent magnets for generating high voltages, *esp* the ignition spark in an internal combustion engine.

magnetoelectricity /mæg͵niːtɔːɪlɛk'trɪsɪti/ *n* electric phenomena produced by magnetism.

magnetometer /͵mægnə'tɒmɪtər/ *n* an instrument for measuring and comparing magnetic fields.

magneton /'mægnɪ͵tɒn/ *n* one of two units of magnetic moment.

magnet school *n* a school in which resources are devoted to developing excellence in one particular field, *eg* science.

Magnificat /mæg'nɪfɪ͵kæt/ *n* the hymn of the Virgin Mary (Luke 1:46-55); a musical setting of this; (*without cap*) any hymn of praise.

magnification /͵mægnɪfɪ'keɪʃən/ *n* magnifying or being magnified; the degree of enlargement of something by a lens, microscope, etc.

magnificence /mæg'nɪfɪsəns/ *n* grandeur of appearance; splendour; pomp.

magnificent /mæg'nɪfɪsənt/ *adj* splendid, stately or sumptuous in appearance; superb, of very high quality.—**magnificently** *adv*.

magnifico /mæg'nɪfɪ͵kɔː/ *n* (*pl* **magnificoes**) a person of importance or high rank; (*formerly*) a title of a Venetian nobleman.

magnify /'mægnɪ͵faɪ/ *vt* (**magnifying, magnified**) to exaggerate; to increase the apparent size of (an object) as (with) a lens.—**magnifiable** *adj*.—**magnifier** *n*.

magniloquent /mæg'nɪləkwənt/ *adj* pompous in style or speech, bombastic.—**magniloquence** *n*.—**magniloquently** *adv*.

magnitude /'mægnɪ͵tuːd/ or /-͵tjuːd/ *n* greatness of size, extent, etc; importance; (*astron*) the apparent brightness of a star.

magnolia /mæg'nɔːliə/ *n* a spring-flowering shrub or tree with evergreen or deciduous leaves and showy flowers.

magnum /'mægnəm/ *n* (*pl* **magnums**) a wine bottle that holds twice the normal quantity.

magnum opus /͵mægnəm'ɔːpəs/ *n* (*pl* **magna opera**) the great or chief work of an artist or author.

magpie /'mægpaɪ/ *n* a black and white bird of the crow family; a person who chatters; an acquisitive person.

maguey /'mægweɪ/ *n* any of several species of a tropical American plant, *esp* one from which fibre is obtained or that is used in the production of alcoholic drinks; the fibre from such a plant.

magus /'meɪgəs/ *n* (*pl* **magi**) a Zoroastrian priest; (*with cap*) any of the three wise men who paid homage to Christ at His birth; a magician, sorcerer.—**magian** *adj, n*.

Magyar /'mægjɑr/ *adj* pertaining to the Hungarian or Magyar race or language; (*sleeve*) cut as part of the bodice, with no armhole seam.

Mahabharata /mə'hɒ͵bɑrətə/ *n* a great Hindu epic that narrates the dynastic wars of ancient India.

maharajah, maharaja /͵mɒhə'rɒdʒə/ *n* the former title of an Indian prince.

maharani, maharanee /͵mɒhə'rɒni/ *n* the wife of a maharajah.

mahatma /mə'hætmə/ *n* (*Hinduism, Buddhism*) a wise man, a sage; (*with cap*) (*Hinduism*) a title or respect for a man of great spirituality.

mahi-mahi /'mɒhiː͵mɒhi/ *n* either of two dolphin fish (genus *Coryphaena*) of the Pacific Ocean, a food fish.

mahjong, mah-jongg /mɒˈdʒɒŋ/ *n* an orig Chinese game for four people played with decorative tiles.

mahlstick /ˈmɒl stɪk/ or /ˈmɔl-/ *see* **maulstick**.

mahogany /məˈhɒgəni/ *n* (*pl* **mahoganies**) the hard, reddish-brown wood of a tropical tree; a reddish-brown colour.

Mahometan /məˈhɒmɪtən/ *see* **Muhammedan**.

mahout /məˈhaʊt/ *n* (*India*) an elephant driver.

maid /meɪd/ *n* a maiden; a woman servant.

maiden /ˈmeɪdən/ *n* a girl or young unmarried woman. • *adj* unmarried or virgin; untried; first.—**maidenhood** *n*.

maidenhair (fern) /ˈmeɪdənˌheər/ *n* a delicate-leafed fern with small light green leaflets.

maidenhead /ˈmeɪdənˌhed/ *n* the hymen.

maidenly /ˈmeɪdənli/ *adj* like or suitable to a maiden; modest; gentle.—**maidenliness** *n*.

maiden name *n* the surname of a woman before marriage.

maiden over *n* (*cricket*) an over during which no runs are scored.

maid of honour *n* the principal unmarried attendant of a bride; a small almond-flavoured tart.

maidservant /ˈmeɪd ˌsərvənt/ *n* a female servant.

maieutic /meɪˈuːtɪk/ *adj* of the Socratic method of teaching by means of questions.

mail[1] /meɪl/ *n* a body armour made of small metal rings or links.

mail[2] *n* letters, packages, etc transported and delivered by the post office; a postal system. • *vt* to send by mail.—**mailable** *adj*.

mailbox /ˈmeɪlbɒks/ *n* a receptacle into which mail is delivered; (*comput*) within the electronic mail system, a disk file or memory area in which messages for a particular destination (or person) are placed.

mailman /ˈmeɪlmən/ or /-mæn/ *n* (*pl* **mailmen**) a person who collects or delivers mail.—*also* **postman**.

mail order *n* an order for goods to be sent by post.

maim /meɪm/ *vt* to cripple; to mutilate.

main /meɪn/ *adj* chief in size, importance, etc; principal. • *n* (*often pl but used a sing*) a principal pipe in a distribution system for water, gas, etc; the essential point.

mainframe /ˈmeɪnfreɪm/ *n* a large computer that can handle multiple tasks concurrently.

mainland /-lənd/ *n* the principal land mass of a continent, as distinguished from nearby islands.

mainline /-laɪn/ *n* the principal road, course, etc.

mainly /-li/ *adv* chiefly, principally.

mainmast /-mæst/ *n* (*naut*) the principal mast of a sailing ship with more than one mast.

mainsail /-seɪl/ or /-səl/ *n* (*naut*) the principal lowermost sail on the mainmast.

mainsheet /-ʃiːt/ *n* (*naut*) one of the ropes by which the mainsail is extended and fastened, controlling its angle.

mainspring /-sprɪŋ/ *n* the principal spring in a clock, watch, etc; the chief incentive, motive, etc.

mainstay /-steɪ/ *n* a chief support.

mainstream /-striːm/ *n* a major trend, line of thought, etc.—*also adj*.

mainstreet /ˈmeɪnstriːt/ *v* ✠ (*Cdn*) to campaign in an election on the main streets of towns and cities.—**mainstreeter** *n*.—**mainstreeting** *n*.

maintain /meɪnˈteɪn/ *vt* to preserve; to support, to sustain; to keep in good condition; to affirm.—**maintainable** *adj*.—**maintainer** *n*.

maintenance /ˈmeɪntənəns/ *n* upkeep; (*financial*) support, *esp* of a spouse after a divorce.

maintop /ˈmeɪntɒp/ *n* (*naut*) the platform on top of the mainmast.

maisonette /ˌmeɪzəˈnet/ *n* a small house; self-contained living quarters, *usu* on two floors with its own entrance, as part of a larger house.

maître d'hôtel /ˌmeɪtrədoːˈtel/ or /ˌmet-/ *n* (*pl* **maîtres d'hôtel**) *n* a head waiter; a hotel manager or owner; a house steward.

maize /meɪz/ *n* corn; a light yellow colour.

Maj *abbr* (*mil*) = major.

majestic /məˈdʒestɪk/ *adj* dignified; imposing.—**majestically** *adv*.

majesty /ˈmædʒəsti/ *n* (*pl* **majesties**) grandeur; (*with cap*) a title used in speaking to or of a sovereign.

majolica /məˈdʒɒlɪkə/ or /məˈjɒl-/ *n* a fine, soft, enamelled kind of pottery of Italian origin, with a glaze of bright metallic oxides.

major /ˈmeɪdʒər/ *adj* greater in size, importance, amount, etc; (*surgery*) very serious, life-threatening; (*mus*) higher than the corresponding minor by half a tone. • *vi* to specialize (in a field of study). • *n* in US, an officer ranking just above a captain, in UK, a lieutenant-colonel; (*mus*) a major key, chord or scale.

major-domo /ˌmeɪdʒərˈdoːmoː/ *n* (*pl* **major-domos**) a head steward; a butler.

majority /məˈdʒɒrɪti/ *n* (*pl* **majorities**) the greater number or part of; the excess of the larger number of votes cast for a candidate in an election; full legal age; the military rank of a major.

major penalty *n* ✠ a five-minute penalty, given for major infractions such as fighting.

majuscule /ˈmædʒə ˌskjuːl/ *n* a capital letter used in printing or in writing. • *adj* of, pertaining to or written in such letters.—**majuscular** *adj*.

make /meɪk/ *vb* (**making, made**) *vt* to cause to exist, occur, or appear; to build, create, produce, manufacture, etc; to prepare for use; to amount to; to have the qualities of; to acquire, earn; to understand; to do, execute; to cause or force; to arrive at, reach; (*with* **believe**) to imagine, pretend; (*with* **good**) to make up for, pay compensation; (*with* **out**) to write out; to complete (a form, etc) in writing; to attempt to understand; to discern, identify; (*with* **up**) to invent, fabricate, *esp* to deceive; to prepare; to make complete; to put together; to settle differences between. • *vi* (*with* **do**) to manage with what is available; (*with* **for**) to go in the direction of; to bring about; (*with* **good**) to become successful or wealthy; (*with* **off**) to leave in haste; (*with* **out**) to pretend; to fare, manage; (*with* **up**) to become reconciled; to compensate for; to put on make-up for the stage. • *n* style, brand, or origin; manner of production.—**maker** *n*.

make-believe /ˈmeɪkbəˈliːv/ *adj* imagined, pretended.—*also n*.

makeshift /ˈmeɪkʃɪft/ *adj* being a temporary substitute.—*also n*.

make-up /ˈmeɪkʌp/ *n* the cosmetics, etc used by an actor; cosmetics generally; the way something is put together, composition; nature, disposition.

makeweight /-weɪt/ *n* something added to make up the required weight; anything of little value added to fill a lack.

making /-ɪŋ/ *n* the act or process of making, creation; (*pl*) earnings; (*pl*) potential; (*sl*) the materials for rolling a cigarette.

Makkah /ˈmɒkə/ *see* **mecca**.

mal- /mæl/ *prefix* = bad or badly, wrong, ill.

malacca /məˈlækə/ *n* the tough stem of a species of climbing palm, rattan; a brown walking stick made of this.—*also* **malacca cane**.

malachite /ˈmæləˌkaɪt/ *n* copper carbonate occurring as a green mineral, used as an ore and for making ornaments.

malacology /ˌmæləˈkɒlədʒi/ *n* the science of molluscs.—**malacological** *adj*.—**malacologist** *n*.

malacostracan /ˌmæləˈkɒstrəkən/ *adj* (*crustacean*) soft-shelled.

maladjusted /ˌmæləˈdʒʌstəd/ *adj* poorly adjusted, *esp* to the social environment.—**maladjustment** *n*.

maladministration /ˌmælədmɪnɪˈstreɪʃən/ *n* corrupt or incompetent management of public affairs.—**maladminister** *vb*.

maladroit /ˌmæləˈdrɔɪt/ *adj* clumsy.—**maladroitness** *n*.

malady /ˈmælədi/ *n* (*pl* **maladies**) a disease, illness.

Malaga /ˈmæləgə/ *n* a sweet, white dessert wine from the Spanish port of Malaga.

Malagasy /ˌmæləˈgæsi/ *n* (*pl* **Malagasy, Malagasies**) a native of Madagascar; the language of Madagascar. • *adj* pertaining to Madagascar, its language or people.

malaise /məˈleɪz/ *n* a feeling of discomfort or of uneasiness.

malamute /ˈmæləˌmjuːt/ *n* a powerful Alaskan dog with a dense grey coat used to pull sledges.—*also* **malemute**.

malanders /ˈmæləndərz/ *n sing* a disease in horses, the main symptom of which is an eczema-like patch on the horse's leg.

malapert /ˈmæləˌpert/ *adj* (*arch*) impudent; pert; saucy.

malapropism /ˈmæləprɒˌpɪzəm/ *n* a ludicrous misuse of words.—**malapropian** *adj*.

malapropos /ˌmæləprəˈpoː/ *adj* out of place, ill-timed. • *adv* in an inappropriate way; unseasonably.

malar /ˈmeɪlər/ *adj* of or relating to the cheek or cheekbone. • *n* the cheekbone.

malaria /məˈleəriə/ *n* an infectious disease caused by mosquito bites, and characterized by recurring attacks of fevers and chills.—**malarial** *adj*.

malcontent /ˈmælkənˌtent/ *adj* discontented and potentially rebellious.—*also n*.

mal de mer /ˌmældəˈmer/ *n* seasickness.

male /meɪl/ *adj* denoting or of the sex that fertilizes the ovum; of, like, or suitable for men and boys; masculine. • *n* a male person, animal or plant.—**maleness** *n*.

malediction /ˌmælə'dɪkʃən/ *n* a curse, an imprecation; a denunciation of evil; a slander.—**maledictory** *adj*.

malefactor /'mælə,fæktər/ *n* a criminal, an evildoer.—**malefaction** *n*.

maleficent /mə'lɛfɪsənt/ *adj* harmful, causing evil; mischiefmaking.—**maleficently** *adv*.—**maleficence** *n*.

malemute /'mælə'mjuːt/ *see* **malamute**.

malevolent /mə'lɛvələnt/ *adj* ill-disposed toward others; spiteful, malicious.—**malevolence** *n*.—**malevolently** *adv*.

malfeasance /mæl'fiːzəns/ *n* (*law*) an illegal action, official misconduct.—**malfeasant** *adj, n*.

malformation /ˌmælfɔr'meɪʃən/ *n* faulty or abnormal formation of a body or part.—**malformed** *adj*.

malfunction /mæl'fʌŋkʃən/ *n* faulty functioning. • *vi* to function wrongly.

malgré lui *Fr.* /'mælgreɪ,luːi/ *adv* against one's wishes, despite oneself.

malic acid /'mælɪk/ *adj* a colourless crystalline acid derived from fruit, *esp* apples.

malice /'mælɪs/ *n* active ill will, intention to inflict injury upon another.—**malicious** *adj*.—**maliciously** *adv*.—**maliciousness** *n*.

malign /mə'laɪn/ *adj* harmful; evil. • *vt* to slander; to defame.—**malignity** *n*.—**malignly** *adv*.

malignant /mə'lɪgnənt/ *adj* having a wish to harm others; injurious; (*disease*) rapidly spreading, resistant to treatment, *esp* of a tumour.—**malignancy** *n*.—**malignantly** *adv*.

malignity /-nɒti/ *n* (*pl* **malignities**) the state of being malignant or deadly; (*often pl*) (an act of) malice; virulence.

malinger /mə'lɪŋgər/ *vi* to feign illness in order to evade work, duty.—**malingerer** *n*.

malison /'mɒliːzən/ *or* /-sən/ *n* (*arch*) a curse, execration.

mall /mɒl/ *n* a shaded avenue, open to the public; a shopping street for pedestrians only; an enclosed shopping centre.

mallard /'mælərd/ *or* /-ɒrd/ *n* (*pl* **mallard, mallards**) a common wild duck, the ancestor of domestic breeds of duck.

malleable /'mæliəbəl/ *adj* pliable; capable of being shaped.—**malleability** *n*.

mallee /'mæli/ *n* a dwarf eucalyptus found in Australia; (*with the*) a sparsely populated area in Australia, the bush.

mallemuck /'mælə,mʌk/ *n* any of various sea birds, incl the fulmar and petrel.

malleolar /mə'liəlɔr/ *adj* pertaining to the ankle.

mallet /'mælət/ *n* a small, *usu* wooden-headed, short-handled hammer; a long-handled version for striking the ball in the games of polo and croquet.

mallow /'mæloː/ *n* any of a widely found genus of plants with pink flowers and palm-shaped leaves; a similar plant, *eg* marshmallow.

malm /mɒm/ *n* soft friable limestone rock; a loamy soil derived from this; a clay and chalk mixture used as an ingredient in brickmaking.

malmsey /'mɒmzi/ *n* (*pl* **malmseys**) a strong, full-flavoured sweet wine orig from Greece but now also made in Madeira, Spain, etc.

malnutrition /ˌmælnuː'trɪʃən/ *or* /ˌmælnjuː-/ *n* lack of nutrition.

malodorous /mæl'oːdərəs/ *adj* having a foul smell, badsmelling.—**malodorously** *adv*.—**malodorousness** *n*.

Malpighian /mæl'pɪgiən/ *adj* (*anat*) pertaining to various structures, such as the capillary system, discovered by the Italian anatomist Marcello Malpighi (1628-94).

malpractice /mæl'præktəs/ *n* professional misconduct, *esp* by a medical practitioner.

malt /mɒlt/ *n* a cereal grain, such as barley, which is soaked and dried and used in brewing; (*inf*) malt liquor, malt whisky.—**malty** *adj*.

maltha /'mɒlθə/ *n* a natural black bitumen; a mineral wax.

Malthusian /mæl'θuːziən/ *adj* of or pertaining to the British political economist Thomas Malthus (1766-1834) or his theory, which maintains that population tends to outgrow its means of subsistence and should be checked by means of birth control. • *n* an advocate of this theory.—**Malthusianism** *n*.

maltose /'mɒltoːz/ *n* a sugar obtained from starch by the action of diatase or malt and used in bacteriological cultures and baby foods.

maltreat /mæl'triːt/ *vt* to treat roughly or badly.—**maltreatment** *n*.

maltster /'mɒltstər/ *n* a maker of or dealer in malt.

malvoisie /'mɒlvwɒziː/ *n* a French dessert wine similar to malmsey.

mama /'mɒmə/ *n* (*inf*) mother.—*also* **mamma**.

mamba /'mæmbə/ *n* a partly tree-living green or black poisonous snake of tropical and southern Africa.

Mameluke /'mæmə,luːk/ *n* (*formerly*) a member of the ruling class in Egypt.

mamma¹ /'mɒmə/ *see* **mama**.

mamma² /'mæmə/ *n* (*pl* **mammae**) the milk-secreting organ of female mammals, such as the udder of a cow, or breast of a woman.—**mammary** *adj*.

mammal /'mæməl/ *n* any member of a class of warm-blooded vertebrates that suckle their young with milk.—**mammalian** *adj*.

mammalogy /mæ'mɒlədʒi/ *n* the branch of zoology involving the study of mammals.—**mammalogical** *adj*.—**mammalogist** *n*.

mammee /mæ'miː/ *n* a tropical American tree with edible fruit; the large red-skinned fruit from this tree.—*also* **mamee apple**.

mammiferous /mæ'mɪfərəs/ *or* /mə-/ *adj* having breasts.

mammilla /mæ'mɪlə/ *or* /mə-/ *n* (*pl* **mammillae**) a nipple; a nipple-shaped thing.

mammillary /'mæmə,lɛri/ *adj* of or like the breast or a nipple.

mammock /'mæmək/ *vt* (*inf*) to break in pieces; to shred. • *n* a small piece.

mammon /'mæmən/ *n* riches regarded as an object of worship and greedy pursuit; (*with cap*) (*Bible*) the pursuit of wealth personified as a false god.—**mammonism** *n*.—**mammonist** *n*.

mammoth /'mæməθ/ *n* an extinct elephant with long, curved tusks. • *adj* enormous.

mammy /'mæmi/ *n* (*pl* **mammies**) (*inf*) mother, as used by a child.

Man. *abbr* ✦ = Manitoba.

man /mæn/ *n* (*pl* **men**) a human being, *esp* an adult male; the human race; an adult male with manly qualities, *eg* courage, virility; a male servant; an individual person; a person with specific qualities for a task, etc; an ordinary soldier, as opposed to an officer; a member of a team, etc; a piece in games such as chess, draughts, etc; a husband. • *vt* (**manning, manned**) to provide with men for work, defence, etc.

manacle /'mænəkəl/ *n* (*usu pl*) a handcuff. • *vt* to handcuff; to restrain.

manage /'mænɪdʒ/ *vt* to control the movement or behaviour of; to have charge of; to direct; to succeed in accomplishing. • *vi* to carry on business; to contrive to get along.—**manageable** *adj*.

management /'mænɪdʒmənt/ *n* those carrying out the administration of a business; the managers collectively; the technique of managing or controlling.

manager /'mænɪdʒər/ *n* a person who manages a company, organization, etc; an agent who looks after the business affairs of an actor, writer, etc; a person who organizes the training of a sports team; a person who manages efficiently.

manageress /ˌmænɪdʒə'rɛs/ *n* a woman who manages a business, shop, etc.

managerial /ˌmænɪ'dʒiːriəl/ *adj* of or pertaining to a manager or management.—**managerially** *adv*.

manakin /'mænəkɪn/ *n* any of a genus of small South American birds with bright plumage and short beaks; a manikin.

mañana /mæn'jɒnə/ *adv* tomorrow; by and by. • *n* an unspecified time in the future.

man-at-arms /'mænæt'ɑrmz/ *n* (*pl* **men-at-arms**) an armed soldier, *esp* of medieval times.

manatee /ˌmænə'tiː/ *n* a large aquatic animal resembling a whale found in tropical seas, the sea cow.

manchineel /ˌmæntʃɪ'niːl/ *n* a poisonous tropical American tree.

manciple /'mænsɪpəl/ *n* in UK, a catering official or steward, *esp* in a monastery, college, or Inn of Court.

Mancunian /mæŋ'kjuːniən/ *adj* of Manchester. • *n* a citizen of Manchester.

mandamus /mæn'deɪməs/ *n* (*pl* **mandamuses**) (*law*) (*formerly*) a writ issued by a superior court directing the person or inferior court to whom it is issued to perform some specified act or public duty.

mandarin /'mændərɪn/ *n* (*formerly*) a high-ranking bureaucrat of the Chinese empire; any high-ranking official, *esp* one given to pedantic sometimes obscure public pronouncements; (*with cap*) the Beijing dialect that is the official pronunciation of the Chinese language; the fruit of a small spiny Chinese tree that has been developed in cultivation.—*also* **tangerine**.

mandarin collar *n* a narrow, stand-up collar, open in front.

mandatary /'mændə,tɛri/ *n* (*pl* **mandataries**) a person or nation to whom a mandate is given.

mandate /'mændeɪt/ n an order or command; the authority to act on the behalf of another, *esp* the will of constituents expressed to their representatives in legislatures; ✳ (*Cdn*) the period during which a government is in power. • *vt* to entrust by mandate.

mandatory /'mændə,tɒri/ *adj* of, containing, or having the nature of a mandate; required by mandate; compulsory; (*nation*) holding a mandate. • *n* a mandatary.—**mandatorily** *adv*.

mandatory supervision *n* ✳ (*Cdn*) supervision by a parole officer of an inmate for the last third of a prison sentence after the inmate's release on the grounds of good behaviour.

mandible /'mændɪbəl/ *n* the lower jaw of a vertebrate; the mouth parts of an insect; either jaw of a beaked animal.—**mandibular** *adj*.

mandolin /,mændə'lɪn/ or /'mæn-/, /-dɒ:-/ *n* a stringed instrument similar to a lute, with four or five pairs of strings.

mandragora /mæn'drægərə/ *n* (*poet*) mandrake; a narcotic obtained from it.

mandrake /'mændreɪk/ *n* a plant of the nightshade family with narcotic properties that, in folklore, shrieked when uprooted; the May apple.

mandrel, mandril /'mændrəl/ *n* the shank of a lathe, to which work is fixed while turned; the revolving arbor of a circular saw or other machine tool; the spindle that drives the headstock of a lathe.

mandrill /'mændril/ *n* a large baboon of West Africa, the male having a red and blue backside.

manducate /'mændjʊ,keɪt/ *vt* (*poet*) to chew, eat.

mane /meɪn/ *n* long hair that grows on the back of the neck of the horse, lion, etc.

man-eater /'mæni:tər/ *n* an animal that eats human flesh.

manège, manege /mæ'neɪʒ/ *n* a school for training horses and teaching horsemanship; the movements of a trained horse.

manes /'mɒneɪz/ or /'meɪni:z/ *n* (*pl: often cap*) in Ancient Rome, ancestral spirits, shades; gods of the lower world: *sing* the spirit of a dead person.

maneuver /mə'nu:vər/ or /-'nju:-/ *see* **manoeuvre**.

manful /'mænfʊl/ *adj* showing courage and resolution.—**manfully** *adv*.

mangabey /'mæŋgə,beɪ/ *n* (*pl* **mangabeys**) a large, slender, arboreal, African monkey.

manganate /'mæŋgə,neɪt/ *n* a salt of manganic acid.

manganese /'mæŋgə,ni:z/ *n* a hard brittle metallic element; its oxide.

manganic /mæn'gænɪk/ *adj* pertaining to, resembling, or containing manganese in the trivalent state.

mange /meɪndʒ/ *n* a skin disease affecting mainly domestic animals, which causes itching.

mangel-wurzel /'mæŋgəl'wɜːzəl/ *n* a variety of beet used as cattle-fodder.

manger /'meɪndʒər/ *n* a trough in a barn or stable for livestock fodder.

mangle[1] /'mæŋgəl/ *vt* to crush, mutilate; to spoil, ruin.

mangle[2] *n* a machine for drying and pressing sheets, etc between rollers. • *vt* to smooth through a mangle.

mango /'mæŋgoʊ/ *n* (*pl* **mangoes**) a yellow-red fleshy tropical fruit with a firm central stone.

mangonel /'mæŋgənəl/ *n* an ancient military engine for hurling stones.

mangosteen /'mæŋgə,sti:n/ *n* a tropical Indian tree; its red-brown, sweet, juicy fruit about the size of an orange.

mangrove /'mæŋgroʊv/ *n* a tropical tree or shrub with root-forming branches.

mangy /'meɪndʒi/ *adj* (**mangier, mangiest**) having mange; scruffy, shabby.—**manginess** *n*.

manhandle /'mæn,hændəl/ *vt* to handle roughly; to move by human force.

manhole /'mænhoʊl/ *n* a hole through which one can enter a sewer, drain, etc.

manhood /'mænhʊd/ *n* the state or time of being a man; virility; courage, etc.

man-hour /-aʊr/ *n* the time unit equal to one hour of work done by one person.

manhunt /'mænhʌnt/ *n* a hunt for a fugitive.—**manhunter** *n*.

mania /'meɪniə/ *n* a mental disorder displaying sometimes violent behaviour and great excitement; great excitement or enthusiasm; a craze.

maniac /'meɪni,æk/ *n* a madman; a person with wild behaviour; a person with great enthusiasm for something.—**maniacal** *adj*.

manic /'mænɪk/ *adj* affected with, characterized by, or relating to mania.

manic-depressive /-dɪ'presɪv/ *adj* of a mental disorder characterized by alternating periods of mania and deep depression. • *n* a person suffering from this.

Manichaeism, Manicheism /'mænɪ'ki:ɪzəm/ *n* the doctrine of the Manicheans, who held the dualistic theory of two eternal equal beings or principles, light (God), the author of all good, and darkness (Evil or Satan), the author of all evil, locked in a constant struggle for ascendancy; any similar doctrine.—**Manichaean, Manichean** *n, adj*.

Manichee /'mænɪki:/ *n* one of the sect of Manicheans.

manicure /'mænɪ,kjʊr/ *n* trimming, polishing etc of fingernails.—*also vt*.—**manicurist** *n*.

manifest /'mænɪ,fest/ *adj* obvious, clearly evident. • *vt* to make clear; to display, to reveal. • *n* a list of a ship's or aircraft's cargo; a list of passengers on an aircraft.—**manifestation** *n*.—**manifestly** *adv*.

manifestation /-'steɪʃən/ *n* the act of manifesting; the state of being manifested; the demonstration of the reality or existence of a quality, person, etc; the form of revelation of an idea, divine being, etc.

manifesto /,mænɪ'festoʊ/ *n* (*pl* **manifestoes, manifestos**) a public printed declaration of intent and policy issued by a government or political party.

manifold /'mænɪ,foʊld/ *adj* having many forms, parts, etc; of many sorts. • *n* a pipe (*eg* in an engine) with many inlets and outlets. • *vt* to make copies of.—**manifolder** *n*.

manikin /'mænɪkɪn/ *n* a little man, a dwarf; an anatomical model of the body; a mannequin.—*also* **mannikin**.

manila, manilla /mə'nɪlə/ *n* a strong, buff-coloured paper originally made from hemp from the Philippines.

manioc /'mænɪ,ɒk/ *n* cassava, a tropical plant from the roots of which tapioca and cassava are prepared.

maniple /'mænɪpəl/ *n* (*formerly*) a band worn on the left arm by a priest at mass; a company of a Roman legion.

manipulate /mə'nɪpjʊ,leɪt/ *vt* to work or handle skilfully; to manage shrewdly or artfully, often in an unfair way.—**manipulation** *n*.—**manipulative** *adj*.—**manipulator** *n*.

manipulation /-'leɪʃən/ *n* the act or process of manipulating; the state of being manipulated; the movement of bones, etc, by a physiotherapist; shrewd or knowing management of others for one's own ends.—**manipulatory** *adj*.

Manitoba maple *n* ✳ a fast-growing North American maple found east of the Rocky Mountains.

Manitoban /,mænə'toʊbən/ *n* ✳ (*Cdn*) a person who lives in or is from Manitoba.

manitou /,mænɪ'tu:/ *n* ✳ among some Indian peoples of northeast North America, a good or evil spirit.

mankind /mæn'kaɪnd/ *n* the human race.

manly /'mænli/ *adj* (**manlier, manliest**) appropriate in character to a man; strong; virile.—**manliness** *n*.

man-made /-'meɪd/ *adj* manufactured or created by man; artificial, synthetic.

manna /'mænə/ *n* (*Bible*) the food miraculously given to the ancient Israelites in the wilderness; any help that comes unexpectedly.

manned /mænd/ *adj* performed by a person; (*spacecraft, etc*) having a human crew.

mannequin /'mænəkɪn/ *n* a model in a fashion show; a life-size model of the human body, used to fit or display clothes.

manner /'mænər/ *n* a method of way of doing something; behaviour; type or kind; habit; (*pl*) polite social behaviour.

mannered /'mænərd/ *adj* full of mannerisms; artificial, stylized, etc.

mannerism /'mænə,rɪzəm/ *n* an idiosyncracy; an affected habit or style in dress, behaviour or gesture; (*with cap*) a post-Reformation movement in art that held that beauty should be represented as an ideal and used exaggeration and distortion of naturalistic forms to attain this.—**mannerist** *adj, n*.

mannerless /-ləs/ *n* rude, bad-mannered.

mannerly /'mænərli/ *adj* polite; respectful. • *adv* politely; respectfully.—**mannerliness** *n*.

mannikin /'mænɪkɪn/ *see* **manikin**.

mannish /'mænɪʃ/ *adj* like or pertaining to a man; (*woman*) masculine, aping men.—**mannishly** *adv*.—**mannishness** *n*.

manoeuvre /mə'nu:vər/ *n* a planned and controlled movement of troops, warships, etc; a skilful or shrewd move; a stratagem. • *vti* to perform or cause to perform manoeuvres; to manage or plan skilfully; to move, get, make, etc by some scheme.—*also* **maneuver.**—**maneuverable, manoeuvrable** *adj.*—**maneuverer, manoeuvrer** *n.*

man-of-war /ˌmænəv'wɔr/ or /-ə'wɔr/ *n* (*pl* **men-of-war**) a (sailing) warship.

manometer /mə'nɒmɪtər/ *n* an instrument for measuring the pressure of gases and liquids.—**manometric, manometrical** *adj.*

manor /'mænər/ *n* a landed estate; the main house on such an estate; (*sl*) a police district.—**manorial** *adj.*

manpower /'mænpaʊr/ *n* power furnished by human strength; the collective availability for work of people in a given area.

manqué /'mɒŋkeɪ/ *adj* potential; unsuccessful, failed.

mansard (roof) /'mænsɑrd/ *n* a roof with a break in its slope, the lower part being steeper than the upper.

manse /mæns/ *n* a nonconformist clergyman's house; (*Scot*) the house of a minister, *esp* a Church of Scotland parish minister; (*arch*) a large house.

manservant /'mæn,sɜrvənt/ *n* (*pl* **menservants**) a male servant, *esp* a valet.

mansion /'mænʃən/ *n* a large, imposing house.

manslaughter /'mæn,slɒtər/ *n* the killing of a human being by another, *esp* when unlawful but without malice.

mansuetude /'mænswɪ,tjuːd/ *n* (*arch*) gentleness, mildness.

manta (ray) /'mæntə/ *n* a very large fish with a flattened body and wing-like fins.

mantel /'mæntəl/ *n* the facing above a fireplace; the shelf above a fireplace.—*also* **mantelpiece.**

mantelet /'mæntələt/ *n* a woman's short cape of the mid-19th century; a movable, protective screen, formerly used by besiegers, gunners, pioneers, etc.—*also* **mantlet.**

mantic /'mæntɪk/ *adj* of, having the power of, or pertaining to divination.

manticore /'mæntɪkɔr/ *n* a fabulous beast with a human head, the body of a lion, and the tail of a scorpion.

mantilla /mæn'tɪlə/ *n* a scarf, *usu* of lace, worn as a headdress in Spain and South America; a woman's light cloak or hood.

mantis /'mæntɪs/ *n* (*pl* **mantises, mantes**) an insect that preys on other insects.—*also* **praying mantis.**

mantissa /mæn'tɪsə/ *n* (*math*) the decimal part of a logarithm.

mantle /'mæntəl/ *n* a loose cloak; anything that envelops or conceals; a fine mesh cover on a gas or oil lamp that emits light by incandescence. • *vt* to cover as with a mantle. • *vi* to be or become covered.

mantlet /'mæntələt/ *see* **mantelet.**

mantra /'mæntrə/ *n* (*Hinduism, Buddhism*) a devotional incantation used in prayer, meditation and in certain forms of yoga.

mantua /'mæntjuə/ *n* a woman's loose gown of the 17th and 18th centuries, worn with the front of the skirt caught up or back to show an underskirt.

manual /'mænjuəl/ *adj* of the hands; operated, done, or used by the hand; involving physical skill or hard work rather than the mind. • *n* a handy book for use as a guide, reference, etc; a book of instructions.—**manually** *adv.*

manufactory /ˌmænju'fæktəri/ *n* (*pl* **manufactories**) (*obs*) a factory, workshop.

manufacture /ˌmænju'fæktʃər/ *vt* to make, *esp* on a large scale, using machinery; to invent, fabricate. • *n* the production of goods by manufacturing.—**manufacturer** *n.*

manumit /ˌmænju'mɪt/ *vt* (**manumitting, manumitted**) to release from slavery; to free.—**manumission** *n.*—**manumitter** *n.*

manure /mə'nʊr/ or /-'njʊr/ *n* animal dung used to fertilize soil. • *vt* to spread manure on.

manus /'meɪnəs/ *n* (*pl* **manus**) (*zool*) the hand or that part of the anatomy corresponding to the hand; in ancient Roman law, the fact of a woman's legal subjugation to her husband.

manuscript /'mænjuskrɪpt/ *n* a book or document that is handwritten or typewritten as opposed to printed; an author's original handwritten or typewritten copy as submitted to a publisher before typesetting and printing.

many /'mɛni/ *adj* (**more, most**) numerous. • *n* a large number of persons or things.

manyplies /'mɛni,plaɪz/ *n sing* a ruminant's third stomach, the omasum.

many-sided /-,saɪdɪd/ *adj* with many aspects; versatile.—**many-sidedness** *n.*

Maori /'maʊri/ *n* (*pl* **Maoris, Maori**) a member of the indigenous peoples of New Zealand; their language.—*also adj.*

map /mæp/ *n* a representation of all or part of the earth's surface, showing either natural features as continents and seas, etc or man-made features as roads, railways etc. • *vt* (**mapping, mapped**) to make a map of.

maple /'meɪpəl/ *n* a tree with two-winged fruits, grown for shade, wood, or sap; its hard light-coloured wood; the flavour of the syrup or sugar made from the sap of the sugar maple.

maple butter *n* ✤ (*Cdn*) a creamy spread made from maple syrup.

maple leaf *n* ✤ the leaf of the maple tree, considered as an emblem of Canada.

Mar. *abbr* = March.

mar /mɒr/ *vt* (**marring, marred**) to blemish, to spoil, to impair.

marabout[1], **marabou** /'mærə,buː/ *n* a large African stork with handsome feathers and a short neck; its down, used as trimming, etc; a material produced from a fine raw silk.

marabout[2], /'mærə,buːt/ *n* in North Africa, a Muslim hermit or saint; the shrine or burial place of a marabout.

maraca /mə'rɒkə/ or /-rækə/ *n* a dried gourd or plastic shell filled with beans, pebbles, etc and shaken as a rhythm instrument.

maraschino /ˌmærə'ʃiːnoː/ or /-'skiːnoː/, /ˌmɛrə-/ *n* a strong sweet liqueur made from a type of wild cherry.

maraschino cherry *n* a cherry preserved in maraschino.

marasmus /mə'ræzməs/ *n* emaciation or atrophy, *esp* in babies.—**marasmic** *adj.*

marathon /'mɛrəθɒn/ *n* a foot race of 26 miles, 385 yards (42.195 km); any endurance contest.

maraud /mə'rɒd/ *vi* to roam in search of plunder.—**marauder** *n.*—**marauding** *adj.*

marble /'mɑrbəl/ *n* a hard limestone rock that takes a high polish; a block or work of art made of marble; a little ball of stone, glass, etc; (*pl*) a children's game played with such balls; (*pl*) (*sl*) wits. • *adj* of or like marble.—**marbly** *adj.*

marbled /'mɑrbəld/ *adj* veined or mottled like marble; (*meat*) streaked with fat.

marc /mɑrk/ *n* (*winemaking*) the refuse from pressed fruit; a brandy derived from this.

marcasite /'mɑrkə,saɪt/ *n* white iron pyrites; a white metal, *esp* steel, cut and polished for use in jewellery.

marcel (wave) /mɑr'sɛl/ *n* a style of artificially waving the hair, popular in the 1920s and 1930s. • *vt* (**marcelling, marcelled**) to style in regular waves.

marcescent /mɑr'sesənt/ *adj* (*bot*) withering without falling off.—**marcescence** *n.*

March /mɑrtʃ/ *n* the third month of the year having 31 days.

march *vi* to walk with regular steps, as in military formation; to advance steadily. • *vt* to make a person or group march. • *n* a steady advance; a regular, steady step; the distance covered in marching; a piece of music for marching.—**marcher** *n.*

marching orders *npl* official orders for infantry to move to a particular destination; (*inf*) a notice of dismissal.

marchioness /ˌmɑrʃə'nes/ or /'mɑr-/ *n* the wife or widow of a marquess; a woman of the rank of marquess.

Mardi gras /'mɑrdi,grɒ/ *n* the last day before Lent, Shrove Tuesday, a day of carnival in some cities, *esp* New Orleans.

mare /mer/ *n* a mature female horse, mule, donkey.

mare clausum /'mɒreɪ'klaʊsum/ or /-ri-/ *n* (*law*) a body of water under one country's jurisdiction and closed to foreign ships.

mare liberum /-'liːbərəm/ *n* (*law*) a body of water open to ships of all countries.

maremma /mə'remə/ *n* (*pl* **maremme**) an unhealthy marshy coastal district, *esp* in Italy.

mare's-tail /'mɛrz,teɪl/ *n* an aquatic plant with tiny flowers and tapering leaves; a wisp of trailing alto-cirrus cloud indicating strong winds at high altitude.

margaric /mɑr'gærɪk/ or /-'gɑr-/, /'mɑrgərɪk/ *adj* pertaining to, or like, a pearl.

margarine /'mɑrdʒərɪn/ *n* a butter substitute made from vegetable and animal fats, etc.

margarite /'mɑrgə,raɪt/ *n* a pearly translucent mineral related to mica; a bead-like rock formation.

margay /'mɑrgeɪ/ *n* a South American tiger cat.

margin /'mɑrdʒɪn/ *n* a border, edge; the blank border of a printed or written page; an amount beyond what is needed; provision for increase, error, etc; (*commerce*) the difference between cost and selling price.

marginal /-əl/ *adj* written in the margin; situated at the margin or border; close to the lower limit of acceptability; very slight, insignificant; (*Brit politics*) denoting a constituency where the sitting MP has only a small majority. • *n* a marginal constituency.—**marginally** *adv*.

marginalia /ˌmɑrdʒɪˈneɪliə/ *npl* notes written in the margin of a book, etc.

marginalize /ˈmɑrdʒɪnəˌlaɪz/ *vt* to transfer someone away from the centre of affairs in order to render them powerless.

marginate /ˈmɑrdʒɪˌneɪt/ *adj* (*biol*) having a margin. • *vt* to border something with a margin.—**margination** *n*.

margrave /ˈmɑrgreɪv/ *n* (*formerly*) a German nobleman, one rank above a count.

margraviate, margravate /ˈmɑrgrəvət/ *n* the domain or jurisdiction of a margrave.

margravine /ˈmɑrgrəˌviːn/ *n* a female margrave; a margrave's wife or widow.

marguerite /ˌmɑrgrəˈriːt/ *n* a large daisy with white or yellow flowers.

Marian /ˈmeriən/ *adj* pertaining to the Virgin Mary, or to Mary, Queen of England, or to Mary, Queen of Scots. • *n* one who worships the Virgin Mary; a partisan of Mary, Queen of England or Mary, Queen of Scots.

marigold /ˈmerɪˌgoːld/ *n* a plant with a yellow or orange flower.

marijuana, marihuana /ˌmerɪˈwɒnə/ *n* a narcotic obtained by smoking the dried flowers and leaves of the hemp plant.—*also* **cannabis, pot.**

marimba /məˈrɪmbə/ *n* a South American xylophone.

marina /məˈriːnə/ *n* a small harbour with pontoons, docks, services, etc for yachts and pleasure craft.

marinade /ˈmerɪneɪd/ or /-ˈneɪd/ *n* a seasoning liquid ir which meat, fish, etc is soaked to enhance flavour or to tenderize it before cooking. • *vt* to soak in a marinade.—*also* **marinate**.

marine /məˈriːn/ *adj* of, in, near, or relating to the sea; maritime; nautical; naval. • *n* a soldier trained for service on land or sea; naval or merchant ships.

mariner /ˈmærɪnər/ *n* a seaman, sailor.

Mariolatry /ˌmeriˈɒlətri/ *n* the exaggerated worship of the Virgin Mary.

marionette /ˌmeriəˈnet/ *n* a little jointed doll or puppet moved by strings or wires.

marital /ˈmerɪtəl/ *adj* of marriage, matrimonial.

maritime /ˈmerɪˌtaɪm/ *adj* on, near, or living near the sea; of navigation, shipping, etc.

Maritime Command *n* ✤ the Canadian navy.

marjoram /ˈmɑrdʒərəm/ *n* a fragrant herb used in cooking and salads.

mark[1] /mɑrk/ *n* a spot, scratch, etc on a surface; a distinguishing sign or characteristic; a cross made instead of a signature; a printed or written symbol, as a punctuation mark; a brand or label on an article showing the maker, etc; an indication of some quality, character, etc; a grade for academic work; a standard of quality; impression, influence, etc; a target; (*sl*) a potential victim for a swindle. • *vt* to make a mark or marks on; to identify as by a mark; to show plainly; to heed; to grade, rate; (*Brit football*) to stay close to an opponent so as to hinder his play.

mark[2] *n* the former monetary unit of Germany, now replaced by the euro.

marked /mɑrkt/ *adj* having a mark or marks; noticeable; obvious.—**markedly** *adv*.

marker /ˈmɑrkər/ *n* one that marks; something used for marking.

market /ˈmɑrkət/ *n* a meeting of people for buying and selling merchandise; a space or building in which a market is held; the chance to sell or buy; demand for (goods, etc); a region where goods can be sold; a section of the community offering demand for goods. • *vti* to offer for sale; to sell, buy domestic provisions.—**marketability** *n*.—**marketable** *adj*.

marketing /ˈmɑrkətɪŋ/ *n* act of buying or selling; all the processes involved in moving goods from the producer to the consumer.

market-making *n* the activity of buying and selling stocks, shares, bonds, securities, etc.—**market-maker** *n*.

marketplace /ˈmɑrkətˌpleɪs/ *n* a market in a public square; the world of economic trade and activity; a sphere in which ideas, opinions, etc compete for acceptance.

market research *n* the gathering of factual information from consumers concerning their preferences for goods and services.

marking /ˈmɑrkɪŋ/ *n* the conferring of a mark or marks; the characteristic arrangement of marks, as on fur or feathers.

marksman /ˈmɑrksmən/ *n* (*pl* **marksmen**) one who is skilled at shooting.—**marksmanship** *n*.

markup /ˈmɑrkʌp/ *n* a selling at an increased price; the amount of increase.—*also vt*.

marl[1] /mɑrl/ *n* a mixture of clay and carbonate of lime, used as a manure. • *vt* to manure w th marl.—**marly** *adj*.

marl[2] *vt* (*naut*) to wind with marlines, securing with a hitch at each turn.

marline, marlin, marling /ˈmɑrlɪn/ *n* (*naut*) a two-stranded cord, often tarred, used for winding round ropes, splicing, etc.

marlinespike, marlinspike, marlingspike /ˈmɑrlɪnˌspaɪk/ *n* a pointed piece of iron used for opening the strands of a rope in splicing, etc.

marmalade /ˈmɑrməˌleɪd/ *n* a jam-like preserve made from oranges, sugar and water.

marmoreal /mɑrˈmɔriəl/, **marmorean** /-ən/ *adj* of or like marble.

marmoset /ˈmɑrməˌzet/ *n* a small monkey of South and Central America.

marmot /ˈmɑrmət/ *n* a widely distributed rodent with rough fur, a bushy tail and short legs.

maroon[1] /məˈruːn/ *n* a dark brownish red.—*also adj*; a type of distress rocket.

maroon[2] *vt* to abandon alone, *esp* on a desolate island; to leave helpless and alone.

marque /mɑrk/ *n* a brand of a product, *esp* a car.

marquee /mɑrˈkiː/ *n* a large tent used for entertainment; a canopy over an entrance, as to a theatre.

marquess /ˈmɑrkwɪs/ *n* In UK, a title of nobility ranking between a duke and an earl.

marquetry, marqueterie /ˈmɑrkɪtri/ *n* (*pl* **marquetries, marqueteries**) decorative inlaid veneers of wood, ivory, etc used *esp* in furniture.

marquis /mɑrˈkiː/ *n* (*pl* **marquises, marquis**) (*Europe*) a nobleman equivalent in rank to a British marquess.

marquisate /-sət/ *n* the estate, dignity, or lordship of a marquis.

marquise /mɑrˈkiːz/ *n* a marchioness; a gemstone or ring setting cut in an oval pointed form.

marriage /ˈmerɪdʒ/ or /ˈmæ-/ *n* the legal contract by which a woman and man become wife and husband; a wedding, either religious or civil; a close union.

marriageable /ˈmerɪdʒəbə/ or /ˈmæ-/ *adj* of an age to marry.—**marriageability** *n*.

marron glacé /ˌmæˌrɒɡlæˈseɪ/ *n* (*pl* **marrons glacés**) a cooked chestnut coated with sugar.

marrow /ˈmerɒ/ or /ˈmæ-/ *n* the fatty tissue in the cavities of bones; the best part or essence of anything; a widely grown green fruit eaten as a vegetable.

marrowbone /-ˌboːn/ *n* a bone containing marrow used in cooking.

marrowfat /-ˌfæt/, **marrow pea** *n* a late variety of pea that has large seeds; the seed of one of these.

marry[1] /ˈmeri/ or /ˈmæri/ *vb* (**marrying, married**) *vt* to join as wife and husband; to take in marriage; to unite. • *vi* to get married.

marry[2] *interj* (*arch*) indeed, forsooth.

Mars /mɑrz/ *n* the Roman god of war; the planet next to Earth, further away from the sun; (*alchemy*) iron.

Marsala /mɑrˈsælə/ or /-ˈsɑlə/ *n* a sweet fortified wine from Sicily.

Marseillaise /ˌmɑrseɪˈjez/ *adj* pertaining to the city of Marseilles in France or to its inhabitants. • *n* the French national anthem, orig a well-known song of the French Revolution, composed in 1792.

marsh /mɑrʃ/ *n* an area of boggy, poorly drained land.—**marshiness** *n*.—**marshy** *adj*.

marshal /ˈmɑrʃəl/ *n* in some armies, a general officer of the highest rank; an official in charge of ceremonies, parades, etc. • *vt* (**marshalling, marshalled** *or* **marshaling, marshaled**) (*ideas, troops*) to arrange in order; to guide.—**marshaller** *n*.

marsh mallow /ˈmɑrʃˌmeloː/ or /-ˌmæloː/ *n* a perennial plant with a pink flower and a mucilaginous root used in confectionery and medicine.

marshmallow *n* a soft spongy confection made of sugar, gelatin, etc; (*formerly*) a sweet paste made from the root of the marsh mallow.

marsupial /mɑrˈsuːpiəl/ *adj* of an order of mammals that carry their young in a pouch. • *n* an animal of this kind, as a kangaroo, opossum.

marsupium /-əm/ *n* (*pl* **marsupia**) in female marsupials, an external pouch for carrying and nurturing young.

mart /mɑrt/ *n* a market.

martagon /ˈmɑrtəgən/ *n* a variety of lily with purple-red flowers found in Europe and Asia; a Turk's-cap lily.

Martello tower /mɑrˈtɛloː/ *n* (*formerly*) a small round fort used for coastal defence.

marten /ˈmɑrtən/ *n* (*pl* **martens, marten**) a carnivorous tree-dwelling weasel-like mammal.

martial /ˈmɑrʃəl/ *adj* warlike; military.—**martially** *adv.*

martial arts *npl* systems of self-defence, *usu* from the Orient, practised as sports, as karate or judo.

martial law *n* rule by military authorities over civilians, as during a war or political emergency.

Martian /ˈmɑrʃən/ *adj* of or relating to the planet Mars. • *n* an inhabitant of Mars.

martin /ˈmɑrtɪn/ *n* one of various types of bird similar to the swallow, with a characteristic shape of tail; the house martin.

martinet /ˌmɑrtɪˈnɛt/ *n* one who exerts strong discipline.—**martinetish, martinettish** *adj.*

martingale, martingal /ˈmɑrtɪŋˌgeɪl/ *n* a broad strap passing from the noseband to the girth of a horse between its forelegs to keep its head down and prevent it from rearing; a gambling system of doubling successive stakes; (*naut*) a short spar under the bowsprit used as a lower stay for the jib boom or flying jib boom.

martini /mɑrˈtiːni/ *n* (*trademark*) (*often with cap*) Italian vermouth; a cocktail of gin and vermouth.

Martinmas /ˈmɑrtɪnməs/ *n* St Martin's Day, November 11, a Christian festival; one of the Scottish quarter days.

martlet /ˈmɑrtlət/ *n* (*arch*) a martin; (*her*) a bird without legs or beak.

martyr /ˈmɑrtər/ *n* a person tortured for a belief or cause; a person who suffers from an illness. • *vt* to kill as a martyr; to make a martyr of.—**martyrdom** *n.*

martyrize /-ˌraɪz/ *vt* to martyr.

martyrology /ˌmɑrtəˈrɒlədʒi/ *n* (*pl* **martyrologies**) a register or history of martyrs; the study of the lives of the martyrs.—**martyrological, martyrologic** *adj.*—**martyrologist** *n.*

martyry /ˈmɑrtəri/ *n* (*pl* **martyries**) a shrine in honour of a martyr.

marvel /ˈmɑrvəl/ *n* anything wonderful; a miracle. • *vti* (**marvelling, marvelled** *or* **marveling, marveled**) to become filled with wonder, surprise, etc.—**marvellous, marvelous** *adj.*

Marxian /ˈmɑrksɪən/ *n* a student or advocate of Marxism.—*also adj.*

Marxism /ˈmɑrksɪzəm/ *n* the theory and practice developed by Karl Marx and Friedrich Engels advocating public ownership of the means of production and the dictatorship of the proletariat until the establishment of a classless society.—**Marxist** *adj, n.*

marzipan /ˈmɑrzɪˌpæn/ *or* /-ˈpæn/ *n* a paste made from ground almonds, sugar and egg white, used to coat cakes or make confectionery.

mascara /mæˈskɛrə/ *n* a cosmetic for darkening the eyelashes.

mascle /ˈmæsəl/ *n* (*her*) a lozenge perforated with a lozenge shape; a voided lozenge.

mascot /ˈmæskɒt/ *n* a person, animal or thing thought to bring good luck.

masculine /ˈmæskjʊlɪn/ *adj* having characteristics of or appropriate to the male sex; (*gram*) of the male gender.—**masculinity** *n.*

MASH *abbr* = mobile army surgical hospital.

mash /mæʃ/ *n* any soft, pulpy mass; crushed malt and hot water for brewing; (*inf*) mashed potatoes. • *vt* to crush into a mash.

mashie /ˈmæʃi/ *n* (*formerly*) an iron golf club with a deep, short blade, more or less lofted.

mask[1] /mɑːsk/ *n* a covering to conceal or protect the face; a moulded likeness of the face; anything that conceals or disguises; a respirator placed over the nose and mouth to aid or prevent inhalation of a gas; (*surgery*) a protective gauze placed over the nose and mouth to prevent the spread of germs; (*photog*) a screen used to cover part of a sensitive surface to prevent exposure by light. • *vt* to cover or conceal as with a mask; to disguise one's intentions or character.—**masked** *adj.*

mask[2] *see* **masque.**

masker /ˈmæskər/ *n* a masked person; a participant in a masque or masquerade.—*also* **masquer.**

masochism /ˈmæsəˌkɪzəm/ *n* abnormal pleasure, *esp* sexual, obtained from having physical or mental pain inflicted on one by another person.—**masochist** *n.*—**masochistic** *adj.*

mason /ˈmeɪsən/ *n* a person skilled in working or building with stone; (*with cap*) a Freemason.

masonic /məˈsɒnɪk/ *adj* (*often cap*) relating to Freemasonry.

masonry /ˈmeɪsənri/ *n* (*pl* **masonries**) stonework.

Masora, Masorah /məˈsɔrə/ *or* /ˈmæsəˈrɒ/ *n* a critical work in Hebrew by the rabbis of the 6-10th cents., indicating how the verbal text of the Bible is to be written in accordance with ancient rules; the critical notes and commentaries of this.—**Masoretic** *adj.*

masque /mæsk/ *n* a poetic drama with pageantry, pantomime, dance, song, etc, popular in 16th and 17th-century England; the words and music for one of these; a masquerade.—*also* **mask.**

masquer /ˈmæskər/ *see* **masker.**

masquerade /ˌmæskəˈreɪd/ *n* a ball or party at which fancy dress and masks are worn; a pretence, false show. • *vi* to take part in a masquerade; to pretend to be what one is not.—**masquerader** *n.*

Mass. *abbr* = Massachusetts.

Mass /mæs/ *n* (*RC Church*) the celebration of the Eucharist.

mass /mæs/ *n* (*pl* **masses**) a quantity of matter of indefinite shape and size; a large quantity or number; bulk; size; the main part; (*physics*) the property of a body expressed as a measure of the amount of material contained in it; (*pl*) the common people, *esp* the lower social classes. • *adj* of or for the masses or for a large number. • *vti* to gather or form into a mass.

massacre /ˈmæsəkər/ *n* the cruel and indiscriminate killing of many people or animals. • *vt* to kill in large numbers.

massage /məˈsɒʒ/ *or* /-ˈsɒdʒ/ *n* a kneading and rubbing of the muscles to stimulate the circulation of the blood. • *vt* to give a massage to.

massé shot /mæˈseɪ/ *n* in billiards, a stroke with the cue held upright, *usu* to cause the ball to curve round another ball before it hits the intended ball.

masseur /məˈsər/ *n* a man who gives a massage professionally.—**masseuse** *nf.*

massif /mæˈsiːf/ *or* /ˈmæsif/ *n* a central mountain mass; a large plateau with distinct edges.

massive /ˈmæsɪv/ *adj* big, solid, or heavy; large and imposing; relatively large in comparison to normal; extensive.—**massively** *adv.*—**massiveness** *n.*

mass media *npl* newspapers, radio, television, and other means of communication with large numbers of people.

mass production *n* quantity production of goods, *esp* by machinery and division of labour.

massy /ˈmæsi/ *adj* (**massier massiest**) (*arch*) massive.

mast /mæst/ *n* a tall vertical pole used to support the sails on a ship; a vertical pole from which a flag is flown; a tall structure supporting a television or radio aerial.

mastaba, mastabah /ˈmæstəbə/ *n* an early Egyptian tomb with a flat roof, the prototype of the pyramids.

mast cell *n* a large blood-borne cell that has a fast-acting role in the body's immune system in fighting inflammation.

mastectomy /mæsˈtɛktəmi/ *n* the removal of a breast by surgery.

master /ˈmæstər/ *n* a man who rules others or has control over something, *esp* the head of a household; an employer; an owner of an animal or slave; the captain of a merchant ship; a male teacher in a private school; an expert craftsman; a writer or painter regarded as great; an original from which a copy can be made, *esp* a phonograph record or magnetic tape; (*with cap*) a title for a boy; one holding an advanced academic degree. • *adj* being a master; chief; main; controlling. • *vt* to be or become master of; (*in art, etc*) to become expert.—**mastership** *n.*

master-at-arms /-ətˈɑrmz/ *n* (*pl* **masters-at-arms**) a ship's chief petty officer with responsibility for policing, administration, etc.

master corporal *n* ✦ a noncommissioned officer in the Canadian army or air force, ranking just below sergeant.

masterful /ˈmæstərˌfʊl/ *adj* acting the part of a master; domineering; expert; skilful.—**masterfully** *adv.*—**masterfulness** *n.*

masterly /-li/ *adj* expert; skilful.—**masterliness** *n.*

mastermind /-ˌmaɪnd/ *n* a very clever person, *esp* one who plans or directs a project. • *vt* to be the mastermind of.

masterpiece /-ˌpiːs/ *n* a work done with extraordinary skill; the greatest work of a person or group.

master seaman *n* ✦ a noncommissioned officer in the Canadian navy, equivalent to a master corporal.

masterstroke /-ˌstroːk/ *n* brilliant stroke of policy, skill, etc.

master warrant officer *n* ✦ a noncommissioned officer in the Canadian army or air force, ranking just below chief warrant officer.

masterwork /-ˌwərk/ *n* a masterpiece.

mastery /ˈmæstəri/ *or* /-tri/ *n* control as by a master; victory; expertise.

masthead /'mæsthed/ *n* the top of a mast; the title and ownership details, etc of a newspaper or periodical printed on the front page.

mastic /'mæstɪk/ *n* an aromatic resin from mastic trees used chiefly in varnishes; a type of putty used for sealing wood, plaster, etc.

masticate /'mæstɪˌkeɪt/ *vt* to chew food before swallowing to reduce to a pulp.—**mastication** *n.*—**masticator** *n.*

masticatory /-kətɔrɪ/ *adj* adapted for, or pertaining to, chewing. • *n* (*pl* **masticatories**) (*med*) something chewed in order to promote the flow of saliva.

mastiff /'mæstɪf/ *n* a breed of large, thickset dogs used chiefly as watchdogs.

mastitis /mæ'staɪtɪs/ *n* an inflammation of a female breast or an udder.

mastodon /'mæstəˌdɒn/ *n* any of an extinct genus of mammals allied to the elephant.—**mastodonic** *adj.*

mastoid /'mæstɔɪd/ *n* the bony prominence behind the ear.

masturbate /'mæstərˌbeɪt/ *vi* to manually stimulate one's sexual organs to achieve orgasm without sexual intercourse.—**masturbation** *n.*

mat[1] /mæt/ *n* a piece of material of woven fibres, etc, used for protection, as under a vase, etc, or on the floor; a thick pad used in wrestling, gymnastics, etc; anything interwoven or tangled into a thick mass. • *vti* (**matting, matted**) to cover as with a mat; to interweave or tangle into a thick mass.

mat[2] *adj* without lustre, dull.—*also* **matt.**

matador /'mætəˌdɔr/ *n* the bullfighter who kills the bull with a sword.

match[1] /mætʃ/ *n* a thin strip of wood or cardboard tipped with a chemical that ignites under friction.

match[2] *n* any person or thing equal or similar to another; two persons or things that go well together; a contest or game; a mating or marriage. • *vt* to join in marriage; to put in opposition (with, against); to be equal or similar to; (*one thing*) to suit to another. • *vi* to be equal, similar, suitable, etc.

matchboard /'mætʃbɔrd/ *n* one of a number of thin planks tongued and grooved to fit together, used for panelling, etc.

matchbox /-bɒks/ *n* a small box for holding matches.

matchless /-ləs/ *adj* unequalled.—**matchlessly** *adv.*

matchmaker /-ˌmeɪkər/ *n* a person who arranges marriages for people; one who schemes to bring about the marriage of two others; a maker of matches.

match play *n* (*golf*) scoring by the number of holes won as opposed to strokes played.

match point *n* (*tennis, badminton, etc*) the situation where the winner of the next point wins the match.

matchwood /'mætʃwʊd/ *n* wood suitable for making matches; wood splinters or fragments.

maté /'mæteɪ/ *n* an evergreen South American shrub, related to holly; an infusion of its dried leaves which makes a mildly stimulating tea,.—*also* **Paraguay tea.**

mate[1] /meɪt/ *n* an associate or colleague; (*inf*) a friend; one of a matched pair; a marriage partner; the male or female of paired animals; an officer of a merchant ship, ranking below the master. • *vti* to join as a pair; to couple in marriage or sexual union.

mate[2] *vt* to checkmate.

matelote /'mætloː/ *n* a stew of fish cooked with wine, etc.

mater /'meɪtər/ *n* (*sl*) mother.

materfamilias /ˌmeɪtərfə'mɪliˌæs/ *n* (*pl* **matresfamilias**) the mother of a family or mistress of a household.

material /mə'tiːriəl/ *adj* of, derived from, or composed of matter, physical; of the body or bodily needs, comfort, etc, not spiritual; important, essential, etc. • *n* what a thing is, or may be made of; elements or parts; cloth, fabric; (*pl*) tools, etc needed to make or do something; a person regarded as fit for a particular task, position, etc.

materialism /mə'tiːriəˌlɪzəm/ *n* concern with money and possessions rather than spiritual values; the doctrine that everything in the world, including thought, can be explained only in terms of matter.—**materialist** *n.*—**materialistic** *adj.*

materiality /məˌtiːri'ælətɪ/ *n* (*pl* **materialities**) the quality or state of being material; material existence; substance.

materialize /mə'tiːriəˌlaɪz/ *vt* to give material form to. • *vi* to become fact; to make an unexpected appearance.—**materialization** *n.*

materially /mə'tiːriəli/ *adv* physically; to a great extent; substantially.

materia medica /mæˌtiːriə 'medikə/ *n* the science of substances used in medicine incl pharmacology, pharmacy, etc; a substance employed as a medicine or in making drugs.

materiel, matériel /məˌtiːri'el/ *n* the baggage, munitions, and provisions of an army or of any other organization.

maternal /mə'tərnəl/ *adj* of, like, or from a mother; related through the mother's side of the family.—**maternally** *adv.*

maternity /mə'tərnɪtɪ/ *n* motherhood; motherliness. • *adj* relating to pregnancy.

matey /'meɪtɪ/ *n* a crony or companion (often used when directly addressing such). • *adj* (**matier, matiest**) (*inf*) friendly, sociable.—**mateyness, matiness** *n.*—**matily** *adv.*

math /mæθ/ *n* (*inf*) mathematics.

mathematical /ˌmæθə'mætɪkəl/, **mathematic** /ˌmæθə'mætɪk/ *adj* of, like or concerned with mathematics; exact and precise.—**mathematically** *adv.*

mathematics /ˌmæθə'mætɪks/ *n* (*used as sing*) the science dealing with quantities, forms, space, etc and their relationships by the use of numbers and symbols; (*sing or pl*) the mathematical operations or processes used in a particular problem, discipline, etc. —**mathematician** *n.*

maths /mæθs/ *n* (*inf*) mathematics.

matin /'mætn/, **matinal** /-nəl/ *adj* of or pertaining to the morning or to matins.

matinée /'mætɪˌneɪ/ *n* a daytime, *esp* an afternoon performance of a play, etc.

matins /'mætɪnz/ *n* (*sing or pl*) (*Anglican Church*) a morning prayer; (*RC Church*) one of the canonical hours of prayer; (*poet*) a bird's morning song.

matriarch /'meɪtriˌɑrk/ *n* a woman who heads or rules her family or tribe.—**matriarchal, matriarchic** *adj.*

matriarchy /'meɪtriˌɑrkɪ/ *n* (*pl* **matriarchies**) form of social organization in which the mother is the ruler of the family or tribe and in which descent is traced through the mother.

matrices /'meɪtriˌsiz/ or /'meɪ-/ *see* **matrix.**

matricide /'mætriˌsaɪd/ or /'meɪt-/ *n* a person who kills his (her) mother; the killing of one's mother.—**matricidal** *adj.*

matriculate /mə'trɪkjʊˌleɪt/ *vti* to enrol, *esp* as a student.—**matriculation** *n.*

matrimony /'mætriˌmoːnɪ/ *n* (*pl* **matrimonies**) the act or rite of marriage; the married state.—**matrimonial** *adj.*—**matrimonially** *adv.*

matrix /'meɪtrɪks/ *n* (*pl* **matrices, matrixes**) the place, substance, etc from which something originates; a mould; the connective intercellular substance in bone, cartilage, or other tissue; (*math*) a rectangular grid of quantities in rows and columns used in solving certain problems.

matron /'meɪtrən/ *n* a wife or widow, *esp* one of mature appearance and manner; a woman in charge of domestic and nursing arrangements in a school, hospital or other institution.—**matronal** *adj.*

matronly /'meɪtrənli/ *adj* pertaining to or suitable for a matron; sedate, dignified; (*figure*) plump.—**matronliness** *n.*

matronymic /ˌmætrə'nɪmɪk/ *see* **metronymic.**

matt /mæt/ *see* **mat**[2].

matter /'mætər/ *n* what a thing is made of; material; whatever occupies space and is perceptible to the senses; any specified substance; content of thought or expression; a quantity; a thing or affair; significance; trouble, difficulty; pus. • *vi* to be of importance.

matter-of-fact *adj* relating to facts, not opinions, imagination, etc.

matting /'mætɪŋ/ *n* a coarse material, such as woven straw or hemp, used for making mats.

mattock /'mætək/ *n* a pick with one head like an axe, the other like an adze.

mattress /'mætrɪs/ *n* a casing of strong cloth filled with cotton, foam rubber, coiled springs, etc, used on a bed.

maturate /'mætʃəˌreɪt/ *vti* (*med*) to discharge pus, to fester; (*arch*) to bring or come to maturation.—**maturative** *adj.*

maturation /ˌmætʃə'reɪʃən/ *n* the process of ripening or coming to maturity; (*biol*) the progressive generation of cells already present in the ovary and testis, mitosis; (*rare*) the act of discharging pus, suppuration.

mature /mə'tʃʊr/ or /-'tʃər/ *adj* mentally and physically well-developed, grown-up; (*fruit, cheese, etc*) ripe; (*bill*) due; (*plan*) completely worked out. • *vti* to make or become mature; to become due.—**maturely** *adv.*—**matureness** *n.*

maturity /-əti/ *n* the state of being mature; full development; the date a loan becomes due.

matutinal /ˌmætjuːˈtaɪnəl/ *adj* of, happening during, or pertaining to the morning; early.—**matutinally** *adv*.

maud /mɒd/ *n* (*Scot*) a grey-striped woollen plaid worn by shepherds.

maudlin /ˈmɔːdlɪn/ *adj* foolishly sentimental; tearfully drunk.

maul /mɒl/ *vt* to bruise or lacerate; to paw.

maulstick /ˈmɒlˌstɪk/ *n* a long stick used by painters as a rest for the hand while painting.—*also* **mahlstick**.

maund /mɒnd/ *n* any of various Asian units of weight, varying from 25 pounds (11 kilograms) to 82 pounds (37 kilograms), according to locality.

maunder /ˈmɒndər/ *vi* to speak, act or move listlessly or purposelessly.—**maunderer** *n*.

Maundy Thursday the Thursday before Good Friday, in remembrance of the Last Supper.

mausoleum /ˌmɒzəˈliːəm/ or /ˌmɒsə-/ *n* (*pl* **mausoleums, mausolea**) a large tomb.

mauve /moːv/ *n* any of several shades of pale purple. • *adj* of this colour.

maverick /ˈmævrɪk/ *n* an independent-minded or unorthodox individual; an unbranded animal, *eg* a stray calf.

mavis /ˈmeɪvɪs/ *n* the song thrush.

mavourneen, mavournin /məˈvɔːrnɪn/ *n* (*Irish*) my darling.

maw /mɒ/ *n* the stomach, crop or throat of animals, *esp* those who require large quantities of food; (*inf*) the throat and stomach of a person who eats food indiscriminately and in large quantities.

mawkish /ˈmɒkɪʃ/ *adj* maudlin; insipid.—**mawkishly** *adv*.—**mawkishness** *n*.

max. /mæks/ *abbr* = maximum.

maxilla /mækˈsɪlə/ *n* (*pl* **maxillae, maxillas**) the upper jawbone; in some insects, any of several parts of the mouth used as a secondary jaw.—**maxillar, maxillary** *adj*.

maxim /ˈmæksɪm/ *n* a concise rule of conduct; a precept.

maxima /ˈmæksɪmə/ *see* **maximum**.

maximal /ˈmæksɪməl/ *adj* of, consisting of, or pertaining to a maximum; (*math*) last in order. • *n* (*math*) in an ordered set, the member last in order.—**maximally** *adv*.

maximalist /ˈmæksɪməlɪst/ *n* one who insists on maximum demands without compromise; (*often with cap*) one who advocates direct action as a means of accomplishing something, *esp* social and political ends.

maximize /ˈmæksɪˌmaɪz/ *vt* to increase to a maximum.—**maximization** *n*.

maximum /ˈmæksɪməm/ *n* (*pl* **maxima, maximums**) the greatest quantity, number, etc. • *adj* highest; greatest possible reached.

maxixe /məˈʃiʃə/ *n* a Brazilian round dance similar to the tango, and like the two-step in rhythm.

maxwell /ˈmækswel/ *n* a unit of magnetic flux in the cgs system.

May /meɪ/ *n* the fifth month of the year having 31 days.

may /meɪ/ *vb aux* (*past* **might**) expressing possibility; permission; wish or hope.

maya /ˈmaɪjə/ *n* (*Hinduism*) illusion, *esp* that of the world as experienced by the senses as non-material.

May apple /ˈmeɪæpəl/ *n* an American plant with an egg-shaped edible fruit; its fruit.

maybe /ˈmeɪbiː/ *adv* perhaps.

May Day *n* the first day of May, celebrated as a traditional spring festival; observed in many countries as a labour holiday.

Mayday /ˈmeɪdeɪ/ *n* the international radio-telephone signal indicating a ship or aircraft in distress.

mayhem /ˈmeɪhem/ *n* violent destruction, confusion.

mayn't /ˈmeɪənt/ = may not.

mayonnaise /ˌmeɪəˈneɪz/ *n* a salad dressing made from egg yolks whisked with oil and lemon juice or vinegar.

mayor /ˈmeɪər/ or /ˈmer/ *n* the chief administrative officer of a municipality.—**mayoral** *adj*.—**mayorship** *n*.

mayoralty /ˈmeɪərəlti/ or /ˈmer-/ *n* (*pl* **mayoralties**) the office or term of office of a mayor.

mayoress /ˈmeɪərəs/ *n* the wife of a mayor; a female mayor.

maypole /ˈmeɪpoːl/ *n* a flower-decked pole hung with ribbons around which May Day festivities are held.

Mazdaism /ˈmæzdəˌɪzəm/ *n* Zoroastrianism.

maze /meɪz/ *n* a confusing, intricate network of pathways, *esp* one with high hedges in a garden; a labyrinth; a confused state.—*adj* **maze like**.

mazer /ˈmeɪzər/ *n* (*arch*) a large drinking cup of hard wood or metal.

mazuma /məˈzuːmə/ *n* (*sl*) money.

mazurka, mazourka /məˈzɜːrkə/ *n* a Polish folk dance in triple time; a musical composition for or imitating this.

mazy /ˈmeɪzi/, **mazier** /-ər/, **maziest** /-əst/ *adj* intricate, winding; perplexing.—**mazily** *adv*.—**maziness** *n*.

MB *abbr* = Bachelor of Medicine; megabyte; ✦ Manitoba.

MBA *abbr* = Master of Business Administration.

McIntosh /ˈmækˌɪntɒʃ/ *n* ✦ a red, medium-sized cooking and eating apple.

MCpl *abbr* ✦ (*Cdn*) = Master Corporal.

McJob /mækˈjɒb/ *n* ✦ (*inf*) a low-paying job with little prospects for advancement.

MD *abbr* = Maryland; Doctor of Medicine; Managing Director.

Md (*chem symbol*) mendelevium.

MDMA *abbr* = methylene dioxymethamphetamine, a synthetic drug used as the stimulant Ecstasy.

MDT /ˈɛmdiːˈtiː/ *abbr* ✦ = Mountain Daylight Time.

me /miː/ *pers pron* the objective case of I.

ME[1] *abbr* = myalgic encephalomyelitis.

ME[2], **Me** *abbr* = Maine.

mead /miːd/ *n* a wine made from a fermented solution of honey and spices.

meadow /ˈmedoː/ *n* a piece of land where grass is grown for hay; low, level, moist grassland.

meadowlark /ˈmedoːlɑːrk/ *n* one of two North American yellow-breasted songbirds related to the Baltimore oriole; any of several birds of South, Central and North America.

meadowsweet /ˈmedoːˌswiːt/ *n* a fragrant white-flowered plant of Europe and Asia.

meagre, meager /ˈmiːgər/ *adj* thin, emaciated; lacking in quality or quantity.—**meagerly, meagrely** *adv*.—**meagerness, meagreness** *n*.

meal[1] /miːl/ *n* any of the times for eating, as lunch, dinner, etc; the food served at such a time.

meal[2] *n* any coarsely ground edible grain; any substance similarly ground.—**mealiness** *n*.—**mealy** *adj*.

mealy-mouthed /ˈmiːliˈmaʊðd/ *adj* not outspoken and blunt; euphemistic; devious in speech.

mean[1] /miːn/ *adj* selfish, ungenerous; despicable; shabby; bad-tempered; (*sl*) difficult; (*sl*) expert.—**meanly** *adv*.—**meanness** *n*.

mean[2] *adj* halfway between extremes; average. • *n* what is between extremes.

mean[3] *vb* (**meaning, meant**) *vt* to have in mind; to intend; to intend to express; to signify. • *vi* to have a (specified) degree of importance, effect, etc.

meander /miːˈændər/ *n* a winding path *esp* a labyrinth; a winding of a stream or river. • *vi* (*river*) to wind; to wander aimlessly.—**meandering** *adj*.

meanie /ˈmiːni/ *n* (*inf*) one who is mean, selfish, etc.—*also* **meanie** (*pl* **meanies**).

meaning /ˈmiːnɪŋ/ *n* sense; significance; import. • *adj* significant.—**meaningful** *adj*.—**meaningless** *adj*.

means /miːnz/ *npl* that by which something is done; resources; wealth.

meant /ment/ *see* **mean**[3].

meantime /ˈmiːntaɪm/, **meanwhile** /ˈmiːnwaɪl/ *adv* in or during the intervening time; at the same time. • *n* the intervening time.

meany /ˈmiːni/ *see* **meanie**.

measles /ˈmiːzəlz/ *n* (*used as sing*) an acute, contagious viral disease, characterized by small red spots on the skin.

measly /ˈmiːzli/ *adj* (**measlier, measliest**) (*inf*) slight, worthless; having measles.

measure /ˈmeʒər/ *n* the extent, dimension, capacity, etc of anything; a determining of this, measurement; a unit of measurement; any standard of valuation; an instrument for measuring; a definite quantity measured out; a course of action; a statute, law; a rhythmical unit. • *vt* to find out the extent, dimensions etc of, *esp* by a standard; to mark off by measuring; to be a measure of. • *vi* to be of specified measurements.—**measurable** *adj*.—**measurably** *adv*.

measured /ˈmeʒərd/ *adj* set or marked off by a standard; rhythmical, regular; carefully planned or considered.

measureless /ˈmeʒərləs/ *adj* infinite, without limit.—**measurelessly** *adv*.

measurement /'mɛʒərmənt/ n a measuring or being measured; an extent or quantity determined by measuring; a system of measuring or of measures.

meat /miːt/ n animal flesh; food as opposed to drink; the essence of something.

meatball /'miːtbɒl/ n a small ball of ground meat usu mixed with breadcrumbs and spices; (inf) a stupid or foolish person.

meatus /mɪ'eɪtəs/ n (pl **meatuses, meatus**) any passage in the body, eg the ear canal.

meaty /'miːti/ adj (**meatier, meatiest**) full of meat; full of substance.

mecca /'mɛkə/ n a place of pilgrimage or a goal of aspiration; a resort or attraction that is visited by a large number of people; (with cap) Islam's holiest city, the birthplace of Muhammad (c. AD570).—also **Makkah**.

mechanic /mə'kænɪk/ n a person skilled in maintaining or operating machines, cars, etc.

mechanical /mə'kænɪkəl/ adj of or using machinery or tools; produced or operated by machinery; done as if by a machine, lacking thought or emotion; of the science of mechanics.—**mechanically** adv.

mechanician /ˌmɛkə'nɪʃən/ n a person skilled in mechanics or machinery; a technician; a mechanist.

mechanics /mə'kænɪks/ n (used as sing) the science of motion and the action of forces on bodies; knowledge of machinery; (pl) the technical aspects of something.

mechanism /'mɛkənɪzəm/ n the working parts of a machine; any system of interrelated parts; any physical or mental process by which a result is produced.

mechanist /'mɛkənɪst/ n an expert in mechanics, a mechanician; an advocate of mechanistic philosophy.

mechanistic /-'nɪstɪk/ adj of or pertaining to mechanics; of or relating to mechanism; attributing phenomena to physical or biological causes.—**mechanistically** adv.

mechanize /'mɛkə,naɪz/ vt to make mechanical; to equip with machinery or motor vehicles.—**mechanization** n.—**mechanized** adj.

meconium /mɪ'kɔːniəm/ n the first faeces of a baby; the juice of the poppy; opium.

MEd abbr = Master of Education.

medal /'mɛdəl/ n a small, flat piece of inscribed metal, commemorating some event or person or awarded for some distinction.—**medallic** adj.

medallion /mə'dæljən/ n a large medal; a design, portrait, etc shaped like a medal; a medal worn on a chain around the neck.

medallist, medalist /'mɛdəlɪst/ n one awarded a medal.

meddle /'mɛdəl/ vi to interfere in another's affairs.—**meddler** n.—**meddlesome** adj.

Mede /miːd/ n an inhabitant of Media, an ancient country in southwest Asia to the south of the Caspian Sea.—**Median** n, adj.

media /'miːdiə/ see **medium**.

mediaeval /mɪ:d'iːvəl/ or /mɛd-/, /ˌmɛdi-/ see **medieval**.

mediaevalism /-,lɪzəm/, **mediaevalist** /-lɪst/ see **medievalism**.

medial /'miːdiəl/ adj of or in the middle; mean, average; (math) pertaining to or denoting an average; median; (phonetics) denoting a sound made by using an average amount of muscular tension, neither strongly vocalized nor gently pronounced.

median /'miːdiən/ adj middle; intermediate. • n a median number, point, line, etc.

mediant /'miːdiənt/ n (mus) the third of any scale.—also adj.

mediastinum /ˌmiːdiə'staɪnəm/ n (pl **mediastina**) (anat) a membranous partition, esp that between the lungs; the part of the body between the lungs containing the heart and associated valves, etc.—**mediastinal** adj.

mediate /'miːdi,eɪt/ vt to intervene (in a dispute); to bring about agreement. • vi to be in an intermediate position; to be an intermediary. • adj involving an intermediary, not direct or immediate.—**mediately** adv.—**mediative** adj.

mediation /ˌmiːdi'eɪʃən/ n the act of mediating; reconciliation; intervention, esp by a neutral nation seeking a settlement between warring nations.

mediatize /'miːdiə,taɪz/ vt to annex (a state) while leaving its ruler his title.—**mediatization** n.

mediator /'miːdi,eɪtər/ n one who or that which mediates; a person who acts as an intermediary; an intercessor.—**mediatory** adj.

medic /'mɛdɪk/ n (inf) a medical student; (inf) a physician or surgeon.

medicable /'mɛdɪkəbəl/ adj potentially curable.

medical /'mɛdɪkəl/ adj relating to the practice or study of medicine. • n (inf) a medical examination.—**medically** adv.

medicament /mə'dɪkəmənt/ or /'mɛdɪ-/ n a medicine or healing application.

medicare /'mɛdɪkeɪr/ n ✻ a system of public health insurance financed by taxes.

medicate /'mɛdɪ,keɪt/ vt to treat with medicine; to impregnate (soap, shampoo, etc) with medication.—**medicative** adj.

medication /ˌmɛdɪ'keɪʃən/ n a treatment with drugs, medicines, etc; a drug, medicine, or remedy.

medicine /'mɛdsɪn/ n any substance used to treat or prevent disease; the science of preventing, treating or curing disease.—**medicinal** adj.—**medicinally** adv.

medico /'mɛdɪ,koː/ n (inf) a doctor or medical student.

medieval /ˌmɪd'iːvəl/ or /mɛd-/, /ˌmɛdi-/ adj of or like the Middle Ages.—also **mediaeval**.

medievalism /-,lɪzəm/ n the spirit, esp in religion and art, customs, etc, characteristic of the Middle Ages; a study of these; any one of these extant since the Middle Ages, or a contemporary imitation of it.—also **mediaevalism**—**medievalist, mediaevalist** n.

medigap /'mɛdɪ,gæp/ n health insurance taken out by an individual to pay for treatment excluded by government schemes.

mediocre /'miːdi'oːkər/ adj average; ordinary; inferior.—**mediocrity** n.

meditate /'mɛdɪ,teɪt/ vi to think deeply; to reflect; to empty the mind in order to concentrate on nothing or on one thing, esp as a religious exercise.—**meditator** n.

meditation /-'teɪʃən/ n the act of meditating; contemplation of spiritual or religious matters.

meditative /'mɛdɪtətɪv/ or /-,teɪtɪv/ adj expressing or characterized by meditation; thoughtful.—**meditatively** adv.—**meditativeness** n.

Mediterranean /ˌmɛdɪtə'reɪniən/ n the Mediterranean Sea. • adj of, or relating to (the area around) the Mediterranean Sea; denoting a subdivision of the Caucasian race characterized by a slender build and dark complexion; (climate) characterized by hot, dry summers and warm, wet winters.

medium /'miːdiəm/ n (pl **media, mediums**) the middle state or condition; a substance for transmitting an effect; any intervening means, instrument, or agency; (pl **media**) a means of communicating information (eg newspapers, television, radio); (pl **mediums**) a person claiming to act as an intermediary between the living and the dead. • adj midway; average.

medlar /'mɛdlər/ n a small fruit tree of Europe and Asia; its apple-like fruit; any one of several trees similar to this; the fruit from one of these.

medley /'mɛdli/ n (pl **medleys**) a miscellany; a musical piece made up of various tunes or passages.

Médoc /'meɪ'dɒk/ or /'mɛdɒk/ n a red wine from the Bordeaux region of France.

medulla /mə'dɛlə/ n (pl **medullas, medullae**) (anat) the marrow of bones; inner tissue; (bot) the pith of plants.—**medular, medullary** adj.

medulla oblongata /ˌɒblɒŋ'gætə/ n (pl **medulla oblongatas, medullae oblongatae**) the nervous tissue of the lower part of the cranium, which governs respiration, the action of the heart, etc.

medusa /mə'djuːsə/ or /-'dʒuː-/ n (pl **medusas, medusae**) a jellyfish; one of two coelenterate life cycles, when it has a sac-like, umbrella-shaped body that is capable of moving freely in water. —also **medusan, medusoid**.—**medusan** adj.

meed /miːd/ n (poet) recompense, reward.

meek /miːk/ adj patient, long-suffering; submissive.—**meekly** adv.—**meekness** n.

meerschaum /'miːrʃəm/ or /-ʃɒm/ n a creamy claylike silicate of magnesium from which pipe bowls and building stones are made; a tobacco pipe with a bowl made of this.

meet[1] /miːt/ vb (**meeting, met**) vt to encounter, to come together; to make the acquaintance of; to contend with, deal with; to experience; to be perceived by (the eye, etc); (demand, etc) to satisfy; (bill, etc) to pay. • vi to come into contact with; to be introduced. • n a meeting to hunt or for an athletics competition.

meet[2] adj (arch) fit, suitable.

meeting /'miːtɪŋ/ n a coming together; a gathering.

mega- /'mɛgə/ prefix great, large; a million of; (inf) greatest.

megabyte /'mɛgəbəɪt/ n (*comput*) a unit of information, approximately equal to one million bytes.

megacephalic /ˌmɛgəsə'fælɪk/ *see* **macrocephalic**.

megacycle /'mɛgəˌsaɪkəl/ n a megahertz.

megahertz /'mɛgəhərts/ n a unit of frequency equal to one million hertz.

megalith /'mɛgəlɪθ/ n a huge stone, *esp* part of a prehistoric monument.—**megalithic** *adj*.

megalomania /ˌmɛgələ'meɪnɪə/ n a mental illness characterized by delusions of grandeur; (*inf*) a lust for power.—**megalomaniac** n, *adj*.—**megalomaniacal** *adj*.

megaphone /'mɛgəˌfoːn/ n a device to amplify and direct the voice.

megapode /'mɛgəˌpoːd/ n any of a family of birds of Australia and the South Pacific that builds mounds of sand, etc, to incubate its eggs.

megaspore /'mɛgəˌspɔr/ n the protective covering containing the embryo in flowering plants.—*also* **macrospore**; the larger spore of certain mosses, ferns and fungi, which forms the female gametophyte.

megass, megasse /mə'gæs/ or /-'gɒs/ n a type of paper produced from the residue left after the extraction of sugar from cane.

megathere /ˌmɛgə'θiːr/ n a huge extinct animal allied to the sloth.—**megatherian** *adj*.

megaton /'mɛgəˌtɛn/ n a unit of explosive force equivalent to one million tons of TNT.

megavolt /'mɛgəvoːlt/ n a million volts.

megawatt /'mɛgəwɒt/ n one million watts.

megilp /mə'gɪlp/ n a mixture of linseed oil and mastic varnish or turpentine, used as a base in oil colours.

megohm /'mɛgoːm/ n a million ohms.

megrim /'miːgrɪm/ n (*arch*) a sick or neuralgic headache, *usu* of one side of the head, a migraine; a whim, caprice; (*pl*) a disease of horses or cattle, characterized by vertigo, the staggers.

meiosis /maɪ'oːsɪs/ n (*pl* **meioses**) (*biol*) the process of cell division where a nucleus splits into four, each new nucleus having half the number of chromosomes that the orig one had; a rhetorical understatement, *esp* one where a negative is used instead of its opposite, *eg* "a not inconsiderable amount" instead of "a large amount"; litotes; (*rare*) any division or separation.—**meiotic** *adj*.—**meiotically** *adv*.

Meistersinger /'mɒɪstərˌsɪŋər/ n (*pl* **Meistersinger, Meistersingers**) a member of one of the various guilds in German cities of the 14th-16th cents., which instituted the development of poetry and music by establishing competitive standards.

melamine /'mɛləˌmiːn/ n a resinous material used for adhesives, coatings, and laminated products.

melancholy /'mɛlənkɒli/ n gloominess or depression; sadness. • *adj* sad; depressed.—**melancholia** n.—**melancholic** *adj*.

mélange /meɪ'lõʒ/ n a (confused) mixture; a medley; (*geol*) a hotchpotch of variously shaped rocks of different periods and sizes.

melanin /'mɛlənɪn/ n a dark brown pigment in the skin, hair, and eyes of humans and animals.

melanism /'mɛlənɪzəm/, **melanosis** /-noːsɪs/ n dark coloration of the skin in pale-skinned people or dark-coloured feathers, etc, in birds and animals, caused by abnormal deposits of black or dark pigment in skin tissue, the opposite of albinism.—**melanistic, melanotic** *adj*.

melanoma /ˌmɛlə'noːmə/ n (*pl* **melanomas, melanomata**) a skin tumour composed of darkly pigmented cells.

melee, mêlée /'meɪleɪ/ or /'mɛleɪ/, /meˈleɪ/ n a confused, noisy struggle.

melic /'mɛlɪk/ *adj* (*poem*) meant to be sung, often used of ancient Greek lyric poetry.

melilot /'mɛləlɒt/ n a species of sweet-scented trefoil or clover, with clusters of small yellow or white flowers.—*also* **sweet clover**.

melinite /'mɛlɪˌnaɪt/ n a high explosive similar to lyddite.

meliorate /'miːlɪəˌreɪt/ vti to improve; to grow better; to make (something) better.—**meliorable** *adj*.—**meliorative** *adj*, n.—**meliorator** n.

melioration /-'reɪʃən/ n the process of improving; the state of being improved; an improvement.

meliorism /'miːlɪəˌrɪzəm/ n the doctrine that in nature there is a tendency to gradual improvement and this may be accelerated by human effort.

melliferous /mə'lɪfərəs/ *adj* forming or yielding honey.

mellifluous /mə'lɪfluːəs/, **mellifluent** /-uːənt/ *adj* (*voice, sounds*) sweetly flowing, smooth.—**mellifluously** *adv*.—**mellifluousness** n.

mellow /'mɛloː/ *adj* (*fruit*) sweet and ripe; (*wine*) matured; (*colour, light, sound*) soft, not harsh; kind-hearted and understanding. • *vti* to soften through age; to mature.—**mellowness** n.

melodeon /mə'loːdɪən/ n a kind of accordion; a small reed organ.

melodic /mə'lɒdɪk/ *adj* pertaining to or having melody.—**melodically** *adv*.

melodious /mə'loːdɪəs/ *adj* full of melody, tuneful, musical; sweet-sounding.—**melodiously** *adv*.—**melodiousness** n.

melodist /'mɛlədɪst/ n a singer; a composer of melodies.

melodize /'mɛləˌdaɪz/ vti to make (something) melodious; to compose a melody (for something); to sing a melody.

melodrama /'mɛləˌdræmə/ or /-drɒmə/ n a play, film, etc filled with overdramatic emotion and action; drama of this genre; sensational events or emotions.—**melodramatic** *adj*.—**melodramatically** *adv*.—**melodramatist** n.

melody /'mɛlədɪ/ n (*pl* **melodies**) a tune; a pleasing series of sounds.—**melodic** *adj*.—**melodious** *adj*.

melon /'mɛlən/ n the large juicy many-seeded fruit of trailing plants, as the watermelon, cantaloupe.

melt /mɛlt/ vti (**melting, melted**, *pp* **molten**) to make or become liquid; to dissolve; to fade or disappear; to soften or be softened emotionally.—**melting** *adj*.—**meltingly** *adv*.

meltdown /'mɛltdaun/ n the melting of the fuel core of a nuclear reactor; the drastic collapse of almost anything.

melting point /'mɛltɪŋ/ n the temperature at which a solid melts.

melting pot n a place, situation, or product of mixing many different races, traditions, cultures, etc.

melton /'mɛltən/ n a kind of thick woollen cloth, with a surface nap, often used for overcoats.

meltwater /'mɛltwɒtər/ n water derived from the melting of snow or ice.

member /'mɛmbər/ n a person belonging to a society or club; a part of a body, such as a limb; a representative in a legislative body; a distinct part of a complex whole.

membership /'mɛmbərʃɪp/ n the state of being a member; the number of members of a body; the members collectively.

membrane /'mɛmbreɪn/ n a thin pliable sheet or film; the fibrous tissue that covers or lines animal organs.—**membranous, membranaceous** *adj*.

memento /mə'mɛntoː/ n (*pl* **mementos, mementoes**) a reminder, *esp* a souvenir.

memento mori /-'mɔri/ or /-raɪ/ n (*pl* **memente mori**) (an object that serves as) a reminder of death.

memo /'mɛmoː/ n (*pl* **memos**) a memorandum.

memoir /'mɛmwɑr/ n an historical account based on personal experience; (*pl*) an autobiographical record.

memorabilia /ˌmɛmərə'biːlɪə/ or /-biːljə/ npl (*sing* **memorabile**) things worthy of remembrance or record; clothing, letters, manuscripts, notes, etc, once belonging to or written by famous people or connected with famous events and thought worthy of collection.

memorable /'mɛmərəbəl/ *adj* worth remembering; easy to remember.—**memorably** *adv*.

memorandum /ˌmɛmə'rændəm/ n (*pl* **memorandums**) an informal written communication as within an office; (*pl* **memoranda**) a note to help the memory.

memorial /mə'mɔrɪəl/ *adj* serving to preserve the memory of the dead. • n a remembrance; a monument.

memorialist /-ɪst/ n one who prepares, signs or presents a memorial; one who writes memoirs.

memorialize /mɪ'mɔrɪəˌlaɪz/ vt to commemorate; to honour by means of a memorial.—**memorialization** n.—**memorializer** n.

memorize /'mɛməˌraɪz/ vt to learn by heart, to commit to memory.—**memorization** n.

memory /'mɛmərɪ/ or /'mɛmrɪ/ n (*pl* **memories**) the process of retaining and reproducing past thoughts and sensations; the sum of things remembered; an individual recollection; commemoration; remembrance; the part of a computer that stores information.—*also* **store**.

memsahib /'mɛmˌsæɪb/ or /-sɒɪb/ n (*formerly*) a form of address for a European married woman in India.

men /mɛn/ *see* **man**.

menace /'mɛnəs/ n a threat; (*inf*) a nuisance. • vt to threaten.—**menacing** *adj*.—**menacingly** *adv*.

menad /'miːˌnæd/ *see* **maenad**.

ménage /meɪ'næʒ/ *or* /-nɒʒ/ *n* a household.

ménage à trois *Fr.* /meɪˌnɑʒɑ'trwɑ/ *n* (*pl* **ménages à trois**) a relationship in which a married couple and a lover of one of them live together.

menagerie /mə'næʒəri/ *or* /-'nædʒ-/, /-'nɒʒ-/ *n* a place where wild animals are kept for exhibition; a collection of wild animals.

mend /mend/ *vt* to repair; (manners, etc) to reform, improve. • *vi* to become better. • *n* the act of mending; a repaired area in a garment, etc.

mendacity /men'dæsɪti/ *n* (*pl* **mendacities**) telling lies; a falsehood.—**mendacious** *adj.*—**mendaciously** *adv*.

mendelevium /ˌmendə'liːviəm/ *n* an artificially produced radioactive metallic element.

Mendelism /'mendəˌlɪzəm/ *n* the theories of the Austrian monk and geneticist Gregor Mendel (1822–84) respecting heredity, as set out in Mendel's laws with later modifications.—**Mendelian** *adj*.

mendicant /'mendɪkənt/ *adj* begging; (*religious orders*) reliant on alms. • *n* a mendicant friar.—**mendicancy, mendicity** *n*.

mending /'mendɪŋ/ *n* garments requiring to be repaired.

menhaden /men'heɪdən/ *n* (*pl* **menhadens, menhaden**) an inedible American fish, yielding a valuable oil.

menhir /'menhiːr/ *n* a tall, monolithic obelisk, sometimes crudely carved, dating from the Bronze Age in the UK or the Neolithic Age in Europe.

menial /'miːniəl/ *adj* consisting of work of little skill; servile. • *n* a domestic servant; a servile person.

meninges /mɪ'nɪndʒiːz/ *npl* (*sing* **meninx**) the three membranes covering and protecting the brain and the spinal cord.—**meningeal** *adj*.

meningitis /ˌmenɪn'dʒaɪtɪs/ *n* inflammation of the membranes enveloping the brain or spinal cord.

meniscus /mə'nɪskəs/ *n* (*pl* **menisci, meniscuses**) a crescent; the crescent-shaped surface of a liquid contained in a tube; a lens convex on one side and concave on the other; (*anat*) the cartilage between the bones of joints, *esp* at the knee.

menology /mɪ'nɒlədʒi/ *n* (*pl* **menologies**) an ecclesiastical calendar; a calendar of saints, *esp* in the Orthodox Church.

menopause /'menəˌpɒz/ *n* the time of life during which a woman's menstrual cycle ceases permanently.—**menopausal** *adj*.

menorrhagia /ˌmenə'reɪdʒiə/ *n* an excessive menstrual flow.

menses /'mensiːz/ *n* (*pl* **menses**) menstruation; the monthly discharge of blood, etc, from the uterus; the days during which this occurs.

Menshevik /'menʃəˌvɪk/ *n* (*pl* **Mensheviks, Mensheviki**) (*hist*) a member of the more moderate Russian socialist party (1903-17) or of a liberal opposition party set up after the Revolution.—**Menshevism** *n*.—**Menshevist** *adj, n*.

menstruation /ˌmen'streɪʃən/ *n* the monthly discharge of blood from the uterus.—**menstrual** *adj.*—**menstruate** *vi*.

menstruum /'menstrʊm/ *n* (*pl* **menstruums, menstrua**) a solvent, *esp* if used in making drugs.

mensurable /'mensərəbəl/ *adj* measurable; (*mus*) of a fixed rhythm.—**mensurability** *n*.

mensuration /ˌmenʃʊ'reɪʃən/ *n* the science of measurement; the act or process of measuring or taking the dimensions of anything; measurement.

mental /'mentəl/ *adj* of, or relating to the mind; occurring or performed in the mind; having a psychiatric disorder; (*inf*) crazy, stupid.—**mentally** *adv*.

mentality /men'tæliti/ *n* (*pl* **mentalities**) intellectual power; disposition, character.

menthol /'menθɒl/ *n* peppermint oil.—**mentholated** *adj*.

mention /'menʃən/ *n* a brief reference to something in speech or writing; an official recognition or citation. • *vt* to refer to briefly; to remark; to honour officially.—**mentionable** *adj*.

mentor /'mentɔr/ *n* a wise and trusted adviser.

menu /'menjuː/ *n* the list of dishes served in a restaurant; a list of options on a computer display.

meow /miː'aʊ/ *n* the cry of a cat; a spiteful remark.—*also vi*.

Mephistophelean, Mephistophelian /ˌmefɪstə'fiːliən/ *adj* pertaining to or like Mephistopheles, the devil of the Faust legend; fiendish, cynical; diabolic.

mephitis /mɪ'faɪtɪs/ *n* a noxious gas emitted from the ground; a foul stench.—**mephitic, mephitical** *adj*.

mercantile /'mɔːkənˌtaɪl/ *adj* of merchants or trade.

mercantilism /'mɔːkəntiˌlɪzəm/ *n* a theory popular in 17th and 18th century Europe suggesting that the wealth of a nation

increases in proportion to the level of the foreign trade surplus, therefore trade and commerce with other countries, the founding of colonies, a merchant navy etc should be encouraged; (*rare*) commercialism—**mercantilist** *n, adj*.

mercenary /'mɔːsəˌneri/ *adj* working or done for money only. • *n* (*pl* **mercenaries**) a soldier hired to fight for a foreign army.—**mercenarily** *adv.*—**mercenariness** *n*.

mercer /'mɔːsər/ *n* a dealer in textiles, *esp* silk and velvet.

mercerize /'mɔːsəˌraɪz/ *vt* to treat cotton thread so as to strengthen it and make it resemble silk.—**mercerization** *n*.

merchandise /'mɔːtʃənˌdaɪs/ *or* /-daɪz/ *n* commercial goods. • *vti* to sell, to trade; to promote sales by display or advertising.—**merchandiser** *n*.

merchandising /-ɪŋ/ *n* the display of goods in a store, etc; the exploitation of a fictional character, pop group, etc, by the production of goods with their image, name, etc.

merchant /'mɔːtʃənt/ *n* a trader; a retailer; (*sl*) a person fond of a particular activity.

merchantable /'mɔːtʃəntəbəl/ *adj* marketable.

merchantman /'mɔːtʃəntmər/ *n* (*pl* **merchantmen**) a trading ship.

merchant marine, merchant navy *n* commercial shipping.

merciful /'mɔːsɪfʊl/ *adj* compassionate, humane.—**mercifulness** *n*.

mercifully /'mɔːsɪfʊli/ *adv* in a merciful way; (*inf*) thank goodness.

merciless /'mɔːsɪləs/ *adj* cruel, pitiless; without mercy.—**mercilessly** *adv.*—**mercilessness** *n*.

mercurial /mɔː'kjʊriəl/ *adj* of, containing, or caused by mercury; lively, sprightly; volatile.—**mercurially** *adv*.

mercuric /mɔː'kjʊrɪk/ *adj* (*chem*) of or containing bivalent mercury.

mercurous /mɔː'kjuːrəs/ *or* /'mɔːkjʊrəs/ *adj* (*chem*) of or containing monovalent mercury.

Mercury /'mɔːkjʊri/ *n* the innermost planet, and the smallest; the Roman god of thieves, traders etc; in ancient Rome, the messenger of the gods.

mercury *n* a heavy silvery liquid metallic element used in thermometers etc.

mercy /'mɔːsi/ *n* clemency; compassion; kindness; pity.

mere /miːr/ *adj* nothing more than; simple, unmixed.

merely /'miːrli/ *adv* simply; solely.

meretricious /ˌmerə'trɪʃəs/ *adj* tawdry, superficially attractive; insincere.

merganser /mɔː'gænsər/ *n* (*pl* **mergansers, merganser**) a large, diving fish-eating duck with a long narrow bill with serrated edges; a sawbill.

merge /mɔːdʒ/ *vti* to blend or cause to fuse together gradually; to (cause to) combine, unite.

merger /'mɔːdʒər/ *n* a combining together, *esp* of two or more commercial organizations.

meridian /mə'rɪdiən/ *n* the imaginary circle on the surface of the earth passing through the north and south poles.

meridional /mə'rɪdiənəl/ *adj* of a meridian; of the south.—**meridionally** *adv*.

meringue /mə'ræŋ/ *n* a mixture of egg whites beaten with sugar and baked; a small cake or shell made from this, *usu* filled with cream.

merino /mə'riːnoː/ *n* (*pl* **merinos**) a breed of sheep with fine silky wool; the wool or the cloth made from it.

merit /'merit/ *n* excellence; worth; (*pl*) (*of a case*) rights and wrongs; a deserving act. • *vt* to be worthy of, to deserve.

meritocracy /ˌmerɪ'tɒkrəsi/ *n* (*pl* **meritocracies**) rule by those most skilled or talented; a social system or government based on this; the most talented group in a society.

meritorious /ˌmerɪ'tɔriəs/ *adj* deserving of merit or honour.—**meritoriously** *adv.*—**meritoriousness** *n*.

merle /mɔːrl/ *n* (*Scot*) a blackbird. • *adj* (*dog, esp a collie*) having blue-grey fur with black tinges or streaks.

merlin /'mɔːrlɪn/ *n* a small dark-coloured falcon, often used in falconry.

merlon /'mɔːrlɒn/ *n* the part of a parapet or battlement between two embrasures.

mermaid /'mɔːrmeɪd/ *n* (*legend*) a woman with a fish's tail.—**merman** *nm* (*pl* **mermen**).

meroblastic /ˌmeroː'blæstɪk/ *adj* (*biol*) (*fertilized egg*) of or pertaining to the splitting of cells in the white only and not the entire ovum.

Merovingian /ˌmeroː'vɪndʒiən/ *adj* pertaining to the first Frankish dynasty of French kings (*c.*500-751). • *n* a member or adherent of this dynasty.

merry /'meri/ *adj* (**merrier, merriest**) cheerful; causing laughter; lively; (*inf*) slightly drunk.—**merrily** *adv.*—**merriment** *n*.

merry-go-round /ˈmɛrɪgoːˌraʊnd/ *n* a revolving platform of hobbyhorses, etc, a carousel.

merrymaking /ˈmɛrɪˌmeɪkɪŋ/ *n* festivity, fun.—**merrymaker** *n*.

merrythought /ˈmɛrɪˌθɔt/ *n* (*rare*) the forked bone of a chicken's breast, the wishbone.

mes-, meso- /ˈmɛsoː/ or /ˈmɛz-/ *prefix* middle.

mesa /ˈmeɪsə/ *n* a rocky plateau with steep sides *usu* found in arid regions.

mésalliance /meɪˈzælɪˌɒs/, *Fr*. /meɪzaliˈɒs/ *n* a misalliance; a marriage with one of lower social position.

mescaline /ˈmɛskəˌliːn/ *n* a hallucinogenic drug derived from the mescal cactus.

mesdames /meɪˈdɒm/, *Fr*. /meɪˈdam/ *see* **madame**.

mesdemoiselles *Fr*. /meɪdmwaˈzɛl/ *see* **mademoiselle**.

mesembryanthemum /mɪˌzɛmbrɪˈænθɪməm/ *n* one of a genus of flowering, succulent plants with thick and fleshy leaves and showy flowers.

mesentery /ˈmɛsənˌtɛri/ *n* (*pl* **mesenteries**) the membrane attaching the small intestines to the abdominal wall.—**mesenteric** *adj*.

mesh /mɛʃ/ *n* an opening between cords of a net, wires of a screen, etc; a net; a network; a snare; (*geared wheels, etc*) engagement. • *vt* to entangle, ensnare. • *vi* to become entangled or interlocked.

mesial /ˈmiːzɪəl/ *adj* (*anat*) in or toward the middle line of the body.—**mesially** *adv*.

mesmerism /ˈmɛzməˌrɪzəm/ *n* hypnotism.—**mesmerist** *n*.

mesmerize /ˈmɛzməˌraɪz/ *vt* to hypnotize; to fascinate.—**mesmeric** *adj*.—**mesmerizer** *n*.

mesne /miːn/ *adj* (*law*) intervening, intermediate.

meso-, mes- /ˈmɛsoː/ or /ˈmɛz-/ *prefix* middle.

mesoblast /ˈmɛsoːˌblæst/ *n* (*biol*) the middle germinal layer of an ovum, the basis of muscles, bones, blood etc.—*also* **mesoderm**.

mesocarp /ˈmɛsoːˌkarp/ *n* the middle layer of the seed vessel of a fruit.

mesocephalic /ˌmɛsoːsəˈfælɪk/ or /ˌmɛz-/ *adj, n* (*person*) with a head or skull of medium proportions.

mesoderm /ˈmɛsoːˌdərm/ *see* **mesoblast**.

mesogastrium /ˌmɛsoːˈgæstrɪəm/ or /ˌmɛz-/ *n* the membrane that supports the embryonic stomach.—**mesogastric** *adj*.

Mesolithic /ˌmɛzoːˈlɪθɪk/ *n, adj* of or pertaining to the archaeological era between the Palaeolithic and Neolithic (*c*.12000-3000BC).

meson /ˈmɛzɒn/ or /ˈmiːzɒn/ *n* an unstable elementary particle having a mass between that of proton and an electron.

mesophyll /ˈmɛsoːfɪl/ *n* the internal tissues of a leaf that are between the upper and lower epidermal layers and contain chlorophyll.—**mesophyllic, mesophyllous** *adj*.

mesophyte /ˈmɛsoːˌfəɪt/ *n* a plant requiring an average water supply.—**mesophytic** *adj*.

mesothorax /-ˈθɔræks/ *n* (*pl* **mesothoraxes, mesothoraces**) the middle ring of an insect's thorax, with the second pair of walking legs and the front pair of wings.

Mesozoic /ˌmɛsoːˈzoːɪk/ or /ˌmɛz-/ *adj* pertaining to the era of geological time lasting from about 248 to 65 million years ago. • *n* this era.

mesquite, mesquit /ˈmɛskiːt/ *n* a small pod-bearing tree of the southwest US whose pods are used as fodder.

mess /mɛs/ *n* a state of disorder or untidiness, *esp* if dirty: a muddle; an unsightly or disagreeable mixture; a portion of soft and pulpy or semi-liquid food; a building where service personnel dine; a communal meal. • *vti* to make a mess (of), bungle; to eat in company; to potter (about).

message /ˈmɛsɪdʒ/ *n* any spoken, written, or other form of communication; the chief idea that the writer, artist, etc seeks to communicate in a work.

messenger /ˈmɛsɪndʒər/ *n* a person who carries a message.

Messiah /məˈsaɪə/ *n* the promised saviour of the Jews; Jesus Christ.—**Messianic** *adj*.

messieurs /ˈmɛsərz/, *Fr*. /mɛsjø/ *see* **monsieur**.

Messrs /ˈmɛsərz/ *pl* of Mr.

messuage /ˈmɛswɪdʒ/ *n* (*law*) a dwelling house with its adjacent buildings and land for the use of the household.

messy /ˈmɛsi/ *adj* (**messier, messiest**) dirty; confused; untidy.—**messily** *adv*.—**messiness** *n*.

mestizo /mɛˈstiːzoː/ *n* (*pl* **mestizos, mestizoes**) a person of mixed parentage, *esp* the child of a Spanish American and an American Indian.

met /mɛt/ *see* **meet**.

meta- /ˈmɛtə/, **met-** /mɛt/ *prefix* after, with, or implying change.

metabolism /məˈtæbəˌlɪzəm/ *n* the total processes in living organisms by which tissue is formed, energy produced and waste products eliminated.—**metabolic** *adj*.

metabolize /məˈtæbəˌlaɪz/ *vt* to process by metabolism; to assimilate.

metacarpal /ˌmɛtəˈkɑrpəl/ *adj* pertaining to the metacarpus. • *n* a bone of the metacarpus.

metacarpus /ˌmɛtəˈkɑrpəs/ *n* (*pl* **metacarpi**) the bones of that part of the hand that is between the wrist and the fingers, or the corresponding part in other animals.

metacenter, metacentre /ˈmɛtəˌsɛntər/ *n* the point in a floating body where the verticals intersect when the body is tilted and on the position of which its equilibrium or stability depends.—**metacentric** *adj*.

metage /ˈmiːtɪdʒ/ *n* the official weighing or measuring of the contents of something; the fee paid for this.

metagenesis /ˌmɛtəˈdʒɛnəsɪs/ *n* the alternation of sexual and asexual generations.—**metagenetic** *adj*.—**metagenetically** *adv*.

metal /ˈmɛtəl/ *n* any of a class of chemical elements which are often lustrous, ductile solids, and are good conductors of heat, electricity, etc, such as gold, iron, copper, etc; any alloy of such elements as brass, bronze, etc; anything consisting of metal.—**metalled** *adj*.

metallic /məˈtælɪk/ *adj* of, relating to, or made of metal; similar to metal.

metalliferous /ˌmɛtəˈlɪfərəs/ *adj* yielding metal or metallic ores.

metalline /ˈmɛtəlɪn/ or /-ˌlaɪn/ *adj* metallic; impregnated with or yielding metal.

metallize, metalize /ˈmɛtəˌlaɪz/ *vt* to give metallic qualities to; to coat or treat with metal.

metallography /ˌmɛtəˈlɒgrəfi/ *n* the science or description of the structure of metals and alloys; (*print*) lithography using metal plates to print an image.

metalloid /ˈmɛtəˌlɔɪd/ *n* a nonmetallic element that possesses some of the chemical properties associated with metals. • *adj* of or having the properties of a metalloid; resembling a metal.—*also* **metalloidal**.

metallurgy /ˈmɛtəˌlərdʒi/ or /məˈtælərdʒi/ *n* the science of separating metals from their ores and preparing them for use by smelting, refining, etc.—**metallurgical** *adj*.—**metallurgist** *n*.

metamere /ˈmɛtəˌmiːr/ *n* a segment of a body, as in earthworms, crayfish, etc.

metameric /ˌmɛtəˈmɛrɪk/ *adj* (*zool*) of or having metameres; (*chem*) having the same elements and molecular weight but different properties.—**metamerism** *n*.

metamorphism /ˌmɛtəˈmɔrˌfɪzəm/ *n* the change in the structure of rocks through heat, pressure, etc.

metamorphosis /ˌmɛtəˈmɔrfəsɪs/ *n* (*pl* **metamorphoses**) a complete change of form, structure, substance, character, appearance, etc; transformation; the marked change in some animals at a stage in their growth, *eg* chrysalis to butterfly.—**metamorphic** *adj*.—**metamorphose** *vi*.

metaphor /ˈmɛtəfər/ *n* a figure of speech in which a word or phrase is used for another of which it is an image.—**metaphoric, metaphorical** *adj*.—**metaphorically** *adv*.

metaphrase /ˈmɛtəˌfreɪz/ *n* a word-for-word translation, the opposite of paraphrase. • *vt* to alter the wording of something, *esp* to alter the meaning; to translate literally.

metaphrast /ˌmɛtəˈfræstɪk/ *n* one who alters text, *esp* one who changes the form, as from verse to prose.—**metaphrastic, metaphrastical** *adj*.

metaphysical /ˌmɛtəˈfɪzɪkəl/ *adj* of or pertaining to metaphysics; abstruse, abstract; supernatural; (*poetry*) fantastic or oversubtle in style.—**metaphysically** *adv*.

metaphysics /ˌmɛtəˈfɪzɪks/ *n sing* the branch of philosophy that seeks to explain the nature of being and reality; speculative philosophy in general.—**metaphysician** *n*.

metaplasm /ˈmɛtəˌplæzəm/ *n* (*biol*) that part of the contents of a cell consisting of inert matter; (*gram*) a change in a word by the adding or dropping of a letter.—**metaplasmic** *adj*.

metastasis /məˈtæstəsɪs/ *n* (*pl* **metastases**) a change or shift in the location of a disease, often used of the spreading of cancer cells; a transformation or change; (*rare*) metabolism.—**metastatic** *adj*.

metatarsal /ˌmɛtəˈtɑːsəl/ adj pertaining to the metatarsus. • n one of the bones of the metatarsus.

metatarsus /ˌmɛtəˈtɑːsəs/ n (pl **metatarsi**) (anat) in humans, the instep, the middle part of the foot between the tarsus and the toes; in other animals, the part corresponding to this.

metathesis /məˈtæθəsɪs/ n (pl **metatheses**) the transposition of the letters or syllables of a word; (chem) a reaction between two compounds in which the first and second parts of one unite with the second and first parts of the other.—**metathetic, metathetical** adj.

metathorax /ˌmɛtəˈθɔːræks/ n (pl **metathoraxes, metathoraces**) the hindmost segment of an insect's thorax, with the third pair of walking legs and the second pair of wings.

metazoan /ˌmɛtəˈzəʊən/ n an animal belonging to a division of the animal kingdom in which the body is made up of a large number of cells, ie all animals except sponges and protozoans.

mete /miːt/ vt to allot; to portion (out).

metempsychosis /ˌmɛtəmsaɪˈkəʊsɪs/ n (pl **metempsychoses**) the transmigration of the soul after the death of the body to another body or form.

meteor /ˈmiːtɪər/ or /-ɔːr/ n a small particle of matter which travels at great speed through space and becomes luminous through friction as it enters the earth's atmosphere; a shooting star.

meteoric /ˌmiːtiˈɒrɪk/ adj of or relating to a meteor; dazzling, transitory.

meteorite /ˈmiːtɪəˌraɪt/ n a meteor that has fallen to earth without being completely vaporized.—**meteoritic** adj.

meteorograph /ˈmiːtɪərəgræf/ or /ˌmiːtiˈɔrəgræf/ n an instrument for recording various meteorological conditions simultaneously.

meteoroid /ˈmiːtɪəˌrɔɪd/ n a small body moving through space, often orbiting the sun which can be seen as a meteor if it enters the earth's atmosphere.

meteorology /ˌmiːtɪəˈrɒlədʒi/ n a study of the earth's atmosphere, particularly weather and climate.—**meteorological** adj.—**meteorologist** n.

-meter /mɪtər/ or /miːtər/ suffix denoting a device for measuring; metre(s) in length.

meter[1] /ˈmiːtər/ n a device for measuring and recording a quantity of gas, water, time, etc supplied; a parking meter. • vt to measure using a meter.

meter[2] see **metre**[1], **metre**[2].

methane /ˈmɛθeɪn/ n a colourless, odourless, flammable gas formed by the decomposition of vegetable matter, as in marshes.

methinks /mɪˈθɪŋks/ vb (pt **methought**) (arch) it appears or seems to me.

method /ˈmɛθəd/ n the mode or procedure of accomplishing something; orderliness of thought; an orderly arrangement or system.

methodical /məˈθɛdɪkəl/ adj orderly, systematic.—**methodically** adv.

Methodist /ˈmɛθədɪst/ n a member of a Christian denomination founded by John Wesley.—**Methodism** n.

methodize /ˈmɛθəˌdaɪz/ vt to reduce to method; systematize.

methodology /ˌmɛθəˈdɒlədʒi/ n (pl **methodologies**) the methods and procedures used by a science or discipline; the philosophical analysis of method and procedure.

methought /mɪˈθɔt/ see **methinks**.

meths /mɛθs/ n (inf) methylated spirit.

Methuselah /məˈθuːzələ/ or /-ˈθjuːzələ/ n a wine bottle eight times the size of an ordinary bottle; (Old Testament) a patriarch reputed to have been 969 years old when he died; a very old person.

methyl /ˈmɛθəl/ n a compound composed of organic material and metals in which metal groups are bound directly to a metal atom.

methylated spirit n a form of alcohol, adulterated to render it undrinkable, used as a solvent.

methylene /ˈmɛθəˌliːn/ n a bivalent organic radical found in unsaturated hydrocarbons; an inflammable liquid obtained from the distillation of wood.

meticulous /məˈtɪkjʊləs/ adj very precise about small details.—**meticulously** adv.—**meticulousness** n.

métier /ˈmeɪtjeɪ/ or /ˈmeɪ-/ n a person's calling or trade, esp if that person has a natural leaning toward it; a strong point, forte.

métis /meɪˈtiː/ n (pl **métis**) (often cap) an offspring of mixed parentage; in Canada, one who is the child or a descendant of a French Canadian and an American Indian; one of a group of

such people forming a political and national entity, who settled in Manitoba and Saskatchewan.—**métisse** nf.

Metol /ˈmiːtɒl/ or /-ˌtoʊl/ n (trademark) a colourless, soluble organic substance used as a photographic developer.

metonymy /mɪˈtɒnəmi/ n (**metonymies**) a figure of speech in which a thing is replaced by its attribute, eg "the pen is mightier than the sword."—**metonym** n.—**metonymical, metonymic** adj.

metope /ˈmɛtəpi/ or /ˈmɛtoʊpɪ/ n (archit) the space between two triglyphs of a Doric frieze

metre[1] /ˈmiːtər/ n rhythmic pattern in verse, the measured arrangement of syllables according to stress; rhythmic pattern in music.—also **meter**.

metre[2] n the basic unit of length in the metric system, consisting of 100 centimetres and equal to 39.37 inches.—also **meter**.

metric /ˈmɛtrɪk/ adj based on the metre as a standard of measurement; of, relating to, or using the metric system.

metrical /ˈmɛtrɪkəl/ adj of, relating to, or composed in rhythmic metre.—**metrically** adv.

metrication /ˌmɛtrɪˈkeɪʃən/ n conversion of an existent system of units into the metric system.

metrics /ˈmɛtrɪks/ n sing the study of verse form; the art of composing verse.

metric system n a decimal system of weights and measures based on the metre, litre and the kilogram.

metro /ˈmɛtroʊ/ n (pl **metros**) an urban underground railway system, such as in Paris and other cities; ✣ a metropolis.

metrology /mɪˈtrɒlədʒi/ n (pl **metrologies**) the science of weights and measures or units of measurement; any of the various systems of units.

metronome /ˈmɛtrəˌnoʊm/ n an instrument that beats musical tempo.—**metronomic** adj.

metronymic /ˌmɛtrəˈnɪmɪk/ adj (name) derived from one's mother or a female ancestor. • n such a name.—also **matronymic**.

metropolis /məˈtrɒpəlɪs/ n the main city, often a capital of a country, state, etc; any large and important city.—**metropolitan** adj.

mettle /ˈmɛtəl/ n courage, spirit.

mettled /-əd/ adj mettlesome

mettlesome /ˈmɛtəlsəm/ adj high-spirited, full of courage.

meunière /mʊnˈjɛr/ adj (fish) coated with flour, cooked in butter and served with parsley and lemon juice.

mew[1] /mjuː/ vi (cat) to emit a high-pitched cry. • n the cry of a cat.

mew[2] n a gull found in northern areas.

mew[3] n a cage for hawks. • vti (hawk) to shed (feathers), to moult; to put in a mew, to confine.

mewl /mjuːl/ vi (baby) to cry feebly, to whimper; to mew. • n a whimper.

mews /mjuːz/ n sing or pl a yard or road lined with buildings formerly used stables and later converted into living accommodation.

mezzanine /ˈmɛzəniːn/ or /ˈmɛzəˈniːn/ n an intermediate storey between others; a theatre balcony.

mezzanine debt see **junk debt**.

mezzo /ˈmɛtsoʊ/ adv (mus) moderately; quite. • n (pl **mezzos**) a mezzo-soprano.

mezzo-relievo /ˈmɛtsoʊrɪˈliːvoʊ/ or /ˈmɛzoʊ/ n (pl **mezzo-relievos**) a carving in half-relief, where the figures project in neither high relief nor low relief from the background.

mezzo-soprano /-səˈprænoʊ/ or /-ˈproʊnoʊ/ n (pl **mezzo-sopranos**) (mus) a singer, or a part, between soprano and contralto.

mezzotint /ˈmɛtsoʊˌtɪnt/ or /ˈmɛzoʊ-/ n a method of engraving on copper in which lights are made by scraping a roughened surface; a print so made. • vt to engrave a copper plate using this method.

mfr abbr = manufacture; manufacturer.

Mg (chem symbol) magnesium.

mg abbr = milligram.

Mgr abbr = manager.

MHA abbr ✣ = Member of the House of Assembly.

MHR abbr = Member of the House of Representatives.

MHz abbr = megahertz.

MI abbr = Michigan; military intelligence; myocardial infarction.

mi. abbr = mile; mill.

MIA abbr = missing in action.

miasma /miˈæzmə/ or /maɪ-/ n (pl **miasmas, miasmata**) an unwholesome, foreboding atmosphere; an unpleasant vapour, as from decaying swamp matter.—**miasmal, miasmatic, miasmic** adj.

mica /'maɪkə/ *n* a mineral that crystallizes in thin, flexible layers, resistant to heat.—**micaceous** *adj*.

mice /maɪs/ *see* **mouse**.

Mich. *abbr* = Michigan.

Michaelmas /'maɪkəlməs/ *n* a church festival commemorating the archangel Michael, celebrated on September 29.

mickey /'mɪkɪ/ *n* ✴ (*inf*) a half-bottle of alcoholic liquor.

micra /'maɪkrə/ *see* **micron**.

micro /'maɪkrəʊ/ *n* (*pl* **micros**) a microwave oven; (*comput*) a microcomputer, a microprocessor.

micro- /'maɪkrəʊ/, **micr-** /'maɪkr/ *prefix* small.

microbe /'maɪkrəʊb/ *n* a microscopic organism, *esp* a disease-causing bacterium.—**microbial, microbic** *adj*.

microbiology /ˌmaɪkrəʊbaɪ'ɒlədʒɪ/ *n* the biology of bacteria and other microorganisms and their effects.—**microbiological, microbiologic** *adj*.—**microbiologically** *adv*.—**microbiologist** *n*.

microbus /-'bʌs/ *n* (*pl* **microbuses, microbusses**) a station wagon that resembles a small bus.

microcephalic /-'sefælɪk/, **microcephalous** /-ləs/ *adj* having an unusually small head.—**microcephaly** *n*.

microchip /'maɪkrəʊtʃɪp/ *n* a small wafer of silicon, etc, containing electronic circuits.—*also* **chip**.

microcircuit /-ˌsɜːkɪt/ *n* a miniature electronic circuit, *esp* an integrated circuit.—**microcircuitry** *n*.

microclimate /-ˌklaɪmət/ *n* the climate of a restricted specific place within an area as opposed to the climate of the area.—**microclimatic** *adj*.

micrococcus /ˌmaɪkrəʊ'kɒkəs/ *n* (**micrococci**) a round bacterium, a source of fermentation and of zymotic disease.—**micrococcal** *adj*.

microcomputer /'maɪkrəʊkəmˌpjuːtər/ *n* a computer in which the central processing unit is contained in one or more microprocessors.

microcosm /ˌmaɪkrəʊ'kɒzəm/ *n* a miniature universe or world.—**microcosmic, microcosmical** *adj*.—**microcosmically** *adv*.

microcyte /'maɪkrəʊsaɪt/ *n* an unusually small red blood corpuscle, often present in disease.—**microcytic** *adj*.

microdot /-ˌdɒt/ *n* a photographic reproduction of a document, plan, etc reduced to a tiny dot, *esp* for reasons of espionage.

microeconomics /-iːkə'nɒmɪks/ *n sing* the branch of economics concerned with the activities of consumers, firms, and commodities.—**microeconomic** *adj*.

microfiche /-ˌfiːtʃ/ *n* (*pl* **microfiche, microfiches**) a sheet of microfilm containing pages of printed matter.—*also* **film card**.

microfilm /-film/ *n* film on which documents, etc, are recorded in reduced scale. • *vt* to record on microfilm.

microfloppy /-ˌflɒpɪ/ *n* (*pl* **microfloppies**) a floppy disk of 3.5 inches diameter contained in a hard covering.

micrograph /-ˌɡræf/ *n* a photograph of something as seen through a microscope; a device for executing minute engraving or writing.

micrography /maɪ'krɒɡrəfɪ/ *n* the description, study or representation of microscopic objects; the process of writing in miniature.—**micrographic** *adj*.

micrometer[1] /maɪ'krɒmɪtər/ *n* any of various instruments for measuring minute distances, angles, thicknesses, or apparent diameters, sometimes used with a microscope.

micrometer[2], **micrometre** /'maɪkrəʊˌmiːtər/ *n* a unit of length of one thousandth of a millimetre, a micron.

micrometry *n* the measurement of tiny objects, distances, etc, by a micrometer.—**micrometric, micrometrical** *adj*.—**micrometrically** *adv*.

micron /'maɪkrɒn/ *n* (*pl* **microns, micra**) one millionth of a metre, a micrometer.

microorganism /ˌmaɪkrəʊ'ɔːɡæˌnɪzəm/ *n* an organism visible only through a microscope.

microphone /'maɪkrəfəʊn/ *n* an instrument for transforming sound waves into electric signals, *esp* for transmission, or recording.—**microphonic** *adj*.

microphotograph /ˌmaɪkrəʊ'fəʊtəˌɡræf/ *n* a photograph taken through a microscope or of microscopic size, in which the details cannot be distinguished by the naked eye; a photomicrograph.—**microphotographic** *adj*.—**microphotography** *n*.

microphyte /'maɪkrəʊfaɪt/ *n* a microscopic vegetable growth, *esp* a parasitic one.—**microphytic** *adj*.

microprocessor /ˌmaɪkrəʊ'prəʊsesər/ *n* a computer processor contained on one or more integrated circuits.

microscope /'maɪkrəˌskoːp/ *n* an optical instrument for making magnified images of minute objects by means of a lens or lenses.

microscopic /ˌmaɪkrəˌskɒpɪk/ *adj* of, with, like, a microscope; visible only through a microscope; very small.—**microscopically** *adv*.

microscopy /maɪ'krɒskəpɪ/ *n* (*pl* **microscopies**) the use of microscopes; microscopic investigation.—**microscopist** *n*.

microseism /'maɪkrəʊˌsiːzəm/ *n* a faint earth tremor, probably not related to earthquakes.—**microseismic** *adj*.

microtome /'maɪkrəʊˌtoːm/ *n* an instrument for cutting thin sections for microscopic examination, used particularly in biology.

microwave /'maɪkrəʊˌweɪv/ *n* an electromagnetic wave between 1 and 100 centimetres in length; (*inf*) a microwave oven. • *vt* to cook (food) in a microwave oven.—**microwavable, microwaveable** *adj*.

microwave oven *n* a cooker in which food is cooked or heated by microwaves.

micturate /'mɪktʃʊreɪt/ *vi* to urinate.—**micturition** *n*.

mid /mɪd/ *adj* middle. • *prep* amid.

mid. /mɪd/ *abbr* = middle.

mid- /mɪd/ *prefix* middle.

midday /'mɪddeɪ/ *n* the middle of the day, noon.

midden /'mɪdən/ *n* a dunghill, a refuse heap.

middle /'mɪdəl/ *adj* halfway between two given points, times, etc; intermediate; central. • *n* the point halfway between two extremes; something intermediate; the waist. • *vt* to put in the middle; (*naut*) to fold (a sail) in the middle.

middle age *n* the time between youth and old age, *c*.40-60.—**middle-aged** *adj*.

Middle Ages *npl* the period of European history between about AD 500 and 1500.

middle class *n* the class between the lower and upper classes, mostly composed of professional and business people.—**middle-class** *adj*.

Middle East *n* a general term applied currently to an area extending from the eastern Mediterranean to the Gulf of Arabia; (formerly) that part of Southern Asia from the Tigris and Euphrates to Burma.

middleman /'mɪdəlmən/ *n* (*pl* **middlemen**) a dealer between producer and consumer; an intermediary.

middle-of-the-road *adj* avoiding extremes, *esp* political extremes.—**middle-of-the-roader** *n*.

middleweight /'mɪdəlˌweɪt/ *n* an professional boxer weighing 154-160 pounds (70-72.5 kilograms); a wrestler weighing *usu* 172-192 pounds (78-87 kilograms).

middling /'mɪdəlɪŋ/ *adj* of medium quality, size, etc; second-rate. • *adv* moderately.—**middlingly** *adv*.

middy /'mɪdɪ/ *n* (*pl* **middies**) (*inf*) a midshipman; a middy blouse; (*Austral*) a glass of beer, *usu* containing half a pint.

middy blouse *n* a loose blouse with a sailor collar.

midge /mɪdʒ/ *n* a small gnat-like insect with a painful bite.

midget /'mɪdʒət/ *n* a very small person, a dwarf; something small of its kind.—*also adj*.

midi /'mɪdɪ/ *n* a coat or skirt that reaches to mid calf.

midland /'mɪdlənd/ *n* the middle part of a country; (*pl*) (*with cap*) central England; the industrial and manufacturing area of that part of England. • *adj* of or in midland; inland.

midlife /'mɪdəlˌlaɪf/ *n* (*pl* **midlives**) middle age.—*also adj*.

midmost *adj* in or nearest the middle. • *adv* in the middle.

midnight /'mɪdnaɪt/ *n* twelve o'clock at night.

Midrash /'mɪdræʃ/ *n* (*pl* **Midrashim**) a critical exposition of or a sermon on the Jewish scriptural law or some portion of it; one of the various collections of these originating between AD 400 and 1200.

midrib /'mɪdrɪb/ *n* the principal central vein of a leaf.

midriff /-rɪf/ *n* the middle part of the torso between the abdomen and the chest.—*also adj*.

midship /-ʃɪp/ *adj* (*naut*) of or pertaining to the middle part of a ship.

midshipman /-ʃɪpmən/ *n* (*pl* **midshipmen**) in some navies, a noncommissioned officer ranking immediately below a sublieutenant; this naval rank; (*formerly*) a naval cadet officer; an American fish with light-producing organs.

midships /-ʃɪps/ *adv* (*naut*) at, near or toward the middle of a ship, amidships.

midst /mɪdst/ *n* middle. • *prep* amidst, among.

midsummer /mɪd'sʌmər/ or /'mɪd-/ n the middle of summer.—also adj.

Midsummer Day n June 24, celebrated as the summer solstice or in commemoration of the birth of St John the Baptist.

Midsummer Eve n the day before Midsummer Day, June 23.

midway /'mɪdweɪ/ adv halfway. • n a middle course of action; the area of a carnival where the sideshows are.

midwife /-waɪf/ n (pl **midwives**) a person trained to assist women before, during, and after childbirth.—**midwifery** n.

mien /miːn/ n the expression of the face; demeanour.

miff /mɪf/ n (inf) a petty quarrel, a tiff; a sulky mood. • vt: to take offence; to offend.

miffy /mɪfi/ adj (**miffier, miffiest**) (inf) touchy, huffy; over-sensitive.—**miffiness** n.

might[1] /maɪt/ see **may**.

might[2] n power, bodily strength.

mightn't /'maɪtənt/ = might not.

mighty /maɪti/ adj (**mightier, mightiest**) powerful, strong; massive; (inf) very.—**mightily** adv.—**mightiness** n.

mignonette /ˌmɪnjə'nɛt/ n a sweet-scented plant with spikes of small green- white flowers; a greyish-green colour; a delicate bobbin lace.

migraine /'maɪgreɪn/ n an intense, periodic headache, usu limited to one side of the head.

migrant /'maɪgrənt/ n a person or animal that moves from one region or country to another; an itinerant agricultural labourer. • adj migrating.

migrate /'maɪgreɪt/ vi to settle in another country or region; (birds, animals) to move to another region with the change in season.—**migration** n.—**migratory** adj.

mikado /mɪ'kɒdoː/ n (sl **mikados**) (arch) (often with cap) the Japanese emperor.

mike /maɪk/ n (inf) a microphone. • vt to provide with a microphone; to transmit by microphone.

Mi'kmaq, Micmac /'mɪkmæk/ n ✤ a member a First Nations people mainly of the Maritime Provinces of Canada; the language of this people. • adj of or pertaining to this people or their language.

mil /mɪl/ n a unit of length of one thousandth of an inch; (gunnery) an angle of one sixty-four-hundredth of a circumference; a milliliter.

mil. abbr = military; militia.

milady /mɪ'leɪdi/ n (pl **miladies**) (formerly) a word used in Europe for an aristocratic Englishwoman.

milage /'maɪlɪdʒ/ see **mileage**.

milch /mɪltʃ/ adj yielding milk, used esp of cattle.

milch cow n a cow from which milk is obtained for human consumption; a ready source of gain.

mild /maɪld/ adj (temper) gentle; (weather) temperate; bland; feeble.—**mildly** adv.—**mildness** n.

mildew /'mɪldu:/ or /-dju:/ n a fungus that attacks some plants or appears on damp cloth, etc as a whitish coating. • vti to affect or be affected with mildew.—**mildewy** adj.

mile /maɪl/ n a unit of linear measure equal to 5,280 feet (1.61 km); the nautical mile is 6,075 feet (1.85 km).

mileage /'maɪlɪdʒ/ n total miles travelled; an allowance per mile for travelling expenses; the average number of miles that can be travelled, as per litre of fuel.—also **milage**.

milestone /'maɪlstoːn/ n a stone marking the number of miles to a place; an important event in life, history, etc.

milfoil /mɪlfɔɪl/ n a yarrow plant; one of various pond plants with feather-like leaves and small flowers.

miliaria /ˌmɪli'ɛriə/ n a skin disease resulting from blocked sweat glands and characterized by an acute itchiness, heat rash.—**miliarial** adj.

miliary /'mɪliˌɛri/ or /-ˌəri/ adj (growth, lesion) very small; (skin disease) marked by small lesions resembling millet seeds.

milieu /mɪl'juː/ or /-'juː/ n (pl **milieus, milieux**) environment, esp social setting.

militant /'mɪlɪtənt/ adj ready to fight, esp for some cause; combative.—also n.—**militance, militancy** n.—**militantly** adv.

militarism /'mɪlɪtəˌrɪzəm/ n military spirit; a policy of aggressive military preparedness.

militarist /'mɪlɪtərɪst/ n a believer in militarism; a student of military science.—**militaristic** adj.—**militaristically** adv.

militarize /-ˌraɪz/ vt to equip and prepare for war.—**militarization** n.

military /'mɪlɪtɛri/ adj relating to soldiers or to war; warlike. • n (pl **militaries**) the armed forces.

militate /'mɪlɪteɪt/ vt to have influence or force; to produce an effect or change.

militia /mɪ'lɪʃə/ n an army composed of civilians called out in time of emergency.—**militiaman** n (pl **militiamen**)

milk /mɪlk/ n a white nutritious liquid secreted by female mammals for feeding their young. • vt to draw milk from; to extract money, etc, from; to exploit.—**milker** n.

milkmaid /mɪlkmeɪd/ n a girl or woman who milks cows or works in a dairy.

milkman /-mæn/ n (pl **milkmen**) a person who sells or delivers milk to homes.

milk run n (sl) a routine journey.

milksop /'mɪlksɒp/ n a weak cowardly man or boy.—**milksoppy** adj.

milk store ✤ (Cdn) a convenience store.

milk toast n toasted bread soaked in warm milk, often eaten by babies and invalids.

milk tooth n any of the first teeth of a mammal.

milkweed /'mɪlkwiːd/ n a plant found mainly in North America yielding a milky sap and with pointed pods containing tufted seeds; any plant with a milky sap.—also **silkweed**.

milkwort /-wərt/ n a kind of plant with small blue, pink or white flowers.

milky /'mɪlki/ adj (**milkier, milkiest**) of, filled with, consisting of, yielding, or resembling milk; timid.—**milkily** adv.—**milkiness** n.

Milky Way n (with the) the galaxy to which the Earth belongs; the system of stars, nebulae, etc, that can be seen in the night sky as a trailing ribbon of light and forms part of the Galaxy.

mill[1] /mɪl/ n an apparatus for grinding by crushing between rough surfaces; a building where grain is ground into flour; a factory. • vt to produce or grind in a mill; (coins) to put a raised edge on. • vi to move around confusedly.—**miller** n.

mill[2] n a unit of money equal to one tenth of a cent.

millboard /'mɪlbɔrd/ n a thick pasteboard, often black or grey, that forms the front and back covers and spine of a book, usu covered by the book binding.

millenarian /ˌmɪlɪ'nɛriən/ adj consisting of or pertaining to a thousand years; pertaining to the millennium or to millenarianism. • n a believer in the millennium; an advocate of millenarianism.

millenarianism n (Christianity) the belief that the Second Coming of Christ will be preceded or followed by a thousand years of holiness.

millenary /'mɪlənˌɛri/ or /mɪ'lɛnəri/ adj of or pertaining to a thousand; millenarian. • n (pl **millenaries**) a thousandth anniversary; one thousand as a total, esp one thousand years; a millenarian.

millennium /mɪ'lɛniəm/ n (pl **millennia, millenniums**) a period of a thousand years; (Christianity) a period of a thousand years of holiness preceding or following the Second Coming of Christ; a coming time of happiness.—**millennial** adj.—**millennially** adv.

millepede /'mɪlɪpiːd/ see **millipede**.

millepore /-pɔr/ n a tropical coelenterate resembling a coral, with a smooth surface perforated with very small pores.

miller /'mɪlər/ n one who or that which mills; an owner of a mill; a moth with a floury appearance.

millesimal /mɪ'lɛsɪməl/ adj pertaining to a thousandth. • n a thousandth.

millet /'mɪlət/ n a cereal grass used for grain and fodder.

milli- /'mɪli/ prefix a thousandth part.

milligram /'mɪlɪˌgræm/ n a thousandth of a gramme.

milliliter, millilitre /mɪlɪˌliːtər/ n a thousandth (.001) of a litre.

millimetre, millimeter /'mɪlɪˌmiːtər/ n a thousandth (.001) of a metre.

milliner /'mɪlɪnər/ n a designer or seller of women's hats.—**millinery** n.

milling /'mɪlɪŋ/ n the act of grinding in or passing through a dressing mill; the process of making a serrated edge on a coin, etc; the serrated edge of such a coin; a stratagem to stop cattle stampeding.

million /'mɪljən/ n (pl **million, millions**) a thousand thousands, the number one followed by six zeros: 1,000,000; (inf) a very large number.—**millionth** adj.

millionaire /ˈmɪljəˌnɛr/ or /ˌmɪljəˈnɛr/ *n* a person who owns at least a million of money; one who is extremely rich.

millipede /ˈmɪlɪpiːd/ *n* a wormlike arthropod with many legs and a segmented body.—*also* **millepede**.

millpond /ˈmɪlpɒnd/ *n* a reservoir of water for driving a mill; any stretch of calm water.

millrace /ˈmɪlreɪs/ *n* a current of water that drives a mill; the channel in which this flows.

mill rate *n* ✤ the rate at which a property is taxed, expressed as the number of mills of tax for every dollar of assessed value.

millstone /ˈmɪlstoːn/ *n* a stone used for grinding corn; a heavy burden.

millwright /ˈmɪlraɪt/ *n* a person who designs, builds, and repairs mills or mill parts.

milord /mɪˈlɔrd/ *n* (*formerly*) a word used in Europe for an aristocratic or rich Englishman.

milt /mɪlt/ *n* the sperm of a male fish; its reproductive glands when filled with this; the spleen of some animals. • *vt* to fertilize (the roe of female fish), *esp* artificially.

milter /ˈmɪltər/ *n* a male fish in the breeding season.

Miltonic /mɪlˈtɒnɪk/, **Miltonian** /mɪlˈtoːnɪən/ *adj* pertaining to, characteristic of, or resembling the writings of the English poet John Milton (1608–74).

mime /maɪm/ *n* a theatrical technique using action without words; a mimic. • *vi* to act or express using gestures alone; (*singers, musicians*) to perform as if singing or playing live to what is actually a prerecorded piece of music.—**mimer** *n*.

mimeograph /ˈmɪmɪəˌɡræf/ *n* a machine for making multiple copies of a letter, drawing, etc, by means of a stencil fixed to an inked drum, and masking the non-printing areas; a copy produced from this machine. • *vti* to produce copies (of something) by using this machine.

mimesis /mɪˈmiːsɪs/ or /maɪ-/ *n* (*art, literature, etc*) the realistic representation of objects, people, everyday life, etc; (*biol*) mimicry; (*med*) a condition characterized by symptoms that occur in other diseases but that cannot be found by objective medical testing; a disease that mimics the symptoms of another disease.

mimetic /maɪˈmɛtɪk/ *adj* of or given to imitation or mimicry; (*biol*) pertaining to or having the ability to mimic.—**mimetically** *adv*.

mimic /ˈmɪmɪk/ *n* a person who imitates, *esp* an actor skilled in mimicry. • *adj* related to mimicry; make-believe; sham. • *vt* (**mimicking, mimicked**) to imitate or ridicule.—**mimicker** *n*.

mimicry /ˈmɪmɪkri/ *n* (*pl* **mimicries**) practice, art, or way of mimicking; (*biol*) the resemblance of an animal to its environment, another animal, etc, to provide protection from predators, mimesis.

mimosa /mɪˈmoːzə/ *n* any of a genus of leguminous plants, *usu* with clustered yellow flowers, whose leaves and stems fold when touched or when exposed to light; the sensitive plant; any of several related or similar plants.

Min. *abbr* = Minister; Ministry.

min. *abbr* = minimum; minute(s).

mina[1] /ˈmaɪnə/ *n* (*pl* **minas, minae**) a weight and coin, current in ancient Anatolia, equal to one sixtieth of a talent.

mina[2] *see* **myna**.

minaret /ˌmɪnəˈrɛt/ or /ˈmɪnəˌrɛt/ *n* a high, slender tower on a mosque from which the call to prayer is made.

minatory /ˈmɪnətəri/, **minatorial** /-rɪəl/ *adj* threatening.—**minatorily** *adv*.

mince /mɪns/ *vt* to chop or cut up into small pieces; to diminish or moderate one's words. • *vi* to speak or walk with affected daintiness.—**mincer** *n*.—**mincing** *adj*.—**mincingly** *adv*.

mincemeat /ˈmɪnsmiːt/ *n* a mixture of chopped apples, raisins, etc, used as a pie filling; finely chopped meat.

mind /maɪnd/ *n* the faculty responsible for intellect, thought, feelings, speech; memory; intellect; reason; opinion; sanity. • *vt* to object to, take offence to; to pay attention to; to obey; to take care of; to be careful about; to care about. • *vi* to pay attention; to be obedient; to be careful; to object.

mind-bending *adj* (*inf*) (*drugs, etc*) unbalancing the mind; (*inf*) stretching credibility to the limits.—**mind-bender** *n*.—**mind-bendingly** *adv*.

mind-blowing *adj* (*inf*) (*drugs*) hallucinatory.

mind-boggling *adj* (*inf*) astonishing, bewildering.—**mind-boggler** *n*.

minded /ˈmaɪndəd/ *adj* disposed, inclined; (in compounds) having a mind as described, *eg* small-minded.—**mindedness** *n*.

minder /ˈmaɪndər/ *n* a person who looks after or protects another.

mind-expanding *adj* producing awareness; psychedelic, distorting.

mindful /ˈmaɪndfʊl/ *adj* heedful, not forgetful.—**mindfully** *adv*.—**mindfulness** *n*.

mindless /-ləs/ *adj* unthinking, stupid; requiring little intellectual effort.—**mindlessly** *adv*.—**mindlessness** *n*.

mindset /-sɛt/ *n* attitude, *esp* when fixed or rigid; a habit.

mind's eye *n* the visual memory or imagination.

mine[1] /maɪn/ *poss pron* belonging to me.

mine[2] *n* an excavation from which minerals are dug; an explosive device concealed in the water or ground to destroy enemy ships, personnel, or vehicles that pass over or near them; a rich supply or source. • *vt* to excavate; to lay explosive mines in an area. • *vi* to dig or work a mine.

mine detector *n* a device for indicating the whereabouts of explosive mines.—**mine detection** *n*.

minefield /ˈmaɪnfiːld/ *n* an area sown with explosive mines; a situation containing hidden problems.

minelayer /ˈmaɪnˌleɪər/ *n* a ship or aircraft for laying mines.

miner /ˈmaɪnər/ *n* a person who works in a mine.

mineral /ˈmɪnərəl/ *n* an inorganic substance, found naturally in the earth; any substance neither vegetable nor animal. • *adj* relating to or containing minerals.

mineralize /ˈmɪnərəˌlaɪz/ *vt* to convert (something) into a mineral; to impregnate (something) with mineral matter; to change something into a fossil-like object. • *vi* (*gases, etc, in molten rock*) to transform a metal into an ore.—**mineralization** *n*.

mineral kingdom *n* the group of natural substances that consist of only inorganic matter.

mineralogy /ˌmɪnəˈrɒlədʒi/ *n* the science of minerals.—**mineralogical** *adj*.—**mineralogically** *adv*.—**mineralogist** *n*.

mineral water *n* water containing mineral salts or gases, often with medicinal properties.

minestrone /ˌmɪnəˈstroːni/ *n* a soup of vegetables with pieces of pasta.

minesweeper /ˈmaɪnˌswiːpər/ *n* a ship for clearing away explosive mines.—**minesweeping** *n*.

mingle /ˈmɪŋɡəl/ *vti* to mix; to combine.—**mingler** *n*.

mingy /ˈmɪndʒi/ *adj* (**mingier, mingiest**) (*inf*) meagre in quantity; miserly, mean.

mini /ˈmɪni/ *n* (*pl* **minis**) something smaller than others of its type; a miniskirt.

mini- /ˈmɪni/ *prefix* small.

miniature /ˈmɪnɪtʃər/ or /-nɪətʃ-/ *adj* minute, on a small scale. • *n* a painting or reproduction on a very small scale.—**miniaturist** *n*.

miniaturize /ˈmɪnɪtʃəˌraɪz/ or /-nɪətʃ-/ *vt* to greatly reduce the size of.—**miniaturization** *n*.

minibar /ˈmɪnɪbɑr/ *n* a small refrigerator in a hotel bedroom, stocked with alcoholic drinks.

minibus /-ˌbʊs/ *n* (*pl* **minibuses, minibusses**) a small bus for carrying up to twelve passengers.

minicab /-ˌkæb/ *n* a saloon car used as a taxi, which can be booked by telephone but not hailed.

minicar /-ˌkɑr/ *n* a very small car.

minicomputer /-kəmˌpjuːtər/ *n* a computer intermediate in size and processing power between a mainframe and a microcomputer.

minim /ˈmɪnɪm/ *n* a unit of fluid measure of one sixtieth of a fluid dram (0.0616ml) in the US and one twentieth of a scruple (0.592ml) in the UK; (*mus*) a half note.

minima /ˈmɪnɪmə/ *see* **minimum**.

minimal /ˈmɪnɪməl/ *adj* very minute; least possible.—**minimality** *n*.—**minimally** *adv*.

minimalism /ˌmɪnɪməˈlɪzəm/ *n* a style in the creation of art, music, etc, that uses the fewest possible elements to achieve the greatest effect.—**minimalist** *n, adj*.

minimize /ˈmɪnɪmaɪz/ *vt* to reduce to or estimate at a minimum.—**minimization** *n*.

minimum /ˈmɪnɪməm/ *n* (*pl* **minimums, minima**) the least possible amount; the lowest degree or point reached.

mining /ˈmaɪnɪŋ/ *n* the act, process, or industry of excavating from the earth; (*mil*) the laying of explosive mines.

mining recorder *n* ✤ (*Cdn*) a government official who registers mining claims.

minion /ˈmɪnɪən/ *n* a servile flatterer or dependant; an obsequious person acting on behalf of or carrying out the wishes of another. • *adj* dainty, graceful.

miniseries /'mɪnɪˌsiːriːz/ *n* (*pl* **miniseries**) (*TV*) the dramatization of a novel, etc, shown in several episodes; (*sport*) a short series.

miniskirt /'mɪnɪˌskərt/ *n* a very short skirt.

minister /'mɪnɪstər/ *n* a clergyman serving a church; an official heading a government department; a diplomat. • *vi* to serve as a minister in a church; to give help (to).—**ministerial** *adj.*—**ministerially** *adv.*

Minister's Permit *n* ♣ (*Cdn*) a permit issued by the federal government that permits a person who is otherwise ineligible for immigrant status to remain in the country for a fixed period.

ministrant /'mɪnɪstrənt/ *adj* serving as a minister. • *n* a person who ministers.

ministration /ˌmɪnɪ'streɪʃən/ *n* the act or process of giving aid; the act of ministering religiously.

ministry /'mɪnɪstri/ *n* (*pl* **ministries**) the act of ministering; the clergy; the profession of a clergyman; a government department headed by a minister; the building housing a government department.

minium /'mɪniəm/ *n* red oxide of lead, used as a pigment in paints; red lead.

miniver /'mɪnɪvər/ *n* a white fur, orig from the Siberian squirrel, used as a trimming on ceremonial robes, etc.

mink /'mɪŋk/ *n* (*pl* **mink, minks**) any of several carnivorous weasel-like mammals valued for its durable soft fur.

Minn. *abbr* = Minnesota.

minnesinger /'mɪnɪˌsɪŋər/ *n* any of the German lyric poets and musicians of the 12th-14th centuries who sang about love and beauty.

minnow /'mɪnoʊ/ *n* (*pl* **minnow, minnows**) a small, slender freshwater fish.

minor /'maɪnər/ *adj* lesser in size, importance, degree, extent, etc; (*mus*) lower than the corresponding major by a half step. • *n* (*law*) a person under full legal age; (*education*) a secondary area of study requiring fewer credits; (*mus*) a minor key, interval, or scale; (*sport*) a minor league. *esp* in baseball. • *vi* (*with* **in**) to take a subject requiring fewer credits.

Minorite /'maɪnəˌraɪt/, **Minorist** /-rɪst/ *n* a Franciscan friar, *esp* one of the order of the Friars Minor.

minority /maɪ'nɒrɪti/ or /mɪ-/ *n* (*pl* **minorities**) the smaller part or number; a political or racial group smaller than the majority group; the state of being under age.

minor penalty *n* ♣ a two-minute penalty in ice hockey, given for minor infractions such as holding.

Minotaur /'mɪnətər/ or /'maɪ-/ *n* (*Greek myth*) a monster with the head of a bull and the body of a man, which ate human flesh.

minster /'mɪnstər/ *n* a large and important church, often with cathedral status.

minstrel /'mɪnstrəl/ *n* a travelling entertainer and musician in the Middle Ages; a performer in a minstrel show.

minstrel show *n* a variety show with performers singing and dancing wearing black face make-up.

minstrelsy /-trəlsi/ *n* (*pl* **minstrelsies**) the art or occupation of minstrels; minstrels collectively; a collection of ballad poetry.

mint[1] /mɪnt/ *n* the place where money is coined; a large amount of money; a source of supply. • *adj* unused, in perfect condition. • *vt* (*coins*) to imprint; to invent.—**minter** *n*.

mint[2] *n* an aromatic plant whose leaves are used for flavouring.—**minty** *adj*.

mintage /'mɪntɪdʒ/ *n* a coin, etc, produced in a mint; the process of producing coins, etc, in a mint; the fee paid to a mint for coining gold or silver; an official mark on a coin.

mint julep *n* a tall drink of bourbon or brandy and sugar over crushed ice, garnished with mint.

minuend /'mɪnjuˌend/ *n* (*math*) the number from which another number is to be subtracted.

minuet /ˌmɪnju'et/ *n* (the music for) a slow, graceful dance in triple time.

minus /'maɪnəs/ *prep* less; (*inf*) without. • *adj* involving subtraction; negative; less than. • *n* a sign (-), indicating subtraction or negative quantity.

minute[1] /'mɪnɪt/ *n* the sixtieth part of an hour or a degree; a moment; (*pl*) an official record of a meeting. • *vt* to record or summarize the proceedings (of).

minute[2] /maɪ'njuːt/ *adj* tiny; detailed; exact.—**minuteness** *n*.

minutely[1] /'mɪnɪtli/ *adj* occurring every minute. • *adv* every minute.

minutely[2] /maɪ'njuːtli/ *adv* in a minute manner; precisely.

minuteman /'mɪnɪtmæn/ *n* (*pl* **minutemen**) (*sometimes cap*) a member of the militia in the War of American Independence, ready to fight at a minute's notice.

minutiae /mɪ'njuːʃeɪɪ/ or /-'nju:-/, /maɪ-/, /-ʃiə/, /-ʃə/ *npl* (*sing* **minutia**) small or unimportant details.

minx /mɪŋks/ *n* a pert, forward girl; (*arch*) a prostitute.—**minxish** *adj*.

Miocene /'maɪəˌsiːn/ *adj* pertaining to the middle division of the Tertiary formation after the Oligocene and before the Pliocene eras, marked by the appearance of grasses and grazing mammals. • *n* this division or rock formation.

miosis /maɪ'oʊsɪs/ *n* abnormal contraction of the pupil of the eye.—*also* **myosis**.—**miotic** *adj*, *n*.

miracle /'mɪrəkəl/ *n* an extraordinary event attributed to the supernatural; an unusual or astounding event; a remarkable example of something.

miraculous /mɪ'rækjʊləs/ *adj* supernatural; wonderful; able to work miracles.—**miraculously** *adv*.—**miraculousness** *n*.

mirage /mɪ'rɒdʒ/ *n* an optical illusion in which a distant object or expanse of water seems to be nearby, caused by light reflection from hot air; anything illusory or fanciful.

mire /maɪr/ *n* an area of wet, soggy, or muddy ground. • *vt* to sink in mire; to dirty; to embroil in difficulties.

mirk /mərk/ *see* **murk**.

mirky /'mərki/ *see* **murky**.

mirror /'mɪrər/ *n* a smooth surface that reflects images; a faithful depiction. • *vt* (**mirroring, mirrored**) to reflect or depict faithfully.

mirth /mərθ/ *n* merriment, *esp* with laughter.

mirthful /'mərθfʊl/ *adj* full of merriment.—**mirthfully** *adv*.—**mirthfulness** *n*.

mirthless /-ləs/ *adj* lacking laughter; miserable.—**mirthlessly** *adv*.—**mirthlessness** *n*.

mis-[1] /mɪs/ *prefix* wrong(ly); bad(ly); no. not.

mis-[2] *see* **miso-**.

misadventure /ˌmɪsəd'ventʃər/ *n* an unlucky accident; bad luck.

misalliance /ˌmɪsə'laɪəns/ *n* an unsuitable alliance, *usu* by marriage with a person of lower social status; a mésalliance.

misanthrope /ˌmɪsən'θroʊp/ or /ˌmɪz-/, **misanthropist** /mɪ'sænθrəpɪst/ or /-'zæn-/ *n* a person who hates or distrusts mankind.

misanthropic /ˌmɪsən'θrɒpɪk/ or /ˌmɪz-/ *adj* of or characterized by hatred of his or her fellow human beings.—**misanthropically** *adv*.—**misanthropy** *n*.

misapprehend /ˌmɪsæpri'hend/ *vt* to misunderstand; to misconceive.—**misapprehension** *n*.

misappropriate /ˌmɪsə'proʊpriˌeɪt/ *vt* to appropriate wrongly or dishonestly; to use illegally; to embezzle.—**misappropriation** *n*.

misbehave /ˌmɪsbi'heɪv/ *vi* to behave badly. • *vt* to behave (oneself) badly.—**misbehavior, misbehaviour** *n*.

misc. *abbr* = miscellaneous.

miscalculate /ˌmɪs'kælkjuˌleɪt/ *vti* to calculate wrongly.—**miscalculation** *n*.

miscarriage /'mɪsˌkærɪdʒ/ *n* the spontaneous expulsion of a foetus prematurely; mismanagement or failure.

miscarry /'mɪsˌkæri/ *vi* (**miscarrying, miscarried**) to spontaneously expel a foetus from the uterus; to be unsuccessful; to fail.

miscellaneous /ˌmɪsə'leɪniəs/ *adj* consisting of various kinds; mixed.—**miscellaneously** *adv*.—**miscellaneousness** *n*.

miscellany /'mɪsələni/ *n* (*pl* **miscellanies**) a mixed collection; a book comprising miscellaneous writings, etc.

mischance /'mɪstʃæns/ *n* bad luck; an unlucky event.

mischief /'mɪstʃɪf/ *n* wayward behaviour; damage.

mischievous /'mɪstʃɪvəs/ *adj* harmful, prankish.—**mischievously** *adv*.—**mischievousness** *n*.

miscible /'mɪsɪbəl/ *adj* (*chem*) (*liquids*) capable of being mixed.—**miscibility** *n*.

misconceive /ˌmɪskən'siːv/ *vt* to conceive wrongly; to misjudge; to misapprehend; to misunderstand.—**misconceiver** *n*.

misconception /ˌmɪskən'sepʃən/ *n* a mistaken idea; misunderstanding.

misconduct /mɪs'kɒndʌkt/ *n* dishonest management; improper behaviour. • *vt* to conduct (oneself) badly; to manage dishonestly.

misconstrue /ˌmɪskən'struː/ *vt* (**misconstruing, misconstrued**) to misinterpret.—**misconstruction** *n*.

miscreant /'mɪskriənt/ *n* an unscrupulous villain; (*arch*) a heretic. • *adj* unscrupulous; (*arch*) heretical.

misdeed /mɪs'diːd/ *n* a wrong or wicked act; crime; sin, etc.

misdemeanour, misdemeanor /ˌmɪsdə'miːnər/ *n* (*law*) a minor offence, a misdeed.

miser /'maɪzər/ *n* a greedy, stingy person who hoards money for its own sake.

miserable /'mɪzrəbəl/ or /'mɪzər-/ *adj* wretched; unhappy; causing misery; bad, inadequate; pitiable.—**miserableness** *n*.—**miserably** *adv*.

Miserere /ˌmɪze'rereɪ/ *n* the 51st Psalm, appointed for penitential acts; a musical setting of this psalm; (*without cap*) a misericord in a choir stall.

misericord, misericorde /'mɪzərɪˌkɔːrd/ *n* a small ledge, often carved, on the underside of a folding seat in the stall of a church against which a worshipper can lean when standing; in the Middle Ages, a small dagger for giving a death thrust to a seriously wounded person, *esp* a knight; (*Christianity*) the relaxation of monastic rules for elderly or infirm monks or nuns; a room in a monastery for those with such a dispensation.

miserly /'maɪzərli/ *adj* like a miser; tending to hoard; very mean.—**miserliness** *n*.

misery /'mɪzəri/ *n* (*pl* **miseries**) extreme pain, unhappiness, or poverty; a cause of such suffering.

misfeasance /mɪs'fiːzəns/ *n* (*law*) the wrong performance of something that is itself legal.—**misfeasor** *n*.

misfire /mɪs'faɪr/ *vi* (*engine, etc*) to fail to ignite, start; to fail to succeed.—*also n*.

misfit /'mɪsfɪt/ *n* something that fits badly; a maladjusted person.

misfortune /mɪs'fɔːrtʃən/ *n* ill luck; trouble; a mishap; bad luck.

misgiving /mɪs'gɪvɪŋ/ *n* a feeling of misapprehension, mistrust.

misguided /mɪs'gaɪdəd/ *adj* foolish; mistaken.—**misguidedly** *adv*.

mishap /'mɪshæp/ *n* an unfortunate accident.

mishmash /'mɪʃmæʃ/ *n* a confused mixture, hotchpotch.

Mishnah, Mishna /'mɪʃnə/ *n* (*Judaism*) the oral law; the written form of this, which was collected in the 2nd century and forms the text of the earlier part of the Talmud.

misinform /ˌmɪsɪn'fɔːrm/ *vt* to supply with wrong information.—**misinformant, misinformer** *n*.—**misinformation** *n*.

misjudge /mɪs'dʒʌdʒ/ *vt* to judge wrongly, to form a wrong opinion.—**misjudgment** *n*.

mislay /mɪs'leɪ/ *vt* (**mislaying, mislaid**) to lose something temporarily; to put down or install improperly.—**mislayer** *n*.

mislead /mɪs'liːd/ *vt* (**misleading, misled**) to deceive; to give wrong information to; to lead into wrongdoing.—**misleader** *n*.

misleading /mɪs'liːdɪŋ/ *adj* deceptive; confusing.—**misleadingly** *adv*.

misnomer /mɪs'noʊmər/ *n* an incorrect or unsuitable name or description.—**misnomered** *adj*.

miso- /'mɪsoʊ/, **mis-** /mɪs/ *prefix* hatred of.

misogamy /mɪ'sɒgəmi/ *n* hatred of marriage.—**misogamic** *adj*.—**misogamist** *n*.

misogynist /ˌmɪsə'dʒɪnɪst/ *n* a hater or distruster of women. •—**misogynistic** *adj*.

misogyny /mɪ'sɒdʒɪni/ *n* hatred of women.—**misogynic** *adj*.

misplace /mɪs'pleɪs/ *vt* to put in a wrong place; (*trust, etc*) to place unwisely.—**misplacement** *n*.

misprint /mɪs'prɪnt/ *vt* to print incorrectly. • *n* an error in printing.

misprision /mɪs'prɪʒən/ *n* (*law*) the concealment of a seriously criminal act; the knowledge of the commission of treason and the failure to report this; (*arch*) contempt; the disparagement or undervaluing of something.

mispronounce /ˌmɪsprə'naʊns/ *vt* to pronounce wrongly.—**mispronunciation** *n*.

misquote /mɪs'kwoʊt/ *vt* to quote wrongly.—**misquotation** *n*.

misread /mɪs'riːd/ *vt* (**misreading, misread**) to read or to interpret wrongly.

misrepresent /ˌmɪsreprɪ'zent/ *vt* to represent falsely; to give an untrue idea of.—**misrepresentation** *n*.—**misrepresentative** *adj*.

misrule *n* bad government. • *vt* to govern badly; to govern in an inhumane manner or with injustice.

miss[1] /mɪs/ *n* (*pl* **misses**) a girl; (*with cap*) a title used before the surname of an unmarried woman or girl.

miss[2] *vt* to fail to reach, hit, find, meet, hear; to omit; to fail to take advantage of; to regret or discover the absence or loss of. • *vi* to fail to hit; to fail to be successful; to misfire, as an engine. • *n* a failure to hit, reach, obtain, etc.

Miss. *abbr* = Mississippi.

missal /'mɪsəl/ *n* a book containing the prayers for Mass.

misshapen /mɪ'ʃeɪpən/ *adj* badly shaped; deformed.

missile /'mɪsəl/ or /-saɪl/ *n* an object, as a rock, spear, rocket, etc, to be thrown, fired, or launched.

missing /'mɪsɪŋ/ *adj* absent; lost; lacking.

missing link *n* something required to complete a series; a hypothetical animal supposedly intermediate between the anthropoid apes and man.

mission /'mɪʃən/ *n* a group of people sent by a church, government, etc to carry out a special duty or task; the sending of an aircraft or spacecraft on a special assignment; a vocation. • *adj* of a mission; (*archit*) of a style of church building established by Spanish missioners in the southwest USA.

missionary /'mɪʃəˌneri/ *n* (*pl* **missionaries**) a person who tries to convert unbelievers to his or her religious faith, *esp* abroad; one sent on a mission. • *adj* of a religious mission; tending to propagandize.

missionary position *n* (*inf*) a position for sexual intercourse with the partners face to face and the man on top.

mission control *n* a command centre that controls space flights from the ground.

missioner *n* a missionary; a person in charge of a parochial mission.

missis /'mɪsɪz/ *n* (*inf*) (*usu with* **the**) one's wife; (*inf*) a name used when directly addressing a woman.—*also* **missus**.

missive /'mɪsɪv/ *n* (*formal*) a letter or message, often official. • *adj* (*rare*) sent specially, or intended to be sent.

misspent /mɪs'spent/ *adj* wasted, frittered away.

missus /'mɪsəz/ *see* **missis**.

mist /mɪst/ *n* a large mass of water vapour, less dense than a fog; something that dims or obscures. • *vti* to cover or be covered, as with mist.

mistake /mɪ'steɪk/ *vb* (**mistaking, mistook**, *pp* **mistaken**). • *vt* to misunderstand; to misinterpret. • *vi* to make a mistake. • *n* a wrong idea, answer, etc; an error of judgment; a blunder; a misunderstanding.—**mistakable** *adj*.—**mistakably** *adv*.

mistaken /mɪ'steɪkən/ *adj* erroneous, ill-judged.—**mistakenly** *adv*.

mister /'mɪstər/ *n* (*inf*) sir; (*with cap*) the title used before a man's surname.

mistime /mɪs'taɪm/ *vt* to do or say at the wrong time; to time wrongly.

mistletoe /'mɪsəlˌtoʊ/ *n* an evergreen parasitic plant with white berries used as a Christmas decoration.

mistreat /mɪs'triːt/ *vt* to treat wrongly or badly.—**mistreatment** *n*.

mistress /'mɪstrəs/ *n* a woman who is head of a household; a woman with whom a man is having a prolonged affair; a female schoolteacher; (*with cap*) the title used before a married woman's surname.

mistrust /mɪs'trʌst/ *n* lack of trust. • *vti* to doubt; to suspect.—**mistrustfully** *adv*

misty /'mɪsti/ *adj* (**mistier, mistiest**) full of mist; dim, obscure.—**mistily** *adv*.—**mistiness** *n*.

misunderstand /ˌmɪsʌndər'stænd/ *vt* (**misunderstanding, misunderstood**) to fail to understand correctly.

misunderstanding /ˌmɪsʌndər'stændɪŋ/ *n* a mistake as to sense; a quarrel or disagreement.

misunderstood /ˌmɪsʌndər'stʊd/ *adj* not fully understood; not appreciated properly.

misuse /mɪs'juːz/ *vt* to use for the wrong purpose or in the wrong way; to ill-treat, abuse. • *n* improper or incorrect use.

mite /maɪt/ *n* any of numerous very small parasitic or free-living insects; (*money, etc*) a very small amount.

miter /'maɪtər/ *see* **mitre**.

mitigate /'mɪtɪˌgeɪt/ *vti* to become or make less severe.—**mitigable** *adj*.—**mitigation** *n*.—**mitigator** *n*.

mitosis /mɪ'toʊsɪs/ or /maɪ-/ *n* (*pl* **mitoses**) a process by which plant or animal cells divide, in which the nucleus of a somatic cell splits into nuclei, each with the same number of chromosomes as there were in the orig cell.—**mitotic** *adj*, *adv*.

mitral /'maɪtrəl/ *adj* of or like a mitre; (*anat*) pertaining to the mitral valve.

mitral valve *n* a valve of the heart between the left atrium and the left ventricle.

mitre, miter /'maɪtər/ *n* the headdress of a bishop; a diagonal joint between two pieces of wood to form a corner. • *vt* to join with a mitre corner.—**miterer** *n*.

mitt /mɪt/ *n* a glove covering the hand but only the base of the fingers; (*sl*) a hand; a boxing glove; a baseball glove.

mitten /'mɪtən/ *n* a glove with a thumb but no separate fingers.

mix /'mɪks/ *vt* to blend together in a single mass; to make by blending ingredients, as a cake; to combine; (*with* **up**) to make into a mixture; to make disordered; to confuse or mistake. • *vi* to be mixed or blended; to get along together. • *n* a mixture.—**mixable** *adj*.

mixed /mɪkst/ *adj* blended; made up of different parts, classes, races, etc; confused.

mixed bag *n* (*inf*) a collection of diverse things or people.

mixed economy *n* an economic system containing both state-owned industries and private enterprise.

mixed-up *adj* (*inf*) perplexed, mentally confused.

mixer /'mɪksər/ *n* a device that blends or mixes; a person considered in terms of their ability (good or bad) to get on with others; a soft drink added to an alcoholic beverage.

mixture /'mɪkstʃər/ *n* the process of mixing; a blend made by mixing.

mix-up *n* a mistake; confusion, muddle; (*inf*) a fight.

mizzen, mizen /'mɪzən/ *n* (*naut*) the lowest sail on the mizzenmast of a vessel; the mizzenmast. • *adj* pertaining to something used with the mizzenmast.

mizzenmast, mizenmast *n* (*naut*) the aftermost mast when there are three masts on a ship; the aftermast on other ships.

mizzle /'mɪzəl/ *vi* to rain in very minute drops, to drizzle. • *n* a very fine rain.

mkt *abbr* = market.

ml *abbr* = mile; milliliter.

MLA /'ɛm'ɛl'eɪ/ *abbr* ✚ = Member of the Legislative Assembly.

Mlle(s) *abbr* = mademoiselle, mesdemoiselles.

MM *abbr* = Messieurs.

mm *abbr* = millimeter.

MN *abbr* = Minnesota.

Mn (*chem symbol*) manganese.

MNA /'ɛm'ɛn'eɪ/ *abbr* ✚ (*Cdn*) = Member of the National Assembly.

mnemonic /nɪ'mɒnɪk/ *adj* of or aiding memory.—*n* a device to aid the memory.—**mnemonically** *adv*.

mnemonics /nɪ'mɒnɪks/ *n sing* a technique of assisting the memory by using formulae to remember things.

Mnemosyne /niː'mɒzɪnɪ/ *n* (*Greek myth*) the goddess of memory.

MO *abbr* = Missouri.

Mo (*chem symbol*) molybdenum.

moa /'moːə/ *n* any one of several extinct species of large, wingless birds of New Zealand.

Moabite /'moːəˌbaɪt/ *adj* pertaining to the ancient kingdom of Moab, now part of Jordan. • *n* an inhabitant of Moab.

moan /moːn/ *n* a low mournful sound as of sorrow or pain. • *vti* to utter a moan; to complain.—**moaner** *n*.—**moaningly** *adv*.

moat /moːt/ *n* a deep ditch surrounding a fortification or castle, *usu* filled with water.

mob /mɒb/ *n* a disorderly or riotous crowd; a contemptuous term for the masses; (*sl*) a gang of criminals. • *vt* (**mobbing, mobbed**) to attack in a disorderly group; to surround.—**mobbish** *adj*.

mobcap /'mɒbkæp/ *n* a plain cap, *usu* surrounded with a frill, worn indoors by women in the 18th century.

mobile /'moːbaɪl/ or /'moːbəl/ *adj* movable, not fixed; easily changing; characterized by ease in change of social status; capable of moving freely and quickly; (*inf*) having transport. • *n* a suspended structure of wood, metal, etc with parts that move in air currents.—**mobility** *n*.

Mobile Command *n* ✚ the Canadian army.

mobilize /'moːbɪˌlaɪz/ *vt* to prepare for action, *esp* war by readying troops for active service; to organize for a particular reason; to put to use.—**mobilization** *n*.

mobocracy /mɒ'bɒkrəsɪ/ *n* (*pl* **mobocracies**) political rule or ascendancy of the mob; a ruling mob.—**mobocrat** *n*.—**mobocratic** *adj*.—**mobocratically** *adv*.

mobster /'mɒbstər/ *n* (*sl*) a gangster.

moccasin /'mɒkəsɪn/ *n* a flat shoe based on Amerindian footwear; any soft, flexible shoe resembling this.

mocha /'moːkə/ *n* a type of coffee, orig from Arabia; a flavouring made from coffee and chocolate.—*also adj*.

mock /mɒk/ *vt* to imitate or ridicule; to behave with scorn; to defy; (*with* **up**) to make a model of. • *n* ridicule; an object of scorn. • *adj* false, sham, counterfeit.—**mocker** *n*.—**mockingly** *adv*.

mockery /'mɒkərɪ/ *n* (*pl* **mockeries**) derision, ridicule, or contempt; imitation, *esp* derisive; someone or something that is mocked; an inadequate person, thing, or action.

mock-heroic *adj* parodying the heroic style of literature or, particularly, poetry, *esp* when the subject matter is unheroic. • *n* a burlesque imitation of an epic poem or of the heroic style in general.—**mock-heroically** *adv*.

mockingbird /'mɒkɪŋˌbɜrd/ *n* a grey American bird with the ability to imitate with exactness the call of other birds.

mockup, mock-up *n* a full-scale working model of a machine, etc.

mod /mɒd/ *n* (*often with* **cap**) a member of a British youth group of the mid-1960s who were highly fashionable clothes and opposed the rockers, another youth group; a member of a revival of this group, in the late 1970s and early 1980s, whose opposition was to skinheads.

mod. *abbr* = moderate, moderato, modern.

modal /'moːdəl/ *adj* of mode or form, not substance; (*gram*) expressing mood; (*philos*) asserting with qualification; (*mus*) of or composed in a mode.—**modality** *n*.—**modally** *adv*.

mode /moːd/ *n* a way of acting, doing or existing; a style or fashion; form; (*mus*) any of the scales used in composition; (*statistics*) the predominant item in a series of items; (*gram*) mood.

model /'mɒdəl/ *n* a pattern; an ideal; a standard worth imitating; a representation on a smaller scale, *usu* three-dimensional; a person who sits for an artist or photographer; a person who displays clothes by wearing them. • *adj* serving as a model; representative of others of the same style. • *vb* (**modelling, modelled** *or* **modeling, modeled**) *vt* (*with* **after, on**) to create by following a model; to display clothes by wearing. • *vi* to serve as a model for an artist, etc.—**modeler, modeller** *n*.

modem /'moːdəm/ *n* a device that links two computers via the telephone network for transmitting data.

moderate /'mɒdərət/ *vti* to make or become moderate; to preside over. • *adj* having reasonable limits; avoiding extremes; mild, calm of medium quality, amount, etc. • *n* a person who holds moderate views.—**moderately** *adv*.—**moderateness** *n*.

moderation /ˌmɒdə'reɪʃən/ *n* moderateness; freedom from excess; equanimity.

moderato /ˌmɒdə'rɒtoː/ *adv* (*mus*) moderately.

moderator /'mɒdəˌreɪtər/ *n* a mediator; (*physics*) a substance that slows the speed of neutrons in a nuclear reactor; (*Presbyterian Church*) a minister who presides at a court, assembly, synod, etc.

modern /'mɒdərn/ *adj* of the present or recent times; up-to-date.—**modernity** *n*.—**modernly** *adv*.

modernism /'mɒdərˌnɪzəm/ *n* modern view, methods or usage; the theory or practice of modern art, literature, etc; (*Christianity*) rationalistic theology.—**modernist** *adj*, *n*.—**modernistic** *adj*.—**modernistically** *adv*.

modernize /'mɒdərˌnaɪz/ *vti* to make or become modern.—**modernization** *n*.

modest /'mɒdəst/ *adj* moderate; having a humble opinion of oneself; unpretentious.—**modestly** *adv*.

modesty /'mɒdəstɪ/ *n* (*pl* **modesties**) the quality or state of being modest; propriety of behaviour or manner; diffidence; moderation.

modicum /'mɒdɪkəm/ *n* (*pl* **modicums, modica**) a small quantity.

modification /ˌmɒdɪfɪ'keɪʃən/ *n* a modifying or being modified; the result of this; a modified form; an adjustment, alteration; (*biol*) a change in an organism caused by environmental factors but not passed on.—**modificator** *n*.—**modificatory, modificative** *adj*.

modifier /'mɒdɪˌfaɪr/ *n* one who or that which modifies; (*gram*) a word, clause or phrase that qualifies or limits the meaning of another word, etc, a qualifier.

modify /'mɒdɪˌfaɪ/ *vt* (**modifying, modified**) to lessen the severity of; to change or alter slightly; (*gram*) to limit in meaning, to qualify.—**modifiable** *adj*.—**modifiability** *n*.

modillion /mə'dɪljən/ *n* (*archit*) an ornamental bracket under a cornice in the Corinthian order.

modiolus /mə'daɪələs/ (*pl* **modioli**) *n* (*anat*) the pillar of the cochlea of the internal ear

modish /'moːdɪʃ/ *adj* fashionable, stylish.—**modishly** *adv*.—**modishness** *n*.

modiste /mɒ'diːst/ *n* a person who makes fashionable dresses or hats.

modulate /'mɒdjuˌleɪt/ or /-dʒəˌleɪt/ *vti* to adjust; to regulate; to vary the pitch, intensity, frequency, etc, of.—**modulator** *n*.—**modulatory** *adj*.

modulation /-ˈleɪʃən/ *n* a modulating or being modulated; a change in pitch or intensity of the voice; (*gram*) inflection, *esp* to change meaning; (*mus*) a transition from one key to another by progression; (*electronics*) the variation of amplitude, frequency or phase of a signal or wave in response to another signal or wave, *esp* in the transfer to carrier waves.

module /ˈmɒdjuːl/ *n* a unit of measurement; a self-contained unit, *esp* in a spacecraft; (*archit*) a semi-diameter of a shaft, etc, used as a standard for regulating other proportions; (*education*) one of a set of learning units making up a course of study.—**modular** *adj*.

modulus /ˈmɒdjʊləs/ *n* (*pl* **moduli**) a quantity expressing the measure of some function or property, *eg* elasticity.

modus operandi /ˈmoːdəsˌɒpəˈrændi/ *n* (*pl* **modi operandi**) a method of operating, procedure.

modus vivendi /ˈmoːdəsvɪˈvɛndi/ *n* (*pl* **modi vivendi**) a compromise, as between two parties in dispute; a way of living.

mofette, moffette /məˈfɛt/ *n* a fissure in an almost extinct volcano from which carbon dioxide and other gases issue; the gases.

mogul, moghul /ˈmoːɡəl/ *n* (*inf*) an important person, a magnate; (*with cap*) a ruler of the former Moghul Empire in India.

mohair /ˈmoːheər/ *n* the long, fine hair of the Angora goat; the silk cloth made from it.

Mohammedan *n, adj* (*offensive*) a former word for Muslim.

Mohave /moːˈhɑːvi/ *n* (*pl* **Mohaves, Mohave**) one of a North American Indian people who occupied the land along the Colorado river.—*also* **Mojave**.

Mohawk /ˈmoːhɒk/ *n* (*pl* **Mohawks, Mohawk**) one of a North American Indian people who occupied the area from the St Lawrence to the Mohawk river. • *n* the language of the Mohawk people.

Mohican /moːˈhiːkən/ *see* **Mahican**.

mohican /moːˈhiːkən/ *n* a hairstyle in which the sides of the head are shaved, leaving a central band of hair, often dyed or in spikes, from the forehead to the nape of the neck.

moidore /ˈmɔɪdɔːr/ *n* an ancient Portuguese gold coin.

moiety /ˈmɔɪəti/ *n* (*pl* **moieties**) one of two parts or shares; a half.

moiré /ˈmɔːreɪ/ or /ˈmwɔːr/ *n* a fabric, *usu* silk, that has a surface pattern suggesting rippling water; such a pattern impressed on a fabric.

moiré effect *n* a pattern created when the same pattern is superimposed on another version of itself.

moist /mɔɪst/ *adj* damp; slightly wet.—**moistly** *adv*.—**moistness** *n*.

moisten /ˈmɔɪsən/ *vti* to make or become moist.—**moistener** *n*.

moisture /ˈmɔɪstʃər/ *n* liquid in a diffused, absorbed, or condensed state.

moisturize /ˈmɔɪstʃəˌraɪz/ *vt* (*skin, air, etc*) to add moisture to.—**moisturizer** *n*.

Mojave /moːˈhɑːvi/ *see* **Mohave**.

moke *n* /moːk/ (*sl*) a boring person; (*Brit*) a donkey; (*Austral*) a horse not of the top class.

molar[1] /ˈmoːlər/ *n* a back tooth, used for grinding food.

molar[2] *adj* of or in the whole mass of matter as distinguished from the properties or motions of atoms or molecules.

molasses /məˈlæsɪz/ or /-sɪz/ *n* (*pl* **molasses**) the thick brown sugar that is produced during the refining of sugar; treacle.

mold[1] /moːld/ *n* a fungus producing a furry growth on the surface of organic matter. • *vi* to become moldy.—*also* **mould**.

mold[2] *n* a hollow form in which something is cast; a pattern; something made in a mold; distinctive character. • *vt* to make in or on a mold; to form, shape, guide.—*also* **mould**.—**moldable** *adj*.—**molder** *n*.

molder /ˈmoːldər/ *vi* to decay to rot, to crumble to dust.

molding /ˈmoːldɪŋ/ *n* anything made in a mould; a shaped strip of wood or plaster, as around the upper walls of a room.—*also* **moulding**.

moldy /ˈmoːldi/ *adj* (**moldier, moldiest**) containing or covered with mould; musty, stale; antiquated; (*sl*) dull, boring.—*also* **mouldy**.—**moldiness** *n*.

mole[1] /moːl/ *n* a spot on the skin, *usu* dark-coloured and raised.

mole[2] *n* a small burrowing insectivore with soft dark fur; a spy within an organization.

mole[3] *n* a large breakwater.

mole[4] *n* the basic SI unit of substance.

molecular /məˈlɛkjʊlər/ *adj* of or inherent in molecules.

molecular biology *n* the branch of biology dealing with the molecular basis of heredity and of protein synthesis.

molecular formula *n* the chemical formula that indicates both the number and type of any atom present in a molecular substance.

molecular weight *n* the total of the atomic weights of all the atoms present in a molecule; the average mass per molecule of any substance relative to one-twelfth the mass of an atom of carbon-12.

molecule /ˈmɒləˌkjuːl/ *n* the simplest unit of a substance, retaining the chemical properties of that substance; a small particle.

molehill /ˈmoːlhɪl/ *n* a mound of earth thrown up by a burrowing mole.

moleskin /-skɪn/ *n* the fur of a mole; a twilled cotton cloth with a soft surface resembling a mole's fur, used for work clothes; (*pl*) trousers made of moleskin.

molest /ˈmɒləst/ *vt* to annoy; to attack or assault, *esp* sexually.—**molestation** *n*.—**molester** *n*.

moll /mɒl/ *adj* (*sl*) a female partner of a thief or other criminal; a prostitute.

mollify /ˈmɒləˌfaɪ/ *vt* (**mollifying, mollified**) to make less severe or violent; to soften.—**mollification** *n*.—**mollifier** *n*.—**mollifyingly** *adv*.

mollusk, mollusc /ˈmɒləsk/ *n* an invertebrate animal *usu* enclosed in a shell, as oysters, etc.—**molluscan, molluskan** *adj, n*.

mollycoddle /ˈmɒliˌkɒdəl/ *vti* to care for someone in an indulgent way; to coddle, pamper. • *n* someone so treated.—**mollycoddler** *n*.

moloch /ˈmoːlɒk/ or /ˈmɒlək/ *n* a spiny Australian lizard with a horned head, found in desert areas; (*with cap*) (*Old Testament*) an ancient Semitic fire god to whom children were offered as a sacrifice.

molt /moːlt/ *vi* to shed hair, skin, horns, etc prior to replacement of new growth. • *n* a moulting.—*also* **moult**.—**molter** *n*.

molten /ˈmoːltən/ *adj* melted by heat.

molto /ˈmoːltoː/ *adj* (*mus*) very (modifying another musical direction).

moly /ˈmoːli/ *n* (*pl* **molies**) (*Greek myth*) a herb with a black root and a white flower with the power of counteracting the spells of Circe.

molybdenum /məˈlɪbdənəm/ *n* a metallic element used in alloys, *esp* strengthening steel.—**molybdous, molybdic** *adj*.

mom /mɒm/ *n* (*inf*) mother.

moment /ˈmoːmənt/ *n* an indefinitely brief period of time; a definite point in time; a brief time of importance.

momenta /moːˈmɛntə/ *see* **momentum**.

momentarily /ˌmoːmənˈtɛrɪli/ *adv* for a short time; in an instant; at any moment.

momentary /ˈmoːmənˌtɛri/ *adj* lasting only for a moment.—**momentariness** *n*.

momentous /moːˈmɛntəs/ *adj* very important.—**momentously** *adv*.—**momentousness** *n*.

momentum /moːˈmɛntəm/ *n* (*pl* **momenta, momentums**) the impetus of a moving object, equal to the product of its mass and its velocity.

momma /ˈmɒmə/ *n* mama.

mommy /ˈmɛmi/ or /ˈmɒmi/ *n* (*pl* **mommies**) (*inf*) mother.

Mon. *abbr* = Monday.

monachism /ˈmɒnəˌkɪzəm/ *n* monasticism; the monastic life or system.—**monachal** *adj*.

monad /ˈmɒnæd/ or /ˈmoː-/ *n* a unit, number one; (*philos*) the ultimate unit of being or evolution in Leibniz's theory; (*chem*) a radical or atom with a valency of one; (*biol*) a single-celled organism.—**monadic, monadical** *adj*.—**monadically** *adv*.

monadelphous /ˌmɒnəˈdɛlfəs/ *adj* (*bot*) having stamens in one bundle of filaments wrapped around the style.

monadism /ˈmɒnæˌdɪzəm/ or /ˈmoː-/ *n* (*philos*) the theory, *esp* as propounded by Leibniz, that the real universe is composed of monads.

monandrous /məˈnædrəs/ *adj* having only one husband or male partner at a time; (*flowers*) having one stamen only; (*plants*) having flowers with only one stamen.

monandry /məˈnædri/ *n* the custom of having only one husband at a time; (*bot*) a being monandrous.

monarch /ˈmɒnərk/ *n* a sovereign who rules by hereditary right; a powerful or dominant thing or person.—**monarchal, monarchic, monarchical** *adj*.—**monarchically** *adv*.

monarchism /ˈmɒnərˌkɪzəm/ *n* the principles of, or devotion to, monarchy.—**monarchist** *n, adj*.—**monarchistic** *adj*.

monarchy /ˈmɒnərki/ n (pl **monarchies**) a government headed by a monarch; a kingdom.

monastery /ˈmɒnəstəri/ n (pl **monasteries**) the residence of a group of monks, or nuns.—**monasterial** adj.

monastic /məˈnæstik/, **monastical** /-əl/ adj of monks or monasteries. • n a monk; a recluse.—**monastically** adv.—**monasticism** n.

Monday /ˈmʌndeɪ/ or /-di/ n the second day of the week.

monecious /məˈniːʃəs/ see **monoecious**.

monetarism /ˈmɒnətəˌrizəm/ n (economics) the theory that control of the money supply is the key to achieving low inflation and economic growth.—**monetarist** n, adj.

monetary adj of the coinage or currency of a country; of or relating to money.—**monetarily** adv.

monetize /ˈmɒnətaɪ/ vt to convert into money; to give a standard of current value to.—**monetization** n.

money /ˈmʌni/ n (pl **moneys, monies**) coins or paper notes authorized by a government as a medium of exchange; property; wealth.

moneychanger n one who changes money into other coinage at fixed rate; a machine that dispenses coins.

moneyed /ˈmʌniːd/ adj rich.—also **monied**.

moneylender n a person who lends money for interest, esp as a business.—**moneylending** n.

monger /ˈmʌŋɡər/ n a dealer.

mongoose /ˈmɒŋɡuːs/ n (pl **mongooses**) a small predatory mammal of Africa and Asia.

mongrel /ˈmʌŋɡrəl/ n an animal or plant of mixed or unknown breed, esp a dog. • adj of mixed breed or origin.—**mongrelism** n.—**mongrelly** adj.

mongrelize /ˈmʌŋɡrəˌlaɪz/ vt to render mongrel.—**mongrelization** n.

monied /ˈmʌniːd/ see **moneyed**.

monies /ˈmʌniːz/ see **money**.

moniker, monicker /ˈmɒnikər/ n (sl) a name; a nickname.

moniliform /məˈniliˌfɔːm/ adj (biol) shaped like a necklace.

monism /ˈmɒnizəm/ or /ˈmoʊn-/ n (philos) the theory that there is only one kind of being and that matter and mind are ultimately identical.—**monist** n, adj.—**monistic** adj.—**monistically** adv.

monition /məˈniʃən/ n an admonition; a formal notice from an ecclesiastical court to an offender; a summons; a warning.

monitor /ˈmɒnitər/ n a student chosen to help the teacher; any device for regulating the performance of a machine, aircraft, etc; a screen for viewing the image being produced by a television camera; a display screen connected to a computer. • vti (TV or radio transmissions, etc) to observe or listen to for political or technical reasons; to watch or check on; to regulate or control, a machine, etc.—**monitorial** adj.

monitory /ˈmɒnitəri/ adj conveying a warning. • n (pl **monitories**) a letter containing an admonition or warning, esp a papal letter.

monk /mʌŋk/ n a male member of a religious order living in a monastery.

monkey /ˈmʌŋki/ n any of the primates except man and the lemurs, esp the smaller, long-tailed primates; a mischievous child; (sl) £500 or $500. • vi (**monkeying, monkeyed**) (inf) to play, trifle, or meddle.

monkey business n (inf) mischief; underhand dealings.

monkey wrench n a large wrench with an adjustable jaw.

monkfish /ˈmʌŋkfiʃ/ n (pl **monkfish, monkfishes**) an angelfish.

monkhood /ˈmʌŋkhʊd/ n the character or condition of a monk; monks collectively.

monkish /ˈmʌŋkiʃ/ adj pertaining to or resembling a monk; monastic.—**monkishly** adv.—**monkishness** n.

monkshood, monk's-hood /ˈmʌŋkshʊd/ n a poisonous plant, aconite.

mono /ˈmɒnoʊ/ adj (inf) monophonic. • n (pl **monos**) (inf) monophonic sound.

mono- /ˈmɒnoʊ/, **mon-** /ˈmɒn/ prefix alone, sole, single.

monobasic /ˌmɒnoʊˈbeɪsɪk/ adj (chem) having one base or atom of a base.

monocarp /ˌmɒnoʊˈkɑːp/ n a monocarpic plant.

monocarpic /ˌmɒnoʊˈkɑːpɪk/, **monocarpous** /-ˈkɑːpəs/ adj (bot) bearing fruit only once.

monochord /ˈmɒnoʊˌkɔːd/ n a one-stringed musical instrument with a sound box for determining musical intervals.

monochromatic /ˌmɒnoʊkrəˈmætɪk/ adj consisting of one colour.—**monochromatically** adv.

monochrome /ˌmɒnoʊˈkroʊm/ n a painting, drawing, or print in a single colour. • adj in one colour or shades of one colour; black and white—**monochromic** adj.

monocle /ˈmɒnoʊkəl/ n a single eyeglass held in place by the face muscles.—**monocled** adj.

monocline /ˈmɒnoʊklaɪn/ n a geological formation in which the strata are tilted one way only.—**monoclinal** adj.

monocotyledon /ˌmɒnoʊˌkɒtɪˈliːdən/ n any plant with one seed leaf and three-part flowers, incl grasses, lilies and orchids.—**monocotyledonous** adj

monocrat /ˈmɒnoʊkræt/ n one who governs alone; an advocate of autocracy or monarchy.—**monocracy** n.

monocular /məˈnɒkjʊlər/ adj pertaining to, for, or with one eye only; adapted for use with one eye.

monodrama /ˈmɒnoʊˌdræmə/ or /-drɒmə/ n a dramatic piece for one actor.—**monodramatic** adj.

monody /ˈmɒnoʊdi/ n (pl **monodies**) in Greek tragedy, a lyrical poem sung by one actor alone; a plaintive poem or song for one voice, a dirge, an elegy; (mus) a composition for one voice, usu accompanied—**monodic, monodical** adj.—**monodist** n.

monoecious /məˈniːʃəs/ adj (bot) having stamens and pistils on the same plant but on different flowers; (zool) hermaphroditic.—also **monecious**.—**monoeciously** adv.

monogamy /məˈnɒɡəmi/ n the practice of being married to only one person at a time.—**monogamist** n.—**monogamous** adj.

monogenesis /ˌmɒnoʊˈdʒenəsɪs/ n derivation from a single cell, resulting in an organism like the adult of the species; asexual reproduction from a single cell; the supposed descent of all organisms from one orig cell; the supposed descent of all human beings from one orig pair.—**monogenous** adj.

monogenetic /-ˈdʒenətɪk/ adj pertaining to or having the property of monogenesis; (animals) born, living and dying on a single host; (rocks) originating from a single source or by a single process.

monogram /ˈmɒnoʊˌɡræm/ n the embroidered or printed initials of one's name on clothing, stationery, etc.—**monogrammed** adj.—**monogrammatic** adj.

monograph /-ˌɡræf/ n a learned paper written on one particular subject. • vt to write such a paper on.—**monographer** n.—**monographic** adj.—**monographically** adv.

monolith /-lɪθ/ n a single large block of stone; any massive, unyielding structure.—**monolithic** adj.—**monolithically** adv.

monologue, monolog /-ˌlɒɡ/ n a long speech; a soliloquy, a skit, etc for one actor only.—**monologuist, monologist** n.

monomania /ˌmɒnoʊˈmeɪniə/ n an irrational obsession with a single subject, object, idea, etc.—**monomaniac** n.—**monomaniacal** adj.

monometallic adj containing only one metal; of monometallism.

monometallism /ˌmɒnoʊˈmetlɪzəm/ n the use of a single metal, often gold or silver, as a standard of currency; the economic system underpinning such a standard.—**monometallist** n.

monomial /məˈnoʊmiəl/ n (math) an expression consisting of one term; (biol) a taxonomic classification consisting of one term.—also adj.

monomorphic /ˌmɒnoʊˈmɔːfɪk/, **monomorphous** /-ˈmɔːfəs/ adj (species) of one type or structure or with parts that have only one type or structure; (individual organism) unchanging in shape throughout its life cycle; (chem) denoting a chemical compound with a single crystalline form.

monopetalous adj (bot) (flowers) having the corolla in one piece; possessing a single petal.

monophobia /ˌmɒnoʊˈfoʊbiə/ n an overwhelming fear of being alone.—**monophobic** adj.

monophonic /ˌmɒnoʊˈfɒnɪk/ adj (sound reproduction) using one channel only for transmission.—**monophonically** adv.

monophthong /ˈmɒnəfˌθɒŋ/ n a simple single vowel sound; two different written vowels pronounced as a single sound.—**monophthongal** adj.

monoplane /ˈmɒnoʊˌpleɪn/ n an aeroplane with a single pair of wings.

monoplegia /ˌmɒnoʊˈpliːdʒə/ or /-dʒiə/ n paralysis affecting one limb or one group of muscles only.—**monoplegic** adj, n.

monopolize /məˈnɒpəˌlaɪz/ vt to get, have, or exploit a monopoly of; to get full control of.—**monopolization** n.—**monopolizer** n.

monopoly /məˈnɒpəli/ n (pl **monopolies**) exclusive control in dealing in a particular commodity or supplying a service; exclusive use or possession; that which is exclusively controlled;

such control granted by a government.—**monopolism** *n.*—**monopolist** *n.*—**monopolistic** *adj.*—**monopolistically** *adv.*

monorail /ˈmɒnəˌreɪl/ *n* a single track railway, often with suspended carriages.

monosepalous /ˌmɒnəˈsɛpələs/ *adj* (*bot*) (*flowers*) having the calyx undivided; possessing a single sepal.

monosodium glutamate /ˌmɒnəˈsoːdiəmˈɡluːtəˌmeɪt/ *n* a chemical additive used to give food a meaty taste.

monospermous /ˌmɒnəˈspɜːməs/, **monospermal** /-ˈspɜːməl/ *adj* (*plants*) one-seeded.

monostich /ˈmɒnəˈstɪk/ *n* a poem in one line.—**monostichic** *adj.*

monosyllabic /ˌmɒnəsɪˈlæbɪk/ *adj* (*word*) having one syllable; characterized by or made up of one syllable; terse; curt.—**monosyllabically** *adv.*

monosyllable /ˈmɒnəˌsɪləbəl/ *n* a word of one syllable.

monotheism /ˈmɒnəˌθiːɪzəm/ *n* the doctrine of or belief in the existence of only one God.—**monotheist** *n.*—**monotheistic** *adj.*—**monotheistically** *adv.*

monotone /ˈmɒnəˌtoːn/ *n* an utterance or musical tone without a change in pitch; a tiresome sameness of style, colour, etc.—**monotonic** *adj.*—**monotonically** *adv.*

monotonous /məˈnɒtənəs/ *adj* unvarying in tone; with dull uniformity, wearisome.—**monotonously** *adv.*—**monotonousness** *n.*

monotony /məˈnɒtəni/ *n* (*pl* **monotonies**) lack of variety; irksome sameness.

monotreme *n* one of a primitive order of Australian egg-laying mammals, with a single vent for digestive, urinary and genital organs.—**monotrematous** *adj.*

Monotype *n* (*trademark*) a hot-metal typesetting machine that casts each character separately; type so cast.

monotype /ˈmɒnəˌtaɪp/ *n* (*print*) one print from a metal or glass plate with a painted image; (*biol*) a genus or species that has only a single type.—**monotypic** *adj.*

monovalent /ˌmɒnəˈveɪlənt/ *adj* (*chem*) with a valency of one; univalent.—**monovalence, monovalency** *n.*

monoxide /məˈnɒksaɪd/ *n* an oxide with one oxygen atom in each molecule.

Monseigneur /mɒsenˈjər/, *Fr.* /mɔ̃sɛˈnjœr/ *n* (*pl* **Messeigneurs**) a French title given to princes, prelates and bishops.

monsieur /məˈsjuː/, *Fr.* /məˈsjø/ *n* (*pl* **messieurs**) the French equivalent of sir in address and of Mr with a name.

Monsignor /mɛnˈsiːnjər/ or /mɒn-/ *n* (*pl* **Monsignors, Monsignore**) (*RC Church*) a title given, *usu* by the Pope, to some prelates or offices.

monsoon /mɒnˈsuːn/ *n* a seasonal wind of southern Asia; the rainy season.

monster /ˈmɒnstər/ *n* any greatly malformed plant or animal; an imaginary beast; a very wicked person; a very large animal or thing. • *adj* very large, huge.

monstrance /ˈmɒnstrəns/ *n* (*RC Church*) a transparent vessel, *usu* set in a gold or silver frame, in which the consecrated Host is carried in procession or exhibited.

monstrosity /mɒnˈstrɒsiti/ *n* (*pl* **monstrosities**) the state or quality of being monstrous; an ugly, unnatural or monstrous thing or person.

monstrous /ˈmɒnstrəs/ *adj* abnormally developed; enormous; horrible.—**monstrously** *adv.*—**monstrousness** *n.*

montage /ˈmɒntɪdʒ/ *n* a rapid sequence of film shots, often superimposed; the art or technique of assembling various elements, *esp* pictures or photographs; such an assemblage.

montane /ˈmɒnteɪn/ *adj* of or inhabiting mountains or mountainous terrain.

monte (bank) /ˈmɒnti/ *n* a gambling card game orig played with dice or cards in Spain.

Montessori method /ˌmɒntəˈsɔːri/ *n* a system of educating very young children, through play, based on free discipline, with each child developing at his own pace.

month /mʌnθ/ *n* any of the twelve divisions of the year; a calendar month.

monthly /ˈmʌnθli/ *adj* continuing for a month; done, happening, payable, etc every month. • *n* a monthly periodical. • *adv* once a month; every month.

monticule /ˈmɒntiˌkjuːl/ *n* a hillock; a small mound resulting from a volcanic eruption.

monument /ˈmɒnjumənt/ *n* an obelisk, statue or building that commemorates a person or an event; an exceptional example.

monumental /ˌmɒnjuˈmɛntəl/ *adj* of, like, or serving as a monument; colossal; lasting.—**monumentality** *n.*—**monumentally** *adv.*

moo /muː/ *n* the long deep sound made by a cow. • *vi* (*cattle*) to low; to make a deep long noise like a cow.

mooch /muːtʃ/ *vt* (*sl*) to wander around aimlessly; (*sl*) to cadge, steal.—**moocher** *n.*

mood /muːd/ *n* a temporary state of mind or temper; a gloomy feeling; a predominant feeling or spirit; (*gram*) that form of a verb indicating mode of action; (*mus*) mode.

moody /ˈmuːdi/ *adj* (**moodier, moodiest**) gloomy; temperamental.—**moodily** *adv.*—**moodiness** *n.*

moon /muːn/ *n* the natural satellite that revolves around the earth and shines by reflected sunlight; any natural satellite of another planet; something shaped like the moon. • *vi* to behave in an idle or abstracted way.

moonbeam /ˈmuːnbiːm/ *n* a ray of moonlight.

mooncalf /-kæf/ *n* (*pl* **mooncalves**) a born fool; an idler; (*arch*) a monster.

moonflower /-flaʊr/ *n* any of a family of climbing or creeping plants with trumpet-shaped flowers that bloom at night; a tropical plant, orig found in Mexico, with white flowers that bloom at night.

moonlight /-laɪt/ *n* the light of the moon. • *vi* (*inf*) to have a secondary (*usu* night-time) job.—**moonlighter** *n.*

moonlit /-lɪt/ *adj* lit by the moon.

moonraker, moonsail *n* (*naut*) a small sail carried above a skysail.

moonshine /-ʃaɪn/ *n* moonlight; (*inf*) nonsense, foolish talk; (*sl*) illegally distilled spirits.

moonshiner /-ˌʃaɪnər/ *n* (*sl*) a distiller of illicit whiskey; a whiskey smuggler.

moonstone /-stoːn/ *n* a translucent yellowish or yellowish-white stone that exhibits pearly blue-tinged reflections, used as a gemstone.

moonstruck /-strʌk/, **moonstricken** /-ˌstrɪkən/ *adj* besotted with love or sentiment; demented.

moonwort /-wərt/ *n* a fern with crescent-shaped fronds, grape fern; honesty.

moony /ˈmuːni/ *adj* (**moonier, mooniest**) of or like the moon; crescent-shaped; round; listless, dreamy; absent-minded.

Moor /mʊr/ or /mɔr/ *n* a North African Muslim of mixed Arab and Berber ancestry.

moor[1] /mʊr/ or /mɔr/ *n* a tract of open wasteland, *usu* covered with heather and often marshy.

moor[2] *vti* (*a ship*) to secure or be secured by cable or anchor.

moorage /ˈmʊrɪdz/ *n* the act of mooring a vessel; a place or charge for mooring.

moorcock /ˈmʊrkɒk/ or /ˈmɔr-/ *n* the male red grouse.

moorfowl /-faʊl/ *n* (*arch*) red grouse collectively.

moorhen /-hɛn/ *n* an aquatic dark-coloured bird with a red bill and a characteristic red mark above the bill, found in ponds and lakes; the female red grouse.

mooring /ˈmʊrɪŋ/ or /ˈmɔr-/ *n* the act of mooring; the place where a ship is moored; (*pl*) the lines, cables, etc by which a ship is moored.

Moorish /ˈmʊrɪʃ/ or /ˈmɔr/ *adj* pertaining to the Moors; denoting a Spanish architectural style of the 13th-16th centuries, one of the distinguishing features of which is the horseshoe arch.

moorland /ˈmʊrlænd/ or /ˈmɔr/ *n* a stretch of moors.

moose /muːs/ *n* (*pl* **moose**) the largest member of the deer family, native to North America.

moose pasture *n* ✷ (*Cdn*) (*sl*) a piece of land that is promoted as having valuable mineral deposits but in fact is worthless.

moot /muːt/ *adj* debatable; hypothetical. • *vt* (**mooting, mooted**) to propose for discussion.

mop /mɒp/ *n* a rag, sponge, etc fixed to a handle for washing floors or dishes; a thick or tangled head of hair. • *vt* (**mopping, mopped**) to wash with a mop.

mope /moːp/ *vi* to be gloomy and apathetic. • *n* a person who mopes, a moper.—**moper** *n.*—**mopey** *adj.*—**mopingly** *adv.*

moped /ˈmoːped/ *n* a light, motor-assisted bicycle.

moppet /ˈmɒpət/ *n* a pet name for a small child, *esp* a girl; (*arch*) a rag doll.

moquette /ˈmɒkət/ *n* a material with short velvety pile used for carpets and upholstery.

MOR *abbr* = middle-of-the-road.

moraine /mə'reɪn/ *n* a mass of earth, stones, etc, deposited by a glacier.—**morainal, morainic** *adj*.

moral /'mɒrəl/ *adj* of or relating to character and human behaviour, particularly as regards right and wrong; virtuous *esp* in sexual conduct; capable of distinguishing right from wrong; probable, although not certain; psychological, emotional. • *n* a moral lesson taught by a fable, event, etc; (*pl*) principles; ethics.

morale /mə'rɑːl/ *n* moral or mental condition with respect to courage, discipline, confidence, etc.

moralism /'mɒrə,lɪzəm/ *n* moralizing; a moral attitude or maxim; the practice of or belief in a system of morals independent of religion.

moralist /'mɒrəlɪst/ *n* a teacher or student of morals; one for whom morality needs no religious sanction; one concerned with the morals of others.—**moralistic** *adj*.—**moralistically** *adv*.

morality /mə'rælɪti/ *n* (*pl* **moralities**) virtue; moral principles; a particular system of moral principles.

morality play *n* a medieval allegorical play.

morality squad *n* ✷ (*Cdn*) a unit of a police force dealing with offences related to prostitution, pornography, drugs, or gambling.

moralize, moralise /'mɒrə,laɪz/ *vt* to explain or interpret morally; to give a moral direction to. • *vi* to make moral pronouncements.—**moralization, moralisation** *n*.—**moralizer, moraliser** *n*.

morally /'mɒrəli/ *adv* in a moral manner, ethically; virtually, practically.

moral philosophy *n* ethics.

Moral Rearmament *n* an international evangelical movement, founded in the US by Frank Buchman (1938), that seeks moral and spiritual revival following conservative Christian principles.—*also* **Buchmanism**.

morass /mə'ræs/ *n* a bog, marsh.

moratorium /,mɒrə'tɔːriəm/ *n* (*pl* **moratoria, moratoriums**) a legally authorized delay in the payment of money due; an authorized delay or suspension of any activity.—**moratory** *adj*.

morbid /'mɔːbɪd/ *adj* diseased, resulting as from a diseased state of mind; gruesome.—**morbidly** *adv*.—**morbidness** *n*.

morbidity /'mɔːbɪdɪti/ *n* the state of being morbid; the relative incidence of disease.

morbific /mɔː'bɪfɪk/ *adj* causing or producing disease.

morceau *Fr.* /mɔːr'so:/ *n* (*pl* **morceaux**) a small piece, a morsel; a short work, *usu* a musical one.

mordacious /mɔː'deɪʃəs/ *adj* biting; sarcastic; cutting.—**mordaciously** *adv*.—**mordacity** *n*.

mordant /'mɔːdənt/ *adj* biting, caustic; corrosive. • *n* a chemical fixative; a corrosive substance.—**mordancy** *n*.—**mordantly** *adv*.

mordent /'mɔːdənt/ *n* (*mus*) a trill created by one note rapidly alternating with another one degree below it, used as an ornament.

more /mɔː/ *adj* (*superl* **most**) greater; further; additional.—*also compar of* **many, much.** • *adv* to a greater extent or degree; again; further.

moreen /mə'riːn/ *or* /mɔː-/ *n* a stout woollen fabric used *esp* for furnishings, often embossed or figured with a watered pattern.

morel[1] /mɒ'rel/ *n* an edible mushroom with a brownish cap.

morel[2] *n* a nightshade, *esp* the black nightshade.

morello /mə'reloː/ *n* (*pl* **morellos**) a small dark-red cherry with a tart flavour.

moreover /mɔːr'oːvər/ *adv* in addition to what has been said before; besides.

mores /'mɔːrz/ *npl* customs so fundamentally established that they have the force of law.

Moresque /mɔː'resk/ *adj* (*archit*) Moorish style. • *n* an example of such decoration or architecture; a design in this style.

morganatic /,mɔːrgə'nætɪk/ *adj* (*marriage*) between a royal person and one of lower rank the children of which are legitimate but neither they nor the morganatic wife or husband share royal rank or property.—**morganatically** *adv*.

morgue /mɔːrg/ *n* a place where the bodies of unknown dead or those dead of unknown causes are temporarily kept prior to burial; a collection of reference materials, *eg* newspaper clippings.

MORI /'mɔːri/ *abbr* = Market and Opinion Research Institute.

moribund /'mɒrɪbʌnd/ *adj* in a dying state; near death.—**moribundity** *n*.

morion /'mɒriˌɒn/ *or n* a 16th-century hat-shaped helmet without beaver or visor.

Mormon /'mɔːmən/ *n* a member of the Church of Latter-Day Saints whose authority is the Bible and the Book of Mormon, revelations to Joseph Smith in 1827.—**Mormonism** *n*.

morn /mɔːn/ *n* (*poet*) dawn, morning; (*Scot*) tomorrow.

mornay /'mɔːneɪ/ *n* a white sauce flavoured with cheese. • *adj* (*eggs, etc*) cooked with this sauce.

morning /'mɔːnɪŋ/ *n* the part of the day from midnight or dawn until noon; the early part of anything. • *adj* of or in the morning.

morning coat *n* a tailcoat, *usu* grey, with a cutaway front.

morning-glory *n* (*pl* **morning-glories**) any of various twining plants with showy blue bell-shaped flowers.

morning sickness *n* a period of nausea and vomiting in the early stages of pregnancy.

morning star *n* a planet, *esp* Venus, rising before the sun.

morning suit *n* a man's formal suit of a morning coat and striped trousers.

morning watch *n* (*naut*) a watch on board ship from 4 am to 8 am.

morocco /mə'rɒkoː/ *n* (*pl* **moroccos**) a fine kind of grained leather of goatskin or sheepskin, used in bookbinding and for shoes.

moron /'mɔːrɒn/ *n* an adult mentally equal to a 8 to 12-year-old child; (*inf*) a very stupid person.—**moronic** *adj*.—**moronically** *adv*.—**moronism, moronity** *n*.

morose /mə'roːs/ *adj* sullen, surly; gloomy.—**morosely** *adv*.—**moroseness** *n*.

morpheme /'mɔːfiːm/ *n* the smallest meaningful unit of language as a base, prefix or suffix.—**morphemic** *adj*.—**morphemically** *adv*.

Morpheus /'mɔːfiəs/ *n* (*Greek myth*) the god of dreams and of sleep.

morphine /'mɔːfiːn/, **morph a** /'mɔːfiə/ *n* an alkaloid derived from opium, used as an anaesthetic and sedative.—**morphinic** *adj*.

morphinism /'mɔːfɪˌnɪzəm/ *n* addiction to morphine; poisoning caused by the excessive use of morphine.

morphogen /'mɔːfəˌdʒen/ *n* that substance in an embryo that determines what the structure will become.

morphology /mɔːr'fɒlədʒi/ *n* a branch of biology dealing with the form and structure of organisms; the study of word formation in a language.—**morphological** *adj*.—**morphologist** *n*.

morris (dance) /'mɒrɪs/ *n* a traditional English dance accompanied by tambourines, bells, castanets, violin, concertina, etc, and *usu* performed by men in costumes representing the Robin Hood legend or other characters from English folklore.

morrow /'mɒroː/ *n* (*arch, poet*) morning; the following day.

morse /mɔːrs/ *n* a jewelled clasp on a cope.

Morse code /mɔːrs/ *n* a code in which letters are represented by dots and dashes or long and short sounds, and are transmitted by visual or audible signals.

morsel /'mɔːsəl/ *n* a small quantity of food; a small piece of anything.

mort[1] /mɔːrt/ *n* a note or notes sounded on a hunting horn to notify a kill.

mort[2] *n* (*dial*) a great amount or number (of).

mort[3] *n* a salmon in its third year.

mortal /'mɔːrtəl/ *adj* subject to death; causing death, fatal; hostile; very intense. • *n* a human being.—**mortally** *adv*.

mortality /mɔːr'tælɪti/ *n* (*pl* **mortalities**) state of being mortal; death on a large scale, as from war; number or frequency of deaths in a given period relative to population.

mortality rate *n* the yearly proportion of deaths to population.—*also* **death rate**.

mortar /'mɔːrtər/ *n* a mixture of cement or lime with sand and water used in building; an artillery piece that fires shells at low velocities and high trajectories; a bowl in which substances are pounded with a pestle.

mortarboard /'mɔːrtərˌbɔːrd/ *n* a small square board for holding mortar; a square black college or university cap with a tassel.

mortgage /'mɔːrgɪdʒ/ *n* a transfer of rights to a piece of property *usu* as security for the payment of a loan or debt that becomes void when the debt is paid • *vt* to make over as a security or pledge; to put an advance claim on.

mortgagee /,mɔːrgɪ'dʒiː/ *n* one to whom a mortgage is made or given.

mortgagor /'mɔːrgɪdʒər/, **mortgager** /-dʒər/ *n* one who grants a mortgage.

mortician /mɔr'tɪʃən/ n a person who manages funerals.

mortification /ˌmɔrtɪfɪ'keɪʃən/ n the act of mortifying; gangrene; (Christianity) subjugation of passions and appetite by abstinence; humiliation; vexation, chagrin caused by something that injures one's pride; (Scots law) a charitable bequest of lands.

mortify /'mɔrtɪˌfaɪ/ vti (**mortifying, mortified**) to subdue by repression or penance; to humiliate or shame; to become gangrenous.—**mortifier** n.—**mortifyingly** adv.

mortise, mortice /'mɔrtɪs/ n a hole in a piece of wood to receive a projection of another piece made to fit.

mortise lock n a lock fitted into a mortise in the frame of a door.

mortmain /'mɔrtmeɪn/ n (law) a tenure of land held by a corporation, ecclesiastical or other, which cannot transfer ownership.

mortuary /'mɔrtʃuˌɛri/ n (pl **mortuaries**) a place of temporary storage for dead bodies.

morula /'mɔrʊlə/ n (pl **morulas, morulae**) the spherical mass of cells produced by the splitting of the ovum in its primary stage.—**morular** adj.

Mosaic /moˈzeɪɪk/, **Mosaical** /-kəl/ adj pertaining to Moses, the lawgiver of the Bible, or to the law, institutions, etc. given through him, or to his writings.

mosaic /moˈzeɪɪk/ n a surface decoration made by inlaying small pieces (of glass, stone, etc) to form figures or patterns; a design made in mosaic. • adj of or made of mosaic. • vt (**mosaicking, mosaicked**) to adorn with or make into mosaic.—**mosaicist** n.

moschatel /'mɒskətəl/ n a plant with a pale-green flower and a musky smell.

Moselle, Mosel /mozəl/ n a German dry white wine from the Moselle valley.

mosey /'moːzi/ vi (inf) (often with **along, on down**) to go, to saunter, to amble.

Moslem /'mɒzləm/ or /'mɒs-/ see **Muslim**.

mosque /mɒsk/ n a place of worship for Muslims.

mosquito /mɒs'kiːtoː/ n (pl **mosquitoes, mosquitos**) a small two-winged bloodsucking insect.

moss /mɒs/ n a very small green plant that grows in clusters on rocks, moist ground, etc.

mossback /'mɒsbæk/ n (sl) a turtle or a crab, lobster, oyster, etc, that is so old that it has moss growing on its back; (inf) an out-of-date or provincial person.

mosstrooper n one of a gang of marauders that ravaged the borderland of England and Scotland in the mid-17th century.

mossy /'mɒsi/ adj (**mossier, mossiest**) overgrown with, or like, moss.—**mossiness** n.

most /moːst/ adj (compar **more**) greatest in number; greatest in amount or degree; in the greatest number of instances.—also superl of **many, much**. • adv in or to the greatest degree or extent. • n the greatest amount or degree; (with pl) the greatest number (of).

-most /moːst/ adj suffix forming a superlative, eg hindmost.

mostly /'moːstli/ adv for the most part; mainly, usually.

mot juste /'moːˌʒʊst/ n (pl **mots justes**) exactly the right word.

mote¹ /moːt/ n a very small particle, a speck (of dust); a mite.

mote² vi (arch) might, must.

motel /moː'tel/ n an hotel for motorists with adjacent parking.

motet /moː'tet/ n (mus) (RC Church) a short sacred vocal composition, an anthem, usu unaccompanied.

moth /mɒθ/ n a four-winged chiefly night-flying insect related to the butterfly.

mothball /'mɒθbɒl/ n a small ball of camphor or naphthalene used to protect stored clothes from moths.

moth-eaten adj eaten into by moths; dilapidated; outmoded.

mother /'mɛðər/ n a female who has given birth to offspring; an origin or source. • adj of or like a mother; native. • vt to be the mother of or a mother to.

motherhood /'mɛðərhʊd/ n the state of being a mother; the qualities of feelings of being a mother; mothers collectively.

mother-in-law n (pl **mothers-in-law**) the mother of one's spouse.

motherland /'mɛðərlænd/ n a person's native land or the country of a person's forebears.

motherly /'mɛðərli/ adj of, proper to a mother; like a mother.—**motherliness** n.

mother-of-pearl n the iridescent lining of the shell of the pearl oyster.

motif /moː'tiːf/ n a recurrent theme in a musical composition — also **motive**.

motile /'moːtaɪl/ adj (biol) able to move without outside aid; exhibiting movement. • n (psychol) a person whose perception of the material world comprises, to a very strong degree, the imagery of movement, esp his own.—**motility** n.

motion /'moːʃən/ n activity, movement; a formal suggestion made in a meeting, law court, or legislative assembly; evacuation of the bowels. • vti to signal or direct by a gesture.

motionless /moːʃənləs/ adj not moving, still.—**motionlessness** n.

motion picture n a film, movie.

motivate /'moːtɪˌveɪt/ vt to supply a motive to; to instigate.—**motivator** n.

motivation /ˌmoːtɪ'veɪʃən/ n a motivating or being motivated; incentive; (psychol) the mental function or instinct that produces, sustains and regulates behaviour in humans and animals.—**motivational** adj.

motive /'moːtɪv/ n something (as a need or desire) that causes a person to act; a motif in music. • adj moving to action; of or relating to motion.—**motiveless** adj.—**motivity** n.

motley /'mɒtli/ adj multicoloured; composed of diverse elements.

motmot /'mɒtmɒt/ n any of various tropical American blue and brownish-green, long-tailed birds similar to the jay, of the same family as the kingfisher.

motor /'moːtər/ n anything that produces motion; a machine for converting electrical energy into mechanical energy; a motor car. • adj producing motion; of or powered by a motor; of, by or for motor vehicles; of or involving muscular movements. • vi to travel by car.

motorbike /'moːtərˌbəɪk/ n a motorcycle.

motorboat /'moːtərˌboːt/ n a boat propelled by an engine or motor.

motorbus /'moːtərˌbəs/ n (pl **motorbuses, motorbusses**) a bus driven by a motor engine.

motorcade /'moːtərˌkeɪd/ n a procession of motor vehicles.

motorcar n a usu four-wheeled vehicle powered by an internal combustion engine.—also **automobile**.

motorcycle /'moːtərsəɪkəl/ n a two-wheeled motor vehicle.—**motorcyclist** n.

motorist /'moːtərɪst/ n a person who drives a car.

motorize /'moːtərəɪz/ vt to equip with a motor; to equip with motor vehicles.—**motorization** n.

motorman /'moːtərˌmæn/ n (pl **motormen**) the driver of a tram or an underground train, or other vehicle powered by electricity; a person who operates a motor.

motor scooter n a small-wheeled motorcycle with an enclosed engine.

motorway /'moːtərˌweɪ/ n a road with controlled access for fast-moving traffic.—also **freeway**.

mottle /'mɒtəl/ vt to mark with coloured blotches or spots, to variegate. • n a pattern of coloured blotches of spots, as on marble; one of the coloured blotches in such a pattern.

mottled /'mɒtəld/ adj marked with blotches of various colours.

motto /'mɒtoː/ n (pl **mottoes, mottos**) a short saying adopted as a maxim or ideal; a slogan on a heraldic crest; a quotation prefixed to a book, etc; verses, etc, in a Christmas cracker.

mouflon, moufflon /'muːflɒn/ n (pl **mouflons, mouflon, moufflons, moufflon**) a wild large-horned sheep with a short fleece, found in Corsica and Sardinia.

Mouillé /muː'jeɪ/ adj softened in sound, palatalized, eg gl in seraglio.

moujik see **muzhik**.

mould /moːld/ see **mold**¹, **mold**².

moulder /'moːldər/ see **molder**.

moulding /-ɪŋ/ see **molding**.

mouldy /'moːldi/ see **moldy**.

moulin /moːlin/ n a deep crack in a glacier through which water and debris drain.

moult /moːlt/ see **molt**.

mound /maʊnd/ n an artificial bank of earth or stones; a heap or bank of earth. • vt to form into a mound.

mount¹ /maʊnt/ n a high hill.

mount² vi to increase. • vt to climb, ascend; to get up on (a horse, platform, etc); to provide with horses; (a jewel) to fix on a support; (a picture) to frame. • n a horse for riding; (for a picture) a backing.—**mountable** adj.—**mounter** n.

mountain /'maʊntən/ n a land mass higher than a hill; a vast number or quantity. • adj of or in mountains.

mountaineer /ˌmauntəˈniːr/ n one who climbs mountains.

mountaineering /-ɪŋ/ n the technique of climbing mountains.

mountainous /ˈmauntənəs/ adj having many mountains; very high; huge.—**mountainously** adv.—**mountainousness** n.

mountebank /ˈmauntəˌbæŋk/ n (formerly) an itinerant quack doctor; a boastful pretender, a charlatan, an impostor.

mounted /ˈmauntəd/ adj seated on horseback or on a bicycle, etc; serving on horseback, as a policeman; placed on a suitable support.

Mountie /ˈmaunti/ n ✦ (Cdn) (inf) a member of the Royal Canadian Mounted Police.

mourn /mɔrn/ vti (someone dead) to grieve for; (something regrettable) to feel or express sorrow for.—**mourner** n.

mournful /ˈmɔrnful/ adj expressing grief or sorrow; causing sorrow.—**mournfully** adv.—**mournfulness** n.

mourning /ˈmɔrnɪŋ/ adj grieving. • n the expression of grief; dark clothes worn by mourners.

mousaka see **moussaka**.

mouse /maus/ n (pl **mice**) a small rodent with a pointed snout, long body and slender tail; a timid person; a hand-held device used to position the cursor and control software on a computer screen.

mouser /-ər/ n an animal that is skilled at catching mice, esp a cat.

moussaka, mousaka /muˈspkə/ n a Greek dish comprising aubergines, minced lamb and tomatoes topped with a cheese or white sauce.

mousse /muːs/ n a chilled dessert made of fruit, eggs, and whipped cream; a similar savoury dish made with meat or fish; a foamy substance applied to the hair to help it keep its style.

mousseline /ˈmuːsliːn/ or /muːsˈliːn/ n a sheer fabric resembling muslin, made of rayon or silk; mousseline sauce.

mousseline sauce n a white sauce to which whipped cream or the white of an egg has been added.

moustache /ˈmʌstæʃ/ or /məˈstæʃ/ see **mustache**.

mousy, mousey /ˈmausi/ adj (**mousier, mousiest**) mouse-like; grey-brown in colour; quiet, stealthy; timid, retiring.—**mousily** adv.—**mousiness** n.

mouth /mauθ/ n (pl **mouths**) the opening in the head through which food is eaten, sound uttered or words spoken; the lips; opening, entrance, as of a bottle, etc. • vt to say, esp insincerely; to form words with the mouth without uttering sound. • vi to utter pompously; to grimace.—**mouther** n.

mouthful /ˈmauθful/ n (pl **mouthfuls**) as much (food) as fills the mouth; a word or phrase that is difficult to say correctly; (sl) a pertinent remark.

mouth organ n a harmonica.

mouthpiece /-piːs/ n the part of a musical instrument placed in the mouth; a person, periodical, etc that expresses the views of others.

mouth-to-mouth resuscitation n a method of artificial respiration in which air is forced into the victim's lungs by blowing into the mouth.

mouthwash /-wɒʃ/ n a flavoured, often antiseptic liquid for rinsing the mouth.

mouthwatering adj appetizing; tasty.

movable, moveable /ˈmuːvəbəl/ adj that may be moved. • npl personal property.—**movably** adv.—**movability** n.

move /muːv/ vt (**moving, moved**) to shift or change place; to set in motion; to rouse the emotions; to put (a motion) formally. • vi to go from one place to another; to walk, to carry oneself; to change place; to evacuate the bowels; to propose a motion as in a meeting; to change residence; (chess, draughts, etc) to change the position of a piece on the board. • n the act of moving; a movement, esp in board games; one's turn to move; a premeditated action.

movement /ˈmuːvmənt/ n act of moving; the moving part of a machine, esp a clock; the policy and activities of a group; a trend, eg in prices; a division of a musical work; tempo.

mover /ˈmuːvər/ n one who moves; (inf) a driving force, an innovator; a proposer of a motion.

movie /ˈmuːvi/ n a cinema film, motion picture; (pl, the showing of a motion picture; the motion-picture medium or industry.

moving /ˈmuːvɪŋ/ adj arousing the emotions; changing position; causing motion.—**movingly** adv.

mow /moː/ vti (**mowing, mowed** pp **mowed** or **mown**) (grass, etc) to cut from with a sickle or lawn mower; (with **down**) to cause to fall like cut grass.—**mower** n.

moxa /ˈmɒksə/ n down obtained from plants, used in Oriental medicine as a counterirritant or for cauterizing by burning on the skin; any plant that yields such down.

mozzarella /ˌmɒtsəˈrɛlə/ or /ˌmɒt-/ n a moist curd cheese noted for its elasticity when melted.

MP abbr = Member of Parliament; Military Police.

mpg abbr = miles per gallon.

mph abbr = miles per hour.

MPP /ˈɛmˈpiːˈpiː/ abbr ✦ (Cdn) = Member of the Provincial Parliament.

Mr /ˈmɪstər/ n (pl **Messrs**) used as a title before a man's name or an office he holds.

MRI abbr = magnetic resonance imaging.

MRM abbr = mechanically removed meat.

Mrs /ˈmɪsɪz/ n (pl **Mrs** or **Mesdames**) used as a title before a married woman's name.

MS abbr = (pl **MSS**) manuscript; multiple sclerosis.

Ms /mɪz/ or /məz/ n the title used before a woman's name instead of Miss or Mrs.

MSc abbr = Master of Science.

MSG abbr = monosodium glutamate.

MT abbr = Montana.

Mt abbr = mount.

Mtl. abbr ✦ = Montreal.

MUC /ˈɛm juːˈsiː/ abbr ✦ = Montreal Urban Community.

much /mʌtʃ/ adj (compar **more**, superl **most**) plenty. • adv considerably; to a great extent.

muchness /ˈmʌtʃnəs/ n (arch) bulk, greatness; **much of a muchness** just about the same.

mucilage /ˈmjuːsɪlɪdʒ/ n an adhesive prepared for use; a sticky substance obtained from some plants.—**mucilaginous** adj.

muck /mʌk/ n moist manure; black earth with decaying matter; mud, dirt, filth. • vt to spread manure; to make dirty; (with **out**) to clear of muck. • vi to move or load muck; (with **about**, **around**) to engage in useless activity.

muckamuck, muckymuck /ˈmʌkəˌmʌk/ n ✦ (inf) an important or self-important person.—also **high muckamuck**.

mucker /ˈmʌkər/ n (mining) a person who clears broken rocks or other waste; (Brit sl) a friend; (US sl) a coarse person.

muckworm n a grub or larva bred in manure or mud; (inf) a skinflint, a hoarder.

mucky /ˈmʌki/ adj (**muckier, muckiest**) of or like muck; muddy; filthy.—**muckily** adv.—**muckiness** n.

mucous /ˈmjuːkəs/ adj slimy, sticky; like mucus.—**mucosity** n.

mucous membrane n the mucus-secreting lining of body cavities.

mucus /ˈmjuːkəs/ n the slimy secretion that keeps mucous membranes moist.

mud /mʌd/ n soft, wet earth. • vt (**muds, mudding, mudded**) to muddy; to throw mud at; to vilify.

muddle /ˈmʌdəl/ vt to confuse; to mix up. • n confusion, mess.

muddleheaded adj silly; confused; absent-minded.—**muddleheadedness** n.

muddy /ˈmʌdi/ adj (**muddier, muddiest**) like or covered with mud; not bright or clear; confused. • vti (**muddying, muddied**) to make or become dirty or unclear.—**muddily** adv.—**muddiness** n.

mudguard /ˈmʌdɡɑrd/ n a screen on a wheel to catch mud splashes.

mudlark n (formerly) a person who worked or dabbled in mud, esp a scavenger on the banks of tidal rivers; (arch sl) a mischievous, poorly dressed child who frequented city streets. (Austral sl) a horse that performs well on wet, muddy ground.

muesli /ˈmjuːzli/ n a mixture of rolled oats, dried fruit, nuts, etc eaten with milk.

muezzin /muːˈɛzɪn/ n a Muslim official who proclaims from the minaret of a mosque the hour of prayer, and summons the faithful to worship.

muff¹ /mʌf/ n a warm soft fur cover for warming the hands.

muff² n a bungling performance; failure to hold a ball when trying to catch it. • vti to bungle.

muffin /ˈmʌfɪn/ n a baked yeast roll.

muffle /ˈmʌfəl/ vt to wrap up for warmth or to hide; (sound) to deaden by wrapping up.

muffler /ˈmʌflər/ n a long scarf; any means of deadening sound; a device for reducing the noise of a vehicle exhaust.

Mufti /ˈmʌfti/ n (pl **Muftis**) an official expounder of Muslim law.

mufti /ˈmʌfti/ n civilian dress worn by a naval or military officer when off duty.

mug /mʌg/ n a cylindrical drinking cup, *usu* of metal or earthenware; its contents; (*sl*) the face; (*sl*) a fool. • *vb* (**mugging, mugged**) *vt* to assault, *usu* with intent to rob.

mugger[1] /'mʌgər/ n a person who assaults with intent to rob.

mugger[2], **muggar, muggur** /'mʌgər/ n a broad-snouted Asian crocodile that lives in marshes and pools.

muggins /'mʌgɪnz/ n (*sl*) an idiot. • *pron* oneself (used deprecatingly).

muggy /'mʌgi/ adj (**muggier, muggiest**) (*weather*) warm, damp and close.—**mugginess** n.

mugwump /'mʌgwʌmp/ n an independent in politics; (*formerly*) a chief, a bigwig.

mujik see **muzhik**.

mukluk /'mʌklʌk/ n ❧ a laced winter boot with a heavy rubber sole and a fabric upper portion, modelled after a traditional Inuit boot.

mulatto /mə'lætoː/ or /-'lɒtoː/, /mjuː-/ n (*pl* **mulattos, mulattoes**) a person with one black parent and one white parent.

mulberry /'mʌl,beri/ or /'mʌlbəri/ n (*pl* **mulberries**) a tree on whose leaves silkworms feed; its berry.

mulch /mʌltʃ/ n loose, organic, strawy dung providing a protective covering around the roots of plants. • *vt* to spread mulch.

mulct /mʌlkt/ *vt* to punish with a fine; to acquire money, etc, by fraud or deception. • n a fine, *esp* for some misdemeanour.

mule[1] /mjuːl/ n the offspring of a male donkey and a female horse; a machine for spinning cotton; an obstinate person; (*sl*) a person used to smuggle drugs.

mule[2] n a slipper without a heel.

muleteer /,mjuːlə'tiːr/ n a mule driver.

muliebrity /,mjuːli'ebrəti/ n (*formal*) womanhood; the qualities of womanhood.

mulish /'mjuːlɪʃ/ adj like a mule; stubborn, intractable, wilful.—**mulishly** adv.—**mulishness** n.

mull[1] /mʌl/ *vti* (*inf*) to ponder (over).

mull[2] *vt* (*wine, etc*) to heat, sweeten and spice.—**mulled** adj.

mullah, mulla /'mʌlə/ or /'mʊlə/ (*formerly*) a Muslim theologian or teacher; a Muslim title of respect.

muller /'mʌlər/ n a flat-bottomed pestle for grinding (drugs, paints) on a slab.

mullet /'mʌlət/ n (*pl* **mullets, mullet**) any of various types of food fish.

mulligatawny /,mʌlɪgə'tɒni/ n a curry-flavoured meat soup.

mullion /'mʌljən/ n an upright bar or division between the panes of a window or the panels of a screen, etc, *esp* in a Gothic arch; a projecting ridge on a rock face. • *vt* to provide with or divide by mullions.

mullock n (*Austral*) a rock containing no gold or from which gold has been extracted, rubbish; (*dial*) disorder.

mult-, multi- /'mʌlti/ *prefix* much, many.

multangular, multiangular adj many-angled.

multeity /mʌl'teɪəti/ n multiplicity.

multicolored, multicoloured /'mʌlti,kʌlərd/ adj many-coloured.

multifarious /,mʌlti'feːriəs/ adj multiform; diversified; of great variety; manifold.—**multifariously** adv.—**multifariousness** n.

multifid /'mʌltifɪd/, **multifidous** /-fɪdəs/ adj (*bot*) cleft into many parts or lobe-like elements.

multifoil /-fɔɪl/ n (*archit*) an ornament with over five leaf-like divisions.—*also adj.*

multiform /-,fɔrm/ adj having many shapes; of many kinds.—**multiformity** n.

multilateral /,mʌlti'lætərəl/ adj having many sides; with several nations or participants.—**multilaterally** adv.

multilingual /-'lɪŋgwəl/ or /-'lɪŋgjuəl/ adj speaking or in more than two languages.—**multilingually** adv.

multimedia n, adj the process of combining computer data, sound and video images to create an environment similar to television.

multimillionaire n a person with two or more millions of money.

multinational /,mʌlti'næʃənəl/ n a business operating in several countries.—*also adj.*

multinomial /,mʌlti'noːmiəl/ n (*math*) an expression that consists of the sum of several terms, a polynomial.—*also adj.*

multiplane /,mʌlti'pleɪn/ n an aeroplane with two or more pairs of wings.

multiple /'mʌltɪpəl/ adj of many parts; manifold; various; complex. • n (*math*) a number exactly divisible by another.

multiple sclerosis n a disease of the nervous system with loss of muscular coordination, etc.

multiplex /'mʌlti,pleks/ adj (*radio, telecommunications*) the use of a single channel of communication to transmit more than one signal; in map-making, the use of three or more cameras so that the end product appears to be rendered in three dimensions; manifold, multiple. • *vi* to transmit messages or send signals in a multiplex system. • *vt* to send (several signals) simultaneously on one frequency.

multipliable /'mʌlti,plaɪəbəl/, **multiplicable** /-,plɪkəbəl/ adj able to be multiplied.

multiplicand /,mʌltɪplɪ'kænd/ n a number to be multiplied by another.

multiplicate /'mʌltɪplɪ,keɪt/ adj (*rare*) consisting of many.

multiplication /,mʌltɪplɪ'keɪʃən/ n the act of multiplying; the process of repeatedly adding a quantity to itself a certain number of times, or any other process which has the same result.—**multiplicational** adj.

multiplicative /'mʌltɪplɪ,keɪtɪv/ adj relating to the mathematical operation of mutiplication; tending to multiply; able to multiply.

multiplicity /,mʌltɪ'plɪsɪti/ n (*pl* **multiplicities**) a great number or variety (of).

multiplier /'mʌlti,plaɪər/ n a thing or person that multiplies; the number by which another is to be multiplied.

multiply /'mʌlti,plaɪ/ *vti* (**multiplying, multiplied**) to increase in number, degree, etc; to find the product (of) by multiplication.

multitude /'mʌlti,tuːd/ or /-,tjuːd/ n a large number (of people).

multitudinous /,mʌlti'tuːdɪnəs/ or /-'tjuːdɪnəs/ adj of a multitude; very many; having innumerable elements.—**multitudinously** adv.—**multitudinousness** n.

mum[1] /mʌm/ n (*inf*) mother.

mum[2] adj silent, not speaking. • n silence. • *vi* (**mumming, mummed**) to act as a mummer.—*also* **mumm**.

mumble /'mʌmbəl/ *vti* to speak indistinctly, mutter. • n a mumbled utterance.—**mumbler** n.—**mumblingly** adv.

mumbo jumbo /,mʌmboː'dʒʌmboː/ n (*pl* **mumbo jumbos**) meaningless ritual, talk, etc.

mumchance /'mʌm,tʃæns/ adj (*arch*) silent; tongue-tied.

mumm see **mum**[2].

mummer /'mʌmər/ n a person who acts in a play without words; an actor.

mummery /'mʌməri/ n (*pl* **mummeries**) performance by mummers; ridiculous ceremonial, pretentious display.

mummify /'mʌmɪ,faɪ/ *vt* (**mummifying, mummified**) to embalm (a body) as a mummy; to shrivel, to desiccate.—**mummification** n.

mummy[1] /'mʌmi/ n (*pl* **mummies**) (*inf*) mother.

mummy[2] n (*pl* **mummies**) a carefully preserved dead body, *esp* an embalmed corpse of ancient Egypt.

mumps /mʌmps/ n *sing* or *pl* an acute contagious virus disease characterized by swelling of the salivary glands.

munch /mʌntʃ/ *vti* to chew steadily.—**muncher** n.

mundane /mʌn'deɪn/ adj routine, everyday; banal; worldly.—**mundanely** adv.

mungo /'mʌŋgoː/ n (*pl* **mungos**) a cheap woollen material made from cloth waste.

municipal /mjuː'nɪsɪpəl/ or /,mjuːnɪ'sɪpəl/ adj of or concerning a city, town, etc or its local government.—**municipally** adv.

municipality /mjuː,nɪsɪ'pæliti/ n (*pl* **municipalities**) a city or town having corporate status and powers of self-government; the governing body of a municipality.

municipalize /mjuː'nɪsɪpə,laɪz/ *vt* to bring under municipal control; to constitute a place as a municipality.—**municipalization** n.

munificent /mjuː'nɪfɪsənt/ adj extremely generous, bountiful.—**munificence** n.—**munificently** adv.

muniment /'mjuːnɪmənt/ n (*rare*) a defence, a fortification; (*pl*) (*law*) deeds, charters, and other papers for proving title to land.

munition /mjuː'nɪʃən/ *vt* to equip with arms. • n (*pl*) war supplies, *esp* weapons and ammunition.

muntjac, muntjak /'mʌntdʒæk/ n any of various small, brown Asian deer with small antlers and a cry similar to that of a dog.

mural /'mjuːrəl/ adj relating to a wall. • n a picture or design painted directly onto a wall.—**muralist** n.

murder /'mʌrdər/ n the intentional and unlawful killing of one person by another; (*inf*) something unusually difficult or dangerous to do or deal with. • *vti* to commit murder (upon), to kill; to mangle, to mar.—**murderer** n.—**murderess** nf.

murderball /'mərdərbɒl/ n ✿ (Cdn) a game in which players attempt to hit their opponents with a large, inflated ball.

murderous /'mərdərəs/ adj capable of or bent on murder; deadly.—**murderously** adv.—**murderousness** n.

murex /'mjʊrəks/ n (pl **murices, murexes**) any of a genus of marine gasteropods, one species of which yields a purple dye used in ancient Greece and Rome.

murine /'mjʊˌraɪn/ adj pertaining to or resembling a mouse or rat; affected, caused or transmitted by rats or mice. • n any animal belonging to the same family as rats and mice.

murk /mərk/ n indistinct gloom, darkness. • adj (arch) dark, obscured by fog or mist.—also **mirk**.

murky /'mərki/ adj (**murkier, murkiest**) dark, gloomy; darkly vague or obscure.—also **mirky**.—**murkily** adv.—**murkiness** n.

murmur /'mərmər/ n a continuous low, indistinct sound; a mumbled complaint; (med) an abnormal sound made by the heart. • vti to make a murmur; to say in a murmur.—**murmurer** n.—**murmurous** adj.

murphy /'mərfi/ n (pl **murphies**) (inf) a potato.

murrain /'mʌrɪn/ n any infectious disease of cattle, such as foot-and-mouth disease; (arch) a plague.

murrhine, murrine /'mɒˌraɪn/ n of or pertaining to an unknown substance (possibly jade or porcelain) used to make delicate pottery in ancient Rome. • n this substance.—also **murra**.

murther /'mərðər/ n (arch) murder.—**murtherer** n.

muscadine /'mʌskədɪn/ or /-ˌdaɪn/ n a type of woody plant that produces a grape used to make wine.

muscat /'mʌskæt/ n any of various types of sweet white grapes used to make wine; muscatel.

muscatel, muscadel /ˌmʌskə'tel/ n a sweet wine made from muscat grapes.

muscle /'mʌsəl/ n fibrous tissue that contracts and relaxes, producing bodily movement; strength; brawn; power. • vi (inf) to force one's way (in).

muscle-bound adj having some of the muscles abnormally enlarged and lacking in elasticity as from too much exercise; inflexible, rigid.

muscovado, muscavado /ˌmʌskə'vɒdoː/ n raw sugar left after the molasses has evaporated from sugar cane.

Muscovite /'mʌskəˌvaɪt/ n a person who lives in, or or ginates from, Moscow; (arch) a Russian. • adj (arch) Russian.

muscovite /'mʌskəˌvaɪt/ n a type of mica often found in granite and sedimentary rocks.

Muscovy (duck) /'mʌskəvi/ n a green-brown duck with white markings and a characteristic red fleshy growth on its beak.—also **musk duck**.

muscular /'mʌskjʊlər/ adj of or done by a muscle; having well-developed muscles; strong, brawny.—**muscularity** n.—**muscularly** adv.

musculature /'mʌskjʊlətʃər/ n the entire system of muscles in a living thing; the system of muscles in an organ or a part of this system.

muse /mjuːz/ vti to ponder, meditate; to be lost in thought. • n a fit of abstraction.—**muser** n.

museum /mjuː'zɪəm/ n a building for exhibiting objects of artistic, historic or scientific interest.

mush /mʌʃ/ n a thick porridge of boiled meal; any thick, soft mass; (inf) sentimentality.

mushroom /'mʌʃruːm/ n a fleshy fungus with a capped stalk, some varieties of which are edible. • vi to gather mushrooms; to spread rapidly, to increase.

mushy /'mʌʃi/ adj (**mushier, mushiest**) soft, pulpy; (st) sentimental, soppy.—**mushily** adv.—**mushiness** n.

music /'mjuːzɪk/ n the art of combining tones into a composition having structure and continuity; vocal or instrumental sounds having rhythm, melody or harmony; an agreeable sound.

musical /'mjuːzɪkəl/ adj of or relating to music or musicians; having the pleasant tonal qualities of music; having an interest in or talent for music. • n a play or film incorporating dialogue, singing and dancing.—**musicality** n.—**musically** adv.

musicale /ˌmjuːzɪ'kæl/ n a musical party.

musical ride n ✿ (Cdn) a display in which police officers demonstrate choreographed movements to music while on horseback.

musician /mjuː'zɪʃən/ n one skilled in music, esp a performer.—**musicianly** adj.—**musicianship** n.

musicology /ˌmjuːzɪ'kɒlədʒi/ n the study of the history, forms, etc of music.—**musicological** adj.—**musicologist** n.

musing /'mjuːzɪŋ/ adj meditative; lost in thought.—**musingly** adv.

musk /mʌsk/ n an animal secretion with a strong odour, used in perfumes; the odour of musk; a plant with a similar odour.

musk duck see Muscovy.

muskeg /'mʌskeg/ n ✿ a swamp or bog in northern North America, consisting of water-saturated vegetation, often covered with a layer of mosses.

muskellunge /'mʌskəˌlʌndʒ/ n (pl **muskellunges, muskellunge**) a large North American game fish similar to the pike.

musket /'mʌskət/ n a long-barrelled, smoothbore shoulder gun formerly used by infantrymen.

musketeer /ˌmʌskə'tɪːr/ n (formerly) a soldier armed with a musket.

musketry /'mʌskətri/ n small-arm fire; practice in this; muskets or musketeers collectively.

muskmelon /'mʌskmelən/ ✿ any of several varieties of widely cultivated melon with a netted or ribbed skin and sweet light-coloured or green flesh and a musky smell; any one of several types of melon related to the honeydew and cantaloupe.

muskrat /'mʌskræt/ n (pl **muskrats, muskrat**) a large North American aquatic rodent, related to the vole, that emits a musky secretion; the fur from this.—also **musquash**.

musky /'mʌski/ adj (**muskier, muskiest**) like or smelling of musk; sweet-smelling.—**muskiness** n.

Muslim /'mʌzlɪm/ or /-ləm/ n an adherent of Islam. • adj of Islam, its adherents and culture.—also **Moslem**.

muslin /'mʌzlɪn/ n a fine cotton cloth.

musquash /'mʌskwɒʃ/ n the fur of the muskrat; the muskrat.

muss /mʌs/ vt (often with **up**) (inf) to disarrange, to rumple. • n a state of disorder.

mussel /'mʌsəl/ n an edible marine bivalve shellfish.

must[1] /mʌst/ aux vb expressing: necessity; probability; certainty. • n (inf) something that must be done, had, etc.

must[2] n newly pressed grape juice, unfermented or partially fermented wine; the pulp and skin of crushed grapes.

must[3] see musth.

must[4] see musty.

mustache n the hair on the upper lip.—also **moustache**.

mustachio /mə'stæʃɪoː/ n (pl **mustachios**) (often pl) a moustache, usu bushy or shaped.

mustang /'mʌstæŋ/ n a small hardy semi-wild horse of the American prairies.

mustard /'mʌstərd/ n the powdered seeds of the mustard plant used as a condiment; a brownish-yellow colour; (sl) zest.

muster /'mʌstər/ vt to assemble or call together, as troops for inspection or duty; to gather. • vi to be assembled, as troops. • n gathering; review; assembly.

musth, must /mʌst/ n a state of sexual frenzy in the males of elephants and certain other large mammals. • adj denoting an animal in musth.

musty /'mʌsti/ adj (**mustier, mustiest**) mouldy, damp; stale.—**mustily** adv.—**mustiness, must** n.

mutable /'mjuːtəbəl/ adj able or tending to change or be changed; fickle, inconstant.—**mutability** n.—**mutably** adv.

mutant /'mjuːtənt/ n a mutation; an organism whose structure has undergone mutation • adj mutating.

mutate /mjuː'teɪt/ vti to experience or cause to experience change or alteration.

mutation /mjuː'teɪʃən/ n the act or process of mutating; alteration; (biol) a sudden change in some inheritable characteristic of a species; (linguistics) a change in a vowel sound when assimilated with another, esp an umlaut.—**mutational** adj.

mutatis /mjuː'tɑːtɪs/, **mutandis** /mjuː'tændɪs/ (Latin) with the necessary changes.

mute /mjuːt/ adj silent; dumb; (colour) subdued. • n a person who is unable to speak; a device that softens the sound of a musical instrument. • vt to lessen the sound of a musical instrument.—**mutely** adv.—**muteness** n.

mutilate /'mjuːtɪˌleɪt/ vt to maim; to damage by removing an essential part of.—**mutilation** n.—**mutilative** adj.—**mutilator** n.

mutineer /ˌmjuːtɪ'nɪːr/ n a person who takes part in a mutiny.

mutinous /'mjuːtɪnəs/ adj threatening mutiny, rebellious; taking part in a mutiny.—**mutinously** adv.

mutiny /'mjuːtɪni/ vi (**mutinying, mutinied**) to revolt against authority, esp in military service. • n (pl **mutinies**) a rebellion against authority, esp by soldiers and sailors against officers.

mutism /'mjuːtɪzəm/ n the inability to speak; dumbness; silence; (*psychiatry*) a state in which a person remains silent although there is no physical cause for this.

mutt /mʌt/ n (*sl*) a fool; a mongrel dog.

mutter /'mʌtər/ vti to utter in a low tone or indistinctly; to grumble.—**mutterer** n.—**mutteringly** adv.

mutton /'mʌtən/ n the edible flesh of sheep.

muttonchops n whiskers on the side of the face, narrow at the top, broad at the bottom.

mutual /'mjuːtʃʊəl/ adj given and received in equal amount; having the same feelings one for the other; shared in common.—**mutuality** n.—**mutually** adv.

mutule /'mjuːtʃuːl/ n (*archit*) a projecting block under the corona of the Doric cornice.

muzhik /'muːʒɪk/ n a peasant in pre-Revolutionary Russia.—*also* **mujik, moujik.**

muzz /mʌz/ vt (*inf*) to make (anything) muzzy.

muzzle /'mʌzəl/ n the projecting nose or mouth of an animal; a strap fitted over the jaws to prevent biting; the open end of a gun barrel. • vt to put a muzzle on; to silence or gag.—**muzzler** n.

muzzy /'mʌzi/ adj (**muzzier, muzziest**) confused, dazed; dizzy; blurred; dull.—**muzzily** adv.—**muzziness** n.

MVA abbr ✱ = market value assessment (for purposes of property taxes).

MW abbr = medium wave; megawatt.

Mx abbr = maxwell.

my /maɪ/ poss adj of or belonging to me.

myalgia /maɪˈældʒə/ or /-dʒɪə/ n pain, stiffness or cramp in the voluntary muscles or in one muscle.

myalgic encephalomyelitis n a viral condition affecting the nervous system, characterized by fatigue and muscle pains.—*also* **post-viral syndrome.**

mycelium /maɪˈsiːliəm/ n (pl **mycelia**) a cellular spawn of fungi.

mycetoma /ˌmaɪsəˌtoːmə/ n (pl **mycetomas, mycetomata**) a fungoid disease, usu of feet, often caused by a wound.

mycology /maɪˈkɒlədʒi/ n the science of fungi or mushrooms; the fungi found in a particular area.—**mycologist** n.

mycosis /maɪˈkoːsɪs/ n (pl **mycoses**) the presence of, or a disease caused by, a parasitic fungus.

mydriasis /mɪˈdraɪəsɪs/ n excessive dilatation of the pupil of the eye.

mydriatic /-tɪk/ adj causing mydriasis. • n a drug that induces mydriasis.

myelitis /maɪəˈlaɪtɪs/ n inflammation of the spinal cord or of bone marrow.

myna (bird) /'maɪnə/ n any of several Asian birds resembling the starling, some species of which can imitate speech.—*also* **mina (bird).**

Mynheer /'maɪˌniːr/ n a Dutch title used before a name, as "Mister" as a term of respect.

myocarditis /ˌmaɪoːkɑːrˈdaɪtɪs/ n an inflammation of the myocardium.

myocardium /ˌmaɪoːˈkɑːrdiəm/ n (pl **myocardia**) the muscular parts of the heart.—**myocardial** adj.

myology /maɪˈɒlədʒi/ n a branch of medicine concerned with studying the muscles or the diseases affecting them.

myope /maɪˈoːp/ n a short-sighted person.

myopia /maɪˈoːpiə/ n short-sightedness.—**myopic** adj.—**myopically** adv.

myosis see **miosis.**

myosotis, myosote /ˌmaɪəˈsoːtɪs/ n any of various small plants with blue, pink, or white flowers, incl the forget-me-not.

myriad /'mɪriəd/ n a great number of persons or things. • adj innumerable.

myriapod /'mɪriəˌpɒd/ n an arthropod with many legs and a segmented body, incl millipedes and centipedes.—**myriapodan** adj, n.—**myriapodous** adj.

myrica /'maɪrɪkə/ n the root bark of the candleberry or wax myrtle.

myrmecology /'maɪrmeˌkɒlədʒi/ or /'mɪr-/ n the scientific study of ants.—**myrmecological** adj.—**myrmecologist** n.

myrmecophagous /'maɪrmeˌkɒfəgəs/ adj feeding on ants; (*jaws, etc*) adapted for eating ants.

Myrmidon /'mɜːrmɪdən/ n (pl **Myrmidons, Myrmidones**) (*Greek myth*) one of a tribe of Thracian warriors formed by Zeus from an anthill who accompanied Achilles to the Trojan war; a brutal, unprincipled or unquestioning follower or subordinate.—*also* adj.

myrobalan /maɪˈrɒbələn/ n any of several tropical trees containing tannin and bearing a fruit that when dried was used medicinally and in dyeing and tanning; the dye from such a fruit.

myrrh /mɜːr/ n a fragrant gum resin used in perfume, incense, etc.

myrtaceous /maɪrˈteɪʃəs/ adj of the myrtle family, incl eucalyptus, clove and guava, with leaves that secrete oil.

myrtle /'mɜːrtəl/ n an evergreen shrub with fragrant leaves; a trailing periwinkle.

myself /maɪˈsɛlf/ pron emphatic and reflexive form of I; in my normal state.

mystagogue /'mɪstəˌgɒg/ n an initiator into or interpreter of mysteries—**mystagogic** adj.—**mystagogy** n.

mysterious /mɪˈstiːriəs/ adj difficult to understand or explain, obscure; delighting in mystery.—**mysteriously** adv.—**mysteriousness** n.

mystery /'mɪstəri/ n (pl **mysteries**) something unexplained and secret; a story about a secret crime, etc; secrecy.

mystic /'mɪstɪk/ n one who seeks direct knowledge of God or spiritual truths by self-surrender. • adj mystical.

mystical /-kəl/ adj having a meaning beyond normal human understanding; magical.—**mystically** adv.

mysticism /-ˌsɪzəm/ n the beliefs or practices of a mystic; belief in a reality accessible by intuition, not the intellect; obscurity of thought or doctrine.

mystify /'mɪstɪˌfaɪ/ vt (**mystifying, mystified**) to puzzle, bewilder, to confuse.—**mystification** n.—**mistifier** n.—**mistifyingly** adv.

myth /mɪθ/ n a fable; a fictitious event; a traditional story of gods and heroes, taken to be true.—**mythic** adj.

mythical /'mɪθɪkəl/ adj imaginary, unreal, untrue; having to do with myths, mythic.—**mythically** adv.

mythicize /'mɪθɪˌsaɪz/ vt to treat as myth; to interpret mythically; to turn (something) into myth.

mythologist /mɪˈθɒləˌdʒɪst/ n a student of myths; a writer of myths.

mythology /mɪˈθɒlədʒi/ n (pl **mythologies**) myths collectively; the study of myths.—**mythological** adj.

mythopoeic /ˌmɪθəpoːˈɛtɪk/ adj producing or creating myths.—**mythopoeia, mythopoeisis** n.

myxedema, myxoedema /ˌmɪksəˈdiːmə/ n an illness leading to physical and mental degeneration due to underactivity of the thyroid gland and thus severe thyroxine deficiency

myxomycete /ˌmɪksoːmaɪˈsiːt/ n any of various organisms forming a network of creamy filaments on decaying wood, leaves, etc, and displaying characteristics of both plants and animals.

N

N (*chem symbol*) nitrogen. • *abbr* = North.

N, n /ɛn/ *n* the 14th letter of the English alphabet; an indefinite number.

n/a *abbr* (*in commerce*) = no account.

NA *abbr* = North America.

Na (*chem symbol*) sodium.

nab /næb/ *vt* (**nabbing, nabbed**) (*sl*) to catch, arrest.

nabob /'neɪbɒb/ *n* in India, a deputy or administrator under the Mogul Empire; one who has amassed wealth in India; a very wealthy man.

nacelle /nə'sɛl/ *n* the car of an aircraft.

nacho /'nɒtʃoː/ or /'nætʃoː/ *n* a Mexican snack consisting of a tortilla chip often served grilled with melted cheese, chilli, etc.

nacre /'neɪkər/ *n* mother-of-pearl; the shellfish that yields it.

nacreous /'neɪkrɪəs/ *adj* having an iridescent lustre; resembling mother of pearl.

nadir /'neɪdiːr/ or /-dər/, /'næd-/ *n* the point opposite the zenith; the lowest point; the depths of despair.

naevus /'niːvəs/ *see* **nevus**.

NAFTA /'næftə/ *abbr* ✤ = North American Free Trade Agreement.

nag[1] /næg/ *vti* (**nagging, nagged**) to scold constantly; to harass; to be felt persistently. • *n* a person who nags.

nag[2] *n* (*inf*) a horse.

Naga /'nɒgə/ *n* (*pl* **Nagas, Naga**) (*Hindu myth*) a deified serpent, *esp* the cobra; a member of the Naga tribes; a class of mendicant Hindus. • *adj* pertaining to an ancient race who invaded India about the 6th century BC, or to certain Burmese border tribes.

nagana /nə'gɒnə/ *n* a disease caused by the tsetse-fly.

Nagari /'nɒgəri/ *n* the name of the Sanskrit alphabet.

nagelflue /'næɡəl,fluː/ *n* a peculiar alpine conglomerate rock, interspersed with nail-like pebbles.

nagor /'næɡɔr/ *n* a Senegal antelope.

Nahum /'neɪhəm/ *n* one of the prophetical books of the Old Testament.

naiad /'naɪæd/ *n* (*pl* **naiads, naiades**) a water nymph; (*pl*) an order of aquatic plants; a family of freshwater bivalves.

naiant /'neɪənt/ *adj* (*her*) representing fishes swimming in a horizontal position.

naif, naïf /nɒ'iːf/ *adj* naive.

nail /neɪl/ *n* a horny plate covering the end of a human finger or toe; a thin pointed metal spike for driving into wood as a fastening or hanging device. • *vt* to fasten with nails; to fix, secure; (*inf*) to catch or hit; (*inf*) to arrest.

nailfile *n* a small metal file or strip of cardboard coated with emery used for trimming and shaping the nails.

nail polish *n* a lacquer for giving a clear or coloured shiny surface to nails.

nainsook /'neɪnsʊk/ *n* a kind of closely woven muslin originally Indian.

naissant /'neɪzənt/ *adj* (*her*) issuing forth or rising from some ordinary, and showing only the foreparts of the body.

naive, naïve /naɪ'iːv/ *adj* inexperienced; unsophisticated; (*argument*) simple.—**naively, naïvely** *adv*.

naiveté, naïveté /naɪ,iːvə'teɪ/ or /naɪ'iːvəti/, **naivety** *n* natural, unaffected simplicity or ingenuousness.

naked /'neɪkəd/ *adj* bare, without clothes; without a covering; without addition or ornament; (*eye*) without optical aid.—**nakedness** *n*.

namby-pamby /,næmbi'pæmbi/ *adj* weakly sentimental or affectedly pretty or fine. • *n* (*pl* **namby-pambies**) an affected person.

name /neɪm/ *n* a word or term by which a person or thing is called; a title; reputation; authority. • *vt* to give a name to; to call by name; to designate; to appoint to an office; (*a date, price, etc*) to specify.

name-calling /-,kɔlɪŋ/ *n* verbal abuse, *esp* in place of reasoned debate.

name-dropping /-,drɒpɪŋ/ *n* the practice of mentioning the names of famous or important people as if they were friends, in order to impress others.—**name-dropper** *n*.

nameless /'neɪmləs/ *adj* without a name; obscure; anonymous; unnamed; indefinable; too distressing or horrifying to be described.

namely /'neɪmli/ *adv* that is to say.

nameplate /'neɪmpleɪt/ *n* a small plate on a door of a room, house, etc displaying the name of the occupant.

namesake /'neɪmseɪk/ *n* a person or thing with the same name as another.

Nanaimo bar *n* ✤ (*Cdn*) a piece of confectionary with a crust of chocolate and cookie crumbs topped by a creamy layer and a chocolate glaze.

nan bread, naan bread *n* a type of slightly leavened Indian bread in a flattened oval shape.

nankeen, nankin /næŋ'kiːn/ or /næn-/ *n* a buff-coloured cotton cloth, originally from China.

nanny /'næni/ *n* (*pl* **nannies**) a child's nurse.

nannyberry /'næniberi/ *n* ✤ a large shrub of northwest North America with dark blue edible fruit.

nanny goat *n* a female domestic goat.

nano- /'nænoː/ or /'neɪnoː/ *prefix* one thousand millionth (10-9) part of, *eg nanosecond*.

nanosecond (ns) *n* one billionth of a second.

nap[1] /næp/ *n* a short sleep, doze. • *vi* (**napping, napped**) to take a nap.

nap[2] *n* a hairy surface on cloth or leather; such a surface.

napalm /'neɪpɒm/ *n* a substance added to petrol to form a jelly-like compound used in firebombs and flame-throwers. • *vt* to attack or burn with napalm.

nape /neɪp/ *n* the back of the neck.

napery /'neɪpəri/ *n* household linen, *esp* for the table.

naphtha /'næpθə/ or /'næf-/ *n* a clear, volatile, inflammable bituminous liquid hydrocarbon exuding from the earth or distilled from coal tar, etc; rock oil.

naphthalene /'næfθə,liːn/ *n* a white crystalline hydrocarbon distilled from coal tar, used in making dyes, explosives and in mothballs.

napiform /'neɪpə,fɔrm/ *adj* turnip-shaped.

napkin /'næpkɪn/ *n* a square of cloth or paper for wiping fingers or mouth or protecting clothes at table, a serviette.

napoleon /nə'poːliən/ *n* a gold coin formerly current in France, value 20 francs.

Napoleonic /nə,poːli'ɒnɪk/ *adj* of or like Emperor Napoleon I.

nappy[1] /'næpi/ *adj* (**nappier nappiest**) covered with nap or pile.

nappy[2] *n* (*pl* **nappies**) a diaper.

narceine /'nɑrsiːn/ or /-ɪn/ *n* an alkaloid obtained from opium and used as a sedative.

narcissism /'nɑrsɪ,sɪzəm/ *n* excessive interest in one's own body or self.—**narcissistic** *adj*.

narcissus /nɑr'sɪsəs/ *n* (*pl* **narcissi, narcissuses**) a spring-flowering bulb plant, *esp* the daffodil.

narco- /nɑrkoː/ *prefix* indicating torpor or narcotics.

narcodollars *npl* (*sl*) US dollars earned by a country by the export of illegal drugs.

narcosis /nɑr'koːsɪs/ *n* (*pl* **narcoses**) a state of unconsciousness or drowsiness produced by narcotics.

narcotic /nɑr'kɒtɪk/ *adj* inducing sleep. • *n* a drug, often addictive, used to relieve pain and induce sleep.

narcotism /-ɪzəm/ *n* a morbid dependence on narcotics.

narcotize /'nɑrkə,taɪz/ *vt* to use a narcotic upon.—**narcotization** *n*.

nard /nɑrd/ *n* spikenard, an aromatic plant; an aromatic unguent prepared from it.

nardoo /nɑr'duː/ *n* a genus of Australian acotyledonous aquatic plants, Australian pillwort, the spore cases of which are used as bread.

narghile /'nɑrɡəli/ *n* a small hookah pipe.

narrate /'nereɪt/ or /nə'reɪt/ *vt* (*a story*) to tell, relate; to give an account of; (*film, TV*) to provide a spoken commentary for.

narration /nə'reɪʃən/ *n* the act of narrating; a statement, written or verbal.

narrative /'nɒrətɪv/ n a spoken or written account of a sequence of events, experiences, etc; the art or process of narration.—*also adj.*

narrator /'nɛrˌeɪtər/ or /nə'reɪt-/ n one who narrates.

narrow /'nɛroː/ or /'nær-/ adj small in width; limited; with little margin; (*views*) prejudiced or bigoted. • n (*usu pl*) the narrow part of a pass, street, or channel. • *vti* to make or grow narrow; to decrease; to contract.—**narrowly** *adv.*—**narrowness** n.

narrow gauge adj denoting the distance of less than standard gauge (4 feet, 8.5 inches/1.44 metres) between rail metals.

narrow-minded /'nɛroː'maɪndɪd/ or /'nær-/ adj prejudiced, bigoted; illiberal.—**narrow-mindedness** n.

narthex /'nɑrθeks/ n in Early Christian churches the western portico, railed off for catechumens and penitents.

narwhal /'nɑrwəl/ n an Arctic whale, the male of which has a long spiral tusk.

nary /'neri/ = never a, ne'er a.

NASA /'næsɒ/ or /'næsə/ abbr = National Aeronautics and Space Administration.

nasal /'neɪzəl/ adj of the nose; sounded through the nose. • n a sound made through the nose.—**nasally** adv.

nascent /'neɪsənt/ or /'næs-/ adj just starting to grow or develop.

naseberry /'neɪzbɛri/ n (pl **naseberries**) sapodilla plum tree.

naso- /'neɪzoː/ prefix nose.

nasturtium /nə'stɜrʃəm/ n an ornamental garden plant with bright flowers, a pungent odour, and edible leaves.

nasty /'næsti/ adj (**nastier, nastiest**) unpleasant; offensive; ill-natured; disagreeable; (*problem*) hard to deal with; (*illness*) serious or dangerous.—**nastily** adv.—**nastiness** n.

Nat. abbr = national; native; natural.

natal /'neɪtəl/ adj pertaining to one's birth or birthday; indigenous.—**natality** n.

natant /'neɪtɒnt/ adj swimming; (*her*) (*fish*) floating on the surface.

natation /nə'teɪʃən/ n the act or art of swimming.—**natational** adj.

natatorial /ˌneɪtə'tɔriəl/, **natatory** adj swimming or adapted for swimming.

nates /'neɪtiːz/ npl (*sing* **natis**) the buttocks.

nation /'neɪʃən/ n people of common territory, descent, culture, language, or history; people united under a single government.

national /'næʃnəl/ adj of a nation; common to a whole nation, general. • n a citizen or subject of a specific country.—**nationally** adv.

national anthem n a patriotic song or hymn adopted officially by a nation for ceremonial and public occasions.

national debt n the total money currently on loan to the government of a nation.

National Guard n in US, state militia that can be called into federal service.

nationalism /'næʃnəˌlɪzəm/ n patriotic sentiments, principles, etc; a policy of national independence or self-government; fanatical patriotism, chauvinism.—**nationalist** n.—**nationalistic** adj.

nationality /ˌnæʃə'næliti/ n (pl **nationalities**) the status of belonging to a nation by birth or naturalization; a nation or national group.

nationalize /'næʃnəˌlaɪz/ vt to make national; to convert into public or government property.—**nationalization** n.

national park n an area designated by a government as of important scenic, historical, or environmental value.

nation-state n ✦ an independent state, most of whose citizens have a common history and culture.

native /'neɪtɪv/ adj inborn; natural to a person; innate; (*language, etc*) of one's place of birth; relating to the indigenous inhabitants of a country or area; occurring naturally. • n a person born in the place indicated; a local inhabitant; an indigenous plant or animal; an indigenous inhabitant, esp a non-White under colonial rule.

Native American n a member of an Indian people in the United States. • adj of or pertaining to such a people or community.

nativism /'neɪtɪˌvɪzəm/ n (*philos*) the doctrine of innate ideas; in US, the advocacy of the claim of native as opposed to that of naturalized Americans.—**nativist** adj, n.—**nativistic** adj.

nativity /nə'tɪvɪti/ n (pl **nativities**) birth; a horoscope at the time of one's birth; (*with cap*) the birth of Christ.

NATO /'neɪtoː/ abbr = North Atlantic Treaty Organization.

natrolite /'nætrəˌlaɪt/ or /'neɪtrə-/ n a hydrated silicate of aluminium and soda.

natron /'neɪtrɒn/ or /-trən/ n a native carbonate of soda.

natter /'nætər/ vi (*inf*) to chat, talk aimlessly.—*also n.*

natty /'næti/ adj (**nattier, nattiest**) tidy, neat, smart.—**nattily** adv.—**nattiness** n.

natural /'nætʃərəl/ adj of or produced by nature; not artificial; innate, not acquired; true to nature; lifelike; normal; at ease; (*mus*) not flat or sharp. • n (*inf*) a person or thing considered to have a natural aptitude (for) or to be an obvious choice (for); (*inf*) a certainty; (*mus*) a natural note or a sign indicating one.—**naturalness** n.

natural childbirth n giving birth using techniques of relaxation, controlled breathing, etc rather than with anaesthetics.

natural gas n gas trapped in the earth's crust, a combustible mixture of methane and hydrocarbons extracted for fuel.

natural history n the study of nature, esp the animal, mineral, and vegetable world.

naturalism /'nætʃərəˌlɪzəm/ or /'nætʃrə-/ n (*art, literature*) the theory or practice of describing nature, character, etc in realistic detail; (*philos*) a theory of the world based on scientific as opposed to spiritual or supernatural explanations.—**naturalistic** adj.

naturalist /'nætʃərəlɪst/ or /'nætʃrə-/ n a person who studies natural history; a person who advocates or practises naturalism.

naturalization /nætʃərəlaɪ'zeɪʃən/ n the act of investing a foreigner with the rights and privileges of a natural-born citizen.

naturalize /'nætʃərəˌlaɪz/ or /'nætʃrə-/ vt to confer citizenship upon (a person of foreign birth); (*plants*) to become established in a different climate. • vi to become established as if native.

natural law n law based on innate moral sense.

naturally /'nætʃərəli/ or /'nætʃrə-/ adv in a natural manner, by nature; of course.

natural number n any of the whole numbers starting with 1.

natural philosophy n physics.

natural resource n a naturally occurring source of wealth as in land, oil, coal, water power, etc.

natural science n the study of material things.

natural selection n the principle that evolution is determined by the survival of the fittest.

nature /'neɪtʃər/ n the phenomena of physical life not dominated by man; the entire material world as a whole, or forces observable in it; the essential character of anything; the innate character of a person, temperament; kind, class; vital force or functions; natural scenery.

nature worship n the worship of the deified forces of nature.

naught /nɒt/ see **nought**.

naughty /'nɒti/ adj (**naughtier, naughtiest**) mischievous or disobedient; titillating.—**naughtily** adv.—**naughtiness** n.

naumachia /nɔ'meɪkiə/, **naumachy** /'nɔməki/ n (pl **naumachias** or **naumachiae, naumachies**) a sea fight; a show representing a sea fight.

nausea /'nɒziə/ n a desire to vomit; disgust.

nauseate /'nɒziˌeɪt/ vti to arouse feelings of disgust; to feel nausea or revulsion.—**nauseating** adj.

nauseous /'nɒʃəs/ or /'nɒziəs/ adj causing nausea; disgusting.—**nauseously** adv.—**nauseousness** n.

nautch /nɒtʃ/ n in India, a dance performed by girls; a dancing exhibition.

nautical /'nɒtɪkəl/ adj of ships, sailors, or navigation.

nautically /-li/ adv in a nautical manner.

nautical mile n an international unit of measure for air and sea navigation equal to 6,075 feet (1.85 km).

nautilus /'nɒtɪləs/ n (pl **nautiluses, nautili**) a genus of cephalopods, including those furnished with a chambered spinal univalve shell; a shellfish with webbed arms once supposed to sail upon the sea; a kind of diving bell.

naval /'neɪvəl/ adj of the navy; of ships.

nave[1] /neɪv/ n the central space of a church, distinct from the chancel and aisles.

nave[2] n the central block of a wheel, the hub.

navel /'neɪvəl/ n the small scar in the abdomen caused by severance of the umbilical cord; a central point.

navigability /nævɪgə'bɪlɪti/ n the quality or state of being navigable.

navigable /'nævɪgəbəl/ adj (*rivers, seas*) that can be sailed upon or steered through.—**navigably** adv.

navigate /'nævɪgeɪt/ vti to steer or direct a ship, aircraft, etc; to travel through or over (*water, air, etc*) in a ship or aircraft; to find a way through, over, etc, and to keep to a course.

navigation /ˌnævɪˈgeɪʃən/ *n* the act, art or science of navigating; the method of calculating the position of a ship, aircraft, etc.—**navigational** *adj*.

navigator /ˈnævɪˌgeɪtər/ *n* one who navigates; one skilled in the science of navigation.

navvy /ˈnævɪ/ *n* (*pl* **navvies**) (*Brit*) a labourer, *esp* one who works on roads or railways.

navy /ˈneɪvɪ/ *n* (*pl* **navies**) (*often with cap*) the warships of a nation; a nation's entire sea force, including ships, men, stores, etc; navy blue.

navy blue *n* an almost black blue.

nawab /nəˈwæb/ or /-ˈwɒb/ *n* an Indian viceroy; a nabob.

nay /neɪ/ *adv* (*arch*) no; not only so; yet more; or rather, and even. • *n* a refusal or denial.

Nazarene /ˌnæzəˈriːn/ *n* a native of Nazareth, applied to Jesus Christ, his followers, and the early Christians as a term of contempt; in the early Church, one of a sect of Judaising Christians.

Nazarite, Nazirite /ˈnæzəˌraɪt/ *n* a native of Nazareth; a Jew devoted by vow to God to a life of abstinence and purity (Numbers 6).

Nazi /ˈnɒtsi/ or /ˈnætsi/ *n* (*pl* **Nazis**) a member of the German National Socialist party (1930s).—*also adj*.

NB *abbr* = nota bene (note well); New Brunswick.

Nb (*chem symbol*) niobium.

NBC *abbr* = National Broadcasting Company.

NC *abbr* = North Carolina.

NCC /ˈɛnˈsiːˈsiː/ *abbr* ♣ (*Cdn*) = National Capital Commission.

NCdt *abbr* ♣ (*Cdn*) = Naval Cadet.

NCO *abbr* = noncommissioned officer.

NCM *abbr* ♣ (*mil*) = noncommissioned member.

ND *abbr* = North Dakota.

Nd (*chem symbol*) neodymium.

NDT /ˈɛnˈdiːˈtiː/ *abbr* ♣ = Newfoundland Daylight Time.

NDP /ˈɛnˈdiːˈpiː/ *abbr* ♣ = New Democratic Party.

NE *abbr* = Nebraska; northeast, northeastern.

Ne (*chem symbol*) neon.

Neanderthal /nɪˈændərˌθɒl/ or /-ˌtɒl/ *adj* denoting or characteristic of Neanderthal man; primitive.

Neanderthal man *n* a type of primitive human inhabiting Europe in Palaeolithic times.

neap /niːp/ *adj* of either of the lowest high tides in the month. • *n* a neap tide.

Neapolitan /nɪəˈpɒlɪtən/ *adj* pertaining to Naples or to its inhabitants.

Neapolitan ice cream *n* brick ice cream in layers of different colours and flavours.

near /nɪər/ *adj* (**nearer, nearest**) close, not distant in space or time; closely knit, intimate; approximate; (*escape, etc*) narrow. • *adv* to or at a little distance; close by; almost • *prep* close to. • *vti* to approach; to draw close to.—**nearness** *n*.

nearby /nɪərˈbaɪ/ *adj* neighbouring; close by in position.

Near East *n* Southeast Europe; (formerly) included Turkey, the Balkans and the area of the Ottoman Empire.

nearly /ˈnɪərlɪ/ *adv* almost, closely.

near miss *n* a bomb, mortar, etc that just fails to hit the target; any type of shot that misses its target; a situation in which two aircraft narrowly avoid a midair collision.

Near North *n* ♣ (*Cdn*) the southern edge of subarctic Canada, north of heavily settled areas.

near-sighted /ˈnɪərˌsaɪtəd/ *adj* short-sighted, myopic.—**near-sightedness** *n*.

neat /niːt/ *adj* clean and tidy; skilful; efficiently done; well made; (*alcoholic drink*) undiluted; (*sl*) nice, pleasing, etc.—**neatly** *adv*.—**neatness** *n*.

neat[2] *n* cattle of the bovine genus. • *adj* pertaining to bovine animals.

neaten /ˈniːtən/ *vt* to make tidy and neat.

neath /niːθ/ *prep* (*poet*) beneath.

neb /nɛb/ *n* (*Scot*) a bird's beak; a mouth; a nose or snout; a projecting part, a point.

nebula /ˈnɛbjʊlə/ *n* (*pl* **nebulae, nebulas**) a gaseous mass or star cluster in the sky appearing as a hazy patch of light.—**nebular** *adj*.

nebular hypothesis *n* the theory that the solar system in its primal condition existed in the form of a nebula, from which the sun, planets, and satellites were produced by condensation.

nebulosity /ˌnɛbjʊˈlɒsɪtɪ/ *n* (*pl* **nebulosities**) the state or quality of being nebulous.

nebulous /ˈnɛbjʊləs/ *adj* indistinct; formless.

necessarily /ˌnɛsəˈsɛrɪlɪ/ *adv* as a natural consequence.

necessary /ˈnɛsəˌsɛrɪ/ *adj* indispensable; required; inevitable. • *n* (*pl* **necessaries**) something necessary; (*pl*) essential needs.

necessitarianism /nəˌsɛsɪˈtɛərɪəˌnɪzəm/ *n* (*philos*) the doctrine of necessity, or that man cannot control his actions by his own free will; fatalism.—**necessitarian** *n*.

necessitate /nəˈsɛsɪˌteɪt/ *vt* to make necessary; to compel.

necessitous /nəˈsɛsɪtəs/ *adj* urgent; pressing; needy.

necessity /nəˈsɛsɪtɪ/ *n* (*pl* **necessities**) a prerequisite; something that cannot be done without; compulsion; need.

neck /nɛk/ *n* the part of the body that connects the head and shoulders; that part of a garment nearest the neck; a neck-like part, *esp* a narrow strip of land; the narrowest part of a bottle; a strait. • *vti* (*sl*) to kiss and caress.

neckerchief /ˈnɛkərtʃɪf/ or /-tʃiːf/ *n* a cloth square worn around the neck.

necklace /ˈnɛkləs/ *n* a string or band, often of precious stones, beads, or pearls, worn around the neck.

neckline /ˈnɛklaɪn/ *n* the line traced by the upper edge of a garment below the neck.

necktie /ˈnɛktaɪ/ *n* a man's tie.

necro-, necr- /ˈnɛkrɒ/ *prefix* corpse.

necrobiosis /ˌnɛkrəʊbaɪˈəʊsɪs/ *n* the decay of living tissue.—**necrobiotic** *adj*.

necrology /nəˈkrɒlədʒɪ/ *n* (*pl* **necrologies**) a register or account of the dead.—**necrological** *adj*.

necromancer /ˈnɛkrəˌmænsər/ *n* one who practises necromancy; a conjurer; a wizard.

necromancy /ˈnɛkrəˌmænsɪ/ *n* predicting the future by alleged communication with the dead; sorcery.—**necromantic** *adj*.

necrophagous /nɛˈkrɒfəgəs/ *adj* (*animal*) feeding on carrion.

necrophilia /ˌnɛkrəˈfɪlɪə/ *n* erotic interest in or copulation with corpses.—*also* **necromania.**—**necrophile** *n*.—**necrophiliac** *n*.

necropolis /nəˈkrɒpəlɪs/ *n* (*pl* **necropolises, necropoleis**) a cemetery.

necropsy /ˈnɛkrɒpsɪ/ *n* (*pl* **necropsies**) a post-mortem examination.

necrosis /nəˈkrəʊsɪs/ *n* mortification and death of a bone; gangrene; a disease in plants characterized by small black spots.—**necrotic** *adj*.

nectar /ˈnɛktər/ *n* a sweetish liquid in many flowers, used by bees to make honey; any delicious drink.

nectareous, nectarous /-ˈtɛrɪəs/ *adj* producing, or sweet, like nectar.

nectarine /nɛktəˈriːn/ or /ˈrɛk-/ *n* a smooth-skinned peach.

nectary /ˈnɛktərɪ/ *n* (*pl* **nectaries**) that part of a flower which secretes a saccharine fluid.

nee, née /neɪ/ *adj* (*literally* born: indicating the maiden name of a married woman.

need /niːd/ *n* necessity; a lack of something; a requirement; poverty. • *vt* to have a need for; to require; to be obliged.

needful /ˈniːdfʊl/ *adj* necessary, required, vital. • *n* (*inf*) what is required, *esp* money.—**needfulness** *n*.

needle /ˈniːdəl/ *n* a small pointed piece of steel for sewing; a larger pointed rod for knitting or crocheting; a stylus; the pointer of a compass, gauge, etc; the thin, short leaf of the pine, spruce, etc; the sharp, slender metal tube at the end of a hypodermic syringe. • *vt* to goad, prod, or tease.

needlepoint /ˈniːdəlpoint/ *n* a type of embroidery worked on canvas; point lace.

needless /ˈniːdləs/ *adj* not needed, unnecessary; uncalled for, pointless.—**needlessly** *adv*.—**needlessness** *n*.

needlework /ˈniːdəlˌwɜːk/ *n* sewing, embroidery.

needn't /ˈniːdənt/ = need not.

needs /niːdz/ *adv* necessarily; indispensably.

needy /ˈniːdɪ/ *adj* (**needier, neediest**) in need, very poor.

neep /niːp/ *n* (*Scot*) a turnip.

ne'er /nɛr/ *adv* (*poet*) never.

ne'er-do-well /ˈnɛrduːˌwɛl/ *adj* good-for-nothing; improvident; lazy. • *n* an irresponsible person.

nefarious /nəˈfɛrɪəs/ *adj* wicked, evil.

neg. *abbr* = negative(ly).

negate /nəˈgeɪt/ *vt* to nullify; to deny.

negation /nəˈgeɪʃən/ *n* a negative statement, denial; the opposite or absence of something; a contradiction.

negative /'nɛgətɪv/ *adj* expressing or meaning denial or refusal; lacking positive attributes; (*math*) denoting a quantity less than zero, or one to be subtracted; (*photog*) reversing the light and shade of the original subject, or having the colours replaced by complementary ones; (*elect*) of the charge carried by electrons; producing such a charge. • *n* a negative word, reply, etc; refusal; something that is the opposite or negation of something else; (*in debate, etc*) the side that votes or argues for the opposition; (*photog*) a negative image on transparent film or a plate. • *vt* to refuse assent, contradict; to veto.—**negatively** *adv*.

neglect /nə'glɛkt/ or /ni-/ *vt* to pay little or no attention to; to disregard; to leave uncared for; to fail to do something. • *n* disregard; lack of attention or care.

neglectful /-fʊl/ *adj* careless; heedless; slighting.—**neglectfully** *adv*.

negligee /'nɛglɪ,ʒeɪ/ *n* a woman's loosely fitting dressing gown.

negligence /'nɛglɪdʒəns/ *n* lack of attention or care; an act of carelessness; a carelessly easy manner.

negligent /'nɛglɪdʒənt/ *adj* careless, heedless.—**negligently** *adv*.

negligible /'nɛglɪdʒɪbəl/ *adj* that need not be regarded; unimportant; trifling.

negotiable /nə'go:ʃəbəl/ *adj* able to be legally negotiated; (*bills, drafts, etc*) transferable.—**negotiability** *n*.

negotiate /nə'go:ʃi,eɪt/ *vti* to discuss, bargain in order to reach an agreement or settlement; to settle by agreement; (*fin*) to obtain or give money value for (a bill); (*obstacle, etc*) to overcome.

negotiation /nə,go:ʃi'eɪʃən/ or /-sɪ'eɪʃən/ *n* the act of negotiating or transacting business; a treaty.

negotiator /-tər/ *n* one who negotiates.

Negrillo /nə'grɪlo:/ *n* (*pl* **Negrillos, Negrilloes**) one of a pigmy Negroid race found in Africa.

Negrito /nə'gri:to:/ *n* (*pl* **Negritos, Negritoes**) one of a diminutive Negroid race of the Philippines and Polynesia.

Negro /'ni:gro:/ *n* (*pl* **Negroes**) (*old fashioned*) a member of the dark-skinned, indigenous peoples of Africa; a member of the Negroid group; a person with some Negro ancestors.—*also* *adj*.—**Negress** *nf*.

Negroid /'ni:grɔɪd/ *adj* denoting, or of, one of the major groups of humankind, including most of the peoples of Africa south of the Sahara.

Negus /'ni:gəs/ *n* (*pl* **Neguses**) a title of the ruler of Ethiopia.

negus *n* (*pl* **neguses**) a beverage of hot water and wine, sweetened and spiced.

neigh /neɪ/ *vi* (**neighing, neighed**) to whinny; to make a sound like the cry of a horse. • *n* the cry of a horse; a whinny.

neighbour, neighbor /'neɪbər/ *n* a person who lives near another; a person or thing situated next to another; a fellow human being. • *vt* to be near, to adjoin.

neighbourhood, neighborhood /-,hʊd/ *n* a particular community, area, or district; the people in an area.

neighbouring, neighboring /-ɪŋ/ *adj* adjoining, nearby.

neighbourly, neighborly /-li/ *adj* characteristic of a neighbour, friendly. • *adv* in a neighbourly or social manner.—**neighbourliness, neighborliness** *n*.

neither /'naɪðər/ or /'ni:ð-/ *adj, pron* not one or the other (of two); not either. • *conj* not either; also not.

nek /nɛk/ *n* (*S Africa*) a depression or pass in a mountain range.

nekton /'nɛktən/ *n* a collective term for minute forms of organic life found at various depths in seas and lakes.—**nektonic** *adj*.

nelson /'nɛlsən/ *n* (*wrestling*) a type of hold in which the arms are placed under an opponent's arms from behind so that pressure can be exerted by the palms on the back of the opponent's neck.

nemato-, nemat- /'nɛməto:/ or /-tə/ *prefix* thread, fibre.

nematode /'nɛmə,to:d/ *adj* thread-like. • *n* a threadworm.

nem. con. *adv* no one contradicting.

nem. diss. *adv* no one dissenting.

Nemean /nɪ'mɪən/ or /'ni:mi-/ *adj* pertaining to the Nemea valley of ancient Greece or to the games held there.

nemesis /'nɛməsɪs/ *n* (*pl* **nemeses**) retribution; just punishment; an agent of defeat.

neo- /'ni:o:/ *prefix* new, newly.

neodymium /,ni:ə'dɪmɪəm/ *n* a silvery-white metallic element used in alloys, etc.

Neolithic /,ni:ə'lɪθɪk/ *adj* of the later Stone Age, marked by the use of polished stone implements.

neologism /ni:'ɒlədʒ,ɪzəm/ *n* a new word; the coining of new words, neology; the introduction of new doctrines.—**neologistic, neological** *adj*.

neologist /-,dʒɪst/ *n* an innovator in language or religion, *esp* one who holds doctrinal views opposed to the orthodox interpretation of revealed religion.

neologize /-,dʒaɪz/ *vt* to introduce new words, phrases, or religious doctrines.

neology /-dʒi/ *n* neologism; doctrines or rationalistic theological interpretation at variance with orthodox belief.

neon /'ni:ɒn/ *n* an inert gaseous element that gives off a bright orange glow, used in lighting and advertisements.

neophyte /'ni:ə,faɪt/ *n* a novice; one recently baptised; a convert. • *adj* recently entered.

neoplasm /'ni:ə,plæzəm/ *n* tissue growth more or less distinct from that in which it occurs.

neoplastic /,ni:ə'plæstɪk/ *adj* newly formed.

neoplasty /'ni:ə,plæsti/ *n* the restoration of tissue by plastic surgery.

NeoPlatonism /,ni:o:'pleɪtə,nɪzəm/ *n* a system of eclectic philosophy combining the doctrines of Plato with Oriental mysticism in the 3rd century AD.—**NeoPlatonist** *n*.

neoteric /,ni:ə'tɛrɪk/ *adj* recent in origin; newfangled, modern.—**neoterically** *adv*.

Neotropical /,ni:o:'trɒpɪkəl/ *adj* of tropical or South America.

Neozoic /,ni:o:'zo:ɪk/ *adj* noting rocks from the Trias to the present time.

Nepalese /,nɛpə'li:z/ *n, adj* (a) Nepali.

Nepali /nə'pɒli/ *n* (*pl* **Nepali, Nepalis**) a native or inhabitant of Nepal; the language of Nepal.—*also adj*.

nepenthe /ni:'pɛnθi/ or /nɪ-/ *n* a drug supposed by the ancient Greeks to have the power of causing forgetfulness of sorrow.—**nepenthean** *adj*.

nephew /'nɛfju:/ *n* the son of a brother or sister.

nephology /ni:'fɒlədʒi/ or /nɪ-/ *n* the study of clouds.—**nephological** *adj*.—**nephologist** *n*.

nephralgia /nə'frældʒiə/ or /-'frældʒə/ *n* pain or disease in the kidneys.—**nephralgic** *adj*.

nephrite /'nɛfraɪt/ *n* jade.

nephritic /nɪ'frɪtɪk/ *adj* of or pertaining to the kidneys or kidney disease; affected with disease of the kidneys.

nephritis /nɪ'fraɪtɪs/ *n* inflammation of the kidneys.

nephro- or **nephr-** /'nɛfro:/ *prefix* kidney; kidneys.

nephrology /nə'frɒlədʒi/ *n* study of the kidneys.

nephrotomy /nə'frɒtəmi/ *n* (*pl* **nephrotomies**) incision into the kidney.

ne plus ultra /,neɪplʊs'ʊltrɒ/ *n* (*Latin*) the farthest attainable point; the acme, the perfect state.—*also* **non plus ultra**.

nepotism /'nɛpə,tɪzəm/ *n* undue favouritism shown to relatives, *esp* in securing jobs.

Neptune /'nɛptu:n/ or /-tju:n/ *n* the Roman god of the sea; the sea personified; the 8th planet from the sun.

Neptunian /nɛp'tju:niən/ or /-'tu:-/ *adj* pertaining to the classical deity Neptune, god of the sea, or to the sea; deposited by the agency of the sea.

neptunium /nɛp'tju:niəm/ *n* a radioactive metallic element.

nerd /nərd/ *n* (*sl*) a boring, straight-laced person; a creep.

Nereid /'ni:riɪd/ *n* (*pl* **Nereides**) (*Greek myth*) a sea nymph.

nereis /'ni:riɪs/ *n* (*zool*) a sea worm.

neroli /'ni:rɒli/ *n* the essential oil of orange flowers.

nervate /'nər,veɪt/ *adj* (*bot*) ribbed.

nervation /nər'veɪʃən/ *n* (*bot*) the arrangement of veins, venation.

nerve /nərv/ *n* any of the fibres or bundles of fibres that transmit impulses of sensation or of movement between the brain and spinal cord and all parts of the body; courage, coolness in danger; (*inf*) audacity, boldness; (*pl*) nervousness, anxiety. • *vt* to give strength, courage, or vigour to.

nerve cell *n* a cell transmitting impulses in nerve tissue.—*also* **neuron, neurone**.

nerve centre, nerve center *n* a group of closely connected cells; (*mil, etc*) a centre of control from which instructions are sent out.

nerve gas *n* a poison gas that affects the nervous system.

nerveless /'nərvləs/ *adj* calm, cool; weak, feeble.—**nervelessly** *adv*.

nerve-racking, nerve-wracking /-,rækɪŋ/ *adj* straining the nerves, stressful.

nervous /'nərvəs/ *adj* excitable, highly strung; anxious, apprehensive; affecting or acting on the nerves or nervous system.

nervous breakdown *n* (*inf*)a (*usu* temporary) period of mental illness resulting from severe emotional strain or anxiety.

nervous system *n* the brain, spinal cord, and nerves collectively.

nervure /'nɜrvjʊr/ *n* the veins of leaves; the horny ribs supporting the membranous wings of an insect.

nervy /'nɜrvi/ *adj* (**nervier, nerviest**) (*inf*) anxious, agitated; (*inf*) impudent, cheeky.

nescience /'nɛɪʃəns/ *n* ignorance; agnosticism.—**nescient** *adj*.

ness /nɛs/ *n* a headland or cape, a promontory.

-ness /nəs/ *suffix* state, quality of being.

nest /nɛst/ *n* a structure or place where birds, fish, mice, etc. lay eggs or give birth to young; a place where young are nurtured; a swarm or brood; a lair; a cosy place; a set of boxes, tables. etc of different sizes, designed to fit together. • *vi* to make or occupy a nest.

nest egg *n* money put aside as a reserve or to establish a fund.

nestle /'nɛsəl/ *vti* to rest snugly; to lie snugly, as in a nest; to lie sheltered or half-hidden.

nestling /'nɛslɪŋ/ or /'nɛst-/ *n* a young bird that has not left the nest.

Nestor /'nɛstər/ *n* (*Greek myth*) a Greek sage of the Trojan war; a wise old man.

Nestorianism /nɛs'tɔːrɪənˌɪzəm/ *n* the 5th-century doctrine of Nestorius, Bishop of Constantinople, who taught that there were two natures in Christ, one human and one divine, which did not unit and form one person; also that the Virgin Mary was not the Mother of God.—**Nestorian** *n, adj*.

net[1] /nɛt/ *n* an openwork material of string, rope, or twine knotted into meshes; a piece of this used to catch fish, to divide a tennis court, etc; a snare. • *vti* (**netting, netted**) to snare or enclose as with a net; to hit (a ball) into a net or goal.

net[2], **nett** *adj* clear of deductions, allowances or charges. • *n* a net amount, price, weight, profit, etc. • *vt* (**netting, netted**) to clear as a profit.

nether /'nɛðər/ *adj* lower or under.

nether world /'nɛðərwɜrld/ *n* the underworld, hell.

nethermost /-ˌmoːst/ *adj* lowest.

netizen *n* literally 'net citizen', someone who uses the Internet.

netsuke /'nɛtsuki/ *n* a Japanese ornamental toggle for fastening the front of a garment.

netting /'nɛtɪŋ/ *n* netted fabric.

nettle /'nɛtəl/ *n* a wild plant with stinging hairs. • *vt* to irritate, annoy.

nettle rash *n* a cutaneous skin eruption resembling the effects of a nettle sting.

network /'nɛtwɜrk/ *n* an arrangement of intersecting lines; a group of people who co-operate with each other; a chain of interconnected operations, computers, etc; (*radio, TV*) a group of broadcasting stations connected to transmit the same programme simultaneously. • *vt* to broadcast on a network; (*comput*) to interconnect systems so that information, software, and peripheral devices, such as printers, can be shared.

networking /-ɪŋ/ *n* the making of contacts and trading information as for career advancement; the interconnection of computer systems.

neural /'njʊrəl/ or /'nɔrəl/ *adj* of or pertaining to the nerves.

neuralgia /nju'rældʒə/ or /nə'ræl-/ *n* pain along a nerve.—**neuralgic** *adj*.

neuralgic /-ɪk/ *adj* pertaining to neuralgia.

neurasthenia /ˌnjʊrəs'θiːniə/ or /ˌnərəs-/ *n* brain and nerve exhaustion, as from influenza, etc.

neurectomy /nu'rɛktəmi/ or /njʊ-/ *n* (*pl* **neurectomies**) excision of a nerve.

neuritis /nju'raɪtɪs/ or /nə'raɪt-/ *n* inflammation of a nerve.

neuro-, neur- /'njʊro:/ or /'nɔro:/ *prefix* nerve.

neuroglia /nju'rɒɡliə/ or /nə'rɒ-/ *n* the delicate connective tissue between the nerve fibres of the brain and spinal cord.

neurology /nju'rɒlədʒi/ or /nə'rɒ-/ *n* the branch of medicine studying the nervous system and its diseases.—**neurological** *adj*.—**neurologist** *n*.

neuroma /nju'roːmə/ or /nə'ro:-/ *n* (*pl* **neuromas, neuromata**) a fibrous tumour occuring in nerve tissue.

neuron, neurone /'njʊrɒn/ or /'nɔrɒn/ *see* **nerve cell**.

neuropathic /ˌnʊro:'pæθɪk/ or /ˌnjʊr-/ *adj* pertaining to, or suffering from, nervous disease; affecting the nerves.—**neuropath** *n*.—**neuropathically** *adv*.

neuropathology /ˌnjʊro:pə'θɒlədʒi/ or /ˌnero:-/ *n* the study of diseases of the nervous system.—**neuropathologist** *adj*.

neuropathy /nju'rɒpəθi/ or /nə'rɒ-/ *n* disease of the nervous system.

neuropteran /nju'rɒptərən/ or /nə'rɒ-/ *n* (*pl* **neuropterans**) any of an order of insects characterized by four transparent, finely

reticulated, membranous wings. • *adj* with four wings marked with a network of nerves—*also* **neuropterous**.

neurosis /nju'ro:sɪs/ or /nə'ro:-/ *n* (*pl* **neuroses**) a mental disorder with symptoms such as anxiety and phobia.

neurosurgery /ˌnjʊro:'sɜrdʒəri/ or /ˌnər-/ *n* the branch of surgery dealing with the nervous system.—**neurosurgical** *adj*.

neurotic /nju'rɒtɪk/ or /nə'rɒ-/ *adj* suffering from neurosis; highly strung; of or acting upon the nerves. • *n* someone with neurosis.

neurotomy /nju'rɒtəmi/ or /nə'rɒ-/ *n* (*pl* **neurotomies**) dissection of the nerves.

neurotransmitter /'njʊro:ˌrænsˌmɪtər/ or /'nər-/ *n* a chemical by which nerves cells communicate with each other or with muscles.

neuter /'nu:tər/ or /'nju:-/ *adj* (*gram*) of gender, neither masculine nor feminine; (*biol*) having no sex organs; having undeveloped sex organs in the adult. • *n* a neuter person, word, plant, or animal. • *vt* to castrate or spay.

neutral /'nu:trəl/ or /'nju:-/ *adj* nonaligned; not taking sides with either party in a dispute or war; having no distinctive characteristics; (*colour*) dull; (*chem*) neither acid nor alkaline; (*physics*) having zero charge. • *n* a neutral state, person, or colour; a position of a gear mechanism in which power is not transmitted.

neutrality /nu:'trælɪti/ or /'nju:-/ *n* the state of being neutral.

neutralize /'nu:trəˌlaɪz/ or /'nju:-/ *vt* to render ineffective; to counterbalance; to declare neutral.—**neutralization** *n*.—**neutralizer** *n*.

neutrally /'nu:trəli/ or /'nju:-/ *adv* in a neutral manner.

neutrino /nu:'tri:no:/ or /nju:-/ *n* (*pl* **neutrinos**) (*physics*) a stable elementary particle with almost zero mass and spin 1/2.

neutron /'nu:tron/ or /'nju:-/ *n* an elementary particle with no electric charge and the same mass approximately as a proton.

neutron bomb *n* a nuclear bomb with a small blast that releases neutrons, destroying life but leaving property undamaged.

neutron number *n* the number of neutrons in the nucleus of an atom.

neutron star *n* a star composed solely of densely packed neutrons that has collapsed under its own gravity.

névé /neɪveɪ/ *n* the granular compressed snow that forms glacier ice.

never /'nɛvər/ *adv* at no time, not ever; not at all; in no case; (*inf*) surely not.

nevermore /ˌnɛvər'mɔr/ *adv* never again.

never-never /ˌnɛvər'nɛvər/ *adj* imaginary, ideal.

nevertheless /ˌnɛvərðə'lɛs/ *adv* all the same, notwithstanding; in spite of, however.

nevus /'ri:vəs/ *n* (*pl* **nevi**) a birthmark, a mole.—*also* **naevus**.—**nevoid** *adj*.

new /nu:/ or /nju:/ *adj* recently made, discovered, or invented; seen, known, or used for the first time; different, changed; recently grown, fresh; unused; unaccustomed; unfamiliar; recently begun. • *adv* again; newly; recently.

new blood *n* a recent arrival in an organization expected to bring new ideas and revitalize the system.

newborn /'nu:bɔrn/ or /'nju:-/ *adj* newly born; reborn.

New Brunswicker *n* ✲ (*Cdn*) a person who lives in or is from New Brunswick.

newcomer /'nu:ˌkʌmər/ or /'nju:-/ *n* a recent arrival.

New Deal *n* the economic and social measures introduced into the USA by President Roosevelt in 1933 to combat the great economic crisis that began in 1929.

New Democrat *n* ✲ (*Cdn*) a member or supporter of the New Democratic Party.

newel /'nu:əl/ or /'nju:əl/ *n* the central pillar of a spiral staircase; the end post of a banister.

New England *n* six northeastern states of the USA.

newfangled /ˌnu:'fæŋɡəld/ or /'nju:-/, /-'fæŋɡəld/ *adj* (*contemptuous*) new; novel, very modern.

Newfie /'nu:fi:/ or /'nju:fi:/ *n* ✲ (*Cdn*) (*inf*) a Newfoundlander.

Newfoundland /ˌnu:fənd'ænd/ or /'nu:fəndlənd/, /'nu:fəndlænd/, /nju:'faʊndlənd/ *n* a large variety of dog, originally from Newfoundland.

Newfoundlander *n* ✲ a person who lives in or is from Newfoundland.

newly /'nu:li/ or /'nju:-/ *adv* recently, lately.

newlywed /'nu:liwɛd/ or /'nju:-/ *n* a recently married person.

new moon *n* the moon when first visible as a crescent.

news /nu:z/ or /nju:z/ *npl* current events; recent happenings; the mass media's coverage of such events; a programme of news on television or radio; information not known before.

newscast /'nu:zkæst/ or /'nju:z-/ *n* radio or television news broadcast.—**newscaster** *n*.

newsdealer /-di:l,ər/, **newsagent** /-,eɪdʒənt/ or /'nju:-/ *n* a retailer of newspapers, magazines, etc.

newsflash /-,flæʃ/ *n* an important news item broadcast separately and often interrupting other programmes.

newsgroup *n* on the Internet, a group of people who use an on-line service to discuss a particular topic.

newsletter /-,letər/ or /'nju:z-/ *n* a bulletin regularly distributed among the members of a group, society, etc, containing information and news of activities, etc.

newspaper /-,peɪpər/ or /'nu:s-/, /nju:-/ *n* a printed periodical containing news published daily or weekly.

newsprint /-prɪnt/ or /'nu:z-/ *n* an inexpensive paper on which newspapers are printed.

newsreel /-ri:l/ or /'nju:z-/ *n* a short film presenting news of current events with a commentary.

newsroom /-ru:m/ or /'nju:z-/ *n* the department of a newspaper or broadcasting system that prepares news for publication or broadcasting; a room, etc, where news for publication or broadcasting; a room, etc, where newspapers, magazines, etc, may be read.

New Style calendar *n* the Gregorian or present style of computing the calendar, which replaced the Julian calendar.

newsworthy /'nju:z,wərði/ or /'nu:z-/ *adj* timely and important or interesting.

newt /nu:t/ or /'nju:t/ *n* any of various small amphibious lizard-like creatures.

New Testament *n* the second part of the Bible including the story of the life and teachings of Christ.

newton /'nu:tən/ or /'nju:-/ *n* the SI unit of force that when acting for 1 second on a mass of 1 kilogram imparts an acceleration of 1 metre per second.

Newtonian /nu:'to:niən/ *adj* pertaining to, discovered by, or invented by, Sir Isaac Newton, the philosopher, or to his system.

new town *n* in UK, any of various towns built since 1946 as planned units sponsored by government to house overspill population from nearby cities, aid urban redevelopment, etc.

New World *n* the Americas.

New Year's (Day) *n* the first day of a new year; 1 January, a legal holiday in many countries.

New Year's Eve *n* the evening of the last day of the year; 31 December.—*also* **Hogmanay**.

next /nekst/ *adj* nearest; immediately preceding or following; adjacent. • *adv* in the nearest time, place, rank, etc; on the first subsequent occasion.

next of kin *n* the nearest relative of a person.

nexus /'neksəs/ *n* (*pl* **nexus, nexuses**) a connecting principle or link.

NF *abbr* ✤ = Newfoundland.

NFB *abbr* ✤ (*Cdn*) = National Film Board.

Nfld *abbr* ✤ = Newfoundland.

NH *abbr* = New Hampshire.

NHL /'ɛn'eɪtʃ'ɛl/ *abbr* ✤ = National Hockey League.

NI *abbr* = Northern Ireland.

Ni (*chem symbol*) nickel.

nib /nɪb/ *n* a pen point. • *vt* (**nibbing, nibbed**) to furnished with a nib; to cut or insert a pen nib.

nibble /'nɪbəl/ *vti* to take small bites at (food, etc); to bite (at) lightly and intermittently.—**nibbler** *n*.

Nibelungenlied /'ni:bə,luŋənli:d/ *n* a medieval German epic poem.

niblick /'nɪblɪk/ *n* a golf club with a heavy head, used for lofting.

nice /naɪs/ *adj* pleasant, attractive, kind, good, etc; particular, fastidious; delicately sensitive.—**nicely** *adv*.

nice-looking *adj* pretty, handsome.

Nicene Creed /'naɪsi:n/ or /'naɪ-/, /-'si:n/ *n* the creed, one of the three held by the Anglican Church, drawn up by the Ecumenical Council of the Early Christian Church at the Council of Nicaea in Asia Minor in 325AD, with additions made at the Council of Constantinople 381.

niceness /'naɪsnəs/ *n* the state or quality of being nice; delicacy of perception or touch.

nicety /'naɪsəti/ *n* (*pl* **niceties**) a subtle point of distinction; refinement.

niche /ni:ʃ/ or /nɪtʃ/ *n* a shallow recess in a wall for a statue, etc; a place, use, or work for which a person or thing is best suited.

nick /nɪk/ *n* a small cut, chip, etc, made on a surface; (*Brit sl*) a police station, prison. • *vt* to make a nick in; to wound superficially; (*Brit sl*) to steal; (*Brit sl*) to arrest.

nickel /'nɪkəl/ *n* a silvery-white metallic element used in alloys and plating; ✤ a US or Canadian coin worth five cents.

nickelodeon /nɪkə'lo:dɪən/ *n* (*US*) an early type of jukebox.

nickel silver *n* an alloy of nickel, copper and zinc.—*also* **German silver**.

nicker /'nɪkər/ *vi* to neigh, to snigger.—*also n*.

nicknack /'nɪk,næk/ *see* **knickknack**.

nickname /'nɪkneɪm/ *n* a substitute name, often descriptive, given in fun; a familiar form of a proper name. • *vt* to give as a nickname.

nicotiana /,nɪko:ti'ænə/ or /-ʃi'ænə/ *n* any of the *Nicotiana* genus of plants of Australia and America, *eg* tobacco.

nicotine /'nɪkə,ti:n/ or /,nɪkə'ti:n/ *n* a poisonous alkaloid present in tobacco.

Nictitate /'nɪktɪ,teɪt/, **nictate** /'nɪk,teɪt/ *vi* to wink.—**nictitation, nictation** *n*.

nictitating membrane *n* a membrane that can be drawn over the eye beneath the eyelid present in many birds, reptiles, fish and some mammals.

nidificate /'nɪdɪfɪ,keɪt/ *vi* to build a nest.

nidification /,nɪdɪfɪ'keɪʃən/ *n* the act of building a nest, rearing young, etc.

nidify /'nɪdɪ,faɪ/ *vi* (**nidifying, nidified**) to nidificate.

nidus /'naɪdəs/ *n* (*pl* **nidi, niduses**) the developing place of spores, seeds, germs, insects' eggs, etc; an accumulation of eggs, tubercles, etc; a nest or hatching place.

niece /ni:s/ *n* the daughter of a brother or sister.

niello /ni'ɛlo:/ *n* (*pl* **nielli, niellos**) an ornamental engraving in black on silver, gold, brass, etc; a black alloy used in this. • *vt* (**nielloing, nielloed**) to engrave or decorate with niello.

Niflheim /'nɪvəlheɪm/ or /-haɪm/ *n* (*Scandinavian myth*) the region of eternal mist and cold.

nifty /'nɪfti/ *adj* (**niftier, niftiest**) (*sl*) neat, stylish.—**niftily** *adv*.—**niftiness** *n*.

niggard /'nɪgərd/ *adj* meanly covetous; parsimonious; miserly; niggardly. • *n* one who is meanly covetous; a stingy person, a miser.

niggardliness /'nɪgərdlinəs/ *n* the state of being niggardly; stinginess.

niggardly /'nɪgərdli/ *adj* giving grudgingly, ungenerous. • *adv* like a niggard.

niggle /'nɪgəl/ *vi* to waste time on petty details; to be finicky.

niggler /-ər/ *n* one who trifles at handiwork.

niggling /-ɪŋ/ *adj* finicky, fussy; petty; gnawing, irritating.—**nigglingly** *adv*.

nigh /naɪ/ *adj, adv, prep* near.

night /naɪt/ *n* the period of darkness from sunset to sunrise; nightfall; a specified or appointed evening.

night blindness *n* poor vision in near darkness.

nightcap /'naɪtkæp/ *n* a cap worn in bed; (*inf*) an alcoholic drink taken just before going to bed.

nightclothes /-klo:ðz/ *npl* clothes for wearing in bed, as a nightgown, pyjamas, etc.

nightclub /-klʌb/ *n* a place of entertainment for drinking, dancing, etc, at night.

nightdress /-dres/ *n* a loose garment worn in bed by women and girls.

nightfall /-fɔl/ *n* the close of the day.

nightflower /-flaʊr/ *n* a flower that opens at night.

nightglass /-glæs/ *n* a short telescope for night use.

nightgown /-gaʊn/ *n* a nightdress.

nightie /'naɪti/ *n* (*inf*) a nightdress, nightgown.—*also* **nighty**.

nightingale /'naɪtɪŋ,geɪl/ *n* a songbird celebrated for its musical song at night.

nightjar /'naɪtdʒər/ *n* a nocturnal bird with dull mottled plumage.

night life /'naɪtlaɪf/ *n* social entertainment at night, *esp* in towns.

night-light /-laɪt/ *n* a dim light kept burning at night.

nightlong /-lɒŋ/ *adj* lasting through the night.

nightly /'naɪtli/ *adj, adv* done or happening by night or every night.

nightmare /'naɪtmer/ *n* a frightening dream; any horrible experience.—**nightmarish** *adj*.

night owl *n* (*inf*) a person who stays up late at night.

night school *n* an educational institution where classes are held in the evening.

nightshade /'naɪtʃeɪd/ *n* a flowering plant related to the potato and tomato, *esp* deadly nightshade (belladonna).

nightshirt /-ʃərt/ *n* a long shirt for sleeping in.

nightspot /-spɒt/ *n* (*inf*) a nightclub.

nightstick /-stɪk/ *n* (*US*) a short club carried by a policeman or policewoman; a truncheon.

nighttime /-taɪm/ *n* night.

night watch *n* a watch by night or the person keeping it; (*pl*) night-time.

night watchman *n* the person who guards a building at night.

nighty /'naɪti/ *n* (*pl* **nighties**) (*inf*) a nightie.

nigrescent /nɪ'grɛsənt/ *adj* blackish, growing black.—**nigrescence** *n*.

nihil /'naɪhɪl/ or /'niː-/ *n* (*Latin*) nothing, nil.

nihil ad rem /ni:lædrɛm/ *adj* (*Latin*) irrelevant.

nihilism /'naɪɪlɪzəm/ or /'naɪhɪlɪzəm/, /'niː-/ *n* the belief that nothing has real existence, scepticism; the rejection of customary beliefs in morality, religion, etc.

nihilist /'nɪhɪlɪst/ *n* a supporter of nihilism.—**nihilisitic** *adj*.

nihility /naɪ'hɪləti/ *n* nonexistence.

nil /nɪl/ *n* nothing.

Nilgai /'niːlgaɪ/, **nilgau** /-gɔ/ *n* (*pl* **nilgai, nilgais, nilgau, nilgaus**) a large short-horned Indian antelope.

Nilometer /naɪ'lɒmətər/ *n* a graduated pillar for measuring the rise of water in the river Nile during its floods; a river gauge.

Nilotic /naɪ'lɒtɪk/ *adj* pertaining to the River Nile.

nimble /'nɪmbəl/ *adj* agile; quick.—**nimbly** *adv*.

nimbus /'nɪmbəs/ *n* (*pl* **nimbi, nimbuses**) (*art*) the halo or cloud of light surrounding the heads of divinities, saints, and sovereigns; a rain cloud.

nimby /'nɪmbi/ *abbr* = not in my back yard.

niminy-piminy /ˌnɪmɪni'pɪmɪni/ *adj* mincing, prim.

Nimrod /'nɪmrɒd/ *n* a distinguished hunter, from Nimrod, "the mighty hunter" (Genesis 10.9).

nincompoop /'nɪnkəmˌpuːp/ or /'nɪŋ-/ *n* a stupid, silly person.

nine /naɪn/ *adj, n* one more than eight. • *n* the symbol for this (9, IX, ix); the ninth in a series or set; something having nine units as members.

ninefold /'naɪnfoːld/ *adj* having nine units or members; being nine times as great or as many.

ninepins /'naɪnpɪnz/ *see* **skittles**.

nineteen /naɪn'tiːn/ or /'naɪn-/ *adj, n* one more than eighteen. • *n* the symbol for this (19, XIX, xix).—**nineteenth** *adj*.

nineteenth /-'tiːnθ/ *adj* being one of 19 equal parts. • *n* a nineteenth part.

nineteenth hole *n* (*golf*) (*sl*) the bar in the clubhouse.

ninetieth /'naɪntiːθ/ *adj* next after 89. • *n* a ninetieth part.

ninety /'naɪnti/ *adj, n* nine times ten. • *n* the symbol for this (90, XC, xc); (*in pl*) **nineties**; the numbers from 90 to 99; the same numbers in a life or century.

ninja /'nɪndʒə/ *n* a Japanese warrior trained in ninjutsu.—*also adj*.

ninjutsu /nɪn'dʒʊtsu:/ *n* an ancient Japanese martial art which practises techniques of stealth or invisibility, orig for the purpose of espionage and political assassination.

ninny /'nɪni/ *n* (*pl* **ninnies**) a person of weak character or mind, a simpleton.

ninon /ni'nɒn/, *Fr.* /ni'nõ:/ *n* a light silk material.

ninth /naɪnθ/ *adj, n* next after eighth; one of nine equal parts of a thing.

Niobe /'naɪəbi/ *n* an inconsolable bereaved woman; (*Greek myth*) a heroine who was turned to stone while weeping for her slain children.—**Niobean** *adj*.

niobic /naɪ'oːbɪk/ *adj* of or containing pentavalent niobium.

niobium /naɪ'oːbiəm/ *n* a metallic element used in alloys.

nip[1] /nɪp/ *vt* (**nipping, nipped**) to pinch, pinch off; to squeeze between two surfaces; (*dog*) to give a small bite; to prevent the growth of; (*plants*) to have a harmful effect on because of cold. • *n* a pinch; a sharp squeeze; a bite; severe frost or biting coldness.

nip[2] *n* a small drink of spirits. • *vti* (**nipping, nipped**) to drink in nips.

nipa /'niːpə/ *n* an East Indian palm.

nipper /'nɪpər/ *n* a person or thing that nips; the pincer of a crab or lobster; (*pl*) pliers, pincers, etc; (*Brit inf*) a small child.

nipple /'nɪpəl/ *n* the small protuberance on a breast or udder through which the milk passes, a teat; a teat-like rubber part on the cap of a baby's bottle; a projection resembling a nipple.

nippy /'nɪpi/ *adj* (**nippier, nippiest**) (*weather*) frosty; (*Brit inf*) quick, nimble.

nirvana /nər'vɒnə/ or /-'vænə/ *n* (*Buddhism*) the highest religious state, when all desire of existence and worldly good is extinguished, and the soul is absorbed into the Deity.

nisi /'naɪsaɪ/ *adj* (*decree, order, rule, etc*) valid unless cause is shown be the contrary by a fixed date, at which it is made absolute.

nisi prius /-'praɪəs/ *n* (*law*) a writt, beginning with these words, direc ing a sheriff to empanel a jury; the name of certain courts for the trial of civil actions in the counties. / a trial of civil causes by judges of assize.

nit /nɪt/ *n* the egg of a louse or other parasitic insect.

niter /'naɪtər/ *see* **nitre**.

niton /'naɪtɒn/ *n* a gaseous radioactive element, radon.

nit-picking /'nɪtˌpɪkɪŋ/ *n* (*inf*) concern with petty details in order to find fault.—*also adj*.

nitrate /'naɪtreɪt/ *n* a salt of nitric acid; a fertilizer made of this.—**nitration** *n*.

nitre /'naɪtər/ *n* potassium nitrate, saltpetre.—*also* **niter**.

nitric /'naɪtrɪk/ *adj* containing nitrogen.

nitric acid *n* a corrosive, caustic liquid used to make explosives, fertilizers, etc.

nitride /'naɪtraɪd/ *n* a compound of nitrogen with a metal, also with phosphorus, silicon or boron.

nitrification /ˌnaɪtrɪfɪ'keɪʃən/ *n* the process of converting into nitre.

nitrify /'naɪtrɪˌfaɪ/ *vti* (**nitrifying, nitrified**) to make or become nitrous.

nitrite /'naɪtraɪt/ *n* a salt of nitrous acid.

nitro-, nitr- /'naɪtro/ *prefix* containing nitrogen; made with nitric acid.

nitrogen /'naɪtrədʒən/ *n* a gaseous element forming nearly 78 per cent of air.

nitrogenize /naɪ'trɒdʒəˌnaɪz/ or /'naɪtrədʒəˌnaɪz/ *vt* to impregnate with nitrogen.—**nitrogenization** *n*.

nitrogenous /naɪ'trɒdʒɪnəs/ *adj* pertaining to, or containing, nitrogen.

nitroglycerin, nitroglycerine /ˌnaɪtro'glɪsərɪn/ *n* a powerful explosive made by adding glycerine to a mixture of nitric and sulphuric acids.

nitrous /'naɪtrəs/ *adj* resembling, obtained from, or impregnated with, nitre.

nitrous acid *n* a compound of four volumes of nitrogen and one of oxygen.

nitrous oxide *n* a compound of one volume of oxygen and two volumes of nitrogen; laughing gas.

nitty-gritty /ˌnɪti'grɪti/ *n* (*sl*) basic elements; harsh realities; practical details.

nitwit /'nɪtwɪt/ *n* (*inf*) a stupid person.

nival /'naɪvəl/ *adj* of or pertaining to snow.

niveous /'nɪviəs/ *adj* resembling snow, snow-like.

nix[1] /nɪks/ *n* (*German myth*) a water sprite; (*Scot*) a kelpie.—**nixie** *nf*.

nix[2] *n* (*sl*) nothing. • *interj* (*sl*) look out! be careful!

nizam /'nɪzɒm/ or /naɪ'zæm/ *n* (*with cap*) a title of the ruler of Hyderabad, India; a Turkish army soldier.

NJ *abbr* = New Jersey.

NLQ *abbr* = (*comput*) near letter quality.

NM *abbr* = New Mexico.

No[1] (*chem symbol*) nobelium.

No[2] *abbr* = number.

No[3], **Noh** /no:/ *n* (*pl* **No, Noh**) Japanese classic dance-drama.

no *adv* (*used to express denial or disagreement*) not so, not at all, by no amount. • *adj* not any; not a; not one, none; not at all; by no means. • *n* (*pl* **noes, nos**) a denial; a refusal; a negative vote or voter.

Noachian /no:'eɪkiən/, **Noachic** /-'ækɪk/ *adj* pertaining to the patriarch Noah, the deluge, or his times.

nob[1] /nɒb/ *n* a knob; (*sl*) the head.

nob[2] *n* (*at cribbage*) knave of suit of turn-up card.

nob[3] *n* (*Brit sl*) a member of the upper classes; a wealthy person.

nobble /'nɒbəl/ *vt* (*Brit sl*) to tamper with (a racehorse) to prevent its winning; to obtain (money) by dishonest means; to suborn (a juror, etc) by bribes or threats; to defeat by underhand methods; to steal; to kidnap.

nobelium /noːˈbiːliəm/ *n* a radioactive metallic element.

Nobel prize /ˈnoːbel/ *n* an annual international prize given for distinction in one of six areas: physics, chemistry, physiology and medicine, economics, literature, and promoting peace.

nobility /noːˈbɪlɪti/ *n* (*pl* **nobilities**) nobleness of character, mind, birth, or rank; the class of people of noble birth.

noble /ˈnoːbəl/ *adj* famous or renowned; excellent in quality or character; of high rank or birth. • *n* a person of high rank in society.

nobleman /-mən/ *n* (*pl* **noblemen**) a peer.—**noblewoman** *nf* (*pl* **noblewomen**).

nobleness /-nəs/ *n* the state of quality of being noble.

noblesse oblige /noːˈblesɒˈbliːʒ/ *n* rank has its obligations.

nobly /ˈnoːbli/ *adv* in a noble manner; of noble rank.

nobody /ˈnoːbədi/ *or* /-bedi/, /-bɒdi/ *n* (*pl* **nobodies**) a person of no importance. • *pron* no person.

nock /nɒk/ *n* a notch in a bow or arrow for the string; (*naut*) the forward upper corner of some sails. • *vt* to fit (an arrow) to string.

nocti-, noct- /ˈnɒkti/ *or* /-tə/ *prefix* night.

noctiluca /ˌnɒktəˈluːkə/ *n* (*pl* **noctilucae**) a phosphorescent animalcule.

noctule /ˈnɒktjuːl/ *n* the largest British kind of bat.

nocturn /ˈnɒktərn/ *n* (*RC Church*) a part of matins.

nocturnal /nɒkˈtərnəl/ *adj* of, relating to, night; active by night.—**nocturnally** *adv*.

nocturne /ˈnɒktərn/ *n* a picture of a night scene; a musical composition appropriate to the night; a lullaby.

nocuous /ˈnɒkjuːəs/ *adj* hurtful.

nod /nɒd/ *vti* (**nodding, nodded**) to incline the head quickly, *esp* in agreement or greeting; to let the head drop, be drowsy; to indicate by a nod; (*with* **off**) (*inf*) to fall asleep. • *n* a quick bob of the head; a sign of assent or command.

nodal /ˈnoːdəl/ *adj* pertaining to nodes.

noddy /ˈnɒdi/ *n* (*pl* **noddies**) a simpleton; a tropical sea bird; a four-wheeled carriage with a door at the back.

node /noːd/ *n* a knob; a knot; a point of intersection; (*med*) a swelling; (*bot*) the joint of a stem and leaf or leaves; (*astron*) two points at which the orbit of a planet intersects he ecliptic; (*math*) the point at which a curve crosses itself; the point of rest in a vibrating body.

nodical /ˈnɒdɪkəl/ *or* /ˈnoːdɪ-/ *adj* (*astron*) pertaining to nodes.

nodose /nəˈdoːs/ *adj* having knots or nodes, knotty, knobbed.—**nodosity** *n*.

nodular /ˈnɒdʒʊlər/, **nodulose** /-ˌloːs/, **nodulous** /-dʒələs/ *adj* pertaining to, or like, a nodule.

nodule /ˈnɒdjuːl/ *n* a small lump or tumour.—**nodular** *adj*.

nodus /ˈnoːdəs/ *n* (*pl* **nodi**) a knotty point, a complication in the plot of a story, etc.

noel, noël /noːˈel/ *n* Christmas, *esp* in carols.

noetic /noːˈetɪk/ *or* /noːˈiːtɪk/ *adj* pertaining to, performed by, or originating in, the mind or intellect, intellectual, abstract. • *n* the science of the intellect.—*also* **noemics**.

no-fault /noːˈfɔlt/ *adj* (*insurance*) providing damages without blame being fixed; (*divorce*) concluded without blame being charged.

nog[1] /nɒg/ *n* a wooden peg or block; a stump. • *vt* (**nogging, nogged**) to secure with nogs.

nog[2] *n* an East Anglian strong beer.

nog[3] *n* (an) eggnog.

noggin /ˈnɒgɪn/ *n* a small quantity of alcoholic drink; (inf) the head.

nogging /ˈnɒgɪŋ/ *n* a partition formed of timber scantlings filled up with bricks.

no-go area /noːˈgoː/ *n* an area that certain individuals or groups are forbidden to enter.

nohow /ˈnoːhau/ *adv* in no way, by no means.

noil /nɔɪl/ *n* a short wool-combing.

noise /nɔɪz/ *n* a sound, *esp* a loud, disturbing or unpleasant one; a din; unwanted fluctuations in a transmitted signal; (*pl*) conventional sounds, words, etc made in reaction, such as sympathy. • *vt* to make public.

noiseless /ˈnɔɪzləs/ *adj* making no sound, silent.—**noiselessly** *adv*.—**noiselessness** *n*.

noisette /nwɒˈzet/ *n* a small round piece of meat.

noisome /ˈnɔɪsəm/ *adj* harmful, noxious; foul-smelling.

noisy /ˈnɔɪzi/ *adj* (**noisier, noisiest**) making much noise; turbulent, clamorous.—**noisily** *adv*.—**noisiness** *n*.

nolens volens /ˌnoːlenzˈvoːlenz/ *adv* (*Latin*) willingly or unwillingly, willy-nilly.

noli me tangere /ˌnoːlaɪmiˈtændʒəri/ *n* (*Latin*) a warning not to meddle; an erosive ulcer, lupus; a wild cucumber; a picture of Christ as he appeared to Mary Magdalen at the sepulchre.

nolle prosequi /ˌnɒliˈprɒsɪˌkwaɪ/ *n* an English legal term indicating the plaintiff's abandonment of his suit.

nolo episcopari /ˌnoːloːˈepəskoːˌpɑri/ *n* (*Latin*) unwillingness to accept office.

nomad /ˈnoːmæd/ *n* one of a people or tribe who move in search of pasture; a wanderer.—**nomadic** *adj*.

nomadic /noːˈmædɪk/ *adj* wandering; leading a wandering life; pastoral.—**nomadically** *adv*.

no-man's-land *n* an unclaimed piece of land; a strip of land, *esp* between armies, borders; an ambiguous area, subject, etc.

nombril /ˈnɒmbrɪl/ *n* (*her*) the centre of an escutcheon.

nom de guerre /ˌnɒmdəˈgɛr/ *or* /nɜ̃-/ *n* (*pl* **noms de guerre**) a pseudonym, an assumed name.

nom de plume /ˌnɒmdəˈpluːm/ *or* /nɜ̃-/ *n* (*pl* **noms de plume**) a pseudonym.

nome /noːm/ *n* a province of modern Greece; a territorial division in ancient Egypt.

nomenclator /ˈnoːmənˌkleɪtər/ *n* an ancient Roman slave who named persons met; one who gives names to things, an inventor of names.

nomenclature /ˈnoːmənˌkleɪtʃər/ *or* /ˈnɒm-/, /noːˈmenklətʃər/ *n* a system of names, terminology, used in a science, etc, or for parts of a device, etc.

nominal /ˈnɒmɪnəl/ *adj* of or like a name; existing in name only; having minimal real worth, token.

nominalism /ˈnɒmɪnəˌlɪzəm/ *n* (*philos*) the doctrine that general notions exist only in the mind or in name, opposite to realism.

nominalist /ˈnɒmɪnəˈlɪst/ *n* one who holds the doctrine of nominalism.—**nominalistic** *adj*.

nominally /ˈnɒmɪnəli/ *adv* in name only.

nominate /ˈnɒmɪˌneɪt/ *vt* to appoint to an office or position; (*candidate*) to propose for election.—**nominator** *n*.

nomination /ˌnɒmɪˈneɪʃən/ *n* the act or right of nominating; the state of being nominated.

nominative /ˈnɒmɪnətɪv/ *adj* (*gram*) denoting the case of the subject of a verb; appointed, not elected. • *n* (*gram*) the nominative case or a word in it.

nominee /ˌnɒmɪˈniː/ *n* a person who is nominated.

nomo-, nom- /ˈnoːmoː/ *or* /-mə/, /ˈnɒmoː/, /-ə/ *prefix* law.

nomography /nəˈmɒgrəfi/ *n* (*pl* **nomographies**) the art of drawing up laws.—**nomographic, nomographical** *adj*.

nomology /noːˈmɒlədʒi/ *n* the science of the laws of the mind.—**nomological** *adj*.—**nomologist** *n*.

nomothetic /ˌnɒməˈθetɪk/ *or* /ˌnoːm-/, **nomothetical** /-əl/ *adj* legislative, founded on a system of laws.

non- /nɒn/ *prefix* not, reversing the meaning of a word.

nonage /ˈnoːnɪdʒ/ *or* /ˈnɒn-/ *n* minority, legal infancy; an early stage.

nonagenarian /ˌnoːnədʒəˈnerɪən/ *or* /ˌnɒn-/ *n* a person who is in his or her nineties.

nonagon /ˈnɒnəgɒn/ *n* a plane figure with 9 sides and 9 angles.—**nonagonal** *adj*.

nonalcoholic /ˌnɒnælkəˈhɒlɪk/ *adj* (*drinks, etc*) containing little or no alcohol.

nonaligned /ˌnɒnəˈlaɪnd/ *adj* not in alliance with any side, *esp* in power politics.

nonce /nɒns/ *n* **for the nonce** for this time only.

nonce word *n* a word coined for one occasion.

nonchalance /ˌnɒnʃəˈlɒns/ *or* /ˈnɒnʃəˌlɒns/, /-ləns/ *n* coolness; indifference.

nonchalant /ˌnɒnʃəˈlɒnt/ *or* /ˈnɒnʃəˌlɒnt/, /-lənt/ *adj* calm; cool, unconcerned, indifferent.—**nonchalantly** *adv*.

noncombatant /ˌnɒnˈkɒmˈbætənt/ *or* /nɒnkəm-/, /-ˈkɒmbætənt/, /-ˈkʌm-/ *n* a member of the armed forces whose duties do not include fighting, as a doctor or chaplain; a civilian during wartime.

noncommissioned officer /ˌnɒnkəˈmɪʃənd/ *n* (*mil*) a subordinate officer, as a corporal, sergeant, etc, appointed from the ranks.

noncommittal /ˌnɒnkəˈmɪtəl/ *adj* not revealing one's opinion.—**noncommittally** *adv*.

non compos mentis /ˌnɒnkɒmpəsˈmentɪs/ *adj* (*Latin*) of unsound mind, not responsible.

nonconductor /ˌnɒnkənˈdʌktər/ *n* a substance that will not conduct electricity or heat.

non-confidence, no-confidence *adj* ✤ pertaining to a motion or vote in a legislature expressing a lack of majority support for the governing party.

nonconformist /ˌnɒnkənˈfɔrmɪst/ *n* a person who does not conform to prevailing attitudes, behaviour, etc; (*with cap*) in Britain, a Protestant who does not belong to the established church.—*also adj*.

nonconformity /ˌnɒnkənˈfɔrmɪti/ *n* (*with cap*) refusal to conform to the established church; a want of conformity, irregularity.

noncooperation /ˌnɒnkoːˌɒpərˈeɪʃən/ *n* refusal to cooperate, *esp* with government decree, etc.—**noncooperative** *adj*.

nondescript /ˈnɒndɪskrɪpt/ *adj* hard to classify, indeterminate; lacking individual characteristics. • *n* a nondescript person or thing.

none /nʌn/ *pron* no one; not anyone; (*pl verb*) not any; no one. • *adv* not at all.

noneffective /ˌnɒnəˈfɛktɪv/ *adj* not effective; (*soldier, sailor*) not qualified for active service.—*also n*.

nonentity /nɒnˈɛntɪti/ *n* (*pl* **nonentities**) a person or thing of no significance.

nones /noːnz/ *npl* in the ancient Roman calendar the ninth day before the Ides, reckoned inclusively, ie 7th of March, May, July, October, and the 5th of the other months; (*RC Church*) the devotional office for the ninth hour or 3 p.m.

nonesuch /ˈnʌnˌsʌtʃ/ *n* an unrivalled person or thing, a nonpareil; a plant like clover used for fodder.—*also* **nonsuch**.

nonet /noːˈnet/ *n* a group of nine connected objects or people; (*mus*) a piece for nine players.

nonetheless /ˌnʌnðəˈles/ or /ˌnʌnðəˌles/ *conj* nevertheless.

nonevent /ˌnɒnɪˈvent/ *n* an event or experience that is unexpectedly disappointing.

nonfeasance /nɒnˈfiːzəns/ *n* (*law*) the omission of an obligatory act.

nonferrous /nɒnˈferəs/ *adj* containing no iron.

nonflammable /nɒnˈflæməbəl/ *adj* not easily set on fire.

nonillion /noːˈnɪljən/ *n* in the US and France, tenth power of a thousand (1 followed by 30 ciphers); in Britain, the ninth power of one million (1 followed by 54 ciphers).—**nonillionth** *adj*.

nonintervention /ˌnɒnɪntərˈvenʃən/ *n* the policy of refusing to interfere in the affairs of others, *esp* nations.—**noninterventionist** *adj*.

nonjuror /nɒnˈdʒʊrər/ *n* one who refused to take the oath of allegiance to William and Mary in 1689.

non-lethal /nɒnˈliːθəl/ *adj* (*international affairs*) pertaining to foreign aid given to provide medicine, clothing or food rather than weapons.

nonmetal /nɒnˈmetəl/ *n* a chemical element (*eg* carbon) that is not a metal.

nonmoral /nɒnˈmɒrəl/ *adj* unconcerned with morality; without moral standards.

nonpareil /ˈnɒnpərəl/ or /ˌnɒnpəˈreɪl/ *adj* without an equal; (*person or thing*) unrivalled, matchless, unsurpassed. • *n* unequalled excellence; (*print*) a 6-point type; a variety of apple; a kind of bird, moth, wheat, etc.

nonpartisan /ˌnɒnˈpɑrtɪzən/ or /ˌnɒnpɑrtɪˈzæn/ *adj* not aligned to one particular political party.

nonparty /nɒnˈpɑrti/ *adj* free from party obligations.

nonplus /nɒnˈplʌs/ *vt* (**nonplusses, nonplussing, nonplussed** or **nonpluses, nonplusing, nonplused**) to cause to be so perplexed that one cannot, go, speak, act further. • *n* (*pl* **nonpluses**) a state of perplexity, a standstill.

non plus ultra *see* **ne plus ultra**.

non-profit /nɒnˈprɒfɪt/ *adj* (*organization*) not conducted for the purpose of making money.

nonproliferation /ˌnɒnprəˌlɪfəˈreɪʃən/ *n, adj* (*placing*) restriction on the acquisition or production of, *esp* nuclear weapons.

nonrepresentational /ˌnɒnˌreprɪzənˈteɪʃənəl/ *adj* (*art*) abstract.

nonsense /ˈnɒnsens/ or /-səns/ *n* words, actions, etc, that are absurd and have no meaning.—*also adj*. • *interj* absurd!

nonsensical /ˌnɒnˈsensɪkəl/ *adj* absurd; unmeaning.—**nonsensically** *adv*.

non sequitur /nɒnˈsekwɪtər/ *n* a statement that has no relevance to what has preceded it.

nonstarter /nɒnˈstɑrtər/ *n* a person who is unlikely to succeed; (*horse, racing car, etc*) withdrawn at the last moment.

non-status Indian *n* ✤ (*Cdn*) a person who is not officially registered as a member of a First Nations community.—*see* **status Indian**.

nonstick /nɒnˈstɪk/ *adj* (*saucepans*) coated with a surface that prevents food from sticking.

nonstop /ˌnɒnˈstɒp/ *adj* (*train, plane, etc*) not making any intermediate stops; not ceasing. • *adv* without stopping or pausing.

nonsuch /ˈnʌnsʌtʃ/ *see* **nor esuch**.

nonsuit /nɒnˈsuːt/ or /-ˈsjuːt/ *n* the withdrawal of a suit during trial either voluntarily or by judgment of the court on the discovery of error or defect in the pleadings. • *vt* to pronounce a nonsuit against.

nonunion /nɒnˈjuːniən/ *adj* not belonging to a trade union.

nonviolence /nɒnˈvaɪələns/ *n* the abstaining from physical force to achieve civil rights.—**nonviolent** *adj*.

noodle[1] /ˈnuːdəl/ *n* (*often pl*) pasta formed into a strip.

noodle[2] *n* (*inf*) a foolish person; (*sl*) the head.

nook /nʊk/ *n* a secluded corner, a retreat; a recess.

noon /nuːn/ *n* midday; twelve o'clock in the day. • *adj* pertaining to noon.

noonday /ˈnuːndeɪ/, **noontide** /ˈnuːntaɪd/, **noontime** /ˈnuːntaɪm/ *adj* pertaining to noon, or midday. • *n* noon.

no one /ˈnoːwʌn/ *pron* nobody.

noose /nuːs/ *n* a loop of rope with a slipknot, used for hanging, snaring, etc. • *vt* to tie in a noose; to make a noose in or of.

nopal /ˈnoːpəl/ *n* an American cactus, the food of the cochineal insect.

nope /noːp/ *adv* (*sl*) no.

nor /nɔr/ or /nər/ *conj* and not; not either.

Nor *abbr* = Norman; north; Norway; Norwegian.

Nordic /ˈnɔrdɪk/ *adj* (*physical type*) characterized by tall stature, long head, light skin and hair, and blue eyes; (skiing) including cross-country runs and jumping.

Norfolk jacket /ˈnɔrfək/ *n* a man's loose jacket with a belt.

noria /ˈnɔriə/ *n* a water-raising apparatus in Spain, etc, a waterwheel.

norm /nɔrm/ *n* a standard or model, *esp* the standard of achievement of a large group.—**normative** *adj*.

normal /ˈnɔrməl/ *adj* regular; usual; stable mentally. • *n* anything normal; the usual state, amount, etc.—**normalcy** *n*.—**normality** *n*.—**normally** *adv*.

normalize /ˈnɔrməˌlaɪz/ *vti* to make or become normal.—**normalization** *n*.

normal school *n* (*US*) a school for the training of teachers for elementary schools.

Norman /ˈnɔrmən/ *n* any of the people of Normandy who conquered England in 1066; a native or inhabitant of Normandy in France. • *adj* pertaining to the Normans or Normandy; (*archit*) of a style introduced into England by the Normans, characterized by rounded arches and massive square towers.—*also* **Normanesque**.

Norn /nɔrn/ *n* (*Scand myth*) one of the three fates, Urd, Verdande and Skuld, representing the past, the present and the future.

Norse /nɔrs/ *adj* of ancient Scandinavia or its inhabitants; of Norway. • *n* the language of Norway.

Norseman /ˈnɔrsmən/ *n* (*pl* **Norsemen**) any of the ancient Scandinavian people, the Vikings.

north /nɔrθ/ *n* one of the four points of the compass, opposite the sun at noon, to the right of a person facing the sunset; the direction in which a compass needle points; (*often with cap*) the northern part of one's country or the earth. • *adj* in, of, or towards the north; from the north. • *adv* in or towards the north.

northeast /nɔrθˈiːst/ *adj, n* (of) the direction midway between north and east.

northeaster /-ər/ *n* a northeast wind.

northeasterly /-ərli/ *adj* towards or coming from the northeast. • *n* (*pl* **northeasterlies**) a northeast wind or storm.

northeastern /-ərn/ *adj* belonging to the northeast, or in that direction.

northeastward /nɔrθˈiːstwərd/ *adj* towards or in the northeast.—*also adv*.—**northeastwards** *adv*.

norther /ˈnɔrðər/ *n* a strong wind or storm from the north, *esp* a strong gale that prevails in the Gulf of Mexico from September to March.

northerly /ˈnɔrðərli/ *adj* in, from, or towards the north. • *n* (*pl* **northerlies**) a northerly wind.

northern /ˈnɔrðərn/ *adj* of or in the north.

northerner /-ər/ *n* a native or inhabitant of the north.

Northern Hemisphere *n* the half of the earth north of the Equator.

northern lights *npl* the aurora borealis.

northernmost /ˈnɔrðərnˌmoːst/ *adj* farthest north.

northing /'nɔrθɪŋ/ n distance northward.

North Pole n the northern end of the axis of the earth at a latitude of 90 degrees north.

north star n the polar star.

northward /'nɔrθwərd/ adj towards or in the north.—*also adv*.—**northwards** adv.

northwest /nɔrθ'west/ adj, n (of) the direction midway between north and west.

northwester /-ər/ n a northwest wind.

northwesterly /-ərli/ adj towards or coming from the northwest. • n (pl **northwesterlies**) a northwest wind or storm.

northwestern /-ərn/ adj belonging to the northwest, or in that direction.

northwestward /nɔrθ'westwərd/ adj towards or in the northwest.—*also adv*.—**northwestwards** adv.

Norwegian /nɔr'wi:dʒən/ adj, n (of or relating to) the language, people, etc, of Norway.

nose /no:z/ n the part of the face above the mouth, used for breathing and smelling, having two nostrils; the sense of smell; anything like a nose in shape or position. • vt to discover as by smell; to nuzzle; to push (away, etc) with the front forward. • vi to sniff for; to inch forwards; to pry.

nosebag /'no:zbæg/ n a bag containing fodder hung from a horse's head.

noseband /-bænd/ n the part of a bridle that covers the horse's nose.

nosebleed /-bli:d/ n a bleeding from the nose.

nose dive n a swift downward plunge of an aircraft, nose first; any sudden sharp drop, as in prices.—**nose-dive** vi.

nosegay /'no:zgeɪ/ n a bouquet.

nose job n (sl) cosmetic plastic surgery to reshape the nose.

nosey /'no:zi/ see **nosy**.

nosh /nɒʃ/ n (sl) food, a meal. • vt to chew. • vi to eat.

nosing /'no:zɪŋ/ n the rounded edge of a step, etc, or the metal shield for it.

noso- /'no:so:/ or /'no:sə/ prefix disease.

nosography /nə'sɒɡrəfi/ n the systematic description of diseases.

nosology /nə'sɒlədʒi/ n the classification of the diseases of animals and plants.—**nosological** adv.—**nosologically** adv.—**nosologist** n.

nostalgia /nɒ'stældʒə/ or /-dʒɪə/, /nə-/ n yearning for past times or places.

nostalgic /nɒ'stældʒɪk/ adj feeling or expressing nostalgia; longing for one's youth.—**nostalgically** adv.

nostology /nɒ'stɒlədʒi/ n the study of senility or ageing, gerontology.—**nostologic** adj.

nostril /'nɒstrəl/ n one of the two external openings of the nose for breathing and smelling.

nostrum /'nɒstrəm/ n a quack remedy, patent medicine.

nosy /'no:zi/ adj (**nosier, nosiest**) (inf) inquisitive, snooping.—**nosily** adv.—**nosiness** n.—*also* **nosey**.

nosy parker /-'pɑrkər/ n (inf) a prying person, busybody.

not /nɒt/ adv expressing denial, refusal, or negation.

nota bene /,no:tə'beneɪ/ note this.—*abbr* • **NB**.

notabilia /,no:tə'bɪliə/ npl things worthy of note.

notability /,no:tə'bɪlɪti/ n (pl **notabilities**) the quality of being notable; a notable person or thing.

notable /'no:təbəl/ adj worthy of being noted or remembered; remarkable, eminent. • n an eminent or famous person.—**notably** adv.

notandum /no:'tændəm/ n (pl **notanda**) a thing to be noted.

notarial /no:'terɪəl/ adj pertaining to, or done by, a notary.

notary /'no:təri/ n (pl **notaries**) a notary public.

notary public n (pl **notaries public**) a public official authorized to certify deeds, contracts, etc.

notation /no:'teɪʃən/ n a system of symbols or signs to represent quantities, etc, esp in mathematics, music, etc.

notch /nɒtʃ/ n a V-shaped cut in an edge or surface; (inf) a step, degree; a narrow pass with steep sides. • vt to cut notches in.

note /no:t/ n a brief summary or record, written down for future reference; a memorandum; a short letter; notice, attention; an explanation or comment on the text of a book; a musical sound of a particular pitch; a sign representing such a sound; a piano or organ key; the vocal sound of a bird. • vt to notice, observe; to write down; to annotate.

notebook /'no:tbʊk/ n a book with blank pages for writing in.

noted /-ɪd/ adj celebrated, well-known.

note paper /-,peɪpər/ n paper for writing letters.

noteworthy /-,wərði/ adj outstanding; remarkable.

nothing /'nʌθɪŋ/ n no thing; not anything; nothingness; a zero; a trifle; a person or thing of no importance or value. • adv in no way, not at all.

nothingness /-nəs/ n the state of being nothing; unconsciousness; worthlessness.

notice /'no:tɪs/ n an announcement; a warning; a placard giving information; a short article about a book, play, etc; attention, heed; a formal warning of intention to end an agreement at a certain time. • vt to observe; to remark upon. • vi to be aware of.

noticeable /-əbəl/ adj easily noticed or seen.—**noticeably** adv.

notice board n a board on which notices are posted.

notifiable /'no:tɪ,faɪəbəl/ adj (infectious diseases) that must be reported to health authorities.

notification /,no:tɪfɪ'keɪʃən/ n the act of notifying; a notice or paper bearing it.

notify /'no:tɪ,faɪ/ vt (**notifying, notified**) to inform; to report, give notice of.

notion /'no:ʃən/ n a general idea; an opinion; a whim.

notional /-əl/ adj hypothetical, abstract; imaginary.

notions /'no:ʃənz/ npl small useful articles, as thread, needles, etc; haberdashery.

noto- /'no:to:/ or /'no:tə/ prefix back.

notochord /'no:tə,kɔrd/ n the rudimentary form of the vertebral column; a band forming the basis of the spinal column.—**notochordal** adj.

notoriety /no:tə'raɪti/ n the state of being notorious; disrepute, infamy; public exposure.

notorious /no:'tɔrɪəs/ or /nə-/ adj widely known, esp unfavourably.—**notoriously** adv.

notornis /no:'tɔrnɪs/ n the gigantic short-winged coot of New Zealand.

nototherium /'no:to:,θɪrɪəm/ n (pl **nototheria**) an extinct gigantic marsupial of Australia.

notwithstanding /,nɒtwɪθ'stændɪŋ/ or /-wɪð-/ prep in spite of. • adv nevertheless. • conj although.

notwithstanding clause n ✦ (Cdn) a section of the Canadian constitution that allows Parliament or a provincial legislature to override certain clauses concerning rights and freedoms.

nougat /'nu:gət/ n a chewy sweet consisting of sugar paste with nuts.

nought /nɒt/ n nothing; a zero. • adv in no degree.—*also* **naught**.

noughts and crosses see **tick-tack-toe**.

noumenon /'nu:mə,nɒn/ or /'naʊ-/ n (pl **noumena**) an object of purely intellectual intuition; (philos) the substance or real existing under the phenomenal.—**noumenal** adj.

noun /naʊn/ n (gram) a word that names a person, a living being, an object, action etc; a substantive.

nourish /'nʌrɪʃ/ vt to feed; to encourage the growth of; to raise, bring up.

nourishing /-ɪŋ/ adj containing nourishment; health-giving; beneficial.

nourishment /-mənt/ n food; the act of nourishing.

nous /naʊs/ n pure intellect; common sense.

nouveau riche /,nu:vo:'ri:ʃ/ n (pl **nouveaux riches**) the new rich, a parvenu.—*also adj*.

Nov abbr = November.

nova /'no:və/ n (pl **novas, novae**) a new star that explodes into bright luminosity before subsiding.

Nova Scotian n ✦ (Cdn) a person who lives in or is from Nova Scotia.

Novatian /'nɑ:veɪʃən/ adj pertaining to the doctrines of the Novatians, a 3rd-century sect who held that the Church should not re-admit the lapsed, and that second marriages were of the nature of sin.

novel /'nɒvəl/ n a relatively long prose narrative that is usually fictitious and in the form of a story. • adj new and unusual.

novelette /,nɒvə'let/ n a short novel.—**novelettish** adj.

novelist /'nɒvəlɪst/ n a writer of novels.

novelize /'nɒvə,laɪz/ vt to turn (a play, film, etc) into a novel.—**novelization** n.

novella /nə'velə/ n (pl **novellas, novelle**) a short novel.

novelty /'nɒvəlti/ n (pl **novelties**) a novel thing or occurrence; a new or unusual thing; (pl) cheap, small objects for sale.

November /no:'vembər/ *n* the eleventh month, having 30 days.

novena /no:'vi:nə/ *n* (*pl* **novenae**) (*RC Church*) a prayer made for nine days to obtain a request through intercession of the Virgin or saint.

novice /'nɒvɪs/ *n* a person on probation in a religious order before taking final vows; a beginner.

novitiate, noviciate /no:'vɪʃiət/ or /-ieɪt/ *n* a probationary period, initiation; a novice; a place where novices live.

now /nau/ *adv* at the present time; by this time; at once; nowadays. • *conj* since; seeing that. • *n* the present time. • *adj* of the present time.

nowadays /'nauə,deɪz/ *adv* in these days; at the present time.

noway /'no:weɪ/ *adv* not at all. • *interj* (**no way**) used to express emphatic denial or refusal.

nowhere /'no:wer/ *adv* not in, at, or to anywhere.

nowise /'no:waɪz/ *adv* not in any manner or degree.

noxious /'nɒkʃəs/ *adj* harmful, unhealthy.—**noxiously** *adv*.—**noxiousness** *n*.

noyade /nwɒ'jɒd/ *n* execution by drowning, *esp* that system of capital punishment for political offenders employed by the French revolutionists of 1789.

noyau /'nɒjɒ/ *n* (*pl* **noyaux**) a liqueur flavoured with bruised bitter almonds.

nozzle /'nɒzəl/ *n* the spout at the end of a hose, pipe, etc.

Np (*chem symbol*) neptunium.

NRC /'en'ɑr'si:/ *abbr* ✦ (*Cdn*) = National Research Council.

NS *abbr* ✦ = Nova Scotia.

NST /'en'es'ti:/ *abbr* ✦ = Newfoundland Standard Time.

NT *abbr* = New Testament; ✦ Newfoundland Time.

-n't /ənt/ = not.

nth /ɛnθ/ *adj* (*maths*) of or having an unspecified number; (*inf*) utmost, extreme.

nu /nju:/ *n* the 13th letter of the Greek alphabet.

nuance /'nu:ɒns/ or /'nju:-/ *n* a subtle difference in meaning, colour, etc.

nub /nʌb/ *n* a lump or small piece; (*inf*) the central point or gist of a matter.

nubbin /'nʌbɪn/ *n* a small or imperfect ear of maize; undeveloped fruit.

nubecula /nju'bekjulə/ *n* (*pl* **nubeculae**) the Magellanic clouds, a small galaxy; cloudy appearance; a light film on the eye.

nubile /'nu:baɪl/ or /'nju:-/ *adj* (*girl*) marriageable; attractive.

nuclear /'nu:kliər/ or /'nju:-/ *adj* of or relating to a nucleus; using nuclear energy; having nuclear weapons.

nuclear bomb *n* a bomb whose explosive power derives from uncontrolled nuclear fusion or fission.

nuclear energy *n* energy released as a result of nuclear fission or fusion.

nuclear family *n* father, mother and children.

nuclear fission *n* the splitting of a nucleus of an atom either spontaneously or by bombarding it with particles.

nuclear fusion *n* the combining of two nuclei into a heavier nucleus, releasing energy in the process.

nuclear power *n* electrical or motive power produced by a nuclear reactor.

nuclear reactor *n* a device in which nuclear fission is maintained and harnessed to produce energy.

nuclear waste *n* radioactive waste.

nucleate /'nu:kliət/ or /'nju:-/ *adj* having a nucleus.

nucleic acid /nu:'kleɪk/ or /-'kli:k/, /nju:-/ *n* DNA, RNA or similar complex acid present in all living cells.

nucleo-, nucle- /'nu:klio:/ or /'nju:-/ *prefix* nucleus; nucleic acid.

nucleolus /,nu:kli'o:ləs/ or /,nju:-/ *n* (*pl* **nucleoli**) a minute body inside a nucleus.

nucleonics /,nu:kli'ɒnɪks/ or /,nju:-/ *n* (*used as sing*) the physics and technology of the applications of nuclear energy.

nucleus /'nu:kliəs/ or /'nju:-/ *n* (*pl* **nuclei**, **nucleuses**) the central part or the core around which something may develop, or be grouped or concentrated; the centrally positively charged portion of an atom; the part of an animal or plant cell that contains genetic material.

nude /nu:d/ or /nju:d/ *adj* naked; bare; undressed. • *n* a naked human figure, *esp* in a work of art; the state of being nude.—**nudity** *n*.

nudge /nʌdʒ/ *vt* to touch gently with the elbow to attract attention or urge into action; to push slightly. • *n* a gentle touch, as with the elbow.

nudibranch /'nu:dɪbræŋk/ or /'nju:-/ *n* any of the order Nudibranchia of shell-less molluscs with naked gills.

nudism /'nu:dɪzəm/ or /'nju:-/ *n* the practice of going nude, *esp* in groups at designated places and times.

nudist /'nu:dɪst/ or /'nju:-/ *n* one who believes in going nude.—*also adj*.

nudity /'nu:diti/ or /'nju:-/ *n* (*pl* **nudities**) nakedness.

nugatory /'nu:gə,tori/ or /'nju:-/ *adj* trifling, worthless; inoperative, not valid; useless.

nugget /'nʌgət/ *n* a small lump, *esp* of gold in its natural state.

nuisance /'nu:səns/ or /'nju:-/ *n* a person or thing that annoys or causes trouble.

nuke /nu:k/ or /nju:k/ *vt* (*sl*) to attack and destroy with a nuclear weapon; (*sl*) to cook or heat (food) in microwave oven. • *n* a nuclear weapon.

null /nʌl/ *adj* without legal force; invalid.

nullah /'nʌlə/ *n* in the East Indes, a watercourse or canal; a ravine.

nulla-nulla /'nʌlə,nʌlə/ *n* (*Austral*) a hard wooden club.

nullifier /'nʌlɪ,faɪər/ *n* one who nullifies.

nullify /'nʌlɪ,faɪ/ *vt* (**nullifying, nullified**) to make null, to cancel out.—**nullification** *n*.

nullipara /nʌ'lɪpərə/ *n* (*pl* **nulliparae**) a woman who has never given birth to a child, *esp* if not a virgin.

nullipore /'nʌlɪ,por/ *n* a marine coral-like plant with calcareous fronds.

nullity /'nʌlti/ *n* (*pl* **nullities**) the state of being null; a legally invalid document or act; something ineffectual, worthless, etc.

Num *abbr* = number; numeral.

numb /nʌm/ *adj* deadened; having no feeling (due to cold, shock, etc.). • *vt* to make numb.—**numbness** *n*.

number /'nʌmbər/ *n* a symbol or word indicating how many; a numeral identifying a person or thing by its position in a series; a single issue of a magazine; a song or piece of music, *esp* as an item in a performance; (*inf*) an object singled out; a total of persons or things; (*gram*) the form of a word indicating singular or plural; a telephone number; (*pl*) arithmetic; (*pl*) numerical superiority. • *vti* to count; to give a number to; to include or be included as one of a group; to limit the number of; to total.

numbered company *n* ✦ (*Cdn*) a corporation whose name is a number, followed by the name of the province in which it is registered.

numberless /-ləs/ *adj* too many to count.

number one *n* the first in a list, series, etc; (*inf*) oneself or one's own interests; (*inf*) the most important person or thing; (*inf*) a best-selling pop record. • *adj* most important, urgent, etc.

numberplate *n* a license plate.

Number Ten *n* 10 Downing Street, the London residence of the British prime minister.

numbles /'nʌmbəlz/ *npl* humbles, entrails, *esp* of a deer.

numbskull /'nʌmskəl/ *see* **numskull**.

numerable /'nu:mərəbəl/ or /'nju:-/ *adj* countable.—**numerably** *adv*.

numeral /'nu:mərəl/ or /'nju:-/ *n* a symbol or group of symbols used to express a number (*eg* two = 2 or II, etc).

numerate /'nu:mərət/ or /'nju:-/ *adj* having a basic understanding of arithmetic. • *vt* to reckon or enumerate; to point or read, as figures.

numerati /,njumə'ræti/ or /-'roti/ *npl* people, *esp* financiers, who are proficient at arithmetic.

numeration /,nu:mə'reɪʃən/ or /,nju:-/ *n* the act of numbering; the art of reading in words numbers expressed by symbols.

numerator /'nu:mə,reɪtər/ or /'nju:-/ *n* the number above the line in a fraction.

numeric, numerical /nu:'merɪkəl/ or /nju:-/, *adj* of or relating to numbers; expressed in numbers.

numerology /,nu:mə'rolədʒi/ or /,nju:-/ *n* the study of the supposed occult meaning of numbers.

numerous /'nu:mərəs/ or /'nju:-/ *adj* many, consisting of many items.

numismatics /,nu:mɪz'mætɪks/ or /,nju:-/ *n* (*used as sing*) the study of coins, medals, etc.—*also* **numismatology**.—**numismatic** *adj*.

numismatist /-'mɪzmətɪst/ *n* one skilled in numismatics; a student of coins.

nummular /'nʌmjulər/ *adj* pertaining to, or like, coins.

nummulite /'nʌmju,laɪt/ *n* a many-chambered fossil foraminifer resembling a coin.—**nummulitic** *adj*.

numskull /'nʌmskʌl/ n a dolt, a blockhead.—*also* **numbskull**.

nun /nʌn/ n a woman belonging to a religious order.

Nunc Dimittis /ˌnʌŋkdɪ'mɪtɪs/ n a canticle.

nunciature /'nʌnsɪəˌtʃər/ n the office of a nuncio; the tenure of it.

nuncio /'nʌnsɪoʊ/ or /nʊn-/ n (pl **nuncios**) the pope's ambassador at a foreign court.

nuncupate /'nʌŋkjuːˌpeɪt/ vt to declare, to make a will verbally, not in writing.

nuncupative /'nʌŋkjuːˌpeɪtɪv/ adj (law) verbal, not written; nominal.

nunnery /'nʌnərɪ/ n (pl **nunneries**) a convent of nuns.

nuptial /'nʌpʃəl/ adj relating to marriage. • npl a wedding ceremony; marriage.

nurse /nɜrs/ n a person trained to care for the sick, injured or aged; a person who looks after another person's child or children. • vt to tend, to care for; (baby) to feed at the breast; (hatred) to foster; to tend with an eye to the future.

nursemaid /'nɜrsmeɪd/ n a woman in charge of children, a nanny.

nursery /'nɜrsrɪ/ or /-ərɪ/ n (pl **nurseries**) a room set aside for children; a place where children may be left in temporary care; a place where young trees and plants are raised for transplanting.

nurseryman /'nɜrsərɪmən/ n (pl **nurserymen**) a person who owns or works in a plant nursery.

nursery rhyme n a short traditional poem or song for children.

nursery school n a school for young children, usu under five.

nursery slope n a gently inclined slope for novice skiers.

nursing /'nɜrsɪŋ/ n the profession of a nurse.

nursing home n an establishment providing care for convalescent, chronically ill, or disabled people.

nursling, nurseling /'nɜrslɪŋ/ n an infant; one who is nursed.

nurture /'nɜrtʃər/ vt to feed; to bring up, educate. • n the act of bringing up a child; nourishment.

nut /nʌt/ n a kernel (sometimes edible) enclosed in a hard shell; a usu metallic threaded block screwed on the end of a bolt; (sl) a mad person; (sl) a devotee, fan. • vt (**nutting, nutted**) to gather nuts.

nutant /'nuːtənt/ or /'njuː-/ adj (bot) having the top bent downward.

nutation /nuː'teɪʃən/ or /njuː-/ n nodding; the periodic vibratory movement of the axis of the earth; (bot) the turning of flowers towards the sun.—**nutational** adj.

nut-brown adj coloured like a ripe hazelnut.

nut case /'nʌtkeɪs/ n (sl) a crazy or foolish person.

nutcracker /'nʌtˌkrækər/ n (usu pl) a tool for cracking nuts; a bird with speckled plumage.

nuthatch /'nʌthætʃ/ n a small climbing bird feeding on nuts.

nutmeg /'nʌtmeg/ n the aromatic kernel produced by a tree, grated and used as a spice.

nutria /'nuːtrɪə/ or /'njuː-/ n the fur or skin of the coypu, a South American beaver.

nutrient /'nuːtrɪənt/ or /'njuː-/ n a substance that nourishes. • adj promoting growth.

nutriment /'nuːtrɪmənt/ or /'njuː-/ n nourishing food, nourishment.

nutrition /nuː'trɪʃən/ or /njuː-/ n the act or process by which plants and animals take in and assimilate food in their systems; the study of the human diet.—**nutritional** adj.

nutritionist /nuː'trɪʃənɪst/ or /njuː-/ n a specialist who studies and advises on the human diet.

nutritious /nuː'trɪʃəs/ or /njuː-/ adj efficient as food; health-giving, nourishing.

nutritive /'nuːtrɪtɪv/ or /'njuː-/ adj serving as good. • n an article of food.—**nutritively** adv.

nuts /nʌts/ adj (inf) very keen (on); (inf) crazy.

nuts and bolts npl (inf) the basic facts or details.

nutshell /'nʌtʃel/ n the hard covering of a nut; a tiny receptacle; a compact way of expression.

nutting /'nʌtɪŋ/ n nut-gathering.

nutty /nʌtɪ/ adj (**nuttier, nuttiest**) tasting of or containing nuts; (sl) very enthusiastic; (sl) crazy, mad, etc.

nux vomica /nʌks'vɒmɪkə/ n the fruit of an East Indian plant (Strychnos Nux vomica), which yields the deadly poison strychnine.

nuzzle /'nʌzəl/ vti to push (against) or rub with the nose or snout; to nestle, snuggle.

NV abbr = Nevada.

NW abbr = northwest, northwestern.

NWT abbr ✦ = Northwest Territories.

NY abbr = New York.

nyctalopia /ˌnɪktə'loʊpɪə/ n night blindness; the inability to see clearly except at night.

nyctitropism /ˌnɪktɪ'troʊpɪzəm/ n (bot) the so-called sleep of plants, turning in certain direction at night.—**nyctitropic** adj.

nylon /'naɪlɒn/ n any of numerous strong, tough, elastic, synthetic materials used esp in plastics and textiles; (pl) stockings made of nylon.

nymph /nɪmf/ n (myth) a spirit of nature envisaged as a maiden; (poet) a lovely young maiden; the chrysalis of an insect.—**nymphean** adj.

nymphet /nɪm'fet/ or /'nɪmfət/ n a sexually desirable pre-adolescent girl.

nympho /'nɪmfoʊ/ n (pl **nymphos**) (inf) a nymphomaniac.

nympholepsy /'nɪmfəˌlepsɪ/ n (pl **nympholepsies**) frenzy caused by desire of the unattainable.

nympholept /'nɪmfəˌlept/ n one inspired by violent enthusiasm for an ideal.—**nympholeptic** adj.

nymphomania /ˌnɪmfə'meɪnɪə/ n uncontrollable sexual desire in women.—**nymphomaniac** adj, n.—**nymphomaniacal** adj.

nystagmus /nɪ'stægməs/ n a condition of the eye, with spasmodic movement of the eyeballs.—**nystagmic** adj.

NZ abbr = New Zealand.

O

O, o /o:/ *n* the 15th letter of the English alphabet; something shaped like the letter O; nought, nothing, zero.

O., o. *abbr* = octavo; old; only.

O (*chem symbol*) oxygen. • *interj* an exclamation of wonder, pain, etc.

O' *prefix* (in Irish *urnames*) descendant of.

o' *prep* (*inf, arch*) short for of or on.

-o /o:/ *n, adj suffix* (*inf*) indicating a diminutive, *cheapo* (*inf*) forming an interjection, *cheerio*.

oaf /o:f/ *n* (*pl* **oafs**) a loutish or stupid person.—**oafish** *adj.*—**oafishly** *adv.*

oak /o:k/ *n* a tree with a hard durable wood, having acorns as fruits.

oak apple *n* a spongy excrescence growing on the leaves or young branches of the oak, caused by the gallfly.

oaken /-ən/ *adj* made of or consisting of oak.

oakum /'o:kəm/ *n* a loose fibre obtained by unpicking old rope and used for caulking.

O & M *abbr* = organization and method(s).

OAP *abbr* = (*Brit*) Old age pensioner, senior citizen.

oar /ɔr/ *n* a pole with a flat blade for rowing a boat; an oarsman.

oarlock /'ɔrlɒk/ *n* (*US*) a rowlock.

oarsman /'ɔrzmən/ *n* (*pl* **oarsmen**) a person who rows a boat.—**oarsmanship** *n.*

OAS *abbr* = Organization of American States.

oasis /o:'eisis/ *n* (*pl* **oases**) a fertile place in a desert; a refuge.

oast /o:st/ *n* a kiln for drying hops or barley.

oatcake /'o:tkeik/ *n* a thin broad cake of oatmeal.

oaten /-ən/ *adj* made of oats.

oath /o:θ/ *n* (*pl* **oaths**) a solemn declaration to a god or a higher authority that one will speak the truth or keep a promise; a swear word; a blasphemous expression.

oatmeal /'o:tmi:l/ *n* ground oats; a porridge of this; a pale greyish-brown colour.

oats /o:ts/ *npl* a cereal grass widely cultivated for its edible grain; the seeds.

OAU *abbr* = Organization of African Unity.

ob. *abbr* = (*Latin*) obiit, died.

ob- /ɒb/ *prefix* before, against, toward, in front of, reversed.

obbligato /ɒbli'gɒto/ *adj* (*mus*) forming an integral part of a musical composition. • *n* (*pl* **obbligatos, obbligati**) an indispensable instrumental part or accompaniment written especially for the instrument named.—*also* **obligato** (*pl* **obligatos, obligati**).

obcordate /ɒb'kɔrdeit/ *adj* (*bot*) inversely cordate.

obdurate /'ɒbdʒurət/ or /-dur-/ *adj* hard-hearted; unyielding, stubborn.—**obduracy** *n.*—**obdurately** *adv.*

OBE *abbr* = Order of the British Empire.

obeah /'o:biə/ *see* obi.

obedience /o:'bi:diəns/ *n* the condition of being obedient; observance of orders, instructions, etc; respect for authority

obedient /o:'bi:diənt/ *adj* obeying; compliant; submissive to authority, dutiful.—**obediently** *adv.*

obeisance /o:'beisəns/ or /-bi:-/ *n* a bow or curtsey; an act of reverence or homage.

obelisk /'ɒbəlisk/ *n* a four-sided tapering pillar *usu* with a pyramidal top; a reference mark used in printing (†).—*also* **dagger**.

obelize /'ɒbə,laiz/ *vt* to mark with an obelus.

obelus /'ɒbələs/ *n* (*pl* **obeli**) a mark (— *or* ÷ *or* †) used in old MSS to indicate a doubtful or spurious reading; in modern writing, a break (—).

obese /o:'bi:s/ *adj* very fat.—**obesity** *n.*

obey /o:'bei/ *vti* (**obeying, obeyed**) to carry out (orders, instructions); to comply (with); to submit (to).

obfuscate /'ɒbfʌ,skeit/ *vt* to bewilder or confuse, to darken.—**obfuscation** *n.*

ob-gyn *abbr* = obstetrician and gynaecologist.

obi[1] /'o:bi/ *n* (*pl* **obis, obi**) a Japanese woman's sash.

obi[2] *n* (*pl* **obis**) in the West Indies and Africa, a system of secret sorcery or magical rites.—*also* **obeah**.

obit /'o:bit/ *n* (*inf*) an obituary.

obiter dictum /,ɒbitər 'diktəm/ *n* (*pl* **obiter dicta**) (*Latin*) a casual remark or opinion expressed incidentally, as by a judge or writer.

obituary /o:'bitʃuəri/ or /ə'titʃ-/ *n* (*pl* **obituaries**) an announcement of a person's death, often with a short biography.—**obituarist** *n.*

object /'ɒbdʒekt/ or /-dʒikt/ *n* something that can be recognized by the senses; a person or thing toward which action, feeling, etc, is directed; a purpose or aim; (*gram*) a noun or part of a sentence governed by a transitive verb or a preposition. • *vti* to state or raise an objection; to oppose; to disapprove.—**objector** *n.*

object ball *n* (*billiards*) the ball meant to be hit by the cue ball.

object glass *n* the lens of a microscope or telescope nearest to the object to be observed and forming the image.

objectify /ɒb'dʒekti,fai/ *vt* (**objectifying, objectified**) to render objective; to embody; to materialize.—**objectification** *n.*

objection /əb'dʒekʃən/ *n* the act of objecting; a ground for, or expression of, disapproval.

objectionable /əb'dʒekʃənəbəl/ *adj* causing an objection; disagreeable.—**objectionably** *adv.*

objective /əb'dʒektv/ *adj* relating to an object; not influenced by opinions or feelings; impartial; having an independent existence of its own, real; (*gram*) of, or appropriate to an object governed by a verb or a preposition. • *n* the thing or placed aimed at; (*gram*) the objective case.—**objectively** *adv.*

objectivism /əɒ'dʒekti,vizəm/ *n* (*philos*) the doctrine that the knowledge of the non-ego is anterior to that of the ego; (*art, literature*) the representation of persons and incidents as they really appear.—**objectivist** *adj, n.*—**objectivistic** *adj.*

objectivity /,ɒbdʒek'tiviti/ *n* the state or quality of being objective.

object lesson *n* a convincing practical illustration of some principle

object program *n* (*compu*) a computer program derived from the conversion of a source program into machine code by a compiler or assembler.

objet d'art /ɒbʒei'dɑr/ *n* (*pl* **objets d'art**) a small decorative object.

objurgate /'ɒbdʒər,geit/ *vt* to chide or reprove, to scold.—**objurgation** *n.*

objurgatory /ɒb'dʒərgə,tɔri/ *adj* containing reproof or censure.

oblanceolate /ɒb'lænsiələt/ *adj* (*bot*) lanceolate in the reversed order.

oblate /'ɒblet/ or /o:-/ *n* (*RC Church*) a secular priest who has devoted himself and his property to the monastery he has entered. *adj* dedicated to a monastic or religious life.

oblate *adj* (*spheroid*) depressed or flattened at the poles; orange-shaped.

oblation /o:'bleiʃən/ *n* an offering or sacrifice; anything presented in religious worship, *esp* the Eucharist.—**oblatory, oblational** *adj.*

obligate /'ɒbli,geit/ *vt* to bind by a contract, promise, sense of duty etc.

obligation /,ɒbli'geiʃən/ *n* the act of obligating; a moral or legal requirement; a debt; a favour; a commitment to pay a certain amount of money; the amount owed under such an obligation.

obligato *see* **obbligato**.

obligatory /ə'bligətori/ *adj* binding, not optional; compulsory.

oblige /ə'blaidʒ/ *vt* to compel by moral, legal, or physical force; (*person*) to make grateful for some favour; to do a favour for.

obligee /,ɒbli'dʒi:/ *n* (*law*) a person in whose favour a bond is made; a creditor.

obliging /ə'blaidʒiŋ/ *adj* ready to do favours, agreeable.—**obligingly** *adv.*

obligor /,ɒbli'gɔr/ *n* (*law*) a person who is bound by a bond; a debtor.

oblique /ə'bli:k/ or /o:-/ *adj* slanting, at an angle; diverging from the straight; indirect, allusive. • *n* an oblique line.—**obliquely** *adv.*

oblique angle *n* an angle greater or less than a right angle.

oblique case *n* (*gram*) any case except the nominative and vocative.

obliquity /ə'blɪkwɪtɪ/ *n* (*pl* **obliquities**) obliqueness; a slanting direction; deviation from a moral code.

obliterate /ə'blɪtə,reɪt/ *vt* to wipe out, to erase, to destroy.—**obliteration** *n*.

oblivion /ə'blɪvɪən/ *n* a state of forgetting or being forgotten; a state of mental withdrawal.

oblivious /ə'blɪvɪəs/ *adj* forgetful, unheeding; unaware (of).

oblong /'ɒblɒŋ/ *adj* rectangular. • *n* any oblong figure.

obloquy /'ɒbləkwɪ/ *n* (*pl* **obloquies**) reproachful language, detraction; calumny; slander, disgrace.

obnoxious /ɒb'nɒkʃəs/ or /əb-/ *adj* objectionable; highly offensive.—**obnoxiously** *adv*.—**obnoxiousness** *n*.

oboe /'oːboː/ *n* an orchestral woodwind instrument having a mouthpiece with a double reed.—**oboist** *n*.

obolus /'ɒbələs/, **obol** *n* (*pl* **oboli, obols**) an ancient Greek silver coin; a modern Greek weight = 1/10th of a gram.

obovate /ɒb'oːveɪt/ *adj* (*bot*) inversely ovate.

obs *abbr* = observation; obsolete.

obscene /ɒb'siːn/ or /əb-/ *adj* indecent, lewd; offensive to a moral or social standard.—**obscenely** *adv*.

obscenity /ɒb'senɪtɪ/ or /əb-/ *n* (*pl* **obscenities**) the state or quality of being obscene; an obscene act, word, etc.

obscurant /əb'skjʊrənt/ *adj, n* (a person) opposed to enlightenment, reactionary.—**obscurantism** *n*.—**obscurantist** *adj, n*.

obscure /ɒb'skjʊr/ or /əb-/ *adj* not clear; dim; indistinct; remote, secret; not easily understood; inconspicuous; unimportant, humble. • *vt* to make unclear, to confuse; to hide.—**obscurely** *adv*.

obscurity /ɒb'skjʊrɪtɪ/ or /əb-/ *n* (*pl* **obscurities**) the state or quality of being obscure; an obscure thing or person.

obsequies /'ɒbsɪkwiːz/ *npl* (*sing* **obsequy**) funeral rites, a funeral.

obsequious /ɒb'siːkwɪəs/ or /əb-/ *adj* subservient; fawning.—**obsequiously** *adv*.

observable /ɒb'zɜrvəbəl/ or /əb-/ *adj* worthy of observation; remarkable.—**observably** *adv*.

observance /ɒb'zɜrvəns/ or /əb-/ *n* the observing of a rule, duty, law, etc; a ceremony or religious rite.

observant /ɒb'zɜrvənt/ or /əb-/ *adj* watchful; attentive, mindful.—**observantly** *adv*.

observation /ɒbzər'veɪʃən/ *n* the act or faculty of observing; a comment or remark; careful noting of the symptoms of a patient, movements of a suspect, etc prior to diagnosis, analysis or interpretation.—**observational** *adj*.—**observationally** *adv*.

observatory /ɒb'zɜrvə,tɔrɪ/ or /əb-/ *n* (*pl* **observatories**) a building for astronomical observation; an institution whose primary purpose is making such observations.

observe /ɒb'zɜrv/ or /əb-/ *vt* to notice; to perceive; (*a law, etc*) to keep to or adhere to; to arrive at as a conclusion; to examine scientifically. • *vi* to take notice; to make a comment (on).—**observable** *adj*.

observer /-ər/ *n* a person who observes; a delegate who attends a formal meeting but may not take part; an expert analyst and commentator in a particular field.

obsess /ɒb'ses/ or /əb-/ *vt* to possess or haunt the mind of; to preoccupy.—**obsessive** *adj, n*.—**obsessively** *adv*.

obsession /ɒb'seʃən/ or /əb-/ *n* a fixed idea, often associated with mental illness; a persistent idea or preoccupation; the condition of obsessing or being obsessed.

obsidian /ɒb'sɪdɪən/ or /əb-/ *n* a hard glassy dark-coloured volcanic lava.

obsolescent /,ɒbsə'lesənt/ *adj* becoming obsolete, going out of date.—**obsolescence** *n*.

obsolete /,ɒbsə'liːt/ or /'ɒbsə,liːt/ *adj* disused, out of date.

obstacle /'ɒbstəkəl/ *n* anything that hinders something; an obstruction.

obstetrics /ɒb'stetrɪks/ or /əb-/ *n sing* the branch of medicine concerned with the care and treatment of women during pregnancy and childbirth.—**obstetric, obstetrical** *adj*.—**obstetrician** *n*.

obstinate /'ɒbstənət/ *adj* stubborn, self-willed; intractable; persistent.—**obstinacy** *n*.—**obstinately** *adv*.

obstreperous /ɒb'strepərəs/ or /əb-/ *adj* unruly, turbulent, noisy.

obstruct /ɒb'stʌkt/ or /əb-/ *vt* to block with an obstacle; to impede; to prevent, hinder; to keep (light, etc) from.

obstruction /ɒb'strʌkʃən/ or /əb-/ *n* that which obstructs; the act or an example of obstructing; a hindrance, obstacle.

obstructionism /-,nɪzəm/ *n* the systematic hindering of political business, etc.—**obstructionist** *adj, n*.

obstructive /ɒb'strʌktɪv/ or /əb-/ *adj* tending to obstruct; preventing, hindering.—**obstructively** *adv*.—**obstructiveness** *n*.

obtain /ɒb'teɪn/ or /əb-/ *vt* to get, to acquire, to gain. • *vi* to be prevalent, hold good.—**obtainable** *adj*.—**obtainment** *n*.

obtect /ɒb'tekt/ *adj* (*pupa*) protected by a hard outer case.

obtrude /ɒb'truːd/ or /əb-/ *vti* to push (an opinion, oneself) on others uninvited; to intrude.—**obtruding** *adj*.

obtrusion /ɒb'truːʒən/ *n* the act of obtruding; an unwelcome intrusion.

obtrusive /ɒb'truːsɪv/ *adj* apt to obtrude, pushy; protruding, sticking out.—**obtrusively** *adv*.—**obtrusiveness** *n*.

obtund /ɒb'tʌnd/ or /əb-/ *vt* (*med*) to blunt, to deaden.

obturate /'ɒbtʃʊrət/ *vt* to stop, to block or seal up; (*gun breech*) to close.—**obturation** *n*.—**obturator** *n*.

obtuse /ɒb'tuːs/ or /əb-/, /-tjuːs/ *adj* mentally slow; not pointed; dull, stupid; (*geom*) greater than a right angle.—**obtusely** *adv*.—**obtuseness** *n*.

obverse /'ɒbvɜrs/ or /ɒb'vɜrs/ *n* the front or top side; (*coin*) the head; a counterpart. • *adj* facing the viewer; with the top wider than the base.—**obversely** *adv*.

obversion /ɒb'vɜrʃən/ *n* (*logic*) the immediate inference by which we deny the opposite of anything affirmed.

obvert /ɒb'vɜrt/ or /əb-/ *vt* (*logic*) to infer by obversion; to turn toward, to face.

obviate /'ɒbvɪ,eɪt/ *vt* to make unnecessary; (*danger, difficulty*) to prevent, clear away.—**obviation** *n*.

obvious /'ɒbvɪəs/ *adj* easily seen or understood; evident.—**obviously** *adv*.—**obviousness** *n*.

obvolute /'ɒbvə,luːt/ *adj* arranged so as to overlap, as the margins of an organ or part of a plant.

OC /'oː'siː/ *abbr* ✤ = Officer of the Order of Canada.

oc- /ɒk/ *prefix* the form of *ob-* before *c*.

ocarina /,ɒkə'riːnə/ *n* an egg-shaped wind instrument played like a flute.

occasion /ə'keɪʒən/ *n* a special occurrence or event; a time when something happens; an opportunity; reason or grounds; a subsidiary cause. • *vt* to cause; to bring about.

occasional /ə'keɪʒənəl/ *adj* infrequent, not continuous; intermittent; produced for an occasion; (*a cause*) incidental.

occasionalism /-,nɪzəm/ *n* (*philos*) the Cartesian theory of occasional causes, that bodily actions are caused and controlled by divine agency and not by the human will / the Cartesian doctrine that apparent action of mind on matter is due to the invervention of God.

occasionally /-lɪ/ *adv* intermittently; now and then; infrequently.

occident /'ɒksɪdənt/ *n* the west; (*with cap*) specifically Europe and America; the countries west of Asia and Turkey in Europe.—**Occidental, occidental** *adj*.

occipital /ɒk'sɪpɪtəl/ *adj* of or pertaining to the occiput.

occiput /'ɒksɪ,pʌt/ *n* (*pl* **occipita, occiputs**) (*anat*) the back part of the skull or head.

occlude /ə'kluːd/ *vti* to shut out or in; to stop up, close; (*chem*) to absorb and retain.

occluded front *n* (*meteorol*) the phenomenon formed by a cold front overtaking a warm front and lifting the warm air above the earth's surface.

occlusion /ə'kluːʒən/ *n* the act of occluding; (*dentistry*) the position of the teeth when the jaws are closed; an occluded front.

occult /ɒ'kʌlt/ *adj* supernatural, magical; secret.—*also n*.

occultation /-'teɪʃən/ *n* (*astron*) a temporary disappearance or obscuration, as the eclipse of a star or planet by the moon, etc.

occulted /ɒ'kʌltəd/ *adj* (*astron*) hidden from the vision, as a star, etc.

occultism /-,tɪzəm/ *n* mysticism, spiritualism, theosophy, etc.—**occultist** *n*.

occult sciences *npl* magic, alchemy and astrology.

occupancy /'ɒkjʊpənsɪ/ *n* (*pl* **occupancies**) the act of taking and holding in possession; the time of possession.

occupant /'ɒkjʊpənt/ *n* a person who occupies, resides in, holds a position or place, etc.

occupation /,ɒkjʊ'peɪʃən/ *n* the act of occupying; the state of being occupied; employment or profession; a pursuit.—**occupational** *adj*.

occupational therapy *n* therapy by means of work in the arts and crafts, to aid recovery from disease or injury.—**occupational therapist** *n*.

occupier /'ɒkjʊ,paɪər/ *n* an occupant.

occupy /'ɒkjuˌpaɪ/ *vt* (**occupying, occupied**) to live in; (*room, office*) to take up or fill; (*a position*) to hold; to engross (one's mind); (*city, etc*) to take possession of.

occur /ə'kər/ or /ɒ:-/ *vi* (**occurring, occurred**) to happen; to exist; to come into the mind of.

occurrence /ə'kərəns/ *n* a happening, an incident, an event; the act or fact of occurring.

ocean /'ɔ:ʃən/ *n* a large stretch of sea, *esp* one of the earth's five oceans; a huge quantity or expanse.

oceangoing *adj* (*vessel*) designed and equipped for travelling on the open ocean.

oceanarium /ˌoˌʃə'neriəm/ *n* (*pl* **oceanariums, oceanaria**) a large seawater aquarium for displays of marine life.

Oceania /ˌoˌʃɪ'æniə/ or /ˌoˌsi-/ *n* the Pacific islands.—**Oceanic** *adj*.

oceanic /ˌoˌʃɪ'ænɪk/ or /ˌoˌsi-/ *adj* of or relating to the ocean; formed or found in the ocean.

Oceanid /o'si:ənɪd/ *n* (*pl* **Oceanids, Oceanides**) (*Greek myth*) a sea nymph.

oceanography /ˌoˌʃə'nɒgrəfi/ *n* the study of the oceans including their physical and chemical make-up, marine biology, and their exploitation.—**oceanographer** *n*.

ocellate, ocellated /'ɒsɪlət/ *adj* marked with small spots or eyes.

ocellus /o'sɛləs/ *n* (*pl* **ocelli**) the facet of a compound eye an eye-like spot, as on a peacock's tail, etc.

ocelot /'ɒsəˌlɒt/ or /'oː-/ *n* a medium-sized spotted wildcat of North and South America.

och /ɒx/ *interj* (*Scot, Irish*) expressing of surprise, contempt, disagreement, disappointment, etc.

ocher, ochre /'oːkər/ *n* a yellow to orange-coloured clay used as a pigment.

ochlo-, ochl- /ɒklɒ/ *prefix* mob.

ochlocracy /ɒk'lɒkrəsi/ *n* (*pl* **ochlocracies**) mob rule.—**ochlocrat** *n*.—**ochlocratic** *adj*.

o'clock /ə'klɒk/ *adv* indicating the hour; indicating a relative direction or position, twelve o'clock being directly ahead or above.

OCR /ˌoːsiː'ɑr/ *abbr* = optical character reader; optical character recognition.

Oct *abbr* = October.

octa- /'ɒktə/ *prefix* eight.

octachord /'ɒktəˌkɔrd/ *n* an eight-stringed musical instrument; a series of eight notes, diatonic scale.—**octachordal** *adj*.

octad /'ɒktæd/ *n* a group of eight; the number eight; (*chem*) an element or radical with a valency of eight.—**octadic** *adj*.

octagon /'ɒktəgɒn/ *n* a plane figure having eight equal sides.—**octagonal** *adj*.

octahedral /ˌɒktə'hiːdrəl/ *adj* having eight equal sides.

octahedron /ˌɒktə'hiːdrən/ *n* (*pl* **octahedrons, octahedra**) a solid figure contained by eight equal equilateral triangles.

octal /'ɒktəl/ *n* (*comput*) a number system with 8 as its base, one digit being equivalent to three bits.

octameter /ɒk'tæmɪtər/ *n* an eight-foot verse.

octane /'ɒktæn/ *n* a hydrocarbon found in petrol.

octane number, octane rating *n* a measure of the anti-knock quality of a liquid motor fuel expressed as a percentage.

octant /'ɒktənt/ *n* the eighth part of a circle; an instrument for measuring angles; (*astron*) an aspect of two planets, etc, when 45 degrees apart.

octave /'ɒktɪv/ *n* (*mus*) the eighth full tone above or below a given tone, the interval of eight degrees between a tone and either of its octaves, or the series of tones within this interval.

octavo /ɒk'tɒvoː/ or /ɒk'teɪvoː/ *n* (*pl* **octavos**) a sheet of printing paper folded in eight leaves or 16 pages (8vo); this size, average $9\frac{1}{2}$ x 6ins). • *adj* having eight leaves or 16 pages to the sheet.

octennial /ɒk'teniəl/ *adj* recurring every eighth year; continuing eight years.—**octennially** *adv*.

octet, octette /ɒk'tet/ *n* a group of eight (performers, lines of a sonnet); a composition for eight instruments or voices.

octillion /'ɒktɪliən/ *n* the eighth power of a million (1 with 48 ciphers) in US and France, the ninth power of a thousand (1 with 27 ciphers).—**octillionth** *adj*.

octo- /'ɒktoː/ *prefix* eight.

October /ɒk'toːbər/ *n* the tenth month of the year, having 31 days.

October surprise *n* (*US*) a political act aimed at generating voting support prior to a November election in the U.S.

octodecimo /ˌɒktoː'desɪˌmoː/ *adj* consiting of 18 leaves or 36 pages to a sheet. • *n* (*pl* **octodecimos**) a book of such size (18mo).

octogenarian /ˌɒktədʒə'neriən/ *n* a person who is in his or her eighties.

octopod /'ɒktəˌpɒd/ *n* an animal with eight feet; an eight-armed mollusc.—*also adj*.

octopus /'ɒktəpəs/ *n* (*pl* **octopuses, octopi**) a mollusc having a soft body and eight tentacles covered with suckers.

octoroon /ˌɒktə'ruːn/ *n* the offspring of a white person and a quadroon.

octosyllable /ˌɒktə'sɪləbəl/ *n* a word or verse of eight syllables.—**octosyllabic** *adj*.

octroi /'ɒktrwɑ/ *n* in France and Belgium, a tax levied upon articles brought into the gates of a city; duty on goods.

octuple /ɒk'tʉpəl/ *adj* eight-fold.

ocular /'ɒkjʊlər/ *adj* of, by, or relating to the eye; resembling an eye in form or function.

oculist /'ɒkjʊlɪst/ *n* (*formerly*) an opththalmologist.

OD /oː'diː/ *n* (*inf*) an overdose of a drug, *esp* a narcotic. • *vi* (**OD'ing, OD'd**) to take an overdose.

od /ɒd/ *n* a hypothetical natural force once used to explain magnetism, mesmerism, etc.

odalisque, odalisk /'oːdəlɪsk/ *n* a female slave or concubine in the harem of a sultan; (*art*) the depiction of a woman in eastern garments reclining.

odd /ɒd/ *adj* eccentric; peculiar; occasional; not divisible by two; with the other of the pair missing; extra or left over. • *npl* probability; balance of advantage in favour of one against another; excess of one number over another, *esp* in betting; likelihood; disagreement; strife; miscellaneous articles, scraps.—**oddly** *adv*.—**oddness** *n*.

oddball /'ɒdbɔːl/ *n* (*sl*) an eccentric person. • *adj* bizarre.

Odd Fellow /'ɒdfeloː/ *n* a member of the order of the benevolent society of the Odd Fellows, a friendly society similar to freemasons.

oddity /'ɒdɪti/ *n* (*pl* **oddities**) the state of being odd; an odd thing or person; peculiarity.

odd man out *n* a person left when others pair off.

oddment /'ɒdmənt/ *n* an odd piece left over, *esp* of fabric.

odds and ends *npl* miscellaneous articles, scraps.

odds-on *adj* (*horse, etc*) (judged to be) having a better than even chance of winning; likely to happen, succeed, win, etc.

ode /oːd/ *n* a lyric poem marked by lofty feeling and dignified style.

odeum /'oːdiəm/ or /-'diːər/ *n* (*pl* **odeums, odea**) a hall for musical performances.

odious /'oːdiəs/ *adj* causing hatred or offence; disgusting.—**odiously** *adv*.—**odiousness** *n*.

odium /'oːdiəm/ *n* general dislike.

odometer /oː'dɒmətər/ *n* an instrument attached to the axle of a vehicle to measure the distance it travels.

odonto-, odont- /ɒ'dɒntɒ/ *prefix* tooth.

odontoglossum /oːdɒntə'glɒsəm/ *n* a tropical orchid.

odontoid /oː'dɒntɔɪd/ *adj* tooth-shaped, tooth-like.

odontology /oːdɒn'tɒlədʒi/ *n* dental science.—**odontological** *adj*.—**odontologist** *n*.

odor /'oːdər/ *n* smell; scent; aroma; a characteristic or predominant quality— *also* **odour**.

odoriferous /oːdə'rɪfərəs/ *adj* diffusing fragrance; (*sl*) smelly.

odorless /-ləs/ *adj* without odour.

odorous /'oːdərəs/ *adj* having or emitting a scent; smelly; fragrant.

odour *see* **odor**.

odyssey /'ɒdɪsi/ *n* (*pl* **odysseys**) a long adventurous journey; an intellectual or spiritual quest.

Oe (*symbol*) oersted.

OECD *abbr* = Organization for Economic Cooperation and Development.

oecumenical /ˌekjʊ'menəkəl/ *adj* a rare spelling of **ecumenical**.

OED *abbr* = Oxford English Dictionary.

oedema /ɪ'diːmə/ *n* (*pl* **oedemata**) a swelling in a body or plant caused by excess fluid.—*also* **edema**.—**oedematous** *adj*.

Oedipus complex /'iːdɪpəs/ *n* (*psychoanal*) a complex arising from the relationship of a son to his parents.

oeil de boeuf *Fr.* /ɪyldi'bœf/ *n* a small round or oval window in the roof or frieze of a large building.

oeillade *Fr.* /ɪ'leɪd/ *n* a suggestive glance or ogle.

oeno- /'iːnoː/, **oen-** *prefix* wine.

oenology /iː'nɒlədʒi/ *n* the science of wines.—*also* **enology**.—**oenological, enological** *adj*.—**oenologist, enologist** *n*.

o'er /'oːər/ *prep, adv* (*poet*) over.

oersted /'ɜrstəd/ *n* the cgs unit of magnetic field strength.

oesophagus *n* (*pl* **oesophagi**) that part of the alimentary canal that takes food, etc, from the pharynx to the stomach.—*also* **esophagus**.

oestrogen *n* a hormone that develops and maintains female characteristics of the body.—*also* **estrogen**.

oestrus, oestrum *n* violent desire, frenzy; the period of ovulation of mammals, heat.—**oestrous** *adj.*—*also* **estrus, estrum**.

oeuvre /ˈɜːvrə/ *n* (*pl* **oeuvres**) a work of art, literature, music, etc; the life's work of an artist, writer or composer.

of /əv/ or /ɒv/ *prep* from; belonging or relating to; concerning; among; by; during; owing to.

of- /ɒf/ *prefix* the form of *ob-* before *f*.

off /ɒf/ *adv* away, from; detached, gone; unavailable; disconnected; out of condition; entirely. • *prep* away from; not on. • *adj* distant; no longer operating; cancelled; (*food or drink*) having gone bad; on the right-hand side; (*runners, etc*) having started a race.

offal /ˈɒfəl/ *n* the entrails of an animal eaten as food.

offbeat *adj* unconventional, eccentric.

off-Broadway *adj* denoting a type of small scale, experimental and generally noncommercial theatre situated outside theatrical Broadway in New York.

off-colour *adj* unwell; risqué.

offend /əˈfend/ *vt* to affront, displease; to insult. • *vi* to break a law.—**offender** *n*.

offense, offence /əˈfens/ *n* an illegal action, crime; a sin; an affront, insult; a cause of displeasure or anger.

offensive /əˈfensɪv/ *adj* causing offence; repulsive, disagreeable; insulting; aggressive. • *n* an attack; a forceful campaign for a cause, etc.—**offensively** *adv.*—**offensiveness** *n*.

offer /ˈɒfər/ *vt* to present for acceptance or rejection; to show willingness (to do something); to present for consideration; to bid; (*a prayer*) to say. • *vi* to present itself; to declare oneself willing. • *n* something offered; a bid or proposal.

offering /ˈɒfərɪŋ/ *n* a gift, present; a sacrifice.

offertory /ˈɒfərˌtɔːri/ or /ˈɒfrə-/ *n* (*pl* **offertories**) (*Anglican Church*) the sentences read in the Communion service during the collection of the alms; the alms collecting; (*RC Church*) an anthem chanted during Mass while the priest prepares the elements a church collection; the part of the service when it is taken.

offhand /ɒfˈhænd/ or /ˈɒfhænd/ *adv* impromptu; without thinking. • *adj* inconsiderate; curt, brusque; unceremonious.

office /ˈɒfɪs/ *n* a room or building where business is carried out; the people there; (*with cap*) the location, staff, of authority of a Government department, etc; a task or function; a position of authority; a duty; a religious ceremony, rite.

officer /ˈɒfɪsər/ *n* an official; a person holding a position of authority in a government, business, club, military services, etc; a policeman.

official /əˈfɪʃəl/ *adj* of an office or its tenure; properly authorized; formal. • *n* a person who holds a public office.—**officially** *adv*.

officialdom /-dəm/ *n* a body of officials.

officialese /əˈfɪʃəˈliːz/ *n* the jargon of official documents or as expressed by officials.

officiant /əˈfɪʃiənt/ *n* an officiating clergyman.

officiate /əˈfɪʃiˌeɪt/ *vi* to conduct a ceremony; to act in an official capacity; to perform the functions of a priest, minister, rabbi, etc.

officious /əˈfɪʃəs/ *adj* interfering, meddlesome; offering unwanted advice.—**officiously** *adv.*—**officiousness** *n*.

offing /ˈɒfɪŋ/ *n* the near or foreseeable future.

offish /ˈɒfɪʃ/ *adj* (*inf*) distant, stiff.

off-key *adj* sung or played in the wrong key; out of tune; out of step.

off-licence *n* in UK, a licence to sell alcohol for consumption off the premises; a place so licensed.—*also* **liquor store, package store**.

off-line *adj* (*comput*) not connected to the central processor; disconnected.

off-load *vt* to unload; to get rid off.

off-piste *adj* pertaining to skiing in areas away from the normal runs.

offprint /ˈɒfprɪnt/ *n* a separately printed copy or part of a publication.

off-putting *adj* discouraging, daunting.

off-roading *n* the sport or hobby of driving on dirt tracks or other rugged terrain.—**off-roader** *n*.

offscourings *npl* refuse, dregs.

offset /ˈɒfset/ *vt* (**offsetting, offset**) to compensate for, counterbalance. • *n* compensation; a method of printing in which an image is transferred from a plate to a rubber surface and then to paper; a sloping ledge on the face of a wall.

offset printing *n* printing in which the impression is transferred from a plate to a rubber surface and then to paper.

offshoot /ˈɒfʃuːt/ *n* a branch or shoot growing from the main stem; something derivative.

offshore /ˈɒfʃɔːr/ *adv* at sea some distance from the shore.

offside /ɒfˈsaɪd/ *adj, adv* illegally in advance of the ball.

offspring /ˈɒfsprɪŋ/ *n* a child, progeny; a result.

offstage /ɒfˈsteɪdʒ/ or /ˈɒf-/ *adj, adv* out of sight of the audience; behind the scenes.

off-the-peg *adj* (*clothes*) produced ready to wear in standard sizes.

off-the-wall *adj* (*sl*) innovative, unusual, unexpected.

off-white *n, adj* (a) white tinged with yellow or grey.

oft /ɒft/ *adv* (*poet*) often.

often /ˈɒfən/ or /ˈɒftən/ *adv* many times, frequently.

ogdoad /ˈɒɡdoʊˈæd/ *n* eight, a set of eight.

ogee /ˈoʊˈdʒiː/ or /-ˈdʒiː/ *n* an architectural wave-like moulding shaped like an S.

ogen melon *n* a type of small melon similar to a cantaloupe with sweel orange flesh.

ogham, ogam /ˈɒɡəm/ *n* an ancient British alphabet, the letters formed by notches; a character in it.

ogive /ˈoʊˈdʒaɪv/ or /-ˈdʒaɪv/ *n* a diagonal groin of a vault; a pointed arch.—**ogival** *adj*.

ogle /ˈoʊɡəl/ *vti* (**ogling, ogled**) to gape at; to make eyes at; to look at lustfully.—**ogler** *n*.

Ogpu /ˈɒɡpuː/ *n* the secret police of Soviet Russia (1923–34).

ogre /ˈoʊɡər/ *n* a man-eating giant; a hideous person.

OH *abbr* = Ohio.

oh /oʊ/ *interj* expressing surprise, delight, pain, etc.

OHIP /ˈoʊˈeɪtʃˈaɪˈpiː/ *abbr* ✹ = Ontario Health Insurance Plan.

ohm /oʊm/ *n* a unit of electrical resistance.

ohmmeter /ˈoʊmˌmiːtər/ *n* an instrument for measuring electrical resistance.

oho /oʊˈhoʊ/ *interj* an exclamation of surprise.

-oid /ɔɪd/ *suffix* like, as in *spheroid*.

oil /ɔɪl/ *n* any of various greasy, combustible liquid substances obtained from animal, vegetable, and mineral matter; petroleum; an oil painting; (*pl*) paint mixed by grinding a pigment in oil • *vt* to smear with oil, lubricate.—**oiled** *adj*.

oilcake /ˈɔɪlkeɪk/ *n* a cattle food of linseed.

oilcan *n* a container with a long spout for releasing oil for lubricating in individual drops.

oilcloth /ˈɔɪlklɒθ/ *n* a waterproof fabric impregnated with oil or synthetic resin.

oil color *n* a colour in which oil is used as a vehicle for pigement.

oiler /ˈɔɪlər/ *n* an oilcan; a greaser.

oil field *n* an area on land or under the sea that produces petroleum.

oilman /ˈɔɪlmən/ *n* (*pl* **oilmen**) a dealer in oils.

oil painting *n* a painting in oils; the art of painting in oils.

oil palm *n* an African palm whose fruit yields an edible oil.

oil rig *n* a drilling rig for extracting oil or natural gas.

oilskin /ˈɔɪlskɪn/ *n* fabric made waterproof by treatment with oil; a waterproof garment of oilskin or a plastic-coated fabric.

oil slick *n* a mass of oil floating on the surface of water.

oil well *n* a well from which petroleum is extracted.

oily /ˈɔɪli/ *adj* (**oilier, oiliest**) like or covered with oil; greasy; too suave or smooth, unctuous.—**oiliness** *n*.

oink /ɔɪŋk/ *n* (*inf*) the grunt of a pig.—*also vi*.

ointment /ˈɔɪntmənt/ *n* a fatty substance used on the skin for healing or cosmetic purposes; a salve.

Oireachtas /ˈɛrəktəs/ *n* the legislature of Ireland, consisting of the president, the Dáil Eireann (the Chamber of Deputies) and the Seanad Eireann (the Senate).

Ojibwa or **Ojibway** /oʊˈdʒɪbweɪ/ *n* ✹ a member of an Indian people of North America mainly living near Lake Superior; the language of this people. • *adj* of or pertaining to this people or their language.

OK[1] *abbr* = Oklahoma.

OK[2], **okay** /oʊˈkeɪ/ *adj, adv* (*inf*) all right; correct(ly). • *n* (*pl* **OK's, okays**) approval. • *vt* (**OK'ing, OK'ed** *or* **okaying, okayed**) to approve, sanction as OK.

oka /ˈoʊkə/ *n* ✹ (*Cdn*) a cured, semi-soft cheese made in Quebec.

okapi /oʊˈkæpi/ *n* (*pl* **okapis, okapi**) an African animal allied to the giraffe but smaller and with a shorter neck.

okay *see* **OK**.

okra /ˈoːkrə/ n a tall annual plant yielding long seed-pods used as a vegetable.

old /oːld/ adj aged; elderly, not young; having lived or existed for a long time; long used, not new; former; of the past, not modern; experienced; worn out; of long standing.

old age security n ✸ (Cdn) a system of pensions paid by the federal government to people who are 65 or older.

Old Bailey n the central criminal court of England.

old boy n a former pupil of a school; (inf) a friendly form of address; an old person.—**old girl** nf.

old boy network n (inf) the monopoly of power by a privileged elite who attended the best public schools and universities.

Old Catholic n one of a body of Roman Catholics who refused to accept the dogma of papal infallibility (1870).

old country n the birthplace of an immigrant or an immigrant's ancestors.

olden /ˈoːldən/ adj relating to a bygone era.

Old English n the English language during the 7th to the 11th centuries.—also Anglo-Saxon.

Old English sheepdog n a breed of sheepdog with an extremely long shaggy coat.

old-fashioned adj out of date; in a fashion of an older time.

Old French n the French language from the 7th to the early 14th centuries.

Old Glory n the Stars and Stripes.

old gold adj of the colour of tarnished gold.

old guard n the (original) conservative elements within a political party or other organization.

old hat adj old-fashioned, cliched.

old lady n (inf) one's wife or mother.

old maid n (derog) a woman, esp an older woman who has never married; a prim, prudish, fussy person.

old man n (inf) father, husband; (inf) someone in charge, esp the captain of a ship.

old master n a painting by one of the best painters working in Europe in ther 16th and 17th centuries; one of these painters.

Old Nick n (inf) the Devil.

old school n supporters of traditional or conservative values and practices.

old school tie n a distinctive tie which indicates which school one attended; the elitism and solidarity use associated with British public schools and their products.

Old Style n the old mode of reckoning time acording to the Julian year of 365 and a quarter days.

Old Testament n the Christian designation for the Holy Scriptures of Judaism, the first of the two general divisions of the Christian Bible.

old-time adj of an earlier period; old-fashioned.

old-timer n an old man; a veteran; a person who has been in the same job, position, etc, for many years.

old wives' tale n a belief sustained by tradition, not accuracy.

Old World n Europe, Asia, and Africa.

old-world adj traditional, quaint; antiquated.

oleaginous /ˌoːliˈædʒənəs/ adj oily; unctuous.

oleander /ˌoːliˈændər/ n a poisonous evergreen shrub with handsome fragrant flowers.

oleaster /ˌoːliˈæstər/ n the wild olive; a yellow-flowered shrub like it.

oleate /ˈoːliːˌeɪt/ n a salt of oleic acid.

olefin, olefine /ˈoːləfɪn/ n a hydrocarbon containing two atoms of hydrogen and one atom of carbon.—**olefinic** adj.

oleic /oːˈliːɪk/ adj obtained from oil.

oleic acid n an oily acid obtained from the saponification of linseed and other oils, or in the making of soap.

olein /ˈoːliːɪn/ n the pure liquid part of oil or fat.

oleo- /ˈoːlio/ prefix oil.

oleograph /ˈoːlioˌɡræf/ n a lithograph in oil colours.

olfactory /oːlˈfæktəri/ or /ɒl-/ adj relating to the sense of smell. • n (pl olfactories) (usu pl) an organ of smell.

olibanum /oːˈlɪbənəm/ n a gum resin used in incense; the frankincense of the ancients.

oligarch /ˈɒlɪˌɡɑːk/ n a member of an oligarchy.

oligarchy /ˈɒlɪˌɡɑːki/ n (pl oligarchies) government by a small group of people; the members of such a government; a state ruled in this way.—**oligarchic, oligarchical** adj.

oligo-, olig- /ˈɒlɪɡo/ prefix few, small.

Oligocene /ˈɒlɪɡəˌsiːn/ n (geol) a term used to denote certain strata intermediate between the Eocene and Miocene.

olio /ˈoːlio/ n (pl olios) a hotchpotch, a stew; a miscellany.

olivaceous /ˌɒlɪ veɪʃəs/ adj olive-green.

olivary /ˈɒlɪvəri/ adj olive-shaped, oval.

olive /ˈɒlɪv/ n an evergreen tree cultivated for its edible hardstoned fruit and oil; its fruit; a yellow-green colour. • adj of a yellow-green colour.

olive branch n a gesture of reconciliation of desire to make peace.

olive drab n the colour of the US service uniform.

olive oil n an edible yellow oil obtained from the fruit of the olive by pressing.

olivine /ˈɒlɪˌviːn/ n a variety of chrysolite.

olla podrida /ˌɒləpəˈdriːdə/ n a mixed stew or hash of meat and vegetables, a favourite Spanish dish; any incongruous mixture.

ology /ˈɒlədʒi/ n (pl ologies) (sl) a branch of knowledge, a science.

Olympiad /əˈlɪmpiˌæd/ n in ancient Greece, the interval (four years) between the celebration of the Olympic games; a system of chronology reckoning from the first Olympiad, 776 BC.

Olympian /əˈlɪmpiən/ adj of Olympus, home of the Greek gods; Olympic; stately; condescending. • n a great person.

Olympic /əˈlɪmpɪk/ adj pertaining to Olympia in Elis, where the Olympic games were celebrated.

Olympic Games n sing or pl an ancient athletic contest revived in 1896 as an international meeting held every four years in a different country.—also Olympics.

OM abbr = Order of Merit.

om /oːm/ n (Hinduism) the mystic name of the supreme being uttered when invoking Brahma; (modern occultism) spiritual essence, supreme truth and virtue.

-oma /ˈoːmə/ n suffix indicating a tumour.

omasum /oːˈmeɪsəm/ n (pl omasa) the third stomach of ruminant animals.

omber ombre /ˈɒmbər/ n an old card game for three players.

ombudsman /ˈɒmbədzmən/ or /-budz-/, /-ˈbudz-/ n (pl ombudsmen) an official appointed to investigate citizens' or consumers' complaints.

omega /oːˈmeɪɡə/ or /-ˈmeɡə/ n the last letter of the Greek alphabet.

omelet, omelette /ˈɒmlət/ or /-ələt/ n eggs beaten and cooked flat in a pan.

omen /ˈoːmən/ n a sign or warning of impending happiness or disaster.

omentum /oːˈmentəm/ n (pl omenta, omentums) (anat) the caul or adipose membrane attached to the stomach.

omerta /ɔːˈmɜːtə/ n a conspiracy of silence, esp as practised by the Mafia.

omicron /ˈɒməkrɒn/ or /ˈoː-/ n the 15th letter of the Greek alphabet.

ominous /ˈɒmənəs/ adj relating to an omen; foreboding evil; threatening.—**ominously** adv.

omission /oːˈmɪʃən/ n something that has been left out or neglected; the act of omitting.

omit /oːˈmɪt/ vt (omitting, omitted) to leave out; to neglect to do, leave undone.

omni- /ˈɒmni/ prefix all; universally.

omnibus /ˈɒmnɪbəs/ n (pl omnibuses) (formal) a bus; a book containing several works usu by one author.

omnifarious /ˌɒmnɪˈferiəs/ adj of all kinds.

omnipotent /ɒmˈnɪpətənt/ adj all-powerful, almighty; having very great power.—**omnipotence** n.

omnipresent /ˌɒmnɪˈprezənt/ adj present everywhere, ubiquitous.—**omnipresence** n.

omniscient /ɒnˈnɪsiənt/ or /-ʃənt/ adj knowing all things.—**omnisciently** adv.—**omniscience** n.

omnium-gatherum /ˌɒmnɪəmˈɡæðərəm/ n a miscellaneous collection of persons or things.

omnivore /ˈɒmnɪˌvɔː/ n an omnivorous animal or person.

omnivorous /ɒmˈnɪvərəs/ adj eating any sort of food; taking in everything indiscriminately.

omophagic /omoˈfæɡɪk/, **omophagous** /-ɡəs/ adj eating raw flesh.—**omophagia** n.

omphalos /ˈɒmfəˌlɒs/ n centre, hub; (ancient Greece) a boss on a shield.

ON abbr ✸ = Ontario.

on /ɒn/ prep in contact with the upper surface of; supported by, attached to, or covering; directed toward; at the time of; concerning, about; using as a basis, condition or principle; immediately after; (sl) using; addicted to. • adv (so as to be) covering or in contact with something; forward; (device) switched on; continuously in progress; due to take place; (actor) on stage; on duty.

• *adj* (*cricket*) designating the part of the field on the batsman's side in front of the wicket. • *n* (*cricket*) the on side.

onager /ˈɒnəgər/ *n* (*pl* **onagri, onagers**) the wild ass.

onanism /ˈoːnəˌnɪzəm/ *n* masturbation; coitus interruptus.—**onanist** *n*, *adj*.

once /wʌns/ *adv* on one occasion only; formerly; at some time. • *conj* as soon as. • *n* one time.

once-over *n* a preliminary survey.

onco- /ˈɒnkoː/ *prefix* swelling, tumour.

oncology /ɒŋˈkɒlədʒɪ/ *n* the branch of medicine dealing with tumours.—**oncologist** *n*.

oncoming /ˈɒnˌkʌmɪŋ/ *adj* approaching.

one /wʌn/ *adj* single; undivided, united; the same; a certain unspecified (time, etc). • *n* the first and lowest cardinal number; an individual thing or person; (*inf*) a drink; (*inf*) a joke. • *pron* an indefinite person, used to apply to many people; someone.

one-armed bandit *n* (*inf*) a slot machine for gambling, operated by pulling down a lever on its side.

one-horse *adj* (*sl*) paltry.

oneiro- /əˈnaɪroː/ *prefix* dream.

one-liner *n* (*inf*) a brief joke or witty comment.

oneness /ˈwʌnnəs/ *n* unity, singleness, concord.

one-night stand *n* a performance given for one night only in a certain place; (*inf*) (a partner in) a sexual liaison that lasts one night only.

one-off *n*, *adj* (*Brit*) (something) performed or made only once.

onerous /ˈɒnərəs/ or /ˈoːn-/ *adj* oppressive, burdensome; troublesome.

oneself /wʌnˈself/ *pron reflex form of* one.

one-sided *adj* favouring one side; unequal.

one-time *adj* sometime, former.

one-track *adj* with a single line of rails; with room for only one idea at a time.

one-upmanship /wʌnˈʌpmənʃɪp/ *n* the skill of being one jump ahead of or going one better than someone or something else.

one-way *adj* (*traffic*) restricted to one direction; requiring no reciprocal action or obligation.

ongoing /ˈɒnˌgoːɪŋ/ *adj* progressing, continuing.

onion /ˈʌnjən/ *n* an edible bulb with a pungent taste and odour.

on-line *adj* referring to equipment that is connected to and controlled by the central processor of a computer.

onlooker /ˈɒnˌlʊkər/ *n* a spectator.

only /ˈoːnlɪ/ *adj* alone of its kind; single, sole. • *adv* solely, merely; just; not more than. • *conj* except that, but.

onoma- /ˈɒnoːmə/ *prefix* name.

onomastic /ˌɒnəˈmæstɪk/ *adj* of or pertaining to a name or names.

onomastics /ˌɒnəˈmæstɪks/ *n sing* the study of proper names.

onomatopoeia /ˌɒnəˌmætəˈpiːə/ *n* the formation of a word to imitate a sound.—**onomatopoeic** *adj*.

onrush /ˈɒnrʌʃ/ *n* a powerful rushing forwards.

onset /ˈɒnset/ *n* a beginning; an assault, attack.

onshore /ˈɒnʃɔr/ *adj*, *adv* towards the land; on land, not the sea.

onslaught /ˈɒnslɒt/ *n* a fierce attack.

Ont. *abbr* ✦ = Ontario.

Ontarian *n* ✦ a person who lives in or is from Ontario.

onto /ˈɒntuː/ *prep* to a position on.

onto- /ɒntə-/ *prefix* being.

ontogeny, ontogenesis /ɒnˈtɒdʒənɪ/ *n* (*biol*) the history of the evolution of individual organisms.—**ontogenic, ontogenetic** *adj*.

ontology /ɒnˈtɒlədʒɪ/ *n* (*philos*) the logic of pure being or reality; metaphysics.—**ontological** *adj*.—**ontologically** *adv*.

onus /ˈoːnəs/ *n* (*pl* **onuses**) responsibility, duty; burden.

onward /ˈɒnwərd/ *adj* advancing, forward. • *adv* to the front, ahead, forward.

onwards /ˈɒnwərdz/ *adv* onward.

onyx /ˈɒnɪks/ *n* a limestone similar to marble with layers of colour.

oo- /ˈoːə/ *prefix* egg.

oodles /ˈuːdəlz/ *npl* (*sl*) an abundance.

oogamous /oːˈɒgəməs/ *adj* heterogamous.

oogenesis /ˌoːəˈdʒenɪsɪs/ *n* the formation of an ovum.—**oogenetic** *adj*.

ooh /uː/ *interj* expressing surprise, delight, pain, etc.

oolite /ˈoːəˌlaɪt/ *n* a limestone composed of grains like the roe of a fish.—**oolitic** *adj*.

oology /oːˈɒlədʒɪ/ *n* the scientific study of birds' eggs; a treatise on birds' eggs.—**oological** *adj*.—**oologist** *n*.

oolong /ˈuːlɒŋ/ *n* a Chinese black tea the flavour of which resembles green tea.

oomiak *see* **umiak**.

oompah /ˈuːmpɒ/ *n* an imitation of the deep sound of a brass instrument such as the tuba.

oomph /ˈuːmf/ *n* (*inf*) energy, verve; sex appeal.

oops /uːps/ or /ʊps/ *interj* expressing surprise or apology, *esp* when making a mistake.

oosperm /ˈuːspɔrm/ *n* a fertilized ovum.

ootheca /ˈuːθəkə/ *n* (*pl* **oothecae**) the egg case of certain molluscs and insects containing the eggs.—**oothecal** *adj*.

ooze /uːz/ *vti* to flow or leak out slowly; to seep; to exude. • *n* soft mud or slime.

op. *abbr* = opera; operation; operator; optical; opposite; opus.

op- /ɒp/ *prefix* form of *ob-* before *p*.

opacity /oːˈpæsɪtɪ/ *n* (*pl* **opacities**) the state of being opaque; obscurity.

opah /ˈoːpə/ *n* a bright-coloured sea fish like the mackerel, the kingfish.

opal /ˈoːpəl/ *n* a white or bluish stone with a play of iridescent colours.

opalescent /ˌoːpəˈlesənt/ *adj* resembling opal in its reflection of light, iridescent.—**opalescence** *n*.

opaline /ˈoːpəˌlaɪn/ *adj* pertaining to or resembling the opal.

opaque /oːˈpeɪk/ *adj* not letting light through; neither transparent nor translucent.—**opaquely** *adv*.—**opaqueness** *n*.

op. cit. *abbr* = (*Latin*) in the work cited.

OPEC /ˈoːpek/ *abbr* = Organization of Petroleum Exporting Countries.

open /ˈoːpən/ *adj* not closed; accessible; uncovered, unprotected; not fenced; free from trees; spread out, unfolded; public; lacking reserve; (*a person*) forthcoming; generous; readily understood; liable (to); unrestricted; (*syllable*) ending with a vowel; (*consonant*) made without stopping the stream of breath. • *vti* to make or become accessible; to unfasten; to begin; to expand, unfold; to come into view. • *n* a wide space; (*sport*) a competition that any player can enter.—**openness** *n*.

open air *n* outdoors.

open-and-shut *adj* easily solved; straightforward.

opencast mining *see* **strip mining**.

open-ended *adj* with no fixed limit of time or amount.

open-eyed *adj* vigilant.

opener /ˈoːpənər/ or /ˈoːpnər/ *n* a device for opening cans or bottles.

openhanded *adj* generous.—**openhandedness** *n*.

openhearted *adj* responsive to emotional appeal, frank.—**openheartedness** *n*.

open-heart surgery *n* surgery on the heart whilst its function is performed temporarily by a heart-lung machine.

opening /ˈoːpənɪŋ/ or /ˈoːpnɪŋ/ *n* a gap, aperture; a beginning; a chance; a job opportunity. • *adj* initial.

open letter *n* a letter addressed to an individual but published in a newspaper for all to see.

openly /ˈoːpənlɪ/ *adv* frankly; publicly.

open-minded *adj* unprejudiced.—**open-mindedness** *n*.

open-mouthed *adj* having the mouth open in surprise; gaping, expectant.

open secret *n* a supposed secret which is actually widely known.

open sesame *n* a way of getting into something usually inaccessible.

openwork /ˈoːpənˌwɜrk/ *n* a pattern with interstices.

opera /ˈɒpərə/ or /ˈɒprə/ *n* a dramatic work represented through music and song; plural form of **opus**.

operable /ˈɒpərəbəl/ *adj* capable of being put into action, practicable; (*med*) capable of being operated upon.

opera bouffe /ˌɒpərəˈbuːf/ *n* a comic or farcical opera.

opera glasses *n* a small binocular telescope used in theatres, etc.

opera hat *n* a man's collapsible top hat.

opera house *n* a theatre for opera.

operate /ˈɒpəˌreɪt/ *vi* to work, to function; to produce a desired effect; to carry out a surgical operation. • *vt* (*a machine*) to work or control; to carry on, run.

operatic /ˌɒpəˈrætɪk/ *adj* of or relating to opera; exaggerated, overacting.

operating system *n* the software in a computer which controls basic operations such as accepting keyboard input, printing, file handling and displaying error messages.

operation /ˌɒpəˈreɪʃən/ *n* a method of operating; a procedure; a military action; a surgical procedure.

operational /ˌɒpəˈreɪʃənəl/ *adj* of or relating to an operation; functioning; ready for use; involved in military activity.—**operationally** *adv*.

operations research, operational research *n* the application of mathematical techniques to the analysis of business methods.

operative /ˈɒpərətɪv/ or /ˈɒprətɪv/ *adj* functioning; in force, effective; of, by surgery. • *n* a mechanic; a secret agent; a private detective.

operator /ˈɒpəˌreɪtər/ *n* a person who operates or works a machine, *esp* a telephone switchboard; a person who owns or runs a business; a person who manipulates.

operculum /əˈpɜrkjʊləm/ or /oːˈp-/ *n* (*pl* **opercula, operculums**) (*biol*) a cap, lid, or cover; the plate closing the orifice of a univalve; a shell; the gill cover of a fish.—**opercular, operculate** *adj*.

operetta /ˌɒpəˈretə/ *n* a light opera.

ophidian /oːˈfɪdiən/ *n* any of the Ophidia, an order of reptiles including the snakes.—*also adj*.

ophiology /ˌɒfɪˈɒlədʒi/ *n* that branch of natural history which treats of snakes.—**ophiological** *adj*.—**ophiologist** *n*.

ophite /oːˈfaɪt/ *n* serpentine marble.

ophthalmia /ɒfˈθælmiə/ or /ɒp-/ *n* inflammation of the eye.

ophthalmic /ɒfˈθælmɪk/ or /ɒp-/ *adj* of, relating to, or situated near, the eye.

ophthalmo-, ophthalm- /ɒfˈθælmoː/ or /ɒp-/ *prefix* eye or eyeball.

ophthalmology /ˌɒpθælˈmɒlədʒi/ or /ɒf-/ *n* the branch of medicine dealing with diseases of the eye.—**ophthalmologist** *n*.

ophthalmoscope /ɒfˈθælməˌskoːp/ or /ɒp-/ *n* an instrument for examining the interior of the eye.

ophthalmoscopy /-i/ *n* examination of the eye.—**ophthalmoscopic** *adj*.

-opia /ˈoːpiə/ *n suffix* indicating a visual defect.

opiate /ˈoːpiət/ *n* a narcotic drug that contains opium; something that induces sleep or calms feelings.

opine /oːˈpaɪn/ *vt* to hold or express the opinion (that).

opinicus /oːˈpɪnɪkəs/ *n* (*her*) a fabulous winged animal with the head and wings of a griffin, the body of a lion, and the tail of a camel.

opinion /əˈpɪnjən/ *n* a belief that is not based on proof; judgment; estimation, evaluation; a formal expert judgment; professional advice.

opinionated /əˈpɪnjəˌneɪtəd/ *adj* unduly confident in one's opinions, dogmatic.

opinionative /-tɪv/ *adj* fond of preconceived ideas; self-conceited.—**opinionatively** *adv*.

opium /ˈoːpiəm/ *n* a narcotic drug produced from an annual Eurasian poppy.

opossum /əˈpɒsəm/ *n* (*pl* **opossums, opossum**) a small nocturnal and arboreal marsupial.

OPP *abbr* ✦ = Ontario Provincial Police.

oppidan /ˈɒpɪdæn/ *adj* urban, town-dwelling.

oppilate /ˈɒpəˌleɪt/ *vt* (*med*) to block up, to obstruct.—**oppilation** *n*.

opponent /əˈpoːnənt/ *n* a person who opposes another; an adversary, antagonist. • *adj* opposing.

opportune /ˌɒpərˈtuːn/ or /-tjuːn/ *adj* well-timed; convenient.—**opportunely** *adv*.

opportuneness /-nəs/ *n* seasonableness.

opportunist /-ɪst/ *n* a person who forms or adapts his or her views or principles to benefit from opportunities; to seize opportunities as they may arise.—**opportunism** *n*.

opportunity /ˌɒpərˈtuːnəti/ or /-ˈtjuːn-/ *n* (*pl* **opportunities**) chance; a favourable combination of circumstances.

opposable /əˈpoːzəbəl/ *adj* that may be opposed.—**opposability** *n*.—**opposably** *adv*.

oppose /əˈpoːz/ *vt* to put in front of or in the way of; to place in opposition; to resist; to fight against; to balance against.—**opposer** *n*.

opposite /ˈɒpəzɪt/ *adj* placed on opposed sides of; face to face; diametrically different; contrary. • *n* a person or thing that is opposite; an antithesis. • *prep, adv* across from.

opposite number *n* a person in a corresponding position on the other side; a counterpart.

opposition /ˌɒpəˈzɪʃən/ *n* the act of opposing or the condition of being opposed; resistance; antithesis; hostility; a political party opposing the government; (*astron*) the diametrically opposite position of two heavenly bodies, when 180 degrees apart.

oppress /əˈpres/ *vt* to treat unjustly; to subjugate; to weigh down in the mind.—**oppressor** *n*.

oppression /əˈpreʃən/ *n* the act of oppressing; the state of being oppressed; persecution; physical or mental distress.

oppressive /əˈpresɪv/ *adj* tyrannical; burdensome; (*weather*) sultry, close.—**oppressively** *adv*.—**oppressiveness** *n*.

opprobrious /əˈproːbriəs/ *adj* abusive; infamous.

opprobrium /əˈproːbriəm/ *n* a reproach with disdain or contempt; disgrace, ignominy.

oppugn /əˈpjuːn/ *vt* to reason against, to controvert; to resist.—**oppugnant** *adj, n*.—**oppugner** *n*.

opsonin /ˈɒpsənɪn/ *n* a chemical agent in blood serum, which makes bacteria vulnerable to phagocytic activity.—**opsonic** *adj*.

opt /ɒpt/ *vi* to choose, to exercise an option; (*with* **in**) to choose to participate in something; (*with* **out**) to choose not to participate in something.

optative /ˈɒptətɪv/ or /ɒpˈteɪtɪv/ *adj* (*gram*) expressing a desire or wish. • *n* an optative mood or form of a verb.

optic /ˈɒptɪk/ *adj* relating to the eye or sight. • *n* (*inf*) the eye; a device for dispensing a standard measure of spirits, etc.

optical /ˈɒptɪkəl/ *adj* of or relating to the eye or light; optic; aiding or correcting vision; visual.—**optically** *adv*.

optical character reader *n* a device that allows printed characters, figures, etc to be scanned and input to a computer, by a process of optical character recognition, the identification of printed text by photoelectric means.

optical disc *n* a compact disc used as a high-capacity storage medium for computers.

optical fiber *n* thin glass fiber through which light can be transmitted.

optician /ɒpˈtɪʃən/ *n* a person who makes or sells optical aids.

optics /ˈɒptɪks/ *n sing* the branch of physics dealing with light and vision.

optimal /ˈɒptɪməl/ *adj* optimum.—**optimally** *adv*.

optimism /ˈɒptɪˌmɪzəm/ *n* a tendency to take the most cheerful view of things; hopefulness; the belief that good must ultimately prevail.—**optimist** *n*.—**optimistic** *adj*.—**optimistically** *adv*.

optimum /ˈɒptɪməm/ *n* (*pl* **optima, optimums**) the best, most favourable condition.—*also adj*.

option /ˈɒpʃən/ *n* the act of choosing; the power to choose; a choice; the right to buy, sell or lease at a fixed price within a specified time.

optional /ˈɒpʃənəl/ *adj* left to choice; not compulsory.—**optionally** *adv*.

optometer /ˈɒptəˌmɪtər/ *n* an instrument for measuring the limits of distinct vision.

opulent /ˈɒpjʊlənt/ *adj* wealthy; luxuriant.—**opulence** *n*.

opuntia /oːˈpʌnʃiə/ *n* any of a genus of cacti; the Indian fig.

opus /ˈoːpəs/ *n* (*pl* **opuses, opera**) an artistic or literary work; a musical composition, *esp* any of the numbered works of a composer.

OR *abbr* = Oregon.

or[1] /ɔr/ or /ər/ *conj* denoting an alternative; the last in a series of choices.

or[2] *n* (*her*) gold, denoted by small engraved dots.

ora *see* **os**[1].

orach, orache /ˈɒrɪtʃ/ *n* mountain spinach.

oracle /ˈɔrəkəl/ or /ˈɒ-/ *n* a place in ancient Greece where a deity was consulted; the response given (often ambiguous); a wise adviser; sage advice.—**oracular** *adj*.

oral /ˈɔrəl/ *adj* of the mouth; spoken, not written; (*drugs*) taken by mouth. • *n* a spoken examination.—**orally** *adv*.

oral history *n* the history of past events as recorded from interviews with people living at the time.

orange /ˈɔrɪndʒ/ or /ˈɒ-/ *n* a round, reddish-yellow, juicy, edible citrus fruit; the tree bearing it; its colour. • *adj* orange-coloured.

orangeade /ˌɔrɪndʒˈeɪd/ or /ˈɒ-/ *n* a drink made with the juice of oranges.

Orangeman /ˈɒrɪndʒmən/ *n* (*pl* **Orangemen**) a member of an Irish protestant political party named after William of Orange.

orangery /ˈɔrɪndʒəri/ or /-dʒri/, /ˈɒ-/ *n* (*pl* **orangeries**) a hothouse for the cultivation of oranges; an orange garden.

orange stick *n* a small thin pointed stick, orig orangewood, used in manicuring the nails.

orangutan, orangoutang /oːˌræŋuːˈtæn/ *n* a large, long-armed, herbivorous anthropoid ape.

orate /ɔ'reɪt/ or /'ɒr-/ *vi* to make an oration; (*inf*) to hold forth.

oration /ɔ'reɪʃən/ or /ər-/ *n* a formal or public speech.

orator /'ɔrətər/ or /'ɒ-/ *n* an eloquent public speaker.—**oratorical** *adj.*

oratorio /ˌɔrə'tɔriː/ or /ˌɒ-/ *n* (*pl* **oratorios**) a sacred story set to music for voices and instruments.

oratory /'ɔrəˌtɔri/ or /'ɒ-/ *n* (*pl* **oratories**) the art of public speaking; eloquence; a place for prayer.

orb /ɔrb/ *n* a sphere or globe; an ornamental sphere surmounted by a cross, *esp* as carried by a sovereign at a coronation.

orbicular, orbiculate, orbiculated /ɔr'bɪkjulər/ *adj* orb-shaped, spherical.—**orbicularity** *n.*

orbit /'ɔrbɪt/ *n* (*astron*) a curved path along which a planet or satellite moves; a field of action or influence; the eye socket; (*physics*) the path of an electron around the nucleus of an atom. • *vti* to put (a satellite, etc) into orbit; to circle round.—**orbital** *adj.*

orca /'ɔrkə/ *n* a grampus; the killer whale; a sea monster.

orchard /'ɔrtʃərd/ *n* an area of land planted with fruit trees.

orchestra /'ɔrkəstrə/ *n* a group of musicians playing together under a conductor; their instruments; the space (or pit) in a theatre where they sit; the stalls of a theatre.—**orchestral** *adj.*

orchestrate /'ɔrkəˌstreɪt/ *vt* to arrange music for performance by an orchestra; to arrange, organize to best effect.—**orchestration** *n.*—**orchestrator** *n.*

orchestrion /ɔr'kestriən/ *n* a large automatic barrel organ.

orchid /'ɔrkɪd/ *n* a plant with unusually shaped flowers in brilliant colours comprising three petals of uneven size.

orchil /'ɔrtʃɪl/ *n* a red or violet dye obtained from lichen; the lichen.—*also* **archil.**

orchis /'ɔrtʃɪs/ *n* a genus of wild orchid with curiously shaped roots and flowers.

orcinol, orcin /'ɔrsɪn/ *n* a substance obtained from lichens yielding dye.

ordain /ɔr'deɪn/ *vti* to confer holy orders upon; to appoint; to decree; to order, to command.—**ordainer** *n.*—**ordainment** *n.*

ordeal /ɔr'diːl/ *n* a severe trial or test; an exacting experience.

order /'ɔrdər/ *n* arrangement; method; relative position; sequence; an undisturbed condition; tidiness; rules of procedure; an efficient state; a class, group, or sort; a religious fraternity; a style of architecture; an honour or decoration; an instruction or command; a rule or regulation; a state or condition, *esp* with regard to functioning; a request to supply something; the goods supplied; (*zool*) divisions between class and family or genus. • *vti* to put or keep (things) in order; to arrange; to command; to request (something) to be supplied.

ordered /'ɔrdərd/ *adj* marked by regularity and discipline; being arranged or identifiable according to a rule; being labelled by ordinal numbers.

orderly /'ɔrdərli/ *adj* in good order; well-behaved; methodical. • *n* (*pl* **orderlies**) a hospital attendant; a soldier attending an officer.—**orderliness** *n.*

ordinal /'ɔrdɪnəl/ *adj* showing position in a series. • *n* an ordinal number.

ordinal number *n* a number denoting its order in a sequence, as first, second, etc.

ordinance /'ɔrdɪnəns/ *n* a decree, a law; a rite.

ordinary /'ɔrdɪneri/ *adj* normal, usual; common; plain, unexceptional. • *n* (*pl* **ordinaries**) a meal for all comers at fixed charges and a fixed time, an inn providing this; archbishop in province, bishop in diocese; prescribed form of service; an ecclesiastical judge; a prison chaplain; (*her*) that part of the escutcheon contained between straight and other lines one of the simple charges.—**ordinarily** *adv.*

ordinary seaman *n* a seaman of the lowest rank, below able-bodied seaman

ordinate /'ɔrdɪnət/ *n* (*geom*) one of the co-ordinates of a point; a straight line in a curve terminated on both sides by the curve and bisected by the diameter.

ordination /ˌɔrdɪ'neɪʃən/ *n* the act of ordaining or being ordained; admission to the ministry.

ordnance /'ɔrdnəns/ *n* military stores; artillery.

Ordovician /ˌɔrdə'vɪʃiən/ or /ˌɔrdə'vɪʃiən/ *adj* (*geol*) of the period between the Cambrian and Silurian.

ordure /'ɔrdjur/ *n* excrement; dung.

ore /ɔr/ *n* a substance from which minerals can be extracted.

öre /'ʊrə/ or /'ərə/ *n* (*pl* **öre**) a monetary unit in Sweden, (Øre) Denmark and Norway.

oread /'ɔriˌæd/ *n* a mountain nymph (Greek).

Oreg. *abbr* = Oregon.

oregano /ɔ'regənoː/ *n* an aromatic herb whose leaves, either fresh of dried, are used to flavour food.

organ /'ɔrgən/ *n* a *usu* large and complex musical wind instrument with pipes, stops, and a keyboard; a part of an animal or plant that performs a vital or natural function; the means by which anything is done; a medium of information or opinion, a periodical.

organdy, organdie /'ɔrgəndi/ *n* (*pl* **organdies**) a light transparent, *usu* stiffened cotton fabric.

organ grinder *n* the player of a barrel organ.

organic /ɔr'gænɪk/ *adj* of or relating to bodily organs; (disease) affecting a bodily organ; of, or derived from, living organisms; systematically arranged; structural; (*chem*) of the class of compounds that are formed from carbon; (vegetables, etc) grown without the use of artificial fertilizers or pesticides.—**organically** *adv.*

organism /'ɔrgəˌnɪzəm/ *n* an animal or plant, any living thing; an organized body.

organist /'ɔrgənɪst/ *n* a person who plays an organ.

organization /ˌɔrgənaɪ'zeɪʃən/ or /-nɪ-/, /-nə-/ *n* the act or process of organizing; the state of being organized; arrangement, structure; an organized body or association.

organize /'ɔrgəˌnaɪz/ *vt* to arrange in an orderly way; to establish; to institute; to persuade to join a cause, group, etc; to arrange for.—**organizer** *n.*

organogenesis /ˌɔrgənoː'dʒenɪsɪs/ or /ɔr'gænoː-/ *n* organic development.—**organogenetic** *adj.*—**organogenetically** *adv.*

organography /ˌɔrgə'nɒgrəfi/ *n* a scientific description of the organs of animals or plants.—**organographic** *adj.*

organology /ˌɔrgə'nɒlədʒi/ *n* that branch of physiology which treats of animal organs.—**organological** *adj.*—**organologist** *n.*

organon /'ɔrgəˌnɒn/ *n* (*pl* **organa, organons**) a body of rules for regulating scientific or philosophical investigation; a method of thought, a logical system.

organotherapy /ˌɔrgənoː'θerəpi/ *n* the treatment of disease with organic extracts.

organzine /'ɔrgənˌzaɪn/ *n* a strong silk thread of a very fine texture; a fabric made from it.

orgasm /'ɔrgæzəm/ *n* the climax of sexual excitement.—**orgasmic** *adj.*

orgeat /'ɔrdʒiət/ or /-ʒæt/ *n* a drink made of barley water flavoured with almonds.

orgy /'ɔrgi/ *n* (*pl* **orgies**) a wild party or gathering of people, with excessive drinking and indiscriminate sexual activity; over-indulgence in any activity.—**orgiastic** *adj.*

oriel /'ɔriəl/ *n* a projecting angular recess with a window; the window.

orient /'ɔriˌent/ or /'ɒr-/, /-ənt/ *n* the East, or Asia, *esp* the Far East.

orient, orientate /'ɔriˌent/ or /'ɒr-/, /ˌɔriɛnˌteɪt/ *vti* to adjust (oneself) to a particular situation; to arrange in a direction, *esp* in relation to the points of the compass; to face or turn in a particular direction.

oriental /ˌɔri'entəl/ or /ˌɒr-/ *adj* (*often cap*) of the Orient, its people or languages.

Orientalism /ɔri'entəlɪzəm/ or /ˌɒr-/ *n* an idiom or custom characteristic of the East.

Orientalist /-ɪst/ *n* an expert in Oriental languages, history, etc.

orientation /ˌɔriɛn'teɪʃən/ or /ˌɒr-/ *n* arrangement; alignment; position relative to a compass direction; one's way of thinking or direction of interest.

orienteering /ˌɔriɛn'tiːrɪŋ/ or /ˌɒr-/ *n* the sport of racing on foot over difficult country using a map and compass.

orifice /'ɔrɪfɪs/ or /'ɒr-/ *n* an opening or mouth of a cavity.

oriflamme /'ɔrɪˌflæm/ or /'ɒr-/ *n* the ancient royal standard of France, a red flag split at one end and forming flame-shaped streamers; a party symbol; a blaze of colour.

orig. *abbr* = origin; original(ly).

origami /ˌɔrɪ'gæmi/ or /ˌɒr/ *n* the Japanese art of paper folding to make complicated shapes.

origin /'ɔrɪdʒɪn/ or /'ɒr-/ *n* the source or beginning of anything; ancestry or parentage.

original /ə'rɪdʒɪnəl/ *adj* relating to the origin or beginning; earliest, primitive; novel; unusual; inventive, creative. • *n* an original work, as of art or literature; something from which copies are made; a creative person; an eccentric.—**originality** *n.*—**originally** *adv.*

original sin *n* the inherent tendency of mankind to sin, derived from Adam and imputed to his descendants.

originate /ə'rɪdʒɪˌneɪt/ *vti* to initiate or begin; to bring or come into being.—**origination** *n*.—**originator** *n*.

orinasal /ˌɒrɪ'neɪzəl/ *adj* (*vowel*) sounded with both the mouth and nose.—*also n*.

oriole /'ɔːrɪəl/ or /-ɔːl/ *n* kinds of yellow, black-winged bird.

orison /'ɒrɪzən/ or /'ɒr-/ *n* (*arch*) a prayer.

orle /ɔːl/ *n* (*her*) an ordinary in the form of a fillet round a shield; (*archit*) a fillet under the capital of a column.

Orlon /'ɔːlɒn/ *n* (*trademark*) an acrylic fibre.

orlop /'ɔːlɒp/ *n* the lowest deck of a ship with three or more decks.

ormer /'ɔːmər/ *n* a mollusc, sea ear.

ormolu /'ɔːməluː/ *n* an imitation gold made of copper and tin alloy, used for decoration.

ornament /'ɔːnəmənt/ *n* anything that enhances the appearance of a person or thing; a small decorative object. • *vt* to adorn, to decorate with ornaments.

ornamental /ˌɔːnə'mentəl/ *adj* serving as an ornament; decorative, not useful.—**ornamentally** *adv*.

ornamentation /-'teɪʃən/ *n* the act or process of ornamenting; something that decorates.

ornate /ɔː'neɪt/ *adj* richly adorned; (*style*) highly elaborate.—**ornately** *adv*.—**ornateness** *n*.

ornery /'ɔːnəri/ *adj* (*sl*) of a bad disposition, hard to manage.

ornitho- /'ɔːnɪθɒː/, **ornith-** /'ɔːnɪθ/ *prefix* bird.

ornithology /ˌɔːnɪ'θɒlədʒi/ *n* the study of birds.—**ornithological** *adj*.—**ornithologically** *adv*.—**ornithologist** *n*.

ornithopter /'ɔːnɪθɒptər/ *n* an aircraft with flapping wings.

ornithorhynchus /ˌɔːnɪθəˈræŋkəs/ *n* an Australian genus of monotremes, including the platypus.

oro- /'ɔːrɒ/ *prefix* mountain.

orogeny /oːˈrɒdʒɪni/, **orogenesis** /ˌɔːrɒˈdʒɛnɪsɪs/ *n* the formation of mountains.—**orogenic, orogenetic** *adj*.

orography, orology /oːˈrɒɡrəfi/ *n* the geography of mountains and mountain systems, their mapping, etc.—**orographic, orological** *adj*.

oroide /oːˈrɔɪd/ *n* a gold-coloured alloy of tin and copper.

orotund /'ɒrəˌtend/ or /'ɔːr-/ *adj* (*voice*) full, resonant; (*style*) pompous, high-flown.

orphan /'ɔːfən/ *n* a child whose parents are dead. • *vt* to cause to become an orphan.—*also adj*.

orphanage /'ɔːfənɪdʒ/ *n* a residential institution for the care of orphans.

Orphean /'ɔːfɪən/ *adj* of or pertaining to Orpheus, the celebrated bard of Classic mythology, or his music; melodious, enchanting.

Orphic /'ɔːfɪk/ *adj* of Orpheus or his cult; mystical.

orphrey /'ɔːfri/ *n* an embroidered band or bands of gold or silver on the front of an ecclesiastical vestment from the neck downward, *esp* on a cope.

orpiment /'ɔːpɪmənt/ *n* a yellow compound of arsenic, used as a pigment.

orpine /'ɔːpɪn/ *n* a succulent plant with fleshy leaves and purple flowers.

orrery /'ɒrəri/ *n* (*pl* **orreries**) a moving model of the solar system, which illustrates by balls mounted on rods the motions, magnitudes, and positions of the planets.

orris /'ɒrɪs/ or /'ɒr-/ *n* a kind of iris.

orrisroot /'ɒrɪsˌruːt/ or /'ɒr-/ *n* the dried roots of the Florentine orris, used in perfumery and medicine.

ortho- /'ɔːθɒ/ *prefix* straight, right, true.

orthocephalic /ˌɔːθɒseˈfælɪk/, **orthocephalous** /-fæləs/ *adj* (*anat*) with a skull of medium proportions, between brachycephalic and dolichocephalic.

orthochromatic /ˌɔːθɒkrɒ'mætɪk/ *adj* (*photog*) giving the correct relative tones to colours, isochromatic.

orthoclase /'ɔːθɒˌkleɪs/ *n* potash feldspar.

orthodontics /ˌɔːθə'dɒntɪks/ *n sing* the branch of dentistry dealing with the correction of irregularities in the teeth.—**orthodontic** *adj*.—**orthodontist** *n*.

orthodox /'ɔːθəˌdɒks/ *adj* conforming with established behaviour or opinions; not heretical; generally accepted, conventional; (*with cap*) of or relating to a conservative political or religious group.

orthodoxy /'ɔːθəˌdɒksi/ *n* (*pl* **orthodoxies**) the state or quality of being orthodox; an orthodox practice or belief.

orthoepy /'ɔːθəˌepi/ or /ɔːˈθoʊɪpi/ *n* the science of correct pronunciation.—**orthoepic** *adj*.—**orthepist** *n*.

orthogenesis /ˌɔːθɒ'dʒenɪsɪs/ *n* evolution following a definite line, determinate variation.—**orthogenetic** *adj*.

orthognathous /ˌɔːrˈθɒːˈnæθəs/ *adj* having an upright jaw, neither receding nor protruding.—**orthognathism** *n*.

orthogonal /ɔːˈθɒɡənəl/ *adj* rectangular.—**orthogonally** *adv*.

orthography /ɔːˈθɒɡrəfi/ *n* (*pl* **orthographies**) the art of spelling and writing words with grammatical correctness; a map projection with a point of sight supposedly infinitely distant.—**orthographer** *n*.—**orthographic, orthographical** *adj*.

orthopedics, orthopaedics /ˌɔːθə'piːdɪks/ *n* the study and surgical treatment of bone and joint disorders.—**orthopedic** *adj*.—**orthopedist** *n*.

orthopteran /ɔːˈθɒptərən/ *n* (*pl* **orthopterans, orthoptera**) any of the Orthoptera order of insects, having their two outer wings overlapping at the top when shut, as in grasshoppers.—**orthopterous** *adj*.

orthoptic /ɔːˈθɒptɪk/ *adj* of correct seeing. • *n* the peep-sight of a rifle.

orthotropism /ˌɔːθɒːˈtrɒpɪzəm/ *n* vertical growth in plants.—**orthotropic** *adj*.—**orthotropous** *adj*.

ortolan /'ɔːtələn/ *n* a small bird, allied to the bunting, much esteemed for its flesh.

oryx /'ɒrɪks/ *n* (*pl* **oryxes, oryx**) a straight-horned African antelope.

OS *abbr* = ordinary seaman; Ordnance Survey (national mapping agency in the UK).

Os (*chem symbol*) osmium.

os[1] *n* (*pl* **ossa**) (*anat*) bone.

os[2] *n* (*pl* **ora**) (*anat*) the mouth.

OSC /'ɒːˈɛsˈsiː/ *abbr* ✦ = Ontario Securities Commision.

Oscar /'ɒskər/ *n* any of several small gold statuettes awarded annually by the US Academy of Motion Picture Arts and Sciences for outstanding achievements.

oscillate /'ɒsɪˌleɪt/ *vi* to swing back and forth as a pendulum; to waver, vacillate between extremes of opinion, etc.—**oscillation** *n*.

oscillator /-tər/ *n* a device for producing alternating current.

oscillatory /ə'sɪlətəri/ or /'ɒsɪˌleɪtəri/ *adj* swinging; vibrating.

oscilloscope /ə'sɪləˌskoʊp/ *n* a device for viewing oscillations on a display screen of a cathode-ray tube.

osculate /'ɒskjuˌleɪt/ *vti* (*species*) to have features in common; (*geom*) to make contact (with); (*humorous*) to kiss, to touch.—**osculation** *n*.

osculatory /'ɒskjulətəri/ *adj* pertaining to kissing. • *n* a tablet or board on which the picture of Christ or the Virgin Mary are painted for worshippers to kiss.

-ose /oːs/ or /oːz/ *suffix* full of.

osier /'oːzɪər/ *n* a willow, the twigs of which are used in basketmaking.

Osiris /oːˈsaɪrɪs/ *n* the best loved of the Egyptian gods, husband of Iris and father of Horus.

-osis /'ɒsɪs/ *n suffix* indicating a particular state, *esp* a diseased condition, *thrombosis*; increase, development of, *fibrosis*.

Osmanli /ɒzˈmænli/ or /ɒs-/ *adj* of or pertaining to the Ottoman Empire.—*also n*.

osmium /'ɒzmɪəm/ *n* a hard bluish-white metallic element used in alloys.

osmometry /ɒsˈmɒmətri/ *n* the measurement of smells.

osmosis /ɒzˈmoʊsɪs/ or /ɒs-/ *n* (*pl* **osmoses**) the percolation and intermixture of fluids separated by a porous membrane.—**osmotic** *adj*.—**osmotically** *adv*.

osmunda, osmund /ɒzˈmʌndə/ *n* the flowering fern of the genus Osmunda.

osnaburg /'ɒznəˌbɜːɡ/ *n* a coarse linen cloth.

osprey /ˌɒsprei/ or /-pri/ *n* (*pl* **ospreys**) a large fish-eating bird of prey.

ossa *see* **os**[2].

ossein /'ɒsiɪn/ *n* gelatinous tissue in bone.

osseous /'ɒsɪəs/ *adj* pertaining to, consisting of, or like, bone.

ossicle /'ɒsɪkəl/ *n* a little bone, *esp* of the ear; (*pl*) hard structures of small size, as the calcareous plates of the starfish.—**ossicular** *adj*.

ossiferous /'ɒsɪfərəs/ *adj* producing or containing bone.

ossification /ˌɒsɪfɪ'keɪʃən/ *n* conversion of soft animal tissue into bone.

ossifrage /ˌɒsɪfreɪdʒ/ *n* an old name for the osprey or lammergeier.

ossify /ˈɒsɪˌfaɪ/ *vb* (**ossifying, ossified**) *vt* to convert into bone or into a bone-like substance; to harden. • *vi* to become bone; to grow rigid and unprogressive.

ossuary /ˈɒsjʊri/ *n* (*pl* **ossuaries**) an urn for bones.

osteal /ˈɒstiːl/ *adj* osseous.

osteitis /ˌɒstiˈaɪtɪs/ *n* inflammation of the bone.

ostensible /ɒˈstɒnsɪbəl/ *adj* apparent; seeming; pretended.—**ostensibly** *adv*.

ostensive /-sɪv/ *adj* showing, exhibiting.

ostentation /ˌɒstenˈteɪʃən/ *n* a showy, pretentious display.—**ostentatious** *adj*.—**ostentatiously** *adv*.

osteo-, oste- /ˈɒstiɔ:/ *prefix* bone.

osteoarthritis /ˌɒstiɔ:ɑːˈθraɪtɪs/ *n* painful inflammation of the joints, *esp* the hips, knees and olhers that bear weight.—**osteoarthritic** *adj*.

osteology /ˌɒstiˈɒlədʒi/ *n* that part of anatomy treating of bones, their structure, etc; a bony structure.—**osteological** *adj*.—**osteologist** *n*.

osteoma /ˌɒstiˈəʊmə/ *n* (*pl* **osteomas, osteomata**) a bone tumour.

osteomalacia /ˌɒstiɔ:məˈleɪʃə/ *n* softening of the bones.

osteomyelitis /ˌɒstiɔ:maɪˈlaɪtɪs/ *n* an infectious disease causing inflammation of the bone marrow.

osteopathy /ˌɒstiˈɒpəθi/ *n* the treatment of disease by manipulation of the bones and muscles, often as an adjunct to medical and surgical measures.—**osteopath** *n*.

osteophyte /ˌɒstiəˈfaɪt/ *n* an abnormal growth from a bone.—**osteophytic** *adj*.

osteoplasty /ˌɒstiəˈplæsti/ *n* (*pl* **osteoplasties**) surgery involving bone replacement and grafting.—**osteoplastic** *adj*.

osteoporosis /ˌɒstiɔ:pəˈrəʊsɪs/ *n* the development of brittle bones due to a calcium deficiency in the bone matrix.—**osteoporotic** *adj*.

osteotome /ˌɒstiəˈtəʊm/ *n* an instrument used in dissecting bones.—**osteotomy** *n*.

ostiary /ˈɒstʃəri/ *n* (*pl* **ostiaries**) (*RC Church*) a church doorkeeper.

ostler /ˈɒslər/ *n* (*formerly*) a man who attended to horses at an inn, a hostler.

ostracize /ˈɒstrəˌsaɪz/ *vt* to exclude, banish from a group, society, etc.—**ostracism** *n*.

ostrich /ˈɒstrɪtʃ/ *n* (*pl* **ostriches, ostrich**) a large, flightless, swift-running African bird.

Ostrogoth /ˈɒstrəˌgɒθ/ *n* an eastern Goth.

OT *abbr* = Old Testament.

otalgia /əˈtældʒiə/ *n* earache.

other /ˈʌðər/ *adj* second; remaining; different; additional. • *pron* the other one; some other one.

other-directed *adj* guided primarily by the influence or example of others.

otherness /-nəs/ *n* diversity.

otherwhere /-wer/ *adv* (*arch*) elsewhere.

otherwhile /-ˌhwaɪl/ or /-ˌwaɪl/ *adv* (*arch*) at another time.

otherwise /-ˌwaɪz/ *adv* if not, or else; differently.

otherworldly /ˌʌðərˈwərldli/ *adj* spiritual; unworldly.—**otherworldliness** *n*.

otic /ˈɒtɪk/ or /ˈəʊ-/ *adj* of the ear.

otiose /ˈəʊtiɒs/ or /ˈəʊʃ-/, /-əʊz/ *adj* superfluous, serving no practical purpose; futile; at leisure.—**otiosity** *n*.

otitis /əʊˈtaɪtɪs/ *n* inflammation of the ear.

oto- /ˈəʊtəʊ:/ *prefix* ear.

otolith /ˈəʊtəlɪθ/ *n* a chalky concretion in the ear.—**otolithic** *adj*.

otology /əʊˈtɒlədʒi/ *n* that part of anatomy which treats of the ear, its structure, etc.—**otological** *adj*.—**otologist** *n*.

otoscope /-ˌskəʊp/ *n* an instrument for examining the interior of the ear.

OTT *abbr* = over the top.

ottava rima /ɒˌtævəˈriːmə/ *n* (*poet*) an Italian stanza of eight lines of five accents each with three rhymes, the seventh and eighth forming a couplet; a stanza of eight five-foot lines rhyming ababab cc.

otter /ˈɒtər/ *n* (*pl* **otters, otter**) a fish-eating mammal with smooth fur and a flat tail.

ottoman /ˈɒtəmən/ *n* an upholstered, backless chair or couch. • *adj* (*with cap*) of or relating to a former Turkish dynasty and empire; Turkish.

ouaniche /ˈwɒnɪʃ/ *n* ✺ a landlocked form of Atlantic salmon found in lakes in Eastern Canada.

oubliette /ˌuːbliˈɛt/ *n* an underground dungeon with its entrance in the roof in which prisoners condemned to perpetual imprisonment or secret death were confined.

ouch[1] /aʊtʃ/ *interj* an exclamation of pain or annoyance.

ouch[2] *n* a clasp, a jewel; the setting of a gem.

ought[1] /ɒt/ *aux vb* expressing obligation or duty; to be bound, to be obliged (to); a variant spelling of **aught**.

ought[2] *see* **aught**.

Ouija /ˈwiːdʒɪ/ or /-dʒə/ *n* (*trademark*) a board with letters and symbols used to obtain messages at seances.

ounce[1] /aʊns/ *n* a unit of weight, equal to one sixteenth of a pound or 28.34 grams; one sixteenth of a pint, one fluid ounce.

ounce[2] *n* the snow leopard; (*poet*) the lynx or an animal like it.

our /aʊr/ or /ɑːr/ *poss adj*, *pron* relating or belonging to us.

ours /ˈaʊrz/ or /ɑːrz/ *pron* belonging to us.

ourselves /aʊrˈselvz/ or /ɑːr-/ *pron* emphatic and reflexive form of we.

-ous /əs/ *suffix* full of, as in *joyous*; (*chem*) containing in lower proportion, as in *ferrous* as opposed to *ferric*.

ousel *see* **ouzel**.

oust /aʊst/ *vt* to eject, expel, *esp* by underhand means; to remove forcibly.

out /aʊt/ *adv* not in; outside; in the open air; to the full extent; beyond bounds; no longer holding office; ruled out, no longer considered; loudly and clearly; no longer included (in a game, fashion, etc); in error; on strike; at an end; extinguished; into the open; published; revealed; (*radio conversation*) transmission ends. • *prep* out of; out through; outside. • *adj* external; outward. • *n* an exit; means of escape.

out- *prefix* out, outside, away from; external; separate; more, longer.

out-and-out *adj* thoroughgoing; absolute; complete.

outback /ˈaʊtbæk/ *n* a remote area inland, *esp* in Australia.

outbalance *vt* to exceed in weight.

outbid /aʊtˈbɪd/ *vt* (**outbidding, outbid**, *pp* **outbidden** *or* **outbid**) to bid higher than.

outboard /ˈaʊtbɔːrd/ *adj* (*engine*) outside a ship, etc. • *n* an engine attached to the outside of a boat.

outbrave /aʊtˈbreɪv/ *vt* to excel in bravery; to defy.

outbreak /ˈaʊtbreɪk/ *n* a sudden eruption (of disease, strife, etc).

outbuilding /ˈaʊtˌbɪldɪŋ/ *n* a detached subsidiary building.

outburst /ˈaʊtbɜːrst/ *n* a bursting out; a spurt; an explosion of anger, etc.

outcast /ˈaʊtkæst/ *n* a person who is rejected by society.

outcaste /ˈaʊtkæst/ *n* one who has lost caste, a pariah. • *vt* to expel from a caste.

outclass /aʊtˈklæs/ *vt* to surpass or excel greatly.

outcome /ˈaʊtkʌm/ *n* the result, consequence.

outcrop /ˈaʊtkrɒp/ *n* an exposed rock surface. • *vi* (**outcropping, outcropped**) to crop out at the surface.

outcry /ˈaʊtkraɪ/ *n* (*pl* **outcries**) protest; uproar.

outdated /aʊtˈdeɪtəd/ *n* obsolete, old-fashioned.

outdistance /aʊtˈdɪstəns/ *vt* to get well ahead of.

outdo /aʊtˈduː/ *vt* (**outdoing, outdid**, *pp* **outdone**) to surpass, to do more than, to excel.

outdoor /ˈaʊtdɔːr/ *adj* existing, taking place, or used in the open air.

outdoors /aʊtˈdɔːrz/ *adv* in or into the open air; out of doors. • *n* the open air, outside world.

outer /ˈaʊtər/ *adj* further out or away.

outermost /ˈaʊtərˌməʊst/ *adj* furthest out; most distant.

outer space *n* any region of space beyond the earth's atmosphere.

outface /aʊtˈfeɪs/ *vt* to stare down or out of countenance; to defy.

outfall /ˈaʊtfɔːl/ *n* the lower end of a watercourse; a point of discharge.

outfield /ˈaʊtfiːld/ *n* the outer part of a cricket or baseball field.

outfit /ˈaʊtfɪt/ *n* the equipment used in an activity; clothes worn together, an ensemble; a group of people associated in an activity. • *vt* (**outfitting, outfitted**) to provide with an outfit or equipment.

outfitter /ˈaʊtˌfɪtər/ *n* a supplier of equipment or clothes.

outflank /aʊtˈflæŋk/ *vt* to get round the side of (an enemy); to circumvent.

outflow /ˈaʊtfləʊ/ *n* a flowing out; something that flows out.

outfox /aʊtˈfɒks/ *vt* to outwit by superior cunning.

outgeneral /aʊtˈdʒenərəl/ *vt* to outdo in strategy.

outgo /aʊtˈgəʊ/ *vt* (**outgoing, outwent**, *pp* **outgone**) to go beyond; to surpass.

outgoing /ˈaʊtˌgəʊɪŋ/ *adj* departing; retiring; sociable, forthcoming. • *n* an outlay; (*pl*) expenditure.

outgrow /aʊtˈgrəʊ/ *vt* (**outgrowing, outgrew**, *pp* **outgrown**) to become too big for; to grow taller than; to grow out of.

outgrowth /'ʊʊtgroːθ/ *n* an offshoot.

outgun /ʊʊt'gʊn/ *vt* (**outgunning, outgunned**) to defeat by greater firepower; (*inf*) to surpass.

outhouse /'ʊʊthʊʊs/ *n* a shet, etc, adjoining a main house.

outing /'ʊʊtɪŋ/ *n* a pleasure trip; an excursion.

outlandish /ʊʊt'lændɪʃ/ *adj* unconventional; strange; fantastic.

outlast /ʊʊt'læst/ *vt* to endure longer than.

outlaw /'ʊʊtlɒ/ *vt* to declare illegal. • *n* an outlawed person; a habitual or notorious criminal.

outlay /'ʊʊtleɪ/ *n* a spending (of money); expenditure.

outlet /'ʊʊtlet/ or /-lət/ *n* an opening or release; a means of expression; a market for goods or services.

outlier /'ʊʊt,laɪər/ *n* a part of a rock or stratum detached at some distance from the principal mass.

outline /'ʊʊtlaɪn/ *n* a profile; a general indication; a rough sketch or draft.—*also vt.*

outlive /ʊʊt'lɪv/ *vt* to live longer than, outlast; to live through; to survive.

outlook /'ʊʊtlʊk/ *n* mental attitude; view; prospect.

outlying /'ʊʊt,laɪŋ/ *adj* detached; remote, distant.

outmaneuver, outmanoeuvre /,ʊʊtmə'nuːvər/ *vt* to outwit in tactics.

outmatch /ʊʊt'mætʃ/ *vt* to be more than a match for.

outmoded /ʊʊt'moːdəd/ *adj* old-fashioned.

outmost /'ʊʊtmoːst/ *adj* outermost.

outnumber /ʊʊt'nʊmbər/ *vt* to exceed in number.

out-of-date *adj* no longer valid, unfashionable; outmoded.

out-of-pocket *adj* (*expenses*) paid for in cash; having lost money.
  outpoint *vt* to accumulate more points than.

out-of-province *adj* ✹ (*Cdn*) in, from, or pertaining to another province.

out-of-the-way *adj* uncommon; secluded.

outpatient /'ʊʊt,peɪʃənt/ *n* a person treated at, but not resident in, a hospital.

outpoint /'ʊʊt'pɒɪnt/ *vt* to accumulate more points than.

outport /'ʊʊtpɔːt/ *n* ✹ a part of harbour at some distance from the chief port.

outpost /'ʊʊtpoːst/ *n* (*mil*) a post or detachment at a distance from a main force.

outpouring /'ʊʊt,pɔːrɪŋ/ *n* an effusion, an emotional speech.

output /'ʊʊtpʊt/ *n* the quantity (of goods, etc) produced, *esp* over a given period; information delivered by a computer, *esp* to a printer; (*elect*) the useful voltage, current, or power delivered.—*also vt.*

outrage /'ʊʊtreɪdʒ/ *n* an extremely vicious or violent act; a grave insult or offence; great anger, etc, aroused by this.—*also vt.*—**outrageous** *adj.*

outrageous /ʊʊt'reɪdʒəs/ *adj* flagrant; atrocious; violent; excessive.—**outrageously** *adv.*—**outrageousness** *n.*

outrank /ʊʊt'ræŋk/ *vt* to be of a higher rank than; to be of a higher priority.

outré /'uːtreɪ/ *adj* outraging decorum; eccentric, unconventional; extravagant.

outride /ʊʊt'raɪd/ *vt* (**outriding, outrode**, *pp* **outridden**) to ride faster or farther than; to keep afloat through (a storm).

outrider /'ʊʊt,raɪdər/ *n* a mounted escort who goes in advance of a carriage, car, etc.

outrigger /'ʊʊt,rɪgər/ *n* a projecting spar for a sail, etc; a projection with a float extending from a canoe to prevent capsizing; a canoe of this type; a projecting frame to support the elevator or tail of an aircraft or the rotor of a helicopter.

outright /'ʊʊtraɪt/ or /ʊʊt'raɪt/ *adj* complete, downright, direct. • *adv* at once; without restrictions.

outrun /ʊʊt'rʊn/ *vt* (**outrunning, outran**, *pp* **outran**) to run faster than; to exceed, to go beyond; to escape by running.

outset /'ʊʊtset/ *n* the start, beginning.

outshine /ʊʊt'ʃaɪn/ *vt* (**outshining, outshone**) to outdo in brilliance, ability; to shine longer and brighter than.

outside /ʊʊt'saɪd/ or /'ʊʊtsaɪd/ *n* the outer part or surface, the exterior. • *adj* outer; outdoor; (*chance, etc*) slight. • *adv* on or to the outside. • *prep* on or to the exterior of; beyond.

outsider /ʊʊt'saɪdər/ *n* a person or thing not included in a set, group, etc, a non-member; a contestant, *esp* a horse, not thought to have a chance in a race.

outsize /'ʊʊtsaɪz/ *adj* of a larger than usual size.

outskirts /'ʊʊtskərts/ *npl* districts remote from the centre, as of a city.

outsmart /ʊʊt'smart/ *vt* to outwit.

outspan /ʊʊt'spæn/ *vt* (**outspanning, outspanned**) (*S Africa*) to unyoke ox teams from a wagon; to encamp. • *n* a halting place.

outspoken /ʊʊt'spoːkən/ *adj* candid in speech, frank, blunt.

outstanding /ʊʊt'stændɪŋ/ *adj* excellent; distinguished, prominent; unpaid; unresolved, still to be done.

outstation /'ʊʊt,steɪʃən/ *n* a distant post or station.

outstay /ʊʊt'steɪ/ *vt* to stay longer than or too long.

outstrip /ʊʊt'strɪp/ *vt* (**outstripping, outstripped**) to surpass; to go faster than.

outtalk /ʊʊt'tɒk/ *vt* to talk down.

outvote /ʊʊt'voːt/ *vt* to defeat by a higher number of votes.

outward /'ʊʊtwərd/ *adj* directed toward the outside; external; clearly apparent. • *adv* toward the outside.

Outward Bound movement *n* (in UK) an educational scheme to promote youth adventure training.

outwardly /-lɪ/ *adv* externally.

outwards /-z/ *adv* outward.

outwear /ʊʊt'wer/ *vt* (**outwearing, outwore**, *pp* **outworn**) to outlast; to wear out.

outweigh /ʊʊt'weɪ/ *vt* to count for more than, to exceed in value, weight, or importance.

outwent *see* **outgo**.

outwit /ʊʊt'wɪt/ *vt* (**outwitting, outwitted**) to get the better of, defeat, by wit or cunning.

outwork /'ʊʊtwərk/ *n* a defence constructed beyond the main body of a fort, etc; work done outside a factory.

ouzel /'uːzəl/ *n* kinds of small bird; a blackbird.—*also* **ousel**.

ouzo /'uːzoː/ *n* a Greek aniseed-flavoured spirit.

ova *see* **ovum**.

oval /'oːvəl/ *adj* egg-shaped; elliptical. • *n* anything oval.

ovariotomy /,oːværɪ'ɒtəmɪ/ *n* (*pl* **ovariotomies**) the surgical operation of removing a tumour from the ovary.

ovaritis /'oːvə'raɪtɪs/ *n* inflammation of the ovary.

ovary /'oːvərɪ/ *n* (*pl* **ovaries**) one of the two female reproductive organs producing eggs.—**ovarian** *adj.*

ovate /'oːveɪt/ *adj* (*bot*) oval, egg-shaped.

ovation /oː'veɪʃən/ *n* enthusiastic applause or public welcome.

oven /'ʊvən/ *n* an enclosed, heated compartment for baking or drying.

ovenbird /'ʊvən,bərd/ *n* a kind of bird with a dome-shaped nest; a fowl for cooking.

oven-ready *adj* (*food*) prepared for immediate cooking in the oven.

ovenware /'ʊvən,wer/ *n* attractive heat-resistant dishes in which food can be cooked and served.

over /'oːvər/ *prep* higher than; on top of; across; to the other side of; above; more than; concerning. • *adv* above; across; in every part; completed; from beginning to end; up and down; in addition; too. • *adj* upper; excessive; surplus; finished; remaining. • *n* (*cricket*) the number of balls bowled before changing ends.

over- *prefix* in excess, too much; above.

overact /,oːvər'ækt/ *vti* to act in an exaggerated manner, to overdo a part.

overactive /,oːvər'æktɪv/ *adj* abnormally or excessively active.— **overactivity** *n.*

overall /'oːvər,ɒl/ *adj* including everything. • *adv* as a whole; generally. • *n* a loose protective garment; (*pl*) a one-piece protective garment covering body and legs.

overarch /,oːvər'artʃ/ *vti* to form an arch (over).

overarm /'oːvər,arm/ *adj*, *adv* (*sport*) bowled, thrown, performed, etc with the arm raised above the shoulder.

overawe /,oːvər'ɒ/ *vt* to restrain by awe, daunt.

overbalance /,oːvər'bæləns/ *vti* to fall over; to upset; to outweigh. • *n* a surplus.

overbear /,oːvər'ber/ *vt* (**overbearing, overbore**, *pp* **overborne**) to dominate, to repress, to bear down.

overbearing /-ɪŋ/ *adj* domineering; overriding.—**overbearingly** *adv.*

overblown /,oːvər'bloːn/ *adj* excessive, pretentious.

overboard /'oːvər,bɒrd/ *adv* over the side of a ship, etc; (*inf*) to extremes of enthusiasm.

overbook /,oːvər'bʊk/ *vti* to sell tickets (for) in excess of the available seats or space.

overburden /,oːvər'bərdən/ *vt* to load too heavily.

overcall /,oːvər'kɒl/ *vti* (*bridge*) to bid more on (a hand) than it is worth; to take a bid away from (a partner).

overcame *see* **overcome**.

overcapitalize /ˌoːvərˈkæpɪtəˌlaɪz/ *vt* to float (a company) with too great a capital.—**overcapitalization** *n*.

overcast /ˈoːvərˌkæst/ *adj* clouded over.

overcharge /ˌoːvərˈtʃɑːrdʒ/ *vt* (*battery*) to overload; to fill to excess; to demand too high a price (from). • *n* an excessive or exorbitant charge or load.

overcloud /ˌoːvərˈklaʊd/ *vti* to cover or become covered with clouds; to make or become dark or depressed.

overcoat /ˈoːvərˌkoːt/ *n* a warm, heavy topcoat.

overcome /ˌoːvərˈkʌm/ *vti* (**overcoming, overcame**, *pp* **overcome**) to get the better of, to prevail; to render helpless or powerless, as by tears, laughter, emotion, etc; to be victorious; to surmount obstacles, etc.

overcompensation /ˈoːvərˌkʌmpənˈseɪʃən/ *n* (*psychoanal*) an excess of compensation, often resulting in an overbearing manner.—**overcompensatory** *adj*.

overcrop /ˌoːvərˈkrɒp/ *vt* (**overcropping, overcropped**) to exhaust (land) by excessive cultivation.

overcrowd /ˌoːvərˈkraʊd/ *vti* to make or become too crowded.

overdo /ˌoːvərˈduː/ *vt* (**overdoing, overdid,** *pp* **overdone**) to do to excess; to overact; to cook (food) too much.—**overdone** *adj*.

overdose /ˈoːvərˌdoːs/ *n* an excessive dose —*also vti*.

overdraft /ˈoːvərˌdræft/ *n* an overdrawing, an amount overdrawn, at a bank.

overdraw /ˌoːvərˈdrɒ/ *vti* (**overdrawing, overdrew,** *pp* **overdrawn**) to draw in excess of a credit balance; to exaggerate in describing; to make an overdraft.

overdress /ˌoːvərˈdrɛs/ *vti* to dress too warmly, too showily, or too formally.

overdrive /ˈoːvərˌdraɪv/ *n* a high gear in a motor vehicle to reduce wear for travelling at high speed. • *vt* (**overdriving, overdrove,** *pp* **overdriven**) to drive too hard, overtax.

overdue /ˌoːvərˈduː/ or /-ˈdjuː/ *adj* past the time for payment, return, performance, etc; in arrears; delayed.

overeat /ˌoːvərˈiːt/ *vi* (**overeating, overate,** *pp* **overeaten**) to eat too much.

overestimate /ˌoːvərˈɛstɪˌmeɪt/ *vt* to set too high an estimate on or for. • *n* an excessive estimate.—**overestimation** *n*.

overexpose /ˌoːvərɪkˈspoːz/ or /ˌoːvərɛk-/ *vt* (*phot*) to expose (a film) to light for too long.—**overexposure** *n*.

overflow /ˌoːvərˈfloː/ *vti* (**overflowing, overflowed,** *pp* **overflown**) to flow over, flood; to exceed the bounds (of); to abound (with emotion, etc). • *n* that which overflows; surplus, excess; an outlet for surplus water, etc.

overgrow /ˌoːvərˈgroː/ *vti* (**overgrowing, overgrew,** *pp* **overgrown**) to cover with growth; to grow too big or fast (for); to outgrow.—**overgrowth** *n*.

overgrown /ˌoːvərˈgroːn/ *adj* grown beyond the normal size; rank; ungainly.

overhand /ˈoːvərˌhænd/ *adj, adv* (*sport*) bowled, thrown, performed, etc with the hand above the shoulder.

overhang /ˌoːvərˈhæŋ/ *vti* (**overhanging, overhung**) to hang or project over. • *n* a projecting part.

overhaul /ˌoːvərˈhɒl/ *vt* to examine for, or make, repairs; to overtake.—*also n*.

overhead /ˌoːvərˈhɛd/ *adj, adv* above the head; in the sky. • *n* (often *pl*) the general, continuing costs of a business, as of rent, light, etc.

overhear /ˌoːvərˈhiːr/ *vt* (**overhearing, overheard**) to hear without the knowledge of the speaker.

overheat /ˌoːvərˈhiːt/ *vti* to make or become excessively hot; to stimulate unduly.

overjoyed /ˌoːvərˈdʒɔɪd/ *adj* highly delighted.

overkill /ˈoːvərˌkɪl/ *n* the capability to employ more weapons, etc than are necessary to destroy an enemy; excess capacity for a task.

overland /ˈoːvərˌlænd/ or /ˌoːvərˈlænd/ *adj, adv* by, on, or across land.

overlap /ˌoːvərˈlæp/ *vt* (**overlapping, overlapped**) to extend over (a thing or each other) so as to coincide in part.—*also n*.

overlay /ˌoːvərˈleɪ/ *vt* (**overlaying, overlaid**) to cover with a coating, to spread over. • *n* a coating.

overleaf /ˌoːvərˈliːf/ *adv* on the other side of the leaf of a book.

overlie /ˌoːvərˈlaɪ/ *vt* (**overlying, overlay,** *pp* **overlain**) to lie on top of; to stifle thus.

overload /ˌoːvərˈloːd/ *vt* to put too great a burden on; (*elect*) to charge with too much current.

overlong /ˌoːvərˈlɒŋ/ *adj, adv* too long.

overlook /ˌoːvərˈlʊk/ *vt* to fail to notice; to look at from above; to excuse.

overlord /ˈoːvərˌlɔrd/ *n* a lord ranking above other lords; an absolute or supreme ruler.

overman /ˌoːvərˈmæn/ *vt* (**overmanning, overmanned**) to supply with too many workers.

overmaster /ˌoːvərˈmæstər/ *vt* to dominate wholly, to overpower.

overmuch /ˌoːvərˈmʌtʃ/ *adj, adv* too much.

overnice /ˌoːvərˌnaɪs/ *adj* too particular.

overnight /ˌoːvərˈnaɪt/ *adv* for the night; in the course of the night; suddenly. • *adj* done in the night; lasting the night.

overpass /ˈoːvərˌpæs/ *n* a road crossing another road, path, etc, at a higher level; the upper level of such a crossing. • *vt* (**overpassing, overpassed,** *pp* **overpast**) to pass beyond, to overstep; to surpass.

overplay /ˌoːvərˈpleɪ/ *vt* to place too much emphasis on; to behave in an exaggerated or affected manner.

overplus /ˈoːvərˌplʌs/ *n* a surplus, an excess.

overpower /ˌoːvərˈpaʊər/ *vt* to overcome by superior force, to subdue; to overwhelm.

overpowering /-ɪŋ/ *adj* overwhelming; compelling; unbearable.

overproduction /ˌoːvərprəˈdʌkʃən/ *n* supply in excess of the demand.

overqualified /ˌoːvərˈkwɒlɪˌfaɪd/ *adj* having more qualifications or experience that required for a particular job.

overrate /ˌoːvərˈreɪt/ *vt* to value or assess too highly.

overreach /ˌoːvərˈriːtʃ/ *vt* to extend beyond; to circumvent, outwit; to fail by trying too much or being too subtle.

overreact /ˌoːvərriˈækt/ *vi* to show an excessive reaction to something.

override /ˌoːvərˈraɪd/ *vt* (**overriding, overrode,** *pp* **overridden**) to ride over; to nullify; to prevail.

overrule /ˌoːvərˈruːl/ *vt* to set aside by higher authority; to prevail over.

overrun /ˌoːvərˈrʌn/ *vt* (**overrunning, overran,** *pp* **overrun**) to attack and defeat; to swarm over; to exceed (a time limit, etc).

overseas /ˌoːvərˈsiːz/ *adj, adv* across or beyond the sea; abroad.

oversee /ˌoːvərˈsiː/ *vt* (**overseeing, oversaw,** *pp* **overseen**) to supervise; to superintend. • *n* **overseer** *n*.

oversell /ˌoːvərˈsɛl/ *vt* (**overselling, oversold**) to sell more than can be delivered, *esp* stocks.

overset /ˈoːvərˌsɛt/ *vti* (**oversetting, overset**) to upset, to disturb; to overthrow.

oversew /ˈoːvərˌsoː/ *vt* (**oversewing, oversewed,** *pp* **oversewn**) to stitch over again to reinforce; to stitch over an edge to prevent fraying.

overshadow /ˌoːvərˈʃædoː/ *vt* to throw a shadow over; to appear more prominent or important than.

overshoe /ˈoːvərˌʃuː/ *n* a galosh.

overshoot /ˌoːvərˈʃuːt/ *vt* (**overshooting, overshot**) to shoot or send beyond (a target, etc); (*aircraft*) to fly or taxi beyond the end of a runway when landing or taking off.—*also n*.

oversight /ˈoːvərˌsaɪt/ *n* a careless mistake or omission; supervision.

oversize /ˈoːvərˌsaɪz/, **oversized** /-ˌsaɪzd/ *adj* of larger than average size.

overslaugh /ˌoːvərslɒ/ *n* (*mil*) the passing over of an ordinary duty because of a special one.

oversleep /ˌoːvərˈsliːp/ *vi* (**oversleeping, overslept**) to sleep beyond the intended time.

overspend /ˌoːvərˈspɛnd/ *vt* (**overspending, overspent**) to spend more than necessary; to wear out, tire. • *vi* to spend more than one can afford.

overstate /ˌoːvərˈsteɪt/ *vt* to state too strongly, to exaggerate.—**overstatement** *n*.

overstay /ˌoːvərˈsteɪ/ *vt* to remain longer than or beyond the limits of.

overstep /ˌoːvərˈstɛp/ *vt* (**overstepping, overstepped**) to exceed; (*a limit*) to step beyond.

overstock /ˌoːvərˈstɒk/ *vt* to lay in too large a stock of or for, to glut.—*also n*.

overstrung /ˌoːvərˈstrʌŋ/ *adj* too highly strung; too sensitive.

oversubscribe /ˌoːvərsəbˈskraɪb/ *vt* to apply for more shares in (an issue) than can be allotted.

overt /oːˈvɜrt/ or /ˈoːvɜrt/ *adj* openly done, unconcealed; (*law*) done with evident intent, deliberate.—**overtly** *adv*.

overtake /ˌoːvərˈteɪk/ *vt* (**overtaking, overtook,** *pp* **overtaken**) to catch up with and pass; to come upon suddenly.

overtax /ˌoːvərˈtæks/ *vt* to make too great demands on; to tax too heavily.

overthrow /ˌoːvərˈθroː/ *vt* (**overthrowing, overthrew,** *pp* **overthrown**) to throw over, overturn; (*government, etc*) to bring down by force.—*also n.*

overtime /ˈoːvərˌtaɪm/ *adv* beyond regular working hours. • *n* extra time worked; payment for this.

overtone /ˈoːvərˌtoːn/ *n* an additional subtle meaning; an implicit quality; (*mus*) a harmonic; the colour of light reflected (as by a paint).

overtook *see* **overtake**.

overtop /ˌoːvərˈtɒp/ *vt* (**overtopping, overtopped**) to be higher than, to tower above.

overtrain /ˌoːvərˈtreɪn/ *vti* to train too hard.

overtrump /ˌoːvərˈtrʌmp/ *vt* to play a higher trump than (the card that has trumped another).

overture /ˈoːvərˌtʃər/ *n* an initiating of negotiations; a formal offer, proposal; (*mus*) an instrumental introduction to an opera, etc.

overturn /ˌoːvərˈtərn/ *vti* to upset, turn over; to overthrow

overview /ˈoːvərˌvjuː/ *n* a general survey.

overweening /ˌoːvərˈwiːnɪŋ/ *adj* arrogant, presumptuous, conceited.

overweight /ˌoːvərˈweɪt/ *adj* weighing more than the proper amount. • *n* excess weight.

overwhelm /ˌoːvərˈwelm/ *vt* to overcome totally; to submerge; to crush; to overpower with emotion.

overwhelming /-ɪŋ/ *adj* irresistible; uncontrollable; vast vastly superior; extreme.

overwork /ˌoːvərˈwərk/ *vti* to work or use too hard or too long.

overwrite /ˌoːvərˈraɪt/ *vt* (**overwriting, overwrote, overwritten**) to write in an overly elaborate style; to write too much; to write data to a computer disk thereby erasing the existing contents.

overwrought /ˌoːvərˈrɒt/ *adj* over-excited; too elaborate.

ovi- /ˈoːvi/ *prefix* egg.

oviduct /ˈoːviˌdʌkt/ *n* the tube which conducts the ovum from the ovary to the uterus.

oviferous /ˈoːvɪˌfərəs/ *adj* egg-carrying.

oviform /ˈoːvɪˌfɔrm/ *adj* egg-shaped.

ovine /ˈoːvaɪn/ *adj* pertaining to sheep.

oviparous /oːˈvɪpərəs/ *adj* producing young by eggs.—**oviparity** *n*.

oviposit /ˌoːvɪˈpɒzɪt/ *vi* to lay or deposit eggs.—**oviposition** *n*.

ovipositor /ˌoːvɪˈpɒzɪtər/ *n* the organ in certain insects by which its eggs are deposited.

ovisac /ˈoːvɪˌsæk/ *n* the cavity in the ovary which contains the ovum.

ovoid /ˈoːvɔɪd/ *adj* egg-shaped.

ovolo /ˈoːvəˌloː/ *n* (*pl* **ovoli**) (*archit*) a round or convex egg-shaped moulding.

ovoviviparous /ˌoːvoːvɪˈvɪpərəs/ *adj* producing eggs containing the young in a living state, as certain animals.—**ovoviviparity** *n*.

ovulate /ˈɒvjuˌleɪt/ *vi* to discharge or produce eggs from an ovary.—**ovulation** *n*.

ovule /ˈoːvjuːl/ *n* the germ borne by the placenta of a plant and subsequently developing into a seed.—**ovular** *adj*.

ovum /ˈoːvəm/ *n* (*pl* **ova**) an unfertilized female egg cell.

owe /oː/ *vti* to be in debt; to be obliged to pay; to feel the need to give, do, etc, as because of gratitude.

owing /ˈoːɪŋ/ *adj* due, to be paid; owed; (*with* **to**) because of, on account of.

owl /aul/ *n* a nocturnal bird of prey with a large head and eyes; a person of nocturnal habits, solemn appearance, etc.—**owlish** *adj*.

owlet /ˈaulət/ *n* a young owl.

own¹ /oːn/ *vti* to possess; to acknowledge, admit; to confess to.

own² *adj* belonging to oneself or itself, often used reflexively (*my own, their own*).

owner /ˈoːnər/ *n* one who owns, a possessor, a proprietor.—**ownership** *n*.

ox /ɒks/ *n* (*pl* **oxen**) a cud-chewing mammal of the cattle family; a castrated bull.

oxalate /ˈɒksəˌleɪt/ *n* a salt of oxalic acid.

oxalic acid /ɒkˈsælɪk/ *n* a poisonous acid obtained from oxalis.

oxalis /ˈɒksəlɪs/ *n* wood sorrel.

oxbow /ˈɒksboː/ *n* a horseshoe loop in a stream; the U-shaped collar of a yoke.

Oxbridge /ˈɒksbrɪdʒ/ *n, adj* (of) the British universities of Oxford and Cambridge.

oxen *see* **ox**.

ox-eye /ˈɒksaɪ/ *n* a kind of flower; a large eye.

Oxfam (*abbr*) the Oxford Committee for Famine Relief.

Oxford Group *n* a former name of Moral Rearmament.

Oxford movement *n* an Anglican high-church movement begun in Oxford in 1833.

oxidation /ɒksɪˈdeɪʃən/ *n* the operation of converting into an oxide.

oxide /ˈɒksaɪd/ *n* a compound of oxygen with another element.

oxidize /ˈɒksɪdaɪz/ *vti* to cause to undergo a chemical reaction with oxygen; to rust.—**oxidization** *n*.

oxlip /ˈɒkslɪp/ *n* a variety of primula; a hybrid between primrose and cowslip.

Oxon. /ˈɒksən/ *abbr* = (*degrees, etc*) of Oxford.

Oxonian /ɒkˈsoːniən/ *adj* pertaining to Oxford. • *n* a graduate or member of Oxford University.

oxtail /ˈɒksteɪl/ *n* the tail of an ox, *esp* skinned and used for stews, soups, etc.

oxy- /ɒksi/ *prefix* sharp; oxygen.

oxyacetylene /ˌɒksiəˈsetɪˌliːn/ *n* a mixture of oxygen with acetylene used in a blowlamp to cut or weld metal.—*also adj*.

oxygen /ˈɒksɪdʒən/ *n* a colourless, odourless, tasteless, highly reactive gaseous element forming part of air, water, etc, and essential to life and combustion.—**oxygenic, oxygenous** *adj*.

oxygenate /ˈɒksɪdʒəˌneɪt/ *or* /ɒkˈsɪ-/ *vt* to combine or supply with oxygen.—**oxygenation** *n*.

oxygenize /ˈɒksɪdʒəˌnaɪz/ *vt* to oxygenate.—**oxygenizer** *n*.

oxygen tent *n* a canopy over a hospital bed, etc, within which a supply of oxygen is maintained.

oxyhemoglobin, oxyhaemoglobin /ˌɒksiˌhiːməˈgloːbɪn/ *n* a loose compound of oxygen and haemoglobin.

oxyhydrogen /ˌɒksiˈhaɪdrədʒən/ *n* a mixture of oxygen with acetylene and hydrogen, as in a blowlamp, by which an intense heat is produced by the combination of gases.

oxymoron /ˌɒksiˈmɔrɒn/ *n* (*pl* **oxymora**) a figure of speech combining contradictory words, "faith unfaithful kept him falsely true."

oxytone /ˈɒksiˌtoːn/ *adj* (*linguistics*) having an acute sound; having the last syllable accented. • *n* an acute sound; a word with the acute accent on the last syllable.

oyez, oyes /oːˈjes/ *or* /-ˈjez/ *interj* the introductory cry of an official or public crier demancing attention or silence.

oyster /ˈɔɪstər/ *n* an edible marine bivalve shellfish.

oystercatcher /ˈɔɪstərˌkætʃər/ *n* a wading sea bird.

oz *abbr* = ounce(s).

Oz /ɒz/ *n* (*Austral sl*) Australia.

ozokerite, ozocerite /oːˈzoːkəˌraɪt/ *or* /-sərəɪt/, /ˌoːzoːˈsiːrəɪt/ *n* a waxy fossil resin used for candles.

ozone /ˈoːzoːn/ *n* a condensed form of oxygen; (*inf*) bracing seaside air.—**ozonic, ozonous** *adj*.

ozone layer *n* a layer of ozone in the stratosphere that absorbs ultraviolet rays from the sun.

ozonize /-ˌnaɪz/ *vt* to charge with ozone.—**ozonization** *n*.—**ozonizer** *n*.

P

P¹ /piː/ *abbr* = parking; (*chess*) pawn.

P² (*chem symbol*) phosphorus.

p *abbr* = page; penny, pence.

PA *abbr* = Panama; Pennsylvania; personal assistant; public address (system).

Pa (*chem symbol*) protactinium.

pa /pɒ/ or /pɑ/ *n* (*inf*) father, papa.

p.a. *abbr* = per annum.

Pablum /ˈpæbləm/ *n* ✹ (*trademark*) a soft cereal for infants.

paca /ˈpækə/ *n* a burrowing rodent found in Central and South America.

pace¹ /peɪs/ *n* a single step; the measure of a single stride; speed of movement. • *vti* to measure by paces; to walk up and down; to determine the pace in a race; to walk with regular steps.—**pacer** *n*.

pace² *prep* with the permission of; with due respect to.

pacemaker /ˈpeɪsmeɪkər/ *n* a person who sets the pace in a race; an electronic device inserted in the heart, used to regulate heartbeat.

pacer /ˈpeɪsər/ *n* a horse trained to pace; a pacemaker.

pacha /ˈpæʃə/ *see* **pasha**.

pachinko /pəˈtʃɪŋkɒ/ *n* a Japanese variation on pinball.

pachisi /pəˈtʃiːzi/ *n* an Indian game, similar to backgammon.

pachouli /pəˈtʃuːli/ *see* **patchouli**.

pachyderm /ˈpækɪˌdɜːrm/ *n* any large thick-skinned mammal, *esp* an elephant.—**pachydermatous** *adj*.

pacific /pəˈsɪfɪk/ *adj* promoting peace; mild, conciliatory.—**pacifically** *adv*.

Pacific salmon *n* ✹ a salmon of the coastal North Pacific Ocean and its tributaries.

pacifier /ˈpæsəˌfaɪr/ *n* a person or thing that pacifies; a baby's dummy.

pacifism /ˈpæsəˌfɪzəm/ *n* opposition to the use of force under any circumstances, specifically the refusal to participate in war.—**pacifist** *n*.

pacify /ˈpæsəˌfaɪ/ *vt* (**pacifying, pacified**) to soothe; to calm; to restore peace to.—**pacification** *n*.

pack /pæk/ *n* a load or bundle (*esp* one carried on the back); a set of playing cards; a group or mass; a number of wild animals living together; an organized troop (as of Cub Scouts); a compact mass (as of snow); a small package used as a container for goods for sale. • *vt* to put together in a bundle or pack; (*suitcase*) to fill; to crowd; to press tightly so as to prevent leakage; to carry in a pack; to send (off); (*sl: gun, etc*) to carry; (*sl: punch*) to deliver with force. • *vi* (*snow, ice*) to form into a hard mass; to assemble one's belongings in suitcases or boxes. • *adj* used for carrying packs, loads, etc.—**packer** *n*.

package /ˈpækɪdʒ/ *n* a parcel, a wrapped bundle; several items, arrangements, etc offered as a unit. • *vt* to make a parcel of; to group together several items, etc.—**packager** *n*.

package holiday, package tour *n* a holiday or tour with all the fares, accommodation, food, etc, arranged for an all-inclusive price.

package store *n* (*US*) a place where alcohol is sold for consumption off the premises.—*also* **liquor store.**

packaging /ˈpækɪdʒɪŋ/ *n* the wrapping round a product offered for sale; the presentation of a product.

pack animal *n* an animal, such as a mule or camel, used for carrying loads.

packed out *adj* (*inf*) crowded.

packet /ˈpækət/ *n* a small box or package; (*sl*) a considerable sum; a vessel carrying mail, etc, between one port and another.

packhorse *n* a horse used for carrying goods.

pack ice *n* sea ice formed into a mass by the crushing together of floes, etc.

packing /ˈpækɪŋ/ *n* material for protecting packed goods or for making airtight or watertight; the act of filling a suitcase, box, etc.

packsaddle /ˈpæksædəl/ *n* a saddle for carrying goods.

pact /pækt/ *n* an agreement or treaty.

PA day *n* ✹ (*Cdn*) professional development day.

pad¹ /pæd/ *n* the dull sound of a footstep. • *vi* (**padding, padded**) to walk, *esp* with a soft step.

pad² *n* a piece of a soft material or stuffing; several sheets of paper glued together at one edge; the cushioned thickening of an animal's sole; a piece of folded absorbent material used as a surgical dressing; a flat concrete surface; (*sl*) one's own home or room. • *vt* (**padding, padded**) to stuff with soft material; to fill with irrelevant information.

padding /ˈpædɪŋ/ *n* stuffing; anything unimportant or false added to achieve length or amount.

paddle¹ /ˈpædəl/ *vi* to wade about or play in shallow water.

paddle² *n* a short oar with a wide blade at one or both ends; a implement shaped like this, used to hit, beat or stir. • *vti* (*canoe, etc*) to propel by a paddle; to beat as with a paddle; to spank.—**paddler** *n*.

paddock /ˈpædək/ *n* an enclosed field in which horses are exercised.

paddy¹ /ˈpædi/ *n* (*pl* **paddies**) threshed unmilled rice; a rice field.

paddy² *n* (*pl* **paddies**) (*sl*) rage, a fit of temper.

pademelon, paddymelon /ˈpædəˌmɛlən/ *n* (*Austral*) a small wallaby.

padlock /ˈpædlɒk/ *n* a detachable lock used to fasten doors etc. • *vt* to secure with a padlock.

padre /ˈpɒdreɪ/ or /ˈpæd-/ *n* a military chaplain.

padrone /pəˈdroːni/ or /-neɪ/ *n* an innkeeper, *esp* in Italy.

paduasoy /ˈpædjuːəˌsɔɪ/ or /ˈpædʒuː-/ *n* a silk fabric.

paean /ˈpiːən/ *n* a song of triumph or thanks; praise.—*also* **pean**.

paediatrics /ˌpiːdiˈætrɪks/ *n sing* the branch of medicine dealing with children and their diseases.—*also* **pediatrics**.—**paediatric** *adj*.—**paediatrician** *n*.

paedo- /ˈpiːdoː/ *prefix* child.—*also* **pedo-**.

paedology /piˈdɒlədʒi/ *n* the study of children.—*also* **pedology**.—**paedologic, paedological** *adj*.—**paedologically** *adv*.—**paedologist** *n*.

paedophilia /ˌpiːdəˈfiːliə/ or /ˌpedə-/ *n* sexual attraction towards children.—*also* **pedophilia**.—**paedophiliac, paedophilic** *adj*.—**paedophile** *n*.

paeon /ˈpiːən/ *n* a four-syllabled metrical foot, comprising, in any order, three short and one long syllable.

pagan /ˈpeɪɡən/ *n* a heathen; a person who has no religion.• *adj* irreligious; heathen, non-Christian.—**paganism** *n*.—**paganist** *adj*, *n*.

paganize /ˈpeɪɡəˌnaɪz/ *vt* to make pagan. • *vi* to become pagan.

page¹ /peɪdʒ/ *n* a boy attendant at a formal function (as a wedding); a uniformed boy employed to run errands. • *vt* to summon by messenger, loudspeaker, etc.

page² *n* a sheet of paper in a book, newspaper etc. • *vt* (*a book*) to number the pages of.—*also* **paginate**.

pageant /ˈpædʒənt/ *n* a spectacular procession or parade; representation in costume of historical events; a mere show.

pageantry /ˈpædʒəntri/ *n* (*pl* **pageantries**) grand or formal display; pomp.

pageboy /ˈpeɪdʒbɔɪ/ *n* a page; a medium-length hairstyle with the ends of the hair turned under.

pager /ˈpeɪdʒər/ *n* a device carried on a person so he or she can be summoned.—*also* **bleeper**.

paginal /ˈpædʒənəl/ *adj* consisting of pages; page for page.

paginate /ˈpædʒəˌneɪt/ *see* **page²**.

pagination /-ˈneɪʃən/ *n* the act of numbering the pages of a book; the arrangement and number of pages.

pagoda /pəˈɡoːdə/ *n* an oriental temple in the form of a tower.

Pahlavi /ˈpɒləvi/ *n* the Persian dialect in which Zoroastrian scriptures were written.

paid /peɪd/ *see* **pay**.

pail /peɪl/ *n* a bucket.

pain /peɪn/ *n* physical or mental suffering; hurting; (*pl*) trouble, exertion. • *vt* to cause distress to.

pained /peɪnd/ *adj* hurt, offended.

painful /'peɪnfʊl/ *adj* giving pain, distressing.—**painfully** *adv.*—**painfulness** *n.*

painkiller /'peɪnˌkɪlər/ *n* a drug that relieves pain.

painless /'peɪnləs/ *adj* without pain.—**painlessly** *adv.*

painstaking /'peɪnˌsteɪkɪŋ/ or /'peɪnzˌteɪkɪŋ/ *adj* very careful, laborious.—**painstakingly** *adv.*

paint /peɪnt/ *vt* (*a picture*) to make using oil pigments, etc; to depict with paints; to cover or decorate with paint; to describe. • *vi* to make a picture. • *n* a colouring pigment; a dried coat of paint.

painter[1] /'peɪntər/ *n* a person who paints, *esp* an artist.

painter[2] *n* a bow rope for tying up a boat.

painting /'peɪntɪŋ/ *n* the act or art of applying paint; a painted picture.

pair /per/ *n* a set of two things that are equal, suited, or used together; any two persons or animals regarded as a unit. • *vti* to form a pair (of); to mate.

paisley /'peɪzli/ *n* an intricate pattern of curved shapes; a soft woollen fabric with this design; a shawl made of this material. • *adj* of this pattern or material.

pajamas /pə'dʒɑːməz/ or /-'dʒæməz/ *see* **pyjamas**.

pakeha /'pækɪhə/ *n* (*New Zealand*) a non-Maori, *esp* a white person.

pal /pæl/ *n* a close friend. • *vi* (**palling, palled**) (*with* **up**) (*inf*) to make friends (with).

palace /'pælɪs/ *n* the official residence of a sovereign, president or bishop; a large stately house or public building.

paladin /'pælədɪn/ *n* a knight-errant, *esp* of the court of Charlemagne.

palatable /'pælətəbəl/ *adj* (*taste*) pleasant; (*fig*) pleasant or acceptable.—**palatability** *n.*—**palatably** *adv.*

palate /'pælət/ *n* the roof of the mouth; taste; mental relish.

palatial /pə'leɪʃəl/ *adj* of or like a palace.—**palatially** *adv.*—**palatialness** *n.*

palaver /pə'lævər/ *n* idle chatter; flattery; cajolery. • *vt* to flatter, cajole. • *vi* to talk idly.

palaeo- /'peɪliːə/ or /-ə/, *Brit.* /'pæliːə/ or /-ə/ *prefix* old; ancient; prehistoric.

palaeobotany /ˌpeɪliːə'bɒtəni/ or /ˌpæliː-/ *n* the study of fossil plants.—*also* (*US*) **paleobotany**.

palaeography /ˌpeɪli'ɒgrəfi/ *n* the study of ancient writing and manuscripts.—*also* (*US*) **paleography**.—**palaeographic, palaeographical** *adj.*—**palaeographer** *n.*

Palaeolithic /ˌpeɪliːə'lɪθɪk/ *adj* pertaining to the early Stone Age.—*also* (*US*) **Paleolithic**.

palaeontology /ˌpeɪliːən'tɒlədʒi/ or /-liən-/ *n* the study of fossils.—*also* (*US*) **paleontology**.—**palaeontological** *adj.*—**palaeontologist** *n.*

Palaeozoic /ˌpeɪliːə'zoʊɪk/ *adj* pertaining to the geological period in which fossils of the earliest forms of life appear which began 600 million years ago and ended 225 million years ago.—*also* (*US*) **Paleozoic**.

palaeozoology /ˌpeɪliːəzuː'ɒlədʒi/ *n* the study of fossil animals.—*also* (*US*) **paleozoology**.—**palaeozoological** *adj.*—**palaeozoologist** *n.*

pale[1] /peɪl/ *n* a fence stake; a boundary; (*her*) a vertical stripe in the middle of a shield.

pale[2] *adj* (*complexion*) with less colour than usual; (*colour, light*) faint, wan, dim. • *vti* to make or become pale.—**palely** *adv.*—**paleness** *n.*

paleface /'peɪlfeɪs/ *n* (*derog*) a term for a white person, supposedly used by Native Americans.

paleo- /'peɪliːə/ or /'pæliːə/ *see* **palaeo-**.

paleobotany /ˌpeɪliːə'bɒtəni/ or /ˌpæliːə-/ *see* **palaeobotany**.

paleography /ˌpeɪli'ɒgrəfi/ *see* **palaeography**.

Paleolithic /ˌpeɪliːə'lɪθɪk/ *see* **Palaeolithic**.

Paleozoic /ˌpeɪliːə'zoʊɪk/ *see* **Palaeozoic**.

paleozoology /ˌpeɪliːəzuː'ɒlədʒi/ *see* **palaeozoology**.

palette /'pælət/ *n* a small, wooden board on which coloured paints are mixed.

palette knife *n* (*pl* **palette knives**) a thin knife used for mixing colours; a round-ended, flexible knife used in cookery.

palfrey /'pɒlfri/ *n* (*arch*) a saddle horse, *esp* for a woman.

palimony /'pælɪmoʊni/ *n* (*inf*) the payment of alimony from one partner in a formal long-term sexual relationship to the other.

palimpsest /'pælɪmpˌsest/ *n* a manuscript which has been written on more than once, the former writing being still discernible in spite of erasure.

palindrome /'pælɪnˌdroʊm/ *n* a word or sentence reading the same forwards as backwards, *eg* "Able was I ere I saw Elba".—**palindromic** *adj.*

paling /'peɪlɪŋ/ *n* a row of stakes in a fence; a railing.

palingenesis /ˌpælɪn'dʒenɪsɪs/ *n* (*pl* **palingeneses**) (*theology*) spiritual rebirth through baptism.—**palingenetic** *adj.*

palinode /'pælɪˌnoʊd/ *n* a poem retracting a former poem.

palisade /ˌpælɪ'seɪd/ *n* a fence made of pointed stakes driven into the ground; a pointed stake used in a fence of this kind.

palish /'peɪlɪʃ/ *adj* somewhat pale.

pall[1] /pɔːl/ *n* a heavy cloth over a coffin; (*of smoke*) a mantle.

pall[2] *vi* to become boring; to become satiated.

Palladian /pə'leɪdiən/ *adj* (*archt*) in the pseudo-classical style of the architect Andrea Palladio (1518–80).

palladium /pə'leɪdiəm/ *n* a rare greyish-white metal found with platinum.

pallbearer /'pɔːlˌberər/ *n* someone who carries the coffin at a funeral.

pallet[1] /'pælət/ *n* a portable platform for lifting and stacking goods.

pallet[2] *n* a straw bed.

palletize, palletise /'pælətaɪz/ *vt* to stack, transport or store on pallets.—**palletization, palletisation** *n.*

palliasse /'pæliˌæs/ *n* a straw mattress.—*also* **paillasse**.

palliate /'pæliˌeɪt/ *vt* to extenuate, to excuse; to alleviate without curing.—**palliation** *n.*—**palliator** *n.*

palliative /'pæliətɪv/ *adj* alleviating without curing; excusing, extenuating. • *n* a thing that palliates.

pallid /'pælɪd/ *adj* wan, pale.—**pallidness** *n.*

pallium /'pæliəm/ *n* (*pl* **pallia, palliums**) a white woollen scarf worn by an archbishop; (*anat*) the cerebral cortex and surrounding matter; (*zool*) a mollusc's outer fold of skin.

pallor /'pælər/ *n* paleness, *esp* of the face.

pally /'pæli/ *adj* (**pallier, palliest**) friendly with; intimate.

palm[1] /pɑːm/ or /pɑːlm/ *n* the underside of the hand between fingers and wrist. • *vt* to conceal in or touch with the palm; (*with* **off**) to pass off by fraud, foist.

palm[2] *n* a tropical branchless tree with fan-shaped leaves; a symbol of victory.

palmaceous /pæl'meɪʃəs/ *adj* of the palm family.

palmar /'pælmər/ *adj* of or in the palm of the hand.

palmate /'pælmeɪt/ or **palmated** *adj* like an open hand; (*bot*) having leaves with lobes radiating from a common point; (*zool*) web-footed.—**palmation** *n.*

palmer /'pɑːmər/ *n* (*formerly*) a pilgrim returning from the Holy Land, carrying a palm branch as a token of the pilgrimage.

palmetto /pæl'metoʊ/ or /pɒl-/ *n* (*pl* **palmettos, palmettoes**) a species of small palm tree.

palmistry /'pɑːmɪstri/ or /'pɒlm-/ *n* foretelling the future from lines of the hand.—**palmist** *n.*

Palm Sunday *n* the Sunday before Easter.

palm-top /'pɑːmtɒp/ or /'pɒlm-/ *n* a portable computer small enough to fit in the palm of the hand.

palmy /'pɑːmi/ or /'pɒlmi/ *adj* (**palmier, palmiest**) abounding in palm trees; (*fig*) flourishing, prosperous.

palmyra /pæl'maɪrə/ *n* a palm found in Asia, the leaves of which are used for matting and thatching.

palomino /ˌpælə'miːnoʊ/ *n* (*pl* **palominos**) a horse with a golden or cream-coloured coat and a white mane and tail.

palp /pælp/, **palpus** /'pælpəs/ *n* (*pl* **palps, palpi**) a jointed feeler attached to the mouth parts of an insect.

palpable /'pælpəbəl/ *adj* tangible; easily perceived, obvious.—**palpability** *n.*—**palpably** *adj.*

palpate /'pælpeɪt/ *vt* to examine by touch, *esp* medically.—**palpation** *n.*

palpebral /pæl'piːbrəl/ *adj* of the eyelids.

palpitate /'pælpɪˌteɪt/ *vi* (*heart*) to beat abnormally fast; to tremble, flutter.—**palpitation** *n.*

palsy /'pɒlzi/ *n* (*pl* **palsies**) paralysis; a condition marked by an uncontrollable tremor of a part of the body. • *vt* (**palsying, palsied**) to paralyse; to make helpless.

palter /'pɒltər/ *vi* to be insincere.

paltry /'pɒltri/ *adj* (**paltrier, paltriest**) almost worthless; trifling.—**paltrily** *adv.*—**paltriness** *n.*

pampas /'pæmpəs/ *npl* the treeless, grassy plains of South America.

pampas grass *n* a tall-stemmed South American grass growing in thick tussocks.

pamper /'pæmpər/ *vt* to overindulge; to coddle, spoil.—**pamperer** *n.*

pampero /pæm'peɪrɔː/ or /-'perɔː/ n (pl **pamperos**) a cold south or south west wind which blows across the pampas.

pamphlet /'pæmflət/ n a thin, unbound booklet, esp one attacking or advocating a cause, etc; a brochure.—**pamphleteer** n.

Pan /pæn/ n (Greek myth) the god of woods and fields.—**Pandean** adj.

pan[1] /pæn/ n a wide metal container, a saucepan; (of scales) a tray; a depression in the earth filled with water; severe criticism; the bowl of a lavatory. • vb (**panning, panned**) •vi (with **out**) (inf) to turn out, esp to turn out well; to succeed. • vt to wash gold-bearing gravel in a pan; (inf) to disparage, find fault with.

pan[2] n a betel leaf; a mixture of betel nuts and lime wrapped in a betel leaf used for chewing.

pan[3] vti (**panning, panned**) (film camera) to move horizontally to follow an object or provide a panoramic view.—also n.

pan- /pæn/ prefix all; general.

panacea /ˌpænə'siːə/ n a cure-all, universal remedy.—**panacean** adj.

panache /pə'næʃ/ n flair; sense of style.

panada /pə'nndə/ or /-'neɪ-/ n (cooking) bread boiled to a pulp and flavoured, used as a sauce base or as stuffing.

panama /'pænəˌmn/ n a hat of a fine, straw-like material.

Pan-American /ˌpænə'merɪkən/ adj of or pertaining to North, South and Central America collectively; advocating unity among American countries.

panatella /ˌpænə'tɛlə/ n a long, slim cigar.

pancake /'pænkeɪk/ or /'pæŋ-/ n a round, thin cake made from batter and cooked on a griddle; a thing shaped thus. • vi (aircraft) to descend vertically in a level position.

panchromatic /ˌpænkrɔː'mætɪk/ adj (photog) sensitive to light of all colours.

pancreas /'pæŋkrɪəs/ n a large gland secreting a digestive juice into the intestine and also producing insulin.—**pancreatic** adj.

pancreatin /'pæŋkrɪətɪn/ n a clear fluid secreted by the pancreas, often extracted from animals and used in medicine.

panda /'pændə/ n a large black and white bear-like herbivore (also **giant panda**); a related reddish-brown raccoon-like animal with a ringed tail —also **lesser panda**.

Pandean /pæn'diən/ adj pertaining to the god Pan.

pandemic /pæn'demɪk/ adj epidemic over a large region, universal.

pandemonium /ˌpændə'mɔːnɪəm/ n (pl **pandemoniums**) uproar; chaos.

pander /'pændər/ n a go-between in sexual liaisons; a pimp. • vi (usu with **to**) to gratify or exploit a person's desires or weaknesses, etc.—**panderer** n.

pandit /'pʊndɪt/ see **pundit**.

P & L abbr = profit and loss.

pane /peɪn/ n a sheet of glass in a frame of a window, door, etc.—**paned** adj.

panegyric /ˌpænɪ'dʒaɪrɪk/ n an ovation or eulogy in praise of a person or event.—**panegyrical** adj.—**panegyrist** n.

panegyrize /'pænɪdʒɪˌraɪz/ vti to compose a panegyric (about); to praise highly.

panel /'pænəl/ n a usu rectangular section or division forming part of a wall, door, etc; a board for instruments or controls; a lengthwise strip in a skirt, etc; a group of selected persons for judging, discussing, etc. • vt (**panelling, panelled** or **paneling, paneled**) to decorate with panels.

panelling, paneling /'pænəlɪŋ/ n panels collectively; sheets of wood, plastic, etc used for panels.

panellist, panelist /'pænəlɪst/ n a member of a panel.

panelology /'pænəˌlɒdʒɪ/ n the collection of comic books as a hobby.

pang /pæŋ/ n a sudden sharp pain or feeling.

pangenesis /pæn'dʒenəsɪs/ n (formerly) the theory that reproductive cells contain particles from all parts of the parents.—**pangenetic** adj.

pangolin /pæŋ'gɔːlɪn/ n an insectivorous mammal, also known as the spiny anteater, found in Africa and Asia.

panhandle[1] /'pæn,hændəl/ n a narrow, projecting tongue of land.

panhandle[2] vi (inf) to beg, esp from passers-by. • vt (inf) to obtain by begging.

panic /'pænɪk/ n a sudden overpowering fright or terror.—also adj. • vti (**panicking, panicked**) to affect or be affected with panic.—**panicky** adj.

panic button n a switch for setting off an alarm; (sl) a frenzied response.

panicle /'pænɪkəl/ n (bot) an irregularly bunched flower cluster.

panic-stricken, panic-struck adj affected by panic.

paniculate /'pænɪkjulət/, **paniculated** /-əd/ adj (bot) arranged in panicles.

panjandrum /pæn'dʒændrəm/ n a pompous official.

panne /pæn/ n a soft, velvet-like fabric.

pannier /'pænjər/ n a large basket for carrying loads on the back of an animal or the shoulders of a person; a bag or case slung over the rear wheel of a bicycle or motorcycle.

pannikin /'pænɪkɪn/ n a small metal drinking-cup.

panoply /'pænəplɪ/ n (pl **panoplies**) a complete array; a full suit of armour.—**panoplied** adj.

panorama /ˌpænə'ræmə/ n a complete view in all directions; a comprehensive presentation of a subject; a constantly changing scene.—**panoramic** adj.—**panoramically** adv.

panpipes /'pæn,paɪp/ npl a wind instrument consisting of short hollow tubes of different lengths, originally of reed, bound together.

pansy /'pænzɪ/ n (pl **pansies**) a garden flower of the violet family, with velvety petals; (sl) an effeminate boy or man.

pant /pænt/ vi to breathe noisily, gasp; to yearn (for or after something). • vt to speak while gasping.

pantalets, pantalettes /ˌpæntə'lets/ npl a woman's long ruffled drawers.

pantaloon /pæntə'luːn/ n (pantomine) a foolish old man on whom the clown plays tricks.

pantaloons /pæntə'luːn/ npl (hist) a man's tight breeches fastened at the calf or the foot; (inf) baggy trousers.

pantheism /'pænθɪ,zəm/ n the doctrine that the universe in its totality is God; willingness to worship all, or several gods.—**pantheist** n.—**pantheistic, pantheistical** adj.

pantheon /'pænθɪɒn/ n a temple to all the gods; a building in which the famous dead of a nation are buried or remembered; a group of famous persons.

panther /'pænθər/ n (pl **panther, panthers**) a leopard, esp one with a black unspotted coat; a puma.

pantihose /'pæntɪ,hoːz/ n women's tights.—also **panty hose**.

panties /'pæntɪz/ npl (inf) short underpants.

pantile /'pæntaɪl/ n a roof tile with an S-shaped cross-section.

panto /'pæntɔː/ n (pl **pantos**) (Brit inf) a pantomime.

pantograph /'pæntə,græf/ n an instrument for copying drawings, maps, etc, to scale.

pantomime /'pæntə,maɪm/ n (Brit) a Christmas theatrical entertainment with music and jokes; a drama without words, using only actions and gestures; mime. • vti to mime.—**pantomimic** adj.

pantomimist /'pæntə,maɪmɪst/ n a person who performs in a pantomime; one who composes a pantomime.

pantoum /pæntaʊm/ n a verse form of four-lined rhyming stanzas.

pantry /'pæntrɪ/ n (pl **pantries**) a small room or cupboard for storing cooking ingredients and utensils, etc.

pants /pænts/ npl trousers; underpants.

panty hose /'pæntɪhoːz/ see **pantihose**.

panzer /'pænzər/ adj (division) armoured. • n a tank, or other armoured vehicle, from a panzer division; (pl) armoured troops.

panzerotto /pænzə'rɒtɔː/ n ✲ (Cdn) a large baked turnover with a pizza-like filling of tomato sauce, cheese, and other ingredients.

pap /pæp/ n soft, bland food for infants, invalids, etc; any oversimplified or insipid writing, ideas, etc.

papa /'pʊpə/ or /pə'pɒ/ n (inf) father.

papacy /'peɪpəsɪ/ n (pl **papacies**) the office or authority of the pope; papal system of government.

papal /'peɪpəl/ adj of the pope or the papacy.—**papally** adv.

paparazzo /ˌpæpə'rætsɔː/ n (pl **paparazzi** /-tsiː/) a freelance photographer who pursues celebrities for sensational or candid shots for publication in newspapers and magazines.

papaveraceous /ˌpæpəvə'reɪʃəs/ adj (bot) pertaining or belonging to the poppy family.

papaw /pə'pɔː/ or /'pɔ,pɔː/ n (the small edible fruit of) a North American tree of the custard-apple family.—also **pawpaw**.

papaya /pə'paɪjə/ n (a West Indian tree bearing) an elongated melon-like fruit with edible yellow flesh and small black seeds.

paper /'peɪpər/ n the thin, flexible material made from pulped rags, wood, etc which is used to write on, wrap in, or cover walls; a single sheet of this; an official document; a newspaper; an essay or lecture; a set of examination questions; (pl) personal documents. • adj like or made of paper. • vt to cover with wallpaper.

paperback /ˈpeɪpərˌbæk/ n a book bound in a flexible paper cover. • adj pertaining to such a book or the publication of such books.

papering /ˈpeɪpərɪŋ/ n the process of covering with paper; paper so used.

paperknife n (pl **paperknives**) a blunt knife for opening letters or cutting folded paper.

paper money n banknotes; paper currency authorized by a government as representing value.

paperweight /ˈpeɪpərˌweɪt/ n a small heavy object for keeping papers in place.

paperwork /ˈpeɪpərˌwɜrk/ n clerical work of any kind.

papery /ˈpeɪpərɪ/ adj like paper in appearance or consistency.— **paperiness** n.

papeterie /ˈpæpətrɪ/ n a case containing paper and writing materials.

papier-mâché /ˈpeɪpər məˈʃeɪ/ n a substance made of paper pulp mixed with size, glue, etc and moulded into various objects when moist.

papilla /pəˈpɪlə/ n (pl **papillae**) a small, nipple-like protuberance.— **papillary, papillate, papillose** adj.

papoose /pəˈpuːs/ n an American Indian young child.

pappus /ˈpæpəs/ n (pl **pappi**) (bot) the feathery substance on the seeds of some plants, eg dandelion, thistle.

pappy /ˈpæpɪ/ adj (**pappier, pappiest**) semi-liquid, like pap.

paprika /ˈpæprɪkə/ or /pəˈpriːkə/ n a mild red condiment ground from the fruit of certain peppers.

Pap test, Pap smear /pæp-/ n a technique for the early detection of cancer by examining specially stained cells from the cervix, etc.

papule /ˈpæpjuːl/, **papula** /-juːlə/ n (pl **papules, papulae** /-juːliː/) a small, solid elevation of the skin.— **papular** adj.

papyrology /ˌpæpɪˈrɒlədʒɪ/ n the study of papyri.— **papyrologist** n.

papyrus /pəˈpaɪrəs/ n (pl **papyri, papyruses**) an aquatic plant; paper made from this plant, as used in ancient times.

par /pɑr/ n the standard or normal level; the established value of a currency in foreign-exchange rates; the face value of stocks, shares, etc; (golf) the score for a hole required by an expert player; equality.

par- /pɑr/ or /pər/, **para-** prefix beside; against; irregular; abnormal; associated in a subsidiary or accessory capacity.

para /ˈpærə/ n (pl **paras**) (inf) a paragraph; a paratrooper.

parabasis /ˈpærəbəsɪs/ n (pl **parabases**) (classical Greek comedy) an address to the audience by the chorus.

parable /ˈpærəbəl/ or /ˈpæ-/ n a short story used to illustrate a religious or moral point.— **parabolist** n.

parabola /pəˈræbələ/ n (pl **parabolas**) (maths) the curve formed by the cutting of a cone by a plane parallel to its side.

parabolic[1] /ˌpærəˈbɒlɪk/ or /ˌpæ-/ adj of or like a parabola; parabolical.

parabolic[2], **parabolical** adj of or expressed in a parable.— **parabolically** adv.

paraboloid /pəˈræbəˌlɔɪd/ n (geom) a solid formed by the revolution of a parabola on its axis.

parachronism /pəræˈkrɒnɪzəm/ n an error in chronology, esp in postdating an event.

parachute /ˈpærəˌʃuːt/ or /ˈpæ-/ n a fabric umbrella-like canopy used to retard speed of fall from an aircraft. • vti to drop, descend by parachute.— **parachutist** n.

paraclete /ˈpærəˌkliːt/ or /ˈpæ-/ n a mediator.

parade /pəˈreɪd/ n a ceremonial procession; an assembly of troops for review; ostentatious display; public walk, promenade. • vti to march or walk through, as for display; to show off; to assemble in military order.

paradigm /ˈpærəˌdaɪm/ n a pattern or model; a list of grammatical inflexions of a word.— **paradigmatic** adj.— **paradigmatically** adv.

paradise /ˈpærəˌdaɪs/ n heaven; (Bible) the Garden of Eden; any place of perfection.

paradisiacal /-ˈdɪsɪəl/, **paradisiac** adj like, or pertaining to, paradise.

paradox /ˈpærəˌdɒks/ n a self-contradictory statement that may be true; an opinion that conflicts with common beliefs; something with seemingly contradictory qualities or phases.— **paradoxical** adj.— **paradoxically** adv.

paraesthesia /pɛˌrəsˈθɪsɪə/ n (med) an abnormal tickling sensation on the skin.— also **paresthesia.**— **paraesthetic** adj.

paraffin /ˈpærəfɪn/ n a white waxy tasteless substance obtained from shale, wood, etc; a distilled oil used as fuel, kerosene.— **paraffinic** adj.

paragenesis /ˌpærəˈdʒɛnəsɪs/, **paragenesia** n (geol) the sequence of formation of the various minerals in a mass of rock— **paragenetic** adj.

paragoge /ˌpærəˈɡoʊdʒɪ/, **paragogue** n (linguistics) the addition of a letter or a syllable to a word.

paragon /ˈpærəɡɒn/ n a model of excellence or perfection.

paragraph /ˈpærəˌɡræf/ n a subdivision in a piece of writing used to separate ideas, marked by the beginning of a new line; a brief ment on in a newspaper. • vt to divide into paragraphs.— **paragraphic** adj.— **paragraphically** adv.

Paraguay tea /ˈpærəˌɡweɪ/ or /-waɪ/ n an infusion of the dried leaves of maté, which makes a mildly stimulating tea.— also **yerba maté**.

parakeet /ˈpærəˌkiːt/ n a small parrot.

paraldehyde /pəˈrældəˌhaɪd/ n a colourless liquid used as a sedative.

paraleipsis /ˌpærəˈlaɪpsɪs/, **paralipsis** /ˌpærəˈlɪpsɪs/ n (pl **paraleipses, paralipses**) (rhetoric) drawing attention to something by deliberately understating it.

parallax /ˈpærəˌlæks/ n the apparent angular shifting of an object caused by a change in position of the observer; (astron) the difference in the apparent position of a heavenly body and its true place.

parallel /ˈpærəˌlɛl/ adj equidistant at every point and extended in the same direction; side by side; never intersecting; similar, corresponding. • n a parallel line, surface, etc; a likeness, counterpart; comparison; a line of latitude. • vt (**paralleling, paralleled**) to make or be parallel; to compare.

parallelepiped /ˌpærəlɛlˈɛpɪˌpɛd/ or /-ləˈpaɪpɪd/ n a regular solid figure bounded by six parallelograms, of which the opposite pairs are equal and parallel.

parallelism /ˈpærəlɛlˌɪzəm/ n the state or quality of being parallel.

parallelogram /ˌpærəˈlɛləˌɡræm/ n a four-sided plane figure whose opposite sides are parallel.

paralogism /pəˈræləˌdʒɪzəm/ n (logic) a fallacy in reasoning made unconsciously by the reasoner.

paralyse, paralyze /ˈpærəˌlaɪz/ vt to affect with paralysis; to bring to a stop.— **paralysation** n.

paralysis /pəˈrælɪsɪs/ n (pl **paralyses** /-ˌsiːz/) a partial or complete loss of voluntary muscle function or sensation in any part of the body; a condition of helpless inactivity.— **paralytic** adj, n.

paramatta /ˌpærəˈmætə/ n a light fabric of cotton and wool.— also **parramatta**.

paramedic /ˌpærəˈmedɪk/ n a person trained to provide emergency medical treatment and to support professional medical staff.

paramedical /ˌpærəˈmedɪkəl/ adj (services) supplementing and assisting the work of professional medical staff.

parameter /pəˈræmətər/ n (math) an arbitrary constant, the value of which influences the content but not the structure of an expression; (inf) a limit or condition affecting action, decision, etc.— **parametric** adj.— **parametrically** adv.

paramilitary /ˌpærəˈmɪlɪtərɪ/ or /-trɪ/ adj (forces) organized on a military pattern and ancillary to military forces.

paramo /ˈpærəˌmoʊ/ n (pl **paramos**) a high bleak plateau in the Andes.

paramount /ˈpærəˌmaunt/ adj of great importance.

paramour /ˈpærəˌmʊr/ n an illicit lover.

parang /ˈpæræŋ/ n a heavy Malay sheath knife.

paranoia /ˌpærəˈnɔɪə/ n a mental illness characterized by delusions of grandeur and persecution; (inf) unfounded fear, suspicion.— **paranoiac** adj, n.

paranoic /ˈpærəˌnɔɪk/ adj of or like paranoia; (inf) highly suspicious or fearful.— also n.

paranormal /ˌpærəˈnɔrməl/ adj beyond the scope of normal experience or scientific explanation.— **paranormally** adv.

parapet /ˈpærəpət/ n a low, protective wall along the edge of a roof, balcony, or bridge, etc.— **parapeted** adj.

paraph /ˈpærəf/ n a mark or flourish after a signature.

paraphernalia /ˌpærəfəˈneɪljə/ npl personal belongings; accessories; (law) what a wife possesses in her own right.

paraphrase /ˈpærəˌfreɪz/ n expression of a passage in other words in order to clarify meaning. • vt to restate.— **paraphrastic** adj.

paraplegia /ˌpærəˈpliːdʒə/ n paralysis of the lower half of the body.— **paraplegic** adj.

parasailing /'pærəseɪlɪŋ/ *n* the sport of gliding through the air attached to an open parachute and towed by a speedboat.—**parasailer, parasailor** *n*.

parascending /ˌpærə'sɛndɪŋ/ *n* a form of parachuting in which participants wearing open parachutes are towed into the air by a vehicle or speedboat and then released to glide to the ground.—**parascender** *n*.

paraselene /ˌpærəsɪ'liːni/ *n* (*pl* **paraselenae** /-niː/) (*astron*) a bright spot on a lunar halo.

parasite /'pærəˌsəɪt/ *n* an organism that lives on and feeds off another without rendering any service in return; a person who sponges off another.—**parasitic** *adj*.—**parasitically** *adv*.

parasiticide /-'sɪtɪˌsəɪd/ *n* a substance which kills parasites.

parasitism /'pærəsɪtˌɪzəm/ *n* the parasite-host relationship; the state or behaviour of a parasite.

parasitize /'pærəsɪˌtəɪz/ *n* to infest with parasites.

parasitology /-'tɒlədʒɪ/ *n* the study of parasites.—**parasitologist** *n*.

parasol /'pærəˌsɒl/ *n* a lightweight umbrella used as a sunshade.

parasynthesis /ˌpærə'sɪnθəsɪs/ *n* (*gram*) derivation from a compound plus affix, *eg* faint-hearted, which is made up from faint + heart + -ed.

parataxis /ˌpærə'tæksɪs/ *n* (*gram*) use of successive clauses without connecting words.

parathyroid /ˌpærə'θaɪrɔɪd/ *adj* (*anat*) lying near the thyroid gland. • *n* a gland near the thyroid that secretes a hormone that regulates the body's calcium levels.

paratroops /'pærətruːps/ *npl* troops dropped by parachute into the enemy area.—**paratrooper** *n*.

paravane /'pærəˌveɪn/ *n* a device shaped like a torpedo, with serrated teeth for destroying the moorings of sea mines.

parboil /'parˌbɔɪl/ *vt* to boil briefly as a preliminary cooking procedure.

parbuckle /'parˌbʌkəl/ *n* a rope sling for raising or lowering casks.

parcel /'parsəl/ *n* a tract or plot of land; a wrapped bundle; a package; a collection or group of persons, animals, or things. • *vt* (**parcelling, parcelled** *or* **parceling, parceled**) to wrap up into a parcel; (*with* **out**) to apportion.

parcenary /'parsəˌnɛri/ *n* joint heirship.

parcener /'parsənər/ *n* a coheir.

parch /partʃ/ *vti* to make or become hot and dry, thirsty; to scorch, roast.—**parched** *adj*.

parchment /'partʃmənt/ *n* the skin of a sheep, etc prepared as a writing material; paper like parchment.

pard /pard/ *n* (*arch*) a leopard.

pardon /'pardən/ *vt* to forgive; to excuse; to release from penalty. • *n* forgiveness; remission of penalty.—**pardonable** *adj*.—**pardonably** *adv*.

pardoner /'pardənər/ *n* one who pardons; (*hist*) a person licensed to sell papal indulgences.

pare /pɛr/ *vt* to cut or shave; to peel; to diminish.

paregoric /ˌpɛrɪ'gɒrɪk/ *n* (*formerly*) an opium-based drug used to treat diarrhoea and coughs.

parenchyma /pə'rɛŋkɪmə/ *n* (*bot*) the soft cellular tissue or pith of plants; (*anat*) the soft tissue of the glandular organs of the body.—**parenchymatous, parenchymal** *adj*.

parent /'pɛrənt/ *n* a father or a mother; an organism producing another; a source.—**parental** *adj*.—**parentally** *adv*.—**parenthood** *n*.

parentage /'pɛrəntɪdʒ/ *n* descent, extraction from parents.

parenthesis /pə'rɛnθəsɪs/ *n* (*pl* **parentheses**) an explanatory comment in a sentence contained within brackets and set in a sentence, independently of grammatical sequence; the brackets themselves ().—**parenthetic, parenthetical** *adj*.—**parenthetically** *adv*.

parenthesize, parenthesise /pə'rɛnθəˌsəɪz/ *vt* to insert as a parenthesis; to enclose in parentheses.

parenting /'pɛrəntɪŋ/ *n* the act of being a parent; the role of a parent in relation to a child; that role in relation to someone who is not the child of a parent.

paresis /pə'riːsɪs/ *or* /'pɛrɪsɪs/ *n* partial or slight paralysis.—**paretic** *adj*.

par excellence /ˌpar ɛksə'lãs/ *or* /par 'ɛksəˌlãs/ *adv* pre-eminently; to the highest degree.

parfait /par'feɪ/ *n* a rich iced dessert of whipped cream, eggs, etc served in a tall glass; layers of ice cream served in a tall glass.

parget /'pardʒət/ *n* a type of plaster. • *vt* to cover with parget.

parhelion /par'hiːliən/ *n* (*pl* **parhelia**) a bright spot on a solar halo.

pariah /pə'raɪə/ *n* a social outcast; a member of a low caste in southern India and Burma.

parietal /pə'raɪətəl/ *adj* (*anat*) pertaining to the wall of a cavity of the body; pertaining to the large lateral bones of the skull.

paring /'pɛrɪŋ/ *n* the act of paring; what is pared off, rind.

pari-mutuel /ˌpariː'mjuːtʃuːˌɛl/ *n* (*pl* **pari-mutuels, parismutuels**) a mechanical betting system in which the losers' stakes, less a deduction for the management, are divided among the winners.

pari passu /ˌparɪ 'pæsuː/ *or* /ˌpɛri/ *adv* (*law*) with equal pace, together; in equal degree.

parish /'pɛrɪʃ/ *n* an ecclesiastical area with its own church and clergy; the inhabitants of a parish; ✽ (*Cdn*) in Quebec and New Brunswick, a subdivision of a county functioning as a political unit.

parishioner /pə'rɪʃənər/ *n* an inhabitant of a parish.

parisyllabic /ˌpærɪsɪ'læbɪk/ *adj* (*inflected noun or verb*) having an equal number of syllables in all or most inflected forms.

parity /'pɛrɪti/ *n* (*pl* **parities**) equality; equality of value at a given ratio between different kinds of money, etc; being at par.

park /park/ *n* land kept as a game preserve or recreation area; a piece of ground in an urban area kept for ornament or recreation; an enclosed stadium, *esp* for ball games; a large enclosed piece of ground attached to a country house. • *vti* (*vehicle*) to leave in a certain place temporarily; to manoeuvre into a parking space.

parka /'parkə/ *n* a warm hooded garment, often of fur, for wear in arctic conditions.

parkade /par'keɪd/ *n* ✽ (*Cdn*) a multilevel structure for parking motor vehicles.

park belt *n* ✽ parkland.

parkette /par'kɛt/ *n* ✽ (*Cdn*) a small urban park.

parking lot /'parkɪŋ/ *n* a car park.

parking meter *n* a coin-operated machine that registers the purchase of parking time for a motor vehicle.

Parkinsonism /'parkɪnsəˌnɪzəm/ *n* Parkinson's disease.

Parkinson's disease *n* a progressive nervous disease resulting in tremor, muscular rigidity, partial paralysis and weakness.

Parkinson's Law *n* any of various humorous observations on human behaviour framed as economic laws, *esp* the notion that work expands to fill the time available for its completion (named after the English writer C N Parkinson b.1909).

parlance /'parləns/ *n* a manner of speech, idiom.

parkland /'parklənd/ *n* ✽ *esp* in Canada, open grassland with widely scattered groves of trees.—*also* **park belt**.

parley /par'leɪ/ *or* /'parleɪ/, /'parli/ *n* a conference, *esp* with an enemy. • *vi* to discuss, *esp* with an enemy with a view to bringing about a peace.

parliament /'parləmənt/ *n* a legislative assembly made up of representatives of a nation or part of a nation; (*with cap*) the supreme governing and legislative body of various countries, *esp* the UK.

parliamentarian /ˌparləmən'tɛriən/ *n* a skilled parliamentary debater; an expert on parliamentary rules; (*with cap*) (*hist*) a supporter of the English Parliament against Charles I.

parliamentary /ˌparlə'mɛntri/ *or* /-'mɛntəri/ *adj* of, used in, or enacted by a parliament; conforming to the rules of a parliament; having a parliament.

Parliament Hill *n* ✽ (*Cdn*) the low hill in Ottawa, Ontario where the parliament of Canada is located; the Canadian federal government.

parlour /'parlər/ *n* a room in a house used primarily for conversation or receiving guests; a room or a shop used for business.

parlour game *n* a game usually played indoors.

parlous /'parləs/ *adj* (*arch*) dangerous; shrewd.—**parlously** *adv*.—**parlousness** *n*.

parmales /par'mæləs/ *n* any of the order Parmales of single-celled algae found in the polar regions.

Parmesan /'parmɪˌzɒn/ *or* /-zən/, /-zæn/, /-ʒɒn/, /-ʒæn/, /-'zɒn/, /-'ʒɒn/ *n* a hard cheese with a sharp flavour used, *esp* grated, as a garnish.

parochial /pə'roːkiəl/ *adj* of or relating to a parish; narrow; provincial in outlook.—**parochially** *adv*.

parochialism /pə'roːkiəlɪzəm/ *n* narrow-mindedness.

parody /'pɛrədi/ *or* /'pæ-/ *n* (*pl* **parodies**) a satirical or humorous imitation of a literary or musical work or style. • *vt* (**parodying, parodied**) to make a parody of.—**parodic** *adj*.—**parodist** *n*.

paroicous /pə'rɔɪʃəs/, **paroecious** /ˌpɛrə'iːʃəs/ *adj* (*bot*) with the two sexes developing in close proximity.

parole /pə'roːl/ n word of honour; the release of a prisoner before his sentence has expired, on condition of future good behaviour. • vt to release on parole.

parolee /-'liː/ n a person on parole.

paronomasia /ˌpɛrənə'meɪzɪə/ n a pun or play on words.

paronym /'pɛrənɪm/ n (gram) a paronymic word.

paronymic, paronymous /pə'rɒnɪməs/ adj (gram) with the same derivation; with the same sound but different spelling and meaning.

parotid /pə'rɒtɪd/ adj (anat) situated near the ear. • n a parotid gland.

parotitis /ˌpɛrə'taɪtɪs/, **parotiditis** n mumps.

paroxysm /'pɛrəkˌsɪzəm/ n a sudden attack of a disease; a violent convulsion of pain or emotion; an outburst of laughter.—**paroxysmal** adj.

parquet /par'keɪ/ or /'par-/ n an inlaid hard wood flooring; the stalls of a theatre below the balcony. • vt to furnish (a room) with a parquet floor.

parquetry /'parkɪtrɪ/ n mosaic woodwork used to cover floors.

parr /par/ n (pl **parrs, parr**) a young salmon.

parramatta /ˌpɛrə'mætə/ see **paramatta**.

parrot /'pɛrət/ n a tropical or subtropical bird with brilliant plumage and the ability to mimic human speech; one who repeats another's words without understanding. • vt to repeat mechanically.

parrotfish /'pɛrətˌfɪʃ/ n (pl **parrotfish, parrotfishes**) a brightly coloured tropical fish, with mouth parts resembling a parrot's beak.

parry /'pɛrɪ/ vt (**parrying, parried**) to ward off, turn aside. • n (pl **parries**) a defensive movement in fencing.

parse /pars/ or /parz/ vti (words) to classify; (sentences) to analyse in terms of grammar; to give a grammatical description of a word or group of words.

parsec /'parsek/ n (astron) a unit of measure for stellar distances equal to 3.26 light years, approx 19 million miles

Parsee /par'siː/ n an Indian adherent of the Zoroastrian religion.—**Parseeism** n.

parsimony /'parsɪˌmoːnɪ/ n extreme frugality; meanness, stinginess.—**parsimonious** adj.

parsley /'parslɪ/ n a bright green herb used to flavour or garnish some foods.

parsnip /'parsnɪp/ n a biennial plant cultivated for its long tapered root used as a vegetable.

parson /'parsən/ n an Anglican clergyman in charge of a parish; (inf) any, esp Protestant, clergyman.

parsonage /'parsənɪdʒ/ n the house provided for a parson by his church.

part /part/ n a section; a portion (of a whole); an essential, separable component of a piece of equipment or a machine; the role of an actor in a play; a written copy of his/her words; (mus) one of the melodies of a harmony; the music for it; duty, share; one of the sides in a conflict; a parting of the hair; (pl) qualities, talent; the genitals; a region, land or territory. • vt to separate; to comb the hair so as to leave a parting. • vi to become separated; to go different ways.

partake /par'teɪk/ vi (**partaking, partook**; pp **partaken**) to participate (in); (food or drink) to have a portion of.

partan /'partən/ n (Scot) a crab.

parterre /par'tɛr/ n an ornamental flower garden; the area of a ground floor of a theatre that lies underneath the balconies.

parthenocarpy /'parθənoːˌkarpɪ/ n (bot) the formation of fruit without seeds having been formed or fertilized.

parthenogenesis /ˌparθənoː'dʒɛnəsɪs/ n reproduction without sexual union; virgin birth.—**parthenogenetic** adj.

partial /'parʃəl/ adj incomplete; biased, prejudiced; (with **to**) having a liking or preference for.—**partially** adv.

partiality /ˌparʃɪ'ælɪtɪ/ n (pl **partialities**) biased judgment; (with **for**) liking, fondness.

partible /'partəbəl/ adj able to be divided or separated.

participant /par'tɪsəpənt/ n one who participates; a sharer.

participate /par'tɪsəpeɪt/ vi to join in or take part with others (in some activity).—**participator** n.—**participatory** adj.

participation /-'peɪʃən/ n the act of participating; the state of being related to a larger whole.

participle /'partɪˌsɪpəl/ or /par'tɪsəpəl/ n (gram) a verb form used in compound forms or as an adjective.—**participial** adj.—**participially** adv.

particle /'partɪkəl/ n a tiny portion of matter; a speck; a very small part; (gram) a word that cannot be used alone, a prefix, a suffix.

parti-coloured adj differently coloured in different parts, variegated.

particular /par'tɪkjulər/ or /pər-/ adj referring or belonging to a specific person or thing; distinct; exceptional; careful; fastidious. • n a detail, single item; (pl) detailed information.

particularism /par'tɪkjuləˌrɪzəm/ or /pər-/, /pə-/ n exclusive devotion to one party or sect; the principle of political freedom for each state in a federation; the theological doctrine that salvation is only for the elect.—**particularist** n.

particularity /parˌtɪkju'lɛrɪtɪ/ or /pər-/, /pə-/ n (pl **particularities**) the quality of being particular, as distinguished from universal; exactness; fastidiousness.

particularize /par'tɪkjuləˌraɪz/ or /pər-/, /pə-/ vt to describe in detail; to mention one by one.—**particularization** n.

particularly /par'tɪkjulərlɪ/ or /pər-/, /pə-/ adv very; especially; in detail.

parting /'partɪŋ/ n a departure; a breaking or separating; a dividing line in combing hair. • adj departing, esp dying; separating; dividing.

partisan, partizan /'partɪˌzæn/ or /-təz-/, /-ən/, /-'zæn/ n a strong supporter of a person, party, or cause.—also adj.—**partisanship, partizanship** n.

partite /'partaɪt/ adj (bot) divided almost to the base.

partition /par'tɪʃən/ n division into parts; that which divides into separate parts; a dividing wall between rooms. • vt to divide.

partitive /'partɪtɪv/ adj (gram) denoting a part or partition. • n a partitive word.

partizan /'partɪˌzæn/ see **partisan**.

partly /'partlɪ/ adv in part; to some extent.

partner /'partnər/ n one of two or more persons jointly owning a business who share the risks and profits; one of a pair who dance or play a game together; either member of a married or non-married couple. • vt to be a partner (in or of); to associate as partners.

partnership /'partnərʃɪp/ n a contract between two or more people involved in a joint business venture; the state of being a partner.

part of speech n each of the categories (eg verb, noun, adjective) into which words are divided according to their grammatical and semantic functions.

partook /par'tuk/ see **partake**.

partridge /'partrɪdʒ/ n (pl **partridge, partridges**) a stout-bodied game bird of the grouse family.

part song n a song with two or more voice parts.

part-time adj working fewer than the full number of hours.—**part-timer** n.—**part time** adv.

parturient /par'turɪənt/ or /-'tjur-/ adj pertaining to childbirth; about to give birth, in labour.

parturition /ˌpartu'rɪʃən/ or /-tjur-/, /-tʃur/ n the act of childbirth.

party /'partɪ/ n (pl **parties**) a group of people united for political or other purpose; a social gathering; a person involved in a contract or lawsuit; a small company, detachment; a person consenting, accessory; (inf) an individual. • vb (**partying, partied**) vi to attend social parties. • vt to give a party for. • adj of or for a party.

party line n a telephone line shared by two or more subscribers; the policies of a political body.

parvenu /'parvənˌuː/ n someone regarded as vulgar or an upstart, following a rise in his social or economic status.—**parvenue** nf.

pas /pɒ/ n (pl **pas**) (ballet) a step or series of steps; a dance sequence.

PASCAL /'pæskəl/ n a high-level computer programming language used esp for teaching.

pascal /'pæskəl/ n the SI unit of pressure.

pas de deux /pa də 'dœ/ n (pl **pas de deux**) a ballet sequence for two dancers.

pasha /'pæʃə/ n a Turkish title given to a high official; (formerly) a provincial governor in the Ottoman Empire.—also **pacha**.

pasque-flower /'pæsk ˌflauər/ n a type of anemone which flowers around Easter.

pasquinade /ˌpæskwɪ'neɪd/ n a lampoon or rude satire.

pass /pæs/ vb (**passing, passed**) vi to go past; to go beyond or exceed; to move from one place or state to another; (time) to elapse; to go; to die; to happen; (with **for**) to be considered as; (in exam) to be successful; (cards) to decline to make a bid; (law) to be approved by a legislative assembly. • vt to go past, through, over, etc; (*time*) to spend; to omit; (*law*) to enact; (*judgment*) to pronounce; to excrete; (*in test, etc*) to gain the required marks; to approve. • *n* a narrow passage or road; a permit; (*in a test, etc*) success; transfer of (a ball) to another player; a gesture of the hand; (*inf*) an uninvited sexual approach.

passable /ˈpæsəbəl/ *adj* fairly good, tolerable; (*a river, etc*) that can be crossed.—**passably** *adv*.

passage /ˈpæsɪdʒ/ *n* act or right of passing; transit; transition; a corridor; a channel; a route or crossing; a lapse of time; a piece of text or music.

passageway /-ˌweɪ/ *n* a narrow way, *esp* flanked by walls, that allows passage; a corridor.

passbook /ˈpæsbʊk/ *n* a bankbook.

passé /pæˈseɪ/ *adj* past its best; outdated.

passementerie /pæsˈmentri/ *n* a decorative trimming of gold or silver lace, braid, beads, etc.

passenger /ˈpæsəndʒər/ *n* a traveller in a public or private conveyance; one who does not pull his/her weight.

passe-partout /ˌpæspɑrˈtuː/ *n* a frame for a picture in which the picture, glass and backing are held together by gummed paper; a master key.

passer-by /ˌpæsərˈbaɪ/ *n* (*pl* **passers-by**) one who happens to pass or go by.

passerine /ˈpæsəˌriːn/ *adj* pertaining to the order of birds which perch.—*also n*.

passim /ˈpæsɪm/ *adv* here and there; throughout.

passing /ˈpæsɪŋ/ *adj* transient; casual. • *n* departure, death.

passion /ˈpæʃən/ *n* compelling emotion, such as love, hate, envy; ardent love, *esp* sexual desire; (*with cap*) the suffering of Christ on the cross; the object of any strong desire.—**passionless** *adj*.

passional /-əl/ *adj* pertaining to passion; due to passion.

passionate /-ət/ *adj* moved by, showing, strong emotion or desire; intense; sensual.—**passionately** *adv*.

passion flower *n* a chiefly tropical climbing vine.

passion fruit *n* the edible fruit of a passion flower.

Passion play *n* a play representing Christ's Passion.

Passion Sunday *n* the second Sunday before Easter.

passive /ˈpæsɪv/ *adj* acted upon, not acting; submissive; (*gram*) denoting the voice of a verb whose subject receives the action.—**passively** *adv*.—**passivity** *n*.

passive resistance *n* nonviolent noncooperation with the authorities.

passive smoking *n* the involuntary inhalation of smoke from others' cigarettes.

Passover /ˈpæsˌoʊvər/ *n* (*Judaism*) a spring holiday, celebrating the liberation of the Israelites from slavery in Egypt.

passport /ˈpæspɔrt/ *n* an official document giving the owner the right to travel abroad; something that secures admission or acceptance.

password /ˈpæswɔrd/ *n* a secret term by which a person is recognized and allowed to pass; any means of admission; a sequence of characters required to access a computer system.

past /pæst/ *adj* completed; ended; in time already elapsed. • *adv* by. • *prep* beyond (in time, place, or amount). • *n* time that has gone by; the history of a person, group, etc; a personal background that is hidden or questionable.

pasta /ˈpæstə/ or /ˈpɒstə/ *n* the flour paste from which spaghetti, noodles, etc is made; any dish of cooked pasta.

paste /peɪst/ *n* a soft plastic mixture; flour and water forming dough or adhesive; a fine glass used for artificial gems. • *vt* to attach with paste; (*sl*) to beat, thrash.

pasteboard /ˈpeɪstbɔrd/ *n* a stiff board made from sheets of paper pasted together. • *adj* flimsy.

pastel /pæˈstɛl/ *n* a dried mixture of chalk, pigments and gum used for drawing; a drawing made with such; a soft, pale colour. • *adj* delicately coloured.

pastelist /-ɪst/ *n* an artist who uses pastels.

pastern /ˈpæstərn/ *n* the part of a horse's foot between the fetlock and the hoof.

Pasteur treatment *n* (*med*) a method of inoculation against rabies by successive injections of vaccine.

pasteurize /ˈpæstʃəˌraɪz/ or /-təˌraɪz/ *vt* (*milk, etc*) to sterilize by heat or radiation to destroy harmful organisms.—**pasteurization** *n*.

pastiche /pæˈstiːʃ/ *n* (*pl* **pastiches**) a literary, musical, or artistic work in imitation of another's style, or consisting of pieces from other sources.—*also* **pasticcio** (*pl* **pasticci**).

pastille /pæˈstiːl/, **pastil** /pæˈstɪl/ *n* an aromatic or medicated lozenge.

pastime /ˈpæstaɪm/ *n* a hobby; recreation, diversion.

pastor /ˈpæstər/ *n* a clergyman in charge of a congregation.

pastoral /ˈpæstərəl/ *adj* of shepherds or rural life; pertaining to spiritual care, *esp* of a congregation.—**pastorally** *adv*.

pastorale /ˌpæstəˈræl/ or /ˈpæstəˌræli/ *n* a musical composition with a pastoral subject.

pastorate /ˈpæstərət/ *n* the office or jurisdiction of a pastor; a collective term for pastors.

pastrami /pəˈstɒmi/ *n* highly seasoned smoked beef.

pastry /ˈpeɪstri/ *n* (*pl* **pastries**) dough made of flour, water, and fat used for making pies, tarts, etc; (*pl*) baked foods made with pastry.

pasturage /ˈpæstərɪdʒ/ *n* the right to graze animals; pasture.

pasture /ˈpæstʃər/ *n* land covered with grass for grazing livestock; the grass growing on it. • *vt* (*cattle, etc*) to put out to graze in a pasture.

pasty[1] /ˈpeɪsti/ *n* (*pl* **pasties**) meat, etc enclosed in pastry and baked.

pasty[2] *adj* (**pastier, pastiest**) like paste; pallid and unhealthy in appearance.—**pastily** *adv*.—**pastiness** *n*.

pat[1] /pæt/ *vti* (**patting, patted**) to strike gently with the palm of the hand or a flat object; to shape or apply by patting. • *n* a light tap, *usu* with the palm of the hand; a light sound; a small lump of shaped butter.

pat[2] *adj* apt; exact; glib.—*also adv*.

patagium /pəˈteɪdʒiəm/ *n* (*pl* **patagia**) (*zool*) the wing membrane of a bat.

patch /pætʃ/ *n* a piece of cloth used for mending; a scrap of material; a shield for an injured eye; a black spot of silk, etc worn on the face; an irregular spot on a surface; a plot of ground; a bandage; an area or spot. • *vt* to repair with a patch; to piece together; to mend in a makeshift way.—**patchable** *adj*.—**patcher** *n*.

patchouli, patchouly /pəˈtʃuːli/ *n* an Asian plant which yields an essential oil from which a perfume is made.

patchwork /ˈpætʃwɜrk/ *n* needlework made of pieces sewn together; something made of various bits.

patchy /ˈpætʃi/ *adj* (**patchier, patchiest**) irregular; uneven; covered with patches.—**patchily** *adv*.—**patchiness** *n*.

pate /peɪt/ *n* the head.

pâté /pæˈteɪ/ or /ˈpæteɪ/ *n* a rich spread made of meat, fish, herbs, etc.

pâté de foie gras /pæteɪˌdəfwɒˈɡrɒ/ *n* (*pl* **pâtés de foie gras**) a rich paste made from goose liver.

patella /pəˈtɛlə/ *n* (*pl* **patellae**) (*anat*) the kneecap.—**patellar** *adj*.

paten /ˈpætən/ *n* (*Christian Church*) a plate used for the bread at the Eucharist.

patent /ˈpætənt/ or /ˈpeɪ-/ *adj* plain; apparent; open to public inspection; protected by a patent. • *n* a government document, granting the exclusive right to produce and sell an invention, etc for a certain time; the right so granted; the thing protected by such a right. • *vt* to secure a patent for.—**patentable** *adj*.

patentee /ˌpætənˈtiː/ or /ˌpeɪt-/ *n* a holder of a patent.

patent leather *n* leather with a hard, glossy finish.

patent medicine *n* a medicine made and sold under patent and available without a prescription.

patent office *n* an office which issues patents.

patently /ˈpeɪtəntli/ *adv* obviously, openly.

patentor /ˈpætəntər/ or /ˈpeɪt-/ *n* the grantor of a patent.

paterfamilias *n* (*pl* **patresfamilias**) the (male) head of a family.

paternal /pəˈtɜrnəl/ *adj* fatherly in disposition; related through the father.—**paternally** *adv*.

paternalism /pəˈtɜrnəˌlɪzəm/ *n* a system that provides for human needs but allows no individual responsibility.—**paternalist** *adj, n*.—**paternalistic** *adj*.—**paternalistically** *adv*.

paternity /pəˈtɜrnɪti/ *n* fatherhood; origin or descent from a father.

paternity suit *n* a lawsuit to determine whether a particular man is the father of a particular child.

paternity test *n* a blood test to establish whether a man is or is not the father of a particular child.

paternoster /ˌpætərˈnɒstər/ *n* the Lord's Prayer in Latin; every eleventh bead in a rosary; a fishing line with hooks at intervals; an elevator consisting of a continuously revolving belt of linked compartments.

path /pæθ/ *n* (*pl* **paths**) a way worn by footsteps; a track for people on foot; a direction; a course of conduct.

-path *n suffix* denoting an expert in a specific area of medicine; denoting a person suffering from a specified disorder.

pathetic /pəˈθetɪk/ *adj* inspiring pity; (*sl*) uninteresting, inadequate.—**pathetically** *adv*.

pathetic fallacy *n* the attribution of human emotions to inanimate objects.

pathfinder /ˈpæθˌfaɪndər/ *n* a person who discovers a way a person who explores untraversed regions to mark out a new route; a person or thing that marks a spot; a radar device for homing on to a target or navigating.—**pathfinding** *n*.

patho- /ˈpæθəː/ *prefix* disease.

pathogen /ˈpæθədʒən/ *n* an agent, such as a microorganism, that causes disease.—**pathogenic** *adj*.

pathogenesis /ˌpæθəˈdʒenəsɪs/, **pathogeny** /pəˈθɒdʒənɪ/ *n* the origin and development of a disease.—**pathogenetic** *adj*.

pathognomonic /ˌpæθənəˈmɒnɪk/ *adj* characteristic of a particular disease.

pathological /ˌpæθəˈlɒdʒɪkəl/, **pathologic** /ˈpæθə lɒdʒɪk/ *adj* of pathology; of the nature of, caused or altered by disease; (*inf*) compulsive.—**pathologically** *adv*.

pathologist /ˈpæθəˌlɒdʒɪst/ or /ˌpəθɒləˈdʒɪst/ *n* a medical specialist who diagnoses by interpreting the changes in tissue and body fluid caused by a disease.

pathology /pəˈθɒlədʒɪ/ *n* (*pl* **pathologies**) the branch of medicine that deals with the nature of disease, *esp* its functional and structural effects; any abnormal variation from a sound condition.

pathos /ˈpeɪθɒs/ *n* a quality that excites pity or sadness; an expression of deep feeling.

pathway /ˈpæθweɪ/ *n* a path; (*chem*) a sequence of enzyme-catalyzed reactions.

-pathy /ˈpæθɪ/ or /ˈpəθɪ/ *n suffix* feeling; disease; medical treatment.

patience /ˈpeɪʃəns/ *n* the capacity to endure or wait calmly; a card game for one—*also* **solitaire**.

patient /ˈpeɪʃənt/ *adj* even-tempered; able to wait or endure calmly; persevering. • *n* a person receiving medical, dental, etc treatment.—**patiently** *adv*.

patina /pəˈtiːnə/ or /ˈpætɪnə/ *n* a green incrustation on old bronze; a surface appearance of something grown beautiful by age or use; a superficial covering or exterior.

patio /ˈpætiɔː/ *n* (*pl* **patios**) an inner, *usu* roofless, courtyard; a paved area adjoining a house, for outdoor lounging, dining, etc.

patisserie /pəˈtiːsərɪ/ *n* a pastry shop; pastries.

patois /ˈpætwɒ/ or /ˈpætwɒ/ *n* (*pl* **patois**) a dialect.

patriarch /ˈpeɪtrɪˌɑːk/ *n* the father and head of a family or tribe; a man of great age and dignity.—**patriarchal** *adj*.

patriarchate /-ət/ *n* the office, rank or jurisdiction of a patriarch; people ruled by a patriarch.

patriarchy /-ɪ/ *n* (*pl* **patriarchies**) government by the head of a family, tribe, etc; a community ruled in this way.

patriate /ˈpætrɪˌeɪt/ *vt* ✸ (*Cdn*) bring a piece of legislation, especially a constitution, under the authority of an independent country that was formerly under the jurisdiction of another.—**patriation** *n*.

patrician /pəˈtrɪʃən/ *n* (*ancient Rome*) a member of the nobility. • *adj* aristocratic; oligarchic.

patricide /ˈpætrɪsaɪd/ *n* the unlawful killing of one's father; a person who kills his or her father.—**patricidal** *adj*.

patrimony /ˈpætrɪˌmoːnɪ/ *n* (*pl* **patrimonies**) an estate or right inherited from a father or one's ancestors; an ecclesiastical endowment or estate.—**patrimonial** *adj*.

patriot /ˈpeɪtrɪət/ *n* one who strongly supports and serves his or her country.—**patriotic** *adj*.—**patriotically** *adv*.

patriotism /ˈpeɪtrɪˌbtɪzəm/ *n* love for or loyalty to one's country.

patristic /pəˈtrɪstɪk/, **patristical** /-əl/ *adj* pertaining to the theology and writings of the fathers of the early Christian church.

patrol /pəˈtroːl/ *vti* (**patrolling, patrolled**) to walk around a building or area in order to watch, guard, inspect. • *n* the act of going the rounds; a unit of persons or vehicles employed for reconnaissance, security, or combat; a subdivision of a Scout or Guide group.—**patroller** *n*.

patrolman /-mən/ *n* (*pl* **patrolmen**) (*chiefly US*) a policeman who patrols a particular area.

patron /ˈpeɪtrən/ *n* a regular client or customer; a person who sponsors and supports the arts, charities, etc; a protector.—**patronal** *adj*.

patronage /ˈpeɪtrənɪdʒ/ or /ˈpæt-/ *n* the support given or custom brought by a patron; clientele; business; trade; the power to grant political favours; such favours.

patronize /ˈpeɪtrənaɪz/ or /ˈpæt-/ *vt* to treat with condescension; to sponsor or support; to be a regular customer of.—**patronization** *n*.

patronizing /-ɪŋ/ *adj* condescending.—**patronizingly** *adv*.

patronymic /ˌpætrəˈnɪmɪk/ *adj* derived from the name of an ancestor. • *n* a name derived from an ancestor.

patsy /ˈpætsɪ/ *n* (*pl* **patsies**) (*sl*) a gullible person; a sucker.

patten /ˈpætən/ *n* a wooden shoe on a metal ring, worn as a protection from the damp.

patter[1] /ˈpætər/ *vi* to make quick tapping sounds, as if by striking something; to run with light steps. • *n* the sound of tapping or quick steps.

patter[2] *vi* to talk rapidly and glibly; to mumble (prayers, etc) mechanically • *vt* to repeat speech mechanically, to gabble. • *n* rapid speech *esp* that of a salesman, comedian, etc; glib speech; chatter; jargon.

pattern /ˈpætən/ *n* a decorative arrangement; a model to be copied; instructions to be followed to make something; a regular way of acting or doing; a predictable route, movement, etc. • *vt* to make or do in imitation of a pattern.—**patterned** *adj*.

patty /ˈpætɪ/ *n* (*pl* **patties**) a small pie; a flat cake of ground meat, fish, etc, *usu* fried.

patulous /ˈpætjʊləs/ *adj* (*bot*) spreading, extended.

paucity /ˈpɔːsɪtɪ/ *n* fewness; lack of; scarcity.

paulownia /pɔːˈloːnɪə/ *n* a member of a Japanese genus of trees, with heart-shaped leaves and purple flowers.

paunch /pɔːntʃ/ *n* the belly, *esp* a potbelly.

paunchy /ˈpɔːntʃɪ/ *adj* (**paunchier, paunchiest**) having a big belly.—**paunchiness** *n*.

pauper /ˈpɔːpər/ *n* a very poor person; (*formerly*) a person dependent on charity.—**pauperism** *n*.

pauperize, pauperise /ˈpɔːpəraɪz/ *vt* to reduce to pauperism.

pause /pɔːz/ *n* a temporary stop, *esp* in speech, action or music. • *vi* to cease in action temporarily, wait; to hesitate.

pavage /ˈpeɪvɪdʒ/ *n* a tax paid for paving streets.

pavane, pavan /pəˈvɒn/ *n* (the music for) an old stately dance.

pave /peɪv/ *vt* (*a road, etc*) to cover with concrete to provide a hard level surface; **pave the way** to prepare a smooth easy way; to facilitate development.—**paving** *n*.

pavement /ˈpeɪvmənt/ *n* flat slabs, tiles, etc forming a surface, *esp* on a public thoroughfare.

pavilion /pəˈvɪljən/ *n* an annexe; a temporary building for exhibitions; a large ornate tent.

pavonine /ˈpævəˌnaɪn/ *adj* pertaining to peacocks; resembling a peacock.

paw /pɔː/ *n* a foot of a mammal with claws; (*sl*) a hand. • *vti* to touch, dig, hit, etc with paws; to maul; to handle clumsily or roughly.

pawky /ˈpɔːkɪ/ *adj* (**pawkier, pawkiest**) (*Scot*) having a dry sense of humour.

pawn[1] /pɔːn/ *n* the piece of lowest value in chess; a person used to advance another's purpose.

pawn[2] *vt* to deposit an article as security for a loan; to wager or risk. • *n* a thing pawned; the state of being given as a pawn.—**pawner** *n*.

pawnbroker /ˈpɔːnˌbroːkər/ *n* a person licensed to lend money at interest on personal property left with him as security.—**pawnbroking** *n*.

pawnshop /ˈpɔːnʃɒp/ *n* a pawnbroker's shop.

pawpaw /ˈpɔːpɔː/ *see* **papaw**

paxwax /ˈpæksˌwæks/ *n* a strong tendon in an animal's neck.

pay /peɪ/ *vti* (**paying, paid**) to give (money) to in payment for a debt, goods or services; to give in compensation; to yield a profit; to bear a cost; to suffer a penalty; (*homage, attention*) to give. • *n* payment for services or goods; salary, wages.—**paying** *adj*.—**payer** *n*.

payable /ˈpeɪəbəl/ *adj* that must be paid, due; to be paid on a specified date.

pay dirt *n* soil, gravel, etc worth mining for minerals; (*inf*) a source of wealth.

PAYE *abbr* = pay-as-you-earn; the deduction of income tax from wages or salaries at source.

payee /peɪˈiː/ *n* one to whom money is paid.

payload /ˈpeɪloːd/ *n* cargo that earns revenue; the total load of an aircraft, spacecraft, satellite, etc.

paymaster /'peɪmæstər/ *n* a person in charge of paying wages and salaries.

payment /'peɪmənt/ *n* the act of paying; amount paid; reward.

paynim /'peɪnɪm/ *n* (*arch*) a heathen; a Muslim.

payola /peɪ'oːlə/ *n* a bribe paid for the clandestine promotion of a product, *esp* one paid to a disc jockey to play a particular record; a system of such bribes.

payphone /'peɪfoːn/ *n* a coin-operated telephone.

payroll /'peɪroːl/ *n* a list of employees and their wages; the actual money for paying wages.

Pb (*chem symbol*) lead.

PBX *abbr* = private branch exchange.

PBS (*US*) *abbr* = Public Broadcasting System.

PC /piː'siː/ *abbr* = personal computer; police constable; political correctness, politically correct; ✹ (*Cdn*) postal code; ✹ (*Cdn*) Progressive Conservative.

pc, p.c. *abbr* = per cent; postcard.

PCB *abbr* = polychlorinated biphenyl; printed circuit board.

PCO /piː'siː'oː/ *abbr* ✹ (*Cdn*) = Privy Council Office.

P.D. (*US*) *abbr* = Police Department; postal district.

Pd (*chem symbol*) palladium.

pd *abbr* = paid.

PD day *n* ✹ (*Cdn*) professional development day.

PDF /piː'diː'ef/ *abbr* = (*comput*) Portable Document Format, a file transfer system that renders a document viewable even without the software program which was initially used to create it.

p.d.q. *abbr* = pretty damn quick.

PDT /'piː'diː'tiː/ *abbr* ✹ = Pacific Daylight Time.

PE *abbr* = Prince Edward Island; physical education.

pea /piː/ *n* the edible, round, green seed of a climbing leguminous annual plant.

peace /piːs/ *n* tranquillity, stillness; freedom from contention, violence or war; a treaty that ends a war.

peaceable /'piːsəbəl/ *adj* inclined to peace.—**peaceably** *adv*.—**peaceableness** *n*.

Peace Corps *n* a US government organization that sends volunteers to work on social, educational, agricultural, etc projects in developing countries.

peace dividend *n* a benefit to a nation generated from the reduction in defence spending when a conflict is ended, to be used for purposes other than armaments etc.

peaceful /'piːsful/ *adj* having peace; tranquil; quiet.—**peacefully** *adv*.—**peacefulness** *n*.

peacemaker /'piːsˌmeɪkər/ *n* one who makes or restores peace; one who reconciles enemies.—**peacemaking** *adj*, *n*.

peace offering *n* a conciliatory gift.

peace pipe *n* a tobacco pipe smoked by American Indians as a sign of peace.

peace process *n* the sequence or progress of negotiations towards the settlement of conflict.

peach /piːtʃ/ *n* a round, sweet, juicy, downy-skinned stone-fruit; the tree bearing it; a yellowish pink colour; (*sl*) a well-liked person or thing.

peachy /'piːtʃi/ *adj* (**peachier, peachiest**) of or resembling a peach; (*inf*) great, excellent.—**peachily** *adv*.—**peachiness** *n*.

peacock /'piːkɒk/ *n* (**peacocks, peacock**) a male peafowl with a large brilliantly coloured fan-like tail; a person who is a show-off.

peafowl /'piːfaʊl/ *n* (**peafowls, peafowl**) a peacock or a peahen.

pea-green *adj* bright green.

peahen /'piːhen/ *n* a female peafowl.

peak /piːk/ *n* the summit of a mountain; the highest point; the pointed end of anything; maximum value; the eyeshade of a cap, visor. • *vti* (*politician, actor, etc*) to reach or cause to reach the height of power, popularity; (*prices*) to reach and stay at the highest level.

peaked /piːkd/ *adj* pointed; having a peak; peaky.

peaky /'piːki/ *adj* (**peakier, peakiest**) drawn, emaciated; sickly; peaked.

peal /piːl/ *n* a reverberating sound as of thunder, laughter, bells, etc; a set of bells, the changes rung on them. • *vti* to sound in peals, ring out.

pean /'piːən/ *see* **paean**.

peameal bacon /'piːmiːl/ *n* ✹ (*Cdn*) back bacon rolled in a coating of fine cornmeal.

peanut /'piːnʌt/ *n* a leguminous plant with underground pods containing edible seeds; the pod or any of its seeds; (*pl*) (*sl*) a trifling thing or amount.

peanut butter *n* a food paste made by grinding roasted peanuts.

pear /pɛr/ *n* a common juicy fruit of tapering oval shape; the tree bearing it.

pearl /pɜrl/ *n* the lustrous white round gem produced by oysters; mother-of-pearl; anything resembling a pearl intrinsically or physically; one that is choice and precious; a bluish medium grey. • *vti* to fish for pearls; to form drops (on), to bespangle.—**pearler** *n*.—**pearliness** *n*.

pearl button *n* a button covered with mother-of-pearl.

pearl diver *n* a person who dives for pearl oysters.

pearl oyster *n* any of various marine bivalve molluscs that yield pearls.

pearly /'pɜrli/ *adj* (**pearlier, pearliest**) clear, lustrous, like a pearl; covered with pearls; bluish grey. • *n* (*pl* **pearlies**) (*pl*) a London costermonger's dress covered with pearl buttons.

Pearly Gates *npl* (*inf*) the gates of Heaven.

pearmain /'pɛrmeɪn/ *n* a variety of apple.

Peary caribou *n* ✹ a small caribou of the Arctic islands of Canada.

peasant /'pezənt/ *n* (*inf*) a countryman or countrywoman; an agricultural labourer; (*derog*) a lout.

peasantry /-ri/ *n* peasants as a class.

pease /piːz/ *n* (*arch*) a pea.

peashooter /'piːˌʃuːtər/ *n* a toy blowpipe through which peas, etc, are blown.

peasouper /'piːˌsuːpər/ *n* (*sl*) a thick yellow fog.

peat /piːt/ *n* decayed vegetable matter from bogs, which is dried and cut into blocks for fuel or used as a fertilizer.—**peaty** *adj*.

pebble /'pebəl/ *n* a small rounded stone; an irregular, grainy surface.—**pebbled** *adj*.—**pebbly** *adj*.

pecan /pi'kæn/ or /'piːkæn/, /pi'kɒn/ *n* a hickory tree widely grown in the US and Mexico for its edible nuts; its wood; its thin-shelled nut.

peccable /'pekəbəl/ *adj* liable to sin.—**peccability** *n*.

peccadillo /ˌpekə'dɪloː/ *n* (*pl* **peccadilloes, peccadillos**) a trifling misdeed, indiscretion.

peccary /'pekəri/ *n* (*pl* **peccaries, peccary**) an American wild piglike mammal.

peccavi /pe'kɑːvi/ *n* (*pl* **peccavis**) a confession of guilt.

peck /pek/ *vt* to strike with the beak or a pointed object; to pick at one's food; (*inf*) to kiss lightly; to nag.—*also n*.

pecker /'pekər/ *n* something, *esp* a bird, that pecks; (*sl*) penis.

pecking order *n* a social hierarchy in groups of some birds (*esp* hens), characterized by the pecking of those lower in the scale and submitting to being pecked by those higher; any social hierarchy.

peckish /'pekɪʃ/ *adj* (*inf*) hungry; irritable.—**peckishly** *adv*.—**peckishness** *n*.

pecten /'pektɪn/ *n* (*pl* **pectens, pectines**) (*zool*) a comblike membrane on the eyes of birds and some reptiles.

pectin /'pektɪn/ *n* a carbohydrate found in fruits and vegetables, yielding a gel that is used to set jellies.—**pectic** *adj*.

pectoral /'pektərəl/ *adj* of or relating to the breast, chest. • *n* the muscle in the chest; something worn on the breast.

peculate /'pekjuˌleɪt/ *vt* to appropriate money entrusted to one's care, to embezzle.—**peculation** *n*.—**peculator** *n*.

peculiar /pə'kjuːliːər/ *adj* belonging exclusively (to); special; distinct; characteristic; strange.—**peculiarly** *adv*.

peculiarity /pəˌkjuːlɪ'erɪti/ *n* (*pl* **peculiarities**) an idiosyncrasy; a characteristic; an oddity.

pecuniary /pə'kjuːniˌeri/ *adj* of or consisting of money.—**pecuniarily** *adv*.

pedagogue /'pedəˌɡɒɡ/ *n* a schoolteacher.—**pedagogic, pedagogical** *adj*.

pedagogy /'pedəˌɡɒdʒi/ *n* the art or science of teaching.

pedal[1] /'pedəl/ *n* a lever operated by the foot. • *vt* (**pedalling, pedalled** *or* **pedaling, pedaled**) to operate or propel by pressing pedals with the foot.—**pedaller, pedaler** *n*.

pedal[2] *adj* (*zool*) pertaining to the foot or feet.

pedalo /'pedəˌloː/ *n* (*pl* **pedalos**) a small pedal-operated pleasure boat.

pedant /'pedənt/ *n* a person who attaches too much importance to insignificant details.

pedantic /pə'dæntɪk/ *adj* of, relating to, or being a pedant; narrowly learned.—**pedantically** *adv*.

pedantry /'pedəntri/ *n* (*pl* **pedantries**) an ostentatious display of learning; the state of being a pedant.

pedate /'pɛdeɪt/ adj (bot) having lateral sections divided into lobes; (zool) having, or resembling, feet.

peddle /'pedəl/ vt to go from place to place selling small items; to sell (drugs, etc) illegally.

peddler /'pedlər/ n a person who peddles goods; a person who sells drugs illegally.

pederast /'pedə,ræst/ n a person who practises pederasty.

pederasty /-i/ n sex between a man and a boy.

pedestal /'pedəstəl/ n the base that supports a column, statue, etc. • vt to set on a pedestal; to serve as a pedestal for.

pedestrian /pə'destrian/ adj on foot; dull, commonplace. • n a person who walks.

pedestrianism /-ɪzəm/ n walking, or a fondness for walking; the quality of being dull or commonplace.

pedestrianize /-aɪz/ vti to convert (an area) for use by pedestrians only.—**pedestrianization** n.

pedicab /'pedi,kæb/ n a pedal-driven rickshaw.

pedicular /pə'dɪkjulər/, **pediculous** /-ləs/ adj pertaining to lice; infested with lice.—**pediculosis** n.

pedicure /'pedi,kjur/ n cosmetic care of the feet, toes, and nails; a person trained to care for feet in this way.

pediform /'pedi,fɔrm/ adj foot-shaped.

pedigree /'pedi,gri:/ n a line of descent of an animal; a recorded purity of breed of an individual; a genealogy; lineage; derivation. • adj having a known ancestry.—**pedigreed** adj.

pediment /'pedimənt/ n a triangular ornament crowning the front of a classical building, esp a Greek temple.—**pedimental, pedimented** adj.

pedometer /pə'dɒmɪtər/ n an instrument for measuring the distance walked by recording the number of steps taken.

peduncle /pə'dʌŋkəl/ n a flower stalk.—**peduncular** adj.

pedunculate /pə'dʌŋkjulət/, **pedunculated** /-leɪtəd/ adj having, or growing upon, a peduncle.

pee /pi:/ vi (sl) to urinate. • n urination; urine.

peek /pi:k/ vi to look quickly or furtively.—also n.

peekaboo /'pi:kə,bu:/ n a child's game in which one person hides behind his or her hands then peeps out suddenly, shouting, "peekaboo!".

peel /pi:l/ vt to remove skin or rind from; to bare. • vi to flake off, as skin or paint. • n rind, esp that of fruit and vegetables.—**peeling** n.

peeler /'pi:lər/ n a device for peeling; (sl) a stripteaser.

peen /pi:n/ n the pointed or thin end of a hammer-head.

peep¹ /pi:p/ vi to make shrill noises as a young bird. • n a peeping sound.

peep² vi to look hastily or furtively; to look through a slit or narrow opening; to be just showing. • n a furtive or hurried glance, a glimpse; (of day) the first appearance.

peeper /'pi:pər/ n one who peeps; (sl) the eye; (sl) a private detective.

peephole /'pi:phoʊl/ n a small hole, esp in a door, to spy through.

peeping Tom n a person who peeps furtively, a voyeur.

peepshow /'pi:pʃoʊ/ n a small show, esp of erotic pictures, viewed through a hole with a lens; a live show with a nude model, viewed from a booth.

peepul /'pi:pəl/ n an Indian fig tree, sacred to Buddhists.—also **pipal**.

peer¹ /piːr/ vi to look closely; to look with difficulty; to peep out.

peer² n an equal in rank, ability, etc; a nobleman.—**peeress** nf.

peerage /'piːrɪdʒ/ n the rank or title of a peer; peers collectively; a book with a list of peers.

peer group n a group of people of the same age, background, education, interests, etc.

peerless /'piːrləs/ adj having no equal, matchless.

peeve /pi:v/ vt (inf) to annoy.

peeved /'pi:vd/ adj annoyed, resentful.

peevish /'pi:vɪʃ/ adj fretful, irritable.—**peevishly** adv.—**peevishness** n.

peg /peg/ n a tapered piece (of wood) for securing or hanging things on, for marking position; a predetermined level at which (a price) is fixed; (mus) one of the movable parts for tuning the string of an instrument. • vti (**pegging, pegged**) to fasten or mark with a peg; (a price) to keep steady; (with **away at**) to work steadily, persevere.

Pegasus /'pegəsəs/ n (Greek myth) the winged horse ridden by Bellerophon.

PEI abbr ♦ = Prince Edward Island.

peignoir /'peɪnwar/ n a woman's dressing gown.

pejorative /pɪ'dʒɔrətɪv/ adj (word, etc) disparaging, derogatory. • n a disparaging word.—**pejoratively** adv.

peke /pi:k/ n (sl) a Pekingese dog.

Pekingese, Pekinese /,pi:kɪŋ'i:z/ n (pl **Pekingese, Pekinese**) a breed of small dog with long, silky hair, short legs, and a pug nose.

pekoe /'pi:koʊ/ n a scented black Chinese tea.

pelage /'pelɪdʒ/ n the hair, wool or fur of an animal.

pelagian /pə'leɪdʒiən/ adj (marine life) of or inhabiting the open sea.—also n.—**pelagic** adj.

pelargonium /,pelɑr'goʊniəm/ n a member of a widely cultivated genus of flowering plants, including geraniums.

pelf /pelf/ n (derog) money, wealth.

pelican /'pelɪkən/ n a large fish-eating waterbird with an expandable pouched bill.

pelisse /pə'li:s/ n a woman's long cloak, usu trimmed with fur.

pellagra /pə'lægrə/ or /-leɪgrə/, /-lɒgrə/ n a disease affecting the skin and nervous system caused by a deficiency of nicotinic acid.—**pellagrous** adj.

pellet /'pelət/ n a small ball of paper, bread, etc; a pill; a small ball of hair, bones, etc regurgitated by a bird of prey; a piece of shot. • vt to form into pellets.

pellicle /'pelɪkəl/ n a thin skin or film.—**pellicular** adj.

pellitory /'pelɪtɔri/ n (pl **pellitories**) a European flowering plant, growing in walls.

pell-mell /pel'mel/ adv, adj in a disorderly rush; confusedly; headlong.

pellucid /pə'lu:sɪd/ or /-'lju-/ adj (water, etc) transparent; (speech, writing, etc) clear, lucid.—**pellucidity, pellucidness** n.

pelmet /'pelmət/ n a canopy for a window frame to hide a curtain rail, etc; a valance.

pelota /pə'loʊtə/ or /-'loʊtɑ/ n a Basque ball game similar to tennis, played with basket-shaped rackets against a wall.

pelt¹ /pelt/ vt to throw missiles, or words, at. • vi (rain) to fall heavily; to hurry, rush. • n a rush.—**pelter** n.

pelt² n a usu undressed skin of an animal with its hair, wool, or fur.

peltry /'peltri/ n (pl **peltries**) a collective term for the pelts of animals.

pelvis /'pelvɪs/ n (pl **pelvises, pelves**) the bony cavity that joins the lower limbs to the body; the bones forming this.—**pelvic** adj.

pemmican, pemican /'pemɪkən/ n a cake of dried lean meat formerly used by North American Indians; a mixture of beef and suet used as emergency rations.

pemphigus /'pemfɪgəs/ n a rare skin disease, characterized by watery blisters.—**pemphigoid, pemphigous** adj.

pen¹ /pen/ n an implement used with ink for writing or drawing. • vt (**penning, penned**) to write, compose.

pen² n a small enclosure for cattle, poultry, etc; a small place of confinement. • vt (**penning, penned**) to enclose in a pen, shut up.

pen³ n a female swan.

pen⁴ n (sl) a penitentiary.

penal /'pi:nəl/ adj relating to, liable to, or prescribing punishment; punitive.—**penally** adv.

penal code n a code of laws concerning crimes and offences and their punishment.

penalize /-aɪz/ vt to impose a penalty; to put under a disadvantage.—**penalization** n.

penalty /'penəlti/ n (pl **penalties**) a punishment attached to an offence; suffering or loss as a result of one's own mistake; a disadvantage imposed for breaking a rule as in sports; a fine.

penalty area n (soccer) the area in front of goal in which a foul by a defending player results in the award of a penalty kick.

penalty box n (ice hockey) an area of the ice where players are sent as a penalty.

penalty killer n ♦ a player in ice hockey who specializes in preventing an opposing team from scoring while a teammate has been sent off the ice because of a penalty.

penalty shot n ♦ a single shot on goal by a player in ice hockey who has been allowed it as a result of an infraction by a member of the opposing team.

penance /'penəns/ n voluntary suffering to atone for a sin; a sacramental rite consisting of confession, absolution, and penance. • vt to impose a penance on.

pence /pens/ see **penny**.

penchant /'penʃənt/ or /'pɑ̃ʃɑ̃/ n inclination, strong liking (for).

pencil /'pɛnsəl/ *n* a pointed rod-shaped instrument with a core of graphite or crayon for writing, drawing, etc; a set of convergent light rays or straight lines; a fine paintbrush. • *vt* (**pencilling, pencilled** *or* **penciling, penciled**) to write, draw, or colour with a pencil; (*with* **in**) to commit tentatively.—**penciller, penciler** *n*.

pendant, pendent /'pɛndənt/ *n* a hanging ornament, *esp* a jewel on a necklace, bracelet, etc; a light-fitting suspended from a ceiling. • *adj* (*usu* **pendent**) hanging; projecting; undecided.—**pendency** *n*.

pendentive /pɛn'dɛntɪv/ *n* (*archit*) a portion of a dome supported by a single pillar.

pending /'pɛndɪŋ/ *adj* undecided; unfinished; imminent. • *prep* during; until, awaiting.

pendragon /pɛn'drægən/ *n* (*hist*) a chief of the ancient Britons or Welsh.

pendulous /'pɛndjuləs/ *adj* hanging downwards and swinging freely.—**pendulously** *adv*.

pendulum /'pɛndjuləm/ *n* a weight suspended from a fixed point so as to swing freely; such a device used to regulate the movement of a clock; something that swings to and fro.

peneplain, peneplane /'piːnəˌpleɪn/ *n* (*geol*) a tract of land which is almost a plain.

penetrable /'pɛnətrəbəl/ *adj* able to be penetrated.—**penetrability** *n*.

penetralia /ˌpɛnə'treɪlɪə/ *npl* the inner parts of a temple, etc; mysteries.

penetrant /'pɛnətrənt/ *adj* penetrating. • *n* something which, or someone who, penetrates.

penetrate /'pɛnəˌtreɪt/ *vti* to thrust, force a way into or through something; to pierce; to permeate; to understand.—**penetrator** *n*.—**penetrative** *adj*.

penetrating /-ɪŋ/ *adj* acute, discerning; (*voice*) easily heard through other sounds.—**penetratingly** *adv*.

penetration /-treɪʃən/ *n* the capability, act, or action of penetrating; acute insight.

penguin /'pɛŋgwɪn/ *n* a flightless, marine bird with black and white plumage, *usu* found in the Antarctic.

penicillate /'pɛnɪsɪlət/ *or* /pɛnɪ'sɪlət/ *adj* (*biol*) having, or forming, small tufts.

penicillin /ˌpɛnɪ'sɪlən/ *n* an antibiotic produced naturally and synthetically from moulds.

penile /'piːnaɪl/ *adj* of, like, or affecting the penis.

peninsula /pə'nɪnsjələ/ *or* /-sə-/ *n* a piece of land almost surrounded by sea.—**peninsular** *adj*.

penis /'piːnəs/ *n* (*pl* **penises, penes**) the male copulative and urinary organ in mammals.

penitence /'pɛnɪtəns/ *n* sorrow for committing a sin, repentance.

penitent /'pɛnɪtənt/ *adj* feeling regret for sin, repentant, contrite. • *n* a person who atones for sin.—**penitently** *adv*.

penitential /ˌpɛnɪ'tɛnʃəl/ *adj* of or expressing penance; being penitent.—**penitentially** *adv*.

penitentiary /ˌpɛnɪ'tɛnʃəri/ *n* (*pl* **penitentiaries**) (*US*) a state or federal prison. • *adj* pertaining to penance; pertaining to the reformatory treatment of prisoners.

penknife /'pɛnnaɪf/ *n* (*pl* **penknives**) a small knife, *usu* with one or more folding blades, that fits into the pocket.

penman /'pɛnmən/ *n* (*pl* **penmen**) a writer.

penmanship /'pɛnmənʃɪp/ *n* the art, or style, of writing.

Penn, Penna /pɛn/ *abbr* = Pennsylvania.

pen name *n* a literary pseudonym.—*also* **nom de plume**.

pennant /'pɛnənt/ *n* a long tapering flag used for identifying vessels and for signalling; such a flag symbolizing a championship.

penniless /'pɛnɪləs/ *adj* having no money; poor.—**pennilessly** *adv*.—**pennilessness** *n*.

pennon /'pɛnən/ *n* a small, pointed or swallow-tailed flag of a medieval knight; a long tapering streamer on a ship.

penny /'pɛni/ *n* (*pl* **pence** *denoting sum*, **pennies** *denoting separate coins*) a bronze coin of the UK worth one hundredth of a pound; (*formerly*) a bronze coin of the UK worth one twelfth of a shilling, or one two hundred and fortieth of a pound; (*US*) a one cent coin.

pennyroyal /ˌpɛni'rɔɪəl/ *n* an aromatic plant of the mint family.

pennyweight /'pɛniˌweɪt/ *n* a weight, equivalent to 24 grains or $\frac{1}{20}$ of an ounce (troy).

pennywort /'pɛniˌwɜrt/ *n* a kind of round-leafed plant, growing variously in walls or in marshes.

pennyworth /'pɛniˌwɜrθ/ *n* a penny's worth (of a purchase); a small amount.

penology /piː'nɒlədʒi/ *n* the study of the punishment and prevention of crime.—*also* **poenology**.—**penological** *adj*.—**penologist** *n*.

pen pal *n* a friend with whom one is in contact only through correspondence.

pensile /'pɛnsaɪl/ *adj* suspended; pendulous.

pension /'pɛnʃən/ *n* a periodic payment to a person beyond retirement age, or widowed, or disabled; a periodic payment in consideration of past services. • *vt* to grant a pension to; (*with* **off**) to dismiss or retire from service with a pension.—**pensionable** *adj*.

pensionary /-ɛri/ *adj* by way of pension. • *n* (*pl* **pensionaries**) a pensioner.

pensioner /-ər/ *n* a person who receives a pension; a senior citizen.

pensive /'pɛnsɪv/ *adj* thoughtful, musing; wistful, melancholic.—**pensively** *adv*.—**pensiveness** *n*.

pentacle /'pɛntəkəl/ *see* **pentagram**.

pentad /'pɛntæd/ *n* a group of five; the number five.

pentadactyl /ˌpɛntə'dæktəl/ *adj* (*zool*) having five fingers or toes.

pentagon /'pɛntəgɒn/ *n* (*geom*) a polygon with five sides; (*with cap*) the pentagonal headquarters of the US defence establishment; the US military leadership collectively.—**pentagonal** *adj*.

pentagram /'pɛntəˌgræm/ *n* a five-pointed star, often used as a magic symbol.—*also* **pentacle**.

pentahedron /ˌpɛntə'hiːdrən/ *n* (*pl* **pentahedrons, pentahedra**) a solid figure with five faces.

pentamerous /pɛn'tæmərəs/ *adj* (*bot, zool*) with five parts.

pentameter /pɛn'tæmətər/ *n* a verse of five metrical feet.

pentangle /'pɛnˌtæŋgəl/ *n* a pentagram.

Pentateuch /'pɛntəˌtuːk/ *or* /-tjuːk/ *n* the collective name for the first five books of the Old Testament.

pentathlon /pɛn'tæθlɒn/ *n* an athletic contest involving participation by each contestant in five different events.—**pentathlete** *n*.

pentatonic /ˌpɛntə'tɒnɪk/ *adj* (*mus*) of five notes.

pentavalent /ˌpɛntə'veɪlənt/ *adj* (*chem*) with a valency of five.

Pentecost /'pɛntəˌkɒst/ *n* a Christian festival on the seventh Sunday after Easter; Whit Sunday.

Pentecostal /ˌpɛntə'kɒstəl/ *adj* denoting a mainly Protestant Christian movement, now with various organized forms, emphasizing the immediate presence of God in the Holy Spirit; of Pentecost or the influence of the Holy Spirit. • *n* a member of a Pentecostal church.—**Pentecostalist** *adj*, *n*.

penthouse /'pɛnthʊs/ *n* an apartment on the roof or in the top floor of a building.

pentstemon /pɛnt'stiːmən/ *n* a flowering garden plant of the family including the beard-tongues.—*also* (*chiefly US*) **penstemon**.

pent-up *adj* (*emotion*) repressed, confined.

penult /pə'nɛlt/ *or* /piː'nɛlt/ *n* the penultimate syllable of a word. • *adj* last but one.

penultimate /pə'nɛltɪmət/ *adj* last but one.—*also adj*.

penumbra /pə'nʌmbrə/ *n* (*pl* **penumbrae, penumbras**) a shaded region around the shadow of an opaque object, *esp* the shadow of the moon or earth in an eclipse; the lighter outer part of a sunspot; (*art*) the boundary of light and shade in a picture.—**penumbral** *adj*.

penurious /pə'njʊriəs/ *adj* grudging with money, stingy; poor; scanty.—**penuriously** *adv*.—**penuriousness** *n*.

penury /'pɛnjuri/ *n* (*pl* **penuries**) extreme poverty; want.

peon /'piːɒn/ *n* a Spanish American labourer; (*formerly*) a Spanish American labourer compelled to work to pay off debts.

peonage /'piːɒnɪdʒ/, **peonism** /'piːɒnɪzəm/ *n* the condition of being a peon; the system of compelling someone to work for a creditor to pay off debts.

peony /'piːəni/ *n* (*pl* **peonies**) a plant with large, showy, red, pink or white flowers.

people /'piːpəl/ *n* the body of enfranchised citizens of a state; a person's family, relatives; the persons of a certain place, group, or class; persons considered indefinitely; human beings; (*pl*) all the persons of a racial or ethnic group, typically having a common language, institutions, homes, and culture. • *vt* to populate with people.

pep /pɛp/ *n* (*inf*) energy, vigour; bounce. • *vt* (**pepping, pepped**) (*usu with* **up**) to enliven by injecting with pep.

pepper /'pɛpər/ *n* a sharp, hot condiment made from the fruit of various plants; the fruit of the pepper plant, which can be red, yellow, or green, sweet or hot, and is eaten as a vegetable. • *vt* to sprinkle or flavour with pepper; to hit with small shot; to pelt; to beat.

peppercorn /'pepər,kɔrn/ *n* a dried pepper berry.

pepper mill *n* hand mill for grinding peppercorns.

peppermint /'pepər,mɪnt/ *n* a pungent and aromatic mint plant; its oil used for flavouring; a sweet flavoured with peppermint.

pepperoni /,pepə'roːni/ *n* a spicy beef and pork sausage.

pepper squash *n* ✦ (*Cdn*) a winter squash with ridged, dark green to orange skin and orange flesh.

pepperwort /'pepərwərt/ *n* a form of aquatic or marsh fern; a type of cress.

peppery /'pepəri/ *adj* of, like, full of, pepper; fiery; hot-tempered.—**pepperiness** *n*.

peppy /'pepi/ *adj* (**peppier, peppiest**) full of bounce; lively.—**peppiness** *n*.

pepsin, pepsine /'pepsɪn/ *n* a digestive enzyme contained in gastric juice.

pep talk *n* (*inf*) a vigorous talk made with the intention of arousing enthusiasm, increasing confidence, etc.

peptic /'peptɪk/ *adj* of or promoting digestion; of, producing, or caused by the action of the digestive juices.

peptic ulcer *n* an ulcer of the stomach lining or duodenum.

peptone /'peptoːn/ *n* a product of the action of pepsin on proteins.

peptonize /'peptə'naɪz/ *vt* to convert into peptone.

Péquiste /peɪ'kiːst/ *n* ✦ (*Cdn*) in Quebec, a member or supporter of the Parti Québécois.

per /pər/ *prep* for or in each; through, by, by means of; (*inf*) according to.

peradventure /pərəd'ventʃər/ or /,per-/ *adv* (*arch*) by chance; perhaps.

perambulate /pə'ræmbju,leɪt/ *vti* to walk around.—**perambulation** *n*.—**perambulatory** *adj*.

perambulator /-ər/ *n* one who or that which perambulates; (*Brit formal*) a pram.

per annum *adv* yearly; each year.

percale /pər'keɪl/ *n* a cotton fabric, often used for sheets.

per capita *adj, adv* of or for each person.

perceive /pər'siːv/ *vt* to become aware of, apprehend, through the senses; to recognize.—**perceivable** *adj*.—**perceivably** *adv*.

per cent, percent /pər'sent/ *adv* in, for each hundred. • *n* a percentage.

percentage /pər'sentədʒ/ *n* rate per hundred parts; a proportion; (*inf*) profit, gain.

percept /'pərsept/ *n* something which is perceived.

perceptible /pər'septɪbəl/ *adj* able to be perceived; discernible.—**perceptibility** *n*.—**perceptibly** *adv*.

perception /pər'sepʃən/ *n* the act or faculty of perceiving; discernment; insight; a way of perceiving, view.—**perceptional** *adj*.

perceptive /pər'septɪv/ *adj* able to perceive; observant.—**perceptively** *adv*.—**perceptivity, perceptiveness** *n*.

perch[1] /pərtʃ/ *n* (*pl* **perch, perches**) a spiny-finned chiefly freshwater edible fish.

perch[2] *n* a pole on which birds roost or alight; an elevated seat or position. • *vti* to alight, rest, on a perch; to balance (oneself) on; to set in a high position.

perchance /pər'tʃæns/ *adv* (*arch*) by chance; perhaps.

Percheron /'pərtʃə,rɒn/ *n* a sturdy breed of draughthorse.

percipient /pər'sɪpiənt/ *adj* perceiving; perceptive. • *n* a person who perceives.—**percipience** *n*.

percolate /'pərkə,leɪt/ *vt* (*liquid*) to pass through a filter or pores; to brew coffee. • *vi* to ooze through; to spread gradually.—**percolation** *n*.

percolator /-ər/ *n* a coffeepot in which boiling water is forced through ground coffee beans.

percuss /pər'kʌs/ *vt* to tap sharply; (*med*) to tap (the patient's body) gently to find out the condition of an internal organ by sound.

percussion /pər'kʌʃən/ *n* impact, collision; musical instruments played by striking with sticks or hammers, *eg* cymbals, drums, etc; such instruments regarded as a section of an orchestra; (*med*) tapping the body to discover the condition of an organ by the sounds.—**percussive** *adj*.

percussionist /-ɪst/ *n* a person who plays a percussion instrument.

percutaneous /,pərkju'teɪniəs/ *adj* (*med*) done through the skin.

per diem /pər'diːem/ *adv, adj* every day. • *n* a daily allowance, as for expenses.

perdition /pər'dɪʃən/ *n* utter loss of the soul; eternal damnation; (*arch*) total destruction, ruin.

peregrinate /'perəgrɪ,neɪt/ *vti* to travel, roam about.—**peregrinator** *n*.—**peregrination** *n*.

peregrine /'perəgrən/ *n* a type of falcon common to most areas of the world.

peremptory /pə'remptəri/ *adj* urgent; absolute; dogmatic; dictatorial.—**peremptorily** *adv*.—**peremptoriness** *n*.

perennial /pə'reniəl/ *adj* perpetual; lasting throughout the year. • *n* (*bot*) a plant lasting more than two years.—**perennially** *adv*.

perestroika /,peres'trɔɪkə/ *n* the Russian word for "reform, reconstruction," applied to the policy, initiated by President Gorbachev of the former USSR, of dismantling the monolithic state institutions and replacing them with democratic forms of legislation and administration.—**perestroikan** *adj*.

perfect /'pərfekt/ *adj* faultless; exact; excellent; complete. • *n* (*gram*) a verb form expressing completed action or designating a present state that is the result of an action in the past. • *vt* to improve; to finish; to make fully accomplished in anything.—**perfecter** *n*.—**perfectness** *n*.

perfectible /pər'fektɪbəl/ *adj* capable of being made perfect.—**perfectibility** *n*.

perfection /pər'fekʃən/ *n* the act of perfecting; the quality or condition of being perfect; great excellence; faultlessness; the highest degree; a perfect person or thing.

perfectionist /-ɪst/ *n* one who demands the highest standard.—**perfectionism** *n*.

perfectly /-li/ *adv* thoroughly, completely; quite well; in a perfect manner.

perfecto /pər'fekto:/ *n* (*pl* **perfectos**) a large cigar, tapered at both ends.

perfervid /pər'fərvɪd/ *adj* (*arch*) very fervid, ardent.

perfidious /pər'fɪdiəs/ *adj* treacherous, faithless; deceitful.—**perfidiously** *adv*.—**perfidiousness** *n*.

perfidy /'pərfɪdi/ *n* (*pl* **perfidies**) breach of faith; treachery.

perfoliate /pər'foːliət/ *adj* (*bot*) with a stalk which apparently passes through the leaf.

perforate /'pərfə,reɪt/ *vt* to pierce; to make a hole or row of holes, by boring through. • *adj* perforated.—**perforatory** *adj*.—**perforator** *n*.

perforation /,pərfə'reɪʃən/ *n* the act of perforating; the condition of being perforated; a hole a row of holes to facilitate tearing.

perforce /pər'fɔrs/ *adv* (*arch*) by necessity.

perform /pər'fɔrm/ *vti* to carry out, do; to put into effect; to act; to execute; to act before an audience; to play a musical instrument.—**performable** *adj*.—**performing** *adj*.

performance /-əns/ *n* the act of performing; a dramatic or musical production; an act or action; (*inf*) a fuss; the capabilities of a vehicle, aircraft, etc. • *adj* high-performance.

performer /-ər/ *n* a person who performs, *esp* one who entertains an audience.

perfume /'pərfjuːm/ or /pər'fjuːm/ *n* a pleasing odour; fragrance; a mixture containing fragrant essential oils and a fixative. • *vt* to scent; to put perfume on.—**perfumer** *n*.

perfumery /pər'fjuːməri/ *n* (*pl* **perfumeries**) a place where perfume is sold; perfume in general.

perfunctory /pər'fʌŋktəri/ *adj* superficial, hasty; done merely as a matter of form, half-hearted; performed carelessly; indifferent.—**perfunctorily** *adv*.—**perfunctoriness** *n*.

perfuse /pər'fjuːz/ *vt* (*with* **with**) to suffuse, permeate.—**perfusion** *n*.—**perfusive** *adj*.

pergola /'pərgələ/ *n* an arbour or walk arched by a latticework structure supporting climbing plants.

perhaps /pər'hæps/ *adv* possibly, maybe.

peri- /'peri/ *prefix* around; near.

perianth /'peri,ænθ/ *n* the outer part of a flower, comprising the calyx and corolla together.

periapt /'peri,æpt/ *n* an amulet.

pericarditis /,perɪkɑr'daɪtɪs/ *n* inflammation of the pericardium.

pericardium /,perɪ'kɑrdiəm/ *n* (*pl* **pericardia**) the membrane enclosing the heart.—**pericardiac, pericardial** *adj*.

pericarp /'peri,kɑrp/ *n* the part of a fruit developed from the wall of the ovary.—**pericarpial** *adj*.

perichondrium /,peri'kɒndriəm/ *n* (*pl* **perichondria**) the membrane covering a cartilage.

periclase /'peri,kleɪs/ *n* magnesium oxide as a mineral in crystal or grain form.

pericranium /,peri'kreɪniəm/ *n* (*pl* **pericrania**) the membrane surrounding the cranium.

peridot /'peri,dɒt/ *n* a pale green semi-precious form of olivine.

perigee /'perɪ,dʒiː/ *n* the point of the moon's, or a planet's, orbit, when it is nearest the earth.—**perigean** *adj.*

perihelion /,perɪ'hiːliən/ *n* (*pl* **perihelia**) the point of a planet's or comet's orbit when it is nearest the sun.

peril /'perɪl/ *n* danger, jeopardy; risk, hazard.

perilous /-əs/ *adj* dangerous.—**perilously** *adv.*

perimeter /pə'rɪmɪtər/ *n* a boundary around an area; (*math*) the curve or line bounding a closed figure; the length of this.—**perimetric** *adj.*—**perimetry** *n.*

perineum /,perɪ'niːəm/ *n* the area between the genitals and the anus.—**perineal** *adj.*

period /'piːrɪəd/ *n* a portion of time; menstruation; an interval of time as in an academic day, playing time in a game, etc; an age or era in history, epoch; a stage in life; (*gram*) a full stop (.); (*astron*) a planet's time of revolution.— *interj* an exclamation used for emphasis.

periodic /,piːrɪ'ɒdɪk/ *adj* relating to a period; recurring at regular intervals, cyclic; intermittent.—**periodically** *adv.*—**periodicity** *n.*

periodical /-əl/ *adj* periodic. • *n* a magazine, etc issued at regular intervals.

periodic table *n* a list of chemical elements tabulated by their atomic number.

periodontics /,periə'dɒntɪks/ *n sing* the branch of dentistry dealing with disorders of the gums and tissues around the teeth.—**periodontal** *adj.*—**periodontist** *n.*

periosteum /,peri'ɒstiəm/ *n* (*pl* **periostea**) the membrane covering the bones.

periostitis /,periɒs'taɪtɪs/ *n* inflammation of the periosteum.

peripatetic /,peripə'tetɪk/ *adj* itinerant; (*teacher*) travelling from one school to another.—*also* **n.**

peripheral /pə'rɪfərəl/ *adj* incidental, superficial; relating to a periphery; (*equipment*) for connection to a computer. • *n* a device such as a printer, scanner, etc used with a computer.—**peripherally** *adv.*

periphery /pə'rɪfəri/ *n* (*pl* **peripheries**) the outer surface or boundary of an area; the outside surface of anything.

periphrasis /pə'rɪfrəsɪs/ *n* (*pl* **periphrases**) a roundabout way of speech; circumlocution.

periphrastic /,peri'fræstɪk/ *adj* using periphrasis; circumlocutory.—**periphrastically** *adv.*

peripteral /pə'rɪptərəl/ *adj* (*archit*) with a row of columns on every side.

periscope /'perə,skoːp/ *n* a device with mirrors that enables the viewer to see objects above or around an obstacle or above water, as from a submarine.

periscopic /,perə'skɒpɪk/ *adj* (*lens*) with a view around; of a periscope.—**periscopically** *adv.*

perish /'perɪʃ/ *vi* to be destroyed or ruined; to die, *esp* violently; (*rubber, etc*) to deteriorate, rot. • *vt* to cause to rot or perish.

perishable /-əbəl/ *adj* liable to spoil or decay. • *n* something perishable, *esp* food.—**perishability** *n.*

peritoneum /,peritə'niːəm/ *n* (*pl* **peritoneums, peritonea**) a membrane that lines the walls of the abdomen.—**peritoneal** *adj.*

peritonitis /,peritə'naɪtɪs/ *n* inflammation of the peritoneum.—**peritonitic** *adj.*

periwinkle[1] /'perɪ,wɪŋkəl/ *n* any of various edible small marine gastropods with spiralled shells.

periwinkle[2] *n* any of various evergreen trailing plants with blue or white flowers.

perjure /'pərdʒər/ *vt* to commit perjury, swear falsely.—**perjurer** *n.*

perjury /'pərdʒəri/ *n* (*pl* **perjuries**) (*law*) the crime of giving false witness under oath, swearing to what is untrue.

perk[1] /pərk/ *n* (*usu pl*) (*inf*) a perquisite.

perk[2] *vti* (*usu with* **up**) to recover self-confidence; to become lively or cheerful; to prick up, as of a dog's ears; to smarten up.

perky /'pərki/ *adj* (**perkier, perkiest**) pert, cheeky; lively, jaunty.—**perkily** *adv.*—**perkiness** *n.*

perm /pərm/ *n* a straightening or curling of hair by use of chemicals or heat lasting through many washings. •*vt* (*hair*) to give a perm to.—*also* **permanent wave.**

permafrost /'pərmə,frɒst/ *n* subsoil that is permanently frozen.

permanence /'pərmənəns/ *n* the condition or quality of being permanent.

permanency /-i/ *n* (*pl* **permanencies**) permanence; a person or thing that is permanent.—**permanently** *adv.*

permanent /'pərmənənt/ *adj* lasting, or intended to last, indefinitely.

permanent wave *n* a perm.

permanganate /pər'mæŋgəneɪt/ or /-nət/ *n* a salt of an acid of manganese, *esp* permanganate of potash.

permeable /'pərmiəbəl/ *adj* admitting the passage of a fluid.—**permeability** *n.*—**permeably** *adv.*

permeate /'pərmi,eɪt/ *vti* to fill every part of, saturate; to pervade, be diffused (through); to pass through by osmosis.—**permeation** *n.*

permissible /pər'mɪsɪbəl/ *adj* allowable.—**permissibility** *n.*

permission /pər'mɪʃən/ *n* authorization; consent.

permissive /pər'mɪsɪv/ *adj* allowing permission; lenient; sexually indulgent.—**permissively** *adv.*—**permissiveness** *n.*

permit /pər'mɪt/ *vti* (**permitting, permitted**) to allow to be done; to authorize; to give opportunity. • *n* a licence.—**permitter** *n.*

permutation /,pərmjʊ'teɪʃən/ *n* any radical alteration; a change in the order of a series; any of the total number of groupings within a group; an ordered arrangement of a set of objects.—**permutational** *adj.*

permute /pər'mjuːt/ *vt* to put into a different order.

pernicious /pər'nɪʃəs/ *adj* destructive; very harmful.—**perniciously** *adv.*—**perniciousness** *n.*

pernickety /pər'nɪkɪti/ *see* **persnickety.**

perorate /'perə,reɪt/ *vi* to speak at length.

peroration /,perə'reɪʃən/ *n* the final part of a speech or discourse.

peroxide /pə'rɒksaɪd/ *n* hydrogen peroxide; a colourless liquid used as an antiseptic and as a bleach.

perpendicular /,pərpən'dɪkjʊlər/ *adj* upright, vertical; (*geom*) at right angles (to). • *n* a perpendicular line, position or style.—**perpendicularity** *n.*—**perpendicularly** *adv.*

perpetrate /'pərpə,treɪt/ *vt* (*something evil, criminal, etc*) to do; (*a blunder, etc*) to commit.—**perpetration** *n.*—**perpetrator** *n.*

perpetual /pər'petʃʊəl/ *adj* continuous; everlasting; (*plant*) blooming continuously throughout the season.—**perpetually** *adv.*

perpetuate /pər'petʃʊeɪt/ *vt* to cause to continue; to make perpetual.—**perpetuation** *n.*—**perpetuator** *n.*

perpetuity /,pərpə'tʃuːɪti/ or /-'tjuː-/, /-'tuː-/ *n* (*pl* **perpetuities**) endless duration, eternity; perpetual continuance; an annuity payable forever.

perplex /pər'pleksɪ/ *vt* to puzzle, bewilder, confuse; to complicate.

perplexity /-ɪti/ *n* (*pl* **perplexities**) bewilderment, a being at a loss; a perplexing thing, a dilemma.

perquisite /'pərkwəzɪt/ *n* an expected or promised privilege, gain, or profit incidental to regular wages or salary; a tip, gratuity; something claimed as an exclusive right.—*also* **perk.**

perron /'perən/ *n* a flight of steps outside a building, leading to the first floor.

perry /'peri/ *n* (*pl* **perries**) a cider-like drink made from pears.

per se /pər'seɪ/ *adv* by itself; by its very nature, intrinsically.

persecute /'pərsə,kjuːt/ *vt* to harass, oppress, *esp* for reasons of race, religion, etc; to worry persistently.—**persecutor** *n.*

persecution /,pərsə'kjuːʃən/ *n* a persecuting or being persecuted; unfair or cruel treatment for reasons of race, religion, etc; a time of persecution.

perseverance /,pərsə'vərəns/ *n* persisting efforts of belief, *esp* in the face of opposition; steadfastness; (*Christianity*) continuance in grace.—**perseverant** *adj.*

persevere /,pərsə'viːr/ *vi* to persist, maintain effort, steadfastly, *esp* in face of difficulties.—**perseveringly** *adv.*

persiennes /,pərsi:'enz/, *Fr.* /pər'sjen/ *npl* outside window shutters with horizontal louvres.

persiflage /'pərsə,flɒʒ/ *n* frivolous talk, banter.

persimmon /pər'sɪmən/ *n* one of a species of tropical American trees; the fruit of such a tree.

persist /pər'sɪst/ *vi* to continue in spite of obstacles or opposition; to persevere; to last.—**persister** *n.*

persistence /pər'sɪstəns/, **persistency** /-tənsi/ *n* a persisting; tenacity of purpose.

persistent /pər'sɪstənt/ *adj* persevering; stubborn.—**persistently** *adv.*

persnickety /pər'snɪkɪti/ *adj* (*inf*) fussy, fastidious; over-attentive to detail.—*also* **pernickety.**

person /'pərsən/ *n* (*pl* **persons**) a human being, individual; the body (including clothing) of a human being; (*in a play*) a character; one who is recognized by law as the subject of rights and duties; (*gram*) one of the three classes of personal pronouns and verb forms, referring to the person(s) speaking, spoken to, or spoken of.

persona /pər'soːnə/ n (pl **personae**) a person; a character in a play, etc; (pl) public role or image.

personable /'pərsənəbəl/ adj pleasing in personality and appearance.—**personableness** n.—**personably** adv.

personage /'pərsənɪdʒ/ n a distinguished person.

persona grata /pər'soːnə,graːtə/ n (pl **personae gratae**) a person who is acceptable or welcome, esp a diplomat to a foreign government.

personal /'pərsənəl/ adj concerning a person's private affairs, or his or her character, habits, body, etc; done in person; (law) of property that is movable; (gram) denoting person.

personality /pərsə'nælɪti/ n (pl **personalities**) one's individual characteristics; excellence or distinction of social and personal traits; a person with such qualities; a celebrity.

personalize /'pərsənə,laɪz/ vt to mark with name, initials etc; to endow with personal characteristics; to take personally; to personify.—**personalization** n.

personally /'pərsənəli/ adv in person; in one's own opinion; as though directed to oneself.

personalty /'pərsənəlti/ n (pl **personalties**) (law) personal property.

persona non grata /pər'soːnə,non'graːtə/ n (pl **personae non gratae**) a person who is not acceptable or welcome, esp to a foreign government.

personate /'pərsə,neɪt/ vt to play the part of (in a play etc); (law) to pretend to be (someone else) for fraudulent purposes.—**personation** n.—**personator** n.

personification /pər,sɒnəfɪ'keɪʃən/ n representation of an abstract idea or a thing as a person; an embodiment, a type; a perfect example.

personify /pər'sɒnə,faɪ/ vt (**personifying, personified**) to think of, represent, as a person; to typify.—**personifier** n.

personnel /pərsə'nɛl/ n the employees of an organization or company; the department that hires them.

perspective /pər'spɛktɪv/ n objectivity; the art of drawing so as to give an impression of relative distance or solidity; a picture so drawn; relation, proportion, between parts of a subject; vista, prospect. • adj of or in perspective.

perspicacious /,pərspɪ'keɪʃəs/ adj of clear understanding; shrewd; discerning.—**perspicaciously** adv.—**perspicacity** n.

perspicuous /pər'spɪkjuːəs/ adj clearly expressed, lucid.—**perspicuity** n.

perspiration /,pərspə'reɪʃən/ n the salty fluid excreted on to the surface of the skin, sweat; the act of perspiring.

perspire /pər'spaɪr/ vti to excrete (moisture) through the pores of the skin to cool the body, to sweat.—**perspiringly** adv.

persuadable /pər'sweɪdəbəl/, **persuasible** /pər'sweɪsɪbəl/ adj able to be persuaded.—**persuadability, persuasibility** n.

persuade /pər'sweɪd/ vt to convince; to induce by argument, reasoning, advice, etc.—**persuader** n.

persuasion /pər'sweɪʒən/ n the act of persuading; a conviction or opinion; a system of religious beliefs; a group adhering to such a system.

persuasive /pər'sweɪsɪv/ adj able to persuade; influencing the mind or emotions.—**persuasively** adv.—**persuasiveness** n.

pert /pərt/ adj impudent, cheeky; sprightly.—**pertly** adv.—**pertness** n.

pertain /pər'teɪn/ vi to belong to; to be appropriate to; to have reference to.

pertinacious /,pərtɪ'neɪʃəs/ adj persistent; unyielding; obstinate.—**pertinacity, pertinaciousness** n.

pertinent /'pərtɪnənt/ adj relevant, apposite; to the point.—**pertinence** n.—**pertinently** adv.

perturb /pər'tərb/ vt to trouble; to agitate; to throw into confusion; (astron) to cause to undergo perturbation.—**perturbable** adj.—**perturbably** adv.—**perturbingly** adv.

perturbation /,pərtər'beɪʃən/ n the state of being troubled, mental agitation; (astron) an irregularity or deviation in a regular orbit produced by some additional force.

peruse /pə'ruːz/ vt to read carefully, to examine.—**perusal** n.

pervade /pər'veɪd/ vt to permeate or spread through; to be rife among.—**pervasion** n.

pervasive /pər'veɪsɪv/ adj able or tending to pervade.—**pervasively** adv.—**pervasiveness** n.

perverse /pər'vərs/ adj deviating from right or truth; persisting in error; wayward; contrary.—**perversely** adv.—**perverseness** n.

perversion /pər'vərʒən/ n an abnormal way of obtaining sexual gratification, eg sadism; a perverted form or usage of something.

perversity /pər'vərsɪti/ n (pl **perversities**) a being perverse; a disposition to thwart or annoy; a perverse act.

pervert /pər'vərt/ vt to corrupt; to misuse; to distort. • n a person who is sexually perverted—**perverter** n.—**pervertible** adj.

perverted /-əd/ adj wrong; harmful; unnatural; sexually deviant.—**pervertedly** adv

pervious /'pərvɪəs/ adj giving passage, permeable; open to new ideas.

pesade /pə'seɪd/ or /-'zɒd/ n (dressage) a position in which the horse is standing on its hind legs and raises its forelegs.

peseta /pə'seɪtə/ n the former unit of currency in Spain, now replaced by the euro.

pesky /'pɛski/ adj (**peskier, peskiest**) (inf) troublesome, annoying.

peso /'peɪsoː/ n (pl **pesos**) a unit of currency in several Latin American countries and the Philippines.

pessary /'pɛsəri/ n (pl **pessaries**) (med) a surgical appliance or suppository inserted into the vagina.

pessimism /'pɛsə,mɪzəm/ n a tendency to see in the world what is bad rather than good; a negative outlook that always expects the worst.—**pessimist** n.—**pessimistic** adj.—**pessimistically** adv.

pest /pɛst/ n anything destructive, esp a plant or animal detrimental to man as rats, flies, weeds, etc; a person who pesters or annoys.

pester /'pɛstər/ vt to annoy or irritate persistently.—**pesterer** n.

pesticide /'pɛstɪsaɪd/ n any chemical for killing pests.—**pesticidal** adj.

pestiferous /pɛ'stɪfərəs/ adj spreading infection; (fig) physically or morally noxious.

pestilence /'pɛstɪləns/ n an outbreak of a fatal epidemic disease; anything regarded as harmful.

pestilent /'pɛstɪlənt/ adj irritating; likely to cause a fatal epidemic.—**pestilently** adv.

pestilential /,pɛstɪlɛnʃəl/ adj of the nature of or conveying pestilence; harmful; annoying.—**pestilentially** adv.

pestle /'pɛsəl/ n a usu club-shaped tool for pounding or grinding substances in a mortar. • vt to beat, pound, or pulverize with a pestle.

pet /pɛt/ n a domesticated animal kept as a companion; a person treated as a favourite. • adj kept as a pet; spoiled, indulged; favourite; particular. • vti (**petting, petted**) to stroke or pat gently; to caress; (inf) to kiss, embrace, etc in making love.

petal /'pɛtəl/ n any of the leaf-like parts of a flower's corolla.—**petaline** adj.—**petalled** adj.

petard /pɪ'tɑrd/ n (formerly) a small bomb used to blow in a door, etc.

peter /'piːtər/ vi (with out) to come to an end; to dwindle to nothing.

petersham /'piːtərʃəm/ n a thick corded ribbon used in dressmaking as a stiffening; a thick woollen fabric used for overcoats, etc.

Peter's Pence n (RC Church) voluntary contributions to the papal treasury; (formerly) in England, an annual tax, until its abolishment by Henry VIII of one penny levied on every house and paid to the Pope.

petiolate /'pɛtiˌoːlət/ adj (bot) growing on a petiole.

petiole /'pɛtiˌoːl/ n (bot) a leaf stalk.

petit /'pɛti/ adj (esp law) of lesser importance.

petite /pə'tiːt/ adj (woman) small and trim in figure.

petition /pə'tɪʃən/ n a formal application or entreaty to an authority; a written demand for action by a government, etc, signed by a number of people. • vi to present a petition to; to ask humbly.—**petitionary** adj—**petitioner** n.

petit mal /,pɛti'mæl/ or /,pəti-/ n a mild form of epilepsy.

petit point /'pɛtipɔɪnt/ n a fine stitch used in needlepoint.

petrel /'pɛtrəl/ n a dark-coloured sea bird capable of flying far from land.

petrifaction /,pɛtrɪ'fækʃən/, **petrification** /,pɛtrɪ'fɪkeɪʃən/ n the process of changing animal or vegetable material into stone.

petrify /'pɛtrɪfaɪ/ vti (**petrifying, petrified**) to turn or be turned into stone; to stun or be stunned with fear, horror, etc.

petro- /'pɛtroː/ prefix rock, stone; petroleum.

petrochemical /,pɛtroː'kɛmɪkəl/ n any chemical obtained from natural gas or petroleum.

petrodollar /'pɛtroːˌdɒlər/ n a notional unit of money earned by the export of petroleum.

petroglyph /'pɛtroːglɪf/ n a rock carving or drawing.

petrography /pɛ'trɒgrəfi/ *n* the scientific description and classification of rocks.—**petrographer** *n*.—**petrographic, petrographical** *adj*.

petrol /'pɛtrəl/ *n* fuel obtained from petroleum; (*US*) gasoline.

petrolatum /ˌpɛtrə'lɒtəm/ *n* a greasy, jelly-like substance obtained from petroleum and used for ointments, etc.

petroleum /pə'troːliəm/ *n* a crude oil consisting of hydrocarbons occurring naturally in certain rock strata and distilled to yield petrol, paraffin, etc.

petrology /pɪ'trɒlədʒi/ *n* (*pl* **petrologies**) the study of rocks and their structure.

petrous /'pɛtrəs/ *adj* of, or like, rock.

petticoat /'pɛtiˌkoːt/ *n* an underskirt; a slip; (*inf*) woman.

pettifog /'pɛtifɒg/ *vi* to be, or behave like, a pettifogger.

pettifogger /-ər/ *n* an inferior or crooked lawyer; someone who quibbles over details.

pettish /'pɛtiʃ/ *adj* peevish, sulky.

pettitoes /'pɛtitoːz/ or /'pɛti-/ *npl* pig's trotters, *esp* as food.

petty /'pɛti/ *adj* (**pettier, pettiest**) trivial; small-minded; minor.—**pettily** *adv*.—**pettiness** *n*.

petty officer *n* a noncommissioned officer in the navy.

petulant /'pɛtjulənt/ or /-tu-/ *adj* showing impatience or irritation; bad-humoured.—**petulance** *n*.—**petulantly** *adv*.

petunia /pə'tuːniə/ or /-tjuː-/ *n* a plant with funnel-shaped purple or white flowers.

petuntse /pə'tʌntseɪ/ or /-'tɛnseɪ/ *n* a fine white clay used with kaolin in the manufacture of porcelain.

pew /pjuː/ *n* a wooden, bench-like seat in a church, often enclosed; (*sl*) a chair.

pewit /'piːwɪt/ *n* the lapwing.—*also* **peewit**.

pewter /'pjuːtər/ *n* an alloy of tin and lead with a silvery-grey colour; dishes, etc, made of pewter.—**pewterer** *n*.

PFC (*US*) *abbr* = private first class.

pfennig /'fɛnɪg/, *Ger*. /pfɛnɪʃ/ *n* (*pl* **pfennigs, pfennige**) a former unit of currency in Germany worth one hundredth of a Deutschmark.

PG *abbr* = parental guidance: denoting a motion-picture suitable for all ages, but advising parental guidance.

PGA *abbr* = Professional Golfers' Association.

phaeton /'feɪtən/ or /'feɪə-/ *n* a light, open, four-wheeled horse-drawn carriage.

phagocyte /'fægəˌsaɪt/ *n* a white corpuscle which devours harmful micro-organisms and other foreign bodies.

phagocytosis /ˌfægəˈsaɪtoːsɪs/ *n* the process by which a phagocyte devours foreign bodies.

phalange /'fælændʒ/ or /fə'lændʒ/ *see* **phalanx**.

phalangeal /fə'lændʒiəl/ *adj* (*anat*) of or pertaining to a phalanx.

phalanger /fə'lændʒər/ *n* a small tree-living marsupial of Australasia, with a long tail and bushy fur.

phalanx /'fælæŋks/ or /'feɪ-/ *n* (*pl* **phalanxes, phalanges**) a massed body or rank of people; (*pl* **phalanges**) a bone of a finger or toe.

phalarope /'fæləˌroːp/ *n* a small wading bird, with a straight bill and webbed feet.

phallic /'fælɪk/ *adj* pertaining to, or resembling, a phallus.

phallicism /'fælɪsɪzəm/, **phallism** /'fælɪzəm/ *n* the worship of the phallus as the emblem of the generative power in nature.

phallus /'fæləs/ *n* (*pl* **phalli, phalluses**) the male reproductive organ.

phanerogam /'fænərəˌgæm/ *n* (*bot*) a flowering plant.—**phanerogamic, phanerogamous** *adj*.

phantasm /'fæn,tæzəm/ *n* a phantom; a vision of an absent person.

phantasmagoria /ˌfænˌtæzmə'gɒriə/, **phantasmagory** /ˌfænˌtæzmə'gɒri/ *n* a series of shifting images, like those seen in a dream.—**phantasmagoric, phantasmagorical** *adj*.

phantom /'fæntəm/ *n* a spectre or apparition. • *adj* illusionary.

pharaoh /'fɛroː/ *n* (*also with cap*) the title of the kings of ancient Egypt.—**pharaonic** *adj*.

Pharisaic /ˌfɛrɪ'seɪɪk/, **Pharisaical** /-əl/ *adj* pertaining to, or characteristic of, the Pharisees; (*fig*) hypocritical.

Pharisee /'fɛrisiː/ *n* a member of a Jewish religious sect, characterized by its strict observance of the letter of the law; (*fig*) a self-righteous person, a hypocrite.

pharmacare /'fɑrməˌkɛr/ *n* ✤ (*Cdn*) a system of health insurance to cover the cost of prescribed drugs, especially a public system financed by taxes.

pharmaceutical /ˌfɑrmə'suːtɪkəl/ or /-'sjuː-/ *adj* of, relating to pharmacy or drugs. • *n* a medicinal drug.

pharmaceutics /ˌfɑrmə'suːtɪks/ or /-'sjuː-/ *n sing* the science of pharmacy.

pharmacist /'fɑrməsɪst/ *n* one licensed to practise pharmacy.

pharmacology /ˌfɑrmə'kɒlədʒi/ *n* the science dealing with the effects of drugs on living organisms.—**pharmacological** *adj*.—**pharmacologist** *n*.

pharmacopoeia /ˌfɑrməkə'piːə/ *n* a book containing a list of drugs with directions for their use.—**pharmacopoeial** *adj*.

pharmacy /'fɑrməsi/ *n* (*pl* **pharmacies**) the preparation and dispensing of drugs and medicines; a drugstore.

pharyngeal /fə'rɪndʒiəl/, **pharyngal** /fə'rɪŋgəl/ *adj* pertaining to, or situated near, the pharynx.

pharyngitis /ˌfɛrɪn'dʒaɪtɪs/ *n* inflammation of the pharynx.

pharyngology /ˌfɛrɪŋ'gɒlədʒi/ *n* the medical study of the pharynx.

pharyngoscope /ˌfɛrɪŋgə'skoːp/ *n* an instrument used for looking at the pharynx.

pharyngotomy /ˌfɛrɪŋ'gɒtəmi/ *n* (*pl* **pharynotomies**) the surgical operation of making an incision into the pharynx.

pharynx /'fɛrɪŋks/ *n* (*pl* **pharynges, pharynxes**) the cavity leading from the mouth and nasal passages to the larynx and oesophagus.

phase *n* (*pl* **phases**) an amount of the moon's or a planet's surface illuminated at a given time; a characteristic period in a regularly recurring sequence of events or stage in a development. • *vt* to do by stages or gradually; (*with* **out**) (*making, using, etc*) to stop gradually.—**phasic** *adj*.

PhD /ˌpiːeɪtʃ'diː/ *abbr* = Doctor of Philosophy.

pheasant /'fɛzənt/ *n* a richly coloured game bird.

phellem /'fɛləm/ or /'fɛləm/ *n* (*bot*) cork.

phenacetin /fi'næsətɪn/ *n* a drug used for the relief of pain and fever.

Phenobarbital /ˌfiːnoː'bɑrbɪˌtɒl/ *n* (*trademark*) a crystalline barbiturate used as a hypnotic and sedative.

phenol /'fiːnɒl/ *n* carbolic acid.

phenology /finɒ'lədʒi/ *n* the study of the influence of climate on certain recurrent phenomena of animal and plant life.

phenomenal /fə'nɒmənəl/ *adj* perceptible through the senses; remarkable; outstanding.—**phenomenally** *adv*.

phenomenalism /-ɪzəm/ *n* (*philos*) the doctrine that all knowledge is derived from sense impressions.—**phenomenalist** *n*.

phenomenon /fə'nɒmənɒn/ or /-nən/ *n* (*pl* **phenomena, phenomenons**) anything perceived by the senses as a fact; a fact or event that can be scientifically described; a remarkable thing or person.

phenyl /'fɛnəl/ or /'fiː-/ *n* the hydrocarbon radical of phenol.

pheromone /'fɛrəˌmoːn/ *n* a molecule that functions as a chemical communication signal between individuals of the same species.

phew /fjuː/ *interj* an exclamation of relief, surprise, etc.

phi /faɪ/ *n* the 21st letter of the Greek alphabet.

phial /'faɪəl/ *n* a small glass bottle; a vial.

Phi Beta Kappa /ˌfaɪbeɪtə'kæpə/ *n* (*US*) (a member of) the oldest college fraternity.

phil- /fɪl/, **philo-** /'fɪlə/ or /'fɪlɒ/ *prefix* loving.

philander /fi'lændər/ *vi* (*man*) to flirt with women for amusement.—**philanderer** *n*.

philanthropist /fi'lænθrəpɪst/ *n* a person who tries to benefit others.

philanthropy /fi'lænθrəpi/ *n* (*pl* **philanthropies**) love of mankind, *esp* as demonstrated by benevolent or charitable actions.—**philanthropic, philanthropical** *adj*.—**philanthropically** *adv*.

philatelist /fi'lætəlɪst/ *n* a person who collects or studies stamps.

philately /fi'lætəli/ *n* the study and collecting of postage and imprinted stamps; stamp collecting.—**philatelic** *adj*.—**philatelically** *adv*.

philharmonic /ˌfɪlhɑr'mɒnɪk/ or /ˌfɪlər-/ *adj* loving music.

philhellene /fɪlhe'liːn/ *n* a lover or supporter of Greece.

philippic /fi'lɪpɪk/ *n* a bitter denunciation, an invective.

philistine /'fɪlɪˌstiːn/ or /-staɪn/ *n* a person with no feeling for culture; an uncultured, conventional person; (*with cap*) a member of a warlike race hostile to ancient Israel. • *adj* uncultured.—**philistinism** *n*.

philogyny /fi'lɒdʒəni/ *n* fondness for women.—**phylogynous** *adj*.—**phylogynist** *n*.

philology /fi'lɒlədʒi/ *n* the study, *esp* comparative, of languages and their history and structure.—**philological** *adj*.—**philologist, philologer** *n*.

philomel /'fɪləˌmɛl/ *n* (*poet*) a nightingale.

philosopher /fɪˈlɒsəfər/ n a person who studies philosophy; a person who acts calmly and rationally.

philosophic /ˌfɪləˈsɒfɪk/, **philosophical** /ˌfɪləˈsɒfɪkəl/ adj of, relating to, or according to philosophy; serene; temperate; resigned.—**philosophically** adv.

philosophize /fɪˈlɒsəfaɪz/ vi to reason like a philosopher; to speculate, moralize.—**philosophizer** n.

philosophy /fɪˈlɒsəfi/ n (pl **philosophies**) the study of the principles underlying conduct, thought, and the nature of the universe; general principles of a field of knowledge; a particular system of ethics; composure; calmness.

philtre, philter /ˈfɪltər/ n a love potion.

phlebitis /fləˈbaɪtɪs/ n (med) an inflammation of a vein.—**phlebitic** adj.

phlebotomize /fləˈbɒtəˌmaɪz/ vti (med) to practise phlebotomy (on).

phlebotomy /fləˈbɒtəmi/ n (pl **phlebotomies**) a surgical incision into a vein to let blood.—**phlebotomist** n.

phlegm /flem/ n a thick mucus discharged from the throat, as during a cold; sluggishness; apathy.

phlegmatic /flegˈmætɪk/, **phlegmatical** /-əl/ adj unemotional, composed; sluggish.—**phlegmatically** adv.

phloem /ˈfləʊɛm/ n (bot) the tissue which carries food around a plant.

phlogiston /flɒˈdʒɪstən/ or /-stɒn/ n (chem) an inflammable element once believed to exist in all combustible bodies.

phlox /flɒks/ n (pl **phlox, phloxes**) a North American flowering plant.

phobia /ˈfəʊbiə/ n an irrational, excessive, and persistent fear of some thing or situation.—**phobic** adj, n.

phoenix /ˈfiːnɪks/ n a mythical bird that set fire to itself and rose from its ashes every 500 years; a symbol of immortality.

phon /fɒn/ n a unit of loudness.

phonate /ˈfəʊneɪt/ vi to utter vocal sounds.—**phonation** n.

phone /fəʊn/ n, vti (inf) (to) telephone.

phone book n (inf) telephone book.

phone-in n a radio programme in which questions or comments by listeners are broadcast.

phonetic /fəˈnetɪk/ adj relating to, or representing, speech sounds.—**phonetically** adv.

phonetician /ˌfəʊnəˈtiːʃən/ n a student of, or expert in, phonetics.

phonetics /fəˈnetɪks/ n sing the science concerned with pronunciation and the representation of speech sounds.

phonetist /fəˈnetɪst/ n a phonetician; an advocate of phonetic spelling.

phoney, phony /ˈfəʊni/ adj (**phonier, phoniest**) (inf) not genuine. • n (pl **phoneys, phonies**) a fake; an insincere person.—**phoneyness, phoniness** n.

phonics /ˈfɒnɪks/ n sing a phonetics-based method of teaching reading.—**phonic** adj.

phonogram /ˈfəʊnəˌgræm/ n (phonetics) a written character representing a particular sound.

phonograph /ˈfəʊnəˌgræf/ n a device for reproducing sounds from a vinyl disc.

phonography /fəˈnɒɡrəfi/ n spelling based on pronunciation; a system of shorthand writing based on sound.

phonology /fəˈnɒlədʒi/ n (pl **phonologies**) the study of speech sounds and their development, and of the sound systems of language.—**phonological** adj.—**phonologist** n.

phony see **phoney**.

phosgene /ˈfɒzdʒiːn/ n a poisonous gas used in chemical warfare and in industry.

phosphate /ˈfɒsfeɪt/ n a compound of phosphorus.—**phosphatic** adj.

phosphene /ˈfɒsfiːn/ n the sensation of luminous rings seen when a closed eye is pressed.

phosphide /ˈfɒsfaɪd/ n a compound of phosphorus with another element.

phosphite /ˈfɒsfaɪt/ n a salt of phosphorous acid.

phosphorescence /ˌfɒsfəˈresəns/ n the property of giving off light without noticeable heat, as phosphorus does; such light.—**phosphorescent** adj.

phosphorous /ˈfɒsfərəs/ adj containing phosphorus in lower or higher proportions.

phosphorus /ˈfɒsfərəs/ n a highly reactive, poisonous nonmetallic element; a phosphorescent substance or body, esp one that glows in the dark.

photic /ˈfəʊtɪk/ adj of, or pertaining to, light.

photo /ˈfəʊtəʊ/ n (pl **photos**) a photograph.

photo- prefix light; a photographic process.

photocell /ˈfəʊtəʊˌsel/ n a photoelectric cell.

photochemical /ˌfəʊtəʊˈkem kəl/ adj of or relating to the effect of radiant energy, esp light.

photochemistry /ˌfəʊtəʊˈkemɪstri/ n the branch of chemistry concerned with the effect of radiant energy in producing chemical changes; photochemical properties or processes.

photocopy /ˈfəʊtəʊˌkɒpi/ n (pl **photocopies**) a photographic reproduction of written or printed work. • vt (**photocopying, photocopied**) to copy in this way.—**photocopier** n.

photoelectric cell /ˌfəʊtəʊɪˈlektrɪk-/ n a cell whose electrical properties are affected by light; any device in which light controls an electric circuit that operates a mechanical device, as for opening doors.—also **photocell**.

photoengraving /ˌfəʊtəʊɪnˈgreɪvɪŋ/ or /-ˈɛngreɪv-/ n any photomechanical process of making printing plates.

photo finish n the finish of a race where the decision on the winner has to be determined by a photograph as the contestants are so close; any race where the winning margin is small.

photogenic /ˌfəʊtəʊˈdʒenɪk/ or /-ˈdʒiːnɪk/ adj likely to look attractive in photographs; (biol) generating light.—**photogenically** adv.

photograph /ˈfəʊtəˌgræf/ n an image produced by photography.—also **photo**.

photographic adj of or like a photograph; minutely accurate like a photograph; (memory) capable of retaining facts, etc, after reading for only a brief time.—**photographically** adv.

photography /fəˈtɒgrəfi/ n the art or process of recording images permanently and visibly by the chemical action of light on sensitive material, producing prints, slides or film.—**photographer** n.

photogravure /ˌfəʊtəʊgrəˈvjʊr/ n a printing process using an intaglio plate photographically produced; printed matter so produced.

photojournalism /ˌfəʊtəʊˈdʒɜːnəˌlɪzəm/ n a form of news reporting in which the story is presented mainly through photographs.—**photojournalist** n.

photolithograph /ˌfəʊtəʊˈlɪθəˌgræf/ n a picture produced by photolithography.

photolithography /ˌfəʊtəʊlɪˈθɒgrəfi/ n (print) lithography using plates made from photographs.

photomechanical /ˌfəʊtəʊməˈkænɪkəl/ adj of or relating to a printing process that utilizes photography in plate-making.—**photomechanically** adv.

photometer /fəʊˈtɒmɪtər/ n an instrument for measuring the intensity of light.

photometry /fəʊˈtɒmɪtri/ n the area of physics concerned with the measurement of light; the use of a photometer.

photomicrograph /ˌfəʊtəʊˈmaɪkrəˌgræf/ n a photograph taken through a microscope.—**photomicrography** n.

photophobia /ˌfəʊtəʊˈfəʊbiə/ n (med) oversensivity (of the eyes) to light; (psychol) fear or, or aversion to, sunlight.

photosphere /ˈfəʊtəʊˌsfɪr/ n the surface of a star, esp the sun.

Photostat /ˈfəʊtəʊˌstæt/ n (trademark) a device for making photographic copies of documents, etc; a copy made in this way. • vt (often without cap) to copy in this way.—**Photostatic** adj.

photosynthesis /ˌfəʊtəʊˈsɪnθəsɪs/ n (bot) the process by which a green plant manufactures sugar from carbon dioxide and water in the presence of light.—**photosynthetic** adj.—**photosynthetically** adv.

photosynthesize /ˌfəʊtəʊˈsɪnθəsaɪz/ vti (plants, etc) to produce by or carry on photosynthesis.

phototelegraphy /ˌfəʊtəʊtɪˈlegrəfi/ n the telegraphic transmission of photographs and drawings.

phrasal /ˈfreɪzəl/ adj of or consisting of a phrase or phrases.—**phrasally** adv.

phrasal verb n (gram) a usu simple verb that combines with a preposition or adverb, or both, to convey a meaning more than the sum of its parts, eg come out.

phrase /freɪz/ n a group of words that does not contain a finite verb but which expresses a single idea by itself; a pointed saying; a high-flown expression; (mus) a short, distinct musical passage. • vt to express orally, put in words; (mus) to divide into melodic phrases.

phrase book n a book containing idiomatic expressions of a foreign language and their translations.

phraseogram /'freɪzɪəˌgræm/ *n* a shorthand symbol representing a phrase.

phraseology /ˌfreɪzɪ'ɒlədʒi/ *n* (*pl* **phraseologies**) mode of expression, wording; phrases used by a particular group.—**phraseological** *adj*.

phrasing /'freɪzɪŋ/ *n* the wording of a speech or a piece of writing; (*mus*) the division of a melodic line, etc, into musical phrases.

phrenetic *see* **frenetic**.

phrenic /'frenɪk/ *adj* (*anat*) of, or pertaining to, the diaphragm.

phrenology /frə'nɒlədʒi/ *n* the belief that intelligence and ability may be judged from the shape of a person's skull; study of the shape of the skull based on this belief.—**phrenological** *adj*.—**phrenologist** *n*.

phthisis /'fθaɪsɪs/ or /'θaɪsɪs/ *n* a wasting disease, *esp* tuberculosis of the lungs.

phycology /faɪ'kɒlədʒi/ *n* the study of algae.

phylactery /fɪ'læktəri/ *n* (*pl* **phylacteries**) (*Judaism*) a small case containing Hebrew texts, worn by Jewish men during prayers.

phyletic /faɪ'letɪk/ *adj* relating to the racial development of an animal or plant type.

phyllode /'fɪloːd/ *n* (*bot*) a flattened petiole with the functions of a leaf.

phyllotaxy /ˌfɪlo'tæksɪ/, **phyllotaxis** /-'tæksɪs/ *n* (*pl* **phyllotaxies, phyllotaxes**) (*bot*) the arrangement of leaves on a stem.

phylloxera /ˌfɪlɒk'siːrə/ or /fɪ'lɒksərə/ *n* (*pl* **phylloxeras, phylloxerae**) an insect which attacks vines.

phylogeny /faɪ'lɒdʒəni/, **phylogenesis** /ˌfaɪlo'dʒenəsɪs/ *n* (*pl* **phylogenies, phylogeneses**) (*biol*) the racial evolution of an animal or plant type.—**phylogenic, phylogenetic** *adj*.

phylum /'faɪləm/ *n* (*pl* **phyla**) a major division of the animal or plant kingdom.

physic /'fɪzɪk/ *vt* (**physicking, physicked**) (*arch*) to administer medicine to.

physical /'fɪzɪkəl/ *adj* relating to the world of matter and energy, the human body, or natural science. • *n* a general medical examination.—**physically** *adv*.

physical chemistry *n* the branch of chemistry concerned with the effect of chemical structure on physical properties and of physical changes brought about by chemical reactions.

physical education *n* education in fitness and cure of the body, stressing athletics and hygiene.

physical therapy *n* the treatment of disorders and disease by physical and mechanical means (as massage, exercise, water, heat, etc).—*also* **physiotherapy**.

physician /fɪ'zɪʃən/ *n* a doctor of medicine.

physicist /'fɪzɪsɪst/ *n* a specialist in physics.

physics /'fɪzɪks/ *n* the branch of science concerned with matter and energy and their interactions in the fields of mechanics, acoustics, optics, heat, electricity, magnetism, radiation, atomic structure and nuclear phenomena; the physical processes and phenomena of a particular system.

physio- /'fɪzɪoː/ *prefix* nature.

physiocrat /'fɪzɪoːˌkræt/ *n* a supporter of the doctrine of government according to a natural order based on land as the sole form of wealth.

physiognomy /ˌfɪzɪ'ɒnəmi/ *n* (*pl* **physiognomies**) the art of judging character from facial features; facial expression, face; physical features generally.—**physiognomic, physiognomical** *adj*.—**physiognomist** *n*.

physiography /ˌfɪzɪ'ɒgrəfi/ *n* the study of the earth's natural features, physical geography.—**physiographer** *n*.

physiology /ˌfɪzɪ'ɒlədʒi/ *n* the science of the functioning and processes of living organisms.—**physiological** *adj*.—**physiologist** *n*.

physiotherapy /ˌfɪzɪoː'θerəpi/ *n* physical therapy.—**physiotherapist** *n*.

physique /fɪ'ziːk/ *n* bodily structure and appearance; build.

phytogenesis /ˌfaɪto'dʒenəsɪs/, **phytogeny** /-'tɒdʒɪni/ *n* the study of plant evolution.

phyton /'faɪtən/ or /-tɒn/ *n* (*bot*) the smallest unit of a plant capable of growing into a new plant.

pi¹ /paɪ/ *n* the 16th letter of the Greek alphabet; (*math*) the Greek letter (π) used as a symbol for the ratio of the circumference to the diameter of a circle, approx. 3.14159.

pi² *n* (*pl* **pis**) (*print*) a jumble of type; any disorder. • *vt* to mix, disarrange (type). • *vi* to become mixed up.—*also* **pie**.

piacular /paɪ'ækjʊlər/ *adj* expiatory; sinful.

piaffe /piː'æf/ *n* (*dressage*) a slow trot.

pia mater /ˌpaɪə'meɪtər/ or /ˌpiːə-/ *n* (*anat*) the inner membrane enclosing the brain.

pianissimo /ˌpiəˈnɪsɪˌmoː/ *adv* (*mus*) very softly.

pianist /'piənɪst/ or /pi'ænɪst/, /'pjænɪst/ *n* a person who plays the piano.

piano /pi'ænoː/ or /'pjænoː/ *n* (*pl* **pianos**) a large stringed keyboard instrument in which each key operates a felt-covered hammer that strikes a corresponding steel wire or wires.

pianoforte /ˌpiænoː'fɔrteɪ/ *n* (*pl* **pianofortes**) a piano.

piastre, piaster /pi'æstər/ *n* a unit of currency in Egypt, Lebanon, Sudan, Syria and South Vietnam.

piazza /pi'ætsə/ or /pi'ɒtsə/ *n* in Italy, a public square; a covered walkway or gallery; a veranda.

pibroch /'piːbrɒx/ or /-brɒk/ *n* a kind of music composed for Scottish bagpipes.

pica /'paɪkə/ *n* (*print*) a standard measurement, equal to 12 points.

picaresque /ˌpɪkə'resk/ *adj* pertaining to a genre of fiction describing the exploits of rogues.

picaroon /ˌpɪkə'ruːn/ *n* (*arch*) a robber, pirate or marauder.

picayune /ˌpɪkə'juːn/ *adj* (*inf*) of little value.

piccalilli /ˌpɪkə'lɪli/ *n* a kind of pickle made with cauliflower, onions, etc.

piccolo /'pɪkəˌloː/ *n* (*pl* **piccolos**) a small shrill flute.

pick /pɪk/ *n* a heavy tool with a shaft and pointed crossbar for breaking ground; a tool for picking, such as a toothpick or icepick; a plectrum; right of selection; choice; best (of). • *vti* to break up or remove with a pick; to pluck at; to nibble (at), eat fussily; to contrive; to choose; (*fruit, etc*) to gather; to steal from a pocket; (*lock*) to force open; (*with* **up**) to lift; to acquire; to call for; to recover; (*inf*) to make the acquaintance of casually; to learn gradually; to resume; to give a lift to; to increase speed.

pickaback /'pɪkəˌbæk/ *see* **piggyback**.

pickaxe, pickax /'pɪkæks/ *n* (*pl* **pickaxes**) a pick with a long pointed head for breaking up hard ground, etc.

pickerel /'pɪkərəl/ or /'pɪkrəl/ *n* (*pl* **pickerel, pickerels**) a North American freshwater fish of the pike family.

picket /'pɪkət/ *n* a pointed stake; a patrol or group of men selected for a special duty; a person posted by strikes outside a place of work to persuade others not to enter. • *vt* (**picketing, picketed**) to tether to a picket; to post as a military picket; to place pickets, or serve as a picket (at a factory, etc).

pickings /'pɪkɪŋz/ *npl* gleanings, perquisites.

pickle /'pɪkəl/ *n* vegetables preserved in vinegar; (*inf*) a plight, mess. • *vt* to preserve in vinegar.

pickled /-d/ *adj* preserved in pickle; (*sl*) drunk.

picklock /'pɪklɒk/ *n* an instrument for picking locks; someone, *esp* a thief, who picks locks.

pick-me-up *n* a tonic.

pickpocket /'pɪkˌpɒkət/ *n* a person who steals from pockets.

pick-up /'pɪkʌp/ *n* the act of picking up; a person or thing picked up; (*elect*) a device for picking up current; the power to accelerate rapidly; the balanced arm of a record player; a pickup truck.

pickup truck *n* a light truck with an enclosed cab and open body.

picnic /'pɪknɪk/ *n* a *usu* informal meal taken on an excursion and eaten outdoors; an outdoor snack; the food so eaten; an easy or agreeable task. • *vi* (**picnicking, picnicked**) to have a picnic.—**picnicker** *n*.

picot /'piːkoː/ *n* a small loop of thread used as an edging to lace.

picotee /ˌpɪkəˌtiː/ or /ˌpɪkə'tiː/ *n* a type of small carnation.

picric acid *n* a toxic acid used as a dye and an explosive.

pictograph /'pɪktəˌgræf/ *n* a picture representing a word or idea.

pictorial /pɪk'tɔrɪəl/ *adj* relating to pictures, painting, or drawing; containing pictures; expressed in pictures; graphic.—**pictorially** *adv*.

picture /'pɪktʃər/ *n* drawing, painting, photography, or other visual representation; a scene; an impression or mental image; a vivid description; a cinema film. • *vt* to portray, describe in a picture; to visualize.

picturesque /ˌpɪktʃə'resk/ *adj* striking, vivid, usually pleasing; making an effective picture.—**picturesquely** *adv*.—**picturesqueness** *n*.

piddle /'pɪdəl/ *vt* to squander. • *vi* (*inf*) to idle; to urinate.

piddling /'pɪdlɪŋ/ *adj* (*inf*) trifling, insignificant.

piddock /'pɪdək/ *n* a bivalve, boring, shellfish.

pidgin /'pɪdʒɪn/ *n* a jargon for trade purposes, using words and grammar from two or more different languages.

pie¹ /paɪ/ *n* a baked dish of fruit, meat, etc, with an under or upper crust of pastry, or both.

pie² *see* **pi²**.

piebald /'paɪbɒld/ *adj* covered with patches of two colours. • *n* a piebald horse, etc.

piece /piːs/ *n* a distinct part of anything; a single object; a literary, dramatic, artistic, or musical composition; (*sl*) a firearm; a man in chess or draughts; an opinion, view; a short distance. • *vt* to fit together, join.—**piecer** *n*.

pièce de résistance /ˌpjɛsdəreɪ'ziːstãs/ *n* (*pl* **pièces de résistance**) the most important item or dish.

piecemeal /'piːsmiːl/ *adv* gradually; bit by bit.

piecework /'piːswɜrk/ *n* work paid for according to the quantity produced.

pied /paɪd/ *adj* of mixed colours, mottled

pied-à-terre /ˌpjeɪdə'teər/ *n* (*pl* **pieds-à-terre**) a flat for occasional use; a second home.

pier /piːr/ *n* a structure supporting the spans of a bridge; a structure built out over water and supported by pillars, used as a landing place, promenade, etc; a heavy column used to support weight.

pierce /piːrs/ *vt* to cut or make a hole through; to force a way into; (*fig*) to touch or move. • *vi* to penetrate.

piercing /'piːrsɪŋ/ *adj* penetrating; keen; (*cold, pain*) acute.—**piercingly** *adv*.

Pierrot /'pjeroː/ *n* (*pantomime*) a male character, *usu* in a loose white costume with a whitened face; a clown in such a costume.

Pietà /ˌpiːe'tɒ/ *n* a picture or sculpture of the Virgin mourning over the dead Christ.

piety /'paɪəti/ *n* (*pl* **pieties**) religious devoutness; the characteristic of being pious.

piezoelectricity /paɪˌiːzoːˌɪlɛk'trɪsɪti/ *n* the production of electricity in certain types of crystal through the application of mechanical stress.—**piezoeletric, piezoelectrical** *adj*.—**piezoelectrically** *adv*.

piffle /'pɪfəl/ *n* (*inf*) silly stuff, nonsense. • *vi* to talk nonsense.

pig /pɪg/ *n* a domesticated animal with a broad snout and fat body raised for food; a hog; a greedy or filthy person; an oblong casting of metal poured from the smelting furnace; (*sl*) a policeman. • *vi* (**pigging, pigged**) (*sow*) to give birth; (*inf*) to live in squalor.

pigeon /'pɪdʒən/ *n* a bird with a small head and a heavy body; (*inf*) a person who is easily conned.

pigeonhole /'pɪdʒən,hoːl/ *n* a small compartment for filing papers, etc; a category *usu* failing to reflect actual complexities. • *vt* to file, classify; to put aside for consideration, shelve.

pigeon-toed *adj* having the toes turned inward.

piggery /'pɪgəri/ *n* (*pl* **piggeries**) a place where pigs are reared; a pigsty.

piggish /'pɪgɪʃ/ *adj* greedy, dirty, selfish, like a pig.—**piggishly** *adv*.—**piggishness** *n*.

piggy /'pɪgi/ *n* (*pl* **piggies**) a child's name for a young or little pig. • *adj* (**piggier, piggiest**) piggish.

piggyback /'pɪgi,bæk/ *n* a ride on the shoulders or back of a person. • *adv* carried on the shoulders or back; transported on top of a larger object.—*also* **pickaback**.

piggy bank *n* a container for coins, often shaped like a pig.

pigheaded /pɪg'hedəd/ *adj* stupidly stubborn.—**pigheadedly** *adv*.—**pigheadedness** *n*.

piglet /'pɪglət/ *n* a young pig.

pigment /'pɪgmənt/ *n* paint; a naturally occurring substance used for colouring.—**pigmentary** *adj*.

pigmentation /ˌpɪgmən'teɪʃən/ *n* (*biol*) coloration of the tissues of plants and animals caused by pigment; the depositing of pigments by cells.

pigmy /'pɪgmi/ *see* **pygmy**.

pignut /'pɪgnʌt/ *n* an earthnut.

pigskin /'pɪgskɪn/ *n* leather made from the skin of a pig.

pigsticker /'pɪg,stɪkər/ *n* a person who goes pigsticking.

pigsticking /'pɪg,stɪkɪŋ/ *n* the hunting of wild boar with a spear, *usu* on horseback.

pigsty /'pɪgstaɪ/ *n* (*pl* **pigsties**) a pen for pigs; a dirty hovel.

pigtail /'pɪgteɪl/ *n* a tight braid of hair.—**pigtailed** *adj*.

pika /'paɪkə/ *n* ✸ a small rodent of mountains and deserts of western North America that has small ears and no tail.

pike¹ /paɪk/ *n* a sharp point or spike; the top of a spear. • *vt* to pierce or kill with a pike.

pike² *n* (*pl* **pike, pikes**) a long-snouted fish, important as a food and game fish.

pike perch *n* (**pike perch, pike perches**) any of various fishes of the perch family resembling the pike.

pike pole *n* ✸ (*Cdn*) a long pole with a pointed, hooked metal tip used for moving logs.

pikestaff /'paɪkstæf/ *n* the shaft of a pike.

pilaf, pilaff /'piːlæf/ *or* /pɪ'læf/ *n* a dish of spiced rice cooked in stock with, optionally, meat or fish.—*also* **pilau**.

pilaster /pɪ'læstər/ *n* a rectangular pillar, *usu* set in a wall.

pilch /pɪltʃ/ *n* (*arch*) a triangular flannel wrap for a baby.

pilchard /'pɪltʃərd/ *n* a fish of the herring family.

pile¹ /paɪl/ *n* a heap or mound of objects; a large amount; a lofty building; a pyre; (*sl*) a fortune. • *vt* (*with* **up, on**) to heap or stack; to load; to accumulate. • *vi* to become heaped up; (*with* **up, out, on**) to move confusedly in a mass.

pile² *n* a vertical beam driven into (the ground) as a foundation for a building, etc. • *vt* to support with piles; to drive piles into.

pile³ *n* the nap of a fabric or carpet; soft, fine fur or wool.

pileate /'pɪliːˌeɪt/, **pileated** /ˌpɪliːˌeɪtəd/ *adj* (*biol*) crested.

piledriver /'paɪl,draɪvər/ *n* a machine for driving in piles.

piles /paɪlz/ *npl* haemorrhoids.

pile-up /'paɪlʌp/ *n* an accumulation of tasks, etc; (*inf*) a collision of several vehicles.

pilfer /'pɪlfər/ *vti* to steal in small quantities.—**pilferage** *n*.—**pilferer** *n*.

pilgrim /'pɪlgrɪm/ *n* a person who makes a pilgrimage.

pilgrimage /-ɪdʒ/ *n* a journey to a holy place as an act of devotion; any long journey; a life's journey.

piliferous /pɪ'lɪfərəs/ *adj* (*esp bot*) hairy.

piliform /'pɪlɪfɔrm/ *adj* (*bot*) in the form of or like a hair.

pill /pɪl/ *n* medicine in round balls or tablet form; (*with cap*) an oral contraceptive.

pillage /'pɪlɪdʒ/ *n* looting, plunder. • *vti* to plunder, *esp* during war.—**pillager** *n*.

pillar /'pɪlər/ *n* a slender, vertical structure used as a support or ornament; a column; a strong supporter of a cause.

pillar box *n* in UK, a mailbox in the shape of a pillar.

pillbox /'pɪlbɒks/ *n* a box for pills, *esp* a decorative one; a small round hat without a brim; (*mil*) a small, fortified, concrete shelter.

pillion /'pɪljən/ *n* a seat behind the driver for a passenger on a motorcycle, etc.

pillory /'pɪləri/ *n* (*pl* **pillories**) (*formerly*) stocks in which criminals were put as punishment. • *vt* (**pillorying, pilloried**) to expose to public scorn and ridicule.

pillow /'pɪloː/ *n* a cushion that supports the head during sleep; something that supports to equalize or distribute pressure. • *vti* to rest on, serve as, a pillow.

pillowcase /-ˌkeɪs/, **pillowslip** /-ˌslɪp/ *n* a removable cover for a pillow.

pilose /'paɪloːz/ *adj* (*biol*) hairy.

pilot /'paɪlət/ *n* a person who operates an aircraft; one who directs ships in and out of harbour; a guide; a television show produced as a sample of a proposed series. • *vt* to direct the course of, act as pilot; to lead or guide.

pilotage /-ɪdʒ/ *n* the work or fee of a pilot.

pilot light *n* a burning gas flame used to light a larger jet; an electric indicator light.

pilule /'pɪljuːl/ *n* a small pill.—**pilular** *adj*.

pimento /pɪ'mentoː/ *n* (*pl* **pimentos**) allspice; a pimiento.

pimiento /ˌpɪmi'entoː/ *or* /pɪ'mjentoː/ *n* a sweet red pepper (*capsicum*) used in salads and cooked dishes.

pimp /pɪmp/ *n* a prostitute's agent.—*also* *vt*.

pimpernel /'pɪmpər,nɛl/ *n* a primulaceous plant with small scarlet, blue or white flowers.

pimple /'pɪmpəl/ *n* a small, raised, inflamed swelling of the skin.—**pimpled** *adj*.

pimply /'pɪmpli/ *adj* (**pimplier, pimpliest**) covered with pimples.

PIN /pɪn/ *abbr* = Personal Identification Number (issued by a bank to a customer to validate electronic transactions).

pin /pɪn/ *n* a piece of metal or wood used to fasten things together; a small piece of pointed wire with a head; an ornament or badge with a pin or clasp for fastening to clothing; (*bowling*) one of the clubs at which the ball is rolled. • *vt* (**pinning, pinned**) to fasten with a pin; to hold, fix; (*with* **down**) to get (someone) to commit himself or herself as to plans, etc; (*a fact, etc*) to establish.

pinafore /ˈpɪnəˌfɔr/ n a sleeveless garment worn over a dress, blouse, etc.

pinaster /ˈpɪnæstər/ n a Southern European pine tree.

pince-nez /ˈpænsneɪ/ or /ˈpæsˈneɪ/ n (pl **pince-nez**) eyeglasses clipped to the nose by a spring.

pincers /ˈpɪnsərz/ npl a tool with two handles and jaws used for gripping and drawing out nails, etc; a grasping claw, as of a crab.

pinch /pɪntʃ/ vti to squeeze or compress painfully; to press between the fingers; to nip; (sl) to steal; (sl) to arrest. • n a squeeze or nip; what can be taken up between the finger and thumb, a small amount; a time of stress; an emergency.

pinchbeck /ˈpɪntʃbek/ n a copper and zinc alloy, used as imitation gold.

pinched /ˈpɪntʃt/ adj appearing to be squeezed; drawn by cold or stress.

pincushion /ˈpɪnˌkʊʃən/ n a pad for holding pins.

Pindaric /pɪnˈdærɪk/ adj (ode) associated with the poet Pindar.

pine¹ /paɪn/ n an evergreen coniferous tree with long needles and well-formed cones; a tree of the pine family; its wood.

pine² vi to languish, waste away through longing or mental stress; (with **for**) to yearn.

pineal gland /ˈpɪniəl/ or /ˈpaɪniəl/ n a pea-sized gland in the brain.

pineapple /ˈpaɪnˌæpəl/ n a tropical plant; its juicy, fleshy, yellow fruit.

pinfold /ˈpɪnfoːld/ n a pound for stray cattle. • vt to shut into, or as if into, such a pound.

ping /pɪŋ/ n a high-pitched ringing sound. • vti to strike with a ping, emit a ping.—**pinger** n.

ping-pong /ˈpɪŋpɒŋ/ n a name for table tennis; (with caps) (trademark) table tennis equipment.

pingo /ˈpɪŋgoː/ n ✷ (pl **pingos**) a dome-shaped mound of ice covered by soil found in the Arctic.

pinion¹ /ˈpɪnjən/ n the outer joint of a bird's wing; a wing feather. • vt to cut off a pinion; to bind arms to sides, restrain.

pinion² n a cogwheel.

pink¹ /pɪŋk/ n any of various garden plants with a fragrant flower, including carnations; a pale red colour; a huntsman's red coat; the highest type. • adj pink-coloured; (inf) radical in political views.

pink² vt to stab, pierce; (cloth, etc) to cut a zigzag edge on; to perforate with pinking shears.

pinkeye /ˈpɪŋkaɪ/ n an inflammation of the conjunctiva, affecting animals and humans.

pinkie, pinky /ˈpɪŋki/ n (pl **pinkies**) the little finger on the human hand.

pinking shears npl shears with notched edges for pinking edges of cloth.

pin money n money given to a woman by her husband for personal expenses.

pinna /ˈpɪnə/ n (pl **pinnae, pinnas**) (biol) the fin of a fish; the feather or wing of a bird; the leaflet of a pinnate leaf.

pinnace /ˈpɪnəs/ n (naut) a small light schooner-rigged vessel with oars; an eight-oared small boat belonging to a warship.

pinnacle /ˈpɪnəkəl/ n a slender tower crowning a roof, etc; a rocky peak of a mountain; the highest point, climax.

pinnate /ˈpɪneɪt/, **pinnated** /-əd/ adj shaped like a feather; (leaf) divided into leaflets.

pinniped /ˈpɪnɪˌped/ adj (zool) with fin-like feet or flippers.

pinny /ˈpɪni/ n (pl **pinnies**) (sl) a pinafore.

pinochle, pinocle /ˈpiːˌnʊkəl/ n a card game.—also **pinuchle**.

pinpoint /ˈpɪnpɔɪnt/ vt to locate or identify very exactly.

pinprick /ˈpɪnprɪk/ n a small puncture as made by a pin; a trivial annoyance.

pins and needles npl a tingling feeling in the fingers, toes, etc, caused by impeded blood circulation returning to normal; (with **on**) in an anxious or expectant state.

pinstripe /ˈpɪnstraɪp/ n a very narrow stripe in suit fabrics, etc.

pint /paɪnt/ n a liquid measure equal to half a quart or one eighth of a gallon (0.47 litres); (inf) a drink of beer.

pintail /ˈpɪnteɪl/ n (pl **pintails, pintail**) a type of duck.

pintle /ˈpɪntəl/ n a bolt or pin esp comprising a pivot.

pinto /ˈpɪntoː/ n (pl **pintos**) a piebald horse.

pinuchle see **pinochle**.

pin-up n (sl) a photograph of a naked or partially naked person; a person who has been so photographed; a photograph of a famous person.

pioneer /ˌpaɪəˈniːr/ n a person who initiates or explores new areas of enterprise, research, etc; an explorer; an early settler; (mil) one who prepares roads, sinks mines, etc. • vti to initiate or take part in the development of; to act as a pioneer (to); to explore (a region).

pious /ˈpaɪəs/ adj devout; religious; sanctimonious.—**piously** adv.—**piousness** n.

pip¹ /pɪp/ n the seed in a fleshy fruit, eg apple, orange.

pip² n a spot with a numerical value on a playing card, dice, etc; (inf) insignia on a uniform showing an officer's rank; a signal on a radar screen.

pip³ vi (**pipping, pipped**) (bird) to chirp, to peep; (hatching bird) to pierce (its shell).

pipal see **peepul**.

pipe /paɪp/ n a tube of wood, metal etc for making musical sounds; (pl) the bagpipes; a stem with a bowl for smoking tobacco; a long tube or hollow body for conveying water, gas, etc. • vt to play on a pipe; (gas, water, etc) to convey by pipe; to lead, summon with the sound of a pipe(s); to trim with piping. • vi (sl) to take the drug crack.

pipeclay /ˈpaɪpkleɪ/ n a white clay, used to make tobacco pipes and to whiten leather, etc. • vt to whiten using pipeclay.

pipeline /ˈpaɪplaɪn/ n a pipe (often underground) used to convey oil, gas, etc; a direct channel for information; the processes through which supplies pass from source to user.

piper /ˈpaɪpər/ n a person who plays a pipe, esp bagpipes.

pipette, pipet /paɪˈpet/ or /pɪ-/ n a hollow glass tube into which liquids are sucked for measurement.

piping /ˈpaɪpɪŋ/ n a length of pipe, pipes collectively; a tube-like fold of material used to trim seams; a strip of icing, cream, for decorating cakes, etc; the art of playing a pipe or bagpipes; a high-pitched sound. • adj making a high-pitched sound.

piping hot adj very hot.

pipistrelle, pipistrel /ˌpɪpɪˈstrel/ n a small brown bat.

pipit /ˈpɪpɪt/ n a type of songbird.

pipkin /ˈpɪpkɪn/ n a small earthenware pot.

pippin /ˈpɪpɪn/ n one of several types of eating apple.

pipsqueak /ˈpɪpskwiːk/ n (inf) a contemptible or insignificant person.

piquant /piːˈkænt/ or /-ˈkɒnt/, /ˈpiːkænt/ adj strong-tasting; pungent, sharp; stimulating.—**piquancy** n.—**piquantly** adv.

pique /piːk/ n resentment, ill-feeling. • vt (**piquing, piqued**) to cause resentment in; to offend.

piqué /piːˈkeɪ/ n a corded cotton fabric.

piquet /pɪˈket/ n a card game for two.

piracy /ˈpaɪrəsi/ n (pl **piracies**) robbery at sea; the hijacking of a ship or aircraft; infringement of copyright; unauthorized use of patented work.

piragua /pɪˈrɒgwə/ or /-ˈrægwə/ see **pirogue**.

piranha /pɪˈrɒnə/ or /-ˈrænə/ n a small voracious freshwater fish of tropical America with sharp teeth and a strong jaw.

pirate /ˈpaɪrət/ n a person who commits robbery at sea; a hijacker; one who infringes copyright. • vti to take by piracy; to publish or reproduce in violation of a copyright.—**piratical, piratic** adj.

pirogue /pɪˈroːg/ n a dugout canoe.—also **piragua**.

pirouette /ˌpɪruˈet/ n a spin on the toes in ballet.—also vi.

piscatorial /ˌpɪskəˈtɔriəl/, **piscatory** /ˈpɪskətɒri/ adj of, or pertaining to, fish or fishing.

Pisces /ˈpaɪsiːz/ n the Fishes, in astrology the twelfth sign of the zodiac, operative from 19 February-20 March.—**Piscean** adj, n.

pisciculture /ˈpɪsɪˌkʌltʃər/ n the controlled rearing and breeding of fish.—**piscicultural** adj.—**pisciculturist** n.

piscina /pɪˈsiːnə/ or /-ˈsaɪnə/ n (pl **piscinae, piscinas**) (RC Church) a basin with a drain in a church wall, used for rinsing sacred vessels after Mass.

piscine /ˈpɪsaɪn/ adj pertaining to fish.

piscivorous /pɪˈsɪvərəs/ adj fish-eating.

pisiform /ˈpɪsɪˌfɔrm/ adj pea-shaped.

pismire /ˈpɪsˌmaɪr/ n an ant.

piss /pɪs/ vi (vulg sl) to urinate. • n urine.

pistachio /pɪˈstæʃioː/ n (pl **pistachios**) a tree found in Mediterranean countries and West Asia; the edible nut of this tree.

piste /piːst/ n a ski trail of packed snow; (fencing) the rectangular area where a bout takes place.

pistil /ˈpɪstɪl/ n the seed-bearing part of a flower.

pistillate /ˈpɪstɪlət/ adj (bot) having a pistil; with a pistil but no stamens.

pistol /'pɪstəl/ n a small, short-barrelled handgun. • vt (**pistolling, pistolled** or **pistoling, pistoled**) to shoot with a pistol.

pistole /pɪ'stoːl/ n (formerly) a gold coin used in Europe.

piston /'pɪstən/ n a disc that slides to and fro in a close-fitting cylinder, as in engines, pumps.

pit /pɪt/ n a deep hole in the earth; a (coal) mine; a scooped-out place for burning something; a sunken or depressed area below the adjacent floor area; a space at the front of the stage for the orchestra; the area in a securities or commodities exchange in which members do the trading; the scar left by smallpox, etc; the stone of a fruit; a place where racing cars refuel • vti (**pitting, pitted**) to set in competition; to mark or become marked with pits; to make a pit stop.

pit-a-pat /'pɪtə,pæt/ adv with quick, light steps or beats. • n quick, light steps or beats. • vi (**pit-a-patting, pit-a-patted**) to make quick, light steps or beats.

pitch[1] /pɪtʃ/ vti (tent, etc) to erect by driving pegs, stakes, etc, into the ground; to set the level of; (mus) to set in key; to express in a style; to throw, hurl; to fall heavily, plunge, esp forward. • n a throw; height, intensity; a musical tone; a place where a street trader or performer works; distance between threads (of a screw); amount of slope; a sound wave frequency; a sports field; (cricket) the area between the wickets; sales talk.

pitch[2] n the black, sticky substance from distillation of tar, etc; any of various bituminous substances. • vt to smear with pitch.

pitch-black /'pɪtʃ'blæk/ adj black, or extremely dark.

pitchblende /'pɪtʃblend/ n a black mineral, composed largely of uranium oxide, that also yields radium.

pitch-dark /'pɪts'dark/ adj completely dark.

pitcher /'pɪtʃər/ n a large water jug; (baseball) the player who pitches the ball.

pitchfork /'pɪtʃfork/ n a long-handled fork for tossing hay, etc. • vt to lift with this; to thrust suddenly or willy-nilly into.

pitchy /'pɪtʃi/ adj (**pitchier, pitchiest**) resembling, or smeared with, pitch.

piteous /'pɪtɪəs/ adj arousing pity; heart-rending.—**piteously** adv.—**piteousness** n.

pitfall /'pɪtfɔːl/ n concealed danger; unexpected difficulty.

pith /pɪθ/ n the soft tissue inside the rind of citrus fruits; the gist, essence; importance.

pithy /'pɪθi/ adj (**pithier, pithiest**) like or full of pith; concise and full of meaning.—**pithily** adv.—**pithiness** n.

pitiable /'pɪtɪəbəl/ adj deserving pity, lamentable, wretched.—**pitiableness** n.—**pitiably** adv.

pitiful /'pɪtɪ,ful/ adj causing pity, touching; contemptible, paltry.—**pitifully** adv.—**pitifulness** n.

pitiless /'pɪtɪləs/ or /'pɪtɪ-/ adj without pity, ruthless.—**pitilessly** adv.—**pitilessness** n.

pitman /'pɪtmən/ n (pl **pitmen**) a miner.

pittance /'pɪtəns/ n a very small quantity or allowance of money.

pituitary /pɪ'tuːɪterɪ/ or /-'tjuː-/ adj of or pertaining to the pituitary gland; (arch) of or secreting mucus. • n (pl **pituitaries**) the pituitary gland.

pituitary gland n a ductless gland at the base of the brain that affects growth and sexual development.

pity /'pɪti/ n (pl **pities**) sympathy with the distress of others; a cause of grief; a regrettable fact. • vt (**pitying, pitied**) to feel pity for.—**pityingly** adv.

pityriasis /,pɪtə'raɪəsɪs/ n (pl **pityriases**) a skin disease characterized by scaly, pink eruptions.

pivot /'pɪvət/ n a pin on which a part turns, fulcrum; a key person upon whom progress depends; a cardinal point or factor. • vt to turn or hinge (on) a pivot; to attach by a pivot. • vi to run on, or as if on, a pivot.—**pivotal** adj.

pixel /'pɪksəl/ n any of the tiny units that form an image (as on a television screen, computer monitor).

pixie, pixy /'pɪksi/ n (pl **pixies**) a fairy or elf.

pixilated /'pɪksə,leɪtɪd/ adj acting as if influenced by pixies; unconventional, eccentric, whimsical; (sl) drunk.

pizza /'piːtsə/ n a baked dough crust covered with cheese, tomatoes, etc.

pizzeria /,piːtsə'riːə/ n a pizza restaurant.

pizzicato /,pɪtsɪ'kæto:/ or /-'koto:/ n (pl **pizzicati, pizzicatos**) (mus) a note or passage played by plucking the string of a violin or other bowed instrument.—also adj.

placable /'plækəbəl/ adj easily to placate.—**placability** n.

placard /'plækɑːd/ or /-kərd/ n a poster or notice for public display.

placate /plə'keɪt/ or /'plæ-/, "pleɪ-/ vt to appease; to pacify.—**placation** n.—**placatory** adj.

place /pleɪs/ n a locality, spot; a town or village; a building, residence; a short street, a square; space, room; a particular point, part, position, etc; the part of space occupied by a person or thing; a position or job; a seat; rank, precedence; a finishing position in a race. • vt to put; to put in a particular place; to find a place or seat for; to identify; to estimate; to rank; (order) to request material from a supplier. • vi to finish second or among the first three in a race.

placebo /plə'siːboː/ n (pl **placebos, placeboes**) something harmless given by a doctor to fool a patient into thinking he is undergoing treatment.

place mat /'pleɪsmæt/ n a small mat serving as an individual table cover for a person at a meal.

placement /'pleɪsmənt/ n a placing or being placed; location or arrangement.

place name n the name of a geographical locality.

placenta /plə'sentə/ n (pl **placentas, placentae**) the organ in the uterus of a female mammal that nourishes the foetus.—**placental** adj.

placer /'plæsər/ n a deposit containing a valuable mineral found in a river, etc.

placid /'plæsɪd/ adj calm, tranquil.—**placidity** n.—**placidly** adv.

placket /'plækət/ n a slit at the waist of a dress or skirt to make it easy to put on or take off.

placoid /'plækɔɪd/ adj platelike.

plafond Fr. /pla'fɔ̃:/ n a ceiling, esp one of elaborate design; a card game.

plagal /'pleɪgəl/ adj (musical composition) having its principal notes between the fifth of the key and its octave.

plagiarism /'pleɪdʒə,rɪzəm/ n the act of stealing from another author's work, literary theft; that which is plagiarized.—**plagiarist** n.—**plagiaristic** adj.

plagiarize /'pleɪdʒə,raɪz/ vt to appropriate writings from another author.—**plagiarizer** n.

plague /pleɪg/ n a highly contagious and deadly disease; (inf) a person who is a nuisance. • vt (**plaguing, plagued**) to afflict with a plague; (inf) to annoy, harass.

plaguy, plaguey /'pleɪgi/ adj (arch) (inf) troublesome, vexatious.

plaice /pleɪs/ n (pl **plaice, plaices**) any of various flatfishes, esp a flounder.

plaid /plæd/ n a long wide piece of woollen cloth used as a cloak in Highland dress; cloth with a tartan or chequered pattern.

plain /pleɪn/ adj level, flat; understandable; straightforward; manifest, obvious; blunt; unadorned; not elaborate; not coloured or patterned; not beautiful; ugly; pure; unmixed. • n a large tract of level country.—**plainness** n.

plain clothes npl ordinary clothes, not uniform, as worn by a policeman on duty.—also adj.

plainly /-li/ adv clearly, intelligibly.

plain sailing n easy progress over an unobstructed course.

plainsman /'pleɪnzmən/ n (pl **plainsmen**) an inhabitant of a plain.

plainsong /'pleɪnsɒŋ/ n an old, plain kind of church music chanted in unison.

plain-spoken /'pleɪn'spoːkən/ adj frank, outspoken.

plaint /pleɪnt/ n (poet) lamentation, sad song; (law) formal statement of grievance.

plaintiff /'pleɪntɪf/ n (law) a person who brings a civil action against another.

plaintive /'pleɪntɪv/ adj sad, mournful.—**plaintively** adv.—**plaintiveness** n.

plait /plæt/ n intertwined strands of hair, straw, etc; a pigtail. • vti (**plaiting, plaited**) to twist strands (of hair) together into a plait.

plan /plæn/ n a scheme or idea; a drawing to scale of a building; a diagram, map; any outline or sketch. • vti (**planning, planned**) to make a plan of; to design; to arrange beforehand; intend; to make plans.

planar /'pleɪnər/ adj of or located in a plane; flat.

planarian /plə'neriən/ n a type of flatworm.

planchet /'plænʃət/ n a plain metal disc from which a coin is made.

planchette /plæn'ʃet/ n a heart-shaped board on wheels, holding a pencil which is supposed to write automatically, giving messages from spirits, when a hand is rested upon it.

plane[1] /pleɪn/ n a tall tree with large broad leaves.

plane² n a tool with a steel blade for smoothing level wooden surfaces. • vt to smooth with a plane.

plane³ n any level or flat surface; a level of attainment; one of the main supporting surfaces of an aeroplane; an aeroplane. • adj flat or level. • vi to fly while keeping the wings motionless; to skim across the surface of water; to travel by aeroplane.

planet /'plænət/ n a celestial body that orbits the sun or other star.

planetarium /,plænə'teriəm/ n (pl **planetariums, planetaria**) a machine used to exhibit the planets, their motions around the sun and their relative distances and magnitudes; a building for housing this instrument; a model of the solar system.

planetary /'plænə,teri/ adj (astrol) under the influence of one of the planets; terrestrial; wandering, erratic.

planetoid /'plænə,tɔɪd/ n an asteroid.

plangent /'plændʒənt/ adj (sound) loud and deep; resounding.— **plangency** n.

planimeter /plə'nɪmɪtər/ n an instrument for measuring the area of an irregular plane figure.

planimetry /-tri/ n the measurement of plane figures.

planish /'plænɪʃ/ vt (metal) to smooth and flatten with a hammer or between rollers.

planisphere /'plænɪ,sfiːr/ n a sphere projected on a plane or a map of the heavens.

plank /plæŋk/ n a long, broad, thick board; one of the policies forming the platform of a political party. • vt to cover with planks.

planking /'plæŋkɪŋ/ n planks collectively; the act of laying boards.

plankton /'plæŋktən/ n the microscopic organisms that float on seas, lakes, etc.

planner /'plænər/ n a person who plans; in UK, an official who plans architectural development and land use.—**planning** n.

planoconcave /,pleɪnoː'kɒnkeɪv/ or /-'keɪv/ adj (lens) with one side flat and the other concave.

planoconvex /,pleɪnoː'kɒnveks/ or /-'veks/ adj (lens) with one side flat and the other convex.

plant /plænt/ n a living organism with cellulose cell walls, which synthesizes its food from carbon dioxide, water and light; a soft-stemmed organism of this kind, as distinguished from a tree or shrub; the machinery, buildings, etc of a factory, etc; (sl) an act of planting; (sl) something or someone planted. • vt (seeds, cuttings) to put into the ground to grow; to place firmly in position; to found or establish; (sl) to conceal something in another's possession in order to implicate.

plantain¹ /'plæn'teɪn/ or /'plæn-/ n a low-growing weed with tough leaves.

plantain² n a tropical broad-leaved tree yielding an edible fruit similar to the banana.

plantar /'plæntər/ adj (anat) pertaining to the sole of the foot.

plantation /plæn'teɪʃən/ n a large cultivated planting of trees; an estate where tea, rubber, cotton, etc, is grown, cultivated by local labour.

planter /'plæntər/ n a person who owns or runs a plantation; a machine that plants; a decorative container for plants.

plantigrade /'plæntɪ,greɪd/ adj (zool) walking on the sole of the foot. • n a plantigrade animal.

plaque /plæk/ n an ornamental tablet or disc attached to or inserted in a surface; a film of mucus on the teeth that harbours bacteria.

plash /plæʃ/ n a splash; a marshy pool or puddle.—**plashy** adj (**plashier, plashiest**).

plasm /'plæzəm/ n a kind of protoplasm; plasma.

plasma /'plæzmə/ n the colourless liquid part of blood, milk, or lymph; a collection of charged particles resembling gas but conducting electricity and affected by a magnetic field.

plasmodium /plæz'moːdiəm/ n (pl **plasmodia**) (biol) a mass of protoplasm formed by the union of single-cell organisms; (med) any of a genus of parasitic protozoa which cause malaria.

plasmolysis /plæz'mɒlɪsɪs/ n (biol) the shrinkage of the protoplasm of a plant cell occurring as a result of loss of water.

plasmolyze /'plæzmoː,laɪz/ vt to subject to plasmolysis.

plaster /'plæstər/ n an adhesive dressing for cuts; a mixture of sand, lime and water that sets hard and is used for covering walls and ceilings. • vt to cover as with plaster; to apply like a plaster; to make lie smooth and flat; to load to excess.—**plasterer** n.

plasterboard /'plæstər,bɔrd/ n a thin board formed by layers of plaster and paper, used in wide sheets for walls, etc.

plaster cast n a rigid dressing of gauze impregnated with plaster of Paris; a sculptor's model in plaster of Paris.

plastered /'plæstərd/ adj (sl) intoxicated.

plaster of Paris n gypsum and water made into a quick-setting paste.

plastic¹ /'plæstɪk/ adj able to be moulded; pliant; made of plastic; (art) relating to modelling or moulding. • n any of various non-metallic compounds, synthetically produced, that can be moulded, cast, squeezed, drawn, or laminated into objects, films, or filaments.—**plastically** adv.

plastic² n colloquial term for charge cards, store cards, credit cards etc. used to pay for goods and services instead of cash.

plasticity /-'stɪsɪti/ n the ability to be moulded or altered; the ability to retain a shape attained by pressure deformation.

plastic surgery n surgery to repair deformed or destroyed parts of the body.

plastron /'plæstrən/ n a breastplate; a trimming on a dress front; a shirt front; a bony plate on the underside of a tortoise or turtle.

plat /plæt/ n (US) a small plot of ground; a map, esp of land divided into lots for building. • vt (**platting, platted**) to make a map of.

platan /'plætən/ n a plane tree.

plate /pleɪt/ n a flat sheet of metal on which an engraving is cut; an illustration printed from it; a full-page illustration separate from text; a sheet of metal photographically prepared with text, etc, for printing from; a sheet of glass with sensitized film used as a photographic negative; a trophy as prize at a race; a coating of metal on another metal; utensils plated in silver or gold; plated ware; a flat shallow dish from which food is eaten; a helping of food; the part of a denture that fits the palate; (inf) a denture. • vt (a metal) to coat with a thin film of another metal; to cover with metal plates.

plateau /plæ'toː/ n (pl **plateaus, plateaux**) a flat, elevated area of land; a stable period; a graphic representation showing this.

plated /'pleɪtɪd/ adj coated with metal, esp silver or gold.

plate glass n rolled, ground, and polished sheet glass.

platelet /'pleɪtlət/ n a small disc-shaped cell in the blood involved in the process of blood clotting.

platen /'plætən/ n the roller on a typewriter; (print) a plate which presses the paper against the type.

plater /'pleɪtər/ n someone who, or something which, plates; a mediocre racehorse.

platform /'plætfɔrm/ n a raised floor for speakers, musicians, etc; a stage; a place or opportunity for public discussion; the raised area next to a railway line where passengers board trains; a statement of political aims.

plating /'pleɪtɪŋ/ n the act or process of plating; a thin coating of metal; a coating of metal plates.

platinize /'plætɪ,naɪz/ vt to coat with platinum.

platinum /'plætɪnəm/ n a valuable, silvery-white metal used for jewellery, etc.

platinum-blond adj (hair) silvery blond. • n someone with hair of this colour.—**platinum-blonde** nf.

platitude /'plætɪtuːd/ or /-'tjuːd/ n a dull truism; a commonplace remark.—**platitudinous** adj.

platitudinize /-'tuːdɪ,naɪz/ or /-'tjuːdɪ-/ vi to utter platitudes.

platonic /plə'tɒnɪk/ adj (love) spiritual and free from physical desire; (with cap) relating to Plato, the Greek philosopher, or his teachings.—**platonically** adv.

platoon /plə'tuːn/ n a military unit divided into squads or sections.

platter /'plætər/ n an oval flat serving dish.

platy /'plæti/ - prefix flat.

platyhelminth /,plæti'helmɪnθ/ n a type of flatworm.

platypus /'plætɪpəs/ or /-pʊs/ n (pl **platypuses**) a small aquatic egg-laying mammal of Australia and Tasmania, with webbed feet, a bill like a duck's, dense fur, and a broad flat tail.—also **duck-billed platypus**.

platyrrhine /'plætɪ,raɪn/ **platyrrhinian** adj (zool) broad-nosed.

plaudit /'plɔdɪt/ n (usu pl) a commendation; a round of applause.

plausible /'plɔzɪbəl/ adj apparently truthful or reasonable.— **plausibility** n.—**plausibly** adv.

play /pleɪ/ vi to amuse oneself (with toys, games, etc); to act carelessly or trifle (with somebody's feelings); to gamble; to act on the stage or perform on a musical instrument; (light) to flicker, shimmer; (water) to discharge or direct on. • vt to participate in a sport; to be somebody's opponent in a game; to perform a dramatic production; (instrument) to produce music on; (hose) to direct; (fish) to give line to; to bet on. • n fun, amusement; the playing of, or manner of playing, a game; the duration of a game; a literary work for performance by actors; gambling; scope, freedom to move.—**playable** adj.

playact /'pleɪ,ækt/ *vi* to behave affectedly or overdramatically; to make believe, pretend; to act in a play.—**playacting** *n.*—**playactor** *n.*

playback /'pleɪbæk/ *n* the act of reproducing recorded sound or pictures, *esp* soon after they are made; a mechanism in an audio or video recorder for doing this.—*also vt.*

playbill /'pleɪbɪl/ *n* a poster advertising a theatrical performance.

playboy /'pleɪbɔɪ/ *n* a person who lives for pleasure

player /'pleɪər/ *n* a person who plays a specified game or instrument; an actor.

playfellow /'pleɪ,fɛloː/ *see* **playmate**.

playful /'pleɪful/ *adj* full of fun; humorous; sportive; fond of sport or amusement.—**playfully** *adv.*—**playfulness** *n.*

playgoer /'pleɪ,goːər/ *n* a person who goes to the theatre, *esp* one who attends frequently or regularly.—**playgoing** *adj, n.*

playground /'pleɪgraʊnd/ *n* an area outdoors for children's recreation.

playhouse /'pleɪhaʊs/ *n* a theatre.

playing card *n* one of a set of 52 cards used for playing games, each card having an identical pattern on one side and its own symbol on the reverse.

playing field *n* a place for playing sport.

playlet /'pleɪlət/ *n* a short play.

playmate /'pleɪmeɪt/ *n* a friend in play.—*also* **playfellow**.

playpen /'pleɪpən/ *n* a portable *usu* collapsible enclosure in which a young child may be left to play safely.

plaything /'pleɪθɪŋ/ *n* a toy; a thing or person treated as a toy.

playtime /'pleɪtaɪm/ *n* a time for recreation, *esp* at a school.

playwright /'pleɪraɪt/ *n* a writer of plays.

plaza /'plæzə/ *n* a public square in a town or city; (*US*) an area for the parking and servicing of cars.

plea /pliː/ *n* (*law*) an answer to a charge, made by the accused person; a request; an entreaty.

plead /pliːd/ *vti* (**pleading, pleaded, plead** *or* **pled**) to beg, implore; to give as an excuse; to answer (guilty or not guilty) to a charge; to argue (a law case).—**pleadable** *adj.*—**pleader** *n.*

pleading /'pliːdɪŋ/ *n* advocacy of a cause in a court of law; one of the allegations and counter allegations made alternately, *usu* in writing, by the parties in a legal action; the act or instance of making a plea; a sincere entreaty. • *adj* begging, imploring.—**pleadingly** *adv.*

pleasant /'plɛzənt/ *adj* agreeable; pleasing.—**pleasantly** *adv.*—**pleasantness** *n.*

pleasantry /'plɛzəntri/ *n* (*pl* **pleasantries**) a polite or amusing remark.

please /pliːz/ *vti* to satisfy; to give pleasure to; to be willing; to have the wish. • *adv* as a word to express politeness or emphasis in a request; an expression of polite affirmation.

pleased /pliːzd/ *adj* gratified.

pleasing /'pliːzɪŋ/ *adj* giving pleasure; agreeable.—**pleasingly** *adv.*

pleasurable /'plɛʒərəbəl/ *adj* gratifying, delightful.—**pleasurably** *adv.*

pleasure /'plɛʒər/ *n* enjoyment, recreation; gratification of the senses; preference.

pleat /pliːt/ *n* a double fold of cloth, etc pressed or stitched in place. • *vt* to gather into pleats.

pleb /plɛb/ *n* a plebeian; (*sl*) a common person.

plebeian /plɪ'biːən/ *adj* relating to the common people; base, vulgar. • *n* a commoner of ancient Rome; a vulgar, coarse person.—**plebeianism** *n.*

plebiscite /'plɛbɪsaɪt/ *n* a direct vote of the electorate on a political issue such as annexation, independent nationhood, etc.

plectrum /'plɛktrəm/ *n* (*pl* **plectra, plectrums**) a thin piece of metal, etc for plucking the strings of a guitar, etc.

pledge /plɛdʒ/ *n* a solemn promise; security for payment of a debt; a token or sign; a toast. • *vt* to give as security; to pawn; to bind by solemn promise; to drink a toast to.

pledgee /plɛ'dʒiː/ *n* someone to whom a pledge is given.

pledget /'plɛdʒɪt/ *n* a small pad of lint, etc, used to apply pressure to wounds.

pleiad /'plaɪəd/ *n* a brilliant group (of people).

Pleiades /'plaɪə,diːz/ *npl* a cluster of seven stars in the constellation Taurus.

plein-air /pleɪn'ɛr/ *adj* (*art*) depicting the effects of light and atmosphere outdoors.

Pleistocene /'pleɪstə,siːn/ *adj* (*geol*) pertaining to the earliest division of the Quaternary Period.

plenary /'plenəri/ *or* /'pliːn-/ *adj* full, complete; (*assembly, etc*) attended by all the members.—**plenarily** *adv.*

plenipotentiary /,plɛnɪpə'tɛnʃɪeri/ *adj* possessing full powers. • *n* (*pl* **plenipotentiaries**) an envoy with authority to act at his own discretion.

plenitude /'plɛnɪtuːd/ *or* /-tjuːd/ *n* abundance.

plenteous /'plɛntɪəs/ *adj* abundant.

plentiful /'plɛntɪful/ *adj* abundant, copious.—**plentifully** *adv.*—**plentifulness** *n.*

plenty /'plɛnti/ *n* an abundance; more than enough; a great number. • *adv* (*sl*) quite.

plenum /'pliːnəm/ *n* (*pl* **plenums, plena**) a full assembly; a space filled with matter.

pleonasm /'pliːə,næzəm/ *n* (*rhetoric*) the use of unnecessary words, *eg* "he is blind and cannot see".—**pleonastic** *adj.*

plesiosaurus, plesiosaur /'pliːsiəsɔːr/ *n* a large, extinct, long-necked swimming reptile.

plessor /'plɛsər/ *see* **plexor**.

plethora /'plɛθərə/ *n* overabundance, glut; (*med*) an excess of red corpuscles in the blood.—**plethoric** *adj.*

pleura /'plʊərə/ *or* /'plʊrə/ *n* (*pl* **pleurae**) the membrane enclosing the lungs.—**pleural** *adj.*

pleurisy /'plʊərɪsi/ *or* /'plʊrɪsi/ *n* inflammation of the membranes enclosing the lungs.—**pleuritic** *adj.*

pleuropneumonia /,plʊərɒnjuː'moʊniə/ *or* /,plʊr-/, /-njuː-/ *n* an inflammation of both the pleura and the lung.

Plexiglas /'plɛksɪ,glæs/ *n* (*trademark*) a transparent thermoplastic.

plexor /'plɛksər/ *n* (*med*) a small hammer used in percussion and for testing reflexes.—*also* **plessor**.

plexus /'plɛksəs/ *n* (*pl* **plexuses, plexus**) a network, *esp* of nerves or blood vessels.

pliable /'plaɪəbəl/ *adj* easily bent or moulded; easily influenced.—**pliability** *n.*—**pliably** *adv.*

pliant /'plaɪənt/ *adj* easily bent or influenced; supple; flexible; yielding.—**pliancy** *n.*—**pliantly** *adv.*

plicate /'plaɪkeɪt/, **plicated** /plɪ'keɪtɪd/ *adj* pleated; folded in the form of a fan.

pliers /'plaɪərz/ *npl* a tool with hinged arms and jaws for cutting, shaping wire.

plight[1] /plaɪt/ *n* a dangerous situation; a predicament.

plight[2] *vt* to pledge, vow solemnly. • *n* a pledge; an engagement.—**plighter** *n.*

Plimsoll line /'plɪmsəl/ *n* a system of markings on the hull of ships to ensure there is no overloading and that cargo is balanced.—*also* **load line**.

plimsolls /'plɪmsəlz/, **plimsoles** /-soːlz/ *npl* (*Brit*) rubber-soled canvas shoes, sneakers.

Pliocene /'plaɪə,siːn/ *adj* (*geol*) pertaining to the latest division of the Tertiary Period.

PLO *abbr* = Palestine Liberation Organization.

plod /plɒd/ *vi* (**plodding, plodded**) to walk heavily and slowly, to trudge; to work or study slowly and laboriously.—**plodder** *n.*—**ploddingly** *adv.*

plop /plɒp/ *vti* (**plopping, plopped**) to fall into water without a splash. • *n* the sound of this • *adv* with a plop.

plot /plɒt/ *n* a small piece of land; a secret plan or conspiracy; the story in a play or novel, etc. • *vt* (**plotting, plotted**) to conspire; (*route*) to mark on a map; (*points*) to mark (on a graph) with coordinates.—**plotter** *r.*

plough /plaʊ/, **plow** *n* a farm implement for turning up soil; any implement like this, as a snowplough. • *vt* to cut and turn up with a plough; to make a furrow (in), to wrinkle; to force a way through; to work at laboriously; (*with* **into**) to run into; (*with* **back**) to reinvest; (*sl*) to fail an examination.—**ploughable** *adj.*—**plougher** *n.*

ploughman, plowman /'plaʊmən/ *n* (*pl* **ploughmen, plowmen**) one who ploughs; a farmworker.

ploughshare, plowshare /'plaʊʃər/ *n* the part of a plough which cuts the soil.

plover /'plʌvər/ *n* a wading bird with a short tail and a straight bill.

ploy /plɔɪ/ *n* a tactic or manoeuvre to outwit an opponent; an occupation or job; an escapade.

pluck /plʌk/ *vt* to pull off or at, to snatch; to strip off feathers; (*fruit, flowers, etc*) to pick; (*person*) to remove from one situation in life and transfer to another. • *vi* to make a sharp pull or twitch. • *n* a pull or tug; heart, courage; dogged resolution.—**plucker** *n.*

plucky /ˈplʌki/ *adj* (**pluckier, pluckiest**) brave, spirited.—**pluckily** *adv.*—**pluckiness** *n.*

plug /plʌg/ *n* a stopper used for filling a hole; a device for connecting an appliance to an electricity supply; a cake of tobacco; a kind of fishing lure; (*inf*) a free advertisement *usu* incorporated in other matter. • *vti* (**plugging, plugged**) to stop up with a plug; (*sl*) to shoot or punch; (*inf*) to seek to advertise by frequent repetition; (*with* **at**) (*inf*) to work doggedly.

plug-in *adj* able to be connected by a plug. • *n* a device or unit able to be connected by a plug; ✹ (*Cdn*) an electrical outlet in a garage for plugging in a block heater.

plum /plʌm/ *n* an oval smooth-skinned sweet stone-fruit; a tree bearing it; a reddish-purple colour; a choice thing.

plumage /ˈpluːmɪdʒ/ *n* a bird's feathers.

plumb /plʌm/ *n* a lead weight attached to a line, used to determine how deep water is or whether a wall is vertical; any of various weights. • *adj* perfectly vertical. • *adv* vertically; in a direct manner; (*inf*) entirely. • *vt* to test by a plumb line; to examine minutely and critically; to weight with lead; to seal with lead; to supply with or install as plumbing. • *vi* to work as a plumber.

plumbago /plʌmˈbeɪgoʊ/ *n* (*pl* **plumbagos**) graphite; one of a genus of flowering plants.

plumber /ˈplʌmər/ *n* a person who installs and repairs water or gas pipes.

plumbing /ˈplʌmɪŋ/ *n* the system of pipes used in water or gas supply, or drainage; the plumber's craft.

plumbism /ˈplʌmbɪzəm/ *n* lead poisoning.

plume /pluːm/ *n* a large or ornamental bird's feather; a feathery ornament or thing; something resembling a feather in structure or density. • *vt* (*feathers*) to preen; to adorn with feathers; to indulge (oneself) with an obvious display of self-satisfaction.

plummet /ˈplʌmət/ *n* a plumb. • *vi* (**plummeting, plummeted**) to fall in a perpendicular manner; to drop sharply and abruptly.

plummy /ˈplʌmi/ *adj* (**plummier, plummiest**) like, full of, plums; (*inf*) rich, desirable; (*inf*) (*voice*) deep, drawling, richsounding.

plump[1] /plʌmp/ *adj* rounded, chubby. • *vti* to make or become plump; to swell.—**plumply** *adv.*—**plumpness** *n.*

plump[2] *vti* to fall, drop or sink, or come into contact suddenly and heavily; (*someone, something*) to favour or give support. • *n* a sudden drop or plunge or the sound of this. • *adv* straight down, straight ahead; abruptly; bluntly.

plum pudding *n* a rich boiled or steamed pudding with suet, dried fruit, spices, etc.

plumule /ˈpluːmjuːl/ *n* (*zool*) a down feather; (*bot*) the embryonic stem of a plant.

plumy /ˈpluːmi/ *adj* (**plumier, plumiest**) feathery; feathered.

plunder /ˈplʌndər/ *vt* to steal goods by force, to loot. • *n* plundering; booty.—**plunderer** *n.*

plunge /plʌndʒ/ *vti* to immerse, dive suddenly; to penetrate quickly; to hurl oneself or rush; (*horse*) to start violently forward.

plunger /ˈplʌndʒər/ *n* a solid cylinder that operates with a plunging motion, as a piston; a larger rubber suction cup used to free clogged drains.

plunk /plʌŋk/ *vt* (*mus*) to pluck. • *vti* to throw or fall heavily. *n* the sound produced by something being plucked, or falling in this way.

pluperfect /pluːˈpɜːfɪkt/ *adj, n* (*gram*) (a tense) denoting an action completed before a past point of time.

plural /ˈplʊrəl/ *adj* more than one; consisting of or containing more than one kind or class. • *n* (*gram*) the form referring to more than one person or thing.—**plurally** *adv.*

pluralism /ˈplʊrəˌlɪzəm/ *n* the simultaneous holding of more than one office or benefice; a theory that reality is composed of a plurality of entities; a theory that there are at least two levels of ultimate reality; the coexistence in society of people of distinct ethnic, cultural or religious groups, each preserving their own traditions; a doctrine or policy advocating this condition.—**pluralist** *n.*—**pluralistic** *adj.*—**pluralistically** *adv.*

plurality /plʊˈrælɪti/ *n* (*pl* **pluralities**) being plural; a majority; a large number; another term for pluralism.

plus /plʌs/ *prep* added to; in addition to. • *adj* indicating addition; positive. • *n* the sign (+) indicating a value greater than zero; an advantage or benefit; an extra.

plush /plʌʃ/ *n* a velvet-like fabric with a nap. • *adj* made of plush; (*inf*) luxurious.

Pluto /ˈpluːtoʊ/ *n* (*Greek myth*) the god of the underworld; (*astron*) the planet farthest from the sun, discovered in 1930.

plutocracy /pluːˈtɒkrəsi/ *n* (*pl* **plutocracies**) government or rule by the wealthy; a wealthy class.—**plutocratic** *adj.*—**plutocratically** *adv.*

plutocrat /ˈpluːtəˌkræt/ *n* a person who has power through wealth; a rich person.

Plutonian /pluːˈtoʊniən/ *adj* pertaining to Pluto or the underworld; infernal.

plutonic /pluːˈtɒnɪk/ *adj* (*geol*) formed from magma cooling beneath the earth's surface.

plutonium /pluːˈtoʊniəm/ *n* a highly toxic transuranic element used as fuel in nuclear power stations and in nuclear weapons.

pluvial /ˈpluːviəl/ *adj* caused by the action of rain; rainy.

pluviometer /ˌpluːviˈɒmətər/ *n* an instrument used to measure rainfall.—*also* **rain gauge.**

ply[1] /plaɪ/ *vti* (**plying, plied**) to work at diligently and energetically; to wield; to subject to persistently; (*goods*) to sell; to go to and fro, run regularly; to keep busy.

ply[2] *n* (*pl* **plies**) a layer or thickness, as of cloth, plywood, etc; any of the twisted strands in a yarn, etc. • *vt* (**plying, plied**) to twist together.

plywood /ˈplaɪwʊd/ *n* a building material consisting of several thin layers of wood glued together.

PM *abbr* = post-mortem; Prime Minister.

Pm (*chem symbol*) promethium.

p.m. *abbr* = post meridiem.

PMS *abbr* = premenstrual syndrome.

PMT *abbr* = premenstrual tension.

pneumatic /nuːˈmætɪk/ or /njuː-/ *adj* concerning wind, air, or gases; operated by or filled with compressed air.—**pneumatically** *adv.*

pneumatics /nuːˈmætɪks/ or /njuː-/ *n sing* the science dealing with the mechanical properties of air.

pneumatology /ˌnuːməˈtɒlədʒi/ or /ˌnjuː-/ *n* the theological study of the Holy Spirit.

pneumatometer /ˌnuːməˈtɒmətər/ or/ˌnjuː-/ *n* an instrument for measuring the amount of air exhaled in one breath.

pneumatophore /ˈnuːmətəˌfɔːr/ or /ˈnjuː-/ *n* the breathing organ of a marsh plant.

pneumonia /nuːˈmoʊniə/ or /njuː-/, /nə-/ *n* acute inflammation of the lungs.—**pneumonic** *adj.*

PO *abbr* = Personnel Officer; Petty Officer; Pilot Officer; post office; postal order.

Po (*chem symbol*) polonium.

poach[1] /poʊtʃ/ *vt* to cook (an egg without its shell, fish, etc) in or over boiling water.

poach[2] *vti* to catch game or fish illegally; to trespass for this purpose; to encroach on, usurp another's rights, etc; to steal another's idea, employee, etc.—**poaching** *n.*

poacher[1] /-ər/ *n* a pan with shallow cups for poaching eggs; a dish for poaching fish, etc.

poacher[2] *n* a person who poaches another's property.

pochard /ˈpoʊtʃərd/ or /-kərd/ *n* (*pl* **pochards, pochard**) a redheaded European duck.

pock /pɒk/ *n* an eruptive pustule on the skin, *esp* as a result of smallpox.

pocket /ˈpɒkət/ *n* a small bag or pouch, *esp* in a garment, for carrying small articles; an isolated or enclosed area; a deposit (as of gold, water, or gas). • *adj* small enough to put in a pocket. • *vt* to put in one's pocket, to steal; (*ball*) to put in a pocket; to envelop; to enclose; (*money*) to take dishonestly; to suppress.

pocketbook /ˈpɒkətˌbʊk/ *n* a small folder or case for letters, money, credit cards, etc; a woman's purse, a handbag; monetary resources; a small *esp* paperback book.

pocketful /ˈpɒkɪtˌfuːl/ *n* (*pl* **pocketfuls**) as much as a pocket holds.

pocketknife /ˈpɒkɪtˌnaɪf/ *n* (*pl* **pocketknives**) a small knife with one or more blades that fold into the handle.

pocket money *n* money for occasional expenses; a child's allowance.

poco /ˈpoʊkoʊ/ *adv* (*mus*) a little.

pococurante /ˌpoʊkoʊkuːˈrænti/ or /-kjuː-/ *n, adj* (someone who is) indifferent.

pod /pɒd/ *n* a dry fruit or seed vessel, as of peas, beans, etc; a protective container or housing; a detachable compartment on a spacecraft. • *vi* (**podding, podded**) to remove the pod from.

podagra /pəˈdægrə/ or /ˈpædəgrə/ *n* gout, *esp* in the feet.—**podagral, podagric, podagrous** *adj.*

podgy /'pɒdʒi/ *adj* (**podgier, podgiest**) short and fat, squat.— *also* **pudgy.—podginess** *n*.

podium /'pəʊdiəm/ *n* (*pl* **podiums, podia**) a platform used by lecturers, etc; a low wall around the arena of an amphitheatre.

podophyllin /ˌpɒdə'fɪlɪn/ *n* a purgative resin obtained from the root of the May apple and mandrake.

poem /'pəʊəm/ *or* /'pəʊm/ *n* an arrangement of words, *esp* in metre, often rhymed, in a style more imaginative than ordinary speech; a poetic thing.

poesy /'pəʊəzi/ *n* (*pl* **poesies**) the art of writing poetry.

poet /'pəʊət/ *n* the writer of a poem; a person with imaginative power and a sense **of beauty.—poetess** *nf*.

poetaster /ˌpəʊət'æstər/ *n* an inferior poet.

poetic /pəʊ'etɪk/, **poetical** *adj* of poets or poetry; written in verse; imaginative, romantic, like poetry.—**poetically** *adv*.

poetic justice *n* an outcome in which vice is punished and virtue rewarded in an appropriate manner.

poetic licence *n* latitude allowed to a poet in grammar, facts, etc.

poetics /pəʊ'etɪks/ *n sing* the theory, or study, of poetry.

poetize /'pəʊəˌtaɪz/ *vt* to make poetic; to compose poetry about. • *vi* to compose poetry.

poet laureate *n* (*pl* **poets laureate**) a poet officially appointed by the British sovereign to write poems celebrating national events, etc.

poetry /'pəʊətri/ *n* the art of writing poems; poems collectively; poetic quality or spirit.

pogey, pogy /'pəʊgi/ *n* ♣ (*Cdn*) unemployment insurance or welfare benefits.

pogo stick /'pəʊgəʊ/ *n* a stilt with a powerful spring used to hop along the ground.

pogrom /pəʊ'grɒm/ *or* /'pɒgrəm/ *n* an organized extermination of a minority group.

poignant /'pɔɪnjənt/ *adj* piercing; incisive; deeply moving.—**poignancy** *n*.—**poignantly** *adv*.

poinsettia /pɔɪn'setə/ *or* /-setiə/ *n* a South American plant, widely cultivated as a house plant for its red bracts, which resemble petals.

point /pɔɪnt/ *n* a dot or tiny mark used in writing or printing (*eg* a decimal point, a full stop); a location; a place in a cycle, course, or scale; a unit in scoring or judging; the sharp end of a knife or pin; a moment of time; one of thirty-two divisions of the compass; a fundamental reason or aim; the tip; a physical characteristic; a railway switch; a unit of size in printing equal to one seventy-second of an inch; a unit used in quoting the prices of stocks, bonds and commodities; a headland or cape. • *vti* to give point to; to sharpen; to aim (at); to extend the finger (at or to); to indicate something; to call attention (to).

point-blank /pɔɪnt'blæŋk/ *adj* aimed straight at a mark; direct, blunt.—*also adv*.

point blanket *n* ♣ (*Cdn*) a Hudson's Bay blanket with markings of short black lines.

pointed /'pɔɪntəd/ *adj* having a point; pertinent; aimed at a particular person or group; conspicuous.—**pointedly** *adv*.—**pointedness** *n*.

pointer /'pɔɪntər/ *n* a rod or needle for pointing; an indicator; a breed of hunting dog.

pointillism /'pwæntɪˌlɪzəm/ *n* in painting, the practice of applying small strokes or dots of colour to a surface so that from a distance they blend together.—**pointillist** *n, adj*.

pointless /'pɔɪntləs/ *adj* without a point; irrelevant, aimless.—**pointlessly** *adv*.—**pointlessness** *n*.

poise[1] /pɔɪz/ *vt* to balance; to hold supported without motion; (*the head*) to hold in a particular way; to put into readiness. • *vi* to become drawn up into readiness; to hover. • *n* a balanced state; self-possessed assurance of manner; gracious tact; bearing, carriage.

poise[2] *n* a centimetre-gram-second unit of viscosity equivalent to one dyne-second per square metre.

poison /'pɔɪzən/ *n* a substance that through its chemical action *usu* destroys or injures an organism; any corrupt influence; an object of aversion or abhorrence. • *vt* to administer poison in order to kill or injure; to put poison into; to influence wrongfully.—**poisoner** *n*.

poison gas *n* a poisonous gas, or a liquid or solid giving off poisonous vapours, used in warfare.

poison ivy *n* a climbing plant with ivory-coloured berries and an acutely irritating oil that causes an intensely itchy skin rash; the rash caused by poison ivy.

poisonous /'pɔɪzənəs/ *adj* being or containing poison; toxic; having a harmful influence; (*inf*) unpleasant.—**poisonously** *adv*.—**poisonousness** *n*.

poke /pəʊk/ *vt* to thrust (at), jab or prod; (*hole, etc*) to make by poking; (*sl*) to hit. • *vi* to jab (at); to pry or search (about or around). • *n* a jab; a prod or nudge; a thrust.

poker[1] /'pəʊkər/ *n* a metal rod for poking or stirring fire.

poker[2] *n* a card game in which a player bets that the value of his hand is higher than that of the hands held by others.

poker face *n* an expressionless face, concealing a person's thoughts or feelings.—**poker-faced** *adj*.

poky, pokey /'pəʊki/ *adj* (**pokier, pokiest**) small and uncomfortable.—**pokily** *adv*.—**pokiness** *n*.

polar /'pəʊlər/ *adj* of or near the North or South Pole; of a pole; having positive and negative electricity; directly opposite.

polar angle *n* the angle between the positive (polar) axis and the radius vector in polar coordinates.

polar bear *n* a large creamy-white bear that inhabits arctic regions.

polar coordinates *npl* either of a pair of coordinates that determine the position of points in space by measuring their distance along a fixed line from the origin or other given point and their angle, which lies between the fixed line and a single axis.

polarimeter /ˌpəʊlə'rɪmɪtər/ *n* an instrument for measuring the polarization of light.

Polaris /pəʊ'lɑrəs/ *or* /pə-/ *n* (*astron*) the brightest star in the Ursa Minor constellation, also known as the Pole Star.

polariscope /pəʊ'leɪrɪˌskəʊp/ *n* an instrument used to detect polarized light.

polarity /pə'lerɪti/ *n* (*pl* **polarities**) the condition of being polar; the magnet's property of pointing north; attraction towards a particular object or in a specific direction; (*elect*) the state, positive or negative, of a body; diametrical opposition; an instance of such opposition.

polarization /ˌpəʊlərɪ'zeɪʃən/ *n* the production or acquirement of polarity; (*optics*) the process of causing light waves to vibrate in a uniform circular, elliptical or linear pattern; (*elect*) the separation of positive and negative charges; the grouping about opposing factions.

polarize /'pəʊləˌraɪz/ *vt* (*light waves*) to cause to vibrate in a definite pattern; to give physical polarity to; to break up into opposing factions; to concentrate.—**polarizable** *adj*.—**polarizer** *n*.

Polaroid /'pəʊləˌrɔɪd/ *n* (*trademark*) a transparent material used *esp* in sunglasses and lamps to prevent glare; a camera that produces a print in seconds.

polder /'pəʊldər/ *n* (*Netherlands*) a piece of land reclaimed from the sea.

pole[1] /pəʊl/ *n* a long slender piece of wood, metal, etc; a flagstaff. • *vt* to propel, support with a pole.

pole[2] *n* either end of an axis, *esp* of the earth; either of two opposed forces, parts, etc, as the ends of a magnet, terminals of a battery, etc; either of two opposed principles.

poleaxe /'pəʊlæks/, **poleax** *n* a long-handled battle axe; a type of axe used to slaughter cattle. • *vt* to hit or knock down with, or as if with, such an axe.

pole bean *n* a climbing plant that produces long green edible pods, a runner bean.

polecat /'pəʊlkæt/ *n* (*pl* **polecats, polecat**) a small, dark-brown animal, found in Europe, North Africa and Asia, related to the weasel and known for its unpleasant smell.

polemic /pə'lemɪk/ *n* a controversy or argument over doctrine; strong criticism; a controversialist. • *adj* involving dispute; controversial.—*also* **polemical.—polemically** *adv*.—**polemicist** *n*.

polemics /pəʊ'lemɪks/ *or* /pə-/ *n sing* the art of controversial debate.

polenta /pə'lentə/ *n* an Italian porridge of maize, barley or chestnut meal.

pole vault *n* a field event in which competitors jump over a high bar using a long flexible pole.—**pole-vault** *vi*.—**pole-vaulter** *n*.

police /pə'lis/ *n* the government department for keeping order, detecting crime, law enforcement, etc; (*pl*) the members of such a department; any similar organization. • *vt* to control, protect, etc with police or a similar force.

policeman /pə'lismən/ *n* (*pl* **policemen**) a member of a police force.—**policewoman** *nf* (*pl* **policewomen**).

police officer *n* a policeman or policewoman.

policy[1] /'pɒləsi/ *n* (*pl* **policies**) a written insurance contract.

policy[2] *n* (*pl* **policies**) political wisdom, statecraft; a course of action selected from among alternatives; a high-level overall plan embracing the general principles and aims of an organization, *esp* a government.

policyholder /'pɒləsiˌhoːldər/ *n* a person who has an insurance policy.

polio /'poːlioː/ *n* poliomyelitis.

poliomyelitis /ˌpoːlioːˌmaiəˈləitis/ *n* an acute infectious virus disease marked by inflammation of nerve cells in the spinal cord, causing paralysis.

Polish /'poːliʃ/ *adj* of or pertaining to Poland, its inhabitants, language or culture. • *n* the Slavic language of Poland.

polish /'pɒliʃ/ *vti* to make or become smooth and shiny by rubbing (with a cloth and polish); to give elegance or culture to; (*with* **off**) (*inf*) to finish completely. • *n* smoothness; elegance of manner; a finish or gloss; a substance, such as wax, used to polish.—**polisher** *n*.

polished /'pɒliʃt/ *adj* accomplished; smoothly or professionally done or performed; (*rice*) having had the husk removed.

polite /pəˈlait/ *adj* courteous; well-bred; refined.—**politely** *adv*.—**politeness** *n*.

politesse /ˌpɒliˈtɛs/ *n* (excessively) formal politeness.

politic /'pɒlətik/ *adj* expedient; shrewdly tactful; prudent.

political /pəˈlitikəl/ *adj* relating to politics or government; characteristic of political parties or politicians.—**politically** *adv*.

political correctness *n* a movement aimed at removing discrimination against women, ethnic minorities, gays and lesbians, etc by combating sexist and racist language or policies in education, the arts, media and government.—**politically correct** *adj*.

political economy *n* the former name for the science of economics.

politician /ˌpɒliˈtiʃən/ *n* a person engaged in politics, often used with implications of seeking personal or partisan gain, scheming, etc.

politico /pəˈlitiˌkoː/ *n* (*sl*) a politician.

politics /'pɒlitiks/ *n* (*sing or pl*) the science and art of government; political activities, beliefs or affairs; factional scheming for power.

polity /'pɒliti/ *n* (*pl* **polities**) the form or constitution of the government of a state; a constitution.

polka /'poːlkə/ or /'poːkə/ *n* a lively dance; the music for this. • *vi* to dance the polka.

polka dot *n* any of a pattern of small round dots forming a pattern on cloth.

poll /poːl/ *n* a counting, listing, etc of persons, *esp* of voters; the number of votes recorded; an opinion survey; (*pl*) a place where votes are cast. • *vti* to receive the votes (of); to cast a vote; to canvass or question in a poll.—**poller** *n*.

pollack /'pɒlək/ *n* (*pl* **pollacks, pollack**) a type of food fish.—*also* **pollock** (*pl* **pollocks, pollock**).

pollan /'pɒlən/ *n* an Irish freshwater fish.

pollard /'pɒlərd/ *n* a tree with its branches pruned to encourage growth; an animal which has cast its horns or antlers, or had them removed.

poll captain *n* ✷ (*Cdn*) a person responsible for an electoral campaign in one part of a constituency.

pollen /'pɒlən/ *n* the yellow dust, containing male spores, that is formed in the anthers of flowers.—**pollinic** *adj*.

pollex /'pɒlɛks/ *n* (*pl* **pollices**) a thumb or similar first digit.

pollinate /'pɒliˌneit/ *vti* to fertilize by uniting pollen with seed.—**pollinator** *n*.

pollination /ˌpɒliˈneiʃən/ *n* the transfer of pollen from the anthers of a flower to the stigma, *esp* by insects.

polliwog, pollywog /'pɒliˌwɒg/ or /-ˌwɔg/ *n* a tadpole.

pollock /'pɒlək/ *see* **pollack**.

pollster /'poːlstər/ *n* a person who conducts a poll or compiles data obtained from a poll.

poll tax *n* a tax of a fixed amount per person levied on adults.

pollute /pəˈluːt/ *vt* to contaminate with harmful substances; to make corrupt; to profane.—**polluter** *n*.

pollution /pəˈluːʃən/ *n* the act of polluting; the state of being polluted; contamination by chemicals, noise, etc.

polo /'poːloː/ *n* a game played on horseback by two teams, using a wooden ball and long-handled mallets.

polonaise /ˌpɒləˈneiz/ *n* a slow, stately dance in three-four time; the music for such a dance; an outfit with a one-piece bodice and a skirt looped up at the sides.

polo shirt *n* a sports shirt made of a knitted fabric.

polonium /pəˈloːniəm/ *n* a radioactive element.

poltergeist /'poːltərˌgaist/ *n* a spirit believed to move heavy objects about and to make noises.

poltroon /pɒlˈtruːn/ *n* (*arch*) a coward.

poly- /'pɒli/ *prefix* many.

polyandry /'pɒliˌændri/ *n* the practice of a woman having more than one husband at the same time.—**polyandrous** *adj*.

polyanthus /ˌpɒliˈænθəs/ *n* (*pl* **polyanthuses**) a hybrid garden primrose; a narcissus with small yellow or white flowers in clusters.

polyatomic /ˌpɒliəˈtɒmik/ *adj* with more than two atoms in the molecule.

polybasic /ˌpɒliˈbeisik/ *adj* (*chem*) having more than two bases or atoms of a base.

polychaete /'pɒliˌkiːt/, **poltchete** *n* a type of marine worm. • *adj* pertaining to this type of worm.—*also* **polychaetous**.

polychromatic /ˌpɒlikroˈmætik/ **polychromic, polychromous** *adj* having many colours; exhibiting a play of colours; (*physics*) (*light, etc*) having a mixture of wavelengths.—**polychromatism** *n*.

polychrome /'pɒliˌkroːm/ *adj* made with, or decorated in, many colours. • *n* a work of art in several colours; a painted statue.

polyclinic /'pɒliˌklini/ *n* a general hospital.

polydactyl /ˌpɒliˈdæktil/ *n, adj* (an animal or person) with more than the normal number of fingers or toes.

polyester /ˌpɒliˈɛstər/ *n* any of a number of synthetic polymeric resins used for adhesives, plastics, and textiles.

polyethylene /ˌpɒliˈɛθiˌliːn/ *n* a light, plastic, multipurpose synthetic material resistant to moisture and chemicals.—*also* **polythene**.

polygamist /pəˈligəməst/ *n* a person who advocates or practises polygamy.

polygamy /pəˈligəmi/ or /poː-/ *n* the practice of being married to more than one person at a time; (*bot*) the condition of having staminate, pistillate and hermaphrodite flowers on one plant; (*zool*) the practice of having more than one mate.—**polygamous** *adj*.—**polygamously** *adv*.

polygenesis /ˌpɒliˈdʒɛnisis/ *n* the derivation of a species or race from many origins.—**polygenetic** *adj*.

polyglot /'pɒliˌglɒt/ *adj* having command of many languages; composed of numerous languages; containing matter in several languages; composed of elements from different languages. • *n* a person who speaks several languages.

polygon /'pɒliˌgɒn/ *n* a closed plane figure bound by three or more straight lines.—**polygonal** *adj*.

polygonum /pəˈligənəm/ *n* one of a family of flowering plants including knotgrass.

polygraph /'pɒliˌgræf/ *n* an instrument for detecting and measuring involuntary changes in blood pressure, breathing, etc, often used as a lie detector.—**polygraphic** *adj*.

polygyny /pəˈlidʒini/ *n* the practice of a man having more than one wife at the same time.—**polygynous** *adj*.

polyhedron /ˌpɒliˈhiːdrən/ or /-ˈhɛdrən/ *n* (*pl* **polyhedrons, polyhedra**) a solid with many (*usu* more than six) plane faces.—**polyhedral** *adj*.

polymath /'pɒliˌmæθ/ *n* someone learned in many subjects.

polymer /'pɒləmər/ *n* (*chem*) a compound that has large molecules composed of many simpler molecules.—**polymeric** *adj*.—**polymerism** *n*.

polymerize /-aiz/ *vti* to (cause to) form a polymer.

polymorph /'pɒliˈmɔrf/ *n* a polymorphous organism.

polymorphous /ˌpɒliˈmɔrfəs/, **polymorphic** *adj* having, or assuming, many different forms.

polynomial /ˌpɒliˈnoːmiəl/ *n* (*math*) an expression consisting of a sum of terms each of which is a product of a constant and one or more variables raised to a positive or zero integral power; (*biol*) a species name of more than two terms. • *adj* composed of or expressed as one or more polynomials.

polyp /'pɒlip/ *n* a small water animal with tentacles at the top of a tube-like body; a growth on mucous membrane.—**polypoid** *adj*.

polyphagous /pəˈlifəgəs/ *adj* voracious; (*zool*) feeding on various kinds of food.

polyphone /'pɒliˌfoːn/ *n* (*linguistics*) a polyphonic letter or symbol

polyphonic /ˌpɒliˈfɒnik/ *adj* many-voiced; (*mus*) contrapuntal; (*phonetics*) representing more than one sound.

polyphony /pə'lıfəni/ *n* (*pl* **polyphonies**) being polyphonic; using polyphones; (*mus*) counterpoint.

polypod /'pɒli,pɒd/ *n adj* (an animal) with many legs.

polypody /'pɒli,pɔːdi/ *n* (*pl* **polypodies**) a type of fern.

polypus /'pɒlıpəs/ *n* (*pl* **polypi**) (*med*) a tumour with branching roots, found in the nose or womb.

polystyrene /,pɒli'staı,riːn/ *n* a rigid plastic material used for packing, insulating, etc.

polysyllable /'pɒli,sıləbəl/ *n* a word of many syllables.—**polysyllabic** *adj.*—**polysyllabically** *adv.*

polytechnic /,pɒli'teknık/ *n* an institution that provides instruction in many applied sciences and technical subjects.

polytheism /'pɒliθiː,ızəm/ *n* belief in many gods, or more than one god.—**polytheist** *n.*—**polytheistic** *adj.*

polythene /'pɒli,θiːn/ *see* **polyethylene**.

polyunsaturated /,pɒlien'sætʃə,reıtəd/ or /-tjʊ,re:təd/ *adj* denoting any of certain plant and animal fats and oils with a low cholesterol content.

polyurethane /,pɒli'jʊərə,θeın/ *n* any of various polymers that are used *esp* in flexible and rigid foams, resins, etc.

pomace /'pʌmıs/ *n* crushed apples for making cider; the crushed apples left after making cider.

pomaceous /pɔː'meıʃəs/ *adj* pertaining to pomes.

pomade /pə'meıd/ or /-'mɒd/ *n* a scented ointment for the hair.

pomander /pə'mændər/ *n* an aromatic ball or powder formerly carried for its pleasant smell or as protection against infection; a container for this.

pome /poːm/ *n* the stoneless fruit of the apple and related plants.

pomegranate /'pɒmə,grænıt/ or /'pɒm,grænıt/ *n* an edible fruit with many seeds; the widely cultivated tropical tree bearing it.

Pomeranian /,pɒmə'reınıə/ *n* a breed of small dog.

pomiculture /'pɒmı,kʌltʃər/ *n* fruit growing.

pommel /'pʌməl/ *n* the rounded, upward-projecting front part of a saddle; a knob on the hilt of a sword. • *vt* (**pomme ling, pommelled** or **pommeling, pommeled**) to pummel.

pommy, pommie /'pɒmi/ *n* (*pl* **pommies**) (*Austral sl*) a British person.

pomology /pə'mɒlədʒi/ *n* the study of fruit growing.—**pomological** *adj.*—**pomologist** *n*.

Pomona /pə'moːnə/ *n* (*Roman myth*) the goddess of fruit trees.

pomp /pɒmp/ *n* stately ceremony; ostentation.

pompadour /'pɒmpə,dɔr/ or /-dʊr/ *n* an 18th century hairstyle.

pompano /'pɒmpəno:/ *n* (*pl* **pompano, pompanos**) an edible American sea fish.

pom-pom /'pɒmpɒm/ *n* a quick-firing automatic anti-aircraft gun.

pompon, pompom /'pɒmpɒm/ *n* an ornamental ball or tuft of fabric strands used on clothing as an ornament; a small tufted flower on some varieties of chrysanthemum and dahlia.

pomposity /pɒm'pɒsıti/ *n* (*pl* **pomposities**) the state of being pompous; self-importance; a pompous utterance or act.

pompous /'pɒmpəs/ *adj* stately; self-important.—**pompously** *adv.*—**pompousness** *n*.

poncho /'pɒntʃoː/ *n* (*pl* **ponchos**) a blanket-like cloak with a hole in the centre for the head.

pond /pɒnd/ *n* a body of standing water smaller than a lake.

ponder /'pɒndər/ *vti* to think deeply; to consider carefully.

ponderable /-əbəl/ *adj* capable of being evaluated; capable of being weighed.—**ponderability** *n*.

ponderous /'pɒndərəs/ *adj* heavy; awkward; dull; lifeless.—**ponderously** *adv.*—**ponderousness** *n*.

pond hockey *n* ✹ (*Cdn*) informal ice hockey played on a frozen pond.

pone /poːn/ *n* (*US*) corn pone; maize bread.

pong /pɒŋ/ *n* (*Brit sl*) an unpleasant smell. • *vi* (*Brit sl*) to stink.

pongee /pɒn'dʒiː/ *n* a thin, unbleached, Chinese silk.

pontifex /'pɒnti,feks/ *n* (*pl* **pontifices**) (*ancient Rome*) a pontiff or high priest.

pontiff /'pɒntıf/ *n* the Pope; a bishop; a pontifex.

pontifical /pɒn'tıfıkəl/ *adj* of a pontiff; pompous. • *npl* a bishop's robes.—**pontifically** *adv*.

pontificate /pɒn'tıfı,keıt/ *vi* to speak sententiously, pompously or dogmatically; to officiate at a pontifical mass.—**pontificator** *n*.

pontoon[1] /pɒn'tuːn/ *n* a boat or cylindrical float forming a support for a bridge.

pontoon[2] *n* a card game.

pony /'poːni/ *n* (*pl* **ponies**) a small horse, a bronco, mustang, etc; (*inf*) a racehorse.

ponytail /'poːni,teıl/ *n* a style of arranging hair to resemble a pony's tail.

poodle /'puːdəl/ *n* a breed of dog of various sizes with a curly coat.

pool[1] /puːl/ *n* a small pond; a puddle; a small collection of liquid; a swimming pool.

pool[2] *n* a game played on a billiards table with six pockets; a combination of resources, funds, supplies, people, etc for some common purpose; the parties forming such a combination. • *vti* to contribute to a common fund, to share.

poop /puːp/ *n* (*naut*) the stern of a ship; the raised deck in the stern of a ship.

poor /pʊr/ or /pɔr/ *adj* having little money, needy; deserving pity, unfortunate; deficient; disappointing; inferior. • *n* those who have little.—**poorness** *n*.

poorhouse /'pʊrhʌʊs/ *n* (*formerly*) a public institution housing poor people.

poorly /'pʊrli/ *adv* insufficiently, badly. • *adj* not in good health.

pop[1] /pɒp/ *n* a short, explosive sound, a shot; any carbonated, nonalcoholic beverage. • *vti* (**popping, popped**) to make or cause a pop; to shoot; to go or come quickly (in, out, up); (*corn, maize*) to roast until it pops; to put suddenly; (*eyes*) to bulge.

pop[2] *adj* in a popular modern style. • *n* pop music; pop art; pop culture.

pop[3] *n* (*inf*) father; (*inf*) a name used to address an old man.

pop art *n* a realistic art style using techniques and subjects from commercial art, comic strips, posters, etc.

popcorn /'pɒpkɔrn/ *n* a kind of corn or maize, which when heated pops or puffs up.

pope /poːp/ *n* the bishop of Rome, head of the RC Church.—**popedom** *n*.

pop-eyed /'pɒpaıd/ *adj* with bulging eyes; (*fig*) astonished.

popgun /'pɒpgʌn/ *n* a toy gun firing pellets with a popping noise.

popinjay /'pɒpın,dʒeı/ *n* a conceited person.

poplar /'pɒplər/ *n* a slender, quick-growing tree of the willow family.

poplin /'pɒplın/ *n* a sturdy corded fabric.

poppet /'pɒpət/ *n* a term of endearment.

poppet valve *n* a valve opened by being lifted from its seat.

poppy /'pɒpi/ *n* (*pl* **poppies**) an annual or perennial plant with showy flowers, one of which yields opium; a strong reddish colour.

poppycock /'pɒpi,kɒk/ *n* (*inf*) nonsense.

populace /'pɒpjʊləs/ *n* the common people; the masses; all the people in a country, region, etc.

popular /'pɒpjʊlər/ *adj* of the people; well liked; pleasing to many people; easy to understand.—**popularly** *adv*.

popularity /-'lerıti/ *n* the condition or quality of being popular.

popularize /'pɒpjʊlə,raız/ *vt* to make popular; to make generally accepted or understood.—**popularization** *n.*—**popularizer** *n*.

populate /'pɒpjʊ,leıt/ *vt* to inhabit; to supply with inhabitants.

population /,pɒpjʊ'leıʃən/ *n* all the inhabitants or the number of people in an area.

populism /,pɒpjʊ'lızəm/ *n* any movement based on belief in the rights, wisdom, or virtue of the common people.

populist /'pɒpjʊlıst/ *n* an advocate of populism; one who claims to represent the people; (*with cap*) a member of the Populist or People's Party in the US (1891–1904) aiming at public control of utilities, etc.

populous /'pɒpjʊləs/ *adj* densely inhabited.—**populously** *adv.*—**populousness** *n*.

porbeagle /'pɔr,biːgəl/ *n* a type of shark.

porcelain /'pɔrsələn/ *n* a hard, white, translucent variety of ceramic ware. • *adj* made of porcelain.—**porcellaneous** *adj*.

porch /pɔrtʃ/ *n* a covered entrance to a building; an open or enclosed gallery or room on the outside of a building.

porcupine /'pɔrkjʊ,paın/ *n* a large rodent covered with protective quills.

pore[1] /pɔr/ *n* a tiny opening, as in the skin, plant leaves, stem, etc, for absorbing and discharging fluids.

pore[2] *vti* (*with* **over**) to look with steady attention; to study closely.

porgy /'pɔrgi/ *n* (*pl* **porgy, porgies**) an edible sea fish.

pork /pɔrk/ *n* the flesh of a pig used as food.

porker /'pɔrkər/ *n* a pig, *esp* a fattened one.

porky /'pɔrki/ *adj* (**porkier, porkiest**) of or like pork; (*sl*) impertinent; (*sl*) obese, fat.—**porkiness** *n*.

porno /'pɔrnə/ *n* (*sl*) pornography—*also* **porn**. • *adj* pornographic.

pornography /pɔr'nɒgrəfi/ *n* writings, pictures, films, etc, intended primarily to arouse sexual desire.—**pornographer** *n.*—**pornographic** *adj.*—**pornographically** *adv.*

porous /'pɔrəs/ *adj* having pores; able to absorb air and fluids, etc.—**porously** *adv.*—**porousness** *n.*

porphyry /'pɔrfiri/ *n* (*pl* **porphyry**) a reddish igneous rock, containing crystals of feldspar.

porpoise /'pɔrpəs/ *n* (*pl* **porpoise, porpoises**) any of several small whales, *esp* a black blunt-nosed whale of the north Atlantic and Pacific; any of several bottle-nosed dolphins.

porridge /'pɒridʒ/ *or* /'pɒr-/ *n* a thick food, *usu* made by boiling oats or oatmeal in water or milk.

porringer /'pɒrindʒər/ *n* a small dish for porridge, etc.

port[1] /pɔrt/ *n* a harbour; a town with a harbour where ships load and unload cargo; airport; a place where goods may be cleared through customs.

port[2] *n* a porthole; an opening, as in a valve face, for the passage of steam, etc; a hole in an armoured vehicle for firing a weapon; a circuit in a computer for inputting or outputting data.

port[3] *n* the left of an aircraft or ship looking forward.—*also adj.*

port[4] *n* a strong, sweet, fortified dark red wine.

portable /'pɔrtəbel/ *adj* capable of being carried or moved about easily.—**portability** *n.*

portage /'pɔrtɒdʒ/ *n* a carrying of boats and supplies overland between navigable rivers, lakes, etc; any route over which this is done. • *vti* (*boats, etc*) to carry over a portage.

portal /'pɔrtəl/ *n* an impressive gate or doorway.

portamento /ˌpɔrtə'mɛntoː/ *n* (*mus*) a continuous glide from one note to another.

portcullis /pɔrt'kʌlis/ *n* a grating that can be lowered to bar entrance to a castle.

portend /pɔr'tɛnd/ *vt* to give warning of, to foreshadow.

portent /'pɔrtɛnt/ *or* /-tənt/ *n* an omen, warning.

portentous /pɔr'tɛntəs/ *adj* ominous; pompous, self-important.—**portentously** *adv.*—**portentousness** *n.*

porter[1] /'pɔrtər/ *n* a doorman or gatekeeper.

porter[2] *n* a person who carries luggage, etc, for hire at a station, airport, etc; a railway attendant for passengers; a dark brown beer.

porterage /'pɔrtərədʒ/ *n* the hire of a porter; the charge for this.

porterhouse /'pɔrtərˌhəʊs/ *n* a choice cut of beef steak; (*formerly*) an eating place.

portfolio /pɔrt'foːlioː/ *n* (*pl* **portfolios**) a flat case for carrying papers, drawings, etc; a collection of work; the office of a cabinet minister or minister of state; a list of stocks, shares, etc.

porthole /'pɔrthoːl/ *n* an opening (as a window) with a cover or closure *esp* in the side of a ship or aircraft; a port through which to shoot; an opening for intake or exhaust of a fluid.

portico /'pɔrtikoː/ *n* (*pl* **porticoes, porticos**) a covered walkway with columns supporting the roof.

portière /pɔrt'jɛr/ *n* a heavy curtain over a door or doorway.

portion /'pɔrʃən/ *n* a part, a share, *esp* an allotted part; a helping of food; destiny. • *vt* to share out.

portly /'pɔrtli/ *adj* (**portlier, portliest**) dignified; stout.—**portliness** *n.*

portmanteau /pɔrt'mæntoː/ *n* (*pl* **portmanteaus, portmanteaux**) a large oblong travelling case with two compartments.

portmanteau word *n* a word combining the sound and sense of two other words, *eg* brunch.

portrait /'pɔrtrət/ *n* a painting, photograph, etc, of a person, *esp* of the face; (*of person*) a likeness; a vivid description.

portraitist /'pɔrtrətɪst/ *n* a maker of portraits by painting, photography, etc.

portraiture /'pɔrtrətʃər/ *n* the drawing of portraits; a portrait; a description in words; portraits collectively.

portray /pɔr'treɪ/ *vt* to make a portrait of; to depict in words; to play the part of in a play, film, etc.—**portrayable** *adj.*—**portrayer** *n.*

portrayal /pɔr'treɪəl/ *n* the act or process of portraying; a description; a representation.

portress /'pɔrtrɪs/ *n* a female porter.

pose /poːz/ *n* a position or attitude, *esp* one held for an artist or photographer; an attitude deliberately adopted for effect. • *vti* to propound, assert; to assume an attitude for effect; to sit for a painting, photograph; to set oneself up (as).

poser /'poːzər/ *n* a person who poses; a difficult problem.

poseur /poː'zər/ *n* an affected, insincere person.

posh /pɒʃ/ *adj* (*inf*) elegant; fashionable.

posit /'pɒzɪt/ *vt* to assume as fact, postulate.

position /pə'zɪʃən/ *n* place, situation; a position occupied; posture; a job; state of affairs; point of view. • *vt* to place or locate.

positional /-əl/ *adj* related to, or fixed by position; involving little movement; dependent on context, environment or position.

positive /'pɒzɪtɪv/ *adj* affirmative; definite; sure; marked by presence, not absence, of qualities; expressed clearly, or in a confident manner; constructive; empirical; (*elect*) charged with positive electricity; (*math*) greater than zero, plus; (*gram*) of adjective or adverb, denoting the simple form; (*photog*) having light, shade, colour as in the original. • *n* a positive quality or quantity; a photographic print made from a negative.

positively /-li/ *adv* in a positive way; decidedly.

positiveness /-nəs/ *n* the condition or quality of being positive; confidence; certainty.

positivism /'pɒzɪtɪvɪzəm/ *n* a philosophy recognizing only matters of fact and experience; the quality of being positive.—**positivist** *n, adj.*—**positivistic** *adj.*—**positivistically** *adv.*

positron /'pɒzɪˌtrɒn/ *n* (*physics*) a particle of the same size as an electron, but with a positive charge.

posology /pə'sɒlədʒi/ *n* the area of medicine dealing with evaluation of doses.

posse /'pɒsi/ *n* a body of people summoned by a sheriff to assist in keeping the peace, etc; (*sl*) a group of criminals, *usu* of Jamaican origin and in New York.

possess /pə'zɛs/ *vt* to own, have, keep; to dominate or control the mind of.—**possessor** *n.*—**possessory** *adj.*

possessed /pə'zɛst/ *adj* owned; controlled as if by a demon.

possession /pə'zɛʃən/ *n* ownership; something possessed; (*pl*) property.

possessive /pə'zɛsɪv/ *adj* of or indicating possession; (*gram*) denoting a case, form or construction expressing possession; having an excessive desire to possess or dominate.—**possessively** *adv.*—**possessiveness** *n.*

posset /'pɒsət/ *n* a hot drink of milk curdled with wine or ale.

possibility /ˌpɒsɪ'bɪliti/ *n* (*pl* **possibilities**) the state of being possible; a possible occurrence, a contingency.

possible /'pɒsɪbəl/ *adj* that may be or may happen; feasible, practicable.—**possibly** *adv.*

possum /'pɒsəm/ *n* (*inf*) an opossum; a phalanger; **play possum** to pretend to be asleep or dead; to remain silent.

post[1] /poːst/ *n* a piece of wood, metal, etc, set upright to support a building, sign, etc; the starting or finishing point of a race. • *vt* (*poster, etc*) to put up; to announce by posting notices; (*name*) to put on a posted or published list.

post[2] *n* a fixed position, *esp* where a sentry or group of soldiers is stationed; a position or job; a trading post; a settlement. • *vt* to station in a given place.

post[3] *n* the official conveyance of letters and parcels, mail; letters, parcels, etc, so conveyed; collection or delivery of post, mail. • *vt* to send a letter or parcel; to keep informed.—**postal** *adj.*

post- /poːst/ *prefix* after.

postage /'poːstɪdʒ/ *n* the charge for sending a letter, etc, as represented by stamps.

postage stamp *n* an adhesive or imprinted stamp issued or authorized by a government and used on mail as evidence of prepayment of postage.

postal card *n* (*US*) a card with a stamp issued by the government for mailing at low rates; a post card.

postal code *n* ✦ (*Cdn*) a series of six alternating letters and numbers used as part of a postal address to speed the processing of mail.

postcard /'poːstkard/ *n* a card, *usu* decorative, for sending messages by post; a postal card.

post chaise *n* (*formerly*) a light, closed, horse-drawn carriage used for carrying both post and passengers.

postcode /'poːstkoːd/ *n* in UK, letters and digits to denote an address and assist sorting.

postdate /poːst'deɪt/ *vt* to write a future date on a letter or cheque.

postdiluvian /ˌpoːstdə'luːviən/, **postdiluvial** *adj* occurring after the Flood (of the Old Testament).

poster /'poːstər/ *n* a *usu* decorative or ornamental printed sheet for advertising.

poste restante /ˌpoːstrɛ'stɑːt/ *n* the department of a post office that will hold mail until it is called for, general delivery.

posterior /pɒ'stiːriər/ *adj* later in time or order; at the rear. • *n* the buttocks.—**posteriorly** *adv.*

posterity /pɒˈsterɪti/ *n* future generations; all of a person's descendants.

postern /ˈpɒstərn/ *n* a back or side entrance; a small private door.

postfix /poːstˈfɪks/ *vt* to append as a suffix. • *n* a suffix.

post-free /ˈpoːstˈfriː/ *adj* postpaid.

postglacial /poːstˈgleɪʃəl/ or /-sɪəl/ *adj* existing after a glacial period.

postgraduate /ˌpoːstˈɡrædʒuːɪt/ *n* a person pursuing study after graduating from a high school or college. • *adj* (*study*) continued after the taking of a degree.

posthaste /ˈpoːstˈheɪst/ *adv* with all possible speed.

posthumous /ˈpɒstjəməs/ or /-juːməs/, /ˈpɒstʃəməs/ *adj* (*child*) born after its father's death; (*award, etc*) given after one's death.—**posthumously** *adv*.

postiche *Fr.* /poˈstiːʃ/ *adj* artificial; superfluous; inappropriate. • *n* an ornament added, *esp* inappropriately, to finished work; a wig; an imitation.

postilion, postillion /pɒˈstɪljən/ *n* someone who rides one of the horses drawing a carriage and guiding the team.

postimpressionism /ˌpoːstɪmˈpreʃənˌɪzəm/ *n* a 19th-century school of painting which sought to express the artist's conception of things rather than their outward appearance.—**postimpressionist** *n, adj*.

postliminium, postliminy /ˌpoːstlɪˈmɪniəm/ *n* (*law*) the right of a prisoner of war or exile to resume his or her former privileges on return to his or her own country.

postlude /ˈpoːstluːd/ *n* (*mus*) a closing movement.

postman /ˈpoːstmæn/ or /-mən/ *n* (*pl* **postmen**) a mailman.

postmark /ˈpoːstmɑːrk/ *n* the post office mark cancelling the stamp on a letter by showing the date, place of posting.

postmaster /ˈpoːstˌmæstər/ *n* the manager of a post office.

postmeridian /ˌpoːstməˈrɪdiən/ *adj* of or taking place in the afternoon.

post meridiem /ˌpoːstməˈrɪdiəm/ = p.m. (Latin for *after noon*).

postmortem /poːstˈmɔːrtəm/ *n* an examination of a corpse to determine the cause of death; an autopsy.—*also adj*.

postnatal /poːstˈneɪtəl/ *adj* occurring immediately after birth.

post-obit /-ˈoːbɪt/ *adj* (*law*) after death. • *n* a bond in which a borrower undertakes to repay a loan on the death of someone from whom he or she expects to receive a legacy.

post office *n* the building where postage stamps are sold and other postal business conducted; a public department handling the transmission of mail.

postpaid /ˈpoːstpeɪd/ *adj* with a charge for postage, post free.

postpone /poːstˈpoːn/ or /poːsˈpoːn/ *vt* to put off, delay to a future date.—**postponable** *adj*.—**postponement** *n*.—**postponer** *n*.

postprandial /poːstˈprændiəl/ *adj* after-dinner.

postscript /ˈpoːstskrɪpt/ or /ˈpoːskrɪpt/ *n* a note added to a letter after completion.

postulant /ˈpɒstjulənt/ or /ˈpɒstʃu-/ *n* someone making a request; a candidate for admission to a religious order.

postulate /ˈpɒstjuˌleɪt/ or /ˈpɒstʃu-/ *vt* to assume to be true; to demand or claim. • *n* a position taken as self-evident; (*math*) an unproved assumption taken as basic; an axiom.—**postulation** *n*.

posture /ˈpɒstʃər/ *n* a pose; a body position; an attitude of mind; an official stand or position. • *vti* to pose in a particular way; to assume a pose.—**postural** *adj*.—**posturer** *n*.

post-viral syndrome *n* the viral condition myalgic encephalomyelitis that affects the nervous system.

posy /ˈpoːzi/ *n* (*pl* **posies**) a small bunch of flowers.

pot[1] /pɒt/ *n* a deep, round cooking vessel; an earthenware or plastic container for plants; a framework for catching fish or lobsters; (*inf*) a large amount (as of money); (*inf*) all the money bet at a single time. • *vb* (**potting, potted**) *vt* to put or preserve in a pot. • *vi* to take a pot shot, shoot.

pot[2] *n* (*sl*) cannabis.

potable /ˈpoːtəbəl/ *adj* drinkable.

potash /ˈpɒtæʃ/ *n* potassium carbonate.

potassium /pəˈtæsiəm/ *n* a soft silvery-white metallic element.—**potassic** *adj*.

potation /poːˈteɪʃən/ *n* the act of drinking; a draught or drink.

potato /pəˈteɪtoː/ *n* (*pl* **potatoes**) a starchy, oval tuber eaten as a vegetable.

potbelly /-ˌbeli/ *n* (*pl* **potbellies**) a protruding belly—**potbellied** *adj*.

potboiler /ˈpɒtbɔɪlər/ *n* an inferior literary or artistic work done simply to earn money.

potboy /ˈpɒtbɔɪ/ *n* (*formerly*) in UK, an assistant in a public house.

poteen /pɒˈtiːn/ *n* (*Irish*) illicitly distilled whiskey.

potency /ˈpoːtənsi/ *n* (*pl* **potencies**) the quality or condition of being potent; power; strength.

potent /ˈpoːtənt/ *adj* powerful; influential; intoxicating; (*a male*) able to have sexual intercourse.—**potently** *adv*.

potentate /ˈpoːtənˌteɪt/ *n* a person with great power; a ruler; a monarch.

potential /pəˈtenʃəl/ *adj* possible, but not yet actual. • *n* the unrealized ability to do something.—**potentially** *adv*.

potentiality /-ʃiˈælɪti/ *n* (*pl* **potentialities**) latent capacity for development or growth; something with this.

potentiate /pəˈtenʃiˌeɪt/ *vt* to make possible; to give power to.

potentilla /ˌpoːtənˈtɪlə/ *n* a flowering plant of the rose family.

pother /ˈpɒðər/ *n* a bustle or turmoil; a turmoil.

pothole /ˈpɒthoːl/ *n* a hole worn in a road by traffic; (*geol*) a deep hole or cave in rock caused by the action of water.

pothouse /ˈpɒtˌhaus/ *n* (*formerly*) in UK, a public house.

pothunter /ˈpɒtˌhʌntər/ *n* someone who hunts for the sake of the game caught, not for the sport.

potion /ˈpoːʃən/ *n* a mixture of liquids, such as poison.

pot light *n* ✹ (*Cdn*) an interior electrical light enclosed in a cylindrical shell and recessed in a ceiling.

potpourri /poːpuˈriː/ *n* (*pl* **potpourris**) a mixture of scented, dried flower petals; a collection; a medley or miscellany.

potsherd /ˈpɒtʃərd/, **potshard** *n* a piece of broken earthenware.

pot shot /ˈpɒtʃɒt/ *n* a random or easy shot.

pottage /ˈpɒtɪdʒ/ *n* a thick broth.

potted /ˈpɒtəd/ *adj* in a pot; preserved (in a pot); (*version, history*) abridged.

potter[1] /ˈpɒtər/ *n* a person who makes earthenware vessels.

potter[2] *vi* to busy oneself idly; (*US*) to putter.—**potterer** *n*.

pottery /ˈpɒtəri/ *n* (*pl* **potteries**) earthenware vessels; a workshop where such articles are made.

potto /ˈpɒtoː/ *n* (*pl* **pottos**) a West African lemur; a kinkajou.

potty[1] /ˈpɒti/ *adj* (**pottier, pottiest**) (*inf*) slightly crazy; trivial, petty.—**pottiness** *n*.

potty[2] *n* (*pl* **potties**) (*inf*) a chamber pot.

pouch /pautʃ/ *n* a small bag or sack; a bag for mail; a sacklike structure, as that on the abdomen of a kangaroo, etc, for carrying young.—**pouched** *adj*.

poult /poːlt/ *n* a young fowl.

poultice /ˈpoːltɪs/ *n* a hot moist dressing applied to a sore part of the body.

poultry /ˈpoːltri/ *n* domesticated birds kept for meat or eggs.

pounce /pauns/ *vi* to swoop or spring suddenly (upon) in order to seize; to make a sudden assault or approach.—*also n*.

pound[1] /paund/ *n* a unit of weight equal to 16 ounces; a unit of money in the UK and other countries, symbol £.

pound[2] *vt* to beat into a powder or a pulp; to hit hard. • *vi* to deliver heavy blows repeatedly (at or on); to move with heavy steps; to throb; (*with* **away**) to work hard and continuously.—**pounder** *n*.

pound[3] *n* a municipal enclosure for stray animals; a depot for holding impounded personal property until claimed; a place or condition of confinement.

poundage /ˈpaundɪdʒ/ *n* a charge per pound of weight; weight in pounds; the act of impounding; the state of being impounded.

poundal /ˈpaundəl/ *n* a unit of force, giving to a mass of one pound an acceleration of one foot per second per second.

pour /pɔːr/ *vti* to cause to flow in a stream; to flow continuously; to rain heavily; to serve tea or coffee.—**pourer** *n*.

pourboire *Fr.* /puːrˈbwaːr/ *n* a tip or gratuity.

pout /paut/ *vti* to push out (the lips); to look sulky. • *n* a thrusting out of the lips; (*pl*) a fit of pique.—**poutingly** *adv*.

pouter /ˈpautər/ *n* someone who pouts; a breed of pigeon with a prominent crop.

poutine *n* ✹ (*Cdn*) French fries and cheese curds covered with a sauce, usually gravy.

poverty /ˈpɒvərti/ *n* the condition of being poor; scarcity.

poverty-stricken *adj* very poor, impoverished.

POW *abbr* = prisoner of war.

powder /ˈpaudər/ *n* any substance in tiny, loose particles; a specific kind of powder, *esp* for medicinal or cosmetic use; fine dry light snow. • *vti* to sprinkle or cover with powder; to reduce to powder.—**powderer** *n*.

powdered /'paudərd/ *adj* sprinkled or covered with powder; reduced to power.

powdered sugar *n* (*US*) icing sugar.

powdery /'paudəri/ *adj* like powder; easily crumbled.

power /'pauər/ *n* ability to do something; political, social or financial control or force; a person or state with influence over others; legal force or authority; physical force; a source of energy; (*math*) the result of continued multiplication of a quantity by itself a specified number of times. • *adj* operated by electricity, a fuel engine, etc; served by an auxiliary system that reduces effort; carrying electricity. • *vt* to supply with a source of power.—**powered** *adj*.

powerful /'pauər,ful/ *adj* mighty; strong; influential.—**powerfully** *adv*.—**powerfulness** *n*.

powerhouse /'pauər,haus/ *n* a power station; (*inf*) a strong or energetic person, team, etc.

powerless /'pauərləs/ *adj* without power; helpless; feeble.—**powerlessly** *adv*.—**powerlessness** *n*.

power station, power plant *n* a building where electric power is generated.

power-striding *n* brisk walking as a means of improving fitness.

powwow /'pauwau/ *n* an American Indian ceremony (as for invoking victory in war); (*inf*) any conference or get-together. • *vi* to confer, chat.

pox /poks/ *n* a virus disease marked by pustules; (*arch*) smallpox; syphilis; a plague; a curse.

pozzuolana, pozzolana /,potswo:'lonə/ *n* volcanic ashes used in hydraulic cement.

pp *abbr* = past participle; (*mus*) pianissimo.

pp. *abbr* = pages.

p.p. *abbr* = per pro.

ppm *abbr* = (*chem*) parts per million.

PPS *abbr* = post (additional) postscript.

PQ *abbr* ✦ = Parti Québécois; Province of Quebec.

PR *abbr* = public relations; proportional representation.

Pr (*chem symbol*) praseodymium.

practicable /'præktɪkəbəl/ *adj* able to be practised; possible, feasible.—**practicability** *n*.—**practicably** *adv*.

practical /'præktɪkəl/ *adj* concerned with action, not theory; workable; suitable; trained by practice; virtual, in effect.

practicality /-'kælɪti/ *n* (*pl* **practicalities**) the condition of being practical; a practical feature or aspect.

practical joke *n* a prank intended to embarrass or to cause discomfort.

practically /'præktɪkli/ *adv* in a practical manner; virtually.

practice /'præktɪs/ *n* action; habit, custom; repetition and exercise to gain skill; the exercise of a profession.

practise /'præktɪs/ *vti* to repeat an exercise to acquire skill; to put into practice; to do habitually or frequently; (*profession*) to work at.

practised /-tɪst/ *adj* acquired by practice; proficient; experienced.

practitioner /præk'tɪʃənər/ *n* a person who practises a profession.

praedial /'pri:dɪəl/ *adj* pertaining to land or landed property.—*also* **predial**.

praetor /'pri:tər/ or /-tor/ *n* (*ancient Rome*) a magistrate, ranking next to a consul.

pragmatic /præg'mætɪk/ *adj* practical; testing the validity of all concepts by their practical results.—**pragmatically** *adv*.

pragmatics /præg'mætɪks/ *n sing* the study of the relationship of signs and symbols and their use; (*linguistics*) the study of meaning derived from context.

pragmatism /'prægmə,tɪzəm/ *n* the judging of events or actions by their results, *esp* in politics; pragmatic behaviour; (*philos*) a theory that judges the truth of a doctrine by the conduct resulting from belief in it.—**pragmatist** *n*.—**pragmatistic** *adj*.

prairie /'preri/ *n* a large area of level or rolling land predominantly in grass; a dry treeless plateau; ✦ (*pl*) the region of western North America that consists of such land; (*Cdn*) (*cap*) the provinces of Manitoba, Saskatchewan, and Alberta.

prairie chicken *n* ✦ a grouse of the North American prairies.

prairie crocus *n* ✦ (*Cdn*) a plant of the buttercup family covered with silky hairs and with purple or white flowers.

prairie dog *n* a burrowing rodent related to the marmot.

prairie lily *n* ✦ a North American lily with upright, spotted reddish-orange flowers.

prairie wolf *n* the coyote.

prairie wool *n* ✦ (*Cdn*) the natural grassy cover of land on the Prairies.

praise /preɪz/ *vt* to express approval of, to commend; to glorify, to worship. • *vi* to express praise. • *n* commendation; glorification.—**praiser** *n*.

praiseworthy /'preɪz,wərði/ *adj* deserving praise; commendable.—**praiseworthily** *adv*.—**praiseworthiness** *n*.

praline /'preɪli:n/ or /'prɒ-/ *n* a confection made of nuts and sugar.

prance /præns/ *vi* (*horse*) to spring on the hind legs, bound; (*person*) to walk or ride in a showy manner; to swagger. • *n* a prancing; a caper.—**prancer** *n*.—**prancingly** *adv*.

prank[1] /præŋk/ *n* a mischievous trick or joke; a ludicrous act.—**prankster** *n*.

prank[2] *vti* to adorn, to deck; to dress up showily.

prase /preɪz/ *n* a green, transparent form of quartz.

praseodymium /,preɪziə'dɪmiəm/ *n* a silvery-white metallic element.

prate /preɪt/ *vti* to chatter, talk idly.—**prater** *n*.

pratincole /'præntɪŋ,ko:l/ *n* a bird resembling a swallow.

prattle /'prætəl/ *vti* to talk in a childish manner; to babble. • *n* empty chatter.—**prattler** *n*.

prawn /prɒn/ *n* an edible marine shrimp-like crustacean. • *vi* to fish for prawns.—**prawner** *n*.

praxis /'præksɪs/ *n* (*pl* **praxises, praxes**) practice; an example, or set of examples, for an exercise.

pray /preɪ/ *vti* to offer prayers to God; to implore.

prayer[1] /preɪ/ *n supplication*, entreaty, praise or thanks to God; the form of this; the act of praying; (*pl*) devotional services; something prayed for.

prayer[2] *n* one who prays.

prayerful /'preɪ,ful/ *adj* given to prayer; devout.—**prayerfully** *adv*.

pre- /pri:/ *prefix* before, beforehand; previous to; surpassingly.

preach /pri:tʃ/ *vi* to advocate in an earnest or moralizing way. • *vt* to deliver a sermon; (*patience, etc*) to advocate.

preacher /'pri:tʃər/ *n* one who preaches, *esp* a Protestant clergyman.

preachify /'pri:tʃɪ,faɪ/ *vi* (*inf*) to hold forth tediously.—**preachification** *n*.

preachy /'pri:tʃi/ *adj* (**preachier, preachiest**) (*inf*) fond of moralizing or preaching.

preamble /pri:'æmbəl/ or /'pri:-/ *n* an introductory part to a document, speech, or story, stating its purpose.—**preambulary** *adj*.

prearrange /,pri:ə'reɪndʒ/ *vt* to arrange beforehand.—**prearrangement** *n*.

prebend /'prebənd/ *n* a stipend granted to a canon or member of the chapter by a cathedral.—**prebendal** *adj*.

prebendary /'prebəndəri/ *n* (*pl* **prebendaries**) someone who holds a prebend.

precancerous /pri:'kænsərəs/ *adj* likely to become cancerous.

precarious /prɪ'keriəs/ *adj* dependent on chance; insecure; dangerous.—**precariously** *adv*.—**precariousness** *n*.

precatory /'prekə,to:ri/, **precative** /'prekə,tɪv/ *adj* suppliant, expresssing a wish.

precaution /prɪ'kɒʃən/ *n* a preventive measure; care taken beforehand; careful foresight.—**precautionary** *adj*.

precede /prɪ'si:d/ *vti* to be, come or go before in time, place, order, rank, or importance.

precedence /'presɪdəns/ *n* priority; the right of higher rank.

precedent /'presɪdənt/ *n* a previous and parallel case serving as an example; (*law*) a decision, etc, serving as a rule. • *adj* preceding; previous.—**precedented** *adj*.—**precedently** *adv*.

precedential /-ʃəl/ *adj* serving as a precedent; having precedence.

preceding /-ɪŋ/ *adj* coming or going before; former.

precentor /prɪ'sentər/ *n* the leader of a choir in a cathedral or church.

precept /'pri:sept/ *n* a rule of moral conduct; a maxim; an order issued by a legally constituted authority to a subordinate.

preceptive /-tɪv/ *adj* of or using precepts; didactic.—**preceptively** *adv*.

preceptor /-ər/ *n* an instructor or teacher.—**preceptress** *nf*.

precession /prɪ'seʃən/ *n* going before, in advance of—**precessional** *adj*.

precinct /'pri:sɪŋkt/ *n* (*usu pl*) an enclosure between buildings, walls, etc; a limited area; an urban area where traffic is prohibited; (*pl*) environs; (*US*) a police district or a subdivision of a voting ward.

precious /'preʃəs/ *adj* of great cost or value; beloved; very fastidious; affected; thoroughgoing. • *adv* (*sl*) very.—**preciously** *adv*.—**preciousness** *n*.

precious metal *n* gold, silver, or platinum.

precious stone *n* a diamond, emerald, ruby, sapphire, pearl, and sometimes black opal; a gem.

precipice /'presɪpɪs/ *n* a cliff or overhanging rock face.

precipitant /prɪ'sɪpɪtənt/ *adj* falling headlong; hasty, impetuous. • *n* (*chem*) a substance causing precipitation.—**precipitance, precipitancy** *n*.

precipitate /prɪ'sɪpɪteɪt/ *vti* to throw from a height; to cause to happen suddenly or too soon; (*chem*) to separate out; to rain; to fall as rain, snow, dew, etc.—**precipitately** *adv*.—**precipitateness** *n*.—**precipitator** *n*.

precipitation /prɪˌsɪpɪ'teɪʃən/ *n* the act of precipitating; undue haste; rain, snow, etc; the amount of this.

precipitous /prɪ'sɪpɪtəs/ *adj* of or like a precipice; sheer, steep.—**precipitously** *adv*.—**precipitousness** *n*.

précis /'preisiː/ *n* (*pl* **précis**) a summary or abstract • *vt* to make a précis of.

precise /prɪ'saɪs/ *adj* clearly defined, exact; accurate; punctilious; particular.—**precisely** *adv*.—**preciseness** *n*.

precision /prɪ'sɪʒən/ *n* the quality of being precise; accuracy. •*adj* (*machines*) having a high degree of accuracy.

preclude /prɪ'kluːd/ *vt* to rule out in advance; to make impossible.—**preclusion** *n*.—**preclusive** *adj*.

precocious /prɪ'koːʃəs/ *adj* prematurely ripe or developed.—**precociously** *adv*.—**precociousness** *n*.

precocity /-'kɒsɪti/ *n* the condition of being precocious, precociousness; early development, *esp* of a child's mind.

precognition /ˌpriːkɒg'nɪʃən/ *n* the supposed extrasensory perception of a future event; clairvoyance.—**precognitive** *adj*.

pre-Columbian /ˌpriːkə'lʌmbiən/ *adj* of or originating in the Americas before their discovery by Christopher Columbus.

preconceive /ˌpriːkən'siːv/ *vt* to form an idea or opinion of before actual experience.

preconception /ˌpriːkən'sepʃən/ *n* the act of preconceiving; an opinion formed without actual knowledge.

precondition /ˌpriːkən'dɪʃən/ *n* a requirement that must be met beforehand, a prerequisite. • *vt* (*an organism, a patient*) to prepare to behave or react in a certain way under certain conditions.

precursor /prɪ'kɜːrsər/ *n* a predecessor; a substance from which another substance is formed.—**precursory** *adj*.

predacious, predaceous /prɪ'deɪʃəs/ *adj* living on prey.—**predaciousness, predaceousness, predacity** *n*.

predate /priː'deɪt/ *vt* to antedate.

predator /'predətər/ *n* a person who preys, plunders or devours; a carnivorous animal.

predatory /'predətəri/ *adj* living on prey, of or relating to a predator; characterized by hunting or plundering.—**predatorily** *adv*.—**predatoriness** *n*.

predecease /ˌpriːdɪ'siːs/ *vt* to die before (another).

predecessor /'priːdɪˌsesər/ or /'priː-/ *n* a former holder of a position or office; an ancestor.

predella /prɪ'delə/ *n* (*pl* **predellae**) a platform for, or shelf upon, an altar; a painting, or sculpture, on such a platform or shelf.

predestinarian /priːˌdestɪ'neəriən/ *adj* pertaining to predestination. • *n* someone who believes in the doctrine of predestination.

predestinate /prɪ'destɪˌneɪt/ *adj* predestined. • *vt* to predestine.

predestination /priːˌdestɪ'neɪʃən/ *n* a predestining or being predestined; destiny; (*theol*) the doctrine that God has from all eternity decreed the salvation or damnation of each soul.

predestine /prɪ'destɪn/ *vt* to foreordain; to destine beforehand.

predetermine /ˌpriːdɪ'tɜːrmɪnət/ *adj* predetermined.

predetermine /ˌpriːdɪ'tɜːrmɪn/ *vt* to decide beforehand.—**predetermination** *n*.

predicable /'predɪkəbəl/ *adj* which can be predicated.

predicament /prɪ'dɪkəmənt/ *n* a difficult or embarrassing situation.

predicant /'predɪkənt/ *adj* pertaining to preaching. • *n* a preaching friar, *esp* a Dominican.

predicate /'predɪˌkeɪt/ *vt* to state as a quality or attribute; to base (on facts, conditions etc). • *n* (*gram*) that which is stated about the subject.—**predication** *n*.

predicative /prɪ'dɪkətɪv/ *adj* (*gram*) (*adjective, etc*) making a statement about the subject of a verb. • *n* a predicative construction.

predicatory /'prɪdɪkəˌtɔːri/ *adj* of or given to preaching.

predict /prɪ'dɪkt/ *vt* to foretell; to state (what one believes will happen).—**predictor** *n*.

predictable /prɪ'dɪktəbəl/ *adj* able to be predicted or anticipated; lacking originality.—**predictability** *n*.—**predictably** *adv*.

prediction /prɪ'dɪkʃən/ *n* the act of predicting; that which is predicted; a forecast or prophecy.—**predictive** *adj*.—**predictively** *adv*.

predigest /ˌpriːdaɪ'dʒest/ *vt* to treat (food) artificially to make easily digestible.

predilection /ˌpriːdɪ'lekʃən/ *n* partiality, liking for.

predispose /ˌpriːdɪ'spoːz/ *vt* to incline beforehand; (*disease, etc*) to make susceptible to.—**predisposition** *n*.

predominant /prɪ'dɒmɪnən/ *adj* ruling over, controlling; influencing.—**predominance, predominancy** *n*.

predominantly /-li/ *adv* mainly.

predominate /prɪ'dɒmɪˌneɪt/ *vt* to rule over; to have influence or control over; to prevail; to be greater in number, intensity, etc.—**predomination** *n*.—**predominator** *n*.

pre-eminent, preeminent /prɪ'emɪnənt/ *adj* distinguished above others; outstanding.—**pre-eminence, preeminence** *n*.—**pre-eminently, preeminently** *adv*.

pre-empt, preempt /prɪ'empt/ or /-'emt/ *vt* to take action to check other action beforehand; to gain the right to buy (public land) by settling on it; to seize before anyone else can; to replace; (*in bridge*) to bid highly to exclude bids from opponents.—**pre-emptor, preemptor** *n*.—**pre-emptory, preemptory** *adj*.

pre-emption, preemption /prɪ'empʃən/ *n* a pre-empting or being pre-empted; a buying or the right to buy before the opportunity is given to others; such a purchase.

pre-emptive, preemptive /prɪ'emptɪv/ *adj* (*bridge*) denoting a high bid to exclude bids from the opposition.—**pre-emptively, preemptively** *adv*.

preen /priːn/ *vti* (*birds*) to clean and trim the feathers; to congratulate (oneself) for achievement; to groom (oneself); to gloat.—**preener** *n*.

prefab /'priːfæb/ *n* (*inf*) a prefabricated part or building.

prefabricate /priː'fæbrɪˌkeɪt/ *vt* (*house, etc*) to build in standardized sections for shipment and quick assembly; to produce artificially.—**prefabrication** *n*.—**prefabricator** *n*.

preface /'prefəs/ *n* an introduction or preliminary explanation; a foreword or introduction to a book; a preamble. • *vt* to serve as a preface; to introduce.—**prefacer** *n*.

prefatory /'prefəˌtɔːri/ *adj* of or pertaining to a preface; introductory.—**prefatorily** *adv*.

prefect /'priːfekt/ *n* a person placed in authority over others; a student monitor in a school; in some countries, an administrative official.—**prefectoral** *adj*.

prefecture /'priːfektʃur/ *n* the office, district, residence, or tenure of a prefect.—**prefectural** *adj*.

prefer /prə'fɜːr/ *vt* (**preferring, preferred**) to like better; to promote, advance; to put before a court, etc, for consideration.—**preferrer** *n*.

preferable /'prefərəbəl/ or /'prefrəbəl/, /prə'fɜːrəbəl/ *adj* deserving preference; superior; more desirable.—**preferably** *adv*.

preference /'prefərəns/ *n* the act of preferring, choosing, or favouring one above another; that which is chosen or preferred; prior right; advantage given to one person, country, etc, over others.

preferential /ˌprefə'renʃəl/ *adj* giving or receiving preference.—**preferentialism** *n*.—**preferentially** *adv*.

preferment /prɪˌfɜːrmənt/ *n* advancement; promotion to a higher post.

prefiguration /ˌpriːfɪgju'reɪʃən/ *n* the act of prefiguring.—**prefigurative** *adj*.

prefigure /priː'fɪgjur/ *vt* to suggest in advance, foreshadow; to imagine beforehand.

prefix /'priːfɪks/ *vt* to put at the beginning of or before; to put as an introduction. • *n* a syllable or group of syllables placed at the beginning of a word, affecting its meaning.—**prefixal** *adj*.—**prefixally** *adv*.

preglacial /priː'gleɪʃəl/ or /-siəl/ *adj* existing before a glacial period.

pregnable /'pregnəbəl/ *adj* capable of being attacked and captured.

pregnancy /'pregnənsi/ *n* (*pl* **pregnancies**) the state of being pregnant; the period of this.

pregnant /'pregnənt/ *adj* having a foetus in the womb; significant, meaningful; imaginative; filled (with) or rich (in).—**pregnantly** *adv*.

prehensile /pri'hɛnsail/ *adj* capable of grasping, *esp* by wrapping around.—**prehensility** *n*.

prehension /pri'hɛnʃən/ *n* grasping; the ability to grasp.

prehistoric /ˌpriːhɪ'stɒrɪk/, **prehistorical** /-kəl/ *adj* of the period before written records began; (*inf*) old-fashioned.—**prehistorically** *adv*.

prehistory /pri'hɪstəri/ *n* (*pl* **prehistories**) events that took place before recorded history; the study of prehistoric events; the history of the earlier background of an incident, etc.—**prehistorian** *n*.

prejudge /pri'dʒʌdʒ/ *vt* to pass judgment on before a trial; to form a premature opinion.—**prejudger** *n*.—**prejudgment, prejudgement** *n*.

prejudice /'predʒudis/ *n* a judgment or opinion made without adequate knowledge; bias; intolerance or hatred of other races, etc; (*law*) injury or disadvantage due to another's action. • *vt* to affect or injure through prejudice.—**prejudiced** *adj*.

prejudicial /ˌpredʒu'dɪʃəl/ *adj* causing prejudice; detrimental, damaging.—**prejudicially** *adv*.

prelacy /'preləsi/ *n* (*pl* **prelacies**) the office or status of a prelate; prelates collectively; church government by prelates.

prelate /'prelət/ *n* a church dignity with episcopal authority.—**prelatic** *adj*.

prelature /-lətʃər/ *n* the office or status of a prelate.

preliminary /pri'lɪmɪneri/ *adj* preparatory; introductory. • *n* (*pl* **preliminaries**) an event preceding another; a preliminary step or measure; (*in school*) a preparatory examination.—**preliminarily** *adv*.

prelims /'priːlɪmz/ or /pri'lɪmz/ *npl* the front matter of a book, before the main text; preliminary university exams.

prelude /'preilu:d/ or /-lju:d/, /'prɛl-/ *n* an introductory act or event; an event preceding another of greater importance; (*mus*) a movement which acts as an introduction. • *vti* to serve as a prelude to, to usher in; to play a prelude.—**preludial** *adj*.—**prelusion** *n*.—**prelusive, prelusory** *adj*.

premarital /pri'mɛritəl/ *adj* (*sex*) taking place before marriage.

premature /pri:mə'tʃur/ or /'prɛm-/ *adj* occurring before the expected or normal time; too early, hasty.—**prematurely** *adv*.—**prematurity** *n*.

premeditate /pri'mɛditeit/ *vt* (*crime, etc*) to plan in advance.—**premeditatedly** *adv*.—**premeditative** *adj*.—**premeditator** *n*.

premeditation /-'teiʃən/ *n* deliberation or thought before doing something; (*law*) the plotting of a crime beforehand, demonstrating intent to commit it.

premier /'priːmjiːr/ or /'priːmjər/, /'priːmiːr/, /'prɛmjər/ *adj* principal; first. • *n* the head of a government, a prime minister.—**premiership** *n*.

premiere, première /prɛm'jɛr/ or /prə'mjɛr/, /'prɛmjɛr/, /'priːmjiːr/, /-'mjiːr/ *n* the first public performance of a play, film, etc. • *vt* to give a premiere of. • *vi* to have a first performance; to appear for the first time as a star performer.

premise /'prɛmɪs/ *n* a proposition on which reasoning is based; something assumed or taken for granted.—*also* **premiss**; (*pl*) a piece of land and its buildings. • *vt* to state as an introduction; to postulate; to base on certain assumptions.

premium /'priːmiəm/ *n* a reward, *esp* an inducement to buy; a periodical payment for insurance; excess over an original price; something given free or at a reduced price with a purchase; a high value or value in excess of expectation. • *adj* (*goods*) high quality.

premonition /ˌprɛmə'nɪʃən/ *n* a foreboding; a feeling of something about to happen.—**premonitory** *adj*.

prenatal /pri'neitəl/ or /'priː-/ *adj* before birth.

preoccupation /priɒkju'peiʃən/ *n* a concern that prevents thought of other things; mental absorption; business that takes precedence; preoccupancy.

preoccupied /pri'ɒkjupaid/ *adj* absent-minded, lost in thought; (*with* **with**) having one's attention completely taken up by.

preoccupy /pri'ɒkju,pai/ *vt* (**preoccupying, preoccupied**) to take possession of beforehand; to engross, fill the thoughts of.

preordain /ˌpriːɔr'dein/ *vt* to ordain beforehand.—**preordination** *n*.

prep /prɛp/ *abbr* = preparatory school; preparation; preposition.

prep school *see* **preparatory school**.

prepaid *see* **prepay**.

preparation /ˌprɛpə'reiʃən/ *n* the act of preparing; a preparatory measure; something prepared, as a medicine, cosmetic, etc.

preparative /pri'pɛrətiv/ *adj* preparatory. • *n* something that prepares the way.—**preparatively** *adv*.

preparatory /'prɛpərə,tori/ or /prə'pɛrətori/ *adj* serving to prepare; introductory. • *adv* by way of preparation; in a preparatory manner.—**preparatorily** *adv*.

preparatory school *n* a private school that prepares students for an advanced school or college.—*also* **prep (school)**.

prepare /prə'per/ *vt* to make ready in advance; to fit out, equip; to cook; to instruct, teach; to put together. • *vi* to make oneself ready.—**preparedly** *adv*.

prepared /prə'perd/ *adj* subjected to a special process or treatment.

preparedness /-nəs/ *n* the state of being prepared, *esp* for waging war.

prepay /pri'pei/ *vt* (**prepaying, prepaid**) to pay in advance.—**prepayment** *n*.

prepense /pri'pens/ *adj* premeditated.

preponderant /prə'pɒndərənt/ *adj* being greater in number, amount, importance, weight, etc; predominant.—**preponderance, preponderancy** *n*.—**preponderantly** *adv*.

preponderate /pri'pɒndə,reit/ *vi* to be greater in number, amount, influence, etc; to predominate, prevail; to weigh more.—**preponderation** *n*.

preposition /ˌprɛpə'zɪʃən/ *n* a word used before a noun or pronoun to show its relation to another part of the sentence.—**prepositional** *adj*.

prepositive /pri'pɒzitiv/ *adj, n* (*gram*) (a particle or word) which can be attached as a prefix to a word.

prepossess /ˌpriːpə'zɛs/ *vt* to impress favourably; to prejudice.

prepossessing /-ɪŋ/ *adj* impressing favourably; attractive.—**prepossessingly** *adv*.

prepossession /-'zeiʃən/ *n* a prepossessed state; a preconceived opinion or judgement.

preposterous /pri'pɒstərəs/ *adj* ridiculous; laughable; absurd.—**preposterously** *adv*.—**preposterousness** *n*.

prepotency /pri'po:tənsi/ *n* the state of being prepotent; (*biol*) a dominant hereditary influence.

prepotent /pri'po:tənt/ *adj* very or more powerful; (*biol*) having a dominant hereditary influence.

prepuce /'priːpjuːs/ *n* the loose skin at the end of the penis.—*also* **foreskin**.

pre-Raphaelite /pri'ræfiə,lait/ *adj, n* (a member) of a 19th-century school of artists who imitated the Italian style of painting before Raphael, using brilliant colour and minute detail.

prerecord /ˌpriːri'kord/ *vt* (*radio, TV programme*) to record in advance for later broadcasting.—**prerecorded** *adj*.

prerequisite /pri'rɛkwizit/ *n* a condition, etc, that must be fulfilled prior to something else. • *adj* required beforehand.

prerogative /prə'rɒgətiv/ *n* a privilege or right accorded through office or hereditary rank.

presage /'prɛsədʒ/ *n* a foreboding or presentiment; an omen. • *vt* to foretell; to have a presentiment of.

presbyopia /ˌprɛzbi:'opiːə/ *n* a condition of long-sightedness, *usu* progressing with age, in which near objects are seen indistinctly, caused by a change in the refractive power of the eye due to the flattening of the lens.

presbyter /'prɛsbitər/ or /'prɛz-/ *n* in the Presbyterian Church, an elder; in the Episcopal Church, a priest or minister.—**presbyterial** *adj*.

presbyterian /ˌprɛsbi'tiːriən/ or /'prɛz-/ *adj* of or denoting government by presbyteries; (*with cap*) of a Presbyterian Church. • *n* a member of a Presbyterian Church.—**Presbyterianism** *n*.

presbytery /'prɛsbitri/ or /'prɛz-/ *n* (*pl* **presbyteries**) in a Presbyterian Church a court composed of ministers and one elder from each church within a district; a district so represented; the eastern part of the chancel of a church; a Roman Catholic priest's house.

preschool /'priːskuːl/ *adj* of or for a child between infancy and school age.

prescience /'presiəns/ *n* foreknowledge.—**prescient** *adj*.

prescribe /prə'skraib/ *vt* to designate; to ordain; (*rules*) to lay down; (*medicine, treatment*) to order, advise.—**prescriber** *n*.

prescript /'priskript/ *n* an ordnance or decree. • *adj* prescribed, directed.

prescription /prə'skrɪpʃən/ *n* act of prescribing; (*med*) a written instruction by a physician for the preparation of a drug; (*law*) establishment of a right or title through long use.

prescriptive /pri'skriptiv/ *adj* prescribing, ordering, advising; based on long use, traditional.—**prescriptively** *adv*.

preselect /ˌpriːsɪˈlɛkt/ *vt* to select beforehand, *usu* according to a particular criterion.—**preselection** *n*.—**preselective** *adj*.

presence /ˈprɛzəns/ *n* being present; immediate surroundings; personal appearance and bearing; impressive bearing, personality, etc; something (as a spirit) felt or believed to be present.

presence of mind *n* readiness of resource in an emergency, etc; the ability to say the right thing.

present[1] /ˈprɛzənt/ *adj* being at the specified place; existing or happening now; (*gram*) denoting action or state now or action that is always true. • *n* the time being; now; the present tense.

present[2] *n* a gift.

present[3] /prəˈzɛnt/ *vt* to introduce someone, *esp* socially; (*a play, etc*) to bring before the public, exhibit; to make a gift or award; to show; to perform; (*law*) to lay a charge before a court; (*weapon*) to point in a particular direction. • *vi* to present a weapon; to become manifest; to come forward as a patient.

presentable /prɪˈzɛntəbəl/ *adj* of decent appearance; fit to go into company.—**presentability** *n*.—**presentably** *adv*.

presentation /ˌprɛzənˈteɪʃən/ or /ˌpriː-/ *n* act of presenting; a display or exhibition; style of presenting; something offered or given; a description or persuasive account; (*med*) the position of a foetus in the uterus.—**presentational** *adj*.

presentative /-ˈteɪtɪv/ *adj* (*of benefice*) admitting presentation by patron; (*philos*) able to be apprehended directly by the mind

presenter /-ər/ *n* a person who presents someone or something; (*radio, TV*) a person who introduces a show, an announcer.

presentiment /prɪˈzɛntɪmənt/ or /-ˈsɛntɪmənt/ *n* a premonition, apprehension, *esp* of evil.

presently /ˈprɛzəntli/ *adv* in a short while, soon.

presentment /prɪˈzɛntmənt/ *n* the act of presenting; something which is presented; a representation or delineation; the laying of a formal statement before a court or authority.

preservation /ˌprɛzərˈveɪʃən/ *n* the act of preserving or securing; a state of being preserved or repaired.

preservationist /-ɪst/ *n* someone who undertakes or advocates preservation (as of a biological species or a historic landmark).

preservative /prəˈzɜrvətɪv/ *adj* preserving. • *n* something that preserves or has the power of preserving, *esp* an additive.

preserve /prəˈzɜrv/ *vt* to keep safe from danger; to protect; (*food*) to can, pickle, or prepare for future use; to keep or reserve for personal or special use. • *vi* to make preserves; to raise and protect game for sport. • *n* (*usu pl*) fruit preserved by cooking in sugar; an area restricted for the protection of natural resources, *esp* one used for regulated hunting, etc; something regarded as reserved for certain persons.—**preservable** *adj*.—**preserver** *n*.

preset /priːˈsɛt/ *vt* (**presetting, preset**) to set (the controls of an electrical device) in advance.

preside /prɪˈzaɪd/ *vi* to take the chair or hold the position of authority; to take control or exercise authority.—**presider** *n*.

presidency /ˈprɛzɪdənsi/ *n* (*pl* **presidencies**) the office, dignity, term, jurisdiction or residence of a president.

president /ˈprɛzɪdənt/ *n* the head of state of a republic; the highest officer of a company, club, etc.—**presidential** *adj*.—**presidentially** *adv*.

president-elect *n* a president who has been elected to office but has not yet taken up the post.

presidio /prɪˈsɪdiˌoʊ/ *n* (*pl* **presidios**) (*Spain*) a fort or military establishment.

presidium /prɪˈzɪdiəm/ or /-ˈsɪdiəm/ *n* (*pl* **presidiums, presidia**) a presiding committee in a communist organization.

press /prɛs/ *vt* to act on with steady force or weight; to push against, squeeze, compress, etc; to squeeze the juice, etc from; (*clothes, etc*) to iron; to embrace closely; to force, compel; to entreat; to emphasize; to trouble; to urge on; (*record*) to make from a matrix. • *vi* to weigh down; to crowd closely; to go forward with determination. • *n* pressure, urgency, etc; a crowd; a machine for crushing, stamping, etc; a machine for printing; a printing or publishing establishment; the gathering and distribution of news and those who perform these functions; newspapers collectively; any of various pressure devices; an upright closet for storing clothes.

press conference *n* a group interview given to members of the press by a politician, celebrity, etc.

pressing /ˈprɛsɪŋ/ *adj* urgent; calling for immediate attention; importunate. • *n* a number of records made at one time from a master.—**pressingly** *adv*.

pressman /ˈprɛsmən/ *n* (*pl* **pressmen**) a journalist; an operator of a printing press.

pressmark /ˈprɛsˌmɑːrk/ *n* a number showing a book's place in a library.

press secretary *n* a person officially in charge of relations with the press for a *usu* prominent public figure.

press-up *n* an exercise involving raising and lowering the body with the arms.

pressure /ˈprɛʃər/ *n* the act of pressing; a compelling force; a moral force; compression; urgency; constraint; (*physics*) force per unit of area. • *vt* to pressurize.

pressure cooker *n* a strong, sealed pan in which food can be cooked quickly by steam under pressure; (*inf*) a situation beset with emotional or social pressure.

pressure group *n* a group of people organized to alert public opinion, legislators, etc, to a particular area of interest.

pressure point *n* a point on the body where a blood vessel can be compressed to check bleeding.

pressurize /ˈprɛʃəraɪz/ *vt* to keep nearly normal atmospheric pressure inside an aeroplane, etc, as at high altitudes; to exert pressure on; to attempt to compel, press.—**pressurization** *n*.—**pressurizer** *n*.

prestidigitation /ˌprɛstɪˌdɪdʒɪˈteɪʃən/ *n* sleight of hand.—**prestidigitator** *n*.

prestige /prɛˈstiːʒ/ or /-ˈstiːʒ/ *n* standing in the eyes of people; commanding position in people's minds.

prestigious /prɛˈstiːdʒəs/ or /-ˈstɪdʒəs/ *adj* imparting prestige or distinction.

prestissimo /prɛˈstɪsɪˌmoʊ/ *adj, adv* (*mus*) very fast.

presto /ˈprɛstoʊ/ *adj, adv* (*mus*) quick; immediately. • *n* (*pl* **prestos**) (*mus*) a lively passage.

presumable /prɪˈzuːməbəl/ or /-ˈzjuː-/ *adj* that may be presumed or taken to be true.

presumably /-məbli/ *adv* as may be presumed.

presume /prɪˈzuːm/ or /-ˈzjuːn/ *vt* to take for granted, suppose. • *vi* to assume to be true; to act without permission; to take liberties; (*with* **on, upon**) to take advantage of.—**presumedly** *adv*.—**presumer** *n*.

presuming /-ɪŋ/ *adj* venturing without permission; presumptuous.—**presumingly** *adv*.

presumption /prɪˈzɛmpʃən/ *n* a supposition; a thing presumed; a strong probability; effrontery.

presumptive /prɪˈzɛmptɪv/ *adj* assumed in the absence of contrary evidence; probable.—**presumptively** *adv*.

presumptuous /prɪˈzɛmptʃʊəs/ *adj* tending to presume; bold; forward.—**presumptuously** *adv*.—**presumptuousness** *n*.

presuppose /ˌpriːsəˈpoʊz/ *vt* to assume beforehand; to involve as a necessary prior condition.—**presupposition** *n*.

pretence /ˈpriːtɛns/ or /prɪˈtɛrs/ *n* the act of pretending; a hypocritical show; a fraud, a sham.—*also* **pretense**.

pretend /prɪˈtɛnd/ *vti* to claim, represent, or assert falsely; to feign, make believe; to lay claim (to).

pretended /prɪˈtɛndɪd/ *adj* feigned; ostensible; untrue; insincerely asserted or claimed.—**pretendedly** *adv*.

pretender /prɪˈtɛndər/ *n* a person who makes a pretence; a claimant to a title.

pretense *see* **pretence**.

pretension /prɪˈtɛnʃən/ *n* a false claim; affectation; assumption of superiority.

pretentious /prɪˈtɛnʃəs/ *adj* claiming great importance; ostentatious.—**pretentiously** *adv*.—**pretentiousness** *n*.

preterit, preterite /ˈprɛtərɪt/ (*gram*) *adj* denoting past action. • *n* the past tense.

preterition /ˌprɛtəˈrɪʃən/ *n* omission; (*theology*) the doctrine of the passing over of the non-elect by God.

preternatural /ˌpriːtərˈnætʃərəl/ or /-nætʃrəl/ *adj* out of the regular course of things, abnormal.

pretext /ˈpriːtɛkst/ *n* a pretended reason to conceal a true one; an excuse.

prettify /ˈprɪtɪˌfaɪ/ *vt* (**prettifying, prettified**) to make pretty.—**prettifaction** *n*.

pretty /ˈprɪti/ *adj* (**prettier, prettiest**) attractive in a dainty, graceful way. • *adv* (*inf*) fairly, moderately. • *n* (*pl* **pretties**) (*inf*) a pretty or pleasing person or thing. • *vt* (**prettying, prettied**) (*with* **up**) (*inf*) to make pretty.—**prettily** *adv*.—**prettiness** *n*.

pretzel /ˈprɛtsəl/ *n* a hard, brittle, salted biscuit, often formed in a loose knot.

prevail /pri'veɪl/ *vi* to overcome; to predominate; to be customary or in force.

prevailing /-ɪŋ/ *adj* generally accepted, widespread; predominant.—**prevailingly** *adv*.

prevalent /'prevələnt/ *adj* current; predominant; widely practised or experienced.—**prevalence** *n*.—**prevalently** *adv*.

prevaricate /prɪ'verɪˌkeɪt/ *vi* to make evasive or misleading statements.—**prevarication** *n*.—**prevaricator** *n*.

prevenient /prɪ'viːnɪənt/ *adj* preceding; anticipating; aiming at prevention.

prevent /prɪ'vent/ *vt* to keep from happening; to hinder.—**preventable, preventible** *adj*.—**preventably, preventibly** *adv*.—**preventer** *n*.

prevention /prɪ'venʃən/ *n* a preventing or being prevented; a hindrance; a preventive.

preventive /prɪ'ventɪv/, **preventative** /prɪ'ventətɪv/ *adj* serving to prevent, precautionary. • *n* something used to prevent disease.—**preventively** *adv*.—**preventiveness** *n*.

preview /'priːvjuː/ *n* an advance, restricted showing, as of a film; a showing of scenes from a film to advertise it. • *vt* to view or show in advance of public presentation; to give a preliminary survey.

previous /'priːvɪəs/ *adj* coming before in time or order; prior, former.—**previously** *adv*.—**previousness** *n*.

prewar *adj* before a war.

prey /preɪ/ *n* an animal killed for food by another; a victim. • *vi* (*with* **on, upon**) to seize and devour prey; (*person*) to victimize; to weigh heavily on the mind.

priapism /'praɪəˌpɪzəm/ *n* (*med*) abnormally prolonged penile erection.

price /praɪs/ *n* the amount, *usu* in money, paid for anything; the cost of obtaining some benefit; value, worth. • *vt* to set the price of something; to estimate a price; (*with* **out of the market**) to deprive by raising prices excessively.

priceless /-ləs/ *adj* very expensive; invaluable; (*inf*) very amusing, odd, or absurd.—**pricelessly** *adv*.

price war *n* a period of commercial competition marked by repeated cutting of prices among competitors.

pricey /'praɪsi/ *adj* (**pricier, priciest**) (*inf*) expensive.—*also* **pricy**.

prick /prɪk/ *n* a sharp point; a puncture or piercing made by a sharp point; the wound or sensation inflicted; a qualm (of conscience); (*offensive*) a spiteful person *usu* with authority. • *vti* to affect with anguish, grief, or remorse; to pierce slightly; to cause a sharp pain to; to goad, spur; (*the ears*) to erect; (*with* **out**) to transfer seedlings.

pricker /-ər/ *n* a thing that pricks, *esp* a prickle or thorn.

pricket /'prɪkɪt/ *n* a buck in its second year.

prickle /'prɪkəl/ *n* a thorn, spine or bristle; a pricking sensation. • *vti* to feel or cause to feel a pricking sensation.

prickly /'prɪkli/ *adj* (**pricklier, prickliest**) having prickles; tingling; irritable.—**prickliness** *n*.

prickly heat *n* a skin eruption caused by inflammation of the sweat glands.

pride /praɪd/ *n* feeling of self-worth or esteem; excessive self-esteem; conceit; a sense of one's own importance; a feeling of elation due to success; the cause of this; splendour; a herd (of lions). • *vti* (*reflex*) (*with* **in** *or* **on**)to be proud of; to take credit for.—**prideful** *adj*.

priedieu /'priːdjuː/ *or* /-duː/ *n* a desk with a low rest for kneeling upon while working or praying.

prier /'praɪər/ *n* one who pries.—*also* **pryer**.

priest /priːst/ *n* in various churches, a person authorized to perform sacred rites; an Anglican, Eastern Orthodox, or Roman Catholic clergyman ranking below a bishop.

priestcraft /'priːstkræft/ *n* the work of a priest and its related skills; (*derog*) the schemes used by priests to get power and wealth.

priestess /'priːstes/ *n* a priest who is a woman; a woman regarded as a leader (as of a movement).

priesthood /'priːsthʊd/ *n* the office of priest; priests collectively.

priestly /'priːstli/ *adj* (**priestlier, priestliest**) of or befitting a priest.—**priestliness** *n*.

prig /prɪg/ *n* a smug, self-righteous person.—**priggery, priggism** *n*.

priggish /-ɪʃ/ *adj* tiresomely precise; strait-laced.—**priggishly** *adv*.—**priggishness** *n*.

prim /prɪm/ *adj* (**primmer, primmest**) proper, formal and precise in manner; demure. • *vti* (**primming, primmed**) to make prim; to assume a prim expression.—**primly** *adv*.—**primness** *n*.

prima ballerina /ˌpriːməˌbæləˈriːnə/ *n* (*pl* **prima ballerinas**) the principal female dancer in a ballet company.

primacy /'praɪməsi/ *n* (*pl* **primacies**) the office of primate; the state of being first.

prima donna /ˌpriːməˈdɒnə/ *n* (*pl* **prima donnas**) the leading female singer in an opera; (*inf*) a temperamental person.

prima facie /ˌpraɪməˈfeɪʃi/ *adv* at first sight. • *adj* true, valid, or sufficient at first impression; self-evident; legally sufficient to establish a fact unless disproved.

primal /'praɪməl/ *adj* primeval; original; primitive; fundamental.

primarily /praɪˈmerɪli/ *adv* mainly.

primary /'praɪmeri/ *or* /'praɪmərɪ/ *adj* first; earliest; original; first in order of time; chief; elementary. • *n* (*pl* **primaries**) a person or thing that is highest in rank, importance, etc; a preliminary election at which candidates are chosen for the final election.

primary colour *n* one of the three colours from which all others except black can be obtained: red, blue, and yellow.

primary school *n* a school for children below age 11; a school for children up to the third or fourth grade of elementary school and sometimes kindergarten.

primate[1] /'praɪmeɪt/ *n* any of the highest order of mammals, including man.—**primatial** *adj*.

primate[2] /'praɪmət/ *n* an archbishop or the highest ranking bishop in a province, etc.—**primateship** *n*.

prime[1] /praɪm/ *adj* first in rank, importance, or quality; chief; (*math*) of a number, divisible only by itself and 1. • *n* the best time; the height of perfection; full maturity; full health and strength.—**primeness** *n*.

prime[2] *vt* to prepare or make something ready; to pour liquid into (a pump) or powder into (a firearm); to paint on a primer.

prime minister *n* the head of the government in a parliamentary democracy.

primer[1]/'praɪmər/ *n* a simple book for teaching; a small introductory book on a subject.

primer[2] *n* a detonating device; a first coat of paint or oil.

prime time *n* (*radio, TV*) the hours when the largest audience is available.

primeval /praɪˈmiːvəl/ *adj* of the first age of the world; primitive.

priming /'praɪmɪŋ/ *n* a preliminary coating (of paint); a powder used to explode a charge.

primipara /ˌpraɪˈmɪpərə/ *n* (*pl* **primiparas, primiparae**) (*obstetrics*) a woman due to give birth to her first child, or who has given birth to only one child.—**primiparous** *adj*.

primitive /'prɪmɪtɪv/ *adj* of the beginning or the earliest times; crude; simple; basic. • *n* a primitive person or thing.—**primitively** *adv*.—**primitiveness** *n*.

primo /'priːmoː/ *n* (*pl* **primos, primi**) (*mus*) the leading part in a duet or ensemble.

primogenitor /ˌpraɪmoːˈdʒenɪtər/ *n* an ancestor or forefather; an earliest ancestor.

primogeniture /ˌpraɪmoːˈdʒenɪtʃər/ *n* the condition of being the first-born child; (*law*) the right of inheritance of the eldest child.—**primogenitary** *adj*.

primordial /praɪˈmɔːdɪəl/ *adj* earliest; primeval; fundamental; primitive.—**primordially** *adv*.

primp /prɪmp/ *vti* to dress (oneself) up.

primrose /'prɪmroːz/ *n* a perennial plant with pale yellow flowers.

primula /'prɪmjʊlə/ *n* any of a genus of plants that includes the primrose, cowslip, etc.

primum mobile /ˌpriːmʊmˈmoːbɪli/ *n* the first movement or cause of motion; (*astron*) the tenth and outermost of the imaginary spheres in the Ptolemaic system, which was supposed to revolve from East to West once every 24 hours, carrying the other spheres with it.

prince /prɪns/ *n* the son of a sovereign; a ruler ranking below a king; the head of a principality; any pre-eminent person.—**princedom** *n*.

Prince Edward Islander *n* ✤ (*Cdn*) a person who lives in or is from Prince Edward Island.

princeling /'prɪnslɪŋ/ *n* a young prince; a petty ruler.

princely /'prɪnsli/ *adj* (**princelier, princeliest**) of or like a prince; lavish, generous; regal.—**princeliness** *n*.

princess /'prɪnses/ *or* /-'ses/ *n* a daughter of a sovereign; the wife of a prince; one outstanding in a specified respect.

principal /'prɪnsɪpəl/ *adj* first in rank or importance; chief. • *n* a principal person; a person who organizes; the head of a college or school; the leading player in a ballet, opera, etc; (*law*) the person who commits a crime; a person for whom another acts as agent; a capital sum lent or invested; a main beam or rafter.—**principalship** *n*.

principality /ˌprɪnsɪˈpælɪtɪ/ *n* (*pl* **principalities**) the position of responsibility of a principal; the rank and territory of a prince.

principally /ˈprɪnsɪpælɪ/ *adv* mainly.

Principal Meridian *n* ✤ a geographical meridian chosen to be the reference point for a land survey.

principle /ˈprɪnsɪpəl/ *n* a basic truth; a law or doctrine used as a basis for others; a moral code of conduct; a chemical constituent with a characteristic quality; a scientific law explaining a natural action; the method of a thing's working.

principled /ˈprɪnsɪpəld/ *adj* having, or acting in line with, moral principles.

prink /prɪŋk/ *vti* to dress (oneself) up; to preen oneself.

print /prɪnt/ *vti* to stamp (a mark, letter, etc) on a surface; to produce (on paper, etc) the impressions of inked type, etc; to produce (a book, etc); to write in letters resembling printed ones; to make (a photographic print). • *n* a mark made on a surface by pressure; the impression of letters, designs, etc, made from inked type, a plate, or block; an impression made by a photomechanical process; a photographic copy, *esp* from a negative.

printable /ˈprɪntəbəl/ *adj* able or fit to be printed.—**printability** *n*.

printed circuit *n* an electronic circuit whose connections are printed on metal-coated board.

printer /ˈprɪntər/ *n* a person engaged in printing; a machine for printing from; a device that produces printout.

printing /ˈprɪntɪŋ/ *n* the activity, skill, or business of producing printed matter; a style of writing using capital letters; the total number of books, etc, printed at one time.—*also* **impression**.

printout /ˈprɪntaʊt/ *n* the printed output of a computer.

prior[1] /ˈpraɪr/ *adj* previous; taking precedence (as in importance).

prior[2] *n* the superior ranking below an abbot in a monastery; the head of a house or group of houses in a religious community.—**prioress** *nf*.

priorate /-rət/ *n* the office or status of a prior.

priority /praɪˈɒrɪtɪ/ *n* (*pl* **priorities**) precedence in rank, time, or place; preference; something requiring specified attention.

priory /ˈpraɪərɪ/ *n* (*pl* **priories**) a religious house under a prior or prioress.

prise, prize /praɪz/ *vt* to force (open, up) with a lever etc.

prism /ˈprɪzəm/ *n* (*geom*) a solid whose ends are similar, equal, and parallel plane figures and whose sides are parallelograms; a transparent body of this form *usu* with triangular ends used for dispersing or reflecting light.

prismatic /prɪzˈmætɪk/ *adj* of or like a prism; (*colours*) formed by a prism; brilliant.—**prismatically** *adv*.

prison /ˈprɪzən/ *n* a building used to house convicted criminals for punishment and suspects remanded in custody while awaiting trial; a penitentiary or jail.

prisoner /ˈprɪznər/ *n* a person held in prison or under arrest; a captive; a person confined by a restraint.

prisoner of war *n* a member of a military force taken prisoner by the enemy during combat.

pristine /ˈprɪstiːn/ or /-ˈstiːn/ *adj* pure; in an original, unspoiled condition.

prithee /ˈprɪðiː/ *interj* (*arch*) pray, please (= "I pray thee").

privacy /ˈpraɪvəsɪ/ or /ˈprɪ-/ *n* (*pl* **privacies**) being private; seclusion; secrecy; one's private life.

private /ˈpraɪvət/ *adj* of or concerning a particular person or group; not open to or controlled by the public; for an individual person; not holding public office; secret. • *n* (*pl*) the genitals; an enlisted man of the lowest military rank in the army.—**privately** *adv*.

private enterprise *n* an economic system in which business activity is operated by private individuals or companies under private not state control.

privateer /ˌpraɪvəˈtiːr/ *n* a privately owned ship commissioned by a government to seize and plunder enemy vessels; a captain or crew member of such a ship.

privation /praɪˈveɪʃən/ *n* being deprived; want of comforts or necessities; hardship.

privative /ˈprɪvətɪv/ *adj* depriving; denoting the absence of something.

privatize /ˈpraɪvəˌtaɪz/ *vt* to restore private ownership by buying back publicly owned stock in a company.

privet /ˈprɪvət/ *n* a white-flowered evergreen shrub used for hedges.

privilege /ˈprɪvəlɪdʒ/ or /ˈprɪvlɪdʒ/ *n* a right or special benefit enjoyed by a person or a small group; a prerogative. • *vt* to bestow a privilege on.

privileged /ˈprɪvəlɪdʒd/ or /ˈprɪvlɪdʒd/ *adj* having or enjoying privileges; not subject to disclosure in a court of law.

privity /ˈprɪvɪtɪ/ *n* (*pl* **privities**) private knowledge; (*law*) a legally recognized relationship.

privy /ˈprɪvɪ/ *adj* private; having access to confidential information. • *n* (*pl* **privies**) a latrine; (*law*) a person with an interest in an action.—**privily** *adv*.

Privy Council Office *n* ✤ (*Cdn*) a federal administrative office that advises the prime minister and other senior officials and coordinates the activities of the cabinet.

prize /praɪz/ *n* an award won in competition or a lottery; a reward given for merit; a thing worth striving for. • *adj* given as, rewarded by, a prize. • *vt* to value highly.

prizefight /ˈpraɪzfaɪt/ *n* a professional boxing match.—**prizefighter** *n*.

PRO *abbr* = public relations officer.

pro[1] /proː/ *adv, prep* in favour of. • *n* (*pl* **pros**) an argument for a proposal or motion.

pro[2] *adj* professional. • *n* (*pl* **pros**) a professional.

pro- *prefix* acting; vice-; favouring; before; forth; according to.

proa /ˈproːə/ *n* a long, narrow, Malay boat propelled by oars and sails.

probability /ˌprɒbəˈbɪlɪtɪ/ *n* (*pl* **probabilities**) that which is probable; likelihood; (*math*) the ratio of the chances in favour of an event to the total number.

probable /ˈprɒbəbəl/ *adj* likely; to be expected.

probably /-lɪ/ *adv* without much doubt.

probang /ˈproːbæŋ/ *n* (*med*) a flexible rod with a sponge at the end used to clear obstructions from, or apply medication to, the gullet.

probate /ˈproːbeɪt/ *n* the validating of a will; the certified copy of a will.

probation /proːˈbeɪʃən/ *n* testing of character or skill; release from prison under supervision by a probation officer; the state or period of being on probation.—**probationary, probational** *adj*.

probation officer *n* an official who watches over prisoners on probation.

probationer /proːˈbeɪʃənər/ *n* a person (as a newly admitted student nurse or teacher) whose fitness is being tested during a trial period; a convicted offender on probation.

probe /proːb/ *n* a flexible surgical instrument for exploring a wound; a device, as an unmanned spacecraft, used to obtain information about an environment; an investigation. • *vt* to explore with a probe; to examine closely; to investigate.—**prober** *n*.

probity /ˈproːbɪtɪ/ or /ˈprɒ-/ *n* honesty, integrity, uprightness.

problem /ˈprɒbləm/ *n* a question for solution; a person, thing or matter difficult to cope with; a puzzle; (*math*) a proposition stating something to be done; an intricate unsettled question.

problematical /ˌprɒbləˈmætɪk/, **problematic** /-kəl/ *adj* presenting a problem; questionable; uncertain.—**problematically** *adv*.

proboscidian, proboscidean /ˌprɒbəˈsɪdɪən/ *adj* pertaining to the class of mammals which includes the elephant. • *n* an animal with a proboscis.

proboscis /proːˈbɒskɪs/ or /-ˈbɒsɪs/ *n* (*pl* **proboscises, proboscides**) an elephant's trunk; a long snout; an insect's sucking organ; (*humorous*) a large) nose.

procedure /prəˈsiːdʒər/ *n* an established mode of conducting business, *esp* in law or in a meeting; a practice; a prescribed or traditional course; a step taken as part of an established order of steps.—**procedural** *adj*.—**procedurally** *adv*.

proceed /prəˈsiːd/ or /proː-/ *vi* to go on, *esp* after stopping; to come from; to continue; to carry on; to issue; to take action; to go to law.

proceeding /-ɪŋ/ *n* an advance or going forward; (*pl*) steps, action, in a lawsuit; (*pl*) published records of a society, etc.

proceeds /ˈproːsiːdz/ *npl* the total amount of money brought in; the net amount received.

process /ˈproːses/ or /ˈprɒ-/ *n* a course or state of going on; a series of events or actions; a method of operation; forward movement; (*law*) a court summons; the whole course of proceedings in a legal action. • *vt* to handle something following set procedures; (*food, etc*) to prepare by a special process; (*law*) to take action; (*film*) to develop.

procession /proːˈseʃən/ or /prə-/ n a group of people marching in order, as in a parade.

processional /proːˈseʃənəl/ or /prə-/ adj pertaining to, or used in, processions. • n a processional hymn or hymn book.

processor /ˈproːsesər/ or /prɒ-/ n one who or that which processes; (comput) a central processing unit.

pro-choice /proːˈtʃɔɪs/ adj supporting a woman's right to choose whether or not to have an abortion.

proclaim /prəˈkleɪm/ vt to announce publicly and officially; to tell openly; to praise.—**proclaimer** n.

proclamation /ˈprɒkləmeɪʃən/ n the act of proclaiming; an official notice to the public.—**proclamatory** adj.

proclitic /prəˈklɪtɪk/ n, adj (a word) so closely connected with the following word as to lose its accent.

proclivity /prəˈklɪvɪti/ n (pl **proclivities**) a tendency or inclination.

proconsul /proːˈkɒnsəl/ n a governor of a colony or province.—**proconsular** adj.—**proconsulate, proconsulship** n.

procrastinate /prəˈkræstɪˌneɪt/ vti to defer action, to delay.—**procrastination** n.—**procrastinator** n.

procreate /ˈproːkriˌeɪt/ vt to bring into being, to engender offspring.—**procreation** n.—**procreant, procreative** adj.—**procreator** n.

Procrustean /proːˈkrʌstiən/ adj compelling uniformity by violent means.

proctor /ˈprɒktər/ n a person who supervises dormitories and examinations in a school.—**proctorial** adj.

procumbent /prəˈkʌmbənt/ adj lying face down, prone; (bot) trailing.

procuration /ˌprɒkjʊˈreɪʃən/ n procuring; (law) the authorization to act on behalf of someone else.

procurator /ˈprɒkjʊˌreɪtər/ n an agent; (ancient Rome) a provincial governor or treasurer.

procuratory /ˈprɒkjʊrəˌtɔːri/ n (law) the authorization to act on another person's behalf.

procure /prəˈkjʊr/ vt to obtain by effort; to get and make available for sexual intercourse; to bring about. • vi to procure women.—**procurable** adj.—**procurement** n.

procurer /prəˈkjʊrər/ n one who procures, esp one who supplies prostitutes.—**procuress** nf.

prod /prɒd/ vt (**prodding, prodded**) to poke or jab, as with a pointed stick; to rouse into activity. • n the action of prodding; a sharp object; a stimulus.—**prodder** n.

prodigal /ˈprɒdɪgəl/ adj wasteful; extravagant; open-handed. • n a wastrel; a person who squanders money.—**prodigally** adv.

prodigality /ˌprɒdɪˈgælɪti/ n (pl **prodigalities**) the state or quality of being prodigal; extravagance, wastefulness; lavishness.

prodigious /prəˈdɪdʒəs/ adj enormous, vast; amazing.—**prodigiously** adv.—**prodigiousness** n.

prodigy /ˈprɒdɪdʒi/ n (pl **prodigies**) an extraordinary person, thing or act; a gifted child.

produce /prəˈdjuːs/ vt to bring about; to bring forward, show; to yield; to cause; to manufacture, make; to give birth to; (play, film) to put before the public. • vi to yield something. • n that which is produced, esp agricultural products.—**producible** adj.—**producibility** n.

producer /ˈprɒdjuːsər/ n someone who produces, esp a farmer or manufacturer; a person who finances or supervises the putting on of a play or making of a film; an apparatus or plant for making gas.

product /ˈprɒdʌkt/ n a thing produced by nature, industry or art; a result; an outgrowth; (math) the number obtained by multiplying two or more numbers together.

production /prəˈdʌkʃən/ n the act of producing; a thing produced; a work presented on the stage or screen or over the air.—**productional** adj.

productive /prəˈdʌktɪv/ adj producing or capable of producing; fertile.—**productively** adv.—**productiveness** n.

productivity /-vɪti/ n the state of being productive; the ratio of the output of a manufacturing business to the input of materials, labour, etc.

proem /ˈproːəm/ n a preface or introduction.

Prof. /proːf/ abbr = professor.

profane /prəˈfeɪn/ adj secular, not sacred; showing no respect for sacred things; irreverent; blasphemous; not possessing esoteric or expert knowledge. • vt to desecrate; to debase by a wrong, unworthy or vulgar use.—**profanation** n.—**profanely** adv.—**profaneness** n.—**profaner** n.

profanity /prəˈfænɪti/ n (pl **profanities**) irreverence; a profane act; blasphemy, swearing.

profess /prəˈfes/ vt to affirm publicly, declare; to claim to be expert in; to declare in words or appearance only.

professed /prəˈfest/ adj openly acknowledged.—**professedly** adv.

profession /prəˈfeʃən/ n an act of professing; avowal, esp of religious belief; an occupation requiring specialized knowledge and often long and intensive academic preparation; the people engaged in this; affirmation; entry into a religious order.

professional /-əl/ adj of or following a profession; conforming to the technical or ethical standards of a profession; earning a livelihood in an activity or field often engaged in by amateurs; having a specified occupation as a permanent career; engaged in by persons receiving financial return; pursuing a line of conduct as though it were a profession. • n one who follows a profession; a professional sportsman; one highly skilled in a particular occupation or field.—**professionally** adv.

professional development day n ✻ a scheduled day on which teachers or other employees take part in seminars and other activities related to professional development.

professionalism /-əˌlɪzəm/ n the methods of professionals; the pursuit of an activity, eg a sport, for financial gain.

professor /prəˈfesər/ n a teacher of the highest rank at an institution of higher education; a teacher.—**professorial** adj.—**professorship** n.

professoriate, professorate /-ˌreɪt/ n a body of professors.

proffer /ˈprɒfər/ vt to offer, usu something intangible.

proficiency /prəˈfɪʃənsi/ n (pl **proficiencies**) a being proficient; competence; skill.

proficient /prəˈfɪʃənt/ adj skilled, competent.—**proficiently** adv.

profile /ˈproːfaɪl/ n a side view of the head as in a portrait, drawing, etc; a biographical sketch; a graph representing a person's abilities. • vt to represent in profile; to produce (as by writing, drawing, etc) a profile of.

profit /ˈprɒfɪt/ n gain; the excess of returns over expenditure; the compensation to entrepreneurs resulting from the assumption of risk; (pl) the excess returns from a business; advantage, benefit. • vti to be of advantage (to), benefit; to gain.—**profitless** adj.

profitable /-təbəl/ adj yielding profit, lucrative; beneficial; useful.—**profitably** adv.—**profitability** n.

profit and loss n a statement at the end of an accounting period that summarizes the revenue and expenditure of a business and shows the consequent profit or loss.

profiteer /ˌprɒfɪˈtiːr/ vi to make exorbitant profits, esp in wartime. • n a person who profiteers.—**profiteering** n.

profitless /ˈprɒfɪtləs/ adj without profit; useless.

profit sharing n a system by which employees share in the profits of a business.—**profit-sharing** adj.

profligate /ˈprɒflɪgət/ adj dissolute; immoral; extravagant. • n a profligate person, a libertine.—**profligacy** n.—**profligately** adv.

pro forma /proːˈfɔːmə/ adj made or carried out as a formality; provided in advance to prescribe form or describe items.

profound /prəˈfaʊnd/ adj at great depth; intellectually deep; abstruse, mysterious.—**profoundly** adv.—**profoundness** n.

profundity /prəˈfendɪti/ n (pl **profundities**) great depth of place, knowledge, skill, etc; a profound or abstruse thing.

profuse /prəˈfjuːz/ adj abundant; generous; extravagant.—**profusely** adv.—**profuseness** n.

profusion /prəˈfjuːʒən/ n an abundance.

progenitive /proːˈdʒenɪtɪv/ adj able to bear offspring.

progenitor /proːˈdʒenɪtər/ n an ancestor.

progeny /proːˈdʒeni/ n (pl **progenies**) offspring; descendants; outcome.

prognathous /prɒgˈneɪθəs/ or /ˈprɒgnəθəs/, **prognathic** /prɒgˈnæθɪk/ adj having projecting lower jaw.—**prognathism** n.

prognosis /prɒgˈnoːsɪs/ n (pl **prognoses**) a prediction; (med) a forecast of the course of a disease.

prognostic /prɒgˈnɒstɪk/ adj predictive (of); foretelling. • n a prediction; an omen; a forewarning symptom.

prognosticate /-ˌkeɪt/ vt to predict; to presage.—**prognostication** n.—**prognosticator** n.

programme /ˈproːgræm/ n (US and comput), **program** a printed list containing details of a ceremony, of the actors in a play, etc; a scheduled radio or television broadcast; a curriculum or syllabus for a course of study; a plan or schedule; a sequence of instructions fed into a computer. • *vti* (**programming, programmed** *or* **programing, programed**) to prepare a plan or schedule; to prepare a plan or schedule to feed a program into a computer; to write a programme.—**programmable** *adj.*—**programmer, programer** *adj.*—**programmatic** *adj.*

progress /'progras/ *n* a movement forwards or onwards, advance; satisfactory growth or development; a tour from place to place in stages. • *vi* to move forward, advance; to improve. • *vt* (*project*) to take to completion.

progression /prə'grɛʃən/ *n* progress; advancement by degrees; (*math*) a series of numbers, each differing from the succeeding according to a fixed law; (*mus*) a regular succession of chords.—**progressional** *adj.*

progressive /prə'grɛsɪv/ *adj* advancing, improving; proceeding by degrees; continuously increasing; aiming at reforms; (*with cap*) denoting a broadly liberal Progressive Party. • *n* a person who believes in moderate political change, esp social improvement by government action; (*with cap*) a member of a Progressive Party.—**progressively** *adv.*—**progressiveness** *n.*—**progressivism** *n.*

prohibit /pro'hɪbɪt/ *vt* to forbid by law; to prevent.

prohibition /pro'hɪbɪʃən/ *n* the act of forbidding; an order that forbids; a legal ban on the manufacture and sale of alcoholic drinks; (*with cap*) the period (1920–33) when there was a legal ban of alcohol in the US.

prohibitionist *n* an advocate of legally prohibiting the sale of alcohol; (*with cap*) a member of the Prohibition Party in the US.

prohibitive /pro'hɪbɪtɪv/, **prohibitory** /-ˌtori/ *adj* forbidding; so high as to prevent purchase, use, etc, of something.—**prohibitively** *adv.*

project /pro'dʒɛkt/ *or* /'pro:-/ *n* a plan, scheme; an undertaking; a task carried out by students, etc, involving research. • *vt* to throw forward; (*light, shadow, etc*) to produce an outline of on a distance surface; to make objective or externalize; (*one's voice*) to make heard at a distance; (*feeling, etc*) to attribute to another; to imagine; to estimate, plan, or figure for the future. • *vi* to jut out; to come across vividly; to make oneself heard clearly.

projectile /prə'dʒɛktaɪl/ *or* /-tɪl/ *n* a missile; something propelled by force. • *adj* throwing forward; capable of being thrown forward.

projection /prə'dʒɛkʃən/ *n* the act of projecting or the condition of being projected; a thing projecting; the representation on a plane surface of part of the earth's surface; a projected image; an estimate of future possibilities based on a current trend; a mental image externalized; an unconscious attribution to another of one's own feelings and motives.—**projectional** *adj.*

projectionist *n* a person who operates a projector.

Projective /prə'dʒɛktɪv/ *adj* (*geom*) pertaining to projection.

projector /prə'dʒɛktər/ *n* an instrument that projects images from transparencies or film; an instrument that projects rays of light; a person who promotes enterprises.

prolapse /pro:'læps/ *vi* (*med*) to fall or slip out of place. • *n* a prolapsed condition.

prolate /pro:'leɪt/ *adj* extended; (*spheroid*) elongated at the poles.

prolegomenon /ˌpro:lɛ'gomənən/ *n* (*pl* **prolegomena**) a critical introduction to a text.

proletariat /ˌpro:lə'teriət/ *n* the lowest social or economic class of a community; wage earners; the industrial working class.—**proletarian** *adj, n.*

proliferate /prə'lɪfəreɪt/ *vi* to grow or reproduce rapidly.—**proliferation** *n.*—**proliferative** *adj.*

proliferous /prə'lɪfərəs/ *adj* reproducing by budding; producing many offshoots.

prolific /prə'lɪfɪk/ *adj* producing abundantly; fruitful.—**prolificacy** *n.*—**prolifically** *adv.*

prolix /'pro:lɪks/ *or* /prə'lɪks/ *adj* verbose, long-winded, tedious.—**prolixity, prolixness** *n.*

prolocutor /pro:'lokjutər/ *n* a chairman or speaker at a convocation, *esp* of the Anglican Church.

prologue, prolog /'pro:log/ *n* the introductory lines of a play, speech, or poem; the reciter of these; a preface; an introductory event. • *vt* (**prologuing, prologued** *or* **prologing, prologed**) to provide with a prologue; to usher in.

prolong /pro'lɒŋ/ *vt* to extend or lengthen in space or time; to spin out.—**prolonger** *n.*

prolongation /prə'lɒŋgeɪʃən/ *n* the act of prolonging; an extension or continuation.

prolusion /prə'lju:ʒən/ *n* a preliminary essay or article.—**prolusory** *adj.*

prom /prom/ *n* a dance for a high school or college class.

promenade /'promə'neɪd/ *n* an esplanade; a ball or dance; a leisurely walk. • *vti* to take a promenade (along or through).—**promenader** *n.*

Promethean /prə'mi:θiən/ *adj* (*myth*) pertaining to Prometheus; life-giving.

prominence /'prominəns/, **prominency** /-si/ *n* the state of being prominent; a projection; relative importance; celebrity, fame.

prominent /'prominənt/ *adj* jutting, projecting; standing out, conspicuous; widely and favourably known; distinguished.—**prominently** *adv.*

promiscuity /ˌpromɪ'skju:ɪti/ *n* (*pl* **promiscuities**) the state of being promiscuous; promiscuous sexual behaviour; an indiscriminate mixture.

promiscuous /prə'mɪskjʊəs/ *adj* indiscriminate, *esp* in sexual liaisons.—**promiscuously** *adv.*—**promiscuousness** *n.*

promise /'promɪs/ *n* a pledge; an undertaking to do or not to do something; an indication, as of a successful future. • *vti* to pledge; to undertake; to give reason to expect.—**promiser** *n.*

promisee /ˌpromɪ'si:/ *n* (*law*) someone to whom a promise is made.

promising /'promɪsɪŋ/ *adj* likely to turn out well; hopeful.

promisor /-ər/ *n* (*law*) someone who makes a promise.

promissory /-sori/ *adj* of the nature of or containing a promise.

promontory /'promontori/ *n* (*pl* **promontories**) a peak of high land that juts out into a body of water.

promote /prə'mo:t/ *vt* to encourage; to advocate; to raise to a higher rank; (*employee, student*) to advance from one grade to the next higher grade; (*product*) to encourage sales by advertising, publicity, or discounting.—**promotable** *adj.*

promoter /-ər/ *n* a person who promotes, *esp* one who organizes and finances a sporting event or pop concert; a substance that increases the activity of a catalyst.

promotion /prə'mo:ʃən/ *n* an elevation in position or rank; the furtherance of the sale of merchandise through advertising, publicity, or discounting.—**promotional** *adj.*

prompt /prompt/ *adj* without delay; quick to respond; immediate; of or relating to prompting actors. • *vt* to urge; to inspire; (*actor*) to remind of forgotten words, etc (as in a play). • *n* something that reminds; a time limit for payment of an account; the contract by which this time is fixed.—**promptly** *adv.*

prompter /-ər/ *n* one that prompts, *esp* a person who sits offstage and reminds actors of forgotten lines.

promptitude *n* quickness of decision and action; readiness; alacrity; punctuality.

promptness *n* alacrity in action or decision; quickness; punctuality.

promulgate /'proməlˌgeɪt/ *vt* to publish, spread abroad; to put (a law) into effect; to proclaim as coming into force.—**promulgation** *n.*—**promulgator** *n.*

pronate /'pro:neɪt/ *vt* (*hand, arm*) to turn so that the palm is downwards.—**pronation** *n.*

pronator /-ər/ *n* a pronating muscle.

prone /pro:n/ *adj* face downwards; lying flat, prostrate; inclined or disposed (to).—**pronely** *adv.*—**proneness** *n.*

prong /prɒŋ/ *n* a spike of a fork or other forked object.—**pronged** *adj.*

pronominal /prə'nominəl/ *adj* pertaining to pronouns; acting as a pronoun.

pronoun /'pro:naʊn/ *n* a word used to represent a noun (*eg I, he, she, it*).

pronounce /prə'naʊns/ *vt* to utter, articulate; to speak officially, pass (judgment); to declare formally.—**pronounceable** *adj.*—**pronouncer** *n.*

pronounced /prə'naʊnst/ *adj* marked, noticeable.—**pronouncedly** *adv.*

pronouncement /prə'naʊnsmənt/ *n* a formal announcement, declaration; a confident assertion.

pronto /'pronto:/ *adv* (*inf*) quickly.

pronunciation /prəˌnʌnsi'eɪʃən/ *n* articulation; the way a word is pronounced.

proof /pru:f/ *n* evidence that establishes the truth; the fact, act, or process of validating; test; demonstration; a sample from type, etc, for correction; a trial print from a photographic negative; the relative strength of an alcoholic liquor. • *adj* resistant; impervious, impenetrable. • *vt* to make proof against (water).

proofread /'pru:fri:d/ *vti* (**proofreading, proofread**) to read and correct (printed proofs).—**proofreader** *n*.

prop[1] /prɒp/ *vt* (**propping, propped**) to support by placing something under or against. • *n* a rigid support; a thing or person giving support.

prop[2] *see* **property**.

prop[3] *n* a propeller.

propaedeutic /ˌpro:pɪ'dju:tɪk/ or /-'dju:-/ *adj* pertaining to propaedeutics, the preliminary knowledge or instruction necessary for the study of any art or science.

propagable /'prɒpəgəbəl/ *adj* which can be propagated.

propaganda /ˌprɒpə'gændə/ *n* the organized spread of ideas, doctrines, etc, to promote a cause; the ideas, etc, so spread.—**propagandism** *n*.—**propagandist** *n, adj*.

propagandize /-ˌdaɪz/ *vt* to spread by propaganda; to use propaganda among. • *vi* to spread propaganda; to use propaganda.

propagate /'prɒpəgeɪt/ *vti* to cause (a plant or animal) to reproduce itself; (*plant or animal*) to reproduce; (*ideas, customs, etc*) to spread.—**propagation** *n*.—**propagative** *adj*.

propagator /-ər/ *n* a device consisting of a box with a ventilated lid, used to regulate growing conditions for seeds and young plants.

propane /'pro:peɪn/ *n* a colourless flammable gas obtained from petroleum and used as a fuel.

pro patria /pro:'pætrɪˌiː/ for one's country.

propel /prə'pel/ *vt* (**propelling, propelled**) to drive or move forward.

propellant, propellent /prə'pelənt/ *n* a thing that propels; an explosive charge; rocket fuel; the gas that activates an aerosol spray.

propeller, propellor /prə'pelər/ *n* a mechanism to impart drive; a device having two or more blades in a revolving hub for propelling a ship or aircraft.

propensity /prə'pensɪti/ *n* (*pl* **propensities**) a natural inclination; disposition, tendency.

proper /'prɒpər/ *adj* own, individual, peculiar; appropriate, fit; correct, conventional; decent, respectable; in the most restricted sense; (*sl*) thorough.

properly /-li/ *adv* in the right way; justifiably; (*sl*) thoroughly.

proper noun *n* the name of a particular person, place, etc.

property /'prɒpərti/ *n* (*pl* **properties**) a quality or attribute; a distinctive feature or characteristic; one's possessions; real estate, land; a movable article used in a stage setting.—*also* **prop**.

prophecy /'prɒfəsi/ *n* (*pl* **prophecies**) a message of divine will and purpose; prediction.

prophesy /'prɒfəsaɪ/ *vti* (**prophesying, prophesied**) to predict with assurance or on the basis of mystic knowledge; to foretell.—**prophesier** *n*.

prophet /'prɒfət/ *n* a religious leader regarded as, or claiming to be, divinely inspired; one who predicts the future.—**prophetess** *nf*.

prophetic /prə'fetɪk/, **prophetical** /-əl/ *adj* of a prophet or prophecy; prophesying events.—**prophetically** *adv*.

prophylactic /ˌprɒfə'læktɪk/ *adj* guarding against disease. • *n* a medicine which guards against disease; a condom.

prophylaxis /ˌprɒfə'læksɪs/ *n* preventive treatment.

propinquity /prə'pɪŋkwɪti/ *n* nearness of time, place or relationship.

propitiate /prə'pɪʃɪˌeɪt/ *vt* to appease, conciliate.—**propitiation** *n*.—**propitiator** *n*.

propitious /prə'pɪʃəs/ *adj* favourable, encouraging; auspicious, opportune.—**propitiously** *adv*.—**propitiousness** *n*.

propolis /'prɒpəlɪs/ *n* a resin from tree buds, collected by bees.

proponent /prə'po:nənt/ *n* someone who makes a proposal, or proposition.

proportion /prə'pɔrʃən/ *n* the relationship between things in size, quantity, or degree; ratio; symmetry, balance; comparative part or share; (*math*) the equality of two ratios; a share or quota; (*pl*) dimensions. • *vt* to put in proper relation with something else; to make proportionate (to).—**proportionment** *n*.—**proportionable** *adj*.

proportional /-əl/ *adj* of proportion; aiming at due proportion; proportionate.—**proportionality** *n*.—**proportionally** *adv*.

proportional representation *n* an electoral system arranged so that minorities are represented in proportion to their strength.

proportionate /-nət/ *adj* in due proportion, corresponding in amount. • *vt* to make proportionate.—**proportionately** *adv*.

proposal /prə'po:zəl/ *n* a scheme, plan, or suggestion; an offer of marriage.

propose /prə'po:z/ *vt* to present for consideration; to suggest; to intend; to announce the drinking of a toast to; (*person*) to nominate; to move as a resolution. • *vi* to make an offer (of marriage).—**proposer** *n*.

proposition /ˌprɒpəzɪʃən/ *n* a proposal for consideration; a plan; a request for sexual intercourse; (*inf*) a proposed deal, as in business; (*inf*) an undertaking to be dealt with; (*math*) a problem to be solved.—**propositional** *adj*.

propound /prə'paʊnd/ *vt* to put forward (a question, suggestion, etc).

proprietary /pro:'praɪətəri/ or /prə-/, /-təri/ *adj* characteristic of a proprietor; privately owned and managed and run as a profit-making organization; (*drug*) made and distributed under a tradename. • *n* (*pl* **proprietaries**) proprietors collectively; a drug protected by secrecy, patent, or copyright against free competition.

proprietor /prə'praɪətər/ *n* one with legal title to something; an owner.—**proprietorial** *adj*.—**proprietorially** *adv*.

propriety /prə'praɪəti/ *n* (*pl* **proprieties**) correctness of conduct or taste; fear of offending against rules of behaviour, *esp* between the sexes; (*pl*) the customs and manners of polite society.

proptosis /'prɒpto:sɪs/ *n* (*pl* **proptoses**) (*med*) a prolapse, *esp* of the eyeball.

propulsion /prə'pelʃən/ *n* the act of propelling; something that propels.—**propulsive, propulsory** *adj*.

propylaeum /ˌprɒpɪ'li:əm/, **propylon** /-'lɒn/ *n* (*pl* **propylaea, propylons** *or* **propyla**) a porch or entrance to a temple.

pro rata /'pro:reɪtə/ *adj, adv* in proportion.

prorogue /prə'ro:g/ *vt* to terminate a session (of a parliament, etc) without dissolving it.

prosaic /prə'zeɪk/ or /pro:/ *adj* commonplace, matter-of-fact, dull.—**prosaically** *adv*.—**prosaicness** *n*.

prosaism /'pro:zeɪˌsɪzəm/ *n* the quality of being prosaic; a word, saying, etc demonstrating this.

proscenium /prə'si:nɪəm/ or /pro:-/ *n* (*pl* **prosceniums**) the part of a stage in front of the curtain.

proscribe /prə'skraɪb/ *vt* to outlaw; to denounce; to prohibit the use of.—**proscriber** *n*.

proscription /prə'skrɪpʃən/ *n* the act of proscribing; the condition of being proscribed; outlawry; interdiction.—**proscriptive** *adj*.—**proscriptively** *adv*.

prose /pro:z/ *n* ordinary language, as opposed to verse. • *adj* in prose; humdrum, dull. • *vti* to talk tediously; to turn into prose.

prosecute /'prɒsəˌkju:t/ *vt* to bring legal action against; to pursue. • *vi* to institute and carry on a legal suit or prosecution.—**prosecutable** *adj*.

prosecution /ˌprɒsə'kju:ʃən/ *n* the act of prosecuting, *esp* by law; the prosecuting party in a legal case.

prosecutor /'prɒsəˌkju:tər/ *n* a person who prosecutes, *esp* in a criminal court.

proselyte /'prɒsəˌlaɪt/ *n* a convert, *esp* to Judaism. • *vti* to proselytize.

proselytize /'prɒsələˌtaɪz/ *vti* to try to make a convert (of).—**proselytizer** *n*.

prosenchyma /prɒ'seŋkɪmə/ *n* (*bot*) tissue of elongated cells with little protoplasm.—**prosenchymatous** *adj*.

prose poem *n* a prose work of poetic style.

prosody *n* the study of verse forms and metrical structure; a particular style, system, or theory of versification.—**prosodic** *adj*.—**prosodically** *adv*.—**prosodist** *n*.

prosopopoeia, prosopopeia /ˌprɒsəpe'pi:ə/ *n* (*rhetoric*) a figure of speech in which an absent, dead or inanimate figure is represented as present and speaking.

prospect /'prɒspekt/ *n* a wide view, a vista; (*pl*) measure of future success; future outlook; expectation; a likely customer, candidate, etc. • *vti* to explore or search (for).

prospective /prə'spektɪv/ *adj* likely; anticipated, expected.—**prospectively** *adv*.

prospector /prə'spektər/ *n* one who prospects for gold, etc.

prospectus /prə'spektəs/ *n* (*pl* **prospectuses**) a printed statement of the features of a new work, enterprise, etc; something (as a condition or statement) that forecasts the course or nature of a situation.

prosper /'prɒspər/ *vi* to thrive; to flourish; to succeed.

prosperity /prɒ'sperɪti/ *n* (*pl* **prosperities**) success; wealth.

prosperous /'prɒspərəs/ *adj* successful, fortunate, thriving; favourable.—**prosperously** *adv*.

prostate /'prɒsteɪt/ *n* (*also* **prostate gland**) a gland situated around the neck of a man's bladder.—**prostatic** *adj*.

prosthesis /'prɒs'θiːsɪs/ *n* (*pl* **prostheses**) (*med*) the replacement of a lost limb, tooth, etc with an artificial one; (*gram*) the addition of a letter or syllable at the beginning of a word.—**prosthetic** *adj*.

prostitute /'prɒstɪˌtuːt/ or /-ˌtjuːt/ *n* a person who has sexual intercourse for money; (*fig*) one who deliberately debases his or her talents (as for money). • *vt* to offer indiscriminately for sexual intercourse, *esp* for money; to devote to corrupt or unworthy purposes.—**prostitutor** *n*.

prostitution /ˌprɒstɪ'tuːʃən/ or /-'tjuː-/ *n* the act or activity of being a prostitute; sexual intercourse for money, etc.

prostrate /'prɒstreɪt/ *adj* lying face downwards; helpless overcome; lying prone or supine. • *vt* to throw oneself down; to lie flat; to humble oneself.—**prostration** *n*.

prostyle /'prɒːstaɪl/ *adj* (*archit*) with columns in front. • *n* a building, *esp* a temple, with columns in front.

prosy /'prɒːzi/ *adj* (**prosier, prosiest**) like prose; dull, dry, tedious.—**prosily** *adv*.—**prosiness** *n*.

protactinium /ˌprɒːtæk'tɪniəm/ *n* a rare radioactive element similar to uranium.

protagonist /prɒː'tægənɪst/ *n* the main character in a drama, novel, etc; a supporter of a cause.

protasis /'prɒtəsɪs/ *n* (*pl* **protases**) (*gram*) an introductory clause of a conditional sentence.

protean /'prɒːtiən/ or /-'tiːən/ *adj* able to assume many shapes, versatile; variable.

protect /prɒ'tekt/ *vt* to defend from danger or harm; to guard; to maintain the status and integrity of, *esp* through financial guarantees; to foster or shield from infringement or restriction; to restrict competition through tariffs and trade controls.

protection /prɒ'tekʃən/ *n* the act of protecting; the condition of being protected; something that protects; shelter; defence; patronage; the taxing of competing imports to foster home industry; the advocacy or theory of this.—*also* **protectionism**; immunity from prosecution or attack obtained by the payment of money.

protectionist /-nɪst/ *n* a person who advocates the protection of home trade by taxing competitive imports. • *adj* serving to protect.—**protectionism** *n*.

protective /prɒ'tektɪv/ *adj* serving to protect, defend, shelter.—**protectively** *adv*.—**protectiveness** *n*.

protector /-ər/ *n* a person or thing that protects; (*with cap*) (*formerly*) a regent who ruled during the minority, absence or illness of a monarch.

protectorate /prɒ'tektərət/ *n* the administration of a weaker state by a powerful one; a state so controlled; a regency; (*with cap*) the English government under Oliver and Richard Cromwell (1653–9).

protégé /'prɒːtəˌʒiː/ or /prɒ-/ *n* a person guided and helped in his career by another person.—**protégée** *nf*.

protein /'prɒːtiːn/ *n* a complex organic compound containing nitrogen that is an essential constituent of food.

pro tem /prɒː'tem/, **pro tempore** /prɒː'tempəri/ *adv* for the time being.

proteolysis /ˌprɒːti'ɒlɪsɪs/ *n* the disintegration of protein, *esp* during digestion.—**proteolytic** *adj*.

proteose /'prɒːtiˌoːz/ *n* a compound substance formed by proteolysis.

protest /'prɒːtest/ *vi* to object to; to remonstrate. • *vt* to assert or affirm; to execute or have executed a formal protest against; to make a statement or gesture in objection to. • *n* public dissent; an objection; a complaint; a formal statement of objection.—**protester, protestor** *n*.—**protestingly** *adv*.

Protestant /'prɒːtəstənt/ *n* a member or adherent of one of the Christian churches deriving from the Reformation a Christian not of the Orthodox or Roman Catholic Church, who adheres to the principles of the Reformation.—**Protestantism** *n*.

protestation /ˌprɒːtə'steɪʃən/ *n* a solemn declaration; a strong protest.

prothalamion /ˌprɒːθə'leɪmiən/ *n* (*pl* **prothalamia**) a bridal song, sung before a marriage ceremony.

prothonotary /ˌprɒːθɒː'noːtəri/ or /prɒ'θɒnəˌtəri/ *n* (*pl* **prothonotaries**) (*formerly*) the principal clerk in certain courts.—*also* **protonotary** (*pl* **protonotaries**).

prothorax /prɒː'θɒːræks/ *n* (*pl* **prothoraxes, prothoraces**) the first segment of an insect's thorax.

protist /'prɒːtɪst/ *n* a single-celled organism, neither animal nor plant.

protocol /'prɒːtəˌkɒl/ *n* a note, minute or draft of an agreement or transaction; the ceremonial etiquette accepted as correct in official dealings, as between heads of state or diplomatic officials; the formatting of data in an electronic communications system; the plan of a scientific experiment or treatment.

proton /'prɒːtɒn/ *n* an elementary particle in the nucleus of all atoms, carrying a unit positive charge of electricity.

protonotary *see* **prothonotary**.

protoplasm /'prɒːtəˌplæzəm/ *n* a semi-fluid viscous colloid, the essential living matter of all plant and animal cells.—**protoplasmic** *adj*.

prototype /'prɒːtəˌtaɪp/ *n* an original model or type from which copies are made.—**prototypal, prototypic, prototypical** *adj*.

protozoan /ˌprɒːtə'zoːən/, **protozoon** /-'zoːɒn/ *n* (*pl* **protozoans, protozoa**) a microscopic animal consisting of a single cell or a group of cells.

protozoology *n* the study of protozoans.

protract /prɒ'trækt/ *vt* to draw out or prolong; to lay down the lines and angles of with scale and protractor; to extend forwards and outwards.—**protractible** *adj*.—**protraction** *n*.

protracted /prɒ'træktəd/ *adj* extended, prolonged; long-drawn-out.—**protractedly** *adv*.—**protractedness** *n*.

protractile /prɒ'træktaɪl/ *adj* (*zool*) able to be extended.—**protractility** *n*.

protractive /prɒ'træktɪv/ *adj* delaying; protracted.

protractor /prɒ'træktər/ or /'prɒːtræktər/ *n* an instrument for measuring and drawing angles; a muscle that extends a limb.

protrude /prɒː'truːd/ *vti* to thrust outwards or forwards; to obtrude; to jut out, project.

protrusile /prɒ'truːsaɪl/ *adj* (*zool*) which can be thrust forward.

protrusion /prɒː'truːʒən/ or /prə-/ *n* the act of protruding; something that protrudes; a bulge, a lump; a projection.

protrusive /prɒː'truːzɪv/ or /prə-/ *adj* tending to protrude; bulging out; unduly conspicuous; obtrusive; (*arch*) thrusting or impelling forward.—**protrusively** *adv*.—**protrusiveness** *n*.

protuberance /prɒ'tuːbərəns/ or /-'tjuːb-/, **protuberancy** /prɒ'tuːbərənsi/ or /-'tjuːb-/ *n* (*pl* **protuberance, protuberancies**) something that protrudes; a swelling, prominence.

protuberant /prɒ'tuːbərənt/ or /-'tjuːb-/ *adj* bulging out, prominent.—**protuberantly** *adv*.

proud /praud/ *adj* having too high an opinion of oneself; arrogant, haughty; having proper self-respect; satisfied with one's achievements.—**proudly** *adv*.—**proudness** *n*.

prove /pruːv/ *vti* (**proving, proved** *or* **proven**) to try out, test, by experiment; to establish or demonstrate as true using accepted procedures; to show (oneself) to be worthy or capable; to turn out (to be), *esp* after trial or test; to rise.—**provable** *adj*.—**provably** *adv*.—**prover** *n*.

provenance /'prɒvənəns/ *n* place of origin, source.

provender /'prɒvəndər/ *n* dry fodder for cattle; any food.

proverb /'prɒvərb/ *n* a short traditional saying expressing a truth or moral instruction; an adage.

proverbial /prɒ'vərbiəl/ *adj* of or like, a proverb; generally known.—**proverbially** *adv*.

provide /prə'vaɪd/ *vti* to arrange for; to supply; to prepare; to afford (an opportunity); to make provision for (financially).—**provider** *n*.

provided /-əd/, **providing** /-ɪŋ/ *conj* on condition (that).

providence /'prɒvɪdəns/ *n* foresight, prudence; God's care and protection.

provident /'prɒvɪdənt/ *adj* providing for the future; far-seeing; thrifty.—**providently** *adv*.

providential /ˌprɒvɪ'denʃəl/ *adj* arranged by providence; very opportune or lucky.—**providentially** *adv*.

province /'prɒvɪns/ *n* an administrative district or division of a country; the jurisdiction of an archbishop; (*pl*) the parts of a country removed from the main cities; a department of knowledge or activity.

provincehood /'prɒvɪnsˌhud/ *n* ✷ (*Cdn*) the quality of status of being a province.

provincial /prə'vɪnʃəl/ *adj* of a province or provinces; having the way, speech, etc of a certain province; country-like; rustic; unsophisticated. • *n* an inhabitant of the provinces or country areas; a person lacking sophistication.—**provinciality** *n*.—**provincially** *adv*.

provincialism /prə'vɪnʃə,lɪzəm/ *n* provincial speech, phrases, or point of view; narrowness.

provincialization /prə,vɪnʃə,laɪ'zeɪʃən/ *n* ❦ (*Cdn*) the transfer of government programs or responsibilities to the provinces.

provision /prə'vɪʒən/ *n* a requirement; something provided for the future; a stipulation, condition; (*pl*) supplies of food, stores. • *vt* to supply with stores.—**provisioner** *n*.

provisional /-əl/, **provisionary** /-ɛri/ *adj* temporary; conditional.—**provisionally** *adv*.

proviso /prə'vaɪzo:/ *n* (*pl* **provisos, provisoes**) a condition, stipulation; a limiting clause in an agreement, etc.

provisory /prə'vaɪzəri/ *adj* conditional; making provision; temporary.—**provisorily** *adv*.

provocation /,prɒvə'keɪʃən/ *n* the act of provoking or inciting; a cause of anger, resentment, etc.

provocative /prə'vɒkətɪv/ *adj* intentionally provoking, *esp* to anger or sexual desire; (*remark*) stimulating argument or discussion.—**provocatively** *adv*.—**provocativeness** *n*.

provoke /prə'vo:k/ *vt* to anger, infuriate; to incite, to arouse; to give rise to; to irritate, exasperate.

provoking /-ɪŋ/ *adj* annoying, exasperating.—**provokingly** *adv*.

provost /'prɒvəst/ *n* a high executive official, as in some churches, colleges, or universities; in Scotland, a mayor.

prow /praʊ/ *n* the forward part of a ship, bow.

prowess /prau'ɛs/ or /'praʊɛs/, /-əs/ *n* bravery, gallantry; skill.

prowl /praʊl/ *vi* to move stealthily, *esp* in search of prey.—*also n.*

prowler /-ər/ *n* one that moves stealthily, *esp* an opportunist thief.

proximal /'prɒksɪməl/ *adj* (*anat*) at the inner end, towards the centre of the body.

proximate /'prɒksɪmət/ *adj* nearest, next; approximate.

proximity /prɒk'sɪməti/ *n* nearness in place, time, series, etc.

proximo /'prɒksɪ,mo:/ *adv* next month.

proxy /'prɒksi/ *n* (*pl* **proxies**) the authority to vote or act for another; a person so authorized.—*also adj.*

prude /pru:d/ *n* a person who is overly modest or proper in behaviour, speech, attitudes to sex, etc.—**prudery** *n*.

prudence /'pru:dəns/ *n* the quality of being prudent; caution; discretion; common sense.

prudent /'pru:dənt/ *adj* cautious; sensible; managing carefully; circumspect.—**prudently** *adv*.

prudential /pru:'dɛnʃəl/ *adj* marked by prudence.—**prudentially** *adv*.

prudish /'pru:dɪʃ/ *adj* over-correct in behaviour.—**prudishly** *adv*.—**prudishness** *n*.

pruinose /'pru:ɪ,no:s/ *adj* (*bot*) covered with a whitish dust or bloom.

prune[1] /pru:n/ *n* a dried plum.

prune[2] *vti* (*plant*) to remove dead or living parts from; to cut away what is unwanted or superfluous.—**pruner** *n*.

prunella /pru:'nelə/ *n* a strong silk or worsted fabric, used in shoes.

prurient /'pruriənt/ *adj* tending to excite lust; having lewd thoughts.—**prurience** *n*.—**pruriently** *adv*.

prurigo /pruə'raɪgo:/ *n* a skin disease causing violent itching.

pruritus /pruə'raɪtəs/ *n* a strong sensation of itching.

Prussian blue /'prʌʃən/ *n* a deep blue.

prussic acid /'prʌsɪk/ *n* a solution of hydrogen and cyanide that makes a deadly poison.

pry[1] /praɪ/ *vi* (**prying, pried**) to snoop into other people's affairs; to inquire impertinently. • *n* (*pl* **pries**) close inspection; impertinent peeping; a highly inquisitive person.

pry[2] *vt* (**prying, pried**) to raise with a lever, to prise.

pryer /'praɪər/ *see* **prier**.

PS /,pi:'es/ *abbr* = postscript.

PSAC /,pi:'sæk/ *abbr* ❦ = Public Service Alliance of Canada.

psalm /sɒm/ *n* a sacred song or hymn, *esp* one from the Book of Psalms in the Bible.

psalmist /'sɒmɪst/ *n* a writer of psalms.

psalmody /'sɒmədi/ or /'sæm-/ *n* (*pl* **psalmodies**) the art or practice of singing psalms or hymns.—**psalmodic** *adj*.—**psalmodist** *n*.

Psalter, psalter /'sɒltər/ *n* the Book of Psalms, *esp* as found in a prayer book.

psaltery /-i/ *n* (*pl* **psalteries**) an ancient stringed musical instrument.

Pseudepigrapha /,su:dɪ'pɪɡrəfə/ or /,sju:-/ *npl* spurious writings falsely ascribed to Biblical figures or times; Jewish writings of the first century BC and first century AD, allegedly by various prophets and kings of the Hebrew scriptures.

pseudo /'su:do:/ or /'sju:-/ *adj* false, pretended.

pseudocarp /'su:do:,kɑrp/ or /'sju:-/ *n* (*bot*) a fruit formed from parts other than the ovary.

pseudomorph /'su:də,mɔrf/ or /'sju:-/ *n* (*geol*) a mineral with the crystalline shape of another mineral.—**pseudomorphic, pseudomorphous** *adj*.—**pseudomorphism** *n*.

pseudonym /'su:də,nɪm/ or /'sju:-/ *n* a false name adopted as by an author.—**pseudonymity** *n*.

pseudonymous /su:'dɒnɪməs/ or /sju:-/ *adj* written or writing under an assumed name.—**pseudonymously** *adv*.

pshaw /pʃɔ/ or /ʃɒ/ *interj* an exclamation of disgust, disbelief, etc.

psittacine /'sɪtə,saɪn/ *n* pertaining to parrots.

psittacosis /,sɪtə'ko:sɪs/ *n* a contagious parrot disease transmissible to humans, in whom it causes pneumonia.

psoas /'so:əs/ *n* a muscle in the loin.

psoriasis /sə'raɪəsɪs/ *n* a chronic skin disease marked by red scaly patches.—**psoriatic** *adj*.

PST /'pi:es'ti:/ *abbr* ❦ = Pacific Standard Time; Provincial Sales Tax.

psyche /'saɪki/ *n* the spirit, soul; the mind, *esp* as a functional entity governing the total organism and its interactions with the environment.

psychedelic /,saɪkə'dɛlɪk/ *adj* of or causing extreme changes in the conscious mind; of or like the auditory or visual effects produced by drugs (as LSD). • *n* a psychedelic drug.—**psychedelically** *adv*.

psychiatrist /saɪkɪ'ætrɪst/ or /saɪkaɪ-/ *n* a specialist in psychiatric medicine.

psychiatry /saɪ'kaɪətri/ *n* the branch of medicine dealing with disorders of the mind, including psychoses and neuroses.—**psychiatric** *adj*.—**psychiatrically** *adv*.

psychic /'saɪkɪk/ *adj* of the soul or spirit; of the mind; having sensitivity to, or contact with, forces that cannot be explained by natural laws.—*also* **psychical**. • *n* a person apparently sensitive to nonphysical forces; a medium; psychic phenomena.

psychoanalyse, psychoanalyze /,saɪko:'ænə,laɪz/ *vt* to analyse and treat by psychoanalysis.

psychoanalysis /,saɪko:ə'næləsəs/ *n* a method of treating neuroses, phobias, and some other mental disorders by analysing emotional conflicts, repressions, etc.—**psychoanalytic, psychoanalytical** *adj*.

psychoanalyst /-'ænə,lɪst/ *n* a specialist in psychoanalysis.

psychodynamics /,saɪko:daɪ'næmɪks/ *n sing* the study of interaction of thoughts, motives, etc within an individual.—**psychodynamic** *adj*.

psychological /,saɪko:'lɒdʒɪkəl/ *adj* of or relating to psychology; of, relating to or coming from the mind or emotions; able to affect the mind or emotions.—**psychologically** *adv*.

psychologist /saɪ'kɒlədʒɪst/ *n* a person trained in psychology.

psychology /saɪ'kɒlədʒi/ *n* (*pl* **psychologies**) the science that studies the human mind and behaviour; mental state.

psychometrics /,saɪko:'metrɪks/ *n sing* the scientific measurement and testing of mental powers.—**psychometric, psychometrical** *adj*.—**psychometrician, psychometrist** *n*.

psychomotor /'saɪko:,mo:tər/ *adj* denoting a physical action induced by a mental condition.

psychoneurosis /,saɪko:nju:'ro:sɪs/ *n* (*pl* **psychoneuroses**) neurosis.

psychopath /'saɪko:,pæθ/ or /'saɪkə-/ *n* a person suffering from a mental disorder that results in antisocial behaviour and lack of guilt.—**psychopathic** *adj*.

psychopathology /,saɪko:pə'θɒlədʒi/ *n* the study of mental disorders.

psychopathy /saɪ'kɒpəθi/ *n* mental disorder or disease.

psychophysiology /,saɪko:fɪzɪ'ɒlədʒi/ *n* the study of the relation between psychological and physiological processes.—**psychophysiological** *adj*.—**psychophysiologist** *n*.

psychosis /saɪ'ko:sɪs/ *n* (*pl* **psychoses**) a mental disorder in which the personality is very seriously disorganized and contact with reality is *usu* impaired.

psychosomatic /,saɪko:so'mætɪk/ *adj* of physical disorders that have a psychological or emotional origin.—**psychosomatically** *adv*.

psychotherapy /,saɪko:'θerəpi/ *n* the treatment of mental disorders by psychological methods.—**psychotherapeutic** *adj*.—**psychotherapist** *n*.

psychotic /saɪ'kɒtɪk/ *adj* of or like a psychosis; having a psychosis. • *n* a person suffering from a psychosis.—**psychotically** *adv*.

psychrometer /saɪˈkrɒmɪtər/ *n* a type of hygrometer with both a wet and a dry bulb.

psychrophilic /saɪˈkrɒfɪlɪk/ or /səɪˈkrɒ-/ *adj* (*biol*) thriving in the cold.

PT *abbr* = physical training.

Pt (*chem symbol*) platinum.

Pt. *abbr* = point (in place names).

pt *abbr* = pint.

PTA /ˌpiːtiːˈeɪ/ *abbr* = Parent-Teacher Association.

ptarmigan /ˈtɑrmɪgən/ *n* (*pl* **ptarmigans, ptarmigan**) a species of grouse.

pteridology /ˌteriˈdɒlədʒi/ *n* the study of ferns.

pterodactyl /ˌterəˈdæktɪl/ *n* an extinct flying reptile with batlike wings.

pteropod /ˈterəpɒd/ *n* a small swimming mollusc with winglike lobes on its foot.

pterosaur /ˈterəˌsɔr/ *n* an extinct flying reptile.

pterygoid /ˈterɪˌgɔɪd/ *adj* (*anat*) of or pertaining to either of the two processes in the skull attached like wings to the spheroid bone.

PTO /ˌpiːtiːˈoʊ/ *abbr* = please turn over.

ptomaine, ptomain /ˈtoʊmeɪn/ *n* a kind of alkaloid, often poisonous, found in decaying matter.

ptosis /ˈtoʊsɪs/ *n* (*pl* **ptoses**) drooping of the eyelid.

ptyalin /ˈtaɪəlɪn/ *n* an enzyme found in saliva.

ptyalism /ˈtaɪəˌlɪzəm/ *n* excessive salivation.

pub /pʌb/ *n* a public house, an inn.

puberty /ˈpjuːbərti/ *n* the stage at which the reproductive organs become functional.—**pubertal** *adj*.

pubescent /pjuːˈbesənt/ *adj* arriving at or having reached puberty; of or relating to puberty; covered with fine soft short hairs.—**pubescence** *n*.

pubic /ˈpjuːbɪk/ *adj* related to or situated near the pubis.

pubis /ˈpjuːbɪs/ *n* (*pl* **pubes**) the front part of the bones composing either half of the pelvis.

public /ˈpʌblɪk/ *adj* of, for, or by the people generally; performed in front of people; for the use of all people; open or known to all; acting officially for the people. • *n* the people in general; a particular section of the people, such as an audience, body of readers, etc; open observation.

public-address system *n* a system using microphones and loudspeakers to enable groups of people to hear clearly in an auditorium or out of doors.

publican /-ən/ *n* a person who keeps a public house; in ancient Rome, a collector of taxes.

publication /ˌpʌbləˈkeɪʃən/ *n* public notification; the printing and distribution of books, magazines, etc; something published as a periodical, book, etc.

public health *n* the practice and science of protecting and improving community health by organized effort including sanitation, preventive medicine, etc.

publicist /ˈpʌbləsɪst/ *n* a person who publicizes, *esp* one whose business it is; a political journalist.

publicity /pʌbˈlɪsɪti/ *n* any information or action that brings a person or cause to public notice; work concerned with such promotional matter; notice by the public.

publicize /ˈpʌblɪˌsaɪz/ *vt* to give publicity to.

publicly /ˈpʌblɪkli/ *adv* in a public manner; openly; by the public; with the consent of the public.

public mischief *n* ✤ (*Cdn*) the criminal offence of making a false report or accusation.

public relations *n* relations with the general public of a company, institution, etc, as through publicity.

public school *n* a school maintained by public money and supervised by local authorities; in England, a private secondary school, *usu* boarding.

public service *n* the supply of a commodity (gas, water, etc) or a service (transport, etc) to the community; a service in the public interest; employment in a government department, *esp* the civil service.

publish /ˈpʌblɪʃ/ *vt* to make generally known; to announce formally; (*book*) to issue for sale to the public. • *vi* to put out an edition; to have one's work accepted for publication.—**publishable** *adj*.

publisher /-ər/ *n* a person or company that prints and issues books, magazines, etc.

publishing /-ɪŋ/ *n* the business of the production and distribution of books, magazines, recordings, etc.

puce /pjuːs/ *n, adj* (a) purplish brown.

puck /pʌk/ *n* a hard rubber disc used in ice hockey.

pucker /ˈpʌkər/ *vti* to draw together in creases, to wrinkle; (*with up*) to contract the lips ready to kiss. • *n* a wrinkle or fold.

puckish /ˈpʌkɪʃ/ *adj* impish, irresponsible.—**puckishly** *adv*.—**puckishness** *n*.

pudding /ˈpʊdɪŋ/ *n* a dessert; a steamed or baked dessert; a suet pie.

puddle /ˈpʌdəl/ *n* a small pool of water, *esp* stagnant, spilled, or muddy water; a rough cement of kneaded clay. • *vti* to dabble in mud, to make muddy; to make or line with puddle; to stir (molten iron) to free it from carbon.—**puddler** *n*.

pudency /ˈpjuːdənsi/ *n* modesty, sense of shame.

pudendum /pjuːˈdendəm/ *n* (*pl* **pudenda**) (*usu pl*) the external reproductive organs, *esp* of a woman.—**pudendal** *adj*.

pudgy /ˈpʌdʒi/ *adj* (**pudgier, pudgiest**) short and fat, squat.—**pudginess** *n*.

pueblo /ˈpweblo/ *n* an Indian settlement in Mexico and the South West United States.

puerile /ˈpjʊəraɪl/ *adj* juvenile; childish.—**puerilely** *adv*.—**puerility** *n*.

puerilism /pjʊəˈrɪlɪzəm/ *n* a psychiatric condition of adults characterized by infantile or childish behaviour.

puerperal /pjuːˈɜrpərəl/ *adj* pertaining to, or following, childbirth.

puff /pʌf/ *n* a sudden short blast or gust; an exhalation of air or smoke; a light pastry; a pad for applying powder; a flattering notice, advertisement. • *vti* to emit a puff; to breathe hard, pant; to put out of breath; to praise with exaggeration; to swell; to blow, smoke, etc, with puffs.

puffball /ˈpʌfbɒl/ *n* a round fungus which emits dustlike spores when broken.

puffer /ˈpʌfər/ *n* someone who, or something which puffs; a tropical fish with a spiny body which can be puffed up to form a globe.

puffin /ˈpʌfɪn/ *n* a sea bird that has a short neck and a brightly coloured laterally compressed bill.

puffiness /ˈpʌfiˌnes/ *n* the state of being puffy or swollen.

puffy /ˈpʌfi/ *adj* (**puffier, puffiest**) inflated, swollen; panting.—**puffily** *adv*.

pug /pʌg/ *n* a breed of small dog with a face and nose like a bulldog. • *vt* (**pugging, pugged**) to mix (clay) for making bricks; to fill (a space) with clay or mortar.

pug nose *n* a nose having a slightly concave bridge and flattened nostrils.—**pug-nosed** *adj*

pugilism /ˌpjuːdʒɪˈlɪzəm/ *n* the practice of fighting with the fists; boxing; skill in doing this.

pugilist /ˈpjuːdʒɪlɪst/ *n* a boxer; a prizefighter.—**pugilistic** *adj*.—**pugilistically** *adv*.

pugnacious /pʌɡˈneɪʃəs/ *adj* fond of fighting, belligerent.—**pugnacity, pugnaciousness** *n*.

puisne /ˈpjuːni/ *adj* (*judge*) lower in rank.

puissance /ˈpjuːɪsəns/ or /ˈpwɪs-/ *n* (*arch*) power; (*showjumping*) an event in which a horse attempts particularly large jumps.—**puissant** *adj*.

puke /pjuːk/ *vti* (*inf*) to vomit.—*also n*.

pukka /ˈpʌkə/ *adj* (*Anglo-Indian*) genuine, real; reliable, sound.

pulchritude /ˈpʌlkrɪˌtjuːd/ *n* beauty.

pule /pjuːl/ *vi* to whine, whimper.

pull /pʊl/ *vt* to tug at; to pluck; to move or draw towards oneself; to drag; to rip; to tear; (*muscle*) to strain; (*inf*) to carry out, perform; (*inf*) to restrain; (*inf: gun, etc*) to draw out; (*inf*) to attract. • *vi* to carry out the action of pulling something; to be capable of being pulled; to move (away, ahead, etc). • *n* the act of pulling or being pulled; a tug; a device for pulling; (*inf*) influence; (*inf*) drawing power.

pullet /ˈpʊlət/ *n* a young hen.

pulley /ˈpʊli/ *n* a wheel with a grooved rim for a cord, etc, used to raise weights by downward pull or change of direction of the pull; a group of these used to increase applied force; a wheel driven by a belt.

pullman /ˈpʊlmən/ *n* (*pl* **Pullmans**) a railway carriage offering luxury accommodation, *usu* with sleeping berths.

pullover /ˈpʊlˌoʊvər/ *n* a buttonless garment with or without sleeves pulled on over the head.

pullulate /ˈpʌljʊˌleɪt/ *vi* to sprout, grow; to multiply quickly; to spring up.—**pullulation** *n*.

pulmonary /ˈpʌlmənəri/ *adj* of, relating to or affecting the lungs; having lungs; denoting the artery that conveys deoxygenated blood directly to the lungs from the right ventricle of the heart.

pulp /pʌlp/ *n* a soft, moist, sticky mass; the soft, juicy part of a fruit or soft pith of a plant stem; ground-up, moistened fibres of wood, rags, etc, used to make paper; a book or magazine printed on cheap paper and often dealing with sensational material. • *vti* to make or become pulp or pulpy; to produce or reproduce (written matter) in pulp form.

pulpit /'pʊlpɪt/ or /'pʌl-/ *n* a raised enclosed platform, *esp* in a church, from which a clergyman preaches; preachers as a group.

pulpy /'pʌlpi/ *adj* (**pulpier, pulpiest**) consisting of or like pulp; soft.—**pulpiness** *n*.

pulque /'puːlkeɪ/ *n* a Mexican alcoholic drink made from the fermented juice of the agave.

pulsar /'pʌlsɑr/ *n* any of several very small stars that emit radio pulses at regular intervals.

pulsate /'pʌlseɪt/ *vi* to beat or throb rhythmically; to vibrate, quiver.—**pulsative** *adj*.

pulsation /'pʌlseɪʃən/ *n* a pulsating; a single beat or throb; rhythmic throbbing.

pulsatory /'pʌlsətəri/ *adj* pertaining to pulsation; pulsating.

pulse¹ /pʌls/ *n* a rhythmic beat or throb, as of the heart; a place where this is felt; an underlying opinion or sentiment or an indication of it; a short radio signal. • *vti* to throb, pulsate.

pulse² *n* the edible seeds of several leguminous plants, such as beans, peas and lentils; the plants producing them.

pulsimeter, pulsometer /pʌl'sɪmətər/ *n* (*med*) an instrument used to measure pulse rate and strength.

pulverize /'pʌlvəˌraɪz/ *vti* to reduce to a fine powder; to demolish, smash; to crumble.—**pulverization** *n*.—**pulverizer** *n*.

pulverulent /pʌl'verjuːlənt/ or /-jə-/ *adj* covered with dust; powdery; crumbling to dust.

pulvinate /'pʌlvəˌneɪt/ or /-nɪt/ **pulvinated** *adj* (*archit*) curved convexly; (*bot*) having a cushionlike pad or swelling.

puma /'pjuːmə/ *n* a mountain lion.

pumice /'pʌmɪs/ *n* a light, porous volcanic rock, used for scrubbing, polishing, etc.—**pumiceous** *adj*.

pummel /'pʌməl/ *vt* (**pummelling, pummelled** *or* **pummeling, pummeled**) to strike repeatedly with the fists, to thump.

pump¹ /pʌmp/ *n* a device that forces a liquid or gas into, or draws it out of, something. • *vti* to move (fluids) with a pump; to remove water, etc, from; to drive air into with a pump; to draw out, move up and down, pour forth, etc, as a pump does; (*inf*) to obtain information through questioning.

pump² *n* a light low shoe or slipper; a rubber-soled shoe.

pumpernickel /'pʌmpərˌnɪkəl/ *n* a coarse rye bread.

pumpkin /'pʌmpkɪn/ *n* a large, round, orange fruit of the gourd family widely cultivated as food.

pun /pʌn/ *n* a play on words of the same sound but different meanings, *usu* humorous. • *vi* (**punning, punned**) to make a pun.—**punningly** *adv*.

punch¹ /pʌntʃ/ *vt* to strike with the fist; to prod or poke; to stamp, perforate with a tool; (*US*) (*cattle*) to herd. • *n* a blow with the fist; (*inf*) vigour; a machine or tool for punching.

punch² *n* a hot, sweet drink made with fruit juices, often mixed with wine or spirits.

punchbowl *n* a bowl for mixing punch; a bowl-shaped hollow.

punch card, punched card *n* in data processing, a card with a series of holes representing data.

puncheon /'pʌntʃən/ *n* a large cask holding between 70 and 120 gallons.

Punchinello /ˌpʌntʃɪ'nelo/ *n* the figure of the clown in Italian puppet theatre; a grotesque character.

punch line /'pʌntʃlaɪn/ *n* the last line of a joke or story, that conveys its humour or point.

punctate /'pʌŋkteɪt/ **punctated** *adj* marked with dots or points.—**punctation** *n*.

punctilio /pʌŋk'tɪlio/ *n* (*pl* **punctilios**) a fine point of etiquette; petty formality.

punctilious /pʌŋk'tɪliəs/ *adj* very formal in conduct; scrupulously exact.

punctual /'pʌŋktʃʊəl/ *adj* being on time; prompt.—**punctuality** *n*.—**punctually** *adv*.

punctuate /'pʌŋktʃʊˌeɪt/ *vt* to use certain standardized marks in (written matter) to clarify meaning; to interrupt; to emphasize. • *vi* to use punctuation marks.—**punctuator** *n*.

punctuation /ˌpʌŋktʃʊ'eɪʃən/ *n* the act of punctuating; the state of being punctuated; a system of punctuation.

punctuation mark *n* one of the standardized symbols used in punctuation, as the period, colon, semicolon, comma, etc.

puncture /'pʌŋktʃər/ *n* a small hole made by a sharp object; the deflation of a tyre caused by a puncture. • *vt* to make useless or ineffective as if by a puncture; to deflate. • *vi* to become punctured.—**puncturable** *adj*.

pundit /'pʌndɪt/ *n* a learned person; an expert; a critic, *esp* one who writes in a daily newspaper.—*also* **pandit**.

pung /pʌŋ/ *n* (*US*) a horse-drawn sleigh.

pungent /'pʌndʒənt/ *adj* having an acrid smell or a sharp taste; caustic; bitter.—**pungency** *n*.—**pungently** *adv*.

punish /'pʌnɪʃ/ *vt* to subject a person to a penalty for a crime or misdemeanour; to chastise; to handle roughly. —**punisher** *n*.

punishable /'pʌnɪʃəbəl/ *adj* liable to legal punishment.—**punishability** *n*.

punishing /-ɪŋ/ *adj* causing retribution; (*inf*) arduous, gruelling, exhausting.—**punishingly** *adv*.

punishment /'pʌnɪʃmənt/ *n* a penalty for a crime or misdemeanour; rough treatment; the act of punishing or being punished.

punitive /'pjuːnɪtɪv/ **punitory** *adj* involving the inflicting of punishment.—**punitively** *adv*.—**punitiveness** *n*.

punk /pʌŋk/ *adj* (*sl*) inferior, of low quality. • *n* (*US*) a young gangster; a follower of punk rock.

punka, punkah /'pʌŋkə/ *n* a palm-leaf fan; (*Anglo-Indian*) a large swinging fan suspended from the ceiling of a room and worked by an attendant.

punk rock *n* an aggressive form of rock music *usu* performed in a coarse, offensive way.

punster /'pʌnstər/ **punner** *n* a person who makes puns.

punt¹ /pʌnt/ *n* a long flat-bottomed square-ended river boat *usu* propelled with a pole. • *vti* to propel or convey in a punt.

punt² *vt* to kick a dropped ball before it reaches the ground. • *n* such a kick.

punter /'pʌntər/ *n* a person who gambles; (*sl*) a consumer; a customer.

punty /'pʌnti/ *n* (*pl* **punties**) an iron rod used in glass-blowing.

puny /'pjuːni/ *adj* (**punier, puniest**) of inferior size, strength, or importance; feeble.—**puniness** *n*.

pup /pʌp/ *n* a young dog, a puppy; a young fox, seal, rat, etc. • *vi* (**pupping, pupped**) to give birth to pups.

pupa /'pjuːpə/ *n* (*pl* **pupae, pupas**) an insect at the quiescent stage between the larva and the adult.—**pupal** *adj*.

pupate /'pjuːpeɪt/ *vi* (*entomology*) to become a pupa.—**pupation** *n*.

pupil¹ /'pjuːpəl/ *n* a child or young person taught under the supervision of a teacher or tutor; a person who has been taught or influenced by a famous or distinguished person.

pupil² *n* the round, dark opening in the centre of the iris of the eye through which light passes.

pupillage, pupilage /'pjuːpəlɪdʒ/ *n* the state of being a pupil; the period of time during which someone is a pupil.

pupillary /'pjuːpəˌleri/ *adj* pertaining to a pupil, or to a legal ward.

pupiparous /pjuː'pɪpərəs/ *adj* (*entomology*) producing young in the pupal state.

puppet /'pʌpɪt/ *n* a doll moved by strings attached to its limbs or by a hand inserted in its body; a person controlled by another. • *adj* of or relating to puppets; acting in response to the controls of another while appearing independent.

puppeteer /pʌpɪ'tiːr/ *n* a person who controls and entertains with puppets.

puppetry /'pʌpətri/ *n* the art of making and entertaining with puppets; stilted presentation.

puppy /'pʌpi/ *n* (*pl* **puppies**) a young domestic dog less than a year old.—**puppyhood** *n*.—**puppyish** *adj*.

Purana /puː'rɒnə/ *n* a book of Hindu scriptures, written in Sanskrit.

purblind /'pɜrblaɪnd/ *adj* half-blind; (*fig*) obtuse, dull.

purchase /'pɜrtʃəs/ *vt* to buy; to obtain by effort or suffering. • *n* the act of purchasing; an object bought; leverage for raising or moving loads; means of achieving advantage.—**purchasable** *adj*.—**purchaser** *n*.

purdah /'pɜrdə/ *n* the custom among Muslims and some Hindus of secluding women from public observation.

pure /pjʊr/ or /pjər/ *adj* clean; not contaminated; not mixed; chaste, innocent; free from taint or defilement; mere; that and that only; abstract and theoretical; (*mus*) not discordant, perfectly in tune.—**pureness** *n*.

purée /pjʊrˈeɪ/ or /ˈpjʊr/ *n* cooked food sieved or pulped in a blender; a thick soup of this. • *vt* (**puréeing, puréed**) to prepare food in this way.

pure laine /pjʊrˈleɪn/ *adj* ✤ (*Cdn*) descended as a French-speaking Quebecer from the original settlers of French Canada; of or pertaining to such a person. • *n* a person of such descent.

purely /ˈpjʊrli/ or /ˈpjɜrli/ *adv* in a pure way; solely, entirely.

purgation /pərˈgeɪʃən/ *n* a purging or purifying.

purgative /ˈpərgətɪv/ *adj* purging, cleansing; • *n* a drug or agent that purges the bowels.

purgatorial /-ˈtɔriəl/ *adj* of, relating to or like purgatory; serving to purify of sin.

purgatory /ˈpərgəˌtɔri/ *n* a place of suffering or purification; (*with cap*: *RC church*) the intermediate place between death and heaven, where venial sins are purged.

purge /pərdʒ/ *vt* to cleanse, purify; (*nation, party, etc*) to rid of troublesome people; to clear (oneself) of a charge; to clear out the bowels of. • *n* the act or process of purging; a purgative; the removal of persons believed to be disloyal from an organization, *esp* a political party.—**purger** *n*.

purificator /ˈpjʊrəfɪˌkeɪtər/ *n* (*Christian Church*) a cloth used to wipe the chalice during Holy Communion.

purify /ˈpjʊrɪˌfaɪ/ *vti* (**purifying, purified**) to make or become pure; to cleanse; to make ceremonially clean; to free from harmful matter.—**purification** *n*.—**purificatory** *adj*.—**purifier** *n*.

Purim /ˈpʊrɪm/ or /puˈriːm/ *n* a Jewish holiday celebrated yearly in February or March, to commemorate the deliverance of the Jews from massacre at the hands of Haman.

purine /ˈpʊriːn/ *n* a white crystalline compound found in uric acid.

purism /ˈpjʊrˌɪzəm/ *n* insistence on correctness in language, form, style, etc.

purist /ˈpjʊrɪst/ *n* someone who is a stickler for correctness in language, style, etc.—**purism** *n*.—**puristic** *adj*.—**puristically** *adv*.

puritan /ˈpjʊrɪtən/ or /ˈpjər/ *adj* a person who is extremely strict in religion or morals; (*with cap*) an extreme English Protestant of Elizabethan or Stuart times. • *adj* of or like a puritan; (*with cap*) of the Puritans.—**puritanism, Puritanism** *n*.

puritanical /ˌpjʊrɪˈtænɪkəl/ or /ˌpjər/ *adj* rigorously strict in religious or moral matters; (*with cap*) of the Puritans or Puritanism.—**puritanically** *adv*.—**puritanicalness** *n*.

purity /ˈpjʊrɪti/ *n* the state of being pure.

purl /pərl/ *vt* to knit a stitch by drawing its base loop from front to back of the fabric. • *n* a stitch made in this way.

purlieu /ˈpərljuː/ *n* (*usu pl*) adjacent or outlying areas.

purlin /ˈpərlɪn/ or **purline** *n* a piece of timber lying horizontally to support rafters.

purloin /pərˈlɔɪn/ *vt* to steal.—**purloiner** *n*.

purple /ˈpərpəl/ *n* a dark, bluish red; crimson cloth or clothing, *esp* as a former emblem of royalty. • *adj* purple-coloured; royal; (*writing style*) over-elaborate. • *vti* to make or become purple.

purport /pərˈpɔrt/ *vt* to claim to be true; to imply; to be intended to seem. • *n* significance; apparent meaning.—**purportedly** *adv*.

purpose /ˈpərpəs/ *n* objective; intention; aim; function; resolution, determination. • *vti* to intend, design.

purposeful /ˈpərpəsˌfʊl/ *adj* determined, resolute; intentional.—**purposefully** *adv*.—**purposefulness** *n*.

purposeless /ˈpərpəsləs/ *adj* lacking purpose; pointless.—**purposelessly** *adv*.—**purposelessness** *n*.

purposely /ˈpərpəsli/ *adv* deliberately; on purpose.

purposive /ˈpərpəsɪv/ *adj* having or serving a purpose.—**purposively** *adv*.

purpura /ˈpərpjʊrə/ *n* a blood disease causing the eruption of small purple spots.

purr /pər/ *vi* (*cat*) to make a low, murmuring sound of pleasure.—**purring** *n*.

purse /pərs/ *n* a small pouch or bag for money; finances, money; a sum of money for a present or a prize; (*US*) a woman's handbag. • *vt* to pucker, wrinkle up.

purser /ˈpərsər/ *n* an officer on a passenger ship in charge of accounts, tickets, etc; an airline official responsible for the comfort and welfare of passengers.

purslane /ˈpərsleɪn/ *n* a flowering plant with fleshy leaves, used in salads.

pursuance /pərˈsuːəns/ or /-ˈsjuːəns/ *n* the pursuing or performance of an action.

pursuant /pərˈsuːənt/ or /-ˈsjuːənt/ *adj* (*law*) according to; (*arch*) pursuing.

pursue /pərˈsuː/ or /-ˈsjuː/ *vb* (**pursuing, pursued**) *vt* to follow; to chase; to strive for; to seek to attain; to engage in; to proceed with. • *vi* to follow in order to capture.—**pursuer** *n*.

pursuit /pərˈsuːt/ or /-ˈsjuːt/ *n* the act of pursuing; an occupation; a pastime.

pursuivant /ˈpərsɪvənt/ or /-swɪ-/ *n* a low-ranking officer of the British College of Heralds; (*formerly*) an attendant or state messenger.

purulent /ˈpjʊrʊlənt/ or /ˈpjʊrju-/ *adj* pertaining to pus.—**purulence, purulency** *adj*.—**purulently** *adv*.

purvey /ˈpərveɪ/ *vti* to procure and supply (provisions).

purveyance /pərˈveɪəns/ *n* the procuring of provisions; the provisions provided; (*formerly*) the right accorded to royalty to buy up provisions without the owner's consent.

purveyor /-ər/ *n* a person who, or an organization which, supplies provisions.

pus /pʌs/ *n* a yellowish fluid produced by infected sores.

push /pʊʃ/ *vti* to exert pressure so as to move; to press against or forward; to impel forward, shove; to urge the use, sale, etc, of; (*inf*) to approach an age; (*inf*) to sell drugs illegally; to make an effort. • *n* a thrust, shove; an effort; an advance against opposition; (*inf*) energy and drive.

push button *n* a knob that activates an electrical switch which opens or closes a circuit to operate a radio, bell, etc.

pushchair /ˈpʊˌtʃer/ *n* a wheeled metal and canvas chair for a small child.—*also* **stroller**.

pusher /ˈpʊʃər/ *n* that which pushes; (*inf*) a person who sells illegal drugs.

pushing /ˈpʊʃɪŋ/ *adj* go-ahead, energetic; ambitious; assertive.

pushover /ˈpʊʃ ˌoʊvər/ *n* (*inf*) something easily done, as a victory over an opposing team; (*inf*) a person easily taken advantage of.

pushy /ˈpʊʃi/ *adj* (**pushier, pushiest**) (*inf*) assertive; forceful; aggressively ambitious.—**pushily** *adv*.—**pushiness** *n*.

pusillanimous /ˌpjuːsəˈlænəməs/ *adj* faint-hearted, cowardly.—**pusillanimity** *n*.

puss /pʊs/ *n* (*inf*) a cat; (*sl*) a girl.

puss *n* (*sl*) the mouth; the face.

pussy /ˈpʊsi/ *n* (*pl* **pussies**) (*inf*) a cat, a pussycat.

pussy *adj* (*pl* **pussier, pussiest**) like or containing pus.

pussycat /ˈpʊsikæt/ *n* (*inf*) a cat; an amiable person.

pussyfoot /ˈpʊsiˌfʊt/ *vi* to move stealthily; to be evasive.—**pussyfooter** *n*.

pustule /ˈpʌstʃuːl/ *n* a blister or swelling containing pus.—**pustular** *adj*.—**pustulation** *n*.

put /pʊt/ *vti* (**putting, put**) to place, set; to cast, throw; to apply, direct; to bring into a specified state; to add (to); to subject to; to submit; to estimate; to stake; to express; to translate; to propose; (*a weight*) to hurl; (*with* **about**) to change the course of (a ship); to worry; (*with* **across**) to effect successfully; (*with* **away**) to remove; to lay by; (*sl*) to consume; (*arch*) to divorce; (*with* **back**) to replace; to return to land; (*with* **by**) to thrust aside; to store up; (*with* **down**) to suppress; to silence; to kill or have killed; to write or enter; to reckon; to assign; (*with* **forth**) to exert; to bud or shoot; to set out; (*with* **in**) to interpose; to spend (time); to apply (for); to call (at); (*with* **off**) to doff, discard; to postpone; to evade; to get rid of; to discourage, repel; to foist (upon); to leave shore; (*with* **on**) to don; to assume, pretend; to increase; to add; to advance; (*with* **out**) to eject; to extend; to exert; to dislocate; to quench; to publish; to place (money) at interest; to disconcert, to anger; to leave shore; (*with* **over**) to succeed in, to carry through; (*with* **up**) to rouse; to offer (prayer); to propose as a candidate; to pack; to sheathe; to lodge; (*with* **up with**) to endure, to tolerate; (*with* **upon**) to impose upon; (*with* **wise**) to disabuse, to enlighten. • *adj* fixed.

putative /ˈpjuːtətɪv/ *adj* reputed, supposed.—**putatively** *adv*.

putrefy /ˈpjuːtrəˌfaɪ/ *vti* (**putrefying, putrefied**) to make or become putrid; to rot, decompose.—**putrefaction** *n*.—**putrefactive** *adj*.—**putrefier** *n*.

putrescent /pjuːˈtresənt/ *adj* decaying, rotting.—**putrescence** *n*.

putrid /ˈpjuːtrɪd/ *adj* rotten or decayed and foul-smelling.—**putridity** *n*.—**putridly** *adv*.

putsch /pʊtʃ/ *n* an uprising or revolt.

putt /pʊt/ *vti* (*golf*) to hit (a ball) with a putter. • *n* in golf, a stroke to make the ball roll into the hole.

puttee /ˈpʊti/ *n* a legging made from a strip of cloth wound spirally from the ankle to the knee.

putter[1] /'pʊtər/ *n* (*golf*) a straight-faced club used in putting.

putter[2] *vi* (*US*) to busy oneself idly; to spend time, to potter.—**putterer** *n*.

putter[3] *n* one who or that which puts; an athlete who puts the shot.

putto /'pʊtəʊ/ *n* (*pl* **putti**) (*art*) a figure of cupid and representations of children.—*also* **amoretto, amorino**.

putty /'pʌtɪ/ *n* (*pl* **putties**) a soft, plastic mixture of powdered chalk and linseed oil used to fill small cracks, fix glass in window frames, etc. • *vt* (**puttying, puttied**) to fix or fill with putty.

puzzle /'pʌzəl/ *vt* to bewilder; to perplex. • *vi* to be perplexed; to exercise one's mind, as over a problem. • *n* bewilderment; a difficult problem; a toy or problem for testing skill or ingenuity; a conundrum.—**puzzlement** *n*.—**puzzler** *n*.

puzzling /-lɪŋ/ *adj* perplexing, bewildering, inexplicable.—**puzzlingly** *adv*.

PVC *abbr* = polyvinyl chloride.

PWA *abbr* = person with AIDS.

pyaemia, pyemia /paɪ'iːmɪə/ *n* blood poisoning.—**pyaemic** *adj*.

pycnometer /pɪk'nɒmətər/ *n* an instrument for measuring densities or specific gravities.

pygmy /'pɪgmɪ/ *n* (*pl* **pygmies**) an undersized person.—*also* **pigmy** (*pl* **pigmies**).

pyjamas /pə'dʒæməz/ or /-'dʒɒməz/ *npl* a loosely fitting sleeping suit of jacket and trousers.—*also* (*US*) **pajamas**.

pylon /'paɪlɒn/ *n* a tower-like structure supporting electric power lines.

pylorus /paɪ'lɔrəs/ *n* (*pl* **pylori**) (*anat*) the opening from the stomach into the intestine.

pyorrhoea, pyorrhea /ˌpaɪə'riːə/ *n* inflammation of the gums and tooth sockets.

pyracantha /ˌpaɪrə'kænθə/ *n* a small, flowering, evergreen shrub.

pyramid /'pɪrəmɪd/ *n* (*geom*) a solid figure having a polygon as base, and whose sides are triangles sharing a common vertex; a huge structure of this shape, as a royal tomb of ancient Egypt; an immaterial structure built on a broad supporting base and narrowing gradually to an apex.—**pyramidal, pyramidical, pyramidic** *adj*.—**pyramidally, pyramidically** *adv*.

pyre /paɪr/ *n* a pile of wood for cremating a dead body.

pyrethrum /paɪ'riːθrəm/ *n* a type of chrysanthemum with showy flowers; an insecticide made from this plant.

pyretic /paɪ'rɛtɪk/ *adj* pertaining to, or causing, fever.

Pyrex /'paɪrɛks/ *n* (*trademark*) heat-resistant glassware.

pyrexia /paɪ'rɛksɪə/ *n* fever.—**pyrexial, pyrexic** *adj*.

pyrheliometer /paɪrˌhiːli'ɒmətər/ or /pɪr-/ *n* an instrument for measuring the sun's heat.

pyrites /paɪ'raɪtiːz/ or /'paɪraɪts/ *n* (*pl* **pyrites**) a sulphide of a metal, *esp* iron.

pyroelectric /ˌpaɪroʊɪ'lɛktrɪk/ *adj* becoming electric as a result of heat.

pyrogenic /ˌpaɪroʊ'dʒɛnɪk/, **pyrogenous** *adj* caused by, or causing, heat, or fever.

pyrolisis /paɪ'rɒləsɪs/ *n* decomposition by heat.

pyromania /ˌpaɪroʊ'meɪnɪə/ *n* (*psychol*) an uncontrollable urge to set things on fire.

pyrometer /paɪ'rɒmɪtər/ *n* an instrument used to measure very high temperatures.—**pyrometry** *n*.

pyrope /'paɪroʊp/ *n* a deep red variety of garnet.

pyrophoric /ˌpaɪroʊ'fɒrɪk/ *adj* igniting when exposed to air.

pyrosis /paɪ'roʊsɪs/ *n* heartburn.

pyrotechnics /ˌpaɪroʊ'tɛknɪks/ *n sing* the art of making or setting off fireworks; (*sing or pl*) a fireworks display; a brilliant display of virtuosity.—**pyrotechnic, pyrotechnical** *adj*.

pyroxylin /paɪ'rɒksəlɪn/, **pyroxyline** *n* a substance derived from cellulose, used in making plastics.

pyrrhic /'pɪrɪk/ *adj* (*victory*) so costly as to be equal to defeat.

pyrrhic /'pɪrɪk/ *n* a metrical foot of two syllables.

Pythagorean /pɪˌθægə'riːən/ or /paɪ-/ *adj* pertaining to, or characteristic of, the Greek philosopher Pythagoras.

python /'paɪθɒn/ *n* a large, nonpoisonous snake that kills by constriction.—**pythonic** *adj*.

pythoness /'paɪθənəs/ *n* a priestess in the temple of Apollo at Delphi, in ancient Greece; a (female) soothsayer; a witch.

pyuria /paɪ'jʊrɪə/ *n* (*med*) the discharge of pus into the urine.

pyx /pɪks/ *n* (*Christian Church*) a container in which consecrated bread is kept.

pyxidium /pɪk'sɪdɪəm/ *n* (*pl* **pyxidia**) (*bot*) a pyxis.

pyxis /'pɪksɪs/ *n* (*pl* **pyxides**) a seed capsule with a lid that falls off to release the seeds.

Q

QC /'kju:'si:/ *abbr* = Queen's Counsel; ♣ Quebec.
QED /ˌkju:i:'di:/ *abbr* = quod erat demonstratum.
QST *abbr* ♣ = Quebec Sales Tax.
q.t. *abbr* = (*inf*) quiet.
qt *abbr* = quart.
qty *abbr* = quantity.
qua /kweɪ/ or /kwɐ/ *prep* as, in the character of, because.
quack[1] /kwæk/ *n* the cry of a duck. • *vi* to make a sound like a duck.
quack[2] *n* an untrained person who practises medicine fraudulently; a person who pretends to have knowledge and skill he does not have.—*also adj*.
quackery /'kwækəri/ *n* (*pl* **quackeries**) pretence of medical or other skill; imposture.
quacksalver /'kwæksælvər/ *n* (*arch*) a quack who deals in ointments, etc; a charlatan.
quad /kwɒd/ *n* quadrangle; quadruplet.
quadr- /kwɒdr/, **quadri-** /'kwɒdri/, **quadru-** /'kwɒdrʊ/ *prefix* four.
quadragenarian /ˌkwɒdrədʒə'neriən/ *n, adj* (a person) forty to forty-nine years old.
Quadragesima (Sunday) /ˌkwɒdrə'dʒəsımə/ *n* the first Sunday in Lent.
Quadragesimal /ˌkwɒdrə'dʒəsıməl/ *adj* pertaining to, or used in, Lent.
quadrangle /'kwɒd,ræŋgəl/ *n* (*geom*) a plane figure with four sides and four angles, a rectangle; a court enclosed by buildings.—**quadrangular** *adj*.
quadrant /'kwɒdrənt/ *n* (*geom*) a quarter of the circumference of a circle; an arc of 90 degrees; an instrument with such an arc for measuring angles, altitudes, or elevations; a curved street.—**quadrantal** *adj*.
quadraphonic /ˌkwɒdrə'fɒnɪk/ *adj* using four channels to record and reproduce sound.—**quadraphonics, quadraphony** *n*.
quadrate /'kwɒdrət/ *adj* (*zool*) of or pertaining to one of a pair of bones found in the skulls of fishes, reptiles and some birds; (*anat*) of or pertaining to the middle bone of the middle ear in mammals; (*arch*) square or rectangular. • *vt* to square or make rectangular; (*often with* **with**) to cause to conform; to correspond. • *n* a quadrate bone; a square or cube.
quadratic /kwɒ'drætɪk/ *adj* square; (*math*) involving the square but no higher power. • *n* a quadratic equation.
quadratic equation *n* an equation in which the highest power of the unknown is the square.
quadratics /-tɪks/ *n sing* the branch of algebra dealing with quadratic equations.
quadrature /'kwɒdrətʃər/ *n* the act of squaring; the reduction of a figure to a square, exactly or approximately; (*astron*) the position of a heavenly body when distant 90 degrees from another, usually the earth, said *esp* of the position of the moon from the sun; (*math*) the finding of square with an area exactly equal to a circle or other figure or a surface; (*electronics*) the state between two waves of being 90 degrees out of phase.
quadrennial /kwɒ'drənɪəl/ *adj* lasting or occurring every four years.—**quadrennially** *adv*.
quadricentennial /ˌkwɒdrə,sen'ti:nɪəl/ *n* a four hundredth anniversary.—*also adj*.
quadrifid /'kwɒdrɪfɪd/ *adj* with four parts, four-cleft.
quadriga /kwɒ'drɪgə/ *n* (*pl* **quadrigas, quadrigae**) an ancient Roman two-wheeled chariot drawn by four horses abreast.
quadrilateral /ˌkwɒdrə'lætərəl/ *adj* having four sides. • *n* (*geom*) a plane figure of four sides; a combination or group that involves four parts or individuals.
quadrille /kwɒ'drɪl/ *n* a square dance for four or more couples; the music for this.
quadrillion /kwɒ'drɪljən/ *n* in Europe, the fourth power of a million, ie 1 with 24 zeros; in US, the fifth power of a thousand, ie, 1 with 15 zeros.—*also adj*.—**quadrillionth** *adj*.

quadrinomial /ˌkwɒdrə'nɔ:mɪəl/ *n* an algebraic expression consisting of four terms.
quadripartite /ˌkwɒdrə'pɑrtaɪt/ *adj* of four parts; shared by four.
quadriplegia /ˌkwɒdrə'plɛdʒə/ *n* paralysis of all four limbs.—**quadriplegic** *adj, n*.
quadrivalent /ˌkwɒdrə've lənt/ *adj* (*chem*) with four valencies; with a valency of four, tetravalent.— **quadrivalency, quadrivalence**.
quadrivial /ˌkwɒ'drɪvɪəl/ *adj* pertaining to a quadrivium; (*roads, etc*) leading in four ways; coming from four directions and meeting at the same point.
quadrivium /ˌkwɒ'drɪvɪəl/ *n* (*pl* **quadrivia**) a medieval course of study comprising arithmetic, geometry, astronomy, and music.
quadroon /kwɒ'dru:n/ *n* the child of one white and one half Negro parent, a person one quarter black.
quadrumanous /ˌkwɒ'dru:mənəs/, **quadrumanal** /ˌkwɒ'dru:mənəl/ *adj* (*monkeys, apes*) the characterisitic of having four hands that can grasp.
quadruped /'kwɒdru,ped/ *n* a four-footed animal.—**quadrupedal** *adj*.
quadruple /kwɒ'dru:pəl/ or /-'drʊ-/ *adj* four times as much or as many; made up of or consisting of four; having four divisions or parts. • *vti* to make or become four times as many.
quadruplet /kwɒ'dru:plət/ or /-'drʊplət/ *n* one of four children born at one birth.
quadruplicate /kwɒ'dru:plɪ,keɪt/ *vt* to multiply by four; to make four copies of. • *adj* fourfold.—**quadruplication** *n*.
quadruplicity /kwɒ'dru:plɪ,sɪtɪ/ *n* (*pl* **quadruplicities**) four-fold nature.
quaestor, questor /'kwi:stər/ *n* in ancient Rome, the public treasurer, or sometimes one of the other public officials.
quaff /kwɒf/ *vti* to take large drinks (of), drain.—**quaffer** *n*.
quagga /'kwægə/ *n* (*pl* **quaggas, quagga**) an extinct striped South African animal like a sand-coloured zebra.
quaggy /'kwægi/ *adj* (**quaggier, quaggiest**) of or like a bog or marsh.
quagmire /'kwæg,maɪr/ or /'kwɒg-/ *n* soft, wet ground; a difficult situation.
quahog /'kwɒhɒg/ or /'kwæ-/ *n* an edible North American clam, found on the Atlantic coast.
quail[1] /kweɪl/ *vi* to cower, to shrink back with fear.
quail[2] *n* (*pl* **quails, quail**) a small American game bird.
quaint /kweɪnt/ *adj* attractive or pleasant in an odd or old-fashioned style.—**quaintly** *adv*.—**quaintness** *n*.
quake /kweɪk/ *vi* to tremble or shiver, *esp* with fear or cold; to quiver. • *n* a shaking or tremor; (*inf*) an earthquake.
Quaker /'kweɪkər/ *n* a popular name for a member of the Society of Friends, a religious sect advocating peace and simplicity.—**Quakerism** *n*.
quaky /'kweɪki/ *adj* (**quakier, quakiest**) shaky; trembling; unstable.—**quakily** *adv*.—**quakiness** *n*.
qualifiable /'kwɒlɪ,faɪəbəl/ *adj* that may be qualified.
qualification /ˌkwɒləfɪ'keɪʃən/ *n* qualifying; a thing that qualifies; a quality or acquirement that makes a person fit for a post, etc; modification; limitation; (*pl*) academic achievements.
qualifier /'kwɒlɪfaɪr/ *n* one that qualifies; an adjective or adverb.
qualify /'kwɒlɪfaɪ/ *vti* (**qualifying, qualified**) to restrict; to describe; to moderate; to modify, limit; to make or become capable or suitable; to fulfil conditions; to pass a final examination; (*gram*) to limit the meaning of.—**qualificatory** *adj*.—**qualifyingly** *adv*.
qualitative /'kwɒlɪ,teɪtɪv/ *adj* of or depending on quality; determining the nature, not the quality, of components.—**qualitatively** *adv*.
quality /'kwɒlɪti/ *n* (*pl* **qualities**) a characteristic or attribute; degree of excellence; high standard. • *adj* of high quality.
qualm /kwɒm/ or /kwɒlm/ *r* a doubt; a misgiving; a scruple; a sudden feeling of faintness or nausea.—**qualmish** *adj*.
quandary /'kwɒndri/ or /-dəri/ *n* (*pl* **quandaries**) a predicament; a dilemma.

quango /'kwæŋɡoː/ *n* (*pl* **quangos**) (*acronym*) quasi-autonomous non-governmental organization.

quant /'kwænt/ or /'kwɒnt/ *n* a long pole, used in punting, with a disc on the end to prevent it from sinking when pushed into mud etc in a river. • *vt, vi* to punt with a quant.

quantify /'kwɒntɪˌfaɪ/ *vt* (**quantifying, quantified**) to express as a quantity; to determine the amount of.—**quantifiable** *adj*.—**quantification** *n*.

quantitative /'kwɒntɪˌteɪtɪv/ *adj* capable of being measured; relating to size or amount.—**quantitatively** *adv*.

quantity /'kwɒntɪti/ *n* (*pl* **quantities**) an amount that can be measured, counted or weighed; a large amount; the property by which a thing can be measured; a number or symbol expressing this property.

quantum /'kwɒntəm/ *n* (*pl* **quanta**) a quantity, share or portion; a fixed, elemental unit of energy. • *adj* large, significant.

quantum leap *n* an abrupt transition from one energy state to another; a sudden or noticeable change or increase.—*also* **quantum jump**.

quaquaversal /ˌkweɪkwəˈvɜrsəl/ *adj* (*geol*) pointing in every direction.

quarantine /'kwɒrənˌtiːn/ or /ˌkwɒrənˈtiːn/ *n* a period of isolation imposed to prevent the spread of disease; the time or place of this. • *vt* to put or keep in quarantine.

quark /kwɒrk/ or /kwɑrk/ *n* (*physics*) a hypothetical elementary particle.

quarrel /'kwɒrəl/ *n* an argument; an angry dispute; a cause of dispute. • *vi* (**quarrelling, quarrelled** *or* **quarreling, quarreled**) to argue violently; to fall out (with); to find fault (with).—**quarreller, quarreler** *n*.

quarrelsome /-səm/ *adj* contentious; apt to quarrel.

quarrier /'kwɒriər/, **quarryman** /'kwɒrɪmən/ *n* (*pl* **quarriers, quarrymen**) one who works in a quarry.

quarry[1] /'kwɒri/ *n* (*pl* **quarries**) an excavation for the extraction of stone, slate, etc; a place from which stone is excavated; a source of information, etc. • *vti* (**quarrying, quarried**) to excavate (from) a quarry; to research.

quarry[2] *n* (*pl* **quarries**) a hunted animal, prey.

quart /'kwɔrt/ or /kɔrt/ *n* a liquid measure equal to a quarter of a gallon or two pints; a dry measure equal to two pints.

quartan /'kwɔrtən/ *adj* recurring every third day, said of a fever, *esp* malaria.

quarter /'kwɔrtər/ *n* a fourth of something; one fourth of a year; one fourth of an hour; (*US*) 25 cents, or a coin of this value; any leg of a four-legged animal with the adjoining parts; a particular district or section; (*pl*) lodgings; a particular source; an unspecified person or group; a compass point other than the cardinal points; mercy; (*her*) any of four quadrants of a shield. • *vti* to share or divide into four; to provide with lodgings; to lodge; to range over (an area) in search of. • *adj* constituting a quarter.

quarterage /'kwɔrtərɪdʒ/ *n* a quarterly payment; (*rare*) a shelter.

quarterback /'kwɔrtərˌbæk/ *n* (*American football*) a player directly behind forwards and the centre, who directs play. • *vt* to direct the attacking play of (a football team); to manage, direct. • *vi* to play quarterback.

quarterbound /'kwɔrtərˌbaʊnd/ *adj* a book bound on the spine only in leather, or another material more expensive than the rest of the binding.

quarterdeck /'kwɔrtərˌdɛk/ *n* the stern area of the upper deck of a ship.

quartered /'kwɔrtərd/ *adj* divided into four quarters, sawn along two diameters, said of logs; (*her*) a shield divided into four parts, each with different arms, or with two sets of arms repeated at diagonally opposite corners; stationed or billeted, said especially of soldiers in civilian lodgings.

quarterfinal /'kwɔrtərˌfaɪnəl/ *n* one of four matches held before the semifinals in a tournament.—*also adj*.

quartering /'kwɔrtərɪŋ/ *n* the assignment of quarters to soldiers etc; (*her*) the division of a shield that contains several coats, often denoting family's alliances and intermarriages; any coat of arms so treated.

quarterlight /'kwɔrtərˌlaɪt/ *n* a *usu* triangular section within the window of a car.

quarterly /'kwɔrtərli/ *adj* occurring, issued, or spaced at three-month intervals; (*her*) divided into quarters. • *adv* once every three months; (*her*) in quarters. • *n* (*pl* **quarterlies**) a publication issued four times a year.

quartermaster /'kwɔrtərˌmæstər/ *n* (*mil*) an officer in charge of stores; (*naut*) a petty officer in charge of steering, etc.

quarter note *n* (*mus*) a note having one fourth the duration of a whole note.

quarters *npl* lodgings, *esp* for soldiers; action stations, *esp* used in reference to each member of the crew of a battleship; in India, accommodation provided by an employer or by the government; (*sl used by soldiers*) (*sing*) a quartermaster.

quarterstaff /'kwɔrtərˌstæf/ *n* (*pl* **quarterstaves**) a staff 6 to 8 feet long and shod with iron, formerly used as a two-handed weapon of defence; the use of one of these.

quartet, quartette /kwɔr'tɛt/ *n* a set or group of four; a piece of music composed for four instruments or voices; a group of four instrumentalists or voices.

quartic /'kwɑrtɪk/ *adj* (*math*) pertaining to the fourth power, biquadratic. • *n* the fourth power, arising from the multiplication of a square number or quantity by itself, biquadratic.

quartile /'kwɔrtaɪl/ *n* (*statistics*) one of three values of a variable that separates its distribution into four sets with equal frequencies. • *adj* (*statistics*) pertaining, or referring, to a quartile; (*astrol*) referring to an aspect of planets separated by 90 degree longitude.

quarto /'kwɔrtoː/ *n* (*pl* **quartos**) a page size, approx 9 by 12 inches; a book of this size of page.

quartz /kwɔrts/ *n* a crystalline mineral, a form of silica, *usu* colourless and transparent.

quartzite /'kwɔrtsaɪt/ *n* a very hard quartz rock; a light-coloured quartz sandstone.

quasar /'kweɪzɑr/ or /-sɑr/ *n* a distant, starlike, celestial object that emits much light and powerful radio waves.

quash /kwɒʃ/ *vt* (*rebellion etc*) to put down; to suppress; to make void.

quasi /'kwɒzi/ *adv* seemingly; as if. • *prefix* almost, apparently.

quassia /'kwɒʃə/ *n* a South American tree yielding bark and wood of excessive bitterness; the bark and wood from a tree of the same family, used to make furniture; formerly a bitter tonic drug obtained from this, which is now used as an ingredient in insecticides.

quatercentenary /ˌkwætərsən'tɛnəri/ or /-'tiːnəri/ *n* (*pl* **quatercentenaries**) a 400th anniversary, or the entire year of celebrations etc of a 400th anniversary.

quaternary /'kwɒtərˌneri/ or /kwə'tɜrnəri/ *adj* consisting of, arranged in, or by, fours; of the number 4; (*chem*) an atom bound to four other atoms or groups, or containing such an atom; (*math*) with four variables. (*with cap*) denoting strata more recent than the Upper Tertiary, ie the most recent geological period, of less than 1 million years ago. • *n* (*pl* **quaternaries**) (*with* **the**) this geological rock system, consisting of Pleistocene and Holocene (recent) epochs.

quaternion /kwə'tɜrniən/ *n* the number 4; a set of 4; (*maths*) a calculus or method of mathematical investigation using a generalized complex number with four components.

quaternity /kwə'tɜrnɪti/ *n* (*pl* **quaternities**) four persons regarded as one, *esp* in relation to God.

quatrain /'kwɒtreɪn/ *n* a four-line stanza, rhymed alternately.

quatrefoil /'kætrəˌfɔɪl/ *n* a four-leaved plant, such as certain clovers; an ornamental figure in architectural tracery divided by cusps into four leaves.

quattrocento /ˌkwætroː'tʃɛntoː/ *n* the fifteenth century, *esp* in connection with Italian art and literature.

quaver /'kweɪvər/ *vi* to tremble, vibrate; to speak or sing with a quivering voice. • *n* a trembling sound or note; (*mus*) an eighth note.—**quaveringly** *adv*.—**quavery** *adj*.

quay /kiː/ *n* a loading wharf or landing place for vessels.

quayage /'kiːədʒ/ *n* an interconnected network of quays; quay dues.

queasy /'kwiːzi/ *adj* (**queasier, queasiest**) nauseous; easily upset; over-scrupulous.—**queasily** *adv*.—**queasiness** *n*.

Quebecer, Quebecker, Québécois *n* ✹ (*Cdn*) a person who lives in or is from Quebec.

Quebec heater *n* ✹ (*Cdn*) a tall, cylindrical stove that uses coal or wood as cooking or heating fuel.

quebracho /keɪ'brɒtʃoː/ *n* (*pl* **quebrachos**) one of two types of South American tree with a hard timber rich in tannin, and used in tanning and dyeing; the medicinal bark of a South American tree, the alkaloids from the bark of which are also used in tanning; the wood or bark from any of these trees; any South American tree yielding a hard wood.

queen /'kwi:n/ *n* a female sovereign and head of state; the wife or widow of a king; a woman considered pre-eminent; the egg-laying female of bees, wasps, etc; a playing card with a picture of a queen; (*chess*) the most powerful piece; (*sl*) a male homosexual, *esp* one who ostentatiously takes a feminine role. • *vi* (*with* **it**) to act like a queen, *esp* to put on airs. • *vt* (a pawn) to promote to a queen in chess.—**queendom** *n*.

queencake /'kwi:nkeik/ *n* a small currant cake.

queenly /'kwi:nli/ *adj* (**queenlier, queenliest**) like or having the character or attributes of a queen; regal.—**queenliness** *n*.

queen mother *n* a queen dowager who is the mother of a ruling sovereign.

queer /kwi:r/ *adj* strange, odd, curious; (*inf*) eccentric; (*sl*) homosexual. • *n* a (male) homosexual. •*vt* (*sl*) to spoil the success of.—**queerness** *n*.

quell /kwel/ *vt* to suppress; to allay.—**queller** *n*.

quench /kwentʃ/ *vt* (*thirst*) to satisfy or slake; (*fire*) to put out, extinguish; (*steel*) to cool; to suppress.—**quenchable** *adj*.—**quencher** *n*.

quenelle /kə'nel/ *n* a ball of savoury cooked meat, formed into various shapes and boiled in stock or fried.

quercine /'kwər'si:n/ *adj* of the oak.

querist /'kwerist/ *n* one who asks questions.

quern /kwərn/ *n* a kind of stone handmill for grinding corn.

querulous /'kwerulǝs/ *adj* complaining, fretful, peevish.—**querulously** *adv*.

query /'kwi:ri/ or /'kweri/ *n* (*pl* **queries**) a question; a question mark; doubt. • *vti* (**querying, queried**) to question; to doubt the accuracy of.

quest /kwest/ *n* a search, seeking, *esp* involving a journey. • *vti* to search (about) for, seek.—**quester** *n*.—**questingly** *adv*.

question /'kwestʃən/ *n* an interrogative sentence; an inquiry; a problem; a doubtful or controversial point; a subject of debate before an assembly; a part of a test or examination. • *vti* to ask questions (of); to interrogate intensively; to dispute; to subject to analysis.—**questioner** *n*.

questionable /-ǝbǝl/ *adj* doubtful; not clearly true or honest.—**questionability** *n*. —**questionably** *adv*.

question mark *n* a punctuation mark (?) used at the end of a sentence to indicate a question, or to express doubt about something; something unknown.

questionnaire /-ner/ *n* a series of questions designed to collect statistical information; a survey made by the use of questionnaire.

question period *n* ✤ (*Cdn*) a scheduled period of time in a legislature during which members may ask questions of government ministers.

quetzal /'kwetzǝl/ or /'ketsǝl/ *n* a large brilliantly coloured Central or Southern American bird, the male having long tail feathers; a Guatemalan coin.

queue /kju:/ *n* a line of people, vehicles, etc awaiting a turn. • *vi* (**queuing, queued**) to wait in turn.

quibble /'kwibǝl/ *n* a minor objection or criticism. • *vi* to argue about trifling matters.—**quibbler** *n*.—**quibblingly** *adv*.

quiche /ki:ʃ/ *n* a savoury tart filled with onions and a cheese and egg custard.

quick /kwik/ *adj* rapid, speedy; nimble; prompt; responsive; alert; eager to learn. • *adv* (*inf*) in a quick manner. • *n* the sensitive flesh below a fingernail or toenail; the inmost sensibilities.—**quickly** *adv*.—**quickness** *n*.

quicken /'kwikǝn/ *vti* to speed up or accelerate; to make alive; to come to life; to invigorate.—**quickener** *n*.

quickie /'kwiki/ *n* (*inf*) anything done rapidly or in haste.

quicklime /'kwiklaim/ *n* calcium oxide.

quicksand /'kwiksænd/ *n* loose wet sand easily yielding to pressure in which persons, animals, etc may be swallowed up

quicksilver /'kwik,silvǝr/ *n* mercury.

quickstep /'kwikstep/ *n* a ballroom dance in quick time; the music for this. • *vi* (**quickstepping, quickstepped**) to do this dance.

quick-tempered *adj* easily angered.

quick-witted *adj* mentally alert; quick in repartee.—**quick-wittedness** *n*.

quid /kwid/ *n* (*pl* **quid**) (*sl*) a pound (sterling).

quiddity /'kwiditi/ *n* (*pl* **quiddities**) (*philos*) the essence of a thing; captious subtlety, a quibble.

quidnunc /'kwidnʌŋk/ *n* one who is curious to know everything that happens; a gossip, a busybody.

quid pro quo /,kwidpro:'kwo:/ *n* (*pl* **quid pro quos**) something equivalent given in exchange for something else.

quiescent /kwi'esǝnt/ *adj* dormant, inactive, inert; silent.—**quiescence** *n*.

quiet /'kwaiǝt/ *adj* silent, not noisy; still, not moving; gentle, not boisterous; unobtrusive, not showy; placid, calm; monotonous, uneventful; undisturbed. • *n* stillness, peace, repose; an undisturbed state. • *vti* to quieten.—**quietly** *adv*.—**quietness** *n*.

quieten /-ǝn/ *vti* to make or become quiet; to calm, soothe.

quietism /'kwaiǝ,tizǝm/ *n* a mental tranquillity and passive attitude towards life; a form of religious mysticism, founded in 17th-century Spain, in which the cultivation of this attitude with reference to God's will is to be attained.

quietize, quietise /'kwaiǝ taiz/ *vt* to insulate something from sound; to soundproof.

quietness /'kwaiǝtnǝs/ *n* repose.

quietude /'kwaiǝ tu:d/ or /-'tju:d/ *n* repose; tranquillity.

quietus /kwai'i:tǝs/ *n* (*pl* **quietuses**) death; the final settlement or discharge of debts etc; anything that results in death or annihilation.

quiff /kwif/ *n* (*Brit*) a curl plastered up above the forehead.

quill /kwil/ *n* the hollow stem of a feather; anything made of this, as a pen; a stiff, hollow spine of a hedgehog or porcupine.

quilt /kwilt/ *n* a thick, warm bedcover; a bedspread; a coverlet of two cloths sewn together with padding between. • *vti* to stitch together like a quilt; to make a quilt.—**quilter** *n*.—**quilting** *n*.

quin /kwin/ *n* a quintuplet.

quinary /'kwainǝri/ *adj* (*pl* **cuinaries**) consisting of, or arranged in, fives; a number system with a base of the number 5; having five parts; the fifth member of something.

quinate /'kwineit/ *adj* (*bot*) with five leaflets on a petiole; said of a digitate leaf.

quince /kwins/ *n* a hard-fleshed yellow Asian fruit used in preserves; the tree it grows on.

quincentenary /,kwinsen'tenǝri/ or /-'ti:nǝri/ *n* (*pl* **quincentenaries**) a 500th anniversary, or the entire year of celebration, etc, of the 500th anniversary.

quincunx /'kwinkʌŋks/ *n* an arrangement of five things in form of four corners and centre of a square; (*bot*) such an arrangement of petals or sepals in bud; (*astrol*) two planets with an aspect of 150 degrees.

quindecagon /kwin'dekǝgon/ *n* a plane figure with 15 angles and 15 sides.

quinine /'kwinain/ or /'kwainain/, /'kwini:n/ *n* a bitter crystalline alkaloid used in medicine; one of its salts used *esp* as an antimalarial and a bitter tonic.

quinqu-, quinque- /'kwiŋkwi/ *prefix* five.

quinquagenarian /,kwiŋkwǝdʒi'neriǝn/ *adj n* (a person) fifty to fifty-nine years old; relating to such a person.

Quinquagesima (Sunday) /,kwiŋkwǝ dʒesimǝ/ *n* the Sunday before Lent.

quinquennial /kwin'kweniǝl/ *adj* lasting five years or occurring every five years.—**quinquennially** *adv*.

quinquennium /kwin'kwen ǝm/ *n* (*pl* **quinquennia**) a period of five years.

quinquepartite /kwinkwe,partait/ *adj* of five parts; shared by five.

quinquereme /'kwinkwǝ,ri:m/ *n* in ancient Rome, a galley with five banks of oars on each side.

quinquevalent /,kwinkwǝ'veilǝnt/ *adj* (*chem*) having a valency of five, pentavalent.—**quinquevalency, quinquevalence** *n*.

quinsy /'kwinzi/ *n* a severe infection of the throat or adjacent parts causing swelling and fever.

quint /kwint/ *n* (*US*) a quintuplet.

quintain /'kwintin/ *n* a post with a sandbag on a pivot, or other object, used for practising the medieval sport of tilting; tilting at this.

quintal /'kwintǝl/ *n* a measure of weight, 100 lb; a measure of weight of 100 kilograms.

quintan /'kwintǝn/ *adj* said of an intermittent fever which recurs every fourth day.

quintessence /kwin'tesǝns/ *n* the purest form or most typical representation of anything, the embodiment.

quintessential /,kwintǝ'senʃǝl/ *adj* most typical; fundamental.—**quintessentially** *adv*.

quintet, quintette /kwin'tet/ *n* a set or group of five; a piece of music composed for five instruments or voices; a group of five instrumentalists or voices.

quintillion /kwɪnˈtɪljən/ *n* (*pl* **quintillions, quintillion**) in Western Europe, a million raised to the fifth power (1,000,0005), known in North America as a nonillion; in North America the sixth power of thousand, known as a trillion in Britain.—**quintillionth** *adj*.

quintuple /kwɪnˈtjupəl/ *adj* fivefold; having five divisions or parts; five times as much or as many. • *vti* to multiply by five. • *n* a number five times greater than another.

quintuplet /kwɪnˈtʊplət/ *n* one of five offspring produced at one birth.

quintuplicate /kwɪnˈtʊplɪˌkeɪt/ *vt* to multiply by five; to make five copies of.• *adj* five-fold. • *n* a set of five objects.—**quintuplication** *n*.

quip /kwɪp/ *n* a witty remark; a gibe. • *vt* (**quipping, quipped**) to make a clever or sarcastic remark.—**quipster** *n*.

quire /ˈkwaɪr/ *n* a set of 24 sheets of paper; one twentieth of a ream; a section of folded sheets sewn together in bookbinding.

quirk /kwɜrk/ *n* an unexpected turn or twist; a peculiarity of character or mannerism.

quirky /ˈkwɜrki/ *adj* (**quirkier, quirkiest**) odd or unusual in character, behaviour or appearance.—**quirkily** *adv*.—**quirkiness** *n*.

quirt /kwɜrt/ *n* a riding whip of plaited leather with a leather thong at the end. • *vt* to lash with this.

quisling /ˈkwɪzlɪŋ/ *n* a traitor who aids an invading enemy to regularize their conquest of his country; a collaborator.

quit /kwɪt/ *vti* (**quitting, quitted** *or* **quit**) to leave; to stop or cease; to resign; to free from obligation; to admit defeat. • *adj* free from; released from.

quitch (grass) /kwɪtʃ/ *n* couchgrass.

quite /kwaɪt/ *adv* completely; somewhat, fairly; really.

quits /kwɪts/ *adj* even; on equal terms by payment or revenge.

quittance /ˈkwɪtəns/ *n* a release from debt or obligation.

quitter /ˈkwɪtər/ *n* a person who gives up easily.

quiver[1] /ˈkwɪvər/ *vi* to shake; to tremble, shiver. • *n* a shiver, vibration.—**quiveringly** *adv*.—**quivery** *adj*.

quiver[2] *n* a case for holding arrows.—**quiverful** *n*.

qui vive /kiːˈviːv/ *n* **on the qui vive** on the alert.

quixotic /kwɪkˈsɒtɪk/, **quixotical** /-əl/ *adj* chivalrous or romantic to extravagance; unrealistically idealistic.—**quixotically** *adv*.

quixotism /ˈkwɪksəˌtɪzəm/, **quixotry** /-tri/ *n* romantic or extravagant notions or schemes; quixotic conduct or ideals.

quiz /kwɪz/ *n* (*pl* **quizzes**) a form of entertainment where players are asked questions of general knowledge; a short written or oral test. • *vt* (**quizzing, quizzed**) to interrogate; to make fun of.—**quizzer** *n*.

quizmaster /ˈkwɪzˌmæstər/ *n* a person who puts the questions to a contestant in a quiz show.

quiz show *n* an entertainment programme on television or radio in which contestants answer questions to win prizes.

quizzical /ˈkwɪzɪkəl/ *adj* humorous and questioning.—**quizzicality** *n*.—**quizzically** *adv*.

quod erat demonstrandum /kwɒdˌɛrætˌdemənˈstrændʊm/ (*Latin*) that which was to be proved.

quodlibet /ˈkwɒdləˌbet/ *n* a subtle or moot point, *esp* as part of a theological argument; (*mus*) a light musical medley.—**quodlibetical** *adj* **quodlibetically** *adv*.

quoin /kɔɪn/ *n* a wedge of wood or metal used to support and steady something (*esp* formerly a gun or cannon); a keystone; an external angle of a building; the stone forming this, the cornerstone; a wedge-shaped wooden block to tighten the pages of type within a chase.

quoit /kɔɪt/ *n* a ring of metal, plastic, etc thrown in quoits; (*pl*) a game in which rings are thrown at or over a peg.

quondam /ˈkwɒndæm/ *adj* that was, former.

quorum /ˈkwɔrəm/ *n* the minimum number that must be present at a meeting or assembly to make its proceedings valid.

quota /ˈkwoːtə/ *n* a proportional share; a prescribed amount; a part to be contributed.

quotable /ˈkwoːtəbəl/ *adj* worthy or fit to be quoted.—**quotability** *n*.

quotation /kwoːˈteɪʃən/ *n* the act of quoting; the words quoted; an estimated price.

quotation mark *n* a punctuation mark to indicate the beginning (' *or* ") and the end ('*or*") of a quoted passage.

quote /kwoːt/ *vt* to cite; to refer to; to repeat the words of a novel, play, poem, speech, etc exactly; to adduce by way of authority; to set off by quotation marks; to state the price of (something). • *n* (*inf*) something quoted; a quotation mark.

quoth /kwoːθ/ *vt* (*arch*) said, used with nouns and all pronouns except thou and you.

quotidian /kwoːˈtɪdiən/ *adj* daily; recurring every day, occurring every day; belonging to each day; commonplace, routine, everyday, trivial. • *n* a fever, *esp* malaria, recurring every day.

quotient /ˈkwoːʃənt/ *n* (*math*) the result obtained when one number is divided by another.

quo warranto /ˈkwoːwəˈrænto:/ *or* /-ˈræn-/ *n* (*law*) a proceeding set in motion to determine the authority by which someone claims an office or privilege; (*formerly*) the title of a writ issued to a person to try the question of title to any public office or privilege.

qwerty, QWERTY /ˈkwɜrti/ *n* (*inf*) a standard typewriter or computer keyboard.

R

R, r /ɑr/ *n* the 18th letter of the English alphabet.
R. *abbr* = rabbi; Regiment; Regina (*Latin* Queen); Republican; Rex (Latin *King*); River; Royal.
RA *abbr* = (UK) Royal Academy or Royal Academician.
Ra (*chem symbol*) radium.
RAAF *abbr* = Royal Australian Air Force.
rabbet, rebate /ˈræbɪt/ *n* a recess or groove cut in a surface (*eg* wood) to receive another piece. • *vt* to cut a rabbet in; to join (pieces of wood, etc) using a rabbet.
rabbi /ˈræbaɪ/ *n* (*pl* **rabbis**) the religious and spiritual leader of a Jewish congregation.
rabbinate /ˈræbɪneɪt/ *n* the position or tenure of a rabbi; rabbis collectively.
rabbinical /rəˈbɪnɪkəl/ *adj* of or pertaining to rabbis, their office, writings, etc.—**rabbinically** *adv*.
rabbit /ˈræbɪt/ *n* a small burrowing mammal of the hare family with long ears, a short tail, and long hind legs; their flesh as food; their fur.
rabbit punch *n* a sharp blow to the back of the neck.
rabble /ˈræbəl/ *n* a disorderly crowd, a mob; the common herd.
rabble-rouser *n* a person who excites a mob to violent action; a demagogue.
Rabelaisian /ˌræbəˈleɪziən/ *adj* of, pertaining to, or resembling the coarse, satirical humour of the French writer François Rabelais (1494–1553).
rabid /ˈræbɪd/ *adj* infected with rabies; raging; fanatical.
rabies /ˈreɪbiːz/ *n* an acute, infectious, viral disease transmitted by the bite of an infected animal.—*also* **hydrophobia**.
raccoon /rəˈkuːn/ *n* a small nocturnal carnivore of North America that lives in trees; its yellowish grey fur.
race[1] /reɪs/ *n* any of the divisions of humankind distinguished *esp* by colour of skin; any geographical, national, or tribal ethnic grouping; a subspecies of plants or animals; distinctive flavour or taste.
race[2] *n* a contest of speed, as in running, swimming, cycling, etc; a rapid current or channel of water. • *vi* to run at top speed or out of control; to compete in a race; (*engine*) to run without a working load or with the transmission disengaged. • *vt* to cause to race; to contest against.
racecourse /ˈreɪskɔrs/ *n* a track over which races are run, *esp* an oval track for racing horses.—*also* **racetrack**.
racehorse /ˈreɪshɔrs/ *n* a horse bred and trained for racing.
raceme /rəˈsiːm/ *n* (*bot*) an arrangement of flowers directly on a main stem, as in the lily of the valley.
racer /ˈreɪsər/ *n* a person who races; a machine used for racing, *esp* a bicycle; a kind of American snake.
race relations *npl* the relationship between different races in a community or nation; the sociological study of such relations.
racetrack /ˈreɪstræk/ *see* **racecourse**.
rachis, rhachis /ˈreɪkɪs/ *n* (*pl* **rachises, rhachises** *or* **rachides, rhachides**) the main stem of a plant's flower-head; the shaft of a feather; the spinal column.
rachitis /rəˈkaɪtɪs/ *n* rickets.
racial /ˈreɪʃəl/ *adj* of or relating to any of the divisions of humankind distinguished by colour, etc.
racism /ˈreɪsɪzəm/, **racialism** /ˈreɪʃəlɪzəm/ *n* a belief in the superiority of some races over others; prejudice against or hatred of other races; discriminating behaviour towards people of another race.—**racist** *n*.
rack /ræk/ *n* a framework for holding or displaying articles; an instrument for torture by stretching; the triangular frame for setting up balls in snooker; a toothed bar to engage with the teeth of a wheel pinion or worm gear; extreme pain or anxiety. • *vt* (*person*) to stretch on a rack; to arrange in or on a rack; to torture, torment; to move parts of machinery with a toothed rack.
racket[1] /ˈrækət/ *n* a bat strung with nylon, for playing tennis, etc. (*pl*) a game for two or four players played in a four-walled court (—*also* **racquet**).
racket[2] *n* noisy confusion; din; an obtaining of money illegally; any fraudulent business.

racketeer /ˌrækəˈtiːr/ *n* a person who extorts money by threat or engages in an illegal profit-making enterprise.
rack railway *n* a railway or a steep incline that has a rack or cog between the rails to engage with a pinion on a locomotive.
rack-rent *n* an extortionate rent.—*also vt*.—**rack-renter** *n*.
raconteur /ˌrækɒnˈtɜr/ *n* a person who excels in relating anecdotes.
racquet *see* **racket**[1].
racy /ˈreɪsi/ *adj* (**racier, raciest**) lively, spirited; risqué.—**racily** *adv*.
rad[1] /ræd/ *n* a unit of absorbed dose of ionizing radiation.
rad[2] (*symbol*) radian.
radar /ˈreɪdɑr/ *n* a system or device for detecting objects such as aircraft by using the reflection of radio waves.
radar beacon *n* a fixed radio transmitter that sends out a signal which allows a ship or an aircraft to determine its own position.
radarscope /-ˌskoːp/ *n* a cathode-ray oscilloscope which displays radar signals.
radial /ˈreɪdiəl/ *adj* like a radius; branching from a common centre.
radial ply *adj* (*tyre*) having the fabric cords of the outer casing lying radial to the hub for greater flexibility.
radial symmetry *n* the state of having similar parts arranged symmetrically around a common axis.
radian /ˈreɪdiən/ *n* the SI unit of plane angle, equal to the angle at the centre of a circle formed by radii of an arc equal in length to the radius.
radiance /ˈreɪdiəns/ *n* the condition of being radiant; brilliant light; dazzling beauty.
radiant /ˈreɪdiənt/ *adj* shining; beaming with happiness; sending out rays; transmitted by radiation.—**radiantly** *adv*.
radiant energy *n* energy in the form of electromagnetic radiation, such as heat or light.
radiant heat *n* heat conveyed by electromagnetic radiation rather than conduction or convection.
radiate /ˈreɪdiˌeɪt/ *vt* (*light, heat, etc*) to emit in rays; (*happiness, love, etc*) to give forth. • *vi* to spread out as if from a centre; to shine; to emit rays.
radiation /ˌreɪdiˈeɪʃən/ *n* radiant particles emitted as energy; rays emitted in nuclear decay; (*med*) treatment using a radioactive substance.
radiation sickness *n* an illness caused by excessive exposure to radiation from radioactive materials.
radiator /ˈreɪdiˌeɪtər/ *or* /ˈræd-/ *n* an apparatus for heating a room; a cooling device for a vehicle engine.
radical /ˈrædɪkəl/ *adj* of or relating to the root or origin; fundamental; favouring basic change. • *n* a person who advocates fundamental political or social change.—**radicalism** *n*.
radically /-li/ *adv* fundamentally.
radical sign *n* the symbol √ placed before a number to show that the square root (or a higher root denoted by an index number over the sign) is to be extracted.
radicchio /rəˈdiːkioː/ *n* (*pl* **radicchios**) a type of Italian chicory with white-veined purple leaves eaten raw in salads.
radices /ˈrædɪsəz/ *see* **radix**.
radicle /ˈrædɪkəl/ *n* the part of a seed that develops into a root; a root-like subdivision of a nerve or vein.
radii /ˈreɪdiˌaɪ/ *see* **radius**.
radio- /ˈreɪdioː/ *prefix* radial; radio; using radiant energy.
radio *n* the transmission of sounds or signals by electromagnetic waves through space, without wires, to a receiving set; such a set; broadcasting by radio as an industry, entertainment, etc. • *adj* of, using, used in, or sent by radio. • *vti* to transmit, or communicate with, by radio.
radioactive /ˌreɪdioːˈæktɪv/ *adj* giving off radiant energy in the form of particles or rays caused by the disintegration of atomic nuclei.—**radioactivity** *n*.
radioactive decay *n* the disintegration of a nucleus as the result of electron capture.
radioactive waste *n* any waste products that contain radioactive materials.—*also* **nuclear waste**.

radio astronomy *n* astronomy dealing with radio waves in space in order to obtain information about the universe.

radio beacon *n* a radio transmitter that sends out signals as an aid to navigation.

radiocarbon /ˌreɪdioˈkɑːbən/ *n* a radioisotope of carbon used in carbon dating.

radiocarbon dating *n* carbon dating.

radio compass *n* a navigational device which can determine the direction of radio waves from a specific radio beacon.

radio control *n* remote control using radio signals.—**radio-controlled** *adj*.

radioelement /ˌreɪdioˈɛləmənt/ *n* a radioactive chemical element.

radio frequency *n* a frequency intermediate between audio frequencies and infrared frequencies used *esp* in radio and television transmission.

radiogram /ˈreɪdioˌɡræm/ *n* a combined radio and record player.

radiograph /ˈreɪdioˌɡræf/ *n* an image produced on sensitive photographic film or plate by radiation other than light, *esp* X-rays.

radiography /ˌreɪdiˈɒɡrəfi/ *n* the production of X-ray photographs for use in medicine, industry, etc.—**radiographer** *n*.

radioisotope /ˌreɪdioˈaɪsətoʊp/ *n* a radioactive isotope.

radiology /ˌreɪdiˈɒlədʒi/ *n* a branch of medicine concerned with the use of radiant energy (as X-rays and radium) in the diagnosis and treatment of disease.—**radiologist** *n*.

radiometer /ˌreɪdiˈɒmɪtər/ *n* an instrument for measuring radiant energy.—**radiometric** *adj*.

radiopaging /ˌreɪdioˈpeɪdʒɪŋ/ *n* a system for alerting a person using a small radio transmitter which beeps in response to a signal from a distance.

radiosonde /ˈreɪdioˌsɒnd/ *n* a small radio transmitter carried by a probe for sending back data on atmospheric conditions.

radio source *n* any celestial object, such as a supernova, that emits radio waves.

radio spectrum *n* that range of frequencies, between 10 kHz and 300,000 MHz, used in radio transmission.

radiotelegraphy /ˌreɪdioˈtɛləɡrəfi/ *n* telegraphy that uses radio waves to transmit messages.—**radiotelegraph** *n*.—**radiotelegraphic** *adj*.

radiotelephone /ˌreɪdioˈtɛləfoʊn/ *n* a device for transmitting telephone messages using radio waves. • *vt* to transmit by radiotelephone. • *vi* to operate a radiotelephone.—**radiotelephony** *n*.

radio telescope *n* an instrument used in radio astronomy to receive and analyse radio waves.

radiotherapy *n* the medical treatment of disease, *esp* cancer, by X-rays or other radioactive substances.—**radiotherapist** *n*.

radio wave *n* an electromagnetic wave having radio frequency.

radish /ˈrædɪʃ/ *n* a pungent root eaten raw as a salad vegetable.

radium /ˈreɪdiəm/ *n* a highly radioactive metallic element.

radium therapy *n* the treatment of cancer by exposure to radiation from radium.

radius /ˈreɪdiəs/ *n* (*pl* **radii**) (*geom*) a straight line joining the centre of a circle or sphere to its circumference; a thing like this, a spoke; a sphere of activity; (*anat*) the thicker of the two bones of the forearm.

radix /ˈreɪdɪks/ *n* (*pl* **radices, radixes**) (*maths*) a number that is the base of a number system or for computation of logarithms.

radome /ˈreɪdoʊm/ *n* a protective housing for a radar antenna constructed from material which is transparent to radio waves.

radon /ˈreɪdɒn/ *n* a gaseous radioactive element.—*also* **niton**.

radula /ˈrædjʊlə/ *n* (*pl* **radulae**) a horny strip covered with minute teeth on the tongue of certain molluscs.

RAF /ræf/ or /ˌɑːrˈeɪˈɛf/ *abbr* = Royal Air Force.

raffia /ˈræfiə/ *n* a kind of palm; fibre from its leaves used in basket-making, etc.

raffish /ˈræfɪʃ/ *adj* untidy, disreputable, rakish; vulgarly flashy.

raffle /ˈræfəl/ *n* a lottery with prizes. • *vt* to offer as a prize in a raffle.

raft /ræft/ *n* a platform of logs, planks, etc strapped together to float on water.

rafter /ˈræftər/ *n* one of the inclined, parallel beams that support a roof.

rag¹ /ræɡ/ *n* a torn or waste scrap of cloth; a shred; (*inf*) a sensationalist newspaper; (*pl*) tattered or shabby clothing.

rag² *vt* (**ragging, ragged**) to tease; to play practical jokes on. • *n* a practical joke; a series of boisterous stunts staged by British students to raise money for charity.

rag³ *n* ragtime music.

raga /ˈrɑːɡə/ *n* (a composition based on) any of various conventional melodic or rhythmic patterns in Indian music used as the basis for improvisation.

ragamuffin /ˈræɡəmʌfɪn/ *n* an unkempt dirty person, *esp* a child.

rag and bone man *n* a junkman.

ragbag /ˈræɡbæɡ/ *n* a bag for scraps; a miscellaneous collection, jumble.

rage /reɪdʒ/ *n* violent anger; passion; frenzy; fashion, craze. • *vi* to behave with violent anger; to storm; to spread rapidly; to be prevalent.

ragged /ˈræɡɪd/ *adj* jagged; uneven; irregular; worn into rags; tattered.—**raggedly** *adv*.—**raggedness** *n*.

ragged robin *n* a Eurasian plant of the pink family with tattered looking pink or white flowers.

raggedy /ˈræɡədi/ *adj* (*inf*) tattered.

ragi, raggee /ˈrɑːɡi/ *n* a cereal grass cultivated in Asia and Africa.

raging /ˈreɪdʒɪŋ/ *adj* violent; intense.

raglan /ˈræɡlən/ *n* a type of loose sleeve cut in one piece with the shoulder of a garment.

ragout /ræˈɡuː/ *n* a stew of meat and vegetables, highly seasoned.

ragtime /ˈræɡtaɪm/ *n* quick tempo jazz piano music.

ragwort /ˈræɡwɜːt/ *n* a European composite plant with yellow flowers.

rah /rɒ/ *interj* hurrah.

raid /reɪd/ *n* a sudden attack to assault or seize. • *vt* to make a raid on; to steal from.—**raider** *n*.

rail¹ /reɪl/ *n* a horizontal bar extending from one post to another, as in a fence, etc; one of a pair of parallel steel lines forming a track for the wheels of a train; a railroad.

rail² *vi* to speak angrily.

railhead /ˈreɪlhɛd/ *n* the furthest point reached by the tracks of an uncompleted railway; a terminus.

railing /ˈreɪlɪŋ/ *n* a fence of rails and posts; rails collectively.

raillery /ˈreɪləri/ *n* (*pl* **railleries**) good-humoured banter, mockery.

railroad /ˈreɪlroʊd/ *n* railway. • *vt* to force unduly; (*bill, etc*) to push forward fast; to imprison hastily, *esp* unjustly.

railway /ˈreɪlweɪ/ *n* a track of parallel steel rails along which carriages are drawn by locomotive engines; a complete system of such tracks.

raiment /ˈreɪmənt/ *n* (*poet*) clothing.

rain /reɪn/ *n* water that falls from the clouds in the form of drops; a shower; a large quantity of anything falling like rain; (*pl*) the rainy season in the tropics. • *vti* (*of rain*) to fall; to fall like rain; (*rain, etc*) to pour down.

rainbow /ˈreɪnboʊ/ *n* the arc containing the colours of the spectrum formed in the sky by the refraction of the sun's rays in falling rain or in mist. • *adj* many-coloured.

rainbow trout *n* a large freshwater trout of Europe and North America with bright markings.

rain check *n* a ticket stub allowing future admission to an event in the case of it being rained off; the postponement of acceptance of an offer or invitation.

raincoat /ˈreɪnkoʊt/ *n* a waterproof coat.

raindrop /-drɒp/ *n* a drop of rain.

rainfall /-fɔːl/ *n* a fall of rain; the amount of rain that falls on a given area in a specified time.

rain forest *n* a dense, evergreen forest in a tropical area with much rainfall.

rain gauge *n* an instrument for measuring rainfall.

rainproof /-pruːf/ *adj* rain-resisting.

rain shadow *n* the leeward side of a hill or mountain where the rain is relatively lighter.

rainy /ˈreɪni/ *adj* (**rainier, rainiest**) full of rain; wet.

rainy day *n* a future need, *esp* financial.

raise /reɪz/ *vt* to elevate; to lift up; to set or place upright; to stir up, rouse; to increase in size, amount, degree, intensity, etc; to breed, bring up; (*question, etc*) to put forward; to collect or levy; (*siege*) to abandon. • *n* a rise in wages.

raisin /ˈreɪzən/ *n* a sweet, dried grape.

raison d'être *Fr.* /ˌreɪzɔːˈdɛtr/ *n* (*pl* **raisons d'être**) reason for existence; justification.

raj /rɑːdʒ/ or /rɒʒ/, /rædʒ/ *n* the period of British rule in India.

rajah, raja /ˈrɑːdʒə/ or /ˈrɒʒə/, /ˈrædʒə/ *n* (*formerly*) an Indian ruler; an Indian or Malayan chief or prince.

rake¹ /reɪk/ *n* a tool with a row of teeth and a handle for gathering together, scraping (leaves, hay, etc) or for smoothing gravel, etc. • *vt* to scrape, gather as with a rake; to sweep with gaze or gunshot; (*with* **in**: *money, etc*) to gather a great amount rapidly; (*with* **up**: *past misdemeanours, etc*) to bring to light.

rake[2] *n* the incline or slope of a mast, stern, etc.

rake[3] *n* a dissolute, debauched man, a libertine.

raki, rakee /rə'kiː/ or /'ræki/ *n* a strong aromatic spirit distilled from grain in Turkey.

rakish /'reɪkɪʃ/ *adj* jaunty, dashing; dissolute.—**rakishly** *adv*.—**rakishness** *n*.

rale /ræl/ *n* a wheezing rattle detectable with a stethoscope in the chest of patients with lung disorders.

rallentando /ˌrælən'tændoː/ *adv* (*mus*) gradually slower.

rally /'ræli/ *vti* (**rallying, rallied**) to bring or come together; to recover strength, revive; to take part in a motor rally; (*with* **round**) to help (a person); to support financially or morally. • *n* (*pl* **rallies**) a large assembly of people for a political purpose; a recovery (after illness); (*stock exchange*) a sharp increase in price after a decline; (*tennis*) a lengthy exchange of shots; a competitive test of driving and navigational skills.

RAM /ræm/ *abbr* = random-access memory.

ram /ræm/ *n* a male sheep; a battering device; a piston; (*with cap*) Aries, the first sign of the zodiac. • *vt* (**ramming, rammed**) to force or drive; to crash; to cram; to thrust violently.

Ramadan /'ræmə,dæn/ *n* the ninth month of the Islamic year; the great fast during it.

ramble /'ræmbəl/ *vi* to wander or stroll about for pleasure; (*plant*) to straggle; to write or talk aimlessly. • *n* a leisurely walk in the countryside.

rambler /'ræmblər/ *n* a person who rambles; a climbing rose.

rambling /-ɪŋ/ *adj* spread out, straggling; circuitous; disconnected; disjointed.

Ramboesque /'ræmboˌɛsk/ *adj* in the aggressive, mindless style of the fictional character Rambo, an indestructible one-man army who featured in several violent action films in the 1980s.

rambunctious /ræm'bʌŋkʃəs/ *adj* (*inf*) boisterous, unruly.—**rambunctiously** *adv*.—**rambunctiousness** *n*.

rambutan /ræm'buːtən/ *n* (a Malaysian tree bearing) a hairy red edible fruit.

ramekin /'ræmkɪn/ *n* a baked dish of cheese, breadcrumbs, etc; the small pot in which this is cooked.

ramification /ˌræməfɪ'keɪʃən/ *n* a branching out; an offshoot; a consequence.

ramify /'ræmə,faɪ/ *vti* to (cause to) divide into branches or constituent parts.

ramjet /'ræmdʒɛt/ *n* (an aircraft having) a type of jet engine that uses compressed air from the forward movement to burn the fuel.

ramose /'reɪmoːs/ or /rə'moːs/ *adj* composed of or having branches.—**ramosely** *adv*.

ramp /ræmp/ *n* a sloping walk or runway joining different levels; a wheeled staircase for boarding a plane; a sloping runway for launching boats, as from trailers.

rampage /'ræmpeɪdʒ/ *n* angry or violent behaviour • *vi* to rush about in an angry or violent manner.

rampant /'ræmpənt/ *adj* dominant; luxuriant, unrestrained; violent; rife, prevalent; (*her*) (of a beast) standing on its hind legs.

rampart /'ræmpɑrt/ *n* an embankment surrounding a fortification; a protective wall; ✦ (*Cdn*) steep rock walls, *esp* in a river gorge.

rampion /'ræmpiən/ *n* a Eurasian plant with bell-shaped red or purple flowers whose root is sometimes used in salads.

ramrod /'ræmrɒd/ *n* a rod for ramming home a charge in a muzzle-loading gun. • *adj* denoting a stiff, inflexible person.

ramshackle /'ræmʃækəl/ *adj* dilapidated.

RAN *abbr* = Royal Australian Navy.

ran /ræn/ *see* **run**.

ranch /ræntʃ/ *n* a large farm for raising cattle, horses, or sheep; a style of house with all the rooms on one floor. • *vi* to own, manage, or work on a ranch.—**rancher** *n*.

rancherie /'ræntʃeri/ *n* a settlement of North American Indians in a reserve in British Columbia, Canada.

rancid /'rænsɪd/ *adj* having an unpleasant smell and taste, as stale fats or oil.—**rancidity, rancidness** *n*.

rancour, rancor /'ræŋkər/ *n* bitter hate or spite.—**rancorous** *adj*.—**rancorously** *adv*.

rand /rænd/ *n* a unit of money in South Africa, divided into 100 cents.

R & B *abbr* = rhythm and blues.

R & D /ˌɑrənd'diː/ *abbr* = research and development.

random /'rændəm/ *adj* haphazard; left to chance.

random-access *adj* (*comput*) direct access to data in any desired order.

randomize /'rændəmaɪz/ *vt* to arrange (*eg* a survey, samples) in a random way to obtain unbiased statistical results.—**randomization** *n*.—**randomizer** *n*.

R and R /ˌɑrənd'ɑr/ *abbr* = rest and recreation.

randy /'rændi/ *adj* (**randier, randiest**) (*sl*) lustful, sexually aroused.

ranee *see* **rani**.

rang /ræŋ/ *see* **ring**[2].

range /reɪndʒ/ *n* a row; a series of mountains, etc; scope, compass; the distance a ship, aircraft, or motor vehicle can travel without refuelling; the distance a gun, etc can fire, a projectile can be thrown, or from gun to target; fluctuation; a large open area for grazing livestock; a place for testing rockets in flight; a place for shooting or golf practice; a cooking stove. • *vt* to place in order or a row; to establish the range of; (*livestock*) to graze on a range. • *vi* to be situated in a line; to rank or classify; (*gun*) to point or aim; to vary (inside limits).

range finder *n* an instrument for determining the range of a target.

ranger /'reɪndʒər/ *n* a forest or park warden.

rangy /'reɪndʒi/ *adj* (**rangier, rangiest**) tall and slim; long-limbed.—**ranginess** *n*.

rani, ranee /'ræni/ *n* in India, a queen or princess; the wife of a rajah.

rank[1] /ræŋk/ *n* a line of objects; a line of soldiers standing abreast; high standing or position; status; (*pl*) ordinary members of the armed forces. • *vti* to arrange in a line; to have a specific position in an organization or on a scale; to outrank; (*with* **with**) to be counted among.

rank[2] *adj* growing uncontrollably; utter, flagrant; offensive in odour or flavour.

rank and file *n* ordinary soldiers; ordinary members, as distinguished from their leaders.

ranking /'ræŋkɪŋ/ *n* a listing of things or people in order of importance. • *adj* of the highest rank; outstanding.

rankle /'ræŋkəl/ *vi* to fester; to cause continuous resentment or irritation.

ransack /'rænsæk/ *vt* to plunder; to search thoroughly.

ransom /'rænsəm/ *n* the release of a captured person or thing; the price paid for this. • *vt* to secure release by payment.

rant /rænt/ *vi* to speak loudly or violently; to preach noisily. • *n* loud, pompous talk.

ranunculus /rə'nʌŋjʊləs/ *n* (*pl* **ranunculuses, ranunculi**) a common genus of *usu* yellow-flowered plants including the buttercup.

rap[1] /ræk/ *n* a sharp blow; a knock; (*inf*) talk, conversation; (*sl*) arrest for a crime; (*sl*) rap music. • *vti* (**rapping, rapped**) to strike lightly or sharply; to knock; (*sl*) to criticize sharply; (*with* **out**) to utter abruptly; (*sl*) to speak in a fast and rhythmic manner to a musical backing.

rap[2] *n* a style of popular music in which (*usu* rhyming) words and phrases are spoken in a rhythmic chant over an instrumental backing.—**rapper** *n*.

rapacious *adj* grasping; extortionate.—**rapaciously** *adv*.—**rapacity** *n*.

rape[1] /reɪp/ *n* the act of forcing a person to have sexual intercourse against his or her will; the plundering (of a city, etc) as in warfare. • *vti* to commit rape (upon).

rape[2] *n* a bright yellow plant of the mustard family grown for its leaves and oily seeds.

rape-shield *adj* ✦ (*Cdn*) pertaining to laws that limit what questions may be asked an alleged victim of a sexual assault on matters of personal, *esp* sexual, history.

rapid /'ræpɪd/ *adj* at great speed; fast; sudden; steep. • *npl* a part of a river where the current flows swiftly.—**rapidity** *n*.—**rapidly** *adv*.

rapid eye movement *n* the rapid jerky movements of the eyeballs associated with dreaming while asleep.

rapier /'reɪpiər/ *n* a straight, two-edged sword with a narrow pointed blade.

rapine /'reɪpaɪn/ or /-pɪn/ *n* plunder, pillage.

rapist /'reɪpɪst/ *n* a person who commits rape.

rap music *n* a song that is rapidly spoken and accompanied by an insistent electronic rhythm

rappel /ræ'pɛl/ *vi* to abseil.

rapport /rə'pɔr/ *n* a sympathetic relationship; accord.

rapprochement *Fr.* /raprɒʃ'mã/ *n* re-establishment of cordial relations; reconciliation.

rapscallion /ræp'skæljən/ *n* a rascal.

rapt /ræpt/ *adj* carried away, enraptured; absorbed, intent.

raptor /'ræptər/ *n* a bird of prey.

raptorial /ræp'tɔriəl/ *adj* of or pertaining to birds of prey; (*birds' feet*) adapted for seizing prey.

rapture /'ræptʃər/ *n* the state of being carried away with love, joy, etc; intense delight, ecstasy.—**rapturous** *adj.*—**rapturously** *adv.*

rara avis /ˌrerə'eɪvɪs/ or /ˌrɑrə'ævɪs/ *n* a rare or unique person or thing.

rare[1] /rer/ *adj* unusual; seldom seen; exceptionally good; (*gas*) of low density, thin. *adv.*—**rareness** *n.*

rare[2] *adj* not completely cooked, partly raw; underdone.

rare earth *n* (an oxide of) any of the lanthanide series of chemical elements.

rarefy /'rerɪfaɪ/ *vti* (**rarefying, rarefied**) to make or become less dense; to thin out; to expand without the addition of matter; to make more spiritual, abstruse or refined.—**rarefied** *adj.*

rare gas *n* an inert gas.

rarely /'rerli/ *adv* almost never, seldom; exceptionally, unusually.

raring /'rerɪŋ/ *adj* (*inf*) eager, enthusiastic.

rarity /'rerɪti/ *n* (*pl* **rarities**) rareness; a rare person or thing.

rasbora /'ræsbərə/ *n* any of various small brightly-coloured tropical fishes popular for aquariums.

rascal /'ræskəl/ *n* a rogue; a villain; a mischievous person.

rase /reɪs/ *see* **raze**.

rash[1] /ræʃ/ *adj* reckless; impetuous.—**rashly** *adv.*—**rashness** *n.*

rash[2] *n* a skin eruption of spots, etc.

rasher /'ræʃər/ *n* a thin slice of bacon or ham.

rasp /ræsp/ *n* a coarse file; a grating sound. • *vt* to scrape with a rasp. • *vi* to produce a grating sound.

raspberry /'ræz,beri/ or /-bəri/, /-bri/ *n* (*pl* **raspberries**) a shrub with white flowers and red berry-like fruits; the fruit produced; (*inf*) a sound of dislike or derision.

Rastafarian /ˌræstə'feriən/, **Rasta** /'ræstə/ *n* a member of a largely Jamaican religious and political movement that worships Ras Tafari, the former Emperor of Ethiopia, Haile Selassie, as God.—*also adj.*

raster /'ræstər/ *n* a grid of lines scanned by an electron beam to make up an image, *esp* on a television screen.

rat /ræt/ *n* a long-tailed rodent similar to a mouse but larger; (*sl*) a sneaky, contemptible person, *esp* an informer; a scab. • *vi* (**ratting, ratted**) to hunt or catch rats; to betray or inform on someone; to work as a scab.

ratafia /ˌrætə'fiːə/ *n* a liqueur flavoured with fruit kernels, such as cherry, peach or almond; a sweet biscuit flavoured with coconut and almond.

ratatouille /ˌrætə'tuːi/ or /-'twiː/ *n* a dish consisting of a thick stew of roughly chopped vegetables such as onions, peppers, courgettes, aubergine, and tomatoes.

ratchet /'rætʃət/ *n* a device with a toothed wheel that moves in one direction only.

rate /reɪt/ *n* the amount, degree, etc of something in relation to units of something else; price, *esp* per unit; degree. • *vt* to fix the value of; to rank; to regard or consider; (*sl*) to think highly of. • *vi* to have value or status.

ratel /'reɪtəl/ *n* a carnivorous nocturnal mammal of Africa and Asia resembling the badger.

ratepayer /'reɪtpeɪər/ *n* a person who pays rates, a householder.

rather /'ræðər/ *adv* more willingly; preferably; somewhat; more accurately; on the contrary; (*inf*) yes, certainly.

ratify /'rætɪˌfaɪ/ *vt* (**ratifying, ratified**) to approve formally; to confirm.

rating /'reɪtɪŋ/ *n* an assessment; an evaluation, an appraisal, as of credit worthiness; classification by grade, as of military personnel; (*radio, TV*) the relative popularity of a programme according to sample polls.

ratio /'reɪʃiɔː/ or /-ʃoː/ *n* (*pl* **ratios**) the number of times one thing contains another; the quantitative relationship between two classes of objects; proportion.

ratiocinate /ˌrætiˈɒsɪˌneɪt/ or /ˌræʃi-/ *vi* to reason or argue systematically.—**ratiocination** *n.*

ration /'ræʃən/ *n* (*food, petrol*) a fixed amount or portion; (*pl*) food supply. • *vt* to supply with rations; (*food, petrol*) to restrict the supply of.

rational /'ræʃənəl/ *adj* of or based on reason; reasonable; sane.—**rationally** *adv.*

rationale /ˌræʃə'næl/ *n* the reason for a course of action; an explanation of principles.

rationalism /'ræʃənəˌlɪzəm/ *n* dependence on reason and rejection of intuition or the supernatural to justify ideas and beliefs, *esp* with regard to religion; the belief that reason can supply knowledge independently of personal experience.

rationality /ˌræʃə'næliti/ *n* (*pl* **rationalities**) the condition of being rational; the practice of being reasonable.

rationalize /'ræʃənəˌlaɪz/ *vti* to make rational; to justify one's reasons for an action; to cut down on personnel or equipment; to substitute a natural for a supernatural explanation.—**rationalization** *n.*

rational number *n* a number that can be expressed as the ratio of two integers.

ratline /'rætlɪn/ *n* any of the short ropes fastened between the shrouds of a sailing ship to form rungs.

ratoon, rattoon /rə'tuːn/ *n* a new shoot sprouting from the root of a perennial plant, *esp* sugarcane, after it has been cut back. • *vt* to encourage growth in this way.

rat race *n* continual hectic competitive activity.

rattan /rə'tæn/ *n* a climbing palm with a jointed stem; cane made of this.

rattle /'rætəl/ *vt* to clatter. • *vt* to make a series of sharp, quick noises; to clatter; to recite rapidly; to chatter; (*inf*) to disconcert, fluster. • *n* a rattling sound; a baby's toy that makes a rattling sound; a voluble talker; the rings on the tail of a rattlesnake.

rattler /'rætlər/ or /'rætələr/ *n* a rattlesnake.

rattlesnake /'rætəlˌsneɪk/ *n* a venomous American snake with a rattle in its tail.

rattling /'rætlɪŋ/ or /'rætəlɪŋ/ *adj* brisk, vigorous; first-rate. • *adv* to an extreme degree; very.

ratty /'ræti/ *adj* (**rattier, rattiest**) like or full of rats; (*sl*) angry, irritable, snappish.

raucous /'rɒkəs/ *adj* hoarse and harsh-sounding; loud and rowdy.

raunchy /'rɒntʃi/ *adj* (**raunchier, raunchiest**) (*sl*) coarse, earthy; careless, slovenly; cheap, inferior.

rauwolfia /rɔ'wʊlfiə/ or /roː-/ *n* a tropical flowering shrub of Southeast Asia; an extract from the root of this used in various drugs.

ravage /'rævɪdʒ/ *vt* to ruin, destroy; to plunder, lay waste. • *n* destruction; ruin; (*pl*) the effects of this.

rave /reɪv/ *vi* to speak wildly or as if delirious; (*inf*) to enthuse. • *n* enthusiastic praise.—**raving** *adj.*

ravel /'rævəl/ *vti* (**ravelling, ravelled** *or* **raveling, raveled**) to entangle or disentangle; to fray; to unwind; to make or become complicated.

raven /'reɪvən/ *n* a large crow-like bird with glossy black feathers. • *adj* of the colour or sheen of a raven.

ravenous /'rævənəs/ *adj* famished; voracious.—**ravenously** *adv.*

ravine /rə'viːn/ *n* a deep, narrow gorge, a large gully.

ravioli /ˌrævi'oːli/ *n* small cases of pasta filled with highly seasoned chopped meat or vegetables.

ravish /'rævɪʃ/ *vt* to violate; to rape; to enrapture.

ravishing /'rævɪʃɪŋ/ *adj* charming, captivating.

raw /rɒ/ *adj* uncooked; unrefined; in a natural state, crude; untrained, inexperienced; sore, skinned; damp, chilly; (*inf*) harsh or unfair.—**rawness** *n.*

rawhide /'rɒhaɪd/ *n* (a whip made from strips of) untanned leather.

raw material *n* something out of which a finished article is made; something with a potential for development, improvement, etc.

ray[1] /reɪ/ *n* a beam of light that comes from a bright source; any of several lines radiating from a centre; a beam of radiant energy, radioactive particles, etc; a tiny amount.

ray[2] *n* any of various fishes with a flattened body and the eyes on the upper surface.

rayon /'reɪɒn/ *n* a textile fibre made from a cellulose solution; a fabric of such fibres.

raze /reɪz/ *vt* to demolish; to erase; to level to the ground.—*also* **rase.**

razor /'reɪzər/ *n* a sharp-edged instrument for shaving.

razorbill /'reɪzərbɪl/ *n* a North Atlantic auk with a flattened sharp-edged bill.

razor clam, razor-shell *n* any of various bivalve marine molluscs with curved sharp shells.

razz /ræz/ vt (inf) to deride, heckle.

razzle-dazzle /'ræzəl,dæzəl/, **razzmatazz** /'ræzmə,tæz/ n (inf) exciting, exuberant or colourful activity or atmosphere.

Rb (chem symbol) rubidium.

RC abbr = Roman Catholic.

RCA abbr = Radio Corporation of America.

RCAF abbr = Royal Canadian Air Force.

RCCh abbr = Roman Catholic Church.

RCL /'ɑr'si:'el/ abbr ✤ = Royal Canadian Legion.

RCMP abbr = Royal Canadian Mounted Police.

RCN abbr = Royal Canadian Navy.

RCP abbr = Royal College of Physicians.

RCS abbr = Royal College of Surgeons.

Rd abbr = road.

Re (chem symbol) rhenium.

re- /ri:/ prefix again, anew; back.

re[1] /ri:/ prep concerning, with reference to.

re[2] n the second note of a major scale in solmization.

reach /ri:tʃ/ vti to arrive at; to extend as far as; to make contact with; to pass, hand over; to attain, realize; to stretch out the hand; to extend in influence, space, etc; to carry, as sight, sound, etc; to try to get. • n the act or power of reaching; extent; mental range; scope; a continuous extent, esp of water.

react /ri:'ækt/ vi to act in response to a person or stimulus; to have a mutual or reverse effect; to revolt; (chem) to undergo a chemical reaction.

reaction /ri'ækʃən/ n an action in response to a stimulus; a revulsion of feeling; exhaustion after excitement, etc; opposition to new ideas; (chem) an action set up by one substance in another.

reactionary /-,ɛri/ adj, n (a person) opposed to political or social change.

reactive /ri:'æktɪv/ adj of or relating to reaction; reacting to stimuli; caused by stress.

reactor /ri'æktər/ n a person or substance that undergoes a reaction; (chem) a vessel in which a reaction occurs; a nuclear reactor.

read /ri:d/ vti (**reading, read**) to understand something written; to speak aloud (from a book); to study by reading; to interpret, divine; to register, as a gauge; to foretell; (of a computer) to obtain (information) from; (sl) to hear and understand (a radio communication, etc); (with **about, of**) to learn by reading; to be phrased in certain words. • adj well-informed.

readable /'ri:dəbəl/ adj legible; pleasantly written.

readdress /,ri:ə'dres/ vt to address again; (letter) to change the address when forwarding.

reader /'ri:dər/ n a person who reads; one who reads aloud to others; a proofreader; a person who evaluates manuscripts; a textbook, esp on reading; a unit that scans material for computation or storage; a senior lecturer.

readership /'ri:dərʃɪp/ n all the readers of a certain publication, author, etc.

readily /'redɪli/ adv in a ready manner; willingly, easily.

reading /'ri:dɪŋ/ n the act of one who reads; any material to be read; the amount measured by a barometer, meter, etc; a particular interpretation of a play, etc.

readjust /,ri:ə'dʒʌst/ vt to adjust again.

read-only memory n a small computer memory that cannot be changed by the computer and that contains a special-purpose program.

read-out /'ri:daut/ n the retrieval of information from a computer memory; the information retrieved.

read-write head n (comput) an electromagnetic head that can read and write data on a magnetic disc.

ready /'redi/ adj (**readier, readiest**) prepared; fit for use; willing; inclined, apt; prompt, quick; handy. • n the state of being ready, esp the position of a firearm aimed for firing. • vt (**readying, readied**) to make ready.—**readiness** n.

ready-made adj made in standard sizes, not to measure.

reagent /ri:'eɪdʒənt/ n (chem) a substance used to detect, measure, or react with other substances.

real /ri:l/ adj existing, actual, not imaginary; true, genuine, not artificial; (law) immovable, consisting of land or houses. • adv (sl) very; really.

real estate n property; land.

realgar /ri'ælgər/ n a reddish mineral composed of arsenic sulphide.

realign /,ri:ə'laɪn/ vti to align again; (politics, diplomacy) to readjust alliances, policies, etc.—**realignment** n.

realism /'ri:ə,lɪzəm/ n practical outlook; (art, literature) the ability to represent things as they really are without concealment; (philos) the doctrine that the physical world has an objective existence; the doctrine that general ideas have an objective existence.—**realist** n.

realistic /riə'lɪstɪk/ adj matter-of-fact, not visionary; lifelike; of or relating to realism.—**realistically** adv.

reality /ri'ælɪti/ n (pl **realities**) the fact or condition of being real; an actual fact or thing; truth.

realization /'riəlaɪ'zeɪʃən/ n the action of realizing; something comprehended or achieved.

realize /'riəlaɪz/ vt to become fully aware of; (ambition, etc) to make happen; to cause to appear real; to convert into money, be sold for.

really /'ri:li/ adv in fact, in reality; positively, very. • interj indeed.

realm /relm/ n a kingdom, country; domain, region; sphere.

real number n any rational or irrational number.

real tennis n an early form of tennis played in a walled indoor court.

real-time adj involving the continual processing, manipulation and presentation of data by a computer as it is generated.

realtor /'ri:əltər/ n a person whose business is selling and leasing property, an estate agent.

realty /'ri:əlti/ n real estate.

ream /ri:m/ n a quantity of paper varying from 480 to 516 sheets; (pl: inf) a great amount.

reap /ri:p/ vti to harvest; to gain (a benefit).

reaper /'ri:pər/ n a person who or a machine that reaps.

rear[1] /rɪr/ n the back part or position, esp of an army; (sl) the rump. • adj of, at, or in the rear.

rear[2] vt to raise; (children) to bring up; to educate, nourish, etc. • vi (horse) to stand on the hind legs.

rear guard n a military detachment assigned to guard the rear of a body of troops. • adj relating to determined defensive resistance.

rear admiral n a naval officer next below in rank to a vice admiral.

rear light, rear lamp n a taillight.

rearm /ri:'ɑrm/ vti to arm or become armed again, esp with better weapons.—**rearmament** r.

rearview mirror n a mirror in a motor vehicle that allows the driver to see following traffic.

rearward /'ri:rwərd/ adj, adv at or towards the rear.—**rearwards** adv.

reason /'ri:zən/ n motive or justification (of an action or belief); the mental power to draw conclusions and determine truth; a cause; moderation; sanity; intelligence. • vti to think logically (about); to analyse; to argue or infer.

reasonable /-əbəl/ adj able to reason or listen to reason; rational; sensible; not expensive; moderate, fair.—**reasonableness** n.—**reasonably** adv.

reasoned /'ri:zənd/ adj convincingly argued.

reassure /,ri:ə'ʃər/ or /-'ʃur/ vt to hearten; to give confidence to; to free from anxiety.—**reassurance** n.

rebate[1] /'ri:beɪt/ n a refund of part of an amount paid; discount.

rebate[2] see **rabbet**.

rebec, rebeck /'ri:bek/ n a medieval stringed instrument shaped like a lute and played with a bow.

rebel /'rebəl/ n a person who refuses to conform with convention. • vi (**rebelling, rebelled** or **rebeling, rebeled**) (army) to rise up against the authorities or the government; to dissent.

rebellion /rə'beljən/ or /rɪ-/ n armed resistance to an established government, insurrection; defiance of authority.

rebellious /rə'beljəs/ or /rɪ-/ adj of or engaged in rebellion; tending to rebel; stubborn.—**rebelliously** adv.

rebirth /ri:'bɔrθ/ or /'ri:-/ n a second or new birth; a revival, renaissance; spiritual regeneration.

rebound /'ri:baund/ or /ri'baund/ vi to spring back after impact; to bounce back; to recover. • n a recoil; an emotional reaction.

rebounder /-ər/ n a small trampoline used for keep-fit exercises.

rebuff /ri:'bʌf/ or /rə'bʌf/ vt to snub, repulse; to refuse unexpectedly.—also n.

rebuke /rə'bju:k/ or /ri:-/ vt to reprimand, chide. • n a reproof, reprimand.

rebus /'ri:bəs/ n (pl **rebuses**) a puzzle using images to represent the sound of words or syllables.

rebut /ri'bʌt/ or /ri:-/ vt (**rebutting, rebutted**) to disprove or refute by argument, etc.—**rebuttal** n.

rec abbr = receipt; recipe; record.

recalcitrant /rəˈkælsɪtrənt/ or /ri-/ *adj* refusing to obey authority, etc; actively disobedient.—**recalcitrance** *n*.

recall /rəˈkɒl/ or /ri-/ *vt* to call back; to bring back to mind, remember; to revoke. • *n* remembrance; a summons to return; the removal from office by popular vote.

recant /rəˈkænt/ or /ri-/ *vti* to repudiate or retract a former opinion, declaration, or belief.—**recantation** *n*.

recap /ˈriːkæp/ *vti* (**recapping, recapped**) to recapitulate. • *n* (*inf*) recapitulation.

recapitulate /ˌriːkəˈpɪtʃuˌleɪt/ *vt* to restate the main points of, to summarize.—**recapitulation** *n*.

recapture /riːˈkæptʃər/ *vt* to capture again; (*a lost feeling, etc*) to discover anew, regain. • *n* the act of recapturing; a thing or feeling recaptured.

recd, rec'd *abbr* = received.

recede /rəˈsiːd/ or /ri-/ *vi* to move back; to withdraw, retreat; to slope backwards; to grow less; to decline in value.

receding /-ɪŋ/ *adj* sloping backwards; disappearing from view; (*hair*) ceasing to grow at the temples.

receipt /rəˈsiːt/ or /ri-/ *n* the act of receiving; a written proof of this; (*pl*) amount received from business. • *vt* to acknowledge and mark as paid; to write a receipt for.

receive /rəˈsiːv/ or /ri-/ *vt* to acquire, be given; to experience, be subjected to; to admit, allow; to greet on arrival; to accept as true; (*stolen goods*) to take in; to transfer electrical signals. • *vi* to be a recipient; to convert radio waves into perceptible signals.

received /rəˈsiːvd/ or /ri-/ *adj* accepted, recognized.

Received Pronunciation *n* the unlocalized accent of British English, regarded as standard.

receiver /rəˈsiːvər/ or /ri-/ *n* a person who receives; equipment that receives electronic signals, *esp* on a telephone; (*law*) a person appointed to manage or hold in trust property in bankruptcy or pending a lawsuit.

receivership /-ʃɪp/ *n* the status of a business in the hands of a receiver.

recent /ˈriːsənt/ *adj* happening lately, fresh; not long established, modern.—**recently** *adv*.

receptacle /rəˈsəptəkəl/ or /ri-/ *n* a container.

reception /rəˈsepʃən/ or /ri-/ *n* the act of receiving or being received; a welcome; a social gathering, often to extend a formal welcome; a response, reaction; the quality of the sound or image produced by a radio or television set.

receptionist /-ɪst/ *n* a person employed to receive visitors to an office, hotel, hospital, etc.

receptive /rəˈseptɪv/ or /ri-/ *adj* able or quick to take in ideas or impressions.

recess /ˈriːses/ *n* a temporary halting of work, a vacation; a hidden or inner place; an alcove or niche. • *vti* to place in a recess; to form a recess in; to take a recess.

recession /rəˈseʃən/ or /ri-/ *n* the act of receding; a downturn in economic activity; an indentation.

recharge /rəˈtʃɑrdʒ/ or /ri-/ *vt* to renew the electric charge in (a battery, etc); to recover one's energies.

recherché /rəˈʃɛrʃeɪ/ *adj* uncommon, choice; refined, precious.

recidivism /rəˈsɪdɪvɪzəm/ *n* inevitable relapse into crime.—**recidivist** *n*.

recipe /ˈresɪpiː/ *n* a list of ingredients and directions for preparing food; a method for achieving an end.

recipient /rəˈsɪpiənt/ or /ri-/ *n* a person who receives.

reciprocal /rəˈsɪprəkəl/ or /ri-/ *adj* done by each to the other; mutual; complementary; interchangeable; (*gram*) expressing a mutual relationship. • *n* (*math*) an expression so related to another that their product is 1.—**reciprocally** *adv*.—**reciprocity** *n*.

reciprocate /rəˈsɪprəˌkeɪt/ or /ri-/ *vti* to give in return; to repay; (*mech*) to move alternately backwards and forwards.—**reciprocating** *adj*.—**reciprocation** *n*.

recital /rəˈsaɪtəl/ or /ri-/ *n* the act of reciting; a detailed account, narrative; a statement of facts; (*mus*) a performance given by an individual musician.

recitation /ˌresəˈteɪʃən/ *n* the act of reciting; something recited, as a poem, etc.

recitative /ˌresətəˈtiːv/ *n* a narrative part of an opera sung in the rhythms of ordinary speech.

recite /rəˈsaɪt/ or /ri-/ *vti* to repeat aloud from memory, declaim; to recount, enumerate; to repeat (a lesson).

reckless /ˈrekləs/ *adj* rash, careless, incautious.—**recklessly** *adv*.—**recklessness** *n*.

reckon /ˈrekən/ *vti* to count; to regard or consider; to think; to calculate; (*with* **with**) to take into account.

reckoning /-ɪŋ/ *n* a calculation; the settlement of an account.

reclaim /rəˈkleɪm/ or /ri-/ *vt* to recover, win back from a wild state or vice; (*wasteland*) to convert into land fit for cultivation; (*plastics, etc*) to obtain from waste materials.—**reclaimable** *adj*.—**reclamation** *n*.

recline /rəˈklaɪn/ *vti* to cause or permit to lean or bend backwards; to lie down on the back or side.—**reclinable** *adj*.

recluse /rəˈkluːs/ or /ri-/ *n* a person who lives in solitude; a hermit.

recognition /ˌrekəgˈnɪʃən/ *n* the act of recognizing; identification; acknowledgment, admission; the sensing and encoding of printed and written data by a machine.

recognizance /rəˈkɒɡnɪzəns/ or /-ˈkɒn-/ *n* (*law*) a bond by which a person undertakes before a court to observe some condition; the sum pledged as surety for this.

recognize /ˈrekəɡˌnaɪz/ *vt* to know again, identify; to greet; to acknowledge formally; to accept, admit.—**recognizable** *adj*.

recoil /rəˈkɔɪl/ or /ri-/ *vti* to spring back, kick, as a gun; to shrink or flinch. • *n* the act of recoiling, a rebound.

recollect /ˌrekəˈlekt/ *vti* to recall; to remind (oneself) of something temporarily forgotten; to call something to mind.

recollection /ˌrekəˈlekʃən/ *n* the act of recalling to mind; a memory, impression; something remembered; tranquillity of mind; religious contemplation.

recombinant DNA /riːˈkɒmbɪnənt-/ *n* molecules of DNA from different sources spliced together in the laboratory.

recombination /riːˌkɒmbəˈneɪʃən/ *n* the combination of genetic material from different sources.

recommend /ˌrekəˈmend/ *vt* to counsel or advise; to commend or praise; to introduce favourably.—**recommendable** *adj*.—**recommendation** *n*.

recompense /ˈrekəmpens/ *n* to reward or pay an equivalent; to compensate. • *n* reward; repayment; compensation.

reconcile /ˈrekənˌsaɪl/ *vt* to re-establish friendly relations; to bring to agreement; to make compatible; to resolve; to settle; to make resigned (to); (*financial account*) to check with another account for accuracy.—**reconcilable** *adj*.—**reconciliation** *n*.

recondite /ˈrekənˌdaɪt/ or /rɪˈkɒn-/ *adj* needing specialized training or knowledge; complex, obscure.

recondition /riːkənˈdɪʃən/ *vt* to repair and restore to good working order.

reconnaissance /rəˈkɒnəsəns/ or /ri-/ *n* a survey of an area, *esp* for obtaining military information about an enemy.

reconnoitre, reconnoiter /ˌrekəˈnɔɪtər/ *vti* to make a reconnaissance (of).

reconsider /ˌriːkənˈsiːdər/ *vt* to consider afresh, review; to modify.—**reconsideration** *n*.

reconstitute /riːˈkɒnstɪˌtuːt/ or /-ˌtjuːt/ *vt* (*a dried or condensed substance*) to constitute again, *esp* to restore to its original form by adding water.—**reconstitution** *n*.

reconstruct /ˌriːkənˈstrʌkt/ *vt* to build again; to build up, as from remains, an image of the original; to supply missing parts by conjecture.—**reconstruction** *n*.

record /ˈrekərd/ or /ˈrekɔrd/ *vt* to preserve evidence of; to write down; to chart; to register, enrol; to register permanently by mechanical means; (*sound or visual images*) to register on a disc, tape, etc for later reproduction; to celebrate; to make a recording. • *vi* to record something. • *adj* being the best, largest, etc. • *n* a written account; a register; a report of proceedings; the known facts about anything or anyone; an outstanding performance or achievement that surpasses others previously recorded; a grooved vinyl disc for playing on a record player; (*comput*) data in machine-readable form.

recorder /-ər/ *n* an official who keeps records; a machine or device that records; a tape recorder; a wind instrument of the flute family.

recording /-ɪŋ/ *n* what is recorded, as on a disc or tape; the record.

recordist /-ɪst/ *n* a person who records sound.

record player *n* an instrument for playing records through a loudspeaker.

recount[1] /rəˈkaʊnt/ or /ri-/ *vt* to narrate the details of; to narrate.

recount[2] /riːˈkaʊnt/ or /ˈri-/ *vt* to count again. • *n* a second counting of election votes.

recoup /rəˈkuːp/ or /ri-/ *vti* to make good (financial losses); to regain; to make up for something lost.

recourse /ˈriːkɔrs/ or /rɪˈkɔrs/ *n* a resort for help or protection when in danger; that to which one turns when seeking help.

re-cover /riːˈkʌvər/ *vt* to put a new cover on.

recover /rəˈkʌvər/ or /ri-/ *vti* to regain after losing; to reclaim; to regain health or after losing emotional control.—**recoverable** *adj.*

recovery /rəˈkʌvəri/ or /ri-/ *n* (*pl* **recoveries**) the act or process of recovering; the condition of having recovered; reclamation; restoration; a retrieval of a capsule, etc after a space flight.

recovery room *n* a hospital room where patients are kept for close observation or care following surgery.

recreate /ˌriːkriˈeɪt/ *vt* to create over again, *esp* mentally.

recreation /ˌrɒkriˈeɪʃən/ *n* relaxation of the body or mind; a sport, pastime or amusement.—**recreational** *adj.*

recreational vehicle *n* a vehicle for camping out such as a motor home, camper, etc.

recreation room *n* a room used for relaxation, recreation, or social activities, *esp* in a hospital, etc.

recriminate /rəˈkrɪmɪˌneɪt/ or /ri-/ *vi* to return an accusation, make a counter-charge.—**recrimination** *n.*—**recriminatory** *adj.*

recrudesce /ˌriːkruːˈdes/ or /ˌrɛk-/ *vi* (*esp disease*) to reappear again.—**recrudescence** *n.*

recruit /rəˈkruːt/ or /ri-/ *n* a soldier newly enlisted; a member newly joined; a beginner. • *vti* to enlist (military personnel); to enlist (new members) for an organization; to increase or maintain the numbers of; to restore, reinvigorate.—**recruitment** *n.*

rectal /ˈrɛktəl/ *adj* of, for, or near the rectum.

rectangle /ˈrɛkˌtæŋgəl/ *n* a parallelogram with all its angles right angles.

rectangular /rɛkˈtæŋgjʊlər/ *adj* having the shape of a rectangle; crossing, meeting, or lying at a right angle; having faces or surfaces shaped like right angles.

rectifier /ˈrɛktəˌfaɪr/ *n* a device that converts alternating current to direct current.

rectify /ˈrɛktəˌfaɪ/ *vt* (**rectifying, rectified**) to put right, correct; to amend; (*chem*) to refine by repeated distillation; (*elect*) to convert to direct current.—**rectifiable** *adj.*

rectilinear /ˌrɛktɪˈlɪniər/, **rectilineal** /-niəl/ *adj* of or bounded by straight lines; straight.

rectitude /ˈrɛktɪˌtuːd/ or /-ˌtjuːd/ *n* moral uprightness; probity; a being correct in judgment or procedure.

recto /ˈrɛktoʊ/ *n* (*pl* **rectos**) the right-hand page of an open book.

rector /ˈrɛktər/ *n* in some churches, a clergyman in charge of a parish; the head of certain schools, colleges, etc.—**rectorial** *adj.*

rectory /-ri/ *n* (*pl* **rectories**) the house of a minister or priest.

rectrix /ˈrɛktrɪks/ *n* (*pl* **rectrices**) any of the tail feathers of a bird, used for controlling the direction of flight.

rectum /ˈrɛktəm/ *n* (*pl* **rectums, recta**) the part of the large intestine leading to the anus.

rectus /ˈrɛktəs/ *n* (*pl* **recti**) any of various straight muscles, *esp* of the abdomen.

recumbent /rəˈkʌmbənt/ or /ri-/ *adj* leaning, resting; lying down.

recuperate /rəˈkuːpəˌreɪt/ or /ri-/ *vti* to get well again; to recover (losses, etc).—**recuperation** *n.*

recur /rəˈkər/ or /ri-/ *vi* (**recurring, recurred**) to be repeated in thought, talk, etc; to occur again or at intervals.—**recurrence** *n.*—**recurrent** *adj.*

recycle /riːˈsaɪkəl/ *vti* (*a substance*) to pass through a process again; (*used matter*) to process to regain re-usable material; to save from loss and restore to usefulness.—**recyclable** *adj.*

red /rɛd/ *adj* (**redder, reddest**) of the colour of blood; politically left-wing. • *n* the colour of blood; any red pigment; a communist.

redact /rəˈdækt/ or /ri-/ *vt* to edit (a manuscript, etc) for publication.—**redaction** *n.*—**redactor** *n.*

red admiral *n* a common butterfly of Europe and North America with black and red markings.

redback /ˈrɛdbæk/ *n* (*Austral*) a poisonous spider with red spots on its back.

red blood cell *n* any blood cell containing haemoglobin that conveys oxygen to the tissues.

red-blooded *adj* (*inf*) vigorous, virile.

redbreast /ˈrɛdˌbrɛst/ *n* a robin.

redbrick /ˈrɛdbrɪk/ *adj, n* (a British university) founded after 1945.

redcap /ˈrɛdkæp/ *n* in US, a porter at a railway station or airport; in UK, a military policeman.

red card *n* (*soccer*) a red card held up by the referee indicating that a player is to be sent off.

red carpet *n* a strip of red carpet for dignitaries to walk on; a grand or impressive welcome or entertainment.

red cedar *n* (the reddish wood of) a North American juniper tree.

red cent *n* (*inf*) a trivial quantity of money.

Red Chamber *n* ✤ (*Cdn*) the Canadian House of Commons.

red corpuscle *n* a red blood cell.

Red Crescent *n* the Red Cross in Muslim countries.

Red Cross *n* a red cross on a white ground, the symbol of the International Red Cross, a society for the relief of suffering in time of war and disaster.

red deer *n* a large deer with a reddish brown coat.

redden /ˈrɛdən/ *vti* to make or become red; to blush.

reddish /ˈrɛdɪʃ/ *adj* tinged with red.—**reddishness** *n.*

red dwarf *n* a star with a relatively small mass and low luminosity.

redeem /rəˈdiːm/ or /ri-/ *vt* to recover by payment; to regain; to deliver from sin; to pay off; to restore to favour; to make amends for.—**redeemable** *adj.*—**redeemer** *n.*

redemption /rəˈdempʃən/ or /ri-/ *n* the act of redeeming or the state of being redeemed; recovery; repurchase; salvation.

redeploy /ˌriːdɪˈplɔɪ/ *vt* (*troops, workers*) to assign to new positions or activities.—**redeployment** *n.*

redeye /ˈrɛdaɪ/ *n* (*sl*) cheap whiskey; ✤ Calgary redeye.

red flag *n* a symbol of communism or revolution; a sign of danger.

red fox *n* the common European fox with reddish fur.

red giant *n* a giant star with a relatively low surface temperature that emits a red glow.

red-handed *adj* caught in the act of committing a crime.

redhead /ˈrɛdhɛd/ *n* a person having red hair.—**redheaded** *adj.*

red herring *n* a herring cured to a dark brown colour; something that diverts attention from the real issue.

red-hot *adj* glowing with heat; extremely hot; very excited, angry, etc; very new.

redirect /ˌriːdɪˈrɛkt/ or /-daɪˈrɛkt/ *vt* to change the direction or course of; to readdress.—**redirection** *n.*

red lead *n* a poisonous red oxide of lead used as a pigment.

red-letter *adj* of special significance.

red light *n* a warning signal, a cautionary sign; a deterrent.

red-light *adj* (*of a district*) containing brothels.

red mullet *n* a food fish of European waters, a goatfish.

redneck /ˈrɛdnɛk/ *n* (*derog*) a poor white farm labourer in the US South. • *adj* racist, reactionary.

redo /riːˈduː/ *vt* (**redoing, redid**, *pp* **redone**) to do again; to redecorate.

red ochre *n* any of several types of reddish earth used as pigments.

redolent /ˈrɛdələnt/ *adj* having a strong scent, fragrant; reminiscent (of).—**redolence** *n.*

redouble /riːˈdʌbəl/ *vti* to do ble again; to make or become twice as much.

redoubt /rɪˈdaʊt/ *n* a detached outpost of a fortification.

redoubtable /rɪˈdaʊtəbəl/ *adj* formidable.

redound /rəˈdaʊnd/ or /ri-/ *vi* to have a directly positive or negative effect (on); to rebound (on or upon).

red pepper *n* a variety of pepper grown for its spicy red fruit, capsicum; its fruit; the fruit of the sweet pepper when ripe and red; cayenne pepper.

red pine *n* ✤ a pine with reddish wood, *esp* of northeast North America.

redress /rəˈdrɛs/ or /ri-/ *vt* to put right, adjust; to compensate, make up for. • *n* remedy; compensation.

red salmon *n* any salmon with pinkish flesh, *esp* the sockeye.

redshank /ˈrɛdʃæŋk/ *n* a type of large European sandpiper.

red squirrel *n* a squirrel with reddish-brown fur of Europe, North America and Asia.

red tape *n* rigid adherence to bureaucratic routine and regulations, causing delay.

reduce /rəˈduːs/ or /ri-/, /-ˈdjuːs/ *vt* to diminish or make smaller in size, amount, extent, or number; to lower in price; to simplify; to make thin; to subdue; to bring or convert (to another state or form).—**reducible** *adj.*

reductio ad absurdum /rɪˌdʌktioːædæbˈzərdəm/ *n* a proof of the falsity of a proposition by demonstrating the absurdity of its logical consequences.

reduction /rəˈdʌkʃən/ or /ri-/ *n* the act or process of reducing or being reduced; something reduced; the amount by which a thing is reduced; (*math*) the conversion of a fraction into decimal form.—**reductional** *adj.*—**reductive** *adj.*

redundant /rɪˈdʌndənt/ or /ri-/ adj surplus to requirements; (Brit person) deprived of one's job as being no longer necessary; excessive, wordy; (words) unnecessary to the meaning.—**redundancy** n.

reduplicate /rəˈduːplɪˌkeɪt/ or /ri-/, /-ˈdjuː-/ vt to make double, to repeat; (gram) to repeat (syllable or letter), to form (word) thus. • adj doubled, repeated.—**reduplication** n.—**reduplicative** adj.

red wine n wine made from black grapes with the skins left on.

redwood /ˈrɛdwʊd/ n an important timber tree of California that can reach a height of 360 feet; any of various trees yielding a red dye or reddish wood.

reed /riːd/ n a tall grass found in marshes; a thin piece of cane in the mouthpiece of a musical instrument; a person or thing too weak to rely on; one easily swayed or overcome.

reedbird /ˈriːdbərd/ see **bobolink**.

re-educate, reeducate /ˌriːeˈdʒʊkeɪt/ or /-ˈdʒuː-/ vt to educate again in order to adapt to changing circumstances.—**re-education, reeducation** n.

reedy /ˈriːdi/ adj (**reedier, reediest**) filled with reeds; resembling a reed; shrill, piping, as in the sound of a reed.—**reedily** adv.—**reediness** n.

reef /riːf/ n a ridge of rocks, sand, or coral at or just below the surface of water; a hazardous obstruction; a lode or vein of ore.

reefer /ˈriːfər/ n a thick double-breasted jacket, formerly worn by sailors; (inf) a cigarette containing cannabis.

reef knot n a symmetrical double knot.

reek /riːk/ n a strong smell. • vi to give off smoke, fumes or a strong or offensive smell.

reel[1] /riːl/ n a winding device; a spool or bobbin; thread wound on this; a length of film, about 300m (1,000ft). • vt to wind on to a reel; (with **in**) to draw in by means of a reel; (with **off**) to tell, write, etc with fluency; (with **out**) to unwind from a reel.

reel[2] vi to stagger or sway about; to be dizzy or in a whirl. • n a staggering motion.

reel[3] n a lively Scottish or Irish dance; the music for it. • vi to dance a reel.

re-enter /riːˈɛntər/ vti to enter again.

re-entry /riːˈɛntri/ n (pl **re-entries**) the act of entering or possessing again; the return of a spacecraft to the earth's atmosphere.

reeve /riːv/ n ✤ (Cdn) an elected leader of a town or municipal council.—**reeveship** n.

ref /rɛf/ n (inf) a referee.

ref. abbr = with reference to.

refectory /rəˈfɛktəri/ or /ri-/ n (pl **refectories**) the dining hall of a monastery, college, etc.

refer /rɪˈfər/ vti (**referring, referred**) to attribute, assign (to); (with **to**) to direct, have recourse (to); to relate to; to mention or allude to; to direct attention (to).—**referable** adj.

referee /ˌrɛfəˈriː/ n an adjudicator, arbitrator; an umpire; a judge.

reference /ˈrɛfərəns/ n the act of referring; a mention or allusion; a testimonial; a person who gives a testimonial; a direction to a passage in a book; a passage in a book referred to.

reference book n a book for reference rather than general reading, eg a yearbook, directory.

reference library n a library whose books may be consulted but not borrowed.

referendum /ˌrɛfəˈrɛndəm/ n (pl **referendums, referenda**) the submission of an issue directly to the vote of the electorate, a plebiscite.

referral /rəˈfɜːrəl/ or /ri-/ n the act of referring or instance of being referred.

refill /riːˈfɪl/ vt to fill again. • n a replacement pack for an empty permanent container; a providing again.

refine /rəˈfaɪn/ or /ri-/ vti to purify; to make free from impurities or coarseness; to make or become cultured.

refined /riˈfaɪnd/ adj polished, cultured; affected.

refinement /rəˈfaɪnmənt/ or /ri-/ n fineness of manners or taste; an improvement; a fine distinction.

refinery /rəˈfaɪnəri/ or /ri-/ n (pl **refineries**) a plant where raw materials, eg sugar, oil, are refined.

refit /riːˈfɪt/ vti (**refitting, refitted**) to make or become functional again by repairing, re-equipping, etc.—also n.

reflation /riːˈfleɪʃən/ n the restoration of deflated prices to a desirable level.—**reflationary** adj.

reflect /rəˈflɛkt/ or /ri-/ vt (light, heat, etc) to throw back; to bend aside or back; to show an image of, as a mirror; to express. • vi to reproduce to the eye or mind; to mirror; to meditate; (with **upon**) to ponder; (with **on**) to discredit, disparage.

reflected /-əd/ adj thrown or cast back; mirrored; bent or folded back.

reflecting telescope n a telescope operated by a series of mirrors.

reflection /rəˈflɛkʃən/ or /ri-/ n a reflecting back, turning aside; the action of changing direction when a ray strikes and is thrown back; reflected heat, light or colour; a reflected image; meditation, thought; reconsideration; reproach.—also **reflexion**.

reflective /rəˈflɛktɪv/ or /ri-/ adj meditative; concerned with ideas.—**reflectively** adv.—**reflectiveness** n.

reflector /rəˈflɛktər/ or /ri-/ n a disc, instrument, strip or other surface that reflects light or heat.

reflex /ˈriːflɛks/ n an involuntary response to a stimulus. • adj (angle) of more than 180 degrees; (camera) with a full-size viewfinder using the main lens.

reflex camera n a camera in which the image from the lens is conveyed by an angled mirror to a viewfinder for composition and focusing.

reflexion see **reflection**.

reflexive /rəˈflɛksɪv/ or /ri-/ adj (pron, verb) referring back to the subject.—**reflexively** adv.

reflexology /ˌriːflɛkˈsɒlədʒi/ n (alternative medicine) a technique of applying pressure to specific points on the hands and feet to stimulate the blood supply to other areas of the body and help relieve stress.—**reflexologist** n.

reform /rəˈfɔːrm/ or /ri-/ vti to improve; to make or become better by the removal of faults; to amend; to abolish abuse. • n improvement or transformation, esp of an institution; removal of social ills.—**reformed** adj.

re-form /riːˈfɔːrm/ vti to form again.

reformation /ˌrɛfərˈmeɪʃən/ n the act of reforming or the state of being reformed; improvement; (with cap) the 16th-century religious revolt that resulted in the formation of Protestant churches.

reformatory /ˌrəˈfɔːrmətəri/ or /ri-/ adj reforming. • n (pl **reformatories**) an institution for reforming young criminals; a prison for women.

reformer /rɪˈfɔːrmər/ n a person who advocates or works for reform; an apparatus for changing the molecular structure of a hydrocarbon to form specialized products.

reform school n a reformatory for young people.

refract /rəˈfrækt/ or /ri-/ vt to cause (a ray of light, etc) to undergo refraction.

refracting telescope n a type of telescope in which the image is formed by a series of lenses.

refraction /rəˈfrækʃən/ or /ri-/ n the bending of a ray or wave of light, heat, or sound as it passes from one medium into another.

refractory /rəˈfræktəri/ or /ri-/ adj obstinate; (disease, etc) resistant to treatment; (muscle) unresponsive to stimuli; able to withstand high temperatures. • n (pl **refractories**) a heat-resistant material.

refrain[1] /rəˈfreɪn/ vi to abstain (from).

refrain[2] n recurring words in a song or poem, esp at the end of a stanza; a chorus.

refrangible /rəˈfrændʒəbəl/ or /ri-/ adj able to be refracted.

refresh /rəˈfrɛʃ/ or /ri-/ vt to revive; to give new energy to; to make cool; to take a drink.

refresher /-ər/ n something that refreshes, esp a drink; a reminder; a training course to renew one's skill or knowledge.

refresher course n a course designed to keep professionals informed of recent developments in their field of knowledge or expertise.

refreshing /-ɪŋ/ adj invigorating, reviving; pleasing because unsophisticated.

refreshment /rɪˈfrɛʃmənt/ n the act of refreshing; a restorative; (pl) food and drink; a light meal.

refrigerate /rəˈfrɪdʒəˌreɪt/ or /ri-/ vti to make, become, or keep, cold; to preserve by keeping cold.—**refrigeration** n.

refrigerator /-ər/ n something that refrigerates; a chamber for keeping food, etc, cool; an apparatus for cooling.—also **fridge, icebox**.

refuel /riːˈfjuːəl/ vti (**refuelling, refuelled** or **refueling, refueled**) to supply with or take on fresh fuel.

refuge /rɛˈfjuːdʒ/ n a protection or shelter from danger; a retreat, sanctuary.

refugee /ˌrəfjuːˈdʒiː/ n a person who flees to another country to escape political or religious persecution.

refund /rə'fɛnd/ or /ri-/ *vti* to repay; to reimburse. • *n* a refunding or the amount refunded.

refurbish /ri'fɜrbɪʃ/ *vt* to renovate or re-equip.—**refurbishment** *n*.

refusal /rə'fju:zəl/ or /ri-/ *n* the act or process of refusing; the choice of refusing or accepting.

refuse¹ /'rɛfju:s/ *n* garbage, waste, rubbish.

refuse² *vt* to decline, reject; to withhold, deny. • *vi* (*horse*) to decline to jump.

refute /rə'fju:t/ or /ri-/ *vt* to rebut; to disprove.—**refutable** *adj*.—**refutably** *adv*.—**refutation** *n*.

regain /rə'geɪn/ or /ri-/ *vt* to get back, recover; to reach again.

regal /'ri:gəl/ *adj* royal; relating to a king or queen.

regale /rə'geɪl/ or /ri-/ *vt* to entertain, as with a feast; to delight.

regalia /rə'geɪliə/ or /-'geɪljə/ *npl* royal insignia or prerogatives; the insignia of an order, office, or membership; finery.

regard /rə'gɑrd/ or /ri-/ *vt* to gaze at, observe; to hold in respect; to consider; to heed, take into account. • *n* a look; attention; reference; respect, esteem; (*pl*) good wishes, greetings.

regarding /-ɪŋ/ *prep* with reference to, about.

regardless /-ləs/ *adj* having no regard to. • *adv* (*inf*) in spite of everything; without heeding the cost, consequences, etc.

regatta /rə'gætə/ or /ri-/ *n* a meeting for yacht or boat races.

regency /'ri:dʒənsi/ *n* (*pl* **regencies**) the status or authority of a regent; a regent's period of office; a body entrusted with the duties of a regent; rule; (*with cap*) in British history, the period 1810-20.

regenerate /ri'dʒɛnəreɪt/ *vti* to renew, give new life to; to be reborn spiritually; to reorganize; to produce anew.—**regeneration** *n*.

regent /'ri:dʒənt/ *n* a person who rules or administers a country during the sovereign's minority, absence, or incapacity; a member of a governing board (as of a university).

reggae /'reɡeɪ/ *n* a strongly accented West Indian musical form with four beats to the bar.

regicide /'redʒɪsaɪd/ *n* the killer or the killing or a king.

regime, régime /reɪ'ʒi:m/ *n* a political or ruling system.

regimen /'redʒɪmen/ *n* a system of diet, exercise, etc, for improving the health; a regular course of training.

regiment /'redʒɪmənt/ *n* a military unit, smaller than a division, consisting *usu* of a number of battalions. • *vt* to organize in a strict manner; to subject to order or conformity.—**regimental** *adj*.

regimentation /,redʒɪmən'teɪʃən/ *n* the act of regimenting; excessive orderliness.

Regina /rə'dʒaɪnə/ or /re'dʒi:nə/ *n* a reigning queen.

region /'ri:dʒən/ *n* a large, indefinite part of the earth's surface; one of the zones into which the atmosphere is divided; an administrative area of a country; a part of the body.—**regional** *adj*.

register /'redʒɪstər/ *n* an official list; a written record, as for attendance; the book containing such a record or list; a tone of voice; a variety of language appropriate to a subject or occasion; (*comput*) a device in which data can be stored and operated on; (*print*) exact alignment; a device for indicating speed, etc; a plate regulating draught. • *vti* to record; to enter in or sign a register; to correspond exactly; to entrust a letter to the post with special precautions for safety; to express emotion facially; to make or convey an impression.

registered /-stərd/ *adj* recorded officially; qualified formally or officially.

registrar /'redʒɪs,trɑr/ *n* a person who keeps records, *esp* one in an educational institution in charge of student records; a hospital doctor below a specialist in rank.

registration /,redʒɪ'streɪʃən/ *n* the act of registering; the condition of having registered.

registry /'redʒɪstri/ *n* (*pl* **registries**) registration; a place where records are kept; an official record book.

regius professor *n* in UK, a person appointed to a university chair founded by the Crown.

regnal /'regnəl/ *adj* pertaining to a sovereign or reign, *esp* designating a year of a reign calculated from the date of accession.

regress /rə'gres/ or /ri-/ *vi* to move backwards; to revert to a former condition.—**regressive** *adj*.—**regressively** *adv*.

regression /rə'greʃən/ or /ri-/ *n* the act of regressing; a relapse, reversion; a return to an earlier time or stage; (*psychoanal*) a retreat of the personality.

regret /rə'gret/ or /ri-/ *vt* (**regretting, regretted**) to feel sorrow, grief, or loss; to remember with longing; (*with* **that**) to repent of. • *n* disappointment; sorrow; grief; (*pl*) polite refusal.—**regretful** *adj*.—**regretfully** *adv*.

regrettable /-əbəl/ *adj* to be regretted; deserving reproof.—**regrettably** *adv*.

regroup /ri'gru:p/ *vti* to group again; (*mil*) to reorganize (troops, etc) following action.

regular /'reɡjulər/ *adj* normal; habitual, not casual; at fixed intervals; according to rule, custom, or the accepted practice; uniform, consistent; symmetrical; fully qualified; belonging to a standing army; (*inf*) thorough, complete; (*inf*) pleasant, friendly. • *n* a professional soldier; (*inf*) a person who attends regularly.—**regularity** *n*.—**regularly** *adv*.

regular army *n* a permanent army; (*with caps*) the United States army.

regularize /-,raɪz/ *vt* to make regular or correct.—**regularization** *n*.

regulate /'reɡjuleɪt/ *vt* to control according to a rule; to cause to conform to a standard or needs; to adjust so as to put in good order.—**regulatory** *adj*.

regulation /,reɡju'leɪʃən/ *n* the act of regulating or state of being regulated; a prescribed rule, ordinance. • *adj* normal, standard.

regulator /'reɡjuleɪtər/ *n* one who or that which regulates; a regulating device; a lever in a watch that adjusts its speed.

regurgitate /ri'gɜrdʒɪ,teɪt/ *vti* to pour back, cast up again, *esp* from the stomach to the mouth.—**regurgitation** *n*.

rehabilitate /,ri:hə'bɪlɪteɪt/ *vt* (*prisoner etc*) to help adapt to society after a stay in an institution; to put back in good condition; to restore to rights or privileges; (*sick person etc*) to help to adjust to normal conditions after illness.—**rehabilitation** *n*.

rehash /'ri:hæʃ/ *n* old materials put in a new form. • *vt* to dish up again.

rehearse /rɪ'hɜrs/ *vti* to practise repeatedly before public performance; to recount, narrate in detail.—**rehearsal** *n*.

rehoboam /,ri:hə'boːm/ *n* a wine bottle that holds six times the amount of a standard bottle.

reify /'ri:faɪ/ *vt* (**reifying, reified**) to make (something abstract) real or concrete.

reign /reɪn/ *n* the rule of a sovereign; the period of this; influence; domination. • *vi* to rule; to prevail.

reimburse /,ri:m'bɜrs/ *vt* to repay; to refund (for expense or loss).—**reimbursable** *adj*—**reimbursement** *n*.

rein /reɪn/ *n* the strap of a bridle for guiding or restraining a horse; (*pl*) a means of control or restraint. • *vt* to control with the rein; to restrain.

reincarnation /,ri:ɪnkɑr'neɪʃən/ *n* the incarnation of the soul after death in another body.—**reincarnate** *adj, vt*.

reindeer /'reɪndɪr/ *n* a large deer with branched antlers found in northern regions.

reindeer moss *n* a lichen of northern regions that provides food for reindeer.

reinforce /ri:n'fɔrs/ *vt* (*army etc*) to strengthen with fresh troops; (*a material*) to add to the strength of.

reinforced concrete *n* concrete with metal bars, wire, etc inserted in it for strength.

reinforcement /,ri:n'fɔrsmənt/ *n* the act of reinforcing; additional support; (*pl*) additional troops.

reinstate /,ri:ɪn'steɪt/ *vt* to restore to a former position, rank, or condition.—**reinstatement** *n*.

reinterpret /,ri:ɪntər'prət/ *vt* to interpret again; to give a new explanation of.—**reinterpretation** *n*.

reissue /ri'ɪʃu:/ *vt* to issue again; to republish. • *n* a new issue; a reprint.

reiterate /ri:'ɪtəreɪt/ *vt* to repeat; to say or do again or many times.—**reiteration** *n*.

reject /rə'dʒekt/ or /ri-/ *vt* to throw away, to discard; to refuse to accept, to decline; to rebuff. • *n* a thing or person rejected.—**rejection** *n*.

rejoice /rə'dʒɔɪs/ or /ri-/ *vi* to feel joyful or happy.

rejoin /ri'dʒɔɪn/ or /'ri:-/ *vt* to join again; to return to.

rejoinder /rə'dʒɔɪndər/ or /ri-/ *n* a retort, a reply.

rejuvenate /rɪ'dʒu:və,neɪt/ or /ri-/ *vt* to give youthful vigour to.—**rejuvenation** *n*.

relapse /rɪ'læps/ *vi* to fall back into a worse state after improvement; to return to a former vice, to backslide. • *n* the recurrence of illness after apparent recovery.

relate /rə'leɪt/ or /ri-/ *vt* to narrate, recount; to show a connection (between two or more things). • *vi* to have a formal relationship (with).

related /-əd/ *adj* connected, allied; akin.

relation /rə'leɪʃən/ or /ri-/ n the way in which one thing stands in respect to another, footing; reference, regard; connection by blood or marriage; a relative; a narration, a narrative; (pl) the connections between or among persons, nations, etc; (pl) one's family and in-laws.

relationship /rɪ'leɪʃənʃɪp/ n the tie or degree of kinship or intimacy; affinity; (inf) an affair.

relative /'relətɪv/ adj having or expressing a relation; corresponding; pertinent; comparative, conditional; respective; meaningful only in relationship; (gram) referring to an antecedent. • n a person related by blood or marriage.—**relatively** adv.

relative molecular mass n the total of the atomic weights of all the atoms present in a molecule; the average mass per molecule of any substance relative to one-twelfth the mass of an atom of carbon-12.—also **molecular weight**.

relative pronoun n a pronoun that is used to connect a dependent clause to a main clause and that refers to a noun in the main clause.

relativity /ˌrelə'tɪvɪti/ n the state of being relative; the relation between one thing and another; (physics) the theory of the relative, rather than absolute, character of motion, velocity, mass, etc, and the interdependence of time, matter, and space.

relax /rə'læks/ or /ri-/ vti to slacken; to make or become less severe or strict; to make (the muscles) less rigid; to take a rest.

relaxant /-ənt/ n a drug that relieves muscular tension.

relaxation /ˌriːlæk'seɪʃən/ n the act of relaxing; the condition of being relaxed; recreation.

relay /'riːleɪ/ n a team of fresh horses, men, etc to relieve others; a race between teams, each member of which goes a part of the distance; (elect) a device for enabling a weak current to control others; a relayed broadcast. • vt (**relaying, relayed**) (news, etc) to spread in stages; to broadcast signals.

relay race n a race between teams in which each member does part of the distance.

release /rɪ'liːs/ vt to set free; to let go; to relinquish; (film, etc) to issue for public exhibition; (information) to make available; (law) to make over to another. • n a releasing, as from prison, work, etc; a device to hold or release a mechanism; a news item, etc, released to the public; (law) a written surrender of a claim.

relegate /'relə,geɪt/ vt to move to an inferior position; to demote; to banish.—**relegation** n.

relent /rə'lent/ or /ri-/ vi to soften in attitude; to become less harsh or severe.

relentless /-ləs/ adj pitiless; unremitting.

relevant /'reləvənt/ adj applying to the matter in hand, pertinent; to the point.—**relevance, relevancy** n.

reliable /rə'laɪəbəl/ or /ri-/ adj dependable, trustworthy.—**reliability** n.—**reliably** adv.

reliance /rə'laɪəns/ or /ri-/ n trust; dependence; a thing relied on.—**reliant** adj.

relic /'relɪk/ n an object, fragment, or custom that has survived from the past; part of a saint's body or belongings; (pl) remains of the dead.

relief /rə'liːf/ or /ri-/ n the sensation following the easing or lifting of discomfort or stress; release from a duty by another person; a person who takes the place of another on duty; that which relieves; aid; assistance to the needy or victims of a disaster; the projection of a carved design from its ground; distinctness, vividness. • adj providing relief in disasters etc.

relief map n a map in which topographic relief is represented by shading, colours, etc.

relieve /rə'liːv/ or /ri-/ vt to bring relief or assistance to; to release from obligation or duty; to ease; (with **oneself**) to empty the bladder or bowels. • vi to give relief; to break the monotony of; to bring into relief, to stand out.

relieved /rə'liːvd/ or /ri-/ adj having or showing relief, esp from anxiety or repressed emotions.

religion /rɪ'lɪdʒən/ n a belief in God or gods; a system of worship and faith; a formalized expression of belief.

religiosity /rɪ,lɪdʒɪ'ɒsɪti/ n the condition of being religious, esp excessively or sentimentally so.—**religiose** adj.

religious /rɪ'lɪdʒəs/ or /ri-/ adj of or conforming to religion; devout, pious; scrupulously and conscientiously faithful.—**religiously** adv.

relinquish /rə'lɪŋkwɪʃ/ or /ri-/ vt to give up; to renounce or surrender.—**relinquishment** n.

reliquary /'relɪkwəri/ n (pl **reliquaries**) a container or shrine for sacred relics.

relish /'relɪʃ/ n an appetizing flavour; a distinctive taste; enjoyment of food or an experience; a spicy accompaniment to food; gusto, zest. • vt to like the flavour of; to enjoy, appreciate.

relocate /'riːlo:,keɪt/ or /,riːlo:'keɪt/, /riːlo:keɪt/ vti to set up in a new place; to place (an employee) in a different job; (business) to move to a new location.—**relocation** n.

reluctant /rə'lʌktənt/ or /ri-/ adj unwilling, loath; offering resistance.—**reluctance** n.—**reluctantly** adv.

rely /rə'laɪ/ or /ri-/ vi (**relying, relied**) to depend on; to trust.

REM /rem/ abbr = rapid eye movement.

remain /rə'meɪn/ or /ri-/ vi to stay behind or in the same place; to continue to be; to survive, to last; to be left over. • npl anything left after use; a corpse.

remainder /-dər/ n what is left, the rest; (math) the result of subtraction; the quantity left over after division; unsold stock, esp of books; (law) the residual interest in an estate.

remake /ri'meɪk/ or /'riːmeɪk/ vt (**remaking, remade**) to make again. • n a new version of an old film.

remand /rə'mænd/ vt to send back into custody for further evidence.—also n.

remark /rə'mɑːrk/ or /ri-/ vti to notice; to observe; to pass a comment (upon). • n a brief comment.

remarkable /-əbəl/ adj unusual; extraordinary; worthy of comment.—**remarkably** adv.

remaster /ri:'mæstər/ vt to make a new (digital) master recording from an original (analogue) recording to provide improved sound quality on vinyl records or compact discs.

remedial /ri'miːdɪəl/ adj providing a remedy; corrective; relating to the teaching of people with learning difficulties.

remedy /'remɪdi/ n a medicine or any means to cure a disease; anything that puts something else to rights. • vt (**remedying, remedied**) to cure; to put right.

remember /rə'membər/ or /ri-/ vti to recall; to bear in mind; to mention (a person) to another as sending regards; to exercise or have the power of memory.

remembrance /rə'membrəns/ or /ri-/ n a reminiscence; a greeting or gift recalling or expressing friendship or affection; the extent of memory; an honouring of the dead or a past event.

Remembrance Day n in Canada, a day, November 11, on which the dead of the two World Wars are commemorated.

Remembrance Sunday n in UK, the Sunday nearest November 11, on which the dead of the two World Wars are commemorated.

remind /rə'maɪnd/ or /ri-/ vt to cause to remember.

reminder /-ər/ n a thing that reminds, esp a letter from a creditor.

reminisce /,remɪ'nɪs/ vi to think, talk, or write about past events.

reminiscence /-əns/ n the recalling of a past experience; (pl) memoirs.

reminiscent /-ənt/ adj reminding, suggestive (of); recalling the past.

remiss /rə'mɪs/ or /ri-/ adj negligent, slack.

remission /rə'mɪʃən/ or /ri-/ n the act of remitting; the reduction in length of a prison term; the lessening of the symptoms of a disease; pardon, forgiveness.

remit /rə'mɪt/ or /ri-/ vti (**remitting, remitted**) to forgive; to refrain from inflicting (a punishment) or exacting (a debt); to abate, moderate; to send payment (by post); (law) to refer to a lower court for reconsideration. • n the act of referring; an area of authority.

remittance /rə'mɪtəns/ or /ri-/ n the sending of money or a payment (by post); the payment or money sent.

remix /'riːmɪks/ or /ri'mɪks/ vt to adjust the balance and separation of a recording.—also n.

remnant /'remnənt/ n a small remaining fragment or number; an oddment or scrap; a trace; an unsold or unused end of piece goods.

remodel /ri:'mɒdəl/ vt (**remodelling, remodelled** or **remodeling, remodeled**) to fashion afresh; to recast.

remonstrate /'remən,streɪt/ vi to protest, to make a complaint (against).—**remonstrance** n.

remorse /rə'mɔːrs/ n regret and guilt for a misdemeanour; compassion.—**remorseful** adj.—**remorsefully** adv.

remorseless /-ləs/ adj ruthless, cruel; relentless.—**remorselessly** adv.—**remorselessness** n.

remote /rə'mo:t/ adj far apart or distant in time or place; out of the way; not closely related; secluded; aloof; vague, faint.—**remotely** adv.

remote control *n* the control of a device or activity from a distance, *usu* by means of an electric circuit or the making or breaking of radio waves.

removal /rɪ'muːvəl/ *n* the act of removing; a change of home or office; dismissal.

remove /rɪ'muːv/ or /rə-/ *vti* to take away and put elsewhere; to dismiss, as from office; to get rid of; to kill; to go away. • *n* a stage in gradation; a degree in relationship.—**removable** *adj.*

removed /rɪ'muːvd/ or /rə-/ *adj* remote; separated by a specified degree, as of relationship; of a younger or older relationship.

remunerate /rɪ'mjuːnə,reɪt/ *vt* to pay for a service; to reward.—**remuneration** *n.*

renaissance /'renə,sɒns/ or /rə'neɪ-/, *Fr.* /ʀɛnɛˈsɔ̃s,/ *n* a rebirth or revival; (*with cap*) the revival of European art and literature under the influence of classical study during the 14th-16th centuries.—*also adj.*

renal /'riːnəl/ *adj* relating to or near the kidneys.

renascent /rɪ'neɪsənt/ or /rɪ'næsənt/ *adj* becoming active again, reviving.

rend /rend/ *vti* (**rending, rent**) to tear, to wrench (apart); to be torn apart.

render /'rendər/ *vt* (*payments, accounts, etc*) to submit, as for approval; to give back; to pay back; to perform; to represent as by drawing; to translate, interpret; to cause to be; (*fat*) to melt down.

rendering /-ɪŋ/ *n* interpretation, translation.

rendezvous /'rɒndeɪ,vuː/ *n* (*pl* **rendezvous**) an arranged meeting; a place to meet; a popular haunt; the process of bringing two spacecraft together. • *vi* to meet by appointment.

rendition /ren'dɪʃən/ *n* an interpretation; performance.

renegade /'renə,geɪd/ *n* a deserter; a person who is faithless to a principle, party, religion, or cause.

renege /rə'neg/ or /rɪ-/, /-'neɪg/ *vti* to go back on, or fail to keep, a promise or agreement.

renegotiate /,riːnɪ'goʊʃɪ,eɪt/ *vti* to negotiate again, *esp* to improve the terms of a contract.—**renegotiable** *adj.*—**renegotiation** *n.*

renew /rɪ'nuː/ or /-'njuː/ *vti* to restore to freshness or vigour; to begin again; to make or get anew; to replace; to grant or obtain an extension of.—**renewable** *adj.*—**renewal** *n.*

rennet /'renət/ *n* an extract from the stomach of calves, etc, used to curdle milk.

reno /'renoʊ/ *n* ♣ (*Cdn*) (*inf*) a renovated house; renovation.

renounce /rə'naʊns/ or /rɪ-/ *vt* to abandon formally; to give up; to disown.

renovate /'renə,veɪt/ *vt* to renew; to restore to good condition; to do up, repair.—**renovation** *n.*—**renovator** *n.*

renown /rɪ'naʊn/ or /rə-/ *n* fame, celebrity.

renowned /rɪ'naʊnd/ or /rə-/ *adj* famous, illustrious.

rent[1] /rent/ *see* **rend**.

rent[2] *n* regular payment to another for the use of a house, machinery, etc. • *vti* to occupy as a tenant; to hire; to let for rent.

rental /rentəl/ *n* an amount paid or received as rent; a house, car, etc, for rent; an act of renting; a business that rents something.

rent boy *n* a young male prostitute.

renunciation /rə,nʌnsɪ'eɪʃən/ *n* the act of renouncing; formal abandonment; repudiation.

re-offer /riː'ɒfər/ *n* ♣ (*Cdn*) be a candidate for re-election.

reopen /riː'oʊpən/ *vti* to open again; to resume.

reorganize /riː'ɔːrgə,naɪz/ *vti* to organize again; to bring about a reorganization.—**reorganization** *n.*

Rep. *abbr* = Representative; Republic; Republican.

rep /rep/ *abbr* = repeat; report; reporter.

repair /rɪ'peər/ or /rə-/ *vt* to mend; to restore to good working order; to make amends for. • *n* the act of repairing; a place repaired; condition as to soundness.

reparable /rɪ'perəbəl/ or /rə-/ *adj* capable of being repaired.

reparation /,repə'reɪʃən/ *n* amends; (*pl*) compensation, as for war damage.

repartee /,repɑː'teɪ/ or /-'tiː/ *n* a witty reply; skill in making such replies.

repast /rɪ'pæst/ *n* a meal.

repatriate /riː'peɪtrɪ,eɪt/ *vt* to send back or restore to one's country of origin or citizenship.—**repatriation** *n.*

repay /rɪ'peɪ/ *vt* (**repaying, repaid**) to pay back; to refund.—**repayable** *adj.*—**repayment** *n.*

repeal /rɪ'piːl/ *vt* to annul, to rescind; to revoke.—*also n.*

repeat /rɪ'piːt/ *vti* to say, write, or do again; to reiterate; to recite after another or from memory; to reproduce; to recur. • *n* a

repetition, encore; anything said or done again, as a re-broadcast of a television programme; (*mus*) a passage to be repeated; the sign for this.—**repeatable** *adj.*

repeated /rɪ'piːtəd/ *adj* frequent; done, seen, etc, again.

repeatedly /-lɪ/ *adv* many times, over and over again.

repeater /rɪ'piːtər/ *n* a clock or watch with a striking mechanism; a device for receiving and amplifying electronic communication signals; a firearm that has a repeating mechanism for reloading; a habitual violator of the laws.

repeating firearm *n* a firearm designed to load cartridges from a magazine.

repel /rə'pel/ *vt* (**repelling, repelled**) to drive back; to beat off, repulse; to reject; to hold off; to cause distaste; (*water, dirt*) to be resistant to.

repellent /rə'pelənt/ *adj* distasteful, unattractive; capable of repelling; impermeable. • *n* a substance that repels, *esp* a spray for protection against insects.

repent /rə'pent/ *vi* to wish one had not done something; to feel remorse or regret (for); to regret and change from evil ways.—**repentant** *adj.*

repentance /rə'pentəns/ *n* penitence; contrition.

repercussion /,riːpər'kʌʃən/ or /,rep/ *n* a rebound; a reverberation; a far-reaching, often indirect reaction to an event.

repertoire /'repər,twɑːr/ or /,repər'twɑːr/ *n* the stock of plays, songs, etc, that a company singer, etc, can perform.

repertory /'repərtɔːri/ or /'repətɔːri/ *n* (*pl* **repertories**) a repertoire; the system of alternating several plays through a season with a permanent acting group.

repetition /,repə'tɪʃən/ *n* the act of repeating; something repeated, a copy.—**repetitive** *adj.*

repetitious /,repə'tɪʃəs/ *adj* full of repetition; boring.—**repetitiously** *adv.*—**repetitiousness** *n.*

rephrase /riː'freɪz/ *vt* to phrase (a statement) in a different way.

replace /riː'pleɪs/ *vt* to put back; to take the place of, to substitute for; to supersede.—**replaceable** *adj.*

replacement /riː'pleɪsmənt/ *n* the act or process of replacing; a person or thing that replaces another.

replenish /rə'plenɪʃ/ *vt* to stock again, refill.—**replenishment** *n.*

replete /rə'pliːt/ *adj* filled, well provided; stuffed, gorged.

repletion /rə'pliːʃən/ *n* complete fullness; satisfaction.

replica /'replɪkə/ *n* an exact copy; a reproduction.

reply /rə'plaɪ/ or /rɪ-/ *vti* (**replying, replied**) to answer, respond; to give as an answer. • *n* an answer.

repo-man /'riːpoʊ/ *n* (*pl* **repo-men**) (*sl*) a person who repossesses (*eg* a motor car).

report /rə'pɔːrt/ or /rɪ-/ *vti* to give an account of; to tell as news; to take down and describe for publication; to make a formal statement of; to complain about or against; to inform against; to present oneself (for duty). • *n* an account of facts; the formal statement of the findings of an investigation; a newspaper, radio or television account of an event; a rumour; a sharp, loud noise, as of a gun.

reportage /'reportɪdʒ/ *n* the art of reporting on current events; an accurate, observant and well-written account of an event.

report card *n* a report on a pupil or student that is periodically given to his or her parent; an evaluation of performance.

reportedly /rə'pɔːrtədli/ *adv* as reported, not directly.

reporter /rə'pɔːrtər/ *n* a person who gathers and reports news for a newspaper, radio or television; a person authorized to make statements concerning law decisions or legislative proceedings.

repose /rɪ'poʊz/ *n* rest, sleep; stillness, peace; composure, serenity. • *vti* to lie down or lay at rest; to place (trust, etc) in someone; to rest; to lie dead.

reposition /,riːpə'zɪʃən/ *vt* to place in a different or new position.

repository /rɪ'pɒzɪtəri/ *n* (*pl* **repositories**) a receptacle; a storehouse, warehouse; a confidant.

repossess /,riːpə'zes/ *vt* to possess again; to restore possession of (property), *esp* for nonpayment of debt.—**repossession** *n.*

reprehend /repri'hend/ *vt* to rebuke, to find fault with, to criticize.

reprehensible /,repri'hensɪbəl/ *adj* blameworthy, culpable.

reprehension /,repri'henʃən/ *n* blame, censure.

re-present /,riːprə'zent/ *vt* to present again.

represent /,repri'zent/ *vt* to portray; to describe; to typify; to stand for, symbolize; to point out; to perform on the stage; to act as an agent for; to deputize for; to serve as a specimen, example, etc, of.—**representable** *adj.*

representation /ˌreprɪzenˈteɪʃən/ *n* the act of representing or being represented, as in a parliamentary assembly; a portrait, reproduction; (*pl*) a presentation of claims, protests, views, etc.

representative /ˌreprɪˈzentətɪv/ *adj* typical; portraying; consisting of or based on representation of the electorate by delegates. • *n* an example or type; a person who acts for another; a delegate, agent, salesman, etc.

repress /rɪˈpres/ *vt* to suppress, restrain; (*emotions*) to keep under control; to exclude involuntarily from the conscious mind.—**repressive** *adj*.—**represser, repressor** *n*.

repression /rɪˈpreʃən/ *n* the act of repressing; the condition of being repressed; domination, tyranny.

reprieve /rɪˈpriːv/ *vt* to postpone or commute the punishment of; to give respite to.—*also n*.

reprimand /ˈreprɪˌmænd/ *n* a formal rebuke. • *vt* to reprove formally.

reprint /rɪˈprɪnt/ *vt* to print again. • *n* a book or article that has appeared in print before.

reprisal /rɪˈpraɪzəl/ *n* an act of retaliation for an injury done.

reprise /rɪˈpraɪz/ or /-priːz/ *n* (*mus*) the repetition of an earlier theme or passage.—*also vt*.

reproach /rɪˈprəʊtʃ/ *vt* to accuse of a fault; to blame. • *n* a reproof; a source of shame or disgrace.—**reproachful** *adj*.

reprobate /ˈreprəˌbeɪt/ *n* a depraved person; a hardened sinner; a scoundrel.

reproduce /ˌriːprəˈdjuːs/ or /-proː-/, /-ˈdjuːs/ *vti* to make a copy, duplicate, or likeness of; to propagate; to produce offspring; to multiply.

reproduction /ˌriːprəˈdʌkʃən/ *n* the act of reproducing; the process by which plants and animals breed; a copy or likeness; a representation.—**reproductive** *adj*.

reprography /rɪˈprɒɡrəfɪ/ *n* the process of reproducing printed material, as by photocopying.—**reprographic** *adj*.

reproof /rɪˈpruːf/ *n* a rebuke, blame.

reprove /rɪˈpruːv/ *vt* to rebuke, censure.—**reprovingly** *adv*.

reptile /ˈreptaɪl/ *n* any of a class of cold-blooded, air-breathing vertebrates with horny scales or plates, as turtles, crocodiles, snakes, lizards, etc; a grovelling or despised person.—**reptilian** *adj*.

Repub *abbr* = Republican.

republic /rəˈpʌblɪk/ *n* a government in which the people elect the head of state, *usu* called president, and in which the people and their elected representatives have supreme power; a country governed in this way; a body of persons freely engaged in a specified activity.

republican /rəˈpʌblɪkən/ *adj* of, characteristic of, or supporting a republic. • *n* an advocate of republican government; (*with cap*) a member of the US Republican party.—**republicanism** *n*.

republish /riːˈpʌblɪʃ/ *vt* to publish again; to issue a new edition of (a book).—**republication** *n*.

repudiate /rəˈpjuːdɪeɪt/ or /rɪ-/ *vt* to reject, disown; to refuse to acknowledge or pay; to deny; (a treaty, etc) to disavow.—**repudiation** *n*.

repugnant /rəˈpʌɡnənt/ *adj* distasteful, offensive; contradictory; incompatible.—**repugnance** *n*.

repulse /rəˈpʌls/ *vt* to drive back; to repel; to reject. • *n* a rebuff, rejection; a defeat, check.

repulsion /rəˈpʌlʃən/ or /rɪ-/ *n* a feeling of disgust; aversion; (*physics*) the tendency of bodies to repel each other.

repulsive /rəˈpʌlsɪv/ *adj* disgusting; loathsome; exercising repulsion.—**repulsively** *adv*.

reputable /ˈrepjuːtəbəl/ *adj* of good repute, respectable.—**reputably** *adv*.

reputation /ˌrepjuˈteɪʃən/ *n* the estimation in which a person or thing is held; good name, honour.

repute /rəˈpjuːt/ *vt* to consider to be, to deem. • *n* reputation.

reputed /rəˈpjuːtəd/ *adj* generally reported; supposed, putative.

reputedly *adv* in common estimation; by repute.

request /-lɪ/ *n* an asking for something; a petition; a demand; the thing asked for. • *vt* to ask for earnestly.

request stop *n* a place where a bus, etc stops only if signalled to do so.—*also* **flag stop**.

requiem *n* a mass for the dead; music for this.

require /ˈrɪqwɪəm/ or /-ɪəm/ *vt* to demand; to need, call for; to order, command.

requirement /rəˈkwaɪrmənt/ *n* a need or want; an essential condition.

requisite /ˈrekwəzɪt/ *adj* needed; essential, indispensable. • *n* something required or indispensable.

requisition /ˈrekwəzɪʃən/ *n* a formal request, demand, or order, as for military supplies; the taking over of private property, etc, for military use. • *vt* to order; to take by requisition.

reredos /ˈriːrdɒs/ or /ˈriːrɪ-/ *n* a screen or partition separating the altar from the choir.

rerun /riːˈrʌn/ *vt* to run (a race, etc) again; to show a television programme, film, etc again.—*also n*.

res /res/ *n* ♣ (*Cdn*) (*inf*) a school or university residence for students.

resale /riːˈseɪl/ *n* the selling again (of something) *usu* to a new buyer; a repeat sale to a customer; a second-hand sale.

reschedule /riːˈskedʒuəl/ or /-ˈskedʒuːl/, /-ˈʃedjuːl/, /-ˈʃedʒuːl/ *vt* (*debt*) to postpone or extend repayment terms.

rescind /rəˈsɪnd/ or /rɪ-/ *vt* to annul, cancel.

rescue /ˈreskjuː/ *vt* to save (a person, thing) from captivity, danger, or harm; to free forcibly from legal custody.—*also n*.—**rescuer** *n*.

research /ˈriːsɜːtʃ/ or /rɪˈsɜːtʃ/ *n* a diligent search; a systematic and careful investigation of a particular subject; a scientific study. • *vi* to carry out an investigation; to study.—**researcher** *n*.

resemble /rəˈzembəl/ *vt* to be like, to have a similarity to.—**resemblance** *n*.

resent /rəˈzent/ or /rɪ-/ *vt* to be indignant about; to begrudge; to take badly.—**resentful** *adj*.—**resentfully** *adv*.—**resentment** *n*.

reserpine /ˈrezərpiːn/ *n* an alkaloid extracted from the roots of a rauwolfia, used to treat high blood pressure and as a sedative.

reservation /ˌrezərˈveɪʃən/ *n* the act of reserving; (*of tickets, accommodation, etc*) a holding until called for; a limitation or proviso; (*pl*) doubt, scepticism; land set aside for a special purpose.

reserve /rəˈzɜːrv/ or /rɪ-/ *vt* to hold back for future use; to retain; to have set aside; (*tickets, hotel room, etc*) to book. • *n* something put aside for future use; land set aside for wild animals; ♣ (*Cdn*) an area of land set apart for the use of a First Nations community; (*sport*) a substitute; (*mil*) a force supplementary to a regular army; a restriction or qualification; reticence of feelings; caution.

reserved /rəˈzɜːrvd/ or /rɪ-/ *adj* set apart, booked; uncommunicative, lacking cordiality.—**reservedly** *adv*.

reservist /-vɪst/ *n* a member of a military reserve force.

reservoir /ˈrezərˌvwɑːr/ or /ˈrezəˌvwɑːr/ *n* a tank or artificial lake for storing water; an extra supply or store.

reset[1] /riːˈset/ *vt* (**resetting, reset**) to set (a bone, gem, type) over again; to place in a new setting; to change the reading of.

reset[2] *vt* (**resetting, reset**) (*Scots law*) to receive (stolen goods).—*also n*.

reshape /riːˈʃeɪp/ *vti* to shape anew.

reside /rəˈzaɪd/ or /rɪ-/ *vi* to live in a place permanently; to be vested or present in.

residence /ˈrezɪdəns/ *n* the act of living in a place; the period of residing; the house where one lives permanently; the status of a legal resident; a building used as a home.

residency /ˈrezɪdənsi/ *n* (*pl* **residencies**) a *usu* official place of residence, *eg* of a governor; a period of advanced training in medicine.

resident /ˈrezɪdənt/ *adj* residing; domiciled; living at one's place of work. • *n* a permanent inhabitant; a doctor who is serving a residency.

residential /ˌrezɪˈdenʃəl/ *adj* of or relating to residence; used for private homes.

residential school *n* ♣ (*Cdn*) a boarding school for First Nations or Inuit students.

residual /reˈzɪdʒuəl/ *adj* left over; remaining as a residue.

residuary /ˈrezɪdʒuərɪ/ *adj* of or relating to the residue of an estate.

residue /ˈrezɪˌduː/ or /-ˌdjuː/ *n* a remainder; a part left over; what is left of an estate after payment of debts and legacies.

resign /rəˈzaɪn/ or /rɪ-/ *vti* to give up (employment, etc); to relinquish; to yield to; to reconcile (oneself).

resignation /ˌrezɪɡˈneɪʃən/ *n* the resigning of office, etc; the written proof of this; patient endurance.

resigned /rəˈzaɪnd/ *adj* submissive, acquiescent; accepting the inevitable.

resilience /rəˈzɪljəns/, or /rɪ-/, /-iəns/, **resiliency** /-si/ *n* the quality of being resilient; physical or mental stamina.

resilient /rəˈzɪljənt/, or /rɪ-/, /-iənt/ *adj* elastic, springing back; buoyant; (*person*) capable of carrying on after suffering hardship.

resin /ˈrezɪn/ *n* a sticky substance exuded in the sap of trees and plants and used in medicines, varnishes, etc; rosin; a similar synthetic substance used in plastics.—**resinous** *adj*.

resist /rə'zɪst/ or /ri-/ *vti* to fight against; to be proof against; to oppose or withstand.

resistance /rə'zɪstəns/ or /ri-/ *n* the act of resisting; the power to resist, as to ward off disease; opposition, *esp* to an occupying force; hindrance; (*elect*) non-conductivity, opposition to a steady current.

resistant /rə'zɪstənt/ or /ri-/ *adj* capable of resisting; (*with* **to**) immune to.

resistor /rə'zɪstər/ or /ri-/ *n* an electrical device that resists current in a circuit.

resolute /'rezə,lu:t/ *adj* determined; firm of purpose, steadfast.—**resolutely** *adv*.—**resoluteness** *n*.

resolution /,rezə'lu:ʃən/ *n* the act of resolving or the state of being resolved; determination; a fixed intention; the formal decision or opinion of a meeting; analysis, disintegration; (*med*) the dispersion of a tumour, etc; the picture definition in a TV; (*mus*) the relieving of a discord by a following concord; (*physics*) the process or capability of making distinguishable closely adjacent optical images or sources of light.

resolve /rə'zɒlv/ *vt* to break into component parts, dissolve; to convert or be converted (into); to analyse; to determine, make up one's mind; to solve, settle; to vote by resolution; to dispel (doubt); to explain; to conclude; (*med: tumour*) to disperse; (*mus: discord*) to convert into concord. • *n* a fixed intention; resolution; courage.

resolving power *n* the ability of a microscope or telescope to produce distinct images of objects in close proximity.

resonance /'rezənəns/ *n* resounding quality; vibration.

resonant /'rezənənt/ *adj* ringing; resounding, echoing.

resonator /,rezə'neɪtər/ *n* a device that produces or increases sound by resonance.

resort /rə'zɔrt/ or /ri-/ *n* a popular holiday location; a source of help, support, etc; recourse. • *vi* to have recourse to; to turn (to) for help, etc.

resound /rə'zaund/ or /ri-/ *vti* to echo; to reverberate; to go on sounding; to be much talked of; to spread (fame).

resounding /-ɪŋ/ *adj* echoing; notable; thorough.

resource /ri:'zɔrs/ or /rɪ-/, /-sɔrs/ *n* source of help; an expedient; the ability to cope with a situation; a means of diversion; (*pl*) wealth; assets; raw materials.

resourceful /-fʊl/ *adj* able to cope in difficult situations; ingenious.—**resourcefulness** *n*.

respect /rə'spekt/ or /ri-/ *n* esteem; consideration; regard; (*pl*) good wishes; reference; relation. • *vt* to feel or show esteem or regard to; to treat considerately.

respectable /rə'spektəbəl/ or /ri-/ *adj* worthy of esteem; well-behaved; proper, correct, well-conducted; of moderate quality or size.—**respectability** *n*.—**respectably** *adv*.

respectful /-fʊl/ *adj* deferential.—**respectfully** *adv*.

respecting /-ɪŋ/ *prep* concerning.

respective /-tɪŋ/ *adj* proper to each, several.

respectively /-tɪvli/ *adv* in the indicated order.

respiration /,respə'reɪʃən/ *n* the act or process of breathing.

respirator /,respə'reɪtər/ *n* an apparatus to maintain breathing by artificial means; a device or mask to prevent the inhalation of harmful substances.

respiratory /'resprə,tɔri/ or /'respərə-/ *adj* of or for respiration.

respire /rə'spaɪr/ *vti* to breathe.

respite /rə'spaɪt/ *n* a temporary delay; a period of rest or relief; a reprieve.

resplendent /rə'splendənt/ *adj* dazzling, shining brilliantly; magnificent.

respond /rə'spɒnd/ or /ri-/ *vti* to answer; to reply; to show a favourable reaction; to be answerable; (*with* **to**) to react.

respondent /rə'spɒndənt/ or /ri-/ *n* a defendant, *esp* in a divorce suit; one who answers.

response /rə'spɒns/ or /ri-/ *n* an answer; a reaction to stimulation.

responsibility /rə,spɒnsə'bɪlɪti/ or /ri-/ *n* (*pl* **responsibilities**) being responsible; a moral obligation or duty; a charge or trust; a thing one is responsible for.

responsible /rə'spɒnsəbəl/ or /ri-/ *adj* having control (over); (*with* **for**) accountable (for); capable of rational conduct; trustworthy; involving responsibility.—**responsibly** *adv*.

responsive /rə'spɒnsɪv/ or /ri-/ *adj* responding; sensitive to influence or stimulus; sympathetic.

rest[1] /rest/ *n* stillness, repose, sleep; inactivity; the state of not moving; relaxation; tranquillity; a support or prop; a pause in music, metre, etc; a place of quiet. • *vti* to take a rest; to give

rest to; to be still; to lie down; to relax; to be fixed (on); to lean, support or be supported; to put one's trust (in).

rest[2] *n* the remainder; the others. • *vi* to remain.

restate /ri:'steɪt/ *vt* to state over again; to put differently.—**restatement** *n*.

restaurant /'restə,rɒnt/ or /'restrɒnt/ *n* a place where meals can be bought and eaten.

restaurateur /,restərə'tɔr/ *n* the keeper of a restaurant.

restful /'restfʊl/ *adj* peaceful.—**restfully** *adv*.—**restfulness** *n*.

rest home *n* an old people's home; a convalescent home.

restitution /,restə'tu:ʃən/ or /-'tju:-/ *n* the restoring of something to its owner; a reimbursement, as for loss.

restive /'restɪv/ *adj* impatient; fidgety.

restless /'restləs/ *adj* unsettled; agitated.—**restlessly** *adv*.—**restlessness** *n*.

restoration /,restɔr'eɪʃən/ *n* the act of restoring; reconstruction; renovation; (*with cap*) the re-establishment of the monarchy in Britain in 1660 under Charles II.

restorative /rə'stɔrətɪv/ *adj* tending to restore health and strength. • *n* a medicine or food that reinvigorates.

restore /rə'stɔr/ or /ri-/ *vt* to give or put back; to re-establish; to repair; to renovate; to bring back to the original condition.—**restorer** *n*.

restrain /rə'straɪn/ or /ri-/ *v* to hold back; to restrict; (*person*) to deprive of freedom.

restrained /rə'straɪnd/ or /ri-/ *adj* moderate; self-controlled; without exuberance.

restraint /rə'straɪnt/ or /ri-/ *n* the ability to hold back; something that restrains; control of emotions, impulses, etc.

restrict /rə'strɪkt/ or /ri-/ *vt* to keep within limits, circumscribe.

restricted /rə'strɪktəd/ or /ri-/ *adj* affected by restriction; limited; not generally available.

restriction /rə'strɪkʃən/ or /ri-/ *n* restraint; limitation; a limiting regulation.—**restrictive** *adj*.

restroom /'restruːm/ *n* a room equipped with toilets, washbowls, etc for the use of the public.

result /rə'zʌlt/ or /ri-/ *vi* to have as a consequence; to terminate in. • *n* a consequence; an outcome; a value obtained by mathematical calculation; (*sport*) the final score; (*pl*) a desired effect.

resultant /rə'zʌltənt/ or /ri-/ *adj* derived from or resulting from something else.

resume /rə'zu:m/ or /-'zju:m/, /ri-/ *vti* to begin again; to continue after a stop or pause; to proceed after interruption.—**resumption** *n*.

résumé /'rezə,meɪ/ or /-zju-/ *n* a summary, *esp* of employment experience; a curriculum vitae.

resurgence /rə'sɜrdʒəns/ or /ri-/ *n* a revival; a renewal of activity.—**resurgent** *adj*.

resurrect /,rezə'rekt/ *vt* to bring back into use; (*a custom*) to revive; to restore to life.

resurrection *n* a revival; a rising from the dead; (*with cap*) the rising of Christ from the dead.

resuscitate /rə'sʌsə,teɪt/ or /ri-/ *vti* to revive when apparently dead or unconscious.—**resuscitation** *n*.

resuscitator /-,teɪtər/ *n* an apparatus for forcing oxygen into the lungs; a person who resuscitates.

retable /rə'teɪbəl/ or /ri-/ *n* a step or ledge behind the altar of a church, slightly raised above it for the reception of lights, flowers, and other symbolical ornaments.

retail /rə'teɪl/ or /ri-/ *n* selling directly to the consumer in small quantities. • *adv* at a retail price. • *vti* to sell or be sold by retail.—*also adj*.—**retailer** *n*.

retain /rə'teɪl/ or /ri-/ *vt* to keep possession of; to keep in the mind, to remember; to keep in place, support; to hire the services of.

retainer /rə'teɪnər/ or /ri-/ *n* that which returns; (*formerly*) a servant to a family, a dependant; a fee to retain the services of.

retaining wall *n* a wall built to hold back earth or water.

retake /rə'teɪk/ or /ri-/ *vt* (**retaking, retook,** *pp* **retaken**) to capture again; to shoot a film scene again. • *n* a scene that has been reshot.

retaliate /rə'tæli,eɪt/ or /ri-/ *vti* to revenge oneself, *usu* by returning like for like; to strike back; to cast back (an accusation).—**retaliation** *n*.—**retaliatory** *adj*.

retard /rə'tɑrd/ or /ri-/ *vti* to slow down, to delay; to make slow or late.—**retardation** *n*.

retardant /rə'tɑrdənt/ or /ri-/ *n* a substance that retards, *esp* a chemical reaction. • *adj* retarding.

retarded /rə'tɑrdəd/ or /ri-/ *adj* slow in physical or mental development.

retch /retʃ/ *vi* to heave as if to vomit.

retention /rə'tenʃən/ or /ri-/ *n* the act of retaining; the capacity to retain; memory; (*med*) the abnormal retaining of fluid in a body cavity.

retentive /rə'tentɪv/ or /ri-/ *adj* capable of retaining; keeping, holding. • *n* one who retains.—**retentiveness** *n*.

rethink /ri:'θɪŋk/ *vt* (**rethinking, rethought**) to consider or think about again, *esp* with a change in mind.

reticent /'retɪsənt/ *adj* reserved in speech; uncommunicative.— **reticence** *n*.

reticle /'retɪkəl/ *n* a network of fine wires, threads, etc placed in the focal plane of an optical instrument.

reticulate /rɪtɪ'kju,leɪt/ *adj* resembling a network.—*also* **reticular**. • *vti* to arrange or be arranged into a network.—**reticulation** *n*.

retina /'retɪnə/ *n* (*pl* **retinas, retinae**) the innermost part of the eye, on which the image is formed.

retinue /'retə,nju:/ or /-,nu:/ *n* a body of attendants.

retire /rə'taɪr/ or /ri-/ *vi* to give up one's work when pensionable age is reached; to withdraw; to retreat; to go to bed. • *vt* (*troops*) to withdraw from use; to compel to retire from a position, work, etc.

retirement /rə'taɪrmənt/ or /ri-/ *n* the act of retiring or the state of being retired; seclusion; privacy.

retiring /rə'taɪrɪŋ/ or /ri-/ *adj* unobtrusive; shy.

retort /rə'tɔrt/ or /ri-/ *vi* to reply sharply or wittily. • *n* a sharp or witty reply; a vessel with a funnel bent downwards used in distilling; a receptacle used in making gas and steel.

retouch /ri:'tʌtʃ/ *vt* (*photograph, etc*) to improve or change by touching up; (*new growth of hair*) to colour to match other hair.

retrace /ri:'treɪs/ *vt* to go back over; to trace back to a source.— **retraceable** *adj*.

retract /rə'trækt/ or /ri-/ *vti* to draw in or back; to withdraw (a statement, opinion, etc); to recant.—**retractable** *adj*.—**retraction** *n*.

retreat /rə'tri:t/ or /ri-/ *vi* to withdraw, retire; to recede. • *n* a withdrawal, *esp* of troops; a sign for retiring; a quiet or secluded place, refuge; seclusion for religious devotion.

retrench /rə'trentʃ/ or /ri-/ *vti* to cut down (*esp* expenses); to economize.—**retrenchment** *n*.

retrial /ri:'traɪəl/ *n* a second trial.

retribution /,retrə'bju:ʃən/ *n* deserved reward; something given or exacted in compensation, *esp* punishment.

retrieve /rə'tri:v/ or /ri-/ *vt* to recover; to revive; (*a loss*) to make good; (*comput*) to obtain information from data stored in a computer. • *vi* (*dogs*) to retrieve game.—**retrievable** *adj*.— **retrieval** *n*.

retriever /rə'tri:vər/ or /ri-/ *n* any of several breeds of dogs capable of being trained for retrieving.

retro /'retro:/ *n* (*pl* **retros**) a retrorocket. • *adj* denoting a fashion or style (in music, clothes, etc) that pays homage to the past.

retro- /'retro:/ *prefix* backwards; behind.

retroactive /,retro:'æktɪv/ *adj* having an effect on things that are already past.

retrograde /,retrə'greɪd/ *adj* going backwards; passing from better to worse.

retrogression /,retrə'greʃən/ *n* going backwards, *usu* a return to a former, less complex, level of development.

retrorocket /,retro:'rɒkət/ *n* a small rocket on an aircraft or spacecraft that produces thrust in the opposite direction to the line of flight to slow it down.

retrospect /'retrə,spekt/ *n* a looking back; a mental review of the past.—**retrospection** *n*.

retrospective /,retrə'spektɪv/ *adj* looking backwards; relating to the past. • *n* an exhibition of an artist's lifetime work.—**retrospectively** *adv*.

retroussé /,retru:'seɪ/ *adj* turned upwards (*esp* of the nose).

retroversion /'retro:,vərʒən/ *n* the act of turning or state of being turned backwards.—**retroverted** *adj*.

Retrovir *n* (*trademark*) AZT.

retrovirus /'retro:,vaɪrəs/ *n* any of various viruses that use RNA to synthesize DNA, reversing the normal process in cells of transcription from DNA to RNA, which includes HIV.

retsina /ret'si:nə/ *n* a Greek white wine flavoured with resin.

return /rə'tərn/ or /rɪ-/ *vi* to come or go back; to reply; to recur. • *vt* to give or send back; to repay; to yield; to answer; to elect. • *n* something returned; a recurrence; recompense; (*pl*) yield, revenue; a form for computing (income) tax.

returnable /rə'tərnəbəl/ or /rɪ-/ *adj* required to be returned; capable of being returned (for reuse).

return ticket *n* (*Brit etc*) a ticket whose price includes the cost of the journey to and back from a destination.

reunion /ri:'ju:niən/ *n* a meeting following separation; a social gathering of former colleagues.

reunite /ri:'ju:naɪt/ *vt* to unite again; to reconcile. • *vi* to become reunited.

reusable /ri:'ju:zəbəl/ *adj* able to be used again; renewable.

Rev. *abbr* = Reverend.

rev /rev/ *vt* (**revving, revved**) (*inf*) (*with* up) to increase the speed of an engine. • *n* revolution per minute.

revaluate /ri:'vælju:,eɪt/ *vt* to reassess the value of; to change (*esp* increase) the exchange value of (a currency).

revamp /ri:'væmp/ *vt* to renovate, to rework, remodel; to transform. • *n* the process of revamping; something revamped.

revanchism /rə'væntʃɪzəm/ or /ri-/ *n* (support for) a policy aimed at regaining lost territory or possessions.—**revanchist** *n*, *adj*.

RevCan /'revkæn/ *n* ✹ (*Cdn*) (*inf*) Revenue Canada.

reveal /rə'vi:l/ or /ri-/ *vt* (*something hidden or secret*) to make known; to expose; to make visible.

reveille /'revəli/ *n* a morning bugle call to wake soldiers.

revel /'revəl/ *vi* (**reveling, revelled** *or* **reveling, reveled**) (*with* in) to take pleasure or delight in; to make merry. • *n* (*pl*) merrymaking; entertainment.—**reveler, reveller** *n*.

revelry /'revəlri/ *n* (*pl* **revelries**) the act of revelling; noisy festivity.

revelation /,revə'leɪʃən/ *n* the act of revealing; the disclosure of something secret; a communication from God to man; an illuminating experience.

revenge /'rəvendʒ/ or /ri-/ *vt* to inflict punishment in return for; to satisfy oneself by retaliation; to avenge. • *n* the act of revenging; retaliation; a vindictive feeling.—**revenger** *n*.

revengeful /'rəvendʒfʊl/ or /ri-/ *adj* keen for revenge; vindictive.

revenue /'revə,nju:/ or /-,nu:/ *n* the total income produced by taxation; gross income from a business or investment.

Revenue Canada *n* ✹ (*Cdn*) the federal government department responsible for collecting taxes.

reverb /ri'vərb/ or /'ri:vərb/ *n* (*mus*) an electronic device for producing an artificial echo.

reverberate /ri'vərbə,reɪt/ *vi* to rebound, recoil; to be reflected in; to resound, to echo.—**reverberation** *n*.

revere /rə'vi:r/ *vt* to regard with great respect or awe; to venerate.

reverence /'revərəns/ *n* profound respect; devotion; a gesture of respect (such as a bow). • *vt* to hold in respect.

reverend /'revərənd/ *adj* worthy of reverence; of or relating to the clergy; (*with cap*) a title for a member of the clergy.

reverent /'revərənt/ *adj* feeling or expressing reverence.—**reverently** *adv*.

reverie /'revəri/ *n* a daydream; (*mus*) a dreamy piece.—*also* **revery** (*pl* **reveries**).

revers /ri'vi:rz/ *n* (*pl* **revers**) a lapel, *esp* on a woman's garment.

reversal /rə'vərsəl/ *n* the act or process of reversing.

reverse /rə'vərs/ *vti* to turn in the opposite direction; to turn outside in, upside down, etc; to move backwards; (*law*) to revoke or annul. • *n* the contrary or opposite of something; the back, *esp* of a coin; a setback; a mechanism for reversing. • *adj* opposite, contrary; causing movement in the opposite direction.

reverse video *n* a technique for highlighting on a computer monitor by reversing the normal text and background colours.

reversible /rə'vərsəbəl/ *adj* with both sides usable; wearable with either side out; able to undergo a series of changes either backwards or forwards. • *n* a reversible cloth or article of clothing.

reversing falls *n* ✹ (*Cdn*) a set of rapids on a tidal river, the flow of which reverses at intervals because of the pressure of the incoming tide.

reversion /rə'vərʒən/ or /ri-/ *n* return to a former condition or type; right to future possession; the return of an estate to the grantor or his heirs.—**reversionary** *adj*.

revert /rə'vərt/ or /ri-/ *vi* to go back (to a former state); to take up again (a former subject); (*biol*) to return to a former or primitive type; (*law*) to go back to a former owner or his heirs.—**revertible** *adj*.

revery /'revəri/ *see* **reverie**.

review /rə'vju:/ *n* an evaluation; a survey; a reconsideration; a critical assessment, a critique; a periodical containing critical essays; an official inspection of ships or troops. • *vt* to re-examine; to inspect formally; to write a critique on.

reviewer /rə'vjuːər/ *n* a person who writes a review, *esp* for a newspaper, a critic.

revile /rə'vaɪl/ *vti* to use abusive language (to or about).

revise /rə'vaɪz/ *vt* to correct and amend; to prepare a new, improved version of; to study again (for an examination).—**revision** *n*.

revitalize /riː'vaɪtə,laɪz/ *vt* to put new life into.—**revitalization** *n*.

revival /rɪ'vaɪvəl/ *n* the act of reviving; recovery from a neglected or depressed state; renewed performance (of a play); renewed interest in; religious awakening.

revivalist /rɪ'vaɪvə,lɪst/ *n* a person who encourages religious practice.—**revivalism** *n*.

revive /rɪ'vaɪv/ *vti* to return to life; to make active again; to take up again.—**reviver** *n*.

revivify /ri'vɪvɪ,faɪ/ *vt* to put new life into; to reanimate; to re-vive.—**revification** *n*.—**revivifier** *n*.

revoke /rɪ'voːk/ or /ri-/ *vt* to cancel; to rescind. • *vi* (*cards*) to fail to follow suit.—**revocable** *adj*.—**revocation** *n*.

revolt /rɪ'voːlt/ or /ri-/ *vt* to rebel; to overturn; to shock. • *vi* to feel great disgust. • *n* rebellion; uprising; loathing.

revolting /rɪ'voːltɪŋ/ or /ri-/ *adj* extremely offensive.—**revolt-ingly** *adv*.

revolution /,revə'luːʃən/ *n* the act of revolting; a motion round a centre or axis; a single completion of an orbit or rotation; a great change; an overthrow of a government, social system, etc.

revolutionary *adj* of or advocating revolution; radically new. • *n* a person who takes part in, or favours, revolution.

revolutionize /,revə'luːʃə,naɪz/ *vt* to cause a complete change in.

revolve /rɪ'vɒlv/ or /ri-/ *vt* to travel or cause to travel in a circle or orbit; to rotate.

revolver /rɪ'vɒlvər/ or /ri-/ *n* a handgun with a magazine that re-volves to reload.

revolving door *n* a door of two or four panels rotating around a central axis within a round chamber and operated electrically or manually.

revue /rɪ'vjuː/ or /ri-/ *n* a musical show with skits, dances, etc, often satirizing recent events.

revulsion /rɪ'vʌlʒən/ or /ri-/ *n* disgust; aversion; a sudden change or reversal of feeling, *esp* withdrawal with a sense of utter distaste.

reward /rɪ'wɔrd/ or /ri-/ *n* something that is given in return for something done; money offered, as for the capture of a crimi-nal. • *vt* to give a reward.

rewarding /rɪ'wɔrdɪŋ/ or /ri-/ *adj* (*experience, activity, etc*) pleasing, profitable.

rewind /ri'waɪnd/ *vt* to wind again; to wind (an audiotape, etc) back to the beginning. • *n* the act of rewinding.

rewire /ri'waɪr/ *vt* to put new wiring into an electrical system.

reword /ri'wɜrd/ *vt* to change the wording of.

rework /ri'wɜrk/ *vt* to use again in a different form; to rewrite; to remodel.

rewrite /ri'raɪt/ *vt* to write again; to revise. • *n* something rewrit-ten; revision.

Rex /reks/ *n* a reigning king.

rf *abbr* = radio frequency.

Rh *abbr* = rhesus.

rhachis /'reɪkɪs/ *see* rachis.

rhapsodize /'ræpsə,daɪz/ *vi* to speak or write (about) with enthu-siasm or emotion.—**rhapsodist** *n*.

rhapsody /'ræpsədi/ *n* (*pl* **rhapsodies**) an enthusiastic speech or writing; (*mus*) an irregular instrumental composition of an epic, heroic or national character.

rhea /'riːə/ *n* any of several large flightless birds of South America resembling ostriches but smaller.

rhenium /'riːniəm/ *n* a hard heat-resistant metallic element.

rheo- /'riːoː/ *prefix* flow, current.

rheology /riː'ɒlədʒi/ *n* the physics of the flow and deformation of matter.—**rheologist** *n*.—**rheological** *adj*.

rheostat /'riːə,stæt/ *n* a device that regulates electric current by varying the resistance to it.—**rheostatic** *adj*.

rhesus factor /'riːsəs/ *n* a substance usually present in the red blood cells of humans and higher animals.

rhesus monkey *n* a type of southern Asian macaque with light brown fur.

rhesus negative *adj* lacking the rhesus factor in the blood.

rhesus positive *adj* containing the rhesus factor in the blood.

rhetoric /'retərɪk/ *n* the art of effective speaking and writing; skill in using speech; insincere language.

rhetorical /rɪ'tɒrɪkəl/ *adj* of or relating to rhetoric; high-flown; bombastic.—**rhetorically** *adv*.

rhetorical question *n* a question asked for effect, to which no answer is expected.

rheum /'ruːm/ *n* a watery discharge from the mucous membranes of the nose, eyes, etc.—**rheumy** *adj*.

rheumatic /ruː'mætɪk/ *adj* of, relating to or suffering from rheumatism. • *n* a person who has rheumatism.

rheumatic fever *n* a disease characterized by inflammation and pain in the joints.

rheumatism /'ruːmə,tɪzəm/ *n* a disorder causing pain in muscles and joints.

rheumatoid /'ruːmə,tɔɪd/ *adj* of or like rheumatism.

rheumatoid arthritis *n* a *usu* chronic disease characterized by inflammation, pain, and swelling of the joints.

rheumatology /,ruːmə'tɒlədʒi/ *n* the study of rheumatic dis-eases.—**rheumatologist** *n*.

rhinal /'raɪnəl/ *adj* of or pertaining to the nose.

rhinestone /'raɪnstoːn/ *n* a colourless imitation precious stone made from paste, glass, or quartz.

Rhine wine *n* any of several wines from the valley of the River Rhine in Germany; a light dry wine from the Rhine valley or elsewhere.

rhinitis /raɪ'naɪtɪs/ *n* inflammation of the mucous membrane of the nose.

rhino- /'raɪnoː/, **rhin-** /raɪn/ *prefix* nose.

rhino /'raɪnoː/ *n* (*pl* **rhinos, rhino**) (*inf*) a rhinoceros.

rhinoceros /raɪ'nɒsərəs/ *n* (*pl* **rhinoceroses, rhinoceros**) a large, thick-skinned mammal with one or two horns on the nose.

rhinology /raɪ'nɒlədʒi/ *n* the branch of medicine dealing with the nose.—**rhinologist** *n*.

rhinoplasty /'raɪno,plæsti/ *n* plastic surgery of the nose.—**rhinoplastic** *adj*.

rhizo- /'raɪzoː/, **rhiz-** /'raɪz/ *prefix* root.

rhizome /'raɪzoːm/ *n* a stem on or below ground that produces roots below and shoots above; a rootstock.

rho /roː/ *n* (*pl* **rhos**) the 17th letter of the Greek alphabet.

Rhode Island Red *n* an American breed of domestic fowl with reddish-brown plumage.

rhodium /'roːdiəm/ *n* a hard white metallic element similar to platinum.

rhododendron /,roːdə'dendrən/ *n* an evergreen shrub with large flowers.

rhomb /rɒm/ *n* a rhombus.

rhombohedron /,rɒmbə'hedrən/ *n* (*pl* **rhombohedrons, rhombohedra**) a six-sided solid figure whose sides are rhom-buses.—**rhombohedral** *adj*.

rhomboid /'rɒmbɔɪd/ *n* a parallelogram whose adjacent sides are unequal and whose angles are not right angles.—*also adj*.

rhombus /'rɒmbəs/ *n* (*pl* **rhombuses, rhombi**) a diamond shape.

rhubarb /'ruːbɑːb/ *n* a plant with large leaves and edible (when cooked) pink stalks; (*inf*) a noisy quarrel.

rhumb /rʌm/ *n* an imaginary line crossing all meridians at the same angle; a course navigated by a ship or aircraft that main-tains a fixed compass bearing.—*also* **rhumb line**.

rhyme /raɪm/ *n* the repetition of sounds *usu* at the ends of lines in verse; such poetry or verse; a word corresponding with another in end sound. • *vti* to form a rhyme (with); to versify, put into rhyme.

rhyming slang *n* a type of slang that substitutes the original (often indecent) word with a word or phrase that rhymes with it, *eg loaf of bread* = *head*.

rhythm /'rɪðəm/ *n* a regular recurrence of beat, accent or silence in the flow of sound, *esp* with words and music; a measured flow; cadence.—**rhythmic, rhythmical** *adj*.—**rhythmically** *adv*.

rhythm and blues *n* a type of music that fuses elements of folk, blues and rock.

rhythm method *n* a method of contraception that relies on ab-stinence from sexual intercourse during the period when ovu-lation is most likely to occur.

rhythm section *n* those instruments in a band or group whose main role is to supply the rhythm, such as the double bass and drums.

RI *abbr* = Rhode Island.

rib /rɪb/ *n* one of the curved bones of the chest attached to the spine; any rib-like structure; a leaf vein; a vein of an insect's wing; a ridge or raised strip, as of knitting; a ridge of a mountain. • *vt* (**ribbing, ribbed**) to provide with ribs; to form vertical ridges in knitting; (*inf*) to tease or ridicule.

ribald /rɪˈbəld/ or /raɪ-/ *adj* irreverent; humorously vulgar.

riband /ˈrɪbənd/ *n* a ribbon.

ribbon /ˈrɪbən/ *n* silk, satin, velvet, etc, woven into a narrow band; a piece of this; a strip of cloth, etc, inked for use, as in a typewriter; (*pl*) torn shreds.

rib cage *n* the bony framework of ribs enclosing the wall of the chest.

riboflavin /ˌraɪbəˈfleɪvɪn/ *n* a factor of the vitamin B complex found in milk, eggs, fruits, etc.

ribonuclease /ˌraɪbəˈnuːklɪˌeɪs/ or /-ˈnjuː-/ *n* any of several enzymes that act as catalytic triggers of RNA hydrolosis.

ribonucleic acid /ˌraɪbəˈnuːkliːɪk/ or /-njuː-/, /-kleɪɪk/ *n* any of a group of nucleic acids found in all living cells, where they are essential to protein development.—**RNA** *abbr*.

ribose /ˈraɪbəʊs/ *n* a sugar occurring in RNA and riboflavin.

ribosome /ˈraɪbəˌsəʊm/ *n* any of the tiny particles containing RNA and protein in cells where protein synthesis takes place.—**ribosomal** *adj*.

rice /raɪs/ *n* an annual cereal grass cultivated in warm climates; its starchy food grain.

ricebird /ˈraɪsˌbɜːd/ *see* **bobolink**.

rice paper *n* a delicate paper prepared from pith.

rich /rɪtʃ/ *adj* having much money, wealthy; abounding in natural resources, fertile; costly, fine; (*food*) sweet or oily, highly flavoured; deep in colour; (*inf*) full of humour. • *n* wealthy people collectively; (*pl* **riches**) wealth, abundance.—**richly** *adv*.—**richness** *n*.

Richter scale /ˈrɪktər/ *n* a scale ranging from 1 to 10 for measuring the intensity of an earthquake.

rick[1] /rɪk/ *n* a stack or large pile of hay, etc, in the open.

rick[2] *vt* (*Brit etc*) to sprain or strain slightly. • *n* such an injury.—*also* **wrick**.

rickets /ˈrɪkɪts/ *n* a children's disease marked by softening of the bones, caused by vitamin D deficiency.

rickettsia /rɪˈketsɪə/ *n* (*pl* **rickettsiae, rickettsias**) any of a genus of microorganisms that inhabit mites, ticks, etc and cause serious diseases, such as typhus.—**rickettsial** *adj*.

rickety /ˈrɪkɪtɪ/ *adj* shaky, unsteady.

rickrack /ˈrɪkræk/ *n* a zigzag braid for trimming clothing.

rickshaw, ricksha /ˈrɪkʃɒ/ *n* a light, two-wheeled man-drawn vehicle, orig used in Japan.

ricochet /ˈrɪkəˌʃeɪ/ *vi* (**ricocheting, ricocheted** *or* **ricochetting, ricochetted**) (*bullet*) to rebound or skip along ground or water. • *n* a rebound or glancing off; (*bullet*) a hit made after ricocheting.

ricotta /rɪˈkɒtə/ *n* a mildly-flavoured soft white cheese made from sheep's milk.

rictus /ˈrɪktəs/ *n* (*pl* **rictus, rictuses**) the gap in an open mouth or beak; a fixed grimace, *esp* in horror.—**rictal** *adj*.

rid /rɪd/ *vt* (**ridding, rid** *or* **ridded**) to free from; to dispose (of).

riddance /ˈrɪdəns/ *n* clearance; disposal.

ridden[1] /ˈrɪdən/ *see* **ride**.

ridden[2] *adj* oppressed by; full of.

riddle[1] /ˈrɪdəl/ *n* a puzzling question; an enigma; a mysterious person or thing.

riddle[2] *n* a coarse sieve. • *vt* to sieve or sift; to perforate with holes; to spread through, permeate.

ride /raɪd/ *vb* (**riding, rode,** *pp* **ridden**) *vti* to be carried along or travel in a vehicle or on an animal, bicycle, etc; to be supported or move on the water; to lie at anchor; to travel over a surface; to move on the body; (*inf*) to continue undisturbed. • *vt* (*horse, bicycle etc*); to sit on and control; to oppress, dominate; (*inf*) to torment. • *n* a trip or journey in a vehicle or on horseback, on a bicycle, etc; a thing to ride at a fairground.

Rideau Hall /ˈriːdəʊ/ ♣ the official residence and office of the Governor General of Canada.

rider /ˈraɪdər/ *n* a person who rides; an addition to a document, amending a clause; an additional statement; something used to move along another piece.

ridge /rɪdʒ/ *n* a narrow crest or top; the ploughed earth thrown up between the furrows; a line where two slopes meet; (*of land etc*) a raised strip or elevation; a range of hills. • *vti* to form into ridges, wrinkle.—**ridged** *adj*.

ridgepole /ˈrɪdʒpəʊl/ *n* the horizontal pole along the top of a tent.

ridicule /ˈrɪdɪˌkjuːl/ *n* mockery, derision. • *vt* to make fun of, to mock.

ridiculous /rɪˈdɪkjʊləs/ *adj* deserving ridicule; preposterous, silly.—**ridiculously** *adv*.—**ridiculousness** *n*.

riding /ˈraɪdɪŋ/ *n* ♣ (*Cdn*) a constituency that elects a member of a legislature.

riesling /ˈriːzlɪŋ/ or /-slɪŋ/ *n* (the grape that produces) a dry white wine.

rife /raɪf/ *adj* widespread; prevalent.

riff /rɪf/ *n* (*jazz, rock*) a musical phrase played repeatedly, *esp* as the background to an extended solo improvisation.—*also vi.*

riffle /ˈrɪfəl/ *vt* to leaf or flick rapidly through (pages, files, etc); to shuffle cards by dividing the deck and then flicking the corners together with the thumbs. • *vi* to flick cursorily (through). • *n* (the sound of) an act or instance of riffling; a ripple in a stream or the small obstruction causing this; grooves, etc at the bottom of a sluice to trap gold particles.

riffraff /ˈrɪfræf/ *n* disreputable persons; refuse, rubbish.

rifle[1] /ˈraɪfəl/ *n* a shoulder gun with a spirally grooved bore.

rifle[2] *vti* to steal; to look through (a person's papers or belongings).

rifling /ˈraɪflɪŋ/ *n* (the cutting of) spiral grooves in the bore of a firearm that spin the projectile.

rift /rɪft/ *n* a split; a cleft; a fissure. • *vti* to split.

rift valley *n* a narrow valley caused by land subsiding between two parallel faults.

rig /rɪg/ *vt* (**rigging, rigged**) (*naut*) to equip with sails and tackle; to set up in working order; to manipulate fraudulently. • *n* the way sails, etc, are rigged; equipment or gear for a special purpose, such as oil drilling; a type of truck.

rigging /ˈrɪgɪŋ/ *n* the ropes for supporting masts and sails; (*in theatre*) a network of ropes and pulleys to support and maintain scenery.

right /raɪt/ *adj* correct, true; just or good; appropriate; fit, recovered; opposite to left; conservative; designating the side meant to be seen. • *adv* straight; directly; completely, exactly; correctly, properly; to or on the right side. • *n* that which is just or correct; truth; fairness; justice; privilege; just or legal claim; (*pl*) the correct condition. • *vti* to set or become upright; to correct; to redress.—**rightness** *n*.

right angle *n* an angle of 90 degrees.

righteous /ˈraɪtʃəs/ *adj* moral, virtuous.—**righteously** *adv*.—**righteousness** *n*.

rightful /ˈraɪtfʊl/ *adj* legitimate; having a just claim.—**rightfully** *adv*.—**rightfulness** *n*.

right-hand *adj* of or towards the right side of a person or thing; for use by the right hand.

right-handed /raɪtˈhændɪd/ *adj* using the right hand; done or made for use with the right hand. • *adv* with the right hand.

rightist /ˈraɪtɪst/ *adj* politically conservative. • *n* a person belonging to or supporting a conservative political party.

rightly /ˈraɪtlɪ/ *adv* in truth; in the right; with good reason; properly.

right-minded *adj* having principles in accordance with standard notions of what is right.

right of way *n* a public path over private ground; the right to use this; precedence over other traffic.

right-on /ˈraɪtˌɒn/ *adj* (*inf*) fashionable, trendy.

right-thinking *adj* holding generally acceptable views.

right-wing *adj* of or relating to the conservative faction of a political party, organization, etc.—**right-winger** *n*.

rigid /ˈrɪdʒɪd/ *adj* stiff, inflexible; severe, strict.—**rigidity** *n*.—**rigidly** *adv*.—**rigidness** *n*.

rigmarole /ˈrɪgməˌrəʊl/ *n* nonsense; a foolishly involved procedure.

rigor /ˈrɪgər/ *n* harsh inflexibility; severity; strictness.—*also* **rigour**.

rigor mortis /ˌrɪgərˈmɔːtɪs/ *n* the stiffening of the body after death.

rigorous *adj* stern, severe, strict.—**rigorously** *adv*.—**rigorousness** *n*.

rigour /ˈrɪgər/ *see* **rigor**.

rile /raɪl/ *vt* (*inf*) to irritate, to annoy, to anger.

rill /rɪl/ *n* a small brook or stream.

rim /rɪm/ *n* a border or raised edge, *esp* of something circular; the outer part of a wheel. • *vt* (**rimming, rimmed**) to supply or surround with a rim; to form a rim.

rimless /ˈrɪmləs/ *adj* lacking a rim; (*glasses*) without a frame.

rind /ˈrɪnd/ *n* crust; peel; bark.

rinderpest /'rɪndər,pest/ *n* an acute viral disease of cattle.

ring[1] /rɪŋ/ *n* a circular band, *esp* of metal, worn on the finger, in the ear, etc; a hollow circle; a round enclosure; an arena for boxing, etc; a group of people engaged in secret or criminal activity to control a market, etc. • *vt* (**ringing, ringed**) to encircle, surround; to fit with a ring.

ring[2] *vti* (**ringing, rang** *or* **rung**, *pp* **rung**) to emit a bell-like sound; to resound; to peal; to sound a bell; to telephone; (*with* **up**) to total and record *esp* by means of a cash register; to achieve. • *n* a ringing sound; a resonant note; a set of church bells.

ringdove *n* a wood pigeon.

ringed /rɪŋd/ *adj* wearing rings; forming rings; having ring-like markings; surrounded by.

ringer /'rɪŋər/ *n* a person that rings bells; (*sl*) a person or thing closely resembling another; a horse entered into a race under a false name, weight, etc.

ringette /rɪŋˈet/ *n* ✹ (*Cdn*) a game resembling hockey that is played with a straight stick and a rubber ring.

ring finger *n* the third finger, *esp* of the left hand, on which a wedding ring is traditionally worn.

ringhals /'rɪŋhælz/ *n* a poisonous African snake that spits venom at its victims.

ringleader /'rɪŋˌliːdər/ *n* a person who takes the lead in mischievous or unlawful behaviour.

ringlet /'rɪŋlət/ *n* a curling lock of hair.

ringmaster /'rɪŋˌmæstər/ *n* a master of ceremonies in a circus.

ringworm /'rɪŋwərm/ *n* a contagious skin infection.

rink /rɪŋk/ *n* an expanse of ice for skating; a smooth floor for roller skating; an alley for bowling.

rink rat *n* ✹ (*Cdn*) (*sl*) a young person who frequents a hockey rink, *esp* one who does chores in exchange for being allowed to skate.

rinse /rɪns/ *vt* to wash lightly; to flush under clean water to remove soap. • *n* the act of rinsing; a preparation for tinting the hair.

rioja /rɪˈoːhə/ *n* a type of Spanish red or white wine.

riot /'raɪət/ *n* violent public disorder; uproar; unrestrained profusion; (*inf*) something very funny. • *vi* to participate in a riot.—**rioter** *n*.—**rioting** *n*.

riotous /'raɪətəs/ *adj* disorderly, tumultuous, seditious luxurious, wanton.—**riotously** *adv*.—**riotousness** *n*.

RIP *abbr* = rest in peace.

rip[1] /rɪp/ *vti* (**ripping, ripped**) to cut or tear apart roughly; to split; (*with* **off, out**) to remove in a violent or rough manner; (*inf*) to rush, speed; (*with* **into**) to attack, *esp* verbally. • *n* a tear; a split.

rip[2] *n* a stretch of broken water caused by currents and tides.

rip cord *n* a cord for releasing a parachute.

ripe /raɪp/ *adj* ready to be eaten or harvested; fully developed; mature.—**ripely** *adv*.—**ripeness** *n*.

ripen /'raɪpən/ *vt* to grow or make ripe.

rip-off *n* (*sl*) the act or a means of stealing; plagiarizing, cheating, etc.

riposte, ripost /rɪˈpɒst/ *n* a counterstroke; a retort; a retaliatory manoeuvre. • *vi* to make a riposte.

ripple /'rɪpəl/ *n* a little wave or undulation on the surface of water; the sound of this. • *vti* to have or form little waves on the surface (of).

rip-roaring /'rɪpˌrɔːrɪŋ/ *adj* (*inf*) exuberant, boisterous, thrilling.

ripsaw /'rɪpsɔː/ *n* a handsaw for cutting wood in the direction of the grain.

riptide *n* a powerful current flowing outwards from the shore.

RISC /rɪsk/ (*abbr*) = Reduced Instruction Set Computer: a computer with advanced yet simplified internal circuitry that allows a significant increase in processing speed over standard designs.

rise /raɪz/ *vi* (**rising, rose**, *pp* **risen**) to get up; to stand up; to ascend; to increase in value or size; to swell; to revolt; to be provoked; to originate; to tower; to slope up; (*voice*) to reach a higher pitch; to ascend from the grave; (*fish*) to come to the surface. • *n* an ascent; origin; an increase in price, salary, etc; an upward slope.

risible /'rɪzɪbəl/ *adj* tending to laugh; provoking laughter, derisory.—**risibility** *n*.

rising /'raɪzɪŋ/ *n* a revolt, insurrection. • *adj* ascending; approaching.

risk /rɪsk/ *n* chance of loss or injury; hazard; danger, peril. • *vt* to expose to possible danger or loss; to take the chance of.

risk capital *n* venture capital.

risky /'rɪski/ *adj* (**riskier, riskiest**) dangerous; uncertain; not secure.

risotto /rɪˈzɒtoː/ *n* (*pl* **risottos**) a dish of onions, rice, butter, etc, cooked in meat stock.

risqué /rɪskeɪ/ *adj* verging on indecency; slightly offensive.

rissole /'rɪsoːl/ *n* a fried cake of minced meat, egg, and breadcrumbs.

rite /raɪt/ *n* a ceremonial practice or procedure, *esp* religious.

rite of passage *n* a ritual indicating a change in an individual's status, as at puberty or marriage.

ritual /'rɪtʃuəl/ *adj* relating to rites or ceremonies. • *n* a fixed (religious) ceremony.—**ritually** *adv*.

ritzy /'rɪtsi/ *adj* (**ritzier, ritziest**) (*sl*) luxurious, smart.

rival /'raɪvəl/ *n* one of two or more people, organizations or teams competing with each other for the same goal. • *adj* competing; having comparable merit or claim. • *vt* (**rivalling, rivalled**) to strive to equal or excel; to be comparable to; to compete.

rivalry /'raɪvəlri/ *n* (*pl* **rivalries**) emulation; competition.

river /'rɪvər/ *n* a large natural stream of fresh water flowing into an ocean, lake, etc; a copious flow.

river basin *n* land drained by a river and its tributaries.

riverbed /'rɪvərbed/ *n* the channel formed by a river.

riverfront /'rɪvərˌfrʌnt/ *n* the land or an area along a river.

riverine /'rɪvəraɪn/ *adj* of, like, or produced by a river; living or located on the banks of a river.

riverside /'rɪvərsaɪd/ *n* the bank of a river.

rivet /'rɪvɪt/ *n* a short, metal bolt for holding metal plates together, the headless end being hammered flat. • *vt* to join with rivets; to fix one's eyes upon immovably; to engross one's attention.

riveter /'rɪvətər/ *n* a person who rivets; a machine that rivets.

Riviera /ˌrɪviˈerə/ *n* the coast of the northern Mediterranean from southeast France to northwest Italy.

rivulet /'rɪvjulət/ *n* a little stream.

riyal /'riːɒl/ *or* /'raɪɒl/ *n* the standard currency unit of Saudi Arabia, Yemen, Qatar, or Dubai.

RM *abbr* ✹ (*Cdn*) = Rural Municipality; Regional Municipality.

RMA /'ar em'eɪ/ *abbr* = Royal Military Academy.

rms *abbr* = root mean square.

RN *abbr* = Registered Nurse; Royal Navy.

Rn (*chem symbol*) radon.

RNA /'ar'en'eɪ/ *abbr* = ribonucleic acid.

roach /roːtʃ/ *n* a small silvery freshwater fish.

road /roːd/ *n* a track, surfaced with tarmac or concrete, made for travelling; a highway; a street; a way or route; an anchorage for ships.

road block /'roːdblɒk/ *n* a barrier erected across a road to halt traffic.

road hockey *n* ✹ (*Cdn*) an informal game of hockey played on a road in which a ball rather than a puck is used.—*also* **street hockey**.

road hog *n* a car driver who obstructs other vehicles by encroaching on the others' traffic lane.

roadhouse /-haus/ *n* a tavern *usu* outside city limits providing meals, etc.

roadie /'roːdi/ *n* (*inf*) a person with responsibility for transporting and setting up stage equipment for a rock group, etc on tour.

road map *n* a map for motorists that gives information on the roads of a particular area.

road metal *n* broken stone and cinders used in making road and railway foundations.

road movie *n* a film genre in which the main characters are on a journey, both in a real and figurative sense.

road runner /'roːdˌrʌnər/ *n* a long-tailed, swift-running, terrestrial North American cuckoo.

roadshow *n* a group of touring entertainers; a radio or television show presented from a touring outside-broadcasting unit.

roadside /-saɪd/ *n* the border of a road.—*also adj*.

road-test *vt* to test (a vehicle) under practical operating conditions.—**road test** *n*.

roadway /'roːdweɪ/ *n* the strip of land over which a road passes; the main part of a road, used by vehicles.

roadwork /'roːdwərk/ *n* conditioning for an athletic contest consisting mainly of long runs.

roam /roːm/ *vti* to wander about, to rove.

roan /roːn/ *adj* having a base colour thickly sprinkled with white or grey. • *n* a horse with a roan coat, *esp* when the base colour is red.

roar /rɔr/ *vti* to make a loud, full, growling sound, as a lion, wind, fire, the sea; to utter loudly, as in a rage; to bellow; to guffaw.—*also n.*

roaring /'rɔrɪŋ/ *adj* boisterous, noisy; brisk.

roast /rɔːst/ *vti* (*meat, etc*) to cook with little or no moisture, as before a fire or in an oven; (*coffee, etc*) to process by exposure to heat; to expose to great heat; (*inf*) to criticize severely; to undergo roasting. • *n* roasted meat; a cut of meat for roasting; a picnic at which food is roasted.

rob /rɒb/ *vb* (**robbing, robbed**) *vt* to seize forcibly; to steal from; to plunder. • *vi* to commit robbery.—**robber** *n*.

robbery /'rɒbəri/ *n* (*pl* **robberies**) theft from a person by intimidation or by violence.

robe /rəʊb/ *n* a long flowing outer garment; the official dress of a judge, academic, etc; a bathrobe or dressing gown; a covering or wrap; (*pl*) ceremonial vestments. • *vti* to put on or dress in robes.

robin /'rɒbɪn/ *n* a songbird with a dull red breast.

robot /rəʊ'bɒt/ *n* a mechanical device that acts in a seemingly human way; a mechanism guided by automatic controls.

robotics /rəʊ'bɒtɪks/ *n* (*used as sing*) the science of designing and using robots.

robust *adj* strong, sturdy; vigorous.—**robustly** *adv*.—**robustness** *n*.

roc /rɒk/ *n* (*Arabian legend*) a giant bird of enormous strength.

rock[1] /rɒk/ *n* a large stone or boulder; a person or thing providing foundation or support; ♣ a curling stone; (*geol*) a natural mineral deposit including sand, clay, etc; a hard sweet; (*inf*) a diamond, ice.

rock[2] *vti* to move to and fro, or from side to side; to sway strongly; to shake. • *n* a rocking motion; rock and roll.

rockabilly /'rɒkəˌbɪli/ *n* a type of fast-paced rock and country music originating in the US South in the 1950s.

rock-and-roll *n* popular music that incorporates country and blues elements and is *usu* played on electronic instruments with a heavily accented beat.

rock bottom *n* the lowest or most fundamental part or level. • *adj* very lowest.

rock crystal *n* transparent colourless quartz used in electronic and optical equipment.

rocker /'rɒkər/ *n* a rocking chair; a curved support on which a cradle, etc, rocks.

rockery /'rɒkəri/ *n* (*pl* **rockeries**) a garden among rocks for alpine plants.—*also* **rock garden**.

rocket /'rɒkət/ *n* any device driven forward by gases escaping through a rear vent, such as a firework, distress signal, or the propulsion mechanism of a spacecraft. • *vi* to move in or like a rocket; to soar.

rocket launcher *n* a device for launching rockets; an aircraft or motor vehicle equipped to launch rockets.

rocketry /'rɒkətri/ *n* the science of building and launching rockets.

rock garden *see* **rockery**.

rock house *n* (*sl*) a place where the drug crack is made available by dealers.

rocking chair *n* a chair mounted on rockers.

rocking horse *n* a toy horse fixed on rockers or springs.

rock salt *n* common salt in solid form or in large crystals.

rocky /'rɒki/ *adj* (**rockier, rockiest**) having many rocks; like rock; rugged, hard; shaky, unstable.

rococo /rə'kəʊkəʊ/ *adj* (*often cap*) elaborately ornate, as in an architectural style of 18th-century Europe.—*also n.*

rod /rɒd/ *n* a stick; a thin bar of metal or wood; a staff of office; a wand; a fishing rod; (*sl*) a pistol.

rode /rəʊd/ *see* **ride**.

rodent /'rəʊdənt/ *n* any of several relatively small gnawing animals with two strong front teeth.

rodeo /'rəʊdɪəʊ/ *n* (*pl* **rodeos**) the rounding up of cattle; a display of cowboy skill.

roe[1] /rəʊ/ *n* the eggs of fish.

roe[2] *n* a small reddish brown deer.—*also* **roe deer**; the female red deer.

roebuck /'rəʊbʌk/ *n* the male roe deer.

roe deer /ˌrəʊ'dɪːr/ *n* a small graceful deer of European and Asian woodlands.

roentgen /'rɒntdʒən/ *n* the unit of measuring X-rays or gamma rays.—*also* **röntgen**.

roger /'rɒdʒər/ *interj* used in radio communications, etc to indicate message received and understood.

rogue /rəʊg/ *n* a scoundrel; a rascal; a mischievous person; a wild animal that lives apart from the herd.—**roguish** *adj*.—**roguishly** *adv*.

role, rôle /rəʊl/ *n* a part in a film or play taken by an actor; a function.

role model *n* a person who inspires others to emulate him or her.

role-playing *n* (*psychol*) a technique in which participants take on and act out roles in order to rehearse a situation or resolve a conflict.

roll /rəʊl/ *n* a scroll; anything wound into cylindrical form; a list or register; a turned-over edge; a rolling movement; a small cake of bread; a trill of some birds; an undulation; the sound of thunder; the beating of drumsticks. • *vi* to move by turning over or from side to side; to move like a wheel; to curl; to move in like waves; to flow. • *vt* to cause to roll; to turn on its axis; to move on wheels; to press with a roller; (*dice*) to throw; to beat rapidly, as a drum.

roll bar *n* a bar that reinforces the frame of a racing or sports car to protect the driver should the vehicle overturn.

roll call *n* the reading aloud of a list of names to check attendance.

roller /'rəʊlər/ *n* a revolving cylinder used for spreading paint, flattening surfaces, moving paper, etc; a large wave.

roller coaster *n* an elevated amusement ride in which small cars move on tracks that curve and dip sharply.—*also* **big dipper**.

roller skate *n* a four-wheeled skate strapped on to shoes.—**roller skating** *n*.

roller towel *n* a towel without ends on a roller.

rolling pin *n* a wooden, plastic or stone cylinder for rolling out pastry.

rolling stock *n* all the vehicles of a railway.

rolling stone *n* a person who cannot settle in one place; a free spirit.

rollmop /'rəʊlmɒp/ *n* a fillet of herring rolled up and pickled in brine or spiced vinegar.

roll-on/roll-off *adj* pertaining to a cargo ship or passenger ferry designed so that vehicles can be driven straight on and off.

roll-top desk /'rəʊltɒp/ *n* a writing desk with a flexible sliding cover of slats.

roly-poly /'rəʊliˌpəʊli/ *n* (*pl* **roly-polies**) a pudding of pastry covered with jam and rolled up; a round and plump person.

ROM /rɒm/ *abbr* (*comput*) = read-only memory.

Roman /'rəʊmən/ *adj* of or relating to the city of Rome or its ancient empire, or the Latin alphabet; Roman Catholic. • *n* an inhabitant or citizen of Rome; a Roman Catholic.

roman /'rəʊmən/ *adj* ordinary type, not italic.

Roman candle *n* a type of cylindrical firework that emits coloured sparks.

Roman Catholic *adj* belonging to the Christian church that is headed by the Pope.—*also n.*

romance /'rəʊmæns/ or /rəʊ'mæns/ *n* a prose narrative; a medieval tale of chivalry; a series of unusual adventures; a novel dealing with this; an atmosphere of awe or wonder; a love story; a love affair; a picturesque falsehood. • *vi* to write romantic fiction; to exaggerate.

Romanesque /ˌrəʊmə'nɛsk/ *adj, n* (in) the style of round-arched and vaulted architecture prevalent between the Classical and Gothic periods.

Roman holiday *n* a holiday or entertainment at the expense of others' suffering.

Roman nose *n* a nose with a slender prominent ridge.

Roman numerals *n* the letters I, V, X, L, C, D, and M used to represent numbers in the manner of the ancient Romans.

romantic /rəʊ'mæntɪk/ *adj* of or given to romance; strange and picturesque; imaginative; sentimental; (*art, literature*) preferring passion and imagination to proportion and finish, subordinating form to content.—**romantically** *adv*.

romanticism /rəʊ'mæntəˌsɪzəm/ *n* a 19th-century philosophical and cultural movement characterized by the desire to bring nature and man into unity through the shaping power of the imagination; romantic approach, quality, or ideals.

romanticize /rəʊ'mæntəˌsaɪz/ *vt* to imbue (a person, concept, etc) with a romantic character. • *vi* to have romantic ideas.—**romanticization** *n*.

Romany /'rɒməni/ or /'rɒː-/ *n* a Gypsy; the Indic language of Gypsies.

romp /rɒmp/ *vi* to play boisterously. • *n* a noisy game; a frolic; an easy win.

rompers /'rɒmpərz/ *npl* a child's one-piece garment; a jumpsuit.

rondo /'rɒndo:/ *n* (*pl* **rondos**) a musical form with a leading theme to which return is made.

röntgen /'rɒntdʒən/ *see* **roentgen.**

roof /ru:f/ *n* (*pl* **roofs**) the upper covering of a building; the top of a vehicle; an upper limit. • *vt* to provide with a roof, to cover.

roof garden *n* a garden on a flat roof or balcony; a top floor decorated as a garden, *esp* if used as a restaurant.

roofing /'ru:fɪŋ/ *n* materials for a roof.

rook[1] /ruk/ *n* a crow-like bird.

rook[2] *n* (*chess*) a piece with the power to move horizontally or vertically, a castle.

rookery /'rukəri/ *n* (*pl* **rookeries**) a colony of rooks; a breeding ground or haunt of other birds or mammals; a crowded place.

rookie /'ruki/ *n* (*sl*) an inexperienced army recruit; any novice.— *also adj.*

room /ru:m/ *n* space; unoccupied space; adequate space; a division of a house, a chamber; scope or opportunity; those in a room; (*pl*) lodgings. • *vi* to lodge.

room clerk *n* a receptionist in a hotel who books in guests and allocates rooms, etc.

rooming house *n* a house with individual rooms to let.

roommate *n* a person with whom one shares a room or rooms.

roomy /'ru:mi/ *adj* (**roomier, roomiest**) having ample space; wide.—**roominess** *n.*

roost /ru:st/ *n* a bird's perch or sleeping-place; a place for resting. • *vi* to rest or sleep on a roost; to settle down, as for the night.

rooster /'ru:stər/ *n* an adult male domestic fowl, a cockerel.

root[1] /ru:t/ *n* the part of a plant, *usu* underground, that anchors the plant, draws water from the soil, etc; the embedded part of a tooth, a hair, etc; a supporting or essential part; something that is an origin or source; (*math*) the factor of a quantity which multiplied by itself gives the quantity; (*mus*) the fundamental note of a chord; (*pl*) plants with edible roots. • *vti* to take root; to become established; (*with* **out**) to tear up, to eradicate.

root[2] *vti* to dig up with the snout; to search about, rummage; (*with* **for**) (*inf*) to encourage a team by cheering.

root beer *n* a carbonated drink flavored with extracts of certain roots and barks.

root crop *n* a crop, such as turnips, sugar beet, cultivated for its edible roots.

rooted /'ru:təd/ *adj* firmly fixed; planted.

root mean square *n* the square root of the average of the squares of a set of numbers.

rootstock /'ru:tstɒk/ *n* an underground stem, rhizome; a stock for grafting, having a root or a piece of root.

rope /ro:p/ *n* a thick cord or thin cable made of twisted fibres or wires; a string or row of things braided, intertwined or threaded together; a viscous thickening in a liquid. • *vt* to tie, bind, divide or enclose with a rope; to lasso; (*liquid*) to become ropy.—**ropy** *adj.*

Roquefort /'rɒkfər/ or /ro:k-/, /-fərt/ *n* a French blue-veined cheese with a strong flavour.

rorqual /'rɔrkwəl/ *n* any of several large whalebone whales with dorsal fins and deep furrows on the skin of the throat and chest.—*also* **finback.**

rosaceous /ro:'zeɪʃəs/ *adj* of or belonging to the large family of plants that includes the rose; resembling a rose; rose-coloured.

rosary /'ro:zəri/ *n* (*pl* **rosaries**) a string of beads for keeping count of prayers; a series of prayers.

rose[1] /ro:z/ *see* **rise.**

rose[2] *n* a prickly-stemmed plant with fragrant flowers of many delicate colours; its flower; a rosette; a perforated nozzle; a pinkish red or purplish red.

rosé /ro:'zeɪ/ *n* a pink wine made from skinless red grapes or by mixing white and red wine.

rose-coloured *adj* rosy; overly optimistic.

rosemary /'ro:z,meri/ *n* a fragrant shrubby mint used in cookery and perfumery.

rosette /ro:'zet/ *n* a rose-shaped bunch of ribbon; a carving, etc, in the shape of a rose.

rosewater /'ro:zwɒtər/ *n* water scented with rose petals.

rose window *n* a circular window filled with tracery.

rosewood /'ro:zwud/ *n* (any of various tropical trees yielding) a fragrant dark wood used in making furniture.

rosin /'rɒzɪn/ *n* a pine-wood resin, *esp* in solid form, used in varnishes, etc, and for waxing the bows of stringed instruments.

roster /'rɒstər/ *n* a list or roll, as of military personnel; a list of duties.

rostrum /'rɒstrəm/ *n* (*pl* **rostrums, rostra**) a platform or stage for public speaking.

rosy /'ro:zi/ *adj* (**rosier, rosiest**) of the colour of roses; having pink, healthy cheeks; optimistic, hopeful.

rot /rɒt/ *vti* (**rotting, rotted**) to decompose; to decay; to become degenerate. • *n* decay; corruption; several different diseases affecting timber or sheep; (*inf*) nonsense.

rota /ro:tə/ *n* a turn in succession; a list or roster of duties.

rotary /'ro:təri/ *adj* revolving; turning like a wheel.

Rotary Club *n* a club belonging to an international organization of business people for promoting community service.—**Rotarian** *n.*

rotate /'ro:teɪt/ or /ro:'teɪt/ *vti* to turn around an axis like a wheel; to follow a sequence.

rotation /ro:'teɪʃən/ *n* the action of rotating; a regular succession, as of crops to avoid exhausting the soil.

rote /ro:t/ *n* a fixed, mechanical way of doing something.

rotgut /'rɒtgət/ *n* (*sl*) a cheap or inferior whiskey or other spirit.

rotisserie /ro:'tɪsəri/ *n* a large rotating spit on which poultry is roasted; a place where such food is prepared.

rotor /'ro:tər/ *n* a rotating part of a machine or engine.

rotten /'rɒtən/ *adj* decayed, decomposed; corrupt; (*inf*) bad, nasty.—**rottenness** *n.*

rotund /ro:'tʌnd/ *adj* rounded; spherical; plump.

rotunda /ro:'tʌndə/ *n* a circular, *esp* domed, building or chamber.

rouble /'ru:bəl/ *n* a coin and monetary unit of Russia.—*also* **ruble.**

rouge /ru:ʒ/ *n* a red cosmetic for colouring the cheeks; a red powder for polishing jewellery, etc. • *vti* to colour (the face) with rouge.

rough /rʌf/ *adj* uneven; not smooth; ill-mannered; violent, rude, unpolished; shaggy; coarse in texture; unrefined; violent, boisterous; stormy; wild; harsh, discordant; crude, unfinished; approximate; (*inf*) difficult. • *n* rough ground; (*golf*) any part of a course with grass, etc, left uncut; a first sketch. • *vt* to make rough; to sketch roughly; (*with* **up**) (*inf*) to injure violently, beat up. • *adv* in a rough manner.—**roughly** *adv.*—**roughness** *n.*

roughage /'rʌfɪdʒ/ *n* rough or coarse food or fodder, as bran, etc.

rough-and-ready *adj* unfinished but sufficient; prepared hastily.

rough-and-tumble *n* a scuffle; confusion.

roughcast /'rʌfkæst/ *n* a mixture of lime and gravel for coating buildings; a rough surface finish. • *vt* (**roughcasting, roughcast**) to coat with roughcast.

rough-cut *n* an early version of a film with the scenes edited together in sequence and a soundtrack added.

roughen /'rʌfən/ *vti* to make or become rough.

roughhouse /'rʌfhəus/ *n* (*sl*) (an instance of) noisy, boisterous or violent behaviour.

roughing /'rʌfɪŋ/ *n* an infraction in ice hockey for using excessive or unnecessary force.

roughneck /-nek/ *n* (*sl*) a coarse person.

roughshod /-ʃɒd/ *adj* marked by force without consideration.

rough stuff *n* (*inf*) violent behaviour.

rough trade *n* (*sl*) a homosexual partner who is tough and possibly violent.

roulade /ru:'lɒd/ *n* food in the shape of a roll, such as cheese or meat; (*mus*) a run of notes on one syllable.

roulette /ru:'let/ *n* a gambling game played with a revolving disc and a ball; a toothed wheel for making dots or perforations.

round /raund/ *adj* circular, spherical, or cylindrical in form; curved; plump; (*math*) expressed to the nearest ten, hundred, etc, not fractional; considerable; candid; (*style*) flowing, balanced; (*vowel*) pronounced with rounded lips. • *adv* circularly; on all sides; from one side to another; in a ring; by indirect way; through a recurring period of time; in circumference; in a roundabout way; about; near; here and there; with a rotating movement; in the opposite direction; around. • *prep* encircling; on every side of; in the vicinity of; in a circuit through; around. • *n* anything round; a circuit; (*shots*) a volley; a unit of ammunition; a series or sequence; a bout, turn; (*golf*) a circuit of a course; a stage of a contest; (*mus*) a kind of canon. • *vt* to make or become round or plump; (*math*) to express as a round number; to complete; to go or pass around. • *vi* to make a circuit; to turn; to reverse direction.—**roundly** *adv.*—**roundness** *n.*

roundabout /'raundə,baut/ *adj* indirect, circuitous. • *n* a circuitous route; a merry-go-round; (*Brit*) a traffic circle.

rounded /'raundəd/ *adj* curved or round; flowing, not angular.

roundhouse /'raʊndhɛʊs/ *n* a circular building for repairing and servicing railway locomotives.

round robin *n* a document with signatures in a circle to conceal their order.

round-shouldered *adj* with bent shoulders; stooping.

round-table conference *n* a conference with all the parties on an equal footing.

round trip *n* a journey to a place and back again.

round-trip ticket *n* a ticket whose price includes the cost of the journey to and back from a destination.

roundup /'raʊndʌp/ *n* a driving together of livestock; (*inf*) the detention of several prisoners; a summary, as of news.

roundworm /'raʊndwɔrm/ *n* a nematode parasitic in people and pigs.

rouse /raʊz/ *vti* to provoke; to stir up; to awaken; to wake up; to become active.

rousing /'raʊzɪŋ/ *adj* stirring; vigorous.

rout[1] /raʊt/ *n* a noisy crowd, a rabble; a disorderly retreat. • *vt* to defeat and put to flight.

rout[2] *vti* to grub up, as a pig; to search haphazardly; to gouge out or make a furrow in (as wood or metal); to cause to emerge, *esp* from bed; to come up with; to uncover.

route /ruːt/ *n* a course to be taken; the roads travelled on a journey. • *vt* to plan the route of; to send (by a specified route).

routine /ruːˈtiːn/ *n* a procedure that is regular and unvarying; a sequence of set movements, as in a dance, skating, etc.—*also adj.*

roux /ruː/ *n* a mixture of equal quantities of flour and melted fat used as the basis for sauces.

rove /roːv/ *vti* to wander about, roam (over).

rover /'roːvər/ *n* a wanderer; a fickle person; a senior Scout.

row[1] /roː/ *n* a line of persons or things; a line of seats (in a theatre, etc).

row[2] *vti* to propel with oars; to transport by rowing. • *n* an act or instance of rowing.—**rower** *n*.

row[3] *n* a noisy quarrel or dispute; a scolding; noise, disturbance. • *vi* to quarrel; to scold.

rowan /'roːən/ or /'raʊ-/ *n* a tree producing white flowers followed by small red berries.

rowboat /roːboːt/, **rowing boat** *n* a small boat made for rowing.

rowdy /'raʊdi/ *adj* (**rowdier, rowdiest**) rough and noisy, disorderly. • *n* (*pl* **rowdies**) a rowdy person, a hooligan.—**rowdiness, rowdyism** *n*.

rowel /'raʊəl/ *n* a spiked revolving disc at the end of a spur.

rowing machine *n* an exercise machine with oars and a sliding seat that simulates a rowing action.

rowlock /'rɒlək/ or /'rʌ-/ *n* a fitting on the side of a boat that holds an oar in place and serves as its fulcrum.

royal /'rɔɪəl/ *adj* relating to or fit for a king or queen; regal; under the patronage of a king or queen; founded by a king or queen; of a kingdom, its government, etc. • *n* a type of topsail; a stag with a head of twelve points; (*inf*) a member of a royal family.—**royally** *adv*.

royal blue *n*, *adj* deep blue.

royal flush *n* (*poker*) a straight flush headed by an ace.

royalist /'rɔɪəlɪst/ *n* a person who advocates monarchy.

royal jelly *n* a nutritious secretion of the honeybee which is fed to larvae, *esp* those destined to become queens; a preparation of this sold as a health product.

royalty /'rɔɪəlti/ *n* (*pl* **royalties**) the rank or power of a king or queen; a royal person or persons; a share of the proceeds from a patent, book, song, etc, paid to the owner, author, composer, etc.

rpm /'ɑrˈpiːˈɛm/ *abbr* = revolutions per minute.

-rrhagia *n suffix* denoting an abnormal discharge.

-rrhoea, -rrhea *n suffix* a flow.

RRIF *abbr* ♣ (*Cdn*) = Registered Retirement Income Fund.

RRSP *abbr* ♣ = Registered Retirement Savings Plan.

RSP *abbr* (*Cdn*) ♣ = Retirement Savings Plan.

RSVP /'ɑrˈɛsˈviːˈpiː/ *abbr* = répondez s'il vous plaît.

Ru (*chem symbol*) ruthenium.

rub /rʌb/ *vti* (**rubbing, rubbed**) to move (a hand, cloth, etc) over the surface of with pressure; to wipe, scour; to clean or polish; (*with* **away, off, out**) to remove or erase by friction; to chafe, grate; to fret; to take a rubbing of; (*with* **along**) to manage somehow; (*with* **down**) to rub vigorously with a towel; to smooth down. • *n* the act or process of rubbing; a drawback, difficulty.

rubber[1] /'rʌbər/ *n* an elastic substance made synthetically or from the sap of various tropical plants; an eraser; (*pl*) galoshes.

rubber[2] *n* a group of three games at whist, bridge, etc; the deciding game.

rubberize /'rʌbəraɪz/ *vt* to coat with rubber to make waterproof.

rubberneck /'rʌbərˌnɛk/ *n* (*sl*) a person who gapes, *esp* intrusively; a sightseer.—*also vi.*

rubber plant *n* an Asian plant related to the fig with shiny leaves, popular as a houseplant.

rubber-stamp *vt* (*inf*) to give automatic approval without investigation.

rubber tree *n* a tree native to South America and widely cultivated in the tropics as a source of latex to make rubber.

rubbing /'rʌbɪŋ/ *n* an impression of an inscribed brass plate, etc, obtained by rubbing a wax substance on paper laid over it.

rubbish /'rʌbɪʃ/ *n* refuse; garbage, trash; nonsense. —**rubbishy** *adj*.

rubble /'rʌbəl/ *n* rough broken stone or rock; builders' rubbish.

rubby /'rʌbi/ *n* (*pl* **rubbies**) ♣ a drunkard who consumes rubbing alcohol, aftershave lotion, or some other cheap intoxicating substance.

rubella /ruːˈbɛlə/ *n* a mild contagious viral disease that may cause damage to an unborn child; German measles.

Rubenesque /ˌruːbəˈnɛsk/ *adj* of, like or pertaining to the art of the Florentine painter Peter Paul Rubens (1577-1640); opulent, colourful; (*woman's figure*) full-breasted and shapely.

rubidium /ruːˈbɪdiəm/ *n* a soft radioactive metallic element.

ruble /'ruːbəl/ *see* **rouble**.

rubric /'ruːbrɪk/ *n* a heading or line marked out in red; any rule, explanatory comment, etc.

ruby /'ruːbi/ *n* (*pl* **rubies**) a deep red, transparent, valuable precious stone. • *adj* of the colour of a ruby.

ruby orange *n* an orange with red juice.

ruche /ruːʃ/ *vt* to pleat, gather, or flute fabric for use as a trimming. • *n* ruched fabric.

rucksack /'rʊksæk/ *n* a bag worn on the back by hikers, used to carry camping or climbing equipment.

ruction /'rʌkʃən/ *n* (*inf*) a disturbance, a row, uproar.

rudder /'rʌdər/ *n* a flat vertical piece of wood or metal hinged to the stern of a ship or boat or the rear of an aircraft to steer by; a guiding principle.

ruddy /'rʌdi/ *adj* (**ruddier, ruddiest**) reddish pink; (*complexion*) of a healthy, red colour.

rude /ruːd/ *adj* uncivil, ill-mannered; uncultured, coarse; harsh, brutal; crude, roughly made; in a natural state, primitive; vigorous, hearty.—**rudely** *adv*.—**rudeness** *n*.

rudiment /'ruːdɪmənt/ *n* a first stage; a first slight beginning of something; an imperfectly developed organ; (*pl*) elements, first principles.

rudimentary /'ruːdɪməntri/ or /-təri/ *adj* elementary; imperfectly developed or represented only by a vestige.

rue /ruː/ *vti* (**rueing, rued**) to feel remorse for (a sin, fault, etc); to regret (an act, etc). • *n* (*arch*) sorrow.

rueful /'ruːfʊl/ *adj* regretful; dejected; showing good-humoured self-pity.—**ruefully** *adv*.

ruff /rʌf/ *n* a pleated collar or frill worn round the neck; a fringe of feathers or fur round the neck of a bird or animal.

ruffian /'rʌfiən/ *n* a brutal lawless person; a villain.

ruffle /'rʌfəl/ *vti* to disturb the smoothness of, disarrange; to irritate; to agitate; to upset; to swagger about; to be quarrelsome; to flutter. • *n* pleated material used as a trim; a frill; a bird's ruff; a dispute, quarrel.

rug /rʌg/ *n* a thick heavy fabric used as a floor covering; a thick woollen wrap or coverlet.

rugby /'rʌgbi/ *n* a football game for two teams of 15 players played with an oval ball.

rugged /'rʌgəd/ *adj* rocky; rough, uneven; strong; stern; robust.—**ruggedly** *adv*.—**ruggedness** *n*.

rugger /'rʌgər/ *n* (*Brit inf*) rugby.

ruin /'ruːɪn/ *n* destruction; downfall, wrecked state; the cause of this; a loss of fortune; (*pl*) the remains of something destroyed, decayed, etc. • *vti* to destroy; to spoil; to bankrupt; to come to ruin.

ruinous /'ruːɪnəs/ *adj* in ruins, tumbledown; causing ruin, disastrous.

rule /ruːl/ *n* a straight-edged instrument for drawing lines and measuring; government; the exercise of authority; a regulation, an order; a principle, a standard; habitual practice; the code of a religious order; a straight line. • *vti* to govern, to exercise authority over; to manage; to draw (lines) with a ruler; (*with* **out**) to exclude, to eliminate; to make impossible.

rule of thumb *n* a rough commonsense approach as opposed to a precise or theoretical one.

ruler /'ru:lər/ *n* a person who governs; a strip of wood, metal, etc, with a straight edge, used in drawing lines, measuring etc.

ruling /'ru:lər/ *adj* governing; reigning; dominant. • *n* an authoritative pronouncement.

rum /rʌm/ *n* a spirit made from sugar cane.

rumba /'rʌmbə/ *n* a dance of Cuban origin with a complex rhythm. • *vi* to dance the rumba.

rumble /'rʌmbəl/ *vti* to make a low heavy rolling noise (as thunder); to move with such a sound; (*sl*) to see through, find out. • *n* the dull deep vibrant noise of thunder, etc.

rumbustious /rʌm'bʌstʃəs/ *adj* unruly, boisterous.

rumen /'ru:mən/ *n* (*pl* **rumens, rumina**) the first compartment of the stomach of a ruminant mammal.

ruminant /'ru:mənənt/ *n* a cud-chewing animal, such as cattle, deer, camels, etc. • *adj* chewing the cud; thoughtful.

ruminate /'ru:mɪˌneɪt/ *vi* to regurgitate food after it has been swallowed, chew cud; to ponder deeply, muse (on).

rummage /'rʌmɪdʒ/ *n* odds and ends; a search by ransacking. • *vti* to search thoroughly; to ransack; to fish (out).

rummage sale *n* a sale of second-hand clothes, books, etc to raise money for charity.—*also* **jumble sale**.

rummy /'rʌmi/ *n* a card game whose object is to form sets and sequences.

rumour, rumor /'ru:mər/ *n* hearsay, gossip; common talk not based on definite knowledge; an unconfirmed report, story. • *vt* to report by way of rumour.

rump /rʌmp/ *n* the hindquarters of an animal's body; the buttocks; the back end.

rumple /'rʌmpəl/ *n* a crease or wrinkle. • *vti* to crease; to disarrange, tousle.

rumpus /'rʌmpəs/ *n* (*pl* **rumpuses**) a commotion; a din.

run /rʌn/ *vi* (**running, ran** *or* **run**, *pp* **run**) to go by moving the legs faster than in walking; to hurry; to flee; to flow; to operate; to be valid; to compete in a race, election, etc; (*colours*), to merge; (*with* **across**) to meet by accident; (*with* **around** *vi* (*inf*) to associate (with); to behave evasively or promiscuously; (*with* **away** *vi* to take flight, escape; to go out of control; (*with* **away with**) to abscond, elope; to steal; to win easily; (*with* **down**) (*engine, etc*) to cease to operate through lack of power; to become tired or exhausted; (*with* **off**) to leave hastily; to decide (a race) with a run-off; (*with* **through**) to use up (money, etc) completely; to read quickly. • *vt* (*a car, etc*) to drive; (*a business, etc*) to manage; (*a story*) to publish in a newspaper; (*temperature*) to suffer from a fever; (*with* **down**) to knock down with a moving vehicle; to collide with and cause to sink; to chase and capture; to tire, exhaust; to investigate, find; to criticize persistently; (*engine, etc*) to allow to gradually lose power; to reduce in quantity; (*with* **in**) to run a new car engine gently to start with; (*inf*) to arrest; (*with* **off**) to compose and talk glibly; to produce quickly, as copies on a photocopier; (*liquid*) to drain off; (*with* **out**) to exhaust a supply; (*inf*) to desert; (*with* **over**) (*vehicle*) to knock down a person or animal; to overflow; to exceed a limit; to rehearse quickly; (*with* **through**) to pierce with a sword or knife; to rehearse; (*with* **up**) to incur or amass. • *n* an act of running; a trip; a flow; a series; prevalence; a trend; an enclosure for chickens, etc; free and unrestricted access to all parts; (*in tights, etc*) a hole, a ladder.

run-around *n* deceitful or evasive behaviour towards someone.

runaway /'rʌnəweɪ/ *n* a person or thing that runs away; a fugitive. • *adj* out of control; (*inflation*) rising uncontrollably; (*race, etc*) easily won.

run-down /'rʌndaʊn/ *adj* dilapidated; ill; tired.

rundown /'rʌndaʊn/ *n* a brief summary; the process of going into a decline.

rune /ru:n/ *n* a letter of a primitive Teutonic alphabet; a magic mark or sign.—**runic** *adj*.

run-in /'rʌnɪn/ *n* (*inf*) a quarrel.

rung[1] /rʌŋ/ *see* **ring**[2].

rung[2] *n* the step of a ladder; the crossbar of a chair.

runner /'rʌnər/ *n* an athlete; a person who runs; a smuggler; a groove or strip on which something glides.

runner bean *n* (*Brit*) a climbing plant that produces long green edible pods.

runner-up *n* (*pl* **runners-up**) the competitor who finishes second in a race, contest, etc.

running /'rʌnɪŋ/ *n* the act of moving swiftly; that which runs or flows; a racing, managing, etc. • *adj* moving swiftly; kept for a race; being in motion; continuous; discharging pus. • *adv* in succession.

running commentary *n* a verbal description on TV or radio of an event as it happens, *esp* sport.

running mate *n* the candidate in a US election standing for the less important of two positions in a linked office.

runny /'rʌni/ *adj* (**runnier, runniest**) tending to flow.

run-off /'rʌnɒf/ *n* a final deciding race, contest, etc.

run-of-the-mill *adj* average, mediocre.

runt /rʌnt/ *n* an unusually small animal, *esp* the smallest of a litter of pigs; a person of small stature.

run-through *n* a rehearsal; a cursory reading.

run-up *n* a preliminary period.

runway /'rʌnweɪ/ *n* a landing strip for aircraft.

rupee /ru:'pi:/ *n* a unit of money in India, Pakistan, Sri Lanka, Seychelles, Mauritius, and Nepal.

rupiah /ru:'pi:ə/ *n* (*pl* **rupiah, rupiahs**) the standard currency unit of Indonesia.

rupture /'rʌptʃər/ *n* a breach; a severance, quarrel; the act of bursting or breaking; hernia. • *vti* to cause or suffer a rupture.

rural /'ru:rəl/ *adj* relating to the country or agriculture, rustic.— **rurally** *adv*.

ruse /ru:z/ *n* a trick or stratagem.

rush[1] /rʌʃ/ *vti* to move, push, drive, etc, swiftly or impetuously; to make a sudden attack (on); to do with unusual haste; to hurry. • *adj* marked by or needing extra speed or urgency. • *n* a sudden surge; a sudden demand; a press, as of business, requiring unusual haste; an unedited film print.

rush[2] *n* a marsh plant; its slender pithy stem; a worthless thing.

rush hour *n* the time at the beginning and end of the working day when traffic is at its heaviest.

rusk /rʌsk/ *n* a sweet or plain bread sliced and rebaked until dry and crisp.

russet /'rʌsət/ *adj* reddish-brown. • *n* a russet colour; a winter apple with a rough russet skin; a homespun russet cloth.

Russian /'rʌʃən/ *n* a native or inhabitant of Russia; the Slavonic language of Russians.—*also adj*.

Russian roulette *n* an act of bravado in which the cylinder of a revolver loaded with a single bullet is spun and the muzzle then pointed at the head and fired.

Russo- /'rʌsəʊ/ *prefix* Russia; Russian.

rust /rʌst/ *n* a reddish oxide coating formed on iron or steel when exposed to moisture; a reddish brown colour; a red mould on plants; the fungus causing this. • *vti* to form rust (on); to deteriorate, as through disuse.

rustic /'rʌstɪk/ *n* pertaining to or characteristic of the country; rural; simple, unsophisticated. • *n* a person from the country; a simple country dweller.

rustle /'rʌsəl/ *n* a crisp, rubbing sound as of dry leaves, paper, etc. • *vti* to make or move with a rustle; to hustle; to steal (cattle); (*with* **up**) (*inf*) to collect or get together.

rustler /'rʌslər/ *n* a person who steals livestock, *esp* cattle; a hustler.

rusty /'rʌsti/ *adj* (**rustier, rustiest**) coated with rust; rust-coloured, faded; out of practice; antiquated.—**rustiness** *n*.

rut[1] *n* a track worn by wheels; an undeviating mechanical routine. • *vt* (**rutting, rutted**) to mark with ruts.

rut[2] *n* the seasonal period of sexual excitement in male ruminants, such as deer. • *vi* (**rutting, rutted**) to be in rut.

rutabaga /'ru:təˌbeɪgə/ *n* a swede.

ruthenium *n* a rare metallic element of the platinum group.

ruthless /'ru:θləs/ *adj* cruel; merciless.—**ruthlessly** *adv*.—**ruthlessness** *n*.

RV /'ɑr'vi:/ *abbr* = recreational vehicle.

rye /raɪ/ *n* a hardy annual grass; its grain, used for making flour and whiskey; a whiskey made from rye.

S

S *abbr* = Saint; siemens; small; South, Southern; (*chem symbol*) sulphur.

S, s /ɛs/ *n* the 19th letter of the English alphabet; something shaped like an S.

SA *abbr* = South Africa; South America; Salvation Army.

Sabbatarian /ˌsæbəˈtɛriən/ *n* a strict observer of the sabbath.— **Sabbatarianism** *n*.

Sabbath /ˈsæbəθ/ *n* a day of rest and worship observed on a Saturday by Jews, Sunday by Christians and Friday by Muslims.

Sabbatical /səˈbætɪkəl/ *adj* of, pertaining to, or resembling the Sabbath.

sabbatical *n* a year's leave from a teaching post, often paid, for research or travel.

SABC *abbr* = South African Broadcasting Corporation.

saber *see* **sabre**.

sabin /ˈseɪbɪn/ *n* (*physics*) a unit of acoustic absorption.

Sabine /ˈsæbaɪn/ *n* a member of an ancient people who lived in the central Apennines in Italy.—*also adj*.

sable /ˈseɪbəl/ *n* a carnivorous mammal of arctic regions valued for its luxuriant dark brown fur; its fur.

sabot /ˈsæˈboː/ or /ˈsæboː/ *n* a shoe made from a single piece of wood; a shoe with a wooden sole and cloth upper.

sabotage /ˈsæbəˌtɒʒ/ *n* deliberate damage of machinery, or disruption of public services, by enemy agents, disgruntled employees, etc, to prevent their effective operation. • *vt* to practise sabotage on; to spoil, disrupt.

saboteur /ˌsæbəˈtər/ *n* a person who engages in sabotage.

sabra /ˈsæbrə/ *n* a Jew born in Israel.

sabre /ˈseɪbər/ *n* a cavalry sword with a curved blade; a light fencing sword.—*also* **saber**.

sabre-rattling *n* (*inf*) a conspicuous display of military power or aggression.

sabre-toothed tiger *n* an extinct species of large cat with long curved upper canine teeth.

sac /sæk/ *n* a bag-like part or cavity in a plant or animal.

saccate /ˈsækət/ *adj* in the shape of a sac or pouch.

saccharide /ˈsækəˌraɪd/ *n* a sugar.

saccharimeter /səˈkærɪmətər/ *n* an instrument for measuring the concentration of sugar solutions.

saccharin /ˈsækərɪn/ or /ˈsækrɪn/ *n* a non-fattening sugar substitute.

saccharine /ˈsækəˌrɪn/ or /ˈsækrɪn/ *adj* containing sugar; excessively sweet.

saccharo-, sacchar- /ˈsækəro/ *prefix* sugar.

sacerdotal /ˌsæsərˈdoːtəl/ *adj* relating to priests or the priesthood.—**sacerdotalism** *n*.—**sacerdotally** *adv*.

sachem /ˈseɪtʃəm/ *n* an American Indian chief of certain tribes; a political boss.

sachet /sæˈʃeɪ/ *n* a sealed envelope or packet; a small perfumed bag or pad used to perfume clothes.

sack[1] /sæk/ *n* a large bag made of coarse cloth used as a container; the contents of this; a loose-fitting dress or coat; (*baseball*) a bag serving as a base; (*sl: with* **the**) dismissal. • *vt* to put into sacks; (*sl*) to dismiss.

sack[2] *n* the plunder or destruction of a place. • *vt* to plunder or loot.

sackbut /ˈsækbʌt/ *n* a type of medieval trombone.

sackcloth /ˈsækklɒθ/ *n* a coarse fabric for sacks, etc; penitential clothing.

sacking /ˈsækɪŋ/ *n* the coarse cloth used for sacks; the storming and plundering of a place.

sack race *n* a jumping race in which the participants' legs and lower bodies are enclosed in sacks.

sacra *see* **sacrum**.

sacrament /ˈsækrəmənt/ *n* a religious ceremony forming outward and visible sign of inward and spiritual grace, *esp* baptism and the Eucharist; the consecrated elements in the Eucharist, *esp* the bread; a sacred symbol or pledge.

sacramental /ˌsækrəˈmentəl/ *adj* of, pertaining to, or like a sacrament. • *n* (*RC Church*) a rite recognized as similar to a sacrament, *eg* the use of holy water.—**sacramentally** *adv*.

sacred /ˈseɪkrəd/ *adj* regarded as holy; consecrated to a god or God; connected with religion; worthy of or regarded with reverence, sacrosanct.

sacred cow *n* (*inf*) a person or thing regarded as above criticism.

sacrifice /ˈsækrɪˌfaɪs/ *n* the act of offering ceremonially to a deity; the slaughter of an animal (or person) to please a deity; the surrender of something valuable for the sake of something more important or worthy; loss without return; something sacrificed, an offering. • *vt* to slaughter or give up as a sacrifice; to give up for a higher good; to sell at a loss.—**sacrificial** *adj*.

sacrilege /ˈsækrɪlɪdʒ/ *n* violation of anything holy or sacred.

sacrilegious /-ˈlɪdʒəs/ *adj* guilty of sacrilege; irreverent.—**sacrilegiously** *adv*.—**sacrilegiousness** *n*.

sacristan /ˈsækrɪstən/ *n* a person in charge of the contents of a church; a sexton.

sacristy /ˈsækrɪsti/ *n* (*pl* **sacristies**) a room in a church where the sacred vessels, etc are kept.

sacrosanct /ˈsækroˌsæŋkt/ *adj* inviolable; very holy.

sacrum /ˈsækrəm/ or /ˈseɪkrəm/ *n* (*pl* **sacra**) a compound bone at the base of the spine forming the back of the pelvis.

sad /sæd/ *adj* (**sadder, saddest**) expressing grief or unhappiness; sorrowful; deplorable.—**sadly** *adv*.—**sadness** *n*.

sadden /ˈsædən/ *vti* to make or become sad.

saddle /ˈsædəl/ *n* a seat, *usu* of leather, for a rider on a horse, bicycle, etc; a ridge connecting two mountain peaks; a joint of mutton or venison consisting of the two loins; in **the saddle** mounted on a saddle; in control. • *vt* to put a saddle on; to burden, encumber.

saddlebag /ˈsædəlˌbæg/ *n* a bag hung from the saddle of a horse or bicycle.

saddlebow /-ˌboː/ *n* the arched front of a saddle.

saddlecloth /-ˌklɒθ/ or /-ˌklɒθ/ *n* a piece of cloth placed under a horse's saddle to prevent chafing.

saddler /ˈsædlər/ *n* a person who makes or sells saddles, harness, etc.

saddlery /ˈsædləri/ *n* (*pl* **saddleries**) articles made by a saddler; the business or premises of a saddler.

saddle soap *n* an oily soap for cleaning and preserving leather.

saddletree /ˈsædˌltriː/ *n* the frame of a saddle.

sadhu, saddhu /ˈsɒduː/ *n* a Hindu holy man.

sadism /ˈseɪdɪzəm/ *n* sexual pleasure obtained from inflicting cruelty upon another; extreme cruelty.—**sadist** *n*.—**sadistic** *adj*.—**sadistically** *adv*.

sadomasochism /ˌseɪdoːˈmæsəˌkɪzəm/ *n* sexual pleasure obtained from inflicting cruelty upon oneself and receiving it from another.—**sadomasochist** *n*.—**sadomasochistic** *adj*.

s.a.e. *abbr* = stamped addressed envelope.

safari /səˈfɑri/ *n* (*pl* **safaris**) a journey or hunting expedition, *esp* in Africa.

safari jacket *n* a belted shirt jacket with pleated pockets.

safari suit *n* a safari jacket and matching trousers or skirt made from denim or similar hard-wearing material.

safe /seɪf/ *adj* unhurt; out of danger; reliable; secure; involving no risk; trustworthy; giving protection; prudent; sure; incapable of doing harm. • *n* a locking metal box or compartment for valuables.—**safely** *adv*.

safe-conduct *n* written permission for the holder to travel safely through hostile country.

safecracker *n* a person who opens and robs safes.—*also* **safebreaker**.—**safecracking** *n*.

safe-deposit *adj* (*box, room, etc*) designed for the protective storage of valuables, deeds, etc. • *n* a building with safes for renting—*also* **safety deposit**.

safeguard /ˈseɪfgɑrd/ *n* anything that protects against injury or danger; a proviso against foreseen risks. • *vt* to protect.

safe house *n* a refuge for victims of domestic violence, sexual abuse, etc run by social welfare organizations; a clandestine place used by intelligence services, terrorists, etc as a refuge.

safekeeping /ˌseɪfˈkiːpɪŋ/ *n* the act or process of keeping safely; protection.

safe period *n* the time in a woman's menstrual cycle when she is least likely to conceive.

safe seat *n* a parliamentary constituency in which the sitting MP enjoys a substantial majority and can be assured of re-election.

safe sex *n* sex in which precautions are taken to lessen the risk of catching AIDS or other sexually transmitted diseases.

safety /'seɪftɪ/ *n* (*pl* **safeties**) freedom from danger; the state of being safe.

safety belt *n* a belt worn by a person working at a great height to prevent falling; a seatbelt in a car.

safety curtain *n* a fireproof curtain that can be lowered to separate a theatre stage from the auditorium.

safety deposit *see* **safe-deposit**.

safety glass *n* shatterproof glass.

safety lamp *n* a miner's lamp in which the flame is enclosed by a protective gauze to prevent it igniting combustible gases.

safety match *n* a match that will only ignite on a particular surface.

safety net *n* a net suspended beneath acrobats, etc; any protection against loss.

safety pin *n* a pin with a guard to cover the point.

safety razor *n* a razor with a guard that covers the blade to protect the skin from accidental cuts.

safety valve *n* an automatic valve for relieving excess pressure of steam, etc; a harmless outlet for emotion.

saffian /'sæfɪən/ *n* a brightly dyed leather made from the skin of goats or sheep.

safflower /'sæflaʊr/ *n* (a red dye and oil derived from) a thistle-like plant with large orange or red flowers.

saffron /'sæfrən/ *n* a crocus whose bright yellow stigmas are used as a food colouring and flavouring; an orange-yellow colour.

sag /sæg/ *vi* (**sagging, sagged**) to droop downward in the middle; to sink or hang down unevenly under pressure.

saga /'sægə/ or /'sɒgə/ *n* a long story of heroic deeds.

sagacious /sə'geɪʃəs/ *adj* mentally acute, shrewd; wise.—**sagaciously** *adv*.—**sagaciousness** *n*.

sagacity /sə'gæsɪtɪ/ *n* (*pl* **sagacities**) readiness of apprehension; discriminating intelligence; acute practical judgment.

sagamore /'sægə,mɔr/ *n* an American Indian chief of certain tribes.

sage[1] /seɪdʒ/ *adj* wise through reflection and experience. • *n* a person of profound wisdom.—**sagely** *adv*.—**sagely** *adv*.

sage[2] *n* a herb with leaves used for flavouring food; sagebrush.

sagebrush /'seɪdʒbrʌʃ/ *n* a low shrub of the alkaline plains of North America.

sagger, saggar /'sægər/ *n* a fireproof clay case in which procelain is put for baking.

sagittate /'sædʒɪ,teɪt/ *adj* (*leaf*) shaped like an arrowhead.

Sagittarius /sædʒɪ'terɪəs/ *n* the Archer, ninth sign of the zodiac; in astrology, operative November 22–December 20.—**Sagittarian** *adj, n*.

sago /'seɪgəʊ/ *n* (*pl* **sagos**) a type of Asian palm; its starchy pith used in puddings.

saguaro /sə'gwɑrəʊ/ *n* (*pl* **saguaros**) a large cactus of North American and Mexican desert areas bearing white flowers and edible fruit.

sahib /'sɑhɪb/ or /'sɑɪb/ *n* a form of polite address formerly used by Indians to European men.

said /sed/ *see* **say**.

saiga /'saɪgə/ or /'seɪ–/ *n* a stocky antelope of the Russian steppes.

sail /seɪl/ *n* a piece of canvas used to catch the wind to propel or steer a vessel; sails collectively; anything like a sail; an arm of a windmill; a voyage in a sailing vessel; **under sail** with the sails set; under way. • *vt* to navigate a vessel; to manage (a vessel); **to set sail** to spread the sails; to begin a voyage. • *vi* to be moved by sails; to travel by water; to glide or pass smoothly; to walk in a stately manner.

sailboard /'seɪlbɔrd/ *n* a type of large surfboard with a sail used in windsurfing.

sailboat /'seɪlboʊt/ *n* a sailing boat.

sailcloth /'seɪlklɒθ/ *n* canvas used for sails; a strong durable fabric for clothing.

sailer /'seɪlər/ *n* a sailing vessel.

sailfish /'seɪlfɪʃ/ *n* (*pl* **sailfish, sailfishes**) a large game fish of tropical waters with a long sail-like dorsal fin.

sailing /'seɪlɪŋ/ *n* the act of sailing; the motion or direction of a ship, etc on water; a departure from a port.

sailing boat *n* a boat that is propelled by a sail or sails.

sailor /'seɪlər/ *n* a person who sails; one of a ship's crew.

sailoring /'seɪlərɪŋ/ *n* a sailor's life.

sailplane *n* a type of light glider. • *vi* to fly a sailplane.

sain /seɪn/ *vt* (*arch*) to make the sign of the cross on; to bless in order to protect from evil.

sainfoin /'seɪnfoɪn/ or /'sæn–/ *n* a Eurasian leguminous plant with pink flowers, grown for fodder.

saint /seɪnt/ *n* a person who is very patient, charitable, etc; a person who is canonized by the Roman Catholic church; one of the blessed in heaven.—**sainthood** *n*.

Saint Bernard *n* a breed of large dog with a reddish brown coat, often used as a rescue dog.

sainted /'seɪntəd/ *adj* canonized; holy; dead; much admired.

St Jean Baptist Day *n* ✹ (*Cdn*) in Quebec, common and formerly official name of a public holiday celebrated on June 24.

saintly /'seɪntlɪ/ *adj* (**saintlier, saintliest**) of, like, or relating to a saint.—**saintliness** *n*.

Saint Patrick's Day *n* March 17, observed by the Irish in honour of the patron saint of Ireland.

saint's day *n* a day in the church calender which is devoted to the commemoration of a particular saint.

sake[1] /seɪk/ *n* behalf; purpose; benefit; interest.

sake[2] /'sɒki/ **saké, saki** *n* a Japanese alcoholic drink made from fermented rice and drunk warm.

sal /sɒl/ *n* (*chem*) a salt.

salaam /sə'lɒm/ *n* a form of ceremonial greeting in Muslim countries. • *vti* to make a salaam (to).

salable *adj* marketable; in good demand.—*also* **saleable**.

salacious /sə'leɪʃəs/ *adj* lustful; obscene.—**salaciously** *adv*.—**salaciousness** *n*.

salad /'sæləd/ *n* a dish, *usu* cold, of vegetables, fruits, meat, eggs, etc; lettuce, etc, used for this.

salad bar *n* a buffet in a restaurant at which diners choose their own salads.

salad days *npl* a time of youth and inexperience.

salad dressing *n* a cooked or uncooked sauce of oil, vinegar, spices, etc, to put on a salad.

salade niçoise *n* a salad of various ingredients, including tomatoes, hard-boiled eggs, and anchovy fillets or tuna fish.

salal /sə'læl/ *n* ✹ a shrub of western North America with pink or white flowers and edible purple-black berries.

salamander /'sælə,mændər/ *n* any of various lizard-like amphibians; a mythical lizard-like creature that was supposedly impervious to fire.

salami /sə'lɒmi/ *n* a highly seasoned Italian sausage.

salaried /'sælərɪd/ *adj* receiving a salary.

salary /'sælərɪ/ *n* (*pl* **salaries**) fixed, regular payment for non-manual work, *usu* paid monthly.

salchow /'saʊkaʊ/ *n* (*ice-skating*) a jump incorporating turns in the air.

sale /seɪl/ *n* the act of selling; the exchange of goods or services for money; the market or opportunity of selling; an auction; the disposal of goods at reduced prices; the period of this.

saleable /'seɪləbəl/ *see* **salable**.

salep /'sæləp/ *n* (food made from) the starchy dried roots of various orchidaceous plants.

saleratus /sælə'rætəs/ *n* sodium bicarbonate used in cooking.

saleroom /'seɪlruːm/ *n* a salesroom; an auction room.

salesclerk /'seɪlzˌklɑrk/ *n* a person who sells goods in a store.

salesman /'seɪlzmən/ *n* (*pl* **salesmen**) a person who sells either in a given territory or in a store.—**saleswoman** *nf* (*pl* **saleswomen**).

salesmanship /-ʃɪp/ *n* the art or skill of selling.

salesperson /'seɪlzˌpɜrsən/ *n* (*pl* **salespeople**) a salesman or saleswoman.

sales representative *n* a person who travels to sell within a given territory.

salesroom /'seɪlzruːm/ *n* a place where goods are displayed for sale; a saleroom.

sales talk *n* talk aimed at selling something; any talk to persuade.

sales tax *n* a tax levied (*usu* as a percentage) on the price of an object bought by a consumer.

Salic /'sælɪk/ or /'seɪ–/ *adj* of or pertaining to the Franks; relating to the Salic law.

Salic law *n* the law of the Franks excluding females from the succession to the French throne.

salicin /'sælɪsɪn/ *n* a bitter compound obtained from the bark of willows and poplars, used in medicine.

salient /'seɪlɪənt/ *adj* projecting outward; conspicuous; noteworthy; leaping, gushing.—**salience, saliency** *n*.—**saliently** *adv*.

salify /'sælɪ.faɪ/ *vt* to make salty; (*chem*) to convert into a salt.—**salification** *n*.

salimeter /'sælɪ.mɪtər/ *n* a device for measuring the amount of salt in a solution.

saline /'seɪliːn/ *adj* of or impregnated with salt or salts; salty. • *n* a solution of salt and water.—**salinity** *n*.

Salishan /'sælɪʃən/ *n* ✹ a speaker of one of a grouping of Indian languages in the Pacific Northwest coast of North America; the language spoken by a people using one of these languages. • *adj* of or pertaining to this people or their language.

saliva /sə'laɪvə/ *n* the liquid secreted by glands in the mouth that aids digestion.—**salivary** *adj*.

salivate /'sælɪveɪt/ *vi* to secrete saliva, *esp* excessively.—**salivation** *n*.

sallenders /'sælɪndərz/ *npl* an eczematous rash on a horse's hock.

sallet /'sælət/ *n* a light helmet of the 15th century.

sallow /'sælo:/ *adj* (*complexion*) an unhealthy yellow colour, a pale brown colour.—**sallowness** *n*.

sally /'sæli/ *n* (*pl* sallies) a sudden attack; an outburst; a lively remark, quip. • *vi* (**sallying, sallied**) to make a sally; to go (forth).

salmagundi /ˌsælmə'gʊndi/ *n* a mixed dish of chopped meat, anchovies, eggs, vegetables, etc; a miscellany.

salmi /'sɒlmi/ *n* (*pl* salmis) a casserole of game-birds in a rich wine sauce.

salmon /'sæmən/ *n* (*pl* salmon, salmons) a large silvery edible fish that lives in salt water and spawns in fresh water; salmon pink.

salmonella /ˌsælmə'nelə/ *n* (*pl* salmonellae, salmonella, salmonellas) any of a genus of bacteria that causes food poisoning and diseases of the genital tract.

salmon ladder *n* a series of steps (*eg* in a waterfall or dam) to allow salmon to swim upstream to their breeding grounds.

salmon pink *adj* a yellowish pink colour.

salmon trout *n* a large trout resembling a salmon.

salon /sə'lɒn/ *n* a large reception hall or drawing room for receiving guests; the shop of a hairdresser, beautician, or couturier; an art gallery.

saloon /sə'luːn/ *n* a large reception room; a large cabin for the social use of a ship's passengers; a four-seater car with a boot; a place where alcoholic drinks are sold and consumed.

saloon bar *n* a comfortably furnished bar.

salopettes /ˌsælə'pets/ *npl* thick quilted trousers with shoulder straps, worn for skiing.

salsa /'sælsə/ *n* (the music for) a type of Puerto Rican dance.

salsify /'sælsə.fi/ *n* (*pl* salsifies) a purple-flowered plant with an edible root.

SALT /sɒlt/ *abbr* = Strategic Arms Limitation Talks *or* Treaty.

salt /sɒlt/ *n* a white crystalline substance (sodium chloride) used as a seasoning or preservative; piquancy, wit; (*chem*) a compound of an acid and a base; (*pl*) mineral salt as an aperient. • *adj* containing or tasting of salt; preserved with salt; pungent. • *vt* to flavour, pickle or sprinkle with salt; to give flavour or piquancy to (as a story); (*with* away) to hoard; to keep for the future.

saltbush /'sɒltbʊʃ/ *n* a shrub-like plant which provides grazing in dry regions.

salt cellar /'sɒlt.selər/ *n* a vessel for salt at the table; a saltshaker.

saltchuck /'sɒlttʃek/ *n* ✹ on the Pacific Northwest coast of North America, the ocean or one of its outlets.

salter /'sɒltər/ *n* ✹ someone who or something that salts; (*Cdn*) a truck that dispenses salt on roads to melt snow and ice.

saltire /'sɒl.taɪr/ *n* an X-shaped cross dividing a shield, flag, etc, into four compartments.

salt lick *n* an area where animals go to lick salt residue; a block of salt for animals to lick.

salt marsh *n* an area regularly flooded by seawater.

saltpan *n* a hollow or depression where salt is deposited by evaporating seawater.

saltpetre, saltpeter /ˌsɒlt'piːtər/ *n* a white powder (potassium nitrate) used in making gunpowder, etc.

saltshaker *n* a container for salt with a perforated top.

saltwater *adj* of or living in salt water or the sea.

salty /'sɒlti/ *adj* (**saltier, saltiest**) of, containing or tasting of salt; witty; earthy, coarse.

salubrious /sə'luːbrɪəs/ *adj* health-giving; wholesome.—**salubriously** *adv*.—**salubriousness** *n*.

saluki /sə'luːki/ *n* a breed of tall, slender hounds with long silky coats.

salutary /'sælju.tərɪ/ *adj* beneficial, wholesome.—**salutarily** *adv*.—**salutariness** *n*.

salutation /ˌsælju:'teɪʃən/ *n* a greeting; the words used in it.

salute /sə'luːt/ *n* a gesture of respect or greeting; (*mil*) a motion of the right hand to the head, or to a rifle; a discharge of guns, etc, as a military mark of honour. • *vti* to make a salute (to); to greet; to kiss; to praise or honour.

salvable /'sælvəbəl/ *adj* able to be salvaged.

salvage /'sælvɪdʒ/ *n* the rescuing of a ship or property from loss at sea, by fire, etc; the reward paid for this; the thing salvaged; waste material intended for further use. • *vt* to save from loss or danger.—**salvageable** *adj*.—**salvager** *n*.

salvation /sæl'veɪʃən/ *n* the act of saving or the state of being saved; in Christianity, the deliverance from evil; a means of preservation.—**salvational** *adj*.

Salvation Army *n* an international religious and charitable group organized on military lines founded by William Booth in 1865.—**Salvationist** *n*.

salve[1] /sælv/ *or* /sæv/ *n* a healing ointment or balm; a soothing influence. • *vt* to apply ointment to; to smooth over; to soothe.

salve[2] *vt* to salvage; (*arch*) to save.

salver /'sælvər/ *n* a small tray.

salvia /'sælvɪə/ *n* any of a genus of plants or small shrubs with red or purple flowers.

salvo[1] /'sælvo:/ *n* (**salvoes, salvos**) a firing of several guns or missiles simultaneously; a sudden burst; a spirited verbal attack.

salvo[2] *n* (*pl* salvos) an exception or reservation.

sal volatile /ˌsælvə'lætɪli/ *n* a solution of ammonium carbonate in alcohol used as a remedy for faintness.

salvor /'sælvər/ *n* a person or vessel effecting a salvage at sea.

SAM (*abbr*) surface-to-air missile.

samara /sə'mærə/ *or* /sə'mɑrə/ *n* a dry winged single-seeded fruit produced by the ash, elm, etc.

Samaritan /sə'mærɪtən/ *n* a native or inhabitant of Samaria in ancient Palestine; a compassionate person; a Good Samaritan; a member of a voluntary organization that helps people in distress or despair.

samarium /sə'merɪəm/ *n* a silvery metallic element used in lasers and alloys.

samba /'sæmbə/ *n* a Brazilian dance of African origin; the music for this. • *vi* to dance the samba.

same /seɪm/ *adj* identical; exactly similar; unchanged; uniform, monotonous; previously mentioned. • *pron* the same person or thing. • *adv* in like manner.

sameness /-nəs/ *n* the state of being the same; monotony.

Samian /'seɪmɪən/ *n* a native or inhabitant of the Aegean island of Samos in Greece. • *adj* of or pertaining to Samos or its people.

Samian ware *n* a type of red or black pottery from Samos.

samisen /'sæmɪsɪn/ *n* a Japanese guitar-like instrument with three strings.

samite /'sæmaɪt/ *or* /'seɪ-/ *n* a medieval heavy silken fabric.

samizdat /'sæmɪz.dæt/ *or* /-'dæt/ *n* in the former Soviet Union, a system for the clandestine printing and distribution of banned literature.

Samoan /sə'moːən/ *n* a native or inhabitant of Samoa, a group of islands in the South Pacific; the Polynesian language of Samoa. • *adj* of or pertaining to Samoa, its people or language.

samosa /sə'moːsə/ *n* (*pl* samosas, samosa) an Indian savoury pasty with a spicy meat or vegetable filling.

samovar /'sæmə.vɑr/ *n* a metal urn with an internal element used for boiling water for tea, *esp* in Russia.

Samoyed /'sæmə.jed/ *n* a member of a people of the northern Urals; the language of these people; a breed of sledge-dog with a thick creamy coat and a tightly curled tail.—**Samoyedic** *adj*.

sampan /'sæm.pæn/ *n* a small flat-bottomed Chinese river boat.

samphire /'sæm.faɪr/ *n* a Eurasian coastal rock plant with edible fleshy leaves.

sample /'sæmpəl/ *n* a specimen; a small part representative of the whole; an instance. • *vt* (*food, drink*) to taste a small quantity of; to test by taking a sample.

sampler /'sæmplər/ *n* a person who takes samples; something containing a representative selection (as a record, book); an assortment; a piece of ornamental embroidery showing different stitches and patterns as an example of skill.

sampling /'sæmplɪŋ/ *n* (*mus industry*) the practice of extracting phrases from several recorded songs and putting them together electronically to make a new one.

samurai /'sæmu,raɪ/ *n* (*pl* **samurai**) a member of an ancient Japanese warrior caste.

samurai bond *n* a financial bond issued in yen by a non-Japanese company.

-san *n suffix* a Japanese title of respect similar to Mr, Mrs, etc.

sanatorium /,sænə'tɔːriəm/ *see* **sanitarium**.

sancta *see* **sanctum**.

sanctified /'sæŋktɪ,faɪd/ *adj* hallowed; consecrated; sanctimonious.

sanctify /'sæŋktɪ,faɪ/ *vt* (**sanctifying, sanctified**) to make holy; to purify from sin or evil; (*the Church*) to give official approval.—**sanctification** *n*.—**sanctifier** *n*.

sanctimonious /,sæŋktɪ'məʊniəs/ *adj* pretending to be holy; hypocritically pious or righteous.—**sanctimoniously** *adv*.—sanctimoniousness *n*.

sanctimony /'sæŋktɪ,məʊni/ *n* self-righteousness; hypocrisy.

sanction /'sæŋkʃən/ *n* express permission, authorization; a binding influence; a penalty by which a law is enforced, *esp* a prohibition on trade with a country that has violated international law. • *vt* to permit; to give authority.—**sanctionable** *adj*.

sanctity /'sæŋktɪti/ *n* (*pl* **sanctities**) the condition of being holy or sacred; inviolability.

sanctuary /'sæŋktʃuː,eri/ *n* (*pl* **sanctuaries**) a sacred place; the part of a church around the altar; a place where one is free from arrest or violence, an asylum; a refuge; an animal reserve.

sanctum /'sæŋktəm/ *n* (*pl* **sanctums, sancta**) a holy place; a private room where one is not to be disturbed.

Sanctus /'sæŋktəs/ *n* (*Christianity*) the hymn "Holy, holy, holy" used in communion; an orchestral setting of this.

sand /sænd/ *n* very fine rock particles; (*pl*) a desert; a sandy beach. • *vt* to smooth or polish with sand or sandpaper; to sprinkle with sand. • *adj* reddish yellow.

sandal[1] /'sændəl/ *n* a shoe consisting of a sole strapped to the foot; a low slipper or shoe.—**sandalled, sandaled** *adj*.

sandal[2] *n* sandalwood.

sandalwood /'sændəl,wʊd/ *n* the yellow, scented wood of an Asian tree; the tree.

sandbag /'sændbæg/ *n* a bag of sand used for ballast or to protect against floodwater. • *vt* (**sandbagging, sandbagged**) to protect by laying sandbags; to hit with a sandbag; (*inf*) to coerce; (*sl*) to deceive.—**sandbagger** *n*.

sandbank /'sændbæŋk/ *n* a sand bar; a large deposit of sand forming a hill or mound.

sand bar /'sændbɑr/ *n* a ridge of sand built up in a river, a lake, or coastal waters by currents.

sandblast /'sændblæst/ *vt* (*a building*) to clean by blasting with sand at high velocity.—*also n*.

sand box /'sændbɒks/ *n* a small enclosure filled with sand for children to play in.—*also* **sandpit**.

sand castle /'sænd,kæsəl/ *n* a model of a castle moulded from damp sand, as made at the seaside by children.

sander /'sændər/ *n* a power-driven tool for sanding wood or other surfaces.

sanderling /'sændərlɪŋ/ *n* a small wading bird.

sandglass /'sændglæs/ *n* an instrument that measures time by the running of sand through a narrow aperture.

S & L *abbr* = savings and loan association.

S & M *abbr* = sadomasochism.

sandman /'sændmæn/ *n* (*pl* **sandmen**) (*folklore*) an imaginary being who sends children to sleep by sprinkling sand in their eyes.

sand martin *n* a small European songbird that nests in holes in sandy riverbanks, etc.

sandpaper /'sænd,peɪpər/ *n* a paper coated on one side with sand or another abrasive, used to smooth or polish. • *vt* to rub with sandpaper.

sandpiper /'sænd,paɪpər/ *n* any of numerous small wading birds.

sandpit /'sændpɪt/ *see* **sand box**.

sandstone /'sændstɔːn/ *n* a sedimentary rock of compacted sand.

sandstorm /'sændstɔːm/ *n* a windstorm in a desert carrying clouds of sand.

sand trap *n* (*golf*) a pit of sand forming an obstacle on a golf course, a bunker.

sand wedge *n* (*golf*) a club for hitting the ball out of a sand trap.

sandwich /'sændwɪtʃ/ or /'sænwɪtʃ/, /'sæm-/ *n* two slices of bread with meat, cheese, or other filling between; anything in a sandwich-like arrangement. • *vt* to place between two things or two layers; to make such a place for.

sandwich board *n* two asu hinged boards hanging from the shoulders, one in front and one at the back, carried by a sandwich man.

sandwich man *n* a person who advertises by wearing a sandwich board.

sandy /'sændi/ *adj* (**sandier, sandiest**) of, like, or sprinkled with sand; yellowish grey.—**sandiness** *n*.

sane /seɪn/ *adj* mentally sound, not mad; reasonable, sensible.—**sanely** *adv*.—**saneness** *n*.

sang *see* **sing**.

sangfroid /sæŋ'frwɒ/ or /sɑ̃-/, /-fwɔ/ *n* coolness in danger, imperturbability.

Sangreal /'sæŋgriəl/ *n* the Holy Grail.

sangria /sæŋ'griːə/ *n* a Spanish drink made with red wine, orange juice and fresh fruit laced with brandy.

sanguinary /'sæŋgwɪnˌeri/ *adj* accompanied by bloodshed; bloodthirsty.—**sanguinarily** *adv*.

sanguine /'sæŋgwɪn/ *adj* confident, hopeful; blood-red; (*complexion*) ruddy.—**sanguineness** *n*.

sanguinely /-li/ *adv* confidently, hopefully.

sanguineous /-nəs/ *adj* of or relating to blood; full-blooded; blood-red; sanguinary; sanguine.

sanies /'seɪniːz/ *n* a watery mixture of blood and pus discharged from a sore or wound.—**sanious** *adj*.

sanitarian /,sænɪ'teriən/ *adj* hygienic. • *n* a specialist in matters of public health.

sanitarium /,sænɪ'teriəm/ *n* (*pl* **sanitariums, sanitaria**) an establishment for the treatment of convalescents or the chronically ill.—*also* **sanatorium**.

sanitary /'sænɪˌteri/ *adj* relating to the promotion and protection of health; relating to the supply of water, drainage, and sewage disposal; hygienic.—**sanitarily** *adv*.—**sanitariness** *n*.

sanitary cordon *n* a cordon sanitaire.

sanitary engineering *n* the design, construction and installation of water and sewage systems.—**sanitary engineer** *n*.

sanitary napkin, sanitary towel *n* an absorbent pad worn externally during menstruation.

sanitation /,sænɪ'teɪʃən/ *n* the science and practice of achieving hygienic conditions; drainage and disposal of sewage.

sanitize /'sænəˌtaɪz/ *vt* to clean or sterilize; to make (language, etc) more respectable or acceptable.

sanity /'sænɪti/ *n* the condition of being sane; mental health; common sense.

sank *see* **sink**.

Sanka /'sæŋkə/ *n* (*trademark*) a decaffeinated coffee.

sannup /'sænəp/ *n* an American Indian warrior, a brave.

Sans. *abbr* = Sanskrit.

sans /sɒnz/ or /sɑ̃/ *prep* without.

sansculotte /,sɑ̃kjuː'lɒt/ *n* in the French Revolution, a man without breeches, a term of contempt applied to a revolutionary who wore pantaloons instead of knee breeches; any revolutionary.

sans doute *Fr.* /sɒn'duːt/ doubtless; certainly.

Sansk. *abbr* = Sanskrit.

Sanskrit /'sænskrɪt/ *n* the ancient language used in Indian and Hindu sacred literature.—**Sanskrit** *adj*.—**Sanskritic** *adj*.

sans-serif, sanserif *n* (*print*) a character or typeface with no serifs.

sans souci *Fr.* /sɒnsuː'siː/ free from care.

Santa /'sæntə/ *n* Santa Claus. • *adj* sainted, holy.

Santa Claus /'sæntə,klɒz/ *n* a legendary fat, white-bearded old man who brings presents to children at Christmas.—*also* **Father Christmas**.

sap[1] /sæp/ *n* the vital juice of plants; energy and health; (*inf*) a fool. • *vt* (**sapping, sapped**) to drain of sap; to exhaust the energy of.

sap[2] *n* a narrow or covered siege trench; the digging of this, undermining. • *vti* (**sapping, sapped**) to attack by or dig a sap; to undermine insidiously.

saphead /'sæp,hed/ *n* (*sl*) a fool, a stupid person.

sapid /'sæpɪd/ *adj* having a pleasing flavour; agreeable.—**sapidity** *n*.

sapient /'seɪpiənt/ *adj* (*often ironical*) wise, discerning.—**sapience** *n*.—**sapiently** *adv*.

sapling /'sæplɪŋ/ *n* a young tree; a youth.

saponify /sə'pɒnɪˌfaɪ/ *vt* (**saponifying, saponified**) (*chem*) to convert (fat, oil, etc) into soap by combination with an alkali. • *vi* to undergo this process.—**saponification** *n*.—**saponifier** *n*.

sapor /'seɪpər/ *n* taste, flavour.

sapper /ˈsæpər/ *n* one who or that which saps; a soldier who lays, detects or disarms mines.

sapphire /ˈsæfaɪr/ *n* a transparent blue precious stone; a deep pure blue.—*also adj.*

sapro-, sapr- /ˈsæproː/ *prefix* dead or decaying matter.

saprogenic /ˌsæprəˈdʒɛnɪk/, **saprogenous** /-ˈdʒɛnəs/ *adj* producing or caused by putrefaction.

saprophagous /sæˈprɒfəgəs/ *adj* feeding on decaying matter.

saprophyte /ˈsæprəˌfaɪt/ *n* a plant or fungus that grows on dead organic matter.—**saprophytic** *adj.*

Saracen /ˈsærəsən/ *n* a member of a nomadic people of the Syrian desert; a Muslim at the time of the Crusades. • *adj* of or pertaining to Saracens.—**Saracenic** *adj.*

sarcasm /ˈsɑrˌkæzəm/ *n* a scornful or ironic remark; the use of this.—**sarcastic** *adj.*—**sarcastically** *adv.*

sarco- /ˈsɑrkoː/, **sarc-** /sɑrk/ *prefix* flesh.

sarcoma /sɑrˈkoːmə/ *n* (*pl* **sarcomas, sarcomata**) a malignant tumour of connective tissue.—**sarcomatous** *adj.*

sarcophagus /sɑrˈkɒfəgəs/ *n* (*pl* **sarcophagi, sarcophaguses**) a large stone coffin or tomb.

sard /sɑrd/ *n* an orange-red variety of chalcedony.

sardine /sɑrˈdiːn/ *n* (*pl* **sardines, sardine**) a small, edible seafish.

sardonic /sɑrˈdɒnɪk/ *adj* (*smile, etc*) derisive, mocking, maliciously jocular.—**sardonically** *adv.*

sardonyx /ˈsɑrdəɑnɪks/ *n* an onyx with alternate layers of white chalcedony and orange sard.

sargasso /sɑrˈgæsoː/ *n* (*pl* **sargassos**) a large mass of floating sargassum.

sargassum /sɑrˈgæsəm/ *n* any of a genus of tropical seaweed with air bladders that form to float in large masses.

sarge /sɑrdʒ/ *n* (*sl*) sergeant.

sari, saree /ˈsɑri/ *n* a Hindu woman's principal garment, consisting of a long piece of cloth wrapped around the waist and across the shoulder.

sark /sɑrk/ *n* (*Scot*) a shirt.

sarong /səˈrɒŋ/ *n* a long strip of cloth wrapped around the lower body, worn *esp* in the Malay archipelago and the Pacific Islands.

sarsaparilla /ˌsɑrspəˈrɪlə/ *n* any of various tropical American trailing plants; the dried roots of these used as a flavouring and (formerly) in medicine; a soft drink flavoured with these roots.

sartorial /sɑrˈtɔriəl/ *adj* of or relating to the making of men's clothing.—**sartorially** *adv.*

sartorius /sɑrˈtɔriəs/ *n* (*pl* **sartorii**) a muscle that helps flex the knee.

SASE *abbr* = self-addressed stamped envelope.

sash[1] /sæʃ/ *n* a band of satin or ribbon worn around the waist or over the shoulder, often as a badge of honour.

sash[2] *n* a frame for holding the glass of a window, *esp* one that slides vertically.

sashay /sæˈʃeɪ/ *n* (*inf*) to walk in a casual manner, saunter; to swagger.

sash cord *n* a cord used to attach a sash weight to a sash.

sashimi /sæˈʃiːmi/ *n* a Japanese dish of thin strips of raw fish.

sash weight *n* a weight used to balance a sliding sash in an open position.

sash window *n* a window with sliding sashes.

Sask. *abbr* ✦ = Saskatchewan.

Saskatchewaner *n* ✦ (*Cdn*) a person who lives in or is from Saskatchewan.

saskatoon /ˌsæskəˈtuːn/ *n* ✦ (*Cdn*) a shrub of western North America; the sweet purple berry of this shrub.

Sasquatch /ˈsæskwɒtʃ/ *n* ✦ a large, hairy, humanlike creature that supposedly inhabits the Pacific Northwest of North America.—*also* **Bigfoot.**

sass /sæs/ *n* (*inf*) rudeness, impudence. • *vt* to talk rudely or impudently to.

sassafras /ˈsæsəˌfræs/ *n* a North American tree of the laurel family; the aromatic dried root of this used as a flavouring.

Sassenach /ˈsæsəˌnæx/ or /-ˌnæk/ *n* (*Scot, Irish*) an English person.

sassy /ˈsæsi/ *adj* (**sassier, sassiest**) (*sl*) rude; cheeky.

Sat *abbr* = Saturday; Saturn.

sat *see* **sit.**

Satan /ˈseɪtən/ *n* the devil, the adversary of God.

satanic /səˈtænɪk/, **satanical** /-kəl/ *adj* of or relating to Satan, devilish; marked by viciousness or cruelty.—**satanically** *adv.*

Satanism /ˈseɪtəˌnɪzəm/ *n* the worship of Satan; the perversion of Christian ceremonial forms associated with this.—**Satanist** *n.*

satay, saté /sæˈteɪ/ or /ˈsæteɪ/ *n* an Indonesian dish of cubed chicken, beef, etc served with a piquant peanut sauce.

satchel /ˈsætʃəl/ *n* a bag with shoulder straps for carrying school books, etc.

sate /seɪt/ *vt* to satisfy to repletion, to satiate.

sateen /sæˈtiːn/ *n* a closely woven fabric with a glossy surface made in imitation of satin.

satellite /ˈsætəˌlaɪt/ *n* a planet orbiting another; a man-made object orbiting the earth, moon, etc, to gather scientific information or for communication; a nation economically dependent on a more powerful one.

satellite broadcasting, satellite television *n* the transmission of television programmes via an orbiting satellite to subscribers in possession of a receiving satellite dish aerial.

sati *see* **suttee.**

satiable /ˈseɪʃəbəl/ *adj* able to be satiated or sated.—**satiability** *n.*—**satiably** *adv.*

satiate /ˈseɪʃiˌeɪt/ *vt* to provide with more than enough so as to weary or disgust; to gorge.—**satiation** *n.*

satiety /səˈtaɪti/ *n* the state of being sated; a feeling of having had too much.

satin /ˈsætən/ *n* a fabric of woven silk with a smooth, shiny surface on one side. • *adj* of or resembling satin.

satinwood /ˈsætɪnˌwʊd/ *n* a smooth yellowish brown hard wood; a tree that yields such wood.

satiny /-ni/ *adj* smooth and lustrous, like satin.

satire /ˈsætaɪr/ *n* a literary work in which folly or evil in people's behaviour are held up to ridicule; trenchant wit, sarcasm.—**satirical** *adj.*—**satirically** *adv.*

satirist /ˈsætərɪst/ *n* a writer of satires.

satirize /ˈsætəraɪz/ *vt* to attack with satire.—**satirizer** *n.*

satisfaction /ˌsætɪsˈfækʃən/ *n* the act of satisfying or the condition of being satisfied; that which satisfies; comfort; atonement, reparation.

satisfactory /ˌsætɪsˈfæktəri/ or /-ˈfæktri/ *adj* giving satisfaction; adequate; acceptable; convincing.—**satisfactorily** *adv.*—**satisfactoriness** *n.*

satisfy /ˈsætəsˌfaɪ/ *vb* (**satisfying, satisfied**) *vi* to be enough for; to fulfil the needs or desires of. • *vt* to give enough to; (*hunger, desire etc.*) to appease; to please; to gratify; to comply with; (*creditor*) to discharge, to pay in full; to convince; to make reparation to; (*guilt, etc*) to atone for.

satori /səˈtɔri/ *n* (*Zen Buddhism*) a state of intuitive enlightenment.

satsuma /ˈsætsʊmə/ or /sæˈtsuːmə/ *n* a loose-skinned, seedless, small orange; (*with cap*) a glazed yellow Japanese pottery.

saturate /ˈsætʃəˌreɪt/ *vt* to soak thoroughly; to fill completely.—**saturator** *n.*

saturated /ˈsætʃəˌreɪt/ *adj* (*chem*) absorbing the maximum amount possible of a substance; pure in colour.

saturation /ˌsætʃəˈreɪʃən/ *n* the act of saturating or the condition of being saturated; the supplying of a market with all the goods it will absorb; an overwhelming concentration of military power.

Saturday /ˈsætərˌdeɪ/ or /-di/ *n* the seventh and last day of the week.

Saturn /ˈsætərn/ *n* (*Roman myth*) the god of agriculture; (*astron*) the second largest planet in the solar system, with three rings revolving about it.—**Saturnian** *adj.*

Saturnalia /ˌsætərˈneɪliə/ *n* (*pl* **Saturnalias, Saturnalia**) in ancient Rome, a festival held in December in honour of Saturn; (*without cap*) a wild, unrestrained celebration.—**Saturnalian** *n.*

saturnine /ˈsætərˌnaɪn/ *adj* sullen, morose.—**saturninely** *adv.*

satyagraha /sʌtˈjɒgrəˌhə/ *n* the principle and practice of passive resistance as adopted by Mahatma Gandhi in opposition to British colonial rule in India.

satyr /ˈsætər/ or /ˈseɪtər/ *n* (*Greek myth*) a woodland god in human form but with goat's ears, tail, and legs; a man with strong sexual appetites; a man with satyriasis.—**satyric** *adj.*

satyriasis /ˌsætɪˈraɪəsɪs/ *n* excessive sexual desire in men.

sauce /sɒs/ *n* a liquid or dressing served with food to enhance its flavour; stewed or preserved fruit eaten with other food or as a dessert; (*inf*) impudence. • *vt* to season with sauce; to make piquant; (*sl*) to cheek.

saucepan /ˈsɒspæn/ *n* a deep cooking pan with a handle and lid.

saucer /ˈsɒsər/ *n* a round shallow dish placed under a cup; a shallow depression; a thing shaped like a saucer.

saucy /'sɔsi/ *adj* (**saucier, sauciest**) rude, impertinent; sprightly.— **saucily** *adv*.—**sauciness** *n*.

sauerkraut /'sauər,kraut/ *n* a German dish of chopped pickled cabbage.

sauna /'sɔnə/ *n* exposure of the body to hot steam, followed by cold water; the room where this is done.

saunter /'sɔntər/ *vi* to walk in a leisurely or idle way. • *n* a stroll.— **saunterer** *n*.

-saur /sɔr/ *n suffix* (*scientific*) reptiles.

saurian /'sɔriən/ *adj* of or resembling a lizard. • *n* (*formerly*) lizard.

sauro- /'sɔrɔ:/ *prefix* lizard.

saury /'sɔri/ *n* (*pl* **sauries**) an Atlantic fish with a long body and elongated jaws.

sausage /'sɔsidʒ/ *n* minced seasoned meat, *esp* pork, packed into animal gut or other casing.

sauté /'sɔtei/ or /-'tei/, /sɔ:-/ *adj* fried quickly and lightly. • *vt* (**sautéing, sautéed**) to fry in a small amount of oil or fat. • *n* a sautéed dish.

sauve qui peut /səuvki'pœ/ *n* a precipitate flight, a general stampede.

savage /'sævidʒ/ *adj* fierce; wild; untamed; uncivilized; ferocious; primitive. • *n* a member of a primitive society; a brutal, fierce person or animal.—**savagely** *adv*.—**savageness** *n*.

savagery /'sævədʒəri/ *n* (*pl* **savageries**) the state of being a savage; an act of violence or cruelty; an uncivilized state.

savanna, savannah /sə'vænə/ *n* a treeless plain; an area of tropical or subtropical grassland.

savant /'sæ'vã/ or /-'vãt/ *n* (pl **savants**) a person with extensive knowledge, *esp* in a certain discipline.

savate /sə'væt/ *n* a form of boxing using both the fists and the feet.

save[1] /seiv/ *vt* to rescue from harm or danger; to keep, to accumulate; to set aside for future use; to avoid the necessity of; (*energy etc*) to prevent waste of; (*theol*) to deliver from sin. • *vi* to avoid waste, expense, etc; to economize; to store up money or goods; (*sports*) to keep an opponent from scoring or winning. • *n* (*sports*) the act of preventing one's opponent from scoring.—**savable, saveable** *adj*.

save[2] *conj, prep* except, but.

saveloy /'sævə,lɔi/ *n* a type of highly-seasoned smoked sausage.

saver /'seivər/ *n* a person who saves money in a bank or building society.

savin, savine /'sævin/ *n* a small Eurasian juniper bush with dark fruit the oil from which was once used medicinally.

saving[1] /'seiviŋ/ *adj* thrifty, economical; (*clause*) containing a reservation; redeeming. • *n* what is saved; (*pl*) money saved for future use.

saving[2] *prep* except; with apology to.

savings and loan association *n* a company that pays interest on deposits and issues loans to enable people to buy their own houses, a building society.

savings account *n* a bank account that earns interest.

savings bank *n* a bank receiving small deposits and holding them in interest-bearing accounts.

saviour, savior /'seivjər/ *n* a person who saves another from harm or danger; (*with cap*) Jesus Christ.

savory /'seivəri/ *n* (*pl* **savories**) any of various Mediterranean aromatic plants used as herbs for flavouring.

savoir-faire *n* the skill of knowing the right thing to do; tact.

savour, savor /'seivjər/ *n* the flavour or smell of something; a distinctive quality. • *vti* to season; to enjoy; to have a specified taste or smell; to smack (of); to appreciate critically.— **savourer, savorer** *n*.

savoury, savory /'seivəri/ *adj* having a good taste or smell; spicy, not sweet; reputable. • *n* (*pl* **savouries, savories**) a savoury dish at the beginning or end of dinner; (*pl*) snacks served with drinks.— **savourily, savorily** *adv*.—**savouriness, savoriness** *n*.

savoy (cabbage) /'sævɔi/ or /sə'vɔi/ *n* a variety of cabbage with wrinkled leaves.

savvy /'sævi/ *vti* (**savvying, savvied**) (*sl*) to understand. • *n* (*sl*) understanding, know-how. • *adj* (**savvier, savviest**) (*sl*) shrewd.

saw[1] *see* **see**[1].

saw[2] /sɔ/ *n* a tool with a toothed edge for cutting wood, etc. • *vti* (**sawing, sawed**, *pp* **sawed** *or* **sawn**) to cut or shape with a saw; to use a saw; to make a to-and-fro motion.—**sawer** *n*.

saw[3] *n* a wise saying, a proverb.

sawbill /'sɔbil/ *n* a large, diving, fish-eating duck with a long narrow bill with serrated edges.

sawbones /'sɔbo:nz/ *n* (*sl*) a doctor or surgeon.

sawbuck /'sɔbʌk/ *n* a sawhorse.

sawdust /'sɔdʌst/ *n* fine particles of wood caused by sawing.

sawed-off *see* **sawn-off**.

sawfish /'sɔfiʃ/ *n* (*pl* **sawfish, sawfishes**) a large ray with a serrated snout.

sawfly /'sɔflai/ *n* (*pl* **sawflies**) any of various insects with a saw-like ovipositor.

sawhorse /'sɔhɔrs/ *n* a trestle, etc on which wood is laid for sawing.

sawmill /'sɔmil/ *n* a mill where timber is cut into logs or planks.

sawn *see* **saw**[2].

sawn-off *adj* (*shotgun*) having the barrel shortened to aid concealment; (*person*) (*sl*) small.—*also* **sawed-off**.

saw-off *n* ✳ a compromise reached by competing persons or groups; a tie or stalemate.

saw set /sɔ'set/ *n* an instrument for setting the teeth of a saw by bending each tooth to the left or right alternately.

sawyer /'sɔiər/ or /'sɔjər/ *n* a person employed to saw timber.

sax /sæks/ *n* saxophone.

saxatile /'sæksə,tail/ or /-t l/ *adj* saxicolous.

saxe blue /,sæks'blu:/ *n* a light greyish-blue.—*also adj*.

saxhorn /'sækshɔrn/ *n* a brass musical instrument resembling a tuba.

saxicolous /sæk'sikə,ləs/, **saxicoline** /sæk'sikə,lain/ *adj* living among or on rocks.

saxifrage /'sæksifreidʒ/ or /-frədʒ/ *n* any of a genus of plants with small flowers and tufted leaves, popular in rock gardens.

Saxon /'sæksən/ *adj, n* (of) a member of a North German people that settled the southern part of Britain in the 5th-6th century.

saxony /'sæksəni/ *n* a fine wool; cloth made from it.

saxophone /'sæksə,fo:n/ *n* a brass wind instrument with a single reed and about twenty finger-keys.—**saxophonic** *adj*.—**saxophonist** *n*.

say /sei/ *vb* (**says, saying, said**) *vt* to speak, to utter; to state in words; to affirm, declare; to recite; to estimate; to assume. • *vi* to tell; to express in words. • *n* (*pl* **says**) the act of uttering; the right or opportunity to speak; a share in a decision. • *adv* for example. • *interj* expressing admiration, surprise, etc.

saying /'seiiŋ/ *n* a common remark; a proverb or adage.

say-so *n* (*inf*) an unfounded assertion; an authorization; the right to authorize.

sayyid, sayid /'seiid/ *n* a Muslim title of respect applied to descendants of Mohammed's daughter Fatima.

Sb (*chem symbol*) antimony.

SBKKV *abbr* = space-based kinetic kill vehicle, a system of missiles launched from a satellite.

'sblood *interj* (*obs*) God's blood.

SC *abbr* = South Carolina; Supreme Court.

Sc (*chem symbol*) scandium.

sc. *abbr* = scene; science; scilicet; (*weight*) scruple; (*print*) small capitals.

scab /skæb/ *n* a dry crust on a wound or sore; a plant disease characterized by crustaceous spots; a worker who refuses to join a strike or who replaces a striking worker. • *vi* (**scabbing, scabbed**) to form a scab; to be covered with scabs; to work as a scab.—**scabby** *adj*.

scabbard /'skæbərd/ *n* a sheath for a sword or dagger. • *vt* to sheathe.

scabies /'skeibi:z/ *n* a contagious, itching skin disease.

scabiosa /skæbi'o:sə/ *n* any of a genus of Mediterranean plants with tightly clustered blue, red or white flowers.—*also* **scabious**.

scabious[1] /'skeibiəs/ *adj* covered with scabs; of or resembling scabies.

scabious[2] *n* a scabiosa.

scabrous /'skæbrəs/ *adj* (*surface*) rough, scaly; indecent, offensive; intractable, difficult to manage.—**scabrously** *adv*.— **scabrousness** *n*.

scaffold /'skæfo:ld/ or /-fəld/ *n* a raised platform for the execution of a criminal; capital punishment; scaffolding.

scaffolding /'skæfo:ldiŋ/ or /-fəldiŋ/ *n* a temporary framework of wood and metal for use by workmen constructing a building, etc; materials for a scaffold.

scalable /'skeiləbəl/ *adj* able to be scaled or climbed.

scalar /'skeilər/ *adj* (*math*) having magnitude but not direction. • *n* a scalar quantity, *eg* time, mass.

scalar product *n* a scalar produced by multiplying together the magnitudes of two vectors and the cosine of the angle between them.

scalawag /ˈskæləˌwæg/ *n* (*inf*) a rascal; a scamp; a Southern white who supported the Republicans after the American Civil War.—*also* **scallawag, scallywag**.

scald /skɒld/ *vt* to burn with hot liquid or steam; to heat almost to boiling point; to immerse in boiling water (to sterilize). • *n* an injury caused by hot liquid or steam.

scale[1] /skeɪl/ *n* (*pl*) a machine or instrument for weighing; one of the pans or the tray of a set of scales; (*pl*) (*with cap*) Libra, the seventh sign of the zodiac. • *vti* to weigh in a set of scales; to have a specified weight on a set of scales.

scale[2] *n* one of the thin plates covering a fish or reptile; a flake (of dry skin); an incrustation on teeth, etc. • *vti* to remove the scales from; to flake off.

scale[3] *n* a graduated measure; an instrument so marked; (*math*) the basis for a numerical system, 10 being that in general use; (*mus*) a series of tones from the keynote to its octave, in order of pitch; the proportion that a map, etc, bears to what it represents; a series of degrees classified by size, amount, etc; relative scope or size. • *vt* (*wall*) to go up or over; (*model*) to make or draw to scale; to increase or decrease in size.

scaled /skeɪld/ *adj* (*reptile, etc*) covered with or having scales.

scale insect *n* any of various small insects that feed on host plants and secrete a waxy covering for protection.

scalene /skeɪˈliːn/ *or* /skeɪˈliːn/ *adj* (*geom*) having three sides of unequal length. • *n* a scalene triangle.

scallawag, scallywag /ˈskæləˌwæg/ *or* /ˈskæliː-/ *see* **scalawag**.

scallion /ˈskæljən/ *n* a young onion with a small bulb and long shoots eaten raw in salads, a spring onion or shallot.

scallop /ˈskæləp/ *or* /ˈskɒləp/ *n* an edible shellfish with two fluted, fan-shaped shells; one of a series of curves in an edging. • *vt* to cut into scallops.—**scalloped** *adj*.

scalp /skælp/ *n* the skin covering the skull, *usu* covered with hair. • *vti* to cut the scalp from; to criticize sharply; (*inf*) (*tickets, etc*) to buy and resell at higher prices.

scalpel /ˈskælpəl/ *n* a short, thin, very sharp knife used *esp* for surgery.

scaly /ˈskeɪli/ *adj* (**scalier, scaliest**) (*reptile etc*) like or covered with scales.—**scaliness** *n*.

scaly anteater *n* a pangolin.

scamp /skæmp/ *n* a rascal; a mischievous child.

scamper /ˈskæmpər/ *vi* to run away quickly or playfully. • *n* a brisk or playful run or movement.

scampi /ˈskæmpi/ *n* a dish of large shrimps or prawns cooked in breadcrumbs or prepared with a flavoured dressing.

scan /skæn/ *vb* (**scanning, scanned**) *vt* (*page etc*) to look through quickly; to scrutinize; (*med*) to examine with a radiological device; (*TV*) to pass an electronic beam over; (*radar*) to detect with an electronic beam; (*poem*) to conform to a rhythmical pattern; to check for recorded data by means of a mechanical or electronic device; (*human body*) to make a scan of in a scanner. • *vi* to analyse the pattern of verse. • *n* the act of scanning or an instance of being scanned.

scandal /ˈskændəl/ *n* a disgraceful event or action; talk arising from immoral behaviour; a feeling of moral outrage; the thing or person causing this; disgrace; malicious gossip.

scandalize /-aɪz/ *vt* to shock the moral feelings of; to defame.—**scandalization** *n*.—**scandalizer** *n*.

scandalmonger /ˈskændəlˌmɒŋgər/ *or* /-ˌmʌŋgər/ *n* a person who spreads scandal or hot malicious gossip.—**scandalmongering** *n*.

scandalous /ˈskændələs/ *adj* causing scandal; shameful; spreading slander.—**scandalously** *adv*.—**scandalousness** *n*.

Scandinavian /ˌskændiˈneɪviən/ *adj* of or pertaining to Scandinavia, the region comprising Norway, Sweden, and Denmark, and sometimes Iceland, or its people. • *n* a native or inhabitant of Scandinavia.

scandium /ˈskændiəm/ *n* a rare metallic element present in small quantities in various minerals.

scanner /ˈskænər/ *n* a person or thing that scans; an electronic device that monitors or scans; a device for receiving or transmitting radar signals; a device for scanning the human body to obtain an image of an internal part.

scanning electron microscope *n* an electron microscope which scans an object to produce a three-dimensional image.

scansion /ˈskænʃən/ *n* the analysis of verse to show its metre.

scant /skænt/ *adj* limited; meagre; insufficient; scanty; grudging.

scantling /ˈskæntlɪŋ/ *n* a small piece of timber; the dimensions of timber and stone for a building or of a component for a ship or aircraft; a small quantity.

scanty /ˈskænti/ *adj* (**scantier, scantiest**) barely adequate; insufficient; small.—**scantily** *adv*.—**scantiness** *n*.

scapegoat /ˈskeɪpgoːt/ *n* a person who bears the blame for others; one who is the object of irrational hostility.

scapegrace /ˈskeɪpgreɪs/ *n* a graceless, hare-brained person; an incorrigible scamp.

scapula /ˈskæpjulə/ *n* (*pl* **scapulae**) the shoulder blade.

scapular /ˈskæpjulər/ *adj* of or relating to the scapula. • *n* a monastic robe worn in various Christian religious orders, consisting of a wide piece of cloth worn over the shoulders and hanging down at the front and back; any of the feathers along the base of a bird's wing.

scar[1] /skar/ *n* a mark left after the healing of a wound or sore; a blemish resulting from damage or wear. • *vti* (**scarring, scarred**) to mark with or form a scar.

scar[2] *n* a protruding or isolated rock; a precipitous crag; a rocky part of a hillside.

scarab /ˈskɛrəb/ *or* /ˈskæ-/ *n* a dung-beetle held to be sacred in ancient Egypt; a gem or seal in the shape of this.

scarabaeid /ˌskærəˈbiːɪd/ *n* any of a family of beetles including the dung beetle.—*also adj*.

scarce /skers/ *adj* not in abundance; hard to find; rare.—**scarceness** *n*.

scarcely /ˈskersli/ *adv* hardly, only just; probably not or certainly not.

scarcity /ˈskersiti/ *n* (**scarcities**) the state of being scarce; a dearth, deficiency.

scare /sker/ *vti* to startle; to frighten or become frightened; to drive away by frightening. • *n* a sudden fear; a period of general fear; a false alarm.

scarecrow /ˈskerkroː/ *n* a wooden figure dressed in clothes for scaring birds from crops; a thin or tattered person; something frightening but harmless.

scaremonger /ˈskerˌmɒŋgər/ *or* /-ˌmʌŋgər/ *n* a person who causes fear or panic by spreading rumours; an alarmist.

scarf /skarf/ *n* (*pl* **scarves**) a rectangular or square piece of cloth worn around the neck, shoulders or head for warmth or decoration.

scarfskin /ˈskarfskɪn/ *n* the outer layer of skin; cuticle.

scarify /ˈskerɪˌfaɪ/ *or* /ˈskæ-/ *vt* (**scarifying, scarified**) to make cuts in, to scratch; to criticize savagely; to loosen the surface of (soil); to hasten germination by softening the wall (of a hard seed).—**scarification** *n*.

scarlatina /ˌskarləˈtiːnə/ *n* scarlet fever.

scarlet /ˈskarlət/ *n* a bright red with a tinge of orange; scarlet cloth or clothes. • *adj* scarlet coloured; immoral or sinful.

scarlet fever *n* an acute contagious disease marked by a sore throat, fever, and a scarlet rash.

scarlet pimpernel *n* a plant with red, purple or white flowers that close in dull weather.

scarlet runner *n* a climbing bean plant with scarlet flowers and elongated edible pods.—*also* **runner bean**.

scarlet woman *n* (*arch*) a prostitute.

scarp /skarp/ *n* a low steep slope; the inner face of a ditch in a fortification.

scarper /ˈskarpər/ *vi* (*inf*) to run away.

scarves *see* **scarf**.

scary /ˈskeri/ *adj* (**scarier, scariest**) frightening, alarming.—**scariness** *n*.

scat[1] /skæt/ *vi* (**scatting, scatted**) (*inf*) to leave hastily.

scat[2] *n* (*jazz*) a form of improvised singing without words. • *vi* (**scatting, scatted**) to sing in this way.

scathing /ˈskeɪðɪŋ/ *adj* bitterly critical; cutting, withering.—**scathingly** *adv*.

scatology /skəˈtɒlədʒi/ *n* the scientific study of fossil and human excrement; a preoccupation with excrement or obscenity.—**scatological** *adj*.

scatter /ˈskætər/ *vti* to throw loosely about; to sprinkle; to dissipate; to put or take to flight; to disperse; to occur at random. • *n* a scattering or sprinkling.

scatterbrain /ˈskætərˌbreɪn/ *n* a frivolous, heedless person.—**scatterbrained** *adj*.

scattered /ˈskætərˌbreɪnd/ *adj* dispersed widely, spaced out; straggling.

scattering /ˈskætərɪŋ/ *n* a small amount spread over a large area; a dispersion.

scatty /'skæti/ *adj* (**scattier, scattiest**) (*inf*) thoughtless, absent-minded, crazy.—**scattily** *adv*.—**scattiness** *n*.

scaup (duck) /skɒp/ *n* a diving duck of Europe and America.

scavenge /'skævəndʒ/ *vi* to gather things discarded by others; (*animal*) to eat decaying matter.—**scavenger** *n*.

ScB *abbr* = Bachelor of Science.

ScD *abbr* = Doctor of Science.

scenario /sə'nɑ:riɔ:/ or /-ɑriɔ/ *n* (*pl* **scenarios**) an outline of events, real or imagined; the plot or script of a film, etc.

scene /si:n/ *n* the place in which anything occurs; the place in which the action of a play or a story occurs; a section of a play, a division of an act; the stage of a theatre; a painted screen, etc, used on this; an unseemly display of strong emotion; a landscape; surroundings; a place of action; (*inf*) an area of interest or activity (*eg the music scene*).

scene dock *n* (*theatre*) a storage area for scenery near the stage.

scenery /'si:nəri/ *n* (*pl* **sceneries**) painted screens, etc, used to represent places, as in a play, film, etc; an aspect of a landscape, *esp* of beautiful or impressive countryside.

scenic /'si:nɪk/ *adj* relating to natural scenery; picturesque; of or used on the stage.—**scenically** *adv*.

scenic railway *n* a miniature railway at an amusement park, etc.

scent /sɛnt/ *n* a perfume; an odour left by an animal, by which it can be tracked; the sense of smell; a line of pursuit or discovery. • *vt* to recognize by the sense of smell; to track by smell; to impart an odour to, to perfume; to get wind of, to detect.

scented /'sɛntəd/ *adj* perfumed.

sceptic *n* a person who questions opinions generally accepted; a person who doubts religious doctrines, an agnostic; an adherent of scepticism.—*also* **skeptic**.

sceptical *adj* doubting; questioning.—*also* **skeptical**.—**sceptically, skeptically** *adv*.

scepticism *n* an attitude of questioning criticism, doubt; (*philos*) the doctrine that absolute knowledge is unattainable.—*also* **skepticism**.

sceptre, scepter /'sɛptər/ *n* the staff of office held by a monarch on a ceremonial occasion; sovereignty.

schedule /'skɛdʒuəl/ or /'skɛdʒu:l/, /'ʃɛdju:l/, /'ʃɛdʒu l/ *n* a timetable; a list, inventory or tabulated statement; a timed plan for a project. • *vt* to make a schedule; to plan.

scheelite /'ʃi:laɪt/ *n* a mineral consisting of calcium tungstate.

schema /'ski:mə/ *n* (*pl* **schemata**) a plan or diagram.

schematic /ski:'mætɪk/ or /skɪ-/ *adj* of or like a scheme or diagram.—**schematically** *adv*.

schematize /'ski:mə,taɪz/ *vt* to form into or express as a scheme.—**schematization** *n*.

scheme /ski:m/ *n* a plan; a project; a systematic arrangement; a diagram; an underhand plot. • *vti* to devise or plot.—**schemer** *n*.

scheming /'ski:mɪŋ/ *adj* cunning; intriguing.

scherzando /skɛrt'sændo:/ *adj, adv* (*mus*) to be performed lightheartedly. • *n* (*pl* **scherzandi**) a piece of music played in this manner.

scherzo /'skɛrtso:/ *n* (*pl* **scherzos, scherzi**) a lively musical passage or movement, *usu* in triple time.

schilling /'ʃɪlɪŋ/ *n* the standard monetary unit of Austria.

schism /'skɪzəm/ *n* a division or separation into two parties, *esp* of a church; the sin of this; discord, disharmony.

schismatic /skɪz'mætɪk/, **schismatical** /-kəl/ *adj* of or creating schism. • *n* a person who creates schism or supports schism.—**schismatically** *adv*.

schist /ʃɪst/ *n* a type of crystalline rock in thin layers.—**schistose** *adj*.

schistosome /'ʃɪstə,so:m/ *n* any of a genus of parasitic worms that infest the blood vessels of humans and animals.

schistosomiasis /,ʃɪstəsɔ:'maɪəsɪs/ *n* a disease caused by infestation with schistosomes.

schizo /'skɪtso:/ *n* (*pl* **schizos**) (*inf*) a schizophrenic person. • *adj* schizophrenic.

schizo- /'skɪtsɔ:/, **schiz-** /skɪts/ *prefix* split, division.

schizocarp /'skɪtsə,kɑrp/ *n* a dry fruit that splits into single-seeded parts.

schizoid /'skɪtsɔɪd/ *adj* mildly schizophrenic.—*also* *n*.

schizomycete /'skɪtsəmɔ,si:t/ *n* any microscopic organism such as a bacterium.

schizophrenia /skɪtsə'fri:niə/ or /-'fri:njə/ *n* a mental disorder characterized by withdrawal from reality and deterioration of the personality; the presence of mutually contradictory qualities or parts.—**schizophrenic** *adj, n*.

schieren /'ʃli:rən/ *n* (*physics*) visible streaks in a transparent medium caused by variations in its density.

schmaltz, schmalz /ʃmɒlts/ *n* overly sentimental music, art, film, etc.—**schmaltzy, schmalzy** *adj*.

schnapps /ʃnæps/ or /ʃnɒps/ *n* (*pl* **schnapps**) a Dutch spirit distilled from potatoes; (*Germany*) any strong spirit.

schnauzer /'ʃnauzər/ or /'ʃnautsər/ *n* an orig German breed of terrier with a short wiry coat.

schnitzel /'ʃnɪtzəl/ *n* a cutlet of veal.

schnorkle *see* **snorkel**.

Schnozzle /'ʃnɒzəl/ *n* (*sl*) nose.

scholar /'skɒlər/ *n* a pupil; a student; a learned person; the holder of a scholarship.

scholarly /-li/ *adj* learned, erudite, academic.

scholarship /'skɒlərʃɪp/ *n* an annual grant to a scholar or student, *usu* won by competitive examination; learning, academic achievement.

scholastic /skə'læstɪk/ *adj* of or relating to schools, scholars, or education; academic.—**scholastically** *adv*.

school[1] /sku:l/ *n* a shoal of porpoises, whales, or other aquatic animals of one kind swimming together.

school[2] *n* an educational establishment; its teachers and students; a regular session of teaching; formal education, schooling; a particular division of a university; a place or means of discipline; a group of thinkers, artists, writers, holding similar principles. • *vt* to train; to teach; to control or discipline.

schoolboy /'sku:lbɔɪ/ *n* a boy who attends school.

schoolchild /'sku:ltʃaɪld/ *n* (*pl* **schoolchildren**) a child who attends school.

schoolgirl /'sku:lgərl/ *n* a girl who attends school.

schoolhouse /'sku:lhaʊs/ *n* a building used as a school.

schooling /'sku:lɪŋ/ *n* instruction in school.

schoolmaster /'sku:l,mæstər/ *n* a man who teaches in school.

schoolmate /'sku:lmeɪt/ *n* a companion at school.—*also* **schoolfellow**.

schoolmistress /'sku:l,mɪstrəs/ *n* a woman who teaches in school.

schoolroom /'sku:lru:m/ *n* a room in which pupils are taught, as in a school.

schoolteacher /'sku:l,ti:tʃər/ *n* a person who teaches in school.

schooner /'sku:nər/ *n* a sailing ship with two or more masts rigged with fore-and-aft sails; a large drinking glass for sherry or beer.

schottische /ʃɒ'ti:ʃ/ *n* (music for) a type of slow dance resembling a polka.

schuss /ʃʊs/ *n* (*skiing*) a fast straight downhill run. • *vi* to ski down this.

sci. *abbr* = science; scientific.

sciatic /saɪ'ætɪk/ *adj* of the hip.

sciatica /saɪ'ætɪkə/ *n* pain along the sciatic nerve, *esp* in the back of the thigh; (*loosely*) pain in the lower back or adjacent parts.

sciatic nerve *n* a long nerve running from the pelvic region to the back of the thigh.

science /'saɪəns/ *n* knowledge gained by systematic experimentation and analysis, and the formulation of general principles; a branch of this; skill or technique.

science fiction *n* highly imaginative fiction typically involving actual or projected scientific phenomena.

science park *n* an area where scientific discoveries are translated into commercial products and applications.

scientific /saɪən'tɪfɪk/ *adj* of or concerned with science; based on or using the principles and methods of science; systematic and exact; having or showing expert skill.—**scientifically** *adv*.

scientism /'saɪən,tɪzəm/ *n* the use of scientific methods; the inappropriate use of or reliance on scientific methods.

scientist /'saɪəntɪst/ *n* a specialist in a branch of science, as in chemistry, etc.

Scientology /,saɪən'tɒlədʒi/ *n* (*trademark*) a religious philosophy founded by L. Ron Hubbard in 1951.

sci-fi /'saɪfaɪ/ or /'saɪ'faɪ/ *n* science fiction.

scilicet /'sɪlə,sɛt/ *adv* namely, that is to say.

scilla /'sɪlə/ *n* any of a genus of plants with small pink, blue or white flowers grown from bulbs.

scimitar /'sɪmɪtər/ *n* an Oriental curved sword, broadest near the point.

scintigraphy /sɪn'tɪgrəfi/ *n* the production of images of internal body parts by detecting high-energy particles from a radioactive tracer administered to a patient.

scintilla /sɪn'tɪlə/ *n* an iota, tiny amount.

scintillate /'sɪntɪˌleɪt/ *vti* to give off sparks; to sparkle.—**scintillation** *n*.

scintillating /-ɪŋ/ *adj* sparkling; amusing.

scintillation counter *n* an instrument for registering the intensity of a radioactive source by recording the flashes of light produced by the impact of emitted photons on a phospor.

scion /'saɪən/ *n* a shoot for grafting; a young member of a family, a descendant.

scirrhus /'sɪrəs/ or /'skɪ-/ *n* (*pl* **scirrhi, scirrhuses**) a cancerous tumour consisting of fibrous tissue.

scission /'sɪʃn/ *n* the act of cutting or dividing; a cut, divide, or split.

scissor /'sɪzər/ *vt* to cut with scissors, to clip. • *npl* a tool for cutting paper, hair, etc, consisting of two fastened pivoted blades whose edges slide past each other; a gymnastic feat in which the leg movements resemble the opening and closing of scissors.

scissors kick *n* (*swimming*) a kick in which the legs move from the hip in a scissoring motion.

sciurine /'saɪəˌrin/ *adj* of or resembling a family of rodents which include squirrels and marmots.

SCLC *abbr* = Southern Christian Leadership Conference.

sclera /'sklɪːrə/ *n* the opaque outer covering of the eyeball excluding the cornea.

sclerenchyma /sklɪˈreŋkɪmə/ *n* a tissue forming the hard fibrous parts of plants.

sclero- /'sklɛro:/, **scler-** /sklɛr/ *prefix* hardness.

scleroderma /sklɪːrəˈdərmə/ or /sklɛr-/ *n* (*med*) a chronic disease in women causing thickening and hardening of the skin.

sclerodermatous /-təs/ *adj* (*zool*) covered with a hard layer of tissue, *eg* scales.

sclerosis /skləˈroːsɪs/ *n* a pathological hardening of body tissue; a disease marked by this.

sclerotic /skləˈrɒtɪk/ *adj* pertaining to the sclera; of or affected by sclerosis. • *n* the sclera.

sclerous /'sklɪːrəs/ or /'sklɛr-/ *adj* hard, bony.

scoff[1] /skɒf/ *vti* to jeer (at) or mock. • *n* an expression or object of derision; mocking words, a taunt.

scoff[2] *vt* (*sl*) to eat quickly and greedily; *n* ✦ (*Cdn*) (*inf*) a big meal.

scold /skoːld/ *vi* to reprove angrily; to tell off.

scolding /-ɪŋ/ *n* a harsh reprimand.

scoliosis /ˌskoːliˈoːsɪs/ *n* (*med*) lateral curvature of the spine.

scollop *see* **scallop**.

scombroid /'skɒmbrɔɪd/ *n* any member of a suborder of spiny-finned marine fishes used for food, such as the mackerel and tuna.—*also adj*.

sconce[1] /skɒns/ *n* a bracket on a wall for holding candles or electric lights.

sconce[2] *n* a defensive fortification, a bulwark.

scone /skuːn/ *n* a small, round cake made from flour and fat which is baked and spread with butter, etc.

scoop /skuːp/ *n* a small shovel-like utensil as for taking up flour, ice cream, etc; the bucket of a dredge, etc; the act of scooping or the amount scooped up at one time; (*inf*) a piece of exclusive news; (*inf*) the advantage gained in being the first to publish or broadcast this. • *vt* to shovel, lift or hollow out with a scoop; (*inf*) to obtain as a scoop; (*inf: rival newspaper etc*) to forestall with a news item.

scoot /skuːt/ *vti* to run quickly; to hurry (off).

scooter /'skuːtər/ *n* a child's two-wheeled vehicle with a footboard and steering handle; a motor scooter.

scope /skoːp/ *n* the opportunity to use one's abilities; extent; range; an instrument for viewing.

scopolamine /skəˈpɒˌləmiːn/ *n* an alkaloid extracted from certain plants, used as a sedative and for travel sickness.—*also* **hyoscine**.

scorbutic /skɔrˈbjuːtɪk/ *adj* of, suffering from, or resembling scurvy.—**scorbutically** *adv*.

scorch /skɔrtʃ/ *vti* to burn or be burned on the surface; to wither from over-exposure to heat; to singe; (*inf*) to drive or cycle furiously.

scorcher /'skɔrtʃər/ *n* (*inf*) a very hot day.

scorching /-ɪŋ/ *adj* (*inf: weather*) very hot; scathing.

score /skɔr/ *n* the total number of points made in a game or examination; a notch or scratch; a line indicating deletion or position; a group of twenty; a written copy of a musical composition showing the different parts; the music composed for a film; a grievance for settling; a reason or motive; (*inf*) the real facts; a bill or reckoning; (*pl*) an indefinite, large number. • *vt* to mark with cuts; (*mus*) to arrange in a score, to orchestrate; to gain or record points, as in a game; to evaluate in testing. • *vi* to make points, as in a game; to keep the score of a game; to gain an advantage, a success, etc; (*sl*) to be successful in seduction; (*with* **off**) to get the better of someone.—**scorer** *n*.

scoreboard /'skɔrbɔrd/ *n* a large manually or electronically operated board showing the score in a game or match.

scorecard /'skɔrkɑrd/ *n* (*golf, etc*) a card on which scores are recorded.

scorn /skɔrn/ *n* extreme contempt or disdain; the object of this. • *vt* to treat with contempt, to despise; to reject or refuse as unworthy.—**scornful** *adj*.—**scornfully** *adv*.

Scorpio /ˌskɔrpioː/ *n* the eighth sign of the zodiac in astrology, operative October 23-November 21.—**Scorpionic** *adj*.

scorpion /'skɔrpiən/ *n* a small, tropical, insect-like animal with pincers and a jointed tail with a poisonous sting.

scorpion fish *n* any of a genus of fish with poisonous spines on the dorsal fins.

Scot /skɒt/ *n* a native or inhabitant of Scotland; a member of a Celtic people from Ireland who settled in northern Britain in the 5th-6th centuries.

scotch /skɒtʃ/ *vt* (*a rumour*) to stamp out.

Scotch *n* whisky made in Scotland.

Scotch broth *n* a thick soup made from beef or mutton with vegetables and pearl barley.

Scotch egg *n* a hard-boiled egg enclosed in sausagemeat, coated in breadcrumbs, and fried.

Scotchman /'skɒtʃmən/ *n* (*pl* **Scotchmen**) a Scotsman.—**Scotchwoman** (*pl* **Scotchwomen**) *nf*.

Scotch mist *n* a dense, wet mist; fine drizzle.

Scotch terrier *n* a Scottish terrier.

scoter /'skoːtər/ *n* (*pl* **scoters, scoter**) a large sea duck with black plumage.

scot-free *adj* without penalty or injury.

Scotland Yard /'skɒtlənd/ *n* the headquarters of the London metropolitan police force.

scotoma /skɒˈtoːmə/ *n* (*pl* **scotomas, scotomata**) a blind spot in the visual field.

Scots /skɒts/ *adj* of or pertaining to Scotland, its law, money, and people, and the Scots language. • *n* the dialect of English developed in Lowland Scotland.

Scotsman /'skɒtsmən/ *n* (*pl* **Scotsmen**) a native or inhabitant of Scotland.—**Scotswoman** *n* (*pl* **Scotswomen**) *nf*.

Scots pine /-paɪn/ *n* (the wood of) a European pine with needlelike leaves.

Scotticism /'skɒtɪˌsɪzəm/ *n* a Scottish word or idiom.

Scottie /'skɒti/ *n* (*inf*) a Scotsman; a Scottish terrier.

Scottish /'skɒtɪʃ/ *adj* of or relating to Scotland and its people.

Scottish deerhound *n* a large rough-haired greyhound, a deerhound.

Scottish National Party *n* a political party seeking independence for Scotland.

Scottish terrier *n* a small terrier with short legs and a wiry coat.

scoundrel /'skaʊndrəl/ *n* a rascal; a dishonest person.

scour[1] /'skaʊr/ *vt* to clean by rubbing with an abrasive cloth; to flush out with a current of water; to purge. • *n* the act or process of scouring; a place scoured by running water; scouring action (as of a glacier); damage done by scouring action.

scour[2] *vt* to hasten over or along, to range over, *esp* in search or pursuit.

scourge /skərdʒ/ *n* a whip; a means of inflicting punishment; a person who harasses and causes widespread and great affliction; a pest. • *vt* to flog; to punish harshly.

Scouse /skaʊs/ *n* (*inf*) a person from Liverpool; the dialect of Liverpool.—*also adj*.

scout /skaʊt/ *n* a person, plane, etc, sent to observe the enemy's strength, etc; a person employed to find new talent or survey a competitor, etc; (*with cap*) a member of the Scouting Association, an organization for young people. • *vti* to reconnoitre; to go in search of (something).

scouting /'skaʊtɪŋ/ *n* the act of one who scouts; (*with cap*) the activities of the Scouting Association.

Scouting Association *n* (*formerly* Boy Scouts, Girl Guides) an organization to develop in young people self-reliance and initiative, moral and physical courage and a courteous spirit.

scoutmaster /'skaʊtˌmæstər/ *n* (*formerly*) the adult leader of a troop of Scouts.

scow /skaʊ/ *n* an unpowered flat-bottomed boat for carrying freight, refuse, etc.

scowl /skaʊl/ *n* a contraction of the brows in an angry or threatening manner; a sullen expression. • *vi* to make a scowl; to look sullen.

Scrabble /'skræbəl/ *n* (*trademark*) a game in which words are formed from individual lettered tiles on a grid.

scrabble *vi* to scratch or grope about; to struggle; to scramble. • *n* a repeated scratching or clawing; a scramble; a scribble.

scrag /skræg/ *n* a scrawny person or animal; the lean end of a neck of mutton or veal; (*loosely*) neck.

scraggly /'skrægli/ *adj* (**scragglier, scraggliest**) untidy, uneven.

scraggy /'skrægi/ *adj* (**scraggier, scraggiest**) thin and bony, gaunt.

scram /skræm/ *vi* (**scramming, scrammed**) (*sl*) to get out, to go away at once.

scramble /'skræmbəl/ *vi* to move or climb hastily on all fours; to scuffle or struggle for something; to move with urgency or panic. • *vt* to mix haphazardly;to stir (slightly beaten eggs) while cooking; (*transmitted signals*) to make unintelligible in transit. • *n* a hard climb or advance; a disorderly struggle; a rapid emergency take-off of fighter planes; a motorcycle rally over rough ground.—**scrambler** *n*.

scrap[1] /skræp/ *n* a small piece; a fragment of discarded material; (*pl*) bits of food. • *adj* in the form of pieces, leftovers, etc; used and discarded. • *vt* (**scrapping, scrapped**) to discard; to make into scraps.

scrap[2] *n* (*inf*) a fight or quarrel. • *vi* (**scrapping, scrapped**) to have a scrap.

scrapbook /'skræpbʊk/ *n* a book for pasting clippings etc, in.

scrape /skreɪp/ *vt* to rub with a sharp or abrasive object so as to clean, smooth or remove; to eke out or to be economical; to amass in small portions; to draw along with a grating or vibration; to get narrowly past, to graze; to draw back the foot in making a bow; (*with* **together**) to save or collect with difficulty. • *vi* (*with* **through**) to manage or succeed with difficulty or by a slim margin. • *n* the act of scraping; a grating sound; an abrasion, scratch; an awkward predicament.

scraper /'skreɪpər/ *n* an instrument for scraping; a grating or edge for scraping mud from boots.

scraperboard /'skræpbɔrd/ *n* a board with a black surface which can be scraped off with a special tool to form a design.

scrapheap *n* a pile of discarded material or things.

scraping /'skreɪpɪŋ/ *n* a piece scraped off.

scrappy /'skræpi/ *adj* (**scrappier, scrappiest**) disjointed; fragmentary; full of gaps.—**scrappily** *adv*.—**scrappiness** *n*.

scratch /skrætʃ/ *vt* to mark with a sharp point; to scrape with the nails or claws; to rub to relieve an itch; to chafe; to write awkwardly; (*writing etc*) to strike out; to withdraw from a race, etc. • *vi* to use nails or claws to tear or dig. • *n* the act of scratching; a mark or sound made by this; a slight injury; a starting line for a race; a scribble. • *adj* taken at random, haphazard, impromptu; without a handicap.

scratch pad *n* a notebook.

scratch video *n* a collage of images from existing television or cinema film.

scratchy /'skrætʃi/ *adj* (**scratchier, scratchiest**) making a scratching noise; uneven, ragged.—**scratchily** *adv*.—**scratchiness** *n*.

scrawl /skrɔl/ *n* careless or illegible handwriting; a scribble. • *vti* to draw or write carelessly.

scrawny /'skrɔni/ *adj* (**scrawnier, scrawniest**) skinny; bony.—**scrawniness** *n*.

scream /skri:m/ *vti* to utter a piercing cry, as of pain, fear, etc; to shout; to shriek. • *n* a sharp, piercing cry; (*inf*) a very funny person or thing.

scree /skri:/ *n* loose shifting stones; a slope covered with these.

screech /skri:tʃ/ *n* a harsh, high-pitched cry; ✶ (*Cdn*) a dark rum bottled in Newfoundland. • *vti* to utter a screech, to shriek.

screed /skri:d/ *n* a long, tedious letter or speech; an informal piece of writing.

screen /skri:n/ *n* a movable partition or framework to conceal, divide, or protect; a shelter or shield from heat, danger or view; an electronic display (as in a television set, computer terminal, etc); a surface on which films, slides, etc are projected; the motion picture industry; a coarse wire mesh over a window or door to keep out insects; a sieve. • *vt* to conceal or shelter; to grade by passing through a screen; to separate according to skill, etc; (*a film*) to show on a screen.

screening /'skri:nɪŋ/ *n* a showing of a film; a metal or plastic mesh, as for window screens; the refuse matter after sieving.

screenplay /'skri:npleɪ/ *n* a story written in a form suitable for a film.

screenwriter /'skri:nraɪtər/ *n* a person who writes screenplays.

screw /skru:/ *n* a metal cylinder or cone with a spiral thread around it for fastening things by being turned; any spiral thing like this; a twist or turn of a screw; a twist of paper; pressure; a propeller with revolving blades on a shaft. • *vt* to fasten, tighten etc with a screw; to oppress; to extort, to cheat out of something due; (*sl, vulg*) to have sexual intercourse with; (*with* **up**) to gather (courage, etc) • *vi* to go together or come apart by being turned like a screw; to twist or turn with a writhing movement; (*sl, vulg*) to have sexual intercourse; (*with* **up**) to bungle.

screwball /'skru:bɔl/ *n* (*sl*) an odd or eccentric person. • *adj* whimsical, zany.

screwdriver /'skru:draɪvər/ *n* a tool like a blunt chisel for turning screws; a drink of vodka and orange juice.

screwed /skru:d/ *adj* (*sl*) drunk.

screw eye *n* a metal screw with a ring instead of a slotted head.

screw pine *n* any of various tropical plants with slender stems and clusters of spiral leaves.

screw propeller *n* an early form of propeller based on the Archimedes screw.

screw top *n* a cap that screws onto the top of a bottle or other container; a bottle, etc having this.

screwy /'skru:i/ *adj* (**screwier, screwiest**) (*sl*) eccentric, odd.—**screwiness** *n*.

scribble /'skrɪbəl/ *vti* to draw or write hastily or carelessly, to scrawl; to be a writer. • *n* hasty writing, a scrawl.—**scribbler** *n*.

scribe /skraɪb/ *n* a person who copies (documents); an author or journalist; (*Bible*) an expounder of Jewish law. • *vt* to draw a line on by cutting with a pointed instrument.

scriber /'skraɪbər/ *n* a pointed tool used to score or mark lines (e.g on metal) as guides for cutting.

scrim /skrɪm/ *n* a light open-weave fabric used in upholstery, lining, and theatre sets.

scrimmage /'skrɪmɪdʒ/ *n* a confused struggle; a skirmish; (*football*) the period between the ball entering play and it being declared dead. • *vi* to engage in a scrimmage.

scrimp /skrɪmp/ *vti* to be sparing or frugal (with); to make too small, to skimp.

scrimshank /'skrɪmʃæŋk/ *vi* (*inf*) to shirk work, *esp* military duties.

scrimshaw /'skrɪmʃɔ/ *n* carvings made from shells, whalebone, ivory, etc, *usu* by sailors; the art of producing such carvings.

scrip /skrɪp/ *n* a written list; a certificate entitling the holder to a share of company stock.

Script. *abbr* = Scripture(s).

script /skrɪpt/ *n* handwriting; a style of writing; the text of a stage play, screenplay or broadcast; a plan of action; (*print*) type that resembles handwriting. • *vt* to write a script (for).

scriptural /'skrɪptʃərəl/ *adj* of or based on the Bible or Scripture.

scripture /'skrɪptʃər/ *n* any sacred writing; (*with cap, often pl*) the Jewish Bible or Old Testament; the Christian Bible or Old and New Testaments. • *adj* contained in or quoted from the Bible.

scriptwriter /'skrɪptraɪtər/ *n* a writer of screenplays for films, TV, etc; a screenwriter.—**scriptwriting** *n*.

scrofula /'skrɒfjʊlə/ *n* tuberculosis of the lymph glands in the neck.—**scrofulous** *adj*.

scroll /skrəʊl/ *n* a roll of parchment or paper with writing on it; an ornament like this; (*her*) a ribbon with a motto; a list. • *vti* (*comput*) to move text across a screen; to decorate with scrolls.

scroll saw *n* a thin saw for cutting intricate designs.

Scrooge /skru:dʒ/ *n* (*also without cap*) a miserly, miserable person (after the character in *A Christmas Carol* by Charles Dickens).

scrotum /'skrəʊtəm/ *n* (*pl* **scrota, scrotums**) the pouch of skin containing the testicles.

scrounge /skraʊndʒ/ *vti* (*inf*) to seek or obtain (something) for nothing.—**scrounger** *n*.

scrub[1] /skrʌb/ *n* an arid area of stunted trees and shrubs; such vegetation; anything small or mean. • *adj* small, stunted, inferior, etc.

scrub[2] *vti* (**scrubbing, scrubbed**) to clean vigorously, to scour; to rub hard; (*inf*) to remove, to cancel. • *n* the act of scrubbing.

scrubber /'skrʌbər/ *n* a person or thing that scrubs; (*sl*) a promiscuous woman.

scrubby /'skrʌbi/ *adj* (**scrubbier, scrubbiest**) stunted; paltry; unkempt.—**scrubbily** *adv*.—**scrubbiness** *n*.

scruff[1] /skrʌf/ *n* the back of the neck, the nape.

scruff[2] *n* (*inf*) a shabbily dressed person.

scruffy /'skrʌfi/ *adj* (**scruffier, scruffiest**) shabby; unkempt.—**scruffily** *adv*.—**scruffiness** *n*.

scrum /skrʌm/ *n* a scrummage; ✹ (*Cdn*) the informal, disorganized questioning of a politician by reporters who crowd around him or her.—*also* **media scrum**.

scrum half *n* (*rugby*) (the position held by) the player who puts the ball into the scrum.

scrummage /'skrʌmɪdʒ/ *n* (*Rugby football*) a play consisting of a tussle between rival forwards in a compact mass for possession of the ball. • *vi* to form a scrum(mage).

scrump /skrʌmp/ *vt* (*dial*) to steal apples from an orchard or garden.

scrumptious /'skrʌmpʃəs/ *adj* (*inf*) delicious; very pleasing.—**scrumptiously** *adv*.—**scrumptiousness** *n*.

scrunch /skrʌntʃ/ *vti* to crumple, *esp* the hair when drying; to crunch; to be crumpled or crunched. • *n* a crunching sound; the act of scrunching.

scruncheon /'skrʌntʃən/ *n* ✹ a small piece of crisply fried pork used as a garnish.

scruple /'skru:pəl/ *n* (*usu pl*) a moral principle or belief causing one to doubt or hesitate about a course of action. • *vti* to hesitate owing to scruples.

scrupulous /'skru:pjuləs/ *adj* careful; conscientious; thorough.—**scrupulously** *adv*.—**scrupulousness** *n*.

scrutineer /skru:tɪ'nɪːr/ *n* a person who scrutinizes, *esp* an inspector of ballot papers.

scrutinize /'skru:tɪˌnaɪz/ *vti* to look closely at, to examine narrowly; to make a scrutiny.—**scrutinizer** *n*.

scrutiny /'skru:tɪni/ *n* (*pl* **scrutinies**) a careful examination; a critical gaze; an official inspection of votes cast in an election.

scuba /'sku:bə/ *n* a diver's apparatus with compressed-air tanks for breathing underwater.

scud /skʌd/ *vti* (**scudding, scudded**) to go along swiftly; to be driven before the wind. • *n* an act of scudding; light clouds, etc, driven by wind; a type of missile.

scuff /skʌf/ *vti* to drag the feet, to shuffle; to wear or mark the surface of by doing this.

scuffle /'skʌfəl/ *n* a confused fight; the sound of shuffling. • *vi* to fight confusedly; to move by shuffling.

scull /skʌl/ *n* an oar worked from side to side over the stern of a boat; a light rowing boat for racing. • *vti* to propel with a scull.

scullery /'skʌləri/ *n* (*pl* **sculleries**) a room for storage or kitchen work, such as washing dishes, etc.

sculpt /skʌlpt/ *vt* to carve, to sculpture.

sculptor /'skʌlptər/ *n* a person skilled in sculpture.

sculptress /'skʌlptrəs/ *n* a woman skilled in sculpture.

sculpture /'skʌlptʃər/ *n* the art of carving wood or forming clay, stone, etc, into figures, statues, etc; a three-dimensional work of art; a sculptor's work. • *vt* to carve, adorn or portray with sculptures; to shape, mould or form like sculpture.—**sculptural** *adj*.

scum /skʌm/ *n* a thin layer of impurities on top of a liquid; refuse; despicable people.

scumbag /'skʌmbæg/ *n* (*sl*) a disgusting or despicable person.

scumble /'skʌmbəl/ *vt* (*drawing and painting*) to soften lines or colours by applying a thin coat of opaque colour. • *n* the upper layer of colour applied for this purpose.

scunner /'skʌnər/ *n* (*Scot*) disgust. • *vti* to feel or cause to feel disgust.—**scunnered** *adj*

scupper /'skʌpər/ *n* a hole in a ship's side that lets water run from the deck into the sea. • *vt* (*sl*) to sink deliberately; to disable.

scurf /skʌrf/ *n* small flakes of dead skin (as dandruff); any scaly coating.

scurrilous /'skʌrɪləs/ *adj* abusive; grossly offensive.

scurry /'skʌri/ *vi* (**scurrying, scurried**) to hurry with quick, short steps, to scamper. • *n* (*pl* **scurries**) a bustle; a flurry (as of snow).

scurvy /'skʌrvi/ *n* a disease caused by a deficiency of vitamin C. • *adj* base; contemptible.

scut /skʌt/ *n* the short tail of certain animals, such as the deer or hare.

scute /skju:t/, **scutum** /-təm/ *n* an external scales or plate on the bodies of animals such as the armadillo, turtle, etc.

scutellum /sku'teləm/ *n* (*pl* **scutella**) any of the small horny scales or plates on a plant or animal.

scuttle[1] /'skʌtəl/ *vi* to run quickly; to hurry away. • *n* a short swift run; a hurried pace.

scuttle[2] *n* a bucket with a lip for storing coal.

scuttle[3] *n* (*naut*) a hatchway, a hole with a cover in a ship's deck or side. • *vt* to sink a ship by making holes in the bottom.

scuttlebut /'skʌtəlˌbʌt/ *n* (*formerly*) a cask containing drinking water on the deck of a ship; (*sl*) gossip.

scuzzy /'skʌzi/ *adj* (**scuzzier, scuzziest**) (*sl*) filthy, squalid.

scythe /saɪð/ *n* a two-handed implement with a large curved blade for cutting grass, etc. • *vti* to cut with a scythe; to mow down.

SD *abbr* = South Dakota.

SDI *abbr* = Strategic Defense Initiative.

SE *abbr* = southeast(ern).

Se (*chem symbol*) selenium.

sea /si:/ *n* the ocean; a section of this; a vast expanse of water; a heavy wave, the swell of the ocean; something like the sea in size; the seafaring life. • *adj* marine, of the sea.

sea anchor *n* a device dragged behind a vessel to slow the rate of drifting or keep it heading into the wind.

sea anemone *n* any of various solitary brightly coloured polyps with a ring of petal-like tentacles surrounding the mouth.

sea bass *n* any of numerous American marine fishes with a long body and a spiny dorsal fin.

seaboard /'si:bɔrd/ *n*, *adj* (land) bordering on the sea.

seaborne /'si:bɔrn/ *adj* conveyed by the sea; carried on a ship.

sea bream *n* any of numerous marine food fishes of European seas.

sea breeze *n* a wind that blows from the sea to the land.

sea change *n* a radical transformation.

seacock /'si:kɒk/ *n* a valve in the hull of a vessel through which water can pass in or out.

sea cow *see* **dugong**.

sea cucumber *n* an echinoderm with an elongated body, leathery skin and an oral ring of tentacles at one end.

sea dog *n* an old sailor.

SeaDoo /'si:du:/ *n* ✹ (*Cdn*) (*trademark*) a narrow, jet-propelled watercraft for one or two persons, ridden like a motorcycle.

sea eagle *n* any of various fish-eating eagles.

seafarer /'si:ˌfɛrər/ *n* a sailor; a person who travels by sea.

seafaring /'si:ˌfɛrɪŋ/ *n* travelling by sea, *esp* the work of a sailor.—*also adj*.

seafood /'si:fu:d/ *n* edible fish or shellfish from the sea.

sea front /'si:frʌnt/ *n* the waterfront of a seaside place.

sea green *adj, n* (a) pale bluish green.

seagoing /-gɔ:ɪŋ/ *adj* (*ship*) made for use on the open sea.

seagull /'si:gʌl/ *n* a gull.

sea holly *n* a European coastal plant with blue flowers.

sea horse *n* a small bony-plated fish with a horselike head and neck and a long tail, that swims in an upright position; in fable, a horse with the tail of a fish.

sea kale /'si:keɪl/ *n* a European coastal plant with fleshy leaves and edible shoots.

seal[1] /si:l/ *n* an engraved stamp for impressing wax, lead, etc; wax, lead, etc, so impressed; that which authenticates or pledges; a device for closing or securing tightly. • *vt* to fix a seal to; to close tightly or securely; to shut up; to mark as settled, to confirm.

seal[2] *n* an aquatic mammal with four webbed flippers; the fur of some seals; a dark brown. • *vi* to hunt seals.

sea lane *n* a route for ships.

sealant /'si:lənt/ *n* a thing that seals, as wax, etc; a substance for stopping a leak, making watertight, etc.

sea lavender *n* any of a genus of coastal plants with white, pink or purple flowers.

sealed-beam *adj* (*car headlight*) having the reflector incorporated in the lamp.

sea legs *npl* (*inf*) the ability to walk steadily on a moving ship and to be free from seasickness.

sealer /'si:lər/ *n* a person or a ship whose business is hunting seals.

sea level *n* the level of the surface of the sea in relation to the land.

sea lily *n* an echinoderm with a thin elongated body topped by petal-like tentacles.

sealing wax *n* a resinous compound that is plastic when warm and used for sealing letters, etc.

sea lion *n* a large seal of the Pacific Ocean that has a loud roar and, in the male, a mane.

sealskin /'si:lskɪn/ *n* the fur of a seal; a coat of this.

Sealyham terrier /'si:lɪhæm/ *n* a breed of wire-haired terrier with short legs and a longish, *usu* white, coat.

seam /siːm/ *n* the line where two pieces of cloth are stitched together; (*geol*) a stratum of coal, oil, etc, between thicker ones; a line or wrinkle. • *vt* to join with a seam; to furrow.

seaman /'siːmən/ *n* (*pl* **seamen**) a sailor; a naval rank.

seamanship /'siːmənʃɪp/ *n* the skill of handling, working and navigating a ship.

sea mile *n* a nautical mile.

sea mouse *n* a marine worm with a broad body covered in hairlike bristles.

seamstress /'siːmstrəs/ or /'sem-/ *n* a woman who sews for a living.

seamy /'siːmi/ *adj* (**seamier, seamiest**) unpleasant or sordid.

seance, séance /'seɪɒns/ or /-ās/ *n* a meeting of spiritualists to try to communicate with the dead.

sea otter *n* a large marine otter of North Pacific coasts that feeds on shellfish.

sea pink *n* the plant thrift.

seaplane /'siːpleɪn/ *n* an aeroplane with floats that allow it to take off from and land on water.

seaport /'siːpɔːt/ *n* a port, harbour or town accessible to oceangoing ships.

sear /siːr/ *vt* to burn or scorch the surface of; to brand with a heated iron; to wither up.

search /sɜːtʃ/ *vi* to look around to find something; to explore. • *vt* to examine or inspect closely; to probe into. • *n* the act of searching; an investigation; a quest.—**searcher** *n*.

search engine *n* (*comput*) a tool that is used to look for and retrieve information on the Web.

searching /'sɜːtʃɪŋ/ *adj* keen, piercing; examining thoroughly.—**searchingly** *adv*.

searchlight /'sɜːtʃlaɪt/ *n* a powerful ray of light projected by an apparatus on a swivel; the apparatus.

search party *n* a group of people organized to locate a missing person or thing.

search warrant *n* a legal document that authorizes a police search.

seascape /'siːskeɪp/ *n* a picture of a scene at sea.

Sea Scout *n* a member of a Scout troop specializing in sailing, canoeing, diving, etc.

sea serpent *n* a legendary sea-dwelling monster resembling a snake or dragon.

seashell /'siːʃel/ *n* the discarded or empty shell of a marine mollusc.

seashore /'siːʃɔːr/ *n* land beside the sea or between high and low water marks; the beach.

seasick /'siːsɪk/ *adj* affected with nausea brought on by the motion of a ship.—**seasickness** *n*.

seaside /'siːsaɪd/ *n* seashore.

sea snail *n* a spiral-shelled marine mollusc, such as a whelk; a small slimy fish with pelvic fins formed into a sucker.

sea snake *n* a venomous snake of tropical waters with an oar-shaped tail.

season /'siːzən/ *n* one of the four equal parts into which the year is divided: spring, summer, autumn, or winter; a period of time; a time when something is plentiful or in use; a suitable time; (*inf*) a season ticket. • *vt* (*food*) to flavour by adding salt, spices, etc; to make mature or experienced; (*wood*) to dry until ready for use. • *vi* to become experienced.

seasonable /'siːzənəbəl/ *adj* suitable for the season; timely, opportune.—**seasonableness** *n*.—**seasonably** *adv*.

seasonal /'siːzənəl/ *adj* of or relating to a particular season.—**seasonally** *adv*.

seasonal affective disorder *n* a state of depression that affects some people in the winter months, thought to be caused by a lack of sunlight.

seasoning /'siːzənɪŋ/ *n* salt, spices, etc, used to enhance the flavour of food; the process of making something fit for use.

season ticket *n* a ticket or set of tickets valid for a number of concerts, games, journeys, etc, during a specified period.

seat /siːt/ *n* a piece of furniture for sitting on, such as a chair, bench, etc; the part of a chair on which one sits; the buttocks, the part of the trousers covering them; a way of sitting (on a horse, etc); the chief location, or centre; a part at or forming a base; the right to sit as a member; a parliamentary constituency; a large country house. • *vt* to place on a seat; to provide with seats; to settle.

seat belt *n* an anchored strap worn in a car or aeroplane to secure a person to a seat.

seated /'siːtəd/ *adj* provided with a seat or seats; fixed, confirmed; located.

seating /'siːtɪŋ/ *n* the arrangement or provision of seats.

SEATO *abbr* = South East Asia Treaty Organization.

seat sale *n* ✷ (*Cdn*) a sale of airline tickets at a discount price.

sea trout *n* a marine variety of brown trout that migrates to fresh water to spawn.

sea urchin *n* a small marine animal with a round body enclosed in a shell covered with sharp spines.

sea wall /'siːwɒl/ *n* a barrier or embankment to prevent erosion by the sea.

seaward /'siːwərd/ *adj* toward the sea. • *adv* toward or in the direction of the sea.—**seawards** *adv*.

seaway /'siːweɪ/ *n* an ocean traffic lane; a waterway for seagoing traffic to an inland port.

seaweed /'siːwiːd/ *n* a mass of plants growing in or under water; a sea plant, *esp* a marine alga.

seaworthy /s'iːˌwɜːði/ *adj* fit to go to sea; able to withstand sea water, watertight.—**seaworthiness** *n*.

sebaceous /sə'beɪʃəs/ *adj* of, secreting, containing, or producing oily or fatty matter.

sebaceous glands *npl* the small skin glands that secrete sebum onto the skin surface.

seborrhoea, seborrhea /ˌsebə'riə/ *n* the excessive secretion of sebum.—**seborrhoeic, seborrheic** *adj*.

sebum /'siːbəm/ *n* a fatty substance secreted by the sebaceous glands to lubricate the hair and skin.

SEC *abbr* = Securities and Exchange Commission.

sec[1] /sek/ *adj* (*wine*) dry; (*champagne*) medium sweet.

sec[2] *n* (*inf*) a second.

sec[3] *abbr* = secant.

sec. *abbr* = second.

secant /'siːkənt/ *n* a trigonometrical function that is the reciprocal of the cosine; a straight line that intersects a curve.

secateurs /'sekəˌtɜːz/ *npl* a pair of small shears with curved blades for pruning, etc.

secede /sə'siːd/ *vi* to withdraw formally one's membership from a society or organization.—**seceder** *n*.

secession /sə'seʃən/ *n* the act or an instance of seceding; a breaking away.—**secessional** *adj*.

seclude /sə'kluːd/ *vt* to keep (a person, etc) separate from others; to remove or screen from view.

secluded /sə'kluːdəd/ *adj* private; sheltered; kept from contact with other people.

seclusion /sə'kluːʒən/ *n* the state of being secluded; privacy, solitude.

second /'sekənd/ *adj* next after first: alternate; another of the same kind; next below the first in rank, value, etc. • *n* a person or thing coming second; another; an article of merchandise not of first quality; an aid or assistant, as to a boxer, duellist; the gear after low gear: one sixtieth of a minute of time or of an angular degree; (*pl*) (*inf*) another helping of food. • *adv* in the second place, group, etc. • *vt* to act as a second (to); (*a motion, resolution, etc*) to support; (*mil*) to place on temporary service elsewhere.

secondary /'sekəndˌeri/ *adj* subordinate; second in rank or importance; in the second stage; derived, not primary; relating to secondary school. • *n* (*pl* **secondaries**) that which is secondary; a delegate, a deputy.—**secondarily** *adv*.

secondary cell *n* a battery that can convert chemical energy to electrical energy by reversible chemical reactions and so be recharged.

secondary colour *n* a colour formed by mixing two primary colours.

secondary emission *n* (*physics*) the emission of secondary electrons from a solid surface due to bombardment by a beam of primary electrons or other elementary particles.

secondary school *n* a school between elementary or primary school and college or university.

secondary sexual characteristic *n* an attribute of a human being or animal that is characteristic of a particular sex but is not directly concerned with reproduction.

second best *adj* next to the best; inferior. • *adv* in second place. • *n* next to the best; an inferior alternative.

second chamber *n* the upper house in a legislative assembly with two chambers.

second childhood *n* dotage, senility.

second class *n* the class next to the first in a classification. • *adj* (second-class) relating to a second class; inferior, mediocre; (*seating, accommodation*) next in price and quality to first class; (*mail*) less expensive and handled more slowly (than first class).

Second Coming n (*Christianity*) the return to earth of Christ at the Last Judgment as prophesied.

second cousin n a child of the first cousin of one's parent.

second-degree burn n a burn which causes blistering of the skin.

second fiddle n (the musical part for) a second violin in an orchestra or string quartet; (*inf*) a person of secondary importance.

second hand n the moving pointer in a clock or watch that indicates the seconds.

second-hand adj bought after use by another; derived, not original.—*also adv.*

secondly adv in the second place.

second nature n a long-established habit, etc, deeply fixed in a person's nature.

second person n that form of a pronoun (as *you*) or verb (as *are*) that refers to the person spoken to.

second-rate adj of inferior quality.

second sight n the supposed faculty of seeing events before they occur.

second string n a reserve or substitute player in a team.

second thought n a change in thought or decision after consideration.

second wind n a return to regular breathing after a bout of exercise; renewed energy or enthusiasm.

secrecy /'si:krəsi/ n (pl **secrecies**) the state of being secret; the ability to keep secret.

secret /'si:krət/ adj not made public; concealed from others; hidden; private; remote. • n something hidden; a mystery; a hidden cause.

secret agent n a spy.

secretaire /ˌsɛkrə'tɛr/ n a writing desk with an upper section for books and documents.

secretariat /ˌsɛkrə'tɛriət/ n an administrative office or staff, as in a government.

secretary /'sɛkrəˌtɛri/ n (pl **secretaries**) a person employed to deal with correspondence, filing, telephone calls of another or of an association; the head of a state department.—**secretarial** adj.

secretary bird n a large long-legged African bird of prey that eats mostly snakes.

Secretary-General n (pl **secretaries-general**) the chief administrator of a large organization (*eg* the United Nations).

Secretary of State n in the UK, any of various ministers in charge of government departments; (*with caps*) in the US, the minister in charge of foreign affairs.

secrete / sə'kri:t/ vt to conceal; to hide; (*cell, gland, etc*) to produce and release (a substance) out of blood or sap.

secretion /sə'kri:ʃən/ n the process of secreting; a substance secreted by an animal or plant.

secretive /'si:krətɪv/ adj given to secrecy; uncommunicative, reticent.—**secretively** adv.—**secretiveness** n.

secretly /-li/ adv in a secret way; unknown to others.

secretory /sɪ'kri:təri/ adj having the function of secreting, as a gland.

secret police n a police force that operates covertly to suppress political dissent rather than criminal activity.

secret service n a government agency that gathers intelligence, infiltrates terrorist or subversive organizations, conducts espionage, etc in the interests of national security.

sect /sɛkt/ n a religious denomination; a group of people united by a common interest or belief; a faction.

sectarian /sɛk'tɛriən/ adj of or confined to a religious sect; bigoted. • n a member or adherent of a sect.

sectarianism /-ɪzəm/ n devotion to a sect; religious narrowness.

section /'sɛkʃən/ n the act of cutting; a severed or separable part; a division; a distinct portion; a slice; a representation of anything cut through to show its interior; (*geom*) the cutting of a solid by a plane; a plane figure formed by this. • vti to cut or separate into sections; to represent in sections; to become separated or cut into parts.

sectional /'sɛkʃənəl/ adj of a section; made up of several sections; local rather than general in character.—**sectionally** adv.

sector /'sɛktər/ n (*geom*) a space enclosed by two radii of a circle and the arc they cut off; a distinctive part (as of an economy); a subdivision; (*mil*) an area of activity.

secular /'sɛkjulər/ adj having no connection with religion or the church; worldly.—**secularly** adv.

secularize /'sɛkjulərˌaɪz/ vt to change from religious to civil use or control.—**secularization** n.

secure /sə'kju:ər/ or /-'kjər/ adj free from danger, safe; stable; firmly held or fixed; confident, assured (of); reliable. • vt to make safe; to fasten firmly; to protect; to confine; to fortify; to guarantee; to gain possession of, to obtain.—**securely** adv.

security /sə'kju:rɪti/ or /-kjər-/ n (pl **securities**) the state of being secure; a financial guarantee, surety; a pledge for repayment, etc; a protection or safeguard; a certificate of shares or bonds.

Security Council n the principal council of the United Nations charged with maintaining world peace.

security guard n a person employed to protect public buildings, banks, offices, etc and to transport large sums of money.

security police n a police force whose function is to prevent espionage; the military police of an air force.

security risk n a person or thing regarded as a potential threat to security.

sedan /sɪ'dæn/ n a car with no division between driver and passengers; a covered chair for one person with poles carried by two bearers.

sedate[1] /sə'deɪt/ adj calm; composed; serious and unemotional.—**sedately** adv.—**sedateness** n.

sedate[2] vti to calm or become calm by the administration of a sedative.

sedation /sə'deɪʃən/ n the act of calming or the condition of being calmed, *esp* by sedatives; the administration of sedatives to calm a patient.

sedative /'sɛdətɪv/ n a drug with a soothing, calming effect. • adj having a soothing, calming effect.

sedentary /'sɛdənˌtɛri/ adj requiring a sitting position; inactive; not migratory.

Seder /'seɪdər/ n a Jewish ceremonial meal held on the first night of Passover.

sedge /sɛdʒ/ n a grass-like plant that grows in marshes or beside water.

sedge warbler n a European songbird that inhabits marshy areas.

sediment /'sɛdəmənt/ n matter that settles at the bottom of a liquid; (*geol*) matter deposited by water or wind.

sedimentary /ˌsɛdə'mɛntəri/ adj relating to or formed by sediment.

sedition /sə'dɪʃən/ n incitement to rebel against the government.—**seditious** adj.—**seditiously** adv.

seduce /sə'du:s/ or /-'dju:s/ vt to lead astray; to corrupt; to entice into unlawful sexual intercourse.—**seducer** n.

seduction /sə'dʌkʃən/ n the act of seducing; temptations; attraction.

seductive /sə'dʌktəv/ adj tending to seduce; enticing, alluring.—**seductively** adv.—**seductiveness** n.

sedulous /'sɛdjuləs/ adj diligent; persevering.—**sedulously** adv.—**sedulousness** n.

see[1] /si:/ vt (**seeing, saw, pp seen**) to perceive with the eyes; to observe; to grasp with the intelligence; to ascertain; to take care (that); to accompany; to visit; to meet; to consult; (*guests*) to receive; (*with* **through**) to persist or endure to the end; to assist (*eg* a friend) during a crisis, difficulty, etc. • vi to have the faculty of sight; to make inquiry; to consider, to reflect; to understand; (*with* **about**) to deal with; to consider in detail; (*with* **off**) to be present when someone leaves on a journey, etc; (*inf*) to repel, get rid of; (*with* **through**) to recognize the true character of.

see[2] n the diocese of a bishop.

seed /si:d/ n the small, hard part (ovule) of a plant from which a new plant grows; such seeds collectively; the source of anything; sperm or semen; descendants; (*tennis*) a seeded tournament player. • vti to sow (seed); to produce or shed seed; to remove seeds from; (*tennis*) to arrange (a tournament) so that the best players cannot meet until later rounds.

seedbed /'si:dbɛd/ n a nursery bed for a plant; a place or source of growth or development.

seed cake /'si:dkeɪk/ n a sweet cake flavoured with aromatic (*usu* caraway) seeds.

seed coral n small pieces of coral used in jewellery.

seed corn n corn reserved for sowing; assets promising future earning potential.

seedless /'si:dləs/ adj without seeds.

seedling /'si:dlɪŋ/ n a young plant raised from seed, not from a cutting; a young tree before it is a sapling.

seed money n money used to start a new project or enterprise.

seed oyster *n* a young oyster ready for transplantation to a new bed.

seed pearl *n* a very small pearl.

seed potato *n* a potato tuber ready for planting.

seed vessel *n* a pericarp.

seedy /'si:di/ *adj* (**seedier, seediest**) full of seeds; out of sorts, indisposed; shabby; rundown.—**seedily** *adv*.—**seediness** *n*.

seeing /'si:ɪŋ/ *n* vision, sight. • *adj* having sight; observant. • *conj* in view of the fact that; since.

seek /si:k/ *vti* (**seeking, sought**) to search for; to try to find, obtain, or achieve; to resort to; (*with* **to**) to try to, to endeavour; (*with* **out**) to search for and locate a person or thing; to try to secure the society of.—**seeker** *n*.

seem /si:m/ *vi* to appear (to be); to give the impression of; to appear to oneself.

seeming /'si:mɪŋ/ *adj* that seems real, true; ostensible, apparent.—**seemingly** *adv*.

seemly /'si:mli/ *adj* (**seemlier, seemliest**) proper, fitting.—**seemliness** *n*.

seen /si:n/ *see* **see**[1].

seep /si:p/ *vi* to ooze gently, to leak through.

seepage /'si:pədʒ/ *n* the act of seeping; the liquid that has seeped.

seer /'si:ər/ or /'si:r/ *n* a person who sees visions, a prophet.

seersucker /'si:r,sʌkər/ *n* a light, *usu* cotton, fabric with a puckered surface.

seesaw /'si:sɔ/ *n* a plank balanced across a central support so that it is tilted up and down by a person sitting on each end; an up-and-down movement like this; vacillation. • *vi* to move up and down; to fluctuate. • *adj, adv* alternately rising and falling.

seethe /si:ð/ *vi* to be very angry inwardly; to swarm (with people).

segment /'segmənt/ *n* a section; a portion; one of the two parts of a circle or sphere when a line is drawn through it. • *vti* to cut or separate into segments.—**segmentation** *n*.

segregate /'segrə,geɪt/ *vti* to set apart from others, to isolate; to separate racial or minority groups.

segregation /,segrə'geɪʃən/ *n* the act of segregating or the condition of being segregated; the policy of compelling racial groups to live apart.

seguidilla /,segə'di:ljə/ or /,seɪgə-/, /'di:jə/ *n* (the music for) a lively Spanish dance in triple time.

seiche /seɪʃ/ *n* an undulation of the surface of a lake, caused by earth tremors or changes in barometric pressure.

seigneur /si:'njər/ *n* a feudal lord; ✤ (*Cdn*) (*hist*) a person in French Canada who rented land to tenant farmers.—**seigneurial** *adj*.

seigneury /'si:njəri/ *n* (*pl* **seigneuries**) the estate or authority of a seigneur.

seine /seɪn/ *n* a large fishing net that hangs vertically by means of floats along the top and weights along the bottom. • *vi* to catch fish with this.

seismic /'saɪzmɪk/ *adj* of or caused by earthquakes.—**seismically** *adv*.

seismo- /'saɪzmɔ:/, **seism-** /'saɪzm/ *prefix* earthquake.

seismograph /'saɪzmə,græf/ *n* an instrument for recording the direction, intensity, and time of an earthquake.—**seismographer** *n*.—**seismographic** *adj*.—**seismography** *n*.

seismology /saɪz'mɒlədʒi/ *n* the scientific study of earthquakes.—**seismologic, seismological** *adj*.—**seismologist** *n*.

seize /si:z/ *vt* to grasp; to capture; to take hold of suddenly or forcibly; to attack or afflict suddenly. • *vi* (*machinery*) to become jammed.—**seizable** *adj*.

seizure /'si:ʒər/ *n* the act of seizing; what is seized; a sudden attack of illness, an apoplectic stroke.

seldom /'seldəm/ *adv* not often, rarely.

select /sə'lekt/ *vti* to choose or pick out. • *adj* excellent; choice; limited (*eg* in membership); exclusive.

select committee *n* a parliamentary committee established to investigate and report on a particular subject.

selection /sə'lekʃən/ *n* the act of selecting; what is or are selected; the process by which certain animals or plants survive while others are eliminated, natural selection.

selective /sə'lektɪv/ *adj* having the power of selection; highly specific in activity or effect.—**selectively** *adv*.—**selectiveness** *n*.

selenium /sə'li:niəm/ *n* a nonmetallic solid chemical element with semiconductive and photoconductive properties that has various uses in electronics.

seleno- /sə'li:nɔ:/, **selen-** /sə'li:n/ *prefix* the moon.

selenography /,si:lə'nɒgrəfi/ *n* the study and mapping of the physical features of the moon.—**selenographer** *n*.—**selenographic** *adj*.

self- /self/ *prefix* of itself or oneself; by, for, in relation to, itself or oneself: automatic.

self *n* (*pl* **selves**) the identity, character, etc, of any person or thing; one's own person as distinct from all others; one's own interests or advantage. • *adj* (*colour*) matching, uniform.

self-abnegation /,self,æbnɪ'geɪʃən/ *n* denial of one's own interests or desires in favour of those of others.

self-absorption /,selfəb'zɔrpʃən/ *n* preoccupation with one's own interests and welfare.

self-abuse /,selfə'bju:s/ *n* masturbation.

self-acting /self'æktɪŋ/ *adj* automatic.

self-addressed /,selfə'drest/ *adj* addressed to return to the sender; intended for oneself.

self-aggrandizement /,selfə'grændaɪzmənt/ or /-dɪzmənt/ *n* acting to increase one's own power and importance at the expense of others.—**self-aggrandizing** *adj*.

self-approbation /selfæprəbeɪʃən/ *n* satisfaction with one's own actions or accomplishments, *esp* to excess.

self-assertion /,selfə'sɜrʃən/ *n* the act of asserting one's own opinions, ideas, or rights, *esp* determinedly.—**self-assertive** *adj*.

self-assured /-ə'ʃʊrd/ *adj* confident.—**self-assurance** *n*.

self-catering /self'keɪtərɪŋ/ *adj* catering for oneself.

self-centred, self-centered /self'sentərd/ *adj* preoccupied with one's own affairs.—**self-centeredly, self-centeredly** *adv*.—**self-centredness, self-centeredness** *n*.

self-coloured, self-colored /self'kʌlərd/ *adj* of a single colour.

self-confessed /,selfkən'fest/ *adj* according to one's own testimony.

self-confident /self'kɒnfɪdənt/ *adj* sure of one's own powers.—**self-confidence** *n*.—**self-confidently** *adv*.

self-conscious /self'kɒnʃəs/ *adj* embarrassed or awkward in the presence of others, ill at ease.—**self-consciously** *adv*.—**self-consciousness** *n*.

self-contained /,selfkən'teɪnd/ *adj* complete in itself; showing self-control; uncommunicative.—**self-containment** *n*.

self control /,selfkən'trəʊl/ *n* control of one's emotions, desires, etc, by the will.—**self-controlled** *adj*.

self-deception /,selfdə'sepʃən/ or /-di-/ *n* the act or state of deceiving oneself.

self-defence, self-defense /,selfdə'fens/ or /-di-/ *n* the act of defending oneself; (*law*) a plea for the justification for the use of force.

self-denial /,selfdə'naɪəl/ or /-di-/ *n* abstention from pleasure, etc; unselfishness.

self-determination /,selfdə,tɜrmə'neɪʃən/ or /-di-/ *n* free will; the choice of action without compulsion; the right of a nation to choose its own form of government.

self-drive /-draɪv/ *adj* (*hired vehicle*) driven by the hirer.

self-educated /self'edjuː,keɪtəd/ *adj* educated without benefit of formal instruction; educated at one's own expense.

self-effacement /,selfə'feɪsɪŋ/ *n* the act of making oneself or one's actions inconspicuous, due to modesty or timidity.

self-employed /,selfɛm'plɔɪd/ *adj* earning one's living in one's own business or profession, not employed by another; working freelance.

self-esteem /,selfə'sti:m/ *n* confidence and respect for oneself; an exaggerated opinion of oneself.

self-evident /self'evɪdənt/ *adj* evident without proof or explanation.—**self-evidently** *adv*.

self-explanatory /,selfɪk'splænətəri/ *adj* easily understood without explanation.

self-expression /,selfɪk'spreʃən/ *n* the expression of one's own personality, as in creative art.

self-governing /self'gʌvərnɪŋ/ *adj* autonomous; (*colony, etc*) having an elective legislation.—**self-government** *n*.

self-help /self'help/ *n* the provision of means to help oneself, instead of relying on others.

self-image /self'ɪmɪdʒ/ *n* one's sense of oneself or one's importance.

self-importance /,selfɪm'pɔrtəns/ *n* an exaggerated estimate of one's own worth; pompousness.—**self-important** *adj*.

self-induced /,selfɪn'dju:st/ or /-'dju:st/ *adj* brought on by oneself or itself.

self-induction /,selfɪn'dekʃən/ *n* the production of an electromotive force in a circuit by a variation in the electric current in the same circuit.

self-indulgence /ˌsɛlfɪnˈdʌldʒəns/ *n* undue gratification of one's desires, appetites, or whims.—**self-indulgent** *adj*.

self-inflicted /ˌsɛlfɪnˈflɪktəd/ *adj* (*wound, etc*) caused to a person by himself.

self-interest /sɛlfˈɪntrəst/ *n* regard to one's own advantage.

selfish /ˈsɛlfɪʃ/ *adj* chiefly concerned with oneself; lacking in consideration for others.—**selfishly** *adv*.—**selfishness** *n*.

self-justification /sɛlfˌdʒʌstɪfɪˈkeɪʃən/ *n* the act or instance of making excuses for one's actions, etc.

selfless /ˈsɛlfləs/ *adj* with no thought of self, unselfish.—**selflessly** *adv*.—**selflessness** *n*.

self-loading /sɛlfˈloʊdɪŋ/ *n* (*firearm*) semiautomatic.—**self-loader** *n*.

self-love /sɛlfˈlʌv/ *n* conceit; selfishness.

self-made /ˈsɛlfmeɪd/ *adj* having achieved status or wealth by one's own efforts.

self-opinionated /sɛlfəˈpɪnjəˌneɪtɪd/ *adj* conceited; stubborn.

self-pity /sɛlfˈpɪti/ *n* pity for oneself.—**self-pitying** *adj*.

self-pollination /sɛlfˌpɒlɪˈneɪʃən/ *n* the transfer of pollen from the anther to the stigma in the same flower.

self-portrait /sɛlfˈpɔrtrət/ *n* an artist or author's painting or account of himself or herself.

self-possessed /sɛlf/ *adj* cool and collected.

self-preservation /sɛlfˌprɛzərˈveɪʃən/ *n* the instinct to protect oneself from injury or death.

self-propelled /ˌsɛlfprəˈpɛld/ *adj* (*vehicle*) moving under its own power.

self-raising /sɛlfˈreɪzɪŋ/ *adj* (*flour*) self-rising.

self-realization /sɛlfˌriːəlaɪˈzeɪʃən/ *n* the understanding or achievement of one's own potential or desires.

self-regard /ˌsɛlfrəˈɡɑrd/ or /-rɪˈɡɑrd/ *n* concern for one's own interests; respect for oneself.

self-reliant /ˌsɛlfrɪˈlaɪənt/ *adj* relying on one's own powers; confident.—**self-reliance** *n*.

self-reproach /ˌsɛlfrɪˈproʊtʃ/ *n* the act of blaming oneself.

self-respect /ˌsɛlfrɪˈspɛkt/ *n* proper respect for oneself, one's standing and dignity.—**self-respecting** *adj*.

self-righteous /sɛlfˈraɪtʃəs/ *adj* thinking oneself better than others; priggish.—**self-righteousness** *n*.

self-rising /sɛlfˈraɪzɪŋ/ *adj* (*flour*) containing a raising agent, self-raising.

self-rule /sɛlfˈruːl/ *n* self-government.

self-sacrifice /sɛlfˈsækrɪˌfaɪs/ *n* the sacrifice of one's own interests, welfare, etc, to secure that of others.

selfsame /ˈsɛlfseɪm/ *adj* identical, the very same.

self-satisfied /sɛlfˈsætɪsˌfaɪd/ *adj* smugly conceited.

self-seeking /ˈsɛlfˌsiːkɪŋ/ *adj* preoccupied with securing one's own well-being or interest; selfish.—**self-seeker** *n*.

self-service /sɛlfˈsɜrvəs/ *adj* serving oneself in a cafe, shop, filling station, etc.

self-serving /sɛlfˈsɜrvɪŋ/ *adj* always seeking to protect or further one's own interests.

self-sown /sɛlfˈsoʊn/ *adj* (*plants*) grown from seeds that were planted or deposited naturally without intervention by humans or animals.

self-starter /sɛlfˈstɑrtər/ *n* an electric device for starting an engine; a motivated employee who requires little supervision.

self-styled /ˈsɛlfstaɪld/ *adj* called by oneself; pretended.

self-sufficient /ˌsɛlfsəˈfɪʃənt/ *adj* independent; supporting oneself (*eg* in growing food) without the help of others.—**self-sufficiency** *n*.

self-supporting /ˌsɛlfsəˈpɔrtɪŋ/ *adj* able to manage without help from others; able to stand unaided.

self-will /sɛlfˈwɪl/ *n* fixed adherence to one's own desires, intentions, etc; obstinacy.

self-winding /sɛlfˈwaɪndɪŋ/ *adj* (*watch*) wound automatically by an internal mechanism.

sell /sɛl/ *vb* (**selling, sold**) *vt* to exchange (goods, services, etc) for money or other equivalent; to offer for sale; to promote; to deal in; (*with* **up**) to sell all the goods of (a debtor) to clear the debt. • *vi* (*with* **off**) to clear out (stock) at bargain prices; (*with* **out**) to sell off, to betray for money or reward; (*inf*) to disappoint, to trick; to make sales; to attract buyers; (*with* **up**) to sell one's house, business, etc. • *n* an act or instance of selling; (*inf*) a disappointment, a trick, a fraud.—**seller** *n*.

Sellotape /ˈsɛləˌteɪp/ *n* (*trademark*) a transparent adhesive tape. • *vt* to seal or stick (something) using adhesive tape.

sellout *n* a show, game, etc, for which all the tickets are sold; (*inf*) a betrayal.

selvage, selvedge /ˈsɛlvɪdʒ/ *n* the edge of cloth so finished as to prevent unravelling.

selves /sɛlvz/ *see* **self**.

Sem *abbr* = Seminary; Semitic.

sem *abbr* = semester; semicolon.

semantic /səˈmæntɪk/ *adj* relating to the meaning of words. • *npl* the study of word meanings and changes.

semaphore /ˈsɛməˌfɔr/ *n* a system of visual signalling using the operator's arms, flags, etc; a signalling device consisting of a post with movable arms.

sematic /sɪˈmætɪk/ *adj* (*animal colouration*) warning of danger.

semblance /ˈsɛmbləns/ *n* likeness, resemblance; an outward, sometimes deceptive appearance.

semen /ˈsiːmən/ *n* the fluid that carries sperm in men and male animals.

semester /sɛˈmɛstər/ *n* an academic or school half-year.

semi /ˈsɛmi/ *n* (*pl* **semis**) (*inf*) a semidetached house; a semifinal.

semi- /ˈsɛmi/ or /-maɪ/ *prefix* half; not fully; twice in a (specified period).

semiannual /ˌsɛmiˈænjʊəl/ *adj* happening twice a year, or lasting for six months.—*also* **semiyearly**.

semiautomatic /ˌsɛmiˌɒtəˈmætɪk/ or /ˌsɛmaɪ-/ *adj* partly automatic; (*firearm*) self-loading but discharging in single shots only as the trigger is pulled.

semibreve /ˈsɛmiˌbriːv/ or /ˈsɛmaɪ-/ *n* (*mus*) a note equal to two minims.—*also* **whole note**.

semicircle /ˈsɛmiˌsɜrkəl/ or /ˈsɛmaɪ-/ *n* half of a circle.—**semicircular** *adj*.

semicircular canal *n* any of the three fluid-filled tubes in the inner ear concerned with maintaining balance.

semicolon /ˌsɛmiˈkoʊlən/ or /ˌsɛmaɪ-/ *n* the punctuation mark (;) of intermediate value between a comma and a full stop.

semiconductor /ˌsɛmikənˈdʌktər/ or /ˌsɛmaɪ-/ *n* a substance in a transmitter, as silicon, used to control the flow of current.

semiconscious /ˌsɛmiˈkɒnʃəs/ or /ˌsɛmaɪ-/ *adj* not fully conscious.—**semiconsciousness** *n*.

semi-detached /ˌsɛmidəˈtætʃt/ or /ˌsɛmaɪ-/ *adj* (*house*) with another joined to it on one side.—*also n*.

semifinal /ˌsɛmiˈfaɪnəl/ or /ˌsɛmaɪ-/ *adj, n* (the match or round) before the final in a knockout tournament.—**semifinalist** *n*.

semifluid /ˌsɛmiˈfluːɪd/ or /ˌsɛmaɪ-/ *n* having qualities between those of a fluid and a solid; viscous.

semiliterate /ˌsɛmiˈlɪtərɪt/ *n* barely able to read or write.

semilunar /ˌsɛmiˈluːnər/ or /ˌsɛmaɪ-/ *adj* in the shape of a crescent.

semilunar valve *n* either one of the two crescent-shaped valves in the heart.

seminal /ˈsɛmənəl/ *adj* of, relating to, or containing semen; promising or contributing to further development; original, influential.—**seminally** *adv*.

seminar /ˈsɛməˌnɑr/ *n* a group of students engaged in study or research under supervision; any group meeting to pool and discuss ideas.

seminary /ˈsɛməˌnɛri/ *n* (*pl* **seminaries**) a training college for priests, ministers, etc; a school for young women.

seminiferous /ˌsɛmiˈnɪfərəs/ *adj* producing or containing semen; (*plants*) bearing seeds.

semiology /ˌsɛmiˈɒlədʒi/ or /ˌsɛm-/ *n* the study of signs and symbols.—**semiologic, semiological** *adj*.—**semiologist** *n*.

semiotics /ˌsɛmiˈɒtɪks/ or /ˌsɛm-/ *n sing* the study of signs and symbols, *esp* their use in language and relationship to the world of things and ideas; the study of the symptoms of disease.—**semiotic, semiotical** *adj*.—**semiotician** *n*.

semiprecious /ˌsɛmiˈprɛʃəs/ or /ˌsɛmaɪ-/ *adj* denoting gems of lower value than precious stones.

semiprofessional /ˌsɛmiprəˈfɛʃənəl/ *adj* taking part in sport for pay, but not on a fulltime basis.—**semiprofessionally** *adv*.

semiquaver /ˈsɛmiˌkweɪvər/ *n* (*mus*) a sixteenth note.

semirigid /ˌsɛmiˈrɪdʒəd/ or /ˌsɛmaɪ-/ *adj* (*airship*) having a flexible gas container attached to a rigid keel.

semiskilled /ˌsɛmiˈskɪld/ or /ˌsɛmaɪ-/ *adj* partly skilled or trained.

semiskimmed /ˈsɛmiˌskɪmd/ *adj* (*milk*) having the cream partially removed.

semisolid /ˌsɛmiˈsɒləd/ or /ˌsɛmaɪ-/ *adj* having the properties between that of a liquid and a solid; extremely viscous.

Semite /'sɛmaɪt/ or /'siːm-/ n a member of the group of peoples including Arabs and Jews.
Semitic /sə'mɪtɪk/ adj of or belonging to Semites; Jewish.
Semitism /'sɛmə,tɪzəm/ n any political or economic policy relating to Jews.
semitone /'sɛmi,toːn/ n (mus) an interval equal to half a tone.
semitrailer /,semi'treɪlər/ or /,semaɪ-/ n a trailer that has wheels at the back but is supported at the front by the towing vehicle.
semivowel /'semi,vaʊəl/ or /,semaɪ-/ n (phon) a consonant that sound like a vowel (eg y or j), a glide.
semiyearly /-,jiːrli/ see **semiannual**.
semolina /,semə'liːnə/ n coarse particles of grain left after the sifting of wheat.
sempre /'sɛmpreɪ/ or /-ri/ adv (mus) always.
Sen abbr = senator; senior.
senate /'sɛnət/ n a legislative or governing body; (with cap) the upper branch of a two-body legislature in France, the US, etc; the governing body of some universities.
senator /'sɛnətər/ n a member of a senate.—**senatoria** adj.
send /send/ vti (**sending, sent**) to cause or enable to go; to have conveyed, to dispatch (a message or messenger); to cause to move, to propel; to grant; to cause to be; (sl) to move (a person) to ecstasy; (with **down**) to expel from university; (with **for**) to order to be brought, to summon; (with **up**) (inf) to send to prison; to imitate or make fun of.—**sender** n.
send-off n a friendly demonstration at a departure; a start given to someone or something.
senescent /sə'nɛsənt/ adj growing old.—**senescence** n.
seneschal /'senəʃəl/ n (hist) a steward in the house of a feudal lord.
senile /'siːnaɪl/ or /'sɛn-/ adj of or relating to old age; weakened, esp mentally, by old age.—**senility** n.
senior /'siːnjər/ adj higher in rank; of or for seniors; longer in service; older (when used to distinguish between father and son with the same first name). • n one's elder or superior in standing; a person of advanced age; a student in the last year of college or high school.
senior citizen n an elderly person, esp a retired one.
senior common room n a staffroom in a British college or university.
seniority /sin'jɔrəti/ or /-'jʌr-/ n (pl **seniorities**) the condition of being senior; status, priority, etc, in a given job.
sensation /sen'seɪʃən/ n awareness due to stimulation of the senses; an effect on the senses; a thrill; a state of excited interest; the cause of this.
sensational /sen'seɪʃənəl/ adj of or relating to sensation; exciting violent emotions; melodramatic.—**sensationally** adv.
sensationalism /sen'seɪʃənə,lɪzəm/ n the use of sensational writing, language, etc; the doctrine that all knowledge is obtained from sense impressions.—**sensationalist** adj.
sense /sɛns/ n one of the five human and animal faculties by which objects are perceived: sight, hearing, smell, taste, and touch; awareness; moral discernment; soundness of judgment; meaning, intelligibility; (pl) conscious awareness. • vt to perceive; to become aware of; to understand; to detect.
senseless /'sɛnsləs/ adj stupid, foolish; meaningless, purposeless; unconscious.—**senselessly** adv.—**senselessness** n.
sense organ n a bodily structure that reacts to stimuli and transmits them to the brain as nerve impulses.
sensibility /,sɛnsə'bɪliti/ n (pl **sensibilities**) the capacity to feel; over-sensitiveness; susceptibility; (pl) sensitive awareness or feelings.
sensible /'sɛnsəbəl/ adj having good sense or judgment; reasonable; practical; perceptible by the senses, appreciable; conscious (of); sensitive.—**sensibleness** n.—**sensibly** adv.
sensitive /'sɛnsɪtɪv/ adj having the power of sensation; feeling readily and acutely, keenly perceptive; (skin) delicate, easily irritated; (wound etc) still in a painful condition; easily hurt or shocked, tender, touchy; highly responsive to slight changes; sensory; (photog) reacting to light.—**sensitively** adj.—**sensitiveness** n.
sensitive plant n a tropical American plant whose leaves and stems fold when touched.
sensitivity /,sɛnsə'tɪvəti/ n (pl **sensitivities**) the condition of being sensitive; awareness of changes or differences; responsiveness to stimuli or feelings, esp to excess.
sensitize /'sɛnsə,taɪz/ vt to make or become sensitive; (person) to render sensitive to an antigen, etc; (photog: paper etc) to render sensitive to light.—**sensitization** n.—**sensitizer** n.

sensitometer /,sɛnsə'tɒmɪtər/ n a device for measuring the sensitivity to light of a photographic medium.
sensor /'sɛnsər/ n a device for detecting, recording, or measuring physical phenomena, as heat, pulse, etc; a sense organ.
sensorium /sɛn'sɔriəm/ n (pl **sensoriums, sensoria**) the area of the brain regarded as responsible for receiving and processing external stimuli; the body's entire sensory apparatus.
sensory /'sɛnsəri/ adj of or relating to the senses, sensation, or the sense organs; conveying nerve impulses to the brain.
sensual /'sɛnʃʊəl/ adj bodily, relating to the senses rather than the mind; arousing sexual desire.—**sensuality** n.—**sensually** adv.
sensuous /'sɛnʃʊəs/ adj giving pleasure to the mind or body through the senses.—**sensuously** adv.—**sensuousness** n.
sent /sɛnt/ see **send**.
sentence /'sɛntəns/ n a court judgment; the punishment imposed; (gram) a series of words conveying a complete thought. • v (a convicted person) to pronounce punishment upon; to condemn (to).
sententious /sɛn'tɛnʃəs/ adj terse, pithy; making frequent use of axioms and maxims; exhibiting a pompous, moralizing tone.—**sententiously** adv.—**sententiousness** n.
sentient /'sɛnʃənt/ adj making use of the senses, conscious.—**sentiently** adv.
sentiment /'sɛntəmənt/ n a feeling, awareness, or emotion; the thought behind something; an attitude of mind; a tendency to be swayed by feeling rather than reason; an exaggerated emotion.
sentimental /,sɛntə'mɛntəl/ adj of or arising from feelings; foolishly emotional; nostalgic.—**sentimentally** adv.
sentimentality /-'tæliti/ n (pl **sentimentalities**) the quality or state of being sentimental; an affected or extreme tenderness.
sentinel /'sɛntɪnəl/ n a sentry or guard.
sentry /'sɛntri/ n (pl **sentries**) a soldier on guard to give warning of danger and to prevent unauthorized access.
sentry box n a shelter for a sentry.
senza /'sɛnzə/ prep (mus) without.
señor /se'njɔr/ n (pl **señors, señores**) the title of a Spanish-speaking man, equivalent to Mr or sir.
señora /se'njɔrə/ n (pl **señoras**) the title of a Spanish-speaking married woman, equivalent to Mrs or madam.
señorita /,senjə'riːtə/ n. (pl **señoritas**) the title of a Spanish-speaking unmarried woman, equivalent to Miss or madam.
Sep. abbr = September; Septuagint.
sepal /'siːpəl/ or /'sɛp-/ n any of the individual parts of the calyx of a flower.
separable /'sɛpərəbəl/ adj able to be separated or parted.—**separability** n.—**separably** adv.
separate /'sɛprət/ or /'sɛpərət/ vt to divide or part; to sever; to set or keep apart; to sort into different sizes. • vi to go different ways; to cease to live together as man and wife. • adj divided; distinct, individual; not shared. • n (pl) articles of clothing designed to be interchangeable with others to form various outfits.—**separately** adv.—**separateness** n.
separate school n ✣ (Cdn) a publicly funded school for members of a religious minority, esp Roman Catholics.
separation /,sɛpə'reɪʃən/ n the act of separating or the state of being separate; a formal arrangement of husband and wife to live apart.
separatist /'sɛprətɪst/ or /'sɛpə-/ n a person who advocates or practises separation from an organization, church, or government; a person who advocates racial or political separation.—also adj.—**separatism** n.
separator /'sɛpə,reɪtər/ n one who separates; a machine that separates liquids from solids or liquids of different specific gravities.
Sephardi /sə'fɑrdi/ n (pl **Sephardim**) a Jew of Spanish, Portuguese or North African descent.—**Sephardic** adj.
sepia /'siːpiə/ adj, n (a) dark reddish brown.
sepoy /'siːpɔɪ/ n (formerly) an Indian soldier employed by the British.
seppuku /sə'puːkuː/ n harakiri.
sepsis /'sɛpsɪs/ n a septic state or agency; blood poisoning.
Sept. abbr = September.
septa /'sɛptə/ see **septum**.
September /sep'tembər/ n the ninth month of the year, having 30 days.
septennial /sep'tɛniəl/ adj occuring every, or lasting, seven years. • n a seven-year period.—**septennially** adv.

septet /sɛpˈtɛt/ *n* a set of seven singers or players; a musical composition for seven instruments or voices.

septic /ˈsɛptɪk/ *adj* infected by microorganisms; causing or caused by putrefaction.—**septically** *adv.*—**septicity** *n*.

septicaemia, septicemia /ˌsɛptəˈsiːmiə/ *n* a disease caused by poisonous bacteria in the blood.—**septicaemic, septicemic** *adj*.

septic tank *n* an underground tank in which sewage is decomposed by the action of bacteria.

septuagenarian /ˌsɛptuːədʒəˈnɛriən/ or /ˌsɛptəgəˈnɛriən/, /ˌsɛptʃuːə-/ *n* a person in his or her seventies.

Septuagesima /ˌsɛptjuːəˈdʒɛsɪmə/ *n* the third Sunday before Lent.

Septuagint /ˈsɛptuːəˌdʒɪnt/ or /ˌsɛpˈtuːəˌdʒɪnt/, /ˈsɛptʃuː-/ *n* the Greek version of the Old Testament including the Apocrypha (said to have been translated by 70 scholars).

septum /ˈsɛptəm/ *n* (*pl* **septa**) a dividing membrane between two bodily cavities or parts.—**septal** *adj*.

septuplet /sɛpˈtʊplɪt/ or /-ˈtuːplɪt/, /ˈsɛptəˌplɛt/ *n* one of seven offspring produced at one birth.

sepulchral /sɪˈpʌlkrəl/ *adj* of or like a sepulchre; dismal, funereal; (*sound*) deep and hollow.

sepulchre, sepulcher /ˈsɛpəlkər/ *n* a tomb, a burial vault.

sequel /ˈsiːkwəl/ *n* something that follows, the succeeding part; a consequence; the continuation of a story begun in an earlier literary work, film, etc.

sequela /sɪˈkwiːlə/ *n* (*pl* **sequelae**) (*med*) a condition arising from an existing disease; any complication of a disease or injury.

sequence /ˈsiːkwəns/ *n* order of succession; a series of succeeding things; a single, uninterrupted episode, as in a film.

sequential /sɪˈkwɛnʃəl/ *adj* arranged in a sequence; following in sequence; consecutive.—**sequentially** *adv*.

sequester /sɪˈkwɛstər/ *vt* to place apart; to retire in seclusion; (*law*) to remove from one's possession until the claims of one's creditors are satisfied.

sequestrate /sɪˈkwɛstreɪt/ *vt* to sequester.—**sequestration** *n*.

sequin /ˈsiːkwɪn/ *n* a shiny round piece of metal or foil sewn on clothes for decoration.

sequoia /səˈkwɔɪə/ *n* a lofty coniferous Californian tree.

sera /ˈsɪrə/ *see* **serum**.

sérac /seˈræk/ *n* a pinnacle or tower-shaped mass of ice among the crevasses of a glacier.

seraglio /səˈræliɔː/ *n* (*pl* **seraglios**) a harem in a Muslim household or palace.

seraph /ˈsɛrəf/ *n* (*pl* **seraphs, seraphim**) (*theol*) a member of the highest order of angels.—**seraphic** *adj*.

Serb /sɜːb/, **Serbian** /ˈsɜːbiən/ *n* a native or inhabitant of Serbia; the Serbo-Croatian language of Serbia.—*also adj*.

Serbo-Croatian /ˌsɜːboˈkrɔːˈeɪʃən/, **Serbo-Croat** /ˌsɜːboˈkrɔːæt/ *n* the Slavonic language of the Serbs and Croatians.—*also adj*.

serenade /ˌsɛrəˈneɪd/ *n* music sung or played at night beneath a person's window, *esp* by a lover. • *vt* to entertain with a serenade.

serendipity /ˌsɛrənˈdɪpɪti/ *n* the faculty of making fortunate finds by chance.

serene /səˈriːn/ *adj* calm; untroubled; tranquil; clear and unclouded; (*with cap*) honoured (used as part of certain royal titles).—**serenely** *adv.*—**serenity** *n*.

serf /sɜːf/ *n* (*pl* **serfs**) a labourer in feudal service who was bound to, and could be sold with, the land he worked; a drudge.—**serfdom** *n*.

serge /sɜːdʒ/ *n* a hard-wearing twilled woollen fabric.

sergeant /ˈsɑːdʒənt/ *n* a noncommissioned officer ranking above a corporal in the army, air force, and marine corps; a police officer ranking above a constable.

sergeant-at-arms *n* (*pl* **sergeants-at-arms**) an official in various legislative assemblies responsible for enforcing discipline.

sergeant major *n* a noncommissioned officer in the army, air force, marine corps serving as chief administrative assistant in a headquarters.

Sergt. *abbr* = Sergeant.

serial /ˈsiːriəl/ *adj* of or forming a series; published, shown or broadcast by instalments at regular intervals. • *n* a story presented in regular instalments with a connected plot.

serialism /ˈsiːriəlɪsm/ *n* (*mus*) the use of the twelve notes of the chromatic scale in a fixed order in a composition.

serialize /ˈsiːriəˌlaɪz/ *vt* to arrange, publish or broadcast in serial form.—**serialization** *n*.

serial killer *n* one who commits over a period of time a number of killings often with a trademark method or pattern.

serial number *n* one of a series of numbers given for identification.

seriatim /ˌsiːriˈeɪtɪm/ or /ˌsɛr-/ *adv* consecutively.

sericeous /sɪˈrɪʃəs/ *adj* (*bot*) covered in fine hairs

sericulture /ˈsɛrɪˌkʌltʃər/ *n* the breeding of silkworms to produce raw silk.—**sericultural** *adj.*—**sericulturist** *n*.

series /ˈsiːriːz/ *n sing, pl* a succession of items or events; a succession of things connected by some likeness; a sequence, a set; a radio or television serial whose episodes have self-contained plots; a set of books issued by one publisher; (*math*) a progression of numbers or quantities according to a certain law.

serif /ˈsɛrɪf/ *n* (*print*) a small line at the top or the bottom of the main stroke of a letter.

serigraph /ˈsɛrɪgræf/ *n* a print made using the silk-screen technique.—**serigraphy** *n*.

serin /ˈsɛrɪn/ *n* any of various small European finches related to the canary.

seriocomic /ˌsiːrioˈkɒmɪk/ *adj* combining humour and seriousness.—**seriocomically** *adv*.

serious /ˈsiːriəs/ *adj* grave, solemn, not frivolous; meaning what one says, sincere, earnest; requiring close attention or thought; important; critical.—**seriously** *adv.*—**seriousness** *n*.

sermon /ˈsɜːmən/ *n* a speech on religion or morals, *esp* by a clergyman; a long, serious talk of reproof, *esp* a tedious one.

sermonize /ˈsɜːməˌnaɪz/ *vti* to compose sermons; to preach at or to at length.—**sermonizer** *n*.

sero- /sɪːroː/ *prefix* serum.

serology /sɪˈrɒlədʒi/ *n* the scientific study of serums.—**serological** *adj.*—**serologist** *n*.

seropositive /ˌsiːroːˈpɒzɪtɪv/ *adj* having a particular disease (*eg* AIDS) for which one's blood has been tested.

serotinin /ˌsɛroːˈtɪnɪn/ *n* a substance occurring in various body tissues that induces vasoconstriction.

serous /ˈsiːrəs/ *n* of or producing serum.

serous membrane *n* a thin membrane lining a body cavity that secretes a thin lubricant.

serpent /ˈsɜːpənt/ *n* a snake; a venomous or treacherous person.

serpentine /ˈsɜːpənˌtaɪn/ or /-ˈtiːn/ *adj* like a serpent; twisting, tortuous; crooked, treacherous.

serpigo /sɜːˈpaɪgoː/ *n* a spreading skin complaint such as ringworm or herpes.

SERPS (*abbr*) state earnings-related pension scheme.

serrate /seˈreɪt/ *adj* (*leaves, etc*) having toothed edges; notched like a saw. • *vt* to make serrate.

serrated /-əd/ *adj* having an edge notched like the teeth of a saw.

serration /seˈreɪʃən/ *n* the state of being serrated; a saw-like edge; a single notch in a serrated edge.

serried /ˈsɛriːd/ *adj* packed closely, in compact order.

serum /ˈsiːrəm/ *n* (*pl* **serums, sera**) the watery part of bodily fluid, *esp* liquid that separates out from the blood when it coagulates; such fluid taken from the blood of an animal immune to a disease, used as an antitoxin.

serum albumin *n* the principal blood protein.

serum hepatitis *n* a viral disease, characterized by acute inflammation of the liver and jaundice, transmitted by contact with infected blood.

serval /ˈsɜːvəl/ *n* (*pl* **servals, serval**) an African cat with long legs and a tawny coat with black spots.

servant /ˈsɜːvənt/ *n* a personal or domestic attendant; one in the service of another.

serve /sɜːv/ *vt* to work for; to do military or naval service (for); to be useful to; to meet the needs (of), to suffice; (*a customer*) to wait upon; (*food, etc*) to hand round; (*a sentence*) to undergo; to be a soldier, sailor, etc; (*of a male animal*) to copulate with; (*law*) to deliver (a summons, etc); (*naut*) to bind (a rope) with thin cord to prevent fraying; (*tennis*) to put (the ball) into play. • *vi* to be employed as a servant; to be enough. • *n* the act of serving in tennis, etc.

server /ˈsɜːvər/ *n* one who serves, *esp* at tennis; something used in serving food and drink; a person who serves legal processes on another; the celebrant's assistant at mass; (*comput*) a computer used in a local area network that is the main source of programs or shared data.

service /ˈsɜːvɪs/ *n* the act of serving; the state of being a servant; domestic employment; a department of state employ; the people engaged in it; military employment or duty; work done for others; use, assistance; attendance in a hotel, etc: a facility providing a regular supply of trains, etc; a set of dishes; any religious ceremony; an overhaul of a vehicle; (tennis) the act or manner of seving; (pl) friendly help or professional aid; a system of providing a utility, as water, gas, etc. • vt to provide with assistance; to overhaul.

serviceable /'sərvisəbəl/ adj useful; durable.—**serviceably** adv.—**serviceableness** n.

service area n a place offering a range of services such as restaurants, toilet facilities, and petrol.

service charge n a sum added to a restaurant or hotel bill, etc for service.

serviceman /'sərvismən/ n (pl **servicemen**) a member of the armed services; a person whose work is repairing something.—**servicewoman** nf (pl **servicewomen**).

service road n a minor road beside a main route that provides access to local shops, housing, etc.

service station n a place selling fuel, etc, for motor vehicles; a place at which some service is offered.

serviette /,sərvi'et/ n a small napkin.

servile /'sərvail/ adj of or like a slave; subservient; submissive; menial.—**servilely** adv.—**servility** n.

serving /'sərviŋ/ n a portion of food or drink.

servitude /'sərvi,tuːd/ or /-,tjuːd/ n slavery, bondage; work imposed as punishment for a crime.

servo /'sərvoː/ n (pl **servos**) (inf) a servomotor or servomechanism. • adj activated by a servomechanism.

servomechanism /,sərvoː'mekə,nizəm/ n an automatic device which uses small amounts of power to control a system of much greater power.

servomotor /'sərvoː,moːtər/ n a motor that supplies power to a servomechanism.

sesame /'sesəmi/ n an Asian plant that yields oil-bearing seeds; its seeds, also used for flavouring.

sesamoid /'sesə,moid/ adj of or pertaining to the small bones or lumps of cartilage in a tendon.

sesqui- /'seskwi/ or /-kwə/ prefix one and a half; (chem.) a ratio of two to three.

sesquicentenniel /,seskwisen'teniəl/ or /,seskwə-/ n a period of 150 years; (the celebration of) a 150th anniversary.—also adj.

sessile /'sesail/ adj (leaves) without a stalk; permanently attached.

session /'seʃən/ n the meeting of a court, legislature, etc; a series of such meetings; a period of these; a period of study, classes, etc; a university year; a period of time passed in an activity.

sesterce /'sestərs/, **sestertius** /se'stərʃəs/ or /-'stərtiəs/ n in ancient Rome, a coin worth a quarter of a denarius.

sestet /ses'tet/ n a poem or stanza of six lines, esp the last six lines of a sonnet.

set /set/ vb (**setting, set**) vt to put in a specified place, condition, etc; (trap for animals) to fix; (clock etc) to adjust; (table) to arrange for a meal; (hair) to fix in a desired style; (bone) to put into normal position, etc; to make settled, rigid, or fixed; (gems) to mount; to direct; to furnish (an example) for others; to fit (words to music or music to words); (type) to arrange for printing; (with against) to weigh up, compare; to cause to be opposed to; (with aside) to discard; to reserve for a particular reason; (with down) to place (something) on a surface; to record, put in writing; to regard; to attribute (to); to allow to alight from (a vehicle); (with out) to present or display; to explain in detail; to plan, lay out. • vi to become firm, hard or fixed; to begin to move (out, forth, off, etc); (sun) to sink below the horizon; (with about) to begin; to abuse physically or verbally; (with in) to stitch (a sleeve) within a garment; to become established; (with off) to show up by contrast; to set in motion; to cause to explode; (with on) to urge (as a dog) to attack or pursue; to go on, advance; (with out) to begin a journey, career, etc; (with to) to start working, esp eagerly; to start fighting; (with up) to erect; to establish, to found; (with upon) to attack, usu with violence. • adj fixed, established; intentional; rigid, firm; obstinate; ready. • n a number of persons or things classed or belonging together; a group, a clique; the way in which a thing is set; direction; the scenery for a play, film, etc; assembled equipment for radio or television reception, etc; (math) the totality of points, numbers, or objects that satisfy a given condition; (tennis) a series of games forming a unit of a match; a rooted cutting of a plant ready for transplanting; a badger's burrow.—also **sett**.

seta /'siːtə/ n (pl **setae**) a bristle or similar appendage of an animal or plant.

setback /'setbæk/ n misfortune; a reversal.

setline /'setlain/ n a long fishing line with hooked shorter lines attached at regular intervals.

set piece n a formal or elaborate performance, esp of a work of art, music, etc; an elaborate fireworks display; (sport) a carefully rehearsed team move usu aimed at gaining the ball when play resumes.

setscrew /'set,skruː/ n a screw which when tightened prevents parts of a machine from moving relative to one another.

set-square n a flat triangular instrument for drawing angles.

settee /se'tiː/ n a sofa for two people.

setter /'setər/ n a large breed of gundog trained to stand rigid when spotting game.

set theory n the branch of mathematics concerned with the relations and properties of sets.

setting /'setiŋ/ n a background, scene, surroundings, environment; a mounting, as for a gem; the music for a song, etc.

settle /'setəl/ vti to put in order; to pay (an account); to clarify; to decide, to come to an agreement; to make or become quiet or calm; to make or become firm; to establish or become established in a place, business, home, etc; to colonize (a country); to take up residence; to come to rest; (dregs) to fall to the bottom; to stabilize; to make or become comfortable (for resting); (bird) to alight; to bestow legally for life; (with for) to be content with.

settlement /'setəlmənt/ n the act of settling; a sum settled, esp on a woman at her marriage; an arrangement; a small village; a newly established colony; subsidence (of buildings).

settler /'setlər/ n a person who settles; an early colonist.

set-to n (inf) a squabble, fight.

set-up n the plan, makeup, etc, of equipment used in an organization; the details of a situation, plan, etc; (inf) a contest, etc, arranged to result in an easy win.

seven /'sevən/ adj, n one more than six. • n the symbol for this (7, VII, vii); the seventh in a series or set; something having seven units as members.

sevenfold /'sevən,foːld/ adj having seven units or members; being seven times as great or as many.

seven seas npl all the world's oceans.

seventeen /,sevən'tiːn/ adj, n one more than sixteen. • n the symbol for this (17, XVII, xvii).—**seventeenth** adj.

seventh /'sevənθ/ adj, n next after sixth; one of seven equal parts of a thing. • n (mus) an interval of seven diatonic degrees; the leading note.

seventh heaven n perfect happiness.

seventy /'sevənti/ adj, n seven times ten. • n the symbol for this (70, LXX, lxx); (in pl) **seventies** (70s) the numbers for 70 to 79; the same numbers in a life or century.—**seventieth** adj.

sever /'sevər/ vti to separate, to divide into parts; to break off.—**severance** n.

several /'sevrəl/ adj more than two but not very many; various; separate, distinct; respective. • pron (with pl vb) a few. • n (with pl vb) a small number (of).

severe /si'viːr/ adj harsh, not lenient; very strict; stern; censorious; exacting, difficult; violent, not slight; (illness) critical; (art) plain, not floric.—**severely** adv.—**severity** n.

Seville orange /'sevil/ n (an orange tree bearing) a fruit with bitter flesh used to make marmalade.

Sèvres /sevr/ n a type of fine porcelain made in France.

sew /soː/ vti (**sewing, sewn** or **sewed**) to join or stitch together with needle and thread; to make, mend, etc, by sewing; (with up) to get full control of; (inf) to make sure of success in.—**sewing** n.

sewage /'suːidʒ/ n waste matter carried away in a sewer.

sewage farm n a place where sewage is treated for use as manure.

sewer [1] /'suːər/ n one who sews.

sewer [2] n an underground pipe or drain for carrying off liquid waste matter, etc; a main drain.

sewerage /'suːəridʒ/ n a system of drainage by sewers; sewage.

sewing machine n a machine for sewing or stitching usu driven by an electric motor.

sewn /soːn/ see **sew**.

sex /seks/ n the characteristics that distinguish male and female organisms on the basis of their reproductive function; either of the two categories (male and female) so distinguished; males or females collectively; the state of being male or female; the attraction between the sexes; (inf) sexual intercourse.

sex- *prefix* six.

sexagenarian /ˌseksədʒɪˈneriən/ *n* a person in the age range 60–69.—*also adj.*

Sexagesima /ˌseksəˈdʒesɪmə/ *n* the second Sunday before Lent.

sexagesimal /ˌseksəˈdʒesɪməl/ *adj* of or based on the number 60.

sex appeal *n* what makes a person sexually desirable.

sex chromosome *n* a chromosome that determines the sex of an animal.

sexed /sekst/ *adj* having a certain amount of sex or sexuality.

sex hormone *n* a hormone affecting the development of sexual organs and characteristics.

sexism /ˈseksɪzəm/ *n* exploitation and domination of one sex by the other, *esp* of women by men.—**sexist** *adj*, *n*.

sexless /ˈsekslɒs/ *adj* without sexual intercourse; sexually unappealing.—**sexlessly** *adv*.—**sexlessness** *n*.

sex object *n* a person regarded solely in terms of their sexual attractiveness.

sexology /sekˈsɒlədʒi/ *n* the study of human sexuality.—**sexologist** *n*.—**sexological** *adj*.

sex shop *n* a shop specializing in sex aids, pornographic magazines, etc.

sextant /ˈsekstənt/ *n* a navigator's instrument for measuring the altitude of the sun, etc, to determine position at sea.

sextet /sekˈstet/ *n* a set of six singers or players; a musical composition for six instruments or voices.

sexton /ˈsekstən/ *n* an officer in charge of the maintenance of church property.

sextuple /ˈseks̩tʊpəl/ *adj* having six units or members; being six times as much or as many.—*also n*.

sextuplet /ˈseks̩tʊplət/ *n* one of six offspring produced at one birth.

sexual /ˈsekʃʊəl/ *adj* of sex or the sexes; having sex.—**sexually** *adj*.

sexual harassment *n* frequent unwelcome attention from the opposite sex in the form of suggestive remarks, fondling, etc.

sexual intercourse *n* the act of copulating.

sexuality /ˌsekʃʊˈælɪti/ *n* sexual activity; expression of sexual interest, *esp* when excessive.

sexually transmitted disease *n* any of various diseases, such as syphilis or AIDS, transmitted by sexual contact.—*also* **venereal disease**.

sexy /ˈseksi/ *adj* (**sexier, sexiest**) (*inf*) exciting, or intending to excite, sexual desire; attractive, entertaining; fashionable or stylish and as a result worthwhile.—**sexily** *adv*.—**sexiness** *n*.

SF *abbr* = science fiction.

sf, sfz *abbr* = sforzando.

sforzando /sfɔrˈtsændoː/, **sforzato** /-ˈtsɒtoː/ *adv* (*mus*) with vigour at the start. • *n* a notation indicating this.

sgd *abbr* = signed.

SGM *abbr* = Sergeant Major.

sgraffito /sgrɒˈfiːtoː/ *n* (*pl* **sgraffiti**) (an example of) a technique in ceramic or mural design in which the surface layer (of glaze, plaster, etc) is scraped away to expose a contrasting background.

Sgt *abbr* = sergeant

Sgt Maj *abbr* = sergeant major.

sh /ʃ/ *interj* used to command silence.

shabby /ˈʃæbi/ *adj* (**shabbier, shabbiest**) (*clothes*) threadbare, worn, or dirty; run-down, dilapidated; (*act, trick*) mean, shameful.—**shabbily** *adv*.—**shabbiness** *n*.

shack /ʃæk/ *n* a small, crudely built house or cabin; a shanty. • *vi* (*with* **up**) (*sl*) to cohabit (with); to spend the night (with), *esp* a person of the opposite sex.

shackle /ˈʃækəl/ *n* a metal fastening, *usu* in pairs, for the wrists or ankles of a prisoner; a staple; anything that restrains freedom; (*pl*) fetters. • *vt* to fasten or join by a shackle; to hamper, to impede.

shad /ʃæd/ *n* (*pl* **shad, shads**) any of various fishes of the herring family used as food.

shade /ʃeɪd/ *n* relative darkness; dimness; the darker parts of anything; shadow; a shield or screen protecting from bright light; a ghost; a place sheltered from the sun; degree of darkness of a colour, *esp* when made by the addition of black; a minute difference; a blind; (*pl*) the darkness of approaching night; (*pl: sl*) sunglasses. • *vti* to screen from light; to overshadow; to make dark; to pass by degrees into another colour; to change slightly or by degrees.

shading /ˈʃeɪdɪŋ/ *n* the fine gradations of colour, line, tone, etc, creating light and dark in a painting, etc; a shielding against light; nuances.

shadow /ˈʃædoː/ *n* a patch of shade; darkness, obscurity; the dark parts of a painting, etc; shelter, protection; the dark shape of an object produced on a surface by intercepted light; an inseparable companion; a person (as a detective, etc) who shadows; an unsubstantial thing, a phantom; a mere remnant, a slight trace; gloom, affliction. • *vt* to cast a shadow over; to cloud; to follow and watch, *esp* in secret. • *adj* having an indistinct pattern or darker section; (*opposition party*) matching a function or position of the party in power.

shadow-box *vi* (*boxing*) to practice blows against an invisible opponent.

shadowy /ˈʃædoːi/ *adj* full of shadows; dim, indistinct; unsubstantial.

shady /ˈʃeɪdi/ *adj* (**shadier, shadiest**) giving or full of shade; sheltered from the sun; (*inf*) of doubtful honesty, disreputable.

SHAEF (*abbr*) Supreme Headquarters Allied Expeditionary Forces.

shaft /ʃæft/ *n* a straight rod, a pole; a stem, a shank; the main part of a column; an arrow or spear, or its stem; anything hurled like a missile; a ray of light, a stroke of lightning; a revolving rod for transmitting power, an axle; one of the poles between which a horse is harnessed; a hole giving access to a mine; a vertical opening through a building, as for a lift; a critical remark or attack; (*sl*) harsh or unfair treatment.

shag /ʃæg/ *n* a coarse tobacco cut into long pieces; a rough mop of hair, etc; a crested cormorant. • *adj* (*carpet*) having long, thick, woollen threads.

shaggy /ˈʃægi/ *adj* (**shaggier, shaggiest**) (*hair, fur, etc*) long and unkempt; rough; untidy.—**shagginess** *n*.

shaggy-dog story *n* (*inf*) a long joke with a punch line that is a deliberate anticlimax.

shagreen /ʃæˈgriːn/ *n* the rough skin of certain sharks and rays; a type of leather with a gritty surface made from the hides of certain animals.

shah /ʃɒ/ *n* the title of the former ruler of Iran.

shake /ʃeɪk/ *vti* (**shaking, shook,** *pp* **shaken**) to move to and fro with quick short motions, to agitate; to tremble or vibrate; to jar or jolt; to brandish; to make or become unsteady; to weaken; to unsettle; to unnerve or become unnerved; to clasp (another's hand) as in greeting; (*with* **down**) to cause to subside by shaking; to obtain makeshift accommodation; (*sl*) to extort money from; (*with* **off**) to get rid of; (*with* **out**) to empty by shaking; to spread (a sail); (*with* **up**) to shake together, to mix; to upset. • *n* the act of shaking or being shaken; a jolt; a shock; a milkshake; (*inf*) a deal; (*pl inf*) a convulsive trembling.

shakedown /ˈʃeɪkdaʊn/ *n* a makeshift or improvised bed; (*sl*) an extortion of money, as by blackmail; a thorough search.

shaker /ˈʃeɪkər/ *n* a container for holding condiments; a container in which cocktail ingredients are mixed.

shakers /-kərz/ *see* **movers and shakers**.

Shakespearean, Shakespearian /ʃeɪkˈspiːriən/ *adj* of, pertaining to, or characteristic of William Shakespeare (1564-1616) or his works.

shako /ˈʃeɪkoː/ *n* (*pl* **shakos, shakoes**) a cylindrical military cap with a high crown and tall plume.

shake-up /ˈʃeɪkʌp/ *n* an extensive reorganization.

shaky /ˈʃeɪki/ *adj* (**shakier, shakiest**) unsteady; infirm; unreliable.—**shakily** *adv*.—**shakiness** *n*.

shale /ʃeɪl/ *n* a kind of clay rock like slate but softer.

shall /ʃæl/ or /ʃəl/ *vb aux* (*pt* **should**) used formally to express the future in the 1st person and determination, obligation or necessity in the 2nd and 3rd person; the more common form is **will**.

shallot /ˈʃælət/ or /ʃəˈlɒt/ *n* a small onion.

shallow /ˈʃæloː/ *adj* having little depth; superficial, trivial. • *n* a shallow area in otherwise deep water.—**shallowness** *n*.

shalt /ʃælt/ (*arch*) *the 2nd person sing of* **shall**.

sham /ʃæm/ *n* a pretence; a person or thing that is a fraud. • *adj* counterfeit; fake.

shaman /ˈʃeɪmən/ *n* a priest of shamanism believed to possess magical powers which allow him to communicate with and influence the spirit world.

shamanism /-ˌɪzəm/ *n* a religion of northern Asia which views the world as dominated by good and evil spirits that can be influenced only by the shamans.

shamateur /ˈʃæməˌtʃər/ or /-tər/ *n* (*sport*) a player, athlete, etc who is officially classed as an amateur but who accepts payment.

shamble /'ʃæmbəl/ *vi* to walk with an ungainly stumbling gait.—also *n*.

shambles /'ʃæmbəlz/ *npl* a scene of great disorder; a slaughterhouse.

shambolic /ʃæm'bɒlɪk/ *adj* (*inf*) disorganized; utterly confused.

shame /ʃeɪm/ *n* a painful emotion arising from guilt or impropriety; modesty; disgrace, dishonour; the cause of this; (*s!*) a piece of unfairness. • *vti* to cause to feel shame; to bring disgrace on; to force by shame (into); to humiliate by showing superior qualities.

shamefaced /'ʃeɪmfeɪst/ *adj* bashful or modest; sheepish; showing shame; ashamed.—**shamefacedly** *adv*.—**shamefacedness** *n*.

shameful /'ʃeɪmfʊl/ *adj* disgraceful; outrageous.—**shamefully** *adv*.—**shamefulness** *n*.

shameless /'ʃeɪmləs/ *adj* immodest; impudent; brazen.—**shamelessly** *adv*.—**shamelessness** *n*.

shammy (leather) /'ʃæmi/ *see* **chamois leather**.

shampoo /ʃæm'pu:/ *n* a liquid cleansing agent for washing the hair; the process of washing the hair or a carpet, etc. • *vt* to wash with shampoo.—**shampooer** *n*.

shamrock /'ʃæmrɒk/ *n* a three-leaved cloverlike plant, the national emblem of Ireland.

shan't /ʃænt/ = shall not.

shandy /'ʃændi/ *n* (*pl* **shandies**) beer diluted with a non-alcoholic drink (as lemonade).

shanghai /ʃæŋ'haɪ/ *vt* (**shanghaiing, shanghaied**) to force (a sailor, etc) to join a ship's crew, *esp* by kidnapping or drugging; to trick or force (a person) into doing something.—**shanghaier** *n*.

Shangri-la /ˌʃæŋgrɪ'lɑ/ *n* an imaginary utopia.

shank /ʃæŋk/ *n* the leg from the knee to the ankle, the shin; a shaft, stem, or handle.

shanks's pony, shanks's mare *n* one's own legs as used for walking.

shantung /ʃæn'tʊŋ/ *n* a coarse kind of silk.

shanty[1] /'ʃænti/ *n* (*pl* **shanties**) a crude hut built from corrugated iron or cardboard.

shanty[2] *n* (*pl* **shanties**) (*formerly*) a song sung by sailors in the rhythm of their work, a chantey.

shantytown /'ʃænti,taʊn/ *n* a community of poor people living in shanties.

SHAPE /ʃeɪp/ (*abbr*) Supreme Headquarters Allied Powers Europe.

shape /ʃeɪp/ *n* the external appearance, outline or contour of a thing; a figure; a definite form; an orderly arrangement; a mould or pattern; (*inf*) condition. • *vt* to give shape to; to form; to model, to mould; to determine; (*with* **up**) to develop to a definite or satisfactory form.

shapeless /'ʃeɪpləs/ *adj* lacking definite form; baggy.—**shapelessly** *adv*.—**shapelessness** *n*.

shapely /'ʃeɪpli/ *adj* (**shapelier, shapeliest**) well-proportioned.—**shapeliness** *n*.

shard /ʃɑrd/ *n* a fragment or broken piece, *esp* of pottery.

share /ʃeə/ *n* an allotted portion, a part; one of the parts into which a company's capital stock is divided, entitling the holder to a share of profits. • *vti* to distribute, to apportion (out); to have or experience in common with others; to divide into portions; to contribute or receive a share of; to use jointly.

sharecropper /'ʃeə,krɒpər/ *n* a tenant farmer who hands over a portion of the crop as rent.—**sharecrop** *vi*.

shareholder /'ʃeəhoʊldər/ *n* a holder of shares in a property, *esp* a company.

share option *n* an option open to employees to buy shares in the company they work for.

shark /ʃɑrk/ *n* a large voracious marine fish; an extortioner, a swindler; (*sl*) an expert in a given activity.

sharkskin /'ʃɑrkskɪn/ *n* a rayon fabric with a smooth shiny finish.

sharp /ʃɑrp/ *adj* having a keen edge or fine point; pointed, not rounded; clear-cut; distinct; intense, piercing; cutting, severe; keen, biting; clever, artful; alert, mentally acute; (*mus*) raised a semitone in pitch; out of tune by being too high; (*sl*) smartly dressed. • *adv* punctually; quickly; (*mus*) above the right pitch. • *n* (*mus*) a note that is a semitone higher than the note denoted by the same letter; the symbol for this.—**sharply** *adv*.—**sharpness** *n*.

sharpen /'ʃɑrpən/ *vti* to make or become sharp or sharper.

sharpener /-ər/ *n* something that sharpens.

sharpshooter /'ʃɑrp,ʃu:tər/ *n* a marksman.

sharp-tongued /-,tʊŋd/ *adj* sarcastic; quick to criticize.

sharp-witted /ʃɑrp'wɪtɪd/ *adj* thinking quickly and effectively.—**sharp-wittedly** *adv*.—**sharp-wittedness** *n*.

shatter /'ʃætər/ *vti* to reduce to fragments suddenly; to smash; to damage or be damaged severely.

shatterproof /'ʃætərpru:f/ *adj* resistant to shattering.

shave /ʃeɪv/ *vti* to remove facial or body hair with a razor; to cut away thin slices, to pare; to miss narrowly, to graze. • *n* the act or process of shaving; a narrow escape or miss; a paring.

shaven /'ʃeɪvən/ *adj* shaved.

shaver /'ʃeɪvər/ *n* one who shaves; an instrument for shaving, *esp* an electrical one.

Shavian /'ʃeɪvɪən/ *adj* of, relating to, or resembling the works of the writer George Bernard Shaw (1856–1950).

shaving /'ʃeɪvɪŋ/ *n* the act of using a razor or scraping; a thin slice of wood, metal, etc, shaved off.

shawl /ʃɔl/ *n* a large square or oblong cloth worn as a covering for the head or shoulders or as a wrapping for a baby.

shawm /ʃɔm/ *n* a medieval woodwind instrument resembling an oboe.

she /ʃi:/ *pron* (*obj* **her**, *poss* **her, hers**) the female person or thing named before or in question. • *n* a female person or animal.

shea /ʃi:/ *or* /'ʃi:ə/ *n* a tropical African tree with seeds that yield a butter-like fat used as food.

sheaf /ʃi:f/ *n* (*pl* **sheaves**) a bundle of reaped corn bound together; a collection of papers, etc, tied in a bundle.

shear /ʃi:r/ *vti* (**shearing, sheared** *or* **shorn**) to clip or cut (through); to remove (a sheep's fleece) by clipping; to divest; (*metal*) to break off because of a heavy force or twist. • *n* a stress acting sideways on a rivet and causing a break, etc; a machine for cutting metal (*pl*) large scissors; (*pl*) a tool for cutting hedges, etc.

shearling /'ʃi:rlɪŋ/ *n* (the fleece of) a sheep after its first shearing.

shearwater /'ʃi:r,wɔtər/ *n* any of various seabirds that often glide close to the water.

sheath /ʃi:θ/ *n* (*pl* **sheaths**) a close-fitting cover, *esp* for a blade; a condom; a closefitting dress *usu* worn without a belt.

sheathe /ʃi:ð/ *vt* to put into a sheath; to encase, to protect with a casing; (*cat*) to withdraw its claws.

sheath-knife *n* a knife with a fixed blade covered by a sheath.

sheave[1] /ʃi:v/ *vt* to gather into sheaves.

sheave[2] *n* a grooved wheel, *esp* in a pulley.

sheaves /ʃi:vz/ *see* **sheaf**.

shebang /ʃə'bæŋ/ *n* (*inf*) affair, business.

shebeen /ʃə'bi:n/ *n* an unlicensed or illegal drinking den.

she'd /ʃi:d/ = she had; she would.

shed[1] /ʃed/ *n* a hut for storing garden tools; a large roofed shelter often with one or more sides open; a warehouse.

shed[2] *vt* (**shedding, shed**) (*tears*) to let fall; (*skin, etc*) to lose or cast off; to allow or cause to flow; to diffuse, radiate. • *n* a parting in the hair.

sheen /ʃi:n/ *n* a gloss, lustre; brightness.

sheep /ʃi:p/ *n* (*pl* **sheep**) a cud-chewing four-footed animal with a fleece and edible flesh called mutton; a bashful, submissive person.

sheepcote /-,koʊt/ *n* a sheepfold.

sheep-dip /-,dɪp/ *n* a liquid disinfectant or insecticide into which sheep are plunged to destroy parasites.

sheepdog /'ʃi:pdɒg/ *n* a dog trained to tend, drive, or guard sheep.

sheepfold /'ʃi:pfoʊld/ *n* an enclosure for sheep.

sheepish /'ʃi:pɪʃ/ *adj* bashful, embarrassed.—**sheepishly** *adv*.—**sheepishness** *n*.

sheep's eyes *npl* (*arch*) amorous glances.

sheepshank /'ʃi:pʃæŋk/ *n* a knot in a rope to shorten it temporarily.

sheepskin /'ʃi:pskɪn/ *n* the skin of a sheep, *esp* with the fleece; a rug, parchment, or leather made from it; a garment made of or lined with sheepskin.

sheepwalk /'ʃi:pwɒk/ *n* an area of pasture for sheep.

sheer[1] /ʃi:r/ *adj* pure, unmixed; downright, utter; perpendicular, extremely steep; (*fabric*) delicately fine, transparent. • *adv* outright; perpendicularly, steeply.

sheer[2] *vti* to deviate or cause to deviate from a course; to swerve. • *n* the act of sheering; the upward curve of a deck toward bow or stern; a change in a ship's course.

sheerlegs /'ʃi:rlegz/ *n sing* a hoisting device comprising two or more upright poles crossed at the top from which lifting gear is suspended.

sheet[1] /ʃiːt/ *n* a broad thin piece of any material, as glass, plywood, metal, etc; a large rectangular piece of cloth used as inner bed clothes; a single piece of paper; (*inf*) a newspaper; a broad, flat expanse; a suspended or moving expanse (as of fire or rain).

sheet[2] *n* a rope that controls the angle of a sail in relation to the wind.

sheet anchor *n* a large anchor used only in emergencies; a support in extremity.

sheet bend *n* a knot for joining ropes of different thicknesses.

sheet glass *n* glass made in large sheets directly from the furnace or by making a cylinder and then flattening it.

sheeting /ʃiːtɪŋ/ *n* fabric for sheets.

sheet lightning *n* lightning that has the appearance of a broad sheet due to reflection and diffusion by the clouds and sky.

sheet metal *n* metal rolled out in the form of a thin sheet.

sheet music *n* music printed on unbound sheets of paper.

sheikh /ʃiːk/ or /ʃeɪk/ *n* an Arab chief.

sheila /ˈʃiːlə/ *n* (*Austral, NZ sl*) a girl or woman.

shekel /ˈʃekəl/ *n* the unit of money in Israel; an old Jewish weight or silver coin; (*pl*) (*sl*) money.

shelduck /ˈʃeldʌk/, **sheldrake** /-ˌdreɪk/ *n* any of several Old World brightly plumaged ducks.

shelf /ʃelf/ *n* (*pl* **shelves**) a board fixed horizontally on a wall or in a cupboard for holding articles; a ledge on a cliff face; a reef, a shoal.

shelf life *n* the length of time for which something may be stored without deterioration.

shell /ʃel/ *n* a hard outside covering of a nut, egg, shellfish, etc; an explosive projectile; an external framework; a light racing boat; outward show; a cartridge. • *vt* to remove the shell from; to bombard (with shells); (*with* **out**) (*inf*) to pay out (money).

she'll /ʃiːl/ or /ʃɪl/ = she will; she shall.

shellac, shellack /ʃəˈlæk/ *n* a resin *usu* produced in thin, flaky layers or shells; a thin varnish containing this and alcohol.

shellfish /ˈʃelfɪʃ/ *n* an aquatic animal, *esp* an edible one, with a shell.

shellproof /ˈʃelˌpruːf/ *adj* impervious to artillery shells, rockets and bombs.

shell shock *n* a nervous disorder caused by the shock of being under fire.—**shell-shocked** *adj*.

shelter /ˈʃeltər/ *n* a structure that protects, *esp* against weather; a place giving protection, a refuge; protection. • *vti* to give shelter to, to shield, to cover; to take shelter.

sheltie, shelty /ˈʃelti/ *n* (*pl* **shelties**) a Shetland pony or Shetland sheepdog.

shelve /ʃelv/ *vti* to place on a shelf; to defer consideration, to put aside; to slope gently, to incline.

shelves /ʃelvz/ *see* **shelf**.

shelving /ˈʃelvɪŋ/ *n* material for making shelves; shelves collectively.

shemozzle /ʃəˈmɒzəl/ *n* (*inf*) a scene of confusion; a brawl.

shenanigan /ʃəˈnænɪɡən/ *n* (*often pl*) trickery, deception; mischief, boisterous high spirits.

shepherd /ˈʃepərd/ *n* a person who looks after sheep; a pastor. • *vt* to look after, as a shepherd; to manoeuvre or marshal in a particular direction.—**shepherdess** *nf*.

shepherd dog *n* a sheepdog.

shepherd's pie *n* a dish of minced meat covered with a mashed potato crust.

shepherd's purse *n* an annual plant with small white flowers and heart-shaped seed pods.

sherbet /ˈʃɔːbət/ *n* a fruit-flavoured powder that can be used to make a slightly sparkling drink; a sorbet.

sheriff /ˈʃerɪf/ *n* in US, the chief law enforcement officer of a county; in Scotland, a judge in an intermediate law court; in England and Wales, the chief officer of the Crown, a ceremonial post.

sheriff court *n* (*Scot*) the court dealing with the majority of criminal and civil cases.

Sherpa /ˈʃɔːpə/ *n* (*pl* **Sherpas, Sherpa**) a member of a people living on the southern slopes of the Himalayas on the borders of Nepal and Tibet.

sherry /ˈʃeri/ *n* (*pl* **sherries**) a fortified wine originally made in Spain.

she's /ʃiːz/ = she is; she has.

Shetland pony /ˈʃetlənd/ *n* a breed of small sturdy pony with a shaggy mane.

Shetland sheepdog *n* a breed of dog resembling a collie but smaller.

SHF, shf *abbr* = superhigh frequency.

Shiah, Shia /ˈʃiə/ *n* a member of the main branch of Islam who acknowledge Muhammad's cousin Ali and his successors as the true imams.—*also adj*.

shibboleth /ˈʃɪbəˌleθ/ *n* a slogan or catchword, *esp* that regarded as outmoded or identified with a particular group or culture; a custom or linguistic usage which identifies members of a particular group, party, class, etc.

shied /ʃaɪd/ *see* **shy**[1], **shy**[2].

shield /ʃiːld/ *n* a broad piece of armour carried for defence, *usu* on the left arm; a protective covering or guard; a thing or person that protects; a trophy in the shape of a shield. • *vti* to defend; to protect; to screen.

shier /ˈʃaɪər/, **shiest** /-əst/ *see* **shy**[1].

shift /ʃɪft/ *vti* to change position (of); to contrive, to manage; to remove, to transfer; to replace by another or others; (*gears*) to change the arrangement of. • *n* a change in position; an expedient; a group of people working in relay with others; the time worked by them; a change or transfer; a straight dress.

shiftless /ˈʃɪftləs/ *adj* incapable; feckless.—**shiftlessly** *adv*.—**shiftlessness** *n*.

shifty /ˈʃɪfti/ *adj* (**shiftier, shiftiest**) artful, tricky; evasive.—**shiftily** *adv*.—**shiftiness** *n*.

shigella /ʃɪˈɡelə/ *n* any of a genus of rod-shaped bacteria causing dysentery in humans and animals.

Shiite /ˈʃiːaɪt/, **Shiah** /ˈʃiːə/ *n* a follower of Shiah.—*also adj*.

shillelagh /ʃɪˈleɪlə/ *n* an Irish club or cudgel.

shilling /ˈʃɪlɪŋ/ *n* a former unit of currency of the UK and other countries, worth one twentieth of a pound.

shillyshally /ˈʃɪliˌʃæli/ *vi* (**shillyshallying, shillyshallied**) to vacillate, to hesitate. • *n* (*pl* **shillyshallies**) the inability to make up one's mind.

shim /ʃɪm/ *n* a thin washer or spacer used to tighten or space out joints, etc. • *vt* (**shimming, shimmed**) to space out, etc using shims.

shimmer /ˈʃɪmər/ *vi* to glisten softly, to glimmer.—*also n*.—**shimmery** *adj*.

shimmy /ˈʃɪmi/ *n* (*pl* **shimmies**) a jazz dance involving rapid movements of the upper body; an abnormal vibration in a vehicle or aircraft. • *vi* (**shimmying, shimmied**) to dance a shimmy; to vibrate.

shin /ʃɪn/ *n* the front part of the leg from the knee to the ankle; the shank. • *vi* (*with* **up**) to climb (a pole, etc) by gripping with legs and hands.

shinbone /ˈʃɪnˌbəʊn/ *n* the tibia.

shindig /ˈʃɪndɪɡ/ *n* (*inf*) a lively, noisy celebration; an uproar.

shine /ʃaɪn/ *vti* (**shining, shone**) to emit light; to be bright, to glow; to be brilliant or conspicuous; to direct the light of; to cause to gleam by polishing. • *n* a lustre, a gloss; (*sl*) a liking.

shiner /ˈʃaɪnər/ *n* (*inf*) a black eye.

shingle[1] /ˈʃɪŋɡəl/ *n* a thin wedge-shaped roof tile; a small signboard.

shingle[2] *n* waterworn pebbles as on a beach; an area covered with these.—**shingly** *adj*.

shingles /ˈʃɪŋɡəlz/ *npl* a virus disease marked by a painful rash of red spots on the skin.

shinny /ˈʃɪni/ *n* ❋ (*Cdn*) an informal game of ice hockey, *usu* played without a referee or a net.

Shinto /ˈʃɪntəʊ/ *n* the indigenous religion of Japan, involving veneration of the emperor, and the worship of ancestors and various natural deities.—**Shintoism** *n*.—**Shintoist** *n*.

shinty /ˈʃɪnti/ *n* a game similar to hockey and hurling, played with a ball and curved sticks.

shiny /ˈʃaɪni/ *adj* (**shinier, shiniest**) glossy, polished; worn smooth.

ship /ʃɪp/ *n* a large vessel navigating deep water; its officers and crew; a spacecraft. • *vti* (**shipping, shipped**) to transport by any carrier; to take in (water) over the side; to lay (oars) inside a boat; to go on board; to go or travel by ship.

shipboard /ˈʃɪpbɔːrd/ *n* the side of a ship.

shipbuilder /ˈʃɪpˌbɪldər/ *n* a person or company that designs or constructs ships.—**shipbuilding** *n*.

ship chandler *n* an individual or business that provides essential supplies for ships.

shipload /ˈʃɪpləʊd/ *n* as much as a ship can carry.

shipmaster /ˈʃɪpˌmæstər/ *n* the captain or master of a ship.

shipmate /ˈʃɪpmeɪt/ *n* a fellow sailor.

shipment /ˈʃɪpmənt/ *n* goods shipped; a consignment.

ship of the line *n* (*formerly*) a warship large enough to fight in the first line of battle.

shipowner /'ʃɪpˌoːnər/ *n* a person who owns (or has shares in) a ship.

shipper /'ʃɪpər/ *n* an individual or company that ships goods.

shipping /'ʃɪpɪŋ/ *n* the business of transporting goods; ships collectively.

ship's biscuit *n* a type of hard biscuit that was formerly part of a sailor's diet.

shipshape /'ʃɪpˌʃeɪp/ *adj* in good order, tidy.

shipworm /'ʃɪpwɜrm/ *n* any of a genus of worm-like molluscs that burrow in submerged wood.

shipwreck /'ʃɪprɛk/ *n* the loss of a vessel at sea; the remains of a wrecked ship; ruin, destruction. • *vti* to destroy by or suffer shipwreck; to ruin.

shipwright /'ʃɪpraɪt/ *n* a person skilled in constructing and repairing ships.

shipyard /'ʃɪpjɑrd/ *n* a yard or shed where ships are built or repaired.

shire /ʃaɪr/ *n* in the UK, a county; a large powerful breed of draught horse.

shirk /ʃɜrk/ *vti* to neglect or avoid work; to refuse to face (duty, danger, etc).—**shirker** *n*.

shirr /ʃɜr/ *vt* to gather (fabric) with parallel threads run through it; to bake (eggs) in buttered dishes.

shirring /'ʃɜrɪŋ/ or /ʃɜrɪŋ/ *n* a gathering made in cloth by drawing the material up on parallel rows of short stitches.

shirt /ʃɜrt/ *n* a sleeved garment of cotton, etc, for the upper body, typically having a fitted collar and cuffs and front buttons; (*inf*) one's money or resources.

shirtdress /'ʃɜrtˌdrɛs/ *n* a long shirt worn as a dress.

shirting /-ɪŋ/ *n* a fabric suitable for men's shirts.

shirtsleeve /-ˌsliːv/ *n* the sleeve of a shirt.

shirt-tail /-ˌteɪl/ *n* the flap of material at the back of a shirt below the waist.

shirtwaister, shirtwaist /-ˌweɪst/ *n* a woman's dress tailored in front in style similar to a shirt.

shirty /'ʃɜrti/ *adj* (**shirtier, shirtiest**) (*sl*) irritable, rude.

shish kebab /ˌʃɪʃkəˈbɒb/ or /-bæb/ *n* a kebab.

shit[1] **shite,** /ʃɪt/ *n* (*vulg*) waste matter from humans or animals; excrement; heroin; something that is worthless. • *vti* to defecate (on). • *interj* (*sl*) an expression of strong disgust or disapproval.

shit[2] *n* (*sl*) something that is good.

shivaree /'ʃɪvəri/ *see* **charivari**.

shiver[1] /'ʃɪvər/ *n* a small fragment, a splinter.

shiver[2] *vi* to shake or tremble, as with cold or fear, to shudder.— *also n.*—**shivery** *adj*.

shoal[1] /ʃoːl/ *n* a large number of fish swimming together; a large crowd. • *vi* to form shoals.

shoal[2] *n* a submerged sandbank, *esp* one that shows at low tide; a shallow place; a hidden danger. • *vti* to come to a less deep part; to become shallower.

shock[1] /ʃɒk/ *n* a shaggy mass of hair.

shock[2] *n* a violent jolt or impact; a sudden disturbance to the emotions; the event or experience causing this; the nerve sensation caused by an electrical charge through the body; a disorder of the blood circulation, produced by displacement of body fluids (due to injury); (*sl*) a paralytic stroke. • *vt* to outrage, horrify. • *vi* to experience extreme horror, outrage, etc.

shock absorber *n* a device, as on the springs of a car, that absorbs the force of bumps and jars.

shocker /'ʃɒkər/ *n* a sensational novel, play, etc; anything that shocks; (*sl*) a very bad specimen.

shock-jock *n* a disc-jockey at a radio station deliberately provocative in presentation, particularly when airing controversial issues.

shocking /'ʃɒkɪŋ/ *adj* revolting; scandalous, improper; very bad.—**shockingly** *adv*.

shockproof /'ʃɒkpruːf/ *adj* capable of withstanding shock without damage.

shock therapy, shock treatment *n* the treatment of certain mental illnesses by inducing convulsions using drugs or by passing electricity through the brain.

shock troops *npl* a highly disciplined force trained to lead an attack.

shock wave *n* the violent effect in the vicinity of an explosion caused by the change in atmospheric pressure; the compressed wave built up when the speed of a body or fluid exceeds

that at which sound can be transmitted in the medium in which it is travelling.

shod /ʃɒd/ **shodden** *see* **shoe**.

shoddy /'ʃɒdi/ *adj* (**shoddier, shoddiest**) made of inferior material; cheap and nasty, trashy.—**shoddily** *adv*.—**shoddiness** *n*.

shoe /ʃuː/ *n* an outer covering for the foot not enclosing the ankle; a thing like a shoe, a partial casing; a horseshoe; a drag for a wheel; a device to guide movement, provide contact, or protect against wear or slipping; a dealing box that holds several decks of cards. • *vt* (**shoeing, shod** *or* **shoed,** *pp* **shod, shoed** *or* **shodden**) to provide with shoes; to cover for strength or protection.

shoehorn /'ʃuːhɔrn/ *n* a curved piece of plastic, metal, or horn used for easing the heel into a shoe.

shoelace /'ʃuːleɪs/ *n* a cord that passes through eyelets in a shoe and is tied to keep the shoe on the foot.

shoemaker /'ʃuːˌmeɪkər/ *n* a person who makes or mends shoes.

shoestring /'ʃuːstrɪŋ/ *n* a shoelace; (*inf*) a small amount of money.

shoetree /'ʃuːtriː/ *n* a block of wood, plastic or metal for preserving the shape of a shoe.

shogun /'ʃoːgən/ *n* the hereditary commander of the army in feudal Japan.

shone /ʃɒn/ *see* **shine**.

shoo /ʃuː/ *interj* used to frighten (animals, people) away. • *vt* (**shooing, shooed**) to frighten away (as if) by shouting "shoo". • *vi* to cry "shoo".

shoo-in /'ʃuːˌɪn/ *n* (*inf*) a person or thing certain to win or succeed.

shook /ʃʊk/ *see* **shake**.

shoot /ʃuːt/ *vb* (**shooting, shot**) *vt* to discharge or fire (a gun etc); to hit or kill with a bullet, etc; (*rapids*) to be carried swiftly over; to propel quickly; to thrust out; (*bolt*) to slide home; to variegate (with another colour, etc); (*a film scene*) to photograph; (*sport*) to kick or drive (a ball, etc) at goal; (*with* **down**) to disprove (an argument); (*with* **up**) to grow rapidly, to rise abruptly. • *vi* to move swiftly, to dart; to emit; to put forth buds, to sprout; to attack or kill indiscriminately; • *n* a contest, a shooting trip, etc; a new growth or sprout.

shooting /'ʃuːtɪŋ/ *n* the act of firing a gun or letting off an arrow.

shooting star *n* a meteor.

shooting stick *n* a spiked stick with a handle that folds out into a small seat.

shop /ʃɒp/ *n* a building were retail goods are sold or services provided; a factory; a workshop; the details and technicalities of one's own work, and talk about these. • *vti* (**shopping, shopped**) to visit shops to examine or buy; (*sl*) to inform on (a person) to the police; (*with* **around**) to hunt for the best buy.

shop assistant *n* a person who serves customers in a retail shop.

shop floor *n* the part of a factory where goods are manufactured; the work force employed there, *usu* unionized.

shopkeeper /'ʃɒpˌkiːpər/ *n* a person who owns or runs a shop.— **shopkeeping** *n*.

shoplifter /'ʃɒplɪftər/ *n* a person who steals goods from shops.

shoplifting /-ɪŋ/ *n* stealing from a shop during shopping hours.—**shoplifter** *n*.

shopper /'ʃɒpər/ *n* a person who shops; a bag for carrying shopping.

shopping /'ʃɒpɪŋ/ *n* the act of shopping; the goods bought.—*also adj*.

shopping centre *n* a complex of shops, restaurants, and service establishments with a common parking area.—*also* **shopping plaza**.

shopping mall *n* a large enclosed shopping centre.

shopsoiled /'ʃɒpsɔɪld/ *adj* shopworn.

shoptalk /-ˌtɔk/ *n* the specialized vocabulary of those in the same line of work or sharing an area of interest; talk about work after hours.

shopwalker /-ˌwɔkər/ *n* a person employed in large shop who oversees shop assistants, helps customers, etc.

shopworn /-ˌwɔrn/ *adj* faded, etc, from being on display in a shop.

shore[1] /ʃɔr/ *n* land beside the sea or a large body of water; beach.

shore[2] *n* a prop or beam used for support. • *vt* to prop (up), to support with a shore.

shoreline /'ʃɔrlaɪn/ *n* the edge of an expanse of water.

shorn /ʃɔrn/ *see* **shear**.

short /ʃɔrt/ *adj* not measuring much; not long or tall; not great in range or scope; brief; concise; not retentive; curt; abrupt; less than the correct amount; below standard; deficient, lacking; (*pastry*) crisp or flaky; (*vowel*) not prolonged, unstressed;

(*drink*) undiluted, neat. • *n* something short; (*pl*) trousers not covering the knee; (*pl*) an undergarment like these; a short circuit. • *adv* abruptly; concisely; without reaching the end. • *vti* to give less than what is needed; to short-change; to short-circuit.—**shortness** *n*.

shortage /'ʃɔrtədʒ/ *n* a deficiency.

shortbread /'ʃɔrtbred/ *n* a rich, crumbly cake or biscuit made with much shortening.

short-change /-,tʃeɪndʒ/ *vt* to give back less than the correct change; (*sl*) to cheat.

short-circuit /-'sərkɪt/ *n* the deviation of an electric current by a path of small resistance; an interrupted electric current. • *vti* to establish a short-circuit in; to cut off electric current; to provide with a short cut.

shortcoming /'ʃɔrt,kʌmɪŋ/ *n* a defect or inadequacy.

shortcrust pastry *n* a firm but crumbly pastry made with half as much fat as flour.

short cut /'ʃɔrtkʌt/ *n* a shorter route; any way of saving time, effort, etc.

shorten /'ʃɔrtən/ *vt* to make or become short or shorter; to reduce the amount of (sail) spread; to make (pastry, etc) crisp and flaky by adding fat.

shortening /'ʃɔrtənɪŋ/ *n* the act of shortening; the state of becoming shortened; a fat used for making pastry, etc, crisp and flaky.

shortfall /'ʃɔrtfɔl/ *n* (the amount or degree of) a deficit or deficiency.

shorthand /'ʃɔrthænd/ *n* a method of rapid writing using signs or contractions.—*also adj.*

short-handed /-ɪd/ *adj* not having the usual number of assistants.

shorthand typist *n* a person who produces typewritten documents from shorthand notes.—*also* **stenographer.**

short head /'ʃɔrt,hed/ *n* (*horse racing*) a distance less than a horse's head.

shorthorn /'ʃɔrthɔrn/ *n* one of a breed of large heavy cattle with short curved horns.

short list /'ʃɔrt,lɪst/ *n* a selected list of qualified applicants from which a choice must be made.

short-list *vt* to place (a person) on a short list.

short-lived /'ʃɔrt'laɪvd/ or /-'lɪvd/ *adj* not lasting or living for long.

shortly /'ʃɔrtli/ *adv* soon, in a short time; briefly; rudely.

short-range *adj* having a limited range in time or distance.

short shrift *n* curt, dismissive treatment.

short-sighted /ʃɔrt'saɪtəd/ or /'ʃɔrt-/ *adj* not able to see well at a distance; lacking foresight.—**short-sightedly** *adv.*—**short-sightedness** *n*.

short-tempered *adj* easily annoyed.

short-term *adj* of or for a limited time.

short time *n* a reduction in working hours due to recession, etc.

short-winded *adj* easily becoming breathless; (*speech, writing*) brief, to the point.

shortwave *n* a radio wave 60 metres or less in length.

shot[1] /ʃɒt/ *see* **shoot.**

shot[2] *n* the act of shooting; range, scope; an attempt; a solid projectile for a gun; projectiles collectively; small lead pellets for a shotgun; a marksman; a photograph or a continuous film sequence; a hypodermic injection, as of vaccine; a drink of alcohol.

shotgun /'ʃɒtgʌn/ *n* a smooth-bore gun for firing small shot at close range.

shotgun wedding *n* (*inf*) an enforced wedding, *usu* because the woman is pregnant.

shot put *n* a field event in which a heavy metal ball is proepelled with an overhand thrust from the shoulder.—**shot-putter** *n*.

shotten /'ʃɒtən/ *adj* (*fish*) having spawned recently.

should /ʃʊd/ *vb aux* used to express obligation, duty, expectation or probability, or a future condition.—*also pt of* **shall.**

shoulder /'ʃoʊldər/ *n* the joint connecting the arm with the trunk; a part like a shoulder; (*pl*) the upper part of the back; (*pl*) the capacity to bear a task or blame; a projecting part; the strip of land bordering a road. • *vti* to place on the shoulder to carry; to assume responsibility; to push with the shoulder, to jostle.

shoulder blade *n* the large flat triangular bone on either side of the back part of the human shoulder.

shoulder strap *n* a strap over the shoulders to hold up a garment, bag, etc.

shouldn't /ʃʊdənt/ = should not.

shout /ʃaʊt/ *n* a loud call; a yell. • *vti* to call loudly, to yell; (*with* **down**) to drown out or silence (a person speaking) by shouting.

shove /ʃʌv/ *vti* to drive forward; to push; to jostle; (*with* **off**) to push (a boat) off from the shore; (*inf*) to depart, leave. • *n* a forceful push.

shove-halfpenny *n* a game in which coins or discs are slid across a board marked with a scoring grid.

shovel /'ʃʌvəl/ *n* a broad tool like a scoop with a long handle for moving loose material. • *vt* (**shovelling, shovelled** *or* **shoveling, shoveled**) to move or lift with a shovel.

shoveller, shoveler /'ʃʌvələr/ *n* any of several pond and marsh ducks with a broad beak.

shovelhead *n* a breed of shark with a shovel-shaped head.

show /ʃoʊ/ *vti* (**showing, showed** *or* **shown**) to present to view, to exhibit; to demonstrate, to make clear; to prove; to manifest, to disclose; to direct, to guide; to appear, to be visible; to finish third in a horse race; (*inf*) to arrive; (*with* **off**) to display to advantage; to try to attract admiration; to behave pretentiously; (*with* **up**) to put in an appearance, to arrive; to expose to ridicule. • *n* a display, an exhibition; an entertainment; a theatrical performance; a radio or television programme; third place at the finish (as a horse race).

show business, show biz /'ʃoʊbɪz/ *n* the entertainment industry.

showcase /'ʃoʊkeɪs/ *n* a glass case or cabinet for displaying items in a shop or museum; a setting or situation designed to exhibit something to best advantage.—*also vt.*

showdown /'ʃoʊdaʊn/ *n* (*inf*) a final conflict; a disclosure of cards at poker.

shower /ʃaʊr/ *n* a brief period of rain, hail, or snow; a similar fall, as of tears, meteors, arrows, etc; a great number; a method of cleansing in which the body is sprayed with water from above; a wash in this; a party for the presentation of gifts, *esp* to a bride. • *vt* to pour copiously; to sprinkle; to bestow (with gifts). • *vi* to cleanse in a shower.

showgirl /'ʃoʊgərl/ *n* a girl who appears in a chorus line, variety act, etc.

show house *n* a house on a new housing estate used as a sample for prospective buyers.

showjumping *n* the competitive riding of horses to demonstrate their skill in jumping.

showman /'ʃoʊmən/ *n* (*pl* **showmen**) a man who manages or presents a theatrical show, circus, etc; a person skilled in presentation.

shown /ʃoʊn/ *see* **show.**

showpiece /'ʃoʊpiːs/ *n* an exhibit; a perfect example of something.

showplace /-pleɪs/ *n* a place (*eg* tourist attraction, historic site) regarded as of exemplary interest or beauty.

showroom /-ruːm/ *n* a room where goods for sale are displayed.

showy /'ʃoʊi/ *adj* (**showier, showiest**) bright, colourful; ostentatious.—**showily** *adv.*—**showiness** *n*.

shrank /ʃræŋk/ *see* **shrink.**

shrapnel /'ʃræpnəl/ *n* an artillery shell filled with small pieces of metal that scatter on impact.

shred /ʃred/ *n* a strip cut or torn off; a fragment, a scrap. • *vt* (**shredding, shredded**) to cut or tear into small pieces.

shrew /ʃruː/ *n* a small, brown, nocturnal mouse-like animal with a long snout; a bad-tempered, nagging woman.

shrewd /ʃruːd/ *adj* astute, having common sense; keen, penetrating.—**shrewdly** *adv.*—**shrewdness** *n*.

shrewish /'ʃruːɪʃ/ *adj* sharp-tongued, nagging.

shriek /ʃriːk/ *n* a loud, shrill cry, a scream. • *vti* to screech, to scream.

shrieval /'ʃriːvəl/ *adj* of or pertaining to a sheriff.

shrievalty /'ʃriːvəlti/ *n* (*pl* **shrievalties**) the office, term of office or jurisdiction of a sheriff.

shrike /ʃraɪk/ *n* a bird with a hooked beak that impales its prey, mainly insects and small animals, on thorns.

shrill /ʃrɪl/ *adj* high-pitched and piercing in sound; strident.

shrimp /ʃrɪmp/ *n* a small edible shellfish with a long tail; (*sl*) a small or unimportant person. • *vt* to fish for shrimps.

shrine /ʃraɪn/ *n* a container for sacred relics; a saint's tomb; a place of worship; a hallowed place.

shrink /ʃrɪŋk/ *vti* (**shrinking, shrank** *or* **shrunk**, *pp* **shrunk** *or* **shrunken**) to become smaller, to contract as from cold, wetting, etc; to recoil (from), to flinch; to cause (cloth, etc) to contract by soaking. • *n* (*sl*) a psychiatrist.—**shrinkable** *adj*.

shrinkage /'ʃrɪŋkɪdʒ/ *n* contraction; diminution.

shrinking violet *n* a very shy or unassuming person.

shrink-wrap /'ʃrɪŋkˌræp/ vt (**shrink-wrapping, shrink-wrapped**) (book etc) to wrap in plastic film that is then shrunk by heat to form a tightly fitting package.

shrive /ʃraɪv/ vb (**shriving, shrived** or **shrove**, pp **shriven** or **shrived**) vt (arch) to hear the confession of; to impose penance on and absolve. • vi to confess, do penance and receive absolution.

shrivel /'ʃrɪvəl/ vti (**shrivelling, shrivelled** or **shriveling, shriveled**) to dry up or wither and become wrinkled; to curl up with heat, etc.

shroud /ʃraʊd/ n a burial cloth; anything that envelops or conceals; (naut) a supporting rope for a mast. • vt to wrap in a shroud; to envelop or conceal.

shrove /ʃroːv/ see **shrive**.

Shrovetide /'ʃroːvtaɪd/ n the three days before Ash Wednesday.

Shrove Tuesday n the last day before Lent.

shrub /ʃrʌb/ n a woody plant smaller than a tree with several stems rising from the same root; a bush.—**shrubby** adj.

shrubbery /'ʃrʌbəri/ n (pl **shrubberies**) an area of land planted with shrubs.

shrug /ʃrʌg/ vti (**shrugging, shrugged**) to draw up and contract (the shoulders) as a sign of doubt, indifference, etc; (with **off**) to brush aside; to shake off; (a garment) to remove by wriggling out. • n the act of shrugging.

shrunk /ʃrʌŋk/ see **shrink**.

shrunken /'ʃrʌŋkən/ adj shrivelled, pinched; reduced.

shtoom /ʃtuːm/ n (sl) silent, dumb.

shuck /ʃʌk/ n a husk, pod or shell. • vt to remove the shucks from.

shucks /ʃʌks/ interj used to express disappointment, irritation, etc.

shudder /'ʃʌdər/ vi to tremble violently, to shiver; to feel strong repugnance. • n a convulsive shiver of the body; a vibration.

shuffle /'ʃʌfəl/ vt to scrape (the feet) along the ground; to walk with dragging steps; (playing cards) to change the order of, to mix; to intermingle, to mix up; (with **off**) to get rid of.—also n.

shuffleboard /'ʃʌfəlbɔrd/ n a game in which players propel plastic or wooden discs into numbered scoring areas marked on a large flat surface.

shufty, shufti /'ʃʌfti/ n (pl **shufties**) (sl) a peek, a glance.

shun /ʃʌn/ vt (**shunning, shunned**) to avoid scrupulously; to keep away from.

shunt /ʃʌnt/ vti to move to a different place to put aside, to shelve; (trains) to switch from one track to another; (sl) to collide.—also n.

shush /ʃʊʃ/ or /ʃʌʃ/ interj used to demand silence; peace, silence. • vt to demand silence (as if) by saying "shush".

shut /ʃʌt/ vti (**shutting, shut**) to close; to lock, to fasten; to close up parts of, to fold together; to bar; (with **down**) to (cause to) stop working or operating; (with **in**) to confine; to enclose; to block the view from; (with **off**) to check the flow of; to debar; (with **out**) to exclude; (with **up**) to confine; (inf) to stop talking; (inf) to silence.

shutdown /'ʃʌtdaʊn/ n a stoppage of work or activity, as in a factory.

shuteye /-aɪ/ n (inf) sleep.

shutter /'ʃʌtər/ n a movable cover for a window; a flap device for regulating the exposure of light to a camera lens.

shuttle /'ʃʌtəl/ n a device in a loom for holding the weft thread and carrying it between the warp threads; a bus, aircraft, etc, making back-and-forth trips over a short route. • vti to move back and forth rapidly.

shuttlecock[1] /'ʃʌtəlˌkɒk/ n a cork stuck with feathers, or a plastic imitation, hit with a racket in badminton.

shuttlecock[2] see **battledore**.

shy[1] /ʃaɪ/ adj (**shyer, shyest** or **shier, shiest**) very self-conscious, timid; bashful; wary, suspicious (of); (sl) lacking. • vi (**shying, shied**) to move suddenly, as when startled; to be or become cautious, etc. • n (pl **shies**) a sudden movement.—**shyly** adv.—**shyness** n.

shy[2] vt (**shying, shied**) to throw (something). • n (pl **shies**) a throw; (inf) an attempt, try.

shyster /'ʃaɪstər/ n (inf) a person, esp a lawyer, who is manipulative and disreputable.

SI n (Système International d'Unités) the universally used system of units based on the metre, second, kilogram, ampere, kelvin, candela, siemens, tesla, weber and mole.

Si (chem symbol) silicon.

si /siː/ n (mus) ti.

sial /'saɪæl/ n the outer layer of the earth's crust composed mostly of rock rich in silicon and aluminium.

Siamese cat /saɪ'miːz/ or /ˌsaɪə'miːz/ n a breed of domestic shorthaired cat with a fawn or grey coat, darker ears, paws, tail and face, and blue eyes.

Siamese fighting fish n an aggressive brightly coloured freshwater fish.

Siamese twins npl twin babies born with the bodies joined together at some point, esp the hip.

sib /sɪb/ n a sibling.

sibilant /'sɪbɪlənt/ adj hissing. • n a sibilant letter, eg s, z.—**sibilance** n.

sibling /'sɪblɪŋ/ n a brother or sister.

sibyl /'sɪbəl/ n in ancient Greece and Rome, a female prophet or oracle.

sic /sɪk/ adv as written (used in text to indicate that an error or doubtful usage is reproduced from the original).

sick /sɪk/ adj unhealthy, ill; having nausea, vomiting; thoroughly tired (of); disgusted by or suffering from an excess; (inf) of humour, sadistic, gruesome.—**sickness** n.

sick bay n an area in a ship used as a hospital or dispensary; a room used for the treatment of the sick.

sickbed /'sɪkbɛd/ n the bed where one lies sick.

sick building syndrome n a collection of symptoms, thought to be caused by micro-organisms found in humidifiers and including lethargy, headache and eye irritation, that affect those who work in totally air-conditioned buildings.—also **humidifier fever**.

sicken /'sɪkən/ vti to make or become sick or nauseated; to show signs of illness; to nauseate.

sickening /'sɪkənɪŋ/ adj disgusting.—**sickeningly** adv.

sickle /'sɪkəl/ n a tool with a crescent-shaped blade for cutting tall grasses; anything shaped like this.

sick leave n absence from work due to illness.

sickle cell anaemia n a form of anaemia that is hereditary and marked by the presence of sickle-shaped red blood cells.

sick list n a list of employees, soldiers, etc who are absent due to illness.

sickly /'sɪkli/ adj (**sicklier, sickliest**) inclined to be ill; unhealthy; causing nausea; mawkish; pale, feeble.—**sickliness** n.

sick-making adj (inf) nauseating, galling.

sick pay n wages or salaries paid to an employee while he or she is off sick.

sickroom /'sɪkruːm/ n the room to which a patient is confined while sick.

side /saɪd/ n a line or surface bounding anything; the left or right part of the body; the top or underneath surface; the slope of a hill; an aspect, a direction; a party or faction; a cause; a team; a line of descent; (sl) conceit. • adj toward or at the side, lateral; incidental. • vi to associate with a particular faction.

side arms /saɪdɑrmz/ n weapons (eg a pistol, dagger) worn in a belt or holster at the side of the waist.

sideboard /-bɔrd/ n a long table or cabinet for holding cutlery, crockery, etc; (pl) two strips of hair growing down a man's cheeks.—also **sideburns**.

sidecar /-kɑr/ n a small car attached to the side of a motor cycle; a cocktail of brandy, liqueur, and lemon juice.

sided /'saɪdəd/ adj having sides of a specified number or kind.

side dish n food accompanying a main course at a meal.

side drum n a small double-headed drum with snares, carried and played at the side

side effect n a secondary and usu adverse effect, as of a drug or medical treatment.

side-glance n a look directed to one side; a slight reference.

sidekick /'saɪdkɪk/ n (sl) a confederate; a partner; a close friend.

sidelight /-laɪt/ n light coming from the side; a light on the side of a car, etc; incidental information.

sideline /-laɪn/ n a line marking the side limit of a playing area; a minor branch of business; a subsidiary interest.

sidelong /-lɒŋ/ adj oblique, not direct. • adv obliquely.

sidereal /saɪ'dɪəriəl/ adj of or by reference to stars and constellations.

siderite /'saɪdəˌraɪt/ n a mineral composed mainly of ferrous carbonate used as a source of iron.

sidero-, sider- /'saɪdərɔ/ or /'saɪ-/ prefix iron.

siderosis /ˌsaɪdə'rɔːsɪs/ n a lung disease caused by inhalation of iron or other types of metallic particles.

side-saddle /ˈsaɪdsædəl/ *n* a saddle that enables a rider to sit with both feet on the same side of a horse. • *adv* as if sitting on a side-saddle.

sideshow /-ʃoː/ *n* a minor attraction at a fair, etc; a subsidiary event.

sidesman /ˈsaɪdzmən/ *n* (*pl* **sidesmen**) (*Anglican Church*) an officer assisting the churchwardens.

side-splitting /ˈsaɪdˌsplɪtɪŋ/ *adj* uproariously funny.

sidestep /-stɛp/ *vti* to take a step to one side; to avoid or dodge.—*also n*.

sidestroke /-ˌstroːk/ *n* (*swimming*) a stroke used while swimming on one's side.

sideswipe /-ˌswaɪp/ *n* a glancing blow; (*inf*) an incidental jibe or criticism.

sidetrack /-træk/ *vt* to prevent action by diversionary tactics; to shunt aside, to shelve. • *n* a railroad siding.

sidewalk /-wɒk/ *n* a path, *usu* paved, at the side of a street.

sidewall /-wɔl/ *n* either of the sides of a pneumatic tyre.

Sideward /ˈsaɪdwərd/, **sidewards** /-wərdz/ *adj*, *adv* sideways.

Sideways /ˈsaɪdweɪz/, **sideway** /-weɪ/ *adj*, *adv* toward or from one side; facing to the side.

side whiskers *n* sideboards or sideburns.

sidewinder /ˈsaɪdˌwaɪndər/ *n* a North American rattlesnake that moves in a twisting sideways motion.

sidewise /ˈsaɪdwaɪz/ *adv* sideways.

siding /ˈsaɪdɪŋ/ *n* a short line beside a main railway track for use in shunting; a covering as of boards for the outside of a frame building.

sidle /ˈsaɪdəl/ *vi* to move sideways, *esp* to edge along.

SIDS /sɪdz/ *abbr* = sudden infant death syndrome.

siege /siːdʒ/ *n* the surrounding of a fortified place to cut off supplies and compel its surrender; the act of besieging; a continued attempt to gain something.

siemens /ˈsiːmənz/ *n* (*pl* **siemens**) the SI unit of electrical conductance.

sienna /siːˈɛnə/ *n* an earthy pigment, either yellowish brown (raw sienna) or reddish brown (burnt sienna).

sierra /sɪˈɛrə/ *n* a range of mountains with jagged peaks.

siesta /siːˈɛstə/ *n* a midday nap, *esp* in hot countries.

sieve /sɪv/ *n* a utensil with a meshed wire bottom for sifting and straining; a person who cannot keep secrets. • *vt* to put through a sieve, to sift.

sift /sɪft/ *vti* to separate coarser parts from finer with a sieve; to sort out; to examine critically; to pass as through a sieve.

sigh /saɪ/ *vti* to draw deep audible breath as a sign of weariness, relief, etc; to make a sound like this; to pine or lament (for); to utter with a sigh.—*also n*.

sight /saɪt/ *n* the act or faculty of seeing; what is seen or is worth seeing, a spectacle; a view or glimpse; range of vision; a device on a gun etc to guide the eye in aiming it; aim taken with this; (*inf*) anything that looks unpleasant, odd, etc. • *vti* to catch sight of; to aim through a sight.

sighted /ˈsaɪtəd/ *adj* having sight, *esp* of a particular character, *eg* shortsighted.

sightless /-ləs/ *adj* without sight, blind.—**sightlessly** *adv*.—**sightlessness** *n*.

sightly /-li/ *adj* (**sightlier, sightliest**) pleasing to the eye; comely.—**sightliness** *n*.

sight-read /-riːd/ *vt* (**sight-reading, sight-read**) to play or sing from a piece of printed music without previous preparation. • *vi* to read at sight.

sightseeing /-ˌsiːŋ/ *n* the viewing or visiting of places of interest.—**sightseer** *n*.

sigma /ˈsɪɡmə/ *n* the 18th letter of the Greek alphabet; (*math*) the symbol S indicating summation.

Sigmoid /ˈsɪɡmɔɪd/, **sigmoidal** /-əl/ *adj* curved like the letter S.

sign /saɪn/ *n* a mark or symbol; a gesture; an indication, token, trace, or symptom (of); an omen; (*math*) a conventional mark used to indicate an operation to be performed; a board or placard with publicly displayed information. • *vi* to append one's signature; to ratify thus. • *vt* to engage by written contract; to write one's name on; to make or indicate by a sign; to signal; to communicate by sign language; (*with* **away**) to relinquish by signing a deed, etc; (*with* **on**) to accept employment; to register; (*with* **off**) to complete a broadcast.

signal /ˈsɪɡnəl/ *n* a sign, device or gesture to intimate a warning or to give information, *esp* at a distance; a message so conveyed; a semaphore system used by railways; in radio, etc, the electrical impulses transmitted or received; a sign or event that initiates action. • *vti* (**signalling, signalled** *or* **signaling, signaled**) to make a signal or signals (to); to communicate by signals. • *adj* striking, notable.—**signaller, signaler** *n*.

signalize /ˈsɪɡnəˌlaɪz/ *vt* to point out; distinguish.—**signalization** *n*.

signally /ˈsɪɡnəli/ *adv* remarkably; notably.

signalman /ˈsɪɡnəlmən/ *n* (*pl* **signalmen**) a person who works signals or transmits signals.

signatory /ˈsɪɡnəˌtɔri/ *n* (*pl* **signatories**) a party or state that has signed an agreement or treaty; the person who signs on behalf of their government.

signature /ˈsɪɡnətʃər/ *n* a person's name written by himself or herself; the act of signing one's own name; a characteristic mark; (*mus*) the flats and sharps after the clef showing the key; (*print*) a mark on the first pages of each sheet of a book as a guide to the binder; such a sheet when folded.

signature tune *n* a tune associated with a performer or a TV, radio programme, etc.

signboard /ˈsaɪnbɔrd/ *n* a board with a sign or inscription in front of a business, shop, etc.

signet /ˈsɪɡnət/ *n* a small seal, *esp* one set in a ring; an official seal used in lieu of a signature in authenticating documents; the impression made by this.

signet ring *n* a ring with a seal set in it.

significant /sɪɡˈnɪfɪkənt/ *adj* full of meaning, *esp* a special or hidden one; momentous, important; highly expressive; indicative (of).—**significance** *n*.—**significantly** *adv*.

signify /ˈsɪɡnəˌfaɪ/ *vti* (**signifying, signified**) to mean; to be a sign of; to indicate; to represent; to matter, to be important; to make a sign.—**signification** *n*.

sign language *n* a system of manual signs and gestures for conveying meaning, used *esp* by the deaf.

signor, signior /siˈnjɔr/ *n* (*pl* **signors, signori**) an Italian man—equivalent to Mr.

signora /siˈnjɔrə/ *n* (*pl* **signoras, signore**) a married Italian woman—equivalent to Mrs or madam.

signore /-ˈnjɔːre/ *n* (*pl* **signori**) an Italian man—equivalent to sir.

signorina /ˌsiːnjəˈriːnə/ *n* (*pl* **signorinas, signorine**) an unmarried Italian woman—equivalent to Miss.

signpost /ˈsaɪnpoːst/ *n* a post with signs on it to direct travellers; a beacon, a guide.—*also vt*.

Sikh /siːk/ *n* a member of an Indian sect, founded in the 16th century, that teaches monotheism and rejects idolatry and caste. • *adj* of or pertaining to the Sikhs or their beliefs.

silage /ˈsaɪlədʒ/ *n* green fodder preserved for the winter in a silo.

sild /sɪld/ *n* (*pl* **silds, sild**) a young herring, *esp* when canned in Norway.

silence /ˈsaɪləns/ *n* absence of sound; the time this lasts; refusal to speak or make a sound; secrecy. • *vt* to cause to be silent. • *interj* be silent!

silencer /ˈsaɪlənsər/ *n* a device for reducing the noise of a vehicle exhaust or gun, a muffler.

silent /ˈsaɪlənt/ *adj* not speaking; taciturn; noiseless; still.—**silently** *adv*.

silent majority *n* those who rarely assert their views but are presumed to be moderates.

silhouette /ˌsɪluːˈɛt/ *n* the outline of a shape against light or a lighter background; a solid outline drawing, *usu* in solid black on white, *esp* of a profile. • *vt* to show up in outline; to depict in silhouette.

silica /ˈsɪləkə/ *n* a hard mineral, a compound of oxygen and silicon, found in quartz and flint.

silicate /ˈsɪləˌkət/ *n* a salt containing silicon.

siliceous, silicious /sɪˈlɪʃəs/ *adj* of containing silica.

silicon /ˈsɪlɪkən/ *n* a metalloid element occuring in silica and used extensively in transistors, etc, and as a compound in glass, etc. • *adj* of an area in which there are a number of computer software and hardware companies.

silicon chip *n* a microchip.

silicone /ˈsɪləˌkoːn/ *n* an organic polymer compound with good lubricating and insulating properties, used widely as a repellent, resin, etc.

silicosis /ˌsɪləˈkoːsɪs/ *n* a disease of the lungs caused by prolonged inhalation of silica particles.

silk /sɪlk/ *n* a fibre produced by silkworms; lustrous textile cloth, thread or a garment made of silk; (*pl*) silk garments; (*pl*) the colours of a racing stable, worn by a jockey, etc. •*adj* of, relating to or made of silk.

silk cotton *n* kapok.

silken /'sɪlkən/ *adj* made of or like silk; silky.

silk hat *n* a top hat covered in silk.

silk screen /'sɪlkskriːn/ *n* a stencil method of printing a colour design through the meshes of a fabric, as silk; a print so produced.—**silk-screen** *vt*.

silkweed /-wiːd/ *see* milkweed.

silkworm /'sɪlkwɜːm/ *n* a caterpillar of various moths that feeds on mulberry leaves and produces a strong fibre to construct its cocoon.

silky /'sɪlki/ *adj* (**silkier, silkiest**) soft and smooth like silk; glossy; suave.—**silkiness** *n*.

sill /sɪl/ *n* a heavy, horizontal slab of wood or stone at the bottom of a window frame or door.

sillabub /'sɪləˌbʌb/ *see* syllabub.

silly /'sɪli/ *adj* (**sillier, silliest**) foolish, stupid; frivolous; lacking in sense or judgment; being stunned or dazed. • *n* (*pl* **sillies**) a silly person.—**silliness** *n*.

silo /'saɪloʊ/ *n* (*pl* **silos**) an airtight pit or tower for storing fodder in a green compressed state; a deep pit for storing cement, coal, etc; an underground structure from which a missile can be fired.

silt /sɪlt/ *n* a fine-grained sandy sediment carried or deposited by water. • *vti* to fill or choke up with silt.

Silurian /sə'lʊriən/ *adj* (*geol*) of or pertaining to the division of Palaeozoic rocks between Ordovician and Devonian. • *n* this period.

silver /'sɪlvər/ *n* a ductile, malleable, greyish-white metallic element used in jewellery, cutlery, tableware, coins, etc; a lustrous, greyish white. • *adj* made of or plated with silver; silvery; (*hair*) grey; marking the 25th in a series. • *vt* to coat with silver or a substance resembling silver; to make or become silvery or grey.

silver birch *n* a Eurasian birch tree with silvery bark.

silver fox *n* (the pelt of) a red fox in a colour phase when its fur is black with silver-tipped hairs.

silver-gilt *n* gilded silver.

silver lining *n* a more favourable aspect of an otherwise hopeless situation.

silver paper *n* a metallic paper coated or laminated to resemble silver, tinfoil.

silver plate *n* a plating of silver; domestic utensils made of silver or of silver-plated metal.—**silver-plate** *vt*.

silver screen *n* (*inf*) (*with* **the**) the film industry; the screen on which a film is projected.

silver service *n* (*in restaurants*) a manner of serving food using a spoon and fork in one hand.

silverside /'sɪlvərsaɪd/ *n* a joint of beef cut from the upper haunch.

silversmith /-smɪθ/ *n* a worker in silver.

silver thaw *n* ✹ (*Cdn*) a glassy coating of ice on trees or other surfaces caused by freezing rain or a sudden frost.

silver-tongued /-tʌŋd/ *adj* plausible, eloquent.

silverware /-ˌwer/ *n* items, such as serving plates, cutlery, etc made from silver or silver plate.

silver wedding *n* the 25th anniversary of a marriage.

silverweed /'sɪlvərwiːd/ *n* any of various plants with silvery leaves or hairs.

silvery /'sɪlvəri/ *adj* white and lustrous like silver; covered with silver; resembling silver in colour; (*sound*) soft and clear.

silviculture /'sɪlvəˌkʌltʃər/ *n* the branch of forestry dealing with the care and development of forests.

simian /'sɪmiən/ *adj* of or like an ape or monkey.

simian immunodeficiency virus *n* a virus, similar to human immunodeficiency virus, that interferes with the ability of the immune system of monkeys to resist disease.

similar /'sɪmələr/ *adj* having a resemblance to, like; nearly corresponding; (*geom*) corresponding exactly in shape if not size.—**similarity** *n*.—**similarly** *adv*.

simile /'sɪmɪli/ *n* a figure of speech likening one thing to another by the use of like, as, etc.

similitude /sɪ'mɪləˌtuːd/ or /-tjuːd/ *n* the state of being similar; guise, likeness.

simmer /'sɪmər/ *vti* to boil gently; to be or keep on the point of boiling; to be in a state of suppressed rage or laughter; (*with* **down**) to abate. • *n* the state of simmering.

simnel cake /'sɪmnəl/ *n* a rich fruit cake with marzipan and decorations traditionally eaten during Lent or Easter.

simony /'saɪməni/ or /'sɪm-/ *n* the buying and selling of ecclesiastical offices.

Simoom /sə'muːm/, **simoon** /-muːn/ *n* a strong, hot, dry wind of the Arabian and North African deserts.

simpatico /sɪm'pætɪˌkoʊ/ *adj* (*inf*) agreeable, sympathetic.

simper /'sɪmpər/ *vi* to smile in a silly or self-conscious way.—*also n*.

simple /'sɪmpəl/ *adj* single, uncompounded; plain, not elaborate; clear, not complicated; easy to do, understand, or solve; artless, not sophisticated; weak in intellect; unsuspecting, credulous; sheer, mere.—**simpleness** *n*.

simple fraction *n* a fraction in which both the numerator and denominator are whole numbers.

simple-hearted /-'hɑːrtɪd/ *adj* sincere, honest.

simple interest *n* interest paid on the principal of a loan only.

simple-minded /-'maɪndɪd/ *adj* foolish; mentally retarded.

simpleton /'sɪmpəltən/ *n* a foolish, weak-minded person.

simplicity /sɪm'plɪsɪti/ *n* (*pl* **simplicities**) the quality or state of being simple; absence of complications; easiness; lack of ornament, plainness, restraint; artlessness; directness; guilelessness, openness, naivety.

simplification /ˌsɪmplɪfɪ'keɪʃən/ *n* the act or result of making less complicated.

simplify /'sɪmplɪˌfaɪ/ *vt* (**simplifying, simplified**) to make simple or easy to understand.

simplistic /sɪm'plɪstɪk/ *adj* oversimplified; uncomplicated.—**simplistically** *adv*.

simply /'sɪmpli/ *adv* in a simple way; plainly; merely; absolutely.

simulacrum /ˌsɪmju'leɪkrəm/ *n* (*pl* **simulacra**) a likeness or representation, *esp* a superficial one.

simulate /'sɪmjuleɪt/ *vt* to pretend to have or feel, to feign; (*conditions*) to reproduce in order to conduct an experiment; to imitate.—**simulation** *n*.

simulator /'sɪmjuˌleɪtər/ *n* a device that simulates specific conditions in order to test actions or reactions.

simulcast /'saɪməlˌkæst/ or /'sɪm-/ *n* a simultaneous radio and television broadcast.—*also vt*.

simultaneous /ˌsaɪməl'teɪniəs/ or /ˌsɪm-/ *adj* done or occurring at the same time.—**simultaneity** *n*.—**simultaneously** *adv*.

SIN /sɪn/ *abbr* ✹ (*Cdn*) = Social Insurance Number.

sin[1] /sɪn/ *n* an offence against a religious or moral principle; transgression of the law of God; a wicked act, an offence; a misdeed, a fault. • *vi* (**sinning, sinned**) to commit a sin; to offend (against).

sin[2] *abbr* = sine.

sin bin /'sɪn bɪn/ *n* (*ice hockey, etc*) (*sl*) an enclosure off the playing area where players guilty of fouls are temporarily sent.

since /sɪns/ *adv* from then until now; subsequently; ago. • *prep* during, or continuously from (then) until now; after. • *conj* from the time that; because, seeing that.

sincere /sɪn'sɪːr/ *adj* genuine, real, not pretended; honest, straightforward.—**sincerely** *adv*.

sincerity /-'serɪti/ *n* the quality or state of being sincere; genuineness, honesty, seriousness.

sinciput /'sɪnsɪˌpʊt/ *n* (*pl* **sinciputs, sincipita**) the front part of the skull; forehead.

sine /saɪn/ *n* (*trig*) a function that in a right-angled triangle is equal to the ratio of the length of the side opposite the angle to that of the hypotenuse.

sinecure /'sɪnəˌkjʊr/ *n* a position or office that provides an income without involving duties.

sine die /ˌsaɪni'daɪi/ or /ˌsɪneɪ'diːeɪ/ *adv* without a date, indefinitely.

sine qua non /ˌsɪneɪkwɒ'nɒn/ or /-noːn/ *n* an essential condition, a necessity.

sinew /'sɪnjuː/ *n* a cord of fibrous tissue, a tendon; (*usu pl*) the chief supporting force, a mainstay; (*pl*) muscles, brawn.

sinewy /'sɪnjuːi/ *adj* having a lean body and strong muscles; tough, stringy.

sinfonia /ˌsɪnfə'niːə/ or /sɪn'foʊniə/ *n* (*pl* **sinfonie, sinfonias**) a symphony.

sinfonietta /ˌsɪnfə'njetə/ *n* a short symphony; a small orchestra.

sinful /'sɪnfəl/ *adj* guilty of sin, wicked.—**sinfully** *adv*.—**sinfulness** *n*.

sing /sɪŋ/ *vti* (**singing, sang**, *pp* **sung**) to utter (words) with musical modulations; (*a song*) to perform; to hum, to ring; to write poetry (about), to praise; (*with* **out**) to shout, call out.—**singer** *n*.—**singing** *n*.

sing. *abbr* = singular.

singe /sɪndʒ/ *vt* (**singeing, singed**) to burn slightly; to scorch, *esp* to remove feathers, etc.—*also n.*

Singhalese /ˌsɪŋɡəˈliːz/ or /-ˈliːs/ *see* **Sinhalese**.

singing /ˈsɪŋɪŋ/ *n* the art or an act of singing.

singing telegram *n* (a service that provides) a greetings message delivered in song, *usu* by a person in fancy dress.

single /ˈsɪŋɡəl/ *adj* one only, not double; individual; composed of one part; alone, sole; separate; unmarried; for one; with one contestant on each side; simple; whole, unbroken; (*tennis*) played between two persons only; (*ticket*) for the outward journey only. • *n* a single ticket; a game between two players; a hit scoring one; a record with one tune on each side. • *vt* (*with* **out**) to pick out, to select.

single blessedness *n* the unmarried state.

single-breasted /ˈsɪŋɡəlˈbrɛstɪd/ *adj* (*suit, etc*) fastening in the centre with a single row of buttons.

single cream *n* cream with a low fat content.

single-decker *n* a bus with only one level of passenger accommodation.

single entry *n* (*book-keeping*) a system in which transactions are kept in one account only.

single figures *npl* the numbers less than 10, ie 1 to 9.

single file *n* a single column of persons or things, one behind the other.

single-handed /-ˈhændɪd/ *adj, adv* without assistance, unaided.—**single-handedly** *adv.*—**single-handedness** *n.*

single-lens reflex *n* a camera whose lens allows the photographer to see the same image as it exposes.

single-minded /-ˈmaɪndɪd/ *adj* having only one aim in mind.—**single-mindedly** *adv.*—**single-mindedness** *n.*

singles bar *n* a bar or social club for single people only.

singlestick /-ˌstɪk/ *n* fencing with wooden sticks instead of swords; the stick used for this.

singlet /ˈsɪŋɡlət/ *n* an undervest.

single ticket *n* a ticket for a one-way journey only.

singleton /ˈsɪŋɡəltən/ *n* a playing card that is the only one of its suit in a hand.

singly /ˈsɪŋɡli/ *adv* alone; one by one.

singsong /ˈsɪŋsɒŋ/ *n* a droning monotonous utterance; a verse with a regular, marked rhythm and rhyme; (*inf*) a party where everyone sings. • *adj* having a regular or monotonous rhythm.

singular /ˈsɪŋjʊlər/ *adj* remarkable; exceptional; unusual; eccentric, odd; (*gram*) referring to only one person or thing. • *n* (*gram*) the singular number or form of a word.

singularity /ˌsɪŋɡjʊˈlɛrɪti/ or /-ˈlæ-/ *n* (*pl* **singularities**) the state of being singular; uniqueness; an odd trait, a peculiarity.

singularly /ˈsɪŋjʊlərli/ *adv* unusually; exceptionally.

Sinhalese /ˌsɪnhəˈliːz/ or /ˌsɪnəˈliːz/ *n* a member of a people who form the largest community in Sri Lanka; the language of these people.—*also adj.*—*also* **Singhalese**.

sinister /ˈsɪnɪstər/ *adj* inauspicious; ominous; ill-omened; evil-looking; malignant; wicked; left; (*her*) on the left side of the shield.

sinistral /ˈsɪnɪstrəl/ *adj* of or on the left; left-handed.—**sinistrally** *adv.*

sink /sɪŋk/ *vti* (**sinking, sank** or **sunk, pp sunk**) to go under the surface or to the bottom (of a liquid); to submerge in water; to go down slowly; (*wind*) to subside; to pass to a lower state; to droop, to decline; to grow weaker; to become hollow; to lower, to degrade; to cause to sink; to make by digging out; to invest; (*with* **in**) to penetrate; to thrust into; (*inf*) to be understood or in full. • *n* a basin with an outflow pipe, *usu* in a kitchen; a cesspool; an area of sunken land.—**sinking** *n.*

sinker /ˈsɪŋkər/ *n* a weight used to submerge a fishing line.

sinkhole /-hoːl/ *n* a hole in rock strata, *esp* limestone, though which water sinks or runs underground; a hole into which foul waste matter is discharged.

sinking fund *n* money put aside for gradual payment of a debt.

Sinn Fein /ʃɪnˈfeɪn/ *n* a republican party in Ireland which is the political wing of the IRA.

sinner /ˈsɪnər/ *n* a person who sins.

Sino- /ˈsaɪnoː/ *prefix* Chinese.

Sino-Tebetan /ˌsaɪnoːtɪˈbɛtən/ *n* a family of languages that includes all the Chinese languages, Burmese and Tibetan.—*also adj.*

Sinology /saɪˈnɒlədʒi/ or /sɪ-/ *n* the study of Chinese language, history, society, etc.—**Sinologist** *n.*—**Sinological** *adj.*

sinsemilla /sɪnsəˈmɪlə/ *n* (a plant which produces) a highly potent type of marijuana.

sinter /ˈsɪntər/ *n* a white silicious deposit formed by the evaporation of hot mineral waters. • *vt* to form (metal or glass powder) into lumps by the application of heat and pressure.

sinuate /ˈsɪnjʊət/ *adj* (*leaf*) having a wavy edge.—**sinuately** *adv.*

sinuous /ˈsɪnjʊəs/ *adj* curving; winding; tortuous.—**sinuously** *adv.*—**sinuousness** *n.*

sinus /ˈsaɪnəs/ *n* (*pl* **sinuses**) an air cavity in the skull that opens in the nasal cavities.

sinusitis /ˌsaɪnəˈsaɪtɪs/ *n* inflammation of a sinus.

Siouan /ˈsuːən/ *n* a family of North American Indian languages.

Sioux /suː/ *n* (*pl* **Sioux**) a member of various North American Indian peoples who speak Siouan.

sip /sɪp/ *vti* (**sipping, sipped**) to drink in small mouthfuls. • *n* the act of sipping; the quantity sipped.

siphon /ˈsaɪfən/ *n* a bent tube for drawing off liquids from a higher to a lower level by atmospheric pressure; a bottle with an internal tube and tap at the top for aerated water. • *vti* to draw off, or be drawn off, with a siphon.—*also* **syphon**.

siphon bottle *n* a soda siphon.

sir /sər/ *n* a title of respect used to address a man in speech or correspondence; (*with cap*) a title preceding the first name of a knight or baronet. • *vt* to address as "sir".

sire /ˈsaɪr/ *n* a father; a male ancestor; the male parent of an animal; a form of address to a king. • *vt* (*animal*) to beget.

siren /ˈsaɪrən/ *n* a device producing a loud wailing sound as a warning signal; a fabled sea nymph who lured sailors to destruction with a sweet song; a seductive or alluring woman.

sirenian /saɪˈriːnɪən/ *n* a member of an order of plant-eating mammals that live in water, comprising the dugong and the manatee.—*also adj.*

sirloin /ˈsərlɔɪn/ *n* the upper part of a loin of beef.

sirocco /sɪˈrɒkoː/ *n* a hot, oppressive wind that blows across southern Europe from North Africa.

sirree /səˈriː/ *interj* (*inf*) sir – used for emphasis, *esp* after *yes* or *no*.

sis /sɪs/ *n* (*inf*) sister.

sisal /ˈsaɪsəl/ *n* (a tropical agave plant whose leaves yield) a tough fibre used to make rope.

siskin /ˈsɪskɪn/ *n* a Eurasian songbird with greenish plumage related to the goldfinch.

sissy /ˈsɪsi/ *n* (*pl* **sissies**) an effeminate, feeble or cowardly boy or man.—*also adj.*

sister /ˈsɪstər/ *n* a female sibling, a daughter of the same parents; a female member or associate of the same race, creed, trade union, etc; a member of a religious sisterhood; one of the same kind, model, etc; a senior nurse. • *adj* (*ship, etc*) belonging to the same type.

sisterhood /-hʊd/ *n* a female religious or charitable order; the state of being a sister.

sister-in-law /-ɪnˌlɔ/ *n* (*pl* **sisters-in-law**) the sister of a husband or wife; the wife of a brother.

sisterly /-li/ *adj* like a sister, kind, affectionate.

sistrum /ˈsɪstrəm/ *n* (*pl* **sistra**) an ancient Egyptian metal rattle used as a percussion instrument.

sit /sɪt/ *vti* (**sitting, sat**) to rest oneself on the buttocks, as on a chair; (*bird*) to perch; (*hen*) to cover eggs for hatching; (*legislator, etc*) to occupy a seat; (*court*) to be in session; to pose, as for a portrait; to ride (a horse); to press or weigh (upon); to be located; to rest or lie; to take an examination; to take care of a child, pet, etc, while the parents or owners are away; to cause to sit; to provide seats or seating room for; (*with* **down**) to take a seat; (*with* **for**) to represent in parliament; (*with* **in**) to attend a discussion or a musical session; to participate in a sit-in; (*with* **on**) to hold a meeting to discuss; to delay action on something; (*inf*) to suppress; to rebuke; (*with* **out**) to sit through the whole; to abstain from dancing; (*with* **up**) to straighten the back while sitting; not to go to bed; (*inf*) to be astonished.

sitar /ˈsɪtɑr/ or /ˈsɪtɑr/ *n* an Indian musical instrument similar to a lute with a long neck.

sitcom /ˈsɪtkɒm/ *see* **situation comedy**.

site /saɪt/ *n* a space occupied or to be occupied by a building; a situation; the place or scene of something. • *vt* to locate, to place.

sit-in /ˈsɪtɪn/ *n* a strike in which the strikers refuse to leave the premises; civil disobedience in which demonstrators occupy a public place and refuse to leave voluntarily.

sitka spruce /'sɪtkə/ n a tall North American spruce tree.

sitter /'sɪtər/ n a person who looks after a child, dog, house, etc, while the parents or owners are away.

sitting /'sɪtɪŋ/ n the state of being seated; a period of being seated, as for a meal, a portrait; a session, as of a court; a clutch of eggs. • adj that is sitting; being in a judicial or legislative seat; used in or for sitting; performed while sitting.

sitting duck, sitting target n (inf) a person or thing that is an easy target for attack, criticism, etc.

sitting room /-ruːm/ n a room other than a bedroom or kitchen; a parlour.

sitting tenant n a tenant in occupation of a property.

situate /'sɪtʃʊeɪt/ vt to place in a site, situation, or category.

situated /-ɪd/ adj having a site, located; placed; provided with money, etc.

situation /sɪtʃʊ'eɪʃən/ n a place, a position; a state of affairs, circumstances; a job or post.

situation comedy n a comic television or radio series made up of episodes involving the same group of characters.—also **sitcom**.

sit-up /'sɪt ʌp/ n an exercise of sitting up from a prone position without using hands or legs.

SIV abbr = simian immunodeficiency virus.

Siwash /'saɪwɒʃ/ n ♣ (Cdn) a thick woollen sweater with designs taken from the mythology of First Nations peoples of the northwest coast of North America.

six /sɪks/ adj, n one more than five. • n the symbol for this (6, VI, vi); the sixth in a series or set; something having six units as members.

sixer /'sɪksər/ n a leader of a group of six Brownies or Cub Scouts.

sixfold /'sɪksfoːld/ adj having six units or members being six times as great or as many.

six-pack /-pæk/ n a pack of six units, as of cans of beer, etc, sold together.

sixpence /-pəns/ n (formerly) a British coin worth six old pennies.

six-shooter /-ʃuːtər/ n (inf) a six-chambered revolver.

sixteen /ˌsɪks'tiːn/ or /'sɪks-/ adj, n one more than fifteen. • n the symbol for this (16, XVI, xvi).—**sixteenth** adj, n.

sixteenth note n a musical note with a sixteenth the time value of a whole note, a semiquaver.

sixth /sɪksθ/ n one of six equal parts of a thing; (mus) an interval of six diatonic degrees; the sixth tone of a diatonic scale.—also adv. • adj next after fifth.—**sixthly** adv.

sixth sense n intuitive power.

sixty /'sɪksti/ n six times ten. • n (pl **sixties**) the symbol for this (60, LX, lx); (in pl) sixties (60s), the numbers for 60 to 69; the same numbers in a life or century.—**sixtieth** adj, adv.

sixty-fourth note n a musical note with the time value of one sixty-fourth of a whole note; a hemidemisemiquaver.

sixty-nine /ˌsɪksti'naɪn/ n soixante-neuf.

sizable, sizeable /'saɪzəbəl/ adj of some size; large.—**sizably, sizeably** adv.—**sizableness, sizeableness** n.

size[1] /saɪz/ n magnitude; the dimensions or proportions of something; a graduated measurement, as of clothing or shoes. • vt to sort according to size; to measure; (with **up**) (inf) to make an estimate or judgment of; to meet requirements.

size[2] n a thin pasty substance used to glaze paper, stiffen cloth, etc. • vt to treat with size.

sized /'saɪzd/ adj having a specified size.

sizzle /'sɪzəl/ vti to make a hissing spluttering noise, as of frying; to be extremely hot; to be very angry; to scorch, sear or fry with a sizzling sound. • n a hissing sound.

SJ abbr = Society of Jesus.

sjambok /'ʃæmbɒk/ n (in S Africa) a heavy whip made from rhinoceros hide.

SK abbr ♣ = Saskatchewan.

ska /skɒ/ n a form of West Indian pop music, a precursor of reggae.

skate[1] /skeɪt/ n a steel blade attached to a boot for glicing on ice; a boot with such a runner; a roller skate. • vi to move on skates; (with **over**) to avoid dealing with (an issue, problem, etc) directly.—**skater** n.

skate[2] n an edible fish of the ray family with a broad, flat body and short, spineless tail.

skateboard /'skeɪtbɔrd/ n a short, oblong board with two wheels at each end for standing on and riding.—also vi.

skean-dhu /skiːn'duː/ or /'skiːən-/ n (Scot) a dagger worn in the stocking as part of Highland dress.

skedaddle /skɪ'dædəl/ vi (inf) to run away.—also n.

skeet /skiːt/ n a type of clay-pigeon shooting in which clay targets are hurled into range at varying speeds and trajectories from two traps.

skein /skeɪn/ n a folded coil of yarn, thread, etc; a tangle; a flight of wild fowl, esp geese.

skeleton /'skelətən/ n the bony framework of the body of a human, an animal or plant; the bones separated from flesh and preserved in their natural position; a supporting structure, a framework; an outline, an abstract; a very thin person; something shameful kept secret. • adj (staff, crew, etc) reduced to the lowest possible level.—**skeletal** adj.

skeleton key n a key with a slender bit that can open many simple locks.

skeptic /'skeptɪk/ see **sceptic**.

skeptical /-əl/ see **sceptical**.

skepticism /'skeptɪˌsɪzəm/ see **scepticism**.

skerry /'skeri/ n (pl **skerries**) a rocky isle or reef.

sketch /sketʃ/ n a rough drawing, quickly made; a preliminary draft; a short literary piece or essay; a short humorous item for a revue, etc; a brief outline. • vi to make a sketch (of); to plan roughly.

sketchy /'sketʃi/ adj (**sketchier, sketchiest**) incomplete; vague; inadequate.—**sketchi** y adv.—**sketchiness** n.

skew /skjuː/ adj slanting oblique, set at an angle. • adv at a slant. • vti to slant or set at a slant; to swerve.

skewbald /'skjuːbɒld/ adj marked with patches of white and another colour except black. • n an animal, esp a horse, with such markings.

skewer /'skjuːər/ n a long wooden or metal pin on which pieces of meat and vegetables are cooked. • vt to pierce and fasten on a skewer; to transfix.

skewwhiff /skjuːwɪf/ adj (inf) askew, not straight.

ski /skiː/ n (pl **skis**) a long narrow runner of wood, metal or plastic that is fastened to a boot for moving across snow; a water-ski. • vi (**skiing, skied**) to travel on skis.—**skier** n.

skibob /-bɒb/ n a snow vehicle similar to a bicycle with a low seat and steering handle mounted on two skis instead of wheels.

skid /skɪd/ vti (**skidding, skidded**) to slide without rotating; to slip sideways; (vehicle) to slide sideways out of control; to cause (a vehicle) to skid. • n the act of skidding; a drag to reduce speed; a ship's fender; a movable support for a heavy object; a runner on an aircraft's landing gear.

Ski-Doo /skɪ'duː/ n ♣ (Cdn) (trademark) a snowmobile.

skid row, skid road n (sl) a shabby district where vagrants, etc, live.

skied /skiːd/ see **ski**.

skiff /skɪf/ n a small light boat for rowing.

skiffle /'skɪfəl/ n a type of music using guitars and makeshift instruments (eg washboards) which became popular in the 1950s.

ski jump n a long ramp surmounting a slope from which skiers jump in competition.—**ski-jump** vi.

skilful, skillful /'skɪlfʊl/ adj having skill; proficient, adroit.—**skilfully, skillfully** adv.—**skilfulness, skillfulness** n.

ski lift n any of various devices for conveying skiers up a slope, such as a chair lift.

skill /skɪl/ n proficiency; expertness, dexterity; a developed aptitude or ability; a type of work or craft requiring specialist training.

skilled /skɪld/ adj fully trained, expert.

skillet /'skɪlət/ n a frying pan.

skim /skɪm/ vti (**skimming, skimmed**) to remove (cream, scum) from the surface of; to glide lightly over, to brush the surface of; to read superficially.

skimmer /'skɪmər/ n that which skims, esp a perforated utensil for skimming milk.

skimmia /'skɪmiə/ n any of a genus of evergreen shrubs with red berries.

skim milk, skimmed milk n milk from which the cream has been removed.

skimp /skɪmp/ vti to give scant measure (of), to stint; to be sparing or frugal (with).

skimpy /'skɪmpi/ adj (**skimpier, skimpiest**) small in size; inadequate, scant, meagre.—**skimpily** adv.—**skimpiness** n.

skin /skɪn/ n the tissue forming the outer covering of the body; a hide; the rind of a fruit; an outer layer or casing; a film on the surface of a liquid; a vessel for water, etc, made of hide. • vti (**skinning, skinned**) to remove the skin from, to peel; to injure by scraping (the knee, etc); to cover or become covered with skin; (inf) to swindle.

skin-deep *adj* superficial.

skin diving *n* the sport of swimming underwater with scuba equipment.—**skin-diver** *n*.

skinflint /-flɪnt/ *n* a stingy person.

skinful /-fʊl/ *n* (*pl* **skinfuls**) (*sl*) as much alcoholic drink as one can take.

skin graft *n* a piece of skin taken from one part of the body to replace damaged skin elsewhere.

skinhead /-hed/ *n* a British youth with cropped hair, large boots and braces, often belonging to an aggressive gang.

skink /skɪŋk/ *n* a small lizard of tropical Asia and Africa.

skinned /'skɪnd/ *adj* having skin of a specified kind.

skinny /'skɪni/ *adj* (**skinnier, skinniest**) very thin; emaciated.—**skinniness** *n*.

skint /skɪnt/ *adj* (*sl*) having no money.

skintight /'skɪn,taɪt/ *adj* (*clothing*) fitting tightly; clinging.

skip[1] /skɪp/ *vti* (**skipping, skipped**) to leap or hop lightly over; to keep jumping over a rope as it is swung under one; to make omissions, to pass over, *esp* in reading; (*inf*) to leave (town) hurriedly, to make off; (*inf*) to miss deliberately. • *n* a skipping movement; a light jump.

skip[2] *n* a large metal container for holding building debris; a cage or bucket for hoisting workers or materials in a mine, quarry, etc.

ski pants *npl* fashion trousers worn tight with a strap that fits under the foot.

skipjack /'skɪpdʒæk/ *n* (*pl* **skipjack, skipjacks**) any of various food fishes including two varieties of tuna, one striped (skipjack) and the other spotted (black skipjack).

skiplane /'ski:,pleɪn/ *n* a light aircraft fitted with skis for taking off and landing on snow.

ski pole *n* one of a pair of pointed metal sticks used by skiers to provide forward thrust and to aid stability.—*also* **ski stick**.

skipper /'skɪpər/ *n* the captain of a boat, aircraft, or team. • *vt* to act as skipper; to captain.

skipping rope *n* a light rope, *usu* with a handle at each end, that is swung over the head and under the feet while jumping.

skirl /skərl/ *n* (*Scot*) the shrill wailing sound characteristic of bagpipes.—*also vi*.

skirmish /'skərmɪʃ/ *n* a minor fight in a war; a conflict or clash. • *vi* to take part in a skirmish.

skirt /skərt/ *n* a woman's garment that hangs from the waist; the lower part of a dress or coat; an outer edge, a border; (*sl*) a woman. • *vti* to border; to move along the edge (of); to evade.

skirting /'skərtɪŋ/ *n* a border, an edging; fabric for skirts.

skirting board *n* a narrow panel of wood at the foot of an interior wall.

ski stick *see ski pole*.

skit /skɪt/ *n* a short humorous sketch, as in the theatre.

ski tow *n* a motor-driven device that pulls skiers uphill.

skitter /'skɪtər/ *vti* to move or cause to move quickly or to skim across a surface.

skittish /'skɪtɪʃ/ *adj* (*animal*) frisky, easily frightened; (*person*) playful, frivolous, lively.—**skittishly** *adv*.—**skittishness** *n*.

skittles /'skɪtəls/ *n* a game in which a wooden or plastic bottle-shaped pin is knocked down by a ball.—*also* **ninepins**.

skive /skaɪv/ *vi* (*inf*) to avoid work or duties because of laziness.

skivvy /'skɪvi/ *n* (*pl* **skivvies**) a female domestic servant. • *vi* (**skivvying, skivvied**) to perform menial domestic duties.

skol, skoal /skɒl/ or /skoːl/ *interj* good health, cheers (*used in a toast*).

skookum /'sku:kəm/ *adj* ♣ in the Pacific Northwest of North America, strong or brave.

skua /'skju:ə/ *n* any of various large predatory seabirds with dark plumage.

skulduggery, skullduggery /skʌl'dʌgəri/ *n* (*inf*) deceit, underhand dealing.

skulk /skʌlk/ *vi* to move in a stealthy manner; to lurk.

skull /skʌl/ *n* the bony casing enclosing the brain; the cranium.

skull and crossbones *n* (*pl* **skulls and crossbones**) an image of a human skull and crossed thighbones used as a warning of danger.

skunk /skʌŋk/ *n* a small black-and-white mammal that emits a foul-smelling liquid when frightened; its fur; (*sl*) an obnoxious or mean person.

skunky /'skʌŋki/ *adj* ♣ (*Cdn*) tasting foul, *esp* in beer that has been exposed to air too long.

sky /skaɪ/ *n* (*pl* **skies**) the apparent vault over the earth; heaven; the upper atmosphere; weather, climate.

sky-blue *adj, n* (of) a bright pure blue, azure.

sky-diving /'skaɪ,daɪvɪŋ/ *n* the sport of parachute jumping involving free-fall manoeuvres.—**sky-diver** *n*.

Skye terrier /skaɪ/ *n* a breed of short-legged terrier with long hair and a long body.

sky-high /'skaɪ'haɪ/ *adj, adv* very high; in an enthusiastic manner; extremely expensive.

skyjack /-dʒæk/ *vt* to hijack an aircraft.

skylark /-lɑrk/ *n* a lark famous for its song as it soars.

skylight /-laɪt/ *n* a window in the roof or ceiling.

skyline /-laɪn/ *n* the visible horizon; the outline, as of mountains, buildings, etc, seen against the sky.

skyrocket /-rɒkət/ *n* a rocket. • *vi* to rise rapidly (*eg* in price, status, etc).

skyscraper /-,skreɪpər/ *n* a very tall building.

skyward /-wərd/ *adj, adv* toward the sky.—**skywards** *adv*.

skywriting /-,raɪtɪŋ/ *n* (the act of creating) writing in the sky formed by smoke or vapour emitted from an aircraft.

slab /slæb/ *n* a flat, broad, thick piece (as of stone, wood, or bread, etc); something resembling this. • *vt* to cut or form into slabs; to cover or support with slabs; to put on thickly.

slack /slæk/ *adj* loose, relaxed, not tight; (*business*) slow, not brisk; sluggish; inattentive, careless. • *n* the part (of a rope, etc) that hangs loose; a dull period; a lull; (*pl*) trousers for casual wear. • *vti* to neglect (one's work, etc), to be lazy; (*with off*) to slacken (a rope, etc).—**slackness** *n*.

slacken /'slækən/ *vti* to make or become less active, brisk, etc; to loosen or relax, as a rope; to diminish, to abate.—**slackening** *n, adj*.

slacker /'slækər/ *n* a lazy person; a person who shirks.

slack water *n* the turn of the tide; a slow-moving stretch of water.

slag /slæg/ *n* the waste product from the smelting of metals; volcanic lava.

slain /sleɪn/ *see* **slay**.

slake /sleɪk/ *vt* to quench or satisfy (thirst, etc); to mix (lime) with water.

slalom /'slɒləm/ *n* downhill skiing in a zigzag course between upright markers; (*skiing, canoeing, etc*) a timed race over a slalom course. • *vi* to move over a zigzag course.

slam /slæm/ *vti* (**slamming, slammed**) to shut with a loud noise, to bang; to throw (down) violently; (*inf*) to criticize severely. • *n* a sound or the act of slamming, a bang; (*inf*) severe criticism; (*bridge*) the taking of 12 or 13 tricks.

slammer /'slæmər/ *n* (*sl*) a prison or jail.

slander /'slændər/ *n* a false and malicious statement about another; the uttering of this. • *vt* to utter a slander about, to defame.—**slanderous** *adj*.

slang /slæŋ/ *n* words or expressions used in familiar speech but not regarded as standard English; jargon of a particular social class, age group, etc. • *adj* relating to slang.

slant /slænt/ *vti* to incline, to slope; to tell in such a way as to have a bias. • *n* a slope; an oblique position; a bias, a point of view. • *adj* sloping.—**slantly** *adv*.

slanted /'slæntɪŋ/ *adj* prejudiced, biased; sloping.

slantwise /-waɪz/ *adv* at a slant.

slap /slæp/ *n* a smack with the open hand; an insult; a rebuff. • *vt* (**slapping, slapped**) to strike with something flat; to put, hit, etc, with force. • *adv* directly, full.

slapdash /'slæpdæʃ/ *adj* impetuous; hurried; careless; haphazard. • *adv* carelessly.

slaphappy *adj* (**slaphappier, slaphappiest**) casually or cheerfully irresponsible; giddy, punch-drunk.

slapstick /-stɪk/ *n* boisterous humour of a knockabout kind.

slap-up *adj* (*inf*) (*meals, entertainment*) lavish, luxury.

slash /slæʃ/ *vti* to cut gashes in, to slit; to strike fiercely (at) with a sword, etc; to reduce (prices) sharply. • *n* a cutting blow; a long slit, a gash.

slat /slæt/ *n* a thin, flat, narrow strip of wood, etc.

slate[1] /sleɪt/ *vt* to criticize or punish severely.

slate[2] *n* a fine-grained rock easily split into thin layers; a flat plate of this or other material used in roofing; a tablet (as of slate) for writing on; a list of proposed candidates. • *adj* the colour of slate, a deep bluish-grey colour; made of slate. • *vt* to cover with slates; to suggest as a political candidate.

slater /'sleɪtər/ *n* a person trained in roofing with slates; a wood louse.

slatted /'slætəd/ *adj* having slats.

slattern /'slætərn/ *n* a slovenly woman; a slut.

slaughter /'slɒtər/ n the butchering of animals for food; a whole-sale killing, a massacre.—*also vt.*—**slaughterer** n.

slaughterhouse /-ˌhaʊs/ n a place where animals are slaugh-tered, an abattoir.

Slav /slæv/ n any person who speaks a Slavonic language.

slave /sleɪv/ n a person without freedom or personal rights, who is legally owned by another; a person under domination, *esp* of a habit or vice; a person who works like a slave, a drudge. • *vti* to toil hard, as a slave.

slave driver n a supervisor of slaves at work; a hard taskmaster.

slaveholder /'sleɪvˌhoʊldər/ n a person who owns slaves.

slaver[1] /'sleɪvər/ n a person engaged in the buying and selling of slaves.

slaver[2] /'slævər/ *vti* to dribble, to cover with saliva; to fawn upon, to flatter.

slavery /'sleɪvəri/ n the condition of being a slave; bondage; drudgery; slave-owning as an institution.

slave ship n a ship used in the slave trade.

Slave State n (*hist*) any of the Southern states of the US where slavery was legal until the Civil War.

slave trade n commercial traffic in slaves, *esp* the transport of Black Africans to Europe and America in the 16th to 19th centuries.

Slavic /'slævɪk/ *see* **Slavonic**.

slavish /'sleɪvɪʃ/ *adj* servile; abject; unoriginal.—**slavishly** *adv.*—**slavishness** n.

Slavonic /slə'vɒnɪk/, **Slavic** *adj* of or characteristic of the Slavs. • n a branch of the Indo-European family of languages, includ-ing Russian, Bulgarian, Polish and Czech.

slaw /slɔ/ n coleslaw.

slay /sleɪ/ *vti* (**slaying, slew**, *pp* **slain**) to kill in great numbers; to murder; (*sl*) to overwhelm, to affect in a powerful way.—**slayer** n.

sleaze /sli:z/ n (*inf*) sleaziness.

sleazy /'sli:zi/ *adj* (**sleazier, sleaziest**) disreputable, squalid.—**sleaziness** n.

sled /sled/, **sledge** /sledʒ/ n a framework on runners for travel-ling over snow or ice; a toboggan; a sleigh. • *vti* to go or convey by sledge.

sledgehammer /'sledʒˌhæmər/ n a large, heavy hammer for two hands.

sleek /sli:k/ *adj* smooth, glossy; having a prosperous or well-groomed appearance; plausible.

sleep /sli:p/ n a natural, regularly recurring rest for the body, with little or no consciousness; a period spent sleeping; a state of numbness followed by tingling. • *vti* (**sleeping, slept**) to rest in a state of sleep; to be inactive; to provide beds for; (*with* **around**) (*inf*) to be sexually promiscuous; (*with* **in**) to sleep on the premises; to sleep too long in the morning; (*with* **on**) to have a night's rest before making a decision; (*with* **off**) to get rid of by sleeping; (*with* **over**) to pass the night in someone else's house; (*with* **with**) to have sexual relations with.

sleeper /'sli:pər/ n a person or thing that sleeps; a horizontal beam that carries and spreads a weight; a sleeping car; some-thing that suddenly attains prominence or value.

sleeping bag n a padded bag for sleeping in, *esp* outdoors.

sleeping car n a railway carriage with berths.

sleeping partner n a partner in a business who takes no part in its management.

sleeping pill n a pill that induces sleep.

sleeping platform n ✤ a bench or ledge for sleeping inside an igloo.

sleeping sickness n a serious infectious disease marked by lethargy, coma.

sleepless /'sli:pləs/ *adj* without sleep; unable to sleep.

sleepwalker /-ˌwɔkər/ n a person who walks while asleep, a som-nambulist.—**sleepwalking** n.

sleepy /'sli:pi/ *adj* (**sleepier, sleepiest**) drowsy; tired; lazy, not alert.—**sleepily** *adv.*—**sleepiness** n.

sleepyhead /-ˌhed/ n a tired or lazy person.

sleet /sli:t/ n snow or hail mixed with rain. • *vi* to rain in the form of sleet.

sleeve /sli:v/ n the part of a garment enclosing the arm; (*mech*) a tube that fits over a part; an open-ended cover, *esp* a paper-board envelope for a record.

sleeveless /'sli:vlɪs/ *adj* (*garment*) without sleeves.

sleigh /sleɪ/ n a light vehicle on runners for travelling over snow; a sledge.

sleight of hand n manual dexterity, such as in conjuring or jug-gling; a deception.

slender /'slendər/ *adj* thin; slim; slight; scanty.—**slenderly** *adv.*—**slenderness** n

slept /slept/ *see* **sleep**.

sleuth /slu:θ/ n (*inf*) a detective.

sleuthhound n a bloodhound; (*inf*) a detective.

slew[1] /slu:/ *see* **slay**.

slew[2], **slue** *vti* to twist or be twisted sideways.

slew[3], **slue** n (*inf*) a great quantity.

slice /slaɪs/ n a thin flat piece cut from something (as bread, etc); a wedge-shaped piece (of cake, pie, etc); a portion, a share; a broad knife for serving fish, cheese, etc; (*golf*) a stroke that makes the ball curl to the right. • *vti* to divide into parts; to cut into slices; to strike (a ball) so that it curves.—**slicer** n.—**slic-ing** *adj, n*.

slick /slɪk/ *adj* clever, deft; smart but unsound; insincere; wily; (*inf*) smooth but superficial, tricky, etc. • n a patch or area of oil floating on water. • *vt* to make glossy; (*with* **up**) (*inf*) to make smart, neat, etc.

slicker /'slɪkər/ n a loose waterproof coat.

slide /slaɪd/ *vti* (**sliding, slid**) to move along in constant contact with a smooth surface, as on ice, to glide; to coast over snow and ice; to pass gradually (into); to move (an object) unobtru-sively. • n the act of sliding, a glide; a strip of smooth ice for sliding on; a chute; the glass plate of a microscope; a photo-graphic transparency; a landslide.

slide rule n a ruler with a graduated sliding part for making cal-culations.

sliding scale /'slaɪdɪŋ/ n a schedule for automatically varying one thing (*eg* wages) according to the fluctuations of another thing (*eg* cost of living); a flexible scale.

Slier /slaɪər/, **sliest** /-əst/ *see* **sly**.

slight /slaɪt/ *adj* small; inconsiderable; trifling; slim; frail, flimsy. • *vt* to disregard as insignificant; to treat with disrespect, to snub. • n intentional indifference or neglect, discourtesy.

slighting /'slaɪtɪŋ/ *adj* disparaging; hurtful.

slightly /-li/ *adv* to a small degree; slenderly.

slightness /-nəs/ n frailness or slenderness; lack of weight, solid-ity, importance, or thoroughness.

slim[1] /slɪm/ *adj* slender, not stout; small in amount, degree, etc; slight. • *vti* (**slimming, slimmed**) to make or become slim; to reduce one's weight by diet, etc.—**slimness** n.

slim[2] n the name used in Africa for AIDS.

slime /slaɪm/ n a sticky slippery, half-liquid substance; a gluti-nous mud; mucus secreted by various animals (*eg* slugs).

slimmer /'slɪmər/ n a person who controls their diet to lose weight.

slimming /-ɪŋ/ n the process of losing weight by dieting.

slimy /'slaɪmi/ *adj* (**slimier, slimiest**) like or covered with slime; repulsive; fawning.—**sliminess** n.

sling[1] /slɪŋ/ n a loop of leather with a string attached for hurling stones; a rope for lifting or hoisting weights; a bandage sus-pended from the neck for supporting an injured arm. • *vt* (**sling-ing, slung**) to throw, lift, or suspend (as) with a sling; to hurl.

sling[2] n a drink of sweetened water mixed with a spirit such as gin.

slingback /'slɪŋbæk/ n a shoe whose back consists of a strap.

slingshot /'slɪŋʃɒt/ n a contraption with elastic for shooting small stones, a catapult.

slink /slɪŋk/ *vi* (**slinking, slinked** *or* **slunk**) to move stealthily or furtively, to sneak.

slinky /'slɪŋki/ *adj* (**slinkier, slinkiest**) (*inf*) sinuous in line or movement; (*clothes*) hugging the figure.

slip[1] /slɪp/ *vti* (**slipping, slipped**) to slide, to glide; to lose one's foothold and slide; to go or put quietly or quickly; to let go, to release; to escape from; (*with* **up**) to make a slight mistake. • n the act of slipping; a mistake, a lapse; a woman's undergar-ment; a pillowcase; a slipway.

slip[2] n a small piece of paper; a young, slim person; a long seat or narrow pew; a shoot for grafting, a cutting; a descendant, an offspring.

slip[3] n a mixture of watery clay used for coating or decorating pot-tery.

slipcase /'slɪpkeɪs/ n a protective case for one or more books with an open end to reveal the spines.

slipknot /-nɒt/ n a knot that slips along the rope around which it is tied; a knot that can be undone at a pull.

slip-on /-ˌɒn/ *adj* (*garment or shoe*) easy to put on or take off.—*also n.*

slippage /ˈslɪpədʒ/ *n* a slipping, as of one gear past another.

slipped disc *n* a ruptured cartilaginous disc between vertebrae.

slipper /ˈslɪpər/ *n* a light, soft, shoe worn in the house.

slippery /-i/ or /-pri/ *adj* so smooth as to cause slipping; difficult to hold or catch; evasive, unreliable, shifty.

slippy /ˈslɪpi/ *adj* (**slippier, slippiest**) slippery.

slip road *n* a road that gives access to a main road or motorway.

slipshod /ˈslɪpʃɒd/ *adj* having the shoes down at heel; slovenly, careless.

slip stitch /-stɪtʃ/ *n* a concealed stitch used for hemming; an unworked stitch in knitting.—**slipstitch** *vt.*

slipstream /-striːm/ *n* a stream of air driven astern by the engine of an aircraft; an area of forward suction immediately behind a rapidly moving racing car.

slip-up /-ʌp/ *n* (*inf*) an error, a lapse.

slipway /-weɪ/ *n* an inclined surface for launching or repairing ships; a sloped landing stage.

slit /slɪt/ *vt* (**slitting, slit**) to cut open or tear lengthways; to slash or tear into strips. • *n* a long cut, a slash; a narrow opening.—**slitter** *n.*

slither /ˈslɪðər/ *vi* to slide, as on a loose or wet surface; to slip or slide like a snake.—**slithery** *adj.*

slit trench *n* a narrow trench to provide shelter during battle.

sliver /ˈslɪvər/ *n* a small narrow piece torn off, a splinter; a thin slice.

slivovitz, slivowitz /ˈslɪvəvɪts/ *n* plum brandy.

slob /slɒb/ *n* (*sl*) a coarse or sloppy person.

slobber /ˈslɒbər/ *vti* to drool; to run at the mouth; to smear with dribbling saliva or food. • *n* dribbling saliva; maudlin talk.

slob ice *n* ✦ (*Cdn*) a sludgy mass of densely packed sea ice.

sloe /sloː/ *n* (the dark fruit of the) blackthorn.

sloe-eyed /ˈsloːˌaɪd/ *adj* having almond-shaped dark or black eyes.

sloe gin /-ˌdʒɪn/ *n* a gin flavoured with sloes.

slog /slɒg/ *vti* (**slogging, slogged**) to hit hard and wildly; to work laboriously; to trudge doggedly. • *n* a hard, boring spell of work; a strenuous walk or hike; a hard, random hit.—**slogger** *n.*

slogan /ˈsloːgən/ *n* a catchy phrase used in advertising or as a motto by a political party, etc.

sloop /sluːp/ *n* a small sailing vessel with one mast and a jib.

slop /slɒp/ *n* a puddle of spilled liquid; unappetizing semi-liquid food; (*pl*) liquid kitchen refuse. • *vti* (**slopping, slopped**) to spill or be spilled; (*with* **out**) (*prisoners*) to empty slop from chamber pots in the morning.

slope /sloːp/ *n* rising or falling ground; an inclined line or surface; the amount or degree of this. • *vti* to incline, to slant; (*inf*) to make off, to go.

sloppy /ˈslɒpi/ *adj* (**sloppier, sloppiest**) slushy; (*inf*) maudlin, sentimental; (*inf*) careless, untidy.—**sloppily** *adv.*—**sloppiness** *n.*

slosh /slɒʃ/ *n* watery snow, slush; (*inf*) a heavy blow; the sound of liquid splashing. • *vi* to walk (through) or splash (around) in liquid, mud, etc; (*of liquid*) to splash. • *vt* to throw or splash liquid, etc at someone or something; (*inf*) to hit somebody.

sloshed /slɒʃd/ *adj* (*inf*) drunk.

slot /slɒt/ *n* a long narrow opening in a mechanism for inserting a coin, a slit. • *vt* (**slotting, slotted**) to fit into a slot; to provide with a slot; (*inf*) to place in a series.

sloth /slɒθ/ *n* laziness, indolence; a slow-moving South American animal.—**slothful** *adj.*

slot machine *n* a machine operated by the insertion of a coin, used for gambling or dispensing drinks, etc.

slouch /slaʊtʃ/ *vti* to sit, stand or move in a drooping, slovenly way. • *n* a drooping slovenly posture or gait; the downward droop of a hat brim; (*inf*) a poor performer, a lazy or incompetent person.

slouch hat *n* a hat with a soft wide brim that can be pulled down to cover the ears.

slough[1] /slaʊ/ *n* a bog; deep, hopeless dejection.

slough[2] *n* the dead, outer skin of a snake. • *vti* to cast off, as a dead skin.

Slovak /ˈsloːvæk/ *n* a native or inhabitant of Slovakia in Czechoslovakia; the language of Slovakia.—*also adj.*

Slovene /ˌsləˈviːn/ *n* a native or inhabitant of Slovenia, formerly part of Yugoslavia; the Slavonic language of Slovenia.—*also adj.*

slovenly /ˌslʌvənli/ or /ˈslʌv-/ *adj* untidy, dirty; careless.—**slovenliness** *n.*

slow /sloː/ *adj* moving at low speed, not fast; gradual; not quick in understanding; reluctant, backward; dull, sluggish; not progressive; (*clock*) behind in time; tedious, boring; (*surface*) causing slowness. • *vti* (*also with* **up, down**) to reduce the speed (of).—**slowly** *adv.*—**slowness** *n.*

slowcoach /ˈsloːkoːtʃ/ *n* (*inf*) a person who moves, works or thinks slowly.

slow handclap *n* slow regular clapping expressive of audience dissatisfaction.

slow match, slow fuse *n* a slow-burning match or fuse for igniting explosives.

slow-motion /-ˈmoːʃən/ *adj* moving slowly; denoting a filmed or taped scene with the original action slowed down.

slowpoke /-poːk/ *see* **slowcoach**.

slowworm /-wɔːm/ *n* a legless European lizard with a greyish elongated body and very small eyes.

SLR *abbr* = single-lens reflex.

slub /slʌb/ *n* a lump in a piece of yarn or thread.

sludge /slʌdʒ/ *n* soft mud or snow; sediment; sewage.

slue /sluː/ *see* **slew**[2].

slug[1] /slʌg/ *n* a mollusc resembling a snail but with no outer shell.

slug[2] *n* a small bullet; a disc for inserting into a slot machine; a line of type; (*inf*) a hard blow; a drink of spirits. • *vt* (**slugging, slugged**) (*inf*) to hit hard with a fist or a bat.

sluggard /ˈslʌgərd/ *n* a lazy person. • *adj* lazy.

sluggish /ˈslʌgɪʃ/ *adj* slow, inactive; unresponsive.—**sluggishly** *adv.*—**sluggishness** *n.*

sluice /sluːs/ *n* a gate regulating a flow of water; the water passing through this; an artificial water channel. • *vti* to draw off through a sluice; to wash with a stream of water; to stream out as from a sluice.

slum /slʌm/ *n* a squalid, rundown house; (*usu pl*) an overcrowded area characterized by poverty, etc. • *vi* (**slumming, slummed**) to make do with less comfort.

slumber /ˈslʌmbər/ *vi* to sleep. • *n* a light sleep.

slump /slʌmp/ *n* a sudden fall in value or slackening in demand; (*sport*) a period of poor play. • *vi* to fall or decline suddenly; to sink down heavily; to collapse; to slouch.

slung /slʌŋ/ *see* **sling**.

slunk /slʌŋk/ *see* **slink**.

slur /slɜr/ *vti* (**slurring, slurred**) to pronounce or speak indistinctly; (*letters, words*) to run together; (*mus*) to produce by gliding without a break; to make disparaging remarks. • *n* the act of slurring; a stigma, an imputation of disgrace; (*mus*) a curved line over notes to be slurred.

slurp /slɜrp/ *vti* (*sl*) to drink or eat noisily. • *n* a loud sipping or sucking sound.

slurry /ˈslɜri/ *n* (*pl* **slurries**) a liquid mixture of insoluble matter (as mud, lime, etc).

slush /slʌʃ/ *n* liquid mud; melting snow; (*inf*) sentimental language.—**slushy** *adj.*

slush fund *n* a fund of money used secretly to bribe, etc.

slut /slʌt/ *n* a slovenly or immoral woman.—**sluttish** *adj.*

sly /slaɪ/ *adj* (**slyer, slyest** *or* **slier, sliest**) secretively cunning, wily; underhand; knowing.—**slyly** *adv.*—**slyness** *n.*

SM *abbr* = master of science; sergeant major.

Sm (*chem symbol*) samarium.

S/M, S-M *abbr* = sadomasochism.

smack[1] /smæk/ *n* a taste; a distinctive smell or flavour; small quantity, a trace. • *vi* to have a smell or taste (of); to have a slight trace of something.

smack[2] *vt* to strike or slap with the open hand; to kiss noisily; to make a sharp noise with the lips.—*also n.*

smack[3] *n* a small fishing vessel used in coastal waters.

smacker /ˈsmækər/ *n* (*sl*) a noisy kiss; (*sl*) a pound note or dollar bill.

small /smɒl/ *adj* little in size, number, importance, etc; small, humble; operating on a minor scale; young; petty. • *adv* in small pieces. • *n* the narrow, curving part of the back.

small arms *npl* portable firearms, such as handguns.

small beer *n* (*inf*) people or things regarded as trivial.

small change *n* coins of low value.

small fry *npl* people or things of little significance.

smallholding /ˈsmɒlˌhoːldɪŋ/ *n* in UK, a small piece of agricultural land, *usu* between one and fifty acres.—**smallholder** *n.*

small hours *npl* the period between midnight and dawn.

small intestine *n* the section of the alimentary canal between the stomach and the colon.

small-minded /-ˌmaɪndɪd/ *adj* intolerant, narrow-minded; mean, vindictive.—**small-mindedly** *adv.*—**small-mindedness** *n*.

smallpox /-pɒks/ *n* an acute contagious viral disease, now rare, causing the eruption of pustules which leave the skin scarred and pitted.

small print *n* small type that is difficult to read in a contract or other document, *esp* conditions and limitations made deliberately inconspicuous.

small-scale /-skeɪl/ *adj* small in size or scope.

small screen *n* a television.

small talk *n* light, social conversation.

small-time /-taɪm/ *adj* (*inf*) unimportant.

smalt /smɒlt/ *n* a blue pigment used in colouring glass and ceramics.

smarmy /'smɑrmi/ *adj* (**smarmier, smarmiest**) (*inf*) obsequious, unpleasantly smooth and flattering.

smart /smɑrt/ *n* a sudden, stinging pain. • *vi* to have or cause a sharp, stinging pain (as by a slap); to feel distress. • *adj* stinging; astute; clever, witty; fashionable; neatly dressed; (*equipment, etc*) capable of seemingly intelligent action through computer control; (*bombs, missiles*) guided to the target by lasers ensuring pinpoint accuracy.—**smartly** *adv.*—**smartness** *n*.

smart aleck /'smɑrtˌælək/ *n* (*inf*) an annoyingly clever person, a know-all.

smart card *n* a credit card containing a memory chip that records transactions made with the card.

smarten /'smɑrtən/ *vti* to make or become smart.

smart money *n* money invested or bet by experienced gamblers or financiers; money paid to secure release from an unpleasant situation, or obligation, *esp* military service.

smart set *n sing* or *pl* fashionable people or society.

smash /smæʃ/ *vti* to break into pieces with noise or violence; to hit, collide, or move with force; to destroy or be destroyed. • *n* a hard, heavy hit; a violent, noisy breaking; a violent collision; total failure, *esp* in business; (*inf*) a popular success.

smashed /smæʃd/ *adj* (*sl*) drunk or under the influence of drugs.

smasher /'smæʃər/ *n* (*inf*) an attractive or excellent person or thing.

smashing /-ɪŋ/ *n* (*inf*) excellent.

smash-up /-ʌp/ *n* (*inf*) a serious collision, a crash.

smattering /'smætərɪŋ/ *n* a slight superficial knowledge; a small number.

smear /smɪr/ *vt* to cover with anything greasy or sticky to make a smudge; to slander. • *n* a smudge; a slanderous attack; a deposit of blood, secretion, etc on a glass slide for examination under a microscope.

smear test *n* microscopic analysis of a smear of bodily cells, *esp* from the cervix, for cancer.

smegma /'smegmə/ *n* a sebaceous secretion which accumulates as solid matter in the folds of the skin, *esp* under the foreskin.

smell /smel/ *n* the sense by which odours are perceived with the nose; a scent, odour, or stench; a trace. • *vti* (**smelling, smelt** *or* **smelled**) to have or perceive an odour.—**smelly** *adj*.

smelling salts *npl* a preparation of ammonia used as a stimulant in cases of faintness, etc.

smelt[1] /smelt/ *vt* to extract ore from metal by melting.

smelt[2] *n* any of various small marine or freshwater food fishes related to the salmon.

smelt[3] *see* smell.

smidgen, smidgin /'smɪdʒən/ *n* (*inf*) a small amount.

smilax /'smaɪlæks/ *n* any of a genus of climbing plants bearing red berries that includes the sarsaparilla; an African vine cultivated for its decorative green leaves.

smile /smaɪl/ *vti* to express amusement, friendship, pleasure, etc, by a slight turning up of the corners of the mouth. • *n* the act of smiling; a bright aspect.—**smilingly** *adv*.

smirch /smɜrtʃ/ *vt* to dishonour; to soil, stain, or sully. • *n* a stain on reputation; a smudge, smear.

smirk /smɜrk/ *vi* to smile in an expression of smugness or scorn. • *n* a smug or scornful smile.—**smirkingly** *adv*.

smite /smaɪt/ *vb* (**smiting, smote,** *pp* **smitten** *or* **smote**) *vt* (*arch*) to strike hard; to kill or injure; to have a powerful affect on. • *vi* to strike, beat or come down (on) with force.—**smiter** *n*.

smith /'smɪθ/ *n* a person who works in metal; a blacksmith.

smithereens /smɪðə'riːnz/ *npl* (*inf*) fragments.

smithery /'smɪθəri/ *n* the trade of a blacksmith.

smithy /'smɪθi/ or /'smɪði/ *n* (*pl* **smithies**) a blacksmith's workshop.

smitten /'smɪtən/ *see* smite.

smock /smɒk/ *n* a loose shirtlike outer garment to protect the clothes.

smocking /'smɒkɪŋ/ *n* ornamental stitching in a honeycomb pattern.

smog /smɒg/ *n* a mixture of fog and smoke; polluted air.—**smoggy** *adj*.

smoke /smoːk/ *n* a cloud or plume of gas and small particles emitted from a burning substance; any similar vapour; an act of smoking tobacco, etc; (*inf*) a cigar or cigarette. • *vi* to give off smoke; to (habitually) draw in and exhale the smoke of tobacco, etc. • *vt* to fumigate; to cure food by treating with smoke; to darken (*eg* glass) using smoke; (*with* **out**) to flush out using smoke; to bring into public view.—**smokable, smokeable** *adj*.

smoke and mirrors *n pʰr* a presentation, demonstration or explanation seen to be unclear and deceptive, involving an intent to confuse.

smoke detector *n* an electrical device that sets off an alarm when smoke is detected.

smokeless /'smoːkləs/ *adj* giving off little or no smoke.

smoker /-ər/ *n* a person who habitually smokes tobacco; a smoking car; (*formerly*) a gathering of men to smoke.

smoke screen /-skriːn/ *n* dense smoke used to conceal military movements, etc; something designed to obscure, conceal, or disguise the truth.

smokestack /-stæk/ *n* a tall chimney or funnel which discharges smoke or exhaust gases into the air.

smoking car *n* a train compartment where smoking is permitted.

smoky /'smoːki/ *adj* (**smokier, smokiest**) emitting smoke, *esp* excessively; filled with smoke; resembling smoke in appearance, flavour, smell, colour, etc.—**smokily** *adv.*—**smokiness** *n*.

smoky quartz *n* cairngorm.

smolder /'smoːldər/ *see* smoulder.

smolt /smoːlt/ *n* a young salmon, about two years old, at the stage where it migrates to the sea for the first time.

smooch /smuːtʃ/ *vi* (*sl*) to kiss and cuddle, *esp* while dancing as a couple. • *n* (*sl*) a long kiss, an embrace.—**smoochy** *adj*.

smooth /smuːð/ *adj* having an even or flat surface; silky; not rough or lumpy; hairless; of even consistency; calm, unruffled; gently flowing in rhythm or sound. • *vti* to make smooth; to calm; to make easier.—**smoothly** *adv.*—**smoothness** *n*.

smoothbore /'smuːðbɔr/ *n* (*firearm*) not rifled. • *n* such a gun.

smoothen /'smuːðən/ *vt* to make or become smooth.

smooth-faced /'smuːðˌfeɪst/ *adj* shaven; having a smooth surface; hypocritical.

smoothie /'smuːði/ *n* (*sl*) a person, *esp* a man, who is excessively suave and self-assured in speech and appearance.

smooth muscle *n* a muscle capable of regular involuntary contractions, as in the walls of the stomach and gut.

smooth-tongued /-ˌtʌŋd/ *adj* persuasive in speech.

smoothy /'smuːði/ *n* (*pl* **smoothies**) (*sl*) a smoothie.

smorgasbord, smörgåsbord /'smɔrgəsbɔrd/ *n* a type of buffet or hors d'œuvres of various cold dishes of cheese, fish, salads, etc, served in Scandinavia; a restaurant specializing in this.

smote /smoːt/ *see* smite

smother /'smʌðər/ *vt* to stifle, to suffocate; to put out a fire by covering it to remove the air supply; to cover over thickly; to hold back, suppress. • *vi* to undergo suffocation.—*also n*.

smoulder /'smoːldər/ *vi* to burn slowly or without flame; (*feelings*) to linger on in a suppressed state; to have concealed feelings of anger, jealousy, etc.—*also* **smolder**.

smudge /smʌdʒ/ *n* a dirty or blurred spot or area; a fire made to produce dense smoke. • *vt* to make a smudge; to smear; to blur; to produce smoke to protect against insects, etc. • *vi* to become smudged.

smudgy /'smʌdʒi/ *adj* blurred or dirty, smeared.—**smudgily** *adv.*—**smudginess** *n*.

smug /smʌg/ *adj* (**smugger, smuggest**) complacent, self-satisfied.—**smugly** *adv.*—**smugness** *n*.

smuggle /'smʌgəl/ *vt* to import or export (goods) secretly without paying customs duties; to convey or introduce secretly.—**smuggler** *n*.

smut /smʌt/ *n* a speck or smudge of dirt, soot, etc; indecent talk, writing, or pictures; a fungal disease of crop plants that covers the leaves in sooty spores. • *vti* (**smutting, smutted**) to stain or become stained with smut; (*crops, etc*) to infect or become infected with smut.

smut disease *n* a disease of wheat caused by fungi.

smutty /'smʌti/ *adj* (**smuttier, smuttiest**) soiled with smuts; obscene, filthy.—**smuttily** *adv.*—**smuttiness** *n.*

Sn (*chem symbol*) tin.

snack /snæk/ *n* a light meal between regular meals.

snaffle /'snæfəl/ *n* a jointed bit for a bridle.—*also* **snaffle bit**. • *vt* (*inf*) to snatch or steal for oneself.

snafu /snæ'fuː/ *or* /'snæfuː/ *n* (*sl*) (*situation normal all fucked up*) a state of utter confusion. • *adj* confused, chaotic. • *vt* (**snafuing, snafued**) to cause a state of confusion or chaos.

snag /snæg/ *n* a sharp point or projection; a tear, as in cloth, made by a snag, etc; an unexpected or hidden difficulty. • *vti* (**snagging, snagged**) to tear, etc, on a snag; to clear of snags.

snail /sneɪl/ *n* a mollusc having a wormlike body and a spiral protective shell; a slow-moving or sluggish person or thing.

snail-paced /'sneɪlˌpeɪst/ *adj* moving very slowly.

snail's pace *n* a very slow speed or rate of progress.

snake /sneɪl/ *n* a limbless, scaly reptile with a long, tapering body and with salivary glands often modified to produce venom; a sly, treacherous person. • *vt* to twist along like a snake. • *vi* to crawl silently and stealthily.

snake charmer *n* a person who entertains by appearing to mesmerize venomous snakes by playing music.

snake fence *n* ✿ (*Cdn*) a fence of roughly split logs arranged in a zigzag pattern.

snakeroot /'sneɪkruːt/ *n* any of various North American plants whose roots have been used to treat snakebites.

snakes and ladders *n* a British board game in which counters are moved on a grid of squares, some of which have ladders leading nearer the finish, and others snakes leading back toward the start.

snakeskin /-skɪn/ *n* the skin of a snake as used to make handbags, shoes, etc.

snakestone /-stoːn/ *n* an ammonite twisted like a ram's horn.

snakeweed /-wiːd/ *n* a herb with twisted roots, bistort.

snaky /'sneɪki/ *adj* (**snakier, snakiest**) like or full of snakes; treacherous looking.—**snakily** *adv.*—**snakiness** *n.*

snap /snæp/ *vti* (**snapping, snapped**) to break suddenly; to make or cause to make a sudden, cracking sound; to close, fasten, etc with this sound; (*with* **at**) to bite or grasp suddenly; to speak or utter sharply. • *adj* sudden. • *n* a sharp, cracking sound; a fastener that closes with a snapping sound; a crisp biscuit; a snapshot; a sudden spell of cold weather; (*inf*) vigour, energy.

snapdragon /'snæpˌdrægən/ *n* any of several plants of the figwort family with showy white, red or yellow flowers shaped like small jaws.

snap fastener *n* a press stud.

snapper /-ər/ *n* one who or that which snaps; (*pl* **snapper, snappers**) any of various sea fishes used as food; a snapping turtle.

snapping turtle *n* a large North American turtle with powerful jaws, a snapper.

snappy /'snæpi/ *adj* (**snappier, snappiest**) speaking sharply; brisk; lively; smart, fashionable.—**snappily** *adv.*—**snappiness** *n.*

snapshot /-ʃɒt/ *n* a photograph taken casually with a simple camera.

snare /sneɪr/ *n* a loop of string or wire for trapping birds or animals; something that catches one unawares, a trap; a loop of gut wound with wire stretched around a snare drum that produces a rattling sound. • *vt* to trap using a snare.

snare drum *n* a double-headed drum with snares.

snarl[1] /snɑrl/ *vi* to growl with bared teeth; to speak in a rough, angry manner. • *vt* to express in a snarling manner. • *n* the act of snarling; the sound of this.

snarl[2] *vti* to make or become entangled or complicated. • *n* a tangle; disorder.

snarl-up /'snɑrlʌp/ *n* (*inf*) an instance or state of blockage or disorder, *esp* a traffic jam.

snatch /snætʃ/ *vt* to seize or grasp suddenly; to take as opportunity occurs. • *n* the act of snatching; a brief period; a fragment; (*inf*) a robbery.

snazzy /'snæzi/ *adj* (**snazzier, snazziest**) (*inf*) stylish, fashionable; flashy.

sneak /sniːk/ *vti* (**sneaking, sneaked**, *pp* (*sl*) **snuck**) to move, act, give, put, take, etc, secretly or stealthily. • *n* a person who acts secretly or stealthily; (*inf*) a person who tells or informs on others. • *adj* without warning.

sneaker /'sniːkər/ *n* one who or that which sneaks; a shoe with a cloth upper and soft rubber sole, worn informally.

sneaking /-ɪŋ/ *adj* underhand; secret; (*suspicion, admiration, etc*) felt or thought, but not openly expressed.—**sneakingly** *adv.*

sneaky /'sniːki/ *adj* (**sneakier, sneakiest**) like a sneak; furtive; underhand.—**sneakily** *adv.*—**sneakiness** *n.*

sneer /sniːr/ *vi* to show scorn or contempt by curling up the upper lip. • *n* a derisive look or remark.—**sneerer** *n.*—**sneeringly** *adv.*

sneeze /sniːz/ *vi* to expel air through the nose violently and audibly. • *n* the act of sneezing.—**sneezy** *adj.*

snick /snɪk/ *n* a tiny cut or notch; (*cricket*) a stroke of the edge of the bat. • *vt* to make a tiny cut or notch in something; to hit (a ball) with a snick.

snicker /'snɪkər/ *vi* to laugh furtively and slyly, to snigger; to neigh, to whinny. • *n* a half-suppressed laugh, a giggle.—**snickeringly** *adv.*

snide /snaɪd/ *adj* malicious; superior in attitude; sneering.—**snidely** *adv.*—**snideness** *n.*

sniff /snɪf/ *vti* to inhale through the nose audibly; to smell by sniffing; to scoff; (*with* **at**) to express dislike or contempt for. • *n* the act of sniffing; the sound of this; a smell.—**sniffer** *n.*

sniffer dog *n* a police dog trained to locate hidden drugs or explosives by smell.

sniffle /'snɪfəl/ *vi* to sniff repeatedly. • *n* the act or sound of sniffling.

sniffy /'snɪfi/ *adj* (**sniffier, sniffiest**) (*inf*) disdainful, dismissive.—**sniffily** *adv.*—**sniffiness** *n.*

snifter /'snɪftər/ *n* a glass with a wide body and narrow top to preserve the aroma of brandy or other spirits; (*inf*) a small amount of alcoholic drink.

snigger /'snɪgər/ *vti* to laugh disrespectfully, to snicker.—*also* **n.**

snip /snɪp/ *vti* (**snipping, snipped**) to cut or clip with a single stroke of the scissors, etc. • *n* a small piece cut off; the act or sound of snipping; (*inf*) a bargain; (*inf*) a certainty, cinch.

snipe /snaɪp/ *n* (*pl* **snipes, snipe**) any of various birds with long straight flexible bills. • *vi* to shoot snipe; to shoot at individuals from a hidden position; to make sly criticisms of.—**sniper** *n.*

snippet /'snɪpət/ *n* a scrap of information.

snitch /snɪtʃ/ *vi* (*sl*) to inform, betray. • *vt* (*sl*) to steal, pilfer. • *n* (*sl*) an informer; the nose.—**snitcher** *n.*

snivel /'snɪvəl/ *vi* (**snivelling, snivelled** *or* **sniveling, sniveled**) to whine or whimper; to have a runny nose.—**sniveler, sniveller** *n.*

snob /snɒb/ *n* a person who wishes to be associated with those of a higher social status, whilst acting condescendingly to those whom he or she regards as inferior.

snobbery /'snɒbəri/ *n* (*pl* **snobberies**) snobbish behaviour or attitude; a snobbish act.

snobbish /-ɪʃ/ *adj* pertaining to, characteristic of, or like a snob.—**snobbishly** *adv.*—**snobbishness** *n.*

SNOBOL /'snoːbɒl/ *n* (*comput*) String Orientated Symbolic Language: a programming language used for text (ie strings of characters) retrieval and manipulation.

Sno-cat *n* (*trademark*) a vehicle designed for travelling on snow.

snog /snɒg/ *vi* (**snogging, snogged**) (*Brit sl*) to kiss and cuddle.—*also* n.

snood /snuːd/ *n* a small net or fabric pouch for holding a woman's hair at the back of the head; (*Scot*) a ribbon around the hair formerly worn by unmarried girls.

snook /snuːk/ *n* (*sl*) a gesture of contempt with the thumb to the nose and fingers spread.

snooker /'snʊkər/ *or* /'snuːk-/ *n* a game played on a billiard table with 15 red balls, 6 variously coloured balls, and a white cue ball; a position in the game where a ball lies directly between the cue ball and target ball. • *vt* to place in a snooker; (*inf*) to obstruct, thwart.

snoop /snuːp/ *vi* (*inf*) to pry about in a sneaking way. • *n* an act of snooping; a person who pries into other people's business.—**snooper** *n.*

snooperscope /'snuːpərˌskoːp/ *n* an infrared night-vision device used by the police and military services.

snoot /snuːt/ *n* (*sl*) the nose.

snooty /'snuːti/ *adj* (**snootier, snootiest**) haughty, snobbish.—**snootily** *adv.*—**snootiness** *n.*

snooze /snuːz/ *vi* (*inf*) to sleep lightly. • *n* (*inf*) a nap.

snore /snɔr/ *vi* to breathe roughly and noisily while asleep. • *n* the act or sound of snoring.

snorkel /'snɔrkəl/ *n* a breathing tube extending above the water, used in swimming just below the surface. • *vi* (**snorkelling, snorkelled** *or* **snorkeling, snorkeled**) to swim using a snorkel.—**snorkeler** *n.*

snort /snɔːt/ *vi* to exhale noisily through the nostrils, *esp* as an expression of contempt or scorn. • *vt* to inhale (a drug) through the nose.

snorter /ˈsnɔːtər/ *n* (*sl*) something remarkable for its size, strength, difficulty, etc.

snot /snɒt/ *n* (*sl*) nasal mucus; (*sl*) a snotty person.

snotty /ˈsnɒti/ *adj* (**snottier, snottiest**) covered with snot; (*sl*) irritatingly unpleasant; snobbish.—**snottily** *adv.*—**snottiness** *n.*

snout /snaʊt/ *n* the nose or muzzle of an animal.

snow /snoʊ/ *n* frozen water vapour in the form of white flakes; a snowfall; a mass of snow. • *vi* to fall as snow; to deceive with smooth talk.

snow apple *n* ♣ (*Cdn*) a white-fleshed eating apple first grown in Quebec.

snowball /ˈsnoʊbɔːl/ *n* snow pressed together in a ball for throwing; a drink made with advocaat and lemonade. • *vi* to throw snowballs; to increase rapidly in size.

snowberry /-beri/ *n* (*pl* **snowberries**) any of various shrubs bearing white berries.

snowbird /ˈsnoʊbɜːd/ *n* ♣ (*Cdn*) a small, mainly white bird of the finch or junco family, *esp* the snow bunting; a person from Canada or northern America who lives in a southern US state during the winter.

snow-blind /-blaɪnd/ *adj* temporarily blinded or dazzled by the intense glare of sunlight reflected from snow.—**snow-blindness** *n.*

snowblower /-bloʊər/ *n* a machine for clearing snow from roads by sucking it up and blowing it off to the side.

snowboard /-bɔːd/ *n* a board shaped like a large ski on which a person can stand to slide across snow.

snowbound /-baʊnd/ *adj* trapped by or covered in snow.

snowcap /-kæp/ *n* a covering of snow, as on a mountain peak.—**snowcapped** *adj.*

snowdrift /-drɪft/ *n* a bank of drifted snow.

snowdrop /-drɒp/ *n* a Eurasian plant of the daffodil family with white flowers that appears in early spring.

snowfall /-fɔːl/ *n* a fall of snow; the amount of snow in a given time or area.

snowflake /-fleɪk/ *n* a fragile cluster of ice crystals.

snow goose *n* a large white North American goose with black-tipped wings.

snow leopard *n* a large cat of the central Asian mountains with a tawny coat that becomes white in winter.

snow line, snow limit *n* the lowest limit in altitude of permanent snow.

snowman /-mæn/ *n* (*pl* **snowmen**) snow piled into the shape of a human figure.

snowmobile /-moʊbiːl/ *n* a motor vehicle for travelling at speed over snow.

snowplough, snowplow /-plaʊ/ *n* a vehicle designed for clearing away snow.

snow route *n* ♣ (*Cdn*) a major urban road that gets priority in the removal of snow.

snowshoe /-ʃuː/ *n* footwear in the shape of a racket-like frame with thongs for walking on soft snow. • *vi* (**snowshoeing, snowshoed**) to walk on snow using snowshoes.

snowstorm /-stɔːm/ *n* a storm with heavy snow.

snow tyre *n* a heavy tyre with deep treads for improved traction on snow and ice.

snow-white /-ˈwaɪt/ or /-ˈhwaɪt/ *adj* pure white.

snowy /ˈsnoʊi/ *adj* (**snowier, snowiest**) covered with snow; white or pure, like snow.—**snowily** *adv.*—**snowiness** *n.*

snowy owl *n* a large owl with white plumage of northern regions.

Snr, snr *abbr* = senior.

snub /snʌb/ *vt* (**snubbing, snubbed**) to insult by ignoring or making a cutting remark. • *n* the act of snubbing; an intentional slight.

snub-nosed /ˈsnʌbˌnoʊzd/ *adj* having a short upturned nose; (*pistol*) having a very short barrel.

snuck /snʌk/ *see* **sneak**.

snuff[1] /snʌf/ *n* a powdered preparation of tobacco inhaled through the nostrils.

snuff[2] *n* the charred portion of a wick. • *vt* to extinguish (a candle flame).

snuffbox /ˈsnʌfbɒks/ *n* a small box for snuff.

snuffer /ˈsnʌfər/ *n* a cone-shaped device for putting out a candle.

snuffle /ˈsnʌfəl/ *vi* to make sniffing noises, as when suffering from a cold or crying. • *n* the act of snuffling; (*pl*) a form of catarrh.

snuff movie *n* a pornographic film which ends by depicting the brutal murder of an unsuspecting participant.

snug /snʌg/ *adj* (**snugger, snuggest**) cosy; warm; close-fitting.—**snugly** *adv.*—**snugness** *n.*

snuggle /ˈsnʌgəl/ *vi* to nestle, cuddle. • *vt* to cuddle.

snye /snaɪ/ *n* ♣ (*Cdn*) a side channel of a river, *esp* one that diverges from a river and then rejoins it.

so[1] /soʊ/ *adv* in this way; as shown; as stated; to such an extent; very; (*inf*) very much; therefore; more or less; also, likewise; then.

so[2] *see* **sol**.

soak /soʊk/ *vt* to submerge in a liquid; to take in, absorb; (*sl*) to extract large amounts of money from. • *vi* to become saturated; to penetrate. • *n* the act or process of soaking.

so-and-so /ˈsoʊənˌsoʊ/ *n* (*pl* **so-and-sos**) an unspecified person or thing; (*inf*) (*euphemism*) an unpleasant or disliked person or thing.

soap /soʊp/ *n* a substance used with water to produce suds for washing; (*inf*) a soap opera. • *vt* to rub with soap.—**soapy** *adj.*

soapberry /ˈsoʊpˌberi/ *n* (*pl* **soapberries**) any of various tropical American trees bearing fruit which are rich in saponin.

soapbox /-bɒks/ *n* a temporary platform from which to deliver informal speeches.

soap opera *n* (*inf*) a daytime radio or television serial melodrama.

soapstone /-stoʊn/ *n* a type of soft grey-green stone with a soapy texture.—*also* **steatite**.

soapwort /-wɔːt/ *n* a Eurasian herbaceous plant of the pink family whose leaves form a soapy lather with water.

soapy /ˈsoʊpi/ *adj* (**soapier, soapiest**) like or full of soap; flattering, unctuous.—**soapily** *adv.*—**soapiness** *n.*

soar /sɔːr/ *vi* to rise high in the air; to glide along high in the air; to increase; to rise in status.—**soarer** *n.*

sob /sɒb/ *vb* (**sobbing, sobbed**) *vi* to weep with convulsive gasps. • *vt* to speak while sobbing.

sober /ˈsoʊbər/ *adj* not drunk; serious and thoughtful; realistic, rational; subdued in colour. • *vt* (*often with* **up** *or* **down**) to make or become sober.—**soberly** *adv.*—**soberness** *n.*

sobriety /səˈbraɪəti/ *n* soberness; temperance; seriousness.

sobriquet /ˌsoʊbrɪˈkeɪ/ *or* /ˈsoʊbrɪˌkeɪ/, /-ˈkɛt/ *n* a nickname.—*also* **soubriquet**.

sob story *n* (*inf*) a tale of distress intended to arouse sympathy.

Soc., soc. *abbr* = socialist; society.

so-called /ˈsoʊˈkoʊld/ *adj* commonly named or known as.

soccer /ˈsɒkər/ *n* a football game played on a field by two teams of 11 players with a round inflated ball, association football.

sociable /ˈsoʊʃəbəl/ *adj* friendly; companionable.—**sociability** *n.*—**sociably** *adv.*

social /ˈsoʊʃəl/ *adj* living or organized in a community, not solitary; relating to human beings living in society; of or intended for communal activities; sociable. • *n* an informal gathering of people, such as a party.—**socially** *adv.*

social anthropology *n* the branch of anthropology that studies social and cultural systems and beliefs.

social climber *n* a person who strives to attain a higher social position.

social contract, social compact *n* a tacit agreement between individuals in society and between individuals and the government which defines the rights and duties of each.

Social Democratic Party *n* a political party that advocates the transition from capitalism to socialism in a gradual manner.—**Social Democrat** *n.*—**Social Democratic** *adj.*

social disease *n* venereal disease.

social insurance number *n* ♣ (*Cdn*) a nine-digit number issued by the federal government to individuals and used for identification purposes.

socialism /ˈsoʊʃəˌlɪzəm/ *n* (a system based on) a political and economic theory advocating state ownership of the means of production and distribution.—**socialist** *n, adj.*—**socialistic** *adj.*—**socialistically** *adv.*

socialite /-laɪt/ *n* a person active or prominent in fashionable society.

socialize /-laɪz/ *vt* to meet other people socially.—**socialization** *n.*—**socializer** *n.*

social science *n* the study of human social organization and relationships using scientific methods.

social security *n* financial assistance for the unemployed, the disabled, etc to alleviate economic distress.

social service *n* a welfare service provided by the state, such as housing, education, and health.—**social-service** *adj*.

social work *n* any of various professional welfare services to aid the underprivileged in society.—**social worker** *n*.

society /sə'saɪtɪ/ *n* (*pl* **societies**) the social relationships between human beings or animals organized collectively; the system of human institutional organization; a community with the same language and customs; an interest group or organization; the fashionable or privileged members of a community; companionship.—**societal** *adj*.

Society of Friends *n* the official name for the Quakers.

Society of Jesus *n* the Roman Catholic religious order of the Jesuits.

socio- /-'səʊsɪəʊ/ or /-ʃɪəʊ/ *prefix* society; social.

socioeconomic /ˌsəʊsɪəʊˌiːkə'nɒmɪk/ or /ˌsəʊʃɪəʊ-/ *adj* of or involving social and economic aspects.

sociolinguistics /-lɪŋ'ɡwɪstɪk/ *n sing* the study of the social and cultural context of language.—**sociolinguist** *n*.

sociology /ˌsəʊsɪ'ɒlədʒɪ/ or /ˌsəʊʃɪ-/ *n* the study of the development and structure of society and social relationships.—**sociological** *adj*.—**sociologically** *adv*.—**sociologist** *n*.

sociometry /-'ɒmɪtrɪ/ or /ˌsəʊʃɪ-/ *n* the study of social relations within small groups.—**sociometric** *adj*.

sociopath /'səʊsɪəˌpæθ/ or /'səʊsɪəʊ-/, /'səʊʃɪ-/ *n* a person suffering from a mental disorder that results in antisocial behaviour and lack of guilt.—**sociopathic** *adj*.

sociopolitical /ˌsəʊsɪəʊpə'lɪtɪkəl/ *adj* of or involving social and political aspects.

sock[1] /sɒk/ *n* a kind of short stocking covering the foot and lower leg.

sock[2] *vt* (*sl*) to punch hard. • *n* a blow.

socket /'sɒkət/ *n* a hollow part into which something is inserted, such as an eye, a bone, a tooth, an electric plug, etc.

sockeye /'sɒkaɪ/ *n* a Pacific salmon valued as a food fish.—*also* **red salmon.**

Socratic /sə'krætɪk/ *adj* of or relating to Socrates (*c*.470-399BC), the Greek philosopher, or his methods. • *n* an adherent of Socrates or his philosophy.

Socratic irony *n* feigning ignorance when posing questions to expose the real ignorance of the person responding.

Socratic method *n* philosophical instruction by means of question and answer.

sod[1] /sɒd/ *n* a lump of earth covered with grass; turf. • *vt* (**sodding, sodded**) to cover with turf.

sod[2] *n* (*sl*) an obnoxious person; (*loosely*) a person, man. • *vi* (**sodding, sodded**) (*Brit sl*) to damn; (*with* **off**) (*sl*) to go away.—*also interj*.

soda /'səʊdə/ *n* sodium bicarbonate; sodium carbonate; soda water.

soda bread *n* bread made with baking soda instead of yeast.

soda fountain *n* a counter selling soft drinks, ice cream, snacks, etc; a device that dispenses soda water.

soda siphon *n* a pressurized container that dispenses soda water.

soda water *n* a fizzy drink made by charging water with carbon dioxide under pressure.

sodden /'sɒdən/ *adj* completely soaked through.—**soddenly** *adv*.

sodium /'səʊdɪəm/ *n* a metallic element.

sodium bicarbonate *n* a white soluble alkaline powder used in baking powder, fire extinguishers and in antacid medicines.

sodium chloride *n* salt.

sodium hydroxide *n* a white alkaline solid used in the manufacture of soap, paper and rayon.

sodium nitrate *n* a white crystalline compound used in fertilizers, matches and explosives, and as a food preservative.

sodium-vapour lamp *n* an electric lamp using sodium vapour through which a current is passed to produce an orange light, *esp* used for street lighting.

Sodom /'sɒdəm/ *n* (*Bible*) a wicked city destroyed by God; a wicked and depraved place.

sodomite /'sɒdəˌmaɪt/ *n* a person who practises sodomy.

sodomy /'sɒdəmɪ/ *n* anal sexual intercourse between males or between a man and woman.

sofa /'səʊfə/ *n* an upholstered couch or settee with fixed back and arms.

soffit /'sɒfɪt/ *n* the underside of a structural element, such as an arch, stairway, balcony, etc.

soft /sɒft/ *adj* malleable; easily cut, shaped, etc; not as hard as normal, desirable, etc; smooth to the touch; (*drinks*) nonalcoholic; mild, as a breeze; lenient; (*sl*) easy, comfortable; (*colour, light*) not bright; (*sound*) gentle, low; (*drugs*) non-addictive.—**softly** *adv*.—**softness** *n*.

softball /'sɒftbɔl/ *n* a game similar to baseball, but played with a larger, softer ball.

soft-boiled /-bɔɪld/ *adj* (*egg*) boiled so that the white hardens while the yolk remains soft.

soft-core /'sɒftkɔr/ *adj* (*pornography*) not sexually explicit.

softcover /-kʌvər/ *adj* paperback. • *n* a paperback book.

soft drink *n* a nonalcoholic drink.

soften /'sɒfən/ *vti* to make or become soft or softer.—**softener** *n*.

soft-focus *adj* (*lens*) designed to produce a slightly blurred image.

soft furnishings *npl* items such as curtains, carpets, rugs, etc.

soft goods /'sɒftɡʊdz/ *npl* textile and clothing products.

softheaded /-ˌhɛdɪd/ *adj* stupid, feeble-minded.—**softheadedly** *adv*.—**softheadedness** *n*.

softhearted /-ˌhɑrtɪd/ *adj* kind; sentimental.—**softheartedly** *adv*.—**softheartedness** *n*.

soft landing *n* a landing by a spacecraft which leaves the vehicle and occupants undamaged.

soft option *n* the easiest choice in a range of alternatives.

soft palate *n* the fleshy area at the back of the roof of the mouth.

soft paste *n* a type of translucent porcelain made from refined clay, ground glass, bone ash, etc.

soft-pedal /-pɛdəl/ *n* a pedal on a piano for muting the tone. • *vt* (*inf*) (**soft-pedalling, soft-pedalled** *or* **soft-pedaling, soft-pedaled**) to avoid direct reference to, *esp* something embarrassing or unpleasant.

soft porn *n* (*inf*) soft-core pornography.

soft sell *n* selling by gentle persuasion.—**soft-sell** *adj*.

soft soap *n* a type of semisolid or liquid soap; (*inf*) flattery.

soft-soap *vt* (*inf*) to flatter.—**soft-soaper** *n*.

soft spot *n* a sentimental fondness (for).

soft touch *n* (*inf*) a person who is easily persuaded or exploited.

software /-wɛr/ *n* the programs used in computers.

softwood /-wʊd/ *n* the wood of any coniferous tree.

softy /'sɒftɪ/ *n* (*pl* **softies**) (*inf*) a person regarded as sentimental or physically weak.

soggy /'sɒɡɪ/ *adj* (**soggier, soggiest**) soaked with water; moist and heavy.—**soggily** *adv*.—**sogginess** *n*.

soi-disant *Fr.* /swediː'zɑ̃/ *adj* self-styled.

soigné, soignée /'swɒnjeɪ/ *adj* well-groomed; elegant.

soil[1] /sɔɪl/ *n* the ground or earth in which plants grow; territory.

soil[2] *vt* to make or become dirty or stained.

soil pipe *n* a sewage or waste-water pipe.

soiree, soirée /swɑr'eɪ/ or /'swɑr/ *n* an evening party of music in a private house.

soixante-neuf /ˌswɛsɑ̃'nəf/ *n* a sexual position that facilitates mutual cunnilingus and fellatio; sixty-nine.

sojourn /'sɒdʒɜrn/ *n* a temporary stay. • *vi* to stay for a short time.—**sojourner** *n*.

sol[1] /sɒl/ *n* (*mus*) the name for the fifth note of the diatonic scale—*also* **so.**

sol[2] *n* liquid in which a colloid is dissolved or suspended.

sol. *abbr* = soluble; solution.

solace /'sɒləs/ *n* comfort in misery; consolation. • *vt* to bring solace to.

solar /səʊlər/ *adj* of or from the sun; powered by light or heat from the sun; reckoned by the sun.

solar cell *n* a cell that converts the sun's rays into electricity.

solar constant *n* the quantity of sun's energy radiated onto a given area of the earth's surface in a prescribed period.

solar day *n* the period of time during which the earth makes a complete revolution relative to the sun.

solar flare *n* a sudden brief eruption of intense energy from the sun's surface.

solarium /sə'lɛrɪəm/ *n* (*pl* **solariums, solaria**) a glass-enclosed room for sunbathing or exposure to the sun for medical treatment.

solar month *n* the period of time taken for the moon to make one complete revolution around the earth (approx. 27 days).

solar panel *n* a large thin panel that absorbs energy from sunlight and regenerates it.

solar plexus *n* the network of nerves behind the stomach; (*inf*) the pit of the stomach.

solar pond *n* a shallow artificial pond of salt water covered by fresh water, which absorbs heat from the sun's rays and converts it to electricity.

solar system *n* the sun and those bodies moving about it under the attraction of gravity.

solar wind *n* the constant flow of charged particles from the sun into outer space.

solar year *n* the period of time taken for the earth to make one revolution around the sun.

sold /sold/ *see* **sell**.

solder /'sɒdər/ *n* a metal alloy used when melted to join or patch metal parts, etc. • *vti* to join or be joined with solder.

soldering iron *n* an electrically heated tool for melting and applying solder.

soldier /'soldʒər/ *n* a person who serves in an army, *esp* a non-commissioned officer or private. • *vi* to serve as a soldier; *(with on)* to continue regardless of difficulties or dangers.—**soldierly** *adj*.

soldier of fortune *n* a man in constant search of military adventure; a mercenary.

soldiery /'soldʒəri/ *n (pl* **soldieries)** soldiers collectively; a body of soldiers; the profession of being a soldier.

sole[1] /sol/ *n* the underside of the foot or shoe. • *vt* to put a new sole on (a shoe).

sole[2] *n (pl* **sole, soles)** a type of flatfish used as food.

sole[3] *adj* only, being the only one; exclusive.—**solely** *adv*.

solecism /'sɒləˌsɪzəm/ *n* an error in speech or writing; a breach of etiquette or good manners.

solemn /'sɒləm/ *adj* serious; formal; sacred; performed with religious ceremony.—**solemnly** *adv*.—**solemnness** *n*.

solemnity /sə'lɛmnɪti/ *n (pl* **solemnities)** solemness; a formal rite.

solenoid /'sɒləˌnɔɪd/ or /'sɒl-/ *n* a coil of wire that produces a magnetic field when an electric current is passed through it.—**solenoidal** *adj*.

sol-fa /sol'fɒ/ *see* tonic sol-fa.

sol-fa syllable *n* any of the syllables *(do, re, mi,* etc) used to represent the notes of the musical scale in tonic sol-fa or solmization.

solfatara /ˌsolfə'tɑːrə/ *n* a volcanic outlet that emits only (sulphurous) gases and (water) vapours.

solfeggio /sɒl'fedʒɪoː/ *n (pl* **solfeggi, solfeggios)** *(singing using)* the application of the sol-fa syllables to musical scales or melody.

solicit /sə'lɪsɪt/ *vti* to make a request or application to (a person for something); *(prostitute)* to offer sexual services for money.—**solicitation** *n*.

solicitor /-ər/ *n* a lawyer.

solicitous /-əs/ *adj* showing concern or attention.—**solicitously** *adv*.—**solicitousness** *n*.

solicitude /sə'lɪsɪˌtuːd/ or /-ˌtjuːd/ *n* the state of being solicitous; concern; anxiety; carefulness.

solid /'sɒlɪd/ *adj* firm; compact; not hollow; strongly constructed; having three dimensions; neither liquid nor gaseous; unanimous. • *n* a solid substance (not liquid or gas); a three-dimensional figure.—**solidly** *adv*.—**solidness** *n*.

solidarity /ˌsɒlɪ'dɛrɪti/ *n (pl* **solidarities)** unity of interest and action.

solid geometry *n* geometry of three-dimensional figures.

solidi /'sɒlɪdi/ *see* **solidus**.

solidify /sə'lɪdəˌfaɪ/ *vti* **(solidifying, solidified)** to make or become solid, compact, hard, etc.—**solidification** *n*.

solidity /sə'lɪdɪti/ *n* the state of being solid; density; compactness; stability; truth; moral firmness.

solid-state *adj (electronic devices)* using components, such as transistors, in which the current flow is through solid materials as opposed to a vacuum; of or relating to solids or their properties and characteristics.

solid-state physics *n sing* the physics of the properties of solids.

solidus /'sɒlɪdəs/ *n (pl* **solidi)** an oblique stroke (/) used to separate items of text as in dates, alternative words, lists, or the terms of fractions.

soliloquize /sə'lɪləˌkwaɪz/ *vt* to utter a soliloquy. • *vi* to talk to oneself.—**soliloquist** *n*.

soliloquy /sə'lɪləkwi/ *n (pl* **soliloquies)** the act of talking to oneself; an act or speech in a play that takes this form.

solipsism /'sɒlɪpˌsɪzəm/ *n (philos)* the theory that the only possible true knowledge is of self-existence.—**solipsistic** *adj*.—**solipsist** *n*.

solitaire /'sɒlɪˌter/ *n* a single gemstone, *esp* a diamond; a card game for one, patience.

solitary /'sɒlɪtəri/ *adj* alone; only; single; living alone; lonely. • *n (pl* **solitaries)** a recluse.—**solitarily** *adv*.—**solitariness** *n*.

solitude /'sɒlɪˌtuːd/ or /-ˌtjuːd/ *n* the state of being alone; lack of company; a lonely place.—**solitudinous** *adj*.

solmization /ˌsɒlmə'zeɪʃən/ *n (mus)* the use of syllables to name the notes or degrees of a musical scale.

solo /'soːloː/ *n (pl* **solos)** a musical composition for one voice or instrument; a flight by a single person in an aircraft, *esp* a first flight. • *vi* to perform by oneself. • *adv* alone. • *adj* unaccompanied.—**soloist** *n*.

so long *interj (inf)* goodbye, farewell.

solo whist *n* a form of whist in which any player may bid independently to win or lose a prescribed number of tricks.

solstice /'sɒlstɪs/ or /'sɒl-/ *n* either of the two times in the year at which the sun is farthest from the equator (June 21 and December 21).—**solsticial** *adj*.

soluble /'sɒljubəl/ *adj* capable of being dissolved *(usu* in water); capable of being solved or answered.—**solubility** *n*.—**solubly** *adv*.

solute /-juːt/ *n* a dissolved substance in a solution.

solution /sə'luːʃən/ *n* the act or process of answering a problem; the answer found; the dispersion of one substance in another, *usu* a liquid, so as to form a homogeneous mixture.

solvable /'sɒlvəbəl/ or /-sɒl-/ *adj* capable of being solved.—**solvability** *n*.

solve /sɒlv/ *vt* to work out the answer to; to clear up, resolve.

solvent /'sɒlvənt/ *adj* capable of dissolving a substance; able to pay all debts. • *n* a liquid that dissolves substances.—**solvency** *n*.

solvent abuse *n* the deliberate inhalation of fumes from solvents (such as in glue and polish) to become intoxicated.

soma /'soːmə/ *n (pl* **somatas, somas)** all of an organism except the germ cells.

Somali /sə'mɒli/ or /-'mæli/ *n (pl* **Somalis, Somali)** a native or inhabitant of Somalia; the Somali language.—*also adj*.—**Somalian** *adj*.

somatic /sə'mætɪk/ *adj* of or relating to the body, as opposed to the mind.—**somatically** *adv*.

somato-, somat- *prefix* body.

somatotype /'soːmətoːˌtɔɪp/ *n* physical build, body type.

sombre, somber /'sɒmbər/ *adj* dark, gloomy or dull; dismal; sad.—**sombrely, somberly** *adv*.—**sombreness, somberness** *n*.

sombrero /sɒm'breroː/ *n (pl* **sombreros)** a wide-brimmed hat with a high crown, worn *esp* in Spanish-speaking countries.

some /sʌm/ *adj* certain but not specified or known; of a certain unspecified quantity, degree, etc; a little; *(inf)* remarkable, striking, etc. • *pron* a certain unspecified quantity, number, etc.

-some /-səm/ *adj suffix* apt to, *eg* tiresome. • *n suffix* a group of, *eg* foursome.

somebody /'sʌmˌbɒdi/ or /-bədi/ *n (pl* **somebodies)** an unspecified person; an important person. • *pron* someone.

someday /-deɪ/ *adv* at some future day or time.

somehow /-haʊ/ *adv* in a way or by a method not known or stated.

someone /-wʌn/ *n* somebody.—*also pron*.

someplace /-pleɪs/ *adv* somewhere.

somersault /'sʌmərˌsɒlt/ *n* a forward or backward roll head over heels along the ground or in mid-air.—*also vi*.

something /-θɪŋ/ *n pron* a thing not definitely known, understood, etc; an important or notable thing. • *adv* to some degree.

sometime /-taɪm/ *adj* former. • *adv* at some unspecified future date. • *adj* having been formerly; being so occasionally or in only some respects.

sometimes /-taɪmz/ *adv* at times, now and then.

someway /-weɪ/ *adv* in a certain unspecified manner.

somewhat /-wɒt/ or /-wɒt/ *adv* to some extent, degree, etc; a little.

somewhere /-wer/, **somewheres** /-werz/ *adv* in, to or at some place not known or specified.

sommelier /ˌsɒməl'jeɪ/ *n* a wine waiter.

somnambulate /sɒm'næmbjuˌleɪt/ *vi* to get up and walk while asleep.—**somnambulant** *adj*.—**somnambulation** *n*.

somnambulism /sɒm'næmbjuˌlɪzəm/ *n* the practice of walking in one's sleep.—**somnambulist** *n*.—**somnambulistic** *adj*.

somnolent /'sɒmnələnt/ *adj* sleepy, drowsy.—**somnolence, somnolency** *n*.

son /sʌn/ *n* a male offspring or descendant.

sonar /'soːnɑr/ *n* an apparatus that detects underwater objects by means of reflecting sound waves.

sonata /sə'nɒtə/ or /-'nætə/ n (mus) a composition for a solo instrument, usu the piano.

sondage /'sɒndɒdʒ/ n (archaeol) a deep inspection trench.

sonde /sɒnd/ n a device for collecting scientific data in the upper atmosphere.

sone /soːn/ n a unit of loudness equivalent to 40 phons.

son et lumière /,sɒneɪ'luːmjer/ n an evening entertainment staged at historical sites and buildings using lighting displays, music and recorded speech to illuminate the history of the place.

song /sɒŋ/ n a piece of music composed for the voice; the act or process of singing; the call of certain birds.

song and dance n (inf) a fuss; a long involved story.

songbird /'sɒŋbərd/ n a bird with a musical call.

songster /'sɒŋstər/ n a singer; a songbird—**songstress** nf.

sonic /'sɒnɪk/ adj of, producing, or involving sound waves.—**sonically** adv.

sonic barrier n the increase in air resistance experienced by objects travelling close to the speed of sound, the sound barrier.

sonic boom n an explosive sound produced by the shockwave when an aircraft, etc reaches supersonic speed.

son-in-law /'sɒnɪnˌlɔ/ n (pl **sons-in-law**) a daughter's husband.

sonnet /'sɒnɪt/ n a rhyming poem in a single stanza of fourteen lines.

sonneteer /,sɒnə'tiːr/ n a composer of sonnets.

sonny /'sʌnɪ/ n (pl **sonnies**) a patronizing form of address to a boy.

sonobuoy /'sɒnəˌbɔɪ/ n a buoy used to detect underwater sounds and transmit them by radio to surface vessels.

sonorous /'sɒnərəs/ or /'soːn-/, /sə'nɔrəs/ adj giving out sound; full, rich, or deep in sound.—**sonorously** adv.—**sonorousness** n.

soon /suːn/ adv in a short time; before long; **sooner** or **later** at some future unspecified time, eventually.

soot /sʊt/ n a black powder produced from flames.—**sooty** adj.

soothe /suːð/ vt to calm or comfort; to alleviate; to relieve (pain, etc).—**soothing** adj.—**soothingly** adv.

soothsayer /'suːθˌseɪər/ n a person who predicts events.

SOP abbr = standard operating procedure.

sop /sɒp/ n a piece of bread or other food dipped in liquid before being eaten; a concession, bribe offered to appease or cajole. • vt (**sopping, sopped**) to dip (bread, etc) into liquid. • vi to be soaked.

sop. abbr = soprano.

soph abbr = sophomore.

sophism /'sɒfɪzəm/ n a clever but fallacious argument.—**sophistry** n.—**sophist** n.—**sophistic, sophistical** adj.

sophisticated /sə'fɪstəkeɪtəd/ adj refined; worldly-wise; intelligent; complex.—**sophistication** n.

sophomore /'sɒfmɔr/ or /'sɒfəˌmɔr/ n in US, a second-year student at college or high school.—**sophomoric** adj.

soporific /,sɒpə'rɪfɪk/ adj inducing sleep; sleepy.

sopping /'sɒpɪŋ/ adj wet through.

soppy /'sɒpɪ/ adj (**soppier, soppiest**) wet; (inf) sickly sentimental.—**soppily** adv.—**soppiness** n.

sopranino /,sɒprə'niːnɔ/ n (pl **sopraninos**) a musical instrument of the highest pitch in its class.

soprano /sə'prænɔ/ n (pl **sopranos, soprani**) the highest singing voice of females or boys; a person who sings soprano.

sorbet /sɔr'beɪ/ or /'sɔrbət/ n a flavoured water ice; sherbet.

sorcerer /'sɔrsərər/ n person who uses magic powers; a magician or wizard.—**sorceress** nf.

sorcery /-rɪ/ n (pl **sorceries**) the practice of magic, esp with the assistance of evil spirits.

sordid /'sɔrdɪd/ adj filthy, squalid; vile; base; selfish.—**sordidly** adv.—**sordidness** n.

sordino /sɔr'diːnɔ/ n (pl **sordini**) a mute for a stringed or brass musical instrument.

sore /sɔr/ n a painful or tender injury or wound; an ulcer or boil; grief; a cause of distress. • adj painful; tender; distressed.—**soreness** n.

sorehead /'sɔrhed/ n (inf) an angry, disgruntled person.

sorely /'sɔrlɪ/ adv seriously, urgently.

sorghum /-gəm/ n any of a genus of tropical cereal grasses grown for fodder.

sorority /sə'rɔrɪtɪ/ n (pl **sororities**) a society of women university students.

sorrel[1] /'sɑrəl/ n a colour between orange-brown and light brown; an animal, esp a horse, of this colour.

sorrel[2] n a herb with bitter leaves used in salads.

sorrow /'sɔrɔ/ or /'sɒ-/ n sadness; regret; an expression of grief. • vi to mourn, to grieve.

sorrowful /-fʊl/ adj full of, showing or causing sorrow.—**sorrowfully** adv.—**sorrowfulness** n.

sorry /'sɒrɪ/ or /'sɔ-/ adj (**sorrier, sorriest**) feeling pity, sympathy, remorse or regret; pitiful; poor.—**sorrily** adv.—**sorriness** n.

sort /sɔrt/ n a class, kind, or variety; quality or type. • vt to arrange according to kind; to classify; (with out) to find a solution to, resolve; to disentangle; to organize, discipline; (inf) to punish, to attack violently.—**sorter** n.

sorted /-ɪd/ adj (sl) the state of being fully prepared or organized; put in order.

sortie /'sɔrtɪ/ n a sudden attack by troops from a besieged position; one mission by a single military plane.

SOS /,ɛsoː'ɛs/ n an international signal code of distress; an urgent call for help or rescue.

so-so adj not good but not bad, middling. • adv average, indifferently.

sot /sɒt/ n a habitual drunkard.

soteriology /sɔ,tiːri:'ɒlədʒɪ/ or /sɒ-/ n (theol) the doctrine of salvation, esp through Jesus Christ.—**soteriological** adj.

sotto voce /,sɒtoː'voːtʃɪ/ adv in an undertone.

sou /suː/ n (pl **sous**) (formerly) a French coin of little value; a very small sum of money.

soubrette /suː'brɛt/ n a minor female role in a comedy, esp a pert lady's maid; a saucy girl.

soubriquet /,soː'brɪkeɪ/ or /'soːbrɪˌkeɪ/, /-'kɛt/ see **sobriquet**.

soufflé /'suːfleɪ/ n a baked dish made light and puffy by adding beaten egg whites before baking.—also adj.

sough /saʊ/ or /sʌf/ vi to make a moaning sound like the wind.—also n.

sought /sɔt/ see **seek**.

souk /suːk/ n an open-air market in Muslim countries.

soul /soːl/ n a person's spirit; the seat of the emotions, desires; essence; character; a human being. • adj characteristic of American Blacks.

soul-destroying adj extremely boring, depressing.

soul food n (inf) traditional food (eg yams, chitterlings) eaten by Blacks of the Southern US.

soulful /'soːlfʊl/ adj expressing profound sentiment.—**soulfully** adv.—**soulfulness** n.

soulless /'soːlləs/ adj devoid of emotion; bleak; dull.

soul mate /'soːlmeɪt/ n a person, such as a lover or close friend, with whom one bonds deeply.

soul music n music derived from Afro-American gospel singing marked by intensity of feeling and closely related to rhythm and blues.

soul-searching n close examination of one's conscience, motives, etc.

sound[1] /saʊnd/ adj healthy; free from injury or damage; substantial; stable; deep (as sleep) solid; thorough.—**soundly** adv.—**soundness** n.

sound[2] n a narrow channel of water connecting two seas or between a mainland and an island.

sound[3] n vibrations transmitted through the air and detected by the ear; the sensation of hearing; any audible noise; the impression given by something. • vi to make a sound; to give a summons by sound. • vt to cause to make a sound; to voice; to make a signal or order by sound; (with off) (inf) to complain loudly.

sound[4] vt to measure the depth of; (often with out) to attempt to discover the opinions and intentions of (someone).

sound barrier n the increase in air resistance experienced by objects travelling close to the speed of sound, the sonic barrier.

sound board n a thin board in certain musical instruments that resonates to enhance the sound; a sounding board.

soundbox n the hollow resonating cavity of a musical instrument such as a guitar or violin.

sound effects npl artificial sounds used for dramatic purposes in plays, television programmes, films, etc.

sounding[1] /'saʊndɪŋ/ n measurement of the depth of water; a test, sampling, eg of public opinion.

sounding[2] adj resounding.

sounding board *n* a thin board placed behind a platform to direct the sound at the audience; a sound board; a person or thing used to test reaction to a new idea or plan.

sounding line *n* a line marked at regular intervals for sounding.

soundproof /'saundpruːf/ *adj* unable to be penetrated by sound. • *vt* to make soundproof by insulation, etc.

soundtrack /'saundtræk/ *n* the sound accompanying a film; the area on cinema film that carries the sound recording.

soup /suːp/ *n* a liquid food made from boiling meat, fish, vegetables, etc, in water; (*inf*) a difficult or embarrassing **situation**. • *vt* (with up (*inf*) to increase the power and performance of an engine.—**soupy** *adj*.

soupçon /'suːpsɔ̃/ *n* a slight flavour; a trace.

soup kitchen *n* a place where soup and other food is dispensed to the homeless and destitute.

sour /'sauər/ *adj* having a sharp, biting taste; spoiled by fermentation; cross; bad-tempered; distasteful or unpleasant; (*soil*) acid in reaction. • *vti* to make or become sour.—**sourly** *adv.*—**sourness** *n.*

source /sɔrs/ *n* a spring forming the head of a stream; an origin or cause; a person, book, etc, that provides information. • *vti* (*inf*) to find a supplier; to identify a source.

source program *n* (*comput*) an original program that has been translated into machine code.

sour cream *n* cream deliberately soured by bacteria and used in sauces, dressings, etc.

sourdough /'saurdoʊ/ *n* dough used in more than one baking to save on fresh yeast; a prospector in North America who lived on bread made from sourdough.

sour grapes *n sing* pretending to dislike something because it cannot be obtained or achieved by oneself.

sourpuss /'saur.pus/ *n* (*inf*) a gloomy person.

souse /sɐus/ *vt* to immerse in water or other liquid; to saturate; to pickle or steep in a marinade; (*sl*) to make drunk. • *vi* to become saturated or immersed. • *n* the act of sousing; something pickled; pickling liquid; (*sl*) a drunkard.

soutane /suː'tæn/ *n* a cassock.

south /saʊθ/ *n* the direction to one's right when facing the direction of the rising sun; the region, country, continent, etc, lying relatively in that direction. • *adj, adv* facing toward or situated in the south.

Southdown *n* a breed of hornless sheep that yields wool and *esp* meat.

southeast /saʊθ'iːst/ *n* the point on a compass midway between south and east. • *adj, adv* at, toward, or from the southeast.

southeasterly /saʊθ'iːstərli/ *adj, adv* toward or from the southeast. • *n* (*pl* **southeasterlies**) a wind from the southeast.

southeastern /saʊθ'iːstərn/ *adj* in, toward, or from the southeast; inhabiting or characteristic of the southeast.—**southeasterner** *n.*

southerly /'sʌðərli/ *adj* in, toward, or from the south. • *n* (*pl* **southerlies**) a wind from the south.

southern /'sʌðərn/ *adj* in, toward, or from the south; inhabiting or characteristic of the south.—**southernmost** *adj.*

southerner /'sʌðərnər/ *n* an inhabitant of the south.

southern lights *npl* the aurora australis.

southpaw /'sʌθpɔ/ *n* (*inf*) a left-handed boxer; a left-handed person.—*also adj.*

South Pole *n* the most southerly point on the earth's axis; the most southerly point on the celestial sphere; (*without caps*) the pole of a magnet that points south.

southward /'saʊθwərd/ *adj* toward the south.—**southwards** *adv.*

southwest /'saʊθwest/ *n* the point on a compass midway between south and west. • *adj, adv* at, toward, or from the southwest.

southwester /'saʊθwestərnər/ *n* a strong wind from the southwest.

southwesterly *adj, adv* toward or from the southwest. • *n* (*pl* **southwesterlies**) a wind from the southwest.

southwestern *adj* in, toward, or from the southwest; inhabiting or characteristic of the southwest.—**southwesterner** *n.*

souvenir /ˌsuːvə'niːr/ *n* a keepsake, a memento.

sou'wester /sau'westər/ *n* a waterproof hat with a wide brim at the back worn by sailors.

sovereign /'sɒvrən/ *adj* supreme in authority or rank; (*country, state, etc*) independent. • *n* a supreme ruler; a monarch.—**sovereignty** *n.*

sovereignist /'sɒvrənɪst/, **sovereigntist** /-tɪst/ *n* ✹ (*Cdn*) a person who supports greater self-government for Quebec, *esp* its political independence. • of or pertaining to the movement for the political independence of Quebec.

soviet /'soːvɪət/ *n* a workers' council in the former USSR.

sovietism /-ɪzəm/ *n* a political system of which the soviet is the unit.

sow[1] /sau/ *n* an adult female pig.

sow[2] /soː/ *vt* (**sowing, sowed,** *pp* **sown** *or* **sowed**) to plant or scatter seed on or in the ground; to disseminate; to implant.—**sower** *n.*

soya bean, soybean /'sɔɪbiːn/ *n* a type of bean (orig from Asia) used as a source of food and oil.

soy sauce, soya sauce *n* a dark, salty sauce made from fermented soybeans.

sozzled /'sɒzəld/ *adj* (*in*) drunk.

sp *abbr* = species.

Sp. *abbr* = Spain; Spaniard; Spanish.

spa /spɒ/ *n* a mineral spring; a resort where there is a mineral spring.

space /speɪs/ *n* the limitless three-dimensional expanse within which all objects exist outer space; a specific area; an interval, empty area; room; an unoccupied area or seat. • *vt* to arrange at intervals.

Space Age *n* the era when space exploration has become possible.

space-age *adj* of or pertaining to the Space Age; modern.

space bar *n* the long bar on a typewriter or computer keyboard for inserting spaces.

spacecraft /'speɪskræft/ *n* a vehicle for travel in outer space.

spaced-out, spaced /speɪst/ *adj* (*sl*) high on drugs.

spaceman /'speɪsmæn/ *r* (*pl* **spacemen**) a person who travels in outer space; an alien.—**spacewoman** (*pl* **spacewomen**) *nf.*

space probe *n* an unmanned rocket equipped for exploring outer space.

spaceship /'speɪsʃɪp/ *n* a crewed spacecraft.

space shuttle *n* a manned spacecraft designed as a reusable ferry between the earth and a space station.

space station, space platform *n* a manned artificial satellite designed to orbit the earth and serve as a permanent base for space exploration.

spacesuit /'speɪsuːt/ *n* a sealed and pressurized suit worn by astronauts in space.

space-time (continuum) *n* (*physics*) the four-dimensional coordinate system comprising the three spatial and one temporal coordinates which together define a continuum in which any particle or event may be located.

spacewalk /'speɪswɔk/ *n* a period of time spent by an astronaut floating in space outside a spacecraft. • *vi* to walk in space.—**spacewalker** *n.*

spacious /'speɪʃəs/ *adj* large in extent; roomy.—**spaciously** *adv.*—**spaciousness** *n.*

spade[1] /speɪd/ *n* a tool with a broad blade and a handle, used for digging.

spade[2] *n* a black symbol resembling a stylized spearhead marking one of the four suits of playing cards; a card of this suit.

spadework /'speɪdwɜːk/ *n* routine preliminary work.

spadix /'speɪdɪks/ *n* (*pl* **spadixes, spadices**) a spike of flowers clustered around a fleshy stem and enclosed in a spathe.

spaghetti /spə'geti/ *n* pasta made in thin, solid strings.

spaghetti western *n* a type of violent cowboy film, *usu* shot on location in Italy or Spain, which became popular in the 1960s.

spake /speɪk/ (*arch*) *pt of* **speak.**

Spam /spæm/ *n* (*trademark*) tinned pork luncheon meat.

spam *n* the term given to junk mail in email transmissions.

span /spæn/ *n* a unit of length equal to a hand's breadth (about 9 inches/23 cm); the full extent between any two limits, such as the ends of a bridge or arch. • *vt* (**spanning, spanned**) to extend across.

Span. *abbr* = Spanish.

spandrel /'spændrəl/ *n* the space between the right or left shoulder of an arch and the rectangular wall or moulding enclosing it.

spangle /'spæŋɡəl/ *n* a sequin or other small piece of shiny decoration; any small glittering particle. • *vt* to decorate with spangles. • *vi* to sparkle with or like spangles.—**spangly** *adj.*

Spaniard /'spænjərd/ *n* a native or inhabitant of Spain.

spaniel /'spænjəl/ *n* any of various breeds of dog with large drooping ears and a long silky coat.

Spanish /'spænɪʃ/ *adj* of or pertaining to Spain. • *n* the language of Spain and Spanish Americans; the people of Spain.

Spanish-American *adj* of or pertaining to the countries in America where Spanish is spoken. • *n* a native or inhabitant of a Spanish-American country.

Spanish fly *n* a European blister beetle; a substance prepared from dried Spanish fly (cantharides) which purportedly acts as an aphrodisiac.

Spanish guitar *n* a type of classical acoustic guitar music; the guitar used to play this.

Spanish omelette *n* an omelette containing chopped vegetables such as onions, tomatoes, pimentoes, etc.

spank /spæŋk/ *vt* to slap with the flat of the hand, *esp* on the buttocks.—*also n.*

spanking /'spæŋkɪŋ/ *adj* (*inf*) very impressive, large, smart, etc; (*inf*) brisk, lively.—*also adv.*

spanner /'spænər/ *n* a tool with a hole or (often adjustable) jaws to grip and turn nuts or bolts, a wrench.

spar¹ /spɑr/ *n* a pole supporting the rigging of a ship; one of the main structural members of the wing of an airplane.

spar² *vi* to box using gentle blows, as in training; to argue.—*also n.*

spare /sper/ *vt* to refrain from harming or killing; to afford; to make (something) available (*eg* time). • *adj* kept as an extra, additional; scanty. • *n* a spare part; a spare tyre.—**sparely** *adv.*—**spareness** *n.*

sparerib /'sperrɪb/ *n* a pork rib with most of the meat cut away.

spare tyre *n* (*inf*) a roll of excess fat around the waist.

sparing /'sperɪŋ/ *adj* frugal, economical.—**sparingly** *adv.*—**sparingness** *n.*

spark /spɑrk/ *n* a fiery or glowing particle thrown off by burning material or by friction; a flash of light from an electrical discharge; a trace. • *vt* to stir up; to activate. • *vi* to give off sparks.

sparking plug /'spɑrkɪŋ/ *n* sa spark plug.

sparkle /'spɑrkəl/ *n* a spark; vivacity. • *vi* to shine; to glitter; (*water, wine*) to effervesce; to be lively or witty.

sparkler /'spɑrklər/ *n* a handheld firework that throws off brilliant sparks; (*inf*) a diamond.

spark plug *n* a device that produces a spark to ignite the explosive mixture in an internal combustion engine.—*also* **sparking plug.**

sparring partner *n* (*boxing*) a partner who stands in as an opponent for training purposes; a person with whom one regularly argues.

sparrow /'spero:/ or /'spæro:/ *n* any of various small brownish songbirds related to the finch.

sparse /spɑrs/ *adj* spread out thinly; scanty.—**sparsely** *adv.*—**sparseness, sparsity** *n.*

Spartan /'spɑrtən/ *adj* of or pertaining to Sparta in ancient Greece; rigourously severe. • *n* ✽ (*Cdn*) a crisp medium-sized red cooking or eating apple.

spasm /'spæzəm/ *n* a sudden, involuntary muscular contraction; any sudden burst (of emotion or activity).—**spasmodic** *adj* intermittent; of or like a spasm.—**spasmodically** *adv.*

spastic /'spæstɪk/ *n* a person who suffers from cerebral palsy. • *adj* affected by muscle spasm.—**spasticity** *n.*

spat¹ *see* **spit²**.

spat² /spæt/ *n* a gaiter covering the ankle and instep and fastening under the shoe.

spat³ *n* a young oyster or other bivalve mollusc.

spat⁴ *n* a petty argument, or quarrel. • *vi* to have a petty argument.

spate /speɪt/ *n* a large amount; a sudden outburst (as of words); a sudden flood.

spathe /speɪð/ *n* a leafy part that encloses the floral spikes of certain flowers.

spatial /'speɪʃəl/ *adj* relating to space.—**spatially** *adv.*

spatiotemporal /ˌspeɪʃioˈtempərəl/ *adj* of, involving, or occurring in both space and time; of or pertaining to space-time.

spatter /'spætər/ *vti* to scatter or spurt out in drops; to splash.—*also n.*

spatula /'spætʃulə/ *n* a tool with a broad, flexible blade for spreading or mixing foods, paints, etc.

spatulate /'spætʃulət/ *adj* shaped like a spatula.

spawn /spɒn/ *n* a mass of eggs deposited by fish, frogs, or amphibians; offspring. • *vti* to lay eggs; to produce, *esp* in great quantity.

spay /speɪ/ *vt* (*female animals*) to sterilize by removing the ovaries from.

SPCA *abbr* = Society for the Prevention of Cruelty to Animals.

SPCC *abbr* = Society for the Prevention of Cruelty to Children.

speak /spiːk/ *vi* (**speaking, spoke,** *pp* **spoken**) to utter words; to talk; to converse with; to deliver a speech; to be suggestive of something; to produce a characteristic sound; (*with* **out, up**) to speak loudly; to express an opinion frankly.—**speakable** *adj.*

speakeasy /'spiːkˌiːzi/ *n* (*pl* **speakeasies**) a club where alcoholic drink was sold illegally during the Prohibition era in the US in the 1920s.

speaker /'spiːkər/ *n* a person who speaks, *esp* before an audience; the presiding official in a legislative assembly; a loudspeaker.

speaking clock *n* a recorded telephone message which gives the time.

spear /spiːr/ *n* a weapon with a long shaft and a sharp point; a blade or shoot (of grass, broccoli, etc). • *vt* to pierce with a spear.

spearhead /'spiːrhɛd/ *n* the pointed head of a spear; the leading person or group in an attack or other action. • *vt* to serve as a leader of.

spearing /'spiːrɪŋ/ *n* ✽ an infraction in ice hockey for jabbing or poking an opponent with one's stick.

spearmint /'spiːrmɪnt/ *n* a common mint plant which yields an oil used for flavouring.

special /'spɛʃəl/ *adj* distinguished; uncommon; designed for a particular purpose; peculiar to one person or thing.—**specially** *adv.*

Special Branch *n* the division of the British police force that deals with political security.

specialist /'spɛʃəlɪst/ *n* a person who concentrates on a particular area of study or activity, *esp* in medicine.

speciality /ˌspɛʃiˈælɪti/ *n* (*pl* **specialities**) a special skill or interest; a special product.—*also* **specialty**.

specialize /'spɛʃəlaɪz/ *vi* to concentrate on a particular area of study or activity. • *vt* to adapt to a particular use or purpose.—**specialization** *n.*

special licence *n* in the UK, a licence allowing a marriage to take place without regard to the normal legal requirements.

special pleading *n* (*law*) the allegation of new facts in an action as opposed to a direct denial or admission of the opposition evidence; arguments that concentrate on the positive as opposed to the negative aspects of a case.

specialty /'spɛʃəlti/ *see* **speciality**.

speciation /ˌspiːʃiˈeɪʃən/ or /ˌspiːs-/ *n* the evolution of a species.—**speciate** *vi.*

specie /'spiːʃi/ *n* money in coin.

species /'spiːsiːz/ or /'spiːʃ-/ *n* (*pl* **species**) a class of plants or animals with the same main characteristics, enabling interbreeding; a distinct kind or sort.

specific /spəˈsɪfɪk/ *adj* explicit; definite; of a particular kind. • *n* a characteristic quality or influence; a drug effective in treating a particular disease.—**specifically** *adv.*—**specificity** *n.*

specification /ˌspɛsɪfɪˈkeɪʃən/ *n* a requirement; (*pl*) detailed description of dimensions, materials, etc of something.

specific gravity *n* the ratio of the density of a substance to that of the same volume of water.

specific heat capacity *n* the heat required to raise the temperature of a unit of mass of a given substance by one degree.

specify /'spɛsɪˌfaɪ/ *vt* (**specifying, specified**) to state specifically; to set down as a condition.—**specifier** *n.*

specimen /'spɛsɪmən/ *n* (*plant, animal, etc*) an example of a particular species; a sample; (*inf*) a person.

specious /'spiːʃəs/ *adj* apparently true, but in fact false.—**speciously** *adv.*—**speciousness** *n.*

speck /spɛk/ *n* a small spot; a fleck.

speckle /'spɛkəl/ *n* a small mark of a different colour. • *vt* to mark with speckles.

specs /spɛks/ *npl* specifications; (*inf*) spectacles.

spectacle /'spɛktəkəl/ *n* an unusual or interesting scene; a large public show; an object of derision or ridicule; (*pl*) a pair of glasses.—**spectacled** *adj.*

spectacular /spɛkˈtækjulər/ *adj* impressive; astonishing.—**spectacularly** *adv.*

spectate /'spɛkteɪt/ *vi* to be a spectator.

spectator /'spɛkˌteɪtər/ *n* an onlooker.

specter *see* **spectre**.

spectra *see* **spectrum**.

spectral /'spɛktrəl/ *adj* of or like a spectre; of or produced by a spectrum.—**spectrality** *adv.*—**spectrally** *adv.*

spectre /'spɛktər/ *n* an apparition or ghost; a haunting mental image.—*also* **specter**.

spectro- /'spɛktrɔ:/ *prefix* spectrum.

spectrograph /'spɛktrɔ:,grɑːf/ *n* a device for producing and recording spectra.—**spectrographic** *adj*.

spectrometer /spɛk'trɒmətər/ *n* a spectroscope used to measure spectra.—**spectrometric** *adj*.—**spectrometry** *n*.

spectroscope /'spɛktrɔ:,skoʊp/ *n* an instrument for generating and examining spectra.—**spectroscopic** *adj*.—**spectroscopically** *adv*.—**spectroscopy** *n*.

spectrum /'spɛktrəm/ *n* (*pl* **spectra**) the range of colour which is produced when a white light is passed through a prism; any similar distribution of wave frequencies; a broad range.

speculate /'spɛkjʊ,leɪt/ *vi* to theorize, to conjecture; to make investments in the hope of making a profit.—**speculation** *n*.—**speculator** *n*.

speculative /'spɛkjʊlətɪv/ *adj* of or based on speculation; engaging in speculation in finance, etc.—**speculatively** *adv*.

speculum /'spɛkjʊləm/ *n* (*pl* **specula, speculums**) a medical instrument for dilating and examining a bodily passage or cavity; a mirror used as a reflector in an optical instrument such as a telescope.

sped *see* **speed**.

speech /spiːtʃ/ *n* the action or power of speaking; a public address or talk; language, dialect.

speechify /'spiːtʃɪ,faɪ/ *vi* (**speechifying, speechified**) to make a speech or speeches, *esp* in a dull or pompous manner.—**speechifier** *n*.

Speech from the Throne *n* ✦ (*Cdn*) a speech read on behalf of a government by a sovereign or the sovereign's representative that outlines proposed measures.—*also* **Throne Speech**.

speechless /'spiːtʃləs/ *adj* unable to speak; silent, as from shock; impossible to express in words.—**speechlessly** *adv*.—**speechlessness** *n*.

speed /spiːd/ *n* quickness; rapidity or rate of motion; (*photog*) the sensitivity of film to light; (*sl*) an amphetamine drug. • *vi* (**speeding, sped** *or* **speeded**) to go quickly, to hurry; to drive (a vehicle) at an illegally high speed.

speeding /'spiːdɪŋ/ *n* the driving of a vehicle at an illegally high or dangerous speed.

speedometer /spə'dɒmətər/ *n* an instrument in a motor vehicle for measuring its speed.

speedway /'spiːdweɪ/ *n* the sport of racing light motorcycles around dirt or cinder tracks; a stadium for motorcycle racing; in US, a road reserved for fast traffic.

speedwell /'spiːdwɛl/ *n* any of various plants of the figwort family with small blue or white flowers.

speedy /'spiːdi/ *adj* (**speedier, speediest**) quick; prompt.—**speedily** *adv*.—**speediness** *n*.

speleology /,spiːli'ɒlədʒi/ *n* the scientific study of caves.—**speleological** *adj*.—**speleologist** *n*.

spell[1] /spɛl/ *n* a sequence of words used to perform magic; fascination.

spell[2] *vb* (**spelling, spelt** *or* **spelled**) *vt* to name or write down in correct order the letters to form a word; (*letters*) to form a word when placed in the correct order; to indicate; (*with* **out**) to read slowly and painstakingly; to explain in detail; to discern, realize the meaning of. • *vi* to spell words.

spell[3] *n* a *usu* indefinite period of time; a period of duty in a certain occupation or activity. • *vt* to relieve, stand in for

spellbound /'spɛlbaʊnd/ *adj* entranced, enthralled.

spelling bee *n* a spelling contest.

spelt *see* **spell**[2].

spelunker /spɪ'lʌŋkər/ *n* a person whose hobby is exploring caves.—**spelunking** *n*.

spend /spɛnd/ *vb* (**spending, spent**) *vt* to pay out (money); to concentrate (one's time or energy) on an activity; to pass, as time; to use up. • *vi* to pay out money.—**spender** *n*.

spendthrift /'spɛndθrɪft/ *n* a person who spends money wastefully or extravagantly.

spent[1] *see* **spend**.

spent[2] *adj* consumed, used up; physically drained, exhausted.

sperm /spɜːrm/ *n* semen; the male reproductive cell.

spermaceti /,spɜːrmə'sɛti/ *n* a waxy substance derived from the oil in the head of a sperm whale.

spermat(o)-, sperm(o)- /spər'mætoʊ/ *prefix* sperm.

spermatic /spər'mætɪk/ *adj* pertaining to, consisting of, or conveying, sperm.

spermatid /'spɜːrmətɪd/ *n* any of the four male gametes that form into a spermatozoon.

spermatocyte /spər'mætoʊ,saɪt/ *n* a cell that develops into a male germ cell.

spermatogenesis /spər,mætoʊ'dʒɛnɪsɪs/ *n* the formation and development of spermatozoa in the testis.—**spermatogenetic** *adj*.

spermatogonium /spər,mætoʊ'goʊniəm/ *n* (*pl* **spermatogonia**) an immature male germ cell.

spermatophyte /spər'mætoʊ,faɪt/ *n* a plant that produces seeds.—**spermatophytic** *adj*.

spermatozoon /spər,mætoʊ'zoʊɒn/ *n* (*pl* **spermatozoa**) any of the male reproductive cells present in the semen.

spermicide /'spɜːrmə,saɪd/ *n* a substance that destroys sperm.—**spermicidal** *adj*.

sperm oil *n* oil obtained from the head of the sperm whale.

sperm whale *n* a large whale with a blunt head which is hunted for its oil and spermaceti.

spew /spjuː/ *vti* to vomit; to flow or gush forth. • *n* something spewed.

sphagnum /'sfægnəm/ *or* /'spæg/ *n* a genus of moss which grows in bogs and is a major constituent of peat.

sphalerite /'sfælə,raɪt/ *see* **blende**.

sphenoid /'sfiːnɔɪd/ *adj* wedge-shaped; of or pertaining to the sphenoid bone. • *n* a sphenoid bone.

sphenoid bone *n* a wedge-shaped bone at the base of the skull.

sphere /sfɪːr/ *n* a ball, globe or other perfectly round object; a field of activity or interest; a social class.—**spherical, spheric** *adj*.—**spherically** *adv*.

spheroid /'sfɪːrɔɪd/ *n* a figure that is nearly a sphere.

spherometer /sfɪ'rɒmətər/ *n* an instrument for measuring the curvature of spherical surfaces.

spherule /'sfɛruːl/ *n* a small sphere.

sphincter /'sfɪŋktər/ *n* a ring-shaped muscle controlling the opening and closing of an orifice.

sphinx /sfɪŋks/ *n* (*with cap*) (*Greek myth*) a monster with a lion's body and human head which killed travellers who gave the wrong answer to a riddle; (*without cap*) any of various massive statues with a lion's body and human head erected by the ancient Egyptians; a mysterious or enigmatic person.

sphygmograph /,sfɪɡmoʊ'ɡrɑːf/ *n* a device that records variations in blood pressure and pulse.—**sphygmographic** *adj*.—**sphygmography** *n*.

sphygmomanometer /'sfɪɡmoʊmə'nɒmətər/ *n* a device for measuring arterial blood pressure.

spicate /'spɪkeɪt/ *adj* (*flowers, leaves*) spiked, pointed.

spicatto /spɪ'kætoʊ/ *or* /-'kɒtoʊ/ *n* (*pl* **spicattos**) (*mus*) (a musical piece or passage played using) a technique in which the bow is made to rebound lightly off the strings of an instrument.—*also* *adj*.

spice /spaɪs/ *n* an aromatic vegetable substance used for flavouring and seasoning food; these substances collectively; something that adds zest or interest. • *vt* to flavour with spice; to add zest to.

spicebush /'spaɪsbʊʃ/ *n* an aromatic North American plant.

spick-and-span *adj* scrupulously clean and tidy.

spicule /'spɪkjuːl/ *n* a small needle-like body in the skeleton of sponges, corals, etc; a jet of hot gas erupting from the surface of the sun.

spicy /'spaɪsi/ *adj* (**spicier, spiciest**) flavoured with spice; pungent; (*inf*) somewhat scandalous or indecent.—**spicily** *adv*.—**spiciness** *n*.

spider /'spaɪdər/ *n* a small wingless creature (arachnid) with eight legs, and abdominal spinnerets for spinning silk threads to make webs.

spider crab *n* any of various crabs with triangular bodies and very long legs.

spider monkey *n* a monkey of South and Central America with a slender body and long limbs.

spiderwort /'spaɪdər,wɜːrt/ *n* tradescantia.

spidery /'spaɪdəri/ *adj* thin, and angular, like a spider's legs.

spied *see* **spy**.

spiel /ʃpiːl/ *or* /spiːl/ *n* glib talk intended to cajole or persuade.—*also* *vi*.

spiffing /'spɪfɪŋ/ *n* (*sl*) (*arch*) excellent.

spiffy /'spɪfi/ *adj* (**spiffier, spiffiest**) smart, elegant.

spigo /'spɪɡət/ *n* a small stopper or tap for a cask; a tap.

spike /spaɪk/ *n* long heavy nail; a sharp-pointed projection, as on a shoe to prevent slipping; an ear of corn, etc; a cluster of stalkless flowers arranged on a long stem. • *vt* to pierce with a spike.—**spiky** *adj*

spikenard /'spaɪknɑrd/ *n* (a fragrant oil derived from) an Indian aromatic plant.

spilikin /'spɪlɪkɪn/ *see* **spillikin**

spill[1] /spɪl/ *vti* (**spilling, spilled** *or* **spilt**) to cause, *esp* unintentionally, to flow out of a container; to shed (blood). • *n* something spilled.—**spillage** *n*.

spill[2] *n* a splinter or thin strip of wood or twisted paper for lighting a fire, etc.

spillikin *n* a sliver of wood, cardboard or plastic.—*also* **spilikin**.

spillway /'spɪlweɪ/ *n* a channel for surplus water from a dam, etc.

spilt *see* **spill**[1].

spin /spɪn/ *vb* (**spinning, spun**) *vt* to rotate rapidly; to draw out and twist fibres into thread or yarn; (*spiders, silkworm, etc*) to make a web or cocoon; to draw out (a story) to a great length; (*with* **out**) to prolong, extend; to cause to last longer, *eg* money. • *vi* to seem to be spinning from dizziness; (*wheels*) to turn rapidly without imparting forward motion. • *n* a swift rotation; (*inf*) a brief, fast ride in a vehicle; an emphasis or slant imparted to information, proposals or policies.

spina bifida /ˌspaɪnəˈbɪfɪdə/ *n* a congenital abnormality in the formation of the spine causing the meninges to protrude, and associated with partial paralysis.

spinach /'spɪnɪtʃ/ *n* a plant with large, green edible leaves.

spinal /'spaɪnəl/ *adj* of or relating to the spine or spinal cord.—**spinally** *adv*.

spinal column *n* the skeleton of jointed vertebrae and interconnecting cartilaginous tissue that surrounds and protects the spinal cord.—*also* **spine, backbone**.

spinal cord *n* the cord of nerves enclosed by the spinal column.

spindle /'spɪndəl/ *n* the notched rod by which thread is twisted in spinning; a pin around which machinery turns.

spindly /'spɪndli/ *adj* (**spindlier, spindliest**) tall and slender; frail.

spindrift /'spɪndrɪft/ *n* sea spray.

spine /spaɪn/ *n* a sharp, stiff projection, as a thorn of the cactus or quill of a porcupine; a spinal column; the backbone of a book.

spine-chiller *n* a book, film, etc that inspires terror.—**spine-chilling** *adj*.

spineless /'spaɪnləs/ *adj* lacking a spine; weak-willed; irresolute.—**spinelessly** *adv*.—**spinelessness** *n*.

spinet /'spɪnət/ *or* /spɪ'nət/ *n* a type of small harpsichord.

spinifex /'spɪnɪˌfɛks/ *n* any of several coarse Australian grasses with spiny seed heads or spiked leaves.

spinnaker /'spɪnəkər/ *n* a large triangular sail sometimes carried by racing yachts.

spinner /'spɪnər/ *n* a revolving fishing lure; (*cricket*) a ball bowled with a spin, or a bowler who does this.

spinneret /'spɪnəˌrɛt/ *n* an organ in spiders and other insects for producing silk threads.

spinning wheel *n* a small household machine with a wheel-driven spindle for spinning yarn from fibre.

spin-off /'spɪnɒf/ *n* a product or benefit derived incidentally from existing research and development.

spinose /'spaɪnoːs/ *adj* (*plants*) spiny.

spinster /'spɪnstər/ *n* an unmarried woman.

spiny /spaɪni/ *adj* (**spinier, spiniest**) covered with spines or thorns; troublesome.

spiny anteater *n* the echidna.

spiny lobster *n* any of several large edible crustaceans with a spiny shell.

spiracle /'spaɪrəkəl/ *n* a respiratory aperture in various insects and some fishes; the blowhole in whales.

spiraea, spirea /ˌspaɪ'riːə/ *n* any of various plants of the rose family having clusters of small white or pink flowers.

spiral /'spaɪrəl/ *adj* winding round in a continuous curve up or down a centre or pole. • *n* a helix; a spiral line or shape; a continuous expansion or decrease, *eg* in inflation. • *vi* (**spiralling, spiralled** *or* **spiraling, spiraled**) to move up or down in a spiral curve; to increase or decrease steadily.

spiral galaxy *n* a galaxy in which two arms consisting of new stars spiral outward from an ellipsoidal nucleus of old stars.

spire /'spaɪr/ *n* the tapering point of a steeple.

spirillum /ˌspaɪ'rɪləm/ *n* (*pl* **spirilla**) a bacterium with a curved or spiral body.

spirit /'spiːrɪt/ *or* /'spɪrɪt/ *n* soul; a supernatural being, as a ghost, angel, etc; (*pl*) disposition; mood; vivacity, courage, etc; real meaning; essential quality; (*usu pl*) distilled alcoholic liquor. • *vt* to carry (away, off, etc) secretly and swiftly.

spirited /'spɪrɪtəd/ *adj* full of life; animated.—**spiritedly** *adv*.—**spiritedness** *n*.

spirit level *n* a glass tube filled with liquid containing an air bubble and mounted in a frame, used for testing whether a surface is level.

spiritual /'spɪrɪtʃʊəl/ *adj* of the soul; religious; sacred. • *n* an emotional religious song, originating among the Black slaves in the American South.—**spirituality** *n*.—**spiritually** *adv*.

spiritualism /'spɪrɪtʃʊəˌlɪzəm/ *n* the belief that the spirits of the dead can communicate with the living, as through mediums.—**spiritualist** *n*.

spirochaete, spirochete /'spaɪrəˌkiːt/ *n* any of a genus of slender spiral-shaped bacteria that includes those causing syphilis.

spirograph /'spaɪrəˌgræf/ *n* a device that records respiratory movements.—**spirographic** *adj*.

spirt *see* **spurt**.

spit[1] /spɪt/ *n* a pointed iron rod on which meat is roasted; a long narrow strip of land projecting into the water. • *vt* (**spitting, spitted**) to fix as on a spit, impale.

spit[2] *vb* (**spitting, spat** *or* **spit**) *vt* to eject from the mouth; to utter with scorn. • *vi* to expel saliva from the mouth; (*hot fat*) to splutter; to rain lightly. • *n* saliva.

spit and polish *n* (*inf*) obsession with neatness and cleanliness, *esp* in the military services.

spite /spaɪt/ *n* ill will; malice. • *vt* to annoy spitefully, to vex.—**spiteful** *adj*.

spitting image *n* (*inf*) a person who almost exactly resembles another.

spittle /'spɪtəl/ *n* saliva ejected from the mouth.

spittoon /spɪ'tuːn/ *n* a *usu* metal pan for spitting into, a cuspidor.

spiv /spɪv/ *n* (*sl*) a person of smart appearance who lives by shady dealings, *esp* on the black market.

splake /spleɪk/ *n* ✦ a hybrid cross between a lake trout and a brook trout.

splanchnic /'splæŋknɪk/ *adj* of or pertaining to the viscera.

splash /splæʃ/ *vti* to spatter with liquid; to move with a splash; to display prominently; (*with* **down**) to land (a spacecraft) on water. • *n* something splashed; a patch of colour; a small amount, *esp* of a mixer added to an alcoholic drink.—**splashy** *adj*.

splashdown /'splæʃdaʊn/ *n* (the scheduled time of) the landing of a spacecraft on the ocean.

splatter /'splætər/ *vti* to splash, spatter.—*also n*.

splay /spleɪ/ *vti* to turn out at an angle; to spread out.

spleen /spliːn/ *n* a large lymphatic organ in the upper left part of the abdomen which modifies the blood structure; spitefulness; ill humour.

splendid /'splɛndɪd/ *adj* brilliant; magnificent; (*inf*) very good.—**splendidly** *adv*.—**splendidness** *n*.

splendiferous /splɛn'dɪfərəs/ *adj* (*inf*) splendid.

splendour, splendor /'splɛndər/ *n* brilliance; magnificence; grandeur.—**splendorous, splendrous** *adj*.

splenetic /splɪ'nɛtɪk/ *adj* of or pertaining to the spleen; spiteful; irritable.—**splenetically** *adv*.

splenic /'splinɪk/ *or* /'splɛnɪk/ *n* of, pertaining to, or in the spleen.

splenius /'spliːnɪəs/ *n* (*pl* **splenii**) either of the two muscles at either side of the back of the neck that move the head.—**splenial** *adj*.

splenomegaly /ˌspliːnoʊ'mɛgəli/ *n* distension of the spleen.

splice /splaɪs/ *vt* to unite (two ends of a rope) by intertwining the strands; to connect (two pieces of timber) by overlapping.—*also n*.

spline /splaɪn/ *n* a key or slot in a shaft that fits into grooves in a surrounding sleeve and locks the two together.

splint /splɪnt/ *n* a rigid structure used to immobilize and support a fractured limb; a splinter of wood for lighting fires. • *vt* to put in splints.

splinter /'splɪntər/ *n* a thin, sharp piece of wood, glass, or metal broken off. • *vti* to break off into splinters.—**splintery** *adj*.

splinter group *n* a small group that has split off from the main body.

split /splɪt/ *vti* (**splitting, split**) to break apart (*usu* into two pieces); to separate into factions; to divide into shares; to burst or tear. • *n* the act or process of splitting; a narrow gap made (as if) by splitting; a dessert consisting of sliced fruit, *esp* banana, with ice cream, nuts, etc; (*often pl*) the act of extending the legs in opposite directions and lowering the the body to the floor. • *adj* divided; torn; fractured.

split infinitive *n* (*gram*) an infinitive with another word between *to* and the verb.

split-level /-'levəl/ *adj* (*building*) having rooms or areas in one part less than a full story higher than another that adjoins them.

split personality *n* unstable in mood or behaviour; having two or more distinct personalities.

split-screen *n* (*cinema, television*) a technique involving the simultaneous projection of different images onto separate areas of the screen.

split second *n* a very brief moment, an instant.—**split-second** *adj*.

split shift *n* a shift in which the working hours are divided into two distinct periods.

splodge /splɒdʒ/, **splotch** *n* a large irregular spot, stain or smear. • *vt* to mark with a splodge or splotch.—**splodgy, splotchy** *adj*.

splurge /splɜrdʒ/ *vi* to spend lavishly (on); to show off. • *n* an extravagant display, *esp* of wealth.

splutter /'splʌtər/ *vi* to spit out food or drops of liquid noisily; to utter words confusedly and hurriedly.—*also n*.

spoil /spɔɪl/ *vb* (**spoiling, spoiled** *or* **spoilt**) *vt* to damage as to make useless, etc; to impair the enjoyment, etc, of; to overindulge (a child). • *vi* to become spoiled; to decay, etc, as food. • *npl* booty, valuables seized in war; the opportunities for financial gain from holding public office.

spoiler /'spɔɪlər/ *n* a projecting structure on an aircraft wing that increases drag to reduce lift; any similar structure for increasing the stability of vehicles at high speed.

spoil-sport /'spɔɪlspɔrt/ *n* (*inf*) a person who spoils the fun of others.

spoilt /spɔɪlt/ *see* **spoil**.

spoke¹ /spoːk/ **spoken** *see* **speak**.

spoke² *n* any of the braces extending from the hub to the rim of a wheel.

spokeshave /'spoːkʃeɪv/ *n* a small two-handled plane used for smoothing curved surfaces.

spokesman /'spoːksmən/ *n* (*pl* **spokesmen**) a person authorized to speak on behalf of others.—**spokeswoman** *nf* (*pl* **spokeswomen**).

spondylitis /ˌspɒndɪ'laɪtɪs/ *n* inflammation of the vertebrae.

sponge /spʌndʒ/ *n* a plantlike marine animal with an internal skeleton of elastic interlacing horny fibres; a piece of natural or manmade sponge for washing or cleaning. • *vt* to wipe with a sponge. • *vi* (*inf*) to scrounge.—**sponginess** *n*.—**spongy** *adj*.

sponge bag *n* a small waterproof bag for toilet articles, a washbag.

sponge cake *n* a sweet cake with a light porous texture.

sponson /'spɒnsən/ *n* a projecting gun-mounting on a ship or tank, etc to allow forward fire; an air-filled projection on the hull of a seaplane to provide stability.

sponsor /'spɒnsər/ *n* a person or organization that pays the expenses connected with an artistic production or sports event in return for advertising; in US, a business firm, etc that pays for a radio or TV programme advertising its product. • *vt* to act as sponsor for.—**sponsorship** *n*.

spontaneity /ˌspɒntə'neɪɪtiː/ *n* (*pl* **spontaneities**) the quality of being spontaneous; a spontaneous action, etc.

spontaneous /spɒn'teɪnɪəs/ *adj* arising naturally; unpremeditated.—**spontaneously** *adv*.—**spontaneousness** *n*.

spontaneous combustion *n* the self-igniting of a substance through internal chemical processes such as oxidation.

spontaneous generation *n* abiogenesis.

spoof /spuːf/ *n* (*sl*) a hoax or joke; a light satire.—*also vti*.

spook /spuːk/ *n* (*inf*) a ghost; (*inf*) a spy. • *vt* to frighten.—**spooky** *adj*.

spool /spuːl/ *n* a cylinder, bobbin, or reel, upon which thread, photographic film, etc, are wound. • *vt* to wind on a spool.

spoon /spuːn/ *n* utensil with a shallow bowl and a handle, for eating, stirring, etc.—**spoonful** *n*.

spoonbill /'spuːnbɪl/ *n* any of various wading birds with flattened bills.

spoonerism /'spuːnəˌrɪzəm/ *n* the accidental transposition of the initial letters or opening syllables of two or more words with amusing results, *eg half-warmed fish* for *half-formed wish*.

spoor /spʊr/ *n* a trail, *esp* of a wild animal. • *vti* to track (something) by a spoor.

sporadic /spə'rædɪk/ *adj* occurring here and there; intermittent.—**sporadically** *adv*.

sporangium /spə'rændʒəm/ *n* (*pl* **sporangia**) (*in fungi, etc*) an organ or part in which asexual spores are produced.

spore /spɔr/ *n* an asexual reproductive body produced by algae, fungae and ferns capable of giving rise to new individuals.

sporogenesis /ˌspɔrə'dʒenəsɪs/ *n* the formation of spores in plants and animals.—**sporogenous** *adj*.

sporozoan /ˌspɔrə'zoːən/ *n* any of a group of spore-producing parasitic protozoans that includes the malaria parasite.

sporran /'spɒrən/ *n* an ornamental pouch worn in front of the kilt as part of traditional Highland dress in Scotland.

sport /spɔrt/ *n* an athletic game or pastime, often competitive and involving physical capability; good-humoured joking; (*inf*) a person regarded as fair and abiding by the rules. • *vi* to play, to frolic. • *vt* (*inf*) to display, flaunt.

sporting /'spɔrtɪŋ/ *adj* interested in, concerned with, or suitable for sport; exhibiting sportsmanship; willing to take a risk.—**sportingly** *adv*.

sportive /'spɔrtɪv/ *adj* playful.—**sportively** *adv*.—**sportiveness** *n*.

sportscast /'spɔrtskæst/ *n* a sports broadcast.—**sportscaster** *n*.

sportsman /'spɔrtsmən/ *n* (*pl* **sportsmen**) a person engaged in sport; a person who plays by the rules, is fair, is a good loser, etc.—**sportswoman** *nf* (*pl* **sportswomen**).—**sportsman-like, sportsmanly** *adj*.—**sportsmanship** *n*.

sports medicine *n* the branch of medicine dealing with sports injuries.

sporty /'spɔrti/ *adj* (**sportier, sportiest**) (*inf*) fond of sport; flashy, ostentatious.—**sportily** *adv*.—**sportiness** *n*.

sporule /'spɔruːl/ *n* a tiny spore.

spot /spɒt/ *n* a small area differing in colour, etc, from the surrounding area; a stain, speck, etc; a taint on character or reputation; a small quantity or amount; a locality; (*inf*) a difficult or embarrassing situation; a place on an entertainment programme; a spotlight. • *vt* (**spotting, spotted**) to mark with spots; (*inf*) to identify or recognise; to glimpse.

spot check /'spɒt'tʃek/ *n* a sudden random examination.—**spot-check** *vt*.

spotless /'spɒtləs/ *adj* immaculate.—**spotlessly** *adv*.—**spotlessness** *n*.

spotlight /'spɒtlaɪt/ *n* a powerful light used to illuminate a small area; intense public attention. • *vt* (**spotlighting, spotlighted** *or* **spotlit**) to illuminate with a spotlight; to focus attention on.

spot on *adj* (*inf*) absolutely right.

spotted dick /'spɒtɪd/ *n* a steamed pudding made with suet and currants.

spotty /'spɒti/ *adj* (**spottier, spottiest**) marked with spots, *esp* on the skin; intermittent, uneven.—**spottily** *adv*.—**spottiness** *n*.

spot-weld *vt* to join two pieces of metal with circular welds.—**spot-welder** *n*.—**spot welding** *n*.

spouse /spaʊs/ *n* (one's) husband or wife.

spout /spaʊt/ *vti* to eject in a strong jet or spurts; (*inf*) to drone on boringly. • *n* a projecting lip or tube for pouring out liquids.

spp *abbr* = species (*pl*).

SPQR *abbr* = *Senatus Populusque Romanus* (the Senate and People of Rome).

sprain /spreɪn/ *n* a wrenching of a joint by sudden twisting or tearing of ligaments.—*also vt*.

sprang /spræŋ/ *see* **spring**.

sprat /spræt/ *n* a small food fish related to the herring; a small or young herring.

sprawl /sprɔl/ *vi* to lie down with the limbs stretched out in an untidy manner; to spread out in a straggling way. • *n* a sprawling position.

spray¹ /spreɪ/ *n* fine particles of a liquid; mist; an aerosol or atomizer. • *vti* to direct a spray (on); to apply as a spray.

spray² *n* a number of flowers on one branch; a decorative flower arrangement; an ornament resembling this.

spray gun *n* a device for applying paint, varnish, etc in the form of a spray.

spread /spred/ *vt* (**spreading, spread**) to extend; to unfold or open; to disseminate; to distribute; to apply a coating (*eg* butter).

• *vi* to expand in all directions. • *n* an expanse; (*inf*) a feast; food which can be spread on bread; a bed cover.

spread eagle *n* an emblem of an eagle with wings and legs stretched out.

spread-eagle /'spred,i:gəl/ *vt* to stand or lie with the limbs outstretched.—**spread-eagled** *adj*.

spreadsheet /'spredʃi:t/ *n* a computer program that allows easy entry and manipulation of text and figures, used for accounting and financial planning.

spree /spri:/ *n* (*inf*) excessive indulgence, *eg* in spending money, alcohol consumption, etc.

spree killer *n* one who kills a group or number of people in an unpremeditated at a single site or location.

sprier /spraɪər/ *see* spry.

sprig /sprɪg/ *n* a twig with leaves on it.

sprightly /'spraɪtli/ *adj* (**sprightlier, sprightliest**) full of life or energy.—**sprightliness** *n*.

spring /sprɪŋ/ *vb* (**springing, sprang** *or* **sprung,** *pp* **sprung**) *vi* to move suddenly, as by elastic force; to arise suddenly; to originate. • *vt* to cause to spring up, to cause to operate suddenly. • *n* a leap; the season between winter and summer; a coiled piece of wire that springs back to its original shape when stretched; the source of a stream.

spring balance *n* a device that measures weight by the tension of a spring linked to a pointer on a calibrated scale.—*also* **spring scale**.

springboard /'sprɪŋbɔrd/ *n* a flexible board used by divers and in gymnastics to provided added height or impetus.

springbok /'sprɪŋbɒk/ *n* a South African gazelle.

spring break-up *n* ✤ (*Cdn*) the breakup of solid ice in a body of water in the spring.

spring chicken *n* a young chicken from two to ten months old; (*inf*) a young inexperienced person.

spring-clean /-'kli:n/ *vi* to clean (a house, etc) thoroughly.—**spring clean** *n*.

springe /sprɪndʒ/ *n* a snare for catching small animals.

spring onion *n* a scallion.

spring roll *n* a Chinese savoury snack comprising a mixture of beansprouts, chopped meat, etc rolled in a thin pancake and fried.

spring scale *see* **spring balance**.

springtail /'sprɪŋteɪl/ *n* any of various small wingless leaping insects.

spring tide *n* a high tide that occurs at the full or new moon.

springtime /'sprɪŋtaɪm/ *n* the season of spring; the earliest and most promising period in the life of something or someone.

springy /'sprɪŋi/ *adj* (**springier, springiest**) elastic, resilient; light, spongy.—**springily** *adv*.—**springiness** *n*.

sprinkle /'sprɪŋkəl/ *vt* to scatter in droplets or particles (on something).—*also* *n*.

sprinkler /'sprɪŋklər/ *n* a nozzle for spraying water; a fire-extinguishing system that operates automatically on detection of smoke or heat.

sprinkling /'sprɪŋklɪŋ/ *n* a small quantity scattered randomly.

sprint /sprɪnt/ *n* a short run or race at full speed. • *vi* to go at top speed.—**sprinter** *n*.

sprit /sprɪt/ *n* a small spar which runs from the mast to the outer upper corner of a sail.

sprite /spraɪt/ *n* an elf or imp; a dainty person.

spritsail /'sprɪtsəl/ *or* /-seɪl/ *n* a sail extended by a sprit.

spritzer /'sprɪtsər/ *n* a drink made with wine, *usu* white, and soda water.

sprocket /'sprɒkət/ *n* a wheel with a row of teeth which engage the holes in a chain, or a reel of film, in order to turn it.

sprout /spraʊt/ *n* a new shoot on a plant; a small cabbage-like vegetable. • *vt* to put forth (shoots). • *vi* to begin to grow.

spruce[1] /spru:s/ *adj* smart, neat, trim. • *vt* to smarten.

spruce[2] *n* an evergreen tree of the pine family with a conical head and soft light wood.

spruce grouse *n* ✤ a grouse of North American softwood forests.

sprung /sprʌŋ/ *see* **spring**.

spry /spraɪ/ *adj* (**sprier, spriest** *or* **spryer, spryest**) vigorous, agile.—**spryly** *adv*.—**spryness** *n*.

spud /spʌd/ *n* a small narrow digging tool; (*inf*) a potato. • *vt* (**spudding, spudded**) to dig with a spud.—**spudder** *n*.

spume /spju:m/ *n* foam; surf; froth.

spun /spʌn/ *see* **spin**.

spunk /spʌŋk/ *n* a spark, a match; (*sl*) pluck, courage.

spunky /'spʌŋki/ *adj* (**spunkier, spunkiest**) full of courage; spirited.—**spunkily** *adv*.—**spunkiness** *n*.

spun silk *n* a shiny material made from silk waste.

spur /spər/ *n* a small metal wheel on a rider's heel, with sharp points for urging on the horse; encouragement, stimulus; a hard sharp projection. • *vt* (**spurring, spurred**) to urge on.

spurge /spərdʒ/ *n* any of various plants that produce a bitter milky juice.

spurious /'spəriəs/ *or* /'spjʊr-/ *adj* not legitimate or genuine; false.—**spuriously** *adv*.—**spuriousness** *n*.

spurn /spərn/ *vt* to reject with disdain. • *n* disdainful rejection.

spurt /spərt/ *vt* to gush forth in a sudden stream or jet. • *n* a sudden stream or jet; a burst of activity.—*also* **spirt**.

sputnik /'spʊtnɪk/ *or* /'sput-/ *n* the name used for series of artificial satellites launched by the former Soviet Union in the 1950s and 1960s (Russian for *travelling companion*).

sputter /'spʌtər/ *vi* to splutter.—*also* *n*.

sputum /'spju:təm/ *n* (*pl* **sputa**) saliva and mucus.

spy /spaɪ/ *n* (*pl* **spies**) a secret agent employed to collect information on rivals. • *vb* (**spying, spied**) *vi* to keep under secret surveillance, act as a spy (*usu with* **on**). • *vt* to catch sight of.

spyglass /'spaɪglæs/ *n* a small telescope.

sq *abbr* = sequence; squadron; square.

squab /skwɒb/ *n* (*pl* **squabs, squab**) a young bird, *esp* a pigeon; a stuffed cushion; a short fat person. • *adj* (*birds*) unfledged; short and fat.

squabble /'skwɒbəl/ *vi* to quarrel noisily. • *n* a noisy, petty quarrel.—*also* *n*.

squad /skwɒd/ *n* a small group of soldiers which form a working unit; a section of a police force; (*sport*) a group of players from which a team is selected.

squadron /'skwɒdrən/ *n* a unit of warships, cavalry, military aircraft, etc.

squalid /'skwɒlɪd/ *adj* filthy; neglected, sordid; degrading.—**squalidly** *adv*.—**squalidness** *n*.

squall /skwɔl/ *vi* to cry out loudly (like a baby). • *n* a loud cry; a violent gust of wind.

squalor /'skwɒlər/ *n* foulness; dirt, filth.

squama /'skweɪmə/ *n* (*pl* **squamae**) (*biol*) (something resembling) a scale.

squander /'skwɒndər/ *vt* to spend extravagantly or wastefully.

square /skwɛr/ *n* a shape with four sides of equal length and four right angles; an open space in a town, surrounded by buildings; (*inf*) an old-fashioned person; an instrument for drawing right angles; the product of a number multiplied by itself. • *adj* square-shaped; forming a square; forming a right angle (with); (*financial account*) settled; fair, honest; equal in score; (*inf*) old-fashioned. • *vt* to make square; to multiply (a quantity) by itself; (*with* **away**) (*inf*) to put in order, tidy up. • *vi* to agree.—**squarely** *adv*.—**squareness** *n*.

square bracket *n* either of a pair of written or printed characters [ ] used to enclose text or in mathematical expressions.

square dance *n* any of various dances in which the participants join hands to form squares.—**square-dance** *vi*.

square meal *n* a meal of satisfying quantity.

square measure *n* the measure of an area; the square of a lineal measure.

square root *n* a number that when multiplied by itself produces a given number (2 is the square root of 4).

square timber *n* ✤ (*Cdn*) (*hist*) logs cut into lengths with the round sides cut flat in order to be shipped more compactly.

squash[1] /skwɒʃ/ *vt* to squeeze, press, or crush; to suppress. • *vi* to squelch; to crowd. • *n* a crushed mass; a crowd of people pressed together; a fruit-flavoured drink; a game played in a walled court with rackets and rubber ball.—**squashy** *adj*.

squash[2] *n* (*pl* **squashes, squash**) a marrow or gourd eaten as a vegetable.

squat /skwɒt/ *vi* (**squatting, squatted**) to crouch down upon the heels; to occupy land or property, without permission or title. • *adj* short and dumpy. • *n* the act of squatting; a house that is occupied by squatters.

squatter /'skwɒtər/ *n* a person who squats.

squaw /skwɒ/ *n* a North American Indian woman.

squawk /skwɒk/ *n* a loud, raucous call or cry, as of a bird; (*inf*) a loud protest.—*also vi*.

squeak /skwi:k/ *vi* to make a high-pitched cry. • *n* a squeaky noise.—**squeaker** *n*.—**squeaky** *adj*.

squeaky-clean /'skwi:ki/ *adj* spotless; above reproach.

squeal /skwi:l/ *vi* to make a shrill and prolonged cry or sound; (*sl*) to be an informer; to protest.

squeamish /'skwi:mɪʃ/ *adj* easily nauseated; easily shocked or disgusted.—**squeamishly** *adv*.—**squeamishness** *n*.

squeegee /'skwi:dʒi:/ *n* a tool with a rubber-edged blade for scraping away excess water from a surface, *esp* a window. • *vt* (**squeegeeing, squeegeed**) to wipe clean with a squeegee.

squeeze /skwi:z/ *vt* to press firmly, compress; to grasp tightly; to hug; to force (through, into) by pressing; to extract liquid, juice, from by pressure; to obtain (money, etc) by force, to harass. • *n* squeezing or being squeezed; a hug; a small amount squeezed from something; a crowding together; financial pressure or hardship.—**squeezable** *adj*.

squelch /skwɛltʃ/ *vi* to walk through soft, wet ground, making a sucking noise. • *vt* to crush or squash completely. • *n* a squelching sound.

squib /skwɪb/ *n* a small firework that fizzes then explodes; a short, witty attack in speech or writing, a lampoon.

squid /skwɪd/ *n* (*pl* **squids, squid**) an edible mollusc, related to the cuttlefish, with a long body and ten arms.

squid jigger *n* ✲ (*Cdn*) in Newfoundland, a weighted line with many hooks, used to catch squid for use as bait.—**squid jigging** *n*.

squiffy /'skwɪfi/ *adj* (**squiffier, squiffiest**) slightly drunk.

squiggle /'skwɪgəl/ *n* a short wavy line, *esp* handwritten. • *vi* to squirm; to wriggle.—**squiggly** *adj*.

squill /skwɪl/ *n* a Mediterranean plant of the lilly family; a seashore variety of this whose bulbs were formerly used medicinally.

squint /skwɪnt/ *vi* to half close or cross the eyes; to glance sideways. • *n* crossed eyes, as caused by a visual disorder; a glance sideways; (*inf*) a look. • *adj* squinting; (*inf*) crooked.

squire /'skwaɪr/ *n* a country gentleman, *esp* the leading landowner in a district.

squirm /skwɜrm/ *vi* to writhe; to wriggle; to feel embarrassed or ashamed.

squirrel /'skwɜrəl/ *n* (*pl* **squirrels, squirrel**) a bushy tailed rodent with grey or reddish fur which lives in trees and feeds on nuts. • *vt* (**squirrelling, squirrelled** *or* **squirreling, squirreled**) (*usu with* **away**) to hoard.

squirrel cage *n* a small cylindrical cage which is rotated by a small animal running inside; the rotor of an induction motor with cylindrically arranged copper bars.

squirt /skwɜrt/ *vt* to eject liquid in a jet. • *vi* to spurt. • *n* a jet of liquid; (*inf*) an insignificant person.

squish /skwɪʃ/ *vt* to crush, *esp* so as to produce a squelching sound. • *vi* to make or move with a squelching sound. • *n* a soft squelching sound.—**squishy** *adj*.

Sr[1] (*chem symbol*) strontium.

Sr[2] *abbr* = Senior; Señor.

SRO *abbr* = standing room only.

SS[1] *abbr* = Saints; steamship;

SS[2] *abbr* = *Schutzstaffel*, the Nazi paramilitary police force elite guard.

St *abbr* = Saint.

St. *abbr* = Street.

stab /stæb/ *vt* (**stabbing, stabbed**) to injure with a knife or pointed weapon; to pain suddenly and sharply. • *vi* to thrust at (as if) with a pointed weapon. • *n* an act or instance of stabbing; a wound made by stabbing; a sudden sensation, as of emotion, pain, etc; (*inf*) an attempt.

stabile /'steɪbaɪl/ *n* an abstract sculpture resembling a mobile but stationary.

stabilize /'steɪbɪlaɪz/ *vti* to make or become stable or steady.—**stabilization** *n*.

stabilizer /'steɪbɪlaɪzər/ *n* a device for stabilizing (an aircraft, ship, bicycle, etc).

stable[1] /'steɪbəl/ *adj* steady or firm; firmly established; permanent; not decomposing readily.—**stability** *n*.

stable[2] *n* a building where horses or cattle are kept; a group of racehorses belonging to one owner; a group of people working for or trained by a specific establishment, as writers performers, etc. • *vti* to put, keep, or live in a stable.

staccato /stə'kætoː/ *or* /-'kptoː/ *adj* (*musical notes*) short, abrupt; (*speech*) sharp, abrupt, disconnected. • *adv* in a staccato manner.

stack /stæk/ *n* a large neatly arranged pile (of hay, papers, records, etc); a chimney stack; (*inf*) a large amount of; a number of aircraft circling an airport waiting for permission to land. • *vt* to pile, arrange in a stack.

stadia /'steɪdiə/ *see* **stadium**.

stadium /'steɪdiəm/ *n* (*pl* **stadium, stadia**) a sports ground surrounded by tiers of seats.

staff[1] /stæf/ *n* (*pl* **staves**) a strong stick or pole; (*mus*) one of the five horizontal lines upon which music is written.—*also* **stave**; (*pl* **staffs**) a body of officers who help a commanding officer, or perform special duties; the workers employed in an establishment; the teachers or lecturers of an educational institution. • *vt* to provide with staff.

stag /stæg/ *n* a full-grown male deer. • *adj* (*party*) for men only.

stag beetle *n* any of various beetles with large pincer-like mandibles.

stage /steɪdʒ/ *n* a degree or step in a process; a raised platform, *esp* for acting on; (*with* **the**) the theatre, the theatrical calling; any field of action or setting; a portion of a journey; a propulsion unit of a space rocket discarded when its fuel is spent. • *vt* to perform a play on the stage; to plan, organize (an event).

stagecoach /'steɪdʒkoːtʃ/ *n* a four-wheeled vehicle drawn by horses, that formerly carried passengers or mail.

stagecraft /'steɪdʒkræft/ *n* skill in writing or staging plays.

stage direction *n* an instruction in the text of a play (regarding characterization, movement, lighting, etc) for an actor or director.

stage door *n* the back entrance to a theatre used by the staff and players.

stage fright *n* nervousness at appearing before an audience.

stage left *n* the area of a stage to the left of an actor facing the audience.

stage-manage *vt* to act as a stage-manager; to organize or direct from behind the scenes.

stage manager *n* a person responsible for the stage arrangements prior to and during the performance of a play.

stage right *n* the area of a stage to the right of an actor facing the audience.

stage-struck *adj* obsessed with theatre and the idea of becoming an actor.

stage whisper *n* a loud whisper made by an actor and intentionally audible to the audience.

stagflation /stæg'fleɪʃən/ *n* an economic situation characterized by a combination of high inflation and stagnant or declining output and employment.

stagger /'stægər/ *vi* to walk unsteadily, to totter. • *vt* to astound; to give a shock to; to arrange so as not to overlap; to alternate.

staggering /'stægərɪŋ/ *adj* astounding.—**staggeringly** *adv*.

staging /'steɪdʒɪŋ/ *n* a temporary platform, *esp* horizontal planking supported by scaffolding.

staging area *n* an assembly point for troops in transit.

staging post *n* a regular stopover point on a long route.

stagnant /'stægnənt/ *adj* (*water*) not flowing, standing still with a revolting smell; unchanging, dull.—**stagnancy** *n*.

stagnate /'stægneɪt/ *vi* to be, or become, stagnant.—**stagnation** *n*.

stag party *n* a party for men only, *usu* given for one who is due to be married shortly.

stagy /'steɪdʒi/, **stagey** *adj* (**stagier, stagiest**) theatrical, dramatic.

staid /steɪd/ *adj* sober; sedate; old-fashioned.—**staidly** *adv*.—**staidness** *n*.

stain /steɪn/ *vt* to dye; to discolour with spots of something which cannot be removed. • *vi* to become stained; to produce stains. • *n* a discoloured mark; a moral blemish; a dye or liquid for staining materials, *eg* wood.

stained glass *n* coloured glass used in windows.

stainless /'steɪnləs/ *adj* free from stain; (materials) resistant to staining.—**stainlessly** *adv*.

stainless steel *n* a type of steel resistant to tarnishing and corrosion.

stair /'stɛr/ *n* a flight of stairs; a single step; (*pl*) a stairway.

staircase /'stɛrkeɪs/ *n* a flight of stairs with banisters.

stairway /'stɛrweɪ/ *n* a staircase.

stairwell /'stɛrwɛl/ *n* the vertical shaft for a staircase.

stake[1] /steɪk/ *n* a sharpened metal or wooden post driven into the ground, as a marker or fence post; a post to which persons were tied for execution by burning; this form of execution. • *vt* to support with, tie or tether to a stake; to mark out (land) with stakes; (*with* **out**) to put under surveillance.

stake[2] *vt* to bet; (*inf*) to provide with money or resources. • *n* a bet; a financial interest; (*pl*) money risked on a race; (*pl*) the prize in a race.

stakeout /'steɪkʊaʊt/ *n* surveillance, *esp* by police; premises under surveillance.

stalactite /stə'læk,taɪt/ or /'stælək-/ *n* an icicle-like calcium deposit hanging from the roof of a cave.

stalag /'stælæg/ *n* a German prisoner-of-war camp in World War II.

stalagmite /stə'læg,maɪt/ or /'stæ-/ *n* a cylindrical deposit projecting upward from the floor of a cave, caused by the dripping of water and lime from the roof.

stale /steɪl/ *adj* deteriorated from age; tainted; musty; stagnant; jaded.—**staleness** *n*.

stalemate /'steɪlmeɪt/ *n* (*chess*) a situation in which a king can only be moved in and out of check, thus causing a draw; a deadlock.—*also vt*.

Stalinism /'stælɪ,nɪzəm/ *n* the theory and practice of authoritarian rule associated with the Soviet dictator Joseph Stalin (1879–1953).—**Stalinist** *n, adj*.

stalk[1] /stɔk/ *n* the stem of a plant.

stalk[2] *vi* to stride in a stiff or angry way; to hunt (game, prey) stealthily.—**stalker** *n*.

stalking-horse *n* a means of concealing true intentions; a candidate standing in an election to confuse the opposition or test the amount of prospective support for the real candidate in whose favour the stand-in then withdraws.

stall[1] /stɔl/ *n* a compartment for one animal in a stable; a table or stand for the display or sale of goods; a stalling of an engine; (*aircraft*) a loss of lift and downward plunge due to an excessive decrease in airspeed; (*pl*) the seats on the ground floor of a theatre. • *vti* (*car engine*) to stop or cause to stop suddenly, *eg* by misuse of the clutch; (*aircraft*) to lose or cause to lose lift because of an excessive reduction in airspeed.

stall[2] *vti* to play for time; to postpone or delay. • *n* (*inf*) any action used in stalling.

stallion /'stæljən/ *n* an uncastrated male horse, *esp* one kept for breeding.

stalwart /'stɔlwərt/ *adj* strong, sturdy; resolute; dependable. • *n* a loyal, hardworking supporter.

stamen /'steɪmən/ *n* (*pl* **stamens, stamina**) the pollen-bearing part of a flower.

stamina /'stæmɪnə/ *n* strength; staying power.

staminate /'stæmɪnət/ or /-neɪt/ *adj* (*plants*) having or producing stamens.

stammer /'stæmər/ *vti* to pause or falter in speaking; to stutter.—*also n*.—**stammerer** *n*.

stamp /stæmp/ *vt* to put a mark on; to imprint with an official seal; to affix a postage stamp; (*with* **out**) to extinguish by stamping; to suppress, eradicate, by force. • *vi* to bring the foot down heavily (on). • *n* a postage stamp; the mark cancelling a postage stamp; a block for imprinting.

stamp duty, stamp tax *n* a tax on some types of legal documents.

stampede /stæm'piːd/ *n* an impulsive rush of a panic-stricken herd; a rush of a crowd.—*also vti*.

stamping ground *n* (*inf*) a favourite or habitual meeting place.

stance /stæns/ *n* posture; the attitude taken in a given situation.

stanch /stæntʃ/ see **staunch**[2].

stanchion /'stæntʃən/ *n* an upright post, pillar, rod or similar support. • *vt* to provide with a stanchion.

stand /stænd/ *vb* (**standing, stood**) *vi* to be in an upright position; to be on, or rise to one's feet; to make resistance; to remain unchanged; to endure, tolerate; to reach a deadlock; (*with* **by**) to look on without interfering; to be available for use if required; (*with* **down**) to withdraw, resign; to leave a witness box after testifying in court; (*soldier*) to go off duty; (*with* **off**) to remain at a distance; to reach a stalemate; (*with* **up**) to rise to one's feet. • *vt* to put upright; to endure, tolerate; (*with* **by**) to remain loyal to, to defend; (*with* **off**) to (cause to) keep at a distance; to lay off (employees) temporarily; (*with* **up**) to resist; to withstand criticism, close examination, etc; (*inf*) to fail to keep an appointment with. • *n* a strong opinion; a standing position; a standstill; a place for taxis awaiting hire; (*pl*) a structure for spectators; the place taken by a witness for testifying in court; a piece of furniture for hanging things from; a stall or booth for a small retail business.

standard /'stændərd/ *n* a flag, banner, or emblem; an upright pole, pillar; an authorized weight or measure; a criterion; an established or accepted level of achievement; (*pl*) moral principles. • *adj* serving as a standard; typical.

standard-bearer *n* a person who carries a standard; the leader of a particular cause or party.

standardize /'standardaɪz/ *vt* to make standard; to reduce to a standard.—**standardization** *n*.—**standardizer** *n*.

standard of living *n* the level of material comforts enjoyed by an individual, family, group or community.

stand-by /'stændbaɪ/ *n* (*pl* **stand-bys**) a person or thing held in readiness for use in an emergency, etc.—*also adj*.

stand-in *n* a substitute; a person who takes the place of an actor during the preparation of a scene or in stunts.—*also vi*.

standing /'stændɪŋ/ *n* status or reputation; length of service, duration. • *adj* upright; permanent; (*jump*) performed from a stationary position.

standing army *n* a permanent body of paid soldiers as maintained by a nation.

standing order *n* an instruction to a bank by a depositor to pay fixed amounts at regular intervals (for bills, etc); a regulation governing conduct, procedure, etc in an organization or assembly.

standoff /'stændɒf/ *n* a deadlock, stalemate.

standoffish /stænd'ɒfɪʃ/ *adj* aloof, reserved.

standpipe /'stændpaɪp/ *n* a vertical pipe with a tap providing an external water supply.

standpoint /'stændpɔɪnt/ *n* a point of view, opinion.

stand-up *adj* (*collar*) upright; (*fight*) furious; (*comedian*) telling jokes standing alone in front of an audience.

standstill /'stændstɪl/ *n* a complete halt.

stank /stæŋk/ *see* **stink**.

stannic /'stænɪk/ *adj* of or containing (tetravalent) tin.

stannous /'stænəs/ *adj* of or containing (bivalent) tin.

stanza /'stænzə/ *n* a group of lines which form a division of a poem.

staple[1] /'steɪpəl/ *n* a principal commodity of trade or industry of a region or nation; a main constituent. • *adj* chief.

staple[2] *n* a U-shaped thin piece of wire for fastening. • *vt* to fasten with a staple.

star /stɑr/ *n* any one of the celestial bodies, *esp* those visible by night which appear as small points of light, including planets, comets, meteors, and less commonly the sun and moon; a figure with five points; an exceptionally successful or skilful person; a famous actor, actress, musician, etc. • *vti* (**starring, starred**) to feature or be featured as a star.

starboard /'stɑrbərd/ or /-bərd/ *n* the right side of a ship or aircraft when facing the bow.

starch /stɑrtʃ/ *n* a white, tasteless, food substance found in potatoes, cereal, etc; a fabric stiffener based on this. • *vt* to stiffen with starch.—**starchy** *adj*.

star-crossed /'stɑr,krɒst/ *adj* ill-fated; unfortunate.

stardom /-dəm/ *n* the fame and status enjoyed by celebrities or stars.

stardust /'stɑrdʌst/ *n* a large cluster of distant stars appearing as dust; a feeling of romance.

stare /ster/ *vi* to gaze fixedly, as in horror, astonishment, etc; to glare. • *n* a fixed gaze.

starfish /'stɑrfɪʃ/ *n* (*pl* **starfish, starfishes**) an echinoderm consisting of a central disc from which five arms radiate outward.

stargaze /'stɑrgeɪz/ *vi* to look at the stars; to daydream.

stark /stɑrk/ *adj* bare; plain; blunt; utter. • *adv* completely.—**starkly** *adv*.—**starkness** *n*.

starkers /'stɑrkərz/ *adj* (*inf*) completely naked.

starlet /'stɑrlət/ *n* a young actress regarded as a potential star.

starling /'stɑrlɪŋ/ *n* any of a family of small songbirds, *esp* a common European bird with black plumage tinged with green that congregates in large groups.

Star of David a six-pointed star formed by two intersecting triangles, a hexagram.

starry-eyed /'stɑriaɪd/ *adj* dreamy, impractical, overly optimistic.

Stars and Stripes *n sing* (*with* **the**) the national flag of the USA consisting of 13 alternate red and white stripes and a blue square filled with white stars representing the individual states.—*also* **Star-Spangled Banner**.

Star Spangled Banner *n* (*with* **the**) the national anthem of the USA; the Stars and Stripes.

star-studded *adj* featuring many celebrities.

start /stɑrt/ *vi* to commence, begin; to jump involuntarily, from fright. • *vt* to begin. • *n* a beginning; a slight involuntary body movement; a career opening.

starter /'stɑrtər/ n a person who starts something, *esp* an official who signals the beginning of a race; a competitor in a race; the first course of a meal; a small electric motor used to start an internal combustion engine.—*also* **self-starter**.

starting block n one of a pair of angled wooden or metal pads or blocks against which a sprinter braces the feet in crouch starts.

starting gate n (*horseracing*) a removable barrier holding each horse in line and which is raised to start a race.

starting grid n (*motor racing*) the numbered grid where drivers line up at the start of a race, position being determined by the times gained in practice laps.

starting price n (*esp horseracing*) the final odds on a horse offered by bookmakers at the start of a race.

starting stalls npl the metal enclosures for horses at the starting line with gates that spring open simultaneously to start the race.

startle /'stɑrtəl/ vti to be, or cause to be, frightened or surprised.—**startling** adj.

starve /stɑrv/ vi to die or suffer from a lack of food. • vt deprive (a person) of food; to deprive (of) anything necessary.—**starvation** n.

star warrior n one who advocates the US's Strategic Defense Initiative.

Star Wars n sing the popular name for the Strategic Defense Initiative.

stash /stæʃ/ vt to hide (money, etc) for future use. • n a hiding place; something hidden; (sl) drugs hidden for personal consumption.

state /steɪt/ n condition; frame of mind; position in society; ceremonious style; (*with cap*) an area or community with its own government, or forming a federation under a sovereign government. • adj of the state or State; public; ceremonial. • vt to express in words; to specify, declare officially.

statecraft /'steɪtkræft/ n the art of government; statesmanship.

state department n the government department that handles foreign affairs; foreign office.

statehouse /'steɪthʊs/ n the building which houses a state legislature in the US.

stateless /'steɪtləs/ adj not having a nationality.—**statelessness** n.

stately /'steɪtli/ adj (**statelier, stateliest**) dignified; majestic.—**stateliness** n.

stately home n a large country mansion, *usu* of historical interest, which is open to the public.

statement /'steɪtmənt/ n a formal announcement; a declaration; a document showing one's bank balance.

statement of claim ✹ (*Cdn*) a legal document that states what a plaintiff seeks to establish as the outcome of a civil suit.

state-of-the-art adj using the most advanced technology yet possible.

stateroom /'steɪtruːm/ n a luxury private cabin in a ship; a large room in a palace used for state occasions.

States n sing or pl the USA.

state school n any school funded by the state which provides free education.

stateside /'steɪtsaɪd/ adj of, in, or to the US.—*also adv*.

statesman /'steɪtsmən/ n (pl **statesmen**) a well-known and experienced politician.—**statesmanship** n.

static /'stætɪk/ adj fixed; stationary; at rest. • n electrical interference causing noise on radio or TV.

statics /'stætɪks/ n sing the branch of mechanics dealing with the forces that produce a state of equilibrium.

static electricity n electricity which is stationary as opposed to flowing in a current.

station /'steɪʃən/ n a railway or bus terminal or stop; headquarters (of the emergency services); military headquarters; (*inf*) a TV channel; position in society, standing. • vt to assign to a post, place, office.

stationary /'steɪʃənɛri/ adj not moving.

stationer /'steɪʃənər/ n a dealer in stationery, office supplies, etc.

stationery /'steɪʃənɛri/ or /'steɪʃənriː/ n writing materials, *esp* paper and envelopes.

station house n a building that houses police or fire services.

stationmaster /'steɪʃənmæstər/ or /-ˌmɒstər/ n the senior official in charge of a railway station.

station wagon n a car with extra carrying space reached through a rear door.

statism /'steɪtɪzəm/ n the concentration of economic and political power in the state.—**statist** n.

statistic /stə'tɪstɪk/ n a fact obtained from analysing information expressed in numbers.

statistics /stə'tɪstɪks/ n sing the branch of mathematics dealing with the collection, analysis and presentation of numerical data.—**statistical** adj.—**statistician** n.

stator /'steɪtər/ n the stationary part of a motor or generator.

statoscope /'stætəˌskoʊp/ n a sensitive aneroid barometer for indicating minute fluctuations in pressure, used in altimeters in aircraft.

statuary /'stætʃuˌɛri/ n (pl **statuaries**) statues collectively.

statue /'stætʃuː/ n a representation of a human or animal form that is carved or moulded.

statuesque /ˌstætʃuˈɛsk/ adj like a statue.—**statuesquely** adv.—**statuesqueness** n.

statuette /ˌstætʃuˈɛt/ n a small statue, figurine.

stature /'stætʃər/ n the standing height of a person; level of attainment.

status /'stætəs/ or /'steɪt-/ n (pl **statuses**) social or professional position or standing; prestige; condition or standing from the point of view of the law; position of affairs.

status Indian n ✹ (*Cdn*) a person who is officially registered as a member of a First Nations community.

status quo /ˌsteɪtəs 'kwoʊ/ or /ˌsteɪt-/ n the existing state of affairs.

status symbol n a possession that indicates high social standing, wealth, etc.

statute /'stætʃuːt/ n a law enacted by a legislature; a regulation.

statute book n a register of statutes enacted by a legislature.

statute law n law enacted by a legislature.

statute mile n (*formal*) a mile.

statute of limitations n a statute that restricts the period of time in which proceedings may be brought to enforce a right or punish an offence.

statutory /'stætʃətɔri/ or /'stætʃuːtɔri/ adj established, regulated, or required by statute.

staunch[1] /stɔntʃ/ adj loyal; dependable.—**staunchly** adv.—**staunchness** n.

staunch[2] vt to stem the flow of, as blood. • vi to cease to flow.—*also* **stanch**.

stave /steɪv/ n a piece of wood of a cask or barrel; (*mus*) a staff. • vt (**staving, staved** or **stove**) (*usu with* **in**) to smash or dent inward.

staves /steɪvz/ see **staff**.

stay[1] /steɪ/ n a rope supporting a mast.

stay[2] vi to remain in a place; to wait; to reside temporarily. • vt to support; to endure; to stop, restrain. • n a suspension of legal proceedings; a short time spent as a visitor or guest.

stay-at-home n a quiet, placid, unadventurous person.—*also adj*.

staying power n stamina.

St Bernard n a Saint Bernard dog.

STD abbr = sexually transmitted disease; subscriber trunk dialling.

steadfast /'stedfæst/ or /'stedfəst/ adj firm, fixed; resolute.—**steadfastly** adv.—**steadfastness** n.

steady /'stedi/ adj (**steadier, steadiest**) firm, stable; regular, constant; calm, unexcitable. • n (pl **steadies**) (*inf*) a regular boyfriend or girlfriend • vti (**steadying, steadied**) to make or become steady.—**steadily** adv.—**steadiness** n.

steady-state theory n the theory that the universe remains in a steady equilibrium as matter is continuously created as it expands.

steak /steɪk/ n a slice of meat, *esp* beef or fish, for grilling or frying.

steakhouse /'steɪkˌhaʊs/ n a restaurant that specializes in steaks.

steal /stiːl/ vt (**stealing, stole,** pp **stolen**) to take (from someone) dishonestly; to obtain secretly. • n (*inf*) an unbelievable bargain.

stealth /stelθ/ n a manner of moving quietly and secretly.

Stealth technology n the development, in great secrecy, of a new type of military aircraft.

stealthy /'stelθi/ adj (**stealthier, stealthiest**) acting or performed in a quiet, secret manner; unobtrusive, furtive.—**stealthily** adv.—**stealthiness** n.

steam /stiːm/ n the hot mist or vapour created by boiling water. • vi to give off steam; to move by steam power; to cook with steam; (sl) to take part in illegal steaming; (*with* **up**) (*glasses, windows*) to become covered in condensation. • adj driven by steam.

steamboat /'stiːmboʊt/ n a boat powered by steam.

steam engine *n* a stationary or locomotive engine powered by steam.

steamer /ˈstiːmər/ *n* a pan with a perforated bottom for cooking by steam; a ship propelled by steam engines; (*sl*) one who takes part in steaming.

steamie /ˈstiːmi/ *n* ✹ (*Cdn*) in Quebec, a steamed hot dog.

steaming /ˈstiːmɪŋ/ *n* (*sl*) the practice of multiple mugging by a gang of youths who move rapidly down a street, mugging and shiplifting.

steam iron *n* an electric iron that can heat water to use as steam which is emitted through the face to improve pressing.

steamroller /ˈstiːmˌroːlər/ *n* a vehicle with heavy rollers for pressing down road surfaces; an overpowering person or thing. • *vt* to crush (as if) with a steamroller; to obtain or influence by overpowering force.

steamy /ˈstiːmi/ *adj* (**steamier, steamiest**) full of steam; (*inf*) erotic.—**steamily** *adv*.—**steaminess** *n*.

stearic acid /ˈstiːrɪk/ or /stiːˈɑrɪk/ *n* a fatty acid derived from solid fats and used for making candles and soap.

steatite /ˈstiːətaɪt/ *n* soapstone.

steato- /ˈstiːtoː/ *prefix* fat.

steed /stiːd/ *n* (*arch, poet*) a horse.

steel /stiːl/ *n* an alloy of iron and carbon; strength or courage. • *adj* of, or like, steel. • *vt* to cover with steel; to harden; to nerve (oneself).

steel band *n* a band that uses percussion instruments made from oil drums.

steel grey *n* a bluish-grey colour.

steel wool *n* a compact mass of steel fibres used for scouring and polishing.

steely /ˈstiːli/ *adj* (**steelier, steeliest**) of or like steel; hard, relentless.—**steeliness** *n*.

steelyard /ˈstiːljɑrd/ *n* a balance using a pivoted graduated arm along which a weight slides.

steenbok /ˈstiːnbɒk/ or /ˈsteɪn-/ *n* (*pl* **steenboks, steenbok**) any of a genus of small antelopes of central and southern Africa.

steep¹ /stiːp/ *adj* sloping sharply; (*inf*) excessive, exorbitant.—**steeply** *adv*.—**steepness** *n*.

steep² *vti* to soak or be soaked in a liquid; to saturate; to imbue.—*also n*.

steepen /-ən/ *vti* to make or become steeper.

steeple /ˈstiːpəl/ *n* a tower of a church, with or without a spire; the spire alone.

steeplechase /ˈstiːpəlˌtʃeɪs/ *n* a horse race across country or on a course over jumps; a track race over hurdles and water jumps.—**steeplechaser** *n*.

steeplejack /ˈstiːpəlˌdʒæk/ *n* a person who climbs and repairs tall chimneys.

steer¹ /stiːr/ *n* a castrated male of the cattle family.

steer² *vti* to direct (a vehicle, ship, bicycle, etc) in the correct direction of travel.

steerage /ˈstiːrɪdʒ/ *n* the cheapest berths on a passenger ship.

steerageway /-ˌweɪ/ *n* a rate of forward motion that allows a vessel to be steered.

steering *n* the mechanism that controls the direction of a ship, vehicle, etc; the practice of manoeuvring non-white house buyers or tenants away from white areas.

steering committee *n* a committee that organizes the content and order of business for a legislative assembly.

stegosaur, stegosaurus /ˌstegəˈsɔrəs/ *n* (*pl* **stegosaurs, stegosauri**) any of various plant-eating dinosaurs with armoured body plates.

stein /staɪn/ *n* an earthenware beer mug, often with a hinged lid.

stele /stiːl/ or /ˈstiːli/ *n* (*pl* **stelae, steles**) an upright slab of stone with inscriptions dating from prehistoric times; an inscribed commemorative slab placed on the front of a building; the vascular tissue in the stems and roots of plants.

stellar /ˈstelər/ *adj* of, or composed of stars.

stellate /ˈsteleɪt/ or /-lət/ **stellated** *adj* of, resembling or composed of stars.

Steller's jay /ˈstelərz/ *n* ✹ a blue jay with a dark crest found in central and western North America.

stellular /ˈsteljʊlər/ *adj* filled with or composed of small stars; star-shaped.

St Elmo's fire *n* a flame-like electric discharge from a ship's mast and rigging in thundery weather, St Elmo's fire.—*also* **corposant**.

stem¹ /stem/ *n* a plant stalk; the upright slender part of anything, such as a wineglass; the root of a word. • *vi* (**stemming, stemmed**) to originate (from).

stem² *vt* (**stemming, stemmed**) to stop, check (the flow or tide).

stench /stentʃ/ *n* a foul odour.

stencil /ˈstensəl/ *n* a pierced sheet of card or metal for reproducing letters by applying paint; a design so made. • *vti* (**stencilling, stencilled** or **stenciling, stenciled**) to produce (letters, etc) or designs using a stencil.—**stenciller, stenciler** *n*.

Sten gun /stengən/ *n* a light sub-machine gun.

stenography /stəˈnɒɡrəfi/ *n* shorthand.—**stenographer** *n*.

stenosis /stɪˈnoːsɪs/ *n* (*pl* **stenoses**) an abnormal narrowing of a bodily passage or orifice.—**stenotic** *adj*.

stentorian /stenˈtɔriən/ *adj* (*voice*) loud, booming.

step /step/ *n* one movement of the foot ahead in walking, running, or dancing; a pace; a grade or degree; a stage toward a goal; one tread of a stair, rung of a ladder. • *vti* (**stepping, stepped**) to take a step or a number of paces.

step- /step/ *prefix* related by remarriage of a spouse or parent.

stepbrother /ˈstepˌbrʌðər/ *n* a son of one's step-parent from a former marriage.

stepchild /ˈsteptʃaɪld/ *n* (*pl* **stepchildren**) a stepson or stepdaughter.

stepdaughter /ˈstepˌdɒtər/ *n* the daughter of one's spouse from a former marriage.

stepfather /ˈstepˌfʊðər/ *n* the husband of one's remarried mother.

stephanotis /ˌstefəˈnoːtɪs/ *n* a tropical climbing plant with fragrant white flowers.

stepladder /ˈstepˌlædər/ *n* a short portable ladder with flat steps fixed within a frame.

stepmother /ˈstepˌmʌðər/ *n* the wife of one's remarried father.

step-parent *n* stepfather or stepmother.

steppe /step/ *n* a vast grassy treeless plain.

stepping stone *n* a stone or stones allowing a stream, puddle, etc to be crossed by foot; a means of advancing toward some end.

stepsister /ˈstepˌsɪstər/ *n* the daughter of one's step-parent from a former marriage.

stepson /ˈstepsən/ *n* the son of one's spouse from a former marriage.

steradian /stəˈreɪdiən/ *n* a unit of solid angular measurement.

stere /stiːr/ *n* a unit equal to one cubic metre (35.3 cubic feet), used for measuring timber.

stereo /ˈsterioː/ *n* (*pl* **stereos**) a hi-fi or record player with two loudspeakers; stereophonic sound. • *adj* stereophonic.

stereochemistry /ˌsterioːˈkemɪstri/ *n* the study of the composition and properties of matter in relation to the spatial arrangement of atoms in molecules.

stereograph /ˈsterioːˌgræf/ *n* two almost identical images that when superimposed and viewed through a stereoscope produce a three-dimensional picture.

stereophonic /ˌsterioːˈfɒnɪk/ *adj* (*sound reproduction system*) using two separate channels for recording and transmission to create a spatial effect.—**stereophonically** *adv*.—**stereophony** *n*.

stereoscope /ˈsterioˌskoːp/ *n* an optical device which blends two images viewed from a slightly different aspect into a single three-dimensional picture.—**stereoscopic** *adj*.

stereoscopy /-ˈɒskəpi/ *n* viewing objects in three dimensions.

stereotype /ˈsterioˌtaɪp/ *n* a fixed, general image of a person or thing shared by many people.—*also vt*.

steric /ˈstiːrɪk/ *adj* of or pertaining to the spatial arrangement of atoms in a molecule.

sterile /ˈsteraɪl/ or /ˈsterɪl/ *adj* unable to produce offspring, fruit, seeds, or spores; fruitless; free from germs.—**sterility** *n*.

sterilize /ˈsterəˌlaɪz/ *vt* to render incapable of reproduction; to free from germs.—**sterilization** *n*.—**sterilizer** *n*.

sterling /ˈstɜrlɪŋ/ *n* the British system of money. • *adj* of excellent character.

stern¹ /stɜrn/ *adj* severe; austere, harsh.—**sternly** *adv*.—**sternness** *n*.

stern² *n* the rear part of a boat or ship.

sternum /ˈstɜrnəm/ *n* (*pl* **sterna, sternums**) the breastbone.

sternutation /ˌstɜrnjuːˈteɪʃən/ *n* sneezing.

sternutator /ˈstɜrnjuːˌteɪtər/ *n* a substance that induces sneezing, tears, etc, such as a gas used in riot control.

steroid /ˈsterɔɪd/ or /ˈstiːrɔɪd/ *n* any of a large number of compounds sharing the same chemical structure, including sterols and many hormones.

sterol /'sterɒl/ n any of various solid steroid alcohols, such as cholesterol, found in plants and animals.

stertorous /'stɔrtərəs/ adj characterized by heavy breathing or snoring sounds.—**stertorously** adv.—**stertorousness** n.

stet /stet/ vt a proofreading direction meaning that deleted matter marked by a row of dots should remain. • vt (**stetting, stetted**) to mark (text) in this way.

stethoscope /'steθə,skəʊp/ n an instrument used to detect body sounds.—**stethoscopic** adj.

stetson /'stetsən/ n a man's felt hat with a broad brim and high crown.

stevedore /'stiːvə,dɔr/ n a labourer who loads and unloads ships.

stew /stuː/ or /stjuː/ n a meal of cooked meat with vegetables. • vt to cook slowly.

steward /'stuːərd/ or /'stjuː-/ n a manager (of property); a race organizer; a person who serves food on an aircraft or ship and looks after passengers.

stewardess /'stuːərdes/ or /'stjuː-/ n a woman steward on an aircraft or ship.

stick[1] /stɪk/ vb (**sticking, stuck**) vt to pierce or stab to attach with glue, adhesive tape, etc; (with **up**) (inf) to rob at gunpoint. • vi to cling to, to adhere; to stay close to; to be held up; (with **around**) (inf) to wait in the vicinity, to linger; (with **by**) to remain faithful to; to stay close to.

stick[2] n a broken off shoot or branch of a tree; a walking stick; a hockey stick; a rod.

sticker /'stɪkər/ n an adhesive label or poster.

sticking plaster n a thin strip of cloth with an adhesive backing for covering small cuts and abrasions.

stick insect n a wingless insect with a long thin body resembling a twig.

stick-in-the-mud /'stɪk'nðə,mʌd/ n (inf) a person who feels threatened by new ideas or situations.

stickleback /'stɪkəl,bæk/ n any of various small freshwater fishes with sharp spines on the back.

stickler /'stɪklər/ n a person who is scrupulous or obstinate about something.

stick-up /'stɪkʌp/ n (inf) a robbery at gunpoint.

sticky /'stɪki/ adj (**stickier, stickiest**) covered with adhesive or something sweet; (weather) warm and humid; (inf) difficult.—**stickily** adv.—**stickiness** n.

sticky end n (inf) an unpleasant death.

sticky wicket n (cricket) a damp wicket that is difficult to bat on; (inf) an awkward or unpleasant situation.

stiff /stɪf/ adj not flexible or supple; rigid; firm; moving with difficulty; having aching joints and muscles; formal, unfriendly; (drink) potent; (breeze) strong; (penalty) severe. • n (sl) a corpse. • adv utterly.—**stiffly** adv.—**stiffness** n.

stiffen /'stɪfən/ vti to make or become stiff.—**stiffener** n.

stiff-necked /'stɪf,nekt/ adj stubborn, aloof.

stifle /'staɪfəl/ vt to suffocate; to smother; to suppress, hold back.

stifling /'staɪfəlɪŋ/ adj excessively hot and stuffy.

stigma /'stɪgmə/ n (pl **stigmas, stigmata**) a social disgrace; the part of a flower that receives pollen; (Christianity) marks resembling the wounds of Christ thought to appear on the bodies of saintly people.

stigmatize /'stɪgmə,taɪz/ vt to brand as bad or disgraceful.—**stigmatization** n.

stile /staɪl/ n a step, or set of steps, for climbing over a wall or fence.

stiletto /stɪ'letəʊ/ n (pl **stilettos**) a small slender dagger; a pointed tool for piercing holes in leather, etc; a high heel tapering to a point on a woman's shoe. • vt (**stilettoeing, stilettoed**) to stab with a stiletto.

still[1] /stɪl/ adj motionless; calm; silent; (drink) not carbonated. • n a single photograph taken from a cinema film. • vti to make or become still. • adv continuously; nevertheless.—**stillness** n.

still[2] n an apparatus for distilling liquids, esp spirits.

stillborn /'stɪlbɔrn/ adj born dead; (idea, project, etc) a failure from the start, abortive.

still life n (pl **still lives**) a painting of inanimate objects, such as flowers, fruit, etc.

stilt /stɪlt/ n either of a pair of poles with footrests on which one can walk, as in a circus; a supporting column.

stilted /'stɪltɪd/ adj (speech, writing) pompous, unnaturally formal; (conversation) forced, intermittent.

Stilton /'stɪltən/ n a blue-veined cheese with a strong flavour.

stimulant /'stɪmjʊlənt/ n a drug, drink, or food that increases one's heart rate and body activity.

stimulate /'stɪmjʊleɪt/ vt to excite, arouse.—**stimulation** n.

stimulus /'stɪmjʊləs/ n (pl **stimuli**) something that acts as an incentive; an agent that arouses or provokes a response in a living organism.

sting /stɪŋ/ n a sharp pointed organ of a bee, wasp, etc, or hair on a plant, used for injecting poison; a skin wound caused by injected poison from an insect or plant; (sl) a swindle. • vt to wound with a sting; to cause to suffer mentally; to goad, incite; (sl) to cheat by overcharging. • vi to feel a sharp pain.

stingray /'stɪŋreɪ/ n any of various rays with a whiplike tail bearing sharp venomous spines.

stingy /'stɪndʒi/ adj (**stingier, stingiest**) miserly, mean.—**stingily** adv.—**stinginess** n.

stink /stɪŋk/ vi (**stinking, stank** or **stunk, pp stunk**) to give out an offensive smell; (sl) to possess something in an excessive amount; (sl) to be extremely bad in quality. • n a foul smell.

stink bomb n a small glass capsule which releases a foul smell when broken, used for practical jokes.

stinker /'stɪŋkər/ n (inf) an offensive person or thing; (inf) something difficult or unpleasant.

stinkhorn /'stɪŋkhɔrn/ n a type of foul-smelling fungus.

stinko /'stɪŋkəʊ/ adj (sl) drunk.

stinkweed /'stɪŋkwiːd/ n any of various plants with pungent scents.

stint /stɪnt/ vt to be frugal in the supply or allowance of something. • vi to be frugal, miserly. • n a fixed period or quantity of work; a limitation, restriction.

stipe /staɪp/ n a short stalk or stem of a plant, esp of a mushroom.

stipend /'staɪpend/ n a regular payment of money as wages or for expenses, esp to a clergyman.

stipendiary /stɪ'pendjəri/ or /-iːeri/, /staɪ-/ adj of or receiving a stipend. • n (pl **stipendiaries**) a person who receives a stipend.

stipple /'stɪpəl/ vt to engrave, paint, draw, etc, in tiny dots.

stipulate /'stɪpjʊleɪt/ vt to specify as a condition of an agreement.—**stipulation** n.

stir[1] /stɜr/ vb (**stirring, stirred**) vt to mix, as with a spoon; to rouse; to stimulate or excite; (with **up**) to agitate, instigate. • vi to be disturbed; to move oneself; to be active. • n a stirring movement; tumult.

stir[2] n (sl) prison.

stir-fry /'stɜr,fraɪ/ vt to cook (chopped vegetables, etc) by stirring rapidly in hot oil in a wok or frying pan.

stirring /'stɜrɪŋ/ adj rousing, exciting.—**stirringly** adv.

stirrup /'stɜrəp/ n a strap and flat-bottomed ring hanging from a saddle, for a rider's foot.

stirrup cup n a farewell drink, orig given to a rider on horseback before departure.

stirrup pump n a small portable water pump held steady by a stirrup-shaped foot bracket, used for fire-fighting.

stitch /stɪtʃ/ n a single in-and-out movement of a threaded needle in sewing; a single loop of a yarn in knitting or crocheting; a sudden, sharp pain, esp in the side. • vti to sew.

stoat /stəʊt/ n a small European mammal related to the weasel.

stochastic /stə'kæstɪk/ adj random; involving chance or probability.

stock /stɒk/ n raw material; goods on hand; shares of corporate capital, or the certificates showing such ownership; lineage, family, race; a store; the cattle, horses, etc, kept on a farm; the broth obtained by boiling meat, bones, and vegetables as a foundation for soup, etc. • vt to supply; to keep in store. • adj standard; hackneyed.

stockade /stɒ'keɪd/ n a defensive enclosure or barrier of stakes fixed in the ground.

stockbroker /'stɒk,brəʊkər/ n a person who deals in stocks.

stock car n a standard production saloon car modified for racing.

stockholder /'stɒk,həʊldər/ n an owner of corporate stock.

stocking filler n a gift suitable for a Christmas stocking.

stocking /'stɒkɪŋ/ n a sock; a nylon covering for a woman's leg, supported by suspenders.

stock market, stock exchange n the market for dealing in stocks and shares.

stockpile /'stɒkpaɪl/ n a reserve supply of essentials.—also vt.

stock-still /'stɒk'stɪl/ adv motionless.

stocktaking /'stɒk,teɪkɪŋ/ n making an inventory of goods on hand (in a shop, warehouse, etc); evaluating one's present condition, resources, etc.

stocky /'stɒki/ *adj* (**stockier, stockiest**) short and sturdy.—**stockily** *adv.*—**stockiness** *n.*

stockyard /'stɒkjɑːd/ *n* a yard for holding cattle, sheep, pigs, etc before they are sold, transported, or slaughtered.

stodge /stɒdʒ/ *n* (*inf*) heavy, starchy food.

stodgy /'stɒdʒi/ *adj* (**stodgier, stodgiest**) (*food*) thick, heavy and indigestible; uninteresting.—**stodgily** *adv.*—**stodginess** *n.*

stoic /'stoɪk/ *n* a person who suffers hardship without showing emotion.—**stoical** *adj.*—**stoically** *adv.*—**stoicism** *n.*

stoke /stoːk/ *vt* to stir and feed (a fire) with fuel.

STOL /stɒl/ *abbr* = short take-off and landing, a system that allows an aircraft to take off and land within a short distance.

stole[1] /stoːl/ *see* **steal**.

stole[2] *n* a long scarf or piece of fur worn on the shoulders.

stolen /'stoːlən/ *see* **steal**.

stolid /'stɒlɪd/ *adj* impassive; unemotional.—**stolidity** *n.*—**stolidly** *adv.*

stoma /'stoːmə/ *n* (*pl* **stomata**) a minute aperture in the epidermis of a plant for the passage of gases; an orifice or mouthlike opening; a permanent surgical opening, *esp* in the abdominal wall.

stomach /'stʌmək/ *n* the organ where food is digested; the belly. • *vt* to put up with.

stomach pump *n* a suction pump that empties the contents of the stomach through a long tube inserted orally.

stomata /'stoːmætə/ *see* **stoma**.

stomatitis /ˌstoːmə'taɪtəs/ *n* inflammation of the mouth.

stomatology /ˌstoːmə'tɒlədʒi/ *n* the branch of medicine concerned with the mouth.—**stomatological** *adj.*

stomp /stɒmp/ *vti* to walk with heavy steps; to stamp. • *n* an early jazz dance.

stone /stoːn/ *n* a small lump of rock; a precious stone or gem; the hard seed of a fruit; (*pl* **stone**) a unit of weight (14 lb./6.35 kg). • *vt* to throw stones at; to remove stones from (fruit).

Stone Age *n* the prehistoric age of human culture characterized by the use of stone tools and weapons.

stoned /stoːnd/ *adj* (*inf*) under the influence of drink or drugs.

stonefish /'stoːnfɪʃ/ *n* (*pl* **stonefish, stonefishes**) a venomous tropical fish with markings that resemble a stone on the seabed.

Stone sheep *n* ✤ a wild, thin-horned sheep of the mountainous parts othe Yukon and northern Brtish Columbia.

stone's throw *n* a short distance.

stonewall /'stoːnwɒl/ *vi* to obstruct or hinder, *esp* in politics and government.

stonewashed /'stoːnwɒʃd/ *adj* (*clothes*) made to appear worn and faded by the abrasive action of pumice particles.

stony, stoney /'stoːni/ *adj* (**stonier, stoniest**) of, like, or full of stones; unfeeling, heartless.—**stonily** *adv.*—**stoniness** *n.*

stony-broke *adj* (*inf*) completely without money.

stony-hearted *adj* unfeeling, cruel.—**stony-heartedness** *n.*

stood /stuːd/ *see* **stand**.

stooge /stuːdʒ/ *n* (*sl*) a performer who feeds lines to a comedian; a person subordinate to or dominated by another; a stool pigeon. • *vi* to act as a stooge.

stool /stuːl/ *n* a seat or a support for the back when sitting, with no back or arms; matter evacuated from the bowels.

stool pigeon *n* a police informer.

stoop[1] /stuːp/ *vti* to bend the body forward and downward; to degrade oneself; to deign.—*also n.*

stoop[2] *n* a porch or small landing with stairs at the entrance to a house or building.

stooped /stuːpt/ *adj* hunched.

stop /stɒp/ *vb* (**stopping, stopped**) *vt* to halt; to prevent; to intercept; to plug or block. • *vi* to cease; to come to an end; to stay. • *n* an act or instance of stopping; an impediment; (a knob controlling) a set of organ pipes; any of the standard settings of the aperture in a camera lens, f-stop; a regular stopping place for a bus or train; a punctuation mark, *esp* full stop.

stop bath *n* a mildly acidic solution used to halt the development of a negative print, plate, etc.

stopcock /'stɒpkɒk/ *n* a device for regulating the flow of liquid in a pipe.

stopgap /'stɒpˌgæp/ *n* a temporary substitute, expedient.

stoplight /'stɒplaɪt/ *n* a red light on a traffic signal warning vehicles to halt; a brake light.

stopover /'stɒpˌoːvər/ *n* a short break in a journey.

stoppage /'stɒpɪdʒ/ *n* stopping or being stopped; an obstruction; a deduction from pay; a concerted cessation of work by employees, as during a strike.

stopper /'stɒpər/ *n* a cork or bung.

stop press *n* (the space reserved for) an item of last minute news added to a newspaper after printing has begun.

stopwatch /'stɒpwɒtʃ/ *n* a watch that can be started and stopped, used for timing sporting events.

storage /'stoːrɪdʒ/ *n* storing or being stored; an area reserved for storing; (*comput*) the storing of data in a computer memory or on disk, tape, etc.

storage battery *n* an accumulator.

storage capacity *n* the maximum amount of information that can be held in computer memory or a storage device.

storage device *n* a piece of computer equipment, such as a hard disk, used to store data.

storage heater *n* a radiator which accumulates heat during periods of off-peak electricity.

store /stoːr/ *n* a large supply of goods for future use; a warehouse; a shop. • *vt* to set aside; to put in a warehouse, etc; (*comput*) to put (data) into a computer memory or onto a storage device.

store card *n* a charge card issued by a store or chain of stores for the purchase of goods there only.

storehouse /'stoːrhəʊs/ *n* a place for storing things; a rich source or supply.

storey /'stoːri/ *n* (*pl* **storeys**) a horizontal division of a building, a story.

stork /stoːrk/ *n* a long-necked and long-legged wading bird.

storksbill /'stoːrksˌbɪl/ *n* any of several plants of the geranium family with pink or purple flowers.

storm /stoːrm/ *n* a heavy fall of rain, snow, etc with strong winds; a violent commotion; a furore; (*mil*) an attack on a fortified place. • *vt* to rush, invade. • *vi* to be angry; to rain, snow hard.—**stormy** *adj.*

stormbound /'stoːrmbaʊnd/ *adj* affected or confined by storms.

storm-stayed *adj* ✤ (*Cdn*) stranded in a place because of severe weather conditions, *esp* a snowstorm.

storm trooper *n* a member of the Sturmabteilung, a semi-military group of the German Nazi party (1924–45) notorious for its violence; a member of a shock troop.

Storting /'stoːrtɪŋ/, **Storthing** *n* the parliament of Norway.

story[1] /'stoːri/ *n* (*pl* **stories**) a narrative of real or imaginary events; a plot of a literary work; an anecdote; an account; (*inf*) a lie; a news article.

story[2] *n* (*pl* **stories**) a horizontal division of a building, a storey; a set of rooms occupying this space.

storyboard /'stoːriˌbɔːrd/ *n* (*films, television*) a sequence of drawings or photographs showing the images to be shot to film for a particular story.

stout /staʊt/ *adj* strong; short and plump; sturdy. • *n* strong dark beer.—**stoutly** *adv.*—**stoutness** *n.*

stouthearted /-ˌhɑrtɪd/ *adj* brave.—**stoutheartedly** *adv.*

stove[1] /stoːv/ *n* a cooker; heating apparatus.

stove[2] *see* **stave**.

stow /stoː/ *vt* to store, pack, in an orderly way.

stowage /'stoːɪdʒ/ *n* stowing or being stowed; goods in storage; a place for storage or the charge for this.

stowaway /'stoːəˌweɪ/ *n* a person who hides on a ship, car, aircraft etc to avoid paying the fare.

St Patrick's Day *abbr* = Saint Patrick's Day.

strabismus /strə'bɪzməs/ *n* a squint.

straddle /'strædəl/ *vt* to have one leg or support on either side of something.

strafe /streɪf/ *vt* to machine-gun (troops, vehicles, etc) from the air.—*also n.*

straggle /'strægəl/ *vi* to stray; to wander.—**straggler** *n.*—**straggly** *adj.*

straight /streɪt/ *adj* (*line*) continuing in one direction, not curved or bent; direct; honest; (*sl*) heterosexual; (*alcoholic drinks*) neat, not diluted. • *adv* directly; without delay. • *n* being straight; a straight line, form, or position; a straight part of a racetrack; (*poker*) a hand containing five cards in sequence.—**straightness** *n.*

straight and narrow *n* (*inf*) the honest and virtuous way of life.

straight angle *n* an angle of 180°.

straightaway /'streɪtəˌweɪ/ *adv* without delay.

straightedge /'streɪtedʒ/ *n* a length of wood, metal, etc used to rule or test for accurate straight lines.

straighten /'streɪtən/ *vti* to make or become straight; (*with* **out**) to make or become less confused or entangled; to resolve.

straight face *n* a face betraying no signs of emotion, *esp* amusement.—**straight-faced** *adj*.

straight fight *n* a contest between only two candidates.

straight flush *n* (*poker*) five cards of the same suit in sequence.

straightforward /streɪt'fɔrwərd/ *adj* honest, open; simple; easy.—**straightforwardly** *adv*.—**straightforwardness** *n*.

straightjacket /'streɪt,dʒækɪt/ *see* **straitjacket**.

straight-laced /-'leɪst/ *see* **strait-laced**.

straight man *n* a person who acts as a stooge to a comedian.

straight-out *adj* (*inf*) honest, direct; thorough.

strain[1] /streɪn/ *vt* to tax; to stretch; to overexert; to stress; to injure (a muscle) by overstretching; (food) to drain or sieve. • *n* overexertion; tension; an injury from straining.

strain[2] *n* a plant or animal within a species having a common characteristic; a trait; a trace.

strained /streɪnd/ *adj* (*action, behaviour*) produced by excessive effort; (*mood, atmosphere*) tense, worried.

strainer /'streɪnər/ *n* a sieve or colander used for straining liquids, pasta, tea, etc.

strait /streɪt/ *n* a channel of sea linking two larger seas (*usu pl*) difficulty, distress.

straitjacket /'streɪt,dʒækət/ *n* a coatlike device for restraining violent people; something that restricts or limits.—*also vt.* — *also* **straightjacket**.

strait-laced /'streɪt,leɪsd/ *adj* prim, morally strict.—*also* **straight-laced**.

strand[1] /strænd/ *vt* to run aground; to leave helpless, without transport or money.

strand[2] *n* a single piece of thread or wire twisted together to make a rope or cable; a tress of hair.—*also vt.*

strange /streɪndʒ/ *adj* peculiar; odd; unknown; unfamiliar.—**strangely** *adv*.—**strangeness** *n*.

stranger /'streɪndʒər/ *n* a person who is unknown; a new arrival to a place, town, social gathering, etc; a person who is unfamiliar with or ignorant of something.

strangle /'stræŋgəl/ *vt* to kill by compressing the windpipe, to choke; to stifle, suppress.—**strangler** *n*.

stranglehold /'stræŋgəl,hoːld/ *n* (*wrestling*) a grip that presses an opponent's windpipe; a powerful restrictive force or influence.

strangles /'stræŋgəlz/ *n sing* an infectious bacterial disease of horses that inflames the respiratory tract, equine distemper.

strangulate /'stræŋgjʊ,leɪt/ *vt* to strangle; to compress (*eg* a blood vessel or the intestine) so as to cause a blockage. • *vi* to become strangulated.—**strangulatation** *n*.

strangury /'stræŋgjʊri/ *n* slow, painful urination.

strap /stræp/ *n* a narrow strip of leather or cloth for carrying or holding (a bag, etc); a fastening, as on a shoe, wristwatch. • *vti* (**strapping, strapped**) to fasten with a strap; to beat with a strap.

straphanger /'stræp,hæŋər/ *n* (*inf*) a standing passenger in a bus or train, etc.

strapping /'stræpɪŋ/ *adj* tall, well-built.

strata /strætə/ *see* **stratum**.

stratagem /'strætədʒəm/ *n* a clever action planned to deceive or outwit an enemy.

strategic /strə'tiːdʒɪk/ **strategical** *adj* of, relating to, or important in strategy; (*weapons*) designed to strike at the enemy's homeland, not for use on the battlefield.—**strategically** *adv*.

Strategic Defense Initiative *n* the US government's proposed deployment of satellites armed with laser devices to destroy enemy missiles.

strategy /'strætədʒi/ *n* (*pl* **strategies**) the planning and conduct of war; a political, economic, or business policy.—**strategist** *n*.

strath /stræθ/ *n* (*Scot*) a wide, flat river valley.

strathspey /stræθ'speɪ/ *n* (the music for) a type of Scottish dance with slow gliding steps.

straticulate /stræti'kjuːleɪt/ *n* (*rocks*) having thin strata.

stratified /'stræti,faɪd/ *adj* arranged or deposited in strata or layers.—**stratification** *n*.

stratigraphy /strə'tɪgrəfi/ *n* (the scientific study of) the composition and order of rock strata.—**stratigraphic** *adj*.

stratocumulus /,stræto:'kjuːmjʊləs/ *n* (*pl* **stratocumuli**) layers of dark cloud in dense round masses.

stratosphere /'stræto,sfiːr/ *n* a layer of the earth's atmosphere above 10 km (6 miles) in which temperature increases with height.—**stratospheric** *adj*.

stratum /'strætəm/ *n* (*pl* **strata, stratums**) a layer of sedimentary rock; a level (of society).

stratus /'strætəs/ *n* (*pl* **strati**) a continuous horizontal layer of cloud.

straw /strɒ/ *n* the stalks of threshed grain; a tube for sucking up a drink.

strawberry /'strɔbəri/ or /-bəri/ *n* (*pl* **strawberries**) a soft red fruit used in desserts and jam.

strawberry blonde *adj* (*hair*) reddish blonde. • *n* a woman with hair of this colour.

strawberry mark *n* an irregular blood-coloured birth mark.

strawberry tree *n* a European evergreen tree bearing fruit resembling strawberries.

straw poll *n* an unofficial poll to assess public opinion.

stray /streɪ/ *vi* to wander; to deviate; to digress. • *n* a domestic animal that has become lost. • *adj* random.

streak /striːk/ *n* a line or long mark of contrasting colour; a flash of lightning; a characteristic, a trace. • *vti* to mark with or form streaks; to run naked in public as a prank.—**streaker** *n*.

streaky /'striːki/ *adj* (**streakier, streakiest**) marked with streaks; (*bacon*) having alternate layers of fat and lean.

stream /striːm/ *n* a small river, brook, etc; a flow of liquid; anything flowing and continuous. • *vi* to flow, gush.

streamer /'striːmər/ *n* a banner; a long decorative ribbon.

streamline /'striːmlaɪn/ *v* to shape (a car, boat, etc) in a way that lessens resistance through air or water; to make more efficient, to simplify.—**streamlined** *adj*.

street /striːt/ *n* a public road in a town or city lined with houses; such a road with its buildings and pavements; the people living working, etc, along a given street. • *adj* pertaining to urban youth culture.

streetcar /'striːtkər/ *n* an electrically powered vehicle for public transport, which travels along rails set into the ground, a tram.

street cred, street credibility *n* the mastery of the style and ways or urban culture.

street fighter *n* (*sl*) a person who is tough and combative.

street hockey *n* ✦ (*Cdn*) road hockey.

street value *n* the value of a commodity, *esp* an illegal drug, in terms of the price charged to the ultimate users.

streetwalker /'striːt,wɔkər/ *n* a prostitute who solicits in the streets.

streetwise /'striːt,twaɪz/ *adj* (*inf*) experienced in surviving or avoiding the potential dangers of urban life.

strength /streŋθ/ or /streŋkθ/ *n* the state or quality of being physically or mentally strong; power of exerting or withstanding pressure, stress, force; potency; effectiveness.

strengthen /'streŋθən/ or /'streŋkθən/ *vti* to make or become stronger.

strenuous /'strenjʊəs/ *adj* vigorous; requiring exertion.—**strenuously** *adv*.—**strenuousness** *n*.

strep /strep/ *n* (*inf*) a streptococcus.

strepitoso /,strepɪ'toːsoː/ *adv* (*mus*) in a boisterous manner.

streptococcus /,strepto:'kɒkəs/ *n* (*pl* **streptococci**) any of a genus of spherical bacteria occurring in chains of different length.

streptomycin /,strepto:'maɪsɪn/ *n* an antibiotic derived from a soil bacterium, used in the treatment of infections such as tuberculosis.

stress /stres/ *n* pressure; mental or physical tension or strain; emphasis; (*physics*) a system of forces producing or sustaining a strain. • *vt* to exert pressure on; to emphasize.

stretch /stretʃ/ *vt* to extend, to draw out. • *vi* to extend, spread; to extend (the limbs, body); to be capable of expanding, as in elastic material. • *n* the act of stretching or instance of being stretched; the capacity for being stretched; an expanse of time or space; (*sl*) a period of imprisonment.—**stretchy** *adj*.

stretcher /'stretʃər/ *n* a portable frame for carrying the sick or injured.

strew /struː/ *vt* (**strewing, strewed**, *pp* **strewn** *or* **strewed**) to scatter; to spread.

strewth /struːθ/ *interj* used to express surprise or alarm.

striation /straɪ'eɪʃən/ *n* any of a series of parallel grooves, scratches, ridges or lines on a surface.—**striated** *adj*.

stricken /'strɪkən/ *adj* suffering (from an illness); afflicted, as by something painful.

strict /strɪkt/ *adj* harsh, firm; enforcing rules rigorously; rigid.—**strictly** *adv*.—**strictness** *n*.

stricture /'strɪktʃər/ *n* harsh criticism, censure.
stride /straɪd/ *vi* (**striding, strode**, *pp* **stridden**) to walk with long steps. • *vt* to straddle.—*also n.*
strident /'straɪdənt/ *adj* loud and harsh.—**stridency** *n.*—**stridently** *adv.*
stridulate /'strɪdjʊˌleɪt/ *vi* (of insects) to make a chirping or scraping sound.
strife /straɪf/ *n* a fight, quarrel; struggle.
strike /straɪk/ *vb* (**striking, struck**) *vt* to hit; to crash into; (*mil*) to attack; to ignite (a match) by friction; (*disease, etc*) to afflict suddenly; to come upon, *esp* unexpectedly; to delete; (*clock*) to indicate by sounding; to assume (*eg* an attitude); to occur to; (*medal, coin*) to produce by stamping; (*flag, tent*) to lower, take down; to come upon (oil, ore, etc) by drilling or excavation; (*with* **down**) to afflict or cause to die suddenly; (*with* **off**) to delete or erase from (a list, etc); to prevent from continuing in a profession, *esp* due to malpractice; to sever or separate from (as if) with a blow; (*with* **out**) to erase or delete; (*with* **up**) to cause to begin, to bring about. • *vi* to cease work to enforce a demand (for higher wages or better working conditions). • *n* a stoppage of work; a military attack; (*with* **out**) to begin on a journey; (*baseball*) to be put out on strikes; (*inf*) to be completely unsuccessful; (*with* **up**) (*orchestra, band*) to begin to play or sing.
strikebound /'straɪkbaʊnd/ *adj* (*factory, etc*) closed or paralysed by striking workers.
strikebreaker /'straɪkˌbreɪkər/ *n* a person who continues work whilst colleagues are on strike; a person hired to replace a striking worker.—**strikebreaking** *n, adj.*
strike pay *n* money paid to workers on strike from trade union funds.
striker /'straɪkər/ *n* a worker who is on strike; a mechanism that strikes, as in a clock; (*soccer*) a forward player whose primary role is to score goals.
striking /'straɪkɪŋ/ *adj* impressive.—**strikingly** *adv.*
Strine /straɪn/ *n* Australian English (a humorous rendering of the Australian for *Australian*).
string /strɪŋ/ *n* a thin length of cord or twine used for tying, fastening, etc; a stretched length of catgut, wire, or other material in a musical instrument; (*pl*) the stringed instruments in an orchestra; their players; a line or series of things. • *vt* (**stringing, strung**) to thread on a string; (*with* **up**) (*sl*) to kill by hanging. • *vi* (*with* **along**) (*inf*) to appear to agree (with); to accompany; to deceive, *esp* to gain time.
stringed /strɪŋd/ *adj* (*musical instruments*) having strings.
stringent /'strɪndʒənt/ *adj* strict.—**stringently** *adv.*—**stringency** *n.*
stringer /'strɪŋər/ *n* a horizontal support in a structure; a long horizontal brace to strengthen a framework, as in an aircraft fuselage; a journalist or photographer temporarily employed by a newspaper, magazine or news service to cover a particular area.
string quartet *n* (a piece of music written for) a musical ensemble comprising two violins, one viola, and one cello.
string tie *n* a narrow tie.
stringy /'strɪŋi/ *adj* (**stringier, stringiest**) of or resembling string; (*meat, etc*) fibrous, chewy; (*physique*) sinewy.
strip /strɪp/ *vb* (**stripping, stripped**) *vt* to peel off; to divest; to take away removable parts. • *vi* to undress. • *n* a long, narrow piece of cloth, land, etc); an airstrip or runway.
strip cartoon *n* a series of drawings in a newspaper, etc which tell a story.
strip club *n* a nightclub which features striptease artists.
stripe /straɪp/ *n* a narrow band of a different colour from the background; a chevron worn on a military uniform to indicate rank. • *vt* to mark with a stripe.—**striped** *adj.*—**stripy** *adj.*
strip lighting *n* lighting using long fluorescent tubes.
stripling /'strɪplɪŋ/ *n* a youth, boy.
strip mining *n* mining by surface excavation, opencast mining.
stripper /'strɪpər/ *n* a striptease artist; a device or solvent that removes paint.
striptease /'strɪptiːz/ *n* an erotic show where a person removes their clothes slowly and seductively to music.
strive /straɪv/ *vi* (**striving, strove**, *pp* **striven**) to endeavour earnestly, labour hard, to struggle, contend.
strobe /stroːb/ *n* (*inf*) a stroboscope.
strobe lighting *n* (the equipment used to produce) high-intensity flashing light.

stroboscope /'stroːbəˌskoːp/ *n* a device for observing motion by making the subject visible at prescribed intervals using a synchronized flashing light.
strode /stroːd/ *see* **stride**.
stroganoff /'stroːgəˌnɒf/ *n* sliced beef cooked with mushrooms and onions in a sour cream sauce.
stroke[1] /stroːk/ *n* a blow or hit; (*med*) a seizure; the sound of a clock; (*sport*) an act of hitting a ball; a manner of swimming; the sweep of an oar in rowing; a movement of a pen, pencil, or paintbrush.
stroke[2] *vt* to caress; to do so as a sign of affection.
stroke play *n* (*golf*) scoring by the number of strokes taken.
stroll /stroːl/ *vi* to walk leisurely, to saunter. • *n* a leisurely walk for pleasure.
stroller /'stroːlər/ *n* a wheeled metal and canvas chair for a small child, a pushchair.
strong /strɒŋ/ *adj* physically or mentally powerful; potent; intense; healthy; convincing; powerfully affecting the sense of smell or taste, pungent. • *adv* effectively, vigorously.—**strongly** *adv.*
strong-arm *adj* using unwarranted physical force.
strongbox /'strɒŋbɒks/ *n* a solid, secure container for valuables.
strong drink *n* alcoholic drink.
stronghold /'strɒŋhoːld/ *n* a fortress; a centre of strength or support.
strong-minded *adj* resolute, determined.—**strong-mindedly** *adv.*—**strong-mindedness** *n.*
strong point *n* something at which one excels.
strongroom /'strɒŋruːm/ *n* a room specially designed to keep money and valuables secure from theft or fire, etc.
strontium /'strɒnʃiəm/ or /-ʃəm/, /-tiəm/ *n* a soft metallic element.
strop /strɒp/ *n* a strip of leather for sharpening a razor. • *vt* (**stropping, stropped**) to sharpen using a strop.
strophe /'stroːfi/ *n* a stanza or movement of a Greek chorus alternating with the antistrophe sung when moving to the left.—**strophic** *adj.*
stroppy /'strɒpi/ *adj* (**stroppier, stroppiest**) (*inf*) surly, angry; quarrelsome.
strove /stroːv/ *see* **strive**.
struck /strʌk/ *see* **strike**.
structuralism /'strʌktʃərəˌlɪzəm/ *n* a view of the social sciences, literature, linguistics, etc, which stresses the importance of inherent underlying hierarchical structures, interrelationships and patterns of organization.—**structuralist** *n.*
structure /'strʌktʃər/ *n* organization; construction; arrangement of parts in an organism, or of atoms in a molecule of a substance; system, framework; order. • *vt* to organize, to arrange; to build up.—**structural** *adj.*—**structurally** *adv.*
strudel /'struːdəl/ *n* very thin pastry rolled up with a fruit filling and baked.
struggle /'strʌgəl/ *vi* to move strenuously so as to escape; to strive; to fight; to exert strength; to make one's way (along, through, up, etc) with difficulty. • *n* a violent effort; a fight.
strum /strʌm/ *vt* (**strumming, strummed**) to play on (a guitar, etc), by moving the thumb across the strings.
struma /'struːmə/ *n* (*pl* **strumae**) enlargement of the thyroid gland; goitre.
strumpet /'strʌmpət/ *n* (*arch*) a prostitute.
strung /strʌŋ/ *see* **string**.
strung-up *adj* (*inf*) tense, anxious.
strut[1] /strʌt/ *vi* (**strutting, strutted**) to walk in a proud or pompous manner.
strut[2] *n* a brace or structural support. • *vt* to brace.
struthious /'struːθiəs/ *adj* (*birds*) related to or resembling the ostrich.
strychnine /'strɪknaɪn/ or /-niːn/, /-nɪn/ *n* a poison used in very small quantities as a stimulant.
stub /stʌb/ *n* a short piece left after the larger part has been removed or used; the counterfoil of a cheque, receipt, etc. • *vt* (**stubbing, stubbed**) to knock (one's toe or foot) painfully; to extinguish (a cigarette).
stubble /'stʌbəl/ *n* the stubs or stumps left in the ground when a crop has been harvested; any short, bristly growth, as of beard.—**stubbly** *adj.*
stubborn /'stʌbərn/ *adj* obstinate; persevering; determined, inflexible.—**stubbornly** *adv.*—**stubbornness** *n.*
stubby /'stʌbi/ *adj* (**stubbier, stubbiest**) short and thick; (*Austral sl*) a small bottle of beer.

stucco /'stɛkoː/ n (pl **stuccoes, stuccos**) a type of cement or plaster used to coat and decorate outside surfaces of walls. • vt (**stuccoing, stuccoed**) to decorate or finish with stucco.

stuck /stɛk/ see **stick**.

stuck-up adj (inf) conceited; proud; snobbish.

stud[1] /stʌd/ n a male animal, esp a horse, kept for breeding; a collection of horses and mares for breeding; a farm or stable for stud animals.

stud[2] n a large-headed nail; an ornamental fastener. • vt (**studding, studded**) to cover with studs.

studbook n a written record of the pedigree of a thoroughbred horse, dog, etc.

student /'stuːdənt/ or /'stjuː-/ n a person who studies or investigates a particular subject; a person who is enrolled for study at a school, college, university, etc.

studied /'stʌdiːd/ adj carefully planned.—**studiedly** adv.—**studiedness** n.

studio /'stuːdioː/ or /'stjuː-/ n (pl **studios**) the workshop of an artist, photographer or musician; (pl) a building where motion pictures are made; a room where television or radio programmes are recorded.

studio couch n a couch resembling a divan that can be converted into a bed.

studio flat n a small flat with one main room, a kitchen and a bathroom.

studious /'stuːdiəs/ or /'stjuː-/ adj given to study; careful.—**studiously** adv.—**studiousness** n.

study /'stʌdiː/ vt (**studying, studied**) to observe and investigate (eg phenomena) closely; to learn (eg a language); to scrutinize; to follow a course (at college, etc). • n (pl **studies**) the process of studying; a detailed investigation and analysis of a subject; the written report of a study of something; a room for studying.

stuff /stʌf/ n material; matter; textile fabrics; cloth, esp when woollen; personal possessions generally. • vt to cram or fill.

stuffed shirt n (inf) a pretentious or pompous person.

stuffing /'stʌfɪŋ/ n material used to stuff or fill anything; a seasoned mixture put inside poultry, meat, vegetables etc before cooking.

stuffy /'stʌfiː/ adj (**stuffier, stuffiest**) badly ventilated; lacking in fresh air; dull, uninspired.—**stuffily** adv.—**stuffiness** n.

stultify /'stɛltɪfaɪ/ vt (**stultifying, stultified**) to make ineffectual or futile.—**stultification** n.

stumble /'stɛmbəl/ vi to trip up or lose balance when walking; to falter; to discover by chance (with **across** or **on**). • n a trip; a blunder.

stumbling block n an obstacle to further progress.

stump /stɛmp/ n the part of a tree remaining in the ground after the trunk has been felled; the part of a limb, tooth, that remains after the larger part is cut off or destroyed. • vi (inf) to confuse, baffle; to campaign for an election.

stumpy /'stɛmpiː/ adj (**stumpier, stumpiest**) short and thick.—**stumpiness** n.

stun /stɛn/ vt (**stunning, stunned**) to render unconscious due to a fall or heavy blow; to surprise completely; to shock.

stung /stɛŋ/ see **sting**.

stun gun n a type of gun that emits high-voltage electricity to stun victims.

stunk /stɛŋk/ see **stink**.

stunner /'stɛnər/ n (inf) a strikingly attractive or impressive person or thing.

stunning /'stɛnɪŋ/ adj (inf) strikingly attractive.—**stunningly** adv.

stunt[1] /stɛnt/ vt to prevent the growth of, to dwarf.

stunt[2] n a daring or spectacular feat; a project designed to attract attention. • vi to carry out stunts.

stupa /'stuːpə/ n a domed shrine holding Buddhist relics.

stupefy /'stuːpəfaɪ/ or /'stjuː-/ vt (**stupefying, stupefied**) to dull the senses of.—**stupefaction** n.

stupendous /stuː'pɛndəs/ or /'stjuː-/ adj wonderful, astonishing.—**stupendously** adv.

stupid /'stuːpɪd/ or /'stjuː-/ adj lacking in understanding or common sense; silly; foolish; stunned.—**stupidity** n.—**stupidly** adv.

stupor /'stuːpər/ or /'stjuː-/ n extreme lethargy; mental dullness.

sturdy /'stɛrdiː/ adj (**sturdier, sturdiest**) firm; strong, robust.—**sturdily** adv.—**sturdiness** n.

sturgeon /'stɛrdʒən/ n any of various large food fishes whose roe is also eaten as caviare.

Sturmabteilung see **storm trooper**.

stutter /'stɛtər/ vi to stammer.—also n.

sty[1] /staɪ/, **stye** n (pl **sties**) an inflamed swelling on the eyelid.

sty[2] n (pl **sties**) a pen for pigs; any filthy place.

style /staɪl/ n the manner of writing, painting, composing music peculiar to an individual or group; fashion, elegance. • vt to design or shape (eg hair).—**styler** n.

stylish /'staɪlɪʃ/ adj having style; fashionable.—**stylishly** adv.—**stylishness** n.

stylist /'staɪlɪst/ n a person who writes, paints, etc, with attention to style; a designer; a hairdresser.

stylistic /staɪ'lɪstɪk/ adj of literary or artistic style.—**stylistically** adv.

stylize /'staɪlaɪz/ vt to give a conventional style to.—**stylization** n.—**stylizer** n.

stylus /'staɪləs/ n (pl **sty uses, styli**) the device attached to the cartridge on the arm of a record-player that rests in the groove of a record and transmits the vibrations that are converted to sound.

stymie /'staɪmi/ n (pl **stymies**) (golf) a situation in which a ball is obstructed by another ball between it and the hole. • vt (**stymieing, stymied**) to obstruct, hinder.

styptic /'stɪptɪk/ adj acting to stop bleeding by contracting the blood vessels. • n a styptic drug.

styrene /'staɪriːn/ n a liquid hydrocarbon used in making rubber and plastics.

suave /swɒv/ adj charming, polite.—**suavely** adv.—**suaveness** n.

suavity /-vɪt/ n (pl **suavities**) politeness; urbanity; a suave action, comment, etc.

sub /sɛb/ n (inf) a submarine; a substitute; a subscription; a subeditor.

sub- /sɛb/ or /sɒb/ prefix under, below; subordinate, next in rank to.

subaltern /sɛb'ɒltərn/ or /'sɒbəltərn/ n a commissioned officer in the British army ranking below captain. • adj inferior in rank or status.

subaqua /ˌsɛbə'kwɒ/ adj of or pertaining to underwater sports.

subatomic /ˌsɛbə'tɒmɪk/ adj smaller than an atom; occurring within an atom.

subconscious /sɛb'kɒnʃəs/ adj happening without one's awareness. • n the part of the mind that is active without one's conscious awareness.—**subconsciously** adv.—**subconsciousness** n.

subcontinent /'sɛbˌkɒnt nənt/ n a land mass having great size but smaller than any of the usu recognized continents.

subcontract /'sɛbˌkɒntrækt/ or /ˌsɛb'kɒn-/ n a secondary contract, under which work or supply of materials is let out to a firm other than the main party of the contract.—also vt.—**subcontractor** n.

subculture /'sɛbˌkʌltʃər/ n a distinct group with its own customs, language, dress, etc within an existing culture.

subcutaneous /ˌsɛbkju:'teɪniəs/ adj under the skin.—**subcutaneously** adv.

subdivide /ˌsɛbdɪ'vaɪd/ vt to further divide what has already been divided. • vi to divide or be divided into parts.—**subdivision** n.

subdue /sɒb'duː/ or /-'djuː/ vt to dominate; to render submissive; to repress (eg a desire, impulse); to soften, tone down (eg colour, etc).

subeditor /sɛb'edɪtər/ n a person who checks and corrects newspaper articles.—**subedit** vt.

subhead /'sɛbhed/, **subheading** /'sɛbhedɪŋ/ n a heading associated with a subdivision of a text.

subhuman /ˌsɛb'hjuːmən/ adj (animals) lower down the evolutionary scale than mankind; less than human.

subject /'sɛbdʒɪkt/ adj under the power of; liable. • n a person under the power of another; a citizen; a topic; a theme; the scheme or idea of a work of art. • vt to bring under control; to make liable; to cause to undergo something.—**subjection** n.

subjective /sɒb'dʒektɪv/ adj determined by one's own mind or consciousness; relating to reality as perceived and not independent of the mind; arising from one's own thoughts and emotions, personal.—**subjectively** adv.—**subjectivity** n.

sub judice /sɛb 'dʒuːdəs/ or /sɒb 'juːdɪˌkeɪ/ adv being decided by a court.

subjugate /'sɛbdʒʊˌgeɪt/ vt to overpower, to conquer.—**subjugation** n.

subjunctive /səb'dʒʌŋktɪv/ *adv* denoting that mood of a verb which expresses doubt, condition, wish, or hope. • *n* the subjunctive mood.

sublet /sʌb'let/ *vt* (**subletting, sublet**) to let (a property which one is renting) to another.

sublime /sə'blaɪm/ *adj* noble; exalted.—**sublimely** *adv*.—**sublimity** *n*.

subliminal /səb'lɪmənəl/ *adj* beneath or beyond the conscious awareness.—**subliminally** *adv*.

subliminal advertising *n* advertising using subliminal images to influence the viewer unconsciously.

sub-machine gun /ˌsʌbmə'ʃiːn/ *n* a light automatic or semiautomatic gun designed to be fired from the hip or shoulder.

submarine /ˌsʌbmə'riːn/ or /'sʌb-/ *adj* underwater, *esp* under the sea. • *n* a naval vessel capable of being propelled under water, *esp* for firing torpedoes or missiles.

submerge /səb'mɜːdʒ/, **submerse** *vt* to plunge or sink under water; to cover, hide.—**submergence, submersion** *n*.

submersible /səb'mɜːsɪbəl/ *adj* capable of being submerged. • *n* an underwater vessel used for exploration or construction work.

submission /səb'mɪʃən/ *n* an act of submitting; something submitted, as an idea or proposal; the state of being submissive, compliant; the act of referring something for another's consideration, criticism, etc.—**submissively** *adv*.—**submissiveness** *n*.

submit /səb'mɪt/ *vb* (**submitting, submitted**) *vt* to surrender (oneself) to another person or force; to refer to another for consideration or judgment; to offer as an opinion. • *vi* to yield, to surrender.

subnormal /sʌb'nɔːməl/ *adj* less than normal; having low intelligence.—**subnormality** *n*.—**subnormally** *adv*.

subordinate /sə'bɔːdənət/ *adj* secondary; lower in order, rank. • *n* a subordinate person. • *vt* to put in a lower position or rank.—**subordination** *n*.

suborn /sə'bɔːn/ *vt* to persuade to commit perjury or some other illegal act.

subpoena /sə'piːnə/ *n* a written legal order requiring the attendance of a person in court. • *vt* (**subpoenaing, subpoenaed**) to serve with a subpoena.

sub rosa /sʌb'rəʊzə/ *adv* in secret.

subroutine /'sʌbruːˌtiːn/ *n* a self-contained section of a computer program that performs a particular task as many times as required by the main program.

subscribe /səb'skraɪb/ *vt* to pay to receive regular copies (of a magazine, etc); to donate money (to a charity, campaign); to support or agree with (an opinion, faith).—**subscriber** *n*.—**subscription** *n*.

subscriber trunk dialling *n* a service that allows users to dial long-distance calls directly.

subscript /'sʌbskrɪpt/ *n* a character written or printed below another character.—*also adj*.

subsequent /'sʌbsəkwent/ *adj* occurring or following after.—**subsequently** *adv*.

subservient /səb'sɜːvɪənt/ *adj* obsequious; servile; subordinate.—**subservience** *n*.—**subserviently** *adv*.

subside /səb'saɪd/ *vi* to sink or fall to the bottom; to settle; to diminish; to abate.—**subsidence** *n*.

subsidiarity /səb'sɪdieriti/ or /səb'sɪdʒəriti/ *n* the devolution of decision making or control to the lowest effective level.

subsidiary /səb'sɪdieri/ or /səb'sɪdʒəri/ *adj* secondary; supplementary; (*company*) owned or controlled by another. • *n* (*pl* subsidiaries) an accessory, an auxiliary; a business owned by another.—**subsidiarily** *adv*.

subsidize /'sʌbsɪˌdaɪz/ *vt* to aid or support with a subsidy.—**subsidization** *n*.—**subsidizer** *n*.

subsidy /'sʌbsɪdi/ *n* (*pl* subsidies) government financial aid to a private person or company to assist an enterprise.

subsist /səb'sɪst/ *vi* to exist; to continue; to manage to keep oneself alive (on).

subsistence /səb'sɪstəns/ *n* existence; livelihood.—**subsistent** *adj*.

subsoil /'sʌbsɔɪl/ *n* the layer of soil lying immediately beneath the surface soil.

subsonic /sʌb'sɒnɪk/ *adj* travelling at a speed less than that of sound.

substance /'sʌbstəns/ *n* matter (such as powder, liquid); the essential nature or part; significance.

substantial /səb'stænʃəl/ *adj* of considerable value or size; important; strongly built.—**substantiality** *n*.—**substantially** *adv*.

substantiate /səb'stænʃiˌeɪt/ *vt* to prove, to verify.—**substantiation** *n*.

substitute /'sʌbstɪˌtuːt/ or /-ˌtjuːt/ *vt* to put or act in place of another person or thing (*with* **for**); to replace (by). • *n* a person or thing that serves in place of another.—*also adj*.—**substitution** *n*.

substructure /'sʌbˌstrʌktʃər/ *n* a foundation or supporting framework.

subsume /səb'suːm/ or /-'sjuːm/ *vt* to include in a larger group or category.

subterfuge /'sʌbtəˌfjuːdʒ/ *n* a trick employed to conceal something.

subterranean /ˌsʌbtə'reɪnɪən/ *adj* below the surface of the earth; concealed.

subtitle /'sʌbˌtaɪtəl/ *n* an explanatory, *usu* secondary, title to a book; a printed translation superimposed on a foreign language film.—*also vt*.

subtle /'sʌtəl/ *adj* delicate; slight; not noticeable; difficult to define, put into words; ingenious.—**subtleness** *n*.—**subtly** *adv*.

subtlety /'sʌtəlti/ *n* (*pl* subtleties) subtleness; a fine distinction.

subtotal /'sʌbˌtoːtəl/ *n* the sum of part of a series of figures. • *vt* (**subtotalling, subtotalled** *or* **subtotaling, subtotaled**) to sum in part.

subtract /səb'trækt/ *vti* to take away or deduct, as one quantity from another.—**subtraction** *n*.

subtropical /sʌb'trɒpɪkəl/ *adj* of, characteristic of, the regions bordering on the tropics.

suburb /'sʌbɜːb/ *n* a residential district on the outskirts of a large town or city.—**suburban** *adj*.—**suburbia** *n*.

suburbanite /-ənaɪt/ *n* a person who lives in a suburb.

subversion /səb'vɜːʒən/ *n* the act of undermining the authority of a government, institution, etc; collapse, ruin.

subversive /səb'vɜːsɪv/ *adj* liable to subvert established authority. • *n* a person who engages in subversive activities.—**subversively** *adv*.—**subversiveness** *n*.

subvert /səb'vɜːt/ *vt* to overthrow, to ruin (something established); to corrupt, as in morals.

subway /'sʌbweɪ/ *n* a passage under a street; an underground metropolitan electric railway.

succeed /sək'siːd/ *vt* to come after, to follow; to take the place of. • *vi* to accomplish what is attempted; to prosper.

success /sək'ses/ *n* the gaining of wealth, fame, etc; the favourable outcome (of anything attempted); a successful person or action.

successful /-fʊl/ *adj* having success.—**successfully** *adv*.—**successfulness** *n*.

succession /sək'seʃən/ *n* following in sequence; a number of persons or things following in order; the act or process of succeeding to a title, throne, etc; the line of descent to succeed to something.

successive /sək'sesɪv/ *adj* following in sequence.—**successively** *adv*.—**successiveness** *n*.

successor /sək'sesər/ *n* a person who succeeds another, as to an office.

succinct /sə'sɪŋkt/ or /sək-/ *adj* clear, concise.—**succinctly** *adv*.—**succinctness** *n*.

succotash /sɛ'kəˌtæʃ/ *n* a cooked mixture of sweetcorn and lima beans.

succour, succor /sɛ'kər/ *n* (a person or thing that provides) help, support, *esp* in time of need. • *vt* to provide such help.

succubus /'sɛkjʊbəs/, **succuba** *n* (*pl* succubi, succubae) a female demon thought to have sexual intercourse with sleeping men.

succulent /'sɛkjʊlənt/ *adj* juicy; moist and tasty; (*plant*) having fleshy tissue. • *n* a succulent plant (as a cactus).—**succulence, succulency** *n*.—**succulently** *adv*.

succumb /sə'kʌm/ *vi* to yield to superior strength or overpowering desire; to die.

such /sʌtʃ/ *adj* of a specified kind (*eg* such people, such a film); so great. • *adv* so; very.

suchlike /'sʌtʃlaɪk/ *adj* of similar kind.

suck /sʌk/ *vt* to draw (a liquid, air) into the mouth; to dissolve or roll about in the mouth (as a sweet); to draw in as if by sucking (*with* **in, up**, etc).—*also n*.

sucker /'sʌkər/ *n* (*sl*) a person who is easily taken in or deceived; a cup-shaped piece of rubber that adheres to surfaces.

suckle /'sʌkəl/ vt to feed at the breast or udder.

suckling /'sʌklɪŋ/ n a young animal that is not yet weaned.

sucks /sʌks/ interj (sl) used to express disappointment.

sucre /'suːkər/ n the monetary unit of Ecuador.

sucrose /'suːkroːs/ n sugar.

suction /'sʌkʃən/ n the act or process of sucking; the exertion of a force to form a vacuum.

sudden /'sʌdən/ adj happening quickly and unexpectedly, abrupt.—**suddenly** adv.—**suddenness** n.

sudden death n (sport) extra time in a tied match, the winner being the next to score or take a point.

suds /sʌds/ npl the bubbles or foam on the surface of soapy water.—**sudsy** adj.

sue /suː/ vt (**suing, sued**) to bring a legal action against.

suede, suède /sweɪd/ n leather finished with a soft nap.

suet /'suːət/ n white, solid fat in animal tissue, used in cooking.

suffer /'sʌfər/ vt to undergo; to endure; to experience. • vi to feel pain or distress.—**sufferer** n.—**suffering** n.

sufferable /-əbəl/ adj endurable.—**sufferably** adv.

sufferance /-rəns/ n reluctant tolerance, tacit permission; endurance.

suffice /sə'faɪs/ vi to be sufficient, adequate (for some purpose).

sufficient /sə'fɪʃənt/ adj enough; adequate.—**sufficiency** n.—**sufficiently** adv.

suffix /'sʌfɪks/ n (pl **suffixes**) a letter, syllable, or syllables added to the end of a word to modify its meaning or to form a new derivative.

suffocate /'sʌfəkeɪt/ vti to kill or be killed by depriving of oxygen, or by inhaling a poisonous gas; to feel hot and uncomfortable due to lack of air; to prevent from developing.—**suffocation** n.

suffrage /'sʌfrɪdʒ/ n the right to vote.

suffuse /sə'fjuːz/ vt to spread over or fill, as with colour or light.—**suffusion** n.

sugar /'ʃʊgər/ n a sweet white, crystalline substance obtained from sugar cane and sugar beet. • vi to sweeten.

sugar beet n a type of beet from which sugar is extracted.

sugar cane n a tall grass with stout canes grown as a source of sugar.

sugar daddy n a wealthy and usu elderly man who lavishes gifts on an attractive young woman.

sugar maple n ❀ a North American maple from which sap is tapped to make maple syrup.

sugar shack n ❀ (Cdn) a building in which maple sap is boiled to make maple syrup.

sugary /'ʃʊgəri/ adj resembling or containing sugar; cloyingly sweet in manner, content, etc.—**sugariness** n.

suggest /sə'dʒest/ vt to put forward for consideration; to bring to one's mind; to evoke.—**suggestion** n.

suggestible /sə'dʒestəbəl/ adj easily influenced by others.—**suggestibility** n.

suggestive /-tɪv/ adj evocative; rather indecent, risqué.—**suggestively** adv.—**suggestiveness** n.

suicidal /ˌsuːɪ'saɪdəl/ adj of, pertaining to, suicide liable to commit suicide; destructive of one's own interests.—**suicidally** adv.

suicide /'suːɪˌsaɪd/ n a person who kills himself intentionally; the act or instance of killing oneself intentionally; ruin of one's own interests.

suicide gene n a gene having bacteria that end its life cycle.

sui generis /ˌsuːɪ'dʒenərɪs/ adj unique.

suit /suːt/ n a set of matching garments, such as a jacket and trousers or skirt; one of the four sets of thirteen playing cards; a lawsuit. • vt to be appropriate; to be convenient or acceptable to.

suitable /'suːtəbəl/ adj fitting; convenient (to, for).—**suitably** adv.—**suitability** n.

suitcase /-keɪs/ n a portable, oblong travelling case.

suite /swiːt/ n a number of followers or attendants; a set, esp of rooms, furniture, pieces of music.

suitor /'suːtər/ n a man who courts a woman; (law) a person who brings a lawsuit.

sukiyaki /ˌsʊkɪ'joki/ n a Japanese dish of thinly sliced beef, vegetables and seafood cooked rapidly in soy sauce, saké, etc, at the table.

sulfa /'sʌlfə/ see **sulpha**.

sulfate /'sʌlfeɪt/ see **sulphate**.

sulfonamide /ˌsʌl'fɒnəˌmaɪd/ see **sulphonamide**.

sulfur /'sʌlfər/ see **sulphur**.

sulfuric /'sʌlfjʊrɪk/ see **sulphuric**.

sulk /sʌlk/ vi to be sullen.

sulky /'sʌlki/ adj (**sulkier, sulkiest**) bad-tempered, quiet and sullen, because of resentment.—**sulkily** adv.—**sulkiness** n.

sullen /'sʌlən/ adj moody and silent; gloomy, dull.—**sullenly** adv.—**sullenness** n.

sully /'sʌli/ vt (**sullying, sullied**) to blemish, to defile the purity of • n (pl **sullies**) a tarnish or stain.

sulph-, sulf- /sʌlf/ prefix sulphur.

sulpha drug n any of various sulphonamide drugs used for treating bacterial infections.

sulphate /'sʌlfeɪt/ n a salt of sulphuric acid.—also **sulfate**.

sulphonamide /ˌsʌl'fɒnəˌmaɪd/ n any of a group of compounds that are amides of sulphonic acid, such as the sulfa drugs.—also **sulfonamide**.

sulphonic acid n any of a group strong organic acids used in the manufacture of drugs, dyes and detergents.

sulphur /'sʌlfər/ n a yellow nonmetallic element that is inflammable and has a strong odour.—also **sulfur**.—**sulphuric, sulfuric** adj.

sulphur dioxide n a pungent toxic gas used in various industrial processes that is a major air pollutant.

sulphuric acid n a powerfully corrosive acid.

sultan /'sʌltən/ n a ruler, esp of a Muslim state.

sultana /sʌl'tɑːnə/ n a dried, white grape used in cooking; the wife or female relative of a sultan.

sultanate /'sʌltənət/ n a country or region ruled by a sultan; the office or authority of a sultan.

sultry /'sʌltri/ adj (**sultrier, sultriest**) (weather) very hot, humid and close; sensual; passionate.—**sultrily** adv.—**sultriness** n.

sum /sʌm/ n the result of two or more things added together; the total, aggregate; a quantity of money; essence, gist. • vt (**summing, summed**) to add (usu with **up**); to encapsulate; to summarize.

summarize /'sʌməˌraɪz/ vt to make or be a summary of.—**summarization** n.—**summarizer** n.

summary /'sʌməri/ adj concise; performed quickly, without formality. • n (pl **summaries**) a brief account of the main points of something.—**summarily** adv.—**summariness** n.

summation /sʌ'meɪʃən/ n the act of finding a sum or total; the result of summation; a summary; the summing up of an argument, esp by a lawyer before a jury.

summer /'sʌmər/ n the warmest season of the year, between spring and autumn.—**summery** adj.

summerhouse n a small building in a garden used as a shady retreat in summer.

summer school n an academic course held during the summer.

summer student n ❀ (Cdn) a student who works at a job in the summer.

summing-up n a concluding summary of the points in a speech, argument, etc; a review of the main evidence made by a judge to the jury before it considers its verdict.

summit /'sʌmɪt/ n the highest point, the peak; a meeting of world leaders.

summitry /-ri/ n the practice of convening, or style of conducting, summit conferences.

summon /'sʌmən/ vt to order to appear, esp in court; to convene; to gather (strength, enthusiasm, etc).

summons /'sʌmənz/ n (pl **summonses**) a call to appear (in court). • vt to serve with a summons.

sumo /'suːmoː/ n traditional Japanese wrestling.

sump /sʌmp/ n a section of the crankcase under an engine for the oil to drain into to form a reservoir.

sumptuous /'sʌmptʃuːəs/ adj lavish; luxurious.—**sumptuously** adv.—**sumptuousness** n.

sun /sʌn/ n the star around which the earth and other planets revolve which gives light and heat to the solar system; the sunshine. • vi (**sunning, sunned**) to expose oneself to the sun's rays.

Sun. abbr = Sunday.

sunbaked adj baked hard by exposure to the sun.

sunbathe /'sʌnbeɪð/ vi to lie in the rays of the sun or a sun lamp to get a suntan.—**sunbather** n.

sunbeam /-biːm/ n a ray of sunlight.

sunburn /-bɜːrn/ n inflammation of the skin from exposure to sunlight.—also vti.

sunburst /-bɜːrst/ n a sudden flash of sunlight; a pattern resembling the sun surrounded by rays; a brooch with a design resembling this.

sundae /'sʌndeɪ/ n a serving of ice cream covered with a topping of fruit, syrup, nuts, etc.

Sunday /'sʌndeɪ/ n the day of the week after Saturday, regarded as a day of worship by Christians; a newspaper published on a Sunday.

Sunday best n best clothes kept for wearing on Sundays.

Sunday school n a class for religious instruction held on Sundays.

sundew n any of various bog plants with sticky hairs that trap insects.

sundial n a device that shows the time by casting a shadow on a graduated dial.

sundown /'sʌndaʊn/ n sunset.

sundry /'sʌndrɪ/ adj miscellaneous, various. • n (pl **sundries**) (pl) miscellaneous small things.

sunflower /'sʌn‚flaʊr/ n a tall plant with large yellow flowers whose seeds yield oil.

sung /sʌŋ/ see **sing**.

sunglasses /'sʌn‚glæsəz/ npl tinted glasses to protect the eyes from sunlight.

sunk /sʌŋk/ see **sink**.

sunlamp n an electric lamp that produces ultra-violet rays for tanning the skin.

Sunna /'sʌnə/ n the body of Islamic doctrine accepted by orthodox Muslims as based on the life and teachings of Mohammed.

Sunni /'sʌni/ n the branch of Islam that accepts the orthodoxy of the Sunna.—**Sunnite** n.

sunny /'sʌni/ adj (**sunnier, sunniest**) (weather) bright with sunshine; (person, mood) cheerful.—**sunnily** adv.—**sunniness** n.

sunrise/'sʌnraɪz/ n dawn.

sunrise industry n a high-technology industry with a bright future.

sunroof /'sʌnruːf/ n a panel in the roof of a car that slides open.

sunset /-sɛt/ n dusk.

sunshine /-ʃaɪn/ n the light and heat from the sun.

sunspot /-spɒt/ n a dark patch sometimes visible on the sun's surface; (inf) a holiday resort with guaranteed sunshine.

sunstroke /-strok/ n illness caused by exposure to the sun.

suntan /-tæn/ n browning of the skin by the sun.—**suntanned** adj.

suntrap /-træp/ n a sunny sheltered spot.

super /'suːpər/ adj (inf) fantastic, excellent; (inf) a superintendent, as in the police. • n a variety of high-octane petrol.

super- /'suːpər/ prefix above, on the top of; extremely, excessively; greater in size, quality, etc.

superable adj able to be overcome.—**superably** adv.

superannuate /‚suːpər'ænjʊ‚eɪt/ vt to pension off on account of old age or illness.

superannuation /‚suːpər‚ænjʊ'eɪʃən/ n regular contributions from employees' wages toward a pension scheme.

superb /'suːpərb/ adj grand; excellent; of the highest quality.—**superbly** adv.

supercharge /'suːpər‚tʃɑrdʒ/ vt to increase the power of an engine by using a device that supplies air or fuel in increased quantities by raising the intake pressure; to charge (the atmosphere, a conversation, etc) with excess tension or emotion.—**supercharger** n.

supercilious /‚suːpər'sɪliəs/ adj arrogant; haughty, disdainful.—**superciliously** adv.—**superciliousness** n.

superconductivity /‚suːpər‚kɒndʌk'tɪvɪti/ n (physics) the complete loss of electrical resistance exhibited by certain materials at very low temperatures.—**superconducting, superconductive** adj.—**superconduction** n.—**superconductor** n.

supercool /'suːpər‚kuːl/ vt to cool (a liquid, etc) below freezing without solidification or crystallization.

superdelegate n in US, a delegate to a Democratic party convention, appointed rather than elected.

superego /‚suːpər'iː‚goː/ n (pl **superegos**) (psychol) the division of the unconscious mind that functions as a conscience.

superficial /‚suːpər'fɪʃəl/ adj near the surface; slight, not profound; (person) shallow in nature.—**superficiality** n.—**superficially** adv.

superfluous /suː'pərfluəs/ adj exceeding what is required; unnecessary.—**superfluity** n.

supergiant /'suːpər‚dʒaɪənt/ n a star of enormous size and brightness with a low density.

superglue /'suːpər‚gluː/ n an adhesive that forms strong bonds instantly.

supergrass n an informer who incriminates a large number of people.

superheat /‚suːpər'hiːt/ vt to heat above boiling point without vaporization; to heat a vapour above boiling point without boiling occurring.

superhigh frequency n a radio frequency between 30,000 and 3,000 megahertz.

superhuman /-'hjuːmən/ adj surpassing normal human strength or abilities; divine.

superimpose /-ɪm'poːz/ vt to put or lay upon something else.

superintend /-ɪn'tɛnd/ vt to have the charge and direction of; to control, manage.

superintendent /-ɪn'tɛndənt/ n a person who manages or supervises; a director; a British police officer next above the rank of inspector.

superior /suː'piːriər/ or /sʊ-/ adj higher in place, quality, rank, excellence; greater in number, power. • n a person of higher rank.—**superiority** n.

superiority complex n an inflated opinion of one's own abilities and merits.

superl. abbr = superlative.

superlative /suː'pərlətɪv/ adj of outstanding quality; (gram) denoting the extreme degree of comparison of adjectives and adverbs.—**superlatively** adv.

superman /'suːpər‚mæn/ n (pl **supermen**) a person of outstanding abilities and achievements.

supermarket /‚suːpər'mɑrkət/ n a large self-service, shop selling food and household goods.

supernatural /-'nætʃərəl/ adj relating to things that cannot be explained by nature; involving ghosts, spirits, etc.—**supernaturally** adv.

supernova /-'noːvə/ n (pl **supernovae, supernovas**) a star that explodes temporarily burning with an intensity one hundred million times that of the sun.

supernumerary /‚suːpər'nuːmər‚ɛri/ or /-njuː-/ adj extra; beyond the usual number. • n (pl **supernumeraries**) an extra person or thing.

superpose /‚suːpər'poːz/ vt to place (a geometric figure) on top of another so that their outlines coincide; to lay on top of.—**superposition** n.

superpower /'suːpər‚paʊər/ n a nation with great economic and military strength.

superscript /'suːpərskrɪpt/ n a character written or printed above another character.—also adj.

supersede /‚suːpər'siːd/ vt to take the place of, replace.

supersmart card n a smart card equipped with a screen and a keyboard, allowing interaction with the user.

supersonic /‚suːpər'sɒnɪk/ adj faster than the speed of sound.—**supersonically** adv.

superstar /'suːpər‚stɑr/ n (inf) a sporting celebrity; a famous film actor or musician.

superstition /‚suːpər'stɪʃən/ n irrational belief based on ignorance or fear.—**superstitious** adj.

superstore /'suːpər‚stɔr/ n a very large supermarket.

superstructure /-‚strʌktʃər/ n a structure above or on something else, as above the base or foundation, as above the main deck of a ship.

Super Tuesday n the Tuesday, usu in March, on which a number of states, with over half of all the delegates, hold primary elections for the selection of Presidential candidates.

supervise /-‚vaɪz/ vti to have charge of, direct, to superintend.—**supervision** n.

supervisor /-‚vaɪzər/ n one who supervises; an overseer, an inspector.—**supervisory** adj.

supine /'suːpaɪn/ adj lying on the back; lazy, indigent.—**supinely** adv.

supper /'sʌpər/ n a meal taken in the evening, esp when dinner is eaten at midday; an evening social event; the food served at a supper; a light meal served late in the evening.

supplant /sə'plænt/ vt to replace; to remove in order to replace with something else.

supple /'sʌpəl/ adj flexible, easily bent; lithe; (mind) adaptable.—**suppleness** n.

supplement /'sʌpləmənt/ n an addition or extra amount (usu of money); an additional section of a book, periodical or newspaper. • vt to add to.—**supplemental** adj.

supply /'sʌplaɪ/ vt (**supplying, supplied**) to provide, meet (a deficiency, a need); to fill (a vacant place). • n (pl **supplies**) a stock; (pl) provisions.—**supplier** n.

support /sə'pɔrt/ vt to hold up, bear; to tolerate, withstand; to assist; to advocate (a cause, policy); to provide for (financially). • n a means of support; maintenance.

supporter /-ər/ n a person who backs a political party, sports team, etc.

suppose /sə'poːz/ vt to assume; to presume as true without definite knowledge; to think probable; to expect. • vi to conjecture.

supposed /sə'poːzd/ adj believed to be on available evidence.

supposedly /sə'poːzədli/ adv allegedly.

supposition /ˌsʌpə'zɪʃən/ n an assumption, hypothesis.

suppositious /ˌsʌpə'zɪʃəs/ adj hypothetical.

suppository /sə'pɒzɪˌtɔri/ n (pl **suppositories**) a cone or cylinder of medicated soluble material for insertion into the rectum or vagina.

suppress /sə'pres/ vt to crush, put an end to (eg a rebellion); to restrain (a person); to subdue.—**suppression** n.—**suppressor** n.

suppurate /'sʌpjəˌreɪt/ vi to form or discharge pus.—**suppuration** n.—**suppurative** adj.

supra /'suːprə/ prefix above, situated above; over; beyond.

supranational /ˌsuːprə'næʃənəl/ adj transcending national boundaries or interests.

supremacist /sə'preməsɪst/ or /suː-/ n a person who advocates the supremacy of a particular group.

supreme /suː'priːm/ or /sə-/ adj of highest power; greatest; final; ultimate.—**supremacy** n.

Supreme Court n the highest judicial body in a nation or state.

supremo /sə'priːmoː/ or /suː-/ n (pl **supremos**) (inf) the person in overall charge, a boss.

Supt abbr = superintendent.

surcharge /sər'tʃɑrdʒ/ vt to overcharge (a person); to charge an additional sum; to overload. • n an additional tax or charge; an additional or excessive load.

surd /sərd/ n (math) a number containing an irrational root; an irrational number.

sure /ʃər/ or /ʃʊr/ adj certain; without doubt; reliable, inevitable; secure; safe; dependable. • adv certainly.

sure-fire /'ʃərfaɪr/ or /'ʃʊr-/ adj (inf) certain to succeed.

sure-footed adj not liable to slip or fall; unlikely to make a mistake.

surely /'ʃərli/ or /'ʃʊr-/ adv certainly; securely; it is to be hoped or expected that.

sure thing n (inf) something assured of success. • interj yes, of course.

surety /'ʃərəti/ or /'ʃʊr-/ n (pl **sureties**) a person who undertakes responsibility for the fulfilment of another's debt; security given as a guarantee of payment of a debt.

surf /sərf/ n the waves of the sea breaking on the shore or a reef.

surface /'sərfəs/ n the exterior face of an object; any of the faces of a solid; the uppermost level of sea or land; a flat area, such as the top of a table; superficial features. • adj superficial; external. • vt to cover with a surface, as in paving. • vi to rise to the surface of water.

surfboard /'sərfbɔrd/ n a long, narrow board used in the sport of surfing.

surfeit /'sərfiːt/ n an excessive amount.

surfing /'sərfɪŋ/ n the sport of riding in toward shore on the crest of a wave, esp on a surfboard.

surg. abbr = surgeon; surgery; surgical.

surge /sərdʒ/ n the rolling of the sea, as after a large wave; a sudden, strong increase, as of power.—also vi.

surgeon /'sərdʒən/ n a medical specialist who practises surgery.

surgery /'sərdʒəri/ n (pl **surgeries**) the treatment of diseases or injuries by manual or instrumental operations; the consulting room of a doctor or dentist; the daily period when a doctor is available for consultation; the regular period when an MP, lawyer, etc is available for consultation.—**surgical** adj.—**surgically** adv.

surgical spirit n methylated spirit used for sterilizing.

surly /'sərli/ adj (**surlier, surliest**) ill-tempered or rude.—**surlily** adv.—**surliness** n.

surmise /sər'maɪz/ n guess, conjecture. • vt to infer the existence of from partial evidence.

surmount /sər'maʊnt/ vt to overcome; to rise above.

surname /'sərneɪm/ n the family name. • vt to give a surname to.

surpass /sər'pæs/ vt to outdo, to outshine; to excel; to exceed.

surpassing /-ɪŋ/ adj exceptional; greatly exceeding others.—**surpassingly** adv.

surplice /'sərplɪs/ or /-pləs/ n a loose, white, wide-sleeved clerical garment worn by clergymen and choristers

surplus /'sərpləs/ n (pl **surpluses**) an amount in excess of what is required; an excess of revenues over expenditure in a financial year.

surprise /'sərpraɪz/ n the act of catching unawares; an unexpected gift, event; astonishment. • vt to cause to feel astonished; to attack unexpectedly; to take unawares.—**surprising** adj.—**surprisingly** adv.

surreal /sə'riːəl/ adj bizarre.

surrealism /-ˌlɪzm/ n a movement in art characterized by the expression of the activities of the unconscious mind and dream elements.—**surrealist** n.—**surrealistic** adj.

surrender /sə'rendər/ vt to relinquish or give up possession or power. • vi to give oneself up (to an enemy).—also n.

surreptitious /ˌsʌrep'tɪʃəs/ adj done by stealth; clandestine, secret.—**surreptitiously** adv.

surrogacy /'sʌrəgəsi/, **surrogate motherhood** n a practice in which a woman bears a child for a childless couple.—**surrogate mother** n.

surrogate /'sʌrəgət/ n a person or thing acting as a substitute for another person or thing.—also adj.

surrogate mother n a woman who bears a child on behalf of a childless couple.

surround /sə'raʊnd/ vt to encircle on all or nearly all sides; (mil) to encircle. • n a border around the edge of something.

surroundings /-ɪŋz/ npl the conditions, objects, etc around a person or thing; the environment.

surtax /'sərtæks/ n an additional tax, esp on income above a prescribed level.—also vt.

surtitle /'sərˌtaɪtəl/ n a caption projected onto a screen above the stage during an opera as a translation of the libretto or to explain some detail of the action.—also vt.

surveillance /sər'veɪləns/ n a secret watch kept over a person, esp a suspect.

survey /'sərveɪ/ vt (**surveying, surveyed**) to take a general view of; to appraise; to examine carefully; to measure and make a map of an area. • n (pl **surveys**) a detailed study, as by gathering information and analysing it, a general view; the process of surveying an area or a house.

surveyor /sər'veɪər/ or /'sər-/ n a person who surveys land or buildings.

survival /sər'vaɪvəl/ n surviving; a person or thing that survives; a relic.

survive /sər'vaɪv/ vt to live after the death of another person; to continue, endure; to come through alive. • vi to remain alive (after experiencing a dangerous situation).—**survivor** n.

susceptible /sə'septəbəl/ adj ready or liable to be affected by; impressionable.—**susceptibility** n.—**susceptibly** adv.

sushi /'suːʃi/ n a Japanese dish of small cakes of cold rice with various toppings, esp raw fish.

suspect /sə'spekt/ vt to mistrust; to believe to be guilty; to think probable. • n a person under suspicion. • adj open to suspicion.

suspend /sə'spend/ vt to hang; to discontinue, or cease temporarily; to postpone; to debar temporarily from a privilege, etc.

suspended animation n a cessation of the vital functions in an organism, esp though freezing.

suspended sentence n a sentence that does not come into force unless a further offence is committed.

suspender /-ər/ n a fastener for holding up stockings; (pl) braces.

suspender belt n a belt with suspenders to hold up a woman's stockings.

suspense /sə'spens/ n mental anxiety or uncertainty; excitement.

suspension /sə'spenʃən/ n suspending or being suspended; a temporary interruption or postponement; a temporary removal from office, privileges, etc; the system of springs, shock absorbers, etc that support a vehicle on its axles; (chem) a dispersion of fine particles in a liquid.

suspension bridge n a bridge carrying a roadway suspended by cables anchored to towers at either end.

suspicion /sə'spɪʃən/ n act of suspecting; a belief formed or held without sure proof; mistrust; a trace.—**suspicious** adj.—**suspiciously** adv.

sustain /sə'steɪn/ vt hold up, support; to maintain; to suffer (eg an injury); to nourish.

sustenance /'sʌstənəns/ n nourishment.

suttee /sʌ'tiː/ or /'sʌti/ n (Hinduism) (formerly) the practice of a widow throwing herself on her husband's funeral pyre; this custom.—also **sati**.

suture /'suːtʃər/ *n* a stitch holding together a wound after surgery.—*also vt*.

svelte /svɛlt/ *adj* slim and elegant.

SW *abbr* = southwest(ern); short wave.

swab /swɒb/ *n* a wad of absorbent material, *usu* cotton, used to clean wounds, take specimens, etc; a mop.—*also vt*.

swaddle /'swɒdəl/ *vt* to bind tightly, envelop; to wrap a baby in swaddling clothes.

swaddling clothes *npl* narrow strips of cloth used to wrap and restrain an infant.

swag /swæg/ *n* (*sl*) loot.

swagger /'swægər/ *vi* to strut; to brag loudly. • *n* boastfulness; swinging gait.

Swahili /swəˈhiːli/ or /swɒ-/ *n* a language spoken in Kenya, Tanzania and other parts of east Africa; (*pl* **Swahilis, Swahili**) a member of a people speaking this language who live mainly in Zanzibar.

swain /sweɪn/ *n* (*poet*) a male suitor or lover.

swallow[1] /'swɒloʊ/ *n* a small migratory bird with long wings and a forked tail.

swallow[2] *vt* to cause food and drink to move from the mouth to the stomach; to endure; to engulf; (*inf*) to accept gullibly; (*emotion, etc*) to repress.—*also n*.

swallow dive *n* a dive executed with the back arched and arms outstretched at the start.

swam /swæm/ *see* **swim**.

swami /'swɒmi/ *n* (*pl* **swamies, swamis**) a Hindu religious teacher.

swamp /swæmp/ *n* wet, spongy land; bog. • *vt* to overwhelm; to flood as with water.—**swampy** *adj*.

swan /swɒn/ *n* a large, *usu* white, bird with a very long neck that lives on rivers and lakes. • *vi* (**swanning, swanned**) (*inf*) to wander aimlessly.

swan dive *n* a swallow dive.

swank /swæŋk/ *vi* (*inf*) to show off.—*also n*.—**swanky** *adj*.

swan song *n* a final appearance, performance, etc by a person facing retirement or death.

swap /swɒp/ *vti* (**swapping, swapped**) (*inf*) to trade, barter. • *n* (*inf*) the act of exchanging one thing for another.—*also* **swop**.

SWAPO, Swapo /'swɒpoʊ/ (*abbr*) South West Africa People's Organization.

sward /swɔːd/ *n* (an area of land with) a surface of short grass.

swarm /swɔːrm/ *n* a colony of migrating bees; a moving mass, crowd or throng. • *vi* to move in great numbers; to teem.

swarthy /'swɔːrði/ *adj* (**swarthier, swarthiest**) dark-complexioned.—**swarthiness** *n*.

swashbuckling /'swɒʃbʌklɪŋ/ *adj* swaggering; exciting, adventurous.—**swashbuckler** *n*.

swastika /swəsˈtiːkə/ or /'swɒstɪkə/ *n* an ancient symbol formed by a cross with the ends of the arms bent at right-angles, used by Nazi Germany.

swat /swɒt/ *vt* (**swatting, swatted**) (*inf*) to hit with a sharp blow; to swipe.—*also n*.—**swatter** *n*.

swath /swɒθ/ *n* the width of one sweep of a scythe or other mowing device; a strip, row, etc, mowed; a broad strip.

swathe /swɒθ/ or /sweɪð/ *vt* to bind or wrap round, as with a bandage; to envelop, enclose.

sway /sweɪ/ *vi* to swing or move from one side to the other or to and fro; to lean to one side; to vacillate in judgment or opinion. • *n* influence; control.

swear /swɛr/ *vi* (**swearing, swore**, *pp* **sworn**) to make a solemn affirmation, promise, etc, calling God as a witness; to give evidence on oath; to curse, blaspheme or use obscene language; to vow; (*with* **off**) to promise abstinence from. • *vt* (*with* **in**) to appoint to an office by the administration of an oath.

swearword *n* a profane or obscene expression.

sweat /swɛt/ *n* perspiration; (*inf*) hard work; (*inf*) a state of eagerness, anxiety.—*also vti*.—**sweaty** *adj*.

sweatband /'swɛtbænd/ *n* a strip of material in a hat, or worn on the wrist or around the forehead, to absorb sweat.

sweat lodge *n* ✤ a structure used by North American Indians inside which water is poured on hot stones to induce sweating for religious or healing purposes.

sweater /'swɛtər/ *n* a knitted pullover.

sweatshirt /-ʃərt/ *n* a loose, collarless, heavy cotton jersey.

sweatshop /-ʃɒp/ *n* a small factory or workshop where employees work long hours at low wages in poor conditions.

Swede /swiːd/ *n* a native of Sweden.

swede /swiːd/ *n* a round root vegetable with yellow flesh.

swede saw *n* ✤ (*Cdn*) a hand saw with a bow-like tubular frame and many teeth.

Swedish /'swiːdɪʃ/ *adj* pertaining to Sweden, its people or language. • *n* the language of Sweden.

sweep /swiːp/ *vb* (**sweeping, swept**) *vt* to clean with a broom; to remove (rubbish, dirt) with a brush. • *vi* to pass by swiftly. • *n* a movement, *esp* in an arc; a stroke; scope; range; a sweepstake.

sweeper /'swiːpər/ *n* a person who sweeps, *esp* the roads; (*soccer*) (*inf*) a player positioned before the goalkeeper to collect loose balls, tackle attacking players, etc.

sweeping /-ɪŋ/ *adj* wide-ranging; indiscriminate.—**sweepingly** *adv*.

sweepstake /-steɪk/, **sweepstakes** /-steɪks/ *n* a lottery in which the prize constitutes all the money staked; a horserace, etc in which the winner receives the entire prize.

sweet /swiːt/ *adj* having a taste like sugar; pleasing to other senses; gentle; kind. • *n* a small piece of confectionery; a dessert.—**sweetly** *adv*.—**sweetness** *n*.

sweet-and-sour *adj* (*food*) cooked in a sauce containing sugar and vinegar or lemon juice.

sweet brier *n* a Eurasian rose with pink flowers.

sweetbread /'swiːtbrɛd/ *n* the pancreas or thymus gland of an animal, cooked as food.

sweet cicely *n* an aromatic European plant with small white flowers; the aniseed-flavoured leaves of this once used in cookery.

sweet clover *n* a species of sweet-scented trefoil or clover, with clusters of small yellow or white flowers; melilot.

sweetcorn /'swiːtkɔːrn/ *n* maize, corn on the cob.

sweeten /'swiːtən/ *vti* to make or become sweet or sweeter; to mollify.

sweetener /-ər/ *n* a sweetening substance that contains no sugar; (*sl*) a bribe.

sweetheart /'swiːthɑːrt/ *n* a lover.

sweetie /'swiːti/ *n* (*inf*) a sweet; (*inf*) sweetheart, darling; a kindly, pleasant person.

sweetmeat /'swiːtmiːt/ *n* a sweet, preserve, small cake, or other sugary delicacy.

sweet pea *n* a climbing garden plant cultivated for its large fragrant blooms.

sweet pepper *n* (a plant bearing) a large fruit with thick fleshy walls eaten ripe (red) or unripe (green).

sweet potato *n* (a tropical climbing plant with) a large edible tuberous root.

sweet-talk *vt* (*inf*) to flatter, cajole.—**sweet talk** *n*.

sweet william *n* a widely grown Eurasian plant with clusters of white, red, pink, or purple flowers.

swell /swɛl/ *vi* (**swelling, swelled**, *pp* **swollen** *or* **swelled**) to increase in size or volume; to rise into waves; to bulge out. • *n* the movement of the sea; a bulge; a gradual increase in the loudness of a musical note; (*inf*) a socially prominent person. • *adj* excellent.

swelling /'swɛlɪŋ/ *n* inflammation.

swelter /'swɛltər/ *vi* to suffer from heat. • *n* humid, oppressive heat.

sweltering /-ɪŋ/ *adj* uncomfortably hot.

swept /swɛpt/ *see* **sweep**.

sweptback *adj* (*aircraft wing*) slanting backward.

sweptwing *adj* (*aircraft*) having sweptback wings.

swerve /swɜːrv/ *vi* to turn aside suddenly from a line or course; to veer.—*also n*.

swift /swɪft/ *adj* moving with great speed; rapid. • *n* a swallow-like bird.—**swiftly** *adv*.—**swiftness** *n*.

swig /swɪg/ *vt* (*inf*) to take a long drink, *esp* from a bottle.—*also n*.

swill /swɪl/ *vti* to drink greedily; to guzzle; to rinse with a large amount of water. • *n* liquid refuse fed to pigs.

swim /swɪm/ *vi* (**swimming, swam**, *pp* **swum**) to move through water by using limbs or fins; to be dizzy; to be flooded with. • *n* the act of swimming.—**swimmer** *n*.

swimming costume, swimsuit /'swɪmsuːt/ *n* a one-piece garment for swimming in.

swimmingly /'swɪmɪŋli/ *adv* (*inf*) easily, without effort.

swindle /'swɪndəl/ *vti* to cheat (someone) of money or property.—*also n*.—**swindler** *n*.

swindle sheet *n* (*sl*) an expenses form.

swine /swaɪn/ *n* (*pl* **swine**) a pig; (*inf*) an contemptible person; (*inf*) an unpleasant thing.

swine fever *n* a viral infection of pigs.

swineherd /'swaɪnhərd/ *n* a person who looks after pigs.

swing /swɪŋ/ *vb* (**swinging, swung**) *vi* to sway or move to and fro, as an object hanging in the air; to pivot; to shift from one mood or opinion to another; (*music*) to have a lively rhythm; (*sl*) to be hanged. • *vt* to whirl; to play swing music; to influence; to achieve, bring about. • *n* a swinging, curving or rhythmic movement; a suspended seat for swinging in; a shift from one condition to another; a type of popular jazz played by a large band and characterized by a lively, steady rhythm.

swingeing /'swɪndʒɪn/ *adj* drastic, severe.

swinging /'swɪŋɪŋ/ *adj* (*inf*) up-to-date; lively.

swing riding *n* ✦ (*Cdn*) a constituency in which more than one candidate in an election has a good chance of winning.

swing-wing *adj* of or pertaining to an aircraft with movable wings that are swept back at high speeds and moved forward for approach and landing.—*also n.*

swipe /swaɪp/ *n* (*inf*) a hard, sweeping blow. • *vt* (*inf*) to hit with a swipe; (*sl*) to steal.

swirl /swərl/ *vti* to turn with a whirling motion.—*also n.*

swish /swɪʃ/ *vi* to move with a soft, whistling, hissing sound. • *n* a swishing sound. • *adj* (*inf*) smart, fashionable.

Swiss /swɪs/ *adj* of or belonging to Switzerland. • *n* (*pl* **Swiss**) a native of Switzerland.

swiss roll *n* a thin sponge cake spread with a layer of jam and rolled up.

switch /swɪtʃ/ *n* a control for turning on and off an electrical device; a sudden change; a swap. • *vt* to shift, change, swap; to turn on or off (as of an electrical device).

switchback /'swɪtʃbæk/ *n* a zigzag road in a mountain region; a roller coaster.

switchblade /-bleɪd/ *n* a flick knife.

switchboard /-bɔrd/ *n* an installation in a building where telephone calls are connected.

swivel /'swɪvəl/ *n* a coupling that permits parts to rotate. • *vi* (**swivelling, swivelled** *or* **swiveling, swiveled**) to turn (as if) on a pin or pivot.

swollen /'swoːlən/ *see* **swell**.

swoon /swuːn/ *vt* to faint.—*also n.*

swoop /swuːp/ *vt* to carry off abruptly. • *vi* to make a sudden attack (*usu with* **down**) as a bird in hunting.—*also n.*

swop /swɒp/ *see* **swap**.

sword /sɔrd/ *n* a weapon with a long blade and a handle at one end.

sword dance *n* a dance in which swords are brandished or placed on the ground and stepped between.

swordfish /'sɔrdfɪʃ/ *n* a large marine fish with a sword-like upper jaw.

swordplay /'sɔrdpleɪ/ *n* fighting with swords; verbal combat.

swordsman /'sɔrdsmən/ *n* (*pl* **swordsmen**) a person skilled in the use of a sword.

swordstick *n* a walking stick concealing a sword.

swore /swoːr/ *see* **swear**.

sworn /swɔrn/ *see* **swear**.

swot /swɒt/ *vi* (*inf*) to study hard for an examination. • *n* (*inf*) a person who studies hard.

swum /swʌm/ *see* **swim**.

swung /swʌŋ/ *see* **swing**.

sycamore /'sɪkəˌmɔr/ *n* a Eurasian maple tree; an American plane tree; a tree of Africa and Asia bearing a fruit resembling a fig.

sycophant /'sɪkəˌfænt/ *or* /'saɪk-, /-fənt/ *n* a person who flatters and praises powerful people to win their favour.—**sycophancy** *n.*—**sycophantic** *adj.*

syllabi /'sɪləˌbaɪ/ *see* **syllabus**.

syllabic /sɪ'læbɪk/ *adj* consisting of syllables; articulated in syllables.

syllable /'sɪləbəl/ *n* word or part of a word uttered in a single sound; one or more letters written to represent a spoken syllable.

syllabub, sillabub /'sɪləˌbʌb/ *n* a cold dessert made with sweetened whipped cream flavoured with sherry, wine, lemon juice, etc.

syllabus /'sɪləbəs/ *n* (*pl* **syllabuses, syllabi**) a summary or outline of a course of study or of examination requirements; the subjects studied for a particular course.

syllogism /'sɪlɒdʒɪzəm/ *n* a form of reasoning consisting of a major premise, a minor premise and a conclusion. *eg All men must die; I am a man; therefore I must die.*

sylph /sɪlf/ *n* a slim girl or woman.

symbiosis /ˌsɪmbaɪ'oːsɪs/ *n* a mutually advantageous partnership between two interdependent plant or animal species.—**symbiotic** *adj.*

symbol /'sɪmbəl/ *n* a representation; an object used to represent something abstract; an arbitrary or conventional sign standing for a quality, process, relation, etc as in music, chemistry, mathematics, etc.

symbolic /sɪm'bɒlɪk/, **symbolical** /-əl/ *adj* of, using, or constituting a symbol.—**symbolically** *adv.*

symbolism /-'bɒlɪzəm/ *n* the use of symbols; a system of symbolic representation.—**symbolist** *n.*

symbolize /ˌsɪmbəˌlaɪz/ *vt* to be a symbol; to represent by a symbol.—**symbolization** *n.*—**symbolizer** *n.*

symmetrical /sɪ'metrɪkəl/, **symmetric** /sɪ'metrɪk/ *adj* having symmetry.—**symmetrically** *adv.*

symmetry /'sɪmətri/ *n* (*pl* **symmetries**) the corresponding arrangement of one part to another in size, shape and position; balance or harmony of form resulting from this.

sympathetic /ˌsɪmpə'θetɪk/ *adj* having sympathy; compassionate.—**sympathetically** *adv.*

sympathize /'sɪmpəˌθaɪz/ *vi* feel sympathy for; to commiserate; to be in sympathy (with).—**sympathizer** *n.*—**sympathizingly** *adv.*

sympathy /'sɪmpəθi/ *n* (*pl* **sympathies**) agreement of ideas and opinions; compassion; (*pl*) support for an action or cause.

symphony /'sɪmfəni/ *n* (*pl* **symphonies**) an orchestral composition in several movements; a large orchestra for playing symphonic works.—**symphonic** *adj.*—**symphonically** *adv.*

symposium /sɪm'poːzɪəm/ *n* (*pl* **symposiums, symposia**) a conference at which several specialists deliver short addresses on a topic; an anthology of scholarly essays.

symptom /'sɪmptəm/ *n* a bodily sensation experienced by a patient indicative of a particular disease; an indication.

symptomatic /ˌsɪmptə'mætɪk/ *adj* of, being, or relating to symptoms; indicative.—**symptomatically** *adv.*

syn /sɪn/ *prefix* together.

synagogue /'sɪnəgɒg/ *n* the building where Jews assemble for worship and religious study.

synapse /'sɪnæps/ *or* /-'næps/, /'saɪn-/ *n* the point at which a nerve impulse is transmitted between neurons.

sync, synch /sɪŋk/ *n* (*inf*) synchronization. • *vti* (*inf*) to synchronize.

synchromesh /'sɪŋkroˌmeʃ/ *adj* (*gear system*) incorporating a device that regulates the revolving parts in a gear so that they are at the same speed when brought into contact. • *n* a gear system using this.

synchronize /'sɪŋkrənaɪz/ *vti* to occur at the same time and speed; (*watches*) to adjust to show the same time.—**synchronization** *n.*—**synchronizer** *n.*

synchronous /sɪn'krɒnəs/ *adj* occurring at the same time.—**synchronously** *adv.*—**synchronousness** *n.*

syncopate /'sɪŋkəpeɪt/ *vt* (*mus*) to modify beats (in a musical piece) by displacing the rhythmical accents from strong beats to weak ones and vice versa.—**syncopation** *n.*

syndicate /'sɪndɪkət/ *n* an association of individuals or corporations formed for a project requiring much capital; any group, as of criminals, organized for some undertaking; an organization selling articles or features to many newspapers, etc. • *vt* to manage as or form into a syndicate; to sell (an article, etc) through a syndicate. • *vi* to form a syndicate.—**syndication** *n.*

syndrome /'sɪndroːm/ *or* /-drəm/ *n* a characteristic pattern of signs and symptoms of a disease.

synergist /'sɪnərdʒɪst/ *n* a muscle that works in conjunction with another muscle; a drug that combines with another drug, the two having a greater effect when taken together than separately.—**synergism** *n.*—**synergistic** *adj.*

synergy /'sɪnərdʒi/ *n* synergism; in business, the possibility that the merger of two individual companies will produce a combined operation of greater productivity and efficiency.—**synergetic, synergistic** *adj.*

synesis /'sɪnəsɪs/ *n* (*gram*) a construction in harmony with its sense rather than with strict syntax, *eg* "a large number were present."

synod /'sɪnəd/ *n* a council of members of a church that meets to discuss religious issues.

synonym /'sɪnənɪm/ *n* a word that has the same, or similar, meaning as another or others in the same language.

synonymous /sɪ'nɒnɪməs/ *adj* having the same meaning; equivalent.—**synonymously** *adv.*

synonymy /sɪ'nɒnɪmɪ/ *n* (*pl* **synonymies**) the condition of being synonymous; a system or collection of synonyms; the use of synonyms for emphasis, *eg* "in any shape or form".

synopsis /sɪ'nɒpsɪs/ *n* (*pl* **synopses**) a summary or brief review of a subject.

synovia /saɪ'noːvɪə/ or /sɪn-/ *n* a thick fluid that lubricates the joints and tendons.—**synovial** *adj.*

synovitis /ˌsaɪnə'vaɪtɪs/ *n* inflammation of the membrane around a joint.

syntax /'sɪntæks/ *n* (*gram*) the arrangement of words in the sentences and phrases of language; the rules governing this.—**syntactic** *adj.*—**syntactically** *adv.*

synth /sɪnθ/ *n* a synthesizer.

synthesis /'sɪnθəsɪs/ *n* (*pl* **syntheses**) the process of combining separate elements of thought into a whole; the production of a compound by a chemical reaction.

synthesize /'sɪnθəˌsaɪz/ *vti* to combine into a whole.

synthesizer /-ər/ *n* an electronic device producing music and sounds by using a computer to combine individual sounds previously recorded.

synthetic /sɪn'θetɪk/ *adj* produced by chemical synthesis; artificial.—**synthetically** *adv.*

syphilis /'sɪfɪlɪs/ *n* a contagious, infectious venereal disease.—**syphilitic** *adj.*

syphon /'saɪfən/ *see* **siphon**.

Syrian /'sɪrɪən/ *n* a native or inhabitant of Syria; the Arabic dialect spoken there.—*also adj.*

syringe /sɪ'rɪndʒ/ or /'sɪr-/ *n* a hollow tube with a plunger at one end and a sharp needle at the other by which liquids are injected or withdrawn, *esp* in medicine. • *vt* to inject or cleanse with a syringe.

syrinx /'sɪrɪŋks/ *n* (*pl* **syringes**) the vocal organ in birds.

syrup /'sɪrəp/ *n* a thick sweet substance made by boiling sugar with water; the concentrated juice of a fruit or plant.—**syrupy** *adj.*

systaltic /sɪ'stæltɪk/ or /-'stɒl-/ *adj* (*heart, etc*) alternately expanding and contracting; pulsating.

system /'sɪstəm/ *n* a method of working or organizing by following a set of rules; routine; organization; structure; a political regime; an arrangement of parts fitting together.

systematic /ˌsɪstə'mætɪk/ *adj* constituting or based on a system; according to a system.—**systematically** *adv.*

systematize /ˌsɪstəmə'taɪz/ *vt* to arrange according to a system.—**systematization** *n.*—**systematizer** *n.*

systemic /sɪ'stemɪk/ *adj* (*poison, infection, etc*) of or affecting the entire body; (*insecticide, etc*) designed to be taken up into the plant tissues.—**systemically** *adv.*

systemize /ˌsɪstə'maɪz/ *vt* to systematize.—**systemization** *n.*

systems analysis *n* analysis of a particular task or operation to determine how computer hardware and software may best perform it.—**systems analyst** *n.*

systole /'sɪstəlɪ/ *n* the regular contractions of the chambers of the heart by which the circulation of blppd is maintained.—**systolic** *adj.*

T

T (*chem symbol*) tritium.

T, t /tiː/ *n* the 20th letter of the English alphabet; something shaped like a T.

t *abbr* = ton.

T4 slip /'tiːfɔːr/ *n* ✺ (*Cdn*) an official statement of employment income and deductions for the year, used to calculate the amount of income taxes owed to the government.

TA /tiːˈeɪ/ *abbr* = teaching assistant.

Ta (*chem symbol*) tantalum.

tab[1] /tæb/ *n* tabulator; tablet. • *vt* (**tabbing, tabbed**) to tabulate.

tab[2] *n* a small tag, label or flap; (*inf*) a bill, as for expenses. • *vt* (**tabbing, tabbed**) to fix a tab on.

tabard /'tæbərd/ *n* a short armless tunic, *esp* one bearing a coat of arms and worn by a herald or by a knight over his armour; a sleeveless garment shaped like this worn by women.

Tabasco /tə'bæskoː/ *n* (*trademark*) a very hot red pepper sauce.

tabbouleh /tə'buːleɪ/ *n* an Arabic salad made with vegetables, spices, lemon juice and cracked wheat.

tabby /'tæbi/ *n* (*pl* **tabbies**) a domestic cat with a striped coat, *esp* a female; a heavy watered silk. • *adj* striped in brown or grey. • *vt* (**tabbying, tabbied**) to pattern (silk) with a wavy pattern.

tabernacle /'tæbər,nækəl/ *n* (*Bible*) the portable tent carried by Jews through the desert containing their sacred writings; a place of worship.—**tabernacular** *adj*.

tabes /'teɪbiːz/ *n* (*pl* **tabes**) wasting caused by chronic disease.—**tabetic** *adj, n*.

tabes dorsalis /-'dɔːrsəlɪs/ *n* paralysis caused by syphilis at an advanced stage when it attacks the spinal cord.

tablature /'tæblətʃər/ *n* musical notation indicating the strings, frets, fingering, rhythm, etc, to be used, *esp* for the lute.

table /'teɪbəl/ *n* a piece of furniture consisting of a slab or board on legs; the people seated round a table; supply of food; a flat surface; a level area; a slab or tablet in a wall; an inscription on this; a list of facts and figures arranged in columns for reference or comparison; a folding leaf of a backgammon board; **at table** having a meal; **on the table** (*legislative bill, etc*) postponed, often indefinitely; **to turn the tables on** to put (an opponent) in a position of disadvantage previously held by oneself. • *vt* to submit, to put forward; to postpone indefinitely; to lay on a table. • *adj* of, on or at a table.

tableau /'tæbloː/ *n* (*pl* **tableaux, tableaus**) a dramatic or graphic representation of a group or scene; a tableau vivant.

tableau vivant /,tæbloː'viːvã/ *n* (*pl* **tableaux vivants**) a representation of an historical scene by people in costume posed silently and motionless.

tablecloth /'teɪbəl,klɒθ/ *n* a cloth for covering a table.

table d'hôte /,tæblə'doːt/ *n* (*pl* **tables d'hôte**) a meal at a fixed price for a set number of courses.—*also adj*.

tableland /'teɪbəl,lænd/ *n* an expanse of flat elevated land, a plateau.

tablespoon /'teɪbəl,spuːn/ *n* a large serving spoon; a unit of measure in cooking.

tablespoonful /-fʊl/ *n* (**tablespoonfuls**) the amount a tablespoon holds.

tablet /'tæblət/ *n* a pad of paper; a medicinal pill; a cake of solid substance, such as soap; a slab of stone.

table tennis *n* a game like tennis played on a table with small bats and a ball.

tableware /'teɪbəl,wer/ *n* dishes, cutlery, etc for use at mealtimes.

tabloid /'tæblɔɪd/ *n* a small-format newspaper characterized by emphasis on photographs and news in condensed form.

taboo, tabu /tə'buː/ or /tæ-/ *n* (*pl* **taboos, tabus**) a religious or social prohibition of the use or practice of something; the thing prohibited. • *adj* forbidden from use, mention, etc. • *vt* (**tabooing, tabooed** *or* **tabuing, tabued**) to forbid by social or personal influence the use, practice or mention of something or contact with someone.

tabor, tabour /'teɪbər/ *n* a small drum formerly used to accompany a pipe, both instruments being played by the same person.

tabular /'tæbjʊlər/ *adj* like a table, flat; arranged in the form of a table; calculated with a table.—**tabularly** *adv*.

tabula rasa /,tæbjʊlə'raːzə/ *n* (*pl* **tabulae rasae**) the mind when regarded as in its original state and clear of impressions; a fresh start.

tabulate /'tæbjʊ,leɪt/ *vt* to arrange (written material) in tabular form.—**tabulation** *n*.

tabulator /-ər/ *n* a device that sets stops to locate columns on a typewriter or word processor.

TAC /tæk/ *abbr* = Tactical Air Command.

tacamahac /'tækmə,hæk/ *n* (any tree yielding) any of various pungent gum resins used *esp* in incense.

tacet /'tæsət/ or /'teɪ-/ *vi* a direction on a musical score indicating that from this point a particular instrument is not to play.

tachism /'tæʃɪzəm/ *n* a form of action painting using random blobs of colour.

tachistoscope /tə'kɪstə,skoːp/ *n* a device for projecting visual information onto a screen for a split second only, used in the study of perception and learning.

tacho- /'tækoː/ *prefix* speed.

tachograph /'tækə,græf/ *n* a device in motor vehicles, *esp* lorries, to record speed and time of travel.

tachometer /tə'kɒmətər/ *n* an instrument for measuring the speed of rotation of a shaft, as in a vehicle engine.

tachy- /'tæki/ *prefix* rapid or accelerated.

tachycardia /,tæki'kɑːrdiə/ *n* an abnormally fast heartbeat.

tachygraphy /tə'kɪgrəfi/ *n* shorthand, *esp* as used in ancient Greece and Rome.

tachymeter /tə'kɪmətər/ *n* a surveying instrument for measuring long distances rapidly.

tachyon /'tækiɒn/ *n* (*physics*) a theoretical elementary particle that can travel faster than light.

tacit /'tæsɪt/ *adj* implied without really being spoken; understood.—**tacitly** *adv*.—**tacitness** *n*.

taciturn /'tæsɪ,tɜːrn/ *adj* habitually silent and reserved.—**taciturnity** *n*.

tack[1] /tæk/ *n* a short, flat-headed nail; the course of a sailing ship; a course of action, approach; adhesiveness. • *vt* to fasten with tacks. • *vi* to change direction.

tack[2] *n* (*inf*) food.

tack[3] *n* riding equipment for horses.

tackle /'tækəl/ *n* a system of ropes and pulleys for lifting; equipment; rigging; (*sport*) an act of grabbing and stopping an opponent. • *vt* (*task, etc*) to attend to, undertake; (*a person*) to confront; (*sport*) to challenge with a tackle.

tacky[1] /'tæki/ *adj* (**tackier, tackiest**) (*paint, etc*) sticky.

tacky[2] *adj* (**tackier, tackiest**) (*inf*) shabby; ostentatious and vulgar; seedy.—**tackiness** *n*.

tact /tækt/ *n* discretion in managing the feelings of others.—**tactful** *adj*.—**tactless** *adj*.

tactical voting *n* the strategy in elections of voting for the candidate most likely to defeat the favourite, rather than voting for one's preferred choice.

tactics /'tæktɪks/ *n sing* stratagem; ploy; the science or art of manoeuvring troops in the presence of the enemy.—**tactical** *adj*.—**tactician** *n*.

tactile /'tæktaɪl/ *adj* re ating to, or having a sense of touch.

tad /tæd/ *n* (*inf*) a small boy; (*inf*) a tiny quantity; a bit.

tadpole /'tædpoːl/ *n* the larva of a frog or toad, *esp* at the stage when the head and tail have developed.

taeniasis /tiː'naɪəsɪs/ *n* infestation with tapeworms.—*also* **teniasis**.

taffeta /'tæfətə/ *n* a thin glossy fabric with a silky lustre.

taffrail /'tæfreɪl/ *n* the rail at the stern of a ship.

tag[1] /tæg/ *n* a strip or label for identification. • *vt* to attach a tag; to mark with a tag. • *vi* (*with* **onto, after, along**) to trail along (behind).

tag² *n* a children's chasing game; (*baseball*) the putting out of a runner by touching him with the ball. • *vt* (**tagging, tagged**) to touch another player in a game of tag; to put a runner out by touching him with the ball.

tag end *n* the final part of something.

tagliatelle /ˌtæljəˈteli/ *n* pasta in narrow ribbons.

tahini /təˈhiːni/ *n* a thick paste of ground sesame seeds.

tahr /tɑr/ *n* a type of Himalayan wild goat.

Tahitian /təˈhiːʃən/ or /-tiən/ *adj* of or pertaining to the South Pacific island of Tahiti, its people or language. • *n* a native of Tahiti; the Polynesian language spoken in Tahiti.

t'ai chi ch'uan /taɪˈtʃiːˌtʃwɒn/ *n* a Chinese form of exercise using movements designed to improve balance and coordination.—*also* **t'ai chi.**

taiga /ˈtaɪgə/ *n* coniferous forests dominated by spruces and firs extending across the subarctic regions of Eurasia and North America.

tail /teɪl/ *n* the appendage of an animal growing from the rear, generally hanging loose; the rear part of anything; (*pl*) the side of a coin without a head on it; (*inf*) a person who keeps another under surveillance, *esp* a detective. • *vti* to follow closely, to shadow; (*with* **off, away**) to (cause to) dwindle.

tailback /ˈteɪlbæk/ *n* a long queue of traffic behind an obstruction; (*football*) the offensive back farthest from the line of scrimmage.

tailboard /ˈteɪlbɔrd/ *n* a hinged or removable section at the rear of a motor vehicle.

tail coat *n* a man's black or grey coat cut horizontally just below the waist at the front with two long tails at the back.

tail-end *adj* tardy; being the last in line. • *n* the last.

tailgate /ˈteɪlgeɪt/ *n* the hinged board at the rear of a truck which can be let down or removed. • *vti* to drive dangerously close behind (another vehicle).—**tailgater** *n*.

taillight /ˈteɪllaɪt/ *n* a red warning light at the rear of a motor vehicle.

tailor /ˈteɪlər/ *n* a person who makes and repairs outer garments, *esp.* men's suits. • *vi* to work as a tailor. • *vt* to adapt to fit a particular requirement.

tailor-made *adj* specially designed for a particular purpose or person.

tailpipe /ˈteɪlpaɪp/ *n* a pipe at the rear of jet engine or motor vehicle for discharging exhaust gases.

tailplane /ˈteɪlpleɪn/ *n* a small stabilizing wing at the rear of an aircraft, a horizontal stabilizer.

tail rotor *n* the small propeller at the rear of a helicopter that counteracts the tendency of the body to spin in the opposite direction to the main rotor blades.

tailspin /ˈteɪlspɪn/ *n* a spiralling nose dive; (*inf*) a state of chaos.

tailstock /ˈteɪlstɒk/ *n* the adjustable part of a lathe that supports the free end of a workpiece.

tailwind /ˈteɪlwɪnd/ *n* a wind in the same direction as a ship or aircraft is travelling.

taint /teɪnt/ *vt* to contaminate; to infect. • *vi* to be corrupted or disgraced. • *n* a stain; corruption.

taipan¹ /ˈtaɪpæn/ *n* a powerful businessman operating in Hong Kong or China.

taipan² *n* a venomous Australian snake.

take /teɪk/ *vb* (**taking, took,** *pp* **taken**) *vt* to lay hold of; to grasp or seize; to gain, win; to choose, select; (*attitude, pose*) to adopt; to understand; to consume; to accept or agree to; to lead or carry with one; to use as a means of travel; (*math*) to subtract (from); to use; to steal; (*gram*) to be used with; to endure calmly; (*with* **apart**) to dismantle; to criticize; (*with* **back**) to retract, withdraw (a promise, etc); (*with* **down**) to write down; to dismantle; to humiliate; (*with* **for**) (*inf*) to mistakenly believe to be; (*with* **in**) to understand, perceive; to include; to make a garment smaller by altering seams, etc; to offer accommodation to; (*inf*) to swindle, deceive; (*with* **on**) to employ as labour; to assume or acquire; to agree to do (something); to fight against; (*with* **out**) to extract; to obtain, procure; to escort; (*sl*) to kill; (*with* **up**) to begin as a business or hobby; to accept an offer or invitation; to occupy (time or space); to act as a patron to; to shorten (a garment); to interrupt or criticize; to absorb. • *vi* (*plant, etc*) to start growing successfully; to become effective; to catch on; to have recourse to; to go to; (*with* **after**) to resemble in appearance, character, etc; (*with* **on**) (*inf*) to become upset or distraught; (*with* **to**) to escape to as a refuge; to acquire a liking for; to adopt as a habit; (*with* **up**) to resume, continue further. • *n* (*film, TV*) the amount of film used without stopping the camera when shooting.

takeaway /ˈteɪkəˌweɪ/ *n* a takeout.

take-home pay *n* pay remaining after all deductions, such as income tax, have been made.

taken /ˈteɪkən/ *see* **take.**

takeoff /ˈteɪkɒf/ *n* the process of an aircraft becoming airborne; (*inf*) an amusing impression or caricature of another person.

takeout, take-out /ˈteɪkaʊt/ *n* a cooked meal that is sold for consumption outside the premises; a shop or restaurant that provides such meals.—*also adj.*

takeover /ˈteɪkoːvər/ *n* the taking over of control, as in business.—*also adj.*

taking /ˈteɪkɪŋ/ *adj* attractive, charming; (*inf*) catching, contagious. • *n* the act of one that takes; (*pl*) earnings; profits.

talc /tælk/ *n* a type of smooth mineral used in ceramics and talcum powder; talcum powder.

talcum powder /ˈtælkəm/ *n* perfumed powdered talc for the skin.

tale /teɪl/ *n* a narrative or story; a fictitious account, a lie; idle or malicious gossip.

talent /ˈtælənt/ *n* any innate or special aptitude.—**talented** *adj*.

talent scout *n* a person employed to recruit talented people for professional careers in sport, entertainment, etc.

talent show *n* a show which gives amateurs a chance to perform in the hope of attracting interest from professionals for permanent engagements.

talipot /ˈtælɪˌpɒt/ *n* a palm tree of the East Indies with large leaves used for roofing, umbrellas, etc.

talisman /ˈtælɪzmən/ or /ˈtælɪs-/ *n* (*pl* **talismans**) an object or charm supposed to ward off evil and bring good luck; an amulet.

talk /tɒk/ *vt* to speak; to know how to speak (a language); to discuss or speak of (something); to influence by talking; (*with* **down**) to silence or override (a speaker, argument, etc) by talking loudly; to radio instructions to (an aircraft) so that it may land safely; (*with* **into**) to persuade by argument or talking; (*with* **out**) to resolve by discussion; (*with* **round**) to persuade by talking. • *vi* to converse; to discuss; to gossip; to divulge information; (*with* **back**) to reply impudently; (*with* **down**) to speak in a condescending manner (to); (*with* **round**) to discuss (a subject) without reaching any conclusion; (*with* **shop**) to discuss work, *esp* after working hours. • *n* a discussion; a lecture; gossip; (*pl*) negotiations.

talkative /ˈtɒkətɪv/ *adj* given to talking a great deal.

talkie /ˈtɒki/ *n* (*inf*) an early motion-picture film with sound.

talking book *n* a recording of a book for the blind.

talking head *n* the head and shoulders of a person on television talking directly to the camera without using visual material.

talking picture *n* a talkie.

talking point *n* a subject for conversation or discussion; something that lends support to an argument.

talking-to *n* a reprimand, lecture.

talk show *n* a television or radio programme with informal interviews and conversation, a chat show.

tall /tɒl/ *adj* above average in height; (*inf*) (*story*) exaggerated.—**tallness** *n*.

tallboy /ˈtɒlbɔɪ/ *n* a high chest of drawers on legs, a highboy.

tallith /ˈtæliθ/ *n* (*pl* **tallithim**) a fringed shawl worn by Jewish men during religious services.

tall order *n* (*inf*) a request that is difficult to fulfil.

tallow /ˈtæloː/ *n* solid animal fat used to make soap, candles, etc.

tall ship *n* a square-rigged sailing vessel.

tall story *n* (*inf*) an exaggerated or unbelievable account.

tally /ˈtæli/ *n* (*pl* **tallies**) reckoning, account; one score in a game. • *vi* (**tallying, tallied**) to correspond; to keep score.

tally-ho *n* the cry of a person at a fox hunt when sighting the quarry.—*also vti.*

Talmud /ˈtælmʊd/ or /-məd/ *n* the body of Jewish law.—**Talmudic** *adj.*

talon /ˈtælən/ *n* a claw of an animal, *esp* a bird of prey.

talus¹ /ˈteɪləs/ *n* (*pl* **tali**) the anklebone.

talus² *n* (*pl* **taluses**) scree; the sloping side of a wall.

tamale /təˈmɒli/ or /-ˈmæli/ *n* a Mexican dish of minced meat with crushed maize and seasonings.

tamandua /təˈmændjuːə/ *n* a small tree-dwelling anteater of Central and South America.

tamarack /ˈtæməˌræk/ *n* (the wood of) any of various North American larches.

tamarin /'tæmərin/ *n* any of numerous small monkeys of South America resembling marmosets.

tamarind /'tæmərind/ *n* a tropical evergreen tree bearing a pulpy fruit used for food, in beverages and in laxative preparations.

tamarisk /'tæmərisk/ *n* any of a genus of evergreen trees and shrubs of Mediterranean and tropical regions with tiny leaves and numerous clusters of pink or white flowers.

tambour /'tæmbur/ *n* a drum; (an embroidery produced on) a circular frame for holding fabric taut during embroidery; a rolling top on a desk or cabinet made from thin strips of wood on a canvas backing. • *vt* to embroider using a tambour.

tamboura, tambura /tæm'burə/ *n* an Indian stringed instrument used to provide a drone as accompaniment to singing.

tambourin /,tæmbə'ri:n/ *n* a dance of Provence in France; the music for this; a long drum used in Provence.

tambourine *n* a percussion hand instrument made of skin stretched over a circular frame with small jingling metal discs around the edge.

tambura *see* **tamboura**.

tame /teim/ *adj* (*animal*) not wild, domesticated; compliant; dull, uninteresting. • *vt* (*animal*) to domesticate; to subdue; to soften.

Tamil /'tæmil/ *n* a member of a people inhabiting southeastern India and Sri Lanka; the language they speak.—*also adj.*

tam-o'-shanter /'tæmə,ʃæntər/ *n* a tight-fitting Scottish woollen or cloth beret with a full crown and a pompom on top.

tamp /tæmp/ *vt* to pack down firmly with a series of blows; to pack (a blast-hole) with sand or earth above the explosive charge.

tamper /'tæmpər/ *vi* to meddle (with); to interfere (with).

tampion /'tæmpiən/ *n* a plug for the muzzle of a gun.

tampon /'tæmpɒn/ *n* a firm plug of cotton wool inserted in the vagina during menstruation.

tam-tam /'tæmtæm/ *n* a gong.

tan¹ /tæn/ *n* a yellowish-brown colour; suntan. • *vti* (**tanning, tanned**) to acquire a suntan through sunbathing; (*skin, hide*) to convert into leather using tannin; (*inf*) to thrash.

tan² *abbr* = tangent.

tanager /'tænədʒər/ *n* any of numerous American woodland songbirds, the male of which has vividly coloured plumage.

tanbark /'tænbɑrk/ *n* bark, *esp* from the oak, used as a source of tannin.

tandem /'tændəm/ *n* a bicycle for two riders, sitting one behind the other.

tandoori /tæn'duri/ *n* an Indian method of cooking meat, vegetables and bread using a large clay oven.

tang /tæŋ/ *n* sharp smell or a strong taste.—**tangy** *adj.*

tangent /'tændʒənt/ *n* a line that touches a curve or circle at one point, without crossing it. • *adj* touching at one point.

tangential /tæn'dʒenʃəl/ *adj* of superficial relevance; digressive.

tangerine /tændʒə'ri:n/ *n* a small, sweet orange with a loose skin; the colour of this.—*also adj.*

tangible /'tændʒibəl/ *adj* capable of being felt, seen or noticed; substantial; real.—**tangibility** *n.*

tangle /'tæŋgəl/ *n* a mass of hair, string or wire knotted together confusedly; a complication. • *vt* to intertwine in a mass, to snarl; to entangle, complicate. • *vi* to become tangled or complicated; (*with* **with**) to become involved in argument with.

tango /'tæŋgo:/ *n* (*pl* **tangos**) a Latin American ballroom dance. • *vi* (**tangoing, tangoed**) to dance the tango.

tangram /'tæŋgræm/ *n* a Chinese puzzle made from a square cut into a rhomboid, a square and five triangles, which can be combined to produce different figures.

tank /tæŋk/ *n* a large container for storing liquids or gases; an armoured combat vehicle, mounted with guns and having caterpillar tracks.

tanka /'tæŋkə/ *n* (*pl* **tankas, tanka**) a Japanese verse form with five lines.

tankage /'tæŋkidʒ/ *n* the capacity of a tank; the storing of oil, etc in tanks.

tankard /'tæŋkərd/ *n* a tall, one-handled drinking mug, often with a hinged lid.

tanked /'tæŋkt/ *adj* (*sl*) extremely drunk.

tank engine *n* a steam locomotive that carries its own water supplies instead of using a tender.

tanker /'tæŋkər/ *n* a large ship or truck for transporting oil and other liquids.

tank top *n* a sleeveless pullover with a low neck.

tanner /'tænər/ *n* a person who tans skins.

tannery /-i/ *n* (*pl* **tanneries**) a place where hides are tanned.

tannic /'tænik/ *adj* of, resembling, or derived from tan or tannin.

tannic acid *n* tannin.

tannin /'tænin/ *n* a yellow or brown chemical found in plants or tea, used in tanning.

tansy /'tænzi/ *n* (*pl* **tansies**) any of numerous aromatic plants with yellow flowers and finely-divided leaves, once used for seasoning and as a medicine.

tantalize /'tæntə,laiz/ *vt* to tease or torment by presenting something greatly desired, but keeping it inaccessible.

tantalum /'tæntələm/ *n* a hard metallic element of the vanadium family, *esp* used for hardening alloys.

tantalus /'tæntələs/ *n* a cabinet or case where bottles of spirit may be locked up yet remain visible.

tantamount /'tæntə,maunt/ *adj* equivalent (to) in effect; as good as.

tantara /'tæntərə/ *n* the sound of a horn or trumpet playing a fanfare.

tantrum /'tæntrəm/ *n* a childish fit of bad temper.

Tao /tau/ *or* /dau/ *n* (*Taoism*) the spirit of creative harmony in the universe; the path of virtuous conduct in harmony with the natural order.

Taoiseach /'ti:ʃəx/ *n* the Prime Minister of the Republic of Ireland.

Taoism /'tauizəm/ *or* /'dau-/ *n* a Chinese religious and philosophical system advocating a simple passive life in harmony with the natural order.

tap¹ /tæp/ *n* a quick, light blow or touch; a piece of metal attached to the heel or toe of a shoe for reinforcement or to tap-dance. • *vti* (**tapping, tapped**) to strike lightly; to make a tapping sound.

tap² *n* a device controlling the flow of liquid through a pipe or from a container, a faucet. • *vt* (**tapping, tapped**) to pierce in order to draw fluid from; to connect a secret listening device to a telephone; (*inf*) to ask for money from; (*resources, etc*) to draw on.

tap-dance *vi* to perform a step dance in shoes with taps.—**tap-dancer** *n.*—**tap-dancing** *n.*

tape /teip/ *n* a strong, narrow strip of cloth, paper, etc, used for tying, binding, etc; tape measure; magnetic tape, as in a cassette or videotape. • *vt* to wrap with tape; to record on magnetic tape.

tape deck *n* a tape recorder in a hi-fi system.

tape measure *n* a tape marked in inches or centimetres for measuring.

tape player *n* a self-contained tape recorder.

tape recorder *n* a machine used for recording and reproducing sounds or music on magnetic tape, *esp* as part of a hi-fi system, a tape deck.

tape recording *n* a recording made on magnetic tape.

taper /'teipər/ *n* a long thin candle. • *vti* to make or become gradually narrower toward one end.—**tapering** *adj.*

tapestry /'tæpəstri/ *n* (*pl* **tapestries**) a heavy fabric woven with patterns or figures, used for wall hangings and furnishings.

tapeworm /'teipwɔrm/ *n* a tape-like, parasitic, intestinal worm.

tapioca /,tæpi'o:kə/ *n* a glutinous starch extracted from the root of the cassava and used in puddings, etc.

tapir /'teipər/ *or* /-pi:r/ *n* (*pl* **tapirs, tapir**) a South American hoofed mammal with a short flexible proboscis.

tappet /'tæpət/ *n* a projecting arm or lever (*eg* a cam) that moves or is moved by another part in a machine.

taproom /'tæpru:m/ *n* a bar.

taps /tæps/ *n sing* a call on a bugle at a military camp signalling lights out; any similar signal, as at a military funeral.

tar¹ /tɑr/ *n* a thick, dark, viscous substance obtained from wood, coal, peat, etc., used for surfacing roads. • *vt* to coat with tar.—**tarry** *adj.*

tar² *n* a (*inf*) a sailor.

taramasalata /,tærəməsə'lætə/ *n* a pale pink fish-roe paste served as a starter.

tarantella /,tærən'telə/ *n* (the music for) a lively peasant dance of southern Italy.

tarantula /tə'ræntʃulə/ *n* (*pl* **tarantulas, tarantulae**) a large, hairy spider with a poisonous bite that is painful but not deadly.

tarboosh, tarbush /tɑ'bu:ʃ/ *n* a brimless red cap resembling a fez worn by Muslim men.

tardy /'tɑrdi/ *adj* (**tardier, tardiest**) slow; later than expected.—**tardily** *adv.*—**tardiness** *n.*

tare¹ /ter/ *n* (the seed of) a type of vetch plant.

tare² *n* (an allowance for) the weight of the wrapping or container in which goods are packed; the weight of an unloaded goods vehicle. • *vt* to weigh in order to calculate the tare.

target /'tɑrgət/ *n* a mark to aim at, *esp* in shooting; an objective or ambition.

tariff /'tɛrɪf/ or /'tærɪf/ *n* a tax on imports or exports; (*in a hotel*) a list of prices; the rate of charge for public services, such as gas or electricity.

tarlatan, tarletan /'tɑrlətən/ *n* a type of thin stiff cotton fabric.

tarmac /'tɑrmæk/, **tarmacadam** /ˌtɑrmə'kædəm/ *n* a material for surfacing roads made from crushed stones and tar; an airport runway. • *vti* (**tarmacking, tarmacked**) to lay down a tarmac surface.

tarn /tɑrn/ *n* a small mountain lake.

tarnish /'tɑrnɪʃ/ *vi* (*metal*) to lose its lustre or discolour due to exposure to the air. • *vt* (*reputation*) to taint.—*also n.*

taro /'tɑroʊ/ *n* (*pl* **taros**) (the edible root of) a tropical Asian plant.

tarot /'tæroʊ/ *n* a game played with 22 pictorial cards, which are also used for fortune-telling.

tarpaulin /tɑr'pɔlən/ *n* canvas cloth coated with a waterproof substance.

tarragon /'tɛrəˌgɒn/ *n* an aromatic herb used for flavouring.

tarry /'tɛri/ *vi* (**tarrying, tarried**) to delay or dawdle; to linger; to wait briefly.

tarsus /'tɑrsəs/ *n* (*pl* **tarsi**) the small bones of the ankle and the heel in vertebrates; the plate of tissue that stiffens the eyelid.— **tarsal** *adj, n.*

tart[1] /tɑrt/ *adj* having a sour, sharp taste; (*speech*) sharp, severe. —**tartly** *adv.*—**tartness** *n.*

tart[2] *n* an open pastry case containing fruit, jam or custard; (*inf*) a prostitute. • *vt* (*with* **up**) (*inf*) to dress cheaply and gaudily; to decorate, *esp* cheaply.

tartan /'tɑrtən/ *n* a woollen cloth with a chequered pattern, having a distinctive design for each Scottish clan.

tartar /'tɑrtər/ *n* a hard, yellow, crusty deposit which forms on the teeth; a salty deposit on the sides of wine casks.

tartaric acid *n* an organic acid obtained from grapes and many other fruits.

tartar sauce *n* a mayonnaise sauce with chopped capers, herbs, etc, eaten *esp* with fish.

task /tæsk/ *n* a specific amount of work to be done; a chore.

task force *n* a small unit with a specific mission, *usu* military.

taskmaster /'tæskˌmæstər/ *n* a person who demands constant hard work.

Tasmanian devil *n* a burrowing flesh-eating marsupial of Tasmania with a black coat and long tail.

tassel /'tɛsəl/ *n* an ornamental tuft of silken threads decorating soft furnishings, clothes, etc; a growth that looks like this, *esp* on corn. • *vb* (**tasselling, tasseled** *or* **tasseling, tasseled**) *vt* to decorate with tassels. • *vi* (*plant*) to grow tassels.

taste /teɪst/ *vt* to perceive (a flavour) by taking into the mouth; to try by eating and drinking a little; to sample; to experience. • *vi* to try by the mouth; to have a specific flavour. • *n* the sense by which flavours are perceived; a small portion; the ability to recognize what is beautiful, attractive, etc; liking; a brief experience.

taste bud *n* any of the small projecting sensory organs on the tongue's surface by which taste is perceived.

tasteful /'teɪstfʊl/ *adj* showing good taste.—**tastefully** *adv.*—**tastefulness** *n.*

tasteless /'teɪstləs/ *adj* without taste, bland; in bad taste.—**tastelessly** *adv.*

taster /'teɪstər/ *n* a person skilled in determining the balance of flavours in a product, *esp* tea, wine; a device for tasting or sampling; (*formerly*) a person who tasted food before it was served to a king, etc.

tasty /'teɪsti/ *adj* (**tastier, tastiest**) savoury; having a pleasant flavour.

ta-ta /tæ'tɒ/ *interj* (*Brit inf*) goodbye.

tatami /tə'tɒmi/ *n* (*pl* **tatamis, tatami**) straw matting used as a floor covering, *esp* in Japan.

tatter /'tætər/ *n* a torn or ragged piece of cloth.—**tattered** *adj.*

tatterdemalion /ˌtætərdɪ'mæljən/ or /-meɪl-/ *n* a person wearing ragged clothes, a ragamuffin.—*also adj.*

tatting /'tætɪŋ/ *n* (the process of making) a type of delicate handmade lace.

tattle /'tætəl/ *vi* to gossip. • *vt* to reveal (secrets, etc) by gossiping. • *n* (a) gossip.

tattletale /'tætəlˌteɪl/ *n* a gossip. • *adj* telltale.

tattoo[1] /tæ'tuː/ *n* (*pl* **tattoos**) a continuous beating of a drum; a military display of exercises and music.

tattoo[2] *vt* (**tattooing, tattooed**) to make permanent patterns or pictures on the skin by pricking and marking with dyes. • *n* (*pl* **tattoos**) marks made on the skin in this way.

tatty /'tæti/ *adj* (**tattier, tattiest**) shabby, ragged.

tau /taʊ/ or /tɔ/ *n* the 19th letter of the Greek alphabet.

taught /tɒt/ *see* **teach**.

taunt /tɒnt/ *vt* to provoke with mockery or contempt; to tease. • *n* an insult.

taupe /toːp/ *n, adj* (a) brownish-grey.

taurine /'tɔriːn/ or /-raɪn/ *n* of or like a bull.

tauromachy /tɔ'rɒməki/ *n* the art or practice of bullfighting.

Taurus /'tɔrəs/ *n* the Bull, the second sign of the zodiac.—**Taurean** *adj.*

taut /tɒt/ *adj* stretched tight; tense; stressed.

tauten /'tɒt'n/ *vti* to make or become taut.

tauto-, taut- /'tɒtoʊ/ *prefix* same.

tautog /tɒ'tɒg/ *n* a large North American food fish related to the wrasse.

tautology /tɒ'tɒlədʒi/ *n* (*pl* **tautologies**) a statement which uses different words to repeat the same thing.—**tautological, tautologous** *adj.*

tavern /'tævərn/ *n* a place licensed to sell alcoholic drinks; an inn.

taverna /tə'vɑrnə/ *n* a Greek hotel with its own bar; a Greek restaurant.

tawdry /'tɒdri/ *adj* (**tawdrier, tawdriest**) showy, cheap, and of poor quality.

tawny /'tɒni/ *adj* yellowish brown.

tawny owl *n* a European owl with brown plumage.

tawse /tɒz/ *n* (*Scot*) a leather strap with a slit end formerly used for punishing schoolchildren.

tax /tæks/ *n* a rate imposed by the government on property or persons to raise revenues; a strain. • *vt* to impose a tax (upon); to strain.

taxa /'tæksə/ *see* **taxon**.

taxable /'tæksəbəl/ *adj* able or liable to be taxed.

taxation /tæk'seɪʃən/ *n* the act of levying taxes; the amount raised as tax.

tax avoidance *n* avoiding paying tax using legal means.

tax-deductible *adj* (*expenses, etc*) legitimately deducted from income before tax assessment.

tax evasion *n* avoiding paying tax using illegal methods.

tax exile *n* a person who lives abroad to avoid paying high taxes.

tax haven *n* a place where taxes are lower than average.

taxi /'tæksi/ *n* (*pl* **taxis**) a taxicab. • *vi* (**taxiing** *or* **taxying, taxied**) (*aircraft*) to move along the runway before takeoff or after landing.

taxicab /'tæksikæb/ *n* a car, *usu* fitted with a taximeter, that may be hired to transport passengers.

taxidermy /'tæksiˌdɜrmi/ *n* the art of preparing and stuffing the skins of animals ready for exhibiting.—**taxidermist** *n.*

taximeter /'tæksiˌmiːtər/ *n* a meter fitted into a taxi to record the time taken for a journey.

taxis /'tæksɪs/ *n* a movement in a simple organism (*eg* a bacterium) in response to certain external stimulii; (*surgery*) the restoration of a displaced part by manual pressure.

taxiway /'tæksiweɪ/ *n* a marked route from a terminal to a runway along which an aircraft taxis.

taxon /'tæksən/ *n* (*pl* **taxa**) any taxonomic group or category.

taxonomy /tæk'sɒnəmi/ *n* (the science of) the classification of living things into groups based on similarities of biological origin, design, function, etc.

taxpayer /'tæksˌpeɪər/ *n* a person who or an organization that pays taxes.

tax return *n* a statement of a person's income for the purposes of tax assessment.

tax shelter *n* a financial arrangement to minimize tax liability.

tax therapist *n* a tax adviser who helps with the completion of income tax forms.

TB *abbr* = tuberculosis.

Tb (*chem symbol*) terbium.

T-bone steak *n* a large sirloin steak containing a T-shaped bone.

tbs., tbsp. *abbr* = tablespoon; tablespoonful.

Tc (*chem symbol*) technetium.

T-cell *n* a lymphocyte that kills cells infected with a virus.—*also* **T-lymphocyte**.

Te (*chem symbol*) tellurium.

tea /tiː/ *n* a shrub growing in China, India, Sri Lanka, etc; its dried, shredded leaves, which are infused in boiling water for a beverage; in UK, a light meal taken in mid-afternoon; a main meal taken in the early evening.

tea bag *n* a small porous bag containing tea leaves for infusing.

tea ball *n* a perforated metal ball which holds tea leaves to make tea.

tea biscuit *n* ✹ (*Cdn*) a small baked cake leavened with baking powder or soda, often containing raisins or currants; (*Brit*) a semi-sweet, plain biscuit.

tea caddy *n* an airtight container for storing tea.

teach /tiːtʃ/ *vb* (**teaching, taught**) *vt* to impart knowledge to; to give lessons (to); to train; to help to learn. • *vi* to give instruction, *esp* as a profession.—**teachable** *adj*.

tea chest *n* a large wooden box used to transport tea.

teacher /ˈtiːtʃər/ *n* a person who instructs others, *esp* as an occupation.

teach-in *n* an informal conference at a university or college with lectures and discussions on a topical issue.

teaching /ˈtiːtʃɪŋ/ *n* the profession or practice of being a teacher; the act of giving instruction.

tea cloth *n* a tea towel for drying dishes; a dishtowel.

tea cosy *n* a cover for a teapot to keep the contents warm.

teacup /ˈtiːkʌp/ *n* a small cup for drinking tea.

teak /tiːk/ *n* a type of hard wood from an East Indian tree.

teal /tiːl/ *n* (*pl* **teal, teals**) a small freshwater duck; a dark greenish blue.

team /tiːm/ *n* a group of people participating in a sport together; a group of people working together; two or more animals pulling a vehicle. • *vi* (*with* **up**) to join in cooperative activity.

team-mate /ˈtiːmmeɪt/ *n* a colleague, a fellow team member.

team spirit *n* willingness to work harmoniously within a group.

teamster /ˈtiːmstər/ *n* a truck driver.

teamwork /ˈtiːmwɜːk/ *n* cooperation of individuals for the benefit of the team; the ability of a team to work together.

teapot /ˈtiːpɒt/ *n* a vessel in which tea is made.

teapoy /ˈtiːpɔɪ/ *n* a three-legged stand or table.

tear[1] /tɛr/ *n* a drop of salty liquid appearing in the eyes when crying or when the eyes are smarting; anything tear-shaped.

tear[2] *vb* (**tearing, tore,** *pp* **torn**) *vt* to pull apart by force; to split; to lacerate; (*with* **down**) to destroy, demolish. • *vi* to move with speed; (*with* **into**) (*inf*) to attack physically or verbally. • *n* a hole or split.

tearaway /ˈtɛrəweɪ/ *n* an impetuous, violent person.

tearful /ˈtɪrful/ *adj* weeping; sad.—**tearfully** *adv*.

tear gas *n* gas that irritates the eyes and nasal passages, used in riot control.

tearing /ˈtɛrɪŋ/ *adj* overwhelming, violent.

tear-jerker /ˈtɪrˌdʒɜːkər/ *n* a strongly sentimental book, film, play, etc.

tearoom /ˈtiːˌruːm/ *n* **teashop** *n* a restaurant where tea and light refreshments are served.

tea rose *n* any of numerous garden bush roses descended from a Chinese rose and valued for their large tea-scented blooms.

tease /tiːz/ *vt* to separate the fibres of; to torment or irritate; to taunt playfully. • *n* a person who teases or torments; (*inf*) a flirt.—**teaser** *n*.

teasel, teazel, teazle /ˈtiːzəl/ *n* any of various plants with prickly leaves and flower heads formerly dried and used to raise a nap on woollen cloth; an implement used for this purpose.

tea service, tea set *n* the set of cups and saucers, etc for serving tea.

teashop *n* a tearoom.

teaspoon /ˈtiːspuːn/ *n* a small spoon for use with a teacup or as a measure; the amount measured by this.—**teaspoonful** *n*.

teat /tiːt/ or /tɪt/ *n* the nipple on a breast or udder; the mouthpiece of a baby's feeding bottle.

tea towel, tea cloth *n* a towel for drying dishes; a dishtowel.

tech. /tɛk/ *abbr* = technical; technology.

technetium /tɛkˈniːʃɪəm/ or /-ʃəm/ *n* an artificially produced metallic element whose radioisotope is used in radiotherapy.

technical /ˈtɛknɪkəl/ *adj* relating to, or specializing in practical, industrial, mechanical or applied sciences; (*expression, etc*) belonging to or peculiar to a particular field of activity.—**technically** *adv*.

technicality /ˌtɛknɪˈkælɪtɪ/ *n* (*pl* **technicalities**) a petty formality or technical point.

technical knockout *n* (*boxing*) a decision by a referee to end a fight because a boxer is too badly hurt to continue.

technician /tɛkˈnɪʃən/ *n* a person skilled in the practice of any art, *esp* in practical work with scientific equipment.

Technicolor /ˈtɛknɪˌkʌlər/ *n* (*trademark*) the production of colour film by combining identical scenes with different primary colours into a single print.

technique /tɛkˈniːk/ *n* method of performing a particular task; knack.

techno- /ˈtɛknəʊ/ *prefix* technical; technological.

technocracy /tɛkˈnɒkrəsɪ/ *n* (*pl* **technocracies**) government by technical experts.—**technocrat** *n*.—**technocratic** *adj*.

technology /tɛkˈnɒlədʒɪ/ *n* (*pl* **technologies**) the application of mechanical and applied sciences to industrial use.—**technological** *adj*.—**technologist** *n*.

techy /ˈtɛtʃɪ/ *see* **tetchy**.

tectonic /tɛkˈtɒnɪk/ *adj* of or relating to building or construction; (*geological structures or forces*) resulting from deformation of the earth's crust.

tectonics /tɛkˈtɒnɪks/ *n sing* the art or science of constructing buildings, etc; the study of the forces which shape the earth's geological structure.

teddy /ˈtɛdɪ/ *n* (*pl* **teddies**) a woman's one-piece undergarment.

teddy bear *n* a stuffed toy bear.

Te Deum /tiːˈdiːəm/ or /teɪ ˈdeɪəm/ *n* a Latin hymn used in services of thanksgiving to God.

tedious /ˈtiːdɪəs/ *adj* monotonous; boring.—**tediously** *adv*.—**tedium** *n*.

tee /tiː/ *n* (*golf*) the place from where the first stroke is played at each hole; a small peg from which the ball is driven. • *vti* to position (the ball) on the tee; (*with* **off**) to hit a golf ball from a tee.

teem[1] /tiːm/ *vi* (*with* **with**) to be prolific or abundant in.

teem[2] *vi* to pour (with rain).

teen /tiːn/ *n* a teenager. • *adj* teenage.

teenager /ˈtiːnˌeɪdʒər/ *n* (*inf*) a person who is in his or her teens.

teens /tiːnz/ *npl* the years of one's life from thir*teen* to nine*teen*.—**teenage, teer aged** *adj*.

teeny /ˈtiːnɪ/ *adj* (**teenier, teeniest**) (*inf*) tiny.

teenybopper /ˈtiːnɪˌbɒpər/ *n* a young girl who avidly follows the latest fashions in clothes and pop music.

teepee /ˈtiːpiː/ *see* **tepee**.

tee-shirt *see* **T-shirt**.

teeter /ˈtiːtər/ *vi* to move or stand unsteadily.

teeth /tiːθ/ *see* **tooth**.

teethe /tiːð/ *vi* to cut one's first teeth.

teething /ˈtiːðɪŋ/ *n* the condition in babies of the first growth of teeth.

teething ring *n* a hard ring for a teething baby to chew on.

teething troubles *npl* problems encountered in the early stages of a project, etc; pain caused by growing teeth.

teetotaller, teetotaler /ˌtiːˈtəʊtələr/ *n* a person who abstains from alcoholic drinks.—**teetotal** *adj*.

TEFL /ˈtɛfəl/ *abbr* = Teaching English as a Foreign Language.

Teflon /ˈtɛflɒn/ *n* (*trademark*) polytetrafluoroethylene, a coating for pots and pans that prevents food sticking. • *adj* (*inf*) able to avoid (political) scandal by claiming ignorance or blaming others.

tegument /ˈtɛɡjʊmənt/ *n* an outer covering; an integument.

tektite /ˈtɛktaɪt/ *n* a spherical glassy object found in various parts of the world and thought to be of meteoric origin.

tel. *abbr* = telephone.

tel-, tele- /ˈtɛlɪ/ *prefix* at a distance; television.

telaesthesia /ˌtɛləsˈθiːsɪə/ *n* supposed perception of objects or events beyond the normal range of the senses.—*also* **telesthesia**.—**telaesthetic, telesthetic** *adj*.

telamon /ˈtɛləmən/ or /-mon/ *n* (*archit*) a figure or half-figure of a man, used in place of a column or pilaster to support an entablature, an atlas.

telecast /ˈtɛləˌkæst/ *vt* to broadcast by television. • *n* a television broadcast.—**telecaster** *n*.

telecom /ˈtɛləkɒm/ **telecoms** *n* short for telecommunications.

telecommunication /ˌtɛləkəˌmjuːnɪˈkeɪʃən/ *n* communication of information over long distances by telephone and radio; (*pl*) the technology of telephone and radio communication.

teledu /ˈtɛləˌduː/ *n* a mammal of Java and Sumatra resembling the badger and related to the skunk, which releases a foul-smelling liquid when threatened.

telefilm /ˈtɛləfɪlm/ *n* a motion picture produced for television.

telegenic /ˌtɛləˈdʒɛnɪk/ *adj* suitable for television in content or appearance.

telegram /ˈtelɪˌgræm/ *n* a message sent by telegraph.

telegraph /ˈtelɪˌgræf/ *n* a system for transmitting messages over long distances using electricity, wires and a code. • *vt* to transmit by telegraph.—**telegraphic** *adj.*—**telegraphy** *n.*

telekinesis /ˌtelɪkɪˈniːsɪs/ *n* the movement of objects using pure thought without the application of physical force.—**telekinetic** *adj.*

telemark /ˈtelɪˌmɑːk/ *n* (*skiing*) a turn in which one ski is placed ahead of the other and then angled gradually inward.

telemeter /ˈtelɪˌmiːtər/ or /təˈlemɪtər/ *n* any instrument that measures or records events and transmits the data to a distant receiver; (*surveying*) a device for measuring distances. • *vt* to gather and transmit data from a distance.

telemetry /tɪˈlemətri/ *n* the use of radio waves to transmit, register and record the readings of an instrument at a distance.

telencephalon /ˌtelenˈsefəˌlɒn/ *n* the frontal brain including the cerebrum, parts of the hypothalamus and the third ventricle.—**telencephalic** *adj.*

teleology /ˌteliˈɒlədʒi/ or /ˌtiː-/ *n* the philosophical doctrine that explains nature or natural processes in terms of purpose or design.—**teleological** *adj.*—**teleologist** *n.*

telepathy /təˈlepəθi/ *n* the communication between people's minds of thoughts and feelings, without the need for speech or proximity.—**telepathic** *adj.*

telephone /ˈtelɪˌfəʊn/ *n* an instrument for transmitting speech at a distance, *esp* by means of electricity. • *vt* (*someone*) to call by telephone.

telephone book *n* a book listing the names, addresses and telephone numbers of subscribers in a given area.

telephone booth *n* a cubicle for paid public use of a telephone.

telephone directory *n* a telephone book.

telephone operator, telephonist *n* a person who operates a telephone switchboard.

telephony /tɪˈlefəni/ *n* the system by which sounds are transmitted by telephone.—**telephonic** *adj.*

telephotography /ˌtelɪfəˈtɒgrəfi/ *n* the use of a telephoto lens to photograph distant objects.

telephoto lens /ˌtelɪˈfəʊtəʊlens/ *n* a camera lens that magnifies distant objects.

teleprinter /ˈtelɪˌprɪntər/ *n* a teletypewriter.

Teleprompter /ˈtelɪˌprɒmptər/ *n* (*trademark*) a prompting device used in TV, etc, which provides speakers with a script that remains invisible to the audience, an autocue.

telesales /ˈtelɪˌseɪlz/ *npl* selling products and services by telephone.

telescope /ˈtelɪˌskəʊp/ *n* a tubular optical instrument for viewing objects at a distance.

telescopic /ˌtelɪˈskɒpɪk/ *adj* of or like a telescope; that can be viewed by through a telescope.—**telescopically** *adv.*

telesthesia /ˌteles'θiːʒə/ or /-ziə/ *see* **telaesthesia**.

Teletext /ˈtelɪˌtekst/ *n* (*trademark*) written information transmitted non-interactively to television viewers.

telethon /ˈtelɪˌθɒn/ *n* a long television extravaganza which encourages viewers to send in money for a charitable cause.

Teletype /ˈtelɪˌtaɪp/ *n* (*trademark*) a teleprinter.

teletypewriter /ˌtelɪˈtaɪpˌraɪtər/ *n* a telegraph apparatus with a keyboard that transmits and a printer that receives messages over a distance.

televangelist /teleˈvændʒəlɪst/ *n* a person, *usu* a minister of the Christian Pentecostal church, who conducts television shows to preach the church's message and seek donations.

televise /ˈtelɪˌvaɪz/ *vt* (*a programme*) to transmit by television.

television /ˈtelɪˌvɪʒən/ *n* the transmission of visual images and accompanying sound through electrical and sound waves; a television receiving set; television broadcasting.

telex /ˈteleks/ *n* a communication system whereby subscribers hire teletypewriters for transmitting messages. • *vt* to transmit by telex.

tell /tel/ *vb* (**telling, told**) *vt* to narrate; to disclose; to inform; to notify; to instruct; to distinguish; (*with* **off**) (*inf*) to reprimand; to count off and assign to a duty. • *vi* to tell tales, to inform on; to produce a marked effect.

teller /ˈtelər/ *n* a bank clerk; a person appointed to count votes in an election.

telling /ˈtelɪŋ/ *adj* having great impact.

telltale /ˈtelˌteɪl/ *n* a person who tells tales about others. • *adj* revealing what is meant to be hidden.

tellurian /teˈlʊəriən/ or /tə-/ *adj* of the earth. • *n* an inhabitant of the earth.

telluric /teˈlʊərɪk/ *adj* of or in the earth or soil; of or containing (high valency) tellurium.

tellurium /teˈlʊəriəm/ *n* a brittle nonmetallic element related to sulphur and selenium.

tellurometer /teˈlʊərəˌmiːtər/ *n* (*surveying*) an electronic instrument for measuring distances using microwaves.

telly /ˈteli/ *n* (*pl* **tellies**) (*Brit inf*) television.

telo- /ˈtelə/ or /-ɔː/, **tel-** *prefix* end.

temerity /təˈmeriti/ *n* rashness.

temp /temp/ *n* (*inf*) a temporary employee.

temp. /temp/ *abbr* = temperature.

temper /ˈtempər/ *n* a frame of mind; a fit of anger. • *vt* to tone down, moderate; (*steel*) to heat and cool repeatedly to bring to the correct hardness.

tempera /ˈtempərə/ *n* (a method of painting using) powdered pigments mixed with an emulsion, *esp* egg yolk and water; a painting done in tempera; opaque watercolour used for posters.

temperament /ˈtemprəmənt/ or /-pərmənt/ *n* one's disposition.

temperamental /ˌtemprəˈmentəl/ or /-pər-/ *adj* easily irritated; erratic.—**temperamentally** *adv.*

temperance /ˈtemprəns/ or /-pərəns/ *n* moderation; abstinence from alcohol.

temperate /ˈtemprət/ or /-pərət/ *adj* mild or moderate in temperature; (*behaviour*) moderate, self-controlled.

temperature /ˈtemprətʃər/ or /-pərtʃər/ *n* degree of heat or cold; body heat above the normal.

tempest /ˈtempəst/ *n* a violent storm.

tempestuous /temˈpestʃʊəs/ *adj* stormy; violent; passionate.

tempi /ˈtempi/ *see* **tempo**.

template /ˈtempleɪt/ or /-plət/ *n* a pattern, gauge or mould used as a guide *esp* in cutting metal, stone or plastic.

temple[1] /ˈtempəl/ *n* a place of worship.

temple[2] *n* the region on either side of the head above the cheekbone.

tempo /ˈtempəʊ/ *n* (*pl* **tempos, tempi**) (*mus*) the speed at which music is meant to be played; rate of any activity.

temporal[1] /ˈtempərəl/ *adj* relating to time; secular, civil.

temporal[2] *adj* of or relating to the temples of the head.

temporality /ˌtempəˈræliti/ *n* (*pl* **temporalities**) the state or condition of being temporal; a secular or civil authority or power.

temporal lobe *n* a lobe on each side of the cerebral hemisphere associated with hearing and speech.

temporary /ˈtempəreri/ *adj* lasting or used for a limited time only; not permanent.—**temporarily** *adv.*

temporize /ˈtempəˌraɪz/ *vi* to delay in order to gain time; to act to fit the occasion.—**temporization** *n.*—**temporizer** *n.*

tempt /tempt/ *vt* to entice to do wrong; to invite, attract, induce.—**tempter** *n.*—**temptress** *nf.*

temptation /tempˈteɪʃən/ *n* the act of tempting or the state of being tempted; something or someone that tempts.

tempting /ˈtemptɪŋ/ *adj* attractive, inviting.

tempura /temˈpʊərə/ *n* a Japanese dish of seafood or vegetables fried in batter.

ten /ten/ *adj, n* the cardinal number next above nine. • *n* the symbol for this (10, X, x).

tenable /ˈtenəbəl/ *adj* capable of being believed, held, or defended.

tenacious /təˈneɪʃəs/ *adj* grasping firmly; persistent; retentive; adhesive.

tenacity /təˈnæsiti/ *n* the state or quality of being tenacious; doggedness, obstinacy; adhesiveness, stickiness.

tenaculum /təˈnækjʊləm/ *n* (*pl* **tenacula**) a hooked surgical instrument for seizing and holding parts, such as arteries.

tenancy /ˈtenənsi/ *n* (*pl* **tenancies**) the temporary possession by a tenant of another's property; the period of this.

tenant /ˈtenənt/ *n* a person who pays rent to occupy a house or flat or for the use of land or buildings; an occupant.

tenant farmer *n* a farmer who works land owned by someone else to whom he pays rent.

tench /tentʃ/ *n* (*pl* **tench**) a freshwater fish of the carp family.

tend[1] /tend/ *vt* to take care of; to attend (to).

tend[2] *vi* to be inclined; to move in a specific direction.

tendency /ˈtendənsi/ *n* (*pl* **tendencies**) an inclination or leaning.

tendentious, tendencious /tenˈdenʃəs/ *adj* showing bias, not impartial.—**tendentiousness, tendenciousness** *n.*

tender[1] /'tɛndər/ *n* a railroad car attached to locomotives to carry fuel and water; a small ship that brings stores to a larger one.

tender[2] *vt* to present for acceptance; to offer as payment. • *vi* to make an offer. • *n* an offer to provide goods or services at a fixed price.

tender[3] *adj* soft, delicate; fragile; painful, sore; sensitive; sympathetic.—**tenderly** *adv.*—**tenderness** *n*.

tenderfoot /'tɛndər,fʊt/ *n* a newcomer to rough, outdoor life; an inexperienced beginner.

tenderhearted *n* having a compassionate, loving or sensitive disposition.—**tenderheartedly** *adv.*—**tenderheartedness** *n*.

tenderize /'tɛndə,raɪz/ *vt* (*meat*) to make more tender by pounding or by adding a substance that softens.—**tenderization** *n*.—**tenderizer** *n*.

tenderloin /'tɛndər,lɔɪn/ *n* a cut of meat from between the ribs and sirloin.

tendon /'tɛndən/ *n* fibrous tissue attaching a muscle to a bone.

tendril /'tɛndrɪl/ *n* a thread-like shoot of a climbing plant by which it attaches itself for support.

tenement /'tɛnəmənt/ *n* a building divided into flats, each occupied by a separate owner or tenant.

tenesmus /tə'nɛzməs/ *n* (*med*) an urgent but ineffectual attempt to urinate or void the bowels.

tenet /'tɛnət/ *n* any belief or doctrine.

tenfold /'tɛnfoːld/ *adj*, *adv* 10 times as much or as many; composed of 10 parts.

ten-gallon hat /'tɛn'gælən/ *n* a wide-brimmed hat with a high crown, *esp* worn by cowboys.

teniasis /'tiːniəsɪs/ *see* **taeniasis**.

Tenn. *abbr* = Tennessee.

tenner /'tɛnər/ *n* (*inf*) a ten-pound note; a ten-dollar bill.

tennis /'tɛnɪs/ *n* a game for two or four people, played by hitting a ball over a net with a racket.

tennis court *n* a court surfaced with clay, asphalt or grass on which tennis is played.

tennis elbow *n* stiffness and pain in the elbow joint due to excessive exercise, such as playing tennis.

tenon /'tɛnən/ *n* a projection on the end of a piece of wood for connecting with a mortise. • *vt* to form a tenon; to connect using a tenon and mortise.

tenon saw *n* a fine-toothed saw with a sturdy back used for cutting tenons, etc.

tenor /'tɛnər/ *n* a general purpose or intent; the highest regular adult male voice, higher than a baritone and lower than an alto; a man who sings tenor.

tenor clef *n* a C clef placed so as to designate the fourth line of the staff as middle C.

tenosynovitis /,tɛnoʊ,saɪnoʊ'vaɪtɪs/ *n* inflammation of the tendons in a joint through repetitive movements of the joint concerned.

tenpin /'tɛnpɪn/ *n* a bowling pin used in tenpins.

tenpin bowling *n* in UK, tenpins.

tenpins /'tɛnpɪnz/ *n sing* a bowling game involving the rolling of a large bowl along a lane to knock over as many as possible of tenpins.

tenrec /'tɛnrɛk/ *n* any of various related mammals of Madagascar resembling shrews.

tense[1] /tɛns/ *n* (*gram*) the verb form that indicates the time of an action or the existence of a state.

tense[2] *adj* stretched, taut; apprehensive; nervous and highly strung. • *vti* to make or become tense.—**tensely** *adv.*—**tenseness** *n*.

tensile /'tɛnsaɪl/ or /-səl/ *adj* of or relating to tension; stretchable.

tensile strength *n* the greatest stress a material can bear without breaking.

tensimeter /tɛn'sɪmətər/ *n* an instrument that measures differences in vapour pressures.

tensiometer /,tɛnsi'ɒmətər/ *n* an instrument for measuring tensile strength; an instrument for comparing vapour pressures in different liquids; an instrument for measuring the surface tension of a liquid; an instrument for measuring the moisture content of soil.

tension /'tɛnʃən/ *n* the act of stretching; the state of being stretched; (*between forces, etc*) opposition; stress; mental strain.

tensor /'tɛnsər/ *n* any muscle that stretches or tightens a body part.

tent /tɛnt/ *n* a portable shelter of canvas, plastic or other waterproof fabric, which is erected on poles and fixed to the ground by ropes and pegs.

tentacle /'tɛntəkəl/ *n* a long, slender, flexible growth near the mouth of invertebrates, used for feeling, grasping or handling.

tentative /'tɛntətɪv/ *adj* provisional; not definite.—**tentatively** *adv.*—**tentativeness** *n*.

tenterhook /'tɛntər,hʊk/ *n* one of a series of hooks on which cloth is stretched to dry; (*pl.*) (*with* **on**) in a tense or anxious state.

tenth /tɛnθ/ *adj* the last of ten; being one of ten equal parts. • *n* one of ten equal parts.

tent ring *n* ✸ (*Cdn*) a ring of stones used to hold down a tent or other temporary structure.

tenuous /'tɛnjuəs/ *adj* slight, flimsy, insubstantial.—**tenuousness** *n*.

tenure /'tɛnjər/ *n* the holding of property or a position; the period of time which a position lasts; a permanent position, *usu* granted after holding a job for a number of years.—**tenured** *adj*.

tenuto /tə'nuːtoː/ *adv*, *adj* (*mus*) (*note*) sustained for its full time value.

teocalli /,tiːə'kælɪ/ *n* (*pl* **teocallis**) the pyramid-shaped bases supporting Aztec temples.

tepee /'tiːpi/ *n* a cone-shaped, North American Indian tent formed of skins; a wigwam.—*also* **teepee**.

tepid /'tɛpɪd/ *adj* slightly warm, lukewarm.

tequila /tə'kiːlə/ *n* a spirit distilled from a Mexican agave plant; the plant itself.

ter. *abbr* = terrace; territory.

ter- /tər/ *prefix* three times; third; three.

tera- /'tɛrə/ *prefix* ten to the power of 12.

terbium /'tɜrbiəm/ *n* a metallic element of the rare earth group.

tercel /'tɜrsəl/ *see* **tiercel**.

tercentenary /,tɜrsən'tɛnəri/ *n* (*pl* **tercentenaries**) a three hundredth anniversary.—*also adj*.

terebene /'tɛrə,biːn/ *n* a liquid hydrocarbon derived from oil of turpentine and sulphuric acid used in making varnishes, as an antiseptic and in medicines.

terebinth /'tɛrəbɪnθ/ *n* a European tree that yields a resinous liquid.

terebinthine /,tɛrə'bɪnθɪn/ or /-,θɪn/, /-,θaɪn/ *n* or or pertaining to the terebinth; of or like turpentine.

teredo /tə'riːdoː/ *n* (*pl* **teredos, teredines**) a burrowing mollusc, the shipworm.

terete /tə'riːt/ *adj* (*plant, animal part*) having a smooth cylindrical shape.

tergiversate /'tɜrdʒɪvərseɪt/ *vi* to switch allegiances; to be evasive, to equivocate.

term /tɜrm/ *n* a limit; any prescribed period of time; a division of an academic year; a word or expression, *esp* in a specialized field of knowledge; (*pl*) mutual relationship between people; (*pl*) conditions of a contract, etc. • *vt* to call, designate.

termagant /'tɜrməgənt/ *n* (*arch*) a shrewish, nagging woman.

terminal /'tɜrmɪnəl/ *adj* being or situated at the end or extremity; (*disease*) fatal, incurable. • *n* a bus, coach or railroad station at the end of the line; the point at which an electrical current enters or leaves a device; a device with a keyboard and monitor for inputting or viewing data from a computer.—**terminally** *adv*.

terminate /'tɜrmɪneɪt/ *vti* to bring or come to an end.—**termination** *n*.

terminology /,tɜrmɪ'nɒlədʒɪ/ *n* (*pl* **terminologies**) the terms used in any specialized subject.

terminus /'tɜrmɪnəs/ *n* (*pl* **termini, terminuses**) the final part; a limit; end of a transportation line.

termitarium /,tɜrmɪ'tɛriəm/ *n* (*pl* **termitaria**) a termites' nest.

termite /'tɜrmaɪt/ *n* a wood-eating, white, ant-like insect.

tern /tɜrn/ *n* a small, black and white sea bird.

ternary /'tɜrnəri/ *adj* in three parts; (*number system*) using three as a base.

terpene /'tɜrpiːn/ *n* any of various hydrocarbons present in the essential oils of plants, *esp* conifers.

Terpsichorean /,tɜrpsɪ'koriən/ or /-kə'riːən/ *adj* pertaining to dancing, or to Terpsichore, the Muse of dancing and choral song in classical myth.

terrace /'tɛrəs/ *n* a raised level area of earth, often part of a slope; an unroofed paved area adjoining a house; a row of houses; a patio or balcony. • *vt* to make into a terrace.

terracotta /,tɛrə'kɒtə/ *n* a brownish-red clay used for making flower pots and statues, which is baked but not glazed; a brown-red colour.

terra firma /,tɛrə'fɜrmə/ *n* solid ground; the earth.

terrain /tə'reɪn/ *n* the surface features of a tract of land; (*fig*) field of activity.

terra incognita /ˌterəɪŋkɒgˈniːtə/ or /ɪnˈkɒgnɪtə/ *n* an unexplored or unknown area or country.

terrapin /ˈterəpɪn/ *n* an aquatic North American turtle.

terrarium /təˈreriəm/ *n* (*pl* **terraria, terrariums**) an enclosure for small land animals; a glass container for plants.

terrazzo /teˈrætsoː/ or /-ˈræzoː/ *n* mosaic flooring in the form of marble chips set in mortar and highly polished.

terrestrial /təˈrestriəl/ *adj* relating to, or existing on, the earth; earthly; representing the earth.

terrible /ˈterɪbəl/ *adj* causing great fear; dreadful; (*inf*) very unpleasant.

terribly /ˈterɪbli/ *adv* frighteningly; (*inf*) very.

terrier /ˈteriər/ *n* a type of small, active dog.

terrific /təˈrɪfɪk/ *adj* of great size; (*inf*) excellent.

terrify /ˈterɪfaɪ/ *vt* (**terrifying, terrified**) to fill with terror, to frighten greatly.

terrine /təˈriːn/ *n* an earthenware dish for pâté; pâté or similar food served in this.

territorial /ˌterəˈtɔriəl/ *adj* relating to or owned by a territory. • *n* (*with cap*) a member of the Territorial Army, a British volunteer reserve force.

territorial waters *npl* the coastal and inland waters under the jurisdiction of a nation.

territory /ˈterətəri/ *n* (*pl* **territories**) an area under the jurisdiction of a city or state; a wide tract of land; an area assigned to a salesman; an area of knowledge.

terror /ˈterər/ *n* great fear; an object or person inspiring fear or dread.

terrorism /ˈterərˌɪzəm/ *n* the use of terror and violence to intimidate.— **terrorist** *n*.

terrorize /ˈterəˌraɪz/ *vt* to terrify; to control by terror.—**terrorization** *n*.

terry /ˈteri/ *n* (*pl* **terries**) a cloth with an uncut pile made of looped threads.

terse /tɜrs/ *adj* abrupt, to the point, concise.—**tersely** *adv*.

tertian /ˈtɜrʃən/ *adj* (*fever*) occurring on alternate days.

tertiary /ˈtɜrʃəri/ *adj* third.

TESOL /ˈtesɒl/ *abbr* = Teachers of English to Speakers of Other Languages.

tesla /ˈteslə/ *n* the SI unit of magnetic flux density.

tessellated /ˈtesəˌleɪtəd/ *adj* resembling mosaic.

tessera /ˈtesərə/ *n* (*pl* **tesserae**) a piece of marble, glass, etc used in a mosaic.

tessitura /ˌtesəˈtʊrə/ *n* (*mus*) the natural pitch of a voice or instrument.

test /test/ *n* an examination; trial; a chemical reaction to test a substance or to test for an illness; a series of questions or exercises. • *vt* to examine critically.

testament /ˈtestəmənt/ *n* a will; proof; tribute; (*arch*) a covenant made by God with men; (*with cap*) one of the two main parts of the Bible.

testate /ˈtesteɪt/ *adj* having made and left a will.

testator /təˈsteɪtər/ *n* a person who leaves a will.

test ban *n* an agreement between nations to limit or abandon tests of nuclear weapons.

test-bed *n* an area designed for testing machinery.

test case *n* a legal action that establishes a precedent.

testes /ˈtesˌtiːz/ *see* **testis**.

testicle /ˈtestɪkəl/ *n* either of the two male reproductive glands that produce sperm, a testis.

testify /ˈtestəˌfaɪ/ *vb* (**testifying, testified**) *vi* to give evidence under oath; to serve as witness (to); (*with* **to**) to be evidence of. • *vt* to be evidence of.

testimonial /ˌtestəˈmoːniəl/ *adj* relating to a testimony. • *n* a recommendation of one's character or abilities.

testimony /ˈtestəˌmoːni/ *n* (*pl* **testimonies**) evidence; declaration of truth or fact.

testis /ˈtestɪs/ *n* (*pl* **testes**) a testicle.

test match *n* one of a series of international cricket or Rugby football matches.

testosterone /teˈstɒstəˌroːn/ *n* a steroid hormone secreted by the testes.

test pilot *n* someone who flies new types of aircraft to test their performance and characteristics.

test tube *n* a cylinder of thin glass closed at one end, used in scientific experiments.

test-tube baby *n* a baby which develops from an ovum fertilized outside the mother's body and replaced in the womb.

testy /ˈtesti/ *adj* (**testier, testiest**) touchy, irritable.

tetanus /ˈtetnəs/ or /ˈtetənəs/ *n* an intense and painful spasm of muscles, caused by the infection of a wound by bacteria; lockjaw.

tetchy /ˈtetʃi/ *adj* (**tetchier, tetchiest**) irritable, touchy.—*also* **techy**.—**tetchily** *adv*.—**tetchiness** *n*.

tête-à-tête /ˌtetæˈtet/ *n* (*pl* **tête-à-têtes, tête-à-tête**) a private conversation between two people.

tether /ˈteðər/ *n* a rope or chain for tying an animal; the limit of one's endurance. • *vt* to fasten with a tether; to limit.

tetra- /ˈtetrə/, **tetr-** *prefix* four.

tetrahedron /ˌtetrəˈhiːdrən/ or /-ˈhedrən/ *n* (*pl* **tetrahedrons, tetrahedra**) a solid figure enclosed by four plane faces of triangular shape.

tetrahydroamino-acridine /ˌtetrəˌhaɪdroːəˌmiːnoˈækrɪˌdiːn/ *n* a drug currently being tried out for use in the treatment of Alzheimer's disease.

tetrahydrocannabinol /ˌtetrəˌhaɪdrəkəˈnæbɪnɒl/ *n* a natural compound that is the main intoxicant in cannabis and can also be produced synthetically.

tetralogy /teˈtrælədʒi/ or /-ˈtrɒlədʒi/ *n* (*pl* **tetralogies**) a series of four related works, such as novels or plays.

tetravalent /ˌtetrəˈveɪlənt/ *adj* (*chem*) having a valency of four.

Teutonic /tuːˈtɒnɪk/ or /tjuː-/ *adj* of Germanic peoples or their language.

Tex. *abbr* = Texas.

Tex-Mex /teksˈmeks/ *adj* of or pertaining to a Texan version of something Mexican, such as food or music.

text /tekst/ *n* the main part of a printed work; the original or exact wording; a passage from the Bible forming the basis of a sermon; a subject or topic; a textbook.

textbook /ˈtekstbʊk/ *n* a book used as a basis for instruction.

textile /ˈtekstaɪl/ *n* a woven fabric or cloth. • *adj* relating to the making of fabrics.

textual /ˈtekstʃʊəl/ *adj* of or relating to a text; contained in or based on a text; (*operation, etc*) exactly as planned according to theory or calculation.

textual criticism *n* the study of a written work (*eg* the Bible) to establish the original text; the close reading and analysis of any literary work.

texture /ˈtekstʃər/ *n* the characteristic appearance, arrangement or feel of a thing; the way in which threads in a material are interwoven.—**textural** *adj*.

TGIF *abbr* = thank God it's Friday.

Th (*chem symbol*) thorium.

Th. *abbr* = Thursday.

THA *abbr* = tetrahydroamino-acridine.

Thai /taɪ/ *n* (*pl* **Thais, Thai**) a native or inhabitant of Thailand; the language of Thailand.—*also adj*.

thalamus /ˈθæləməs/ *n* (*pl* **thalami**) either of the two masses of tissue which sit close together at the base of the brain.

thalidomide /θəˈlɪdəˌmaɪd/ *n* a sedative drug withdrawn from use when it was discovered to cause malformation in unborn babies.

thallium /ˈθæliəm/ *n* a soft white poisonous metallic element.

than /ðən/ or /ðæn/ *conj* introducing the second element of a comparison.

thanatology /ˌθænəˈtɒlədʒi/ *n* the scientific study of death.

thank /θæŋk/ *vt* to express gratitude to or appreciation for. • *npl* an expression of gratitude.—**thankful** *adj*.—**thankfully** *adv*.

thankless /ˈθæŋkləs/ *adj* without thanks; unappreciated; fruitless, unrewarding.—**thanklessness** *n*.

thanksgiving /ˌθæŋksˈgɪvɪŋ/ *n* the act of giving thanks; a prayer of gratitude to God; (*with cap*) Thanksgiving Day.

Thanksgiving Day *n* a legal holiday observed on the fourth Thursday of November in the US, and on the second Monday of October in Canada.

thank-you *n* an expression of gratitude.

that /ðæt/ or /ðət/ *demons adj, pron* (*pl* **those**) the (one) there or then, *esp* the latter or more distant thing. • *rel pron* who or which. • *conj* introducing noun clause or adverbial clause of purpose or consequence; because; in order that; (*preceded by* **so, such**) as a result.

thatch /θætʃ/ *n* roofing straw. • *vt* to cover a roof with thatch.

thaumaturgy /ˌθɔːməˈtɒlədʒi/ *n* (*pl* **thaumatologies**) the study of miracles; a discourse on miracles.

thaumaturge /ˈθɔːməˌtɜrdʒ/, **thaumaturgist** /ˈθɔːməˌtɜrdʒəst/ *n* a miracle-worker; a magician.—**thaumaturgy** *n*.

thaw /θɒ/ *vi* to melt or grow liquid; to become friendly. •*vt* to cause to melt. • *n* the melting of ice or snow by warm weather.

THC *abbr* = tetrahydrocannabinol.

the /ði/ (before vowels) or /ðə/ (before consonants), /'ði:/ *demons adj* denoting a particular person or thing. • *adv* used before comparative adjectives or adverbs for emphasis.

theatre, theater /'θiətər/ *n* a building where plays and operas are performed; the theatrical world as a whole; a setting for important events; field of operations.

theatre-in-the-round *n* a theatre with seats arranged in a circle around the stage area.

theatrical /θi:'ætrɪkəl/ *adj* relating to the theatre; melodramatic, affected.—**theatrically** *adv.*

theatricals /θi:'ætrɪkəlz/ *npl* performances of drama, *esp* by amateurs.

thee /ði:/ *pron* the objective case of **thou.**

theft /θeft/ *n* act or crime of stealing.

theine /'θi:i:n/ *n* caffeine.

their /ðer/ *poss adj* of or belonging to them; his, hers, its.

theirs /ðerz/ *poss pron* of or belonging to them; his, hers, its.

theism /'θi:ɪzəm/ *n* belief in the existence of a God or gods, *esp* God as the supernatural Creator of the universe.—**theist** *n.*—**theistic** *adj.*

them /ðem/ or /ðəm/ *pron* the objective case of **they.**

theme /θi:m/ *n* the main subject of a discussion; an idea or motif in a work; a short essay; a leading melody; a style adopted for an exhibition, activity, etc.—**thematic** *adj.*

theme park *n* a leisure area in which the buildings and settings follow a particular theme, *eg* a period in history.

theme song *n* a recurring melody in a film score or musical that is associated with the work or a particular character; a signature tune.

themselves /ðəm'selvz/ *pron* the reflexive form of **they** or **them.**

then /ðen/ *adv* at that time; afterward; immediately; next in time. • *conj* for that reason; in that case.

thenar /'θi:nər/ or /'θi:nɑr/ *n* the ball of the thumb; the palm of the hand.

thence /ðens/ *adv* from that time or place; for that reason.

thenceforth /ðens'fɔrθ/ *adv* from that time on; thereafter.

thenceforward, thenceforwards *adv* thenceforth.

theo- /'θi:o:/, **the-** *prefix* god.

theobromine /θiə'bro:mi:n/ *n* an alkaloid similar to caffeine present in cacao beans and tea, used in treating heart disease.

theocracy /θi:'ɒkrəsi/ *n* (*pl* **theocracies**) (a state having) government by a deity or priesthood.—**theocrat** *n.*—**theocratic** *adj.*

theodolite /θi:'ɒdəlaɪt/ *n* a surveying instrument for measuring angles.

theol. *abbr* = theologian; theological; theology.

theologian /θiə'lo:dʒən/ *n* a person who studies and interprets religious texts, etc; a teacher of theology.

theology /θi:'ɒlədʒi/ *n* (*pl* **theologies**) the study of God and of religious doctrine and matters of divinity.—**theological, theologic** *adj.*—**theologically** *adv.*

theorem /'θi:rəm/ or /'θi:ərəm/ *n* a proposition that can be proved from accepted principles; law or principle.

theoretical /θiə'retɪkəl/, **theoretic** /θiə'retɪk/ *adj* of or based on theory, not practical application; hypothetical; conjectural.—**theoretically** *adv.*

theoretician /ˌθi:rə'tɪʃən/ *n* a person who concentrates on the theoretical basis of a subject.

theoretics /θiə'retɪks/ *npl* the speculative parts of a science.

theorize /'θi:əraɪz/ or /'θi:raɪz/ *vi* to form theories; to speculate.—**theorist, theorizer** *n.*—**theorization** *n.*

theory /'θi:ri/ or /θi:əri/ *n* (*pl* **theories**) an explanation or system of anything; ideas and abstract principles of a science or art; speculation; a hypothesis.

therapeutic /ˌθerə'pju:tɪk/, **therapeutical** *adj* relating to the treatment of disease; beneficial.—**therapeutically** *adv.*

therapeutics /ˌθerə'pju:tɪks/ *npl* the curative branch of medicine.

therapy /'θerəpi/ *n* (*pl* **therapies**) the treatment of physical or mental illness.—**therapist** *n.*

there /ðer/ *adv* in, at or to, that place or point; in that respect; in that matter.

thereabout, thereabouts /'ðerəˌbʊts/ or /-'bʊts/ *adv* at or near that place or number.

thereafter /ðer'æftər/ *adv* after that; according to that.

thereagainst /ˌðerə'genst/ *adv* in opposition to; contrary to.

thereat /ðer'æt/ *adv* at that place; at such time.

thereby /'ðerbaɪ/ or /-'baɪ/ *adv* by that means.

therefore /'ðerfɔr/ *adv* for that or this reason; consequently.

therein /ðer'ɪn/ *adv* in that place or respect.

thereof /ðer'ɒv/ *adv* of this or that; because of that.

thereon /ðer'ɒn/ *adv* on that or it; immediately following that.

thereupon /'θerəpɒn/ or /ˌðerə'pɒn/ *adv* immediately after that.

therm /θɜrm/ *n* a measurement of heat.

thermal /'θɜrməl/, **thermic** /'θɜrmɪk/ *adj* generating heat; hot; warm; (*underwear*) of a knitted material with air spaces for insulation. • *n* a rising current of warm air.

thermion /'θɜrmiˌɒn/ *n* an electron emitted by a material at high temperature.

thermionic /ˌθɜrmiɒ'nɪk/ *adj* of, pertaining to, or worked by thermions, *esp* a tube.

thermistor /θɜr'mɪstər/ *n* a semiconductor device whose resistance varies inversely with a change in temperature.

thermo- /'θɜrmo:/, **therm-** *prefix* heat.

thermocouple /'θɜrmo:ˌkʌpəl/ *n* a device which generates a thermoelectric effect between two dissimilar semiconductors, used in measuring temperature differences.

thermodynamics /ˌθɜrmo:daɪ'næmɪks/ *n sing* the branch of physics concerned with the relationship between heat and other forms of energy.

thermoelectric /ˌθɜrmo:ɪ'lektrɪk/, **thermoelectrical** /-kəl/ *adj* of or derived from electricity generated by difference of temperature.—**thermoelectricity** *n.*

thermometer /θɜr'mɒmɪtər/ *n* an instrument for measuring temperature.

thermonuclear /ˌθɜrmo:'nju:kliər/ or /-'nju:-/ *adj* of or relating to nuclear fusion or using nuclear weapons that utilize fusion reactions.

thermoplastic /ˌθɜrmo:'plæstɪk/ *adj* becoming soft and malleable when heated. • *n* a resin or synthetic plastic that can be heated, moulded and cooled without appreciable change of its properties.

Thermos /'θɜrmɒs/ *n* (*trademark*) a brand of vacuum bottle.

thermostat /'θɜrmoˌstæt/ *n* an automatic device for regulating temperatures.

thesaurus /θə'sɔrəs/ *n* (*pl* **thesauri, thesauruses**) a reference book of synonyms and antonyms.

these /ði:z/ *see* **this.**

thesis /'θi:sɪs/ *n* (*pl* **theses**) a dissertation written as part of an academic degree; a theory expressed as a statement for discussion.

thespian /'θespiən/ *adj* of or pertaining to drama. • *n* an actor or actress.

theta /'θeɪtə/ *n* the eighth letter of the Greek alphabet.

they /ðeɪ/ *pers pron, pl of* **he, she** *or* **it.**

they'd /ðeɪd/ = they would; they had.

they'll /ðeɪl/ or /ðel/ = they will; they shall.

they're /ðer/ = they are

they've /ðeɪv/ = they have.

thiamine, thiamin /'θaɪəmɪn/ *n* vitamin B, present in a wide variety of plants and animals and essential for normal metabolism and nerve function.

thick /θɪk/ *adj* dense; viscous; fat, broad; abundant, closely set; in quick succession; crowded; (*inf*) stupid. • *adv* closely; frequently.

thicken /'θɪkən/ *vti* to make or become thick.—**thickener** *n.*

thicket /'θɪkət/ *n* a small group of trees or shrubs growing thickly and closely together.

thickhead /'θɪkhed/ *n* (*inf*) an ignorant person, an idiot.—**thickheaded** *adj.*

thickness /'θɪknəs/ *n* being thick; the dimension other than length or width; a layer.

thickset /θɪk'set/ *adj* having a short, stocky body.

thick-skinned /'θɪk'skɪnd/ *adj* not sensitive; not easily offended.

thick-witted /'θɪkˌwɪtɪd/ *adj* stupid.

thief /θi:f/ *n* (*pl* **thieves**) a person who steals.

thieve /θi:v/ *vti* to steal.

thigh /θaɪ/ *n* the thick fleshy part of the leg from the hip to the knee.

thighbone /'θaɪbo:n/ *n* the femur.

thimble /'θɪmbəl/ *n* a cap or cover worn to protect the finger when sewing.

thimbleful /'θɪmbəlˌfʊl/ *n* what a thimble contains, a tiny amount.

thin /θɪn/ *adj* (**thinner, thinnest**) narrow; slim; lean; sparse, weak, watery; (*material*) fine; not dense. • *vt* to make thin; to make less crowded; to water down.—**thinly** *adv*.—**thinness** *n*.

thine /ðaɪn/ *pron* an old-fashioned word for **yours**.

thing /θɪŋ/ *n* an inanimate object; an event; an action; (*pl*) possessions; (*inf*) an obsession.

thingamabob, thingumabob /ˈθɪŋəməˌbɒb/ *n* (*inf*) something or someone the name of which has been forgotten, is unknown or is hard to categorize, etc.—*also* **thingamajig, thingumajig, thingummy, thingie**.

think /θɪŋk/ *vb* (**thinking, thought**) *vi* to exercise the mind in order to make a decision; to revolve ideas in the mind, to ponder; to remember; to consider. • *vt* to judge, to believe or consider; (*with* up) to concoct, devise; (*with* over) to ponder, to consider the costs and benefits of.—**thinker** *n*.

thinking /ˈθɪŋkɪŋ/ *adj* capable of using thought, rational; intelligent. • *n* the process of using thought; opinion, reasoning.

think-tank /ˈθɪŋktæŋk/ *n* (*inf*) a group of experts convened to analyse and advise on ways of handling a particular problem.

thinner /ˈθɪnər/ *n* a substance, such as turpentine, added to paint, varnish, etc, to thin it.

thin-skinned /ˈθɪnˈskɪnd/ *adj* overly sensitive to criticism; easily offended.

third /θɜrd/ *adj* the last of three; being one of three equal parts. • *n* one of three equal parts.

third class *n* a class of mail in the US and Canadian postal systems that includes all printed matter, except periodicals, weighing below a certain amount and unsealed; the cheapest accommodation on a ship, aircraft, etc.—**third-class** *adj, adv*.

third degree *n* the use of torture, bullying or rough questioning to obtain information.

third-degree burn *n* a severe burn which destroys surface and underlying tissue and may involve loss of fluid and shock.

thirdly /ˈθɜrdli/ *adv* in the third place; as a third point.

third person *n* grammatical forms, such as pronouns and verbs, used when referring to the person or thing spoken or written of, not to the person speaking or writing or to the person or persons addressed.

third-rate *adj* inferior.

Third World *n* the underdeveloped countries of the world (*usu* refers to Africa, Asia and South America).

thirst /θɜrst/ *n* a craving for drink; a longing. • *vi* to feel thirst; to have a longing.

thirsty /ˈθɜrsti/ *adj* (**thirstier, thirstiest**) having a desire to drink; dry, arid; longing or craving for.—**thirstily** *adv*.—**thirstiness** *n*.

thirteen /θɜrˈtiːn/ *adj, n* three and ten.—**thirteenth** *adj, n*.

thirty /ˈθɜrti/ *adj, n* (*pl* **thirties**) three times ten.—**thirtieth** *adj, n*.

thirty-second note *n* (*mus*) a note with a time value of one thirty-secondth of a whole note, a demisemiquaver.

this /ðɪs/ *demons pron* (*pl* **these**) *or adj* denoting a person or thing near, just mentioned, or about to be mentioned.

thistle /ˈθɪsəl/ *n* a wild plant with prickly leaves and a purple flower.

thistledown /ˈθɪsəlˌdaʊn/ *n* the feathery cluster of seeds produced by the thistle.

thither /ˈðɪðər/ *adv* (*arch*) to or toward that place.

tho, tho' /ðoʊ/ *conj, adv* (*inf*) though.

thong /θɒŋ/ *n* a piece or strap of leather to lash things together; the lash of a whip; a sandal held on the foot by a thong passing between the toes and fixed to a strap passing over the top of the foot.

Thor /ˈθɔr/ *n* (*Norse myth*) the god of thunder.

thorax /ˈθɔræks/ *n* (*pl* **thoraxes, thoraces**) the part of the body enclosed by the ribs; the chest; (*in insects*) the middle one of the three chief divisions of the body.—**thoracic** *adj*.

thorium /ˈθɔriəm/ *n* a radioactive metallic element used in industry and as a nuclear fuel.

thorn /θɔrn/ *n* a shrub or small tree having thorns, *esp* hawthorn; a sharp point or prickle on the stem of a plant or the branch of a tree.

thorny /ˈθɔrni/ *adj* (**thornier, thorniest**) prickly; (*problem*) knotty.

thoron /ˈθɔrˌɒn/ *n* a gas that is a radioactive isotope of radon.

thorough /ˈθɜroʊ/ *or* /ˈθɜrə/, /ˈθʌrə/ *adj* complete, very detailed and painstaking, exhaustive.—**thoroughness** *n*.

thoroughbred /ˈθɜroʊˌbred/ *or* /ˈθʌroʊ-/, /ˈθʌrə-/ *adj* bred from pure stock. • *n* a pedigree animal, *esp* a horse.

thoroughfare /ˈθɜroʊˌfer/ *or* /ˈθʌroʊ-/, /ˈθʌrə-/ *n* a way through; a public highway, road; right of passing through.

thoroughgoing /ˈθɜroʊˌɡoʊɪŋ/ *or* /ˈθʌroʊ-/, /ˈθʌrə-/ *adj* very thorough; out-and-out.

thoroughly /-li/ *adv* completely, fully; entirely, absolutely.

those /ðoʊz/ *adj, pron* plural of **that**.

thou[1] /ðaʊ/ *pron* an old-fashioned word for **you**.

thou[2] *n* (*pl* **thous, thou**) (*inf*) a thousand; a thousandth of an inch.

though /ðoʊ/ *conj* yet, even if. • *adv* however; nevertheless.

thought /θɒt/ *n* the act of thinking; reasoning; serious consideration; an idea; opinions collectively; design, intention. • *pt, pp* of **think**.

thoughtful /ˈθɒtfʊl/ *adj* pensive; considerate.

thoughtless /ˈθɒtləs/ *adj* without thought; inconsiderate.

thousand /ˈθaʊzənd/ *adj* ten times one hundred; (*pl*) denoting any large but unspecified number. • *n* the number 1000.—**thousandth** *adj, n*.

thrash /θræʃ/ *vt* to beat soundly; to defeat; (*with* out) to discuss thoroughly, until agreement is reached. • *vi* to thresh grain; to writhe.

thrashing /-ɪŋ/ *n* a beating or flogging; punishment.

thread /θred/ *n* a fine strand or filament; a long thin piece of cotton, silk or nylon for sewing; the spiral part of a screw; (*of reasoning*) a line. • *vt* to pass a thread through the eye of a needle; to make one's way (through).

threadbare /ˈθredber/ *adj* worn, shabby.

threadworm /ˈθredwɜrm/ *n* a long slender worm, parasitic in humans and pigs.

threat /θret/ *n* a declaration of an intention to inflict harm or punishment upon another.

threaten /ˈθretən/ *vti* to utter threats to; to portend.

threatening /ˈθretənɪŋ/ *adj* menacing, intimidating; warning; ominous, sinister.—**threateningly** *adv*.

three /θriː/ *adj, n* the cardinal number next above two. • *n* the symbol (3, III, iii) expressing this.

three-D, 3-D /ˈθriːˌdi/ *n* a three-dimensional effect.

three-dimensional /-dəˈmenʃənəl/ *adj* having three dimensions.

threefold /ˈθriːfoʊld/ *adj, adv* three times as much or as many; composed of three parts.

three-quarter /ˈθriːˈkwɔrtər/ *adj* being three quarters of the normal size or length. • *n* (*Rugby football*) one of *usu* four attacking players used particularly for running with the ball.

three Rs *npl* reading, writing and arithmetic, regarded as the basis of learning.

threescore /ˈθriːˈskɔr/ *n* (*arch*) sixty.—*also adj*.

threesome /ˈθriːsəm/ *n* a group of three; a game for three people.

threnody /ˈθrenədi/, **threnode** *n* (*pl* **threnodies, threnodes**) a song or speech of lamentation, *esp* on a person's death.

thresh /θreʃ/ *or* /θræʃ/ *vti* to beat out (grain) from (husks).

threshold /ˈθreʃoʊld/ *or* /-hoʊld/ *n* the sill at the door of a building; doorway, entrance; the starting point, beginning.

threw /θruː/ *see* **throw**.

thrice /θraɪs/ *adv* three times.

thrift /θrɪft/ *n* careful management of money.—**thrifty** *adj*.

thrift shop *n* a shop that sells used clothing and other items to raise money for charity.

thrill /θrɪl/ *vti* to tingle with pleasure or excitement. • *n* a sensation of pleasure and excitement; a trembling or quiver.

thriller /ˈθrɪlər/ *n* a novel, film or play depicting an exciting story of mystery and suspense.

thrilling /-ɪŋ/ *adj* exciting, gripping.

thrips /θrɪps/ *n* (*pl* **thrips**) any of various small insects with sucking mouthparts that feed on and damage plants.

thrive /θraɪv/ *vi* (**thriving, thrived** *or* **throve, pp thrived** *or* **thriven**) to prosper, to be successful; to grow vigorously.—**thriving** *adj*.

thro', thro /θruː/ *prep, adv* (*inf*) through.

throat /θroʊt/ *n* the front part of the neck; the passage from the back of the mouth to the top part of the tubes into the lungs and stomach; an entrance.

throaty /ˈθroʊti/ *adj* (**throatier, throatiest**) hoarse; guttural; deep, husky.—**throatily** *adv*.

throb /θrɒb/ *vi* (**throbbing, throbbed**) to beat or pulsate rhythmically, with more than usual force; to vibrate, beat.—*also n*.

throes /θroʊz/ *npl* violent pangs or pain.

thrombin /ˈθrɒmbɪn/ *n* an enzyme that contributes to blood clotting.

thrombocyte /ˈθrɒmbəˌsaɪt/ *n* a blood platelet.

thrombosis /θrɒmˈboʊsɪs/ *n* (*pl* **thromboses**) the forming of a blood clot in the heart or in a blood-vessel.

thrombus /ˈθrɒmbəs/ *n* (*pl* **thrombi**) the blood clot that blocks a vessel in thrombosis.

throne /θroʊn/ *n* a chair of state occupied by a monarch; sovereign power. • *vt* to place on a throne.

Throne Speech *n* ✤ speech from the Throne.

throng /θrɒŋ/ *n* a crowd. • *vti* to crowd, congregate.

throstle /ˈθrɒsəl/ *n* any of various Old World thrushes.

throttle /ˈθrɒtəl/ *n* a valve controlling the flow of fuel or steam to an engine. • *vt* to regulate the speed of (an engine) using a throttle; to choke or strangle.

through /θruː/ *prep* from one side or end to the other; into and then out of; covering all parts; from beginning to end of; by means of; in consequence of; up to and including. • *adv* from one end or side to the other; completely. • *adj* going without interruption; unobstructed.

throughout /θruːˈaʊt/ *prep* in every part of; from beginning to end. • *adv* everywhere; at every moment.

throughput /ˈθruːpʊt/ *n* the amount of material processed in a particular period, *esp* by a computer.

throughway /ˈθruːweɪ/ *see* **thruway**.

throve /θroʊv/ *see* **thrive**.

throw /θroʊ/ *vb* (**throwing, threw,** *pp* **thrown**) *vt* to hurl, to fling; to cast off; (*party*) to hold; (*inf*) to confuse or disconcert; (*with* **off**) to cast off, discard, abandon; to distract, elude; to produce in a casual manner; to confuse, disconcert; (*with* **out**) to discard, reject; to dismiss or eject, *esp* forcibly; to emit, give forth; to construct out from a main section; to confuse, distract; (*with* **over**) to abandon, jilt; (*with* **together**) to assemble hurriedly or carelessly; to bring (people) into casual contact; (*with* **up**) to raise quickly; to resign from, abandon; to build hurriedly; to produce; (*inf*) to vomit. • *vi* to cast or hurl through the air (with the arm and wrist); to cast dice; (*with* **up**) (*inf*) to vomit. • *n* the act of throwing; the distance to which anything can be thrown; a cast of dice.

throwaway /ˈθroʊəweɪ/ *adj* disposable.

throwback /ˈθroʊbæk/ *n* a reversion to an earlier or more primitive type.

throw-in *n* (*soccer*) a throw from touch to resume play.

thrown /θroʊn/ *see* **throw**.

thru /θruː/ *prep* (*sl*) through.

thrum /θrʌm/ *vi* (**thrumming, thrummed**) to strum; to beat incessantly.

thrush[1] /θrʌʃ/ *n* a songbird with a brown back and spotted breast.

thrush[2] *n* a fungal infection occurring in the mouths of babies or in women's vaginas.

thrust /θrʌst/ *vti* (**thrusting, thrust**) to push with force; to stab, pierce; to force into a situation. • *n* a forceful push or stab; pressure; the driving force of a propeller; forward movement; the point or basic meaning.

thruway /ˈθruːweɪ/ *n* an expressway.—*also* **throughway.**

thud /θʌd/ *n* a dull, heavy sound, caused by a blow or a heavy object falling. • *vi* (**thudding, thudded**) to make such a sound.

thug /θʌg/ *n* a violent and rough person, *esp* a criminal.

thuggery /ˈθʌgəri/ *n* rough and violent behaviour.

thulium /ˈθuːliəm/ or /ˈθjuː-/ *n* a malleable metallic element of the rare-earth group.

thumb /θʌm/ *n* the first, short, thick finger of the human hand. • *vt* (*book*) to turn (the pages) idly.

thumbed /θʌmd/ *adj* worn by use.

thumb index *n* a series of semicircular notches cut in the edge of a book for easier reference to particular parts.

thumbnail /ˈθʌmneɪl/ *n* the nail of the thumb. • *adj* concise.

thumbnut /ˈθʌmnʌt/ *n* a wing nut.

thumbscrew /ˈθʌmskruː/ *n* an instrument of torture that crushes the thumbs; a screw with a modified head for tightening with the finger and thumb.

thumbtack /ˈθʌmtæk/ *n* a flat-headed pin used for fastening paper, drawings, etc, a drawing pin.

thump /θʌmp/ *n* a heavy blow; a thud. • *vt* to strike with something heavy. • *vi* to throb or beat violently.

thumping /ˈθʌmpɪŋ/ *adj* (*inf*) very great.

thunder /ˈθʌndər/ *n* the deep rumbling or loud cracking sound after a flash of lightning; any similar sound. • *vi* to sound as thunder. • *vt* (*words*) to utter loudly.

thunderbolt /ˈθʌndərboʊlt/ *n* a flash of lightning accompanied by thunder; anything sudden and shocking.

thunderclap /ˈθʌndərklæp/ *n* a loud bang of thunder.

thundering /ˈθʌndərɪŋ/ *adj* (*inf*) unusually great, excessive.

thunderous /ˈθʌndərəs/ *adj* very loud; producing thunder.

thunderstorm /ˈθʌndərstɔrm/ *n* a storm with thunder and lightning.

thunderstruck /ˈθʌndərstrʌk/ *adj* astonished.

thundery /ˈθʌndəri/ *adj* indicating thunder.

Thur., Thurs. *abbr* = Thursday.

thurible /ˈθjʊərəbəl/ *n* a censer.

Thursday /ˈθɜrzdeɪ/ or /-di/ *n* the fifth day of the week.

thus /ðʌs/ *adv* in this or that way; to this degree or extent; so; therefore.

thwack /θwæk/ *vti* to hit hard, whack. • *n* a heavy blow, whack; the sound of this.

thwart /θwɔrt/ *vt* to prevent, to frustrate.

thy /ðaɪ/ *poss adj* an old-fashioned word for **your.**

thyme /taɪm/ *n* a herb with small leaves used for flavouring savoury food.

thymol /ˈθaɪmɒl/ *n* a substance obtained from thyme and used as a fungicide and antiseptic.

thymus /ˈθaɪməs/ *n* (*pl* **thymuses, thymi**) a gland near the base of the neck that shrinks after puberty.

thyristor /θaɪˈrɪstər/ *n* any of various semiconductor devices that act as switches or rectifiers.

thyroid /ˈθaɪrɔɪd/ *n* the gland in the neck affecting growth and metabolism.

thyrotropin /ˌθaɪrəˈtroʊpɪn/ or /θaɪˈrɒtrəpɪn/, **thyrotrophin** *n* a hormone secreted by the pituitary gland that stimulates the thyroid gland.

thyroxin, thyroxine /θaɪˈrɒksən/ *n* the main hormone produced by the thyroid gland.

Tl (*chem symbol*) thallium.

Ti (*chem symbol*) titanium.

ti /tiː/ *n* the seventh note of the scale in solmization.

tiara /tiˈerə/ or /-ˈɑrə/ *n* a semicircular crown decorated with jewels.

tibia /ˈtɪbiə/ *n* (*pl* **tibiae, tibias**) the inner and thicker of the two bones between the knee and the ankle; the shinbone.

tic /tɪk/ *n* any involuntary regularly repeated, spasmodic contraction of a muscle.

tick[1] /tɪk/ *n* a small bloodsucking insect that lives on people and animals.

tick[2] *vi* to make a regular series of short sounds; to beat, as a clock; (*inf*) to work, function; (*with* **over**) (*engine*) to idle; to function routinely. • *n* the sound of a clock; (*sl*) a moment.

tick[3] *vt* (*often with* **off**) to check off, as items in a list. • *n* a check mark (√) to check off items on a list or to indicate correctness.

ticker /ˈtɪkər/ *n* a telegraphic device that receives and outputs stock-market prices on a paper tape; any similar device operated electronically and outputting to a display monitor; (*inf*) the heart; (*inf*) a watch.

ticker tape *n* a continuous length of paper tape output from a telegraphic ticker.

ticket /ˈtɪkət/ *n* a printed card, etc, that gives one a right of travel or entry; a label on merchandise giving size, price, etc.

tickle /ˈtɪkəl/ *vt* to touch lightly to provoke pleasure or laughter; to please or delight.

ticklish /ˈtɪkəlɪʃ/ or /ˈtɪklɪʃ/, **tickly** *adj* sensitive to being tickled; easily offended; difficult or delicate.

tick-tack-toe /tɪktækˈtoʊ/ *n sing* a game in which two players place noughts and crosses into squares on a grid with nine spaces, the winner being the first to form a row of three noughts or crosses, noughts and crosses.

ticktock *n* a ticking sound, *esp* of a clock. • *vi* to make such a sound.

tidal /ˈtaɪdəl/ *adj* relating to, or having, tides.

tidal wave *n* a large wave as a result of high winds with spring tides; a huge destructive wave caused by earthquakes; something overwhelming.

tidbit /ˈtɪdbɪt/ *see* **titbit.**

tiddly /ˈtɪdli/ or /ˈtɪdəli/ *adj* (**tiddlier, tiddliest**) (*inf*) very small; (*inf*) slightly drunk.

tiddlywinks, tiddledywinks /ˈtɪdliwɪŋks/ or /ˈtɪdəli-/ *npl* a game whose object is to flick small plastic discs into a container by snapping them with a larger disc.

tide /taɪd/ *n* the regular rise and fall of the seas, oceans, etc *usu* twice a day; a current of water; a tendency; a flood. • *vt* (*with* **over**) to help along temporarily.

tidemark /ˈtaɪdmɑːk/ *n* the highest or lowest point reached by the sea.

tide rip *n* a rip current.

tidewater /ˈtaɪdˌwɒtər/ *n* water overflowing land at flood tide; water that is affected by the tide.

tidings /ˈtaɪdɪŋz/ *npl* news, information.

tidy /ˈtaɪdi/ *adj* (**tidier, tidiest**) neat; orderly. • *vt* to make neat; to put things in order.—**tidily** *adv*.—**tidiness** *n*.

tie /taɪ/ *vb* (**tying, tied**) *vt* to bind; to fasten with a string or thread; to make a bow or knot in; to restrict; (*with* **in**) to link with something; (*with* **up**) to fasten tightly (as if) with cord, string, etc; to connect, link; to invest money, etc, so as to make it unavailable for alternative uses; to preoccupy, distract. • *vi* to score the same number of points (as an opponent); (*with* **in**) to be linked in a certain way; (*with* **up**) to dock (a vessel). • *n* a knot, bow, etc; a bond; a long narrow piece of cloth worn with a shirt; necktie; an equality in score.

tiebreaker /ˈtaɪˌbreɪkər/, **tiebreak** /ˈtaɪbreɪk/ *n* any means of deciding a contest which has ended in a draw, such as an extra game, hole, question, etc.

tie-dyeing, tie-dye *n* a method of producing patterns on textiles by tying or knotting parts of the fabric to limit the amount of dye absorbed.

tie-in *n* a link or connection; a book linked to a film or TV series.

tie line *n* a telephone link between two private branch exchanges.

tiepin *n* a decorative pin used to secure the ends of a tie to a shirt.

tier /tɪr/ *n* a row or rank in a series when several rows are placed one above another.

tiercel /ˈtɪrsəl/ *n* a male of various hawks, *esp* as used in falconry.—*also* **tercel**.

tie-up *n* a link, connection; a standstill.

tiff /tɪf/ *n* a petty quarrel or disagreement. • *vi* to quarrel; to be in a huff.

tiger /ˈtaɪɡər/ *n* a large, fierce carnivorous animal of the cat family, having orange and black stripes.—**tigress** *nf*.

tiger beetle *n* any of numerous predatory beetles with powerful mandibles and spotted wing cases.

tiger cat *n* an ocelot or similar medium-sized wildcat with a striped coat.

tiger lily *n* a lily of China and Japan cultivated for its dark-spotted orange flowers.

tiger moth *n* any of various large moths marked with stripes or spots.

tiger's eye, tigereye *n* a brownish-yellow gemstone.

tiger shark *n* a large shark of warm waters with a striped or spotted skin.

tiger snake *n* an aggressive poisonous Australian snake with striped markings.

tight /taɪt/ *adj* taut; fitting closely; not leaky; constricted; miserly; difficult; providing little space or time for variance; (*contest*) close; (*inf*) drunk.

tighten /ˈtaɪtən/ *vti* to make or grow tight or tighter.

tightfisted /ˈtaɪtˌfɪstɪd/ *adj* miserly.

tightknit /ˈtaɪtˌnɪt/ *adj* tightly integrated.

tight-lipped /ˈtaɪtˈlɪpt/ *adj* having the lips firmly pressed together, as from annoyance; taciturn.

tightrope /ˈtaɪtroʊp/ *n* a taut rope on which acrobats walk.

tights /taɪts/ *npl* a one-piece garment covering the legs and lower body; panty hose.

tigon /ˈtaɪɡən/, **tiglon** /ˈtaɪɡlən/ *n* the hybrid offspring of a tiger and a lioness.

tike /taɪk/ *see* **tyke**.

tilde /ˈtɪldə/ *n* a sign ~ placed above a letter to indicate a nasal sound, as in Spanish *señor*.

tile /taɪl/ *n* a thin slab of baked clay used for covering roofs, floors, etc. • *vt* to cover with tiles.

till[1] /tɪl/ *n* a drawer inside a cash register for keeping money.

till[2] *prep* until. • *conj* until.

till[3] *vt* (*land*) to cultivate for raising crops, as by ploughing.

tiller /ˈtɪlər/ *n* the handle or lever for turning a rudder in order to steer a boat.

tilt /tɪlt/ *vi* to slope, incline, slant. • *vt* to raise one end of. • *n* a slope or angle.

timbale *Fr.* /tɑˈbæl/ *n* a mixture of meat or fish with cream cooked in a mould lined with vegetables or pastry.

timber /ˈtɪmbər/ *n* wood when used as building material; a beam; trees collectively. • *vt* to provide with timber or beams.

timbered /ˈtɪmbərd/ *adj* (*building*) having wooden beams on the exterior.

timber hitch *n* a knot used to tie a rope, etc to a log or spar.

timber line /ˈtɪmbərˌlaɪn/ *see* **tree line**.

timber wolf *n* a type of large grey North American wolf.

timbre /ˈtæmbər/ or *Fr.* /ˈtæbrə/ *n* the quality of sound of a voice or musical instrument.

time /taɪm/ *n* the past, present and future; a particular moment; hour of the day; an opportunity; the right moment; duration; occasion; musical beat. • *vt* to regulate as to time; to measure or record the duration of.

time and motion study *n* the study of working procedures to improve efficiency.

time bomb *n* a bomb designed to explode at a predetermined time; something with a potentially delayed reaction.

time clock *n* a device that records the times of arrival and departure of an employee on a card.

time-consuming *adj* using up or taking a lot of time.

time exposure *n* exposure of a photographic film for *usu* several seconds; a photograph taken in this way.

time-honoured *adj* traditional, in accordance with venerable customs.

time immemorial *n* the far distant past beyond memory or record.

timekeeper /ˈtaɪmˌkiːpər/ *n* a person or instrument that records or keeps time; an employee who records the hours worked by others.—**timekeeping** *n*.

time lag *n* the interval between two connected events.

time-lapse photography *n* a technique of filming very slow action, such as plant growth, by taking single frames at fixed intervals and then running them at normal speed.

timeless /ˈtaɪmləs/ *adj* eternal; ageless.

timely /ˈtaɪmli/ *adj* at the right time, opportune.—**timeliness** *n*.

time-out *n* (*sport*) a suspension of play to rest, discuss tactics, etc; a brief rest period.

timepiece /ˈtaɪmpiːs/ *n* a clock or watch.

timer /ˈtaɪmər/ *n* a device for measuring, recording or controlling time; a device for controlling lights, heating, etc by setting an electrical clock to regulate their operations.

timeserver *n* a person whose opinions, behaviour, etc, follow current fashions.—**timeserving** *adj, n*.

timeshare *n* joint ownership of holiday accommodation by several people with each occupying the same premises in turn for short periods.

time signature *n* a sign on a musical staff indicating the number of beats per bar and time value of each beat.

timetable /ˈtaɪmˌteɪbəl/ *n* a list of times of arrivals and departures of trains, aeroplanes, etc; a schedule showing a planned order or sequence.

timeworn *adj* dilapidated; old-fashioned, hackneyed.

time zone *n* a geographical region throughout which the same standard time is used.

timid /ˈtɪmɪd/ *adj* shy; lacking confidence.—**timidity** *n*.—**timidly** *adv*.

timing /ˈtaɪmɪŋ/ *n* the control and expression of speech or actions to create the best effect, *esp* in the theatre, etc.

timocracy /taɪˈmɒkrəsi/ *n* (*pl* **timocracies**) a form of government in which ownership of property is required to hold office.

timorous /ˈtɪmərəs/ *adj* timid, fearful.—**timorously** *adv*.—**timorousness** *n*.

timpani /ˈtɪmpəni/ *npl* a set of kettledrums.—**timpanist** *n*.—*also* **tympani, tympany**.

tin /tɪn/ *n* a malleable metallic element; a container of tin, a can. • *adj* made of tin or tin plate. • *vt* (**tinning, tinned**) to put food into a tin.

tinctorial /tɪŋkˈtɔːrɪəl/ *adj* pertaining to colouring, dyeing or staining.

tincture /ˈtɪŋktʃər/ *n* an extract of a substance in a solution of alcohol for medicinal use; a colour, hue, tint; a hint of flavour or aroma; an heraldic colour. • *vt* to tint with a colour.

tinder /ˈtɪndər/ *n* dry wood for lighting a fire from a spark.

tinderbox /ˈtɪndərbɒks/ *n* a metal box with tinder, flint and steel for making a spark; an unstable or potentially explosive person, thing or situation.

tine /taɪn/ *n* a slender projecting point, as the prong of a fork or point of an antler.

tinea /ˈtɪnɪə/ *n* a fungal skin condition, *esp* ringworm.

tinfoil /ˈtɪnfɔɪl/ *n* baking foil for wrapping food; silver paper.

ting /tɪŋ/ *n* a high sharp ringing sound. • *vi* to make this sound.

tinge /tɪndʒ/ *vt* to tint or colour. • *n* a slight tint, colour or flavour.

tingle /'tɪŋgəl/ *vi* to feel a prickling, itching or stinging sensation. • *n* a prickling sensation; a thrill.—**tinglingly** *adv*.—**tingly** *adj*.

tin god *n* a self-important person; a person who is undeservedly venerated.

tinker /'tɪŋkər/ *n* (*formerly*) a travelling mender of pots and pans. • *vi* to fiddle with; to attempt to repair.

tinkle /'tɪŋkəl/ *vi* to make a sound like a small bell ringing; to clink, to jingle; to clink repeatedly. • *n* a tinkling sound; (*inf*) a telephone call.

tinnitus /tɪ'naɪtəs/ *n* a continuous ringing or roaring sound in the ears caused by an infection, etc.

tinny /'tɪni/ *adj* (**tinnier, tinniest**) of or resembling tin; flimsy in construction or appearance; (*food*) having a metallic taste; having a high metallic sound.

tin plate *n* thin sheets of iron or steel plated with tin.—**tin-plate** *adj*.

tinsel /'tɪnsəl/ *n* a shiny Christmas decoration made of long pieces of thread wound round with thin strips of metal or plastic foil; something showy but of low value. • *adj* cheaply showy, flashy. • *vt* (**tinselling, tinselled** *or* **tinseling, tinseled**) to adorn with tinsel.

Tinseltown /'tɪnsəl,taun/ *n* (*inf*) Hollywood.

tint /tɪnt/ *n* a shade of any colour, *esp* a pale one; a tinge; a hair dye. • *vt* to colour or tinge.

tintinnabulation /,tɪntɪ,næbju'leɪʃən/ *n* (the sound of) a ringing of bells.

tiny /'taɪni/ *adj* (**tinier, tiniest**) very small.

tip[1] /tɪp/ *n* the pointed end of anything; the end, as of a billiard cue, etc. • *vt* (**tipping, tipped**) to put a tip on.

tip[2] *vti* (**tipping, tipped**) to tilt or cause to tilt; to overturn; to empty (out, into, etc); to give a gratuity to, as a waiter, etc; (*rubbish*) to dump; to give a helpful hint or inside information to. • *n* a light tap; a gratuity; a rubbish dump; an inside piece of information; a helpful hint.

tip-off /'tɪpɒf/ *n* a warning based on inside information.

tipple /'tɪpəl/ *vi* to drink alcohol regularly in small quantities. • *n* an alcoholic drink.

tipster /'tɪpstər/ *n* a person who gives horse-racing tips.

tipsy /'tɪpsi/ *adj* (**tipsier, tipsiest**) slightly drunk.

tiptoe /'tɪptəʊ/ *vi* (**tiptoeing, tiptoed**) to walk very quietly or carefully.

tiptop /'tɪptɒp/ *adj* excellent. • *adv* at the peak of condition. • *n* the best; the highest point.

tirade /'taɪreɪd/ *n* a long angry speech of censure or criticism.

tire[1] /taɪr/ *vt* to exhaust the strength of, to weary. • *vi* to become weary; to lose patience; to become bored.

tire[2] /taɪr/ *n* a protective, *usu* rubber, covering around the rim of a wheel.—*also* **tyre**.

tired /taɪrd/ *adj* weary, sleepy; hackneyed, conventional, flat; (*with* **of**) exasperated by, bored with.

tireless /'taɪrləs/ *adj* never wearying.—**tirelessly** *adv*.—**tirelessness** *n*.

tiresome /'taɪrsəm/ *adj* tedious.

tiro /'taɪrəʊ/ *see* **tyro**.

'tis /tɪz/ (*poet*) = it is.

tissue /'tɪʃuː/ *or* /'tɪʃjuː/ *n* thin, absorbent paper used as a disposable handkerchief, etc; a very finely woven fabric; a mass of organic cells of a similar structure and function.

tit[1] /tɪt/ *n* a songbird such as a blue tit or great tit.

tit[2] *n* (*vulg*) a woman's breast.

titan /'taɪtən/ *n* a person of enormous strength, size or ability.

titanic /taɪ'tænɪk/ *adj* monumental; huge.

titanium /taɪ'teɪniəm/ *or* /tɪ-/ *n* a strong metallic element used to make lightweight alloys.

titanium dioxide *n* a white powder used chiefly as a pigment.

titbit /'tɪtbɪt/ *n* a tasty morsel of food; a choice item of information.—*also* **tidbit**.

titer /'taɪtər/ *or* /'tiːt-/ *see* **titre**.

tit for tat *n* an equivalent given in retaliation.

tithe /taɪð/ *n* a tenth part of agricultural produce, formerly allotted for the maintenance of the clergy and other church purposes. • *vti* to pay a tithe.

titillate /'tɪtə,leɪt/ *vt* to tickle; to arouse or excite pleasurably.

titillation /-'leɪʃən/ *n* the act of titillating; the condition of being titillated; a pleasurable feeling, *esp* sexual.

titivate, tittivate /'tɪtɪ,veɪt/ *vti* to smarten up.

title /'taɪtəl/ *n* the name of a book, play, piece of music, work of art, etc; the heading of a section of a book; a name denoting nobility or rank or office held, or attached to a personal name; (*law*) that which gives a legal right (to possession).

titled /'taɪtəld/ *adj* having a title.

title deed *n* a deed or document proving a title or right to possession.

title page *n* the page of a book containing its title and usually the author's and publisher's names.

title role *n* the character in a play, film, etc after whom it is named.

titrate /'taɪtreɪt/ *vt* to measure by titration.

titration /-'treɪʃən/ *n* a method of determining the amount of a constituent in a solution by adding a known quantity of a reagent.

titre /'taɪtər/ *n* the concentration of a substance in a solution as determined by titration.

titter /'tɪtər/ *vi* to giggle, snigger. • *n* a suppressed laugh.

tittle-tattle /'tɪtəl,tætəl/ *n* idle chat, empty gossip.

titular /'tɪtjʊlər/ *adj* having, or relating to, a title; existing in name or title only.

tizzy /'tɪzi/ *n* (*inf*) a state of confusion or agitation.

TKO /tiː keɪəʊ/ *abbr* = technical knockout.

TLC *abbr* = tender loving care.

T-lymphocyte /'tiː,lɪmfəsaɪt/ *see* **T-cell**.

TM *abbr* = trademark; transcendental meditation.

Tm (*chem symbol*) thulium.

TN *abbr* = Tennessee.

TNT *abbr* = trinitrotoluene.

to /tuː/ *prep* in the direction of; toward; as far as; expressing the purpose of an action; indicating the infinitive; introducing the indirect object; in comparison with. • *adv* toward.

TO *abbr* ✻ (*Cdn*) = Toronto.

toad /təʊd/ *n* an amphibious reptile, like a frog, but having a drier skin and spending less time in water.

toadflax /'təʊdflæks/ *n* a common perennial plant with yellow and orange flowers.

toadstool /'təʊdstuːl/ *n* a mushroom, *esp* a poisonous or inedible one.

toady /'təʊdi/ *n* (*pl* **toadies**) a person who flatters insincerely, a sycophant. • *vi* (**toadying, toadied**) (*with* **to**) to act in a servile manner.

to and fro *adj* forward and backward; here and there.—**toing and froing** *n*.

toast /təʊst/ *vt* to brown over a fire or in a toaster; to warm; to drink to the health of. • *n* toasted bread; the sentiment or person to which one drinks.

toaster /'təʊstər/ *n* a person who toasts; a thing that toasts, *esp* an electrical appliance for toasting.

toastmaster /'təʊst,mæstər/ *n* the proposer of toasts at public dinners.—**toastmistress** *nf*.

tobacco /tə'bækəʊ/ *n* (*pl* **tobaccos, tobaccoes**) a plant whose dried leaves are used for smoking, chewing or snuff.

tobacconist /tə'bækənɪst/ *n* a person or shop that sells cigarettes, etc.

toboggan /tə'bɒgən/ *n* a sledge, sled.

toby jug /'təʊbi/ *n* (*pl* **tobies, toby jugs**) a mug in the shape of a man with a three-cornered hat.

toccata /tə'kɑːtə/ *n* a piece of music for keyboard in a free style with rapid runs.

tocopherol /,təʊkɒ'fərɒl/ *n* vitamin E, present in wheat-germ oil, egg yolk, etc.

tocsin /'tɒksɪn/ *n* an alarm bell; a warning signal.

today /tə'deɪ/ *n* this day; the present age. • *adv* on this day; nowadays.

toddle /'tɒdəl/ *vi* to walk with short, unsteady, steps, as a child who is learning to walk.

toddler /'tɒdlər/ *n* a young child.

toddy /'tɒdi/ *n* (*pl* **toddies**) a drink of whisky or brandy, sugar, and hot water.

to-do /tə'duː/ *n* (*pl* **to-dos**) (*inf*) a fuss, commotion, quarrel.

toe /təʊ/ *n* one of the five digits on the foot; the part of the shoe or sock that covers the toes.

toe cap /'təʊkæp/ *n* a reinforced covering on the toe of a shoe or boot.

toehold /'təʊhəʊld/ *n* a small ledge, crack, etc used in climbing; any slight means of support or access; (*wrestling*) a hold in which an opponent's foot is twisted.

toenail /'təʊneɪl/ *n* the thin, hard covering on the end of the toes.

toe rubbers *npl* ✸ (*Cdn*) low rubber overshoes that extend from the heel of a man's shoe, under the sole and over the tip of the toe.

toffee, toffy /'tɒfi/ *n* (*pl* **toffees, toffies**) a sweet of brittle but tender texture made by boiling sugar and butter together.

toffee apple *n* an apple coated with toffee and eaten from a stick.

toffee-nosed *adj* (*inf*) pretentious, patronizing, arrogant.

tofu /'toːfuː/ *n* unfermented soya bean curd, used in cooking.

tog[1] /tɒg/ *n* (*pl*) (*inf*) clothes. • *vt* (**togging, togged**) (*inf*) to dress.

tog[2] *n* in UK, an official measurement of the warmth of a quilt, etc.

toga /'toːgə/ *n* a piece of cloth draped around the body, as worn by citizens in ancient Rome.

together /tə'gɛðər/ *adv* in one place or group; in cooperation with; in unison; jointly.

toggle /'tɒgəl/ *n* a peg attached to a rope to prevent it from passing through a loop or knot; a button of this form; (*comput*) a software instruction for starting or stopping a style, etc. • *vt* to fasten with a toggle.

toggle switch *n* an electrical device for opening or closing a circuit.

toil /tɔil/ *vi* to work strenuously; to move with great effort. • *n* hard work.

toilet /'tɔilət/ *n* a lavatory; the room containing a lavatory; the act of washing and dressing oneself.

toilet paper, toilet tissue *n* an absorbent paper for cleansing after urination, etc, *usu* wound around a cardboard cylinder.

toiletry /'tɔilətri/ *n* (*pl* **toiletries**) a lotion, perfume, etc used in washing and dressing oneself.

toilet water *n* a diluted perfume.

token /'toːkən/ *n* a symbol, sign; an indication; a metal disc for a slot machine; a souvenir; a gift voucher. • *adj* nominal; symbolic.

tokenism /'toːkən,izəm/ *n* the making of only a token effort.

tolbooth /'tɒl,buːθ/ *n* (*Scot*) a town hall; a jail.

told /toːld/ *see* **tell**.

tolerable /'tɒlərəbəl/ *adj* bearable; fairly good.—**tolerably** *adv*.

tolerance /'tɒlərəns/ *n* open-mindedness; forbearance; (*med*) ability to resist the action of a drug, etc; ability of a substance to endure heat, stress, etc without damage.

tolerant /'tɒlərənt/ *adj* able to put up with the beliefs, actions, etc of others; broad-minded; showing tolerance to a drug, etc; capable of enduring stress, etc.

tolerate /'tɒlə,reit/ *vt* to endure, put up with, suffer.

toll[1] /toːl/ *n* money levied for passing over a bridge or road; a charge for a service, such as a long-distance telephone call; the number of people killed in an accident or disaster.

toll[2] *vt* (*bell*) to ring slowly and repeatedly, as a funeral bell. • *vi* to sound, as a bell. • *n* the sound of a bell when tolling.

tollbooth *n* a booth where money is paid to pass over a , road, etc.—*also* **tolbooth**.

toll call *n* a telephone call charged at higher than the standard or local rate.

tollgate /'toːlgeit/ *n* a gate where money is paid to pass over a bridge, road, etc.

toluene /'tɒljuːˌiːn/ *n* a flammable hydrocarbon derived from petroleum and coal tar used as a solvent and in organic synthesis.

tom /tɒm/ *n* a male animal, *esp* a cat.

tomahawk /'tɒmə,hɒk/ *n* a light axe used by North American Indians.

tomato /tə'meitoː/ or /-'mætoː/ *n* (*pl* **tomatoes**) a plant with red pulpy fruit used as a vegetable.

tomb /tuːm/ *n* a vault in the earth for the burial of the dead.

tomboy /'tɒmbɔi/ *n* a girl who likes rough outdoor activities.

tombstone /'tuːmstoːn/ *n* a memorial stone over a grave.

tomcat /'tɒmkæt/ *n* a male cat.

Tom, Dick and Harry /ˌtɒm dik ənd 'hɛri/ *n* an ordinary person, anybody taken at random.

tome /toːm/ *n* a large, heavy book, *esp* a scholarly one.

-tome /toːm/ *n suffix* a cutting instrument.

tomfool /tɒm'fuːl/ *n* a fool.

tomfoolery /tɒm'fuːləri/ *n* (*pl* **tomfooleries**) foolish behaviour; nonsense.

Tommy /'tɒmi/ *n* (*pl* **Tommies**) (*inf*) a private in the British army.

tommy gun *n* a (Thompson) sub-machine gun.

tommyrot /'tɒmi,rɒt/ *n* complete nonsense.

tomography /tə'mɒgrəfi/ *n* a process which produces an x-ray photograph of a plane section of the body or other object.

tomorrow /tə'mɒroː/ or /-mɒroː/ *n* the day after today; the future.— *also adv*.

tomtit /tɒm'tit/ or /'tɒmˌtit/ *n* any of various small tits, *esp* a blue tit.

tom-tom /'tɒmˌtɒm/ *n* a long small-headed drum usually beaten with the hands.

-tomy /təmi/ *n suffix* surgical incision.

ton /tʌn/ *n* a unit of weight equivalent to 2,000 pounds in US or 2,240 pounds in UK; (*pl*) (*inf*) a great quantity.

tonal /'toːnəl/ *n* of or pertaining to tone; having a key.

tonality /toː'næliti/ *n* (*pl* **tonalities**) the character of a musical composition in relation to scale or key; a system of tones; the scheme of colours and tones in a painting.

tone /toːn/ *n* the quality of a sound; pitch or inflection of the voice; colour, shade; body condition. • *vti* to give tone to; to harmonize (with); (*with* **down**) to (become) moderate in tone; (*with* **up**) to make or become healthier, tighter, etc.

tone arm *n* the tracking arm in a record player that holds the cartridge and stylus.

tone-deaf *adj* insensitive to differences in musical pitch.

tone poem *n* a symphonic poem.

toner /'toːnər/ *n* a cosmetic used on the skin for various effects; a chemical used to alter the tone of a photograph; the ink particles used in various reprographic devices such as laser printers and photocopiers.

tong /tɒŋ/ *n* a Chinese-American secret society.

tongs /'tɒŋgz/ *npl* an instrument consisting of two arms that are hinged, used for grasping and lifting.

tongue /tʌŋ/ *n* the soft, moveable organ in the mouth, used in tasting, swallowing, and speech; the ability to speak; a language; (*shoe*) a piece of leather under the laces; a jet of flame; the tongue of an animal served as food; the catch of a buckle.

tongue-lash /'tʌŋˌlæʃ/ *vt* to scold, rebuke severely.—**tongue lashing** *n*.

tongue-tied /-ˌtaid/ *adj* speechless.

tongue-twister *n* a sequence of words that it is difficult to pronounce quickly and clearly.

tonic /'tɒnik/ *n* a medicine that improves physical well-being; something that imparts vigour; a carbonated mineral water with a bitter taste. • *adj* relating to tones or sounds.

tonic sol-fa *n* the system of sol-fa or solmization syllables used to represent the notes of the musical scale.

tonight /tə'nait/ *n* this night; the night or evening of the present day.—*also adv*.

tonnage /'tʌnidʒ/ *n* a merchant ship's capacity measured in tons; the weight of its cargo; the amount of shipping of a country or port; merchant ships collectively; a duty levied on ships based on tonnage or capacity.

tonne /tʌn/ *n* metric ton, 1,000 kg.

tonometer /toː'nɒmətər/ *n* a device, such as a tuning fork, for measuring the pitch of tones.

tonsil /'tɒnsil/ *n* one of the two oval organs of soft tissue situated one on each side of the throat.

tonsillectomy /ˌtɒnsə'lɛktəmi/ *n* (*pl* **tonsillectomies**) a surgical operation to remove the tonsils.

tonsillitis /ˌtɒnsə'laitis/ *n* inflammation of the tonsils.

tonsure /'tɒnʃər/ *n* shaving part of the head to denote a clerical state in certain churches and religious orders; the shaved area itself. • *vt* to give a tonsure to (a monk, etc).—**tonsured** *adj*.

Tony /'toːni/ *n* (*pl* **Tonys, Tonies**) an annual award for excellence in the theatre.

too /tuː/ *adv* in addition; also, likewise; extremely; very.

took /tʊk/ *see* **take**.

tool /tuːl/ *n* an implement that is used by hand; a means for achieving any purpose.

tooling /'tuːliŋ/ *n* a design or decoration made with a tool, as on leather.

tool-maker /'tuːlˌmeikər/ *n* a person who repairs and maintains precision machine tools.

toolroom /-ˌruːm/ *n* an area in a factory, machine shop, etc where tools are kept or repaired.

toonie /'tuːni/ *n* ✸ (*Cdn*) (*inf*) the Canadian two-dollar coin.

toot /tuːt/ *vi* to hoot a car horn, whistle, etc in short blasts. • *n* a hoot.—*also vt*.

tooth /tuːθ/ *n* (*pl* **teeth**) one of the white, bone-like structures arranged in rows in the mouth, used in biting and chewing; the palate; a tooth-like projection on a comb, saw, or wheel.

toothache /'tuːθeik/ *n* a pain in a tooth.

toothbrush /-brʌʃ/ *n* a small brush for cleaning teeth.

toothed whale *n* any of various whales with simple teeth, such as dolphins.

toothpaste /-peɪst/ *n* a paste for cleaning teeth, used with a toothbrush.

toothpick /-pɪk/ *n* a sliver of wood or plastic for removing food particles from between the teeth.

tooth powder *n* a powder used for cleaning the teeth.

toothsome /-səm/ *adj* appetizing.

toothy /'tu:θɪ/ *adj* (**toothier, toothiest**) having or revealing prominent teeth.

top[1] /tɒp/ *n* the highest, or uppermost, part or surface of anything; the highest in rank; the crown of the head; the lid. • *adj* highest; greatest. • *vt* to cover on the top; to remove the top of or from; to rise above; to surpass; (*with* **up**) to raise up to the full capacity or amount.

top[2] *n* a child's toy, which is spun on its pointed base.

topaz /'tɒ:pæz/ *n* any of various yellow gems.

top brass *npl* (*inf*) the highest-ranking military or other officials.

topcoat /'tɒpkoːt/ *n* an overcoat.

top dog *n* (*inf*) the leader, the most important person.

top drawer *n* the most prominent people in society.

tope[1] /toːp/ *vi* to consume alcoholic drink in excessive quantities.—**toper** *n*.

tope[2] *n* a small grey European shark.

topee /'toːpi/ *n* a pith helmet.—*also* **topi**.

top flight *adj* excellent, of the highest quality.

topgallant /tɒp'gælənt/ or /tə'gælənt/ *n* a mast or sail above a topmast.—*also adj*.

top gear *n* the highest gear in a motor vehicle; maximum speed or activity.

top hat *n* a man's tall, silk hat.

top-heavy *adj* having an upper part too heavy for the lower, causing instability.

topi /'toːpi/ *see* **topee**.

topiary /'toːpɪˌɛri/ *adj* pertaining to the art or practice of trimming bushes and trees into ornamental shapes. • *n* (**topiaries**) a tree or bush shaped in this way.

topic /'tɒpɪk/ *n* a subject for discussion; the theme of a speech or writing.

topical /-əl/ *adj* of current interest.

topknot /'tɒpnɒt/ *n* a tuft of hair or knot of ribbons on the head.

topless /-ləs/ *adj* lacking a top; (*garment*) revealing the breasts; wearing such a garment.

topmast /-mæst/ *n* a mast next above the lowest mast.

topmost /moːst/ *adj* nearest the top, highest.

topnotch /-nɒtʃ/ *adj* (*inf*) excellent.

topo- /'toːpoː/, **top-** /tɒp/ *prefix* place; locality.

topography /tə'pɒgrəfɪ/ *n* (*pl* **topographies**) the study or description of surface features of a place on maps or charts.—**topographer** *n*.—**topographical** *adj*.

topology /tə'pɒlədʒɪ/ *n* the study of the properties of geometric figures that are unaffected by distortion.—**topological** *adj*.—**topologist** *n*.

topping /'tɒpɪŋ/ *n* a top layer, *esp* a sauce for food.

topple /'tɒpəl/ *vi* to fall over. • *vt* to cause to overbalance and fall; (*government*) to overthrow.

topsail /'tɒpseɪl/ or /-səl/ *n* a square sail next above the lowest sail on a mast.

top secret *adj* highly confidential.

topside /-saɪd/ *n* the upper side; a boneless cut of beef; the open or upper decks of a ship. • *adv* on top.

topsoil /-soɪl/ *n* the surface layer of soil.

topspin /-spɪn/ *n* a spin imparted to a ball that makes it travel faster or higher.

topsy-turvy /'tɒpsɪˌtɜrvɪ/ *adj*, *adv* turned upside down; in confusion.

toque /tuːk/ *n* a small brimless hat for women; ✳ (*Cda*) a close-fitting, stretchable knitted hat.

tor /tɔr/ *n* a high, rocky hill.

Torah /'tɔrə/ *n* (a scroll containing) the Pentateuch; Jewish sacred writings and teachings collectively.

torch /tɔrtʃ/ *n* a flashlight; a device for giving off a hot flame.—**torchlight** *n*.

torchbearer /'tɔrtʃˌbɛrər/ *n* a person carrying a torch; a leader, source of inspiration.

torch song /tɔrtʃsɒŋ/ *n* a sentimental song about the sufferings of love.—**torch singer** *n*.

tore /tɔr/ *see* **tear**.

toreador /'tɔrɪəˌdɔr/ *n* a bullfighter, *esp* on horseback.

torero /tə'rɛrɔ/ *n* (*pl* **toreros**) a bullfighter, *esp* one who fights on foot.

torii /'tɔriɪ/ *n* (*pl* **torii**) a gateway to a Japanese Shinto temple.

torment /'tɔrment/ *n* torture, anguish; a source of pain. • *vt* to afflict with extreme pain, physical or mental.—**tormentor, tormenter** *n*.

torn /tɔrn/ *see* **tear**[2].

tornado /tɔr'neɪdɔ/ *n* (*pl* **tornadoes, tornados**) a violently whirling column of air seen as a funnel-shaped cloud that *usu* destroys everything in its narrow path.

toroid /'tɔrɔɪd/ *n* (a solid enclosed by) a surface generated by a circle rotated about a line in the same plane as but not intersecting the circle.—**toroidal** *adj*.

torpedo /tɔr'piːdɔ/ *n* (*pl* **torpedoes**) a self-propelled submarine offensive weapon, carrying an explosive charge. • *vt* to attack, hit, or destroy with torpedo(es).

torpedo boat *n* a small high-speed warship from which torpedoes are launched.

torpid /'tɔrpɪd/ *adj* lethargic, sluggish.—**torpidity** *n*.

torpor /'tɔrpər/ *n* a state of lethargy.

torque /'tɔrk/ *n* (*physics*) a force that causes rotation around a central point, such as an axle.

torr /tɔr/ *n* (*pl* **torr**) a unit of pressure equal to 133.322 newtons per square metre.

torrent /'tɒrənt/ *n* a rushing stream; a flood of words.—**torrential** *adj*.

torrid /'tɒrɪd/ *adj* burning, parched or scorched with heat; passionate.—**torridity, torridness** *n*.

torsi /'tɔrsɪ/ *see* **torso**.

torsion /'tɔrʃən/ *n* a twisting effect on an object when equal forces are applied at both ends but in opposite directions.

torsk /tɔrsk/ *n* (*pl* **torsk, torsks**) a large marine food fish related to the cod.

torso /'tɔrsɔ/ *n* (*pl* **torsos, torsi**) the trunk of the human body.

tort /tɔrt/ *n* (*law*) a private or civil wrong.

torte /tɔrt/ *n* a rich cake or tart filled with cream, fruit, etc.

tortellini /ˌtɔrtə'liːni/ *n* small stuffed pasta shapes.

tortilla /tɔr't:ə/ *n* a round thin maize pancake usually eaten hot with a topping or filling.

tortoise /'tɔrtəs/ *n* a slow-moving reptile with a dome-shaped shell into which it can withdraw.

tortoiseshell /'tɔrtəsˌʃɛl/ *n* a brown and yellow colour.

tortricid /'tɔrtrɪsɪd/ *n* any of a family of moths whose larvae live in nests of rolled-up leaves.

tortuous /'tɔrtʃəs/ *adj* full of twists, involved.—**tortuously** *adv*.

torture /'tɔrtʃər/ *n* subjection to severe physical or mental pain to extort a confession, or as a punishment. —*also vt*.—**torturer** *n*.

torus /'tɔrəs/ *n* a convex semicircular moulding, *esp* at the base of a column; a toroid.—**toric** *adj*.

Tory /'tɔrɪ/ *n* (*pl* **Tories**) a member of the Conservative Party in UK politics; an American supporter of the British during the American Revolution; ✳ a member or supporter of the Progressive Conservative Party of Canada.—*also adj*.

tosh /'tɒʃ/ *n* (*sl*) nonsense.

toss /tɒs/ *vt* to throw up; to pitch; to fling; (*head*) to throw back; (*with* **off**) to produce, write, perform, etc, quickly and easily; to drink in one gulp. • *v* to be tossed about; to move restlessly; (*with* **up**) to spin a coin to decide a question by the side that falls uppermost. • *n* the act of tossing or being tossed; a pitch; a fall.

toss-up *n* the throwing of a coin to decide a question; an even chance.

tot[1] /tɒt/ *n* anything little, *esp* a child; a small measure of spirits.

tot[2] *vt* (**totting, totted**) (*with* **up**) to add up or total.

total /'toːtəl/ *adj* whole, complete; absolute. • *n* the whole sum; the entire amount. • *vt* (**totalling, totalled** *or* **totaling, totaled**) to add up.—**totally** *adv*.

totalitarian /toːˌtælɪ'tɛrɪən/ *adj* relating to a system of government in which one political group maintains complete control, *esp* under a dictator. —**totalitarianism** *n*.

totality /toː'tælɪtɪ/ *n* (*pl* **totalities**) the whole amount.

totalizator /'toːtəlaɪˌzeɪtər/ *n* a machine for registering bets and computing the odds and payoff, as at a racetrack.

tote[1] /toːt/ *n* (*inf*) totalizator.

tote[2] *vt* to carry.

tote bag *n* (*inf*) a large bag for shopping or other items.

totem /'to:təm/ *n* an object regarded as a symbol and treated with respect by a particular group of people.

totem pole *n* a large pole carved with totemic symbols used in rituals by certain North American Indian tribes.

totter /'tɒtər/ *vi* to walk unsteadily; to shake or sway as if about to fall.—**tottery** *adj*.

toucan /'tu:kən/ *n* a fruit-eating South American bird with an immense, brightly coloured beak.

touch /tʌtʃ/ *vt* to come in contact with, *esp* with the hand or fingers; to reach; to affect with emotion; to tinge or tint; to border on; (*sl*) to ask for money (from); (*with* **off**) to cause to explode, as with a lighted match; to cause (violence, a riot, etc) to start; (*with* **up**) to improve by making minor alterations or additions to. • *vi* to be in contact; to be adjacent; to allude to. • *n* the act of touching; the sense by which something is perceived through contact; a trace; understanding; a special quality or skill.

touch-and-go *adj* precarious, risky.

touchdown /'tʌtʃdaun/ *n* the moment when an aircraft or spaceship lands; (*Rugby football, American football*) a placing of the ball on the ground to score.

touché /tu:'ʃeɪ/ *interj* (*fencing*) used to acknowledge an opponent's hit; an acknowledgement of a valid or accomplished reply, remark, witty comment, etc.

touched /tʌtʃt/ *adj* emotionally affected; mentally disturbed.

touching /'tʌtʃɪŋ/ *adj* affecting, moving.

touch judge *n* a linesman in Rugby football.

touchline /'tʌtʃlaɪn/ *n* (*football, etc*) the side boundary of a pitch.

touchmark /-mark/ *n* a maker's distinguishing mark on pewter.

touchpaper /-peɪpər/ *n* paper impregnated with a slow-burning substance used to ignite fireworks.

touchstone /-sto:n/ *n* a siliceous stone used to test gold and silver from the marks they make on it; any test or standard of genuineness.

touch-type *vi* to type quickly and accurately without looking at the keyboard.—**touch-typist** *n*.

touchwood /-wud/ *n* dry rotten wood useful for tinder.

touchy /'tʌtʃi/ *adj* (**tochier, touchiest**) irritable; very risky.

tough /tʌf/ *adj* strong; durable; hardy; rough and violent; difficult; (*inf*) unlucky.—**toughen** *vti*.—**toughness** *n*.

tough-minded *adj* realistic; unsentimental.

toupee /tu:'piː/ *n* a wig or section of hair to cover a bald spot, *esp* worn by men.

tour /tur/ *n* a turn, period, etc as of military duty; a long trip, as for sightseeing. • *vti* to go on a tour (through).

touraco /'turə,ko:/ *n* (*pl* **touracos**) any of a family of brightly coloured crested birds native to Africa.

tour de force /turdə'fors/ *n* (*pl* **tours de force**) an outstanding achievement or performance.

tourism /'turizəm/ *n* travelling for pleasure; the business of catering for people who do this; the encouragement of touring.

tourist /'turizəm/ *n* one who makes a tour, a sightseer, travelling for pleasure.—*also adj*.

tourist class *n* economy accommodation, as on a ship, aircraft, etc.

touristy /'turisti/ *adj* (*inf*) full of or designed for tourists.

tourmaline /'turmə,liːn/ *n* a silicate mineral of various colours used in jewellery and electronic equipment.

tournament /'tɜrnəmənt/ or /'tur-/ *n* a sporting event involving a number of competitors and a series of games.

tournedos /'tʊrnə,do:/ *n* (*pl* **tournedos**) a thick round fillet of beef steak.

tourniquet /'tɜrnəkət/ or /'tur-/, /-,keɪ/, /-,kiː/ *n* a device for compressing a blood vessel to stop bleeding.

tour operator *n* a company that specializes in offering package tours.

tourtière /tor'tjɛr/ *n* ✤ (*Cdn*) a French-Canadian pie of ground pork and spices.

tousle /'tɒzəl/ or /-zəl/ *vt* to make untidy, ruffle, make tangled (*esp* hair).

tout /'taut/ *vti* (*inf*) to praise highly; (*inf*) to sell betting tips on (race horses); (*inf*) to solicit business in a brazen way. • *n* (*inf*) a person who does so.

tovarish, tovarich /tə'varɪʃ/ *n* a comrade.

tow /tau/ *vt* to pull or drag with a rope. • *n* the act of towing; a towrope.

towage /'to:ɪdʒ/ *n* the act of towing; the charge made for it.

toward /tə'wɔrd/ or /twɔrd/, **towards** /-wɔrdz/ *prep* in the direction of; concerning; just before; as a contribution to.

towel /'tauəl/ *n* an absorbent cloth for drying the skin after it is washed, and for other purposes; **to throw in the towel** to admit defeat. • *vti* (**towelling, towelled** *or* **toweling, toweled**) to rub (oneself) with a towel.

towelette /'tauəl,ɛt/ *n* a small moistened tissue for cleaning the face, etc.

towelling, toweling /'tauəlɪŋ/ *n* cloth for towels; a rubbing with a towel.

tower /'tauər/ *n* a tall, narrow building, standing alone or forming part of another; a fortress. • *vi* (*with* **over**) to rise above; to loom.

tower block *n* a skyscraper.

towering /'tauərɪŋ/ *adj* immensely tall; powerful, impressive; intense.

town /taun/ *n* a densely populated urban centre, smaller than a city and larger than a village; the people of a town.

townie /'tauni/ *n* (*pl* **townies**) a person who lives in a city or town as opposed to the countryside.—*also* **towny**.

town hall *n* a large building housing the offices of the town council, often with a hall for public meetings.

town house /'taunhous/ *n* a two or three-story house with a garage below, *usu* one of a row; a house in a fashionable area; one's house in town.

township /'taunʃɪp/ *n* a division of a county in many US states, constituting a unit of local government; in South Africa, an urban area reserved for Blacks.

towny /'tauni/ *see* **townie**.

towpath /'to:pæθ/ *n* the footpath beside a river or canal.

towrope, towline *n* a strong rope or cable for towing a wheeled vehicle, ship, etc.

tox- /tɒks/, **toxic-** /'tɒksɪk/, **toxico-** /'tɒksɪko:/ *prefix* poison.

toxaemia, toxemia /tɒk'si:miə/ *n* a type of blood poisoning.—**toxaemic, toxemic** *adj*.

toxic /'tɒksɪk/ *adj* poisonous; harmful; deadly.—**toxicity** *n*.

toxicant /-ənt/ *n* a poison. • *adj* poisonous.

toxicology /tɒksɪ'kɒlədʒi/ *n* the scientific study of poisons, their effects and antidotes.—**toxicologic, toxicological** *adj*.—**toxicologist** *n*.

toxin /'tɒksɪn/ *n* a poison produced by microorganisms and causing certain diseases.

toxocariasis /,tɒksə'kærɪeɪsɪs/ *n* a disease in humans caused by the larvae of a parasitic roundworm found in dogs and cats.

toxoid /'tɒksɔɪd/ *n* a toxin of reduced power used in vaccines to stimulate the production of antitoxins.

toxoplasmosis /,tɒkso:plæz'mo:sɪs/ *n* a disease affecting the central nervous system caused by a parasitic worm.

toy /tɔɪ/ *n* an object for children to play with; a replica; a miniature. • *vi* to trifle; to flirt.

toyboy *n* the younger male lover of an older woman.

trace /treɪs/ *n* a mark etc left by a person, animal or thing; a barely perceptible footprint; a small quantity. • *vt* to follow by tracks; to discover the whereabouts of; (*map, etc*) to copy by following the lines on transparent paper.

traceable /'treɪsəbəl/ *adj* able to be traced.—**traceably** *adv*.

trace element *n* a chemical element, as copper, zinc, etc, essential in nutrition but only in minute amounts.

tracer /'treɪsər/ *n* a projectile which glows or leaves a smoke trail allowing its flight to be observed; a radioisotope introduced into the body whose course can be traced by a detector for diagnostic purposes.

trachea /'treɪkɪə/ or /trə'kiːə/ *n* (*pl* **tracheae**) the air passage from the mouth to the lungs, the windpipe.

tracheo- /'treɪkio:/, **trache-** /'treɪki/ *prefix* trachea.

tracheotomy /,treɪki'ɒtəmi/ *n* (*pl* **tracheotomies**) an incision into the trachea, *esp* to bypass a blockage in the air passage.

trachoma /trə'ko:mə/ *n* an infectious eye disease caused by a virus that leads to scarring and eventual blindness.—**trachomatous** *adj*.

trachyte /'treɪkaɪt/ or /'træk-/ *n* a type of light-coloured volcanic rock.

tracing /'treɪsɪŋ/ *n* a copy of a drawing, etc made by tracing.

tracing paper *n* transparent paper used for tracing.

track /træk/ *vt* to follow the tracks of; (*satellite, etc*) to follow by radar and record position; (*with* **down**) to find by tracking. • *n* a mark left; a footprint; parallel steel rails on which trains run; a course for running or racing; sports performed on a track, as running, hurdling; the band on which the wheels of a tractor or tank run; one piece of music on a record; a sound track.

track-and-field *adj* denoting various competitive athletic events (as running, jumping, weight-throwing) performed on a track and adjacent field.

tracker /'trækər/ *n* a person who follows by tracking footprints, etc; a dog that follows a scent.

track event *n* an athletic event that takes place on a running track.

tracking station *n* a place that uses radio or radar antennae to follow the course of objects in space or the atmosphere.

tracklaying *adj* (*vehicle*) having an endless loop of metal track around the wheels.

track record *n* (*inf*) a record of the past achievements or failures of someone or something.

track shoe *n* a spiked running shoe.

tracksuit *n* a loose suit worn by athletes to keep warm.

tract[1] /trækt/ *n* an expanse of land or water; a part of a bodily system or organ.

tract[2] *n* a treatise.

tractable /'træktəbəl/ *adj* easily worked; easily taught; docile.

traction /'trækʃən/ *n* act or state of drawing and pulling; (*med*) the using of weights to pull on a muscle, etc, to correct an abnormal condition.

tractor /'træktər/ *n* a motor vehicle for pulling heavy loads and farming machinery.

trad /træd/ *adj* (*inf*) traditional. • *n* traditional jazz.

trade /treɪd/ *n* buying and selling (of commodities); commerce; occupation; customers; business. • *vi* to buy and sell; to exchange; (*with* **on**) to take advantage of.—**trader** *n*.

trade cycle *n* a recurrent fluctuation in economic activity between boom and slump.

trade gap *n* the amount by which the value of a country's visible imports exceeds its visible exports.

trade-in *n* a used item given in part payment when buying a replacement.

trade-off *n* the exchange or substitution of one thing or priority for another, often as a compromise.

trademark /'treɪdmɑrk/ *n* a name used on a product by a manufacturer to distinguish it from its competitors, *esp* when legally protected.—*also vt.*

tradescantia /ˌtrædə'skæntiə/ *n* any of a genus of common houseplants cultivated for their variegated foliage.

tradesman /'treɪdzmən/ *n* (*pl* **tradesmen**) a shopkeeper; a skilled worker.

trade union, trades union *n* an organized association of employees of any trade or industry for the protection of their income and working conditions.

trade wind *n* a wind that blows toward the equator at either side of it.

trading /'treɪdɪŋ/ *n* the act of buying and selling (goods, etc).—*also adj.*

tradition /trə'dɪʃən/ *n* the handing down from generation to generation of opinions and practices; the belief or practice thus passed on; custom.—**traditional** *adj.*—**traditionally** *adv.*

traduce /trə'duːs/ or /-'djuːs/ *vt* to speak badly of; to misrepresent.

traffic /'træfɪk/ *n* trade; the movement or number of vehicles, pedestrians, etc, along a street, etc. • *vi* (**trafficking, trafficked**) to do business (*esp.* in illegal drugs).

traffic circle *n* a junction of thoroughfares where traffic circulates one way to ease progress, a roundabout.

traffic island *n* a raised area in the centre of a road to guide traffic and provide refuge for pedestrians crossing

traffic light *n* one of a set of coloured lights used to control traffic at street crossings, etc.

traffic pattern *n* a network of airlanes above an airport to which aircraft are restricted.

tragacanth /'trægəˌkænθ/ *n* a gum obtained from a species of spiny leguminous plants used in pharmacy and in calico printing.

tragedian /trə'dʒiːdiən/ *n* an actor who plays mainly tragic roles.—**tragedienne** *nf.*

tragedy /'trædʒədi/ *n* (*pl* **tragedies**) a play or drama that is serious and sad, and the climax a catastrophe; an accident or situation involving death or suffering.—**tragic** *adj.*—**tragically** *adv.*

tragicomedy /ˌtrædʒɪ'kɒmədi/ *n* a dramatic or literary work which combines tragic and comic elements; a situation or event with tragic and comic aspects.

trail /treɪl/ *vt* to drag along the ground; to have in its wake; to follow behind; to advertise a film, event or programme beforehand. • *vi* to hang or drag loosely behind; (*plant*) to climb; (*with* **off** or

away) to grow weaker or dimmer. • *n* a path or track; the scent of an animal; something left in the wake (*eg a trail of smoke*).

trailblazer /'treɪlˌbleɪzər/ *n* a person who blazes a trail; a pioneer in a particular field.

trailer /-ər/ *n* a large vehicle designed to be towed by a truck, etc; a motor home; an advertisement for a film or television programme.

trailer park *n* an area available for rent to motor homes, caravans, etc, *usu* with electricity, water, etc, piped in.

trailing edge *n* the rear edge of an aerofoil.

train /treɪn/ *vt* to teach, to guide; to tame for use, as animals; to prepare for racing, etc; (*gun, etc*) to aim. • *vi* to do exercise or preparation. • *n* a series of railroad cars pulled by a locomotive; a sequence; the back part of a dress that trails along the floor; a retinue.

trained /treɪnd/ *adj* skilled.

trainee /treɪ'niː/ *n* a person who is being trained.

trainer /'treɪnər/ *n* a coach or instructor in sports; a person who prepares horses for racing.

training /-ɪŋ/ *n* practical instruction; a course of physical exercises.

training school *n* an institution for training in vocational subjects, *eg* teaching, nursing.

training ship *n* a moored vessel on which people are taught seamanship.

train oil *n* oil obtained from whale blubber.

train surfing *n* the practice of clinging onto the outside of a moving train for kicks.—**train surfer** *n*.

traipse /treɪps/ *vi* to walk wearily, trudge about. • *n* a tiring walk, a trudge.

trait /treɪt/ *n* a characteristic feature.

traitor /'treɪtər/ *n* a person who commits treason or betrays his country, friends, etc.—**traitorous** *adj*.

trajectory /trə'dʒɛktəri/ *n* (*pl* **trajectories**) the path of an object, such as a bullet, moving through space.

tram[1] /træm/ *n* a small wagon running on rails in a mine; a streetcar; a cable car.

tram[2] *n* a double twisted thread used in some silks.

trammel /'træməl/ *n* a type of net for catching birds or fish; (*often pl*) a hindrance to freedom of movement or action; an instrument for drawing ellipses. • *vt* (**trammelling, trammelled** or **trammeling, trammeled**) to trap, catch; to hinder, restrict.

tramp /træmp/ *vti* to walk heavily; to tread or trample; to wander about as a tramp. • *n* a vagrant; (*sl*) a prostitute.

trample /'træmpəl/ *vti* to tread under foot.

trampoline /ˌtræmpə'liːn/ *n* a sheet of strong canvas stretched tightly on a frame, used in acrobatic tumbling.

trance /træns/ *n* a state of unconsciousness, induced by hypnosis, in which some of the powers of the waking body, such as response to commands, may be retained.

tranche /trɑːnʃ/ *n* a portion of something, *esp* a sum of money or issue of shares.

tranquil /'træŋkwɪl/ *adj* quiet, calm, peaceful.—**tranquilly** *adv*.

tranquillize, tranquilize /'træŋkwɪˌlaɪz/ *vt* to make tranquil, *esp* by administering a drug.—**tranquillization, tranquillization** *n*.

tranquillizer, tranquilizer /ˌtræŋkwɪ'laɪzər/ *n* a drug that calms.

tranquility, tranquillity /træŋ'kwɪlɪti/ *n* the state of being tranquil; calmness.

trans. *abbr* = transitive; translated; translation; translator.

trans- /trænz/ *prefix* through; across; on the other side of.

transact /træn'zækt/ *vt* (*business*) to conduct or carry out.

transaction /træn'zækʃən/ *n* the act of transacting; something transacted, *esp* a business deal; (*pl*) a record of the proceedings of a society.

transalpine /trænz'ælpaɪn/ *adj* beyond (*usu* north) of the Alps.

transatlantic /ˌtrænzət'læntɪk/ *adj* crossing the Atlantic Ocean; across, beyond the Atlantic.

trans-Canada *adj* ✸ (*Cdn*) across, including, or involving all of Canada.

transceiver /træn'siːvər/ *n* a combined radio transmitter and receiver.

transcend /træn'sɛnd/ *vt* to rise above or beyond; to surpass.—**transcendent** *adj*.

transcendental /ˌtrænsɛn'dɛntəl/ *adj* beyond physical experience; surpassing; supernatural.—**transcendentally** *adv*.

transcendental meditation *n* a technique for emptying and refreshing the mind by repeating a mantra.

transcontinental /ˌtrænskɒntɪˈnɛntəl/ *adj* extending or travelling across a continent.—**transcontinentally** *adv*.

transcribe /trænˈskraɪb/ *vt* to write out fully from notes or a tape recording; to make a phonetic transcription; to arrange a piece of music for an instrument other than the one it was written for.

transcript /trænˈskrɪpt/ *n* a written or printed copy made by transcribing; an official copy of proceedings, etc.

transcription /trænˈskrɪpʃən/ *n* the act of transcribing; something transcribed, *esp* a piece of music; a transcript; a recording made for broadcasting.

transducer /trænsˈduːsər/ or /-ˈdjuːs/ *n* a device that converts energy from one form into another.

transept /trænˈsept/ *n* one of the two wings of a church, at right angles to the nave.

transfer /ˈtrænsfər/ *vb* (**transferring, transferred**) *vt* to carry, convey, from one place to another; (*law*) to make over (property) to another; (*money*) to move from the control of one institution to another. • *vi* to change to another bus, etc. • *n* the act of transferring; the state of being transferred; someone or something that is transferred; a design that can be moved from one surface to another.—**transferable** *adj*.

transference /ˈtrænsfərəns/ *n* the act of transferring; the state of being transferred; (*psychoanal*) the redirection of emotion under analysis, *usu* toward the analyst.

transfer RNA *n* a form of RNA that carries an amino acid to a ribosome in protein synthesis.

transfiguration /ˌtrænsfɪɡəˈreɪʃən/ *n* a change in appearance, *esp* to a more spiritual or exalted form; (*with cap*) (the festival commemorating) the change in the appearance of Christ as described in the Gospels.

transfigure /ˈtrænsfɪɡər/ *vt* to transform or become transformed in appearance, *esp* for the better.

transfix /ˈtrænsfɪks/ *vt* to impale with a sharp weapon; to paralyse with shock or horror.

transform /ˈtrænsfɔrm/ *vti* to change the shape, appearance, or condition of; to convert.—**transformation** *n*.

transformer /-ər/ *n* a device for changing alternating current with an increase or decrease of voltage.

transfusion /trænsˈfjuːʒən/ *n* the injection of blood into the veins of a sick or injured person.—**transfuse** *vt*.

transgress /-ˈɡrɛs/ *vti* to break or violate (a moral law or code of behaviour); to overstep (a limit).—**transgressor** *n*.

transgression /-ˈɡrɛʃən/ *n* the act of transgressing; infringement of a rule, etc; a sin.

transhumance /-ˈhjuːməns/ *n* the seasonal movement of livestock to new grazing areas.

transient /ˈtrænzɪənt/ *adj* temporary; of short duration, momentary.—**transience** *n*.

transistor /trænˈzɪstɪv/ *n* a device using a semiconductor to amplify sound, as in a radio or television; a small portable radio.

transit /ˈtrænzɪt/ *n* a passing over or through; conveyance of people or goods.

transit camp *n* temporary accommodation for soldiers, refugees, etc.

transition /trænˈzɪʃən/ *n* passage from one place or state to another; change.—**transitional** *adj*.

transitive /ˈtrænzɪtɪv/ *adj* (*gram*) denoting a verb that requires a direct object; of or relating to transition.—**transitively** *adv*.—**transitivity** *n*.

transitory /ˈtrænzɪˌtɔri/ *adj* lasting only a short time.—**transitorily** *adv*.—**transitoriness** *n*.

translate /ˈtrænzleɪt/ or /-ˈleɪt/ *vti* to express in another language; to explain, interpret.—**translator** *n*.

translation /trænzˈleɪʃən/ *n* the act of translating; something translated into another language or state; an interpretation.

transliterate /-ˈlɪtəˌreɪt/ *vt* to convert a word, etc into the corresponding characters of another alphabet.—**transliteration** *n*.

translucent /-ˈluːsənt/ *adj* allowing light to pass through, but not transparent.—**translucence** *n*.

transmigrate /ˌtrænzmaɪˈɡreɪt/ *vi* (*soul*) to pass into the body of another person after death; to migrate.

transmission /trænzˈmɪʃən/ *n* the act of transmitting; something transmitted; a system using gears, etc, to transfer power from an engine to a moving part, *esp* wheels of a vehicle; a radio or television broadcast.

transmit /ˈtrænzmɪt/ *vt* (**transmitting, transmitted**) to send from one place or person to another; to communicate; to convey; (*radio or television signals*) to send out.

transmitter /-ər/ *n* an apparatus for broadcasting television or radio programmes.

transmogrify /trænzˈmɒɡrɪˌfaɪ/ *vt* (**transmogrifying, transmogrified**) to change shape, *esp* in a bizarre or comic manner.—**transmogrification** *n*.

transmute /-ˈmjuːt/ *vt* to change into a different form or substance.—**transmutation** *n*.

transnational /-ˈnæʃənəl/ *n* extending beyond national boundaries.

transoceanic /-ˌoʊʃɪˈænɪk/ *adj* on or from the other side of ocean; crossing the ocean.

transom /ˈtrænsəm/ *n* a horizontal bar across a window or between a door and a window over it; a fanlight; any of several transverse beams supporting and strengthening the stern of a vessel.

transparency /ˈtrænspərənsi/ *n* (*pl* **transparencies**) the state of being transparent; (*photog*) a slide.

transparent /trænsˈpɛrənt/ *adj* that may be easily seen through; clear, easily understood.—**transparently** *adv*.—**transparentness** *n*.

transpire /trænˈspaɪr/ *vti* to emit, to pass off through the pores of the skin; to exhale (moisture); (*news*) to become known, to leak out; (*inf*) to happen.—**transpiration** *n*.

transplant /-ˈplænt/ *vt* (*plant*) to remove and plant in another place; (*med*) to remove an organ from one person and transfer it to another.—*also n*.

transport /-ˈpɔrt/ *vt* to convey from one place to another; to enrapture. • *n* the system of transporting goods or passengers; the conveyance of troops and their equipment by sea or land; a vehicle for this purpose.—**transportable** *adj*.—**transportation** *n*.

transpose /-ˈpoʊz/ *vt* to put into a different order; to interchange; (*mus*) to change the key of.—**transposition** *n*.

transputer /-ˈpjuːtər/ *n* (*comput*) a fast microchip comprising a 32-bit microprocessor which is used as a component in compact supercomputers.

transsexual /-ˈsɛkʃuəl/ *n* a person born of one sex who identifies psychologically with the opposite sex.—**transsexualism** *n*.

transubstantiation /ˌtrænsəbˌstænʃɪˈeɪʃən/ *n* (*esp in RC Church*) the doctrine that the bread and wine of the communion are wholly transformed into the body and blood of Christ when consecrated, although their appearance remains unchanged.

transuranic /-juːˈrænɪk/ *adj* (*element*) having an atomic number greater than that of uranium.

transverse /ˈtrænzvərs/ *adj* crosswise.—**transversely** *adv*.

transvestite /trænzˈvɛstaɪt/ *n* a person who gains sexual pleasure from wearing the clothes of the opposite sex.—**transvestism** *n*.

trap /træp/ *n* a mechanical device or pit for snaring animals; an ambush; a trick to catch someone out; a two-wheeled horse-drawn carriage. • *vt* (**trapping, trapped**) to catch in a trap; to trick.

trapdoor *n* a hinged or sliding door in a roof, ceiling or floor.

trapeze /trəˈpiːz/ *n* a gymnastic apparatus consisting of a horizontal bar suspended by two parallel ropes.

trapezium /trəˈpiːzɪəm/ *n* (*pl* **trapeziums, trapezia**) a quadrilateral in which two of the sides are parallel; in US, a quadrilateral in which none of the sides are parallel.—**trapezial** *adj*.

trapezoid /ˈtræpəˌzɔɪd/ *n* a quadrilateral in which none of the sides are parallel. In US, a quadrilateral with two sides parallel.

trapper /ˈtræpər/ *n* a person who traps animals, *esp* for their skins.

trappings /-ɪŋz/ *npl* trimmings; additions; ornaments.

trash /træʃ/ *n* nonsense; refuse; rubbish.

trash can *n* a container for household refuse, a dustbin, garbage can.

trashy /ˈtræʃi/ *adj* (**trashier, trashiest**) of poor quality.—**trashiness** *n*.

trattoria /ˌtrætəˈriːə/ *n* (*pl* **trattorias, trattorie**) an Italian restaurant.

trauma /ˈtrɔmə/ *n* an emotional shock that may cause long-term psychological damage; an upsetting experience.—**traumatic** *adj*.

travel /ˈtrævəl/ *vb* (**travelling, travelled** *or* **traveling, traveled**) *vi* to journey or move from one place to another. • *vt* to journey across, through. • *n* journey.

travel agency *n* an agency through which one can book travel.—**travel agent** *n*.

traveller, traveler /-ər/ *n* a person who travels; a salesman who travels for a company.

traveller's cheque *n* a draft purchased from a bank, etc signed at the time of purchase and signed again at the time of cashing.

travelogue, travelog /-lɒg/ *n* a film or illustrated lecture on travel.

traverse /trə'vərs/ or /'trævərs/ *n* a horizontal move in rock climbing, skiing, etc. • *vt* to cross.

travertine /'trævər,ti:n/ *n* a mineral comprising mostly calcium carbonate, used for building.

travesty /'trævəsti/ *n* (*pl* **travesties**) a misrepresentation; a poor imitation; a parody.

trawl /trɒl/ *vti* to fish by dragging a large net behind a fishing boat.

trawler /-ər/ *n* a boat used for trawling.

tray /treɪ/ *n* a flat board, or sheet of metal or plastic, surrounded by a rim, used for carrying food or drink.

treacherous /'tretʃərəs/ *adj* untrustworthy, disloyal; unstable, dangerous.

treachery /-ri/ *n* (*pl* **treacheries**) disloyalty, betrayal of trust.

treacle /'tri:kəl/ *n* a thick sticky substance obtained during the refining of sugar.—**treacly** *adj*.

tread /tri:d/ *vti* (**treading, trod**, *pp* **trodden**) to step or walk on, along, in, over or across; to crush or squash (with the feet); to trample (on). • *n* a step, way of walking; the part of a shoe, wheel, or tire that touches the ground.

treadle /'tri:dəl/ *n* a foot lever or pedal on a machine.

treadmill /'tredmɪl/ *n* a grind; a monotonous routine.

treas. *abbr* = treasurer, treasury.

treason /'tri:zən/ *n* the crime of betraying one's government or attempting to overthrow it; treachery.—**treasonable** *adj*.

treasure /'treʒər/ *n* wealth and riches hoarded up; a person or thing much valued. • *vt* to hoard up; to prize greatly.

treasurer /-ər/ *n* a person appointed to take charge of the finances of a society, government or city.

treasure hunt *n* a game in which players follow clues to locate a hidden object.

treasure-trove *n* (*law*) valuable items such as gold and silver found buried and of unknown ownership; any valuable find

treasury /-ri/ *n* (*pl* **treasuries**) a place where valuable objects are deposited; the funds or revenues of a government.

Treasury Board *n* ✤ (*Cdn*) a government department responsible for reviewing planned expenditures.

treat /tri:t/ *vt* to deal with or regard; to subject to the action of a chemical; to apply medical treatment to; to pay for another person's entertainment; to deal with in speech or writing. • *n* an entertainment paid for by another person; a pleasure seldom indulged; a unusual cause of enjoyment.

treatise /'tri:tɪs/ *n* a formal essay in which a subject is treated systematically.

treatment /'tri:tmənt/ *n* the application of drugs, etc, to a patient; the manner of dealing with a person or thing, *esp* in a novel or painting; behaviour toward someone.

treaty /'tri:ti/ *n* (*pl* **treaties**) a formal agreement between states.

treble /'trebəl/ *adj* triple, threefold; (*mus*) denoting the treble. • *n* the highest range of musical notes in singing. • *vti* to make or become three times as much.

treble clef *n* (*mus*) a clef that places G above middle C on the second line of the staff.

trebuchet /'trebju,ʃet/ or /-bəʃet/ *n* a type of medieval military catapult used in sieges.

trecento /treɪ'tʃento:/ *n* the 14th century, *esp* in reference to Italian art and literature.

tree /tri:/ *n* a tall, woody, perennial plant having a single trunk, branches and leaves.

tree creeper /'tri:,kri:pər/ *n* any of various small songbirds with curved beaks for prising insects from tree trunks.

tree fern *n* a large tropical fern with a woody stem.

tree frog *n* any of various frogs that inhabit trees.

tree line /'tri:laɪn/ *n* the height or latitude beyond which no trees grow on mountains or in cold regions.—*also* **timber line**.

tree surgeon *n* a person skilled in saving diseased or damaged trees.—**tree surgery** *n*.

tree toad *n* a tree frog.

trefoil /'trefɔɪl/ *n* any of various plants with three leaflets; an ornament or design resembling this.

trek /trek/ *vi* (**trekking, trekked**) to travel slowly or laboriously; (*inf*) to go on foot (to). • *n* a long and difficult journey; a migration.

trellis /'trelɪs/ *n* a structure of latticework, for supporting climbing plants, etc.—**trelliswork** *n*.

tremble /'trembəl/ *vi* to shake, shiver from cold or fear; to quiver.—*also* *n*.

trembler /'tremblər/ *n* a device that makes or breaks an electric circuit when subject to vibration.

tremendous /trɪ'mendəs/ *adj* awe-inspiring; very large or great; (*inf*) wonderful; marvellous.

tremolo /'tremo:lo:/ *n* (*pl* **tremolos**) a tremulous effect in playing or singing; a device that produces this effect, as in an organ.

tremor /'tremər/ *n* a vibration; an involuntary shaking.

tremulous /'tremjuləs/ *adj* quivering; agitated.

trench /trentʃ/ *n* a long narrow channel in the earth, used for drainage; such an excavation made for military purposes.

trenchant /'trentʃənt/ *adj* keen; incisive; effective.

trench coat *n* a waterproof coat.

trencher /'trentʃər/ *n* a wooden board formerly used for serving food.

trencherman /-mən/ *n* a person who eats heartily.

trench fever *n* an infectious disease characterized by fever and muscular pains that is transmitted by lice.

trench foot *n* a degenerative condition of the feet caused by prolonged immersion in cold water.

trend /trend/ *n* tendency; a current style or fashion.

trendsetter *n* a person who starts a new fashion.

trendy /'trendi/ *adj* (**trendier, trendiest**) (*inf*) fashionable. • *n* (*pl* **trendies**) (*inf*) a person who tries to be fashionable.— **trendily** *adv*.—**trendiness** *n*.

trepan /trɪ'pæn/ *n* a primitive form of trephine. • *vt* (**trepanning, trepanned**) to cut with a trepan.

trepang /trɪ'pæŋ/ *n* a type of large sea cucumber dried and used in Chinese cookery, bêche-de-mer.

trephine /trɪ'faɪn/ *n* a surgical saw for removing circular sections of bone, *esp* from the skull. • *vt* to cut with a trephine.

trepidation /,trepɪ'deɪʃən/ *n* a state of fear or anxiety.

trespass /'trespəs/ *vi* to intrude upon another person's property without their permission; to encroach upon, or infringe, another's rights. • *n* act of trespassing.—**trespasser** *n*.

tress /tres/ *n* a lock, braid, or plait of hair.

trestle /'tresəl/ *n* a wooden framework for supporting a table top or scaffold boards.

trews /tru:z/ *npl* tight-fitting tartan trousers.

trey /tre/ *n* three spots or the number three on a dice, domino or playing card.

tri- /traɪ/ *prefix* having, made up of, or containing three or three parts; every third.

triactor /traɪ'æktər/ *n* ✤ (*Cdn*) a bet on the first three finishers in a horse race, specifying the order of their finish.

triad /'traɪæd/ *n* a group or set of three, a trio.

triage /'triæʒ/ or /trɪ'æʒ/, /-'ɑːʒ/, /-'ɒʒ/ *n* the sorting and treatment of the wounded according to chance of survival.

trial /'traɪəl/ *n* a test or experiment; judicial examination; an attempt; a preliminary race, game in a competition; suffering; hardship; a person causing annoyance.

trial and error *n* solving problems through trying various solutions and rejecting the least successful.

trial run *n* an opportunity to test something before purchase, as a vehicle; a rehearsal.

triangle /'traɪ,æŋgəl/ *n* (*math*) a plane figure with three angles and three sides; a percussion instrument consisting of a triangular metal bar beaten with a metal stick.—**triangular** *adj*.

triangulate /traɪ'æŋgju,leɪt/ *vt* to divide into triangles; to make triangular; to survey by dividing an area into a network of triangles.—**triangulation** *n*.

triathlon /traɪ'æθlən/ *n* an athletic event in which all contestants compete in swimming, cycling and running.

triatomic /,traɪə'tɒmɪk/ *adj* (*chem*) having three atoms in the molecule.

tribadism /'traɪbədɪzəm/ *n* simulated heterosexual intercourse by lesbians with one partner lying on top of the other.

tribe /traɪb/ *n* a group of people of the same race, sharing the same customs, religion, language or land.—**tribal** *adj*.—**tribesman** *n*.

tribo- /'traɪbo/ *prefix* friction.

triboelectricity /,traɪbo:,i lek'trɪsɪti/ *n* electricity generated by friction.

tribology /traɪ'bɒlədʒi/ *n* the study of friction, wear and lubrication between moving surfaces, as gearing systems.

triboluminescence /ˌtraɪboˌluːmɪˈnesəns/ *n* luminescence caused by friction.—**triboluminescent** *adj*.

tribulation /ˈtrɪbjʊleɪʃən/ *n* distress, difficulty, hardship.

tribunal /traɪˈbjuːnəl/ or /trɪ-/ *n* a court of justice; a committee that investigates and decides on a particular problem.

tribune[1] /trɪˈbjuːn/ *n* in ancient Rome, a magistrate appointed to protect the rights of common people; a champion of the people.

tribune[2] *n* a raised platform or dais from which speeches are delivered.

tributary /trɪˈbjuːˌteri/ *n* (*pl* **tributaries**) a stream or river flowing into a larger one.

tribute /trɪˈbjuːt/ *n* a speech, gift or action to show one's respect or thanks to someone; a payment made at certain intervals by one nation to another in return for peace.

tricentenary /traɪˌsentəˈneri/ *n* (*pl* **tricentenaries**) a tricentennial.—*also adj*.

tricentennial /ˌtraɪsenˈteniəl/ *adj* lasting, or happening every, 300 years. • *n* an anniversary of 300 years; a period of 300 years.

triceps /ˈtraɪseps/ *n* (*pl* **tricepses, triceps**) any three-headed muscle, *esp* the large muscle that extends the forearm.

trichiasis /trɪˈkaɪəsɪs/ *n* a condition of having in-growing eyelashes which irritate the eyeball.

trichina /trɪˈkiːnə/ *n* (*pl* **trichinae**) a hair-like parasitic worm that infests the intestines and muscles of pigs and humans.

trichinosis /ˌtrɪkəˈnoːsɪs/ *n* a disease in humans caused by infestation of muscular tissues by trichinae.

tricho- /ˈtrɪkoː/, **trich-** /trɪk/ *prefix* hair; filament.

trichology /trɪˈkɒlədʒi/ *n* the medical study and treatment of hair diseases.—**trichologist** *n*.

trichosis /trɪˈkoːsɪs/ *n* any disease of the hair.

trichotomy /trɪˈkɒtəmi/ *n* (*pl* **trichotomies**) a division into three parts or categories.—**trichotomous** *adj*.

trichromatic /ˌtraɪkrəˈmætɪk/ *adj* of, involving, or combining three colours; of or having normal colour vision.—**trichromatism** *n*.

trick /trɪk/ *n* fraud; deception; a mischievous plan or joke; a magical illusion; a clever feat; skill, knack; the playing cards won in a round. • *adj* using fraud or clever contrivance to deceive. • *vt* to deceive, cheat.—**trickster** *n*.

trickery /ˈtrɪkəri/ *n* (*pl* **trickeries**) the practice or an act of using underhand methods to achieve an aim; deception.

trickle /ˈtrɪkəl/ *vti* to flow or cause to flow in drops or in a small stream.—*also n*.

trickle-down *adj* denoting a theory in economics that financial incentives to big business will percolate through to small businesses and individuals.

trick or treat *n* a Halloween tradition in which children dress in costumes, call on their neighbours and threaten to do mischief if refused presents of sweets, apples, nuts, money, etc.

tricky /ˈtrɪki/ *adj* (**trickier, trickiest**) complicated, difficult to handle; risky; cunning, deceitful.—**trickily** *adv*.—**trickiness** *n*.

tricolour, tricolor /ˈtraɪˌkələr/ *n* a flag with three stripes of different colours.

tricorn /ˈtraɪkɔrn/ *adj* having three horns or corners. • *n* a three-cornered hat.

tricuspid /traɪˈkʌspɪd/ *adj* having three cusps, flaps, points, or segments. • *n* a tooth with three cusps.

tricycle /ˈtraɪsaɪkəl/ *n* a three-wheeled pedal cycle, *esp* for children.

trident /ˈtraɪdənt/ *n* three-pronged spear.

tridentate /traɪˈdenteɪt/, **tridental** /-ˈdentəl/ *adj* having three teeth or prongs.

tried[1] /traɪd/ *see* **try**.

tried[2] *adj* tested; trustworthy.

triennial /traɪˈeniəl/ *adj* happening every third year; lasting for three years.

triennium /traɪˈeniəm/ *n* (*pl* **trienniums, triennia**) a period of three years.

trier /ˈtraɪər/ *n* one who tries.

trifle /ˈtraɪfəl/ *vi* to treat lightly; to dally. • *n* anything of little value; a dessert of whipped cream, custard, sponge cake, sherry, etc.

trifling /ˈtraɪflɪŋ/ *adj* insignificant.

trifocal /traɪˈfoːkəl/ *adj* having three focuses or focal lengths. • *npl* glasses with trifocal lenses.

trifurcate /traɪˈfɜrkət/, **trifurcated** /-əd/ *adj* having three branches or forks.

trig. *abbr* = trigonometrical; trigonometry.

trigeminal /traɪˈdʒemɪnəl/ *adj* pertaining to the trigeminal nerve.

trigeminal nerve *n* either of a pair of cranial nerves that supply various facial muscles.

trigger /ˈtrɪgər/ *n* a catch that when pulled activates the firing mechanism of a gun. • *vt* (*with* **off**) to initiate; to set (off).

trigger-happy *adj* too eager to resort to firearms or violence; rash, aggressive.

trigonometric function *n* any of various functions (*eg* sine, cosine, tangent) expressed as ratios of the sides of a right-angled triangle.

trigonometry /ˌtrɪgəˈnɒmətri/ *n* the branch of mathematics concerned with calculating the angles of triangles or the lengths of their sides.

trike /traɪk/ *n* (*inf*) a tricycle.

trilateral /traɪˈlætərəl/ *adj* having three sides.

trilby /ˈtrɪlbi/ *n* (*pl* **trilbies**) a soft felt hat with a fold in the crown.

trilingual /traɪˈlɪŋgwəl/ or /-juːəl/ *adj* speaking three languages; written in three languages.—**trilingualism** *n*.

trill /trɪl/ *vti* to sing or play with a tremulous tone; (*a bird*) to make a shrill, warbling sound.—*also n*.

trillion /ˈtrɪliən/ *n* a million million (1012); (*formerly*) in UK, a million million million (1018); (*inf*) (*pl*) a very large number.

trilobite /ˈtraɪləˌbaɪt/ *n* any of a group of extinct Palaeozoic marine arthropods each with a body in three sections.

trilogy /ˈtrɪlədʒi/ *n* (*pl* **trilogies**) any series of three related literary or operatic works.

trim /trɪm/ *adj* (**trimmer, trimmest**) in good condition; tidy, neat; slim. • *vt* to neaten; to cut or prune; to decorate; (*ship, aircraft*) to balance the weight of cargo in. • *n* a decorative edging; a haircut that tidies.

trimaran /ˈtraɪməˌræn/ *n* a boat with three hulls.

trimester /ˈtraɪˌmestər/ or /traɪˈmestər/ *n* a period of three months; a division of the academic year in certain North American colleges and universities.

trimming /ˈtrɪmɪŋ/ *n* decorative part of clothing; (*pl*) accompaniments.

trinitrotoluene /traɪˌnaɪtrəˈtɒljuːˌiːn/ *n* a solid yellow chemical substance used as a high explosive.

trinity /ˈtrɪnɪti / *n* (*pl* **trinities**) a group of three; (*with cap*) in Christianity, the union of Father, Son and Holy Spirit in one God.

trinket /ˈtrɪŋkət/ *n* a small or worthless ornament.

trinomial /traɪˈnoːmiəl/ *adj* having three terms. • *n* (*math*) a polynomial consisting of three terms.

trio /ˈtriːoː/ *n* (*pl* **trios**) a set of three; (*mus*) a group of three singers or instrumentalists.

triode /ˈtraɪoːd/ *n* an electronic valve or semiconductor device with three electrodes.

trip /ˈtrɪp/ *vb* (**tripping, tripped**) *vi* to move or tread lightly; to stumble and fall; to make a blunder. • *vt* (*often with* **up**) to cause to stumble; to activate a trip. • *n* a stumble; a journey, tour, or voyage; a slip; a mistake; a light step; a mechanical switch; (*sl*) a hallucinatory experience under the influence of a drug.

tripartite /traɪˈpɑrtaɪt/ *adj* made up of or divided into three parts; involving or binding three parties.

tripe /traɪp/ *n* the stomach lining of a ruminant, prepared for cooking; (*inf*) rubbish, nonsense.

triplane /ˈtraɪˌpleɪn/ *n* an aircraft with three wings positioned one above the other.

triple /ˈtrɪpəl/ *adj* threefold; three times as many. • *vti* to treble.

triple jump *n* an athletic event in which a competitor makes a hop, step and jump in succession.

triplet /ˈtrɪplət/ *n* one of three children born at one birth.

triplicate /ˈtrɪplɪkət/ *adj* threefold.

tripod /ˈtraɪpɒd/ *n* a three-legged stand, as for supporting a camera.

tripper /ˈtrɪpər/ *n* a tourist; a trip switch.

triptych /ˈtrɪptɪk/ *n* a picture consisting of three panels fixed or hinged side by side.

tripwire /ˈtrɪpwaɪr/ *n* a concealed wire that sets off a bomb, booby trap, etc when tripped over.

trireme /ˈtraɪriːm/ *n* an ancient Greek galley with three banks of oars.

trisect /ˈtraɪsekt/ *vt* to divide into three (equal) parts.—**trisection** *n*.

trishaw /ˈtraɪʃɒ/ *n* a rickshaw.

triskelion /traɪˈskɛlɪən/ *n* (*pl* **triskelia**) a symbol consisting of three bent limbs or branches radiating from a centre.

trismus /ˈtrɪzməs/ *n* lockjaw.

trisyllable /ˌtraɪˈsɪləbəl/ *n* a word of three syllables.

trite /traɪt/ *adj* dull; hackneyed.

tritium /ˈtrɪtɪəm/ *n* a radioactive isotope of hydrogen.

triton /ˈtraɪtən/ *n* any of various marine gastropod molluscs having a heavy spiral shell; (*with cap*) (*Greek myth*) a sea-god depicted as half man and half fish blowing a spiral shell.

triturate /ˈtrɪtʃəˌreɪt/ *vt* to crush or grind into a fine powder.—**trituration** *n*.

triumph /ˈtraɪəmf/ *n* a victory; success; a great achievement. • *vi* to win a victory or success; to rejoice over a victory.—**triumphal** *adj*.

triumphant /traɪˈæmfənt/ *adj* feeling or showing triumph; celebratory; victorious.—**triumphantly** *adv*.

triumvir /traɪˈæmvər/ *n* (*pl* **triumvirs, triumviri**) a member of a ruling body of three persons.

triumvirate /traɪˈæmvərət/ *n* the office of a triumvir; joint rule by three persons.

trivalent /traɪˈveɪlənt/ *adj* having a valency of three.

trivet /ˈtrɪvət/ *n* a three-legged metal stand for supporting hot dishes.

trivia /ˈtrɪvɪə/ *npl* unimportant details.

trivial /-əl/ *adj* unimportant; commonplace.

triviality /ˌtrɪvɪˈælɪtɪ/ *n* (*pl* **trivialities**) a trifle, detail; the state of being trivial.

Trivial Pursuit *n* ✤ (*Cdn*) (*trademark*) a board game in which players advance by answering questions taken from general subject areas.

-trix /trɪks/ *n suffix* female.

t-RNA *abbr* = transfer RNA.

trocar /ˈtroːkɑr/ *n* a pointed instrument for inserting drainage tubes into bodily cavities.

trochal /ˈtroːkəl/ *adj* wheel-shaped.

troche /ˈtroːki/ *n* a medicinal lozenge.

trochee /ˈtroːki/ *n* a metrical foot comprising one long syllable followed by one short syllable.

trod /trɒd/, **trodden** /ˈtrɒdn/ *see* **tread**.

troglodyte /ˈtrɒɡləˌdaɪt/ *n a cave dweller*.

troika /ˈtrɔɪkə/ *n* (a Russian vehicle drawn by) three horses harnessed abreast; a triumvirate.

troll /troːl/ *n* a supernatural creature, dwelling in a cave, hill, etc.

trolley /ˈtrɒlɪ/ *n* (*pl* **trolleys**) a table on wheels for carrying or serving food; a cart for transporting luggage; a cart for carrying shopping in a supermarket; a device that transmits electric current from an overhead wire to a motor vehicle, such as a trolleybus.

trolleybus, trolley car *n* a bus that sometimes runs on rails and is powered by electricity from overhead wires.

trollop /ˈtrɒləp/ *n* a slovenly woman; a prostitute.—**trollopy** *adj*.

trombone /trɒmˈboːn/ *n* brass musical wind instrument whose length is varied with a U-shaped sliding section.

troop /truːp/ *n* a crowd of people; a group of soldiers within a cavalry regiment; (*pl*) armed forces; soldiers. • *vi* to go in a crowd.

trooper /ˈtruːpər/ *n* a cavalryman; a mounted policeman or a state policeman.

troopship /ˈtruːpʃɪp/ *n* a ship used to transport military forces.

trope /troːp/ *n* a word or phrase used in a figurative sense.

-trope /troːp/ *n suffix* turning, being attracted toward.

trophic /ˈtroːfɪk/ or /ˈtrɒfɪk/ *adj* pertaining to nutrition.

tropho- /ˈtrɒfoː/, **troph-** *prefix* nutrition.

trophy /ˈtroːfɪ/ *n* (*pl* **trophies**) a cup or shield won as a prize in a competition or contest; a memento, as taken in battle or hunting.

-trophy /ˈtroːfɪ/ *n suffix* growth, nutrition.

tropic /ˈtrɒpɪk/ *n* one of the two parallel lines of latitude north and south of the equator; (*pl*) the regions lying between these lines.

-tropic /ˈtrɒpɪk/ *adj suffix* turning to or responding to an external stimulus.

tropical /ˈtrɒpɪkəl/ *adj* relating to the tropics; (*weather*) hot and humid.

tropism /ˈtroːpɪzəm/ *n* the involuntary direction of growth of a plant due to an external stimulus.

-tropism /trəˌpɪzəm/, **-tropy** *n suffix* turning or developing in response to an external stimulus.

tropo- /trɒpə/ *prefix* turning or changing.

-tropous /ˈtrɒpoːz/ *adj suffix* turning away.

tropopause /ˈtrɒpəˌpɒz/ or /ˈtroː-/ *n* the region between the troposphere and stratosphere.

troposphere /ˈtrɒpəˌsfiːr/ or /ˈtroː-/ *n* the region of the atmosphere below the stratosphere which varies in temperature and in which clouds form.

trot /trɒt/ *vb* (**trotting, trotted**) *vi* (*horse*) to go, lifting the feet higher than in walking and moving at a faster rate. • *vt* (*with* **out**) (*inf*) to produce or display repeatedly, *esp* for others' approval; to produce in a trite or careless manner. • *n* the gait of a horse; a brisk pace.

trotter /ˈtrɒtər/ *n* a horse trained for fast trotting; the foot of an animal, *esp* a pig.

troubadour /ˈtruːbəˌdɔr/ *n* a minstrel; a poet or singer.

trouble /ˈtrʌbəl/ *vti* to cause trouble to; to worry; to pain; to upset; to cause inconvenience; to take pains (to). • *n* an anxiety; a medical condition causing pain; a problem; unrest or disturbance.—**troublesome** *adj*.

troubleshooter /ˈtrʌbəlˌʃuːtər/ *n* a person whose work is to locate and eliminate a source of trouble or conflict.—**troubleshooting** *n*.

trough /trɒf/ *n* a long, narrow container for water or animal feed; a channel in the ground; an elongated area of low barometric pressure.

trounce /traʊns/ *vt* to defeat completely.

troupe /truːp/ *n* a travelling company, *esp* of actors, dancers or acrobats.—**trouper** *n*.

trousers /ˈtraʊzərz/ *npl* an item of clothing covering the body from waist to ankle, with two tubes of material for the legs; pants.

trousseau /ˈtruːsoː/ or /truːˈsoː/ *n* (*pl* **trousseaux, trousseaus**) the clothes and linen a bride collects for her marriage.

trout /traʊt/ *n* (*pl* **trout**) a game fish of the salmon family living in fresh water.

trove /troːv/ *see* **treasure trove**.

trowel /traʊəl/ *n* a hand tool for gardening; a flat-bladed tool for spreading cement, etc.

troy (weight) /trɔɪ/ *n* a system for weighing precious stones and metals, in which one pound = 12 ounces and one ounce = 20 pennyweights or 480 grains.

truant /ˈtruːənt/ *n* a pupil who is absent from school without permission. • *vi* to play truant.—*also adj*.—**truancy** *n*.

truce /truːs/ *n* an agreement between two armies or states to suspend hostilities.

truck /trʌk/ *n* a heavy motor vehicle for transporting goods; a vehicle open at the back for moving goods or animals. • *vt* (*goods*) to convey by truck. • *vi* to drive a truck.

trucker /ˈtrʌkər/ *n* a truck driver.

truculent /ˈtrʌkjʊlənt/ *adj* sullen; aggressive.—**truculence** *n*.—**truculently** *adv*.

trudge /trʌdʒ/ *vti* to travel on foot, heavily or wearily. • *n* a tiring walk.

true /truː/ *adj* (**truer, truest**) conforming with fact; correct, accurate; genuine; loyal; perfectly in tune. • *adv* truthfully; rightly.

true-blue /ˈtruːˈbluː/ *adj* staunchly loyal or committed.—**true blue** *n*.

truelove /ˈtruːˌlʌv/ *n* a sweetheart.

truffle /ˈtrʌfəl/ *n* a round edible underground fungus; a sweet made with chocolate, butter and sugar.

truism /ˈtruːɪzəm/ *n* a self-evident truth.

truly /ˈtruːlɪ/ *adv* completely; genuinely; to a great degree.

trump /trʌmp/ *n* (*cards*) the suit that is chosen to have the highest value in one game. • *vt* to play a trump card on; (*with* **up**) to invent maliciously, fabricate (an accusation, etc).

trumpery /ˈtrʌmpərɪ/ *adj* worthless. • *n* (*pl* **trumperies**) foolish talk, nonsense; a worthless article.

trumpet /ˈtrʌmpət/ *n* a brass wind instrument consisting of a long tube with a flared end and three buttons. • *vti* to proclaim loudly.—**trumpeter** *n*.

trumpeter swan *n* a rare wild North American swan with a black bill.

truncate /ˈtrʌŋkeɪt/ or /trʌŋˈkeɪt/ *vt* to cut the top end off; to shorten.—**truncation** *n*.

truncheon /ˈtrʌntʃən/ *n* a short, thick club carried by a policeman.

trundle /ˈtrʌndəl/ *vt* (*an object*) to push or pull on wheels. • *vi* to move along slowly.

trunk /trʌŋk/ *n* the main stem of a tree; the torso; the main body of anything; the proboscis of an elephant; a strong box or chest for clothes, etc, *esp* on a journey; storage space at the rear of an automobile; (*pl*) a man's short, light pants for swimming.

trunk line *n* a transportation system handling through traffic; a communications system.

trunk road *n* a main road.

truss /trʌs/ *n* a supporting framework for a roof or bridge; a hernia brace. • *vt* to bind (up).

trust /trʌst/ *n* firm belief in the truth of anything, faith in a person; confidence in; custody; a financial arrangement of investing money for another person; a business syndicate. • *adj* held in trust. • *vti* to have confidence in; to believe.—**trustful** *adj*.

trustee /trʌs'ti:/ *n* a person who has legal control of money or property that they are keeping or investing for another person, or for an organization or institution.—**trusteeship** *n*.

trustworthy /'trʌst,wərði/ *adj* reliable, dependable.

trusty /'trʌsti/ *adj* (**trustier, trustiest**) trustworthy, faithful. • *n* a prisoner granted special privileges as a trustworthy person.—**trustily** *adv*.—**trustiness** *n*.

truth /tru:θ/ *n* that which is true, factual or genuine; agreement with reality.

truthful /'tru:θfʊl/ *adj* telling the truth; accurate, realistic; honest, frank.—**truthfulness** *n*.

try /traɪ/ *vb* (**trying, tried**) *vt* to test the result or effect by experiment; to determine judicially; to put strain on; (*with* **on**) to put (a garment) on to check the fit, etc; (*inf*) to attempt to deceive somebody; (*with* **out**) to test (someone) for a job, etc. • *vi* to attempt; to make an effort; (*with* **out**) to undergo a test (for a job, team, etc). • *n* (*pl* **tries**) an attempt, an effort; (*Rugby football*) a score made with a touchdown.

trying /'traɪɪŋ/ *adj* causing annoyance, exasperating.—**tryingly** *adv*.—**tryingness** *n*.

try-on /'traɪɒn/ *n* (*inf*) a trying on of clothes to check the fit; an attempt to deceive.

tryout /'traɪaʊt/ *n* an experimental test; an audition for a theatrical part; (*sports, etc*) a test for a position in a team.

trypanosome /'trɪpənə,soʊm/ or /trɪ'pænə-/ *n* any of genus of parasitic worms that infest the blood of animals and humans and can cause sleeping sickness.

trypanosomiasis /,trɪpənəsə'maɪəsɪs/ or /trɪ'pænə-/ *n* (a disease caused by) infection with trypanosomes.

trypsin /'trɪpsɪn/ *n* an enzyme in the pancreas involved in digestion.—**tryptic** *adj*.

tryptophan /'trɪptə,fæn/, **tryptophane** *n* an amino acid found in proteins which is essential to life.

try square *n* an L-shaped instrument for drawing and testing right angles.

tryst /trɪst/ *n* an appointment to meet secretly.

tsar /tsɑr/ or /zɑr/ *n* (*formerly*) the title of the emperors of Russia (until 1917) and sovereigns of certain other Slav nations; a powerful person.—*also* **czar**.

tsarevitch /'tsɑrəvɪtʃ/ or /'zɑr-/ *n* the eldest son of a tsar.—*also* **czarevitch**.

tsarina /tsɑ'ri:nə/ or /zɑ-/, **tsaritsa** /tsɑ'ri:tzə/ or /zɑ-/ *n* the wife of a tsar; an empress.—*also* **czarina**.

TSE /'ti:'es'i:/ *abbr* ✺ = Toronto Stock Exchange.

tsetse fly /'tsi:tsi/ or /'ti:tsi/ *n* a fly that feeds on blood and transmits diseases.

T-shirt /'ti:ʃərt/ *n* a short-sleeved casual cotton top.—*also* **tee-shirt**.

tsp. *abbr* = teaspoon.

T-square /'ti:skwer/ *n* a T-shaped instrument for drawing and determining right angles.

Tu. *abbr* = Tuesday.

tub /tʌb/ *n* a circular container, made of staves and hoops; a bathtub.

tuba /'tu:bə/ or /'tju:bə/ *n* a large brass instrument of bass pitch.

tubby /'tʌbi/ *adj* (**tubbier, tubbiest**) plump.

tube /tu:b/ or /'tju:b/ *n* a long, thin, hollow pipe; a soft metal or plastic cylinder in which thick liquids or pastes, such as toothpaste, are stored; (*inf*) in UK, the underground railway system.—**tubular** *adj*.

tubeless tire /'tu:blɪs/ or /'tju:b-/ *n* a tire that remains airtight without requiring an inner tube.

tuber /'tu:bər/ or /'tju:bər/ *n* the swollen, fleshy root of a plant where reserves of food are stored up, as a potato.

tubercle /'tu:bərkəl/ or /'tju:-/ *n* a small round swelling or nodule, *esp* on bone, skin or a plant; an abnormal lump, *esp* one characteristic of tuberculosis.

tubercle bacillus *n* a bacterium that causes tuberculosis.

tuberculate /tu:'bərkju,leɪt/ or /-lɪt/ *adj* affected with tubercles.—**tuberculation** *n*.

tuberculin /tu'bərkjulɪn/ *n* a sterile liquid prepared with weakened tubercle bacillus and used in the diagnosis of tuberculosis.

tuberculosis /tu,bərkju'loːsɪs/ *n* an infectious disease of the lungs.—**tubercular** *adj*.

tuberose /'tu:bə,roːz/ or /'tu:broːz/, /'tju:-/ *n* a bulbous Mexican plant with fragrant white flowers.

tuberous /'tu:bərəs/ or /'tju:bərəs/ *adj* (*plants*) forming or resembling tubers.

tubing /'tu:bɪŋ/ or /'tju:bɪŋ/ *n* tubes collectively; a length of tube; the material from which tubes are made; a circular fabric.

tub-thumper /'tʌb,θʌmpər/ *n* a passionate or aggressive public speaker.

tubular bells /'tu:bjələr/ or /'tju:-/ *npl* an orchestral percussion instrument consisting of a set of long metal tubes played with a mallet to simulate the sounds of bells.

tuck /tʌk/ *vt* to draw or gather together in a fold; (*with* up) to wrap snugly. • *vi* (*inf*) (*with* into) to eat greedily. • *n* a fold in a garment.

tucker /'tʌkər/ *vt* (*inf*) to exhaust, tire (out).

Tue., Tues. *abbr* = Tuesday.

Tuesday /'tu:zdeɪ/ or /'tju:z-/, /-di/ *n* the third day of the week.

tufa /'tu:fə/ or /'tju:-/ *n* a type of porous rock deposited from springs.

tuff /tʌf/ *n* a type of volcanic rock composed of fused lava ash.

tuffet /'tʌfɪt/ *n* a small low seat; a clump of grass.

tuft /tʌft/ *n* a bunch of grass, hair or feathers held together at the base; a clump.

tug /tʌg/ *vti* (**tugging, tugged**) to pull with effort or to drag along. • *n* a strong pull; a tugboat.

tugboat /'tʌgboːt/ *n* a small powerful boat for towing ships.

tug of love *n* a conflict over the custody of a child between separated parents, etc.

tug of war *n* a contest in which two teams tug on opposite ends of a rope to pull the opposing team over a central line; a struggle for supremacy between two opponents.

tuition /tu:'ɪʃən/ or /tju:-/ *n* teaching, instruction.

tulip /'tu:lɪp/ or /'tju:-/ *n* a highly-coloured cup-shaped flower grown from bulbs.

tulip tree *n* a North American tree with large tulip-shaped flowers.

tulipwood /'tu:lɪp,wʊd/ *n* the soft white wood of the tulip tree used in making furniture.

tulle /tu:l/ *n* a delicate semi-transparent fabric of rayon, silk, etc, used for scarfs and veils.

tullibee /'tɛlɪbi/ *n* ✺ (*Cdn*) a North American whitefish.

tumble /'tʌmbəl/ *vi* to fall over; to roll or to twist the body, as an acrobat; (*with* to) (*inf*) to discover (a secret, etc); to understand. • *vt* to push or cause to fall. • *n* a fall; a somersault.

tumbledown /'tʌmbəldaʊn/ *adj* dilapidated, crumbling.

tumble-dry *vt* (*clothes*) to dry by rotating with warm air in a machine.—**tumble dryer** *n*.

tumbler /'tʌmblər/ *n* a large drinking glass without a handle or stem; an acrobat.

tumbler switch *n* a simple electrical switch used in lighting.

tumbleweed /'tʌmbəl,wi:d/ *n* a plant that detaches from its roots and is blown around by the wind.

tumbrel /'tʌmbrəl/, **tumbril** /-rɪl/ *n* a farm cart that tips up to deposit its load; a cart of similar design used to carry prisoners to the guillotine during the French Revolution.

tumescent /tju:'mesənt/ or /tju:-/ *adj* swollen or beginning to swell.

tumid /'tu:mɪd/ or /'tju:-/ *adj* swollen, distended; pompous, bombastic.—**tumidly** *adv*.—**tumidity** *n*.

tummy /'tʌmi/ *n* (*pl* **tummies**) (*inf*) stomach.

tumour, tumor /'tu:mər/ or /'tju:-/ *n* an abnormal growth of tissue in any part of the body.

tumult /'tju:mʌlt/ or /'tu:-/, /-məlt/, /'tʌməlt/ *n* a commotion; an uproar.

tumultuous /tə'mʌltʃʊəs/ or /tu:-/, /tju:-/, /-tjʊəs/ *adj* disorderly; rowdy, noisy; restless.—**tumultuously** *adv*.—**tumultuousness** *n*.

tun /tʌn/ *n* a large wine or beer cask; a unit of capacity equal to about 252 wine gallons (954 litres).

tuna /'tuːnə/ *or* /'tjuː-/ *n* (*pl* **tuna, tunas**) a large ocean fish of the mackerel group.

tundra /'tʌndrə/ *n* a vast treeless arctic plain.

tune /tuːn/ *or* /tjuːn/ *n* a melody; correct musical pitch; harmony. • *vt* (*musical instrument*) to adjust the notes of; (*radio, TV etc*) to adjust the resonant frequency, etc, to a particular value; (*with* **up**) to adjust an engine to improve its performance. • *vi* (*with* **up**) to adjust (musical instruments) to a common pitch before playing.—**tuneful** *adj*.—**tunefully** *adv*.

tune-up /tuːnʌp/ *or* /tjuː-/ *n* an adjustment of a musical instrument to correct pitch or of an engine to improve its performance.

tungsten /'tʌŋstən/ *n* a hard malleable greyish white metallic element used in lamps, etc, and in alloys with steel.

tunic /'tuːnɪk/ *or* /'tjuː-/ *n* a hip or knee-length loose, *usu* belted blouse-like garment; a close-fitting jacket worn by soldiers and policemen.

tunicate /'tuːnɪkət/ *or* /'tjuː-/, /-ˌkeɪt/ *n* any of a group of small primitive marine animals with sac-shaped bodies enclosed in a thick membrane. • *adj* having or enclosed in a membrane; (*bulbs*) made up from concentric layers of tissue.

tuning fork *n* a two-pronged steel fork that produces a fixed note when struck and is used to tune musical instruments or set a pitch for singing.

tunnel /'tʌnəl/ *n* an underground passage, *esp* one for cars or trains underneath a river or town centre. • *vb* (**tunnelling, tunnelled** *or* **tunneling, tunneled**) *vt* to make a way through. • *vi* to make a tunnel.

tunnel vision *n* a condition in which peripheral vision is impaired; a narrowness of viewpoint due to preoccupation with a single idea, plan, etc.

tunny /'tʌni/ *n* (*pl* **tunnies, tunny**) tuna.

tuppence /'tʌpəns/ *n* twopence.

turban /'tɜːbən/ *n* a headdress consisting of cloth wound in folds around the head worn by men; a woman's hat of this shape.

turbid /'tɜːbɪd/ *adj* muddy; dense; thick.—**turbidity** *n*.—**turbidly** *adv*.

turbine /'tɜːbaɪn/ *n* a machine in which power is produced when the forced passage of steam, water, etc causes the blades to rotate.

turbo- /'tɜːbo/ *prefix* of, driven or powered by a turbine.

turbofan /'tɜːboˌfæn/ *n* a jet engine with a large fan that forces air out with the exhaust gases to increase thrust; an aircraft with such engines; the fan in such an engine.

turbojet /'tɜːboˌdʒet/ *n* (an aircraft with) a turbojet engine.

turbojet engine *n* a gas turbine that provides propulsive power from a jet of hot exhaust gases.

turboprop /'tɜːboˌprɒp/ *n* a jet aircraft engine that also operates a turbine-driven air compressor.

turbot /'tɜːbət/ *n* (*pl* **turbot, turbots**) a large, flat, round edible fish.

turbulence /'tɜːbjuləns/ *n* a state of confusion and disorder; (*weather*) instability causing gusty air currents.

turbulent /'tɜːbjulənt/ *adj* disturbed, in violent commotion.

turd /tɜːd/ *n* (*vulg*) a piece of excrement; (*vulg sl*) a despicable person.

tureen /tə'riːn/ *or* /tjuː-/ *n* a large dish for serving soup, etc.

turf /tɜːf/ *n* (*pl* **turfs, turves**) the surface layer of grass and its roots; (*with* **the**) horse racing; a racetrack. • *vt* to cover with turf; (*with* **out**) (*inf*) to eject forcibly, throw out.

turf war *n* a dispute over an area, or land claimed by one party as being under control in the face of the claims of another individual or group.

turgid /'tɜːdʒɪd/ *adj* swollen; pompous, bombastic.—**turgidity** *n*.—**turgidly** *adv*.

Turk /tɜːk/ *n* a native or inhabitant of Turkey; any speaker of a Turkic language.

Turk. /tɜːk/ *abbr* = Turkey; Turkish.

turkey /'tɜːki/ *n* (*pl* **turkeys, turkey**) a large bird farmed for its meat.

turkey buzzard *n* an American vulture.

turkey cock /'tɜːkiˌkɒk/ *n* a male turkey.

Turkey red *n* (a cotton fabric of) a bright red colour.

Turki /'tɜːki/ *adj* of, being or pertaining to the Turkic languages or speakers of these languages; the Turkic languages collectively.

Turkic /'tɜːkɪk/ *n* a branch of the Altaic family of languages including Turkish, Tartar, etc.

Turkish /'tɜːkɪʃ/ *adj* pertaining to Turkey, its people or their language. • *n* the official language of Turkey.

Turkish bath *n* a bath with steam rooms, showers, massage, etc.

Turkish coffee *n* strong black (*usu* sweetened) coffee.

Turkish delight *n* a jelly-like flower-flavoured sweet covered with icing sugar.

Turk's-cap lily *n* a variety of lily with purple-red flowers found in Europe and Asia, martagon lily.

turmeric /'tɜːmərɪk/ *n* a tropical Indian plant; the powdered stem of this plant used as a yellow colouring agent and curry spice.

turmoil /'tɜːmɔɪl/ *n* agitation; disturbance, confusion.

turn /tɜːn/ *vi* to revolve; to go in the opposite direction; to depend on; to appeal (to) for help; to direct (thought or attention) away from; to change in character; to be shaped on the lathe; (*with* **off**) to leave or deviate from a road, etc; (*with* **in**) (*inf*) to retire to bed for the night; (*with* **on**) to depend on; (*with* **to**) to begin a task; (*with* **up**) to appear, arrive; to find unexpectedly; to happen without warning. • *vt* to change the position or direction of by revolving; to reverse; to transform; (*age, etc*) to have just passed; to change or convert; to invert; (*with* **off**) to cause to cease operating (as if) by flicking a switch, turning a knob, etc; (*inf*) to cause a person to lose interest in or develop a dislike for something; (*with* **down**) to reduce the volume or intensity of (sound, brightness, etc); to refuse, decline; to fold down (sheets, a collar, etc) (*with* **in**) to deliver; to produce, record (a performance, score, etc); (*with* **on**) to cause to begin operating (as if) by flicking a switch, turning a knob, etc; (*sl*) to arouse or excite, *esp* sexually; (*with* **up**) to discover, uncover; to increase the volume or intensity of (sound, brightness, etc). • *n* a rotation; new direction or tendency; a place in sequence; a turning point, crisis; performer's act; an act of kindness or malice; a bend.

turnabout /'tɜːnəbaʊt/ *n* a reversal of position, opinion, attitude, etc.

turncoat /'tɜːnkoːt/ *n* a deserter, renegade.

turner /'tɜːnər/ *n* a person who operates a lathe.

turning /'tɜːnɪŋ/ *n* a road, path, etc that leads off from a main way; the point where it leads off; a bend; the art of shaping objects on a lathe; an object so made; (*pl*) waste produced on a lathe.

turning point *n* the point at which a significant change occurs.

turnip /'tɜːnəp/ *or* /-nɪp/ *n* a plant with a large white or yellow root, cultivated as a vegetable.

turnout /'tɜːnaʊt/ *n* a gathering of people.

turnover /'tɜːnˌoːvər/ *n* the volume of business transacted in a given period; a fruit or meat pasty; the rate of replacement of workers.

turnpike /'tɜːnpaɪk/ *n* a toll road, *esp* one that is an expressway.

turnround /'tɜːnraʊnd/ *n* (the time required to complete) the unloading and reloading of a ship, aircraft, etc.

turnstile /'tɜːnstaɪl/ *n* a mechanical gate across a footpath or entrance which admits only one person at a time.

turntable /'tɜːnˌteɪbəl/ *n* a circular, horizontal revolving platform, as in a record player.

turn-up /'tɜːnˌʌp/ *n* the cuff of a trouser; (*inf*) a surprise.

turpentine /'tɜːpəntaɪn/ *n* an oily resin secreted by coniferous trees, used as a solvent and thinner for paints.—*also* **turps**.

turpentine tree *n* a terebinth or related tree that yields a turpentine.

turpitude /'tɜːpɪˌtuːd/ *or* /-ˌtjuːd/ *n* depravity; wickedness.

turps /tɜːps/ *n sing* (*inf*) turpentine.

turquoise /'tɜːkɔɪz/ *or* /-kwɔɪz/ *n* an opaque greenish-blue mineral, valued as a gem; the colour of turquoise.—*also adj*.

turret /'tʌrɪt/ *n* a small tower on a building rising above it; a dome or revolving structure for guns, as on a warship, tank or aeroplane.—**turreted** *adj*.

turtle /'tɜːtəl/ *n* any of an order of land, freshwater or marine reptiles having a soft body encased in a hard shell; **to turn turtle** to turn upside down.

turtledove /'tɜːtəlˌdʌv/ *n* a brown dove with speckled wings and a dark tail, noted for its cooing and its care for its partner and young.

turtleneck /'tɜːtəlnek/ *n* a high close-fitting neckline on a sweater.

turves /tɜːvz/ *see* **turf**.

tusk /tʌsk/ *n* a long, projecting tooth on either side of the mouth, as of the elephant.—**tusked** *adj*.

tusker /'tʌskər/ *n* an animal with tusks.

tussle /'tʌsəl/ *n* a scuffle.

tussock /'tʌsək/ n a dense tuft of grass.

tutelage /'tu:təlɔdʒ/ or /'tju:-/ n guardianship; guidance by a tutor.

tutor /'tu:tər/ or /'tju:-/ n a private teacher who instructs pupils individually; a member of staff responsible for the supervision and teaching of students in a British university. • vt to instruct; to act as a tutor.

tutorial /tu:'tɔriəl/ or /tju:-/ n a period of tuition by a tutor to an individual or a small group. • adj of or pertaining to a tutor.

tutti /'tu:ti/ adj, adv (mus) all together, to be performed by the whole orchestra. • n a musical piece or passage so performed.

tutti-frutti /ˌtu:ti'fru:ti/ n (pl **tutti-fruttis**) a type of ice cream containing pieces of chopped candied fruits.

tut-tut /tʌt'tʌt/ interj an exclamation of impatience or mild disapproval. • vi (**tut-tutting, tut-tutted**) to express disapproval or impatience by uttering "tut-tut".

tutu /'tu:tu:/ n a short, projecting, layered skirt worn by a ballerina.

tu-whit tu-whoo /tuˌwɪttu'wu:/ interj an imitation of the cry of an owl.

tuxedo /tʌk'si:do:/ n a man's semi-formal suit with a tailless jacket.—also **dinner jacket**.

TV /ti:'vi:/ abbr = television.

TVA abbr = Tennessee Valley Authority.

TVP abbr = textured vegetable protein; a meat substitute used in vegetarian dishes.

twaddle /'twɒdəl/ n utter rubbish in speech or writing. • vi to speak or write twaddle.

twain /tweɪn/ adj, n (arch) two.

twang /twæŋ/ n a sharp, vibrant sound, as of a taut string when plucked; a nasal tone of voice. • vt to make a twanging sound.

'twas /twɒz/ or /twɒz/ (poet) = it was.

tweak /twi:k/ vt to twist, pinch or pull with sudden jerks. • n a sharp pinch or twist.

twee /twi:/ adj (inf) excessively quaint, affected.

tweed /twi:d/ n a twilled woollen fabric used in making clothes.

'tween /twi:n/ prep (arch) between.

tweet /twi:t/ interj an imitation of the chirp of a small bird. • vi to make this sound.

tweeter /'twi:tər/ n a small loudspeaker for reproducing high-frequency sounds.

tweezers /'twi:zərz/ n sing small pincers used for plucking.

twelfth /twelfθ/ or /twelθ/ adj the last of twelve; being one of twelve equal parts.

Twelfth Day n Epiphany.

twelfth man n the reserve member of a cricket team.

Twelfth Night n the evening of Epiphany, the twelfth day after Christmas, 6 January; the eve of Epiphany, 5th January.

twelve /twelv/ adj the cardinal number next after eleven. • n the symbol for this (12, XII, xii).

twelve-tone /twelv'to:n/ adj pertaining to a type of serial music using only the twelve semitones of the chromatic scale as a tone row for compositions.

twelvemo /'twelvmo:/ n a book of sheets folded into twelve leaves; this book size.—also **duodecimo**.

twenty /'twenti/ adj, n two times ten. • n (pl **twenties**) the symbol for this (20, XX, xx).—**twentieth** adj.

twenty-one /'twenti'wʌn/ n pontoon (card game); blackjack.

twenty-twenty, 20/20 /ˌtwenti'twenti/ adj (vision) normal.

'twere /twər/ (poet) = it were.

twerp /twərp/ n (inf) a foolish or contemptible person.—also **twirp**.

twice /twɒɪs/ adv two times; two times as much; doubly.

twiddle /'twɪdəl/ vt to twirl or fiddle with idly.

twig[1] /twɪg/ n a small branch or shoot of a tree.—**twiggy** adj.

twig[2] vti (**twigging, twigged**) (inf) to grasp the meaning of.

twilight /'twaɪlaɪt/ n the dim light just after sunset and before sunrise; the final stages of something.

twilit /'twaɪlɪt/ adj lit by twilight.

twill /twɪl/ n a cloth woven in such a way as to produce diagonal lines across it.—**twilled** adj.

twin /twɪn/ n either of two persons or animals born at the same birth; one thing resembling another. • adj double; very like another; consisting of two parts nearly alike. • vt (**twinning, twinned**) to pair together.

twin bed n one of a pair of single beds.

twine /twaɪn/ n a string of twisted fibres or hemp. • vti to twist together; to wind around.

twin-engined /'twɪn'endʒənd/ adj (aircraft) having two engines.

twinge /twɪndʒ/ n a sudden, stabbing pain; an emotional pang.

twinkle /'twɪŋkəl/ vi to sparkle; to flicker.

twinkling /'twɪŋklɪŋ/ n a wink; an instant; the shining of the stars.

twin-screw /'twɪn'skru:/ adj (vessel) having two propellers.

twinset n a jumper and cardigan designed to be worn together.

twin-tub n a washing machine with two drums, one for washing and the other for spin-drying.

twirl /twərl/ vt to whirl; to rotate; to wind or twist. • vi to turn around rapidly.

twirp /twərp/ see **twerp**.

twist /twɪst/ vt to unite by winding together; to coil; to confuse or distort (the meaning of); to bend. • vi to revolve; to writhe. • n the act or result of twisting; a twist of thread; a curve or bend; an unexpected event; a wrench.

twister /'twɪstər/ n a tornado; (inf) a dishonest person, a swindler.

twisty /'twɪsti/ adj (**twistier, twistiest**) winding.

twit[1] /twɪt/ vt (**twitting, twitted**) to tease or reproach. • n a nervous state.

twit[2] n (Brit inf) a silly or foolish person.

twitch /twɪtʃ/ vt to pull with a sudden jerk. • vi to be suddenly jerked. • n a sudden muscular spasm.

twitter /'twɪtər/ n a chirp, as of a bird. • vi to chirp.

two /tu:/ adj, n the cardinal number next above one. • n the symbol for this (2, II, ii).

two-cycle /'tu:'saɪkəl/ see **two-stroke**.

two-dimensional /'tu:də'menʃənəl/ adj of or having two dimensions; lacking (the illusion of) depth.

two-edged /'tu:'edʒd/ adj having two cutting edges; (remark, etc) double-edged.

two-faced /'tu:ˌfeɪst/ adj deceitful, hypocritical.

twofold /'tu:fo:ld/ adj multiplied by two; double. • adv doubly.

two-four n ✤ (Cdn) (inf) a case of twenty-four bottles of beer.

two-handed /'tu:'hændɪd/ adj having or needing two hands; ambidextrous; requiring two people.

twopence /'tʌpəns/ n the sum of two pence; in UK, a coin of this value; something of little value.—also **tuppence**.

two-piece /'tu:'pi:s/ n a garment consisting of two separate matching bits.—also adj.

two-ply /'tu:'plaɪ/ adj made of two thicknesses or strands.

two solitudes npl ✤ (Cdn) the French- and English-speaking peoples of Canada, considered as being independent and isolated from each other.

twosome /'tu:səm/ n a group of two; a game for two people.

two-step /'tu:'step/ n (the music for) a ballroom dance in duple time.

two-stroke /'tu:'stro:k/ n, adj (an internal combustion engine) having a piston which makes two strokes for every explosion.—also **two-cycle**.

two-time /'tu:'taɪm/ vti (sl) to be unfaithful to (a lover, etc); to double-cross.—**two-timer** n.

two-tone /'tu:'to:n/ adj of two colours or shades of the same colour; (sirens, etc) having two notes.

two-way /'tu:'weɪ/ adj allowing movement or operation in two (opposite) directions; involving two participants; involving mutual obligation; (radio, telephone) capable of transmitting and receiving messages.

two-way mirror n a sheet of glass that reflects as a mirror on one side but can be seen through from the other.

'twould /twud/ (poet) = it would.

TX abbr = Texas.

tycoon /taɪ'ku:n/ n a powerful industrialist, etc.

tyke /təɪk/ n a (mongrel) dog; (inf) a cheeky child.—also **tike**.

tympani, tympany /'tɪmpəni/ see **timpani**.

tympanic bone n a bone enclosing part of the middle ear and supporting the tympanic membrane.

tympanic membrane n the eardrum.

tympanites /ˌtɪmpə'naɪti:z/ n distension of the abdomen caused by the accumulation of gas in the intestine.—**tympanitic** adj.

tympanitis /ˌtɪmpə'naɪtɪs/ n inflammation of the eardrum.

tympanum /'tɪmpənəm/ n (pl **tympanums, tympana**) the cavity of the middle ear; the tympanic membrane, eardrum; the space between the lintel of a doorway and the enclosing arch; the (recessed) triangular face of a pediment.

type /təɪp/ n a kind, class or group; sort; model; a block of metal for printing letters; style of print. • vt to write by means of a typewriter; to classify.

-type /təɪp/ n suffix of the form specified; printing process.

typecast /'təɪpkæst/ vt (**typecasting, typecast**) (actœr) to cast in the same role repeatedly because of physical appearance, etc.

typeface /'təɪpfeɪs/ n the printing surface of a type character; a particular design of a set of type characters.

typescript /'təɪpskrɪpt/ n a typed copy of a book, document, etc.

typeset /'təɪp‚set/ vt (**typesetting, typeset**) to set in type.—**typesetter** n.

typewriter /'təɪp‚rəɪtər/ n a keyboard machine for printing characters.

typhoid /'təɪfɔɪd/ n typhoid fever. • adj of or pertaining to typhoid fever.—also **typhoidal**.

typhoid fever n an acute infectious disease acquired by ingesting contaminated food or water.

typhoon /taɪ'fuːn/ n a violent tropical cyclone originating in the western Pacific.

typhus /'təɪfəs/ n a highly contagious acute disease spread by body lice and characterized by fever, a rash and headache.—**typhous** adj.

typical /'tɪpɪkəl/ adj representative of a particular type; characteristic.—**typicality** n.—**typically** adv.

typify /'tɪpɪ‚faɪ/ vt (**typifying, typified**) to characterize.—**typification** n.

typist /'təɪpɪst/ n a person who types or uses a typewriter, esp as a job.

typo /'təɪpoː/ n (pl **typos**) (inf) a typographical error.

typography /taɪ'pɒgrəfi/ n the way in which printed material is designed or set for printing.—**typographic, typographical** adj.

tyrannicide /ti'ræn‚saɪd/ or /tə-/, /taɪ-/ n (a person responsible for) the killing of a tyrant.

tyrannize /'tɪrə‚naɪz/ vi to exercise power (over) in a vicious and oppressive manner. • v to crush, oppress.—**tyrannizer** n.

tyrannosaur /tə'rænəsɔr/ or /taɪ-/, /ti-/, **tyrannosaurus** ‚-‚rænə'sɔrəs/ n a large carnivorous dinosaur of the Cretaceous period which stood on powerful hind legs.

tyranny /'tɪrəni/ n (pl **tyrannies**) the government or authority of a tyrant; harshness; oppression.

tyrant /'taɪrənt/ n a person who uses his or her power arbitrarily and oppressively; a despot.—**tyrannical** adj.

tyre see **tire**.

tyro /'taɪ‚roː/ n (pl **tyros**) a novice, a beginner.—also **tiro**.

tzar /tsɑr/ or /zɑr/ n a czar.—**tzarevitch** n.—**tzarina** n.

tzatsiki /tsæt'siːkiː/ n a Greek dip made from plain yogurt, shredded cucumber, and mint.

U

U /juː/ *abbr* = uranium; (*cinema*) universal (suitable for all age groups).

U, u *n* the 21st letter of the English alphabet; something shaped like a U.

UAE *abbr* = United Arab Emirates.

ubiety /juːˈbaɪətɪ/ *n* the state of being in a specific place.

ubiquitous /juːˈbɪkwɪtəs/ *adj* existing, or seeming to exist everywhere at once.—**ubiquity** *n*.

U-boat /ˈjuːbəʊt/ *n* a German submarine.

uc *abbr* = upper case.

udder /ˈʌdər/ *n* a milk-secreting organ containing two or more teats, as in cows.

UEL /ˈjuːˈiːˈɛl/ *abbr* ✤ (*Cdn*) = United Empire Loyalist.

UFO *abbr* = unidentified flying object.

ufology /juːˈfɒlədʒɪ/ *n* the study of UFOs.—**ufologist** *n*.

ugh /ə/ or /ʌɡ/, /ʌx/ *interj* an expression of disgust, dislike or horror.

ugli /ˈʌɡlɪ/, **ugli fruit** *n* (*pl* **uglis, uglies**) a citrus fruit that is a cross between a grapefruit and a tangerine.

ugly /ˈʌɡlɪ/ *adj* (**uglier, ugliest**) unsightly; unattractive; repulsive; ill tempered.—**ugliness** *n*.

ugly duckling *n* an initially unpromising person or thing that turns out successfully.

UHF *abbr* = ultrahigh frequency.

uh-huh /əˈhʌ/ *interj* used to indicate assent or agreement.

UHT *abbr* = ultra-heat treated (milk or cream).

UI *abbr* ✤ (*Cdn*) = Unemployment Insurance.

UK *abbr* = United Kingdom.

ukelele, ukulele /juːkəˈleɪlɪ/ *n* a small, four-stringed guitar.

ulcer /ˈʌlsər/ *n* an open sore on the surface of the skin or a mucous membrane.—**ulcerous** *adj*.

ulcerate /ˈʌlsəˌreɪt/ *vti* to make or become ulcerous.

-ule /juːl/ or /jʊl/ *n suffix* smallness.

ulema /ˈuːlɪmə/ *n* (a member of) a body of Muslim theologians and religious scholars.

-ulent /jʊlənt/ *adj suffix* abundant.

ullage /ˈʌlɪdʒ/ *n* the amount by which a container (*eg.* a barrel) is less than full.

ulna /ˈʌlnə/ *n* (*pl* **ulnas, ulnae**) the longer and thinner of the two bones in the human forearm; the corresponding bone in the forelimb of other vertebrates.—**ulnar** *adj*.

ulnar nerve /ˈʌlnər/ *n* a nerve in the forearm that passes close to the skin surface at the elbow.

ulotrichous /juːˈlɒtrɪkəs/ *adj* having woolly or curly hair.

ulster /ˈʌlstər/ *n* a long heavy double-breasted overcoat with a belt.

Ulsterman /ˈʌlstərmən/ *n* (*pl* **Ulstermen**) a native or inhabitant of Ulster (a former province of Ireland now divided between Northern Ireland and the Republic of Ireland).—**Ulsterwoman** (*pl* **Ulsterwomen**) *nf*.

ulterior /ʌlˈtiːrɪər/ *adj* (*motives*) hidden, not evident; subsequent.

ultima /ˈʌltɪmə/ *n* the last syllable of a word.

ultimate /ˈʌltɪmət/ *adj* last; final; most significant; essential. • *n* the most significant thing.—**ultimately** *adv*.

ultimatum /ʌltɪˈmeɪtəm/ *n* (*pl* **ultimatums, ultimata**) the final proposal, condition or terms in negotiations.

ultimogeniture /ˌʌltɪmɒˈdʒɛnɪtʃər/ *n* (*law*) inheritance by the youngest son.

ultra /ˈʌltrə/ *adj* extreme, uncompromising. • *n* an extremist.

ultra- /ˈʌltrə/ *prefix* beyond.

ultraconservative /ˌʌltrəkənˈsɜːvətɪv/ *adj* deeply conservative or reactionary. • *n* a reactionary person.

ultrafiche /ˈʌltrəˌfiːʃ/ *n* a type of high-density microfiche containing a very large number of microcopies.

ultrahigh frequency /ˌʌltrəˈhaɪ/ *n* a radio frequency in the range between 300 megahertz and 3000 megahertz.

ultraism /ˈʌltraɪzəm/ *n* the advocacy of extreme action.—**ultraist** *n*.

ultramarine /ˌʌltrəməˈriːn/ *adj* deep blue. • *n* a blue pigment; a vivid, deep blue.

ultramicroscope /ˌʌltrəˈmaɪkrəˌskəʊp/ *n* an optical device for viewing tiny particles undetectable by a conventional microscope.—**ultramicroscopic** *adj*.

ultrashort /ˌʌltrəˈʃɔːt/ *adj* (*radio wave*) having a wavelength less than 10 metres.

ultrasonic /ˌʌltrəˈsɒnɪk/ *adj* (*waves, vibrations*) having a frequency beyond the human ear's audible range.

ultrasound /ˈʌltrəˌsaʊnd/ *n* ultrasonic waves used in medical diagnosis and therapy.

ultraviolet /ʌltrəˈvaɪələt/ *adj* of light waves, shorter than the wavelengths of visible light and longer than X-rays.

ultraviolet light /ʌltrəˈvaɪələt laɪt/ *n* ultraviolet radiation.

ultravirus /ˌʌltrəˈvaɪrəs/ *n* a virus small enough to pass through the finest filter.

ulu /ˈuːluː/ *n* ✤ a traditional large knife used by the Inuit.

ululate /ˈʌljʊˌleɪt/ or /ˈjuːl-/ *vi* to howl or wail, as with pain or grief.—**ululant** *adj*.—**ululation** *n*.

umbel /ˈʌmbəl/ *n* a flower-cluster characteristic of plants of the carrot family, in which the stalks grow from the same place on the main stem producing an umbrella effect.—**umbellate** *adj*.

umbelliferous /ʌmbəˈlɪfərəs/ *adj* of or pertaining to a family of plants and shrubs bearing umbels, including carrots, parsley and fennel.—**umbellifer** *n*.

umber /ˈʌmbər/ *n* a brown pigment. • *adj* dark brown.

umbilical /ʌmˈbɪlɪkəl/ *n* of, pertaining to, near, or resembling the navel.

umbilical cord *n* the vascular tube connecting a foetus with the placenta through which oxygen and nutrients are passed.

umbilicate /ʌmˈbɪlɪkət/, **umbilicated** *n* depressed or shaped like a navel; having an umbilicus.—**umbilication** *n*.

umbilicus /ʌmˈbɪlɪkəs/ or /ˌʌmbɪˈlaɪkəs/ *n* (*pl* **umbilici**) the navel; a navel-shaped depression on a plant or animal.

umbo /ˈʌmbəʊ/ *n* (*pl* **umbones, umbos**) the boss in the centre of a shield; a rounded anatomical protrusion.

umbra /ˈʌmbrə/ *n* (*pl* **umbrae, umbras**) an area of total shadow, *esp* during an eclipse; the dark centre of a sunspot.—**umbral** *adj*.

umbrage /ˈʌmbrɪdʒ/ *n* resentment; offence.

umbrella /ʌmˈbrɛlə/ *n* a cloth-covered collapsible frame carried in the hand for protection from rain or sun; a general protection.

umiak /ˈuːmɪˌæk/ *n* an Eskimo boat made from hide stretched over a wooden frame; ✤ a large, open, flat-bottomed boat used by the Inuit.—*also* **oomiak**.

umlaut /ˈʊmlaʊt/ *n* the mark (¨) placed over a vowel in German and other languages to modify its sound; the change of a vowel brought about by its assimilation to another vowel.

umpire /ˈʌmpaɪr/ *n* an official who enforces the rules in sport; an arbitrator.—*also vti*.

umpteen /ˈʌmptiːn/ or /-ˈtiːn/ *adj* (*inf*) an undetermined large number.—**umpteenth** *adj*.

UN *abbr* = United Nations.

un- /ʌn/ *prefix* not; opposite of; contrary to; reversal of an action or state.

'un, un /ən/ *pron* (*dial*) one.

unable /ʌnˈeɪbəl/ *adj* not able; lacking the strength, skill, power or opportunity (to do something).

unaccountable /ˌʌnəˈkaʊntəbəl/ *adj* inexplicable, puzzling; not to be called to account for one's actions.

unaccustomed /ˌʌnəˈkʌstəmd/ *adj* (*with* **to**) not used (to); not usual or familiar.

una corda /ˈuːnəˈkɔːdə/ *adj, adv* (*mus*) (*piano*) to be played with the soft pedal depressed.

unadulterated /ˌʌnəˈdʌltəˌreɪtəd/ *adj* pure, unmixed.

unadvised /ˌʌnədˈvaɪzd/ *adj* unwise, imprudent; not advised.—**unadvisedly** *adv*.

unaffected /ˌʌnəˈfɛktəd/ *adj* sincere, frank, without pretension; not influenced or affected.—**unaffectedly** *adv*.

un-American *adj* contrary to US customs, ideals or interests.—**un-Americanism** *n*.

unanimous /ju:'nænɪməs/ *adj* showing complete agreement.—**unanimity** *n*.—**unanimously** *adv*.

unapproachable /ˌʌnə'prəʊtʃəbəl/ *adj* aloof, unfriendly; impossible to reach; not to be equalled or rivalled.

unarmed /ʌn'ɑrmd/ *adj* not in possession of weapons; defenceless.

unasked /ʌn'æskt/ *adj* not asked or asked for; not invited or requested; spontaneous. • *adv* of one's own accord; without prompting.

unassailable /ˌʌnə'seɪləbəl/ *adj* not open to attack; not open to criticism or doubt.

unassuming /ˌʌnə'su:mɪŋ/ or /-sju:-/ *adj* unpretentious; modest.

unattached /ˌʌnə'tætʃt/ *adj* unmarried, not engaged to be married; not belonging to a particular group, organization, etc.

unattended /ˌʌnə'tendəd/ *adj* not supervised; not accompanied.

unauthorized /ʌn'ɔθəˌraɪzd/ *adj* not endorsed by authority.

unavailing /ˌʌnə'veɪlɪŋ/ *adj* futile, hopeless.—**unavailingly** *adv*.

unavoidable /ˌʌnə'vɔɪdəbəl/ *adj* bound to happen, inevitable; necessary, compulsory.—**unavoidably** *adv*.

unaware /ˌʌnə'wɛr/ *adj* not conscious or aware (of); ignorant (of).

unawares /ˌʌnə'wɛrz/ *adv* by surprise; unexpectedly without warning.

unbalanced /ʌn'bælənsd/ *adj* mentally unstable; having bias or over-representing a particular view, group, interest, etc; (*bookkeeping*) not having equal debit and credit totals.

unbearable /ʌn'bɛrəbəl/ *adj* intolerable, not able to be endured.—**unbearably** *adv*.

unbeatable /ʌn'bi:təbəl/ *adj* impossible to beat; outstanding, excellent.

unbeaten /ʌn'bi:tən/ *adj* not beaten, unsurpassed.

unbecoming /ˌʌnbɪ'kʌmɪŋ/ *adj* (*clothes, make-up, etc*) not enhancing the wearer's appearance; (*behaviour*) not suitable or seemly.

unbeknown /ˌʌnbɪ'nəʊn/ *adj* (*with* **to**) happening without (a person's) knowledge.

unbelief /ʌnbɪ'li:f/ *n* disbelief, scepticism, *esp* in religious matters.

unbelievable /ˌʌnbɪ'li:vəbəl/ *adj* not able to be believed; incredible.—**unbelievably** *adv*.

unbeliever /ˌʌnbɪ'li:vər/ *n* a person who does not believe, *esp* in a religion.

unbelieving /ˌʌnbɪ'li:vɪŋ/ *adj* lacking belief; sceptical.—**unbelievingly** *adv*.

unbend /ʌn'bend/ *vb* (**unbending, unbent**) *vt* to straighten from a bent shape; to release or untie (*eg* a rope). • *vi* to become more relaxed, affable or informal in manner.

unbending /ʌn'bendɪŋ/ *adj* severe, stern; inflexible, unchanging; rigid in behaviour or attitude.

unbiased, unbiassed /ʌn'baɪəst/ *adj* without prejudice or bias; impartial, even-handed, disinterested.

unbidden /ʌn'bɪdən/ *adj* not commanded, asked for or invited.

unblushing /ʌn'blʌʃɪŋ/ *adj* shameless, impudent.—**unblushingly** *adv*.

unborn /ʌn'bɔrn/ *adj* not yet born; still to appear or happen in the future.

unbosom /ʌn'bʊzəm/ *vt* to reveal the thoughts or feelings of (oneself).

unbounded /ʌn'baʊndəd/ *adj* without limits.

unbowed /ʌn'baʊd/ *adj* not bowed; not subdued, free.

unbridled /ʌn'braɪdəld/ *adj* unrestrained; (*horse*) having no bridle.

unbroken /ʌn'brəʊkən/ *adj* whole, in one piece; continuous, uninterrupted; (*record*) not yet beaten; (*horses, etc*) wild, untamed; organized, disciplined.

unburden /ʌn'bɔrdən/ *vt* to reveal or confess one's troubles, secrets, etc to another in order to relieve the mind; to take off a burden.

unbutton /ʌn'bʌtən/ *vt* to unfasten the buttons of (a garment).

unbuttoned /ʌn'bʌtənd/ *adj* unfastened; (*inf*) free, uninhibited.

uncalled-for /ʌn'kɔld fɔr/ *adj* unnecessary, unwanted, unwarranted.

uncanny /ʌn'kæni/ *adj* (**uncannier, uncanniest**) odd; unexpected; suggestive of supernatural powers; unearthly.

unceremonious /ˌʌnserə'məʊniəs/ *adj* without ceremony, informal; abrupt, rude.—**unceremoniously** *adv*.

uncertain /ʌn'sɜrtən/ *adj* not knowing accurately, doubtful; (*with* **of**) not confident or sure; not fixed, variable, changeable.—**uncertainty** *n*.

uncertainty principle *n* (*phys*) the principle that it is impossible to determine accurately both the position and momentum of an elementary particle simultaneously.—*also* **Heisenberg uncertainty principle.**

uncharted /ʌn'tʃɑrtəd/ *adj* not marked on a map; unsurveyed, unexplored.

unchristian /ʌn'krɪstʃən/ *adj* contrary to Christian belief or principle; savage, pagan.

uncial /'ʌnsiəl/ or /-ʃəl/ *adj* written in or resembling large rounded capital letters as used in early medieval Greek and Latin manuscripts. • *n* an uncial character or manuscript.

uncinate /'ʌnsɪnət/ *adj* (*plant, animal*) having a hook-shaped part.

uncircumcised /ʌn'sɜrkəmˌsaɪzd/ *adj* not circumcised; not Jewish; impure.—**uncircumcision** *n*.

uncivil /ʌn'sɪvəl/ *adj* lacking in manners, impolite.—**uncivility** *n*.

uncivilized /ʌn'sɪvəˌlaɪzd/ *adj* not civilized, unsophisticated; remote, wild.

uncle /'ʌŋkəl/ *n* the brother of one's father or mother; the husband of one's aunt.

unclean /ʌn'kli:n/ *adj* not clean, contaminated; ceremonially defiled.

Uncle Sam *n* the government of the US personified.

unclothe /ʌn'kləʊð/ *vt* (**unclothing, unclothed** *or* **unclad**) to remove the clothes from; to uncover.

uncoil /ʌn'kɔɪl/ *vti* to (cause to) unwind.

uncomfortable /ʌn'kʌmftərbəl/ or /-fərtəbəl/, /-frtəbəl/ *adj* causing discomfort; feeling discomfort or unease.

uncommitted /ˌʌnkə'mɪtəd/ *adj* not bound to a particular cause, belief or course of action.

uncommon /ʌn'kɒmən/ *adj* rare, unusual; extraordinary.

uncommonly /-li/ *adv* hardly ever; exceptionally, particularly.

uncommunicative /ˌʌnkə'mju:nɪkətɪv/ *adj* not willing to talk or express an opinion, etc; reserved.

uncompromising /ʌn'kɒmprəˌmaɪzɪŋ/ *adj* not prepared to compromise; inflexible, obstinate.

unconcern /ˌʌnkən'sɜrn/ *n* indifference.

unconcerned /-d/ *adj* not involved in or concerned with; not troubled.

unconditional /ˌʌnkən'dɪʃənəl/ *adj* without restrictions or conditions, absolute.

unconscionable /ʌn'kɒnʃənəbəl/ *adj* unscrupulous; unreasonable.—**unconscionably** *adv*.

unconscious /ʌn'kɒnʃəs/ *adj* not aware (of); lacking normal perception by the senses, insensible; unintentional. • *n* the deepest level of mind containing feelings and emotions of which one is unaware and unable to control.—**unconsciously** *adv*.

unconsciousness /-nəs/ *n* the state of being without the senses, as when knocked out.

unconstitutional /ˌʌnkɒnstɪ'tu:ʃənəl/ or /-'tju:-/ *adj* contrary to the constitution of a country.—**unconstitutionality** *n*.

unconventional /ˌʌnkən'venʃənəl/ *adj* not bound by social rules or conventions.—**unconventionally** *adv*.

uncork /ʌn'kɔrk/ *vt* to pull the cork from a bottle; (*emotions, desires, etc*) to unleash, give vent to.

uncouple /ʌn'kʌpəl/ *vti* to disconnect or become disconnected.

uncouth /ʌn'ku:θ/ *adj* lacking in manners; rough; rude.—**uncouthness** *n*.

uncover /ʌn'kʌvər/ *vt* to remove the cover from; to reveal or expose; to remove one's hat in greeting or out of respect.

uncovered /ʌn'kʌvərd/ *adj* not having a cover; revealed; not having any insurance or security; with one's hat removed out of respect, etc.

UNCTAD /'ju:ˌenˌsiˌtiːˌæˌdiː/ *abbr* = United Nations Conference on Trade and Development.

unction /'ʌŋkʃən/ *n* an anointing, as for medical or religious purposes; anything that soothes or comforts; affected sincerity.

unctuous /'ʌŋktʃʊəs/ *adj* oily; smarmy; too suave; insincerely charming.—**unctuously** *adv*.—**unctuousness** *n*.

uncurl /ʌn'kɜrl/ *vti* to straighten; to straighten up, relax.

uncut /ʌn'kʌt/ *adj* not cut; (*book*) not having the folds of the leaves trimmed or slit; (*gemstone*) not cut into shape; not abridged.

undaunted /ʌn'dɒntəd/ *adj* fearless; not discouraged.—**undauntedly** *adv*.

undecagon /ʌn'dekəˌgɒn/ *n* a polygon with eleven sides.

undeceive /ˌʌndɪ'siːv/ *vt* to free from deception or error.

undecided /ˌʌndɪ'saɪdəd/ *adj* doubtful, hesitant; (*solution, etc*) not determined.—**undecidedly** *adv*.

undeniable /ʌndəˈnaɪəbəl/ *adj* readily apparent, obviously true; unquestionably excellent.

under /ˈʌndər/ *prep* lower than; beneath the surface of; below; covered by; subject to; less than, falling short of. • *adv* beneath, below, lower down. • *adj* lower in position, degree or rank; subordinate.

under- /ˈʌndər/ *prefix* beneath, below.

underachieve /ˌʌndərəˈtʃiːv/ *vi* to perform less well than expected given one's potential.—**underachiever** *n*.

underact /ˌʌndərˈækt/ *vt* to perform (a dramatic role) without proper conviction or emphasis.

underage /ˌʌndərˈeɪdʒ/ *adj* below the normal or legal age.

underarm /ˈʌndərɑrm/ *adj*, of, for, in, or used on the area under the arm, or armpit; done with the hand below the level of the elbow or shoulder.

underbelly /ˈʌndərˌbeli/ *n* (*pl* **underbellies**) the underside of an animal, etc; the most vulnerable part of something.

underbid /ˌʌndərˈbɪd/ *vb* (**underbidding, underbid**) *vt* to bid a lower amount than (rivals); (*bridge, etc*) to bid less than the strength of the hand merits. • *vi* to bid too low.

undercapitalized /ʌndərˈkæpɪtəlaɪz/ *adj* (*business*) having insufficient capital to operate efficiently.

undercarriage /ˈʌndərˌkerɪdʒ/ *n* the landing gear of an aeroplane; a car's supporting framework.

undercharge /ˌʌndərˈtʃɑrdʒ/ *vt* to charge below the fair price.

underclass /ˈʌndərˌklæs/ *n* those least privileged people in society who fall outside the normal social scale, characterized by poverty, unemployment, poor education, social instability, etc.

underclothes /ˈʌndərˌkloːz/ or /-ˌkloːðz/ *npl* underwear.—*also* **underclothing**.

undercoat /ˈʌndərˌkoːt/ *n* a coat of paint, etc, applied as a base below another; a growth of hair or fur under another; a coat worn under an overcoat.

undercover /ˌʌndərˈkʌvər/ or /ˈʌn-/ *adj* done or operating secretly.

undercurrent /ˈʌndərˌkʌrənt/ *n* a hidden current under water; an emotion, opinion, etc, not apparent.

undercut /ˌʌndərˈkʌt/ *vt* (**undercutting, undercut**) to charge less than a competitor; to undermine.

underdeveloped /ˌʌndərdəˈveləpt/ *adj* not fully grown, immature; (*societies*) having an inadequate social and political infrastructure for sustained economic growth; (*film*) not processed long enough to form a proper image.

underdog /ˈʌndərˌdɒg/ *n* the loser in an encounter, contest, etc; a person in an inferior position.

underdone /ˌʌndərˈdʌn/ *adj* not sufficiently or completely cooked.

underdressed /ˌʌndərˈdrest/ *adj* wearing clothes that are too informal for a particular occasion.

underemployed /ˌʌndərəmˈplɔɪd/ *adj* not fully or most efficiently employed.

underestimate /ˌʌndərˈestəˌmeɪt/ *vti* to set too low an estimate on or for. • *n* too low an estimate.

underexpose /ˌʌndərəkˈspoːz/ *vt* (*photog*) to fail to expose (film) to light sufficiently long to produce a good image.—**underexposed** *adj*.—**underexposure** *n*.

underfelt /ˈʌndərˌfelt/ *n* a layer of thick felt between a carpet and floor.

underfoot /ˌʌndərˈfut/ *adv* underneath the foot or feet; on the ground.

undergarment /ˈʌndərˌgɑrmənt/ *n* a piece of underwear or clothing worn beneath other outer clothing.

undergo /ˌʌndərˈgoː/ *vt* (**undergoing, underwent,** *pp* **undergone**) to experience, suffer, endure.

undergraduate /ˌʌndərˈgrædʒuət/ *n* a student at a college or university studying for a first degree.

underground /ˌʌndərˈgraund/ *adj* situated under the surface of the ground; secret; (of noncommercial newspapers, movies, etc that are unconventional, radical, etc. • *n* a secret group working for the overthrow of the government or the expulsion of occupying forces; an underground railway system; a subway.

undergrowth /ˈʌndərˌgroːθ/ *n* shrubs, plants, etc growing beneath trees.

underhand /ˈʌndərˌhænd/ *adv* (*sport*) with an underarm motion; underhandedly.

underhanded /ˈʌndərˌhændəd/ *adj* sly, secret, deceptive.—**underhandedly** *adv*.

underlay /ˌʌndərˈleɪ/ *n* a material, lining laid beneath another for support; felt or rubber laid beneath a carpet for insulation, etc.

underlie /ˌʌndərˈlaɪ/ *vt* (**underlying, underlay,** *pp* **underlain**) to be situated under; to form the basis of.

underline /ˈʌndərˌlaɪn/ *vt* to put a line underneath; to emphasize.

underling /ˈʌndərlɪŋ/ *n* a person of inferior rank or status to someone else; a subordinate.

underlying /ˈʌndərˌlaɪɪŋ/ *adj* existing, but hard to detect; fundamental, supporting.

undermentioned /ˈʌndərˌmenʃənd/ *adj* mentioned below or later in the text.

undermine /ˈʌndərˌmaɪn/ *vt* to wear away, or weaken; to injure or weaken, *esp* by subtle or insidious means.

underneath /ˌʌndərˈniːθ/ *adv* under. • *adj* lower. • *n* the underside.—*also prep*.

undernourished /ˌʌndərˈnərɪʃt/ *adj* consuming or supplied with less than the minimum quantity of food necessary for normal health and growth.

underpants /ˈʌndərˌpænts/ *npl* pants worn as an undergarment by men and boys.

underpass /ˈʌndərˌpæs/ *n* a section of road running beneath another road, a railway, etc.

underpin /ˌʌndərˈpɪn/ *vt* to strengthen or support from beneath.

underpinning /ˈʌndərˌpɪnɪŋ/ *n* the material used to support a structure, the foundation.

underplay /ˈʌndərˌpleɪ/ *vt* to perform (a dramatic role) with restraint; to play down the importance of.

underprivileged /ˌʌndərˈprɪvɪlɪdʒd/ or /-ˈprɪvəlɪdʒd/ *adj* lacking the basic rights of other members of society; poor.

underproof /ˈʌndərˈpruːf/ *adj* containing less alcohol per volume than proof spirit.

underrate /ˌʌndərˈreɪt/ *vt* to undervalue, to underestimate.

underscore /ˈʌndərˌskor/ *vt* to draw a line under; to emphasize.

undersea /ˈʌndərˌsiː/ *adj, adv* below the surface of the sea.

underseal /ˈʌndərˌsiːl/ *n* a protective layer of tar, etc applied to the underside of a vehicle. • *vt* to apply this protective layer.

undersecretary /ˌʌndərˈsekrəˌteri/ *n* (*pl* **undersecretaries**) a senior civil servant in Great Britain; in US, a secretary immediately subordinate to a principal.

undersell /ˌʌndərˈsel/ *vt* (**underselling, undersold**) to sell at a reduced price; to sell at a price lower than (someone else); to promote with moderation.

undersexed /ˌʌndərˈseksd/ *adj* having a weaker than normal sex drive.

undershirt /ˌʌndərˈʃərt/ *n* a vest.

undershoot /ˌʌndərˈʃuːt/ *vti* (**undershooting, undershot**) to (cause to) land short of a runway; to shoot short of a target.

underside /ˈʌndərˌsaɪd/ *n* the lower surface.

undersigned /ˈʌndərˌsaɪnd/ *adj* signed at the end. • *n* a person who signs his or her name at the end of a document.

undersized /ˈʌndərˌsaɪzd/ *adj* less than usual size.

underskirt /ˈʌndərˌskərt/ *n* a woman's undergarment worn beneath the skirt, a petticoat.

underslung /ˈʌndərˌslʌŋ/ *adj* suspended from above; (*vehicle chassis*) suspended below the axles.

understand /ˌʌndərˈstænd/ *vb* (**understanding, understood**) *vt* to comprehend; to realize; to believe; to assume; to know thoroughly (*eg* a language); to accept; to be sympathetic with. • *vi* to comprehend; to believe.—**understandable** *adj*.

understanding /ˌʌndərˈstændɪŋ/ *n* comprehension; compassion; sympathy; personal opinion, viewpoint; mutual agreement. • *adj* sympathetic.

understate /ˌʌndərˈsteɪt/ *vt* to state something in restrained terms; to represent as less than is the case.—**understatement** *n*.

understudy /ˈʌndərˌstʌdi/ *vti* (**understudying, understudied**) to learn a role or part so as to be able to replace (the actor playing it); to act as an understudy (to).—*also n*.

undertake /ˌʌndərˈteɪk/ *vt* (**undertaking, undertook,** *pp* **undertaken**) to attempt to; to agree to; to commit oneself to; promise; to guarantee.

undertaker /ˈʌndərˌteɪkər/ *n* a funeral director.

undertaking /ˈʌndərˌteɪkɪŋ/ *n* enterprise; task; promise; obligation.

underthings /ˈʌndərˌθɪŋz/ *npl* underwear.

undertone /ˈʌndərˌtoːn/ *n* a hushed tone of voice; an undercurrent of feeling; a pale colour.

undertow /ˈʌndərˌtoː/ *n* the backwash from a breaking wave; an undercurrent moving in a different direction from the surface current.

undervalue /ˌʌndər'vælju:/ vt (**undervaluing, undervalued**) to put too low a price or value on.—**undervaluation** n.

underwater /ˌʌndər'wɒtər/ adj being carried on under the surface of the water, esp the sea; submerged; below the water line of a vessel.—also adv.

under way /ˌʌndər'weɪ/ adv in or into motion or progress.

underwear /'ʌndərˌwer/ n garments worn underneath one's outer clothes, next to the skin.

underweight /ˌʌndər'weɪt/ adj weighing less than normal or necessary.

underwent /ˌʌndər'went/ see **undergo**.

underwhelm /ˌʌndər'welm/ vt to disappoint.

underworld /'ʌndərˌwɜrld/ n criminals as an organized group; (myth) Hades.

underwrite /'ʌndərˌraɪt/ or /ˌʌn-/ vt to agree to finance (an undertaking, etc); to sign one's name to (an insurance policy), thus assuming liability. • vi to work as an underwriter.—**underwriter** n.

undesirable /ˌʌndə'zaɪrəbəl/ adj not desirable; not pleasant; objectionable.—**undesirability** n.—**undesirably** adv.

undetermined /ˌʌndə'tɜrmənd/ adj not yet decided; not discovered.

undies /'ʌndiːz/ npl (inf) women's underwear.

undo /ʌn'duː/ vt (**undoing, undid,** pp **undone**) to untie or unwrap; to reverse (what has been done); to bring ruin on.

undone /ʌn'dʌn/ adj not done; not fastened or tied.

undoubted /ʌn'daʊtəd/ adj without doubt; definite, certain.—**undoubtedly** adv.

undreamed /ʌn'driːmd/, **undreamt** /ʌn'dremt/ n (with **of**) not thought of or imagined.

undress /ʌn'dres/ vt to remove the clothes from. • vi to take off one's clothes.

undressed /ʌn'dresd/ adj not dressed, partially or informally clothed; (wound) not bandaged; (food) not prepared for serving; (hides) not processed.

undue /ʌn'duː/ adj or /-djuː/ adj improper; excessive.

undulate /'ʌndjuˌleɪt/ or /-dʒuˌleɪt/ vti to move or cause to move like waves; to have or cause to have a wavy form or surface.

undulation /ˌʌndjuˈleɪʃən/ or /-dʒu-/ n a wavelike form or motion.

unduly /ʌn'duːli/ or /-djuː-/ adv too; excessively; improperly.

undying /ʌn'daɪɪŋ/ adj eternal.

unearned /ʌn'ɜrnd/ adj (income) not earned by labour or skill; undeserved.

unearth /ʌn'ɜrθ/ vt to dig up from the earth; to discover; to reveal.

unearthly /ʌn'ɜrθli/ adj mysterious; eerie; supernatural; absurd, unreasonable.

uneasy /ʌn'iːzi/ adj uncomfortable; restless; anxious; disquieting.—**uneasily** adv.—**uneasiness** n.

uneatable /ʌn'iːtəbəl/ adj (food) not edible, esp because of its condition or appearance.

uneconomic /ˌʌnekə'nɒmɪk/ or /ˌʌniːk-/ adj wasteful; unprofitable.

unemployable /ˌʌnəm'plɔɪəbəl/ adj not fit or acceptable for work.

unemployed /ˌʌnəm'plɔɪd/ adj not having a job, out of work.—**unemployment** n.

unequal /ʌn'iːkwəl/ adj not equal; not regular or uniform; not sufficiently strong or able.—**unequally** adv.

unequalled, unequaled /ʌn'iːkwəld/ adj not equalled; supreme.

unequivocal /ˌʌnə'kwɪvəkəl/ adj unambiguous; plain; clear.—**unequivocally** adv.

unerring /ʌn'erɪŋ/ or /-'ərɪŋ/ adj sure, unfailing.

UNESCO /juː'neskoː/ abbr = United Nations Educational, Scientific and Cultural Organization.

uneven /ʌn'iːvən/ adj not level or smooth; variable; not divisible by two without leaving a remainder.—**unevenness** n.

uneventful /ˌʌnə'ventfʊl/ adj ordinary, routine.—**uneventfully** adv.

unexampled /ˌʌnəg'zæmpəld/ adj without precedent or comparison.

unexceptionable /ˌʌnɪk'sepʃənəbəl/ adj irreproachable.

unexceptional /ˌʌnək'sepʃənəl/ adj ordinary, normal.

unexpected /ˌʌnək'spektəd/ adj not looked for, unforeseen.—**unexpectedly** adv.

unfailing /ʌn'feɪlɪŋ/ adj not failing or giving up; persistent; constant, dependable.—**unfailingly** adv.

unfair /ʌn'fer/ adj unjust; unequal; against the rules.—**unfairly** adv.—**unfairness** n.

unfaithful /ʌn'feɪθfʊl/ adj disloyal; not abiding by a promise; adulterous.—**unfaithfully** adv.—**unfaithfulness** n.

unfamiliar /ˌʌnfə'mɪljər/ adj not known, strange; (with **with**) not familiar.

unfasten /ʌn'fæsən/ vt to open or become opened; to undo or become undone; to loose loosen.

unfathomable /ʌn'fæðəməbəl/ adj not able to be measured; incomprehensible.

unfavourable, unfavorable /ʌn'feɪvərəbəl/ adj negative, disapproving; adverse.

unfeeling /ʌn'fiːlɪŋ/ adj callous, hardhearted.—**unfeelingly** adv.

unfinished /ʌn'fɪnɪʃt/ adj not finished, incomplete; in the making; crude, sketchy.

unfit /ʌn'fɪt/ adj unsuitable; in bad physical condition.

unflappable /ʌn'flæpəbəl/ adj (inf) calm, not easily agitated.

unflinching /ʌn'flɪntʃɪŋ/ adj calm, steadfast.—**unflinchingly** adv.

unfold /ʌn'fəʊld/ vti to open or spread out; to become revealed; to develop.

unforeseen /ˌʌnfɔr'siːn/ adj unsuspected.

unforgettable /ˌʌnfɔr'getəbəl/ or /-fɔr-/ adj never to be forgotten; fixed in the mind; impressive, exceptional.—**unforgettably** adv.

unfortunate /ʌn'fɔrtʃənət/ adj unlucky; disastrous; regrettable. • n an unlucky person.

unfortunately /ʌn'fɔrtʃənətli/ adv regrettably, unluckily, unhappily.

unfounded /ʌn'faʊndəd/ adj groundless; baseless.

unfreeze /ʌn'friːz/ vti (**unfreezing, unfroze, unfrozen**) to (cause to) thaw; to remove restrictions on (wage or price rises, etc).

unfrock /ʌn'frɒk/ vt to remove (a person in holy orders) from ecclesiastical office.

unfurl /ʌn'fɜrl/ vti to open; to unfold.

ungainly /ʌn'geɪnli/ adj (**ungainlier, ungainliest**) awkward; clumsy.—**ungainliness** n.

ungodly /ʌn'gɒdli/ adj (**ungodlier, ungodliest**) not religious; sinful; wicked; (inf) outrageous.

ungovernable /ʌn'gʌvərnəbəl/ adj not able to be controlled or restrained.

unguarded /ʌn'gɑrdəd/ adj without protection, vulnerable; open to attack; careless; candid, frank.—**unguardedly** adv.

unguent /'ʌŋgwənt/ n a lubricant or ointment.

ungulate /'ʌŋgjʊlət/ n adj (an animal) having hooves.

unhallowed /ʌn'hæloːd/ adj not consecrated; sinful.

unhappy /ʌn'hæpi/ adj (**unhappier, unhappiest**) not happy or fortunate; sad; wretched; not suitable.—**unhappily** adv.—**unhappiness** n.

unhealthy /ʌn'helθi/ adj (**unhealthier, unhealthiest**) not healthy or fit, sick; encouraging or resulting from poor health; harmful, degrading; dangerous.—**unhealthily** adv.—**unhealthiness** n.

unheard /ʌn'hɜrd/ adj not heard; not listened to.

unheard-of adj not known before; without precedent.

unhinge /ʌn'hɪndʒ/ vt to make crazy, derange.

unholy /ʌn'hoːli/ adj (**unholier, unholiest**) wicked; (inf) outrageous, enormous.

unhook /ʌn'hʊk/ vt to remove from a hook; to unfasten the hooks of (a garment).

uni /'juːni/ n (inf) university.

uni- /juːni/ prefix one; single.

unicameral /ˌjuːnɪ'kæmərəl/ adj of or having only one legislative chamber.—**unicameral y** adv.

UNICEF /'juːnəˌsef/ abbr = United Nations International Children's Emergency Fund, now United Nations Children's Fund.

unicellular /ˌjuːnɪ'seljələr/ adj (microorganisms, etc) consisting of a single cell.—**unicellularity** n.

unicorn /'juːnɪkɔrn/ n an imaginary creature with a body like a horse and a single horn on the forehead.

unicycle /'juːnɪˌsaɪkəl/ n a pedal-driven cycle with a single wheel, used by circus and street entertainers.

unidirectional /ˌjuːnɪdɪ'rekʃənəl/ or /ˌjuːnɪdaɪ-/ adj involving, going in, or operating in one direction only.

uniform /'juːnɪˌfɔrm/ adj unchanging in form; consistent; identical. • n the distinctive clothes worn by members of the same organization, such as soldiers, schoolchildren.—**uniformly** adv.

uniformity /ˌjuːnɪ'fɔrmɪti/ n (pl **uniformities**) the state of being consistent or the same; dullness, monotony.

unify /'juːnɪˌfaɪ/ *vt* (**unifying, unified**) to make into one; to unite.—**unification** *n*.

unilateral /ˌjuːnɪˈlætərəl/ *adj* involving one only of several parties; not reciprocal.—**unilateralism** *n*.—**unilaterally** *adv*.

unimpeachable /ˌʌnɪmˈpiːtʃəbəl/ *adj* completely honest, truthful, etc; irreproachable.—**unimpeachably** *adv*.

uninhibited /ˌʌnɪnˈhæbɪtəd/ *adj* not repressed or restrained; relaxed, spontaneous.—**uninhibitedly** *adv*.

uninterested /ʌnˈɪntrəstəd/ or /-təˈrestəd/ *adj* lacking interest; not concerned, indifferent.—**uninterestedly** *adv*.

union /'juːnjən/ *n* the act of uniting; a combination of several things; a confederation of individuals or groups; marriage; a trades union.

unionist /'juːnjənɪst/ *n* an advocate or supporter of union or unionism.—**unionism** *n*.

unionize /'juːnjəˌnaɪz/ *vt* to organize (employees) into a trade union.—**unionization** *n*.

Union Jack *n* the national flag of the UK.

unipolar /ˌjuːnɪˈpoːlər/ *adj* of, produced by, or having a single electric or magnetic pole.—**unipolarity** *n*.

unique /juːˈniːk/ *adj* without equal; the only one of its kind.—**uniquely** *adv*.

unisex /'juːnɪˌseks/ *adj* of a style that can be worn by both sexes.

unisexual /ˌjuːnɪˈseksʊəl/ *adj* of one sex only; having male or female sex organs but not both.—**unisexually** *adv*.—**unisexuality** *n*.

unison /'juːnɪsən/ *n* accordance of sound, concord, harmony; **in unison** simultaneously, in agreement, in harmony.

unit /'juːnɪt/ *n* the smallest whole number, one; a single or whole entity; (*measurement*) a standard amount; an establishment or group of people who carry out a specific function; a piece of furniture fitting together with other pieces.—**unitary** *adj*.

unite /juˈnaɪt/ or /juː-/ *vti* to join into one, to combine; to be unified in purpose.

United Kingdom *n* Great Britain and Northern Ireland.

United Nations *n sing or pl* an international organization of nations for world peace and security formed in 1945.

United States *n* a federation of states, *esp* the United States of America.

unit trust /'juːnɪt trʌst/ *n* a company that manages a range of investments on behalf of members of the public whose interests are looked after by an independent trust.

unity /'juːnɪti/ *n* (*pl* **unities**) oneness; harmony; concord.

Univ. *abbr* = university.

universal /ˌjuːnɪˈvɜːsəl/ *adj* widespread; general; relating to all the world or the universe; relating to or applicable to all mankind.—**universally** *adv*.—**universality** *n* (*pl* **universalities**).

universe /'juːnɪˌvɜːs/ *n* all existing things; (*astron*) the totality of space, stars, planets and other forms of matter and energy; the world.

university /ˌjuːnɪˈvɜːsɪti/ *n* (*pl* **universities**) an institution of higher education which confers bachelors' and higher degrees; the campus or staff of a university.

unjust /ʌnˈdʒʌst/ *adj* not characterized by justice; not fair.—**unjustly** *adv*.—**unjustness** *n*.

unkempt /ʌnˈkempt/ *adj* uncombed; slovenly, dishevelled.

unkind /ʌnˈkaɪnd/ *adj* lacking in kindness or sympathy; harsh; cruel.—**unkindly** *adv*.—**unkindness** *n*.

unknown /ʌnˈnoːn/ *adj* not known; not famous; not understood; with an unknown value. • *n* an unknown person or thing.

unleaded /ʌnˈledəd/ *adj* (*petrol*) not mixed with tetraethyl lead.

unleash /ʌnˈliːʃ/ *vt* to release from a leash; to free from restraint.

unleavened /ʌnˈlevənd/ *adj* (*bread, etc*) made without yeast or other raising agent.

unless /ʌnˈles/ or /ənˈles/ *conj* if not; except that.

unlettered /ʌnˈletərd/ *adj* illiterate.

unlike /ʌnˈlaɪk/ *adj* not the same, dissimilar. • *prep* not like; not characteristic of.—**unlikeness** *n*.

unlikely /ʌnˈlaɪkli/ *adj* improbable; unpromising.

unlimited /ʌnˈlɪmɪtəd/ *adj* without limits; boundless; not restricted.—**unlimitedly** *adv*.

unlisted /ʌnˈlɪstəd/ *adj* not on a list; ex-directory.

unload /ʌnˈloːd/ *vti* to remove a load, discharge freight from a truck, ship, etc; to relieve of or express troubles, etc; to dispose of, dump; to empty, *esp* a gun.

unlock /ʌnˈlɒk/ *vt* (*door, lock, etc*) to unfasten; to let loose; to reveal; to release.

unloose /ʌnˈluːs/, **unloosen** /ʌnˈluːsən/ *vt* to relax (a grip, etc); to release, free; to untie.

unlovely /ʌnˈlʌvli/ *n* ugly, unpleasant.—**unloveliness** *n*.

unlucky /ʌnˈlʌki/ *adj* (**unluckier, unluckiest**) not lucky, not fortunate; likely to bring misfortune; regrettable.

unman /ʌnˈmæn/ *vt* (**unmanning, unmanned**) to weaken the nerve or courage of; to make effeminate.

unmanly /ʌnˈmænli/ *adj* weak, cowardly; effeminate.—**unmanliness** *n*.

unmanned /ʌnˈmænd/ *adj* (*spacecraft, etc*) not manned, operated by remote control.

unmannerly /ʌnˈmænərli/ *adj* lacking good manners; rude.—**unmannerliness** *n*.

unmask /ʌnˈmæsk/ *vti* to remove the mask from; to expose, show up.

unmentionable /ʌnˈmenʃənəbəl/ *adj* too bad, shocking, embarrassing, etc to be mentioned.

unmentionables /ʌnˈmenʃənəbəls/ *npl* underwear.

unmistakable, unmistakeable /ˌʌnmɪˈsteɪkəbəl/ *adj* obvious, clear.—**unmistakably, unmistakeably** *adv*.

unmitigated /ʌnˈmɪtɪˌɡeɪtəd/ *adj* unqualified, absolute.

unmoved /ʌnˈmuːvd/ *adj* not touched by emotion, calm.

unnatural /ʌnˈnætʃərəl/ *adj* abnormal; contrary to nature; artificial; affected; strange; wicked.—**unnaturally** *adv*.

unnecessary /ʌnˈnesəseri/ *adj* not necessary.—**unnecessarily** *adv*.—**unnecessariness** *n*.

unnerve /ʌnˈnɜːv/ *vt* to cause to lose courage, strength, confidence; to frighten.

unnumbered /ʌnˈnembərd/ *adj* countless; not having a number.

UNO /'juːnoː/ *abbr* = United Nations Organization.

unobtrusive /ˌʌnəbˈtruːsɪv/ *adj* modest, staying in the background.

unoccupied /ʌnˈɒkjuˌpaɪd/ *adj* not occupied, empty; unemployed.

unpack /ʌnˈpæk/ *vti* (*suitcase, etc*) to remove the contents of; (*container, etc*) to take things out of; to unload.

unparalleled /ʌnˈpærəˌleld/ *adj* having no equal, unmatched.

unparliamentary /ˌʌnpɑːləˈmentri/ *adj* contrary to parliamentary procedure or practice.

unperson /'ʌnˌpɜːsən/ *n* a person (*eg*. a political dissident) whose existence is officially ignored or denied.

unpick /ʌnˈpɪk/ *vt* to undo the stitching of.

unplaced /ʌnˈpleɪst/ *adj* not placed; not among the first three at the end of a race.

unpleasant /ʌnˈplezənt/ *adj* not pleasing or agreeable; nasty; objectionable.—**unpleasantly** *adv*.—**unpleasantness** *n*.

unplumbed /ʌnˈplʌmd/ *adj* not plumbed; not fully investigated or explored.

unpopular /ʌnˈpɒpjʊlər/ *adj* disliked; lacking general approval.—**unpopularity** *n*.

unprecedented /ʌnˈpresəˌdentəd/ *adj* having no precedent; unparalleled.

unprejudiced /ʌnˈpredʒʊdɪst/ *adj* not prejudiced, impartial.

unprepossessing /ˌʌnpriːpəˈzesɪŋ/ *adj* unattractive, repellent.

unpretentious /ˌʌnprəˈtenʃəs/ *adj* modest, not boasting.

unprincipled /ʌnˈprɪnsɪpəld/ *adj* lacking scruples.

unprintable /ʌnˈprɪntəbəl/ *adj* too bad, libellous, obscene, etc to be printed.

unprofessional /ˌʌnprəˈfeʃənəl/ *adj* contrary to professional etiquette.—**unprofessionally** *adv*.

unputdownable /ˌʌnpʊtˈdaʊnəbəl/ *adj* (*book*) grippingly readable.

unqualified /ʌnˈkwɒlɪfaɪd/ *adj* lacking recognized qualifications; not equal to; not restricted, complete.

unquestionable /ʌnˈkwestʃənəbəl/ *adj* certain, not disputed.—**unquestionably** *adv*.

unquestioned /ʌnˈkwestʃənd/ *adj* not called into question; indisputable.

unquiet /ʌnˈkwaɪət/ *adj* turbulent, disordered; nervous, agitated.—**unquietly** *adv*.—**unquietness** *n*.

unquote /'ʌnkwoːt/ *interj* used when speaking to indicate the end of a direct quotation.

unravel /ʌnˈrævəl/ *vt* (**unravelling, unravelled** *or* **unraveling, unraveled**) to disentangle; to solve.

unread /ʌnˈred/ *adj* not read (yet); unfamiliar with a specified subject; illiterate.

unreadable /ʌnˈriːdəbəl/ *adj* illegible; not worth reading.

unreal /ʌnˈriːl/ *adj* not real; imaginary, fanciful; false, insincere.

unreason /ʌnˈriːzən/ *n* absence of reason in thought or action.

unreasonable /ʌnˈriːzənəbəl/ *adj* contrary to reason; lacking reason; immoderate; excessive.—**unreasonably** *adv*.

unreasoning /ʌnˈriːzənɪŋ/ *adj* lacking reason, irrational.

unrelenting /ˌʌnrɪˈlentɪŋ/ *adj* relentless; continuous.—**unrelentingly** *adv*.

unremitting /ˌʌnrɪˈmɪtɪŋ/ *adj* incessant.

unrequited /ˌʌnrɪˈkwaɪtəd/ *adj* not reciprocated, not returned.

unreserved /ˌʌnrɪˈzɜːvd/ *adj* not reserved; frank, demonstrative; absolute, entire; not booked.

unreservedly /-vədli/ *adv* without conditions; openly.

unrest /ʌnˈrest/ *n* uneasiness; anxiety; angry discontent verging on revolt.

unrighteous /ʌnˈraɪtʃəs/ *adj* sinful, wicked.

unrivalled, unrivaled /ʌnˈraɪvəld/ *adj* without equal, peerless.

unroll /ʌnˈroːl/ *vti* to open out or down from a roll; to unfold; to straighten out; to reveal or become revealed.

unruffled /ʌnˈrʌfəld/ *adj* cool and calm; still, smooth.

unruly /ʌnˈruːli/ *adj* (**unrulier, unruliest**) hard to control, restrain, or keep in order; disobedient.

unsaddle /ʌnˈsædəl/ *vt* to take the saddle from; to unseat. • *vi* to remove the saddle from a horse.

unsaid /ʌnˈsed/ *adj* not said or expressed.

unsaturated /ʌnˈsætʃəˌreɪtəd/ or /-tjuˌreɪtəd/ *adj* (*chemical substance*) having double or triple bonds and therefore able to form products by chemical addition; (*vegetable fats*) containing fatty acids with double bonds.—**unsaturation** *n*.

unsavoury, unsavory /ʌnˈseɪvəri/ *adj* distasteful; disagreeable; offensive.

unscathed /ʌnˈskeɪðd/ *adj* unharmed.

unscramble /ʌnˈskræmbəl/ *vt* to disentangle; (*a scrambled message*) to make intelligible.

unscrew /ʌnˈskruː/ *vti* to remove a screw from; (*lid, etc*) to loosen by turning.

unscrupulous /ʌnˈskruːpjʊləs/ *adj* without principles.

unseasonable /ʌnˈsiːzənəbəl/ *n* (*weather*) unusual for the season of the year; untimely.—**unseasonableness** *n*.—**unseasonably** *adv*.

unseat /ʌnˈsiːt/ *vt* to dislodge from a seat, saddle, etc; to remove from office.

unseeded /ʌnˈsiːdəd/ *adj* (*tennis players, etc*) not ranked among the top players in the preliminary rounds of a competition.

unseemly /ʌnˈsiːmli/ *adj* unbecoming; inappropriate.

unseen /ʌnˈsiːn/ *adj* concealed, hidden; not seen or read beforehand.

unselfish /ʌnˈselfɪʃ/ *adj* not selfish; thinking of others before oneself.—**unselfishly** *adv*.—**unselfishness** *n*.

unsettle /ʌnˈsetəl/ *vti* to disturb, disrupt, or disorder.

unsettled /ʌnˈsetəld/ *adj* changeable; lacking stability; unpredictable; not concluded.

unsheathe /ʌnˈʃiːð/ *vt* to draw (a weapon) from a sheath.

unsightly /ʌnˈsaɪtli/ *adj* unattractive; ugly.

unskilful, unskillful /ʌnˈskɪlfʊl/ *adj* clumsy, awkward

unskilled /ʌnˈskɪld/ *adj* without special skill or training.

unsociable /ʌnˈsoːʃəbəl/ *n* antisocial; reserved.

unsocial /ʌnˈsoːʃəl/ *n* averse to social activities; (*working hours*) outwith the normal working day.

unsolicited /ˌʌnsəˈlɪsɪtəd/ *adj* not asked for.

unsophisticated /ˌʌnsəˈfɪstɪˌkeɪtəd/ *adj* naïve, inexperienced; simple; pure, unadulterated.

unsound /ʌnˈsaʊnd/ *adj* flimsy, not stable; defective, flawed; in poor health; not sane.—**unsoundly** *adv*.—**unsoundness** *n*.

unsparing /ʌnˈspeərɪŋ/ *adj* profuse, lavish; severe.

unspeakable /ʌnˈspiːkəbəl/ *adj* bad beyond words, indescribable.

unstable /ʌnˈsteɪbəl/ *adj* easily upset; mentally unbalanced; irresolute.

unsteady /ʌnˈstedi/ *adj* (**unsteadier, unsteadiest**) shaky, reeling; vacillating.—**unsteadily** *adv*.

unstop /ʌnˈstɒp/ *vt* (**unstopping, unstopped**) to remove the stopper from; to free from an obstruction.

unstrung /ʌnˈstrʌŋ/ *adj* emotionally distressed.

unstudied /ʌnˈstʌdid/ *adj* natural; unaffected in manner.

unsubstantial /ˌʌnsəbˈstænʃəl/ *adj* lacking weight, flimsy; of doubtful factual validity.

unsullied /ʌnˈsʌlid/ *adj* not stained, pure.

unsung /ʌnˈsʌŋ/ *adj* not acclaimed or celebrated.

unswerving /ʌnˈswɜːvɪŋ/ *adj* not deviating; constant, unchanging.

untangle /ʌnˈtæŋgəl/ *vt* to rid of tangles, unravel; to sort out.

untaught /ʌnˈtɒt/ *adj* not educated or trained; not acquired by teaching.

untenable /ʌnˈtenəbəl/ *adj* not able to be justified or defended.—**untenability** *n*.

unthinkable /ʌnˈθɪŋkətəl/ *adj* inconceivable; out of the question; improbable.—**unthinkably** *adv*.

unthinking /ʌnˈθɪŋkɪŋ/ *adj* unable to think; thoughtless, inconsiderate.—**unthinkingly** *adv*.

untidy /ʌnˈtaɪdi/ *adj* (**untidier, untidiest**) not neat, disordered. • *vt* (**untidying, untidied**) to make untidy.—**untidily** *adv*.

untie /ʌnˈtaɪ/ *vt* (**untying, untied**) to undo a knot in, unfasten.

until /ʌnˈtɪl/ or /ən-/ *prep* up to the time of; before. • *conj* up to the time when or that; to the point, degree, etc that; before.

untimely /ʌnˈtaɪmli/ *adj* premature; inopportune.

unto /ˈʌntuː/ or /ˈʌntə/ *prep* (*arch*) to.

untold /ʌnˈtoːld/ *adj* not told; too great to be counted; immeasurable.

untouchable /ʌnˈtʌtʃəbəl/ *adj* unable to be touched or handled; exempt from criticism or control; lying beyond reach.

untoward /ˌʌntəˈwoːd/ *adj* unseemly; unfavourable; adverse.

untrue /ʌnˈtruː/ *adj* incorrect, false; not faithful, disloyal; inaccurate.

untruth /ʌnˈtruːθ/ *n* falsehood; a lie.

untruthful /ʌnˈtruːθfʊl/ *adj* telling lies; false.

untutored /ʌnˈtuːtəd/ or /-ˈtjuːtəd/ *adj* lacking (refined) education.

unused /ʌnˈjuːzd/ *adj* not (yet) used; (*with to*) not accustomed (to something).

unusual /ʌnˈjuːʒuəl/ *adj* uncommon; rare.

unutterable /ʌnˈʌtərəbəl/ *adj* impossible to express in words.—**unutterably** *adv*.

unvarnished /ʌnˈvɑːnɪʃt/ *adj* not varnished; plain, direct; not embellished.

unveil /ʌnˈveil/ *vt* to reveal; to disclose.

unwaged /ʌnˈweɪdʒd/ *adj* not paid a wage; unemployed.

unwarrantable /ʌnˈwɒrəntəbəl/ *adj* indefensible.

unwarranted /ʌnˈwɒrəntəd/ *adj* not authorized.

unwary /ʌnˈweəri/ *adj* lacking caution; heedless, gullible; unguarded.—**unwarily** *adv*.

unwelcome /ʌnˈwelkəm/ *adj* not welcome, not invited; disagreeable; unpleasant.

unwell /ʌnˈwel/ *adj* ill, not well; (*inf*) suffering from a hangover.

unwholesome /ʌnˈhoːlsəm/ *adj* harmful to physical, mental or moral health and well-being; ill-looking; (*food*) of poor quality.—**unwholesomeness** *n*.

unwieldy /ʌnˈwiːldi/ *adj* not easily moved or handled, as because of large size; awkward.—**unwieldily** *adv*.—**unwieldiness** *n*.

unwilling /ʌnˈwɪlɪŋ/ *adj* not willing, reluctant; said or done with reluctance.—**unwillingly** *adv*.—**unwillingness** *n*.

unwind /ʌnˈwaɪnd/ *vt* to untangle; to undo. • *vi* to relax.

unwise /ʌnˈwaɪz/ *adj* lacking wisdom; imprudent.—**unwisely** *adv*.

unwitting /ʌnˈwɪtɪŋ/ *adj* not knowing; unintentional.—**unwittingly** *adv*.

unworldly /ʌnˈwɜːldli/ *adj* spiritual, not concerned with the material world.

unworthy /ʌnˈwɜːði/ *adj* (**unworthier, unworthiest**) not deserving.

unwritten /ʌnˈrɪtən/ *adj* not written or printed; traditional; oral.

unwritten law *n* law based on custom or mores rather than legislative enactment.

up /ʌp/ *adv* to, toward, in or on a higher place; to a later period; so as to be even with in time, degree, etc. • *prep* from a lower to a higher point on or along. • *adj* moving or directed upward; at an end; (*inf*) well-informed. • *vt* (**upping, upped**) to raise; to increase; to take up. • *n* ascent; high point.

upalong /ˈʌpəlɒŋ/ *adv* ✹ (*Cdn*) in Newfoundland, to or on a distant location, *esp* to or on the mainland of Canada. • *n* such a location.

up-and-coming *adj* promising for the future; likely to succeed.

upas /ˈjuːpəs/ *n* a Javanese tree that yields a poisonous sap.

upbeat /ˈʌpbiːt/ *n* (*mus*) an unaccented beat in the last bar. • *adj* (*inf*) cheerful, optimistic.

upbraid /ʌpˈbreɪd/ *vt* to rebuke severely; to reproach.

upbringing /ˈʌpˌbrɪŋɪŋ/ *n* the process of educating and nurturing (a child).

upcountry /ʌp'kʌntri/ or /'ʌp-/ *adv* towards the interior of a country, inland.

update /'ʌpdeɪt/ *vt* to bring up to date.

updraught, updraft /'ʌpdrɑːft/ *n* a upward flow of air or other gas.

upend /ʌp'ɛnd/ *vti* to turn or become turned on end; to upset or transform completely.

upfront /ʌp'frʌnt/ or /'ʌp-/ *adj* honest, open. • *adv* (*money*) paid in advance.

upgrade /'ʌpgreɪd/ *vt* to improve, raise to a higher grade.

upheaval /ʌp'hiːvəl/ *n* radical or violent change.

uphill /'ʌphɪl/ *adj* ascending, rising; difficult, arduous. • *adv* up a slope or hill; against difficulties.

uphold /ʌp'hoːld/ *vt* (**upholding, upheld**) to support, sustain; to defend.

upholster /ʌp'oːlstər/ or /ʌp'hoːl-/ *vt* (*furniture*) to fit with stuffing, springs, covering, etc.—**upholsterer** *n*.

upholstery /ʌp'oːlstəri/ or /ʌp'hoːl-/ *n* (*pl* **upholsteries**) materials used to make a soft covering *esp* for a seat.

upkeep /'ʌpkiːp/ *n* maintenance; the cost of it.

upland /'ʌplænd/ or /-lənd/ *n* an area of high ground. • *adj* of or pertaining to uplands.

uplift /ʌp'lɪft/ *vt* to raise, lift up; to improve the moral, cultural, spiritual, etc standard or condition of. • *n* a moral, cultural, spiritual, etc improvement.

upmarket /'ʌpmɑrkət/ *adj* of or appealing to wealthier buyers.

upmost /'ʌp‚moːst/ *see* **uppermost**.

upon /ə'pɒn/ *prep* on, on top of.

upper /'ʌpər/ *adj* farther up; higher in position, rank, status. • *n* the part of a boot or shoe above the sole; (*sl*) a drug used as a stimulant.

upper case *n* capital letters.—**upper-case** *adj*.

upper class *n* people occupying the highest social rank.—*also adj*.

upper crust *n* (*inf*) the aristocracy.

uppercut /'ʌpərkʌt/ *n* an upward swinging punch to the chin.— *also vb*.

upper hand *n* the position of control, advantage.

upper house, chamber *n* one of the two houses of a bicameral legislature, such as the British House of Lords or US Senate.

uppermost /'ʌpər‚moːst/ *adj* at the top; highest in importance. • *adv* into the highest position, etc.—*also* **upmost**.

uppity /'ʌpiti/ *adj* (*inf*) snobbish, arrogant.

upright /'ʌpraɪt/ *adj* vertical, in an erect position; righteous, honest, just. • *n* a vertical post or support. • *adv* vertically.

uprising /'ʌp‚raɪzɪŋ/ *n* a revolt; a rebellion.

uproar /'ʌprɔːr/ *n* a noisy disturbance; a commotion; an outcry.

uproarious /ʌp'rɔːriəs/ *adj* making or marked by an uproar; extremely funny; (*laughter*) boisterous.—**uproariously** *adv*.

uproot /ʌp'ruːt/ or /'ʌp-/ *vt* to tear out by the roots; to remove from established surroundings.

upset[1] /ʌp'sɛt/ or /'ʌp-/ *vt* (**upsetting, upset**) to overturn; to spill; to disturb; to put out of order; to distress; to overthrow; to make physically sick.

upset[2] *n* an unexpected defeat; distress or its cause. • *adj* distressed; confused; defeated.

upshot /'ʌpʃɒt/ *n* the conclusion; the result.

upside down /‚ʌpsaɪd'daʊn/ *adj* inverted; the wrong way up; (*inf*) topsy turvy.

upsilon /'juːpsɪ‚lɒn/ or /ʌp'saɪlən/ *n* the 20th letter of the Greek alphabet.

upstage /ʌp'steɪdʒ/ *vt* to draw attention to oneself. • *adv* to the rear of the stage.

upstairs /ʌp'stɛrz/ or /'ʌp-/ *adv* up the stairs; to an upper level or storey. • *n* an upper floor.

upstanding /ʌp'stændɪŋ/ *adj* honest; of good character; in a standing position.

upstart /'ʌpstɑrt/ *n* a person who has suddenly risen to a position of wealth and power; an arrogant person.

upstate /'ʌpsteɪt/ *n* the mostly northern areas of a US state. • *adv, adj* towards, in, or pertaining to this area of a US state.

upstream /'ʌpstriːm/ *adv, adj* in the direction from which a stream is flowing.

upstroke /'ʌp‚strok/ *n* an upward stroke, as of a pen, paintbrush, piston, etc.

upsurge /'ʌpsərdʒ/ *n* a sudden rise or swell.

upswing /'ʌpswɪŋ/ *n* an upward swing or movement; an improvement, *esp* in the state of the economy.

uptake /'ʌpteɪk/ *n* a taking up; a shaft or pipe for carrying smoke upwards; (*inf*) understanding.

uptight /ʌp'taɪt/ or /'ʌptaɪt/ *adj* (*inf*) very tense, nervous, etc.

up-to-date /‚ʌptə'deɪt/ *adj* modern; fashionable.

upturn /'ʌptərn/ *n* an upward trend; an (economic) improvement. • *vt* to turn upside down.

upward /'ʌpwərd/, **upwards** /-z/ *adj* from a lower to a higher place.—*also adv*.

upwardly-mobile *adj* aspiring to improve one's social and economic status.—**upward mobility** *n*.

upwind /'ʌpwɪnd/ or /-'wɪnd/ *adj, adv* in the direction from which the wind is blowing.

uraemia, uremia /juˈriːmiə/ *n* the accumulation of waste products in the blood that are normally passed in the urine.

uranium /juˈreɪniəm/ *n* a metallic element used as a source of nuclear energy.

urano- /'jurənoː/ *prefix* sky; the heavens.

uranography /‚jurə'nɒgrəfi/ *n* the description and mapping of the stars, etc by astronomers.—**uranographer** *n*.—**uranographic** *adj*.

Uranus /ju'reɪnəs/ or /'jurən-/ *n* the seventh planet from the sun.

urate /'jureɪt/ *n* a salt or ester of uric acid.—**uratic** *adj*.

urban /'ərbən/ *adj* of or relating to a city.—**urbanization, urbanisation** *n*.

urbane /ər'beɪn/ *adj* sophisticated; refined.—**urbanity** *n*.

urban guerrilla *n* a terrorist who operates in a town or city.

urbanite /'ərbə‚naɪt/ *n* a person who lives in a town or city.

urban renewal *n* rehabilitation of dilapidated city areas, as by housing construction and slum clearance.

urchin /'ərtʃɪn/ *n* a raggedly dressed mischievous child; a sea urchin.

urea /ju'riːə/ *n* a soluble crystalline compound present in urine produced by protein metabolism.

ureter /ju'riːtər/ *n* a tube that carries urine from the kidney to the bladder or cloaca.

urethra /ju'riːθrə/ *n* the duct carrying urine out of the bladder.

urethritis /jurɪ'θraɪtɪs/ *n* inflammation of the urethra.

uretic /ju'rɛtɪk/ *adj* of or pertaining to the urine.

urge /ərdʒ/ *vt* to drive forward; to press, plead with. • *n* an impulse, yearning.

urgency /'ərdʒənsi/ *n* (*pl* **urgencies**) the quality or condition of being urgent; compelling need; importance.

urgent /'ərdʒənt/ *adj* impelling; persistent; calling for immediate attention.—**urgently** *adv*.

-urgy /ərdʒi/ *n suffix* technology; technique.

-uria /'juri/ *n suffix* diseased condition of the urine.

uric /'jurik/ *adj* of, present in, or derived from urine.

uric acid *n* a white odourless substance found in the urine of birds, reptiles and some mammals.

urinal /'jurənəl/ *n* a bowl or trough for urination in public lavatories.

urinalysis /‚juri'nælɪsɪs/ *n* (*pl* **urinalyses**) the chemical analysis of urine for signs of disease.

urinate /'jurə‚neɪt/ *vi* to pass urine.

urine /'jurɪn/ *n* a yellowish fluid excreted by the kidneys and conveyed to the bladder.—**urinary** *adj*.

urinogenital /‚jurəno:'dʒɛnɪtəl/ *adj* urogenital.

urn /ərn/ *n* a vase or large vessel; a receptacle for preserving the ashes of the dead; a large metal container for boiling water for tea or coffee.

uro- /'juroː/, **ur-** *prefix* urine; urinary tract.

urogenital /‚juroː'dʒɛnɪtəl/, **urinogenital** *adj* of or pertaining to the urinary and reproductive organs.—*also* **genitourinary**.

urology /ju'rɒlədʒi/ *n* the medical study and treatment of urogenital diseases.—**urologist** *n*.—**urological** *adj*.

uroscopy /ju'rɒskəpi/ *n* the diagnosis of diseases by the examination of the patient's urine.

ursine /'ərsaɪn/ *adj* of or resembling a bear.

urticaria /‚ərtɪ'kɛriə/ *n* an allergic reaction which produces raised itchy whitish patches on the skin.—*also* **hives, nettle rash**.

us /ʌs/ or /əs/ *pron* the objective case of **we**.

US *abbr* = United States.

USA *abbr* = United States of America.

USAF *abbr* = United States Air Force.

usage /'juːsədʒ/ *n* customary use; practice, custom; use of language.

use[1] /juːz/ *vt* to put to some purpose; to utilize; to exploit (a person); to partake of (drink, drugs, tobacco, etc).—**usable, useable** *adj*.

use[2] *n* act of using or putting to a purpose; usage; usefulness; need (for); advantage; practice, custom.

used /ju:zd/ *adj* not new; second-hand.

useful /'ju:sful/ *adj* able to be used to good effect; (*inf*) capable, commendable.—**usefully** *adv*.

useless /'ju:sləs/ *adj* having no use.—**uselessly** *adv*.—**uselessness** *n*.

user /'ju:zər/ *n* one who uses; (*inf*) a drug addict.

user-friendly *adj* easy to understand and operate.

usher /'ʌʃər/ *n* one who shows people to their seats in a theatre, church, etc; a doorkeeper in a law court. • *vt* to escort to seats, etc.

usherette /ʌʃər'ɛt/ *nf* a woman who directs people to their seats in a cinema.

USN *abbr* = United States Navy.

USSR *abbr* = (*formerly*) Union of Soviet Socialist Republics.

usual /'ju:ʒuəl/ *adj* customary; ordinary; normal.—**usually** *adv*.

usurer /'ju:ʒərər/ *n* a person who lends money at an excessively high rate of interest.

usurp /ju'sɔrp/ or /-zɔrp/ *vt* to seize or appropriate unlawfully.—**usurper** *n*.

usury /'ju:ʒəri/ *n* (*pl* **usuries**) the practice of taking excessive interest on a loan; an excessive interest rate.

UT *abbr* = Utah.

utensil /ju:'tɛnsəl/ *n* an implement or container, *esp* one for use in the kitchen.

uterus /'ju:tərəs/ *n* (*pl* **uteri**) the female organ in which offspring are developed until birth, the womb.—**uterine** *adj*.

utilitarian /ju:tɪlɪ'tɛriər/ *adj* designed to be of practical use.

utility /ju:'tɪlɪti/ *n* (*pl* **utilities**) usefulness; a public service, such as telephone, electricity, etc; a company providing such a service.

utility room *n* a room containing laundry appliances, heating equipment, etc.

utilize /'ju:tə,laɪz/ *vt* to make practical use of.—**utilization** *n*.

utmost /'ʌtmo:st/ *adj* of the greatest degree or amount; furthest. • *n* the most possible.

utopia /ju:'to:piə/ *n* a imaginary society or place considered to be ideal or perfect.—**utopian** *adj, n*.

utter[1] /'ʌtər/ *adj* absolute; complete.

utter[2] *vt* to say; to speak —**utterance** *n*.

utterly /-li/ *adv* completely.

UV *abbr* = ultraviolet.

uvula /'ju:vjulə/ *n* (*pl* **uvulas, uvulae**) the fleshy tissue suspended in the back of the throat over the back part of the tongue.

uxorious /ʌk'zɔriəs/ *adj* excessively fond of one's wife; doting.—**uxoriously** *adv*.—**uxoriousness** *n*.

V

V *abbr* = volt(s).

V, v /viː/ *n* the 22nd letter of the English alphabet; something shaped like a V.

v *abbr* = velocity; *versus* against; *vide* see; verb.

VA *abbr* = Veterans Administration; Virginia.

vac /væk/ *abbr* = vacuum.

vac /væk/ *n* (*inf*) a vacation.

vacancy /ˈveɪkənsi/ *n* (*pl* **vacancies**) emptiness; an unoccupied job or position.

vacant /ˈveɪkənt/ *adj* empty; unoccupied; (*expression*) blank.—**vacantly** *adv*.—**vacantness** *n*.

vacate /ˈveɪkeɪt/ or /vəˈkeɪt/ *vt* to leave empty; to give up possession of.

vacation /veɪˈkeɪʃən/ *n* a holiday; a period of the year when universities, colleges and law courts are closed. • *vi* to go on holiday.

vacationer /-ər/, **vacationist** /-ɪst/ *n* a person on vacation, a holiday-maker.

vacation pay *n* ✤ (*Cdn*) the wages to which an employee is legally entitled to receive as a paid vacation, or a sum of money equivalent to it.

vaccinal /ˈvæksɪnəl/ *adj* pertaining to or caused by a vaccine or vaccination.

vaccinate /ˈvæksɪˌneɪt/ *vt* to inoculate with vaccine as a protection against a disease.—**vaccinator** *n*.

vaccination /ˌvæksɪˈneɪʃən/ *n* inoculation with a vaccine; the resulting scar.

vaccine /ˈvæksiːn/ or /ˈvæksiːn/ *n* a modified and hence harmless virus or other microorganism used for inoculation to give immunity from certain diseases by stimulating antibody production; cowpox virus used in this way against smallpox.

vaccinia /vækˈsɪniə/ *n* (*med*) cowpox.—**vaccinial** *adj*.

vacillate /ˈvæsɪˌleɪt/ *vi* to waver, to show indecision; to fluctuate.—**vacillation** *n*.—**vacillator** *n*.

vacuity /vəˈkjuːɪti/ *n* (*pl* **vacuities**) emptiness; a vacant state of mind or expression; absence of matter; a vacuum; idleness; lack; an inane remark.

vacuole /ˈvækjuːˌɒl/ *n* (*biol*) a small cell or cavity filled with fluid in the interior of organic cells or protoplasm.—**vacuolate, vacuolated** *adj*.

vacuous /ˈvækjuːəs/ *adj* empty; lacking intelligence, mindless.—**vacuously** *adv*.—**vacuousness** *n*.

vacuum /ˈvækjuːm/ *n* (*pl* **vacuums, vacua**) a region devoid of all matter; a region in which gas is present at low pressure; a vacuum cleaner. • *vt* to clean with a vacuum cleaner. • *adj* of, having or creating a vacuum; working by suction or maintenance of a partial vacuum.

vacuum cleaner *n* an electrical appliance for removing dust from carpets, etc, by suction.—**vacuum-clean** *vt*.

vacuum bottle, vacuum flask *n* a container for keeping liquids hot or cold.

vacuum-packed /ˈvækjuːmˌpækt/ *adj* sealed in an airtight packet from which the air has been removed.

vade mecum /ˌvædiˈmiːkəm/ or /ˌveɪdiˈmeɪkəm/ *n* (*pl* **vade mecums**) a handbook or manual, etc, for ready reference, *usu* of a size to fit in a pocket.

vagabond /ˈvægəˌbɒnd/ *n* a vagrant; a wandering, homeless person.—**vagabondage** *n*.—**vagabondism** *n*.

vagal /ˈveɪgəl/ *adj* of, pertaining to, affected or controlled by the vagus nerve.

vagary /ˈveɪgəri/ *n* (*pl* **vagaries**) unpredictable or erratic behaviour or actions; a whim.—**vagarious** *adj*.

vagina /vəˈdʒaɪnə/ *n* (**vaginas, vaginae**) in female mammals and humans, the canal connecting the uterus and the external sex organs.—**vaginal** *adj*.

vaginate /ˈvædʒənɪt/ or /-ˌneɪt/, **vaginated** *adj* (*bot*) (*plant parts*) sheathed; with a vagina or sheath.

vagrancy /ˈveɪgrənsi/ (*pl* **vagrancies**) the habits and life of a vagrant; a wandering without a settled home.

vagrant /ˈveɪgrənt/ *n* a person who has no settled home, a tramp. • *adj* wandering, roaming; wayward.—**vagrantly** *adv*.

vague /veɪg/ *adj* unclear; indistinct, imprecise; (*person*) absent-minded.—**vaguely** *adv*.—**vagueness** *n*.

vagus /ˈveɪgəs/ *n* (*pl* **vagi**) vagus nerve.

vagus nerve *n* either of a pair of cranial nerves supplying the larynx, heart, lungs, etc.

vail[1] /veɪl/ *vti* (*arch*) to lower, to let fall; to take off (a hat) in respect.

vail[2] *n* (*arch*) a gratuity, a tip.

vain /veɪn/ *adj* conceited; excessively concerned with one's appearance; senseless; futile; worthless; **in vain** to no purpose.—**vainly** *adv*.—**vainness** *n*.

vainglorious /veɪnˈglɔːriəs/ *adj* elated by one's achievements; boastful; showy.—**vaingloriously** *adv*.—**vaingloriousness** *n*.

vainglory /ˈveɪnglɔːri/ or /-ˈglɔːri/ *n* (*pl* **vainglories**) excessive vanity; boastfulness; showiness.

vair /veər/ *n* a fur trimming on medieval robes, probably of Russian squirrel; (*her*) fur represented by small shields, coloured white and blue alternately.

valance /ˈvæləns/ or /ˈveɪl-/ *n* a decorative cover for the base of a bed; a canopy for a window frame to hide rods, etc; a pelmet.—**valanced** *adj*.

vale[1] /veɪl/ *n* a valley.

vale[2] *interj*, *n* (*arch*) farewell.

valediction /ˌvælɪˈdɪkʃən/ *n* a saying farewell; a taking leave; an instance of this; a speech made at this time.

valedictorian /ˌvælədɪkˈtɔːriən/ *n* a college student appointed on grounds of merit to deliver the valedictory oration on Commencement day.

valedictory /ˌvælədɪkˈtɔːri/ *adj* uttered or bestowed on saying farewell; shown, performed or done by way of valediction. • *n* (*pl* **valedictories**) a valedictory oration; a statement or speech made on leaving a position, etc.

valence /ˈveɪləns/, **valency** /-si/ *n* (*pl* **valences, valencies**) (*chem*) the power of elements to combine; the number of atoms of hydrogen that an atom or group can combine with to form a compound.

valence electron, valency electron *n* (*chem*) one of the electrons present in the outermost shell of an atom of a corresponding element.

Valenciennes (lace) /væˌlãsiˈɛn/ *n* an ornate type of bobbin lace, formerly made of linen, now *usu* of cotton.

-valent /ˈveɪlənt/ *adj suffix* having a specified number of valences, *eg univalent*.

valentine /ˈvælənˌtaɪn/ *n* a lover or sweetheart chosen on St Valentine's Day, February 14; a card or gift sent on that day.

valerian /vəˈliːriən/ *n* a herb with a root formerly used for medicinal purposes; the root of this used as a sedative.

valet /ˈvæˈleɪ/ or /ˈvæ-/ *n* a manservant; a steward in a hotel or on board ship. • *vt* to attend (someone) as a valet. • *vi* to work as a valet.

valetudinarian /ˌvælɪˌtjuːdɪˈneəriən/, **valetudinary** /-ri/ *n* (*pl* **valetudinarians, valetudinaries**) a person who is overly preoccupied with his or her own health, a hypochondriac; a chronic invalid. • *adj* of ill health; sickly; seeking to recover health—**valetudinarianism** *n*.

valgus /ˈvælgəs/ *adj* (*med*) deviating outwards from the vertical middle line of the body. • *n* (*pl* **valguses**) a deformity caused by a twisting from the middle line of the body, *eg* bow-legs.

Valhalla /vælˈhælə/ *n* (*Scandinavian myth*) the palace or hall of immortality in which the souls of heroes slain in battle dwell.—*also* **Walhalla**.

valiant /ˈvæljənt/ *adj* courageous; brave.—**valiance, valiancy** *n*.—**valiantly** *adv*.

valid /ˈvælɪd/ *adj* based on facts; (*objection, etc*) sound; legally acceptable; binding.—**validity** *n*.—**validly** *adv*.

validate /ˈvælɪˌdeɪt/ *vt* to corroborate; to legalize.—**validation** *n*.

valine /ˈvæliːn/ or /ˈveɪ-/ *n* an amino acid formed by the digestion of protein.

valise /vəˈliːs/ *n* a small case, *usu* of a size large enough to carry what is needed for an overnight visit.

Valkyrie /vælˈkiːriː/ or /ˈvælkɪri/ *n* (*Scandinavian myth*) one of the twelve Norse war goddesses, handmaidens of Odin, who selected those who were worthy to be slain in battle and led them to Valhalla.—*also* **Walkyrie**.

vallation /væˈleɪʃən/ *n* a defensive wall; a rampart; the act of building this.

vallecula /vəˈlɛkjulə/ *n* (*pl* **valleculae**) (*anat*) a cleft or depressed area; (*bot*) a groove, a deep wrinkle.—**vallecular**, **valleculate** *adj*.

valley /ˈvæli/ *n* (*pl* **valleys**) low land between hills or mountains *usu* with a river or stream flowing along its bottom; something resembling a valley, *eg* the angle where two sloping sides of a roof meet.

valonia /vəˈloːniə/ *n* a large, dried acorn cup, or unripened acorn, from a particular kind of oak tree, used in tanning, dyeing, ink-making, etc.

valor /ˈvælər/ *see* **valour**.

valorize /ˈvæləˌraɪz/ *vt* to give an arbitrary price to (something) under government control.—**valorization** *n*.

valorous /ˈvælərəs/ *adj* (*person*) valiant, courageous; (*action*) characterized by valour.—**valorously** *adv*.—**valorousness** *n*.

valour /ˈvælər/ *n* courage; bravery (in battle).—*also* **valor**.

valse *Fr.* /vals/ *n* a waltz, often used in the titles of musical compositions.

valuable /ˈvæljuːəbəl/ or /ˈvæljəbəl/ *adj* having considerable importance or monetary worth. • *n* a personal possession of value, *esp* jewellery; (*pl*) valuable possessions.—**valuably** *adv*.

valuate /ˈvæljuːeɪt/ *vt* to estimate the worth of, to value.—**valuator** *n*.

valuation /ˌvæljuːˈeɪʃən/ *n* the act of valuing or valuating; an estimated price or worth; an estimation.—**valuational** *adj*.

value /ˈvæljuː/ *n* worth, merit, importance; market value; purchasing power; relative worth; (*pl*) moral principles. • *vt* (**valuing**, **valued**) to estimate the worth of; to regard highly; to prize.—**valuer** *n*.

value-added tax *n* a tax levied on the difference between the production cost of an item and its selling price.

valued /ˈvæljuːd/ *adj* estimated; esteemed, prized.

value judgment *n* a subjective or unwarranted judgment.

valueless /ˈvæljuːləs/ *adj* without value; worthless.—**valuelessness** *n*.

valuta /vəluːtə/ *n* the value of one currency in terms of another.

valvar /ˈvælvjulər/ *see* **valvular**.

valvate /ˈvælˌveɪt/ *adj* having, resembling, or operating by means of a valve or valves; (*bot*) (*petals*) meeting at the edges without overlapping.

valve /vælv/ *n* a device for controlling the flow of a gas or liquid through a pipe; (*anat*) a tube allowing blood to flow in one direction only; (*mus*) a device on a brass instrument for increasing the length of the tube and thus altering the pitch being played.

valvular /ˈvælvjulər/ *adj* of, affecting a valve or valves, *esp* of the heart; acting like a valve; shaped like a valve; operating by means of a valve or valves.

valvule /ˈvælˌvjuːl/, **valvelet** /ˈvælvələt/ *n* a little valve; anything resembling this.

valvulitis /ˌvælvjəlaɪtəs/ *n* inflammation of the valves, *esp* of the heart.

vambrace /ˈvæmbreɪs/ *n* plate armour for the forearm.

vamoose, vamose /væˈmuːs/ *vi* (*sl*) to make off quickly, to decamp.

vamp[1] /væmp/ *n* the part of a sock, boot or shoe covering the front of the foot; anything patched up or refurbished; an improvised musical accompaniment made up of chords. • *vt* to provide with a (new) vamp; to mend or repair; (*with* **up**) to renovate; (*mus*) to improvise.—**vamper** *n*.

vamp[2] *n* a seductive woman. • *vt* to fascinate or exploit by seducing. • *vi* to act as a vamp.

vampire /ˈvæmpaɪr/ *n* (*folklore*) a dead creature that by night leaves its grave to suck the blood of living people; a person who preys on others, an extortioner; a vampire bat.—**vampiric** *adj*.

vampire bat *n* a tropical American blood-sucking bat.

vampirism /ˈvæmpaɪrˌɪzəm/ *n* belief in vampires; bloodsucking, or other acts associated with vampires.

van[1] /væn/ *n* a covered motor vehicle for transporting goods, etc.

van[2] *n* the vanguard.

vanadium /vəˈneɪdiəm/ *n* a rare soft white metallic element used in steel alloys.—**vanadic** *adj*.

Vancouverite /vænˈkuːvəraɪt/ *n* ♣ a person who lives in or is from Vancouver, British Columbia.

vandal /ˈvændəl/ *n* a person who wilfully or ignorantly damages property; (*with cap*) a member of a Germanic tribe that sacked Rome (455AD). • *adj* of of acting like a vandal; characterized by vandalism or lack of culture.

vandalism /ˈvændəˌlɪzm/ *n* the ruthless destruction or spoiling of anything beautiful or venerable; barbarous, ignorant or inartistic treatment.—**vandalistic** *adj*.

vandalize /ˈvændəˌlaɪz/ *vt* to carry out an act of vandalism.—**vandalization** *n*.

Van de Graaf generator /ˌvændəˈgræf/ *n* a machine that continuously separates electrostatic charges and in so doing produces a very high voltage.

van der Waals' force /ˌvændərˈwɒls/ *n* a weak attractive force between two neighbouring atoms.

Vandyke beard /vænˈdaɪk/ *n* a small pointed beard.

Vandyke collar *n* a wide, white collar of lace or sewed work, with a deeply indented edge.

vane /veɪn/ *n* a blade at the top of a spire, etc to show wind direction; a weather vane; a blade on a windmill or propeller.

vang /væŋ/ *n* (*naut*) a guy rope from the end of a gaff to the deck, used for steadying the extremity of the peak of a gaff to the side of a ship; a rope running from the boom of a mainsail to the deck, used to keep the boom lowered.

vanguard /vænɡɑːrd/ *n* the front part of an army; the leading position of any movement.

vanilla /vəˈnɪlə/ or /-ˈnɛlə/ *n* extract from the orchid pod used as a flavouring.—**vanillic** *adj* from vanilla.

vanish /ˈvænɪʃ/ *vi* to disappear from sight, to become invisible, *esp* in a rapid and mysterious manner; to fade away; to cease to exist; (*math*) (*numbers, quantities*) to become zero.—**vanisher** *n*.

vanishing cream *n* a cleansing or foundation cream for make-up that is colourless when applied to the face.

vanity /ˈvænɪti/ *n* (*pl* **vanities**) a fruitless endeavour; worthlessness; empty pride or conceit; love of indiscriminate admiration; an idle matter or show; a worthless or unfounded idea or statement; emptiness, lightness.

vanity case, vanity box *n* a small case used for carrying cosmetics, etc.

vanquish /ˈvæŋkwɪʃ/ *vt* to conquer; to defeat; to overcome, to subdue.—**vanquisher** *n*.—**vanquishment** *n*.

vantage /ˈvæntɪdʒ/ *n* a favourable position; a position allowing a clear view or understanding.

vanward /ˈvænwərd/ *adj* towards the front, in the van. • *adv* forward, towards the front.

vapid /ˈvæpɪd/ *adj* flavourless, flat, insipid; dull, lifeless.—**vapidity** *n*.—**vapidly** *adv*.

vapor /ˈveɪpər/ *see* **vapour**.

vaporish /-ɪʃ/ *see* **vapourish**.

vaporize /ˈveɪpəˌraɪz/ *vt* to change into vapour.—**vaporization** *n*.—**vaporizer** *n*.

vaporous /ˈveɪpərəs/ *adj* in the form of or like vapour; foggy, steamy; unreal, fanciful.—**vaporously** *adv*.—**vaporosity** *n*.

vapour /ˈveɪpər/ *n* the gaseous state of a substance normally liquid or solid; particles of water or smoke in the air; (*pl*) hysteria. • *vi* to pass off in vapour, vaporize; to boast.—*also* **vapor**.

vapourish /-ɪʃ/ *adj* like vapour; full of vapour; (*arch*) in a state of depression and lethargy.—*also* **vaporish**.—**vapourishness**, **vapurishness** *n*.

vapour trail *n* condensed vapour left in the wake of an aircraft exhaust appearing as a white trail in the sky.

varec /ˈværek/ *n* the ash left after burning kelp.

variable /ˈvɛriəbəl/ *adj* 1 able to change; not constant. • *n* (*math*) a changing quantity that can have different values, as opposed to a constant.—**variability** *n*.—**variably** *adv*.

variance /ˈvɛriəns/ *n* disagreement, dissension; variation; tendency to vary; (*law*) a discrepancy between two statements or documents; **at variance** in conflict.

variant /ˈvɛriənt/ *adj* different; differing from an accepted or normal type, text, etc. • *n* a variant form or reading.

variation /ˌvɛriˈeɪʃən/ *n* a varying or being varied; alteration; deviation from a standard or type; diversity; deviation of the magnetic needle from true north; the measure of this; (*gram*) inflexion; (*mus*) repetition of a theme or melody with modifications.—**variational** *adj*.

varicella /ˌværɪˈsɛlə/ *n* (*med*) chickenpox.—**varicelloid** *adj*.

varices /'væra,si:z/ *see* **varix**.

varicocele /'værɪkə,si:l/ *n* a swelling of the veins of the scrotum or of the spermatic cord.

varicoloured, varicolored /'verɪ,kələrd/ *adj* variegated, particoloured; of several colours.

varicose /'verɪ,ko:s/ *adj* (*veins*) abnormally swollen and dilated.—**varicosis** *n*.—**varicosity** *n*.

varied /'verɪd/ *adj* showing variety, changing; partially changed; various; variegated.—**variedly** *adv*.

variegate /'verə,geɪt/ *or* /-riə,geɪt/ *vt* to mark with different colours or tints; to dapple, streak; to cause to diversify.

variegated /'verə,geɪtəd/ *or* /-riə,geɪtəd/ *adj* marked with different colours.

variegation /,verə'geɪʃən/ *n* the condition of being variegated; diversity of colours.

variety /və'raɪəti/ *n* (*pl* **varieties**) diversity; an assortment.—**varietal** *adj*.

variety show *n* an entertainment made up of various acts, such as songs, comedy turns, etc.

variform /'verɪ,fɔrm/ *adj* having various forms.

variola /və'raɪələ/ *n* (*med*) smallpox.—**variolar** *adj*.

variolate /və'raɪəleɪt/ *adj* having shallow, pitted depressions similar to those left on the skin after smallpox. • *vt* to inoculate with smallpox virus.—**variolation** *n*.

variole /'verɪ,o:l/ *n* a whitish spot or round mass consisting of radiating threads of crystal.

variolite /'verɪə,laɪt/ *n* a kind of igneous rock with whitish spots, made up of clustered varioles.—**variolitic** *adj*.

varioloid /'verɪə,lɔɪd/ *n* smallpox modified by vaccination or other means of acquired partial immunity. • *adj* like smallpox.

variorum /,verɪ'ɔrəm/ *n* an edition of the works of an author with notes by various commentators.—*also adj*.

various /'verɪəs/ *adj* varied, different; several.—**variously** *adv*.

varix /'verɪks/ *n* (*pl* **varices**) (*med*) a varicose vein; a twisted, dilated artery.

varlet /'varlət/ *n* a scoundrel; (*arch*) a servant, attendant, or page of a knight.

varmint /'varmɪnt/ *n* (*dial*) a rascal; an offensive or trying person or animal; (*hunting sl*) the fox.

varnish /'varnɪʃ/ *n* a sticky liquid which dries and forms a hard, glossy coating. • *vt* to coat with varnish.—**varnisher** *n*.

varsity /'varsɪti/ *n* (*pl* **varsities**) (*Brit, NZ inf*) university.

varus /'verəs/ *n* (*pl* **varuses**) a deformity caused by a turning in towards the vertical midline of the body, *eg* pigeon toes.

vary /'verɪ/ *vti* (**varying, varied**) to change, to diversify, modify; to become altered.—**varyingly** *adv*.

vascular /'væskjʊlər/ *adj* (*biol*) of, consisting of, or containing vessels as part of a structure of animal and vegetable organisms for conveying blood, sap, etc.—**vascularity** *n*.

vasculum /'væskjʊləm/ *n* (*pl* **vascula, vasculums**) a botanist's specimen box.

vas deferens /væs'defə,renz/ *n* (*pl* **vasa deferentia**) the spermatic duct.

vase /vɒz/ *or* /veɪz/, /veɪs/ *n* a vessel for displaying flowers.

vasectomy /və'sektəmi/ *n* (*pl* **vasectomies**) male sterilization involving the cutting of the sperm-carrying tube.

Vaseline /'væsə,li:n/ *n* (*trademark*) petroleum jelly used as a lubricant.

vasoconstrictor /,veɪzo:kən'strɪktər/ *n* a nerve, drug, etc, that constricts blood vessels.—**vasoconstrictive** *adj*.

vasodilator /,veɪzo:daɪ'leɪtər/ *n* a nerve, drug etc that dilates blood vessels.—**vasodilative** *adj*.

vasomotor /'veɪzo:,mo:tər/ *adj* (*nerve, drug, etc*) pertaining to or controlling the diameter of blood vessels.

vassal /'væsəl/ *n* a servant, dependant; subordinate.

vassalage /'væsəlɪdʒ/ *n* the state of being a vassal; the obligations associated with such a state; servitude; dependence; (*rare*) vassals collectively.

vast /væst/ *adj* immense.—**vastly** *adv*.—**vastness** *n*.

vasty (**vastier, vastiest**) /'væsti/ *adj* (*arch*) vast.

VAT /,vi:eɪ'ti:/ *or* /væt/ *abbr* = value added tax.

vat /væt/ *n* a large barrel or tank. • *vt* (**vatting, vatted**) to put in a vat; to treat in a vat.

vatic /'vætɪk/, **vatical** /'vætɪkəl/ *adj* of or relating to a prophet or prophecy.

Vatican /'vætɪkən/ *n* the residence of the pope in Rome; papal authority.

Vaticanism /'vætɪkən,ɪzəm/ *n* (*often derog*) the doctrine of Papal supremacy and infallibility.

vaticination /væ,tɪsɪ'neɪʃən/ *n* a prophecy.

vaudeville /'vɒdvɪl/ *or* /'vɒdə,vɪl/ *n* a stage show consisting of various acts, such as singing, dancing and comedy.

vault[1] /vɒlt/ *n* an arched ceiling or roof; a burial chamber; a strongroom for valuables; a cellar.—**vaulted** *adj*.

vault[2] *vti* to leap or jump over an obstacle. • *n* a leap.—**vaulter** *n*.

vaulting[1] /'vɒltɪŋ/ *n* (*arch*) arched work in a building, etc.

vaulting[2] *adj* overly confident; to an exaggerated degree; used in the act of leaping over.

vaunt /vɒnt/ *vti* to display boastfully; to brag. • *n* a boast.—**vaunter** *n*.—**vauntingly** *adv*.

vavasour, vavasor, vavassor /'vævə,sʊr/ *n* (*feudalism*) the tenant of a baron or lord who is that lord's vassal and who in turn has several vassals under him.

VC *abbr* = Victoria Cross; vice-chairman; Vietcong.

VCR *abbr* = video cassette recorder.

VD *abbr* = venereal disease.

VDU *abbr* = video display unit.

veal /vi:l/ *n* the edible flesh of a calf.

vector /'vektər/ *n* (*physics*) a physical quantity having both direction and magnitude, *eg* displacement, acceleration, etc; an aircraft's or missile's course; (*biol*) a piece of DNA that transmits a parasitic disease.—**vectorial** *adj*.

Veda /'veɪdə/ *or* /'vi:-/ *n* (any of) the oldest sacred books or collection of hymns of the Hindus, written in old Sanskrit and of great antiquity.—**Vedic** *adj*.

Vedanta /vɪ'dænt/ *or* /ve'dɒ-/ *n* a Hindu philosophy based on the Veda, postulating that the world of the senses is based on an illusion.—**Vedantic** *adj*.

vedette /ve'det/ *n* a small patrol boat.—*also* **vedette boat**; a mounted sentry in advance of an outpost.—*also* **vidette**.

Vedic /'veɪdɪk/ *or* /'vi:-/ *adj* pertaining to the Veda, or to the old Sanskrit in which these were written; pertaining to the original Indo-Europeans of India.

veer /vi:r/ *vi* (*wind*) to change direction; to swing around; to change from one mood or opinion to another.—**veeringly** *adv*.

veery /'vi:ri/ *n* (*pl* **veeries**) a tawny North American thrush.

veg. /vedʒ/ *abbr* = vegetable(s).

vegan /'vi:gən/ *or* /'veɪ-/, /'vedʒən/ *n* a strict vegetarian who consumes no animal or dairy products.

vegetable /'vedʒtəbəl/ *or* /'vedʒətəbəl/ *n* a herbaceous plant grown for food. • *adj* of, relating to or derived from plants.

vegetal /'vedʒətəl/ *adj* of growth and vital functions; vegetable.

vegetarian /,vedʒə'terɪən/ *n* a person who consumes a diet that excludes meat and fish. • *adj* of vegetarians; consisting wholly of vegetables.

vegetarianism /-,ɪzəm/ *n* the doctrine or practice of vegetarians; abstention from meating meat, fish, or other animal products.

vegetate /'vedʒə,teɪt/ *vi* to grow like a plant; to sprout; to lead a mentally inactive, aimless life.

vegetation /,vedʒə'teɪʃən/ *n* vegetable growth; plants in general.—**vegetational** *adj*.

vegetative /'vedʒə,teɪtɪv/, **vegetive** /'vedʒətɪv/ *adj* (*plants*) growing or having the power of growing, or producing growth in; (*way of life*) dull, passive, uneventful; (*reproduction*) asexual; referring to functions other than sexual reproduction.

vehement /'vi:əmənt/ *adj* passionate; forceful; furious.—**vehemence, vehemency** *n*.—**vehemently** *adv*.

vehicle /'vi:əkəl/ *n* a conveyance, such as a car, bus or truck, for carrying people or goods on land; a means of transmission for ideas, impressions, etc, a medium; (*med*) a substance in which a strong medicine can be administered palatably.—**vehicular** *adj*.

veil /veɪl/ *n* a thin fabric worn over the head or face of a woman; a nun's headdress; anything that conceals; a velum. • *vt* to put on a veil; to cover; to conceal, dissemble.

veiled /'veɪld/ *adj* covered with or wearing a veil; shrouded in a veil; concealed, hidden; covert; not openly declared; (*sound, voice*) indistinct, muffled.

vein /veɪn/ *n* (*anat*) one of the vessels that convey the blood back to the heart; (*geol*) a seam of a mineral within a rock; (*bot*) a branching rib in a leaf; a streak of different colour, as in marble, cheese, etc; a style or mood (*serious vein*). • *vt* to streak.—**veiny** *adj*.

veinlet /'veɪnlɪt/ *n* a small vein.

veinprint /'veɪn,prɪnt/ *n* the pattern of veins on the back of the hand, which is unique to an individual.

velamen /vɪˈleɪmən/ n (pl **velamina**) (anat) an outer membrane or epidermis; a velum; (bot) a thick, moisture-absorbing aerial root, consisting of dead cells, found on some plants.

velar /ˈviːlər/ adj of the velum or soft palate; (phonetics) pronounced with the back of the tongue touching the soft palate. • n a velar sound.

velarium /vəˈlɛəriəm/ n (pl **velaria**) in ancient Rome the great awning that stretched over open theatres.

Velcro /ˈvelkroʊ/ n (trademark) a nylon material made of matching strips of tiny hooks and pile that are easily pressed together or pulled apart.

veld, veldt /velt/ n in South Africa, open grass country.

velites /ˈviːlɪˌtiːz/ n in ancient Rome, a lightly armed soldier, usu from the poorer section of society.

velleity /vəˈliːəti/ n (pl **velleities**) (arch) the lowest degree of desire, mere inclination.

vellum /ˈveləm/ n fine parchment; a good quality writing paper.

veloce /ˈveloʊs/ adv (mus) very quickly.

velocipede /vəˈlɒsɪˌpiːd/ n an early form of bicycle, propelled by striking the toes on the road; any early form of bicycle or tricycle.

velocity /vəˈlɒsɪti/ n (pl **velocities**) the rate of change of position of any object; speed.

velour /vəˈlʊr/, **velours** /vəˈlʊrz/ n a velvet-like fabric.

velouté /vəluːˈteɪ/ n a rich white sauce or soup, with a basis of egg yolks, cream and stock.

velum /ˈviːləm/ n (pl **vela**) (anat) the soft palate; any body structure resembling a veil; (bot, zool) a membranous covering or organ, such as the membranous covering of certain molluscs or that covering a developing mushroom.

velure /vəˈlʊr/ n a kind of plush or velvet-like material; a velvet pad for smoothing a silk hat.

velutinous /vəˈluːtɪnəs/ adj (bot) thickly covered with short hairs, velvety.

velvet /ˈvelvət/ n a fabric made from silk, rayon, etc with a soft, thick pile; anything like velvet in texture.

velveteen /ˌvelvəˈtiːn/ n a cotton cloth with a pile like velvet.

velvety /ˈvelvəti/ adj soft to the touch; mellow.

vena /ˈviːnə/ n (pl **venae**) (anat) a vein.

vena cava /ˌviːnəˈkeɪvə/ n (pl **venae cavae**) one of the two major veins that empty blood into the right chamber of the heart in air-breathing vertebrates.

venal /ˈviːnəl/ adj corrupt; willing to accept bribes.—**venality** n.—**venally** adv.

venatic /vɪˈnætɪk/, **venatical** /vɪˈnætɪkəl/ adj of or pertaining to hunting; (people) likely to engage in hunting.

venation /vɪˈneɪʃən/ n the arrangement of veins in a leaf or an insect's wing; these veins collectively.—**venational** adj.

vend /vend/ vt to sell, to offer for sale; to peddle; (rare) to state or disseminate (an opinion, etc).

vendace /ˈvenˌdeɪs/ n (pl **vendaces, vendace**) either of two types of small European freshwater fish.

vendee /venˈdiː/ n (law) a buyer; someone to whom something has been sold.

vendetta /venˈdetə/ n the taking of private vengeance; a feud.—**vendettist** n.

vendible /ˈvendəbəl/ adj saleable; (arch) venal. • n (usu pl) something that is saleable.

vending machine n a coin-operated machine which dispenses goods.

vendor, vender /ˈvendər/ or /-dɔr/ n a seller; a machine that ejects goods, etc, after a required amount of coins has been inserted.

veneer /vəˈniːr/ n an overlay of fine wood or plastic; a superficial appearance. • vt to cover with veneer.

venerable /ˈvenərəbəl/ adj worthy of reverence or respect.—**venerability** n.—**venerably** adv.

venerate /ˈvenəˌreɪt/ vt to revere; to respect.—**venerator** n.

veneration /ˌvenəˈreɪʃən/ n a venerating or being venerated; respect mingled with awe, deep reverence.

venereal /vəˈnɪːriəl/ adj (disease) resulting from sexual intercourse.

venereal disease n any of various diseases, such as syphilis or AIDS, transmitted by sexual contact.—also **sexually transmitted disease**.

venery[1] /ˈvenəri/ n (arch) hunting, usu with hounds, the chase.

venery[2] n (arch) sexual indulgence, the pursuit of sexual gratification.

venesection /ˈviːnəˌsekʃən/ n the operation of opening a vein; phlebotomy.

Venetian blind n a window blind formed of long thin horizontal slips of wood that can be pivoted.

vengeance /ˈvendʒəns/ n the act of taking revenge; retribution; **with a vengeance** to a high degree; and no mistake.

vengeful /ˈvendʒful/ adj bent on vengeance; vindictive.—**vengefully** adv **vengefulness** n.

venial /ˈviːniəl/ adj (sin) forgivable, excusable, not very wrong; (sin) not entailing damnation.—**veniality** n.—**venially** adv.

venison /ˈvenɪsən/ or /-zən/ n the edible flesh of the deer.

Venite /vɪˈnaɪti/ n (Anglican church) the 95th Psalm, used as a canticle at Matins; the music for this.

venom /ˈvenəm/ n the poison of a snake, wasp, etc; spite, malice, rancour.

venomous /ˈvenəməs/ adj secreting venom; malicious, spiteful.—**venomously** adv.—**venomousness** n.

venose /ˈviːnoʊs/ adj having many veins, veiny; venous; (plant) with a surface of vein-like ridges.

venosity /vɪˈnɒsəti/ n the state of being abnormally venose; (blood vessels, organs) the condition of containing too much blood.

venous /ˈviːnəs/ adj pertaining to, contained in, or consisting of veins or blood.—**venously** adv.—**venousness** n.

vent[1] /vent/ n a small opening or slit; an outlet or flue for the escape of fumes. • vt to release; (temper) to give expression to.—**venter** n

vent[2] n a slit in the back of a coat, often forming a flap; an opening in a battlemented wall.

ventage /ˈventɪdʒ/ n a finger-hole of a flute or similar instrument; a small opening, an outlet.

ventail /ˈvenˌteɪl/ n the part of a helmet protecting the lower part of the face.

venter /ˈventər/ n (anat, zool) the belly or abdomen of vertebrates; the part of a muscle that swells outwards; (bot) the swollen base of that part of some plants containing the egg cell; (law) the womb.

ventilate /ˈventɪˌleɪt/ vt to supply with fresh air; to oxygenate (the blood); to make public to submit to discussion.—**ventilative** adj.

ventilation /ˌventɪˈleɪʃən/ n the act of ventilating; the state of being ventilated; free discussion.

ventilator /ˈventɪˌleɪtər/ n an appliance for ventilating a room, etc; (med) a device for enabling a patient to breathe normally.

ventral /ˈventrəl/ adj (anat) of or on the belly, abdominal; (bot) of, pertaining to, or located on that part of a plant facing towards the stem, esp a leaf.

ventricle /ˈventrɪkəl/ n a small cavity; one of the lower chambers of the heart, which pumps blood; one of the four cavities of the brain.—**ventricular** adj.

ventricose, ventricous /ˈventrɪˌkoʊs/ adj (biol) swelling, esp on one side only.—**ventricosity** n.

ventriloquism /venˈtrɪləˌkwɪzəm/, **ventriloquy** /venˈtrɪləkwi/ n the act or art of speaking so that the sounds appear to come from a source other than the actual speaker.—**ventriloquial** adj.—**ventriloquist** n.—**ventriloquistic** adj.

ventriloquize /venˈtrɪləˌkwaɪz/ vi to practise ventriloquism.

venture /ˈventʃər/ n a dangerous expedition; a risky undertaking. • vti to risk; to dare.—**venturer** n.

venture capital n capital available for investment in risky but potentially very profitable enterprises and repayable at higher than normal interest rates, risk capital.

venturesome /ˈventʃərsəm/ adj daring, rash; risky, hazardous.—**venturesomely** adv.—**venturesomeness** n.

venue /ˈvenjuː/ n the place of an action or event.

Venus /ˈviːnəs/ n (Roman myth) the goddess of love; (astron) the planet second from the sun, that can sometimes be seen as a bright star in the morning or evening; a beautiful woman.

veracious /vəˈreɪʃəs/ adj observant of the truth, truthful; honest; true, accurate.—**veraciously** adv.—**veraciousness** n.

veracity /vəˈræsɪti/ n (pl **veracities**) habitual observance of the truth; correspondence with the truth or facts; a truthful statement, a truth.

veranda, verandah /vəˈrændə/ n a roofed porch, supported by light pillars.

veratrine /ˈverəˌtriːn/ or /-trɪn/ n a poisonous mixture of alkaloids from plants of the hellebore family, formerly used medically, to relieve neuralgia or as a counter-irritant.

verb /vərb/ n (gram) the part of speech that expresses an action, a process, state or condition or mode of being.

verbal /'vərbəl/ adj of, concerned with or expressed in words; spoken, not written; literal; (gram) of, pertaining to or characteristic of a verb.—**verbally** adv.

verbalism /'vərbə,lızəm/ n something expressed in words; a word or phrase; excessive attention to wording rather than content; meaningless phrases or sentences resulting from this.

verbalist /,vərbə'lıst/ n one skilled with words; one who concentrates on words rather than content.—**verbalistic** adj.

verbalize /'vərbə,laız/ vt to put into words; to make into a verb.—**verbalization** n.

verbatim /vər'beıtım/ adj, adv word for word.

verbena /vər'bi:nə/ n any of various kinds of ornamental fragrant plant, usu found in America, with red, white or purple flowers; any similar type of plant.

verbiage /'vərbiədʒ/ n more words than are needed for clarity, wordiness; the use of too many words.

verbify /'vərbə,faı/ vti (**verbifying, verbified**) to convert (a noun, etc) into a verb; to be verbose.

verbose /vər'bo:s/ adj using more words than are necessary; overloaded with words.—**verbosely** adv.—**verbosity** n.

verdant /'vərdənt/ adj (grass, foliage) green and fresh; covered with grass; inexperienced, gullible.—**verdancy** n.—**verdantly** adv.

verderer /'vərdərər/ n (formerly) in England, an official who had charge of the royal forests and was responsible for maintaining peace in them.

verdict /'vərdıkt/ n the decision of a jury at the end of a trial; decision, judgment.

verdigris /'vərdıgrıs/ or /-,gri:s/ n a greenish deposit that forms on copper or brass.

verdure /'vərdjər/ or /-dʒər/ n green vegetation; greenness; freshness; the freshness and healthy growth of vegetation.—**verdurous** adj.—**verdurousness** n.

verge[1] /vərdʒ/ n the brink; the extreme edge or margin; a grass border beside a road; a staff or wand as an emblem of office; the spindle of a watch balance; (archit) a projecting edge of roof tiles or slates.

verge[2] vi to incline, descend; (with **on**) to border on, to be on the verge of.

verger /'vərdʒər/ n an official who has care of the interior of a church; a staff bearer of a bishop, etc.

veridical /və'rıdıkəl/ adj truthful, veracious; (psychol) of or pertaining to events in dreams that in retrospect appear to have foretold the future.

verifiable /,verı'faıəbəl/ adj capable of being verified.—**verifiability** n.

verification /,verıfı'keıʃən/ n the act of proving to be true; confirmation; the state of being verified; a marshalling of facts, etc that proves the truth of, eg a theory; (law) (formerly) a short affidavit at the end of a pleading indicating that the pleader is willing to supply proof.

verify /'verıfaı/ vt (**verifying, verified**) to confirm the truth of, to check; to substantiate, to bear out; (law) to authenticate or support by proofs.—**verifiable** adj.—**verification** n.—**verifier** n.

verily /'verıli/ adv (arch) in truth, certainly.

verisimilitude /,verısı'mılı,tu:d/ or /-,tju:d/ n the appearance of truth, probability.—**verisimilar** adj.

verismo /ve'rızmo:/ n a type of opera concerned with representing contemporary life of ordinary people in an honest and realistic way.

veritable /'verıtəbəl/ adj real, genuine.—**veritably** adv.

verity /'verıti/ n (pl **verities**) the quality or state of being true; a truth; a true fact, reality.

verjuice /'vərdʒu:s/ n an acidic liquor expressed from unripe grapes, apples, etc, formerly used in sauces; sourness, tartness.

vermeil /'vərmeıl/ or /-mıl/ n silver-gilt, or any other metal gilded; (poet) vermilion. • adj of a bright red colour.

vermicelli /,vərmı'tʃeli/ n a pasta similar to spaghetti but in finer strings.

vermicide /'vərmı,saıd/ n a substance for killing worms.—**vermicidal** adj.

vermicular /vərmıkjulər/ adj vermiform; vermiculate; wormlike; pertaining to or caused by worms.

vermiculate /vər'mıkjulət/ adj moving like a worm; worm-eaten; adorned with wavy lines; (thoughts) constantly recurring, casuistic. • vt to mark with close wavy lines.—**vermiculation** n.

vermiform /'vərmı,fɔrm/ adj worm-shaped.

vermiform appendix n the worm-shaped structure attached to the caecum vestigially in humans and certain other mammals, the appendix.

vermifuge /'vərmı,fju:dʒ/ n a drug, etc, that expels intestinal worms.

vermilion, vermillion /vər'mıljən/ n a bright scarlet colour. • adj of this colour.

vermin /'vərmın/ n (used as pl) pests, such as insects and rodents; persons dangerous to society.

vermination /,vərmı'neıʃən/ n the breeding or spread of vermin, worms or larvae; infestation with vermin, worms or larvae.

verminous /'vərmınəs/ adj infested with, caused by, or like vermin.

vermouth /vər'mu:θ/ n a white wine flavoured with herbs, used in cocktails and as an aperitif.

vernacular /vər'nækjulər/ n the commonly spoken language or dialect of a country or region. • adj native.—**vernacularly** adv.

vernacularism /-ızəm/ n vernacular usage; a vernacular word or expression.

vernal /'vərnəl/ adj of, appearing in, relating to, or suggestive of the spring.—**vernally** adv.

vernation /vər'neıʃən/ n (bot) the arrangement of leaves within a bud.

vernier /'vərniər/ n a small sliding scale attached to a larger fixed scale, with gradations to indicate minute subdivisions of the smallest divisions on the main fixed scale; an additional apparatus used to finetune or adjust an instrument. • adj of, pertaining to, or having a vernier.

Veronal /'verənəl/ (trademark) n a sedative or hypnotic drug; barbitone.

veronica[1] /və'rɒnıkə/ n any of several plants with blue, pink or white flowers, incl speedwell.

veronica[2] n (RC Church) the image of Christ's face that in legend appeared on a handkerchief given to him by St Veronica as he went to his crucifixion; this handkerchief; any similar image of Christ's face on a cloth.

veronica[3] n (bullfighting) a manoeuvre by a matador in which he swings the cape slowly before the bull while standing still.

verruca /və'ru:kə/ n (pl **verrucae, verrucas**) a wart on the hand or foot; (biol) a wart-like excrescence.—**verrucose, verrucous** adj.

versatile /'vərsə,taıl/ adj turning readily from one occupation to another, adaptable; talented in many different ways; variable, fickle, changeable; (biol) able to move or turn freely.—**versatilely** adv.—**versatility** n.

verse /vərs/ n a line of poetry; a stanza of a poem; a metrical composition, esp of a light nature; a short section of a chapter in the Bible. • vti to make verses (about).

versed /vərst/ adj skilled or learned in a subject.

versicle /'vərsıkəl/ n a short verse or text sung by priest and congregation alternately in a liturgical service.

versicolour, versicolor /'vərsı,kələr/ adj parti-coloured; changeable in colour, iridescent.

versification /,vərsıfı'keıʃən/ n verse-making; the metre or verses of a poem; the conversion of prose into verse.

versify /'vərsı,faı/ vti (**versifying, versified**) to write poetry or verse; to turn into verse.—**versifier** n.

version /'vərʒən/ n a translation from one language into another; a particular account or description.—**versional** adj.

vers libre /ver'li:brə/ n verse with no regular metrical system; free verse.

verso /'vərso:/ n (pl **versos**) a left-hand, even-numbered page of a book, the back of the recto; the back of a printed sheet; the reverse of a coin.

versus /'vərsəs/ prep against; in contrast to.

vert /vərt/ n (English law) (formerly) the right to collect whatever grows and bears a green leaf in a forest; green vegetation; (her) green.

vert. /vərt/ abbr = vertical.

vertebra /'vərtəbrə/ n (pl **vertebrae, vertebras**) one of the interconnecting bones of the spinal column.—**vertebral** adj.

vertebrate /'vərtə,breıt/ or /-brət/ n an animal with a backbone. • adj having a backbone; of the vertebrates.

vertebration /,vərtə'breıʃən/ n division into vertebrae or vertebrae-like segments.

vertex /'vərteks/ n (pl **vertexes, vertices**) the topmost point; apex; (anat) the crown of the head; (geom) the point at which two sides of a polygon or the planes of a solid intersect.

vertical /'vɜrtɪkəl/ adj perpendicular to the horizon; upright. • n a vertical line or plane.—**verticality** n.—**vertically** adv.

verticil /'vɜrtɪsɪl/ n a whorl-like arrangement of leaves or flowers around a stem.

verticillate /ˌvɜr'tɪsɪlət/ adj (biol) arranged in a whorl-like pattern.—**verticillately** adv.—**verticillation** n.

vertiginous /vɜr'tɪdʒɪnəs/ adj revolving, rotary; giddy; causing giddiness; whirling.—**vertiginously** adv.—**vertiginousness** n.

vertigo /'vɜrtɪgoʊ/ n (pl vertigoes, vertigines) a sensation of dizziness and sickness caused by a disorder of the sense of balance.—**vertiginous** adj.

vertu /vɜr'tuː/ or /'vɜr,tuː/ see virtu.

vervain /'vɜrveɪn/ n a perennial European with clusters of tiny bluish-purple flowers.

verve /vɜrv/ n enthusiasm; liveliness; energy.

vervet /'vɜrvət/ n a small African monkey with dark hands and feet and yellowish or greenish coat.

very /'vɛri/ adj complete; absolute; same. • adv extremely; truly; really.

Very light n a coloured flare fired from a Very pistol as a signal at sea or to give temporary light.

vesica /'vɛsɪkə/ n (pl vesicae) (anat) the bladder, esp the urinary bladder; (art) a pointed oval halo used as an aureole in medieval sculpture or painting.—**vesical** adj.

vesicant /'vɛsɪkənt/, vesicatory /'vɛsɪkəˌtɔri/ n (pl vesicants, vesicatories) a substance (eg mustard gas) that causes blistering, with applications in chemical warfare. • adj raising blisters.

vesicate /'vɛsɪˌkeɪt/ vt to raise blisters on. • vi to become blistered.—**vesication** n.

vesicle /'vɛsɪkəl/ n a small blister; a small cyst or sac; (anat) a bladder-like vessel or cavity, esp one filled with serous fluid; (geol) a cavity in rock formed by gases during solidification; (bot) a small sac found in some seaweeds and aquatic plants.—**vesicular** adj.

vesper /'vɛspər/ n (arch) evening; (with cap) the evening star; (Anglican Church) evensong; (RC Church) the sixth of the canonical hours. • adj pertaining to evening or vespers.

vespertine /'vɛspərˌtaɪn/ or /-tɪn/, vespertinal /-əl/ adj of evening; (bot) opening in the evening; (zool) active in the evening; (astron) setting about sunset.

vespiary /'vɛspiˌɛri/ n (pl vespiaries) a nest of wasps or hornets.

vespine /'vɛspaɪn/ adj of, pertaining to, or like a wasp or wasps.

vessel /'vɛsəl/ n a container; a ship or boat; a tube in the body along which fluids pass.

vest /vɛst/ n a sleeveless undergarment worn next to the skin, a singlet; a waistcoat. • vt to place or settle (power, authority, etc.); (with in) to confer or be conferred on; to invest with a right to.

Vesta /'vɛstə/ n (astron) a bright asteroid; (Roman myth) the goddess of the hearth and the household fire.

vesta /'vɛstə/ n a short match of wax or wood, lit by friction.

vestal /'vɛstəl/ adj pertaining to or sacred to the goddess Vesta; vowed to chastity, pure. • n a vestal virgin; a virgin.

vestal virgin n one of the six virgin priestesses who tended the sacred fire on the altar of the temple of Vesta, in ancient Rome.

vested /'vɛstəd/ adj (law) having permanent entitlement to the possession or use of property, now and in the future, ratified by law or custom; (priest, etc) clothed in ecclesiastical vestments.

vested interest n (law) a permanent entitlement to the possession and use of property, now and in the future; a strong reason for acting in a certain way, usu for personal gain; (usu pl) people in such a state.

vestibule /'vɛstɪˌbjuːl/ n an entrance hall or lobby; a covered entrance at the end of a rail carriage; (anat) a communicating channel.—**vestibular** adj.

vestige /'vɛstɪdʒ/ n a hint; a trace; a rudimentary survival of a former organ; a particle.—**vestigial** adj.—**vestigially** adv.

vestment /'vɛstmənt/ n a garment or robe, esp that worn by a priest or official.—**vestmental** adj.

vestry /'vɛstri/ n (pl vestries) a room in a church where vestments, etc, are kept and parochial meetings held; a meeting for parish business.—**vestral** adj.

vestryman /'vɛstrimən/ n (pl vestrymen) a member of a vestry elected by the parishioners.

vesture /'vɛstʃər/ n (arch) clothing; something that clothes, a covering; (law) everything growing on someone's land apart from trees; something obtained from land, such as wheat. • (arch) vt to clothe.

vesuvianite /və'suːviəˌnaɪt/ n a mineral of a green, brown or yellow colour, similar to the garnet, idocrase.

vet /vɛt/ n a veterinary surgeon. • vt (vetting, vetted) to examine, check for errors, etc.

vetch /vɛtʃ/ n a common leguminous climbing plant with blue or purple flowers and a stem with tendrils, found in temperate climates and used for green fodder; any similar plant.

vetchling /'vɛtʃlɪŋ/ n a climbing plant like a vetch mainly found in northern temperate regions with angled or winged stems with tendrils and gaudy flowers.

veteran /'vɛtərən/ or /'vɛtrən/ adj old, experienced; having served in the armed forces. • n a person who has served in the armed forces; a person who has given long service in a particular activity.

veterinary /'vɛtrɪˌnɛri/ or /'vɛtərɪ-/ adj of or dealing with diseases of domestic animals.

veterinarian /ˌvɛtrɪ'nɛriən/ or /ˌvɛtərɪ-/, veterinary surgeon n a person trained in treating sick or injured animals.

veto /'viːtoʊ/ n (pl vetoes) the right of a person or group to prohibit an action or legislation; a prohibition. • vt (vetoing, vetoed) to refuse to agree to; to prohibit.—**vetoer** n.

vex /vɛks/ vt to annoy; to puzzle, confuse.—**vexer** n.—**vexingly** adv.

vexation /vɛk'seɪʃən/ n a vexing or being vexed; an annoying thing; irritation, distress.

vexatious /vɛk'seɪʃəs/ adj causing vexation; annoying; troublesome; harassing; (litigation) designed merely to annoy.—**vexatiously** adv.

vexed /vɛkst/ adj annoyed; (question) much debated.—**vexedly** adv.—**vexedness** n.

vexillum /vɛk'sɪləm/ n (pl vexilla) (bot) the largest petal found on flowers of the plant family to which the sweet pea and similar plants belong; (zool) the vane of a feather.

VHF abbr = very high frequency.

via /'viːə/ or /'vaɪə/ prep by way of.

viable /'vaɪəbəl/ adj capable of growing or developing; workable; practicable.—**viability** n.—**viably** adv.

viaduct /'vaɪəˌdʌkt/ n a road or railway carried by a bridge with arches over a valley, river, etc.

vial /'vaɪəl/ n a small bottle for medicines, etc; a phial.

via media /ˌviːə'miːdiə/ or /-'miːdiə/, /ˌvaɪə-/ n a middle course between extremes; a compromise.

viand /'vaɪənd/ n an article of food. (pl) meat ready to be cooked; food.

viaticum /vaɪ'ætɪkəm/ n (pl viatica, viaticums) (RC Church) the Eucharist administered to someone whose death is or might be imminent; (rare) an allowance or provisions given to a person setting out on a journey.

vibes /vaɪbz/ npl (sl) vibrations; vibraphone.

vibraculum /vaɪ'brækjʊləm/ n (pl vibracula) (zool) a whip-like appendage by which some polyzoans ward off parasites.

vibrant /'vaɪbrənt/ adj vibrating; resonant; bright; lively.—**vibrancy** n.—**vibrantly** adv.

vibraphone /'vaɪbrəˌfoʊn/ n a percussion instrument that produces a vibrato by resonating metal bars.—**vibraphonist** n.

vibrate /'vaɪbreɪt/ vti to shake; to move quickly backwards and forwards; to quiver; to oscillate; to resound.—**vibratingly** adv.

vibratile /'vaɪbrəˌtaɪl/ adj capable of or characterized by vibrating.—**vibratility** n.

vibration /vaɪ'breɪʃən/ n a vibrating or being vibrated; oscillation; resonance; vacillation; (usu pl) an emotional reaction instinctively sensed; (physics) the rapid alternating of particles caused by the disturbance of equilibrium.—**vibrational** adj.

vibrative /'vaɪbrəˌtɪv/ adj vibratory.

vibrato /vɪ'brɑːtoʊ/ n (pl vibratos) (mus) a pulsating effect obtained by rapid variation of emphasis on the same tone.

vibrator /'vaɪbreɪtər/ n the vibrating part in various instruments; a dildo.

vibratory /'vaɪbrəˌtɔri/ adj vibrating; consisting of or causing vibrations.

vibrio /'vɪbrioʊ/ n (pl vibrios) a spiral or curved, rod-like bacillus.—**vibrioid** adj.

vibrissa /vaɪ'brɪsə/ n (pl vibrissae) a sensitive whisker on an animal's face; any of the bristle-like feathers found in the beak area of certain insect-eating birds.

viburnum /vaɪ'bɜrnəm/ n any of several shrubs or trees, incl the guelder rose, with red or black berry-like fruits, found in various temperate and sub-tropical regions; the dried bark from some of these, sometimes used medicinally.

vicar /ˈvɪkər/ *n* a parish priest; a clergyman in charge of a chapel.

vicarage /ˈvɪkərɪdʒ/ *n* the residence of a vicar.

vicarial /vəˈkɛrɪəl/ *adj* of, pertaining to, or acting as a vicar, vicars or a vicariate; (*ecclesiastical functions*) delegated, vicarious.

vicariate, vicarate /vəˈkɛrɪət/ *n* the rank, office, or district of a vicar.

vicarious /vɪˈkɛrɪəs/ or /vaɪ-/ *adj* substitute; obtained second-hand by listening to or watching another person's experiences.—**vicariously** *adv.*—**vicariousness** *n.*

vice[1] /vaɪs/ *n* an evil action or habit; a grave moral fault; great wickedness; a serious defect, a blemish.

vice[2] *n* a clamping device with jaws, used for holding objects firmly.—*also* **vise.**

vice- /vaɪs/ *prefix* one who acts in place of or as a deputy to another.

vice admiral /vaɪsˈædmərəl/ *n* a rank of naval officer next below admiral.

vice-chairman *n* (*pl* **vice-chairmen**) one who takes the chair in a chairman's absence.

vice chancellor /vaɪsˈtʃænsələr/ *n* the chief executive officer of a university.

vice consul *n* a person who acts in place of a consul in a subordinate district, etc.

vicegerent /vaɪsˈdʒɛrənt/ *n adj* a person holding delegated power or ruling as another's deputy.—*also adj.*—**vicegerency** *n.*

vicennial /vaɪˈsɛnɪəl/ *adj* lasting twenty years; happening every twenty years.

vice president /vaɪsˈprɛzɪdənt/ *n* a deputy or assistant president.

viceregal /vaɪsˈriːgəl/ *adj* of or relating to a viceroy; (*Austral, NZ*) of or relating to a governor general.

vicereine /ˈvaɪsreɪn/ *n* a viceroy's wife.

viceroy /ˈvaɪsrɔɪ/ *n* one who rules a country or province as a representative of a king or queen.

viceroyalty /-ˈrɔɪəlti/, **viceroyship** /-ʃɪp/ *n* (*pl* **viceroyalties, viceroyships**) the office or term of a viceroy.

vice versa /ˌvaɪsˈvɜrsə/ or /ˌvaɪsə-/ *adv* conversely; the other way round.

vichyssoise /ˌviːʃiːˈswɒz/ or /ˈvɪ-/ *n* leek and potato soup consumed cold.

Vichy water /ˈviːʃiː/ *n* a mineral water from Vichy in France.

vicinage /ˈvɪsɪnədʒ/ *n* a surrounding district, a neighbourhood; the people of a neighbourhood; proximity.

vicinal /ˈvɪsɪnəl/ *adj* neighbouring; adjacent; (*chem*) resembling or substituting for a crystal face or form; denoting substituted atoms on adjacent atoms in a molecule.

vicinity /vəˈsɪnɪti/ *n* (*pl* **vicinities**) a nearby area; proximity.

vicious /ˈvɪʃəs/ *adj* cruel; violent; malicious; ferocious.—**viciously** *adv.*—**viciousness** *n.*

vicissitude /vɪˈsɪsɪˌtuːd/ or /-ˌtjuːd/ *n* a change of circumstances or fortune; (*pl*) ups and downs.—**vicissitudinary, vicissitudinous** *adj.*

victim /ˈvɪktəm/ or /-tɪm/ *n* a person who has been killed or injured by an action beyond his or her control; a dupe.

victimize /-ˌaɪz/ or /-tɪm-/ *vt* to make a victim of, to cause to suffer.—**victimization** *n.*—**victimizer** *n.*

victor /ˈvɪktər/ *n* a winner; a conqueror.

victoria /vɪkˈtɔːrɪə/ *n* a light, open, four-wheeled, two-seater carriage; a giant South American water-lily; a victoria plum.

Victoria Day *n* ✤ (*Cdn*) a public holiday celebrated on the Monday on or preceding May 25.

Victorian /vɪkˈtɔːrɪən/ *adj* of or living in the reign of Queen Victoria; old-fashioned; prudish.

victoria plum *n* a large purplish-red sweet variety of plum.

victorious /vɪkˈtɔːrɪəs/ *adj* having won in battle or contest; emblematic of victory; triumphant.—**victoriously** *adv.*

victory /ˈvɪktəri/ *n* (*pl* **victories**) triumph in battle; success; achievement.

victual /ˈvɪtəl/ *n* (*usu pl*) food, provisions. • *vt* (**victualling, victualled** *or* **victualing, victualed**) to supply with food; to take in provisions.

victualler, victualer /ˈvɪtlər/ *n* (*formerly*) a supplier of provisions, *esp* to an army; a provision ship; an innkeeper.

vicuña, vicuna /vɪˈkjuːnə/ *n* a South American animal similar to the llama with a fine, long, reddish silky fleece; cloth made from this fleece.

vide /ˈviːdeɪ/ (*Latin*) see.

vide infra /ˈɪnfrə/ (*Latin*) see later (in this book).

videlicet /vəˈdɛlɪˌsɛt/ *adv* that is to say, namely.

video /ˈvɪdɪoː/ *n* (*pl* **videos**) the transmission or recording of television programmes or films, using a television set and a video recorder and tape. • *vt* (**videoing, videoed**) to record on video tape.

video cassette *n* a cassette containing video tape.

video recorder *n* the machine on which video cassettes are played or recorded.

video tape /ˈvɪdɪoːteɪp/ *n* a magnetic tape on which images and sounds can be recorded for reproduction on television.—**video-tape** *vt.*

vide supra /ˈviːdeɪˈsuːprə/ (*Latin*) see earlier (in this book).

vidette /vɪˈdɛt/ *see* **vedette.**

vidkid /ˈvɪdˈkɪd/ *n* a child who is addicted to watching television or video.

vie /vaɪ/ *vi* (**vying, vied**) to contend or strive for superiority.—**vier** *n.*

view /vjuː/ *n* sight; range of vision; inspection, examination; intention; scene; opinion. • *vt* to see; to consider; to examine intellectually.

viewer /ˈvjuːər/ *n* a person who views, *esp* television; an optical device used in viewing.

viewfinder /ˈvjuːˌfaɪndər/ *n* a device in a camera showing the view to be photographed.

viewless /ˈvjuːləs/ *adj* without a view; (*poet*) invisible, unseen.

viewpoint /ˈvjuːpɔɪnt/ *n* opinion; a place from which something can be viewed, *esp* a scenic panorama.

vigil /ˈvɪdʒəl/ *n* keeping watch at night.

vigilance /ˈvɪdʒələns/ *n* a being vigilant; watchfulness; alertness.

vigilant /ˈvɪdʒələnt/ *adj* on the watch to discover and avoid danger, watchful; alert; cautious.—**vigilantly** *adv.*

vigilante /vɪdʒəˈlænti/ *n* a self-appointed law enforcer.

vignette /vɪnˈjɛt/ *n* a small picture or design in a book without a line framing it; a picture, the edges of which shade off gradually into the background; a short word sketch. • *vt* to depict in vignette; to shade off into the background.—**vignettist** *n.*

vigor /ˈvɪgər/ *see* **vigour.**

vigoroso /ˌvɪgəˈroːsoː/ or It. /ˌvɪgəˈrosə/ *adv* (*mus*) with vigour.

vigorous /ˈvɪgərəs/ *adj* full of vigour; powerful; lusty.—**vigorously** *adv.*—**vigorousness** *n.*

vigour /ˈvɪgər/ *n* physical or mental strength; vitality.—*also* **vigor.**

Viking /ˈvaɪkɪŋ/ *n* one of the Norse pirates who ravaged the coasts of Europe from the 8th–10th centuries.

vilayet /ˈviːləˌjɛt/ *n* a province of Turkey.

vile /vaɪl/ *adj* wicked; evil; offensive; very bad.—**vilely** *adv.*—**vileness** *n.*

vilify /ˈvɪləˌfaɪ/ *vt* (**vilifying, vilified**) to malign.—**vilification** *n.*—**vilifier** *n.*

villa /ˈvɪːlə/ *n* a large country or suburban house.

village /ˈvɪlədʒ/ *n* a collection of houses smaller than a town.

villager /-ər/ *n* an inhabitant of a village.

villain /ˈvɪlən/ *n* a scoundrel; the main evil character in a play, film or novel; (*arch*) a boor.

villainous /-əs/ *adj* depraved, evil, wicked; very bad, wretched.—**villainously** *adv.*—**villainousness** *n.*

villainy /-i/ *n* (*pl* **villainies**) great wickedness; an atrocious crime.

villanella /ˌvɪləˈnɛlə/ *n* (*pl* **villanelle**) a popular part-song of 17th-century Italy.

villanelle /ˌvɪləˈnɛl/ *n* a poem of 19 lines in six stanzas rhymed aba aba aba aba aba abaa, the 6th, 12th and 18th lines being the same as the first, and the 9th, 15th and 19th the same as the third.

villein /ˈvɪlən/ *n* (*hist*) a feudal tenant of the lowest class, a serf.

villi /ˈvɪlˌaɪ/ *see* **villus.**

villous, villose /ˈvɪləus/ *adj* covered with villi; (*bot*) covered with long, thin, soft hairs.

villus /ˈvɪləs/ *n* (*pl* **villi**) (*biol*) the velvety fibre of the mucous membrane of the intestine; (*bot*) the soft hair covering a fruit or flower.—**villosity.**

vim /vɪm/ *n* (*sl*) energy, force.

vimineous /vəˈmɪnɪəs/ *adj* (*bot*) of or producing long flexible shoots.

vina /ˈviːˌnɒ/ *n* a seven-stringed Indian musical instrument.

vinaceous /vaɪˈneɪʃəs/ *adj* of the colour of wine; wine-red.

vinaigrette /ˌvɪnəˈgrɛt/ *n* a salad dressing made from oil, vinegar and seasoning.

vincible /'vɪnsəbəl/ *adj* capable of being conquered or overcome.—**vincibility** *n*.

vinculum /'vɪŋkjʊləm/ *n* (*pl* **vincula**) (*anat*) a ligament; (*math*) a horizontal line over quantities having the effect of a parenthesis; (*print*) a brace; a bond of union, a tie.

vindicate /'vɪndɪˌkeɪt/ *vt* to establish the existence or truth of, to justify; to clear of charges, to absolve from blame.—**vindicable** *adj*.—**vindicator** *n*.—**vindicatory** *adj*.

vindication /-'keɪʃən/ *n* a vindicating or being vindicated; an event, fact, evidence, etc, that justifies a deed or claim.

vindictive /vɪn'dɪktɪv/ *adj* vengeful; spiteful; (*damages*) exemplary, punitive.—**vindictively** *adv*.—**vindictiveness** *n*.

vine /'vaɪn/ *n* any climbing plant, or its stem; a grapevine; a sphere of activity, *esp* spiritual or mental endeavour.

vinedresser /'vaɪnˌdresər/ *n* a person who cultivates vines.

vinegar /'vɪnəgər/ *n* a sour-tasting liquid containing acetic acid, used as a condiment and preservative.

vinegary /'vɪnəgəri/ *adj* of or like vinegar; sour; ill-tempered.

vinery /'vaɪnəri/ *n* (*pl* **vineries**) a place where grapes are grown or wine is made.

vineyard /'vɪnjərd/ *n* a plantation of grapevines.

vingt-et-un *Fr.* /vætei'œ̃/ *n* a gambling game with cards in which players try to obtain points better than the banker's but not more than 21.—*also* **blackjack, pontoon, twenty-one**.

vinic /'vaɪnɪk/ or /'vɪnɪk/ *adj* contained in or obtained from wine.

viniculture /'vɪnɪˌkeltʃər/ *n* the cultivation of vines and manufacture of wine, viticulture.—**vinicultural** *adj*.—**viniculturist** *n*.

viniferous /vaɪ'nɪfərəs/ *adj* wine-producing.

vinificator /ˌvɪnəfɪ'keɪtər/ *n* in winemaking, an apparatus for collecting alcoholic vapours.

vin ordinaire *Fr.* /ˌvæ ɔrdɪ'ner/ *n* (*pl* **vins ordinaires**) the ordinary table wine of France.

vinous /'vaɪnəs/ *adj* of, pertaining to, or having the qualities of wine; like wine; wine-coloured; inspired by wine.—**vinosity** *n*.

vintage /'vɪntədʒ/ *n* the grape harvest of one season; wine, *esp* of good quality, made in a particular year; wine of a particular region; the product of a particular period. • *adj* (*cars*) classic; (*wine*) of a specified year and of good quality; (*play*) characteristic of the best.

vintager /'vɪntədʒər/ *n* a gatherer of grapes in a wine harvest.

vintner /'vɪntnər/ *n* a wine merchant.

vinyl /'vaɪnl/ *n* a strong plastic used in floor coverings, furniture and records, etc.

viol /'vaɪəl/ *n* a family of medieval six-stringed instruments played with a bow, similar to a violin but with a softer sound.

viola[1] /vɪ'oːlə/ *n* a stringed instrument of the violin family, and tuned a fifth below it.

viola[2] /vaɪoːlə/ or /vi:-/ *n* any of several plants of the genus that includes violets and pansies.

violable /'vaɪələbəl/ *adj* capable of being violated or broken.

violaceous /ˌvaɪə'leɪʃəs/ *adj* of violet colour or family.

viola da gamba /vi:ələ'gæmbə/ *n* the bass viol.

viola d'amore /vi:oːlədæ'mɔreɪ/ *n* a tenor viol with seven strings and a sweet tone.

violate /'vaɪəˌleɪt/ *vt* to break or infringe (an agreement); to rape; to disturb (one's privacy).—**violative** *adj*.—**violator** *n*.

violation /-'leɪʃən/ *n* the act of violating, infringing, or injuring; rape; outrage; an act of irreverence or profanation.

violence /'vaɪələns/ *n* physical force intended to cause injury or destruction; natural force; passion, intensity.

violent /'vaɪələnt/ *adj* urged or driven by force; vehement; impetuous; forcible; furious; severe.—**violently** *adv*.

violet /'vaɪələt/ or /'vaɪlət/ *n* a small plant with bluish-purple flowers; a bluish-purple colour.

violin /ˌvaɪə'lɪn/ *n* a four-stringed musical instrument, played with a bow.

violinist /-ɪst/ *n* a person who plays the violin.

violist /vi'oːləst/ *n* a player of a viol or viola.

violoncellist /ˌvi:ə,lɒn'tʃelɪst/ or /ˌvaɪə-/ *n* a performer on the violoncello.

violoncello /ˌvi:ələn'tʃeloː/ *n* (*pl* **violoncellos**) the full name for a **cello**.

violone /vjo:'lo:neɪ/ *n* the largest type of viol, corresponding to the double-bass.

VIP /ˌvi:aɪ'pi:/ *abbr* = Very Important Person.

viper /'vaɪpər/ *n* a common European venomous snake.—**viperine** *adj*.

viperous /-əs/, **viperish** /-ɪʃ/ *adj* viper-like; malignant.

virago /vɪ'rɑːgoː/ or /-'reɪgoː/ *n* (*pl* **viragoes, viragos**) a bad-tempered woman.

viral /'vaɪrəl/ *adj* of or caused by a virus.

virelay, virelai /'vɪrəˌleɪ/ *n* an old French form of poem with short lines and two rhymes variously arranged.

vireo /'vɪrioː/ *n* (*pl* **vireos**) a small greenish American singing bird.

virescence /vɪr'esəns/ *n* the state of being virescent, *esp* in place of the normal colour of petals.

virescent /vaɪ'resənt/ or /vɪ-/ *adj* beginning to be green; greenish.

virgate[1] /'vərgət/ *adj* (*bot*) slim and straight.

virgate[2] *n* an old English unit of land equal to approx 30 acres.

virgin /'vərdʒɪn/ *n* a person (*esp* a woman) who has never had sexual intercourse; (*with cap*) Mary, the mother of Christ; a painting or statue of her. • *adj* chaste; pure; untouched.

virginal[1] /-əl/ *adj* of or pertaining to a virgin or virginity; befitting a virgin; chaste, pure, innocent; fresh, unsullied, untouched.

virginal[2] *n* a small rectangular keyed musical instrument resembling a harpsichord but without legs.

virginity /vər'dʒɪnɪti/ *n* the state of being a virgin; the state of being chaste, untouched, etc.

Virgo /'vərgoː/ *n* the Virgin, the 6th sign of the zodiac.—**Virgoan** *adj*.

virgo intacta *n* (*pl* **virgines intactae**) (*law*) a girl or woman who is a virgin.

virgulate /'vərgju:lɪt/ or /-ˌleɪt/ *adj* rod-shaped.

virgule /'vərgju:l/ *n* a small rod; a slanting punctuation mark (/), a solidus.

viridescent /ˌvɪrə'desənt/ *adj* greenish; turning green.— **viridescence** *n*.

viridity /və'rɪdəti/ *n* greenness; freshness.

virile /'vɪraɪl/ or /-əl/ *adj* of a mature man, manly; strong, forceful; sexually potent.—**virility** *n*.

virtu /vər'tu:/ *n* a love or knowledge of the fine arts, connoisseurship; artistic excellence, fine workmanship; the quality of appealing to a collector; artistic objects, antiques, curios, etc, collectively.—*also* **vertu**.

virtual /'vərtʃuəl/ *adj* in effect or essence, though not in fact or strict definition; (*comput*) denoting memory, making use of an external memory to increase capacity.

virtually /-i/ or /-tju:-/ *adv* to all intents and purposes, practically.

virtue /'vərtʃu:/ *n* moral excellence; any admirable quality; chastity; merit.

virtuoso /ˌvərtʃu:'oːsoː/ or /-tju:-/, /-zoː/ *n* (*pl* **virtuosos, virtuosi**) a person highly skilled in an activity, *esp* in playing a musical instrument. • *adj* skilled, masterly in technique.—**virtuosic** *adj*.—**virtuosity** *n*.

virtuous /-əs/ or /-tju:əs-/ *adj* righteous; upright; pure.—**virtuously** *adv*.—**virtuousness** *n*.

virulent /'vɪrulənt/ or /'vɪrju/ *adj* (*disease*) deadly; extremely poisonous; hostile; vicious.—**virulence** *n*.—**virulently** *adv*.

virus /'vaɪrəs/ *n* a microorganism capable of causing ill-health; illness caused by virus; (*comput*) an unauthorized computer program which inserts itself into computer systems and causes disruption to existing software.

visa /'vi:zə/ *n* an endorsement on a passport allowing the bearer to travel in the country of the government issuing it. • *vt* (**visaing, visaed**) to mark with a visa; to grant a visa to.

visage /'vɪzɪdʒ/ *n* the face; the countenance; appearance.

visard /'vɪzərd/ *see* **vizard**.

vis-à-vis /ˌvi:zə'vi:/ *prep* opposite to; in face of. • *adj, adv* facing. • *n* the person opposite; a counterpart.

viscacha /vɪs'kæʃə/ *n* a South American burrowing rodent, that looks like a large chinchilla.—*also* **vizcacha**.

viscera /'vɪsərə/ *npl* (*sing* **viscus**) the large internal organs of the animal body, the entrails.

visceral /-l/ *adj* of, pertaining to, or affecting the viscera; pertaining to or touching deeply inward feelings.—**viscerally** *adv*.

viscid /'vɪsɪd/ *adj* (*leaves*) covered with a sticky layer; (*fluids*) thick, glutinous.—**viscidity** *n*.—**viscidly** *adv*.

viscometer /vɪs'kɒmɪtər/, **viscosimeter** /vɪ'skɒsɪ-/ *n* an instrument for measuring viscosity.

viscose /'vɪskoːs/ or /-koːz/ *n* a form of cellulose used in making artificial silk.

viscosity /vɪ'skɒsɪti/ *n* (*pl* **viscosities**) the property or state of being sticky or glutinous; (*physics*) a property of fluids that indicates their resistance to flow.

viscount /'vaɪkaunt/ *n* in Britain, a title of nobility next below an earl.—**viscountess** *nf*.

viscountcy /-si/ *n* (*pl* **viscountcies**) the rank of a viscount.

viscous /'vɪskəs/ *adj* sticky, thick; having viscosity.—**viscously** *adv*.—**viscousness** *n*.

viscus /'vɪskəs/ *see* **viscera**.

vise /vaɪs/ *see* **vice**.

visibility /ˌvɪzɪ'bɪlɪti/ *n* (*pl* **visibilities**) clearness of seeing or being seen; the degree of clearness of the atmosphere.

visible /'vɪzɪbəl/ *adj* able to be seen, perceptible; apparent, evident.—**visibleness** *n*.—**visibly** *adv*.

visible speech *n* a phonetic alphabet representing the actual movements of the vocal organs and used in teaching the deaf.

vision /'vɪʒən/ *n* the power of seeing, sight; a supernatural appearance; a revelation; foresight; imagination; a mental concept; a person, scene, etc of unusual beauty; something seen in a dream or trance.—**visional** *adj*.

visionary /-ˌeri/ *adj* imaginative; having foresight; existing in imagination only, not real. • *n* (*pl* **visionaries**) an imaginative person; a dreamer; an idealist, a mystic.

visit /'vɪzɪt/ *vt* to go to see; to pay a call upon a person or place; to stay with or at; to punish or reward with. • *vi* to see or meet someone regularly. • *n* the act of going to see, a call.—**visitable** *adj*.

visitant /'vɪzɪtənt/ *n* a migratory bird; a visitor, *esp* a pilgrim; a ghost. • *adj* (*arch*) visiting.

visitation /ˌvɪzɪ'teɪʃən/ *n* a visit by a superior; a punitive act of God; an official visit; right of access of a divorced parent to his or her children; a large migration of animals; (*with cap*) the visit paid by the Virgin Mary to Elizabeth (Luke 1:39*ff*); a picture representing the event; the day on which this is commemorated, 2 July.—**visitational** *adj*.

visiting card *n* a small card with a person's name on it, left when paying visits.

visitor /'vɪzɪtər/ *n* a person who visits; a caller; a tourist; a migratory bird pausing in transit; an official acting as an inspector and adviser.

visor /'vaɪzər/ *n* a movable part of a helmet protecting the face; the peak of a cap.—*also* **vizor**.—**visored** *adj*.

vista /'vɪstə/ *n* a view, as from a high place; a mental picture.—**vistaed, vista'd** *adj*.

visual /'vɪʒuəl/ or /'vɪʒj-/ *adj* having, producing, or relating to vision or sight; perceptible, visible; (*knowledge*) attained by sight or vision; (*impressions, etc*) based upon something seen; of the nature of, producing or conveying a picture in the mind; (*physics*) optical. • *n* a piece of graphic material used for display or to convey a concept, etc; (*pl*) the visual aspect of a film, etc.—**visually** *adv*.

visual aid *n* a film, slide or overhead projector, etc used to aid teaching.

visualize /'vɪʒuəˌlaɪz/ *vt* to form a mental picture of; to make visible to the mind or imagination. • *vi* to construct a visual image in the mind.—**visualization** *n*.—**visualizer** *n*.

vital /'vaɪtəl/ *adj* of, connected with or necessary to life; essential; lively, animated; fundamental; (*wound, error*) fatal. • *n* (*pl*) the bodily organs essential for life.—**vitally** *adv*.

vitalism /'vaɪtəˌlɪzəm/ *n* the belief that life cannot be explained as resulting wholly from physical and chemical processes, but must include some other vital non-material force or process.—**vitalist** *n*.—**vitalistic** *adj*.

vitality /vaɪ'tælɪti/ *n* (*pl* **vitalities**) vigour, hold on life; spirits; animation; capacity to last, durability.

vitalize /'vaɪtəˌlaɪz/ *vt* to give life to; to animate; to make vigorous.—**vitalization** *n*.

vital statistics *npl* data recording births, deaths, marriages, etc used in compiling population statistics; (*inf*) the measurements of a woman's figure.

vitamin /'vaɪtəmɪn/ *n* one of several organic substances occurring naturally in foods, which are essential for good health.—**vitaminic** *adj*.

vitellin /vɪ'telɪn/ or /vaɪ-/ *n* a protein forming the major component in the yolk of birds' eggs.

vitelline /vɪ'telaɪn/ or /vaɪ-/, /-lɪn/ *adj* of or pertaining to egg yolk; of a yellow colour close to the shade of egg yolk.

vitiate /'vɪʃiˌeɪt/ *vt* to make faulty or ineffective; to taint; to deprave; to invalidate or annul (a legal document, etc).—**vitiation** *n*.—**vitiator** *n*.

viticulture /'vɪtɪˌkʌltʃər/ *n* the science of grapes and grape-growing.—**viticulturer, viticulturist** *n*.—**viticultural** *adj*.

vitreous /'vɪtriəs/ *adj* of like or obtained from glass; of the vitreous body.—**vitreousness** *n*.

vitreous body, vitreous humour *n* the transparent tissue of the eyeball.

vitrescence /vɪ'tresəns/ *n* the quality of being vitrescent; the process of changing something, such as a crystalline material, into glass.

vitrescent /-ənt/ *adj* capable of being made into or becoming like glass.

vitric /vɪ'trɪk/ *adj* glass-like.

vitrify /'vɪtrɪˌfaɪ/ *vt* (**vitrifying, vitrified**) to convert into glass or a glass-like substance.—**vitrifiable** *adj*.—**vitrification, vitrifaction** *n*.

vitriol /'vɪtriˌɒl/ or /'vɪtriəl/ *n* sulphuric acid; savage criticism. • *vt* (**vitrioling, vitrioled** or **vitriolling, vitriolled**) to throw vitriol over, to poison with vitriol.

vitriolic /ˌvɪtrɪ'ɒlɪk/ *adj* of or relating to vitriol; scathing, bitter.

vitriolize /'vɪtriəˌlaɪz/ *vt* to harm by throwing vitriol over; to change into vitriol; to use vitriol in or as a part of the processing of something.—**vitriolization** *n*.

vitta /'vɪtə/ *n* (*pl* **vittae**) (*bot*) an oil tube in the fruit of some plants, *eg* parsley; (*zool*) a coloured stripe.—**vittate** *adj*.

vituline /'vɪtə/ *adj* of, like, calves or veal.

vituperate /vɪtu:pəˌreɪt/ or /-'tju:/, /vaɪ-/ *vt* to berate; to abuse verbally.—**vituperative** *adj*.—**vituperator** *n*.

vituperation /-'reɪʃən/ *n* the act of vituperating; blame, censure, reproof; the expression of this in abusive or violent language.

viva[1] /'vi:və/ *interj* long live, hurrah for.

viva[2] /'vaɪvə/ *n* in UK, an oral examination, a viva voce. • *vt* (**vivas** or **viva's, vivaing, vivaed** or **viva'd**) to examine orally.

vivace /vɪ'vɒtʃeɪ/ *adv* (*mus*) in a lively manner; with spirit.

vivacious /vɪ'veɪʃəs/ or /vaɪ-/ *adj* lively; animated; spirited.—**vivaciously** *adv*.—**vivaciousness** *n*.

vivacity /vɪ'væsɪti/ *n* (*pl* **vivacities**) vivaciousness; animation of the mind or disposition; liveliness of conception or perception; spirited conduct, manner or speech; brilliancy of light or colour.

vivarium /vaɪ'veriəm/ or /vɪ-/ *n* (*pl* **vivariums, vivaria**) a place for keeping animals in their natural state for research or observation.

viva voce /ˌvi:və'vɒtʃeɪ/ or /'vo:tʃeɪ/ *adj, adv* orally, by word of mouth. • *n* an oral examination, a viva.

vivid /'vɪvɪd/ *adj* brightly coloured; graphic; lively; intense.—**vividly** *adv*.—**vividness** *n*.

vivify /'vɪvɪˌfaɪ/ *vt* (**vivifying, vivified**) to give life to; to make more lively or more vivid.—**vivification** *n*.—**vivifier** *n*.

viviparous /vɪ'vɪpərəs/ *adj* (*zool*) giving birth to young that have developed inside the body, as do most mammals.—**viviparity** *n*.—**viviparously** *adv*.

vivisect /'vɪvɪˌsekt/ or /-'sekt/ *vt* to subject to vivisection.—**vivisector** *n*.

vivisection /ˌvɪvɪ'sekʃən/ *n* the practice of performing surgical operations on living animals for scientific research.—**vivisectional** *adj*.

vivisectionist /-ɪst/ *n* a person who practises or approves of vivisection.

vixen /'vɪksən/ *n* a female fox; a malicious or shrewish woman.—**vixenish** *adj*.

viz. /vɪz/ *abbr* = **videlicet** namely.

vizard /'vɪzərd/ *n* (*arch*) a mask or other object that disguises; a visor.—*also* **visard**.

vizcacha /vɪs'kɒtʃə/ *see* **vischacha**.

vizier, vizir /'vɪziːər/ or /vɪ'ziːr/ *n* a minister of state or high official in Muslim countries, *esp* in the Ottoman Empire.

vizierate /-rət/ *n* the status, authority or (term of) office of a vizier.

vizor /vaɪ'zər/ *see* **visor**.

vocable /'vo:kəbəl/ *n* (*linguistics*) a word looked on as a pattern of characters or sounds with no regard to meaning; a sound; a vowel. • *adj* able to be spoken.

vocabulary /və'kæbjuˌleri/ *n* (*pl* **vocabularies**) an alphabetical list of words with their meanings; the words of a language; an individual's command or use of particular words.

vocal /'vo:kəl/ *adj* of, for, endowed with, relating to, or produced by the voice; outspoken, noisy; (*phonetics*) having a vowel function. • *n* a vowel; (*pl*) music for the voice, not another instrument.—**vocally** *adv*.

vocal chords *npl* either of two pairs of elastic membranous folds in the larynx, *esp* the lower pair, which vibrate and produce sound.

vocalic /vo'kælɪk/ *adj* of, like or containing vowels.

vocalise /vo:kə'li:z/ *n* a vocal exercise to improve flexibility and control of the voice in which a singer sings to one vowel sound.

vocalist /'vo:kəlɪst/ *n* a singer.

vocalize /'vo:kə,laɪz/ *vti* to express with the voice; to articulate, utter distinctly; to use the singing voice; to sing to vowel sounds; to write with vowels or vowel points.—**vocalization** *n*.—**vocalizer** *n*.

vocation /vo'keɪʃən/ *n* a calling to a particular career or occupation, *esp* to a religious life; a sense of fitness for a particular career.

vocational /-əl/ *adj* of or relating to a vocation or occupation; providing special training for a particular career.—**vocationally** *adv*.

vocative /'vɒkətɪv/ *adj* used, involved in or pertaining to loud utterances to attract attention; (*gram*) denoting the case of a noun, adjective, or pronoun used in addressing a person in some inflected languages, *eg* Latin. • *n* (*gram*) a vocative case or form.

vociferant /vo'sɪfər,ənt/ *adj* clamorous, noisy • *n* a clamorous, noisy person.

vociferate /və'sɪfə,reɪt/ *vti* to speak loudly and insistently, to clamour; to shout, to bawl.—**vociferation** *n*.—**vociferator** *n*.

vociferous /vo'sɪfərəs/ *adj* clamorous, noisy.—**vociferously** *adv*.—**vociferousness** *n*.

vodka /'vɒdkə/ *n* a spirit distilled from rye, potatoes, etc.

vogue /vo:g/ *n* the fashion at a specified time; popularity. • *adj* fashionable, in vogue.—**voguish** *adj*.

voice /vɔɪs/ *n* sound from the mouth; sound produced by speaking or singing; the quality of this; the power of speech; utterance; expressed opinion, vote; (*gram*) the forms of a verb showing the relation of subject to action; (*phonetics*) a sound uttered with vibration of the vocal chords not with mere breath. • *vt* to express; to speak; (*mus*) to regulate so as to give the correct tone; (*phonetics*) to utter with the voice, to make sonant.—**voicer** *n*.

voiced /-t/ *adj* having a voice, *esp* of a specified kind, quality or tone; (*phonetics*) uttered with the voice or vibration of the vocal chords, sonant.

voiceful /'vɔɪsful/ *adj* (*poet*) having a voice; sonorous

voiceless /'vɔɪsləs/ *adj* speechless, dumb; (*phonetics*) not voiced.—**voicelessly** *adv*.—**voicelessness** *n*.

voice-over *n* the voice of an unseen narrator, *esp* in a film, TV commercial, etc.

void /vɔɪd/ *adj* unoccupied, empty; not legally binding; having no cards of a particular suit. • *n* an empty space, a vacuum; vacancy, sense of loss. • *vt* to discharge, to emit; empty; to make invalid.—**voidable** *adj*.—**voider** *n*.

voidance /'vɔɪdəns/ *n* the act of voiding or evacuating; emptiness; the annulment of a legal deed.

voided /-'vɔɪdɪd/ *adj* (*her*) having the inner part of a figure cut away, leaving only the outer edges; being, or having been caused to be, empty.

voile /vɔɪl/ or /vwɒl/ *n* a light, sheer fabric of silk, rayon, etc, used for dresses, scarves, etc.

volant /'vo:lənt/ *adj* flying; able to fly; (*her*) appearing to fly; (*poet*) nimble.

Volapuk, Volapük /'vo:lə,puk/ or /'vɒlə-/ *n* an artificial language taking elements from English, French, German, Latin. etc, invented in 1880 and intended for international commercial use.—**Volapukist, Volapükist** *n*.

volar /'vo:lər/ *adj* (*anat*) of the palm of the hand or sole of the foot.

volatile /'vɒlə,taɪl/ *adj* evaporating very quickly; changeable, fickle; unstable; light-hearted, mercurial; flighty; (*comput*) having a memory that loses data when power is disconnected.—**volatility** *n*.

volatilize /və'lætɪ,laɪz/ *vti* to turn into vapour, to (cause to) evaporate.—**volatilization** *n*.

vol-au-vent /'vɒlo:,vɒ̃/ *n* a case of light puff pastry filled with a savoury sauce.

volcanic /vɒl'kænɪk/ *adj* of, like or due to the action of a volcano; violent, intense.—**volcanically** *adv*.

volcanism /'vɒlkənɪzəm/ *n* volcanic action.—*also* **vulcanism**.

volcanize /'vɒlkə,naɪz/ *vt* to subject to volcanic heat; to cause to change by means of volcanic heat.—**volcanization** *n*.

volcano /vɒl'keɪno:/ *n* (*pl* **volcanoes, volcanos**) a hill or mountain formed by ejection of lava, ashes, etc through an opening in the earth's crust.

volcanology /,vɒlkə'nɒlədʒi/ *n* the science of volcanoes and the occurrences associated with them.—*also* **vulcanology**.—**volcanological, vulcanological** *adj*.—**volcanologist, vulcanologist** *n*.

vole[1] /vo:l/ *n* a small rat-like rodent with a short tail.

vole[2] *vt* to win all the tricks in a deal. • *n* a slam.

volitant /'vɒlɪtənt/ *adj* able to fly, volant; flying, or otherwise moving about, in a rapid, nimble fashion.

volition /və'lɪʃən/ *n* the exercise of the will; choice.—**volitional** *adj*.

volitive /'vɒlɪtɪv/ *adj* pertaining to or having the power of will; (*gram*) desiderative; expressing a wish or intention.

volley /'vɒli/ *n* (*pl* **volleys**) the multiple discharge of many missiles or small arms; a barrage; (*tennis, volleyball*) the return of the ball before it reaches the ground. • *vt* (**volleying, volleyed**) to return (a ball) before it hits the ground.—**volleyer** *n*.

volleyball /-,bɔl/ *n* a team game played by hitting a large inflated ball over a net with the hands; the ball used.

volt[1] /vo:lt/ *n* the circular gait of a horse in dressage; (*fencing*) a leap to avoid a thrust.

volt[2] *n* the unit of measure of the force of an electrical current.

volta /'vo:ltə/ or /'vɒl/ *n* (*pl* **volte**) a lively 16th-century Italian dance; (*mus*) music in triple time, originally written to accompany such a dance; (*mus*) a particular time as specified.

voltage /'vo:ltɪdʒ/ *n* electrical energy that moves a charge around a circuit, measured in volts.

voltaic /vɒl'teɪɪk/ *adj* pertaining to electricity generated by chemical action or galvanism; galvanic.

voltaism /'vɒltə,ɪzəm/ *n* galvanism; electricity generated by chemical action.

voltameter /vɒl'tæmɪtər/ *n* an instrument for measuring an electric charge; a coulombmeter.

volte-face /vo:ltə'fæs/ *n* (*pl* **volte-faces, volte-face**) a change to an opposite opinion or direction.

voltmeter /'vo:lt,mi:tər/ *n* an instrument for measuring voltage.

voluble /'vɒljubəl/ *adj* speaking with a great flow of words, fluent; (*arch*) revolving, rotating; (*bot*) twining.—**volubility** *n*.—**volubly** *adv*.

volubleness /'vɒljubəlnəs/ *n* excessive fluency of speech.

volume /'vɒlju:m/ *n* the amount of space occupied by an object; quantity, amount; intensity of sound; a book; one book of a series.—**volumed** *adj*.

volumeter /vo:'lju:mətər/ *n* an instrument for measuring the volume of a gas, liquid, or solid.

volumetric /,vɒlju'metrɪk/ *adj* of or relating to measurement by volume.—**volumetrically** *adv*.

voluminous /və'lu:mɪnəs/ *adj* of great size or bulk; (*writings*) capable of filling many volumes; (*clothes*) ample, loose.—**voluminosity** *n*.—**voluminously** *adv*.

voluntarism /'vɒləntə,rɪzəm/ *n* the theory that the will is dominant over the intellect; a belief in voluntary participation not compulsion in a course of action; voluntaryism.—**voluntaryist** *n*.

voluntary /'vɒlən,teri/ *adj* spontaneous, deliberate; without remuneration; supported by voluntary effort; having free will; (*law*) acting gratuitously or from choice, not because of any legal compulsion or argument; (*muscles*) controlled by conscious effort; designed; pertaining to voluntaryism. • *n* (*pl* **voluntaries**) an organ solo, often improvised, played before or after a church service; (*arch*) a volunteer.—**voluntarily** *adv*.—**voluntariness** *n*.

voluntaryism /-təri,ɪzəm/ *n* the theory that churches, schools, etc, should depend on voluntary contributions, not state aid.—**voluntarist** *n*.—**voluntaristic** *adj*.

volunteer /,vɒlən'ti:r/ *n* a person who carries out work voluntarily; a person who freely undertakes military service. • *vti* to offer unasked; to come forward, enlist or serve voluntarily.

voluptuary /və'lʌptʃu,eri/ *n* (*pl* **voluptuaries**) a person given up to bodily pleasures or the enjoyment of luxury, a sensualist. • *adj* exciting sensual desire; devoted to pleasures of the senses; voluptuous; luxurious.

voluptuous /və'lʌptʃuəs/ *adj* excessively fond of pleasure; having an attractive figure; luxurious; exciting sensual desire.—**voluptuously** *adv*.—**voluptuousness** *n*.

volute /'vɒlju:t/ or /və'lju:t/, /-'lu:t/ *n* a spiral; a whorl; anything shaped to resemble a spiral or otherwise convoluted form; a spiral, scroll-shaped ornament, *esp* on an Ionic capital, a helix; a tropical shellfish with a spiral shell; any of the whorls found on the shells of snails; an auxiliary curved part of an engine that collects waste gases or liquids from that engine. • *adj* spiral-shaped; (*machinery*) moving spirally; (*bot*) rolled up.—*also* **voluted**.

volution /vəˈluːʃən/ *n* a spiral; a convoluted or turning shape or movement; any of the whorls of a shell.

volvox /ˈvɒlˌvɒks/ *n* a genus of round, hollow microscopic plants having a rotatory motion, found in ponds, etc.

vomer /ˈvoːmər/ *n* the flat, slender bone separating the nostrils in mammals.

vomit /ˈvɒmɪt/ *vi* to eject the contents of the stomach through the mouth, to spew. • *n* matter ejected from the stomach when vomiting.—**vomiter** *n*.

vomitive /ˈvɒmətɪv/ *adj* of or causing vomiting. • *n* an emetic.

vomitory /ˈvɒmɪtəri/ *adj* vomitive. • *n* (*pl* **vomitories**) an emetic; an aperture for vomited matter; any opening through which something is ejected; in ancient Rome, a corridor from a street entrance to a tier of seats in an amphitheatre.—*also* **vomitorium**.

vomiturition /ˌvɒmɪtjuˈrɪʃən/ *n* violent retching; repeated vomiting.

voodoo /ˈvuːduː/ *n* (*pl* **voodoos**) a religious cult in the West Indies, based on a belief in sorcery, etc; one who practises voodoo. • *vt* (**voodooing, voodooed**) to affect by voodoo.

voodooism /-ˌɪzəm/ *n* the beliefs and practices of voodoo.—**voodooist** *n*.—**voodooistic** *adj*.

voracious /vəˈreɪʃəs/ *adj* eager to devour (food, literature etc); very greedy.—**voraciously** *adv*.—**voracity** *n*.

vortex /ˈvɔrteks/ *n* (*pl* **vortexes, vortices**) a whirlpool; a powerful eddy; a whirlwind; a whirling motion or mass.—**vortical** *adj*.—**vortically** *adv*.

vorticella /ˌvɔrtɪˈsɛlə/ *n* (*pl* **vorticellae**) any of a genus of ciliated, bell-shaped animalcules.

vorticism /ˈvɔrtəˌsɪzəm/ *n* an art movement in which cubist techniques were amalgamated with that aspect of futurism expressing reservations about the quality of contemporary life, and its reliance on machines, so that objects were presented so as to give the effect of an assemblage of vortices.—**vorticist** *n*.

vortiginous /vɔrˈtɪdʒənəs/ *adj* whirling, vortical; vortex-like.

votary /ˈvoːtəri/ *n* (*pl* **votaries**) a person vowed to religious service or worship; an ardent follower, a devotee of a person, religion, occupation, idea, etc.—*also* **votarist**. • *adj* ardently devoted to a deity or saint.

vote /voːt/ *n* an indication of a choice or opinion as to a matter on which one has a right to be consulted; a ballot; decision by a majority; the right to vote; franchise. • *vi* to cast one's vote. • *vt* to elect (to office).—**votable, voteable** *adj*.

voter /ˈvoːtər/ *n* a person with a right to vote, *esp* one who uses it.

votive /ˈvoːtɪv/ *adj* given, consecrated, or promised by vow; (*RC Church*) voluntary, given by free will not by prescription.

vouch /vaʊtʃ/ *vt* to provide evidence or proof of. • *vi* to give assurance; to guarantee.

voucher /ˈvaʊtʃər/ *n* a written record of a transaction; a receipt; a token that can be exchanged for something else.

vouchsafe /-ˈseɪf/ *vt* to give, to grant; to condescend (to).—**vouchsafement** *n*.

voussoir /ˈvuːswɔr/ *n* any of the wedge-shaped stones forming the arch of a bridge or vault.

vow /vaʊ/ *n* a solemn or binding promise. • *vt* to promise; to resolve.—**vower** *n*.

vowel /ˈvaʊəl/ *n* an open speech sound produced by continuous passage of the breath; a letter representing such a sound, as *a, e, i, o, u*. • *adj* of or constituting a vowel.—**vowelless** *adj*.

vowelize /ˈvaʊəlˌaɪz/ *vt* to insert vowel points in (*usu* something written in Hebrew).—**vowelization** *n*.

vowel point *n* a diacritical mark indicating a vowel in Hebrew, Arabic, etc.

vox /vɒks/ *n* (*pl* **voces**) a voice; a sound.

vox humana *n* an organ stop with tones like the human voice.

vox populi /ˌvɒksˈpɒpjuˌli/ *n* popular opinion; the voice of the people.

voyage /ˈvɔɪədʒ/ *n* a long journey, *esp* by ship or spacecraft. • *vi* to journey.—**voyager** *n*.

voyageur /ˌvɔɪəˈdʒər/ or /ˌvwɒjæˈʒər/ *n* ✾ (*Cdn*) (*hist*) a French-speaking paddler of a canoe employed to transport goods to and from trading posts in the interior of the country; any boatman, trapper or guide, *esp* in Northern Canada.

voyeur /vɔɪˈjər/ *n* a person who is sexually gratified from watching sexual acts or objects; a peeping Tom.—**voyeurism** *n*.—**voyeuristic** *adj*.

VP *abbr* = vice-president.

vraisemblance /vəˈraɪsɛmˌblɒns/ *n* an appearance of truth, verisimilitude.

vs *abbr* = *versus* against.

VSO *abbr* = Voluntary Service Overseas.

VT *abbr* = Vermont.

vug, vugh /vʌg/ *n* (*mining*) a small cavity, often crystal-lined, in a lode or rock.

Vulcan /ˈvʌlkən/ *n* (*Roman myth*) the god of fire and smiths; (*arch*) a planet once thought to orbit Mercury.

vulcanism /ˈvʌlkəˌnɪsm/ *see* **volcanism**.

vulcanite /ˈvʌlkəˌnaɪt/ *n* a hard, vulcanized rubber, which is resistant to the effects of chemicals, ebonite.

vulcanize /ˈvʌlkəˌnaɪz/ *vt* to treat (rubber) with sulphur, white lead and other substances at high temperatures under pressure to improve its strength and elasticity or render it hard and non-elastic; to change the properties of (any material) in a similar way.—**vulcanization** *n*.

vulcanology /ˌvʌlkəˈnɒlədʒi/ *see* **volcanology**.

vulgar /ˈvʌlgər/ *adj* of the common people; vernacular; unrefined, in bad taste; coarse; offensive, indecent.—**vulgarly** *adv*.—**vulgarness** *n*.

vulgarian /vʌlˈgeriən/ *n* a vulgar pretentious person, *esp* one who shows of his or her wealth.

vulgarism /ˈvʌlgəˌrɪzəm/ *n* a crude expression; coarseness.

vulgarity /vʌlˈgeriti/ *n* (*pl* **vulgarities**) coarseness of manners or language; a vulgar phrase, expression, act, etc.

vulgarize /ˈvʌlgəˌraɪz/ *vt* to debase; to popularize.—**vulgarization** *n*.—**vulgarizer** *n*.

Vulgate /ˈvʌlgeɪt/ *n* a 4th-century Latin version of the Bible made by St Jerome, by combining text from the original language material and an earlier Latin text derived from the Greek; (*RC Church*) a revised form of this used as the authorized version. • *adj* pertaining to, or contained in, the Vulgate.

vulnerable /ˈvʌlnərəbəl/ *adj* capable of being wounded physically or mentally; open to persuasion; easily influenced; open to attack, assailable; (*contract bridge*) having won one game and liable to doubled penalties.—**vulnerability** *n*.—**vulnerably** *adv*.

vulnerary /ˈvʌlnərˌeri/ *adj* used for healing wounds. • *n* (*pl* **vulneraries**) a drug, ointment, etc, used in this way.

vulpine /ˈvʌlpaɪn/, **vulpecular** /vʌlˈpekjuˌlər/ *adj* pertaining to, like, or characteristic of a fox; cunning.

vulture /ˈvʌltʃər/ *n* a large bird of prey having no feathers on the neck or head and feeding chiefly on carrion; a rapacious person.

vulturine /-ˌriːn/, **vulturous** /-əs/ *adj* vulture-like.

vulva /ˈvʌlvə/ *n* (*pl* **vulvae, vulvas**) the external genitals of human females.—**vulval, vulvar, vulvate** *adj*.

vulviform /ˈvʌlvəˌfɔrm/ *adj* like a cleft with projecting edges.

vulvitis /vʌlˈvaɪtɪs/ *n* inflammation of the vulva.

vying /ˈvaɪɪŋ/ *see* **vie**.

W

W (*chem symbol*) tungsten.

w *abbr* = watt(s); west.

W, w *n* the 23rd letter of the English alphabet.

WA *abbr* = Washington.

WAC *abbr* = Women's Army Corps.

wacky /'wæki/ *adj* (**wackier, wackiest**) (*sl*) crazy, eccentric.—**wackily** *adv*.—**wackiness** *n*.

wad /wɒd/ *n* a small, soft mass, as of cotton or paper; a bundle of paper money.

wadding /'wɒdɪŋ/ *n* any soft material for use in padding, packing, etc.

waddle /'wɒdəl/ *vi* to walk with short steps and sway from side to side, as a duck.—*also n*.

waddy /wɒdi:/ *n* (*pl* **waddies**) a club with a thickened head used as a weapon by Australian Aborigines. • *vt* (**waddying, waddied**) to hit with a waddy.

wade /weɪd/ *vti* to walk through water; to pass (through) with difficulty.

wader /'weɪdər/ *n* a bird that wades, *eg* the heron; (*pl*) high waterproof boots worn by anglers.

wadi, wady /'wɒdi/ *n* a channel of a stream in North Africa which is dry except in the rainy season.

WAF *abbr* = Women in the Air Force.

wafer /'weɪfər/ *n* a thin crisp cracker or biscuit; (*Christianity*) the disc of unleavened bread used in the Eucharist.

waferboard /'weɪfər,bɔrd/ *n* ✳ (*Cdn*) a rigid sheet or panel composed of wood chips.

waffle[1] /'wɒfəl/ *n* a thick, crisp pancake baked in a waffle iron.

waffle[2] *vi* (*esp Brit inf*) to speak or write at length without saying anything substantial.

waffle iron *n* a metal cooking utensil with two hinged metal parts that close and impress a square pattern on a waffle.

waft /wɒft/ or /wæft/ *vt* to drift or float through the air. • *n* a breath, scent or sound carried through the air.

wag[1] /wæg/ *vti* (**wagging, wagged**) to move rapidly from side to side or up and down (as of a finger, tail).—*also n*.

wag[2] *n* a joker, a wit.

wage /weɪdʒ/ *vt* to carry on, *esp* war. • *n* (*often pl*) payment for work or services.

wage earner *n* a person who works for wages.

wager /'weɪdʒər/ *n* a bet. • *vti* to bet.

waggle /'wægəl/ *vti* to wag.—*also n*.

Wagnerian /vɒg'neɪriən/ *n* of or resembling the music of Richard Wagner (1813–83), characterized by dramatic grandeur and emotional intensity.

wagon /'wægən/ *n* a four-wheeled vehicle pulled by a horse or tractor, for carrying heavy goods.

wagoner /-ər/ *n* a driver of a wagon.

wagon-lit /-lɪt/ *n* (*pl* **wagons-lits**) a sleeping-car on a European train.

wagtail /'wægteɪl/ *n* any of numerous small birds with tails that jerk constantly.

wah-wah /'wɒwɒ/ *n* the sound of a trumpet, etc when alternately muted and unmuted; a pedal or lever used with an electric guitar, etc to imitate this sound.

waif /weɪf/ *n* a homeless, neglected child.

wail /weɪl/ *vi* to make a long, loud cry of sorrow or grief; to howl, to moan.—*also n*.

wain /weɪn/ *n* (*poet*) a farm wagon.

wainscot /'weɪnskɒt/ *n* wooden panelling on the interior of a wall.—*also* **wainscoting**. • *vt* to line (a wall) with a wainscot.

wainwright /-raɪt/ *n* a person who builds wagons.

waist /weɪst/ *n* the narrowest part of the human trunk, between the ribs and the hips; the narrow part of anything that is wider at the ends; the part of a garment covering the waist.

waistband /'weɪstbænd/ *n* a band of material (on a skirt, trousers, etc) that strengthens and completes the waist.

waistcoat /-kout/ *n* a waist-length, sleeveless garment worn immediately under a suit jacket; a vest.

waistline /-laɪn/ *n* the narrowest part of the waist; its measurement; the seam that joins the bodice and skirt of a dress, etc; the level of this.

wait /weɪt/ *vti* to stay, or to be, in expectation or readiness; to defer or to be postponed; to remain; (*with* **at** *or* **on**) to serve food at a meal. • *n* act or period of waiting.

waiter /'weɪtər/ *n* a man or woman who serves at table, as in a restaurant.—**waitress** *nf*.

waiting /-ɪŋ/ *n* the act of remaining inactive or stationary; a period of waiting. • *adj* of or pertaining to a wait; in attendance.

waiting game *n* a delay in acting or deciding in order to benefit from more favourable circumstances later.

waiting list *n* a list of people applying for or waiting to obtain something.

waiting room *n* a room for people to wait in at a station, hospital, etc.

waive /weɪv/ *vt* to refrain from enforcing; to relinquish voluntarily.

waiver /'weɪvər/ *n* (*law*) a waiving of a right, claim etc.

wake[1] /weɪk/ *vb* (**waking, woke**, *pp* **woken**) *vi* to emerge from sleep; to become awake. • *vt* to rouse from sleep. • *n* a watch or vigil beside a corpse, on the eve of the burial.—**wakeful** *adj*.—**waken** *vti*.

wake[2] *n* the waves or foamy water left in the track of a ship; a trail.

wale /weɪl/ *n* a ridge or mark on the body, a weal; a ridge on a ribbed material such as corduroy; a heavy plank along a ship's side.

Walhalla /væl'hæl'ə/ or /'vɒlhɒl'ə/ *see* **Valhalla**.

walk /wɔk/ *vi* to travel on foot with alternate steps; (*with* **out**) to leave suddenly; to go on strike; (*with* **on**) to abandon, jilt. • *vt* to pass through or over; (*a dog*) to exercise; to escort on foot. • *n* the act of walking; distance walked over; gait; a ramble or stroll; a profession.—**walker** *n*.

walkabout /'wɔkəbaut/ *n* a ceremonial wander through the Australian bush made periodically by an Aborigine; an informal stroll through a crowd by a politician, celebrity, etc.

walkie-talkie, walky-talky /ˌwɔki'tɔki/ *n* (*pl* **walkie-talkies, walky-talkies**) a portable two-way radio transmitter and receiver.

walk-in *adj* (*cupboard*) large enough to enter and move around in.

walking /'wɔkɪŋ/ *adj* able to walk; appearing to walk; ambulatory; marked by travelling on foot (*walking holiday*); intended for walkers (*walking boots*); in animate form (*walking bomb*). • *n* the act of walking; gait; the condition of a track, etc.

walking papers *n* (*sl*) notice of dismissal.

walking stick *n* a stick used in walking, a cane.

walkman /'wɔkmən/ *n* (*trademark*) a small portable cassette player (and sometimes radio) used with earphones.

walk-on *n* a small (*esp* non-speaking) part in a play.

walkout /'wɔkaut/ *n* a strike; a sudden departure.

walkover /-ˌouvər/ *n* an unopposed or easy victory; a horse race with only one starter.

walk-through *n* a rehearsal.

walkway /'wɔkweɪ/ *n* road, path, etc, for pedestrians only.

Walkyrie /væl'kɪri/ or /'vælkəri/ *see* **Valkyrie**.

wall /wɒl/ *n* a vertical structure of brick, stone, etc for enclosing, dividing or protecting. • *vt* to enclose with a wall; to close up with a wall.

wallaby /'wɒləbi/ *n* (*pl* **wallabies, wallaby**) a small kangaroo-like animal.

wallah, walla /'wɒlə/ *n* (*inf*) a person with a specified job or responsibility.

wallaroo /ˌwɒlə'ruː/ *n* (*pl* **wallaroos, wallaroo**) a type of large kangaroo.

walled /wɒld/ *adj* having walls; surrounded or protected as if by walls; fortified.

wallet /'wɒlət/ *n* a flat pocketbook for paper money, cards etc.

walleye /'wɒlaɪ/ *n* an eye with an opaque cornea; any eye with a pale or white iris; a squint in which an eye turns outward; ✳ a large North American freshwater fish with prominent eyes.

wallflower /'wɒlˌflauər/ *n* a fragrant plant with red or yellow flowers; a person who does not dance for lack of a partner.

Walloon /wɒˈluːn/ *n* a member of a French-speaking people of southern Belgium and adjacent areas of France; the French dialect of Walloons.—*also adj.*

wallop /ˈwɒləp/ *vt* (*inf*) to beat or defeat soundly; (*inf*) to strike hard. • *n* (*inf*) a hard blow.

walloping /-ɪŋ/ *adj* (*inf*) large, massive. • *n* (*inf*) a thrashing, a defeat.

wallow /ˈwɒloː/ *vi* (*animal*) to roll about in mud; to indulge oneself in emotion.—*also n.*

wallpaper /ˈwɒlˌpeɪpər/ *n* decorated paper for covering the walls of a room.

Wall Street *n* a street in New York where the Stock Exchange is situated; the centre of American finance.

wall-to-wall /ˈwɒltuːˈwɒl/ *adj* (*carpet*) covering the whole area of a room; (*inf*) nonstop, continuous.

wally /ˈwɒli/ *n* (*pl* **wallies**) (*Brit sl*) an idiot.

walnut /-nʌt/ *n* a tree producing an edible nut with a round shell and wrinkled seed; its nut; its wood used for furniture.

walrus /-rəs/ *n* (*pl* **walruses, walrus**) a large, thick-skinned aquatic animal, related to the seals, having long canine teeth and coarse whiskers.

walrus moustache *n* a thick drooping moustache.

waltz /wɒlts/ *n* a piece of music with three beats to the bar; a whirling or slowly circling dance. • *vi* to dance a waltz.

wampum /ˈwɒmpəm/ *n* polished shells strung like beads formerly used as money by North American Indians.

wan /wɒn/ *adj* (**wanner, wannest**) pale and sickly; feeble or weak.—**wanly** *adv.*—**wanness** *n.*

wand /wɒnd/ *n* a magician's rod.

wander /ˈwɒndər/ *vi* to ramble with no definite destination; to go astray; to lose concentration.—*also n.*

wandering Jew *n* any of various trailing or climbing plants; (*with cap*) a legendary figure condemned by Christ to roam the world until the Day of Judgement as punishment for an insult.

wanderlust /-ˌlʌst/ *n* a compelling desire for travel.

wane /weɪn/ *vi* to decrease, *esp* of the moon; to decline. • *n* decrease, decline.

wangle /ˈwæŋɡəl/ *vti* (*inf*) to achieve (something) by devious means.

wannabe, wannabee /ˈwɒnəbi/ *n* someone who aspires to be like someone else (who is *usu* successful or famous) perhaps in appearance, mode of dress etc. • *adj* would-be, aspiring.

want /wɒnt/ *n* lack; poverty. • *vt* to need; to require; to lack; to wish (for).

want ad *n* (*inf*) a newspaper or magazine advertisement requesting an item, job, etc.

wanted /ˈwɒntəd/ *adj* sought after.

wanting /-ɪŋ/ *adj* lacking.

wanton /-ən/ *adj* malicious; wilful; sexually provocative.

wapiti /ˈwɒpɪti/ *n* (*pl* **wapitis**) a large deer of North America.

war /wɔr/ *n* military conflict between nations or parties; a conflict; a contest. • *vi* (**warring, warred**) to make war.

warble /ˈwɔrbəl/ *vi* to sing with trills and runs; to sing like a bird.

warble fly *n* a species of fly the larvae of which burrow under the skin of cattle causing painful lumps.

warbler /wɔrblər/ *n* any of a family of small Old World songbirds which includes the nightingale and robin.

war crime *n* a crime committed in wartime (such as mistreatment of prisoners) which violates conventional notions of decency.

war cry *n* a rallying call in battle; a party catchword.

ward /wɔrd/ *n* a section of a hospital; an electoral district; a division of a prison; a child placed under the supervision of a court. • *vt* (*with* **off**) to repel; to fend off.—**wardship** *n.*

-ward /wərd/, **-wards** /-z/ *adj suffix* indicating a certain direction.

war dance *n* a ritual dance before or after battle as practised by certain North American Indian tribes.

warden /ˈwɔrdən/ *n* an official; a person in charge of a building or home; a prison governor.

warder /-ər/ *n* (*Brit*) a prison officer.

ward heeler *n* (*sl*) a local political hanger-on for a politician.

wardrobe /-roːb/ *n* a cupboard for clothes; one's clothes.

wardroom /-ruːm/ *n* a room in a warship for use by officers with the exception of the captain.

ware /wer/ *n* (*pl*) merchandise, goods for sale; pottery.

warehouse /ˈwerhɐʊs/ *n* a building for storing goods.

warehouse club *n* a large scale members-only retail outlet which offers product discount.

warfare /ˈwɔrfer/ *n* armed hostilities; conflict.

warfarin /-fərɪn/ *n* a crystalline substance used in medicine as an anticoagulant and also as a poison to kill rodents.

war game *n* a simulated battle or tactical exercise using models or computers for military training; a re-enactment of a battle using model soldiers.

warhead /-hed/ *n* the section of a missile containing the explosive.

warhorse /-hɔrs/ *n* a horse used in battle; (*inf*) a veteran of military or political conflict.

warlike /-laɪk/ *adj* hostile.

warlock /-lɒk/ *n* a sorcerer, a magician.

warlord /-lɔrd/ *n* a military leader or ruler of (part of) a country.

warm /wɔrm/ *adj* moderately hot; friendly, kind; (*colours*) rich; enthusiastic. • *vt* to make warm. • *vi* to become enthusiastic (about). —**warmly** *adv.*—**warmth** *n.*

warm-blooded /-blʌdɪd/ *adj* having a constant and relatively high temperature; passionate.

warm front *n* the edge of an advancing mass of warm air.

warm-hearted /-ˈhɑrtəd/ *adj* kind, sympathetic; affectionate.

warming pan *n* a long-handled (*usu* copper) pan filled with hot coals and formerly used to warm a bed.

warmonger /ˈwɔrˌmɒŋɡər/ or /-ˌmʌŋɡər/ *n* a person who incites war, *esp* for personal gain; warrior, a fighting soldier.

warm-up /-ʌp/ *n* a period of exercise or practice before a race, etc.

warn /wɔrn/ *vt* to notify of danger; to caution or advise (against).—**warning** *n.*

warp /wɔrp/ *vti* to twist out of shape; to distort; to corrupt. • *n* the threads arranged lengthwise on a loom across which other threads are passed.

war paint *n* paint smeared on the face and body by North American Indians before entering battle; (*inf*) formal or ceremonial dress, regalia; (*inf*) cosmetics.

warpath /ˈwɔrpæθ/ *n* the route used by a war party of North American Indians; (*with* **on the**) on a hostile expedition; (*with* **on the**) (*inf*) angry.

warped /wɔrpt/ *adj* distorted, twisted; embittered.

warplane /ˈwɔrpleɪn/ *n* an aircraft for use in combat.

warrant /ˈwɒrənt/ *vt* to guarantee; to justify. • *n* a document giving authorization; a writ for arrest.

warrantee /ˌwɒrənˈtiː/ *n* somebody to whom a warrant is given.

warrant officer *n* a person in the armed services holding a rank between commissioned officers and NCOs.

warrantor /-ər/ *n* a person or company that offers a warranty.

warranty /ˈwɒrənti/ *n* (*pl* **warranties**) a pledge to replace something if it is not as represented, a guarantee.

warren /ˈwɒrən/ *n* an area in which rabbits breed.

warring /-ɪŋ/ *adj* engaged in war.

warrior /-ɪər/ *n* a soldier, fighter.

warship /-ʃɪp/ *n* a ship equipped for war.

wart /wɔrt/ *n* a small, hard projection on the skin.—**warty** *adj.*

wart hog /ˈwɔrthɒɡ/ *n* an African wild pig with warty lumps on the face, large tusks and thick coarse hair.

wartime /-taɪm/ *adj, n* (of) a period or time of war.

wary /ˈweri/ *adj* (**warier, wariest**) watchful; cautious.—**warily** *adv.*—**wariness** *n.*

was /wɒz/ or /wəz/ *see* **be.**

wash /wɒʃ/ *vti* to cleanse with water and soap; to flow against or over; to sweep along by the action of water; to separate gold, etc, from earth by washing; to cover with a thin coat of metal or paint; (*with* **down**) to wash thoroughly from top to bottom; to take a drink of liquid to help in swallowing food. • *n* a washing; the break of waves on the shore; the waves left behind by a boat; a liquid used for washing.

washable /ˈwɒʃəbəl/ *adj* able to be washed without damage.—**washability** *n.*

washboard /-bɔrd/ *n* a corrugated board used (*esp* formerly) for scrubbing clothes.

washbowl /ˈwɒʃboːl/, **washbasin** /-beɪsɪn/ *n* a basin or bowl, *esp* a bathroom fixture, for use in washing one's hands, etc.—*also* **wash-hand basin.**

washcloth /-klɒθ/ *n* a flannel.

washed-out *adj* faded in colour; fatigued.

washed-up *adj* unsuccessful, ineffective; unpromising.

washer /-ər/ *n* a flat ring of metal, rubber, etc, to give tightness to joints; a washing machine.

washing /-ɪŋ/ *n* the act of cleansing with water; a number of items washed together.

washing machine *n* a device for washing clothes.

washing powder *n* a powdered detergent formulated for washing fabrics.

washing soda *n* sodium carbonate dissolved in water used for washing and cleaning.

washing-up *n* (*Brit*) the washing of dishes and cutlery after a meal; the dishes and cutlery waiting to be washed.

washout /-ʊt/ *n* (*sl*) a failure.

washroom /-ruːm/ *n* cloakroom, lavatory.

washstand /-stænd/ *n* a piece of furniture for holding a bowl and jug of water used for washing.

washtub /-tʌb/ *n* a large tub used for washing clothes.

washy /-i/ *adj* (**washier, washiest**) weak, watery; pale; lacking in strength or vigour.—**washiness** *n*.

wasn't /'wɒzənt/ = was not.

wasp /wɒsp/ *n* a winged insect with a black and yellow striped body, which can sting.

Wasp, WASP *n* an American of northern European, *esp* British, descent and Protestant upbringing, regarded as belonging to the most privileged group in American society (*White Anglo-Saxon Protestant*).

waspish /'wɒspɪʃ/ *adj* sharp in speech or manner, irritable.

wasp waist *n* a very slender waist.

wassail /'wɒseɪl/ or /'wɒsəl/ *n* (*formerly*) a toast made at festivities; a festive celebration with a lot of drinking and merriment; spiced ale or mulled wine served (*esp* formerly) at Christmas or other festive occasions. • *vi* to make merry.

Wassermann test /'wɒsərmən/ *n* a blood test used to diagnose syphilis.

wastage /'weɪstɪdʒ/ *n* anything lost by use or natural decay; wasteful or avoidable loss of something valuable.

waste /weɪst/ *adj* useless; left over; uncultivated or uninhabited. • *vt* to ravage; to squander; to use foolishly; to fail to use. • *vi* to lose strength, etc as by disease. • *n* uncultivated or uninhabited land; discarded material, garbage, excrement.—**wasteful** *adj*.—**wastefully** *adv*.—**wastefulness** *n*.

wasted /'weɪstəd/ *adj* ravaged, devastated; not used to best advantage; weak, emaciated; (*sl*) dead, killed; (*sl*) showing the effects of alcohol or drug abuse.

wasteland /-lænd/ *n* a piece of barren or uncultivated land; a desolate region; something (*eg* a period of time, relationship) lacking in moral, spiritual, emotional, etc vitality.

wastepaper /-peɪpər/ *n* paper discarded as waste.

wastepipe /-paɪp/ *n* a pipe carrying off used water from sinks, baths, etc.

waster /-ər/ *n* a wasteful person or thing; a good-for-nothing.

wasting asset *n* a non-renewable resource such as a coal mine.

wastrel /-rəl/ *n* a vagabond; a waster, idler.

watch /wɒtʃ/ *n* surveillance; close observation; vigil; guard; a small timepiece worn on the wrist, etc; a period of duty on a ship. • *vi* to look with attention; to wait for; to keep vigil. • *vt* to keep one's eyes fixed on; to guard; to tend; to observe closely; (*chance, etc*) to wait for.—**watcher** *n*.—**watchful** *adj*.—**watchfully** *adv*.—**watchfulness** *n*.

watchband /'wɒtʃbænd/ *n* a strap of leather, etc, for securing a watch to the wrist.

watchcase /'wɒtʃkeɪs/ *n* a protective metal casing for a watch mechanism.

watchdog /-dɒg/ *n* a dog that guards property; a person or group that monitors safety, standards, etc.

watchmaker /-meɪkər/ *n* a person who makes and repairs watches.

watchman /-mən/ *n* (*pl* **watchmen**) a person who guards a building or other property.

watch night *n* a religious service on New Year's Eve.

watchtower /-tauər/ *n* a tower for a sentry to keep watch from.

watchword /-wərd/ *n* a password.

water /'wɒtər/ *n* the substance H₂O, a clear, thin liquid, lacking taste or smell, and essential for life; any body of it, as the ocean, a lake, river, etc; bodily secretions such as tears, urine. • *vt* to moisten with water; to irrigate; to dilute with water; (*with* **down**) to dilute; to reduce in strength or effectiveness. • *vi* (*eyes*) to smart; to salivate; to take in water.

water bed /-bɛd/ *n* a bed with a water-filled mattress.

water bird *n* any swimming or wading bird.

water biscuit *n* a thin, crisp biscuit, *usu* served with cheese.

water blister *n* a blister on the skin filled with watery fluid instead of blood.

water boatman *n* any of various aquatic bugs adapted for swimming.

water bomber *n* ✦ (*Cdn*) an aircraft used to drop water on a forest fire.

waterborne /-bɔːn/ *adj* floating on or travelling by water.

waterbuck /-bʌk/ *n* an African antelope which lives in swampy areas.

water buffalo *n* a common domesticated Asian buffalo.

water cannon *n* an apparatus for pumping water at high pressure to disperse crowds.

water chestnut *n* an Asian aquatic plant with edible nutlike fruit; (the edible tuber of) a Chinese plant with a succulent root.

water clock *n* a clock with a mechanism operated by flowing or dripping water.

water-closet *n* a lavatory.

watercolour, watercolor /-kʌlər/ *n* a water-soluble paint; a picture painted with watercolours.

water-cooled *adj* (*engine etc*) cooled by the circulation of water.

watercourse /-kɔːs/ *n* (a channel for) a stream, river or canal.

watercraft /-kræft/ *n* skill in handling boats and other vessels; a vessel travelling by water.

watercress /-krɛs/ *n* a plant growing in ponds and streams, used in a salad.

water cure *n* hydropathy.

water diviner *n* a person who searches for water using a divining rod.

waterfall /-fɔːl/ *n* a fall of water over a precipice or down a hill.

water flea *n* any of numerous tiny freshwater crustaceans.

waterfowl /-faʊl/ *n* (*pl* **waterfowl**) a bird that frequents lakes, rivers, etc, *esp* a duck.

waterfront /-frʌnt/ *n* an area alongside a body of water, *esp* a docks.

water gas *n* a toxic inflammable mixture of carbon monoxide and hydrogen produced by passing steam over hot carbon, used as a fuel.

water glass /-glæs/ *n* a solution of sodium or potassium silicate in water used as a protective coating and to preserve eggs.

water hammer *n* (the sound of) the concussion of water in a pipe when a blockage is suddenly dislodged.

water hole *n* a water-filled hollow where animals drink.

water hyacinth *n* a floating aquatic plant of tropical America that often blocks waterways with its dense growth.

water ice *n* an iced dessert made from frozen water, sugar and a flavouring.

watering can *n* a container with a spout for watering plants.

watering hole *n* (*inf*) a bar or pub.

watering place *n* a place where animals or people can obtain water; a spa resort.

water jacket *n* a casing filled with water used for cooling machinery.

water jump *n* a ditch filled with water used as an obstacle in a steeplechase and other sporting contests.

water level *n* the surface level of water in a reservoir, etc.

water lily *n* any of a family of plants with large floating leaves and showy flowers.

waterline /-laɪn/ *n* a line up to which a ship's hull is submerged.

waterlogged /-lɒgd/ *adj* soaked or saturated with water.

water main *n* a main pipe or conduit for carrying water.

watermark /-mɑːk/ *n* a line marking the height to which water has risen; a mark impressed on paper which can only be seen when held up to the light.

watermelon /-mɛlən/ *n* a large fruit with a hard green rind and edible red watery flesh.

water mill /-mɪl/ *n* a mill operated by a water wheel.

water pistol *n* a toy gun that shoots a stream of water.

water polo *n* a game played in water by two teams of seven swimmers with the aim of scoring by hitting a ball into the opponents' goal.

water power *n* the power of falling or moving water used to operate machinery or generate electricity.

waterproof /-pruːf/ *adj* impervious to water; watertight.—*also vt*.

water-repellent *adj* (*fabrics, etc*) treated with a substance that prevents penetration by water.

water-resistant *adj* (*fabrics, etc*) designed to resist water penetration as long as possible.

watershed /-ʃɛd/ *n* a turning point.

waterside /-saɪd/ *n* the edge of a body of water.

water-skiing *n* the sport of planing on water by being towed by a motorboat.—**water-skier** *n*.

water softener *n* a device or chemical designed to counteract chemicals that cause hardness in water.

water-soluble *adj* capable of dissolving in water.

water spaniel *n* a breed of large curly-coated spaniel used in hunting waterfowl.

waterspout /-ˌspeʊt/ *n* a pipe for draining water; a tall column of water formed by a whirlwind and reaching from the sea to the clouds.

water table *n* the level below which the ground is saturated with water.

watertight /-ˌtəɪt/ *adj* not allowing water to pass through; foolproof.

water tower *n* an elevated tank or reservoir to allow water to be supplied under pressure.

waterway /-ˌweɪ/ *n* a navigable channel of water.

water wheel *n* a wheel designed to be turned by running water and used to drive machinery; a wheel used for raising water.

water wings *npl* inflatable rubber floats worn on the arms of those learning to swim.

waterworks /-ˌwɜːks/ *n* (*as sing*) an establishment that supplies water to a district; (*pl: inf*) the urinary system; (*inf*) tears.

waterworn /-ˌwɔːn/ *adj* rubbed smooth by the action of water.

watery /-i/ *adj* thin, diluted.

watt /ˈwɒt/ *n* a unit of electrical power.

wattage /-ɪdʒ/ *n* amount of electrical power.

wattle /ˈwɒtəl/ *n* (material for) a framework of stakes or poles interwoven with thin branches, twigs, etc formerly used for fencing and building; a loose flap of skin hanging from the necks of certain birds and lizards; an Australian acacia tree with small brightly-coloured flowers. • *vt* to build of or with wattle; to interweave or interlace (with sticks, etc) to make a light frame.

wave /weɪv/ *n* an undulation travelling on the surface of water; the form in which light and sound are thought to travel; an increase or upsurge (*eg* of crime); a hair curl; a movement of the hand in greeting or farewell. • *vti* to move freely backward and forward; to flutter; to undulate; to move the hand to and fro in greeting, farewell, etc; (*with* **down**) to signal (a vehicle, etc) to stop with a wave.—**wavy** *adj*.

wave band /ˈweɪvbænd/ *n* a range of radio frequencies or wavelengths.

waveguide /-gaɪd/ *n* a metal tube used to guide microwaves along a particular path.

wavelength /-leŋθ/ or /-leŋkθ/ *n* the distance between the crests of successive waves of light or sound; radio frequency.

wavelet /-lət/ *n* a small wave.

wave mechanics *n sing* (*physics*) the theory in quantum mechanics that describes the behaviour of elementary particles in terms of their wave properties.

waver /ˈweɪvər/ *vi* to hesitate; to falter.—**waverer** *n*.

wax[1] /wæks/ *n* beeswax; an oily substance used to make candles, polish, etc. • *vt* to rub, polish, cover or treat with wax.

wax[2] *vi* to increase in strength, size, etc.

waxen /ˈwæksən/ *adj* made of wax; pale and smooth like wax.

wax paper *n* paper that has been rendered moistureproof by treating with wax.

waxwork /-wɜːk/ *n* a figure or model formed of wax; (*pl*) an exhibition of such figures.

waxy /-i/ *adj* (**waxier, waxiest**) consisting of or like wax; adhesive.—**waxily** *adv*.—**waxiness** *n*.

way /weɪ/ *n* path, route; road; distance; room to advance; direction; state; means; possibility; manner of living; (*pl*) habits.

waybill /ˈweɪbɪl/ *n* a document with list of goods and shipping instructions accompanying a shipment.

wayfarer /-ˌfeɪrər/ *n* a traveller.

waylay /weɪˈleɪ/ *vt* (**waylaying, waylaid**) to lie in wait for; to accost.

way-out /-aʊt/ *adj* (*inf*) unconventional, unusual; amazing.

-ways /-z/ *adv suffix* indicating a certain direction or manner.

ways and means *npl* the methods used to accomplish something; the revenues and means of raising revenues for the use of government.

wayside /ˈweɪsaɪd/ *n* the side of or land adjacent to a road.

wayward /-wərd/ *adj* wilful, stubborn; unpredictable.—**waywardness** *n*.

WBA *abbr* = World Boxing Association.

WBC *abbr* = World Boxing Council.

WC *abbr* = (*Brit*) water-closet.

WCB *abbr* ✸ (*Cdn*) = Workers' Compensation Board.

we /wiː/ *pron pl* of I; I and others.

weak /wiːk/ *adj* lacking power or strength; feeble; ineffectual.—**weakness** *n*.

weaken /ˈwiːkən/ *vti* to make or grow weaker.

weak interaction *n* (*physics*) an interaction between elementary particles that is responsible for certain particle decay processes.

weak-kneed /ˈwiːkˌniːd/ *adj* (*inf*) submissive, easily intimidated.

weakling /-lɪŋ/ *n* a person who lacks strength of character.

weakly /-li/ *adj* (**weaklier, weakliest**) not robust; sickly. • *adv* in a weak manner, feebly.

weak-minded /-ˌmaɪndɪd/ *adj* lacking in determination; feeble-minded.

weal /wiːl/ *n* a raised mark on the skin left by a blow with a lash.

wealth /welθ/ *n* a large amount of possessions or money; affluence; an abundance (of).—**wealthy** *adj*.

wean /wiːn/ *vt* (*baby, animal*) to replace the mother's milk with other nourishment; to dissuade (from indulging a habit).

weapon /ˈwepən/ *n* any instrument used in fighting.

weaponry /-ri/ *n* weapons collectively.

wear /weɪr/ *vb* (**wearing, wore,** *pp* **worn**) *vt* to have on the body as clothing; (*hair, etc*) to arrange in a particular way; to display; to rub away; to impair by use; to exhaust, tire; (*with* **down**) to overcome gradually through persistent pressure; (*with* **out**) to tire or exhaust. • *vi* to be impaired by use or time; to be spent tediously; (*with* **off**) to become gradually weaker in effect; (*with* **out**) to make or become worthless through prolonged use. • *n* deterioration from frequent use; articles worn.—**wearer** *n*.

wearable /ˈweɪrəbəl/ *adj* suitable to be worn.

wear and tear *n* deterioration or depreciation from everyday use.

wearing /-ɪŋ/ *adj* exhausting, tiresome, oppressive.

weary /ˈwiːri/ *adj* (**wearier, weariest**) tired; bored. • *vti* (**wearying, wearied**) to make or become tired.—**weariness** *n*.—**wearisome** *adj*.

weasel /ˈwiːzəl/ *n* a small carnivorous animal with a long slender body and reddish fur.

weasel words *npl* (*inf*) evasive or misleading talk.

weather /ˈweðər/ *n* atmospheric conditions, such as temperature, rainfall, cloudiness, etc. • *vt* to expose to the action of the weather; to survive. • *vi* to withstand the weather.

weather-beaten /-ˌbiːtən/ *adj* worn or damaged by the weather; hardened or bronzed through exposure to the weather.

weatherboard /-ˌbɔːd/ *n* a sloping, *usu* overlapping, timber board used as external cladding for a wall or roof.—**weatherboarding** *n*.

weather-bound /-ˌbaʊnd/ *adj* delayed or postponed due to bad weather.

weathercock /-ˌkɒk/ *n* a weather vane in the form of a cock to show the wind direction.

weathered /ˈweðərd/ *adj* affected or seasoned by exposure to the weather; (*rocks*) altered in shape by erosion; (*roof*) having a sloped surface to allow rainwater to escape.

weather eye *n* an eye trained to observe changes in the weather; (*inf*) an alert or watchful gaze.

weatherglass *n* a barometer.

weathering /-ɪŋ/ *n* the erosion of rocks through the action of the wind, rain, frost, etc.

weatherman /-ˌmæn/ *n* (*pl* **weathermen**) a weather forecaster on radio or television who is usually also a professional meteorologist.

weather map *n* a chart showing weather conditions over a particular area for a specified period.

weatherproof /-pruːf/ *adj* designed to withstand exposure to weather without damage or deterioration.—*also vt*.

weather station *n* a meteorological post for collecting, recording and transmitting data on weather conditions.

weather vane *n* a device attached to a tall structure to indicate wind direction.

weave /wiːv/ *vb* (**weaving, wove,** *pp* **woven**) *vt* to interlace threads in a loom to form fabric; to construct. • *vi* to make a way through (*eg* a crowd), to zigzag.—**weaver** *n*.

weaverbird /ˈwiːvərbərd/ *n* any of various Old World songbirds that build nests of interwoven grass, twigs, etc, including the house sparrow.

Web *n* short for Worldwide Web.

web /wɛb/ *n* a woven fabric; the fine threads spun by a spider; the membrane joining the digits of birds, animals.

webbed /-d/ *adj* (*ducks, etc*) having the digits connected by a fold of skin.

webbing /'wɛbɪŋ/ *n* a strong narrow woven fabric of jute, cotton, etc, used for straps and belts; anything forming a web.

weber /'veɪbər/ *n* the SI unit of magnetic flux.

wed /wɛd/ *vti* (**wedding, wedded** *or* **wed**) to marry; to join closely.

Wed *abbr* = Wednesday.

we'd /wiːd/ = we had; we would.

wedded /'wɛdɪd/ *adj* of or resulting from marriage; devoted (to art, etc).

wedding /-ɪŋ/ *n* marriage; the ceremony of marriage.

wedding cake *n* an ornately decorated rich fruit cake, *usu* in three tiers, served at a wedding.

wedding ring *n* a band of gold or platinum used at a wedding and worn to show marital status.

wedge /wɛdʒ/ *n* a v-shaped block of wood or metal for splitting or fastening; a wedge-shaped object. • *vti* to split or secure with a wedge; to thrust (in) tightly; to become fixed tightly.

wedlock /'wɛdlɒk/ *n* marriage.

Wednesday /'wɛnzdeɪ/ *or* /-di/ *n* fourth day of the week, between Tuesday and Thursday.

wee[1] /wiː/ *adj* (*Scot*) small, tiny.

wee[2] *n* (*inf*) the act of passing urine; urine. • *vt* (*inf*) to pass urine.—*also* **wee-wee**.

weed /wiːd/ *n* any undesired plant, *esp* one that crowds out desired plants; (*sl*) marijuana; (*pl*) a widow's black mourning clothes. • *vt* to remove weeds; (*with* **out**) to remove or eliminate (something superfluous or harmful).

weedkiller /'wiːdkɪlər/ *n* a chemical or hormonal substance used to kill weeds.

weedy /'wiːdi/ *adj* (**weedier, weediest**) full of weeds; (*inf*) thin and scrawny.

week /wiːk/ *n* the period of seven consecutive days, *esp* from Sunday to Sunday.

weekday /'wiːkdeɪ/ *n* a day of the week other than Saturday or Sunday.

weekend, week-end /-ɛnd/ *or* /-'ɛnd/ *n* the period from Friday night to Sunday night.—*also adj*.

weekly /-li/ *adj* happening once a week or every week.

weeknight /-naɪt/ *n* the evening or night of a weekday.

weeny /'wiːni/ *adj* (**weenier, weeniest**) (*inf*) tiny, minute.

weep /wiːp/ *vti* (**weeping, wept**) to shed tears, to cry; (*wound*) to ooze.

weepie /'wiːpi/ *n* (*inf*) a sentimental film.

weeping /-ɪŋ/ *n* the act of weeping. • *adj* shedding tears; exuding moisture; (*tree*) with drooping branches.—**weepingly** *adv*.

weeping willow *n* a Chinese willow tree with slender drooping branches.

weepy /'wiːpi/ *adj* (**weepier, weepiest**) tearful; prone to crying.—**weepily** *adv*.—**weepiness** *n*.

weevil /'wiːvəl/ *n* a beetle which feeds on plants and crops.

wee-wee /'wiːwiː/ *see* **wee**[2].

weft /wɛft/ *n* the yarn woven across the lengthwise threads in a loom.—*also* **woof**.

weigh /weɪ/ *vt* to measure the weight of; to consider carefully; (*with* **down**) to weight; to oppress; (*with* **up**) to assess, make a judgment about (a person, thing, etc). • *vi* to have weight; to be burdensome; (*with* **in**) (*boxer, wrestler*) to be weighed before a bout; (*jockey*) to be weighed after a race; (*inf*) to make a contribution to (*eg* an argument).

weighbridge *n* a large scale consisting of a metal plate set into the road onto which vehicles are driven to be weighed.

weigh-in /'weɪɪn/ *n* (*sports*) the checking of the weight of a contestant, *esp* of a jockey after a race or of a boxer before a bout.

weight /weɪt/ *n* the amount which anything weighs; influence; any unit of heaviness. • *vt* to attach a weight to.

weightlessness /'weɪtləsnəs/ *n* the state of having no or little reaction to gravity, *esp* in space travel.

weight lifting /-ˌlɪftɪŋ/ *n* the sport of lifting weights of a specific amount in a particular way.—**weight lifter** *n*.

weight training *n* physical exercise involving lifting heavy weights.

weight watcher *n* a person on a diet to lose weight.

weighty /'weɪti/ *adj* (**weightier, weightiest**) heavy; serious.—**weightily** *adv*.

weir /wɪər/ *n* a low dam across a river which controls the flow of water.

weird /wɪrd/ *adj* unearthly, mysterious; eerie; bizarre.—**weirdly** *adv*.

Weirdo /'wɪrdoː/, **weirdie** /'wɪrdi/ *n* (*pl* **weirdos, weirdies**) (*inf*) an eccentric person.

welch /wɛlʃ/ *see* **welsh**.

welcome /'wɛlkəm/ *adj* gladly received; pleasing. • *n* reception of a person or thing. • *vt* to greet kindly.

weld /wɛld/ *vt* to unite, as metal by heating until fused or soft enough to hammer together; to join closely. • *n* a welded joint.

welfare /'wɛlfer/ *n* wellbeing; health; assistance or financial aid granted to the poor, the unemployed, etc.

welfare state *n* a state in which the government assumes responsibility for the health and social security of its citizens.

well[1] /wɛl/ *n* a spring; a hole bored in the ground to provide a source of water, oil, gas, etc; the open space in the middle of a staircase. • *vi* to pour forth.

well[2] *adj* (**better, best**) agreeable; comfortable; in good health. • *adv* in a proper, satisfactory, or excellent manner; thoroughly; prosperously; with good reason; to a considerable degree; fully. • *interj* an expression of surprise, etc.

we'll /wiːl/ *or* /wɪl/ = we will; we shall.

well-advised /ˌwɛləd'vaɪzd/ *adj* acting with good sense; carefully thought out.

well-appointed /-ə'pɔɪntɪd/ *adj* fully equipped or furnished.

well-balanced /'wɛl'bælənst/ *adj* sensible, sane.

well-being /-ˌbiːɪŋ/ *n* condition of being well or contented; welfare.

well-bred /-'brɛd/ *adj* well brought up; of good stock.

well-connected /-'kənɛktɪd/ *adj* having powerful friends or relatives.

well-disposed /-dɪs'poːzd/ *adj* favourable, feeling kindly (toward).

well-done /-'dʌn/ *adj* performed with skill; thoroughly cooked, as meat.

well-favoured, well-favored /-feɪvərd/ *adj* attractive.

well-found /-'faund/ *adj* fully equipped.

well-founded /-'faundɪd/ *adj* borne out by facts.

well-groomed /-ˈgruːmd/ *adj* clean and tidy in dress and appearance.

well-grounded /-'graundɪd/ *adj* well instructed in a subject.

wellhead /-hɛd/ *n* the source of a stream, spring, etc; a source, origin.

well-heeled /-'hiːld/ *adj* (*inf*) wealthy.

wellies /'wɛliːz/ *npl* (*Brit inf*) wellingtons.

well-informed /-ɪn'fɔːmd/ *adj* knowledgeable on a wide range of subjects; possessing reliable information on a specific matter.

wellington (boot) /'wɛlɪŋtən/ *n* a rubber, waterproof boot.

well-intentioned /-ɪn'tɛnʃənd/ *adj* having good intentions (but often without producing good results).

well-knit /'wɛl'nɪt/ *adj* firm, compact.

well-known /-'noːn/ *adj* widely known, famous; known fully.

well-mannered /-mænərd/ *adj* having or showing good manners; polite.

well-meaning /-'miːnɪŋ/ *adj* having good intentions (but often without producing good results).

well-nigh /- naɪ/ *adv* almost.

well-off /-'ɒf/ *adj* in comfortable circumstances; prosperous.

well-preserved /-pri'zɔːrvd/ *adj* well looked after; remaining youthful in appearance.

well-read /'wɛl'rɛd/ *adj* having read widely and deeply.

well-rounded /-'raundɪd/ *adj* having a pleasantly curved or rounded shape; full, complete.

well-spoken /-'spoːkən/ *adj* spoken clearly and eloquently; spoken in a pleasing manner.

well-thought-of /-'θɔt,ɒv/ *adj* having a good reputation.

well-thumbed *adj* (*book*) marked by frequent handling.

well-to-do /-tə'duː/ *adj* prosperous.

well-wisher /-ˌwɪʃər/ *n* a person who is sympathetic to another person, cause, etc.

well-worn /-'wɔrn/ *adj* showing signs of wear; (*phrase, etc*) trite, hackneyed.

Welsh /wɛlʃ/ *adj* relating to the people of Wales or their language.—*also n*.

welsh *vti* to avoid paying a gambling debt; to run off without paying.—*also* **welch**.—**welsher, welcher** *n*.

Welsh corgi /-'kɔrgiː/ *n* a corgi.

Welsh dresser *n* a dresser with drawers and cupboards below and open shelves above.

Welsh rabbit, Welsh rarebit *n* melted cheese on toast.

welt /welt/ *n* a band or strip to strengthen a seam; a weal.

welter /'weltər/ *vi* to roll or wallow. • *n* a jumble.

welterweight /-ˌweɪt/ *n* a professional boxer weighing 140–147 pounds; a wrestler weighing 154–172 pounds.

wench /wentʃ/ *n* (*used facetiously*) a girl or young woman.

wend /wend/ *vt* to amble, to saunter.

Wendy house /'wendihəus/ *n* (*Brit*) a toy house for children to play in.

Wensleydale /'wenzliˌdeɪl/ *n* a mild crumbly English cheese.

went /went/ *see* **go**.

wept /wept/ *see* **weep**.

were /wər/ *see* **be**.

we're /wiːr/ = we are.

weren't /wərnt/ = were not.

werewolf /'werwʊlf/ or /'wiːr-/ *n* (*pl* **werewolves**) an imaginary person able to transform himself for a time into a wolf.

west /west/ *n* the direction of the sun at sunset; one of the four points of the compass; the region in the west of any country; (*with cap*) Europe and the Western Hemisphere. • *adj* situated in, or toward the west. • *adv* in or to the west.

westerly /'westərli/ *adj* toward the west; blowing from the west. • *n* (*pl* **westerlies**) a wind blowing from the west.—*also adv*.

western /'westərn/ *adj* of or in the west. • *n* a film, novel, etc about the *usu* pre-20th century American West.

Western Canadian *n* ❧ a person who lives in or is from Manitoba, or one of the provinces west of it. • *adj* of or pertaining to such a person.

westerner /-ər/ *n* a person from the west.

Western Hemisphere *n* that half of the earth containing North and South America.

westernize /'westərˌnaɪz/ *vti* to make or become familiar with the ideas, institutions, customs, etc of the West.—**westernization** *n*.

westernmost /'westərnˌmoːst/ *adj* farthest west.

westward /-wərd/ *adj* toward the west.—*also adv*.—**westwards** *adv*.

wet /wet/ *adj* (**wetter, wettest**) covered or saturated with water or other liquid; rainy; misty; not yet dry. • *n* water or other liquid; rain or rainy weather. • *vti* (**wetting, wet** *or* **wetted**) to soak; to moisten.—**wetness** *n*.

wet blanket *n* (*inf*) a person who dampens the enthusiasm of others.

wet dream *n* (*inf*) an erotic dream causing orgasm.

wet nurse *n* a woman employed to care for or suckle another's child.

wet-nurse /-ˌnərs/ *vt* to act as a wet nurse; (*inf*) to devote constant attention to (a person).

wet rot *n* (*Brit*) decay in timber caused by a fungus; any of various fungi that cause rot in damp timber.

wet suit /'wetsuːt/ *n* a close-fitting suit worn by divers, etc, to retain body heat.

we've /wiːv/ = we have.

whack /wæk/ *vti* (*inf*) to strike sharply, *esp* making a sound. • *n* (*inf*) a sharp blow.

whacking /'wækɪŋ/ *adj* (*Brit inf*) enormous. • *adv* (*inf*) very, extremely.

whale /weɪl/ *n* a very large sea mammal that breathes through a blowhole, and resembles a fish in shape. • *vi* to hunt whales.

whalebone /'weɪlboːn/ *n* a horny substance forming plates in the upper jaws of toothless whales; a piece of this formerly used for stiffening undergarments.

whalebone whale *n* any of various large whales that have whalebone plates instead of teeth which are used to filter plankton for food.

whaler /'weɪlər/ *n* a person or a ship employed in hunting whales.

whaling /-ɪŋ/ *n* the practice of hunting whales for food, oil, etc.

wham /wæm/ *n* (the sound of) a heavy blow. • *vti* (**whamming, whammed**) to hit or cause to hit with a loud noise.

whang /wæŋ/ *n* (the sound of) a forceful blow. • *vti* to hit or cause to hit with force.

wharf /wɔrf/ *n* (*pl* **wharfs, wharves**) a platform for loading and unloading ships in harbour.

wharfage /'wɔrfɪdʒ/ *n* (the charge for) the use of a wharf; wharves collectively.

wharfinger /-fɪndʒər/ *n* the owner or manager of a wharf.

what /wet/ or /wɒt/ *adj* of what sort, how much, how great. • *relative pron* that which; as much or many as. • *interj* used as an expression of surprise or astonishment.

whatever /wet'evər/ or /wɒt-/ *pron* anything that; no matter what.

whatnot /'wetnɒt/ or /wɒt-/ *n* (*inf*) something or someone the name of which has been forgotten, is unknown or is hard to categorize; a set of open shelves for ornaments, photographs, etc.

whatsit /'wetzɪt/ or /wɒt-/ *n* (*inf*) something or someone the name of which has been forgotten, is unknown or is hard to categorize.

whatsoever /ˌwetso:'evər/ or /wɒt-/ *adj* whatever.

wheat /wiːt/ *n* a cereal grain *usu* ground into flour for bread.

wheatear /'wiːtiːr/ *n* a small grey and white migratory thrush.

wheaten /'wiːtən/ *adj* made from the grain or flour of wheat; pale yellow in colour.

wheat germ *n* the kernel of a grain of wheat, high in nutritive value.

wheatmeal /-miːl/ *adj*, *n* (made from) brown flour with a high proportion of wheat grain.

wheat pool *n* ❧ (*Cdn*) a farmer's cooperative in western Canada for the sale of wheat and other cereal crops.

whee /wiː/ *interj* used to express joy or delight.

wheedle /'wiːdəl/ *vt* to persuade, to cajole (into); to coax with flattery.

wheel /wiːl/ *n* a solid disc or circular rim turning on an axle; a steering wheel; (*pl*) the moving forces. • *vt* to transport on wheels. • *vi* to turn round or on an axis; to move in a circular direction, as a bird.

wheelbarrow /'wiːlˌbero:/ *n* a cart with one wheel in front and two handles and legs at the rear.

wheelbase /-beɪs/ *n* the distance between the front and rear axles of a vehicle.

wheelchair /-tʃer/ *n* a chair with large wheels for invalids.

wheel clamp *n* (*Brit*) a device that prevents an illegally parked car from being driven away until a fine is paid to release it.—*also vt*.

wheeler-dealer /-ər'diːlər/ *n* (*inf*) a shrewd operator in business, politics, etc.

wheelie /'wiːli/ *n* a stunt in which a bicycle or motorcycle is ridden for a distance with the front wheel off the ground.

wheelwright /-raɪt/ *n* a person who makes and repairs wheels for a living.

wheeze /wiːz/ *vi* to breathe with a rasping sound; to breathe with difficulty.—*also n*.

wheezy /'wiːzi/ *adj* (**wheezier, wheeziest**) making a wheezing sound.—**wheezily** *adv*.—**wheeziness** *n*.

whelk /welk/ *n* a shellfish with a snail-like shell.

whelp /welp/ *n* the young of various animals, *esp* a dog; an impudent child. • *vt* to give birth to (a puppy, etc). • *vi* (*bitch*) to bring forth young.

when /wen/ *adv* at what or which time. • *conj* at the time at which; although; *relative pron* at which.

whence /wens/ *adv* from what place.—*also conj*.

whenever /wen'evər/ *adv*, *conj* at whatever time.

whensoever /ˌwenso:'evər/ *conj*, *adv* whenever.

where /wer/ *adv* at which or what place; to which place; from what source; *relative pron* in or to which.

whereabouts /'werə'bauts/ *adv* near or at what place; about where. • *n* approximate location.

whereas /wer'æz/ *conj* since; on the contrary.

whereby /-'baɪ/ *adv* by which.—*also conj*.

wherein /-'ɪn/ *adv* (*formal*) in what; how. • *conj* in which; where.

whereof /-ɛv/ *adv*, *conj* (*arch*) of what or which.

whereon /-'ɒn/ *adv*, *conj* (*arch*) on what or which.

wheresoever /ˌwerso:'evər/ *adv* (*emphatic*) wherever.

whereto /wer'tuː/ *adv*, *conj* (*formal*) to what or which.

whereupon /'werə'pɒn/ or /ˌwerə'pɒn/ *adv* at which point; upon which.

wherever /wer'evər/ *adv* at or to whatever place.

wherewithal /'werwɪˌθɒl/ or /-ˌðɒl/ *n* the means or resources.

whet /wet/ *vt* (**whetting, whetted**) to sharpen by rubbing, to stimulate.

whether /'weðər/ *conj* introducing an alternative possibility or condition.

whetstone /'wetsto:n/ *n* a stone for sharpening the edges of tools; something that sharpens or stimulates.

whew /hwjuː/ *interj* an exclamation of astonishment, amazement, relief, etc.

whey /weɪ/ *n* the watery part of milk that is separated from the curds in sour milk.

which /wɪtʃ/ *adj* what one (of). • *pron* which person or thing; that. • *relative pron* person or thing referred to.

whichever /-ˈɛvər/ *pron* whatever one that; whether one or the other; no matter which.—*also adj.*

whichsoever /ˌwitʃsoːˈɛvər/ *adj, pron* (*arch*) whichever.

whiff /wif/ *n* a sudden puff of air, smoke or odour.

while /wail/ *n* a period of time. • *conj* during the time that; whereas; although. • *vt* to pass (the time) pleasantly.

whilst /wailst/ *conj* (*esp Brit*) while.

whim /wim/ *n* a fancy; an irrational thought.

whimper /ˈwimpər/ *vi* to make a low, unhappy cry.—*also n.*

whimsical /-zəkəl/ *adj* unusual, odd, fantastic.—**whimsicality** *n.*

whimsy, whimsey /-zi/ *n* (*pl* whimsies, whimseys) a fanciful notion, a whim.

whine /wain/ *vi* (*dog*) to make a long, high-pitched cry; (*person*) to complain childishly. • *n* a plaintive cry.

whinge /windʒ/ *vi* to moan, complain.—*also n.*

whinny /ˈwini/ *vi* (**whinnying, whinnied**) to neigh softly.—*also n.*

whip /wip/ *n* a piece of leather attached to a handle used for punishing people or driving on animals; an officer in parliament who maintains party discipline. • *vb* (**whipping, whipped**) *vt* to move, pull, throw, etc suddenly; to strike, as with a lash; (*eggs, etc*) to beat into a froth; (*with* **up**) to stir into action, excite; (*inf*) to produce in a hurry. • *vi* to move rapidly.

whipcord /ˈwipkord/ *n* a strong cord of tightly twisted strands used for whips; a cotton or worsted fabric with diagonal ridges.

whip hand *n* (*usu with* **the**) the dominant position.

whiplash /-læʃ/ *n* a stroke with a whip; a neck injury when the head is jerked forward and backward.

whipped cream *n* cream that has been stiffened by beating, used as a topping for desserts, etc.

whippersnapper /ˈwipərˌsnæpər/ *n* an insignificant but impudent young person.

whippet /ˈwipit/ *n* a small racing dog like a greyhound.

whipping boy *n* a person who is constantly punished for the mistakes of others, a scapegoat.

whippoorwill /-ərˌwil/ *n* a nocturnal American bird with a distinctive call.

whip-round *n* (*Brit inf*) an appeal among friends for contributions.

whipsaw /-so/ *n* any of various types of saw with a long flexible blade.

whipstock /-stɒk/ *n* the handle of a whip.

whir, whirr /wər/ or /hwər/ *n* a humming or buzzing sound. • *vti* (**whirring, whirred**) to revolve with a buzzing noise.

whirl /wərl/ *n* a swift turning; confusion, commotion; (*inf*) an attempt or try. • *vti* to turn around rapidly; to spin.

whirligig /ˈwərligig/ *n* a spinning top.

whirlpool /-puːl/ *n* a circular current or vortex of water.

whirlpool bath *n* a bath with a device that swirls water.

whirlwind /-wind/ *n* a whirling column of air; rapid activity.

whisk /wisk/ *vt* to make a quick sweeping movement; (*eggs, cream*) to beat, whip. • *vi* to move nimbly and efficiently. • *n* a kitchen utensil for whisking; (*inf*) a small amount.

whisker /ˈwiskər/ *n* any of the sensory bristles on the face of a cat, etc; (*pl*) the hair growing on a man's face, *esp* the cheeks.—**whiskered** *adj.*

whiskey /-ki/ *n* whisky distilled in the US or Ireland.

whisky *n* (*pl* **whiskies**) a spirit distilled from barley or rye.

whisper /ˈwispər/ *vti* to speak softly; to spread a rumour. • *n* a hushed tone; a hint, trace.

whist /wist/ *n* a card game for four players in two sides, each side attempting to win the greater number of the 13 tricks.

whistle /ˈwisəl/ *vti* to make a shrill sound by forcing the breath through the lips; to make a similar sound with a whistle; (*wind*) to move with a shrill sound; (*with* **for**) (*inf*) to demand or hope for in vain. • *n* a whistling sound; a musical instrument; a metal tube that is blown to make a shrill warning sound.

whistle stop *n* a minor railroad station where trains stop only on signal; a brief appearance by a candidate on tour during an election campaign.

Whit /wit/ *see* **Whitsuntide.**

whit *n* the tiniest possible amount.

white /ˈwait/ *adj* of the colour of snow; pure; bright; (*skin*) light-coloured. • *n* the colour white; the white part of an egg or the eye.

white ant *n* a termite.

whitebait /-beit/ *n* (*pl* **whitebait**) the edible young of the herring and sprat.

white blood cell *n* a leucocyte.

whitecap /-kæp/ *n* a wave with a white foamy crest.

white-collar /-kɒlər/ *adj* of office and professional workers.

white dwarf *n* a small faint star of high density.

white elephant *n* a thing of little use.

white feather *n* a symbol of cowardice.

whitefish *n* ✷ (*pl* same or **whitefishes**) a freshwater fish of the trout family in northern North America.

white flag *n* a flag of plain white material used to signify surrender or arrange a truce.

whitefly /ˈwaitflai/ *n* (*pl* **whiteflies**) any of various small insects that feed on and injure plants.

white gold *n* a pale alloy of gold chiefly with platinum and palladium.

white goods *npl* household appliances, as refrigerators, etc; household linen, as sheets, towels, etc.

Whitehall /-hɒl/ *n* the British government; departmental government.

white heat *n* an intense heat accompanied by the emission of white light from a substance; (*inf*) intense excitement or emotion.

white-hot /-hɒt/ *adj* of a temperature so hot that white light is emitted; intensely passionate.

White House *n* the official residence of the president of the US; the US presidency.

white lead *n* a white solid of mostly lead carbonate, *esp* used in pigments.

white lie *n* a harmless lie, *esp* as uttered out of politeness.

white light *n* light, *eg* sunlight, that contains approximately equal proportions of the whole spectrum of visible radiation.

white matter *n* whitish tissue in the brain and spinal cord composed of nerve fibres.

white meat *n* a light-coloured meat such as poultry or veal.

white metal *n* an alloy, *esp* of tin, used in bearings, domestic utensils, etc.

whiten /ˈwaitən/ *vti* to make or become white; to bleach.

white noise *n* sound that contains approximately equal proportions of all the audible frequencies.

whiteout /-aut/ *n* a weather condition when heavy cloud and snow reflect most of the available light and greatly reduce visibility.

white paper *n* a government document detailing proposed legislation.

white sauce *n* a sauce made with butter, flour and seasonings mixed with milk, cream or stock.

white slave *n* a woman or girl held against her will and forced into prostitution.

white spirit *n* (*Brit*) a colourless inflammable liquid distilled from petroleum and used as a solvent and thinner for paint.

white tie *n* a white bow tie worn as part of a man's formal evening dress.—**white-tie** *adj.*

whitewash /ˈwaitwɒʃ/ *n* a mixture of lime and water, used for whitening walls; concealment of the truth.—*also vt.*

white water *n* water with a foaming surface, as in rapids.

white whale *n* the beluga.

white wine *n* wine made from green grapes or from skinned black grapes.

whitewood /-wʊd/ *n* (any of various trees yielding) a light-coloured wood.

whither /ˈwiðər/ *adv* to what or which place.

whiting /ˈwaitiŋ/ *n* (*pl* **whitings, whiting**) an edible saltwater fish of the cod family.

whitlow /ˈwitloː/ *n* a painful inflammation at the end of a finger or toe.

Whitsun /-sən/ *adj* (*Christianity*) of, observed on, or pertaining to Whit Sunday or Whitsuntide. • *n* Whitsuntide.

Whit Sunday *n* (*Christianity*) the seventh Sunday after Easter, Pentecost.

Whitsuntide /ˈwitsənˌtaid/ *n* (*Christianity*) the week beginning with Whit Sunday.—*also* **Whit.**

whittle /-əl/ *vt* to pare or cut thin shavings from (wood); (*with* away *or* down) to reduce.

whiz, whizz /wiz/ *vi* (**whizzing, whizzed**) to make a humming sound. • *n* (*pl* **whizzes**) a humming sound; (*inf*) an expert.

whiz kid, whizz kid *n* (*inf*) a person of extraordinary achievements given their relatively young age.

WHO *abbr* = World Health Organization.

who /huː/ *pron* what or which person; that.

whoa /woː/ *interj* a command given, *esp* to a horse, to slow down or come to a halt.

who'd /huːd/ = who would.

whodunit, whodunnit /huːˈdʌnɪt/ *n* (*inf*) a detective novel, play, etc.

whoever /huːˈɛvər/ *pron* anyone who; whatever person.

whole /hoːl/ *adj* not broken, intact; containing the total amount, number, etc.; complete. • *n* the entire amount; a thing complete in itself.

wholefood *n* unrefined food, free from additives.

wholehearted /ˈhoːlˌhɑrtəd/ *adj* sincere, single-minded, enthusiastic.—**wholeheartedly** *adv*.

whole hog /ˈhoːlˈhɒg/ *n* (*inf*) the complete amount or extent.

wholemeal /ˈhoːlmiːl/ *adj* (*Brit*) *see* **wholewheat**.

whole note *n* (*mus*) a note with a time value equal to two half notes.—*also* **semibreve**.

whole number *n* a number without fractions; an integer.

wholesale /-seɪl/ *n* selling of goods, *usu* at lower prices and in quantity, to a retailer.

wholesome /-səm/ *adj* healthy; mentally beneficial.—**wholesomeness** *n*.

wholewheat /-wiːt/ or /hwiːt/ *adj* (*esp US flour*) made from the entire wheat kernel.—*also* **wholemeal**.

who'll /huːl/ or /ˈhuːəl/ = who will; who shall.

wholly /ˈhoːlli/ *adv* completely.

whom /huːm/ *pron* objective case of **who**.

whomever /-ˈɛvər/ *pron* the objective form of **whoever**.

whoop /wuːp/ or /wʊp/, /huːp/ *n* a loud cry of excitement.

whoopee /ˈhuːpiː/ or /ˈwʊpiː/, /wuːpiː/ *interj* used to express wild excitement. • *n* boisterous fun.

whoopee cushion *n* a joke cushion that emits a rude noise when sat on.

whooping cough /ˈwuːpɪŋ/ or /ˈhuːpɪŋ/ *n* an infectious disease, *esp* of children, causing coughing spasms.

whoops /wʊps/ *interj* (*inf*) an exclamation of surprise or apology.

whoosh /wuːʃ/ or /wʊʃ/ *n* a rushing or hissing sound. • *vi* to make or move with such a sound.

whop /wɒp/ or /hwɒp/ *vt* (**whopping, whopped**) to beat, thrash; to defeat completely.

whopper /ˈwɒpər/ *n* (*inf*) a large specimen.—**whopping** *adj*.

whore /hɔr/ or /hʊr/ *n* a prostitute.

whorehouse /ˈhɔrhəʊs/ or /ˈhʊr-/ *n* a brothel.

whoremonger /-ˌmʌŋɡər/ or /-mʊŋɡər/, /ˈhʊr-/ *n* a person who uses the services of whores.—*also* **whoremaster**.

whorl /wɔrl/ or /wərl/ *n* a ring of leaves or petals round a stem; a single turn of a spiral; something shaped like a spiral; the central ridges of a fingerprint forming a complete circle.

whortleberry /ˈwɔrtəlˌberi/ *n* a bilberry.

who's /huːz/ = who is.

whose /huːz/ *pron* the possessive case of **who** or **which**.

whosoever /ˌhuːsoˈɛvər/ *pron* (*arch*) whoever.

who's who *n* a reference book containing the names and brief biographical details of famous or important people.

why /waɪ/ *adv* for what cause or reason? • *interj* exclamation of surprise. • *n* (*pl* **whys**) a cause.

whydah /ˈwɪdə/ *n* any of various African weaverbirds with black and white plumage.

WI *abbr* = Wisconsin; West Indies; (*esp Brit*) Women's Institute.

wick /wɪk/ *n* a cord, as in a candle or lamp, that supplies fuel to the flame.

wicked /ˈwɪkɪd/ *adj* evil, immoral, sinful.—**wickedly** *adv*.—**wickedness** *n*.

wicker /-ər/ *n* a long, thin, flexible twig; such twigs woven together, as in making baskets.—**wickerwork** *n*.

wicket /-ɪt/ *n* a small door or gate; (*croquet*) any of the small wire arches through which the balls must be hit; (*cricket*) the stumps at which the bowler aims the ball; the area between the bowler and the batsman; a batsman's innings.

wicketkeeper /ˈwɪkɪtˌkiːpər/ *n* (*cricket*) the fielder standing immediately behind the wicket.

widdershins /ˈwɪdərˌʃɪnz/ *see* **withershins**.

wide /waɪd/ *adj* broad; extensive; of a definite distance from side to side; (*with* **of**) far from the aim; open fully. • *n* (*cricket*) a ball bowled beyond the reach of the batsman.—**widely** *adv*.

wide-angle /ˈwaɪdˌæŋɡəl/ *adj* (*photog*) with an angle of view of 60 degrees or more.

wide-awake /-əˌweɪk/ *adj* fully awake; ready, alert.

wide-eyed /-ˌaɪd/ *adj* astonished; innocent.

widen /ˈwaɪdən/ *vti* to make or grow wide or wider.

widespread /-spred/ or /-ˈspred/ *adj* widely extended; general.

widget /ˈwɪdʒɪt/ *n* (*inf*) a small device or gadget the name of which is lost or forgotten; a whatsit.

widow /ˈwɪdoː/ *n* a woman whose husband has died. • *vt* to cause to become a widow.—**widowhood** *n*.

widower /-ər/ *n* a man whose wife has died.

widow's peak *n* a pointed growth of hair in the middle of the forehead.

width /wɪdθ/ or /wɪtθ/ *n* breadth.

wield /wiːld/ *vt* (*a weapon, etc*) to brandish; to exercise power.

wife /wəɪf/ *n* (*pl* **wives**) a married woman.

wig /wɪɡ/ *n* an artificial covering of real or synthetic hair for the head.

wigeon, widgeon /ˈwɪdʒən/ *n* a Eurasian wild duck the male of which has a gingery head.

wigging /ˈwɪɡɪŋ/ *n* (*Brit inf*) a severe reprimand.

wiggle /ˈwɪɡəl/ *vti* to move from side to side with jerky movements.

wigwag /-wæɡ/ *vb* (**wigwagging, wigwagged**) *vi* to move back and forth; to send a signal by means of flag semaphore. • *vt* to signal by wigwagging; to cause (something) to move back and forth. • *n* (the message sent using) a system of signalling with flags.

wigwam /-wæm/ *n* a North American Indian conical shelter.

wilco /ˈwɪlkoː/ *interj* used in telecommunications to indicate that a message is received and being acted upon.

wild /waɪld/ *adj* in its natural state; not tamed or cultivated; uncivilized; lacking control; disorderly; furious.—**wildly** *adv*.—**wildness** *n*.

wild boar *n* a wild pig with tusks, of Europe and Asia.

wild card *n* (*card games*) a card with an arbitrary value determined by the holder; (*sport*) a team that has not qualified for a competition but is allowed to take part; (*sl*) an unpredictable element.

wildcat /ˈwaɪldkæt/ *adj* (*strike*) unofficial. • *n* a fierce, undomesticated cat.

wildebeest /ˈwɪldəˌbiːst/ or /ˈvɪl-/ *n* (*pl* **wildebeests, wildebeest**) a gnu.

wilderness /-ərnəs/ *n* an uncultivated and desolate place.

wild-eyed /ˈwaɪdˌaɪd/ *adj* staring angrily or crazily.

wildfire /-ˌfaɪr/ *n* a fire that spreads fast and is hard to put out.

wildfowl /-faʊl/ *n* any bird that is hunted for game, *esp* waterbirds such as ducks and geese.

wild-goose chase *n* a futile pursuit of something.

wilding /ˈwaɪldɪŋ/ *n* (the fruit of) any uncultivated plant; a wild animal; (*sl*) a violent rampage though the streets by a teenage gang.

wildlife /-ləɪf/ *n* animals in the wild.

wild oat *n* (*usu pl*) a Eurasian grass related to cultivated oats; (*pl*) youthful excesses.

wild rice *n* a North American grass that bears edible grains; its grain.

Wild West *n* the western US during the lawless period of early settlement.

wile /waɪl/ *n* a trick, craftiness.

wilful /ˈwɪlfʊl/ *adj* stubborn; done intentionally.—*also* **willful**.—**wilfully, willfully** *adv*.—**wilfulness, willfulness** *n*.

will¹ /wɪl/ *n* power of choosing or determining; desire; determination; attitude, disposition; a legal document directing the disposal of one's property after death. • *vt* to bequeath; to command.

will² *aux vb* used in constructions with 2nd and 3rd persons; used to show futurity, determination, obligation.

willful /ˈwɪlfəl/ *see* **wilful**.

willies /ˈwɪliːz/ *npl* (with **the**) nervousness, jumpiness.

willing /-ɪŋ/ *adj* ready, inclined; eager.—**willingly** *adv*.—**willingness** *n*.

will-o'-the-wisp /ˌwɪləðəˈwɪsp/ *n* a pale phosphorescent glow sometimes seen over marshy areas and thought to be caused by combustion of gas from decaying organic matter; an elusive person or thing.

willow /ˈwɪloː/ *n* a tree or shrub with slender, flexible branches; the wood of the willow.

willowherb /-hərb/ or /-ərb/ *n* any of various plants of the evening-primrose family with pink or white flowers.

willow pattern *n* a traditional oriental-style design on china tableware consisting of a scene with figures and a willow tree, *usu* in blue on a white background.

willowy /-i/ *adj* flexible, graceful.

willpower /'wɪlˌpaʊər/ *n* the ability to control one's emotions and actions.

willy-nilly /ˌwɪlɪ'nɪlɪ/ *adv* whether desired or not.

wilt /wɪlt/ *vi* to become limp, as from heat; (*plant*) to droop; to become weak or faint.

wily /'waɪlɪ/ *adj* (**wilier, wiliest**) crafty; sly.—**wiliness** *n*.

WIMP, Wimp /wɪmp/ (*acronym*) (*comput*) a graphical interface using Windows, Icons, Mice and Pull-down menus that makes a computer easier to use.

wimp *n* (*inf*) a weak or ineffectual person.

wimple /'wɪmpəl/ *n* a linen or silk cloth draped round the head and neck but leaving the face uncovered, worn by women in medieval times and still used by some nuns.

win /wɪn/ *vti* (**winning, won**) to gain with effort; to succeed in a contest; to gain *eg* by luck; to achieve influence over; (*with* **over**) to gain the support or affection of (someone). • *n* a success.

wince /wɪns/ *vi* to shrink back; to flinch (as in pain).—*also n*.

winch /wɪntʃ/ *n* a hoisting machine. • *vt* to hoist or lower with a winch.

wind[1] /wɪnd/ *n* a current of air; breath; scent of game; (*inf*) flatulence; tendency; (*mus*) wind instrument(s). • *vt* (**winding, winded**) to cause to be short of breath; to perceive by scent.

wind[2] *vb* (**winding, wound**) *vt* to turn by cranking; to tighten the spring of a clock; to coil around something else; to encircle or cover, as with a bandage; (*with* **down**) to lower by winding a handle, etc. • *vi* to turn, to twist, to meander; (*with* **down**) to diminish in power or intensity; to slacken; to relax.

windage /'wɪndɪdʒ/ *n* the difference between the bore of a gun and the diameter of the projectile; (an allowance for) the deflection of a projectile caused by the wind.

windbag /-bæg/ *n* (*inf*) a person who talks a lot of rubbish.

windblown /-bloːn/ *adj* blown or shaped by the wind.

windbreak /-breɪk/ *n* a shelter that breaks the force of the wind, as a line of trees.

windburn /-bɜrn/ *n* redness and soreness of the skin due to the wind.

windcheater /-ˌtʃiːtər/ *n* a warm hooded jacket of windproof material.

wind-chill /-ˌtʃɪl/ *n* a measure of the effect of low temperature combined with wind.

winded /'wɪndɪd/ *adj* out of breath.

winder /-ər/ *n* one who or that which winds; a winding apparatus; a key for winding a spring-driven mechanism; a step in a spiral staircase.

windfall /-fɔl/ *n* fruit blown off a tree; any unexpected gain, *esp* financial.

winding /-ɪŋ/ *adj* meandering.

winding sheet *n* a sheet used to wrap a body for burial.

wind instrument *n* a musical instrument played by blowing into it or passing an air current through it.

windjammer /'wɪndˌdʒæmər/ *n* a large fast merchant sailing vessel.

windlass /-ləs/ *n* any of various devices for hoisting, hauling or lifting using a rope or chain wound round a motorized drum. • *vt* to hoist, etc using a windlass.

wind machine *n* a device used in film and theatre to produce realistic wind effects.

windmill /-mɪl/ *n* a machine operated by the force of the wind turning a set of sails.

window /'wɪndoː/ *n* a framework containing glass in the opening in a wall of a building, or in a vehicle, etc, for air and light.

window box *n* a narrow box on a windowsill for growing flowers, etc.

windowdressing *n* the arrangement of goods in a shop window; ornamentation intended to disguise the true nature of something.

windowpane /-peɪn/ *n* the glass in a window.

window-shopping /-ˌʃɒpɪŋ/ *n* the occupation of looking at goods for sale without buying them.—**window-shopper** *n*.

windowsill /-sɪl/ *n* a sill beneath a window.

windpipe /'wɪndpaɪp/ *n* the air passage from the mouth to the lungs, the trachea.

windrow /'wɪndroː/ *n* a row of leaves or pile of soil heaped up by or as if by the wind; ✤ a large pile of snow or gravel heaped up at the side of a road by a snow plough or grader.

windscreen /-skriːn/, **windshield** /-ʃiːld/ *n* a protective shield of glass in the front of a vehicle.

windscreen wiper, windshield wiper *n* a metal blade with a rubber edge that removes rain, etc, from a windscreen.

windsock /-sɒk/ *n* a canvas cylinder flown from an airport mast to show the direction of the wind.—*also* **drogue**.

windsurfing /-ˌsɜrfɪŋ/ *n* the sport of skimming along the surface of the water standing on a surfboard fitted with a sail.

windswept /-swept/ *adj* exposed to the wind; dishevelled.

wind tunnel *n* an apparatus for maintaining a constant force of air current to test the aerodynamics of an aircraft, etc.

wind-up /'waɪndʌp/ *n* the conclusion.

windward /'wɪndwərd/ *adv*, *adj* toward the direction where the wind blows from.

windy /'wɪndɪ/ or /'waɪndɪ/ *adj* (**windier, windiest**) exposed to the winds; stormy; verbose.

wine /waɪn/ *n* fermented grape juice used as an alcoholic beverage; the fermented juice of other fruits or plants.

wine bar *n* a bar that serves wine and food.

wine box *n* wine sold in a box with a small tap for pouring.

wine cellar *n* a place for storing wines, ideally a cool cellar; a stock of stored wines.

wine-coloured /waɪnˌkʌlərd/ *adj* dark purplish-red.

wine cooler *n* a vessel that is filled with ice for cooling wine bottles.

wineglass /-glæs/ *n* a glass, *usu* with a stem, for drinking wine.

winegrower /-groːə r/ *n* a person who grows vines and makes wine.

wine press /-pres/ *n* (a place containing) equipment for squeezing juice from grapes to make wine.

winery /'waɪnərɪ/ *n* (*pl* **wineries**) a place where wine is made.

wineskin /-skɪn/ *n* the skin of an animal, *esp* a goat, sewn into a bag for holding wine.

wing /wɪŋ/ *n* the forelimb of a bird, bat or insect, by which it flies; the main lateral surface of an aeroplane; a projecting part of a building; the side of a stage; a section of a political party. • *vti* to make one's way swiftly; to wound without killing.

wing chair *n* an armchair with high sides for excluding draughts.

wing collar *n* a stiff upturned shirt collar with the points turned down.

wing ding /'wɪŋdɪŋ/ *n* (*inf*) a wild party; a real or pretended fit.

wing nut *n* a nut that is tightened manually using flat wings that project on each side.

wingspan /-spæn/, **wingspread** /-spred/ *n* the width of a bird or aeroplane between the tips of the wings.

wink /wɪŋk/ *vi* to quickly open and close one's eye; to give a hint by winking; (*with* **at**) to disregard; to allow (something normally prohibited) to happen. • *n* the act of winking; an instant.

winkle[1] /'wɪŋkəl/ *n* a periwinkle.

winkle[2] *n* an edible sea snail. • *vt* (*with* **out**) (*inf*) to extract, prise out; to uncover, disclose.

winkle-pickers /-ˌpɪkərs/ *npl* shoes or boots with sharp pointed toes.

winner /'wɪnər/ *n* one that wins; (*inf*) a person or thing that is assured of success.

winning /-ɪŋ/ *n* a victory; (*pl*) money won in gambling. • *adj* charming.

Winnipeg goldeye *n* ✤ goldeye.

winnow /'wɪnoː/ *vt* to separate out the chaff from (the grain) by blowing air across it; to analyze.

wino /'waɪnoː/ *n* (*pl* **winos**) (*inf*) a down-and-out addicted to cheap wine.

winsome /'wɪnsəm/ *adj* charming, pleasing.

winter /-tər/ *n* the coldest season of the year: in the northern hemisphere from November or December to January or February. • *vi* to spend the winter.

wintergreen /'wɪntərˌgriːn/ *n* any of various evergreen plants or shrubs; an aromatic essential oil from these formerly used in medicine.

winterize /-ˌaɪz/ *vt* to prepare something (*eg* a car) to withstand winter weather.—**winterization** *n*.

winter road *n* ✤ (*Cdn*) a road made of compacted snow or ice over a frozen lake or land impassable in warmer weather.

winter sports *npl* sports that take place on ice or snow, such as skiing.

wintry, wintery /-rɪ/ *adj* (**wintrier, wintriest**) typical of winter, cold, stormy, snowy; unfriendly, frigid.

winy /'waɪnɪ/ *adj* (**winier, winiest**) tasting like or resembling wine.

wipe /waɪp/ *vt* to rub a surface with a cloth in order to clean or dry it; (*with* **out**) to remove; to erase; to kill off; to destroy. • *n* a wiping.

wiper /'waɪpər/ n a person or thing that wipes; a windscreen wiper.

wire /waɪr/ n a flexible thread of metal; a length of this; (*horse racing*) the finish line of a race; a telegram. • *adj* formed of wire. • *vt* to fasten, furnish, connect, etc, with wire; to send a telegram.

wired /-d/ *adj* (*sl*) wearing a hidden electronic recording or listening device; (*sl*) nervous or edgy, *esp* as a result of taking a stimulating drug.

wire-haired /'waɪr,herd/ *adj* (*dogs, etc*) having a coat of stiff hairs.

wireless /-ləs/ n (*formerly*) a radio.

wire service n in US, a news agency that sends out news to television and radio stations.

wiretap /-tæp/ *vb* (**wiretapping, wiretapped**) *vi* to connect to a telephone wire in order to listen in to a private conversation. • *vt* to tap (a telephone).—**wiretapper** n.

wireworm /-wərm/ n the filament-like larva of certain beetles which infest and destroy plant roots.

wiring /-ɪŋ/ n a system of wires used in an electrical device or circuit.

wiry /'waɪri/ *adj* (**wirier, wiriest**) lean, supple and sinewy.—**wiriness** n.

wisdom /'wɪzdəm/ n the ability to use knowledge; sound judgment.

wisdom tooth n one of four teeth set at the end of each side of the upper and lower jaw in humans and grown last.

wise /waɪz/ *adj* having knowledge or common sense; learned; prudent. • *vti* (*with* **up**) (*inf*) (to cause) to become informed or aware.— **wisely** *adv*.

-wise /waɪz/ *adv suffix* direction or manner; concerning.

wiseacre /'waɪz,eɪkər/ n a person who pretends to be clever or wise, a know-all.

wisecrack /-kræk/ n (*inf*) a witty or sarcastic remark.—*also vi.*

wise guy /-gaɪ/ n (*inf*) a person who is always making critical or sarcastic comments.

wise use n a policy designed to protect the use of natural resources and promote environmental awareness.

wish /wɪʃ/ *vti* to long for; to express a desire. • n desire; thing desired.

wishbone /'wɪʃbo:n/ n the forked bone at the front of the breastbone of a bird consisting of the fused clavicles.

wishful /-fʊl/ *adj* having a wish; hopeful.

wishful thinking n the mistaken belief that one's wishes correspond to reality.

wishy-washy /'wɪʃiˌwɒʃi/ *adj* weak, thin, feeble.

wisp /wɪsp/ n a thin strand; a small bunch, as of hay; anything slender.—**wispy** *adj*.

wisteria, wistaria /wɪ'sti:riə/ n a purple-flowered climbing plant.

wistful /'wɪstfʊl/ *adj* pensive; sad; yearning.—**wistfully** *adv*.—**wistfulness** n.

wit /wɪt/ n (*speech, writing*) the facility of combining ideas with humorous effect; a person with this ability; (*pl*) ability to think quickly.

witch /wɪtʃ/ n a woman who practises magic and is considered to a have dealings with the devil.

witchcraft /wɪtʃkræft/ n the practice of magic.

witch doctor n a man in certain tribes who appears to be able to cure sickness or cause harm to people.

witchery /-əri/ n (*pl* **witcheries**) witchcraft; fascination.

witch hazel n any of a genus of North American shrubs with yellow flowers; a soothing lotion made from the bark of this applied to lumps, bruises, skin rashes, etc.

witch hunt n a campaign of harassment of those with dissenting opinions; the search for and persecution of those accused of witchcraft.

witching /-ɪŋ/ *adj* of or suitable for witchcraft.

with /wɪθ/ or /wɪð/ *prep* denoting nearness or agreement; in the company of; in the same direction as; among; by means of; possessing.

withal /wɪ'ðɒl/ *adv* (*arch*) as well; moreover.

withdraw /wɪθ'drɔ/ or /wɪð-/ *vb* (**withdrawing, withdrew,** *pp* **withdrawn**) *vt* to draw back or away; to remove; to retract. • *vi* to retire; to retreat.—**withdrawal** n.

withdrawn /wɪθdrɒn/ or /wɪð/ *adj* introverted, reserved; remote.

wither /'wɪðər/ *vi* to fade or become limp or dry, as of a plant. • *vt* to cause to dry up or fade.

withers /-z/ *npl* the ridge between the shoulder blades of a horse.

withershins /-ʃɪnz/ *adv* counter-clockwise.—*also* **widdershins**.

withhold /wɪθ'ho:ld/ *vt* (**withholding, withheld**) to hold back; to deduct; to restrain; to refuse to grant.

within /wɪθɪn/ or /-ðɪn/ *prep* inside; not exceeding; not beyond.

without /wɪ'θɐʊt/ or /-ðɐʊt/ *prep* outside or out of, beyond; not having, lacking. • *adv* outside.

withstand /wɪθ'stænd/ or /wɪð-/ *vt* (**withstanding, withstood**) to oppose or resist, *esp* successfully; to endure.

witless /'wɪtləs/ *adj* foolish, stupid; not witty.

witness /-nəs/ n a person who gives evidence or attests a signing; testimony (of a fact). • *vt* to have first-hand knowledge of; to see; to be the scene of; to serve as evidence of; to attest a signing. • *vi* to testify.

witness stand, witness box n an enclosure for witnesses in a court of law.

witticism /'wɪtɪsɪzəm/ n a witty remark.

wittingly /'wɪtɪŋli/ *adv* knowingly.

witty /'wɪti/ *adj* (**wittier, wittiest**) full of wit.—**wittily** *adv*.—**wittiness** n.

wives /waɪvz/ *see* **wife**.

wizard /'wɪzərd/ n a magician; a man who practises witchcraft or magic; an expert.—**wizardry** n.

wizened /-ənd/ *adj* dried up, wrinkled, shrivelled.

wk *abbr* = week.

woad /wo:d/ n (a blue dye obtained from the leaves of) a European plant of the mustard family.

wobble /'wɒbəl/ *vi* to sway unsteadily from side to side; to waver, to hesitate.—**wobbly** *adj*.

wodge /wɒdʒ/ n (*Brit inf*) a thick slice or chunk of something.

woe /wo:/ n grief, misery; (*pl*) misfortune.—**woeful** *adj*.—**woefully** *adv*.

woebegone /'wo:bəˌgɒn/ *adj* sorrowful.

wok /wɒk/ n a large, metal, hemispherical pan used for Chinese-style cooking.

woke /wo:k/, **woken** /'wo:kən/ *see* **wake**[1].

wolf /wʊlf/ n (*pl* **wolves**) a wild animal of the dog family that hunts in packs; a flirtatious man.

wolfcall /'wʊlfkɒl/ n a whistle made by a man when seeing an attractive woman.—*also* **wolf whistle**.

wolfhound /'wʊlfhaʊnd/ n any of several types of large dog formerly used to hunt wolves.

wolfram /-rəm/ n tungsten; wolframite.

wolframite /-rəˌmaɪt/ n a mineral that is the chief ore of tungsten and also contains iron and manganese.

wolf whistle *see* **wolf call**.

wolverine /ˌwʊlvər'i:n/ or /'wʊlvərˌi:n/ n a voracious carnivorous animal of northern forests of Europe, North America and Asia with thick black fur.

wolves /wʊlvz/ *see* **wolf**.

woman /'wʊmən/ n (*pl* **women**) an adult human female; the female sex.

womanhood /-ˌhʊd/ n the state of being a woman.

womanish /-ɪʃ/ n resembling a woman; suitable for women.

womanize /'wʊməˌnaɪz/ *vi* to pursue women for sex.—**womanizer** n.

womankind /'wʊmənˌkaɪnd/ n female human beings; women collectively, *esp* as distinct from men.

womanly /-li/ *adj* having the qualities of a woman.

womb /wu:m/ n the female organ in which offspring are developed until birth, the uterus; any womb-like cavity; a place where something is produced.

wombat /'wɒmbæt/ n an Australian marsupial mammal resembling a small bear.

women /'wɪmɪn/ *see* **woman**.

womenfolk /-ˌfo:k/ *npl* women collectively; the female members of a family, group or community.

Women's Institute n (*esp Brit*) an organization for women which engages in various social and cultural activities.

Women's Movement n a feminist movement seeking to end male domination of women in society.

won /wɒn/ *see* **win**.

wonder /'wʌndər/ n a feeling of surprise or astonishment; something that excites such a feeling; a prodigy. • *vi* to feel wonder; to be curious; to speculate; to marvel.

wonderful /-ˌfʊl/ *adj* marvellous.—**wonderfully** *adv*.

wonderland /-ˌlænd/ n a land full of marvels.

wonderment /-mənt/ n astonishment, awe; curiosity.

wondrous /-əs/ *adj* (*poet*) wonderful, marvellous.

wonky /'wɒŋki/ *adj* (**wonkier, wonkiest**) (*sl*) crooked, unsteady.

wont /wɒnt/ *adj* accustomed; inclined. • *n* habit.

won't /wo:nt/ = will not.

woo /wu:/ *vt* (**wooing, wooed**) to seek to attract with a view to marriage; to court; to solicit eagerly.—**wooer** *n*.

wood /wʊd/ *n* the hard fibrous substance under the bark of trees; trees cut or sawn, timber; a thick growth of trees.

wood alcohol *n* methanol.

woodbine /'wʊdbaɪn/ *n* wild honeysuckle.

woodchuck /-tʃʊk/ *n* a North American marmot with thick reddish-brown fur.—*also* **groundhog**.

woodcock /-kɒk/ *n* a game bird related to the snipe.

woodcraft /-kræft/ *n* skill in living and surviving in the forest, *esp* hunting; skill at woodwork.

woodcut /-kʌt/ *n* an engraving made on wood; a print made from this.

woodcutter /-ˌkʌtər/ *n* a person whose job is to cut down trees.

wooded /'wʊdɪd/ *adj* covered with trees.

wooden /-ən/ *adj* made of wood; stiff.

wood engraving *n* the art of engraving illustrations on wood; (a print taken from) a piece of engraved wood.

woodenhead /'wʊdənˌhed/ *n* (*inf*) a foolish person.

woodland /-lənd/ *n* land covered with trees.

woodlot /'wʊdlɒt/ *n* ❀ an area of treed land, *esp* on a far, from which firewood can be cut.

woodlouse /-laʊs/ *n* (*pl* **woodlice**) a small ground-dwelling wingless crustacean with a segmented body that can roll itself into a ball.

woodman /-mən/ *n* (*pl* **woodmen**) a forester or woodcutter.

wood nymph *n* (*Greek myth*) a nymph of the woods, a dryad.

woodpecker /-ˌpekər/ *n* a bird that pecks holes in trees to extract insects.

wood pigeon *n* a large European wild pigeon with white patches of feathers on the body and neck.

woodpile /-paɪl/ *n* a pile of wood, *esp* firewood.

wood pulp *n* wood that has been pulped and treated for paper-making.

wood screw *n* a pointed metal screw with an external thread and slotted head designed to be driven into wood with a screwdriver.

woodshed /-ʃed/ *n* a small shed for storing wood (*eg* firewood), tools, gardening equipment, etc.

woodsman /'wʊdzmən/ *n* (*pl* **woodsmen**) a person who lives and works in a wood; a woodman.

woodwind /-wɪnd/ *n* section of an orchestra in which wind instruments, originally made of wood, are played.

woodwork /-wɜrk/ *n* carpentry.

woodworm /-wɜrm/ *n* (*esp Brit*) an insect larva that bores into wood; the damage in furniture so caused.

woody /-wʊdi/ *adj* (**woodier, woodiest**) covered in trees.

woof[1] /wʊf/ *n* the horizontal threads crossing the warp in a woven fabric.

woof[2] /wʊf/ *or* /wu:f/ *interj* a noise like the bark of a dog. • *vi* to make this sound.

woofer /'wu:fər/ *n* a loudspeaker.

wool /wʊl/ *n* the fleece of sheep and other animals; thread or yarn spun from the coats of sheep; cloth made from this yarn.

woollen, woolen /'wʊlən/ *adj* made of wool.

woolly bear *n* a large furry caterpillar produced by the tiger moth.

woolly, wooly /'wʊli/ *adj* (**woollier, woolliest** *or* **woolier, wooliest**) of, like or covered with wool; indistinct, blurred; muddled. • *n* (*pl* **woollies**) (*inf*) a woollen garment.—**woolliness, wooliness** *n*.

woolsack /-sæk/ *n* the official seat of the Lord Chancellor in the British House of Lords (formerly made from a large sack of wool).

woozy /'wu:zi/ *adj* (**woozier, wooziest**) (*inf*) mentally confused, dazed; dizzy, nauseous.

word /wɜrd/ *n* a single unit of language in speech or writing; talk, discussion; a message; a promise; a command; information; a password; (*pl*) lyrics; (*pl*) a quarrel. • *vt* to put into words, to phrase; to flatter.

word blindness *n* alexia or dyslexia.

word for word /'wɜrdfər'wɜrd/ *adj, adv* (a *translation*, etc) using exactly the same words, verbatim.

wording /'wɜrdɪŋ/ *n* the way in which words are used, *esp* in written form; a choice of words.

word-perfect *adj* able to repeat something without mistake.—*also* **letter-perfect**.

wordplay /-pleɪ/ *n* verbal wit or repartee.

word processor *n* computer software that allows the input, formatting, storage and printing of text electronically; the hardware, including microprocessor, monitor, keyboard and printer, required to operate word-processing software.

wordy /'wɜrdi/ *adj* (**wordier, wordiest**) verbose.

wore /wɔ:r/ *see* **wear**.

work /wɜrk/ *n* employment, occupation; a task; the product of work; manner of working; place of work; a literary composition; (*pl*) a factory, plant. • *vi* to be employed, to have a job; to operate (a machine, etc); to produce effects; (*with* **on**) to (attempt to) persuade by persistent effort; (*with* **out**) to undertake a regular, planned series of exercises. • *vt* to effect, to achieve; (*with* **off**) to eliminate though effort; (*with* **over**) to examine closely; (*inf*) to assault violently. —**workable** *adj*.—**worker** *n*.

workaday /'wɜrkəˌdeɪ/ *adj* suited for working days; ordinary, mundane.

workaholic /ˌwɜrkə'hɒlɪk/ *n* a person with a compulsive need to work.

workbench /'wɜrkbentʃ/ *n* a bench designed for woodworking, metalworking, etc.

workbook /-bʊk/ *n* an exercise book with spaces for answers to set questions.

workbox /-bɒks/ *n* a box for holding material and tools for work.

workday /-deɪ/ *see* **working day**.

work force /-fɔrs/ *n* the number of workers who are engaged in a particular industry; the total number of workers who are potentially available.

workhorse /-hɔrs/ *n* a horse used for work on a farm; (*inf*) a person or thing that works the hardest in an organization, business, etc.

workhouse /-haʊs/ *n* (*formerly*) in UK, a public institution for paupers; in US, a prison for petty offenders whose sentences are served by manual labour.

working /'wɜrkɪŋ/ *adj* spent in or used for work; functioning. • *n* operation; mode of operation; (*pl*) the manner of functioning or operating; (*pl*) the parts of a mine that are worked.

working capital *n* liquid capital available for the daily operation of a business.

working class *n* people who work for wages, *esp* manual workers; proletariat —*also adj*.

working day, workday *n* a day for working as opposed to a holiday; the number of hours spent working during the day.

working drawing *n* a plan or drawing used to guide a builder, engineer, etc during the actual construction.

working party *n* (*esp Brit*) a committee established to investigate a particular problem.

workload /-loːd/ *n* the amount of work done or required to be done in a particular period.

workman /-mən/ *n* (*pl* **workmen**) a person employed in manual labour; a person who works in a particular manner.

workmanlike /-mənˌlaɪk/ *adj* skilful.

workmanship /-mənʃɪp/ *n* technical skill; the way a thing is made, style.

workmate /-meɪt/ *n* (*Brit*) a colleague with whom one works.

work of art *n* a fine painting, sculpture, building, etc; something that has the aesthetic qualities of a work of art.

work-out /'wɜrkaʊt/ *n* a session of strenuous physical exercises.

workroom /-ru:m/ *n* a room for work, a workshop.

workshop /-ʃɒp/ *n* a room or building where work is done; a seminar for specified intensive study, work, etc.

workshy /-ʃaɪ/ *adj* (*Brit*) disinclined to work.

work station /-ˌsteɪʃən/ *n* a place in an office, *esp* a desk equipped with a computer terminal, where a single person works.

work-to-rule *n* (*Brit*) industrial action in which employees adhere strictly to rules and regulations in the workplace with the aim of slowing production.—**work to rule** *vi*.

worktop /-tɒp/ *n* (*Brit*) an area in a kitchen, *usu* with a laminated surface, where food is prepared.

world /wɜrld/ *n* the planet earth and its inhabitants; mankind; the universe; a sphere of existence; the public.

worldbeater /'wɜrldˌbiːtər/ *n* someone or something surpassing all others, a champion.—**worldbeating** *adj*.

world-class /-'klæs/ *adj* of the highest quality in the world.

worldly /-li/ *adj* (**worldlier, worldliest**) earthly, rather than spiritual; material; experienced.

world music *n* popular music of or combining ethnic styles from various different countries around the world.

world power *n* a country that is powerful enough to influence international politics.

World Series *n* an annual competition (best of seven games) between the winning teams of the two major North American baseball leagues.

world-shaking *adj* of momentous significance.

World War I *n* a war (1914–18) in which Belgium, France, Italy, Japan, Russia, UK, US, and other allies defeated Germany, Austria, Bulgaria, and Turkey.

World War II *n* a war (1939–45) in which France, UK, US, USSR, and other allies defeated Germany, Italy, and Japan.

world-weary /-ˌwɪriː/ *adj* tired of life.

worldwide /-waɪd/ or /-ˈwaɪd/ *adj* universal.

WORM *abbr* (*comput*) = Write Once Read Many Times: an optical disk that stores information which cannot then be overwritten, used for data archiving and backup.

worm /wɜrm/ *n* an earthworm; an insect larva; the thread of a screw. • *vt* to work (oneself into a position) slowly or secretly; to extract information by slow and persistent means.

worm-eaten /ˈwɜrmˌiːtən/ *adj* eaten into (as if) by worms; decayed; antiquated.

worms /-z/ or /ˈvɔrmz/ *n sing* any disease or condition caused by infestation with parasitic worms.

worm's-eye view /ˈwɜrmzˌaɪ/ *n* the view from the very bottom or humblest position.

wormwood /-wʊd/ *n* a European plant that yields a bitter oil used in making absinthe; (something causing) bitterness.

wormy /ˈwɜrmiː/ *adj* (**wormier, wormiest**) infested with or eaten by worms; resembling a worm; full of holes caused by burrowing worms.

worn /wɔrn/ *see* **wear**.

worn-out /-aʊt/ *adj* (*machine, etc*) past its useful life; (*person*) depressed, tired.

worriment /ˈwɜrimənt/ *n* (*inf*) worry, anxiety.

worrisome /-səm/ *adj* causing worry; prone to anxiety.

worry /ˈwɜriː/ *vb* (**worrying, worried**) *vt* to bother, pester, harass. • *vi* to be uneasy or anxious; to fret. • *n* (*pl* **worries**) a cause or feeling of anxiety.—**worrier** *n*.

worry beads *npl* a string of beads fiddled with for comfort or to relieve tension.

worse /wɜrs/ *adj* (*compar of* **bad** *and* **ill**) less favourable; not so well as before. • *adv* with great severity.—**worsen** *vti*.

worship /ˈwɜrʃɪp/ *n* religious adoration; a religious ritual, *eg* prayers; devotion. • *vb* (**worshipping, worshipped** *or* **worshiping, worshiped**) *vt* to adore or idolize. • *vi* to participate in a religious service.—**worshipper, worshiper** *n*.

worshipful /-ˌfʊl/ *adj* feeling or displaying worship or respect; (*with cap*) in UK, used as a title of respect for various high-ranking officials.

worst /wɜrst/ *adj* (*superl of* **bad** *or* **ill**; *see also* **worse**) bad or ill in the highest degree; of the lowest quality. • *adv* to the worst degree. • *n* the least good part.

worst-case /ˈwɜrstˌkeɪs/ *adj* being, or taking account of, the worst possible situation or outcome (*worst-case scenario*).

worsted /- əd/ *n* twisted thread or yarn made from long, combed wool.

worth /wɜrθ/ *n* value; price; excellence; importance. • *adj* equal in value to; meriting.

worthless /ˈwɜrθləs/ *adj* valueless; useless; of bad character.—**worthlessness** *n*.

worthwhile /-waɪl/ or /-ˈwaɪl/ *adj* important or rewarding enough to justify the effort.

worthy /ˈwɜrðiː/ *adj* (**worthier, worthiest**) virtuous; deserving. • *n* (*pl* **worthies**) a worthy person, a local celebrity.—**worthily** *adv*.

would /wʊd/ or /wəd/ *see* **will²**.

would-be /ˈwʊdbiː/ *adj* aspiring or professing to be.

wouldn't /-ənt/ = would not.

wound¹ /wuːnd/ *n* any cut, bruise, hurt, or injury caused to the skin; hurt feelings. • *vt* to injure.

wound² *see* **wind²**.

wove /woːv/, **woven** /ˈwoːvən/ *see* **weave**.

wow /waʊ/ *interj* exclamation of astonishment. • *n* (*sl*) a success.

wp, WP *abbr* = word processing; word processor.

Wpg. *abbr* ✤ = Winnipeg.

wpm *abbr* = words per minute.

wrack¹ /ræk/ *n* destruction; **wrack and ruin** (the remains of) something destroyed.

wrack² *n* seaweed deposited on the shore.

wraith /reɪθ/ *n* an apparition of a living person, supposedly a sign of impending death; any ghost.

wrangle /ˈræŋgəl/ *vi* to argue; to dispute noisily. • *n* a noisy argument.

wrap /ræp/ *vt* (**wrapping, wrapped**) to fold (paper) around (a present, purchase etc); to wind (around); to enfold; (*with* **up**) to enclose in paper; (*inf*) to make the final arrangements for. • *vi* (*with* **up**) to put warm clothes on; (*inf*) to be quiet. • *n* a shawl.

wrapper /ˈræpər/ *n* one who or that which wraps; a book jacket; a light dressing gown.

wrasse /ræs/ *n* a marine food fish with thick lips and brilliant colouration.

wrath /ræθ/ *n* intense anger; rage.—**wrathful** *adj*.

wreak /riːk/ *vt* to inflict or exact (*eg* vengeance, havoc).

wreath /riːθ/ *n* (*pl* **wreaths**) a twisted ring of leaves, flowers, etc; something like this in shape.

wreathe /riːð/ *vti* to form into a wreath; to decorate with wreaths; to move or coil in wreaths.

wreck /rɛk/ *n* accidental destruction of a ship; a badly damaged ship; a run-down person or thing. • *vt* to destroy; to ruin.

wreckage /ˈrɛkɪdʒ/ *n* the process of wrecking; remnants from a wreck.

wrecked /-t/ *adj* (*sl*) intoxicated by alcohol or drugs; exhausted.

wrecker /ˈrɛkər/ *n* a person who causes a wreck; a demolition worker; a breakdown van.

wren /rɛn/ *n* small brownish songbird, with a short erect tail.

wrench /-tʃ/ *vt* to give something a violent pull or twist; to injure with a twist, to sprain; to distort. • *n* a forceful twist; a sprain; a spanner; emotional upset caused by parting.

wrest /rɛst/ *vt* to take with force (from); to seize; to obtain by toil.

wrestle /ˈrɛsəl/ *vti* to fight by holding and trying to throw one's opponent down; to struggle. • *n* a contest in which the opponents wrestle.—**wrestler** *n*.

wrestling /-ɪŋ/ *n* the skill or sport of fighting by grappling and trying to throw each other to the ground.

wretch /rɛtʃ/ *n* a miserable or pitied person; a despised and scorned person.

wretched /ˈrɛtʃəd/ *adj* very miserable; in poor circumstances; despicable.—**wretchedly** *adv*.—**wretchedness** *n*.

wrier /raɪər/, **wriest** /-əst/ *see* **wry**.

wriggle /ˈrɪgəl/ *vi* to move with a twisting motion; to squirm, to writhe; to use evasive tricks.—*also n*.—**wriggler** *n*.—**wriggly** *adj*.

wright /raɪt/ *n* a maker (*eg* playwright), a builder (*eg* shipwright).

wring /rɪŋ/ *vt* (**wringing, wrung**) to twist; to compress by twisting in order to squeeze water from; to pain; to obtain forcibly.

wrinkle /ˈrɪŋkəl/ *n* a small crease or fold on a surface. • *vti* to make or become wrinkled.

wrist /rɪst/ *n* the joint connecting the hand with the forearm.

wristband /ˈrɪstbænd/ *n* the cuff of a sleeve that covers the wrist; a band round the wrist that absorbs sweat.

wristwatch /-wɒtʃ/ *n* a watch worn on a bracelet or strap around the wrist.

writ /rɪt/ *n* (*law*) a written court order.

write /raɪt/ *vb* (**writing, wrote,** *pp* **written**) *vt* to form letters on paper with a pen or pencil; to express in writing; to compose (a letter, music, literary work, etc); to communicate by letter; (*with* **off**) to cancel a bad debt as a loss; (*inf*) to damage (a vehicle) beyond repair; (*with* **down**) *vt* to put in writing; to harm or demean (a person) in writing; (*with* **up**) to describe, update, or put into finished form by writing; to praise or publicize in writing. • *vi* to be a writer; (*with* **down to** *or* **for**) to write in a simplified style for a less educated taste.

write-off /ˈraɪtˌɒf/ *n* a debt cancelled as a loss; (*inf*) a badly damaged car.

writer /ˈraɪtər/ *n* an author; a scribe or clerk.

writer's cramp *n* painful spasms or paralysis in the thumb and fingers from excessive writing.

write-up *n* a published report or review, *esp* a favourable one.

writhe /raɪð/ *vi* to twist the body violently, as in pain; to squirm (under, at).

writing /ˈraɪtɪŋ/ *n* the act of forming letters on paper, etc; a written document; authorship; (*pl*) literary works.

writing paper *n* paper treated to accept ink and used *esp* for letters.

written /'rɪtən/ *see* **write**.

wrong /rɒŋ/ *adj* not right, incorrect; mistaken, misinformed; immoral. • *n* harm; injury done to another. • *adv* incorrectly. • *vt* to do wrong to.—**wrongly** *adv*.

wrongdoer /'rɒŋ‚duːər/ *n* a person who breaks (moral) laws.—**wrongdoing** *n*.

wrongful /-ful/ *adj* unwarranted, unjust.—**wrongfully** *adv*.

wrong-headed /-'hedɪd/ *adj* stubborn; of poor judgment.

wrote /rəʊt/ *see* **write**.

wrought /rɔːt/ *adj* formed; made; (*metals*) shaped by hammering, etc.

wrought iron *n* iron that is forged or rolled, not cast.

wrung /rʌŋ/ *see* **wring**.

wry /raɪ/ *adj* (**wryer, wryest** *or* **wrier, wriest**) twisted, contorted; ironic.—**wryly** *adv*.—**wryness** *n*.

wt *abbr* = weight.

wunderkind /'vʊndər‚kɪnd/ *n* (*pl* **wunderkinder, wunderkinds**) a child prodigy; a whizz kid.

wurst /wɜːst/ *or* /wʊrst/ *n* any of various types of spicy sausage from Germany or Austria.

WWI *abbr* = World War I.

WWII *abbr* = World War II.

WWF *abbr* = World Wildlife Fund for Nature.

WWW *abbr* = World Wide Web.

WY *abbr* = Wyoming.

WYSIWYG /'wɪzɪ‚wɪg/ *adj* (*acronym*) (*comput*) what you see is what you get: meaning that the layout and style of text, etc, on screen will be exactly as printed out.

X

X, x /ɛks/ n the 24th letter of the English alphabet; something shaped like an X; the mark used by an illiterate person to represent a signature; a mark (on a map) to show a particular spot.

X, x symbol (math) unknown quantity; the figure 10. • n an unknown or mysterious factor.

xanth- /zænθ/, **xantho-** /zænθo:/ or /-θə/ prefix yellow.

xanthein /ˈzænθiin/ n a soluble yellow pigment found in plant tissue.

xanthic /-ɪk/ adj yellowish; of or relating to xanthine.

xanthine /-ɪːn/ n an insoluble yellow pigment found in plant tissue; a yellowish-white crystalline compound allied to uric acid; a derivative of this.

Xanthippe /zænˈθɪpi/ n the wife of Socrates (fl 5th century BC); a quarrelsome scolding wife.

xantho-, xanth- /ˈzænθo:/ or /-θə/ prefix yellow.

xanthochroid /ˈzænθəˌkrɔɪd/ adj blond and blue-eyed with fair white skin. • n an xanthochroid person.

xanthoma /zænˈθoːmə/ n (pl **xanthomas, xanthomata**) a small yellow tumour in the skin caused by deposits of lipids.—**xanthomatous** adj.

xanthophyll /ˈzænθə fɪl/ n (bot) an orange or yellow pigment in autumn leaves.—**xanthophyllous** adj.

xanthopsia /ˈzænθoːpsɪə/ n a disturbance in vision causing everything to appear yellow.

xanthosis /ˈzænθosɪs/ n a yellow pigmentation of the skin in diabetes, etc.

xanthous /ˈzænθəs/ adj yellow.

x-axis /ˈɛksˌæksɪs/ n (pl **x-axes**) the reference axis of a graph along which the x coordinate is measured.

X-chromosome n one of the pair (with the Y-chromosome) of sex chromosomes that occur in females.

Xe (chem symbol) xenon.

xebec /ˈziːbɛk/ n a small three-masted Mediterranean sailing vessel with lateen sails.

xeno- /ˈzɛno:/ or /ˈziːnoː/, **xen-** /ˈzɛn/ or /ziːn/ prefix strange; foreign.

xenolith /ˈzɛnəlɪθ/ or /ˈziːn-/ n (geol) a rock occuring in a system of rocks to which it does not belong.

xenomorphic /ˈzɛnoˌmɔrfɪk/ adj (mineral grain) abnormal in shape owing to the pressure of adjacent minerals in rock.

xenon /ˈzɛnɒn/ n a heavy inert colourless odourless gaseous element found in tiny quantities in the atmosphere.

xenophobia /ˌzɛnəˈfoːbiə/ or /ˌziːn-/ n fear or dislike of strangers or foreigners.—**xenophobe** n.—**xenophobic** adj.

xer-, xero- /ˈziːro:/ or /ˈzɛro:/ prefix dryness.

xeroderma /ˌziːrəˈdɜrmə/, **xerodermia** /ˌziːrəˈdɜrmiə/ n dryness of the skin caused by a deficiency in secretions from the sebaceous glands.

xerography /ziːˈrɒgrəfi/ or /zɛ-/ n photocopying by using light to form an electrostatic image on a photoconductive plate to which toner powder adheres, the particles then being fused by heat and the image transferred onto paper.—**xerographic** adj.—**xerographically** adv.

xerophilous /ziːˈrɒfɪləs/ or /zɛ-/ adj (plant) drought-loving; adapted to a dry climate.—**xerophily** n.

xerophthalmia /ˌzɪrɒfˈθælmiə/ n a disease of the eye with dryness and ulceration of the cornea, caused by vitamin deficiency.—**xerophthalmic** adj.

xerophyte /ˈziːrəˌfɔɪt/ or /zɛ-/ n a xerophilous plant, eg cactus, that has adapted for growth with a limited water supply.—**xerophytic** adj.

xerostomia /ziːˈrɒsˌtəmiə/ n abnormal dryness of the mouth caused by failure of the salivary glands.

Xerox /ˈziːrɒks/ n (trademark) a photocopying process using xerography; the copy produced by this. • vt to produce a copy in this way.

x-height n (print) the height of the letter x in lowercase.

xi /saɪ/ or /gzaɪ/, /zaɪ/ n (pl **xis**) the 14th letter of the Greek alphabet.

xiphisternum /ˌzɪfəˈstɜrnəm/ n (pl **xiphisterna**) (anat, zool) the lowest part of the breastbone, the xiphoid process.—**xiphisternal** adj.

xiphoid /ˈzɪfɔɪd/ adj sword-shaped. • n the xiphoid process.

xiphoid process n the xiphisternum.

Xmas /ˈkrɪsməs/ or /ˈɛksməs/ abbr = Christmas.

X-ray, x-ray /ˈɛksreɪ/ n radiation of very short wavelengths, capable of penetrating solid bodies, and printing on a photographic plate a shadow picture of objects not permeable by light rays. • vt to photograph by x-rays.

XST abbr = experimental Stealth technology.

xylem /ˈzaɪlɛm/ n the woody vegetable tissue in plants that conducts water and gives support.

xylo- /ˈzaɪloː/, **xyl-** /ˈzaɪl/ prefix wood.

xylograph /ˈzaɪləˌgræf/ n a wood engraving; an impression made from a wood block.

xylography /zaɪˈlɒgrəfi/ n the art of making wood engravings or making woodcuts; the art of printing from wood blocks.—**xylographer** n.—**xylographic** adj.—**xylographically** adv.

xyloid /ˈzaɪˌlɔɪd/ adj like wood.

xylophagous /zaɪˈlɒfəgəs/ adj (insects) wood-eating.

xylophone /ˈzaɪləˌfoːn/ n a percussion instrument consisting of a series of wooden bars which are struck with small hammers.—**xylophonic** adj.

xylophonist /ˈzaɪləˌfoːnɪst/ n a performer on a xylophone.

xylotomous /zaɪˈlɒtəməs/ adj (insects) boring into or cutting wood.

Y

Y (*chem symbol*) yttrium.

Y /waɪ/ *abbr* = yen (Japanese currency).

Y, y *n* the 25th letter of the English alphabet; something shaped like a Y.

Y, y *symbol* (*math*) the second unknown quantity.

y *abbr* = year; yard.

yabber /ˈjæbər/ *n* (*Austral sl*) talk, *esp* in broken English. • *vti* to talk.

yacht /jɒt/ *n* a sailing or mechanically driven vessel, used for pleasure cruises or racing. • *vi* to race or cruise in a yacht.—**yachting** *n*.—**yachtsman** *n* (*pl* **yachtsmen**).—**yachtswoman** *nf* (*pl* **yachtswomen**).

yackety-yak (var. of **yak**²) *n* (*sl*) persistent trivial chatter.

yah /jæ/ *interj* expressing derision.

yahoo /ˈjæhuː/ *n* (*pl* **yahoos**) a crude, vicious person.

Yahweh, Yahveh /ˈjɒweɪ/ *n* Jehovah.

yak¹ /jæk/ *n* a domesticated species of ox found in Tibet having horns and long hair.

yak² *n* (*sl*) persistent trivial talk or chatter. • *vi* (**yakking, yakked**) to talk in this way.

Yale lock *n* (*trademark*) a type of cylinder lock for doors.

yam /jæm/ *n* the edible, starchy tuberous root of a tropical climbing plant; sweet potato.

yamen /ˈjɑmən/ *n* (*formerly*) the official residence of a Chinese madarin.

yammer /ˈjæmər/ *vi* (*inf*) to whimper or whine constantly; (*inf*) to complain loudly and persistently. • *n* (*inf*) a whining or complaining sound.

Yank /jæŋk/ *n* (*inf*) a Yankee.

yank *vti* to pull suddenly, to jerk. • *n* a sudden sharp pull.

Yankee /ˈjæŋki/ *n* (*inf*) a citizen of the US, an American.

yap /jæp/ *vi* (**yapping, yapped**) to yelp, bark; (*sl*) to talk constantly, *esp* in a noisy or irritating manner.

yapok, yapock /ˈjæpɒk/ *n* a tropical American aquatic marsupial with webbed hind feet, thick fur, and a long tail.

yard¹ /jɑrd/ *n* a unit of measure of three feet and equivalent to 0.9144 metres; (*naut*) a spar hung across a mast to support a sail.

yard² *n* an enclosed concrete area, *esp* near a building; an enclosure for a commercial activity (*eg* a shipyard); an area of ground for growing herbs, fruits, flowers, or vegetables, *usu* attached to a house, a garden; an area with tracks for the making up of trains, servicing of locomotives, etc.

yardage¹ /ˈjɑrdɪdʒ/ *n* a length measured in yards.

yardage² *n* the use of a yard; the charge made for this.

yardarm /ˈjɑrdɑrm/ *n* (*naut*) either half of a yard.

yardman /ˈjɑrdmən/ *n* (*pl* **yardmen**) a worker in a railroad yard.

yardmaster /-mæstər/ *n* the manager of a railroad yard.

yardstick /-stɪk/ *n* a standard used in judging.

yare /jər/ *adj* ready; active, brisk; (*yacht*, *etc*) easily handled.

Yarmulke /ˈjɑrməlkə/ *n* a skullcap worn by Jewish men at prayer and by Orthodox male Jews at all times.

yarn /jɑrn/ *n* fibres of wool, cotton etc spun into strands for weaving, knitting, etc; (*inf*) a tale or story. • *vi* to tell a yarn; to talk at length.

yarrow /ˈjæroʊ/ *n* a strongly scented astringent herb with clusters of small flowers.

yashmak, yashmac /ˈjæʃmæk/ *n* a veil worn by Muslim women, showing only the eyes.

yataghan, yatagan /ˈjætə,gæn/ or /-gən/ *n* a short curved Turkish sword without a guard.

yatter /ˈjætər/ *vi* (*sl*) to gabble, to chatter.—*also n*.

yauld /jɔːd/ or /jɒd/, /jɒld/ *adj* (*Scot*) active; alert.

yaupon /ˈjɔːpən/ *n* an American evergreen shrub with the holly family.

yaw /jɒ/ *vi* (*ship*, *aircraft*) to deviate from a course; (*aircraft*) to turn from side to side about the vertical axis. • *vt* to cause to yaw. • *n* a yawing movement or course.

yawl /jɒl/ *n* a two-masted sailing vessel with its aftermast at the stern.

yawn /jɒn/ *vi* to open the jaws involuntarily and inhale, as from drowsiness; to gape.—*also n*.

yawning /ˈjɒnɪŋ/ *adj* gaping; wide-open; drowsy.—**yawningly** *adv*.

yawp /jɒp/ *vi* to cry harshly, to scream; (*sl*) to speak foolishly. • *n* such a cry or talk.

yaws /jɒz/ *n sing* a tropical disease causing ulceration of the skin, framboesia.

y-axis /ˈwaɪ,æksɪs/ *n* (*pl* **y-axes**) the reference axis of a graph along which the y coordinate is measured.

Yb (*chem symbol*) ytterbium.

Y-chromosome *n* one of the pair (with the X-chromosome) of sex chromosomes that occur in males.

yclept /ɪˈklept/ *adj* (*arch*) named.

yd., yds *abbr* = yard(s).

ye¹ /jiː/ *pron* (*arch*) you (the person addressed and others) the old method of printing the.

ye² *definite article* (*arch*) the.

yea /jeɪ/ *adv*, *n* (*arch*) yes

yeah /jæ/ or /jeɪ/ *adv* (*inf*) yes.

yean /jiːn/ *vi* (*sheep*, *goat*) to bring forth (a lamb or kid).

yeanling /ˈjiːlɪŋ/ *n* a lamb or kid.

year /jiːr/ *n* a period of twelve months, or 365 or 366 days, beginning with 1 January and ending with 31 December; a period of approximately twelve months.

yearbook /ˈjiːrbʊk/ *n* an annual publication reviewing the events of the previous year or bringing information up to date.

yearling /-lɪŋ/ *n* an animal a year old or in its second year.

yearlong /-lɒŋ/ *adj* lasting a year.

yearly /-li/ *adj* occurring every year; lasting a year. • *adv* once a year; from year to year.

yearn /jɜrn/ *vi* to feel desire (for); to long for.—**yearning** *n*.

yeast /jiːst/ *n* a fungus that causes alcoholic fermentation, used in brewing and baking.

yeasty /ˈjiːsti/ *adj* (**yeastier, yeastiest**) smelling of or containing yeast.—**yeastiness** *n*.

yegg /jeg/, **yegman** /-mən/ *n* (*pl* **yeggs, yegmen**) (*sl*) a safecracker, a criminal.

yeld /jeld/ *adj* (*Scot*) barren, giving no milk.

yell /jel/ *vti* to shout loudly; to scream; to emit a yell. • *n* a loud shout; a concerted cheer by supporters, students, etc, at a game.

yellow /ˈjeloʊ/ *adj* of the colour of lemons, egg yolk, etc; having a yellowish skin; (*inf*) cowardly. • *n* the colour yellow. • *vi* to become or turn yellow.

yellow-belly /-beli/ *n* (*pl* **yellow-bellies**) (*sl*) a coward.—**yellow-bellied** *adj*.

yellow fever *n* an infectious tropical fever caused by a virus transmitted by certain mosquitoes.

yellowhammer /-,hæmər/ *n* a small European bird with a yellow head, neck and breast.

yellow jacket *n* an American hornet or wasp with yellow markings.

yellow pages *npi* (*part of*) a telephone directory that lists business subscribers under different categories according to the type of service offered.

yellow spot *n* (*anat*) the point of acutest vision in the retina.

yellow streak *n* (*inf*) a cowardly nature.

Yellow Transparent *n* ✤ (*Cdn*) an early yellow-skinned cooking and eating apple.

yellowwood /-wʊd/ *n* an American tree; its wood, which yields a yellow dye.

yelp /jelp/ *vti* to utter a sharp, shrill cry or bark.—*also n*.

yen¹ /jen/ *n* (*pl* **yen**) the monetary unit of Japan.

yen² *n* (*inf*) a yearning, an ambition.

yeoman /ˈjoːmən/ *n* (*pl* **yeomen**) (*formerly*) a farmer who cultivated his own land; a non-commissioned officer in the navy, marines.

yeomanly /-li/ *adj* of or like a yeoman; workmanlike.—*also adv*.

yeoman of the guard *n* a member of the British sovereign's veteran bodyguard.

yeomanry /-ri/ *n* yeomen collectively; in UK, a volunteer cavalry force raised from country districts as a home guard (1761–1907) now part of the Territorial Army.

yeoman service *n* effective assistance.

yep /jɛp/ *adv* (*inf*) yes.

yerba (maté) /'jɛrbə/ *n* an infusion of dried leaves of the maté, which makes a mildly stimulating tea.

yes /jɛs/ *adv* a word of affirmation or consent.

yes man *n* a servile, fawning, sycophantic person.

yester /'jɛstər/ *adv* (*rare*) of yesterday.

yesterday /'jɛstərdeɪ/ *n* the day before today; the recent past. • *adv* on the day before today; recently.

yet /jɛt/ *adv* still; so far; even. • *conj* nevertheless; however; still.

yeti /'jeti/ *n* a mysterious animal thought to live high in the Himalayan mountains but never seen.—*also* **abominable snowman.**

yew /juː/ *n* an evergreen tree or shrub with thin, sharp leaves and red berries.

Y-fronts /'wɔɪfrʌnts/ *npl* (*trademark*) men's underpants with an inverted Y-shaped opening at the front.

Ygdrasil, Yggdrasil /'ɪgdrəsɪl/ *n* (*Norse myth*) an ash tree whose roots and branches bind together earth, heaven, and hell.

yid /jɪd/ *n* (*derog*) a Jew.

Yiddish /'jɪdɪʃ/ *n* a mixed German and Hebrew dialect spoken by European Jews.

yield /jiːld/ *vt* to resign; to give forth, to produce, as a crop, result, profit, etc. • *vi* to submit; to give way to physical force, to surrender. • *n* the amount yielded; the profit or return on a financial investment.

yip /jɪp/ *n* a cry, an exclamation. • *vi* (**yipping, yipped**) to utter a yip.

yippee /'jɪpiː/ or /-'piː/ *interj* used to express exuberant delight.

ylang-ylang /'iːlæŋˌiːlæŋ/ *n* a Malaysian tree with fragrant flowers; a perfume made from the flowers.

YMCA *abbr* = Young Men's Christian Association.

YMHA *abbr* = Young Men's Hebrew Association.

yob /jɒb/, **yobbo** /'jɒbo:/ *n* (*pl* **yobs, yobbos**) (*sl*) a young lout, a hooligan.

yodel /'jo:dəl/ *vti* (**yodelling, yodelled** or **yodeling, yodeled**) to sing, alternating from the ordinary voice to falsetto.—**yodeller, yodeler** *n*.

yoga /'jo:gə/ *n* a system of exercises for attaining bodily and mental control and well-being.—**yogic** *adj*.

yogi /'jo:gi/ *n* (*pl* **yogis, yogin**) a person skilled in yoga.

yogurt, yoghurt /'jɒgərt/ *n* a semi-liquid food made from milk curdled by bacteria.

yo-heave-ho /'jo:hi:vˌho:/ *interj* (*formerly*) a cry made by sailors while heaving anchor, etc.

yoicks /jɔɪks/ *interj* a foxhunting cry urging on the hounds.

yoke /jo:k/ *n* a bond or tie; slavery; the wooden frame joining oxen to make them pull together; part of a garment that is fitted below the neck. • *vt* to put a yoke on; to join together.

yokel /'jo:kəl/ *n* (*derog*) country people who are regarded as unsophisticated and simple-minded.

yolk /jo:k/ *n* the yellow part of an egg.

yolk sac *n* the membrane enclosing an egg yolk.

Yom Kippur /jɒmkɪ'pʊr/ *n* an annual Jewish holiday marked by fasting and prayer.—*also* **Day of Atonement**.

yomp /jɒmp/ *vi* to march laboriously carrying heavy equipment, *esp* over rough terrain.

yon /jɒn/ *adj, adv* (*dial*) yonder, over there.

yonder /'jɒndər/ *adv* over there.

yore /jɔr/ *n* time long past.

Yorkist /'jɔrkɪst/ *n* an adherent of the royal house of York in England, *esp* during the Wars of the Roses (1455–85).—*also adj*.

Yorkshire pudding *n* a baked pudding made from batter and traditionally eaten with roast beef.

Yorkshire terrier *n* a small shaggy breed of terrier with a long coat of bluish grey and tan hair.

you /juː/ *pron* (*gram*) 2nd person singular or plural; the person or persons spoken to.

you'd /ju:d/ or /jud/ = you would; you had.

you'll /ju:l/ or /jul/ = you will; you shall.

young /jɛŋ/ *adj* in the early period of life; in the first part of growth; new; inexperienced. • *n* young people; offspring.

youngling /-lɪŋ/ *n* (*poet*) a young child or animal.

youngster /jɛŋ'stər/ *n* a young person; a youth.

your /jɔr/ or /jur/ *poss adj* of or belonging to or done by you.

you're /jur/ or /jɔr/, /jɔr/ = you are.

yours /jurz/ or /jɔrz/ *poss pron* of or belonging to you.

yourself /jɔrˌsɛlf/ or /jur-/ *pron* (*pl* **yourselves**) the emphatic and reflexive form of **you**.

youth /ju:θ/ *n* the period between childhood and adulthood; young people collectively; the early stages of something; a young man or boy.—**youthful** *adj*.—**youthfully** *adv*.

youth hostel *n* a supervised lodging for *usu* young travellers.

you've /ju:v/ or /juv/ = you have.

yowl /jaul/ *n* a loud mournful cry, *esp* from pain.—*also vi*.

yo-yo /'jo:jo:/ *n* (*pl* **yo-yos**) a hand-held toy made of a flat spool which can be made to wind up and down a piece of string.

yr *abbr* = year; younger; your.

yrs *abbr* = years; yours.

YST /'waɪˌɛs'tiː/ *abbr* ✹ = Yukon Standard Time.

YT /'waɪ'tiː/ *abbr* ✹ = Yukon Territories; Yukon Time.

ytterbium /ɪ'tɜrbiəm/ *n* a soft metallic element of the lanthanide series.

yttrium /'ɪtriəm/ *n* a metallic element used in alloys and lasers.

yuan /ju:'ɒn/ *n* (*pl* **yuan**) the monetary unit of the People's Republic of China.

yucca /'jʌkə/ *n* a plant with stiff, spear-like leaves and white flowers.

yuck /jʌk/ *interj* (*sl*) expressing disgust.

yucky /'jʌki/ *adj* (**yuckier, yuckiest**) (*sl*) disgusting.

Yukoner *n* ✹ (*Cdn*) a person who lives in or is from Manitoba.

Yukon Gold *n* ✹ (*Cdn*) a smooth-skinned, yellow-fleshed, early-maturing variety of potato.

yule /ju:l/ *n* Christmas.

Yule log /'ju:llɒg/ *n* a large log traditionally burnt in the fire on Christmas Eve.

yuletide /'ju:ltaɪd/ *n* the Christmas festival or season.

yummy /'jʌmi/ *adj* (**yummier, yummiest**) (*inf*) tasty, pleasing. • *interj* yum-yum.

yum-yum /'jʌmˌjʌm/ *interj* used to express pleasure, *esp* when eating.

yup /jɛp/ *adv* (*inf*) yes.

yuppie /'jʌpi/ *n* (*inf*) any young professional regarded as affluent, ambitious, materialistic, etc.

yurt /jurt/ or /jərt/ *n* a circular portable tent of skins used by the Mongolian nomads of Siberia.

YWCA *abbr* = Young Women's Christian Association.

YWHA *abbr* = Young Women's Hebrew Association.

Z

Z /zɛd/ or /ziː/ (*symbol*) (*physics*) impedance; (*chem*) atomic number.

z /zɛd/ (*symbol*) (*math*) an algebraic variable; the z-axis.

Z, z /zɛd/ *n* the 26th letter of the English alphabet; something shaped like a Z; (*math*) the third unknown quantity.

z. *abbr* = zero; zone.

zabaglione /ˌzɒbɒˈloːneɪ/ *n* a dessert of whipped egg yolks, sugar and marsala wine.

Zaïrese /zaɪrˈiːz/ *n* a native or inhabitant of the African republic of Zaïre.—*also adj*.

zamindar /zəˈmiːndər/ *n* (*hist*) in India, a district tax collector under the Mogul empire; a landowner paying land tax.—*also* **zemindar**.

zany /ˈzeɪnɪ/ *adj* (**zanier, zaniest**) comical; eccentric.—**zanily** *adv*.—**zaniness** *n*.

zap /zæp/ *vb* (**zapping, zapped**) *vt* to attack; to kill; to bombard; (*comput*) to get rid of data. • *vi* to rush around.

zappy /ˈzæpɪ/ *adj* (**zappier, zappiest**) (*sl*) energetic, snappy.

zareba, zariba /zəˈriːbə/ *n* in northern East Africa, a stockade made of thorn hedges as a protection against wild animals or enemies; a place so protected.

zarf /zɑrf/ *n* an ornamental holder for a coffee cup used in Arab countries.

zarzuela /zɑrˈzweɪlə/ *n* a traditional Spanish one-act comic opera with a satirical theme and including dialogue.

z-axis /ˈziːæksɪs/ *n* the reference axis of a three-dimensional coordinate system, along which the z-coordinate is measured.

zeal /ziːl/ *n* fervent devotion; fanaticism.

zealot /ˈzɛlət/ *n* an extreme partisan, a fanatic.

zealous /ˈzɛləs/ *adj* full of zeal; ardent.—**zealously** *adv*.—**zealousness** *n*.

zebra /ˈziːbrə/ or /ˈzɛb-/ *n* (*pl* **zebras, zebra**) a black and white striped wild animal related to the horse.—**zebrine** *adj*.

zebra crossing *n* a street crossing for pedestrians marked by black and white strips on the road.

zebu /ˈziːbuː/ *n* (*pl* **zebus, zebu**) an Asian and African ox with a prominent hump and a large dewlap.

zed /zɛd/ *n* ✠ the letter z.

zee /ziː/ *n* (*pl* **zees**) in US, the letter z.

zedoary /ˈzɛdoːˌɛrɪ/ *n* an aromatic substance like ginger made from the root stock of an Indian plant.

Zeitgeist /ˈtsaɪtˌɡaɪst/ *n* the spirit of the time; the beliefs, attitudes, tastes, etc, of a particular period.

zemindar /ˈzɪˌmiːnˈdɑr/ *see* **zamindar**.

zemstvo /ˈzɛmstvoː/ *n* (*pl* **zemstvos, zemstva**) a local elective assembly in the old Russian empire.

Zen /zɛn/ *n* a Japanese Buddhist sect that emphasizes self-awareness and self-mastery as the means to enlightenment.

zenana /zɛˈnɒnə/ *n* the part of the house reserved for women and girls in a Muslim household.

Zend-Avesta /ˌzɛndəˈvɛstə/ *n* the sacred writings of the Zoroastrians.

zenith /ˈziːnɪθ/ or /ˈzɛn/ *n* the point at which the sun or moon appears to be exactly overhead; peak, summit (of ambition, etc).

zephyr /ˈzɛfər/ *n* a soft, gentle breeze; a very thin woollen material; a garment made of this.

zeppelin /ˈzɛpəlɪn/ *n* a rigid, cigar-shaped airship.

zero /ˈziːroː/ *n* (*pl* **zeros, zeroes**) the symbol 0; nothing; the lowest point; freezing point, 0 degrees Celsius. • *vi* (*with* **in**) (*inf*) to focus attention on (a problem, subject, etc); (*inf*) to converge upon; (*with* **in on**) to concentrate fire (from a weapon) on a specific target.

zero gravity *n* weightlessness.

zero hour *n* the time at which something is scheduled to begin.

zest /zɛst/ *n* the outer part of the skin of an orange or lemon used to give flavour; enthusiasm; excitement.—**zestful** *adj*.—**zestfully** *adv*.—**zestfulness** *n*.

zeta /ˈziːtə/ *n* the sixth letter of the Greek alphabet.

zeugma /ˈzuːɡmə/ or /ˈzjuː-/ *n* a figure of speech in which a word is used with two others, to only one of which it properly applies.—**zeugmatic** *adj*.

Zeus /ˈzuːs/ or /ˈzjuːs/ *n* (*Greek myth*) the king of the gods.

zigzag /ˈzɪɡzæɡ/ *n* a series of short, sharp angles in alternate directions. • *adj* having sharp turns. • *vti* (**zigzagging, zigzagged**) to move or form in a zigzag.

zilch /zɪltʃ/, **zilcho** *n* (*sl*) nothing.

zillah /ˈzɪlə/ *n* (*hist*) an administrative district in India during British rule.

zillion /ˈzɪljən/ *n* (*pl* **zillion, zillions**) (*inf*) an indefinitely large number or quantity.

Zimb *abbr* = Zimbabwe.

Zimbabwean /zɪmˈbɒbwiən/ or /-weɪən/ *n* a native or inhabitant of the African republic of Zimbabwe.—*also adj*.

Zimmer /ˈzɪmər/ *n* (*trade-mark*) a frame of tubular metal used by the infirm as a walking aid.

zinc /zɪŋk/ *n* a bluish-white metallic element used in alloys and batteries. • *vt* (**zincing, zinced** *or* **zincking, zincked**) to coat with zinc.—**zincic** *adj*.

zincograph /ˈzɪŋkəˌɡræf/ *n* a design in relief on a zinc plate; a print made from this. • *vti* to etch on zinc; to reproduce in this way.—**zincographer** *n*.—**zincographic** *adj*.—**zincography** *n*.

zing /zɪŋ/ *n* (*inf*) a high-pitched buzz; (*inf*) vitality, exuberance. • *vi* (*inf*) to move with a zinging sound.

zinnia /ˈzɪnjə/ *n* a tropical American plant with showy flowers.

Zionism /ˈzaɪəˌnɪzəm/ *n* a movement formerly to resettle Jews in Palestine as their national home, now concerned with the development of Israel.—**Zionist** *n, adj*.—**Zionistic** *adj*.

zip /zɪp/ *n* a light whizzing sound of a bullet, etc; (*sl*) brisk energy; a slide fastener on clothing, bags, etc with interlocking teeth, a zipper. • *vb* (**zipping, zipped**) *vi* to move at high speed, to dart. • *vt* to fasten with a zip.

ZIP Code /zɪp/ *n* (*trade-mark*) a postcode that uses digits to denote an area.

zipper /ˈzɪpər/ *n* a zip.

zippy /-ɪ/ *adj* (**zippier, zippiest**) speedy; energetic.

zircon /ˈzɜrkɒn/ *n* a variously coloured hard translucent mineral, some varieties of which are cut as gemstones.

zirconium /zɜrˈkoːniəm/ *n* a metallic element found in zircon and used in alloys.

zit /zɪt/ *n* (*sl*) a pimple, spot.

zither /ˈzɪðər/ *n* a musical instrument with 30–45 strings over a shallow sounding box played by plucking.—**zitherist** *n*.

zloty /ˈzlɒtɪ/ *n* (*pl* **zlotys, zloty**) the monetary unit of Poland.

Zn (*chem symbol*) zinc.

zodiac /ˈzoːdiˌæk/ *n* an imaginary belt in the heavens along which the sun, moon, and chief planets appear to move, divided crosswise into twelve equal areas, called "signs of the zodiac," each named after a constellation; a diagram representing this.—**zodiacal** *adj*.

zodiacal light *n* a luminous triangular tract of sky sometimes seen before dawn or after dusk, *esp* in the tropics.

zoetrope /ˈzoːɪtrʊp/ *n* a toy with a revolving cylinder showing a series of pictures in apparent motion.

-zoic /ˈzoɪk/ *adj suffix* (*animal*) having a specified kind of existence; (*geol*) belonging to an era with a particular form of life.

Zollverein /ˈtsɒlfəˌraɪn/ *n* in 19th century, a union of German states with common customs tariffs against outside countries and free trade among themselves; any customs union.

zombie, zombi /ˈzɒmbɪ/ *n* (*pl* **zombies**) a person who is lifeless and apathetic; an automaton.

zonate /ˈzoːneɪt/, **zonated** *adj* (*bot, zool*) marked with bands.

zone /zoːn/ *n* a region, area; a subdivision; any area with a specified use or restriction. • *vt* to divide or mark off into zones; to designate as a zone; to encircle with a zone.—**zonal** *adj*.

zonked /zɒŋt/ *adj* (*sl*) intoxicated by drugs or alcohol; (*sl*) exhausted.

zoo /zuː/ *n* (*pl* **zoos**) a place where a collection of living wild animals is kept for public showing.

zoo-, zo- /ˈzoːə/ or /ˈzuːə/ *prefix* animals.

zoochemistry /ˈzoːəˌkɛməstri/ *n* the chemistry of the constituents of animal bodies.—**zoochemical** *adj*.

zoogeography /ˌzoːədʒiˈɒɡrəfi/ or /ˌzuːə-/ *n* the science of the geographical distribution of animals.—**zoogeographer** *n*.—**zoogeographic, zoogeographical** *adj*.

zoography /zoːˈɒɡrəfi/ or /zuː-/ *n* descriptive zoology.—**zoographic, zoographical** *adj*.

zooid /ˈzoːɔɪd/ or /ˈzuː/ *adj* resembling but not completely being an animal or plant. • *n* a zooid organism; an animal organism produced by fission; (*corals, etc*) a member of a compound organism.

zool. *abbr* = zoological; zoology.

zoological garden /ˌzoːəˈlɒdʒɪkəlˈɡɑrdən/ *n* a zoo.

zoologist /zoːˈɒlədʒɪst/ *n* a person who studies animals and animal behaviour.

zoology /-dʒi/ or /zuː/ *n* (*pl* **zoologies**) the study of animals with regard to their classification, structure and habits.—**zoological** *adj*.—**zoologically** *adv*.

zoom /zuːm/ *vi* to go quickly, to speed; to climb upward sharply in an aeroplane; to rise rapidly; (*photog*) to focus in on an object using a zoom lens. • *n* the act of zooming; a zoom lens.

zoom lens *n* (*photog*) a camera lens that makes distant objects appear closer without moving the camera.

zoomorphism /ˌzoːəˈmɔrfɪzəm/ or /ˌzuːə/, /zuːˈmɔrfɪzəm/ *n* the representation (*esp* of a deity) in the form of or with the attributes of an animal.—**zoomorphic** *adj*.

zoophyte /ˈzoːəˌfəɪt/ or /ˈzuːə/ *n* any animal (*eg* coral, a sponge) that resembles a plant.—**zoophytic** *adj*.

zootomy /zoːˈɒtəmi/ *n* animal anatomy; the dissection of animals.—**zootomical** *adj*.—**zootomist** *n*.

zorille, zoril /ˈzɒrɪl/ *n* a small African mammal that resembles and smells like a skunk.

Zoroastrianism /ˌzɔroːˈæstriənizəm/ *n* a religious system founded by the Persian prophet Zoroaster (*c*.628-551BC), based on the recognition of the dual principle of good and evil.—**Zoroastrian** *n, adj*.

Zouave /zuːˈɒv/ or /zwɒv/ *n* (*formerly*) a soldier in a French-Algerian infantry unit characterized by a colourful eastern-style uniform; a soldier in a similiar unit, *esp* a Union Army unit of the American Civil War.

zounds /zaundz/ *interj* (*arch*) expressing anger and astonishment.

Zr (*chem symbol*) zirconium.

zucchetto /zuːˈketoː/ or /tsuː-/ *n* (*pl* **zucchettos**) a skullcap worn by Roman Catholic ecclesiastics, which varies in colour according to rank (black for a priest, purple for a bishop, red for a cardinal, white for the Pope).

zucchini /zuːˈkiːni/ *npl n* a type of small vegetable marrow.—*also* **courgette**.

Zulu /ˈzuːluː/ *n* (*pl* **Zulus, Zulu**) a member of a Negroid people of South Africa, or their language.—*also adj*.

zwieback /ˈzwiːbæk/ *n* a thin rusk.

zyg-, zygo- /ˈzaɪɡoː/ *prefix* yoked, paired.

zygodactyl /ˌzaɪɡoːˈdæktɪl/ *adj* (*bird*) with the toes in pairs, two pointing forward and two backward. • *n* a zygodactyl bird, *eg* the parrot.—**zygodactylous** *adj*.

zygomorphic /ˌzaɪɡəˈmɔrfɪk/, **zygomorphous** /-ˈmɔrfəs/ *adj* (*flowers*) bilaterally symmetrical.—**zygomorphism, zygomorphy** *n*.

zygospore /ˌzaɪɡəˈspoːr/ *n* a spore formed from the fusion of gametes.—**zygosporic** *adj*.

zygote /ˈzaɪɡoːt/ *n* the cell formed by the union of an ovum and a sperm; the developing organism from such a cell.

zymosis /zaɪˈmoːsɪs/ or /zɪ-/ *n* (*pl* **zymoses**) an infectious disease caused by a virus or organism that acts like a ferment; fermentation.

zymotic /zaɪˈmɒtɪk/ or /zɪ-/ *adj* caused by or relating to an infection or an infectious disease; producing fermentation.

zymurgy /ˈzaɪmərdʒi/ *n* the chemistry of fermentation in brewing, etc.

THESAURUS

A

aback *adv* back, backward, rearward, regressively.

abaft *prep* (*naut*) aft, astern, back of, behind.

abandon *vb* abdicate, abjure, desert, drop, evacuate, forsake, forswear, leave, quit, relinquish, yield; cede, forgo, give up, let go, renounce, resign, surrender, vacate, waive. • *n* careless freedom, dash, impetuosity, impulse, wildness.

abandoned *adj* depraved, derelict, deserted, discarded, dropped, forsaken, left, outcast, rejected, relinquished; corrupt, demoralized, depraved, dissolute, graceless, impenitent, irreclaimable, lost, obdurate, profligate, reprobate, shameless, sinful, unprincipled, vicious, wicked.

abandonment *n* desertion, dereliction, giving up, leaving, relinquishment, renunciation, surrender.

abase *vb* depress, drop, lower, reduce, sink; debase, degrade, disgrace, humble, humiliate.

abasement *n* abjection, debasement, degradation, disgrace, humbleness, humiliation, shame.

abash *vb* affront, bewilder, confound, confuse, dash, discompose, disconcert, embarrass, humiliate, humble, shame, snub.

abashment *n* confusion, embarrassment, humiliation, mortification, shame.

abate *vb* diminish, decrease, lessen, lower, moderate, reduce, relax, remove, slacken; allow, bate, deduct, mitigate, rebate, remit; allay, alleviate, appease, assuage, blunt, calm, compose, dull, mitigate, moderate, mollify, pacify, qualify, quiet, quell, soften, soothe, tranquillize.

abatement *n* alleviation, assuagement, decrement, decrease, extenuation, mitigation, moderation, remission; cessation, decline, diminution, ebb, fading, lowering, sinking, settlement; allowance, deduction, rebate, reduction.

abbey *n* convent, monastery, priory.

abbreviate *vb* abridge, compress, condense, contract, cut, curtail, epitomize, reduce, retrench, shorten.

abbreviation *n* abridgment, compression, condensation, contraction, curtailment, cutting, reduction, shortening.

abdicate *vb* abandon, cede, forgo, forsake, give up, quit, relinquish, renounce, resign, retire, surrender.

abdication *n* abandonment, abdicating, relinquishment, renunciation, resignation, surrender.

abdomen *n* belly, gut, paunch, stomach.

abduct *vb* carry off, kidnap, spirit away, take away.

abduction *n* carrying off, kidnapping, removal, seizure, withdrawal.

aberrant *adj* deviating, devious, divergent, diverging, erratic, rambling, wandering; abnormal, anomalistic, anomalous, disconnected, eccentric, erratic, exceptional, inconsequent, peculiar, irregular, preternatural, singular, strange, unnatural, unusual.

aberration *n* departure, deviation, divergence, rambling, wandering; abnormality, anomaly, eccentricity, irregularity, peculiarity, singularity, unconformity; delusion, disorder, hallucination, illusion, instability.

abet *vb* aid, assist, back, help, support, sustain, uphold; advocate, condone, countenance, encourage, favour, incite, sanction.

abettor *n* ally, assistant; adviser, advocate, promoter, accessory, accomplice, associate, confederate.

abeyance *n* anticipation, calculation, expectancy, waiting; dormancy, inactivity, intermission, quiescence, remission, reservation, suppression, suspension.

abhor *vb* abominate, detest, dislike intensely, execrate, hate, loathe, nauseate, view with horror.

abhorrence *n* abomination, antipathy, aversion, detestation, disgust, hatred, horror, loathing.

abhorrent *adj* abominating, detesting, hating, loathing; hateful, horrifying, horrible, loathsome, nauseating, odious, offensive, repellent, repugnant, repulsive, revolting, shocking.

abide *vb* lodge, rest, sojourn, stay, wait; dwell, inhabit, live, reside; bear, continue, persevere, persist, remain; endure, last, suffer, tolerate; (*with* **by**) act up to, conform to, discharge, fulfil, keep, persist in.

abiding *adj* changeless, constant, continuing, durable, enduring, immutable, lasting, permanent, stable, unchangeable.

ability *n* ableness, adroitness, aptitude, aptness, cleverness, dexterity, efficacy, efficiency, facility, might, ingenuity, knack, power, readiness, skill, strength, talent, vigour; competency, qualification; calibre, capability, capacity, expertness, faculty, gift, parts.

abject *adj* base, beggarly, contemptible, cringing, degraded, despicable, dirty, grovelling, ignoble, low, mean, menial, miserable, paltry, pitiful, poor, servile, sneaking, slavish, vile, worthless, wretched.

abjectness *n* abasement, abjection, baseness, contemptibleness, meanness, pitifulness, servility, vileness.

abjuration *n* abandonment, abnegation, discarding, disowning, rejection, relinquishment, renunciation, repudiation; disavowal, disclaimer, disclaiming, recall, recantation, repeal, retraction, reversal, revocation.

abjure *vb* abandon, discard, disclaim, disown, forgo, forswear, give up, reject, relinquish, renounce, repudiate; disavow, disclaim, recall, recant, renounce, repeal, retract, revoke, withdraw.

able *adj* accomplished, adroit, apt, clever, expert, ingenious, practical, proficient, qualified, quick, skilful, talented, versed; competent, effective, efficient, fitted, quick; capable, gifted, mighty, powerful, talented; athletic, brawny, muscular, robust, stalwart, strong, vigorous.

ablution *n* baptism, bathing, cleansing, lavation, purification, washing.

abnegation *n* abandonment, denial, renunciation, surrender.

abnormal *adj* aberrant, anomalous, divergent, eccentric, exceptional, peculiar, odd, singular, strange, uncomfortable, unnatural, unusual, weird.

abnormality *n* abnormity, anomaly, deformity, idiosyncrasy, irregularity, monstrosity, peculiarity, oddity, singularity, unconformity.

aboard *adv* inside, within, on.

abode *n* domicile, dwelling, habitation, home, house, lodging, quarters, residence, residency, seat.

abolish *vb* abrogate, annul, cancel, eliminate, invalidate, nullify, quash, repeal, rescind, revoke; annihilate, destroy, end, eradicate, extirpate, extinguish, obliterate, overthrow, suppress, terminate.

abolition *n* abrogation, annulling, annulment, cancellation, cancelling, nullification, repeal, rescinding, rescission, revocation; annihilation, destruction, eradication, extinction, extinguishment, extirpation, obliteration, overthrow, subversion, suppression.

abominable *adj* accursed, contemptible, cursed, damnable, detestable, execrable, hellish, horrid, nefarious, odious, abhorrent, detestable, disgusting, foul, hateful, loathsome, nauseous, obnoxious, shocking, revolting, repugnant, repulsive; shabby, vile, wretched.

abominate *vb* abhor, detest, execrate, hate, loathe, recoil from, revolt at, shrink from, shudder at.

abomination *n* abhorrence, antipathy, aversion, detestation, disgust, execration, hatred, loathing, nauseation; contamination, corruption, corruptness, defilement, foulness, impurity, loathsomeness, odiousness, pollution, taint, uncleanness; annoyance, curse, evil, infliction, nuisance, plague, torment.

aboriginal *adj* autochthonal, autochthonous, first, indigenous, native, original, primary, prime, primeval, primitive, pristine.

abortion *n* miscarriage, premature labour; disappointment, failure.

abortive *adj* immature, incomplete, rudimental, rudimentary, stunted, untimely; futile, fruitless, idle, ineffectual, inoperative, nugatory, profitless, unavailing, unsuccessful, useless, vain.

abound *vb* flow, flourish, increase, swarm, swell; exuberate, luxuriate, overflow, proliferate, swarm, teem.

about *prep* around, encircling, surrounding, round; near; concerning, referring to, regarding, relating to, relative to, respecting, touching, with regard to, with respect to; all over, over, through. • *adv* around, before; approximately, near, nearly.

above *adj* above-mentioned, aforementioned, aforesaid, foregoing, preceding, previous, prior. • *adv* aloft, overhead; before, previously; of a higher rank. • *prep* higher than, on top of; exceeding, greater than, more than, over; beyond, superior to.

above-board *adj* candid, frank, honest, open, straightforward, truthful, upright. • *adv* candidly, fairly, openly, sincerely.

abrade *vb* erase, erode, rub off, scrape out, wear away.

abrasion *n* attrition, disintegration, friction, wearing down; scrape, scratch.

abreast *adv* aligned, alongside.

abridge *vb* abbreviate, condense, compress, shorten, summarize; contract, diminish, lessen, reduce.

abridgment *n* compression, condensation, contraction, curtailment, diminution, epitomizing, reduction, shortening; abstract, brief, compendium, digest, epitome, outline, précis, summary, syllabus, synopsis; deprivation, limitation, restriction.

abroad *adv* expansively, unrestrainedly, ubiquitously, widely; forth, out of doors; overseas; extensively, publicly.

abrogate *vb* abolish, annul, cancel, invalidate, nullify, overrule, quash, repeal, rescind, revoke, set aside, vacate, void.

abrogation *n* abolition, annulling, annulment, cancellation, cancelling, repeal rescinding, rescission, revocation, voidance, voiding.

abrupt *adj* broken, craggy, jagged, rough, rugged; acclivous, acclivitous, precipitous, steep; hasty, ill-timed, precipitate, sudden, unanticipated, unexpected; blunt, brusque, curt, discourteous; cramped, harsh, jerky, stiff.

abscess *n* boil, fester, pustule, sore, ulcer.

abscond *vb* bolt, decamp, elope, escape, flee, fly, retreat, run off, sneak away, steal away, withdraw.

absence *n* nonappearance, nonattendance; abstraction, distraction, inattention, musing, preoccupation, reverie; default, defect, deficiency, lack, privation.

absent *adj* abroad, away, elsewhere, gone, not present, otherwhere; abstracted, dreaming, inattentive, lost, musing, napping, preoccupied.

absolute *adj* complete, ideal, independent, perfect, supreme, unconditional, unconditioned, unlimited, unqualified, unrestricted; arbitrary, authoritative, autocratic, despotic, dictatorial, imperious, irresponsible, tyrannical, tyrannous; actual, categorical, certain, decided, determinate, genuine, positive, real, unequivocal, unquestionable, veritable.

absolutely *adv* completely, definitely, unconditionally; actually, downright, indeed, indubitably, infallibly, positively, really, truly, unquestionably.

absoluteness *n* actuality, completeness, ideality, perfection, positiveness, reality, supremeness; absolutism, arbitrariness, despotism, tyranny.

absolution *n* acquittal, clearance, deliverance, discharge, forgiveness, liberation, pardon, release, remission, shrift, shriving.

absolutism *n* absoluteness, arbitrariness, autocracy, despotism, tyranny.

absolve *vb* acquit, clear, deliver, discharge, exculpate, excuse, exonerate, forgive, free, liberate, loose, pardon, release, set free, shrive.

absorb *vb* appropriate, assimilate, drink in, imbibe, soak up; consume, destroy, devour, engorge, engulf, exhaust, swallow up, take up; arrest, engage, engross, fix, immerse, occupy, rivet.

absorbent *adj* absorbing, imbibing, penetrable, porous, receptive.

absorption *adj* appropriation, assimilation, imbibing, osmosis, soaking up; consumption, destroying, devouring, engorgement, engulfing, exhaustion, swallowing up; concentration, engagement, engrossment, immersion, occupation, preoccupation.

abstain *vb* avoid, cease, deny oneself, desist, forbear, refrain, refuse, stop, withhold.

abstemious *adj* abstinent, frugal, moderate, self-denying, sober, temperate.

abstinence *n* abstemiousness, avoidance, forbearance, moderation, self-restraint, soberness, sobriety, teetotalism, temperance.

abstinent *adj* abstaining, fasting; abstemious, restraining, self-denying, self-restraining, sober, temperate.

abstract *vb* detach, disengage, disjoin, dissociate, disunite, isolate, separate; appropriate, purloin, seize, steal, take; abbreviate, abridge, epitomize. • *adj* isolated, separate, simple, unrelated; abstracted, occult, recondite, refined, subtle, vague; nonobjective, nonrepresentational. • *n* abridgment, condensation, digest, excerpt, extract, précis, selection, summary, synopsis.

abstracted *adj* absent, absent-minded, dreaming, inattentive, lost, musing, preoccupied; abstruse, refined, subtle.

abstraction *n* absence, absent-mindedness, brown study, inattention, muse, musing, preoccupation, reverie; disconnection, disjunction, isolation, separation; abduction, appropriation, pilfering, purloining, seizure, stealing, taking.

abstruse *adj* abstract, attenuated, dark, difficult, enigmatic, hidden, indefinite, mysterious, mystic, mystical, obscure, occult, profound, recondite, remote, subtle, transcendental, vague.

absurd *adj* egregious, fantastic, foolish, incongruous, ill-advised, ill-judged, irrational, ludicrous, nonsensical, nugatory, preposterous, ridiculous, self-annulling, senseless, silly, stupid, unreasonable.

absurdity *n* drivel, extravagance, fatuity, folly, foolery, foolishness, idiocy, nonsense.

abundance *n* affluence, amplitude, ampleness, copiousness, exuberance, fertility, flow, flood, largeness, luxuriance, opulence, overflow, plenitude, profusion, richness, store, wealth.

abundant *adj* abounding, ample, bountiful, copious, exuberant, flowing, full, good, large, lavish, rich, liberal, much, overflowing, plentiful, plenteous, replete, teeming, thick.

abuse *vb* betray, cajole, deceive, desecrate, dishonour, misapply, misemploy, misuse, pervert, pollute, profane, prostitute, violate, wrong; harm, hurt, ill-use, ill-treat, injure, maltreat, mishandle; asperse, berate, blacken, calumniate, defame, disparage, lampoon, lash, malign, revile, reproach, satirize, slander, traduce, upbraid, vilify. • *n* desecration, dishonour, illuse, misuse, perversion, pollution, profanation; ill-treatment, maltreatment, outrage; malfeasance, malversation; aspersion, defamation, disparagement, insult, invective, obloquy, opprobrium, railing, rating, reviling, ribaldry, rudeness, scurrility, upbraiding, vilification, vituperation.

abusive *adj* calumnious, carping, condemnatory, contumelious, damnatory, denunciatory, injurious, insolent, insulting, offensive, opprobrious, reproachful, reviling, ribald, rude, scurrilous, vilificatory, vituperative.

abut *vb* adjoin, border, impinge, meet, project.

abutment *n* bank, bulwark, buttress, embankment, fortification; abutting, abuttal, adjacency, contiguity, juxtaposition.

abuttal *n* adjacency, boundary, contiguity, juxtaposition, nearness, next, terminus.

abyss *n* abysm, chasm, gorge, gulf, pit.

academic *adj* collegiate, lettered, scholastic. • *n* academician, classicist, doctor, fellow, pundit, savant, scholar, student, teacher.

academy *n* college, high school, institute, school.

accede *vb* accept, acquiesce, agree, assent to, comply with, concur, consent, yield.

accelerate *vb* dispatch, expedite, forward, hasten, hurry, precipitate, press on, quicken, speed, urge on.

acceleration *n* expedition, hastening, hurrying, quickening, pickup, precipitation, speeding up, stepping up.

accent *vb* accentuate, emphasize, stress. • *n* cadence, inflection, intonation, tone; beat, emphasis, ictus.

accentuate *vb* accent, emphasize, mark, point up, punctuate, stress; highlight, overemphasize, overstress, underline, underscore.

accept *vb* acquire, derive, get, gain, obtain, receive, take; accede to, acknowledge, acquiesce in, admit, agree to, approve, assent to, avow, embrace; estimate, construe, interpret, regard, value.

acceptable *adj* agreeable, gratifying, pleasant, pleasing, pleasurable, welcome.

acceptance *n* accepting, acknowledgment, receipt, reception, taking; approbation, approval, gratification, satisfaction.

acceptation *n* construction, import, interpretation, meaning, sense, significance, signification, understanding; adoption, approval, currency, vogue.

access *vb* broach, enter, open, open up. • *n* approach, avenue, entrance, entry, passage, way; admission, admittance, audience, interview; addition, accession, aggrandizement, enlargement, gain, increase, increment; (*med*) attack, fit, onset, recurrence.

accession *n* addition, augmentation, enlargement, extension, increase; succession.

accessory *adj* abetting, additional, additive, adjunct, aiding, ancillary, assisting, contributory, helping, subsidiary, subordinate, supplemental. • *n* abettor, accomplice, assistant, associate, confederate, helper; accompaniment, attendant, concomitant, detail, subsidiary.

accident *n* calamity, casualty, condition, contingency, disaster, fortuity, incident, misadventure, miscarriage, mischance, misfortune, mishap; affection, alteration, chance, contingency, mode, modification, property, quality, state.

accidental *adj* casual, chance, contingent, fortuitous, undesigned, unintended; adventitious, dispensable, immaterial, incidental, nonessential.

acclamation *n* acclaim, applause, cheer, cry, plaudit, outcry, salutation, shouting.

acclimatization, acclimation *n* adaptation, adjustment, conditioning, familiarization, habituation, inurement, naturalization.

acclimatize, acclimate *vb* accustom, adapt, adjust, condition, familiarize, habituate, inure, naturalize, season.

acclivity *n* ascent, height, hill, rising ground, steep, upward slope.

accommodate *vb* contain, furnish, hold, oblige, serve, supply; adapt, fit, suit; adjust, compose, harmonize, reconcile, settle.

accommodation *n* advantage, convenience, privilege; adaptation, agreement, conformity, fitness, suitableness; adjustment, harmonization, harmony, pacification, reconciliation, settlement.

accompaniment *n* adjunct, appendage, attachment, attendant, concomitant.

accompany *vb* attend, chaperon, convoy, escort, follow, go with.

accomplice *n* abettor, accessory, ally, assistant, associate, confederate, partner.

accomplish *vb* achieve, bring about, carry, carry through, complete, compass, consummate, do, effect, execute, perform, perfect; conclude, end, finish, terminate.

accomplished *adj* achieved, completed, done, effected, executed, finished, fulfilled, realized; able, adroit, apt, consummate, educated, experienced, expert, finished, instructed, practised, proficient, qualified, ripe, skilful, versed; elegant, fashionable, fine, polished, polite, refined.

accomplishment *n* achievement, acquirement, attainment, qualification; completion, fulfilment.

accord *vb* admit, allow, concede, deign, give, grant, vouchsafe, yield; agree, assent, concur, correspond, harmonize, quadrate, tally. • *n* accordance, agreement, concord, concurrence, conformity, consensus, harmony, unanimity, unison.

accordant *adj* agreeable, agreeing, congruous, consonant, harmonious, suitable, symphonious.

accordingly *adv* agreeably, conformably, consistently, suitably; consequently, hence, so, thence, therefore, thus, whence, wherefore.

accost *vb* address, confront, greet, hail, salute, speak to, stop.

account *vb* assess, appraise, estimate, evaluate, judge, rate; (*with for*) assign, attribute, explain, expound, justify, rationalize, vindicate. • *n* inventory, record, register, score; bill, book, charge; calculation, computation, count, reckoning, score, tale, tally; chronicle, detail, description, narration, narrative, portrayal, recital, rehearsal, relation, report, statement, tidings, word; elucidation, explanation, exposition, consideration, ground, motive, reason, regard, sake; consequence, consideration, dignity, distinction, importance, note, repute, reputation, worth.

accountable *adj* amenable, answerable, duty-bound, liable, responsible.

accoutre *vb* arm, dress, equip, fit out, furnish.

accredit *vb* authorize, depute, empower, entrust.

accrue *vb* arise, come, follow, flow, inure, issue, proceed, result.

accumulate *vb* agglomerate, aggregate, amass, bring together, collect, gather, grow, hoard, increase, pile, store.

accumulation *n* agglomeration, aggregation, collection, heap, hoard, mass, pile, store.

accuracy *n* carefulness, correctness, exactness, fidelity, precision, strictness.

accurate *adj* close, correct, exact, faithful, nice, precise, regular, strict, true, truthful.

accusation *n* arraignment, charge, incrimination, impeachment, indictment.

accuse *vb* arraign, charge, censure, impeach, indict, tax.

accustom *vb* discipline, drill, familiarize, habituate, harden, inure, train, use.

ace *n* (*cards, dice*) one spot, single pip, single point; atom, bit, grain, iota, jot, particle single, unit, whit; expert, master, virtuoso. • *adj* best, expert, fine, outstanding, superb.

acerbity *n* acidity, acricity, acridness, astringency, bitterness, roughness, sourness, tartness; acrimony, bitterness, harshness, severity, venom.

achieve *vb* accomplish, attain, complete, do, effect, execute, finish, fulfil, perform, realize; acquire, gain, get, obtain, win.

achievement *n* accomplishment, acquirement, attainment, completion, consummation, performance, realization; deed, exploit, feat, work.

acid *adj* pungent, sharp, sour, stinging, tart, vinegary.

acknowledge *vb* recognize; accept, admit, accept, allow, concede, grant; avow, confess, own, profess.

acme *n* apex, climax, height, peak, pinnacle, summit, top, vertex, zenith.

acquaint *vb* familiarize; announce, apprise, communicate, enlighten, disclose, inform, make aware, make known, notify, tell.

acquaintance *n* companionship, familiarity, fellowship, intimacy, knowledge; associate, companion, comrade, friend.

acquiesce *vb* bow, comply, consent, give way, rest, submit, yield; agree, assent, concur, consent.

acquire *vb* achieve, attain, earn, gain, get, have, obtain, procure, realize, secure, win; learn thoroughly, master.

acquirement *n* acquiring, gaining, gathering, mastery; acquisition, accomplishment, attainment.

acquit *vb* absolve, clear, discharge, exculpate, excuse, exonerate, forgive, liberate, pardon, pay, quit, release, set free, settle.

acquittal *n* absolution, acquittance, clearance, deliverance, discharge, exoneration, liberation, release.

acquittance *n* discharge quittance, receipt.

acrid *adj* biting, bitter, caustic, pungent, sharp.

acrimonious *adj* acrid, bitter, caustic, censorious, crabbed, harsh, malignant, petulant, sarcastic, severe, testy, virulent.

acrimony *n* causticity, causticness, corrosiveness, sharpness, abusiveness, acridity, asperity, bitterness, churlishness, harshness, rancour, severity, spite, venom.

act *vb* do, execute, function, make, operate, work; enact, feign, perform, play. • *n* achievement, deed, exploit, feat, performance, proceeding, turn; bill, decree, enactment, law, ordinance, statute; actuality, existence, fact, reality.

acting *adj* interim, provisional, substitute, temporary. • *n* enacting, impersonation, performance, portrayal, theatre; counterfeiting, dissimulation, imitation, pretence.

action *n* achievement, activity, agency, deed, exertion, exploit, feat; battle, combat, conflict, contest, encounter, engagement, operation; lawsuit, prosecution.

active *adj* effective, efficient, influential, living, operative; assiduous, bustling, busy, diligent, industrious, restless; agile, alert, brisk, energetic, lively, nimble, prompt, quick, smart, spirited, sprightly, supple; animated, ebullient, fervent, vigorous.

actual *adj* certain, decided, genuine, objective, real, substantial, tangible, true, veritable; perceptible, present, sensible, tangible; absolute, categorical, positive.

actuate *vb* impel, incite, induce, instigate, move, persuade, prompt.

acumen *n* acuteness, astuteness, discernment, ingenuity, keenness, penetration, sagacity, sharpness, shrewdness.

acute *adj* pointed, sharp; astute, bright, discerning, ingenious, intelligent, keen, quick, penetrating, piercing, sagacious, sage, sharp, shrewd, smart, subtle; distressing, fierce, intense, piercing, pungent, poignant, severe, violent; high, high-toned, sharp, shrill; (*med*) sudden, temporary, violent.

adage *n* aphorism, dictum, maxim, proverb, saw, saying.

adapt *vb* accommodate, adjust, conform, coordinate, fit, qualify, proportion, suit, temper.

add *vb* adjoin, affix, annex, append, attach, join, tag; sum, sum up, total.

addict *vb* accustom, apply, dedicate, devote, habituate. • *n* devotee, enthusiast, fan; head, junkie, user.

addicted *adj* attached, devoted, given up to, inclined, prone, wedded.

addition *n* augmentation, accession, enlargement, extension, increase, supplement; adjunct, appendage, appendix, extra.

address *vb* accost, apply to, court, direct. • *n* appeal, application, entreaty, invocation, memorial, petition, request, solicitation, suit; discourse, oration, lecture, sermon, speech; ability, adroitness, art, dexterity, expertness, skill; courtesy, deportment, demeanour, tact.

adduce *vb* advance, allege, assign, offer, present; cite, mention, name.

adept *adj* accomplished, experienced, practised, proficient, skilled. • *n* expert, master, virtuoso.

adequate *adj* able, adapted, capable, competent, equal, fit, requisite, satisfactory, sufficient, suitable.

adhere *vb* cling, cleave, cohere, hold, stick; appertain, belong, pertain.

adherent *adj* adhering, clinging, sticking. • *n* acolyte, dependant, disciple, follower, partisan, supporter, vassal.

adhesion *n* adherence, attachment, clinging, coherence, sticking.

adhesive *adj* clinging, sticking; glutinous, gummy, sticky, tenacious, viscous. • *n* binder, cement, glue, paste.

adieu *n* farewell, goodbye, parting, valediction.

adipose *adj* fat, fatty, greasy, oily, oleaginous, sebaceous.

adjacent *adj* adjoining, bordering, conterminous, contiguous, near, near to, neighbouring, touching.

adjoin *vb* abut, add, annex, append, border, combine, neighbour, unite, verge.

adjourn *vb* defer, delay, postpone, procrastinate; close, dissolve, end, interrupt, prorogue, suspend.

adjudge *vb* allot, assign, award; decide, decree, determine, settle.

adjunct *n* addition, advantage, appendage, appurtenance, attachment, attribute, auxiliary, dependency, help.

adjure *vb* beg, beseech, entreat, pray, supplicate.

adjust *vb* adapt, arrange, dispose, rectify; regulate, set right, settle, suit; compose, harmonize, pacify, reconcile, settle; accommodate, adapt, fit, suit.

administer *vb* contribute, deal out, dispense, supply; conduct, control, direct, govern, manage, oversee, superintend; conduce, contribute.

admirable *adj* astonishing, striking, surprising, wonderful; excellent, fine, rare, superb.

admiration *n* affection, approbation, approval, astonishment, delight, esteem, pleasure, regard.

admirer *n* beau, gallant, suitor, sweetheart; fan, follower, supporter.

admissible *adj* allowable, lawful, permissible, possible.

admission *n* access, admittance, entrance, introduction; acceptance, acknowledgement, allowance, assent, avowal, concession.

admit *vb* give access to, let in, receive; agree to, accept, acknowledge, concede, confess; allow, bear, permit, suffer, tolerate.

admonish *vb* censure, rebuke, reprove; advise caution, counsel, enjoin, forewarn, warn; acquaint, apprise, inform, instruct, notify, remind.

admonition *n* censure, rebuke, remonstrance; advice, caution, chiding, counsel, instruction, monition.

adolescence *n* minority, nonage, teens, youth.

adolescent *adj* juvenile, young, youthful. • *n* minor, teenager, youth.

adopt *vb* appropriate, assume; accept, approve, avow, espouse, maintain, support; affiliate, father, foster.

adore *vb* worship; esteem, honour, idolize, love, revere, venerate.

adorn *vb* beautify, decorate, embellish, enrich, garnish, gild, grace, ornament.

adroit *adj* apt, dextrous, expert, handy, ingenious, ready, skilful.

adulation *n* blandishment, cajolery, fawning, flattery, flummery, praise, sycophancy.

adult *adj* grown-up, mature, ripe, ripened. • *n* grown-up person.

adulterate *vb* alloy, contaminate, corrupt, debase, deteriorate, vitiate.

advance *adj* beforehand, forward, leading. • *vb* propel, push, send forward; aggrandize, dignify, elevate, exalt, promote; benefit, forward, further, improve, promote; adduce, allege, assign, offer, propose, propound; augment, increase; proceed, progress; grow, improve, prosper, thrive. • *n* march, progress; advancement, enhancement, growth, promotion, rise; offer, overture, proffering, proposal, proposition, tender; appreciation, rise.

advancement *n* advance, benefit, gain, growth, improvement, profit.

advantage *n* ascendancy, precedence, pre-eminence, superiority, upper-hand; benefit, blessing, emolument, gain, profit, return; account, behalf, interest; accommodation, convenience, prerogative, privilege.

advantageous *adj* beneficial, favourable, profitable.

advent *n* accession, approach, arrival, coming, visitation.

adventitious *adj* accidental, extraneous, extrinsic, foreign, fortuitous, nonessential.

adventure *vb* dare, hazard, imperil, peril, risk, venture. • *n* chance, contingency, experiment, fortuity, hazard, risk, venture; crisis, contingency, event, incident, occurrence, transaction.

adventurous *adj* bold, chivalrous, courageous, daring, doughty; foolhardy, headlong, precipitate, rash, reckless; dangerous, hazardous, perilous.

adversary *n* antagonist, enemy, foe, opponent.

adverse *adj* conflicting, contrary, opposing; antagonistic, harmful, hostile, hurtful, inimical, unfavourable, unpropitious; calamitous, disastrous, unfortunate, unlucky, untoward.

adversity *n* affliction, calamity, disaster, distress, misery, misfortune, sorrow, suffering, woe.

advertise *vb* advise, announce, declare, inform, placard, proclaim, publish.

advertisement *n* announcement, information, notice, proclamation.

advice *n* admonition, caution, counsel, exhortation, persuasion, suggestion, recommendation; information, intelligence, notice, notification; care, counsel, deliberation, forethought.

advisable *adj* advantageous, desirable, expedient, prudent.

advise *vb* admonish, counsel, commend, recommend, suggest, urge; acquaint, apprise, inform, notify; confer, consult, deliberate.

adviser *n* counsellor, director, guide, instructor.

advocate *vb* countenance, defend, favour, justify, maintain, support, uphold, vindicate. • *n* apologist, counsellor, defender, maintainer, patron, pleader, supporter; attorney, barrister, counsel, lawyer, solicitor.

aegis *n* defence, protection, safeguard, shelter.

aesthetic *adj* appropriate, beautiful, tasteful.

affable *adj* accessible, approachable, communicative, conversable, cordial, easy, familiar, frank, free, sociable, social; complaisant, courteous, civil, obliging, polite, urbane.

affair *n* business, circumstance, concern, matter, office, question; event, incident, occurrence, performance, proceeding, transaction; battle, combat, conflict, encounter, engagement, skirmish.

affairs *npl* administration, relations; business, estate, finances, property.

affect *vb* act upon, alter, change, influence, modify, transform; concern, interest, regard, relate; improve, melt, move, overcome, subdue, touch; aim at, aspire to, crave, yearn for; adopt, assume, feign.

affectation *n* affectedness, airs, artificiality, foppery, pretension, simulation.

affected *adj* artificial, assumed, feigned, insincere, theatrical; assuming, conceited, foppish, vain.

affection *n* bent, bias, feeling, inclination, passion, proclivity, propensity; accident, attribute, character, mark, modification, mode, note, property; attachment, endearment, fondness, goodwill, kindness, partiality, love.

affectionate *adj* attached, devoted, fond, kind, loving, sympathetic, tender.

affiliate *vb* ally, annex, associate, connect, incorporate, join, unite. • *n* ally, associate, confederate.

affinity *n* connection, propinquity, relationship; analogy, attraction, correspondence, likeness, relation, resemblance, similarity, sympathy.

affirm *vb* allege, assert, asseverate, aver, declare, state; approve, confirm, establish, ratify.

affix *vb* annex, attach, connect, fasten, join, subjoin, tack.

afflict *vb* agonize, distress, grieve, pain, persecute, plague, torment, trouble, try, wound.

affliction *n* adversity, calamity, disaster, misfortune, stroke, visitation; bitterness, depression, distress, grief, misery, plague, scourge, sorrow, trial, tribulation, wretchedness, woe.

affluent *adj* abounding, abundant, bounteous, plenteous; moneyed, opulent, rich, wealthy.

afford *vb* furnish, produce, supply, yield; bestow, communicate, confer, give, grant, impart, offer; bear, endure, support.

affray *n* brawl, conflict, disturbance, feud, fight, quarrel, scuffle, struggle.

affright *vb* affray, alarm, appal, confound, dismay, shock, startle. • *n* alarm, consternation, fear, fright, panic, terror.

affront *vb* abuse, insult, outrage; annoy, chafe, displease, fret, irritate, offend, pique, provoke, vex. • *n* abuse, contumely, insult, outrage, vexation, wrong.

afraid *adj* aghast, alarmed, anxious, apprehensive, frightened, scared, timid.

after *prep* later than, subsequent to; behind, following; about, according to; because of, in imitation of. • *adj* behind, consecutive, ensuing, following, later, succeeding, successive, subsequent; aft, back, hind, rear, rearmost, tail. • *adv* afterwards, later, next, since, subsequently, then, thereafter.

again *adv* afresh, anew, another time, once more; besides, further, in addition, moreover.

against *prep* adverse to, contrary to, in opposition to, resisting; abutting, close up to, facing, fronting, off, opposite to, over; in anticipation of, for, in expectation of; in compensation for, to counterbalance, to match.

age *vb* decline, grow old, mature. • *n* aeon, date, epoch, period, time; decline, old age, senility; antiquity, oldness.

agency *n* action, force, intervention, means, mediation, operation, procurement; charge, direction, management, superintendence, supervision.

agent *n* actor, doer, executor, operator, performer; active element, cause, force; attorney, broker, commissioner, deputy, factor, intermediary, manager, middleman.

agglomeration *n* accumulation, aggregation, conglomeration, heap, lump, pile.

agglutinate *vb* cement, fasten, glue, unite.

aggrandize *vb* advance, dignify, elevate, enrich, exalt, promote.

aggravate *vb* heighten, increase, worsen; colour, exaggerate, magnify, overstate; enrage, irritate, provoke, tease.

aggravation *n* exaggeration, heightening, irritation.

aggregate *vb* accumulate, amass, collect, heap, pile. • *adj* collected, total. • *n* amount, gross, total, whole.

aggressive *adj* assailing, assailant, assaulting, attacking, invading, offensive; pushing, self-assertive.

aggressor *n* assailant, assaulter, attacker, invader.

aggrieve *vb* afflict, grieve, pain; abuse, ill-treat, impose, injure, oppress, wrong.

aghast *adj* appalled, dismayed, frightened, horrified, horror-struck, panic-stricken, terrified; amazed, astonished, startled, thunderstruck.

agile *adj* active, alert, brisk, lively, nimble, prompt, smart, ready.

agitate *vb* disturb, jar, rock, shake, trouble; disquiet, excite, ferment, rouse, trouble; confuse, discontent, flurry, fluster, flutter; canvass, debate, discuss, dispute, investigate.

agitation *n* concussion, shake, shaking; commotion, convulsion, disturbance, ferment, jarring, storm, tumult, turmoil; discomposure, distraction, emotion, excitement, flutter, perturbation, ruffle, tremor, trepidation; controversy, debate, discussion.

agnostic *n* doubter, empiricist, sceptic.

agonize *vb* distress, excruciate, rack, torment, torture.

agony *n* anguish, distress, pangs.

agree *vb* accord, concur, harmonize, unite; accede, acquiesce, assent, comply, concur, subscribe; bargain, contract, covenant, engage, promise, undertake; compound, compromise; chime, cohere, conform, correspond, match, suit, tally.

agreeable *adj* charming, pleasant, pleasing.

agreement *n* accordance, compliance, concord, harmony, union; bargain, compact, contract, pact, treaty.

agriculture *n* cultivation, culture, farming, geoponics, husbandry, tillage.

aid *vb* assist, help, serve, support; relieve, succour; advance, facilitate, further, promote. • *n* assistance, cooperation, help, patronage; alms, subsidy, succour, relief.

ailment *n* disease, illness, sickness.

aim *vb* direct, level, point, train; design, intend, mean, purpose, seek. • *n* bearing, course, direction, tendency; design, object, view, reason.

air *vb* expose, display, ventilate. • *n* atmosphere, breeze; appearance, aspect, manner; melody, tune.

aisle *n* passage, walk.

akin *adj* allied, kin, related; analogous, cognate, congenial, connected.

alacrity *n* agility, alertness, activity, eagerness, promptitude; cheerfulness, gaiety, hilarity, liveliness, vivacity.

alarm *vb* daunt, frighten, scare, startle, terrify. • *n* alarm-bell, tocsin, warning; apprehension, fear, fright, terror.

alert *adj* awake, circumspect, vigilant, watchful, wary; active, brisk, lively, nimble, quick, prompt, ready, sprightly. • *vb* alarm, arouse, caution, forewarn, signal, warn. • *n* alarm, signal, warning.

alertness *n* circumspection, vigilance, watchfulness, wariness; activity, briskness, nimbleness, promptness, readiness, spryness.

alien *adj* foreign, not native; differing, estranged, inappropriate, remote, unallied, separated. • *n* foreigner, stranger.

alienate *vb* (*legal*) assign, demise, transfer; disaffect, estrange, wean, withdraw.

alienation *n* (*legal*) assignment, conveyance, transfer; breach, disaffection, division, estrangement, rupture; (*med*) aberration, delusion, derangement, hallucination, insanity, madness.

alike *adj* akin, analogous, duplicate, identical, resembling, similar • *adv* equally.

aliment *n* diet, fare, meat, nutriment, provision, rations, sustenance.

alive *adj* animate, breathing, live; aware, responsive, sensitive, susceptible; brisk, cheerful, lively, sprightly.

allay *vb* appease, calm, check, compose; alleviate, assuage, lessen, moderate, solace, temper.

allege *vb* affirm, assert, declare, maintain, say; adduce, advance, assign, cite, plead, produce, quote.

allegiance *n* duty, homage, fealty, fidelity, loyalty, obligation.

allegory *n* apologue, fable, myth, parable, story, tale.

alleviate *vb* assuage, lighten, mitigate, mollify, moderate, quell, quiet, quieten, soften, soothe.

alliance *n* affinity, intermarriage, relation; coalition, combination, confederacy, league, treaty, union; affiliation, connection, relationship, similarity.

allot *vb* divide, dispense, distribute; assign, fix, prescribe, specify.

allow *vb* acknowledge, admit, concede, confess, grant, own; authorize, grant, let, permit; bear, endure, suffer, tolerate; grant, yield, relinquish, spare; approve, justify, sanction; abate, bate, deduct, remit.

allude *vb* glance, hint, mention, imply, insinuate, intimate, refer, suggest, touch.

allure *vb* attract, beguile, cajole, coax, entice, lure, persuade, seduce, tempt. • *n* appeal, attraction, lure, temptation.

allusion *n* hint, implication, intimation, insinuation, mention, reference, suggestion.

ally *vb* combine, connect, join, league, marry, unite. • *n* aider, assistant, associate, coadjutor, colleague, friend, partner.

almighty *adj* all-powerful, omnipotent.

alms *npl* benefaction, bounty, charity, dole, gift, gratuity.

alone *adj* companionless, deserted, forsaken, isolated, lonely, only, single, sole, solitary.

along *adv* lengthways, lengthwise; forward, onward; beside, together, simultaneously.

aloud *adv* audibly, loudly, sonorously, vociferously.

alter *vb* change, conform, modify, shift, turn, transform, transmit, vary.

altercation *n* bickering, contention, controversy, dispute, dissension, strife, wrangling.

alternating *adj* intermittent, interrupted.

alternative *adj* another, different, second, substitute. • *n* choice, option, preference.

although *conj* albeit, even if, for all that, notwithstanding, though.

altitude *n* elevation, height, loftiness.

altogether *adv* completely, entirely, totally, utterly.

always *adv* continually, eternally, ever, evermore, perpetually, unceasingly.

amalgamate *vb* blend, combine, commingle, compound, incorporate, mix.

amass *vb* accumulate, aggregate, collect, gather, heap, scrape together.

amateur *n* dilettante, nonprofessional.

amaze *vb* astonish, astound, bewilder, confound, confuse, dumbfound, perplex, stagger, stupefy.

amazement *n* astonishment, bewilderment, confusion, marvel, surprise, wonder.

ambassador *n* deputy, envoy, legate, minister, plenipotentiary.

ambiguous *adj* dubious, doubtful, enigmatic, equivocal, uncertain, indefinite, indistinct, obscure, vague.

ambition *n* aspiration, emulation, longing, yearning.

ambitious *adj* aspiring, avid, eager, intent.

ameliorate *vb* amend, benefit, better, elevate, improve, mend.

amenability *n* amenableness, responsiveness; accountability, liability, responsibility.

amenable *adj* acquiescent, agreeable, persuadable, responsive, susceptible; accountable, liable, responsible.

amend *vb* better, correct, improve, mend, redress, reform.

amends *npl* atonement, compensation, expiation, indemnification, recompense, reparation, restitution.

amenity *n* agreeableness, mildness, pleasantness, softness; affability, civility, courtesy, geniality, graciousness, urbanity.

amiable *adj* attractive, benign, charming, genial, good-natured, harmonious, kind, lovable, lovely, pleasant, pleasing, sweet, winning, winsome.

amicable *adj* amiable, cordial, friendly, harmonious, kind, kindly, peaceable.

amiss *adj* erroneous, inaccurate, incorrect, faulty, improper, wrong. • *adv* erroneously, inaccurately, incorrectly, wrongly.

amnesty *n* absolution, condonation, dispensation, forgiveness, oblivion.

amorous *adj* ardent, enamoured, fond, longing, loving, passionate, tender; erotic, impassioned.

amorphous *adj* formless, irregular, shapeless, unshapen; noncrystalline, structureless; chaotic, characterless, clumsy, disorganized, misshapen, unorganized, vague.

amount *n* aggregate, sum, total.

ample *adj* broad, capacious, extended, extensive, great, large, roomy, spacious; abounding, abundant, copious, generous, liberal, plentiful; diffusive, unrestricted.

amputate *vb* clip, curtail, prune, lop, remove, separate, sever.

amuse *vb* charm, cheer, divert, enliven, entertain, gladden, relax, solace; beguile, cheat, deceive, delude, mislead.

amusement *n* diversion, entertainment, frolic, fun, merriment, pleasure.

analeptic *adj* comforting, invigorating, restorative.

analogy *n* correspondence, likeness, parallelism, parity, resemblance, similarity.

analysis *n* decomposition, dissection, resolution, separation.

anarchy *n* chaos, confusion, disorder, misrule, lawlessness, riot.

anathema *n* ban, curse, denunciation, excommunication, execration, malediction, proscription.

anatomy *n* dissection; form, skeleton, structure.

ancestor *n* father, forebear, forefather, progenitor.

ancestry *n* family, house, line, lineage; descent, genealogy, parentage, pedigree, stock.

anchor *vb* fasten, fix, secure; cast anchor, take firm hold. • *n* (*naut*) ground tackle; defence, hold, security, stay.

ancient *adj* old, primitive, pristine; antiquated, antique, archaic, obsolete.

ancillary *adj* accessory, auxiliary, contributory, helpful, instrumental.

angelic *adj* adorable, celestial, cherubic, heavenly, saintly, seraphic; entrancing, enrapturing, rapturous, ravishing.

anger *vb* chafe, displease, enrage, gall, infuriate, irritate, madden. • *n* choler, exasperation, fury, gall, indignation, ire, passion, rage, resentment, spleen, wrath.

angle *vb* fish. • *n* divergence, flare, opening; bend, corner, crotch, cusp, point; fish-hook, hook.

angry *adj* chafed, exasperated, furious, galled, incensed, irritated, nettled, piqued, provoked, resentful.

anguish *n* agony, distress, grief, pang, rack, torment, torture.

anile *adj* aged, decrepit, doting, imbecile, senile.

animadversion *n* comment, notice, observation, remark; blame, censure, condemnation, reproof, stricture.

animate *vb* inform, quicken, vitalize, vivify; fortify, invigorate, revive; activate, enliven, excite, heat, impel, kindle, rouse, stimulate, stir, waken; elate, embolden, encourage, exhilarate, gladden, hearten. • *adj* alive, breathing, live, living, organic, quick.

animosity *n* bitterness, enmity, grudge, hatred, hostility, rancour, rankling, spleen, virulence.

annals *npl* archives, chronicles, records, registers, rolls.

annex *vb* affix, append, attach, subjoin, tag, tack; connect, join, unite.

annihilate *vb* abolish, annul, destroy, dissolve, exterminate, extinguish, kill, obliterate, raze, ruin.

annotation *n* comment, explanation, illustration, note, observation, remark.

announce *vb* advertise, communicate, declare, disclose, proclaim, promulgate, publish, report, reveal, trumpet.

announcement *n* advertisement, annunciation, bulletin, declaration, manifesto, notice, notification, proclamation.

annoy *vb* badger, chafe, disquiet, disturb, fret, hector, irk, irritate, molest, pain, pester, plague, trouble, vex, worry, wound.

annul *vb* abolish, abrogate, cancel, countermand, nullify, overrule, quash, repeal, recall, reverse, revoke.

anoint *vb* consecrate, oil, sanctify, smear.

anonymous *adj* nameless, unacknowledged, unsigned.

answer *vb* fulfil, rejoin, reply, respond, satisfy. • *n* rejoinder, reply, response, retort; confutation, rebuttal, refutation.

answerable *adj* accountable, amenable, correspondent, liable, responsible, suited.

antagonism *n* contradiction, discordance, disharmony, dissonant, incompatibility, opposition.

antecedent *adj* anterior, foregoing, forerunning, precedent, preceding, previous. • *n* forerunner, precursor.

anterior *adj* antecedent, foregoing, preceding, previous, prior; fore, front.

anticipate *vb* antedate, forestall, foretaste, prevent; count upon, expect, forecast, foresee.

anticipation *n* apprehension, contemplation, expectation, hope, prospect, trust; expectancy, forecast, foresight, foretaste, preconception, presentiment.

antidote *n* corrective, counteractive, counter-poison; cure, remedy, restorative, specific.

antipathy *n* abhorrence, aversion, disgust, detestation, hate, hatred, horror, loathing, repugnance.

antique *adj* ancient, archaic, bygone, old, old-fashioned.

anxiety *n* apprehension, care, concern, disquiet, fear, foreboding, misgiving, perplexity, trouble, uneasiness, vexation, worry.

anxious *adj* apprehensive, restless, solicitous, uneasy, unquiet, worried.

apart *adv* aloof, aside, separately; asunder.

apathetic *adj* cold, dull, impassive, inert, listless, obtuse, passionless, sluggish, torpid, unfeeling.

ape *vb* counterfeit, imitate, mimic; affect. • *n* simian, troglodyte; imitator, mimic; image, imitation, likeness, type.

aperture *n* chasm, cleft, eye, gap, opening, hole, orifice, passage.

aphorism *n* adage, apothegm, byword, maxim, proverb, saw, saying.

apish *adj* imitative, mimicking; affected, foppish, trifling.

aplomb *n* composure, confidence, equanimity, self-confidence.

apocryphal *adj* doubtful, fabulous, false, legendary, spurious, uncanonical.

apologetic *adj* exculpatory, excusatory; defensive, vindictive.

apology *n* defence, justification, vindication; acknowledgement, excuse, explanation, plea, reparation.

apostate *adj* backsliding, disloyal, faithless, false, perfidious, recreant, traitorous, untrue. • *n* backslider, deserter, pervert, renegade, turncoat.

apostle *n* angel, herald, messenger, missionary, preacher; advocate, follower, supporter.

apothegm *n* aphorism, byword, dictum, maxim, proverb, saw, saying.

appal *vb* affright, alarm, daunt, dismay, frighten, horrify, scare, shock.

apparel *n* attire, array, clothes, clothing, dress, garments, habit, raiment, robes, suit, trappings, vestments.

apparent *adj* discernible, perceptible, visible; conspicuous, evident, legible, manifest, obvious, open, patent, plain, unmistakable; external, ostensible, seeming, superficial.

apparition *n* appearance, appearing, epiphany, manifestation; being, form; ghost, phantom, spectre, spirit, vision.

appeal *vb* address, entreat, implore, invoke, refer, request, solicit. • *n* application, entreaty, invocation, solicitation, suit.

appear *vb* emerge, loom; break, open; arise, occur, offer; look, seem, show.

appearance *n* advent, arrival, apparition, coming; form, shape; colour, face, fashion, feature, guise, pretence, pretext; air, aspect, complexion, demeanour, manner, mien.

appease *vb* abate, allay, assuage, calm, ease, lessen, mitigate, pacify, placate, quell, soothe, temper, tranquillize.

appellation *n* address, cognomen, denomination, epithet, style, title.

append *vb* attach, fasten, hang; add, annex, subjoin, tack, tag.

appendix *n* addition, adjunct, appurtenance, codicil; excursus, supplement.

appetite *n* craving, desire, longing, lust, passion; gusto, relish, stomach, zest; hunger.

applaud *vb* acclaim, cheer, clap, compliment, encourage, extol, magnify.

applause *n* acclamation, approval, cheers, commendation, plaudit.

applicable *adj* adapted, appropriate, apt, befitting, fitting, germane, pertinent, proper, relevant.

application *n* emollient, lotion, ointment, poultice, wash; appliance, exercise, practice, use; appeal, petition, request, solicitation, suit; assiduity, constancy, diligence, effort, industry.

apply *vb* bestow, lay upon; appropriate, convert, employ, exercise, use; addict, address, dedicate, devote, direct, engage.

appoint *vb* determine, establish, fix, prescribe; bid, command, decree, direct, order, require; allot, assign, delegate, depute, detail, destine, settle; constitute, create, name, nominate; equip, furnish, supply.

apportion *vb* allocate, allot, allow, assign, deal, disperse, divide, share.

apposite *adj* apt, fit, germane, pertinent, relevant, suitable, pertinent.

appraise *vb* appreciate, estimate, prize, rate, value.

appreciate *vb* appreciate, esteem, estimate, rate, realize, value.

apprehend *vb* arrest, catch, detain, seize, take; conceive, imagine, regard, view; appreciate, perceive, realize see, take in; fear, forebode; conceive, fancy, hold, imagine, presume, understand.

apprehension *n* arrest, capture, seizure; intellect, intelligence, mind, reason; discernment, intellect, knowledge, perception, sense; belief, fancy, idea, notion, sentiment, view; alarm, care, dread, distrust, fear, misgiving, suspicion.

apprise *vb* acquaint, inform, notify, tell.

approach *vb* advance, approximate, come close; broach; resemble. • *n* advance, advent; approximation, convergence, nearing, tendency; entrance, path, way.

approbation *n* approval, commendation, liking, praise; assent, concurrence, consent, endorsement, ratification, sanction.

appropriate *vb* adopt, arrogate, assume, set apart; allot, apportion, assign, devote; apply, convert, employ, use. • *adj* adapted, apt, befitting, fit, opportune, seemly, suitable.

approve *vb* appreciate, commend, like, praise, recommend, value; confirm, countenance, justify, ratify, sustain, uphold.

approximate *vb* approach, resemble. • *adj* approaching, proximate; almost exact, inexact, rough.

apt *adj* applicable, apposite, appropriate, befitting, fit, felicitous, germane; disposed, inclined, liable, prone, subject; able, adroit, clever, dextrous, expert, handy, happy, prompt, ready, skilful.

aptitude *n* applicability, appropriateness, felicity, fitness, pertinence, suitability; inclination, tendency, turn; ability, address, adroitness, quickness, readiness, tact.

arbitrary *adj* absolute, autocratic, despotic, domineering, imperious, overbearing, unlimited; capricious, discretionary, fanciful, voluntary, whimsical.

arcade *n* colonnade, loggia.

arch[1] *adj* cunning, knowing, frolicsome, merry, mirthful, playful, roguish, shrewd, sly; consummate, chief, leading, pre-eminent, prime, primary, principal.

arch[2] *vb* span, vault; bend, curve. • *n* archway, span, vault.

archaic *adj* ancient, antiquated, antique, bygone, obsolete, old.

archives *npl* documents, muniments, records, registers, rolls.

ardent *adj* burning, fiery, hot; eager, earnest, fervent, impassioned, keen, passionate, warm, zealous.

ardour *n* glow, heat, warmth; eagerness, enthusiasm, fervour, heat, passion, soul, spirit, warmth, zeal.

arduous *adj* high, lofty, steep, uphill; difficult, fatiguing, hard, laborious, onerous, tiresome, toilsome, wearisome.

area *n* circle, circuit, district, domain, field, range, realm, region, tract.

argue *vb* plead, reason upon; debate, dispute; denote, evince, imply, indicate, mean, prove; contest, debate, discuss, sift.

arid *adj* barren, dry, parched, sterile, unfertile; dry, dull, jejune, pointless, uninteresting.

aright *adv* correctly, justly, rightly, truly.

arise *vb* ascend, mount, soar, tower; appear, emerge, rise, spring; begin, originate; rebel, revolt, rise; accrue, come, emanate, ensue, flow, issue, originate, proceed, result.

aristocracy *n* gentry, nobility, noblesse, peerage.

arm[1] *n* bough, branch, limb, protection; cove, creek, estuary, firth, fjord, frith, inlet.

arm[2] *vb* array, equip, furnish; clothe, cover, fortify, guard, protect, strengthen.

arms *npl* accoutrements, armour, array, harness, mail, panoply, weapons; crest, escutcheon.

army *n* battalions, force, host, legions, troops; host, multitude, throng, vast assemblage.

around *prep* about, encircling, encompassing, round, surrounding. • *adv* about, approximately, generally, near, nearly, practically, round, thereabouts.

arouse *vb* animate, awaken, excite, incite, kindle, provoke, rouse, stimulate, warm, whet.

arraign *vb* accuse, censure, charge, denounce, impeach, indict, prosecute, tax.

arrange *vb* array, class, classify, dispose, distribute, group, range, rank; adjust, determine, fix upon, settle; concoct, construct, devise, plan, prepare, project.

arrant *adj* bad, consummate, downright, gross, notorious, rank, utter.

array *vb* arrange, dispose, place, range, rank; accoutre, adorn, attire, decorate, dress, enrobe, embellish, equip, garnish, habit, invest. • *n* arrangement, collection, disposition, marshalling, order; apparel, attire, clothes, dress, garments; army, battalions, soldiery, troops.

arrest *vb* check, delay, hinder, hold, interrupt, obstruct, restrain, stay, stop, withhold; apprehend, capture, catch, seize, take; catch, engage, engross, fix, occupy, secure, rivet. • *n* check, checking, detention, hindrance, interruption, obstruction, restraining, stay, staying, stopping; apprehension, capture, detention, seizure.

arrive *vb* attain, come, get to, reach.

arrogance *n* assumption, assurance, disdain, effrontery, haughtiness, loftiness, lordliness, presumption, pride, scornfulness, superciliousness.

arrogate *vb* assume, claim unduly, demand, usurp.

arrow *n* bolt, dart, reed, shaft.

art *n* business, craft, employment, trade; address, adroitness, aptitude, dexterity, ingenuity, knack, readiness, sagacity, skill; artfulness, artifice, astuteness, craft, deceit, duplicity, finesse, subtlety.

artful *adj* crafty, cunning, disingenuous, insincere, sly, tricky, wily.

article *n* branch, clause, division, head, item, member, paragraph, part, point, portion; essay, paper, piece; commodity, substance, thing.

artifice *n* art, chicanery, contrivance, cunning, deception, deceit, duplicity, effort, finesse, fraud, imposture, invention, stratagem, subterfuge, trick, trickery.

artificial *adj* counterfeit, sham, spurious; assumed, affected, constrained, fictitious, forced, laboured, strained.

artless *adj* ignorant, rude, unskilful, untaught; natural, plain, simple; candid, fair, frank, guileless, honest, plain, unaffected, simple, sincere, truthful, unsuspicious.

ascend *vb* arise, aspire, climb, mount, soar, tower.

ascendancy, ascendency *n* authority, control, domination, mastery, power, predominance, sovereignty, superiority, sway.

ascertain *vb* certify, define, determine, establish, fix, settle, verify; discover, find out, get at.

ashamed *adj* abashed, confused.

ask *vb* interrogate, inquire, question; adjure, beg, conjure, crave, desire, dun, entreat, implore, invite, inquire, petition, request, solicit, supplicate, seek, sue.

aspect *n* air, bearing, countenance, expression, feature, look, mien, visage; appearance, attitude, condition, light, phase, position, posture, situation, state, view; angle, direction, outlook, prospect.

asperity *n* ruggedness, roughness, unevenness; acrimony, causticity, corrosiveness, sharpness, sourness, tartness; acerbity, bitterness, churlishness, harshness, sternness, sullenness, severity, virulence.

aspersion *n* abuse, backbiting, calumny, censure, defamation, detraction, slander, vituperation, reflection, reproach.

aspiration *n* aim, ambition, craving, hankering, hope, longing.

aspire *vb* desire, hope, long, yearn; ascend, mount, rise, soar, tower.

assail *vb* assault, attack, invade, oppugn; impugn, malign, maltreat; ply, storm.

assassinate *vb* dispatch, kill, murder, slay.

assault *vb* assail, attack, charge, invade. • *n* aggression, attack, charge, incursion, invasion, onset, onslaught; storm.

assemble *vb* call, collect, congregate, convene, convoke, gather, levy, muster; converge, forgather.

assembly *n* company, collection, concourse, congregation, gathering, meeting, rout, throng; caucus, congress, conclave, convention, convocation, diet, legislature, meeting, parliament, synod.

assent *vb* accede, acquiesce, agree, concur, subscribe, yield. • *n* accord, acquiescence, allowance, approval, approbation, consent.

assert *vb* affirm, allege, aver, asseverate, declare, express, maintain, predicate, pronounce, protest; claim, defend, emphasize, maintain, press, uphold, vindicate.

assertion *n* affirmation, allegation, asseveration, averment, declaration, position, predication, remark, statement, word; defence, emphasis, maintenance, pressing, support, vindication.

assess *vb* appraise, compute, estimate, rate, value; assign, determine, fix, impose, levy.

asseverate *vb* affirm, aver, avow, declare, maintain, protest.

assiduous *adj* active, busy, careful, constant, diligent, devoted, indefatigable, industrious, sedulous, unremitting, untiring.

assign *vb* allot, appoint, apportion, appropriate; fix, designate, determine, specify; adduce, advance, allege, give, grant, offer, present, show.

assist *vb* abet, aid, befriend, further, help, patronize, promote, second, speed, support, sustain; aid, relieve, succour; alternate with, relieve, spell.

associate *vb* affiliate, combine, conjoin, couple, join, link, relate, yoke; consort, fraternize, mingle, sort. • *n* chum, companion, comrade, familiar, follower, mate; ally, confederate, friend, partner, fellow.

association *n* combination, company, confederation, connection, partnership, society.

assort *vb* arrange, class, classify, distribute, group, rank, sort; agree, be adapted, consort, suit.

assuage *vb* allay, alleviate, appease, calm, ease, lessen, mitigate, moderate, mollify, pacify, quell, relieve, soothe, tranquillize.

assume *vb* take, undertake; affect, counterfeit, feign, pretend, sham; arrogate, usurp; beg, hypothesize, imply, postulate, posit, presuppose, suppose, simulate.

assurance *n* assuredness, certainty, conviction, persuasion, pledge, security, surety, warrant; engagement, pledge, promise; averment, assertion, protestation; audacity, confidence, courage, firmness, intrepidity; arrogance, brass, boldness, effrontery, face, front, impudence.

assure *vb* encourage, embolden, hearten; certify, insure, secure against loss, vouch for.

astonish *vb* amaze, astound, confound, daze, dumbfound, overwhelm, startle, stun, stupefy, surprise.

astute *adj* acute, cunning, deep, discerning, ingenious, intelligent, penetrating, perspicacious, quick, sagacious, sharp, shrewd.

asylum *n* refuge, retreat, sanctuary, shelter.

athletic *adj* brawny, lusty, muscular, powerful, robust, sinewy, stalwart, stout, strapping, strong, sturdy.

athletics *npl* aerobics, eurythmics, exercise, exercising, gymnastics, sports, track and field, workout.

atom *n* bit, molecule, monad, particle, scintilla.

atone *vb* answer, compensate, expiate, satisfy.

atonement *n* amends, expiation, propitiation, reparation, satisfaction.

atrocity *n* depravity, enormity, flagrancy, ferocity, savagery, villainy.

attach *vb* affix, annex, connect, fasten, join, hitch, tie; charm, captivate, enamour, endear, engage, win; (*legal*) distress, distrain, seize, take.

attack *vb* assail, assault, charge, encounter, invade, set upon, storm, tackle; censure, criticise, impugn. • *n* aggression, assault, charge, offence, onset, onslaught, raid, thrust.

attain *vb* accomplish, achieve, acquire, get, obtain, secure; arrive at, come to, reach.

attempt *vb* assail, assault, attack; aim, endeavour, seek, strive, try. • *n* effort, endeavour, enterprise, experiment, undertaking, venture; assault, attack, onset.

attend *vb* accompany, escort, follow; guard, protect, watch; minister to, serve, wait on; give heed, hear, harken, listen; be attendant, serve, tend, wait.

attention *n* care, circumspection, heed, mindfulness, observation, regard, watch, watchfulness; application, reflection, study; civility, courtesy, deference, politeness, regard, respect; addresses, courtship, devotion, suit, wooing.

attentive *adj* alive, awake, careful, civil, considerate, courteous, heedful, mindful, observant, watchful.

attenuate *vb* contract, dilute, diminish, elongate, lengthen, lessen, rarefy, reduce, slim, thin, weaken.

attest *vb* authenticate, certify, corroborate, confirm, ratify, seal, vouch; adjure, call to witness, invoke; confess, display, exhibit, manifest, prove, show, witness.

attic *n* garret, loft, upper storey.

Attic *adj* delicate, subtle, penetrating, pointed, pungent; chaste, classic, correct, elegant, polished, pure.

attire *vb* accoutre, apparel, array, clothe, dress, enrobe, equip, rig, robe. • *n* clothes, clothing, costume, dress, garb, gear, habiliment, outfit, toilet, trapping, vestment, vesture, wardrobe.

attitude *n* pose, position, posture; aspect, conjuncture, condition, phase, prediction, situation, standing, state.

attract *vb* draw, pull; allure, captivate, charm, decoy, enamour, endear, entice, engage, fascinate, invite, win.

attraction *n* affinity, drawing, pull; allurement, charm, enticement, fascination, magnetism, lure, seduction, witchery.

attribute *vb* ascribe, assign, impute, refer. • *n* characteristic, mark, note, peculiarity, predicate, property, quality.

attrition *n* abrasion, friction, rubbing.

attune *vb* accord, harmonize, modulate, tune; accommodate, adapt, adjust, attempt.

audacity *n* boldness, courage, daring, fearlessness, intrepidity; assurance, brass, effrontery, face, front, impudence, insolence, presumption, sauciness.

audience *n* assemblage, congregation; hearing, interview, reception.

augment *vb* add to, enhance, enlarge, increase, magnify, multiply, swell.

augmentation *n* accession, addition, enlargement, extension, increase.

augury *n* prediction, prognostication, prophecy, soothsaying; auspice, forerunner, harbinger, herald, omen, precursor, portent, sign.

august *adj* awe-inspiring, awful, dignified, grand, imposing, kingly, majestic, noble, princely, regal, solemn, stately, venerable.

auspicious *adj* fortunate, happy, lucky, prosperous, successful; bright, favourable, golden, opportune, promising, prosperous.

austere *adj* ascetic, difficult, formal, hard, harsh, morose, relentless, rigid, rigorous, severe, stern, stiff, strict, uncompromising, unrelenting.

authentic *adj* genuine, pure, real, true, unadulterated, uncorrupted, veritable; accurate, authoritative, reliable, true, trustworthy.

authority *n* dominion, empire, government, jurisdiction, power, sovereignty; ascendency, control, influence, rule, supremacy, sway; authorization, liberty, order, permit, precept, sanction, warranty; testimony, witness; connoisseur, expert, master.

authorize *vb* empower, enable, entitle; allow, approve, confirm, countenance, permit, ratify, sanction.

auxiliary *adj* aiding, ancillary, assisting, helpful, subsidiary. • *n* ally, assistant, confederate, help.

avail *vb* assist, benefit, help, profit, use, service.

available *adj* accessible, advantageous, applicable, beneficial, profitable, serviceable, useful.

avarice *n* acquisitiveness, covetousness, greediness, penuriousness, rapacity.

avaricious *adj* grasping, miserly, niggardly, parsimonious.

avenge *vb* punish, retaliate, revenge, vindicate.

avenue *n* access, entrance, entry, passage; alley, path, road, street, walk; channel, pass, route, way.

aver *vb* allege, assert, asseverate, avouch, declare, pronounce, protest, say.

averse *adj* adverse, backward, disinclined, indisposed, opposed, unwilling.

aversion *n* abhorrence, antipathy, disgust, dislike, hate, hatred, loathing, reluctance, repugnance.

avid *adj* eager, greedy, voracious.

avocation *n* business, calling, employment, occupation, trade, vocation; distraction, hindrance, interruption.

avoid *vb* dodge, elude, escape, eschew, shun; forebear, refrain from.

avouch *vb* allege, assert, declare, maintain, say.

avow *vb* admit, acknowledge, confess, own.

awaken *vb* arouse, excite, incite, kindle, provoke, spur, stimulate; wake, waken; begin, be excited.

award *vb* adjudge, allot, assign, bestow, decree, grant. • *n* adjudication, allotment, assignment, decision, decree, determination, gift, judgement.

aware *adj* acquainted, apprised, conscious, conversant, informed, knowing, mindful, sensible.

away *adv* absent, not present. • *adj* at a distance; elsewhere; out of the way.

awe *vb* cow, daunt, intimidate, overawe. • *n* abashment, fear, reverence; dread, fear, fearfulness, terror.

awful *adj* august, awesome, dread, grand, inspired; abashed, alarming, appalled, dire, frightful, portentous, tremendous.

awkward *adj* bungling, clumsy, inept, maladroit, unskilful; lumbering, unfit, ungainly unmanageable; boorish; inconvenient, unsuitable.

axiom *n* adage, aphorism, apothegm, maxim, postulation, truism.

axis *n* axle, shaft, spindle.

azure *adj* blue, cerulean, sky-coloured.

B

babble *vb* blather, chatter, gibber, jabber, prate, prattle. • *n* chat, gossip, palaver, prate, tattle.

babel *n* clamour, confusion, din, discord, disorder, hubbub, jargon, pother.

baby *vb* coddle, cosset, indulge, mollycoddle, pamper, spoil. • *adj* babyish, childish, infantile, puerile; diminutive, doll-like, miniature, pocket, pocket-sized, small-scale. • *n* babe, brat, child, infant, suckling, nursling; chicken, coward, milksop, namby-pamby, sad sack, weakling; miniature; innocent.

bacchanal *n* carouse, debauchery, drunkenness, revelry, roisterousness.

back *vb* abet, aid, countenance, favour, second, support, sustain; go back, move back, retreat, withdraw. • *adj* hindmost. • *adv* in return, in consideration; ago, gone, since; aside, away, behind, by; abaft, astern, backwards, hindwards, rearwards. • *n* end, hind part, posterior, rear.

backbite *vb* abuse, asperse, blacken, defame, libel, malign, revile, scandalize, slander, traduce, vilify.

backbone *n* chine, spine; constancy, courage, decision, firmness, nerve, pluck, resolution, steadfastness.

backslider *n* apostate, deserter, renegade.

backward *adj* disinclined, hesitating, indisposed, loath, reluctant, unwilling, wavering; dull, slow, sluggish, stolid, stupid. • *adv* aback, behind, rearward.

bad *adj* baleful, baneful, detrimental, evil, harmful, hurtful, injurious, noxious, pernicious, unwholesome, vicious; abandoned, corrupt, depraved, immoral, sinful, unfair, unprincipled, wicked; unfortunate, unhappy, unlucky, miserable; disappointing, discouraging, distressing, sad, unwelcoming; abominable, mean, shabby, scurvy, vile, wretched; defective, inferior, imperfect, incompetent, poor, unsuitable; hard, heavy, serious, severe.

badge *n* brand, emblem, mark, sign, symbol, token.

badger *vb* annoy, bait, bother, hector, harry, pester, persecute, tease, torment, trouble, vex, worry.

baffle *vb* balk, block, check, circumvent, defeat, foil, frustrate, mar, thwart, undermine, upset; bewilder, confound, disconcert, perplex.

bait *vb* harry, tease, worry. • *n* allurement, decoy, enticement, lure, temptation.

balance *vb* equilibrate, pose, (*naut*) trim; compare, weigh; compensate, counteract, estimate; adjust, clear, equalize, square. • *n* equilibrium, liberation; excess, remainder, residue, surplus.

bald *adj* bare, naked, uncovered, treeless; dull, inelegant, meagre, prosaic, tame, unadorned, vapid.

baleful *adj* baneful, deadly, calamitous, hurtful, injurious, mischievous, noxious, pernicious, ruinous.

balk *vb* baffle, defeat, disappoint, disconcert, foil, frustrate, thwart.

ball *n* drop, globe, orb, pellet, marble, sphere; bullet, missile, projectile, shot; assembly, dance.

balmy *adj* aromatic, fragrant, healing, odorous, perfumed.

ban *vb* anathematize, curse, execrate; interdict, outlaw. • *n* edict, proclamation; anathema, curse, denunciation, execration; interdiction, outlawry, penalty, prohibition

band[1] *vb* belt, bind, cinch, encircle, gird, girdle; ally, associate, combine, connect, join, league; bar, marble, streak, stripe, striate, vein. • *n* crew, gang, horde, society, troop; ensemble, group, orchestra.

band[2] *n* ligament, ligature, tie; bond, chain, cord, fetter, manacle, shackle, trammel; bandage, belt, binding, cincture, girth, tourniquet.

bandit *n* brigand, freebooter, footpad, gangster, highwayman, outlaw, robber.

baneful *adj* poisonous, venomous; deadly, destructive, hurtful, mischievous, noxious, pernicious.

bang *vb* beat, knock, maul, pommel, pound, strike, thrash, thump; slam; clatter, rattle, resound, ring. • *n* clang, clangour, whang; blow, knock, lick, thump, thwack, whack.

banish *vb* exile, expatriate, ostracize; dismiss, exclude, expel.

bank[1] *vb* incline, slope, tilt; embank. • *n* dike, embankment, escarpment, heap, knoll, mound; border, bound, brim, brink, margin, rim, strand; course, row, tier.

bank[2] *vb* deposit, keep, save. • *n* depository, fund, reserve, savings, stockpile.

banner *n* colours, ensign, flag, standard, pennon, standard, streamer.

banter *vb* chaff, deride, jeer, joke, mock, quiz, rally, ridicule. • *n* badinage, chaff, derision, jesting, joking, mockery, quizzing, raillery, ridicule.

bar *vb* exclude, hinder, obstruct, prevent, prohibit, restrain, stop. • *n* grating, pole, rail, rod; barricade, hindrance, impediment, obstacle, obstruction, stop; bank, sand bar, shallow, shoal, spit; (*legal*) barristers, counsel, court, judgement, tribunal.

barbarian *adj* brutal, cruel, ferocious, fierce, fell, inhuman, ruthless, savage, truculent, unfeeling. • *n* brute, ruffian, savage.

barbaric *adj* barbarous, rude, savage, uncivilized, untamed; capricious, coarse, gaudy, riotous, showy, outlandish, uncouth, untamed, wild.

bare *vb* denude, depilate, divest, strip, unsheathe; disclose, manifest, open, reveal, show. • *adj* denuded, exposed, naked, nude, stripped, unclothed, uncovered, undressed, unsheltered; alone, mere, sheer, simple; bald, meagre, plain, unadorned, uncovered, unfurnished; empty, destitute, indigent, poor.

bargain *vb* agree, contract, covenant, stipulate; convey, sell, transfer. • *n* agreement, compact, contract, covenant, convention, indenture, transaction, stipulation, treaty; proceeds, purchase, result.

barren *adj* childless, infecund, sterile; (*bot*) acarpous, sterile; bare, infertile, poor, sterile, unproductive; ineffectual, unfruitful, uninstructive.

barricade *vb* block up, fortify, protect, obstruct. • *n* barrier, obstruction, palisade, stockade.

barrier *n* bar, barricade, hindrance, impediment, obstacle, obstruction, stop.

barter *vb* bargain, exchange, sell, trade, traffic.

base1 *adj* cheap, inferior, worthless; counterfeit, debased, false, spurious; baseborn, humble, lowly, mean, nameless, plebeian, unknown, untitled, vulgar; abject, beggarly, contemptible, degraded, despicable, low, menial, pitiful, servile, sordid, sorry, worthless.

base[2] *vb* establish, found, ground. • *n* foundation, fundament, substructure, underpinning; pedestal, plinth, stand; centre, headquarters, HQ, seat; starting point; basis, cause, grounds, reason, standpoint; bottom, foot, foundation, ground.

bashful *adj* coy, diffident, shy, timid.

basis n base, bottom, foundation, fundament, ground, groundwork.

bastard *adj* adulterated, baseborn, counterfeit, false, illegitimate, sham. • *n* love child.

batch *vb* assemble, bunch, bundle, collect, gather, group. • *n* amount, collection, crowd, lot, quantity.

bathe *vb* immerse, lave, wash; cover, enfold, enwrap, drench, flood, infold, suffuse. • *n* bath, shower, swim.

batter[1] *vb* beat, pelt, smite; break, bruise, demolish, destroy, shatter, shiver, smash; abrade, deface, disfigure, indent, mar; incline, recede, retreat, slope. • *n* batsman, striker.

batter[2] *n* dough, goo, goop, gunk, paste, pulp.

battle *vb* contend, contest, engage, fight, strive, struggle. • *n* action, affair, brush, combat, conflict, contest, engagement, fight, fray.

bauble *n* gewgaw, gimcrack, knick-knack, plaything, toy, trifle, trinket.

bawdy *adj* obscene, filthy, impure, indecent, lascivious, lewd, smutty, unchaste.

bawl *vb* clamour, cry, hoot, howl, roar, shout, squall, vociferate, yell.

bay[1] *vb* bark, howl, wail, yell, yelp.

bay[2] *n* alcove, compartment, niche, nook, opening, recess.

bay[3] *n* bight, cove, gulf, inlet.

bays *npl* applause, chaplet, fame, garland, glory, honour, plaudits, praise, renown.

beach *vb* ground, maroon, strand. • *n* coast, margin, rim, sands, seashore, seaside, shore, shoreline, strand, waterfront.

beacon *vb* brighten, flame, shine, signal; enlighten, illuminate, illumine, guide, light, signal. • *n* lighthouse, pharos, watchtower; sign, signal.

beadle *n* apparitor, church officer, crier, servitor, summoner.

beak *n* bill, mandible, (*sl*) nose; (*naut*) bow, prow, stem.

beam *vb* beacon, gleam, glisten, glitter, shine. • *n* balk, girder, joist, scantling, stud; gleam, pencil, ray, streak.

bear *vb* support, sustain, uphold; carry, convey, deport, transport, waft; abide, brook, endure, stand, suffer, tolerate, undergo; carry on, keep up, maintain; cherish, entertain, harbour; produce; cast, drop, sustain; endure, submit, suffer; act, operate, work. • *n* growler, grumbler, moaner, snarler; speculator.

bearable *adj* endurable, sufferable, supportable, tolerable.

bearing *n* air, behaviour, demeanour, deportment, conduct, carriage, conduct, mien, port; connection, dependency, relation; endurance, patience, suffering; aim, course direction; bringing forth, producing; bed, receptacle, socket.

beastly *adj* abominable, brutish, ignoble, low, sensual, vile.

beat *vb* bang, baste, belabour, buffet, cane, cudgel, drub, hammer, hit, knock, maul, pound, pummel, punch, strke, thrash, thump, thwack, whack, whip; bray, bruise, pound pulverize; batter, pelt; conquer, defeat, overcome, rout subdue, surpass, vanquish; pulsate, throb; dash, strike. • *adj* baffled, bamboozled, confounded, mystified, nonplused, perplexed, puzzled, stumped; done, dog-tired, exhausted, tired out, worn out; beaten, defeated, licked, worsted. • *n* blow, striking, stroke; beating, pulsation, throb; accent, metre, rhythm; circuit, course, round.

beatific *adj* ecstatic, enchanting, enraptured, ravishing, rapt.

beatitude *n* blessing, ecstasy, felicity, happiness.

beau *n* coxcomb, dandy, exquisite, fop, popinjay; admirer, lover, suitor, sweetheart.

beautiful *adj* charming, comely, fair, fine, exquisite, handsome, lovely, pretty.

beautify *vb* adorn, array, bedeck, deck, decorate, embellish, emblazon, garnish, gild, grace, ornament, set.

beauty *n* elegance, grace, symmetry; attractiveness, comeliness, fairness, loveliness, seemliness; belle.

become *vb* change to, get, go, wax; adorn, befit, set off, suit.

becoming *adj* appropriate, apt, congruous, decent, decorous, due, fit, proper, right, seemly, suitable; comely, graceful, neat, pretty.

bed *vb* embed, establish, imbed, implant, infix, inset, plant; harbour, house, lodge. • *n* berth, bunk, cot, couch; channel, depression, hollow; base, foundation, receptacle, support, underlay; accumulation, layer, seam, stratum, vein.

bedim *vb* cloud, darken, dim, obscure.

befall *vb* betide, overtake; chance, happen, occur, supervene.

befitting *adj* appropriate, apt, becoming, decorous, fit, proper, right, suitable, seemly.

befool *vb* bamboozle, beguile, cheat, circumvent, delude, deceive, dupe, fool, hoax, hoodwink, infatuate, stupefy, trick.

befriend *vb* aid, benefit, countenance, encourage, favour, help, patronize.

beg *vb* adjure, ask, beseech, conjure, crave, entreat, implore, importune, petition, pray, request, solicit, supplicate.

beggarly *adj* destitute, needy, poor; abject, base, despicable, grovelling, low, mean, miserable, miserly, paltry, pitiful, scant, servile, shabby, sorry, stingy, vile, wretched.

begin *vb* arise, commence, enter, open; inaugurate, institute, originate, start.

beginning *n* arising, commencement, dawn, emergence, inauguration, inception, initiation, opening, outset, start, rise; origin, source.

beguile *vb* cheat, deceive, delude; amuse, cheer, divert, entertain, solace.

behaviour *n* air, bearing, carriage, comportment, conduct, demeanour, deportment, manner, manners, mien.

behest *n* bidding, charge, command, commandment, direction, hest, injunction, mandate, order, precept.

behind *prep* abaft, aft, following. • *adv* abaft, aft, astern, rearward. • *adj* arrested, backward, checked, detained, retarded; after, behind. • *n* afterpart, rear, stern, tail; back, back side, reverse; bottom, buttocks, posterior, rump.

behold *vb* consider, contemplate, eye, observe, regard, see, survey, view.

behoove *vb* become, befit, suit; be binding, be obligatory.

being *n* actuality, existence, reality, subsistence; core, essence, heart, root.

beleaguer *vb* besiege, blockade, invest; beset, block, encumber, encompass, encounter, obstruct, surround.

belief *n* assurance, confidence, conviction, persuasion, trust; acceptance, assent, credence, credit, currency; creed, doctrine, dogma, faith, opinion, tenet.

bellow *vb* bawl, clamour, cry, howl, vociferate, yell.

belt *n* band, cincture, girdle, girth, zone; region, stretch, strip.

bemoan *vb* bewail, deplore, lament, mourn.

bemused *adj* bewildered, confused, fuddled, muddled, muzzy, stupefied, tipsy.

bend *vb* bow, crook, curve, deflect, draw; direct, incline, turn; bend, dispose, influence, mould, persuade, subdue; (*naut*) fasten, make fast; crook, deflect, deviate, diverge, swerve; bow, lower, stoop; condescend, deign. • *n* angle, arc, arcuation, crook, curvature, curve, elbow, flexure, turn.

beneath *prep* below, under, underneath; unbecoming, unbefitting, unworthy. • *adv* below, underneath.

benediction *n* beatitude, benefit, benison, blessing, boon, grace, favour.

benefaction *n* alms, boon, charity, contribution, donation, favour, gift, grant, gratuity, offering, present.

beneficent *adj* benevolent, bounteous, bountiful, charitable, generous, kind, liberal.

beneficial *adj* advantageous, favourable, helpful, profitable, salutary serviceable, useful, wholesome.

benefit *vb* befriend, help, serve; advantage, avail, profit. • *n* favour, good turn, kindness, service; account, advantage, behalf, gain, good, interest, profit, utility.

benevolence *n* beneficence, benignity, generosity, goodwill, humanity, kindliness, kindness.

benevolent *adj* altruistic, benign, charitable, generous, humane, kind, kind-hearted, liberal, obliging, philanthropic, tender, unselfish.

benign *adj* amiable, amicable, beneficent, benevolent, complaisant, friendly, gentle, good, gracious, humane, kind, kindly, obliging.

bent *adj* angled, angular, bowed, crooked, curved, deflected, embowed, flexed, hooked, twisted; disposed, inclined, prone, minded; (*with* **on**) determined, fixed on, resolved, set on. • *n* bias, inclination, leaning, partiality, penchant, predilection, prepossession, proclivity, propensity.

bequeath *vb* devise, give, grant, leave, will; impart, transmit.

berate *vb* chide, rate, reprimand, reprove, scold.

bereave *vb* afflict, deprive of, despoil, dispossess, divest, rob, spoil, strip.

beseech *vb* beg, conjure, entreat, implore, importune, petition, supplicate; ask, beg, crave, solicit.

beset *vb* besiege, encompass, enclose, environ, encircle, hem in, surround; decorate, embarrass, embellish, entangle, garnish, ornament, perplex, set.

beside[1] *prep* at the side of, by the side of, close to, near; aside from, not according to, out of the course of, out of the way of; not in possession of, out of.

besides[1] *prep* barring, distinct from, excluding, except, excepting, in addition to, other than, over and above, save.

beside[2], **besides**[2] *adv* additionally, also, further, furthermore, in addition, more, moreover, over and above, too, yet.

besiege *vb* beset, blockade, encircle, encompass, environ, invest, surround.

besot *vb* drench, intoxicate, soak, steep; befool, delude, infatuate, stultify, stupefy.

bespatter *vb* bedaub, befoul, besmirch, smear, spatter.

bespeak *vb* accost, address, declare, evince, forestall, imply, indicate, prearrange, predict, proclaim, solicit.

best *vb* better, exceed, excel, predominate, rival, surpass; beat, defeat, outdo, worst. • *adj* chief, first, foremost, highest, leading, utmost. • *adv* advantageously, excellently; extremely, greatly. • *n* choice, cream, flower, pick.

bestial *adj* beast-like, beastly, brutal, degraded, depraved, irrational, low, vile; sensual.

bestow *vb* deposit, dispose, put, place, store, stow; accord, give, grant, impart.

bet *vb* gamble, hazard, lay, pledge, stake, wage, wager. • *n* gamble, hazard, stake, wager.

bethink *vb* cogitate, consider, ponder, recall, recollect, reflect, remember.

betide *vb* befall, happen, occur, overtake.

betimes *adv* beforehand, early, forward, soon.

betoken *vb* argue, betray, denote, evince, imply, indicate, prove, represent, show, signify, typify.

betray *vb* be false to, break, violate; blab, discover, divulge, expose, reveal, show, tell; argue, betoken, display, evince, expose, exhibit, imply, indicate, manifest, reveal; beguile, delude, ensnare, lure, mislead; corrupt, ruin, seduce, undo.

betroth *vb* affiance, engage to marry, pledge in marriage, plight.

better *vb* advance, amend, correct, exceed, improve, promote, rectify, reform. • *adj* bigger, fitter, greater, larger, less ill, preferable. • *n* advantage, superiority, upper hand, victory; improvement, greater good.

between *prep* amidst, among, betwixt.

bewail *vb* bemoan, deplore, express, lament, mourn over, rue, sorrow.

beware *vb* avoid, heed, look out, mind.

bewilder *vb* confound, confuse, daze, distract, embarrass, entangle, muddle, mystify, nonplus, perplex, pose, puzzle, stagger.

bewitch *vb* captivate, charm, enchant, enrapture, entrance, fascinate, spellbind, transport.

beyond *prep* above, before, farther, over, past, remote, yonder.

bias *vb* bend, dispose, incline, influence, predispose, prejudice. • *n* bent, inclination, leaning, partiality, penchant, predilection, prepossession, proclivity, propensity, slant, tendency, turn.

bicker *vb* argue, dispute, jangle, quarrel, spar, spat, squabble, wrangle.

bid *vb* charge, command, direct, enjoin, order, require, summon; ask, call, invite, pray, request, solicit; offer, propose, proffer, tender. • *n* bidding, offer, proposal.

big *adj* bumper, bulking, bulky, great, huge, large, massive, monstrous; important, imposing; distended, inflated, full, swollen, tumid; fecund, fruitful, productive, teeming.

bigoted *adj* dogmatic, hidebound, intolerant, obstinate, narrow-minded, opinionated, prejudiced.

bill[1] *vb* charge, dun, invoice; programme, schedule; advertise, boost, plug, promote, publicize. • *n* account, charges, reckoning, score; advertisement, banner, hoarding, placard, poster; playbill, programme, schedule; bill of exchange, certificate, money; account, reckoning, statement.

bill[2] *n* beak, mandible, (*sl*) nose; billhook, brush-cutter, hedge-bill, hedging knife; caress, fondle, kiss, toy.

billet *vb* allot, apportion, assign, distribute, quarter, station. • *n* accommodation, lodgings, quarters.

billow *vb* surge, wave; heave, roll; bag, baloon, bulge, dilate, swell. • *n* roller, surge, swell, wave.

bin *n* box, bunker, crib, frame, receptacle.

bind *vb* confine, enchain, fetter, restrain, restrict; bandage, tie up, wrap; fasten, lash, pinion, secure, tie, truss; engage, hold, oblige, obligate, pledge; contract, harden, shrink, stiffen.

birth *n* ancestry, blood, descent, extraction, lineage, race; being, creation, creature, offspring, production, progeny.

bit *n* crumb, fragment, morsel, mouthful, piece, scrap; atom, grain, jot, mite, particle, tittle, whit; instant, minute, moment, second.

bite *vb* champ, chew, crunch, gnaw; burn, make smart, sting; catch, clutch, grapple, grasp, grip; bamboozle, cheat, cozen, deceive, defraud, dupe, gull, mislead, outwit, overreach, trick. • *n* grasp, hold; punch, relish, spice, pungency, tang, zest; lick, morsel, sip, taste; crick, nip, pain, pang, prick, sting.

bitter *adj* acrid; dire, fell, merciless, relentless, ruthless; harsh, severe, stern; afflictive, calamitous, distressing, galling, grievous, painful, poignant, sore, sorrowful.

black *adj* dark, ebony, inky, jet, sable, swarthy; dingy, dusky, lowering, murky, pitchy; calamitous, dark, depressing, disastrous, dismal, doleful, forbidding, gloomy, melancholy, mournful, sombre, sullen.

blacken *vb* darken; deface, defile, soil, stain, sully; asperse, besmirch, calumniate, defame, malign, revile, slander, traduce, vilify.

blamable *adj* blameable, blameworthy, censurable, culpable, delinquent. faulty, remiss, reprehensible.

blame *vb* accuse, censure, condemn, disapprove, reflect upon, reprehend, reproach, reprove, upbraid. • *n* animadversion, censure, condemnation, disapproval, dispraise, disapprobation, reprehension, reproach, reproof; defect, demerit, fault, guilt, misdeed, shortcoming, sin, wrong.

blameless *adj* faultless, guiltless, inculpable, innocent, irreproachable, unblemished, undefiled, unimpeachable, unspotted, unsullied, spotless, stainless.

blanch *vb* bleach, fade, etiolate, whiten.

bland *adj* balmy, demulcent, gentle, mild, soothing, soft; affable, amiable, complaisant, kindly, mild, suave.

blandishment *n* cajolery, coaxing, compliment, fascination, fawning, flattery, wheedling.

blank *adj* bare, empty, vacuous, void; amazed, astonished, confounded, confused, dumbfounded, nonplussed; absolute, complete, entire, mere, perfect, pure, simple, unabated, unadulterated, unmitigated, unmixed, utter, perfect.

blare *vb* blazon, blow, peal, proclaim, trumpet. • *n* blast, clang, clangour, peal.

blasphemy *n* impiousness, sacrilege; cursing, profanity, swearing.

blast *vb* annihilate, blight, destroy, kill, ruin, shrivel, wither; burst, explode, kill. • *n* blow, gust, squall; blare, clang, peal; burst, discharge, explosion.

blaze *vb* blazon, proclaim, publish; burn, flame, glow. • *n* flame, flare, flash, glow, light.

bleach *vb* blanch, etiolate, render white, whiten.

bleak *adj* bare, exposed, unprotected, unsheltered, storm-beaten, windswept; biting, chill, cold, piercing, raw; cheerless, comfortless, desolate, dreary, uncongenial.

blemish *vb* blur, injure, mar, spot, stain, sully, taint, tarnish; asperse, calumniate, defame, malign, revile, slander, traduce, vilify. • *n* blot, blur, defect, disfigurement, fault, flaw, imperfection, soil, speck, spot, stain, tarnish; disgrace, dishonour, reproach, stain, taint.

blend *vb* amalgamate, coalesce, combine, commingle, fuse, mingle, mix, unite. • *n* amalgamation, combination, compound, fusion, mix, mixture, union.

bless *vb* beatify, delight, gladden; adore, celebrate, exalt, extol, glorify, magnify, praise.

blessedness *n* beatitude, bliss, blissfulness, felicity, happiness, joy.

blight *vb* blast, destroy, kill, ruin, shrivel, wither; annihilate, annul, crush, disappoint, frustrate. • *n* blast, mildew, pestilence.

blind *vb* blear, darken, deprive of sight; blindfold, hoodwink. • *adj* eyeless, sightless, stone-blind, unseeing; benighted, ignorant, injudicious, purblind, undiscerning, unenlightened; concealed, confused, dark, dim, hidden, intricate, involved, labyrinthine, obscure, private, remote; careless, headlong, heedless, inconsiderate, indiscriminate, thoughtless; blank, closed, shut. • *n* cover, curtain, screen, shade, shutter; blinker; concealment, disguise, feint, pretence, pretext, ruse, stratagem, subterfuge.

blink *vb* nictate, nictitate, wink; flicker, flutter, gleam, glitter, intermit, twinkle; avoid, disregard, evade, gloss over, ignore, overlook, pass over. • *n* glance, glimpse, sight, view, wink; gleam, glimmer, sheen, shimmer, twinkle.

bliss *n* beatification, beatitude, blessedness, blissfulness, ecstasy, felicity, happiness, heaven, joy, rapture, transport.

blithe *adj* airy, animated, blithesome, buoyant, cheerful, debonair, elated, happy, jocund, joyful, joyous, lively, mirthful, sprightly, vivacious.

bloat *vb* dilate, distend, inflate, swell.

block *vb* arrest, bar, blockade, check, choke, close, hinder, impede, jam, obstruct, stop; form, mould, shape; brace, stiffen. • *n* lump, mass; blockhead, dunce, fool, simpleton; pulley, tackle; execution, scaffold; jam, obstruction, pack, stoppage.

blood *n* children, descendants, offspring, posterity, progeny; family, house, kin, kindred, line, relations; consanguinity, descent, kinship, lineage, relationship; courage, disposition, feelings, mettle, passion, spirit, temper.

bloom *vb* blossom, blow, flower; thrive, prosper. • *n* blossom, blossoming, blow, efflorescence, florescence, flowering; delicacy, delicateness, flush, freshness, heyday, prime, vigour; flush, glow, rose.

blossom *vb* bloom, blow, flower. • *n* bloom, blow, efflorescence, flower.

blot *vb* cancel, efface, erase, expunge, obliterate, rub out; blur, deface, disfigure, obscure, spot, stain, sully; disgrace, dishonour, tarnish. • *n* blemish, blur, erasure, spot, obliteration, stain; disgrace, dishonour, stigma.

blow[1] *n* bang, beat, buffet, dab, impact, knock, pat, punch, rap, slam, stroke, thump, wallop, buffet, impact; affliction, calamity, disaster, misfortune, setback.

blow[2] *vb* breathe, gasp, pant, puff; flow, move, scud, stream, waft. • *n* blast, gale, gust, squall, storm, wind.

blue *adj* azure, cerulean, cobalt, indigo, sapphire, ultramarine; ghastly, livid, pallid; dejected, depressed, dispirited, downcast, gloomy, glum, mopey, melancholic, melancholy, sad.

bluff[1] *adj* abrupt, blunt, blustering, coarse, frank, good-natured, open, outspoken; abrupt, precipitous, sheer, steep. • *n* cliff, headland, height.

bluff[2] *vb* deceive, defraud, lie, mislead. • *n* deceit, deception, feint, fraud, lie.

blunder *vb* err, flounder, mistake; stumble. • *n* error, fault, howler, mistake, solecism.

blunt *adj* dull, edgeless, obtuse, pointless, unsharpened; insensible, stolid, thick-witted; abrupt, bluff, downright, plain-spoken, outspoken, unceremonious, uncourtly. • *vb* deaden, dull, numb, weaken.

blur *vb* bedim, darken, dim, obscure; blemish, blot, spot, stain, sully, tarnish. • *n* blemish, blot, soil, spot, stain, tarnish; disgrace, smear.

blush *vb* colour, flush, glow, redden. • *n* bloom, flush, glow, colour, reddening, suffusion.

bluster *vb* boast, brag, bully, domineer, roar, swagger, swell, vaunt. • *n* boisterousness, noise, tumult, turbulence; braggadocio, bravado, boasting, gasconade, swaggering.

board *n* deal, panel, plank; diet, entertainment, fare, food, meals, provision, victuals; cabinet, conclave, committee, council; directorate; panel.

boast *vb* bluster, brag, crack, flourish, crow, vaunt. • *n* blustering, boasting, bombast, brag, braggadocio, bravado, bombast, swaggering, vaunt.

bode *vb* augur, betoken, forebode, foreshadow, foretell, portend, predict, prefigure, presage, prophesy.

bodily *adj* carnal, corporeal, fleshly, physical. • *adv* altogether, completely, entirely, wholly.

body *n* carcass, corpse, remains; stem, torso, trunk; aggregate, bulk, corpus, mass; being, individual, mortal creature, person; assemblage, association, band, company, corporation, corps, coterie, force, party, society, troop; consistency, substance, thickness.

boggle *vb* demur, falter, hang fire, hesitate, shrink, vacillate, waver.

boil[1] *vb* agitate, bubble, foam, froth, rage, seethe, simmer. • *n* ebullience, ebullition.

boil[2] (*med*) gathering, pimple, pustule, swelling, tumour.

boisterous *adj* loud, roaring, stormy; clamouring, loud, noisy, obstreperous, tumultuous, turbulent.

bold *adj* adventurous, audacious, courageous, brave, daring, dauntless, doughty, fearless, gallant, hardy, heroic, intrepid, mettlesome, manful, manly, spirited, stouthearted, undaunted, valiant, valorous; assured, confident, self-reliant; assuming, forward, impertinent, impudent, insolent, push, rude, saucy; conspicuous, projecting, prominent, striking; abrupt, precipitous, prominent, steep.

bolster *vb* aid, assist, defend, help, maintain, prop, stay, support. • *n* cushion, pillow; prop, support.

bolt *vb* abscond, flee, fly. • *n* arrow, dart, missile, shaft; thunderbolt.

bombast *n* bluster, brag, braggadocio, fustian, gasconade, mouthing, pomposity, rant.

bond *vb* bind, connect, fuse, glue, join. • *adj* captive, enslaved, enthralled, subjugated. • *n* band, cord, fastening, ligament, ligature, link, nexus; bondage, captivity, chains, constraint, fetters, prison, shackle; attachment, attraction, connection, coupling, link, tie, union; compact, obligation, pledge, promise.

bondage *n* captivity, confinement, enslavement, enthralment, peonage, serfdom, servitude, slavery, thraldom, vassalage.

bonny *adj* beautiful, handsome, fair, fine, pretty; airy, blithe, buoyant, buxom, cheerful, jolly, joyous, merry, playful, sporty, sprightly, winsome.

bonus *n* gift, honorarium, premium, reward, subsidy.

booby *n* blockhead, dunce, fool, idiot, simpleton.

book *vb* bespeak, engage, reserve; programme, schedule; list, log, record, register. • *n* booklet, brochure, compendium, handbook, manual, monograph, pamphlet, textbook, tract, treatise, volume, work.

bookish *adj* erudite, learned, literary, scholarly, studious.

boon *adj* convivial, jolly, jovial, hearty; close, intimate. • *n* benefaction, favour, grant, gift, present; advantage, benefit, blessing, good, privilege.

boor *n* bumpkin, clodhopper, clown, lout, lubber, peasant, rustic, swain.

boorish *adj* awkward, bearish, clownish, course, gruff, ill-bred, loutish, lubberly, rude, rustic, uncivilized, uncouth, uneducated.

bootless *adj* abortive, fruitless, futile, profitless, vain, worthless, useless.

booty *n* loot, pillage, plunder, spoil.

border *vb* bound, edge, fringe, line, march, rim, skirt, verge; abut, adjoin, butt, conjoin, connect, neighbour. • *n* brim, brink, edge, fringe, hem, margin, rim, skirt, verge; boundary, confine, frontier, limit, march, outskirts.

bore[1] *vb* annoy, fatigue, plague, tire, trouble, vex, weary, worry. • *n* bother, nuisance, pest, worry.

bore[2] *vb* drill, perforate, pierce, sink, tunnel. • *n* calibre, hole, shaft, tunnel.

borrow *vb* take and return, use temporarily; adopt, appropriate, imitate; dissemble, feign, simulate.

boss[1] *vb* emboss, stud. • *n* knob, protuberance, stud.

boss[2] *vb* command, direct, employ, run. • *n* employer, foreman, master, overseer, superintendent.

botch *vb* blunder, bungle, cobble, mar, mend, mess, patch, spoil. • *n* blotch, pustule, sore; failure, miscarriage.

bother *vb* annoy, disturb, harass, molest, perplex, pester, plague, tease, trouble, vex, worry. • *n* annoyance, perplexity, plague, trouble, vexation.

bottom *vb* build, establish, found. • *adj* base, basic, ground, lowermost, lowest, nethermost, undermost. • *n* base, basis, foot, foundation, groundwork; dale, meadow, valley; buttocks, fundament, seat; dregs, grounds, lees, sediment.

bounce *vb* bound, jump, leap, rebound, recoil, spring. • *n* knock, thump; bound, jump, leap, spring, vault.

bound[1] *adj* assured, certain, decided, determined, resolute, resolved; confined, hampered, restricted, restrained; committed, contracted, engaged, pledged, promised; beholden, duty-bound, obligated, obliged.

bound[2] *vb* border, delimit, circumscribe, confine, demarcate, limit, restrict, terminate. • *n* boundary, confine, edge, limit, march, margin, periphery, term, verge.

bound[3] *vb* jump, leap, spring. • *n* bounce, jump, leap, spring, vault.

boundary *n* border, bourn, circuit, circumference, confine, limit, march, periphery, term, verge.

boundless *adj* endless, immeasurable, infinite, limitless, unbounded, unconfined, undefined, unlimited, vast.

bountiful *adj* beneficent, bounteous, generous, liberal, munificent, princely.

bounty *n* beneficence, benevolence, charity, donation, generosity, gift, kindness, premium, present, reward.

bourn *n* border, boundary, confine, limit; brook, burn, rill, rivulet, stream, torrent.

bow[1] *n* (*naut*) beak, prow, stem.

bow[2] *vb* arc, bend, buckle, crook, curve, droop, flex, yield; crush, depress, subdue; curtsy, genuflect, kowtow, submit. • *n* arc, bend, bilge, bulge, convex, curve, flexion; bob, curtsy, genuflection, greeting, homage, obeisance; coming out, debut, introduction; curtain call, encore.

bowels *npl* entrails, guts, insides, viscera; compassion, mercy, pity, sympathy, tenderness.

box[1] *vb* fight, hit, mill, spar. • *n* blow, buffet, fight, hit, spar.

box[2] *vb* barrel, case, pack, parcel. • *n* case, chest, container, crate, portmanteau, trunk.

boy *n* lad, stripling, youth.

brace *vb* make tight, tighten; buttress, fortify, reinforce, shore, strengthen, support, truss. • *n* couple, pair; clamp, girder, prop, shore, stay, support, tie, truss.

brag *vb* bluster, boast, flourish, gasconade, vaunt.

branch *vb* diverge, fork, bifurcate, ramify, spread. • *n* bough, offset, limb, shoot, sprig, twig; arm, fork, ramification, spur; article, department, member, part, portion, section, subdivision.

brand *vb* denounce, stigmatize, mark. • *n* firebrand, torch; bolt, lightning flash; cachet, mark, stamp, tally; blot, reproach, stain, stigma.

brave *vb* dare, defy. • *adj* bold, courageous, fearless, heroic, intrepid, stalwart.

bravery *n* courage, daring, fearlessness, gallantry, valour.

brawl *vb* bicker, dispute, jangle, quarrel, squabble. • *n* broil, dispute, feud, fracas, fray, jangle, quarrel, row, scuffle, squabble, uproar, wrangle.

brawny *adj* athletic, lusty, muscular, powerful, robust, sinewy, stalwart, strapping, strong, sturdy.

bray *vb* clamour, hoot, roar, trumpet, vociferate. • *n* blare, crash, roar, shout.

breach *n* break, chasm, crack, disruption, fissure, flaw, fracture, opening, rent, rift, rupture; alienation, difference, disaffection, disagreement, split.

bread *n* aliment, diet, fare, food, nourishment, nutriment, provisions, regimen, victuals.

break *vb* crack, disrupt, fracture, part, rend, rive, sever; batter, burst, crush, shatter, smash, splinter; cashier, degrade, discard, discharge, dismiss; disobey, infringe, transgress, violate; intermit, interrupt, stop; disclose, open, unfold. • *n* aperture, breach, chasm, fissure, gap, rent, rip, rupture; break-up, crash, debacle.

breast *vb* face, oppose, resist, stem, withstand. • *n* bosom, chest, thorax; affections, conscience, heart; mammary gland, mammary organ, pap, udder.

breath *n* exhaling, inhaling, pant, sigh, respiration, whiff; animation, existence, life; pause, respite, rest; breathing space, instant, moment.

breathe *vb* live, exist; emit, exhale, give out; diffuse, express, indicate, manifest, show.

breed *vb* bear, beget, engender, hatch, produce; bring up, foster, nourish, nurture, raise, rear; discipline, educate, instruct, nurture, rear, school, teach, train; generate, originate. • *n* extraction, family, lineage, pedigree, progeny, race, strain.

brevity *n* briefness, compression, conciseness, curtness, pithiness, shortness, terseness, transiency.

brew *vb* concoct, contrive, devise, excite, foment, instigate, plot. • *n* beverage, concoction, drink, liquor, mixture, potation.

bribe *vb* buy, corrupt, influence, pay off, suborn. • *n* allurement, corruption, enticement, graft, pay-off, subornation.

bridle *vb* check, curb, control, govern, restrain. • *n* check, control, curb.

brief *vb* direct, give directions, instruct; capsulate, summarize, delineate, describe, draft, outline, sketch; (*law*) retain. • *adj* concise, curt, inconsiderable, laconic, pithy, short, succinct, terse; fleeting, momentary, short, temporary, transient. • *n* abstract, breviary, briefing, epitome, compendium, summary, syllabus; (*law*) precept, writ.

brigand *n* bandit, footpad, freebooter, gangster, highwayman, marauder, outlaw, robber, thug.

bright *adj* blazing, brilliant, dazzling, gleaming, glowing, light, luminous, radiant, shining, sparkling, sunny; clear, cloudless, lambent, lucid, transparent; famous, glorious, illustrious; acute, discerning, ingenious, intelligent, keen; auspicious, cheering, encouraging, exhilarating, favourable, inspiring, promising, propitious; cheerful, genial, happy, lively, merry, pleasant, smiling, vivacious.

brilliant *adj* beaming, bright, effulgent, gleaming, glistening, glittering, lustrous, radiant, resplendent, shining, sparkling splendid; admirable, celebrated, distinguished, famous, glorious, illustrious, renowned; dazzling, decided, prominent, signal, striking, unusual.

brim *n* border, brink, edge, rim, margin, skirt, verge; bank, border, coast, margin, shore.

bring *vb* bear, convey, fetch; accompany, attend, conduct, convey, convoy, guide, lead; gain, get, obtain, procure, produce.

brisk *adj* active, alert, agile, lively, nimble, perky, quick, smart, spirited, spry.

brittle *adj* brash, breakable, crisp, crumbling, fragile, frangible, frail, shivery.

broach *vb* open, pierce, set; approach, break, hint, suggest; proclaim, publish, utter.

broad *adj* ample, expansive, extensive, large, spacious, sweeping, vast, wide; enlarged, hospitable, liberal, tolerant; diffused, open, spread; coarse, gross, indecent, indelicate, unrefined, vulgar.

broaden *vb* augment, enlarge, expand, extend, increase, spread, stretch, widen.

broken *adj* fractured, rent, ruptured, separated, severed, shattered, shivered, torn; exhausted, feeble, impaired, shaken, shattered, spent, wasted; defective, halting, hesitating, imperfect, stammering, stumbling; contrite, humble, lowly, penitent; abrupt, craggy, precipitous, rough.

broker *n* agent, factor, go-between, middleman.

brood *vb* incubate, sit. • *n* issue, offspring, progeny; breed, kind, line, lineage, sort, strain.

brook *vb* abide, bear, endure, suffer, tolerate. • *n* burn, beck, creek, rill, rivulet, run, streamlet.

brotherhood *n* association, clan, clique, coterie, fraternity, junta, society.

brotherly *adj* affectionate, amicable, cordial, friendly, kind.

browbeat *vb* bully, intimidate, overawe, overbear.

bruise *vb* contuse, crunch, squeeze; batter, break, maul, pound, pulverize; batter, deface, indent. • *n* blemish, contusion, swelling.

brush¹ *n* brushwood, bush, scrub, scrubwood, shrubs, thicket, wilderness.

brush² *vb* buff, clean, polish, swab, sweep, wipe; curry, groom, rub down; caress, flick, glance, graze, scrape, skim, touch. • *n* besom, broom; action, affair, collision, contest, conflict, encounter, engagement, fight, skirmish.

brutal *adj* barbaric, barbarous, brutish, cruel, ferocious, inhuman, ruthless, savage; bearish, brusque, churlish, gruff, impolite, harsh, rude, rough, truculent, uncivil.

brute *n* barbarian, beast, monster, ogre, savage; animal, beast, creature. • *adj* carnal, mindless, physical; bestial, coarse, gross.

bubble *vb* boil, effervesce, foam. • *n* bead, blob, fluid, globule; bagatelle, trifle; cheat, delusion, hoax.

buccaneer *n* corsair, freebooter, pirate.

buck *vb* jump, leap. • *n* beau, blade, blood, dandy, fop, gallant, spark; male.

bud *vb* burgeon, germinate, push, shoot, sprout, vegetate. • *n* burgeon, gem, germ, gemmule, shoot, sprout.

budget *vb* allocate, cost, estimate. • *n* account, estimate, financial statement; assets, finances, funds, means, resources; bag, bundle, pack, packet, parcel, roll; assortment, batch, collection, lot, set, store.

buffet¹ *vb* beat, box, cuff, slap, smite, strike; resist, struggle against. • *n* blow, box, cuff, slap, strike;

buffet² *n* cupboard, sideboard; refreshment counter.

buffoon *n* antic, clown, droll, fool, harlequin, jester, mountebank.

build *vb* construct, erect, establish, fabricate, fashion, model, raise, rear. • *n* body, figure, form, frame, physique; construction, shape, structure.

building *n* construction, erection, fabrication; edifice, fabric, house, pile, substructure, structure.

bulk *n* dimension, magnitude, mass, size, volume; amplitude, bulkiness, massiveness; body, majority, mass.

bully *vb* browbeat, bulldoze, domineer, haze, hector, intimidate, overbear. • *n* blusterer, browbeater, bulldozer, hector, swaggerer, roisterer, tyrant.

bulwark *n* barrier, fortification, parapet, rampart, wall; palladium, safeguard, security.

bump *vb* collide, knock, strike, thump. • *n* blow, jar, jolt, knock, shock, thump; lump, protuberance, swelling.

bunch *vb* assemble, collect, crowd, group, herd, pack. • *n* bulge, bump, bundle, hump, knob, lump, protuberance; cluster, hand, fascicle; assortment, batch, collection, group, lot, parcel, set; knot, tuft.

bundle *vb* bale, pack, package, parcel, truss, wrap. • *n* bale, batch, bunch, collection, heap, pack, package, packet, parcel, pile, roll, truss.

bungler *n* botcher, duffer, fumbler, lout, lubber, mis-manager, muddler.

burden *vb* encumber, grieve, load, oppress, overlay, overload, saddle, surcharge, try. • *n* capacity, cargo, freight, lading, load, tonnage, weight; affliction, charge, clog, encumbrance, impediment, grievance, sorrow, trial, trouble; drift, point, substance, tenor, surcharge.

bureau *n* chest of drawers, dresser; counting room, office.

burial *n* burying, entombment, inhumation, interment, sepulture.

burlesque *vb* ape, imitate, lampoon, mock, ridicule, satirize. • *n* caricature, extravaganza, parody, send-up, take-off, travesty.

burn¹ *n* beck, brook, gill, rill, rivulet, runnel, runlet, stream water.

burn² *vb* blaze, conflagrate, enflame, fire, flame, ignite, kindle, light, smoulder; cremate, incinerate; scald, scorch, singe; boil, broil, cook, roast, seethe, simmer, stew, swelter, toast; bronze, brown, sunburn, suntan, tan; bake, desiccate, dry, parch, sear, shrivel, wither; glow, incandesce, tingle, warm. • n scald, scorch, singe; sunburn.

burning adj aflame, fiery, hot, scorching; ardent, earnest, fervent, fervid, impassioned, intense.

burnish vb brighten, buff, furbish, polish, shine. • n glaze, gloss, patina, polish, shine.

burst vb break open, be rent, explode, shatter, split open. • adj broken, kaput, punctured, ruptured, shattered, split. • n break, breakage, breach, fracture, rupture; blast, blowout, blowup, discharge, detonation, explosion; spurt; blaze, flare, flash; cloudburst, downpour; bang, crack, crash, report, sound; fusillade, salvo, spray, volley, outburst, outbreak flare-up, blaze, eruption.

bury vb entomb, inearth, inhume, inter; conceal, hide, secrete, shroud.

business n calling, employment, occupation, profession, pursuit, vocation; commerce, dealing, trade, traffic; affair, concern, engagement, matter, transaction, undertaking; duty, function, office, task, work.

bustle vb fuss, hurry, scurry. • n ado, commotion, flurry, fuss, hurry, hustle, pother, stir, tumult.

busy vb devote, employ, engage, occupy, spend, work. • adj employed, engaged, occupied; active, assiduous, diligent, engrossed, industrious, sedulous, working; agile, brisk, nimble, spry, stirring; meddling, officious.

but conj except, excepting, further, howbeit, moreover, still, unless, yet. • adv all the same, even, notwithstanding, still, yet.

butchery n massacre, murder, slaughter.

butt[1] vb bunt, push, shove, shunt, strike; encroach, impose, interfere, intrude, invade, obtrude. • n buck, bunt, push, shove, shunt, thrust.

butt[2] n barrel, cask.

butt[3] n aim, goal, mark, object, point, target; dupe, gull, victim.

butt[4] vb abut, adjoin, conjoin, connect, neighbour. • n end, piece, remainder, stub, stump; buttocks, posterior, rump.

buttonhole vb bore, catch, detain in conversation, importune.

buttress vb brace, prop, shore, stay, support. • n brace, bulwark, prop, stay, support.

buxom adj comely, fresh, healthy, hearty, plump, rosy, ruddy, vigorous.

byword n adage, aphorism, apothegm, dictum, maxim, proverb, saying, saw.

C

cabal *vb* conspire, intrigue, machinate, plot. • *n* clique, combination, confederacy, coterie, faction, gang, junta, league, party, set; conspiracy, intrigue, machination, plot.

cabbalistic, cabalistic *adj* dark, fanciful, mysterious, mystic, occult, secret.

cabaret *n* tavern, inn, public house, wine shop.

cabin *n* berth, bunk, cot, cottage, crib, dwelling, hovel, hut, shack, shanty, shed.

cabinet *n* apartment, boudoir, chamber, closet; case, davenport, desk, escritoire; council, ministry.

cachinnation *n* guffaw, laugh, laughter.

cackle *vb* giggle, laugh, snicker, titter; babble, chatter, gabble, palaver, prate, prattle, titter. • *n* babble, chatter, giggle, prate, prattle, snigger, titter.

cacophonous *adj* discordant, grating, harsh, inharmonious, jarring, raucous.

cadaverous *adj* bloodless, deathlike, ghastly, pale, pallid, wan.

cage *vb* confine, immure, imprison, incarcerate. • *n* coop, pen, pound.

caitiff *adj* base, craven, pusillanimous, rascally, recreant. • *n* coward, knave, miscreant, rascal, rogue, scoundrel, sneak, traitor, vagabond, villain, wretch.

cajole *vb* blandish, coax, flatter, jolly, wheedle; beguile, deceive, delude, entrap, inveigle, tempt.

calamity *n* adversity, affliction, blow, casualty, cataclysm, catastrophe, disaster, distress, downfall, evil, hardship, mischance, misery, misfortune, mishap, reverse, ruin, stroke, trial, visitation.

calculate *vb* cast, compute, count, estimate, figure, rate, reckon, weigh; tell.

calculating *adj* crafty, designing, scheming, selfish; careful, cautious, circumspect, far-sighted, politic, sagacious, wary.

calefaction *n* heating, warming; hotness, incandescence, warmth.

calendar *n* almanac, ephemeris, register; catalogue, list, schedule.

calibre *n* bore, capacity, diameter, gauge; ability, capacity, endowment, faculty, gifts, parts, scope, talent.

call *vb* christen, denominate, designate, dub, entitle, name, phrase, style, term; bid, invite, summons; assemble, convene, convoke, muster; cry, exclaim; arouse, awaken, proclaim, rouse, shout, waken; appoint, elect, ordain. • *n* cry, outcry, voice; appeal, invitation, summons; claim, demand, summons; appointment, election, invitation.

calling *n* business, craft, employment, occupation, profession, pursuit, trade.

callous *adj* hard, hardened, indurated; apathetic, dull, indifferent, insensible, inured, obdurate, obtuse, sluggish, torpid, unfeeling, unsusceptible.

callow *adj* naked, unfeathered, unfledged; green, immature, inexperienced, sappy, silly, soft, unfledged, unsophisticated.

calm *vb* allay, becalm, compose, hush, lull, smooth, still, tranquillize; alleviate, appease, assuage, moderate, mollify, pacify, quiet, soften, soothe, tranquillize. • *adj* halcyon, mild, peaceful, placid, quiet, reposeful, serene, smooth, still, tranquil, unruffled; collected, cool, composed, controlled, impassive, imperturbable, sedate, self-possessed, undisturbed, unperturbed, unruffled, untroubled. • *n* lull; equanimity, peace, placidity, quiet, repose, serenity, stillness, tranquillity.

calorific *adj* heat, heat-producing.

calumniate *vb* abuse, asperse, backbite, blacken, blemish, defame, discredit, disparage, lampoon, libel, malign, revile, slander, traduce, vilify.

calumny *n* abuses, aspersion, backbiting, defamation, detraction, evil-speaking, insult, libel, lying, obloquy, slander, vilification, vituperation.

camarilla *n* cabal, clique, junta, ring.

camber *vb* arch, bend, curve. • *n* arch, arching, convexity.

camp¹ *vb* bivouac, encamp, lodge, pitch, tent. • *n* bivouac, cantonment, encampment, laager; cabal, circle, clique, coterie, faction, group, junta, party, ring, set.

camp² *adj* affected, artificial, effeminate, exaggerated, mannered, theatrical.

canaille *n* mob, populace, proletariat, rabble, ragbag, riffraff, scum.

canal *n* channel, duct, pipe, tube.

cancel *vb* blot, efface, erase, expunge, obliterate; abrogate, annul, countermand, nullify, quash, repeal, rescind, revoke.

candelabrum *n* candlestick, chandelier, lustre.

candid *adj* fair, impartial, just, unbiased, unprejudiced; artless, frank, free, guileless, honest, honourable, ingenuous, naive, open, plain, sincere, straightforward.

candidate *n* applicant, aspirant, claimant, competitor, probationer.

candour *n* fairness, impartiality, justice; artlessness, frankness, guilelessness, honesty, ingenuousness, openness, simplicity, sincerity, straightforwardness, truthfulness.

canker *vb* corrode, erode, rot, rust, waste; blight, consume, corrupt, embitter, envenom, infect, poison, sour. • *n* gangrene, rot; bale, bane, blight, corruption, infection, irritation.

canon *n* catalogue, criterion, formula, formulary, law, regulation, rule, standard, statute.

canorous *adj* musical, tuneful.

cant¹ *vb* whine. • *adj* current, partisan, popular, rote, routine, set; argotic, slangy. • *n* hypocrisy; argot, jargon, lingo, slang.

cant² *vb* bevel, incline, list, slant, tilt, turn. • *n* bevel, inclination, leaning, list, pitch, slant, tilt, turn.

cantankerous *adj* contumacious, crabbed, cross-grained, dogged, headstrong, heady, intractable, obdurate, obstinate, perverse, refractory, stiff, stubborn, wilful, unyielding.

canting *adj* affected, pious, sanctimonious, whining.

canvas *n* burlap, scrim, tarpaulin.

canvass *vb* discuss, dispute; analyze, consider, examine, investigate, review, scrutinize, sift, study; campaign, electioneer, solicit votes. • *n* debate, discussion, dispute; examination, scrutiny, sifting.

canyon *n* gorge, gulch, ravine.

cap *vb* cover, surmount; complete, crown, finish; exceed, overtop, surpass, transcend; match, parallel, pattern. • *n* beret, headcover, head-dress; acme, chief, crown, head, peak, perfection, pitch, summit, top.

capability *n* ability, brains, calibre, capableness, capacity, competency, efficiency, faculty, force, power, scope, skill.

capable *adj* adapted, fitted, qualified, suited; able, accomplished, clever, competent, efficient, gifted, ingenious, intelligent, sagacious, skilful.

capacious *adj* ample, broad, comprehensive, expanded, extensive, large, roomy, spacious, wide.

capacitate *vb* enable, qualify.

capacity *n* amplitude, dimensions, magnitude, volume; aptitude, aptness, brains, calibre, discernment, faculty, forte, genius, gift, parts, power, talent, turn, wit; ability, capability, calibre, cleverness, competency, efficiency, skill; character, charge, function, office, position, post, province, service, sphere.

caparison *vb* accoutre, costume, equip, outfit, rig out. • *n* accoutrements, armour, get-up, harness, housing, livery, outfit, panoply, tack, tackle, trappings, turnout.

caper *vb* bound, caracole, frisk, gambol, hop, leap, prank, romp, skip, spring. • *n* bound, dance, gambol, frisk, hop, jump, leap, prance, romp, skip.

capillary *adj* delicate, fine, minute, slender.

capital *adj* cardinal, chief, essential, important, leading, main, major, pre-eminent, principal, prominent; fatal; excellent, first-class, first-rate, good, prime, splendid. • *n* chief city, metropolis, seat; money, estate, investments, shares, stock.

caprice *n* crotchet, fancy, fickleness, freak, humour, inconstancy, maggot, phantasy, quirk, vagary, whim, whimsy.

capricious *adj* changeable, crotchety, fanciful, fantastical, fickle, fitful, freakish, humoursome, odd, puckish, queer, uncertain, variable, wayward, whimsical.

capsize *vb* overturn, upset.

capsule *n* case, covering, envelope, sheath, shell, wrapper: pericarp, pod, seed-vessel.

captain *vb* command, direct, head, lead, manage, officer, preside. • *n* chief, chieftain, commander, leader, master, officer, soldier, warrior.

captious *adj* carping, caviling, censorious, critical, fault-finding, hypercritical; acrimonious, cantankerous, contentious, crabbed, cross, snappish, snarling, splenetic, testy, touchy, waspish; ensnaring, insidious.

captivate *vb* allure, attract, bewitch, catch, capture, charm, enamour, enchant, enthral, fascinate, gain, hypnotize, infatuate, win.

captivity *n* confinement, durance, duress, imprisonment; bondage, enthralment, servitude, slavery, subjection, thraldom, vassalage.

capture *vb* apprehend, arrest, catch, seize. • *n* apprehension, arrest, catch, catching, imprisonment, seizure; bag, prize.

carcass *n* body, cadaver, corpse, corse, remains.

cardinal *adj* capital, central, chief, essential, first, important, leading, main, pre-eminent, primary, principal, vital.

care *n* anxiety, concern, perplexity, trouble, solicitude, worry; attention, carefulness, caution, circumspection, heed, regard, vigilance, wariness, watchfulness; charge, custody, guardianship, keep, oversight, superintendence, ward; burden, charge, concern, responsibility.

careful *adj* anxious, solicitous, concerned, troubled, uneasy; attentive, heedful, mindful, regardful, thoughtful; cautious, canny, circumspect, discreet, leery, vigilant, watchful.

careless *adj* carefree, nonchalant, unapprehensive, undisturbed, unperplexed, unsolicitous, untroubled; disregardful heedless, inattentive, incautious, inconsiderate, neglectful, negligent, regardless, remiss, thoughtless, unobservant, unconcerned, unconsidered, unmindful, unthinking.

carelessness *n* heedlessness, inadvertence, inattention, inconsiderateness, neglect, negligence, remissness, slackness, thoughtlessness, unconcern.

caress *vb* coddle, cuddle, cosset, embrace, fondle, hug, kiss, pet. • *n* cuddle, embrace, fondling, hug, kiss.

caressing *n* blandishment, dalliance, endearment, fondling.

cargo *n* freight, lading, load.

caricature *vb* burlesque, parody, send-up, take-off, travesty. • *n* burlesque, farce, ludicrous, parody, representation, take-off, travesty.

carious *adj* decayed, mortified, putrid, rotten, ulcerated.

cark *vb* annoy, fret, grieve, harass, perplex, worry.

carnage *n* bloodshed, butchery, havoc, massacre murder, slaughter.

carnal *adj* animal, concupiscent, fleshly, lascivious, lecherous, lewd, libidinous, lubricous, lustful, salacious, sensual, voluptuous; bodily, earthy, mundane. natural, secular, temporal, unregenerate, unspiritual.

carol *vb* chant, hum, sing, warble. • *n* canticle, chorus, ditty, hymn, lay, song, warble.

carousal *n* banquet, entertainment, feast, festival, merry-making, regale; bacchanal, carouse, debauch, jamboree, jollification, orgy, revel, revelling, revelry, saturnalia, spree, wassail.

carp *vb* cavil, censure, criticize, fault.

carping *adj* captious, cavilling, censorious, hypercritical. • *n* cavil, censure, fault-finding, hypercriticism.

carriage *n* conveyance, vehicle; air, bearing, behaviour, conduct, demeanour, deportment, front, mien, port.

carry *vb* bear, convey, transfer, transmit, transport; impel, push forward, urge; accomplish, compass, effect, gain, secure; bear up, support, sustain; infer, involve, imply, import, signify.

cart *n* conveyance, tumbril, van, vehicle, wagon.

carte-blanche *n* authority, power.

carve *vb* chisel, cut, divide, engrave, grave, hack, hew, indent, incise, sculpt, sculpture; fashion, form, mould, shape.

cascade *vb* cataract, descend, drop, engulf, fall, inundate, overflow, plunge, tumble. • *n* cataract, fall, falls, force, linn, waterfall.

case¹ *vb* cover, encase, enclose, envelop, protect, wrap; box, pack. • *n* capsule, covering, sheathe; box, cabinet, container, holder, receptacle.

case² *n* condition, plight, predicament, situation, state; example, instance, occurrence; circumstance, condition, contingency; event; action, argument, cause, lawsuit, process, suit, trial.

case-hardened *adj* hardened, indurated, steeled brazen, brazen-faced, obdurate, reprobate.

cash *n* banknotes, bullion, coin, currency, money, payment, specie.

cashier *vb* break, discard, discharge, dismiss.

cast *vb* fling, hurl, pitch, send, shy, sling, throw, toss; drive, force, impel, thrust; lay aside, put off, shed; calculate, compute, reckon; communicate diffuse, impart, shed, throw. • *n* fling, throw, toss; shade, tinge, tint, touch; air, character, look, manner, mien, style, tone, turn; form, mould.

castaway *adj* abandoned, cast-off, discarded, rejected. • *n* derelict, outcast, reprobate, vagabond.

caste *n* class, grade, lineage, order, race, rank, species, status.

castigate *vb* beat, chastise, flog, lambaste, lash, thrash, whip; chaste, correct, discipline, punish; criticize, flagellate, upbraid.

castle *n* citadel, fortress, stronghold.

castrate *vb* caponize, emasculate, geld; mortify, subdue, suppress, weaken.

casual *adj* accidental, contingent, fortuitous, incidental, irregular, occasional, random, uncertain, unforeseen, unintentional, unpremeditated; informal, relaxed.

casualty *n* chance, contingency, fortuity, mishap, accident, catastrophe, disaster, mischance, misfortune.

cat *n* grimalkin, kitten, puss, tabby, tomcat.

cataclysm *n* deluge, flood, inundation; disaster, upheaval.

catacomb *n* crypt, tomb, vault.

catalogue *vb* alphabetize, categorize, chronicle, class, classify, codify, file, index, list, record, tabulate. • *n* enumeration, index, inventory, invoice, list, record, register, roll, schedule.

cataract *n* cascade, fall, waterfall.

catastrophe *n* conclusion, consummation, denouement, end, finale, issue, termination, upshot; adversity, blow, calamity, cataclysm, debacle, disaster, ill, misfortune, mischance, mishap, trial, trouble.

catch *vb* clutch, grasp, gripe, nab, seize, snatch; apprehend, arrest, capture; overtake; enmesh, ensnare, entangle, entrap, lime, net; bewitch, captivate, charm, enchant, fascinate, win; surprise, take unawares. • *n* arrest, capture, seizure; bag, find, haul, plum, prize; drawback, fault, hitch, obstacle, rub, snag; captive, conquest.

catching *adj* communicable, contagious, infectious, pestiferous, pestilential; attractive, captivating, charming, enchanting, fascinating, taking, winning, winsome.

catechize *adj* examine, interrogate, question, quiz.

catechumen *n* convert, disciple, learner, neophyte, novice, proselyte, pupil, tyro.

categorical *adj* absolute, direct, downright, emphatic, explicit, express, positive, unconditional, unqualified, unreserved, utter.

category *n* class, division, head, heading, list, order, rank, sort.

catenation *n* conjunction, connection, union.

cater *vb* feed, provide, purvey.

cathartic *adj* abstergent. aperient, cleansing, evacuant, laxative, purgative. • *n* aperient, laxative, physic, purgative, purge.

catholic *adj* general, universal, world-wide; charitable, liberal, tolerant, unbigoted, unexclusive, unsectarian.

cause *vb* breed, create, originate, produce; effect, effectuate, occasion, produce. • *n* agent, creator, mainspring, origin, original, producer, source, spring; account, agency, consideration, ground, incentive, incitement, inducement, motive, reason; aim, end, object, purpose; action, case, suit, trial.

caustic *adj* acrid, cathartic, consuming, corroding, corrosive, eating, erosive, mordant, virulent; biting, bitter, burning, cutting, sarcastic, satirical, scathing, severe, sharp, stinging.

caution *vb* admonish, forewarn, warn. • *n* care, carefulness, circumspection, discretion, forethought, heed, heedfulness, providence, prudence, wariness, vigilance, watchfulness; admonition, advice, counsel, injunction, warning.

cautious *adj* careful, chary, circumspect, discreet, heedful, prudent, wary, vigilant, wary, watchful.

cavalier *adj* arrogant, curt, disdainful, haughty, insolent, scornful, supercilious; debonair, gallant, gay. • *n* chevalier, equestrian, horseman, horse-soldier, knight.

cave *n* cavern, cavity, den grot, grotto.

cavil *vb* carp, censure, hypercriticize, object.

cavilling *adj* captious, carping, censorious, critical, hypercritical.

cavity *n* hollow, pocket, vacuole, void.

cease *vb* desist, intermit, pause, refrain, stay, stop; fail; discontinue, end, quit, terminate.

ceaseless *adj* continual, continuous, incessant, unceasing, unintermitting, uninterrupted, unremitting; endless, eternal, everlasting, perpetual.

cede *vb* abandon, abdicate, relinquish, resign, surrender, transfer, yield; convey, grant.

celebrate *vb* applaud, bless, commend, emblazon, extol, glorify, laud, magnify, praise, trumpet; commemorate, honour, keep, observe; solemnize.

celebrated *adj* distinguished, eminent, famed, famous, glorious, illustrious, notable, renowned.

celebrity *n* credit, distinction, eminence, fame, glory, honour, renown, reputation, repute; lion, notable, star.

celerity *n* fleetness, haste, quickness, rapidity, speed, swiftness, velocity.

celestial *adj* empyreal, empyrean; angelic, divine, god-like, heavenly, seraphic, supernal, supernatural.

celibate *adj* single, unmarried. • *n* bachelor, single, virgin.

cellular *adj* alveolate, honeycombed.

cement *vb* attach, bind, join, combine, connect, solder, unite, weld; cohere, stick. • *n* glue, paste, mortar, solder.

cemetery *n* burial-ground, burying-ground, churchyard, god's acre, graveyard, necropolis.

censor *vb* blue-pencil, bowdlerize, cut, edit, expurgate; classify, kill, quash, squash, suppress. • *n* caviller, censurer, faultfinder.

censorious *adj* captious, carping, caviling, condemnatory, faultfinding, hypercritical, severe.

censure *vb* abuse, blame, chide, condemn, rebuke, reprehend, reprimand, reproach, reprobate, reprove, scold, upbraid. • *n* animadversion, blame, condemnation, criticism, disapprobation, disapproval, rebuke, remonstrance, reprehension, reproach, reproof, stricture.

ceremonious *adj* civil, courtly, lofty, stately; formal, studied; exact, formal, punctilious, precise, starched, stiff.

ceremony *n* ceremonial, etiquette, form, formality, observance, solemnity, rite; parade, pomp, show, stateliness.

certain *adj* absolute, incontestable, incontrovertible, indisputable, indubitable, positive, undeniable, undisputed, unquestionable, unquestioned; assured, confident, sure, undoubting; infallible, never-failing, unfailing; actual, existing, real; constant, determinate, fixed, settled, stated.

certainty *n* indubitability, indubitableness, inevitableness, inevitability, surety, unquestionability, unquestionableness; assurance, assuredness, certitude, confidence, conviction, surety.

certify *vb* attest, notify, testify, vouch; ascertain, determine, verify, show.

cerulean *adj* azure, blue, sky-blue.

cessation *n* ceasing, discontinuance, intermission, pause, remission, respite, rest, stop, stoppage, suspension.

cession *n* abandonment, capitulation, ceding, concession, conveyance, grant, relinquishement, renunciation, surrender, yielding.

chafe *vb* rub; anger, annoy, chagrin, enrage, exasperate, fret, gall, incense, irritate, nettle, offend, provoke, ruffle, tease, vex; fret, fume, rage.

chaff *vb* banter, deride, jeer, mock, rally, ridicule. scoff. • *n* glumes, hulls, husks; refuse, rubbish, trash, waste.

chaffer *n* bargain, haggle, higgle, negotiate.

chagrin *vb* annoy, chafe, displease, irritate, mortify, provoke, vex. • *n* annoyance, displeasure, disquiet, dissatisfaction, fretfulness, humiliation, ill-humour, irritation, mortification, spleen, vexation.

chain *vb* bind, confine, fetter, manacle, restrain, shackle, trammel; enslave. • *n* bond, fetter, manacle, shackle, union.

chalice *n* bowl, cup, goblet.

challenge *vb* brave, call out, dare, defy, dispute; demand, require. • *n* defiance, interrogation, question; exception, objection.

chamber *n* apartment, hall, room; cavity, hollow.

champion *vb* advocate, defend, uphold. • *n* defender, promoter, protector, vindicator; belt-holder, hero, victor, warrior, winner.

chance *vb* befall, betide, happen, occur. • *adj* accidental, adventitious, casual, fortuitous, incidental, unexpected, unforeseen. • *n* accident, cast, fortuity, fortune, hap, luck; contingency, possibility; occasion, opening, opportunity; contingency, fortuity, gamble, peradventure, uncertainty; hazard, jeopardy, peril, risk.

change *vb* alter, fluctuate, modify, vary; displace, remove, replace, shift, substitute; barter, commute, exchange. • *n* alteration, mutation, revolution, transition, transmutation, turning, variance, variation; innovation, novelty, variety, vicissitude.

changeable *adj* alterable, inconstant, modifiable, mutable, uncertain, unsettled, unstable, unsteadfast, unsteady, variable,

variant; capricious, fickle, fitful, flighty, giddy, mercurial, vacillating, volatile, wavering.

changeless *adj* abiding, consistent, constant, fixed, immutable, permanent, regular, reliable, resolute, settled, stationary, unalterable, unchanging.

channel *vb* chamfer, cut, flute, groove. • *n* canal, conduit, duct, passage; aqueduct, canal, chute, drain, flume, furrow; chamfer, groove, fluting, furrow, gutter.

chant *vb* carol, sing, warble; intone, recite; canticle, song.

chaos *n* anarchy, confusion, disorder.

chapfallen *adj* blue, crest-fallen, dejected, depressed, despondent, discouraged, disheartened, dispirited, downcast, downhearted, low-spirited, melancholy, sad.

chaplet *n* coronal, garland, wreath.

char *vb* burn, scorch.

character *n* emblem, figure, hieroglyph, ideograph, letter, mark, sign, symbol; bent, constitution, cast, disposition, nature, quality; individual, original, person, personage; reputation, repute; nature, traits; eccentric, trait.

characteristic *adj* distinctive, peculiar, singular, special, specific, typical. • *n* attribute, feature, idiosyncrasy, lineament, mark, peculiarity, quality, trait.

charge *vb* burden, encumber, freight, lade, load; entrust; ascribe, impute, lay; accuse, arraign, blame, criminate, impeach, inculpate, indict, involve; bid, command, exhort, enjoin, order, require, tax; assault, attack bear down. • *n* burden, cargo, freight, lading, load; care, custody, keeping, management, ward; commission, duty, employment, office, trust; responsibility, trust; command, direction, injunction, mandate, order, precept; exhortation, instruction; cost, debit, expense, expenditure, outlay; price, sum; assault, attack, encounter, onset, onslaught.

charger *n* dish, platter; mount, steed, war-horse.

charily *adv* carefully, cautiously, distrustfully, prudently, sparingly, suspiciously, warily.

charitable *adj* beneficial, beneficent, benignant, bountiful, generous, kind, liberal, open-handed; candid, considerate, lenient, mild.

charity *n* benevolence, benignity, fellow-feeling, good-nature, goodwill, kind-heartedness, kindness, tenderheartedness; beneficence, bounty, generosity, humanity, philanthropy. liberality.

charlatan *n* cheat, empiric, impostor, mountebank, pretender, quack.

charm *vb* allure, attract, becharm, bewitch, captivate, catch, delight, enamour, enchain, enchant, enrapture, enravish, fascinate, transport, win. • *n* enchantment, incantation, magic, necromancy, sorcery, spell, witchery; amulet, talisman; allurement, attraction, attractiveness, fascination.

charming *adj* bewitching, captivating, delightful, enchanting, enrapturing, fascinating, lovely.

charter *vb* incorporate; hire, let. • *n* franchise, immunity, liberty, prerogation, privilege, right; bond, deed, indenture, instrument, prerogative.

chary *adj* careful, cautious, circumspect, shy, wary; abstemious, careful, choice, economical, frugal, provident, saving, sparing, temperate, thrifty, unwasteful.

chase *vb* follow, hunt, pursue, track; emboss. • *n* course, field-sport, hunt, hunting.

chasm *n* cavity, cleft, fissure, gap, hollow, hiatus, opening.

chaste *adj* clean, continent, innocent, modest, pure, pureminded, undefiled, virtuous; chastened, pure, simple, unaffected, uncorrupt.

chasten *vb* correct, humble; purify, refine, render, subdue.

chastening *n* chastisement, correction, discipline, humbling.

chastise *vb* castigate, correct, flog, lash, punish, whip; chasten, correct, discipline, humble, punish, subdue.

chastity *n* abstinence, celibacy, continence, innocence, modesty, pure-mindedness, purity, virtue; cleanness, decency; chasteness, refinement, restrainedness, simplicity, sobriety, unaffectedness.

chat *vb* babble, chatter, confabulate, gossip, prate, prattle. • *n* chit-chat, confabulation, conversation, gossip, prattle.

chatter *vb* babble, chat, confabulate, gossip, prate, prattle. • *n* babble, chat, gabble, jabber, patter, prattle.

cheap *adj* inexpensive, low-priced; common, indifferent, inferior, mean, meretricious, paltry, poor.

cheapen *vb* belittle, depreciate.

cheat *vb* cozen, deceive, dissemble, juggle, shuffle; bamboozle, befool, beguile, cajole, circumvent, deceive, defraud, chouse, delude, dupe, ensnare, entrap, fool, gammon, gull, hoax, hoodwink, inveigle, jockey, mislead, outwit, overreach, trick. • *n* artifice, beguilement, blind, catch, chouse, deceit, deception, fraud, imposition, imposture, juggle, pitfall, snare, stratagem, swindle, trap, trick, wile; counterfeit, deception, delusion, illusion, mockery, paste, sham, tinsel; beguiler, charlatan, cheater, cozener, impostor, jockey, knave, mountebank trickster, rogue, render, sharper, seizer, shuffler, swindler, taker, tearer.

check *vb* block, bridle, control, counteract, curb, hinder, obstruct, repress, restrain; chide, rebuke, reprimand, reprove. • *n* bar, barrier, block, brake, bridle, clog, control, curb, damper, hindrance, impediment, interference, obstacle, obstruction, rebuff, repression, restraint, stop, stopper.

cheep *vb* chirp, creak, peep, pipe, squeak.

cheer *vb* animate, encourage, enliven, exhilarate gladden, incite, inspirit; comfort, console, solace; applaud, clap. • *n* cheerfulness, gaiety, gladness, glee, hilarity, jollity, joy, merriment, mirth; entertainment, food, provision, repast, viands, victuals; acclamation, hurrah, huzza.

cheerful *adj* animated, airy, blithe, buoyant, cheery, gay, glad, gleeful, happy, joyful, jocund, jolly, joyous, light-hearted, lightsome, lively, merry, mirthful, sprightly, sunny, animating, cheering, cheery, encouraging, enlivening, glad, gladdening, gladsome, grateful, inspiriting, jocund, pleasant.

cheerless *adj* dark, dejected, desolate, despondent, disconsolate, discouraged, dismal, doleful, dreary, forlorn, gloomy, joyless, low-spirited, lugubrious, melancholy, mournful, rueful, sad, sombre, spiritless, woe-begone.

cherish *vb* comfort, foster, nourish, nurse, nurture, support, sustain; treasure; encourage, entertain, indulge, harbour.

chest *n* box, case, coffer; breast, thorax, trunk.

chew *vb* crunch, manducate, masticate, munch; bite, champ, gnaw; meditate, ruminate.

chicanery *n* chicane, deception, duplicity, intrigue, intriguing, sophistication, sophistry, stratagems, tergiversation trickery, wiles, wire-pulling.

chide *vb* admonish, blame, censure, rebuke, reprimand, reprove, scold, upbraid; chafe, clamour, fret, fume, scold.

chief *adj* first, foremost, headmost, leading, master, supereminent, supreme, top; capital, cardinal, especial, essential, grand, great, main, master, paramount, prime, principal, supreme, vital. • *n* chieftain, commander; head, leader.

chiffonier *n* cabinet, sideboard.

child *n* babe, baby, bairn, bantling, brat, chit, infant, nursling, suckling, wean; issue, offspring, progeny.

childbirth *n* child-bearing, delivery, labour, parturition, travail.

childish *adj* infantile, juvenile, puerile, tender, young; foolish, frivolous, silly, trifling, weak.

childlike *adj* docile, dutiful, gentle, meek, obedient, submissive; confiding, guileless, ingenuous, innocent, simple, trustful, uncrafty.

chill *vb* dampen, depress, deject, discourage, dishearten. • *adj* bleak, chilly, cold, frigid, gelid. • *n* chilliness, cold, coldness, frigidity; ague, rigour, shiver; damp, depression.

chime *vb* accord, harmonize. • *n* accord, consonance.

chimera *n* crochet, delusion, dream, fantasy, hallucination, illusion, phantom.

chimerical *adj* delusive, fanciful, fantastic, illusory, imaginary, quixotic, shadowy, unfounded, visionary, wild.

chink[1] *vb* cleave, crack, fissure, crevasse, incise, split, slit. • *n* aperture, cleft, crack, cranny, crevice, fissure, gap, opening, slit.

chink[2] *vb, n* jingle, clink, ring, ting, tink, tinkle.

chip *vb* flake, fragment, hew, pare, scrape. • *n* flake, fragment, paring, scrap.

chirp *vb* cheep, chirrup, peep, twitter.

chirrup *vb* animate, cheer, encourage, inspirit.

chisel *vb* carve, cut, gouge, sculpt, sculpture.

chivalrous *adj* adventurous, bold, brave, chivalric, gallant, knightly, valiant, warlike; gallant, generous, high-minded, magnanimous.

chivalry *n* knighthood, knight-errantry; courtesy, gallantry, politeness; courage, valour.

choice *adj* excellent, exquisite, precious, rare, select, superior, uncommon, unusual, valuable; careful, chary, frugal, sparing. • *n* alternative, election, option, selection; favourite, pick, preference.

choke *vb* gag, smother, stifle, strangle, suffocate, throttle; overcome, overpower, smother, suppress; bar, block, close, obstruct, stop.

choleric *adj* angry, fiery, hasty, hot, fiery, irascible, irritable, passionate, petulant, testy, touchy, waspish.

choose *vb* adopt, co-opt, cull, designate, elect, pick, predestine, prefer, select.

chop *vb* cut, hack, hew; mince; shift, veer. • *n* slice; brand, quality, chap, jaw.

chouse *vb* bamboozle, beguile, cheat, circumvent, cozen, deceive, defraud, delude, dupe, gull, hoodwink, overreach, swindle, trick, victimize. • *n* cully, dupe, gull, simpleton, tool; artifice, cheat, circumvention, deceit deception, delusion, double-dealing, fraud, imposition, imposture, ruse, stratagem, trick, wile.

christen *vb* baptize; call, dub, denominate, designate, entitle, name, style, term, title

chronic *adj* confirmed, continuing, deep-seated, inveterate, rooted.

chronicle *vb* narrate, record, register. • *n* diary, journal, register; account, annals, history, narration, recital, record.

chuckle *vb* crow, exult, giggle, laugh, snigger, titter. • *n* giggle, laughter, snigger, titter.

chum *n* buddy, companion, comrade, crony, friend, mate, pal.

churl *n* boor, bumpkin, clodhopper, clown, countryman, lout, peasant, ploughman, rustic; curmudgeon, hunks, miser, niggard, scrimp, skinflint.

churlish *adj* brusque, brutish, cynical, harsh, impolite, rough, rude, snappish, snarling, surly, uncivil, waspish; crabbed, ill-tempered, morose, sullen; close, close-fisted, illiberal, mean, miserly, niggardly, penurious, stingy.

churn *vb* agitate, jostle.

cicatrice *n* cicatrix, mark, scar, seam.

cicesbeo *n* beau, escort, gallant, gigolo.

cincture *n* band, belt, cestos, cestus, girdle.

cipher *n* naught, nothing, zero; character, device, monogram, symbol; nobody, nonentity.

circle *vb* compass, encircle, encompass, gird, girdle, ring; gyrate, revolve, rotate, round, turn. • *n* circlet, corona, gyre, hoop, ring, rondure; circumference, cordon, periphery; ball, globe, orb, sphere; compass, enclosure; class, clique, company, coterie, fraternity, set, society; bounds, circuit, compass, field, province, range, region, sphere.

circuit *n* ambit, circumambience, circumambiency, cycle, revolution, turn; bounds, district, field, province, range, region, space, sphere, tract; boundary, compass; course, detour, perambulation, round, tour.

circuitous *adj* ambiguous, devious, indirect, roundabout, tortuous, turning, winding.

circulate *vb* diffuse, disseminate, promulgate, propagate, publish, spread.

circumference *n* bound, boundary, circuit, girth, outline, perimeter, periphery.

circumlocution *n* circuitousness, obliqueness, periphrase, periphrasis, verbosity, wordiness.

circumscribe *vb* bound, define, encircle, enclose, encompass, limit, surround; confine, restrict.

circumspect *adj* attentive, careful, cautious, considerate, discreet, heedful, judicious, observant, prudent, vigilant, wary, watchful.

circumstance *n* accident, incident; condition, detail, event, fact, happening, occurrence, position, situation.

circumstantial *adj* detailed, particular; indirect, inferential, presumptive.

circumvent *vb* check, checkmate, outgeneral, thwart; bamboozle, beguile, cheat, chouse, cozen, deceive, defraud, delude, dupe, gull, hoodwink, inveigle, mislead, outwit, overreach, trick.

circumvention *n* cheat, cheating, chicanery, deceit, deception, duplicity, fraud, guile, imposition, imposture, indirection, trickery, wiles.

cistern *n* basin, pond, reservoir, tank.

citation *n* excerpt, extract, quotation; enumeration, mention, quotation, quoting.

cite *vb* adduce, enumerate, extract, mention, name, quote; call, summon.

citizen *n* burgess, burgher, denizen, dweller, freeman, inhabitant, resident, subject, townsman.

civil *adj* civic, municipal, political; domestic; accommodating, affable, civilized, complaisant, courteous, courtly, debonair, easy, gracious, obliging, polished, polite, refined, suave, urbane, well-bred, well-mannered.

civility *n* affability, amiability, complaisance, courteousness, courtesy, good-breeding, politeness, suavity, urbanity.

civilize *vb* cultivate, educate, enlighten, humanize, improve, polish, refine.

claim *vb* ask, assert, challenge, demand, exact, require. • *n* call, demand, lien, requisition; pretension, privilege, right, title.

clammy *adj* adhesive, dauby, glutinous, gummy, ropy, smeary, sticky, viscid, viscous; close, damp, dank, moist, sticky, sweaty.

clamour *vb* shout, vociferate. • *n* blare, din, exclamation, hullabaloo, noise, outcry, uproar, vociferation.

clan *n* family, phratry, race, sect, tribe; band, brotherhood, clique, coterie, fraternity, gang, set, society, sodality.

clandestine *adj* concealed, covert, fraudulent, furtive, hidden, private, secret, sly, stealthy, surreptitious, underhand.

clap *vb* pat, slap, strike; force, slam; applaud, cheer. • *n* blow, knock, slap; bang, burst, explosion, peal, slam.

clarify *vb* cleanse, clear, depurate, purify, strain.

clash *vb* collide, crash, strike; clang, clank, clatter, crash, rattle; contend, disagree, interfere. • *n* collision; clang, clangour, clank, clashing, clatter, crash, rattle; contradiction, disagreement, interference, jar, jarring, opposition.

clasp *vb* clutch, entwine, grasp, grapple, grip, seize; embrace, enfold, fold, hug. • *n* buckle, catch, hasp, hook; embrace, hug.

class *vb* arrange, classify, dispose, distribute, range, rank. • *n* form, grade, order, rank, status; group, seminar; breed, kind, sort; category, collection, denomination, division, group, head.

classical *adj* first-rate, master, masterly, model, standard; Greek, Latin, Roman; Attic, chaste, elegant, polished, pure, refined.

classify *vb* arrange, assort, categorize, class, dispose, distribute, group, pigeonhole, rank, systematize, tabulate.

clatter *vb* clash, rattle; babble, clack, gabble, jabber, prate, prattle. • *n* clattering, clutter, rattling.

clause *n* article, condition, provision, stipulation.

claw *vb* lacerate, scratch, tear. • *n* talon, ungula.

clean *vb* cleanse, clear, purge, purify, rinse, scour, scrub, wash, wipe. • *adj* immaculate, spotless, unsmirched, unsoiled, unspotted, unstained, unsullied, white; clarified, pure, purified, unadulterated, unmixed; adroit, delicate, dextrous, graceful, light, neat, shapely; complete, entire, flawless, faultless, perfect, unabated, unblemished, unimpaired, whole; chaste, innocent, moral, pure, undefiled. • *adv* altogether, completely, entirely, perfectly, quite, thoroughly, wholly.

cleanse *vb* clean, clear, elutriate, purge, purify, rinse, scour, scrub, wash, wipe.

clear *vb* clarify, cleanse, purify, refine; emancipate, disenthral, free, liberate, loose; absolve, acquit, discharge, exonerate, justify, vindicate; disembarrass, disengage, disentangle, extricate, loosen, rid; clean up, scour, sweep; balance; emancipate, free, liberate. • *adj* bright, crystalline, light, limpid, luminous, pellucid, transparent; pure, unadulterated, unmixed; free, open, unencumbered, unobstructed; cloudless, fair, serene, sunny, unclouded, undimmed, unobscured; net; distinct, intelligible, lucid, luminous, perspicuous; apparent, conspicuous, distinct, evident, indisputable, manifest, obvious, palpable, unambiguous, undeniable, unequivocal, unmistakable, unquestionable, visible; clean, guiltless, immaculate, innocent, irreproachable, sinless, spotless, unblemished, undefiled, unspotted, unsullied; unhampered, unimpeded, unobstructed; euphonious, fluty, liquid, mellifluous, musical, silvery, sonorous.

cleave[1] *vb* crack, divide, open, part, rend, rive, sever, split, sunder.

cleave[2] *vb* adhere, cling, cohere, hold, stick.

cleft *adj* bifurcated, cloven, forked. • *n* breach, break, chasm, chink, cranny, crevice, fissure, fracture, gap, interstice, opening, rent, rift.

clemency *n* mildness, softness; compassion, fellow-feeling, forgivingness, gentleness, kindness, lenience, leniency, lenity, mercifulness, mercy, mildness, tenderness.

clement *adj* compassionate, forgiving, gentle, humane, indulgent, kind, kind-hearted, lenient, merciful, mild, tender, tender-hearted.

clench *vb* close tightly, grip; fasten, fix, rivet, secure.

clergy *n* clergymen, the cloth, ministers.

clever *adj* able, apt, gifted, talented; adroit, capable, dextrous, discerning, expert, handy, ingenious, knowing, quick, ready, skilful, smart, talented.

click *vb* beat, clack, clink, tick. • *n* beat, clack, clink, tick; catch, detent, pawl, ratchet.

cliff *n* crag, palisade, precipice, scar, steep.

climate *n* clime, temperature, weather; country, region.

climax *vb* consummate, crown, culminate, peak. • *n* acme, consummation, crown, culmination, head, peak, summit, top, zenith.

clinch *vb* clasp, clench, clutch, grapple, grasp, grip; fasten, secure; confirm, establish, fix. • *n* catch, clutch, grasp, grip; clincher, clamp, cramp, holdfast.

cling *vb* adhere, clear, stick; clasp, embrace, entwine.

clink *vb, n* chink, jingle, ring, tinkle; chime, rhyme.

clip *vb* cut, shear, snip; curtail, cut, dock, pare, prune, trim. • *n* cutting, shearing; blow, knock, lick, rap, thump, thwack, thump.

clique *n* association, brotherhood, cabal, camarilla, clan, club, coterie, gang, junta, party, ring, set, sodality.

cloak *vb* conceal, cover, dissemble, hide, mask, veil. • *n* mantle, surcoat; blind, cover, mask, pretext, veil.

clock *vb* mark time, measure, stopwatch; clock up, record, register. • *n* chronometer, horologue, timekeeper, timepiece, timer, watch.

clog *vb* fetter, hamper, shackle, trammel; choke, obstruct; burden, cumber, embarrass, encumber, hamper, hinder, impede, load, restrain, trammel. • *n* dead-weight, drag-weight, fetter, shackle, trammel; check, drawback, encumbrance, hindrance, impediment, obstacle, obstruction.

cloister *n* abbey, convent, monastery, nunnery, priory; arcade, colonnade, piazza.

close[1] *adj* closed, confined, snug, tight; hidden, private, secret; incommunicative, reserved, reticent, secretive, taciturn; concealed, retired, secluded, withdrawn; confined, motionless, stagnant; airless, oppressive, stale, stifling, stuffy, sultry; compact, compressed, dense, form, solid, thick; adjacent, adjoining, approaching, immediately, near, nearly, neighbouring; attached, dear, confidential, devoted, intimate; assiduous, earnest, fixed, intense, intent, unremitting; accurate, exact, faithful, nice, precise, strict; churlish, close-fisted, curmudgeonly, mean, illiberal, miserly, niggardly, parsimonious, penurious, stingy, ungenerous. • *n* courtyard, enclosure, grounds, precinct, yard.

close[2] *vb* occlude, seal, shut; choke, clog, estop, obstruct, stop; cease, complete, concede, end, finish, terminate; coalesce, unite; cease, conclude, finish, terminate; clinch, grapple, agree. • *n* cessation, conclusion, end, finish, termination.

closet *n* cabinet, retiring-room; press, store-room.

clot *vb* coagulate, concrete. • *n* coagulation, concretion, lump.

clothe *vb* array, attire, deck, dress, rig; cover,endow, envelop, enwrap, invest with, swathe.

clothes *n* apparel, array, attire, clothing, costume, dress, garb, garments, gear, habiliments, habits, raiment, rig, vestments, vesture.

cloud *vb* becloud, obnubilate, overcast, overspread; befog, darken, dim, obscure, shade, shadow. • *n* cirrus, cumulus, fog, haze, mist, nebulosity, scud, stratus, vapour; army, crowd, horde, host, multitude, swarm, throng; darkness, eclipse, gloom, obscuration, obscurity.

cloudy *adj* clouded, filmy, foggy, hazy, lowering, lurid, murky, overcast; confused, dark, dim, obscure; depressing, dismal, gloomy, sullen; clouded, mottled; blurred, dimmed, lustreless, muddy.

clown *n* churl, clod-breaker, clodhopper, hind, husbandman, lubber; boor, bumpkin, churl, fellow, lout; blockhead, dolt, clodpoll, dunce, dunderhead, numbskull, simpleton, thickhead; buffoon, droll, farceur, fool, harlequin, jack-a-dandy, jack-pudding, jester, merry-andrew, mime, pantaloon, pickle-herring, punch, scaramouch, zany.

clownish *adj* awkward, boorish, clumsy, coarse, loutish, ungainly, rough, rustic; churlish, ill-bred, ill-mannered, impolite, rude, uncivil.

cloy *vb* glut, pall, sate, satiate, surfeit.

club *vb* combine, unite; beat, bludgeon, cudgel. • *n* bat, bludgeon, cosh, cudgel, hickory, shillelagh, stick, truncheon; association, company, coterie, fraternity, set, society, sodality.

clump *vb* assemble, batch, bunch, cluster, group, lump; lumber, stamp, stomp, stump, trudge. • *n* assemblage, bunch, cluster, collection, group, patch, tuft.

clumsy *adj* botched, cumbrous, heavy, ill-made, ill-shaped, lumbering, ponderous, unwieldy; awkward, blundering, bungling, elephantine, heavy-handed, inapt, mal adroit, unhandy, unskilled.

cluster *vb* assemble, batch, bunch, clump, collect, gather, group, lump, throng. • *n* agglomeration, assemblage, batch, bunch, clump, collection, gathering, group, throng.

clutch[1] vb catch, clasp, clench, clinch, grab, grapple, grasp, grip, hold, seize, snatch, squeeze. • n clasp, clench, clinch, grasp, grip, hold, seizure.

clutch[2] n aerie, brood, hatching, nest.

clutches npl claws, paws, talons; hands, power.

clutter vb confuse, disarrange, disarray, disorder, jumble, litter, mess, muss; clatter. • n bustle, clatter, clattering, racket; confusion, disarray, disorder, jumble, litter, mess, muss.

coadjutor n abettor, accomplice, aider, ally, assistant, associate, auxiliary, collaborator, colleague, cooperator, fellow-helper, helper, helpmate, partner.

coagulate vb clot, congeal, concrete, curdle, thicken.

coalesce vb amalgamate, blend, cohere, combine, commix, incorporate, mix, unite; concur, fraternize.

coalition n alliance, association, combination, compact, confederacy, confederation, conjunction, conspiracy, co-partnership, federation, league, union.

coarse adj crude, impure, rough, unpurified; broad, gross, indecent, indelicate, ribald, vulgar; bearish, bluff, boorish, brutish, churlish, clownish, gruff, impolite, loutish, rude, unpolished; crass, inelegant.

coast vb flow, glide, roll, skim, sail, slide, sweep. • n littoral, seaboard, sea-coast, seaside, shore, strand; border.

coat vb cover, spread. • n cut-away, frock, jacket; coating, cover, covering; layer.

coax vb allure, beguile, cajole, cog, entice, flatter, persuade, soothe, wheedle.

cobble vb botch, bungle; mend, patch, repair, tinker.

cobweb adj flimsy, gauzy, slight, thin, worthless. • n entanglement, meshes, snare, toils.

cochleate adj cochlear, cochleary, cochleous, cochleated, spiral, spiry.

cockle vb corrugate, pucker, wrinkle.

coddle vb caress, cocker, fondle, humour, indulge, nurse, pamper, pet.

codger n churl, curmudgeon, hunks, lick-penny, miser, niggard, screw, scrimp, skinflint.

codify vb condense, digest, summarize, systematize, tabulate.

coerce vb check, curb, repress, restrain, subdue; compel, constrain, drive, force, urge.

coercion n check, curb, repression, restraint; compulsion, constraint, force.

coeval adj coetaneous, coexistent, contemporaneous, contemporary, synchronous.

coexistent adj coetaneous, coeval, simultaneous, synchronous.

coffer n box, casket, chest, trunk; money-chest, safe, strongbox; caisson.

cogent adj compelling, conclusive, convincing, effective, forcible, influential, irresistible, persuasive, potent, powerful, resistless, strong, trenchant, urgent.

cogitate vb consider, deliberate, meditate, ponder, reflect, ruminate, muse, think, weigh.

cognate adj affiliated, affined, akin, allied, alike, analogous, connected, kindred, related, similar.

cognizance n cognition, knowing, knowledge, notice, observation.

cohere vb agree, coincide, conform, fit, square, suit.

coherence n coalition, cohesion, connection, dependence, union; agreement, congruity, consistency, correspondence, harmony, intelligibility, intelligible, meaning, rationality, unity.

coherent adj adherent, connected, united; congruous consistent, intelligible, logical.

cohort n band, battalion, line, squadron.

coil vb curl, twine, twirl, twist, wind. • n convolution, curlicue, helix, knot, roll, spiral, tendril, twirl, volute, whorl; bustle, care, clamour, confusion, entanglements, perplexities, tumult, turmoil, uproar.

coin vb counterfeit, create, devise, fabricate, forge, form, invent, mint, originate, mould, stamp. • n coign, corner, quoin; key, plug, prop, wedge; cash, money, specie.

coincide vb cohere, correspond, square, tally; acquiesce, agree, harmonize, concur.

coincidence n corresponding, squaring, tallying; agreeing, concurrent, concurring.

cold adj arctic, biting, bleak, boreal, chill, chilly, cutting, frosty, gelid, glacial, icy, nipping, polar, raw, wintry; frost-bitten, shivering; apathetic, cold-blooded, dead, freezing, frigid, indifferent, lukewarm, passionless, phlegmatic, sluggish, stoical, stony, torpid, unconcerned, unfeeling, unimpressible, unresponsive, unsusceptible, unsympathetic; dead, dull, spiritless, unaffecting, uninspiring, uninteresting. • n chill, chilliness, coldness.

collapse vb break down, fail, fall. • n depression, exhaustion, failure, faint, prostration, sinking, subsidence.

collar vb apprehend, arrest, capture, grab, nab, seize. • n collarette, gorget, neckband, ruff, torque; band, belt, fillet, guard, ring, yoke.

collate vb adduce, collect, compare, compose.

collateral adj contingent, indirect, secondary, subordinate; concurrent, parallel; confirmatory, corroborative; accessory, accompanying, additional, ancillary, auxiliary, concomitant, contributory, simultaneous, supernumerary; consanguineous, related. • n guarantee, guaranty, security, surety, warranty; accessory, extra, nonessential, unessential; consanguinean, relative.

collation n luncheon, repast, meal.

colleague n aider, ally, assistant, associate, auxiliary, coadjutor, collaborator, companion, confederate, confrere, cooperator, helper, partner.

collect vb assemble, compile, gather, muster; accumulate, aggregate, amass, garner.

collected adj calm, composed, cool, placid, self-possessed, serene, unperturbed.

collection n aggregation, assemblage, cluster, crowd, drove, gathering, group, pack; accumulation, congeries, conglomeration, heap, hoard, lot, mass, pile, store; alms, contribution, offering, offertory.

colligate vb bind, combine, fasten, unite.

collision n clash, concussion, crash, encounter, impact, impingement, shock; conflict, crashing, interference, opposition.

collocate vb arrange, dispose, place, set.

colloquy n conference, conversation, dialogue, discourse, talk.

collude vb concert, connive, conspire.

collusion n connivance, conspiracy, coven, craft, deceit.

collusive adj conniving, conspiratorial, , dishonest, deceitful, deceptive, fraudulent.

colossal adj Cyclopean, enormous, gigantic, Herculean, huge, immense, monstrous, prodigious, vast.

colour vb discolour, dye, paint, stain, tinge, tint; disguise, varnish; disguise, distort, garble, misrepresent, pervert; blush, flush, redden, show. • n hue, shade, tinge, tint, tone; paint, pigment, stain; redness, rosiness, ruddiness; complexion; appearance, disguise, excuse, guise, plea, pretence, pretext, semblance.

colourless adj achromatic, uncoloured, untinged; blanched, hueless, livid, pale, pallid; blank, characterless, dull, expressionless, inexpressive, monotonous.

colours n banner, ensign, flag, standard.

column n pillar, pilaster; file, line, row.

coma n drowsiness, lethargy, somnolence, stupor, torpor; bunch, clump, cluster, tuft.

comatose adj drowsy, lethargic, sleepy, somnolent, stupefied.

comb vb card, curry, dress, groom, rake, unknot, untangle; rake, ransack, rummage, scour, search. • n card, hatchel, ripple; harrow, rake.

combat vb contend, contest, fight, struggle, war; battle, oppose, resist, struggle, withstand. • n action, affair, battle, brush, conflict, contest, encounter, fight, skirmish.

combative adj belligerent, contentious, militant, pugnacious, quarrelsome.

combination n association, conjunction, connection, union; alliance, cartel, coalition, confederacy, consolidation, league, merger, syndicate; cabal, clique, conspiracy, faction, junta, ring; amalgamation, compound, mixture.

combine vb cooperate, merge, pool, unite; amalgamate, blend, incorporate, mix.

combustible adj consumable, inflammable.

come vb advance, approach; arise, ensue, flow, follow, issue, originate, proceed, result; befall, betide, happen, occur.

comely adj becoming, decent, decorous, fitting, seemly, suitable; beautiful, fair, graceful, handsome, personable, pretty, symmetrical.

comfort vb alleviate, animate, cheer, console, encourage, enliven, gladden, inspirit, invigorate, refresh, revive, solace, soothe, strengthen. • n aid, assistance, countenance, help, support, succour; consolation, solace, encouragement, relief; ease, enjoyment, peace, satisfaction.

comfortable *adj* acceptable, agreeable, delightful, enjoyable, grateful, gratifying, happy, pleasant, pleasurable, welcome; commodious, convenient, easeful, snug; painless.

comfortless *adj* bleak, cheerless, desolate, drear, dreary, forlorn, miserable, wretched; broken-hearted, desolate, disconsolate, forlorn, heart-broken, inconsolable, miserable, woe-begone, wretched.

comical *adj* amusing, burlesque, comic, diverting, droll, farcical, funny, humorous, laughable, ludicrous, sportive, whimsical.

coming *adj* approaching, arising, arriving, ensuing, eventual, expected, forthcoming, future, imminent, issuing, looming, nearing, prospective, ultimate; emergent, emerging, successful; due, owed, owing. • *n* advent, approach, arrival; imminence, imminency, nearness; apparition, appearance, disclosure, emergence, manifestation, materialization, occurrence, presentation, revelation, rising.

comity *n* affability, amenity, civility, courtesy, politeness, suavity, urbanity.

command *vb* bid, charge, direct, enjoin, order, require; control, dominate, govern, lead, rule, sway; claim, challenge, compel, demand, exact. • *n* behest, bidding, charge, commandment, direction, hest, injunction, mandate, order, requirement, requisition; ascendency, authority, dominion, control, government, power, rule, sway, supremacy.

commander *n* captain, chief, chieftain, commandment, head, leader.

commemorate *vb* celebrate, keep, observe, solemnize.

commence *vb* begin, inaugurate, initiate, institute, open, originate, start.

commend *vb* assign, bespeak, confide, recommend, remit; commit, entrust, yield; applaud, approve, eulogize, extol, laud, praise.

commendation *n* approbation, approval, good opinion, recommendation; praise, encomium, eulogy, panegyric.

commensurate *adj* commeasurable, commensurable; coextensive, conterminous, equal; adequate, appropriate, corresponding, due, proportionate, proportioned, sufficient.

comment *vb* animadvert, annotate, criticize, explain, interpret, note, remark. • *n* annotation, elucidation, explanation, exposition, illustration, commentary, note, gloss; animadversion, observation, remark.

commentator *n* annotator, commentator, critic, expositor, expounder, interpreter.

commerce *n* business, exchange, dealing, trade, traffic; communication, communion, intercourse.

commercial *adj* mercantile, trading.

commination *n* denunciation, menace, threat, threatening.

commingle *vb* amalgamate, blend, combine, commix, intermingle, intermix, join, mingle, mix, unite.

comminute *vb* bray, bruise, grind, levigate, powder, pulverize, triturate.

commiserate *vb* compassionate, condole, pity, sympathize.

commiseration *n* compassion, pitying; condolence, pity, sympathy.

commission *vb* authorize, empower; delegate, depute. • *n* doing, perpetration; care, charge, duty, employment, errand, office, task, trust; allowance, compensation, fee, rake-off.

commissioner *n* agent, delegate, deputy.

commit *vb* confide, consign, delegate, entrust, remand; consign, deposit, lay, place, put, relegate, resign; do, enact, perform, perpetrate; imprison; engage, implicate, pledge.

commix *vb* amalgamate, blend, combine, commingle, compound, intermingle, mingle, mix, unite.

commodious *adj* advantageous, ample, comfortable, convenient, fit, proper, roomy, spacious, suitable, useful.

commodity *n* goods, merchandise, produce, wares.

common *adj* collective, public; general, useful; common-place, customary, everyday, familiar, frequent, habitual, usual; banal, hackneyed, stale, threadbare, trite; indifferent, inferior, low, ordinary, plebeian, popular, undistinguished, vulgar.

commonplace *adj* common, hackneyed, ordinary, stale, threadbare, trite. • *n* banality, cliché, platitude; jotting, memoir, memorandum, note, reminder.

common-sense, common-sensical *adj* practical, sagacious, sensible, sober.

commotion *n* agitation, disturbance, ferment, perturbation, welter; ado, bustle, disorder, disturbance, hurly-burly, pother, tumult, turbulence, turmoil.

communicate *vb* bestow, confer, convey, give, impart, transmit; acquaint, announce, declare, disclose, divulge, publish, reveal, unfold; commune, converse, correspond.

communication *n* conveyance, disclosure, giving, imparting, transmittal; commerce, conference, conversation, converse, correspondence, intercourse; announcement, dispatch, information, message, news.

communicative *adj* affable, chatty, conversable, free, open, sociable, unreserved.

communion *n* converse, fellowship, intercourse, participation; Eucharist, holy communion, Lord's Supper, sacrament.

community *n* commonwealth, people, public, society; association, brotherhood, college, society; likeness, participancy, sameness, similarity.

compact[1] *n* agreement, arrangement, bargain, concordant, contract, covenant, convention, pact, stipulation, treaty.

compact[2] *vb* compress, condense, pack, press; bind, consolidate, unite. • *adj* close, compressed, condensed, dense, firm, solid; brief, compendious, concise, laconic, pithy, pointed, sententious, short, succinct, terse.

companion *n* accomplice, ally, associate, comrade, compeer, confederate, consort, crony, friend, fellow, mate; partaker, participant, participator, partner, sharer.

companionable *adj* affable, conversable, familiar, friendly, genial, neighbourly, sociable.

companionship *n* association, fellowship, friendship, intercourse, society.

company *n* assemblage, assembly, band, bevy, body, circle, collection, communication, concourse, congregation, coterie, crew, crowd, flock, gang, gathering, group, herd, rout, set, syndicate, troop; party; companionship, fellowship, guests, society, visitor, visitors; association, copartnership, corporation, firm, house, partnership.

compare *vb* assimilate, balance, collate, parallel; liken, resemble.

comparison *n* collation, compare, estimate; simile, similitude.

compartment *n* bay, cell, division, pigeonhole, section.

compass *vb* embrace, encompass, enclose, encircle, environ, surround; beleaguer, beset, besiege, block, blockade, invest; accomplish, achieve, attain, carry, consummate, effect, obtain, perform, procure, realize; contrive, devise, intend, meditate, plot, purpose. • *n* bound, boundary, extent, gamut, limit, range, reach, register, scope, stretch; circuit, round.

compassion *n* clemency, commiseration, condolence, fellow-feeling, heart, humanity, kind-heartedness, kindness, kindliness, mercy, pity, rue, ruth, sorrow, sympathy, tenderheartedness, tenderness.

compassionate *adj* benignant, clement, commiserative, gracious, kind, merciful, pitying, ruthful, sympathetic, tender.

compatible *adj* accordant, agreeable to, congruous, consistent, consonant, reconcilable, suitable.

compeer *n* associate, comrade, companion, equal, fellow, mate, peer.

compel *vb* constrain, force, coerce, drive, necessitate, oblige; bend, bow, subdue, subject.

compend *n* abbreviation, abridgement, abstract, breviary, brief, compendium, conspectus, digest, epitome, précis, summary, syllabus, synopsis.

compendious *adj* abbreviated, abridged, brief, comprehensive, concise, short, succinct, summary.

compensate *vb* counterbalance, counterpoise, countervail; guerdon, recompense, reimburse, remunerate, reward; indemnify, reimburse, repay, requite; atone.

compensation *n* pay, payment, recompense, remuneration, reward, salary; amends, atonement, indemnification, indemnity, reparation, requital, satisfaction; balance, counterpoise, equalization, offset.

compete *vb* contend, contest, cope, emulate, rival, strive, struggle, vie.

competence *n* ability, capability, capacity, fitness, qualification, suitableness; adequacy, adequateness, enough, sufficiency.

competent *adj* able, capable, clever, equal, endowed, qualified; adapted, adequate, convenient, fit, sufficient, suitable.

competition *n* contest, emulation, rivalry, rivals.

competitor *n* adversary, antagonist, contestant, emulator, opponent.

compile *vb* compose, prepare, write; arrange, collect, select.

complacency *n* content, contentment, gratification, pleasure, satisfaction; affability, civility, complaisance, courtesy, politeness.

complacent *adj* contented, gratified, pleased, satisfied; affable, civil, complaisant, courteous, easy, gracious, grateful obliging, polite, urbane.

complain *vb* bemoan, bewail, deplore, grieve, groan, grouch, grumble, lament, moan, murmur, repine, whine.

complainant *n* accuser, plaintiff.

complaining *adj* fault-finding, murmuring, querulous.

complaint *n* grievance, gripe, grumble, lament, lamentation, plaint, murmur, wail; ail, ailment, annoyance, disease, disorder, illness, indisposition, malady, sickness; accusation, charge, information.

complete *vb* accomplish, achieve, conclude, consummate, do, effect, effectuate, end, execute, finish, fulfil, perfect, perform, realize, terminate. • *adj* clean, consummate, faultless, full, perfect, perform, thorough; all, entire, integral, total, unbroken, undiminished, undivided, unimpaired, whole; accomplished, achieved, completed, concluded, consummated, ended, finished.

completion *n* accomplishing, accomplishment, achieving, conclusion, consummation, effecting, effectuation, ending, execution, finishing, perfecting, performance, termination.

complex *adj* composite, compound, compounded, manifold, mingled, mixed; complicate, complicated, entangled, intricate, involved, knotty, mazy, tangled. • *n* complexus, complication, involute, skein, tangle; entirety, integration, network, totality, whole; compulsion, fixation, obsession, preoccupation, prepossession; prejudice.

complexion *n* colour, hue, tint.

complexity *n* complication, entanglement, intricacy, involution.

compliance *n* concession, obedience, submission; acquiescence, agreement, assent, concurrence, consent; compliancy, yieldingness.

complicate *vb* confuse, entangle, interweave, involve.

complication *n* complexity, confusion, entanglement, intricacy; combination, complexus, mixture.

compliment *vb* commend, congratulate, eulogize, extol, flatter, laud, praise. • *n* admiration, commendation, courtesy, encomium, eulogy, favour, flattery, honour, laudation, praise, tribute.

complimentary *adj* commendatory, congratulatory, encomiastic, eulogistic, flattering, laudatory, panegyrical.

comply *vb* adhere to, complete, discharge, fulfil, meet, observe, perform, satisfy; accede, accord, acquiesce, agree to assent, consent to, yield.

component *adj* composing, constituent, constituting. • *n* constituent, element, ingredient, part.

comport *vb* accord, agree, coincide, correspond, fit, harmonize, square, suit, tally.

compose *vb* build, compact, compound, constitute, form, make, synthesize; contrive, create, frame, imagine, indite, invent, write; adjust, arrange, regulate, settle; appease, assuage, calm, pacify, quell, quiet, soothe, still, tranquillize.

composed *adj* calm, collected, cool, imperturbable, placid, quiet, sedate, self-possessed, tranquil, undisturbed, unmoved, unruffled.

composite *adj* amalgamated, combined, complex, compounded, mixed; integrated, unitary. • *n* admixture, amalgam blend, combination, composition, compound, mixture, unification.

composition *n* constitution, construction, formation, framing, making; compound, mixture; arrangement, combination, conjunction, make-up, synthesize, union; invention, opus, piece, production, writing; agreement, arrangement, compromise.

compost *n* fertilizer, fertilizing, manure, mixture.

composure *n* calmness, coolness, equanimity, placidity, sedateness, quiet, self-possession, serenity, tranquillity.

compotation *n* conviviality, frolicking, jollification, revelling, revelry, rousing, wassailling; bacchanal, carousal, carouse, debauch, orgy, revel, saturnalia, wassail.

compound[1] *vb* amalgamate, blend, combine, intermingle, intermix, mingle, mix, unite; adjust, arrange, compose, compromise, settle. • *adj* complex, composite. • *n* combination, composition, mixture; farrago, hodgepodge, jumble, medley, mess, olio.

compound[2] *n* enclosure, garden, yard.

comprehend *vb* comprise, contain, embrace, embody, enclose, include, involve; apprehend, conceive, discern, grasp know, imagine, master, perceive, see, understand.

comprehension *n* comprising, embracing, inclusion; compass, domain, embrace, field, limits, province, range, reach, scope, sphere, sweep; connotation, depth, force, intention; conception, grasp, intelligence, understanding; intellect, intelligence, mind, reason, understanding.

comprehensive *adj* all-embracing, ample, broad, capacious, compendious, extensive, full, inclusive, large, sweeping, wide.

compress *vb* abbreviate, condense, constrict, contract, crowd, press, shorten, squeeze, summarize.

compression *n* condensation, confining, pinching, pressing, squeezing; brevity, pithiness, succinctness, terseness.

comprise *vb* comprehend, contain, embody, embrace, enclose, include, involve.

compromise *vb* adjust, arbitrate, arrange, compose, compound, settle; imperil, jeopardize, prejudice; commit, engage, implicate, pledge; agree, compound. • *n* adjustment, agreement, composition, settlement.

compulsion *n* coercion, constraint, force, forcing, pressure, urgency.

compulsory *adj* coercive, compelling, constraining; binding, enforced, imperative, necessary, obligatory, unavoidable.

compunction *n* contrition, misgiving, penitence, qualm, regret, reluctance, remorse, repentance, sorrow.

computable *adj* calculable, numerable, reckonable.

computation *n* account, calculation, estimate, reckoning, score, tally.

compute *vb* calculate, count, enumerate, estimate, figure, measure, number, rate, reckon, sum.

comrade *n* accomplice, ally, associate, chum, companion, compatrio, compeer, crony, fellow, mate, pal.

concatenate *vb* connect, join, link, unite.

concatenation *n* connection; chain, congeries, linking, series, sequence, succession.

concave *adj* depressed, excavated, hollow, hollowed, scooped.

conceal *vb* bury, cover, screen, secrete; disguise, dissemble, mask.

concede *vb* grant, surrender, yield; acknowledge, admit, allow, confess, grant.

conceit *n* belief, conception, fancy, idea, image, imagination, notion thought; caprice, illusion, vagary, whim; estimate, estimation impression, judgement, opinion; conceitedness, egoism, self-complacency, priggishness, priggery, self-conceit, self-esteem, self-sufficiency, vanity; crotchet, point, quip, quirk.

conceited *adj* egotistical, opinionated, opinionative, overweening, self-conceited, vain.

conceivable *adj* imaginable, picturable; cogitable, comprehensible, intelligible, rational, thinkable.

conceive *vb* create, contrive, devise, form, plan, purpose; fancy, imagine; comprehend, fathom, think, understand; assume, imagine, suppose; bear, become pregnant.

concern *vb* affect, belong to, interest, pertain to, regard, relate to, touch; disquiet, disturb, trouble. • *n* affair, business, matter, transaction; concernment, consequence, importance, interest, moment, weight; anxiety, care, carefulness, solicitude, worry; business, company, establishment, firm, house.

concert *vb* combine, concoct, contrive, design, devise, invent, plan, plot, project. • *n* agreement, concord, concordance, cooperation, harmony, union, unison.

concession *n* acquiescence, assent, cessation, compliance, surrender, yielding; acknowledgement, allowance, boon, confession, grant, privilege.

conciliate *vb* appease, pacify, placate, propitiate, reconcile; engage, gain, secure, win, win over.

concise *adj* brief, compact, compendious, comprehensive, compressed, condensed, crisp, laconic, pithy, pointed, pregnant, sententious, short, succinct, summary, terse.

conclave *n* assembly, cabinet, council.

conclude *vb* close, end, finish, terminate; deduce, gather, infer, judge; decide, determine, judge; arrange, complete, settle; bar, hinder, restrain, stop; decide, determine, resolve.

conclusion *n* deduction, inference; decision, determination, judgement close, completion, end, event, finale, issue, termination, upshot; arrangement, closing, effecting, establishing, settlement.

conclusive *adj* clinching, convincing, decisive, irrefutable, unanswerable; final, ultimate.

concoct *vb* brew, contrive, design, devise, frame, hatch, invent, mature, plan, plot, prepare, project.

concomitant *adj* accessory, accompanying, attendant, attending, coincident, concurrent, conjoined. • *n* accessory, accompaniment attendant.

concord *n* agreement, amity, friendship, harmony, peace, unanimity, union, unison, unity; accord, adaptation, concordance, consonance, harmony.

concordant *adj* accordant, agreeable, agreeing, harmonious.

concordat *n* agreement, bargain, compact, convention, covenant, stipulation, treaty.

concourse *n* confluence, conflux, congress; assemblage, assembly, collection, crowd, gathering, meeting, multitude, throng.

concrete *vb* cake, congeal, coagulate, harden, solidify, thicken. • *adj* compact, consolidated, firm, solid, solidified; agglomerated, complex, conglomerated, compound, concreted; completely, entire, individualized, total. • *n* compound, concretion, mixture; cement.

concubine *n* hetaera, hetaira, mistress, paramour.

concupiscence *n* lasciviousness, lechery, lewdness, lust, pruriency.

concupiscent *adj* carnal, lascivious, lecherous, lewd, libidinous, lustful, prurient, rampant, salacious, sensual.

concur *vb* accede, acquiesce, agree, approve, assent, coincide, consent, harmonize; combine, conspire, cooperate, help.

concurrent *adj* agreeing, coincident, harmonizing, meeting, uniting; associate, associated, attendant, concomitant, conjoined, united.

concussion *n* agitation, shaking; clash, crash, shock.

condemn *vb* adjudge, convict, doom, sentence; disapprove, proscribe, reprobate; blame, censure, damn, deprecate, disapprove, reprehend, reprove, upbraid.

condemnation *n* conviction, doom, judgement, penalty, sentence; banning, disapproval, proscription; guilt, sin, wrong; blame, censure, disapprobation, disapproval, reprobation, reproof.

condemnatory *adj* blaming, censuring, damnatory, deprecatory, disapproving, reproachful.

condense *vb* compress, concentrate, consolidate, densify, thicken; abbreviate, abridge, contract, curtail, diminish, epitomize, reduce, shorten, summarize; liquefy.

condescend *vb* deign, vouchsafe; descend, stoop, submit.

condescension *n* affability, civility, courtesy, deference, favour, graciousness, obeisance.

condign *adj* adequate, deserved, just, merited, suitable.

condiment *n* appetizer, relish, sauce, seasoning.

condition *vb* postulate, specify, stipulate; groom, prepare, qualify, ready, train; acclimatize, accustom, adapt, adjust, familiarize, habituate, naturalize; attune, commission, fix, overhaul, prepare, recondition, repair, service, tune. • *n* case, circumstances, plight, predicament, situation, state; class, estate, grade, rank, station; arrangement, consideration, provision, proviso, stipulation; attendant, necessity, postulate, precondition, prerequisite.

condole *vb* commiserate, compassionate, console, sympathize.

condonation *n* forgiveness, overlooking, pardon.

condone *vb* excuse, forgive, pardon.

conduce *vb* contribute, lead, tend; advance, aid.

conducive *adj* conducting, contributing, instrumental, promotive, subservient, subsidiary.

conduct *vb* convoy, direct, escort, lead; administer, command, govern, lead, preside, superintend; manage, operate, regulate; direct, lead. • *n* administration, direction, guidance, leadership, management; convoy, escort, guard; actions, bearing, behaviour, career, carriage, demeanour, deportment, manners.

conductor *n* guide, lead; director, leader, manager; propagator, transmitter.

conduit *n* canal, channel, duct, passage, pipe, tube.

confederacy *n* alliance, coalition, compact, confederation, covenant, federation, league, union.

confer *vb* advise, consult, converse, deliberate, discourse, parley, talk; bestow, give, grant, vouchsafe.

confess *vb* acknowledge, admit, avow, own; admit, concede, grant, recognize; attest, exhibit, manifest, prove, show; shrive.

confession *n* acknowledgement, admission, avowal.

confide *vb* commit, consign, entrust, trust.

confidence *n* belief, certitude, dependence, faith, reliance, trust; aplomb, assurance, boldness, cocksureness, courage, firmness, intrepidity, self-reliance; secrecy.

confident *adj* assured, certain, cocksure, positive, sure: bold, presumptuous. sanguine, undaunted.

confidential *adj* intimate, private, secret; faithful, trustworthy.

configuration *n* conformation, contour, figure, form, gestalt, outline, shape.

confine *vb* restrain, shut in, shut up; immure, imprison, incarcerate, impound, jail, mew; bound, circumscribe, limit, restrict. • *n* border, boundary, frontier, limit.

confinement *n* restraint; captivity, duress, durance, immurement, imprisonment, incarceration; childbed, childbirth, delivery, lying-in, parturition.

confines *npl* borders, boundaries, edges, frontiers, limits, marches, precincts.

confirm *vb* assure, establish, fix, settle; strengthen; authenticate, avouch, corroborate, countersign, endorse, substantiate, verify; bind, ratify, sanction.

confirmation *n* establishment, settlement; corroboration, proof, substantiation, verification.

confiscate *vb* appropriate, forfeit, seize.

conflict *vb* clash, combat, contend, contest, disagree, fight, interfere, strive, struggle. • *n* battle, collision, combat, contention, contest, encounter, fight, struggle; antagonism, clashing, disagreement, discord, disharmony, inconsistency, interference, opposition.

confluence *n* conflux, junction, meeting, union; army, assemblage, assembly, concourse, crowd, collection, horde, host, multitude, swarm.

confluent *adj* blending, concurring, flowing, joining, meeting, merging, uniting.

conform *vb* accommodate, adapt, adjust; agree, comport, correspond, harmonize, square, tally.

conformation *n* accordance, agreement, compliance, conformity; configuration, figure, form, manner, shape, structure.

confound *vb* confuse; baffle, bewilder, embarrass, flurry, mystify, nonplus, perplex, pose; amaze, astonish, astound, bewilder, dumfound, paralyse, petrify, startle, stun, stupefy, surprise; annihilate, demolish, destroy, overthrow, overwhelm, ruin; abash, confuse, discompose, disconcert, mortify, shame.

confront *vb* face; challenge, contrapose, encounter, oppose, threaten.

confuse *vb* blend, confound, intermingle, mingle, mix; derange, disarrange, disorder, jumble, mess, muddle; darken, obscure, perplex; befuddle, bewilder, embarrass, flabbergast, flurry, fluster, mystify, nonplus, pose; abash, confound, discompose, disconcert, mortify, shame.

confusion *n* anarchy, chaos, clutter, confusedness, derangement, disarrangement, disarray, disorder, jumble, muddle; agitation, commotion, ferment, stir, tumult, turmoil; astonishment, bewilderment, distraction, embarrassment, fluster, fuddle, perplexity; abashment, discomfiture, mortification, shame; annihilation, defeat, demolition, destruction, overthrow, ruin.

confute *vb* disprove, oppugn, overthrow, refute, silence.

congeal *vb* benumb, condense, curdle, freeze, stiffen, thicken.

congenial *adj* kindred, similar, sympathetic; adapted, agreeable, natural, suitable, suited; agreeable, favourable, genial.

congenital *adj* connate, connatural, inborn.

congeries *n* accumulation, agglomeration, aggregate, aggregation, collection, conglomeration, crowd, cluster, heap, mass.

congratulate *vb* compliment, felicitate, gratulate, greet, hail, salute.

congregate *vb* assemble, collect, convene, convoke, gather, muster; gather, meet, swarm, throng.

congregation *n* assemblage, assembly, collection, gathering, meeting.

congress *n* assembly, conclave, conference, convention, convocation, council, diet, meeting.

congruity *n* agreement, conformity, consistency, fitness, suitableness.

congruous *adj* accordant, agreeing, compatible, consistent, consonant, suitable; appropriate, befitting, fit, meet, proper, seemly.

conjecture *vb* assume, guess, hypothesize, imagine, suppose, surmise, suspect; dare say, fancy, presume. • *n* assumption, guess, hypothesis, supposition, surmise, theory.

conjoin *vb* associate, combine, connect, join, unite.

conjugal *adj* bridal, connubial, hymeneal, matrimonial, nuptial.

conjunction *n* combination, concurrence, connection; crisis, emergency, exigency, juncture.

conjure *vb* adjure, beg, beseech, crave, entreat, implore, invoke, pray, supplicate; bewitch, charm, enchant, fascinate; juggle.

connect *vb* associate, conjoin, combine, couple, hyphenate, interlink, join, link, unite; cohere, interlock.

connected *adj* associated, coupled, joined, united; akin, allied, related; communicating.

connection *n* alliance, association, dependence, junction, union; commerce, communication, intercourse; affinity, relationship; kindred, kinsman, relation, relative.

connive *vb* collude, conspire, plot, scheme.

connoisseur *n* critic, expert, virtuoso.

connotation *n* comprehension, depth, force, intent, intention, meaning.

connubial *adj* bridal, conjugal, hymeneal, matrimonial nuptial.

conquer *vb* beat, checkmate, crush, defeat, discomfit, humble, master, overcome, overpower, overthrow, prevail, quel l, reduce, rout, subdue, subjugate, vanquish; overcome, surmount.

conqueror *n* humbler, subduer, subjugator, vanquisher; superior, victor, winner.

conquest *n* defeat, discomfiture, mastery, overthrow, reduction, subjection, subjugation; triumph, victor; winning.

consanguinity *n* affinity, kinship, blood-relationship, kin, kindred, relationship.

conscientious *adj* careful, exact, fair, faithful, high-principled, honest, honourable, incorruptible, just, scrupulous, straight-forward, uncorrupt, upright.

conscious *adj* intelligent, knowing, percipient, sentient; intellectual, rational, reasoning, reflecting, self-conscious, thinking; apprised, awake, aware, cognizant, percipient, sensible; self-admitted, self-accusing.

consecrate *vb* dedicate, devote, ordain; hallow, sanctify, venerate.

consecutive *adj* following, succeeding.

consent *vb* agree, allow, assent, concur, permit, yield; accede, acquiesce, comply. • *n* approval, assent, concurrence. permission; accord, agreement, consensus, concord, cooperation, harmony, unison; acquiescence, compliance.

consequence *n* effect, end, event, issue, result; conclusion, deduction, inference; concatenation, connection, consecution; concern, distinction, importance. influence, interest, moment, standing, weight.

consequential *adj* consequent, following, resulting, sequential; arrogant, conceited, inflated, pompous, pretentious, self-important, self-sufficient, vainglorious.

conservation *n* guardianship, maintenance, preservation, protection.

conservative *adj* conservatory, moderate, moderationist; preservative; reactionary, unprogressive. • *n* die-hard, reactionary, redneck, rightist, right-winger; moderate; preservative.

conserve *vb* keep, maintain, preserve, protect, save, sustain, uphold. • *n* confit, confection, jam, preserve, sweetmeat.

consider *vb* attend, brood, contemplate, examine, heed, mark, mind, ponder, reflect, revolve, study, weigh; care for, consult, envisage, regard, respect; cogitate, deliberate, mediate, muse, ponder, reflect, ruminate, think; account, believe, deem, hold, judge, opine.

considerate *adj* circumspect, deliberate, discrete, judicious, provident, prudent, serious, sober, staid, thoughtful; charitable, forbearing, patient.

consideration *n* attention, cogitation, contemplation, deliberation, notice, heed, meditation, pondering, reflection, regard; consequence, importance, important, moment, significant, weight; account, cause, ground, motive, reason, sake, score.

consign *vb* deliver, hand over, remand, resign, transfer, transmit; commit, entrust; ship.

consignor *n* sender, shipper, transmitter.

consistency *n* compactness, consistence, density, thickness; agreement, compatibility, conformableness, congruity, consonance, correspondence, harmony.

consistent *adj* accordant, agreeing, comfortable, compatible, congruous, consonant, correspondent, harmonious, logical.

consolation *n* alleviation, comfort, condolence, encouragement, relief, solace.

console *vb* assuage, calm, cheer, comfort, encourage, solace, relieve, soothe.

consolidate *vb* cement, compact, compress, condense, conduce, harden, solidify, thicken; combine, conjoin, fuse, unite.

consolidation *n* solidification; combination, union.

consonance *n* accord, concord, conformity, harmony; accord, accordance, agreement, congruence, congruity, consistency, unison.

consonant *adj* accordant, according, harmonious; compatible, congruous, consistent. • *n* articulation, letter-sound.

consort *vb* associate, fraternize. • *n* associate, companion, fellow, husband, spouse, partner.

conspectus *n* abstract, brief, breviary, compend, compendium, digest, epitome, outline, precis, summary, syllabus, synopsis.

conspicuous *adj* apparent, clear, discernible, glaring, manifest, noticeable, perceptible. plain, striking, visible; celebrated, distinguished, eminent, famed, famous, illustrious, marked, noted, outstanding. pre-eminent, prominent, remarkable, signal.

conspiracy *n* cabal, collusion, confederation, intrigue, league, machination, plot, scheme.

conspire *vb* concur, conduce, cooperate; combine, compass, contrive, devise, project; confederate, contrive, hatch, plot, scheme.

constancy *n* immutability, permanence, stability, unchangeableness; regularity, unchangeableness; decision, determination, firmness, inflexibility, resolution, steadfastness, steadiness; devotion, faithfulness, fidelity, loyalty, trustiness, truth.

constant *adj* abiding, enduring, fixed, immutable, invariable, invariant, permanent, perpetual, stable, unalterable, unchanging, unvaried; certain, regular, stated, uniform; determined, firm, resolute, stanch, stead fast, steady, unanswering, undeviating, unmoved, unshaken, unwavering; assiduous, diligent, persevering, sedulous, tenacious, unremitting; continual, continuous, incessant, perpetual, sustained, unbroken, uninterrupted; devoted, faithful, loyal, true, trusty.

consternation *n* alarm, amazement, awe, bewilderment, dread, fear, fright, horror, panic, terror.

constituent *adj* component, composing, constituting, forming; appointing, electoral. • *n* component, element, ingredient, principal; elector, voter.

constitute *vb* compose, form, make; appoint, delegate, depute, empower, enact, establish, fix, set up.

constitution *n* establishment, formation, make-up, organization, structure; character, characteristic, disposition, form, habit, humour, peculiarity, physique, quality, spirit, temper, temperament.

constitutional *adj* congenital, connate, inborn, inbred, inherent, innate, natural, organic; lawful, legal, legitimate. • *n* airing, exercise, promenade, stretch, walk.

constrain *vb* coerce, compel, drive, force; chain, confine, curb, enthral, hold, restrain; draw, impel, urge.

constriction *n* compression, constraint, contraction.

construct *vb* build, fabricate, erect, raise, set up; arrange, establish, form, found, frame, institute, invent, make, organize, originate.

construction *n* building erection, fabrication; configuration, conformation, figure, form, formation, made. shape, structure; explanation, interpretation, rendering, version.

construe *vb* analyse, explain, expound, interpret, parse, render, translate.

consult *vb* advise, ask, confer, counsel, deliberate, interrogate, question; consider, regard.

consume *vb* absorb, decay, destroy, devour, dissipate, exhaust, expend, lavish, lessen, spend, squander, vanish, waste.

consummate[1] *vb* accomplish, achieve, compass, complete, conclude, crown, effect, effectuate, end, execute, finish, perfect, perform.

consummate[2] *adj* complete, done, effected, finished, fulfilled, perfect, supreme.

consumption *n* decay, decline, decrease, destruction, diminution, expenditure, use, waste; atrophy, emaciation.

contact *vb* hit, impinge, touch; approach, be heard, communicate with, reach. • *n* approximation, contiguity, junction, juxtaposition, taction, tangency, touch.

contagion *n* infection; contamination, corruption, infection, taint.

contagious *adj* catching, epidemic, infectious; deadly, pestiferous, pestilential. poisonous.

contain *vb* accommodate, comprehend, comprise, embody, embrace, enclose, include; check, restrain.

contaminate *vb* corrupt, defile, deprave, infect, poison, pollute, soil, stain, sully, taint, tarnish, vitiate.

contamination *n* contaminating, defilement, defiling, polluting, pollution; abomination, defilement, impurity, foulness, infection, pollution, stain, taint, uncleanness.

contemn *vb* despise, disdain, disregard, neglect, scorn, scout, slight, spurn.

contemplate *vb* behold, gaze upon, observe, survey; consider, dwell on, meditate on, muse on, ponder, reflect upon, study, survey, think about; design, intend, mean, plan, purpose.

contemplation *n* cogitation, deliberation, meditation, pondering, reflection, speculation, study, thought; prospect, prospective, view; expectation.

contemporaneous *adj* coetaneous, coeval, coexistent, coexisting, coincident, concomitant, contemporary, simultaneous, synchronous.

contemporary *adj* coetaneous, coeval, coexistent, coexisting, coincident, concomitant, concurrent, contemporaneous, current, present, simultaneous, synchronous; advanced, modern, modernistic, progressive, up-to-date. • *n* coeval, coexistent, compeer, fellow.

contempt *n* contumely, derision, despite, disdain, disregard, misprision, mockery, scorn, slight.

contemptible *adj* abject, base, despicable, haughty, insolent, insulting, low, mean, paltry, pitiful, scurvy, sorry, supercilious, vile, worthless.

contemptuous *adj* arrogant, contumelious, disdainful, haughty, insolent, insulting, scornful, sneering, supercilious.

contend *vb* battle, combat, compete, contest, fight, strive, struggle, vie; argue, debate, dispute, litigate; affirm, assert, contest, maintain.

content[1] *n* essence, gist, meaning, meat, stuff, substance; capacity, measure, space, volume.

content[2] *vb* appease, delight, gladden, gratify, humour, indulge, please, satisfy, suffice. • *adj* agreeable, contented, happy, pleased, satisfied. • *n* contentment, ease, peace, satisfaction.

contention *n* discord, dissension, feud, squabble, strife, quarrel, rapture, wrangle, wrangling; altercation, bickering, contest, controversy, debate, dispute, litigation, logomachy.

contentious *adj* belligerent, cross, litigious, peevish, perverse, petulant, pugnacious, quarrelsome, wrangling; captious, caviling, disputatious.

conterminous *adj* adjacent, adjoining, contiguous; co-extensive, coincident, commensurate.

contest *vb* argue, contend, controvert, debate, dispute, litigate, question; strive, struggle; compete, cope, fight, vie. • *n* altercation, contention, controversy, difference, dispute, debate, quarrel; affray, battle, bout, combat, conflict, encounter, fight, match, scrimmage, struggle, tussle; competition, contention, rivalry.

contexture *n* composition, constitution, framework, structure, texture.

contiguous *adj* abutting, adjacent, adjoining, beside, bordering, conterminous, meeting, near, neighbouring, touching.

continent[1] *n* mainland, mass, tract.

continent[2] *adj* abstemious, abstinent, chaste, restrained, self-commanding, self-controlled, moderate, sober, temperate.

contingency *n* accidentalness, chance, fortuity, uncertainty; accident, casualty, event, incident, occurrence.

contingent *adj* accidental, adventitious, casual, fortuitous, incidental; conditional, dependent, uncertain. • *n* proportion, quota, share.

continual *adj* constant, constant, perpetual, unceasing, uninterrupted, unremitting; endless, eternal, everlasting, interminable, perennial, permanent, perpetual, unending; constant, oft-repeated.

continuance *n* abiding, continuation, duration, endurance, lasting, persistence, stay; continuation, extension, perpetuation, prolongation, protraction; concatenation, connection, sequence, succession; constancy, endurance, perseverance, persistence.

continue *vb* endure, last, remain; abide, linger, remain, stay, tarry; endure, persevere, persist, stick; extend, prolong, perpetuate, protract.

continuous *adj* connected, continued, extended, prolonged, unbroken, unintermitted, uninterrupted.

contour *n* outline, profile.

contraband *adj* banned, forbidden, illegal, illicit, interdicted, prohibited, smuggled, unlawful.

contract *vb* abbreviate, abridge, condense, confine, curtail, diminish, epitomize, lessen, narrow, reduce, shorten; absorb, catch, incur, get, make, take; constrict, shrink, shrivel, wrinkle; agree, bargain, covenant, engage, pledge, stipulate. • *n* agreement, arrangement, bargain, bond, compact, concordat, covenant, convention, engagement, pact, stipulation, treaty.

contradict *vb* assail, challenge, controvert, deny, dispute, gainsay, impugn, traverse; abrogate, annul, belie, counter, disallow, negative, contravene, counteract, oppose, thwart.

contradiction *n* controversion, denial, gainsaying; antinomy, clashing, contrariety, incongruity, opposition.

contradictory *adj* antagonistic, contrary, incompatible, inconsistent, negating, opposed, opposite, repugnant.

contrariety *n* antagonism, clashing, contradiction, contrast, opposition, repugnance.

contrary *adj* adverse, counter, discordant, opposed, opposing, opposite; antagonistic, conflicting, contradictory, repugnant, retroactive; forward, headstrong, obstinate, refractory, stubborn, unruly, wayward, perverse. • *n* antithesis, converse, obverse, opposite, reverse.

contrast *vb* compare, differentiate, distinguish, oppose. • *n* contrariety, difference, opposition; comparison, distinction.

contravene *vb* abrogate, annul, contradict, counteract, countervail, cross, go against, hinder, interfere, nullify, oppose, set aside, thwart.

contravention *n* abrogation, contradiction, interference, opposition, transgression, traversal, violation.

contretemps *n* accident, mischance, mishap.

contribute *vb* bestow, donate, give, grant, subscribe; afford, aid, furnish, supply; concur, conduce, conspire, cooperate, minister, serve, tend.

contribution *n* bestowal, bestowment, grant; donation, gift, offering, subscription.

contrite *adj* humble, penitent, repentant, sorrowful.

contrition *n* compunction, humiliation, penitence, regret, remorse, repentance, self-condemnation, self-reproach, sorrow.

contrivance *n* design, inventive, inventiveness; contraption, device, gadget, invention, machine; artifice, device, fabrication, machination, plan, plot, scheme, shift, stratagem.

contrive *vb* arrange, brew, concoct, design, devise, effect, form, frame, hatch, invent, plan, project; consider, plan, plot, scheme; manage, make out.

control *vb* command, direct, dominate, govern, manage, oversee, sway, regulate, rule, superintend; bridle, check, counteract, curb, check, hinder, repress, restrain. • *n* ascendency, command, direction, disposition, dominion, government, guidance, mastery, oversight, regiment, regulation, rule, superintendence, supremacy, sway.

controversy *n* altercation, argument, contention, debate, discussion, disputation, dispute, logomachy, polemics, quarrel, strife; lawsuit.

contumacious *adj* disobedient, cross-grained, disrespectful, haughty, headstrong, intractable, obdurate, obstinate, pertinacious, perverse, rebellious, refractory, stiff-necked, stubborn.

contumacy *n* doggedness, haughtiness, headiness, obduracy, obstinacy, pertinacity, perverseness, stubbornness; contempt, disobedience, disrespect, insolence, insubordination, rebelliousness.

contumelious *adj* abusive, arrogant, calumnious, contemptuous, disdainful, insolent, insulting, opprobrious, overbearing, rude, scornful, supercilious.

contumely *n* abuse, affront, arrogance, contempt, contemptuousness, disdain, indignity, insolence, insult, obloquy, opprobrium, reproach, rudeness, scorn, superciliousness.

contuse *vb* bruise, crush, injure, knock, squeeze, wound.

contusion *n* bruise, crush, injury, knock, squeeze, wound.

convalescence *n* recovery, recuperation.

convene *vb* assemble, congregate, gather, meet, muster; assemble, call, collect, convoke, muster, summon.

convenience *n* fitness, propriety, suitableness; accessibility, accommodation, comfort, commodiousness, ease, handiness, satisfaction, serviceability, serviceableness.

convenient *adj* adapted, appropriate, fit, fitted, proper, suitable, suited; advantageous, beneficial, comfortable, commodious, favourable, handy, helpful, serviceable, timely, useful.

convent *n* abbey, cloister, monastery, priory.

convention *n* assembly, congress, convocation, meeting; agreement, bargain, compact, contract, pact, stipulation, treaty; custom, formality, usage.

conventional *adj* agreed on, bargained for, stipulated; accustomed, approved, common, customary, everyday, habitual, ordinary, orthodox, regular, standard, traditional, usual, wonted.

conversable *adj* affable, communicative, free, open, sociable, social, unreversed.

conversation *n* chat, colloquy, communion, confabulation, conference, converse, dialogue, discourse, intercourse, interlocution, parley, talk.

converse[1] *vb* commune; chat, confabulate, discourse, gossip, parley, talk. • *n* commerce, communication, intercourse; colloquy, conversation, talk.

converse[2] *adj* adverse, contradictory, contrary, counter, opposed, opposing, opposite; *n* antithesis, contrary, opposite, reverse.

conversion *n* change, reduction, resolution, transformation, transmutation; interchange, reversal, transposition.

convert *vb* alter, change, transform, transmute; interchange, reverse, transpose; apply, appropriate, convince. • *n* catechumen, disciple, neophyte, proselyte.

convey *vb* bear, bring, carry, fetch, transmit, transport, waft; abalienate, alienate, cede, consign, deliver, demise, devise, devolve, grant, sell, transfer.

conveyance *n* alienation, cession, transfer, transference, transmission; carriage, carrying, conveying, transfer, transmission.

convict *vb* condemn, confute, convince, imprison, sentence. • *n* criminal, culprit, felon, malefactor, prisoner.

convivial *adj* festal, festive, gay, jolly, jovial, merry, mirthful, social.

convocation *n* assembling, convening, convoking, gathering, summoning; assembly, congress, convention, council, diet, meeting, synod.

convoke *vb* assemble, convene, muster, summon.

convoy *vb* accompany, attend, escort, guard, protect. • *n* attendance, attendant, escort, guard, protection.

convulse *vb* agitate, derange, disorder, disturb, shake, shatter.

convulsion *n* cramp, fit, spasm; agitation, commotion, disturbance, shaking, tumult.

cook *vb* bake, boil, broil, fry, grill, microwave, roast, spit-roast, steam, stir-fry; falsify, garble.

cool *vb* chill, ice, refrigerate; abate, allay, calm, damp, moderate, quiet, temper. • *adj* calm, collected, composed, dispassionate, placid, sedate, self-possessed, quiet, staid, unexcited, unimpassioned, undisturbed, unruffled; cold-blooded, indifferent, lukewarm, unconcerned; apathetic, chilling, freezing, frigid, repellent; bold, impertinent, impudent, self-possessed, shameless. • *n* chill, chilliness, coolness; calmness, composure, coolheadedness, countenance, equanimity, poise, self-possession, self-restraint.

coop *vb* cage, confine, encage, immure, imprison. • *n* barrel, box, cage, pen.

cooperate *vb* abet, aid, assist, co-act, collaborate, combine, concur, conduce, conspire, contribute, help, unite.

cooperation *n* aid, assistance, co-action, concert, concurrence, collaboration, synergy.

coordinate *vb* accord, agree, arrange, equalize, harmonize, integrate, methodize, organize, regulate, synchronize, systematize. • *adj* coequal, equal, equivalent, tantamount; coincident, synchronous. • *n* complement, counterpart, like, pendant; companion, fellow, match, mate.

copartnership *n* association, fraternity, partnership; company, concern, establishment, firm, house.

cope *vb* combat, compete, contend, encounter, engage, strive, struggle, vie.

copious *adj* abundant, ample, exuberant, full, overflowing, plenteous, plentiful, profuse, rich.

copiousness *n* abundance, exuberance, fullness, plenty, profusion, richness.

copse *n* coppice, grove, thicket.

copulation *n* coition, congress, coupling.

copy *vb* duplicate, reproduce, trace, transcribe; follow, imitate, pattern. • *n* counterscript, duplicate, facsimile, off-print, replica, reproduction, transcript; archetype, model, original, pattern; manuscript, typescript.

cord *n* braid, gimp, line, string.

cordate *adj* cordiform, heart-shaped.

cordial *adj* affectionate, ardent, earnest, heartfelt, hearty sincere, warm, warm-hearted; grateful, invigorating, restorative, pleasant, refreshing. • *n* balm, balsam, elixir, tisane, tonic; liqueur.

core *n* centre, essence, heart, kernel.

corner *vb* confound, confuse, nonplus, perplex, pose, puzzle. • *n* angle, bend, crutch, cusp, elbow, joint, knee; niche, nook, recess, retreat.

corollary *n* conclusion, consequence, deduction, induction, inference.

coronal *n* bays, chaplet, crown, garland, laurel, wreath.

corporal *adj* bodily; corporeal, material, physical.

corporeal *adj* bodily, fleshly, substantial; corporal, material, nonspiritual, physical.

corps *n* band, body, company, contingent, division, platoon, regiment, squad, squadron, troop.

corpse *n* body, carcass, corse, remains; ashes, dust.

corpulent *adj* big, burly, fat, fleshy, large, lusty, obese, plump, portly, pursy, rotund, stout.

corpuscle *n* atom, bit, grain, iota, jot, mite, molecule, monad, particle, scintilla, scrap, whit.

correct *vb* adjust, amend, cure, improve, mend, reclaim, rectify, redress, reform, regulate, remedy; chasten, discipline, punish. • *adj* accurate, equitable, exact, faultless, just, precise, proper, regular, right, true, upright.

correction *n* amendment, improvement, redress; chastening, discipline, punishment.

corrective *adj* alternative, correctory, counteractive, emendatory, improving, modifying, rectifying, reformative, reformatory.

correctness *n* accuracy, exactness, faultlessness, nicety, precision, propriety, rectitude, regularity, rightness, truth.

correlate *n* complement, correlative, counterpart.

correspond *vb* accord, agree, answer, comport, conform, fit, harmonize, match, square, suit, tally; answer, belong, correlate; communicate.

correspondence *n* accord, agreement, coincidence, concurrence, conformity, congruity, fitness, harmony, match; correlation, counterposition; communication, letters, writing.

corroborate *vb* confirm, establish, ratify, substantiate, support, sustain, strengthen.

corrode *vb* canker, erode, gnaw; consume, deteriorate, rust, waste; blight, embitter, envenom, poison.

corrosive *adj* acrid, biting, consuming, cathartic, caustic, corroding, eroding, erosive, violent; consuming, corroding, gnawing, mordant, wasting, wearing; blighting, cankerous, carking, embittering, envenoming, poisoning.

corrugate *vb* cockle, crease, furrow, groove, pucker, rumple, wrinkle.

corrupt *vb* putrefy, putrid, render; contaminate, defile, infect, pollute, spoil, taint, vitiate; degrade, demoralize, deprave, pervert; adulterate, debase, falsify, sophisticate; bribe, entice. • *adj* contaminated, corrupted, impure, infected, putrid, rotten, spoiled, tainted, unsound; abandoned, debauched, depraved, dissolute, profligate, reprobate, vicious, wicked; bribable, buyable.

corruption *n* putrefaction, putrescence, rottenness; adulteration, contamination, debasement, defilement, infection, perversion, pollution, vitiation; demoralization, depravation, depravity, immorality, laxity, sinfulness, wickedness; bribery, dishonesty.

corsair *n* buccaneer, picaroon, pirate, rover, sea-robber, sea-rover.

corset *n* bodice, girdle, stays.

cosmonaut *n* astronaut, spaceman.

cosmos *n* creation, macrocosm, universe, world; harmony, order, structure.

cost *vb* absorb, consume, require. • *n* amount, charge, expenditure, expense, outlay, price; costliness, preciousness, richness, splendour, sumptuousness; damage, detriment, loss, pain, sacrifice, suffering.

costly *adj* dear, expensive, high-priced; gorgeous, luxurious, precious, rich, splendid, sumptuous, valuable.

costume *n* apparel, attire, dress, robes, uniform.

cosy, cozy *adj* comfortable, easy, snug; chatty, conversable, social, talkative.

coterie *n* association, brotherhood, circle, club, set, society, sodality.

cottage *n* cabin, chalet, cot, hut, lodge, shack, shanty.

couch *vb* lie, recline; crouch, squat; bend down, stoop; conceal, cover up, hide; lay, level. • *n* bed, davenport, divan, lounge, seat, settee, settle, sofa.

council *n* advisers, cabinet, ministry; assembly, congress, conclave, convention, convocation, diet, husting, meeting, parliament, synod.

counsel *vb* admonish, advise, caution, recommend, warm. • *n* admonition, advice, caution, instruction, opinion, recommendation, suggestion; deliberation, forethought; advocate, barrister, counsellor, lawyer.

count *vb* enumerate, number, score; calculate, cast, compute, estimate, reckon; account, consider, deem, esteem, hold, judge, regard, think; tell. • *n* reckoning, tally.

countenance *vb* abet, aid, approve, assist, befriend, encourage, favour, patronize, sanction, support. • *n* aspect, look, men; aid, approbation, approval, assistance, encouragement, favour, patronage, sanction, support.

counter[1] *n* abacus, calculator, computer, meter, reckoner, tabulator, totalizator; bar, buffet, shopboard, table; (*naut*) end, poop, stern, tail; chip, token.

counter[2] *vb* contradict, contravene, counteract, oppose, retaliate. • *adj* adverse, against, contrary, opposed, opposite. • *adv* contrariwise, contrary. • *n* antithesis, contrary, converse, opposite, reverse; counterblast, counterblow, retaliation.

counteract *vb* check, contrapose, contravene, cross, counter, counterpose, defeat, foil, frustrate, hinder, oppose, resist, thwart, traverse; annul, countervail, counterbalance, destroy, neutralize, offset.

counteractive *adj* antidote, corrective, counteragent, medicine, remedy, restorative.

counterbalance *vb* balance, counterpoise; compensate, countervail.

counterfeit *vb* forge, imitate; fake, feign, pretend, sham, simulate; copy, imitate. • *adj* fake, forged, fraudulent, spurious, supposititious; false, feigned, hypocritical, mock, sham, simulated, spurious; copied, imitated, resembling. • *n* copy, fake, forgery, sham.

countermand *vb* abrogate, annul, cancel, recall, repeal, rescind, revoke.

counterpane *n* coverlet, duvet, quilt.

counterpart *n* copy, duplicate; complement, correlate, correlative, reverse, supplement; fellow, mate, match, tally, twin.

counterpoise *vb* balance, counteract, countervail, counterbalance, equilibrate, offset. • *n* balance, counterweight.

countersign *n* password, watchword.

countervail *vb* balance, compensate, counterbalance.

country *n* land, region; countryside; fatherland, home, kingdom, state, territory; nation, people, population. • *adj* rural, rustic; countrified, rough, rude, uncultivated, unpolished, unrefined.

countryman *n* compatriot, fellow-citizen; boor, clown, farmer, hind, husbandman, peasant, rustic, swain.

couple *vb* pair, unite; copulate, embrace; buckle, clasp, conjoin, connect, join, link, pair, yoke. • *n* brace, pair, twain, two; bond, coupling, lea, link, tie.

courage *n* audaciousness, audacity, boldness, bravery, daring, derring-do, dauntlessness, fearlessness, firmness, fortitude, gallantry, hardihood, heroism, intrepidity, manhood, mettle, nerve, pluck, prowess, resolution, spirit, spunk, valorousness, valour.

courageous *adj* audacious, brave, bold, chivalrous, daring, dauntless, fearless, gallant, hardy, heroic, intrepid, lion-hearted, mettlesome, plucky, resolute, reliant, staunch, stout, undismayed, valiant, valorous.

course *vb* chase, follow, hunt, pursue, race, run. • *n* career, circuit, race, run; road, route, track, way; bearing, direction, path, tremor, track; ambit, beat, orbit, round; process, progress, sequence; order, regularity, succession, turn; behaviour, conduct, deportment; arrangement, series, system.

court *vb* coddle, fawn, flatter, ingratiate; address, woo; seek; invite, solicit. • *n* area, courtyard, patio, quadrangle; addresses, civilities, homage, respects, solicitations; retinue, palace, tribunal.

courteous *adj* affable, attentive, ceremonious, civil, complaisant, courtly, debonair, elegant, gracious, obliging, polished, polite, refined, respected, urbane, well-bred, well-mannered.

courtesan *n* harlot, prostitute, strumpet, vamp, wanton, wench, whore.

courtesy *n* affability, civility, complaisance, courteousness, elegance, good-breeding, graciousness, polish, politeness, refine, urbanity.

courtly *adj* affable, ceremonious, civil, elegant, flattering, lordly, obliging, polished, polite, refined, urbane.

courtyard *n* area, court, patio, quadrangle, yard.

cove[1] *n* anchorage, bay, bight, creek, firth, fjord, inlet.

cove[2] *n* bloke, chap, character, customer, fellow, type.

covenant *vb* agree, bargain, contract, stipulate. • *n* bond, deed; arrangement, bargain, compact, concordat, contract, convention, pact, stipulation, treaty.

cover *vb* overlay, overspread; cloak, conceal, curtain, disguise, hide, mask, screen, secrete, shroud, veil; defend, guard, protect, shelter, shield; case, clothe, envelop, invest, jacket, sheathe; comprehend, comprise, contain, embody, embrace, include. • *n* capsule, case, covering, integument, tegument, top; cloak, disguise, screen, veil; guard, defence, protection, safeguard, shelter, shield; shrubbery, thicket, underbrush, undergrowth, underwood, woods.

covert *adj* clandestine, concealed, disguised, hidden, insidious, private, secret, sly, stealthy, underhand. • *n* coppice, shade, shrubbery, thicket, underwood; asylum; defence, harbour, hiding-place, refuge, retreat, sanctuary, shelter.

covet *vb* aim after, desire, long for, yearn for; hanker after, lust after.

covetous *adj* acquisitive, avaricious, close-fisted, grasping, greedy, miserly, niggardly, parsimonious, penurious, rapacious.

cow[1] *n* bovine, heifer.

cow[2] *vb* abash, break, daunt, discourage, dishearten, frighten, intimidate, overawe, subdue.

coward *adj* cowardly, timid. • *n* caitiff, craven, dastard, milksop, poltroon, recreant, skulker, sneak, wheyface.

cowardly *adj* base, chicken-hearted, coward, craven, dastardly, faint-hearted, fearful, lily-livered, mean, pusillanimous, timid, timorous, white-livered, yellow.

cower *vb* bend, cringe, crouch, fawn, shrink, squat, stoop.

coxcomb *n* beau, dandy, dude, exquisite, fop, jackanapes, popinjay, prig.

coy *adj* backward, bashful, demure, diffident, distant, modest, reserved, retiring, self-effacing, shrinking, shy, timid.

coyness *n* affectation, archness, backwardness, bashfulness, coquettishness, demureness, diffidence, evasiveness, modesty, primness, reserve, shrinking, shyness, timidity.

cozen *vb* beguile, cheat, chouse, circumvent, deceive, defraud, diddle, dupe, gull, overreach, swindle, trick, victimize.

cozy *see* **cosy.**

crabbed *adj* acrid, rough, sore, tart; acrimonious, cantankerous, captious, caustic, censorious, churlish, cross, growling, harsh, ill-tempered, morose, peevish, petulant, snappish, snarling, splenetic, surly, testy, touchy, waspish; difficult, intractable, perplexing, tough, trying, unmanageable.

crabbedness *n* acridity, acridness, roughness, sourness, tartness; acerbity, acrimonious, asperity, churlishness, harshness, ill-tempered, moodiness, moroseness, sullenness; difficulty, intractability, perplexity.

crack *vb* break, chop, cleave, split; snap; craze, madden; boast, brag, bluster, crow, gasconade, vapour, vaunt. • *adj* capital, excellent, first-class, first-rate, tip-top. • *n* breach, break, chink, cleft, cranny, crevice, fissure, fracture, opening, rent, rift, split; burst, clap, explosion, pop, report; snap.

cracked *adj* broken, crackled, split; crack-brained, crazed, crazy, demented, deranged, flighty, insane.

crackle *vb* crepitate, decrepitate, snap.

craft *n* ability, aptitude, cleverness, dexterity, expertness, power, readiness, skill, tact, talent; artifice, artfulness, cunning, craftiness, deceitfulness, deception, guile, shrewdness, subtlety; art, avocation, business, calling, employment, handicraft, trade, vocation; vessel.

crafty *adj* arch, artful, astute, cunning, crooked, deceitful, designing, fraudulent, guileful, insidious, intriguing, scheming, shrewd, sly, subtle, tricky, wily.

crag *n* rock; neck, throat.

craggy *adj* broken, cragged, jagged, rough, rugged, scraggy, uneven.

cram *vb* fill, glut, gorge, satiate, stuff; compress, crowd, overcrowd, press, squeeze; coach, grind.

cramp *vb* convulse; check, clog, confine, hamper, hinder, impede, obstruct, restrain, restrict. • *n* convulsion, crick, spasm; check, restraint, restriction, obstruction.

crank *vb* bend, crankle, crinkle, turn, twist, wind. • *n* bend, quirk, turn, twist, winding.

cranny *n* breach, break, chink, cleft, crack, crevice, fissure, gap, hole, interstice, nook, opening, rift.

crapulous *adj* crapulent, drunk, drunken, inebriated, intoxicated, tipsy.

crash *vb* break, shatter, shiver, smash, splinter. • *adj* emergency, fast, intensive, rushed, speeded-up. • *n* clang, clash, collision concussion, jar.

crass *adj* coarse, gross, raw, thick, unabated, unrefined.

cravat *n* neckcloth, neckerchief, necktie.

crave *vb* ask, beg, beseech, entreat, implore, petition, solicit, supplicate; desire, hanker after, long for, need, want, yearn for.

craven *n* coward, dastard, milk-sop, poltroon, recreant. • *adj* cowardly, chicken-hearted, lily-livered, pusillanimous, yellow.

craving *n* hankering, hungering, longing, yearning.

craw *n* crop, gullet, stomach, throat.

craze *vb* bewilder, confuse, dement, derange, madden; disorder, impair, weaken. • *n* fashion, mania, mode, novelty.

crazy *adj* broken, crank, rickety, shaky, shattered, tottering; crack-brained, delirious, demented, deranged, distracted, idiotic, insane, lunatic, mad, silly.

create *vb* originate, procreate; cause, design, fashion, form, invent, occasion, produce; appoint, constitute, make.

creation *n* formation, invention, origination, production cosmos, universe; appointment, constitution, establishment, nomination.

creator *n* author, designer, inventor, fashioner, maker, originator; god.

creature *n* animal, beast, being, body, brute, man, person; dependant, hanger-on, minion, parasite, retainer, vassal; miscreant, wretch.

credence *n* acceptance, belief, confidence, credit, faith, reliance, trust.

credentials *npl* certificate, diploma, missive, passport, recommendation, testament, testimonial, title, voucher, warrant.

credibility *n* believability, plausibility, tenability, , trustworthiness.

credit *vb* accept, believe, trust; loan, trust. • *n* belief, confidence, credence, faith, reliance, trust; esteem, regard, reputableness, reputation; influence, power; honour, merit; loan, trust.

creditable *adj* estimable, honourable, meritorious, praiseworthy, reputable, respectable.

credulity *n* credulousness, gullibility, silliness, simplicity, stupidity.

credulous *adj* dupable, green, gullible, naive, over-trusting, trustful, uncritical, unsuspecting, unsuspicious.

creed *n* belief, confession, doctrine, dogma, opinion, profession, tenet.

creek *n* bay, bight, cove, fjord, inlet; rivulet, streamlet.

creep *vb* crawl; steal upon; cringe, fawn, grovel, insinuate. • *n* crawl, scrabble, scramble; fawner, groveller, sycophant, toady.

crenate *adj* indented, notched, scalloped.

crepitate *vb* crack, crackle, decrepitate, snap.

crest *n* comb, plume, topknot, tuft; apex, crown, head, ridge, summit, top; arms, badge, bearings.

crestfallen *adj* chap-fallen, dejected, depressed, despondent, discouraged, disheartened, dispirited, downcast, downhearted, low-spirited, melancholy, sad.

crevice *n* chink, cleft, crack, cranny, fissure, fracture, gap, hole, interstice, opening, rent, rift.

crew *n* company, complement, hands; company, corps, gang, horde, mob, party, posse, set, squad, team, throng.

crib *vb* cage, confine, encage, enclose, imprison; pilfer, purloin. • *n* manger, rack; bin, bunker; plagiarism, plunder, theft.

crick *vb* jar, rick, wrench, wrick. • *n* convulsion, cramp, jarring, spasm, rick, wrench, wrick.

crime *n* felony, misdeed, misdemeanour, offence, violation; delinquency, fault, guilt, iniquity, sin, transgression, unrighteousness, wickedness, wrong.

criminal *adj* culpable, felonious, flagitious, guilty, illegal, immoral, iniquitous, nefarious, unlawful, vicious, wicked, wrong. • *n* convict, culprit, delinquent, felon, malefactor, offender, sinner, transgressor.

criminate *vb* accuse, arraign, charge, convict, impeach, indict; implicate, involve.

crimp *vb* crisp, curl.

cringe *vb* bend, bow, cower, crouch, fawn, grovel, kneel, sneak, stoop, truckle.

cripple *vb* cramp, destroy, disable, enfeeble, impair, lame, maim, mutilate, paralyse, ruin, weaken.

crisis *n* acme, climax, height; conjuncture, emergency, exigency, juncture, pass, pinch, push, rub, strait, urgency.

crisp *adj* brittle, curled, friable, frizzled.

criterion *n* canon, gauge, measure, principle, proof, rule, standard, test, touchstone.

critic *n* arbiter, caviller, censor, connoisseur, judge, nit-picker, reviewer.

critical *adj* accurate, exact, nice; captious, carping, cavilling, censorious, exacting; crucial, decisive, determining, important, turning: dangerous, dubious, exigent, hazardous, imminent, momentous, precarious, ticklish.

criticism *n* analysis, animadversion, appreciation, comment, critique, evaluation, judgement, review, strictures.

criticize *vb* appraise, evaluate, examine, judge.

croak *vb* complain, groan, grumble, moan, mumble, repine; die.

crone *n* hag, witch.

crony *n* ally, associate, chum, friend, mate, mucker, pal.

crook *vb* bend, bow, curve, incurvate, turn, wind. • *n* bend, curvature, flexion, turn; artifice, machination, trick; criminal, thief, villain.

crooked *adj* angular, bent, bowed, curved, winding, zigzag; askew, aslant, awry, deformed, disfigured, distorted, twisted, wry; crafty, deceitful, devious, dishonest, dishonourable, fraudulent, insidious, intriguing, knavish, tricky, underhanded, unfair, unscrupulous.

crop *vb* gather, mow, pick pluck, reap; browse, nibble; clip, curtail lop, reduce, shorten. • *n* harvest, produce, yield.

cross *vb* intersect, pass over, traverse; hinder, interfere, obstruct, thwart; interbred, intermix. • *adj* transverse; cantankerous, captious, crabbed, churlish, crusty, cynical, fractious, fretful, grouchy, ill-natured, ill-tempered, irascible, irritable, morose, peevish, pettish, petulant, snappish, snarling, sour, spleeny, splenetic, sulky, sullen, surly, testy, touchy, waspish. • *n* crucifix, gibbet, rood; affliction, misfortune, trial, trouble, vexation; cross-breeding, hybrid, intermixture.

cross-grained *adj* cantankerous, headstrong, obdurate, peevish, perverse, refractory, stubborn, untractable, wayward.

crossing *n* intersection, overpass, traversing, under-pass.

crossways, crosswise *adv* across, over, transversely.

crotchet *n* caprice, fad, fancy, freak, quirk, vagary, whim, whimsy.

crouch *vb* cower, cringe fawn, truckle; crouch, kneel, stoop, squat; bow, curtsy, genuflect.

croup *n* buttocks, crupper, rump.

crow *vb* bluster, boast, brag, chuckle, exult, flourish, gasconade, swagger, triumph, vapour, vaunt.

crowd *vb* compress, cram, jam, pack, press; collect, congregate, flock, herd, huddle, swarm. • *n* assembly, company, concourse, flock, herd, horde, host, jam, multitude, press, throng; mob, pack, populace, rabble, rout.

crown *vb* adorn, dignify, honour; recompense, requite, reward; cap, complete, consummate, finish, perfect. • *n* bays, chaplet, coronal, coronet, garland, diadem, laurel, wreath; monarchy, royalty, sovereignty; diadem; dignity, honour, recompense, reward; apex, crest, summit, top.

crowning *adj* completing, consummating, dignifying, finishing, perfecting

crucial *adj* intersecting, transverse; critical, decisive, searching, severe, testing, trying.

crude *adj* raw, uncooked undressed, unworked; harsh, immature, rough, unripe; crass, coarse, unrefined; awkward, immature, indigestible, rude, uncouth, unpolished, unpremeditated.

cruel *adj* barbarous, blood-thirsty, dire, fell, ferocious, inexorable, hard-hearted, inhuman merciless, pitiless, relentless, ruthless, sanguinary, savage, truculent, uncompassionate, unfeeling, unmerciful, unrelenting; bitter, cold, hard, severe, sharp, unfeeling.

crumble *vb* bruise, crush, decay, disintegrate, perish, pound, pulverize, triturate.

crumple *vb* rumple, wrinkle.

crush *vb* bruise, compress, contuse, squash, squeeze; bray, comminute, crumble, disintegrate, mash; demolish, raze, shatter; conquer, overcome, overpower, overwhelm, quell, subdue.

crust *n* coat, coating, incrustation, outside, shell, surface.

crusty *adj* churlish, crabbed, cross, cynical, fretful, forward, morose, peevish, pettish, petulant, snappish, snarling, surly, testy, touchy, waspish; friable, hard, short.

cry *vb* call, clamour, exclaim; blubber, snivel, sob, wail, weep, whimper; bawl, bellow hoot, roar, shout, vociferate, scream, screech, squawk, squall, squeal, yell; announce, blazon, proclaim, publish. • *n* acclamation, clamour, ejaculation, exclamation, outcry, crying, lament, lamentation, plaint, weeping; bawl, bellow, howl, roar, scream, screech, shriek, yell; announcement, proclamation, publication.

crypt *n* catacomb, tomb, vault.

cuddle *vb* cosset, nestle, snuggle, squat; caress, embrace, fondle, hug, pet. • *n* caress, embrace, hug.

cudgel *vb* bang, baste, batter, beat, cane, drub, thrash, thump. • *n* bastinado, baton, bludgeon, club, shillelagh, stick, truncheon.

cue *vb* intimate, prompt remind, sign, signal. • *n* catchword, hint, intimation, nod, prompting, sign, signal, suggestion.

cuff *vb* beat, box, buffet knock, pummel, punch, slap, smack, strike, thump. • *n* blow, box, punch, slap, smack, strike, thump.

cul-de-sac *n* alley, dead end, impasse, pocket.

cull *vb* choose, elect, pick select; collect, gather, glean, pluck.

culmination *n* acme, apex, climax, completion, consummation, crown, summit, top, zenith.

culpability *n* blame, blameworthiness, criminality, culpableness, guilt, remissness, sinfulness.

culpable *adj* blameable, blameworthy, censurable, faulty, guilty, reprehensible, sinful, transgressive, wrong.

culprit *n* delinquent, criminal, evil-doer, felon, malefactor, offender.

cultivate *vb* farm, fertilize, till, work; civilize, develop, discipline, elevate, improve, meliorate, refine, train; investigate, prosecute, pursue, search, study; cherish, foster, nourish, patronize, promote.

culture *n* agriculture, cultivation, farming, husbandry, tillage; cultivation, elevation, improvement, refinement.

cumber *vb* burden, clog, encumber, hamper, impede, obstruct, oppress, overload; annoy, distract, embarrass, harass, perplex, plague, torment, trouble, worry.

cumbersome *adj* burdensome, clumsy, cumbrous, embarrassing, heavy, inconvenient, oppressive, troublesome, unmanageable, unwieldy, vexatious.

cuneiform *adj* cuneate, wedge-shaped.

cunning *adj* artful, astute, crafty, crooked, deceitful, designing, diplomatic, foxy, guileful, intriguing, machiavellian, sharp, shrewd, sly, subtle, tricky, wily; curious, ingenious. • *n* art, artfulness, artifice, astuteness, craft, shrewdness, subtlety; craftiness, chicane, chicanery, deceit, deception, intrigue, slyness.

cup *n* beaker, bowl, chalice, goblet, mug; cupful, draught, potion.

cupboard *n* buffet, cabinet, closet.

cupidity *n* avidity, greed, hankering, longing, lust; acquisitiveness, avarice, covetousness, greediness, stinginess.

curative *adj* healing, medicinal, remedial, restorative.

curator *n* custodian, guardian, keeper, superintendent.

curb *vb* bridle, check, control, hinder, moderate, repress, restrain. • *n* bridle, check, control, hindrance, rein, restraint.

cure *vb* alleviate, correct, heal, mend, remedy, restore; kipper, pickle, preserve. • *n* antidote, corrective, help, remedy, reparative, restorative, specific; alleviation, healing, restorative.

curiosity *n* interest, inquiringness, inquisitiveness; celebrity, curio, marvel, novelty, oddity, phenomenon, rarity, sight, spectacle, wonder.

curious *adj* interested, inquiring, inquisitive, meddling, peering, prying, scrutinizing; extraordinary, marvellous, novel, queer, rare, singular, strange, unique, unusual; cunning, elegant, fine, finished, neat, skilful, well-wrought.

curl *vb* coil, twist, wind, writhe; bend, buckle, ripple, wave. • *n* curlicue, lovelock, ringlet; flexure, sinuosity, undulation, wave, waving, winding.

curmudgeon *n* churl, lick-penny, miser, niggard, screw, scrimp, skinflint.

currency *n* publicity; acceptance, circulation, transmission; bills, coins, money, notes.

current *adj* common, general, popular, rife; circulating, passing; existing, instant, present, prevalent, widespread. • *n* course, progression, river, stream, tide, undertow. • *adv* commonly, generally, popularly, publicly.

curry *vb* comb, dress; beat, cudgel, drub, thrash.

curse *vb* anathematize, damn, denounce, execrate, imprecate, invoke, maledict; blast, blight, destroy, doom; afflict, annoy, harass, injure, plague, scourge, torment, vex; blaspheme, swear. • *n* anathema, ban, denunciation, execration, fulmination, imprecation, malediction, malison; affliction, annoyance, plague, scourge, torment, trouble, vexation; ban, condemnation, penalty, sentence.

cursed *adj* accursed, banned, blighted, curse-laden, unholy; abominable, detestable, execrable, hateful, villainous; annoying, confounded, plaguing, scourging, tormenting, troublesome, vexatious.

cursory *adj* brief, careless, desultory, hasty, passing, rapid, slight, summary, superficial, transient, transitory.

curt *adj* brief, concise, laconic, short, terse; crusty, rude, snappish, tart.

curtail *vb* abridge, dock, lop, retrench, shorten; abbreviate, contract, decrease, diminish, lessen.

curtain *vb* cloak, cover, drape, mantle, screen, shade, shield, veil. • *n* arras, drape, drop, portière, screen, shade.

curvature *n* arcuation, bend, bending, camber, crook, curve, flexure, incurvation.

curve *vb* bend, crook, inflect, turn, twist, wind. • *n* arcuation, bend, bending, camber, crook, flexure, incurvation.

curvet *vb* bound, leap, vault; caper, frisk.

cushion *vb* absorb, damp, dampen, deaden, dull, muffle, mute, soften, subdue, suppress; cradle, pillow, support. • *n* bolster, hassock, pad, pillow, woolsack.

cusp *n* angle, horn, point.

custodian *n* curator, guardian, keeper, sacristan, superintendent, warden.

custody *n* care, charge, guardianship, keeping, safe-keeping, protection, watch, ward; confinement, durance, duress, imprisonment, prison.

custom *n* consuetude, convention, fashion, habit, manner, mode, practice, rule, usage, use, way; form, formality, observation; patronage; duty, impost, tax, toll, tribute.

customary *adj* accustomed, common, consuetudinary, conventional, familiar, fashionable, general, habitual, gnomic, prescriptive, regular, usual, wonted.

cut *vb* chop, cleave, divide, gash, incise, lance, sever, slice, slit, wound; carve, chisel, sculpture; hurt, move, pierce, touch; ignore, slight; abbreviate, abridge, curtail, shorten. • *n* gash, groove, incision, nick, slash, slice, slit; channel, passage; piece, slice; fling, sarcasm, taunt; fashion, form, mode, shape, style.

cutthroat *adj* barbarous, cruel, ferocious, murderous; competitive, exacting, exorbitant, extortionate, rivalling, ruthless, usurious, vying. • *n* assassin, murderer, ruffian.

cutting *adj* keen, sharp; acid, biting, bitter, caustic, piercing, sarcastic, sardonic, satirical, severe, trenchant, wounding.

cycle *n* age, circle, era, period, revolution, round.

Cyclopean *adj* colossal, enormous, gigantic, Herculean, immense, vast.

cynical *adj* captious, carping, censorious, churlish, crabbed, cross, crusty, fretful, ill-natured, ill-tempered, morose, peevish, pettish, petulant, sarcastic, satirical, snappish, snarling, surly, testy, touchy, waspish; contemptuous, derisive, misanthropic, pessimistic, scornful.

cynosure *n* attraction, centre.

cyst *n* pouch, sac.

D

dab vb box, rap, slap, strike, tap touch; coat, daub, smear. • adj adept, expert, proficient; pat. • n lump, mass, pat.

dabble vb dip, moisten, soak, spatter, splash, sprinkle, wet; meddle, tamper, trifle.

daft adj absurd, delirious, foolish, giddy, idiotic, insane, silly, simple, stupid, witless; frolicsome, merry, mirthful, playful, sportive.

dagger n bayonet, dirk, poniard, stiletto.

dainty adj delicate, delicious, luscious, nice, palatable, savoury, tender, toothsome; beautiful, charming, choice, delicate, elegant, exquisite, fine, neat; fastidious, finical, finicky, over-nice, particular, scrupulous, squeamish. • n delicacy, titbit treat.

dale n bottom, dell, dingle, glen, vale, valley.

dalliance n caressing, endearments, flirtation, fondling

dally vb dawdle, fritter, idle, trifle, waste time; flirt, fondle, toy.

damage vb harm, hurt, impair, injure, mar. • n detriment, harm, hurt, injury, loss, mischief.

damages npl compensation, fine, forfeiture, indemnity, reparation, satisfaction.

dame n babe, baby, broad, doll, girl; lady, madam, matron, mistress.

damn vb condemn, doom, kill, ruin. • n bean, curse, fig, hoot, rap, sou, straw, whit.

damnable adj abominable, accursed, atrocious, cursed, detestable, hateful, execrable, odious, outrageous.

damp vb dampen, moisten; allay, abate, check, discourage, moderate, repress, restrain; chill, cool, deaden, deject, depress, dispirit. • adj dank, humid, moist, wet. • n dampness, dank, fog, mist, moisture, vapour; chill, dejection, depression.

damper n check, hindrance, impediment, obstacle; damp, depression, discouragement, wet blanket.

dandle vb amuse, caress, fondle, pet, toss; dance.

danger n jeopardy, insecurity, hazard, peril, risk, venture.

dangerous adj critical, hazardous, insecure, perilous, risky, ticklish, unsafe.

dangle vb drape, hang, pend, sway, swing; fawn.

dank adj damp, humid, moist, wet.

dapper adj active, agile, alert, brisk, lively, nimble, quick, ready, smart, spry; neat, nice, pretty, spruce, trim.

dapple vb diversify, spot, variegate. • adj dappled, spotted, variegated.

dare vb challenge, defy, endanger, hazard, provoke, risk. • n challenge, defiance, gage.

daring adj adventurous, bold, brave, chivalrous, courageous, dauntless, doughty, fearless, gallant, heroic, intrepid, valiant, valorous. • n adventurousness, boldness, bravery, courage, dauntlessness, doughtiness, fearlessness, intrepidity, undauntedness, valour.

dark adj black, cloudy, darksome, dusky, ebon, inky, lightless, lurid, moonless, murky, opaque, overcast, pitchy, rayless, shady, shadowy, starless, sunless, swart, tenebrous, umbrageous, unenlightened, unilluminated; abstruse, cabbalistic, enigmatical, incomprehensible, mysterious, mystic, mystical, obscure, occult, opaque, recondite, transcendental, unillumined, unintelligible; cheerless, discouraging, dismal, disheartening, funereal, gloomy; benighted, darkened, ignorant, rude, unlettered, untaught; atrocious, damnable, infamous, flagitious, foul, horrible, infernal, nefarious, vile, wicked. • n darkness, dusk, murkiness, obscurity; concealment, privacy, secrecy; blindness, ignorance.

darken vb cloud, dim, eclipse, obscure, shade, shadow; chill, damp, depress, gloom, sadden; benight, stultify, stupefy; obscure, perplex; defile, dim, dull, stain, sully.

darkness n blackness, dimness, gloom, obscurity; blindness, ignorance; cheerlessness, despondency, gloom, joylessness; privacy, secrecy.

darling adj beloved, cherished, dear, loved, precious, treasured. • n dear, favourite, idol, love, sweetheart.

dart vb ejaculate, hurl, launch, propel, sling, throw; emit, shoot; dash, rush, scoot, spring.

dash vb break, destroy, disappoint, frustrate, ruin, shatter, spoil, thwart; abash, confound, disappoint, surprise; bolt, dart, fly, run, speed, rush. • n blow, stroke; advance, onset, rush; infusion, smack, spice, sprinkling, tincture, tinge, touch; flourish, show.

dashing adj headlong, impetuous, precipitate, rushing; brilliant, gay, showy, spirited.

dastardly adj base, cowardly, coward, cowering, craven, pusillanimous, recreant. • n coward, craven, milksop, poltroon, recreant.

data npl conditions, facts, information, premises.

date n age, cycle, day, generation, time; epoch, era, period; appointment, arrangement, assignation, engagement, interview, rendezvous, tryst; catch, steady, sweetheart.

daub vb bedaub, begrime, besmear, blur, cover, deface, defile, grime, plaster, smear, smudge, soil, sully. • n smear, smirch, smudge.

daunt vb alarm, appal, check, cow, deter, discourage, frighten, intimate, scare, subdue, tame, terrify, thwart.

dauntless adj bold, brave, chivalrous, courageous, daring, doughty, gallant, heroic, indomitable, intrepid, unaffrighted, unconquerable, undaunted, undismayed, valiant, valorous.

dawdle vb dally, delay, fiddle, idle, lag, loiter, potter, trifle.

dawn vb appear, begin, break, gleam, glimmer, open, rise. • n daybreak, dawning, cockcrow, sunrise, sun-up.

day n daylight, sunlight, sunshine; age, epoch, generation, lifetime, time.

daze vb blind, dazzle; bewilder, confound, confuse, perplex, stun, stupefy. • n bewilderment, confusion, discomposure, perturbation, pother; coma, stupor, swoon, trance.

dazzle vb blind, daze; astonish, confound, overpower, surprise. • n brightness, brilliance, splendour.

dead adj breathless, deceased, defunct, departed, gone, inanimate, lifeless; apathetic, callous, cold, dull, frigid, indifferent, inert, lukewarm, numb, obtuse, spiritless, torpid, unfeeling; flat, insipid, stagnant, tasteless, vapid; barren, inactive, sterile, unemployed, unprofitable, useless. • adv absolutely, completely, downright, fundamentally, quite; direct, directly, due, exactly, just, right, squarely, straight. • n depth, midst; hush, peace, quietude, silence, stillness.

deaden vb abate, damp, dampen, dull, impair, muffle, mute, restrain, retard, smother, weaken; benumb, blunt, hebetate, obtund, paralyse.

deadly adj deleterious, destructive, fatal, lethal, malignant, mortal, murderous, noxious, pernicious, poisonous, venomous; implacable, mortal, rancorous, sanguinary.

deal vb allot, apportion, assign, bestow, dispense, distribute, divide, give, reward, share; bargain, trade, traffic, treat with. • n amount, degree, distribution, extent, lot, portion, quantity, share; bargain, transaction.

dear adj costly, expensive, high-priced; beloved, cherished, darling, esteemed, precious, treasured. • n beloved, darling, deary, honey, love, precious, sweet, sweetie, sweetheart.

dearth n deficiency, insufficiency, scarcity; famine, lack, need, shortage, want.

death n cessation, decease, demise, departure, destruction, dissolution, dying, end, exit, mortality, passing.

deathless adj eternal, everlasting, immortal, imperishable, undying; boring, dull, turgid.

debacle n breakdown, cataclysm, collapse; rout, stampede.

debar vb blackball, deny, exclude, hinder, prevent, prohibit, restrain, shut out, stop, withhold.

debase vb adulterate, alloy, depress, deteriorate, impair, injure, lower, pervert, reduce, vitiate; abase, degrade, disgrace, dishonour, humble, humiliate, mortify, shame; befoul, contaminate, corrupt, defile, foul, pollute, soil, taint.

debate vb argue, canvass, contest, discuss, dispute; contend, deliberate, wrangle. • n controversy, discussion, disputation; altercation, contention, contest, dispute, logomachy.

debauch vb corrupt, deprave, pollute, vitiate; deflower, ravish, seduce, violate. • n carousal, orgy, revel, saturnalia.

debauchery *n* dissipation, dissoluteness, excesses, intemperance; debauch, excess, intemperance, lewdness, licentiousness, lust; bacchanal, carousal, compotation, indulgence, orgies, potation, revelry, revels, saturnalia, spree.

debilitate *vb* enervate, enfeeble, exhaust, prostrate, relax, weaken.

debility *n* enervation, exhaustion, faintness, feebleness, frailty, imbecility, infirmity, languor, prostration, weakness.

debonair *adj* affable, civil, complaisant, courteous, easy, gracious, kind, obliging, polite, refined, urbane, well-bred.

debris *n* detritus, fragments, remains, rubbish, rubble, ruins, wreck, wreckage.

debt *n* arrears, debit, due, liability, obligation; fault, misdoing, offence, shortcoming, sin, transgression, trespass.

decadence *n* caducity, decay, declension, decline, degeneracy, degeneration, deterioration, fall, retrogression.

decamp *vb* abscond, bolt, escape, flee, fly.

decapitate *vb* behead, decollate, guillotine.

decay *vb* decline, deteriorate, disintegrate, fail, perish, wane, waste, wither; decompose, putrefy, rot. • *n* caducity, decadence, declension, decline, decomposition, decrepitude, degeneracy, degeneration, deterioration, dilapidation, disintegration, fading, failing, perishing, putrefaction, ruin, wasting, withering.

deceased *adj* dead, defunct, departed, gone, late, lost.

deceit *n* artifice, cheating, chicanery, cozenage, craftiness, deceitfulness, deception, double-dealing, duplicity, finesse, fraud, guile, hypocrisy, imposition, imposture, pretence, sham, treachery, tricky, underhandedness, wile.

deceitful *adj* counterfeit, deceptive, delusive, fallacious, hollow, illusive, illusory, insidious, misleading; circumventive, cunning, designing, dissembling, dodgy, double-dealing, evasive, false, fraudulent, guileful, hypocritical, insincere, tricky, underhanded, wily.

deceive *vb* befool, beguile, betray, cheat, chouse, circumvent, cozen, defraud, delude, disappoint, double-cross, dupe, ensnare, entrap, fool, gull, hoax, hoodwink, humbug, mislead, outwit, overreach, trick.

deceiver *n* charlatan, cheat, humbug, hypocrite, knave, impostor, pretender, rogue, sharper, trickster.

decent *adj* appropriate, becoming, befitting, comely, seemly, decorous, fit, proper, seemly; chaste, delicate, modest, pure; moderate, passable, respectable, tolerable.

deception *n* artifice, cheating, chicanery, cozenage, craftiness, deceitfulness, deception, double-dealing, duplicity, finesse, fraud, guile, hoax, hypocrisy, imposition, imposture, pretence, sham, treachery, trick, underhandedness, wile; cheat, chouse, ruse, stratagem, wile.

deceptive *adj* deceitful, deceiving, delusive, disingenuous, fallacious, false, illusive, illusory, misleading.

decide *vb* close, conclude, determine, end, settle, terminate; resolve; adjudge, adjudicate, award.

decided *adj* determined, firm, resolute, unhesitating, unwavering; absolute, categorical, positive, unequivocal; certain, clear, indisputable, undeniable, unmistakable, unquestionable.

deciduous *adj* caducous, nonperennial, temporary.

decipher *vb* explain, expound, interpret, reveal, solve, unfold, unravel; read.

decision *n* conclusion, determination, judgement, settlement; adjudication, award, decree, pronouncement, sentence; firmness, resolution.

decisive *adj* conclusive, determinative, final.

deck *vb* adorn, array, beautify, decorate, embellish, grace, ornament; apparel, attire, bedeck, clothe, dress, robe.

declaim *vb* harangue, mouth, rant, speak, spout.

declamation *n* declaiming, haranguing, mouthing, ranting, spouting.

declamatory *adj* bombastic, discursive, fustian, grandiloquent, high-flown, high-sounding, incoherent, inflated, pompous, pretentious, rhetorical, swelling, turgid.

declaration *n* affirmation, assertion, asseveration, averment, avowal, protestation, statement; announcement, proclamation, publication.

declaratory *adj* affirmative, annunciatory, assertive, declarative, definite, enunciative, enunciatory, expressive; explanatory, expository.

declare *vb* advertise, affirm, announce, assert, asseverate, aver, blazon, bruit, proclaim, promulgate, pronounce, publish, state, utter.

declension *n* decadence, decay, decline, degeneracy, deterioration, diminution; inflection, variation; declination, nonacceptance, refusal.

declination *n* bending, descent, inclination; decadence, decay, decline, degeneracy, degeneration, degradation, deterioration, diminution; aberration, departure, deviation, digression, divagation, divergence; declinature, nonacceptance, refusal.

decline *vb* incline, lean, slope; decay, droop, fail, flag, languish, pine, sink; degenerate, depreciate, deteriorate; decrease, diminish, dwindle, fade, ebb, lapse, lessen, wane; avoid, refuse, reject; inflect, vary. • *n* decadence, decay, declension, declination, degeneracy, deterioration, diminution, wane; atrophy, consumption, marasmus, phthisis; declivity, hill, incline, slope.

declivity *n* declination, descent, incline, slope.

decompose *vb* analyse, disintegrate, dissolve, distil, resolve, separate; corrupt, decay, putrefy, rot.

decomposition *n* analysis, break-up, disintegration, resolution; caries, corruption, crumbling, decay, disintegration, dissolution, putrescence, rotting.

decorate *vb* adorn, beautify, bedeck, deck, embellish, enrich, garnish, grace, ornament.

decoration *n* adorning, beautifying, bedecking, decking, enriching, garnishing, ornamentation, ornamenting; adornment, enrichment, embellishment, ornament.

decorous *adj* appropriate, becoming, befitting, comely, decent, fit, suitable, proper, sedate, seemly, staid.

decorum *n* appropriate behaviour, courtliness, decency, deportment, dignity, gravity, politeness, propriety, sedateness, seemliness.

decoy *vb* allure, deceive, ensnare, entice, entrap, inveigle, lure, seduce, tempt. • *n* allurement, lure, enticement.

decrease *vb* abate, contract, decline, diminish, dwindle, ebb, lessen, subside, wane; curtail, diminish, lessen, lower, reduce, retrench. • *n* abatement, contraction, declension, decline, decrement, diminishing, diminution, ebb, ebbing, lessening, reduction, subsidence, waning.

decree *vb* adjudge, appoint, command, decide, determine, enact, enjoin, order, ordain. • *n* act, command, edict, enactment, fiat, law, mandate, order, ordinance, precept, regulation, statute.

decrement *n* decrease, diminution, lessening, loss, waste.

decrepit *adj* feeble, effete, shattered, wasted, weak; aged, crippled, superannuated.

decry *vb* abuse, belittle, blame, condemn, denounce, depreciate, detract, discredit, disparage, run down, traduce, underrate, undervalue.

dedicate *vb* consecrate, devote, hallow, sanctify; address, inscribe.

deduce *vb* conclude, derive, draw, gather, infer.

deducible *adj* derivable, inferable.

deduct *vb* remove, subtract, withdraw; abate, detract.

deduction *n* removal, subtraction, withdrawal; abatement, allowance, defalcation, discount, rebate, reduction, reprise; conclusion, consequence, corollary, inference.

deed *n* achievement, act, action, derring-do, exploit, feat, performance; fact, truth, reality; charter, contract, document, indenture, instrument, transfer.

deem *vb* account, believe, conceive, consider, count, estimate, hold, imagine, judge, regard, suppose, think; fancy, opine.

deep *adj* abysmal, extensive, great, profound; abstruse, difficult, hard, intricate, knotty, mysterious, recondite, unfathomable; astute, cunning, designing, discerning, intelligent, insidious, penetrating, sagacious, shrewd; absorbed, engrossed; bass, grave, low; entire, great, heartfelt, thorough. • *n* main, ocean, water, sea; abyss, depth, profundity; enigma, mystery, riddle; silence, stillness.

deeply *adv* profoundly; completely, entirely, extensively, greatly, thoroughly; affectingly, distressingly, feelingly, mournfully, sadly.

deface *vb* blotch, deform, disfigure, injure, mar, mutilate, obliterate, soil, spoil, sully, tarnish.

de facto *adj* actual, real. • *adv* actually, in effect, in fact, really, truly.

defalcate *vb* abate, curtail, retrench, lop.

defalcation *n* abatement, deduction, diminution, discount, reduction; default, deficiency, deficit, shortage, shortcoming; embezzlement, fraud.

defamation *n* abuse, aspersion, back-biting, calumny, detraction, disparagement, libel, obloquy, opprobrium, scandal, slander.

defamatory *adj* abusive, calumnious, libellous, slanderous.

defame *vb* abuse, asperse, blacken, belie, besmirch, blemish, calumniate, detract, disgrace, dishonour, libel, malign, revile, slander, smirch, traduce, vilify.

default *vb* defalcate, dishonour, fail, repudiate, welsh. • *n* defalcation, failure, lapse, neglect, offence, omission, oversight, shortcoming ; defect, deficiency, deficit, delinquency, destitution, fault, lack, want.

defaulter *n* delinquent, embezzler, offender, peculator.

defeat *vb* beat, checkmate, conquer, discomfit, overcome, overpower, overthrow, repulse, rout, ruin, vanquish; baffle, balk, block, disappoint, disconcert, foil, frustrate, thwart. • *n* discomfiture, downfall, overthrow, repulse, rout, vanquishment; bafflement, checkmate, frustration.

defect *vb* abandon, desert, rebel, revolt. • *n* default, deficiency, destitution, lack, shortcoming, spot, taint, want; blemish, blotch, error, flaw, imperfection, mistake; failing, fault, foible.

defection *n* abandonment, desertion, rebellion, revolt; apostasy, backsliding, dereliction.

defective *adj* deficient, inadequate, incomplete, insufficient, scant, short; faulty, imperfect, marred.

defence *n* defending, guarding, holding, maintaining, maintenance, protection; buckler, bulwark, fortification, guard, protection, rampart, resistance, shield; apology, excuse, justification, plea, vindication.

defenceless *adj* exposed, helpless, unarmed, unprotected, unguarded, unshielded, weak.

defend *vb* cover, fortify, guard, preserve, protect, safeguard, screen, secure, shelter, shield; assert, espouse, justify, maintain, plead, uphold, vindicate.

defender *n* asserter, maintainer, pleader, upholder; champion, protector, vindicator.

defer[1] *vb* adjourn, delay, pigeonhole, procrastinate, postpone, prorogue, protract, shelve, table.

defer[2] *vb* abide by, acknowledge, bow to, give way, submit, yield; admire, esteem, honour, regard, respect.

deference *n* esteem, homage, honour, obeisance, regard, respect, reverence, veneration; complaisance, consideration; obedience, submission.

deferential *adj* respectful, reverential.

defiance *n* challenge, daring; contempt, despite, disobedience, disregard, opposition, spite.

defiant *adj* contumacious, recalcitrant, resistant; bold, courageous, resistant.

deficiency *n* dearth, default, deficit, insufficiency, lack, meagreness, scantiness, scarcity, shortage, shortness, want; defect, error, failing, falling, fault, foible, frailty, imperfection, infirmity, weakness.

deficient *adj* defective, faulty, imperfect, inadequate, incomplete, insufficient, lacking, scant, scanty, scarce, short, unsatisfactory, wanting.

deficit *n* deficiency, lack, scarcity, shortage, shortness.

defile[1] *vb* dirty, foul, soil, stain, tarnish; contaminate, debase, poison, pollute, sully, taint, vitiate; corrupt, debauch, deflower, ravish, seduce, violate.

defile[2] *vb* file, march, parade, promenade. • *n* col, gorge, pass, passage, ravine, strait.

define *vb* bound, circumscribe, designate, delimit, demarcate, determine, explain, limit, specify.

definite *adj* defined, determinate, determined, fixed, restricted; assured, certain, clear, exact, explicit, positive, precise, specific, unequivocal.

definitive *adj* categorical, determinate, explicit, express, positive, unconditional; conclusive, decisive, final.

deflect *vb* bend, deviate, diverge, swerve, turn, twist, waver, wind.

deflower *vb* corrupt, debauch, defile, seduce.

deform *vb* deface, disfigure, distort, injure, mar, misshape, ruin, spoil.

deformity *n* abnormality, crookedness, defect, disfigurement, distortion, inelegance, irregularity, malformation, misproportion, misshapenness, monstrosity, ugliness.

defraud *vb* beguile, cheat, chouse, circumvent, cozen, deceive, delude, diddle, dupe, embezzle, gull, overreach, outwit, pilfer, rob, swindle, trick.

defray *vb* bear, discharge, liquidate, meet, pay, settle.

deft *adj* adroit, apt, clever, dab, dextrous, expert, handy, ready, skilful.

defunct *adj* dead, deceased, departed, extinct, gone; abrogated, annulled, cancelled, inoperative.

defy *vb* challenge, dare; brave, contemn, despise, disregard, face, flout, provoke, scorn, slight, spurn.

degeneracy *n* abasement, caducity, corruption, debasement, decadence, decay, declension, decline, decrease, degenerateness, degeneration, degradation, depravation, deterioration; inferiority, meanness, poorness.

degenerate *vb* decay, decline, decrease, deteriorate, retrograde, sink. • *adj* base, corrupt, decayed, degenerated, deteriorated, fallen, inferior, low, mean, perverted.

degeneration *n* debasement, decline, degeneracy, deterioration.

degradation *n* deposition, disgrace, dishonour, humiliation, ignominy; abasement, caducity, corruption, debasement, decadence, decline, degeneracy, degeneration, deterioration, perversion, vitiation.

degrade *vb* abase, alloy, break, cashier, corrupt, debase, demote, discredit, disgrace, dishonour, disparage, downgrade, humiliate, humble, lower, pervert, vitiate; deteriorate, impair, lower, sink.

degree *n* stage, step; class, grade, order, quality, rank, standing, station; extent, measure; division, interval, space.

deify *vb* apotheosize, idolize, glorify, revere; elevate, ennoble, exalt.

deign *vb* accord, condescend, grant, vouchsafe.

deject *vb* depress, discourage, dishearten, dispirit, sadden.

dejected *adj* blue, chapfallen, crestfallen, depressed, despondent, disheartened, dispirited, doleful, downcast, downhearted, gloomy, low-spirited, miserable, sad, wretched.

delay *vb* defer, postpone, procrastinate; arrest, detain, check, hinder, impede, retard, stay, stop; prolong, protract; dawdle, linger, loiter, tarry. • *n* deferment, postponement, procrastination; check, detention, hindrance, impediment, retardation, stoppage; prolonging, protraction; dallying, dawdling, lingering, tarrying, stay, stop.

delectable *adj* agreeable, charming, delightful, enjoyable, gratifying, pleasant, pleasing.

delectation *n* delight, ecstasy, gladness, joy, rapture, ravishment, transport.

delegate *vb* appoint, authorize, mission, depute, deputize, transfer; commit, entrust. • *n* ambassador, commissioner, delegate, deputy, envoy, representative.

delete *vb* cancel, efface, erase, expunge, obliterate, remove.

deleterious *adj* deadly, destructive, lethal, noxious, poisonous; harmful, hurtful, injurious, pernicious, unwholesome.

deliberate *vb* cogitate, consider, consult, meditate, muse, ponder, reflect, ruminate, think, weigh. • *adj* careful, cautious, circumspect, considerate, heedful, purposeful, methodical, thoughtful, wary; well-advised, well-considered; aforethought, intentional, premeditated, purposed, studied.

deliberation *n* caution, circumspection, cogitation, consideration, coolness, meditation, prudence, reflection, thought, thoughtfulness, wariness; purpose.

delicacy *n* agreeableness, daintiness, deliciousness, pleasantness, relish, savouriness; bonne bouche, dainty, tidbit; elegance, fitness, lightness, niceness, nicety, smoothness, softness, tenderness; fragility, frailty, slenderness, slightness, tenderness, weakness; carefulness, discrimination, fastidiousness, finesse, nicety, scrupulousness, sensitivity, subtlety, tact; purity, refinement, sensibility.

delicate *adj* agreeable, delicious, pleasant, pleasing, palatable, savoury; elegant, exquisite, fine, nice; careful, dainty, discriminating, fastidious, scrupulous; fragile, frail, slender, slight, tender, delicate; pure, refined.

delicious *adj* dainty, delicate, luscious, nice, palatable, savory; agreeable, charming, choice, delightful, exquisite, grateful, pleasant.

delight *vb* charm, enchant, enrapture, gratify, please, ravish, rejoice, satisfy, transport. • *n* charm, delectation, ecstasy, enjoyment, gladness, gratification, happiness, joy, pleasure, rapture, ravishment, satisfaction, transport.

delightful *adj* agreeable, captivating, charming, delectable, enchanting, enjoyable, enrapturing, rapturous, ravishing, transporting.

delineate *vb* design, draw, figure, paint, sketch, trace; depict, describe, picture, portray.

delineation *n* design, draught, drawing, figure, outline, sketch; account, description, picture, portrayal.

delinquency *n* crime, fault, misdeed, misdemeanour, offence, wrong-doing.

delinquent *adj* negligent, offending. • *n* criminal, culprit, defaulter, malefactor, miscreant, misdoer, offender, transgressor, wrong-doer.

delirious *adj* crazy, demented, deranged, frantic, frenzied, light-headed, mad, insane, raving, wandering.

delirium *n* aberration, derangement, frenzy, hallucination, incoherence, insanity, lunacy, madness, raving, wandering.

deliver *vb* emancipate, free, liberate, release; extricate, redeem, rescue, save; commit, give, impart, transfer; cede, grant, relinquish, resign, yield; declare, emit, promulgate, pronounce, speak, utter; deal, discharge.

deliverance *n* emancipation, escape, liberation, redemption, release.

delivery *n* conveyance, surrender; commitment, giving, rendering, transference, transferral, transmission; elocution, enunciation, pronunciation, speech, utterance; childbirth, confinement, labour, parturition, travail.

dell *n* dale, dingle, glen, valley, ravine.

delude *vb* beguile, cheat, chouse, circumvent, cozen, deceive, dupe, gull, misguide, mislead, overreach, trick.

deluge *vb* drown, inundate, overflow, overwhelm, submerge. • *n* cataclysm, downpour, flood, inundation, overflow, rush.

delusion *n* artifice, cheat, clap-trap, deceit, dodge, fetch, fraud, imposition, imposture, ruse, snare, trick, wile; deception, error, fallacy, fancy, hallucination, illusion, mistake, mockery, phantasm.

delusive *adj* deceitful, deceiving, deceptive, fallacious, illusional, illusionary, illusive.

demand *vb* challenge, exact, require; claim, necessitate, require; ask, inquire. • *n* claim, draft, exaction, requirement, requisition; call, want; inquiry, interrogation, question.

demarcation *n* bound, boundary, confine, distinction, division, enclosure, limit, separation.

demeanour *n* air, bearing, behaviour, carriage, deportment, manner, mien.

demented *adj* crack-brained, crazed, crazy, daft, deranged, dotty, foolish, idiotic, infatuated, insane, lunatic.

dementia *n* idiocy, insanity, lunacy.

demerit *n* delinquency, fault, ill-desert.

demise *vb* alienate, consign, convey, devolve, grant, transfer; bequeath, devise, leave, will. • *n* alienation, conveyance, transfer, transference, transmission; death, decease.

demolish *vb* annihilate, destroy, dismantle, level, over-throw, overturn, pulverize, raze, ruin.

demon *n* devil, fiend, kelpie, goblin, troll.

demoniac, demoniacal *adj* demonic, demonical, devilish, diabolic, diabolical, fiendish, hellish, infernal, Mephistophelean, Mephistophelian, satanic; delirious, distracted, frantic, frenzied, feverish, hysterical, mad, overwrought, rabid.

demonstrate *vb* establish, exhibit, illustrate, indicate, manifest, prove, show.

demonstration *n* display, exhibition, manifestation, show.

demonstrative *adj* affectionate, communicative, effusive, emotional, expansive, expressive, extroverted, open, outgoing, passionate, sentimental, suggestive, talkative, unreserved; absolute, apodictic, certain, conclusive, probative; exemplificative, illustrative.

demoralize *vb* corrupt, debase, debauch, deprave, vitiate; depress, discourage, dishearten, weaken.

demulcent *adj* emollient, lenitive, mild, mollifying, sedative, soothing.

demur *vb* halt, hesitate, pause, stop, waver; doubt, object, scruple. • *n* demurral, hesitance, hesitancy, hesitation, objection, pause, qualm, scruple.

demure *adj* prudish; coy, decorous, grave, modest, priggish, prudish, sedate, sober, staid.

den *n* cavern, cave; haunt, lair, resort, retreat.

denial *n* contradiction, controverting, negation; abjuration, disavowal, disclaimer, disowning; disallowance, refusal, rejection.

denizen *n* citizen, dweller, inhabitant, resident.

denominate *vb* call, christen, designate, dub, entitle, name, phrase, style, term.

denomination *n* appellation, designation, name, style, term, title; class, kind, sort; body, persuasion, school, sect.

denote *vb* betoken, connote, designate, imply, indicate, mark, mean, note, show, signify, typify.

dénouement *n* catastrophe, unravelling; consummation, issue, finale, upshot, conclusion, termination.

denounce *vb* menace, threaten; arraign, attack, brand, censure, condemn, proscribe, stigmatize, upbraid; accuse, inform, denunciate.

dense *adj* close, compact, compressed, condensed, thick; dull, slow, stupid.

dent *vb* depress, dint, indent, pit. • *n* depression, dint, indentation, nick, notch.

dentate *adj* notched, serrate, toothed.

denude *vb* bare, divest, strip.

denunciation *n* menace, threat; arraignment, censure, fulmination, invective; exposure.

deny *vb* contradict, gainsay, oppose, refute, traverse; abjure, abnegate, disavow, disclaim, disown, renounce; disallow, refuse, reject, withhold.

depart *vb* absent, disappear, vanish; abandon, decamp, go, leave, migrate, quit, remove, withdraw; decease, die; deviate, diverge, vary.

department *n* district, division, part, portion, province; bureau, function, office, province, sphere, station; branch, division, subdivision.

departure *n* exit, leaving, parting, removal, recession, removal, retirement, withdrawal; abandonment, forsaking; death, decease, demise, deviation, exit.

depend *vb* hang, hinge, turn.

dependant *n* client, hanger-on, henchman, minion, retainer, subordinate, vassal; attendant, circumstance, concomitant, consequence, corollary.

dependence *n* concatenation, connection, interdependence; confidence, reliance, trust; buttress, prop, staff, stay, support, supporter; contingency, need, subjection, subordination.

dependency *n* adjunct, appurtenance; colony, province.

dependent *adj* hanging, pendant; conditioned, contingent, relying, subject, subordinate.

depict *vb* delineate, limn, outline, paint, pencil, portray, sketch; describe, render, represent.

deplete *vb* drain, empty, evacuate, exhaust, reduce.

deplorable *adj* calamitous, distressful, distressing, grievous, lamentable, melancholy, miserable, mournful, pitiable, regrettable, sad, wretched.

deplore *vb* bemoan, bewail, grieve for, lament, mourn, regret.

deploy *vb* display, expand, extend, open, unfold.

deportment *n* air, bearing, behaviour, breeding, carriage, comportment, conduct, demeanour, manner, mien, port.

depose *vb* break, cashier, degrade, dethrone, dismiss, displace, oust, reduce; avouch, declare, depone, testify.

deposit *vb* drop, dump, precipitate; lay, put; bank, hoard, lodge, put, save, store; commit, entrust. • *n* diluvium, dregs, lees, precipitate, precipitation, sediment, settlement, settlings, silt; money, pawn, pledge, security, stake.

depositary *n* fiduciary, guardian, trustee.

deposition *n* affidavit, evidence, testimony; deposit, precipitation, settlement; dethroning, displacement, removal.

depository *n* deposit, depot, storehouse, warehouse.

depot *n* depository, magazine, storehouse, warehouse.

depravation *n* abasement, corruption, deterioration, impairing, injury, vitiation; debasement, degeneracy, degeneration, depravity, impairment.

depraved *adj* abandoned, corrupt, corrupted, debased, debauched, degenerate, dissolute, evil, graceless, hardened, immoral, lascivious, lewd, licentious, lost, perverted, profligate, reprobate, shameless, sinful, vicious, wicked.

depravity *n* corruption, degeneracy, depravedness; baseness, contamination, corruption, corruptness, criminality, demoralization, immorality, iniquity, license, perversion, vice, viciousness, wickedness.

depreciate *vb* underestimate, undervalue, underrate; belittle, censure, decry, degrade, disparage, malign, traduce.

depreciation *n* belittling, censure, derogation, detraction, disparagement, maligning, traducing.

depredation *n* despoiling, devastation, pilfering, pillage, plunder, rapine, robbery, spoliation, theft.

depress *vb* bow, detrude, drop, lower, reduce, sink; abase, abash, degrade, debase, disgrace, humble, humiliate; chill, damp, dampen, deject, discourage, dishearten, dispirit, sadden; deaden, lower.

depression *n* cavity, concavity, dent, dimple, dint, excavation, hollow, hollowness, indentation, pit; blues, cheerlessness, dejection, dejectedness, despondency, disconsolateness, disheartenment, dispiritedness, dole, dolefulness, downheartedness, dumps, gloom, gloominess, hypochondria, melancholy, sadness, vapours; inactivity, lowness, stagnation; abasement, debasement, degradation, humiliation.

deprivation *n* bereavement, dispossession, loss, privation, spoliation, stripping.

deprive *vb* bereave, denude, despoil, dispossess, divest, rob, strip.

depth *n* abyss, deepness, drop, profundity; extent, measure; middle, midst, stillness; astuteness, discernment, penetration, perspicacity, profoundness, profundity, sagacity, shrewdness.

deputation *n* commission, delegation; commissioners, deputies, delegates, delegation, embassies, envoys, legation.

depute *vb* accredit, appoint, authorize, charge, commission, delegate, empower, entrust.

deputy *adj* acting, assistant, vice, subordinate. • *n* agent, commissioner, delegate, envoy, factor, legate, lieutenant, proxy, representative, substitute, viceregent.

derange *vb* confound, confuse, disarrange, disconcert, disorder, displace, madden, perturb, unsettle; discompose, disconcert, disturb, perturb, ruffle, upset; craze, madden, unbalance, unhinge.

derangement *n* confusion, disarrangement, disorder, irregularity; discomposure, disturbance, perturbation; aberration, alienation, delirium, dementia, hallucination, insanity, lunacy, madness, mania.

derelict *adj* abandoned, forsaken, left, relinquished; delinquent, faithless, guilty, neglectful, negligent, unfaithful. • *n* castaway, castoff, outcast, tramp, vagrant, wreck, wretch.

dereliction *n* abandonment, desertion, relinquishement, renunciation; delinquency, failure, faithlessness, fault, neglect, negligence.

deride *vb* chaff, flout, gibe, insult, jeer, lampoon, mock, ridicule, satirize, scoff, scorn, sneer, taunt.

derision *n* contempt, disrespect, insult, laughter, mockery, ridicule, scorn.

derisive *adj* contemptuous, contumelious, mocking, ridiculing, scoffing, scornful.

derivation *n* descent, extraction, genealogy, etymology; deducing, deriving, drawing, getting, obtaining; beginning, foundation, origination, source.

derive *vb* draw, get, obtain, receive; deduce, follow, infer, trace.

derogate *vb* compromise, depreciate, detract, diminish, disparage, lessen.

derogatory *adj* belittling, depreciative, deprecatory, detracting, dishonouring, disparaging, injurious.

descant *vb* amplify, animadvert, dilate, discourse, discuss, enlarge, expatiate. • *n* melody, soprano, treble; animadversion, commentary, remarks; discourse, discussion.

descend *vb* drop, fall, pitch, plunge, sink, swoop; alight, dismount; go, pass, proceed, devolve; derive, issue, originate.

descendants *npl* offspring, issue, posterity, progeny.

descent *n* downrush, drop, fall; descending; decline, declivity, dip, pitch, slope; ancestry, derivation, extraction, genealogy, lineage, parentage, pedigree; assault, attack, foray, incursion, invasion, raid.

describe *vb* define, delineate, draw, illustrate, limn, sketch, specify, trace; detail; depict, explain, narrate, portray, recount, relate, represent; characterize.

description *n* delineation, tracing; account, depiction, explanation, narration, narrative, portrayal, recital, relation, report, representation; class, kind, sort, species.

descry *vb* behold, discover, discern, distinguish, espy, observe, perceive, see; detect, recognize.

desecrate *vb* abuse, pervert, defile, pollute, profane, violate.

desert[1] *n* due, excellence, merit, worth; punishment, reward.

desert[2] *vb* abandon, abscond, forsake, leave, quit, relinquish, renounce, resign, quit, vacate.

desert[3] *adj* barren, desolate, forsaken, lonely, solitary, uncultivated, uninhabited, unproductive, untilled, waste, wild.

deserted *adj* abandoned, forsaken, relinquished.

deserter *n* abandoner, forsaker, quitter, runaway; apostate, backslider, fugitive, recreant, renegade, revolter, traitor, turncoat.

desertion *n* abandonment, dereliction, recreancy, relinquishment.

deserve *vb* earn, gain, merit, procure, win.

desiderate *vb* desire, lack, miss, need, want.

design *vb* brew, concoct, contrive, devise, intend, invent, mean, plan, project, scheme; intend, mean, purpose; delineate, describe, draw, outline, sketch, trace. • *n* aim, device, drift, intent,

intention, mark, meaning, object, plan, proposal, project, purport, purpose, scheme, scope; delineation, draught, drawing, outline, plan, sketch; adaptation, artifice, contrivance, invention, inventiveness.

designate *vb* denote, distinguish, indicate, particularize, select, show, specify, stipulate; characterize, define, describe; call, christen, denominate, dub, entitle, name, style; allot, appoint, christen.

designation *n* indication, particularization, selection, specification; class, description, kind; appellation, denomination, name, style, title.

designing *adj* artful, astute, crafty, crooked, cunning, deceitful, insidious, intriguing, Machiavellian, scheming, sly, subtle, treacherous, trickish, tricky, unscrupulous, wily.

desirable *adj* agreeable, beneficial, covetable, eligible, enviable, good, pleasing, preferable.

desire *vb* covet, crave, desiderate, fancy, hanker after, long for, lust after, want, wish, yearn for; ask, entreat, request, solicit. • *n* eroticism, lasciviousness, libidinousness, libido, lust, lustfulness, passion; eagerness, fancy, hope, inclination, mind, partiality, penchant, pleasure, volition, want, wish.

desirous *adj* avid, eager, desiring, longing, solicitous, wishful.

desist *vb* cease, discontinue, forbear, pause, stay, stop.

desolate *vb* depopulate, despoil, destroy, devastate, pillage, plunder, ravage, ruin, sack. • *adj* bare, barren, bleak, desert, forsaken, lonely, solitary, unfrequented, uninhabited, waste, wild; companionable, lonely, lonesome, solitary; desolated, destroyed, devastated, ravaged, ruined; cheerless, comfortless, companionless, disconsolate, dreary, forlorn, forsaken, miserable, wretched.

desolation *n* destruction, devastation, havoc, ravage, ruin; barrenness, bleakness, desolateness, dreariness, loneliness, solitariness, solitude, wildness; gloom, gloominess, misery, sadness, unhappiness, wretchedness.

despair *vb* despond, give up, lose hope. • *n* dejection, desperation, despondency, disheartenment, hopelessness.

despatch *see* **dispatch**.

desperado *n* daredevil, gangster, marauder, ruffian, thug, tough.

desperate *adj* despairing, despondent, desponding, hopeless; forlorn, irretrievable; extreme; audacious, daring, foolhardy, frantic, furious, headstrong, precipitate, rash, reckless, violent, wild, wretched; extreme, great, monstrous, prodigious, supreme.

desperation *n* despair, hopelessness; fury, rage.

despicable *adj* abject, base, contemptible, degrading, low, mean, paltry, pitiful, shameful, sordid, vile, worthless.

despise *vb* contemn, disdain, disregard, neglect, scorn, slight, spurn, undervalue.

despite *n* malevolence, malice, malignity, spite; contempt, contumacy, defiance. • *prep* notwithstanding.

despoil *vb* bereave, denude, deprive, dispossess, divest, strip; devastate, fleece, pillage, plunder, ravage, rifle, rob.

despond *vb* despair, give up, lose hope, mourn, sorrow.

despondency *n* blues, dejection, depression, discouragement, gloom, hopelessness, melancholy, sadness.

despondent *adj* dejected, depressed, discouraged, disheartened, dispirited, low-spirited, melancholy.

despot *n* autocrat, dictator; oppressor, tyrant.

despotic *adj* absolute, arrogant, autocratic, dictatorial, imperious; arbitrary, oppressive, tyrannical, tyrannous.

despotism *n* absolutism, autocracy, dictatorship; oppression, tyranny.

destination *n* appointment, decree, destiny, doom, fate, foreordainment, foreordination, fortune, lot, ordination, star; aim, design, drift, end, intention, object, purpose, scope; bourne, goal, harbour, haven, journey's end, resting-place, terminus.

destine *vb* allot, appoint, assign, consecrate, devote, ordain; design, intend, predetermine; decree, doom, foreordain, predestine.

destitute *adj* distressed, indigent, moneyless, necessitous, needy, penniless, penurious, pinched, poor, reduced, wanting.

destitution *n* indigence, need, penury, poverty, privation, want.

destroy *vb* demolish, overthrow, overturn, subvert, raze, ruin; annihilate, dissolve, efface, quench; desolate, devastate, devour, ravage, waste; eradicate, extinguish, extirpate, kill, uproot, slay.

destruction *n* demolition, havoc, overthrow, ruin, subversion; desolation, devastation, holocaust, ravage; annihilation, eradication, extinction, extirpation; death, massacre, murder, slaughter.

destructive *adj* baleful, baneful, deadly, deleterious, detrimental, fatal, hurtful, injurious, lethal, mischievous, noxious, pernicious, ruinous; annihilatory, eradicative, exterminative, extirpative.

desultory *adj* capricious, cursory, discursive, erratic, fitful, inconstant, inexact, irregular, loose, rambling, roving, slight, spasmodic, unconnected, unmethodical, unsettled, unsystematic, vague, wandering.

detach *vb* disengage, disconnect, disjoin, dissever, disunite, divide, part, separate, sever, unfix; appoint, detail, send.

detail *vb* delineate, depict, describe, enumerate, narrate, particularize, portray, recount, rehearse, relate, specify; appoint, detach, send. • *n* account, narration, narrative, recital, relation; appointment, detachment; item, part.

details *npl* facts, minutiae, particulars, parts.

detain *vb* arrest, check, delay, hinder, hold, keep, restrain, retain, stay, stop; confine.

detect *vb* ascertain, catch, descry, disclose, discover, expose, reveal, unmask.

detention *n* confinement, delay, hindrance, restraint, withholding.

deter *vb* debar, discourage, frighten, hinder, prevent, restrain, stop, withhold.

deteriorate *vb* corrupt, debase, degrade, deprave, disgrace, impair, spoil, vitiate; decline, degenerate, depreciate, worsen.

deterioration *n* corruption, debasement, degradation, depravation, vitiation, perversion; caducity, decadence, decay, decline, degeneracy, degeneration, impairment.

determinate *adj* absolute, certain, definite, determined, established, explicit, express, fixed, limited, positive, settled; conclusive, decided, decisive, definitive.

determination *n* ascertainment, decision, deciding, determining, fixing, settlement, settling; conclusion, judgment, purpose, resolution, resolve, result; direction, leaning, tendency; firmness, constancy, effort, endeavour, exertion, grit, persistence, stamina, resoluteness; definition, limitation, qualification.

determine *vb* adjust, conclude, decide, end, establish, fix, resolve, settle; ascertain, certify, check, verify; impel, incline, induce, influence, lead, turn; decide, resolve; condition, define, limit; compel, necessitate.

detest *vb* abhor, abominate, despise, execrate, hate, loathe, nauseate, recoil from.

detestable *adj* abhorred, abominable, accursed, cursed, damnable, execrable, hateful, odious; disgusting, loathsome, nauseating, offensive, repulsive, sickening, vile.

dethrone *vb* depose, uncrown.

detract *vb* abuse, asperse, belittle, calumniate, debase, decry, defame, depreciate, derogate, disparage, slander, traduce, vilify; deprecate, deteriorate, diminish, lessen.

detraction *n* abuse, aspersion, calumny, censure, defamation, depreciation, derogation, disparagement, slander.

detriment *n* cost, damage, disadvantage, evil, harm, hurt, injury, loss, mischief, prejudice.

detrimental *adj* baleful, deleterious, destructive, harmful, hurtful, injurious, mischievous, pernicious, prejudicial.

devastate *vb* desolate, despoil, destroy, lay waste, harry, pillage, plunder, ravage, sack, spoil, strip, waste.

devastation *n* despoiling, destroying, harrying, pillaging, plundering, ravaging, sacking, spoiling, stripping, wasting; desolation, destruction, havoc, pillage, rapine, ravage, ruin, waste.

develop *vb* disentangle, disclose, evolve, exhibit, explicate, uncover, unfold, unravel; cultivate, grow, mature, open, progress.

development *n* disclosure, disentanglement, exhibition, unfolding, unravelling; growth, increase, maturation, maturing; evolution, growth, progression; elaboration, expansion, explication.

deviate *vb* alter, deflect, digress, diverge, sheer off, slew, tack, turn aside, wheel, wheel about; err, go astray, stray, swerve, wander; differ, vary.

deviation *n* aberration, departure, depression, divarication, divergence, turning; alteration, change, difference, variance, variation.

device *n* contraption, contrivance, gadget, invention; design, expedient, plan, project, resort, resource, scheme, shift; artifice, evasion, fraud, manoeuvre, ruse, stratagem, trick, wile; blazon, emblazonment, emblem, sign, symbol, type.

devil *n* archfiend, demon, fiend, goblin; Apollyon, Belial, Deuce, Evil One, Lucifer, Old Harry, Old Nick, Old Serpent, Prince of Darkness, Satan.

devilish *adj* demon, demonic, demonical, demoniac, demoniacal, diabolic, diabolical, fiendish, hellish, infernal, Mephistophelean, Mephistophelian, satanic; atrocious, barbarous, cruel, malevolent, malicious, malign, malignant, wicked.

devilry *n* devilment, diablerie, mischief; devilishness, fiendishness, wickedness.

devious *adj* deviating, erratic, roundabout, wandering; circuitous, confusing, crooked, labyrinthine, mazy, obscure; crooked, disingenuous, misleading, treacherous.

devise *vb* brew, compass, concert, concoct, contrive, dream up, excogitate, imagine, invent, plan, project, scheme; bequeath, demise, leave, will.

devoid *adj* bare, destitute, empty, vacant, void.

devolve *vb* alienate, consign, convey, deliver over, demise, fall, hand over, make over, pass, transfer.

devote *vb* appropriate, consecrate, dedicate, destine; set apart; addict, apply, give up, resign; consign, doom, give over.

devoted *adj* affectionate, attached, loving; ardent, assiduous, earnest, zealous.

devotee *n* bigot, enthusiast, fan, fanatic, zealot.

devotion *n* consecration, dedication, duty; devotedness, devoutness, fidelity, godliness, holiness, piety, religion, religiousness, saintliness, sanctity; adoration, prayer, worship; affection, attachment, love; ardour, devotedness, eagerness, earnestness, fervour, passion, spirit, zeal.

devotional *adj* devout, godly, pious, religious, saintly.

devour *vb* engorge, gorge, gulp down, raven, swallow eagerly, wolf; annihilate, consume, destroy, expend, spend, swallow up, waste.

devout *adj* devotional, godly, holy, pious, religious, saint-like, saintly; earnest, grave, serious, sincere, solemn.

dexterity *n* ability, address, adroitness, aptitude, aptness, art, cleverness, expertness, facility, knack, quickness, readiness, skilfulness, skill, tact.

dexterous, dextrous *adj* able, adept, adroit, apt, deft, clever, expert, facile, handy, nimble-fingered, quick, ready, skilful.

diabolic, diabolical *adj* atrocious, barbarous, cruel, devilish, fiendish, hellish, impious, infernal, malevolent, malign, malignant, satanic, wicked.

diagram *n* chart, delineation, figure, graph, map, outline, plan, sketch.

dialect *n* idiom, localism, provincialism; jargon, lingo, patois, patter; language, parlance, phraseology, speech, tongue.

dialectal *adj* idiomatic, local, provincial.

dialectic, dialectical *adj* analytical, critical, logical, rational, rationalistic.

dialogue *n* colloquy, communication, conference, conversation, converse, intercourse, interlocution; playbook, script, speech, text, words.

diaphanous *adj* clear, filmy, gossamer, pellucid, sheer, translucent, transparent.

diarrhoea *n* (*med*) flux, looseness, purging, relaxation.

diary *n* chronicle, daybook, journal, register.

diatribe *n* disputation, disquisition, dissertation; abuse, harangue, invective, philippic, reviling, tirade.

dictate *vb* bid, direct, command, decree, enjoin, ordain, order, prescribe, require. • *n* bidding, command, decree, injunction, order; maxim, precept, rule.

dictation *n* direction, order, prescription.

dictator *n* autocrat, despot, tyrant.

dictatorial *adj* absolute, unlimited, unrestricted; authoritative, despotic, dictatory, domineering, imperious, overbearing, peremptory, tyrannical.

dictatorship *n* absolutism, authoritarianism, autocracy, despotism, iron rule, totalitarianism, tyranny.

diction *n* expression, language, phraseology, style, vocabulary, wording.

dictionary *n* glossary, lexicon, thesaurus, vocabulary, wordbook; cyclopedia, encyclopedia.

dictum *n* affirmation, assertion, saying; (*law*) award, arbitrament, decision, opinion.

didactic, didactical *adj* educational, instructive, pedagogic, preceptive.

die *vb* decease, demise, depart, expire, pass on; decay, decline, fade, fade out, perish, wither; cease, disappear, vanish; faint, fall, sink.

diet[1] *vb* eat, feed, nourish; abstain, fast, regulate, slim. • *n* aliment, fare, food, nourishment, nutriment, provision, rations, regimen, subsistence, viands, victuals.

diet[2] *n* assembly, congress, convention, convocation, council, parliament.

differ *vb* deviate, diverge, vary; disagree, dissent; bicker, contend, dispute, quarrel, wrangle.

difference *n* contrariety, contrast, departure, deviation, disagreement, disparity, dissimilarity, dissimilitude, divergence, diversity, heterogeneity, inconformity, nuance, opposition, unlikeness, variation; alienation, altercation, bickering, breach, contention, contest, controversy, debate, disaccord, disagreement, disharmony, dispute, dissension, embroilment, falling out, irreconcilability, jarring, misunderstanding, quarrel, rupture, schism, strife, variance, wrangle; discrimination, distinction.

different *adj* distinct, nonidentical, separate, unlike; contradistinct, contrary, contrasted, deviating, disagreeing, discrepant, dissimilar, divergent, diverse, incompatible, incongruous, unlike, variant, various; divers, heterogeneous, manifold, many, sundry.

difficult *adj* arduous, exacting, hard, Herculean, stiff, tough, uphill; abstruse, complex, intricate, knotty, obscure, perplexing; austere, rigid, unaccommodating, uncompliant, unyielding; dainty, fastidious, squeamish.

difficulty *n* arduousness, laboriousness; bar, barrier, crux, deadlock, dilemma, embarrassment, emergency, exigency, fix, hindrance, impediment, knot, obstacle, obstruction, perplexity, pickle, pinch, predicament, stand, standstill, thwart, trial, trouble; cavil, objection; complication, controversy, difference, embarrassment, embroilment, imbroglio, misunderstanding.

diffidence *n* distrust, doubt, hesitance, hesitancy, hesitation, reluctance; bashfulness, modesty, sheepishness, shyness, timidity.

diffident *adj* distrustful, doubtful, hesitant, hesitating, reluctant; bashful, modest, over-modest, sheepish, shy, timid.

diffuse[1] *vb* circulate, disperse, disseminate, distribute, intermingle, propagate, scatter, spread, strew.

diffuse[2] *adj* broadcast, dispersed, scattered, sparse, sporadic, widespread; broad, extensive, liberal, profuse, wide; copious, loose, prolix, rambling, verbose, wordy.

diffusion *n* circulation, dispersion, dissemination, distribution, extension, propagation, spread, strewing.

diffusive *adj* expansive, permeating, wide-reaching; spreading, dispersive, disseminative, distributive, distributory.

dig *vb* channel, delve, excavate, grub, hollow out, quarry, scoop, tunnel. • *n* poke, punch, thrust.

digest[1] *vb* arrange, classify, codify, dispose, methodize, systemize, tabulate; concoct; assimilate, consider, contemplate, meditate, ponder, reflect upon, study; master; macerate, soak, steep.

digest[2] *n* code, system; abridgement, abstract, brief, breviary, compend, compendium, conspectus, epitome, summary, synopsis.

dignified *adj* august, courtly, decorous, grave, imposing, majestic, noble, stately.

dignify *vb* advance, aggrandize, elevate, ennoble, exalt, promote; adorn, grace, honour.

dignity *n* elevation, eminence, exaltation, excellence, glory, greatness, honour, place, rank, respectability, standing, station; decorum, grandeur, majesty, nobleness, stateliness; preferment; dignitary, magistrate; elevation, height.

digress *vb* depart, deviate, diverge, expatiate, wander.

digression *n* departure, deviation, divergence; episode, excursus.

dilapidate *vb* demolish, destroy, disintegrate, ruin, waste.

dilapidated *adj* decayed, ruined, run down, wasted.

dilapidation *n* decay, demolition, destruction, disintegration, disrepair, dissolution, downfall, ruin, waste.

dilate *vb* distend, enlarge, expand, extend, inflate, swell, tend, widen; amplify, descant, dwell, enlarge, expatiate.

dilation *n* amplification, bloating, distension, enlargement, expanding, expansion, spreading, swelling.

dilatory *adj* backward, behind-hand, delaying, laggard, lagging, lingering, loitering, off-putting, procrastinating, slack, slow, sluggish, tardy.

dilemma *n* difficulty, fix, plight, predicament, problem, quandary, strait.

diligence *n* activity, application, assiduity, assiduousness, attention, care, constancy, earnestness, heedfulness, industry, laboriousness, perseverance, sedulousness.

diligent *adj* active, assiduous, attentive, busy, careful, constant, earnest, hard-working, indefatigable, industrious, laborious, notable, painstaking, persevering, persistent, sedulous, tireless.

dilly-dally *vb* dally, dawdle, delay, lag, linger, loiter, saunter, trifle.

dilute *vb* attenuate, reduce, thin, weaken. • *adj* attenuated, diluted, thin, weak, wishy-washy.

dim *vb* blur, cloud, darken, dull, obscure, sully, tarnish. • *adj* cloudy, dark, dusky, faint, ill-defined, indefinite, indistinct, mysterious, obscure, shadowy; dull, obtuse; clouded, confused, darkened, faint, obscured; blurred, dulled, sullied, tarnished.

dimension *n* extension, extent, measure.

dimensions *npl* amplitude, bigness, bulk, capacity, greatness, largeness, magnitude, mass, massiveness, size, volume; measurements.

diminish *vb* abate, belittle, contract, decrease, lessen, reduce; curtail, cut, dwindle, melt, narrow, shrink, shrivel, subside, taper off, weaken.

diminution *n* abatement, abridgement, attenuation, contraction, curtailment, decrescendo, cut, decay, decrease, deduction, lessening, reduction, retrenchment, weakening.

diminutive *adj* contracted, dwarfish, little, minute, puny, pygmy, small, tiny.

din *vb* beat, boom, clamour, drum, hammer, pound, repeat, ring, thunder. • *n* bruit, clamour, clash, clatter, crash, crashing, hubbub, hullabaloo, hurly-burly, noise, outcry, racket, row, shout, uproar.

dingle *n* dale, dell, glen, vale, valley.

dingy *adj* brown, dun, dusky; bedimmed, colourless, dimmed, dulled, faded, obscure, smirched, soiled, sullied.

dint *n* blow, stroke; dent, indentation, nick, notch; force, power.

diocese *n* bishopric, charge, episcopate, jurisdiction, see.

dip *vb* douse, duck, immerse, plunge, souse; bail, ladle; dive, pitch; bend, incline, slope. • *n* decline, declivity, descent, drop, fall; concavity, depression, hole, hollow, pit, sink; bathe, dipping, ducking, sousing, swim.

diplomat *n* diplomatist, envoy, legate, minister, negotiator.

dire *adj* alarming, awful, calamitous, cruel, destructive, disastrous, dismal, dreadful, fearful, gloomy, horrible, horrid, implacable, inexorable, portentous, shocking, terrible, terrific, tremendous, woeful.

direct *vb* aim, cast, level, point, turn; advise, conduct, control, dispose, guide, govern, manage, regulate, rule; command, bid, enjoin, instruct, order; lead, show; address, superscribe. • *adj* immediate, straight, undeviating; absolute, categorical, express, plain, unambiguous; downright, earnest, frank, ingenuous, open, outspoken, sincere, straightforward, unequivocal.

direction *n* aim; tendency; bearing, course; administration, conduct, control, government, management, oversight, superintendence; guidance, lead; command, order, prescription; address, superscription.

directly *adv* absolutely, expressly, openly, unambiguously; forthwith, immediately, instantly, quickly, presently, promptly, soon, speedily.

director *n* boss, manager, superintendent; adviser, counsellor, guide, instructor, mentor, monitor.

direful *adj* awful, calamitous, dire, dreadful, fearful, gloomy, horrible, shocking, terrible, terrific, tremendous.

dirge *n* coronach, elegy, lament, monody, requiem, threnody.

dirty *vb* befoul, defile, draggle, foul, pollute, soil, sully. • *adj* begrimed, defiled, filthy, foul, mucky, nasty, soiled, unclean; clouded, cloudy, dark, dull, muddy, sullied; base, beggarly, contemptible, despicable, grovelling, low, mean, paltry, pitiful, scurvy, shabby, sneaking, squalid; disagreeable, rainy, sloppy, uncomfortable.

disability *n* disablement, disqualification, impotence, impotency, inability, incapacity, incompetence, incompetency, unfitness, weakness.

disable *vb* cripple, enfeeble, hamstring, impair, paralyse, unman, weaken; disenable, disqualify, incapacitate, unfit.

disabuse *vb* correct, undeceive.

disadvantage *n* disadvantageousness, inconvenience, unfavourableness; damage, detriment, disservice, drawback, harm, hindrance, hurt, injury, loss, prejudice.

disadvantageous *adj* inconvenient, inexpedient, unfavourable; deleterious, detrimental, harmful, hurtful, injurious, prejudicial.

disaffect *vb* alienate, disdain, dislike, disorder, estrange.

disaffected *adj* alienated, disloyal, dissatisfied, estranged.

disaffection *n* alienation, breach, disagreement, dislike, disloyalty, dissatisfaction, estrangement, repugnance, ill will, unfriendliness.

disagree *vb* deviate, differ, diverge, vary; dissent; argue, bicker, clash, debate, dispute, quarrel, wrangle.

disagreeable *adj* contrary, displeasing, distasteful, nasty, offensive, unpleasant, unpleasing, unsuitable.

disagreement *n* deviation, difference, discrepancy, dissimilarity, dissimilitude, divergence, diversity, incongruity, unlikeness; disaccord, dissent; argument, bickering, clashing, conflict, contention, dispute, dissension, disunion, disunity, jarring, misunderstanding, quarrel, strife, variance, wrangle.

disallow *vb* forbid, prohibit; disapprove, reject; deny, disavow, disclaim, dismiss, disown, repudiate.

disappear *vb* depart, fade, vanish; cease, dissolve.

disappoint *vb* baffle, balk, deceive, defeat, delude, disconcert, foil, frustrate, mortify, tantalize, thwart, vex.

disappointment *n* baffling, balk, failure, foiling, frustration, miscarriage, mortification, unfulfilment.

disapprobation *n* blame, censure, condemnation, disapproval, dislike, displeasure, reproof.

disapprove *vb* blame, censure, condemn, deprecate, dislike; disallow, reject.

disarrange *vb* agitate, confuse, derange, disallow, dishevel, dislike, dislocate, disorder, disorganize, disturb, jumble, reject, rumple, tumble, unsettle.

disarray *n* confusion, disorder; dishabille.

disaster *n* accident, adversity, blow, calamity, casualty, catastrophe, misadventure, mischance, misfortune, mishap, reverse, ruin, stroke.

disastrous *adj* adverse, calamitous, catastrophic, destructive, hapless, ill-fated, ill-starred, ruinous, unfortunate, unlucky, unpropitious, unprosperous, untoward.

disavow *vb* deny, disallow, disclaim, disown.

disband *vb* break up, disperse, scatter, separate.

disbelief *n* agnosticism, doubt, nonconviction, rejection, unbelief.

disburden *vb* alleviate, diminish, disburden, discharge, disencumber, ease, free, relieve, rid.

disbursement *n* expenditure, spending.

discard *vb* abandon, cast off, lay aside, reject; banish, break, cashier, discharge, dismiss, remove, repudiate.

discern *vb* differentiate, discriminate, distinguish, judge; behold, descry, discover, espy, notice, observe, perceive, recognize, see.

discernible *adj* detectable, discoverable, perceptible.

discerning *adj* acute, astute, clear-sighted, discriminating, discriminative, eagle-eyed, ingenious, intelligent, judicious, knowing, perspicacious, piercing, sagacious, sharp, shrewd.

discernment *n* acumen, acuteness, astuteness, brightness, cleverness, discrimination, ingenuity, insight, intelligence, judgement, penetration, perspicacity, sagacity, sharpness, shrewdness; beholding, descrying, discerning, discovery, espial, notice, perception.

discharge *vb* disburden, unburden, unload; eject, emit, excrete, expel, void; cash, liquidate, pay; absolve, acquit, clear, exonerate, free, release, relieve; cashier, discard, dismiss, sack; destroy, remove; execute, perform, fulfil, observe; annul, cancel, invalidate, nullify, rescind. • *n* disburdening, unloading; acquittal, dismissal, displacement, ejection, emission, evacuation, excretion, expulsion, vent, voiding; blast, burst, detonation, explosion, firing; execution, fulfilment, observance; annulment, clearance, liquidation, payment, satisfaction, settlement; exemption, liberation, release; flow, flux, execration.

disciple *n* catechumen, learner, pupil, scholar, student; adherent, follower, partisan, supporter.

discipline *vb* breed, drill, educate, exercise, form, instruct, teach, train; control, govern, regulate, school; chasten, chastise, punish. • *n* culture, drill, drilling, education, exercise, instruction, training; control, government, regulation, subjection; chastisement, correction, punishment.

disclaim *vb* abandon, disallow, disown, disavow; reject, renounce, repudiate.

disclose *vb* discover, exhibit, expose, manifest, uncover; bare, betray, blab, communicate, divulge, impart, publish, reveal, show, tell, unfold, unveil, utter.

disclosure *n* betrayal, discovery, exposé, exposure, revelation, uncovering. discolour *vb* stain, tarnish, tinge.

discomfit *vb* beat, checkmate, conquer, defeat, overcome, overpower, overthrow, rout, subdue, vanquish, worst; abash, baffle, balk, confound, disconcert, foil, frustrate, perplex, upset.

discomfiture *n* confusion, defeat, frustration, overthrow, rout, vexation.

discomfort *n* annoyance, disquiet, distress, inquietude, malaise, trouble, uneasiness, unpleasantness, vexation.

discommode *vb* annoy, disquiet, disturb, harass, incommode, inconvenience, molest, trouble.

discompose *vb* confuse, derange, disarrange, disorder, disturb, embroil, jumble, unsettle; agitate, annoy, chafe, displease, disquiet, fret, harass, irritate, nettle, plague, provoke, ruffle, trouble, upset, vex, worry; abash, bewilder, disconcert, embarrass, fluster, perplex.

disconcert *vb* baffle, balk, contravene, defeat, disarrange, frustrate, interrupt, thwart, undo, upset; abash, agitate, bewilder, confuse, demoralize, discompose, disturb, embarrass, faze, perplex, perturb, unbalance, worry.

disconnect *vb* detach, disengage, disjoin, dissociate, disunite, separate, sever, uncouple, unlink.

disconsolate *adj* broken-hearted, cheerless, comfortless, dejected, desolate, forlorn, gloomy, heartbroken, inconsolable, melancholy, miserable, sad, sorrowful, unhappy, woeful, wretched.

discontent *n* discontentment, displeasure, dissatisfaction, inquietude, restlessness, uneasiness.

discontinuance *n* cessation, discontinuation, disjunction, disruption, intermission, interruption, separation, stop, stoppage, stopping, suspension.

discontinue *vb* cease, intermit, interrupt, quit, stop.

discord *n* contention, difference, disagreement, dissension, opposition, quarrelling, rupture, strife, variance, wrangling; cacophony, discordance, dissonance, harshness, jangle, jarring.

discordance *n* conflict, disagreement, incongruity, inconsistency, opposition, repugnance; discord, dissonance.

discordant *adj* contradictory, contrary, disagreeing, incongruous, inconsistent, opposite, repugnant; cacophonous, dissonant, harsh, inharmonious, jangling, jarring.

discount *vb* allow for, deduct, lower, rebate, reduce, subtract; disregard, ignore, overlook. • *n* abatement, drawback; allowance, deduction, rebate, reduction.

discourage *vb* abase, awe, damp, daunt, deject, depress, deject, dismay, dishearten, dispirit, frighten, intimidate; deter, dissuade, hinder; disfavour, discountenance.

discouragement *n* disheartening; dissuasion; damper, deterrent, embarrassment, hindrance, impediment, obstacle, wet blanket.

discourse *vb* expiate, hold forth, lucubrate, sermonize, speak; advise, confer, converse, parley, talk; emit, utter. • *n* address, disquisition, dissertation, homily, lecture, preachment, sermon, speech, treatise; colloquy, conversation, converse, talk.

discourteous *adj* abrupt, brusque, curt, disrespectful, ill-bred, ill-mannered, impolite, inurbane, rude, uncivil, uncourtly, ungentlemanly, unmannerly.

discourtesy *n* abruptness, brusqueness, ill-breeding, impoliteness, incivility, rudeness.

discover *vb* communicate, disclose, exhibit, impart, manifest, show, reveal, tell; ascertain, behold, discern, espy, see; descry, detect, determine, discern; contrive, invent, originate.

discredit *vb* disbelieve, doubt, question; depreciate, disgrace, dishonour, disparage, reproach. • *n* disbelief, distrust; disgrace, dishonour, disrepute, ignominy, notoriety, obloquy, odium, opprobrium, reproach, scandal.

discreditable *adj* derogatory, disgraceful, disreputable, dishonourable, ignominious, infamous, inglorious, scandalous, unworthy.

discreet *adj* careful, cautious, circumspect, considerate, discerning, heedful, judicious, prudent, sagacious, wary, wise.

discrepancy *n* contrariety, difference, disagreement, discordance, dissonance, divergence, incongruity, inconsistency, variance, variation.

discrete *adj* discontinuous, disjunct, distinct, separate; disjunctive.

discretion *n* care, carefulness, caution, circumspection, considerateness, consideration, heedfulness, judgement, judicious, prudence, wariness; discrimination, maturity, responsibility; choice, option, pleasure, will.

discrimination *n* difference, distinction; acumen, acuteness, discernment, in-sight, judgement, penetration, sagacity.

discriminatory *adj* characteristic, characterizing, discriminating, discriminative, distinctive, distinguishing.

discursive *adj* argumentative, reasoning; casual, cursory, desultory, digressive, erratic, excursive, loose, rambling, roving, wandering, wave.

discus *n* disk, quoit.

discuss vb agitate, argue, canvass, consider, debate, deliberate, examine, sift, ventilate.

disdain vb contemn, deride, despise, disregard, reject, scorn, slight, scout, spurn. • n arrogance, contempt, contumely, haughtiness, hauteur, scorn, sneer, superciliousness.

disdainful adj cavalier, contemptuous, contumelious, haughty, scornful, supercilious.

disease n affection, affliction, ail, ailment, complaint, disorder, distemper, illness, indisposition, infirmity, malady, sickness.

disembarrass vb clear, disburden, disencumber, disengage, disentangle, extricate, ease, free, release, rid.

disembodied adj bodiless, disincarnate, immaterial, incorporeal, spiritual, unbodied.

disembowel vb degut, embowel, eviscerate.

disengage vb clear, deliver, discharge, disembarrass, disembroil, disencumber, disentangle, extricate, liberate, release; detach, disjoin, dissociate, disunite, divide, separate; wean, withdraw.

disentangle vb loosen, separate, unfold, unravel, untwist; clear, detach, disconnect, disembroil, disengage, extricate, liberate, loose, unloose.

disfavour n disapproval, disesteem, dislike, disrespect; discredit, disregard, disrepute, unacceptableness; disservice unkindness. • vb disapprove, dislike, object, oppose.

disfigure vb blemish, deface, deform, injure, mar, spoil.

disfigurement n blemishing, defacement, deforming, disfiguration, injury, marring, spoiling; blemish, defect, deformity, scar, spot, stain.

disgorge vb belch, cast up, spew, throw up, vomit; discharge, eject; give up, relinquish, surrender, yield.

disgrace vb degrade, humble, humiliate; abase, debase, defame, discredit, disfavour, dishonour, disparage, reproach, stain, sully, taint, tarnish. • n abomination, disrepute, humiliation, ignominy, infamy, mortification, shame, scandal.

disgraceful adj discreditable, dishonourable, disreputable, ignominious, infamous, opprobrious, scandalous, shameful.

disguise vb cloak, conceal, cover, dissemble, hide, mask, muffle, screen, secrete, shroud, veil. • n concealment, cover, mask, veil; blind, cloak, masquerade, pretence, pretext, veneer.

disguised adj cloaked, masked, veiled.

disgust vb nauseate, sicken; abominate, detest, displease, offend, repel, repulse, revolt. • n disrelish, distaste, loathing, nausea; abhorrence, abomination, antipathy, aversion, detestation, dislike, repugnance, revulsion.

dish vb deal out, give, ladle, serve; blight, dash, frustrate, mar, ruin, spoil. • n bowl, plate, saucer, vessel.

dishearten vb cast down, damp, dampen, daunt, deject, depress, deter, discourage, dispirit.

dished adj baffled, balked, disappointed, disconcerted, foiled, frustrated, upset.

dishevelled adj disarranged, disordered, messed, tousled, tumbled, unkempt, untidy, untrimmed.

dishonest adj cheating, corrupt, crafty, crooked, deceitful, deceiving, deceptive, designing, faithless, false, falsehearted, fraudulent, guileful, knavish, perfidious, slippery, treacherous, unfair, unscrupulous.

dishonesty n deceitfulness, faithlessness, falsehood, fraud, fraudulence, fraudulency, improbity, knavery, perfidious, treachery, trickery.

dishonour vb abase, defame, degrade, discredit, disfavour, dishonour, disgrace, disparage, reproach, shame, taint. • n abasement, basement, contempt, degradation, discredit, disesteem, disfavour, disgrace, dishonour, disparagement, disrepute, ignominy, infamy, obloquy, odium, opprobrium, reproach, scandal, shame.

dishonourable adj discreditable, disgraceful, disreputable, ignominious, infamous, scandalous, shameful; base, false, falsehearted, shameless.

disinclination n alienation, antipathy, aversion, dislike, indisposition, reluctance, repugnance, unwillingness.

disinfect vb cleanse, deodorize, fumigate, purify, sterilize.

disingenuous adj artful, deceitful, dishonest, hollow, insidious, insincere, uncandid, unfair, wily.

disintegrate vb crumble, decompose, dissolve, disunite, pulverize, separate.

disinter vb dig up, disentomb, disinhume, exhume, unbury.

disinterested adj candid, fair, high-minded, impartial, indifferent, unbiased, unselfish, unprejudiced; generous, liberal, magnanimous.

disjoin vb detach, disconnect, dissever, dissociate, disunite, divide, part, separate, sever, sunder.

disjointed adj desultory, disconnected, incoherent, loose.

disjunction n disassociation, disconnection, disunion, isolation, parting, separation, severance.

dislike vb abominate, detest, disapprove, disrelish, hate, loathe. • n antagonism, antipathy, aversion, disapproval, disfavour, disgust, disinclination, displeasure, disrelish, distaste, loathing, repugnance.

dislocate vb disarrange, displace, disturb; disarticulate, disjoint, luxate, slip.

dislodge vb dismount, dispel, displace, eject, expel, oust, remove.

disloyal adj disaffected, faithless, false, perfidious, traitorous, treacherous, treasonable, undutiful, unfaithful, unpatriotic, untrue.

disloyalty n faithlessness, perfidy, treachery, treason, undutifulness, unfaithfulness.

dismal adj cheerless, dark, dreary, dull, gloomy, lonesome; blue, calamitous, doleful, dolorous, funereal, lugubrious, melancholy, mournful, sad, sombre, sorrowful.

dismantle vb divest, strip, unrig.

dismay vb affright, alarm, appal, daunt, discourage, dishearten, frighten, horrify, intimidate, paralyse, scare, terrify. • n affright, alarm, consternation, fear, fright, horror, terror.

dismember vb disjoint, dislimb, dislocate, mutilate; divide, separate, rend, sever.

dismiss vb banish, cashier, discard, discharge, disperse, reject, release, remove.

dismount vb alight, descend, dismantle, unhorse; dislodge, displace.

disobedient adj froward, noncompliant, noncomplying, obstinate, rebellious, refractory, uncomplying, undutiful, unruly, unsubmissive.

disobey vb infringe, transgress, violate.

disobliging adj ill-natured, unaccommodating, unamiable, unfriendly, unkind.

disorder vb confound, confuse, derange, disarrange, discompose, disorganize, disturb, unsettle, upset. • n confusion, derangement, disarrangement, disarray, disorganization, irregularity, jumble, litter, mess, topsy-turvy; brawl, commotion, disturbance, fight, quarrel, riot, tumult; riotousness, tumultuousness, turbulence; ail, ailment, complaint, distemper, illness, indisposition, malady, sickness.

disorderly adj chaotic, confused, intemperate, irregular, unmethodical, unsystematic, untidy; lawless, rebellious, riotous, tumultuous, turbulent ungovernable, unmanageable, unruly.

disorganization n chaos, confusion, demoralization, derangement, disorder.

disorganize vb confuse demoralize, derange, disarrange, discompose, disorder, disturb, unsettle, upset.

disown vb disavow, disclaim, reject, renounce, repudiate; abnegate, deny, disallow.

disparage vb belittle, decry, depreciate, derogate from, detract from, doubt, question, run down, underestimate, underpraise, underrate, undervalue; asperse, defame, inveigh against, reflect on, reproach, slur, speak ill of, traduce, vilify.

disparagement n belittlement, depreciation, derogation, detraction, underrating, undervaluing; derogation, detraction, diminution, harm, impairment, injury, lessening, prejudice, worsening; aspersion, calumny, defamation, reflection, reproach, traduction, vilification; blackening, disgrace, dispraise, indignity, reproach.

disparity n difference, disproportion, inequality; dissimilarity, dissimilitude, unlikeness.

dispassionate adj calm, collected, composed, cool, imperturbable, inexcitable, moderate, quiet, serene, sober, staid, temperate, undisturbed, unexcitable, unexcited, unimpassioned, unruffled; candid, disinterested, fair, impartial, neutral, unbiased.

dispatch, despatch vb assassinate, kill, murder, slaughter, slay; accelerate, conclude, dismiss, expedite, finish, forward, hasten, hurry, quicken, speed. • n dispatching, sending; diligence, expedition, haste, rapidity, speed; completion, conduct, doing, transaction; communication, document, instruction, letter, message, missive, report.

dispel vb banish, disperse, dissipate, scatter.

dispensation *n* allotment, apportioning, apportionment, dispensing, distributing, distribution; administration, stewardship; economy, plan, scheme, system; exemption, immunity, indulgence, licence, privilege.

dispense *vb* allot, apportion, assign, distribute; administer, apply, execute; absolve, excuse, exempt, exonerate, release, relieve.

disperse *vb* dispel, dissipate, dissolve, scatter, separate; diffuse, disseminate, spread; disappear, vanish.

dispirit *vb* damp, dampen, depress, deject, discourage, dishearten.

dispirited *adj* chapfallen, dejected, depressed, discouraged, disheartened, down-cast, down-hearted.

displace *vb* dislocate, mislay, misplace, move; dislodge, remove; cashier, depose, discard, discharge, dismiss, oust, replace, unseat.

display *vb* expand, extend, open, spread, unfold; exhibit, show; flaunt, parade. • *n* exhibition, manifestation, show; flourish, ostentation, pageant, parade, pomp.

displease *vb* disgruntle, disgust, disoblige, dissatisfy, offend; affront, aggravate, anger, annoy, chafe, chagrin, fret, irritate, nettle, pique, provoke, vex.

displeasure *n* disaffection, disapprobation, disapproval, dislike, dissatisfaction, distaste; anger, annoyance, indignation, irritation, pique, resentment, vexation, wrath; injury, offence.

disport *vb* caper, frisk, frolic, gambol, play, sport, wanton; amuse, beguile, cheer, divert, entertain, relax, solace.

disposal *n* arrangement, disposition; conduct, control, direction, disposure, government, management, ordering, regulation; bestowment, dispensation, distribution.

dispose *vb* arrange, distribute, marshal, group, place, range, rank, set; adjust, determine, regulate, settle; bias, incline, induce, lead, move, predispose; control, decide, regulate, rule, settle; arrange, bargain, compound; alienate, convey, demise, sell, transfer.

disposed *adj* apt, inclined, prone, ready, tending.

disposition *n* arrangement, arranging, classification, disposing, grouping, location, placing; adjustment, control, direction, disposure, disposal, management, ordering, regulation; aptitude, bent, bias, inclination, nature, predisposition, proclivity, proneness, propensity, tendency; character, constitution, humour, native, nature, temper, temperament, turn; inclination, willingness; bestowal, bestowment, dispensation, distribution.

dispossess *vb* deprive, divest, expropriate, strip; dislodge, eject, oust; disseise, disseize, evict, oust.

dispraise *n* blame, censure; discredit, disgrace, dishonour, disparagement, opprobrium, reproach, shame.

disproof *n* confutation, rebuttal, refutation.

disproportion *n* disparity, inadequacy, inequality, insufficiency, unsuitableness; incommensurateness.

disprove *vb* confute, rebel, rebut.

disputable *adj* controvertible, debatable, doubtful, questionable.

disputation *n* argumentation, controversy, debate, dispute.

disputatious *adj* argumentative, bickering, captious, caviling, contentious, dissentious, litigious, polemical, pugnacious, quarrelsome.

dispute *vb* altercate, argue, debate, litigate, question; bicker, brawl, jangle, quarrel, spar, spat, squabble, tiff, wrangle; agitate, argue, debate, ventilate; challenge, contradict, controvert, deny, impugn; contest, struggle for. • *n* controversy, debate, discussion, disputation; altercation, argument, bickering, brawl, disagreement, dissension, spat, squabble, tiff, wrangle.

disqualification *n* disability, incapitation.

disqualify *vb* disable, incapacitate, unfit; disenable, preclude, prohibit.

disquiet *vb* agitate, annoy, bother, discompose, disturb, excite, fret, harass, incommode, molest, plague, pester, trouble, vex, worry. • *n* anxiety, discomposure, disquietude, disturbance, restlessness, solicitude, trouble, uneasiness, unrest, vexation, worry.

disquisition *n* dissertation, discourse, essay, paper, thesis, treatise.

disregard *vb* contemn, despise, disdain, disobey, disparage, ignore, neglect, overlook, slight. • *n* contempt, ignoring, inattention, neglect, pretermit, oversight, slight; disesteem, disfavour, indifference.

disrelish *vb* dislike, loathe. • *n* dislike, distaste; flatness, insipidity, insipidness, nauseousness; antipathy, aversion, repugnance.

disreputable *adj* derogatory, discreditable, dishonourable, disgraceful, infamous, opprobrious, scandalous, shameful; base, contemptible, low, mean, vicious, vile, vulgar.

disrepute *n* abasement, degradation, derogation, discredit, disgrace, dishonour, ill-repute, odium.

disrespect *n* disesteem, disregard, irreverence, neglect, slight.

disrespectful *adj* discourteous, impertinent, impolite, rude, uncivil, uncourteous.

dissatisfaction *n* discontent, disquiet, inquietude, uneasiness; disapprobation, disapproval, dislike, displeasure.

dissect *vb* analyze, examine, explore, investigate, scrutinize, sift; cut apart.

dissemble *vb* cloak, conceal, cover, disguise, hide; counterfeit, dissimulate, feign, pretend.

dissembler *n* dissimulator, feigner, hypocrite, pretender, sham.

disseminate *vb* circulate, diffuse, disperse, proclaim, promulgate, propagate, publish, scatter, spread.

dissension *n* contention, difference, disagreement, discord, quarrel, strife, variance.

dissent *vb* decline, differ, disagree, refuse. • *n* difference, disagreement, nonconformity, opposition, recusancy, refusal.

dissentient *adj* disagreeing, dissenting, dissident, factious.

dissertation *n* discourse, disquisition, essay, thesis, treatise.

disservice *n* disadvantage, disfavour, harm, hurt, ill-turn, injury, mischief.

dissidence *n* disagreement, dissent, nonconformity, sectarianism.

dissimilar *adj* different, divergent, diverse, heterogeneous, unlike, various.

dissimilarity *n* dissimilitude, disparity, divergent, diversity, unlikeness, variation.

dissimulation *n* concealment, deceit, dissembling, double-dealing, duplicity, feigning, hypocrisy, pretence.

dissipate *vb* dispel, disperse, scatter; consume, expend, lavish, spend, squander, waste; disappear, vanish.

dissipation *n* dispersion, dissemination, scattering, vanishing; squandering, waste; crapulence, debauchery, dissoluteness, drunkenness, excess, profligacy.

dissociate *vb* disjoin, dissever, disunite, divide, separate, sever, sunder.

dissolute *adj* abandoned, corrupt, debauched, depraved, disorderly, dissipated, graceless, lax, lewd, licentious, loose, profligate, rakish, reprobate, shameless, vicious, wanton, wild.

dissolution *n* liquefaction, melting, solution; decomposition, putrefaction; death, disease; destruction, overthrow, ruin; termination.

dissolve *vb* liquefy, melt; disorganize, disunite, divide, loose, separate, sever; destroy, ruin; disappear, fade, scatter, vanish; crumble, decompose, disintegrate, perish.

dissonance *n* cacophony, discord, discordance, harshness, jarring; disagreement, discrepancy, incongruity, inconsistency.

dissonant *adj* discordant, grating, harsh, jangling, jarring, unharmonious; contradictory, disagreeing, discrepant, incongruous, inconsistent.

distance *vb* excel, outdo, outstrip, surpass. • *n* farness, remoteness; aloofness, coldness, frigidity, reserve, stiffness, offishness; absence, separation, space.

distant *adj* far, far-away, remote; aloof, ceremonious, cold, cool, frigid, haughty, reserved, stiff, uncordial; faint, indirect, obscure, slight.

distaste *n* disgust, disrelish; antipathy, aversion, disinclination, dislike, displeasure, dissatisfaction, repugnance.

distasteful *adj* disgusting, loathsome, nauseating, nauseous, unpalatable, unsavoury; disagreeable, displeasing, offensive, repugnant, repulsive, unpleasant.

distemper *n* ail, ailment, complaint, disease, disorder, illness, indisposition, malady, sickness.

distempered *adj* diseased, disordered; immoderate, inordinate, intemperate, unregulated.

distend *vb* bloat, dilate, enlarge, expand, increase, inflate, puff, stretch, swell, widen.

distil *vb* dribble, drip, drop; extract, separate.

distinct *adj* definite, different, discrete, disjunct, individual, separate, unconnected; clear, defined, manifest, obvious, plain, unconfused, unmistakable, well-defined.

distinction *n* discernment, discrimination, distinguishing; difference; account, celebrity, credit, eminence, fame, name, note, rank, renown, reputation, repute, respectability, superiority.

distinctive *adj* characteristic, differentiating, discriminating, distinguishing.

distinctness n difference, separateness; clearness, explicitness, lucidity, lucidness, perspicuity, precision.

distinguish vb characterize, mark; differentiate, discern, discriminate, perceive, recognize, see, single out, tell; demarcate, divide, separate; celebrate, honour, signalize.

distinguished adj celebrated, eminent, famous, illustrious, noted; conspicuous, extraordinary, laureate, marked, shining, superior, transcendent.

distort vb contort, deform, gnarl, screw, twist, warp, wrest; falsify, misrepresent, pervert.

distortion n contortion, deformation, deformity, twist, wryness; falsification, misrepresentation, perversion, wresting.

distract vb divert, draw away; bewilder, confound, confuse, derange, discompose, disconcert, disturb, embarrass, harass, madden, mystify, perplex, puzzle.

distracted adj crazed, crazy, deranged, frantic, furious, insane, mad, raving, wild.

distraction n abstraction, bewilderment, confusion, mystification, embarrassment, perplexity; agitation, commotion, discord, disorder, disturbance, division, perturbation, tumult, turmoil; aberration, alienation, delirium, derangement, frenzy, hallucination, incoherence, insanity, lunacy, madness, mania, raving, wandering.

distress vb afflict, annoy, grieve, harry, pain, perplex, rack, trouble; distrain, seize, take. • n affliction, calamity, disaster, misery, misfortune, adversity, hardship, perplexity, trial, tribulation; agony, anguish, dolour, grief, sorrow, suffering; gnawing, gripe, griping, pain, torment, torture; destitution, indigence, poverty, privation, straits, want.

distribute vb allocate, allot, apportion, assign, deal, dispense, divide, dole out, give, mete, partition, prorate, share; administer, arrange, assort, class, classify, dispose.

distribution n allocation, allotment, apportionment, assignment, assortment, dispensation, dispensing; arrangement, disposal, disposition, classification, division, dole, grouping, partition, sharing.

district n circuit, department, neighbourhood, province, quarter, region, section, territory, tract, ward.

distrust vb disbelieve, discredit, doubt, misbelieve, mistrust, question, suspect. • n doubt, misgiving, mistrust, question, suspicion.

distrustful adj doubting, dubious, suspicious.

disturb vb agitate, shake, stir; confuse, derange, disarrange, disorder, unsettle, upset; annoy, discompose, disconcert, disquiet, distract, fuss, incommode, molest, perturb, plague, trouble, ruffle, vex, worry; impede, interrupt, hinder.

disturbance n agitation, commotion, confusion, convulsion, derangement, disorder, perturbation, unsettlement; annoyance, discomposure, distraction, excitement, fuss; hindrance, interruption, molestation; brawl, commotion, disorder, excitement, fracas, hubbub, riot, rising, tumult, turmoil, uproar.

disunion n disconnection, disjunction, division, separation, severance; breach, feud, rupture, schism.

disunite vb detach, disconnect, disjoin, dissever, dissociate, divide, part, rend, separate, segregate, sever, sunder; alienate estrange.

disuse n desuetude, discontinuance, disusage, neglect, nonobservance.

ditch vb canalize, dig, excavate, furrow, gouge, trench; abandon, discard, dump, jettison, scrap. • n channel, drain, fosse, moat, trench.

divagation n deviation, digression, rambling, roaming, straying, wandering.

divan n bed, chesterfield, couch, settee, sofa.

divaricate vb diverge, fork, part.

dive vb explore, fathom, penetrate, plunge, sound. • n drop, fall, header, plunge; bar, den, dump, joint, saloon.

diverge vb divide, radiate, separate; divaricate, separate; deviate, differ, disagree, vary.

divers adj different, manifold, many, numerous, several, sundry, various.

diverse adj different, differing, disagreeing, dissimilar, divergent, heterogeneous, multifarious, multiform, separate, unlike, variant, various, varying.

diversion n deflection, diverting; amusement, delight, distraction, enjoyment, entertainment, game, gratification, pastime, play, pleasure, recreation, sport; detour, digression.

diversity n difference, dissimilarity, dissimilitude, divergence, unlikeness, variation; heterogeneity, manifoldness, multifariousness, multiformity, variety.

divert vb deflect, distract, disturb; amuse, beguile, delight, entertain, exhilarate, give pleasure, gratify, recreate, refresh, solace.

divest vb denude, disrobe, strip, unclothe, undress; deprive, dispossess, strip.

divide vb bisect, cleave, cut, dismember, dissever, disunite, open, part, rend, segregate, separate, sever, shear, split, sunder; allocate, allot, apportion, assign, dispense, distribute, dole, mete, portion, share; compartmentalize, demarcate, partition; alienate, disunite, estrange.

divination n augury, divining, foretelling, incantation, magic, sooth-saying, sorcery; prediction, presage, prophecy.

divine vb foretell, predict, presage, prognosticate, vaticinate, prophesy; believe, conjecture, fancy, guess, suppose, surmise, suspect, think. • adj deiform, godlike, superhuman, supernatural angelic, celestial, heavenly, holy, sacred, seraphic, spiritual; exalted, exalting, rapturous, supreme, transcendent. • n churchman, clergyman, ecclesiastic, minister, parson, pastor, priest.

division n compartmentalization, disconnection, disjunction, dismemberment, segmentation, separation, severance; category, class, compartment, head, parcel portion, section, segment; demarcation, partition; alienation, allotment, apportionment, distribution; breach, difference, disagreement, discord, disunion, estrangement, feud, rupture, variance.

divorce vb disconnect, dissolve, disunite, part, put away, separate, sever, split up, sunder, unmarry. • n disjunction, dissolution, disunion, division, divorcement, parting, separation, severance.

divulge vb communicate, declare, disclose, discover, exhibit, expose, impart, proclaim, promulgate, publish, reveal, tell, uncover.

dizzy adj giddy, vertiginous; careless, heedless, thoughtless.

do vb accomplish, achieve, act, commit, effect, execute, perform; complete, conclude, end, finish, settle, terminate; conduct, transact; observe, perform, practice; translate, render; cook, prepare; cheat, chouse, cozen, hoax, swindle; serve, suffice. • n act, action, adventure, deed, doing, exploit, feat, thing; banquet, event, feast, function, party.

docile adj amenable, obedient, pliant, teachable, tractable, yielding.

dock vb clip, curtail, cut, deduct, truncate; lessen, shorten.

dock vb anchor, moor; join, meet. • n anchorage, basin, berth, dockage, dockyard, dry dock, harbour, haven, marina, pier, shipyard, wharf.

doctor vb adulterate, alter, cook, falsify, manipulate, tamper with; attend, minister to, cure, heal, remedy, treat; fix, mend, overhaul, repair, service. • n general practitioner, GP, healer, leech, medic, physician; adept, savant.

doctrinaire adj impractical, theoretical. • n ideologist, theorist, thinker.

doctrine n article, belief, creed, dogma, opinion, precept, principle, teaching, tenet.

dodge vb equivocate, evade, prevaricate, quibble, shuffle. • n artifice, cavil, evasion, quibble, subterfuge, trick.

dogged adj cantankerous, headstrong, inflexible, intractable, mulish, obstinate, pertinacious, perverse, resolute, stubborn, tenacious, unyielding, wilful; churlish, morose, sour, sullen, surly.

dogma n article, belief, creed, doctrine, opinion, precept, principle, tenet.

dogmatic adj authoritative, categorical, formal, settled; arrogant, confident, dictatorial, imperious, magisterial, opinionated, oracular, overbearing, peremptory, positive; doctrinal.

dole vb allocate, allot, apportion, assign, deal, distribute, divide, share. • n allocation, allotment, apportionment, distribution; part, portion, share; alms, donation, gift, gratuity, pittance; affliction, distress, grief, sorrow, woe.

doleful adj lugubrious, melancholy, piteous, rueful, sad, sombre, sorrowful, woebegone, woeful; cheerless, dark, dismal, dolorous, dreary, gloomy.

dolorous adj cheerless, dark, dismal, gloomy; doleful, lugubrious, mournful, piteous, rueful, sad, sorrowful, woeful.

dolt n blockhead, booby, dullard, dunce, fool, ignoramus, simpleton.

domain n authority, dominion, jurisdiction, province, sway; empire, realm, territory; lands, estate; branch, department, region.

domestic n charwoman, help, home help, maid, servant. • adj domiciliary, family, home, household, private; domesticated; internal, intestine.

domesticate vb tame; adopt, assimilate, familiarize, naturalize.

domicile vb domiciliate, dwell, inhabit, live, remain, reside. • n abode, dwelling, habitation, harbour, home, house, residence.

dominant *adj* ascendant, ascending, chief, controlling, governing, influential, outstanding, paramount, predominant, preeminent, preponderant, presiding, prevailing, ruling.

dominate *vb* control, rule, sway; command, overlook, overtop, surmount.

domineer *vb* rule, tyrannize; bluster, bully, hector, menace, swagger, swell, threaten.

dominion *n* ascendancy, authority, command, control, domain, domination, government, jurisdiction, mastery, rule, sovereign, sovereignty, supremacy, sway; country, kingdom, realm, region, territory.

donation *n* alms, benefaction, boon, contribution, dole, donative, gift, grant, gratuity, largess, offering, present, subscription.

done *adj* accomplished, achieved, effected, executed, performed; completed, concluded, ended, finished, terminated; carried on, transacted; rendered, translated; cooked, prepared; cheated, cozened, hoaxed, swindled; (*with* **for**) damned, dished, *hors de combat*, ruined, shelved, spoiled, wound up.

donkey *n* ass, mule; dunce, fool, simpleton.

donor *n* benefactor, bestower, giver; donator.

double *vb* fold, plait; duplicate, geminate, increase, multiply, repeat; return. • *adj* binary, coupled, geminate, paired; dual, twice, twofold; deceitful, dishonest, double-dealing, false, hollow, insincere, knavish, perfidious, treacherous, two-faced. • *adv* doubly, twice, twofold. • *n* doubling, fold, plait; artifice, manoeuvre, ruse, shift, stratagem, trick, wile; copy, counterpart, twin.

doublet *n* jacket, jerkin.

doubt *vb* demur, fluctuate, hesitate, vacillate, waver; distrust, mistrust, query, question, suspect. • *n* dubiety, dubiousness, dubitation, hesitance, hesitancy, hesitation, incertitude, indecision, irresolution, question, suspense, uncertainty, vacillation; distrust, misgiving, mistrust, scepticism, suspicion.

doubtful *adj* dubious, hesitating, sceptical, undecided, undetermined, wavering; ambiguous, dubious, enigmatical, equivocal, hazardous, obscure, problematical, unsure; indeterminate, questionable, undecided, unquestioned.

doubtless *adv* certainly, unquestionably; clearly, indisputably, precisely.

doughty *adj* adventurous, bold, brave, chivalrous, courageous, daring, dauntless, fearless, gallant, heroic, intrepid, redoubtable, valiant, valorous.

douse *see* **dowse**.

dowdy *adj* awkward, dingy, ill-dressed, shabby, slatternly, slovenly; old-fashioned, unfashionable.

dowel *n* peg, pin, pinion, tenon.

dower *n* endowment, gift; dowry; portion, share.

downcast *adj* chapfallen, crestfallen, dejected, depressed, despondent, discouraged, disheartened, dispirited, downhearted, low-spirited, sad, unhappy.

downfall *n* descent, destruction, fall, ruin.

downhearted *adj* chapfallen, crestfallen, dejected, depressed, despondent, discouraged, disheartened, dispirited, downcast, low-spirited, sad, unhappy.

downright *adj* absolute, categorical, clear, explicit, plain, positive, sheer, simple, undisguised, unequivocal, utter; aboveboard, artless, blunt, direct, frank, honest, ingenuous, open, sincere, straightforward, unceremonious.

downy *adj* lanate, lanated, lanose.

dowse, douse *vb* dip, immerse, plunge, souse, submerge.

doxy *n* mistress, paramour; courtesan, drab, harlot, prostitute, strumpet, streetwalker, whore.

doze *vb* drowse, nap, sleep, slumber. • *n* drowse, forty-winks, nap.

dozy *adj* drowsy, heavy, sleepy, sluggish.

draft *vb* detach, select; commandeer, conscript, impress; delineate, draw, outline, sketch. • *n* conscription, drawing, selection; delineation, outline, sketch; bill, cheque, order.

drag *vb* draw, haul, pull, tow, tug; trail; linger, loiter. • *n* favour, influence, pull; brake, check, curb, lag, resistance, retardation, scotch, skid, slackening, slack-off, slowing.

draggle *vb* befoul, bemire, besmirch, dangle, drabble, trail.

dragoon *vb* compel, drive, force, harass, harry, persecute. • *n* cavalier, equestrian, horse-soldier.

drain *vb* milk, sluice, tap; empty, evacuate, exhaust; dry. • *n* channel, culvert, ditch, sewer, sluice, trench, watercourse; exhaustion, withdrawal.

draught *n* current, drawing, pulling, traction; cup, dose, drench, drink, potion; delineation, design, draft, outline, sketch.

draw *vb* drag, haul, tow, tug, pull; attract; drain, suck, syphon; extract, extort; breathe in, inhale, inspire; allure, engage, entice, induce, influence, lead, move, persuade; extend, protract, stretch; delineate, depict, sketch; deduce, derive, infer; compose, draft, formulate, frame, prepare; blister, vesicate, write.

drawback *n* defect, deficiency, detriment, disadvantage, fault, flaw, imperfection, injury; abatement, allowance, deduction, discount, rebate, reduction.

drawing *n* attracting, draining, inhaling, pulling, traction; delineation, draught, outline, picture, plan, sketch.

dread *vb* apprehend, fear. • *adj* dreadful, frightful, horrible, terrible; awful, venerable. • *n* affright, alarm, apprehension, fear, terror; awe, veneration.

dreadful *adj* alarming, appalling, awesome, dire, direful, fearful, formidable, frightful, horrible, horrid, terrible, terrific, tremendous; awful, venerable.

dream *vb* fancy, imagine, think. • *n* conceit, day-dream, delusion, fancy, fantasy, hallucination, illusion, imagination, reverie, vagary, vision.

dreamer *n* enthusiast, visionary.

dreamy *adj* absent, abstracted, fanciful, ideal, misty, shadowy, speculative, unreal, visionary.

dreary *adj* cheerless, chilling, comfortless, dark, depressing, dismal, drear, gloomy, lonely, lonesome, sad, solitary, sorrowful; boring, dull, monotonous, tedious, tiresome, uninteresting, wearisome.

dregs *npl* feculence, grounds, lees, off-scourings, residuum, scourings, sediment, waste; draff, dross, refuse, scum, trash.

drench *vb* dowse, drown, imbrue, saturate, soak, souse, steep, wet; physic, purge.

dress *vb* align, straighten; adjust, arrange, dispose; fit, prepare; accoutre, apparel, array, attire, clothe, robe, rig; adorn, bedeck, deck, decorate, drape, embellish, trim. • *n* apparel, attire, clothes, clothing, costume, garb, guise, garments, habiliment, habit, raiment, suit, toilet, vesture; bedizenment, bravery; frock, gown, rob.

dressing *n* compost, fertilizer, manure; forcemeat, stuffing.

dressy *adj* flashy, gaudy, showy.

driblet *n* bit, drop, fragment, morsel, piece, scrap.

drift *vb* accumulate, drive, float, wander. • *n* bearing, course, direction; aim, design, intent, intention, mark, object, proposal, purpose, scope, tendency; detritus, deposit, diluvium; gallery, passage, tunnel; current, rush, sweep; heap, pile.

drill[1] *vb* bore, perforate, pierce; discipline, exercise, instruct, teach, train. • *n* borer; discipline, exercise, training.

drill[2] *n* channel, furrow, trench.

drink *vb* imbibe, sip, swill; carouse, indulge, revel, tipple, tope; swallow, quaff; absorb. • *n* beverage, draught, liquid, potation, potion; dram, nip, sip, snifter, refreshment.

drip *vb* dribble, drop, leak, trickle; distil, filter, percolate; ooze, reek, seep, weep. • *n* dribble, drippings, drop, leak, leakage, leaking, trickle, tricklet; bore, nuisance, wet blanket.

drive *vb* hurl, impel, propel, send, shoot, thrust; actuate, incite, press, urge; coerce, compel, constrain, force, harass, oblige, overburden, press, rush; go, guide, ride, travel; aim, intend. • *n* effort, energy, pressure; airing, ride; road.

drivel *vb* babble, blether, dote, drool, slaver, slobber. • *n* balderdash, drivelling, fatuity, nonsense, prating, rubbish, slaver, stuff, twaddle.

drizzle *vb* mizzle, rain, shower, sprinkle. • *n* haar, mist, mizzle, rain, sprinkling.

droll *adj* comic, comical, farcical, funny, jocular, ludicrous, laughable, ridiculous; amusing, diverting, facetious, odd, quaint, queer, waggish. • *n* buffoon, clown, comedian, fool, harlequin, jester, punch, Punchinello, scaramouch, wag, zany.

drollery *n* archness, buffoonery, fun, humour, jocularity, pleasantry, waggishness, whimsicality.

drone *vb* dawdle, drawl, idle, loaf, lounge; hum. • *n* idler, loafer, lounger, sluggard.

drool *vb* drivel, slaver.

droop *vb* fade, wilt, wither; decline, fail, faint, flag, languish, sink, weaken; bend, hang.

drop *vb* distil, drip, shed; decline, depress, descend, dump, lower, sink; abandon, desert, forsake, forswear, leave, omit, relinquish, quit; cease, discontinue, intermit, remit; fall, precipitate. • *n* bead, droplet, globule; earring, pendant.

dross *n* cinder, lees, recrement, scoria, scum, slag; refuse, waste.

drought *n* aridity, drouth, dryness, thirstiness.

drove *n* flock, herd; collection, company, crowd.

drown *vb* deluge, engulf, flood, immerse, inundate, overflow, sink, submerge, swamp; overcome, overpower, overwhelm.

drowse *vb* doze, nap, sleep, slumber, snooze. • *n* doze, forty winks, nap, siesta, sleep, snooze.

drowsy *adj* dozy, sleepy; comatose, lethargic, stupid; lulling, soporific.

drub *vb* bang, beat, cane, cudgel, flog, hit, knock, pommel, pound, strike, thrash, thump, whack.

drubbing *n* beating, caning, cudgelling, flagellation, flogging, pommelling, pounding, thrashing, thumping, whacking.

drudge *vb* grub, grind, plod, slave, toil, work. • *n* grind, hack, hard worker, menial, plodder, scullion, servant, slave, toiler, worker.

drug *vb* dose, medicate; disgust, surfeit. • *n* medicine, physic, remedy; poison.

drunk *adj* boozed, drunken, inebriated, intoxicated, maudlin, soaked, tipsy; ablaze, aflame, delirious, fervent, suffused. • *n* alcoholic, boozer, dipsomaniac, drunkard, inebriate, lush, soak; bacchanal, bender, binge.

drunkard *n* alcoholic, boozer, carouser, dipsomaniac, drinker, drunk, inebriate, reveller, sot, tippler, toper.

dry *vb* dehydrate, desiccate, drain, exsiccate, parch. • *adj* desiccated, dried, juiceless, sapless, unmoistened; arid, droughty, parched; drouthy, thirsty; barren, dull, insipid, jejune, plain, pointless, tame, tedious, tiresome, unembellished, uninteresting, vapid; cutting, keen, sarcastic, severe, sharp, sly.

dub *vb* call, christen, denominate, designate, entitle, name, style, term.

dubious *adj* doubtful, fluctuating, hesitant, irresolute, skeptical, uncertain, undecided, unsettled, wavering; ambiguous, doubtful, equivocal, improbable, questionable, uncertain.

duck *vb* dip, dive, immerse, plunge, submerge, souse; bend, bow, dodge, stoop.

duct *n* canal, channel, conduit, pipe, tube; blood-vessel.

ductile *adj* compliant, docile, facile, tractable, yielding; flexible, malleable, pliant; extensible, tensile.

dudgeon *n* anger, indignation, ill will, ire, malice, resentment, umbrage, wrath.

due *adj* owed, owing; appropriate, becoming, befitting, bounden, fit, proper, suitable, right. • *adv* dead, direct, directly, exactly, just, right, squarely, straight. • *n* claim, debt, desert, right.

dulcet *adj* delicious, honeyed, luscious, sweet; harmonious, melodious; agreeable, charming, delightful, pleasant, pleasing.

dull *vb* blunt; benumb, besot, deaden, hebetate, obtund, paralyse, stupefy; dampen, deject, depress, discourage, dishearten, dispirit; allay, alleviate, assuage, mitigate, moderate, quiet, soften; deaden, dim, sully, tarnish. • *adj* blockish, brutish, doltish, obtuse, stolid, stupid, unintelligent; apathetic, callous, dead, insensible, passionless, phlegmatic, unfeeling, unimpassioned, unresponsive; heavy, inactive, inanimate, inert, languish, lifeless, slow, sluggish, torpid; blunt, dulled, hebetate, obtuse; cheerless, dismal, dreary, gloomy, sad, sombre; dim, lack-lustre, lustreless,

matt, obscure, opaque, tarnished; dry, flat, insipid, irksome, jejune, prosy, tedious, tiresome, uninteresting, wearisome.

duly *adv* befittingly, decorously, fitly, properly, rightly; regularly.

dumb *adj* inarticulate, mute, silent, soundless, speechless, voiceless.

dumbfound, dumfound *vb* amaze, astonish, astound, bewilder, confound, confuse, nonplus, pose.

dumps *npl* blues, dejection, depression, despondency, gloom, gloominess, melancholy, sadness.

dun[1] *adj* greyish-brown, brown, drab.

dun[2] *vb* beset, importure, press, urge.

dunce *n* ass, block, blockhead, clodpole, dolt, donkey, dullard, dunderhead, fool, goose, halfwit, ignoramus, jackass, lackwit, loon, nincompoop, numskull, oaf, simpleton, thickhead, witling.

dupe *vb* beguile, cheat, chouse, circumvent, cozen, deceive, delude, gull, hoodwink, outwit, overreach, swindle, trick. • *n* gull, simpleton.

duplicate *vb* copy, double, repeat, replicate, reproduce. • *adj* doubled, twofold. • *n* copy counterpart, facsimile, replica, transcript.

duplicity *n* artifice, chicanery, circumvention, deceit, deception, dishonesty, dissimulation, double-dealing, falseness, fraud, guile, hypocrisy, perfidy.

durable *adj* abiding, constant, continuing, enduring, firm, lasting, permanent, persistent, stable.

duration *n* continuance, continuation, permanency, perpetuation, prolongation; period, time.

duress *n* captivity, confinement, constraint, durance, hardship, imprisonment, restraint; compulsion.

dusky *adj* cloudy, darkish, dim, murky, obscure, overcast, shady, shadowy; dark, swarthy, tawny.

dutiful *adj* duteous, obedient, submissive; deferential, respectful, reverential.

duty *n* allegiance, devoirs, obligation, responsibility, reverence; business, engagement, function, office, service; custom, excise, impost, tariff, tax, toll.

dwarf *vb* lower, stunt. • *n* bantam, homunculus, manikin, midget, pygmy.

dwarfish *adj* diminutive, dwarfed, little, low, pygmy, small, stunted, tiny, undersized.

dwell *vb* abide, inhabit, live, lodge, remain, reside, rest, sojourn, stay, stop, tarry, tenant.

dwelling *n* abode, cot, domicile, dugout, establishment, habitation, home, house, hutch, lodging, mansion, quarters, residence.

dwindle *vb* decrease, diminish, lessen, shrink; decay, decline, deteriorate, pine, sink, waste away.

dye *vb* colour, stain, tinge. • *n* cast, colour, hue, shade, stain, tinge, tint.

dying *adj* expiring; mortal, perishable. • *n* death, decease, demise, departure, dissolution, exit.

dynasty *n* dominion, empire, government, rule, sovereignty.

dyspepsia *n* indigestion.

E

eager *adj* agog, avid, anxious, desirous, fain, greedy, impatient, keen, longing, yearning; animated, ardent, earnest, enthusiastic, fervent, fervid, forward, glowing, hot, impetuous, sanguine, vehement, zealous.

eagerness *n* ardour, avidity, earnestness, enthusiasm, fervour, greediness, heartiness, hunger, impatience, impetuosity, intentness, keenness, longing, thirst, vehemence, yearning, zeal.

eagle-eyed *adj* discerning, hawk-eyed, sharp-sighted.

ear[1] *n* attention, hearing, heed, regard.

ear[2] *n* head, spike.

early *adj* opportune, seasonable, timely; forward, premature; dawning, matutinal. • *adv* anon, beforehand, betimes, ere, seasonably, shortly, soon.

earn *vb* acquire, gain, get, obtain, procure, realize, reap, win; deserve, merit.

earnest *adj* animated, ardent, eager, cordial, fervent, fervid, glowing, hearty, impassioned, importune, warm, zealous; fixed, intent, steady; sincere, true, truthful; important, momentous, serious, weighty. • *n* reality, seriousness, truth; foretaste, pledge, promise; handsel, payment.

earnings *npl* allowance, emoluments, gains, income, pay, proceeds, profits, remuneration, reward, salary, stipend.

earth *n* globe, orb, planet, world; clay, clod, dirt, glebe, ground, humus, land, loam, sod, soil, turf; mankind, world.

earthborn *adj* abject, base, earthly, grovelling, low, mean, unspiritual.

earthly *adj* terrestrial; base, carnal, earthborn, low, gross, grovelling, sensual, sordid, unspiritual, worldly; bodily, material, mundane, natural, secular, temporal.

earthy *adj* clayey, earth-like, terrene; earthly, terrestrial; coarse, gross, material, unrefined.

ease *vb* disburden, disencumber, pacify, quiet, relieve, still; abate, allay, alleviate, appease, assuage, diminish, mitigate, soothe; loosen, release; facilitate, favour. • *n* leisure, quiescence, repose, rest; calmness, content, contentment, enjoyment, happiness, peace, quiet, quietness, quietude, relief, repose, satisfaction, serenity, tranquillity; easiness, facility, readiness; flexibility, freedom, liberty, lightness, naturalness, unconcern, unconstraint; comfort, elbowroom.

easy *adj* light; careless, comfortable, contented, effortless, painless, quiet, satisfied, tranquil, untroubled; accommodating, complaisant, compliant, complying, facile, indolent, manageable, pliant, submissive, tractable, yielding; graceful, informal, natural, unconstrained; flowing, ready, smooth, unaffected; gentle, lenient, mild, moderate; affluent, loose, unconcerned, unembarrassed.

eat *vb* chew, consume, devour, engorge, ingest, ravage, swallow; corrode, demolish, erode; breakfast, dine, feed, lunch, sup.

eatable *adj* edible, esculent, harmless, wholesome.

ebb *vb* abate, recede, retire, subside; decay, decline, decrease, degenerate, deteriorate, sink, wane. • *n* refluence, reflux, regress, regression, retrocedence, retrocession, retrogression, return; caducity, decay, decline, degeneration, deterioration, wane, waning; abatement, decrease, decrement, diminution.

ebullience *n* ebullition, effervescence; burst, bursting, overenthusiasm, overflow, rush, vigour.

ebullition *n* boiling, bubbling; effervescence, fermentation; burst, fit, outbreak, outburst, paroxysm.

eccentric *adj* decentred, parabolic; aberrant, abnormal, anomalous, cranky, erratic, fantastic, irregular, odd, outlandish, peculiar, singular, strange, uncommon, unnatural, wayward, whimsical. • *n* crank, curiosity, original.

eccentricity *n* ellipticity, flattening, flatness, oblateness; aberration, irregularity, oddity, oddness, peculiarity, singularity, strangeness, waywardness.

ecclesiastic[1], **ecclesiastical** *adj* churchish, churchly, clerical, ministerial, nonsecular, pastoral, priestly, religious, sacerdotal.

ecclesiastic[2] *n* chaplain, churchman, clergyman, cleric, clerk, divine, minister, parson, pastor, priest, reverend, shepherd.

echo *vb* reply, resound, reverberate, ring; re-echo, repeat. • *n* answer, repetition, reverberation; imitation.

éclat *n* acclamation, applause, brilliancy, effect, glory, lustre, pomp, renown, show, splendour.

eclipse *vb* cloud, darken, dim, obscure, overshadow, veil; annihilate, annul, blot out, extinguish. • *n* clouding, concealment, darkening, dimming, disappearance, hiding, obscuration, occultation, shrouding, vanishing, veiling; annihilation, blotting out, destruction, extinction, extinguishment, obliteration.

eclogue *n* bucolic, idyl, pastoral.

economize *vb* husband, manage, save; retrench.

economy *n* frugality, husbandry, parsimony, providence, retrenchment, saving, skimping, stinginess, thrift, thriftiness; administration, arrangement, management, method, order, plan, regulation, system; dispensation.

ecstasy *n* frenzy, madness, paroxysm, trance; delight, gladness, joy, rhapsody, rapture, ravishment, transport.

eddy *vb* gurgle, surge, spin, swirl, whirl. • *n* countercurrent; swirl, vortex, whirlpool.

edge *vb* sharpen; border, fringe, rim. • *n* border, brim, brink, bound, crest, fringe, hem, lip, margin, rim, verge; animation, intensity, interest, keenness, sharpness, zest; acrimony, bitterness, gall, sharpness, sting.

edging *n* border, frill, fringe, trimming.

edible *adj* eatable, esculent, harmless, wholesome.

edict *n* act, command, constitution, decision, decree, law, mandate, manifesto, notice, order, ordinance, proclamation, regulation, rescript, statute.

edifice *n* building, fabric, habitation, house, structure.

edify *vb* educate, elevate, enlightenment, improve, inform, instruct, nurture, teach, upbuild.

edition *n* impression, issue, number.

educate *vb* breed, cultivate, develop, discipline, drill, edify, exercise, indoctrinate, inform, instruct, mature, nurture, rear, school, teach, train.

educated *adj* cultured, lettered, literate.

education *n* breeding, cultivation, culture, development, discipline, drilling, indoctrination, instruction, nurture, pedagogics, schooling, teaching, training, tuition.

educe *vb* bring out, draw out, elicit, evolve, extract.

eerie *adj* awesome, fearful, frightening, strange, uncanny, weird.

efface *vb* blot, blot out, cancel, delete, destroy, erase, expunge, obliterate, remove, sponge.

effect *vb* cause, create, effectuate, produce; accomplish, achieve, carry, compass, complete, conclude, consummate, contrive, do, execute, force, negotiate, perform, realize, work. • *n* consequence, event, fruit, issue, outcome, result; efficiency, fact, force, power, reality; validity, weight; drift, import, intent, meaning, purport, significance, tenor.

effective *adj* able, active, adequate, competent, convincing, effectual, sufficient; cogent, efficacious, energetic, forcible, potent, powerful.

effects *npl* chattels, furniture, goods, movables, property.

effectual *adj* operative, successful; active, effective, efficacious, efficient.

effectuate *vb* accomplish, achieve, complete, do, effect, execute, fulfil, perform, secure.

effeminate *adj* delicate, feminine, soft, tender, timorous, unmanly, womanish, womanlike, womanly; camp.

effervesce *vb* bubble, ferment, foam, froth.

effete *adj* addle, barren, fruitless, sterile, unfruitful, unproductive, unprolific; decayed, exhausted, spent, wasted.

efficacious *adj* active, adequate, competent, effective, effectual, efficient, energetic, operative, powerful.

efficacy *n* ability, competency, effectiveness, efficiency, energy, force, potency, power, strength, vigour, virtue.

efficient *adj* active, capable, competent, effective, effectual, efficacious, operative, potent; able, energetic, ready, skilful.

effigy *n* figure, image, likeness, portrait, representation, statue.

effloresce *vb* bloom, flower.

efflorescence *n* blooming, blossoming, flowering.

effluence *n* discharge, efflux, effluvium, emanation, emission, flow, outflow, outpouring.

effort *n* application, attempt, endeavour, essay, exertion, pains, spurt, strain, strife, stretch, struggle, trial, trouble.

effrontery *n* assurance, audacity, boldness, brass, disrespect, hardihood, impudence, incivility, insolence, presumption, rudeness, sauciness, shamelessness.

effulgent *adj* burning, beaming, blazing, bright, brilliant, dazzling, flaming, glowing, lustrous, radiant, refulgent, resplendent, shining, splendid.

effusion *n* discharge, efflux, emission, gush, outpouring; shedding, spilling, waste; address, speech, talk, utterance.

egg *vb* (*with* **on**) encourage, incite, instigate, push, stimulate, urge; harass, harry, provoke.

ego *n* id, self, me, subject, superego.

egotism *n* self-admiration, self-assertion, self-commendation, self-conceit, self-esteem, self-importance, self-praise; egoism, selfishness.

egotistic, egotistical *adj* bumptious, conceited, egoistical, opinionated, self-asserting, self-admiring, self-centred, self-conceited, self-important, self-loving, vain.

egregious *adj* conspicuous, enormous, extraordinary, flagrant, great, gross, huge, monstrous, outrageous, prodigious, remarkable, tremendous.

egress *n* departure, emergence, exit, outlet, way out.

eject *vb* belch, discharge, disgorge, emit, evacuate, puke, spew, spit, spout, spurt, void, vomit; bounce, cashier, discharge, dismiss, disposes, eliminate, evict, expel, fire, oust; banish, reject, throw out.

elaborate *vb* develop, improve, mature, produce, refine, ripen. • *adj* complicated, decorated, detailed, dressy, laboured, laborious, ornate, perfected, studied.

elapse *vb* go, lapse, pass.

elastic *adj* rebounding, recoiling, resilient, springy; buoyant, recuperative.

elated *adj* animated, cheered, elate, elevated excited, exhilarated, exultant, flushed, puffed up, roused.

elbow *vb* crowd, force, hustle, jostle, nudge, push, shoulder. • *n* angle, bend, corner, flexure, joining, turn.

elder *adj* older, senior; ranking; ancient, earlier, older. • *n* ancestor, senior; presbyter, prior, senator.

elect *vb* appoint, choose, cull, designate, pick, prefer, select. • *adj* choice, chosen, picked, selected; appointed, elected; predestinated, redeemed.

election *n* appointment, choice, preference, selection; alternative, freedom, freewill, liberty; predestination.

elector *n* chooser, constituent, selector, voter.

electrify *vb* charge, galvanize; astonish, enchant, excite, rouse, startle, stir, thrill.

elegance, elegancy *n* beauty, grace, propriety, symmetry; courtliness, daintiness, gentility, nicety, polish, politeness, refinement, taste.

elegant *adj* beautiful, chaste, classical, dainty, graceful, fine, handsome, neat, symmetrical, tasteful, trim, well-made, well-proportioned; accomplished, courtly, cultivated, fashionable, genteel, polished, polite, refined.

elegiac *adj* dirgeful, mournful, plaintive, sorrowful.

elegy *n* dirge, epicedium, lament, ode, threnody.

element *n* basis, component, constituent, factor, germ, ingredient, part, principle, rudiment, unit; environment, milieu, sphere.

elementary *adj* primordial, simple, uncombined, uncomplicated, uncompounded; basic, component, fundamental, initial, primary, rudimental, rudimentary.

elevate *vb* erect, hoist, lift, raise; advance, aggrandize, exalt, promote; dignify, ennoble, exalt, greaten, improve, refine; animate, cheer, elate, excite, exhilarate, rouse.

elfin *adj* elflike, elvish, mischievous, weird.

elicit *vb* draw out, educe, evoke, extort, fetch, obtain, pump, wrest, wring; deduce, educe.

eligible *adj* desirable, preferable; qualified, suitable, worthy.

eliminate *vb* disengage, eradicate, exclude, expel, remove, separate; ignore, omit, reject.

ellipsis *n* gap, hiatus, lacuna, omission.

elliptical *adj* oval; defective, incomplete.

elocution *n* declamation, delivery, oratory, rhetoric, speech, utterance.

elongate *vb* draw, draw out, extend, lengthen, protract, stretch.

elope *vb* abscond, bolt, decamp, disappear, leave.

eloquence *n* fluency, oratory, rhetoric.

else *adv* besides, differently, otherwise.

elucidate *vb* clarify, demonstrate, explain, expound, illuminate, illustrate, interpret, unfold.

elucidation *n* annotation, clarification, comment, commentary, elucidating, explaining, explanation, exposition, gloss, scholium.

elude *vb* avoid, escape, evade, shun, slip; baffle, balk, disappoint, disconcert, escape, foil, frustrate, thwart.

elusive *adj* deceptive, deceitful, delusive, evasive, fallacious, fraudulent, illusory; equivocatory, equivocating, shuffling.

Elysian *adj* blissful, celestial, delightful, enchanting, heavenly, ravishing, seraphic.

emaciation *n* attenuation, lankness, leanness, meagreness, tabes, tabescence, thinness.

emanate *vb* arise, come, emerge, flow, issue, originate, proceed, spring.

emancipate *vb* deliver, discharge, disenthral, enfranchise, free, liberate, manumit, release, unchain, unfetter, unshackle.

emancipation *n* deliverance, enfranchisement, deliverance, freedom, liberation, manumission, release.

emasculate *vb* castrate, geld; debilitate, effeminize, enervate, unman, weaken.

embalm *vb* cherish, consecrate, conserve, enshrine, preserve, store, treasure; perfume, scent.

embargo *vb* ban, bar, blockade, debar, exclude, prohibit, proscribe, restrict, stop, withhold. • *n* ban, bar, blockade, exclusion, hindrance, impediment, prohibition, prohibitory, proscription, restraint, restriction, stoppage.

embark *vb* engage, enlist.

embarrass *vb* beset, entangle, perplex; annoy, clog, bother, distress, hamper, harass, involve, plague, trouble, vex; abash, confound, confuse, discomfit, disconcert, dumbfound, mortify, nonplus, pose, shame.

embellish *vb* adorn, beautify, bedeck, deck, decorate, emblazon, enhance, enrich, garnish, grace, ornament.

embellishment *n* adornment, decoration, enrichment, ornament, ornamentation.

embezzle *vb* appropriate, defalcate, filch, misappropriate, peculate, pilfer, purloin, steal.

embitter *vb* aggravate, envenom, exacerbate; anger, enrage, exasperate, madden.

emblem *n* badge, cognizance, device, mark, representation, sign, symbol, token, type.

embody *vb* combine, compact, concentrate, incorporate; comprehend, comprise, contain, embrace, include; codify, methodize, systematize.

embolden *vb* animate, cheer, elate, encourage, gladden, hearten, inspirit, nerve, reassure.

embosom *vb* bury, cherish, clasp, conceal, enfold, envelop, enwrap, foster, hide, nurse, surround.

embrace *vb* clasp; accept, seize, welcome; comprehend, comprise, contain, cover, embody, encircle, enclose, encompass, enfold, hold, include. • *n* clasp, fold, hug.

embroil *vb* commingle, encumber, ensnarl, entangle, implicate, involve; confuse, discompose, disorder, distract, disturb, perplex, trouble.

embryo *n* beginning, germ, nucleus, root, rudiment.

embryonic *adj* incipient, rudimentary, undeveloped.

emendation *n* amendment, correction, improvement, rectification.

emerge *vb* rise; emanate, escape, issue; appear, arise, outcrop.

emergency *n* crisis, difficulty, dilemma, exigency, extremity, necessity, pass, pinch, push, strait, urgency; conjuncture, crisis, juncture, pass.

emigration *n* departure, exodus, migration, removal.

eminence *n* elevation, hill, projection, prominence, protuberance; celebrity, conspicuousness, distinction, exaltation, fame, loftiness, note, preferment, reputation, repute, renown.

eminent *adj* elevated, high, lofty; celebrated, conspicuous, distinguished, exalted, famous, illustrious, notable, prominent, remarkable, renowned.

emissary *n* messenger, scout, secret agent, spy.

emit *vb* breathe out, dart, discharge, eject, emanate, exhale, gust, hurl, jet, outpour, shed, shoot, spurt, squirt.

emollient *adj* relaxing, softening, soothing. • *n* softener.

emolument *n* compensation, gain, hire, income, lucre, pay, pecuniary, profits, salary, stipend, wages; advantage, benefit, profit, perquisites.

emotion *n* agitation, excitement, feeling, passion, perturbation, sentiment, sympathy, trepidation.

emphasis *n* accent, stress; force, importance, impressiveness, moment, significance, weight.

emphatic *adj* decided, distinct, earnest, energetic, expressive, forcible, impressive, intensive, positive, significant, strong, unequivocal.

empire *n* domain, dominion, sovereignty, supremacy; authority, command, control, government, rule, sway.

empirical, empiric *adj* experimental, experiential; hypothetical, provisional, tentative; charlatanic, quackish.

employ *vb* busy, devote, engage, engross, enlist, exercise, occupy, retain; apply, commission, use. • *n* employment, service.

employee *n* agent, clerk, employee, hand, servant, workman.

employment *n* avocation, business, calling, craft, employ, engagement, occupation, profession, pursuit, trade, vocation, work.

emporium *n* market, mart, shop, store.

empower *vb* authorize, commission, permit, qualify, sanction, warrant; enable.

empty *vb* deplete, drain, evacuate, exhaust; discharge, disembogue; flow, embogue. • *adj* blank, hollow, unoccupied, vacant, vacuous, void; deplete, destitute, devoid, hungry; unfilled, unfurnished, unsupplied; unsatisfactory, unsatisfying, unsubstantial, useless, vain; clear, deserted, desolate, exhausted, free, unburdened, unloaded, waste; foolish, frivolous, inane, senseless, silly, stupid, trivial, weak.

empyrean, empyreal *adj* aerial, airy, ethereal, heavenly, refined, sublimated, sublimed.

emulation *n* competition, rivalry, strife, vying; contention, envy, jealousy.

enable *vb* authorize, capacitate, commission, empower, fit, permit, prepare, qualify, sanction, warrant.

enact *vb* authorize, command, decree, establish, legislate, ordain, order, sanction; act, perform, personate, play, represent.

enactment *n* act, decree, law, edict, ordinance.

enamour *vb* bewitch, captivate, charm, enchant, endear, fascinate.

enchain *vb* bind, confine, enslave, fetter, hold, manacle, restrain, shackle.

enchant *vb* beguile, bewitch, charm, delude, fascinate; captivate, catch, enamour, win; beatify, delight, enrapture, rapture, ravish, transport.

enchanting *adj* bewitching, blissful, captivating, charming, delightful, enrapturing, fascinating, rapturous, ravishing.

enchantment *n* charm, conjuration, incantation, magic, necromancy, sorcery, spell, witchery; bliss, delight, fascination, rapture, ravishment, transport.

encase *vb* encircle, enclose, incase, infix, set; chase, emboss, engrave, inlay, ornament.

encage *vb* confine, coop up, impound, imprison, shut up.

encircle *vb* belt, circumscribe, encompass, enclose, engird, enring, environ, gird, ring, span, surround, twine; clasp, embrace, enfold, fold.

enclose, inclose *vb* circumscribe, corral, coop, embosom, encircle, encompass, environ, fence in, hedge, include, pen, shut in, surround; box, cover, encase, envelop, wrap.

encomium *n* applause, commendation, eulogy, laudation, panegyric, praise.

encompass *vb* belt, compass, encircle, enclose, engird, environ, gird, surround; beset, besiege, hem in, include, invest, surround.

encounter *vb* confront, face, meet; attack, combat, contend, engage, strive, struggle. • *n* assault, attack, clash, collision, meeting, onset; action, affair, battle, brush, combat, conflict, contest, dispute, engagement, skirmish.

encourage *vb* animate, assure, cheer, comfort, console, embolden, enhearten, fortify, hearten, incite, inspirit, instigate, reassure, stimulate, strengthen; abet, aid, advance, approve, countenance, favour, foster, further, help, patronize, promote, support.

encroach *vb* infringe, invade, intrude, tench, trespass, usurp.

encumber *vb* burden, clog, hamper, hinder, impede, load, obstruct, overload, oppress, retard; complicate, embarrass, entangle, involve, perplex.

encumbrance *n* burden, clog, deadweight, drag, embarrassment, hampering, hindrance, impediment, incubus, load; claim, debt, liability, lien.

end *vb* abolish, close, conclude, discontinue, dissolve, drop, finish, stop, terminate; annihilate, destroy, kill; cease, terminate. • *n* extremity, tip; cessation, close, denouement, ending, expiration, finale, finis, finish, last, period, stoppage, wind-up; completion, conclusion, consummation; annihilation, catastrophe, destruction, dissolution; bound, limit, termination, terminus; consequence, event, issue, result, settlement, sequel, upshot; fragment, remnant, scrap, stub, tag, tail; aim, design, goal, intent, intention, object, objective, purpose.

endanger *vb* compromise, hazard, imperil, jeopardize, peril, risk.

endear *vb* attach, bind, captivate, charm, win.

endearment *n* attachment, fondness, love, tenderness; caress, blandishment, fondling.

endeavour *vb* aim, attempt, essay, labour, seek, strive, struggle, study, try. • *n* aim, attempt, conatus, effort, essay, exertion, trial, struggle, trial.

endless *adj* boundless, illimitable, immeasurable, indeterminable, infinite, interminable, limitless, unlimited; dateless, eternal, everlasting, never-ending, perpetual, unending; deathless, ever-enduring, ever-living, immortal, imperishable, undying.

endorse, indorse *vb* approve, back, confirm, guarantee, ratify, sanction, superscribe, support, visé, vouch for, warrant; superscribe.

endow *vb* bequeath, clothe, confer, dower, endue, enrich, gift, indue, invest, supply.

endowment *n* bequest, boon, bounty, gift, grant, largesse, present; foundation, fund, property, revenue; ability, aptitude, capability, capacity, faculty, genius, gift, parts, power, qualification, quality, talent.

endurance *n* abiding, bearing, sufferance, suffering, tolerance, toleration; backbone, bottom, forbearance, fortitude, guts, patience, resignation.

endure *vb* bear, support, sustain; experience, suffer, undergo, weather; abide, brook, permit, pocket, swallow, tolerate, stomach; submit, withstand; continue, last, persist, remain, wear.

enemy *n* adversary, foe; antagonist, foeman, opponent, rival.

energetic *adj* active, effective, efficacious, emphatic, enterprising, forceful, forcible, hearty, mettlesome, potent, powerful, strenuous, strong, vigorous.

energy *n* activity, dash, drive, efficacy, efficiency, force, go, impetus, intensity, mettle, might, potency, power, strength, verve, vim; animation, life, manliness, spirit, spiritedness, stamina, vigour, zeal.

enervate *vb* break, debilitate, devitalize, emasculate, enfeeble, exhaust, paralyse, relax, soften, unhinge, unnerve, weaken.

enfeeble *vb* debilitate, devitalize, enervate, exhaust, relax, unhinge, unnerve, weaken.

enfold, infold *vb* enclose, envelop, fold, enwrap, wrap; clasp, embrace.

enforce *vb* compel, constrain, exact, force, oblige, require, urge.

enfranchise *vb* emancipate, free, liberate, manumit, release.

engage *vb* bind, commit, obligate, pledge, promise; affiance, betroth, plight; book, brief, employ, enlist, hire, retain; arrest, allure, attach, draw, entertain, fix, gain, win; busy, commission, contract, engross, occupy; attack, encounter; combat, contend, contest, fight, interlock, struggle; embark, enlist; agree, promise, stipulate, undertake, warrant.

engagement *n* appointment, assurance, contract, obligation, pledge, promise, stipulation; affiancing, betrothment, betrothal, plighting; avocation, business, calling, employment, enterprise, occupation; action, battle, combat, encounter, fight.

engender *vb* bear, beget, breed, create, generate, procreate, propagate; cause, excite, incite, occasion, produce.

engine *n* invention, machine; agency, agent, device, implement, instrument, means, method, tool, weapon.

engorge *vb* bolt, devour, eat, gobble, gorge, gulp, swallow; glut, obstruct, stuff.

engrave *vb* carve, chisel, cut, etch, grave, hatch, incise, sculpt; grave, impress, imprint, infix.

engross *vb* absorb, engage, occupy, take up; buy up, forestall, monopolize.

engrossment n absorption, forestalling, monopoly.

engulf, ingulf vb absorb, overwhelm, plunge, swallow up.

enhance vb advance, aggravate, augment, elevate, heighten, increase, intensify, raise, swell.

enhearten vb animate, assure, cheer, comfort, console, embolden, encourage, hearten, incite, inspirit, reassure, stimulate.

enigma n conundrum, mystery, problem, puzzle, riddle.

enigmatic, enigmatical adj ambiguous, dark, doubtful, equivocal, hidden, incomprehensible, mysterious, mystic, obscure, occult, perplexing, puzzling, recondite, uncertain, unintelligible.

enjoin vb admonish, advise, urge; bid, command, direct, order, prescribe, require; prohibit, restrain.

enjoy vb like, possess, relish.

enjoyment n delight, delectation, gratification, happiness, indulgence, pleasure, satisfaction; possession.

enkindle vb inflame, ignite, kindle; excite, incite, instigate, provoke, rouse, stimulate.

enlarge vb amplify, augment, broaden, develop, dilate, distend, expand, extend, grow, increase, magnify, widen; aggrandize, engreaten, ennoble, expand, exaggerate, greaten; swell.

enlighten vb illume, illuminate, illumine; counsel, educate, civilize, inform, instruct, teach.

enlist vb enrol, levy, recruit, register; enrol, list; embark, engage.

enliven vb animate, invigorate, quicken, reanimate, rouse, wake; exhilarate, cheer, brighten, delight, elate, gladden, inspire, inspirit, rouse.

enmity n animosity, aversion, bitterness, hate, hatred, hostility, ill-will, malevolence, malignity, rancour.

ennoble vb aggrandize, dignify, elevate, engreaten, enlarge, exalt, glorify, greaten, raise.

ennui n boredom, irksomeness, languor, lassitude, listlessness, tedium, tiresomeness, weariness.

enormity n atrociousness, atrocity, depravity, flagitiousness, heinousness, nefariousness, outrageousness, villainy, wickedness.

enormous adj abnormal, exceptional, inordinate, irregular; colossal, Cyclopean, elephantine, Herculean, huge, immense, monstrous, vast, gigantic, prodigious, titanic, tremendous.

enough adj abundant, adequate, ample, plenty, sufficient. • adv satisfactorily, sufficiently. • n abundance, plenty, sufficiency.

enquire see **inquire**.

enrage vb anger, chafe, exasperate, incense, inflame, infuriate, irritate, madden, provoke.

enrapture vb beatify, bewitch, delight, enchant, enravish, entrance, surpassingly, transport.

enrich vb endow; adorn, deck, decorate, embellish, grace, ornament.

enrobe vb clothe, dress, apparel, array, attire, invest, robe.

enrol vb catalogue, engage, engross, enlist, list, register; chronicle, record.

ensconce vb conceal, cover, harbour, hide, protect, screen, secure, settle, shelter, shield, snugly.

enshrine vb embalm, enclose, entomb; cherish, treasure.

ensign n banner, colours, eagle, flag, gonfalon, pennon, standard, streamer; sign, signal, symbol; badge, hatchment.

enslave vb captivate, dominate, master, overmaster, overpower, subjugate.

ensnare vb catch, entrap; allure, inveigle, seduce; bewilder, confound, embarrass, encumber, entangle, perplex.

ensue vb follow, succeed; arise, come, flow, issue, proceed, result, spring.

entangle vb catch, ensnare, entrap; confuse, enmesh, intertwine, intertwist, interweave, knot, mat, ravel, tangle; bewilder, embarrass, encumber, ensnare, involve, nonplus, perplex, puzzle.

enterprise n adventure, attempt, cause, effort, endeavour, essay, project, undertaking, scheme, venture; activity, adventurousness, daring, dash, energy, initiative, readiness, push.

enterprising adj adventurous, audacious, bold, daring, dashing, venturesome, venturous; active, adventurous, alert, efficient, energetic, prompt, resourceful, smart, spirited, stirring, strenuous, zealous.

entertain vb fete, receive, regale, treat; cherish, foster, harbour, hold, lodge, shelter; admit, consider; amuse, cheer, divert, please, recreate.

entertainment n hospitality; banquet, collation, feast, festival, reception, treat; amusement, diversion, pastime, recreation, sport.

enthusiasm n ecstasy, exaltation, fanaticism; ardour, earnestness, devotion, eagerness, fervour, passion, warmth, zeal.

enthusiast n bigot, devotee, fan, fanatic, freak, zealot; castlebuilder, dreamer, visionary.

entice vb allure, attract, bait, cajole, coax, decoy, inveigle, lure, persuade, prevail on, seduce, tempt, wheedle, wile.

enticement n allurement, attraction, bait, blandishment, inducement, inveiglement, lure, persuasion, seduction.

entire adj complete, integrated, perfect, unbroken, undiminished, undivided, unimpaired, whole; complete, full, plenary, thorough; mere, pure, sheer, unalloyed, unmingled, unmitigated, unmixed.

entitle vb call, characterize, christen, denominate, designate, dub, name, style; empower, enable, fit for, qualify for.

entomb vb bury, inhume, inter.

entrails npl bowels, guts, intestines, inwards, offal, viscera.

entrance[1] n access, approach, avenue, incoming, ingress; adit, avenue, aperture, door, doorway, entry, gate, hallway, inlet, lobby, mouth, passage, portal, stile, vestibule; beginning, commencement, debut, initiation, introduction; admission, entrée.

entrance[2] vb bewitch, captivate, charm, delight, enchant, enrapture, fascinate, ravish, transport.

entrap vb catch, ensnare; allure, entice, inveigle, seduce; embarrass, entangle, involve, nonplus, perplex, pose, stagger.

entreat vb adjure, beg, beseech, crave, enjoin, implore, importune, petition, pray, solicit, supplicate.

entreaty n adjuration, appeal, importunity, petition, prayer, request, solicitation, suit, supplication.

entrée n access, admission, admittance.

entrench, intrench vb furrow; circumvallate, fortify; encroach, infringe, invade, trench, trespass.

entrenchment, intrenchment n entrenching; earthwork, fortification; defence, protection, shelter; encroachment, inroad, invasion.

entrust vb commit, confide, consign.

entwine vt entwist, interlace, intertwine, interweave, inweave, twine, twist, weave; embrace, encircle, encumber, interlace, surround.

enumerate vb calculate, cite, compute, count, detail, mention, number, numerate, reckon, recount, specify, tell.

enunciate vb articulate, declare, proclaim, promulgate, pronounce, propound, publish, say, speak, utter.

envelop vb encase, enfold, enwrap, fold, pack, wrap; cover, encircle, encompass, enshroud, hide, involve, surround.

envelope n capsule, case, covering, integument, shroud, skin, wrapper, veil, vesture, wrap.

envenom vb poison, taint; embitter, malign; aggravate, enrage, exasperate, incense, inflame, irritate, madden, provoke.

environ n begird, belt, embrace, encircle, encompass, enclose, engird, envelop, gird, hedge, hem, surround; beset, besiege, encompass, invest.

environs npl neighbourhood, vicinage, vicinity.

envoy n ambassador, legate, minister, plenipotentiary; courier, messenger.

envy vb hate; begrudge, grudge; covet, emulate, desire. • n enviousness, hate, hatred, ill-will, jealousy, malice, spite; grudge, grudging.

enwrap vb absorb, cover, encase, engross, envelop, infold, involve, wrap, wrap up.

ephemeral adj brief, diurnal, evanescent, fleeting, flitting, fugacious, fugitive, momentary, occasional, short-lived, transient, transitory.

epic adj Homeric, heroic, narrative.

epicure n gastronome, glutton, gourmand, gourmet; epicurean, sensualist, Sybarite, voluptuary.

epidemic adj general, pandemic, prevailing, prevalent. • n outbreak, pandemia, pestilence, plague, spread, wave.

epidermis n cuticle, scarf-skin.

epigrammatic adj antithetic, concise, laconic, piquant, poignant, pointed, pungent, sharp, terse.

episcopal adj Episcopalian, pontifical, prelatic.

epistle n communication, letter, missive, note.

epithet n appellation, description, designation, name, predicate, title.

epitome n abbreviation, abridgement, abstract, breviary, brief, comment, compendium, condensation, conspectus, digest, summary, syllabus, synopsis.

epitomize *vb* abbreviate, abridge, abstract, condense, contract, curtail, cut, reduce, shorten, summarize.

epoch *n* age, date, era, period, time.

equable *adj* calm, equal, even, even-tempered, regular, steady, uniform, serene, tranquil, unruffled.

equal *vb* equalize, even, match. • *adj* alike, coordinate, equivalent, like, tantamount; even, level, equable, regular, uniform; equitable, even-handed, fair, impartial, just, unbiased; co-extensive, commensurate, corresponding, parallel, proportionate; adequate, competent, fit, sufficient. • *n* compeer, fellow, match, peer; rival.

equanimity *n* calmness, composure, coolness, peace, regularity, self-possession, serenity, steadiness.

equestrian *adj* equine, horse-like, horsy. • *n* horseman, rider; cavalier, cavalryman, chevalier, horse soldier, knight.

equilibrist *n* acrobat, balancer, funambulist, rope-walker.

equip *vb* appoint, arm, furnish, provide, rig, supply; accoutre, array, dress.

equipage *n* accoutrements, apparatus, baggage, effects, equipment, furniture; carriage, turnout, vehicle; attendance, procession, retinue, suite, train.

equipment *n* accoutrement, apparatus, baggage, equipage, furniture, gear, outfit, rigging.

equipoise *n* balance, equilibrium.

equitable *adj* even-handed, candid, honest, impartial, just, unbiased, unprejudiced, upright; adequate, fair, proper, reasonable, right.

equity *n* just, right; fair play, fairness, impartiality, justice, rectitude, reasonableness, righteousness, uprightness.

equivalent *adj* commensurate, equal, equipollent, tantamount; interchangeable, synonymous. • *n* complement, coordinate, counterpart, double, equal, fellow, like, match, parallel, pendant, quid pro quo.

equivocal *adj* ambiguous; doubtful, dubious, enigmatic, indeterminate, problematical, puzzling, uncertain.

equivocate *vb* dodge, evade, fence, palter, prevaricate, shuffle, quibble.

equivocation *n* evasion, paltering, prevarication, quibbling, shuffling; double entendre, double meaning, quibble.

era *n* age, date, epoch, period, time.

eradicate *vb* extirpate, root, uproot; abolish, annihilate, destroy, obliterate.

erase *vb* blot, cancel, delete, efface, expunge, obliterate, scrape out.

erasure *n* cancellation, cancelling, effacing, expunging, obliteration.

erect *vb* build, construct, raise, rear; create, establish, form, found, institute, plant. • *adj* standing, unrecumbent, uplifted, upright; elevated, vertical, perpendicular, straight; bold, firm, undaunted, undismayed, unshaken, unterrified.

erelong *adv* early, quickly, shortly, soon, speedily.

eremite *n* anchoret, anchorite, hermit, recluse, solitary.

ergo *adv* consequently, hence, therefore.

erode *vb* canker, consume, corrode, destroy, eat away, fret, rub.

erosive *adj* acrid, cathartic, caustic, corroding, corrosive, eating, virulent.

erotic *adj* amorous, amatory, arousing, seductive, stimulating, titillating.

err *vb* deviate, ramble, rove, stray, wander; blunder, misjudge, mistake; fall, lapse, nod, offend, sin, stumble, trespass, trip.

errand *n* charge, commission, mandate, message, mission, purpose.

errant *adj* adventurous, rambling, roving, stray, wandering.

erratic *adj* nomadic, rambling, roving, wandering; moving, planetary; abnormal, capricious, deviating, eccentric, irregular, odd, queer, strange.

erratum *n* correction, corrigendum, error, misprint, mistake.

erroneous *adj* false, incorrect, inaccurate, inexact, mistaken untrue, wrong.

error *n* blunder, fallacy, inaccuracy, misapprehension, mistake, oversight; delinquency, fault, iniquity, misdeed, misdoing, misstep, obliquity, offence, shortcoming, sin, transgression, trespass, wrongdoing.

erudition *n* knowledge, learning, lore, scholarship.

eruption *n* explosion, outbreak, outburst; sally; rash.

escape *vb* avoid, elude, evade, flee from, shun; abscond, bolt, decamp, flee, fly; slip. • *n* flight; release; passage, passing; leakage.

eschew *vb* abstain, avoid, elude, flee from, shun.

escort *vb* convey, guard, protect; accompany, attend, conduct. • *n* attendant, bodyguard, cavalier, companion, convoy, gallant, guard, squire; protection, safe conduct, safeguard; attendance, company.

esculent *adj* eatable, edible, wholesome.

esoteric *adj* hidden, inmost, inner, mysterious, private, recondite, secret.

especial *adj* absolute, chief, distinct, distinguished, marked, particular, peculiar, principal, singular, special, specific, uncommon, unusual; detailed, minute, noteworthy.

espousal *n* affiancing, betrothing, espousing, plighting; adoption, defence, maintenance, support.

espouse *vb* betroth, plight, promise; marry, wed; adopt, champion, defend, embrace, maintain, support.

espy *vb* descry, detect, discern, discover, observe, perceive, spy, watch.

esquire *n* armiger, attendant, escort, gentleman, squire.

essay[1] *vb* attempt, endeavour, try. • *n* aim, attempt, effort, endeavour, exertion, struggle, trial.

essay[2] *n* article, composition, disquisition, dissertation, paper, thesis.

essence *n* nature, quintessence, substance; extract, part; odour, perfume, scent; being, entity, existence, nature.

essential *adj* fundamental, indispensable, important, inward, intrinsic, necessary, requisite, vital; diffusible, pure, rectified, volatile.

establish *vb* fix, secure, set, settle; decree, enact, ordain; build, constitute, erect, form, found, institute, organize, originate, pitch, plant, raise; ensconce, ground, install, place, plant, root, secure; approve, confirm, ratify, sanction; prove, substantiate, verify.

estate *n* condition, state; position, rank, standing; division, order; effects, fortune, possessions, property; interest.

esteem *vb* appreciate, estimate, rate, reckon, value; admire, honour, like, prize, respect, revere, reverence, value, venerate, worship; account, believe, consider, deem, fancy, hold, imagine, suppose, regard, think. • *n* account, appreciation, consideration, estimate, estimation, judgement, opinion, reckoning, valuation; credit, honour, regard, respect, reverence.

estimable *adj* appreciable, calculable, computable; admirable, credible, deserving, excellent, good, meritorious, precious, respectful, valuable, worthy.

estimate *vb* appraise, appreciate, esteem, prise, rate, value; assess, calculate, compute, count, gauge, judge, reckon. • *n* estimation, judgement, valuation; calculation, computation.

estimation *n* appreciation, estimate, valuation; esteem, estimate, judgement, opinion; honour, reckoning, regard, respect, reverence.

estop *vb* bar, impede, preclude, stop.

estrange *vb* withdraw, withhold; alienate, divert; disaffect, destroy.

estuary *n* creek, inlet, fiord, firth, frith, mouth.

etch *vb* corrode, engrave.

eternal *adj* absolute, inevitable, necessary, self-active, self-existent, self-originated; abiding, ceaseless, endless, ever-enduring, everlasting, incessant, interminable, never-ending, perennial, permanent, perpetual, sempiternal, unceasing, unending; deathless, immortal, imperishable, incorruptible, indestructible, never-dying, undying; immutable, unchangeable; constant, continual, continuous, incessant, persistent, unbroken, uninterrupted.

ethereal *adj* aerial, airy, celestial, empyreal, heavenly, unworldly; attenuated, light, subtle, tenuous, volatile; delicate, fairy, flimsy, fragile, rare, refined, subtle.

eulogize *vb* applaud, commend, extol, laud, magnify, praise.

eulogy *n* discourse, eulogium, panegyric, speech; applause, encomium, commendation, laudation, praise.

euphonious *adj* clear, euphonic, harmonious, mellifluous, mellow, melodious, musical, silvery, smooth, sweet-toned.

evacuant *adj* abstergent, cathartic, cleansing, emetic, purgative. • *n* cathartic, purgative.

evacuate *vb* empty; discharge, clean out, clear out, eject, excrete, expel, purge, void; abandon, desert, forsake, leave, quit, relinquish, withdraw.

evade *vb* elude, escape; avoid, decline, dodge, funk, shun; baffle, elude, foil; dodge, equivocate, fence, palter, prevaricate, quibble, shuffle.

evanescence *n* disappearance, evanishing, evanishment, vanishing; transience, transientness, transitoriness.

evanescent *adj* ephemeral, fleeting, flitting, fugitive, passing, short-lived, transient, transitory, vanishing.

evaporate vb distil, volatilize; dehydrate, dry, vaporize; disperse, dissolve, fade, vanish.

evaporation n distillation, volatilization; dehydration, drying, vaporization; disappearance, dispersal, dissolution.

evasion n artifice, avoidance, bluffing, deceit, dodge, equivocation, escape, excuse, funking, prevarication, quibble, shift, subterfuge, shuffling, sophistical, tergiversation.

evasive adj elusive, elusory, equivocating, prevaricating, shuffling, slippery, sophistical.

even vb balance, equalize, harmonize, symmetrize; align, flatten, flush, level, smooth, square. • adj flat, horizontal, level, plane, smooth; calm, composed, equable, equal, peaceful, placid, regular, steady, uniform, unruffled; direct, equitable, fair, impartial, just, straightforward. • adv exactly, just, verily; likewise. • n eve, evening, eventide, vesper.

evening n dusk, eve, even, eventide, nightfall, sunset, twilight.

event n circumstance, episode, fact, happening, incident, occurrence; conclusion, consequence, end, issue, outcome, result, sequel, termination; adventure, affair.

eventful adj critical, important, memorable, momentous, remarkable, signal, stirring.

eventual adj final, last, ultimate; conditional, contingent, possible. • adv always, aye, constantly, continually, eternally, ever evermore, forever, incessantly, perpetually, unceasingly.

everlasting adj ceaseless, constant, continual, endless, eternal, ever-during, incessant, interminable, never-ceasing, never-ending, perpetual, unceasing, unending, unintermitting, uninterrupted; deathless, ever-living, immortal, imperishable, never-dying, undying.

evermore adv always, constantly, continually, eternally, ever, forever, perpetually.

everyday adj accustomed, common, commonplace, customary, habitual, routine, usual, wonted.

evict vb dispossess, eject, thrust out.

evidence vb evince, make clear, manifest, prove, show, testify, vouch. • n affirmation, attestation, averment, confirmation, corroboration, deposition, grounds, indication, proof, testimony, token, trace, voucher, witness.

evident adj apparent, bald, clear, conspicuous, distinct, downright, incontestable, indisputable, manifest, obvious, open, overt, palpable, patent, plain, unmistakable.

evil adj bad, ill; base, corrupt, malicious, malevolent, malign, nefarious, perverse, sinful, vicious, vile, wicked, wrong; bad, deleterious, baleful, baneful, destructive, harmful, hurtful, injurious, mischievous, noxious, pernicious, profane; adverse, calamitous, diabolic, disastrous, unfortunate, unhappy, unpropitious, woeful. • n calamity, disaster, ill, misery, misfortune, pain, reverse, sorrow, suffering, woe; badness, baseness, corruption, depravity, malignity, sin, viciousness, wickedness; bale, bane, blast, canker, curse, harm, injury, mischief, wrong.

evince vb establish, evidence, manifest, prove, show; disclose, display, indicate, reveal.

eviscerate vb disembowel, embowel, gut.

evoke vb arouse, elicit, excite, provoke, rouse.

evolve vb develop, educe, exhibit, expand, open, unfold, unroll.

exacerbate vb aggravate, embitter, enrage, exasperate, excite, inflame, infuriate, irritate, provoke, vex.

exact vb elicit, extort, mulch, require, squeeze; ask, claim, compel, demand, enforce, requisition, take. • adj rigid, rigorous, scrupulous, severe, strict; diametric, express, faultless, precise, true; accurate, close, correct, definite, faithful, literal, undeviating; accurate, critical, delicate, fine, nice, sensitive; careful, methodical, punctilious, orderly, punctual, regular.

exacting adj critical, difficult, exactive, rigid, extortionary.

exaction n contribution, extortion, oppression, rapacity, tribute.

exactness n accuracy, correctness, exactitude, faithfulness, faultlessness, fidelity, nicety, precision, rigour; carefulness, method, precision, regularity, rigidness, scrupulousity, scrupulousness, strictness.

exaggerate vb enlarge, magnify, overcharge, overcolour, overstate, romance, strain, stretch.

exalt vb elevate, erect, heighten, lift up, raise; aggrandize, dignify, elevate, ennoble; bless, extol, glorify, magnify, praise.

exalted adj elated, elevated, high, highflown, lofty, lordy, magnificent.

examination n inspection, observation; exploration, inquiry, inquisition, investigation, perusal, research, search, scrutiny, survey; catechism, probation, review, test, trial.

examine vb inspect, observe; canvass, consider, explore, inquire, investigate, scrutinize, study, test; catechize, interrogate.

example n archetype, copy, model, pattern, piece, prototype, representative, sample, sampler, specimen, standard; exemplification, illustration, instance, precedent, warning.

exanimate adj dead, defunct, inanimate, lifeless; inanimate, inert, sluggish, spiritless, torpid.

exasperate vb affront, anger, chafe, enrage, incense, irritate, nettle, offend, provoke, vex; aggravate, exacerbate, inflame, rouse.

exasperation n annoyance, exacerbation, irritation, pro- vocation; anger, fury, ire, passion, rage, wrath; aggravation, heightening, increase, worsening.

excavate vb burrow, cut, delve, dig, hollow, hollow out, scoop, trench.

exceed vb cap, overstep, surpass, transcend; excel, outdo, outstrip, outvie, pass.

excel vb beat, eclipse, outdo, outrival, outstrip, outvie, surpass; cap, exceed, transcend.

excellence n distinction, eminence, pre-eminence, superiority, transcendence; fineness, fitness, goodness, perfection, purity, quality, superiority; advantage; goodness, probity, uprightness, virtue, worth.

excellent adj admirable, choice, crack, eminent, first-rate, prime, sterling, superior, tiptop, transcendent; deserving, estimable, praiseworthy, virtuous, worthy.

except vb exclude, leave out, omit, reject. • conj unless. • prep bar, but, excepting, excluding, save.

exceptional adj aberrant, abnormal, anomalous, exceptive, irregular, peculiar, rare, special, strange, superior, uncommon, unnatural, unusual.

excerpt vb cite, cull, extract, quote, select, take. • n citation, extract, quotation, selection.

excess adj excessive, unnecessary, redundant, spare, superfluous, surplus. • n disproportion, fulsomeness, glut, oversupply, plethora, redundance redundancy, surfeit, superabundance, superfluity; overplus, remainder, surplus; debauchery, dissipation, dissoluteness, intemperance, immoderation, overindulgence, unrestraint; extravagance, immoderation, overdoing.

excessive adj disproportionate, exuberant, superabundant, superfluous, undue; extravagant, enormous, inordinate, outrageous, unreasonable; extreme, immoderate, intemperate; vehement, violent.

exchange vb barter, change, commute, shuffle, substitute, swap, trade, truck; bandy, interchange. • n barter, change, commutation, dealing, shuffle, substitution, trade, traffic; interchange, reciprocity; bazaar, bourse, fair, market.

excise[1] n capitation, customs, dues, duty, tariff, tax, taxes, toll.

excise[2] vb cancel, cut, delete, edit, efface, eradicate, erase, expunge, extirpate, remove, strike out.

excision n destruction, eradication, extermination, extirpation.

excitable adj impressible, nervous, sensitive, susceptible; choleric, hasty, hot-headed, hot-tempered, irascible, irritable, passionate, quick-tempered.

excite vb animate, arouse, awaken, brew, evoke, impel, incite, inflame, instigate, kindle, move, prompt, provoke, rouse, spur, stimulate; create, elicit, evoke, raise; agitate, discompose, disturb, irritate.

excitement n excitation exciting; incitement, motive, stimulus; activity, agitation, bustle, commotion, disturbance, ferment, flutter, perturbation, sensation, stir, tension; choler, heat, irritation, passion, violence, warmth.

exclaim vb call, cry, declare, ejaculate, shout, utter, vociferate.

exclude vb ban, bar, blackball, debar, ostracize, preclude, reject; hinder, prevent, prohibit, restrain, withhold; except, omit; eject, eliminate, expel, extrude.

exclusive adj debarring, excluding; illiberal, narrow, narrow-minded, selfish, uncharitable; aristocratic, choice, clannish, cliquish, fastidious, fashionable, select, snobbish; only, sole, special.

excommunicate vb anathematize, ban, curse, denounce, dismiss, eject, exclude, expel, exscind, proscribe, unchurch.

excoriate vb abrade, flay gall, scar, scarify, score, skin, strip.

excrement n dejections, dung, faeces, excreta, excretion, ordure, stool.

excrescence n fungus, growth, knob, lump, outgrowth, protuberance, tumour, wart.

excrete vb discharge, eject, eliminate, separate.

excruciate vb agonize, rack, torment, torture.

exculpate vb absolve, acquit, clear, discharge, exonerate, free, justify, release, set right, vindicate.

excursion n drive, expedition, jaunt, journey, ramble, ride, sally, tour, trip, voyage, walk; digression, episode.

excursive adj devious, diffuse, digressive, discursive, erratic, rambling, roaming, roving, wandering.

excusable adj allowable, defensible, forgivable, justifiable, pardonable, venial, warrantable.

excursus n discussion, disquisition, dissertation.

excuse vb absolve, acquit, exculpate, exonerate, forgive, pardon, remit; extenuate, justify; exempt, free, release; overlook. • n absolution, apology, defence, extenuation, justification, plea; colour, disguise, evasion, guise, pretence, pretext, makeshift, semblance, subterfuge.

execrable adj abhorrent, abominable, accursed, cursed, damnable, detestable, hateful, odious; disgusting, loathsome, nauseating, nauseous, obnoxious, offensive, repulsive, revolting, sickening, vile.

execrate vb curse, damn, imprecate; abhor, abominate, detest, hate, loathe.

execute vb accomplish, achieve, carry out, complete, consummate, do, effect, effectuate, finish, perform, perpetrate; administer, enforce, seal, sign; behead, electrocute, guillotine, hang.

execution n accomplishment, achievement, completion, consummation, operation, performance; warrant, writ; beheading, electrocution, hanging.

executive adj administrative, commanding, controlling, directing, managing, ministerial, officiating, presiding, ruling. • n administrator, director, manager.

exegetic, exegetical adj explanatory, explicative, explicatory, expository, hermeneutic, interpretative.

exemplary adj assiduous, close, exact, faithful, punctual, punctilious, rigid, rigorous, scrupulous; commendable, correct, good, estimable, excellent, praiseworthy, virtuous; admonitory, condign, monitory, warning.

exemplify vb evidence, exhibit, illustrate, manifest, show.

exempt vb absolve, except, excuse, exonerate, free, release, relieve. • adj absolved, excepted, excused, exempted, free, immune, liberated, privileged, released.

exemption n absolution, dispensation, exception, immunity, privilege, release.

exercise vb apply, busy, employ, exert, praxis, use; effect, exert, produce, wield; break in, discipline, drill, habituate, school, train; practise, prosecute, pursue; task, test, try; afflict, agitate, annoy, burden, pain, trouble. • n appliance, application, custom, employment, operation, performance, play, plying, practice, usage, use, working; action, activity, effort, exertion, labour, toil, work; discipline, drill, drilling, schooling, training; lesson, praxis, study, task, test, theme.

exert vb employ, endeavour, exercise, labour, strain, strive, struggle, toil, use, work.

exertion n action, exercise, exerting, use; attempt, effort, endeavour, labour, strain, stretch, struggle, toil, trial.

exhalation n emission, evaporation; damp, effluvium, fog, fume, mist, reek, smoke, steam, vapour.

exhale vb breathe, discharge, elect, emanate, emit, evaporate, reek; blow, expire, puff.

exhaust vb drain, draw, empty; consume, destroy, dissipate, expend, impoverish, lavish, spend, squander, waste; cripple, debilitate, deplete, disable, enfeeble, enervate, overtire, prostrate, weaken.

exhaustion n debilitation, enervation, fatigue, lassitude, weariness.

exhibit vb demonstrate, disclose, display, evince, expose, express, indicate, manifest, offer, present, reveal, show; offer, present, propose.

exhibition n demonstration, display, exposition, manifestation, representation, spectacle, show; allowance, benefaction, grant, pension, scholarship.

exhilarate vb animate, cheer, elate, enliven, gladden, inspire, inspirit, rejoice, stimulate.

exhilaration n animating, cheering, elating, enlivening, gladdening, rejoicing, stimulating; animation, cheer, cheerfulness, gaiety, gladness, glee, good spirits, hilarity, joyousness.

exhort vb advise, caution, encourage, incite, persuade, stimulate, urge, warm; preach.

exhume vb disentomb, disinhume, disinter, unbury, unearth.

exigency, exigence n demand, necessity, need, requirement, urgency, want; conjuncture, crisis, difficulty, distress, emergency, extremity, juncture, nonplus, quandary, pass, pinch, pressure, strait.

exiguous adj attenuated, diminutive, fine, small, scanty, slender, tiny.

exile vb banish, expatriate, expel, ostracize, proscribe. • n banishment, expatriation, expulsion, ostracism, proscription, separation; outcast, refugee.

exist vb be, breathe, live; abide, continue, endure, last, remain.

existence n being, subsisting, subsistence; being, creature, entity, essence, thing; animation, continuation, life, living, vitality, vivacity.

exit vb depart, egress, go, leave. • n departure, withdrawal; death, decrease, demise, end; egress, outlet.

exonerate vb absolve, acquit, clear, exculpate, justify, vindicate; absolve, discharge, except, exempt, free, release.

exorbitant adj enormous, excessive, extravagant, inordinate, unreasonable.

exorcise vb cast out, drive away, expel; deliver, purify; address, conjure.

exordium n introduction, opening, preamble, preface, prelude, proem, prologue.

exotic adj extraneous, foreign; extravagant.

expand vb develop, open, spread, unfold, unfurl; diffuse, enlarge, extend, increase, stretch; dilate, distend, enlarge.

expanse n area, expansion, extent, field, stretch.

expansion n expansion, opening, spreading; diastole, dilation, distension, swelling; development, diffusion, enlargement, increase; expanse, extent, stretch.

ex parte adj biased, one-sided, partisan.

expatiate vb amplify, decant, dilate, enlarge, range, rove.

expatriate vb banish, exile, expel, ostracize, proscribe. • adj banished, exiled, refugee. • n displaced person, emigrant, exile.

expect vb anticipate, await, calculate, contemplate, forecast, foresee, hope, reckon, rely.

expectancy n expectance, expectation; abeyance, prospect.

expectation n anticipation, expectance, expectancy, hope, prospect; assurance, confidence, presumption, reliance, trust.

expedient adj advisable, appropriate, convenient, desirable, fit, proper, politic, suitable; advantageous, profitable, useful. • n contrivance, device, means, method, resort, resource, scheme, shift, stopgap, substitute.

expedite vb accelerate, advance, dispatch, facilitate, forward, hasten, hurry, precipitate, press, quicken, urge.

expedition n alacrity, alertness, celerity, dispatch, haste, promptness, quickness, speed; enterprise, undertaking; campaign, excursion, journey, march, quest, voyage.

expeditious adj quick, speedy, swift, rapid; active, alert, diligent, nimble, prompt, punctual, swift.

expel vb dislodge, egest, eject, eliminate, excrete; discharge, eject, evacuate, void; bounce, discharge, exclude, exscind, fire, oust, relegate, remove; banish, disown, excommunicate, exile, expatriate, ostracize, proscribe, unchurch.

expend vb disburse, spend; consume, employ, exert, use; dissipate, exhaust, scatter, waste.

expenditure n disbursement, outlay, outlaying, spending; charge, cost, expenditure, outlay.

expensive adj costly, dear, high-priced; extravagant, lavish, wasteful.

experience vb endure, suffer; feel, know; encounter, suffer, undergo. • n endurance, practice, trial; evidence, knowledge, proof, test, testimony.

experienced adj able, accomplished, expert, instructed, knowing, old, practised, qualified, skilful, trained, thoroughbred, versed, veteran, wise.

experiment vb examine, investigate, test, try. • n assay, examination, investigation, ordeal, practice, proof, test, testimony, touchstone, trial.

expert adj able, adroit, apt, clever, dextrous, proficient, prompt, quick, ready, skilful. • n adept, authority, connoisseur, crack, master, specialist.

expertise n adroitness, aptness, dexterity, facility, promptness, skilfulness, skill.

expiate vb atone, redeem, satisfy.

expiration *n* death, decease, demise, departure, exit; cessation, close, conclusion, end, termination.

expire *vb* cease, close, conclude, end, stop, terminate; emit, exhale; decease, depart, die, perish.

explain *vb* demonstrate, elucidate, expound, illustrate, interpret, resolve, solve, unfold, unravel; account for, justify, warrant.

explanation *n* clarification, description, elucidation, exegesis, explication, exposition, illustration, interpretation; account, answer, deduction, justification, key, meaning, secret, solution, warrant.

explicit *adj* absolute, categorical, clear, definite, determinate, exact, express, plain, positive, precise, unambiguous, unequivocal, unreserved.

explode *vb* burst, detonate, discharge, displode, shatter, shiver; contemn, discard, repudiate, scorn, scout.

exploit *vb* befool, milk, use, utilize. • *n* achievement, act, deed, feat.

explore *vb* examine, fathom, inquire, inspect, investigate, prospect, scrutinize, seek.

explosion *n* blast, burst, bursting, clap, crack, detonation, discharge, displosion, fulmination, pop.

exponent *n* example, illustration, index, indication, specimen, symbol, type; commentator, demonstrator, elucidator, expounder, illustrator, interpreter.

expose *vb* bare, display, uncover; descry, detect, disclose, unearth; denounce, mask; subject; endanger, jeopardize, risk, venture.

exposé *n* exhibit, exposition, manifesto; denouncement, divulgement, exposure, revelation.

exposition *n* disclosure, interpretation; commentary, critique, elucidation, exegesis, explanation, explication, interpretation; display, show.

expound *vb* develop, present, rehearse, reproduce, unfold; clear, elucidate, explain, interpret.

express *vb* air, assert, asseverate, declare, emit, enunciate, manifest, utter, vent, signify, speak, state, voice; betoken, denote, equal, exhibit, indicate, intimate, present, represent, show, symbolize. • *adj* categorical, clear, definite, determinate, explicit, outspoken, plain, positive, unambiguous; accurate, close, exact, faithful, precise, true; particular, special; fast, nonstop, quick, rapid, speedy, swift. • *n* dispatch, message.

expression *n* assertion, asseveration, communication, declaration, emission, statement, utterance, voicing; language, locution, phrase, remark, saying, term, word; air, aspect, look, mien.

expressive *adj* indicative, meaningful, significant; demonstrative, eloquent, emphatic, energetic, forcible, lively, strong, vivid; appropriate, sympathetic, well-modulated.

expulsion *n* discharge, eviction, expelling, ousting; elimination, evacuation, excretion; ejection, excision, excommunication, extrusion, ostracism, separation.

expunge *vb* annihilate, annul, cancel, delete, destroy, efface, erase, obliterate, wipe out.

expurgate *vb* clean, cleanse, purge, purify; bowdlerize, emasculate.

exquisite *adj* accurate, delicate, discriminating, exact, fastidious, nice, refined; choice, elect, excellent, precious, rare, valuable; complete, consummate, matchless, perfect; acute, keen, intense, poignant. • *n* beau, coxcomb, dandy, fop, popinjay.

extant *adj* existent, existing, present, surviving, undestroyed, visible.

extempore *adj* extemporaneous, extemporary, impromptu, improvised. • *adv* offhand, suddenly, unpremeditatedly, unpreparedly.

extend *vb* reach, stretch; continue, elongate, lengthen, prolong, protract, widen; augment, broaden, dilate, distend, enlarge, expand, increase; diffuse, spread; give, impart, offer, yield; lie, range.

extensible *adj* ductile, elastic, extendible, extensile, protractible, protractile.

extension *n* augmentation, continuation, delay, dilatation, dilation, distension, enlargement, expansion, increase, prolongation, protraction.

extensive *adj* broad, capacious, comprehensive, expanded, extended, far-reaching, large, wide, widespread.

extent *n* amplitude, expanse, expansion; amount, bulk, content, degree, magnitude, size, volume; compass, measure, length, proportions, reach, stretch; area, field, latitude, range, scope; breadth, depth, height, width.

extenuate *vb* diminish, lessen, reduce, soften, weaken; excuse, mitigate, palliate, qualify.

exterior *adj* external, outer, outlying, outside, outward, superficial, surface; extrinsic, foreign. • *n* outside, surface; appearance.

exterminate *vb* abolish, annihilate, destroy, eliminate, eradicate, extirpate, uproot.

external *adj* exterior, outer, outside, outward, superficial; extrinsic, foreign; apparent, visible.

extinct *adj* extinguished, quenched; closed, dead, ended, lapsed, terminated, vanished.

extinction *n* death, extinguishment; abolishment, abolition, annihilation, destruction, excision, extermination, extirpation.

extinguish *vb* choke, douse, put out, quell, smother, stifle, suffocate, suppress; destroy, nullify, subdue; eclipse, obscure.

extirpate *vb* abolish, annihilate, deracinate, destroy, eradicate, exterminate, uproot, weed.

extol *vb* celebrate, exalt, glorify, laud, magnify, praise; applaud, commend, eulogize, panegyrize.

extort *vb* elicit, exact, extract, force, squeeze, wrench, wrest, wring.

extortion *n* blackmail, compulsion, demand, exaction, oppression, overcharge, rapacity, tribute; exorbitance.

extortionate *adj* bloodsucking, exacting, hard, harsh, oppressive, rapacious, rigorous, severe; exorbitant, unreasonable.

extra *adj* accessory, additional, auxiliary, collateral; another, farther, fresh, further, more, new, other, plus, ulterior; side, spare, supernumerary, supplemental, supplementary, surplus; extraordinary, extreme, unusual. • *adv* additionally, also, beyond, farthermore, furthermore, more, moreover, plus. • *n* accessory, appendage, collateral, nonessential, special, supernumerary, supplement; bonus, premium; balance, leftover, remainder, spare, surplus.

extract *vb* extort, pull out, remove, withdraw; derive, distil, draw, express, squeeze; cite, determine, derive, quote, select. • *n* citation, excerpt, passage, quotation, selection; decoction, distillation, essence, infusion, juice.

extraction *n* drawing out, derivation, distillation, elicitation, essence, pulling out; birth, descent, genealogy, lineage, origin, parentage.

extraneous *adj* external, extrinsic, foreign; additional, adventitious, external, superfluous, supplementary, unessential.

extraordinary *adj* abnormal, amazing, distinguished, egregious, exceptional, marvellous, monstrous, particular, peculiar, phenomenal, prodigious, rare, remarkable, signal, singular, special, strange, uncommon, unprecedented, unusual, unwonted, wonderful.

extravagance *n* excess, enormity, exorbitance, preposterousness, unreasonableness; absurdity, excess, folly, irregularity, wildness; lavishness, prodigality, profuseness, profusion, superabundance; waste.

extravagant *adj* excessive, exorbitant, inordinate, preposterous, unreasonable; absurd, foolish, irregular, wild; lavish, prodigal, profuse, spendthrift.

extreme *adj* farthest, outermost, remotest, utmost, uttermost; greatest, highest; final, last, ultimate; drastic, egregious, excessive, extravagant, immoderate, intense, outrageous, radical, unreasonable. • *n* end, extremity, limit; acme, climax, degree, height, pink; danger, distress.

extremity *n* border, edge, end, extreme, limb, termination, verge.

extricate *vb* clear, deliver, disembarrass, disengage, disentangle, liberate, release, relieve.

extrinsic *adj* external, extraneous, foreign, outside, outward, superabundance, superfluity.

exuberance *n* abundance, copiousness, flood, luxuriance, plenitude; excess, lavishness, overabundance, overflow, overgrowth, over-luxuriance, profusion, rankness, redundancy, superabundance, superfluity.

exuberant *adj* abounding, abundant, copious, fertile, flowing, luxuriant, prolific, rich; excessive, lavish, overabundant, overflowing, over-luxuriant, profuse, rank, redundant, superabounding, superabundant, wanton.

exude *vb* discharge, excrete, secrete, sweat; infiltrate, ooze, percolate.

exult *vb* gloat, glory, jubilate, rejoice, transport, triumph, taunt, vault.

exultation *n* delight, elation, joy, jubilation, transport, triumph.

eye *vb* contemplate, inspect, ogle, scrutinize, survey, view, watch. • *n* estimate, judgement, look, sight, vision, view; inspection, notice, observation, scrutiny, sight, vigilance, watch; aperture, eyelet, peephole, perforation; bud, shoot.

F

fable *n* allegory, legend, myth, parable, story, tale; fabrication, falsehood, fiction, figment, forgery, untruth.

fabric *n* building, edifice, pile, structure; conformation, make, texture, workmanship; cloth, material, stuff, textile, tissue, web.

fabricate *vb* build, construct, erect, frame; compose, devise, fashion, make, manufacture; coin, fake, feign, forge, invent.

fabrication *n* building, construction, erection; manufacture; fable, fake, falsehood, fiction, figment, forgery, invention, lie.

fabulous *adj* amazing, apocryphal, coined, fabricated, feigned, fictitious, forged, imaginary, invented, legendary, marvellous, mythical, romancing, unbelievable, unreal.

façade *n* elevation, face, front.

face *vb* confront; beard, buck, brave, dare, defy, front, oppose; dress, level, polish, smooth; cover, incrust, veneer. • *n* cover, facet, surface; breast, escarpment, front; countenance, features, grimace, physiognomy, visage; appearance, expression, look, semblance; assurance, audacity, boldness, brass, confidence, effrontery, impudence.

facet *n* cut, face, lozenge, surface.

facetious *adj* amusing, comical, droll, funny, humorous, jocose, jocular, pleasant, waggish, witty; entertaining, gay, lively, merry, sportive, sprightly.

facile *adj* easy; affable, approachable, complaisant, conversable, courteous, mild; compliant, ductile, flexible, fluent, manageable, pliable, pliant, tractable, yielding; dextrous, ready, skilful.

facilitate *vb* expedite, help.

facility *n* ease, easiness; ability, dexterity, expertness, knack, quickness, readiness; ductility, flexibility, pliancy; advantage, appliance, convenience, means, resource; affability, civility, complaisance, politeness.

facsimile *n* copy, duplicate, fax, reproduction.

fact *n* act, circumstance, deed, event, incident, occurrence, performance; actuality, certainty, existence, reality, truth.

faction *n* cabal, clique, combination, division, junta, party, side; disagreement, discord, disorder, dissension, recalcitrance, recalcitrancy, refractoriness, sedition, seditiousness, tumult, turbulence, turbulency.

factious *adj* litigious, malcontent, rebellious, recalcitrant, refractory, seditious. turbulent.

factitious *adj* artful, artificial, conventional, false, unnatural, unreal.

factor *n* agent, bailiff, broker, consignee, go-between, steward, component, element, ingredient; influence, reason.

factory *n* manufactory, mill, work, workshop.

faculty *n* ability, capability, capacity, endowment, power, property, quality; ableness, address, adroitness, aptitude, aptness, clearness, competency, dexterity, efficiency, expertness, facility, forte, ingenuity, knack, qualification, quickness, readiness, skill, skilfulness, talent, turn; body, department, profession; authority, prerogative, license, privilege, right.

fade *vb* disappear, die, evanesce, fall, faint, perish, vanish; decay, decline, droop, fall, languish, wither; bleach, blanch, pale; disperse, dissolve.

faeces *npl* dregs, lees, sediment, settlings; dung, excrement, ordure, settlings.

fag *vb* droop, flag, faint, sink; drudge, toil; fatigue, jade, tire, weary. • *n* drudgery, fatigue, work; drudge, grub, hack; cigarette, smoke.

fail *vb* break, collapse, decay, decline, fade, sicken, sink, wane; cease, disappear; fall, miscarry, miss; neglect, omit; bankrupt, break.

failing *adj* deficient, lacking, needing, wanting; declining, deteriorating, fading, flagging, languishing, sinking, waning, wilting; unsuccessful. • *prep* lacking, needing, wanting. • *n* decay, decline; failure, miscarriage; defect, deficiency, fault, foible, frailty, imperfection, infirmity, shortcoming, vice, weakness; error, lapse, slip; bankruptcy, insolvency.

failure *n* defectiveness, deficiency, delinquency, shortcoming; fail, miscarriage, negligence, neglect, nonobservance, nonperformance, omission, slip; abortion, botch, breakdown, collapse, fiasco, fizzle; bankruptcy, crash, downfall, insolvency, ruin; decay, declension, decline, loss.

fain *adj* anxious, glad, inclined, pleased, rejoiced, well-pleased. • *adv* cheerfully, eagerly, gladly, joyfully, willingly.

faint *vb* swoon; decline, fade, fail, languish, weaken. • *adj* swooning; drooping, exhausted, feeble, languid, listless, sickly, weak; gentle, inconsiderable, little, slight, small, soft, thin; dim, dull, indistinct, perceptible, scarce, slight; cowardly, dastardly, faint-hearted, fearful, timid, timorous; dejected, depressed, discouraged, disheartened, dispirited. • *n* blackout, swoon.

faint-hearted *adj* cowardly, dastardly, faint, fearful, timid, timorous.

fair[1] *adj* spotless, unblemished, unspotted, unstained, untarnished; blond, light, white; beautiful, comely, handsome, shapely; clear, cloudless, pleasant, unclouded; favourable, prosperous; hopeful, promising, propitious; clear, distinct, open, plain, unencumbered, unobstructed; candid, frank, honest, honourable, impartial, ingenuous, just, unbiased, upright; equitable, proper; average, decent, indifferent, mediocre, moderate, ordinary, passable, reasonable, respectful, tolerable.

fair[2] *n* bazaar, carnival, exposition, festival, fete, funfair, gala, kermess.

fairy *n* brownie, elf, demon, fay, sprite.

faith *n* assurance, belief, confidence, credence, credit, dependence, reliance, trust; creed, doctrine, dogma, persuasion, religion, tenet; constancy, faithfulness, fidelity, loyalty, truth, truthfulness.

faithful *adj* constant, devoted, loyal, staunch, steadfast, true; honest, upright, reliable, trustworthy, trusty; reliable, truthful; accurate, close, conscientious, exact, nice, strict.

faithless *adj* unbelieving; dishonest, disloyal, false, fickle, fluctuating, inconstant, mercurial, mutable, perfidious, shifting, treacherous, truthless, unsteady, untruthful, vacillating, variable, wavering.

fall *vb* collapse, depend, descend, drop, sink, topple, tumble; abate, decline, decrease, depreciate, ebb, subside; err, lapse, sin, stumble, transgress, trespass, trip; die, perish; befall, chance, come, happen, occur, pass; become, get; come, pass. • *n* collapse, comedown, descent, downcome, dropping, falling, flop, plop, tumble; cascade, cataract, waterfall; death, destruction, downfall, overthrow, ruin, surrender; comeuppance, degradation; apostasy, declension, failure, lapse, slip; decline, decrease, depreciation, diminution, ebb, sinking, subsidence; cadence, close; declivity, inclination, slope.

fallacious *adj* absurd, deceptive, deceiving, delusive, disappointing, erroneous, false, illusive, illusory, misleading; paralogistic, sophistical, worthless.

fallacy *n* aberration, deceit, deception, delusion, error, falsehood, illusion, misapprehension, misconception, mistake, untruth; non sequitur, paralogism, sophism, sophistry.

fallibility *n* frailty, imperfection, uncertainty.

fallible *adj* erring, frail, ignorant, imperfect, uncertain, weak.

fallow *adj* left, neglected, uncultivated, unsowed, untilled; dormant, inactive, inert.

false *adj* lying, mendacious, truthless, untrue, unveracious; dishonest, dishonourable, disingenuous, disloyal, double-faced, double-tongued, faithless, false-hearted, perfidious, treacherous, unfaithful; fictitious, forged, made-up, unreliable, untrustworthy; artificial, bastard, bogus, counterfeit, factitious, feigned, forged, hollow, hypocritical, make-believe, pretended, pseudo, sham, spurious, suppositious; erroneous, improper, incorrect, unfounded, wrong; deceitful, deceiving, deceptive, disappointing, fallacious, misleading.

false-hearted *adj* dishonourable, disloyal, double, double-tongued, faithless, false, perfidious, treacherous.

falsehood *n* falsity; fabrication, fib, fiction, lie, untruth; cheat, counterfeit, imposture, mendacity, treachery.

falsify *vb* alter, adulterate, belie, cook, counterfeit, doctor, fake, falsely, garble, misrepresent, misstate, represent; disprove; violate.

falsity *n* falsehood, untruth, untruthfulness.

falter *vb* halt, hesitate, lisp, quaver, stammer, stutter; fail, stagger, stumble, totter, tremble, waver; dodder.

fame *n* bruit, hearsay, report, rumour; celebrity, credit, eminence, glory, greatness, honour, illustriousness, kudos, lustre, notoriety, renown, reputation, repute.

familiar *adj* acquainted, aware, conversant, well-versed; amicable, close, cordial, domestic, fraternal, friendly, homely, intimate, near; affable, accessible, companionable, conversable, courteous, civil, friendly, kindly, sociable, social; easy, free and easy, unceremonious, unconstrained; common, frequent, well-known. • *n* acquaintance, associate, companion, friend, intimate.

familiarity *n* acquaintance, knowledge, understanding; fellowship, friendship, intimacy, closeness, friendliness, sociability; freedom, informality, liberty; disrespect, overfreedom, presumption; intercourse.

familiarize *vb* accustom, habituate, inure, train, use.

family *n* brood, household, people; ancestors, blood, breed, clan, dynasty, kindred, house, lineage, race, stock, strain, tribe; class, genus, group, kind, subdivision.

famine *n* dearth, destitution, hunger, scarcity, starvation.

famish *vb* distress, exhaust, pinch, starve.

famous *adj* celebrated, conspicuous, distinguished, eminent, excellent, fabled, famed, far-famed, great, glorious, heroic, honoured, illustrious, immortal, notable, noted, notorious, remarkable, renowned, signal.

fan[1] *vb* agitate, beat, move, winnow; blow, cool, refresh, ventilate; excite, fire, increase, rouse, stimulate. • *n* blower, cooler, punkah, ventilator.

fan[2] *n* admirer, buff, devotee, enthusiast, fancier, follower, pursuer, supporter.

fanatic *n* bigot, devotee, enthusiast, visionary, zealot.

fanatical *adj* bigoted, enthusiastic, frenzied, mad, rabid, visionary, wild, zealous.

fanciful *adj* capricious, crotchety, imaginary, visionary, whimsical; chimerical, fantastical, ideal, imaginary, wild.

fancy *vb* apprehend, believe, conjecture, imagine, suppose, think; conceive, imagine. • *adj* elegant, fine, nice, ornamented; extravagant, fanciful, whimsical. • *n* imagination; apprehension, conceit, conception, impression, idea, image, notion, thought; approval, fondness, inclination, judgement, liking, penchant, taste; caprice, crotchet, fantasy, freak, humour, maggot, quirk, vagary, whim, whimsy; apparition, chimera, daydream, delusion, hallucination, megrim, phantasm, reverie, vision.

fanfaron *n* blatherskite, blusterer, braggadocio, bully, hector, swaggerer, vapourer.

fang *n* claw, nail, talon, tooth; tusk.

fantastic *adj* chimerical, fanciful, imaginary, romantic, unreal, visionary; bizarre, capricious, grotesque, odd, quaint, queer, strange, whimsical, wild.

far *adj* distant, long, protracted, remote; farther, remoter; alienated, estranged, hostile. • *adv* considerably, extremely, greatly, very much; afar, distantly, far away, remotely.

farce *n* burlesque, caricature, parody, travesty; forcemeat, stuffing.

farcical *adj* absurd, comic, droll, funny, laughable, ludicrous, ridiculous.

fardel *n* bundle, burden, load, pack; annoyance, burden, ill, trouble.

fare *vb* go, journey, pass, travel; happen, prosper, prove; feed, live, manage, subsist. • *n* charge, price, ticket money; passenger, traveller; board, commons, food, table, victuals, provisions; condition, experience, fortune, luck, outcome.

farewell *n* adieu, leave-taking, valediction; departure, leave, parting, valedictory.

far-fetched *adj* abstruse, catachrestic, forced, recondite, strained.

farrago *n* gallimaufry, hodgepodge, hotchpotch, jumble, medley, miscellany, mixture, potpourri, salmagundi.

farther *adj* additional; further, remoter, ulterior. • *adv* beyond, further; besides, furthermore, moreover.

farthingale *n* crinoline, hoop, hoop skirt.

fascinate *vb* affect, bewitch, overpower, spellbind, stupefy, transfix; absorb, captivate, catch, charm, delight, enamour, enchant, enrapture, entrance.

fascination *n* absorption, charm, enchantment, magic, sorcery, spell, witchcraft, witchery.

fash *vb* harass, perplex, plague, torment, trouble, vex, worry. • *n* anxiety, care, trouble, vexation.

fashion *vb* contrive, create, design, forge, form, make, mould, pattern, shape; accommodate, adapt, adjust, fit, suit. • *n* appearance, cast, configuration, conformation, cut, figure, form, make, model, mould, pattern, shape, stamp; manner, method, sort, wake; conventionalism, conventionality, custom, fad, mode, style, usage, vogue; breeding, gentility; quality.

fashionable *adj* modish, stylish; current, modern, prevailing, up-to-date; customary, usual; genteel, well-bred.

fast[1] *adj* close, fastened, firm, fixed, immovable, tenacious, tight; constant, faithful, permanent, resolute, staunch, steadfast, unswerving, unwavering; fortified, impregnable, strong; deep, profound, sound; fleet, quick, rapid, swift; dissipated, dissolute, extravagant, giddy, reckless, thoughtless, thriftless, wild. • *adv* firmly, immovably, tightly; quickly, rapidly, swiftly; extravagantly, prodigally, reckless, wildly.

fast[2] *vb* abstain, go hungry, starve. • *n* abstention, abstinence, diet, fasting, starvation.

fasten *vb* attach, bind, bolt, catch, chain, cleat, fix, gird, lace, lock, pin, secure, strap, tether, tie; belay, bend; connect, hold, join, unite.

fastidious *adj* critical, dainty, delicate, difficult, exquisite, finical, hypercritical, meticulous, overdelicate, overnice, particular, precise, precious, punctilious, queasy, squeamish.

fat *adj* adipose, fatty, greasy, oily, oleaginous, unctuous; corpulent, fleshy, gross, obese, paunchy, portly, plump, pudgy, pursy; coarse, dull, heavy, sluggish, stupid; lucrative, profitable, rich; fertile, fruitful, productive, rich. • *n* adipose tissue, ester, grease, oil; best part, cream, flower; corpulence, fatness, fleshiness, obesity, plumpness, stoutness.

fatal *adj* deadly, lethal, mortal; baleful, baneful, calamitous, catastrophic, destructive, mischievous, pernicious, ruinous; destined, doomed, foreordained, inevitable, predestined.

fatality *n* destiny, fate; mortality; calamity, disaster.

fate *n* destination, destiny, fate; cup, die, doom, experience, lot, fortune, portion, weird; death, destruction, ruin.

fated *adj* appointed, destined, doomed, foredoomed, predetermined, predestinated, predestined, preordained.

fatherly *adj* benign, kind, paternal, protecting, tender.

fathom *vb* comprehend, divine, penetrate, reach, understand; estimate, gauge, measure, plumb, probe, sound.

fathomless *adj* abysmal, bottomless, deep, immeasurable, profound; impenetrable, incomprehensible, obscure.

fatigue *vb* exhaust, fag, jade, tire, weaken, weary. • *n* exhaustion, lassitude, tiredness, weariness; hardship, labour, toil.

fatuity *n* foolishness, idiocy, imbecility, stupidity; absurdity, folly, inanity, infatuation, madness.

fatuous *adj* dense, drivelling, dull, foolish, idiotic, stupid, witless; infatuated, mad, senseless, silly, weak.

fault *n* blemish, defect, flaw, foible, frailty, imperfection, infirmity, negligence, obliquity, offence, shortcoming, spot, weakness; delinquency, error, indiscretion, lapse, misdeed, misdemeanour, offence, peccadillo, slip, transgression, trespass, vice, wrong; blame, culpability.

faultless *adj* blameless, guiltless, immaculate, innocent, sinless, spotless, stainless; accurate, correct, perfect, unblemished.

faulty *adj* bad, defective, imperfect, incorrect; blameable, blameworthy, censurable, culpable, reprehensible.

faux pas *n* blunder, indiscretion, mistake.

favour *vb* befriend, countenance, encourage, patronize; approve; ease, facilitate; aid, assist, help, oblige, support; extenuate, humour, indulge, palliate, spare. • *n* approval, benignity, countenance, esteem, friendless, goodwill, grace, kindness; benefaction, benefit, boon, dispensation, kindness; championship, patronage, popularity, support; gift, present, token; badge, decoration, knot, rosette; leave, pardon, permission; advantage, cover, indulgence, protection; bias, partiality, prejudice.

favourable *adj* auspicious, friendly, kind, propitious, well-disposed, willing; conducive, contributing, propitious; adapted, advantage, beneficial, benign, convenient, fair, fit, good, helpful, suitable.

favourite *adj* beloved, darling, dear; choice, fancied, esteemed, pet, preferred.

fawn *vb* bootlick, bow, creep, cringe, crouch, dangle, kneel, stoop, toady, truckle.

fealty *n* allegiance, homage, loyalty, obeisance, submission; devotion, faithfulness, fidelity, honour, loyalty.

fear *vb* apprehend, dread; revere, reverence, venerate. • *n* affright, alarm, apprehension, consternation, dismay, dread, fright, horror, panic, phobia, scare, terror; disquietude, flutter, perturbation, palpitation, quaking, quivering, trembling, tremor, trepidation; anxiety, apprehension, concern, misdoubt, misgiving, qualm, solicitude; awe, dread, reverence, veneration.

fearful *adj* afraid, apprehensive, haunted; chicken-hearted, chicken-livered, cowardly, faint-hearted, lily-livered, nervous, pusillanimous, timid, timorous; dire, direful, dreadful, frightful, ghastly, horrible, shocking, terrible.

fearless *adj* bold, brave, courageous, daring, dauntless, doughty, gallant, heroic, intrepid, unterrified, valiant, valorous.

feasible *adj* achievable, attainable, possible, practicable, suitable.

feast *vb* delight, gladden, gratify, rejoice. • *n* banquet, carousal, entertainment, regale, repast, revels, symposium, treat; celebration, festival, fete, holiday; delight, enjoyment, pleasure.

feat *n* accomplishment, achievement, act, deed, exploit, performance, stunt, trick.

feather *n* plume; kind, nature, species.

featly *adv* adroitly, dextrously, nimbly, skilfully.

feature *vb* envisage, envision, picture, visualize; imagine; specialize; appear in, headline, star. • *n* appearance, aspect, component; conformation, fashion, make; characteristic, item, mark, particularity, peculiarity, property, point, trait; leader, lead item, special; favour, expression, lineament; article, film, motion picture, movie, story; highlight, high spot.

fecund *adj* fruitful, impregnated, productive, prolific, rich.

fecundity *n* fertility, fruitfulness, productiveness.

federation *n* alliance, allying, confederation, federating, federation, leaguing, union, uniting; affiliation, coalition, combination, compact, confederacy, entente, federacy, league, copartnership.

fee *vb* pay, recompense, reward. • *n* account, bill, charge, compensation, honorarium, remuneration, reward, tip; benefice, fief, feud.

feeble *adj* anaemic, debilitated, declining, drooping, enervated, exhausted, frail, infirm, languid, languishing, sickly; dim, faint, imperfect, indistinct.

feed *vb* contribute, provide, supply; cherish, eat, nourish, subsist, sustain. • *n* fodder, food, foodstuff, forage, provender.

feel *vb* apprehend, intuit, perceive, sense; examine, handle, probe, touch; enjoy, experience, suffer; prove, sound, test, try; appear, look, seem; believe, conceive, deem, fancy, infer, opine, suppose, think. • *n* atmosphere, feeling, quality; finish, surface, texture.

feeling *n* consciousness, impression, notion, perception, sensation; atmosphere, sense, sentience, touch; affecting, emotion, heartstrings, impression, passion, soul, sympathy; sensibility, sentiment, susceptibility, tenderness; attitude, impression, opinion.

feign *vb* devise, fabricate, forge, imagine, invent; affect, assume, counterfeit, imitate, pretend, sham, simulate.

feint *n* artifice, blind, expedient, make-believe, pretence, stratagem, trick.

felicitate *vb* complicate, congratulate; beatify, bless, delight.

felicitous *adj* appropriate, apt, fit, happy, ingenious, inspired, opportune, pertinent, seasonable, skilful, well-timed; auspicious, fortunate, prosperous, propitious, successful.

felicity *n* blessedness, bliss, blissfulness, gladness, happiness, joy; appropriateness, aptitude, aptness, felicitousness, fitness, grace, propriety, readiness, suitableness; fortune, luck, success.

fell[1] *vb* beat, knock down, level, prostrate; cut, demolish, hew.

fell[2] *adj* barbarous, bloodthirsty, bloody, cruel, ferocious, fierce, implacable, inhuman, malicious, malign, malignant, pitiless, relentless, ruthless, sanguinary, savage, unrelenting, vandalistic; deadly, destructive.

fellow *adj* affiliated, associated, joint, like, mutual, similar, twin. • *n* associate, companion, comrade; compeer, equal, peer; counterpart, mate, match, partner; member; boy, character, individual, man, person.

fellowship *n* brotherhood, companionship, comradeship, familiarity, intimacy; participation; partnership; communion, converse, intercourse; affability, kindliness, sociability, sociableness.

felon *n* convict, criminal, culprit, delinquent, malefactor, outlaw; inflammation, whitlow.

felonious *adj* atrocious, cruel, felon, heinous, infamous, malicious, malign, malignant, nefarious, perfidious, vicious, villainous.

female *adj* delicate, gentle, ladylike, soft; fertile, pistil-bearing, pistillate.

feminine *adj* affectionate, delicate, gentle, graceful, modest, soft, tender; female, ladylike, maidenly, womanish, womanly; effeminateness, effeminacy, softness, unmanliness, weakness, womanliness.

fen *n* bog, marsh, moor, morass, quagmire, slough, swamp.

fence *vb* defend, enclose, fortify, guard, protect, surround; circumscribe, evade, equivocate, hedge, prevaricate; guard, parry. • *n* barrier, hedge, hoarding, palings, palisade, stockade, wall; defence, protection, guard, security, shield; fencing, swordplay, swordsmanship; receiver.

fenny *adj* boggy, fennish, swampy, marshy.

feral, ferine *adj* ferocious, fierce, rapacious, ravenous, savage, untamed, wild.

ferment *vb* agitate, excite, heat; boil, brew, bubble, concoct, heat, seethe. • *n* barm, leaven, yeast; agitation, commotion, fever, glow, heat, tumult.

ferocious *adj* feral, fierce, rapacious, ravenous, savage, untamed, wild; barbarous, bloody, bloodthirsty, brutal, cruel, fell, inhuman, merciless, murderous, pitiless, remorseless, ruthless, sanguinary, truculent, vandalistic, violent.

ferocity *n* ferociousness, ferocity, fierceness, rapacity, savageness, wildness; barbarity, cruelty, inhumanity.

fertile *adj* bearing, breeding, fecund, prolific; exuberant, fruitful, luxuriant, plenteous, productive, rich, teeming; female, fruit-bearing, pistillate.

fertility *n* fertileness, fertility; abundance, exuberant, fruitfulness, luxuriance, plenteousness, productiveness, richness.

fervent *adj* burning, hot, glowing, melting, seething; animated, ardent, earnest, enthusiastic, fervid, fierce, fiery, glowing, impassioned, intense, passionate, vehement, warm, zealous.

fervour *n* heat, warmth; animation, ardour, eagerness, earnestness, excitement, fervency, intensity, vehemence, zeal.

fester *vb* corrupt, rankle, suppurate, ulcerate; putrefy, rot. • *n* abscess, canker, gathering, pustule, sore, suppination; festering, rankling.

festival *n* anniversary, carnival, feast, fete, gala, holiday, jubilee; banquet, carousal, celebration, entertainment, treat.

festive *adj* carnival, convivial, festal, festival, gay, jolly, jovial, joyful, merry, mirthful, uproarious.

festivity *n* conviviality, festival, gaiety, jollity, joviality, joyfulness, joyousness, merrymaking, mirth.

festoon *vb* adorn, decorate, embellish, garland, hoop, ornament. • *n* decoration, embellishment, garland, hoop, ornament, ornamentation.

fetch *vb* bring, elicit, get; accomplish, achieve, effect, perform; attain, reach. • *n* artifice, dodge, ruse, stratagem, trick.

fetid *adj* foul, malodorous, mephitic, noisome, offensive, rancid, rank, rank-smelling, stinking, strong-smelling.

fetish *n* charm, medicine, talisman.

fetter *vb* clog, hamper, shackle, trammel; bind, chain, confine, encumber, hamper, restrain, tie, trammel. • *n* bond, chain, clog, hamper, shackle.

feud *vb* argue, bicker, clash, contend, dispute, quarrel. • *n* affray, argument, bickering, broil, clashing, contention, contest, discord, dissension, enmity, fray, grudge, hostility, jarring, quarrel, rupture, strife, vendetta.

fever *n* agitation, excitement, ferment, fire, flush, heat, passion.

fey *adj* clairvoyant, ethereal, strange, unusual, whimsical; death-smitten, doomed.

fiasco *n* failure, fizzle.

fiat *n* command, decree, order, ordinance.

fibre *n* filament, pile, staple, strand, texture, thread; stamina, strength, toughness.

fickle *adj* capricious, changeable, faithless, fitful, inconstant, irresolute, mercurial, mutable, shifting, unsettled, unstable, unsteady, vacillating, variable, veering, violate, volatile, wavering.

fiction *n* fancy, fantasy, imagination, invention; novel, romance; fable, fabrication, falsehood, figment, forgery, invention, lie.

fictitious *adj* assumed, fabulous, fanciful, feigned, imaginary, invented, mythical, unreal; artificial, counterfeit, dummy, false, spurious, suppositious.

fiddle *vb* dawdle, fidget, interfere, tinker, trifle; cheat, swindle, tamper. • *n* fraud, swindle; fiddler, violin, violinist.

fiddle-de-dee *interj* fudge, moonshine, nonsense, stuff.

fiddle-faddle *n* frivolity, gabble, gibberish, nonsense, prate, stuff, trifling, trivia, twaddle.

fidelity *n* constancy, devotedness, devotion, dutifulness, faithfulness, fealty, loyalty, true-heartedness, truth; accuracy, closeness, exactness, faithfulness, precision.

fidget *vb* chafe, fret, hitch, twitch, worry. • *n* fidgetiness, impatience, restlessness, uneasiness.

fiduciary *adj* confident, fiducial, firm, steadfast, trustful, undoubting, unwavering; reliable, trustworthy. • *n* depositary, trustee.

field *n* clearing, glebe, meadow; expanse, extent, opportunity, range, room, scope, surface; department, domain, province, realm, region.

fiendish *adj* atrocious, cruel, demoniac, devilish, diabolical, hellish, implacable, infernal, malevolent, malicious, malign, malignant.

fierce *adj* barbarous, brutal, cruel, fell, ferocious, furious, infuriate, ravenous, savage; fiery, impetuous, murderous, passionate, tearing, tigerish, truculent, turbulent, uncurbed, untamed, vehement, violent.

fiery *adj* fervent, fervid, flaming, heated, hot, glowing, lurid; ardent, fierce, impassioned, impetuous, inflamed, passionate, vehement.

fight *vb* battle, combat, war; contend, contest, dispute, feud, oppose, strive, struggle, wrestle; encounter, engage; handle, manage, manoeuvre. • *n* affair, affray, action, battle, brush, combat, conflict, confrontation, contest, duel, encounter, engagement, melée, quarrel, struggle, war; brawl, broil, riot, row, skirmish; fighting, pluck, pugnacity, resistance, spirit, temper.

figment *n* fable, fabrication, falsehood, fiction, invention.

figurative *adj* emblematical, representative, symbolic, representative, typical; metaphorical, tropical; florid, flowery, ornate, poetical.

figure *vb* adorn, diversify, ornament, variegate; delineate, depict, represent, signify, symbolize, typify; conceive, image, imagine, picture; calculate, cipher, compute; act, appear, perform. • *n* configuration, conformation, form, outline, shape; effigy, image, likeness, representative; design, diagram, drawing, pattern; image, metaphor, trope; emblem, symbol, type; character, digit, number, numeral.

filament *n* cirrus, fibre, fibril, gossamer, hair, strand, tendril, thread.

filch *vb* crib, nick, pilfer, purloin, rob, snitch, steal, thieve.

file[1] *vb* order, pigeonhole, record, tidy. • *n* data, dossier, folder, portfolio; column, line, list, range, rank, row, series, tier.

file[2] *vb* burnish, furbish, polish, rasp, refine, smooth.

filibuster *vb* delay, frustrate, obstruct, play for time, stall, temporize. • *n* frustrator, obstructionist, thwarter; adventurer, buccaneer, corsair, freebooter, pirate.

fill *vb* occupy, pervade; dilate, distend, expand, stretch, trim; furnish, replenish, stock, store, supply; cloy, congest, content, cram, glut, gorge, line, pack, pall, sate, satiate, satisfy, saturate, stuff, suffuse, swell; engage, fulfil, hold, occupy, officiate, perform.

film *vb* becloud, cloud, coat, cover, darken, fog, mist, obfuscate, obscure, veil; photograph, shoot, take. • *n* cloud, coating, gauze, membrane, nebula, pellicle, scum, skin, veil; thread.

filter *vb* filtrate, strain; exude, ooze, percolate, transude. • *n* diffuser, colander, riddle, sieve, sifter, strainer.

filth *n* dirt, nastiness, ordure; corruption, defilement, foulness, grossness, impurity, obscenity, pollution, squalor, uncleanness, vileness.

filthy *adj* defiled, dirty, foul, licentious, nasty, obscene, pornographic, squalid, unclean; corrupt, gross, impure, unclean; miry, mucky, muddy.

final *adj* eventual, extreme, last, latest, terminal, ultimate; conclusive, decisive, definitive, irrevocable.

finale *n* conclusion, end, termination.

finances *npl* funds, resources, revenues, treasury; income, property.

find *vb* discover, fall upon; gain, get, obtain, procure; ascertain, notice, observe, perceive, remark; catch, detect; contribute, furnish, provide, supply. • *n* acquisition, catch, discovery, finding, plum, prize, strike.

fine[1] *vb* filter, purify, refine. • *adj* comminuted, little, minute, small; capillary, delicate, small; choice, light; exact, keen, sharp; attenuated, subtle, tenuous, thin; exquisite, fastidious, nice, refined, sensitive, subtle; dandy, excellent, superb, superior; beautiful, elegant, handsome, magnificent, splendid; clean, pure, unadulterated.

fine[2] *vb* amerce, mulct, penalize, punish. • *n* amercement, forfeit, forfeiture, mulct, penalty, punishment.

finery *n* decorations, frippery, gewgaws, ornaments, splendour, showiness, trappings, trimmings, trinkets.

finesse *vb* manipulate, manoeuvre. • *n* artifice, contrivance, cunning, craft, manipulation, manoeuvre, manoeuvring, ruses, stratagems, strategy, wiles.

finger *vb* handle, manipulate, play, purloin.

finical *adj* critical, dainty, dapper, fastidious, foppish, jaunty, overnice, overparticular, scrupulous, spruce, squeamish, trim.

finish *vb* accomplish, achieve, complete, consummate, execute, fulfil, perform; elaborate, perfect, polish; close, conclude, end, terminate. • *n* elaboration, elegance, perfection, polish; close, end, death, termination, wind-up.

finite *adj* bounded, circumscribed, conditioned, contracted, definable, limited, restricted, terminable.

fire *vb* ignite, kindle, light; animate, enliven, excite, inflame, inspirit, invigorate, rouse, stir up; discharge, eject, expel, hurl. • *n* combustion; blaze, conflagration; discharge, firing; animation, ardour, enthusiasm, fervour, fervency, fever, force, heat, impetuosity, inflammation, intensity, passion, spirit, vigour, violence; light, lustre, radiance, splendour; imagination, imaginativeness, inspiration, vivacity; affliction, persecution, torture, trouble.

firm[1] *adj* established, coherent, confirmed, consistent, fast, fixed, immovable, inflexible, rooted, secure, settled, stable; compact, compressed, dense, hard, solid; constant, determined, resolute, staunch, steadfast, steady, unshaken; loyal, robust, sinewy, stanch, stout, sturdy, strong.

firm[2] *n* association, business, company, concern, corporation, house, partnership.

firmament *n* heavens, sky, vault, welkin.

firmness *n* compactness, fixedness, hardness, solidity; stability, strength; constancy, soundness, steadfastness, steadiness.

first *adj* capital, chief, foremost, highest, leading, prime, principal; earliest, eldest, original; maiden; elementary, primary, rudimentary; aboriginal, primal, primeval, primitive, pristine. • *adv* chiefly, firstly, initially, mainly, primarily, principally; before, foremost, headmost; before, rather, rather than, sooner, sooner than. • *n* alpha, initial, prime.

first-rate *adj* excellent, prime, superior.

fissure *n* breach, break, chasm, chink, cleft, crack, cranny, crevice, fracture, gap, hole, interstice, opening, rent, rift.

fit[1] *vb* adapt, adjust, suit; become, conform; accommodate, equip, prepare, provide, qualify. • *adj* capacitated, competent, fitted; adequate, appropriate, apt, becoming, befitting, consonant, convenient, fitting, good, meet, pertinent, proper, seemly, suitable.

fit[2] *n* convulsion, fit, paroxysm, qualm, seizure, spasm, spell; fancy, humour, whim; mood, pet, tantrum; interval, period, spell, turn.

fitful *adj* capricious, changeable, convulsive, fanciful, fantastic, fickle, humoursome, impulsive, intermittent, irregular, odd, spasmodic, unstable, variable, whimsical; checkered, eventful.

fitness *n* adaptation, appropriateness, aptitude, aptness, pertinence, propriety, suitableness; preparation, qualification.

fix *vb* establish, fasten, place, plant, set; adjust, correct, mend, repair; attach, bind, clinch, connect, fasten, lock, rivet, stay, tie; appoint, decide, define, determine, limit, seal, settle; consolidate, harden, solidify; abide, remain, rest; congeal, stiffen. • *n* difficulty, dilemma, quandary, pickle, plight, predicament.

flabbergast *vb* abash, amaze, astonish, astound, confound, confuse, disconcert, dumbfound, nonplus.

flabby *adj* feeble, flaccid, inelastic, limp, soft, week, yielding.

flaccid *adj* baggy, drooping, flabby, inelastic, lax, limber, limp, loose, pendulous, relaxed, soft, weak, yielding.

flag[1] *vb* droop, hang, loose; decline, droop, fail, faint, lag, languish, pine, sink, succumb, weaken, weary; stale, pall.

flag[2] *vb* indicate, mark, semaphore, sign, signal. • *n* banner, colours, ensign, gonfalon, pennant, pennon, standard, streamer.

flagellate *vb* beat, castigate, chastise, cudgel, drub, flog, scourge, thrash, whip.

flagitious *adj* abandoned, atrocious, corrupt, flagrant, heinous, infamous, monstrous, nefarious, profligate, scandalous, villainous, wicked.

flagrant *adj* burning, flaming, glowing, raging; crying, enormous, flagitious, glaring, monstrous, nefarious, notorious, outrageous, shameful, wanton, wicked.

flake *vb* desquamate, scale. • *n* lamina, layer, scale.

flamboyant *adj* bright, gorgeous, ornate, rococo.

flame *vb* blaze, shine; burn, flash, glow, warm. • *n* blaze, brightness, fire, flare, vapour; affection, ardour, enthusiasm, fervency, fervour, keenness, warmth.

flaming *adj* blazing; burning, bursting, exciting, glowing, intense, lambent, vehement, violent.

flap *vb* beat, flutter, shake, vibrate, wave. • *n* apron, fly, lap, lappet, tab; beating, flapping, flop, flutter, slap, shaking, swinging, waving.

flare *vb* blaze, flicker, flutter, waver; dazzle, flame, glare; splay, spread, widen. • *n* blaze, dazzle, flame, glare.

flash *vb* blaze, glance, glare, glisten, light, shimmer, scintillate, sparkle, twinkle. • *n* instant, moment, twinkling.

flashy *adj* flaunting, gaudy, gay, loud, ostentatious, pretentious, showy, tawdry, tinsel.

flat *adj* champaign, horizontal, level; even, plane, smooth, unbroken; low, prostrate, overthrow; dull, frigid, jejune, lifeless, monotonous, pointless, prosaic, spiritless, tame, unanimated, uniform, uninteresting; dead, flashy, insipid, mawkish, stale, tasteless, vapid; absolute, clear, direct, downright, peremptory, positive. • *adv* flatly, flush, horizontally, level. • *n* bar, sandbank, shallow, shoal, strand; champaign, lowland, plain; apartment, floor, lodging, storey.

flatter *vb* compliment, gratify, praise; blandish, blarney, butter up, cajole, coax, coddle, court, entice, fawn, humour, inveigle, wheedle.

flattery *n* adulation, blandishment, blarney, cajolery, fawning, obsequiousness, servility, sycophancy, toadyism.

flaunt *vb* boast, display, disport, flourish, parade, sport, vaunt; brandish.

flaunting *adj* flashy, garish, gaudy, ostentatious, showy, tawdry.

flavour *n* gust, gusto, relish, savour, seasoning, smack, taste, zest; admixture, lacing, seasoning; aroma, essence, soul, spirit.

flaw *n* break, breach, cleft, crack, fissure, fracture, gap, rent, rift; blemish, defect, fault, fleck, imperfection, speck, spot.

flay *vb* excoriate, flay; criticize.

fleck *vb* dapple, mottle, speckle, spot, streak, variegate. • *n* speckle, spot, streak.

flecked *adj* dappled, mottled, piebald, spotted, straked, striped, variegated.

flee *vb* abscond, avoid, decamp, depart, escape, fly, leave, run, skedaddle.

fleece *vb* clip, shear; cheat, despoil, pluck, plunder, rifle, rob, steal, strip.

fleer *vb* mock, jeer, gibe, scoff, sneer.

fleet[1] *n* armada, escadrille, flotilla, navy, squadron; company, group.

fleet[2] *adj* fast, nimble, quick, rapid, speedy, swift.

fleeting *adj* brief, caducous, ephemeral, evanescent, flitting, flying, fugitive, passing, short-lived, temporary, transient, transitory.

fleetness *n* celerity, nimbleness, quickness, rapidity, speed, swiftness, velocity.

flesh *n* food, meat; carnality, desires; kindred, race, stock; man, mankind, world.

fleshly *adj* animal, bodily, carnal, lascivious, lustful, lecherous, sensual.

fleshy *adj* corpulent, fat, obese, plump, stout.

flexibility *n* flexibleness, limbersome, lithesome, pliability, pliancy, suppleness; affability, complaisance, compliance, disposition, ductility, pliancy, tractableness, tractability, yielding.

flexible *adj* flexible, limber, lithe, pliable, pliant, supple, willowy; affable, complaisant, ductile, docile, gentle, tractable, tractile, yielding.

flexose, flexuous *adj* bending, crooked, serpentine, sinuate, sinuous, tortuous, waxy, winding.

flibbertigibbet *n* demon, imp, sprite.

flight[1] *n* flying, mounting, soaring, volition; shower, flight; steps, stairs.

flight[2] *n* departure, fleeing, flying, retreat, rout, stampede; exodus, hegira.

flighty *adj* capricious, deranged, fickle, frivolous, giddy, lightheaded, mercurial, unbalanced, volatile, wild, whimsical.

flimsy *adj* slight, thin, unsubstantial; feeble, foolish, frivolous, light, puerile, shallow, superficial, trashy, trifling, trivial, weak; insubstantial, sleazy.

flinch *vb* blench, flee, recoil, retreat, shirk, shrink, swerve, wince, withdraw.

fling *vb* cast, chuck, dart, emit, heave, hurl, pitch, shy, throw, toss; flounce, wince. • *n* cast, throw, toss.

flippancy *n* volubility, assuredness, glibness, pertness.

flippant *adj* fluent, glib, talkative, voluble; bold, forward, frivolous, glib, impertinent, inconsiderate, irreverent, malapert, pert, saucy, trifling.

flirt *vb* chuck, fling, hurl, pitch, shy, throw, toss; flutter, twirl, whirl, whisk; coquet, dally, philander. • *n* coquette, jilt, philanderer; jerk.

flirtation *n* coquetry, dalliance, philandering.

flit *vb* flicker, flutter, hover; depart, hasten, pass.

flitting *adj* brief, ephemeral, evanescent, fleeting, fugitive, passing, short, transient, transitory.

float *vb* drift, glide, hang, ride, sail, soar, swim, waft; launch, support.

flock *vb* collect, congregate, gather, group, herd, swarm, throng. • *n* collection, group, multitude; bevy, company, convoy, drove, flight, gaggle, herd, pack, swarm, team, troupe; congregation.

flog *vb* beat, castigate, chastise, drub, flagellate, lash, scourge, thrash, whip.

flood *vb* deluge, inundate, overflow, submerge, swamp. • *n* deluge, freshet, inundation, overflow, tide; bore, downpour, eagre, flow, outburst, spate, rush; abundance, excess.

floor *vb* deck, pave; beat, confound, conquer, overthrow, prevail, prostrate, puzzle; disconcert, nonplus. • *n* storey; bottom, deck, flooring, pavement, stage.

florid *adj* bright-coloured, flushed, red-faced, rubicund; embellished, figurative, luxuriant, ornate, rhetorical, rococo.

flounce[1] *vb* fling, jerk, spring, throw, toss, wince. • *n* jerk, spring.

flounce[2] *n* frill, furbelow, ruffle.

flounder *vb* blunder, flop, flounce, plunge, struggle, toss, tumble, wallow.

flourish *vb* grow, thrive; boast, bluster, brag, gasconade, show off, vaunt, vapour; brandish, flaunt, swing, wave. • *n* dash, display, ostentation, parade, show; bombast, fustian, grandiloquence; brandishing, shake, waving; blast, fanfare, tantivy.

flout *vb* chaff, deride, fleer, gibe, insult, jeer, mock, ridicule, scoff, sneer, taunt. • *n* gibe, fling, insult, jeer, mock, mockery, mocking, scoff, scoffing, taunt.

flow *vb* pour, run, stream; deliquesce, liquefy, melt; arise, come, emanate, follow, grow, issue, proceed, result, spring; glide, float, undulate, wave, waver; abound, run. • *n* current, discharge, flood, flux, gush, rush, stream, trickle; abundance, copiousness.

flower *vb* bloom, blossom, effloresce; develop. • *n* bloom, blossom; best, cream, elite, essence, pick; freshness, prime, vigour.

flowery *adj* bloomy, florid; embellished, figurative, florid, ornate, overwrought.

flowing *adj* abundant, copious, fluent, smooth.

fluctuate *vb* oscillate, swing, undulate, vibrate, wave; change, vary; vacillate, waver.

flue *n* chimney, duct; flew, fluff, nap, floss, fur.

fluency *n* liquidness, smoothness; affluence, copiousness; ease, facility, readiness.

fluent *adj* current, flowing, gliding, liquid; smooth; affluent, copious, easy, facile, glib, ready, talkative, voluble.

fluff *vb* blunder, bungle, forget, fumble, mess up, miscue, misremember, muddle, muff. • *n* down, flew, floss, flue, fur, lint, nap; cobweb, feather, gossamer, thistledown; blunder, bungle, fumble, muff.

flume *n* channel, chute, mill race, race.

flummery *n* chaff, frivolity, froth, moonshine, nonsense, trash, trifling; adulation, blandishment, blarney, flattery; brose, porridge, sowens.

flunky, flunkey *n* footman, lackey, livery servant, manservant, valet; snob, toady.

flurry *vb* agitate, confuse, disconcert, disturb, excite, fluster, hurry, perturb. • *n* gust, flaw, squall; agitation, bustle, commotion, confusion, disturbance, excitement, flutter, haste, hurry, hurry-scurry, perturbation, ruffle, scurry.

flush[1] *vb* flow, rush, start; glow, mantle, redden; animate, elate, elevate, erect, excite; cleanse, drench. • *adj* bright, fresh, glowing, vigorous; abundant, affluent, exuberant, fecund, fertile, generous, lavish, liberal, prodigal, prolific, rich, wealthy, well-supplied; even, flat, level, plane. • *adv* evenly, flat, level; full, point-blank, right, square, squarely, straight. • *n* bloom, blush, glow, redness, rosiness, ruddiness; impulse, shock, thrill.

flush[2] *vb* disturb, rouse, start, uncover.

fluster *vb* excite, flush, heat; agitate, disturb, flurry, hurry, perturb; ruffle; confound, confuse, discompose, disconcert. • *n* glow, heat; agitation, flurry, flutter, hurry, hurry-scurry, perturbation, ruffle.

fluted *adj* channelled, corrugated, grooved.

flutter *vb* flap, hover; flirt, flit; beat, palpitate, quiver, tremble; fluctuate, oscillate, vacillate, waver. • *n* agitation, tremor; hurry, commotion, confusion, excitement, flurry, fluster, hurry-scurry, perturbation, quivering, tremble, tumult, twitter.

flux *n* flow, flowing; change, mutation, shifting, transition; diarrhoea, dysentery, looseness; fusing, melting, menstruum, solvent.

fly[1] *vb* aviate, hover, mount, soar; flap, float, flutter, play, sail, soar, undulate, vibrate, wave; burst, explode; abscond, decamp, depart, flee, vanish; elapse, flit, glide, pass, slip.

fly[2] *adj* alert, bright, sharp, smart, wide-awake; astute, cunning, knowing, sly; agile, fleet, nimble, quick, spry.

foal *n* colt, filly.

foam *vb* cream, froth, lather, spume; boil, churn, ferment, fume, seethe, simmer, stew. • *n* bubbles, cream, froth, scum, spray, spume, suds.

fodder *n* feed, food, forage, provender, rations.

foe *n* adversary, antagonist, enemy, foeman, opponent.

fog *vb* bedim, bemist, blear, blur, cloud, dim, enmist, mist; addle, befuddle, confuse, fuddle, muddle. • *n* blear, blur, dimness, film, fogginess, haze, haziness, mist, smog, vapour; befuddlement, confusion, fuddle, maze, muddle.

foggy *adj* blurred, cloudy, dim, dimmed, hazy, indistinct, misty, obscure; befuddled, bewildered, confused, dazed, muddled, muddy, stupid.

foible *n* defect, failing, fault, frailty, imperfection, infirmity, penchant, weakness.

foil[1] *vb* baffle, balk, check, checkmate, circumvent, defeat, disappoint, frustrate, thwart.

foil[2] *n* film, flake, lamina; background, contrast.

foist *vb* impose, insert, interpolate, introduce, palm off, thrust.

fold[1] *vb* bend, cover, double, envelop, wrap; clasp, embrace, enfold, enwrap, gather, infold, interlace; collapse, fail. • *n* double, doubling, gather, plait, plicature

fold[2] *n* cot, enclosure, pen.

foliaceous *adj* foliate, leafy; flaky, foliated, lamellar, lamellate, lamellated, laminated, scaly, schistose.

folk *n* kindred, nation, people.

follow *vb* ensue, succeed; chase, dog, hound, pursue, run after, trail; accompany, attend; conform, heed, obey, observe; cherish, cultivate, seek; practise, pursue; adopt, copy, imitate; arise, come, flow, issue, proceed, result, spring.

follower *n* acolyte, attendant, associate, companion, dependant, retainer, supporter; adherent, admirer, disciple, partisan, pupil; copier, imitator.

folly *n* doltishness, dullness, imbecility, levity, shallowness; absurdity, extravagance, fatuity, foolishness, imprudence, inanity, indiscretion, ineptitude, nonsense, senselessness; blunder, faux pas, indiscretion, unwisdom.

foment *vb* bathe, embrocate, stupe; abet, brew encourage, excite, foster, instigate, promote, stimulate.

fond *adj* absurd, baseless, empty, foolish, senseless, silly, vain, weak; affectionate, amorous, doting, loving, overaffectionate, tender.

fondle *vb* blandish, caress, coddle, cosset, dandle, pet.

fondness *n* absurdity, delusion, folly, silliness, weakness; liking, partiality, predilection, preference, propensity; appetite, relish, taste.

food *n* aliment, board, bread, cheer, commons, diet, fare, meat, nourishment, nutriment, nutrition, pabulum, provisions, rations, regimen, subsistence, sustenance, viands, victuals; feed, fodder, forage, provender.

fool *vb* jest, play, toy, trifle; beguile, cheat, circumvent, cozen, deceive, delude, dupe, gull, hoodwink, overreach, trick. • *n* blockhead, dolt, driveller, idiot, imbecile, nincompoop, ninny, nitwit, simpleton; antic, buffoon, clown, droll, harlequin, jester, merry-andrew, punch, scaramouch, zany, butt, dupe.

foolery *n* absurdity, folly, foolishness, nonsense; buffoonery, mummery, tomfoolery.

foolhardy *adj* adventurous, bold, desperate, harebrained, headlong, hot-headed, incautious, precipitate, rash, reckless, venturesome, venturous.

foolish *adj* brainless, daft, fatuous, idiotic, inane, inept, insensate, irrational, senseless, shallow, silly, simple, thick-skulled, vain, weak, witless; absurd, ill-judged, imprudent, indiscreet, nonsensical, preposterous, ridiculous, unreasonable, unwise; childish, contemptible, idle, puerile, trifling, trivial, vain.

foolishness *n* doltishness, dullness, fatuity, folly, imbecility, shallowness, silliness, stupidity; absurdity, extravagance, imprudence, indiscretion, nonsense; childishness, puerility, triviality.

footing *n* foothold, purchase; basis, foundation, groundwork, installation; condition, grade, rank, standing, state, status; settlement, establishment.

footman *n* footboy, menial, lackey, runner, servant.

footpad *n* bandit, brigand, freebooter, highwayman, robber.

footpath *n* footway, path, trail.

footprint *n* footfall, footmark, footstep, trace, track.

footstep *n* footmark, footprint, trace, track; footfall, step, tread; mark, sign, token, trace, vestige.

fop *n* beau, coxcomb, dandy, dude, exquisite, macaroni, popinjay, prig, swell.

foppish *adj* coxcombical, dandified, dandyish, dressy, finical, spruce, vain.

forage *vb* feed, graze, provender, provision, victual; hunt for, range, rummage, search, seek; maraud, plunder, raid. • *n* feed, fodder, food, pasturage, provender; hunt, rummage, search.

foray *n* descent, incursion, invasion, inroad, irruption, raid.

forbear *vb* cease, desist, hold, pause, stop, stay; abstain, refrain; endure, tolerate; avoid, decline, shun; abstain, omit, withhold.

forbearance *n* abstinence, avoidance, forbearing, self-restraint, shunning, refraining; indulgence, leniency, long-suffering, mildness, moderation, patience.

forbid *vb* ban, debar, disallow, embargo, enjoin, hinder, inhibit, interdict, prohibit, proscribe, taboo, veto.

forbidding *adj* abhorrent, disagreeable, displeasing, odious, offensive, repellant, repulsive, threatening, unpleasant.

force *vb* coerce, compel, constrain, necessitate, oblige; drive, impel, overcome, press, urge; ravish, violate. • *n* emphasis, energy, head, might, pith, power, strength, stress, vigour, vim; agency, efficacy, efficiency, cogency, potency, validity, virtue; coercion, compulsion, constraint, enforcement, vehemence, violence; army, array, battalion, host, legion, phalanx, posse, soldiery, squadron, troop.

forcible *adj* all-powerful, cogent, impressive, irresistible, mighty, potent, powerful, strong, weighty; impetuous, vehement, violent, unrestrained; coerced, coercive, compulsory; convincing, energetic, effective, efficacious, telling, vigorous.

forcibly *adv* mightily, powerfully; coercively, compulsorily, perforce, violently; effectively, energetically, vigorously.

ford *n* current, flood, stream; crossing, wading place.

fore *adj* anterior, antecedent, first, foregoing, former, forward, preceding, previous, prior; advanced, foremost, head, leading.

forebode *vb* augur, betoken, foreshow, foretell, indicate, portend, predict, prefigure, presage, prognosticate, promise, signify.

foreboding *n* augury, omen, prediction, premonition, presage, presentiment, prognostication.

forecast *vb* anticipate, foresee, predict; calculate, contrive, devise, plan, project, scheme. • *n* anticipation, foresight, forethought, planning, prevision, prophecy, provident.

foreclose *vb* debar, hinder, preclude, prevent, stop.

foredoom *vb* foreordain, predestine, preordain.

forego *see* **forgo**.

foregoing *adj* antecedent, anterior, fore, former, preceding, previous, prior.

foregone *adj* bygone, former, past, previous.

foreign *adj* alien, distant, exotic, exterior, external, outward, outlandish, remote, strange, unnative; adventitious, exterior, extraneous, extrinsic, inappropriate, irrelevant, outside, unnatural, unrelated.

foreknowledge *n* foresight, prescience, prognostication.

foremost *adj* first, front, highest, leading, main, principal.

foreordain *vb* appoint, foredoom, predestinate, predetermine, preordain.

forerunner *n* avant-courier, foregoer, harbinger, herald, precursor, predecessor; omen, precursor, prelude, premonition, prognosticate, sign.

foresee *vb* anticipate, forebode, forecast, foreknow, foretell, prognosticate, prophesy.

foreshadow *vb* forebode, predict, prefigure, presage, presignify, prognosticate, prophesy.

foresight *n* foreknowledge, prescience, prevision; anticipation, care, caution, forecast, forethought, precaution, providence, prudence.

forest *n* wood, woods, woodland.

forestall *vb* hinder, frustrate, intercept, preclude, prevent, thwart; antedate, anticipate, foretaste; engross, monopolize, regrate.

foretaste *n* anticipation, forestalling, prelibation.

foretell *vb* predict, prophesy; augur, betoken, forebode, forecast, foreshadow, foreshow, portend, presage, presignify, prognosticate, prophesy.

forethought *n* anticipation, forecast, foresight, precaution, providence, prudence.

forever *adv* always, constantly, continually, endlessly, eternally, ever, evermore, everlastingly, perpetually, unceasingly.

forewarn *vb* admonish, advise, caution, dissuade.

forfeit *vb* alienate, lose. • *n* amercement, damages, fine, forfeiture, mulct, penalty.

forfend *vb* avert, forbid, hinder, prevent, protect.

forge *vb* beat, fabricate, form, frame, hammer; coin, devise, frame, invent; counterfeit, falsify, feign. • *n* furnace, ironworks, smithy.

forgery *n* counterfeit, fake, falsification, imitation.

forgetful *adj* careless, heedless, inattentive, mindless, neglectful, negligent, oblivious, unmindful.

forgive *vb* absolve, acquit, condone, excuse, exonerate, pardon, remit.

forgiveness *n* absolution, acquittal, amnesty, condoning, exoneration, pardon, remission, reprieve.

forgiving *adj* absolutory, absolvatory, acquitting, clearing, excusing, pardoning, placable, releasing.

forgo *vb* abandon, cede, relinquish, renounce, resign, surrender, yield.

fork *vb* bifurcate, branch, divaricate, divide. • *n* bifurcation, branch, branching, crotch, divarication, division.

forked *adj* bifurcated, branching, divaricated, furcate, furcated.

forlorn *adj* abandoned, deserted, forsaken, friendless, helpless, lost, solitary; abject, comfortless, dejected, desolate, destitute, disconsolate, helpless, hopeless, lamentable, pitiable, miserable, woebegone, wretched.

form *vb* fashion model, mould, shape; build, conceive, construct, create, fabricate, make, produce; contrive, devise, frame, invent; compose, constitute, develop, organize; discipline, educate, teach, train. • *n* body, build, cast, configuration, conformation, contour, cut, fashion, figure, format, mould, outline, pattern, shape; formula, formulary, method, mode, practice, ritual; class, kind, manner, model, order, sort, system, type; arrangement, order, regularity, shapeliness; ceremonial, ceremony, conventionality, etiquette, formality, observance, ordinance, punctilio, rite, ritual; bench, seat; class, rank; arrangement, combination, organization.

formal *adj* explicit, express, official, positive, strict; fixed, methodical, regular, rigid, set, stiff; affected, ceremonious, exact, precise, prim, punctilious, starchy. starched; constitutive, essential; external, outward, perfunctory; formative, innate, organic, primordial.

formality *n* ceremonial, ceremony, conventionality, etiquette, punctilio, rite, ritual.

formation *n* creation, genesis, production; composition, constitution; arrangement, combination, disposal, disposition.

formative *adj* creative, determinative, plastic, shaping; derivative, inflectional, nonradical.

former *adj* antecedent, anterior, earlier, foregoing, preceding, previous, prior; late, old-time, quondam; by, bygone, foregone, gone, past.

formidable *adj* appalling, dangerous, difficult, dreadful, fearful, frightful, horrible, menacing, redoubtable, shocking, terrible, terrific, threatening, tremendous.

forsake *vb* abandon, desert, leave, quit; drop, forgo, forswear, relinquish, renounce, surrender, yield.

forsooth *adv* certainly, indeed, really, surely, truly.

forswear *vb* abandon, desert, drop, forsake, leave, quit, reject, renounce; abjure, deny, eschew, perjure, recant, repudiate, retract.

fort *n* bulwark, castle, citadel, defence, fastness, fortification, fortress, stronghold.

forthwith *adv* directly, immediately, instantly, quickly, straightaway.

fortification *n* breastwork, bulwark, castle, citadel, defence, earthwork, fastness, fort, keep, rampart, redoubt, stronghold, tower.

fortify *vb* brace, encourage, entrench, garrison, protect, reinforce, stiffen, strengthen; confirm, corroborate.

fortitude *n* braveness, bravery, courage, determination, endurance, firmness, hardiness, patience, pluck, resolution, strength, valour.

fortuitous *adj* accidental, casual, chance, contingent, incidental.

fortunate *adj* favoured, happy, lucky, prosperous, providential, successful; advantageous, auspicious, favourable, happy, lucky, propitious, timely.

fortune *n* accident, casualty, chance, contingency, fortuity, hap, luck; estate, possessions, property, substance; affluence, felicity, opulence, prosperity, riches, wealth; destination, destiny, doom, fate, lot, star; event, issue, result; favour, success.

forward *vb* advance, aid, encourage, favour, foster, further, help, promote, support; accelerate, dispatch, expedite, hasten, hurry, quicken, speed; dispatch, post, send, ship, transmit. • *adj* ahead, advanced, onward; anterior, front, fore, head; prompt, eager, earnest, hasty, impulsive, quick, ready, willing, zealous; assuming, bold, brazen, brazen-faced, confident, flippant, impertinent, pert, presumptuous, presuming; advanced, early, premature. • *adv* ahead, onward.

foster *vb* cosset, feed, nurse, nourish, support, sustain; advance, aid, breed, cherish, cultivate, encourage, favour, foment, forward, further, harbour, patronize, promote, rear, stimulate.

foul *vb* besmirch, defile, dirty, pollute, soil, stain, sully; clog, collide, entangle, jam. • *adj* dirty, fetid, filthy, impure, nasty, polluted, putrid, soiled, stained, squalid, sullied, rank, tarnished, unclean; disgusting, hateful, loathsome, noisome, odious, offensive; dishonourable, underhand, unfair, sinister; abominable, base, dark, detestable, disgraceful, infamous, scandalous, scurvy, shameful, wile, wicked; coarse, low, obscene, vulgar; abusive, foul-mouthed, foul-spoken, insulting, scurrilous; cloudy, rainy, rough, stormy, wet; feculent, muddy, thick, turbid; entangled, tangled.

foul-mouthed *adj* abusive, blackguardy, blasphemous, filthy, foul, indecent, insolent, insulting, obscene, scurrilous.

found *vb* base, fix, ground, place, rest, set; build, construct, erect, raise; colonize, establish, institute, originate, plant; cast, mould.

foundation *n* base, basis, bed, bottom, footing, ground, groundwork, substructure, support; endowment, establishment, settlement.

founder[1] *n* author, builder, establisher, father, institutor, originator, organizer, planter.

founder[2] *n* caster, moulder.

founder[3] *vb* sink, swamp, welter; collapse, fail, miscarry; fall, stumble, trip.

fountain *n* fount, reservoir, spring, well; jet, upswelling; cause, fountainhead, origin, original, source.

foxy *adj* artful, crafty, cunning, sly, subtle, wily.

fracas *n* affray, brawl, disturbance, outbreak, quarrel, riot, row, uproar, tumult,

fractious *adj* captious, cross, fretful, irritable, peevish, pettish, perverse, petulant, querulous, snappish, splenetic, touchy, testy, waspish.

fracture *vb* break, crack, split. • *n* breaking, rupture; breach, break, cleft, crack, fissure, flaw, opening, rift, rent.

fragile *adj* breakable, brittle, delicate, frangible; feeble, frail, infirm, weak.

fragility *n* breakability, breakableness, brittleness, frangibility, frangibleness; feebleness, frailty, infirmity, weakness.

fragment *vb* atomize, break, fracture, pulverize, splinter. • *n* bit, chip, fraction, fracture, morsel, part, piece, remnant, scrap.

fragrance *n* aroma, balminess, bouquet, odour, perfume, redolence, scent, smell.

fragrant *adj* ambrosial, aromatic, balmy, odoriferous, odorous, perfumed, redolent, spicy, sweet, sweet-scented, sweet-smelling.

frail *adj* breakable, brittle, delicate, fragile, frangible, slight; feeble, infirm, weak.

frailty *n* feebleness, frailness, infirmity, weakness; blemish, defect, failing, fault, foible, imperfection, peccability, shortcoming.

frame *vb* build, compose, constitute, construct, erect, form, make, mould, plan, shape; contrive, devise, fabricate, fashion, forge, invent, plan. • *n* body, carcass, framework, framing, shell, skeleton; constitution, fabric, form, structure, scheme, system; condition, humour, mood, state, temper.

franchise *n* privilege, right; suffrage, vote; exemption, immunity.

frangible *adj* breakable, brittle, fragile.

frank *adj* artless, candid, direct, downright, frank-hearted, free, genuine, guileless, ingenuous, naive, open, outspoken, outright, plain, plain-spoken, point-blank, sincere, straightforward, truthful, unequivocal, unreserved, unrestricted.

frankness *n* candour, ingenuousness, openness, outspokenness, plain speaking, truth, straightforwardness.

frantic *adj* crazy, distracted, distraught, frenzied, furious, infuriate, mad, outrageous, phrenetic, rabid, raging, raving, transported, wild.

fraternity *n* association, brotherhood, circle, clan, club, company, fellowship, league, set, society, sodality; brotherliness.

fraternize *vb* associate, coalesce, concur, consort, cooperate, harmonize, sympathize, unite.

fraud *n* artifice, cheat, craft, deception, deceit, duplicity, guile, hoax, humbug, imposition, imposture, sham, stratagem, treachery, trick, trickery, wile.

fraudulent *adj* crafty, deceitful, deceptive, dishonest, false, knavish, treacherous, trickish, tricky, wily.

fraught *adj* abounding, big, burdened, charged, filled, freighted, laden, pregnant, stored, weighted.

fray[1] *n* affray, battle, brawl, broil, combat, fight, quarrel, riot.

fray[2] *vb* chafe, fret, rub, wear; ravel, shred.

freak *adj* bizarre, freakish, grotesque, monstrous, odd, unexpected, unforeseen. • *n* caprice, crotchet, fancy, humour, maggot, quirk, vagary, whim, whimsey; antic, caper, gambol; abnormality, abortion, monstrosity.

freakish *adj* capricious, changeable, eccentric, erratic, fanciful, humoursome, odd, queer, whimsical.

free *vb* deliver, discharge, disenthral, emancipate, enfranchise, enlarge, liberate, manumit, ransom, release, redeem, rescue, save; clear, disencumber, disengage, extricate, rid, unbind, unchain, unfetter, unlock; exempt, immunize, privilege. • *adj* bondless, independent, loose, unattached, unconfined, unentangled, unimpeded, unrestrained, untrammelled; autonomous, delivered, emancipated, freeborn, liberated, manumitted, ransomed, released, self-governing; clear, exempt, immune, privileged; allowed, permitted; devoid, empty, open, unimpeded, unobstructed, unrestricted; affable, artless, candid, frank, ingenuous, sincere, unreserved; bountiful, charitable, free-hearted, generous, hospitable, liberal, munificent, openhanded; immoderate, lavish, prodigal; eager, prompt, ready, willing; available, gratuitous, spontaneous; careless, lax, loose; bold, easy, familiar, informal, overfamiliar, unconstrained. • *adv* openly, outright, unreservedly, unrestrainedly, unstintingly; freely, gratis, gratuitously.

freebooter *n* bandit, brigand, despoiler, footpad, gangster, highwayman, marauder, pillager, plunderer, robber; buccaneer, pirate, rover.

freedom *n* emancipation, independence, liberation, liberty, release; elbowroom, margin, play, range, scope, swing; franchise, immunity, privilege; familiarity, laxity, license, looseness.

freethinker *n* agnostic, deist, doubter, infidel, sceptic, unbeliever.

freeze *vb* congeal, glaciate, harden, stiffen; benumb, chill.

freight *vb* burden, charge, lade, load. • *n* burden, cargo, lading, load.

frenzy *n* aberration, delirium, derangement, distraction, fury, insanity, lunacy, madness, mania, paroxysm, rage, raving, transport.

frequent *vb* attend, haunt, resort, visit. • *adj* iterating, oft-repeated; common, customary, everyday, familiar, habitual, persistent, usual; constant, continual, incessant.

fresh *adj* new, novel, recent; renewed, revived; blooming, flourishing, green, undecayed, unimpaired, unfaded, unobliterated, unwilted, unwithered, well-preserved; sweet; delicate, fair, fresh-coloured, ruddy, rosy; florid, hardy, healthy, vigorous, strong; active, energetic, unexhausted, unfatigued, unwearied, vigorous; keen, lively, unabated, undecayed, unimpaired, vivid; additional, further; uncured, undried, unsalted, unsmoked; bracing, health-giving, invigorating, refreshing, sweet; brink, stiff, strong; inexperienced, raw, uncultivated, unpracticed, unskilled, untrained, unused.

freshen *vb* quicken, receive, refresh, revive.

fret[1] *vb* abrade, chafe, fray, gall, rub, wear; affront, agitate, annoy, gall, harass, irritate, nettle, provoke, ruffle, tease, vex, wear, worry; ripple, roughen; corrode; fume, peeve, rage, stew. • *n* agitation, fretfulness, fretting, irritation, peevishness, vexation.

fret[2] *vb* diversify, interlace, ornament, variegate. • *n* fretwork, interlacing, ornament; ridge, wale, whelk.

fretful *adj* captious, cross, fractious, ill-humoured, ill-tempered, irritable, peevish, pettish, petulant, querulous, short-tempered, snappish, spleeny, splenetic, testy, touchy, uneasy, waspish.

friable *adj* brittle, crisp, crumbling, powdery, pulverable.

friction *n* abrasion, attrition, grating, rubbing; bickering, disagreement, dissension, wrangling.

friend *adj* benefactor, chum, companion, comrade, crony, confidant, intimate; adherent, ally, associate, confrere, partisan; advocate, defender, encourager, favourer, patron, supporter, well-wisher.

friendly *adj* affectionate, amiable, benevolent, favourable, kind, kind-hearted, kindly, well-disposed; amicable, cordial, fraternal, neighbourly; conciliatory, peaceable, unhostile.

friendship *n* affection, attachment, benevolence, fondness, goodness, love, regard; fellowship, intimacy; amicability, amicableness, amity, cordiality, familiarity, fraternization, friendliness, harmony.

fright *n* affright, alarm, consternation, dismay, funk, horror, panic, scare, terror.

frighten *vb* affright, alarm, appal, daunt, dismay, intimidate, scare, stampede, terrify

frightful *adj* alarming, awful, dire, direful, dread, dreadful, fearful, horrible, horrid, shocking, terrible, terrific; ghastly, grim, grisly, gruesome, hideous.

frigid *adj* cold, cool, gelic; dull, lifeless, spiritless, tame, unanimated, uninterested, uninteresting; chilling, distant, forbidding, formal, freezing, prim, repellent, repelling, repulsive, rigid, stiff.

frill *n* edging, frilling, furbelow, gathering, ruche, ruching, ruffle; affectation, mannerism.

fringe *vb* border, bound, edge, hem, march, rim, skirt, verge. • *n* border, edge, edging, tassel, trimming. • *adj* edging, extra, unofficial.

frisk *vb* caper, dance, frolic, gambol, hop, jump, play, leap, romp, skip, sport, wanton.

frisky *adj* frolicsome, coltish, gay, lively, playful, sportive.

frivolity *n* flummery, folly, fribbling, frippery, frivolousness, levity, puerility, trifling, triviality.

frivolous *adj* childish, empty, flighty, flimsy, flippant, foolish, giddy, idle, light, paltry, petty, puerile, silly, trashy, trifling, trivial, unimportant, vain, worthless.

frolic *vb* caper, frisk, gambol, lark, play, romp, sport. • *n* escapade, gambol, lark, romp, skylark, spree, trick; drollery, fun, play, pleasantry, sport.

frolicsome *adj* coltish, fresh, frolic, gamesome, gay, lively, playful, sportive.

front *vb* confront, encounter, face, oppose. • *adj* anterior, forward; foremost, frontal, headmost. • *n* brow, face, forehead; assurance, boldness, brass, effrontery, impudence; breast, head, van, vanguard; anterior, face, forepart, obverse; facade, frontage.

frontier *n* border, boundary, coast, confine, limits, marches.

frosty *adj* chill, chilly, cold, icy, stinging, wintry; cold, coldhearted, frigid, indifferent, unaffectionate, uncordial, unimpassioned, unloving; dull-hearted, lifeless, spiritless, unanimated; frosted, grey-hearted, hoary, white.

froth *vb* bubble, cream, foam, lather, spume. • *n* bubbles, foam, lather, spume; balderdash, flummery, nonsense, trash, triviality.

frothy *adj* foamy, spumy; empty, frivolous, light, trifling, trivial, unsubstantial, vain.

froward *adj* captious, contrary, contumacious, cross, defiant, disobedient, fractious, impudent, intractable, obstinate, peevish, perverse, petulant, refractory, stubborn, ungovernable, untoward, unyielding, wayward, wilful.

frown *vb* glower, lower, scowl.

frowzy, frowsy *adj* fetid, musty, noisome, rancid, rank, stale; disordered, disorderly, dowdy, slatternly, slovenly.

frugal *adj* abstemious, careful, chary, choice, economical, provident, saving, sparing, temperate, thrifty, unwasteful.

fruit *n* crop, harvest, produce, production; advantage, consequence, effect, good, outcome, product, profit, result; issue, offspring, young.

fruitful *adj* abounding, productive; fecund, fertile, prolific; abundant, exuberant, plenteous, plentiful, rich, teeming.

fruition *n* completion, fulfilment, perfection; enjoyment.

fruitless *adj* acarpous, barren, sterile, infecund, unfertile, unfruitful, unproductive, unprolific; abortive, bootless, futile, idle, ineffectual, profitless, unavailing, unprofitable, useless, vain.

frumpish, frumpy *adj* cross, cross-grained, cross-tempered, dowdy, grumpy, irritable, shabby, slatternly, snappish.

frustrate *vb* baffle, balk, check, circumvent, defeat, disappoint, disconcert, foil, thwart; cross, hinder, outwit.

frustrated *adj* balked, blighted, dashed, defeated, foiled, thwarted; ineffectual, null, useless, vain.

fuddled *adj* befuddled, boozy, corned, crapulous, drunk, groggy, high, inebriated, intoxicated, muddled, slewed, tight, tipsy.

fugacious *adj* evanescent, fleeting, fugitive, transient, transitory.

fugitive *adj* escaping, fleeing, flying; brief, ephemeral, evanescent, fleeting, flitting, fugacious, momentary, short, short-lived, temporal, temporary, transient, transitory, uncertain, unstable, volatile. • *n* émigré, escapee, evacuee, fleer, outlaw, refugee, runaway.

fulfil *vb* accomplish, complete, consummate, effect, effectuate, execute, realize; adhere, discharge, do, keep, obey, observe, perform; answer, fill, meet, satisfy.

full *adj* brimful, filled, flush, replete; abounding, replete, well-stocked; bagging, flowing, loose, voluminous; chock-full, cloyed, crammed, glutted, gorged, overflowing, packed, sated, satiated, saturated, soaked, stuffed, swollen; adequate, complete, entire, mature, perfect; abundant, ample, copious, plenteous, plentiful, sufficient; clear, deep, distinct, loud, rounded, strong; broad, large, capacious, comprehensive, extensive, plump; circumstantial, detailed, exhaustive. • *adv* completely, fully; directly, exactly, precisely.

fullness *n* abundance, affluence, copiousness, plenitude, plenty, profusion; glut, satiety, sating, repletion; completeness, completion, entireness, perfection; clearness, loudness, resonance, strength; dilation, distension, enlargement, plumpness, rotundity, roundness, swelling.

fully *adv* abundantly, amply, completely, copiously, entirely, largely, plentifully, sufficiently.

fulminate *vb* detonate, explode; curse, denounce, hurl, menace, threaten, thunder.

fulsome *adj* excessive, extravagant, fawning; disgusting, nauseous, nauseating, offensive, repulsive; coarse, gross, lustful, questionable.

fumble *vb* bungle, grope, mismanage, stumble; mumble, stammer, stutter.

fume *vb* reek, smoke, vaporize. • *n* effluvium exhalation, reek, smell, smoke, steam, vapour; agitation, fret, fry, fury, passion, pet, rage, storm.

fun *adj* amusing, diverting, droll, entertaining. • *n* amusement, diversion, drollery, frolic, gaiety, humour, jesting, jocularity, jollity, joy, merriment, mirth, play, pranks, sport, pleasantry, waggishness.

function *vb* act, discharge, go, operate, officiate, perform, run, serve, work. • *n* discharge, execution, exercise, operation, performance, purpose, use; activity, business, capacity, duty, employment, occupation, office, part, province, role; ceremony, rite; dependant, derivative.

fund *vb* afford, endow, finance, invest, provide, subsidise, support; garner, hoard, stock, store. • *n* accumulation, capital, endowment, reserve, stock; store, supply; foundation.

fundament *n* bottom, buttocks, seat.

fundamental *adj* basal, basic, bottom, cardinal, constitutional, elementary, essential, indispensable, organic, principal, primary, radical. • *n* essential, principal, rule.

funeral *n* burial, cremation, exequies, internment, obsequies.

funereal *adj* dark, dismal, gloomy, lugubrious, melancholy, mournful, sad, sepulchral, sombre, woeful.

funk *vb* blanch, shrink, quail. • *n* stench, stink; fear, fright, panic.

funny *adj* amusing, comic, comical, diverting, droll, facetious, farcical, humorous, jocose, jocular, laughable, ludicrous, sportive, witty; curious, odd, queer, strange. • *n* jest, joke; cartoon, comic.

furbish *vb* burnish, brighten, polish, renew, renovate, rub, shine.

furious *adj* angry, fierce, frantic, frenzied, fuming, infuriated, mad, raging, violent, wild; boisterous, fierce, impetuous, stormy, tempestuous, tumultuous, turbulent, vehement.

furnish *vb* appoint, endow, provide, supply; decorate, equip, fit; afford, bestow, contribute, give, offer, present, produce, yield.

furniture *n* chattels, effects, household goods, movables; apparatus, appendages, appliances, equipment, fittings, furnishings; decorations, embellishments, ornaments.

furore *n* commotion, craze, enthusiasm, excitement, fad, fury, madness, mania, rage, vogue.

furrow *vb* chamfer, channel, cleave, corrugate, cut, flute, groove, hollow; pucker, seam, wrinkle. • *n* chamfer, channel, cut, depression, fluting, groove, hollow, line, seam, track, trench, rot, wrinkle.

further *vb* advance, aid, assist, encourage, help, forward, promote, succour, strengthen. • *adj* additional. • *adv* also, besides, farther, furthermore, moreover.

furtive *adj* clandestine, hidden, secret, sly, skulking, sneaking, sneaky, stealthy, stolen, surreptitious.

fury *n* anger, frenzy, fit, furore, ire, madness, passion, rage; fierceness, impetuosity, turbulence, turbulency, vehemence; bacchant, bacchante, bedlam, hag, shrew, termagant, virago, vixen.

fuse *vb* dissolve, melt, liquefy, smelt; amalgamate, blend, coalesce, combine, commingle, intermingle, intermix, merge, unite. • *n* match.

fusion *n* liquefaction, melting; amalgamation, blending, commingling, commixture, intermingling, intermixture, union; coalition, merging.

fuss *vb* bustle, fidget; fret, fume, worry. • *n* ado, agitation, bother, bustle, commotion, disturbance, excitement, fidget, flurry, fluster, fret, hurry, pother, stir, worry.

fustian *n* bombast, claptrap, rant, rodomontade; balderdash, inanity, nonsense, stuff, trash, twaddle.

fusty *adj* ill-smelling, malodorous, mildewed, mouldy, musty, rank.

futile *adj* frivolous, trifling, trivial; bootless, fruitless, idle, ineffectual, profitless, unavailing, unprofitable, useless, vain, valueless, worthless.

futility *n* frivolousness, triviality; bootlessness, fruitlessness, uselessness, vanity, worthlessness.

future *adj* coming, eventual, forthcoming, hereafter, prospective, subsequent. • *n* hereafter, outlook, prospect.

G

gabble *vb* babble, chatter, clack, gibber, gossip, prate, prattle. • *n* babble, chatter, clack, gap, gossip, jabber, palaver, prate, prattle, twaddle.

gadabout *n* idler, loafer, rambler, rover, vagrant; gossip, talebearer, vagrant.

gaffer *n* boss, foreman, overseer, supervisor.

gag[1] *n* jape, jest, joke, stunt, wisecrack.

gag[2] *vb* muffle, muzzle, shackle, silence, stifle, throttle; regurgitate, retch, throw up, vomit; choke, gasp, pant. • *n* muzzle.

gage *n* pawn, pledge, security, surety; challenge, defiance, gauntlet, glove.

gaiety *n* animation, blithesomeness, cheerfulness, glee, hilarity, jollity, joviality, merriment, mirth, vivacity.

gain *vb* achieve, acquire, earn, get, obtain, procure, reap, secure; conciliate, enlist, persuade, prevail, win; arrive, attain, reach; clear, net, profit. • *n* accretion, addition, gainings, profits, winnings; acquisition, earnings, emolument, lucre; advantage, benefit, blessing, good, profit.

gainful *adj* advantageous, beneficial, profitable; lucrative, paying, productive, remunerative.

gainsay *vb* contradict, controvert, deny, dispute, forbid.

gait *n* carriage, pace, step, stride, walk.

galaxy *n* assemblage, assembly, cluster, collection, constellation, group.

gale *n* blast, hurricane, squall, storm, tempest, tornado, typhoon.

gall[1] *n* effrontery, impudence; bile; acerbity, bitterness, malice, maliciousness, malignity, rancour, spite.

gall[2] *vb* chafe, excoriate, fret, hurt; affront, annoy, exasperate, harass, incense, irritate, plague, provoke, sting, tease, vex.

gallant *adj* fine, magnificent, showy, splendid, well-dressed; bold, brave, chivalrous, courageous, daring, fearless, heroic, high-spirited, intrepid, valiant, valorous; chivalrous, fine, honourable, high-minded, lofty, magnanimous, noble. • *n* beau, blade, spark; lover, suitor, wooer.

gallantry *n* boldness, bravery, chivalry, courage, courageousness, fearlessness, heroism, intrepidity, prowess, valour; courtesy, courteousness, elegance, politeness.

galling *adj* chafing, irritating, vexing.

gallop *vb* fly, hurry, run, rush, scamper, speed.

gamble *vb* bet, dice, game, hazard, plunge, speculate, wager. • *n* chance, risk, speculation; bet, punt, wager.

gambol *vb* caper, cut, frisk, frolic, hop, jump, leap, romp, skip. • *n* frolic, hop, jump, skip.

game[1] *vb* gamble, sport, stake. • *n* amusement, contest, diversion, pastime, play, sport; adventure, enterprise, measure, plan, project, scheme, stratagem, undertaking; prey, quarry, victim.

game[2] *adj* brave, courageous, dauntless, fearless, gallant, heroic, intrepid, plucky, unflinching, valorous; enduring, persevering, resolute, undaunted; ready, eager, willing.

game[3] *adj* crippled, disabled, halt, injured, lame.

gameness *n* bravery, courage, grit, heart, mettle, nerve, pith, pluck, pluckiness, spirit, stamina.

gamesome *adj* frisky, frolicsome, lively, merry, playful, sportive, sprightly, vivacious.

gammon *vb* bamboozle, beguile, cheat, circumvent, deceive, delude, dupe, gull, hoax, humbug, inveigle, mislead, overreach, outwit. • *n* bosh, hoax, humbug, imposition, nonsense.

gang *n* band, cabal, clique, company, coterie, crew, horde, party, set, troop.

gaol *see* **jail**.

gap *n* breach, break, cavity, chasm, chink, cleft, crack, cranny, crevice, hiatus, hollow, interval, interstice, lacuna, opening, pass, ravine, rift, space, vacancy.

gape *vb* burst open, dehisce, open, stare, yawn.

garb *vb* attire, clothe, dress. • *n* apparel, attire, clothes, costume, dress, garments, habiliment, habit, raiment, robes, uniform, vestment.

garbage *n* filth, offal, refuse, remains, rubbish, trash, waste.

garble *vb* corrupt, distort, falsify, misquote, misrepresent, mutilate, pervert.

gargantuan *adj* big, Brobdingnagian, colossal, enormous, gigantic, huge, prodigious, tremendous.

garish *adj* bright, dazzling, flashy, flaunting, gaudy, glaring, loud, showy, staring, tawdry.

garland *vb* adorn, festoon, wreathe. • *n* chaplet, coronal, crown, festoon, wreath.

garment *n* clothes, clothing, dress, habit, vestment.

garner *vb* accumulate, collect, deposit, gather, hoard, husband, reserve, save, store, treasure.

garnish *vb* adorn, beautify, bedeck, decorate, deck, embellish, grace, ornament, prank, trim. • *n* decoration, enhancement, ornament, trimming.

garrulous *adj* babbling, loquacious, prating, prattling, talkative.

gasconade *n* bluster, boast, brag, bravado, swagger, vaunt, vapouring.

gasp *vb* blow, choke, pant, puff. • *n* blow, exclamation, gulp, puff.

gather *vb* assemble, cluster, collect, convene, group, muster, rally; accumulate, amass, garner, hoard, huddle, lump; bunch, crop, cull glean, pick, pluck, rake, reap, shock, stack; acquire, gain, get win; conclude, deduce, derive, infer; fold, plait, pucker, shirr, tuck; condense, grow, increase, thicken.

gathering *n* acquisition, collecting, earning, gain, heap, pile, procuring; assemblage, assembly, collection, company, concourse, congregation, meeting, muster; abscess, boil, fester, pimple, pustule, sore, suppuration, tumour, ulcer.

gauche *adj* awkward, blundering, bungling, clumsy, inept, tactless, uncouth.

gaudy *adj* bespangled, brilliant, brummagem, cheap, flashy, flaunting, garish, gimcrack, glittering, loud, ostentatious, overdecorated, sham, showy, spurious, tawdry, tinsel.

gauge *vb* calculate, check, determine, weigh; assess, estimate, guess, reckon. • *n* criterion, example, indicator, measure, meter, touchstone, yardstick; bore, depth, height, magnitude, size, thickness, width.

gaunt *adj* angular, attenuated, emaciated, haggard, lank, lean, meagre, scraggy, skinny, slender, spare, thin.

gawky *adj* awkward, boorish, clownish, clumsy, green, loutish, raw, rustic, uncouth, ungainly.

gay *adj* bright, brilliant, dashing, fine, showy; flashy, flaunting, garish, gaudy, glittering, loud, tawdry, tinsel; airy, blithe, blithesome, cheerful, festive, frivolous, frolicsome, gladsome, gleeful, hilarious, jaunty, jolly, jovial, light-hearted, lively, merry, mirthful, sportive, sprightly, vivacious.

gear *vb* adapt, equip, fit, suit, tailor. • *n* apparel, array, clothes, clothing, dress, garb; accoutrements, appliances, appointments, appurtenances, array, harness, goods, movables, subsidiaries; harness, rigging, tackle, trappings; apparatus, machinery, mechanics.

gelid *adj* chill, chilly, cold, freezing, frigid, icy.

gem *n* jewel, stone, treasure.

genealogy *n* ancestry, descent, lineage, pedigree, stock.

general *adj* broad, collective, generic, popular, universal, widespread; catholic, ecumenical; common, current, ordinary, usual; inaccurate, indefinite, inexact, vague.

generally *adv* commonly, extensively, universally, usually.

generate *vb* beget, breed, engender, procreate, propagate, reproduce, spawn; cause, form, make, produce.

generation *n* creation, engendering, formation, procreation, production; age, epoch, era, period, time; breed, children, family, kind, offspring, progeny, race, stock.

generosity *n* disinterestedness, high-mindedness, magnanimity, nobleness; bounteousness, bountifulness, bounty, charity, liberality, openhandedness.

generous *adj* high-minded, honourable, magnanimous, noble; beneficent, bountiful, charitable, free, hospitable, liberal, munificent, open-handed; abundant, ample, copious, plentiful, rich.

genial *adj* cheering, encouraging, enlivening, fostering, inspiring, mild, warm; agreeable, cheerful, cordial, friendly, hearty, jovial, kindly, merry, mirthful, pleasant.

genius *n* aptitude, aptness, bent, capacity, endowment, faculty, flair, gift, talent, turn; brains, creative power, ingenuity, inspiration, intellect, invention, parts, sagacity, wit; adeptness, master, master hand, proficiency; character, disposition, naturalness, nature; deity, demon, spirit.

genteel *adj* aristocratic, courteous, gentlemanly, lady-like, polished, polite, refined, well-bred; elegant, fashionable, graceful, stylish.

gentility *n* civility, courtesy, good breeding, politeness, refinement, urbanity.

gentle *adj* amiable, bland, clement, compassionate, humane, indulgent, kind, kindly, lenient, meek, merciful, mild, moderate, soft, tender, tender-hearted; docile, pacific, peaceable, placid, quiet, tame, temperate, tractable; bland, easy, gradual, light, slight; soft; high-born, noble, well-born; chivalrous, courteous, cultivated, knightly, polished, refined, well-bred.

gentlemanly *adj* civil, complaisant, courteous, cultivated, delicate, genteel, honourable, polite, refined, urbane, well-bred.

genuine *adj* authentic, honest, proper, pure, real, right, true, unadulterated, unalloyed, uncorrupted, veritable; frank, native, sincere, unaffected.

genus *n* class, group, kind, order, race, sort, type.

germ *n* embryo, nucleus, ovule, ovum, seed, seed-bud; bacterium, microbe, microorganism; beginning, cause, origin, rudiment, source.

germane *adj* akin, allied, cognate, related; apposite, appropriate, fitting, pertinent, relevant, suitable.

germinate *vb* bud, burgeon, develop, generate, grow, pollinate, push, shoot, sprout, vegetate.

gesture *vb* indicate, motion, signal, wave. • *n* action, attitude, gesticulation, gesturing, posture, sign, signal.

get *vb* achieve, acquire, attain, earn, gain, obtain, procure, receive, relieve, secure, win; finish, master, prepare; beget, breed, engender, generate, procreate.

gewgaw *n* bauble, gimcrack, gaud, kickshaw, knick-knack, plaything, trifle, toy, trinket.

ghastly *adj* cadaverous, corpse-like, death-like, deathly, ghostly, lurid, pale, pallid, wan; dismal, dreadful, fearful, frightful, grim, grisly, gruesome, hideous, horrible, shocking, terrible.

ghost *n* soul, spirit; apparition, phantom, revenant, shade, spectre, spook, sprite, wraith.

giant *adj* colossal, enormous, Herculean, huge, large, monstrous, prodigious, vast. • *n* colossus, cyclops, Hercules, monster.

gibberish *n* babble, balderdash, drivel, gabble, gobbledygook, jabber, nonsense, prate, prating.

gibe, jibe *vb* deride, fleer, flout, jeer, mock, ridicule, scoff, sneer, taunt. • *n* ridicule, sneer, taunt.

giddiness *n* dizziness, head-spinning, vertigo.

giddy *adj* dizzy, head-spinning, vertiginous; careless, changeable, fickle, flighty, frivolous, hare-brained, headlong, heedless, inconstant, irresolute, light-headed, thoughtless, unsteady, vacillating, wild.

gift *n* alms, allowance, benefaction, bequest, bonus, boon, bounty, contribution, donation, dowry, endowment, favour, grant, gratuity, honorarium, largesse, legacy, offering, premium, present, prize, subscription, subsidy, tip; faculty, talent.

gifted *adj* able, capable, clever, ingenious, intelligent, inventive, sagacious, talented.

gigantic *adj* colossal, Cyclopean, enormous, giant, herculean, huge, immense, prodigious, titanic, tremendous, vast.

giggle *vb*, *n* cackle, grin, laugh, snigger, snicker, titter.

gild *vb* adorn, beautify, bedeck, brighten, decorate, embellish, grace, illuminate.

gimcrack *adj* flimsy, frail, puny; base, cheap, paltry, poor. • *n* bauble, knick-knack, toy, trifle.

gird *vb* belt, girdle; begird, encircle, enclose, encompass, engird, environ, surround; brace, support. • *n* band, belt, cincture, girdle, girth, sash, waistband.

gist *n* basis, core, essence, force, ground, marrow, meaning, pith, point, substance.

give *vb* accord, bequeath, bestow, confer, devise, entrust, present; afford, contribute, donate, furnish, grant, proffer, spare, supply; communicate, impart; deliver, exchange, pay, requite; allow, permit, vouchsafe; emit, pronounce, render, utter; produce,

yield; cause, occasion; apply, devote, surrender; bend, sink, recede, retire, retreat, yield.

glad *adj* delighted, gratified, happy, pleased, rejoicing, well-contented; animated, blithe, cheerful, cheery, elated, gladsome, jocund, joyful, joyous, light, light-hearted, merry, playful, radiant; animating, bright, cheering, exhilarating, gladdening, gratifying, pleasing.

gladden *vb* bless, cheer, delight, elate, enliven, exhilarate, gratify, please, rejoice.

gladiator *n* prize-fighter, sword-player, swordsman.

gladness *n* animation, cheerfulness, delight, gratification, happiness, joy, joyfulness, joyousness, pleasure.

gladsome *adj* airy, blithe, blithesome, cheerful, delighted, frolicsome, glad, gleeful, jocund, jolly, jovial, joyful, joyous, light-hearted, lively, merry, pleased, sportive, sprightly, vivacious.

glamour *n* bewitchment, charm, enchantment, fascination, spell, witchery.

glance *vb* coruscate, gleam, glisten, glister, glitter, scintillate, shine; dart, flit; gaze, glimpse, look, view. • *n* gleam, glitter; gleam, look, view.

glare *vb* dazzle, flame, flare, gleam, glisten, glitter, sparkle; frown, gaze, glower. • *n* flare, glitter.

glaring *adj* dazzling, gleaming, glistening, glittering; barefaced, conspicuous, extreme, manifest, notorious, open.

glassy *adj* brilliant, crystal, crystalline, gleaming, lucent, shining, transparent.

glaze *vb* burnish, calender, furbish, gloss, polish. • *n* coat, enamel, finish, glazing, polish, varnish.

gleam *vb* beam, coruscate, flash, glance, glimmer, glitter, shine, sparkle. • *n* beam, flash, glance, glimmer, glimmering, glow, ray; brightness, coruscation, flashing, gleaming, glitter, glittering, lustre, splendour.

glean *vb* collect, cull, gather, get, harvest, pick, select.

glee *n* exhilaration, fun, gaiety, hilarity, jocularity, jollity, joviality, joy, liveliness, merriment, mirth, sportiveness, verve.

glib *adj* slippery, smooth; artful, facile, flippant, fluent, ready, talkative, voluble.

glide *vb* float, glissade, roll on, skate, skim, slide, slip; flow, lapse, run, roll. • *n* gliding, lapse, sliding, slip.

glimmer *vb* flash, flicker, gleam, glitter, shine, twinkle. • *n* beam, gleam, glimmering, ray; glance, glimpse.

glimpse *vb* espy, look, spot, view. • *n* flash, glance, glimmering, glint, look, sight.

glitter *vb* coruscate, flare, flash, glance, glare, gleam, glisten, glister, scintillate, shine, sparkle. • *n* beam, beaming, brightness, brilliancy, coruscation, gleam, glister, lustre, radiance, scintillation, shine, sparkle, splendour.

gloaming *n* dusk, eventide, nightfall, twilight.

gloat *vb* exult, gaze, rejoice, stare, triumph.

globe *n* ball, earth, orb, sphere.

globular *adj* globate, globated, globe-shaped, globose, globous, round, spheral, spheric, spherical.

globule *n* bead, drop, particle, spherule.

gloom *n* cloud, darkness, dimness, gloominess, obscurity, shade, shadow; cheerlessness, dejection, depression, despondency, downheartedness, dullness, melancholy, sadness.

gloomy *adj* dark, dim, dusky, obscure; cheerless, dismal, lowering, lurid; crestfallen, dejected, depressed, despondent, disheartened, dispirited, downcast, downhearted, glum, melancholy, morose, sad, sullen; depressing, disheartening, dispiriting, heavy, saddening.

glorify *vb* adore, bless, celebrate, exalt, extol, honour, laud, magnify, worship; adorn, brighten, elevate, ennoble, make bright.

glorious *adj* celebrated, conspicuous, distinguished, eminent, excellent, famed, famous, illustrious, pre-eminent, renowned; brilliant, bright, grand, magnificent, radiant, resplendent, splendid; consummate, exalted, high, lofty, noble, supreme.

glory *vb* boast, exult, vaunt. • *n* celebrity, distinction, eminence, fame, honour, illustriousness, praise, renown; brightness, brilliancy, effulgence, lustre, pride, resplendence, splendour; exaltation, exceeding, gloriousness, greatness, grandeur, nobleness; bliss, happiness.

gloss[1] *vb* coat, colour, disguise, extenuate, glaze, palliate, varnish, veneer, veil. • *n* coating, lustre, polish, sheen, varnish, veneer; pretence, pretext.

gloss[2] *vb* annotate, comment, elucidate, explain, interpret. • *n* annotation, comment, commentary, elucidation, explanation, interpretation, note.

glove *n* gantlet, gauntlet, handwear, mitt, mitten; challenge.

glow *vb* incandesce, radiate, shine; blush, burn, flush, redden. • *n* blaze, brightness, brilliance, burning, incandescence, luminosity, reddening; ardour, bloom, enthusiasm, fervency, fervour, flush, impetuosity, vehemence, warmth.

glower *vb* frown, glare, lower, scowl, stare. • *n* frown, glare, scowl.

glum *adj* churlish, crabbed, crestfallen, cross-grained, crusty, depressed, frowning, gloomy, glowering, moody, morose, sour, spleenish, spleeny, sulky, sullen, surly.

glut *vb* block up, cloy, cram, gorge, satiate, stuff. • *n* excess, saturation, surfeit, surplus.

glutinous *adj* adhesive, clammy, cohesive, gluey, gummy, sticky, tenacious, viscid, viscous.

glutton *n* gobbler, gorger, gourmand, gormandizer, greedy-guts, lurcher, pig.

gnarled *adj* contorted, cross-grained, gnarly, knotted, knotty, snaggy, twisted.

go *vb* advance, move, pass, proceed, progress repair; act, operate; be about, extravagate, fare, journey, roam, rove, travel, walk, wend; depart, disappear, cease; elapse, extend, lead, reach, run; avail, concur, contribute, tend, serve; eventuate, fare, turn out; afford, bet, risk, wager. • *n* action, business, case, chance, circumstance, doings, turn; custom, fad, fashion, mode, vogue; energy, endurance, power, stamina, verve, vivacity.

goad *vb* annoy, badger, harass, irritate, sting, worry; arouse, impel, incite, instigate, prod, spur, stimulate, urge. • *n* incentive, incitement, pressure, stimulation.

goal *n* bound, home, limit, mark, mete, post; end, object; aim, design, destination.

gobble *vb* bolt, devour, gorge, gulp, swallow.

goblin *n* apparition, elf, bogey, demon, gnome, hobgoblin, phantom, spectre, sprite.

god *n* almighty, creator, deity, divinity, idol, Jehovah, omnipotence, providence.

godless *adj* atheistic, impious, irreligious, profane, ungodly, wicked.

godlike *adj* celestial, divine, heavenly, supernal.

godly *adj* devout, holy, pious, religious, righteous, saint-like, saintly.

godsend *n* fortune, gift, luck, present, windfall.

golden *adj* aureate, brilliant, bright, gilded, resplendent, shining, splendid; excellent, precious; auspicious, favourable, opportune, propitious; blessed, delightful, glorious, halcyon, happy.

good *adj* advantageous, beneficial, favourable, profitable, serviceable, useful; adequate, appropriate, becoming, convenient, fit, proper, satisfactory, suitable, well-adapted; decorous, dutiful, honest, just, pious, reliable, religious, righteous, true, upright, virtuous, well-behaved, worthy; admirable, capable, excellent, genuine, healthy, precious, sincere, sound, sterling, valid, valuable; benevolent, favourable, friendly, gracious, humane, kind, merciful, obliging, well-disposed; fair, honourable, immaculate, unblemished, unimpeachable, unimpeached, unsullied, untarnished; cheerful, companionable, lively, genial, social; able, competent, dextrous, expert, qualified, ready, skilful, thorough, well-qualified; credit-worthy; agreeable, cheering, gratifying, pleasant. • *n* advantage, benefit, boon, favour, gain, profit, utility; interest, prosperity, welfare, weal; excellence, righteousness, virtue, worth.

good breeding *n* affability, civility, courtesy, good manners, polish, politeness, urbanity.

goodbye *n* adieu, farewell, parting.

goodly *adj* beautiful, comely, good-looking, graceful; agreeable, considerate, desirable, happy, pleasant.

good-natured *adj* amiable, benevolent, friendly, kind, kind-hearted, kindly.

goodness *n* excellence, quality, value, worth; honesty, integrity, morality, principle, probity, righteousness, uprightness, virtue; benevolence, beneficence, benignity, good-will, humaneness, humanity, kindness.

goods *npl* belongings, chattels, effects, furniture, movables; commodities, merchandise, stock, wares.

goodwill *n* benevolence, kindness, good nature; ardour, earnestness, heartiness, willingness, zeal; custom, patronage.

gore[1] *vb* horn, pierce, stab, wound.

gorge[1] *vb* bolt, devour, eat, feed, swallow; cram, fill, glut, gormandize, sate, satiate, stuff, surfeit. • *n* craw, crop, gullet, throat.

gorge[2] *n* canyon, defile, fissure, notch, ravine.

gorgeous *adj* bright, brilliant, dazzling, fine, glittering, grand, magnificent, resplendent, rich, shining, showy, splendid, superb.

Gorgon *n* bugaboo, fright, hobgoblin, hydra, ogre, spectre.

gory *adj* bloody, ensanguined, sanguinary.

gospel *n* creed, doctrine, message, news, revelation, tidings.

gossip *vb* chat, cackle, clack, gabble, prate, prattle, tattle. • *n* babbler, busybody, chatterer, gossipmonger, newsmonger, quidnunc, tale-bearer, tattler, tell-tale; cackle, chat, chit-chat, prate, prattle, tattle.

gourmet *n* connoisseur, epicure, epicurean.

govern *vb* administer, conduct, direct, manage, regulate, reign, rule, superintend, supervise; guide, pilot, steer; bridle, check, command control, curb, restrain, rule, sway.

government *n* autonomy, command, conduct, control, direction, discipline, dominion, guidance, management, regulation, restraint, rule, rulership, sway; administration, cabinet, commonwealth, polity, sovereignty, state.

governor *n* commander, comptroller, director, head, headmaster, manager, overseer, ruler, superintendent, supervisor; chief magistrate, executive; guardian, instructor, tutor.

grab *vb* capture, clutch, seize, snatch.

grace *vb* adorn, beautify, deck, decorate, embellish; dignify, honour. • *n* benignity, concescension, favour, good-will, kindness, love; devotion, efficacy, holiness, love, piety, religion, sanctity, virtue; forgiveness, mercy, pardon, reprieve; accomplishment, attractiveness, charm, elegance, polish, propriety, refinement; beauty, comeliness, ease, gracefulness, symmetry; blessing, petition, thanks.

graceful *adj* beautiful, becoming, comely, easy, elegant; flowing, natural, rounded, unlaboured; appropriate; felicitous, happy, tactful.

graceless *adj* abandoned, corrupt, depraved, dissolute, hardened, incorrigible, irreclaimable, lost, obdurate, profligate, reprobate, repugnant, shameless.

gracious *adj* beneficent, benevolent, benign, benignant, compassionate, condescending, favourable, friendly, gentle, good-natured, kind, kindly, lenient, merciful, mild, tender; affable, civil, courteous, easy, familiar, polite.

grade *vb* arrange, classify, group, order, rank, sort. • *n* brand, degree, intensity, stage, step, rank; gradient, incline, slope.

gradual *adj* approximate, continuous, gentle, progressive, regular, slow, successive.

graduate *vb* adapt, adjust, proportion, regulate. • *n* alumna, alumnus, laureate, postgraduate.

graft *vb* ingraft, inoculate, insert, transplant. • *n* bud, scion, shoot, slip, sprout; corruption, favouritism, influence, nepotism.

grain *n* kernel, ovule, seed; cereals, corn, grist; atom, bit, glimmer, jot, particle, scintilla, scrap, shadow, spark, tittle, trace, whit; disposition, fibre, humour, temper, texture; colour, dye, hue, shade, stain, texture, tincture, tinge.

granary *n* corn-house, garner, grange, store-house.

grand *adj* august, dignified, elevated, eminent, exalted, great, illustrious, lordly, majestic, princely, stately, sublime; fine, glorious, gorgeous, magnificent, pompous, lofty, noble, splendid, superb; chief, leading, main, pre-eminent, principal, superior.

grandee *n* lord, noble, nobleman.

grandeur *n* elevation, greatness, immensity, impressiveness, loftiness, vastness; augustness, dignity, eminence, glory, magnificence, majesty nobility, pomp, splendour, state, stateliness.

grandiloquent *adj* bombastic, declamatory, high-minded, high-sounding, inflated, pompous, rhetorical, stilted, swelling, tumid, turgid.

grant *vb* accord, admit, allow, sanction; cede, concede, give, impart, indulge; bestow, confer, deign, invest, vouchsafe; convey, transfer, yield. • *n* admission, allowance, benefaction, bestowal, boon, bounty, concession, donation, endowment, gift, indulgence, largesse, present; conveyance, cession.

graphic *adj* descriptive, diagrammatic, figural, figurative, forcible, lively, pictorial, picturesque, striking, telling, vivid, well-delineated, well-drawn.

grapple *vb* catch, clutch, grasp, grip, hold, hug, seize, tackle, wrestle.

grasp *vb* catch, clasp, clinch, clutch, grapple, grip, seize; comprehend, understand. • *n* clasp, grip, hold; comprehension, power, reach, scope, understanding.

grasping *adj* acquisitive, avaricious, covetous, exacting, greedy, rapacious, sordid, tight-fisted.

grate *vb* abrade, rub, scrape, triturate; comminute, rasp; creak, fret, grind, jar, vex. • *n* bars, grating, latticework, screen; basket, fire bed.

grateful *adj* appreciative, beholden, indebted, obliged, sensible, thankful; pleasant, welcome.

gratification *n* gratifying, indulgence, indulging, pleasing, satisfaction, satisfying; delight, enjoyment, fruition, pleasure, reward.

gratify *vb* delight, gladden, please; humour, fulfil, grant, indulge, requite, satisfy.

gratifying *adj* agreeable, delightful, grateful, pleasing, welcome.

grating *adj* disagreeable, displeasing, harsh, irritating, offensive. • *n* grate, partition.

gratis *adv* freely, gratuitously.

gratitude *n* goodwill, gratitude, indebtedness, thankfulness.

gratuitous *adj* free, spontaneous, unrewarded, voluntary; assumed, baseless, groundless, unfounded, unwarranted, wanton.

gratuity *n* benefaction, bounty, charity, donation, endowment, gift, grant, largesse, present.

grave[1] *n* crypt, mausoleum, ossuary, pit, sepulchre, sepulture, tomb, vault.

grave[2] *adj* cogent, heavy, important, momentous, ponderous, pressing, serious, weighty; dignified, sage, sedate, serious, slow, solemn, staid, thoughtful; dull, grim, plain, quiet, sober, sombre, subdued; cruel, hard, harsh, severe; despicable, dire, dismal, gross, heinous, infamous, outrageous, scandalous, shameful, shocking; heavy, hollow, low, low-pitched, sepulchral.

grave[3] *vb* engrave, impress, imprint, infix; carve, chisel, cut, sculpt.

gravel *vb* bewilder, embarrass, nonplus, perplex, pose, puzzle, stagger. • *n* grate, grit, sand, shingle.

graveyard *n* burial ground, cemetery, churchyard, god's acre, mortuary, necropolis.

gravity *n* heaviness, weight; demureness, sedateness, seriousness, sobriety, thoughtfulness; importance, moment, momentousness, weightiness.

graze *vb* brush, glance, scrape, scratch; abrade, shave, skim; browse, crop, feed, pasture. • *n* abrasion, bruise, scrape, scratch.

great *adj* ample, big, bulky, Cyclopean, enormous, gigantic, Herculean, huge, immense, large, pregnant, vast; decided, excessive, high, much, pronounced; countless, numerous; chief, considerable, grand, important, leading, main, pre-eminent, principal, superior, weighty; celebrated, distinguished, eminent, exalted, excellent, famed, famous, far-famed, illustrious, noted, prominent, renowned; august, dignified, elevated, grand, lofty, majestic, noble, sublime; chivalrous, generous, high-minded, magnanimous; fine, magnificent, rich, sumptuous.

greatness *n* bulk, dimensions, largeness, magnitude, size; distinction, elevation, eminence, fame, importance, renown; augustness, dignity, grandeur, majesty, loftiness, nobility, nobleness, sublimity; chivalry, generosity, magnanimity, spirit.

greed, greediness *n* gluttony, hunger, omnivorousness, ravenousness, voracity; avidity, covetousness, desire, eagerness, longing; avarice, cupidity, graspingness, grasping, rapacity, selfishness.

greedy *adj* devouring, edacious, gluttonous, insatiable, insatiate, rapacious, ravenous, voracious; desirous, eager; avaricious, grasping, selfish.

green *adj* aquamarine, emerald, olive, verdant, verdure, viridescent, viridian; blooming, flourishing, fresh, undecayed; fresh, new, recent; immature, unfledged, unripe; callow, crude, inexpert, ignorant, inexperienced, raw, unskilful, untrained, verdant, young; unseasoned; conservationist, ecological, environmentalist. • *n* common, grass plot, lawn, sward, turf, verdure.

greenhorn *n* beginner, novice, tyro.

greet *vb* accost, address, complement, hail, receive, salute, welcome.

greeting *n* compliment, salutation, salute, welcome.

grief *n* affliction, agony, anguish, bitterness, distress, dole, heartbreak, misery, regret, sadness, sorrow, suffering, tribulation, mourning, woe; grievance, trial; disaster, failure, mishap.

grievance *n* burden, complaint, hardship, injury, oppression, wrong; affliction, distress, grief, sorrow, trial, woe.

grieve *vb* afflict, aggrieve, agonize, discomfort, distress, hurt, oppress, pain, sadden, wound; bewail, deplore, mourn, lament, regret, sorrow, suffer.

grievous *adj* afflicting, afflictive, burdensome, deplorable, distressing, heavy, lamentable, oppressive, painful, sad, sorrowful; baleful, baneful, calamitous, destructive, detrimental, hurtful, injurious, mischievous, noxious, troublesome; aggravated, atrocious, dreadful, flagitious, flagrant, gross, heinous, iniquitous, intense, intolerable, severe, outrageous, wicked.

grill *vb* broil, griddle, roast, toast; sweat; cross-examine, interrogate, question; torment, torture. • *n* grating, gridiron; cross-examination, cross-questioning.

grim *adj* cruel, ferocious, fierce, harsh, relentless, ruthless, savage, stern, unyielding; appalling, dire, dreadful, fearful, frightful, grisly, hideous, horrid, horrible, terrific.

grimace *vb*, *n* frown, scowl, smirk, sneer.

grime *n* dirt, filth, foulness, smut.

grimy *adj* begrimed, defiled, dirty, filthy, foul, soiled, sullied, unclean.

grind *vb* bruise, crunch, crush, grate, grit, pulverize, rub, triturate; sharpen, whet; afflict, harass, oppress, persecute, plague, trouble. • *n* chore, drudgery, labour, toil.

grip *vb* clasp, clutch, grasp, hold, seize. • *n* clasp, clutch, control, domination, grasp, hold.

grisly *adj* appalling, frightful, dreadful, ghastly, grim, grey, hideous, horrible, horrid, terrible, terrific.

grit *vb* clench, grate, grind. • *n* bran, gravel, pebbles, sand; courage, decision, determination, firmness, perseverance, pluck, resolution, spirit.

groan *vb* complain, lament, moan, whine; creak. • *n* cry, moan, whine; complaint; grouse, grumble.

groom *vb* clean, dress, tidy; brush, tend; coach, educate, nurture, train. • *n* equerry, hostler, manservant, ostler, servant, stablehand, valet, waiter.

groove *n* channel, cut, furrow, rabbet, rebate, recess, rut, scoring; routine.

gross *vb* accumulate, earn, make. • *adj* big, bulky, burly, fat, great, large; dense, dull, stupid, thick; beastly, broad, carnal, coarse, crass, earthy, impure, indelicate, licentious, low, obscene, unbecoming, unrefined, unseemly, vulgar, rough, sensual; aggravated, brutal, enormous, flagrant, glaring, grievous, manifest, obvious, palpable, plain, outrageous, shameful; aggregate, entire, total, whole. • *n* aggregate, bulk, total, whole.

grossness *n* bigness, bulkiness, greatness; density, thickness; coarseness, ill-breeding, rudeness, vulgarity; bestiality, brutality, carnality, coarseness, impurity, indelicacy, licentiousness, sensuality.

grotesque *adj* bizarre, extravagant, fanciful, fantastic, incongruous, odd, strange, unnatural, whimsical, wild; absurd, antic, burlesque, ludicrous, ridiculous.

ground *vb* fell, place; base, establish, fix, found, set; instruct, train. • *n* area, clod, distance, earth, loam, mould, sod, soil, turf; country, domain, land, region, territory; acres, estate, field, property; base, basis, foundation, groundwork, support; account, consideration, excuse, gist, motive, opinion, reason.

groundless *adj* baseless, causeless, false, gratuitous, idle, unauthorized, unfounded, unjustifiable, unsolicited, unsought, unwarranted.

grounds *npl* deposit, dregs, grouts, lees, precipitate, sediment, settlings; accounts, arguments, considerations, reasons, support; campus, gardens, lawns, premises, yard.

group *vb* arrange, assemble, dispose, order. • *n* aggregation, assemblage, assembly, body, combination, class, clump, cluster, collection, order.

grove *n* copse, glade, spinney, thicket, wood, woodland.

grovel *vb* cower, crawl, creep, cringe, fawn, flatter, sneak.

grovelling *adj* creeping, crouching, squat; abject, base, beggarly, cringing, fawning, low, mean, servile, slavish, sneaking, undignified, unworthy, vile.

grow *vb* enlarge, expand, extend, increase, swell; arise, burgeon, develop, germinate, shoot, sprout, vegetate; advance, extend, improve, progress, thrive, wax; cultivate, produce, raise.

growl *vb* complain, croak, find fault, gnarl, groan, grumble, lament, murmur, snarl. • *n* croak, grown, snarl; complaint.

growth *n* augmentation, development, expansion, extension, growing, increase; burgeoning, excrescence, formation, germination, pollution, shooting, sprouting, vegetation; cultivation, produce, product, production; advance, advancement, development, improvement, progress; adulthood, maturity.

grub *vb* clear, dig, eradicate, root. • *n* caterpillar, larvae, maggot; drudge, plodder.

grudge *vb* begrudge, envy, repine; complain, grieve, murmur. • *n* aversion, dislike, enmity, grievance, hate, hatred, ill-will, malevolence, malice, pique, rancour, resentment, spite, venom.

gruff *adj* bluff, blunt, brusque, churlish, discourteous, grumpy, harsh, impolite, rough, rude, rugged, surly, uncivil, ungracious.

grumble *vb* croak, complain, murmur, repine; gnarl, growl, snarl; roar, rumble. • *n* growl, murmur, complaint, roar, rumble.

grumpy *adj* crabbed, cross, glum, moody, morose, sour, sullen, surly.

guarantee *vb* assure, insure, pledge, secure, warrant. • *n* assurance, pledge, security, surety, warrant, warranty.

guard *vb* defend, keep, patrol, protect, safeguard, save, secure, shelter, shield, watch. • *n* aegis, bulwark, custody, defence, palladium, protection, rampart, safeguard, security, shield; keeper, guardian, patrol, sentinel, sentry, warden, watch, watchman; conduct, convoy, escort; attention, care, caution, circumspection, heed, watchfulness.

guarded *adj* careful, cautious, circumspect, reserved, reticent, wary, watchful.

guardian *n* custodian, defender, guard, keeper, preserver, protector, trustee, warden.

guerdon *n* recompense, remuneration, requital, reward.

guess *vb* conjecture, divine, mistrust, surmise, suspect; fathom, find out, penetrate, solve; believe, fancy, hazard, imagine, reckon, suppose, think. • *n* conjecture, divination, notion, supposition, surmise.

guest *n* caller, company, visitant.

guidance *n* conduct, control, direction, escort, government, lead, leadership, pilotage, steering.

guide *vb* conduct, escort, lead, pilot; control, direct, govern, manage, preside, regulate, rule, steer, superintend, supervise. • *n* cicerone, conductor, director, monitor, pilot; adviser, counsellor, instructor, mentor; clew, directory, index, key, thread; guidebook, itinerary, landmark.

guild *n* association, brotherhood, company, corporation, fellowship, fraternity, society, union.

guile *n* art, artfulness, artifice, craft, cunning, deceit, deception, duplicity, fraud, knavery, ruse, subtlety, treachery, trickery, wiles, wiliness.

guileless *adj* artless, candid, frank, honest, ingenuous, innocent, open, pure, simple-minded, sincere, straightforward, truthful, undesigning, unsophisticated.

guilt *n* blame, criminality, culpability, guiltless; ill-desert, iniquity, offensiveness, wickedness, wrong; crime, offence, sin.

guiltless *adj* blameless, immaculate, innocent, pure, sinless, spotless, unpolluted, unspotted, unsullied, untarnished.

guilty *adj* criminal, culpable, evil, sinful, wicked, wrong.

guise *n* appearance, aspect, costume, dress, fashion, figure, form, garb, manner, mode, shape; air, behaviour, demeanour, mien; cover, custom, disguise, habit, pretence, pretext, practice.

gulf *n* abyss, chasm, opening; bay, inlet; whirlpool.

gull *vb* beguile, cheat, circumvent, cozen, deceive, dupe, hoax, overreach, swindle, trick. • *n* cheat, deception, hoax, imposition, fraud, trick; cat's paw, dupe.

gullibility *n* credulity, naiveness, naivety, overtrustfulness, simplicity, unsophistication.

gullible *adj* confiding, credulous, naive, over-trustful, simple, unsophisticated, unsuspicious.

gumption *n* ability, astuteness, cleverness, capacity, common sense, discernment, penetration, power, sagacity, shrewdness, skill; courage, guts, spirit.

gun *n* blunderbuss, cannon, carbine, firearm, musket, pistol, revolver, rifle, shotgun.

gurgle *vb* babble, bubble, murmur, purl, ripple. • *n* babbling, murmur, ripple.

gush *vb* burst, flood, flow, pour, rush, spout, stream; emotionalize, sentimentalize. • *n* flow, jet, onrush, rush, spurt, surge; effusion, effusiveness, loquacity, loquaciousness, talkativeness.

gushing *adj* flowing, issuing, rushing; demonstrative, effusive, sentimental.

gust *vb* blast, blow, puff. • *n* blast, blow, squall; burst, fit, outburst, paroxysm.

gusto *n* enjoyment, gust, liking, pleasure, relish, zest.

gusty *adj* blustering, blustery, puffy, squally, stormy, tempestuous, unsteady, windy.

gut *vb* destroy, disembowel, embowel, eviscerate, paunch. • *n* bowels, entrails, intestines, inwards, viscera.

gutter *n* channel, conduit, kennel, pipe, tube.

guttural *adj* deep, gruff, hoarse, thick, throaty.

guy *vb* caricature, mimic, ridicule. • *n* boy, man, person; dowdy, eccentric, fright, scarecrow.

guzzle *vb* carouse, drink, gorge, gormandize, quaff, swill, tipple, tope.

gyrate *vb* revolve, rotate, spin, whirl.

H

habiliment *n* apparel, attire, clothes, costume, dress, garb, garment, habit, raiment, robes, uniform, vesture, vestment.

habit *vb* accoutre, array, attire, clothe, dress, equip, robe. • *n* condition, constitution, temperament; addiction, custom, habitude, manner, practice, rule, usage, way, wont; apparel, costume, dress, garb, habiliment.

habitation *n* abode, domicile, dwelling, headquarters, home, house, lodging, quarters, residence.

habitual *adj* accustomed, common, confirmed, customary, everyday, familiar, inveterate, ordinary, regular, routine, settled, usual, wonted.

habituate *vb* accustom, familiarize, harden, inure, train, use.

habitude *n* custom, practice, usage, wont.

hack[1] *vb* chop, cut, hew, mangle, mutilate, notch; cough, rasp. • *n* cut, cleft, incision, notch; cough, rasp.

hack[2] *vb* ride. • *adj* hired, mercenary; banal, hackneyed, pedestrian, uninspired, unoriginal. • *n* horse, nag, pony; hireling, mercenary; journalist, scribbler, writer.

hackneyed *adj* banal, common, commonplace, overworked, pedestrian, stale, threadbare, trite.

hag *n* beldame, crone, fury, harridan, jezebel, she-monster, shrew, termagant, virago, vixen, witch.

haggard *adj* intractable, refractory, unruly, untamed, wild, wayward; careworn, emaciated, gaunt, ghastly, lank, lean, meagre, raw, spare, thin, wasted, worn.

haggle *vb* argue, bargain, cavil, chaffer, dispute, higgle, stickle; annoy, badger, bait, fret, harass, tease, worry.

hail[1] *vb* acclaim, greet, salute, welcome; accost, address, call, hallo, signal. • *n* greeting, salute.

hail[2] *vb* assail, bombard, rain, shower, storm, volley. • *n* bombardment, rain, shower, storm, volley.

halcyon *adj* calm, golden, happy, palmy, placid, peaceful, quiet, serene, still, tranquil, unruffled, undisturbed.

hale *adj* hardy, healthy, hearty, robust, sound, strong, vigorous, well.

halfwit *n* blockhead, dunce, moron, simpleton.

halfwitted *adj* doltish, dull, dull-witted, feeble-minded, foolish, sappy, shallow, silly, simple, soft, stolid, stupid, thick.

hall *n* chamber, corridor, entrance, entry, hallway, lobby, passage, vestibule; manor, manor-house; auditorium, lecture-room.

halloo *vb* call, cry, shout. • *n* call, cry, hallo, holla, hollo, shout.

hallow *vb* consecrate, dedicate, devote, revere, sanctify, solemnize; enshrine, honour, respect, reverence, venerate.

hallowed *adj* blessed, holy, honoured, revered, sacred.

hallucination *n* blunder, error, fallacy, mistake; aberration, delusion, illusion, phantasm, phantasy, self-deception, vision.

halo *n* aura, aureole, glory, nimbus.

halt[1] *vb* cease, desist, hold, rest, stand, stop. • *n* end, impasse, pause, standstill, stop.

halt[2] *vb* hesitate, pause, stammer, waver; falter, hobble, limp. • *adj* crippled, disabled, lame. • *n* hobble, limp.

hammer *vb* beat, forge, form, shape; excogitate, contrive, invent.

hammer and tongs *adv* earnestly, energetically, resolutely, strenuously, vigorously, zealously.

hamper *vb* bind, clog, confine, curb, embarrass, encumber, entangle, fetter, hinder, impede, obstruct, prevent, restrain, restrict, shackle, trammel. • *n* basket, box, crate, picnic basket; embarrassment, encumbrance, fetter, handicap, impediment, obstruction, restraint, trammel.

hand *vb* deliver, give, present, transmit; conduct, guide, lead. • *n* direction, part, side; ability, dexterity, faculty, skill, talent; course, inning, management, turn; agency, intervention, participation, share; control, possession, power; artificer, artisan, craftsman, employee, labourer, operative, workman; index, indicator, pointer; chirography, handwriting.

handbook *n* guidebook, manual.

handcuff *vb* bind, fetter, manacle, shackle. • *n* fetter, manacle, shackle.

handful *n* fistful, maniple, smattering.

handicap *vb* encumber, hamper, hinder, restrict. • *n* disadvantage, encumbrance, hampering, hindrance, restriction.

handicraft *n* hand manufacture, handwork, workmanship.

handle *vb* feel, finger, manhandle, paw, touch; direct, manage, manipulate, use, wield; discourse, discuss, treat. • *n* haft, helve, hilt, stock.

handsome *adj* admirable, comely, fine-looking, stately, well-formed, well-proportioned; appropriate, suitable, becoming, easy, graceful; generous, gracious, liberal, magnanimous, noble; ample, large, plentiful, sufficient.

handy *adj* adroit, clever, dextrous, expert, ready, skilful, skilled; close, convenient, near.

hang *vb* attach, swing; execute, truss; decline, drop, droop, incline; adorn, drape; dangle, depend, impend, suspend; rely; cling, loiter, rest, stick; float, hover, pay.

hangdog *adj* ashamed, base, blackguard, low, villainous, scurvy, sneaking.

hanger-on *n* dependant, minion, parasite, vassal.

hanker *vb* covet, crave, desire, hunger, long, lust, want, yearn.

hap *n* accident, chance, fate, fortune, lot.

haphazard *adj* aimless, chance, random.

hapless *adj* ill-fated, ill-starred, luckless, miserable, unfortunate, unhappy, unlucky, wretched.

happen *vb* befall, betide, chance, come, occur.

happily *adv* fortunately, luckily; agreeably, delightfully, prosperously, successfully.

happiness *n* brightness, cheerfulness, delight, gaiety, joy, light-heartedness, merriment, pleasure; beatitude, blessedness, bliss, felicity, enjoyment, welfare, well-being.

happy *adj* blessed, blest, blissful, cheerful, contented, joyful, joyous, light-hearted, merry; charmed, delighted, glad, gladdened, gratified, pleased; fortunate, lucky, prosperous, successful; able, adroit, apt, dextrous, expert, ready, skilful; befitting, felicitous, opportune, pertinent, seasonable, well-timed; auspicious, bright, favourable, propitious.

harangue *vb* address, declaim, spout. • *n* address, bombast, declamation, oration, rant, screed, speech, tirade.

harass *vb* exhaust, fag, fatigue, jade, tire, weary; annoy, badger, distress, gall, heckle, disturb, harry, molest, pester, plague, tantalize, tease, torment, trouble, vex, worry.

harbour *vb* protect, lodge, shelter; cherish, entertain, foster, indulge. • *n* asylum, cover, refuge, resting place, retreat, sanctuary, shelter; anchorage, destination, haven, port.

hard *adj* adamantine, compact, firm, flinty, impenetrable, marble, rigid, solid, resistant, stony, stubborn, unyielding; difficult, intricate, knotty, perplexing, puzzling; arduous, exacting, fatiguing, laborious, toilsome, wearying; austere, callous, cruel, exacting, hard-hearted, incorrigible, inflexible, insensible, insensitive, obdurate, oppressive, reprobate, rigorous, severe, unfeeling, unkind, unsusceptible, unsympathetic, unyielding, untender; calamitous, disagreeable, distressing, grievous, painful, unpleasant; acid, alcoholic, harsh, rough, sour; excessive, intemperate. • *adv* close, near; diligently, earnestly, energetically, incessantly, laboriously; distressfully, painfully, rigorously, severely; forcibly, vehemently, violently.

harden *vb* accustom, discipline, form, habituate, inure, season, train; brace, fortify, indurate, nerve, steel, stiffen, strengthen.

hardened *adj* annealed, case-hardened, tempered, indurated; abandoned, accustomed, benumbed, callous, confirmed, deadened, depraved, habituated, impenitent, incorrigible, inured, insensible, irreclaimable, lost, obdurate, reprobate, seared, seasoned, steeled, trained, unfeeling.

hard-headed *adj* astute, collected, cool, intelligent, sagacious, shrewd, well-balanced, wise.

hardhearted *adj* cruel, fell, implacable, inexorable, merciless, pitiless, relentless, ruthless, unfeeling, uncompassionate, unmerciful, unpitying, unrelenting.

hardihood *n* audacity, boldness, bravery, courage, decision, firmness, fortitude, intrepidity, manhood, mettle, pluck, resolution, stoutness; assurance, audacity, brass, effrontery, impudence.

hardly *adv* barely, scarcely; cruelly, harshly, rigorously, roughly, severely, unkindly.

hardship *n* fatigue, toil, weariness; affliction, burden, calamity, grievance, hardness, injury, misfortune, privation, suffering, trial, trouble.

hardy *adj* enduring, firm, hale, healthy, hearty, inured, lusty, rigorous, robust, rugged, sound, stout, strong, sturdy, tough; bold, brave, courageous, daring, heroic, intrepid, manly, resolute, stout-hearted, valiant.

harebrained *adj* careless, changeable, flighty, gidcy, harumscarum, headlong, heedless, rash, reckless, unsteady, volatile, wild.

hark *interj* attend, hear, hearken, listen.

harlequin *n* antic, buffoon, clown, droll, fool, jester, punch, fool.

harm *vb* damage, hurt, injure, scathe; abuse, desecrate, ill-use, ill-treat, maltreat, molest. • *n* damage, detriment, disadvantage, hurt, injury, mischief, misfortune, prejudice, wrong.

harmful *adj* baneful, detrimental, disadvantageous, hurtful, injurious, mischievous, noxious, pernicious, prejudicial.

harmless *adj* innocent, innocuous, innoxious, inoffensive, safe, unoffending.

harmonious *adj* concordant, consonous, harmonic; dulcet, euphonious, mellifluous, melodious, musical, smooth, tuneful; comfortable, congruent, consistent, correspondent, orderly, symmetrical; agreeable, amicable, brotherly, cordial, fraternal, friendly, neighbourly.

harmonize *vb* adapt, attune, reconcile, unite; accord, agree, blend, chime, comport, conform, correspond, square, sympathize, tally, tune.

harmony *n* euphony, melodiousness, melody; accord, accordance, agreement, chime, concord, concordance, consonance, order, unison; adaptation, congruence, congruity, consistency, correspondence, fairness, smoothness, suitableness; amity, friendship, peace.

harness *vb* hitch, tackle. • *n* equipment, gear, tackle, tackling; accoutrements, armour, array, mail, mounting.

harp *vb* dwell, iterate, reiterate, renew, repeat.

harping *n* dwelling, iteration, reiteration, repetition.

harrow *vb* harass, lacerate, rend, tear, torment torture, wound.

harry *vb* devastate, pillage, plunder, raid, ravage, rob; annoy, chafe, disturb, fret, gall, harass, harrow, incommode, pester, plague, molest, tease, torment, trouble, vex, worry.

harsh *adj* acid, acrid, astringent, biting, caustic, corrosive, crabbed, rough, sharp, sour, tart; cacophonous, discordant, grating, jarring, metallic, raucous, strident, unmelodious; abusive, austere, crabbed, crabby, cruel, disagreeable, hard, ill-natured, ill-tempered, morose, rigorous, severe, stern, unfeeling; bearish, bluff, blunt, brutal, gruff, rude, uncivil, ungracious.

harshness *n* roughness; acerbity, asperity, austerity churlishness, crabbedness, hardness, ill-nature, ill-temper, moroseness, rigour, severity, sternness, unkindness; bluffness, bluntness, churlishness, gruffness, incivility, ungraciousness, rudeness.

harum-scarum *adj* hare-brained, precipitate, rash, reckless, volatile, wild.

harvest *vb* gather, glean, reap. • *n* crops, produce, yield; consequence, effect, issue, outcome, produce, result.

haste *n* alacrity, celerity, dispatch, expedition, nimbleness, promptitude, quickness, rapidity, speed, urgency, velocity; flurry, hurry, hustle, impetuosity, precipitateness, precipitation, press, rashness, rush, vehemence.

hasten *vb* haste, hurry; accelerate, dispatch, expedite, precipitate, press, push, quicken, speed, urge.

hasty *adj* brisk, fast, fleet, quick, rapid, speedy, swift; cursory, hurried, passing, slight, superficial; ill-advised, rash, reckless; headlong, helter-skelter, pell-mell, precipitate; abrupt, choleric, excitable, fiery, fretful, hot-headed, irascible, irritable, passionate, peevish, peppery, pettish, petulant, testy, touchy, waspish.

hatch *vb* brew, concoct, contrive, excogitate, design, devise, plan, plot, project, scheme; breed, incubate.

hate *vb* abhor, abominate, detest, dislike, execrate, loathe, nauseate. • *n* abomination, animosity, antipathy, detestation, dislike, enmity, execration, hatred, hostility, loathing.

hateful *adj* malevolent, malicious, malign, malignant, rancorous, spiteful; abhorrent, abominable, accursed, damnable, detestable, execrable, horrid, odious, shocking; disgusting, foul, loathsome, nauseous, obnoxious, offensive, repellent, repugnant, repulsive, revolting, vile.

hatred *n* animosity, enmity, hate, hostility, ill-will, malevolence, malice, malignity, odium, rancour; abhorrence, abomination, antipathy, aversion, detestation, disgust, execration, horror, loathing, repugnance, revulsion.

haughtiness *n* arrogance, contempt, contemptuousness, disdain, hauteur, insolence, loftiness, pride, self-importance, snobbishness, stateliness, superciliousness.

haughty *adj* arrogant, assuming, contemptuous, disdainful, imperious, insolent, lofty, lordly, overbearing, overweening, proud, scornful, snobbish, supercilious.

haul *vb* drag, draw, lug, pull, tow, trail, tug. • *n* heaving, pull, tug; booty, harvest, takings, yield.

haunt *vb* frequent, resort; follow, importune; hover, inhabit, obsess. • *n* den, resort, retreat.

hauteur *n* arrogance, contempt, contemptuousness, disdain, haughtiness, insolence, loftiness, pride, self-importance, stateliness, superciliousness.

have *vb* cherish, exercise, experience, keep, hold, occupy, own, possess; acquire, gain get, obtain, receive; accept, take.

haven *n* asylum, refuge, retreat, shelter; anchorage, harbour, port.

havoc *n* carnage, damage, desolation, destruction, devastation, ravage, ruin, slaughter, waste, wreck.

hawk-eyed *adj* eagle-eyed, sharp-sighted.

hazard *vb* adventure, risk, venture; endanger, imperil, jeopardize. • *n* accident, casualty, chance, contingency, event, fortuity, stake; danger, jeopardy, peril, risk, venture.

hazardous *adj* dangerous, insecure, perilous, precarious, risky, uncertain, unsafe.

haze *n* fog, har, mist, smog; cloud, dimness, fume, miasma, obscurity, pall.

hazy *adj* foggy, misty, cloudy, dim, nebulous, obscure; confused, indefinite, indistinct, uncertain, vague.

head *vb* command, control, direct, govern, guide, lead, rule; aim, point, tend; beat, excel, outdo, precede, surpass. • *adj* chief, first, grand, highest, leading, main, principal; adverse, contrary. • *n* acme, summit, top; beginning, commencement, origin, rise, source; chief, chieftain, commander, director, leader, master, principal, superintendent, superior; intellect, mind, thought, understanding; branch, category, class, department, division, section, subject, topic; brain, crown, headpiece, intellect, mind, thought, understanding; cape, headland, point, promontory.

headiness *n* hurry, precipitation, rashness; obstinacy, stubbornness.

headless *adj* acephalous, beheaded; leaderless, undirected; headstrong, heady, imprudent, obstinate, rash, senseless, stubborn.

headlong *adj* dangerous, hasty, heady, impulsive, inconsiderate, perilous, precipitate, rash, reckless, ruinous, thoughtless; perpendicular, precipitous, sheer, steep. • *adv* hastily, headfirst, helter-skelter, hurriedly, precipitately, rashly, thoughtlessly.

headstone *n* cornerstone, gravestone.

headstrong *adj* cantankerous, cross-grained, dogged, forward, headless, heady, intractable, obstinate, self-willed, stubborn, ungovernable, unruly, violent, wayward.

heady *adj* hasty, headlong, impetuous, impulsive, inconsiderate, precipitate, rash, reckless, rushing, stubborn, thoughtless; exciting, inebriating, inflaming, intoxicating, spirituous, strong.

heal *vb* amend, cure, remedy, repair, restore; compose, harmonize, reconcile, settle, soothe.

healing *adj* curative, palliative, remedial, restoring, restorative; assuaging, assuasive, comforting, composing, gentle, lenitive, mild, soothing.

health *n* healthfulness, robustness, salubrity, sanity, soundness, strength, tone, vigour.

healthy *adj* active, hale, hearty, lusty, sound, vigorous, well; bracing, healthful, health-giving, hygienic, invigorating, nourishing, salubrious, salutary, wholesome.

heap *vb* accumulate, augment, amass, collect, overfill, pile up, store. • *n* accumulation, collection, cumulus, huddle, lot, mass, mound, pile, stack.

hear *vb* eavesdrop, hearken, heed, listen, overhear; ascertain, discover, gather, learn, understand; examine, judge.

heart *n* bosom, breast; centre, core, essence, interior, kernel, marrow, meaning, pith; affection, benevolence, character, disposition, feeling, inclination, love, mind, passion, purpose, will; affections, ardour, emotion, feeling, love; boldness, courage, fortitude, resolution, spirit.

heartache *n* affliction, anguish, bitterness, distress, dole, grief, heartbreak, sorrow, woe.

heartbroken *adj* broken-hearted, cheerless, comfortless, desolate, disconsolate, forlorn, inconsolable, miserable, woebegone, wretched.

hearten *vb* animate, assure, cheer, comfort, console, embolden, encourage, enhearten, incite, inspire, inspirit, reassure, stimulate.

heartfelt *adj* cordial, deep, deep-felt, hearty, profound, sincere, warm.

hearth *n* fireplace, fireside, forge, hearthstone.

heartily *adv* abundantly, completely, cordially, earnestly, freely, largely, sincerely, vigorously.

heartless *adj* brutal, cold, cruel, hard, harsh, merciless, pitiless, unfeeling, unsympathetic; spiritless, timid, timorous, uncourageous.

heart-rending *adj* affecting, afflicting, anguishing, crushing, distressing.

hearty *adj* cordial, deep, earnest, fervent, heartfelt, profound, sincere, true, unfeigned, warm; active, animated, energetic, fit, vigorous, zealous; convivial, hale, healthy, robust, sound, strong, warm; abundant, full, heavy; nourishing, nutritious, rich.

heat *vb* excite, flush, inflame; animate, rouse, stimulate, stir. • *n* calorie, caloricity, torridity, warmth; excitement, fever, flush, impetuosity, passion, vehemence, violence; ardour, earnestness, fervency, fervour, glow, intensity, zeal; exasperation, fierceness, frenzy, rage.

heath *n* field, moor, wasteland, plain.

heathen *adj* animist, animistic; pagan, paganical, paganish, paganistic, unconverted; agnostic, atheist, atheistic, gentile, idolatrous, infidel, irreligious; barbarous, cruel, inhuman, savage. • *n* atheist, gentile, idolater, idolatress, infidel, pagan, unbeliever; barbarian, philistine, savage.

heave *vb* elevate, hoist, lift, raise; breathe, exhale; cast, fling, hurl, send, throw, toss; dilate, expand, pant, rise, swell; retch, throw up; strive, struggle.

heaven *n* empyrean, firmament, sky, welkin; bliss, ecstasy, elysium, felicity, happiness, paradise, rapture, transport.

heavenly *adj* celestial, empyreal, ethereal; angelic, beatific, beatified, cherubic, divine, elysian, glorious, god-like, sainted, saintly, seraphic; blissful, delightful, divine, ecstatic, enrapturing, enravishing, exquisite, golden, rapturous, ravishing, exquisite, transporting.

heaviness *n* gravity, heft, ponderousness, weight; grievousness, oppressiveness, severity; dullness, languor, lassitude, sluggishness, stupidity; dejection, depression, despondency, gloom, melancholy, sadness, seriousness.

heavy *adj* grave, hard, onerous, ponderous, weighty; afflictive, burdensome, crushing, cumbersome, grievous, oppressive, severe, serious; dilatory, dull, inactive, inanimate, indolent, inert, lifeless, listless, sleepy, slow, sluggish, stupid, torpid; chapfallen, crestfallen, crushed, depressed, dejected, despondent, disconsolate, downhearted, gloomy, low-spirited, melancholy, sad, sobered, sorrowful; difficult, laborious, tedious, tiresome, wearisome, weary; burdened, encumbered, loaded; clammy, clayey, cloggy, ill-raised, miry, muddy, soggy; boisterous, deep, energetic, loud, roaring, severe, stormy, strong, tempestuous, violent; cloudy, dark, dense, gloomy, lowering, overcast.

hebetate *adj* blunt; dull, obtuse, sluggish, stupid, stupefied.

hectic *adj* animated, excited, fevered, feverish, flushed, heated, hot.

hector *vb* bluster, boast, bully, menace, threaten; annoy, fret, harass, harry, irritate, provoke, tease, vex, worry. • *n* blusterer, bully, swaggerer.

hedge *vb* block, encumber, hinder, obstruct, surround; enclose, fence, fortify, guard, protect; disappear, dodge, evade, hide, skulk, temporize. • *n* barrier, hedgerow, fence, limit.

heed *vb* attend, consider, mark, mind, note, notice, observe, regard. • *n* attention, care, carefulness, caution, circumspection,

consideration, heedfulness, mindfulness, notice, observation, regard, wariness, vigilance, watchfulness.

heedful *adj* attentive, careful, cautious, circumspect, mindful, observant, observing, provident, regardful, watchful, wary.

heedless *adj* careless, inattentive, neglectful, negligent, precipitate, rash, reckless, thoughtless, unmindful, unminding, unobserving, unobservant.

heft *n* handle, haft, helve; bulk, weight.

hegemony *n* ascendancy, authority, headship, leadership, predominance, preponderance, rule.

height *n* altitude, elevation, tallness; acme, apex, climax, eminence, head, meridian, pinnacle, summit, top, vertex, zenith; eminence, hill, mountain; dignity, exaltation, grandeur, loftiness, perfection.

heighten *vb* elevate, raise; ennoble, exalt, magnify, make greater; augment, enhance, improve, increase, strengthen; aggravate, intensify.

heinous *adj* aggravated, atrocious, crying, enormous, excessive, flagitious, flagrant, hateful, infamous, monstrous, nefarious, odious, villainous.

heir *n* child, inheritor, offspring, product.

helical *adj* screw-shaped, spiral, winding.

hellish *adj* abominable, accursed, atrocious, curst, damnable, damned, demoniacal, detestable, devilish, diabolical, execrable, fiendish, infernal, monstrous, nefarious, satanic.

helm *n* rudder, steering-gear, tiller, wheel; command, control, direction, rein, rule.

help *vb* relieve, save, succour; abet, aid, assist, back, cooperate, second, serve, support, sustain, wait; alleviate, ameliorate, better, cure, heal, improve, remedy, restore; control, hinder, prevent, repress, resist, withstand; avoid, forbear, control. • *n* aid, assistance, succour, support; relief, remedy; assistant, helper, servant.

helper *adj* aider, abettor, ally, assistant, auxiliary, coadjutor, colleague, helpmate, partner, supporter.

helpful *adj* advantageous, assistant, auxiliary, beneficial, contributory, convenient, favourable, kind, profitable, serviceable, useful.

helpless *adj* disabled, feeble, imbecile, impotent, infirm, powerless, prostrate, resourceless, weak; abandoned, defenceless, exposed, unprotected; desperate, irremediable, remediless.

helpmate *n* companion, consort, husband, partner, wife; aider, assistant, associate, helper.

helter-skelter *adj* disorderly, headlong, irregular, pell-mell, precipitate. • *adv* confusedly, hastily, headlong, higgledy-piggledy, pell-mell, precipitately, wildly.

hem *vb* border, edge, skirt; beset, confine, enclose, environ, surround, sew; hesitate. • *n* border, edge, trim.

henchman *n* attendant, follower, retainer, servant, supporter.

herald *vb* announce, proclaim, publish. • *n* announcer, crier, publisher; harbinger, precursor, proclaimer.

heraldry *n* blazonry, emblazonry.

herbage *n* greenery, herb, pasture, plants, vegetation.

herculean *adj* able-bodied, athletic, brawny, mighty, muscular, powerful, puissant, sinewy, stalwart, strong, sturdy, vigorous; dangerous, difficult, hard, laborious, perilous, toilsome, troublesome; colossal, Cyclopean, gigantic, great, large, strapping.

herd *vb* drive, gather, lead, tend; assemble, associate, flock. • *n* drover, herder, herdsman, shepherd; crowd, multitude, populace, rabble; assemblage, assembly, collection, drove, flock, pack.

hereditary *adj* ancestral, inheritable, inherited, patrimonial, transmitted.

heresy *n* dissent, error, heterodoxy, impiety, recusancy, unorthodoxy.

heretic *n* dissenter, dissident, nonconformist, recusant, schismatic, sectarian, sectary, separatist, unbeliever.

heretical *adj* heterodox, impious, schismatic, schismatical, sectarian, unorthodox.

heritage *n* estate, inheritance, legacy, patrimony, portion.

hermetic *adj* airtight, impervious; cabbalistic, emblematic, emblematical, magical, mysterious, mystic, mystical, occult, secret, symbolic, symbolical.

hermit *n* anchoress, anchoret, anchorite, ascetic, eremite, monk, recluse, solitaire, solitary.

heroic *adj* bold, brave, courageous, daring, dauntless, fearless, gallant, illustrious, intrepid, magnanimous, noble, valiant; desperate, extravagant, extreme, violent.

heroism *n* boldness, bravery, courage, daring, endurance, fearlessness, fortitude, gallantry, intrepidity, prowess, valour.

hesitate *vb* boggle, delay, demur, doubt, pause, scruple, shilly-shally, stickle, vacillate, waver; falter, stammer, stutter.

hesitation *n* halting, misgiving, reluctance; delay, doubt, indecision, suspense, uncertainty, vacillation; faltering, stammering, stuttering.

heterodox *adj* heretical, recusant, schismatic, unorthodox, unsound; apocryphal, uncanonical.

heterogeneous *adj* contrasted, contrary, different, dissimilar, diverse, incongruous, indiscriminate, miscellaneous, mixed, opposed, unhomogeneous, unlike.

hew *vb* chop, cut, fell, hack; fashion, form, shape, smooth.

hiatus *n* blank, break, chasm, gap, interval, lacuna, opening, rift.

hidden *adj* blind, clandestine, cloaked, close, concealed, covered, covert, enshrouded, latent, masked, occult, private, secluded, secret, suppressed, undiscovered, veiled; abstruse, cabbalistic, cryptic, dark, esoteric, hermetic, inward, mysterious, mystic, mystical, obscure, oracular, recondite.

hide *vb* bury, conceal, cover, secrete, suppress, withhold; cloak, disguise, eclipse, hoard, mask, screen, shelter, veil.

hideous *adj* abominable, appalling, awful, dreadful, frightful, ghastly, ghoulish, grim, grisly, horrible, horrid, repulsive, revolting, shocking, terrible, terrifying.

hie *vb* hasten, speed.

hieratic *adj* consecrated, devoted, priestly, sacred, sacerdotal.

hieroglyph *n* picture-writing, rebus, sign, symbol.

hieroglyphic *adj* emblematic, emblematical, figurative, obscure, symbolic, symbolical.

higgle *vb* hawk, peddle; bargain, chaffer, haggle, negotiate.

higgledy-piggledy *adj* chaotic, confused, disorderly, jumbled. • *adv* confusedly, in disorder, helter-skelter, pell-mell.

high *adj* elevated, high-reaching, lofty, soaring, tall, towering; distinguished, eminent, pre-eminent, prominent, superior; admirable, dignified, exalted, great, noble; arrogant, haughty, lordly, proud, supercilious; boisterous, strong, tumultuous, turbulent, violent; costly, dear, pricey; acute, high-pitched, high-toned, piercing, sharp, shrill; tainted, malodorous. • *adv* powerfully, profoundly; eminently, loftily; luxuriously, richly.

high-flown *adj* elevated, presumptuous, proud, lofty, swollen; extravagant, high-coloured, lofty, overdrawn, overstrained; bombastic, inflated, pompous, pretentious, strained, swollen, turgid.

high-handed *adj* arbitrary, despotic, dictatorial, domineering, oppressive, overbearing, self-willed, violent, wilful.

highly strung *adj* ardent, excitable, irascible, nervous, quick, tense; high-spirited, sensitive.

high-minded *adj* arrogant, haughty, lofty, proud; elevated, high-toned; generous honourable, magnanimous, noble, spiritual.

highwayman *n* bandit, brigand, footpad, freebooter, marauder, outlaw, robber.

hilarious *adj* boisterous, cheerful, comical, convivial, riotous, uproarious, jovial, joyful, merry, mirthful, noisy.

hilarity *n* cheerfulness, conviviality, exhilarated gaiety glee, jollity, joviality, joyousness, merriment, mirth.

hill *n* ascent, ben, elevation, eminence, hillock, knoll, mount, mountain, rise, tor.

hind *adj* back, hinder, hindmost, posterior, rear, rearward.

hinder *vb* bar, check, clog, delay, embarrass, encumber, impede, interrupt, obstruct, oppose, prevent, restrain, retard, stop, thwart.

hindrance *n* check, deterrent, encumbrance, hitch, impediment, interruption, obstacle, obstruction, restraint, stop, stoppage.

hinge *vb* depend, hang, rest, turn.

hint *vb* allude, glance, imply, insinuate, intimate, mention, refer, suggest. • *n* allusion, clue, implication, indication, innuendo, insinuation, intimation, mention, reminder, suggestion, taste, trace.

hire *vb* buy, rent, secure; charter, employ, engage, lease, let. • *n* allowance, bribe, compensation, pay, remuneration, rent, reward, salary, stipend, wages.

hireling *n* employee, mercenary, myrmidon.

hirsute *adj* bristled, bristly, hairy, shaggy; boorish, course, ill-bred, loutish, rough, rude, rustic, uncouth, unmannerly.

hiss *vb* shrill, sibilate, whistle, whir, whiz; condemn, damn, ridicule. • *n* fizzle, hissing, sibilant, sibilation, sizzle.

historian *n* annalist, autobiographer, biographer, chronicler, narrator, recorder.

history *n* account, autobiography, annals, biography, chronicle, genealogy, memoirs, narration, narrative, recital, record, relation, story.

hit *vb* discomfit, hurt, knock, strike; accomplish, achieve, attain, gain, reach, secure, succeed, win; accord, fit, suit; beat, clash, collide, contact, smite. • *n* blow, collision, strike, stroke; chance, fortune, hazard, success, venture.

hitch *vb* catch, impede, stick, stop; attach, connect, fasten, harness, join, tether, tie, unite, yoke. • *n* catch, check, hindrance, impediment, interruption, obstacle; knot, noose.

hoar *adj* ancient, grey, hoary, old, white.

hoard *vb* accumulate, amass, collect, deposit, garner, hive, husband, save, store, treasure. • *n* accumulation, collection, deposit, fund, mass, reserve, savings, stockpile, store.

hoarse *adj* discordant, grating, gruff, guttural, harsh, husky, low, raucous, rough.

hoary *adj* grey, hoar, silvery, white; ancient, old, venerable.

hoax *vb* deceive, dupe, fool, gammon, gull, hoodwink, swindle, trick. • *n* canard, cheat, deception, fraud, humbug, imposition, imposture, joke, trick, swindle.

hobble *vb* falter, halt, hop, limp; fasten, fetter, hopple, shackle, tie. • *n* halt, limp; clog, fetter, shackle; embarrassment, difficulty, perplexity, pickle, strait.

hobgoblin *n* apparition, bogey, bugbear, goblin, imp, spectre, spirit, sprite.

hobnail *n* bumpkin, churl, clodhopper, clown, lout, rustic.

hocus-pocus *n* cheater, impostor, juggler, sharper, swindler, trickster; artifice, cheat, deceit, deception, delusion, hoax, imposition, juggle, trick.

hodgepodge *n* farrago, hash, hotchpotch, jumble, medley, miscellany, mixture, ragout, stew.

hog *n* beast, glutton, pig; grunter, porker, swine.

hoggish *adj* brutish, filthy, gluttonish, piggish, swinish; grasping, greedy, mean, selfish, sordid.

hoist *vb* elevate, heave, lift, raise, rear. • *n* elevator, lift.

hold *vb* clasp, clinch, clutch, grasp, grip, seize; have, keep, occupy, possess, retain; bind, confine, control, detain, imprison, restrain, restrict; connect, fasten, fix, lock; arrest, check, stay, stop, suspend, withhold; continue, keep up, maintain, manage, prosecute, support, sustain; cherish, embrace, entertain; account, believe, consider, count, deem, entertain, esteem, judge, reckon, regard, think; accommodate, admit, carry, contain, receive, stow; assemble, conduct, convene; endure, last, persist, remain; adhere, cleave, cling, cohere, stick. • *n* anchor, bite, clasp, control, embrace, foothold, grasp, grip, possession, retention, seizure; prop, stay, support; claim, footing, vantage point; castle, fort, fortification, fortress, stronghold, tower; locker, storage, storehouse.

hole *n* aperture, opening, perforation; abyss, bore, cave, cavern, cavity, chasm, depression, excavation, eye, hollow, pit, pore, void; burrow, cover, lair, retreat; den, hovel, kennel.

holiday *n* anniversary, celebration, feast, festival, festivity, fete, gala, recess, vacation.

holiness *n* blessedness, consecration, devotion, devoutness, godliness, piety, purity, religiousness, righteousness, sacredness, saintliness, sanctity, sinlessness.

hollow *vb* dig, excavate, groove, scoop. • *adj* cavernous, concave, depressed, empty, sunken, vacant, void; deceitful, faithless, false, false-hearted, hollow-hearted, hypocritical, insincere, pharisaical, treacherous, unfeeling; deep, low, muffled, reverberating, rumbling, sepulchral. • *n* basin, bowl, depression; cave, cavern, cavity, concavity, dent, dimple, dint, depression, excavation, hole, pit; canal, channel, cup, dimple, dig, groove, pocket, sag.

holocaust *n* carnage, destruction, devastation, genocide, massacre.

holy *adj* blessed, consecrated, dedicated, devoted, hallowed, sacred, sanctified; devout, godly, pious, pure, religious, righteous, saintlike, saintly, sinless, spiritual.

homage *n* allegiance, devotion, fealty, fidelity, loyalty; court, deference, duty, honour, obeisance, respect, reverence, service; adoration, devotion, worship.

home *adj* domestic, family; close, direct, effective, penetrating, pointed. • *n* abode, dwelling, seat, quarters, residence.

homely *adj* domestic, familiar, house-like; coarse, commonplace, homespun, inelegant, plain, simple, unattractive, uncomely, unpolished, unpretentious.

homespun *adj* coarse, homely, inelegant, plain, rude, rustic, unpolished.

homicide *n* manslaughter, murder.

homily *n* address, discourse, lecture, sermon.

homogeneous *adj* akin, alike, cognate, kindred, similar, uniform.

honest *adj* equitable, fair, faithful, honourable, open, straight, straightforward; conscientious, equitable, reliable, sound, square, true, trustworthy, trusty, uncorrupted, upright, virtuous; above-board, faithful, genuine, thorough, unadulterated; creditable, decent, proper, reputable, respectable, suitable; chaste, decent; candid, direct, frank, ingenuous, sincere, unreserved.

honesty *n* equity, fairness, faithfulness, fidelity, honour, integrity, justice, probity, trustiness, trustworthiness, uprightness; truth, truthfulness, veracity; genuineness, thoroughness; candour, frankness, ingenuousness, openness, sincerity, straightforwardness, unreserve.

honorary *adj* formal, nominal, titular, unofficial, unpaid.

honour *vb* dignify, exalt, glorify, grace; respect, revere, reverence, venerate; adore, hallow, worship; celebrate, commemorate, keep, observe. • *n* civility, deference, esteem, homage, respect, reverence, veneration; dignity, distinction, elevation, nobleness; consideration, credit, fame, glory, reputation; high-mindedness, honesty, integrity, magnanimity, probity, uprightness; chastity, purity, virtue; boast, credit, ornament, pride.

honourable *adj* elevated, famous, great, illustrious, noble; admirable, conscientious, fair, honest, just, magnanimous, true, trustworthy, upright, virtuous, worshipful; creditable, esteemed, estimable, equitable, proper, respected, reputable, right.

honours *npl* dignities, distinctions, privilege, titles; adornments, beauties, decorations, glories; civilities.

hood *n* capuche, coif, cover, cowl, head.

hoodwink *vb* blind, blindfold; cloak, conceal, cover, hide; cheat, circumvent, cozen, deceive, delete, dupe, fool, gull, impose, overreach, trick.

hook *vb* catch, ensnare, entrap, hasp, snare; bend, curve. • *n* catch, clasp, fastener, hasp; snare, trap; cutter, grass-hook, reaper, reaping-hook, sickle.

hooked *adj* aquiline, bent, crooked, curved, hamate, unciform.

hoop *vb* clasp, encircle, enclose, surround. • *n* band, circlet, girdle, ring; crinoline, farthingale.

hoot *vb* boo, cry, jeer, shout, yell; condemn, decry, denounce, execrate, hiss. • *n* boo, cry, jeer, shout, yell.

hop *vb* bound, caper, frisk, jump, leap, skip, spring; dance, trip; halt, hobble, limp. • *n* bound, caper, dance, jump, leap, skip, spring.

hope *vb* anticipate, await, desire, expect, long; believe, rely, trust. • *n* confidence, belief, faith, reliance, sanguineness, sanguinity, trust; anticipation, desire, expectancy, expectation.

hopeful *adj* anticipatory, confident, expectant, fond, optimistic, sanguine; cheerful, encouraging, promising.

hopeless *adj* abject, crushed, depressed, despondent, despairing, desperate, disconsolate, downcast, forlorn, pessimistic, woebegone; abandoned, helpless, incurable, irremediable, remediless; impossible, impracticable, unachievable, unattainable.

horde *n* clan, crew, gang, troop; crowd, multitude, pack, throng.

horn *vb* gore, pierce. • *n* trumpet, wind instrument; beaker, drinking cup, cornucopia; spike, spur; cusp, prong, wing.

horrid *adj* alarming, awful, bristling, dire, dreadful, fearful, frightful, harrowing, hideous, horrible, horrific, horrifying, rough, terrible, terrific; abominable, disagreeable, disgusting, odious, offensive, repulsive, revolting, shocking, unpleasant, vile.

horrify *vb* affright, alarm, frighten, shock, terrify, terrorise.

horror *n* alarm, awe, consternation, dismay, dread, fear, fright, panic; abhorrence, abomination, antipathy, aversion, detestation, disgust, hatred, loathing, repugnance, revulsion; shuddering.

horse *n* charger, cob, colt, courser, filly, gelding, mare, nag, pad, palfrey, pony, stallion, steed; cavalry, horseman; buck, clotheshorse, frame, sawhorse, stand, support.

horseman *n* cavalier, equestrian, rider; cavalryman, chasseur, dragoon, horse-soldier.

hospitable *adj* attentive, bountiful, kind; bountiful, cordial, generous, liberal, open, receptive, sociable, unconstrained, unreserved.

host[1] *n* entertainer, innkeeper, landlord, master of ceremonies, presenter, proprietor, owner, receptionist.

host[2] *n* array, army, legion; assemblage, assembly, horde, multitude, throng.

host[3] *n* altar bread, bread, consecrated bread, loaf, wafer.

hostile *adj* inimical, unfriendly, warlike; adverse, antagonistic, contrary, opposed, opposite, repugnant.

hostilities *npl* conflict, fighting, war, warfare.

hostility *n* animosity, antagonism, enmity, hatred, ill-will, unfriendliness; contrariness, opposition, repugnance, variance.

hot *adj* burning, fiery, scalding; boiling, flaming, heated, incandescent, parching, roasting, torrid; heated, oppressive, sweltering, warm; angry, choleric, excitable, furious, hasty, impatient, impetuous, irascible, lustful, passionate, touchy, urgent, violent; animated, ardent, eager, fervent, fervid, glowing, passionate, vehement; acrid, biting, highly flavoured, highly seasoned, peppery, piquant, pungent, sharp, stinging.

hotchpotch *n* farrago, jumble, hodgepodge, medley, miscellany, stew.

hotel *n* inn, public house, tavern.

hot-headed *adj* furious, headlong, headstrong, hot-brained, impetuous, inconsiderate, passionate, precipitate, rash, reckless, vehement, violent.

hound *vb* drive, incite, spur, urge; bate, chase, goad, harass, harry, hunt, pursue.

house *vb* harbour, lodge, protect, shelter. • *n* abode, domicile, dwelling, habitation, home, mansion, residence; building, edifice; family, household; kindred, race, lineage, tribe; company, concern, firm, partnership; hotel, inn, public house, tavern.

housing *n* accommodation, dwellings, houses; casing, container, covering, protection, shelter.

hovel *n* cabin, cot, den, hole, hut, shed.

hover *vb* flutter; hang; vacillate, waver.

however *adv* but, however, nevertheless, notwithstanding, still, though, yet.

howl *vb* bawl, cry, lament, ululate, weep, yell, yowl. • *n* cry, yell, ululation.

hoyden *n* romp, tomboy.

hoydenish *adj* bad-mannered, boisterous, bold, ill-behaved, illtaught, inelegant, romping, rough, rude, rustic, tomboyish, uncouth, ungenteel, unladylike, unruly.

hubbub *n* clamour, confusion, din, disorder, disturbance, hullabaloo, racket, riot, outcry, tumult, uproar.

huckster *n* hawker, peddler, retailer.

huddle *vb* cluster, crowd, gather; crouch, curl up, nestle, snuggle. • *n* confusion, crowd, disorder, disturbance, jumble, tumult.

hue *n* cast, colour, complexion, dye, shade, tinge, tint, tone.

huff *vb* blow, breathe, exhale, pant, puff. • *n* anger, fume, miff, passion, pet, quarrel, rage, temper, tiff.

hug *vb* clasp, cling, cuddle, embrace, grasp, grip, squeeze; cherish, nurse, retain. • *n* clasp, cuddle, embrace, grasp, squeeze.

huge *adj* bulky, colossal, Cyclopean, elephantine, enormous, gigantic, herculean, immense, stupendous, vast.

huggermugger *adj* clandestine, secret, sly; base, contemptible, mean, unfair; confused, disorderly, slovenly.

hull *vb* husk, peel, shell. • *n* covering, husk, rind, shell.

hullabaloo *n* clamour, confusion, din, disturbance, hubbub, outcry, racket, vociferation, uproar.

hum *vb* buzz, drone, murmur; croon, sing.

humane *adj* accommodating, benevolent, benign, charitable, clement, compassionate, gentle, good-hearted, kind, kindhearted, lenient, merciful, obliging, tender, sympathetic; cultivating, elevating, humanizing, refining, rational, spiritual.

humanity *n* benevolence, benignity, charity, fellow-feeling, humaneness, kind-heartedness, kindness, philanthropy, sympathy, tenderness; humankind, mankind, mortality.

humanize *vb* civilize, cultivate, educate, enlighten, improve, polish, reclaim, refine, soften.

humble *vb* abase, abash, break, crush, debase, degrade, disgrace, humiliate, lower, mortify, reduce, sink, subdue. • *adj* meek, modest, lowly, simple, submissive, unambitious, unassuming, unobtrusive, unostentatious, unpretending; low, obscure, mean, plain, poor, small, undistinguished, unpretentious.

humbug vb cheat, cozen, deceive, hoax, swindle, trick. • n cheat, dodge, gammon, hoax, imposition, imposture, deception, fraud, trick; cant, charlatanism, charlatanry, hypocrisy, mummery, quackery; charlatan, impostor, fake, quack.

humdrum adj boring, dronish, dreary, dry, dull, monotonous, prosy, stupid, tedious, tiresome, wearisome.

humid adj damp, dank, moist, wet.

humiliate vb abase, abash, debase, degrade, depress, humble, mortify, shame.

humiliation n abasement, affront, condescension, crushing, degradation, disgrace, dishonouring, humbling, indignity, mortification, self-abasement, submissiveness, resignation.

humility n diffidence, humbleness, lowliness, meekness, modesty, self-abasement, submissiveness.

humorist n comic, comedian, droll, jester, joker, wag, wit.

humorous adj comic, comical, droll, facetious, funny, humorous, jocose, jocular, laughable, ludicrous, merry, playful, pleasant, sportive, whimsical, witty.

humour vb favour, gratify, indulge. • n bent, bias, disposition, predilection, prosperity, temper, vein; mood, state; caprice, crotchet, fancy, freak, vagary, whim, whimsy, wrinkle; drollery, facetiousness, fun, jocoseness, jocularity, pleasantry, wit; fluid, moisture, vapour.

hunch vb arch, jostle, nudge, punch, push, shove. • n bunch, hump, knob, protuberance; nudge, punch, push, shove; feeling, idea, intuition, premonition.

hungry adj covetous, craving, desirous, greedy; famished, starved, starving; barren, poor, unfertile, unproductive.

hunk n chunk, hunch, lump, slice.

hunt vb chase, drive, follow, hound, pursue, stalk, trap, trail; poach, shoot; search, seek. • n chase, field-sport, hunting, pursuit.

hurl vb cast, dart, fling, pitch, project, send, sling, throw, toss.

hurly-burly n bustle, commotion, confusion, disturbance, hurl, hurly, uproar, tumult, turmoil.

hurricane n cyclone, gale, storm, tempest, tornado, typhoon.

hurried adj cursory, hasty, slight, superficial.

hurry vb drive, precipitate; dispatch, expedite, hasten, quicken, speed; haste, scurry. • n agitation, bustle, confusion, flurry, flutter, perturbation, precipitation; celerity, haste, dispatch, expedition, promptitude, promptness, quickness.

hurt vb damage, disable disadvantage, harm, impair, injure, mar; bruise, pain, wound; afflict, grieve, offend; ache, smart, throb. • n damage, detriment, disadvantage, harm, injury, mischief; ache, bruise, pain, suffering, wound.

hurtful adj baleful, baneful, deleterious, destructive, detrimental, disadvantageous, harmful, injurious, mischievous, noxious, pernicious, prejudicial, unwholesome.

husband vb economize, hoard, save, store.

husbandry n agriculture, cultivation, farming, geoponics, tillage; economy, frugality, thrift.

hush vb quiet, repress, silence, still, suppress; appease, assuage, calm, console, quiet, still. • n quiet, quietness, silence, stillness.

hypocrite n deceiver, dissembler, impostor, pretender.

hypocritical adj deceiving, dissembling, false, insincere, spurious, two-faced.

hypothesis n assumption, proposition, supposition, theory.

hypothetical adj assumed, imaginary, supposed, theoretical.

hysterical adj frantic, frenzied, overwrought, uncontrollable; comical, uproarious.

I

ice *vb* chill, congeal, freeze. • *n* crystal; frosting, sugar.

icy *adj* glacial; chilling, cold, frosty; cold-hearted, distant, frigid, indifferent, unemotional.

idea *n* archetype, essence, exemplar, ideal, model, pattern, plan, model; fantasy, fiction, image, imagination; apprehension, conceit, conception, fancy, illusion, impression, thought; belief, judgement, notion, opinion, sentiment, supposition.

ideal *adj* intellectual, mental; chimerical, fancied, fanciful, fantastic, illusory, imaginary, unreal, visionary, shadowy; complete, consummate, excellent, perfect; impractical, unattainable, utopian. • *n* criterion, example, model, standard.

identical *adj* equivalent, same, selfsame, tantamount.

identity *n* existence, individuality, personality, sameness.

ideology *n* belief, creed, dogma, philosophy, principle.

idiocy *n* fatuity, feebleness, foolishness, imbecility, insanity.

idiosyncrasy *n* caprice, eccentricity, fad, peculiarity, singularity.

idiot *n* blockhead, booby, dunce, fool, ignoramus, imbecile, simpleton.

idiotic *adj* fatuous, foolish, imbecile, irrational, senseless, sottish, stupid.

idle *adj* inactive, unemployed, unoccupied, vacant; indolent, inert, lazy, slothful, sluggish; abortive, bootless, fruitless, futile, groundless, ineffectual, unavailing, useless, vain; foolish, frivolous, trashy, trifling, trivial, unimportant, unprofitable. • *vb* dally, dawdle, laze, loiter, potter, waste; drift, shirk, slack.

idler *n* dawdler, doodle, drone, laggard, lazybones, loafer, lounger, slacker, slowcoach, sluggard, trifler.

idol *n* deity, god, icon, image, pagan, simulacrum, symbol; delusion, falsity, pretender, sham; beloved, darling, favourite, pet.

idolater *n* heathen, pagan; admirer, adorer, worshipper.

idolize *vb* canonize, deify; adore, honour, love, reverence, venerate.

idyll *n* eclogue, pastoral.

if *conj* admitting, allowing, granting, provided, supposing, though, whether. • *n* condition, hesitation, uncertainty.

igneous *adj* combustible, combustive, conflagrative, fiery, molten.

ignite *vb* burn, inflame, kindle, light, torch.

ignoble *adj* base-born, low, low-born, mean, peasant, plebeian, rustic, vulgar; contemptible, degraded, insignificant, mean, worthless; disgraceful, dishonourable, infamous, low, unworthy.

ignominious *adj* discreditable, disgraceful, dishonourable, disreputable, infamous, opprobrious, scandalous, shameful; base, contemptible, despicable.

ignominy *n* abasement, contempt, discredit, disgrace, dishonour disrepute, infamy, obloquy, odium, opprobrium, scandal, shame.

ignoramus *n* blockhead, duffer, dunce, fool, greenhorn, novice, numskull, simpleton.

ignorance *n* benightedness, darkness, illiteracy, nescience, rusticity; blindness, unawareness.

ignorant *adj* blind, illiterate, nescient, unaware, unconversant, uneducated, unenlightened, uninformed, uninstructed, unlearned, unread, untaught, untutored, unwitting.

ignore *vb* disregard, neglect, overlook, reject, skip.

ill *adj* bad, evil, faulty, harmful, iniquitous, naughty, unfavourable, unfortunate, unjust, wicked; ailing, diseased, disordered, indisposed, sick, unwell, wrong; crabbed, cross, hateful, malicious, malevolent, peevish, surly, unkind, ill-bred; ill-favoured, ugly, unprepossessing. • *adv* badly, poorly, unfortunately. • *n* badness, depravity, evil, mischief, misfortune, wickedness; affliction, ailment, calamity, harm, misery, pain, trouble.

ill-advised *adj* foolish, ill-judged, imprudent, injudicious, unwise.

ill-bred *adj* discourteous, ill-behaved, ill-mannered, impolite, rude, uncivil, uncourteous, uncouth.

illegal *adj* contraband, forbidden, illegitimate, illicit, prohibited, unauthorized, unlawful, unlicensed.

illegible *adj* indecipherable, obscure, undecipherable, unreadable.

illegitimate *adj* bastard, misbegotten, natural.

ill-fated *adj* ill-starred, luckless, unfortunate, unlucky.

ill-favoured *adj* homely, ugly, offensive, plain, unpleasant.

ill humour *n* fretfulness, ill-temper, peevishness, petulance, testiness.

illiberal *adj* close, close-fisted, covetous, mean, miserly, narrow, niggardly, parsimonious, penurious, selfish, sordid, stingy, ungenerous; bigoted, narrow-minded, uncharitable, ungentlemanly, vulgar.

illicit *adj* illegal, illegitimate, unauthorized, unlawful, unlegalized, unlicensed; criminal, guilty, forbidden, improper, wrong.

illimitable *adj* boundless, endless, immeasurable, immense, infinite, unbounded, unlimited, vast.

illiterate *adj* ignorant, uneducated, uninstructed, unlearned, unlettered, untaught, untutored.

ill-judged *adj* foolish, ill-advised, imprudent, injudicious, unwise.

ill-mannered *adj* discourteous, ill-behaved, ill-bred, impolite, rude, uncivil, uncourteous, uncouth, unpolished.

ill-natured *adj* disobliging, hateful, malevolent, unamiable, unfriendly, unkind; acrimonious, bitter, churlish, crabbed, cross, cross-grained, crusty, ill-tempered, morose, perverse, petulant, sour, spiteful, sulky, sullen, wayward.

illness *n* ailing, ailment, complaint, disease, disorder, distemper, indisposition, malady, sickness.

illogical *adj* absurd, fallacious, inconsistent, inconclusive, inconsequent, incorrect, invalid, unreasonable, unsound.

ill-proportioned *adj* awkward, ill-made, ill-shaped, misshapen, misproportioned, shapeless.

ill-starred *adj* ill-fated, luckless, unfortunate, unhappy, unlucky.

ill temper *n* bad temper, crabbedness, crossness, grouchiness, ill nature, moroseness, sulkiness, sullenness.

ill-tempered *adj* acrimonious, bad-tempered, crabbed, cross, grouchy, ill-natured, morose, sour, sulky, surly.

ill-timed *adj* inapposite, inopportune, irrelevant, unseasonable, untimely.

ill-treat *vb* abuse, ill-use, injure, maltreat, mishandle, misuse.

illude *vb* cheat, deceive, delude, disappoint, mock, swindle, trick.

illuminate *vb* illume, illumine, light; adorn, brighten, decorate, depict, edify, enlighten, inform, inspire, instruct, make wise.

illusion *n* chimera, deception, delusion, error, fallacy, false appearance, fantasy, hallucination, mockery, phantasm.

illusive, illusory *adj* barmecide, deceitful, deceptive, delusive, fallacious, imaginary, make-believe, mock, sham, unsatisfying, unreal, unsubstantial, visionary, tantalizing.

illustrate *vb* clarify, demonstrate, elucidate, enlighten, exemplify, explain; adorn, depict, draw.

illustration *n* demonstration, elucidation, enlightenment, exemplification, explanation, interpretation; adornment, decoration, picture.

illustrative *adj* elucidative, elucidatory, exemplifying.

illustrious *adj* bright, brilliant, glorious, radiant, splendid; celebrated, conspicuous, distinguished, eminent, famed, famous, noble, noted, remarkable, renowned, signal.

ill will *n* animosity, dislike, enmity, envy, grudge, hate, hatred, hostility, ill nature, malevolence, malice, malignity, rancour, spleen, spite, uncharitableness, unkindness, venom.

image *n* idol, statue; copy, effigy, figure, form, imago, likeness, picture, resemblance, representation, shape, similitude, simulacrum, statue, symbol; conception, counterpart, embodiment, idea, reflection.

imagery *n* dream, phantasm, phantom, vision.

imaginable *adj* assumable, cogitable, conceivable, conjecturable, plausible, possible, supposable, thinkable.

imaginary *adj* chimerical, dreamy, fancied, fanciful, fantastic, fictitious, ideal, illusive, illusory, invented, quixotic, shadowy, unreal, utopian, visionary, wild; assumed, conceivable, hypothetical, supposed.

imagination *n* chimera, conception, fancy, fantasy, invention, unreality; position; contrivance, device, plot, scheme.

imaginative *adj* creative, dreamy, fanciful, inventive, poetical, plastic, visionary.

imagine *vb* conceive, dream, fancy, imagine, picture, pretend; contrive, create, devise, frame, invent, mould, project; assume, suppose, hypothesize; apprehend, assume, believe, deem, guess, opine, suppose, think.

imbecile *adj* cretinous, drivelling, fatuous, feeble, feeble-minded, foolish, helpless, idiotic, imbecilic, inane, infirm, witless. • *n* dotard, driveller.

imbecility *n* debility, feebleness, helplessness, infirmity, weakness; foolishness, idiocy, silliness, stupidity, weak-mindedness.

imbibe *vb* absorb, assimilate, drink, suck, swallow; acquire, gain, gather, get, receive.

imbroglio *n* complexity, complication, embarrassment, entanglement, misunderstanding.

imbrue *vb* drench, embrue, gain, moisten, soak, stain, steep, wet.

imbue *vb* colour, dye, stain, tincture, tinge, tint; bathe, impregnate, infuse, inoculate, permeate, pervade, provide, saturate, steep.

imitate *vb* copy, counterfeit, duplicate, echo, emulate, follow, forge, mirror, reproduce, simulate; ape, impersonate, mimic, mock, personate; burlesque, parody, travesty.

imitation *adj* artificial, fake, man-made, mock, reproduction, synthetic. • *n* aping, copying, imitation, mimicking, parroting; copy, duplicate, likeness, resemblance; mimicry, mocking; burlesque, parody, travesty.

imitative *adj* copying, emulative, imitating, mimetic, simulative; apeish, aping, mimicking.

imitator *n* copier, copycat, copyist, echo, impersonator, mimic, mimicker, parrot.

immaculate *adj* clean, pure, spotless, stainless, unblemished, uncontaminated, undefiled, unpolluted, unspotted, unsullied, untainted, untarnished; faultless, guiltless, holy, innocent, pure, saintly, sinless, stainless.

immanent *adj* congenital, inborn, indwelling, inherent, innate, internal, intrinsic, subjective.

immaterial *adj* bodiless, ethereal, extramundane, impalpable, incorporeal, mental, metaphysical, spiritual, unbodied, unfleshly, unsubstantial; inconsequential, insignificant, nonessential, unessential, unimportant.

immature *adj* crude, green, imperfect, raw, rudimental, rudimentary, unfinished, unformed, unprepared, unripe, unripened, youthful; hasty, premature, unseasonable, untimely.

immaturity *n* crudeness, crudity, greenness, imperfection, rawness, unpreparedness, unripeness.

immeasurable *adj* bottomless, boundless, illimitable, immense, infinite, limitless, measureless, unbounded, vast.

immediate *adj* close, contiguous, near, next, proximate; intuitive, primary, unmeditated; direct, instant, instantaneous, present, pressing, prompt.

immediately *adv* closely, proximately; directly, forthwith, instantly, presently, presto, pronto.

immemorial *adj* ancient, hoary, olden.

immense *adj* boundless, illimitable, infinite, interminable, measureless, unbounded, unlimited; colossal, elephantine, enormous, gigantic, huge, large, monstrous, mountainous, prodigious, stupendous, titanic, tremendous, vast.

immensity *n* boundlessness, endlessness, limitlessness, infiniteness, infinitude, infinity; amplitude, enormity, greatness, hugeness, magnitude, vastness.

immerse *vb* baptize, bathe, dip, douse, duck, overwhelm, plunge, sink, souse, submerge; absorb, engage, engross, involve.

immersion *n* dipping, immersing, plunging; absorption, engagement; disappearance; baptism.

imminent *adj* close, impending, near, overhanging, threatening, alarming, dangerous, perilous.

immobile *adj* fixed, immovable, inflexible, motionless, quiescent, stable, static, stationary, steadfast; dull, expressionless, impassive, rigid, stiff, stolid.

immobility *n* fixedness, fixity, immovability, immovableness, motionlessness, stability, steadfastness, unmovableness; dullness, expressionlessness, inflexibility, rigidity, stiffness, stolidity.

immoderate *adj* excessive, exorbitant, extravagant, extreme, inordinate, intemperate, unreasonable.

immodest *adj* coarse, gross, indecorous, indelicate, lewd, shameless; bold, brazen, forward, impudent, indecent; broad, filthy, impure, indecent, obscene, smutty, unchaste.

immodesty *n* coarseness, grossness, indecorum, indelicacy, shamelessness; impurity, lewdness, obscenity, smuttiness, unchastity; boldness, brass, forwardness, impatience.

immolate *vb* kill, sacrifice.

immoral *adj* antisocial, corrupt, loose, sinful, unethical, vicious, wicked, wrong; bad, depraved, dissolute, profligate, unprincipled; abandoned, indecent, licentious.

immorality *n* corruption, corruptness, criminality, demoralization, depravity, impurity, profligacy, sin, sinfulness, vice, wickedness; wrong.

immortal *adj* deathless, ever-living, imperishable, incorruptible, indestructible, indissoluble, never-dying, undying, unfading; ceaseless, continuing, eternal, endless, everlasting, never-ending, perpetual, sempiternal; abiding, enduring, lasting, permanent. • *n* god, goddess; genius, hero.

immortality *n* deathlessness, incorruptibility, incorruptibleness, indestructibility; perpetuity.

immortalize *vb* apotheosize, enshrine, glorify, perpetuate.

immovable *adj* firm, fixed, immobile, stable, stationary; impassive, steadfast, unalterable, unchangeable, unshaken, unyielding.

immunity *n* exemption, exoneration, freedom, release; charter, franchise, liberty, license, prerogative, privilege, right.

immure *vb* confine, entomb, imprison, incarcerate.

immutability *n* constancy, inflexibility, invariability, invariableness, permanence, stability, unalterableness, unchangeableness.

immutable *adj* constant, fixed, inflexible, invariable, permanent, stable, unalterable, unchangeable, undeviating.

imp *n* demon, devil, elf, flibbertigibbet, hobgoblin, scamp, sprite; graft, scion, shoot.

impact *vb* collide, crash, strike. • *n* brunt, impression, impulse, shock, stroke, touch; collision, contact, impinging, striking.

impair *vb* blemish, damage, deface, deteriorate, injure, mar, ruin, spoil, vitiate; decrease, diminish, lessen, reduce; enervate, enfeeble, weaken.

impale *vb* hole, pierce, puncture, spear, spike, stab, transfix.

impalpable *adj* attenuated, delicate, fine, intangible; imperceptible, inapprehensible, incorporeal, indistinct, shadowy, unsubstantial.

impart *vb* bestow, confer, give, grant; communicate, disclose, discover, divulge, relate, reveal, share, tell.

impartial *adj* candid, disinterested, dispassionate, equal, equitable, even-handed, fair, honourable, just, unbiased, unprejudiced, unwarped.

impassable *adj* blocked, closed, impenetrable, impermeable, impervious, inaccessible, pathless, unattainable, unnavigable, unreachable.

impassioned *adj* animated, ardent, burning, excited, fervent, fervid, fiery, glowing, impetuous, intense, passionate, vehement, warm, zealous.

impassive *adj* calm, passionless; apathetic, callous, indifferent, insensible, insusceptible, unfeeling, unimpressible, unsusceptible.

impassivity *n* calmness, composure, indifference, insensibility, insusceptibility, passionlessness, stolidity.

impatience *n* disquietude, restlessness, uneasiness; eagerness, haste, impetuosity, precipitation, vehemence; heat, irritableness, irritability, violence.

impatient *adj* restless, uneasy, unquiet; eager, hasty, impetuous, precipitate, vehement; abrupt, brusque, choleric, fretful, hot, intolerant, irritable, peevish, sudden, testy, violent.

impeach *vb* accuse, arraign, charge, indict; asperse, censure, denounce, disparage, discredit, impair, impute, incriminate, lessen.

impeachment *n* accusation, arraignment, indictment; aspersion, censure, disparagement, imputation, incrimination, reproach.

impeccable *adj* faultless, immaculate, incorrupt, innocent, perfect, pure, sinless, stainless, uncorrupt.

impede *vb* bar, block, check, clog, curb, delay, encumber, hinder, interrupt, obstruct, restrain, retard, stop, thwart.

impediment *n* bar, barrier, block, check, curb, difficulty, encumbrance, hindrance, obstacle, obstruction, stumbling block.

impel *vb* drive, push, send, urge; actuate, animate, compel, constrain, embolden, incite, induce, influence, instigate, move, persuade, stimulate.

impend *vb* approach, menace, near, threaten.

impending *adj* approaching, imminent, menacing, near, threatening.

impenetrable *adj* impermeable, impervious, inaccessible; cold, dull, impassive, indifferent, obtuse, senseless, stolid, unsympathetic; dense, proof.

impenitence *n* hardheartedness, impenitency, impenitentness, obduracy, stubbornness.

impenitent *adj* hardened, hard-hearted, incorrigible, irreclaimable, obdurate, recusant, relentless, seared, stubborn, uncontrite, unconverted, unrepentant.

imperative *adj* authoritative, commanding, despotic, domineering, imperious, overbearing, peremptory, urgent; binding, obligatory.

imperceptible *adj* inaudible, indiscernible, indistinguishable, invisible; fine, impalpable, inappreciable, gradual, minute.

imperfect *adj* abortive, crude, deficient, garbled, incomplete, poor; defective, faulty, impaired.

imperfection *n* defectiveness, deficiency, faultiness, incompleteness; blemish, defect, fault, flaw, lack, stain, taint; failing, foible, frailty, limitation, vice, weakness.

imperial *adj* kingly, regal, royal, sovereign; august, consummate, exalted, grand, great, kingly, magnificent, majestic, noble, regal, royal, queenly, supreme, sovereign, supreme, consummate.

imperil *vb* endanger, expose, hazard, jeopardize, risk.

imperious *adj* arrogant, authoritative, commanding, compelling, despotic, dictatorial, domineering, haughty, imperative, lordly, magisterial, overbearing, tyrannical, urgent, compelling.

imperishable *adj* eternal, everlasting, immortal, incorruptible, indestructible, never-ending, perennial, unfading.

impermeable *adj* impenetrable, impervious.

impermissible *adj* deniable, insufferable, objectionable, unallowable, unallowed, unlawful.

impersonate *vb* act, ape, enact, imitate, mimic, mock, personate; embody, incarnate, personify, typify.

impersonation *n* incarnation, manifestation, personification; enacting, imitation, impersonating, mimicking, personating, representation.

impertinence *n* irrelevance, irrelevancy, unfitness, impropriety; assurance, boldness, brass, brazenness, effrontery, face, forwardness, impudence, incivility, insolence, intrusiveness, presumption, rudeness, sauciness, pertness.

impertinent *adj* inapplicable, inapposite, irrelevant; bold, forward, impudent, insolent, intrusive, malapert, meddling, officious, pert, rude, saucy, unmannerly.

imperturbability *n* calmness, collectedness, composure, dispassion, placidity, placidness, sedateness, serenity, steadiness, tranquility.

imperturbable *adj* calm, collected, composed, cool, placid, sedate, serene, tranquil, unmoved, undisturbed, unexcitable, unmoved, unruffled.

impervious *adj* impassable, impenetrable, impermeable.

impetuosity *n* force, fury, haste, precipitancy, vehemence, violence.

impetuous *adj* ardent, boisterous, brash, breakneck, fierce, fiery, furious, hasty, headlong, hot, hot-headed, impulsive, overzealous, passionate, precipitate, vehement, violent.

impetus *n* energy, force, momentum, propulsion.

impiety *n* irreverence, profanity, ungodliness; iniquity, sacrilegiousness, sin, sinfulness, ungodliness, unholiness, unrighteousness, wickedness.

impinge *vb* clash, dash, encroach, hit, infringe, strike, touch.

impious *adj* blasphemous, godless, iniquitous, irreligious, irreverent, profane, sinful, ungodly, unholy, unrighteous, wicked.

implacable *adj* deadly, inexorable, merciless, pitiless, rancorous, relentless, unappeasable, unforgiving, unpropitiating, unrelenting.

implant *vb* ingraft, infix, insert, introduce, place.

implement *vb* effect, execute, fulfil. • *n* appliance, instrument, tool, utensil.

implicate *vb* entangle, enfold; compromise, concern, entangle, include, involve.

implication *n* entanglement, involvement, involution; connotation, hint, inference, innuendo, intimation; conclusion, meaning, significance.

implicit *adj* implied, inferred, understood; absolute, constant, firm, steadfast, unhesitating, unquestioning, unreserved, unshaken.

implicitly *adv* by implication, silently, tacitly, unspokenly, virtually, wordlessly.

implore *vb* adjure, ask, beg, beseech, entreat, petition, pray, solicit, supplicate.

imply *vb* betoken, connote, denote, import, include, infer, insinuate, involve, mean, presuppose, signify.

impolicy *n* folly, imprudence, ill-judgement, indiscretion, inexpediency.

impolite *adj* bearish, boorish, discourteous, disrespectful, ill-bred, insolent, rough, rude, uncivil, uncourteous, ungentle, ungentlemanly, ungracious, unmannerly, unpolished, unrefined.

impoliteness *n* boorishness, discourteousness, discourtesy, disrespect, ill-breeding, incivility, insolence, rudeness, unmannerliness.

impolitic *adj* ill-advised, imprudent, indiscreet, inexpedient, injudicious, unwise.

import *vb* bring in, introduce, transport; betoken, denote, imply, mean, purport, signify. • *n* goods, importation, merchandise; bearing, drift, gist, intention, interpretation, matter, meaning, purpose, sense, signification, spirit, tenor; consequence, importance, significance, weight.

importance *n* concern, consequence, gravity, import, moment, momentousness, significance, weight, weightiness; consequence, pomposity, self-importance.

important *adj* considerable, grave, material, momentous, notable, pompous, ponderous, serious, significant, urgent, valuable, weighty; esteemed, influential, prominent, substantial; consequential, pompous, self-important.

importunate *adj* busy, earnest, persistent, pertinacious, pressing, teasing, troublesome, urgent.

importune *vb* ask, beset, dun, ply, press, solicit, urge.

importunity *n* appeal, beseechment, entreaty, petition, plying, prayer, pressing, suit, supplication, urging; contention, insistence; urgency.

impose *vb* lay, place, put, set; appoint, charge, dictate, enjoin, force, inflict, obtrude, prescribe, tax; (*with* **on, upon**) abuse, cheat, circumvent, deceive, delude, dupe, exploit, hoax, trick, victimize.

imposing *adj* august, commanding, dignified, exalted, grand, grandiose, impressive, lofty, magnificent, majestic, noble, stately, striking.

imposition *n* imposing, laying, placing, putting; burden, charge, constraint, injunction, levy, oppression, tax; artifice, cheating, deception, dupery, fraud, imposture, trickery.

impossibility *n* hopelessness, impracticability, inability, infeasibility, unattainability; inconceivability.

impossible *adj* hopeless, impracticable, infeasible, unachievable, unattainable; inconceivable, self-contradictory, unthinkable.

impost *n* custom, duty, excise, rate, tax, toil, tribute.

impostor *n* charlatan, cheat, counterfeiter, deceiver, double-dealer, humbug, hypocrite, knave, mountebank, pretender, quack, rogue, trickster.

imposture *n* artifice, cheat, deceit, deception, delusion, dodge, fraud, hoax, imposition, ruse, stratagem, trick, wile.

impotence *n* disability, feebleness, frailty, helplessness, inability, incapability, incapacity, incompetence, inefficaciousness, inefficacy, inefficiency, infirmity, powerlessness, weakness.

impotent *adj* disabled, enfeebled, feeble, frail, helpless, incapable, incapacitated, incompetent, inefficient, infirm, nerveless, powerless, unable, weak; barren, sterile.

impound *vb* confine, coop, engage, imprison.

impoverish *vb* beggar, pauperize; deplete, exhaust, ruin.

impracticability *n* impossibility, impracticableness, impracticality, infeasibility, unpracticability.

impracticable *adj* impossible, infeasible; intractable, obstinate, recalcitrant, stubborn, thorny, unmanageable; impassable, insurmountable.

impracticality *n* impossibility, impracticableness, impractibility, infeasibility, unpracticability; irrationality, unpracticalness, unrealism, unreality, unreasonableness.

imprecate *vb* anathematize, curse, execrate, invoke, maledict.

imprecation *n* anathema, curse, denunciation, execration, invocation, malediction.

imprecatory *adj* appealing, beseeching, entreating, imploratory, imploring, imprecatory, pleading; cursing, damnatory, execrating, maledictory.

impregnable *adj* immovable, impenetrable, indestructible, invincible, inviolable, invulnerable, irrefrangible, secure, unconquerable, unassailable, unyielding.

impregnate *vb* fecundate, fertilize, fructify; dye, fill, imbrue, imbue, infuse, permeate, pervade, saturate, soak, tincture, tinge.

impress *vb* engrave, imprint, print, stamp; affect, move, strike; fix, inculcate; draft, enlist, levy, press, requisition. • *n* impression, imprint, mark, print, seal, stamp; cognizance, device, emblem, motto, symbol.

impressibility *n* affectibility, impressionability, pliancy, receptiveness, responsiveness, sensibility, sensitiveness, susceptibility.

impressible *adj* affectible, excitable, impressionable, pliant, receptive, responsive, sensitive, soft, susceptible, tender.

impression *n* edition, imprinting, printing, stamping; brand, dent, impress, mark, stamp; effect, influence, sensation; fancy, idea, instinct, notion, opinion, recollection.

impressive *adj* affecting, effective, emphatic, exciting, forcible, moving, overpowering, powerful, solemn, speaking, splendid, stirring, striking, telling, touching.

imprint *vb* engrave, mark, print, stamp; impress, inculcate. • *n* impression, mark, print, sign, stamp.

imprison *vb* confine, jail, immure, incarcerate, shut up.

imprisonment *n* captivity, commitment, confinement, constraint, durance, duress, incarceration, restraint.

improbability *n* doubt, uncertainty, unlikelihood.

improbable *adj* doubtful, uncertain, unlikely, unplausible.

improbity *n* dishonesty, faithlessness, fraud, fraudulence, knavery, unfairness.

impromptu *adj* extempore, improvised, offhand, spontaneous, unpremeditated, unprepared, unrehearsed. • *adv* extemporaneously, extemporarily, extempore, offhand, ad-lib.

improper *adj* immodest, inapposite, inappropriate, irregular, unadapted, unapt, unfit, unsuitable, unsuited; indecent, indecorous, indelicate, unbecoming, unseemly; erroneous, inaccurate, incorrect, wrong.

impropriety *n* inappropriateness, unfitness, unsuitability, unsuitableness; indecorousness, indecorum, unseemliness.

improve *vb* ameliorate, amend, better, correct, edify, meliorate, mend, rectify, reform; cultivate; gain, mend, progress; enhance, increase, rise.

improvement *n* ameliorating, amelioration, amendment, bettering, improving, meliorating, melioration; advancement, proficiency, progress.

improvidence *n* imprudence, thriftlessness, unthriftiness.

improvident *adj* careless, heedless, imprudent, incautious, inconsiderate, negligent, prodigal, rash, reckless, shiftless, thoughtless, thriftless, unthrifty, wasteful.

improvisation *n* ad-libbing, contrivance, extemporaneousness, extemporariness, extemporization, fabrication, invention; (*mus*) extempore, impromptu.

improvise *vb* ad-lib, contrive, extemporize, fabricate, imagine, invent.

imprudence *n* carelessness, heedlessness, improvidence, incautiousness, inconsideration, indiscretion, rashness.

imprudent *adj* careless, heedless, ill-advised, ill-judged, improvident, incautious, inconsiderate, indiscreet, rash, unadvised, unwise.

impudence *n* assurance, audacity, boldness, brashness, brass, bumptiousness, cheek, cheekiness, effrontery, face, flippancy, forwardness, front, gall, impertinence, insolence, jaw, lip, nerve, pertness, presumption, rudeness, sauciness, shamelessness.

impudent *adj* bold, bold-faced, brazen, brazen-faced, cool, flippant, forward, immodest, impertinent, insolent, insulting, pert, presumptuous, rude, saucy, shameless.

impugn *vb* assail, attack, challenge, contradict, dispute, gainsay, oppose, question, resist.

impulse *n* force, impetus, impelling, momentum, push, thrust; appetite, inclination, instinct, passion, proclivity; incentive, incitement, influence, instigation, motive, instigation.

impulsive *adj* impelling, moving, propulsive; emotional, hasty, heedless, hot, impetuous, mad-cap, passionate, quick, rash, vehement, violent.

impunity *n* exemption, immunity, liberty, licence, permission, security.

impure *adj* defiled, dirty, feculent, filthy, foul, polluted, unclean; bawdy, coarse, immodest, gross, immoral, indelicate, indecent, lewd, licentious, loose, obscene, ribald, smutty, unchaste; adulterated, corrupt, mixed.

impurity *n* defilement, feculence, filth, foulness, pollution, uncleanness; admixture, coarseness, grossness, immodesty, indecency, indelicacy, lewdness, licentiousness, looseness, obscenity, ribaldry, smut, smuttiness, unchastity, vulgarity.

imputable *adj* ascribable, attributable, chargeable, owing, referable, traceable, owing.

imputation *n* attributing, charging, imputing; accusation, blame, censure, reproach.

impute *vb* ascribe, attribute, charge, consider, imply, insinuate, refer.

inability *n* impotence, incapacity, incapability, incompetence, incompetency, inefficiency; disability, disqualification.

inaccessible *adj* unapproachable, unattainable.

inaccuracy *n* erroneousness, impropriety, incorrectness, inexactness; blunder, defect, error, fault, mistake.

inaccurate *adj* defective, erroneous, faulty, incorrect, inexact, mistaken, wrong.

inaccurately *adv* carelessly, cursorily, imprecisely, incorrectly, inexactly, mistakenly, unprecisely, wrongly.

inactive *adj* inactive; dormant, inert, inoperative, peaceful, quiet, quiescent; dilatory, drowsy, dull, idle, inanimate, indolent, inert, lazy, lifeless, lumpish, passive, slothful, sleepy, stagnant, supine.

inactivity *n* dilatoriness, idleness, inaction, indolence, inertness, laziness, sloth, sluggishness, supineness, torpidity, torpor.

inadequacy *n* inadequateness, insufficiency; defectiveness, imperfection, incompetence, incompetency, incompleteness, insufficiency, unfitness, unsuitableness.

inadequate *adj* disproportionate, incapable, insufficient, unequal; defective, imperfect, inapt, incompetent, incomplete.

inadmissible *adj* improper, incompetent, unacceptable, unallowable, unqualified, unreasonable.

inadvertence, inadvertency *n* carelessness, heedlessness, inattention, inconsiderateness, negligence, thoughtlessness; blunder, error, oversight, slip.

inadvertent *adj* careless, heedless, inattentive, inconsiderate, negligent, thoughtless, unobservant.

inadvertently *adv* accidently, carelessly, heedlessly, inconsiderately, negligently, thoughtlessly, unintentionally.

inalienable *adj* undeprivable, unforfeitable, untransferable.

inane *adj* empty, fatuous, vacuous, void; foolish, frivolous, idiotic, puerile, senseless, silly, stupid, trifling, vain, worthless.

inanimate *adj* breathless, dead, extinct; dead, dull, inert, lifeless, soulless, spiritless.

inanition *n* emptiness, inanity, vacuity; exhaustion, hunger, malnutrition, starvation, want.

inanity *n* emptiness, foolishness, inanition, vacuity; folly, frivolousness, puerility, vanity, worthlessness.

inapplicable *adj* inapposite, inappropriate, inapt, irrelevant, unfit, unsuitable, unsuited.

inapposite *adj* impertinent, inapplicable, irrelevant, nonpertinent; inappropriate, unfit, unsuitable.

inappreciable *adj* impalpable, imperceptible, inconsiderable, inconspicuous, indiscernible, infinitesimal, insignificant, negligible, undiscernible, unnoticed.

inappropriate *adj* inapposite, unadapted, unbecoming, unfit, unsuitable, unsuited.

inapt *adj* inapposite, unapt, unfit, unsuitable; awkward, clumsy, dull, slow, stolid, stupid.

inaptitude *n* awkwardness, inapplicability, inappropriateness, inaptness, unfitness, unsuitableness.

inarticulate *adj* blurred, indistinct, thick; dumb, mute.

inartificial *adj* artless, direct, guileless, ingenuous, naive, simple, simple-minded, sincere, single-minded.

inasmuch as *conj* considering that, seeing that, since.

inattention *n* absent-mindedness, carelessness, disregard, heedlessness, inadvertence, inapplication, inconsiderateness, neglect, remissness, slip, thoughtlessness, unmindfulness, unobservance.

inattentive *adj* absent-minded, careless, disregarding, heedless, inadvertent, inconsiderate, neglectful, remiss, thoughtless, unmindful, unobservant.

inaudible *adj* faint, indistinct, muffled; mute, noiseless, silent, still.

inaugurate *vb* induct, install, introduce, invest; begin, commence, initiate, institute, originate.

inauguration *n* beginning, commencement, initiation, institution, investiture, installation, opening, origination.

inauspicious *adj* bad, discouraging, ill-omened, ill-starred, ominous, unfavourable, unfortunate, unlucky, unpromising, unpropitious, untoward.

inborn *adj* congenital, inbred, ingrained, inherent, innate, instinctive, native, natural.

incalculable *adj* countless, enormous, immense, incalculable, inestimable, innumerable, sumless, unknown, untold.

incandescence *n* candescence, glow, gleam, luminousness, luminosity.

incandescent *adj* aglow, candent, candescent, gleaming, glowing, luminous, luminant, radiant.

incantation *n* charm, conjuration, enchantment, magic, necromancy, sorcery, spell, witchcraft, witchery.

incapability *n* disability, inability, incapacity, incompetence.

incapable *adj* feeble, impotent, incompetent, insufficient, unable, unfit, unfitted, unqualified, weak.

incapacious *adj* cramped, deficient, incommodious, narrow, scant.

incapacitate *vb* cripple, disable; disqualify, make unfit.

incapacity *n* disability, inability, incapability, incompetence; disqualification, unfitness.

incarcerate *vb* commit, confine, immure, imprison, jail, restrain, restrict.

incarnate *vb* body, embody, incorporate, personify. • *adj* bodied, embodied, incorporated, personified.

incarnation *n* embodiment, exemplification, impersonation, manifestation, personification.

incautious *adj* impolitic, imprudent, indiscreet, uncircumspect, unwary; careless, headlong, heedless, inconsiderate, negligent, rash, reckless, thoughtless.

incendiary *adj* dissentious, factious, inflammatory, seditious. • *n* agitator, firebrand, fire-raiser.

incense[1] *vb* anger, chafe, enkindle, enrage, exasperate, excite, heat, inflame, irritate, madden, provoke.

incense[2] *n* aroma, fragrance, perfume, scent; admiration, adulation, applause, laudation.

incentive *n* cause, encouragement, goad, impulse, incitement, inducement, instigation, mainspring, motive, provocation, spur, stimulus.

inception *n* beginning, commencement, inauguration, initiation, origin, rise, start.

incertitude *n* ambiguity, doubt, doubtfulness, indecision, uncertainty.

incessant *adj* ceaseless, constant, continual, continuous, eternal, everlasting, never-ending, perpetual, unceasing, unending, uninterrupted, unremitting.

inchoate *adj* beginning, commencing, inceptive, incipient, initial.

incident *n* circumstance, episode, event, fact, happening, occurrence. • *adj* happening, belonging, pertaining, appertaining, accessory, relating, natural; falling, impinging.

incidental *adj* accidental, casual, chance, concomitant, contingent, fortuitous, subordinate; adventitious, extraneous, nonessential, occasional.

incinerate *vb* burn, char, conflagrate, cremate, incremate.

incipient *adj* beginning, commencing, inchoate, inceptive, originating, starting.

incised *adj* carved, cut, engraved, gashed, graved, graven.

incision *n* cut, gash, notch, opening, penetration.

incisive *adj* cutting; acute, biting, sarcastic, satirical, sharp; acute, clear, distinct, penetrating, sharp-cut, trenchant.

incite *vb* actuate, animate, arouse, drive, encourage, excite, foment, goad, hound, impel, instigate, prod, prompt, provoke, push, rouse, spur, stimulate, urge.

incitement *n* encouragement, goad, impulse, incentive, inducement, motive, provocative, spur, stimulus.

incivility *n* discourteousness, discourtesy, disrespect, ill-breeding, ill-manners, impoliteness, impudence, inurbanity, rudeness, uncourtliness, unmannerliness.

inclemency *n* boisterousness, cruelty, harshness, rigour, roughness, severity, storminess, tempestuousness, tyranny.

inclement *adj* boisterous, harsh, rigorous, rough, severe, stormy; cruel, unmerciful.

inclination *n* inclining, leaning, slant, slope; trending, verging; aptitude, bent, bias, disposition, penchant, predilection, predisposition, proclivity, proneness, propensity, tendency, turn, twist; desire, fondness, liking, taste, partiality, predilection, wish; bow, nod, obeisance.

incline *vb* lean, slant, slope; bend, nod, verge; tend; bias, dispose, predispose, turn; bow. • *n* ascent, descent, grade, gradient, rise, slope.

inclose *see* **enclose**.

include *vb* contain, hold; comprehend, comprise, contain, cover, embody, embrace, incorporate, involve, take in.

inclusive *adj* comprehending, embracing, encircling, enclosing, including, taking in.

incognito, incognita *adj* camouflaged, concealed, disguised, unknown. • *n* camouflage, concealment, disguise.

incoherent *adj* detached, loose, nonadhesive, noncohesive; disconnected, incongruous, inconsequential, inconsistent, uncoordinated; confused, illogical, irrational, rambling, unintelligible, wild.

income *n* earnings, emolument, gains, interest, pay, perquisite, proceeds, profits, receipts, rents, return, revenue, salary, wages.

incommensurate *adj* disproportionate, inadequate, insufficient, unequal.

incommode *vb* annoy, discommode, disquiet, disturb, embarrass, hinder, inconvenience, molest, plague, trouble, upset, vex.

incommodious *adj* awkward, cumbersome, cumbrous, inconvenient, unhandy, unmanageable, unsuitable, unwieldy; annoying, disadvantageous, harassing, irritating, vexatious.

incommunicative *adj* exclusive, unsociable, unsocial, reserved.

incomparable *adj* matchless, inimitable, peerless, surpassing, transcendent, unequalled, unparalleled, unrivalled.

incompatibility *n* contrariety, contradictoriness, discrepancy, incongruity, inconsistency, irreconcilability, unsuitability, unsuitableness

incompatible *adj* contradictory, incongruous, inconsistent, inharmonious, irreconcilable, unadapted, unsuitable.

incompetence *n* inability, incapability, incapacity, incompetency; inadequacy, insufficiency; disqualification, unfitness.

incompetent *adj* incapable, unable; inadequate, insufficient; disqualified, incapacitated, unconstitutional, unfit, unfitted.

incomplete *adj* defective, deficient, imperfect, partial; inexhaustive, unaccompanied, uncompleted, unexecuted, unfinished.

incomprehensible *adj* inconceivable, inexhaustible, unfathomable, unimaginable; inconceivable, unintelligible, unthinkable.

incomputable *adj* enormous, immense, incalculable, innumerable, prodigious.

inconceivable *adj* incomprehensible, incredible, unbelievable, unimaginable, unthinkable.

inconclusive *adj* inconsequent, inconsequential, indecisive, unconvincing, illogical, unproved, unproven.

incongruity *n* absurdity, contradiction, contradictoriness, contrariety, discordance, discordancy, discrepancy, impropriety, inappropriateness, incoherence, incompatibility, inconsistency, unfitness, unsuitableness.

incongruous *adj* absurd, contradictory, contrary, disagreeing, discrepant, inappropriate, incoherent, incompatible, inconsistent, inharmonious, unfit, unsuitable.

inconsequent *adj* desultory, disconnected, fragmentary, illogical, inconclusive, inconsistent, irrelevant, loose.

inconsiderable *adj* immaterial, insignificant, petty, slight, small, trifling, trivial, unimportant.

inconsiderate *adj* intolerant, uncharitable, unthoughtful; careless, heedless, giddy, hare-brained, hasty, headlong, imprudent, inadvertent, inattentive, indifferent, indiscreet, light-headed, negligent, rash, thoughtless.

inconsistency *n* incoherence, incompatibility, incongruity, unsuitableness; contradiction, contrariety; changeableness, inconstancy, instability, vacillation, unsteadiness.

inconsistent *adj* different, discrepant, illogical, incoherent, incompatible, incongruous, inconsequent, inconsonant, irreconcilable, unsuitable; contradictory, contrary; changeable, fickle, inconstant, unstable, unsteady, vacillating, variable.

inconsolable *adj* comfortless, crushed, disconsolate, forlorn, heartbroken, hopeless, woebegone.

inconstancy *n* changeableness, mutability, variability, variation, fluctuation, faithlessness, fickleness, capriciousness, vacillation, uncertainty, unsteadiness, volatility.

inconstant *adj* capricious, changeable, faithless, fickle, fluctuating, mercurial, mutable, unsettled, unsteady, vacillating, variable, varying, volatile, wavering; mutable, uncertain, unstable.

incontestable *adj* certain, incontrovertible, indisputable, indubitable, irrefrangible, sure, undeniable, unquestionable.

incontinence *n* excess, extravagance, indulgence, intemperance, irrepressibility, lasciviousness, lewdness, licentiousness, prodigality, profligacy, riotousness, unrestraint, wantonness, wildness.

incontinent *adj* debauched, lascivious, lewd, licentious, lustful, prodigal, unchaste, uncontrolled, unrestrained.

incontrovertible *adj* certain, incontestable, indisputable, indubitable, irrefutable, sure, undeniable, unquestionable.

inconvenience *vb* discommode; annoy, disturb, molest, trouble, vex. • *n* annoyance, disadvantage, disturbance, molestation, trouble, vexation; awkwardness, cumbersomeness, incommodiousness, unwieldiness; unfitness, unseasonableness, unsuitableness.

inconvenient *adj* annoying, awkward, cumbersome, cumbrous, disadvantageous, incommodious, inopportune, troublesome, uncomfortable, unfit, unhandy, unmanageable, unseasonable, unsuitable, untimely, unwieldy, vexatious.

incorporate *vb* affiliate, amalgamate, associate, blend, combine, consolidate, include, merge, mix, unite; embody, incarnate. • *adj* incorporeal, immaterial, spiritual, supernatural; blended, consolidated, merged, united.

incorporation *n* affiliation, alignment, amalgamation, association, blend, blending, combination, consolidation, fusion, inclusion, merger, mixture, unification, union, embodiment, incarnation, personification.

incorporeal *adj* bodiless, immaterial, impalpable, incorporate, spiritual, supernatural, unsubstantial.

incorrect *adj* erroneous, false, inaccurate, inexact, untrue, wrong; faulty, improper, mistaken, ungrammatical, unbecoming, unsound.

incorrectness *n* error, inaccuracy, inexactness, mistake.

incorrigible *adj* abandoned, graceless, hardened, irreclaimable, lost, obdurate, recreant, reprobate, shameless; helpless, hopeless, irremediable, irrecoverable, irreparable, irretrievable, irreversible, remediless.

incorruptibility *n* unpurchasableness; deathlessness, immortality, imperishableness, incorruptibleness, incorruption, indestructibility.

incorruptible *adj* honest, unbribable; imperishable, indestructible, immortal, undying, deathless, everlasting.

increase *vb* accrue, advance, augment, enlarge, extend, grow, intensify, mount, wax; multiply; enhance, greaten, heighten, raise, reinforce; aggravate, prolong. • *n* accession, accretion, accumulation, addition, augmentation, crescendo, development, enlargement, expansion, extension, growth, heightening, increment, intensification, multiplication, swelling; gain, produce, product, profit; descendants, issue, offspring, progeny.

incredible *adj* absurd, inadmissible, nonsensical, unbelievable.

incredulity *n* distrust, doubt, incredulousness, scepticism, unbelief.

incredulous *adj* distrustful, doubtful, dubious, sceptical, unbelieving.

increment *n* addition, augmentation, enlargement, increase.

incriminate *vb* accuse, blame, charge, criminate, impeach.

incubate *vb* brood, develop, hatch, sit.

inculcate *vb* enforce, implant, impress, infix, infuse, ingraft, inspire, instil.

inculpable *adj* blameless, faultless, innocent, irreprehensible, irreproachable, irreprovable, sinless, unblamable, unblameable.

inculpate *vb* accuse, blame, censure, charge, incriminate, impeach, incriminate.

inculpatory *adj* criminatory, incriminating.

incumbent *adj* binding, devolved, devolving, laid, obligatory; leaning, prone, reclining, resting. • *n* holder, occupant.

incur *vb* acquire, bring, contract.

incurable *adj* cureless, hopeless, irrecoverable, remediless; helpless, incorrigible, irremediable, irreparable, irretrievable, remediless.

incurious *adj* careless, heedless, inattentive, indifferent, uninquisitive, unobservant, uninterested.

incursion *n* descent, foray, raid, inroad, irruption.

incursive *adj* aggressive, hostile, invasive, predatory, raiding.

incurvate *vb* bend, bow, crook, curve. • *adj* (*bot*) aduncous, arcuate, bowed, crooked, curved, hooked.

indebted *adj* beholden, obliged, owing.

indecency *n* impropriety, indecorum, offensiveness, outrageousness, unseemliness; coarseness, filthiness, foulness, grossness, immodesty, impurity, obscenity, vileness.

indecent *adj* bold, improper, indecorous, offensive, outrageous, unbecoming, unseemly; coarse, dirty, filthy, gross, immodest, impure, indelicate, lewd, nasty, obscene, pornographic, salacious, shameless, smutty, unchaste.

indecipherable *adj* illegible, undecipherable, undiscoverable, inexplicable, obscure, unintelligible, unreadable.

indecision *n* changeableness, fickleness, hesitation, inconstancy, irresolution, unsteadiness, vacillation.

indecisive *adj* dubious, hesitating, inconclusive, irresolute, undecided, unsettled, vacillating, wavering.

indecorous *adj* coarse, gross, ill-bred, impolite, improper, indecent, rude, unbecoming, uncivil, unseemly.

indecorum *n* grossness, ill-breeding, ill manners, impoliteness, impropriety, incivility, indecency, indecorousness.

indeed *adv* absolutely, actually, certainly, in fact, in truth, in reality, positively, really, strictly, truly, verily, veritably. • *interj* really! you don't say so! is it possible!

indefatigable *adj* assiduous, never-tiring, persevering, persistent, sedulous, tireless, unflagging, unremitting, untiring, unwearied.

indefeasible *adj* immutable, inalienable, irreversible, irrevocable, unalterable.

indefensible *adj* censurable, defenceless, faulty, unpardonable, untenable; inexcusable, insupportable, unjustifiable, unwarrantable, wrong.

indefinite *adj* confused, doubtful, equivocal, general, imprecise, indefinable, indecisive, indeterminate, indistinct, inexact, inexplicit, lax, loose, nondescript, obscure, uncertain, undefined, undetermined, unfixed, unsettled, vague.

indelible *adj* fast, fixed, ineffaceable, ingrained, permanent.

indelicacy *n* coarseness, grossness, indecorousness, indecorum, impropriety, offensiveness, unseemliness, vulgarity; immodesty, indecency, lewdness, unchastity; foulness, obscenity.

indelicate *adj* broad, coarse, gross, indecorous, intrusive, rude, unbecoming, unseemly; foul, immodest, indecent, lewd, obscene, unchaste, vulgar.

indemnification *n* compensation, reimbursement, remuneration, security.

indemnify *vb* compensate, reimburse, remunerate, requite, secure.

indent *vb* bruise, jag, notch, pink, scallop, serrate; bind, indenture.

indentation *n* bruise, dent, depression, jag, notch.

indenture *vb* bind, indent. • *n* contract, instrument; indentation.

independence *n* freedom, liberty, self-direction; distinctness, nondependence, separation; competence, ease.

independent *adj* absolute, autonomous, free, self-directing, uncoerced, unrestrained, unrestricted, voluntary; (*person*) self-reliant, unconstrained, unconventional.

indescribable *adj* ineffable, inexpressible, nameless, unutterable.

indestructible *adj* abiding, endless, enduring, everlasting, fadeless, imperishable, incorruptible, undecaying.

indeterminate *adj* indefinite, uncertain, undetermined, unfixed.

index *vb* alphabetize, catalogue, codify, earmark, file, list, mark, tabulate. • *n* catalogue, list, register, tally; indicator, lead, mark, pointer, sign, signal, token; contents, table of contents; forefinger; exponent.

indicate *vb* betoken, denote, designate, evince, exhibit, foreshadow, manifest, mark, point out, prefigure, presage, register, show, signify, specify, tell; hint, imply, intimate, sketch, suggest.

indication *n* hint, index, manifestation, mark, note, sign, suggestion, symptom, token.

indicative *adj* significant, suggestive, symptomatic; (*gram*) affirmative, declarative.

indict *vb* (*law*) accuse, charge, present.

indictment *n* (*law*) indicting, presentment; accusation, arraignment, charge, criminaton, impeachment.

indifference *n* apathy, carelessness, coldness, coolness, heedlessness, inattention, insignificance, negligence, unconcern, unconcernedness, uninterestedness; disinterestedness, impartiality, neutrality.

indifferent *adj* apathetic, cold, cool, dead, distant, dull, easygoing, frigid, heedless, inattentive, incurious, insensible, insouciant, listless, Lukewarm, nonchalant, perfunctory, regardless, stoical, unconcerned, uninterested, unmindful, unmoved; equal; fair, medium, middling, moderate, ordinary, passable, tolerable; mediocre, so-so; immaterial, unimportant; disinterested, impartial, neutral, unbiased.

indigence *n* destitution, distress, necessity, need, neediness, pauperism, penury, poverty, privation, want.

indigenous *adj* aboriginal, home-grown, inborn, inherent, native.

indigent *adj* destitute, distressed, insolvent, moneyless, necessitous, needy, penniless, pinched, poor, reduced.

indigested *adj* unconcocted, undigested; crude, ill-advised, ill-considered, ill-judged; confused, disorderly, ill-arranged, unmethodical.

indigestion *n* dyspepsia, dyspepsy.

indignant *adj* angry, exasperated, incensed, irate, ireful, provoked, roused, wrathful, wroth.

indignation *n* anger, choler, displeasure, exasperation, fury, ire, rage, resentment, wrath.

indignity *n* abuse, affront, contumely, dishonour, disrespect, ignominy, insult, obloquy, opprobrium, outrage, reproach, slight.

indirect *adj* circuitous, circumlocutory, collateral, devious, oblique, roundabout, sidelong, tortuous; deceitful, dishonest, dishonorable, unfair; mediate, remote, secondary, subordinate.

indiscernible *adj* imperceptible, indistinguishable, invisible, undiscernible, undiscoverable.

indiscipline *n* laxity, insubordination.

indiscreet *adj* foolish, hasty, headlong, heedless, imprudent, incautious, inconsiderate, injudicious, rash, reckless, unwise.

indiscretion *n* folly, imprudence, inconsiderateness, rashness; blunder, faux pas, lapse, mistake, misstep.

indiscriminate *adj* confused, heterogeneous, indistinct, mingled, miscellaneous, mixed, promiscuous, undiscriminating, undistinguishable, undistinguishing.

indispensable *adj* essential, expedient, necessary, needed, needful, requisite.

indisputable *adj* certain, incontestable, indubitable, infallible, sure, undeniable, undoubted, unmistakable, unquestionable.

indisposed *adj* ailing, ill, sick, unwell; averse, backward, disinclined, loath, reluctant, unfriendly, unwilling.

indisposition *n* ailment, illness, sickness; aversion, backwardness, dislike, disinclination, reluctance, unwillingness.

indisputable *adj* certain, incontestable, indutitable, infallible, sure, undeniable, undoubted, unmistakable, unquestionable.

indissoluble *adj* abiding, enduring, firm, imperishable, incorruptible, indestructible, lasting, stable, unbreakable.

indistinct *adj* ambiguous, doubtful, uncertain; blurred, dim, dull, faint, hazy, misty, nebulous, obscure, shadowy, vague; confused, inarticulate, indefinite, indistinguishable, undefined, undistinguishable.

indistinguishable *adj* imperceptible, indiscernible, unnoticeable, unobservable; chaotic, confused, dim, indistinct, obscure, vague.

indite *vb* compose, pen, write.

individual *adj* characteristic, distinct, identical, idiosyncratic, marked, one, particular, personal, respective, separate, single, singular, special, unique; peculiar, proper; decided, definite, independent, positive, self-guided, unconventional. • *n* being, character, party, person, personage, somebody, someone; type, unit.

individuality *n* definiteness, indentity, personality; originality, self-direction, self-determination, singularity, uniqueness.

individualize *vb* individuate, particularize, singularize, specify.

indivisible *adj* incommensurable, indissoluble, inseparable, unbreakable, unpartiable.

indocile *adj* cantankerous, contumacious, dogged, froward, inapt, headstrong, intractable, mulish, obstinate, perverse, refractory, stubborn, ungovernable, unmanageable, unruly, unteachable.

indoctrinate *vb* brainwash, imbue, initiate, instruct, rehabilitate, teach.

indoctrination *n* grounding, initiation, instruction, rehabilitation.

indolence *n* idleness, inactivity, inertia, inertness, laziness, listlessness, sloth, slothfulness, sluggishness.

indolent *adj* easy, easy-going, inactive, inert, lazy, listless, lumpish, otiose, slothful, sluggish, supine.

indomitable *adj* invincible, unconquerable, unyielding.

indorse *see* **endorse**.

indubitable *adj* certain, evident, incontestable, incontrovertible, indisputable, sure, undeniable, unquestionable.

induce *vb* actuate, allure, bring, draw, drive, entice, impel, incite, influence, instigate, move, persuade, prevail, prompt, spur, urge; bring on, cause, effect, motivate, lead, occasion, produce.

inducement *n* allurement, draw, enticement, instigation, persuasion; cause, consideration, impulse, incentive, incitement, influence, motive, reason, spur, stimulus.

induct *vb* inaugurate, initiate, install, institute, introduce, invest.

induction *n* inauguration, initiation, institution, installation, introduction; conclusion, generalization, inference.

indue *vb* assume, endow, clothe, endue, invest, supply.

indulge *vb* gratify, license, revel, satisfy, wallow, yield to; coddle, cosset, favour, humour, pamper, pet, spoil; allow, cherish, foster, harbour, permit, suffer.

indulgence *n* gratification, humouring, pampering; favour, kindness, lenience, lenity, liberality, tenderness; (*theol*) absolution, remission.

indulgent *adj* clement, easy, favouring, forbearing, gentle, humouring, kind, lenient, mild, pampering, tender, tolerant.

indurate *vb* harden, inure, sear, strengthen.

induration *n* hardening, obduracy.

industrious *adj* assiduous, diligent, hard-working, laborious, notable, operose, sedulous; brisk, busy, persevering, persistent.

industry *n* activity, application, assiduousness, assiduity, diligence; perseverance, persistence, sedulousness, vigour; effort, labour, toil.

inebriated *adj* drunk, intoxicated, stupefied.

ineffable *adj* indescribable, inexpressible, unspeakable, unutterable.

ineffaceable *adj* indelible, indestructible, inerasable, inexpungeable, ingrained.

ineffectual *adj* abortive, bootless, fruitless, futile, inadequate, inefficacious, ineffective, inoperative, useless, unavailing, vain; feeble, inefficient, powerless, impotent, weak.

inefficacy *n* ineffectualness, inefficiency.

inefficient *adj* feeble, incapable, ineffectual, ineffective, inefficacious, weak.

inelastic *adj* flabby, flaccid, inductile, inflexible, irresilient.

inelegant *adj* abrupt, awkward, clumsy, coarse, constrained, cramped, crude, graceless, harsh, homely, homespun, rough, rude, stiff, tasteless, uncourtly, uncouth, ungainly, ungraceful, unpolished, unrefined.

ineligible *adj* disqualified, unqualified; inexpedient, objectionable, unadvisable, undesirable.

inept *adj* awkward, improper, inapposite, inappropriate, unapt, unfit, unsuitable; null, useless, void, worthless; foolish, nonsensical, pointless, senseless, silly, stupid.

ineptitude *n* inappositeness, inappropriateness, inaptitude, unfitness, unsuitability, unsuitable-ness; emptiness, nullity, uselessness, worthlessness; folly, foolishness, nonsense, pointlessness, senselessness, silliness, stupidity.

inequality *n* disproportion, inequitableness, injustice, unfairness; difference, disparity, dissimilarity, diversity, imparity, irregularity, roughness, unevenness; inadequacy, incompetency, insufficiency.

inequitable *adj* unfair, unjust.

inert *adj* comatose, dead, inactive, lifeless, motionless, quiescent, passive; apathetic, dronish, dull, idle, indolent, lazy, lethargic, lumpish, phlegmatic, slothful, sluggish, supine, torpid.

inertia *n* apathy, inertness, lethargy, passiveness, passivity, slothfulness, sluggishness.

inestimable *adj* incalculable, invaluable, precious, priceless, valuable.

inevitable *adj* certain, necessary, unavoidable, undoubted.

inexact *adj* imprecise, inaccurate, incorrect; careless, crude, loose.

inexcusable *adj* indefensible, irremissible, unallowable, unjustifiable, unpardonable.

inexhaustible *adj* boundless, exhaustless, indefatigable, unfailing, unlimited.

inexorable *adj* cruel, firm, hard, immovable, implacable, inflexible, merciless, pitiless, relentless, severe, steadfast, unbending, uncompassionate, unmerciful, unrelenting, unyielding.

inexpedient *adj* disadvantageous, ill-judged, impolitic, imprudent, indiscreet, injudicious, inopportune, unadvisable, unprofitable, unwise.

inexperience *n* greenness, ignorance, rawness.

inexperienced *adj* callow, green, raw, strange, unacquainted, unconversant, undisciplined, uninitiated, unpractised, unschooled, unskilled, untrained, untried, unversed, young.

inexpert *adj* awkward, bungling, clumsy, inapt, maladroit, unhandy, unskilful, unskilled.

inexpiable *adj* implacable, inexorable, irreconcilable, unappeasable; irremissible, unatonable, unpardonable.

inexplicable *adj* enigmatic, enigmatical, incomprehensible, inscrutable, mysterious, strange, unaccountable, unintelligible.

inexpressible *adj* indescribable, ineffable, unspeakable, unutterable; boundless, infinite, surpassing.

inexpressive *adj* blank, characterless, dull, unexpressive.

inextinguishable *adj* unquenchable.

in extremis *adv* moribund.

inextricable *adj* entangled, intricate, perplexed, unsolvable.

infallibility *n* certainty, infallibleness, perfection.

infallible *adj* certain, indubitable, oracular, sure, unerring, unfailing.

infamous *adj* abominable, atrocious, base, damnable, dark, detestable, discreditable, disgraceful, dishonorable, disreputable, heinous, ignominious, nefarious, odious, opprobrious, outrageous, scandalous, shameful, shameless, vile, villainous, wicked.

infamy *n* abasement, discredit, disgrace, dishonour, disrepute, ignominy, obloquy, odium, opprobrium, scandal, shame; atrocity, detestableness, disgracefulness, dishonorableness, odiousness, scandalousness, shamefulness, villainy, wickedness.

infancy *n* beginning, commencement; babyhood, childhood, minority, nonage, pupillage.

infant *n* babe, baby, bairn, bantling, brat, chit, minor, nursling, papoose, suckling, tot.

infantile *adj* childish, infantine, newborn, tender, young; babyish, childish, weak; babylike, childlike.

infatuate *vb* befool, besot, captivate, delude, prepossess, stultify.

infatuation *n* absorption, besottedness, folly, foolishness, prepossession, stupefaction.

infeasible *adj* impractical, unfeasible.

infect *vb* affect, contaminate, corrupt, defile, poison, pollute, taint, vitiate.

infection *n* affection, bane, contagion, contamination, corruption, defilement, pest, poison, pollution, taint, virus, vitiation.

infectious *adj* catching, communicable, contagious, contaminating, corrupting, defiling, demoralizing, pestiferous, pestilential, poisoning, polluting, sympathetic, vitiating.

infecund *adj* barren, infertile, sterile, unfruitful, unproductive, unprolific.

infecundity *n* unfruitfulness.

infelicitous *adj* calamitous, miserable, unfortunate, unhappy, wretched; inauspicious, unfavourable, unpropitious; ill-chosen, inappropriate, unfitting.

infer *vb* collect, conclude, deduce, derive, draw, gather, glean, guess, presume, reason.

inference *n* conclusion, consequence, corollary, deduction, generalization, guess, illation, implication, induction, presumption.

inferior *adj* lower, nether; junior, minor, secondary, subordinate; bad, base, deficient, humble, imperfect, indifferent, mean, mediocre, paltry, poor, second-rate, shabby.

inferiority *n* juniority, subjection, subordination, mediocrity; deficiency, imperfection, inadequacy, shortcoming.

infernal *adj* abominable, accursed, atrocious, damnable, dark, demoniacal, devilish, diabolical, fiendish, fiendlike, hellish, malicious, nefarious, satanic, Stygian.

infertility *n* barrenness, infecundity, sterility, unfruitfulness, unproductivity.

infest *vb* annoy, disturb, harass, haunt, molest, plague, tease, torment, trouble, vex, worry; beset, overrun, possess, swarm, throng.

infidel *n* agnostic, atheist, disbeliever, heathen, heretic, sceptic, unbeliever.

infidelity *n* adultery, disloyalty, faithlessness, treachery, unfaithfulness; disbelief, scepticism, unbelief.

infiltrate *vb* absorb, pervade, soak.

infinite *adj* boundless, endless, illimitable, immeasurable, inexhaustible, interminable, limitless, measureless, perfect, unbounded, unlimited; enormous, immense, stupendous, vast; absolue, eternal, self-determined, self-existent, unconditioned.

infinitesimal *adj* infinitely small; microscopic, miniscule.

infinity *n* absoluteness, boundlessness, endlessness, eternity, immensity, infiniteness, infinitude, interminateness, self-determination, self-existence, vastness.

infirm *adj* ailing, debilitated, enfeebled, feeble, frail, weak, weakened; faltering, irresolute, vacillating, wavering; insecure, precarious, unsound, unstable.

infirmity *n* ailment, debility, feebleness, frailness, frailty, weakness; defect, failing, fault, foible, weakness.

infix *vb* fasten, fix, plant, set; implant, inculcate, infuse, ingraft, instil.

inflame *vb* animate, arouse, excite, enkindle, fire, heat, incite, inspirit, intensify, rouse, stimulate; aggravate, anger, chafe, embitter, enrage, exasperate, incense, infuriate, irritate, madden, nettle, provoke.

inflammability *n* combustibility, combustibleness, inflammableness.

inflammable *adj* combustible, ignitible; excitable.

inflammation *n* burning, conflagration; anger, animosity, excitement, heat, rage, turbulence, violence.

inflammatory *adj* fiery, inflaming; dissentious, incendiary, seditious.

inflate *vb* bloat, blow up, distend, expand, swell, sufflate; elate, puff up; enlarge, increase.

inflated *adj* bloated, distended, puffed-up, swollen; bombastic, declamatory, grandiloquent, high-flown, magniloquent, overblown, pompous, rhetorical, stilted, tumid, turgid.

inflation *n* enlargement, increase, overenlargement, overissue; bloatedness, distension, expansion, sufflation; bombast, conceit, conceitedness, self-conceit, self-complacency, self-importance, self-sufficiency, vaingloriousness, vainglory.

inflect *vb* bend, bow, curve, turn; (*gram*) conjugate, decline, vary.

inflection *n* bend, bending, crook, curvature, curvity, flexure; (*gram*) accidence, conjugation, declension, variation; (*mus*) modulation.

inflexibility *n* inflexibleness, rigidity, stiffness; doggedness, obstinacy, pertinacity, stubbornness; firmness, perseverance, resolution, tenacity.

inflexible *adj* rigid, rigorous, stiff, unbending; cantankerous, cross-grained, dogged, headstrong, heady, inexorable, intractable, obdurate, obstinant, pertinacious, refractory, stubborn, unyielding, wilful; firm, immovable, persevering, resolute, steadfast, unbending.

inflict *vb* bring, impose, lay on.

infliction *n* imposition, inflicting; judgment, punishment.

inflorescence *n* blooming, blossoming, flowering.

influence *vb* affect, bias, control, direct, lead, modify, prejudice, prepossess, sway; actuate, arouse, impel, incite, induce, instigate, move, persuade, prevail upon, rouse. • *n* ascendancy, authority, control, mastery, potency, predominance, pull, rule, sway; credit, reputation, weight; inflow, inflowing, influx; magnetism, power, spell.

influential *adj* controlling, effective, effectual, potent, powerful, strong; authoritative, momentous, substantial, weighty.

influx *n* flowing in, introduction.

infold *see* enfold.

inform *vb* animate, inspire, quicken; acquaint, advise, apprise, enlighten, instruct, notify, teach, tell, tip, warn.

informal *adj* unceremonious, unconventional, unofficial; easy, familiar, natural, simple; irregular, nonconformist, unusual.

informality *n* unceremoniousness; unconventionality; ease, familiarity, naturalness, simplicity; noncomformity, irregularity, unusualness.

informant *n* advertiser, adviser, informer, intelligencer, newsmonger, notifier, relator; accuser, complainant, informer.

information *n* advice, data, intelligence, knowledge, notice; advertisement, enlightenment, instruction, message, tip, word, warning; accusation, complaint, denunciation.

informer *n* accuser, complainant, informant, snitch.

infraction *n* breach, breaking, disobedience, encroachment, infringement, nonobservance, transgression, violation.

infrangible *adj* inseparable, inviolable, unbreakable.

infrequency *n* rareness, rarity, uncommonness, unusualness.

infrequent *adj* rare, uncommon, unfrequent, unusual; occasional, scant, scarce, sporadic.

infringe *vb* break, contravene, disobey, intrude, invade, transgress, violate.

infringement *n* breach, breaking, disobedience, infraction, nonobservance, transgression, violation.

infuriated *adj* angry, enraged, furious, incensed, maddened, raging, wild.

infuse *vb* breathe into, implant, inculcate, ingraft, insinuate, inspire, instil, introduce; macerate, steep.

infusion *n* inculcation, instillation, introduction; infusing, macerating, steeping.

ingathering *n* harvest.

ingenious *adj* able, adroit, artful, bright, clever, fertile, gifted, inventive, ready, sagacious, shrewd, witty.

ingenuity *n* ability, acuteness, aptitude, aptness, capacity, capableness, cleverness, faculty, genius, gift, ingeniousness, inventiveness, knack, readiness, skill, turn.

ingenuous *adj* artless, candid, childlike, downright, frank, generous, guileless, honest, innocent, naive, open, open-hearted, plain, simple-minded, sincere, single-minded, straightforward, transparent, truthful, unreserved.

ingenuousness *n* artlessness, candour, childlikeness, frankness, guilelessness, honesty, naivety, open-heartedness, openness, sincerity, single-mindedness, truthfulness.

inglorious *adj* humble, lowly, mean, nameless, obscure, undistinguished, unhonoured, unknown, unmarked, unnoted; discreditable, disgraceful, humiliating, ignominious, scandalous, shameful.

ingloriousness *n* humbleness, lowliness, meanness, namelessness, obscurity; abasement, discredit, disgrace, dishonour, disrepute, humiliation, infamy, ignominiousness, ignominy, obloquy, odium, opprobrium, shame.

ingraft *vb* graft, implant, inculcate, infix, infuse, instil.

ingrain *vb* dye, imbue, impregnate.

ingratiate *vb* insinuate.

ingratitude *n* thanklessness, ungratefulness, unthankfulness.

ingredient *n* component, constituent, element.

ingress *n* entrance, entré, entry, introgression.

ingulf *see* **engulf**.

inhabit *vb* abide, dwell, live, occupy, people, reside, sojourn.

inhabitable *adj* habitable, livable.

inhabitant *n* citizen, denizen, dweller, inhabiter, resident.

inhalation *n* breath, inhaling, inspiration; sniff, snuff.

inhale *vb* breathe in, draw in, inbreathe, inspire.

inharmonious *adj* discordant, inharmonic, out of tune, unharmonious, unmusical.

inhere *vb* cleave to, stick, stick fast; abide, belong, exist, lie, pertain, reside.

inherent *adj* essential, immanent, inborn, inbred, indwelling, ingrained, innate, inseparable, intrinsic, native, natural, proper; adhering, sticking.

inherit *vb* get, receive.

inheritance *n* heritage, legacy, patrimony; inheriting.

inheritor *n* heir, (*law*) parcener.

inhibit *vb* bar, check, debar, hinder, obstruct, prevent, repress, restrain, stop; forbid, interdict, prohibit.

inhibition *n* check, hindrance, impediment, obstacle, obstruction, restraint; disallowance, embargo, interdict, interdiction, prevention, prohibition.

inhospitable *adj* cool, forbidding, unfriendly, unkind; bigoted, illiberal, intolerant, narrow, prejudiced, ungenerous, unreceptive; barren, wild.

inhospitality *n* inhospitableness, unkindness; illiberality, narrowness.

inhuman *adj* barbarous, brutal, cruel, fell, ferocious, merciless, pitiless, remorseless, ruthless, savage, unfeeling; nonhuman.

inhumanity *n* barbarity, brutality, cruelty, ferocity, savageness; hard-heartedness, unkindness.

inhume *vb* bury, entomb, inter.

inimical *adj* antagonistic, hostile, unfriendly; adverse, contrary, harmful, hurtful, noxious, opposed, pernicious, repugnant, unfavourable.

inimitable *adj* incomparable, matchless, peerless, unequalled, unexampled, unmatched, unparagoned, unparalleled, unrivalled, unsurpassed.

iniquitous *adj* atrocious, criminal, flagitious, heinous, inequitable, nefarious, sinful, wicked, wrong, unfair, unjust, unrighteous.

iniquity *n* injustice, sin, sinfulness, unrighteousness, wickedness, wrong; crime, misdeed, offence.

initial *adj* first; beginning, commencing, incipient, initiatory, introductory, opening, original; elementary, inchoate, rudimentary.

initiate *vb* begin, commence, enter upon, inaugurate, introduce, open; ground, indoctrinate, instruct, prime, teach.

initiation *n* beginning, commencement, inauguration, opening; admission, entrance, introduction; indoctrinate, instruction.

initiative *n* beginning; energy, enterprise.

initiatory *adj* inceptive, initiative.

inject *vb* force in, interject, insert, introduce, intromit.

injudicious *adj* foolish, hasty, ill-advised, ill-judged, imprudent, incautious, inconsiderate, indiscreet, rash, unwise.

injunction *n* admonition, bidding, command, mandate, order, precept.

injure *vb* damage, disfigure, harm, hurt, impair, mar, spoil, sully, wound; abuse, aggrieve, wrong; affront, dishonour, insult.

injurious *adj* baneful, damaging, deadly, deleterious, destructive, detrimental, disadvantageous, evil, fatal, hurtful, mischievous, noxious, pernicious, prejudicial, ruinous; inequitable, iniquitous, unjust, wrongful; contumelious, detractory, libellous, slanderous.

injury *n* evil, ill, injustice, wrong; damage, detriment, harm, hurt, impairment, loss, mischief, prejudice.

injustice *n* inequity, unfairness; grievance, iniquity, injury, wrong.

inkhorn *n* inkbottle, inkstand.

inkling *n* hint, intimation, suggestion, whisper.

inky *adj* atramentous, black, murky.

inland *adj* domestic, hinterland, home, upcountry; interior, internal.

inlet *n* arm, bay, bight, cove, creek; entrance, ingress, passage.

inmate *n* denizen, dweller, guest, intern, occupant.

inmost *adj* deepest, innermost.

inn *n* hostel, hostelry, hotel, pub, public house, tavern.

innate *adj* congenital, constitutional, inborn, inbred, indigenous, inherent, inherited, instinctive, native, natural, organic.

inner *adj* interior, internal.

innermost *adj* deepest, inmost.

innkeeper *n* host, innholder, landlady, landlord, tavernkeeper.

innocence *n* blamelessness, chastity, guilelessness, guiltlessness, purity, simplicity, sinlessness, stainlessness; harmlessness, innocuousness, innoxiousness, inoffensiveness.

innocent *adj* blameless, clean, clear, faultless, guiltless, immaculate, pure, sinless, spotless, unfallen, upright; harmless, innocuous, innoxious, inoffensive; lawful, legitimate, permitted; artless, guileless, ignorant, ingenuous, simple. • *n* babe, child, ingénue, naif, naive, unsophisticate.

innocuous *adj* harmless, innocent, inoffensive, safe.

innovate *vb* change, introduce.

innovation *n* change, introduction; departure, novelty.

innuendo *n* allusion, hint, insinuation, intimation, suggestion.

innumerable *adj* countless, numberless.

inoculate *vb* infect, vaccinate.

inoffensive *adj* harmless, innocent, innocuous, innoxious, unobjectionable, unoffending.

inoperative *adj* inactive, ineffectual, inefficacious, not in force.

inopportune *adj* ill-timed, inexpedient, infelicitous, mistimed, unfortunate, unhappy, unseasonable, untimely.

inordinate *adj* excessive, extravagant, immoderate, intemperate, irregular.

inorganic *adj* inanimate, unorganized; mineral.

inquest *n* inquiry, inquisition, investigation, quest, search.

inquietude *n* anxiety, disquiet, disquietude, disturbance, restlessness, uneasiness.

inquire, enquire *vb* ask, catechize, interpellate, interrogate, investigate, query, question, quiz.

inquiry, enquiry *n* examination, exploration, investigation, research, scrutiny, study; interrogation, query, question, quiz.

inquisition *n* examination, inquest, inquiry, investigation, search.

inquisitive *adj* curious, inquiring, scrutinizing; curious, meddlesome, peeping, peering, prying.

inroad *n* encroachment, foray, incursion, invasion, irruption, raid.

insalubrious *adj* noxious, unhealthful, unhealthy, unwholesome.

insane *adj* abnormal, crazed, crazy, delirious, demented, deranged, distracted, lunatic, mad, maniacal, unhealthy, unsound.

insanity *n* craziness, delirium, dementia, derangement, lunacy, madness, mania, mental aberration, mental alienation.

insatiable *adj* greedy, rapacious, voracious; insatiate, unappeasable.

inscribe *vb* emblaze, endorse, engrave, enroll, impress, imprint, letter, mark, write; address, dedicate.

inscrutable *adj* hidden, impenetrable, incomprehensible, inexplicable, mysterious, undiscover-able, unfathomable, unsearchable.

inscrutableness *n* impenetrability, incomprehensibility, incomprehensibleness, inexplicability, inscrutability, mysteriousness, mystery, unfathomableness, unsearchableness.

insecure *adj* risky, uncertain, unconfident, unsure; exposed, ill-protected, unprotected, unsafe; dangerous, hazardous, perilous; infirm, shaking, shaky, tottering, unstable, weak, wobbly.

insecurity *n* riskiness, uncertainty; danger, hazardousness, peril; instability, shakiness, weakness, wobbliness.

insensate *adj* dull, indifferent, insensible, torpid; brutal, foolish, senseless, unwise; inanimate, insensible, insentient, nonpercipient, unconscious, unperceiving.

insensibility *n* dullness, insentience, lethargy, torpor; apathy, indifference, insusceptibility, unfeelingness, dullness, stupidity; anaesthesia, coma, stupor, unconsciousness.

insensible *adj* imperceivable, imperceptible, undiscoverable; blunted, brutish, deaf, dull, insensate, numb, obtuse, senseless, sluggish, stolid, stupid, torpid, unconscious; apathetic, callous, phlegmatic, impassive, indifferent, insensitive, insentient, unfeeling, unimpressible, unsusceptible.

insensibly *adv* imperceptibly.

insentient *adj* inert, nonsentient, senseless; inanimate, insensible, insensate, nonpercipient, unconscious, unperceiving.

inseparable *adj* close, friendly, intimate, together; incissoluble, indivisible, inseverable.

insert *vb* infix, inject, intercalate, interpolate, introduce, inweave, parenthesize, place, put, set.

inside *adj* inner, interior, internal; confidential, exclusive, internal, private, secret. • *adv* indoors, within. • *n* inner part, interior; nature.

insidious *adj* creeping, deceptive, gradual, secretive; arch, artful, crafty, crooked, cunning, deceitful, designing, diplomatic, foxy, guileful, intriguing, Machiavellian, sly, sneaky, subtle, treacherous, trickish, tricky, wily.

insight *n* discernment, intuition, penetration, perception, perspicuity, understanding.

insignia *npl* badges, marks.

insignificance *n* emptiness, nothingenss, paltriness, triviality, unimportance.

insignificant *adj* contemptible, empty, immaterial, inconsequential, inconsiderable, inferior, meaningless, paltry, petty, small, sorry, trifling, trivial, unessential, unimportant

insincere *adj* deceitful, dishonest, disingenuous, dissembling, dissimulating, double-faced, double-tongued, duplicitous, empty, faithless, false, hollow, hypocritical, pharisaical, truthless, uncandid, untrue.

insincerity *n* bad faith, deceitfulness, dishonesty, disingenuousness, dissimulation, duplicity, falseness, faithlessness, hypocrisy.

insinuate *vb* hint, inculcate, infuse, ingratiate, instil, intimate, introduce, suggest.

insipid *adj* dead, dull, flat, heavy, inanimate, jejune, lifeless, monotonous, pointless, prosaic, prosy, spiritless, stupid, tame, unentertaining, uninteresting; mawkish, savourless, stale, tasteless, vapid, zestless.

insipidity, insipidness *n* dullness, heaviness, lifelessness, prosiness, stupidity, tameness; flatness, mawkishness, staleness, tastlessness, unsavouriness, vapidness, zestlessness.

insist *vb* demand, maintain, urge.

insistence *n* importunity, solicitousness, urging, urgency.

insnare *see* **ensnare**.

insolence *n* impertinence, impudence, malapertness, pertness, rudeness, sauciness; contempt, contumacy, contumely, disrespect, frowardness, insubordination.

insolent *adj* abusive, contemptuous, contumelious, disrespectful, domineering, insulting, offensive, overbearing, rude, supercilious; cheeky, impertinent, impudent, malapert, pert, saucy; contumacious, disobedient, froward, insubordinate.

insoluble *adj* indissoluble, indissolvable, irreducible; inexplicable, insolvable.

insolvable *adj* inexplicable.

insolvent *adj* bankrupt, broken, failed, ruined.

insomnia *n* sleeplessness, wakefulness.

inspect *vb* examine, investigate, look into, pry into, scrutinize; oversee, superintend, supervise.

inspection *n* examination, investigation, scrutiny; oversight, superintendence, supervision.

inspector *n* censor, critic, examiner, visitor; boss, overseer, superintendent, supervisor.

inspiration *n* breathing, inhalation; afflatus, fire, inflatus; elevation, exaltation; enthusiasm.

inspire *vb* breathe, inhale; infuse, instil; animate, cheer, enliven, inspirit; elevate, exalt, stimulate; fill, imbue, impart, inform, quicken.

inspirit *vb* animate, arouse, cheer, comfort, embolden, encourage, enhearten, enliven, fire, hearten, incite, invigorate, quicken, rouse, stimulate.

instable *see* **unstable**.

instability *n* changeableness, fickleness, inconstancy, insecurity, mutability.

install, instal *vb* inaugurate, induct, introduce; establish, place, set up.

installation *n* inauguration, induction, instalment, investiture.

instalment *n* earnest, payment, portion.

instance *vb* adduce, cite, mention, specify. • *n* case, example, exemplification, illustration, occasion; impulse, incitement, instigation, motive, prompting, request, solicitation.

instant *adj* direct, immediate, instantaneous, prompt, quick; current, present; earnest, fast, imperative, importunate, pressing, urgent; ready cocked. • *n* flash, jiffy, moment, second, trice, twinkling; hour, time.

instantaneous *adj* abrupt, immediate, instant, quick, sudden.

instantaneously *adv* forthwith, immediately, presto, quickly, right away.

instauration *n* reconstitution, reconstruction, redintegration, re-establishment, rehabilitation, reinstatement, renewal, renovation, restoration.

instead *adv* in lieu, in place, rather.

instigate *vb* actuate, agitate, encourage, impel, incite, influence, initiate, move, persuade, prevail upon, prompt, provoke, rouse, set on, spur on, stimulate, stir up, tempt, urge.

instigation *n* encouragement, incitement, influence, instance, prompting, solicitation, urgency.

instil, instill *vb* enforce, implant, impress, inculcate, ingraft; impart, infuse, insinuate.

instillation *n* infusion, insinuation, introduction.

instinct *n* natural impulse.

instinctive *adj* automatic, inherent, innate, intuitive, involuntary, natural, spontaneous; impulsive, unreflecting.

institute[1] *n* academy, college, foundation, guild, institution, school; custom, doctrine, dogma, law, maxim, precedent, principle, rule, tenet.

institute[2] *vb* begin, commence, constitute, establish, found, initial, install, introduce, organize, originate, start.

institution *n* enactment, establishment, foundation, institute, society; investiture; custom, law, practice.

instruct *vb* discipline, educate, enlighten, exercise, guide, indoctrinate, inform, initiate, school, teach, train; apprise, bid, command, direct, enjoin, order, prescribe to.

instruction *n* breeding, discipline, education, indoctrination, information, nurture, schooling, teaching, training, tuition; advice, counsel, precept; command, direction, mandate, order.

instructor *n* educator, master, preceptor, schoolteacher, teacher, tutor.

instrument *n* appliance, apparatus, contrivance, device, implement, musical instrument, tool, utensil; agent, means, medium; charter, deed, document, indenture, writing.

instrumental *adj* ancillary, assisting, auxiliary, conducive, contributory, helpful, helping, ministerial, ministrant, serviceable, subservient, subsidiary.

instrumentality *n* agency, intermediary; intervention, means, mediation.

insubordinate *adj* disobedient, disorderly, mutinous, refractory, riotous, seditious, turbulent, ungovernable, unruly.

insubordination *n* disobedience, insurrection, mutiny, revolt, riotousness, sedition; indiscipline, laxity.

insufferable *adj* intolerable, unbearable, unendurable, insupportable; abominable, detestable, disgusting, execrable, outrageous.

insufficiency *n* dearth, defectiveness, deficiency, lack, inadequacy, inadequateness, incapability, incompetence, paucity, shortage.

insufficient *adj* deficient, inadequate, incommensurate, incompetent, scanty; incapable, incompetent, unfitted, unqualified, unsuited, unsatisfactory.

insular *adj* contracted, illiberal, limited, narrow, petty, prejudiced, restricted; isolated, remote.

insulate *vb* detach, disconnect, disengage, disunite, isolate, separate.

insulation *n* disconnection, disengagement, isolation, separation.

insult *vb* abuse, affront, injure, offend, outrage, slander, slight. • *n* abuse, affront, cheek, contumely, indignity, insolence, offence, outrage, sauce, slight.

insulting *adj* abusive, arrogant, contumelious, impertinent, impolite, insolent, rude, vituperative.

insuperable *adj* impassable, insurmountable.

insupportable *adj* insufferable, intolerable, unbearable, unendurable.

insuppressible *adj* irrepressible, uncontrollable.

insurance *n* assurance, security.

insure *vb* assure, guarantee, indemnify, secure, underwrite.

insurgent *adj* disobedient, insubordinate, mutinous, rebellious, revolting, revolutionary, seditious. • *n* mutineer, rebel, revolter, revolutionary.

insurmountable *adj* impassable, insuperable.

insurrection *n* insurgence, mutiny, rebellion, revolt, revolution, rising, sedition, uprising.

intact *adj* scathless, unharmed, unhurt, unimpaired, uninjured, untouched; complete, entire, integral, sound, unbroken, undiminished, whole.

intangible *adj* dim, impalpable, imperceptible, indefinite, insubstantial, intactile, shadowy, vague; aerial, phantom, spiritous.

intangibility *n* imperceptibility, insubstantiality, intangibleness, shadowiness, vagueness.

integral *adj* complete, component, entire, integrant, total, whole.

integrity *n* goodness, honesty, principle, probity, purity, rectitude, soundness, uprightness, virtue; completeness, entireness, entirety, wholeness.

integument *n* coat, covering, envelope, skin, tegument.

intellect *n* brains, cognitive faculty, intelligence, mind, rational faculty, reason, reasoning, faculty, sense, thought, understanding, wit.

intellectual *adj* cerebral, intelligent, mental, scholarly, thoughtful. • *n* academic, highbrow, pundit, savant, scholar.

intelligence *n* acumen, apprehension, brightness, discernment, imagination, insight, penetration, quickness, sagacity, shrewdness, understanding, wits; information, knowledge; advice, instruction, news, notice, notification, tidings; brains, intellect, mentality, sense, spirit.

intelligent *adj* acute, alert, apt, astute, brainy, bright, clear-headed, clear-sighted, clever, discerning, keen-eyed, keen-sighted, knowing, long-headed, quick, quick-sighted, sagacious, sensible, sharp-sighted, sharp-witted, shrewd, understanding.

intelligibility *n* clarity, comprehensibility, intelligibleness, perspicuity.

intelligible *adj* clear, comprehensible, distinct, evident, lucid, manifest, obvious, patent, perspicuous, plain, transparent, understandable.

intemperate *adj* drunken; excessive, extravagant, extreme, immoderate, inordinate, unbridled, uncontrolled, unrestrained; self-indulgent.

intend *vb* aim at, contemplate, design, determine, drive at, mean, meditate, propose, purpose, think of.

intendant *n* inspector, overseer, superintendent, supervisor.

intense *adj* ardent, earnest, fervid, passionate, vehement; close, intent, severe, strained, stretched, strict; energetic, forcible, keen, potent, powerful, sharp, strong, vigorous, violent; acute, deep, extreme, exquisite, grievous, poignant.

intensify *vb* aggravate, concentrate, deepen, enhance, heighten, quicken, strengthen, whet.

intensity *n* closeness, intenseness, severity, strictness; excess, extremity, violence; activity, energy, force, power, strength, vigour; ardour, earnestness, vehemence.

intensive *adj* emphatic, intensifying.

intent *adj* absorbed, attentive, close, eager, earnest, engrossed, occupied, pre-occupied, zealous; bent, determined, decided, resolved, set. • *n* aim, design, drift, end, import, intention, mark, meaning, object, plan, purport, purpose, purview, scope, view.

intention *n* aim, design, drift, end, import, intent, mark, meaning, object, plan, purport, purpose, purview, scope, view.

intentional *adj* contemplated, deliberate, designed, intended, preconcerted, predetermined, premeditated, purposed, studied, voluntary, wilful.

inter *vb* bury, commit to the earth, entomb, inhume, inurn.

intercalate *vb* insert, interpolate.

intercede *vb* arbitrate, interpose, mediate; entreat, plead, supplicate.

intercept *vb* cut off, interrupt, obstruct, seize.

intercession *n* interposition, intervention, mediation; entreaty, pleading, prayer, supplication.

intercessor *n* interceder, mediator.

interchange *vb* alternate, change, exchange, vary. • *n* alternation.

interchangeableness *n* interchangeability.

interchangeably *adv* alternately.

intercourse *n* commerce, communication, communion, connection, converse, correspondence, dealings, fellowship, truck; acquaintance, intimacy.

interdict *vb* debar, forbid, inhibit, prohibit, prescribe, proscribe, restrain from. • *n* ban, decree, interdiction, prohibition.

interest *vb* affect, concern, touch; absorb, attract, engage, enlist, excite, grip, hold, occupy. • *n* advantage, benefit, good, profit, weal; attention, concern, regard, sympathy; part, participation, portion, share, stake; discount, premium, profit.

interested *adj* attentive, concerned, involved, occupied; biassed, patial, prejudiced; selfish, self-seeking.

interesting *adj* attractive, engaging, entertaining, pleasing.

interfere *vb* intermeddle, interpose, meddle; clash, collide, conflict.

interference *n* intermeddling, interposition; clashing, collision, interfering, opposition.

interim *n* intermediate time, interval, meantime.

interior *adj* inmost, inner, internal, inward; inland, remote; domestic, home. • *n* inner part, inland, inside.

interjacent *adj* intermediate, interposed, intervening, parenthetical.

interject *vb* comment, inject, insert, interpose.

interjection *n* exclamation.

interlace *vb* bind, complicate, entwine, intersperse, intertwine, interweave, inweave, knit, mix, plait, twine, twist, unite.

interlard *vb* difersify, interminate, intersperse, intertwine, mix, vary.

interline *vb* insert, write between.

interlineal *adj* interlinear, interlined.

interlink, interlock *vb* connect, interchain, interrelate, join.

interlocution *n* colloquy, conference, dialogue, interchange.

interlocutor *n* respondent, speaker.

interloper *n* intruder, meddler.

intermeddle *vb* interfere, interpose, meddle.

intermediary *n* go-between, mediator.

intermediate *adj* interjacent, interposed, intervening, mean, median, middle, transitional.

interment *n* burial, entombment, inhumation, sepulture.

interminable *adj* boundless, endless, illimitable, immeasurable, infinite, limitless, unbounded, unlimited; long-drawn-out, tedious, wearisome.

intermingle *vb* blend, commingle, commix, intermix, mingle, mix.

intermission *n* cessation, interruption, interval, lull, pause, remission, respite, rest, stop, stoppage, suspension.

intermit *vb* interrupt, intervene, stop, suspend; discontinue, give over, leave off; abate, subside.

intermittent *adj* broken, capricious, discontinuous, fitful, flickering, intermitting, periodic, recurrent, remittent, spasmodic.

intermix *vb* blend, commingle, commix, intermingle, mingle, mix.

internal *adj* inner, inside, interior, inward; incorporeal, mental, spiritual; deeper, emblematic, hidden, higher, metaphorical, secret, symbolical, under; genuine, inherent, intrinsic, real, true; domestic, home, inland, inside.

international *adj* cosmopolitan, universal.

internecine *adj* deadly, destructive, exterminating, exterminatory, interneciary, internecinal, internecive, mortal.

interpellate *vb* interrogate, question.

interpellation *n* interruption; intercession, interposition; interrogation, questioning.

interplay *n* interaction.

interpolate *vb* add, foist, insert, interpose; (*math*) intercalate, introduce.

interpose *vb* arbitrate, intercede, intervene, mediate; interfere, intermeddle, interrupt, meddle, tamper; insert, interject, put in, remark, sandwich, set between; intrude, thrust in.

interposition *n* intercession, interpellation, intervention, mediation.

interpret *vb* decipher, decode, define, elucidate, explain, expound, solve, unfold, unravel; construe, render, translate.

interpretation *n* meaning, sense, signification; elucidation, explanation, explication, exposition; construction, rendering, rendition, translation, version.

interpreter *n* expositor, expounder, translator.

interrogate *vb* ask, catechize, examine, inquire of, interpellate, question.

interrogation *n* catechizing, examination, examining, interpellation, interrogating, questioning; inquiry, query, question.

interrogative *adj* interrogatory, questioning.

interrupt *vb* break, check, disturb, hinder, intercept, interfere with, obstruct, pretermit, stop; break, cut, disconnect, disjoin, dissever, dissolve, disunite, divide, separate, sever, sunder; break off, cease, discontinue, intermit, leave off, suspend.

interruption *n* hindrance, impediment, obstacle, obstruction, stop, stoppage; cessation, discontinuance, intermission, pause, suspension; break, breaking, disconnecting, disconnection, disjunction, dissolution, disunion, disuniting, division, separation, severing, sundering.

intersect *vb* cross, cut, decussate, divide, interrupt.
intersection *n* crossing.
interspace *n* interlude, interstice, interval.
intersperse *vb* intermingle, scatter, sprinkle; diversify, interlard, mix.
interstice *n* interspace, interval, space; chink, crevice.
interstitial *adj* intermediate, intervening.
intertwine *vb* interlace, intertwine, interweave, inweave, twine.
interval *n* interim, interlude, interregnum, pause, period, recess, season, space, spell, term; interstice, skip.
intervene *vb* come between, interfere, mediate; befall, happen, occur.
intervening *adj* interjacent, intermediate; interstitial.
intervention *n* interference, interposition; agency, mediation.
interview *n* conference, consultation, parley; meeting.
interweave *vb* interlace, intertwine, inweave, weave; intermingle, intermix, mingle, mix.
intestinal *adj* domestic, interior, internal.
intestines *npl* bowels, entrails, guts, insides, inwards, viscera.
intimacy *n* close acquaintance, familiarity, fellowship, friendship; closeness, nearness.
intimate[1] *adj* close, near; familiar, friendly; bosom, chummy, close, dear, homelike, special; confidential, personal, private, secret; detailed, exhaustive, first-hand, immediate, penetrating, profound; cosy, warm. • *n* chum, confidant, companion, crony, friend.
intimate[2] *vb* allude to, express, hint, impart, indicate, insinuate, signify, suggest, tell.
intimately *adv* closely, confidentially, familiarly, nearly, thoroughly.
intimation *n* allusion, hint, innuendo, insinuation, suggestion.
intimidate *vb* abash, affright, alarm, appal, browbeat, bully, cow, daunt, dishearten, dismay, frighten, overawe, scare, subdue, terrify, terrorize.
intimidation *n* fear, intimidating, terror, terrorism.
intolerable *adj* insufferable, insupportable, unbearable, unendurable.
intolerance *n* bigotry, narrowness; impatience, rejection.
intolerant *adj* bigoted, narrow, proscriptive; dictatorial, impatient, imperious, overbearing, supercilious.
intonation *n* cadence, modulation, tone; musical recitation.
in toto *adv* entirely, wholly.
intoxicate *vb* fuddle, inebriate, muddle.
intoxicated *adj* boozy, drunk, drunken, fuddled, inebriated, maudlin, mellow, muddled, stewed, tight, tipsy.
intoxication *n* drunkenness, ebriety, inebriation, inebriety; excitement, exhilaration, infatuation.
intractability *n* cantankerousness, contrariety, inflexibility, intractableness, obduracy, obstinacy, perverseness, perversity, pig-headedness, stubbornness, wilfulness.
intractable *adj* cantankerous, contrary, contumacious, cross-grained, dogged, froward, headstrong, indocile, inflexible, mulish, obdurate, obstinate, perverse, pig-headed, refractory, restive, stubborn, tough, uncontrollable, ungovernable, unmanageable, unruly, unyielding, wilful.
intrench *see* **entrench**.
intrenchment *see* **entrenchment**.
intrepid *adj* bold, brave, chivalrous, courageous, daring, dauntless, doughty, fearless, gallant, heroic, unappalled, unawed, undaunted, undismayed, unterrified, valiant, valorous.
intrepidity *n* boldness, bravery, courage, daring, dauntlessness, fearlessness, gallantry, heroism, intrepidness, prowess, spirit, valour.
intricacy *n* complexity, complication, difficulty, entanglement, intricateness, involution, obscurity, perplexity.
intricate *adj* complicated, difficult, entangled, involved, mazy, obscure, perplexed.
intrigue *vb* connive, conspire, machinate, plot, scheme; beguile, bewitch, captivate, charm, fascinate. • *n* artifice, cabal, conspiracy, deception, finesse, Machiavelianism, machination, manoeuvre, plot, ruse, scheme, stratagem, wile; amour, liaison, love affair.
intriguing *adj* arch, artful, crafty, crooked, cunning, deceitful, designing, diplomatic, foxy, Machiavelian, insidious, politic, sly, sneaky, subtle, tortuous, trickish, tricky, wily.
intrinsic *adj* essential, genuine, real, sterling, true; inborn, inbred, ingrained, inherent, internal, inward, native, natural.
intrinsically *adv* essentially, really, truly; inherently, naturally.

introduce *vb* bring in, conduct, import, induct, inject, insert, lead in, usher in; present; begin, broach, commence, inaugurate, initiate, institute, start.
introduction *n* exordium, preface, prelude, proem; introducing, ushering in; presentation.
introductory *adj* precursory, prefatory, preliminary, proemial.
introspection *n* introversion, self-contemplation.
intrude *vb* encroach, impose, infringe, interfere, interlope, obtrude, trespass.
intruder *n* interloper, intermeddler, meddler, stranger.
intrusion *n* encroachment, infringement, intruding, obtrusion.
intrusive *adj* obtrusive, trespassing.
intuition *n* apprehension, cognition, insight, instinct; clairvoyance, divination, presentiment.
intuitive *adj* instinctive, intuitional, natural; clear, distinct, full, immediate.
intumesce *vb* bubble up, dilate, expand, swell.
intumescence *n* inturgescence, swelling, tumefaction, turgescence.
inundate *vb* deluge, drown, flood, glut, overflow, overwhelm, submerge.
inundation *n* cataclysm, deluge, flood, glut, overflow, superfluity.
inure *vb* accustom, discipline, familiarize, habituate, harden, toughen, train, use.
inutile *adj* bootless, ineffectual, inoperative, unavailing, unprofitable, useless.
invade *vb* encroach upon, infringe, violate; attack, enter in, march into.
invalid[1] *adj* baseless, fallacious, false, inoperative, nugatory, unfounded, unsound, untrue, worthless; (*law*) null, void.
invalid[2] *adj* ailing, bedridden, feeble, frail, ill, infirm, sick, sickly, valetudinary, weak, weakly. • *n* convalescent, patient, valetudinarian.
invalidate *vb* abrogate, annul, cancel, nullify, overthrow, quash, repeal, reverse, undo, unmake, vitiate.
invalidity *n* baselessness, fallaciousness, fallacy, falsity, unsoundness.
invaluable *adj* inestimable, priceless.
invariable *adj* changeless, constant, unchanging, uniform, unvarying; changeless, immutable, unalterable, unchangeable.
invariableness *n* changelessness, constancy, uniformity, unvaryingness; changelessness, immutability, unchangeableness, invariability.
invasion *n* encroachment, incursion, infringement, inroad; aggression, assault, attack, foray, raid.
invective *n* abuse, censure, contumely, denunciation, diatribe, railing, reproach, sarcasm, satire, vituperation.
inveigh *vb* blame, censure, condemn, declaim against, denounce, exclaim against, rail at, reproach, vituperate.
inveigle *vb* contrive, devise; concoct, conceive, create, design, excogitate, frame, imagine, originate; coin, fabricate, forge, spin.
invent *vb* concoct, contrive, design, devise, discover, fabricate, find out, frame, originate
invention *n* creation, discovery, ingenuity, inventing, origination; contrivance, design, device; coinage, fabrication, fiction, forgery.
inventive *adj* creative, fertile, ingenious.
inventor *n* author, contriver, creator, originator.
inventory *n* account, catalogue, list, record, roll, register, schedule.
inverse *adj* indirect, inverted, opposite, reversed.
inversion *n* inverting, reversing, transposal, transposition.
invert *vb* capsize, overturn; reverse, transpose.
invertebrate *adj* invertebral; spineless.
invest *vb* put money into; confer, endow, endue; (*mil*) beset, besiege, enclose, surround; array, clothe, dress.
investigate *vb* canvass, consider, dissect, examine, explore, follow up, inquire into, look into, overhaul, probe, question, research, scrutinize, search into, search out, sift, study.
investigation *n* examination, exploration, inquiry, inquisition, overhauling, research, scrutiny, search, sifting, study.
investiture *n* habilitation, induction, installation, ordination.
investment *n* money invested; endowment; (*mil*) beleaguerment, siege; clothes, dress, garments, habiliments, robe, vestment.
inveteracy *n* inveterateness, obstinacy.
inveterate *adj* accustomed, besetting, chronic, confirmed, deep-seated, habitual, habituated, hardened, ingrained, long-established, obstinate.

invidious *adj* disagreeable, envious, hateful, odious, offensive, unfair.

invigorate *vb* animate, brace, energize, fortify, harden, nerve, quicken, refresh, stimulate, strengthen, vivify.

invincible *adj* impregnable, indomitable, ineradicable, insuperable, insurmountable, irrepressible, unconquerable, unsubduable, unyielding.

inviolable *adj* hallowed, holy, inviolate, sacramental, sacred, sacrosanct, stainless.

inviolate *adj* unbroken, unviolated; pure, stainless, unblemished, undefiled, unhurt, uninjured, unpolluted, unprofaned, unstained; inviolable, sacred.

invisibility *n* imperceptibility, indistinctness, invisibleness, obscurity.

invisible *adj* impalpable, imperceptible, indistinguishable, intangible, unapparent, undiscernable, unperceivable, unseen.

invitation *n* bidding, call, challenge, solicitation, summons.

invite *vb* ask, bid, call, challenge, request, solicit, summon; allure, attract, draw on, entice, lead, persuade, prevail upon.

inviting *adj* alluring, attractive, bewitching, captivating, engaging, fascinating, pleasing, winning; prepossessing, promising.

invocation *n* conjuration, orison, petition, prayer, summoning, supplication.

invoice *vb* bill, list. • *n* bill, inventory, list, schedule.

invoke *vb* adjure, appeal to, beseech, beg, call upon, conjure, entreat, implore, importune, pray, pray to, solicit, summon, supplicate.

involuntary *adj* automatic, blind, instinctive, mechanical, reflex, spontaneous, unintentional; compulsory, reluctant, unwilling.

involve *vb* comprise, contain, embrace, imply, include, lead to; complicate, compromise, embarrass, entangle, implicate, incriminate, inculpate; cover, envelop, enwrap, surround, wrap; blend, conjoin, connect, join, mingle; entwine, interlace, intertwine, interweave, inweave.

invulnerability *n* invincibility, invulnerableness.

invulnerable *adj* incontrovertible, invincible, unassailable, irrefragable.

inward[1] *adj* incoming, inner, interior, internal; essential, hidden, mental, spiritual; private, secret.

inward[2], **inwards** *adv* inwardly, towards the inside, within.

inweave *vb* entwine, interlace, intertwine, interweave, weave together.

iota *n* atom, bit, glimmer, grain, jot, mite, particle, scintilla, scrap, shadow, spark, tittle, trace, whit.

irascibility *n* hastiness, hot-headedness, impatience, irascibleness, irritability, peevishness, petulance, quickness, spleen, testiness, touchiness.

irascible *adj* choleric, cranky, hasty, hot, hot-headed, impatient, irritable, nettlesome, peevish, peppery, pettish, petulant, quick, splenetic, snappish, testy, touchy, waspish.

irate *adj* angry, incensed, ireful, irritated, piqued.

ire *n* anger, choler, exasperation, fury, indignation, passion, rage, resentment, wrath.

ireful *adj* angry, furious, incensed, irate, raging, passionate.

iridescent *adj* irisated, nacreous, opalescent, pavonine, prismatic, rainbow-like.

iris *n* rainbow; (*bot*) fleur-de-lis, flower-de-luce; diaphragm of the eye.

irksome *adj* annoying, burdensome, humdrum, monotonous, tedious, tiresome, wearisome, weary, wearying.

iron *adj* ferric, ferrous.

ironic, ironical *adj* mocking, sarcastic.

irons *npl* chains, fetters, gyves, hampers, manacles, shackles.

irony *n* mockery, raillery, ridicule, sarcasm, satire.

irradiate *vb* brighten, illume, illuminate, illumine, light up, shine upon.

irrational *adj* absurd, extravagant, foolish, injudicious, preposterous, ridiculous, silly, unwise; unreasonable, unreasoning, unthinking; brute, brutish; aberrant, alienated, brainless, crazy, demented, fantastic, idiotic, imbecilic, insane, lunatic.

irrationality *n* absurdity, folly, foolishness, unreasonableness; brutishness.

irreclaimable *adj* hopeless, incurable, irrecoverable, irreparable, irretrievable, irreversible, remediless; abandoned, graceless, hardened, impenitent, incorrigible, lost, obdurate, profligate, recreant, reprobate, shameless, unrepentant.

irreconcilable *adj* implacable, inexorable, inexpiable, unappeasable; incompatible, incongruous, inconsistent.

irrecoverable *adj* hopeless, incurable, irremediable, irreparable, irretrievable, remediless.

irrefragable *adj* impregnable, incontestable, incontrovertible, indisputable, invincible, irrefutable, irresistible, unanswerable, unassailable, undeniable.

irrefutable *adj* impregnable, incontestable, incontrovertible, indisputable, invincible, irrefragable, irresistible, unanswerable, unassailable, undeniable.

irregular *adj* aberrant, abnormal, anomalistic, anomalous, crooked, devious, eccentric, erratic, exceptional, heteromorphous, raged, tortuous, unconformable, unusual; capricious, changeable, desultory, fitful, spasmodic, uncertain, unpunctual, unsettled, variable; disordered, disorderly, improper, uncanonical, unparliamentary, unsystematic; asymmetric, uneven, unsymmetrical; disorderly, dissolute, immoral, loose, wild. • *n* casual, freelance, hireling, mercenary.

irregularity *n* aberration, abnormality, anomaly, anomalousness, singularity; capriciousness, changeableness, uncertainty, variableness; asymmetry; disorderliness, dissoluteness, immorality, laxity, looseness, wildness.

irrelevance, irrelevancy *n* impertinency, inapplicability, nonpertinency.

irrelevant *adj* extraneous, foreign, illogical, impertinent, inapplicable, inapposite, inappropriate, inconsequent, unessential, unrelated.

irreligion *n* atheism, godlessness, impiety, ungodliness.

irreligious *adj* godless, ungodly, undevout; blasphemous, disrespectful, impious, irreverent, profane, ribald, wicked.

irremediable *adj* hopeless, incurable, immedicable, irrecoverable, irreparable, remediless.

irremissible *adj* binding, inexpiable, obligatory, unatonable, unpardonable.

irreparable *adj* irrecoverable, irremediable, irretrievable, remediless.

irreprehensible *adj* blameless, faultless, inculpable, innocent, irreproachable, irreprovable, unblamable.

irrepressible *adj* insuppressible, uncontrollable, unquenchable, unsmotherable.

irreproachable *adj* blameless, faultless, inculpable, innocent, irreprehensible, irreprovable, unblamable.

irresistible *adj* irrefragable, irrepressible, overpowering, overwhelming, resistless.

irresolute *adj* changeable, faltering, fickle, hesitant, hesitating, inconstant, mutable, spineless, uncertain, undecided, undetermined, unsettled, unstable, unsteady, vacillating, wavering.

irrespective *adj* independent, regardless.

irresponsible *adj* unaccountable; untrustworthy.

irretrievable *adj* incurable, irrecoverable, irremediable, irreparable, remediless.

irreverence *n* blasphemy, impiety, profaneness, profanity; disesteem, disrespect.

irreverent *adj* blasphemous, impious, irreligious, profane; disrespectful, slighting.

irreversible *adj* irrepealable, irrevocable, unalterable, unchangeable; changeless, immutable, invariable.

irrevocable *adj* irrepealable, irreversible, unalterable, unchangeable.

irrigate *vb* moisten, wash, water, wet.

irrigation *n* watering.

irritability *n* excitability, fretfulness, irascibility, peevishness, petulance, snappishness, susceptibility, testiness.

irritable *adj* captious, choleric, excitable, fiery, fretful, hasty, hot, irascible, passionate, peppery, peevish, pettish, petulant, snappish, splenetic, susceptible, testy, touchy, waspish.

irritate *vb* anger, annoy, chafe, enrage, exacerbate, exasperate, fret, incense, jar, nag, nettle, offend, provoke, rasp, rile, ruffle, vex; gall, tease; (*med*) excite, inflame, stimulate.

irritation *n* irritating; anger, exacerbation, exasperation, excitement, indignation, ire, passion, provocation, resentment, wrath; (*med*) excitation, inflammation, stimulation; burn, itch.

irruption *n* breaking in, bursting in; foray, incursion, inroad, invasion, raid.

island *n* atoll, isle, islet, reef.

isochronal *adj* isochronous, uniform.

isolate *vb* detach, dissociate, insulate, quarantine, segregate, separate, set apart.

isolated *adj* detached, separate, single, solitary.

isolation *n* detachment, disconnection, insulation, quarantine, segregation, separation; loneliness, solitariness, solitude.

issue *vb* come out, flow out, flow forth, gush, run, rush out, spout, spring, spurt, well; arise, come, emanate, ensue, flow, follow, originate, proceed, spring; end, eventuate, result, terminate; appear, come out, deliver, depart, debouch, discharge, emerge, emit, put forth, send out; distribute, give out; publish, utter. • *n* conclusion, consequence, consummation, denouement, end, effect, event, finale, outcome, result, termination, upshot; antagonism, contest, controversy; debouchment, delivering, delivery, discharge, emergence, emigration, emission, issuance; flux, outflow, outpouring, stream; copy, edition, number; egress, exit, outlet, passage cut, vent, way out; escape, sally, sortie; children, offspring, posterity, progeny.

itch *vb* tingle. • *n* itching; burning, coveting, importunate craving, teasing desire, uneasy hankering.

itching *n* itch; craving, longing, importunate craving, desire, appetite, hankering.

item *adv* also, in like manner. • *n* article, detail, entry, particular, point.

iterate *vb* reiterate, repeat.

itinerant *adj* nomadic, peripatetic, roaming, roving, travelling, unsettled, wandering.

itinerary *n* guide, guidebook; circuit, route.

J

jabber *vb* chatter, gabble, prate, prattle.

jacket *n* casing, cover, sheath; anorak, blazer coat, doublet, jerkin.

jaded *adj* dull, exhausted, fatigued, satiated, tired, weary.

jagged *adj* cleft, divided, indented, notched, serrated, ragged, uneven.

jail, gaol *n* bridewell, (*sl*) clink, dungeon, lockup, (*sl*) nick, penitentiary, prison.

jam *vb* block, crowd, crush, press. • *n* block, crowd, crush, mass, pack, press.

jangle *vb* bicker, chatter, dispute, gossip, jar, quarrel, spar, spat, squabble, tiff, wrangle. • *n* clang, clangour, clash, din, dissonance.

jar¹ *vb* clash, grate, interfere, shake; bicker, contend, jangle, quarrel, spar, spat, squabble, tiff, wrangle; agitate, jolt, jounce, shake. • *n* clash, conflict, disaccord, discord, jangle, dissonance; agitation, jolt, jostle, shake, shaking, shock, start.

jar² *n* can, crock, cruse, ewer, flagon.

jarring *adj* conflicting, discordant, inconsistent, inconsonant, wrangling.

jargon *n* gabble, gibberish, nonsense, rigmarole: argot, cant, lingo, slang; chaos, confusion, disarray, disorder, jumble.

jaundiced *adj* biased, envious, prejudiced.

jaunt *n* excursion, ramble, tour, trip.

jaunty *adj* airy, cheery, garish, gay, fine, fluttering, showy, sprightly, unconcerned.

jealous *adj* distrustful, envious, suspicious; anxious, apprehensive, intolerant, solicitous, zealous.

jealousy *n* envy, suspicion, watchfulness.

jeer *vb* deride, despise, flout, gibe, jape, jest, mock, scoff, sneer, spurn, rail, ridicule, taunt. • *n* abuse, derision, mockery, sneer, ridicule, taunt.

jeopardize *vb* endanger, hazard, imperil, risk, venture.

jeopardy *n* danger, hazard, peril, risk, venture.

jerk *vb*, *n* flip, hitch, pluck, tweak, twitch, yank.

jest *vb* banter, joke, quiz. • *n* fun, joke, pleasantry, raillery, sport.

jester *n* humorist, joker, wag; buffoon, clown, droll, fool, harlequin, punch.

jibe *see* **gibe**.

jiffy *n* instant, moment, second, twinkling, trice.

jilt *vb* break with, deceive, disappoint, discard. • *n* coquette, flirt, light-o'-love.

jingle *vb* chink, clink, jangle, rattle, tinkle. • *n* chink, clink, jangle, rattle, tinkle; chorus, ditty, melody, song.

jocose *adj* comical, droll, facetious, funny, humorous, jesting, jocular, merry, sportive, waggish, witty.

jocund *adj* airy, blithe, cheerful, debonair, frolicsome, jolly, joyful, joyous, lively, merry, playful.

jog *vb* jostle, notify, nudge, push, remind, warn; canter, run, trot. • *n* push, reminder.

join *vb* add, annex, append, attach; cement, combine, conjoin, connect, couple, dovetail, link, unite, yoke; amalgamate, assemble, associate, confederate, consolidate.

joint *vb* fit, join, unite. • *adj* combined, concerted, concurrent, conjoint. • *n* connection, junction, juncture, hinge, splice.

joke *vb* banter, jest, frolic, rally. • *n* crank, jest, quip, quirk, witticism.

jolly *adj* airy, blithe, cheerful, frolicsome, gamesome, facetious, funny, gay, jovial, joyous, merry, mirthful, jocular, jocund, playful, sportive, sprightly, waggish; bouncing, chubby, lusty, plump, portly, stout.

jolt *vb* jar, shake, shock. • *n* jar, jolting, jounce, shaking.

jostle *vb* collide, elbow, hustle, joggle, shake, shoulder, shove.

jot *n* ace, atom, bit, corpuscle, iota, grain, mite, particle, scrap, whit.

journal *n* daybook, diary, log; gazette, magazine, newspapers, periodical.

journey *vb* ramble, roam, rove, travel: fare, go, proceed. • *n* excursion, expedition, jaunt, passage, pilgrimage, tour, travel, trip, voyage.

jovial *adj* airy, convivial, festive, jolly, joyous, merry, mirthful.

joy *n* beatification, beatitude, delight, ecstasy, exultation, gladness, glee, mirth, pleasure, rapture, ravishment, transport; bliss, felicity, happiness.

joyful *adj* blithe, blithesome, buoyant, delighted, elate, elated, exultant, glad, happy, jocund, jolly, joyous, merry, rejoicing.

jubilant *adj* exultant, exulting, rejoicing, triumphant.

judge *vb* conclude, decide, decree, determine, pronounce; adjudicate, arbitrate, condemn, doom, sentence, try, umpire; account, apprehend, believe, consider, deem, esteem, guess, hold, imagine, measure, reckon, regard, suppose, think; appreciate, estimate. • *n* adjudicator, arbiter, arbitrator, bencher, justice, magistrate, moderator, referee, umpire, connoisseur, critic.

judgment, judgement *n* brains, ballast, circumspection, depth, discernment, discretion, discrimination, intelligence, judiciousness, penetration, prudence, sagacity, sense, sensibility, taste, understanding, wisdom, wit; conclusion, consideration, decision, determination, estimation, notion, opinion, thought; adjudication, arbitration, award, censure, condemnation, decree, doom, sentence.

judicious *adj* cautious, considerate, cool, critical, discriminating, discreet, enlightened, provident, politic, prudent, rational, reasonable, sagacious, sensible, sober, solid, sound, staid, wise.

jug *n* cruse, ewer, flagon, pitcher, vessel.

juicy *adj* lush, moist, sappy, succulent, watery; entertaining, exciting, interesting, lively, racy, spicy.

jumble *vb* confound, confuse, disarrange, disorder, mix, muddle. • *n* confusion, disarrangement, disorder, medley, mess, mixture, muddle.

jump *vb* bound, caper, clear, hop, leap, skip, spring, vault. • *n* bound, caper, hop, leak, skip, spring, vault; fence, hurdle, obstacle; break, gap, interruption, space; advance, boost, increase, rise; jar, jolt, shock, start, twitch.

junction *n* combination, connection, coupling, hook-up, joining, linking, seam, union; conjunction, joint, juncture.

junta *n* cabal, clique, combination, confederacy, coterie, faction, gang, league, party, set.

just *adj* equitable, lawful, legitimate, reasonable, right, rightful; candid, even-handed, fair, fair-minded, impartial; blameless, conscientious, good, honest, honourable, pure, square, straightforward, virtuous; accurate, correct, exact, normal, proper, regular, true; condign, deserved, due, merited, suitable.

justice *n* accuracy, equitableness, equity, fairness, honesty, impartiality, justness, right; judge, justiciary.

justifiable *adj* defensible, fit, proper, right, vindicable, warrantable.

justification *n* defence, exculpation, excuse, exoneration, reason, vindication, warrant.

justify *vb* approve, defend, exculpate, excuse, exonerate, maintain, vindicate, support, warrant.

justness *n* accuracy, correctness, fitness, justice, precision, propriety.

juvenile *adj* childish, immature, puerile, young, youthful. • *n* boy, child, girl, youth.

juxtaposition *n* adjacency, contiguity, contact, proximity.

K

keen[1] *adj* ardent, eager, earnest, fervid, intense, vehement, vivid; acute, sharp; cutting; acrimonious, biting, bitter, caustic, poignant, pungent, sarcastic, severe; astute, discerning, intelligent, quick, sagacious, sharp-sighted, shrewd.

keen[2] *vb* bemoan, bewail, deplore, grieve, lament, mourn, sorrow, weep. • *n* coronach, dirge, elegy, lament, lamentation, monody, plaint, requiem, threnody.

keenness *n* ardour, eagerness, fervour, vehemence, zest; acuteness, sharpness; rigour, severity, sternness; acrimony, asperity, bitterness, causticity, causticness, pungency; astuteness, sagacity, shrewdness.

keep *vb* detain, hold, retain; continue, preserve; confine, detain, reserve, restrain, withhold; attend, guard, preserve, protect; adhere to, fulfil; celebrate, commemorate, honour, observe, perform, solemnize; maintain, support, sustain; husband, save, store; abide, dwell, lodge, stay, remain; endure. last. • *n* board, maintenance, subsistence, support; donjon, dungeon, stronghold, tower.

keeper *n* caretaker, conservator, curator, custodian, defender, gaoler, governor, guardian, jailer, superintendent, warden, warder, watchman.

keeping *n* care, charge, custody, guard, possession; feed maintenance, support; agreement, conformity, congruity, consistency, harmony.

keepsake *n* memento, souvenir, token.

ken *n* cognizance, sight, view.

key *adj* basic, crucial, essential, important, major, principal. • *n* lock-opener, opener; clue, elucidation, explanation, guide, solution, translation; (*mus*) keynote, tonic; clamp, lever, wedge.

kick *vb* boot, punt; oppose, rebel, resist, spurn. • *n* force, intensity, power, punch, vitality; excitement, pleasure, thrill.

kidnap *vb* abduct, capture, carry off, remove, steal away.

kill *vb* assassinate, butcher, dispatch, destroy, massacre, murder, slaughter, slay.

kin *adj* akin, allied, cognate, kindred, related. • *n* affinity, consanguinity, relationship; connections, family, kindred, kinsfolk, relations, relatives, siblings.

kind[1] *adj* accommodating, amiable, beneficent, benevolent, benign, bland, bounteous, brotherly, charitable clement, compassionate, complaisant, gentle, good, good-natured, forbearing, friendly, generous, gracious, humane, indulgent, lenient, mild, obliging, sympathetic, tender, tender-hearted.

kind[2] *n* breed, class, family, genus, race, set, species, type; brand, character, colour, denomination, description, form, make, manner, nature, persuasion, sort, stamp, strain, style,

kindle *vb* fire, ignite, inflame, light; animate, awaken, bestir, exasperate, excite, foment, incite, provoke, rouse, stimulate, stir, thrill, warm.

kindliness *n* amiability, benevolence, benignity, charity, compassion, friendliness, humanity, kindness, sympathy; gentleness, mildness, softness.

kindly *adj* appropriate, congenial. kindred, natural, proper; benevolent, considerate, friendly, gracious, humane, sympathetic, well-disposed. • *adv* agreeably, graciously, humanely, politely, thoughtfully.

kindness *n* benefaction, charity, favour; amiability, beneficence, benevolence, benignity, clemency, generosity, goodness, grace, humanity, kindliness, mildness, philanthropy, sympathy, tenderness.

kindred *adj* akin, allied, congenial, connected, related, sympathetic. • *n* affinity, consanguinity, flesh, relationship; folks, kin, kinsfolk, kinsmen, relations, relatives.

king *n* majesty, monarch, sovereign.

kingdom *n* dominion, empire, monarchy, rule, sovereignty, supremacy; region, tract; division, department, domain, province, realm.

kingly *adj* imperial, kinglike, monarchical, regal, royal, sovereign; august, glorious, grand, imperial, imposing, magnificent, majestic, noble, splendid.

kink *n* cramp, crick, curl, entanglement, knot, loop, twist; crochet, whim, wrinkle.

kinsfolk *n* kin, kindred, kinsmen, relations, relatives.

kit *n* equipment, implements, outfit, set, working.

knack *n* ability, address, adroitness, aptitude, aptness, dexterity, dexterousness, expertness, facility, quickness, readiness, skill.

knave *n* caitiff, cheat, miscreant, rascal, rogue, scamp, scapegrace, scoundrel, sharper, swindler, trickster, villain.

knavery *n* criminality, dishonesty, fraud, knavishness, rascality, scoundrelism, trickery, villainy.

knavish *adj* dishonest, fraudulent, rascally, scoundrelly, unprincipled, roguish, trickish, tricky, villainous.

knell *vb* announce, peal, ring, toll. • *n* chime, peal, ring, toll.

knife *vb* cut, slash, stab. • *n* blade, jackknife, lance.

knit *vb* connect, interlace, join, unite, weave.

knob *n* boss, bunch, hunch, lump, protuberance, stud.

knock *vb* clap, cuff, hit, rap, rattle, slap, strike, thump; beat, blow, box. • *n* blow, slap, smack, thump; blame, criticism, rejection, setback.

knoll *n* hill, hillock, mound.

knot *vb* complicate, entangle, gnarl, kink, tie, weave. • *n* complication, entanglement; connection, tie; joint, node, knag; bunch, rosette, tuft; band, cluster, clique, crew, gang, group, pack, set, squad.

knotty *adj* gnarled, hard, knaggy, knurled, knotted, rough, rugged; complex, difficult, harassing, intricate, involved, perplexing, troublesome.

know *vb* apprehend, comprehend, cognize, discern, perceive, recognize, see, understand; discriminate, distinguish.

knowing *adj* accomplished, competent, experienced, intelligent, proficient, qualified, skilful, well-informed; aware, conscious, percipient, sensible, thinking; cunning, expressive, significant.

knowingly *adv* consciously, intentionally, purposely, wittingly.

knowledge *n* apprehension, command, comprehension, discernment, judgment, perception, understanding, wit; acquaintance, acquirement, attainments, enlightenment, erudition, information, learning, lore, mastery, scholarship, science; cognition, cognizance, consciousness, ken, notice, prescience, recognition.

knowledgeable *adj* aware, conscious, experienced, well-informed; educated, intelligent, learned, scholarly.

knuckle *vb* cringe, crouch, stoop, submit, yield.

L

laborious *adj* assiduous, diligent, hardworking, indefatigable, industrious, painstaking, sedulous, toiling; arduous, difficult, fatiguing, hard, Herculean, irksome, onerous, tiresome, toilsome, wearisome.

labour *vb* drudge, endeavour, exert, strive, toil, travail, work. • *n* drudgery, effort, exertion, industry, pains, toil, work; childbirth, delivery, parturition.

labyrinth *n* entanglement, intricacy, maze, perplexity, windings.

labyrinthine *adj* confused, convoluted, intricate, involved, labyrinthian, labyrinthic, perplexing, winding.

lace *vb* attach, bind, fasten, intertwine, tie, twine. • *n* filigree, lattice, mesh, net, netting, network, openwork, web.

lacerate *vb* claw, cut, lancinate, mangle, rend, rip, sever, slash, tear, wound; afflict, harrow, rend, torture, wound.

lack *vb* need, want. • *n* dearth, default, defectiveness, deficiency, deficit, destitution, insufficiency, need, scantiness, scarcity, shortcoming, shortness, want.

lackadaisical *adj* languishing, sentimental, pensive.

laconic *adj* brief, compact, concise, pithy, sententious, short, succinct, terse.

lad *n* boy, schoolboy, stripling, youngster, youth.

lading *n* burden, cargo, freight, load.

ladylike *adj* courtly, genteel, refined, well-bred.

lag *vb* dawdle, delay, idle, linger, loiter, saunter, tarry.

laggard *n* idler, lingerer, loiterer, lounger, saunterer, sluggard.

lair *n* burrow, couch, den, form, resting place.

lambent *adj* flickering, gliding, gleaming, licking, touching, twinkling.

lame *vb* cripple, disable, hobble. • *adj* crippled, defective, disabled, halt, hobbling, limping; feeble, insufficient, poor, unsatisfactory, weak.

lament *vb* complain, grieve, keen, moan, mourn, sorrow, wail, weep; bemoan, bewail, deplore, regret. • *n* complaint, lamentation, moan, moaning, plaint, wailing; coronach, dirge, elegy, keen, monody, requiem, threnody.

lamentable *adj* deplorable, doleful, grievous, lamented, melancholy, woeful; contemptible, miserable, pitiful, poor, wretched.

lamentation *n* dirge, grief, lament, moan, moaning, mourning, plaint, ululation, sorrow, wailing.

lampoon *vb* calumniate, defame, lash, libel, parody, ridicule, satirize, slander. • *n* calumny, defamation, libel, parody, pasquinade, parody, satire, slander.

land *vb* arrive, debark, disembark. • *n* earth, ground, soil; country, district, province, region, reservation, territory, tract, weald.

landlord *n* owner, proprietor; host, hotelier, innkeeper.

landscape *n* prospect, scene, view.

language *n* dialect, speech, tongue, vernacular; conversation; expression, idiom, jargon, parlance, phraseology, slang, style, terminology; utterance, voice.

languid *adj* drooping, exhausted, faint, feeble, flagging, languishing, pining, weak; dull, heartless, heavy, inactive, listless, lukewarm, slow, sluggish, spiritless, torpid.

languish *vb* decline, droop, fade, fail, faint, pine, sicken, sink, wither.

languor *n* debility, faintness, feebleness, languidness, languishment, weakness; apathy, ennui, heartlessness, heaviness, lethargy, listlessness, torpidness, torpor, weariness.

lank *adj* attenuated, emaciated, gaunt, lean, meagre, scraggy, slender, skinny, slim, starveling, thin.

lap[1] *vb* drink, lick, mouth, tongue; plash, ripple, splash, wash; quaff, sip, sup, swizzle, tipple. • *n* draught, dram, drench, drink, gulp, lick, swig, swill, quaff, sip, sup, suck; plash, splash, wash.

lap[2] *vb* cover, enfold, fold, turn, twist, swaddle, wrap; distance, pass, outdistance, overlap. • *n* fold, flap, lappet, lapel, ply, plait; ambit, beat, circle, circuit, cycle, loop, orbit, revolution, round, tour, turn, walk.

lapse *vb* glide, sink, slide, slip; err, fail, fall. • *n* course, flow, gliding; declension, decline, fall; error, fault, indiscretion, misstep, shortcoming, slip.

larceny *n* pilfering, robbery, stealing, theft, thievery.

large *adj* big, broad, bulky, colossal, elephantine, enormous, heroic, great, huge, immense, vast; broad, expanded, extensive, spacious, wide; abundant, ample, copious, full, liberal, plentiful; capacious, comprehensive.

lascivious *adj* concupiscent, immodest, incontinent, goatish, lecherous, lewd, libidinous, loose, lubricious, lustful, prurient, salacious, sensual, unchaste, voluptuous, wanton.

lash[1] *vb* belay, bind, strap, tie; fasten, join, moor, pinion, secure.

lash[2] *vb* beat, castigate, chastise, flagellate, flail, flay, flog, goad, scourge, swinge, thrash, whip; assail, censure, excoriate, lampoon, satirize, trounce. • *n* scourge, strap, thong, whip; cut, slap, smack, stroke, stripe.

lass *n* damsel, girl, lassie, maiden, miss.

lassitude *n* dullness, exhaustion, fatigue, languor, languidness, prostration, tiredness, weariness.

last[1] *vb* abide, carry on, continue, dwell, endure, extend, maintain, persist, prevail, remain, stand, stay, survive.

last[2] *adj* hindermost, hindmost, latest; conclusive, final, terminal, ultimate; eventual, endmost, extreme, farthest, ultimate; greatest, highest, maximal, maximum, most, supreme, superlative, utmost; latest, newest; aforegoing, foregoing, latter, preceding; departing, farewell, final, leaving, parting, valedictory. • *n* conclusion, consummation, culmination, end, ending, finale, finis, finish, termination.

last[3] *n* cast, form, matrix, mould, shape, template.

lasting *adj* abiding, durable, enduring, fixed, perennial, permanent, perpetual, stable.

lastly *adv* conclusively, eventually, finally, ultimately.

late *adj* behindhand, delayed, overdue, slow, tardy; deceased, former; recent. • *adv* lately, recently, sometime; tardily.

latent *adj* abeyant, concealed, hidden, invisible, occult, secret, unseen, veiled.

latitude *n* amplitude, breadth, compass, extent, range, room, scope; freedom, indulgence, liberty; laxity.

latter *adj* last, latest, modern, recent.

lattice *n* espalier, grating, latticework, trellis.

laud *vb* approve, celebrate, extol, glorify, magnify, praise.

laudable *adj* commendable, meritorious, praiseworthy.

laugh *vb* cackle, chortle, chuckle, giggle, guffaw, snicker, snigger, titter. • *n* chortle, chuckle, giggle, guffaw, laughter, titter.

laughable *adj* amusing, comical, diverting, droll, farcical, funny, ludicrous, mirthful, ridiculous.

laughter *n* cackle, chortle, chuckle, glee, giggle, guffaw, laugh, laughing.

launch *vb* cast, dart, dispatch, hurl, lance, project, throw; descant, dilate, enlarge, expiate; begin, commence, inaugurate, open, start.

lavish *vb* dissipate, expend, spend, squander, waste. • *adj* excessive, extravagant, generous, immoderate, overliberal, prodigal, profuse, thriftless, unrestrained, unstinted, unthrifty, wasteful.

law *n* act, code, canon, command, commandment, covenant, decree, edict, enactment, order, precept, principle, statute, regulation, rule; jurisprudence; litigation, process, suit.

lawful *adj* constitutional, constituted, legal, legalized, legitimate; allowable, authorized, permissible, warrantable; equitable, rightful, just, proper, valid.

lawless *adj* anarchic, anarchical, chaotic, disorderly, insubordinate, rebellious, reckless, riotous, seditious, wild.

lawyer *n* advocate, attorney, barrister, counsel, counsellor, pettifogger, solicitor.

lax *adj* loose, relaxed, slow; drooping, flabby, soft; neglectful, negligent, remiss; dissolute, immoral, licentious, seditious, wild.

lay[1] *vb* deposit, establish, leave, place, plant, posit, put, set, settle, spread; arrange, dispose, locate, organize, position; bear, produce; advance, lodge, offer, submit; allocate, allot, ascribe, assign, attribute, charge, impute; concoct, contrive, design, plan, plot, prepare; apply, burden, encumber, impose, saddle, tax; bet, gamble, hazard, risk, stake, wager; allay, alleviate, appease, assuage, calm, relieve, soothe, still, suppress; disclose, divulge, explain, reveal, show, unveil; acquire, grab, grasp, seize; assault, attack, beat up; discover, find, unearth; bless, confirm, consecrate, ordain. • *n* arrangement, array, form, formation; attitude, aspect, bearing, demeanour, direction, lie, pose, position, posture, set.

lay² *adj* amateur, inexpert, nonprofessional; civil, laic, laical, nonclerical, nonecclesiastical, nonreligious, secular, temporal, unclerical.

lay³ *n* ballad, carol, ditty, lied, lyric, ode, poem, rhyme, round, song, verse.

layer *n* bed, course, lay, seam, stratum.

laziness *n* idleness, inactivity, indolence, slackness, sloth, fulness, sluggishness, tardiness.

lazy *adj* idle, inactive, indolent, inert, slack, slothful, slow, sluggish, supine, torpid.

lead *vb* conduct, deliver, direct, draw, escort, guide; front, head, precede; advance, excel, outstrip, pass; allure, entice, induce, persuade, prevail; conduce, contribute, serve, tend. • *adj* chief, first, foremost, main, primary, prime, principal. • *n* direction, guidance, leadership; advance; precedence, priority.

leader *n* conductor, director, guide; captain, chief, chieftain, commander, head; superior, dominator, victor.

leading *adj* governing, ruling; capital, chief, first, foremost, highest, principal, superior.

league *vb* ally, associate, band, combine, confederate, unite. • *n* alliance, association, coalition, combination, combine, confederacy, confederation, consortium, union.

leak *vb* drip, escape, exude, ooze, pass, percolate, spill. • *n* chink, crack, crevice, hole, fissure, oozing, opening; drip leakage, leaking, percolation.

lean¹ *adj* bony, emaciated, gaunt, lank, meagre, poor, skinny, thin; dull, barren, jejune, meagre, tame; inadequate, pitiful, scanty, slender; bare, barren, infertile, unproductive.

lean² *vb* incline, slope; bear, recline, repose, rest; confide, depend, rely, trust.

leaning *n* aptitude, bent, bias, disposition, inclination, liking, predilection, proneness, propensity, tendency.

leap *vb* bound, clear, jump, spring, vault; caper, frisk, gambol, hop, skip. • *n* bound, jump, spring, vault; caper, frisk, gambol, hop, skip.

learn *vb* acquire, ascertain, attain, collect, gain, gather, hear, memorize.

learned *adj* erudite, lettered, literate, scholarly, well-read; expert, experienced, knowing, skilled, versed, well-informed.

learner *n* beginner, novice, pupil, student, tyro.

learning *n* acquirements, attainments, culture, education, information, knowledge, lore, scholarship, tuition.

least *adj* meanest, minutest, smallest, tiniest.

leave¹ *vb* abandon, decamp, go, quit, vacate, withdraw; desert, forsake, relinquish, renounce; commit, consign, refer; cease, desist from, discontinue, refrain, stop; allow, let, let alone, permit; bequeath, demise, desist, will.

leave² *n* allowance, liberty, permission, licence, sufferance; departure, retirement, withdrawal; adieu, farewell, goodbye.

leaven *vb* ferment, lighten, raise; colour, elevate, imbue, inspire, lift, permeate, tinge; infect, vitiate. • *n* barm, ferment, yeast; influence, inspiration.

leavings *npl* bits, dregs, fragments, leftovers, pieces, relics, remains, remnants, scraps.

lecherous *adj* carnal, concupiscent, incontinent, lascivious, lewd, libidinous, lubricious, lustful, wanton, salacious, unchaste.

lechery *n* concupiscence, lasciviousness, lewdness, lubriciousness, lubricity, lust, salaciousness, salacity.

lecture *vb* censure, chide, reprimand, reprove, scold, sermonize; address, harangue, teach. • *n* censure, lecturing, lesson, reprimand, reproof, scolding; address, discourse, prelection.

ledge *n* projection, ridge, shelf.

lees *npl* dregs, precipitate, refuse, sediment, settlings.

leg *n* limb, prop.

legacy *n* bequest, gift, heirloom; heritage, inheritance, tradition.

legal *adj* allowable, authorized, constitutional, lawful, legalized, legitimate, proper, sanctioned.

legalize *vb* authorize, legitimate, legitimatize, legitimize, permit, sanction.

legend *n* fable, fiction, myth, narrative, romance, story, tale.

legendary *adj* fabulous, fictitious, mythical, romantic.

legible *adj* clear, decipherable, fair, distinct, plain, readable; apparent, discoverable, recognizable, manifest.

legion *n* army, body, cohort, column, corps, detachment, detail, division, force, maniple, phalanx, platoon; squad; army, horde, host, multitude, number, swarm, throng. • *adj* many, multitudinous, myriad, numerous.

legislate *vb* enact, ordain.

legitimacy *n* lawfulness, legality; genuineness.

legitimate *adj* authorized, lawful, legal, sanctioned; genuine, valid; correct, justifiable, logical, reasonable, warrantable, warranted.

leisure *n* convenience, ease, freedom, liberty, opportunity, recreation, retirement, vacation.

lend *vb* advance, afford, bestow, confer, furnish, give, grant, impart, loan, supply.

lengthen *vb* elongate, extend, produce, prolong, stretch; continue, protract.

lengthy *adj* diffuse, lengthened, long, long-drawn-out, prolix, prolonged, protracted.

lenience, leniency *n* clemency, compassion, forbearance, gentleness, lenity, mercy, mildness, tenderness.

lenient *adj* assuasive, lenitive, mitigating, mitigative, softening, soothing; clement, easy, forbearing, gentle, humouring, indulgent, long-suffering, merciful, mild, tender, tolerant.

lesion *n* derangement, disorder, hurt, injury.

less *adj* baser, inferior, lower, smaller; decreased, fewer, lesser, reduced, smaller, shorter; • *adv* barely, below, least, under; decreasingly. • *prep* excepting, lacking, minus, sans, short of, without.

lessen *vb* abate, abridge, contract, curtail, decrease, diminish, narrow, reduce, shrink; degrade, lower; dwindle, weaken.

lesson *n* exercise, task; instruction, precept; censure, chiding, lecture, lecturing, rebuke, reproof, scolding.

let¹ *vb* admit, allow, authorize, permit, suffer; charter, hire, lease, rent.

let² *vb* hinder, impede, instruct, prevent. • *n* hindrance, impediment, interference, obstacle, obstruction, restriction.

lethal *adj* deadly, destructive, fatal, mortal, murderous.

lethargic *adj* apathetic, comatose, drowsy, dull, heavy, inactive, inert, sleepy, stupid, stupefied, torpid.

lethargy *n* apathy, coma, drowsiness, dullness, hypnotism, inactiveness, inactivity, inertia, sleepiness, sluggishness, stupefaction, stupidity, stupor, torpor.

letter *n* epistle, missive, note.

lettered *adj* bookish, educated, erudite, learned, literary, versed, well-read.

levee *n* ceremony, entertainment, reception, party, soiree; embankment.

level *vb* equalize, flatten, horizontalize, smooth; demolish, destroy, raze; aim, direct, point. • *adj* equal, even, flat, flush, horizontal, plain, plane, smooth. • *n* altitude, degree, equality, evenness, plain, plane, smoothness; deck, floor, layer, stage, storey, tier.

levity *n* buoyancy, facetiousness, fickleness, flightiness, flippancy, frivolity, giddiness, inconstancy, levity, volatility.

levy *vb* collect, exact, gather, tax; call, muster, raise, summon. • *n* duty, tax.

lewd *adj* despicable, impure, lascivious, libidinous, licentious, loose, lustful, profligate, unchaste, vile, wanton, wicked.

liability *n* accountableness, accountability, duty, obligation, responsibility, tendency; exposedness; debt, indebtedness, obligation.

liable *adj* accountable, amenable, answerable, bound, responsible; exposed, likely, obnoxious, subject.

liaison *n* amour, intimacy, intrigue; connection, relation, union.

libel *vb* calumniate, defame, lampoon, satirize, slander, vilify. • *n* calumny, defamation, lampoon, satire, slander, vilification, vituperation.

liberal *adj* beneficent, bountiful, charitable, disinterested, free, generous, munificent, open-hearted, princely, unselfish; broad-minded, catholic, chivalrous, enlarged, high-minded, honourable, magnanimous, tolerant, unbiased, unbigoted; abundant, ample, bounteous, full, large, plentiful, unstinted; humanizing, liberalizing, refined, refining.

liberality *n* beneficence, bountifulness, bounty, charity, disinterestedness, generosity, kindness, munificence; benefaction, donation, gift, gratuity, present; broad-mindedness, catholicity, candour, impartiality, large-mindedness, magnanimity, toleration.

liberate *vb* deliver, discharge, disenthral, emancipate, free, manumit, ransom, release.

libertine *adj* corrupt, depraved, dissolute, licentious, profligate, rakish. • *n* debauchee, lecher, profligate, rake, roue, voluptuary.

liberty *n* emancipation, freedom, independence, liberation, self-direction, self-government; franchise, immunity, privilege; leave, licence, permission.

libidinous *adj* carnal, concupiscent, debauched, impure, incontinent, lascivious, lecherous, lewd, loose, lubricious, lustful, salacious, sensual, unchaste, wanton, wicked.

licence *n* authorization, leave, permission, privilege, right; certificate, charter, dispensation, imprimatur, permit, warrant; anarchy, disorder, freedom, lawlessness, laxity, liberty.

license *vb* allow, authorize, grant, permit, warrant; suffer, tolerate.

licentious *adj* disorderly, riotous, uncontrolled, uncurbed, ungovernable, unrestrained, unruly, wanton; debauched, dissolute, lax, libertine, loose, profligate, rakish; immoral, impure, lascivious, lecherous, lewd, libertine, libidinous, lustful, sensual, unchaste, wicked.

lick *vb* beat, flog, spank, thrash; lap, taste. • *n* blow, slap, stroke; salt-spring.

lie[1] *vb* couch, recline, remain, repose, rest; consist, pertain.

lie[2] *vb* equivocate, falsify, fib, prevaricate, romance. • *n* equivocation, falsehood, falsification, fib, misrepresentation, prevarication, untruth; delusion, illusion.

lief *adv* freely, gladly, willingly.

life *n* activity, alertness, animation, briskness, energy, sparkle, spirit, sprightliness, verve, vigour, vivacity; behaviour, conduct, deportment; being, duration, existence, lifetime; autobiography, biography, curriculum vitae, memoirs, story.

lifeless *adj* dead, deceased, defunct, extinct, inanimate; cold, dull, flat, frigid, inert, lethargic, passive, pulseless, slow, sluggish, tame, torpid.

lift *vb* elevate, exalt, hoist, raise, uplift. • *n* aid, assistance, help; elevator.

light[1] *vb* alight, land, perch, settle. • *adj* porous, sandy, spongy, well-leavened; loose, sandy; free, portable, unburdened, unencumbered; inconsiderable, moderate, negligible, slight, small, trifling, trivial, unimportant; ethereal, feathery, flimsy, gossamer, insubstantial, weightless; easy, effortless, facile; fickle, frivolous, unsettled, unsteady, volatile; airy, buoyant, carefree, light-hearted, lightsome; unaccented, unstressed, weak.

light[2] *vb* conflagrate, fire, ignite, inflame, kindle; brighten, illume, illuminate, illumine, luminate, irradiate, lighten. • *adj* bright, clear, fair, lightsome, luminous, pale, pearly, whitish. • *n* dawn, day, daybreak, sunrise; blaze, brightness, effulgence, gleam, illumination, luminosity, phosphorescence, radiance, ray; candle, lamp, lantern, lighthouse, taper, torch; comprehension, enlightenment, information, insight, instruction, knowledge; elucidation, explanation, illustration; attitude, construction, interpretation, observation, reference, regard, respect, view.

lighten[1] *vb* allay, alleviate, ease, mitigate, palliate; disburden, disencumber, relieve, unburden, unload.

lighten[2] *vb* brighten, gleam, shine; light, illume, illuminate, illumine, irradiate; enlighten, inform; emit, flash.

light-headed *adj* dizzy, giddy, vertiginous; confused, delirious, wandering; addle-pated, frivolous, giddy, heedless, indiscreet, light, rattle-brained, thoughtless, volatile.

light-hearted *adj* blithe, blithesome, carefree, cheerful, frolicsome, gay, glad, gladsome, gleeful, happy, jocund, jovial, joyful, lightsome, merry.

lightness *n* flightiness, frivolity, giddiness, levity, volatility; agility, buoyancy, facility.

like[1] *vb* approve, please; cherish, enjoy, love, relish; esteem, fancy, regard; choose, desire, elect, list, prefer, select, wish. • *n* liking, partiality, preference.

like[2] *adj* alike, allied, analogous, cognate, corresponding, parallel, resembling, similar; equal, same; likely, probable. • *adv* likely, probably. • *n* counterpart, equal, match, peer, twin.

likelihood *n* probability, verisimilitude.

likely *adj* credible, liable, possible, probable; agreeable, appropriate, convenient, likable, pleasing, suitable, well-adapted, well-suited. • *adv* doubtlessly, presumably, probably.

likeness *n* appearance, form, parallel, resemblance, semblance, similarity, similitude; copy, counterpart, effigy, facsimile, image, picture, portrait, representation.

liking *n* desire, fondness, partiality, wish; appearance, bent, bias, disposition, inclination, leaning, penchant, predisposition, proneness, propensity, tendency, turn.

limb *n* arm, extremity, leg, member; bough, branch, offshoot.

limit *vb* bound, circumscribe, define; check, condition, hinder, restrain, restrict. • *n* bound, boundary, bourn, confine, frontier, march, precinct, term, termination, terminus; check, hindrance, obstruction, restraint, restriction.

limitation *n* check, constraint, restraint, restriction.

limitless *adj* boundless, endless, eternal, illimitable, immeasurable, infinite, never-ending, unbounded, undefined, unending, unlimited.

limp[1] *vb* halt, hitch, hobble, totter. • *n* hitch, hobble, shamble, shuffle, totter.

limp[2] *adj* drooping, droopy, floppy, sagging, weak; flabby, flaccid, flexible, limber, pliable, relaxed, slack, soft.

limpid *adj* bright, clear, crystal, crystalline, lucid, pellucid, pure, translucent, transparent.

line *vb* align, line up, range, rank, regiment; border, bound, edge, fringe, hem, interline, march, rim, verge; seam, stripe, streak, striate, trace; carve, chisel, crease, cut, crosshatch; define, delineate, describe. • *n* mark, streak, stripe; cable, cord, rope, string, thread; rank, row; ancestry, family, lineage, race, succession; course, method; business, calling, employment, job, occupation, post, pursuit.

lineage *n* ancestry, birth, breed, descendants, descent, extraction, family, forebears, forefathers, genealogy, house, line, offspring, progeny, race.

lineament *n* feature, line, outline, trait.

linen *n* cloth, fabric, flax, lingerie.

linger *vb* dally, dawdle, delay, idle, lag, loiter, remain, saunter, stay, tarry, wait.

link *vb* bind, conjoin, connect, fasten, join, tie, unite. • *n* bond, connection, connective, copula, coupler, joint, juncture; division, member, part, piece.

liquefy *vb* dissolve, fuse, melt, thaw.

liquid *adj* fluid; clear, dulcet, flowing, mellifluous, mellifluent, melting, soft. • *n* fluid, liquor.

list[1] *vb* alphabetize, catalogue, chronicle, codify, docket, enumerate, file, index, inventory, record, register, tabulate, tally; enlist, enroll; choose, desire, elect, like, please, prefer, wish. • *n* catalogue, enumeration, index, inventory, invoice, register, roll, schedule, scroll, series, table, tally; border, bound, limit; border, edge, selvedge, strip, stripe; fillet, listel.

list[2] *vb* cant, heel, incline, keel, lean, pitch, tilt, tip. • *n* cant, inclination, incline, leaning, pitch, slope, tilt, tip.

listen *vb* attend, eavesdrop, hark, hear, hearken, heed, obey, observe.

listless *adj* apathetic, careless, heedless, impassive, inattentive, indifferent, indolent, languid, torpid, vacant, supine, thoughtless, vacant.

listlessness *n* apathy, carelessness, heedlessness, impassivity, inattention, indifference, indolence, languidness, languor, supineness, thoughtlessness, torpor, torpidity, vacancy.

literally *adv* actually, really; exactly, precisely, rigorously, strictly.

literary *adj* bookish, book-learned, erudite, instructed, learned, lettered, literate, scholarly, well-read.

literature *n* erudition, learning, letters, lore, writings.

lithe *adj* flexible, flexile, limber, pliable, pliant, supple.

litigation *n* contending, contest, disputing, lawsuit.

litigious *adj* contentious, disputatious, quarrelsome; controvertible, disputable.

litter *vb* derange, disarrange, disorder, scatter, strew; bear. • *n* bedding, couch, palanquin, sedan, stretcher; confusion, disarray, disorder, mess, untidiness; fragments, rubbish, shreds, trash.

little *adj* diminutive, infinitesimal, minute, small, tiny, wee; brief, short, small; feeble, inconsiderable, insignificant, moderate, petty, scanty, slender, slight, trivial, unimportant, weak; contemptible, illiberal, mean, narrow, niggardly, paltry, selfish, stingy. • *n* handful, jot, modicum, pinch, pittance, trifle, whit.

live[1] *vb* be, exist; continue, endure, last, remain, survive; abide, dwell, reside; fare, feed, nourish, subsist, support; continue, lead, pass.

live[2] *adj* alive, animate, living, quick; burning, hot, ignited; bright, brilliant, glowing, lively, vivid; active, animated, earnest, glowing, wide-awake.

livelihood *n* living, maintenance, subsistence, support, sustenance.

liveliness *n* activity, animation, briskness, gaiety, spirit, sprightliness, vivacity.

lively *adj* active, agile, alert, brisk, energetic, nimble, quick, smart, stirring, supple, vigorous, vivacious; airy, animated, blithe, blithesome, buoyant, frolicsome, gleeful, jocund, jolly, merry, spirited, sportive, sprightly, spry; bright, brilliant, clear, fresh, glowing, strong, vivid; dynamic, forcible, glowing, impassioned, intense, keen, nervous, piquant, racy, sparkling, strenuous, vigorous.

living *adj* alive, breathing, existing, live, organic, quick; active, lively, quickening. • *n* livelihood, maintenance, subsistence, support; estate, keeping; benefice.

load *vb* freight, lade; burden, cumber, encumber, oppress, weigh. • *n* burden, freightage, pack, weight; cargo, freight, lading; clog, deadweight, encumbrance, incubus, oppression, pressure.

loafer *n* (*sl*) bum, idler, lounger, vagabond, vagrant.

loath *adj* averse, backward, disinclined, indisposed, reluctant, unwilling.

loathe *vb* abhor, abominate, detest, dislike, hate, recoil.

loathing *n* abhorrence, abomination, antipathy, aversion, detestation, disgust, hatred, horror, repugnance, revulsion.

loathsome *adj* disgusting, nauseating, nauseous, offensive, palling, repulsive, revolting, sickening; abominable, abhorrent, detestable, execrable, hateful, odious, shocking.

local *adj* limited, neighbouring, provincial, regional, restricted, sectional, territorial, topical.

locality *n* location, neighbourhood, place, position, site, situation, spot.

locate *vb* determine, establish, fix, place, set, settle.

lock[1] *vb* bolt, fasten, padlock, seal; confine; clog, impede, restrain, stop; clasp, embrace, encircle, enclose, grapple, hug, join, press. • *n* bolt, fastening, padlock; embrace, grapple, hug.

lock[2] *n* curl, ringlet, tress, tuft.

lodge *vb* deposit, fix, settle; fix, place, plant; accommodate, cover, entertain, harbour, quarter, shelter; abide, dwell, inhabit, live, reside, rest; remain, rest, sojourn, stay, stop. • *n* cabin, cot, cottage, hovel, hut, shed; cave, den, haunt, lair; assemblage, assembly, association club, group, society.

lodging *n* abode, apartment, dwelling, habitation, quarters, residence; cover, harbour, protection, refuge, shelter.

loftiness *n* altitude, elevation, height; arrogance, haughtiness, pride, vanity; dignity, grandeur, sublimity.

lofty *adj* elevated, high, tall, towering; arrogant, haughty, proud; eminent, exalted, sublime; dignified, imposing, majestic, stately.

logical *adj* close, coherent, consistent, dialectical, sound, valid; discriminating, rational, reasoned.

loiter *vb* dally, dawdle, delay, dilly-dally, idle, lag, linger, saunter, stroll, tarry.

loneliness *n* isolation, retirement, seclusion, solitariness, solitude; desolation, dreariness, forlornness.

lonely *adj* apart, dreary, isolated, lonesome, remote, retired, secluded, separate, sequestrated, solitary; alone, lone, companionless, friendless, unaccompanied; deserted, desolate, forlorn, forsaken, withdrawn.

lonesome *adj* cheerless, deserted, desolate, dreary, gloomy, lone, lonely.

long[1] *vb* anticipate, await, expect; aspire, covet, crave, desire, hanker, lust, pine, wish, yearn.

long[2] *adj* drawn-out, extended, extensive, far-reaching, lengthy, prolonged, protracted, stretched; diffuse, long-winded, prolix, tedious, wearisome; backward, behindhand, dilatory, lingering, slack, slow, tardy.

longing *n* aspiration, coveting, craving, desire, hankering, hunger, pining, yearning.

long-suffering *adj* enduring, forbearing, patient. • *n* clemency, endurance, forbearing.

look *vb* behold, examine, notice, see, search; consider, inspect, investigate, observe, study, contemplate, gaze, regard, scan, survey, view; anticipate, await, expect; heed, mind, watch; face, front; appear, seem. • *n* examination, gaze, glance, peep, peer, search; appearance, aspect, complexion; air, aspect, manner, mien.

loophole *n* aperture, crenellation, loop, opening; excuse, plea, pretence, pretext, subterfuge.

loose *vb* free, liberate, release, unbind, undo, unfasten, unlash, unlock, untie; ease, loosen, relax, slacken; detach, disconnect, disengage. • *adj* unbound, unconfined, unfastened, unsewn, untied; disengaged, free, unattached; relaxed; diffuse, diffusive, prolix, rambling, unconnected; ill-defined, indefinite, indeterminate, indistinct, vague; careless, heedless, negligent, lax, slack; debauched, dissolute, immoral, licentious, unchaste, wanton.

loosen *vb* liberate, relax, release, separate, slacken, unbind, unloose, untie.

looseness *n* easiness, slackness; laxity, levity; lewdness, unchastity, wantonness, wickedness; diarrhoea, flux.

loot *vb* pillage, plunder, ransack, rifle, rob, sack. • *n* booty, plunder, spoil.

lop *vb* cut, truncate; crop, curtail, dock, prune; detach, dissever, sever.

loquacious *adj* garrulous, talkative, voluble, wordy; noisy, speaking, talking; babbling, blabbing, tattling, tell-tale.

loquacity *n* babbling, chattering, gabbling, garrulity, loquaciousness, talkativeness, volubility.

lord *n* earl, noble, nobleman, peer, viscount; governor, king, liege, master, monarch, prince, ruler, seigneur, seignior, sovereign, superior; husband, spouse.

lordly *adj* aristocratic, dignified, exalted, grand, lofty, majestic, noble; arrogant, despotic, domineering, haughty, imperious, insolent, masterful, overbearing, proud, tyrannical; large, liberal.

lordship *n* authority, command, control, direction, domination, dominion empire, government, rule, sovereignty, sway; manor, domain, seignory.

lore *n* erudition, knowledge, learning, letters, scholarship; admonition, advice, counsel, doctrine, instruction, lesson, teaching, wisdom.

lose *vb* deprive, dispossess, forfeit, miss; dislodge, displace, mislay, misspend, squander, waste; decline, fall, succumb, yield.

loss *n* deprivation, failure, forfeiture, privation; casualty, damage, defeat, destruction, detriment, disadvantage, injury, overthrow, ruin; squandering, waste.

lost *adj* astray, missing; forfeited, missed, unredeemed; dissipated, misspent, squandered, wasted; bewildered, confused, distracted, perplexed, puzzled; absent, absent-minded, abstracted, dreamy, napping, preoccupied; abandoned, corrupt, debauched, depraved, dissolute, graceless, hardened, incorrigible, irreclaimable, licentious, profligate, reprobate, shameless, unchaste, wanton; destroyed, ruined.

lot *n* allotment, apportionment, destiny, doom, fate; accident, chance, fate, fortune, hap, haphazard, hazard; division, parcel, part, portion.

loth *adj* averse, disinclined, disliking, reluctant, unwilling.

loud *adj* high-sounding, noisy, resounding, sonorous; deafening, stentorian strong, stunning; boisterous, clamorous, noisy, obstreperous, tumultuous, turbulent, uproarious, vociferous; emphatic, impressive, positive, vehement; flashy, gaudy, glaring, loud, ostentatious, showy, vulgar.

lounge *vb* loll, recline, sprawl; dawdle, idle, loaf, loiter.

love *vb* adore, like, worship. • *n* accord, affection, amity, courtship, delight, fondness, friendship, kindness, regard, tenderness, warmth; adoration, amour, ardour, attachment, passion; devotion, inclination, liking; benevolence, charity, goodwill.

lovely *adj* beautiful, charming, delectable, delightful, enchanting, exquisite, graceful, pleasing, sweet, winning; admirable, adorable, amiable.

loving *adj* affectionate, dear, fond, kind, tender.

low[1] *vb* bellow, moo.

low[2] *adj* basal, depressed, profound; gentle, grave, soft, subdued; cheap, humble, mean, plebeian, vulgar; abject, base, baseminded, degraded, dirty, grovelling, ignoble, low-minded, menial, scurvy, servile, shabby, slavish, vile; derogatory, disgraceful, dishonourable, disreputable, unbecoming, undignified, ungentlemanly, unhandsome, unmanly; exhausted, feeble, reduced, weak; frugal, plain, poor, simple, spare; lowly, reverent, submissive; dejected, depressed, dispirited.

lower[1] *vb* depress, drop, sink, subside; debase, degrade, disgrace, humble, humiliate, reduce; abate, decrease, diminish, lessen. • *adj* baser, inferior, less, lesser, shorter, smaller; subjacent, under.

lower[2] *vb* blacken, darken, frown, glower, threaten.

lowering *adj* dark, clouded, cloudy, lurid, murky, overcast, threatening.

lowliness *n* humbleness, humility, meekness, self-abasement, submissiveness.

lowly *adj* gentle, humble, meek, mild, modest, plain, poor, simple, unassuming, unpretending, unpretentious; low-born, mean, servile.

loyal *adj* constant, devoted, faithful, patriotic, true.

loyalty *n* allegiance, constancy, devotion, faithfulness, fealty, fidelity, patriotism.

lubricious *adj* slippery, smooth; uncertain, unstable, wavering; impure, incontinent, lascivious, lecherous, lewd, libidinous, licentious, lustful, salacious, unchaste, wanton.

lucid *adj* beaming, bright, brilliant, luminous, radiant, resplendent, shining, clear, crystalline, diaphanous, limpid, lucent, pellucid, pure, transparent; clear, distinct, evident, intelligible, obvious, perspicuous, plain; reasonable, sane, sober, sound.

luck *n* accident, casualty, chance, fate, fortune, hap, haphazard, hazard, serendipity, success.

luckless *adj* ill-fated, ill-starred, unfortunate, unhappy, unlucky, unpropitious, unprosperous, unsuccessful.

lucky *adj* blessed, favoured, fortunate, happy, successful; auspicious, favourable, propitious, prosperous.

lucrative *adj* advantageous, gainful, paying, profitable, remunerative.

ludicrous *adj* absurd, burlesque, comic, comical, droll, farcical, funny, laughable, odd, ridiculous, sportive.

lugubrious *adj* complaining, doleful, gloomy, melancholy, mournful, sad, serious, sombre, sorrowful.

lukewarm *adj* blood-warm, tepid, thermal; apathetic, cold, dull, indifferent, listless, unconcerned, torpid.

lull *vb* calm, compose, hush, quiet, still, tranquillize; abate, cease, decrease, diminish, subside. • *n* calm, calmness, cessation.

lumber[1] *vb* rumble, shamble, trudge.

lumber[2] *n* refuse, rubbish, trash, trumpery; wood.

luminous *adj* effulgent, incandescent, radiant, refulgent, resplendent, shining; bright, brilliant, clear; clear, lucid, lucent, perspicuous, plain.

lunacy *n* aberration, craziness, dementia, derangement, insanity, madness, mania.

lunatic *adj* crazy, demented, deranged, insane, mad, psychopathic. • *n* madman, maniac, psychopath.

lurch *vb* appropriate, filch, pilfer, purloin, steal; deceive, defeat, disappoint, evade; ambush, lurk, skulk; contrive, dodge, shift, trick; pitch, sway.

lure *vb* allure, attract, decoy, entice, inveigle, seduce, tempt. • *n* allurement, attraction, bait, decoy, enticement, temptation.

lurid *adj* dismal, ghastly, gloomy, lowering, murky, pale, wan; glaring, sensational, startling, unrestrained.

lurk *vb* hide, prowl, skulk, slink, sneak, snoop.

luscious *adj* delicious, delightful, grateful, palatable, pleasing, savoury, sweet.

lush *adj* fresh, juicy, luxuriant, moist, sappy, succulent, watery.

lust *vb* covet, crave, desire, hanker, need, want, yearn. • *n* cupidity, desire, longing; carnality, concupiscence, lasciviousness, lechery, lewdness, lubricity, salaciousness, salacity, wantonness.

lustful *adj* carnal, concupiscent, hankering, lascivious, lecherous, licentious, libidinous, lubricious, salacious.

lustily *adv* strongly, vigorously.

lustiness *n* hardihood, power, robustness, stoutness, strength, sturdiness, vigour.

lustre *n* brightness, brilliance, brilliancy, splendour.

lusty *adj* healthful, lively, robust, stout, strong, sturdy, vigorous; bulky, burly, corpulent, fat, large, stout.

luxuriance *n* exuberance, profusion, superabundance.

luxuriant *adj* exuberant, plenteous, plentiful, profuse, superabundant.

luxuriate *vb* abound, delight, enjoy, flourish, indulge, revel.

luxurious *adj* epicurean, opulent, pampered, self-indulgent, sensual, sybaritic, voluptuous.

luxury *n* epicureanism, epicurism, luxuriousness, opulence, sensuality, voluptuousness; delight, enjoyment, gratification, indulgence, pleasure; dainty, delicacy, treat.

lying *adj* equivocating, false, mendacious, untruthful, untrue.

lyric *adj* dulcet, euphonious, lyrical, mellifluous, mellifluent, melodic, melodious, musical, poetic, silvery, tuneful.

lyrical *adj* ecstatic, enthusiastic, expressive, impassion; dulcet, lyric, mellifluous, mellifluent, melodic, melodious, musical, poetic.

M

macabre *adj* cadaverous, deathlike, deathly, dreadful, eerie, frightening, frightful, ghoulish, grim, grisly, gruesome, hideous, horrid, morbid, unearthly, weird.

mace *n* baton, staff, truncheon.

macerate *vb* harass, mortify, torture; digest, soak, soften, steep.

Machiavellian *adj* arch, artful, astute, crafty, crooked, cunning, deceitful, designing, diplomatic, insidious, intriguing, shrewd, sly, subtle, tricky, wily.

machination *n* artifice, cabal, conspiracy, contrivance, design, intrigue, plot, scheme, stratagem, trick.

machine *n* instrument, puppet, tool; machinery, organization, system; engine.

mad *adj* crazed, crazy, delirious, demented, deranged, distracted, insane, irrational, lunatic, maniac, maniacal; enraged, furious, rabid, raging, violent; angry, enraged, exasperated, furious, incensed, provoked, wrathful; distracted, infatuated, wild; frantic, frenzied, raving.

madden *vb* annoy, craze, enrage, exasperate, inflame, infuriate, irritate, provoke.

madness *n* aberration, craziness, dementia, derangement, insanity, lunacy, mania; delirium, frenzy, fury, rage.

magazine *n* depository, depot, entrepot, receptacle, repository, storehouse, warehouse; pamphlet, paper, periodical.

magic *adj* bewitching, charming, enchanting, fascinating, magical, miraculous, spellbinding. • *n* conjuring, enchantment, necromancy, sorcery, thaumaturgy, voodoo, witchcraft; char, fascination, witchery.

magician *n* conjurer, enchanter, juggler, magus, necromancer, shaman, sorcerer, wizard.

magisterial *adj* august, dignified, majestic, pompous; authoritative, despotic, domineering, imperious, dictatorial.

magnanimity *n* chivalry, disinterestedness, forbearance, high-mindedness, generosity, nobility.

magnificence *n* brilliance, éclat, grandeur, luxuriousness, luxury, majesty, pomp, splendour.

magnificent *adj* elegant, grand, majestic, noble, splendid, superb; brilliant, gorgeous, imposing, lavish, luxurious, pompous, showy, stately.

magnify *vb* amplify, augment, enlarge; bless, celebrate, elevate, exalt, extol, glorify, laud, praise; exaggerate.

magnitude *n* bulk, dimension, extent, mass, size, volume; consequence, greatness, importance; grandeur, loftiness, sublimity.

maid *n* damsel, girl, lass, lassie, maiden, virgin; maidservant, servant.

maiden *adj* chaste, pure, undefiled, virgin; fresh, new, unused. • *n* girl, maid, virgin.

maidenly *adj* demure, gentle, modest, maidenlike, reserved.

maim *vb* cripple, disable, disfigure, mangle, mar, mutilate. • *n* crippling, disfigurement, mutilation; harm, hurt, injury, mischief.

main[1] *adj* capital, cardinal, chief, leading, principal; essential, important, indispensable, necessary, requisite, vital; enormous, huge, mighty, vast; pure, sheer; absolute, direct, entire, mere. • *n* channel, pipe; force, might, power, strength, violence.

main[2] *n* high seas, ocean; continent, mainland.

maintain *vb* keep, preserve, support, sustain, uphold; hold, possess; defend, vindicate, justify; carry on, continue, keep up; feed, provide, supply; allege, assert, declare; affirm, aver, contend, hold, say.

maintenance *n* defence, justification, preservation, support, sustenance, vindication; bread, food, livelihood, provisions, subsistence, sustenance, victuals.

majestic *adj* august, dignified, imperial, imposing, lofty, noble, pompous, princely, stately, regal, royal; grand, magnificent, splendid, sublime.

majesty *n* augustness, dignity, elevation, grandeur, loftiness, stateliness.

majority *n* bulk, greater, mass, more, most, plurality, preponderance, superiority; adulthood, manhood.

make *vb* create; fashion, figure, form, frame, mould, shape; cause, construct, effect, establish, fabricate, produce; do, execute, perform, practice; acquire, gain, get, raise, secure; cause, compel, constrain, force, occasion; compose, constitute; go, journey, move, proceed, tend, travel; conduce, contribute, effect, favour, operate; estimate, judge, reckon, suppose, think. • *n* brand, build, constitution, construction, form, shape, structure.

maker *n* creator, god; builder, constructor, fabricator, framer, manufacturer; author, composer, poet, writer.

maladministration *n* malversation, misgovernment, misrule.

maladroit *adj* awkward, bungling, clumsy, inept, inexpert, unhandy, unskilful, unskilled.

malady *n* affliction, ailment, complaint, disease, disorder, illness, indisposition, sickness.

malcontent *adj* discontented, dissatisfied, insurgent, rebellious, resentful, uneasy, unsatisfied. • *n* agitator, complainer, faultfinder, grumbler, spoilsport.

malediction *n* anathema, ban, curse, cursing, denunciation, execration, imprecation, malison.

malefactor *n* convict, criminal, culprit, delinquent, evildoer, felon, offender, outlaw.

malevolence *n* hate, hatred, ill-will, malice, malignity, rancour, spite, spitefulness, vindictiveness.

malevolent *adj* evil-minded, hateful, hostile, ill-natured, malicious, malignant, mischievous, rancorous, spiteful, venomous, vindictive.

malice *n* animosity, bitterness, enmity, grudge, hate, ill-will, malevolence, maliciousness, malignity, pique, rancour, spite, spitefulness, venom, vindictiveness.

malicious *adj* bitter, envious, evil-minded, ill-disposed, ill-natured, invidious, malevolent, malignant, mischievous, rancorous, resentful, spiteful, vicious.

malign *vb* abuse, asperse, blacken, calumniate, defame, disparage, revile, scandalize, slander, traduce, vilify. • *adj* malevolent, malicious, malignant, ill-disposed; baneful, injurious, pernicious, unfavourable, unpropitious.

malignant *adj* bitter, envious, hostile, inimical, malevolent, malicious, malign, spiteful, rancorous, resentful, virulent; heinous, pernicious; ill-boding, unfavourable, unpropitious; dangerous, fatal.

malignity *n* animosity, hatred, ill-will, malice, malevolence, maliciousness, rancour, spite; deadliness, destructiveness, fatality, harmfulness, malignancy, perniciousness, virulence; enormity, evilness, heinousness.

malpractice *n* dereliction, malversation, misbehaviour, misconduct, misdeed, misdoing, sin, transgression.

maltreat *vb* abuse, harm, hurt, ill-treat, ill-use, injure.

mammoth *adj* colossal, enormous, gigantic, huge, immense, vast.

man *n* crew, garrison, furnish, fortify, reinforce, strengthen. • *n* adult, being, body, human, individual, one, person, personage, somebody, soul; humanity, humankind, mankind; attendant, butler, dependant, liege, servant, subject, valet, vassal; employee, workman.

manacle *vb* bind, chain, fetter, handcuff, restrain, shackle, tie. • *n* bond, chain, handcuff, gyve, hand-fetter, shackle.

manage *vb* administer, conduct, direct, guide, handle, operate, order, regulate, superintend, supervise, transact, treat; control, govern, rule; handle, manipulate, train, wield; contrive, economize, husband, save.

manageable *adj* controllable, docile, easy, governable, tamable, tractable.

management *n* administration, care, charge, conduct, control, direction, disposal, economy, government, guidance, superintendence, supervision, surveillance, treatment.

manager *n* comptroller, conductor, director, executive, governor, impresario, overseer, superintendent, supervisor.

mandate *n* charge, command, commission, edict, injunction, order, precept, requirement.

manful *adj* bold, brave, courageous, daring, heroic, honourable, intrepid, noble, stout, strong, undaunted, vigorous.

mangily *adv* basely, foully, meanly, scabbily, scurvily, vilely.

mangle¹ *vb* hack, lacerate, mutilate, rend, tear; cripple, crush, destroy, maim, mar, spoil.

mangle² *vb* calender, polish, press, smooth.

manhood *n* virility; bravery, courage, firmness, fortitude, hardihood, manfulness, manliness, resolution; human nature, humanity; adulthood, maturity.

mania *n* aberration, craziness, delirium, dementia, derangement, frenzy, insanity, lunacy, madness; craze, desire, enthusiasm, fad, fanaticism.

manifest *vb* declare, demonstrate, disclose, discover, display, evidence, evince, exhibit, express, reveal, show. • *adj* apparent, clear, conspicuous, distinct, evident, glaring, indubitable, obvious, open, palpable, patent, plain, unmistakable, visible.

manifestation *n* disclosure, display, exhibition, exposure, expression, revelation.

manifold *adj* complex, diverse, many, multifarious, multiplied, multitudinous, numerous, several, sundry, varied, various.

manipulate *vb* handle, operate, work.

manliness *n* boldness, bravery, courage, dignity, fearlessness, firmness, heroism, intrepidity, nobleness, resolution, valour.

manly *adj* bold, brave, courageous, daring, dignified, firm, heroic, intrepid, manful, noble, stout, strong, undaunted, vigorous; male, masculine, virile.

manner *n* fashion, form, method, mode, style, way; custom, habit, practice; degree, extent, measure; kind, kinds, sort, sorts; air, appearance, aspect, behaviour, carriage, demeanour, deportment, look, mien; mannerism, peculiarity; behaviour, conduct, habits, morals; civility, deportment.

mannerly *adj* ceremonious, civil, complaisant, courteous, polite, refined, respectful, urbane, well-behaved, well-bred.

manners *npl* conduct, habits, morals; air, bearing, behaviour, breeding, carriage, comportment, deportment, etiquette.

manoeuvre *vb* contrive, finesse, intrigue, manage, plan, plot, scheme. • *n* evolution, exercise, movement, operation; artifice, finesse, intrigue, plan, plot, ruse, scheme, stratagem, trick.

mansion *n* abode, dwelling, dwelling house, habitation, hall, residence, seat.

mantle *vb* cloak, cover, discover, obscure; expand, spread; bubble, cream, effervesce, foam, froth, sparkle. • *n* chasuble, cloak, toga; cover, covering, hood.

manufacture *vb* build, compose, construct, create, fabricate, forge, form, make, mould, produce, shape. • *n* constructing, fabrication, making, production.

manumission *n* deliverance, emancipation, enfranchisement, freedom, liberation, release.

manumit *vb* deliver, emancipate, enfranchise, free, liberate, release.

manure *vb* enrich, fertilize. • *n* compost, dressing, fertilizer, guano, muck.

many *adj* abundant, diverse, frequent, innumerable, manifold, multifarious, multifold, multiplied, multitudinous, numerous, sundry, varied, various. • *n* crowd, multitude, people.

map *vb* chart, draw up, plan, plot, set out, sketch. • *n* chart, diagram, outline, plot, sketch.

mar *vb* blot, damage, harm, hurt, impair, injure, ruin, spoil, stain; deface, deform, disfigure, maim, mutilate.

marauder *n* bandit, brigand, desperado, filibuster, freebooter, outlaw, pillager, plunderer, ravager, robber, rover.

march *vb* go, pace, parade, step, tramp, walk. • *n* hike, tramp, walk; parade, procession; gait, step, stride; advance, evolution, progress.

marches *npl* borders, boundaries, confines, frontiers, limits, precincts.

margin *n* border, brim, brink, confine, edge, limit, rim, skirt, verge; latitude, room, space, surplus.

marine *adj* oceanic, pelagic, saltwater, sea; maritime, naval, nautical. • *n* navy, shipping; sea-dog, sea soldier, soldier; sea piece, seascape.

mariner *n* navigator, sailor, salt, seafarer, seaman, tar.

marital *adj* connubial, conjugal, matrimonial.

maritime *adj* marine, naval, nautical, oceanic, sea, seafaring, seagoing; coastal, seaside.

mark *vb* distinguish, earmark, label; betoken, brand, characterize, denote, designate, engrave, impress, imprint, indicate, print, stamp; evince, heed, note, notice, observe, regard, remark, show, spot. • *n* brand, character, characteristic, impression, impress, line, note, print, sign, stamp, symbol, token,

race; evidence, indication, proof, symptom, trace, track, vestige; badge; footprint; bull's-eye, butt, object, target; consequence, distinction, eminence, fame, importance, notability, position, preeminence, reputation, significance.

marked *adj* conspicuous, distinguished, eminent, notable, noted, outstanding, prominent, remarkable.

marriage *n* espousals, nuptials, spousals, wedding; matrimony, wedlock; union; alliance, association, confederation.

marrow *n* medulla, pith; cream, essence, quintessence, substance.

marsh *n* bog, fen, mire, morass, quagmire, slough, swamp.

marshal *vb* arrange, array, dispose, gather, muster, range, order, rank; guide, herald, lead. • *n* conductor, director, master of ceremonies, regulator; harbinger, herald, pursuivant.

marshy *adj* boggy, miry, mossy, swampy, wet.

martial *adj* brave, heroic, military, soldier-like, warlike.

marvel *vb* gape, gaze, goggle, wonder. • *n* miracle, prodigy, wonder; admiration, amazement, astonishment, surprise.

marvellous *adj* amazing, astonishing, extraordinary, miraculous, prodigious, strange, stupendous, wonderful, wondrous; improbable, incredible, surprising, unbelievable.

masculine *adj* bold, hardy, manful, manlike, manly, mannish, virile; potent, powerful, robust, strong, vigorous; bold, coarse, forward.

mask *vb* cloak, conceal, cover, disguise, hide, screen, shroud, veil. • *n* blind, cloak, disguise, screen, veil; evasion, pretence, plea, pretext, ruse, shift, subterfuge, trick; masquerade; bustle, mummery.

masquerade *vb* cover, disguise, hide, mask, revel, veil. • *n* mask, mummery, revel, revelry.

Mass *n* communion, Eucharist.

mass *vb* accumulate, amass, assemble, collect, gather, rally, throng. • *adj* extensive, general, large-scale, widespread. • *n* cake, clot, lump; assemblage, collection, combination, congeries, heap; bulk, dimension, magnitude, size; accumulation, aggregate, body, sum, total, totality, whole.

massacre *vb* annihilate, butcher, exterminate, kill, murder, slaughter, slay. • *n* annihilation, butchery, carnage, extermination, killing, murder, pogrom, slaughter.

massive *adj* big, bulky, colossal, enormous, heavy, huge, immense, ponderous, solid, substantial, vast, weighty.

master *vb* conquer, defeat, direct, govern, overcome, overpower, rule, subdue, subjugate, vanquish; acquire, learn. • *adj* cardinal, chief, especial, grand, great, main, leading, prime, principal; adept, expert, proficient. • *n* director, governor, lord, manager, overseer, superintendent, ruler; captain, commander; instructor, pedagogue, preceptor, schoolteacher, teacher, tutor; holder, owner, possessor, proprietor; chief, head, leader, principal.

masterly *adj* adroit, clever, dextrous, excellent, expert, finished, skilful, skilled; arbitrary, despotic, despotical, domineering, imperious.

mastery *n* command, dominion, mastership, power, rule, supremacy, sway; ascendancy, conquest, leadership, preeminence, superiority, upper-hand, victory; acquisition, acquirement, attainment; ability, cleverness, dexterity, proficiency, skill.

masticate *vb* chew, eat, munch.

match *vb* equal, rival; adapt, fit, harmonize, proportion, suit; marry, mate; combine, couple, join, sort; oppose, pit; correspond, suit, tally. • *n* companion, equal, mate, tally; competition, contest, game, trial; marriage, union.

matchless *adj* consummate, excellent, exquisite, incomparable, inimitable, peerless, perfect, surpassing, unequalled, unmatched, unparalleled, unrivalled.

mate *vb* marry, match, wed; compete, equal, vie; appal, confound, crush, enervate, subdue, stupefy. • *n* associate, companion, compeer, consort, crony, friend, fellow, intimate; companion, equal, match; assistant, subordinate; husband, spouse, wife.

material *adj* bodily, corporeal, nonspiritual, physical, temporal; essential, important, momentous, relevant, vital, weighty. • *n* body, element, stuff, substance.

maternal *adj* motherlike, motherly.

matrimonial *adj* conjugal, connubial, espousal, hymeneal, marital, nuptial, spousal.

matrimony *n* marriage, wedlock.

matter *vb* import, signify, weigh. • *n* body, content, sense, substance; difficulty, distress, trouble; material, stuff; question, subject, subject matter, topic; affair, business, concern, event; consequence, import, importance, moment, significance; discharge, purulence, pus.

mature vb develop, perfect, ripen. • adj complete, fit, full-grown, perfect, ripe; completed, prepared, ready, well-considered, well-digested.

maturity n completeness, completion, matureness, perfection, ripeness.

mawkish adj disgusting, flat, insipid, nauseous, sickly, stale, tasteless, vapid; emotional, feeble, maudlin, sentimental.

maxim n adage, aphorism, apothegm, axiom, byword, dictum, proverb, saw, saying, truism.

maze vb amaze, bewilder, confound, confuse, perplex. • n intricacy, labyrinth, meander; bewilderment, embarrassment, intricacy, perplexity, puzzle, uncertainty.

mazy adj confused, confusing, intricate, labyrinthian, labyrinthic, labyrinthine, perplexing, winding.

meagre adj emaciated, gaunt, lank, lean, poor, skinny, starved, spare, thin; barren, poor, sterile, unproductive; bald, barren, dry, dull, mean, poor, prosy, feeble, insignificant, jejune, scanty, small, tame, uninteresting, vapid.

mean[1] vb contemplate, design, intend, purpose; connote, denote, express, imply, import, indicate, purport, signify, symbolize.

mean[2] adj average, medium, middle; intermediate, intervening. • n measure, mediocrity, medium, moderation; average; agency, instrument, instrumentality, means, measure, method, mode, way.

mean[3] adj coarse, common, humble, ignoble, low, ordinary, plebeian, vulgar; abject, base, base-minded, beggarly, contemptible, degraded, dirty, dishonourable, disingenuous, grovelling, low-minded, pitiful, rascally, scurvy, servile, shabby, sneaking, sorry, spiritless, unfair, vile; illiberal, mercenary, miserly, narrow, narrow-minded, niggardly, parsimonious, penurious, selfish, sordid, stingy, ungenerous, unhandsome; contemptible, despicable, diminutive, insignificant, paltry, petty, poor, small, wretched.

meaning n acceptation, drift, import, intention, purport, purpose, sense, signification.

means npl instrument, method, mode, way; appliance, expedient, measure, resource, shift, step; estate, income, property, resources, revenue, substance, wealth, wherewithal.

measure vb mete; adjust, gauge, proportion; appraise, appreciate, estimate, gauge, value. • n gauge, meter, rule, standard; degree, extent, length, limit; allotment, share, proportion; means, step; foot, metre, rhythm, tune, verse.

measureless adj boundless, endless, immeasurable, immense, limitless, unbounded, unlimited, vast.

meat n aliment, cheer, diet, fare, feed, flesh, food, nourishment, nutriment, provision, rations, regimen, subsistence, sustenance, viands, victuals.

mechanic n artificer, artisan, craftsman, hand, handicraftsman, machinist, operative, workman.

meddle vb interfere, intermeddle, interpose, intrude.

meddlesome adj interfering, intermeddling, intrusive, officious, prying.

mediate vb arbitrate, intercede, interpose, intervene, settle. • adj interposed, intervening, middle.

mediation n arbitration, intercession, interposition, intervention.

mediator n advocate, arbitrator, interceder, intercessor, propitiator, umpire.

medicine n drug, medicament, medication, physic; therapy.

mediocre adj average, commonplace, indifferent, mean, medium, middling, ordinary.

meditate vb concoct, contrive, design, devise, intend, plan, purpose, scheme; chew, contemplate, ruminate, study cogitate, muse, ponder, think.

meditation n cogitation, contemplation, musing, pondering, reflection, ruminating, study, thought.

meditative adj contemplative, pensive, reflective, studious, thoughtful.

medium adj average, mean, mediocre, middle. • n agency, channel, intermediary, instrument, instrumentality, means, organ; conditions, environment, influences; average, means.

medley n confusion, farrago, hodgepodge, hotchpotch, jumble, mass, melange, miscellany, mishmash, mixture.

meed n award, guerdon, premium, prize, recompense, remuneration, reward.

meek adj gentle, humble, lowly, mild, modest, pacific, soft, submissive, unassuming, yielding.

meekness n gentleness, humbleness, humility, lowliness, mildness, modesty, submission, submissiveness.

meet vb cross, intersect, transact; confront, encounter, engage; answer, comply, fulfil, gratify, satisfy; converge, join, unite; assemble, collect, convene, congregate, forgather, muster, rally. • adj adapted, appropriate, befitting, convenient, fit, fitting, proper, qualified, suitable, suited.

meeting n encounter, interview; assemblage, assembly, audience, company, concourse, conference, congregation, convention, gathering; assignation, encounter, introduction, rendezvous; confluence, conflux, intersection, joining, junction, union; collision.

melancholy adj blue, dejected, depressed, despondent, desponding, disconsolate, dismal, dispirited, doleful, down, downcast, downhearted, gloomy, glum, hypochondriac, low-spirited, lugubrious, moody, mopish, sad, sombre, sorrowful, unhappy; afflictive, calamitous, unfortunate, unlucky; dark, gloomy, grave, quiet. • n blues, dejection, depression, despondency, dismals, dumps, gloom, gloominess, hypochondria, sadness, vapours.

melee n affray, brawl, broil, contest, fight, fray, scuffle.

mellifluous, mellifluent adj dulcet, euphonic, euphonical, euphonious, mellow, silver-toned, silvery, smooth, soft, sweet.

mellow vb mature, ripen; improve, smooth, soften, tone; pulverize; perfect. • adj mature, ripe; dulcet, mellifluous, mellifluent, rich, silver-toned, silvery, smooth, soft; delicate; genial, good-humoured, jolly, jovial, matured, softened; mellowy, loamy, unctuous; perfected, well-prepared; disguised, fuddled, intoxicated, tipsy.

melodious adj arioso, concordant, dulcet, euphonious, harmonious, mellifluous, mellifluent, musical, silvery, sweet, tuneful.

melody n air, descant, music, plainsong, song, theme, tune.

melt vb dissolve, fuse, liquefy, thaw; mollify, relax, soften, subdue; dissipate, waste; blend, pass, shade.

member n arm, leg, limb, organ; component, constituent, element, part, portion; branch, clause, division, head.

memento n memorial, remembrance, reminder, souvenir.

memoir n account, autobiography, biography, journal, narrative, record, register.

memorable adj celebrated, distinguished, extraordinary, famous, great, illustrious, important, notable, noteworthy, remarkable, signal, significant.

memorandum n minute, note, record.

memorial adj commemorative, monumental. • n cairn, commemoration, memento, monument, plaque, record, souvenir; memorandum, remembrance.

memory n recollection, remembrance, reminiscence; celebrity, fame, renown, reputation; commemoration, memorial.

menace vb alarm, frighten, intimidate, threaten. • n danger, hazard, peril, threat, warning; nuisance, pest, troublemaker.

menage n household, housekeeping, management.

mend vb darn, patch, rectify, retit, repair, restore, retouch; ameliorate, amend, better, correct, emend, improve, meliorate, reconcile, rectify, reform; advance, help; augment, increase.

mendacious adj deceitful, deceptive, fallacious, false, lying, untrue, untruthful.

mendacity n deceit, deceitfulness, deception, duplicity, falsehood, lie, untruth.

mendicant n beggar, pauper, tramp.

menial adj base, low, mean, servile, vile. • n attendant, bondsman, domestic, flunkey, footman, lackey, serf, servant, slave, underling, valet, waiter

mensuration n measurement, measuring; survey, surveying.

mental adj ideal, immaterial, intellectual, psychiatric, subjective.

mention vb acquaint, allude, cite, communicate, declare, disclose, divulge, impart, inform, name, report, reveal, state, tell. • n allusion, citation, designation, notice, noting, reference.

mentor n adviser, counsellor, guide, instructor, monitor.

mephitic adj baleful, baneful, fetid, foul, mephitical, noisome, noxious, poisonous, pestilential.

mercantile adj commercial, marketable, trading.

mercenary adj hired, paid, purchased, venal; avaricious, covetous, grasping, mean, niggardly, parsimonious, penurious, sordid, stingy. • n hireling, soldier.

merchandise n commodities, goods, wares.

merchant n dealer, retailer, shopkeeper, trader, tradesman.

merciful adj clement, compassionate, forgiving, gracious, lenient, pitiful; benignant, forbearing, gentle, humane, kind, mild, tender, tender-hearted.

merciless adj barbarous, callous, cruel, fell, hard-hearted, inexorable, pitiless, relentless, remorseless, ruthless, savage, severe, uncompassionate, unfeeling, unmerciful, unrelenting, unrepenting, unsparing.

mercurial *adj* active, lively, nimble, prompt, quick, sprightly; cheerful, light-hearted; changeable, fickle, flighty, inconstant, mobile, volatile.

mercy *n* benevolence, clemency, compassion, gentleness, kindness, lenience, leniency, lenity, mildness, pity, tenderness; blessing, favour, grace; discretion, disposal; forgiveness, pardon.

mere *adj* bald, bare, naked, plain, sole, simple; absolute, entire, pure, sheer, unmixed. • *n* lake, pond, pool.

meretricious *adj* deceitful, brummagem, false, gaudy, make-believe, sham, showy, spurious, tawdry.

merge *vb* bury, dip, immerse, involve, lose, plunge, sink, submerge.

meridian *n* acme, apex, climax, culmination, summit, zenith; midday, noon, noontide.

merit *vb* deserve, earn, incur; acquire, gain, profit, value. • *n* claim, right; credit, desert, excellence, goodness, worth, worthiness.

meritorious *adj* commendable, deserving, excellent, good, worthy.

merriment *n* amusement, frolic, gaiety, hilarity, jocularity, jollity, joviality, laughter, liveliness, mirth, sport, sportiveness.

merry *adj* agreeable, brisk, delightful, exhilarating, lively, pleasant, stirring; airy, blithe, blithesome, buxom, cheerful, comical, droll, facetious, frolicsome, gladsome, gleeful, hilarious, jocund, jolly, jovial, joyous, light-hearted, lively, mirthful, sportive, sprightly, vivacious.

mess *n* company, set; farrago, hodgepodge, hotchpotch, jumble, medley, mass, melange, miscellany, mishmash, mixture; confusion, muddle, perplexity, pickle, plight, predicament.

message *n* communication, dispatch, intimation, letter, missive, notice, telegram, wire, word.

messenger *n* carrier, courier, emissary, envoy, express, mercury, nuncio; forerunner, harbinger, herald, precursor.

metamorphic *adj* changeable, mutable, variable.

metamorphose *vb* change, mutate, transfigure, transform, transmute.

metamorphosis *n* change, mutation, transfiguration, transformation, transmutation.

metaphorical *adj* allegorical, figurative, symbolic, symbolical.

metaphysical *adj* abstract, allegorical, figurative, general, intellectual, parabolic, subjective, unreal.

mete *vb* dispense, distribute, divide, measure, ration, share. • *n* bound, boundary, butt, limit, measure, term, terminus.

meteor *n* aerolite, falling star, shooting star.

method *n* course, manner, means, mode, procedure, process, rule, way; arrangement, classification, disposition, order, plan, regularity, scheme, system.

methodical *adj* exact, orderly, regular, systematic, systematical.

metropolis *n* capital, city, conurbation.

mettle *n* constitution, element, material, stuff; character, disposition, spirit, temper; ardour, courage, fire, hardihood, life, nerve, pluck, sprightliness, vigour.

mettlesome *adj* ardent, brisk, courageous, fiery, frisky, high-spirited, lively, spirited, sprightly.

mew *vb* confine, coop, encase, enclose, imprison; cast, change, mould, shed.

microscopic *adj* infinitesimal, minute, tiny.

middle *adj* central, halfway, mean, medial, mid; intermediate, intervening. • *n* centre, halfway, mean, midst.

middleman *n* agent, broker, factor, go-between, intermediary.

mien *n* air, appearance, aspect, bearing, behaviour, carriage, countenance, demeanour, deportment, look, manner.

might *n* ability, capacity, efficacy, efficiency, force, main, power, prowess, puissance, strength.

mighty *adj* able, bold, courageous, potent, powerful, puissant, robust, strong, sturdy, valiant, valorous, vigorous; bulky, enormous, huge, immense, monstrous, stupendous, vast.

migratory *adj* nomadic, roving, shifting, strolling, unsettled, wandering, vagrant.

mild *adj* amiable, clement, compassionate, gentle, good-natured, indulgent, kind, lenient, meek, merciful, pacific, tender; bland, pleasant, soft, suave; calm, kind, placid, temperate, tranquil; assuasive, compliant, demulcent, emollient, lenitive, mollifying, soothing.

mildness *n* amiability, clemency, gentleness, indulgence, kindness, meekness, moderation, softness, tenderness, warmth.

mildew *n* blight, blast, mould, must, mustiness, smut, rust.

milieu *n* background, environment, sphere, surroundings.

militant *adj* belligerent, combative, contending, fighting.

military *adj* martial, soldier, soldierly, warlike. • *n* army, militia, soldiers.

mill *vb* comminute, crush, grate, grind, levigate, powder, pulverize. • *n* factory, manufactory; grinder; crowd, throng.

mimic *vb* ape, counterfeit, imitate, impersonate, mime, mock, parody. • *adj* imitative, mock, simulated. • *n* imitator, impersonator, mime, mocker, parodist, parrot.

mince[1] *vb* chop, cut, hash, shatter. • *n* forcemeat, hash, mash, mincemeat.

mince[2] *vb* attenuate, diminish, extenuate, mitigate, palliate, soften; pose, sashay, simper, smirk.

mind[1] *vb* attend, heed, mark, note, notice, regard, tend, watch; obey, observe, submit; design, incline, intend, mean; recall, recollect, remember, remind; beware, look out, watch out. • *n* soul, spirit; brains, common sense, intellect, reason, sense, understanding; belief, consideration, contemplation, judgement, opinion, reflection, sentiment, thought; memory, recollection, remembrance; bent, desire, disposition, inclination, intention, leaning, purpose, tendency, will.

mind[2] *vb* balk, begrudge, grudge, object, resent.

mindful *adj* attentive, careful, heedful, observant, regardful, thoughtful.

mindless *adj* dull, heavy, insensible, senseless, sluggish, stupid, unthinking; careless, forgetful, heedless, neglectful, negligent, regardless.

mine *vb* dig, excavate, quarry, unearth; sap, undermine, weaken; destroy, ruin. • *n* colliery, deposit, lode, pit, shaft.

mingle *vb* blend, combine, commingle, compound, intermingle, intermix, join, mix, unite.

miniature *adj* bantam, diminutive, little, small, tiny.

minion *n* creature, dependant, favourite, hanger-on, parasite, sycophant; darling, favourite, flatterer, pet.

minister *vb* administer, afford, furnish, give, supply; aid, assist, contribute, help, succour. • *n* agent, assistant, servant, subordinate, underling; administrator, executive; ambassador, delegate, envoy, plenipotentiary; chaplain, churchman, clergyman, cleric, curate, divine, ecclesiastic, parson, pastor, preacher, priest, rector, vicar.

ministry *n* agency, aid, help, instrumentality, interposition, intervention, ministration, service, support; administration, cabinet, council, government.

minor *adj* less, smaller; inferior, junior, secondary, subordinate, younger; inconsiderable, petty, unimportant, small.

minstrel *n* bard, musician, singer, troubadour.

mint *vb* coin, stamp; fabricate, fashion, forge, invent, make, produce. • *adj* fresh, new, perfect, undamaged. • *n* die, punch, seal, stamp; fortune, (*inf*) heap, million, pile, wad.

minute[1] *adj* diminutive, fine, little, microscopic, miniature, slender, slight, small, tiny; circumstantial, critical, detailed, exact, fussy, meticulous, nice, particular, precise.

minute[2] *n* account, entry, item, memorandum, note, proceedings, record; instant, moment, second, trice, twinkling.

miracle *n* marvel, prodigy, wonder.

miraculous *adj* supernatural, thaumaturgic, thaumaturgical; amazing, extraordinary, incredible, marvellous, unaccountable, unbelievable, wondrous.

mirror *vb* copy, echo, emulate, reflect, show. • *n* looking-glass, reflector, speculum; archetype, exemplar, example, model, paragon, pattern, prototype.

mirth *n* cheerfulness, festivity, frolic, fun, gaiety, gladness, glee, hilarity, festivity, jollity, joviality, joyousness, laughter, merriment, merry-making, rejoicing, sport.

mirthful *adj* cheery, cheery, festive, frolicsome, hilarious, jocund, jolly, merry, jovial, joyous, lively, playful, sportive, vivacious; comic, droll, humorous, facetious, funny, jocose, jocular, ludicrous, merry, waggish, witty.

misadventure *n* accident, calamity, catastrophe, cross, disaster, failure, ill-luck, infelicity, mischance, misfortune, mishap, reverse.

misanthrope *n* cynic, egoist, egotist, man-hater, misanthropist.

misapply *vb* abuse, misuse, pervert.

misapprehend *vb* misconceive, mistake, misunderstand.

misbehaviour *n* ill-behaviour, ill-conduct, incivility, miscarriage, misconduct, misdemeanour, naughtiness, rudeness.

miscarriage *n* calamity, defeat, disaster, failure, mischance, mishap; misbehaviour, misconduct, ill-behaviour.

miscellaneous *adj* confused, diverse, diversified, heterogeneous, indiscriminate, jumbled, many, mingled, mixed, promiscuous, stromatic, stromatous, various.

miscellany *n* collection, diversity, farrago, gallimaufry, hodge-podge, hotchpotch, jumble, medley, mishmash, melange, miscellaneous, mixture, variety.

mischance *n* accident, calamity, disaster, ill-fortune, ill-luck, in-felicity, misadventure, misfortune, mishap.

mischief *n* damage, detriment, disadvantage, evil, harm, hurt, ill, injury, prejudice; ill-consequence, misfortune, trouble; devilry, wrong-doing.

mischievous *adj* destructive, detrimental, harmful, hurtful, inju-rious, noxious, pernicious; malicious, sinful, vicious, wicked; annoying, impish, naughty, troublesome, vexatious.

misconceive *vb* misapprehend, misjudge, mistake, misunder-stand.

misconduct *vb* botch, bungle, misdirect, mismanage. • *n* bad conduct, ill-conduct, misbehaviour, misdemeanour rudeness, transgression; ill-management, mismanagement.

misconstrue *vb* misread, mistranslate; misapprehend, misinter-pret, mistake, misunderstand.

miscreant *adj* corrupt, criminal, evil, rascally, unprincipled, vi-cious, villainous, wicked. • *n* caitiff, knave, ragamuffin, rascal, rogue, ruffian, scamp, scoundrel, vagabond, villain.

misdemeanour *n* fault, ill-behaviour, misbehaviour, misconduct, misdeed, offence, transgression, trespass.

miser *n* churl, curmudgeon, lickpenny, money-grabber, niggard, penny-pincher, pinch-fist, screw, scrimp, skinflint.

miserable *adj* afflicted, broken-hearted, comfortless, disconso-late, distressed, forlorn, heartbroken, unhappy, wretched; calamitous, hapless, ill-starred, pitiable, unfortunate, unlucky; poor, valueless, worthless; abject, contemptible, despicable, low, mean, worthless.

miserly *adj* avaricious, beggarly, close, close-fisted, covetous, grasping, mean, niggardly, parsimonious, penurious, sordid, stingy, tight-fisted.

misery *n* affliction, agony, anguish, calamity, desolation, distress, grief, heartache, heavy-heartedness, misfortune, sorrow, suf-fering, torment, torture, tribulation, unhappiness, woe, wretchedness.

misfortune *n* adversity, affliction, bad luck, blow, calamity, casu-alty, catastrophe, disaster, distress, hardship, harm, ill, inflic-tion, misadventure, mischance, mishap, reverse, scourge, stroke, trial, trouble, visitation.

misgiving *n* apprehension, distrust, doubt, hesitation, suspicion, uncertainty.

mishap *n* accident, calamity, disaster, ill luck, misadventure, mis-chance, misfortune.

misinterpret *vb* distort, falsify, misapprehend, misconceive, mis-construe, misjudge.

mislead *vb* beguile, deceive, delude, misdirect, misguide.

mismanage *vb* botch, fumble, misconduct, mishandle, misrule.

misprize *vb* slight, underestimate, underrate, undervalue.

misrepresent *vb* belie, caricature, distort, falsify, misinterpret, misstate, pervert.

misrule *n* anarchy, confusion, disorder, malad-ministration, mis-government, mismanagement.

miss¹ *vb* blunder, err, fail, fall short, forgo, lack, lose, miscarry, mistake, omit, overlook, trip; avoid, escape, evade, skip, slip; feel the loss of, need, want, wish. • *n* blunder, error, failure, fault, mistake, omission, oversight, slip, trip; loss, want.

miss² *n* damsel, girl, lass, maid, maiden.

misshapen *adj* deformed, ill-formed, ill-shaped, ill-propor-tioned, misformed, ugly, ungainly.

missile *n* projectile, weapon.

mission *n* commission, legation; business, charge, duty, errand, office, trust; delegation, deputation, embassy.

missive *n* communication, epistle, letter, message, note.

mist *vb* cloud, drizzle, mizzle, smog. • *n* cloud, fog, haze; bewil-derment, obscurity, perplexity.

mistake *vb* misapprehend, miscalculate, misconceive, mis-judge, misunderstand; confound, take; blunder, err. • *n* misapprehension, miscalculation, misconception, mistaking, misunderstanding; blunder, error, fault, inaccuracy, oversight, slip, trip.

mistaken *adj* erroneous, inaccurate, incorrect, misinformed, wrong.

mistrust *vb* distrust, doubt, suspect; apprehend, fear, surmise, suspect. • *n* doubt, distrust, misgiving, suspicion.

misty *adj* cloudy, clouded, dark, dim, foggy, obscure, overcast.

misunderstand *vb* misapprehend, misconceive, misconstrue, mistake.

misunderstanding *n* error, misapprehension, misconception, mistake; difference, difficulty, disagreement, discord, dissen-sion, quarrel.

misuse *vb* desecrate, misapply, misemploy, pervert, profane; abuse, ill-treat, maltreat, ill-use; fritter, squander, waste. • *n* abuse, perversion, profanation, prostitution; ill-treatment, ill-use, ill-usage, misusage; misapplication, solecism.

mitigate *vb* abate, alleviate, assuage, diminish, extenuate, lessen, moderate, palliate, relieve; allay, appease, calm, mollify, pacify, quell, quiet, reduce, soften, soothe; moderate, temper.

mitigation *n* abatement, allaying, alleviation, assuagement, diminution, moderation, palliation, relief.

mix *vb* alloy, amalgamate, blend, commingle, combine, com-pound, incorporate, interfuse, interlard, mingle, unite; associ-ate, join. • *n* alloy, amalgam, blend, combination, compound, mixture.

mixture *n* admixture, association, intermixture, union; com-pound, farrago, hash, hodgepodge, hotchpotch, jumble, med-ley, melange, mishmash; diversity, miscellany, variety.

moan *vb* bemoan, bewail, deplore, grieve, groan, lament, mourn, sigh weep. • *n* groan, lament, lamentation, sigh, wail.

mob *vb* crowd, jostle, surround, swarm, pack, throng. • *n* assem-blage, crowd, rabble, multitude, throng, tumult; dregs, canaille, populace, rabble, riffraff, scum.

mobile *adj* changeable, fickle, expressive, inconstant, sensitive, variable, volatile.

mock *vb* ape, counterfeit, imitate, mimic, take off; deride, flout, gibe, insult, jeer, ridicule, taunt; balk, cheat, deceive, defeat, disappoint, dupe, eluce, illude, mislead. • *adj* assumed, clap-trap, counterfeit, fake, false, feigned, make-believe, pretended, spurious. • *n* fake, imitation, phoney, sham; gibe, insult, jeer, scoff, taunt.

mockery *n* contumely, counterfeit, deception, derision, imitation, jeering, mimicry, ridicule, scoffing, scorn, sham, travesty.

mode *n* fashion, manner, method, style, way; accident, affection, degree, graduation, modification, quality, variety.

model *vb* design, fashion, form, mould, plan, shape. • *adj* ad-mirable, archetypal, estimable, exemplary, ideal, meritorious, paradigmatic, perfect, praiseworthy, worthy. • *n* archetype, de-sign, mould, original, pattern, protoplast, prototype, type; dummy, example, form; copy, facsimile, image, imitation, rep-resentation.

moderate *vb* abate, allay, appease, assuage, blunt, dull, lessen, soothe, mitigate, mollify, pacify, quell, quiet, reduce, repress, soften, still, subdue diminish, qualify, slacken, temper; control, govern, regulate. • *adj* abstinent, frugal, sparing, tem-perate; limited, mediocre; abstemious, sober; calm, cool, judi-cious, reasonable, steady; gentle, mild, temperate, tolerable.

moderation *n* abstemiousness, forbearance, frugality, restraint, sobriety, temperance; calmness, composure, coolness, deliber-ateness, equanimity, mildness, sedateness.

modern *adj* fresh, late, latest, new, novel, present, recent, up-to-date.

modest *adj* bashful, coy, diffident, humble, meek, reserved, retir-ing, shy, unassuming, unobtrusive, unostentatious, unpretend-ing, unpretentious; chaste, proper, pure, virtuous; becoming, decent, moderate.

modesty *n* bashfulness, coyness, diffidence, humility, meekness, propriety, prudishness, reserve, shyness, unobtrusiveness; chastity, purity, virtue; decency, moderation.

modification *n* alteration, change, qualification, reformation, variation; form, manner, mode, state.

modify *vb* alter, change, qualify, reform, shape, vary; lower, mod-erate, qualify, soften.

modish *adj* fashionable, stylish; ceremonious, conventional, courtly, genteel.

modulate *vb* attune, harmonize, tune; inflect, vary; adapt, adjust, proportion.

moiety *n* half; part, portion, share.

moil *vb* drudge, labour, toil; bespatter, daub, defile, soil, splash, spot, stain; fatigue, weary, tire.

moist *adj* damp, dank, humid, marshy, muggy, swampy, wet.

moisture *n* dampness, dankness, humidity, wetness.

mole *n* breakwater, dike, dyke, jetty, mound, pier, quay.

molecule *n* atom, monad, particle.

molest *vb* annoy, badger, bore, bother, chafe, discommode, disquiet, disturb, harass, harry, fret, gull, hector, incommode, inconvenience, irritate, oppress, pester, plague, tease, torment, trouble, vex, worry.

mollify *vb* soften; appease, calm, compose, pacify, quiet, soothe, tranquillize; abate, allay, assuage, blunt, dull, ease, lessen, mitigate, moderate, relieve, temper; qualify, tone down.

moment *n* flash, instant, jiffy, second, trice, twinkling, wink; avail, consequence, consideration, force, gravity, importance, significance, signification, value, weight; drive, force, impetus, momentum.

momentous *adj* grave, important, serious, significant, vital, weighty.

momentum *n* impetus, moment.

monarch *n* autocrat, despot; chief, dictator, emperor, king, potentate, prince, queen, ruler, sovereign.

monastery *n* abbey, cloister, convent, lamasery, nunnery, priory.

monastic *adj* coenobitic, coenobitical, conventual, monkish, secluded.

money *n* banknotes, cash, coin, currency, riches, specie, wealth.

moneyed, monied *adj* affluent, opulent, rich, well-off, well-to-do.

monitor *vb* check, observe, oversee, supervise, watch. • *n* admonisher, admonitor, adviser, counsellor, instructor, mentor, overseer.

monomania *n* delusion, hallucination, illusion, insanity, self-deception.

monopolize *vb* control, dominate, engross, forestall.

monotonous *adj* boring, dull, tedious, tiresome, undiversified, uniform, unvaried, unvarying, wearisome.

monotony *n* boredom, dullness, sameness, tedium, tiresomeness, uniformity, wearisomeness.

monster *adj* enormous, gigantic, huge, immense, mammoth, monstrous. • *n* enormity, marvel, prodigy, wonder; brute, demon, fiend, miscreant, ruffian, villain, wretch.

monstrous *adj* abnormal, preternatural, prodigious, unnatural; colossal, enormous, extraordinary, huge, immense, stupendous, vast; marvellous, strange, wonderful; bad, base, dreadful, flagrant, frightful, hateful, hideous, horrible, shocking, terrible.

monument *n* memorial, record, remembrance, testimonial; cairn, cenotaph, gravestone, mausoleum, memorial, pillar, tomb, tombstone.

mood *n* disposition, humour, temper, vein.

moody *adj* capricious, humoursome, variable; angry, crabbed, crusty, fretful, ill-tempered, irascible, irritable, passionate, pettish, peevish, petulant, snappish, snarling, sour, testy; crossgrained, dogged, frowning, glowering, glum, intractable, morose, perverse, spleeny, stubborn, sulky, sullen, wayward; abstracted, gloomy, melancholy, pensive, sad, saturnine.

moonshine *n* balderdash, fiction, flummery, fudge, fustian, nonsense, pretence, stuff, trash, twaddle, vanity.

moor[1] *vb* anchor, berth, fasten, fix, secure, tie.

moor[2] *n* bog, common, heath, moorland, morass, moss, wasteland.

moot *vb* agitate, argue, debate, discuss, dispute. • *adj* arguable, debatable, doubtful, unsettled.

mopish *adj* dejected, depressed, desponding, downcast, downhearted, gloomy, glum, sad.

moral *adj* ethical, good, honest, honourable, just, upright, virtuous; abstract, ideal, intellectual, mental. • *n* intent, meaning, significance.

morals *npl* ethics, morality; behaviour, conduct, habits, manners.

morass *n* bog, fen, marsh, quagmire, slough, swamp.

morbid *adj* ailing, corrupted, diseased, sick, sickly, tainted, unhealthy, unsound, vitiated; depressed, downcast, gloomy, pessimistic, sensitive.

mordacious *adj* acrid, biting, cutting, mordant, pungent, sharp, stinging; caustic, poignant, satirical, sarcastic, scathing, severe.

mordant *adj* biting, caustic, keen, mordacious, nipping, sarcastic.

moreover *adv, conj* also, besides, further, furthermore, likewise, too.

morning *n* aurora, daybreak, dawn, morn, morningtide, sunrise.

morose *adj* austere, churlish, crabbed, crusty, dejected, desponding, downcast, downhearted, gloomy, glum, melancholy, moody, sad, severe, sour, sullen, surly.

morsel *n* bite, mouthful, titbit; bit, fragment, part, piece, scrap.

mortal *adj* deadly, destructive, fatal, final, human, lethal, perishable, vital. • *n* being, earthling, human, man, person, woman.

mortality *n* corruption, death, destruction, fatality.

mortification *n* chagrin, disappointment, discontent, dissatisfaction, displeasure, humiliation, trouble, shame, vexation; humility, penance, self-abasement, self-denial; gangrene, necrosis.

mortify *vb* annoy, chagrin, depress, disappoint, displease, disquiet, dissatisfy, harass, humble, plague, vex, worry; abase, abash, confound, humiliate, restrain, shame, subdue; corrupt, fester, gangrene, putrefy.

mortuary *n* burial place, cemetery, churchyard, graveyard, necropolis; charnel house, morgue.

mostly *adv* chiefly, customarily, especially, generally, mainly, particularly, principally.

mote *n* atom, corpuscle, flaw, mite, particle, speck, spot.

motherly *adj* affectionate, kind, maternal, paternal, tender.

motion *vb* beckon, direct, gesture, signal. • *n* action, change, drift, flux, movement, passage, stir, transit; air, gait, port; gesture, impulse, prompting, suggestion; proposal, proposition.

motionless *adj* fixed, immobile, quiescent, stable, stagnant, standing, stationary, still, torpid, unmoved.

motive *adj* activating, driving, moving, operative. • *n* cause, consideration, ground, impulse, incentive, incitement, inducement, influence, occasion, prompting, purpose, reason, spur, stimulus.

motley *adj* coloured, dappled, mottled, speckled, spotted, variegated; composite, diversified, heterogeneous, mingled, mixed.

mottled *adj* dappled, motley, piebald, speckled, spotted, variegated.

mould[1] *vb* carve, cast, fashion, form, make, model, shape. • *n* cast, character, fashion, form, matrix, pattern, shape; material, matter, substance.

mould[2] *n* blight, mildew, mouldiness, must, mustiness, rot; fungus, lichen, mushroom, puffball, rust, smut, toadstool; earth, loam, soil.

moulder *vb* crumble, decay, perish, waste.

mouldy *adj* decaying, fusty, mildewed, musty.

mound *n* bank, barrow, hill, hillock, knoll, tumulus; bulwark, defence, rampart.

mount[1] *n* hill, mountain, peak.

mount[2] *vb* arise, ascend, climb, rise, soar, tower; escalate, scale; embellish, ornament; bestride, get upon. • *n* charger, horse, ride, steed.

mountain *n* alp, height, hill, mount, peak; abundance, heap, mound, stack.

mountebank *n* charlatan, cheat, impostor, pretender, quack.

mourn *vb* bemoan, bewail, deplore, grieve, lament, sorrow, wail.

mournful *adj* afflicting, afflictive, calamitous, deplorable, distressed, grievous, lamentable, sad, woeful; doleful, heavy, heavy-hearted, lugubrious, melancholy, sorrowful, tearful.

mouth *vb* clamour, declaim, rant, roar, vociferate. • *n* chaps, jaws; aperture, opening, orifice; entrance, inlet; oracle, mouthpiece, speaker, spokesman.

movables *npl* chattels, effects, furniture, goods, property, wares.

move *vb* dislodge, drive, impel, propel, push, shift, start, stir; actuate, incite, instigate, rouse; determine, incline, induce, influence, persuade, prompt; affect, impress, touch, trouble; agitate, awaken, excite, incense, irritate; propose, recommend, suggest; go, march, proceed, walk; act, live; flit, remove. • *n* action, motion, movement.

movement *n* change, move, motion, passage; emotion; crusade, drive.

moving *adj* impelling, influencing, instigating, persuading, persuasive; affecting, impressive, pathetic, touching.

mucous *adj* glutinous, gummy, mucilaginous, ropy, slimy, viscid.

mud *n* dirt, mire, muck, slime.

muddle *vb* confuse, disarrange, disorder; fuddle, inebriate, stupefy; muff, mull, spoil. • *n* confusion, disorder, mess, plight, predicament.

muddy *vb* dirty, foul, smear, soil; confuse, obscure. • *adj* dirty, foul, impure, slimy, soiled, turbid; bothered, confused, dull, heavy, stupid; incoherent, obscure, vague.

muffle *vb* cover, envelop, shroud, wrap; conceal, disguise, involve; deaden, soften, stifle, suppress.

mulish *adj* cross-grained, headstrong, intractable, obstinate, stubborn.

multifarious *adj* different, divers, diverse, diversified, manifold, multiform, multitudinous, various.

multiloquence *n* garrulity, loquacity, loquaciousness, talkativeness.

multiply *vb* augment, extend, increase, spread.

multitude *n* numerousness; host, legion; army, assemblage, assembly, collection, concourse, congregation, crowd, horde, mob, swarm, throng; commonality, herd, mass, mob, pack, populace, rabble.

mundane *adj* earthly, secular, sublunary, temporal, terrene, terrestrial, worldly.

munificence *n* benefice, bounteousness, bountifulness, bounty, generosity, liberality.

munificent *adj* beneficent, bounteous, bountiful, free generous, liberal, princely.

murder *vb* assassinate, butcher, destroy, dispatch, kill, massacre, slaughter, slay; abuse, mar, spoil. • *n* assassination, butchery, destruction, homicide, killing, manslaughter, massacre.

murderer *n* assassin, butcher, cut-throat, killer, manslaughterer, slaughterer, slayer.

murderous *adj* barbarous, bloodthirsty, bloody, cruel, fell, sanguinary, savage.

murky *adj* cheerless, cloudy, dark, dim, dusky, gloomy hazy, lowering, lurid, obscure, overcast.

murmur *vb* croak, grumble, mumble, mutter; hum, whisper. • *n* complaint, grumble, mutter, plaint, whimper, hum, undertone, whisper.

muscular *adj* sinewy; athletic, brawny, powerful, lusty, stalwart, stout, strong, sturdy, vigorous.

muse *vb* brood, cogitate, consider, contemplate, deliberate, dream, meditate, ponder, reflect, ruminate, speculate, think. • *n* abstraction, musing, reverie.

music *n* harmony, melody, symphony.

musical *adj* dulcet, harmonious, melodious, sweet, sweet-sounding, symphonious, tuneful.

musing *adj* absent-minded, meditative, preoccupied. • *n* absent-mindedness, abstraction, contemplation, daydreaming, mediation, muse, reflection, reverie, rumination.

muster *vb* assemble, collect, congregate, convene, convoke, gather, marshal, meet, rally, summon. • *n* assemblage, assembly, collection, congregation, convention, convocation, gathering, meeting, rally.

musty *adj* fetid, foul, fusty, mouldy, rank, sour, spoiled; hackneyed, old, stale, threadbare, trite; ill-favoured, insipid, vapid; dull, heavy, rusty, spiritless.

mutable *adj* alterable, changeable; changeful, fickle, inconstant, irresolute, mutational unsettled, unstable, unsteady, vacillating, variable, wavering.

mutation *n* alteration, change, variation.

mute *vb* dampen, lower moderate, muffle, soften. • *adj* dumb, voiceless silent, speechless, still, taciturn.

mutilate *vb* cripple, damage, disable, disfigure, hamstring, injure, maim, mangle, mar.

mutinous *adj* contumacious, insubordinate, rebellious, refractory, riotous, tumultuous, turbulent, unruly; insurgent, seditious.

mutiny *vb* rebel, revolt, rise, resist. • *n* insubordination, insurrection, rebellion, revolt, revolution, riot, rising, sedition, uprising.

mutter *vb* grumble, muffle, mumble, murmur.

mutual *adj* alternate, common, correlative, interchangeable, interchanged, reciprocal, requited.

myopic *adj* near-sighted, purblind, short-sighted.

myriad *adj* innumerable, manifold, multitudinous, uncounted. • *n* host, million(s), multitude, score(s), sea, swarm, thousand(s).

mysterious *adj* abstruse, cabbalistic, concealed, cryptic, dark, dim, enigmatic, enigmatical, hidden, incomprehensible, inexplicable, inscrutable, mystic, mystical, obscure, occult, puzzling, recondite, secret, sphinx-like, unaccountable, unfathomable, unintelligible, unknown.

mystery *n* enigma, puzzle, riddle, secret; art, business, calling, trade.

mystical *adj* abstruse, cabbalistic, dark, enigmatical, esoteric, hidden, inscrutable, mysterious, obscure, occult, recondite, transcendental; allegorical, emblematic, emblematical, symbolical.

mystify *vb* befog, bewilder, confound, confuse, dumbfound, embarrass, obfuscate, perplex, pose, puzzle.

myth *n* fable, legend, tradition; allegory, fiction, invention, parable, story; falsehood, fancy, figment, lie, untruth.

mythical *adj* allegorical, fabled, fabulous, fanciful, fictitious, imaginary, legendary, mythological.

N

nab *vb* catch, clutch, grasp, seize.

nag[1] *vb* carp, fuss, hector, henpeck, pester, torment, worry. • *n* nagger, scold, shrew, tartar.

nag[2] *n* bronco, crock, hack, horse, pony, scrag.

naive *adj* artless, candid, ingenuous, natural, plain, simple, unaffected, unsophisticated.

naked *adj* bare, nude, uncovered; denuded, unclad, unclothed, undressed; defenceless, exposed, open, unarmed, unguarded, unprotected; evident, manifest, plain, stark, unconcealed, undisguised; mere, sheer, simple; bare, destitute, rough, rude, unfurnished, unprovided; uncoloured, unexaggerated, unvarnished.

name *vb* call, christen, denounce, dub, entitle, phrase, style, term; mention; denominate, designate, indicate, nominate, specify. • *n* appellation, cognomen, denomination, designation, epithet, nickname, surname, sobriquet, title; character, credit, reputation, repute; celebrity, distinction, eminence, fame, honour, note, praise, renown.

narcotic *adj* stupefacient, stupefactive, stupefying. • *n* anaesthetic, anodyne, dope, opiate, sedative, stupefacient, tranquillizer.

narrate *vb* chronicle, describe, detail, enumerate, recite, recount, rehearse, relate, tell.

narration *n* account, description, chronicle, history, narrative, recital, rehearsal, relation, story, tale.

narrow *vb* confine, contract, cramp, limit, restrict, straiten. • *adj* circumscribed, confined, contracted, cramped, incapacious, limited, pinched, scanty, straitened; bigoted, hidebound, illiberal, ungenerous; close, near.

nastiness *n* defilement, dirtiness, filth, filthiness, foulness, impurity, pollution, squalor, uncleanness; indecency, grossness, obscenity, pornography, ribaldry, smut, smuttiness.

nasty *adj* defiled, dirty, filthy, foul, impure, loathsome, polluted, squalid, unclean; gross, indecent, indelicate, lewd, loose, obscene, smutty, vile; disagreeable, disgusting, nauseous, odious, offensive, repulsive, sickening; aggravating, annoying, pesky, pestering, troublesome.

nation *n* commonwealth, realm, state; community, people, population, race, stock, tribe.

native *adj* aboriginal, autochthonal, autochthonous, domestic, home, indigenous, vernacular; genuine, intrinsic, natural, original, real; congenital, inborn, inbred, inherent, innate, natal. • *n* aborigine, autochthon, inhabitant, national, resident.

natty *adj* dandyish, fine, foppish, jaunty, neat, nice, spruce, tidy.

natural *adj* indigenous, innate, native, original; characteristic, essential; legitimate, normal, regular; artless, authentic, genuine, ingenious, unreal, simple, spontaneous, unaffected; bastard, illegitimate.

nature *n* universe, world; character, constitution, essence; kind, quality, species, sort; disposition, grain, humour, mood, temper; being, intellect, intelligence, mind.

naughty *adj* bad, corrupt, mischievous, perverse, worthless.

nausea *n* queasiness, seasickness; loathing, qualm; aversion, disgust, repugnance.

nauseous *adj* abhorrent, disgusting, distasteful, loathsome, offensive, repulsive, revolting, sickening.

naval *adj* marine, maritime, nautical.

navigate *vb* cruise, direct, guide, pilot, plan, sail, steer.

navy *n* fleet, shipping, vessels.

near *vb* approach, draw close. • *adj* adjacent, approximate, close, contiguous, neighbouring, nigh; approaching, forthcoming, imminent, impending; dear, familiar, friendly, intimate; direct, immediate, short, straight; accurate, literal; narrow, parsimonious.

nearly *adv* almost, approximately, well-nigh; closely, intimately, pressingly; meanly, parsimoniously, penuriously, stingily.

neat *adj* clean, cleanly, orderly, tidy, trim, unsoiled; nice, smart, spruce; chaste, pure, simple; excellent, pure, unadulterated; adroit, clever, exact, finished; dainty, nice.

nebulous *adj* cloudy, hazy, misty.

necessary *adj* inevitable, unavoidable; essential, expedient, indispensable, needful, requisite; compelling, compulsory, involuntary. • *n* essential, necessity, requirement, requisite.

necessitate *vb* compel, constrain, demand, force, impel, oblige.

necessitous *adj* destitute, distressed, indigent, moneyless, needy, penniless, pinched, poor, poverty-stricken; narrow, pinching.

necessity *n* inevitability, inevitableness, unavoidability, unavoidableness; compulsion, destiny, fatality, fate; emergency, urgency, exigency, indigence, indispensability, indispensableness, need, needfulness, poverty, want; essentiality, essentialness, requirement, requisite.

necromancy *n* conjuration, divination, enchantment, magic, sorcery, witchcraft, wizardry.

necropolis *n* burial ground, cemetery, churchyard, crematorium, graveyard, mortuary.

need *vb* demand, lack, require, want. • *n* emergency, exigency, extremity, necessity, strait, urgency, want; destitution, distress, indigence, neediness, penury, poverty, privation.

needful *adj* distressful, necessitous, necessary; essential, indispensable, requisite.

needless *adj* superfluous, unnecessary, useless.

needy *adj* destitute, indigent, necessitous, poor.

nefarious *adj* abominable, atrocious, detestable, dreadful, execrable, flagitious, heinous, horrible, infamous, iniquitous, scandalous, vile, wicked.

negation *n* denial, disavowal, disclaimer, rejection, renunciation.

neglect *vb* condemn, despise, disregard, forget, ignore, omit, overlook, slight. • *n* carelessness, default, failure, heedlessness, inattention, omission, remissness; disregard, disrespect, slight; indifference, negligence.

negligence *n* carelessness, disregard, heedlessness, inadvertency, inattention, indifference, neglect, remissness, slackness, thoughtlessness; defect, fault, inadvertence, omission, shortcoming.

negligent *adj* careless, heedless, inattentive, indifferent, neglectful, regardless, thoughtless.

negotiate *vb* arrange, bargain, deal, debate, sell, settle, transact, treat.

neighbourhood *n* district, environs, locality, vicinage, vicinity; adjacency, nearness, propinquity, proximity.

neighbourly *adj* attentive, civil, friendly, kind, obliging, social.

neophyte *n* beginner, catechumen, convert, novice, pupil, tyro.

nerve *vb* brace, energize, fortify, invigorate, strengthen. • *n* force, might, power, strength, vigour; coolness, courage, endurance, firmness, fortitude, hardihood, manhood, pluck, resolution, self-command, steadiness.

nervous *adj* forcible, powerful, robust, strong, vigorous; irritable, fearful, shaky, timid, timorous, weak, weakly.

nestle *vb* cuddle, harbour, lodge, nuzzle, snug, snuggle.

nettle *vb* chafe, exasperate, fret, harass, incense, irritate, provoke, ruffle, sting, tease, vex.

neutral *adj* impartial, indifferent; colourless, mediocre.

neutralize *vb* cancel, counterbalance, counterpoise, invalidate, offset.

nevertheless *adv* however, nonetheless, notwithstanding, yet.

new *adj* fresh, latest, modern, novel, recent, unused; additional, another, further; reinvigorated, renovated, repaired.

news *n* advice, information, intelligence, report, tidings, word.

nice *adj* accurate, correct, critical, definite, delicate, exact, exquisite, precise, rigorous, strict; dainty, difficult, exacting, fastidious, finical, punctilious, squeamish; discerning, discriminating, particular, precise, scrupulous; neat, tidy, trim; fine, minute, refined, subtle; delicate, delicious, luscious, palatable, savoury, soft, tender; agreeable, delightful, good, pleasant.

nicety *n* accuracy, exactness, niceness, precision, truth, daintiness, fastidiousness, squeamishness; discrimination, subtlety.

niggard *n* churl, curmudgeon, miser, screw, scrimp, skinflint.

niggardly *adj* avaricious, close, close-fisted, illiberal, mean, mercenary, miserly, parsimonious, penurious, skinflint, sordid, stingy.

nigh *adj* adjacent, adjoining, contiguous, near; present, proximate. • *adv* almost, near, nearly.

nimble *adj* active, agile, alert, brisk, lively, prompt, quick, speedy, sprightly, spry, swift, tripping.

nobility *n* aristocracy, dignity, elevation, eminence, grandeur, greatness, loftiness, magnanimity, nobleness, peerage, superiority, worthiness.

noble *adj* dignified, elevated, eminent, exalted, generous, great, honourable, illustrious, magnanimous, superior, worthy; choice, excellent; aristocratic, gentle, high-born, patrician; grand, lofty, lordly, magnificent, splendid, stately. • *n* aristocrat, grandee, lord, nobleman, peer.

noctambulist *n* sleepwalker, somnambulist.

noise *vb* bruit, gossip, repeat, report, rumour. • *n* ado, blare, clamour, clatter, cry, din, fuss, hubbub, hullabaloo, outcry, pandemonium, racket, row, sound, tumult, uproar, vociferation.

noiseless *adj* inaudible, quiet, silent, soundless.

noisome *adj* bad, baneful, deleterious, disgusting, fetid, foul, hurtful, injurious, mischievous, nocuous, noxious, offensive, pernicious, pestiferous, pestilential, poisonous, unhealthy, unwholesome.

noisy *adj* blatant, blustering, boisterous, brawling, clamorous, loud, uproarious, riotous, tumultuous, vociferous.

nomadic *adj* migratory, pastoral, vagrant, wandering.

nominal *adj* formal, inconsiderable, minimal, ostensible, pretended, professed, so-called, titular.

nominate *vb* appoint, choose, designate, name, present, propose.

nonchalant *adj* apathetic, careless, cool, indifferent, unconcerned.

nondescript *adj* amorphous, characterless, commonplace, dull, indescribable, odd, ordinary, unclassifiable, uninteresting, unremarkable.

nonentity *n* cipher, futility, inexistence, inexistency insignificance, nobody, nonexistence, nothingness.

nonplus *vb* astonish, bewilder, confound, confuse, discomfit, disconcert, embarrass, floor, gravel, perplex, pose, puzzle.

nonsensical *adj* absurd, foolish, irrational, senseless, silly, stupid.

norm *n* model, pattern, rule, standard.

normal *adj* analogical, legitimate, natural, ordinary, regular, usual; erect, perpendicular, vertical.

notable *adj* distinguished, extraordinary, memorable, noted, remarkable, signal; conspicuous, evident, noticeable, observable, plain, prominent, striking; notorious, rare, well-known. • *n* celebrity, dignitary, notability, worthy.

note *vb* heed, mark, notice, observe, regard, remark; record, register; denote, designate. • *n* memorandum, minute, record; annotation, comment, remark, scholium; indication, mark, sign, symbol, token; account, bill, catalogue, reckoning; billet, epistle, letter; consideration, heed, notice, observation; celebrity, consequence, credit, distinction, eminence, fame, notability, notedness, renown, reputation, respectability; banknote, bill, promissory note; song, strain, tune, voice.

noted *adj* celebrated, conspicuous, distinguished, eminent, famed, famous, illustrious, notable, notorious, remarkable, renowned, well-known.

nothing *n* inexistence, nonentity, nonexistence, nothingness, nullity; bagatelle, trifle.

notice *vb* mark, note, observe, perceive, regard, see; comment on, mention, remark; attend to, heed. • *n* cognizance, heed, note, observation, regard; advice, announcement, information, intelligence, mention, news, notification; communication, intimation, premonition, warning; attention, civility, consideration, respect; comments, remarks.

notify *vb* advertise, announce, declare, publish, promulgate; acquaint, apprise, inform.

notion *n* concept, conception, idea; apprehension, belief, conceit, conviction, expectation, estimation, impression, judgement, opinion, sentiment, view.

notoriety *n* celebrity, fame, figure, name, note, publicity, reputation, repute, vogue.

notorious *adj* apparent, egregious, evident, notable, obvious, open, overt, manifest, patent, well-known; celebrated, conspicuous, distinguished, famed, famous, flagrant, infamous, noted, remarkable, renowned.

notwithstanding *conj* despite, however, nevertheless, yet. • *prep* despite.

nourish *vb* feed, nurse, nurture; maintain, supply, support; breed, educate, instruct, train; cherish, encourage, foment, foster, promote, succour.

nourishment *n* aliment, diet, food, nutriment, nutrition, sustenance.

novel *adj* fresh, modern, new, rare, recent, strange, uncommon, unusual. • *n* fiction, romance, story, tale.

novice *n* convert, proselyte; initiate, neophyte, novitiate, probationer; apprentice, beginner, learner, tyro.

noxious *adj* baneful, deadly, deleterious, destructive, detrimental, hurtful, injurious, insalubrious, mischievous, noisome, pernicious, pestilent, poisonous, unfavourable, unwholesome.

nude *adj* bare, denuded, exposed, naked, uncovered, unclothed, undressed.

nugatory *adj* frivolous, insignificant, trifling, trivial, vain, worthless; bootless, ineffectual, inefficacious, inoperative, null, unavailing, useless.

nuisance *n* annoyance, bore, bother, infliction, offence, pest, plague, trouble.

null *adj* ineffectual, invalid, nugatory, useless, void; characterless, colourless.

nullify *vb* abolish, abrogate, annul, cancel, invalidate, negate, quash, repeal, revoke.

numb *vb* benumb, deaden, stupefy. • *adj* benumbed, deadened, dulled, insensible, paralysed.

number *vb* calculate, compute, count, enumerate, numerate, reckon, tell; account, reckon. • *n* digit, figure, numeral; horde, multitude, numerousness, throng; aggregate, collection, sum, total.

numerous *adj* abundant, many, numberless.

nuncio *n* ambassador, legate, messenger.

nunnery *n* abbey, cloister, convent, monastery.

nuptial *adj* bridal, conjugal, connubial, hymeneal, matrimonial.

nuptials *npl* espousal, marriage, wedding.

nurse *vb* nourish, nurture; rear, suckle; cherish, encourage, feed, foment, foster, pamper, promote, succour; economize, manage; caress, dandle, fondle. • *n* auxiliary, orderly, sister; amah, *au pair*, babysitter, nanny, nursemaid, nurserymaid.

nurture *vb* feed, nourish, nurse, tend; breed, discipline, educate, instruct, rear, school, train. • *n* diet, food, nourishment; breeding, discipline, education, instruction, schooling, training, tuition; attention, nourishing, nursing.

nutriment *n* aliment, food, nourishment, nutrition, pabulum, subsistence, sustenance.

nutrition *n* diet, food, nourishment, nutriment.

nutritious *adj* invigorating, nourishing, strengthening, supporting, sustaining.

nymph *n* damsel, dryad, lass, girl, maid, maiden, naiad.

O

oaf *n* blockhead, dolt, dunce, fool, idiot, simpleton.

oath *n* blasphemy, curse, expletive, imprecation, malediction; affirmation, pledge, promise, vow.

obduracy *n* contumacy, doggedness, obstinacy, stubbornness, tenacity; depravity, impenitence.

obdurate *adj* hard, harsh, rough, rugged; callous, cantankerous, dogged, firm, hardened, inflexible, insensible, obstinate, pigheaded, unfeeling, stubborn, unbending, unyielding; depraved, graceless, lost, reprobate, shameless, impenitent, incorrigible, irreclaimable.

obedience *n* acquiescence, agreement, compliance, duty, respect, reverence, submission, submissiveness, subservience.

obedient *adj* acquiescent, compliant, deferential, duteous, dutiful, observant, regardful, respectful, submissive, subservient, yielding.

obeisance *n* bow, courtesy, curtsy, homage, reverence, salutation.

obelisk *n* column, pillar.

obese *adj* corpulent, fat, fleshy, gross, plump, podgy, portly, stout.

obesity *n* corpulence, corpulency, embonpoint, fatness, fleshiness, obeseness, plumpness.

obey *vb* comply, conform, heed, keep, mind, observe, submit, yield.

obfuscate *vb* cloud, darken, obscure; bewilder, confuse, muddle.

object[1] *vb* cavil, contravene, demur, deprecate, disapprove of, except to, impeach, oppose, protest, refuse.

object[2] *n* particular, phenomenon, precept, reality, thing; aim, butt, destination, end, mark, recipient, target; design, drift, goal, intention, motive, purpose, use, view.

objection *n* censure, difficulty, doubt, exception, protest, remonstrance, scruple.

objurgate *vb* chide, reprehend, reprove.

oblation *n* gift, offering, sacrifice.

obligation *n* accountability, accountableness, responsibility; agreement, bond, contract, covenant, engagement, stipulation; debt, indebtedness, liability.

obligatory *adj* binding, coercive, compulsory, enforced, necessary, unavoidable.

oblige *vb* bind, coerce, compel, constrain, force, necessitate, require; accommodate, benefit, convenience, favour, gratify, please; obligate, bind.

obliging *adj* accommodating, civil, complaisant, considerate, kind, friendly, polite.

oblique *adj* aslant, inclined, sidelong, slanting; indirect, obscure.

obliterate *vb* cancel, delete, destroy, efface, eradicate, erase, expunge.

oblivious *adj* careless, forgetful, heedless, inattentive, mindless, negligent, neglectful.

obloquy *n* aspersion, backbiting, blame, calumny, censure, contumely, defamation, detraction, disgrace, odium, reproach, reviling, slander, traducing.

obnoxious *adj* blameworthy, censurable, faulty, reprehensible; hateful, objectionable, obscene, odious, offensive, repellent, repugnant, repulsive, unpleasant, unpleasing.

obscene *adj* broad, coarse, filthy, gross, immodest, impure, indecent, indelicate, ribald, unchaste, lewd, licentious, loose, offensive, pornographic, shameless, smutty; disgusting, dirty, foul.

obscure *vb* becloud, befog, blur, cloud, darken, eclipse, dim, obfuscate, obnubilate, shade; conceal, cover, equivocate, hide. • *adj* dark, darksome, dim, dusky, gloomy, lurid, murky, rayless, shadowy, sombre, unenlightened, unilluminated; abstruse, blind, cabbalistic, difficult, doubtful, enigmatic, high, incomprehensible, indefinite, indistinct, intricate, involved, mysterious, mystic, recondite, undefined, unintelligible, vague; remote, secluded; humble, inglorious, nameless, renownless, undistinguished, unhonoured, unknown, unnoted, unnoticed.

obsequious *adj* cringing, deferential, fawning, flattering, servile, slavish, supple, subservient, sycophantic, truckling.

observant *adj* attentive, heedful, mindful, perceptive, quick, regardful, vigilant, watchful.

observation *n* attention, cognition, notice, observance; annotation, note, remark; experience, knowledge.

observe *vb* eye, mark, note, notice, remark, watch; behold, detect, discover, perceive, see; express, mention, remark, say, utter; comply, conform, follow, fulfil, obey; celebrate, keep, regard, solemnize.

obsolete *adj* ancient, antiquated, antique, archaic, disused, neglected, old, old-fashioned, obsolescent, out-of-date, past, passé, unfashionable.

obstacle *n* barrier, check, difficulty, hindrance, impediment, interference, interruption, obstruction, snag, stumbling block.

obstinacy *n* contumacy, doggedness, headiness, firmness, inflexibility, intractability, obduracy, persistence, perseverance, perversity, resoluteness, stubbornness, tenacity, wilfulness.

obstinate *adj* cross-grained, contumacious, dogged, firm, headstrong, inflexible, immovable, intractable, mulish, obdurate, opinionated, persistent, pertinacious, perverse, resolute, self-willed, stubborn, tenacious, unyielding, wilful.

obstreperous *adj* boisterous, clamorous, loud, noisy, riotous, tumultuous, turbulent, unruly, uproarious, vociferous.

obstruct *vb* bar, barricade, block, blockade, block up, choke, clog, close, glut, jam, obturate, stop; hinder, impede, oppose, prevent; arrest, check, curb, delay, embrace, interrupt, retard, slow.

obstruction *n* bar, barrier, block, blocking, check, difficulty, hindrance, impediment, obstacle, stoppage; check, clog, embarrassment, interruption, obturation.

obtain *vb* achieve, acquire, attain, bring, contrive, earn, elicit, gain, get, induce, procure, secure; hold, prevail, stand, subsist.

obtrude *vb* encroach, infringe, interfere, intrude, trespass.

obtrusive *adj* forward, interfering, intrusive, meddling, officious.

obtuse *adj* blunt; blockish, doltish, dull, dull-witted, heavy, stockish, stolid, stupid, slow, unintellectual, unintelligent.

obviate *vb* anticipate, avert, counteract, preclude, prevent, remove.

obvious *adj* exposed, liable, open, subject; apparent, clear, distinct, evident, manifest, palatable, patent, perceptible, plain, self-evident, unmistakable, visible.

occasion *vb* breed, cause, create, originate, produce; induce, influence, move, persuade. • *n* casualty, event, incident, occurrence; conjuncture, convenience, juncture, opening, opportunity; condition, necessity, need, exigency, requirement, want; cause, ground, reason; inducement, influence; circumstance, exigency.

occasional *adj* accidental, casual, incidental, infrequent, irregular, uncommon; causative, causing.

occasionally *adv* casually, sometimes.

occult *adj* abstruse, cabbalistic, hidden, latent, secret, invisible, mysterious, mystic, mystical, recondite, shrouded, undetected, undiscovered, unknown, unrevealed, veiled. • *n* magic, sorcery, witchcraft.

occupation *n* holding, occupancy, possession, tenure, use; avocation, business, calling, craft, employment, engagement, job, post, profession, trade, vocation.

occupy *vb* capture, hold, keep, possess; cover, fill, garrison, inhabit, take up, tenant; engage, employ, use.

occur *vb* appear, arise, offer; befall, chance, eventuate, happen, result, supervene.

occurrence *n* accident, adventure, affair, casualty, event, happening, incident, proceeding, transaction.

odd *adj* additional, redundant, remaining; casual, incidental; inappropriate, queer, unsuitable; comical, droll, erratic, extravagant, extraordinary, fantastic, grotesque, irregular, peculiar, quaint, singular, strange, uncommon, uncouth, unique, unusual, whimsical.

odds *npl* difference, disparity, inequality; advantage, superiority, supremacy.

odious *adj* abominable, detestable, execrable, hateful, shocking; hated, obnoxious, unpopular; disagreeable, forbidding, loathsome, offensive.

odium *n* abhorrence, detestation, dislike, enmity, hate, hatred; odiousness, repulsiveness; obloquy, opprobrium, reproach, shame.

odorous *adj* aromatic, balmy, fragrant, perfumed, redolent, scented, sweet-scented, sweet-smelling.

odour *n* aroma, fragrance, perfume, redolence, scent, smell.

offal *n* carrion, dregs, garbage, refuse, rubbish, waste

offence *n* aggression, attack, assault; anger, displeasure, indignation, pique, resentment, umbrage, wrath; affront, harm, injury, injustice, insult, outrage, wrong; crime, delinquency, fault, misdeed, misdemeanour, sin, transgression, trespass.

offend *vb* affront, annoy, chafe, displease, fret, gall, irritate, mortify, nettle, provoke, vex; molest, pain, shock, wound; fall, sin, stumble, transgress.

offender *n* convict, criminal, culprit, delinquent, felon, malefactor, sinner, transgressor, trespasser.

offensive *adj* aggressive, attacking, invading; disgusting, loathsome, nauseating, nauseous, repulsive, sickening; abominable, detestable, disagreeable, displeasing, execrable, hateful, obnoxious, repugnant, revolting, shocking, unpalatable, unpleasant; abusive, disagreeable, impertinent, insolent, insulting, irritating, opprobrious, rude, saucy, unpleasant. • *n* attack, onslaught.

offer *vb* present, proffer, tender; exhibit; furnish, propose, propound, show; volunteer; dare, essay, endeavour, venture. • *n* overture, proffering, proposal, proposition, tender, overture; attempt, bid, endeavour, essay.

offhand *adj* abrupt, brusque, casual, curt, extempore, impromptu, informal, unpremeditated, unstudied. • *adv* carelessly, casually, clumsily, haphazardly, informally, slapdash; ad-lib, extemporaneously, extemporarily, extempore, impromptu.

office *n* duty, function, service, work; berth, place, position, post, situation; business, capacity, charge, employment, trust; bureau, room.

officiate *vb* act, perform, preside, serve.

officious *adj* busy, dictatorial, forward, impertinent, interfering, intermeddling, meddlesome, meddling, obtrusive, pushing, pushy.

offset *vb* balance, counteract, counterbalance, counterpoise. • *n* branch, offshoot, scion, shoot, slip, sprout, twig; counterbalance, counterpoise, set-off, equivalent.

offspring *n* brood, children, descendants, issue, litter, posterity, progeny; cadet, child, scion.

often *adv* frequently, generally, oftentimes, repeatedly.

ogre *n* bugbear, demon, devil, goblin, hobgoblin, monster, spectre.

old *adj* aged, ancient, antiquated, antique, archaic, elderly, obsolete, olden, old-fashioned, superannuated; decayed, done, senile, worn-out; original, primitive, pristine; former, preceding, pre-existing.

oleaginous *adj* adipose, fat, fatty, greasy, oily, sebaceous, unctuous.

omen *n* augury, auspice, foreboding, portent, presage, prognosis, sign, warning.

ominous *adj* inauspicious, monitory, portentous, premonitory, threatening, unpropitious.

omission *n* default, failure, forgetfulness, neglect, oversight.

omit *vb* disregard, drop, eliminate, exclude, miss, neglect, overlook, skip.

omnipotent *adj* almighty, all-powerful.

omniscient *adj* all-knowing, all-seeing, all-wise.

oneness *n* individuality, singleness, unity.

onerous *adj* burdensome, difficult, hard, heavy, laborious, oppressive, responsible, weighty.

one-sided *adj* partial, prejudiced, unfair, unilateral, unjust.

only *adj* alone, single, sole, solitary. • *adv* barely, merely, simply.

onset *n* assault, attack, charge, onslaught, storm, storming.

onus *n* burden, liability, load, responsibility.

ooze *vb* distil, drip, drop, shed; drain, exude, filter, leak, percolate, stain, transude. • *n* mire, mud, slime.

opaque *adj* dark, dim, hazy, muddy; abstruse, cryptic, enigmatic, enigmatical, obscure, unclear.

open *vb* expand, spread; begin, commence, initiate; disclose, exhibit, reveal, show; unbar, unclose, uncover, unlock, unseal, untie. • *adj* expanded, extended, unclosed, spread wide; aboveboard, artless, candid, cordial, fair, frank, guileless, hearty, honest, sincere, open-hearted, single-minded, undesigning, undisguised, undissembling, unreserved; bounteous, bountiful, free, generous, liberal, munificent; ajar, uncovered; exposed, undefended, unprotected; clear, unobstructed; accessible, public, unenclosed, unrestricted; mild, moderate; apparent, debatable, evident, obvious, patent, plain, undetermined.

opening *adj* commencing, first, inaugural, initiatory, introductory. • *n* aperture, breach, chasm, cleft, fissure, flaw, gap, gulf, hole, interspace, loophole, orifice, perforation, rent, rift; beginning, commencement, dawn; chance, opportunity, vacancy.

openly *adv* candidly, frankly, honestly, plainly, publicly.

openness *n* candour, frankness, honesty, ingenuousness, plainness, unreservedness

operate *vb* act, function, work; cause, effect, occasion, produce; manipulate, use, run.

operation *n* manipulation, performance, procedure, proceeding, process; action, affair, manoeuvre, motion, movement.

operative *adj* active, effective, effectual, efficient, serviceable, vigorous; important, indicative, influential, significant. • *n* artisan, employee, labourer, mechanic, worker, workman.

opiate *adj* narcotic, sedative, soporiferous, soporific. • *n* anodyne, drug, narcotic, sedative, tranquillizer.

opine *vb* apprehend, believe, conceive, fancy, judge, suppose, presume, surmise, think.

opinion *n* conception, idea, impression, judgment, notion, sentiment, view; belief, persuasion, tenet; esteem, estimation, judgment.

opinionated *adj* biased, bigoted, cocksure, conceited, dictatorial, dogmatic, opinionative, prejudiced, stubborn.

opponent *adj* adverse, antagonistic, contrary, opposing, opposite, repugnant. • *n* adversary, antagonist, competitor, contestant, counteragent, enemy, foe, opposite, opposer, party, rival.

opportune *adj* appropriate, auspicious, convenient, favourable, felicitous, fit, fitting, fortunate, lucky, propitious, seasonable, suitable, timely, well-timed.

opportunity *n* chance, convenience, moment, occasion.

oppose *vb* combat, contravene, counteract, dispute, obstruct, oppugn, resist, thwart, withstand; check, prevent; confront, counterpoise.

opposite *adj* facing, fronting; conflicting, contradictory, contrary, different, diverse, incompatible, inconsistent, irreconcilable; adverse, antagonistic, hostile, inimical, opposed, opposing, repugnant. • *n* contradiction, contrary, converse, reverse.

opposition *n* antagonism, antinomy, contrariety, inconsistency, repugnance; counteraction, counter-influence, hostility, resistance; hindrance, obstacle, obstruction, oppression, prevention.

oppress *vb* burden, crush, depress, harass, load, maltreat, overburden, overpower, overwhelm, persecute, subdue, suppress, tyrannize, wrong.

oppression *n* abuse, calamity, cruelty, hardship, injury, injustice, misery, persecution, severity, suffering, tyranny; depression, dullness, heaviness, lassitude.

oppressive *adj* close, muggy, stifling, suffocating, sultry.

opprobrious *adj* abusive, condemnatory, contemptuous, damnatory, insolent, insulting, offensive, reproachable, scandalous, scurrilous, vituperative; despised, dishonourable, disreputable, hateful, infamous, shameful.

opprobrium *n* contumely, scurrility; calumny, disgrace, ignominy, infamy, obloquy, odium, reproach.

oppugn *vb* assail, argue, attack, combat, contravene, oppose, resist, thwart, withstand.

option *n* choice, discretion, election, preference, selection.

optional *adj* discretionary, elective, nonobligatory, voluntary.

opulence *n* affluence, fortune, independence, luxury, riches, wealth.

opulent *adj* affluent, flush, luxurious, moneyed, plentiful, rich, sumptuous, wealthy.

oracular *adj* ominous, portentous, prophetic; authoritative, dogmatic, magisterial, positive; aged, grave, wise; ambiguous, blind, dark, equivocal, obscure.

oral *adj* nuncupative, spoken, verbal, vocal.

oration *n* address, declamation, discourse, harangue, speech.

orb *n* ball, globe, sphere; circle, circuit, orbit, ring; disk, wheel.

orbit *vb* circle, encircle, revolve around. • *n* course, path, revolution, track.

ordain *vb* appoint, call, consecrate, elect, experiment, constitute, establish, institute, regulate; decree, enjoin, enact, order, prescribe.

order *vb* adjust, arrange, methodize, regulate, systematize; carry on, conduct, manage; bid, command, direct, instruct, require. • *n* arrangement, disposition, method, regularity, symmetry, system; law, regulation, rule; discipline, peace, quiet; command, commission, direction, injunction, instruction, mandate, prescription; class, degree, grade, kind, rank; family, tribe; brotherhood, community, fraternity, society; sequence, succession.

orderly *adj* methodical, regular, systematic; peaceable, quiet, well-behaved; neat, shipshape, tidy.

ordinance *n* appointment, command, decree, edict, enactment, law, order, prescript, regulation, rule, statute; ceremony, observance, sacrament, rite, ritual.

ordinary *adj* accustomed, customary, established, everyday, normal, regular, settled, wonted, everyday, regular; common, frequent, habitual, usual; average, commonplace, indifferent, inferior, mean, mediocre, second-rate, undistinguished; homely, plain.

organization *n* business, construction, constitution, organism, structure, system.

organize *vb* adjust, constitute, construct, form, make, shape; arrange, coordinate, correlate, establish, systematize.

orgy *n* carousal, debauch, debauchery, revel, saturnalia.

orifice *n* aperture, hole, mouth, perforation, pore, vent.

origin *n* beginning, birth, commencement, cradle, derivation, foundation, fountain, fountainhead, original, rise, root, source, spring, starting point; cause, occasion; heritage, lineage, parentage.

original *adj* aboriginal, first, primary, primeval, primitive, primordial, pristine; fresh, inventive, novel; eccentric, odd, peculiar. • *n* cause, commencement, origin, source, spring; archetype, exemplar, model, pattern, prototype, protoplast, type.

originate *vb* arise, begin, emanate, flow, proceed, rise, spring; create, discover, form, invent, produce.

originator *n* author, creator, former, inventor, maker, parent.

orison *n* petition, prayer, solicitation, supplication.

ornament *vb* adorn, beautify, bedeck, bedizen, decorate, deck, emblazon, garnish, grace. • *n* adornment, bedizenment, decoration, design, embellishment, garnish, ornamentation.

ornate *adj* beautiful, bedecked, decorated, elaborate, elegant, embellished, florid, flowery, ornamental, ornamented.

orthodox *adj* conventional, correct, sound, true.

oscillate *vb* fluctuate, sway, swing, vacillate, vary, vibrate.

ostensible *adj* apparent, assigned, avowed, declared, exhibited, manifest, presented, visible; plausible, professed, specious.

ostentation *n* dash, display, flourish, pageantry, parade, pomp, pomposity, pompousness, show, vaunting; appearance, semblance, showiness.

ostentatious *adj* boastful, dashing, flaunting, pompous, pretentious, showy, vain, vainglorious; gaudy.

ostracize *vb* banish, boycott, exclude, excommunicate, exile, expatriate, expel, evict.

oust *vb* dislodge, dispossess, eject, evict, expel.

outbreak *n* ebullition, eruption, explosion, outburst; affray, broil, conflict, commotion, fray, riot, row; flare-up, manifestation.

outcast *n* exile, expatriate; castaway, pariah, reprobate, vagabond.

outcome *n* conclusion, consequence, event, issue, result, upshot.

outcry *n* cry, scream, screech, yell; bruit, clamour, noise, tumult, vociferation.

outdo *vb* beat, exceed, excel, outgo, outstrip, outvie, surpass.

outlandish *adj* alien, exotic, foreign, strange; barbarous, bizarre, uncouth.

outlaw *vb* ban, banish, condemn, exclude, forbid, make illegal, prohibit. • *n* bandit, brigand, crook, freebooter, highwayman, lawbreaker, marauder, robber, thief.

outlay *n* disbursement, expenditure, outgoings.

outline *vb* delineate, draft, draw, plan, silhouette, sketch. • *n* contour, profile; delineation, draft, drawing, plan, rough draft, silhouette, sketch.

outlive *vb* last, live longer, survive.

outlook *n* future, prospect, sight, view; lookout, watch-tower.

outrage *vb* abuse, injure, insult, maltreat, offend, shock, injure. • *n* abuse, affront, indignity, insult, offence.

outrageous *adj* abusive, frantic, furious, frenzied, mad, raging, turbulent, violent, wild; atrocious, enormous, flagrant, heinous, monstrous, nefarious, villainous; enormous, excessive, extravagant, unwarrantable.

outré *adj* excessive, exorbitant, extravagant, immoderate, inordinate, overstrained, unconventional.

outrun *vb* beat, exceed, outdistance, outgo, outstrip, outspeed, surpass.

outset *n* beginning, commencement, entrance, opening, start, starting point.

outshine *vb* eclipse, outstrip, overshadow, surpass.

outspoken *adj* abrupt, blunt, candid, frank, plain, plainspoken, unceremonious, unreserved.

outstanding *adj* due, owing, uncollected, ungathered, unpaid, unsettled; conspicuous, eminent, prominent, striking.

outward *adj* exterior, external, outer, outside.

outwit *vb* cheat, circumvent, deceive, defraud, diddle, dupe, gull, outmanoeuvre, overreach, swindle, victimize.

overawe *vb* affright, awe, browbeat, cow, daunt, frighten, intimidate, scare, terrify.

overbalance *vb* capsize, overset, overturn, tumble, upset; outweigh, preponderate.

overbearing *adj* oppressive, overpowering; arrogant, dictatorial, dogmatic, domineering, haughty, imperious, overweening, proud, supercilious.

overcast *vb* cloud, darken, overcloud, overshadow, shade, shadow. • *adj* cloudy, darkened, hazy, murky, obscure.

overcharge *vb* burden, oppress, overburden, overload, surcharge; crowd, overfill; exaggerate, overstate, overstrain.

overcome *vb* beat, choke, conquer, crush, defeat, discomfit, overbear, overmaster, overpower, overthrow, overturn, overwhelm, prevail, rout, subdue, subjugate, surmount, vanquish.

overflow *vb* brim over, fall over, pour over, pour out, shower, spill; deluge, inundate, submerge. • *n* deluge, inundation, profusion, superabundance.

overhaul *vb* overtake; check, examine, inspect, repair, survey. • *n* check, examination, inspection.

overlay *vb* cover, spread over; overlie, overpress, smother; crush, overpower, overwhelm; cloud, hide, obscure, overcast. • *n* appliqué, covering, decoration, veneer.

overlook *vb* inspect, oversee, superintend, supervise; disregard, miss, neglect, slight; condone, excuse, forgive, pardon, pass over.

overpower *vb* beat, conquer, crush, defeat, discomfit, overbear, overcome, overmaster, overturn, overwhelm, subdue, subjugate, vanquish.

overreach *vb* exceed, outstrip, overshoot, pass, surpass; cheat, circumvent, deceive, defraud.

override *vb* outride, outweigh, pass, quash, supersede, surpass.

overrule *vb* control, govern, sway; annul, cancel, nullify, recall, reject, repeal, repudiate, rescind, revoke, reject, set aside, supersede, suppress.

oversight *n* care, charge, control, direction, inspection, management, superintendence, supervision, surveillance; blunder, error, fault, inadvertence, inattention, lapse, miss, mistake, neglect, omission, slip, trip.

overt *adj* apparent, glaring, open, manifest, notorious, patent, public, unconcealed.

overthrow *vb* overturn, upset, subvert; demolish, destroy, level; beat, conquer, crush, defeat, discomfit, foil, master, overcome, overpower, overwhelm, rout, subjugate, vanquish, worst. • *n* downfall, fall, prostration, subversion; destruction, demolition, ruin; defeat, discomfiture, dispersion, rout.

overturn *vb* invert, overthrow, reverse, subvert, upset.

overture *n* invitation, offer, proposal, proposition.

overweening *adj* arrogant, conceited, consequential, egotistical, haughty, opinionated, proud, supercilious, vain, vainglorious.

overwhelm *vb* drown, engulf, inundate, overflow, submerge, swallow up, swamp; conquer, crush, defeat, overbear, overcome, overpower, subdue, vanquish.

overwrought *adj* overdone, overelaborate; agitated, excited, overexcited, overworked, stirred.

own[1] *vb* have, hold, possess; avow, confess; acknowledge, admit, allow, concede.

own[2] *adj* particular, personal, private.

owner *n* freeholder, holder, landlord, possessor, proprietor.

P

pace *vb* go, hasten, hurry, move, step, walk. • *n* amble gait, step, walk.

pacific *adj* appeasing, conciliatory, ironic, mollifying, placating, peacemaking, propitiatory; calm, gentle, peaceable, peaceful, quiet, smooth, tranquil, unruffled.

pacify *vb* appease, conciliate, harmonize, tranquillize; allay, appease, assuage, calm, compose, hush, lay, lull, moderate, mollify, placate, propitiate, quell, quiet, smooth, soften, soothe, still.

pack *vb* compact, compress, crowd, fill; bundle, burden, load, stow. • *n* bale, budget, bundle, package, packet, parcel; burden, load; assemblage, assembly, assortment, collection, set; band, bevy, clan, company, crew, gang, knot, lot, party, squad.

pact *n* agreement, alliance, bargain, bond, compact, concordat, contract, convention, covenant, league, stipulation.

pagan *adj* heathen, heathenish, idolatrous, irreligious, paganist, paganistic. • *n* gentile, heathen, idolater.

pageantry *n* display, flourish, magnificence, parade, pomp, show, splendour, state.

pain *vb* agonize, bite, distress, hurt, rack, sting, torment, torture; afflict, aggrieve, annoy, bore, chafe, displease, disquiet, fret, grieve, harass, incommode, plague, tease, trouble, vex, worry; rankle, smart, shoot, sting, twinge. • *n* ache, agony, anguish, discomfort, distress, gripe, hurt, pang, smart, soreness, sting, suffering, throe, torment, torture, twinge; affliction, anguish, anxiety, bitterness, care, chagrin, disquiet, dolour, grief, heartache, misery, punishment, solicitude, sorrow, trouble, uneasiness, unhappiness, vexation, woe, wretchedness.

painful *adj* agonizing, distressful, excruciating, racking, sharp, tormenting, torturing; afflicting, afflictive, annoying, baleful, disagreeable, displeasing, disquieting, distressing, dolorous, grievous, provoking, troublesome, unpleasant, vexatious; arduous, careful, difficult, hard, severe, sore, toilsome.

pains *npl* care, effort, labour, task, toilsomeness, trouble; childbirth, labour, travail.

painstaking *adj* assiduous, careful, conscientious, diligent, hardworking, industrious, laborious, persevering, plodding, sedulous, strenuous.

paint *vb* delineate, depict, describe, draw, figure, pencil, portray, represent, sketch; adorn, beautify, deck, embellish, ornament. • *n* colouring, dye, pigment, stain; cosmetics, greasepaint, make-up.

pair *vb* couple, marry, mate, match. • *n* brace, couple, double, duo, match, twosome.

pal *n* buddy, chum, companion, comrade, crony, friend, mate, mucker.

palatable *adj* acceptable, agreeable, appetizing, delicate, delicious, enjoyable, flavourful, flavoursome, gustative, gustatory, luscious, nice, pleasant, pleasing, savoury, relishable, tasteful, tasty, toothsome.

palaver *vb* chat, chatter, converse, patter, prattle, say, speak, talk; confer, parley; blandish, cajole, flatter, wheedle. • *n* chat, chatter, conversation, discussion, language, prattle, speech, talk; confab, confabulation, conference, conclave, parley, powwow; balderdash, cajolery, flummery, gibberish.

pale *vb* blanch, lose colour, whiten. • *adj* ashen, ashy, blanched, bloodless, pallid, sickly, wan, white; blank, dim, obscure, spectral. • *n* picket, stake; circuit, enclosure; district, region, territory; boundary, confine, fence, limit.

pall[1] *n* cloak, cover, curtain, mantle, pallium, shield, shroud, veil.

pall[2] *vb* cloy, glut, gorge, satiate, surfeit; deject, depress, discourage, dishearten, dispirit; cloak, cover, drape, invest, overspread, shroud.

palliate *vb* cloak, conceal, cover, excuse, extenuate, hide, gloss, lessen; abate, allay, alleviate, assuage, blunt, diminish, dull, ease, mitigate, moderate, mollify, quell, quiet, relieve, soften, soothe, still.

pallid *adj* ashen, ashy, cadaverous, colourless, pale, sallow, wan, whitish.

palm[1] *vb* foist, impose, obtrude, pass off; handle, touch.

palm[2] *n* bays, crown, laurels, prize, trophy, victory.

palmy *adj* flourishing, fortunate, glorious, golden, halcyon, happy, joyous, prosperous, thriving, victorious.

palpable *adj* corporeal, material, tactile, tangible; evident, glaring, gross, intelligible, manifest, obvious, patent, plain, unmistakable.

palpitate *vb* flutter, pulsate, throb; quiver, shiver, tremble.

palter *vb* dodge, equivocate, evade, haggle, prevaricate, quibble, shift, shuffle, trifle.

paltry *adj* diminutive, feeble, inconsiderable, insignificant, little, miserable, petty, slender, slight, small, sorry, trifling, trivial, unimportant, wretched.

pamper *vb* baby, coddle, fondle, gratify, humour, spoil.

panacea *n* catholicon, cure-all, medicine, remedy.

panegyric *adj* commendatory, encomiastic, encomiastical, eulogistic, eulogistical, laudatory, panegyrical. • *n* eulogy, laudation, praise, paean, tribute.

pang *n* agony, anguish, distress, gripe, pain, throe, twinge.

panic *vb* affright, alarm, scare, startle, terrify; become terrified, overreact. • *n* alarm, consternation, fear, fright, jitters, terror.

pant *vb* blow, gasp, puff; heave, palpitate, pulsate, throb; languish; desire, hunger, long, sigh, thirst, yearn. • *n* blow, gasp, puff.

parable *n* allegory, fable, story.

paraclete *n* advocate, comforter, consoler, intercessor, mediator.

parade *vb* display, flaunt, show, vaunt. • *n* ceremony, display, flaunting, ostentation, pomp, show; array, pageant, review, spectacle; mall, promenade.

paradox *n* absurdity, contradiction, mystery.

paragon *n* flower, ideal, masterpiece, model, nonpareil, pattern, standard.

paragraph *n* clause, item, notice, passage, section, sentence, subdivision.

parallel *vb* be alike, compare, conform, correlate, match. • *adj* abreast, concurrent; allied, analogous, correspondent, equal, like, resembling, similar. • *n* conformity, likeness, resemblance, similarity; analogue, correlative, counterpart.

paramount *adj* chief, dominant, eminent, pre-eminent, principal, superior, supreme.

paraphernalia *n* accoutrements, appendages, appurtenances, baggage, belongings, effects, equipage, equipment, ornaments, trappings.

parasite *n* bloodsucker, fawner, flatterer, flunky, hanger-on, leech, spaniel, sycophant, toady, wheedler.

parcel *vb* allot, apportion, dispense, distribute, divide. • *n* budget, bundle, package; batch, collection, group, lot, set; division, part, patch, pierce, plot, portion, tract.

parched *adj* arid, dry, scorched, shrivelled, thirsty.

pardon *vb* condone, forgive, overlook, remit; absolve, acquit, clear, discharge, excuse, release. • *n* absolution, amnesty, condonation, discharge, excuse, forgiveness, grace, mercy, overlook, release.

parentage *n* ancestry, birth, descent, extraction, family, lineage, origin, parenthood, pedigree, stock.

pariah *n* outcast, wretch.

parish *n* community, congregation, parishioners; district, subdivision.

parity *n* analogy, correspondence, equality, equivalence, likeness, sameness, similarity.

parody *vb* burlesque, caricature, imitate, lampoon, mock, ridicule, satirize, travesty. • *n* burlesque, caricature, imitation, ridicule, satire, travesty.

paroxysm *n* attack, convulsion, exacerbation, fit, outburst, seizure, spasm, throe.

parsimonious *adj* avaricious, close, close-fisted, covetous, frugal, grasping, grudging, illiberal, mean, mercenary, miserly, near, niggardly, penurious, shabby, sordid, sparing, stingy, tightfisted.

parson *n* churchman, clergyman, divine, ecclesiastic, incumbent, minister, pastor, priest, rector.

part *vb* break, dismember, dissever, divide, sever, subdivide, sunder; detach, disconnect, disjoin, dissociate, disunite, separate; allot, apportion, distribute, divide, mete, share; secrete. • *n* crumb, division, fraction, fragment, moiety, parcel, piece, portion, remnant, scrap, section, segment, subdivision; component, constituent, element, ingredient, member, organ; lot, share; concern, interest, participation; allotment, apportionment, dividend; business, charge, duty, function, office, work; faction, party, side; character, cue, lines, role; clause, paragraph, passage.

partake *vb* engage, participate, share; consume, eat, take; evince, evoke, show, suggest.

partial *adj* component, fractional, imperfect, incomplete, limited; biased, influential, interested, one-sided, prejudiced, prepossessed, unfair, unjust, warped; fond, indulgent.

participate *vb* engage in, partake, perform, share.

particle *n* atom, bit, corpuscle, crumb, drop, glimmer, grain, granule, iota, jot, mite, molecule, morsel, mote, scrap, shred, snip, spark, speck, whit.

particular *adj* especial, special, specific; distinct, individual, respective, separate, single; characteristic, distinctive, peculiar; individual, intimate, own, personal, private; notable, noteworthy; circumstantial, definite, detailed, exact, minute, narrow, precise; careful, close, conscientious, critical, fastidious, nice, scrupulous, strict; marked, odd, singular, strange, uncommon. • *n* case, circumstance, count, detail, feature, instance, item, particularity, point, regard, respect.

parting *adj* breaking, dividing, separating; final, last, valedictory; declining, departing. • *n* breaking, disruption, rupture, severing; detachment, division, separation; death, departure, farewell, leave-taking.

partisan *adj* biased, factional, interested, partial, prejudiced. • *n* adherent, backer, champion, disciple, follower, supporter, votary; baton, halberd, pike, quarterstaff, truncheon, staff.

partition *vb* apportion, distribute, divide, portion, separate, share. • *n* division, separation; barrier, division, screen, wall; allotment, apportionment, distribution.

partner *n* associate, colleague, copartner, partaker, participant, participator; accomplice, ally, coadjutor, confederate; companion, consort, spouse.

partnership *n* association, company, copartnership, firm, house, society; connection, interest, participation, union.

parts *npl* abilities, accomplishments, endowments, faculties, genius, gifts, intellect, intelligence, mind, qualities, powers, talents; districts, regions.

party *n* alliance, association, cabal, circle, clique, combination, confederacy, coterie, faction, group, junta, league, ring, set; body, company, detachment, squad, troop; assembly, gathering; partaker, participant, participator, sharer; defendant, litigant, plaintiff; individual, one, person, somebody; cause, division, interest, side.

pass[1] *vb* devolve, fall, go, move, proceed; change, elapse, flit, glide, lapse, slip; cease, die, fade, expire, vanish; happen, occur; convey, deliver, send, transmit, transfer; disregard, ignore, neglect; exceed, excel, surpass; approve, ratify, sanction; answer, do, succeed, suffice, suit; express, pronounce, utter; beguile, wile.

pass[2] *n* avenue, ford, road, route, way; defile, gorge, passage, ravine; authorization, licence, passport, permission, ticket; condition, conjecture, plight, situation, state; lunge, push, thrust, tilt; transfer, trick.

passable *adj* admissible, allowable, mediocre, middling, moderate, ordinary, so-so, tolerable; acceptable, current, receivable; navigable, traversable.

passage *n* going, passing, progress, transit; evacuation, journey, migration, transit, voyage; avenue, channel, course, pass, path, road, route, thoroughfare, vennel, way; access, currency, entry, reception; act, deed, event, feat, incidence, occurrence, passion; corridor, gallery, gate, hall; clause, paragraph, sentence, text; course, death, decease, departure, expiration, lapse; affair, brush, change, collision, combat, conflict, contest, encounter, exchange, joust, skirmish, tilt.

passenger *n* fare, itinerant, tourist, traveller, voyager, wayfarer.

passionate *adj* animated, ardent, burning, earnest, enthusiastic, excited, fervent, fiery, furious, glowing, hot-blooded, impassioned, impetuous, impulsive, intense, vehement, warm, zealous; hot-headed, irascible, quick-tempered, tempestuous, violent.

passive *adj* inactive, inert, quiescent, receptive; apathetic, enduring, long-suffering, nonresistant, patient, stoical, submissive, suffering, unresisting.

past *adj* accomplished, elapsed, ended, gone, spent; ancient, bygone, former, obsolete, outworn. • *adv* above, extra, beyond, over. • *prep* above, after, beyond, exceeding. • *n* antiquity, heretofore, history, olden times, yesterday.

pastime *n* amusement, diversion, entertainment, hobby, play, recreation, sport.

pastor *n* clergyman, churchman, divine, ecclesiastic, minister, parson, priest, vicar.

pat[1] *vb* dab, hit, rap, tap; caress, chuck, fondle, pet. • *n* dab, pad, rap, tap; caress.

pat[2] *adj* appropriate, apt, fit, pertinent, suitable. • *adv* aptly, conveniently, fitly, opportunely, seasonably.

patch *vb* mend, repair. • *n* repair; parcel, plot, tract.

patent *adj* expanded, open, spreading; apparent, clear, conspicuous, evident, glaring, indisputable, manifest, notorious, obvious, public, open, palpable, plain, unconcealed, unmistakable. • *n* copyright, privilege, right.

paternity *n* derivation, descent, fatherhood, origin.

path *n* access, avenue, course, footway, passage, pathway, road, route, track, trail, way.

pathetic *adj* affecting, melting, moving, pitiable, plaintive, sad, tender, touching.

patience *n* endurance, fortitude, long-sufferance, resignation, submission, sufferance; calmness, composure, quietness; forbearance, indulgence, leniency; assiduity, constancy, diligence, indefatigability, indefatigableness, perseverance, persistence.

patient *adj* meek, passive, resigned, submissive, uncomplaining, unrepining; calm, composed, contented, quiet; indulgent, lenient, long-suffering; assiduous, constant, diligent, indefatigable, persevering, persistent. • *n* case, invalid, subject, sufferer.

patrician *adj* aristocratic, blue-blooded, highborn, noble, senatorial, well-born. • *n* aristocrat, blue blood, nobleman.

patron *n* advocate, defender, favourer, guardian, helper, protector, supporter.

patronize *vb* aid, assist, befriend, countenance, defend, favour, maintain, support; condescend, disparage, scorn.

pattern *vb* copy, follow, imitate. • *n* archetype, exemplar, last, model, original, paradigm, plan, prototype; example, guide, sample, specimen; mirror, paragon; design, figure, shape, style, type.

paucity *n* deficiency, exiguity, insufficiency, lack, poverty, rarity, shortage.

paunch *n* abdomen, belly, gut, stomach.

pauperism *n* beggary, destitution, indigence, mendicancy, mendicity, need, poverty, penury, want.

pause *vb* breathe, cease, delay, desist, rest, stay, stop, wait; delay, forbear, intermit, stay, stop, tarry, wait; deliberate, demur, hesitate, waver. • *n* break, caesura, cessation, halt, intermission, interruption, interval, remission, rest, stop, stoppage, stopping, suspension; hesitation, suspense, uncertainty; paragraph.

pawn[1] *n* cat's-paw, dupe, plaything, puppet, stooge, tool, toy.

pawn[2] *vb* bet, gage, hazard, lay, pledge, risk, stake, wager. • *n* assurance, bond, guarantee, pledge, security.

pay *vb* defray, discharge, discount, foot, honour, liquidate, meet, quit, settle; compensate, recompense, reimburse, requite, reward; punish, revenge; give, offer, render. • *n* allowance, commission, compensation, emolument, hire, recompense, reimbursement, remuneration, requital, reward, salary, wages.

peace *n* calm, calmness, quiet, quietness, repose, stillness; accord, amity, friendliness, harmony; composure, equanimity, imperturbability, placidity, quietude, tranquillity; agreement, armistice.

peaceable *adj* pacific, peaceful; amiable, amicable, friendly, gentle, inoffensive, mild; placid, quiet, serene, still, tranquil, undisturbed, unmoved.

peaceful *adj* quiet, undisturbed; amicable, concordant, friendly, gentle, harmonious, mild, pacific, peaceable; calm, composed, placid, serene, still.

peak *vb* climax, culminate, top; dwindle, thin. • *n* acme, apex, crest, crown, pinnacle, summit, top, zenith.

peaked *adj* piked, pointed, thin.

peasant *n* boor, countryman, clown, hind, labourer, rustic, swain.

peculate *vb* appropriate, defraud, embezzle, misappropriate, pilfer, purloin, rob, steal.

peculiar *adj* appropriate, idiosyncratic, individual, proper; characteristic, eccentric, exceptional, extraordinary, odd, queer, rare, singular, strange, striking, uncommon, unusual; individual, especial, particular, select, special, specific.

peculiarity *n* appropriateness, distinctiveness, individuality, speciality; characteristic, idiosyncrasy, oddity, peculiarity, singularity.

pedantic *adj* conceited, fussy, officious, ostentatious, over-learned, particular, pedagogical, pompous, pragmatical, precise, pretentious, priggish, stilted.

pedlar *n* chapman, costermonger, hawker, packman, vendor.

pedigree *adj* purebred, thoroughbred. • *n* ancestry, breed, descent, extraction, family, genealogy, house, line, lineage, race, stock, strain.

peer[1] *vb* gaze, look, peek, peep, pry, squinny, squint, appear, emerge.

peer[2] *n* associate, co-equal, companion, compeer, equal, equivalent, fellow, like, mate, match; aristocrat, baron, count, duke, earl, grandee, lord, marquis, noble, nobleman, viscount.

peerless *adj* excellent, incomparable, matchless, outstanding, superlative, unequalled, unique, unmatched, unsurpassed.

peevish *adj* acrimonious, captious, churlish, complaining, crabbed, cross, crusty, discontented, fretful, ill-natured, ill-tempered, irascible, irritable, pettish, petulant, querulous, snappish, snarling, splenetic, spleeny, testy, waspish; forward, headstrong, obstinate, self-willed, stubborn; childish, silly, thoughtless, trifling.

pellucid *adj* bright, clear, crystalline, diaphanous, limpid, lucid, transparent.

pelt[1] *vb* assail, batter, beat, belabour, bombard, pepper, stone, strike; cast, hurl, throw; hurry, rush, speed, tear.

pelt[2] *n* coat, hide, skin.

pen[1] *vb* compose, draft, indite, inscribe, write.

pen[2] *vb* confine, coop, encage, enclose, impound, imprison, incarcerate. • *n* cage, coop, corral, crib, hutch, enclosure, paddock, pound, stall, sty.

penalty *n* chastisement, fine, forfeiture, mulct, punishment, retribution.

penance *n* humiliation, maceration, mortification, penalty, punishment.

penchant *n* bent, bias, disposition, fondness, inclination, leaning, liking, predilection, predisposition, proclivity, proneness, propensity, taste, tendency, turn.

penetrate *vb* bore, burrow, cut, enter, invade, penetrate, percolate, perforate, pervade, pierce, soak, stab; affect, sensitize, touch; comprehend, discern, perceive, understand.

penetrating *adj* penetrative, permeating, piercing, sharp, subtle; acute, clear-sighted, discerning, intelligent, keen, quick, sagacious, sharp-witted, shrewd.

penetration *n* acuteness, discernment, insight, sagacity.

penitence *n* compunction, contrition, qualms, regret, remorse, repentance, sorrow.

penitent *adj* compunctious, conscience-stricken, contrite, regretful, remorseful, repentant, sorrowing, sorrowful. • *n* penance-doer, penitentiary, repentant.

penniless *adj* destitute, distressed, impecunious, indigent, moneyless, pinched, poor, necessitous, needy, pensive, poverty-stricken, reduced.

pensive *adj* contemplative, dreamy, meditative, reflective, sober, thoughtful; grave, melancholic, melancholy, mournful, sad, serious, solemn.

penurious *adj* inadequate, ill-provided, insufficient, meagre, niggardly, poor, scanty, stinted; avaricious, close, close-fisted, covetous, illiberal, grasping, grudging, mean, mercenary, miserly, near, niggardly, parsimonious, sordid, stingy, tightfisted.

penury *n* beggary, destitution, indigence, need, poverty, privation, want.

people *vb* colonize, inhabit, populate. • *n* clan, country, family, nation, race, state, tribe; folk, humankind, persons, population, public; commons, community, democracy, populace, proletariat; mob, multitude, rabble.

perceive *vb* behold, descry, detect, discern, discover, discriminate, distinguish, note, notice, observe, recognize, remark, see, spot; appreciate, comprehend, know, understand.

perceptible *adj* apparent, appreciable, cognizable, discernible, noticeable, perceivable, understandable, visible.

perception *n* apprehension, cognition, discernment, perceiving, recognition, seeing; comprehension, conception, consciousness, perceptiveness, perceptivity, understanding, feeling.

perchance *adv* haply, maybe, mayhap, peradventure, perhaps, possibly, probably.

percolate *vb* drain, drip, exude, filter, filtrate, ooze, penetrate, stain, transude.

percussion *n* collision, clash, concussion, crash, encounter, shock.

perdition *n* damnation, demolition, destruction, downfall, hell, overthrow, ruin, wreck.

peremptory *adj* absolute, authoritative, categorical, commanding, decisive, express, imperative, imperious, positive; determined, resolute, resolved; arbitrary, dogmatic, incontrovertible.

perennial *adj* ceaseless, constant, continual, deathless, enduring, immortal, imperishable, lasting, never-failing, permanent, perpetual, unceasing, undying, unfailing, uninterrupted.

perfect *vb* accomplish, complete, consummate, elaborate, finish. • *adj* completed, finished; complete, entire, full, unqualified, utter, whole; capital, consummate, excellent, exquisite, faultless, ideal; accomplished, disciplined, expert, skilled; blameless, faultless, holy, immaculate, pure, spotless, unblemished.

perfection *n* completeness, completion, consummation, correctness, excellence, faultlessness, finish, maturity, perfection, perfectness, wholeness; beauty, quality.

perfidious *adj* deceitful, dishonest, disloyal, double-faced, faithless, false, false-hearted, traitorous, treacherous, unfaithful, untrustworthy, venal.

perfidy *n* defection, disloyalty, faithlessness, infidelity, perfidiousness, traitorousness, treachery, treason.

perforate *vb* bore, drill, penetrate, pierce, pink, prick, punch, riddle, trepan.

perform *vb* accomplish, achieve, compass, consummate, do, effect, transact; complete, discharge, execute, fulfil, meet, observe, satisfy; act, play, represent.

performance *n* accomplishment, achievement, completion, consummation, discharge, doing, execution, fulfilment; act, action, deed, exploit, feat, work; composition, production; acting, entertainment, exhibition, play, representation, hold; execution, playing.

perfume *n* aroma, balminess, bouquet, fragrance, incense, odour, redolence, scent, smell, sweetness.

perfunctory *adj* careless, formal, heedless, indifferent, mechanical, negligent, reckless, slight, slovenly, thoughtless, unmindful.

perhaps *adv* haply, peradventure, perchance, possibly.

peril *vb* endanger, imperil, jeopardize, risk. • *n* danger, hazard, insecurity, jeopardy, pitfall, risk, snare, uncertainty.

perilous *adj* dangerous, hazardous, risky, unsafe.

period *n* aeon, age, cycle, date, eon, epoch, season, span, spell, stage, term, time; continuance, duration; bound, conclusion, determination, end, limit, term, termination; clause, phrase, proposition, sentence.

periodical *adj* cyclical, incidental, intermittent, recurrent, recurring, regular, seasonal, systematic. • *n* magazine, paper, review, serial, weekly.

periphery *n* boundary, circumference, outside, perimeter, superficies, surface.

perish *vb* decay, moulder, shrivel, waste, wither; decease, die, expire, vanish.

perishable *adj* decaying, decomposable, destructible; dying, frail, mortal, temporary.

perjured *adj* false, forsworn, perfidious, traitorous, treacherous, untrue.

permanent *adj* abiding, constant, continuing, durable, enduring, fixed, immutable, invariable, lasting, perpetual, persistent, stable, standing, steadfast, unchangeable, unchanging, unfading, unmovable.

permissible *adj* admissible, allowable, free, lawful, legal, legitimate, proper, sufferable, unprohibited.

permission *n* allowance, authorization, consent, dispensation, leave, liberty, licence, permit, sufferance, toleration, warrant.

permit *vb* agree, allow, endure, let, suffer, tolerate; admit, authorize, consent, empower, license, warrant. • *n* leave, liberty, licence, passport, permission, sanction, warrant.

pernicious *adj* baleful, baneful, damaging, deadly, deleterious, destructive, detrimental, disadvantageous, fatal, harmful, hurtful, injurious, malign, mischievous, noisome, noxious, prejudicial, ruinous; evil-hearted, malevolent, malicious, malignant, mischief-making, wicked.

perpetrate *vb* commit, do, execute, perform.

perpetual *adj* ceaseless, continual, constant, endless, enduring, eternal, ever-enduring, everlasting, incessant, interminable, never-ceasing, never-ending, perennial, permanent, sempiternal, unceasing, unending, unfailing, uninterrupted.

perplex *vb* complicate, encumber, entangle, involve, snarl, tangle; beset, bewilder, confound, confuse, corner, distract, embarrass, fog, mystify, nonplus, pother, puzzle, set; annoy, bother, disturb, harass, molest, pester, plague, tease, trouble, vex, worry.

persecute *vb* afflict, distress, harass, molest, oppress, worry; annoy, beset, importune, pester, solicit, tease.

perseverance n constancy, continuance, doggedness, indefatigableness, persistence, persistency, pertinacity, resolution, steadfastness, steadiness, tenacity.

persevere vb continue, determine, endure, maintain, persist, remain, resolve, stick.

persist vb continue, endure, last, remain; insist, persevere.

persistent adj constant, continuing, enduring, fixed, immovable, persevering, persisting, steady, tenacious; contumacious, dogged, indefatigable, obdurate, obstinate, pertinacious, perverse, pigheaded, stubborn.

personable adj comely, good-looking, graceful, seemly, well-turned-out.

personal adj individual, peculiar, private, special; bodily, corporal, corporeal, exterior, material, physical.

personate vb act, impersonate, personify, play, represent; disguise, mast; counterfeit, feign, simulate.

perspective n panorama, prospect, view, vista; proportion, relation.

perspicacious adj keen-sighted, quick-sighted, sharp-sighted; acute, clever, discerning, keen, penetrating, sagacious, sharp-witted, shrewd.

perspicacity n acumen, acuteness, astuteness, discernment, insight, penetration, perspicaciousness, sagacity, sharpness, shrewdness.

perspicuity n clearness, distinctness, explicitness, intelligibility, lucidity, lucidness, perspicuousness, plainness, transparency.

perspicuous adj clear, distinct, explicit, intelligible, lucid, obvious, plain, transparent, unequivocal.

perspire vb exhale, glow, sweat, swelter.

persuade vb allure, actuate, entice, impel, incite, induce, influence, lead, move, prevail upon, urge; advise, counsel; convince, satisfy; inculcate, teach.

persuasion n exhortation, incitement, inducement, influence; belief, conviction, opinion; creed, doctrine, dogma, tenet; kind, sort, variety.

persuasive adj cogent, convincing, inducing, inducible, logical, persuading, plausible, sound, valid, weighty.

pert adj brisk, dapper, lively, nimble, smart, sprightly, perky; bold, flippant, forward, free, impertinent, impudent, malapert, presuming, smart, saucy.

pertain vb appertain, befit, behove, belong, concern, refer, regard, relate.

pertinacious adj constant, determined, firm, obdurate, persevering, resolute, staunch, steadfast, steady; dogged, headstrong, inflexible, mulish, intractable, obstinate, perverse, stubborn, unyielding, wayward, wilful.

pertinent adj adapted, applicable, apposite, appropriate, apropos, apt, fit, germane, pat, proper, relevant, suitable; appurtenant, belonging, concerning, pertaining, regarding.

perturb vb agitate, disquiet, distress, disturb, excite, trouble, unsettle, upset, vex, worry; confuse.

pervade vb affect, animate, diffuse, extend, fill, imbue, impregnate, infiltrate, penetrate, permeate.

perverse adj bad, disturbed, oblique, perverted; contrary, dogged, headstrong, mulish, obstinate, pertinacious, perversive, stubborn, ungovernable, intractable, unyielding, wayward, wilful; cantankerous, churlish, crabbed, cross, cross-grained, crusty, cussed, morose, peevish, petulant, snappish, snarling, spiteful, spleeny, surly, testy, touchy, wicked, wrong-headed; inconvenient, troublesome, untoward, vexatious.

perversion n abasement, corruption, debasement, impairment, injury, prostitution, vitiation.

perverted adj corrupt, debased, distorted, evil, impaired, misguiding, vitiated, wicked.

pessimistic adj cynical, dark, dejected, depressed, despondent, downhearted, gloomy, glum, melancholy, melancholic, morose, sad.

pest n disease, epidemic, infection, pestilence, plague; annoyance, bane, curse, infliction, nuisance, scourge, trouble.

pestilent adj contagious, infectious, malignant, pestilential; deadly, evil, injurious, malign, mischievous, noxious, poisonous; annoying, corrupt, pernicious, troublesome, vexatious.

petition vb ask, beg, crave, entreat, pray, solicit, sue, supplicate. • n address, appeal, application, entreaty, prayer, request, solicitation, supplication, suit.

petrify vb calcify, fossilize, lapidify; benumb, deaden; amaze, appal, astonish, astound, confound, dumbfound, paralyse, stun, stupefy.

petty adj diminutive, frivolous, inconsiderable, inferior, insignificant, little, mean, slight, small, trifling, trivial, unimportant.

petulant adj acrimonious, captious, cavilling, censorious, choleric, crabbed, cross, crusty, forward, fretful, hasty, ill-humoured, ill-tempered, irascible, irritable, peevish, perverse, pettish, querulous, snappish, snarling, testy, touchy, waspish.

phantom n apparition, ghost, illusion, phantasm, spectre, vision, wraith.

pharisaism n cant, formalism, hypocrisy, phariseeism, piety, sanctimoniousness, self-righteousness.

phenomenal adj marvellous, miraculous, prodigious, wondrous.

philanthropy n alms-giving, altruism, benevolence, charity, grace, humanitarianism, humanity, kindness.

philosophical, philosophic adj rational, reasonable, sound, wise; calm, collected, composed, cool, imperturbable, sedate, serene, stoical, tranquil, unruffled.

phlegmatic adj apathetic, calm, cold, cold-blooded, dull, frigid, heavy, impassive, indifferent, inert, sluggish, stoical, tame, unfeeling.

phobia n aversion, detestation, dislike, distaste, dread, fear, hatred.

phrase vb call, christen, denominate, designate, describe, dub, entitle, name, style. • n diction, expression, phraseology, style.

phraseology n diction, expression, language, phrasing, style.

physical adj material, natural; bodily, corporeal, external, substantial, tangible, sensible.

physiognomy n configuration, countenance, face, look, visage.

picaroon n adventurer, cheat, rogue; buccaneer, corsair, freebooter, marauder, pirate, plunderer, sea-rover.

pick vb peck, pierce, strike; cut, detach, gather, pluck; choose, cull, select; acquire, collect, get; pilfer, steal. • n pickaxe, pike, spike, toothpick.

picture vb delineate, draw, imagine, paint, represent. • n drawing, engraving, painting, print; copy, counterpart, delineation, embodiment, illustration, image, likeness, portraiture, portrayal, semblance, representation, resemblance, similitude; description.

picturesque adj beautiful, charming, colourful, graphic, scenic, striking, vivid.

piece vb mend, patch, repair; augment, complete, enlarge, increase; cement, join, unite. • n amount, bit, chunk, cut, fragment, hunk, part, quantity, scrap, shred, slice; portion; article, item, object; composition, lucubration, work, writing.

pied adj irregular, motley, mottled, particoloured, piebald, spotted, variegated.

pierce vb gore, impale, pink, prick, stab, transfix; bore, drill, excite, penetrate, perforate, puncture; affect, move, rouse, strike, thrill, touch.

piety n devotion, devoutness, holiness, godliness, grace, religion, sanctity.

pile[1] vb accumulate, amass; collect, gather, heap, load. • n accumulation, collection, heap, mass, stack; fortune, wad; building, edifice, erection, fabric, pyramid, skyscraper, structure, tower; reactor, nuclear reactor.

pile[2] n beam, column, pier, pillar, pole, post.

pile[3] n down, feel, finish, fur, fluff, fuzz, grain, nap, pappus, shag, surface, texture.

pilfer vb filch, purloin, rob, steal, thieve.

pilgrim n journeyer, sojourner, traveller, wanderer, wayfarer; crusader, devotee, palmer.

pilgrimage n crusade, excursion, expedition, journey, tour, trip.

pillage vb despoil, loot, plunder, rifle, sack, spoil, strip. • n depredation, destruction, devastation, plundering, rapine, spoliation; despoliation, plunder, rifling, sack, spoils.

pillar n column, pier, pilaster, post, shaft, stanchion; maintainer, prop, support, supporter, upholder.

pilot vb conduct, control, direct, guide, navigate, steer. • adj experimental, model, trial. • n helmsman, navigator, steersman; airman, aviator, conductor, director, flier, guide.

pinch vb compress, contract, cramp, gripe, nip, squeeze; afflict, distress, famish, oppress, straiten, stint; frost, nip; apprehend, arrest; economize, spare, stint. • n gripe, nip; pang, throe; crisis, difficulty, emergency, exigency, oppression, pressure, push, strait, stress.

pine vb decay, decline, droop, fade, flag, languish, waste, wilt, wither; desire, long, yearn.

pinion vb bind, chain, fasten, fetter, maim, restrain, shackle. • n pennon, wing; feather, quill, pen, plume, wing; fetter.

pinnacle *n* minaret, turret; acme, apex, height, peak, summit, top, zenith.

pious *adj* filial; devout, godly, holy, religious, reverential, righteous, saintly.

piquant *adj* biting, highly flavoured, piercing, prickling pungent, sharp, stinging; interesting, lively, racy, sparkling, stimulating; cutting, keen, pointed, severe, strong, tart.

pique *vb* goad, incite, instigate, spur, stimulate, urge; affront, chafe, displease, fret, incense, irritate, nettle, offend, provoke, sting, vex, wound. • *n* annoyance, displeasure, irritation, offence, resentment, vexation.

pirate *vb* copy, crib, plagiarize, reproduce, steal. • *n* buccaneer, corsair, freebooter, marauder, picaroon, privateer, seadog, sea-robber, sea-rover, sea wolf.

pit *vb* match, oppose; dent, gouge, hole, mark, nick, notch, scar. • *n* cavity, hole, hollow; crater, dent, depression, dint, excavation, well; abyss, chasm, gulf; pitfall, snare, trap: auditorium, orchestra.

pitch *vb* fall, lurch, plunge, reel; light, settle, rest; cast, dart, fling, heave, hurl, lance, launch, send, toss, throw; erect, establish, fix, locate, place, plant, set, settle, station. • *n* degree, extent, height, intensity, measure, modulation, rage, rate; declivity, descent, inclination, slope; cast, jerk, plunge, throw, toss; place, position, spot; field, ground; line, patter.

piteous *adj* affecting, distressing, doleful, grievous, mournful, pathetic, rueful, sorrowful, woeful; deplorable, lamentable, miserable, pitiable, wretched; compassionate, tender.

pith *n* chief, core, essence, heart, gist, kernel, marrow, part, quintessence, soul, substance; importance, moment, weight; cogency, force, energy, strength, vigour.

pithy *adj* cogent, energetic, forcible, powerful; compact, concise, brief, laconic, meaty, pointed, short, sententious, substantial, terse; corky, porous.

pitiable *adj* deplorable, lamentable, miserable, pathetic, piteous, pitiable, woeful, wretched; abject, base, contemptible, despicable, disreputable, insignificant, low, paltry, mean, rascally, sorry, vile, worthless.

pitiably *adv* deplorably, distressingly, grievously, lamentably, miserably, pathetically, piteously, woefully, wretchedly.

pitiful *adj* compassionate, kind, lenient, merciful, mild, sympathetic, tender, tenderhearted; deplorable, lamentable, miserable, pathetic, piteous, pitiable, wretched; abject, base, contemptible, despicable, disreputable, insignificant, mean, paltry, rascally, sorry, vile, worthless.

pitiless *adj* cruel, hardhearted, implacable, inexorable, merciless, unmerciful, relentless, remorseless, unfeeling, unpitying, unrelenting, unsympathetic.

pittance *n* allowance, allotment, alms, charity, dole, gift; driblet, drop, insufficiency, mite, modicum, trifle.

pity *vb* commiserate, condole, sympathize. • *n* clemency, commiseration, compassion, condolence, fellow-feeling, grace, humanity, leniency, mercy, quarter, sympathy, tenderheartedness.

pivot *vb* depend, hinge, turn. • *n* axis, axle, centre, focus, hinge, joint.

place *vb* arrange, bestow, commit, deposit, dispose, fix, install, lay, locate, lodge, orient, orientate, pitch, plant, pose, put, seat, set, settle, situate, stand, station, rest; allocate, arrange, class, classify, identify, order, organize, recognize; appoint, assign, commission, establish, induct, nominate. • *n* area, courtyard, square; bounds, district, division, locale, locality, location, part, position, premises, quarter, region, scene, site, situation, spot, station, tract, whereabouts; calling, charge, employment, function, occupation, office, pitch, post; calling, condition, grade, precedence, rank, sphere, stakes, standing; abode, building, dwelling, habitation, mansion, residence, seat; city, town, village; fort, fortress, stronghold; paragraph, part, passage, portion; ground, occasion, opportunity, reason, room; lieu, stead.

placid *adj* calm, collected, composed, cool, equable, gentle, peaceful, quiet, serene, tranquil, undisturbed, unexcitable, unmoved, unruffled; halcyon, mild, serene.

plague *vb* afflict, annoy, badger, bore, bother, pester, chafe, disquiet, distress, disturb, embarrass, harass, fret, gall, harry, hector, incommode, irritate, molest, perplex, tantalize, tease, torment, trouble, vex, worry. • *n* disease, pestilence, pest; affliction, annoyance, curse, molestation, nuisance, thorn, torment, trouble, vexation, worry.

plain *adj* dull, even, flat, level, plane, smooth, uniform; clear, open, unencumbered, uninterrupted; apparent, certain, con-

spicuous, evident, distinct, glaring, manifest, notable, notorious, obvious, overt, palpable, patent, prominent, pronounced, staring, transparent, unmistakable, visible; explicit, intelligible, perspicuous, unambiguous, unequivocal; homely, ugly; aboveboard, blunt, crude, candid, direct, downright, frank, honest, ingenuous, open, openhearted, sincere, single-minded, straightforward, undesigning, unreserved, unsophisticated: artless, common, natural, simple, unaffected, unearned; absolute, mere, unmistakable; clear, direct, easy; audible, articulate, definite; frugal, homely; unadorned, unfigured, unornamented, unvariegated. • *n* expanse, flats, grassland, pampas, plateau, prairie, steppe, stretch.

plaint *n* complaint, cry, lament, lamentation, moan, wail.

plaintiff *n* accuser, prosecutor.

plaintive *adj* dirge-like, doleful, grievous, melancholy, mournful, piteous, rueful, sad, sorrowful, woeful.

plan *vb* arrange, calculate, concert, delineate, devise, diagram, figure, premeditate, project, represent, study; concoct, conspire, contrive, design, digest, hatch, invent, manoeuvre, machinate, plot, prepare, scheme. • *n* chart, delineation, diagram, draught, drawing, layout, map, plot, sketch; arrangement, conception, contrivance, design, device, idea, method, programme, project, proposal, proposition, scheme, system; cabal, conspiracy, intrigue, machination; custom, process, way.

plane *vb* even, flatten, level, smooth; float, fly, glide, skate, skim, soar. • *adj* even, flat, horizontal, level, smooth. • *n* degree, evenness, level, levelness, smoothness; aeroplane, aircraft; groover, jointer, rabbet, rebate, scraper.

plant *vb* bed, sow; breed, engender; direct, point, set; colonize, furnish, inhabit, settle; establish, introduce; deposit, establish, fix, found, hide. • *n* herb, organism, vegetable; establishment, equipment, factory, works.

plaster *vb* bedaub, coat, cover, smear, spread. • *n* cement, gypsum, mortar, stucco.

plastic *adj* ductile, flexible, formative, mouldable, pliable, pliant, soft.

platitude *n* dullness, flatness, insipidity, mawkishness; banality, commonplace, truism; balderdash, chatter, flummery, fudge, jargon, moonshine, nonsense, palaver, stuff, trash, twaddle, verbiage.

plaudit *n* acclaim, acclamation, applause, approbation, clapping, commendation, encomium, praise.

plausible *adj* believable, credible, probable, reasonable; bland, fair-spoken, glib, smooth, suave.

play *vb* caper, disport, frisk, frolic, gambol, revel, romp, skip, sport; dally, flirt, idle, toy, trifle, wanton; flutter, hover, wave; act, impersonate, perform, personate, represent; bet, gamble, stake, wager. • *n* amusement, exercise, frolic, gambols, game, jest, pastime, prank, romp, sport; gambling, gaming; act, comedy, drama, farce, performance, tragedy; action, motion, movement; elbowroom, freedom, latitude, movement, opportunity, range, scope, sweep, swing, use.

playful *adj* frisky, frolicsome, gamesome, jolly, kittenish, merry, mirthful, rollicking, sportive; amusing, arch, humorous, lively, mischievous, roguish, skittish, sprightly, vivacious.

plead *vb* answer, appeal, argue, reason; argue, defend, discuss, reason, rejoin; beg, beseech, entreat, implore, petition, sue, supplicate.

pleasant *adj* acceptable, agreeable, delectable, delightful, enjoyable, grateful, gratifying, nice, pleasing, pleasurable, prepossessing, seemly, welcome; cheerful, enlivening, good-humoured, gracious, likable, lively, merry, sportive, sprightly, vivacious; amusing, facetious, humorous, jocose, jocular, sportive, witty.

please *vb* charm, delight, elate, gladden, gratify, pleasure, rejoice; content, oblige, satisfy; choose, like, prefer.

pleasure *n* cheer, comfort, delight, delectation, elation, enjoyment, exhilaration, joy, gladness, gratifying, gusto, relish, satisfaction, solace; amusement, diversion, entertainment, indulgence, refreshment, treat; gratification, luxury, sensuality, voluptuousness; choice, desire, preference, purpose, will, wish; favour, kindness.

plebeian *adj* base, common, ignoble, low, lowborn, mean, obscure, popular, vulgar. • *n* commoner, peasant, proletarian.

pledge *vb* hypothecate, mortgage, pawn, plight; affiance, bind, contract, engage, plight, promise. • *n* collateral, deposit, gage, pawn; earnest, guarantee, security; hostage, security.

plenipotentiary *n* ambassador, envoy, legate, minister.

plenitude *n* abundance, completeness, fullness, plenteousness, plentifulness, plenty, plethora, profusion, repletion.

plentiful *adj* abundant, ample, copious, full, enough, exuberant, fruitful, luxuriant, plenteous, productive, sufficient.

plenty *n* abundance, adequacy, affluence, amplitude, copiousness, enough, exuberance, fertility, fruitfulness, fullness, overflow, plenteousness, plentifulness, plethora, profusion, sufficiency, supply.

pleonastic *adj* circumlocutory, diffuse, redundant, superfluous, tautological, verbose, wordy.

plethora *n* fullness, plenitude, repletion; excess, redundance, redundancy, superabundance, superfluity, surfeit.

pliable *adj* flexible, limber, lithe, lithesome, pliable, pliant, supple; adaptable, compliant, docile, ductile, facile, manageable, obsequious, tractable, yielding.

plight¹ *n* case, category, complication, condition, dilemma, imbroglio, mess, muddle, pass, predicament, scrape, situation, state, strait.

plight² *vb* avow, contract, covenant, engage, honour, pledge, promise, propose, swear, vow. • *n* avowal, contract, covenant, oath, pledge, promise, troth, vow, word; affiancing, betrothal, engagement.

plod *vb* drudge, lumber, moil, persevere, persist, toil, trudge.

plot¹ *vb* connive, conspire, intrigue, machinate, scheme; brew, concoct, contrive, devise, frame, hatch, compass, plan, project; chart, map. • *n* blueprint, chart, diagram, draft, outline, plan, scenario, skeleton; cabal, combination, complicity, connivance, conspiracy, intrigue, plan, project, scheme, stratagem; script, story, subject, theme, thread, topic.

plot² *n* field, lot, parcel, patch, piece, plat, section, tract.

pluck¹ *vb* cull, gather, pick; jerk, pull, snatch, tear, tug, twitch.

pluck² *n* backbone, bravery, courage, daring, determination, energy, force, grit, hardihood, heroism, indomitability, indomitableness, manhood, mettle, nerve, resolution, spirit, valour.

plump¹ *adj* bonny, bouncing, buxom, chubby, corpulent, fat, fleshy, full-figured, obese, portly, rotund, round, sleek, stout, well-rounded; distended, full, swollen, tumid.

plump² *vb* dive, drop, plank, plop, plunge, plunk, put; choose, favour, support • *adj* blunt, complete, direct, downright, full, unqualified, unreserved.

plunder *vb* desolate, despoil, devastate, fleece, forage, harry, loot, maraud, pillage, raid, ransack, ravage, rifle, rob, sack, spoil, spoliate, plunge. • *n* freebooting, devastation, harrying, marauding, rapine, robbery, sack; booty, pillage, prey, spoil.

ply¹ *vb* apply, employ, exert, manipulate, wield; exercise, practise; assail, belabour, beset, press; importune, solicit, urge; offer, present.

ply² *n* fold, layer, plait, twist; bent, bias, direction, turn.

pocket *vb* appropriate, steal; bear, endure, suffer, tolerate. • *n* cavity, cul-de-sac, hollow, pouch, receptacle.

poignant *adj* bitter, intense, penetrating, pierce, severe, sharp; acrid, biting, mordacious, piquant, prickling, pungent, sharp, stinging; caustic, irritating, keen, mordant, pointed, satirical, severe.

point *vb* acuminate, sharpen; aim, direct, level; designate indicate, show; punctuate. • *n* apex, needle, nib, pin, prong, spike, stylus, tip; cape, headland, projection, promontory; eve, instant, moment, period, verge; place, site, spot, stage, station; condition, degree, grade, state; aim, design, end, intent, limit, object, purpose; nicety, pique, punctilio, trifle; position, proposition, question, text, theme, thesis; aspect, matter, respect; characteristic, peculiarity, trait; character, mark, stop; dot, jot, speck; epigram, quip, quirk, sally, witticism; poignancy, sting.

point-blank *adj* categorical, direct, downright, explicit, express, plain, straight. • *adv* categorically, directly, flush, full, plainly, right, straight.

pointless *adj* blunt, obtuse; aimless, dull, flat, fruitless, futile, meaningless, vague, vapid, stupid.

poise *vb* balance, float, hang, hover, support, suspend. • *n* aplomb, balance, composure, dignity, equanimity, equilibrium, equipoise, serenity.

poison *vb* adulterate, contaminate, corrupt, defile, embitter, envenom, impair, infect, intoxicate, pollute, taint, vitiate. • *adj* deadly, lethal, poisonous, toxic. • *n* bane, canker, contagion, pest, taint, toxin, venom, virulence, virus.

poisonous *adj* baneful, corruptive, deadly, fatal, noxious, pestiferous, pestilential, toxic, venomous.

poke *vb* jab, jog, punch, push, shove, thrust; interfere, meddle, pry, snoop. • *n* jab, jog, punch, push, shove, thrust; bag, pocket, pouch, sack.

pole¹ *n* caber, mast, post, rod, spar, staff, stick; bar, beam, pile, shaft; oar, paddle, scull.

pole² *n* axis, axle, hub, pivot, spindle.

poles *npl* antipodes, antipoles, counterpoles, opposites.

policy *n* administration, government, management, rule; plan, plank, platform, role; art, address, cunning, discretion, prudence, shrewdness, skill, stratagem, strategy, tactics; acumen, astuteness, wisdom, wit.

polish *vb* brighten, buff, burnish, furbish, glaze, gloss, scour, shine, smooth; civilize, refine. • *n* brightness, brilliance, brilliancy, lustre, splendour; accomplishment, elegance, finish, grace, refinement.

polished *adj* bright, burnished, glossed, glossy, lustrous, shining, smooth; accomplished, cultivated, elegant, finished, graceful, polite, refined.

polite *adj* attentive, accomplished, affable, chivalrous, civil, complaisant, courtly, courteous, cultivated, elegant, gallant, genteel, gentle, gentlemanly, gracious, mannerly, obliging, polished, refined, suave, urbane, well, well-bred, well-mannered.

politic *adj* civic, civil, political; astute, discreet, judicious, long-headed, noncommittal, provident, prudent, prudential, sagacious, wary, wise; artful, crafty, cunning, diplomatic, expedient, foxy, ingenious, intriguing, Machiavellian, shrewd, skilful, sly, subtle, strategic, timeserving, unscrupulous, wily; well-adapted, well-devised.

political *adj* civic, civil, national, politic, public.

pollute *vb* defile, foul, soil, taint; contaminate, corrupt, debase, demoralize, deprave, impair, infect, pervert, poison, stain, tarnish, vitiate; desecrate, profane; abuse, debauch, defile, deflower, dishonour, ravish, violate.

pollution *n* abomination, contamination, corruption, defilement, foulness, impurity, pollutedness, taint, uncleanness, vitiation.

poltroon *n* coward, crave, dastard, milksop, recreant, skulk, sneak.

pomp *n* display, flourish, grandeur, magnificence, ostentation, pageant, pageantry, parade, pompousness, pride, show, splendour, state, style.

pompous *adj* august, boastful, bombastic, dignified, gorgeous, grand, inflated, lofty, magisterial, ostentatious, pretentious, showy, splendid, stately, sumptuous, superb, vainglorious.

ponder *vb* cogitate, consider, contemplate, deliberate, examine, meditate, muse, reflect, study, weigh.

ponderous *adj* bulky, heavy, massive, weighty; dull, laboured, slow-moving; important, momentous; forcible, mighty.

poniard *n* dagger, dirk, stiletto.

poor *adj* indigent, necessitous, needy, pinched, straitened; destitute, distressed, embarrassed, impecunious, impoverished, insolvent, moneyless, penniless, poverty-stricken, reduced, seedy, unprosperous; emaciated, gaunt, spare, lank, lean, shrunk, skinny, spare, thin; barren, fruitless, sterile, unfertile, unfruitful, unproductive, unprolific; flimsy, inadequate, insignificant, insufficient, paltry, slender, slight, small, trifling, trivial, unimportant, valueless, worthless; decrepit, delicate, feeble, frail, infirm, unsound, weak; inferior, shabby, valueless, worthless; bad, beggarly, contemptible, despicable, humble, inferior, low, mean, pitiful, sorry; bald, cold, dry, dull, feeble, frigid, jejune, languid, meagre, prosaic, prosing, spiritless, tame, vapid, weak; ill-fated, ill-starred, inauspicious, indifferent, luckless, miserable, pitiable, unfavourable, unfortunate, unhappy, unlucky, wretched; deficient, imperfect, inadequate, insufficient, mediocre, scant, scanty; faulty, unsatisfactory; feeble.

populace *n* citizens, crowd, inhabitants, masses, people, public, throng.

popular *adj* lay, plebeian, public; comprehensible, easy, familiar, plain; acceptable, accepted, accredited, admired, approved, favoured, liked, pleasing, praised, received; common, current, prevailing, prevalent; cheap, inexpensive.

pore¹ *n* hole, opening, orifice, spiracle.

pore² *vb* brood, consider, dwell, examine, gaze, read, study.

porous *adj* honeycombed, light, loose, open, penetrable, perforated, permeable, pervious, sandy.

porridge *n* broth, gruel, mush, pap, pottage, soup.

port¹ *n* anchorage, harbour, haven, shelter; door, entrance, gate, passageway; embrasure, porthole.

port[2] *n* air, appearance, bearing, behaviour, carriage, demeanour, deportment, mien, presence.

portable *adj* convenient, handy, light, manageable, movable, portative, transmissible.

portend *vb* augur, betoken, bode, forebode, foreshadow, foretoken, indicate, presage, procrastinate, signify, threaten.

portent *n* augury, omen, presage, prognosis, sign, warning; marvel, phenomenon, wonder.

portion *vb* allot, distribute, divide, parcel; endow, supply. • *n* bit, fragment, morsel, part, piece, scrap, section; allotment, contingent, dividend, division, lot, measure, quantity, quota, ration, share; inheritance.

portly *adj* dignified, grand, imposing, magisterial, majestic, stately; bulky, burly, corpulent, fleshy, large, plump, round, stout.

portray *vb* act, draw, depict, delineate, describe, paint, picture, represent, pose, position, sketch.

pose *vb* arrange, place, set; bewilder, confound, dumbfound, embarrass, mystify, nonplus, perplex, place, puzzle, set, stagger; affect, attitudinize. • *n* attitude, posture; affectation, air, facade, mannerism, pretence, role.

position *vb* arrange, array, fix, locate, place, put, set, site, stand. • *n* locality, place, post, site, situation, spot, station; relation; attitude, bearing, posture; affirmation, assertion, doctrine, predication, principle, proposition, thesis; caste, dignity, honour, rank, standing, status; circumstance, condition, phase, place, state; berth, billet, incumbency, place, post, situation.

positive *adj* categorical, clear, defined, definite, direct, determinate, explicit, express, expressed, precise, unequivocal, unmistakable, unqualified; absolute, actual, real, substantial, true, veritable; assured, certain, confident, convinced, sure; decisive, incontrovertible, indisputable, indubitable, inescapable; imperative, unconditional, undeniable; decided, dogmatic, emphatic, obstinate, overbearing, overconfident, peremptory, stubborn, tenacious.

possess *vb* control, have, hold, keep, obsess, obtain, occupy, own, seize.

possession *n* monopoly, ownership, proprietorship; control, occupation, occupancy, retention, tenancy, tenure; bedevilment, lunacy, madness, obsession; (*pl*) assets, effects, estate, property, wealth.

possessor *n* owner, proprietor.

possible *adj* conceivable, contingent, imaginable, potential; accessible, feasible, likely, practical, practicable, workable.

possibly *adv* haply, maybe, mayhap, peradventure, perchance, perhaps.

post[1] *vb* advertise, announce, inform, placard, publish; brand, defame, disgrace, vilify; enter, slate, record, register. • *n* column, picket, pier, pillar, stake, support.

post[2] *vb* establish, fix, place, put, set, station. • *n* billet, employment, office, place, position, quarter, seat, situation, station.

post[3] *vb* drop, dispatch, mail. • *n* carrier, courier, express, mercury, messenger, postman; dispatch, haste, hurry, speed.

posterior *adj* after, ensuing, following, later, latter, postprandial, subsequent. • *n* back, buttocks, hind, hinder, rump.

posterity *n* descendants, offspring, progeny, seed; breed, brood, children, family, heirs, issue.

postpone *vb* adjourn, defer, delay, procrastinate, prorogue, retard.

postscript *n* addition, afterthought, appendix, supplement.

postulate *vb* assume, presuppose; beseech, entreat, solicit, supplicate. • *n* assumption, axiom, conjecture, hypothesis, proposition, speculation, supposition, theory.

posture *vb* attitudinize, pose. • *n* attitude, pose, position; condition, disposition, mood, phase, state.

pot *n* kettle, pan, saucepan, skillet; can, cup, mug, tankard; crock, jar, jug.

potency *n* efficacy, energy, force, intensity, might, power, strength, vigour; authority, control, influence, sway.

potent *adj* efficacious, forceful, forcible, intense, powerful, strong, virile; able, authoritative, capable, efficient, mighty, puissant, strong; cogent, influential.

potentate *n* emperor, king, monarch, prince, sovereign, ruler.

potential *adj* able, capable, inherent, latent, possible. • *n* ability, capability, dynamic, possibility, potentiality, power.

pother *vb* beset, bewilder, confound, confuse, embarrass, harass, perplex, pose, puzzle, tease. • *n* bustle, commotion, confusion, disturbance, flutter, fuss, huddle, hurly-burly, rumpus, tumult, turbulence, turmoil.

pound[1] *vb* beat, strike, thump; bray, bruise, comminute, crush, levigate, pulverize, triturate; confound, coop, enclose, impound.

pound[2] *n* enclosure, fold, pen.

pour *vb* cascade, emerge, flood, flow, gush, issue, rain, shower, stream.

pouting *adj* bad-tempered, cross, ill-humoured, moody, morose, sulky, sullen.

poverty *n* destitution, difficulties, distress, impecuniosity, impecuniousness, indigence, necessity, need, neediness, penury, privation, straits, want; beggary, mendicancy, pauperism, pennilessness; dearth, jejuneness, lack, scantiness, sparingness, meagreness; exiguity, paucity, poorness, smallness; humbleness, inferiority, lowliness; barrenness, sterility, unfruitfulness, unproductiveness.

power *n* ability, ableness, capability, cogency, competency, efficacy, faculty, might, potency, validity, talent; energy, force, strength, virtue; capacity, susceptibility; endowment, faculty, gift, talent; ascendancy, authoritativeness, authority, carte blanche, command, control, domination, dominion, government, influence, omnipotence, predominance, prerogative, pressure, proxy, puissance, rule, sovereignty, sway, warrant; governor, monarch, potentate, ruler, sovereign; army, host, troop.

powerful *adj* mighty, potent, puissant; able-bodied, herculean, muscular, nervous, robust, sinewy, strong, sturdy, vigorous, vivid; able, commanding, dominating, forceful, forcible, overpowering; cogent, effective, effectual, efficacious, efficient, energetic, influential, operative, valid.

practicable *adj* achievable, attainable, bearable, feasible, performable, possible, workable; operative, passable, penetrable.

practical *adj* hardheaded, matter-of-fact, pragmatic, pragmatical; able, experienced, practised, proficient, qualified, trained, skilled, throughbred, versed; effective, useful, virtual, workable.

practice *n* custom, habit, manner, method, repetition; procedure, usage, use; application, drill, exercise, pursuit; action, acts, behaviour, conduct, dealing, proceeding.

practise *vb* apply, do, exercise, follow, observe, perform, perpetrate, pursue.

practised *adj* able, accomplished, experienced, instructed, practical, proficient, qualified, skilled, thoroughbred, trained, versed.

pragmatic *adj* impertinent, intermeddling, interfering, intrusive, meddlesome, meddling, obtrusive, officious, over-busy; earthy, hard-headed, matter-of-fact, practical, pragmatical, realistic, sensible, stolid.

praise *vb* approbate, acclaim, applaud, approve, commend; celebrate, compliment, eulogize, extol, flatter, laud; adore, bless, exalt, glorify, magnify, worship. • *n* acclaim, approbation, approval, commendation; encomium, eulogy, glorification, laud, laudation, panegyric; exaltation, extolling, glorification, homage, tribute, worship; celebrity, distinction, fame, glory, honour, renown; desert, merit, praiseworthiness.

praiseworthy *adj* commendable, creditable, good, laudable, meritorious.

prank *n* antic, caper, escapade, frolic, gambol, trick.

prate *vb* babble, chatter, gabble, jabber, palaver, prattle, tattle. • *n* chatter, gabble, nonsense, palaver, prattle, twaddle.

pray *vb* ask, beg, beseech, conjure, entreat, implore, importune, invoke, petition, request, solicit, supplicate.

prayer *n* beseeching, entreaty, imploration, petition, request, solicitation, suit, supplication; adoration, devotion(s), litany, invocation, orison, praise, suffrage.

preach *vb* declare, deliver, proclaim, pronounce, publish; inculcate, press, teach, urge; exhort, lecture, moralize, sermonize.

preamble *n* foreword, introduction, preface, prelude, prologue.

precarious *adj* critical, doubtful, dubious, equivocal, hazardous, insecure, perilous, unassured, riskful, risky, uncertain, unsettled, unstable, unsteady.

precaution *n* care, caution, circumspection, foresight, forethought, providence, prudence, safeguard, wariness; anticipation, premonition, provision.

precautionary *adj* preservative, preventative, provident.

precede *vb* antedate, forerun, head, herald, introduce, lead, utter.

precedence *n* advantage, antecedence, lead, pre-eminence, preference, priority, superiority, supremacy.

precedent *n* antecedent, authority, custom, example, instance, model, pattern, procedure, standard, usage.

precept *n* behest, bidding, canon, charge, command, commandment, decree, dictate, edict, injunction, instruction, law, mandate, ordinance, ordination, order, regulation; direction, doctrine, maxim, principle, teaching, rubric, rule.

preceptor *n* instructor, lecturer, master, pedagogue, professor, schoolteacher, teacher, tutor.

precinct *n* border, bound, boundary, confine, environs, frontier, enclosure, limit, list, march, neighbourhood, purlieus, term, terminus; area, district.

precious *adj* costly, inestimable, invaluable, priceless, prized, valuable; adored, beloved, cherished, darling, dear, idolized, treasured; fastidious, overnice, over-refined, precise.

precipice *n* bluff, cliff, crag, steep.

precipitate *vb* advance, accelerate, dispatch, expedite, forward, further, hasten, hurry, plunge, press, quicken, speed. • *adj* hasty, hurried, headlong, impetuous, indiscreet, overhasty, rash, reckless; abrupt, sudden, violent.

precipitous *adj* abrupt, cliffy, craggy, perpendicular, uphill, sheer, steep.

precise *adj* accurate, correct, definite, distinct, exact, explicit, express, nice, pointed, severe, strict, unequivocal, well-defined; careful, scrupulous; ceremonious, finical, formal, prim, punctilious, rigid, starched, stiff.

precision *n* accuracy, correctness, definiteness, distinctness, exactitude, exactness, nicety, preciseness.

preclude *vb* bar, check, debar, hinder, inhibit, obviate, prevent, prohibit, restrain, stop.

precocious *adj* advanced, forward, overforward, premature.

preconcert *vb* concoct, prearrange, predetermine, premeditate, prepare.

precursor *n* antecedent, cause, forerunner, predecessor; harbinger, herald, messenger, pioneer; omen, presage, sign.

precursory *adj* antecedent, anterior, forerunning, precedent, preceding, previous, prior; initiatory, introductory, precursive, prefatory, preliminary, prelusive, prelusory, premonitory, preparatory, prognosticative.

predatory *adj* greedy, pillaging, plundering, predacious, rapacious, ravaging, ravenous, voracious.

predestination *n* doom, fate, foredoom, foreordainment, foreordination, necessity, predetermination, preordination.

predicament *n* attitude, case, condition, plight, position, posture, situation, state; corner, dilemma, emergency, exigency, fix, hole, impasse, mess, pass, pinch, push, quandary, scrape.

predict *vb* augur, betoken, bode, divine, forebode, forecast, foredoom, foresee, forespeak, foretell, foretoken, forewarn, portend, prognosticate, prophesy, read, signify, soothsay.

predilection *n* bent, bias, desire, fondness, inclination, leaning, liking, love, partiality, predisposition, preference, prejudice, prepossession.

predisposition *n* aptitude, bent, bias, disposition, inclination, leaning, proclivity, proneness, propensity, willingness.

predominant *adj* ascendant, controlling, dominant, overruling, prevailing, prevalent, reigning, ruling, sovereign, supreme.

predominate *vb* dominate, preponderate, prevail, rule.

pre-eminent *adj* chief, conspicuous, consummate, controlling, distinguished, excellent, excelling, paramount, peerless, predominant, renowned, superior, supreme, surpassing, transcendent, unequalled.

preface *vb* begin, introduce, induct, launch, open, precede. • *n* exordium, foreword, induction, introduction, preamble, preliminary, prelude, prelusion, premise, proem, prologue, prolusion.

prefatory *adj* antecedent, initiative, introductory, precursive, precursory, preliminary, prelusive, prelusory, preparatory, proemial.

prefer *vb* address, offer, present, proffer, tender; advance, elevate, promote, raise; adopt, choose, elect, fancy, pick, select, wish.

preference *n* advancement, choice, election, estimation, precedence, priority, selection.

preferment *n* advancement, benefice, dignity, elevation, exaltation, promotion.

pregnant *adj* big, enceinte, parturient; fraught, full, important, replete, significant, weighty; fecund, fertile, fruitful, generative, potential, procreant, procreative, productive, prolific.

prejudice *vb* bias, incline, influence, turn, warp; damage, diminish, hurt, impair, injure. • *n* bias, intolerance, partiality, preconception, predilection, prejudgement, prepossession, unfairness; damage, detriment, disadvantage, harm, hurt, impairment, injury, loss, mischief.

prejudiced *adj* biased, bigoted, influenced, one-sided, partial, partisan, unfair.

preliminary *adj* antecedent, initiatory, introductory, precedent, precursive, precursory, prefatory, prelusive, prelusory, preparatory, previous, prior, proemial. • *n* beginning, initiation, introduction, opening, preamble, preface, prelude, start.

prelude *n* introduction, opening, overture, prelusion, preparation, voluntary; exordium, preamble, preface, preliminary, proem.

premature *adj* hasty, ill-considered, precipitate, unmatured, unprepared, unripe, unseasonable, untimely.

premeditation *n* deliberation, design, forethought, intention, prearrangement, predetermination, purpose.

premise *vb* introduce, preamble, preface, prefix. • *n* affirmation, antecedent, argument, assertion, assumption, basis, foundation, ground, hypothesis, position, premiss, presupposition, proposition, support, thesis, theorem.

premium *n* bonus, bounty, encouragement, fee, gift, guerdon, meed, payment, prize, recompense, remuneration, reward; appreciation, enhancement.

premonition *n* caution, foreboding, foreshadowing, forewarning, indication, omen, portent, presage, presentiment, sign, warning.

preoccupied *adj* absent, absentminded, abstracted, dreaming, engrossed, inadvertent, inattentive, lost, musing, unobservant.

prepare *vb* adapt, adjust, fit, qualify; arrange, concoct, fabricate, make, order, plan, procure, provide.

preponderant *adj* outweighing, overbalancing, preponderating.

prepossessing *adj* alluring, amiable, attractive, bewitching, captivating, charming, engaging, fascinating, inviting, taking, winning.

preposterous *adj* absurd, excessive, exorbitant, extravagant, foolish, improper, irrational, monstrous, nonsensical, perverted, ridiculous, unfit, unreasonable, wrong.

prerogative *n* advantage, birthright, claim, franchise, immunity, liberty, privilege, right.

presage *vb* divine, forebode; augur, betoken, bode, foreshadow, foretell, foretoken, indicate, portend, predict, prognosticate, prophesy, signify, soothsay. • *n* augury, auspice, boding, foreboding, foreshowing, indication, omen, portent, prognostication, sign, token; foreknowledge, precognition, prediction, premonition, presentiment, prophecy.

prescribe *vb* advocate, appoint, command, decree, dictate, direct, enjoin, establish, institute, ordain, order.

presence *n* attendance, company, inhabitance, inhabitancy, nearness, neighbourhood, occupancy, propinquity, proximity, residence, ubiquity, vicinity; air, appearance, carriage, demeanour, mien, personality.

present[1] *adj* near; actual, current, existing, happening, immediate, instant, living; available, quick, ready; attentive, favourable. • *n* now, time being, today.

present[2] *n* benefaction, boon, donation, favour, gift, grant, gratuity, largesse, offering.

present[3] *vb* introduce, nominate; exhibit, offer; bestow, confer, give, grant; deliver, hand; advance, express, prefer, proffer, tender.

presentiment *n* anticipation, apprehension, foreboding, forecast, foretaste, forethought, prescience.

presently *adv* anon, directly, forthwith, immediately, shortly, soon.

preservation *n* cherishing, conservation, curing, maintenance, protection, support; safety, salvation, security; integrity, keeping, soundness.

preserve *vb* defend, guard, keep, protect, rescue, save, secure, shield; maintain, uphold, sustain, support; conserve, economize, husband, retain. • *n* comfit, compote, confection, confiture, conserve, jam, jelly, marmalade, sweetmeat; enclosure, warren.

preside *vb* control, direct, govern, manage, officiate.

press *vb* compress, crowd, crush, squeeze; flatten, iron, smooth; clasp, embrace, hug; force, compel, constrain; emphasize, enforce, enjoin, inculcate, stress, urge; hasten, hurry, push, rush; crowd, throng; entreat, importune, solicit. • *n* crowd, crush, multitude, throng; hurry, pressure, urgency; case, closet, cupboard, repository.

pressing *adj* constraining, critical, distressing, imperative, importunate, persistent, serious, urgent, vital.

pressure *n* compressing, crushing, squeezing; influence, force; compulsion, exigency, hurry, persuasion, press, stress, urgency; affliction, calamity, difficulty, distress, embarrassment, grievance, oppression, straits; impression, stamp.

prestidigitation *n* conjuring, juggling, legerdemain, sleight-of-hand.

prestige *n* credit, distinction, importance, influence, reputation, weight.

presume *vb* anticipate, apprehend, assume, believe, conjecture, deduce, expect, infer, surmise, suppose, think; consider, presuppose; dare, undertake, venture.

presumption *n* anticipation, assumption, belief, concession, conclusion, condition, conjecture, deduction, guess, hypothesis, inference, opinion, supposition, understanding; arrogance, assurance, audacity, boldness, brass, effrontery, forwardness, haughtiness, presumptuousness; probability.

presumptuous *adj* arrogant, assuming, audacious, bold, brash, forward, irreverent, insolent, intrusive, presuming; foolhardy, overconfident, rash.

pretence *n* affectation, cloak, colour, disguise, mask, semblance, show, simulation, veil, window-dressing; excuse, evasion, fabrication, feigning, makeshift, pretext, sham, subterfuge; claim, pretension.

pretend *vb* affect, counterfeit, deem, dissemble, fake, falsify, feign, sham, simulate; act, imagine, lie, profess; aspire, claim.

pretension *n* assertion, assumption, claim, demand, pretence; affectation, airs, conceit, ostentation, pertness, pretentiousness, priggishness, vanity.

pretentious *adj* affected, assuming, conceited, conspicuous, ostentatious, presuming, priggish, showy, tawdry, unnatural, vain.

preternatural *adj* abnormal, anomalous, extraordinary, inexplicable, irregular, miraculous, mysterious, odd, peculiar, strange, unnatural.

pretext *n* affectation, appearance, blind, cloak, colour, guise, mask, pretence, semblance, show, simulation, veil; excuse, justification, plea, vindication.

pretty *adj* attractive, beautiful, bonny, comely, elegant, fair, handsome, neat, pleasing, trim; affected, foppish. • *adv* fairly, moderately, quite, rather, somewhat.

prevail *vb* overcome, succeed, triumph, win; obtain, predominate, preponderate, reign, rule.

prevailing *adj* controlling, dominant, effectual, efficacious, general, influential, operative, overruling, persuading, predominant, preponderant, prevalent, ruling, successful.

prevalent *adj* ascendant, compelling, efficacious, governing, predominant, prevailing, successful, superior; extensive, general, rife, widespread.

prevaricate *vb* cavil, deviate, dodge, equivocate, evade, palter, pettifog, quibble, shift, shuffle, tergiversate.

prevent *vb* bar, check, debar, deter, forestall, help, hinder, impede, inhibit, intercept, interrupt, obstruct, obviate, preclude, prohibit, restrain, save, stop, thwart.

prevention *n* anticipation, determent, deterrence, deterrent, frustration, hindrance, interception, interruption, obstruction, preclusion, prohibition, restriction, stoppage.

previous *adj* antecedent, anterior, earlier, foregoing, foregone, former, precedent, preceding, prior.

prey *vb* devour, eat, feed on, live off; exploit, intimidate, terrorize; burden, distress, haunt, oppress, trouble, worry. • *n* booty, loot, pillage, plunder, prize, rapine, spoil; food, game, kill quarry, victim; depredation, ravage.

price *vb* assess, estimate, evaluate, rate, value. • *n* amount, cost, expense, outlay, value; appraisal, charge, estimation, excellence, figure, rate, quotation, valuation, value, worth; compensation, guerdon, recompense, return, reward.

priceless *adj* dear, expensive, precious, inestimable, invaluable, valuable; amusing, comic, droll, funny, humorous, killing, rich.

prick *vb* perforate, pierce, puncture, stick; drive, goad, impel, incite, spur, urge; cut, hurt, mark, pain, sting, wound; hasten, post, ride. • *n* mark, perforation, point, puncture; prickle, sting, wound.

pride *vb* boast, brag, crow, preen, revel in. • *n* conceit, egotism, self-complacency, self-esteem, self-exaltation, self-importance, self-sufficiency, vanity; arrogance, assumption, disdain, haughtiness, hauteur, insolence, loftiness, lordliness, pomposity, presumption, superciliousness, vainglory; decorum, dignity, elevation, self-respect; decoration, glory, ornament, show, splendour.

priest *n* churchman, clergyman, divine, ecclesiastic, minister, pastor, presbyter.

prim *adj* demure, formal, nice, precise, prudish, starch, starched, stiff, strait-laced.

primary *adj* aboriginal, earliest, first, initial, original, prime, primitive, primeval, primordial, pristine; chief, main, principal; basic, elementary, fundamental, preparatory; radical.

prime[1] *adj* aboriginal, basic, first, initial, original, primal, primary, primeval, primitive, primordial, pristine; chief, foremost, highest, leading, main, paramount, principal; blooming, early; capital, cardinal, dominant, predominant; excellent, first-class, first-rate, optimal, optimum, quintessential, superlative; beginning, opening. • *n* beginning, dawn, morning, opening; spring, springtime, youth; bloom, cream, flower, height, heyday, optimum, perfection, quintessence, zenith.

prime[2] *vb* charge, load, prepare, undercoat; coach, groom, train, tutor.

primeval *adj* original, primitive, primordial, pristine.

primitive *adj* aboriginal, first, fundamental, original, primal, primary, prime, primitive, primordial, pristine; ancient, antiquated, crude, old-fashioned, quaint, simple, uncivilized, unsophisticated.

prince *n* monarch, potentate, ruler, sovereign; dauphin, heir apparent, infant; chief, leader, potentate.

princely *adj* imperial, regal, royal; august, generous, grand, liberal, magnanimous, magnificent, majestic, munificent, noble, pompous, splendid, superb, titled; dignified, elevated, high-minded, lofty, noble, stately.

principal *adj* capital, cardinal, chief, essential, first, foremost, highest, leading, main, pre-eminent, prime. • *n* chief, head, leader; head teacher, master.

principally *adv* chiefly, essentially, especially, mainly, particularly.

principle *n* cause, fountain, fountainhead, groundwork, mainspring, nature, origin, source, spring; basis, constituent, element, essence, substratum; assumption, axiom, law, maxim, postulation; doctrine, dogma, impulse, maxim, opinion, precept, rule, tenet, theory; conviction, ground, motive, reason; equity, goodness, honesty, honour, incorruptibility, integrity, justice, probity, rectitude, righteousness, trustiness, truth, uprightness, virtue, worth; faculty, power.

prink *vb* adorn, deck, decorate; preen, primp, spruce.

print *vb* engrave, impress, imprint, mark, stamp; issue, publish. • *n* book, periodical, publication; copy, engraving, photograph, picture; characters, font, fount, lettering, type, typeface.

prior *adj* antecedent, anterior, earlier, foregoing, precedent, preceding, precursory, previous, superior.

priority *n* antecedence, anteriority, precedence, pre-eminence, pre-existence, superiority.

priory *n* abbey, cloister, convent, monastery, nunnery.

prison *n* confinement, dungeon, gaol, jail, keep, lockup, penitentiary, reformatory; can, clink, cooler, jug.

pristine *adj* ancient, earliest, first, former, old, original, primary, primeval, primitive, primordial.

privacy *n* concealment, secrecy; retirement, retreat, seclusion, solitude.

private *adj* retired, secluded, sequestrated, solitary; individual, own particular, peculiar, personal, special, unofficial; confidential, privy; clandestine, concealed, hidden, secret. • *n* GI, soldier, tommy.

privation *n* bereavement, deprivation, dispossession, loss; destitution, distress, indigence, necessity, need, want; absence, negation; degradation.

privilege *n* advantage, charter, claim, exemption, favour, franchise, immunity, leave, liberty, licence, permission, prerogative, right.

privy *adj* individual, particular, peculiar, personal, private, special; clandestine, secret; retired, sequestrated.

prize[1] *vb* appreciate, cherish, esteem, treasure, value.

prize[2] *adj* best, champion, first-rate, outstanding, winning. • *n* guerdon, honours, meed, premium, reward; cup, decoration, medal, laurels, palm, trophy; booty, capture, lot, plunder, spoil; advantage, gain, privilege.

probability *n* chance, prospect, likelihood, presumption; appearance, credibility, credibleness, likeliness, verisimilitude.

probable *adj* apparent, credible, likely, presumable, reasonable.

probably *adv* apparently, likely, maybe, perchance, perhaps, presumably, possibly, seemingly.

probation *n* essay, examination, ordeal, proof, test, trial; novitiate.

probe *vb* examine, explore fathom, investigate, measure, prove, scrutinize, search, sift, sound, test, verify. • *n* examination, exploration, inquiry, investigation, scrutiny, study.

probity *n* candour, conscientiousness, equity, fairness, faith, goodness, honesty, honour, incorruptibility, integrity, justice, loyalty, morality, principle, rectitude, righteousness, sincerity, soundness, trustworthiness, truth, truthfulness, uprightness, veracity, virtue, worth.

problem *adj* difficult, intractable, uncontrollable, unruly. • *n* dilemma, dispute, doubt, enigma, exercise, proposition, puzzle, riddle, theorem.

problematic *adj* debatable, disputable, doubtful, dubious, enigmatic, problematical, puzzling, questionable, suspicious, uncertain, unsettled.

procedure *n* conduct, course, custom, management, method, operation, policy, practice, process; act, action, deed, measure, performance, proceeding, step, transaction.

proceed *vb* advance, continue, go, pass, progress; accrue, arise, come, emanate, ensue, flow, follow, issue, originate, result, spring.

proceeds *npl* balance, earnings, effects, gain, income, net, produce, products, profits, receipts, returns, yield.

process *vb* advance, deal with, fulfil, handle, progress; alter, convert, refine, transform. • *n* advance, course, progress, train; action, conduct, management, measure, mode, operation, performance, practice, procedure, proceeding, step, transaction, way; action, case, suit, trial; outgrowth, projection, protuberance.

procession *n* cavalcade, cortege, file, march, parade, retinue, train.

proclaim *vb* advertise, announce, blazon, broach, broadcast, circulate, cry, declare, herald, promulgate, publish, trumpet; ban, outlaw, proscribe.

proclamation *n* advertisement, announcement, blazon, declaration, promulgation, publication; ban, decree, edict, manifesto, ordinance.

proclivity *n* bearing, bent, bias, determination, direction, disposition, drift, inclination, leaning, predisposition, proneness, propensity, tendency, turn; aptitude, facility, readiness.

procrastinate *vb* adjourn, defer, delay, postpone, prolong, protract, retard; neglect, omit; lag, loiter.

procrastination *n* delay, dilatoriness, postponement, protraction, slowness, tardiness.

procreate *vb* beget, breed, engender, generate, produce, propagate.

procurable *adj* acquirable, compassable, obtainable.

procurator *n* agent, attorney, deputy, proctor, proxy, representative, solicitor.

procure *vb* acquire, gain, get, obtain; cause, compass, contrive, effect.

procurer *n* bawd, pander, pimp.

prodigal *adj* abundant, dissipated, excessive, extravagant, generous, improvident, lavish, profuse, reckless, squandering, thriftless, unthrifty, wasteful. • *n* spendthrift, squanderer, waster, wastrel.

prodigality *n* excess, extravagance, lavishness, profusion, squandering, unthriftiness, waste, wastefulness.

prodigious *adj* amazing, astonishing, astounding, extraordinary, marvellous, miraculous, portentous, remarkable, startling, strange, surprising, uncommon, wonderful, wondrous; enormous, huge, immense, monstrous, vast.

prodigy *n* marvel, miracle, phenomenon, portent, sign, wonder; curiosity, monster, monstrosity.

produce *vb* exhibit, show; bear, beget, breed, conceive, engender, furnish, generate, hatch, procreate, yield; accomplish, achieve, cause, create, effect, make, occasion, originate; accrue, afford, give, impart, make, render; extend, lengthen, prolong, protract; fabricate, fashion, manufacture. • *n* crop, fruit, greengrocery, harvest, product, vegetables, yield.

producer *n* creator, inventor, maker, originator; agriculturalist, farmer, greengrocer, husbandman, raiser.

product *n* crops, fruits, harvest, outcome, proceeds, produce, production, returns, yield; consequence, effect, fruit, issue, performance, production, result, work.

production *n* fruit, produce, product; construction, creation, erection, fabrication, making, performance; completion, fruition; birth, breeding, development, growth, propagation; opus, publication, work; continuation, extension, lengthening, prolongation.

productive *adj* copious, fertile, fruitful, luxuriant, plenteous, prolific, teeming; causative, constructive, creative, efficient, life-giving, producing.

proem *n* exordium, foreword, introduction, preface, prelims, prelude, prolegomena.

profane *vb* defile, desecrate, pollute, violate; abuse, debase. • *adj* blasphemous, godless, heathen, idolatrous, impious, impure, pagan, secular, temporal, unconsecrated, unhallowed, unholy, unsanctified, worldly, unspiritual; impure, polluted, unholy.

profanity *n* blasphemy, impiety, irreverence, profaneness, sacrilege.

profess *vb* acknowledge, affirm, allege, aver, avouch, avow, confess, declare, own, proclaim, state; affect, feign, pretend.

profession *n* acknowledgement, assertion, avowal, claim, declaration; avocation, evasion, pretence, pretension, protestation, representation; business, calling, employment, engagement, occupation, office, trade, vocation.

proffer *vb* offer, propose, propound, suggest, tender, volunteer. • *n* offer, proposal, suggestion, tender.

proficiency *n* advancement, forwardness, improvement; accomplishment, aptitude, competency, dexterity, mastery, skill.

proficient *adj* able, accomplished, adept, competent, conversant, dextrous, expert, finished, masterly, practised, skilled, skilful, thoroughbred, trained, qualified, well-versed. • *n* adept, expert, master, master-hand.

profit *vb* advance, benefit, gain, improve. • *n* aid, clearance, earnings, emolument, fruit, gain, lucre, produce, return; advancement, advantage, benefit, interest, perquisite, service, use, utility, weal.

profitable *adj* advantageous, beneficial, desirable, gainful, productive, useful; lucrative, remunerative.

profitless *adj* bootless, fruitless, unprofitable, useless, valueless, worthless.

profligate *adj* abandoned, corrupt, corrupted, degenerate, depraved, dissipated, dissolute, graceless, immoral, shameless, vicious, vitiated, wicked. • *n* debauchee, libertine, rake, reprobate, roué.

profound *adj* abysmal, deep, fathomless; heavy, undisturbed; erudite, learned, penetrating, sagacious, skilled; deeply felt, far-reaching, heartfelt, intense, lively, strong, touching, vivid; low, submissive; abstruse, mysterious, obscure, occult, subtle, recondite; complete, thorough.

profundity *n* deepness, depth, profoundness.

profuse *adj* abundant, bountiful, copious, excessive, extravagant, exuberant, generous, improvident, lavish, overabundant, plentiful, prodigal, wasteful.

profusion *n* abundance, bounty, copiousness, excess, exuberance, extravagance, lavishness, prodigality, profuseness, superabundance, waste.

progenitor *n* ancestor, forebear, forefather.

progeny *n* breed, children, descendants, family, issue, lineage, offshoot, offspring, posterity, race, scion, stock, young.

prognostic *adj* foreshadowing, foreshowing, foretokening. • *n* augury, foreboding, indication, omen, presage, prognostication, sign, symptom, token; foretelling, prediction, prophecy.

prognosticate *vb* foretell, predict, prophesy; augur, betoken, forebode, foreshadow, foreshow, foretoken, indicate, portend, presage.

prognostication *n* foreknowledge, foreshowing, foretelling, prediction, presage; augury, foreboding, foretoken, indication, portent, prophecy.

progress *vb* advance, continue, proceed; better, gain, improve, increase. • *n* advance, advancement, progression; course, headway, ongoing, passage; betterment, development, growth, improvement, increase, reform; circuit, procession.

prohibit *vb* debar, hamper, hinder, preclude, prevent; ban, disallow, forbid, inhibit, interdict.

prohibition *n* ban, bar, disallowance, embargo, forbiddance, inhibition, interdict, interdiction, obstruction, prevention, proscription, taboo, veto.

prohibitive *adj* forbidding, prohibiting, refraining, restrictive.

project *vb* cast, eject, fling, hurl, propel, shoot, throw; brew, concoct, contrive, design, devise, intend, plan, plot, purpose, scheme; delineate, draw, exhibit; bulge, extend, jut, protrude. • *n* contrivance, design, device, intention, plan, proposal, purpose, scheme.

projectile *n* bullet, missile, shell.

projection *n* delivery, ejection, emission, propulsion, throwing; contriving, designing, planning, scheming; bulge, extension, outshoot, process, prominence, protuberance, salience, saliency, salient, spur; delineation, map, plan.

proletarian *adj* mean, plebeian, vile, vulgar. • *n* commoner, plebeian.

proletariat *n* commonality, hoi polloi, masses, mob, plebs, working class.

prolific *adj* abundant, fertile, fruitful, generative, productive, teeming.

prolix *adj* boring, circumlocutory, discursive, diffuse, lengthy, long, long-winded, loose, prolonged, protracted, prosaic, rambling, tedious, tiresome, verbose, wordy.

prologue *n* foreword, introduction, preamble, preface, preliminary, prelude, proem.

prolong *vb* continue, extend, lengthen, protract, sustain; defer, postpone.

promenade *vb* saunter, walk. • *n* dance, stroll, walk; boulevard, esplanade, parade, walkway.

prominent *adj* convex, embossed, jutting, projecting, protuberant, raised, relieved; celebrated, conspicuous, distinguished, eminent, famous, foremost, influential, leading, main, noticeable, outstanding; conspicuous, distinctive, important, manifest, marked, principal, salient.

promiscuous *adj* confused, heterogeneous, indiscriminate, intermingled, mingled, miscellaneous, mixed; abandoned, dissipated, dissolute, immoral, licentious, loose, unchaste. wanton.

promise *vb* covenant, engage, pledge, subscribe, swear, underwrite, vow; assure, attest, guarantee, warrant; agree, bargain, engage, stipulate, undertake. • *n* agreement, assurance, contract, engagement, oath, parole, pledge, profession, undertaking, vow, word.

promising *adj* auspicious, encouraging, hopeful, likely, propitious.

promote *vb* advance, aid, assist, cultivate, encourage, further, help, promote; dignify, elevate, exalt, graduate, honour, pass, prefer, raise.

promotion *n* advancement, encouragement, furtherance; elevation, exaltation, preferment.

prompt *vb* actuate, dispose, impel, incite, incline, induce, instigate, stimulate, urge; remind; dictate, hint, influence, suggest. • *adj* active, alert, apt, quick, ready; forward, hasty; disposed, inclined, prone; early, exact, immediate, instant precise, punctual, seasonable, timely. • *adv* apace, directly, forthwith, immediately, promptly. • *n* cue, hint, prompter, reminder, stimulus.

promptly *adv* apace, directly, expeditiously, forthwith, immediately, instantly, pronto, punctually, quickly, speedily, straightway, straightaway, summarily, swiftly.

promptness *n* activity, alertness, alacrity, promptitude, readiness, quickness.

promulgate *vb* advertise, announce, broadcast, bruit, circulate, declare, notify, proclaim, publish, spread, trumpet.

prone *adj* flat, horizontal, prostrate, recumbent; declivitous, inclined, inclining, sloping; apt, bent, disposed, inclined, predisposed, tending; eager, prompt, ready.

pronounce *vb* articulate, enunciate, frame, say, speak, utter; affirm, announce, assert, declare, deliver, state.

proof *adj* firm, fixed, impenetrable, stable, steadfast. • *n* essay, examination, ordeal, test, trial; attestation, certification, conclusion, conclusiveness, confirmation, corroboration, demonstration, evidence, ratification, substantiation, testimony, verification.

prop *vb* bolster, brace, buttress, maintain, shore, stay, support, sustain, truss, uphold. • *n* support, stay; buttress, fulcrum, pin, shore, strut.

propaganda *n* inculcation, indoctrination, promotion.

propagate *vb* continue, increase, multiply; circulate, diffuse, disseminate, extend, promote, promulgate, publish, spread, transmit; beget, breed, engender, generate, originate, procreate.

propel *vb* drive, force, impel, push, urge; cast, fling, hurl, project, throw.

propensity *n* aptitude, bent, bias, disposition, inclination, ply, proclivity, proneness, tendency.

proper *adj* individual, inherent, natural, original, particular, peculiar, special, specific; adapted, appropriate, becoming, befitting, convenient, decent, decorous, demure, fit, fitting, legitimate, meet, pertinent, respectable, right, seemly, suitable; accurate, correct, exact, fair, fastidious, formal, just, precise, actual, real.

property *n* attribute, characteristic, disposition, mark, peculiarity, quality, trait, virtue; appurtenance, assets, belongings, chattels, circumstances, effects, estate, goods, possessions, resources, wealth; ownership, possession, proprietorship, tenure; claim, copyright, interest, participation, right, title.

prophecy *n* augury, divination, forecast, foretelling, portent, prediction, premonition, presage, prognostication; exhortation, instruction, preaching.

prophesy *vb* augur, divine, foretell, predict, prognosticate.

propinquity *n* adjacency, contiguity, nearness, neighbourhood, proximity, vicinity; affinity, connection, consanguinity, kindred, relationship.

propitiate *vb* appease, atone, conciliate, intercede, mediate, pacify, reconcile, satisfy.

propitious *adj* benevolent, benign, friendly, gracious, kind, merciful; auspicious, encouraging, favourable, fortunate, happy, lucky, opportune, promising, prosperous, thriving, timely, well-disposed.

proportion *vb* adjust, graduate, regulate; form, shape. • *n* arrangement, relation; adjustment, commensuration, dimension, distribution, symmetry; extent, lot, part, portion, quota, ratio, share.

proposal *n* design, motion, offer, overture, proffer, proposition, recommendation, scheme, statement, suggestion, tender.

propose *vb* move, offer, pose, present, propound, proffer, put, recommend, state, submit, suggest, tender; design, intend, mean, purpose.

proposition *vb* accost, proffer, solicit. • *n* offer, overture, project, proposal, suggestion, tender, undertaking; affirmation, assertion, axiom, declaration, dictum, doctrine, position, postulation, predication, statement, theorem, thesis.

proprietor *n* lord, master, owner, possessor, proprietary.

propriety *n* accuracy, adaptation, appropriation, aptness, becomingness, consonance, correctness, fitness, justness, reasonableness, rightness, seemliness, suitableness; conventionality, decency, decorum, demureness, fastidiousness, formality, modesty, properness, respectability.

prorogation *n* adjournment, continuance, postponement.

prosaic *adj* commonplace dull, flat, humdrum, matter-of-fact, pedestrian, plain, prolix, prosing, sober, stupid, tame, tedious, tiresome, unentertaining, unimaginative, uninspired, uninteresting, unromantic, vapid.

proscribe *vb* banish, doom, exile, expel, ostracize, outlaw; exclude, forbid, interdict, prohibit; censure, condemn, curse, denounce, reject.

prosecute *vb* conduct, continue, exercise, follow, persist, pursue; arraign, indict, sue, summon.

prospect *vb* explore, search, seek, survey. • *n* display, field, landscape, outlook, perspective, scene, show, sight, spectacle, survey, view, vision, vista; picture, scenery; anticipation, calculation, contemplation, expectance, expectancy, expectation, foreseeing, foresight, hope, presumption, promise, trust; likelihood, probability.

prospectus *n* announcement, conspectus, description, design, outline, plan, programme, sketch, syllabus.

prosper *vb* aid, favour, forward, help; advance, flourish, grow rich, thrive, succeed; batten, increase.

prosperity *n* affluence, blessings, happiness, felicity, good luck, success, thrift, weal, welfare, well-being; boom, heyday.

prosperous *adj* blooming, flourishing, fortunate, golden, halcyon, rich, successful, thriving; auspicious, booming, bright, favourable, good, golden, lucky, promising, propitious, providential, rosy.

prostrate *vb* demolish, destroy, fell, level, overthrow, overturn, ruin; depress, exhaust, overcome, reduce. • *adj* fallen, prostrated, prone, recumbent, supine; helpless, powerless.

prostration *n* demolition, destruction, overthrow; dejection, depression, exhaustion.

prosy *adj* prosaic, unpoetic, unpoetical; dull, flat, jejune, stupid, tedious, tiresome, unentertaining, unimaginative, uninteresting.

protect *vb* cover, defend, guard, shield; fortify, harbour, house, preserve, save, screen, secure, shelter; champion, countenance, foster patronize.

protector *n* champion, custodian, defender, guardian, patron, warden.

protest *vb* affirm, assert, asseverate, attest, aver, avow, declare, profess, testify; demur, expostulate, object, remonstrate, repudiate. • *n* complaint declaration, disapproval, objection, protestation.

prototype *n* archetype, copy, exemplar, example, ideal, model, original, paradigm, precedent, protoplast, type.

protract *vb* continue, extend, lengthen, prolong; defer, delay, postpone.

protrude *vb* beetle, bulge, extend, jut, project.

protuberance *n* bulge, bump, elevation, excrescence, hump, lump, process, projection, prominence, roundness, swelling, tumour.

proud *adj* assuming, conceited, contended, egotistical, over-weening, self-conscious, self-satisfied, vain; arrogant, boastful, haughty, high-spirited, highly strung, imperious, lofty, lordly, presumptuous, supercilious, uppish, vainglorious.

prove *vb* ascertain, conform, demonstrate, establish, evidence, evince, justify, manifest, show, substantiate, sustain, verify; assay, check, examine, experiment, test, try.

proverb *n* adage, aphorism, apothegm, byword, dictum, maxim, precept, saw, saying.

proverbial *adj* acknowledged, current, notorious, unquestioned.

provide *vb* arrange, collect, plan, prepare, procure; gather, keep, store; afford, contribute, feed, furnish, produce, stock, supply, yield; cater, purvey; agree, bargain, condition, contract, covenant, engage, stipulate.

provided, providing *conj* granted, if, supposing.

provident *adj* careful, cautious, considerate, discreet, farseeing, forecasting, forehanded, foreseeing, prudent; economical, frugal, thrifty.

province *n* district, domain, region, section, territory, tract; colony, dependency; business, calling, capacity, charge, department, duty, employment, function, office, part, post, sphere; department, division, jurisdiction.

provincial *adj* annexed, appendant, outlying; bucolic, countrified, rude, rural, rustic, unpolished, unrefined; insular, local, narrow. • *n* peasant, rustic, yokel.

provision *n* anticipation, providing; arrangement, care, preparation, readiness; equipment, fund, grist, hoard, reserve, resources, stock, store, supplies, supply; clause, condition, prerequisite, proviso, reservation, stipulation.

provisions *npl* eatables, fare, food, provender, supplies, viands, victuals.

proviso *n* clause, condition, provision, stipulation.

provocation *n* incentive, incitement, provocativeness, stimulant, stimulus; affront, indignity, insult, offence; angering, vexation.

provoke *vb* animate, arouse, awaken, excite, impel, incite, induce, inflame, instigate, kindle, move, rouse, stimulate; affront, aggravate, anger, annoy, chafe, enrage, exacerbate, exasperate, incense, infuriate, irritate, nettle, offend, pique, vex; cause, elicit, evoke, instigate, occasion, produce, promote.

provoking *adj* aggravating, annoying, exasperating, irritating, offensive, tormenting, vexatious, vexing.

prowess *n* bravery, courage, daring, fearlessness, gallantry, heroism, intrepidity, valour; aptitude, dexterity, expertness, facility.

proximity *n* adjacency, contiguity, nearness, neighbourhood, propinquity, vicinage, vicinity.

proxy *n* agent, attorney, commissioner, delegate, deputy, lieutenant, representative, substitute.

prudence *n* carefulness, caution, circumspection, common sense, considerateness, discretion, forecast, foresight, judgment, judiciousness, policy, providence, sense, tact, wariness, wisdom.

prudent *adj* cautious, careful, circumspect, considerate, discreet, foreseeing, heedful, judicious, politic, provident, prudential, wary, wise.

prudish *adj* coy, demure, modest, precise, prim, reserved, strait-laced.

prune *vb* abbreviate, clip, cut, dock, lop, thin, trim; dress, preen.

prurient *adj* covetous, craving, desiring, hankering, itching, lascivious, libidinous, longing, lustful.

pry *vb* examine, ferret, inspect, investigate, peep, peer, question, scrutinize, search; force, lever, prise.

public *adj* civil, common, countrywide, general, national, political, state; known, notorious, open, popular, published, well-known. • *n* citizens, community, country, everyone, general public, masses, nation, people, population; audience, buyers, following, supporters.

publication *n* advertisement, announcement, disclosure, divulgement, divulgence, proclamation, promulgation, report; edition, issue, issuance, printing.

publicity *n* daylight, currency, limelight, notoriety, spotlight; outlet, vent.

publish *vb* advertise, air, bruit, announce, blaze, blazon, broach, communicate, declare, diffuse, disclose, disseminate, impart, placard, post, proclaim, promulgate, reveal, tell, utter, vent, ventilate.

pucker *vb* cockle, contract, corrugate, crease, crinkle, furrow, gather, pinch, purse, shirr, wrinkle. • *n* crease, crinkle, fold, furrow, wrinkle.

puerile *adj* boyish, childish, infantile, juvenile, youthful; foolish, frivolous, idle, nonsensical, petty, senseless, silly, simple, trifling, trivial, weak.

puffy *adj* distended, swelled, swollen, tumid, turgid; bombastic, extravagant, inflated, pompous.

pugnacious *adj* belligerent, bellicose, contentious, fighting, irascible, irritable, petulant, quarrelsome.

puissant *adj* forcible, mighty, potent, powerful, strong.

pull *vb* drag, draw, haul, row, tow, tug; cull, extract, gather, pick, pluck; detach, rend, tear, wrest. • *n* pluck, shake, tug, twitch, wrench; contest, struggle; attraction, gravity, magnetism; graft, influence, power.

pulsate *vb* beat, palpitate, pant, throb, thump, vibrate.

pulverize *vb* bruise, comminute, grind, levigate, triturate.

pun *vb* assonate, alliterate, play on words. • *n* assonance, alliteration, clinch, conceit, double-meaning, paranomasia, play on words, quip, rhyme, witticism, wordplay.

punctilious *adj* careful, ceremonious, conscientious, exact, formal, nice, particular, precise, punctual, scrupulous, strict.

punctual *adj* exact, nice, precise, punctilious; early, prompt, ready, regular, seasonable, timely.

puncture *vb* bore, penetrate, perforate, pierce, prick. • *n* bite, hole, sting, wound.

pungent *adj* acid, acrid, biting, burning, caustic, hot, mordant, penetrating, peppery, piercing, piquant, prickling, racy, salty, seasoned, sharp, smart, sour, spicy, stimulating, stinging; acute, acrimonious, cutting, distressing, irritating, keen, painful, peevish, poignant, pointed, satirical, severe, tart, trenchant, waspish.

punish *vb* beat, castigate, chasten, chastise, correct, discipline, flog, lash, scourge, torture, whip.

punishment *n* castigation, chastening, chastisement, correction, discipline, infliction, retribution, scourging, trial; judgment, nemesis, penalty.

puny *adj* feeble, inferior, weak; dwarf, dwarfish, insignificant, diminutive, little, petty, pygmy, small, stunted, tiny, underdeveloped, undersized.

pupil *n* beginner, catechumen, disciple, learner, neophyte, novice, scholar, student, tyro.

pupillage *n* minority, nonage, tutelage, wardship.

puppet *n* doll, image, manikin, marionette; cat's-paw, pawn, tool.

purchase *vb* buy, gain, get, obtain, pay for, procure; achieve, attain, earn, win. • *n* acquisition, buy, gain, possession, property; advantage, foothold, grasp, hold, influence, support.

pure *adj* clean, clear, fair, immaculate, spotless, stainless, unadulterated, unalloyed, unblemished, uncorrupted, undefiled, unpolluted, unspotted, unstained, unsullied, untainted, untarnished; chaste, continent, guileless, guiltless, holy, honest, incorrupt, innocent, modest, sincere, true, uncorrupt, upright, virgin, virtuous; genuine, perfect, real, simple, true, unadorned; absolute, essential, mere, sheer, thorough; classic, classical.

purge *vb* cleanse, clear, purify; clarify, defecate, evacuate; deterge, scour; absolve, pardon, shrive. • *n* elimination, eradication, expulsion, removal, suppression; cathartic, emetic, enema, laxative, physic.

purify *vb* clean, cleanse, clear, depurate, expurgate, purge, refine, wash; clarify, fine.

puritanical *adj* ascetic, narrow-minded, overscrupulous, prim, prudish, rigid, severe, strait-laced, strict.

purity *n* clearness, fineness; cleanness, correctness, faultlessness, immaculacy, immaculateness; guilelessness, guiltlessness, holiness, honesty, innocence, integrity, piety, simplicity, truth, uprightness, virtue; excellence, genuineness; homogeneity, simpleness; chasteness, chastity, continence, modesty, pudency, virginity.

purlieus *npl* borders, bounds, confines, environs, limits, neighbourhood, outskirts, precincts, suburbs, vicinage, vicinity.

purloin *vb* abstract, crib, filch, pilfer, rob, steal, thieve.

purport *vb* allege, assert, claim, maintain, pretend, profess; denote, express, imply, indicate, mean, signify, suggest. • *n* bearing, current, design, drift, gist, import, intent, meaning, scope, sense, significance, signification, spirit, tendency, tenor.

purpose *vb* contemplate, design, intend, mean, meditate; determine, resolve. • *n* aim, design, drift, end, intent, intention, object, resolution, resolve, view; plan, project; meaning, purport, sense; consequence, effect.

pursue *vb* chase, dog, follow, hound, hunt, shadow, track; conduct, continue, cultivate, maintain, practise, prosecute; seek, strive; accompany, attend.

pursuit *n* chase, hunt, race; conduct, cultivation, practice, prosecution, pursuance; avocation, calling, business, employment, fad, hobby, occupation, vocation.

pursy *adj* corpulent, fat, fleshy, plump, podgy, pudgy, short, thick; short-breathed, short-winded; opulent, rich.

purview *n* body, compass, extent, limit, reach, scope, sphere, view.

push *vb* elbow, crowd, hustle, impel, jostle, shoulder, shove, thrust; advance, drive, hurry, propel, urge; importune, persuade, tease. • *n* pressure, thrust; determination, perseverance; emergency, exigency, extremity, pinch, strait, test, trial; assault, attack, charge, endeavour, onset.

pusillanimous *adj* chicken, chicken-hearted, cowardly, dastardly, faint-hearted, feeble, lily-livered, mean-spirited, spiritless, timid, recreant, timorous, weak.

pustule *n* abscess, blain blister, blotch, boil, fester, gathering, pimple, sore, ulcer.

put *vb* bring, collocate, deposit, impose, lay, locate, place, set; enjoin, impose, inflict, levy; offer, present, propose, state; compel, constrain, force, oblige; entice, incite, induce, urge; express, utter.

putative *adj* deemed, reckoned, reported, reputed, supposed.

putrefy *vb* corrupt, decay, decompose, fester, rot, stink.

putrid *adj* corrupt, decayed, decompose, fetid, rank, rotten, stinking.

puzzle *vb* bewilder, confound, confuse, embarrass, gravel, mystify, nonplus, perplex, pose, stagger; complicate, entangle.• *n* conundrum, enigma, labyrinth, maze, paradox, poser, problem, riddle; bewilderment, complication, confusion, difficulty, dilemma, embarrassment, mystification, perplexity, point, quandary, question.

pygmy *adj* diminutive, dwarf, dwarfish, Lilliputian, little, midget, stunted, tiny. • *n* dwarf, Lilliputian, midget.

Q

quack[1] *vb, n* cackle, cry, squeak.

quack[2] *adj* fake, false, sham. • *n* charlatan, empiric, humbug, impostor, mountebank, pretender.

quadruple *adj* fourfold, quadruplicate.

quagmire *n* bog, fen, marsh, morass, slough, swamp; difficulty, impasse, muddle, predicament.

quail *vb* blench, cower, droop, faint, flinch, shrink, tremble.

quaint *adj* antiquated, antique, archaic, curious, droll, extraordinary, fanciful, odd, old-fashioned, queer, singular, uncommon, unique, unusual; affected, fantastic, far-fetched, whimsical; artful, ingenious.

quake *vb* quiver, shake, shiver, shudder; move, vibrate. • *n* earthquake, shake, shudder.

qualification *n* ability, accomplishment, capability, competency, eligibility, fitness, suitability; condition, exception, limitation, modification, proviso, restriction, stipulation; abatement, allowance, diminution, mitigation.

qualified *adj* accomplished, certificated, certified, competent, fitted, equipped, licensed, trained; adapted, circumscribed, conditional, limited, modified, restricted.

qualify *vb* adapt, capacitate, empower, entitle, equip, fit; limit, modify, narrow, restrain, restrict; abate, assuage, ease, mitigate, moderate, reduce, soften; diminish, modulate, temper, regulate, vary.

quality *n* affection, attribute, characteristic, colour, distinction, feature, flavour, mark, nature, peculiarity, property, singularity, timbre, tinge, trait; character, condition, disposition, humour, mood, temper; brand, calibre, capacity, class, description, excellence, grade, kind, rank, sort, stamp, standing, station, status, virtue; aristocracy, gentility, gentry, noblesse, nobility.

qualm *n* agony, pang, throe; nausea, queasiness, sickness; compunction, remorse, uneasiness, twinge.

quandary *n* bewilderment, difficulty, dilemma, doubt, embarrassment, perplexity, pickle, plight, predicament, problem, puzzle, strait, uncertainty.

quantity *n* content, extent, greatness, measure, number, portion, share, size; aggregate, batch, amount, bulk, lot, mass, quantum, store, sum, volume; duration, length.

quarrel *vb* altercate, bicker, brawl, carp, cavil, clash, contend, differ, dispute, fight, jangle, jar, scold, scuffle, spar, spat, squabble, strive, wrangle. • *n* altercation, affray, bickering, brawl, breach, breeze, broil, clash, contention, contest, controversy, difference, disagreement, discord, dispute, dissension, disturbance, feud, fight, fray, imbroglio, jar, miff, misunderstanding, quarrelling, row, rupture, spat, squabble, strife, tiff, tumult, variance, wrangle.

quarrelsome *adj* argumentative, choleric, combative, contentious, cross, discordant, disputatious, dissentious, fiery, irascible, irritable, petulant, pugnacious, ugly, wranglesome.

quarter *vb* billet, lodge, post, station; allot, furnish, share. • *n* abode, billet, dwelling, habitation, lodgings, posts, quarters, stations; direction, district, locality, location, lodge, position, region, territory; clemency, mercy, mildness.

quash *vb* abate, abolish, annul, cancel, invalidate, nullify, overthrow; crush, extinguish, repress, stop, subdue, suppress.

queasy *adj* nauseated, pukish, seasick, sick, squeamish.

queer *vb* botch, harm, impair, mar, spoil. • *adj* curious, droll, extraordinary, fantastic, odd, peculiar, quaint, singular, strange, uncommon, unusual, whimsical; gay, homosexual.

quell *vb* conquer, crush, overcome, overpower, subdue; bridle, check, curb, extinguish, lay, quench, rein in, repress, restrain, stifle; allay, calm, compose, hush, lull, pacify, quiet, quieten, still, tranquillize; alleviate, appease, blunt, deaden, dull, mitigate, mollify, soften, soothe.

quench *vb* extinguish, put out; check, destroy, repress, satiate, stifle, still, suppress; allay, cool, dampen, extinguish, slake.

querulous *adj* bewailing, complaining, cross, discontented, dissatisfied, fretful, fretting, irritable, mourning, murmuring, peevish, petulant, plaintive, touchy, whining.

query *vb* ask, enquire, inquire, question; dispute, doubt. • *n* enquiry, inquiry, interrogatory, issue, problem, question.

quest *n* expedition, journey, search, voyage; pursuit, suit; examination, enquiry, inquiry; demand, desire, invitation, prayer, request, solicitation.

question *vb* ask, catechize, enquire, examine, inquire, interrogate, quiz, sound out; doubt, query; challenge, dispute. • *n* examination, enquiry, inquiry, interpellation, interrogation; enquiry, inquiry, interrogatory, query; debate, discussion, disquisition, examination, investigation, issue, trial; controversy, dispute, doubt; motion, mystery, point, poser, problem, proposition, puzzle, topic.

questionable *adj* ambiguous, controversial, controvertible, debatable, doubtful, disputable, equivocal, problematic, problematical, suspicious, uncertain, undecided.

quibble *vb* cavil, equivocate, evade, prevaricate, shuffle. • *n* equivocation, evasion, pretence, prevarication, quirk, shift, shuffle, sophism, subtlety, subterfuge.

quick *adj* active, agile, alert, animated, brisk, lively, nimble, prompt, ready, smart, sprightly; expeditious, fast, fleet, flying, hurried, rapid, speedy, swift; adroit, apt, clever, dextrous, expert, skilful; choleric, hasty, impetuous, irascible, irritable, passionate, peppery, petulant, precipitate, sharp, unceremonious, testy, touchy, waspish; alive, animate, live, living.

quicken *vb* animate, energize, resuscitate, revivify, vivify; cheer, enliven, invigorate, reinvigorate, revive, whet; accelerate, dispatch, expedite, hasten, hurry, speed; actuate, excite, incite, kindle, refresh, sharpen, stimulate; accelerate, live, take effect.

quickly *adv* apace, fast, immediately, nimbly, quick, rapidly, readily, soon, speedily, swiftly.

quickness *n* celerity, dispatch, expedition, haste, rapidity, speed, swiftness, velocity; agility, alertness, activity, briskness, liveliness, nimbleness, promptness, readiness, smartness; adroitness, aptitude, aptness, dexterity, facility, knack; acumen, acuteness, keenness, penetration, perspicacity, sagacity, sharpness, shrewdness.

quiescent *adj* at rest, hushed, motionless, quiet, resting, still; calm, mute, placid, quiet, serene, still, tranquil, unagitated, undisturbed, unruffled.

quiet *adj* hushed, motionless, quiescent, still, unmoved; calm, contented, gentle, mild, meek, modest, peaceable, peaceful, placid, silent, smooth, tranquil, undemonstrative, unobtrusive, unruffled; patient; retired, secluded. • *n* calmness, peace, repose, rest, silence, stillness.

quieten *vb* arrest, discontinue, intermit, interrupt, still, stop, suspend; allay, appease, calm, compose, lull, pacify, sober, soothe, tranquillize; hush, silence; alleviate, assuage, blunt, dull, mitigate, moderate, mollify, soften.

quip *n* crank, flout, gibe, jeer, mock, quirk, repartee, retort, sarcasm, sally, scoff, sneer, taunt, witticism.

quit *vb* absolve, acquit, deliver, free, release; clear, deliver, discharge from, free, liberate, relieve; acquit, behave, conduct; carry through, perform; discharge, pay, repay, requite; relinquish, renounce, resign, stop, surrender; depart from, leave, withdraw from; abandon, desert, forsake, forswear. • *adj* absolved, acquitted, clear, discharged, free, released.

quite *adv* completely, entirely, exactly, perfectly, positively, precisely, totally, wholly.

quiver *vb* flicker, flutter, oscillate, palpitate, quake, play, shake, shiver, shudder, tremble, twitch, vibrate. • *n* shake, shiver, shudder, trembling.

quixotic *adj* absurd, chimerical, fanciful, fantastic, fantastical, freakish, imaginary, mad, romantic, utopian, visionary, wild.

quiz *vb* examine, question, test; peer at; banter, hoax, puzzle, ridicule. • *n* enigma, hoax, jest, joke, puzzle; jester, joker, hoax.

quota *n* allocation, allotment, apportionment, contingent, portion, proportion, quantity, share.

quotation *n* citation, clipping, cutting, extract, excerpt, reference, selection; estimate, rate, tender.

quote *vb* adduce, cite, excerpt, extract, illustrate, instance, name, repeat, take; estimate, tender.

R

rabble *n* commonality, horde, mob, populace, riffraff, rout, scum, trash.

rabid *adj* frantic, furious, mad, raging, wild; bigoted, fanatical, intolerant, irrational, narrow-minded, rampant.

race[1] *n* ancestry, breed, family, generation, house, kindred, line, lineage, pedigree, stock, strain; clan, folk, nation, people, tribe; breed, children, descendants, issue, offspring, progeny, stock.

race[2] *vb* career, compete, contest, course, hasten, hurry, run, speed. • *n* career, chase, competition, contest, course, dash, heat, match, pursuit, run, sprint; flavour, quality, smack, strength, taste.

rack *vb* agonize, distress, excruciate, rend, torment, torture, wring; exhaust, force, harass, oppress, strain, stretch, wrest. • *n* agony, anguish, pang, torment, torture; crib, manger; neck, crag; dampness, mist, moisture, vapour.

racket *n* clamour, clatter, din, dissipation, disturbance, fracas, frolic, hubbub, noise, outcry, tumult, uproar; game, graft, scheme, understanding.

racy *adj* flavoursome, palatable, piquant, pungent, rich, spicy, strong; forcible, lively, pungent, smart, spirited, stimulating, vigorous, vivacious.

radiance *n* brightness, brilliance, brilliancy, effluence, efflux, emission, glare, glitter, light, lustre, refulgence, resplendence, shine, splendour.

radiant *adj* beaming, brilliant, effulgent, glittering, glorious, luminous, lustrous, resplendent, shining, sparkling, splendid; ecstatic, happy, pleased.

radiate *vb* beam, gleam, glitter, shine; emanate, emit, diffuse, spread.

radical *adj* constitutional, deep-seated, essential, fundamental, ingrained, inherent, innate, native, natural, organic, original, uncompromising; original, primitive, simple, uncompounded, underived; complete, entire, extreme, fanatic, insurgent, perfect, rebellious, thorough, total. • *n* etymon, radix, root; fanatic, revolutionary.

rage *vb* bluster, boil, chafe, foam, fret, fume, ravage, rave. • *n* excitement, frenzy, fury, madness, passion, rampage, raving, vehemence, wrath; craze, fashion, mania, mode, style, vogue.

ragged *adj* rent, tattered, torn; contemptible, mean, poor, shabby; jagged, rough, rugged, shaggy, uneven; discordant, dissonant, inharmonious, unmusical.

raid *vb* assault, forage, invade, pillage, plunder. • *n* attack, foray, invasion, inroad, plunder.

rail *vb* abuse, censure, inveigh, scoff, scold, sneer, upbraid.

raillery *n* banter, chaff, irony, joke, pleasantry, ridicule, satire.

raiment *n* array, apparel, attire, clothes, clothing, costume, dress, garb, garments, habiliment, habit, vestments, vesture.

rain *vb* drizzle, drop, fall, pour, shower, sprinkle, teem; bestow, lavish. • *n* cloudburst, downpour, drizzle, mist, shower, sprinkling.

raise *vb* boost, construct, erect, heave, hoist, lift, uplift, upraise, rear; advance, elevate, ennoble, exalt, promote; aggravate, amplify, augment, enhance, heighten, increase, invigorate; arouse, awake, cause, effect, excite, originate, produce, rouse, stir up; occasion, start; assemble, collect, get, levy, obtain; breed, cultivate, grow, propagate, rear; ferment, leaven, work.

rake[1] *vb* collect, comb, gather, scratch; ransack, scour.

rake[2] *n* debauchee, libertine, profligate, roué.

rakish *adj* debauched, dissipated, dissolute, lewd, licentious; cavalier, jaunty.

ramble *vb* digress, maunder, range, roam, rove, saunter, straggle, stray, stroll, wander. • *n* excursion, rambling, roving, tour, trip, stroll, wandering.

rambling *adj* discursive, irregular; straggling, strolling, wandering.

ramification *n* arborescence, branching, divarication, forking, radiation; branch, division, offshoot, subdivision; consequence, upshot.

ramify *vb* branch, divaricate, extend, separate.

rampant *adj* excessive, exuberant, luxuriant, rank, wanton; boisterous, dominant, headstrong, impetuous, predominant, raging, uncontrollable, unbridled, ungovernable, vehement, violent.

rampart *n* bulwark, circumvallation, defence, fence, fortification, guard, security, wall.

rancid *adj* bad, fetid, foul, fusty, musty, offensive, rank, sour, stinking, tainted.

rancorous *adj* bitter, implacable, malevolent, malicious, malign, malignant, resentful, spiteful, vindictive, virulent.

rancour *n* animosity, antipathy, bitterness, enmity, gall, grudge, hate, hatred, ill-will, malevolence, malice, malignity, spite, venom, vindictiveness.

random *adj* accidental, casual, chance, fortuitous, haphazard, irregular, stray, wandering.

range *vb* course, cruise, extend, ramble, roam, rove, straggle, stray, stroll, wander; bend, lie, run; arrange, class, dispose, rank. • *n* file, line, row, rank, tier; class, kind, order, sort; excursion, expedition, ramble, roving, wandering; amplitude, bound, command, compass, distance, extent, latitude, reach, scope, sweep, view; register.

rank[1] *vb* arrange, class, classify, range. • *n* file, line, order, range, row, tier; class, division, group, order, series; birth, blood, caste, degree, estate, grade, position, quality, sphere, stakes, standing; dignity, distinction, eminence, nobility.

rank[2] *adj* dense, exuberant, luxuriant, overabundant, overgrown, vigorous, wild; excessive, extreme, extravagant, flagrant, gross, rampant, sheer, unmitigated, utter, violent; fetid, foul, fusty, musty, offensive, rancid; fertile, productive, rich; coarse, disgusting.

ransack *vb* pillage, plunder, ravage, rifle, sack, strip; explore, overhaul, rummage, search thoroughly.

ransom *vb* deliver, emancipate, free, liberate, redeem, rescue, unfetter. • *n* money, payment pay-off, price; deliverance, liberation, redemption, release.

rant *vb* declaim, mouth, spout, vociferate. • *n* bombast, cant, exaggeration, fustian.

rapacious *adj* predacious, preying, raptorial; avaricious, grasping, greedy ravenous, voracious.

rapid *adj* fast, fleet, quick, swift; brisk, expeditious, hasty, hurried, quick, speedy.

rapine *n* depredation, pillage, plunder, robbery, spoliation.

rapt *adj* absorbed, charmed, delighted, ecstatic, engrossed, enraptured, entranced, fascinated, inspired, spellbound.

rapture *vb* enrapture, ravish, transport. • *n* delight, exultation, enthusiasm, rhapsody; beatification, beatitude, bliss, ecstasy, felicity, happiness, joy, spell, transport.

rare[1] *adj* sparse, subtle, thin; extraordinary, infrequent, scarce, singular, strange, uncommon, unique, unusual; choice, excellent exquisite, fine, incomparable, inimitable.

rare[2] *adj* bloody, underdone.

rarity *n* attenuation, ethereality, etherealness, rarefaction, rareness, tenuity, tenuousness, thinness; infrequency, scarcity, singularity, sparseness, uncommonness, unwontedness.

rascal *n* blackguard, caitiff, knave, miscreant, rogue, reprobate, scallywag, scapegrace, scamp, scoundrel, vagabond, villain.

rash[1] *adj* adventurous, audacious, careless, foolhardy, hasty, headlong, headstrong, heedless, incautious, inconsiderate, indiscreet, injudicious, impetuous, impulsive, incautious, precipitate, quick, rapid, reckless, temerarious, thoughtless, unguarded, unwary, venturesome.

rash[2] *n* breaking-out, efflorescence, eruption; epidemic, flood, outbreak, plague, spate.

rashness *n* carelessness, foolhardiness, hastiness, heedlessness, inconsideration, indiscretion, precipitation, recklessness, temerity, venturesomeness.

rate[1] *vb* appraise, compute, estimate, value. • *n* cost, price; class, degree, estimate, rank, value, valuation, worth; proportion, ration assessment, charge, impost, tax.

rate[2] *vb* abuse, berate, censure, chide, criticize, find fault, reprimand, reprove, scold.

ratify *vb* confirm, corroborate, endorse, establish, seal, settle, substantiate; approve, bind, consent, sanction.

ration *vb* apportion, deal, distribute, dole, restrict. • *n* allowance, portion, quota, share.

rational *adj* intellectual, reasoning; equitable, fair, fit, just, moderate, natural, normal, proper, reasonable, right; discreet, enlightened, intelligent, judicious, sagacious, sensible, sound, wise.

raucous *adj* harsh, hoarse, husky, rough.

ravage *vb* consume, desolate, despoil, destroy, devastate, harry, overrun, pillage, plunder, ransack, ruin, sack, spoil, strip, waste. • *n* desolation, despoilment, destruction, devastation, havoc, pillage, plunder, rapine, ruin, spoil, waste.

ravenous *adj* devouring, ferocious, gluttonous, greedy, insatiable, omnivorous, ravening, rapacious, voracious.

ravine *n* canyon, cleft, defile, gap, gorge, gulch, gully, pass.

raving *adj* delirious, deranged, distracted, frantic, frenzied, furious, infuriated, mad, phrenetic, raging. • *n* delirium, frenzy, fury, madness, rage.

ravish *vb* abuse, debauch, defile, deflower, force, outrage, violate; captivate, charm, delight, enchant, enrapture, entrance, overjoy, transport; abduct, kidnap, seize, snatch, strip.

raw *adj* fresh, inexperienced, unpractised, unprepared, unseasoned, untried, unskilled; crude, green, immature, unfinished, unripe; bare, chafed, excoriated, galled, sensitive, sore; bleak, chilly, cold, cutting, damp, piercing, windswept; uncooked.

ray *n* beam, emanation, gleam, moonbeam, radiance, shaft, streak, sunbeam.

raze *vb* demolish, destroy, dismantle, extirpate, fell, level, overthrow, ruin, subvert; efface, erase, obliterate.

reach *vb* extend, stretch; grasp, hit, strike, touch; arrive at, attain, gain, get, obtain, win. • *n* capability, capacity, grasp.

readily *adv* easily, promptly, quickly; cheerfully, willingly.

readiness *n* alacrity, alertness, expedition, quickness, promptitude, promptness; aptitude, aptness, dexterity, easiness, expertness, facility, quickness, skill; preparation, preparedness, ripeness; cheerfulness, disposition, eagerness, ease, willingness.

ready *vb* arrange, equip, organize, prepare. • *adj* alert, expeditious, prompt, quick, punctual, speedy; adroit, apt, clever, dextrous, expert, facile, handy, keen, nimble, prepared, prompt, ripe, quick, sharp, skilful, smart; cheerful, disposed, eager, free, inclined, willing; accommodating, available, convenient, near, handy; easy, facile, fluent, offhand, opportune, short, spontaneous.

real *adj* absolute, actual, certain, literal, positive, practical, substantial, substantive, veritable; authentic, genuine, true; essential, internal, intrinsic.

realize *vb* accomplish, achieve, discharge, effect, effectuate, perfect, perform; apprehend, comprehend, experience, recognize, understand; externalize, substantiate; acquire, earn, gain, get, net, obtain, produce, sell.

reality *n* actuality, certainty, fact, truth, verity.

really *adv* absolutely, actually, certainly, indeed, positively, truly, verily, veritably.

reap *vb* acquire, crop, gain, gather, get, harvest, obtain, receive.

rear[1] *adj* aft, back, following, hind, last. • *n* background, reverse, setting; heel, posterior, rear end, rump, stern, tail; path, trail, train, wake.

rear[2] *vb* construct, elevate, erect, hoist, lift, raise; cherish, educate, foster, instruct, nourish, nurse, nurture, train; breed, grow; rouse, stir up.

reason *vb* argue, conclude, debate, deduce, draw from, infer, intellectualize, syllogize, think, trace. • *n* faculty, intellect, intelligence, judgement, mind, principle, sanity, sense, thinking, understanding; account, argument, basis, cause, consideration, excuse, explanation, gist, ground, motive, occasion, pretence, proof; aim, design, end, object, purpose; argument, reasoning; common sense, reasonableness, wisdom; equity, fairness, justice, right; exposition, rationale, theory.

reasonable *adj* equitable, fair, fit, honest, just, proper, rational, right, suitable; enlightened, intelligent, judicious, sagacious, sensible, wise; considerable, fair, moderate, tolerable; credible, intellectual, plausible, well-founded; sane, sober, sound; cheap, inexpensive, low-priced.

rebate *vb* abate, bate, blunt, deduct, diminish, lessen, reduce; cut, pare, rabbet. • *n* decrease, decrement, diminution, lessening; allowance, deduction, discount, reduction.

rebel *vb* mutiny, resist, revolt, strike. • *adj* insubordinate, insurgent, mutinous, rebellious. • *n* insurgent, mutineer, traitor.

rebellion *n* anarchy, insubordination, insurrection, mutiny, resistance, revolt, revolution, uprising.

rebellious *adj* contumacious, defiant, disloyal, disobedient, insubordinate, intractable, obstinate, mutinous, rebel, refractory, seditious.

rebuff *vb* check, chide, oppose, refuse, reject, repel, reprimand, resist, snub. • *n* check, defeat, discouragement, opposition, rejection, resistance, snub.

rebuke *vb* blame, censure, chide, lecture, upbraid, reprehend, reprimand, reprove, scold, silence. • *n* blame, censure, chiding, expostulation, remonstrance, reprimand, reprehension, reproach, reproof, reproval; affliction, chastisement, punishment.

recall *vb* abjure, abnegate, annul, cancel, countermand, deny, nullify, overrule, recant, repeal, repudiate, rescind, retract, revoke, swallow, withdraw; commemorate, recollect, remember, retrace, review, revive. • *n* abjuration, abnegation, annulment, cancellation, nullification, recantation, repeal, repudiation, rescindment, retraction, revocation, withdrawal; memory, recollection, remembrance, reminiscence.

recant *vb* abjure, annul, disavow, disown, recall, renounce, repudiate, retract, revoke, unsay.

recapitulate *vb* epitomize, recite, rehearse, reiterate, repeat, restate, review, summarize.

recede *vb* desist, ebb, retire, regress, retreat, retrograde, return, withdraw.

receive *vb* accept, acquire, derive, gain, get, obtain, take; admit, shelter, take in; entertain, greet, welcome; allow, permit, tolerate; adopt, approve, believe, credit, embrace, follow, learn, understand; accommodate, carry, contain, hold, include, retain; bear, encounter, endure, experience, meet, suffer, sustain.

recent *adj* fresh, new, novel; latter, modern, young; deceased, foregoing, late, preceding, retiring.

reception *n* acceptance, receipt, receiving; entertainment, greeting, welcome; levee, soiree, party; admission, credence; belief, credence, recognition.

recess *n* alcove, corner, depth, hollow, niche, nook, privacy, retreat, seclusion; break, holiday, intermission, interval, respite, vacation; recession, retirement, retreat, withdrawal.

reciprocal *adj* alternate, commutable, complementary, correlative, correspondent, mutual.

recital *n* rehearsal, repetition, recitation; account, description, detail, explanation, narration, relation, statement, telling.

recite *vb* declaim, deliver, rehearse, repeat; describe, mention, narrate, recount, relate, tell; count, detail, enumerate, number, recapitulate.

reckless *adj* breakneck, careless, desperate, devil-may-care, flighty, foolhardy, giddy, harebrained, headlong, heedless, inattentive, improvident, imprudent, inconsiderate, indifferent, indiscreet, mindless, negligent, rash, regardless, remiss, thoughtless, temerarious, uncircumspect, unconcerned, unsteady, volatile, wild.

reckon *vb* calculate, cast, compute, consider, count, enumerate, guess, number; account, class, esteem, estimate, regard, repute, value.

reckoning *n* calculation, computation, consideration, counting; account, bill, charge, estimate, register, score; arrangement, settlement.

reclaim *vb* amend, correct, reform; recover, redeem, regenerate, regain, reinstate, restore; civilize, tame.

recline *vb* couch, lean, lie, lounge, repose, rest.

recluse *adj* anchoritic, anchoritical, cloistered, eremitic, eremitical, hermitic, hermitical, reclusive, solitary. • *n* anchorite, ascetic, eremite, hermit, monk, solitary.

reclusive *adj* recluse, retired, secluded, sequestered, sequestrated, solitary.

recognition *n* identification, memory, recollection, remembrance; acknowledgement, appreciation, avowal, comprehension, confession, notice; allowance, concession.

recognize *vb* apprehend, identify, perceive, remember; acknowledge, admit, avow, confess, own; allow, concede, grant; greet, salute.

recoil *vb* react, rebound, reverberate; retire, retreat, withdraw; blench, fail, falter, quail, shrink. • *n* backstroke, boomerang, elasticity, kick, reaction, rebound, repercussion, resilience, revulsion, ricochet, shrinking.

recollect *vb* recall, remember, reminisce.

recollection *n* memory, remembrance, reminiscence.

recommend *vb* approve, commend, endorse, praise, sanction; commit; advise, counsel, prescribe, suggest.

recommendation *n* advocacy, approbation, approval, commendation, counsel, credential, praise, testimonial.

recompense *vb* compensate, remunerate, repay, requite, reward, satisfy; indemnify, redress, reimburse. • *n* amends, compensation, indemnification, indemnity, remuneration, repayment, reward, satisfaction; requital, retribution.

reconcilable *adj* appeasable, forgiving, placable; companionable, congruous, consistent.

reconcile *vb* appease, conciliate, pacify, placate, propitiate, reunite; content, harmonize, regulate; adjust, compose, heal, settle.

recondite *adj* concealed, dark, hidden, mystic, mystical, obscure, occult, secret, transcendental.

record *vb* chronicle, enter, note, register. • *n* account, annals, archive, chronicle, diary, docket, enrolment, entry, file, list, minute, memoir, memorandum, memorial, note, proceedings, register, registry, report, roll, score; mark, memorial, relic, trace, track, trail, vestige; memory, remembrance; achievement, career, history.

recount *vb* describe, detail, enumerate, mention, narrate, particularize, portray, recite, relate, rehearse, report, tell.

recover *vb* recapture, reclaim, regain; rally, recruit, repair, retrieve; cure, heal, restore, revive; redeem, rescue, salvage, save; convalesce, recuperate.

recreant *adj* base, cowardly, craven, dastardly, faint-hearted, mean-spirited, pusillanimous, yielding; apostate, backsliding, faithless, false, perfidious, treacherous, unfaithful, untrue. • *n* coward, dastard; apostate, backslider, renegade.

recreation *n* amusement, cheer, diversion, entertainment, fun, game, leisure, pastime, play, relaxation, sport.

recreational *adj* amusing, diverting, entertaining, refreshing, relaxing, relieving.

recruit *vb* repair, replenish; recover, refresh, regain, reinvigorate, renew, renovate, restore, retrieve, revive, strengthen, supply. • *n* auxiliary, beginner, helper, learner, novice, tyro.

rectify *vb* adjust, amend, better, correct, emend, improve, mend, redress, reform, regulate, straighten.

rectitude *n* conscientiousness, equity, goodness, honesty, integrity, justice, principle, probity, right, righteousness, straightforwardness, uprightness, virtue.

recumbent *adj* leaning, lying, prone, prostrate, reclining; idle, inactive, listless, reposing.

recur *vb* reappear, resort, return, revert.

recusancy *n* dissent, heresy, heterodoxy, nonconformity.

redeem *vb* reform, regain, repurchase, retrieve; free, liberate, ransom, rescue, save; deliver, reclaim, recover, reinstate; atone, compensate for, recompense; discharge, fulfil, keep, perform, satisfy.

redemption *n* buying, compensation, recovery, repurchase, retrieval; deliverance, liberation, ransom, release, rescue, salvation; discharge, fulfilment, performance.

redolent *adj* aromatic, balmy, fragrant, odoriferous, odorous, scented, sweet, sweet-smelling.

redoubtable *adj* awful, doughty, dreadful, formidable, terrible, valiant.

redound *vb* accrue, conduce, contribute, result, tend.

redress *vb* amend, correct, order, rectify, remedy, repair; compensate, ease, relieve. • *n* abatement, amends, atonement, compensation, correction, cure, indemnification, rectification, repair, righting, remedy, relief, reparation, satisfaction.

reduce *vb* bring; form, make, model, mould, remodel, render, resolve, shape; abate, abbreviate, abridge, attenuate, contract, curtail, decimate, decrease, diminish, lessen, minimize, shorten, thin; abase, debase, degrade, depress, dwarf, impair, lower, weaken; capture, conquer, master, overpower, overthrow, subject, subdue, subjugate, vanquish; impoverish, ruin; resolve, solve.

redundant *adj* copious, excessive, exuberant, fulsome, inordinate, lavish, needless, overflowing, overmuch, plentiful, prodigal, superabundant, replete, superfluous, unnecessary, useless; diffuse, periphrastic, pleonastic, tautological, verbose, wordy.

reel[1] *n* capstan, winch, windlass; bobbin, spool.

reel[2] *vb* falter, flounder, heave, lurch, pitch, plunge, rear, rock, roll, stagger, sway, toss, totter, tumble, wallow, welter, vacillate; spin, swing, turn, twirl, wheel, whirl. • *n* gyre, pirouette, spin, turn, twirl, wheel, whirl.

re-establish *vb* re-found, rehabilitate, reinstall, reinstate, renew, renovate, replace, restore.

refer *vb* commit, consign, direct, leave, relegate, send, submit; ascribe, assign, attribute, impute; appertain, belong, concern, pertain, point, relate, respect, touch; appeal, apply, consult; advert, allude, cite, quote

referee *vb* arbitrate, judge, umpire. • *n* arbiter, arbitrator, judge, umpire.

reference *n* concern, connection, regard, respect; allusion, ascription, citation, hint, intimation, mark, reference, relegation.

refine *vb* clarify, cleanse, defecate, fine, purify; cultivate, humanize improve, polish, rarefy, spiritualize.

refined *adj* courtly, cultured, genteel, polished, polite; discerning, discriminating, fastidious, sensitive; filtered, processed, purified.

refinement *n* clarification, filtration, purification, sublimation; betterment, improvement; delicacy, cultivation, culture, elegance, elevation, finish, gentility, good breeding, polish, politeness, purity, spirituality style.

reflect *vb* copy, imitate, mirror, reproduce; cogitate, consider, contemplate, deliberate, meditate, muse, ponder, ruminate, study, think.

reflection *n* echo, shadow; cogitation, consideration, contemplation, deliberation, idea, meditation, musing, opinion, remark, rumination, thinking, thought; aspersion, blame, censure, criticism, disparagement, reproach, slur.

reflective *adj* reflecting, reflexive; cogitating, deliberating, musing pondering, reasoning, thoughtful.

reform *vb* amend, ameliorate, better, correct, improve, mend, meliorate, rectify, reclaim, redeem, regenerate, repair, restore; reconstruct, remodel, reshape. • *n* amendment, correction, progress, reconstruction, rectification, reformation.

reformation *n* amendment, emendation, improvement, reform; adoption, conversion, redemption; refashioning, regeneration, reproduction, reconstruction.

refractory *adj* cantankerous, contumacious, cross-grained, disobedient, dogged, headstrong, heady, incoercible, intractable, mulish, obstinate, perverse, recalcitrant, self-willed, stiff, stubborn, sullen, ungovernable, unmanageable, unruly, unyielding.

refrain[1] *vb* abstain, cease, desist, forbear, stop, withhold.

refrain[2] *n* chorus, song, undersong.

refresh *vb* air, brace, cheer cool, enliven, exhilarate, freshen, invigorate, reanimate, recreate, recruit, reinvigorate, revive, regale, slake.

refreshing *adj* comfortable, cooling, grateful, invigorating, pleasant, reanimating, restful, reviving.

refuge *n* asylum, covert, harbour, haven, protection, retreat, safety, sanction, security, shelter.

refulgent *adj* bright, brilliant, effulgent, lustrous, radiant, resplendent, shining.

refund *vb* reimburse, repay, restore, return. • *n* reimbursement, repayment.

refuse[1] *n* chaff, discard, draff, dross, dregs, garbage, junk, leavings, lees, litter, lumber, offal, recrement, remains, rubbish, scoria, scum, sediment, slag, sweepings, trash, waste.

refuse[2] *vb* decline, deny, withhold; disallow, disavow, exclude, rebuff, reject, renege, renounce, repel, repudiate, repulse, revoke, veto.

refute *vb* confute, defeat, disprove, overcome, overthrow, rebut, repel, silence.

regain *vb* recapture, recover, re-obtain, repossess, retrieve.

regal *adj* imposing, imperial, kingly, noble, royal, sovereign.

regale *vb* delight, entertain, gratify, refresh; banquet, feast.

regard *vb* behold, gaze, look, notice, mark, observe, remark, see, view, watch; attend to, consider, heed, mind, respect; esteem, honour, revere, reverence, value; account, believe, estimate, deem, hold, imagine, reckon, suppose, think, treat, use. • *n* aspect, gaze, look, view; attention, attentiveness, care, concern, consideration, heed, notice, observance; account, reference, relation, respect; admiration, affection, attachment, deference, esteem, estimation, favour, honour, interest, liking, love, respect, reverence, sympathy, value; account, eminence, note, reputation, repute; condition, matter, point.

regardful *adj* attentive, careful, considerate, deferential, heedful, mindful, observing, thoughtful, watchful.

regarding *prep* concerning, respecting, touching.

regardless *adj* careless, disregarding, heedless, inattentive, indifferent, mindless, neglectful, negligent, unconcerned, unmindful, unobservant. • *adv* however, irrespectively, nevertheless, nonetheless, notwithstanding.

regenerate *vb* reproduce; renovate, revive; change, convert, renew, sanctify. • *adj* born-again, converted, reformed, regenerated.

regime *n* administration, government, rule.

region *n* climate, clime, country, district, division, latitude, locale, locality, province, quarter, scene, territory, tract; area, neighbourhood, part, place, portion, spot, space, sphere, terrain, vicinity.

register *vb* delineate, portray, record, show. • *n* annals, archive, catalogue, chronicle, list, record, roll, schedule; clerk, registrar, registry; compass, range.

regret *vb* bewail, deplore, grieve, lament, repine, sorrow; bemoan, repent, mourn, rue. • *n* concern, disappointment, grief, lamentation, rue, sorrow, trouble; compunction, contrition, penitence, remorse, repentance, repining, self-condemnation, self-reproach.

regular *adj* conventional, natural, normal, ordinary, typical; correct, customary, cyclic, established, fixed, habitual, periodic, periodical, recurring, reasonable, rhythmic, seasonal, stated, usual; steady, constant, uniform, even; just, methodical, orderly, punctual, systematic, unvarying; complete, genuine, indubitable, out-and-out, perfect, thorough; balanced, consistent, symmetrical.

regulate *vb* adjust, arrange, dispose, methodize, order, organize, settle, standardize, time, systematize; conduct, control, direct, govern, guide, manage, rule.

regulation *adj* customary, mandatory, official, required, standard. • *n* adjustment, arrangement, control, disposal, disposition, law, management, order, ordering, precept, rule, settlement.

rehabilitate *vb* reinstate, re-establish, restore; reconstruct, reconstitute, reintegrate, reinvigorate, renew, renovate.

rehearsal *n* drill, practice, recital, recitation, repetition; account, history, mention, narration, narrative, recounting, relation, statement, story, telling.

rehearse *vb* recite, repeat; delineate, depict, describe, detail, enumerate, narrate, portray, recapitulate, recount, relate, tell.

reign *vb* administer, command, govern, influence, predominate, prevail, rule. • *n* control, dominion, empire, influence, power, royalty, sovereignty, power, rule, sway.

reimburse *vb* refund, repay, restore; compensate, indemnify, requite, satisfy.

rein *vb* bridle, check, control, curb, guide, harness, hold, restrain, restrict. • *n* bridle, check, curb, harness, restraint, restriction.

reinforce *vb* augment, fortify, strengthen.

reinstate *vb* re-establish, rehabilitate, reinstall, replace, restore.

reject *vb* cashier, discard, dismiss, eject, exclude, pluck; decline, deny, disallow, despise, disapprove, disbelieve, rebuff, refuse, renounce, repel, repudiate, scout, slight, spurn, veto. • *n* cast-off, discard, failure, refusal, repudiation.

rejoice *vb* cheer, delight, enliven, enrapture, exhilarate, gladden, gratify, please, transport; crow, exult, delight, gloat, glory, jubilate, triumph, vaunt.

rejoin *vb* answer, rebut, respond, retort.

relate *vb* describe, detail, mention, narrate, recite, recount, rehearse, report, tell; apply, connect, correlate.

relation *n* account, chronicle, description, detail, explanation, history, mention, narration, narrative, recital, rehearsal, report, statement, story, tale; affinity, application, bearing, connection, correlation, dependency, pertinence, relationship; concern, reference, regard, respect; alliance, nearness, propinquity, rapport; blood, consanguinity, cousinship, kin, kindred, kinship, relationship; kinsman, kinswoman, relative.

relax *vb* loose, loosen, slacken, unbrace, unstrain; debilitate, enervate, enfeeble, prostrate, unbrace, unstring, weaken; abate, diminish, lessen, mitigate, reduce, remit; amuse, divert, ease, entertain, recreate, unbend.

release *vb* deliver, discharge, disengage, exempt, extricate, free, liberate, loose, unloose; acquit, discharge, quit, relinquish, remit. • *n* deliverance, discharge, freedom, liberation; absolution, dispensation, excuse, exemption, exoneration; acquaintance, clearance.

relentless *adj* cruel, hard, impenitent, implacable, inexorable, merciless, obdurate, pitiless, rancorous, remorseless, ruthless, unappeasable, uncompassionate, unfeeling, unforgiving, unmerciful, unpitying, unrelenting, unyielding, vindictive.

relevant *adj* applicable, appropriate, apposite, apt, apropos, fit, germane, pertinent, proper, relative, suitable.

reliable *adj* authentic, certain, constant, dependable, sure, trustworthy, trusty, unfailing.

reliance *n* assurance, confidence, credence, dependence, hope, trust.

relic *n* keepsake, memento, memorial, remembrance, souvenir, token, trophy; trace, vestige.

relics *npl* fragments, leavings, remainder, remains, remnants, ruins, scraps; body, cadaver, corpse, remains.

relict *n* dowager, widow.

relief *n* aid, alleviation, amelioration, assistance, assuagement, comfort, deliverance, ease, easement, help, mitigation, reinforcement, respite, rest, succour, softening, support; indemnification, redress, remedy; embossment, projection, prominence, protrusion; clearness, distinction, perspective, vividness.

relieve *vb* aid, comfort, help, spell, succour, support, sustain; abate, allay, alleviate, assuage, cure, diminish, ease, lessen, lighten, mitigate, remedy, remove, soothe; indemnify, redress, right, repair; disengage, free, release, remedy, rescue.

religious *adj* devotional, devout, god-fearing, godly, holy, pious, prayerful, spiritual; conscientious, exact, rigid, scrupulous, strict; canonical, divine, theological.

relinquish *vb* abandon, desert, forsake, forswear, leave, quit, renounce, resign, vacate; abdicate, cede, forbear, forgo, give up, surrender, yield.

relish *vb* appreciate, enjoy, like, prefer; season, flavour, taste. • *n* appetite, appreciation, enjoyment, fondness, gratification, gusto, inclination, liking, partiality, predilection, taste, zest; cast, flavour, manner, quality, savour, seasoning, sort, tang, tinge, touch; appetizer, condiment.

reluctance *n* aversion, backwardness, disinclination, dislike, loathing, repugnance, unwillingness.

reluctant *adj* averse, backward, disinclined, hesitant, indisposed, loath, unwilling.

rely *vb* confide, count, depend, hope, lean, reckon, repose, trust.

remain *vb* abide, continue, endure, last; exceed, persist, survive; abide, continue, dwell, halt, inhabit, rest, sojourn, stay, stop, tarry, wait.

remainder *n* balance, excess, leavings, remains, remnant, residue, rest, surplus.

remark *vb* heed, notice, observe, regard; comment, express, mention, observe, say, state, utter. • *n* consideration, heed, notice, observation, regard; annotation, comment, gloss, note, stricture; assertion, averment, comment, declaration, saying, statement, utterance.

remarkable *adj* conspicuous, distinguished, eminent, extraordinary, famous, notable, noteworthy, noticeable, pre-eminent, rare, singular, strange, striking, uncommon, unusual, wonderful.

remedy *vb* cure, heal, help, palliate, relieve; amend, correct, rectify, redress, repair, restore, retrieve. • *n* antidote, antitoxin, corrective, counteractive, cure, help, medicine, nostrum, panacea, restorative, specific; redress, reparation, restitution, restoration; aid, assistance, relief.

remembrance *n* recollection, reminiscence, retrospection; keepsake, memento, memorial, memory, reminder, souvenir, token; consideration, regard, thought.

reminiscence *n* memory, recollection, remembrance, retrospective.

remiss *adj* backward, behindhand, dilatory, indolent, languid, lax, lazy, slack, slow, tardy; careless, dilatory, heedless, idle, inattentive, neglectful, negligent, shiftless, slothful, thoughtless.

remission *n* abatement, decrease, diminution, lessening, mitigation, moderation, reduction, relaxation; cancellation, discharge, release, relinquishment; intermission, interruption, pause, rest, stop, stoppage, suspense, suspension; absolution, acquittal, excuse, exoneration, forgiveness, indulgence, pardon.

remit *vb* replace, restore, return; abate, bate, diminish, relax; release; absolve, condone, excuse, forgive, overlook, pardon; relinquish, resign, surrender; consign, forward, refer, send, transmit. • *n* authorization, brief, instructions, orders.

remnant *n* remainder, remains, residue, rest, trace; fragment, piece, scrap.

remorse *n* compunction, contrition, penitence, qualm, regret, repentance, reproach, self-reproach, sorrow.

remorseless *adj* cruel, barbarous, hard, harsh, implacable, inexorable, merciless, pitiless, relentless, ruthless, savage, uncompassionate, unmerciful, unrelenting.

remote *adj* distant, far, out-of-the-way; alien, far-fetched, foreign, inappropriate, unconnected, unrelated; abstracted, separated; inconsiderable, slight; isolated, removed, secluded, sequestrated.

removal *n* abstraction, departure, dislodgement, displacement, relegation, remove, shift, transference; elimination, extraction, withdrawal; abatement, destruction; discharge, dismissal, ejection, expulsion.

remove *vb* carry, dislodge, displace, shift, transfer, transport; abstract, extract, withdraw; abate, banish, destroy, suppress; cashier, depose, discharge, dismiss, eject, expel, oust, retire; depart, move.

remunerate *vb* compensate, indemnify, pay, recompense, reimburse, repay, requite, reward, satisfy.

remuneration *n* compensation, earnings, indemnity, pay, payment, recompense, reimbursement, reparation, repayment, reward, salary, wages.

remunerative *adj* gainful, lucrative, paying, profitable; compensatory, recompensing, remuneratory, reparative, requiting, rewarding.

rend *vb* break, burst, cleave, crack, destroy, dismember, dissever, disrupt, divide, fracture, lacerate, rive, rupture, sever, shiver, snap, split, sunder, tear.

render *vb* restore, return, surrender; assign, deliver, give, present; afford, contribute, furnish, supply, yield; construe, interpret, translate.

rendition *n* restitution, return, surrender; delineation, exhibition, interpretation, rendering, representation, reproduction; translation, version.

renegade *adj* apostate, backsliding, disloyal, false, outlawed, rebellious, recreant, unfaithful. • *n* apostate, backslider, recreant, turncoat; deserter, outlaw, rebel, revolter, traitor; vagabond, wretch.

renew *vb* rebuild, recreate, re-establish, refit, refresh, rejuvenate, renovate, repair, replenish, restore, resuscitate, revive; continue, recommence, repeat; iterate, reiterate; regenerate, transform.

renounce *vb* abjure, abnegate, decline, deny, disclaim, disown, forswear, neglect, recant, repudiate, reject, slight; abandon, abdicate, drop, forgo, forsake, desert, leave, quit, relinquish, resign.

renovate *vb* reconstitute, re-establish, refresh, refurbish, renew, restore, revamp; reanimate, recreate, regenerate, reproduce, resuscitate, revive, revivify.

renown *n* celebrity, distinction, eminence, fame, figure, glory, honour, greatness, name, note, notability, notoriety, reputation, repute.

renowned *adj* celebrated, distinguished, eminent, famed, famous, honoured, illustrious, remarkable, wonderful.

rent[1] *n* breach, break, crack, cleft, crevice, fissure, flaw, fracture, gap, laceration, opening, rift, rupture, separation, split, tear; schism.

rent[2] *vb* hire, lease, let. • *n* income, rental, revenue.

repair[1] *vb* mend, patch, piece, refit, retouch, tinker, vamp; correct, recruit, restore, retrieve. • *n* mending, refitting, renewal, reparation, restoration.

repair[2] *vb* betake oneself, go, move, resort, turn.

repairable *adj* curable, recoverable, reparable, restorable, retrievable.

reparable *adj* curable, recoverable, repairable, restorable, retrievable.

reparation *n* renewal, repair, restoration; amends, atonement, compensation, correction, indemnification, recompense, redress, requital, restitution, satisfaction.

repay *vb* refund, reimburse, restore, return; compensate, recompense, remunerate, reward, satisfy; avenge, retaliate, revenge.

repeal *vb* abolish, annul, cancel, recall, rescind, reverse, revoke. • *n* abolition, abrogation, annulment, cancellation, rescission, reversal, revocation.

repeat *vb* double, duplicate, iterate; cite, narrate, quote, recapitulate, recite, rehearse; echo, renew, reproduce. • *n* duplicate, duplication, echo, iteration, recapitulation, reiteration, repetition.

repel *vb* beat, disperse, repulse, scatter; check, confront, oppose, parry, rebuff, resist, withstand; decline, refuse, reject; disgust, revolt, sicken.

repellent *adj* abhorrent, disgusting, forbidding, repelling, repugnant, repulsive, revolting, uninviting.

repent *vb* atone, regret, relent, rue, sorrow.

repentance *n* compunction, contriteness, contrition, penitence, regret, remorse, self-accusation, self-condemnation, self-reproach.

repentant *adj* contrite, penitent, regretful, remorseful, rueful, sorrowful, sorry.

repercussion *n* rebound, recoil, reverberation; backlash, consequence, result.

repetition *n* harping, iteration, recapitulation, reiteration; diffuseness, redundancy, tautology, verbosity; narration, recital, rehearsal, relation, retailing; recurrence, renewal.

repine *vb* croak, complain, fret, grumble, long, mope, murmur.

replace *vb* re-establish, reinstate, reset; refund, repay, restore; succeed, supersede, supplant.

replenish *vb* fill, refill, renew, re-supply; enrich, furnish, provide, store, supply.

replete *adj* abounding, charged, exuberant, fraught, full, glutted, gorged, satiated, well-stocked.

repletion *n* abundance, exuberance, fullness, glut, profusion, satiation, satiety, surfeit.

replica *n* autograph, copy, duplicate, facsimile, reproduction.

reply *vb* answer, echo, rejoin, respond. • *n* acknowledgement, answer, rejoinder, repartee, replication, response, retort.

report *vb* announce, annunciate, communicate, declare; advertise, broadcast, bruit, describe, detail, herald, mention, narrate, noise, promulgate, publish, recite, relate, rumour, state, tell; minute, record. • *n* account, announcement, communication, declaration, statement; advice, description, detail, narration, narrative, news, recital, story, tale, talk, tidings; gossip, hearsay, rumour; clap, detonation, discharge, explosion, noise, repercussion, sound; fame, reputation, repute; account, bulletin, minute, note, record, statement.

repose[1] *vb* compose, recline, rest, settle; couch, lie, recline, sleep, slumber; confide, lean. • *n* quiet, recumbence, recumbency, rest, sleep, slumber; breathing time, inactivity, leisure, respite, relaxation; calm, ease, peace, peacefulness, quietness, quietude, stillness, tranquillity.

repose[2] *vb* place, put, stake; deposit, lodge, reposit, store.

repository *n* conservatory, depository, depot, magazine, museum, receptacle, repertory, storehouse, storeroom, thesaurus, treasury, vault.

reprehend *vb* accuse, blame, censure, chide, rebuke, reprimand, reproach, reprove, upbraid.

reprehensible *adj* blameable, blameworthy, censurable, condemnable, culpable, reprovable.

reprehension *n* admonition, blame, censure, condemnation, rebuke, reprimand, reproof.

represent *vb* exhibit, express, show; delineate, depict, describe, draw, portray, sketch; act, impersonate, mimic, personate, personify; exemplify, illustrate, image, reproduce, symbolize, typify.

representation *n* delineation, exhibition, show; impersonation, personation, simulation; account, description, narration, narrative, relation, statement; image, likeness, model, portraiture, resemblance, semblance; sight, spectacle; expostulation, remonstrance.

representative *adj* figurative, illustrative, symbolic, typical; delegated, deputed, representing. • *n* agent, commissioner, delegate, deputy, emissary, envoy, legate, lieutenant, messenger, proxy, substitute.

repress *vb* choke, crush, dull, overcome, overpower, silence, smother, subdue, suppress, quell; bridle, chasten, chastise, check, control, curb, restrain; appease, calm, quiet.

reprimand *vb* admonish, blame, censure, chide, rebuke, reprehend, reproach, reprove, upbraid. • *n* admonition, blame, censure, rebuke, reprehension, reproach, reprobation, reproof, reproval.

reprint *vb* republish. • *n* reimpression, republication; copy.

reproach *vb* blame, censure, rebuke, reprehend, reprimand, reprove, upbraid; abuse, accuse, asperse, condemn, defame, discredit, disparage, revile, traduce, vilify. • *n* abuse, blame, censure, condemnation, contempt, contumely, disapprobation, disapproval, expostulation, insolence, invective, railing, rebuke, remonstrance, reprobation, reproof, reviling, scorn, scurrility, upbraiding, vilification; abasement, discredit, disgrace, dishonour, disrepute, indignity, ignominy, infamy, insult, obloquy, odium, offence, opprobrium, scandal, shame, slur, stigma.

reproachful *adj* abusive, censorious, condemnatory, contemptuous, contumelious, damnatory, insolent, insulting, offensive, opprobrious, railing, reproving, sacrificing, scolding, scornful, scurrilous, upbraiding, vituperative; base, discreditable, disgraceful, dishonourable, disreputable, infamous, scandalous, shameful, vile.

reprobate *vb* censure, condemn, disapprove, discard, reject, reprehend; disallow; abandon, disown. • *adj* abandoned, base, castaway, corrupt, depraved, graceless, hardened, irredeemable, lost, profligate, shameless, vile, vitiated, wicked. • *n* caitiff, castaway, miscreant, outcast, rascal, scamp, scoundrel, sinner, villain.

reproduce *vb* copy, duplicate, emulate, imitate, print, repeat, represent; breed, generate, procreate, propagate.

reproof *n* admonition, animadversion, blame, castigation, censure, chiding, condemnation, correction, criticism, lecture, monition, objurgation, rating, rebuke, reprehension, reprimand, reproach, reproval, upbraiding.

reprove *vb* admonish, blame, castigate, censure, chide, condemn, correct, criticize, inculpate, lecture, objurgate, rate, rebuke, reprimand, reproach, scold, upbraid.

reptilian *adj* abject, crawling, creeping, grovelling, low, mean, treacherous, vile, vulgar.

repudiate *vb* abjure, deny, disavow, discard, disclaim, disown, nullify, reject, renounce.

repugnance *n* contrariety, contrariness, incompatibility, inconsistency, irreconcilability, irreconcilableness, unsuitability, unsuitableness; contest, opposition, resistance, struggle; antipathy, aversion, detestation, dislike, hatred, hostility, reluctance, repulsion, unwillingness.

repugnant *adj* incompatible, inconsistent, irreconcilable; adverse, antagonistic, contrary, hostile, inimical, opposed, opposing, unfavourable; detestable, distasteful, offensive, repellent, repulsive.

repulse *vb* check, defeat, refuse, reject, repel. • *n* repelling, repulsion; denial, refusal; disappointment, failure.

repulsion *n* abhorrence, antagonism, anticipation, aversion, discard, disgust, dislike, hatred, hostility, loathing, rebuff, rejection, repugnance, repulse, spurning.

repulsive *adj* abhorrent, cold, disagreeable, disgusting, forbidding, frigid, harsh, hateful, loathsome, nauseating, nauseous, odious, offensive, repellent, repugnant, reserved, revolting, sickening, ugly, unpleasant.

reputable *adj* creditable, estimable, excellent, good, honourable, respectable, worthy.

reputation *n* account, character, fame, mark, name, repute; celebrity, credit, distinction, eclat, esteem, estimation, glory, honour, prestige, regard, renown, report, respect; notoriety.

repute *vb* account, consider, deem, esteem, estimate, hold, judge, reckon, regard, think.

request *vb* ask, beg, beseech, call, claim, demand, desire, entreat, pray, solicit, supplicate. • *n* asking, entreaty, importunity, invitation, petition, prayer, requisition, solicitation, suit, supplication.

require *vb* beg, beseech, bid, claim, crave, demand, dun, importune, invite, pray, requisition, request, sue, summon; need, want; direct, enjoin, exact, order, prescribe.

requirement *n* claim, demand, exigency, market, need, needfulness, requisite, requisition, request, urgency, want; behest, bidding, charge, command, decree, exaction, injunction, mandate, order, precept.

requisite *adj* essential, imperative, indispensable, necessary, needful, needed, required. • *n* essential, necessity, need, requirement.

requite *vb* compensate, pay, remunerate, reciprocate, recompense, repay, reward, satisfy; avenge, punish, retaliate, satisfy.

rescind *vb* abolish, abrogate, annul, cancel, countermand, quash, recall, repeal, reverse, revoke, vacate, void.

rescue *vb* deliver, extricate, free, liberate, preserve, ransom, recapture, recover, redeem, release, retake, save. • *n* deliverance, extrication, liberation, redemption, release, salvation.

research *vb* analyse, examine, explore, inquire, investigate, probe, study. • *n* analysis, examination, exploration, inquiry, investigation, scrutiny, study.

resemblance *n* affinity, agreement, analogy, likeness, semblance, similarity, similitude; counterpart, facsimile, image, representation.

resemble *vb* compare, liken; copy, counterfeit, imitate.

resentful *adj* angry, bitter, choleric, huffy, hurt, irascible, irritable, malignant, revengeful, sore, touchy.

resentment *n* acrimony, anger, annoyance, bitterness, choler, displeasure, dudgeon, fury, gall, grudge, heartburning, huff, indignation, ire, irritation, pique, rage, soreness, spleen, sulks, umbrage, vexation, wrath.

reservation *n* reserve, suppression; appropriation, booking, exception, restriction, saving; proviso, salvo; custody, park, reserve, sanctuary.

reserve *vb* hold, husband, keep, retain, store. • *adj* alternate, auxiliary, spare, substitute. • *n* reservation; aloofness, backwardness, closeness, coldness, concealment, constraint, suppression, reservedness, retention, restraint, reticence, uncommunicativeness, unresponsiveness; coyness, demureness, modesty, shyness, taciturnity; park, reservation, sanctuary.

reserved *adj* coy, demure, modest, shy, taciturn; aloof, backward, cautious, cold, distant, incommunicative, restrained, reticent, self-controlled, unsociable, unsocial; bespoken, booked, excepted, held, kept, retained, set apart, taken, withheld.

reside *vb* abide, domicile, domiciliate, dwell, inhabit, live, lodge, remain, room, sojourn, stay.

residence *n* inhabitance, inhabitancy, sojourn, stay, stop, tarrying; abode, domicile, dwelling, habitation, home, house, lodging, mansion.

residue *n* leavings, remainder, remains, remnant, residuum, rest; excess, overplus, surplus.

resign *vb* abandon, abdicate, abjure, cede, commit, disclaim, forego, forsake, leave, quit, relinquish, renounce, surrender, yield.

resignation *n* abandonment, abdication, relinquishment, renunciation, retirement, surrender; acquiescence, compliance, endurance, forbearance, fortitude, long-sufferance, patience, submission, sufferance.

resist *vb* assail, attack, baffle, block, check, confront, counteract, disappoint, frustrate, hinder, impede, impugn, neutralize, obstruct, oppose, rebel, rebuff, stand against, stem, stop, strive, thwart, withstand.

resolute *adj* bold, constant, decided, determined, earnest, firm, fixed, game, hardy, inflexible, persevering, pertinacious, relentless, resolved, staunch, steadfast, steady, stout, stouthearted, sturdy, tenacious, unalterable, unbending, undaunted, unflinching, unshaken, unwavering, unyielding.

resolution *n* boldness, disentanglement, explication, unravelling; backbone, constancy, courage, decision, determination, earnestness, energy, firmness, fortitude, grit, hardihood, inflexibility, intention, manliness, pluck, perseverance, purpose, relentlessness, resolve, resoluteness, stamina, steadfastness, steadiness, tenacity.

resolve *vb* analyse, disperse, scatter, separate, reduce; change, dissolve, liquefy, melt, reduce, transform; decipher, disentangle, elucidate, explain, interpret, unfold, solve, unravel; conclude, decide, determine, fix, intend, purpose, will. • *n* conclusion, decision, determination, intention, will; declaration, resolution.

resonant *adj* booming, clangorous, resounding, reverberating, ringing, roaring, sonorous, thundering, vibrant.

resort *vb* frequent, haunt; assemble, congregate, convene, go, repair. • *n* application, expedient, recourse; haunt, refuge, rendezvous, retreat, spa; assembling, confluence, concourse, meeting; recourse, reference.

resound *vb* echo, re-echo, reverberate, ring; celebrate, extol, praise, sound.

resource *n* dependence, resort; appliance, contrivance, device, expedient, instrumentality, means, resort.

resources *npl* capital, funds, income, money, property, reserve, supplies, wealth.

respect *vb* admire, esteem, honour, prize, regard, revere, reverence, spare, value, venerate; consider, heed, notice, observe. • *n* attention, civility, courtesy, consideration, deference, estimation, homage, honour, notice, politeness, recognition, regard, reverence, veneration; consideration, favour, goodwill, kind; aspect, bearing, connection, feature, matter, particular, point, reference, regard, relation.

respects *npl* compliments, greetings, regards.

respectable *adj* considerable, estimable, honourable, presentable, proper, upright, worthy; adequate, moderate; tolerable.

respectful *adj* ceremonious, civil, complaisant, courteous, decorous, deferential, dutiful, formal, polite.

respire *vb* breathe, exhale, live.

respite *vb* delay, relieve, reprieve. • *n* break, cessation, delay, intermission, interval, pause, recess, rest, stay, stop; forbearance, postponement, reprieve.

resplendent *adj* beaming, bright, brilliant, effulgent, lucid, glittering, glorious, gorgeous, luminous, lustrous, radiant, shining, splendid.

respond *vb* answer, reply, rejoin; accord, correspond, suit.

response *n* answer, replication, rejoinder, reply, retort.

responsible *adj* accountable, amenable, answerable, liable, trustworthy.

rest[1] *vb* cease, desist, halt, hold, pause, repose, stop, breathe, relax, unbend; repose, sleep, slumber; lean, lie, lounge, perch, recline, ride; acquiesce, confide, trust; confide, rely, trust; calm, comfort, ease. • *n* fixity, immobility, inactivity, motionlessness, quiescence, quiet, repose; hush, peace, peacefulness, quietness, relief, security, stillness, tranquillity; cessation, intermission, interval, lull, pause, relaxation, respite, stop, stay; siesta, sleep, slumber; death; brace, stay, support; axis, fulcrum, pivot.

rest[2] *vb* be left, remain. • *n* balance, remainder, remnant, residuum; overplus, surplus.

restaurant *n* bistro, café, cafeteria, chophouse, eatery, eating house, pizzeria, trattoria.

restitution *n* restoration, return; amends, compensation, indemnification, recompense, rehabilitation, remuneration, reparation, repayment, requital, satisfaction.

restive *adj* mulish, obstinate, stopping, stubborn, unwilling; impatient, recalcitrant, restless, uneasy, unquiet.

restless *adj* disquieted, disturbed, restive, sleepless, uneasy, unquiet, unresting; changeable, inconstant, irresolute, unsteady, vacillating; active, astatic, roving, transient, unsettled, unstable, wandering; agitated, fidgety, fretful, turbulent.

restoration *n* recall, recovery, re-establishment, reinstatement, reparation, replacement, restitution, return; reconsideration, redemption, reintegration, renewal, renovation repair resuscitation, revival; convalescence, cure, recruitment, recuperation.

restorative *adj* curative, invigorating, recuperative, remedial, restoring, stimulating. • *n* corrective, curative cure, healing, medicine, remedy, reparative, stimulant.

restore *vb* refund, repay, return; caulk, cobble, emend, heal, mend, patch, reintegrate, re-establish, rehabilitate, reinstate, renew, repair, replace, retrieve; cure, heal, recover, revive; resuscitate.

restrain *vb* bridle, check, coerce, confine, constrain, curb, debar, govern, hamper, hinder, hold, keep, muzzle, picket, prevent, repress, restrict, rule, subdue, tie withhold; abridge, circumscribe, narrow.

restraint *n* bridle, check, coercion, control, compulsion, constraint, curb, discipline, repression, suppression; arrest, deterrence, hindrance, inhibition, limitation, prevention, prohibition, restriction, stay, stop; confinement, detention, imprisonment, shackles; constraint, stiffness, reserve, unnaturalness.

restrict *vb* bound, circumscribe, confine, limit, qualify, restrain, straiten.

restriction *n* confinement, limitation; constraint, restraint; reservation, reserve.

result *vb* accrue, arise, come, ensue, flow, follow, issue, originate, proceed, spring, rise; end, eventuate, terminate. • *n* conclusion, consequence, deduction, inference, outcome; corollary, effect, end, event, eventuality, fruit, harvest, issue, product, sequel, termination; decision, determination, finding, resolution, resolve, solution, verdict.

resume *vb* continue, recommence, renew, restart, summarize.

résumé *n* abstract, curriculum vitae, epitome, recapitulation, summary, synopsis.

resuscitate *vb* quicken, reanimate, renew, resurrect, restore, revive, revivify.

retain *vb* detain, hold, husband, keep, preserve, recall, recollect, remember, reserve, save, withhold; engage, maintain.

retainer *n* adherent, attendant, dependant, follower, hanger-on, servant.

retaliate *vb* avenge, match, repay, require, retort, return, turn.

retaliation *n* boomerang, counterstroke, punishment, repayment, requital, retribution, revenge.

retard *vb* check, clog, hinder, impede, obstruct, slacken; adjourn, defer, delay, postpone, procrastinate.

reticent *adj* close, reserved, secretive, silent, taciturn, uncommunicative.

retinue *n* bodyguard, cortege, entourage, escort, followers, household, ménage, suite, tail, train.

retire *vb* discharge, shelve, superannuate, withdraw; depart, leave, resign, retreat.

retired *adj* abstracted, removed, withdrawn; apart, private secret, sequestrated, solitary.

retirement *n* isolation, loneliness, privacy, retreat, seclusion, solitude, withdrawal.

retiring *adj* coy, demure, diffident, modest, reserved, retreating, shy, withdrawing.

retort *vb* answer, rejoin, reply, respond. • *n* answer, rejoinder, repartee, reply, response; crucible, jar, vessel, vial.

retract *vb* reverse, withdraw; abjure, cancel, disavow, recall, recant, revoke, unsay.

retreat *vb* recoil, retire, withdraw; recede. • *n* departure, recession, recoil, retirement, withdrawal; privacy, seclusion, solitude; asylum, cove, den, habitat, haunt, niche, recess, refuge, resort, shelter.

retrench *vb* clip, curtail, cut, delete, dock, lop, mutilate, pare, prune; abridge, decrease, diminish, lessen; confine, limit; economize, encroach.

retribution *n* compensation, desert, judgement, nemesis, penalty, recompense, repayment, requital, retaliation, return, revenge, reward, vengeance.

retrieve *vb* recall, recover, recoup, recruit, re-establish, regain, repair, restore.

retrograde *vb* decline, degenerate, recede, retire, retrocede. • *adj* backward, inverse, retrogressive, unprogressive.

retrospect *n* recollection, re-examination, reminiscence, re-survey, review, survey.

return *vb* reappear, recoil, recur, revert; answer, reply, respond; recriminate, retort; convey, give, communicate, reciprocate, recompense, refund, remit, repay, report, requite, send, tell, transmit; elect. • *n* payment, reimbursement, remittance, repayment; recompense, recovery, recurrence, renewal, repayment, requital, restitution, restoration, reward; advantage, benefit, interest, profit, rent, yield.

reunion *n* assemblage, assembly, gathering, meeting, re-assembly; rapprochement, reconciliation.

reveal *vb* announce communicate, confess, declare, disclose, discover, display, divulge, expose, impart, open, publish, tell, uncover, unmask, unseal, unveil.

revel *vb* carouse, disport, riot, roister, tipple; delight, indulge, luxuriate, wanton. • *n* carousal, feast, festival, saturnalia, spree.

revelry *n* bacchanal, carousal, carouse, debauch, festivity, jollification, jollity, orgy, revel riot, rout, saturnalia, wassail.

revenge *vb* avenge, repay, requite, retaliate, vindicate. • *n* malevolence, rancour, reprisal, requital, retaliation, retribution, vengeance, vindictiveness.

revengeful *adj* implacable, malevolent, malicious, malignant, resentful, rancorous, spiteful, vengeful, vindictive.

revenue *n* fruits, income, produce, proceeds, receipts, return, reward, wealth.

reverberate *vb* echo, re-echo, resound, return.

revere *vb* adore, esteem, hallow, honour, reverence, venerate, worship.

reverence *vb* adore, esteem, hallow, honour, revere, venerate, worship. • *n* adoration, awe, deference, homage, honour, respect, veneration, worship.

reverential *adj* deferential, humble, respectful, reverent, submissive.

reverse *vb* invert, transpose; overset, overthrow, overturn, quash, subvert, undo, unmake; annul, countermand, repeal, rescind, retract, revoke; back, back up, retreat. • *adj* back, converse, contrary, opposite, verso. • *n* back, calamity, check, comedown, contrary, counterpart, defeat, opposite, tail; change, vicissitude; adversity, affliction, hardship, misadventure, mischance, misfortune, mishap, trial.

revert *vb* repel, reverse; backslide, lapse, recur, relapse, return.

review *vb* inspect, overlook, reconsider, re-examine, retrace, revise, survey; analyse, criticize, discuss, edit, judge, scrutinize, study. • *n* reconsideration, re-examination, re-survey, retrospect, survey; analysis, digest, synopsis; commentary, critique, criticism, notice, review, scrutiny, study.

revile *vb* abuse, asperse, backbite, calumniate, defame, execrate, malign, reproach, slander, traduce, upbraid, vilify.

revise *vb* reconsider, re-examine, review; alter, amend, correct, edit, overhaul, polish.

revive *vb* reanimate, reinspire, reinspirit, reinvigorate, resuscitate, revitalize, revivify; animate, cheer, comfort, invigorate, quicken, reawaken, recover, refresh, renew, renovate, rouse, strengthen; reawake, recall.

revocation *n* abjuration, recall, recantation, repeal, retraction, reversal.

revoke *vb* abolish, abrogate, annul, cancel, countermand, invalidate, quash, recall, recant, repeal, repudiate, rescind, retract.

revolt *vb* desert, mutiny, rebel, rise; disgust, nauseate, repel, sicken. • *n* defection, desertion, faithlessness, inconstancy;

disobedience, insurrection, mutiny, outbreak, rebellion, sedition, strike, uprising.

revolting *adj* abhorrent, abominable, disgusting, hateful, monstrous, nauseating, nauseous, objectionable, obnoxious, offensive, repulsive, shocking, sickening; insurgent, mutinous, rebellious.

revolution *n* coup, disobedience, insurrection, mutiny, outbreak, rebellion, sedition, strike, uprising; change, innovation, reformation, transformation, upheaval; circle, circuit, cycle, lap, orbit, rotation, spin, turn.

revolve *vb* circle, circulate, rotate, swing, turn, wheel; devolve, return; consider, mediate, ponder, ruminate, study.

revulsion *n* abstraction, shrinking, withdrawal; change, reaction, reversal, transition; abhorrence, disgust, loathing, repugnance.

reward *vb* compensate, gratify, indemnify, pay, punish, recompense, remember, remunerate, requite. • *n* compensation, gratification, guerdon, indemnification, pay, recompense, remuneration, requital; bounty, bonus, fee, gratuity, honorarium, meed, perquisite, premium, remembrance, tip; punishment, retribution.

rhythm *n* cadence, lilt, pulsation, swing; measure, metre, number.

ribald *adj* base, blue, coarse, filthy, gross, indecent, lewd, loose, low, mean, obscene, vile.

rich *adj* affluent, flush, moneyed, opulent, prosperous, wealthy; costly, estimable, gorgeous, luxurious, precious, splendid, sumptuous, superb, valuable; delicious, luscious, savoury; abundant, ample, copious, enough, full, plentiful, plenteous, sufficient; fertile, fruitful, luxuriant, productive, prolific; bright, dark, deep, exuberant, vivid; harmonious, mellow, melodious, soft, sweet; comical, funny, humorous, laughable.

riches *npl* abundance, affluence, fortune, money, opulence, plenty, richness, wealth, wealthiness.

rickety *adj* broken, imperfect, shaky, shattered, tottering, tumbledown, unsteady, weak.

rid *vb* deliver, free, release; clear, disburden, disencumber, scour, sweep; disinherit, dispatch, dissolve, divorce, finish, sever.

riddance *n* deliverance, disencumberment, extrication, escape, freedom, release, relief.

riddle[1] *vb* explain, solve, unriddle. • *n* conundrum, enigma, mystery, puzzle, rebus.

riddle[2] *vb* sieve, sift, perforate, permeate, spread. • *n* colander, sieve, strainer.

ridge *n* chine, hogback, ledge, saddle, spine, rib, watershed, weal, wrinkle.

ridicule *vb* banter, burlesque, chaff, deride, disparage, jeer, mock, lampoon, rally, satirize, scout, taunt. • *n* badinage, banter, burlesque, chaff, derision, game, gibe, irony, jeer, mockery, persiflage. quip, raillery, sarcasm, satire, sneer, squib, wit.

ridiculous *adj* absurd, amusing, comical, droll, eccentric, fantastic, farcical, funny, laughable, ludicrous, nonsensical, odd, outlandish, preposterous, queer, risible, waggish.

rife *adj* abundant, common, current, general, numerous, plentiful, prevailing, prevalent, replete.

riffraff *n* horde, mob, populace, rabble, scum, trash.

rifle *vb* despoil, fleece, pillage, plunder, ransack, rob, strip.

rift *vb* cleave, rive, split. • *n* breach, break, chink, cleft, crack, cranny, crevice, fissure, fracture, gap, opening, reft, rent.

rig *vb* accoutre, clothe, dress. • *n* costume, dress, garb; equipment, team.

right *vb* adjust, correct, regulate, settle, straighten, vindicate. • *adj* direct, rectilinear, straight; erect, perpendicular, plumb, upright; equitable, even-handed, fair, just, justifiable, honest, lawful, legal, legitimate, rightful, square, unswerving; appropriate, becoming, correct, conventional, fit, fitting, meet, orderly, proper, reasonable, seemly, suitable, well-done; actual, genuine, real, true, unquestionable; dexter, dextral, right-handed. • *adv* equitably, fairly, justly, lawfully, rightfully, rightly; correctly, fitly, properly, suitably, truly; actually, exactly, just, really, truly, well. • *n* authority, claim, liberty, permission, power, privilege, title; equity, good, honour, justice, lawfulness, legality, propriety, reason, righteousness, truth.

righteous *adj* devout, godly, good, holy, honest, incorrupt, just, pious, religious, saintly, uncorrupt, upright, virtuous; equitable, fair, right, rightful.

righteousness *n* equity, faithfulness, godliness, goodness, holiness, honesty, integrity, justice, piety, purity, right, rightfulness, sanctity, uprightness, virtue.

rightful *adj* lawful, legitimate, true; appropriate, correct, deserved, due, equitable, fair, fitting, honest, just, legal, merited, proper, reasonable, suitable.

rigid *adj* firm, hard, inflexible, permanent, stiff, stiffened, unbending, unpliant, unyielding; bristling, erect, precipitous, steep; austere, conventional, correct, exact, formal, harsh, meticulous, precise, rigorous, severe, sharp, stern, strict, unmitigated; cruel.

rigmarole *n* balderdash, flummery, gibberish, gobbledegook, jargon, nonsense, palaver, trash, twaddle, verbiage.

rigour *n* hardness, inflexibility, rigidity, rigidness, stiffness; asperity, austerity, harshness, severity, sternness; evenness, strictness; inclemency.

rile *vb* anger, annoy, irritate, upset, vex.

rim *n* brim, brink, border, confine, curb, edge, flange, girdle, margin, ring, skirt.

ring[1] *vb* circle, encircle, enclose, girdle, surround. • *n* circle, circlet, girdle, hoop, round, whorl; cabal, clique, combination, confederacy, coterie, gang, junta, league, set.

ring[2] *vb* chime, clang, jingle, knell, peal, resound, reverberate, sound, tingle, toll; call, phone, telephone. • *n* chime, knell, peal, tinkle, toll; call, phone call, telephone call.

riot *vb* carouse, luxuriate, revel. • *n* affray, altercation, brawl, broil, commotion, disturbance, fray, outbreak, pandemonium, quarrel, squabble, tumult, uproar; dissipation, excess, luxury, merrymaking, revelry.

riotous *adj* boisterous, luxurious, merry, revelling, unrestrained, wanton; disorderly, insubordinate, lawless, mutinous, rebellious, refractory, seditious, tumultuous, turbulent, ungovernable, unruly, violent.

ripe *adj* advanced, grown, mature, mellow, seasoned, soft; fit, prepared, ready; accomplished, complete, consummate, finished, perfect, perfected.

ripen *vb* burgeon, develop, mature, prepare.

rise *vb* arise, ascend, clamber, climb, levitate, mount; excel, succeed; enlarge, heighten, increase, swell, thrive; revive; grow, kindle, wax; begin, flow, head, originate, proceed, spring, start; mutiny, rebel, revolt; happen, occur. • *n* ascension, ascent, rising; elevation, grade, hill, slope; beginning, emergence, flow, origin, source, spring; advance, augmentation, expansion, increase.

risible *adj* amusing, comical, droll, farcical, funny, laughable, ludicrous, ridiculous.

risk *vb* bet, endanger, hazard, jeopardize, peril, speculate, stake, venture, wager. • *n* chance, danger, hazard, jeopardy, peril, venture.

rite *n* ceremonial, ceremony, form, formulary, ministration, observance, ordinance, ritual, rubric, sacrament, solemnity.

ritual *adj* ceremonial, conventional, formal, habitual, routine, stereotyped. • *n* ceremonial, ceremony, liturgy, observance, rite, sacrament, service; convention, form, formality, habit, practice, protocol.

rival *vb* emulate, match, oppose. • *adj* competing, contending, emulating, emulous, opposing. • *n* antagonist, competitor, emulator, opponent.

rive *vb* cleave, rend, split.

river *n* affluent, current, reach, stream, tributary.

road *n* course, highway, lane, passage, path, pathway, roadway, route, street, thoroughfare, track, trail, turnpike, way.

roam *vb* jaunt, prowl, ramble, range, rove, straggle, stray, stroll, wander.

roar *vb* bawl, bellow, cry, howl, vociferate, yell; boom, peal, rattle, resound, thunder. • *n* bellow, roaring; rage, resonance, storm, thunder; cry, outcry, shout; laugh, laughter, shout.

rob *vb* despoil, fleece, pilfer, pillage, plunder, rook, strip; appropriate, deprive, embezzle, plagiarize.

robber *n* bandit, brigand, desperado, depredator, despoiler, footpad, freebooter, highwayman, marauder, pillager, pirate, plunderer, rifler, thief.

robbery *n* depredation, despoliation, embezzlement, freebooting, larceny, peculation, piracy, plagiarism, plundering, spoliation, theft.

robe *vb* array, clothe, dress, invest. • *n* attire, costume, dress, garment, gown, habit, vestment; bathrobe, dressing gown, housecoat.

robust *adj* able-bodied, athletic, brawny, energetic, firm, forceful, hale, hardy, hearty, iron, lusty, muscular, powerful, seasoned, self-assertive, sinewy, sound, stalwart, stout, strong, sturdy, vigorous.

rock[1] *n* boulder, cliff, crag, reef, stone; asylum, defence, foundation, protection, refuge, strength, support; gneiss, granite, marble, slate, etc.

rock[2] *vb* calm, cradle, lull, quiet, soothe, still, tranquillize; reel, shake, sway, teeter, totter, wobble.

rogue *n* beggar, vagabond, vagrant; caitiff, cheat, knave, rascal, scamp, scapegrace, scoundrel, sharper, swindler, trickster, villain.

roguish *adj* dishonest, fraudulent, knavish, rascally, scoundrelly, trickish, tricky; arch, sportive, mischievous, puckish, waggish, wanton.

role *n* character, function, impersonation, part, task.

roll *vb* gyrate, revolve, rotate, turn, wheel; curl, muffle, swathe, wind; bind, involve, enfold, envelop; flatten, level, smooth, spread; bowl, drive, trundle, wheel; gybe, lean, lurch, stagger, sway, yaw; billow, swell, undulate; wallow, welter; flow, glide, run. • *n* document, scroll, volume; annals, chronicle, history, record, rota; catalogue, inventory, list, register, schedule; booming, resonance, reverberation, thunder; cylinder, roller.

rollicking *adj* frisky, frolicking, frolicsome, jolly, jovial, lively, swaggering.

romance *vb* exaggerate, fantasize. • *n* fantasy, fiction, legend, novel, story, tale; exaggeration, falsehood, lie; ballad, idyll, song.

romantic *adj* extravagant, fanciful, fantastic, ideal, imaginative, sentimental, wild; chimerical, fabulous, fantastic, fictitious, imaginary, improbable, legendary, picturesque, quixotic, sentimental. • *n* dreamer, idealist, sentimentalist, visionary.

romp *vb* caper, gambol, frisk, sport. • *n* caper, frolic, gambol.

room *n* accommodation, capacity, compass, elbowroom, expanse, extent, field, latitude, leeway, play, scope, space, swing; place, stead; apartment, chamber, lodging; chance, occasion, opportunity.

roomy *adj* ample, broad, capacious, comfortable, commodious, expansive, extensive, large, spacious, wide.

root[1] *vb* anchor, embed, fasten, implant, place, settle; confirm, establish. • *n* base, bottom, foundation; cause, occasion, motive, origin, reason, source; etymon, radical, radix, stem.

root[2] *vb* destroy, eradicate, extirpate, exterminate, remove, unearth, uproot; burrow, dig, forage, grub, rummage; applaud, cheer, encourage.

rooted *adj* chronic, confirmed, deep, established, fixed, radical.

roseate *adj* blooming, blushing, rose-coloured, rosy, rubicund; hopeful.

rostrum *n* platform, stage, stand, tribune.

rosy *adj* auspicious, blooming, blushing, favourable, flushed, hopeful, roseate, ruddy, sanguine.

rot *vb* corrupt, decay, decompose, degenerate, putrefy, spoil, taint. • *n* corruption, decay, decomposition, putrefaction.

rotary *adj* circular, rotating, revolving, rotatory, turning, whirling.

rotten *adj* carious, corrupt, decomposed, fetid, putrefied, putrescent, putrid, rank, stinking; defective, unsound; corrupt, deceitful, immoral, treacherous, unsound, untrustworthy.

rotund *adj* buxom, chubby, full, globular, obese, plump, round, stout; fluent, grandiloquent.

roué *n* debauchee, libertine, profligate, rake.

rough *vb* coarsen, roughen; manhandle, mishandle, molest. • *adj* bumpy, craggy, irregular, jagged, rugged, scabrous, scraggy, scratchy, stubby, uneven; approximate, cross-grained, crude, formless, incomplete, knotty, rough-hewn, shapeless, sketchy, uncut, unfashioned, unfinished, unhewn, unpolished, unwrought, vague; bristly, bushy, coarse, disordered, hairy, hirsute, ragged, shaggy, unkempt; austere, bearish, bluff, blunt, brusque, burly, churlish, discourteous, gruff, harsh, impolite, indelicate, rude, surly, uncivil, uncourteous, ungracious, unpolished, unrefined; harsh, severe, sharp, violent; astringent, crabbed, hard, sour, tart; discordant, grating, inharmonious, jarring, raucous, scabrous, unmusical; boisterous, foul, inclement, severe, stormy, tempestuous, tumultuous, turbulent, untamed, violent, wild; acrimonious, brutal, cruel, disorderly, riotous, rowdy, severe, uncivil, unfeeling, ungentle. • *n* bully, rowdy, roughneck, ruffian; draft, outline, sketch, suggestion; unevenness.

round *vb* curve; circuit, encircle, encompass, surround. • *adj* bulbous, circular, cylindrical, globular, orbed, orbicular, rotund, spherical; complete, considerable, entire, full, great, large, unbroken, whole; chubby, corpulent, plump, stout, swelling; continuous, flowing, harmonious, smooth; brisk, quick; blunt, candid, fair, frank, honest, open, plain, upright. • *adv* around, circularly, circuitously. • *prep* about, around. • *n* bout, cycle, game, lap, revolution, rotation, succession, turn; canon, catch, dance; ball, circle, circumference, cylinder, globe, sphere; circuit, compass, perambulation, routine, tour, watch.

roundabout *adj* circuitous, circumlocutory, indirect, tortuous; ample, broad, extensive; encircling, encompassing.

rouse *vb* arouse, awaken, raise, shake, wake, waken; animate, bestir, brace, enkindle, excite, inspire, kindle, rally, stimulate, stir, whet; startle, surprise.

rout *vb* beat, conquer, defeat, discomfit, overcome, overpower, overthrow, vanquish; chase away, dispel, disperse, scatter. • *n* defeat, discomfiture, flight, ruin; concourse, multitude, rabble; brawl, disturbance, noise, roar, uproar.

route *vb* direct, forward, send, steer. • *n* course, circuit, direction, itinerary, journey, march, road, passage, path, way.

routine *adj* conventional, familiar, habitual, ordinary, standard, typical, usual; boring, dull, humdrum, predictable, tiresome. • *n* beat, custom, groove, method, order, path, practice, procedure, round, rut.

rove *vb* prowl, ramble, range, roam, stray, struggle, stroll, wander.

row[1] *n* file, line, queue, range, rank, series, string, tier; alley, street, terrace.

row[2] *vb* argue, dispute, fight, quarrel, squabble. • *n* affray, altercation, brawl, broil, commotion, dispute, disturbance, noise, outbreak, quarrel, riot, squabble, tumult, uproar.

royal *adj* august, courtly, dignified, generous, grand, imperial, kingly, kinglike, magnanimous, magnificent, majestic, monarchical, noble, princely, regal, sovereign, splendid, superb.

rub *vb* abrade, chafe, grate, graze, scrape; burnish, clean, massage, polish, scour, wipe; apply, put, smear, spread. • *n* caress, massage, polish, scouring, shine, wipe; catch, difficulty, drawback, impediment, obstacle, problem.

rubbish *n* debris, detritus, fragments, refuse, ruins, waste; dregs, dross, garbage, litter, lumber, scoria, scum, sweepings, trash, trumpery.

rubicund *adj* blushing, erubescent, florid, flushed, red, reddish, ruddy.

rude *adj* coarse, crude, ill-formed, rough, rugged, shapeless, uneven, unfashioned, unformed, unwrought; artless, barbarous, boorish, clownish, ignorant, illiterate, loutish, raw, savage, uncivilized, uncouth, uncultivated, undisciplined, unpolished, ungraceful, unskilful, unskilled, untaught, untrained, untutored, vulgar; awkward, barbarous, bluff, blunt, boorish, brusque, brutal, churlish, gruff, ill-bred, impertinent, impolite, impudent, insolent, insulting, ribald, saucy, uncivil, uncourteous, unrefined; boisterous, fierce, harsh, severe, tumultuous, turbulent, violent; artless, inelegant, rustic, unpolished; hearty, robust.

rudimentary *adj* elementary, embryonic, fundamental, initial, primary, rudimental, undeveloped.

rue *vb* deplore, grieve, lament, regret, repent.

rueful *adj* dismal, doleful, lamentable, lugubrious, melancholic, melancholy, mournful, penitent, regretful, sad, sorrowful, woeful.

ruffian *n* bully, caitiff, cutthroat, hoodlum, miscreant, monster, murderer, rascal, robber, roisterer, rowdy, scoundrel, villain, wretch.

ruffle *vb* damage, derange, disarrange, dishevel, disorder, ripple, roughen, rumple; agitate, confuse, discompose, disquiet, disturb, excite, harass, irritate, molest, plague, perturb, torment, trouble, vex, worry; cockle, flounce, pucker, wrinkle. • *n* edging, frill, ruff; agitation, bustle, commotion, confusion, contention, disturbance, excitement, fight, fluster, flutter, flurry, perturbation, tumult.

rugged *adj* austere, bristly, coarse, crabbed, cragged, craggy, hard, hardy, irregular, ragged, robust, rough, rude, scraggy, severe, seamed, shaggy, uneven, unkempt, wrinkled; boisterous, inclement, stormy, tempestuous, tumultuous, turbulent, violent; grating, harsh, inharmonious, unmusical, scabrous.

ruin *vb* crush, damn, defeat, demolish, desolate, destroy, devastate, overthrow, overturn, overwhelm, seduce, shatter, smash, subvert, wreck; beggar, impoverish. • *n* damnation, decay, defeat, demolition, desolation, destruction, devastation, discomfiture, downfall, fall, loss, perdition, prostration, rack, ruination, shipwreck, subversion, undoing, wrack, wreck; bane, mischief, pest.

ruination *n* demolition, destruction, overthrow, ruin, subversion.

ruinous *adj* decayed, demolished, dilapidated; baneful, calamitous, damnatory, destructive, disastrous, mischievous, noisome, noxious, pernicious, subversive, wasteful.

rule *vb* bridle, command, conduct, control, direct, domineer, govern, judge, lead, manage, reign, restrain; advise, guide, persuade; adjudicate, decide, determine, establish, settle; obtain, prevail, predominate. • *n* authority, command, control, direction, domination, dominion, empire, government, jurisdiction, lordship, mastery, mastership, regency, reign, sway; behaviour, conduct; habit, method, order, regularity, routine, system; aphorism, canon, convention, criterion, formula, guide, law, maxim, model, precedent, precept, standard, system, test, touchstone; decision, order, prescription, regulation, ruling.

ruler *n* chief, governor, king, lord, master, monarch, potentate, regent, sovereign; director, head, manager, president; controller, guide, rule; straight-edge.

ruminate *vb* brood, chew, cogitate, consider, contemplate, meditate, muse, ponder, reflect, think.

rumour *vb* bruit, circulate, report, tell. • *n* bruit, gossip, hearsay, report, talk; news, report, story, tidings; celebrity, fame, reputation, repute.

rumple *vb* crease, crush, corrugate, crumple, disarrange, dishevel, pucker, ruffle, wrinkle. • *n* crease, corrugation, crumple, fold, pucker, wrinkle.

run *vb* bolt, career, course, gallop, haste, hasten, hie, hurry, lope, post, race, scamper, scour, scud, scuttle, speed, trip; flow, glide, go, move, proceed, stream; fuse, liquefy, melt; advance, pass, proceed, vanish; extend, lie, spread, stretch; circulate, pass, press; average, incline, tend; flee; pierce, stab; drive, force, propel, push, thrust, turn; cast, form, mould, shape; follow, perform, pursue, take; discharge, emit; direct, maintain, manage. • *n* race, running; course, current, flow, motion, passage, progress, way, wont; continuance, currency, popularity; excursion, gallop, journey, trip, trot; demand, pressure; brook, burn, flow, rill, rivulet, runlet, runnel, streamlet.

rupture *vb* break, burst, fracture, sever, split. • *n* breach, break, burst, disruption, fracture, split; contention, faction, feud, hostility, quarrel, schism.

rural *adj* agrarian, bucolic, country, pastoral, rustic, sylvan.

ruse *n* artifice, deception, deceit, fraud, hoax, imposture, manoeuvre, sham, stratagem, trick, wile.

rush *vb* attack, career, charge, dash, drive, gush, hurtle, precipitate, surge, sweep, tear. • *n* dash, onrush, onset, plunge, precipitance, precipitancy, rout, stampede, tear.

rust *vb* corrode, decay, degenerate. • *n* blight, corrosion, crust, mildew, must, mould, mustiness.

rustic *adj* country, rural; awkward, boorish, clownish, countrified, loutish, outlandish, rough, rude, uncouth, unpolished, untaught; coarse, countrified, homely, plain, simple, unadorned; artless, honest, unsophisticated. • *n* boor, bumpkin, clown, countryman, peasant, swain, yokel.

ruthless *adj* barbarous, cruel, fell, ferocious, hardhearted, inexorable, inhuman, merciless, pitiless, relentless, remorseless, savage, truculent, uncompassionate, unmerciful, unpitying, unrelenting, unsparing.

S

sable *adj* black, dark, dusky, ebony, sombre.

sabulous *adj* gritty, sabulose, sandy.

sack[1] *n* bag, pouch.

sack[2] *vb* despoil, devastate, pillage, plunder, ravage, spoil. • *n* desolation, despoliation, destruction, devastation, havoc, ravage, sacking, spoliation, waste; booty, plunder, spoil.

sacred *adj* consecrated, dedicated, devoted, divine, hallowed, holy; inviolable, inviolate; sainted, venerable.

sacrifice *vb* forgo, immolate, surrender. • *n* immolation, oblation, offering; destruction, devotion, loss, surrender.

sacrilege *n* desecration, profanation, violation.

sacrilegious *adj* desecrating, impious, irreverent, profane.

sad *adj* grave, pensive, sedate, serious, sober, sombre, staid.

saddle *vb* burden, charge, clog, encumber, load.

sadly *adv* grievously, miserable, mournfully, sorrowfully; afflictively, badly, calamitously; darkly; gravely, seriously, soberly.

sadness *n* dejection, depression, despondency, melancholy, mournful, sorrow, sorrowfulness; dolefulness, gloominess, grief, mournfulness, sorrow; gravity, sedateness, seriousness.

safe *adj* undamaged, unharmed, unhurt, unscathed; guarded, protected, secure, snug, unexposed; certain, dependable, reliable, sure, trustworthy; good, harmless, sound, whole. • *n* chest, coffer, strongbox.

safeguard *vb* guard, protect. • *n* defence, protection, security; convoy, escort, guard, safe-conduct; pass, passport.

sagacious *adj* acute, apt, astute, clear-sighted, discerning, intelligent, judicious, keen, penetrating, perspicacious, rational, sage, sharp-witted, wise, shrewd.

sagacity *n* acuteness, astuteness, discernment, ingenuity, insight, penetration, perspicacity, quickness, readiness, sense, sharpness, shrewdness, wisdom.

sage *adj* acute, discerning, intelligent, prudent, sagacious, sapient, sensible, shrewd, wise; judicious, well-judged; grave, serious, solemn. • *n* philosopher, pundit, savant.

sailor *n* mariner, navigator, salt, seafarer, seaman, tar.

saintly *adj* devout, godly, holy, pious, religious.

sake *n* end, cause, purpose, reason; account, consideration, interest, regard, respect, score.

saleable *adj* marketable, merchantable, vendible.

salacious *adj* carnal, concupiscent, incontinent, lascivious, lecherous, lewd, libidinous, loose, lustful, prurient, unchaste, wanton.

salary *n* allowance, hire, pay, stipend, wages.

salient *adj* bounding, jumping, leaping; beating, springing, throbbing; jutting, projecting, prominent; conspicuous, remarkable, striking.

saline *adj* briny, salty.

sally *vb* issue, rush. • *n* digression, excursion, sortie, run, trip; escapade, frolic; crank, fancy, jest, joke, quip, quirk, sprightly, witticism.

salt *adj* saline, salted, salty; bitter, pungent, sharp. • *n* flavour, savour, seasoning, smack, relish, taste; humour, piquancy, poignancy, sarcasm, smartness, wit, zest; mariner, sailor, seaman, tar.

salubrious *adj* beneficial, benign, healthful, healthy, salutary, sanitary, wholesome.

salutary *adj* healthy, healthful, helpful, safe, salubrious, wholesome; advantageous, beneficial, good, profitable, serviceable, useful.

salute *vb* accost, address, congratulate, greet, hail, welcome. • *n* address, greeting, salutation.

salvation *n* deliverance, escape, preservation, redemption, rescue, saving.

same *adj* ditto, identical, selfsame; corresponding, like, similar.

sample *vb* savour, sip, smack, sup, taste; test, try; demonstrate, exemplify, illustrate, instance. • *adj* exemplary, illustrative, representative. • *n* demonstration, exemplification, illustration, instance, piece, specimen; example, model, pattern.

sanctify *vb* consecrate, hallow, purify; justify, ratify, sanction.

sanctimonious *adj* affected, devout, holy, hypocritical, pharisaical, pious, self-righteous.

sanction *vb* authorize, countenance, encourage, support; confirm, ratify. • *n* approval, authority, authorization, confirmation, countenance, endorsement, ratification, support, warranty; ban, boycott, embargo, penalty.

sanctity *n* devotion, godliness, goodness, grace, holiness, piety, purity, religiousness, saintliness.

sanctuary *n* altar, church, shrine, temple; asylum, protection, refuge, retreat, shelter.

sane *adj* healthy, lucid, rational, reasonable, sober, sound.

sang-froid *n* calmness, composure, coolness, imperturbability, indifference, nonchalance, phlegm, unconcern.

sanguinary *adj* bloody, gory, murderous; barbarous, bloodthirsty, cruel, fell, pitiless, savage, ruthless.

sanguine *adj* crimson, florid, red; animated, ardent, cheerful, lively, warm; buoyant, confident, enthusiastic, hopeful, optimistic; full-blooded.

sanitary *adj* clean, curative, healing, healthy, hygienic, remedial, therapeutic, wholesome.

sanity *n* normality, rationality, reason, saneness, soundness.

sapient *adj* acute, discerning, intelligent, knowing, sagacious, sage, sensible, shrewd, wise.

sarcastic *adj* acrimonious, biting, cutting, mordacious, mordant, sardonic, satirical, sharp, severe, sneering, taunting.

sardonic *adj* bitter, derisive, ironical, malevolent, malicious, malignant, sarcastic.

satanic *adj* devilish, diabolical, evil, false, fiendish, hellish, infernal, malicious.

satellite *adj* dependent, subordinate, tributary, vassal. • *n* attendant, dependant, follower, hanger-on, retainer, vassal.

satiate *vb* fill, sate, satisfy, suffice; cloy, glut, gorge, overfeed, overfill, pall, surfeit.

satire *n* burlesque, diatribe, invective, fling, irony, lampoon, pasquinade, philippic, ridicule, sarcasm, skit, squib.

satirical *adj* abusive, biting, bitter, censorious, cutting, invective, ironical, keen, mordacious, poignant, reproachful, sarcastic, severe, sharp, taunting.

satirize *vb* abuse, censure, lampoon, ridicule.

satisfaction *n* comfort, complacency, contentment, ease, enjoyment, gratification, pleasure, satiety; amends, appeasement, atonement, compensation, indemnification, recompense, redress, remuneration, reparation, requital, reward.

satisfactory *adj* adequate, conclusive, convincing, decisive, sufficient; gratifying, pleasing.

satisfy *vb* appease, content, fill, gratify, please, sate, satiate, suffice; indemnify, compensate, liquidate, pay, recompense, remunerate, requite; discharge, settle; assure, convince, persuade; answer, fulfil, meet.

saturate *vb* drench, fill, fit, imbue, soak, steep, wet.

saturnine *adj* dark, dull, gloomy, grave, heavy, leaden, morose, phlegmatic, sad, sedate, sombre; melancholic, mournful, serious, unhappy; mischievous, naughty, troublesome, vexatious, wicked.

sauce *n* cheekiness, impudence, insolence; appetizer, compound, condiment, relish, seasoning.

saucy *adj* bold, cavalier, disrespectful, flippant, forward, immodest, impertinent, impudent, insolent, pert, rude.

saunter *vb* amble, dawdle, delay, dilly-dally, lag, linger, loiter, lounge, stroll, tarry. • *n* amble, stroll, walk.

savage *vb* attack, lacerate, mangle, maul. • *adj* rough, uncultivated, wild; rude, uncivilized, unpolished, untaught; bloodthirsty, feral, ferine, ferocious, fierce, rapacious, untamed, vicious; beastly, bestial, brutal, brutish, inhuman; atrocious, barbarous, barbaric, bloody, brutal, cruel, fell, fiendish, hardhearted, heathenish, merciless, murderous, pitiless, relentless, ruthless, sanguinary, truculent; native, rough, rugged. • *n* barbarian, brute, heathen, vandal.

save *vb* keep, liberate, preserve, rescue; salvage, recover, redeem; economize, gather, hoard, husband, reserve, store; hinder, obviate, prevent, spare. • *prep* but, deducting, except.

saviour *n* defender, deliverer, guardian, protector, preserver, rescuer, saver.

savour *vb* affect, appreciate, enjoy, like, partake, relish; flavour, season. • *n* flavour, gusto, relish, smack, taste; fragrance, odour, smell, scent.

savoury *adj* agreeable, delicious, flavourful, luscious, nice, palatable, piquant, relishing.

saw *n* adage, aphorism, apothegm, axiom, byword, dictum, maxim, precept, proverb, sententious saying.

say *vb* declare, express, pronounce, speak, tell, utter; affirm, allege, argue; recite, rehearse, repeat; assume, presume, suppose. • *n* affirmation, declaration, speech, statement; decision, voice, vote.

saying *n* declaration, expression, observation, remark, speech, statement; adage, aphorism, byword, dictum, maxim, proverb, saw.

scale[1] *n* basin, dish, pan; balance.

scale[2] *n* flake, lamina, lamella, layer, plate.

scale[3] *vb* ascend, climb, escalate, mount. • *n* graduation.

scamp *n* cheat, knave, rascal, rogue, scapegrace, scoundrel, swindler, trickster, villain.

scamper *vb* haste, hasten, hie, run, scud, speed, trip.

scan *vb* examine, investigate, scrutinize, search, sift.

scandal *vb* asperse, defame, libel, traduce. • *n* aspersion, calumny, defamation, obloquy, reproach; discredit, disgrace, dishonour, disrepute, ignominy, infamy, odium, opprobrium, offence, shame.

scandalize *vb* offend; asperse, backbite, calumniate, decry, defame, disgust, lampoon, libel, reproach, revile, satirize, slander, traduce, vilify.

scandalous *adj* defamatory, libellous, opprobrious, slanderous; atrocious, disgraceful, disreputable, infamous, inglorious, ignominious, odious, shameful.

scanty *adj* insufficient, meagre, narrow, scant, small; hardly, scarce, short, slender; niggardly, parsimonious, penurious, scrimpy, skimpy, sparing.

scar[1] *vb* hurt, mark, wound. • *n* cicatrice, cicatrix, seam; blemish, defect, disfigurement, flaw, injury, mark.

scar[2] *n* bluff, cliff, crag, precipice.

scarce *adj* deficient, wanting; infrequent, rare, uncommon. • *adv* barely, hardly, scantily.

scarcely *adv* barely, hardly, scantily.

scarcity *n* dearth, deficiency, insufficiency, lack, want; infrequency, rareness, rarity, uncommonness.

scare *vb* affright, alarm, appal, daunt, fright, frighten, intimidate, shock, startle, terrify. • *n* alarm, fright, panic, shock, terror.

scathe *vb* blast, damage, destroy, injure, harm, haste. • *n* damage, harm, injury, mischief, waste.

scatter *vb* broadcast, sprinkle, strew; diffuse, disperse, disseminate, dissipate, distribute, separate, spread; disappoint, dispel, frustrate, overthrow.

scene *n* display, exhibition, pageant, representation, show, sight, spectacle, view; place, situation, spot; arena, stage.

scent *vb* breathe in, inhale, nose, smell, sniff; detect, smell out, sniff out; aromatize, perfume. • *n* aroma, balminess, fragrance, odour, perfume, smell, redolence.

sceptic *n* doubter, freethinker, questioner, unbeliever.

sceptical *adj* doubtful, doubting, dubious, hesitating, incredulous, questioning, unbelieving.

scepticism *n* doubt, dubiety, freethinking, incredulity, unbelief.

schedule *vb* line up, list, plan, programme, tabulate. • *n* document, scroll; catalogue, inventory, list, plan, record, register, roll, table, timetable.

scheme *vb* contrive, design, frame, imagine, plan, plot, project. • *n* plan, system, theory; cabal, conspiracy, contrivance, design, device, intrigue, machination, plan, plot, project, stratagem; arrangement, draught, diagram, outline.

schism *n* division, separation, split; discord, disunion, division, faction, separation.

scholar *n* disciple, learner, pupil, student; don, fellow, intellectual, pedant, savant.

scholarship *n* accomplishments, acquirements, attainments, erudition, knowledge, learning; bursary, exhibition, foundation, grant, maintenance.

scholastic *adj* academic, bookish, lettered, literary; formal, pedantic.

school *vb* drill, educate, exercise, indoctrinate, instruct, teach, train; admonish, control, chide, discipline, govern, reprove, tutor. • *adj* academic, collegiate, institutional, scholastic, schoolish. • *n* academy, college, gymnasium, institute, institution, kindergarten, lyceum, manège, polytechnic, seminary, university; adherents, camarilla, circle, clique, coterie, disciples, followers; body, order, organization, party, sect.

schooling *n* discipline, education, instruction, nurture, teaching, training, tuition.

scintillate *vb* coruscate, flash, gleam, glisten, glitter, sparkle, twinkle.

scoff *vb* deride, flout, jeer, mock, ridicule, taunt; gibe, sneer. • *n* flout, gibe, jeer, sneer, mockery, taunt; derision, ridicule.

scold *vb* berate, blame, censure, chide, rate, reprimand, reprove; brawl, rail, rate, reprimand, upbraid, vituperate. • *n* shrew, termagant, virago, vixen.

scope *n* aim, design, drift, end, intent, intention, mark, object, purpose, tendency, view; amplitude, field, latitude, liberty, margin, opportunity, purview, range, room, space, sphere, vent; extent, length, span, stretch, sweep.

scorch *vb* blister, burn, char, parch, roast, sear, shrivel, singe.

score *vb* cut, furrow, mark, notch, scratch; charge, note, record; impute, note; enter, register. • *n* incision, mark, notch; account, bill, charge, debt, reckoning; consideration, ground, motive, reason.

scorn *vb* condemn, despise, disregard, disdain, scout, slight, spurn. • *n* contempt, derision, disdain, mockery, slight, sneer; scoff.

scornful *adj* contemptuous, defiant, disdainful, contemptuous, regardless.

scot-free *adj* untaxed; clear, unhurt, uninjured, safe.

scoundrel *n* cheat, knave, miscreant, rascal, reprobate, rogue, scamp, swindler, trickster, villain.

scour[1] *vb* brighten, buff, burnish, clean, cleanse, polish, purge, scrape, scrub, rub, wash, whiten; rake; efface, obliterate, overrun.

scour[2] *vb* career, course, range, scamper, scud, scuttle; comb, hunt, rake, ransack, rifle, rummage, search.

scourge *vb* lash, whip; afflict, chasten, chastise, correct, punish; harass, torment. • *n* cord, cowhide, lash, strap, thong, whip; affliction, bane, curse, infliction, nuisance, pest, plague, punishment.

scout *vb* contemn, deride, disdain, despise, ridicule, scoff, scorn, sneer, spurn; investigate, probe, search. • *n* escort, lookout, precursor, vanguard.

scowl *vb* frown, glower, lower. • *n* frown, glower, lower.

scraggy *adj* broken, craggy, rough, rugged, scabrous, scragged, uneven; attenuated, bony, emaciated, gaunt, lank, lean, meagre, scrawny, skinny, thin.

scrap[1] *vb* discard, junk, trash. • *n* bit, fragment, modicum, particle, piece, snippet; bite, crumb, morsel, mouthful; debris, junk, litter, rubbish, rubble, trash, waste.

scrap[2] *vb* altercate, bicker, dispute, clash, fight, hassle, quarrel, row, spat, squabble, tiff, tussle, wrangle. • *n* affray, altercation, bickering, clash, dispute, fight, fray, hassle, melee, quarrel, row, run-in, set-to, spat, squabble, tiff, tussle, wrangle.

scrape *vb* bark, grind, rasp, scuff; accumulate, acquire, collect, gather, save; erase, remove. • *n* difficulty, distress, embarrassment, perplexity, predicament.

scream *vb* screech, shriek, squall, ululate. • *n* cry, outcry, screech, shriek, shrill, ululation.

screen *vb* cloak, conceal, cover, defend, fence, hide, mask, protect, shelter, shroud. • *n* blind, curtain, lattice, partition; defence, guard, protection, shield; cloak, cover, veil, disguise; riddle, sieve.

screw *vb* force, press, pressurize, squeeze, tighten, twist, wrench; oppress, rack; distort. • *n* extortioner, extortionist, miser, scrimp, skinflint; prison guard; sexual intercourse.

scrimmage *n* brawl, melee, riot, scuffle, skirmish.

scrimp *vb* contract, curtail, limit, pinch, reduce, scant, shorten, straiten.

scrimpy *adj* contracted, deficient, narrow, scanty.

scroll *n* inventory, list, parchment, roll, schedule.

scrub[1] *adj* contemptible, inferior, mean, niggardly, scrubby, shabby, small, stunted. • *n* brushwood, underbrush, underwood.

scrub[2] *vb* clean, cleanse, rub, scour, scrape, wash.

scruple *vb* boggle, demur, falter, hesitate, object, pause, stickle, waver. • *n* delicacy, hesitancy, hesitation, nicety, perplexity, qualm.

scrupulous *adj* conscientious, fastidious, nice, precise, punctilious, rigorous, strict; careful, cautious, circumspect, exact, vigilant.

scrutinize *vb* canvass, dissect, examine, explore, investigate, overhaul, probe, search, sift, study.

scrutiny *n* examination, exploration, inquisition, inspection, investigation, search, searching, sifting.

scud *vb* flee, fly, haste, hasten, hie, post, run, scamper, speed, trip.

scuffle *vb* contend, fight, strive, struggle. • *n* altercation, brawl, broil, contest, encounter, fight, fray, quarrel, squabble, struggle, wrangle.

sculpt *vb* carve, chisel, cut, sculpture; engrave, grave.

scurrilous *adj* abusive, blackguardly, contumelious, foul, foul-mouthed, indecent, infamous, insolent, insulting, offensive, opprobrious, reproachful, ribald, vituperative; coarse, gross, low, mean, obscene, vile, vulgar.

scurry *vb* bustle, dash, hasten, hurry, scamper, scud, scutter. • *n* burst, bustle, dash, flurry, haste, hurry, scamper, scud, spurt.

scurvy *adj* scabbed, scabby, scurfy; abject, bad, base, contemptible, despicable, low, mean, pitiful, sorry, vile, vulgar, worthless; malicious, mischievous, offensive.

scuttle[1] *vb* hurry, hustle, run, rush, scamper, scramble, scud, scurry. • *n* dash, drive, flurry, haste, hurry, hustle, race, rush, scamper, scramble, scud, scurry.

scuttle[2] *vb* capsize, founder, go down, sink, overturn, upset. • *n* hatch, hatchway.

seal *vb* close, fasten, secure; attest, authenticate, confirm, establish, ratify, sanction; confine, enclose, imprison. • *n* fastening, stamp, wafer, wax; assurance, attestation, authentication, confirmation, pledge, ratification.

seamy *adj* disreputable, nasty, seedy, sordid, unpleasant.

sear *vb* blight, brand, cauterize, dry, scorch, wither. • *adj* dried up, dry, sere, withered.

search *vb* examine, explore, ferret, inspect, investigate, overhaul, probe, ransack, scrutinize, sift; delve, hunt, forage, inquire, look, rummage. • *n* examination, exploration, hunt, inquiry, inspection, investigation, pursuit, quest, research, seeking, scrutiny.

searching *adj* close, keen, penetrating, trying; examining, exploring, inquiring, investigating, probing, seeking.

seared *adj* callous, graceless, hardened, impenitent, incorrigible, obdurate, shameless, unrepentant.

season *vb* acclimatize, accustom, form, habituate, harden, inure, mature, qualify, temper, train; flavour, spice. • *n* interval, period, spell, term, time, while.

seasonable *adj* appropriate, convenient, fit, opportune, suitable, timely.

seasoning *n* condiment, flavouring, relish, salt, sauce.

seat *vb* establish, fix, locate, place, set, station. • *n* place, site, situation, station; abode, capital, dwelling, house, mansion, residence; bottom, fundament; bench, chair, pew, settle, stall, stool.

secede *vb* apostatize, resign, retire, withdraw.

secluded *adj* close, covert, embowered, isolated, private, removed, retired, screened, sequestrated, withdrawn.

seclusion *n* obscurity, privacy, retirement, secrecy, separation, solitude, withdrawal.

second[1] *n* instant, jiffy, minute, moment, trice.

second[2] *vb* abet, advance, aid, assist, back, encourage, forward, further, help, promote, support, sustain; approve, favour. • *adj* inferior, second-rate, secondary; following, next, subsequent; additional, extra, other; double, duplicate. • *n* another, other; assistant, backer, supporter.

secondary *adj* collateral, inferior, minor, subsidiary, subordinate. • *n* delegate, deputy, proxy.

secrecy *n* clandestineness, concealment, furtiveness, stealth, surreptitiousness.

secret *adj* close, concealed, covered, covert, cryptic, hid, hidden, mysterious, privy, shrouded, veiled, unknown, unrevealed, unseen; cabbalistic, clandestine, furtive, privy, sly, stealthy, surreptitious, underhand; confidential, private, retired, secluded, unseen; abstruse, latent, mysterious, obscure, occult recondite, unknown. • *n* confidence, enigma, key, mystery.

secretary *n* clerk, scribe, writer; escritoire, writing-desk.

secrete[1] *vb* bury, cache, conceal, disguise, hide, shroud, stash; screen, separate.

secrete[2] *vb* discharge, emit, excrete, exude, release, secern.

secretive *adj* cautious, close, reserved, reticent, taciturn, uncommunicative, wary.

sect *n* denomination, faction, schism, school.

section *n* cutting, division, fraction, part, piece, portion, segment, slice.

secular *adj* civil, laic, laical, lay, profane, temporal, worldly.

secure *vb* guard, protect, safeguard; assure, ensure, guarantee, insure; fasten; acquire, gain, get, obtain, procure. • *adj* assured, certain, confident, sure; insured, protected, safe; fast, firm, fixed, immovable, stable; careless, easy, undisturbed, unsuspecting; heedless, inattentive, incautious, negligent, overconfident.

security *n* bulwark, defence, guard, palladium, protection, safeguard, safety, shelter; bond, collateral, deposit, guarantee, pawn, pledge, stake, surety, warranty; carelessness, heedlessness, overconfidence, negligence; assurance, assuredness, certainty, confidence, ease

sedate *adj* calm, collected, composed, contemplative, cool, demure, grave, placid, philosophical, quiet, serene, serious, sober, still, thoughtful, tranquil, undisturbed, unemotional, unruffled.

sedative *adj* allaying, anodyne, assuasive, balmy, calming, composing, demulcent, lenient, lenitive, soothing, tranquillizing. • *n* anaesthetic, anodyne, hypnotic, narcotic, opiate.

sedentary *adj* inactive, motionless, sluggish, torpid.

sediment *n* dregs, grounds, lees, precipitate, residue, residuum, settlings.

sedition *n* insurgence, insurrection, mutiny, rebellion, revolt, riot, rising, treason, tumult, uprising, uproar.

seditious *adj* factious, incendiary, insurgent, mutinous, rebellious, refractory, riotous, tumultuous, turbulent.

seduce *vb* allure, attract, betray, corrupt, debauch, deceive, decoy, deprave, ensnare, entice, inveigle, lead, mislead.

seductive *adj* alluring, attractive, enticing, tempting.

sedulous *adj* active, assiduous, busy, diligent, industrious, laborious, notable, painstaking, persevering, unremitting, untiring.

see *vb* behold, contemplate, descry, glimpse, sight, spot, survey; comprehend, conceive, distinguish, espy, know, notice, observe, perceive, recognize, remark, understand; beware, consider, envisage, regard, visualize; experience, feel, suffer; examine, inspire, notice, observe; discern, look; call on, visit.

seed *n* semen, sperm; embryo, grain, kernel, matured ovule; germ, original; children, descendants, offspring, progeny; birth, generation, race.

seedy *adj* faded, old, shabby, worn; destitute, distressed, indigent, needy, penniless, pinched, poor.

seek *vb* hunt, look, search; court, follow, prosecute, pursue, solicit; attempt, endeavour, strive, try.

seem *vb* appear, assume, look, pretend.

seeming *adj* apparent, appearing, ostensible, specious. • *n* appearance, colour, guise, look, semblance.

seemly *adj* appropriate, becoming, befitting, congruous, convenient, decent, decorous, expedient, fit, fitting, meet, proper, right, suitable; beautiful, comely, fair, good-looking, graceful, handsome, pretty, well-favoured.

seer *n* augur, diviner, foreteller, predictor, prophet, soothsayer.

segment *n* bit, division, part, piece, portion, section, sector.

segregate *vb* detach, disconnect, disperse, insulate, part, separate.

segregation *n* apartheid, discrimination, insulation, separation.

seize *vb* capture, catch, clutch, grab, grapple, grasp, grip, snatch; confiscate, impress, impound; apprehend, comprehend; arrest, take.

seldom *adv* infrequently, occasionally, rarely.

select *vb* choose, cull, pick, prefer. • *adj* choice, chosen, excellent, exquisite, good, picked, rare, selected.

selection *n* choice, election, pick, preference.

self-conscious *adj* awkward, diffident, embarrassed, insecure, nervous.

self-control *n* restraint, willpower.

self-important *adj* assuming, consequential, proud, haughty, lordly, overbearing, overweening.

selfish *adj* egoistic, egotistical, greedy, illiberal, mean, narrow, self-seeking, ungenerous.

self-possessed *adj* calm, collected, composed, cool, placid, sedate, undisturbed, unexcited, unruffled.

self-willed *adj* contumacious, dogged, headstrong, obstinate, pig-headed, stubborn, uncompliant, wilful.

sell *vb* barter, exchange, hawk, market, peddle, trade, vend.

semblance *n* likeness, resemblance, similarity; air, appearance, aspect, bearing, exterior, figure, form, mien, seeming, show; image, representation, similitude.

seminal *adj* important, original; germinal, radical, rudimental, rudimentary, unformed.

seminary *n* academy, college, gymnasium, high school, institute, school, university.

send *vb* cast, drive, emit, fling, hurl, impel, lance, launch, project, propel, throw, toss; delegate, depute, dispatch; forward, transmit; bestow, confer, give, grant.

senile *adj* aged, doddering, superannuated; doting, imbecile.

senior *adj* elder, older; higher.

seniority *n* eldership, precedence, priority, superiority.

sensation *n* feeling, sense, perception; excitement, impression, thrill.

sensational *adj* exciting, melodramatic, startling, thrilling.

sense *vb* appraise, appreciate, estimate, notice, observe, perceive, suspect, understand. • *n* brains, intellect, intelligence, mind, reason, understanding; appreciation, apprehension, discernment, feeling, perception, recognition, tact; connotation, idea, implication, judgment, notion, opinion, sentiment, view; import, interpretation, meaning, purport, significance; sagacity, soundness, substance, wisdom.

senseless *adj* apathetic, inert, insensate, unfeeling; absurd, foolish, ill-judged, nonsensical, silly, unmeaning, unreasonable, unwise; doltish, foolish, simple, stupid, witless, weak-minded.

sensible *adj* apprehensible, perceptible; aware, cognizant, conscious, convinced, persuaded, satisfied; discreet, intelligent, judicious, rational, reasonable, sagacious, sage, sober, sound, wise; observant, understanding; impressionable, sensitive.

sensitive *adj* perceptive, sentient; affected, impressible, impressionable, responsive, susceptible; delicate, tender, touchy.

sensual *adj* animal, bodily, carnal, voluptuous; gross, lascivious, lewd, licentious, unchaste.

sentence *vb* condemn, doom, judge. • *n* decision, determination, judgment, opinion, verdict; doctrine, dogma, opinion, tenet; condemnation, conviction, doom; period, proposition.

sententious *adj* compendious, compact, concise, didactic, laconic, pithy, pointed, succinct, terse.

sentiment *n* judgment, notion, opinion; maxim, saying; emotion, tenderness; disposition, feeling, thought.

sentimental *adj* impressible, impressionable, over-emotional, romantic, tender.

sentinel *n* guard, guardsman, patrol, picket, sentry, watchman.

separate *vb* detach, disconnect, disjoin, disunite, dissever, divide, divorce, part, sever, sunder; eliminate, remove, withdraw; cleave, open. • *adj* detached, disconnected, disjoined, disjointed, dissociated, disunited, divided, parted, severed; discrete, distinct, divorced, unconnected; alone, segregated, withdrawn.

separation *n* disjunction, disjuncture, dissociation; disconnection, disseverance, disseveration, disunion, division, divorce; analysis, decomposition.

sepulchral *adj* deep, dismal, funereal, gloomy, grave, hollow, lugubrious, melancholy, mournful, sad, sombre, woeful.

sepulchre *n* burial place, charnel house, grave, ossuary, sepulture, tomb.

sequel *n* close, conclusion, denouement, end, termination; consequence, event, issue, result, upshot.

sequence *n* following, graduation, progression, succession; arrangement, series, train.

sequestrated *adj* hidden, private, retired, secluded, unfrequented, withdrawn; seized.

seraphic *adj* angelic, celestial, heavenly, sublime; holy, pure, refined.

serene *adj* calm, collected, placid, peaceful, quiet, tranquil, sedate, undisturbed, unperturbed, unruffled; bright, calm, clear, fair, unclouded.

serenity *n* calm, calmness, collectedness, composure, coolness, imperturbability, peace, peacefulness, quiescence, sedateness, tranquillity; brightness, calmness, clearness, fairness, peace, quietness, stillness.

serf *n* bondman, servant, slave, thrall, villein.

serfdom *n* bondage, enslavement, enthralment, servitude, slavery, subjection, thraldom.

series *n* chain, concatenation, course, line, order, progression, sequence, succession, train.

serious *adj* earnest, grave, demure, pious, resolute, sedate, sober, solemn, staid, thoughtful; dangerous, great, important, momentous, weighty.

sermon *n* discourse, exhortation, homily, lecture.

serpentine *adj* anfractuous, convoluted, crooked, meandering, sinuous, spiral, tortuous, twisted, undulating, winding.

servant *n* attendant, dependant, factotum, helper, henchman, retainer, servitor, subaltern, subordinate, underling; domestic, drudge, flunky, lackey, menial, scullion, slave.

serve *vb* aid, assist, attend, help, minister, oblige, succour; advance, benefit, forward, promote; content, satisfy, supply; handle, officiate, manage, manipulate, work.

service *vb* check, maintain, overhaul, repair. • *n* labour, ministration, work; attendance, business, duty, employ, employment, office; advantage, benefit, good, gain, profit; avail, purpose, use, utility; ceremony, function, observance, rite, worship.

serviceable *adj* advantageous, available, beneficial, convenient, functional, handy, helpful, operative, profitable, useful.

servile *adj* dependent, menial; abject, base, beggarly, cringing, fawning, grovelling, low, mean, obsequious, slavish, sneaking, sycophantic, truckling.

servility *n* bondage, dependence, slavery; abjection, abjectness, baseness, fawning, meanness, obsequiousness, slavishness, sycophancy.

servitor *n* attendant, dependant, footman, lackey, retainer, servant, squire, valet, waiter.

servitude *n* bondage, enslavement, enthralment, serfdom, service, slavery, thraldom.

set[1] *vb* lay, locate, mount, place, put, stand, station; appoint, determine, establish, fix, settle; risk, stake, wager; adapt, adjust, regulate; adorn, stud, variegate; arrange, dispose, pose, post; appoint, assign, predetermine, prescribe; estimate, prize, rate, value; embarrass, perplex, pose; contrive, produce; decline, sink; congeal, concern, consolidate, harden, solidify; flow, incline, run, tend; (*with* **about**) begin, commence; (*with* **apart**) appropriate, consecrate, dedicate, devote, reserve, set aside; (*with* **aside**) abrogate, annul, omit, reject; reserve, set apart; (*with* **before**) display, exhibit; (*with* **down**) chronicle, jot down, record, register, state, write down; (*with* **forth**) display, exhibit, explain, expound, manifest, promulgate, publish, put forward, represent, show; (*with* **forward**) advance, further, promote; (*with* **free**) acquit, clear, emancipate, liberate, release; (*with* **off**) adorn, decorate, embellish; define, portion off; (*with* **on**) actuate, encourage, impel, influence, incite, instigate, prompt, spur, urge; attack, assault, set upon; (*with* **out**) display, issue, publish, proclaim, prove, recommend, show; (*with* **right**) correct, put in order; (*with* **to rights**) adjust, regulate; (*with* **up**) elevate, erect, exalt, raise; establish, found, institute; (*with* **upon**) assail, assault, attack, fly at, rush upon. • *adj* appointed, established, formal, ordained, prescribed, regular, settled; determined, fixed, firm, obstinate, positive, stiff, unyielding; immovable, predetermined; located, placed, put. • *n* attitude, position, posture; scene, scenery, setting.

set[2] *n* assortment, collection, suit; class, circle, clique, cluster, company, coterie, division, gang, group, knot, party, school, sect.

setback *n* blow, hitch, hold-up, rebuff; defeat, disappointment, reverse.

set-off *n* adornment, decoration, embellishment, ornament; counterbalance, counterclaim, equivalent.

settle *vb* adjust, arrange, compose, regulate; account, balance, close up, conclude, discharge, liquidate, pay, pay up, reckon, satisfy, square; allay, calm, compose, pacify, quiet, repose, rest, still, tranquillize; confirm, decide, determine, make clear; establish, fix, set; fall, gravitate, sink, subside; abide, colonize, domicile, dwell, establish, inhabit, people, place, plant, reside; (*with* **on**) determine on, fix on, fix upon; establish. • *n* bench, seat, stool.

settled *adj* established, fixed, stable; decided, deep-rooted, steady, unchanging; adjusted, arranged; methodical, orderly, quiet; common, customary, everyday, ordinary, usual, wonted.

set-to *n* combat, conflict, contest, fight.

sever *vb* divide, part, rend, separate, sunder; detach, disconnect, disjoin, disunite.

several *adj* individual, single, particular; distinct, exclusive, independent, separate; different, divers, diverse, manifold, many, sundry, various.

severance *n* partition, separation.

severe *adj* austere, bitter, dour, hard, harsh, inexorable, morose, painful, relentless, rigid, rigorous, rough, sharp, stern, stiff, strait-laced, unmitigated, unrelenting, unsparing; accurate, exact, methodical, strict; chaste, plain, restrained, simple, unadorned; biting, caustic, cruel, cutting, harsh, keen, sarcastic, satirical, trenchant; acute, afflictive, distressing, excruciating, extreme, intense, stringent, violent; critical, exact.

severity *n* austerity, gravity, harshness, rigour, seriousness, sternness, strictness; accuracy, exactness, niceness; chasteness, plainness, simplicity; acrimony, causticity, keenness, sharpness; afflictiveness, extremity, keenness, stringency, violence; cruelty.

sew *vb* baste, bind, hem, stitch, tack.

sex *n* gender, femininity, masculinity, sexuality; coitus, copulation, fornication, love-making.

shabby *adj* faded, mean, poor, ragged, seedy, threadbare, worn, worn-out; beggarly, mean, paltry, penurious, stingy, ungentlemanly, unhandsome.

shackle *vb* chain, fetter, gyve, hamper, manacle; bind, clog, confine, cumber, embarrass, encumber, impede, obstruct, restrict, trammel. • *n* chain, fetter, gyve, hamper, manacle.

shade *vb* cloud, darken, dim, eclipse, obfuscate, obscure; cover, ensconce, hide, protect, screen, shelter. • *n* darkness, dusk, duskiness, gloom, obscurity, shadow; cover, protection, shelter; awning, blind, curtain, screen, shutter, veil; degree, difference, kind, variety; cast, colour, complexion, dye, hue, tinge, tint, tone; apparition, ghost, manes, phantom, shadow, spectre, spirit.

shadow *vb* becloud, cloud, darken, obscure, shade; adumbrate, foreshadow, symbolize, typify; conceal, cover, hide, protect, screen, shroud. • *n* penumbra, shade, umbra, umbrage; darkness, gloom, obscurity; cover, protection, security, shelter; adumbration, foreshadowing, image, prefiguration, representation; apparition, ghost, phantom, shade, spirit; image, portrait, reflection, silhouette.

shadowy *adj* shady, umbrageous; dark, dim, gloomy, murky, obscure; ghostly, imaginary, impalpable, insubstantial, intangible, spectral, unreal, unsubstantial, visionary.

shady *adj* shadowy, umbrageous; crooked.

shaft *n* arrow, missile, weapon; handle, helve; pole, tongue; axis, spindle; pinnacle, spire; stalk, stem, trunk.

shaggy *adj* rough, rugged.

shake *vb* quake, quaver, quiver, shiver, shudder, totter, tremble; agitate, convulse, jar, jolt, stagger; daunt, frighten, intimidate; endanger, move, weaken; oscillate, vibrate, wave; move, put away, remove, throw off. • *n* agitation, concussion, flutter, jar, jolt, quaking, shaking, shivering, shock, trembling, tremor.

shaky *adj* jiggly, quaky, shaking, tottering, trembling.

shallow *adj* flimsy, foolish, frivolous, puerile, trashy, trifling, trivial; empty, ignorant, silly, slight, simple, superficial, unintelligent.

sham *vb* ape, feign, imitate, pretend; cheat, deceive, delude, dupe, impose, trick. • *adj* assumed, counterfeit, false, feigned, mock, make-believe, pretended, spurious. • *n* delusion, feint, fraud, humbug, imposition, imposture, pretence, trick.

shamble *vb* hobble, shuffle.

shambles *npl* abattoir, slaughterhouse; confusion, disorder, mess.

shame *vb* debase, degrade, discredit, disgrace, dishonour, stain, sully, taint, tarnish; abash, confound, confuse, discompose, disconcert, humble, humiliate; deride, flout, jeer, mock, ridicule, sneer. • *n* contempt, degradation, derision, discredit, disgrace, dishonour, disrepute, ignominy, infamy, obloquy, odium, opprobrium; abashment, chagrin, confusion, embarrassment, humiliation, mortification; reproach, scandal; decency, decorousness, decorum, modesty, propriety, seemliness.

shamefaced *adj* bashful, diffident, overmodest.

shameful *adj* atrocious, base, disgraceful, dishonourable, disreputable, heinous, ignominious, infamous, nefarious, opprobrious, outrageous, scandalous, vile, villainous, wicked; degrading, indecent, unbecoming.

shameless *adj* assuming, audacious, bold-faced, brazen, brazen-faced, cool, immodest, impudent, indecent, indelicate, insolent, unabashed, unblushing; abandoned, corrupt, depraved, dissolute, graceless, hardened, incorrigible, irreclaimable, lost, obdurate, profligate, reprobate, sinful, unprincipled, vicious.

shape *vb* create, form, make, produce; fashion, model, mould; adjust, direct, frame, regulate; conceive, conjure up, figure, image, imagine. • *n* appearance, aspect, fashion, figure, form, guise, make; build, cast, cut, model, mould, pattern; apparition, image.

shapeless *adj* amorphous, formless; grotesque, irregular, rude, uncouth, unsymmetrical.

shapely *adj* comely, symmetrical, trim, well-formed.

share *vb* apportion, distribute, divide, parcel out, portion, split; partake, participate; experience, receive. • *n* part, portion, quantum; allotment, allowance, contingent, deal, dividend, division, interest, lot, proportion, quantity, quota.

sharer *n* communicant, partaker, participator.

sharp *adj* acute, cutting, keen, keen-edged, knife-edged, razor-edged, trenchant; acuminate, needle-shaped, peaked, pointed, ridged; apt, astute, carny, clear-sighted, clever, cunning, discerning, discriminating, ingenious, inventive, keen-witted, penetrating, perspicacious, quick, ready, sagacious, sharp-witted, shrewd, smart, subtle, witty; acid, acrid, biting, bitter, burning, high-flavoured, high-seasoned, hot, mordacious, piquant, poignant, pungent, sour, stinging; acrimonious, biting, caustic, cutting, harsh, mordant, sarcastic, severe, tart, trenchant; cruel, hard, rigid; afflicting, distressing, excruciating, intense, painful, piercing, shooting, sore, violent; nipping, pinching; ardent, eager, fervid, fierce, fiery, impetuous, strong; high, screeching, shrill attentive, vigilant; severe; close, exacting, shrewd, cold, crisp, freezing, icy wintry. • *adv* abruptly, sharply, suddenly; exactly, precisely, punctually.

sharp-cut *adj* clear, distinct, well-defined.

sharpen *vb* edge, intensify, point.

sharper *n* cheat, deceiver, defrauder, knave, rogue, shark, swindler, trickster.

sharply *adv* rigorously, roughly, severely; acutely, keenly; vehemently, violently; accurately, exactly, minutely, trenchantly, wittily; abruptly, steeply.

sharpness *n* acuteness, keenness, trenchancy; acuity, spinosity; acumen, cleverness, discernment, ingenuity, quickness, sagacity, shrewdness, smartness, wit; acidity, acridity, piquancy, pungency, sting, tartness; causticness, incisiveness, pungency, sarcasm, satire, severity; afflictiveness, intensity, painfulness, poignancy, ardour, fierceness, violence; discordance, dissonance, highness, screechiness, squeakiness, shrillness.

sharp-sighted *adj* clear-sighted, keen, keen-eyed, keen-sighted.

sharp-witted *adj* acute, clear-sighted, cunning, discerning, ingenious, intelligent, keen, keen-sighted, long-headed, quick, sagacious, sharp, shrewd.

shatter *vb* break, burst, crack, rend, shiver, smash, splinter, split; break up, derange, disorder, overthrow.

shave *vb* crop, cut off, mow, pare; slice; graze, skim, touch.

shaver *n* boy, child, youngster; bargainer, extortioner, sharper.

shear *vb* clip, cut, fleece, strip; divest; break off.

sheath *n* case, casing, covering, envelope, scabbard, sheathing.

sheathe *vb* case, cover, encase, enclose.

shed[1] *n* cabin, cot, hovel, hut, outhouse, shack, shelter.

shed[2] *vb* effuse, let fall, pour out, spill; diffuse, emit, give out, scatter, spread; cast, let fall, put off, slough, throw off.

sheen *n* brightness, gloss, glossiness, shine, spendour.

sheep *n* ewe, lamb, ram.

sheepish *adj* bashful, diffident, overmodest, shamefaced, timid, timorous.

sheer[1] *adj* perpendicular, precipitous, steep, vertical; clear, downright, mere, pure, simple, unadulterated, unmingled, unmixed, unqualified, utter; clear; fine, transparent. • *adv* outright; perpendicularly, steeply.

sheer[2] *vb* decline, deviate, move aside, swerve. • *n* bow, curve.

shelf *n* bracket, console, ledge, mantelpiece.

shell *vb* exfoliate, fall off, peel off; bombard. • *n* carapace, case, covering, shard; bomb, grenade, sharpnel; framework.

shelter *vb* cover, defend, ensconce, harbour, hide, house, protect, screen, shield, shroud • *n* asylum, cover, covert, harbour, haven, hideaway, refuge, retreat, sanctuary; defence, protection, safety, screen, security, shield; guardian, protector.

shelve *vb* dismiss, put aside; incline, slope.

shepherd *vb* escort, guide, marshal, usher; direct, drive, drove, herd, lead; guard, tend, watch over. • *n* drover, grazier, herder, herdsman; chaplain, churchman, clergyman, cleric, divine, ecclesiastic, minister, padre, parson, pastor; chaperon, duenna, escort, guide, squire, usher.

shield *vb* cover, defend, guard, protect, shelter; repel, ward off; avert, forbid, forfend • *n* aegis, buckler, escutcheon, scutcheon, targe; bulwark, cover, defence, guard, palladium, protection, rampart, safeguard, security, shelter.

shift *vb* alter, change, fluctuate, move, vary; chop, dodge, swerve, veer; contrive, devise, manage, plan, scheme, shuffle. • *n* change, substitution, turn; contrivance, expedient, means, resort, resource; artifice, craft, device, dodge, evasion, fraud, mask, ruse, stratagem, subterfuge, trick, wile; chemise, smock.

shiftless *adj* improvident, imprudent, negligent, slack, thriftless, unresourceful.

shifty *adj* tricky, undependable, wily.

shillyshally *vb* hesitate, waver. • *n* hesitation, irresolute, wavering.

shimmer *vb* flash, glimmer, glisten, shine. • *n* blink, glimmer, glitter, twinkle.

shin *vb* climb, swarm. • *n* shinbone, tibia.

shindy *n* disturbance, riot, roughhouse, row, spree, uproar.

shine *vb* beam, blaze, coruscate, flare, give light, glare, gleam, glimmer, glisten, glitter, glow, lighten, radiate, sparkle; excel. • *n* brightness, brilliancy, glaze, gloss, polish, sheen.

shining *adj* beaming, bright, brilliant, effulgent, gleaming, glowing, glistening, glittering, luminous, lustrous, radiant, resplendent, splendid; conspicuous, distinguished, illustrious.

shiny *adj* bright, clear, luminous, sunshiny, unclouded; brilliant, burnished, glassy, glossy, polished.

ship *n* boat, craft, steamer, vessel.

shipshape *adj* neat, orderly, tidy, trim, well-arranged.

shipwreck *vb* cast away, maroon, strand, wreck. • *n* demolition, destruction, miscarriage, overthrow, perdition, ruin, subversion, wreck.

shirk *vb* avoid, dodge, evade, malinger, quit, slack; cheat, shark, trick.

shiver[1] *vb* break, shatter, splinter. • *n* bit, fragment, piece, slice, sliver, splinter.

shiver[2] *vb* quake, quiver, shake, shudder, tremble. • *n* shaking, shivering, shuddering, tremor.

shivery[1] *adj* brittle, crumbly, frangible, friable, shatterable, splintery.

shivery[2] *adj* quaking, quavering, quivering, shaky, trembly, tremulous; chilly, shivering.

shoal[1] *vb* crowd, throng. • *n* crowd, horde, multitude, swarm, throng.

shoal[2] *n* sandbank, shallows; danger.

shock *vb* appall, horrify; disgust, disquiet, disturb, nauseate, offend, outrage, revolt, scandalize, sicken; astound, stagger, stun; collide with, jar, jolt, shake, strike against; encounter, meet. • *n* agitation, blow, offence, stroke, trauma; assault, brunt, conflict; clash, collision, concussion, impact, percussion.

shocking *adj* abominable, detestable, disgraceful, disgusting, execrable, foul, hateful, loathsome, obnoxious, odious, offensive, repugnant, repulsive, revolting; appalling, awful, dire, dreadful, fearful, frightful, ghastly, hideous, horrible, horrid, horrific, monstrous, terrible.

shoot *vb* catapult, expel, hurl, let fly, propel; discharge, fire, let off; dart, fly, pass, pelt; extend, jut, project, protrude, protuberate, push, put forth, send forth, stretch; bud, germinate, sprout; (*with* **up**) grow increase, spring up, run up, start up. • *n* branch, offshoot, scion, sprout, twig.

shop *n* emporium, market, mart, store; workshop.

shore[1] *n* beach, brim, coast, seabord, seaside, strand, waterside.

shore[2] *vb* brace, buttress, prop, stay, support. • *n* beam, brace, buttress, prop, stay, support.

shorn *adj* cut-off; deprived.

short *adj* brief, curtailed; direct, near, straight; compendious, concise, condensed, laconic, pithy, terse, sententious, succinct, summary; abrupt, curt, petulant, pointed, sharp, snappish, uncivil; defective, deficient, inadequate, insufficient, niggardly, scanty, scrimpy; contracted, desitute, lacking, limited, minus, wanting; dwarfish, squat, undersized; brittle, crisp, crumbling, friable. • *adv* abruptly, at once, forthwith, suddenly.

shortcoming *n* defect, deficiency, delinquency, error, failing, failure, fault, imperfection, inadequacy, remissness, slip, weakness.

shorten *vb* abbreviate, abridge, curtail, cut short; abridge, contract, diminish, lessen, retrench, reduce; cut off, dock, lop, trim; confine, hinder, restrain, restrict.

shortening *n* abbreviation, abridgment, contraction, curtailment, diminution, retrenchment, reduction.

shorthand *n* brachygraphy, stenography, tachygraphy.

short-lived *adj* emphemeral, transient, transitory.

shortly *adv* quickly, soon; briefly, concisely, succinctly, tersely.

short-sighted *adj* myopic, nearsighted, purblind; imprudent, indiscreet.

shot[1] *n* discharge; ball, bullet, missile, projectile; marksman, shooter.

shot[2] *adj* chatoyant, iridescent, irisated, moiré, watered; intermingled, interspersed, interwoven.

shoulder *vb* bear, bolster, carry, hump, maintain, pack, support, sustain, tote; crowd, elbow, jostle, press forward, push, thrust. • *n* projection, protuberance.

shoulder blade *n* blade bone, omoplate, scapula, shoulder bone.

shout *vb* bawl, cheer, clamour, exclaim, halloo, roar, vociferate, whoop, yell. • *n* cheer, clamour, exclamation, halloo, hoot, huzza, outcry, roar, vociferation, whoop, yell.

shove *vb* jostle, press against, propel, push, push aside; (*with* **off**) push away, thrust away.

show *vb* blazon, display, exhibit, flaunt, parade, present; indicate, mark, point out; disclose, discover, divulge, explain, make clear, make known, proclaim, publish, reveal, unfold; demonstrate, evidence, manifest, prove, verify; conduct, guide, usher; direct, inform, instruct, teach; expound, elucidate, interpret; (*with* **off**) display, exhibit, make a show, set off; (*with* **up**) expose. • *n* array, exhibition, representation, sight, spectacle; blazonry, bravery, ceremony, dash, demonstration, display, flourish, ostentation, pageant, pageantry, parade, pomp, splendour, splurge; likeness, resemblance, semblance; affectation, appearance, colour, illusion, mask, plausibility, pose, pretence, pretext, simulation, speciousness; entertainment, production.

showy *adj* bedizened, dressy, fine, flashy, flaunting, garish, gaudy, glaring, gorgeous, loud, ornate, smart, swanky, splendid; grand, magnificent, ostentatious, pompous, pretentious, stately, sumptuous.

shred *vb* tear. • *n* bit, fragment, piece, rag, scrap, strip, tatter.

shrew *n* brawler, fury, scold, spitfire, termagant, virago, vixen.

shrewd *adj* arch, artful, astute, crafty, cunning, Machiavellian, sly, subtle, wily; acute, astute, canny, discerning, discriminating, ingenious, keen, knowing, penetrating, sagacious, sharp, sharp-sighted.

shrewdness *n* address, archness, art, artfulness, astuteness, craft, cunning, policy, skill, slyness, subtlety; acumen, acuteness, discernment, ingenuity, keenness, penetration, perspicacity, sagacity, sharpness, wit.

shrewish *adj* brawling, clamorous, froward, peevish, petulant, scolding, vixenish.

shriek *vb* scream, screech, squeal, yell, yelp. • *n* cry, scream, screech, yell.

shrill *adj* acute, high, high-toned, high-pitched, piercing, piping, sharp.

shrine *n* reliquary, sacred tomb; altar, hallowed place, sacred place.

shrink *vb* contract, decrease, dwindle, shrivel, wither; balk, blench, draw back, flinch, give way, quail, recoil, retire, swerve, wince, withdraw.

shrivel *vb* dry, dry up, parch; contract, decrease, dwindle, shrink, wither, wrinkle.

shroud *vb* bury, cloak, conceal, cover, hide, mask, muffle, protect, screen, shelter, veil. • *n* covering, garment; grave clothes, winding sheet.

shrub *n* bush, dwarf tree, low tree.

shrubby *adj* bushy.

shudder *vb* quake, quiver, shake, shiver, tremble. • *n* shaking, shuddering, trembling, tremor.

shuffle *vb* confuse, disorder, intermix, jumble, mix, shift; cavil, dodge, equivocate, evade, prevaricate, quibble, vacillate; struggle. • *n* artifice, cavil, evasion, fraud, pretence, pretext, prevarication, quibble, ruse, shuffling, sophism, subterfuge, trick.

shun *vb* avoid, elude, eschew, escape, evade, get clear of.

shut *vb* close, close up, stop; confine, coop up, enclose, imprison, lock up, shut up; (*with* **in**) confine, enclose; (*with* **off**) bar, exclude, intercept; (*with* **up**) close up, shut; confine, enclose, fasten in, imprison, lock in, lock up.

shy *vb* cast, chuck, fling, hurl, jerk, pitch, sling, throw, toss; boggle, sheer, start aside. • *adj* bashful, coy, diffident, reserved, retiring, sheepish, shrinking, timid; cautious, chary, distrustful, heedful, wary. • *n* start; fling, throw.

sibilant *adj* buzzing, hissing, sibilous.

sick *adj* ailing, ill, indisposed, laid-up, unwell, weak; nauseated, queasy; disgusted, revolted, tired, weary; diseased, distempered, disordered, feeble, morbid, unhealthy, unsound, weak; languishing, longing, pining.

sicken *vb* ail, disease, fall sick, make sick; nauseate; disgust, weary; decay, droop, languish, pine.

sickening *adj* nauseating, nauseous, palling, sickish; disgusting, distasteful, loathsome, offensive, repulsive, revolting.

sickly *adj* ailing, diseased, faint, feeble, infirm, languid, languishing, morbid, unhealthy, valetudinary, weak, weakly.

sickness *n* ail, ailment, complaint, disease, disorder, distemper, illness, indisposition, invalidism, malady, morbidity; nausea, qualmishness, queasiness.

side *vb* border, bound, edge, flank, frontier, march, rim, skirt, verge; avert, turn aside; (*with* **with**) befriend, favour, flock to, join with, second, support. • *adj* flanking, later, skirting; indirect, oblique; extra, odd, off, spare. • *n* border, edge, flank, margin, verge; cause, faction, interest, party, sect.

sideboard *n* buffet, dresser.

side by side abreast, alongside, by the side.

sidelong *adj* lateral, oblique. • *adv* laterally, obliquely; on the side.

sidewalk *n* footpath, footway, pavement.

sideways, sidewise *adv* laterally. • *adv* athwart, crossways, crosswise, laterally, obliquely, sidelong, sidewards.

siesta *n* doze, nap.

sift *vb* part, separate; bolt, screen, winnow; analyse, canvass, discuss, examine, fathom, follow up, inquire into, investigate, probe, scrutinze, sound, try.

sigh *vb* complain, grieve, lament, mourn. • *n* long breath, sough, suspiration.

sight *vb* get sight of, perceive, see. • *n* cognizance, ken, perception, view; beholding, eyesight, seeing, vision; exhibition, prospect, representation, scene, show, spectacle, wonder; consideration, estimation, knowledge; examination, inspection.

sightless *adj* blind, eyeless, unseeing.

sightly *adj* beautiful, comely, handsome.

sign *vb* indicate, signal, signify; countersign, endorse, subscribe. • *n* emblem, index, indication, manifestation, mark, note, proof, signal, signification, symbol, symptom, token; beacon; augury, auspice, foreboding, miracle, omen, portent, presage, prodigy, prognostic, wonder; type; countersign, password.

signal *vb* flag, glance, hail, nod, nudge, salute, sign, signalize, sound, speak, touch, wave, wink. • *adj* conspicuous, eminent, extraordinary, memorable, notable, noteworthy, remarkable. • *n* cue, indication, mark, sign, token.

signalize *vb* celebrate, distinguish, make memorable.

signature *n* mark, sign, stamp; autograph, hand.

significance *n* implication, import, meaning, purport, sense; consequence, importance, moment, portent, weight; emphasis, energy, expressiveness, force, impressiveness.

significant *adj* betokening, expressive, indicative, significative, signifying; important, material, momentous, portentous, weighty; forcible, emphatic, expressive, telling.

signification *n* expression; acceptation, import, meaning, purport, sense.

signify *vb* betoken, communication, express, indicate, intimate; denote, imply, import, mean, purport, suggest; announce, declare, give notice of, impart, make known, manifest, proclaim, utter; augur, foreshadow, indicate, portend, represent; matter, weigh.

silence *vb* hush, muzzle, still; allay, calm, quiet. • *interj* be silent, be still, hush, soft, tush, tut, whist. • *n* calm, hush, lull, noiselessness, peace, quiet, quietude, soundlessness, stillness; dumbness, mumness, muteness, reticence, speechlessness, taciturnity.

silent *adj* calm, hushed, noiseless, quiet, soundless, still; dumb, inarticulate, mum, mute, nonvocal, speechless, tacit; reticent, taciturn, uncommunicative.

silken *adj* flossy, silky, soft.

silkiness *n* smoothness, softness.

silly *adj* brainless, childish, foolish, inept, senseless, shallow, simple, stupid, weak-minded, witless; absurd, extravagant, frivolous, imprudent, indiscreet, nonsensical, preposterous, trifling, unwise. • *n* ass, duffer, goose, idiot, simpleton.

silt *n* alluvium, deposit, deposition, residue, settlement, settlings, sediment.

silver *adj* argent, silvery; bright, silvery, white; clear, mellifluous, soft.

similar *adj* analogous, duplicate, like, resembling, twin; homogeneous, uniform.

similarity *n* agreement, analogy, correspondence, likeness, parallelism, parity, resemblance, sameness, semblance, similitude.

simile *n* comparison, metaphor, similitude.

similitude *n* image, likeness, resemblance; comparison, metaphor, simile.

simmer *vb* boil, bubble, seethe, stew.

simper *vb* smile, smirk.

simple *adj* bare, elementary, homogeneous, incomplex, mere, single, unalloyed, unblended, uncombined, uncompounded, unmingled, unmixed; chaste, plain, homespun, inornate, natural, neat, unadorned, unaffected, unembellished, unpretentious, unstudied, unvarnished; artless, downright, frank, guileless, inartificial, ingenuous, naive, open, simple-hearted, simple-minded, sincere, single-minded, straightforward, true, unconstrained, undesigning, unsophisticated; credulous, fatuous, foolish, shallow, silly, unwise, weak; clear, intelligible, understandable, uninvolved, unmistakable.

simple-hearted *adj* artless, frank, ingenuous, open, simple, single-hearted.

simpleton *n* fool, greenhorn, nincompoop, ninny.

simplicity *n* chasteness, homeliness, naturalness, neatness, plainness, artlessness, frankness, naivety, openness, simplesse, sincerity; clearness; gullibility, folly, silliness, weakness.

simply *adv* artlessly, plainly, sincerely, unaffectedly; barely, merely, of itself, solely; absolutely, alone.

simulate *vb* act, affect, ape, assume, counterfeit, dissemble, feign, mimic, pretend, sham.

simulation *n* counterfeiting, feigning, personation, pretence.

simultaneous *adj* coeval, coincident, concomitant, concurrent, contemporaneous, synchronous.

sin *vb* do wrong, err, transgress, trespass. • *n* delinquency, depravity, guilt, iniquity, misdeed, offence, transgression, unrighteousness, wickedness, wrong.

since *conj* as, because, considering, seeing that. • *adv* ago, before this; from that time. • *prep* after, from the time of, subsequently to.

sincere *adj* pure, unmixed; genuine, honest, inartificial, real, true, unaffected, unfeigned, unvarnished; artless, candid, direct, frank, guileless, hearty, honest, ingenuous, open, plain, single, straightforward, truthful, undissembling, upright, whole-hearted.

sincerity *n* artlessness, candour, earnestness, frankness, genuineness, guilelessness, honesty, ingenuousness, probity, truth, truthfulness, unaffectedness, veracity.

sinew *n* ligament, tendon; brawn, muscle, nerve, strength.

sinewy *adj* able-bodied, brawny, firm, Herculean, muscular, nervous, powerful, robust, stalwart, strapping, strong, sturdy, vigorous, wiry.

sinful *adj* bad, criminal, depraved, immoral, iniquitous, mischievous, peccant, transgressive, unholy, unrighteous, wicked, wrong.

sinfulness *n* corruption, criminality, depravity, iniquity, irreligion, ungodliness, unholiness, unrighteousness, wickedness.

sing *vb* cantillate, carol, chant, hum, hymn, intone, lilt, troll, warble, yodel.

singe *vb* burn, scorch, sear.

singer *n* cantor, caroler, chanter, gleeman, prima donna, minstrel, psalmodist, songster, vocalist.

single *vb* (*with* **out**) choose, pick, select, single. • *adj* alone, isolated, one only, sole, solitary; individual, particular, separate; celibate, unmarried, unwedded; pure, simple, uncompounded, unmixed; honest, ingenuous, sincere, unbiased, uncorrupt, upright.

single-handed *adj* alone, by one's self, unaided, unassisted.

single-minded *adj* artless, candid, guileless, ingenuous, sincere.

singleness *n* individuality, unity; purity, simplicity; ingenuousness, integrity, sincerity, uprightness.

singular *adj* eminent, exceptional, extraordinary, rare, remarkable, strange, uncommon, unusual, unwonted; particular, unexampled, unparalleled, unprecedented; unaccountable; bizarre, curious, eccentric, fantastic, odd, peculiar, queer; individual, single; not complex, single, uncompounded, unique.

singularity *n* aberration, abnormality, irregularity, oddness, rareness, rarity, strangeness, uncommonness; characteristic, idiosyncrasy, individuality, particularity, peculiarity; eccentricity, oddity.

sinister *adj* baleful, injurious, untoward; boding ill, inauspicious, ominous, unlucky; left, on the left hand.

sink *vb* droop, drop, fall, founder, go down, submerge, subside; enter, penetrate; collapse, fail; decay, decline, decrease, dwindle, give way, languish, lose strength; engulf, immerse, merge, submerge, submerse; dig, excavate, scoop out; abase, bring down, crush, debase, degrade, depress, diminish, lessen, lower, overbear; destroy, overthrow, overwhelm, reduce, ruin, swamp, waste. • *n* basin, cloaca, drain.

sinless *adj* faultless, guiltless, immaculate, impeccable, innocent, spotless, unblemished, undefiled, unspotted, unsullied, untarnished.

sinner *n* criminal, delinquent, evildoer, offender, reprobate, wrongdoer.

sinuosity *n* crook, curvature, flexure, sinus, tortuosity, winding.

sinuous *adj* bending, crooked, curved, curvilinear, flexuous, serpentine, sinuate, sinuated, tortuous, undulating, wavy, winding.

sip *vb* drink, suck up, sup; absorb, drink in. • *n* small draught, taste.

sire *vb* father, reproduce; author, breed, conceive, create, generate, originate, produce, propagate. • *n* father, male parent, progenitor; man, male person; sir, sirrah; author, begetter, creator, father, generator, originator.

siren *adj* alluring, bewitching, fascinating, seducing, tempting. • *n* mermaid; charmer, Circe, seducer, seductress, tempter, temptress.

sit *vb* be, remain, repose, rest, stay; bear on, lie, rest; abide, dwell, settle; perch; brood, incubate; become, be suited, fit.

site *vb* locate, place, position, situate, station. • *n* ground, locality, location, place, position, seat, situation, spot, station, whereabouts.

sitting *n* meeting, session.

situation *n* ground, locality, location, place, position, seat, site, spot, whereabouts; case, category, circumstances, condition, juncture, plight, predicament, state; employment, office, place, post, station.

size *n* amplitude, bigness, bulk, dimensions, expanse, greatness, largeness, magnitude, mass, volume.

skeleton *n* framework; draft, outline, sketch.

sketch *vb* design, draft, draw out; delineate, depict, paint, portray, represent. • *n* delineation, design, draft, drawing, outline, plan, skeleton.

sketchy *adj* crude, incomplete, unfinished.

skilful *adj* able, accomplished, adept, adroit, apt, clever, competent, conversant, cunning, deft, dexterous, dextrous, expert, handy, ingenious, masterly, practised, proficient, qualified, quick, ready, skilled, trained, versed, well-versed.

skill *n* ability, address, adroitness, aptitude, aptness, art, cleverness, deftness, dexterity, expertise, expertness, facility, ingenuity, knack, quickness, readiness, skilfulness; discernment, discrimination, knowledge, understanding, wit.

skim *vb* brush, glance, graze, kiss, scrape, scratch, sweep, touch lightly; coast, flow, fly, glide, sail, scud, whisk; dip into, glance at, scan, skip, thumb over, touch upon.

skin *vb* pare, peel; decorticate, excoriate, flay. • *n* cuticle, cutis, derm, epidermis, hide, integument, pellicle, pelt; hull, husk, peel, rind.

skinflint *n* churl, curmudgeon, lickpenny, miser, niggard, scrimp.

skinny *adj* emaciated, lank, lean, poor, shrivelled, shrunk, thin.

skip *vb* bound, caper, frisk, gambol, hop, jump, leap, spring; disregard, intermit, miss, neglect, omit, pass over, skim. • *n* bound, caper, frisk, gambol, hop, jump, leap, spring.

skirmish *vb* battle, brush, collide, combat, contest, fight, scuffle, tussle. • *n* affair, affray, battle, brush, collision, combat, conflict, contest, encounter, fight, scuffle, tussle.

skirt *vb* border, bound, edge, fringe, hem, march, rim; circumnavigate, circumvent, flank, go along. • *n* border, boundary, edge, margin, rim, verge; flap, kilt, overskirt, petticoat.

skittish *adj* changeable, fickle, inconstant; hasty, volatile, wanton; shy, timid, timorous.

skulk *vb* hide, lurk, slink, sneak.

skulker *n* lurker, sneak; shirk, slacker, malingerer.

skull *n* brain pan, cranium.

sky *n* empyrean, firmament, heaven, heavens, welkin.

sky-blue *adj* azure, cerulean, sapphire, sky-coloured.

skylarking *n* carousing, frolicking, sporting.

slab *adj* slimy, thick, viscous. • *n* beam, board, layer, panel, plank, slat, table, tablet; mire, mud, puddle, slime.

slabber *vb* drivel, slaver, slobber; drop, let fall, shed, spill.

slack *vb* ease off, let up; abate, ease up, relax, slacken; malinger, shirk; choke, damp, extinguish, smother, stifle. • *adj* backward, careless, inattentive, lax, negligent, remiss; abated, dilatory, diminished, lingering, slow, tardy; loose, relaxed; dull, idle, inactive, quiet, sluggish. • *n* excess, leeway, looseness, play; coal dust, culm, residue.

slacken *vb* abate, diminish, lessen, lower, mitigate, moderate, neglect, remit, relieve, retard, slack; loosen, relax; flag, slow down; bridle, check, control, curb, repress, restrain.

slackness *n* looseness; inattention, negligence, remissness; slowness, tardiness.

slander *vb* asperse, backbite, belie, brand, calumniate, decry, defame, libel, malign, reproach, scandalize, traduce, vilify; detract from, disparage. • *n* aspersion, backbiting, calumny, defamation, detraction, libel, obloquy, scandal, vilification.

slanderous *adj* calumnious, defamatory, false, libellous, malicious, maligning.

slang *n* argo, cant, jargon, lingo.

slant *vb* incline, lean, lie obliquely, list, slope. • *n* inclination, slope, steep, tilt.

slap *vb* dab, clap, pat, smack, spank, strike. • *adv* instantly, quickly, plumply. • *n* blow, clap.

slapdash *adv* haphazardly, hurriedly, precipitately.

slash *vb* cut, gash, slit. • *n* cut, gash, slit.

slashed *adj* cut, slit; (*bot*) jagged, laciniate, multifid.

slattern *adj* slatternly, slovenly, sluttish. • *n* drab, slut, sloven, trollop.

slatternly *adj* dirty, slattern, slovenly, sluttish, unclean, untidy. • *adv* carelessly, negligently, sluttishly.

slaughter *vb* butcher, kill, massacre, murder, slay. • *n* bloodshed, butchery, carnage, havoc, killing, massacre, murder, slaying.

slaughterer *n* assassin, butcher, cutthroat, destroyer, killer, murderer, slayer.

slave *vb* drudge, moil, toil. • *n* bondmaid, bondservant, bondslave, bondman, captive, dependant, henchman, helot, peon, serf, thrall, vassal, villein; drudge, menial.

slavery *n* bondage, bond-service, captivity, enslavement, enthralment, serfdom, servitude, thraldom, vassalage, villeinage; drudgery, mean labour.

slavish *adj* abject, beggarly, base, cringing, fawning, grovelling, low, mean, obsequious, servile, sycophantic; drudging, laborious, menial, servile.

slay *vb* assassinate, butcher, dispatch, kill, massacre, murder, slaughter; destroy, ruin.

slayer *n* assassin, destroyer, killer, murderer, slaughterer.

sledge *n* drag, sled; cutter, pung, sleigh.

sleek *adj* glossy, satin, silken, silky, smooth.

sleekly *adv* evenly, glossily, nicely, smoothly.

sleep *vb* catnap, doze, drowse, nap, slumber. • *n* dormancy, hypnosis, lethargy, repose, rest, slumber.

sleeping *adj* dormant, inactive, quiescent.

sleepwalker *n* night-walker, noctambulist, somnambulist.

sleepwalking *n* somnambulism.

sleepy *adj* comatose, dozy, drowsy, heavy, lethargic, nodding, somnolent; narcotic, opiate, slumberous, somniferous, somnific, soporiferous, soporific; dull, heavy, inactive, lazy, slow, sluggish, torpid.

sleight *n* adroitness, dexterity, manoeuvring.

sleight of hand *n* conjuring, hocus-pocus, jugglery, legerdemain, prestdigitation.

slender *adj* lank, lithe, narrow, skinny, slim, spindly, thin; feeble, fine, flimsy, fragile, slight, tenuous, weak; inconsiderable, moderate, small, trivial; exiguous, inadequate, insufficient, lean, meagre, pitiful, scanty; abstemious, light, simple, spare, sparing.

slice *vb* cut, divide, part, section; cut off, sever. • *n* chop, collop, piece.

slick *adj* glassy, glossy, polished, sleek, smooth; alert, clever, cunning, shrewd, slippery, unctuous. *vb* burnish, gloss, lacquer, polish, shine, sleek, varnish; grease, lubricate, oil.

slide *vb* glide, move smoothly, slip. • *n* glide, glissade, skid, slip.

sliding *adj* gliding, slippery, uncertain. • *n* backsliding, falling, fault, lapse, transgression.

slight *vb* cold-shoulder, disdain, disregard, neglect, snub; overlook; scamp, skimp, slur. • *adj* inconsiderable, insignificant, little, paltry, petty, small, trifling, trivial, unimportant, unsubstantial; delicate, feeble, frail, gentle, weak; careless, cursory, desultory, hasty, hurried, negligent, scanty, superficial; flimsy, perishable; slender, slim. • *n* discourtesy, disregard, disrespect, inattention, indignity, neglect.

slightingly *adv* contemptuously, disrespectfully, scornfully, slightly.

slightly *adv* inconsiderably, little, somewhat; feebly, slenderly, weakly; cursorily, hastily, negligently, superficially.

slim *vb* bant, diet, lose weight, reduce, slenderize. • *adj* gaunt, lank, lithe, narrow, skinny, slender, spare; inconsiderable, paltry, poor, slight, trifling, trivial, unsubstantial, weak; insufficient, meagre.

slime *n* mire, mud, ooze, sludge.

slimy *adj* miry, muddy, oozy; clammy, gelatinous, glutinous, gummy, lubricious, mucilaginous, mucous, ropy, slabby, viscid, viscous.

sling *vb* cast, fling, hurl, throw; hang up, suspend.

slink *vb* skulk, slip away, sneak, steal away.

slip *vb* glide, slide; err, mistake, trip; lose, omit; disengage, throw off; escape, let go, loose, loosen, release, . • *n* glide, slide, slipping; blunder, lapse, misstep, mistake, oversight, peccadillo, trip; backsliding, error, fault, impropriety, indiscretion, transgression; desertion, escape; cord, leash, strap, string; case, covering, wrapper.

slippery *adj* glib, slithery, smooth; changeable, insecure, mutable, perilous, shaky, uncertain, unsafe, unstable, unsteady; cunning, dishonest, elusive, faithless, false, knavish, perfidious, shifty, treacherous.

slipshod *adj* careless, shuffling, slovenly, untidy.

slit *vb* cut; divide, rend, slash, split, sunder. • *n* cut, gash.

slobber *vb* drivel, drool, slabber, slaver; daub, obscure, smear, stain.

slobbery *adj* dank, floody, moist, muddy, sloppy, wet.

slope *vb* incline, slant, tilt. • *n* acclivity, cant, declivity, glacis, grade, gradient, incline, inclination, obliquity, pitch, ramp.

sloping *adj* aslant, bevelled, declivitous, inclining, oblique, shelving, slanting.

sloppy *adj* muddy, plashy, slabby, slobbery, splashy, wet.

sloth *n* dilatoriness, slowness, tardiness; idleness, inaction, inactivity, indolence, inertness, laziness, lumpishness, slothfulness, sluggishness, supineness, torpor.

slothful *adj* dronish, idle, inactive, indolent, inert, lazy, lumpish, slack, sluggish, supine, torpid.

slouch *vb* droop, loll, slump; shamble, shuffle. • *n* malingerer, shirker, slacker; shamble, shuffle, stoop.

slouching *adj* awkward, clownish, loutish, lubberly, uncouth, ungainly.

slough[1] *n* bog, fen, marsh, morass, quagmire; dejection, depression, despondence, despondency.

slough[2] *vb* cast, desquamate, excuviate, moult, shed, throw off; cast off, discard, divest, jettison, reject. • *n* cast, desquamation.

sloven *n* slattern, slob, slouch, slut.

slovenly *adj* unclean, untidy; blowsy, disorderly, dowcy, frowsy, loose, slatternly, tacky, unkempt, untidy; careless, heedless, lazy, negligent, perfunctory.

slow *vb* abate, brake, check, decelerate, diminish, lessen, mitigate, moderate, modulate, reduce, weaken; delay,detain, retard; ease, ease up, relax, slack, slacken, slack off. • *adj* deliberate, gradual; dead, dull, heavy, inactive, inert, sluggish, stupid; behindhand, late, tardy, unready; delaying, dilatory, lingering, slack.

sludge *n* mire, mud; slosh, slush.

sluggard *n* dawdler, drone, idler, laggard, lounger, slug.

sluggish *adj* dronish, drowsy, idle, inactive, indolent, inert, languid, lazy, listless, lumpish, phlegmatic, slothful, torpid; slow; dull, stupid, supine, tame.

sluice *vb* drain, drench, flood, flush, irrigate. • *n* floodgate, opening, vent.

slumber *vb* catnap, doze, nap, repose, rest, sleep. • *n* catnap, doze, nap, repose, rest, siesta, sleep.

slumberous *adj* drowsy, sleepy, somniferous, somnific, soporific.

slump *vb* droop, drop, fall, flop, founder, sag, sink, sink down; decline, depreciate, deteriorate, ebb, fail, fall away, lose ground, recede, slide, slip, subside, wane. • *n* droop, drop, fall, flop, lowering, sag, sinkage; decline, depreciation, deterioration, downturn, downtrend, subsidence, ebb, falling off, wane; crash, recession, smash.

slur *vb* asperse, calumniate, disparage, depreciate, reproach, traduce; conceal, disregard, gloss over, obscure, pass over, slight. • *n* mark, stain; brand, disgrace, reproach, stain, stigma; innuendo.

slush *n* slosh, sludge.

slushy *vb* plashy, sloppy, sloshy, sludgy.

slut *n* drab, slattern, sloven, trollop.

sluttish *adj* careless, dirty, disorderly, unclean, untidy.

sly *adj* artful, crafty, cunning, insidious, subtle, wily; astute, cautious, shrewd; arch, knowing, clandestine, secret, stealthy, underhand.

smack[1] *vb* smell, taste. • *n* flavour, savour, tang, taste, tincture; dash, infusion, little, space, soupçon, sprinkling, tinge, touch; smattering.

smack[2] *vb* slap, strike; crack, slash, snap; buss, kiss. • *n* crack, slap, slash, snap; buss, kiss.

small *adj* diminutive, Lilliputian, little, miniature, petite, pygmy, tiny, wee; infinitesimal, microscopic, minute; inappreciable, inconsiderable, insignificant, petty, trifling, trivial, unimportant; moderate, paltry, scanty, slender; faint, feeble, puny, slight, weak; illiberal, mean, narrow, narrow-minded, paltry, selfish, scrided, ungenerous, unworthy.

small talk *n* chat, conversation, gossip.

smart[1] *vb* hurt, pain, sting; suffer. • *adj* keen, painful, poignant, pricking, pungent, severe, sharp, stinging.

smart[2] *adj* active, agile, brisk, fresh, lively, nimble, quick, spirited, sprightly, spry; effective, efficient, energetic, forcible, vigorous; adroit, alert, clever, dexterous, dextrous, expert, intelligent, stirring; acute, apt, pertinent, ready, witty; chic, dapper, fine, natty, showy, spruce, trim.

smartness *n* acuteness, keenness, poignancy, pungency, severity, sharpness; efficiency, energy, force, vigour; activity, agility, briskness, liveliness, nimbleness, sprightliness, spryness, vivacity; alertness, cleverness, dexterity, expertise, expertness, intelligence, quickness; acuteness, aptness, pertinency, wit, wittiness; chic, nattiness, spruceness, trimness.

smash *vb* break, crush, cash, mash, shatter. • *n* crash, debacle, destruction, ruin; bankruptcy, failure.

smattering *n* dabbling, smatter, sprinkling.

smear *vb* bedaub, begrime, besmear, daub, plaster, smudge; contaminate, pollute, smirch, smut, soil, stain, sully, tarnish. • *n* blot, blotch, daub, patch, smirch, smudge, spot, stain; calumny, defamation, libel, slander.

smell *vb* scent, sniff, stench, stink. • *n* aroma, bouquet, fragrance, fume, odour, perfume, redolence, scent, stench, stink; sniff, snuff.

smelt *vb* fuse, melt.

smile *vb* grin, laugh, simper, smirk. • *n* grin, simper, smirk.

smite *vb* beat, box, collide, cuff, knock, strike, wallop, whack; destroy, kill, slay; afflict, chasten, punish; blast, destroy.

smitten *adj* attracted, captivated, charmed, enamoured, fascinated, taken; destroyed, killed, slain; smit, struck; afflicted, chastened, punished.

smock *n* chemise, shift, slip; blouse, gaberdine.

smoke *vb* emit, exhale, reek, steam; fumigate, smudge; discover, find out, smell out. • *n* effluvium, exhalation, fume, mist, reek, smother, steam, vapour; fumigation, smudge.

smoky *adj* fuliginous, fumid, fumy, smudgy; begrimed, blackened, dark, reeky, sooty, tanned.

smooth *vb* flatten, level, plane; ease, lubricate; extenuate, palliate, soften; allay, alleviate, assuage, calm, mitigate, mollify. • *adj* even, flat, level, plane, polished, unruffled, unwrinkled; glabrous, glossy, satiny silky, sleek, soft, velvet; euphonious, flowing, liquid, mellifluent; fluent, glib, voluble; bland, flattering, ingratiating, insinuating, mild, oily, smooth-tongued, soothing, suave, unctuous.

smoothly *adv* evenly; eas ly, readily, unobstructedly; blandly, flatteringly, gently, mildly, pleasantly, softly, soothingly.

smooth-tongued *adj* adulatory, cozening, flattering, plausible, smooth, smooth-spoken.

smother *vb* choke, stifle, suffocate; conceal, deaden, extinguish, hide, keep down, repress, suppress; smoke, smoulder.

smudge *vb* besmear, blacken, blur, smear, smut, smutch, soil, spot, stain. • *n* blur, blot, smear, smut, spot, stain.

smug *adj* complacent, self-satisfied; neat, nice, spruce, trim.

smuggler *n* contrabandist, runner.

smut *vb* blacken, smouch, smudge, soil, stain, sully, taint, tarnish. • *n* dirt, smudge, smutch, soot; nastiness, obscenity, ribaldry, smuttiness; pornography.

smutty *adj* coarse, gross, immodest, impure, indecent, indelicate, loose, nasty; dirty, foul, nasty, soiled, stained.

snack *n* bite, light meal, nibble.

snag *vb* catch, enmesh, entangle, hook, snare, sniggle, tangle. • *n* knarl, knob, knot, projection, protuberance, snub; catch, difficulty, drawback, hitch, rub, shortcoming, weakness; obstacle.

snaky *adj* serpentine, snaking, winding; artful, cunning, deceitful, insinuating, sly, subtle.

snap *vb* break, fracture; bite, catch at, seize, snatch at, snip; crack; crackle, crepitate, decrepitate, pop. • *adj* casual, cursory, hasty, offhand, sudden, superficial. • *n* bite, catch, nip, seizure; catch, clasp, fastening, lock; crack, fillip, flick, flip, smack; briskness, energy, verve, vim.

snappish *adj* acrimonious, captious, churlish, crabbed, cross, crusty, froward, irascible, ill-tempered, peevish, perverse, pettish, petulant, snarling, splenetic, surly, tart, testy, touchy, waspish.

snare *vb* catch, ensnare, entangle, entrap. • *n* catch, gin, net, noose, springe, toil, trap, wile.

snarl[1] *vb* girn, gnarl, growl, grumble, murmur. • *n* growl, grumble.

snarl[2] *vb* complicate, disorder, entangle, knot; confuse, embarrass, ensnare. • *n* complication, disorder, entanglement, tangle; difficulty, embarrassment, intricacy.

snatch *vb* catch, clutch, grasp, grip, pluck, pull, seize, snip, twitch, wrest, wring. • *n* bit, fragment, part, portion; catch, effort.

sneak *vb* lurk, skulk, slink, steal; crouch, truckle. • *adj* clandestine, concealed, covert, hidden, secret, sly, underhand. • *n* informer, telltale; lurker, shirk.

sneaky *adj* furtive, skulking, slinking; abject, crouching, grovelling, mean; clandestine, concealed, covert, hidden, secret, sly, underhand.

sneer *vb* flout, gibe, jeer, mock, rail, scoff; (*with* **at**) deride, despise, disdain, laugh at, mock, rail at, scoff, spurn. • *n* flouting, gibe, jeer, scoff.

snicker *vb* giggle, laugh, snigger, titter.

sniff *vb* breathe, inhale, snuff; scent, smell.

snip *vb* clip, cut, nip; snap, snatch. • *n* bit, fragment, particle, piece, shred; share, snack.

snivel *vb* blubber, cry, fret, sniffle, snuffle, weep, whimper, whine.

snivelly *adj* snotty; pitiful, whining.

snob *n* climber, toady.

snooze *vb* catnap, doze, drowse, nap, sleep, slumber. • *n* catnap, nap, sleep, slumber.

snout *n* muzzle, nose; nozzle.

snowy *adj* immaculate, pure, spotless, unblemished, unstained, unsullied, white.

snub[1] *vb* abash, cold-shoulder, cut, discomfit, humble, humiliate, mortify, slight, take down. • *n* check, rebuke, slight.

snub[2] *vb* check, clip, cut short, dock, nip, prune, stunt. • *adj* pug, retroussé, snubbed, squashed, squat, stubby, turned-up.

snuff[1] *vb* breathe, inhale, sniff; scent, smell; snort.

snuff[2] *vb* (*with* **out**) annihilate, destroy, efface, extinguish, obliterate.

snuffle *vb* sniffle; snort, snuff.

snug *adj* close, concealed; comfortable, compact, convenient, neat, trim.

snuggle *vb* cuddle, nestle, nuzzle.

so *adv* thus, with equal reason; in such a manner; in this way, likewise; as it is, as it was, such; for this reason, therefore; be it so, thus be it. • *conj* in case that, on condition that, provided that.

soak *vb* drench, moisten, permeate, saturate, wet; absorb, imbibe; imbue, macerate, steep.

soar *vb* ascend, fly aloft, glide, mount, rise, tower.

sob *vb* cry, sigh convulsively, weep.

sober *vb* (*with* **up**) calm down, collect oneself, compose oneself, control oneself, cool off, master, moderate, simmer down. • *adj* abstemious, abstinent, temperate, unintoxicated; rational, reasonable, sane, sound; calm, collected, composed, cool, dispassionate, moderate, rational, reasonabler, regular, restrained, steady, temperate, unimpassioned, unruffled, well-regulated; demure, grave, quiet, sedate, serious, solemn, sombre, staid; dark, drab, dull-looking, quiet, sad, subdued.

sobriety *n* abstemiousness, abstinence, soberness, temperance; calmness, coolness, gravity, sedateness, sober-mindedness, staidness, thoughtfulness; gravity, seriousness, solemnity.

sobriquet *n* appellation, nickname, nom de plume, pseudonym.

sociability *n* companionableness, comradeship, good fellowship, sociality.

sociable *adj* accessible, affable, communicative, companionable, conversable, friendly, genial, neighbourly, social.

social *adj* civic, civil; accessible, affable, communicative, companionable, familiar, friendly, hospitable, neighbourly, sociable; convivial, festive, gregarious. • *n* conversazione, gathering, gettogether, party, reception, soiree.

society *n* association, companionship, company, converse, fellowship; the community, populace, the public, the world; élite, monde; body, brotherhood, copartnership, corporation, club, fraternity, partnersnip, sodality, union.

sodden *adj* drenched, saturated, soaked, steeped, wet; boiled, decocted, seethed, stewed.

sofa *n* couch, davenport, divan, ottoman, settee.

soft *adj* impressible, malleable, plastic, pliable, yielding; downy, fleecy, velvety, mushy, pulpy, squashy; compliant, facile, irresolute, submissive, undecided, weak; bland, mild, gentle, kind, lenient, soft-hearted, tender; delicate; easy, even, quiet, smooth-going, steady; effeminate, luxurious, unmanly; dulcet, fluty, mellifluous, melodious, smooth. • *interj* hold, stop.

soften *vb* intenerate, mellow, melt, tenderize; abate, allay, alleviate, appease, assuage, attemper, balm, blunt, calm, dull, ease, lessen, make easy, mitigate, moderate, mollify, milden, qualify, quell, quiet, relent, relieve, soothe, still, temper; extenuate, modify, palliate, qualify; enervate, weaken.

soil[1] *n* earth, ground loam, mould; country, land.

soil[2] *vb* bedaub, begrime, bemire, besmear, bespatter, contaminate, daub, defile, dirty, foul, pollute, smirch, stain, sully, taint, tarnish. • *n* blemish, defilement, dirt, filth, foulness; blot, spot, stain, taint, tarnish.

sojourn *vb* abide, dwell, live, lodge, remain, reside, rest, stay, stop, tarry, visit. • *n* residence, stay.

solace *vb* cheer, comfort, console, soothe; allay, assuage, mitigate, relieve, soften. • *n* alleviation, cheer, comfort, consolation, relief.

soldier *n* fighting man, man-at-arms, warrior; GI, private.

soldierly *adj* martial, military, warlike; brave, courageous, gallant, heroic, honourable, intrepid, valiant.

sole *adj* alone, individual, one, only, single, solitary, unique.

solecism *n* barbarism, blunder, error, faux pas, impropriety, incongruity, mistake, slip.

solemn *adj* ceremonial, formal, ritual; devotional, devout, religious, reverential, sacred; earnest, grave, serious, sober; august, awe-inspiring, awful, grand, imposing, impressive, majestic, stately, venerable.

solemnity *n* celebration, ceremony, observance, office, rite; awfulness, sacredness, sanctity; gravity, impressiveness, seriousness.

solemnize *vb* celebrate, commemorate, honour, keep, observe.

solicit *vb* appeal to, ask, beg, beseech, conjure, crave, entreat, implore, importune, petition, pray, press, request, supplicate, urge; arouse, awaken, entice, excite, invite, summon; canvass, seek.

solicitation *n* address, appeal, asking, entreaty, imploration, importunity, insistence, petition, request, suit, supplication, urgency; bidding, call, invitation, summons.

solicitor *n* attorney, law agent, lawyer; asker, canvasser, drummer, petitioner, solicitant.

solicitous *adj* anxious, apprehensive, careful, concerned, disturbed, eager, troubled, uneasy.

solicitude *n* anxiety, care, carefulness, concern, perplexity, trouble.

solid *adj* congealed, firm, hard, impenetrable, rock-like; compact, dense, impermeable, massed; cubic; sound, stable, stout, strong, substantial; just, real, true, valid, weighty; dependable, faithful, reliable, safe, staunch, steadfast, trustworthy, well established.

solidarity *n* communion of interests, community, consolidation, fellowship, joint interest, mutual responsibility.

solidify *vb* compact, congeal, consolidate, harden, petrify.

solidity *n* compactness, consistency, density, firmness, hardness, solidness; fullness; massiveness, stability, strength; dependability, gravity, justice, reliability, soundness, steadiness, validity, weight; cubic content, volume.

soliloquy *n* monologue.

solitariness *n* isolation, privacy, reclusion, retirement, seclusion; loneliness, solitude.

solitary *adj* alone, companionless, lone, lonely, only, separate, unaccompanied; individual, single, sole; desert, deserted, desolate, isolated, lonely, remote, retired, secluded, unfrequented.

solitude *n* isolation, loneliness, privacy, recluseness, retiredness, retirement, seclusion, solitariness; desert, waste, wilderness.

solution *n* answer, clue, disentanglement, elucidation, explication, explanation, key, resolution, unravelling, unriddling; disintegration, dissolution, liquefaction, melting, resolution, separation; breach, disconnection, discontinuance, disjunction, disruption.

solve *vb* clear, clear up, disentangle, elucidate, explain, expound, interpret, make plain, resolve, unfold.

solvent *n* diluent, dissolvent, menstruum.

somatic *adj* bodily, corporeal.

sombre *adj* cloudy, dark, dismal, dull, dusky, gloomy, murky, overcast, rayless, shady, sombrous, sunless; doleful, funereal, grave, lugubrious, melancholy, mournful, sad, sober.

some *adj* a, an, any, one; about, near; certain, little, moderate, part, several.

somebody *n* one, someone, something; celebrity, VIP.

somehow *adv* in some way.

something *n* part, portion, thing; somebody; affair, event, matter.

sometime *adj* former, late. • *adv* formerly, once; now and then, at one time or other, sometimes.

sometimes *adv* at intervals, at times, now and then, occasionally; at a past period, formerly, once.

somewhat *adv* in some degree, more or less, rather, something. • *n* something, a little, more or less, part.

somewhere *adv* here and there, in one place or another, in some place.

somnambulism *n* sleepwalking, somnambulation.

somnambulist *n* night-walker, noctambulist, sleepwalker, somnambulator, somnambule.

somniferous *adj* narcotic, opiate, slumberous, somnific, soporific, soporiferous.

somnolence *n* doziness, drowsiness, sleepiness, somnolency.

somnolent *adj* dozy, drowsy, sleepy.

son *n* cadet, heir, junior, scion.

song *n* aria, ballad, canticle, canzonet, carol, ditty, glee, lay, lullaby, snatch; descant, melody; anthem, hymn, poem, psalm, strain; poesy, poetry, verse.

sonorous *adj* full-toned, resonant, resounding, ringing, sounding; high-sounding, loud.

soon *adv* anon, before long, by and by, in a short time, presently, shortly; betimes, early, forthwith, promptly, quick; gladly, lief, readily, willingly.

soot *n* carbon, crock, dust.

soothe *vb* cajole, flatter, humour; appease, assuage, balm, calm, compose, lull, mollify, pacify, quiet, soften, still, tranquillize; allay, alleviate, blunt, check, deaden, dull, ease, lessen, mitigate, moderate, palliate, qualify, relieve, repress, soften, subdue, temper.

soothsayer *n* augur, diviner, foreteller, necromancer, predictor, prophet, seer, sorcerer, vaticinator.

sooty *adj* black, dark, dusky, fuliginous, murky, sable.

sophism *n* casuistry, fallacy, paralogism, paralogy, quibble, specious argument.

sophist *n* quibbler.

sophistical *adj* casuistical, fallacious, illogical, quibbling, subtle, unsound.

soporific *adj* dormitive, hypnotic, narcotic, opiate, sleepy, slumberous, somnific, somniferous, soporiferous, soporous.

soppy *adj* drenched, saturated, soaked, sopped; emotional, mawkish, sentimental.

soprano *n* (*mus*) descant, discant, treble.

sorcerer *n* charmer, conjurer, diviner, enchanter, juggler, magician, necromancers, seer, shaman, soothsayer, thaumaturgist, wizard.

sorcery *n* black art, charm, divination, enchantment, necromancy, occultism, shamanism, spell, thaumaturgy, voodoo, witchcraft.

sordid *adj* base, degraded, low, mean, vile; avaricious, closefisted, covetous, illiberal, miserly, niggardly, penurious, stingy, ungenerous.

sore *adj* irritated, painful, raw, tender, ulcerated; aggrieved, galled, grieved, hurt, irritable, vexed; afflictive, distressing, severe, sharp, violent. • *n* abscess, boil, fester, gathering, imposthume, pustule, ulcer; affliction, grief, pain, sorrow, trouble.

sorely *adv* greatly, grievously, severely, violently.

sorrily *adv* despicably, meanly, pitiably, poorly, wretchedly.

sorrow *vb* bemoan, bewail, grieve, lament, mourn, weep. • *n* affliction, dolour, grief, heartache, mourning, sadness, trouble, woe.

sorrowful *adj* afflicted, dejected, depressed, grieved, grieving, heartsore, sad; baleful, distressing, grievous, lamentable, melancholy, mournful, painful; disconsolate, dismal, doleful, dolorous, drear, dreary, lugubrious, melancholy, piteous, rueful, woebegone, woeful.

sorry *adj* afflicted, dejected, grieved, pained, poor, sorrowful; distressing, pitiful; chagrined, mortified, pained, regretful, remorseful, sad, vexed; abject, base, beggarly, contemptible, despicable, low, mean, paltry, insignificant, miserable, shabby, worthless, wretched.

sort *vb* arrange, assort, class, classify, distribute, order; conjoin, join, put together; choose, elect, pick out, select; associate, consort, fraternize; accord, agree with, fit, suit. • *n* character, class, denomination, description, kind, nature, order, race, rank, species, type; manner, way.

sortie *n* attack, foray, raid, sally.

so-so *adj* indifferent, mediocre, middling, ordinary, passable, tolerable.

sot *n* blockhead, dolt, dullard, dunce, fool, simpleton; drunkard, tippler, toper.

sottish *adj* doltish, dull, foolish, senseless, simple, stupid; befuddled, besotted, drunken, insensate, senseless, tipsy.

sotto voce *adv* in a low voice, in an undertone, softly.

sough *n* murmur, sigh; breath, breeze, waft.

soul *n* mind, psyche, spirit; being, person; embodiment, essence, personification, spirit, vital principle; ardour, energy, fervour, inspiration, vitality.

soulless *adj* dead, expressionless, lifeless, unfeeling.

sound[1] *adj* entire, intact, unbroken, unhurt, unimpaired, uninjured, unmutilated, whole; hale, hardy, healthy, hearty, vigorous; good, perfect, undecayed; sane, well-balanced; correct, orthodox, right, solid, valid, well-founded; legal; deep, fast, profound, unbroken, undisturbed; forcible, lusty, severe, stout.

sound[2] *n* channel, narrows, strait.

sound[3] *vb* resound; appear, seem; play on; express, pronounce, utter; announce, celebrate, proclaim, publish, spread. • *n* noise, note, tone, voice whisper.

sound[4] *vb* fathom, gauge measure, test; examine, probe, search, test, try.

sounding *adj* audible, resonant, resounding, ringing, sonorous; imposing, significant.

soundless *adj* dumb, noiseless, silent; abysmal, bottomless, deep, profound, unfathomable, unsounded.

soundly *adv* satisfactorily, thoroughly, well; healthily, heartily; forcibly, lustily, severely smartly, stoutly; correctly, rightly, truly; firmly, strongly; deeply, fast, profoundly.

soundness *n* entireness, entirety, integrity, wholeness; healthiness, vigour, saneness, sanity; correctness, orthodoxy, rectitude, reliability, truth, validity; firmness, solidity, strength, validity.

soup *n* broth, consommé, purée.

sour *vb* acidulate; embitter, envenom. • *adj* acetose, acetous, acid, astringent, pricked, sharp, tart, vinegary; acrimonious, crabbed, cross, crusty, fretful, glum, ill-humoured, ill-natured, ill-tempered, peevish, pettish, petulant, snarling, surly; bitter, disagreeable, unpleasant; austere, dismal, gloomy, morose, sad, sullen; bad, coagulated, curdled, musty, rancid, turned.

source *n* beginning, fountain, fountainhead, head, origin, rise, root, spring, well; cause, original.

sourness *n* acidity, sharpness, tartness; acrimony, asperity, churlishness, crabbedness, crossness, discontent, harshness, moroseness, peevishness.

souse *vb* pickle; dip, douse, immerse, plunge, submerge.

souvenir *n* keepsake, memento, remembrance, reminder.

sovereign *adj* imperial, monarchical, princely, regal, royal, supreme; chief, commanding, excellent, highest, paramount, predominant, principal, supreme, utmost; efficacious, effectual. • *n* autocrat, monarch, suzerain; emperor, empress, king, lord, potentate, prince, princess, queen, ruler.

sovereignty *n* authority, dominion, empire, power, rule, supremacy, sway.

sow *vb* scatter, spread, strew; disperse, disseminate, propagate, spread abroad; plant; besprinkle, scatter.

space *n* expanse, expansion, extension, extent, proportions, spread; accommodation, capacity, room, place; distance, interspace, interval.

spacious *adj* extended, extensive, vast, wide; ample, broad, capacious, commodious, large, roomy, wide.

span *vb* compass, cross, encompass, measure, overlay. • *n* brief period, spell; pair, team, yoke.

spank *vb* slap, strike.

spar[1] *n* beam, boom, pole, sprit, yard.

spar[2] *vb* box, fight; argue, bicker, contend, dispute, quarrel, spat, squabble, wrangle.

spare *vb* lay aside, lay by, reserve, save, set apart, set aside; dispense with, do without, part with; forbear, omit, refrain, withhold; exempt, forgive, keep from; afford, allow, give, grant; save; economize, pinch. • *adj* frugal, scanty, sparing, stinted; chary, parsimonious; emaciated, gaunt, lank, lean, meagre, poor, thin, scraggy, skinny, raw-boned; additional, extra, supernumerary.

sparing *adj* little, scanty, scarce; abstemious, meagre, spare; chary, economical, frugal, parsimonious, saving; compassionate, forgiving, lenient, merciful.

spark *vb* scintillate, sparkle; begin, fire, incite, instigate, kindle, light, set off, start, touch off, trigger. • *n* scintilla, scintillation, sparkle; beginning, element, germ, seed.

sparkle *vb* coruscate, flash, gleam, glisten, glister, glitter, radiate, scintillate, shine, twinkle; bubble, effervesce, foam, froth. • *n* glint, scintillation, spark; luminosity, lustre.

sparkling *adj* brilliant, flashing, glistening, glittering, glittery, twinkling; bubbling, effervescing, eloquent, foaming, frothing, mantling; brilliant, glowing, lively, nervous, piquant, racy, spirited, sprightly, witty.

sparse *adj* dispersed, infrequent, scanty, scattered, sporadic, thin.

spartan *adj* bold, brave, chivalric, courageous, daring, dauntless, doughty, fearless, hardy, heroic, intrepid, lion-hearted, undaunted, valiant, valorous; austere, exacting, hard, severe, tough, unsparing; enduring, long-suffering, self-controlled, stoic.

spasm *n* contraction, cramp, crick, twitch; fit, paroxysm, seizure, throe.

spasmodic *adj* erratic, fitful, intermittent, irregular, sporadic; convulsive, paroxysmal, spasmodical, violent.

spat *vb* argue, bicker, dispute, jangle, quarrel, spar, squabble, wrangle.

spatter *vb* bespatter, besprinkle, plash, splash, sprinkle; spit, sputter.

spawn *vb* bring forth, generate, produce. • *n* eggs, roe; fruit, offspring, product.

speak *vb* articulate, deliver, enunciate, express, pronounce, utter; announce, confer, declare, disclose, mention, say, tell; celebrate, make known, proclaim, speak abroad; accost, address, greet, hail; exhibit; argue, converse, dispute, talk; declaim, discourse, hold forth, harangue, orate, plead, spout, treat.

speaker *n* discourse, elocutionist, orator, prolocutor, spokesman; chairman, presiding officer.

speaking *adj* rhetorical, talking; eloquent, expressive; lifelike. • *n* discourse, talk, utterance; declamation, elocution, oratory.

spear *n* dart, gaff, harpoon, javelin, lance, pike; shoot, spire.

special *adj* specific, specifical; especial, individual, particular, peculiar, unique; exceptional, extraordinary, marked, particular, uncommon; appropriate, express.

speciality, specialty *n* particularity; feature, forte, pet subject.

species *n* assemblage, class, collection, group; description, kind, sort, variety; (*law*) fashion, figure, form, shape.

specific *adj* characteristic, especial, particular, peculiar; definite, limited, precise, specified.

specification *n* characterization, designation; details, particularization.

specify *vb* define, designate, detail, indicate, individualize, name, show, particularize.

specimen *n* copy, example, model, pattern, sample.

specious *adj* manifest, obvious, open, showy; flimsy, illusory, ostensible, plausible, sophistical.

speck *n* blemish, blot, flaw, speckle, spot, stain; atom, bit, corpuscle, mite, mote, particle, scintilla.

spectacle *n* display, exhibition, pageant, parade, representation, review, scene, show, sight; curiosity, marvel, phenomenon, wonder.

spectacles *npl* glasses, goggles, shades.

spectator *n* beholder, bystander, observer, onlooker, witness.

spectral *adj* eerie, ghostlike, ghostly, phantomlike, shadowy, spooky, weird, wraithlike.

spectre, specter *n* apparition, banshee, ghost, goblin, hobgoblin, phantom, shade, shadow, spirit, sprite, wraith.

spectrum *n* appearance, image, representation.

speculate *vb* cogitate, conjecture, contemplate, imagine, meditate, muse, ponder, reflect, ruminate, theorize, think; bet, gamble, hazard, risk, trade, venture.

speculation *n* contemplation, intellectualization; conjecture, hypothesis, scheme, supposition, reasoning, reflection, theory, view.

speculative *adj* contemplative, philosophical, speculatory, unpractical; ideal, imaginary, theoretical; hazardous, risky, unsecured.

speculator *n* speculatist, theorist, theorizer; adventurer, dealer, gambler, trader.

speech *n* articulation, language, words; dialect, idiom, locution, tongue; conversation, oral communication, parlance, talk, verbal intercourse; mention, observation, remark, saying; address, declaration, discourse, harangue, oration, palaver.

speechless *adj* dumb, gagged, inarticulate, mute, silent; dazed, dumbfounded, flabbergasted, shocked.

speed *vb* hasten, hurry, rush, scurry; flourish, prosper, succeed, thrive; accelerate, expedite, hasten, hurry, quicken, press forward, urge on; carry through, dispatch, execute; advance, aid, assist, help; favour. • *n* acceleration, celerity, dispatch, expedition, fleetness, haste, hurry, quickness, rapidity, swiftness, velocity; good fortune, good luck, prosperity, success; impetuosity.

speedy *adj* fast, fleet, flying, hasty, hurried, hurrying, nimble, quick, rapid, swift; expeditious, prompt, quick; approaching, early, near.

spell[1] *n* charm, exorcism, hoodoo, incantation, jinx, witchery; allure, bewitchment, captivation, enchantment, entrancement, fascination.

spell[2] *vb* decipher, interpret, read, unfold, unravel, unriddle.

spell[3] *n* fit, interval, period, round, season, stint, term, turn.

spellbound *adj* bewitched, charmed, enchanted, entranced, enthralled, fascinated.

spend *vb* disburse, dispose of, expend, lay out, part with; consume, dissipate, exhaust, lavish, squander, use up, wear, waste; apply, bestow, devote, employ, pass.

spendthrift *n* prodigal, spender, squanderer, waster.

spent *adj* exhausted, fatigued, played out, used up, wearied, worn out.

spew *vb* cast up, puke, throw up, vomit; cast forth, eject.

spheral *adj* complete, perfect, symmetrical.

sphere *n* ball, globe, orb, spheroid; ambit, beat, bound, circle, circuit, compass, department, function, office, orbit, province, range, walk; order, rank, standing; country, domain, quarter, realm, region.

spherical *adj* bulbous, globated, globous, globular, orbicular, rotund, round, spheroid; planetary.

spice *n* flavour, flavouring, relish, savour, taste; admixture, dash, grain, infusion, particle, smack, soupçon, sprinkling, tincture.

spicily *adv* pungently, wittily.

spicy *adj* aromatic, balmy, fragrant; keen, piquant, pointed, pungent, sharp; indelicate, off-colour, racy, risqué, sensational, suggestive.

spill *vb* effuse, pour out, shed. • *n* accident, fall, tumble.

spin *vb* twist; draw out, extend; lengthen, prolong, protract, spend; pirouette, turn, twirl, whirl. • *n* drive, joyride, ride; autorotation, gyration, loop, revolution, rotation, turning, wheeling; pirouette, reel, turn, wheel, whirl.

spindle *n* axis, shaft.

spine *n* barb, prickle, thorn; backbone; ridge.

spinose *adj* briery, spinous, spiny, thorny.

spiny *adj* briery, prickly, spinose, spinous, thorny; difficult, perplexed, troublesome.

spiracle *n* aperture, blowhole, orifice, pore, vent.

spiral *adj* cochlear, cochleated, curled, helical, screw-shaped, spiry, winding. • *n* helix, winding, worm.

spire *n* curl, spiral, twist, wreath; steeple; blade, shoot, spear, stalk; apex, summit.

spirit *vb* animate, encourage, excite, inspirit; carry off, kidnap. • *n* immaterial substance, life, vital essence; person, soul;

angel, apparition, demon, elf, fairy, genius, ghost, phantom, shade, spectre, sprite; disposition, frame of mind, humour, mood, temper; spirits; ardour, cheerfulness, courage, earnestness, energy, enterprise, enthusiasm, fire, force, mettle, resolution, vigour, vim, vivacity, zeal; animation, cheerfulness, enterprise, esprit, glow, liveliness, piquancy, spice, spunk, vivacity, warmth; drift, gist, intent, meaning, purport, sense, significance, tenor; character, characteristic, complexion, essence, nature, quality, quintessence; alcohol, liquor; (*with* **the**) Comforter, Holy Ghost, Paraclete.

spirited *adj* active, alert, animated, ardent, bold, brisk, courageous, earnest, frisky, high-mettled, high-spirited, high-strung, lively, mettlesome, sprightly, vivacious.

spiritless *adj* breathless, dead, extinct, lifeless; dejected, depressed, discouraged, dispirited, low-spirited; apathetic, cold, dull, feeble, languid, phlegmatic, sluggish, soulless, torpid, unenterprising; dull, frigid, heavy, insipid, prosaic, prosy, stupid, tame, uninteresting.

spiritual *adj* ethereal, ghostly, immaterial incorporeal, psychical, supersensible; ideal, moral, unwordly; divine, holy, pure, sacred; ecclesiastical.

spiritualize *vb* elevate, etherealize, purify, refine.

spirituous *adj* alcoholic, ardent, spiritous.

spit[1] *vb* impale, thrust through, transfix.

spit[2] *vb* eject, throw out; drivel, drool, expectorate, salivate, slobber, spawl, splutter. • *n* saliva, spawl, spittle, sputum.

spite *vb* injure, mortify, thwart; annoy, offend, vex. • *n* grudge, hate, hatred, ill-nature, ill-will, malevolence, malice, maliciousness, malignity, pique, rancour, spleen, venom, vindictiveness.

spiteful *adj* evil-minded, hateful, ill-disposed, ill-natured, malevolent, malicious, malign, malignant, rancorous.

spittoon *n* cuspidor.

splash *vb* dabble, dash, plash, spatter, splurge, swash, swish. • *n* blot, daub, spot.

splay *adj* broad, spreading out, turned out, wide.

spleen *n* anger, animosity, chagrin, gall, grudge, hatred, ill-humour, irascibility, malevolence, malice, malignity, peevishness, pique, rancour, spite.

spleeny *adj* angry, fretful, ill-tempered, irritable, peevish, spleenish, splenetic.

splendid *adj* beaming, bright, brilliant, effulgent, glowing, lustrous, radiant, refulgent, resplendent, shining; dazzling, gorgeous, imposing, kingly, magnificent, pompous, showy, sumptuous, superb; celebrated, conspicuous, distinguished, eminent, excellent, famous, glorious, illustrious, noble, preeminent, remarkable, signal; grand, heroic, lofty, noble, sublime.

splendour *n* brightness, brilliance, brilliancy, lustre, radiance, refulgence; display, éclat, gorgeousness, grandeur, magnificence, parade, pomp, show, showiness, stateliness celebrity, eminence, fame, glory, grandeur, renown; grandeur, loftiness, nobleness, sublimity.

splenetic *adj* choleric, cross, fretful, irascible, irritable, peevish, pettish, petulant, snappish, testy, touchy, waspish; churlish, crabbed, morose, sour, sulky, sullen; gloomy, jaundiced.

splice *vb* braid, connect, join, knit, mortise.

splinter *vb* rend, shiver, sliver, split. • *n* fragment, piece.

split *vb* cleave, rive; break, burst, rend, splinter; divide, part, separate, sunder. • *n* crack, fissure, rent; breach, division, separation.

splotch *n* blot, daub, smear, spot, stain.

splutter *vb* sputter, stammer, stutter.

spoil *vb* despoil, fleece, loot, pilfer, plunder, ravage, rob, steal, strip, waste; corrupt, damage, destroy, disfigure, harm, impair, injure, mar, ruin, vitiate; decay, decompose. • *n* booty, loot, pillage, plunder, prey; rapine, robbery, spoliation, waste.

spoiler *n* pillager, plunderer, robber; corrupter, destroyer.

spokesman *n* mouthpiece, prolocutor, speaker.

spoliate *vb* despoil, destroy, loot, pillage, plunder, rob, spoil.

spoliation *n* depradation, deprivation, despoliation, destruction, robbery; destruction, devastation, pillage, plundering, rapine, ravagement.

sponge *vb* cleanse, wipe; efface, expunge, obliterate, rub out, wipe out.

sponger *n* hanger-on, parasite.

spongy *adj* absorbent, porous, spongeous; rainy, showery, wet; drenched, marshy, saturated, soaked, wet.

sponsor *vb* back, capitalize, endorse, finance, guarantee, patronize, promote, support, stake, subsidize, take up, underwrite. • *n* angel, backer, guarantor, patron, promoter, supporter, surety, underwriter; godfather, godmother, godparent.

spontaneity *n* improvisation, impulsiveness, spontaneousness.

spontaneous *adj* free, gratuitous, impulsive, improvised, instinctive, self-acting, self-moving, unbidden, uncompelled, unconstrained, voluntary, willing.

sporadic *adj* dispersed, infrequent, isolated, rare, scattered, separate, spasmodic.

sport *vb* caper, disport frolic, gambol, have fun, make merry, play, romp, skip; trifle display, exhibit. • *n* amusement, diversion, entertainment, frolic, fun, gambol, game, jollity, joviality, merriment, merry-making, mirth, pastime, pleasantry, prank, recreation; jest, joke; derision, jeer, mockery, ridicule; monstrosity.

sportive *adj* frisky, frolicsome, gamesome, hilarious, lively, merry, playful, prankish, rollicking, sprightly, tricksy; comic, facetious, funny, humorous, jocose, jocular, lively, ludicrous, mirthful, vivacious, waggish.

spot *vb* besprinkle, dapple, dot, speck, stud, variegate; blemish, disgrace, soil, splotch, stain, sully, tarnish; detect, discern, espy, make out, observe, see, sight. • *n* blot, dapple, fleck, freckle, maculation, mark, mottle, patch, pip, speck, speckle; blemish, blotch, flaw, pock, splotch, stain, taint; locality, place, site.

spotless *adj* perfect, undefaced, unspotted; blameless, immaculate, innocent, irreproachable, pure, stainless, unblemished, unstained, untainted, untarnished.

spotted *adj* bespeckled, bespotted, dotted, flecked, freckled, maculated, ocellated, speckled, spotty.

spousal *adj* bridal, conjugal, connubial, hymeneal, marital, matrimonial, nuptial, wedded.

spouse *n* companion, consort, husband, mate, partner, wife.

spout *vb* gush, jet, pour out, spirit, spurt, squirt; declaim, mouth, speak, utter. • *n* conduit, tube; beak, nose, nozzle, waterspout.

sprain *vb* overstrain, rick, strain, twist, wrench, wrick.

spray[1] *vb* atomize, besprinkle, douche, gush, jet, shower, splash, splatter, spout, sprinkle, squirt. • *n* aerosol, atomizer, douche, foam, froth, shower, sprinkler, spume.

spray[2] *n* bough, branch, shoot, sprig, twig.

spread *vb* dilate, expand, extend, mantle, stretch; diffuse, disperse, distribute, radiate, scatter, sprinkle, strew; broadcast, circulate, disseminate, divulge, make known, make public, promulgate, propagate, publish; open, unfold, unfurl; cover, extend over, overspread. • *n* compass, extent, range, reach, scope, stretch; expansion, extension; circulation, dissemination, propagation; cloth, cover; banquet, feast, meal.

spree *n* bacchanal, carousal, debauch, frolic, jollification, orgy, revel, revelry, saturnalia.

sprig *n* shoot, spray, twig; lad, youth.

sprightliness *n* animation, activity, briskness, cheerfulness, frolicsomeness, gaiety, life, liveliness, nimbleness, vigour, vivacity.

sprightly *adj* airy, animated, blithe, blithesome, brisk, buoyant, cheerful, debonair, frolicsome, joyous, lively, mercurial, vigorous, vivacious.

spring *vb* bound, hop, jump, leap, prance, vault; arise, emerge, grow, issue, proceed, put forth, shoot forth, stem; derive, descend, emanate, flow, originate, rise, start; fly back, rebound, recoil; bend, warp; grow, thrive, wax. • *adj* hopping, jumping, resilient, springy. • *n* bound, hop, jump, leap, vault; elasticity, flexibility, resilience, resiliency, springiness; fount, fountain, fountainhead, geyser, springhead, well; cause, origin, original, principle, source; seed time, springtime.

springe *n* gin, net, noose, snare, trap.

springiness *n* elasticity, resilience, spring; sponginess, wetness.

springy *adj* bouncing, bounding, elastic, rebounding, recoiling, resilient.

sprinkle *vb* scatter, strew; bedew, besprinkle, dust, powder, sand, spatter; wash, cleanse, purify, shower.

sprinkling *n* affusion, baptism, bedewing, spattering, splattering, spraying, wetting; dash, scattering, seasoning, smack, soupçon, suggestion, tinge, touch, trace, vestige.

sprite *n* apparition, elf, fairy, ghost, goblin, hobgoblin, phantom, pixie, shade, spectre, spirit.

sprout *vb* burgeon, burst forth, germinate, grow, pullulate, push, put forth, ramify, shoot, shoot forth. • *n* shoot, sprig.

spruce *vb* preen, prink; adorn, deck, dress, smarten, trim. • *adj* dandyish, dapper, fine, foppish, jaunty, natty, neat, nice, smart, tidy, trig, trim.

spry *adj* active, agile, alert, brisk, lively, nimble, prompt, quick, ready, smart, sprightly, stirring, supple.

spume *n* foam, froth, scum, spray.

spumy *adj* foamy, frothy, spumous.

spur *vb* gallop, hasten, press on, prick; animate, arouse, drive, goad, impel, incite, induce, instigate, rouse, stimulate, urge forward. • *n* goad, point, prick, rowel; fillip, impulse, incentive, incitement, inducement, instigation, motive, provocation, stimulus, whip; gnarl, knob, knot, point, projection, snag.

spurious *adj* bogus, counterfeit, deceitful, false, feigned, fictitious, make-believe, meretricious, mock, pretended, sham, supposititious, unauthentic.

spurn *vb* drive away, kick; contemn, despise, disregard, flout, scorn, slight; disdain, reject, repudiate.

spurt *vb* gush, jet, spirt, spout, spring out, stream out, well. • *n* gush, jet, spout, squirt; burst, dash, rush.

sputter *vb* spawl, spit, splutter, stammer.

spy *vb* behold, discern, espy, see; detect, discover, search out; explore, inspect, scrutinize, search; shadow, trail, watch. • *n* agent, detective, double agent, mole, scout, undercover agent.

squabble *vb* brawl, fight, quarrel, scuffle, struggle, wrangle; altercate, bicker, contend, dispute, jangle. • *n* brawl, dispute, fight, quarrel, rumpus, scrimmage.

squad *n* band, bevy, crew, gang, knot, lot, relay, set.

squalid *adj* dirty, filthy, foul, mucky, slovenly, unclean, unkempt.

squalidness *n* filthiness, foulness, squalidity, squalor.

squall *vb* bawl, cry, cry out, scream, yell. • *n* bawl, cry, outcry, scream, yell; blast, flurry, gale, gust, hurricane, storm, tempest.

squally *adj* blustering, blustery, gusty, stormy, tempestuous, windy.

squander *vb* dissipate, expend, lavish, lose, misuse, scatter, spend, throw away, waste.

squanderer *n* lavisher, prodigal, spendthrift, waster.

square *vb* make square, quadrate; accommodate, adapt, fit, mould, regulate, shape, suit; adjust, balance, close, make even, settle; accord, chime in, cohere, comport, fall in, fit, harmonize, quadrate, suit. • *adj* four-square, quadrilateral, quadrate; equal, equitable, exact, fair, honest, just, upright; adjusted, balanced, even, settled; true, suitable. • *n* four-sided figure, quadrate, rectangle, tetragon; open area, parade, piazza, plaza.

squash *vb* crush, mash.

squashy *adj* pulpy, soft.

squat *vb* cower, crouch; occupy, plant, settle. • *adj* cowering, crouching; dumpy, pudgy, short, stocky, stubby, thickset.

squeal *vb* creak, cry, howl, scream, screech, shriek, squawk, yell; betray, inform on. • *n* creak, cry, howl, scream, screech, shriek, squawk, yell.

squeamish *adj* nauseated, qualmish, queasy, sickish; dainty, delicate, fastidious, finical, hypercritical, nice, over-nice, particular, priggish.

squeeze *vb* clutch, compress, constrict, grip, nip, pinch, press; drive, force; crush, harass, oppress; crowd, force through; press; (*with* **out**) extract. • *n* congestion, crowd, crush, throng; compression.

squelch *vb* crush, quash, quell, silence, squash, suppress.

squib *n* firework, fuse; lampoon, pasquinade, satire.

squint *vb* look askance, look obliquely, peer. • *adj* askew, aslant, crooked, oblique, skew, skewed, twisted.

squire *vb* accompany, attend, escort, wait on.

squirm *vb* twist, wriggle, writhe.

squirt *vb* eject, jet, splash, spurt.

stab *vb* broach, gore, jab, pierce, pink, spear, stick, transfix, transpierce; wound. • *n* cut, jab, prick, thrust; blow, dagger-stroke, injury, wound.

stability *n* durability, firmness, fixedness, immovability, permanence, stableness, steadiness; constancy, firmness, reliability.

stable *adj* established, fixed, immovable, immutable, invariable, permanent, unalterable, unchangeable; constant, firm, staunch, steadfast, steady, unwavering; abiding, durable, enduring, fast, lasting, permanent, perpetual, secure, sure.

staff *n* baton, cane, pole, rod, stick, wand; bat, bludgeon, club, cudgel, mace; prop, stay, support; employees, personnel, team, workers, work force.

stage *vb* dramatize, perform, present, produce, put on. • *n* dais, platform, rostrum, scaffold, staging, stand; arena, field; boards, playhouse, theatre; degree, point, step; diligence, omnibus, stagecoach.

stagey *adj* bombastic, declamatory, dramatic, melodramatic, ranting, theatrical.

stagger *vb* reel, sway, totter; alternate, fluctuate, overlap, vacillate, vary; falter, hesitate, waver; amaze, astonish, astound, confound, dumbfound, nonplus, pose, shock, surprise.

stagnant *adj* close, motionless, quiet, standing; dormant, dull, heavy, inactive, inert, sluggish, torpid.

stagnate *vb* decay, deteriorate, languish, rot, stand still, vegetate.

staid *adj* calm, composed, demure, grave, sedate, serious, settled, sober, solemn, steady, unadventurous.

stain *vb* blemish, blot, blotch, discolour, maculate, smirch, soil, splotch, spot, sully, tarnish; colour, dye, tinge; contaminate, corrupt, debase, defile, deprave, disgrace, dishonour, pollute, taint. • *n* blemish, blot, defect, discoloration, flaw, imperfection, spot, tarnish; contamination, disgrace, dishonour, infamy, pollution, reproach, shame, taint, tarnish.

stainless *adj* spotless, unspotted, untarnished; blameless, faultless, innocent, guiltless, pure, spotless, uncorrupted, unsullied.

stairs *npl* flight of steps, staircase, stairway.

stake[1] *vb* brace, mark, prop, secure, support. • *n* pale, palisade, peg, picket, post, stick.

stake[2] *vb* finance, pledge, wager; hazard, imperil, jeopardize, peril, risk, venture. • *n* bet, pledge, wager; adventure, hazard, risk, venture.

stale *adj* flat, fusty, insipid, mawkish, mouldy, musty, sour, tasteless, vapid; decayed, effete, faded, old, time-worn, worn-out; common, commonplace, hackneyed, stereotyped, threadbare, trite.

stalk[1] *n* culm, pedicel, peduncle, petiole, shaft, spire, stem, stock.

stalk[2] *vb* march, pace, stride, strut, swagger; follow, hunt, shadow, track, walk stealthily.

stall[1] *n* stable; cell, compartment, recess; booth, kiosk, shop, stand.

stall[2] *vb* block, delay, equivocate, filibuster, hinder, postpone, procrastinate, temporize; arrest, check, conk out, die, fail, halt, stick, stop.

stalwart *adj* able-bodied, athletic, brawny, lusty, muscular, powerful, robust, sinewy, stout, strapping, strong, sturdy, vigorous; bold, brave, daring, gallant, indomitable, intrepid, redoubtable, resolute, valiant, valorous. • *n* backer, member, partisan, supporter.

stamina *n* energy, force, lustiness, power, stoutness, strength, sturdiness, vigour.

stammer *vb* falter, hesitate, stutter. • *n* faltering, hesitation, stutter.

stamp *vb* brand, impress, imprint, mark, print. • *n* brand, impress, impression, print; cast, character, complexion, cut, description, fashion, form, kind, make, mould, sort, type.

stampede *vb* charge, flee, panic. • *n* charge, flight, rout, running away, rush.

stanch *see* **staunch**[1].

stanchion *n* prop, shore, stay, support.

stand *vb* be erect, remain upright; abide, be fixed, continue, endure, hold good, remain; halt, pause, stop; be firm, be resolute, stand ground, stay; be valid, have force; depend, have support, rest; bear, brook, endure, suffer, sustain, weather; abide, admit, await, submit, tolerate, yield; fix, place, put, set upright; (*with* **against**) oppose, resist, withstand; (*with* **by**) be near, be present; aid, assist, defend, help, side with, support; defend, make good, justify, maintain, support, vindicate; (*naut*) attend, be ready; (*with* **fast**) be fixed, be immovable; (*with* **for**) mean, represent, signify; aid, defend, help, maintain, side with, support; (*with* **off**) keep aloof, keep off; not to comply; (*with* **out**) be prominent, jut, project, protrude; not comply, not yield, persist; (*with* **up for**) defend, justify, support, sustain, uphold; (*with* **with**) agree. • *n* place, position, post, standing place, station; halt, stay, stop; dais, platform, rostrum; booth, stall; opposition, resistance.

standard[1] *n* banner, colours, ensign, flag, gonfalon, pennon, streamer.

standard[2] *adj* average, conventional, customary, normal, ordinary, regular, usual; accepted, approved, authoritative, orthodox, received; formulary, prescriptive, regulation. • *n* canon, criterion, model, norm, rule, test, type; gauge, measure, model, scale; support, upright.

standing *adj* established, fixed, immovable, settled; durable, lasting, permanent; motionless, stagnant. • *n* position, stand, station; continuance, duration, existence; footing, ground, hold; condition, estimation, rank, reputation status.

standpoint *n* point of view, viewpoint.

standstill *n* cessation, interruption, stand, stop; deadlock.

stanza *n* measure, staff, stave, strophe, verse.

staple *adj* basic, chief, essential, fundamental, main, primary, principal. • *n* fibre, filament, pile, thread; body, bulk, mass, substance.

star *vb* act, appear, feature, headline, lead, perform, play; emphasize, highlight, stress, underline. • *adj* leading, main, paramount, principal; celebrated, illustrious, well-known. • *n* heavenly body, luminary; asterisk, pentacle, pentagram; destiny, doom, fate, fortune, lot; diva, headliner, hero, heroine, lead, leading lady, leading man, prima ballerina, prima donna, principal, protagonist.

starchy *adj* ceremonious, exact, formal, precise, prim, punctilious, rigid, starched, stiff.

stare *vb* gape, gaze, look intently, watch.

stark *adj* rigid, stiff; absolute, bare, downright, entire, gross, mere, pure, sheer, simple. • *adv* absolutely, completely, entirely, fully, wholly.

starry *adj* astral, sidereal, star-spangled, stellar; bright, brilliant, lustrous, shining, sparkling, twinkling.

start *vb* begin, commence, inaugurate, initiate, institute; discover, invent; flinch, jump, shrink, startle, wince; alarm, disturb, fright, rouse, scare; depart, set off, take off; arise, call forth, evoke, raise; dislocate, move suddenly, spring. • *n* beginning, commencement, inauguration, outset; fit, jump, spasm, twitch; impulse, sally.

startle *vb* flinch, shrink, start, wince; affright, alarm, fright, frighten, scare, shock; amaze, astonish, astound.

startling *adj* abrupt, alarming, astonishing, shocking, sudden, surprising, unexpected, unforeseen, unheard of.

starvation *n* famine, famishment.

starve *vb* famish, perish; be in need, lack, want; kill, subdue.

starveling *adj* attenuated, emaciated, gaunt, hungry, lank, lean, meagre, scraggy, skinny, thin. • *n* beggar, mendicant, pauper.

state *vb* affirm, assert, aver, declare, explain, expound, express, narrate, propound, recite, say, set forth, specify, voice. • *adj* civic, national, public. • *n* case, circumstances, condition, pass, phase, plight, position, posture, predicament, situation, status; condition, guise, mode, quality, rank; dignity, glory, grandeur, magnificence, pageantry, parade, pomp, spendour; body politic, civil community, commonwealth, nation, realm.

statecraft *n* diplomacy, political subtlety, state management, statesmanship.

stated *adj* established, fixed, regular, settled; detailed, set forth, specified.

stately *adj* august, dignified, elevated, grand, imperial, imposing, lofty, magnificent, majestic, noble, princely, royal; ceremonious, formal, magisterial, pompous, solemn.

statement *n* account, allegation, announcement, communiqué, declaration, description, exposition, mention, narration, narrative, recital, relation, report, specification; assertion, predication, proposition, pronouncement, thesis.

statesman *n* politician.

station *vb* establish, fix, locate, place, post, set. • *n* location, place, position, lost, seat, situation; business, employment, function, occupation, office; character, condition, degree, dignity, footing, rank, standing, state, status; depot, stop, terminal.

stationary *adj* fixed, motionless, permanent, quiescent, stable, standing, still.

statuary *n* carving, sculpture, statues.

statue *n* figurine, image, statuette.

stature *n* height, physique, size, tallness; altitude, consequence, elevation, eminence, prominence.

status *n* caste, condition, footing, position, rank, standing, station.

statute *n* act, decree, edict, enactment, law, ordinance, regulation.

staunch[1], **stanch** *vb* arrest, block, check, dam, plug, stem, stop.

staunch[2] *adj* firm, sound, stout, strong; constant, faithful, firm, hearty, loyal, resolute, stable, steadfast, steady, strong, trustworthy, trusty, unwavering, zealous.

stave *vb* break, burst; (*with* **off**) adjourn, defer, delay, postpone, procrastinate, put off, waive.

stay *vb* abide, dwell, lodge, rest, sojourn, tarry; continue, halt, remain, stand still, stop, attend, delay, linger, wait; arrest, check, curb, hold, keep in, prevent, rein in, restrain, withhold; delay, detain, hinder, obstruct; hold up, prop, shore up, support, sustain, uphold. • *n* delay, repose, rest, sojourn; halt, stand, stop; bar, check, curb, hindrance, impediment, interruption, obstacle, obstruction, restraint, stumbling block; buttress, dependence, prop, staff, support, supporter.

stead *n* place, room.

steadfast *adj* established, fast, firm, fixed, stable; constant, faithful, implicit, persevering, pertinacious, resolute, resolved, staunch, steady, unhesitating, unreserved, unshaken, unwavering, wholehearted.

steadiness *n* constancy, firmness, perseverance, persistence, resolution, steadfastness; fixedness, stability.

steady *vb* balance, counterbalance, secure, stabilize, support. • *adj* firm, fixed, stable; constant, equable, regular, undeviating, uniform, unremitting; persevering, resolute, staunch, steadfast, unchangeable, unwavering.

steal *vb* burglarize, burgle, crib, embezzle, filch, peculate, pilfer, plagiarize, poach, purloin, shoplift, thieve; creep, sneak, pass stealthily.

stealing *n* burglary, larceny, peculation, shoplifting, robbery, theft, thievery.

stealth *n* secrecy, slyness, stealthiness.

stealthy *adj* clandestine, furtive, private, secret, skulking, sly, sneaking, surreptitious, underhand.

steam *vb* emit vapour, fume; evaporate, vaporize; coddle, cook, poach; navigate, sail; be hot, sweat. • *n* vapour; effluvium, exhalation, fume, mist, reek, smoke.

steamboat *n* steamer, steamship.

steamy *adj* misty, moist, vaporous; erotic, voluptuous.

steed *n* charger, horse, mount.

steel *vb* case-harden, edge; brace, fortify, harden, make firm, nerve, strengthen.

steep[1] *adj* abrupt, declivitous, precipitous, sheer, sloping, sudden. • *n* declivity, precipice.

steep[2] *vb* digest, drench, imbrue, imbue, macerate, saturate, soak.

steeple *n* belfry, spire, tower, turret.

steer *vb* direct, conduct, govern, guide, pilot, point.

steersman *n* conductor, guide, helmsman, pilot.

stellar *adj* astral, starry, star-spangled, stellary.

stem[1] *vb* (*with* **from**) bud, descend, generate, originate, spring, sprout. • *n* axis, stipe, trunk; pedicel, peduncle, petiole, stalk; branch, descendant, offspring, progeny, scion, shoot; ancestry, descent, family, generation, line, lineage, pedigree, race, stock; (*naut*) beak, bow, cutwater, forepart, prow; helm, lookout; etymon, radical, radix, origin, root.

stem[2] *vb* breast, oppose, resist, withstand; check, dam, oppose, staunch, stay, stop.

stench *n* bad smell, fetor, offensive odour, stink.

stenography *n* brachygraphy, shorthand, tachygraphy.

stentorian *adj* loud-voiced, powerful, sonorous, thundering, trumpet-like.

step *vb* pace, stride, tramp, tread, walk. • *n* footstep, pace, stride; stair, tread; degree, gradation, grade, interval; advance, advancement, progression; act, action, deed, procedure, proceeding; footprint, trace, track, vestige; footfall, gait, pace, walk; expedient, means, measure, method; round, rundle, rung.

steppe *n* pampa, prairie, savannah.

sterile *adj* barren, infecund, unfruitful, unproductive, unprolific; bare, dry, empty, poor; (*bot*) acarpous, male, staminate.

sterility *n* barrenness, fruitlessness, infecundity, unfruitfulness, unproductiveness.

sterling *adj* genuine, positive, pure, real, sound, standard, substantial, true.

stern[1] *adj* austere, dour, forbidding, grim, severe; bitter, cruel, hard, harsh, inflexible, relentless, rigid, rigorous, severe, strict, unrelenting; immovable, incorruptible, steadfast, uncompromising.

stern[2] *n* behind, breach, hind part, posterior, rear, tail; (*naut*) counter, poop, rudderpost, tailpost; butt, buttocks, fundament, rump.

sternness *n* austerity, rigidity, severity; asperity, cruelty, harshness, inflexibility, relentlessness, rigour.

sternum *n* (*anat*) breastbone, sternon.

stertorous *adj* hoarsely breathing, snoring.

stew *vb* boil, seethe, simmer, stive. • *n* ragout; confusion, difficulty, mess, scrape.

steward *n* chamberlain, majordomo, seneschal; maniple, purveyor.

stick[1] *vb* gore, penetrate, pierce, puncture, spear, stab, transfix; infix, insert, thrust; attach, cement, glue, paste; fix in, set; adhere, cleave, cling, hold; abide, persist, remain, stay, stop; doubt, hesitate, scruple, stickle, waver; (*with* **by**) adhere to, be faithful, support. • *n* prick, stab, thrust.

stick[2] *n* birch, rod, switch; bat, bludgeon, club, cudgel, shillelah; cane, staff, walking stick; cue, pole, spar, stake.

stickiness *n* adhesiveness, glutinousness, tenacity, viscosity, viscousness.

stickle *vb* altercate, contend, contest, struggle; doubt, hesitate, scruple, stick, waver.

sticky *adj* adhesive, clinging, gluey, glutinous, gummy, mucilaginous, tenacious, viscid, viscous.

stiff *adj* inflexible, rigid, stark, unbending, unyielding; firm, tenacious, thick; obstinate, pertinacious, strong, stubborn; absolute, austere, dogmatic, inexorable, peremptory, positive, rigorous, severe, straitlaced, strict, stringent, uncompromising; ceremonious, chilling, constrained, formal, frigid, prim, punctilious, stately, starchy, stilted; abrupt, cramped, crude, graceless, harsh, inelegant.

stiff-necked *adj* contumacious, cross-grained, dogged, headstrong, intractable, mulish, obdurate, obstinate, stubborn, unruly.

stiffness *n* hardness, inflexibility, rigidity, rigidness, rigour, starkness; compactness, consistence, denseness, density, thickness; contumaciousness, inflexibility, obstinacy, pertinacity, stubbornness; austerity, harshness, rigorousness, severity, sternness, strictness; constraint, formality, frigidity, precision, primness, tenseness.

stifle *vb* choke, smother, suffocate; check, deaden, destroy, extinguish, quench, repress, stop, suppress; conceal, gag, hush, muffle, muzzle, silence, smother, still.

stigma *n* blot, blur, brand, disgrace, dishonour, reproach, shame, spot, stain, taint, tarnish.

stigmatize *vb* brand, defame, discredit, disgrace, dishonour, post, reproach, slur, villify.

stiletto *n* dagger, dirk, poniard, stylet; bodkin, piercer.

still[1] *vb* hush, muffle, silence, stifle; allay, appease, calm, compose, lull, pacify, quiet, smooth, tranquillize; calm, check, immobilize, restrain, stop, subdue, suppress. • *adj* hushed, mum, mute, noiseless, silent; calm, placid, quiet, serene, stilly, tranquil, unruffled; inert, motionless, quiescent, stagnant, stationary. • *n* hush, lull, peace, quiet, quietness, quietude, silence, stillness, tranquillity; picture, photograph, shot.

still[2] *n* distillery, still-house; distillatory, retort, stillatory.

still[3] *adv, conj* till now, to this time, yet; however, nevertheless, notwithstanding; always, continually, ever, habitually, uniformly; after that, again, in continuance.

stilted *adj* bombastic, fustian, grandiloquent, grandiose, high-flown, high-sounding, inflated, magniloquent, pompous, pretentious, stilty, swelling, tumid, turgid.

stimulant *adj* exciting, stimulating, stimulative. • *n* bracer, cordial, pick-me-up, tonic; fillip, incentive, provocative, spur, stimulus.

stimulate *vb* animate, arouse, awaken, brace, encourage, energize, excite, fire, foment, goad, impel, incite, inflame, inspirit, instigate, kindle, prick, prompt, provoke, rally, rouse, set on, spur, stir up, urge, whet, work up.

stimulus *n* encouragement, fillip, goad, incentive, incitement, motivation, motive, provocation, spur, stimulant.

sting *vb* hurt, nettle, prick, wound; afflict, cut, pain.

stinging *adj* acute, painful, piercing; biting, nipping, pungent, tingling.

stingy *adj* avaricious, close, close-fisted, covetous, grudging, mean, miserly, narrow-hearted, niggardly, parsimonious, penurious.

stink *vb* emit a stench, reek, smell bad. • *n* bad smell, fetor, offensive odour, stench.

stint *vb* bound, confine, limit, restrain; begrudge, pinch, scrimp, skimp, straiten; cease, desist, stop. • *n* bound, limit, restraint; lot, period, project, quota, share, shift, stretch, task, time, turn.

stipend *n* allowance, compensation, emolument, fee, hire, honorarium, pay, remuneration, salary, wages.

stipulate *vb* agree, bargain, condition, contract, covenant, engage, provide, settle terms.

stipulation *n* agreement, bargain, concordat, condition, contract, convention, covenant, engagement, indenture, obligation, pact.

stir *vb* budge, change place, go, move; agitate, bestir, disturb, prod; argue, discuss, moot, raise, start; animate, arouse, awaken, excite, goad, incite, instigate, prompt, provoke, quicken, rouse, spur, stimulate; appear, happen, turn up; get up, rise; (*with* **up**) animate, awaken, incite, instigate, move, provoke, quicken, rouse, stimulate. • *n* activity, ado, agitation, bustle, confusion, excitement, fidget, flurry, fuss, hurry, movement; commotion, disorder, disturbance, tumult, uproar.

stirring *adj* active, brisk, diligent, industrious, lively, smart; animating, arousing, awakening, exciting, quickening, stimulating.

stitch *vb* backstitch, baste, bind, embroider, fell, hem, seam, sew, tack, whip.

stive *vb* stow, stuff; boil, seethe, stew; make close, hot or sultry.

stock *vb* fill, furnish, store, supply; accumulate, garner, hoard, lay in, reposit, reserve, save, treasure up. • *adj* permanent, standard, standing. • *n* assets, capital, commodities, fund, principal, shares; accumulation, hoard, inventory, merchandise, provision, range, reserve, store, supply; ancestry, breed, descent, family, house, line, lineage, parentage, pedigree, race; cravat, neckcloth; butt, haft, hand; block, log, pillar, post, stake; stalk, stem, trunk.

stockholder *n* shareholder.

stocking *n* hose, sock.

stock market *n* stock exchange; cattle market.

stocks *npl* funds, public funds, public securities; shares.

stockstill *adj* dead-still, immobile, motionless, stationary, still, unmoving.

stocky *adj* chubby, chunky, dumpy, plump, short, stout, stubby, thickset.

stoic, stoical *adj* apathetic, cold-blooded, impassive, imperturbable, passionless, patient, philosophic, philosophical, phlegmatic, unimpassioned.

stoicism *n* apathy, coldness, coolness, impassivity, indifference, insensibility, nonchalance, phlegm.

stolen *adj* filched, pilfered, purloined; clandestine, furtive, secret, sly, stealthy, surreptitious.

stolid *adj* blockish, doltish, dull, foolish, heavy, obtuse, slow, stockish, stupid.

stolidity *n* doltishness, dullness, foolishness, obtuseness, stolidness, stupidity.

stomach *vb* abide, bear, brook, endure, put up with, stand, submit to, suffer, swallow, tolerate. • *n* abdomen, belly, gut, paunch, pot, tummy; appetite, desire, inclination, keenness, liking, relish, taste.

stone *vb* cover, face, slate, tile; lapidate, pelt. • *n* boulder, cobble, gravel, pebble, rock; gem, jewel, precious stone; cenotaph, gravestone, monument, tombstone; nut, pit; adamant, agate, flint, gneiss, granite, marble, slate, etc.

stony *adj* gritty, hard, lapidose, lithic, petrous, rocky; adamantine, flinty, hard, inflexible, obdurate; cruel, hard-hearted, inexorable, pitiless, stony-hearted, unfeeling, unrelenting.

stoop *vb* bend forward, bend down, bow, lean, sag, slouch, slump; abase, cower, cringe, give in, submit, succumb, surrender; condescend, deign, descend, vouchsafe; fall, sink. • *n* bend, inclination, sag, slouch, slump; descent, swoop.

stop *vb* block, blockade, close, close up, obstruct, occlude; arrest, check, halt, hold, pause, stall, stay; bar, delay, embargo, hinder, impede, intercept, interrupt, obstruct, preclude, prevent, repress, restrain, staunch, suppress, thwart; break off, cease, desist, discontinue, forbear, give over, leave off, refrain from; intermit, quiet, quieten, terminate; lodge, tarry. • *n* halt, intermission, pause, respite, rest, stoppage, suspension, truce; block, cessation, check, hindrance, interruption, obstruction, repression; bar, impediment, obstacle; full stop, point.

stopcock *n* cock, faucet, tap.

stoppage *n* arrest, block, check, closure, hindrance, interruption, obstruction, prevention.

stopper *n* cork, plug, stopple.

store *vb* accumulate, amass, cache, deposit, garner, hoard, husband, lay by, lay in, lay up, put by, reserve, save, store up, stow away, treasure up; furnish, provide, replenish, stock, supply. • *n* accumulation, cache, deposit, fund, hoard, provision, reserve, stock, supply, treasure, treasury; abundance, plenty; storehouse; emporium, market, shop.

storehouse *n* depository, depot, godown, magazine, repository, store, warehouse.

storm *vb* assail, assault, attack; blow violently; fume, rage, rampage, rant, rave, tear. • *n* blizzard, gale, hurricane, squall, tempest, tornado, typhoon, whirlwind; agitation clamour, commotion, disturbance, insurrection, outbreak sedition, tumult, turmoil; adversity, affliction, calamity, distress; assault, attack, brunt, onset, onslaught; violence.

storminess *n* inclemency, roughness, tempestuousness.

stormy *adj* blustering, boisterous, gusty, squally, tempestuous, windy; passionate, riotous, rough, turbulent, violent, wild; agitated, furious.

story *n* annals, chronicle, history, record; account, narration, narrative, recital, record, rehearsal, relation, report, statement, tale; fable, fiction, novel, romance; anecdote, incident, legend, tale; canard, fabrication, falsehood, fib, figure, invention, lie, untruth.

storyteller *n* bard, chronicler, narrator, raconteur.

stout *adj* able-bodied, athletic, brawny, lusty, robust, sinewy, stalwart, strong, sturdy, vigorous; courageous, hardy, indomitable, stouthearted; contumacious, obstinate, proud, resolute, stubborn; compact, firm, solid, staunch; bouncing, bulky, burly, chubby, corpulent, fat, heavy, jolly, large, obese, plump, portly, stocky, strapping, thickset.

stouthearted *adj* fearless, heroic, redoubtable; bold, brave, courageous, dauntless, doughty, firm, gallant, hardy, indomitable, intrepid, resolute, valiant, valorous.

stow *vb* load, pack, put away, store, stuff.

straddle *vb* bestride.

straggle *vb* rove, wander; deviate, digress, ramble, range, roam, stray, stroll.

straggling *adj* rambling, roving, straying, strolling, wandering; scattered.

straight *adj* direct, near, rectilinear, right, short, undeviating, unswerving; erect, perpendicular, plumb, right, upright, vertical; equitable, fair, honest, honourable, just, square, straightforward. • *adv* at once, directly, forthwith, immediately, straightaway, straightway, without delay.

straightaway, straightway *adv* at once, directly, forthwith, immediately, speedily, straight, suddenly, without delay.

straighten *vb* arrange, make straight, neaten, order, tidy.

straight-laced *see* **strait-laced**.

strain[1] *vb* draw tightly, make tense, stretch, tighten; injure, sprain, wrench; exert, overexert, overtax, rack; embrace, fold, hug, press, squeeze; compel, constrain, force; dilute, distill, drain, filter, filtrate, ooze, percolate, purify, separate; fatigue, overtask, overwork, task, tax, tire. • *n* stress, tenseness, tension, tensity; effort, exertion, force, overexertion; burden, task, tax; sprain, wrench; lay, melody, movement, snatch, song, stave, tune.

strain[2] *n* manner, style, tone, vein; disposition, tendency, trait, turn; descent, extraction, family, lineage, pedigree, race, stock.

strait *adj* close, confined, constrained, constricted, contracted, narrow; rigid, rigorous, severe, strict; difficult, distressful, grievous, straitened. • *n* channel, narrows, pass, sound.

straits *npl* crisis, difficulty, dilemma, distress, embarrassment, emergency, exigency, extremity, hardship, pass, perplexity, pinch, plight, predicament.

straiten *vb* confine, constrain, constrict, contract, limit; narrow; intensify, stretch; distress, embarrass, perplex, pinch, press.

straitened *adj* distressed, embarrassed limited, perplexed, pinched.

strait-laced, straight-laced *adj* austere, formal, prim, rigid, rigorous, stern, stiff, strict, uncompromising.

straitness *n* narrowness, rigour, severity, strictness; difficulty, distress, trouble; insufficiency, narrowness, scarcity, want.

strand[1] *vb* abandon, beach, be wrecked, cast away, go aground, ground, maroon, run aground, wreck. • *n* beach, coast, shore.

strand[2] *n* braid, cord, fibre, filament, line, rope, string, tress.

stranded *adj* aground, ashore, cast away, lost, shipwrecked, wrecked.

strange *adj* alien, exotic, far-fetched, foreign, outlandish, remote; new, novel; curious, exceptional, extraordinary, irregular, odd, particular, peculiar, rare, singular, surprising, uncommon, unusual; abnormal, anomalous, extraordinary, inconceivable,

incredible, inexplicable, marvellous, mysterious, preternatural, unaccountable, unbelievable, unheard of, unique, unnatural, wonderful; bizarre, droll, grotesque, quaint, queer; inexperienced, unacquainted, unfamiliar, unknown; bashful, distant, distrustful, reserved, shy, uncommunicative.

strangeness *n* foreignness; bashfulness, coldness, distance, reserve, shyness, uncommunicativeness; eccentricity, grotesqueness, oddness, singularity, uncommonness, uncouthness.

stranger *n* alien, foreigner, newcomer, immigrant, outsider; guest, visitor.

strangle *vb* choke, contract, smother, squeeze, stifle, suffocate, throttle, tighten; keep back, quiet, repress, still, suppress.

strap *vb* beat, thrash, whip; bind, fasten, sharpen, strop. • *n* thong; band, ligature, strip, tie; razor-strap, strop.

strapping *adj* big, burly, large, lusty, stalwart, stout, strong, tall.

stratagem *n* artifice, cunning, device, dodge, finesse, intrigue, machination, manoeuvre, plan, plot, ruse, scheme, trick, wile.

strategic, strategical *adj* calculated, deliberate, diplomatic, manoeuvering, planned, politic, tactical; critical, decisive, key, vital.

strategy *n* generalship, manoeuvering, plan, policy, stratagem, strategetics, tactics.

stratum *n* band, bed, layer.

straw *n* culm, stalk, stem; button, farthing, fig, penny, pin, rush, snap.

stray *vb* deviate, digress, err, meander, ramble, range, roam, rove, straggle, stroll, swerve, transgress, wander. • *adj* abandoned, lost, strayed, wandering; accidental, erratic, random, scattered.

streak *vb* band, bar, striate, stripe, vein; dart, dash, flash, hurtle, run, speed, sprint, stream, tear. • *n* band, bar, belt, layer, line, strip, stripe, thread, trace, vein; cast, grain, tone, touch, vein; beam, bolt, dart, dash, flare, flash, ray, stream.

streaky *adj* streaked, striped, veined.

stream *vb* course, flow, glide, pour, run, spout; emit, pour out, shed; emanate, go forth, issue, radiate; extend, float, stretch out, wave. • *n* brook, burn, race, rill, rivulet, run, runlet, runnel, trickle; course, current, flow, flux, race, rush, tide, torrent, wake, wash; beam, gleam, patch, radiation, ray, streak.

streamer *n* banner, colours, ensign, flag, pennon, standard.

street *n* avenue, highway, road, way.

strength *n* force, might, main, nerve, potency, power, vigour; hardness, solidity, toughness; impregnability, proof; brawn, grit, healthy, lustiness, muscle, robustness, sinew, stamina, thews, vigorousness; animation, courage, determination, firmness, fortitude, resolution, spirit; cogency, efficacy, soundness, validity; emphasis, energy; security, stay, support; brightness, brilliance, clearness, intensity, vitality, vividness; body, excellence, virtue; impetuosity, vehemence, violence; boldness.

strengthen *vb* buttress, recruit, reinforce; fortify; brace, energize, harden, nerve, steel, stimulate; freshen, invigorate, vitalize; animate, encourage; clench, clinch, confirm, corroborate, establish, fix, justify, sustain, support.

strenuous *adj* active, ardent, eager, earnest, energetic, resolute, vigorous, zealous; bold, determined, doughty, intrepid, resolute, spirited, strong, valiant.

stress *vb* accent, accentuate, emphasize, highlight, point up, underline, underscore; bear, bear upon, press, pressurize; pull, rack, strain, stretch, tense, tug. • *n* accent, accentuation, emphasis; effort, force, pull, strain, tension, tug; boisterousness, severity, violence; pressure, urgency.

stretch *vb* brace, screw, strain, tense, tighten; elongate, extend, lengthen, protract, pull; display, distend, expand, spread, unfold, widen; sprain, strain; distort, exaggerate, misrepresent. • *n* compass, extension, extent, range, reach, scope; effort, exertion, strain, struggle; course, direction.

strict *adj* close, strained, tense, tight; accurate, careful, close, exact, literal, particular, precise, scrupulous; austere, inflexible, harsh, orthodox, puritanical, rigid, rigorous, severe, stern, strait-laced, stringent, uncompromising, unyielding.

stricture *n* animadversion, censure, denunciation, criticism, compression, constrict on, contraction.

strife *n* battle, combat, conflict, contention, contest, discord, quarrel, struggle, warfare.

strike *vb* bang, beat, belabour, box, buffet, cudgel, cuff, hit, knock, lash, pound, punch, rap, slap, slug, smite, thump, whip; impress, imprint, stamp; afflict, chastise, deal, give, inflict, punish; affect, astonish, electrify, stun; clash, collide, dash, touch; surrender, yield; mutiny, rebel, rise.

stringent *adj* binding, contracting, rigid, rigorous, severe, strict.

strip[1] *n* piece, ribbon, shred, slip.

strip[2] *vb* denude, hull, skin, uncover; bereave, deprive, deforest, desolate, despoil, devastate, disarm, dismantle, disrobe, divest, expose, fleece, loot, shave; plunder, pillage, ransack, rob, sack, spoil; disrobe, uncover, undress.

strive *vb* aim, attempt, endeavour, exert, labour, strain, struggle, toil; contend, contest, fight, tussle, wrestle; compete, cope.

stroke[1] *n* blow, glance, hit, impact, knock, lash, pat, percussion, rap, shot, switch, thump; attack, paralysis, stroke; affliction, damage, hardship, hurt, injury, misfortune, reverse, visitation; dash, feat, masterstroke, touch.

stroke[2] *vb* caress, feel, palpate, pet, knead, massage, nuzzle, rub, touch.

stroll *vb* loiter, lounge, ramble, range, rove, saunter, straggle, stray, wander. • *n* excursion, promenade, ramble, rambling, roving, tour, trip, walk, wandering.

strong *adj* energetic, forcible, powerful, robust, sturdy; able, enduring; cogent, firm, valid.

structure *vb* arrange, constitute, construct, make, organize. • *n* arrangement, conformation, configuration, constitution, construction, form, formation, make, organization; anatomy, composition, texture; building, edifice, fabric, framework, pile.

struggle *vb* aim, endeavour, exert, labour, strive, toil, try; battle, contend, contest, fight, wrestle; agonize, flounder, writhe. • *n* effort, endeavour, exertion, labour, pains; battle, conflict, contention, contest, fight, strife; agony, contortions, distress.

stubborn *adj* contumacious, dogged, headstrong, heady, inflexible, intractable, mulish, obdurate, obstinate, perverse, positive, refractory, ungovernable, unmanageable, unruly, unyielding, willful; constant, enduring, firm, hardy, persevering, persistent, steady, stoical, uncomplaining, unremitting; firm, hard, inflexible, stiff, strong, tough, unpliant, studied.

studious *adj* contemplative, meditative, reflective, thoughtful; assiduous, attentive, desirous, diligent, eager, lettered, scholarly, zealous.

study *vb* cogitate, lucubrate, meditate, muse, ponder, reflect, think; analyze, contemplate, examine, investigate, ponder, probe, scrutinize, search, sift, weigh. • *n* exercise, inquiry, investigation, reading, research, stumble; cogitation, consideration, contemplation, examination, meditation, reflection, thought; stun; model, object, representation, sketch; den, library, office, studio.

stunning *adj* deafening, stentorian; dumbfounding, stupefying.

stunted *adj* checked, diminutive, dwarfed, dwarfish, lilliputian, little, nipped, small, undersized.

stupendous *adj* amazing, astonishing, astounding, marvellous, overwhelming, surprising, wonderful; enormous, huge, immense, monstrous, prodigious, towering, tremendous, vast.

stupid *adj* brainless, crass, doltish, dull, foolish, idiotic, inane, inept, obtuse, pointless, prosaic, senseless, simple, slow, sluggish, stolid, tedious, tiresome, witless.

stupor *n* coma, confusion, daze, lethargy, narcosis, numbness, stupefaction, torpor.

sturdy *adj* bold, determined, dogged, firm, hardy, obstinate, persevering, pertinacious, resolute, stiff, stubborn, sturdy; athletic, brawny, forcible, lusty, muscular, powerful, robust, stalwart, stout, strong, thickset, vigorous, well-set.

style *vb* address, call, characterize, denominate, designate, dub, entitle, name, term. • *n* dedication, expression, phraseology, turn; cast, character, fashion, form, genre, make, manner, method, mode, model, shape, vogue, way; appellation, denomination, designation, name, title; chic, elegance, smartness; pen, pin, point, stylus.

stylish *adj* chic, courtly, elegant, fashionable, genteel, modish, polished, smart.

suave *adj* affable, agreeable, amiable, bland, courteous, debonair, delightful, glib, gracious, mild, pleasant, smooth, sweet, oily, unctuous, urbane.

subdue *vb* beat, bend, break, bow, conquer, control, crush, defeat, discomfit, foil, master, overbear, overcome, overpower, overwhelm, quell, rout, subject, subjugate, surmount, vanquish, worst; allay, choke, curb, mellow, moderate, mollify, reduce, repress, restrain, soften, suppress, temper.

subject *vb* control, master, overcome, reduce, subdue, subjugate, tame; enslave, enthral; abandon, refer, submit, surrender. • *adj* beneath, subjacent, underneath; dependent, enslaved, inferior, servile, subjected, subordinate, subservient; conditional, obedient, submissive; disposed, exposed to, liable, obnoxious, prone. • *n* dependent, henchman, liegeman, slave, subordinate; matter, point, subject matter, theme, thesis, topic; nominative, premise; case, object, patient, recipient; ego, mind, self, thinking.

subjoin *vb* add, affix, annex, append, join, suffix.

subjugate *vb* conquer, enslave, enthral, master, overcome, overpower, overthrow, subdue, subject, vanquish.

sublimate *vb* alter, change, repress.

sublime *adj* aloft, *elevated, high,* sacred; eminent, exalted, grand, great, lofty, mighty; august, glorious, magnificent, majestic, noble, stately, solemn, sublunary; elated, elevated, eloquent, exhilarated, raised.

submission *n* capitulation, cession, relinquishment, surrender, yielding; acquiescence, compliance, obedience, resignation; deference, homage, humility, lowliness, obeisance, passiveness, prostration, self-abasement, submissiveness.

submissive *adj* amenable, compliant, docile, pliant, tame, tractable, yielding; acquiescent, long-suffering, obedient, passive, patient, resigned, unassertive, uncomplaining, unrepining; deferential, humble, lowly, meek, obsequious, prostrate, self-abasing.

submit *vb* cede, defer, endure, resign, subject, surrender, yield; commit, propose, refer; offer; acquiesce, bend, capitulate, comply, stoop, succumb.

subordinate *adj* ancillary, dependent, inferior, junior, minor, secondary, subject, subservient, subsidiary. • *n* assistant, dependant, inferior, subject, underling.

subscribe *vb* accede, approve, agree, assent, consent, yield; contribute, donate, give, offer, promise.

subscription *n* aid, assistance, contribution, donation, gift, offering.

subsequent *adj* after, attendant, ensuing, later, latter, following, posterior, sequent, succeeding.

subservient *adj* inferior, obsequious, servile, subject, subordinate; accessory, aiding, auxiliary, conducive, contributory, helpful, instrumental, serviceable, useful.

subside *vb* settle, sink; abate, decline, decrease, diminish, drop, ebb, fall, intermit, lapse, lessen, lower, lull, wane.

subsidence *n* settling, sinking; abatement, decline, decrease, descent, ebb, diminution, lessening.

subsidiary *adj* adjutant, aiding, assistant, auxiliary, cooperative, corroborative, helping, subordinate, subservient.

subsidize *vb* aid, finance, fund, sponsor, support, underwrite.

subsidy *n* aid, bounty, grant, subvention, support, underwriting.

subsist *vb* be, breathe, consist, exist, inhere, live, prevail; abide, continue, endure, persist, remain; feed, maintain, ration, support.

subsistence *n* aliment, food, livelihood, living, maintenance, meat, nourishment, nutriment, provision, rations, support, sustenance, victuals.

substance *n* actuality, element, groundwork, hypostasis, reality, substratum; burden, content, core, drift, essence, gist, heart, import, meaning, pith, sense, significance, solidity, soul, sum, weight; estate, income, means, property, resources, wealth.

substantial *adj* actual, considerable, essential, existent, hypostatic, pithy, potential, real, subsistent, virtual; concrete, durable, positive, solid, tangible, true; corporeal, bodily, material; bulky, firm, goodly, heavy, large, massive, notable, significant, sizable, solid, sound, stable, stout, strong, well-made; cogent, just, efficient, influential, valid, weighty.

substantially *adv* adequately, essentially, firmly, materially, positively, really, truly.

substantiate *vb* actualize, confirm, corroborate, establish, prove, ratify, verify.

subterfuge *n* artifice, evasion, excuse, expedient, mask, pretence, pretext, quirk, shift, shuffle, sophistry, trick.

subtle *adj* arch, artful, astute, crafty, crooked, cunning, designing, diplomatic, intriguing, insinuating, sly, tricky, wily; clever, ingenious; acute, deep, discerning, discriminating, keen, profound, sagacious, shrewd; airy, delicate, ethereal, light, nice, rare, refined, slender, subtle, thin, volatile.

subtlety *n* artfulness, artifice, astuteness, craft, craftiness, cunning, guile, subtleness; acumen, acuteness, cleverness, discernment, intelligence, keenness, sagacity, sharpness, shrewdness; attenuation, delicacy, fitness, nicety, rareness, refinement.

subtract *vb* deduct, detract, diminish, remove, take, withdraw.

suburbs *npl* environs, confines, neighbourhood, outskirts, precincts, purlieus, vicinage.

subversive *adj* destructive, overthrowing, pervasive, ruining, upsetting. • *n* collaborator, dissident, insurrectionist, saboteur, terrorist, traitor.

subvert *vb* invert, overset, overthrow, overturn, reverse, upset; demolish, destroy, extinguish, raze, ruin; confound, corrupt, injure, pervert.

succeed *vb* ensue, follow, inherit, replace; flourish, gain, hit, prevail, prosper, thrive, win.

success *n* attainment, issue, result; fortune, happiness, hit, luck, prosperity, triumph.

successful *adj* auspicious, booming, felicitous, fortunate, happy, lucky, prosperous, victorious, winning.

succession *n* chain, concatenation, cycle, consecution, following, procession, progression, rotation, round, sequence, series, suite; descent, entail, inheritance, lineage, race, reversion.

succinct *adj* brief, compact, compendious, concise, condensed, curt, laconic, pithy, short, summary, terse.

succour *vb* aid, assist, help, relieve; cherish, comfort, encourage, foster, nurse. • *n* aid, assistance, help, relief, support.

succulent *adj* juicy, luscious, lush, nutritive, sappy.

succumb *vb* capitulate, die, submit, surrender, yield.

sudden *adj* abrupt, hasty, hurried, immediate, instantaneous, rash, unanticipated, unexpected, unforeseen, unusual; brief, momentary, quick, rapid.

sue *vb* charge, court, indict, prosecute, solicit, summon, woo; appeal, beg, demand, entreat, implore, petition, plead, pray, supplicate.

suffer *vb* feel, undergo; bear, endure, sustain, tolerate; admit, allow, indulge, let, permit.

sufferable *adj* allowable, bearable, endurable, permissible, tolerable.

sufferance *n* endurance, inconvenience, misery, pain, suffering; long-suffering, moderation, patience, submission; allowance, permission, toleration.

suffice *vb* avail, content, satisfy, serve.

sufficient *adj* adequate, ample, commensurate, competent, enough, full, plenteous, satisfactory; able, equal, fit, qualified, responsible.

suffocate *vb* asphyxiate, choke, smother, stifle, strangle.

suffrage *n* ballot, franchise, voice, vote; approval, attestation, consent, testimonial, witness.

suggest *vb* advise, allude, hint, indicate, insinuate, intimate, move, present, prompt, propose, propound, recommend.

suggestion *n* allusion, hint, indication, insinuation, intimation, presentation, prompting, proposal, recommendation, reminder.

suit *vb* accommodate, adapt, adjust, fashion, fit, level, match; accord, become, befit, gratify, harmonize, please, satisfy, tally. • *n* appeal, entreaty, invocation, petition, prayer, request, solicitation, supplication; courtship, wooing; action, case, cause, process, prosecution, trial; clothing, costume, habit.

suitable *adj* adapted, accordant, agreeable, answerable, apposite, applicable, appropriate, apt, becoming, befitting, conformable, congruous, convenient, consonant, correspondent, decent, due, eligible, expedient, fit, fitting, just, meet, pertinent, proper, relevant, seemly, worthy.

suite *n* attendants, bodyguard, convoy, cortege, court, escort, followers, staff, retainers, retinue, train; collection, series, set, suit; apartment, rooms.

sulky *adj* aloof, churlish, cross, cross-grained, dogged, grouchy, ill-humoured, ill-tempered, moody, morose, perverse, sour, spleenish, spleeny, splenetic, sullen, surly, vexatious, wayward.

sullen *adj* cross, crusty, glum, grumpy, ill-tempered, moody, morose, sore, sour, sulky; cheerless, cloudy, dark, depressing, dismal, foreboding, funereal, gloomy, lowering, melancholy, mournful, sombre; dull, heavy, slow, sluggish; intractable, obstinate, perverse, refractory, stubborn, vexatious; baleful, evil, inauspicious, malign, malignant, sinister, unlucky, unpropitious.

sully *vb* blemish, blot, contaminate, deface, defame, dirty, disgrace, dishonour, foul, smirch, soil, slur, spot, stain, tarnish.

sultry *adj* close, damp, hot, humid, muggy, oppressive, stifling, stuffy, sweltering.

sum *vb* add, calculate, compute, reckon; collect, comprehend, condense, epitomize, summarize. • *n* aggregate, amount, total, totality, whole; compendium, substance, summary; acme, completion, height, summit.

summary *adj* brief, compendious, concise, curt, laconic, pithy, short, succinct, terse; brief, quick, rapid. • *n* abridgement, abstract, brief, compendium, digest, epitome, precis, résumé, syllabus, synopsis.

summit *n* acme, apex, cap, climax, crest, crown, pinnacle, top, vertex, zenith.

summon *vb* arouse, bid, call, cite, invite, invoke, rouse; convene, convoke; charge, indict, prosecute, subpoena, sue.

sumptuous *adj* costly, dear, expensive, gorgeous, grand, lavish, luxurious, magnificent, munificent, pompous, prodigal, rich, showy, splendid, stately, superb.

sunburnt *adj* bronzed, brown, ruddy, tanned.

sunder *vb* break, disconnect, disjoin, dissociate, dissever, disunited, divide, part, separate, sever.

sundry *adj* different, divers, several, some, various.

sunny *adj* bright, brilliant, clear, fine, luminous, radiant, shining, unclouded, warm; cheerful, genial, happy, joyful, mild, optimistic, pleasant, smiling.

superannuated *adj* aged, antle, antiquated, decrepit, disqualified, doting, effete, imbecile, passé, retired, rusty, time-worn, unfit.

superb *adj* august, beautiful, elegant, exquisite, grand, gorgeous, imposing, magnificent, majestic, noble, pompous, rich, showy, splendid, stately, sumptuous.

supercilious *adj* arrogant, condescending, contemptuous, dictatorial, domineering, haughty, high, imperious, insolent, intolerant, lofty, lordly, magisterial, overbearing, overweening, proud, scornful, vainglorious.

superficial *adj* external, flimsy, shallow, untrustworthy.

superfluity *n* excess, exuberance, redundancy, superabundance, surfeit.

superfluous *adj* excessive, redundant, unnecessary.

superintend *vb* administer, conduct, control, direct, inspect, manage, overlook, oversee, supervise.

superintendence *n* care, charge, control, direction, guidance, government, inspection, management, oversight, supervision, surveillance.

superior *adj* better, greater, high, higher, finer, paramount, supreme, ultra, upper; chief, foremost, principal; distinguished, matchless, noble, pre-eminent, preferable, sovereign, surpassing, unrivalled, unsurpassed; predominant, prevalent. • *n* boss, chief, director, head, higher-up, leader, manager, principal, senior, supervisor.

superiority *n* advantage, ascendency, lead, odds, predominance, pre-eminence, prevalence, transcendence; excellence, nobility, worthiness.

superlative *adj* consummate, greatest, incomparable, peerless, pre-eminent, supreme, surpassing transcendent.

supernatural *adj* abnormal, marvellous, metaphysical, miraculous, otherworldly, preternatural, unearthly.

supernumerary *adj* excessive, odd, redundant, superfluous.

supersede *vb* annul, neutralize, obviate, overrule, suspend; displace, remove, replace, succeed, supplant.

supervise *vb* administer, conduct, control, direct, inspect, manage, overlook, oversee, superintend.

supine *adj* apathetic, careless, drowsy, dull, idle, indifferent, indolent, inert, languid, lethargic, listless, lumpish, lazy, negligent, otiose, prostrate, recumbent, sleepy, slothful, sluggish, spineless, torpid.

supplant *vb* overpower, overthrow, undermine; displace, remove, replace, supersede.

supple *adj* elastic, flexible, limber, lithe, pliable, pliant; compliant, humble, submissive, yielding; adulatory, cringing, fawning, flattering, grovelling, obsequious, oily, parasitical, servile, slavish, sycophantic.

supplement *vb* add, augment, extend, reinforce, supply. • *n* addendum, addition, appendix, codicil, complement, continuation, postscript.

suppliant *adj* begging, beseeching, entreating, imploring, precative precatory, praying, suing, supplicating. • *n* applicant, petitioner, solicitor, suitor, supplicant.

supplicate *vb* beg, beseech, crave, entreat, implore, importune, petition, pray, solicit.

supplication *n* invocation, orison, petition, prayer; entreaty, petition, prayer, request, solicitation.

supply *vb* endue, equip, furnish, minister, outfit, provide, replenish, stock, store; afford, accommodate, contribute, furnish, give, grant, yield. • *n* hoard, provision, reserve, stock, store.

support *vb* brace, cradle, pillow, prop, sustain, uphold; bear, endure, undergo, suffer, tolerate; cherish, keep, maintain, nourish, nurture; act, assume, carry, perform, play, represent; accredit, confirm, corroborate, substantiate, verify; abet, advocate, aid, approve, assist, back, befriend, champion, countenance, encourage, favour, float, hold, patronize, relieve, reinforce, succour, vindicate. • *n* bolster, brace, buttress, foothold, guy, hold, prop, purchase, shore, stay, substructure, supporter, underpinning; groundwork, mainstay, staff; base, basis, bed, foundation; keeping, living, livelihood, maintenance, subsistence, sustenance; confirmation, evidence; aid, assistance, backing, behalf, championship, comfort, countenance, encouragement, favour, help, patronage, succour.

suppose *vb* apprehend, believe, conceive, conclude, consider, conjecture, deem, imagine, judge, presume, presuppose, think; assume, hypothesize; imply, posit, predicate, think; fancy, opine, speculate, surmise, suspect, theorize, wean.

supposition *n* conjecture, guess, guesswork, presumption, surmise; assumption, hypothesis, postulation, theory, thesis; doubt, uncertainty.

suppress *vb* choke, crush, destroy, overwhelm, overpower, overthrow, quash, quell, quench, smother, stifle, subdue, withhold; arrest, inhibit, obstruct, repress, restrain, stop; conceal, extinguish, keep, retain, secret, silence, stifle, strangle.

supremacy *n* ascendancy, domination, headship, lordship, mastery, predominance, pre-eminence, primacy, sovereignty.

supreme *adj* chief, dominant, first, greatest, highest, leading, paramount, predominant, pre-eminent, principal, sovereign.

sure *adj* assured, certain, confident, positive; accurate, dependable, effective, honest, infallible, precise, reliable, trustworthy, undeniable, undoubted, unmistakable, well-proven; guaranteed, inevitable, irrevocable; fast, firm, safe, secure, stable, steady.

surely *adv* assuredly, certainly, infallibly, sure, undoubtedly; firmly, safely, securely, steadily.

surety *n* bail, bond, certainty, guarantee, pledge, safety, security.

surfeit *vb* cram, gorge, overfeed, sate, satiate; cloy, nauseate, pall. • *n* excess, fullness, glut, oppression, plethora, satiation, satiety, superabundance, superfluity.

surge *vb* billow, rise, rush, sweep, swell, swirl, tower. • *n* billow, breaker, roller, wave, white horse.

surly *adj* churlish, crabbed, cross, crusty, discourteous, fretful, gruff, grumpy, harsh, ill-natured, ill-tempered, morose, peevish, perverse, pettish, petulant, rough, rude, snappish, snarling, sour, sullen, testy, touchy, uncivil, ungracious, waspish; dark, tempestuous.

surmise *vb* believe, conclude, conjecture, consider, divine, fancy, guess, imagine, presume, suppose, think, suspect. • *n* conclusion, conjecture, doubt, guess, notion, possibility, supposition, suspicion, thought.

surmount *vb* clear, climb, crown, overtop, scale, top, vault; conquer, master, overcome, overpower, subdue, vanquish; exceed, overpass, pass, surpass, transcend.

surpass *vb* beat, cap, eclipse, exceed, excel, outdo, outmatch, outnumber, outrun, outstrip, override, overshadow, overtop, outshine, surmount, transcend.

surplus *adj* additional, leftover, remaining, spare, superfluous, supernumerary, supplementary. • *n* balance, excess, overplus, remainder, residue, superabundance, surfeit.

surprise *vb* amaze, astonish, astound, bewilder, confuse, disconcert, dumbfound, startle, stun. • *n* amazement, astonishment, blow, shock, wonder.

surprising *adj* amazing, astonishing, astounding, extraordinary, marvellous, unexpected, remarkable, startling, strange, unexpected, wonderful.

surrender *vb* cede, sacrifice, yield; abdicate, abandon, forgo, relinquish, renounce, resign, waive; capitulate, comply, succumb. • *n* abandonment, capitulation, cession, delivery, relinquishment, renunciation, resignation, yielding.

surreptitious *adj* clandestine, fraudulent, furtive, secret, sly, stealthy, unauthorized, underhand.

surround *vb* beset, circumscribe, compass, embrace, encircle, encompass, environ, girdle, hem, invest, loop.

surveillance *n* care, charge, control, direction, inspection, management, oversight, superintendence, supervision, surveyorship, vigilance, watch.

survey *vb* contemplate, observe, overlook, reconnoitre, review, scan, scout, view; examine, inspect, scrutinize; oversee, supervise; estimate, measure, plan, plot, prospect. • *n* prospect, retrospect, sight, view; examination, inspection, reconnaissance, review; estimating, measuring, planning, plotting, prospecting, work-study.

survive *vb* endure, last, outlast, outlive.

susceptible *adj* capable, excitable, impressible, impressionable, inclined, predisposed, receptive, sensitive.

suspect *vb* believe, conclude, conjecture, fancy, guess, imagine, judge, suppose, surmise, think; distrust, doubt, mistrust. • *adj* doubtful, dubious, suspicious.

suspend *vb* append, hang, sling, swing; adjourn, arrest, defer, delay, discontinue, hinder, intermit, interrupt, postpone, stay, withhold; debar, dismiss, rusticate.

suspicion *n* assumption, conjecture, dash, guess, hint, inkling, suggestion, supposition, surmise, trace; apprehension, distrust, doubt, fear, jealousy, misgiving, mistrust.

suspicious *adj* distrustful, jealous, mistrustful, suspect, suspecting; doubtful, questionable.

sustain *vb* bear, bolster, fortify, prop, strengthen, support, uphold; maintain, nourish, perpetuate, preserve; aid, assist, comfort, relieve; brave, endure, suffer, undergo; approve, confirm, ratify, sanction, validate; confirm, establish, justify, prove.

sustenance *n* maintenance, subsistence, support; aliment, bread, food, nourishment, nutriment, nutrition, provisions, supplies, victuals.

swagger *vb* bluster, boast, brag, bully, flourish, hector, ruffle, strut, swell, vapour. • *n* airs, arrogance, bluster, boastfulness, braggadocio, ruffling, strut.

swain *n* clown, countryman, hind, peasant, rustic; adorer, gallant, inamorata, lover, suitor, wooer.

swallow *vb* bolt, devour, drink, eat, englut, engorge, gobble, gorge, gulp, imbibe, ingurgitate, swamp; absorb, appropriate, arrogate, devour, engulf, submerge; consume, employ, occupy; brook, digest, endure, pocket, stomach; recant, renounce, retract. • *n* gullet, oesophagus, throat; inclination, liking, palate, relish, taste; deglutition, draught, gulp, ingurgitation, mouthful, taste.

swamp *vb* engulf, overwhelm, sink; capsize, embarrass, overset, ruin, upset, wreck. • *n* bog, fen, marsh, morass, quagmire, slough.

sward *n* grass, lawn, sod, turf.

swarm *vb* abound, crowd, teem, throng. • *n* cloud, concourse, crowd, drove, flock, hive, horde, host, mass, multitude, press, shoal, throng.

swarthy *adj* black, brown, dark, dark-skinned, dusky, tawny.

sway *vb* balance, brandish, move, poise, rock, roll, swing, wave, wield; bend, bias, influence, persuade, turn, urge; control, dominate, direct, govern, guide, manage, rule; hoist, raise; incline, lean, lurch, yaw. • *n* ascendency, authority, command, control, domination, dominion, empire, government, mastership, mastery, omnipotence, predominance, power, rule, sovereignty; bias, direction, influence, weight; preponderance, preponderation; oscillation, sweep, swing, wag, wave.

swear *vb* affirm, attest, avow, declare, depose, promise, say, state, testify, vow; blaspheme, curse.

sweep *vb* clean, brush; graze, touch; rake, scour, traverse. • *n* amplitude, compass, drive, movement, range, reach, scope; destruction, devastation, havoc, ravage; curvature, curve.

sweeping *adj* broad, comprehensive, exaggerated, extensive, extravagant, general, unqualified, wholesale.

sweet *adj* candied, cloying, honeyed, luscious, nectareous, nectarous, sugary, saccharine; balmy, fragrant, odorous, redolent, spicy; harmonious, dulcet, mellifluous, mellow, melodious, musical, pleasant, soft, tuneful, silver-toned, silvery; beautiful, fair, lovely; agreeable, charming, delightful, grateful, gratifying; affectionate, amiable, attractive, engaging, gentle, mild, lovable, winning; benignant, serene; clean, fresh, pure, sound. • *n* fragrance, perfume, redolence; blessing, delight, enjoyment, gratification, joy, pleasure; candy, treat.

swell *vb* belly, bloat, bulge, dilate, distend, expand, inflate, intumesce, puff, swell, tumefy; augment, enlarge, increase; heave, rise, surge; strut, swagger. • *n* swelling; augmentation, excrescence, protuberance; ascent, elevation, hill, rise; force, intensity, power; billows, surge, undulation, waves; beau, blade, buck, coxcomb, dandy, exquisite, fop, popinjay.

swerve *vb* deflect, depart, deviate, stray, turn, wander; bend, incline, yield; climb, swarm, wind.

swift *adj* expeditious, fast, fleet, flying, quick, rapid, speedy; alert, eager, forward, prompt, ready, zealous; instant, sudden.

swiftness *n* celerity, expedition, fleetness, quickness, rapidity, speed, velocity.

swindle *vb* cheat, con, cozen, deceive, defraud, diddle, dupe, embezzle, forge, gull, hoax, overreach, steal, trick, victimize. • *n* cheat, con, deceit, deception, fraud, hoax, imposition, knavery, roguery, trickery.

swindler *n* blackleg, cheat, defaulter, embezzler, faker, fraud, impostor, jockey, knave, peculator, rogue, sharper, trickster.

swing *vb* oscillate, sway, vibrate, wave; dangle, depend, hang; brandish, flourish, whirl; administer, manage. • *n* fluctuation, oscillation, sway, undulation, vibration; elbow-room, freedom, margin, play, range, scope, sweep; bias, tendency.

swoop *vb* descend, pounce, rush, seize, stoop, sweep. • *n* clutch, pounce, seizure; stoop, descent.

sword *n* brand, broadsword, claymore, cutlass, epee, falchion, foil, hanger, rapier, sabre, scimitar.

sybarite *n* epicure, voluptuary.

sycophancy *n* adulation, cringing, fawning, flattery, grovelling, obsequiousness, servility.

sycophant *n* cringer, fawner, flunky, hanger-on, lickspittle, parasite, spaniel, toady, wheedler.

syllabus *n* abridgement, abstract, breviary, brief, compendium, digest, epitome, outline, summary, synopsis.

symbol *n* badge, emblem, exponent, figure, mark, picture, representation, representative, sign, token, type.

symbolic, symbolical *adj* emblematic, figurative, hieroglyphic, representative, significant, typical.

symmetry *n* balance, congruity, evenness, harmony, order, parallelism, proportion, regularity, shapeliness.

sympathetic *adj* affectionate, commiserating, compassionate, condoling, kind, pitiful, tender.

sympathy *n* accord, affinity, agreement, communion, concert, concord, congeniality, correlation, correspondence, harmony, reciprocity, union; commiseration, compassion, condolence, fellow-feeling, kindliness, pity, tenderness, thoughtfulness.

symptom *n* diagnostic, indication, mark, note, prognostic, sign, token.

symptomatic *adj* characteristic, indicative, symbolic, suggestive.

synonymous *adj* equipollent, equivalent, identical, interchangeable, similar, tantamount.

synopsis *n* abridgement, abstract, compendium, digest, epitome, outline, precis, résumé, summary, syllabus.

system *n* method, order, plan.

systematic *adj* methodic, methodical, orderly, regular.

T

tabernacle *n* pavilion, tent; cathedral, chapel, church, minster, synagogue, temple.

table *vb* enter, move, propose, submit, suggest. • *n* plate, slab, tablet; board, counter, desk, stand; catalogue, chart, compendium, index, list, schedule, syllabus, synopsis, tabulation; diet, fare, food, victuals.

tableau *n* picture, scene, representation.

taboo *vb* forbid, interdict, prohibit, proscribe. • *adj* banned, forbidden, inviolable, outlawed, prohibited, proscribed. • *n* ban, interdict, prohibition, proscription.

tacit *adj* implicit, implied, inferred, silent, understood, unexpressed, unspoken.

taciturn *adj* close, dumb, laconic, mum, reserved, reticent, silent, tight-lipped, uncommunicative.

tack *vb* add, affix, append, attach, fasten, tag; gybe, yaw, zigzag. • *n* nail, pin, staple; bearing, course, direction, heading, path, plan, procedure.

tackle *vb* attach, grapple, seize; attempt, try, undertake. • *n* apparatus, cordage, equipment, furniture, gear, harness, implements, rigging, tackling, tools, weapons.

tact *n* address, adroitness, cleverness, dexterity, diplomacy, discernment, finesse, insight, knack, perception, skill, understanding.

tail *vb* dog, follow, shadow, stalk, track. • *adj* abridged, curtailed, limited, reduced. • *n* appendage, conclusion, end, extremity, stub; flap, skirt; queue, retinue, train.

taint *vb* imbue, impregnate; contaminate, corrupt, defile, inflect, mildew, pollute, poison, spoil, touch; blot, stain, sully, tarnish. • *n* stain, tincture, tinge, touch; contamination, corruption, defilement, depravation, infection, pollution; blemish, defect, fault, flaw, spot.

take *vb* accept, obtain, procure, receive; clasp, clutch, grasp, grip, gripe, seize, snatch; filch, misappropriate, pilfer, purloin, steal; abstract, apprehend, appropriate, arrest, bag, capture, ensnare, entrap; attack, befall, smite; capture, carry off, conquer, gain, win; allure, attract, bewitch, captivate, charm, delight, enchant, engage, fascinate, interest, please; consider, hold, interrupt, suppose, regard, understand; choose, elect, espouse, select; employ, expend, use; claim, demand, necessitate, require; bear, endure, experience, feel, perceive, tolerate; deduce, derive, detect, discover, draw; carry, conduct, convey, lead, transfer; clear, surmount; drink, eat, imbibe, inhale, swallow. • *n* proceeds, profits, return, revenue, takings, yield.

tale *n* account, fable, legend, narration, novel, parable, recital, rehearsal, relation, romance, story, yarn; catalogue, count, enumeration, numbering, reckoning, tally.

talent *n* ableness, ability, aptitude, capacity, cleverness, endowment, faculty, forte, genius, gift, knack, parts, power, turn.

talk *vb* chatter, communicate, confer, confess, converse, declaim, discuss, gossip, pontificate, speak. • *n* chatter, communication, conversation, diction, gossip, jargon, language, rumour, speech, utterance.

talkative *adj* chatty, communicative, garrulous, loquacious, voluble.

tally *vb* accord, agree, conform, coincide, correspond, harmonize, match, square, suit. • *n* match, mate; check, counterpart, muster, roll call; account, reckoning.

tame *vb* domesticate, reclaim, train; conquer, master, overcome, repress, subdue, subjugate. • *adj* docile, domestic, domesticated, gentle, mild, reclaimed; broken, crushed, meek, subdued, unresisting, submissive; barren, commonplace, dull, feeble, flat, insipid, jejune, languid, lean, poor, prosaic, prosy, spiritless, tedious, uninteresting, vapid.

tamper *vb* alter, conquer, dabble, damage, interfere, meddle; intrigue, seduce, suborn.

tang *n* aftertaste, flavour, relish, savour, smack, taste; keenness, nip, sting.

tangible *adj* corporeal, material, palpable, tactile, touchable; actual, certain, embodied, evident, obvious, open, perceptible, plain, positive, real, sensible, solid, stable, substantial.

tangle *vb* complicate, entangle, intertwine, interweave, mat, perplex, snarl; catch, ensnare, entrap, involve, catch; embarrass, embroil, perplex. • *n* complication, disorder, intricacy, jumble, perplexity, snarl; dilemma, embarrassment, quandary, perplexity.

tantalize *vb* balk, disappoint, frustrate, irritate, provoke, tease, torment, vex.

tantamount *adj* equal, equivalent, synonymous.

tantrum *n* fit, ill-humour, outburst, paroxysm, temper, whim.

tap[1] *vb* knock, pat, rap, strike, tip, touch. • *n* pat, tip, rap, touch.

tap[2] *vb* broach, draw off, extract, pierce; draw on, exploit, mine, use, utilize; bug, eavesdrop, listen in. • *n* faucet, plug, spigot, spout, stopcock, valve; bug, listening device, transmitter.

tardiness *n* delay, dilatoriness, lateness, procrastination, slackness, slowness.

tardy *adj* slow, sluggish, snail-like; backward, behindhand, dilatory, late, loitering, overdue, slack.

tarn *n* bog, fen, marsh, morass, swamp.

tarnish *vb* blemish, deface, defame, dim, discolour, dull, slur, smear, soil, stain, sully. • *n* blemish, blot, soiling, spot, stain.

tarry *vb* delay, dally, linger, loiter, remain, stay, stop, wait; defer; abide, lodge, rest, sojourn.

tart *adj* acid, acidulous, acrid, astringent, piquant, pungent, sharp, sour; acrimonious, caustic, crabbed, curt, harsh, ill-humoured, ill-tempered, keen, petulant, sarcastic, severe, snappish, testy.

task *vb* burden, overwork, strain, tax. • *n* drudgery, labour, toil, work; business, charge, chore, duty, employment, enterprise, job, mission, stint, undertaking; assignment, exercise, lesson.

taste *vb* experience, feel, perceive, undergo; relish, savour, sip. • *n* flavour, gusto, relish, savour, smack, piquancy; admixture, bit, dash, fragment, hint, infusion, morsel, mouthful, sample, shade, sprinkling, suggestion, tincture; appetite, desire, fondness, liking, partiality, predilection; acumen, cultivation, culture, delicacy, discernment, discrimination, elegance, fine-feeling, grace, judgement, polish, refinement; manner, style.

tasteful *adj* appetizing, delicious, flavoursome, palatable, savoury, tasty, toothsome; aesthetic, artistic, attractive, elegant.

tasteless *adj* flat, insipid, savourless, stale, watery; dull, mawkish, uninteresting, vapid.

tattle *vb* babble, chat, chatter, jabber, prate, prattle; blab, gossip, inform. • *n* gabble, gossip, prate, prattle, tittle-tattle, twaddle.

taunt *vb* censure, chaff, deride, flout, jeer, mock, scoff, sneer, revile, reproach, ridicule, twit, upbraid. • *n* censure, derision, gibe, insult, jeer, quip, quirk, reproach, ridicule, scoff.

taut *adj* strained, stretched, tense, tight.

tautology *n* iteration, pleonasm, redundancy, reiteration, repetition, verbosity, wordiness.

tavern *n* bar, chophouse, hostelry, inn, pub, public house.

tawdry *adj* flashy, gaudy, garish, glittering, loud, meretricious, ostentatious, showy.

tax *vb* burden, demand, exact, load, overtax, require, strain, task; accuse, charge. • *n* assessment, custom, duty, excise, impost, levy, rate, taxation, toll, tribute; burden, charge, demand, requisition, strain; accusation, censure.

teach *vb* catechize, coach, discipline, drill, edify, educate, enlighten, inform, indoctrinate, initiate, instruct, ground, prime, school, train, tutor; communicate, disseminate, explain, expound, impart, implant, inculcate, infuse, instil, interpret, preach, propagate; admonish, advise, counsel, direct, guide, signify, show.

teacher *n* coach, educator, inculcator, informant, instructor, master, pedagogue, preceptor, schoolteacher, trainer, tutor; adviser, counsellor, guide, mentor; pastor, preacher.

tear *vb* burst, slit, rive, rend, rip; claw, lacerate, mangle, shatter, rend, wound; sever, sunder; fume, rage, rant, rave. • *n* fissure, laceration, rent, rip, wrench.

tease *vb* annoy, badger, beg, bother, chafe, chagrin, disturb, harass, harry, hector, importune, irritate, molest, pester, plague, provoke, tantalize, torment, trouble, vex, worry.

tedious *adj* dull, fatiguing, irksome, monotonous, tiresome, trying, uninteresting, wearisome; dilatory, slow, sluggish, tardy.

teem *vb* abound, bear, produce, swarm; discharge, empty, overflow.

teeming *adj* abounding, fraught, full, overflowing, pregnant, prolific, replete, swarming.

tell *vb* compute, count, enumerate, number, reckon; describe, narrate, recount, rehearse, relate, report; acknowledge, announce, betray, confess, declare, disclose, divulge, inform, own, reveal; acquaint, communicate, instruct, teach; discern, discover, distinguish; express, mention, publish, speak, state, utter.

temper *vb* modify, qualify; appease, assuage, calm, mitigate, mollify, moderate, pacify, restrain, soften, soothe; accommodate, adapt, adjust, fit, suit. • *n* character, constitution, nature, organization, quality, structure, temperament, type; disposition, frame, grain, humour, mood, spirits, tone, vein; calmness, composure, equanimity, moderation, tranquillity; anger, illtemper, irritation, spleen, passion.

temperament *n* character, constitution, disposition, habit, idiosyncrasy, nature, organization, temper.

temperate *adj* abstemious, ascetic, austere, chaste, continent, frugal, moderate, self-controlled, self-denying, sparing; calm, cool, dispassionate, mild, sober, sedate.

tempest *n* cyclone, gale, hurricane, squall, storm, tornado; commotion, disturbance, excitement, perturbation, tumult, turmoil.

temporal *adj* civil, lay, mundane, political, profane, secular, terrestrial, worldly; brief, ephemeral, evanescent, fleeting, momentary, short-lived, temporal, transient, transitory.

temporary *adj* brief, ephemeral, evanescent, fleeting, impermanent, momentary, short-lived, transient, transitory.

tempt *vb* prove, test, try; allure, decoy, entice, induce, inveigle, persuade, seduce; dispose, incite, incline, instigate, lead, prompt, provoke.

tempting *adj* alluring, attractive, enticing, inviting, seductive.

tenable *adj* defensible, maintainable, rational, reasonable, sound.

tenacious *adj* retentive, unforgetful; adhesive, clinging, cohesive, firm, glutinous, gummy, resisting, retentive, sticky, strong, tough, unyielding, viscous; dogged, fast, obstinate, opinionated, opinionative, pertinacious, persistent, resolute, stubborn, unwavering.

tenacity *n* retentiveness, tenaciousness; adhesiveness, cohesiveness, glutinosity, glutinousness, gumminess, toughness, stickiness, strength, viscidity; doggedness, firmness, obstinacy, perseverance, persistency, pertinacity, resolution, stubbornness.

tend[1] *vb* accompany, attend, graze, guard, keep, protect, shepherd, watch.

tend[2] *vb* aim, exert, gravitate, head, incline, influence, lead, lean, point, trend, verge; conduce, contribute.

tendency *n* aim, aptitude, bearing, bent, bias, course, determination, disposition, direction, drift, gravitation, inclination, leaning, liability, predisposition, proclivity, proneness, propensity, scope, set, susceptibility, turn, twist, warp.

tender[1] *vb* bid, offer, present, proffer, propose, suggest, volunteer. • *n* bid, offer, proffer, proposal; currency, money.

tender[2] *adj* callow, delicate, effeminate, feeble, feminine, fragile, immature, infantile, soft, weak, young; affectionate, compassionate, gentle, humane, kind, lenient, loving, merciful, mild, pitiful, sensitive, sympathetic, tender-hearted; affecting, disagreeable, painful, pathetic, touching, unpleasant.

tenebrous *adj* cloudy, dark, darksome, dusky, gloomy, murky, obscure, shadowy, shady, sombre, tenebrious.

tenement *n* abode, apartment, domicile, dwelling, flat, house.

tenet *n* belief, creed, position, dogma, doctrine, notion, opinion, position, principle, view.

tenor *n* cast, character, cut, fashion, form, manner, mood, nature, stamp, tendency, trend, tone; drift, gist, import, intent, meaning, purport, sense, significance, spirit.

tense *vb* flex, strain, tauten, tighten. • *adj* rigid, stiff, strained, stretched, taut, tight; excited, highly strung, intent, nervous, rapt.

tentative *adj* essaying, experimental, provisional, testing, toying.

tenure *n* holding, occupancy, occupation, possession, tenancy, tenement, use.

term *vb* call, christen, denominate, designate, dub, entitle, name, phrase, style. • *n* bound, boundary, bourn, confine, limit, mete,

terminus; duration, period, season, semester, span, spell, termination, time; denomination, expression, locution, name, phrase, word.

termagant *n* beldam, hag, scold, shrew, spitfire, virago, vixen.

terminal *adj* bounding, limiting; final, terminating, ultimate. • *n* end, extremity, termination; bound, limit; airport, depot, station, terminus.

terminate *vb* bound, limit; end, finish, close, complete, conclude; eventuate, issue, prove.

termination *n* ending, suffix; bound, extend, limit; end, completion, conclusion, consequence, effect, issue, outcome, result.

terms *npl* conditions, provisions, stipulations.

terrestrial *adj* earthly, mundane, subastral, subcelestial, sublunar, sublunary, tellurian, worldly. • *n* earthling, human.

terrible *adj* appalling, dire, dreadful, fearful, formidable, frightful gruesome, hideous, horrible, horrid, shocking, terrific, tremendous; alarming, awe-inspiring, awful, dread; great, excessive, extreme, severe.

terrific *adj* marvellous, sensational, superb; immense, intense; alarming, dreadful, formidable, frightful, terrible, tremendous.

terrify *vb* affright, alarm, appal, daunt, dismay, fright, frighten, horrify, scare, shock, startle, terrorize.

territory *n* country, district, domain, dominion, division, land, place, province, quarter, region, section, tract.

terror *n* affright, alarm, anxiety, awe, consternation, dismay, dread, fear, fright, horror, intimidation, panic, terrorism.

terse *adj* brief, compact, concise, laconic, neat, pithy, polished, sententious, short, smooth, succinct.

test *vb* assay; examine, prove, try. • *n* attempt, essay, examination, experiment, ordeal, proof, trial; criterion, standard, touchstone; example, exhibition; discrimination, distinction, judgment.

testify *vb* affirm, assert, asseverate, attest, avow, certify, corroborate, declare, depose, evidence, state, swear.

testimonial *n* certificate, credential, recommendation, voucher; monument, record.

testimony *n* affirmation, attestation, confession, confirmation, corroboration, declaration, deposition, profession; evidence, proof, witness.

testy *adj* captious, choleric, cross, fretful, hasty, irascible, irritable, quick, peevish, peppery, pettish, petulant, snappish, splenetic, touchy, waspish.

tetchy *adj* crabbed, cross, fretful, irritable, peevish, sullen, touchy.

tether *vb* chain, fasten, picket, stake, tie. • *n* chain, fastening, rope.

text *n* copy, subject, theme, thesis, topic, treatise.

texture *n* fabric, web, weft; character, coarseness, composition, constitution, fibre, fineness, grain, make-up, nap, organization, structure, tissue.

thankful *adj* appreciative, beholden, grateful, indebted, obliged.

thankfulness *n* appreciation, gratefulness, gratitude.

thankless *adj* profitless, ungracious, ungrateful, unthankful.

thaw *vb* dissolve, liquefy, melt, soften, unbend.

theatre *n* opera house, playhouse; arena, scene, seat, stage.

theatrical *adj* dramatic, dramaturgic, dramaturgical, histrionic, scenic, spectacular; affected, ceremonious, meretricious, ostentatious, pompous, showy, stagy, stilted, unnatural.

theft *n* depredation, embezzlement, fraud, larceny, peculation, pilfering, purloining, robbery, spoliation, stealing, swindling, thieving.

theme *n* composition, essay, motif, subject, text, thesis, topic, treatise.

theoretical *adj* abstract, conjectural, doctrinaire, ideal, hypothetical, pure, speculative, unapplied.

theory *n* assumption, conjecture, hypothesis, idea, plan, postulation, principle, scheme, speculation, surmise, system; doctrine, philosophy, science; explanation, exposition, philosophy, rationale.

therefore *adv* accordingly, afterward, consequently, hence, so, subsequently, then, thence, whence.

thesaurus *n* dictionary, encyclopedia, repository, storehouse, treasure.

thick *adj* bulky, chunky, dumpy, plump, solid, squab, squat, stubby, thickset; clotted, coagulated, crass, dense, dull, gross, heavy, viscous; blurred, cloudy, dirty, foggy, hazy, indistinguishable, misty, obscure, vaporous; muddy, roiled, turbid; abundant, frequent, multitudinous, numerous; close, compact, crowded, set, thickset; confused, guttural, hoarse, inarticulate, indistinct; dim, dull, weak; familiar, friendly, intimate, neighbourly, well-acquainted. • *adv* fast, frequently, quick; closely, densely, thickly. • *n* centre, middle, midst.

thicket *n* clump, coppice, copse, covert, forest, grove, jungle, shrubbery, underbrush, undergrowth, wood, woodland.

thief *n* depredator, filcher, pilferer, lifter, marauder, purloiner, robber, shark, stealer; burglar, corsair, defaulter, defrauder, embezzler, footpad, highwayman, housebreaker, kidnapper, pickpocket, pirate, poacher, privateer, sharper, swindler, peculator.

thieve *vb* cheat, embezzle, peculate, pilfer, plunder, purloin, rob, steal, swindle.

thin *vb* attenuate, dilute, diminish, prune, reduce, refine, weaken. • *adj* attenuated, bony, emaciated, fine, fleshless, flimsy, gaunt, haggard, lank, lanky, lean, meagre, peaked, pinched, poor, scanty, scraggy, scrawny, slender, slight, slim, small, sparse, spindly.

thing *n* being, body, contrivance, creature, entity, object, something, substance; act, action, affair, arrangement, circumstance, concern, deed, event, matter, occurrence, transaction.

think *vb* cogitate, contemplate, dream, meditate, muse, ponder, reflect, ruminate, speculate; consider, deliberate, reason, undertake; apprehend, believe, conceive, conclude, deem, determine, fancy, hold, imagine, judge, opine, presume, reckon, suppose, surmise; design, intend, mean, purpose; account, count, deem, esteem, hold, regard; compass, design, plan, plot. • *n* assessment, contemplation, deliberation, meditation, opinion, reasoning, reflection.

thirst *n* appetite, craving, desire, hunger, longing, yearning; aridity, drought, dryness.

thirsty *adj* arid, dry, parched; eager, greedy, hungry, longing, yearning.

thorn *n* prickle, spine; annoyance, bane, care, evil, infliction, nettle, nuisance, plague, torment, trouble, scourge.

thorny *adj* briary, briery, prickly, spinose, spinous, spiny; acuminate, barbed, pointed, prickling, sharp, spiky; annoying, difficult, harassing, perplexing, rugged, troublesome, trying, vexatious.

thorough, thoroughgoing *adj* absolute, arrant, complete, downright, entire, exhaustive, finished, perfect, radical, sweeping, total unmitigated, utter; accurate, correct, reliable, trustworthy.

though *conj* admitting, allowing, although, granted, granting, if, notwithstanding, still. • *adv* however, nevertheless, still, yet.

thought *n* absorption, cogitation, engrossment, meditation, musing, reflection, reverie, rumination; contemplation, intellect, ratiocination, thinking, thoughtfulness; application, conception, consideration, deliberation, idea, pondering, speculation, study; consciousness, imagination, intellect, perception, understanding; conceit, fancy, notion; conclusion, judgment, motion, opinion, sentiment, supposition, view; anxiety, attention, care, concern, provision, regard, solicitude, thoughtfulness; design, expectation, intention, purpose.

thoughtful *adj* absorbed, contemplative, deliberative, dreamy, engrossed, introspective, pensive, philosophic, reflecting, reflective, sedate, speculative; attentive, careful, cautious, circumspect, considerate, discreet, heedful, friendly, kind-hearted, kindly, mindful, neighbourly, provident, prudent, regardful, watchful, wary; quiet, serious, sober, studious.

thoughtless *adj* careless, casual, flighty, heedless, improvident, inattentive, inconsiderate, neglectful, negligent, precipitate, rash, reckless, regardless, remiss, trifling, unmindful, unthinking; blank, blockish, dull, insensate, stupid, vacant, vacuous.

thraldom *n* bondage, enslavement, enthralment, serfdom, servitude, slavery, subjection, thrall, vassalage.

thrash *vb* beat, bruise, conquer, defeat, drub, flog, lash, maul, pommel, punish, thwack, trounce, wallop, whip.

thread *vb* course, direction, drift, tenor; reeve, trace. • *n* cord, fibre, filament, hair, line, twist; pile, staple.

threadbare *adj* napless, old, seedy, worn; common, commonplace, hackneyed, stale, trite, worn-out.

threat *n* commination, defiance, denunciation, fulmination, intimidation, menace, thunder, thunderbolt.

threaten *vb* denounce, endanger, fulminate, intimidate, menace, thunder; augur, forebode, foreshadow, indicate, portend, presage, prognosticate, warn.

threshold *n* doorsill, sill; door, entrance, gate; beginning, commencement, opening, outset, start.

thrift *n* economy, frugality, parsimony, saving, thriftiness; gain, luck, profit, prosperity, success.

thriftless *adj* extravagant, improvident, lavish, profuse, prodigal, shiftless, unthrifty, wasteful.

thrifty *adj* careful, economical, frugal, provident, saving, sparing; flourishing, prosperous, thriving, vigorous.

thrill *vb* affect, agitate, electrify, inspire, move, penetrate, pierce, rouse, stir, touch. • *n* excitement, sensation, shock, tingling, tremor.

thrilling *adj* affecting, exciting, gripping, moving, sensational, touching.

thrive *vb* advance, batten, bloom, boom, flourish, prosper, succeed.

throng *vb* congregate, crowd, fill, flock, pack, press, swarm. • *n* assemblage, concourse, congregation, crowd, horde, host, mob, multitude, swarm.

throttle *vb* choke, silence, strangle, suffocate.

throw *vb* cast, chuck, dart, fling, hurl, lance, launch, overturn, pitch, pitchfork, send, sling, toss, whirl. • *n* cast, fling, hurl, launch, pitch, sling, toss, whirl; chance, gamble, try, venture.

thrust *vb* clap, dig, drive, force, impel, jam, plunge, poke, propel, push, ram, run, shove, stick. • *n* dig, jab, lunge, pass, plunge, poke, propulsion, push, shove, stab, tilt.

thump *vb* bang, batter, beat, belabour, knock, punch, strike, thrash, thwack, whack. • *n* blow, knock, punch, strike, stroke.

thwart *vb* baffle, balk, contravene, counteract, cross, defeat, disconcert, frustrate, hinder, impede, oppose, obstruct, oppugn; cross, intersect, traverse.

tickle *vb* amuse, delight, divert, enliven, gladden, gratify, please, rejoice, titillate.

ticklish *adj* dangerous, precarious, risky, tottering, uncertain, unstable, unsteady; critical, delicate, difficult, nice.

tide *n* course, current, ebb, flow, stream.

tidings *npl* advice, greetings, information, intelligence, news, report, word.

tidy *vb* clean, neaten, order, straighten. • *adj* clean, neat, orderly, shipshape, spruce, trig, trim.

tie *vb* bind, confine, fasten, knot, lock, manacle, secure, shackle, fetter, yoke; complicate, entangle, interlace, knit; connect, hold, join, link, unite; constrain, oblige, restrain, restrict. • *n* band, fastening, knot, ligament, ligature; allegiance, bond, obligation; bow, cravat, necktie.

tier *n* line, rank, row, series.

tiff *n* fit, fume, passion, pet, miff, rage.

tight *adj* close, compact, fast, firm; taut, tense, stretched; impassable, narrow, strait.

till *vb* cultivate, plough, harrow.

tillage *n* agriculture, cultivation, culture, farming, geoponics, husbandry.

tilt *vb* cant, incline, slant, slope, tip; forge, hammer; point, thrust; joust, rush. • *n* awning, canopy, tent; lunge, pass, thrust; cant, inclination, slant, slope, tip.

time *vb* clock, control, count, measure, regulate, schedule. • *n* duration, interim, interval, season, span, spell, tenure, term, while; aeon, age, date, epoch, eon, era; term; cycle, dynasty, reign; confinement, delivery, parturition; measure, rhythm.

timely *adj* acceptable, appropriate, apropos, early, opportune, prompt, punctual, seasonable, well-timed.

timid *adj* afraid, cowardly, faint-hearted, fearful, irresolute, meticulous, nervous, pusillanimous, skittish, timorous, unadventurous; bashful, coy, diffident, modest, shame-faced, shrinking.

tincture *vb* colour, dye, shade, stain, tinge, tint; flavour, season; imbue, impregnate, impress, infuse. • *n* grain, hue, shade, stain, tinge, tint, tone; flavour, smack, spice, taste; admixture, dash, infusion, seasoning, sprinkling, touch.

tinge *vb* colour, dye, stain, tincture, tint; imbue, impregnate, impress, infuse. • *n* cast, colour, dye, hue, shade, stain, tincture, tint; flavour, smack, spice, quality, taste.

tint *n* cast, colour, complexion, dye, hue, shade, tinge, tone.

tiny *adj* diminutive, dwarfish, Lilliputian, little, microscopic, miniature, minute, puny, pygmy, small, wee.

tip[1] *n* apex, cap, end, extremity, peak, pinnacle, point, top, vertex.

tip[2] *vb* incline, overturn, tilt; dispose of, dump. • *n* donation, fee, gift, gratuity, perquisite, reward; inclination, slant; hint, pointer, suggestion; strike, tap.

tirade *n* abuse, denunciation, diatribe, harangue, outburst.

tire *vb* exhaust, fag, fatigue, harass, jade, weary; bore, bother, irk.

tiresome *adj* annoying, arduous, boring, dull, exhausting, fatiguing, fagging, humdrum, irksome, laborious, monotonous, tedious, wearisome, vexatious.

tissue *n* cloth, fabric; membrane, network, structure, texture, web; accumulation, chain, collection, combination, conglomeration, mass, series, set.

titanic *adj* colossal, Cyclopean, enormous, gigantic, herculean, huge, immense, mighty, monstrous, prodigious, stupendous, vast.

title *vb* call, designate, name, style, term. • *n* caption, legend, head, heading; appellation, application, cognomen, completion, denomination, designation, epithet, name; claim, due, ownership, part, possession, prerogative, privilege, right.

tittle *n* atom, bit, grain, iota, jot, mite, particle, scrap, speck, whit.

tittle-tattle *vb*, *n* babble, cackle, chatter, discourse, gabble, gossip, prattle.

toast *vb* brown, dry, heat; honour, pledge, propose, salute. • *n* compliment, drink, pledge, salutation, salute; favourite, pet.

toil *vb* drudge, labour, strive, work. • *n* drudgery, effort, exertion, exhaustion, grinding, labour, pains, travail, work; gin, net, noose, snare, spring, trap.

toilsome *adj* arduous, difficult, fatiguing, hard, laborious, onerous, painful, severe, tedious, wearisome.

token *adj* nominal, superficial, symbolic. • *n* badge, evidence, index, indication, manifestation, mark, note, sign, symbol, trace, trait; keepsake, memento, memorial, reminder, souvenir.

tolerable *adj* bearable, endurable, sufferable, supportable; fair, indifferent, middling, ordinary, passable, so-so.

tolerance *n* endurance, receptivity, sufferance, toleration.

tolerate *vb* admit, allow, indulge, let, permit, receive; abide, brook, endure, suffer.

toll[1] *n* assessment, charge, customs, demand, dues, duty, fee, impost, levy, rate, tax, tribute; cost, damage, loss.

toll[2] *vb* chime, knell, peal, ring, sound. • *n* chime, knell, peal, ring, ringing, tolling.

tomb *n* catacomb, charnel house, crypt, grave, mausoleum, sepulchre, vault.

tone *vb* blend, harmonize, match, suit. • *n* note, sound; accent, cadence, emphasis, inflection, intonation, modulation; key, mood, strain, temper; elasticity, energy, force, health, strength, tension, vigour; cast, colour, manner, hue, shade, style, tint; drift, tenor.

tongue *n* accent, dialect, language, utterance, vernacular; discourse, parlance, speech, talk; nation, race.

too *adv* additionally, also, further, likewise, moreover, overmuch.

toothsome *adj* agreeable, dainty, delicious, luscious, nice, palatable, savoury.

top *vb* cap, head, tip; ride, surmount; outgo, surpass. • *adj* apical, best, chief, culminating, finest, first, foremost, highest, leading, prime, principal, topmost, uppermost. • *n* acme, apex, crest, crown, head, meridian, pinnacle, summit, surface, vertex, zenith.

topic *n* business, question, subject, text, theme, thesis; division, head, subdivision; commonplace, dictum, maxim, precept, proposition, principle, rule; arrangement, scheme.

topple *vb* fall, overturn, tumble, upset.

torment *vb* annoy, agonize, distress, excruciate, pain, rack, torture; badger, fret, harass, harry, irritate, nettle, plague, provoke, tantalize, tease, trouble, vex, worry. • *n* agony, anguish, pang, rack, torture.

tornado *n* blizzard, cyclone, gale, hurricane, storm, tempest, typhoon, whirlwind.

torpid *adj* benumbed, lethargic, motionless, numb; apathetic, dormant, dull, inactive, indolent, inert, listless, sleepy, slothful, sluggish, stupid.

torpor *n* coma, insensibility, lethargy, numbness, torpidity; inaction, inactivity, inertness, sluggishness, stupidity.

torrid *adj* arid, burnt, dried, parched; burning, fiery, hot, parching, scorching, sultry, tropical, violent.

tortuous *adj* crooked, curved, curvilinear, curvilinear, serpentine, sinuate, sinuated, sinuous, twisted, winding; ambiguous, circuitous, crooked, deceitful, indirect, perverse, roundabout.

torture *vb* agonize, distress, excruciate, pain, rack, torment. • *n* agony, anguish, distress, pain, pang, rack, torment.

toss *vb* cast, fling, hurl, pitch, throw; agitate, rock, shake; disquiet, harass, try; roll, writhe. • *n* cast, fling, pitch, throw.

tota *vb* add, amount to, reach, reckon. • *adj* complete, entire, full, whole; integral, undivided. • *n* aggregate, all, gross, lump, mass, sum, totality, whole.

totter *vb* falter, reel, stagger, vacillate; lean, oscillate, reel, rock, shake, sway, tremble, waver; fail, fall, flag.

touch *vb* feel, graze, hardle, hit, pat, strike, tap; concern, interest, regard; affect, impress, move, stir; grasp, reach, stretch; melt, mollify, soften; afflict, distress, hurt, injure, molest, sting, wound. • *n* hint, smack, suggestion, suspicion, taste, trace; blow, contract, hit, pat tap.

touchiness *n* fretfulness, irritability, irascibility, peevishness, pettishness, petulance snappishness, spleen, testiness.

touching *adj* affecting, heart-rending, impressive, melting, moving, pathetic, pitiable, tender; abutting, adjacent, bordering, tangent.

touchy *adj* choleric, cross, fretful, hot-tempered, irascible, irritable, peevish, petulant quick-tempered, snappish, splenetic, tetchy, testy, waspish.

tough *adj* adhesive, cohesive, flexible, tenacious; coriaceous, leathery; clammy, ropy, sticky, viscous; inflexible, intractable, rigid, stiff; callous, hard, obdurate, stubborn; difficult, formidable, hard, troublesome. • *n* brute, bully, hooligan, ruffian, thug.

tour *vb* journey, perambulate, travel, visit. • *n* circuit, course, excursion, expedition, journey, perambulation, pilgrimage, round.

tow *vb* drag, draw, haul, pull, tug. • *n* drag, lift, pull.

tower *vb* mount, rise, soar, transcend. • *n* belfry, bell tower, column, minaret, spire, steeple, turret; castle, citadel, fortress, stronghold; pillar, refuge, rock, support.

towering *adj* elevated, lofty; excessive, extreme, prodigious, violent.

toy *vb* dally, play, sport, trifle, wanton. • *n* bauble, doll, gewgaw, gimmick, knick-knack, plaything, puppet, trinket; bagatelle, bubble, trifle; play, sport.

trace *vb* follow, track, train; copy, deduce, delineate, derive, describe, draw, sketch. • *n* evidence, footmark, footprint, footstep, impression, mark, remains, sign, token, track, trail, vestige, wake; memorial, record; bit, dash, flavour, hint, suspicion, streak, tinge.

track *vb* chase, draw, follow, pursue, scent, track, trail. • *n* footmark, footprint, footstep, spoor, trace, vestige; course, pathway, rails, road, runway, trace, trail, wake, way.

trackless *adj* pathless, solitary, unfrequented, unused.

tract *n* area, district, quarter, region, territory; parcel, patch, part, piece, plot, portion.

tract *n* discquisition, dissertation, essay, homily, pamphlet, sermon, thesis, tractate, treatise.

tractable *adj* amenable, docile, governable, manageable, submissive, willing, yielding; adaptable, ductile, malleable, plastic, tractile.

trade *vb* bargain, barter chaffer, deal, exchange, interchange, sell, traffic. • *n* bargaining, barter, business, commerce, dealing, traffic; avocation, calling, craft, employment, occupation, office, profession, pursuit, vocation.

traditional *adj* accustomed, apocryphal, customary, established, historic, legendary, old, oral, transmitted, uncertain, unverified, unwritten.

traduce *vb* abuse, asperse, blemish, brand, calumniate, decry, defame, depreciate, disparage, revile, malign, slander, vilify.

traducer *n* calumniator, defamer, detractor, slanderer, vilifier.

traffic *vb* bargain, barter, chaffer, deal, exchange, trade. • *n* barter, business, chaffer, commerce, exchange, intercourse, trade, transportation, truck.

tragedy *n* drama, play; adversity, calamity, catastrophe, disaster, misfortune.

tragic *adj* dramatic; calamitous, catastrophic, disastrous, dreadful fatal, grievous, heart-breaking, mournful, sad, shocking, sorrowful.

trail *vb* follow, hunt, trace track; drag, draw, float, flow, haul, pull. • *n* footmark, footprint footstep, mark, trace, track.

train *vb* drag, draw, haul, trail, tug; allure, entice; discipline, drill, educate, exercise, instruct, school, teach; accustom, break in, familiarize, habituate, inure, prepare, rehearse, use. • *n* trail, wake; entourage, cortege, followers, retinue, staff, suite; chain, consecution, sequel, series, set, succession; course, method, order, process; allure, artifice, device, enticement, lure, persuasion, stratagem, trap.

trait *n* line, mark, stroke, touch; characteristic, feature, lineage, particularity, peculiarity, quality.

traitor *n* apostate, betrayer, deceiver, Judas, miscreant, quisling, renegade, turncoat; conspirator, deserter, insurgent, mutineer, rebel, revolutionary.

traitorous *adj* faithless, false, perfidious, recreant, treacherous; insidious, treasonable.

trammel *vb* clog, confine, cramp, cumber, hamper, hinder, fetter, restrain, restrict, shackle, tie. • *n* bond, chain, fetter, hindrance, impediment, net, restraint, shackle.

tramp *vb* hike, march, plod, trudge, walk. • *n* excursion, journey, march, walk; landloper, loafer, stroller, tramper, vagabond, vagrant.

trample *vb* crush, tread; scorn, spurn.

trance *n* dream, ecstasy, hypnosis, rapture; catalepsy, coma.

tranquil *adj* calm, hushed, peaceful, placid, quiet, serene, still, undisturbed, unmoved, unperturbed, unruffled, untroubled.

tranquillity *n* calmness, peace, peacefulness, placidity, placidness, quiet, quietness, serenity, stillness, tranquilness.

tranquillize *vb* allay, appease, assuage, calm, compose, hush, lay, lull, moderate, pacify, quell, quiet, silence, soothe, still.

transact *vb* conduct, dispatch, enact, execute, do, manage, negotiate, perform, treat.

transaction *n* act, action, conduct, doing, management, negotiation, performance; affair, business, deal, dealing, incident, event, job, matter, occurrence, procedure, proceeding.

transcend *vb* exceed, overlap, overstep, pass, transgress; excel, outstrip, outrival, outvie, overtop, surmount, surpass.

transcendent *adj* consummate, inimitable, peerless, pre-eminent, supereminent, surpassing, unequalled, unparalleled, unrivalled, unsurpassed; metempiric, metempirical, noumenal, super-sensible.

transcript *n* duplicate, engrossment, rescript.

transfer *vb* convey, dispatch, move, remove, send, translate, transmit, transplant, transport; abalienate, alienate, assign, cede, confer, convey, consign, deed, devise, displace, forward, grant, pass, relegate. • *n* abalienation, alienation, assignment, bequest, carriage, cession, change, conveyance, copy, demise, devisal, gift, grant, move, relegation, removal, shift, shipment, transference, transferring, transit, transmission, transportation.

transfigure *vb* change, convert, dignify, idealize, metamorphose, transform.

transform *vb* alter, change, metamorphose, transfigure; convert, resolve, translate, transmogrify, transmute.

transgress *vb* exceed, transcend, overpass, overstep; break, contravene, disobey, infringe, violate; err, intrude, offend, sin, slip, trespass.

transgression *n* breach, disobedience, encroachment, infraction, infringement, transgression, violation; crime, delinquency, error, fault, iniquity, misdeed, misdemeanour, misdoing, offence, sin, slip, trespass, wrongdoing.

transient *adj* diurnal, ephemeral, evanescent, fleeting, fugitive, impertinent, meteoric, mortal, passing, perishable, short-lived, temporary, transitory, volatile; hasty, imperfect, momentary, short.

transitory *adj* brief, ephemeral, evanescent, fleeting, flitting, fugacious, momentary, passing, short, temporary, transient.

translate *vb* remove, transfer, transport; construe, decipher, decode, interpret, render, turn.

translucent *adj* diaphanous, hyaline, pellucid, semi-opaque, semi-transparent.

transmit *vb* forward, remit, send; communicate, conduct, radiate; bear, carry, convey.

transparent *adj* bright, clear, diaphanous, limpid, lucid; crystalline, hyaline, pellucid, serene, translucent, transpicuous, unclouded; open, porous, transpicuous; evident, obvious, manifest, patent.

transpire *vb* befall, chance, happen, occur; evaporate, exhale.

transport *vb* bear, carry, cart, conduct, convey, fetch, remove, ship, take, transfer, truck; banish, expel; beatify, delight, enrapture, enravish, entrance, ravish. • *n* carriage, conveyance, movement, transportation, transporting; beatification, beatitude, bliss, ecstasy, felicity, happiness, rapture, ravishment; frenzy, passion, vehemence, warmth.

transude *vb* exude, filter, ooze, percolate, strain.

trap *vb* catch, ensnare, entrap, noose, snare, springe; ambush, deceive, dupe, trick; enmesh, tangle, trepan. • *n* gin, snare, springe, toil; ambush, artifice, pitfall, stratagem, trepan.

trappings *npl* adornments, decorations, dress, embellishments, frippery, gear, livery, ornaments, paraphernalia, rigging; accoutrements, caparisons, equipment, gear.

trash *n* dregs, dross, garbage, refuse, rubbish, trumpery, waste; balderdash, nonsense, twaddle.

travel *vb* journey, peregrinate, ramble, roam, rove, tour, voyage, walk, wander; go, move, pass. • *n* excursion, expedition, journey, peregrination, ramble, tour, trip, voyage, walk.

traveller *n* excursionist, explorer, globe-trotter, itinerant, passenger, pilgrim, rover, sightseer, tourist, trekker, tripper, voyager, wanderer, wayfarer.

traverse *vb* contravene, counteract, defeat, frustrate, obstruct, oppose, thwart; ford, pass, play, range.

travesty *vb* imitate, parody, take off. • *n* burlesque, caricature, imitation, parody, take-off.

treacherous *adj* deceitful, disloyal, faithless, false, false-hearted, insidious, perfidious, recreant, sly, traitorous, treasonable, unfaithful, unreliable, unsafe, untrustworthy.

treachery *n* betrayal, deceitfulness, disloyalty, double-dealing, faithlessness, foul play, infidelity, insidiousness, perfidiousness, treason, perfidy.

treason *n* betrayal, disloyalty, lèse-majesté, lese-majesty, perfidy, sedition, traitorousness, treachery.

treasonable *adj* disloyal, traitorous, treacherous.

treasure *vb* accumulate, collect, garner, hoard, husband, save, store; cherish, idolize, prize, value, worship. • *n* cash, funds, jewels, money, riches, savings, valuables, wealth; abundance, reserve, stock, store.

treasurer *n* banker, bursar, purser, receiver, trustee.

treat *vb* entertain, feast, gratify, refresh; attend, doctor, dose, handle, manage, serve; bargain, covenant, negotiate, parley. • *n* banquet, entertainment, feast; delight, enjoyment, entertainment, gratification, luxury, pleasure, refreshment.

treatise *n* commentary, discourse, dissertation, disquisition, monograph, tractate.

treatment *n* usage, use; dealing, handling, management, manipulation; doctoring, therapy.

treaty *n* agreement, alliance, bargain, compact, concordat, convention, covenant, entente, league, pact.

tremble *vb* quake, quaver, quiver, shake, shiver, shudder, vibrate, wobble. • *n* quake, quiver, shake, shiver, shudder, tremor, vibration, wobble.

tremendous *adj* colossal, enormous, huge, immense; excellent, marvellous, wonderful; alarming, appalling, awful, dreadful, fearful, frightful, horrid, horrible, terrible.

tremor *n* agitation, quaking, quivering, shaking, trembling, trepidation, tremulousness, vibration.

tremulous *adj* afraid, fearful, quavering, quivering, shaking, shaky, shivering, timid, trembling, vibrating.

trench *vb* carve, cut; ditch, channel, entrench, furrow. • *n* channel, ditch, drain, furrow, gutter, moat, pit, sewer, trough; dugout, entrenchment, fortification.

trenchant *adj* cutting, keen, sharp; acute, biting, caustic, crisp, incisive, pointed, piquant, pungent, sarcastic, sententious, severe, unsparing, vigorous.

trend *vb* drift, gravitate, incline, lean, run, stretch, sweep, tend, turn. • *n* bent, course, direction, drift, inclination, set, leaning, tendency, trending.

trepidation *n* agitation, quaking, quivering, shaking, trembling, tremor; dismay, excitement, fear, perturbation, tremulousness.

trespass *vb* encroach, infringe, intrude, trench; offend, sin, transgress. • *n* encroachment, infringement, injury, intrusion, invasion; crime, delinquency, error, fault, sin, misdeed, misdemeanour, offence, transgression; trespasser.

trial *adj* experimental, exploratory, testing. • *n* examination, experiment, test; experience, knowledge; aim, attempt, effort, endeavour, essay, exertion, struggle; assay, criterion, ordeal, prohibition, proof, test, touchstone; affliction, burden, chagrin, dolour, distress, grief, hardship, heartache, inclination, misery, mortification, pain, sorrow, suffering, tribulation, trouble, unhappiness, vexation, woe, wretchedness; action, case, cause, hearing, suit.

tribe *n* clan, family, lineage, race, sept, stock; class, distinction, division, order.

tribulation *n* adversity, affliction, distress, grief, misery, pain, sorrow, suffering, trial, trouble, unhappiness, woe, wretchedness.

tribunal *n* bench, judgement seat; assizes, bar, court, judicature, session.

tribute *n* subsidy, tax; custom, duty, excise, impost, tax, toll; contribution, grant, offering.

trice *n* flash, instant, jiffy, moment, second, twinkling.

trick *vb* cheat, circumvent, cozen, deceive, defraud, delude, diddle, dupe, fob, gull, hoax, overreach. • *n* artifice, blind, deceit, deception, dodge, fake, feint, fraud, game, hoax, imposture; manoeuvre, shift, ruse, swindle, stratagem, wile; antic, caper, craft, deftness, gambol, sleight; habit, mannerism, peculiarity, practice.

trickle *vb* distil, dribble, drip, drop, ooze, percolate, seep. • *n* dribble, drip, percolation, seepage.

tricky *adj* artful, cunning, deceitful, deceptive, subtle, trickish.

trifle *vb* dally, dawdle, fool, fribble, palter, play, potter, toy. • *n* bagatelle, bauble, bean, fig, nothing, triviality; iota, jot, modicum, particle, trace.

trifling *adj* empty, frippery, frivolous, inconsiderable, insignificant, nugatory, petty, piddling, shallow, slight, small, trivial, unimportant, worthless.

trill *vb* shake, quaver, warble. • *n* quaver, shake, tremolo, warbling.

trim *vb* adjust, arrange, prepare; balance, equalize, fill; adorn, array, bedeck, decorate, dress, embellish, garnish, ornament; clip, curtail, cut, lop, mow, poll, prune, shave, shear; berate, chastise, chide, rebuke, reprimand, reprove, trounce; fluctuate, hedge, shift, shuffle, vacillate. • *adj* compact, neat, nice, shapely, snug, tidy, well-adjusted, well-ordered; chic, elegant, finical, smart, spruce. • *n* dress, embellishment, gear, ornaments, trappings, trimmings; case, condition, order, plight, state.

trinket *n* bagatelle, bauble, bijoux, gewgaw, gimcrack, knick-knack, toy, trifle.

trinkets *npl* bijouterie, jewellery, jewels, ornaments.

trip *vb* caper, dance, frisk, hop, skip; misstep, stumble; bungle, blunder, err, fail, mistake; overthrow, supplant, upset; catch, convict, detect. • *n* hop, skip; lurch, misstep, stumble; blunder, bungle, error, failure, fault, lapse, miss, mistake, oversight; slip; circuit, excursion, expedition, jaunt, journey, ramble, route, stroll, tour.

trite *adj* banal, beaten, common, commonplace, hackneyed, old, ordinary, stale, stereotyped, threadbare, usual, worn.

triturate *vb* beat, bray, bruise, grind, pound, rub, thrash; comminute, levigate, pulverize.

triumph *vb* exult, rejoice; prevail, succeed, win; flourish, prosper, thrive; boast, brag, crow, gloat, swagger, vaunt. • *n* celebration, exultation, joy, jubilation, jubilee, ovation; accomplishment, achievement, conquest, success, victory.

triumphant *adj* boastful, conquering, elated, exultant, exulting, jubilant, rejoicing, successful, victorious.

trivial *adj* frivolous, gimcrack, immaterial, inconsiderable, insignificant, light, little, nugatory, paltry, petty, small, slight, slim, trifling, trumpery, unimportant.

trollop *n* prostitute, slattern, slut, whore.

troop *vb* crowd, flock, muster, throng. • *n* company, crowd, flock, herd, multitude, number, throng; band, body, party, squad, troupe.

trophy *n* laurels, medal, palm, prize.

troth *n* candour, sincerity, truth, veracity, verity; allegiance, belief, faith, fidelity, word; betrothal.

trouble *vb* agitate, confuse, derange, disarrange, disorder, disturb; afflict, ail, annoy, badger, concern, disquiet, distress, fret, grieve, harass, molest, perplex, perturb, pester, plague, torment, vex, worry. • *n* adversity, affliction, calamity, distress, dolour, grief, hardship, misfortune, misery, pain, sorrow, suffering, tribulation, woe; ado, annoyance, anxiety, bother, care, discomfort, embarrassment, fuss, inconvenience, irritation, pains, perplexity, plague, torment, vexation, worry; commotion, disturbance, row; bewilderment, disquietude, embarrassment, perplexity, uneasiness.

troublesome *adj* annoying, distressing, disturbing, galling, grievous, harassing, painful, perplexing, vexatious, worrisome; burdensome, irksome, tiresome, wearisome; importunate, intrusive, teasing; arduous, difficult, hard, inconvenient, trying, unwieldy.

troublous *adj* agitated, disquieted, disturbed, perturbed, tumultuous, turbulent.

trough *n* hutch, manger; channel, depression, hollow, furrow.

truant *vb* be absent, desert, dodge, malinger, shirk, skive. • *n* absentee, deserter, idler, laggard, loiterer, lounger, malingerer, quitter, runaway, shirker, vagabond.

truce *n* armistice, breathing space, cessation, delay, intermission, lull, pause, recess, reprieve, respite, rest.

truck *vb* barter, deal, exchange, trade, traffic. • *n* lorry, van, wagon.

truckle *vb* roll, trundle; cringe, crouch, fawn, knuckle, stoop, submit, yield.

truculent *adj* barbarous, bloodthirsty, ferocious, fierce, savage; cruel, malevolent, relentless; destructive, deadly, fatal, ruthless.

true *adj* actual, unaffected, authentic, genuine, legitimate, pure, real, rightful, sincere, sound, truthful, veritable; substantial, veracious; constant, faithful, loyal, staunch, steady; equitable, honest, honourable, just, upright, trusty, trustworthy, virtuous; accurate, correct, even, exact, right, straight, undeviating. • *adv* good, well.

truism *n* axiom, commonplace, platitude.

trumpery *adj* pinchbeck, rubbishy, trashy, trifling, worthless. • *n* deceit, deception, falsehood, humbug, imposture; frippery, rubbish, stuff, trash, trifles.

truncheon *n* club, cudgel, nightstick, partisan, staff; baton, wand.

trunk *n* body, bole, butt, shaft, stalk, stem, stock, torso; box, chest, coffer.

trundle *vb* bowl, revolve, roll, spin, truckle, wheel.

truss *vb* bind, bundle, close, cram, hang, pack. • *n* bundle, package, packet; apparatus, bandage, support.

trust *vb* confide, depend, expect, hope, rely; believe, credit; commit, entrust. • *n* belief, confidence, credence, faith; credit, tick; charge, deposit; commission, duty, errand; assurance, conviction, expectation, hope, reliance, security.

trustful *adj* confiding, trusting, unquestioning, unsuspecting; faithful, trustworthy, trusty.

trustworthy *adj* confidential, constant, credible, dependable, faithful, firm, honest, incorrupt, upright, reliable, responsible, straightforward, staunch, true, trusty, uncorrupt, upright.

truth *n* fact, reality, veracity; actuality, authenticity, realism; canon, law, oracle, principle; right, truthfulness, veracity; candour, fidelity, frankness, honesty, honour, ingenuousness, integrity, probity, sincerity, virtue; constancy, devotion, faith, fealty, loyalty, steadfastness; accuracy, correctness, exactitude, exactness, nicety, precision, regularity, trueness.

truthful *adj* correct, reliable, true, trustworthy, veracious; artless, candid, frank, guileless, honest, ingenuous, open, sincere, straightforward, trusty.

truthless *adj* canting, disingenuous, dishonest, false, faithless, hollow, hypocritical, insincere, pharisaical, treacherous, unfair, untrustworthy.

try *vb* examine, prove, test; attempt, essay; adjudicate, adjudge, examine, hear; purify, refine; sample, sift, smell, taste; aim, attempt, endeavour, seek, strain, strive. • *n* attempt, effort, endeavour, experiment, trial.

trying *adj* difficult, fatiguing, hard, irksome, tiresome, wearisome; afflicting, afflictive, calamitous, deplorable, dire, distressing, grievous, hard, painful, sad, severe.

tryst *n* appointment, assignation, rendezvous.

tube *n* bore, bronchus, cylinder, duct, hollow, hose, pipe, pipette, worm.

tuft *n* brush, bunch, crest, feather, knot, plume, topknot, tussock; clump, cluster, group.

tug *vb* drag, draw, haul, pull, tow, wrench; labour, strive, struggle. • *n* drag, haul, pull, tow, wrench.

tuition *n* education, instruction, schooling, teaching, training.

tumble *vb* heave, pitch, roll, toss, wallow; fall, sprawl, stumble; topple, trip; derange, disarrange, dishevel, disorder, disturb, rumple, tousle. • *n* collapse, drop, fall, plunge, spill, stumble, trip.

tumbler *n* acrobat, juggler; glass.

tumid *adj* bloated, distended, enlarged, puffed-up, swelled, swollen, turgid; bombastic, declamatory, fustian, grandiloquent, grandiose, high-flown, inflated, pompous, puffy, rhetorical, stilted, swelling.

tumour *n* boil, carbuncle, swelling, tumefaction.

tumult *n* ado, affray, agitation, altercation, bluster, brawl, disturbance, ferment, flurry, feud, fracas, fray, fuss, hubbub, huddle, hurly-burly, melee, noise, perturbation, pother, quarrel, racket, riot, row, squabble, stir, turbulence, turmoil, uproar.

tumultuous *adj* blustery, breezy, bustling, confused, disorderly, disturbed, riotous, turbulent, unruly.

tune *vb* accord, attune, harmonize, modulate; adapt, adjust, attune. • *n* air, aria, melody, strain, tone; agreement, concord, harmony; accord, order.

tuneful *adj* dulcet, harmonious, melodious, musical.

turbid *adj* foul, impure, muddy, thick, unsettled.

turbulence *n* agitation, commotion, confusion, disorder, disturbance, excitement, tumult, tumultuousness, turmoil, unruliness, uproar; insubordination, insurrection, mutiny, rebellion, riot, sedition.

turbulent *adj* agitated, disturbed, restless, tumultuous, wild; blatant, blustering, boisterous, brawling, disorderly, obstreperous, tumultuous, uproarious, vociferous; factious, insubordinate, insurgent, mutinous, raging, rebellious, refractory, revolutionary, riotous, seditious, stormy, violent.

turf *n* grass, greensward, sod, sward; horse racing, racecourse, race-ground.

turgid *adj* bloated, distended, protuberant, puffed-up, swelled, swollen, tumid; bombastic, declamatory, diffuse, digressive, fustian, high-flown, inflated, grandiloquent, grandiose, ostentatious, pompous, puffy, rhetorical, stilted.

turmoil *n* activity, agitation, bustle, commotion, confusion, disorder, disturbance, ferment, flurry, huddle, hubbub, hurly-burly, noise, trouble, tumult, turbulence, uproar.

turn *vb* revolve, rotate; bend, cast, defect, inflict, round, spin, sway, swivel, twirl, twist, wheel; crank, grind, wind; deflect, divert, transfer, warp; form, mould, shape; adapt, fit, manoeuvre, suit; alter, change, conform, metamorphose, transform, transmute, vary; convert, persuade, prejudice; construe, render, translate; depend, hang, hinge, pivot; eventuate, issue, result, terminate; acidify, curdle, ferment. • *n* cycle, gyration, revolution, rotation, round; bending, deflection, deviation, diversion, doubling, flection, flexion, flexure, reel, retroversion, slew, spin, sweep, swing, swirl, swivel, turning, twist, twirl, whirl, winding; alteration, change, variation, vicissitude; bend, circuit, drive, ramble, run, round, stroll; bout, hand, innings, opportunity, shift, spell; act, action, deed, office; convenience, occasion, purpose; cast, fashion, form, guise, manner, mould, phase, shape; aptitude, bent, bias, disposition, faculty, genius, gift, inclination, leaning, proclivity, proneness, propensity, talent, tendency.

turncoat *n* apostate, backslider, deserter, recreant, renegade, traitor, wretch.

turpitude *n* baseness, degradation, depravity, vileness, wickedness.

turret *n* cupola, minaret, pinnacle.

tussle *vb* conflict, contend, contest, scuffle, struggle, wrestle. • *n* conflict, contest, fight, scuffle, struggle.

tutelage *n* care, charge, dependence, guardianship, protection, teaching, tutorage, tutorship, wardship.

tutor *vb* coach, educate, instruct, teach; discipline, train. • *n* coach, governess, governor, instructor, master, preceptor, schoolteacher, teacher.

twaddle *vb* chatter, gabble, maunder, prate, prattle. • *n* balderdash, chatter, flummery, gabble, gibberish, gobbledegook, gossip, jargon, moonshine, nonsense, platitude, prate, prattle, rigmarole, stuff, tattle.

tweak *vb, n* jerk, pinch, pull, twinge, twitch.

twig[1] *n* bough, branch, offshoot, shoot, slip, spray, sprig, stick, switch.

twig[2] *vb* catch on, comprehend, discover, grasp, realize, recognize, see, understand.

twin *vb* couple, link, match, pair. • *adj* double, doubled, duplicate, geminate, identical, matched, matching, second, twain. • *n* corollary, double, duplicate, fellow, likeness, match.

twine *vb* embrace, encircle, entwine, interlace, surround, wreathe; bend, meander, wind; coil, twist. • *n* convolution, coil, twist; embrace, twining, winding; cord, string.

twinge *vb* pinch, tweak, twitch. • *n* pinch, tweak, twitch; gripe, pang, spasm.

twinkle *vb* blink, twink, wink; flash, glimmer, scintillate, sparkle. • *n* blink, flash, gleam, glimmer, scintillation, sparkle; flash, instant, jiffy, moment, second, tick, trice, twinkling.

twinkling *n* flashing, sparkling, twinkle; flash, instant, jiffy, moment, second, tick, trice.

twirl *vb* revolve, rotate, spin, turn, twist, twirl. • *n* convolution, revolution, turn, twist, whirling.

twist *vb* purl, rotate, spin, twine; complicate, contort, convolute, distort, pervert, screw, wring; coil, writhe; encircle, wind, wreathe. • *n* coil, curl, spin, twine; braid, roll; change, complication, development, variation; bend, convolution, turn; defect, distortion, flaw, imperfection; jerk, pull, sprain, wrench; aberration, characteristic, eccentricity, oddity, peculiarity, quirk.

twit[1] *vb* banter, blame, censure, reproach, taunt, upbraid.

twit[2] *n* blockhead, fool, idiot, nincompoop, nitwit.

twitch *vb* jerk, pluck, pull, snatch. • *n* jerk, pull; contraction, pull, quiver, spasm, twitching.

type *n* emblem, mark, stamp; adumbration, image, representation, representative, shadow, sign, symbol, token; archetype, exemplar, model, original, pattern, prototype, protoplast, standard; character, form, kind, nature, sort; figure, letter, text, typography.

typical *adj* emblematic, exemplary, figurative, ideal, indicative, model, representative, symbolic, true.

typify *vb* betoken, denote, embody, exemplify, figure, image, indicate, represent, signify.

tyrannical *adj* absolute, arbitrary, autocratic, cruel, despotic, dictatorial, domineering, high, imperious, irresponsible, severe, tyrannical, unjust; galling, grinding, inhuman, oppressive, overbearing, severe.

tyranny *n* absolutism, autocracy, despotism, dictatorship, harshness, oppression.

tyrant *n* autocrat, despot, dictator, oppressor.

tyro *n* beginner, learner, neophyte, novice; dabbler, smatterer.

U

ubiquitous *adj* omnipresent, present, universal.

udder *n* nipple, pap, teat.

ugly *adj* crooked, homely, ill-favoured, plain, ordinary, unlovely, unprepossessing, unshapely, unsightly; forbidding, frightful, gruesome, hideous, horrible, horrid, loathsome, monstrous, shocking, terrible, repellent, repulsive; bad-tempered, cantankerous, churlish, cross, quarrelsome, spiteful, surly, spiteful, vicious.

ulcer *n* boil, fester, gathering, pustule, sore.

ulterior *adj* beyond, distant, farther; hidden, personal, secret, selfish, undisclosed.

ultimate *adj* conclusive, decisive, eventual, extreme, farthest, final, last. • *n* acme, consummation, culmination, height, peak, pink, quintessence, summit.

ultra *adj* advanced, beyond, extreme, radical.

umbrage *n* shadow, shade; anger, displeasure, dissatisfaction, dudgeon, injury, offence, pique, resentment.

umpire *vb* adjudicate, arbitrate, judge, referee. • *n* adjudicator, arbiter, arbitrator, judge, referee.

unabashed *adj* bold, brazen, confident, unblushing, undaunted, undismayed.

unable *adj* impotent, incapable, incompetent, powerless, weak.

unacceptable *adj* disagreeable, distasteful, offensive, unpleasant, unsatisfactory, unwelcome.

unaccommodating *adj* disobliging, noncompliant, uncivil, ungracious.

unaccomplished *adj* incomplete, unachieved, undone, unperformed, unexecuted, unfinished; ill-educated, uncultivated, unpolished.

unaccountable *adj* inexplicable, incomprehensible, inscrutable, mysterious, unintelligible; irresponsible, unanswerable.

unaccustomed *adj* uninitiated, unskilled, unused; foreign, new, strange, unfamiliar, unusual.

unaffected *adj* artless, honest, naive, natural, plain, simple, sincere, real, unfeigned; chaste, pure, unadorned; insensible, unchanged, unimpressed, unmoved, unstirred, untouched.

unanimity *n* accord, agreement, concert, concord, harmony, union, unity.

unanimous *adj* agreeing, concordant, harmonious, like-minded, solid, united.

unassuming *adj* humble, modest, reserved, unobtrusive, unpretending, unpretentious.

unattainable *adj* inaccessible, unobtainable.

unavailing *adj* abortive, fruitless, futile, ineffectual, ineffective, inept, nugatory, unsuccessful, useless, vain.

unbalanced *adj* unsound, unsteady; unadjusted, unsettled.

unbearable *adj* insufferable, insupportable, unendurable.

unbecoming *adj* inappropriate, indecent, indecorous, improper, unbefitting, unbeseeming, unseemly, unsuitable.

unbelief *n* disbelief, dissent, distrust, incredulity, incredulousness, miscreance, miscreancy, nonconformity; doubt, freethinking, infidelity, scepticism.

unbeliever *n* agnostic, deist, disbeliever, doubter, heathen, infidel, sceptic.

unbending *adj* inflexible, rigid, stiff, unpliant, unyielding; firm, obstinate, resolute, stubborn.

unbiased *adj* disinterested, impartial, indifferent, neutral, uninfluenced, unprejudiced, unwarped.

unbind *vb* loose, undo, unfasten, unloose, untie; free, unchain, unfetter.

unblemished *adj* faultless, guiltless, immaculate, impeccable, innocent, intact, perfect, pure, sinless, spotless, stainless undefiled, unspotted, unsullied, untarnished.

unblushing *adj* boldfaced, impudent, shameless.

unbounded *adj* absolute, boundless, endless, immeasurable, immense, infinite, interminable, measureless, unlimited, vast; immoderate, uncontrolled, unrestrained, unrestricted.

unbridled *adj* dissolute, intractable, lax, licensed, licentious, loose, uncontrolled, ungovernable, unrestrained, violent, wanton.

unbroken *adj* complete, entire, even, full, intact, unimpaired; constant, continuous, fast, profound, sound, successive, undisturbed; inviolate, unbetrayed, unviolated.

unbuckle *vb* loose, unfasten, unloose.

uncanny *adj* inopportune, unsafe; eerie, eery, ghostly, unearthly, unnatural, weird.

unceremonious *adj* abrupt, bluff, blunt, brusque, course, curt, gruff, plain, rough, rude, ungracious; casual, familiar, informal, offhand, unconstrained.

uncertain *adj* ambiguous, doubtful, dubious, equivocal, indefinite, indeterminate, indistinct, questionable, unsettled; insecure precarious, problematical; capricious, changeable, desultory, fitful, fluctuating, irregular, mutable, shaky, slippery, unreliable, variable.

unchaste *adj* dissolute, incontinent, indecent, immoral, lascivious, lecherous, libidinous, lewd, loose, obscene, wanton.

unchecked *adj* uncurbed, unhampered, unhindered, unobstructed, unrestrained, untrammelled.

uncivil *adj* bearish, blunt, boorish, brusque, discourteous, disobliging, disrespectful, gruff, ill-bred, ill-mannered, impolite, irreverent, rough, rude, uncomplaisant, uncourteous, uncouth, ungentle, ungracious, unmannered, unseemly.

unclean *adj* abominable, beastly, dirty, filthy, foul, grimy, grubby, miry, muddy, nasty, offensive, purulent, repulsive, soiled, sullied; improper, indecent, indecorous, obscene, polluted, risqué, sinful, smutty, unholy, uncleanly.

uncomfortable *adj* disagreeable, displeasing, disquieted, distressing, disturbed, uneasy, unpleasant, restless; cheerless, close, oppressive; dismal, miserable, unhappy.

uncommon *adj* choice, exceptional, extraordinary, infrequent, noteworthy, odd, original, queer, rare, remarkable, scarce, singular, strange, unexampled, unfamiliar, unusual, unwonted.

uncommunicative *adj* close, inconversable, reserved, reticent, taciturn, unsociable, unsocial.

uncomplaining *adj* long-suffering, meek, patient, resigned, tolerant.

uncompromising *adj* inflexible, narrow, obstinate, orthodox, rigid, stiff, strict, unyielding.

unconcerned *adj* apathetic, careless, indifferent.

unconditional *adj* absolute, categorical, complete, entire, free, full, positive, unlimited, unqualified, unreserved, unrestricted.

uncongenial *adj* antagonistic, discordant, displeasing, ill-assorted, incompatible, inharmonious, mismatched, unsuited, unsympathetic.

uncouth *adj* awkward, boorish, clownish, clumsy, gawky, inelegant, loutish, lubberly, rough, rude, rustic, uncourtly, ungainly, unpolished, unrefined, unseemly; odd, outlandish, strange, unfamiliar, unusual.

uncover *vb* denude, divest, lay bare, strip; disclose, discover, expose, reveal, unmask, unveil; bare, doff; open, unclose, unseal.

unctuous *adj* adipose, greasy oily, fat, fatty, oleaginous, pinguid, sebaceous; bland, lubricious, smooth, slippery; bland, fawning, glib, obsequious, plausible, servile, suave, sycophantic; fervid, gushing.

uncultivated *adj* fallow, uncultured, unreclaimed, untilled; homely, ignorant, illiterate, rude, uncivilized, uncultured, uneducated, unfit, unlettered, unpolished, unread, unready, unrefined, untaught; rough, savage, sylvan, uncouth, wild.

undaunted *adj* bold, brave, courageous, dauntless, fearless, intrepid, plucky, resolute, undismayed.

undefiled *adj* clean, immaculate, pure, spotless, stainless, unblemished, unspotted, unsullied, untarnished; honest, innocent, inviolate, pure, uncorrupted, unpolluted, unstained.

undemonstrative *adj* calm, composed, demure, impassive, modest, placid, quiet, reserved, sedate, sober, staid, tranquil.

undeniable *adj* certain, conclusive, evident, incontestable, incontrovertible, indisputable, indubitable, obvious, unquestionable.

under *prep* below, beneath, inferior to, lower than, subordinate to, underneath. • *adv* below, beneath, down, lower.

underestimate *vb* belittle, underrate, undervalue.

undergo *vb* bear, endure, experience, suffer, sustain.

underhand *adj* clandestine, deceitful, disingenuous, fraudulent, hidden, secret, sly, stealthy, underhanded, unfair. • *adv* clandestinely, privately, secretly, slyly, stealthily, surreptitiously; fraudulently, unfairly.

underling *n* agent, inferior, servant, subordinate.

undermine *vb* excavate, mine, sap; demoralize, foil, frustrate, thwart, weaken.

understand *vb* apprehend, catch, comprehend, conceive, discern, grasp, know, penetrate, perceive, see, seize, twig; assume, interpret, take; imply, mean.

understanding *adj* compassionate, considerate, forgiving, kind, kindly, patient, sympathetic, tolerant. • *n* brains, comprehension, discernment, faculty, intellect, intelligence, judgement, knowledge, mind, reason, sense.

undertake *vb* assume, attempt, begin, embark on, engage in, enter upon, take in hand; agree, bargain, contract, covenant, engage, guarantee, promise, stipulate.

undertaking *n* adventure, affair, attempt, business, effort, endeavour, engagement, enterprise, essay, move, project, task, venture.

undesigned *adj* spontaneous, unintended, unintentional, unplanned, unpremeditated.

undigested *adj* crude, ill-advised, ill-considered, ill-judged; confused, disorderly, ill-arranged, unmethodical.

undivided *adj* complete, entire, whole; one, united.

undo *vb* annul, cancel, frustrate, invalidate, neutralize, nullify, offset, reverse; disengage, loose, unfasten, unmake, unravel, untie; crush, destroy, overturn, ruin.

undoubted *adj* incontrovertible, indisputable, indubitable, undisputed, unquestionable, unquestioned.

undress *vb* denude, dismantle, disrobe, unclothe, unrobe, peel, strip. • *n* disarray, nakedness, nudity; mufti, negligee.

undue *adj* illegal, illegitimate, improper, unlawful, excessive, disproportionate, disproportioned, immoderate, unsuitable; unfit.

undulation *n* billowing, fluctuation, pulsation, ripple, wave.

undying *adj* deathless, endless, immortal, imperishable.

unearthly *adj* preternatural, supernatural, uncanny, weird.

uneasy *adj* disquieted, disturbed, fidgety, impatient, perturbed, restless, restive, unquiet, worried; awkward, stiff, ungainly, ungraceful; constraining, cramping, disagreeable, uncomfortable.

unending *adj* endless, eternal, everlasting, interminable, never-ending, perpetual, unceasing.

unequal *adj* disproportionate, disproportioned, ill-matched, inferior, irregular, insufficient, not alike, uneven.

unequalled *adj* exceeding, incomparable, inimitable, matchless, new, nonpareil, novel, paramount, peerless, pre-eminent, superlative, surpassing, transcendent, unheard of, unique, unparalleled, unrivalled.

unequivocal *adj* absolute, certain, clear, evident, incontestable, indubitable, positive; explicit, unambiguous, unmistakable.

uneven *adj* hilly, jagged, lumpy, ragged, rough, rugged, stony; motley, unequal, variable, variegated.

uneventful *adj* commonplace, dull, eventless, humdrum, quiet, monotonous, smooth, uninteresting.

unexceptionable *adj* excellent, faultless, good, irreproachable.

unexpected *adj* abrupt, sudden, unforeseen.

unfair *adj* dishonest, dishonourable, faithless, false, hypocritical, inequitable, insincere, oblique, one-sided, partial, unequal, unjust, wrongful.

unfaithful *adj* adulterous, derelict, deceitful, dishonest, disloyal, false, faithless, fickle, perfidious, treacherous, unreliable; negligent; changeable, inconstant, untrue.

unfamiliar *adj* bizarre, foreign, new, novel, outlandish, queer, singular, strange, uncommon, unusual.

unfashionable *adj* antiquated, destitute, disused, obsolete, old-fashioned, unconventional.

unfavourable *adj* adverse, contrary, disadvantageous, discouraging, ill, inauspicious, inimical, inopportune, indisposed, malign, sinister, unfriendly, unlucky, unpropitious, untimely; foul, inclement.

unfeeling *adj* apathetic, callous, heartless, insensible, numb, obdurate, torpid, unconscious, unimpressionable; adamantine, cold-blooded, cruel, hard, merciless, pitiless, stony, unkind, unsympathetic.

unfit *vb* disable, disqualify, incapacitate. • *adj* improper, inappropriate, incompetent, inconsistent, unsuitable; ill-equipped,

inadequate, incapable, unqualified, useless; debilitated, feeble, flabby, unhealthy, unsound.

unflagging *adj* constant, indefatigable, never-ending, persevering, steady, unfaltering, unremitting, untiring, unwearied.

unflinching *adj* firm, resolute, steady, unshrinking.

unfold *vb* display, expand, open, separate, unfurl, unroll; declare, disclose, reveal, tell; decipher, develop, disentangle, evolve, explain, illustrate, interpret, resolve, unravel.

unfortunate *adj* hapless, ill-fated, ill-starred, infelicitous, luckless, unhappy, unlucky, unprosperous, unsuccessful, wretched; calamitous, deplorable, disastrous; inappropriate, inexpedient.

unfrequented *adj* abandoned, deserted, forsaken, lone, solitary, uninhabited, unoccupied.

unfruitful *adj* barren, fruitless, sterile; infecund, unprolific; unprofitable, unproductive.

ungainly *adj* awkward, boorish, clownish, clumsy, gawky, inelegant, loutish, lubberly, lumbering, slouching, stiff, uncourtly, uncouth, ungraceful.

ungentlemanly *adj* ill-bred, impolite, rude, uncivil, ungentle, ungracious, unmannerly.

unhappy *adj* afflicted, disastrous, dismal, distressed, drear, evil, inauspicious, miserable, painful, unfortunate, wretched.

unhealthy *adj* ailing, diseased, feeble, indisposed, infirm, poorly, sickly, toxic, unsanitary, unsound, toxic, venomous.

uniform *adj* alike, constant, even, equable, equal, smooth, steady, regular, unbroken, unchanged, undeviating, unvaried, unvarying. • *n* costume, dress, livery, outfit, regalia, suit.

uniformity *n* constancy, continuity, permanence, regularity, sameness, stability; accordance, agreement, conformity, consistency, unanimity.

unimportant *adj* immaterial, inappreciable, inconsequent, inconsequential, inconsiderable, indifferent, insignificant, mediocre, minor, paltry, petty, small, slight, trifling, trivial.

unintentional *adj* accidental, casual, fortuitous, inadvertent, involuntary, spontaneous, undesigned, unmeant, unplanned, unpremeditated, unthinking.

uninterrupted *adj* continuous, endless, incessant, perpetual, unceasing.

union *n* coalescence, coalition, combination, conjunction, coupling, fusion, incorporation, joining, junction, unification, uniting; agreement, concert, concord, concurrence, harmony, unanimity, unity; alliance, association, club, confederacy, federation, guild, league.

unique *adj* choice, exceptional, matchless, only, peculiar, rare, single, sole, singular, uncommon, unexampled, unmatched.

unison *n* accord, accordance, agreement, concord, harmony.

unite *vb* amalgamate, attach, blend, centralize, coalesce, confederate, consolidate, embody, fuse, incorporate, merge, weld; associate, conjoin, connect, couple, link, marry; combine, join; harmonize, reconcile; agree, concert, concur, cooperate, fraternize.

universal *adj* all-reaching, catholic, cosmic, encyclopedic, general, ubiquitous, unlimited; all, complete, entire, total, whole.

unjust *adj* inequitable, injurious, partial, unequal, unfair, unwarranted, wrong, wrongful; flagitious, heinous, influenced, iniquitous, nefarious, unrighteous, wicked; biased, prejudiced, uncandid.

unjustifiable *adj* indefensible, unjust, unreasonable, unwarrantable; inexcusable, unpardonable.

unknown *adj* unappreciated, unascertained; undiscovered, unexplored, uninvestigated; concealed, dark, enigmatic, hidden, mysterious, mystic; anonymous, incognito, inglorious, nameless, obscure, renownless, undistinguished, unheralded, unnoted.

unladylike *adj* ill-bred, impolite, rude, uncivil, ungentle, ungracious, unmannerly.

unlamented *adj* unmourned, unregretted.

unlimited *adj* boundless, infinite, interminable, limitless, measureless, unbounded; absolute, full, unconfined, unconstrained, unrestricted; indefinite, undefined.

unlucky *adj* baleful, disastrous, ill-fated, ill-starred, luckless, unfortunate, unprosperous, unsuccessful; ill-omened, inauspicious; miserable, unhappy.

unmanageable *adj* awkward, cumbersome, inconvenient, unwieldy; intractable, unruly, unworkable, vicious; difficult, impractical.

unmatched *adj* matchless, unequalled, unparalleled, unrivalled.

unmitigated *adj* absolute, complete, consummate, perfect, sheer, stark, thorough, unqualified, utter.

unnatural *adj* aberrant, abnormal, anomalous, foreign, irregular, prodigious, uncommon; brutal, cold, heartless, inhuman, unfeeling, unusual; affected, artificial, constrained, forced, insincere, self-conscious, stilted, strained; factitious.

unpleasant *adj* disagreeable, displeasing, distasteful, obnoxious, offensive, repulsive, unlovely, ungrateful, unacceptable, unpalatable, unwelcome.

unpremeditated *adj* extempore, impromptu, offhand, spontaneous, undesigned, unintentional, unstudied.

unprincipled *adj* bad, crooked, dishonest, fraudulent, immoral, iniquitous, knavish, lawless, profligate, rascally, roguish, thievish, trickish, tricky, unscrupulous, vicious, villainous, wicked.

unqualified *adj* disqualified, incompetent, ineligible, unadapted, unfit; absolute, certain, consummate, decided, direct, downright, full, outright, unconditional, unmeasured, unrestricted, unmitigated; exaggerated, sweeping.

unreal *adj* chimerical, dreamlike, fanciful, flimsy, ghostly, illusory, insubstantial, nebulous, shadowy, spectral, visionary, unsubstantial.

unreasonable *adj* absurd, excessive, exorbitant, foolish, ill-judged, illogical, immoderate, impractical, injudicious, irrational, nonsensical, preposterous, senseless, silly, stupid, unfair, unreasoning, unwarrantable, unwise.

unreliable *adj* fallible, fickle, irresponsible, treacherous, uncertain, undependable, unstable, unsure, untrustworthy.

unremitting *adj* assiduous, constant, continual, diligent, incessant, indefatigable, persevering, sedulous, unabating, unceasing.

unrepentant *adj* abandoned, callous, graceless, hardened, impenitent, incorrigible, irreclaimable, lost, obdurate, profligate, recreant, seared, shameless.

unrequited *adj* unanswered, unreturned, unrewarded.

unreserved *adj* absolute, entire, full, unlimited; above-board, artless, candid, communicative, fair, frank, guileless, honest, ingenuous, open, sincere, single-minded, undesigning, undissembling; demonstrative, emotional, open-hearted.

unresisting *adj* compliant, long-suffering, non-resistant, obedient, passive, patient, submissive, yielding.

unresponsive *adj* irresponsive, unsympathetic.

unrestrained *adj* unbridled, unchecked, uncurbed, unfettered, unhindered, unobstructed, unreserved; broad, dissolute, incontinent, inordinate, lax, lewd, licentious, loose, wanton; lawless, wild.

unrestricted *adj* free, unbridled, unconditional, unconfined, uncurbed, unfettered, unlimited, unqualified, unrestrained; clear, open, public, unobstructed.

unrevealed *adj* hidden, occult, secret, undiscovered, unknown.

unrewarded *adj* unpaid, uncompensated.

unriddle *vb* explain, expound, solve, unfold, unravel.

unrighteous *adj* evil, sinful, ungodly, unholy, vicious, wicked, wrong; heinous, inequitable, iniquitous, nefarious, unfair, unjust.

unripe *adj* crude, green, hard, immature, premature, sour; incomplete, unfinished.

unrivalled *adj* incomparable, inimitable, matchless, peerless, unequalled, unexampled, unique, unparalleled.

unrobe *vb* disrobe, undress.

unroll *vb* develop, discover, evolve, open, unfold; display, lay open.

unromantic *adj* literal, matter-of-fact, prosaic.

unroot *vb* eradicate, extirpate, root out, uproot.

unruffled *adj* calm, peaceful, placid, quiet, serene, smooth, still, tranquil; collected, composed, cool, imperturbable, peaceful, philosophical, placid, tranquil, undisturbed, unexcited, unmoved.

unruly *adj* disobedient, disorderly, fractious, headstrong, insubordinate, intractable, mutinous, obstreperous, rebellious, refractory, riotous, seditious, turbulent, ungovernable, unmanageable, wanton, wild; lawless, obstinate, rebellious, stubborn, vicious.

unsafe *adj* dangerous, hazardous, insecure, perilous, precarious, risky, treacherous, uncertain, unprotected.

unsaid *adj* tacit, unmentioned, unspoken, unuttered.

unsanctified *adj* profane, unhallowed, unholy.

unsatisfactory *adj* insufficient; disappointing; faulty, feeble, imperfect, poor, weak.

unsatisfied *adj* insatiate, unsated, unsatiated, unstaunched; discontented, displeased, dissatisfied, malcontent; undischarged, unpaid, unperformed, unrendered.

unsavoury *adj* flat, insipid, mawkish, savourless, tasteless, unflavoured, unpalatable, vapid; disagreeable, disgusting, distasteful, nasty, nauseating, nauseous, offensive, rank, revolting, sickening, uninviting, unpleasing.

unsay *vb* recall, recant, retract, take back.

unscathed *adj* unharmed, uninjured.

unschooled *adj* ignorant, uneducated, uninstructed; undisciplined, untrained.

unscrupulous *adj* dishonest, reckless, ruthless, unconscientious, unprincipled, unrestrained.

unsealed *adj* open, unclosed.

unsearchable *adj* hidden, incomprehensible, inscrutable, mysterious.

unseasonable *adj* ill-timed, inappropriate, infelicitous, inopportune, untimely; late, too late; inexpedient, undesireable, unfit, ungrateful, unsuitable, unwelcome; premature, too early.

unseasonably *adv* malapropos, unsuitably, untimely.

unseasoned *adj* inexperienced, unaccustomed, unqualified, untrained; immoderate, inordinate, irregular; green; fresh, unsalted.

unseeing *adj* blind, sightless.

unseemly *adj* improper, indecent, inappropriate, indecorous, unbecoming, uncomely, unfit, unmeet, unsuitable.

unseen *adj* undiscerned, undiscovered, unobserved, unperceived; imperceptible, indiscoverable, invisible, latent.

unselfish *adj* altruistic, devoted, disinterested, generous, high-minded, impersonal, liberal, magnanimous, self-denying, self-forgetful, selfless, self-sacrificing.

unserviceable *adj* ill-conditioned, unsound, useless; profitless, unprofitable

unsettle *vb* confuse, derange, disarrange, disconcert, disorder, disturb, trouble, unbalance, unfix, unhinge, upset.

unsettled *adj* changeable, fickle, inconstant, restless, transient, unstable, unsteady, vacillating, wavering; inequable, unequal; feculent, muddy, roiled, roily, turbid; adrift, afloat, homeless, unestablished, uninhabited; open, tentative, unadjusted, undecided undetermined; due, outstanding, owing, unpaid; perturbed, troubled, unnerved.

unshackle *vb* emancipate, liberate, loose, release, set free, unbind, unchain, unfetter.

unshaken *adj* constant, firm, resolute, steadfast, steady, unmoved.

unshapen *adj* deformed, grotesque, ill-formed, ill-made, ill-shaped, misshapen, shapeless, ugly, uncouth.

unsheltered *adj* exposed, unprotected.

unshrinking *adj* firm, determined, persisting, resolute, unblenching, unflinching.

unshroud *vb* discover, expose, reveal, uncover.

unsightly *adj* deformed, disagreeable, hideous, repellent, repulsive, ugly.

unskilful, unskillful *adj* awkward, bungling, clumsy, inapt, inexpert, maladroit, rough, rude, unhandy, unskilled, unversed.

unskilled *adj* inexperienced, raw, undisciplined, undrilled, uneducated, unexercised, unpractised, unprepared, unschooled; unskilful.

unslaked *adj* unquenched, unslacked.

unsleeping *adj* unslumbering, vigilant, wakeful, watchful.

unsmirched *adj* undefiled, unpolluted, unspotted.

unsociable *adj* distant, reserved, retiring, segregative, shy, solitary, standoffish, taciturn, uncommunicative, uncompanionable, ungenial, unsocial; inhospitable, misanthropic, morose.

unsoiled *adj* clean, spotless, unspotted, unstained, unsullied, untarnished.

unsophisticated *adj* genuine, pure, unadulterated; good, guileless, innocent, undepraved, unpolluted, invitiated; artless, honest, ingenuous, naive, natural, simple, sincere, straightforward, unaffected, undesigning, unstudied.

unsound *adj* decayed, defective, impaired, imperfect, rotten, thin, wasted, weak; broken, disturbed, light, restless; diseased, feeble, infirm, morbid, poorly, sickly, unhealthy, weak; deceitful, erroneous, fallacious, false, faulty, hollow, illogical, incorrect, invalid, ill-advised, irrational, questionable, sophistical, unreasonable, unsubstantial, untenable, wrong; dishonest, false, insincere, unfaithful, untrustworthy, untrue; insubstantial, unreal; heretical, heterodox, unorthodox.

unsparing *adj* bountiful, generous, lavish, liberal, profuse, ungrudging; harsh, inexorable, relentless, rigorous, ruthless, severe, uncompromising, unforgiving.

unspeakable *adj* indescribable, ineffable, inexpressible, unutterable.

unspiritual *adj* bodily, carnal, fleshly, sensual.

unspotted *adj* clean, spotless, unsoiled, unstained, unsullied, untarnished; faultless, immaculate, innocent, pure, stainless, unblemished, uncorrupted, undefiled, untainted.

unstable *adj* infirm, insecure, precarious, top-heavy, tottering, unbalanced, unballasted, unreliable, unsafe, unsettled, unsteady; changeable, erratic, fickle, inconstant, irresolute, mercurial, mutable, vacillating, variable, wavering, weak, volatile.—*also* **instable**.

unstained *adj* colourless, uncoloured, undyed, untinged; clean, spotless, unspotted.

unsteady *adj* fluctuating, oscillating, unsettled; insecure, precarious, unstable; changeable, desultory, ever-changing, fickle, inconstant, irresolute, mutable, unreliable, variable, wavering; drunken, jumpy, tottering, vacillating, wobbly, tipsy.

unstinted *adj* abundant, ample, bountiful, full, large, lavish, plentiful, prodigal, profuse.

unstrung *adj* overcome, shaken, unnerved, weak.

unstudied *adj* extempore, extemporaneous, impromptu, offhand, spontaneous, unpremeditated; inexpert, unskilled, unversed.

unsubdued *adj* unbowed, unbroken, unconquered, untamed.

unsubmissive *adj* disobedient, contumacious, indocile, insubordinate, obstinate, perverse, refractory, uncomplying, ungovernable, unmanageable, unruly, unyielding.

unsubstantial *adj* airy, flimsy, gaseous, gossamery, light, slight, tenuous, thin, vaporous; apparitional, bodiless, chimerical, cloudbuilt, dreamlike, empty, fantastical, ideal, illusory, imaginary, imponderable, moonshiny, spectral, unreal, vague, visionary; erroneous, fallacious, flimsy, groundless, illogical, unfounded, ungrounded, unsolid, unsound, untenable, weak.

unsuccessful *adj* abortive, bootless, fruitless, futile, ineffectual, profitless, unavailing, vain; ill-fated, ill-starred, luckless, unfortunate, unhappy, unlucky, unprosperous.

unsuitable *adj* ill-adapted, inappropriate, malapropos, unfit, unsatisfactory, unsuited; improper, inapplicable, inapt, incongruous, inexpedient, infelicitous, unbecoming, unbeseeming, unfitting.

unsuited *adj* unadapted, unfitted, unqualified.

unsullied *adj* chaste, clean, spotless, unsoiled, unspotted, unstained, untarnished; immaculate, pure, stainless, unblemished, uncorrupted, undefiled, untainted, untouched, virginal.

unsupplied *adj* destitute, unfurnished, unprovided.

unsupported *adj* unaided, unassisted; unbacked, unseconded, unsustained, unupheld.

unsurpassed *adj* matchless, peerless, unequalled, unexampled, unexcelled, unmatched, unparagoned, unparalleled, unrivalled.

unsusceptible *adj* apathetic, cold, impassive, insusceptible, phlegmatic, stoical, unimpressible, unimpressionable.

unsuspecting *adj* confiding, credulous, trusting, unsuspicious.

unsuspicious *adj* confiding, credulous, gullible, simple, trustful, unsuspecting.

unsustainable *adj* insupportable, intolerable; controvertible, erroneous, unmaintainable, untenable.

unswerving *adj* direct, straight, undeviating; constant, determined, firm, resolute, staunch, steadfast, steady, stable, unwavering.

unsymmetrical *adj* amorphous, asymmetric, disproportionate, formless, irregular, unbalanced.

unsystematic, unsystematical *adj* casual, disorderly, haphazard, irregular, planless, unmethodical.

untainted *adj* chaste, clean, faultless, fresh, healthy, pure, sweet, wholesome; spotless, unsoiled, unstained, unsullied, untarnished; immaculate, stainless, unblemished, uncorrupted, undefiled, unspotted.

untamable *adj* unconquerable.

untamed *adj* fierce, unbroken, wild.

untangle *vb* disentangle, explain, explicate.

untarnished *adj* chaste, clean, spotless, unsoiled, unspotted, unstained, unsullied; immaculate, pure, spotless, stainless, unblemished, uncorrupted, undefiled, unspotted, unsullied, untainted, virginal, virtuous.

untaught *adj* illiterate, unenlightened, uninformed, unlettered; ignorant, inexperienced, undisciplined, undrilled, uneducated, uninitiated, uninstructed, untutored.

untenable *adj* indefensible, unmaintainable, unsound; fallacious, hollow, illogical, indefensible, insupportable, unjustifiable, weak.

untenanted *adj* deserted, empty, tenantless, uninhabited, unoccupied.

unterrified *adj* fearless, unappalled, unawed, undismayed, undaunted, unscared.

unthankful *adj* thankless, ungrateful.

unthinking *adj* careless, heedless, inconsiderate, thoughtless, unreasoning, unreflecting; automatic, mechanical.

unthoughtful *adj* careless, heedless, inconsiderate, thoughtless.

unthrifty *adj* extravagant, improvident, lavish, prodigal, profuse, thriftless, wasteful.

untidy *adj* careless, disorderly, dowdy, frumpy, mussy, slatternly, slovenly, unkempt, unneat.

untie *vb* free, loose, loosen, unbind, unfasten, unknot, unloose; clear, resolve, solve, unfold.

until *adv, conj* till, to the time when; to the place, point, state or degree that; • *prep* till, to.

untimely *adj* ill-timed, immature, inconvenient, inopportune, mistimed, premature, unseasonable, unsuitable; ill-considered, inauspicious, uncalled for, unfortunate. • *adv* unseasonably, unsuitably.

untinged *adj* achromatic, colourless, hueless, uncoloured, undyed, unstained.

untiring *adj* persevering, incessant, indefatigable, patient, tireless, unceasing, unfatiguable, unflagging, unremitting, unwearied, unwearying.

untold *adj* countless, incalculable, innumerable, uncounted, unnumbered; unrelated, unrevealed.

untouched *adj* intact, scatheless, unharmed, unhurt, uninjured, unscathed; insensible, unaffected, unmoved, unstirred.

untoward *adj* adverse, froward, intractable, perverse, refractory, stubborn, unfortunate; annoying, ill-timed, inconvenient, unmanageable, vexatious; awkward, uncouth, ungainly, ungraceful.

untrained *adj* green, ignorant, inexperienced, raw, unbroken, undisciplined, undrilled, uneducated, uninstructed, unpractised, unskilled, untaught, untutored.

untrammelled *adj* free, unhampered.

untried *adj* fresh, inexperienced, maiden, new, unassayed, unattempted, unattested, virgin; undecided.

untrodden *adj* pathless, trackless, unbeaten.

untroubled *adj* calm, careless, composed, peaceful, serene, smooth, tranquil, undisturbed, unvexed.

untrue *adj* contrary, false, inaccurate, wrong; disloyal, faithless, perfidious, recreant, treacherous, unfaithful.

untrustworthy *adj* deceitful, dishonest, inaccurate, rotten, slippery, treacherous, undependable, unreliable; disloyal, false; deceptive, fallible, illusive, questionable.

untruth *n* error, faithlessness, falsehood, falsity, incorrectness, inveracity, treachery; deceit, deception, fabrication, fib, fiction, forgery, imposture, invention, lie, misrepresentation, misstatement, story.

untutored *adj* ignorant, inexperienced, undisciplined, undrilled, uneducated, uninitiated, uninstructed, untaught; artless, natural, simple, unsophisticated.

untwist *vb* disentangle, disentwine, ravel, unravel, unwreathe.

unused *adj* idle, unemployed, untried; new, unaccustomed, unfamiliar.

unusual *adj* abnormal, curious, exceptional, extraordinary, odd, peculiar, queer, rare, recherché, remarkable, singular, strange, unaccustomed, uncommon, unwonted.

unutterable *adj* incommunicable, indescribable, ineffable, inexpressible, unspeakable.

unvarnished *adj* unpolished; candid, plain, simple, true, unadorned, unembellished.

unvarying *adj* constant, invariable, unchanging.

unveil *vb* disclose, expose, reveal, show, uncover, unmask.

unveracious *adj* false, lying, mendacious, untruthful.

unversed *adj* inexperienced, raw, undisciplined, undrilled, uneducated, unexercised, unpractised, unprepared, unschooled, unskilful.

unviolated *adj* inviolate, unbetrayed, unbroken.

unwarlike *adj* pacific, peaceful.

unwarped *adj* impartial, unbiased, undistorted, unprejudiced.

unwarrantable *adj* improper, indefensible, unjustifiable.

unwary *adj* careless, hasty, heedless, imprudent, incautious, indiscreet, precipitate, rash, reckless, remiss, uncircumspect, unguarded.

unwavering *adj* constant, determined, firm, fixed, resolute, settled, staunch, steadfast, steady, unhesitating.

unwearied *adj* unfatigued; constant, continual, incessant, indefatigable, persevering, persistent, unceasing, unremitting, untiring.

unwelcome *adj* disagreeable, unacceptable, ungrateful, unpleasant, unpleasing.

unwell *adj* ailing, delicate, diseased, ill, indisposed, sick.

unwept *adj* unlamented, unmourned, unregretted.

unwholesome *adj* baneful, deleterious, injurious, insalubrious, noisome, noxious, poisonous, unhealthful, unhealthy; injudicious, pernicious, unsound; corrupt, tainted.

unwieldy *adj* bulky, clumsy, cumbersome, cumbrous, elephantine, heavy, hulking, large, massy, ponderous, unmanageable, weighty.

unwilling *adj* averse, backward, disinclined, indisposed, laggard, loath, opposed, recalcitrant, reluctant; forced, grudging.

unwind *vb* unravel, unreel, untwine, wind off; disentangle.

unwise *adj* brainless, foolish, ill-advised, ill-judged, impolitic, imprudent, indiscreet, injudicious, inexpedient, senseless, silly, stupid, unwary, weak.

unwitnessed *adj* unknown, unseen, unspied.

unwittingly *adv* ignorantly, inadvertently, unconsciously, undesignedly, unintentionally, unknowingly.

unwonted *adj* infrequent, rare, uncommon, unusual; unaccustomed, unused.

unworthy *adj* undeserving; bad, base, blameworthy, worthless; shameful, unbecoming, vile; contemptible, derogatory, despicable, discreditable, mean, paltry, reprehensible, shabby.

unwrap *vb* open, unfold.

unwrinkled *adj* smooth, unforrowed.

unwritten *adj* oral, traditional, unrecorded; conventional, customary.

unwrought *adj* crude, rough, rude, unfashioned, unformed.

unyielding *adj* constant, determined, indomitable, inflexible, pertinacious, resolute, staunch, steadfast, steady, tenacious, uncompromising, unwavering; headstrong, intractable, obstinate, perverse, self-willed, stiff, stubborn, wayward, wilful; adamantine, firm, grim, hard, immovable, implastic, inexorable, relentless, rigid, unbending.

unyoke *vb* disconnect, disjoin, part, separate.

unyoked *adj* disconnected, separated; licentious, loose, unrestrained.

upbraid *vb* accuse, blame, chide, condemn, criticize, denounce, fault, reproach, reprove, revile, scold, taunt, twit.

upheaval *n* elevation, upthrow; cataclysm, convulsion, disorder, eruption, explosion, outburst, overthrow.

uphill *adj* ascending, upward; arduous, difficult, hard, laborious, strenuous, toilsome, wearisome.

uphold *vb* elevate, raise; bear up, hold up, support, sustain; advocate, aid, champion, countenance, defend, justify, maintain, vindicate.

upland *n* down, fell, ridge, plateau.

uplift *vb* raise, upraise; animate, elevate, inspire, lift, refine. • *n* ascent, climb, elevation, lift, rise, upthrust; exaltation, inspiration, uplifting; improvement, refinement.

upon *prep* on, on top of, over; about, concerning, on the subject of, relating to; immediately after, with.

upper hand *n* advantage, ascendancy, control, dominion, mastership, mastery, pre-eminence, rule, superiority, supremacy, whip hand.

uppermost *adj* foremost, highest, loftiest, supreme, topmost, upmost.

uppish *adj* arrogant, assuming, haughty, perky, proud, smart.

upright *adj* erect, perpendicular, vertical; conscientious, equitable, fair, faithful, good, honest, honourable, incorruptible, just, pure, righteous, straightforward, true, trustworthy, upstanding, virtuous.

uprightness *n* erectness, perpendicularity, verticality; equity, fairness, goodness, honesty, honour, incorruptibility, integrity, justice, probity, rectitude, righteousness, straightforwardness, trustiness, trustworthiness, virtue, worth.

uproar *n* clamour, commotion, confusion, din, disturbance, fracas, hubbub, hurly-burly, noise, pandemonium, racket, riot, tumult, turmoil, vociferation.

uproarious *adj* boisterous, clamorous, loud, noisy, obstreperous, riotous, tumultuous.

uproot *vb* eradicate, extirpate, root out.

upset *vb* capsize, invert, overthrow, overtumble, overturn, spill, tip over, topple, turn turtle; agitate, confound, confuse, discompose, disconcert, distress, disturb, embarrass, excite, fluster, muddle, overwhelm, perturb, shock, startle, trouble, unnerve, unsettle; checkmate, defeat, overthrow, revolutionize, subvert; foil, frustrate, nonplus, thwart. • *adj* disproved, exposed, overthrown; bothered, confused, disconcerted, flustered, mixed-up, perturbed; shocked, startled, unsettled; beaten, defeated, overcome, overpowered, overthrown; discomfited, distressed, discomposed, overexcited, overwrought, shaken, troubled, unnerved. • *n* confutation, refutation; foiling, frustration, overthrow, revolution, revulsion, ruin, subversion, thwarting.

upshot *n* conclusion, consummation, effect, end, event, issue, outcome, result, termination.

upside down *adj* bottom side up, bottom up, confused, head over heels, inverted, topsy-turvy.

upstart *n* adventurer, arriviste, parvenu, snob, social climber, yuppie.

upturned *adj* raised, uplifted; retroussé.

upward *adj* ascending, climbing, mounting, rising, uphill. • *adv* above, aloft, overhead, up; heavenwards, skywards.

urbane *adj* civil, complaisant, courteous, courtly, elegant, mannerly, polished, polite, refined, smooth, suave, well-mannered.

urbanity *n* amenity, civility, complaisance, courtesy, politeness, smoothness, suavity.

urchin *n* brat, child, kid, ragamuffin, rascal, scrap, squirt, tad.

urge *vb* crowd, drive, force on, impel, press, press on, push, push on; beg, beseech, conjure, entreat, exhort, implore, importune, ply, solicit, tease; animate, egg on, encourage, goad, hurry, incite, instigate, quicken, spur, stimulate. • *n* compulsion, desire, drive, impulse, longing, pressure, wish, yearning.

urgency *n* drive, emergency, exigency, haste, necessity, press, pressure, push, stress; clamorousness, entreaty, insistence, importunity, instance, solicitation; goad, incitement, spur, stimulus.

urgent *adj* cogent, critical, crucial, crying, exigent, immediate, imperative, important, importunate, insistent, instant, pertinacious, pressing, serious.

urinal *n* chamber, chamber pot, lavatory, pot, potty, jordan, toilet.

urinate *vb* make water, pee, pee-pee, piddle, piss, stale, wee.

usage *n* treatment; consuetude, custom, fashion, habit, method, mode, practice, prescription, tradition, use.

use *vb* administer, apply, avail oneself of, drive, employ, handle, improve, make use of, manipulate, occupy, operate, ply, put into action, take advantage of, turn to account, wield, work; exercise, exert, exploit, practice, profit by, utilize; absorb, consume, exhaust, expend, swallow up, waste, wear out; accustom, familiarize, habituate, harden, inure, train; act toward, behave toward, deal with, manage, treat; be accustomed, be wont. • *n* appliance, application, consumption, conversion, disposal, exercise, employ, employment, practice, utilization; adaptability, advantage, avail, benefit, convenience, profit, service, usefulness, utility, wear; exigency, necessity, indispensability, need, occasion, requisiteness; custom, habit, handling, method, treatment, usage, way.

useful *adj* active, advantageous, available, availing, beneficial, commodious, conducive, contributory, convenient, effective, good, helpful, instrumental, operative, practical, profitable, remunerative, salutary, suitable, serviceable, utilitarian; available, helpful, serviceable, valuable.

usefulness *n* advantage, profit, serviceableness, utility, value.

useless *adj* abortive, bootless, fruitless, futile, helpless, idle, incapable, incompetent, ineffective, ineffectual, inutile, nugatory, null, profitless, unavailing, unprofitable, unproductive, unserviceable, valueless, worthless; good for nothing, waste.

usher *vb* announce, forerun, herald, induct, introduce, precede; conduct, direct, escort, shepherd, show. • *n* attendant, conductor, escort, shepherd, squire.

usual *adj* accustomed, common, customary, everyday, familiar, frequent, general, habitual, normal, ordinary, prevailing, prevalent, regular, wonted.

usurp *vb* appropriate, arrogate, assume, seize.

usurpation *n* assumption, dispossession, infringement, seizure.

usury *n* interest; exploitation, extortion, profiteering.

utensil *n* device, implement, instrument, tool.

utility *n* advantageousness, avail, benefit, profit, service, use, usefulness; happiness; welfare.

utilize *vb* employ, exploit, make use of, put to use, turn to account, use.

utmost *adj* extreme, farthest, highest, last, main, most distant, remotest; greatest, uttermost. • *n* best, extreme, maximum, most.

Utopian *adj* air-built, air-drawn, chimerical, fanciful, ideal, imaginary, visionary, unreal.

utricle *n* bladder, cyst, sac, vesicle.

utter[1] *adj* complete, entire, perfect, total; absolute, blank, diametric, downright, final, peremptory, sheer, stark, thorough, thoroughgoing, unconditional, unqualified, total.

utter[2] *vb* articulate, breathe, deliver, disclose, divulge, emit, enunciate, express, give forth, pronounce, reveal, speak, talk, tell, voice; announce, circulate, declare, issue, publish.

utterance *n* articulation, delivery, disclosure, emission, expression, pronouncement, pronunciation, publication, speech.

utterly *adv* absolutely, altogether, completely, downright, entirely, quite, totally, unconditionally, wholly.

uttermost *adj* extreme, farthest; greatest, utmost.

V

vacant *adj* blank, empty, unfilled, void; disengaged, free, unemployed, unoccupied, unencumbered; thoughtless, unmeaning, unthinking, unreflective; uninhabited, untenanted.

vacate *vb* abandon, evacuate, relinquish, surrender; abolish, abrogate, annul, cancel, disannul, invalidate, nullify, overrule, quash, rescind.

vacillate *vb* dither, fluctuate, hesitate, oscillate, rock, sway, waver.

vacillation *n* faltering, fluctuation, hesitation, inconstancy, indecision, irresolution, reeling, rocking, staggering, swaying, unsteadiness, wavering.

vacuity *n* emptiness, inanition, vacancy; emptiness, vacancy, vacuum, void; expressionlessness, inanity, nihility.

vacuous *adj* empty, empty-headed, unfilled, vacant, void; inane, unintelligent.

vacuum *n* emptiness, vacuity, void.

vagabond *adj* footloose, idle, meandering, rambling, roving, roaming, strolling, vagrant, wandering. • *n* beggar, castaway, landloper, loafer, lounger, nomad, outcast, tramp, vagrant, wanderer.

vagary *n* caprice, crotchet, fancy, freak, humour, whim.

vagrant *adj* erratic, itinerant, roaming, roving, nomadic, strolling, unsettled, wandering. • *n* beggar, castaway, landloper, loafer, lounger, nomad, outcast, tramp, vagabond, wanderer.

vague *adj* ambiguous, confused, dim, doubtful, indefinite, ill-defined, indistinct, lax, loose, obscure, uncertain, undetermined, unfixed, unsettled.

vain *adj* baseless, delusive, dreamy, empty, false, imaginary, shadowy, suppositional, unsubstantial, unreal, void; abortive, bootless, fruitless, futile, ineffectual, nugatory, profitless, unavailing, unprofitable, trivial, unessential, unimportant, unsatisfactory, unsatisfying, useless, vapid, worthless; arrogant, conceited, egotistical, flushed, high, inflated, opinionated, ostentatious, overweening, proud, self-confident, self-opinionated, vainglorious; gaudy, glittering, gorgeous, showy.

valediction *n* adieu, farewell, goodbye, leave-taking.

valet *n* attendant, flunky, groom, lackey, servant.

valetudinarian *adj* delicate, feeble, frail, infirm, sickly.

valiant *adj* bold, brave, chivalrous, courageous, daring, dauntless, doughty, fearless, gallant, heroic, intrepid, lion-hearted, redoubtable, Spartan, valorous, undaunted.

valid *adj* binding, cogent, conclusive, efficacious, efficient, good, grave, important, just, logical, powerful, solid, sound, strong, substantial, sufficient, weighty.

valley *n* basin, bottom, canyon, dale, dell, dingle, glen, hollow, ravine, strath, vale.

valorous *adj* bold, brave, courageous, dauntless, doughty, intrepid, stout.

valour *n* boldness, bravery, courage, daring, gallantry, heroism, prowess, spirit.

valuable *adj* advantageous, precious, profitable, useful; costly, expensive, rich; admirable, estimable, worthy. • *n* heirloom, treasure.

value *vb* account, appraise, assess, estimate, price, rate, reckon; appreciate, esteem, prize, regard, treasure. • *n* avail, importance, usefulness, utility, worth; cost, equivalent, price, rate; estimation, excellence, importance, merit, valuation.

valueless *adj* miserable, useless, worthless.

vandal *n* barbarian, destroyer, savage.

vandalism *n* barbarism, barbarity, savagery.

vanish *vb* disappear, dissolve, fade, melt.

vanity *n* emptiness, falsity, foolishness, futility, hollowness, insanity, triviality, unreality, worthlessness; arrogance, conceit, egotism, ostentation, self-conceit.

vanquish *vb* conquer, defeat, outwit, overcome, overpower, overthrow, subdue, subjugate; crush, discomfit, foil, master, quell, rout, worst.

vapid *adj* dead, flat, insipid, lifeless, savourless, spiritless, stale, tasteless; dull, feeble, jejune, languid, meagre, prosaic, prosy, tame.

vapour *n* cloud, exhalation, fog, fume, mist, rack, reek, smoke, steam; daydream, dream, fantasy, phantom, vagary, vision, whim, whimsy.

variable *adj* changeable, mutable, shifting; aberrant, alterable, capricious, fickle, fitful, floating, fluctuating, inconstant, mobile, mutable, protean, restless, shifting, unsteady, vacillating, wavering.

variance *n* disagreement, difference, discord, dissension, incompatibility, jarring, strife.

variation *n* alteration, change, modification; departure, deviation, difference, discrepancy, innovation; contrariety, discordance.

variegated *adj* chequered, dappled, diversified, flecked, kaleidoscopic, mottled, multicoloured, pied, spotted, striped.

variety *n* difference, dissimilarity, diversity, diversification, medley, miscellany, mixture, multiplicity, variation; kind, sort.

various *adj* different, diverse, manifold, many, numerous, several, sundry.

varnish *vb* enamel, glaze, japan, lacquer; adorn, decorate, embellish, garnish, gild, polish; disguise, excuse, extenuate, gloss over, palliate. • *n* enamel, lacquer, stain; cover, extenuation, gloss.

vary *vb* alter, metamorphose, transform; alternate, exchange, rotate; diversify, modify, variegate; depart, deviate, swerve.

vassal *n* bondman, liegeman, retainer, serf, slave, subject, thrall.

vassalage *n* bondage, dependence, serfdom, servitude, slavery, subjection.

vast *adj* boundless, infinite, measureless, spacious, wide; colossal, enormous, gigantic, huge, immense, mighty, monstrous, prodigious, tremendous; extraordinary, remarkable.

vaticination *n* augury, divination, prediction, prognostication, prophecy.

vault¹ *vb* arch, bend, curve, span. • *n* cupola, curve, dome; catacomb, cell, cellar, crypt, dungeon, tomb; depository, strongroom.

vault² *vb* bound, jump, leap, spring; tumble, turn. • *n* bound, leap, jump, spring.

vaunt *vb* advertise, boast, brag, display, exult, flaunt, flourish, parade.

veer *vi* change, shift, turn.

vegetate *vb* blossom, develop, flourish, flower, germinate, grow, shoot, sprout, swell; bask, hibernate, idle, stagnate.

vehemence *n* impetuosity, violence; ardour, eagerness, earnestness, enthusiasm, fervency, fervour, heat, keenness, passion, warmth, zeal; force, intensity.

vehement *adj* furious, high, hot, impetuous, passionate, rampant, violent; ardent, burning, eager, earnest, enthusiastic, fervid, fiery, keen, passionate, sanguine, zealous; forcible, mighty, powerful, strong.

veil *vb* cloak, conceal, cover, curtain, envelop, hide, invest, mask, screen, shroud. • *n* cover, curtain, film, shade, screen; blind, cloak, disguise, mask, muffler, visor.

vein *n* course, current, lode, seam, streak, stripe, thread, wave; bent, character, faculty, humour, mood, talent, turn.

velocity *n* acceleration, celerity, expedition, fleetness, haste, quickness, rapidity, speed, swiftness.

velvety *adj* delicate, downy, smooth, soft.

venal *adj* corrupt, mean, purchasable, sordid.

vend *vb* dispose, flog, hawk, retail, sell.

venerable *adj* grave, respected, revered, sage, wise; awful, dread, dreadful; aged, old, patriarchal.

venerate *vb* adore, esteem, honour, respect, revere.

veneration *n* adoration, devotion, esteem, respect, reverence, worship.

vengeance *n* retaliation, retribution, revenge.

venial *adj* allowed, excusable, pardonable, permitted, trivial.

venom *n* poison, virus; acerbity, acrimony, bitterness, gall, hate, ill-will, malevolence, malice, maliciousness, malignity, rancour, spite, virulence.

venomous *adj* deadly, poisonous, septic, toxic, virulent; caustic, malicious, malignant, mischievous, noxious, spiteful.

vent *vb* emit, express, release, utter. • *n* air hole, hole, mouth, opening, orifice; air pipe, air tube, aperture, blowhole, bung-hole, hydrant, plug, spiracle, spout, tap, orifice; effusion, emission, escape, outlet, passage; discharge, expression, utterance.

ventilate *vb* aerate, air, freshen, oxygenate, purify; fan, winnow; canvass, comment, discuss, examine, publish, review, scrutinize.

venture *vb* adventure, dare, hazard, imperil, jeopardize, presume, risk, speculate, test, try, undertake. • *n* adventure, chance, hazard, jeopardy, peril, risk, speculation, stake.

venturesome *adj* adventurous, bold, courageous, daring, doughty, enterprising, fearless, foolhardy, intrepid, presumptuous, rash, venturous.

veracious *adj* reliable, straightforward, true, trustworthy, truthful; credible, genuine, honest, unfeigned.

veracity *n* accuracy, candour, correctness, credibility, exactness, fidelity, frankness, honesty, ingenuousness, probity, sincerity, trueness, truth, truthfulness.

verbal *adj* nuncupative, oral, spoken, unwritten.

verbose *adj* diffusive, long-winded, loquacious, talkative, wordy.

verdant *adj* fresh, green, verdure, verdurous; green, inexperienced, raw, unsophisticated.

verdict *n* answer, decision, finding, judgement, opinion, sentence.

verge *vb* bear, incline, lean, slope, tend; approach, border, skirt. • *n* mace, rod, staff; border, boundary, brink, confine, edge, extreme, limit, margin; edge, eve, point.

verification *n* authentication, attestation, confirmation, corroboration.

verify *vb* attest, authenticate, confirm, corroborate, prove, substantiate.

verily *adv* absolutely, actually, confidently, indeed, positively, really, truly.

verity *n* certainty, reality, truth, truthfulness.

vermicular *adj* convoluted, flexuose, flexuous, meandering, serpentine, sinuous, tortuous, twisting, undulating, waving, winding, wormish, wormlike.

vernacular *adj* common, indigenous, local, mother, native, vulgar. • *n* cant, dialect, jargon, patois, speech.

versatile *adj* capricious, changeable, erratic, mobile, variable; fickle, inconstant, mercurial, unsteady; adaptable, protean, plastic, varied.

versed *adj* able, accomplished, acquainted, clever, conversant, practised, proficient, qualified, skilful, skilled, trained.

version *n* interpretation, reading, rendering, translation.

vertex *n* apex, crown, height, summit, top, zenith.

vertical *adj* erect, perpendicular, plumb, steep, upright.

vertiginous *adj* rotatory, rotary, whirling; dizzy, giddy.

vertigo *n* dizziness, giddiness.

verve *n* animation, ardour, energy, enthusiasm, force, rapture, spirit.

very *adv* absolutely, enormously, excessively, hugely, remarkably, surpassingly. • *adj* actual, exact, identical, precise, same; bare, mere, plain, pure, simple.

vesicle *n* bladder, blister, cell, cyst, follicle.

vest *vb* clothe, cover, dress, envelop; endow, furnish, invest. • *n* dress, garment, robe, vestment, vesture, waistcoat.

vestibule *n* anteroom, entrance hall, lobby, porch.

vestige *n* evidence, footprint, footstep, mark, record, relic, sign, token.

veteran *adj* adept, aged, experienced, disciplined, seasoned, old. • *n* campaigner, old soldier; master, past master, old-timer, old-stager.

veto *vb* ban, embargo, forbid, interdict, negate, prohibit. • *n* ban, embargo, interdict, prohibition, refusal.

vex *vb* annoy, badger, bother, chafe, cross, distress, gall, harass, harry, hector, molest, perplex, pester, plague, tease, torment, trouble, roil, spite, worry; affront, displease, fret, irk, irritate, nettle, offend, provoke; agitate, disquiet, disturb.

vexation *n* affliction, agitation, chagrin, discomfort, displeasure, disquiet, distress, grief, irritation, pique, sorrow, trouble; annoyance, curse, nuisance, plague, torment; damage, troubling, vexing.

vexed *adj* afflicted, agitated, annoyed, bothered, disquieted, harassed, irritated, perplexed, plagued, provoked, troubled, worried.

vibrate *vb* oscillate, sway, swing, undulate, wave; impinge, quiver, sound, thrill; fluctuate, hesitate, vacillate, waver.

vibration *n* nutation, oscillation, vibration.

vicarious *adj* commissioned, delegated, indirect, second-hand, substituted.

vice *n* blemish, defect, failing, fault, imperfection, infirmity; badness, corruption, depravation, depravity, error, evil, immorality, iniquity, laxity, obliquity, sin, viciousness, vileness, wickedness.

vicinity *n* nearness, proximity; locality, neighbourhood, vicinage.

vicious *adj* abandoned, atrocious, bad, corrupt, degenerate, demoralized, depraved, devilish, diabolical, evil, flagrant, hellish, immoral, iniquitous, mischievous, profligate, shameless, sinful, unprincipled, wicked; malicious, spiteful, venomous; foul, impure; debased, faulty; contrary, refractory.

viciousness *n* badness, corruption, depravity, immorality, profligacy.

vicissitude *n* alteration, interchange; change, fluctuation, mutation, revolution, variation.

victim *n* martyr, sacrifice, sufferer; prey; cat's-paw, cull, cully, dupe, gull, gudgeon, puppet.

victimize *vb* bamboozle, befool, beguile, cheat, circumvent, cozen, deceive, defraud, diddle, dupe, fool, gull, hoax, hoodwink, overreach, swindle, trick.

victor *n* champion, conqueror, vanquisher, winner.

victorious *adj* conquering, successful, triumphant, winning.

victory *n* achievement, conquest, mastery, triumph.

victuals *npl* comestibles, eatables, fare, food, meat, provisions, repast, sustenance, viands.

vie *vb* compete, contend, emulate, rival, strive.

view *vb* behold, contemplate, eye, inspect, scan, survey; consider, inspect, regard, study. • *n* inspection, observation, regard, sight; outlook, panorama, perspective, prospect, range, scene, survey, vista; aim, intent, intention, design, drift, object, purpose, scope; belief, conception, impression, idea, judgement, notion, opinion, sentiment, theory; appearance, aspect, show.

vigilance *n* alertness, attentiveness, carefulness, caution, circumspection, observance, watchfulness.

vigilant *adj* alert, attentive, careless, cautious, circumspect, unsleeping, wakeful, watchful.

vigorous *adj* lusty, powerful, strong; active, alert, cordial, energetic, forcible, strenuous, vehement, vivid, virile; brisk, hale, hardy, robust, sound, sturdy, healthy; fresh, flourishing; bold, emphatic, impassioned, lively, nervous, piquant, pointed, severe, sparkling, spirited, trenchant.

vigour *n* activity, efficacy, energy, force, might, potency, power, spirit, strength; bloom, elasticity, haleness, health, heartiness, pep, punch, robustness, soundness, thriftiness, tone, vim, vitality; enthusiasm, freshness, fire, intensity, liveliness, piquancy, strenuousness, vehemence, verve, raciness.

vile *adj* abject, base, beastly, beggarly, brutish, contemptible, despicable, disgusting, grovelling, ignoble, low, odious, paltry, pitiful, repulsive, scurvy, shabby, slavish, sorry, ugly; bad, evil, foul, gross, impure, iniquitous, lewd, obscene, sinful, vicious, wicked; cheap, mean, miserable, valueless, worthless.

vilify *vb* abuse, asperse, backbite, berate, blacken, blemish, brand, calumniate, decry, defame, disparage, lampoon, libel, malign, revile, scandalize, slander, slur, traduce, vituperate.

villain *n* blackguard, knave, miscreant, rascal, reprobate, rogue, ruffian, scamp, scapegrace, scoundrel.

villainous *adj* base, mean, vile; corrupt, depraved, knavish, unprincipled, wicked; atrocious, heinous, outrageous, sinful; mischievous, sorry.

vindicate *vb* defend, justify, uphold; advocate, avenge, assert, maintain, right, support.

vindication *n* apology, excuse, defence, justification.

vindictive *adj* avenging, grudgeful, implacable, malevolent, malicious, malignant, retaliative, revengeful, spiteful, unforgiving, unrelenting, vengeful.

violate *vb* hurt, injure; break, disobey, infringe, invade; desecrate, pollute, profane; abuse, debauch, defile, deflower, outrage, ravish, transgress.

violent *adj* boisterous, demented, forceful, forcible, frenzied, furious, high, hot, impetuous, insane, intense, stormy, tumultuous, turbulent, vehement, wild; fierce, fiery, fuming, heady, heavy, infuriate, passionate, obstreperous, strong, raging, rampant, rank, rapid, raving, refractory, roaring, rough, tearing, towering, ungovernable; accidental, unnatural; desperate, extreme, outrageous, unjust; acute, exquisite, poignant, sharp.

virago *n* amazon, brawler, fury, shrew, tartar, vixen.

virgin *adj* chaste, maidenly, modest, pure, undefiled, stainless, unpolluted, vestal, virginal; fresh, maiden, untouched, unused. • *n* celibate, damsel, girl, lass, maid, maiden.

virile *adj* forceful, manly, masculine, robust, vigorous.

virtual *adj* constructive, equivalent, essential, implicit, implied, indirect, practical, substantial.

virtue *n* chastity, goodness, grace, morality, purity; efficacy, excellence, honesty, integrity, justice, probity, quality, rectitude, worth.

virtuous *adj* blameless, equitable, exemplary, excellent, good, honest, moral, noble, righteous, upright, worthy; chaste, continent, immaculate, innocent, modest, pure, undefiled; efficacious, powerful.

virulent *adj* deadly, malignant, poisonous, toxic, venomous; acrid, acrimonious, bitter, caustic.

visage *n* aspect, countenance, face, guise, physiognomy, semblance.

viscera *n* bowels, entrails, guts, intestines.

viscous *adj* adhesive, clammy, glutinous, ropy, slimy, sticky, tenacious.

visible *adj* observable, perceivable, perceptible, seeable, visual; apparent, clear, conspicuous, discoverable, distinct, evident, manifest, noticeable, obvious, open, palpable, patent, plain, revealed, unhidden, unmistakable.

vision *n* eyesight, seeing, sight; eyeshot, ken; apparition, chimera, dream, ghost, hallucination, illusion, phantom, spectre.

visionary *adj* imaginative, impractical, quixotic, romantic; chimerical, dreamy, fancied, fanciful, fantastic, ideal, illusory, imaginary, romantic, shadowy, unsubstantial, utopian, wild. • *n* dreamer, enthusiast, fanatic, idealist, optimist, theorist, zealot.

vital *adj* basic, cardinal, essential, indispensable, necessary, needful; animate, alive, existing, life-giving, living; paramount.

vitality *n* animation, life, strength, vigour, virility.

vitiate *vb* adulterate, contaminate, corrupt, debase, defile, degrade, deprave, deteriorate, impair, infect, injure, invalidate, poison, pollute, spoil.

vitiation *n* adulteration, corruption, degeneracy, degeneration, degradation, depravation, deterioration, impairment, injury, invalidation, perversion, pollution, prostitution.

vituperate *vb* abuse, berate, blame, censure, denounce, overwhelm, rate, revile, scold, upbraid, vilify.

vituperation *n* abuse, blame, censure, invective, reproach, railing, reviling, scolding, upbraiding.

vivacious *adj* active, animated, breezy, brisk, buxom, cheerful, frolicsome, gay, jocund, light-hearted, lively, merry, mirthful, spirited, sportive, sprightly.

vivacity *n* animation, cheer, cheerfulness, gaiety, liveliness, sprightliness.

vivid *adj* active, animated, bright, brilliant, clear, intense, fresh, lively, living, lucid, quick, sprightly, strong; expressive, graphic, striking, telling.

vivify *vb* animate, arouse, awake, quicken, vitalize.

vixen *n* brawler, scold, shrew, spitfire, tartar, virago.

vocabulary *n* dictionary, glossary, lexicon, wordbook; language, terms, words.

vocation *n* call, citation, injunction, summons; business, calling, employment, occupation, profession, pursuit, trade.

vociferate *vb* bawl, bellow, clamour, cry, exclaim, rant, shout, yell.

vociferous *adj* blatant, clamorous, loud, noisy, obstreperous, ranting, stunning, uproarious.

vogue *adj* fashionable, modish, stylish, trendy. • *n* custom, fashion, favour, mode, practice, repute, style, usage, way.

voice *vb* declare, express, say, utter. • *n* speech, tongue, utterance; noise, notes, sound; opinion, option, preference, suffrage, vote; accent, articulation, enunciation, inflection, intonation, modulation, pronunciation, tone; expression, language, words.

void *vb* clear, eject, emit, empty, evacuate. • *adj* blank, empty, hollow, vacant; clear, destitute, devoid, free, lacking, wanting, without; inept, ineffectual, invalid, nugatory, null; imaginary, unreal, vain. • *n* abyss, blank, chasm, emptiness, hole, vacuum.

volatile *adj* gaseous, incoercible; airy, buoyant, frivolous, gay, jolly, lively, sprightly, vivacious; capricious, changeable, fickle, flighty, flyaway, giddy, harebrained, inconstant, light-headed, mercurial, reckless, unsteady, whimsical, wild.

volition *n* choice, determination, discretion, option, preference, will.

volley *n* fusillade, round, salvo; blast, burst, discharge, emission, explosion, outbreak, report, shower, storm.

voluble *adj* fluent, garrulous, glib, loquacious, talkative.

volume *n* book, tome; amplitude, body, bulk, compass, dimension, size, substance, vastness; fullness, power, quantity.

voluminous *adj* ample, big, bulky, full, great, large; copious, diffuse, discursive, flowing.

voluntary *adj* free, spontaneous, unasked, unbidden, unforced; deliberate, designed, intended, purposed; discretionary, optional, willing.

volunteer *vb* offer, present, proffer, propose, tender.

voluptuary *n* epicure, hedonist, sensualist.

voluptuous *adj* carnal, effeminate, epicurean, fleshy, licentious, luxurious, sensual, sybaritic.

vomit *vb* discharge, eject, emit, puke, regurgitate, spew, throw up.

voracious *adj* devouring, edacious, greedy, hungry, rapacious, ravenous.

vortex *n* eddy, maelstrom, whirl, whirlpool.

votary *adj* devoted, promised. • *n* adherent, devotee, enthusiast, follower, supporter, votarist, zealot.

vote *vb* ballot, elect, opt, return; judge, pronounce, propose, suggest. • *n* ballot, franchise, poll, referendum, suffrage, voice.

vouch *vb* affirm, asseverate, attest, aver, declare, guarantee, support, uphold, verify, warrant.

vouchsafe *vb* accord, cede, deign, grant, stoop, yield.

vow *vb* consecrate, dedicate, devote; asseverate. • *n* oath, pledge, promise.

voyage *vb* cruise, journey, navigate, ply, sail. • *n* crossing, cruise, excursion, journey, passage, sail, trip.

vulgar *adj* base-born, common, ignoble, lowly, plebeian; boorish, cheap, coarse, discourteous, flashy, homespun, garish, gaudy, ill-bred, inelegant, loud, rustic, showy, tawdry, uncultivated, unrefined; general, ordinary, popular, public; base, broad, loose, low, gross, mean, ribald, vile; inelegant, unauthorized.

vulgarity *n* baseness, coarseness, grossness, meanness, rudeness.

vulnerable *adj* accessible, assailable, defenceless, exposed, weak.

W

waddle *vb* toddle, toggle, waggle, wiggle, wobble.

waft *vb* bear, carry, convey, float, transmit, transport. • *n* breath, breeze, draught, puff.

wag[1] *vb* shake, sway, waggle; oscillate, vibrate, waver; advance, move, progress, stir. • *n* flutter, nod, oscillation, vibration.

wag[2] *n* humorist, jester, joker, wit.

wage *vb* bet, hazard, lay, stake, wager; conduct, undertake.

wager *vb* back, bet, gamble, lay, pledge, risk, stake. • *n* bet, gamble, pledge, risk, stake.

wages *npl* allowance, compensation, earnings, emolument, hire, pay, payment, remuneration, salary, stipend.

waggish *adj* frolicsome, gamesome, mischievous, roguish, tricksy; comical, droll, facetious, funny, humorous, jocular, jocose, merry, sportive.

wagon *n* cart, lorry, truck, van, waggon, wain.

wail *vb* bemoan, deplore, lament, mourn; cry, howl, weep. • *n* complaint, cry, lamentation, moan, wailing.

waist *n* bodice, corsage, waistline.

wait *vb* delay, linger, pause, remain, rest, stay, tarry; attend, minister, serve; abide, await, expect, look for. • *n* delay, halt, holdup, pause, respite, rest, stay, stop.

waiter, waitress *n* attendant, lackey, servant, servitor, steward, valet.

waive *vb* defer, forgo, surrender, relinquish, remit, renounce; desert, reject.

wake[1] *vb* arise, awake, awaken; activate, animate, arouse, awaken, excite, kindle, provoke, stimulate. • *n* vigil, watch, watching.

wake[2] *n* course, path, rear, track, trail, wash.

wakeful *adj* awake, sleepless, restless; alert, observant, vigilant, wary, watchful.

wale *n* ridge, streak, stripe, welt, whelk.

walk *vb* advance, depart, go, march, move, pace, saunter, step, stride, stroll, tramp. • *n* amble, carriage, gait, step; beat, career, course, department, field, province; conduct, procedure; alley, avenue, cloister, esplanade, footpath, path, pathway, pavement, promenade, range, sidewalk, way; constitutional, excursion, hike, ramble, saunter, stroll, tramp, turn.

wall *n* escarp, parapet, plane, upright.

wallet *n* bag, knapsack, pocketbook, purse, sack.

wan *adj* ashen, bloodless, cadaverous, colourless, haggard, pale, pallid.

wand *n* baton, mace, truncheon, sceptre.

wander *vb* forage, prowl, ramble, range, roam, rove, stroll; deviate, digress, straggle, stray; moon, rave. • *n* amble, cruise, excursion, ramble, stroll.

wane *vb* abate, decrease, ebb, subside; decline, fail, sink. • *n* decrease, diminution, lessening; decay, declension, decline, failure.

want *vb* crave, desire, need, require, wish; fail, lack, neglect, omit. • *n* absence, defect, default, deficiency, lack; defectiveness, failure, inadequacy, insufficiency, meagreness, paucity, poverty, scantiness, scarcity, shortness, requirement; craving, desire, longing, wish; destitution, distress, indigence, necessity, need, penury, poverty, privation, straits.

wanton *vb* caper, disport, frisk, frolic, play, revel, romp, sport; dally, flirt, toy, trifle. • *adj* free, loose, unchecked, unrestrained, wandering; abounding, exuberant, luxuriant, overgrown, rampant; airy, capricious, coltish, frisky, playful, skittish, sportive; dissolute, irregular, licentious, loose; carnal, immoral, incontinent, lascivious, lecherous, lewd, libidinous, light, lustful, prurient, salacious, unchaste; careless, gratuitous, groundless, heedless, inconsiderate, needless, perverse, reckless, wayward, wilful. • *n* baggage, flirt, harlot, light-o'-love, prostitute, rake, roué, slut, whore.

war *vb* battle, campaign, combat, contend, crusade, engage, fight, strive. • *n* contention, enmity, hostility, strife, warfare.

warble *vb* sing, trill, yodel. • *n* carol, chant, hymn, hum.

ward *vb* guard, watch; defend, fend, parry, protect, repel. • *n* care, charge, guard, guardianship, watch; defender, guardian,

keeper, protector, warden; custody; defence, garrison, protection; minor, pupil; district, division, precinct, quarter; apartment, cubicle.

warehouse *n* depot, magazine, repository, store, storehouse.

wares *npl* commodities, goods, merchandise, movables.

warfare *n* battle, conflict, contest, discord, engagement, fray, hostilities, strife, struggle, war.

warily *adv* carefully, cautiously, charily, circumspectly, heedfully, watchfully, vigilantly.

wariness *n* care, caution, circumspection, foresight, thought, vigilance.

warlike *adj* bellicose, belligerent, combative, hostile, inimical, martial, military, soldierly, watchful.

warm *vb* heat, roast, toast; animate, chafe, excite, rouse. • *adj* lukewarm, tepid; genial, mild, pleasant, sunny; close, muggy, oppressive; affectionate, ardent, cordial, eager, earnest, enthusiastic, fervent, fervid, glowing, hearty, hot, zealous; excited, fiery, flushed, furious, hasty, keen, lively, passionate, quick, vehement, violent.

warmth *n* glow, tepidity; ardour, fervency, fervour, zeal; animation, cordiality, eagerness, earnestness, enthusiasm, excitement, fervency, fever, fire, flush, heat, intensity, passion, spirit, vehemence.

warn *vb* caution, forewarn; admonish, advise; apprise, inform, notify; bid, call, summon.

warning *adj* admonitory, cautionary, cautioning, monitory. • *n* admonition, advice, caveat, caution, monition; information, notice; augury, indication, intimation, omen, portent, presage, prognostic, sign, symptom; call, summons; example, lesson, sample.

warp *vb* bend, bias, contort, deviate, distort, pervert, swerve, turn, twist. • *n* bent, bias, cast, crook, distortion, inclination, leaning, quirk, sheer, skew, slant, slew, swerve, twist, turn.

warrant *vb* answer for, certify, guarantee, secure; affirm, assure, attest, avouch, declare, justify, state; authorize, justify, license, maintain, sanction, support, sustain, uphold. • *n* guarantee, pledge, security, surety, warranty; authentication, authority, commission, verification; order, pass, permit, summons, subpoena, voucher, writ.

warrantable *adj* admissible, allowable, defensible, justifiable, lawful, permissible, proper, right, vindicable.

warrior *n* champion, captain, fighter, hero, soldier.

wary *adj* careful, cautious, chary, circumspect, discreet, guarded, heedful, prudent, scrupulous, vigilant, watchful.

wash *vb* purify, purge; moisten, wet; bathe, clean, flush, irrigate, lap, lave, rinse, sluice; colour, stain, tint. • *n* ablution, bathing, cleansing, lavation, washing; bog, fen, marsh, swamp, quagmire; bath, embrocation, lotion; laundry, washing.

washy *adj* damp, diluted, moist, oozy, sloppy, thin, watery, weak; feeble, jejune, pointless, poor, spiritless, trashy, trumpery, unmeaning, vapid, worthless.

waspish *adj* choleric, fretful, irascible, irritable, peevish, petulant, snappish, testy, touchy; slender, slim, small-waisted.

waste *vb* consume, corrode, decrease, diminish, emaciate, wear; absorb, deplete, devour, dissipate, drain, empty, exhaust, expend, lavish, lose, misspend, misuse, scatter, spend, squander; demolish, desolate, destroy, devastate, devour, dilapidate, harry, pillage, plunder, ravage, ruin, scour, strip; damage, impair, injure; decay, dwindle, perish, wither. • *adj* bare, desolated, destroyed, devastated, empty, ravaged, ruined, spoiled, stripped, void; dismal, dreary, forlorn; abandoned, bare, barren, uncultivated, unimproved, uninhabited, untilled, wild; useless, valueless, worthless; exuberant, superfluous. • *n* consumption, decrement, diminution, dissipation, exhaustion, expenditure, loss, wasting; destruction, dispersion, extravagance, loss, squandering, wanton; decay, desolation, destruction, devastation, havoc, pillage, ravage, ruin; chaff, debris, detritus, dross, excrement, husks, junk, matter, offal, refuse, rubbish, trash, wastrel, worthlessness; barrenness, desert, expanse, solitude, wild, wilderness.

wasteful *adj* destructive, ruinous; extravagant, improvident, lavish, prodigal, profuse, squandering, thriftless, unthrifty.

watch *vb* attend, guard, keep, oversee, protect, superintend, tend; eye, mark, observe. • *n* espial, guard, outlook, wakefulness, watchfulness, watching, vigil, ward; alertness, attention, inspection, observation, surveillance; guard, picket, sentinel, sentry, watchman; pocket watch, ticker, timepiece, wristwatch.

watchful *adj* alert, attentive, awake, careful, circumspect, guarded, heedful, observant, vigilant, wakeful, wary.

watchword *n* catchword, cry, motto, password, shibboleth, word.

waterfall *n* cascade, cataract, fall, linn.

watery *adj* diluted, thin, waterish, weak; insipid, spiritless, tasteful, vapid; moist, wet.

wave *vb* float, flutter, heave, shake, sway, undulate, wallow; brandish, flaunt, flourish, swing; beckon, signal. • *n* billow, bore, breaker, flood, flush, ripple, roll, surge, swell, tide, undulation; flourish, gesture, sway; convolution, curl, roll, unevenness.

waver *vb* flicker, float, undulate, wave; reel, totter; falter, fluctuate, flutter, hesitate, oscillate, quiver, vacillate.

wax *vb* become, grow, increase, mount, rise.

way *n* advance, journey, march, progression, transit, trend; access, alley, artery, avenue, beat, channel, course, highroad, highway, passage, path, road, route, street, track, trail; fashion, manner, means, method, mode, system; distance, interval, space, stretch; behaviour, custom, form, guise, habit, habitude, practice, process, style, usage; device, plan, scheme.

wayfarer *n* itinerant, nomad, passenger, pilgrim, rambler, traveller, walker, wanderer.

wayward *adj* capricious, captious, contrary, forward, headstrong, intractable, obstinate, perverse, refractory, stubborn, unruly, wilful.

weak *adj* debilitated, delicate, enfeebled, enervated, exhausted, faint, feeble, fragile, frail, infirm, invalid, languid, languishing, shaky, sickly, spent, strengthless, tender, unhealthy, unsound, wasted, weakly; accessible, defenceless, unprotected, vulnerable; light, soft, unstressed; boneless, cowardly, infirm; compliant, irresolute, pliable, pliant, undecided, undetermined, unsettled, unstable, unsteady, vacillating, wavering, yielding; childish, foolish, imbecile, senseless, shallow, silly, simple, stupid, weak-minded, witless; erring, foolish, indiscreet, injudicious, unwise; gentle, indistinct, low, small; adulterated, attenuated, diluted, insipid, tasteless, thin, watery; flimsy, frivolous, poor, sleazy, slight, trifling; futile, illogical, inconclusive, ineffective, ineffectual, inefficient, lame, unconvincing, unsatisfactory, unsupported, unsustained, vague, vain; unsafe, unsound, unsubstantial, untrustworthy; helpless, impotent, powerless; breakable, brittle, delicate, frangible; inconsiderable, puny, slender, slight, small.

weaken *vb* cramp, cripple, debilitate, devitalize, enervate, enfeeble, invalidate, relax, sap, shake, stagger, undermine, unman, unnerve, unstring; adulterate, attenuate, debase, depress, dilute, exhaust, impair, impoverish, lessen, lower, reduce.

weakness *n* debility, feebleness, fragility, frailty, infirmity, languor, softness; defect, failing, fault, flaw; fondness, inclination, liking.

weal *n* advantage, good, happiness, interest, profit, utility, prosperity, welfare; ridge, streak, stripe.

wealth *n* assets, capital, cash, fortune, funds, goods, money, possessions, property, riches, treasure; abundance, affluence, opulence, plenty, profusion.

wean *vb* alienate, detach, disengage, withdraw.

wear *vb* bear, carry, don; endure, last; consume, impair, rub, use, waste. • *n* corrosion, deterioration, disintegration, erosion, wear and tear; consumption, use; apparel, array, attire, clothes, clothing, dress, garb, gear.

wearied *adj* apathetic, bored, exhausted, fagged, fatigued, jaded, tired, weary, worn.

weariness *n* apathy, boredom, ennui, exhaustion, fatigue, languor, lassitude, monotony, prostration, sameness, tedium.

wearisome *adj* annoying, boring, dull, exhausting, fatiguing, humdrum, irksome, monotonous, prolix, prosaic, slow, tedious, tiresome, troublesome, trying, uninteresting, vexatious.

weary *adj* debilitate, exhaust, fag, fatigue, harass, jade, tire. • *adj* apathetic, bored, drowsy, exhausted, jaded, spent, tired worn; irksome, tiresome, wearisome.

weave *vb* braid, entwine, interlace, lace, mat, plait, pleat, twine; compose, construct, fabricate, make.

wed *vb* contract, couple, espouse, marry, unite.

wedding *n* bridal, espousal, marriage, nuptials.

wedlock *n* marriage, matrimony.

ween *vb* fancy, imagine, suppose, think.

weep *vb* bemoan, bewail, complain, cry, lament, sob.

weigh *vb* balance, counterbalance, lift, raise; consider, deliberate, esteem, examine, study.

weight *vb* ballast, burden, fill, freight, load; weigh. • *n* gravity, heaviness, heft, tonnage; burden, load, pressure; consequence, efficacy, emphasis, importance, impressiveness, influence, moment, pith, power, significance, value.

weighty *adj* heavy, massive, onerous, ponderous, unwieldy; considerable, efficacious, forcible, grave, important, influential, serious, significant.

weird *adj* eerie, ghostly, strange, supernatural, uncanny, unearthly, witching.

welcome *vb* embrace, greet, hail, receive. • *adj* acceptable, agreeable, grateful, gratifying, pleasant, pleasing, satisfying. • *n* greeting, reception, salutation.

welfare *n* advantage, affluence, benefit, happiness, profit, prosperity, success, thrift, weal, wellbeing.

well[1] *vb* flow, gush, issue, jet, pour, spring. • *n* fount, fountain, reservoir, spring, wellhead, wellspring; origin, source; hole, pit, shaft.

well[2] *adj* hale, healthy, hearty, sound; fortunate, good, happy, profitable, satisfactory, useful. • *adv* accurately, adequately, correctly, efficiently, properly, suitably; abundantly, considerably, fully, thoroughly; agreeably, commendably, favourably, worthily.

wellbeing *n* comfort, good, happiness, health, prosperity, welfare.

welter *vb* flounder, roll, toss, wallow. • *n* confusion, jumble, mess.

wet *vb* dabble, damp, dampen, dip, drench, moisten, saturate, soak, sprinkle, water. • *adj* clammy, damp, dank, dewy, dripping, humid, moist; rainy, showery, sprinkly. • *n* dampness, humidity, moisture, wetness.

whack *vb, n* bang, beat, rap, strike, thrash, thump, thwack.

wharf *n* dock, pier, quay.

wheedle *vb* cajole, coax, flatter, inveigle, lure.

wheel *vb* gyrate, revolve, roll, rotate, spin, swing, turn, twist, whirl, wind. • *n* circle, revolution, roll, rotation, spin, turn, twirl.

whet *vb* grind, sharpen; arouse, awaken, excite, provoke, rouse, stimulate, animate, inspire, kindle, quicken, warm.

whiff *vb, n* blast, gust, puff.

whim *n* caprice, crotchet, fancy, freak, frolic, humour, notion, quirk, sport, vagary, whimsy, wish.

whimsical *adj* capricious, crotchety, eccentric, erratic, fanciful, frolicsome, odd, peculiar, quaint, singular.

whine *vb* cry, grumble, mewl, moan, snivel, wail, whimper. • *n* complaint, cry, grumble, moan, sob, wail, whimper.

whip *vb* beat, lash, strike; flagellate, flog, goad, horsewhip, scourge, slash; hurt, sting; jerk, snap, snatch, whisk. • *n* bullwhip, cane, crop, horsewhip, knout, lash, scourge, switch, thong.

whipping *n* beating, castigation, dusting, flagellation, flogging, thrashing.

whirl *vb* gyrate, pirouette, roll, revolve, rotate, turn, twirl, twist, wheel. • *n* eddy, flurry, flutter, gyration, rotation, spin, swirl, twirl, vortex.

whit *n* atom, bit, grain, iota, jot, mite, particle, scrap, speck, tittle.

white *adj* argent, canescent, chalky, frosty, hoary, ivory, milky, silver, snowy; grey, pale, pallid, wan; candid, clean, chaste, immaculate, innocent, pure, spotless, unblemished.

whole *adj* all, complete, entire, intact, integral, total, undivided; faultless, firm, good, perfect, strong, unbroken, undivided, uninjured; healthy, sound, well. • *adv* entire, in one. • *n* aggregate, all, amount, ensemble, entirety, gross, sum, total, totality.

wholesome *adj* healthy, healthful, invigorating, nourishing, nutritious, salubrious, salutary; beneficial, good, helpful, improving, salutary; fresh, sound, sweet.

wholly *adv* altogether, completely, entirely, fully, totally, utterly.

whoop *vb* halloo, hoot, roar, shout, yell. • *n* bellow, hoot, roar, shout, yell.

whore *n* bawd, courtesan, drab, harlot, prostitute, streetwalker, strumpet.

wicked *adj* abandoned, abominable, depraved, devilish, godless, graceless, immoral, impious, infamous, irreligious, irreverent, profane, sinful, ungodly, unholy, unprincipled, unrighteous, vicious, vile, worthless; atrocious, bad, black, criminal, dark, evil, heinous, ill, iniquitous, monstrous, nefarious, unjust, villainous.

wide *adj* ample, broad, capacious, comprehensive, distended, expanded, large, spacious, vast; distant, remote; prevalent, rife, widespread. • *adv* completely, farthest, fully.

wield *vb* brandish, flourish, handle, manipulate, ply, work; control, manage, sway, use.

wild *adj* feral, undomesticated, untamed; desert, desolate, native, rough, rude, uncultivated; barbarous, ferocious, fierce, savage, uncivilized; dense, luxuriant, rank; disorderly, distracted, frantic, frenzied, furious, impetuous, irregular, mad, outrageous, raving, turbulent, ungoverned, uncontrolled, violent; dissipated, fast, flighty, foolish, giddy, harebrained, heedless, ill-advised, inconsiderate, reckless, thoughtless, unwise; boisterous, rough, stormy; crazy, extravagant, fanciful, grotesque, imaginary, strange. • *n* desert, waste, wilderness.

wilderness *n* desert, waste, wild.

wilful *adj* cantankerous, contumacious, dogged, headstrong, heady, inflexible, intractable, mulish, obdurate, obstinate, perverse, pig-headed, refractory, self-willed, stubborn, unruly, unyielding; arbitrary, capricious, deliberate, intended, intentional, planned, premeditated.

will *vb* bid, command, decree, direct, enjoin, ordain; choose, desire, elect, wish; bequeath, convey, demise, devise, leave. • *n* decision, determination, resoluteness, resolution, self-reliance; desire, disposition, inclination, intent, pleasure, purpose, volition, wish; behest, command, decree, demand, direction, order, request, requirement.

willing *adj* adaptable, amenable, compliant, desirous, disposed, inclined, minded; deliberate, free, intentional, spontaneous, unasked, unbidden, voluntary; cordial, eager, forward, prompt, ready.

willingly *adv* cheerfully, gladly, readily, spontaneously, voluntarily.

wily *adj* arch, artful, crafty, crooked, cunning, deceitful, designing, diplomatic, foxy, insidious, intriguing, politic, sly, subtle, treacherous, tricky.

win *vb* accomplish, achieve, acquire, catch, earn, effect, gain, gather, get, make, obtain, procure, reach, realize, reclaim, recover; gain, succeed, surpass, triumph; arrive, allure, attract, convince, influence, persuade. • *n* conquest, success, triumph, victory.

wind[1] *n* air, blast, breeze, draught, gust, hurricane, whiff, zephyr; breath, breathing, expiration, inspiration, respiration; flatulence, gas, windiness.

wind[2] *vb* coil, crank, encircle, involve, reel, roll, turn, twine, twist; bend, curve, meander, zigzag. • *n* bend, curve, meander, twist, zigzag.

winding *adj* circuitous, devious, flexuose, flexuous, meandering, serpentine, tortuous, turning, twisting. • *n* bend, curve, meander, turn, twist.

windy *adj* breezy, blowy, blustering, boisterous, draughty, gusty, squally, stormy, tempestuous; airy, empty, hollow, inflated.

winning *adj* alluring, attractive, bewitching, brilliant, captivating, charming, dazzling, delightful, enchanting, engaging, fascinating, lovely, persuasive, pleasing, prepossessing; conquering, triumphant, victorious.

winnow *vb* cull, glean, divide, fan, part, select, separate, sift.

winsome *adj* blithe, blithesome, bonny, buoyant, charming, cheerful, debonair, jocund, light-hearted, lively, lovable, merry, pleasant, sportive, winning.

wintry *adj* arctic, boreal, brumal, cold, frosty, icy, snowy.

wipe *vb* clean, dry, mop, rub. • *n* mop, rub, blow, hit, strike; gibe, jeer, sarcasm, sneer, taunt.

wisdom *n* depth, discernment, far-sightedness, foresight, insight, judgement, judiciousness, prescience, profundity, prudence, sagacity, sapience, sense, solidity, understanding, wiseness; attainment, edification, enlightenment, erudition, information, knowledge, learning, lore, scholarship; reason.

wise *adj* deep, discerning, enlightened, intelligent, judicious, penetrating, philosophical, profound, rational, seasonable, sensible, sage, sapient, solid, sound; erudite, informed, knowing, learned, scholarly; crafty, cunning, designing, foxy, politic, sly, subtle, wary, wily.

wish *vb* covet, desire, hanker, list, long; bid, command, desire, direct, intend, mean, order, want. • *n* behest, desire, intention, mind, pleasure, want, will; craving, desire, hankering, inclination, liking, longing, want, yearning.

wistful *adj* contemplative, engrossed, meditative, musing, pensive, reflective, thoughtful; desirous, eager, earnest, longing.

wit *n* genius, intellect, intelligence, reason, sense, understanding; brightness, banter, cleverness, drollery, facetiousness, fun, humour, jocularity, piquancy, point, raillery, satire, sparkle, whim; conceit, epigram, jest, joke, pleasantry, quip, quirk, repartee, sally, witticism; humorist, joker, wag.

witch *n* charmer, enchantress, fascinator, sorceress; crone, hag, sibyl.

witchcraft *n* conjuration, enchantment, magic, necromancy, sorcery, spell.

withdraw *vb* abstract, deduct, remove, retire, separate, sequester, sequestrate, subduct, subtract; disengage, wean; abjure, recall, recant, relinquish, resign, retract, revoke; abdicate, decamp, depart, dissociate, retire, shrink, vacate.

wither *vb* contract, droop, dry, sear, shrivel, wilt, wizen; decay, decline, languish, pine, waste.

withhold *vb* check, detain, hinder, repress, restrain, retain, suppress.

withstand *vb* confront, defy, face, oppose, resist.

witless *adj* daft, dull, foolish, halfwitted, obtuse, senseless, shallow, silly, stupid, unintelligent.

witness *vb* corroborate, mark, note, notice, observe, see. • *n* attestation, conformation, corroboration, evidence, proof, testimony; beholder, bystander, corroborator, deponent, eyewitness, onlooker, spectator, testifier.

witty *adj* bright, clever, droll, facetious, funny, humorous, jocose, jocular, pleasant, waggish; alert, penetrating, quick, sparkling, sprightly.

wizard *n* charmer, diviner, conjurer, enchanter, magician, necromancer, seer, soothsayer, sorcerer.

woe *n* affliction, agony, anguish, bitterness, depression, distress, dole, grief, heartache, melancholy, misery, sorrow, torture, tribulation, trouble, unhappiness, wretchedness.

woeful *adj* afflicted, agonized, anguished, burdened, disconsolate, distressed, melancholy, miserable, mournful, piteous, sad, sorrowful, troubled, unhappy, wretched; afflicting, afflictive, calamitous, deplorable, depressing, disastrous, distressing, dreadful, tragic, tragical, grievous, lamentable, pitiable, saddening.

wonder *vb* admire, gape, marvel; conjecture, ponder, query, question, speculate. • *n* amazement, astonishment, awe, bewilderment, curiosity, marvel, miracle, prodigy, surprise, stupefaction, wonderment.

wonderful *adj* amazing, astonishing, astounding, awe-inspiring, awesome, awful, extraordinary, marvellous, miraculous, portentous, prodigious, startling, stupendous, surprising.

wont *adj* accustomed, customary, familiar, habitual, ordinary, usual. • *n* custom, habit, practice, rule, usage.

wonted *adj* accustomed, common, conventional, customary, everyday, familiar, frequent, habitual, ordinary, regular, usual.

wood *n* coppice, copse, covert, forest, greenwood, grove, spinney, thicket, woodland.

word *vb* express, phrase, put, say, state, term, utter. • *n* expression, name, phrase, term, utterance; account, advice, information, intelligence, message, news, report, tidings; affirmation, assertion, averment, avowal, declaration, statement; conversation, speech; agreement, assurance, engagement, parole, pledge, plight, promise; behest, bidding, command, direction, order, precept; countersign, password, signal, watchword.

wordy *adj* circumlocutory, diffuse, garrulous, inflated, lengthened, long-winded, loquacious, periphrastic, rambling, talkative, tedious, verbose, windy.

work *vb* act, operate; drudge, fag, grind, grub, labour, slave, sweat, toil; move, perform, succeed; aim, attempt, strive, try; effervesce, ferment, leaven, rise; accomplish, beget, cause, effect, engender, manage, originate, produce; exert, strain; embroider, stitch. • *n* exertion, drudgery, grind, labour, pain, toil; business, employment, function, occupation, task; action, accomplishment, achievement, composition, deed, feat, fruit, handiwork, opus, performance, product, production; fabric, manufacture; ferment, leaven; management, treatment.

workman *n* journeyman, employee, labourer, operative, worker, wright; artisan, craftsman, mechanic.

world *n* cosmos, creation, earth, globe, nature, planet, sphere, universe.

worldly *adj* common, earthly, human, mundane, sublunary, terrestrial; carnal, fleshly, profane, secular, temporal; ambitious, grovelling, irreligious, selfish, proud, sordid, unsanctified, unspiritual; sophisticated, worldly-wise.

worry *vb* annoy, badger, bait, beset, bore, bother, chafe, disquiet, disturb, fret, gall, harass, harry, hector, infest, irritate, molest, persecute, pester, plague, tease, torment, trouble, vex. • *n* annoyance, anxiety, apprehensiveness, care, concern, disquiet, fear, misgiving, perplexity, solicitude, trouble, uneasiness, vexation.

worship *vb* adore, esteem, honour, revere, venerate; deify, idolize; aspire, pray. • *n* adoration, devotion, esteem, homage, idolatry, idolizing, respect, reverence; aspiration, exultation, invocation, laud, praise, prayer, supplication.

worst *vb* beat, choke, conquer, crush, defeat, discomfit, foil, master, overpower, overthrow, quell, rout, subdue, subjugate, vanquish.

worth *n* account, character, credit, desert, excellence, importance, integrity, merit, nobleness, worthiness, virtue; cost, estimation, price, value.

worthless *adj* futile, meritless, miserable, nugatory, paltry, poor, trifling, unproductive, unsalable, unserviceable, useless, valueless, wretched; abject, base, corrupt, degraded, ignoble, low, mean, vile.

worthy *adj* deserving, fit, suitable; estimable, excellent, exemplary, good, honest, honourable, reputable, righteous, upright, virtuous. • *n* celebrity, dignitary, luminary, notability, personage, somebody, VIP.

wound *vb* damage, harm, hurt, injure; cut, gall, harrow, irritate, lacerate, pain, prick, stab; annoy, mortify, offend. • *n* blow, hurt, injury; damage, detriment; anguish, grief, pain, pang, torture.

wraith *n* apparition, ghost, phantom, spectre, vision.

wrangle *vb* argue, bicker, brawl, cavil, dispute, jangle, jar, quarrel, squabble, spar, spat. • *n* altercation, argument, bickering, brawl, contest, controversy, jar, quarrel, squabble.

wrap *vb* cloak, cover, encase, envelop, muffle, swathe, wind. • *n* blanket, cape, cloak, cover, overcoat, shawl.

wrath *n* anger, choler, exasperation, fury, heat, resentment, indignation, ire, irritation, offence, passion, rage.

wrathful *adj* angry, enraged, exasperated, furious, hot, indignant, infuriated, irate, mad, passionate, provoked, rageful.

wreak *vb* execute, exercise, indulge, inflict, work.

wreath *n* chaplet, curl, festoon, garland, ring, twine.

wreathe *vb* encircle, festoon, garland, intertwine, surround, twine, twist.

wreck *vb* founder, shipwreck, strand; blast, blight, break, devastate, ruin, spoil. • *n* crash, desolation, destruction, perdition, prostration, ruin, shipwreck, smash, undoing.

wrench *vb* distort, pervert, twist, wrest, wring; sprain, strain; extort, extract. • *n* twist, wring, sprain, strain; monkey wrench, spanner.

wrest *vb* force, pull, strain, twist, wrench, wring.

wrestle *vb* contend, contest, grapple, strive, struggle.

wretch *n* outcast, pariah, pilgarlic, troglodyte, vagabond, victim, sufferer; beggar, criminal, hound, knave, miscreant, rascal, ruffian, rogue, scoundrel, villain.

wretched *adj* afflicted, comfortless, distressed, forlorn, sad, unfortunate, unhappy, woebegone; afflicting, calamitous, deplorable, depressing, pitiable, sad, saddening, shocking, sorrowful; bad, beggarly, contemptible, mean, paltry, pitiful, poor, shabby, sorry, vile, worthless.

wring *vb* contort, twist, wrench; extort, force, wrest; anguish, distress, harass, pain, rack, torture.

wrinkle[1] *vb* cockle, corrugate, crease, gather, pucker, rumple. • *n* cockle, corrugation, crease, crimp, crinkle, crumple, fold, furrow, gather, plait, ridge, rumple.

wrinkle[2] *n* caprice, fancy, notion, quirk, whim; device, tip, trick.

writ *n* decree, order, subpoena, summons.

write *vb* compose, copy, indite, inscribe, pen, scrawl, scribble, transcribe.

writer *n* amanuensis, author, clerk, penman, scribe, secretary.

writhe *vb* contort, distort, squirm, twist, wriggle.

written *adj* composed, indited, inscribed, penned, transcribed.

wrong *vb* abuse, encroach, injure, maltreat, oppress. • *adj* inequitable, unfair, unjust, wrongful; bad, criminal, evil, guilty, immoral, improper, iniquitous, reprehensible, sinful, vicious, wicked; amiss, improper, inappropriate, unfit, unsuitable; erroneous, false, faulty, inaccurate, incorrect, mistaken, untrue. • *adv* amiss, erroneously, falsely, faultily, improperly, inaccurately, incorrectly, wrongly. • *n* foul, grievance, inequity, injury, injustice, trespass, unfairness; blame, crime, dishonesty, evil, guilt, immorality, iniquity, misdeed, misdoing, sin, transgression, unrighteousness, vice, wickedness, wrongdoing; error, falsity.

wroth *adj* angry, enraged, exasperated, furious, incensed, indignant, irate, passionate, provoked, resentful.

wrought *adj* done, effected, performed, worked.

wry *adj* askew, awry, contorted, crooked, distorted, twisted.

XYZ

xanthous *adj* blonde, fair, light-complexioned, xanthic, yellow.

xiphoid *adj* ensiform, gladiate, sword-like, sword-shaped.

Xmas *n* Christmas, Christmastide, Noel, Yule, Yuletide.

X-ray *n* roentgen ray, röntgen ray.

xylograph *n* cut, woodcut, wood engraving.

xylographer *n* wood engraver.

xylophagous *adj* wood-eating, wood-nourished.

yap *vb* bark, cry, yelp. • *n* bark, cry, yelp.

yard *n* close, compound, court, courtyard, enclosure, garden.

yarn *n* anecdote, boasting, fabrication, narrative, story, tale, untruth.

yawn *vb* dehisce, gape, open wide. • *n* gap, gape, gulf.

yearn *vb* crave, desire, hanker after, long for.

yell *vb* bawl, bellow, cry out, howl, roar, scream, screech, shriek, squeal. • *n* cry, howl, roar, scream, screech, shriek.

yellow *adj* aureate, gilded, gilt, gold, golden, lemon, primrose, saffron, xanthic, xanthous.

yelp *vb* bark, howl, yap; complain, bitch, grouse. • *n* bark, sharp cry, howl.

yet *adv* at last, besides, further, however, over and above, so far, still, thus far, ultimately.• *conj* moreover, nevertheless, notwithstanding, now.

yield *vb* afford, bear, bestow, communicate, confer, fetch, furnish, impart, produce, render, supply; accede, accord, acknowledge, acquiesce, allow, assent, comply, concede, give, grant, permit; abandon, abdicate, cede, forgo, give up, let go, quit, relax, relinquish, resign, submit, succumb, surrender, waive. • *n* earnings, income, output, produce, profit, return, revenue.

yielding *adj* accommodating, acquiescent, affable, compliant, complaisant, easy, manageable, obedient, passive, submissive, unresisting; bending, flexible, flexile, plastic, pliant, soft, supple, tractable; fertile, productive.

yoke *vb* associate, bracket, connect, couple, harness, interlink, join, link, unite. • *n* bond, chain, ligature, link, tie, union; bondage, dependence, enslavement, service, servitude, subjection, vassalage; couple, pair.

yokel *n* boor, bumpkin, countryman, peasant, rustic.

yore *adj* ancient, antique, old, olden. • *n* long ago, long since, olden times.

young *adj* green, ignorant, inexperienced, juvenile, new, recent, youthful. • *n* young people, youth; babies, issue, brood, offspring, progeny, spawn.

youngster *n* adolescent, boy, girl, lad, lass, stripling, youth.

youth *n* adolescence, childhood, immaturity, juvenile, juvenility, minority, nonage, pupillage, wardship; boy, girl, lad, lass, schoolboy, schoolgirl, slip, sprig, stripling, youngster.

youthful *adj* boyish, childish, girlish, immature, juvenile, puerile, young.

zany adj comic, comical, crazy, droll, eccentric, funny, imaginative, scatterbrained; clownish, foolish, ludicrous, silly. • *n* buffoon, clown, droll, fool, harlequin, jester, punch.

zeal *n* alacrity, ardour, cordiality, devotedness, devotion, earnestness, eagerness, energy, enthusiasm, fervour, glow, heartiness, intensity, jealousness, passion, soul, spirit, warmth.

zealot *n* bigot, devotee, fanatic, freak, partisan.

zealous *adj* ardent, burning, devoted, eager, earnest, enthusiastic, fervent, fiery, forward, glowing, jealous, keen, passionate, prompt, ready, swift, warm.

zenith *n* acme, apex, climax, culmination, heyday, pinnacle, prime, summit, top, utmost, height.

zero *n* cipher, naught, nadir, nil, nothing, nought.

zest *n* appetite, enjoyment, exhilaration, gusto, liking, piquancy, relish, thrill; edge, flavour, salt, savour, tang, taste; appetizer, sauce.

zone *n* band, belt, cincture, girdle, girth; circuit, clime, region.

zymotic *adj* bacterial, fermentative, germinating.

MAPS OF THE WORLD

Contents

Symbols for maps on pages:
8-22, 27-38, 40-54, 60-62

Inhabitants
More than 5 million   **New York**

1 000 000 - 5 000 000   **Seattle**

250 000 - 1 000 000   **Mexicali**

100 000 - 250 000   Tijuana

25 000 - 100 000   Sparks

Less than 25 000   Monterey

National capital (UPPERCASE)   **OTTAWA**

State capital   **Boise**

International boundary

Disputed international
boundary

State boundary

Disputed state
boundary

Major road

Other road

Road under
construction

Seasonal road

Railway

Canal

Highest peak   ▲
in continent   McKinley

Highest peak   △
in country   Logan

Height in feet   ▲
                                       17000ft

Depth in feet   ▽
                                       185ft

Coral reef

Dam | Ka'inji
                                         Dam

Waterfall | Niagara
                                         Falls

Pass   )(

International airport   ⊕

National airport   ✈

Historical site   ⚲

Scientific site   ⌀

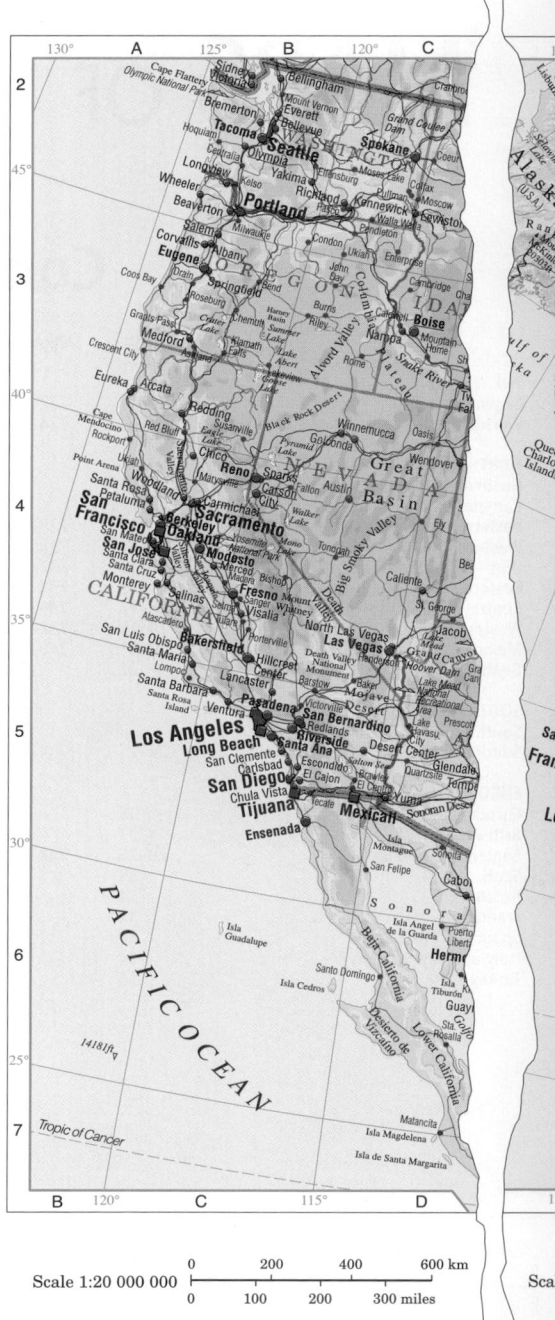

Scale 1:20 000 000

| 0 | 200 | 400 | 600 km |

| 0 | 100 | 200 | 300 miles |

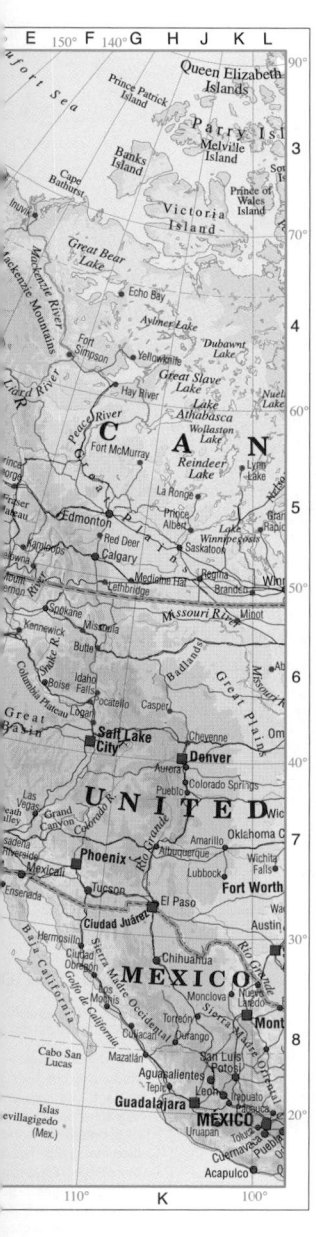

Symbols for maps on pages:
7, 24-25, 56-59

Inhabitants

🔺 **Chicago**   More than 5 million

■ **Columbus**   1 000 000 - 5 000 000

● Quebec   250 000 - 1 000 000

● Halifax   100 000 - 250 000

● ● Anderson   Less than 100 000

NASSAU   National capital (UPPERCASE)

Sacramento   State capital

━━━━━   International boundary

▬ ▬ ▬   Disputed international boundary

────   Major road

- - - -   Road under construction

────   Major railway

⊥⊥⊥⊥   Canal

▲ McKinley   Highest peak in continent

▲ Logan   Highest peak in country

▲ 17000ft   Heights in feet

▼ 185ft   Depths in feet

- - - - -   Coral reef

△   Scientific station

────   Territorial claims in Antarctica

- - - - -   Disputed territorial claims in Antarctica

I *Grand Coulee Dam*   Dam

I *Virginia Falls*   Waterfall

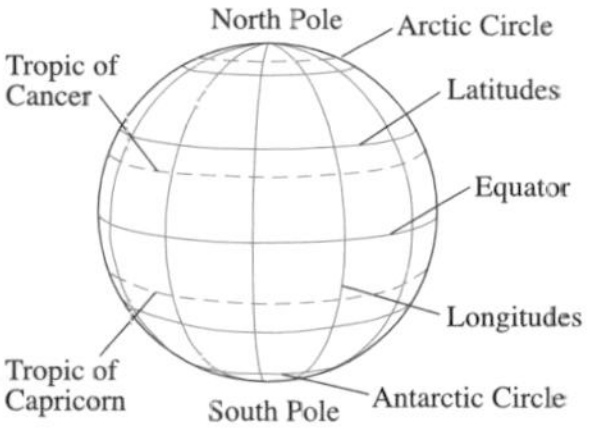

North Pole — Arctic Circle
Tropic of Cancer — Latitudes
— Equator
— Longitudes
Tropic of Capricorn
South Pole — Antarctic Circle

Colour Key for Contours

Glacier/ice cap

6000m

5000m

4000m

3000m

2000m

1000m

500m

200m

0m

▨ Marshland

◍ Salt lake

◌ Seasonal lake

▨ Salt desert

Symbols for Political maps on pages:
5, 6, 23, 26, 39, 55

Inhabitants

● **Lagos**   More than 5 million

● **Ibadan**   1 000 000 - 5 000 000

● Kano   250 000 - 1 000 000

● Gashua   100 000 - 250 000

● Maradi   25 000 - 100 000

■ ■ ■   National Capital

● ●   State Capital

────   International boundary

- - - -   Disputed International boundary

────   State boundary

────   Railway

The letters and numbers in the map edges are there to help you find names. Look for London in the index **29** D4. Turn to page 29 and look top or bottom for number 4 and left or right for letter D. In this blue grid square you will find the city of London.

Scale 1:50 000 000 means that a distance on the map is 50 000 000 times longer than on the Earth's surface e.g. 1 cm on the map represents 500 km on the surface and 1 inch on the map represents 800 miles.

| 0 | 500 | 1000 | 1500 km |
| 0 | 250 | 500 | 750 miles |

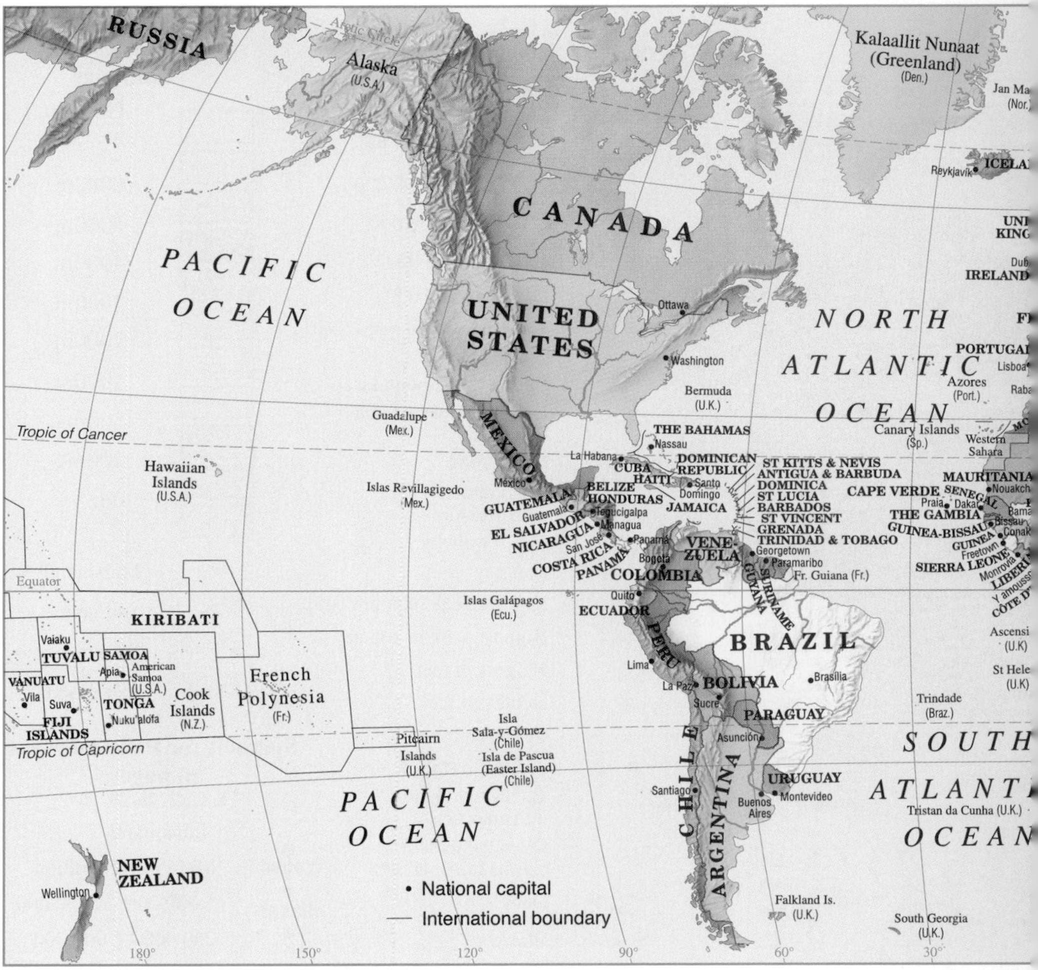

WORLD, POLITICAL MAP

150° 180° 150° 120° 90° 60° 30°

60°

RUSSIA

Alaska (U.S.A.)

Kalaallit Nunaat (Greenland) (Den.)

Jan Ma (Nor.)

Reykjavík   ICELA

CANADA

UNI
KING

Dub
IRELAND

PACIFIC
OCEAN

NORTH

F

UNITED
STATES

Ottawa

PORTUGA

Washington

ATLANTIC

Lisboa

Azores (Port.)

Raba

30°

Bermuda (U.K.)

OCEAN

Tropic of Cancer

Guadalupe (Mex.)

THE BAHAMAS

Canary Islands (Sp.)

Western Sahara

Nassau

Hawaiian
Islands
(U.S.A.)

Islas Revillagigedo
Mex.)

México

DOMINICAN
REPUBLIC

ST KITTS & NEVIS
ANTIGUA & BARBUDA

MAURITANIA

CUBA

La Habana

Nouakc

MEXICO

Santo
Domingo

DOMINICA

CAPE VERDE

SENEG

Dakar

HAITI

BELIZE

Praia

Bamak

GUATEMALA

Guatemala

HONDURAS

JAMAICA

ST LUCIA
BARBADOS

THE GAMBIA

GUINEA-BISSAU

Bissau
Conakr

Tegucigalpa

ST VINCENT

EL SALVADOR

San José

Managua

GRENADA

TRINIDAD & TOBAGO

GUINEA

Freetown

SIERRA LEONE

NICARAGUA

VENE-

Georgetown

LIBERIA

Monrovia

COSTA RICA

Bogotá

ZUELA

Paramaribo

Y

amougo

PANAMA

COLOMBIA

GUYANA

Fr. Guiana (Fr.)

CÔTE D'

Panama

SURINAME

0°

Equator

Islas Galápagos
(Ecu.)

Quito

ECUADOR

BRAZIL

Ascensi
(U.K.)

KIRIBATI

Vaiaku

Lima

PERU

St Hele
(U.K.)

TUVALU   SAMOA

Apia

American
Samoa
(U.S.A.)

French
Polynesia
(Fr.)

La Paz

BOLIVIA

Brasília

Sucre

VANUATU

Vila

Suva

TONGA

Cook
Islands
(N.Z.)

PARAGUAY

Trindade (Braz.)

FIJI
ISLANDS

Nuku'alofa

Tropic of Capricorn

Isla
Sala-y-Gómez
(Chile)

Asunción

SOUTH

Pitcairn
Islands
(U.K.)

Isla de Pascua
(Easter Island)
(Chile)

URUGUAY

ATLANTI

30°

PACIFIC
OCEAN

Santiago

Montevideo

Buenos
Aires

Tristan da Cunha (U.K.)

OCEAN

CHILE

ARGENTINA

NEW
ZEALAND

Wellington

Falkland Is.
(U.K.)

South Georgia
(U.K.)

• National capital
— International boundary

180° 150° 120° 90° 60° 30°

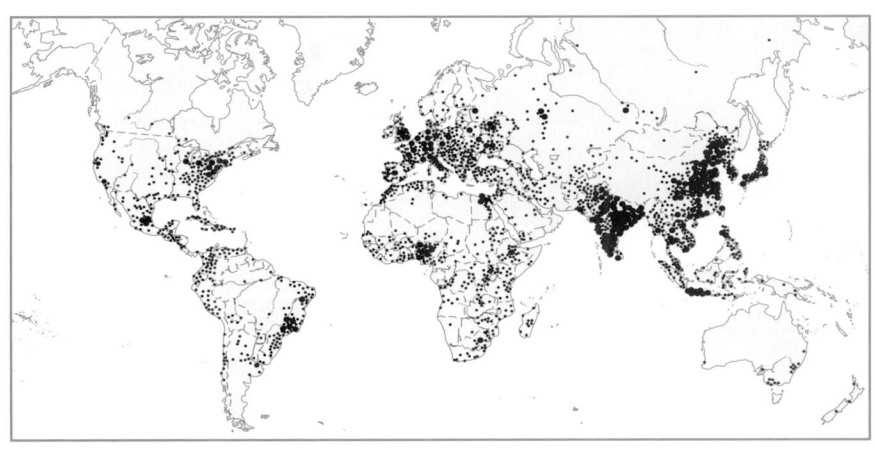

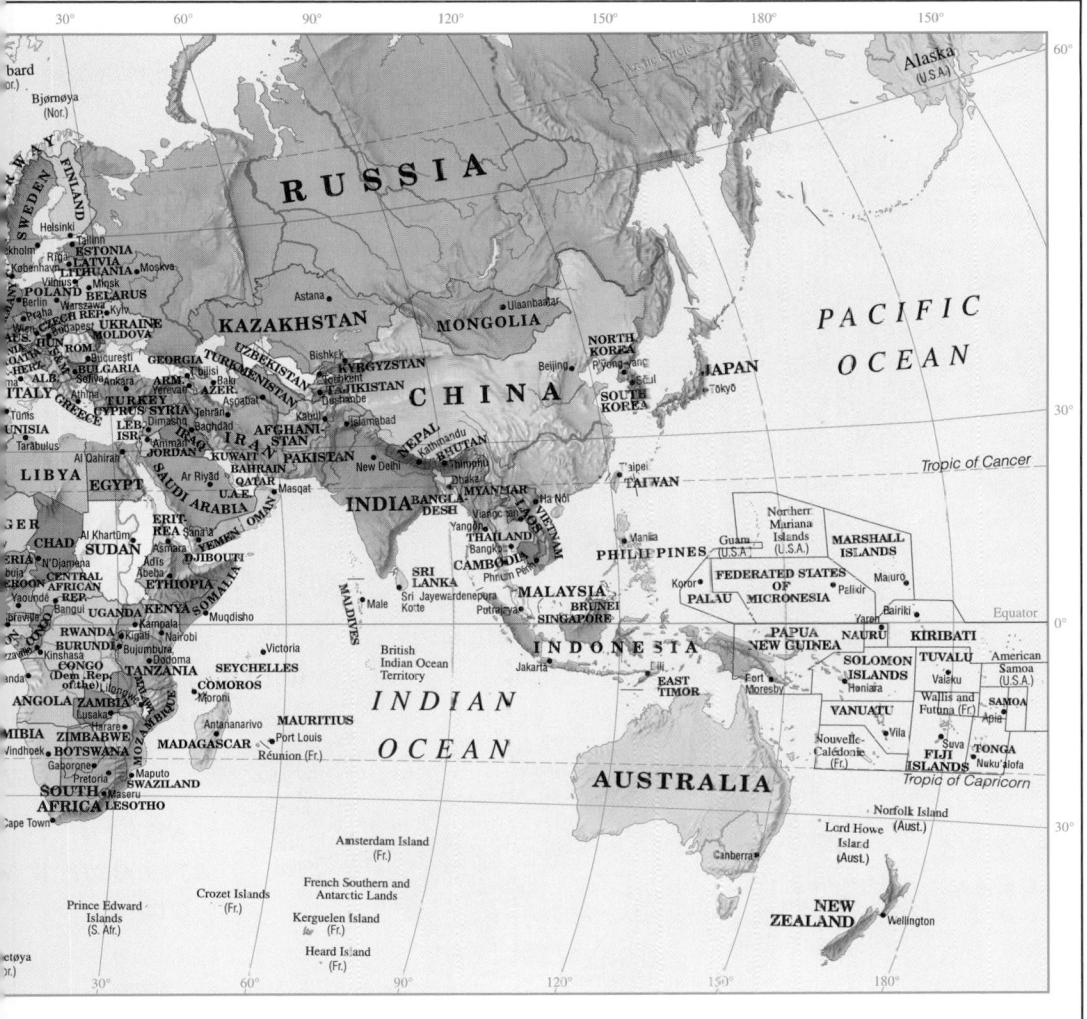

TIME ZONES

The Earth spins around its axis anticlockwise and completes one turn every 24 hours. As the world rotates it is day on the part facing the Sun and night on the side in shadow. As shown on this map, we have divided the Earth into 24 standard time zones. They are based upon lines of longitude at 15 degree intervals but mainly follow country or state boundaries. You can compare times around the world by using the map. For example; when it is 12 noon in London it is 5 hours earlier in New York or 7 am.

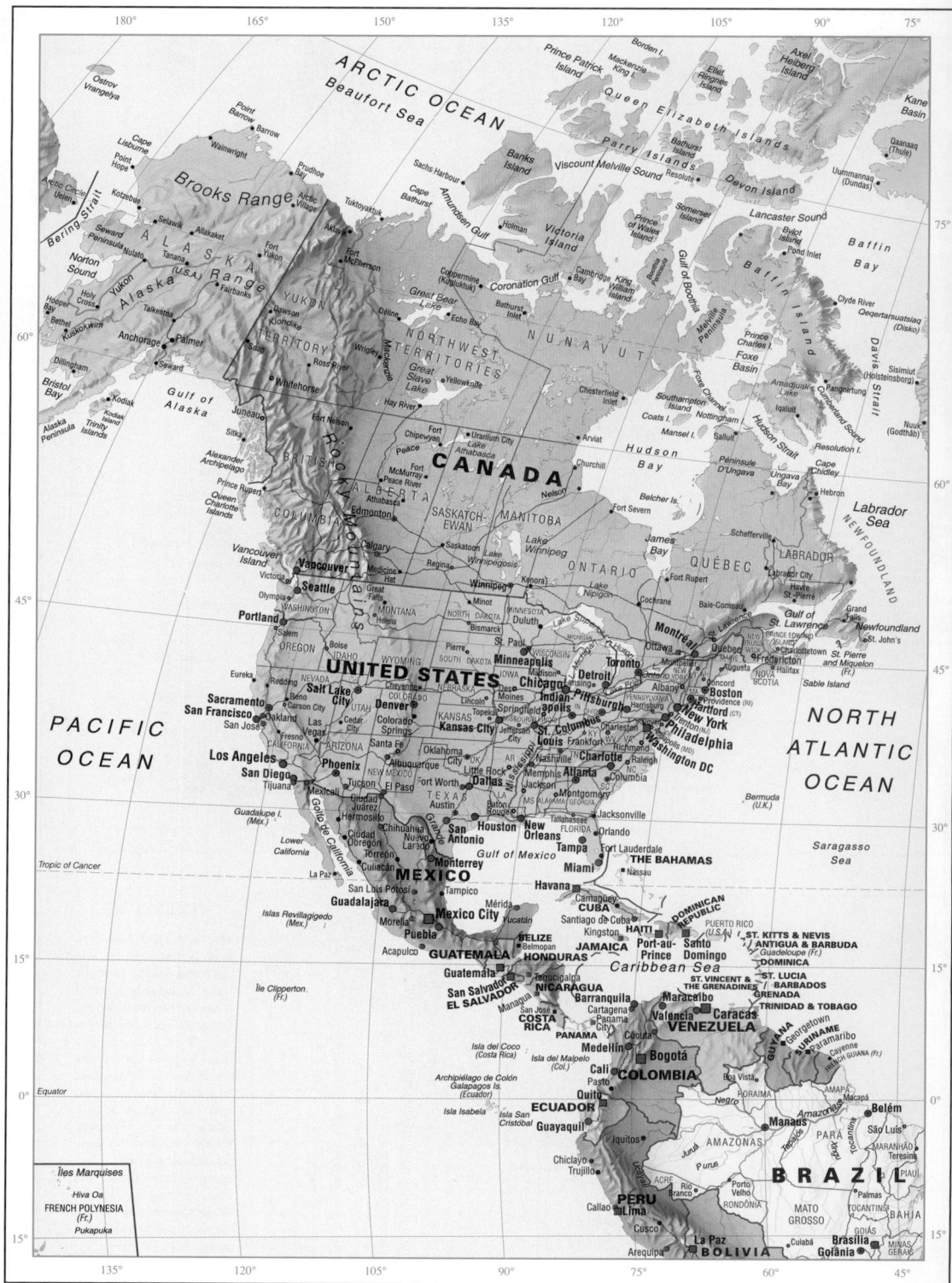

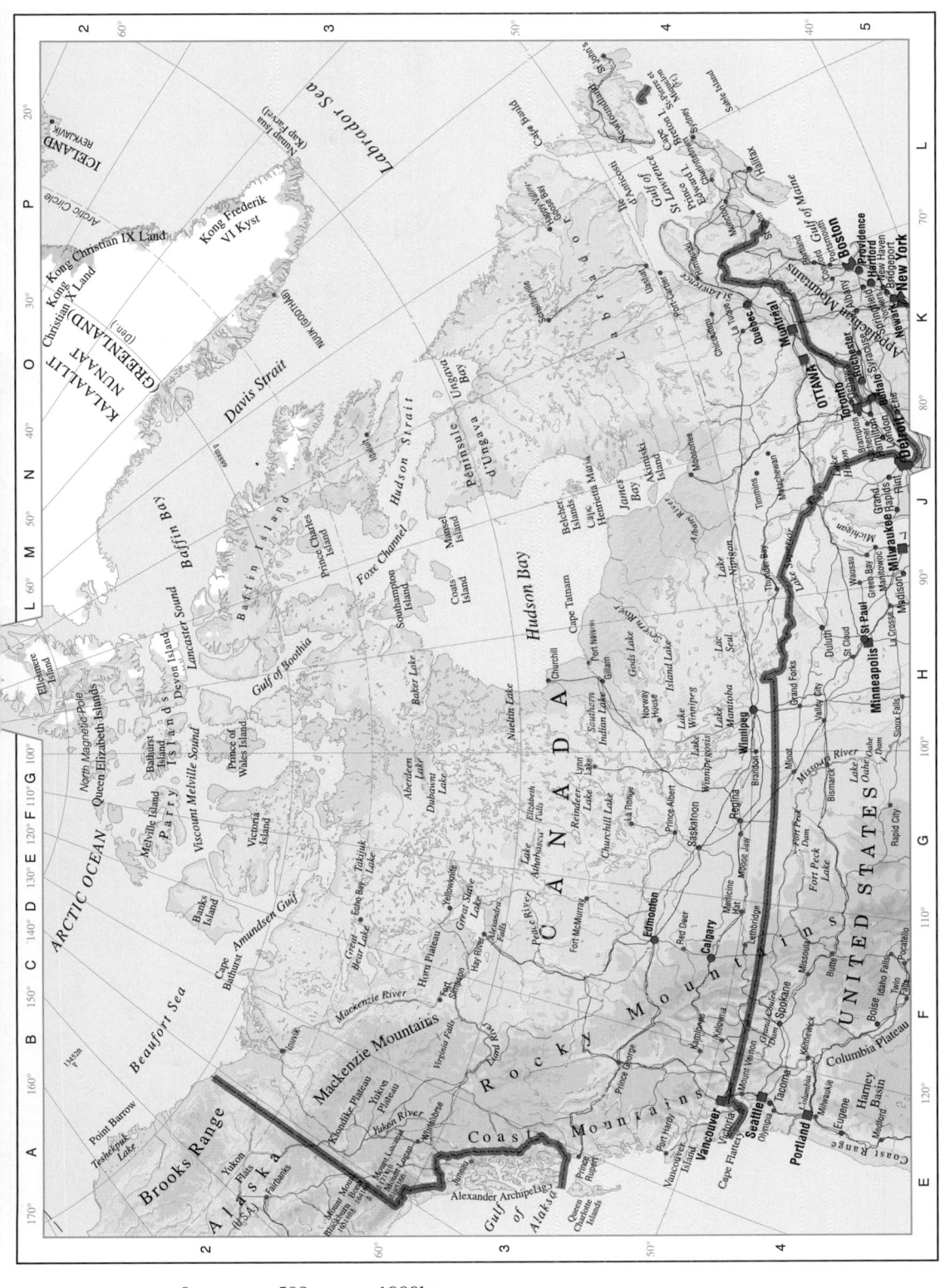

Scale 1: 31 250 000

0 500 1000km

0 300 600miles

© Geddes & Grosset

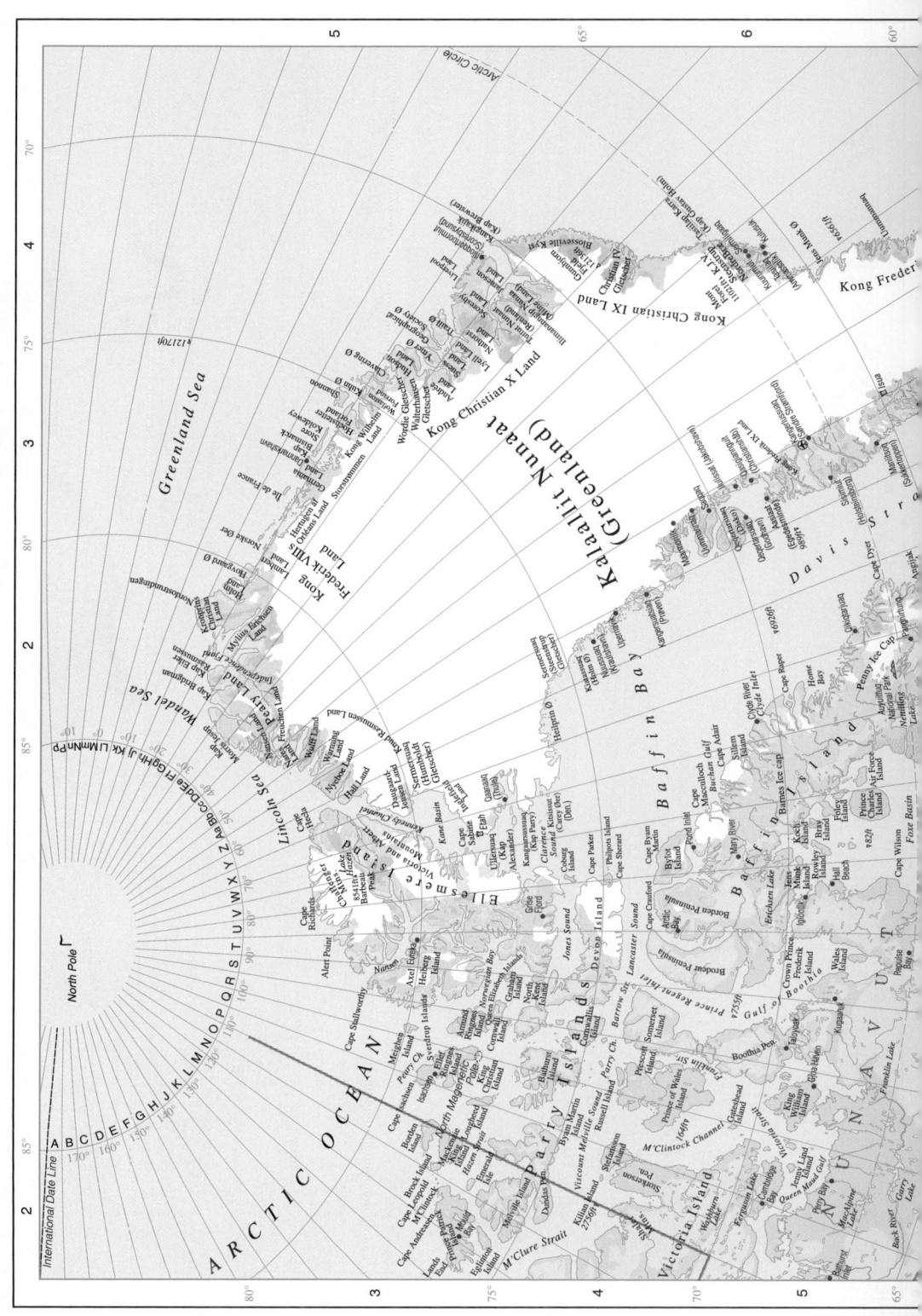

Scale 1: 20 000 000

```
0        250      500km
|--|--|--|----|----|

0       150      300miles
```

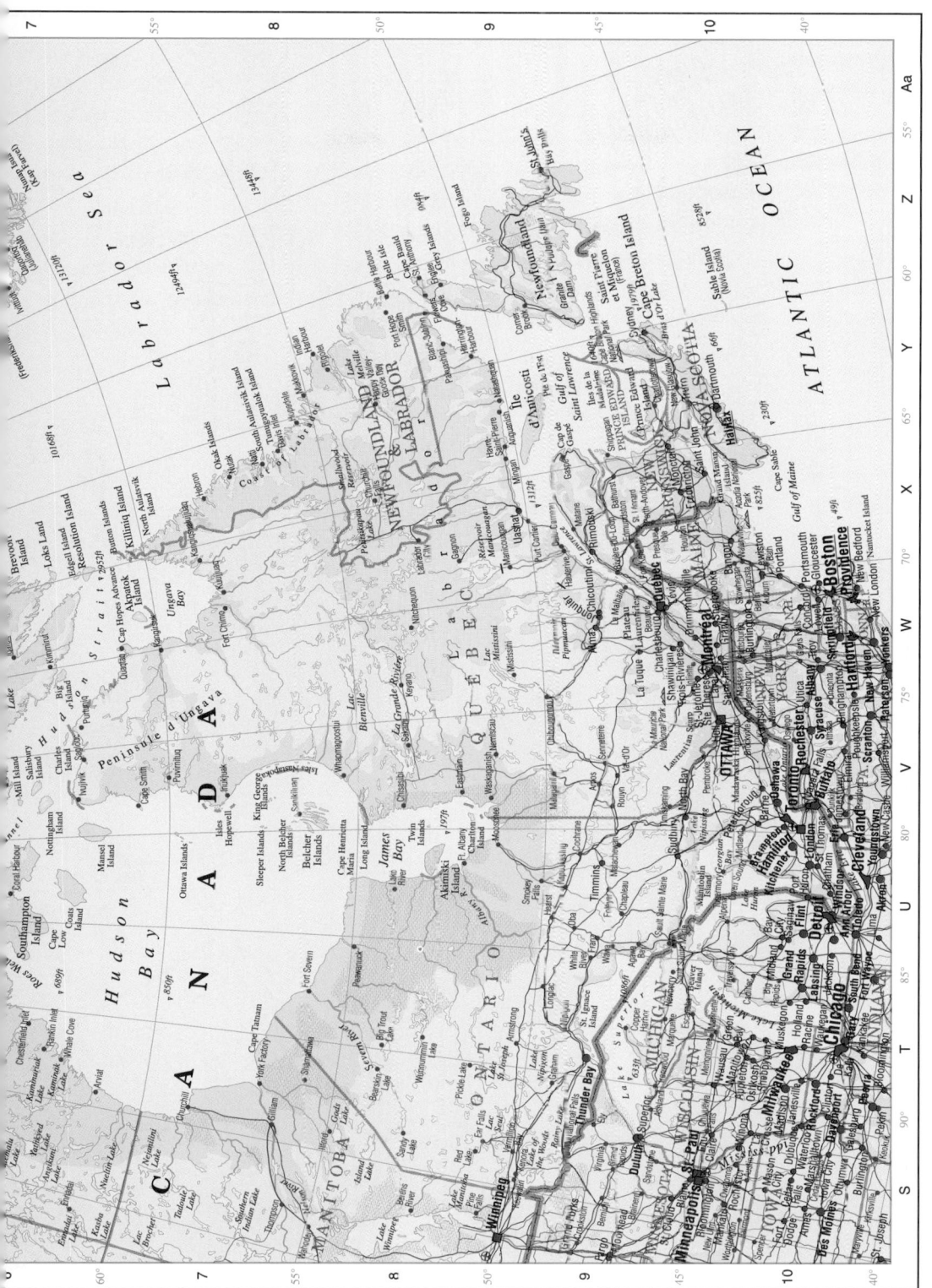

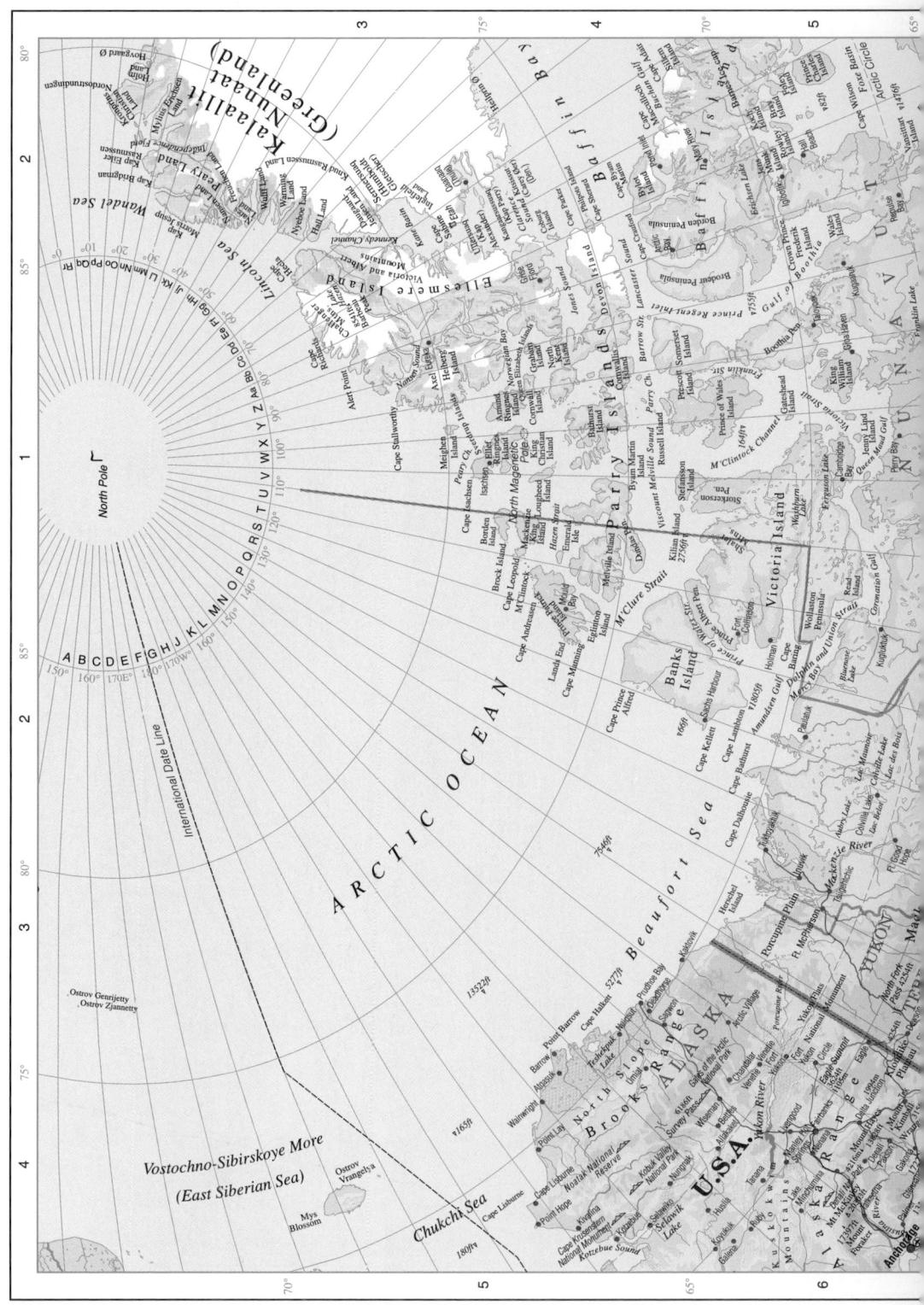

Scale 1: 20 000 000

| 0 | 250 | 500km |
| 0 | 150 | 300miles |

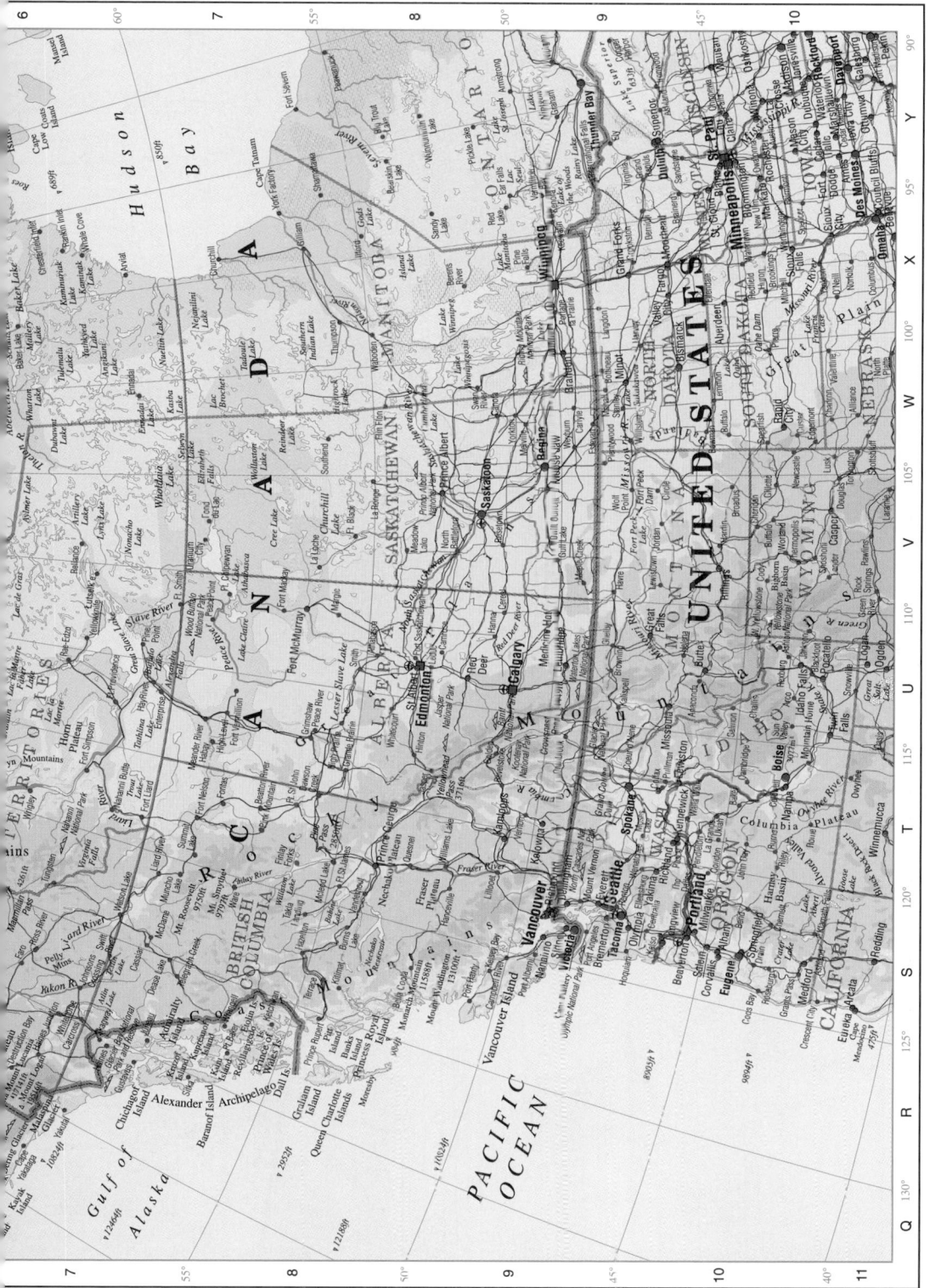

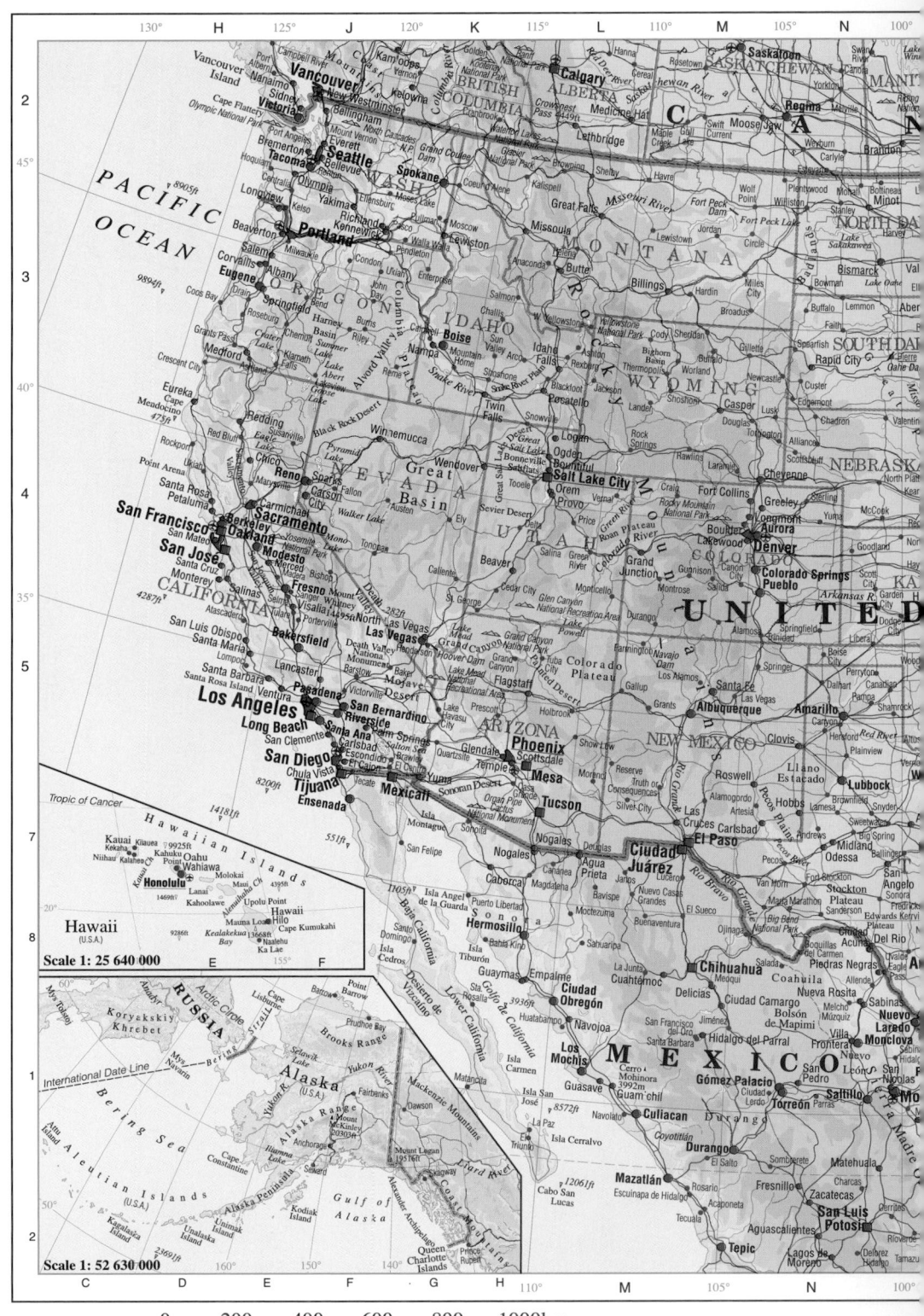

Scale 1: 19 231 000

| 0 | 200 | 400 | 600 | 800 | 1000km |

| 0 | 100 | 200 | 300 | 400 | 500 | 600miles |

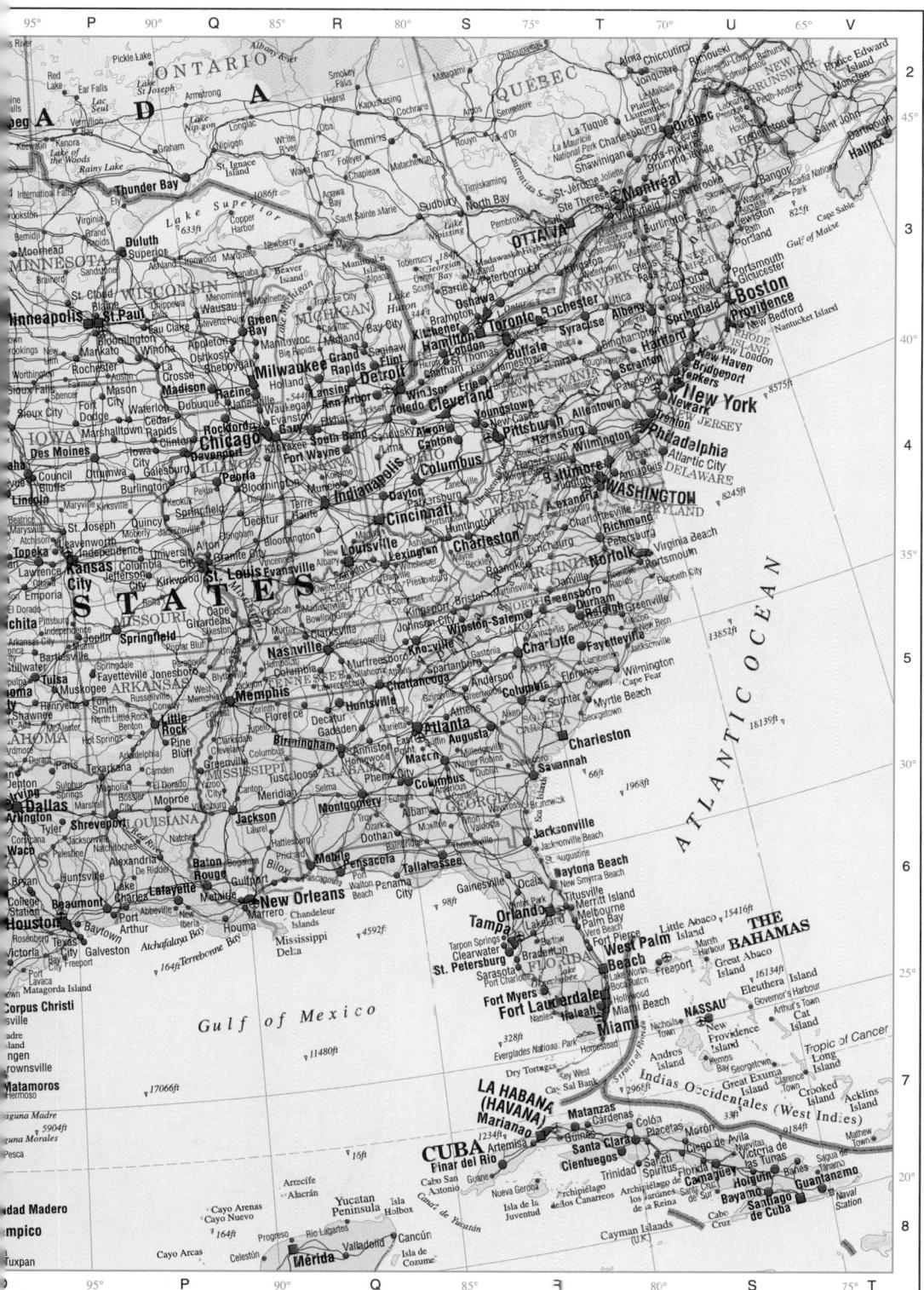

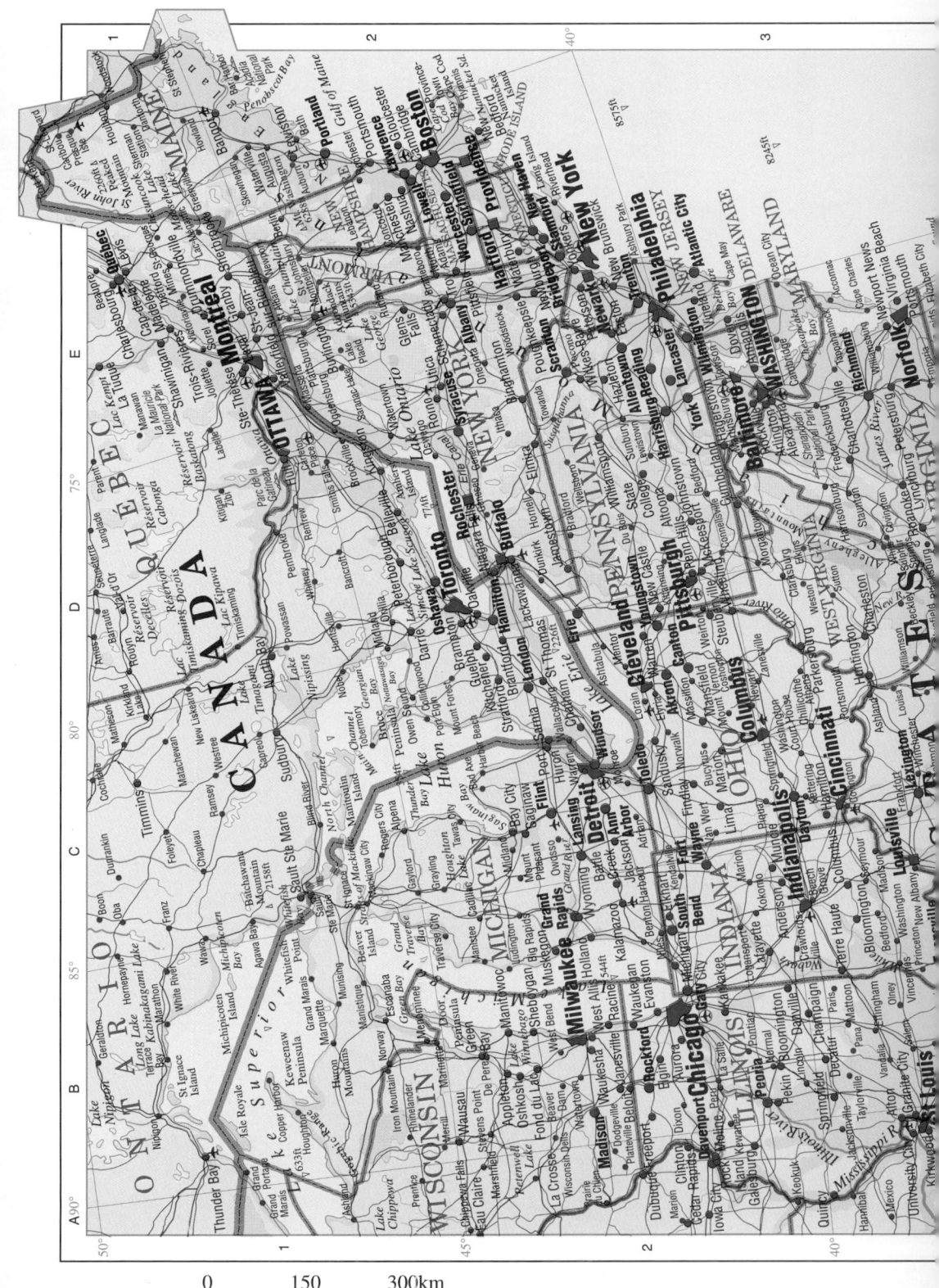

Scale 1: 10 000 000

| 0 | 150 | 300km |

| 0 | 75 | 150miles |

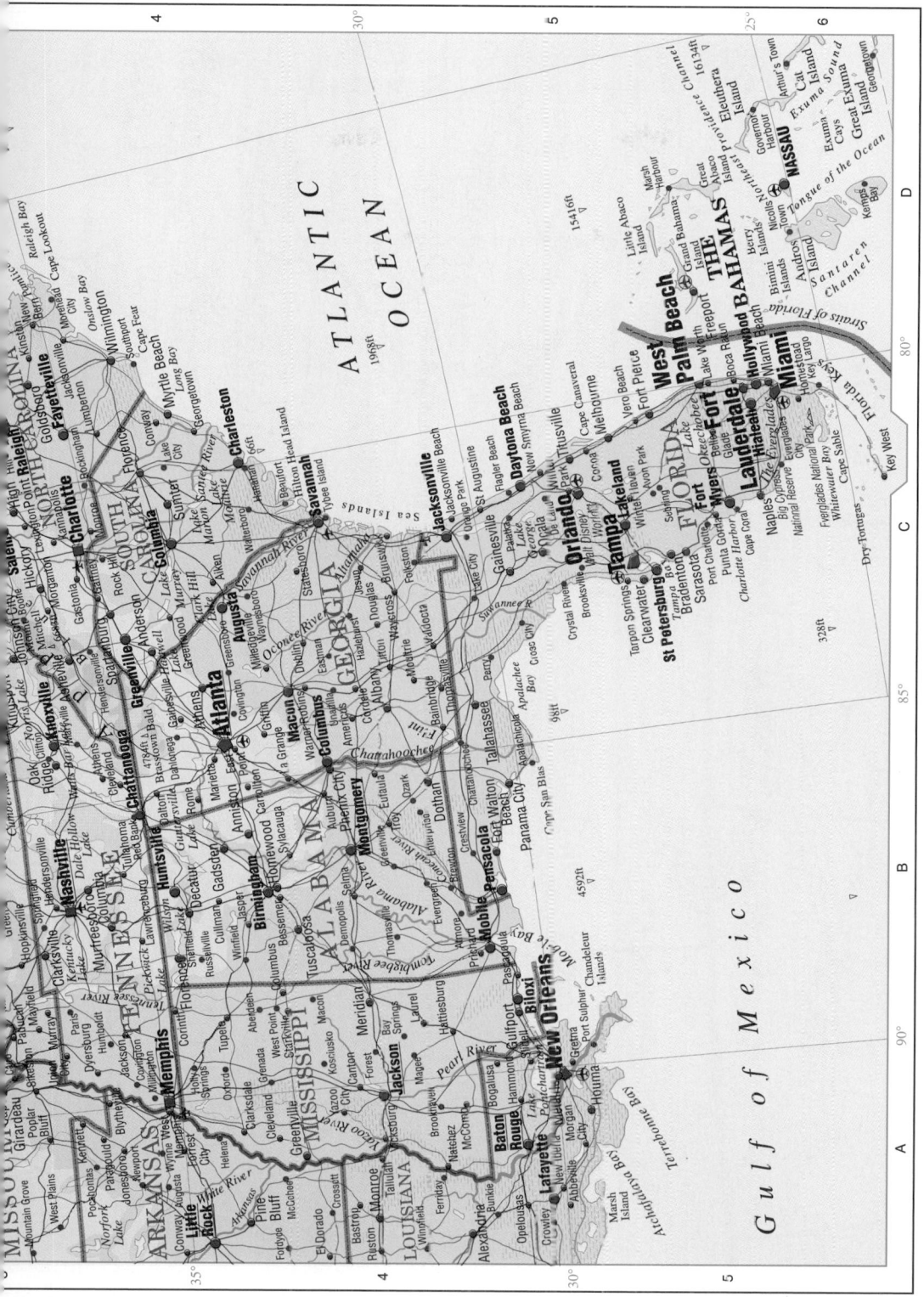

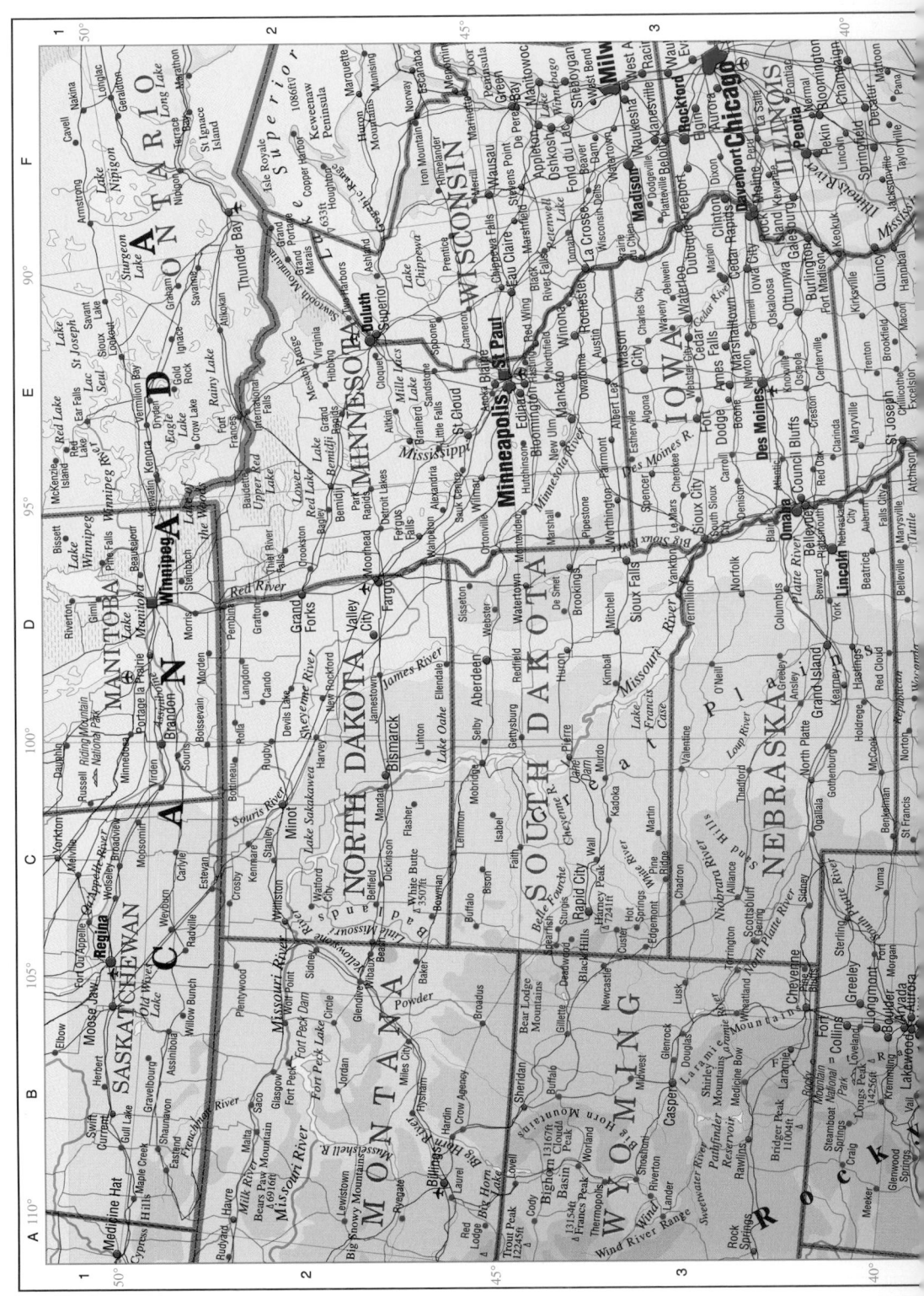

Scale 1: 10 000 000

0   150   300km

0   75   150miles

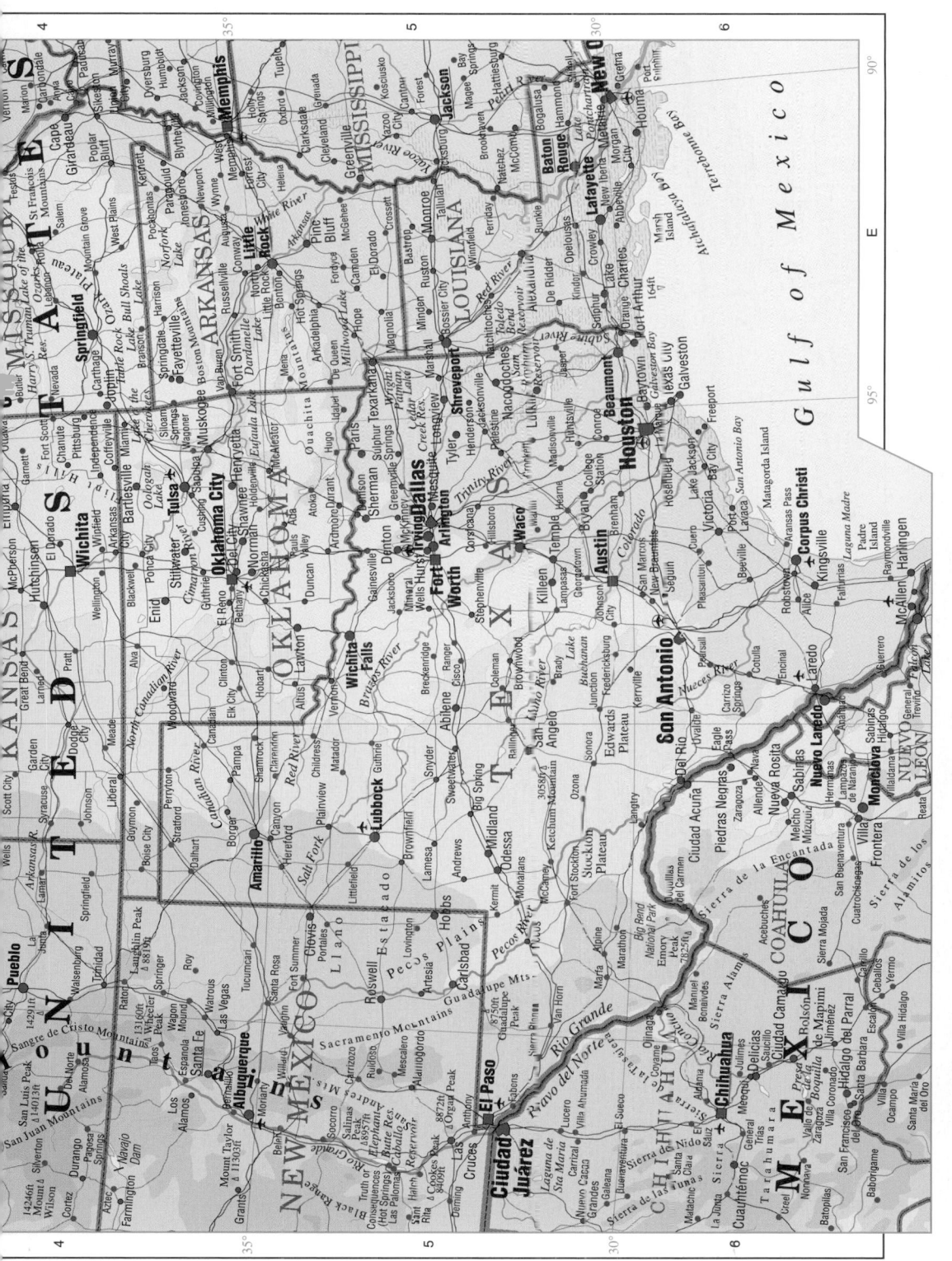

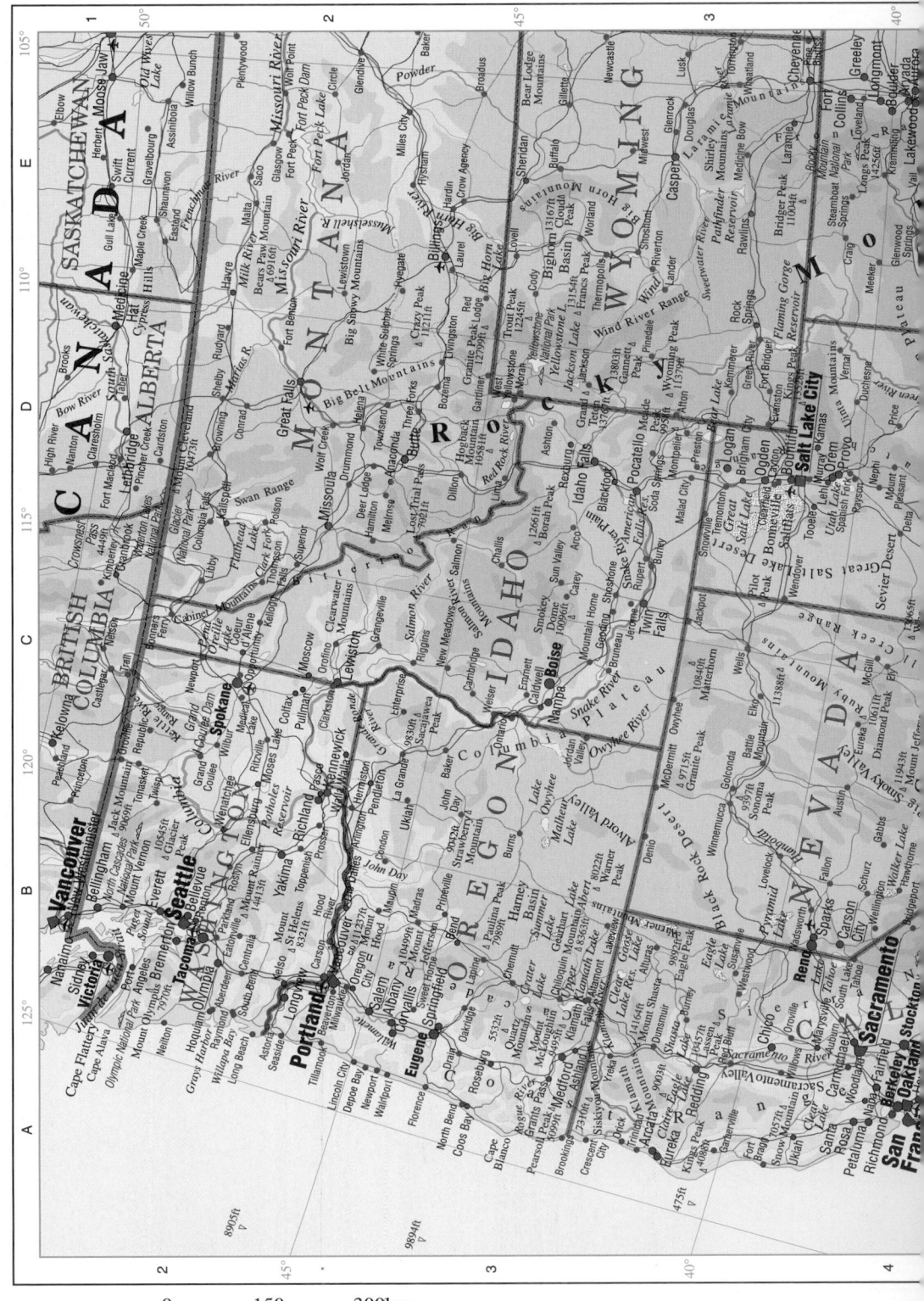

Scale 1: 10 000 000

0   150   300km

0   75   150miles

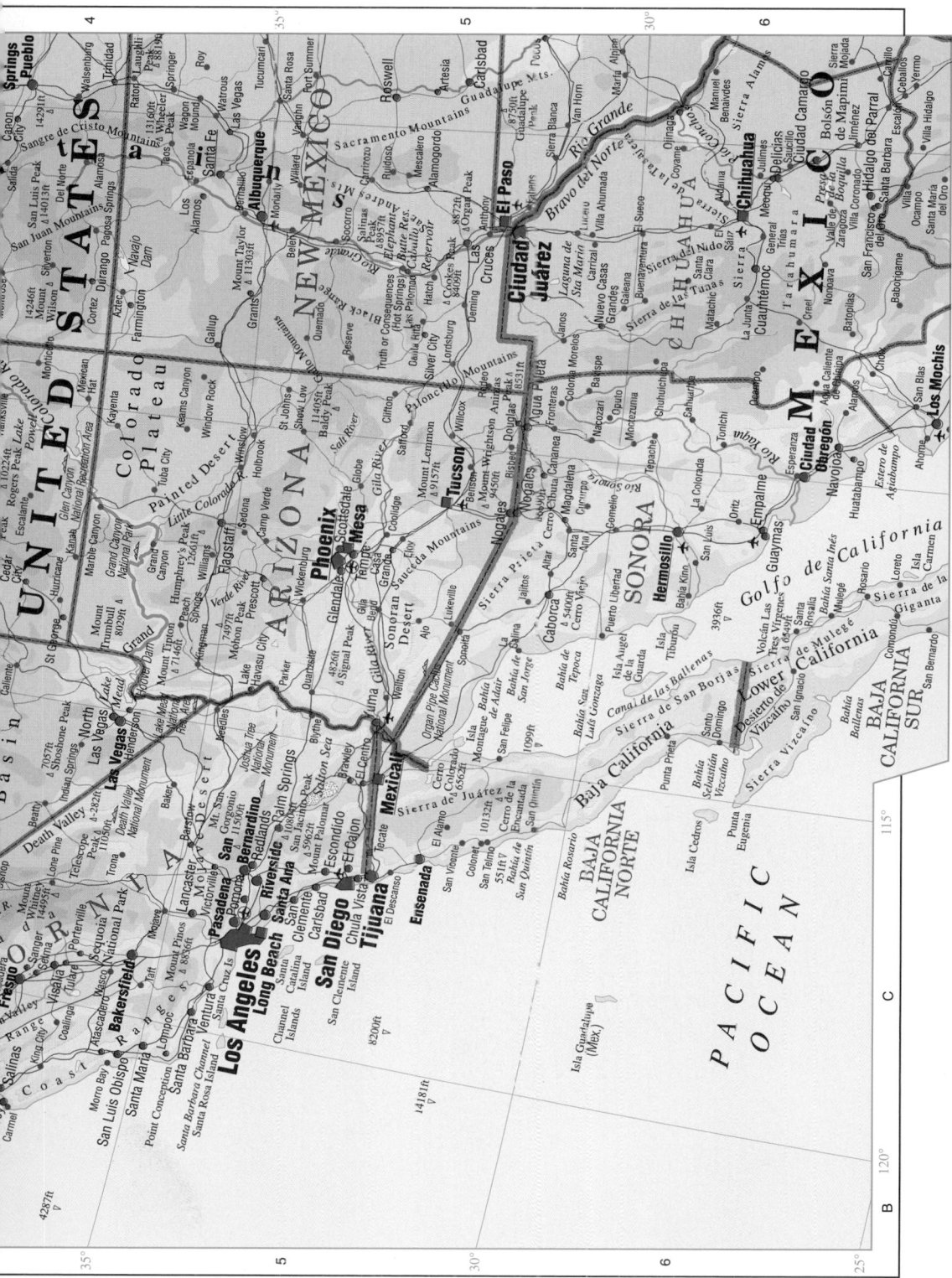

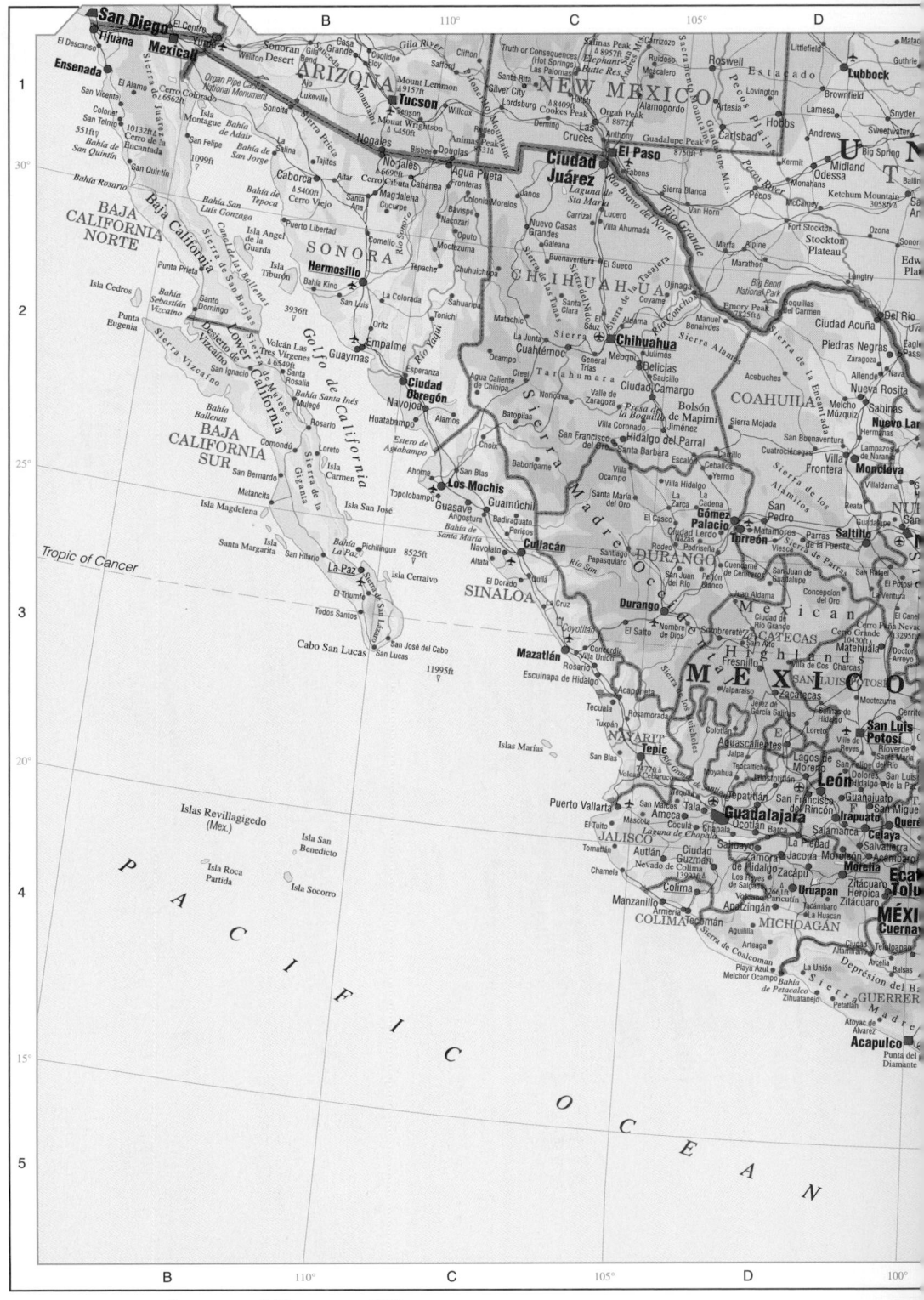

Scale 1: 12 800 000

0   200   400km

0   100   200miles

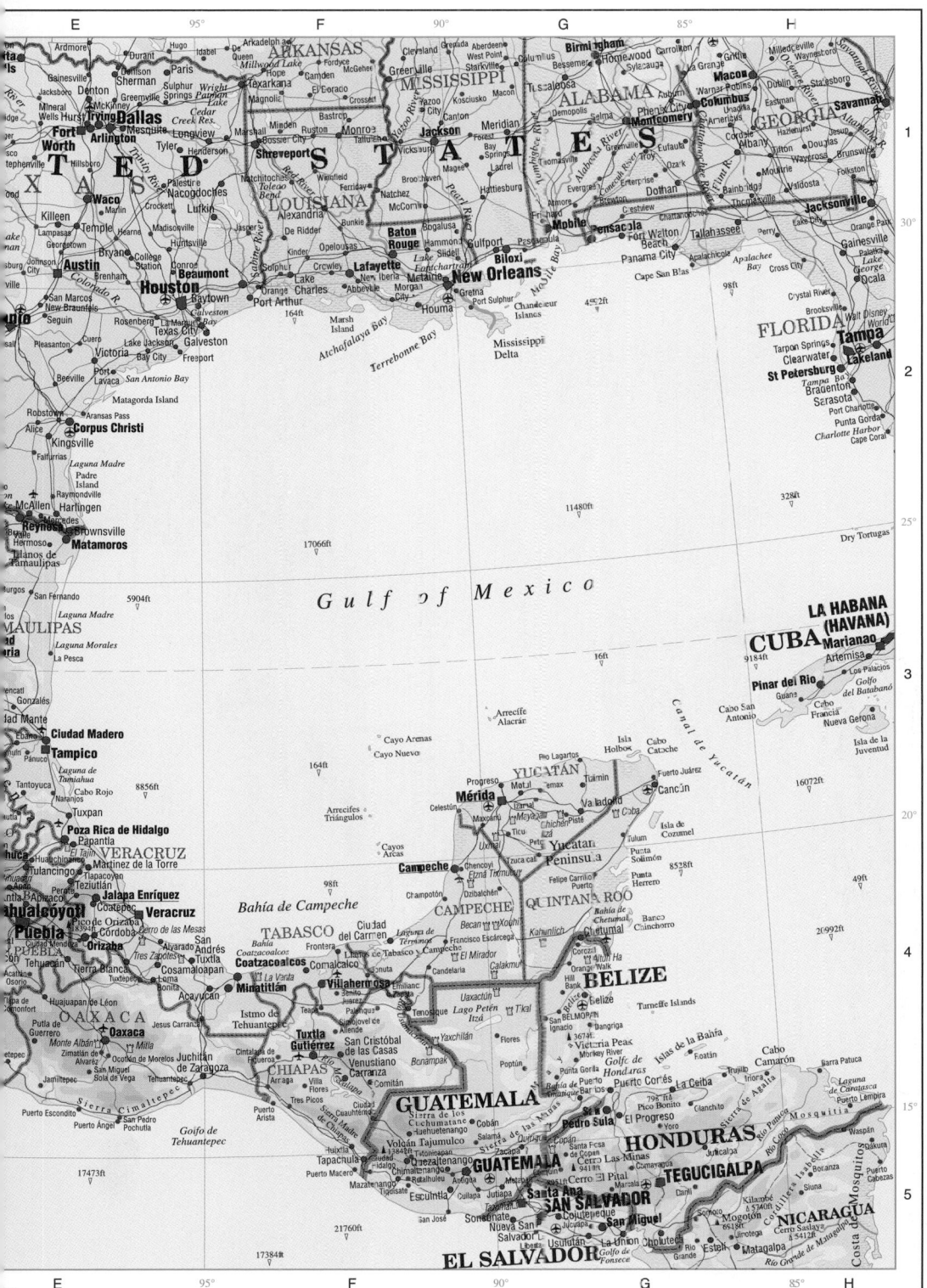

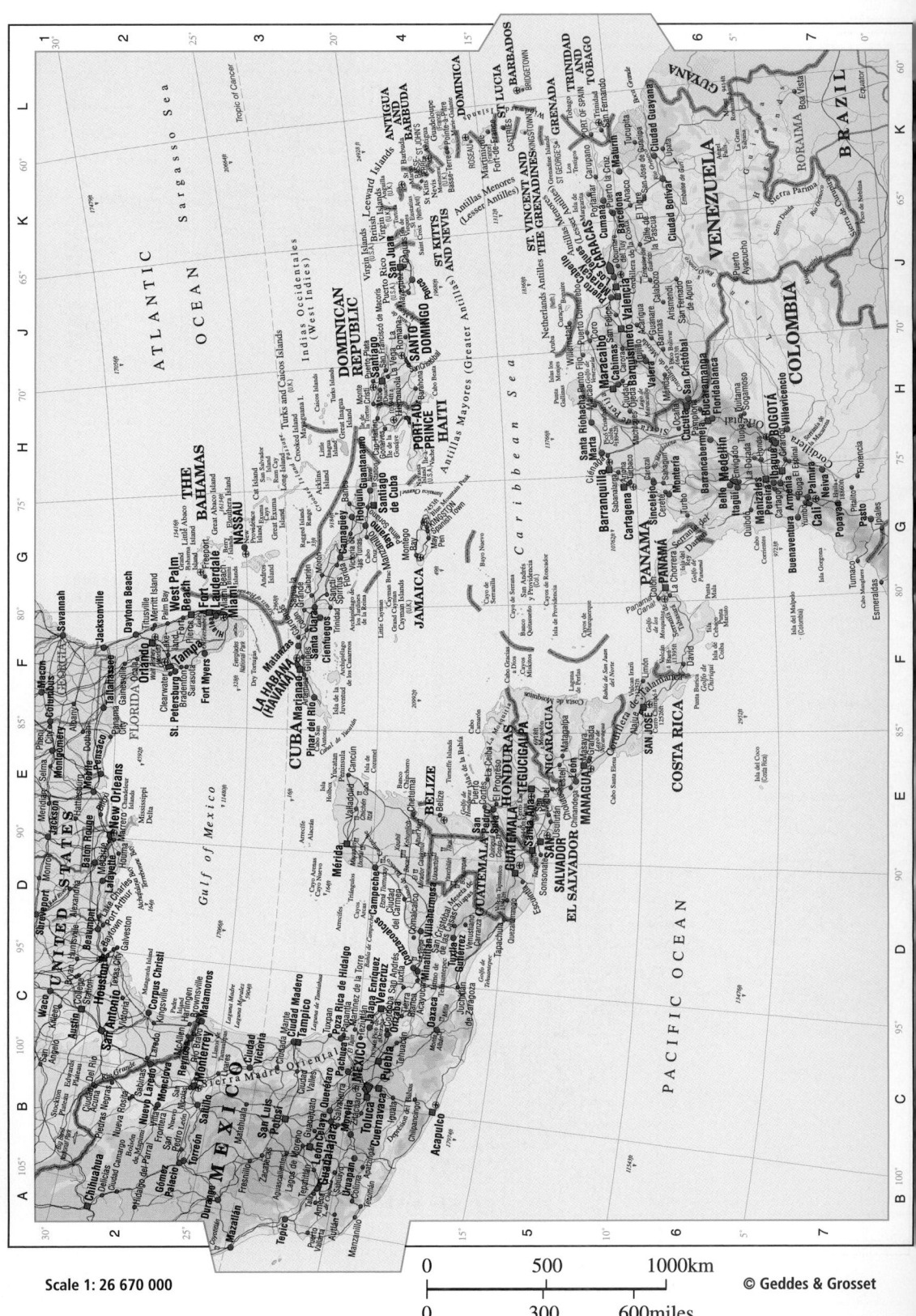

© Geddes & Grosset

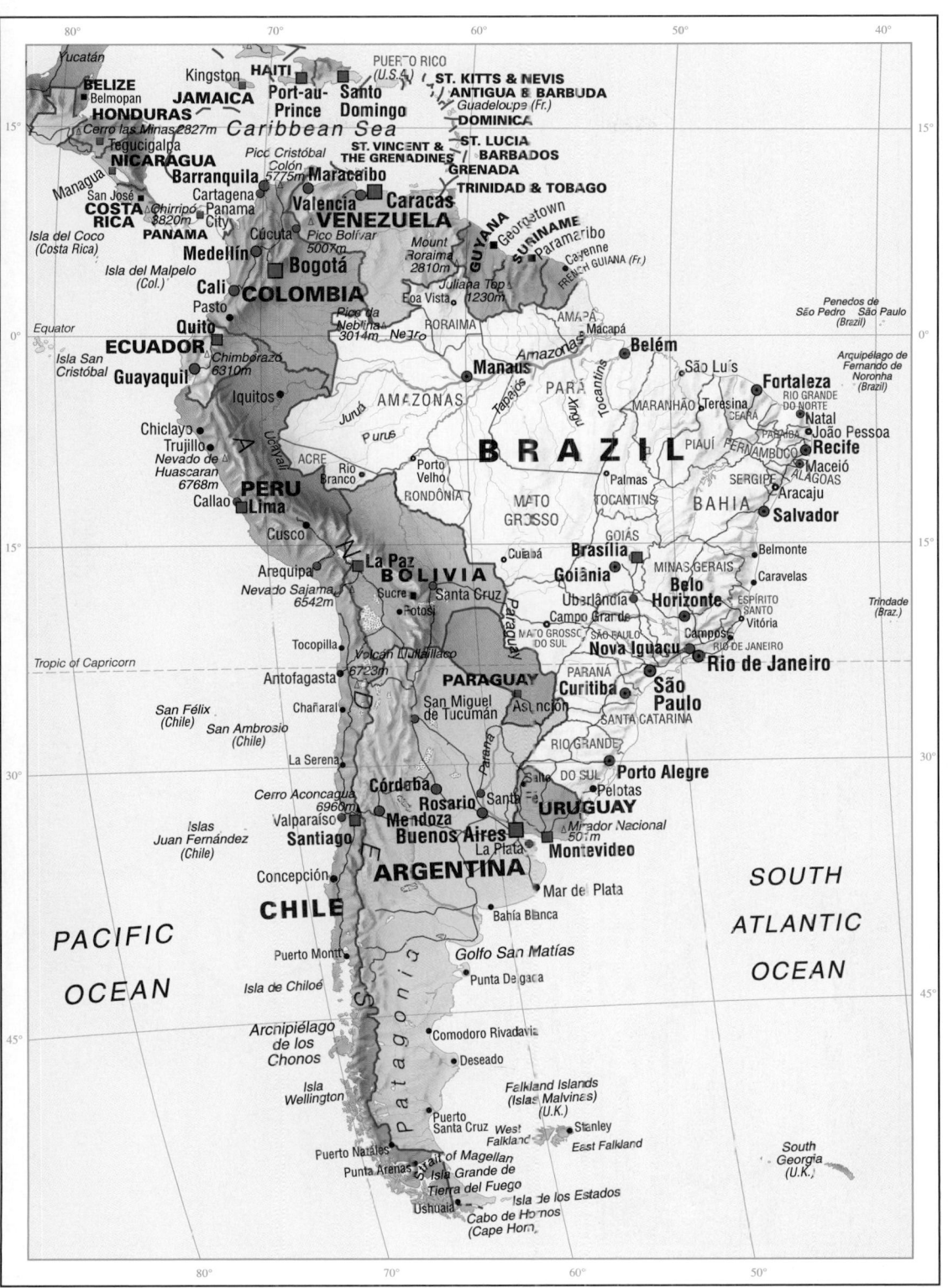

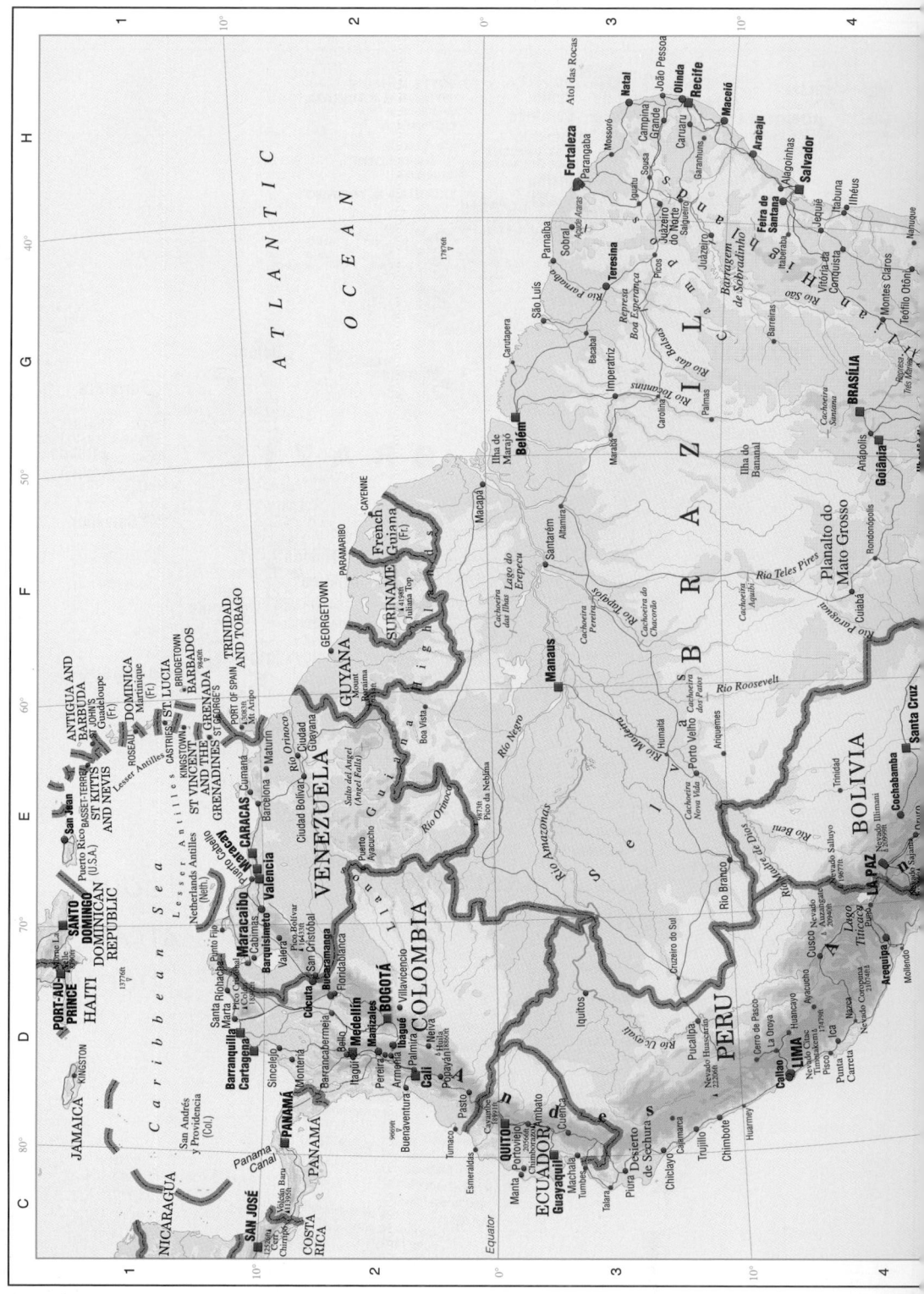

Scale 1: 31 250 000

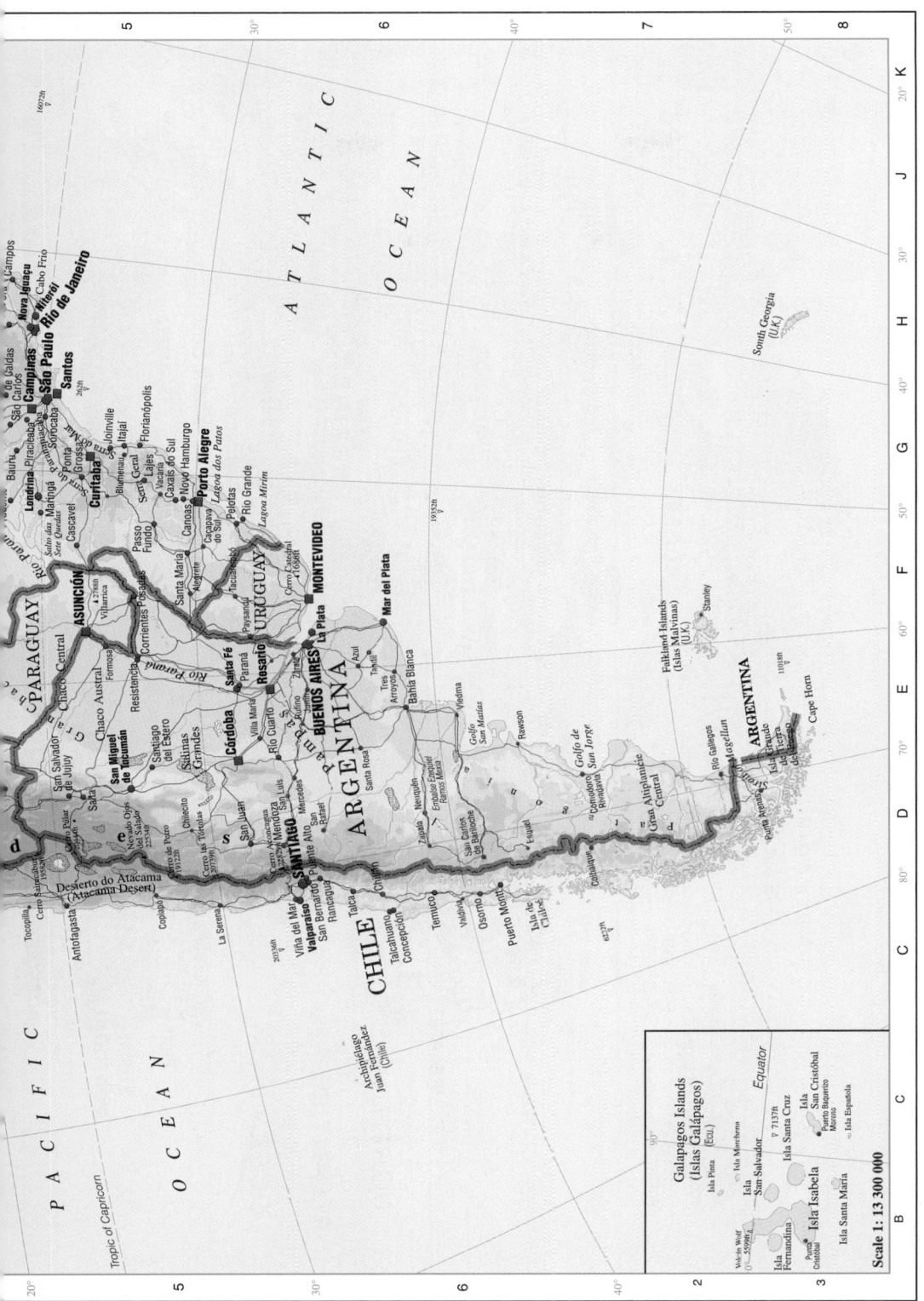

PARAGUAY

ASUNCIÓN

Londrina

Campinas
São Paulo
Nova Iguaçu
Niterói
Rio de Janeiro
Cabo Frio
Santos

Curitiba
Joinville
Florianópolis

Porto Alegre

URUGUAY
MONTEVIDEO
La Plata
Mar del Plata

Santa Fé
Paraná
Rosario
BUENOS AIRES

Córdoba

San Miguel
de Tucumán

ARGENTINA

CHILE

SANTIAGO
Valparaíso

Concepción
Temuco

Puerto Montt

Desierto do Atacama
(Atacama Desert)

Antofagasta

La Serena

Archipiélago
Juan Fernández
(Chile)

PACIFIC

OCEAN

ATLANTIC

OCEAN

Falkland Islands
(Islas Malvinas)
(U.K.)
Stanley

South Georgia
(U.K.)

Cape Horn
ARGENTINA

Golfo de
San Jorge

Golfo
San Matías

Río Gallegos

Tropic of Capricorn

Galapagos Islands
(Islas Galápagos)

Equator

Isla
San Salvador

Isla
Isla Santa Cruz
Isla
San Cristóbal
Puerto Baquerizo
Moreno
Isla Española

Isla
Fernandina
Isla Isabela
Isla Santa María

Scale 1: 13 300 000

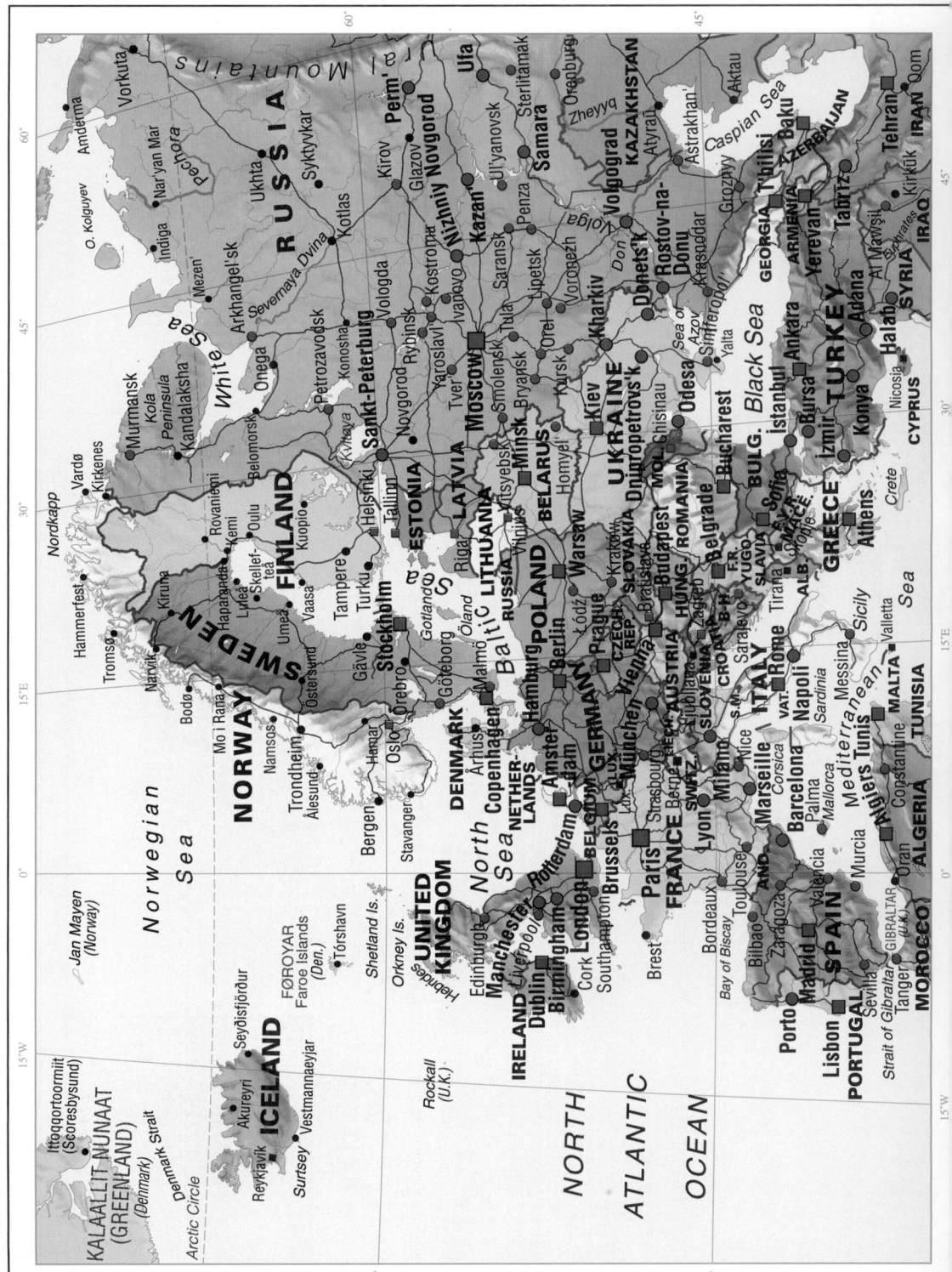

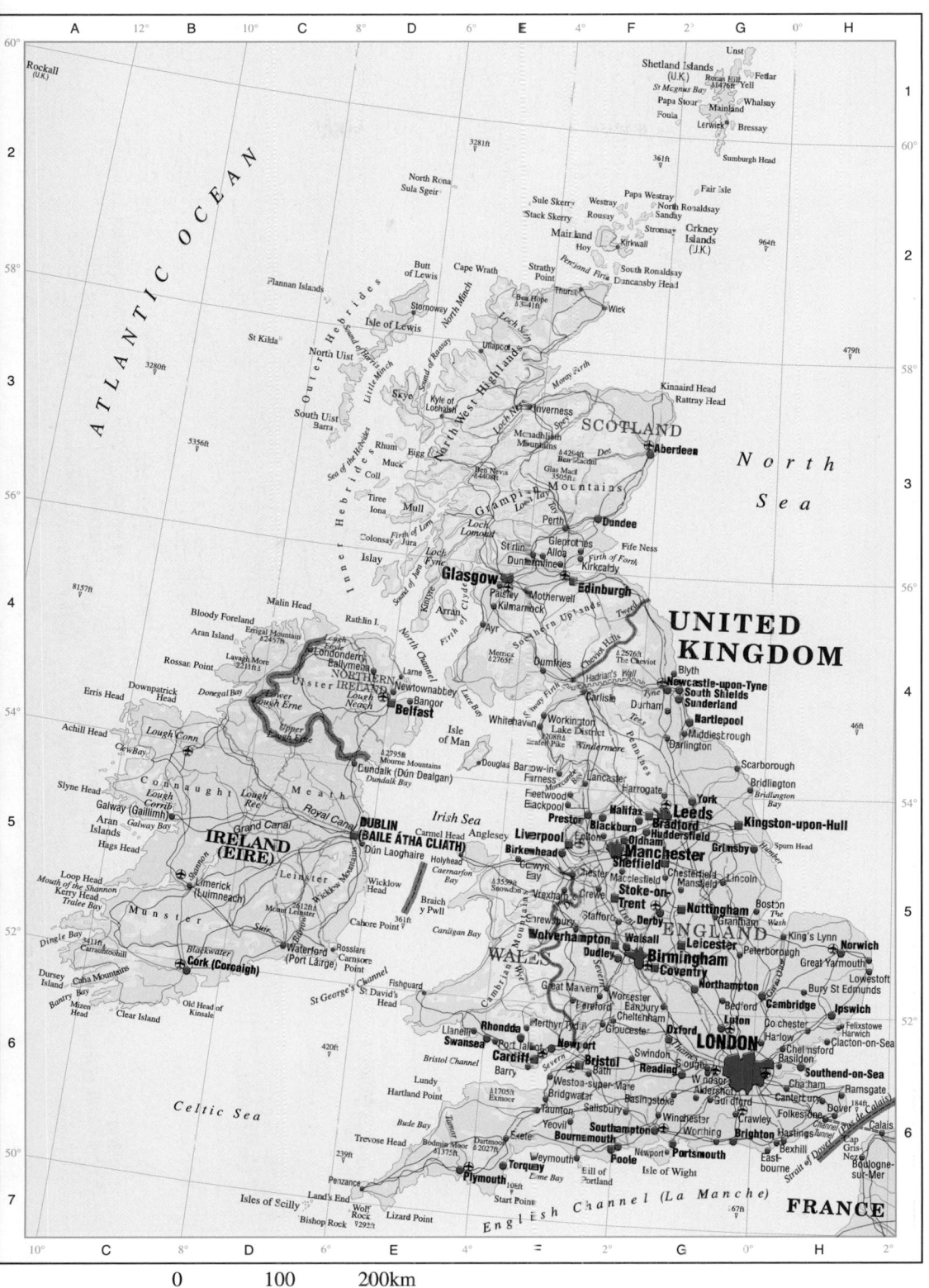

Scale 1: 6 670 000

| 0 | 100 | 200km |

| 0 | 50 | 100miles |

© Geddes & Grosset

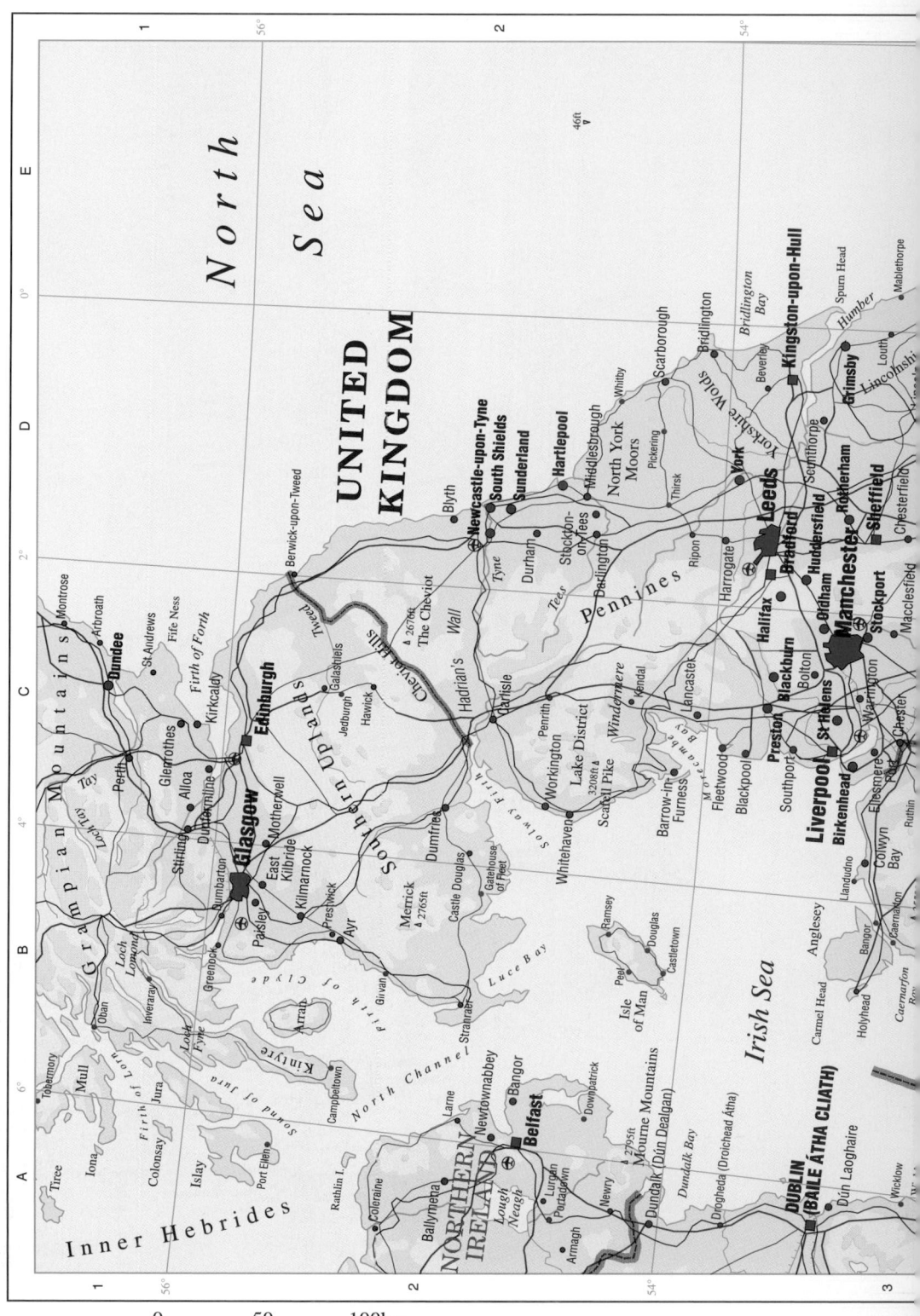

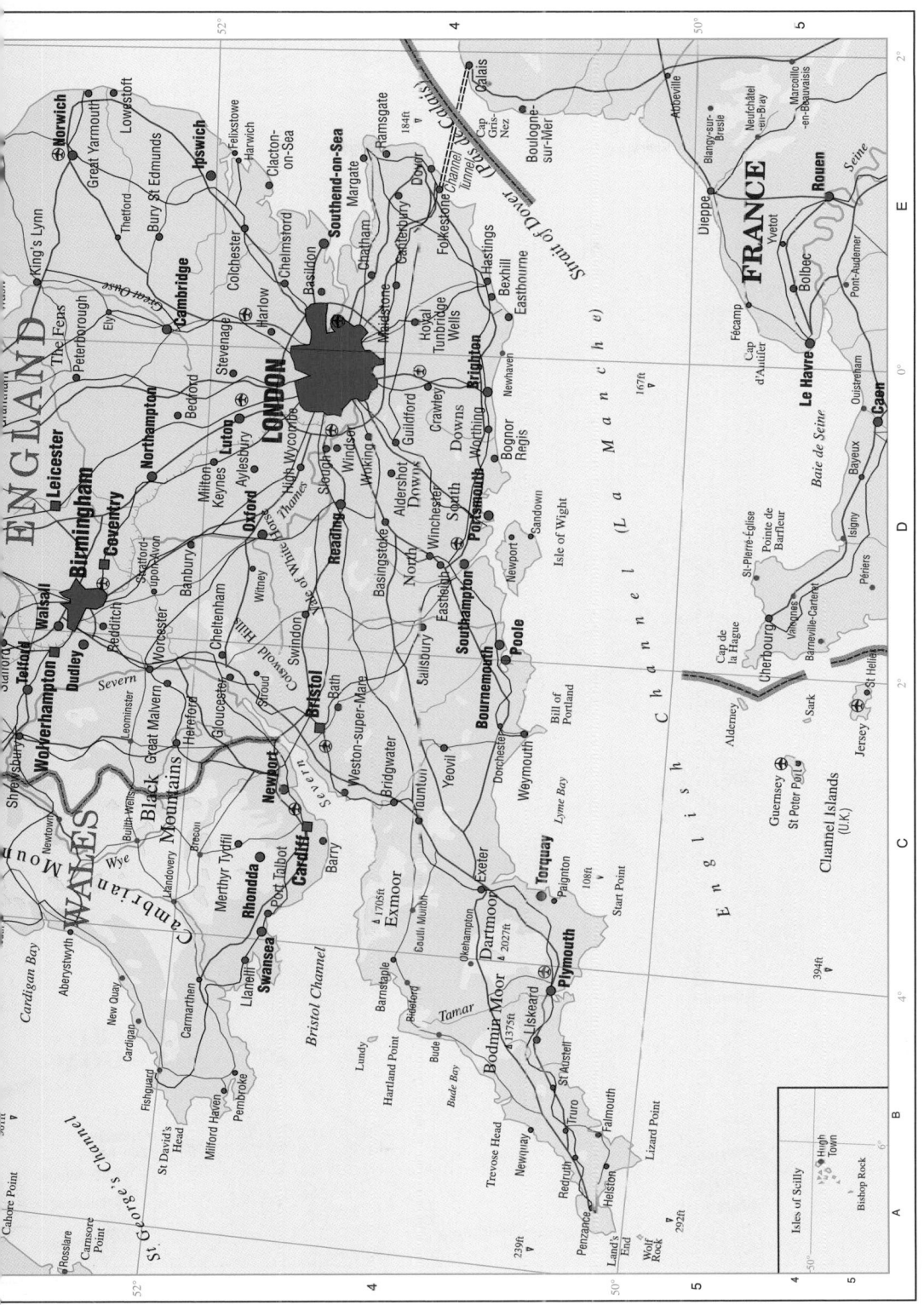

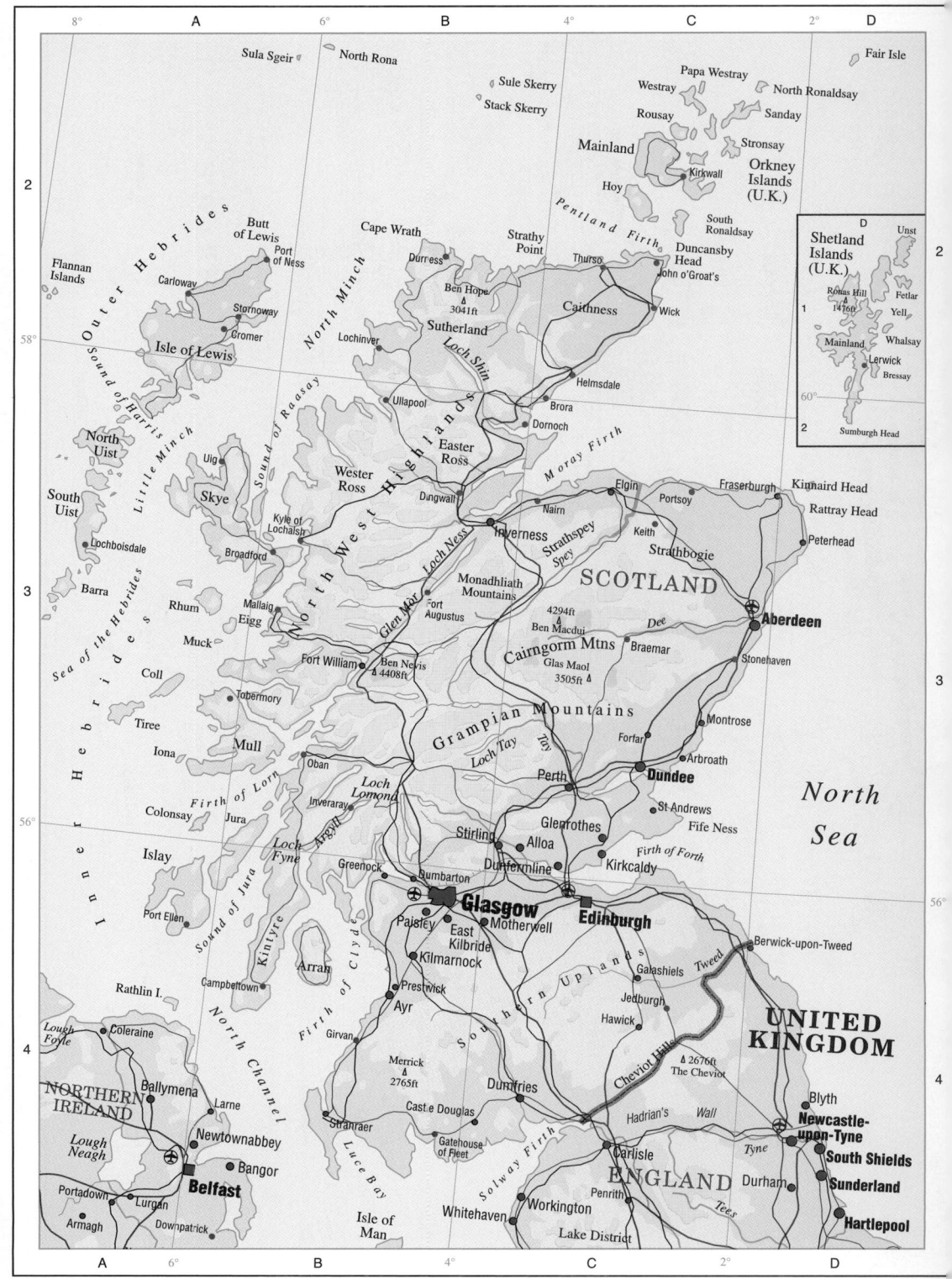

Scale 1: 3 117 000

0 — 50 — 100km

0 — 25 — 50miles

© Geddes & Grosset

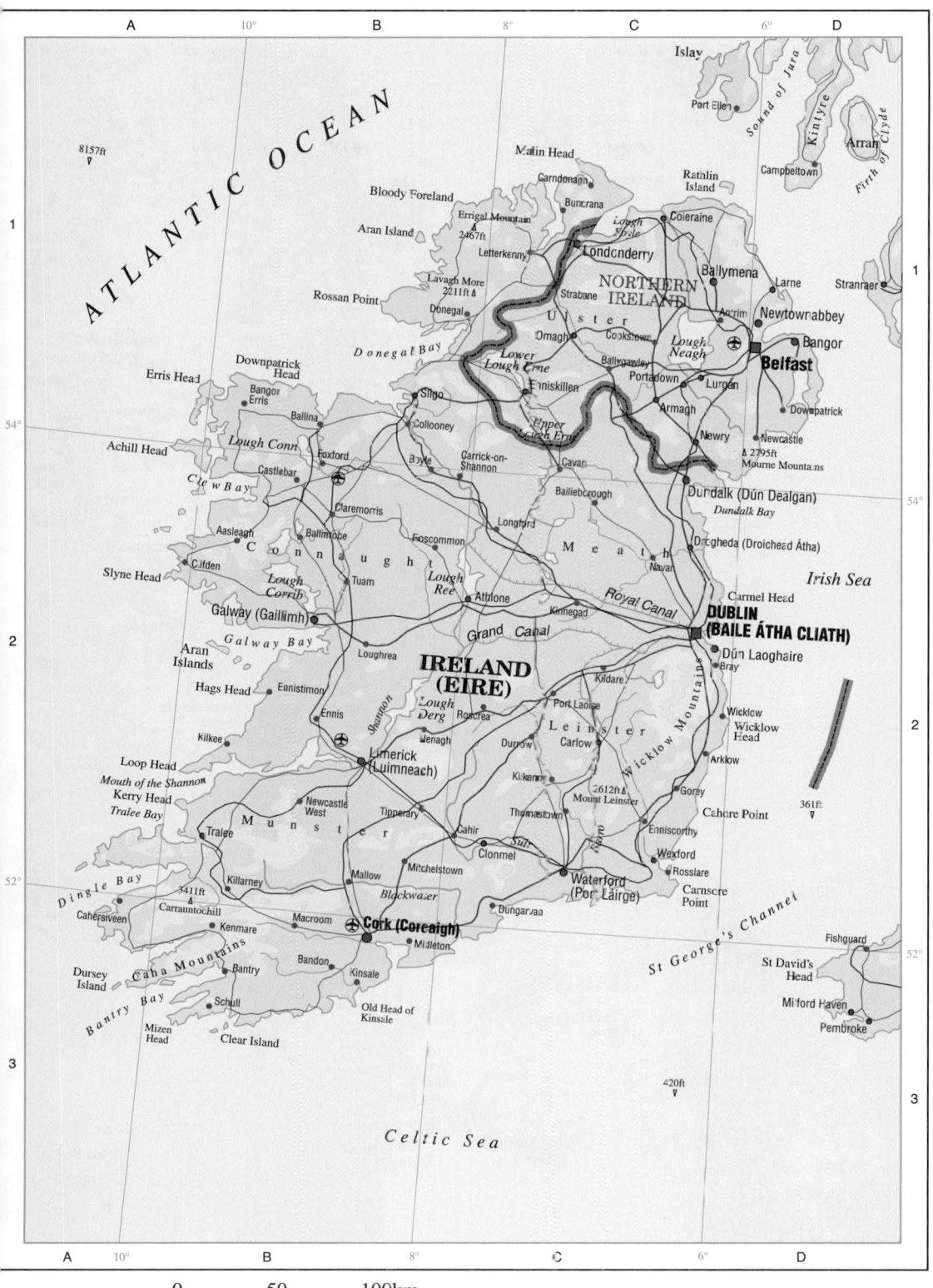

Scale 1: 3 335 000   0   50   100km

0   25   50miles

© Geddes & Grosset

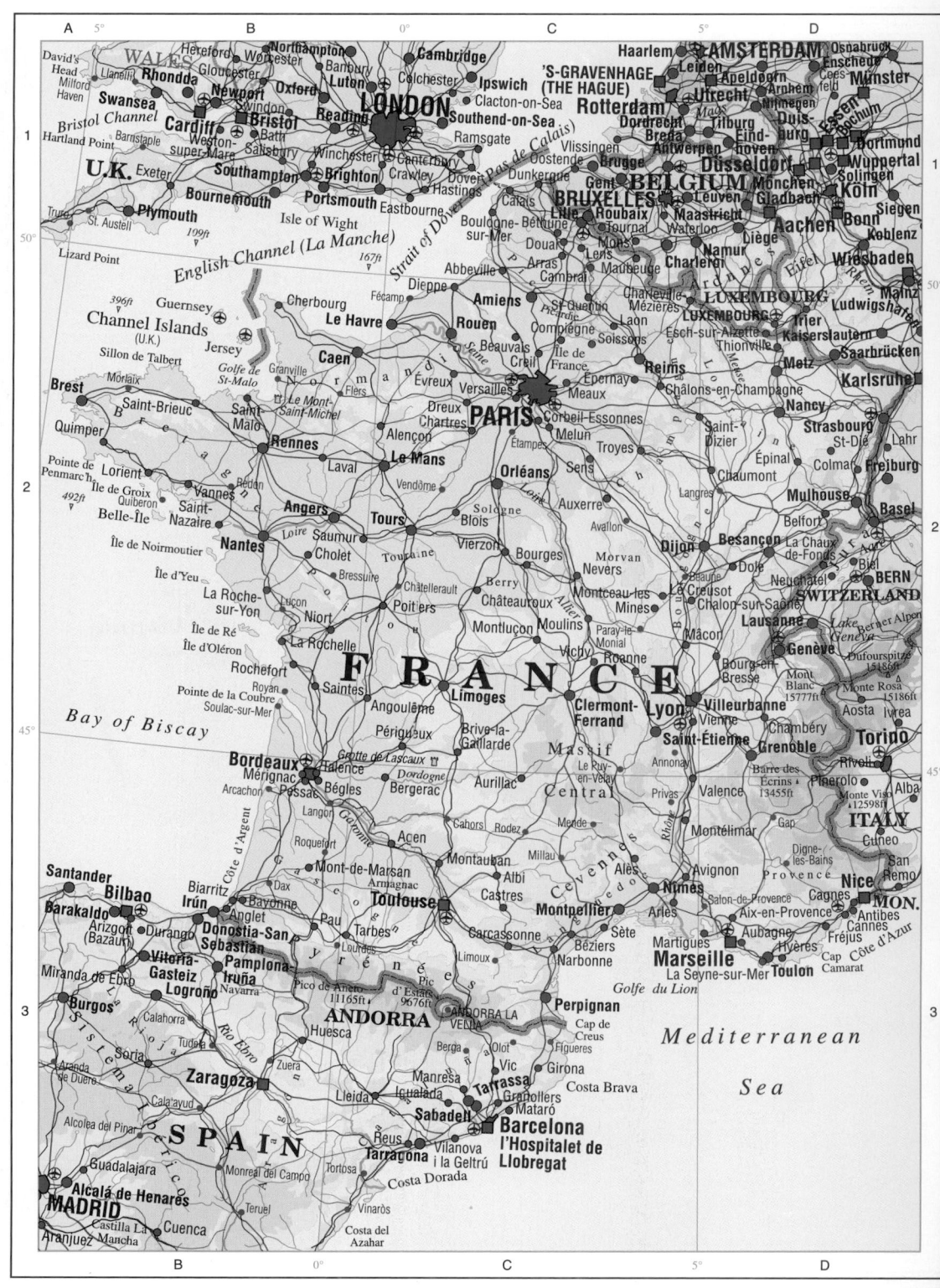

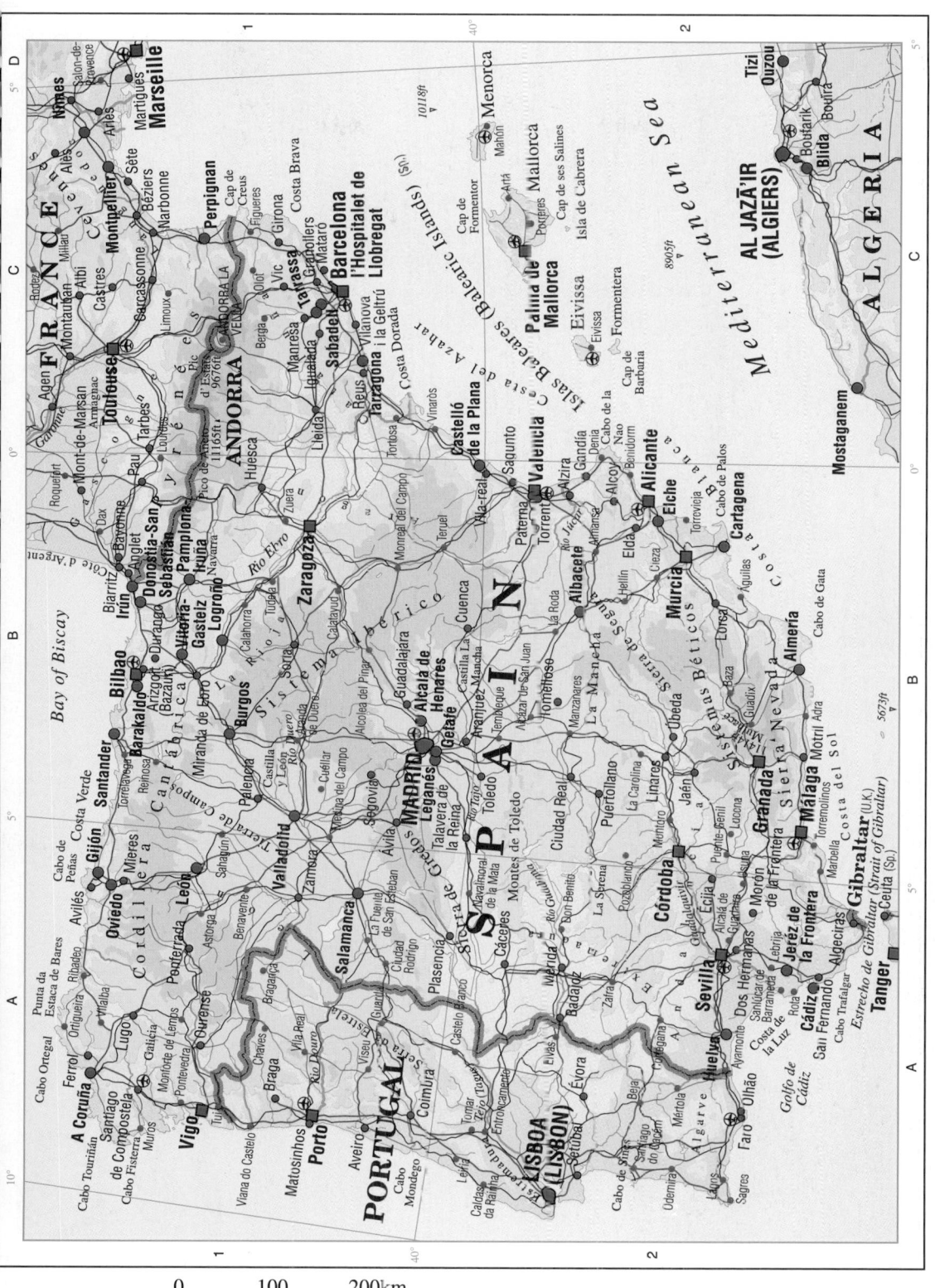

Scale 1: 7 143 000

0   100   200km

0   50   100miles

© Geddes & Grosset

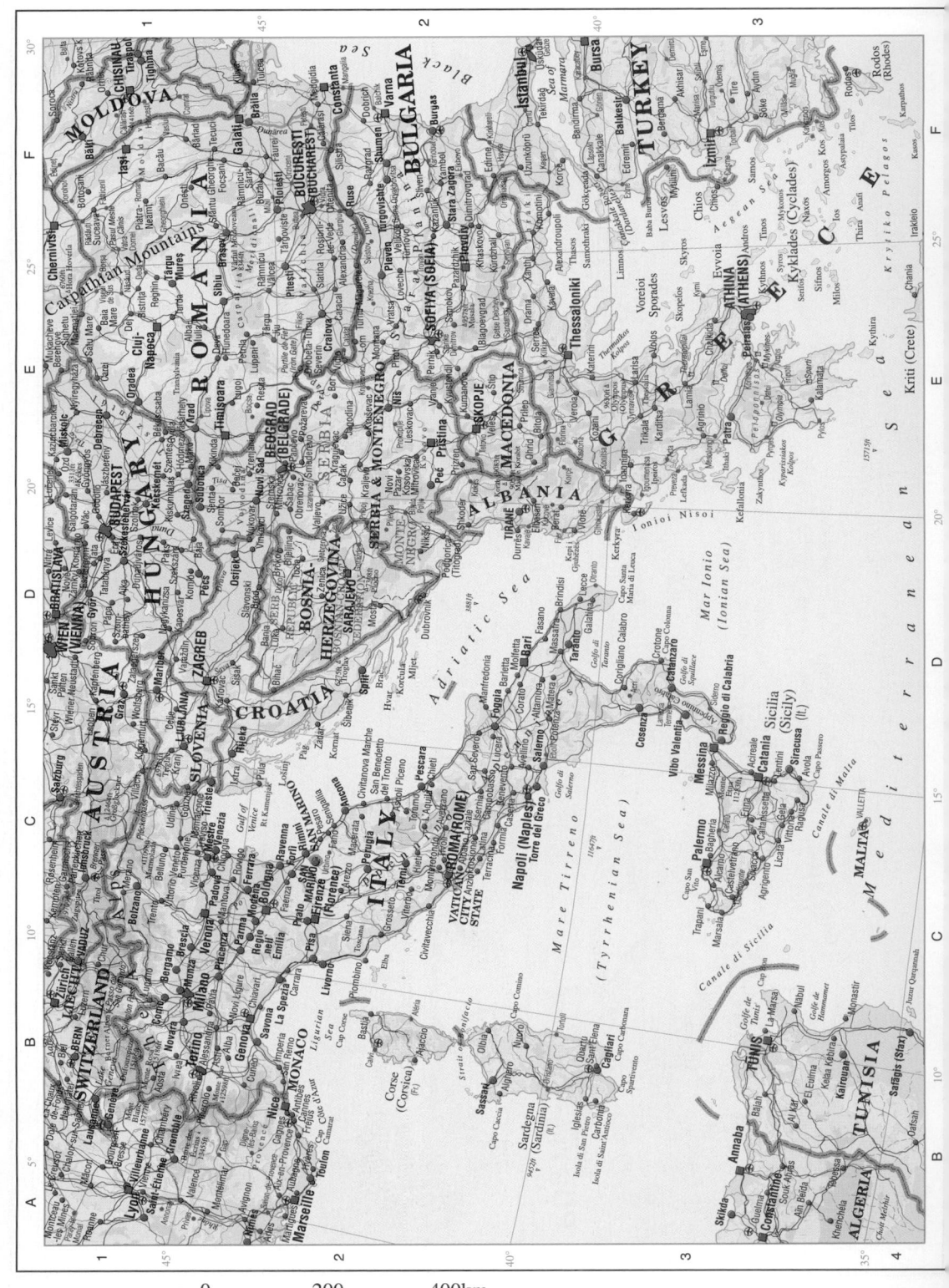

Scale 1: 10 893 000

0   200   400km

0   100   200miles

© Geddes & Grosset

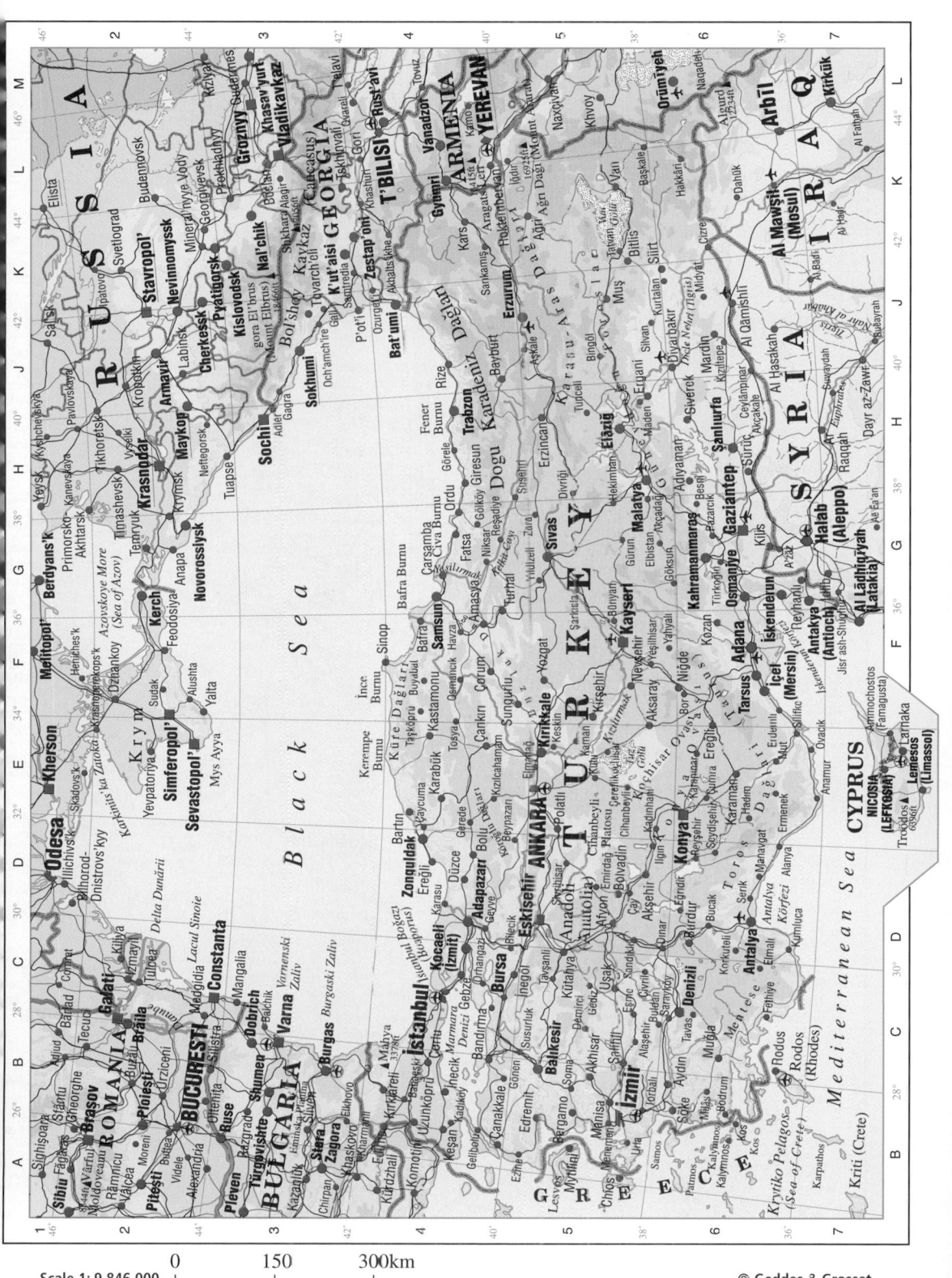

Scale 1: 9 846 000

0   150   300km

0   75   150miles

© Geddes & Grosset

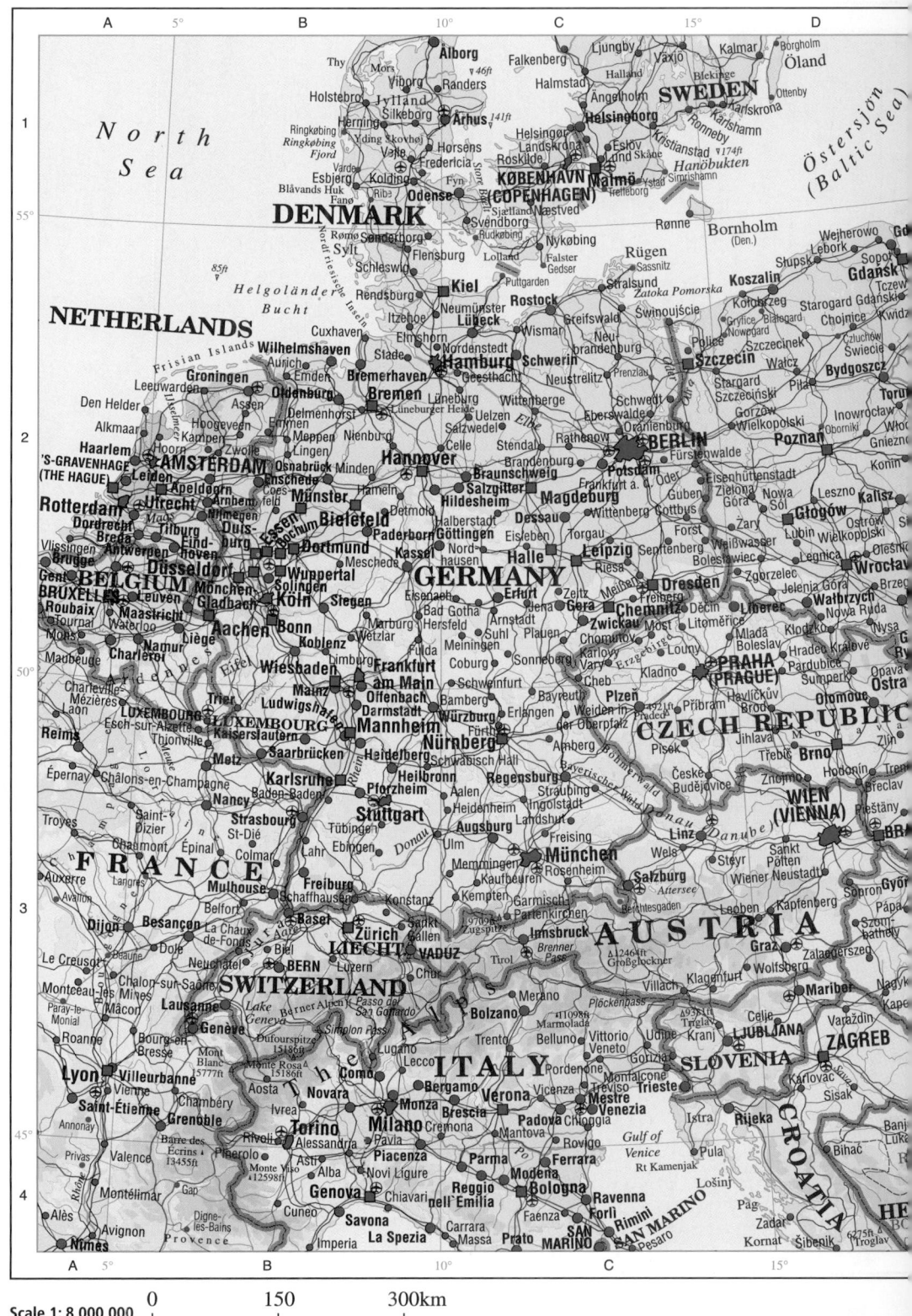

Scale 1: 8 000 000

| 0 | 150 | 300km |

| 0 | 75 | 150miles |

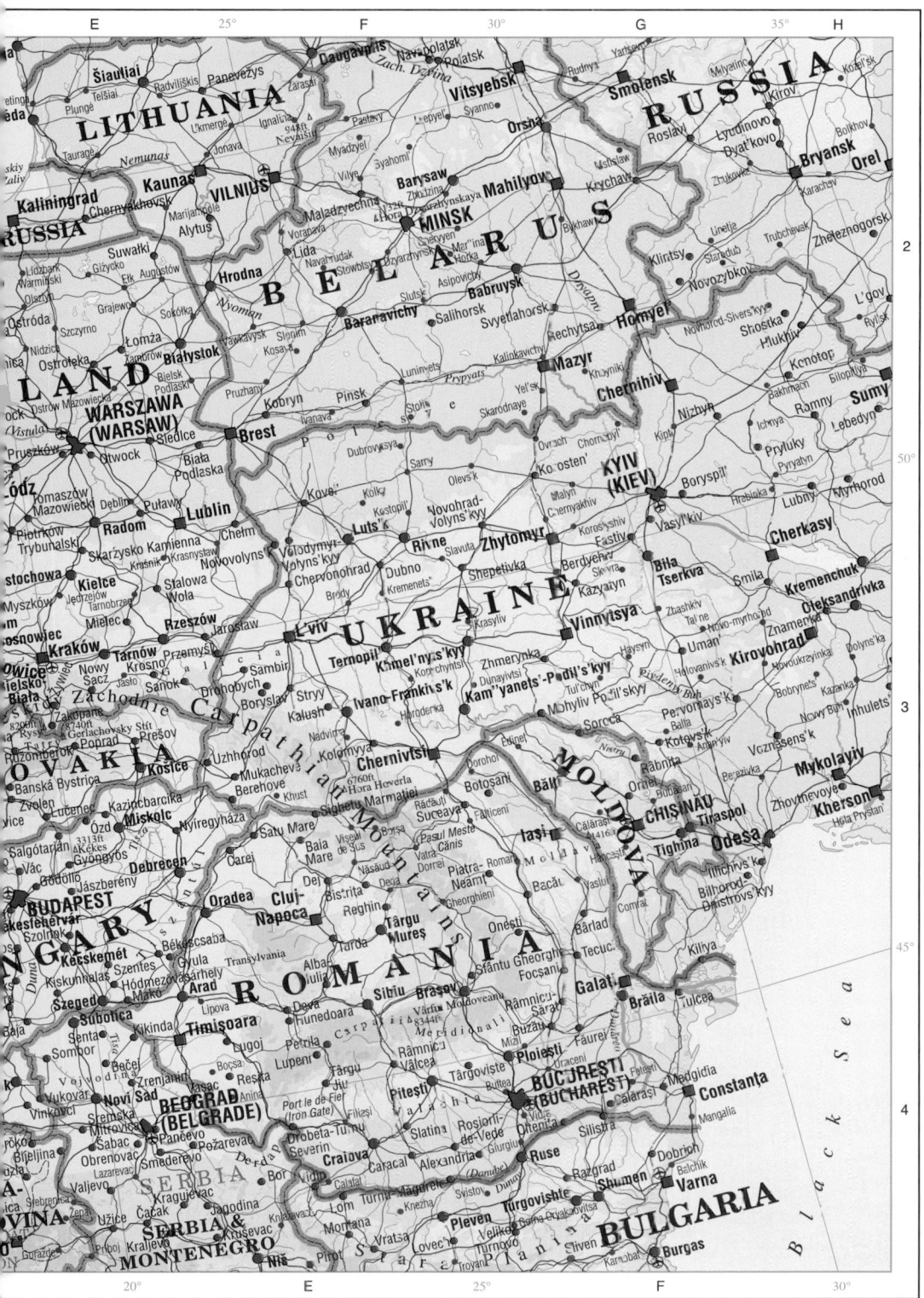

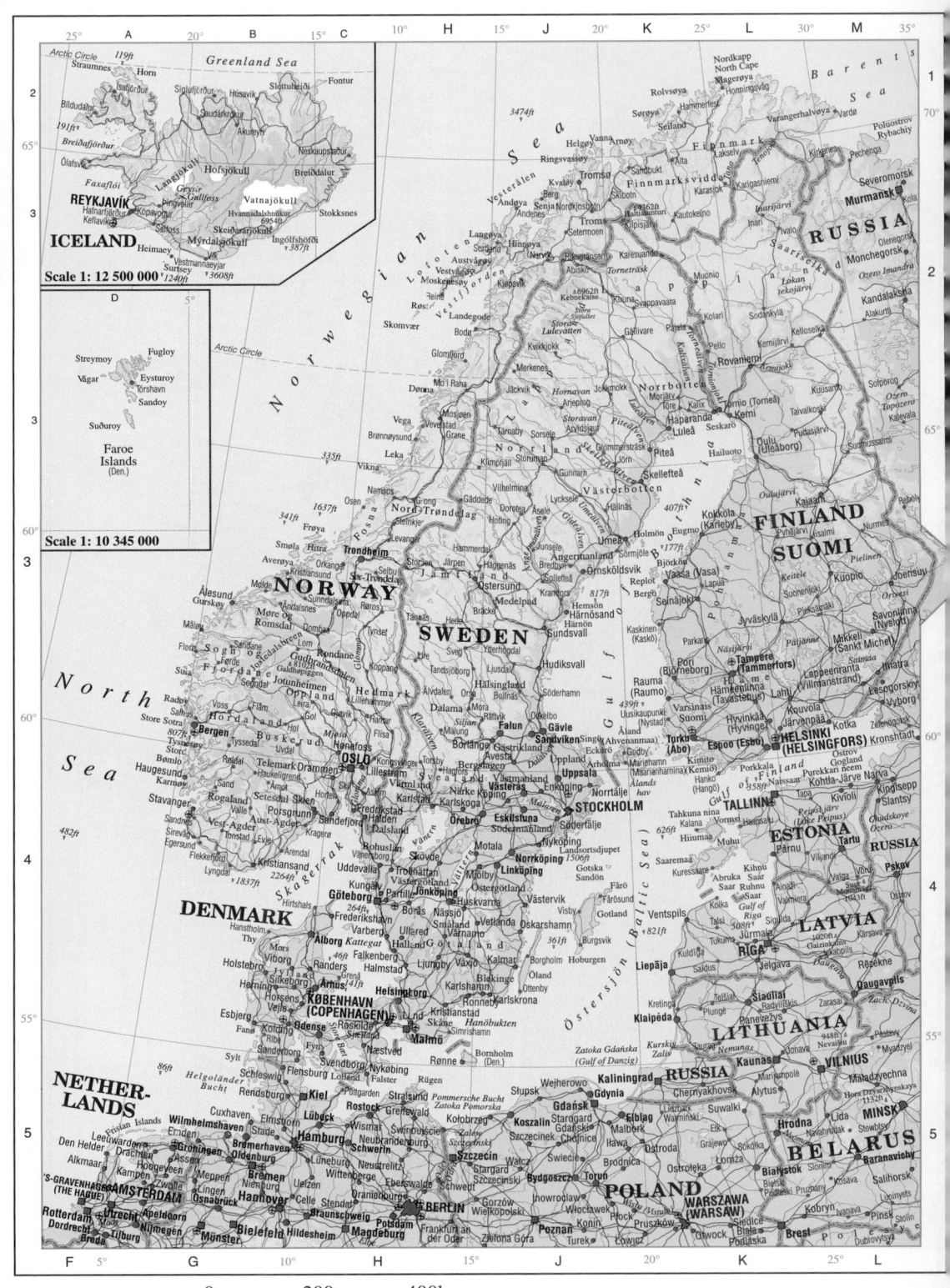

Scale 1: 12 500 000

0   200   400km

0   100   200miles

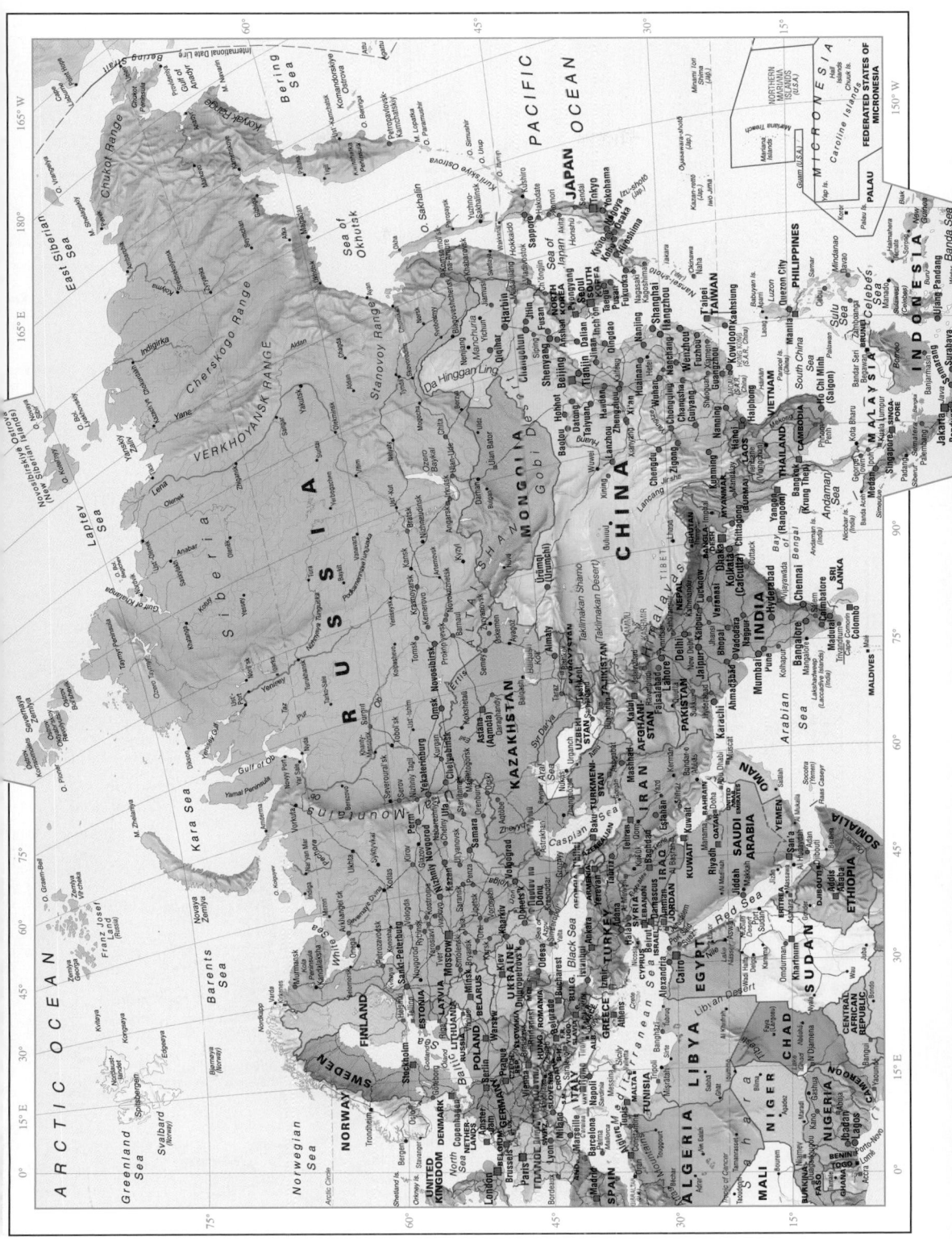

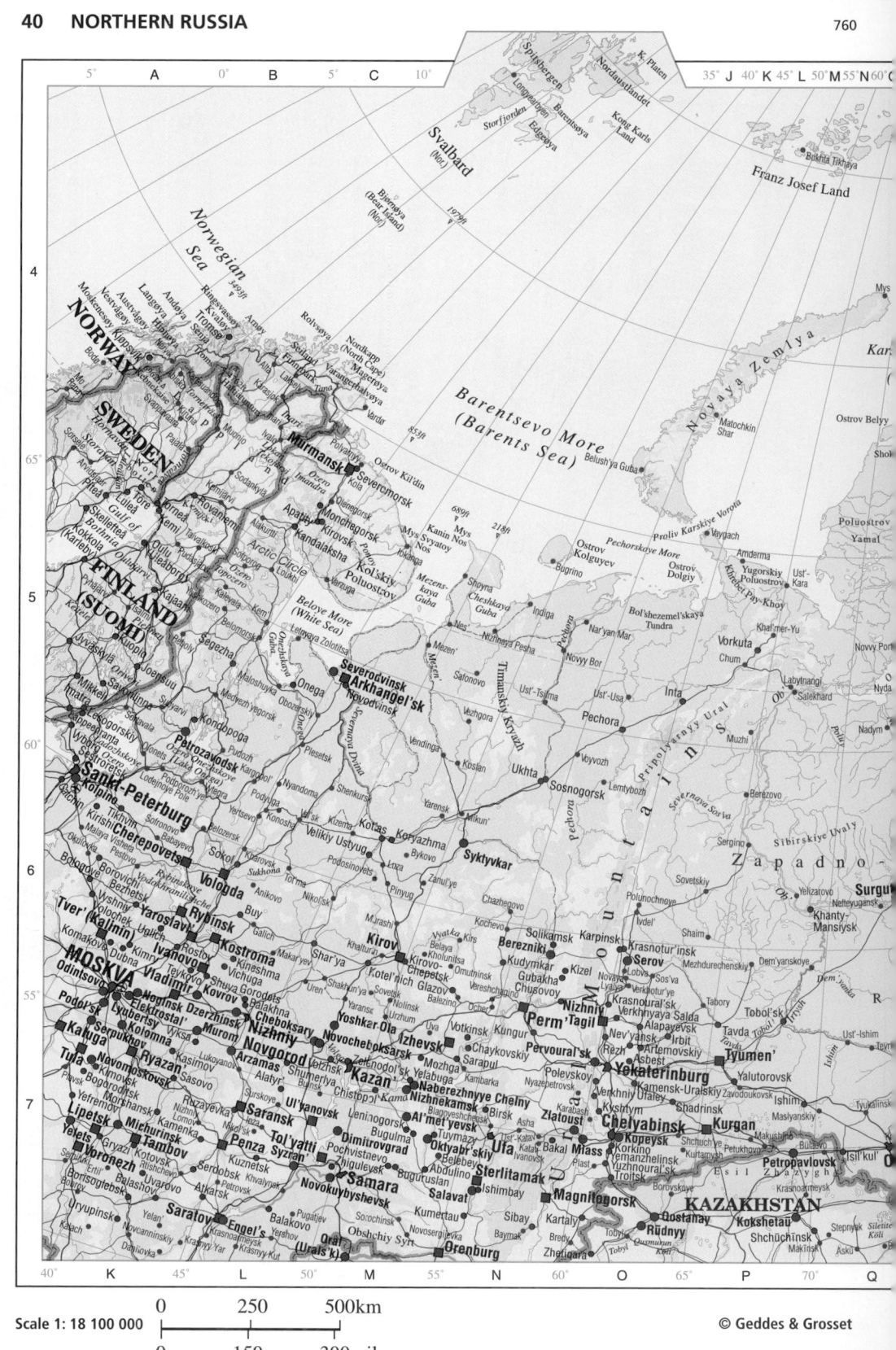

0   250   500km

0   150   300miles

© Geddes & Grosset

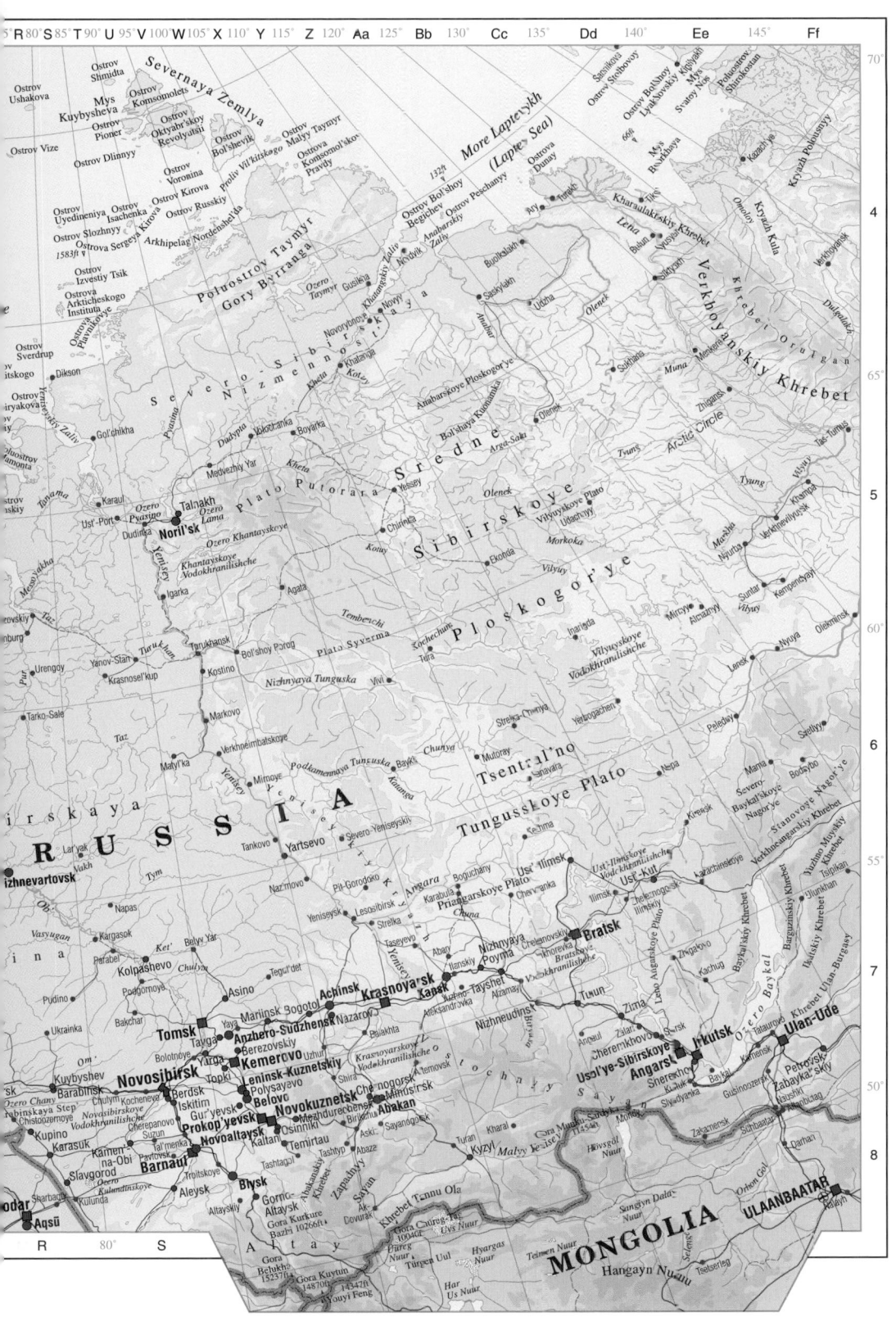

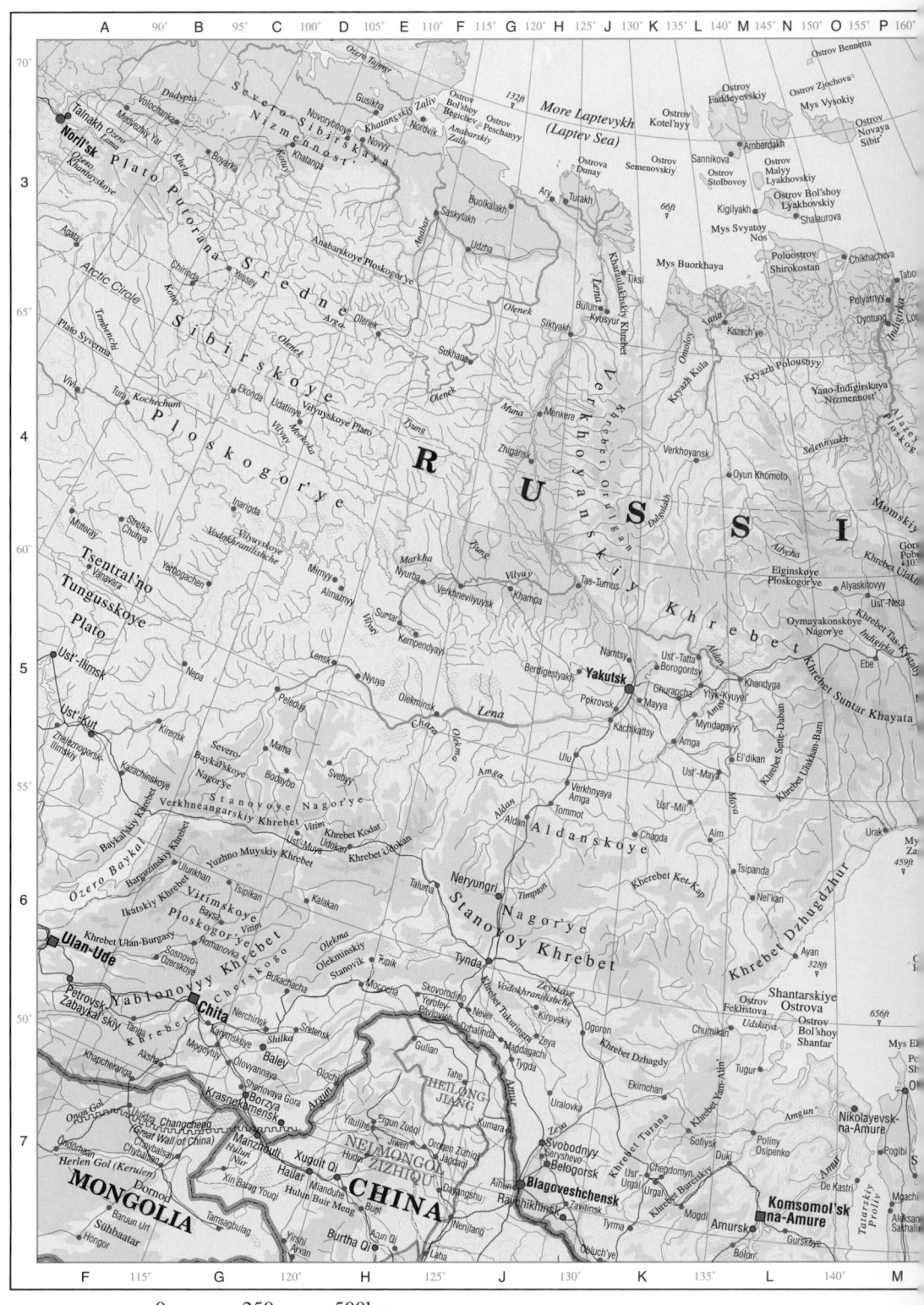

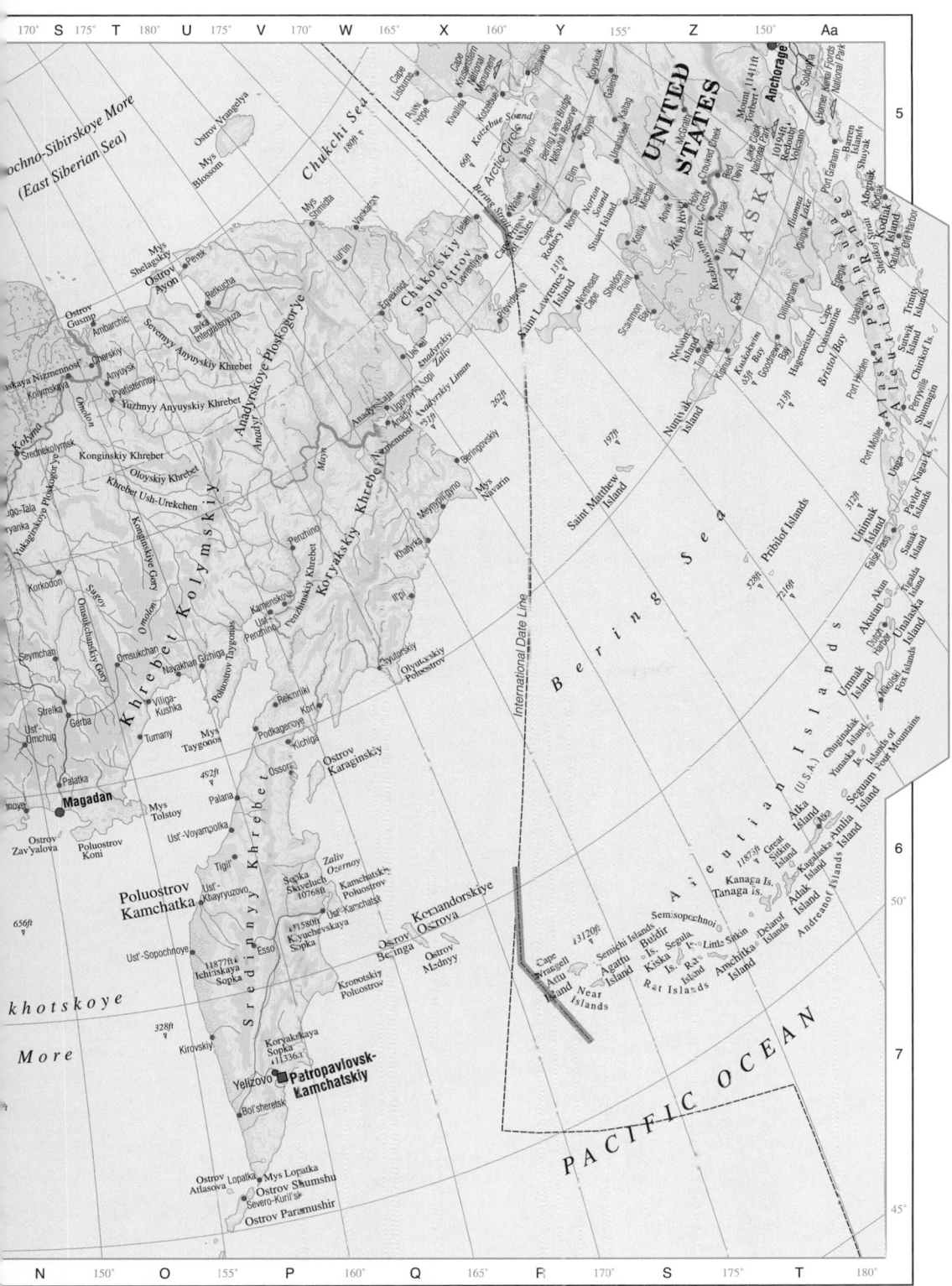

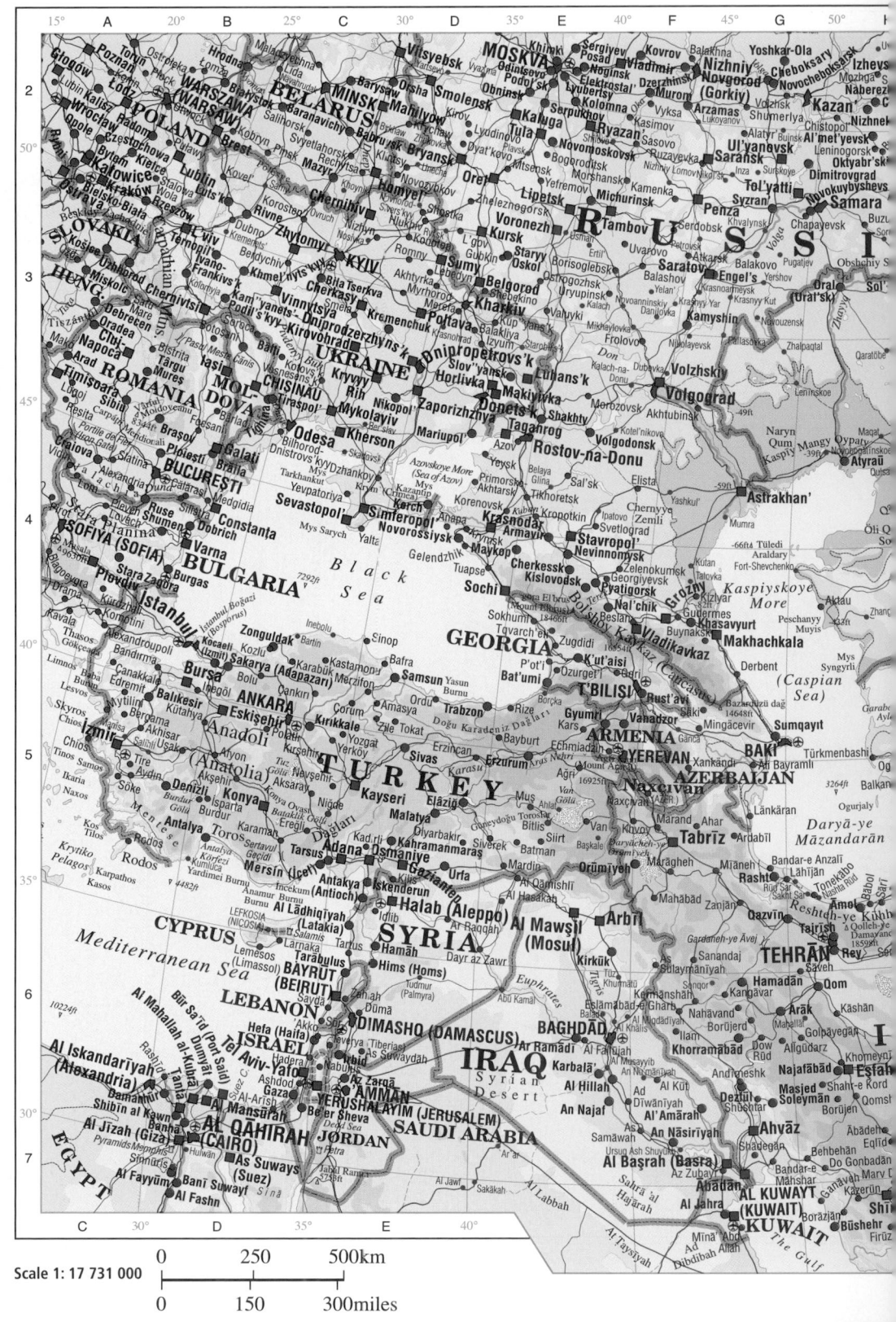

Scale 1: 17 731 000

0   250   500km

0   150   300miles

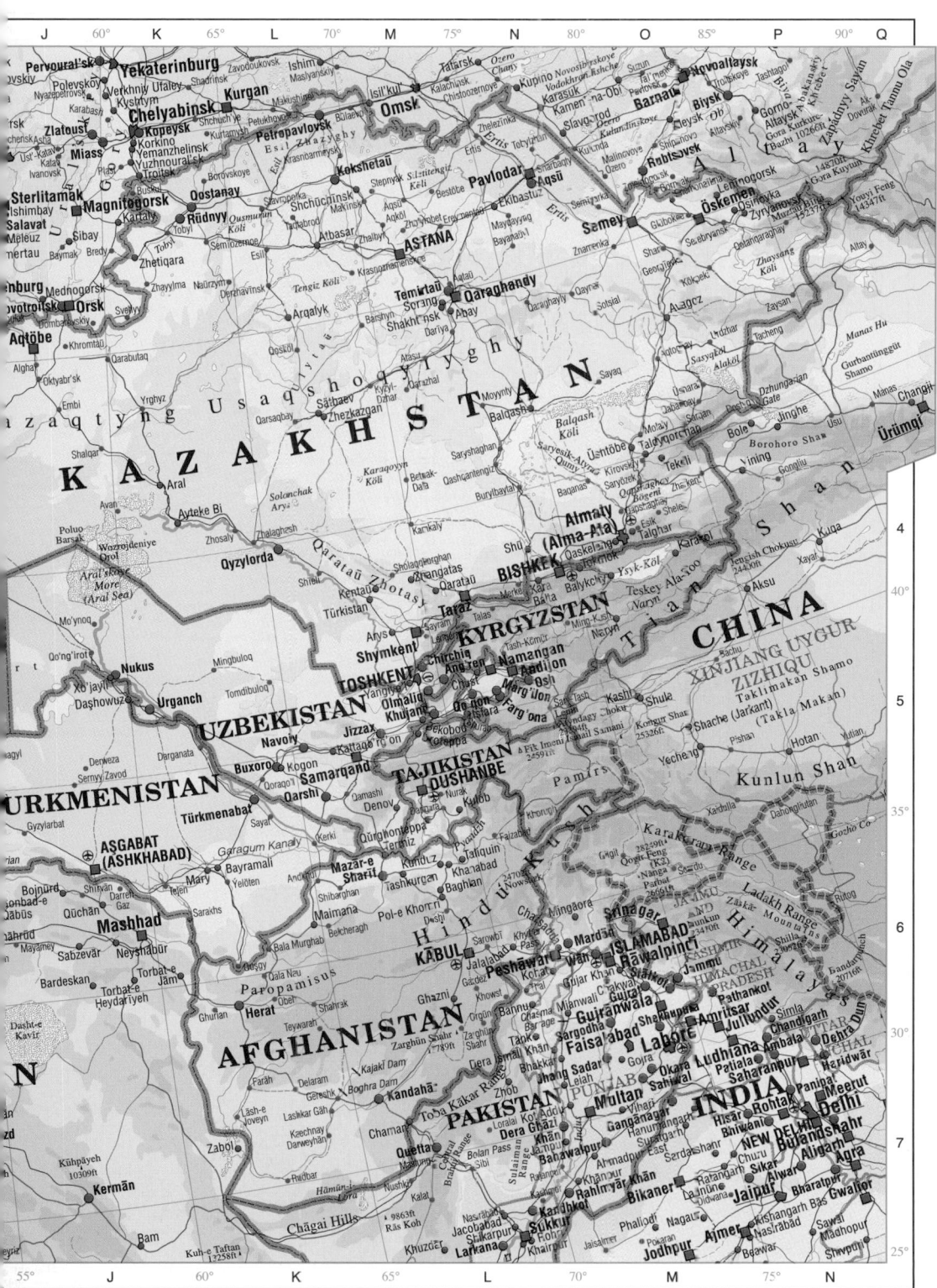

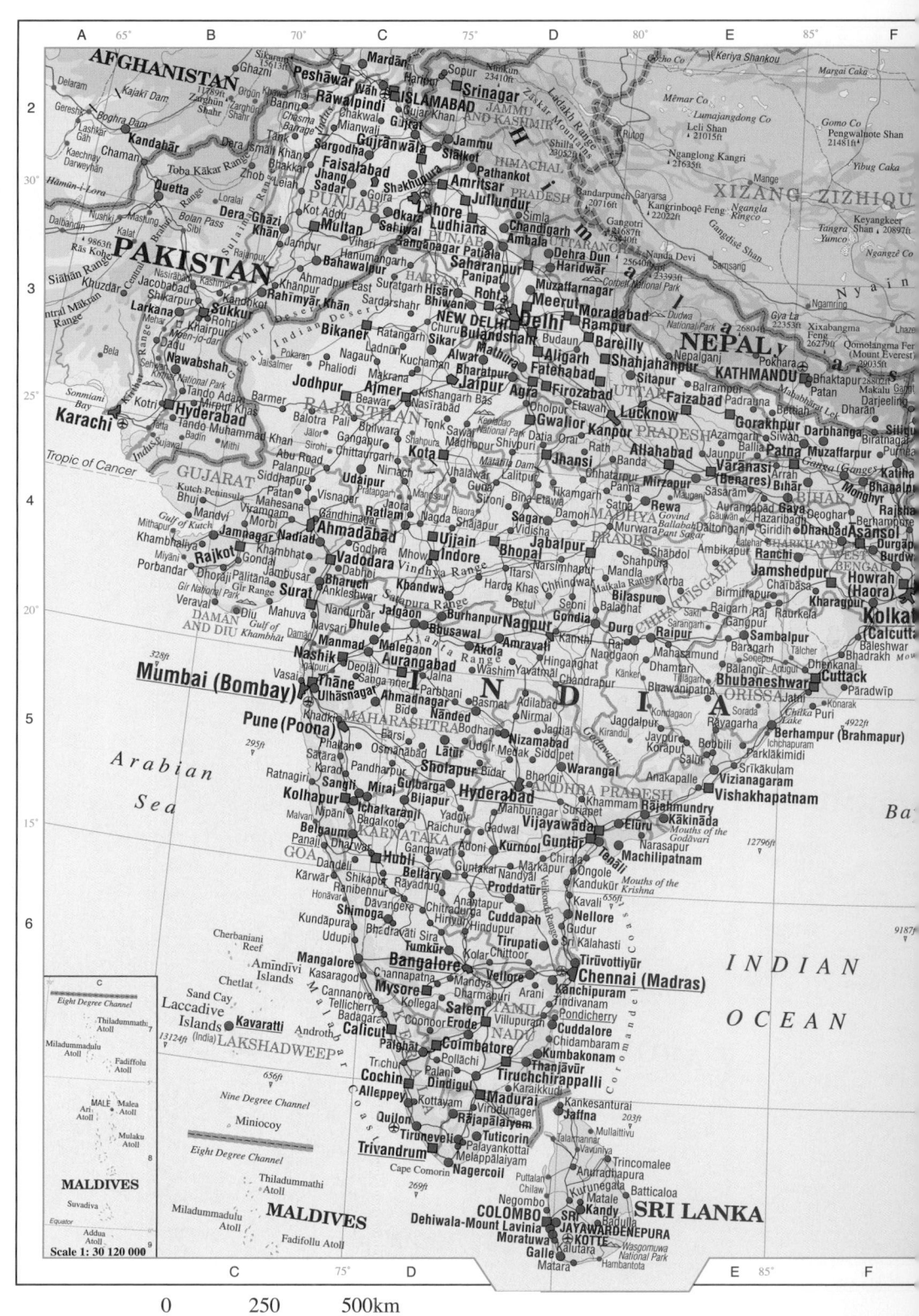

Scale 1: 30 120 000

Scale 1: 17 705 000

0   250   500km

0   150   300miles

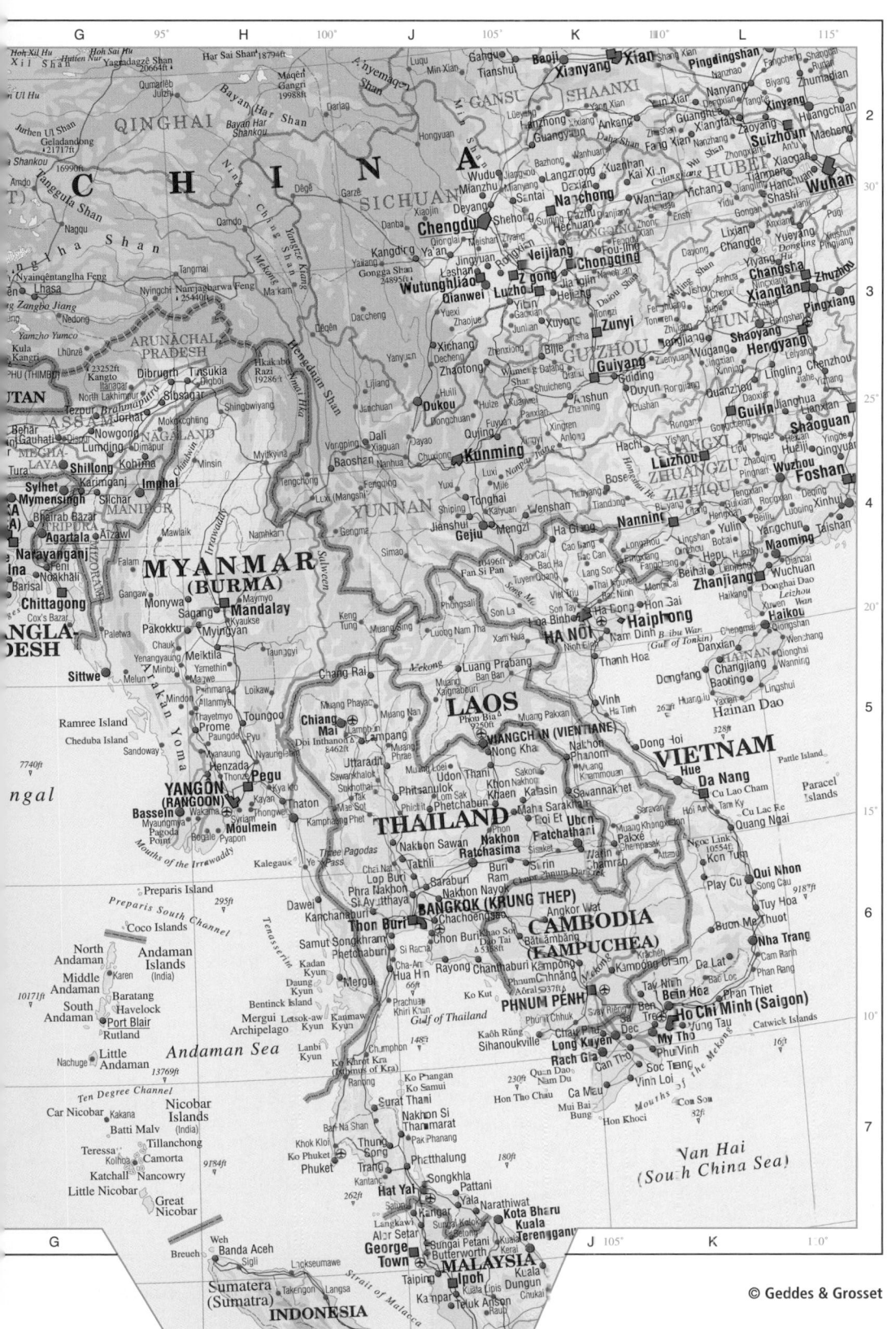

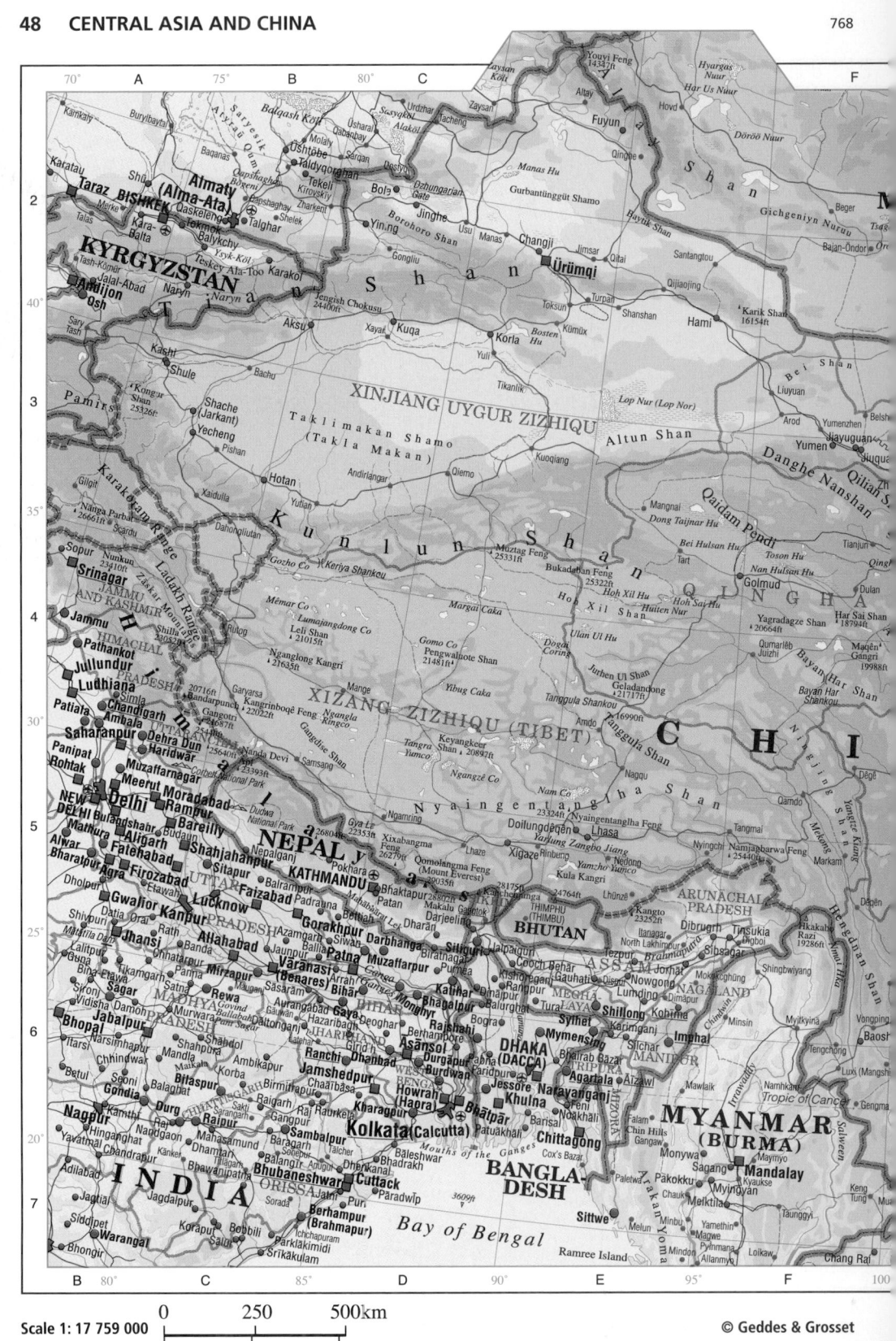

Scale 1: 17 759 000

0   250   500km

0   150   300miles

© Geddes & Grosset

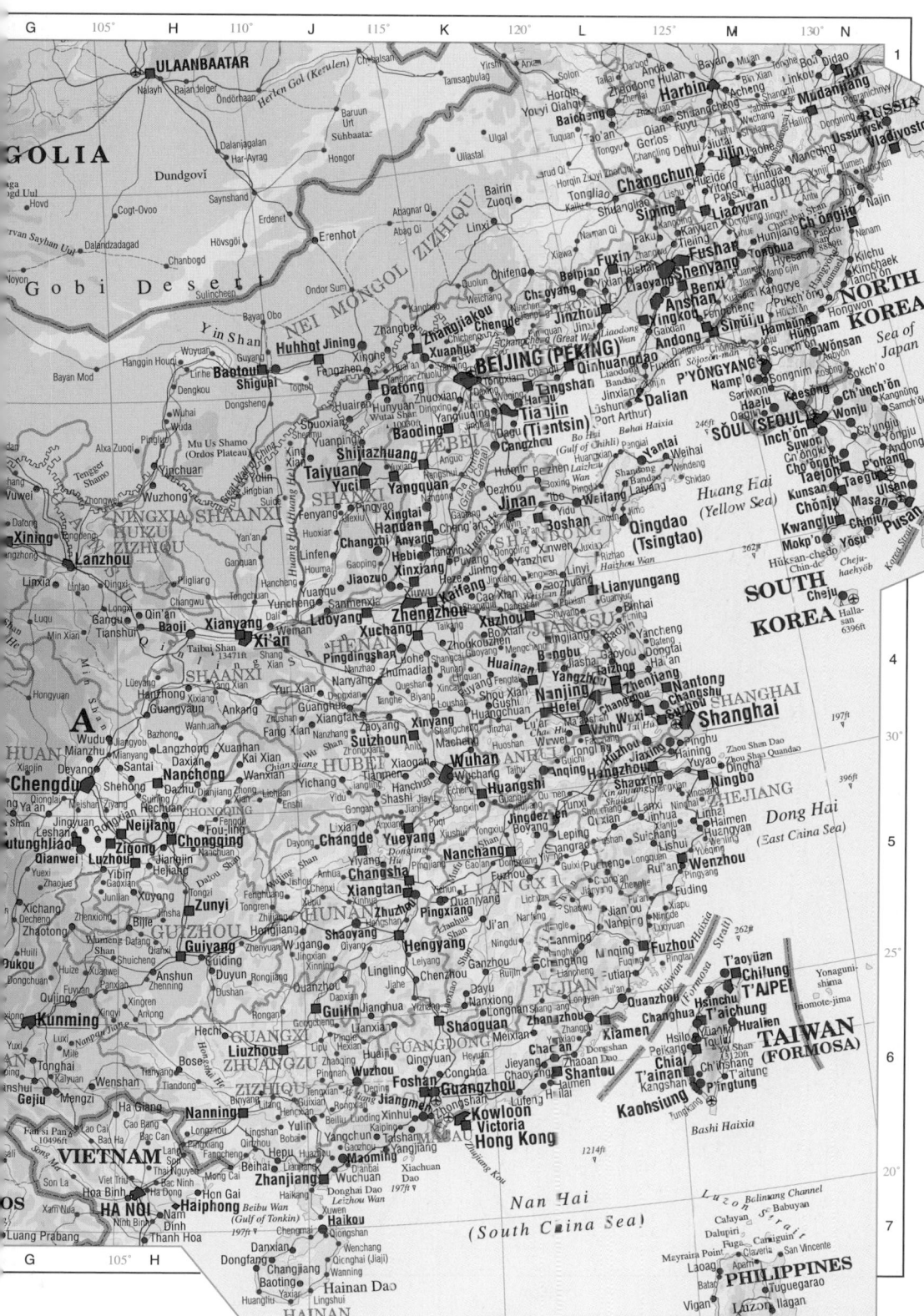

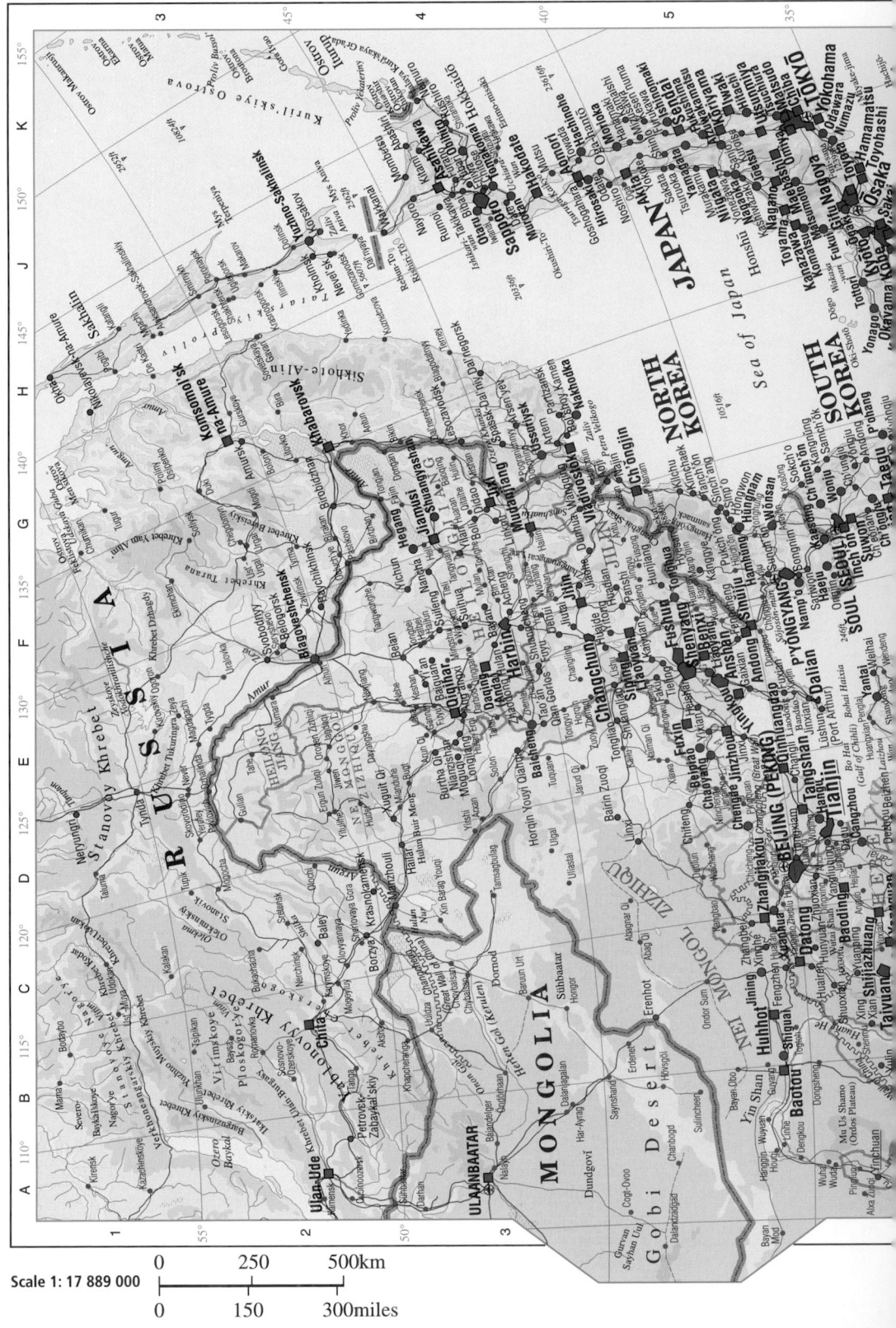

Scale 1: 17 889 000

0   250   500km

0   150   300miles

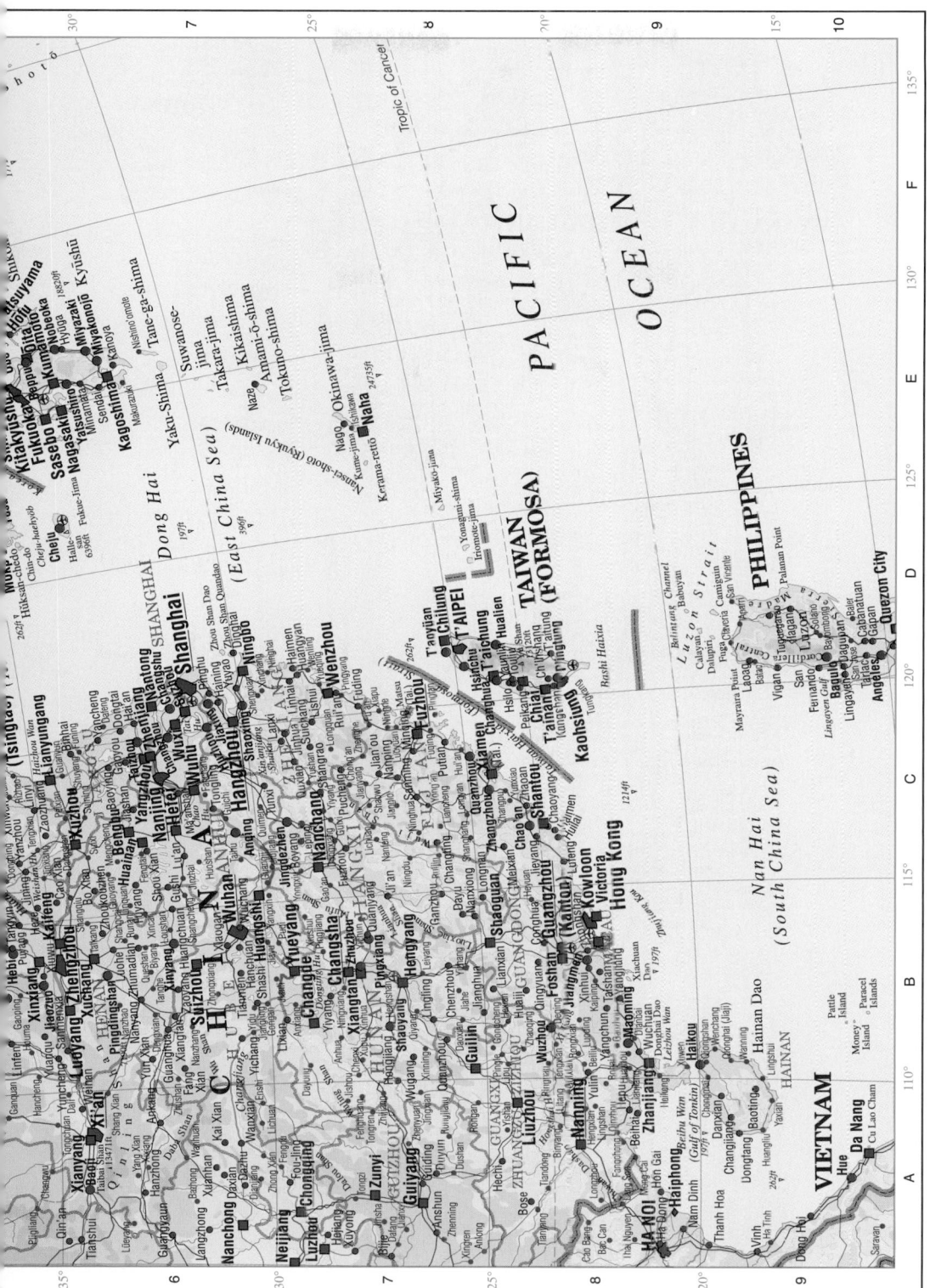

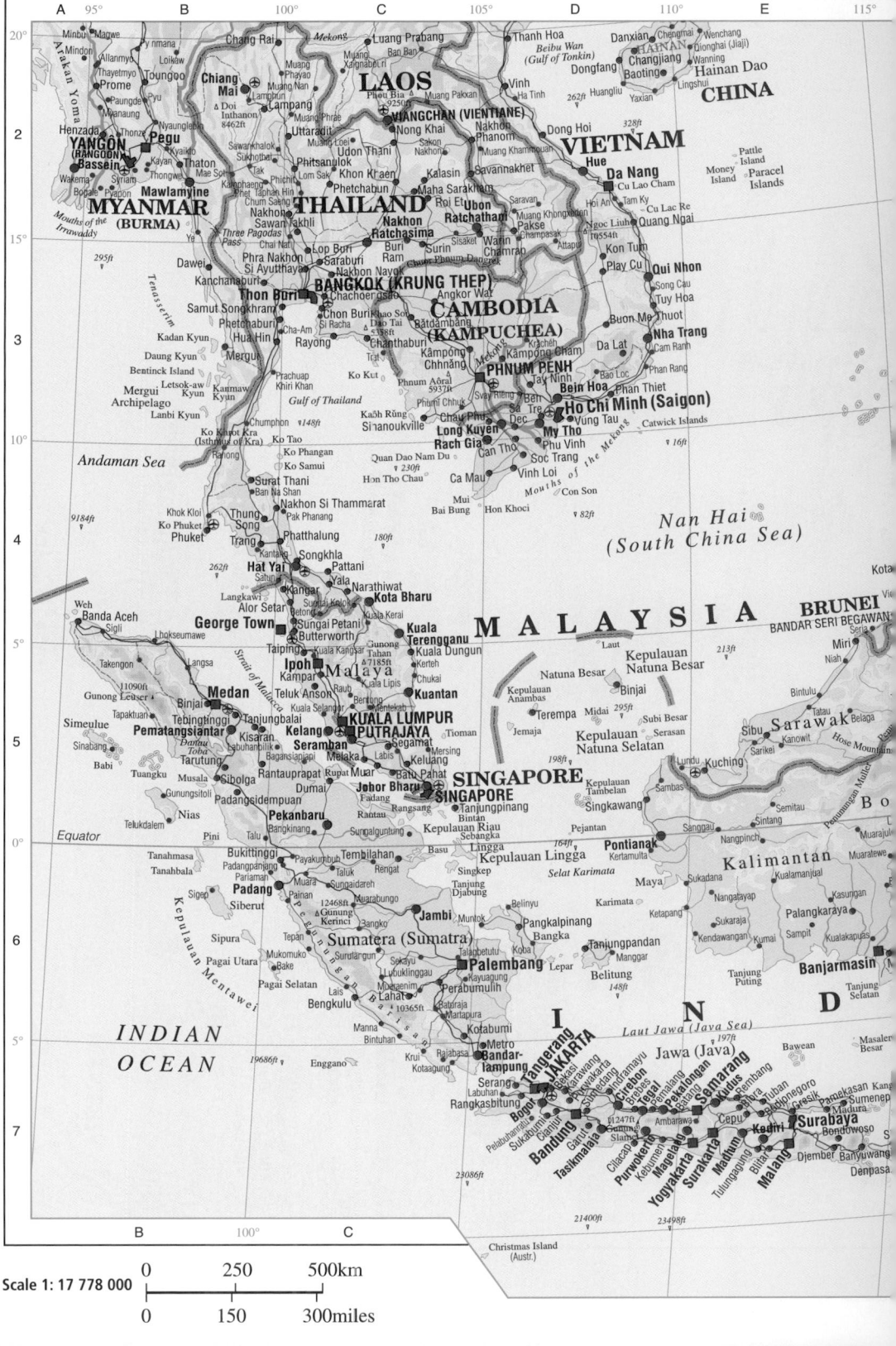

Scale 1: 17 778 000

| 0 | 250 | 500km |

| 0 | 150 | 300miles |

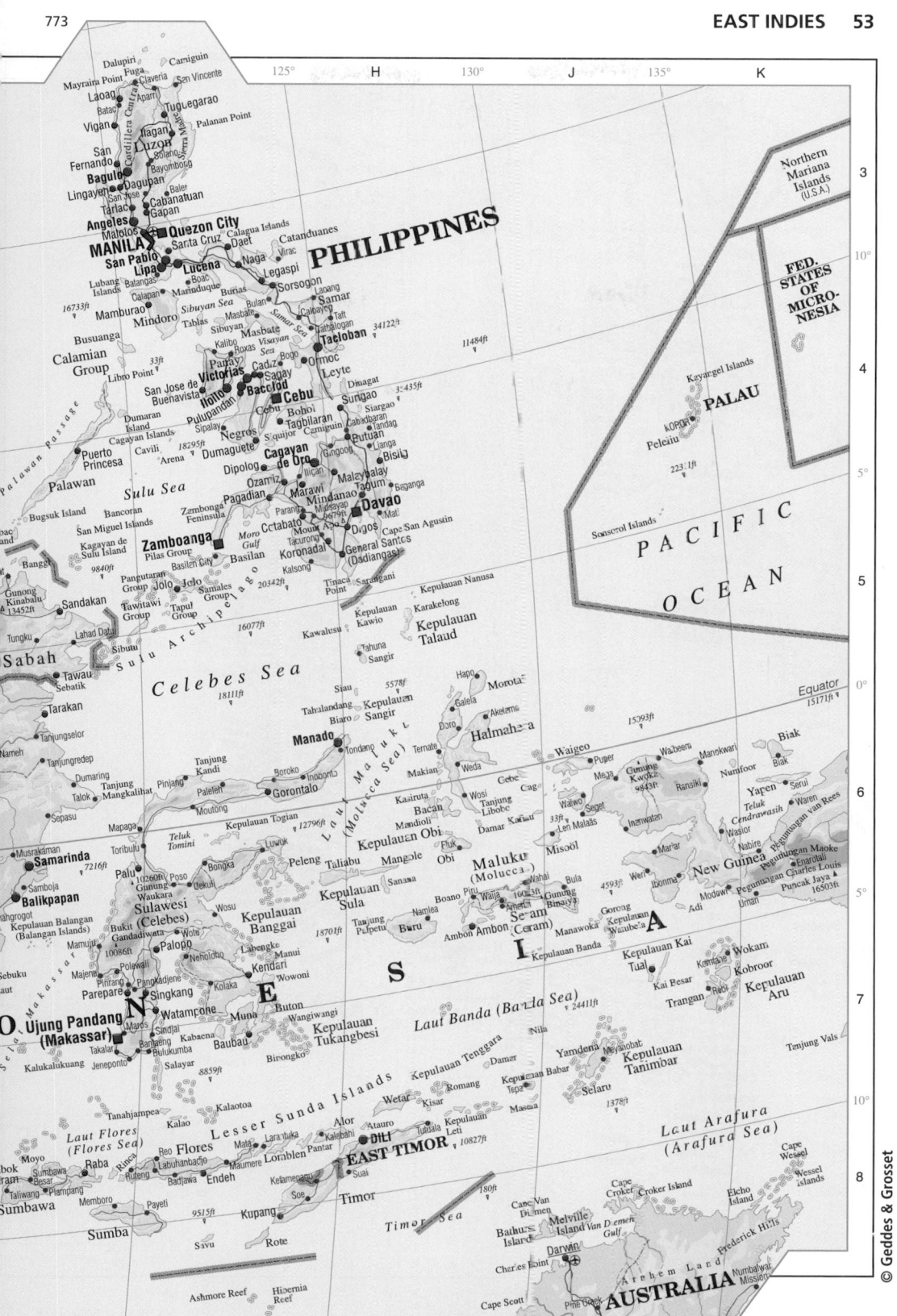

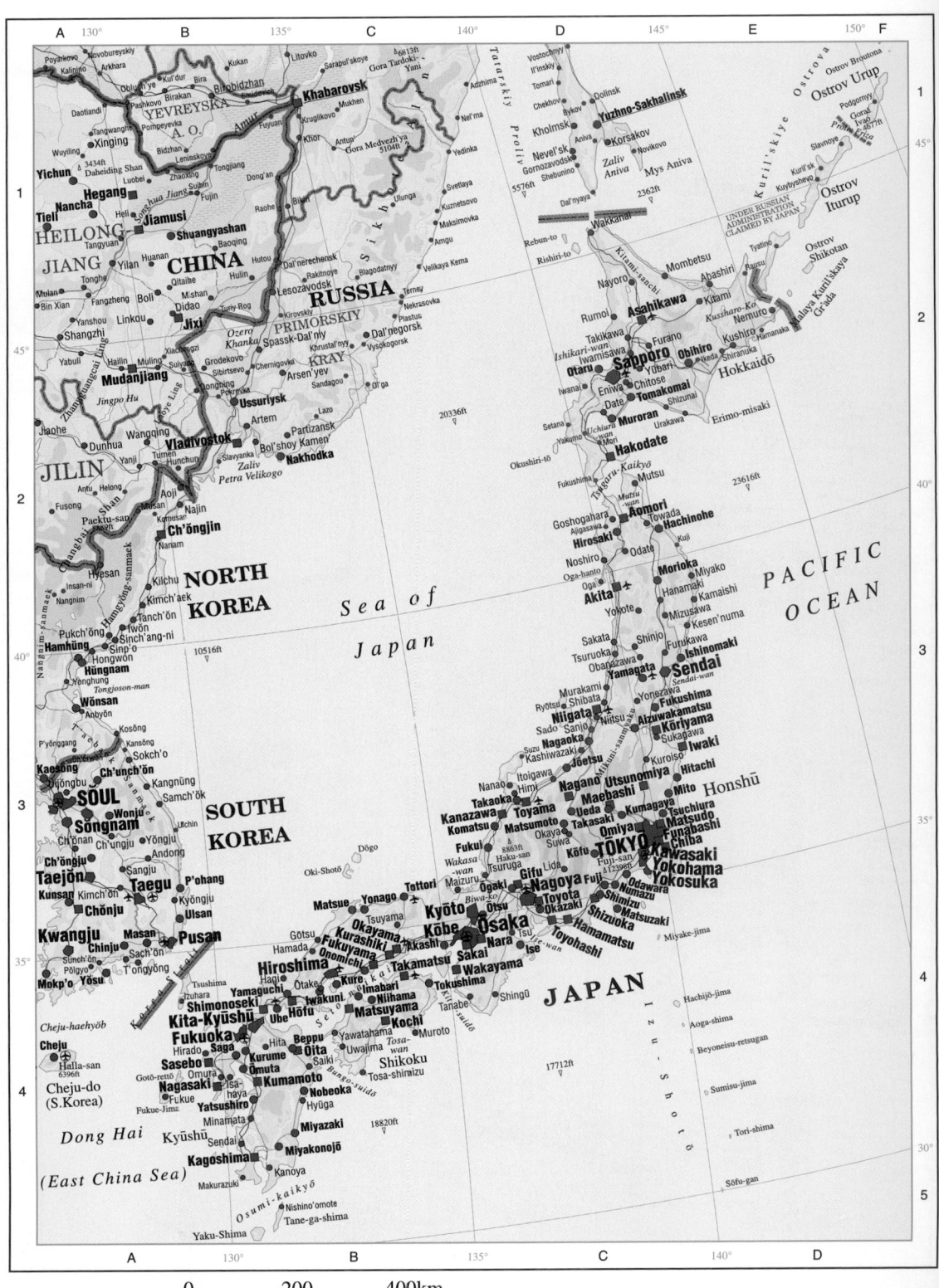

Scale 1: 12 500 000

0   200   400km

0   100   200miles

© Geddes & Grosset

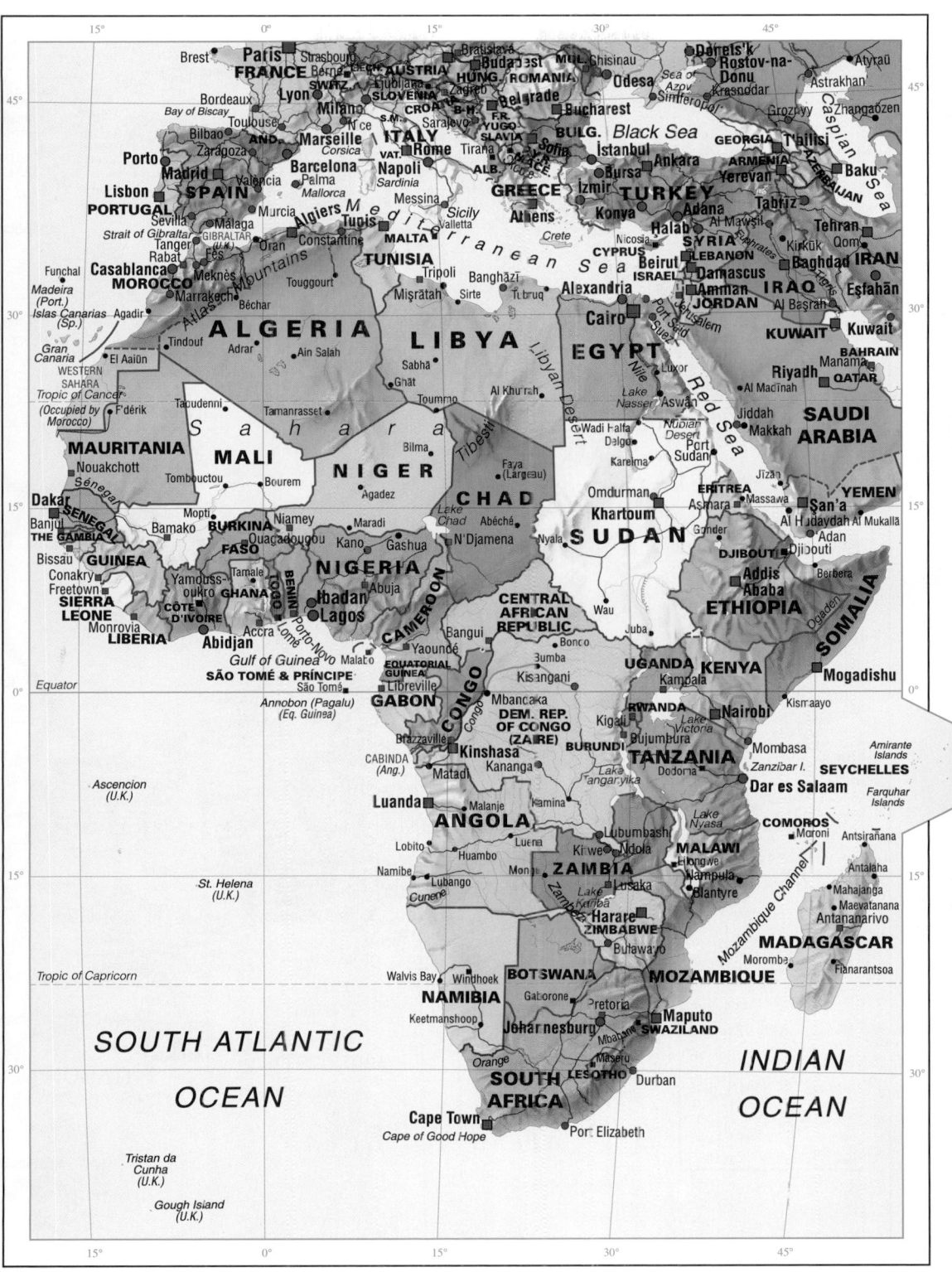

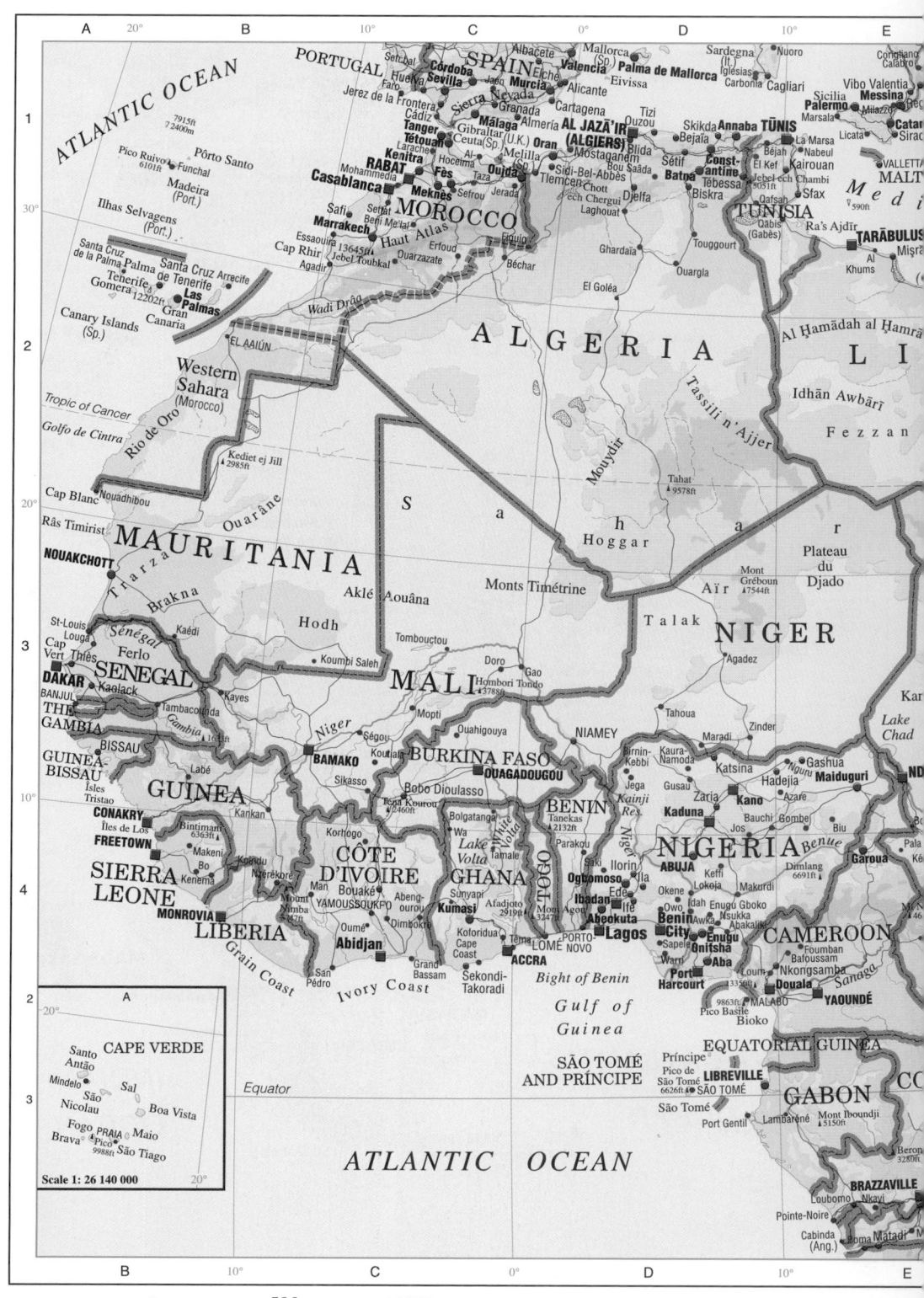

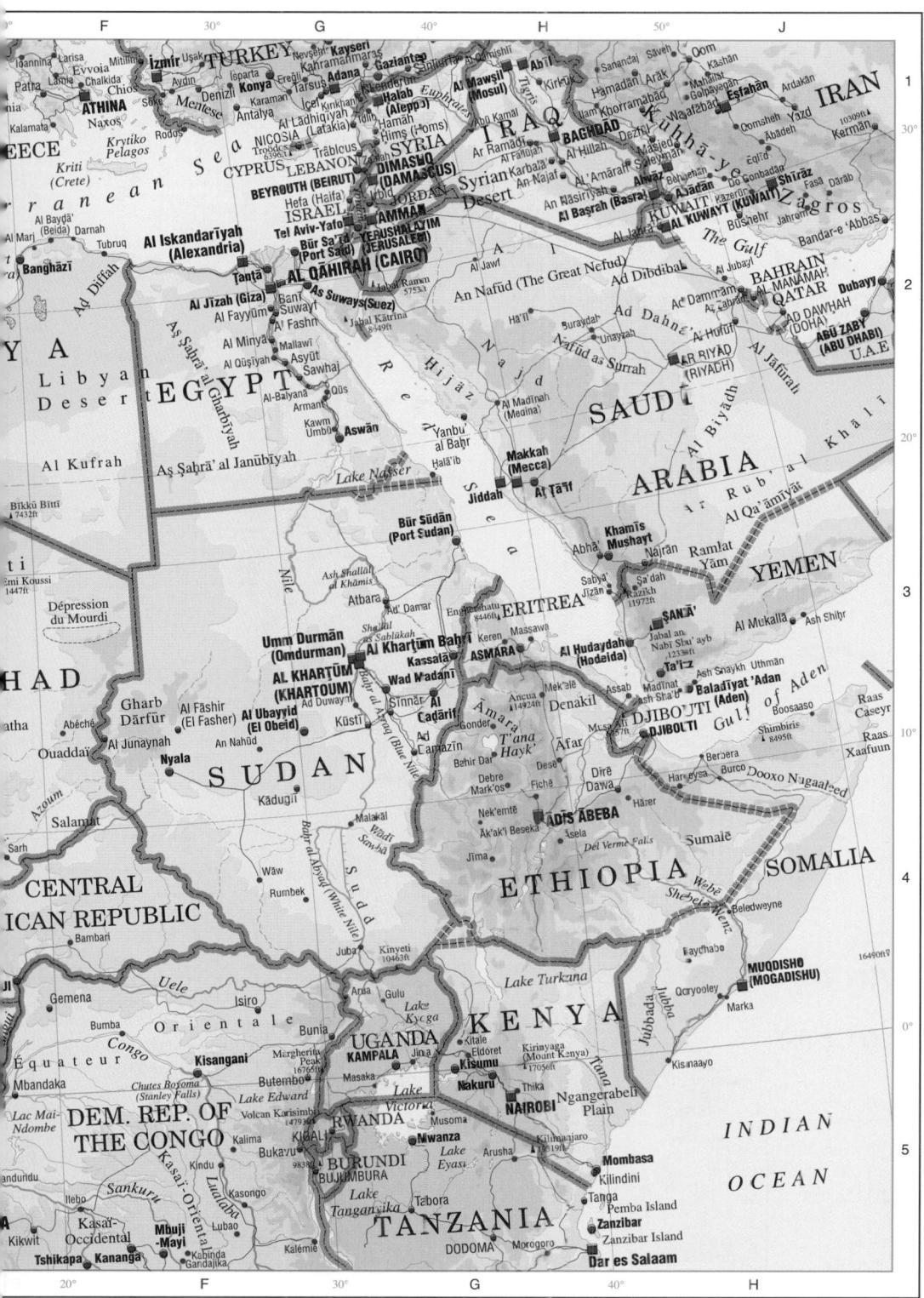

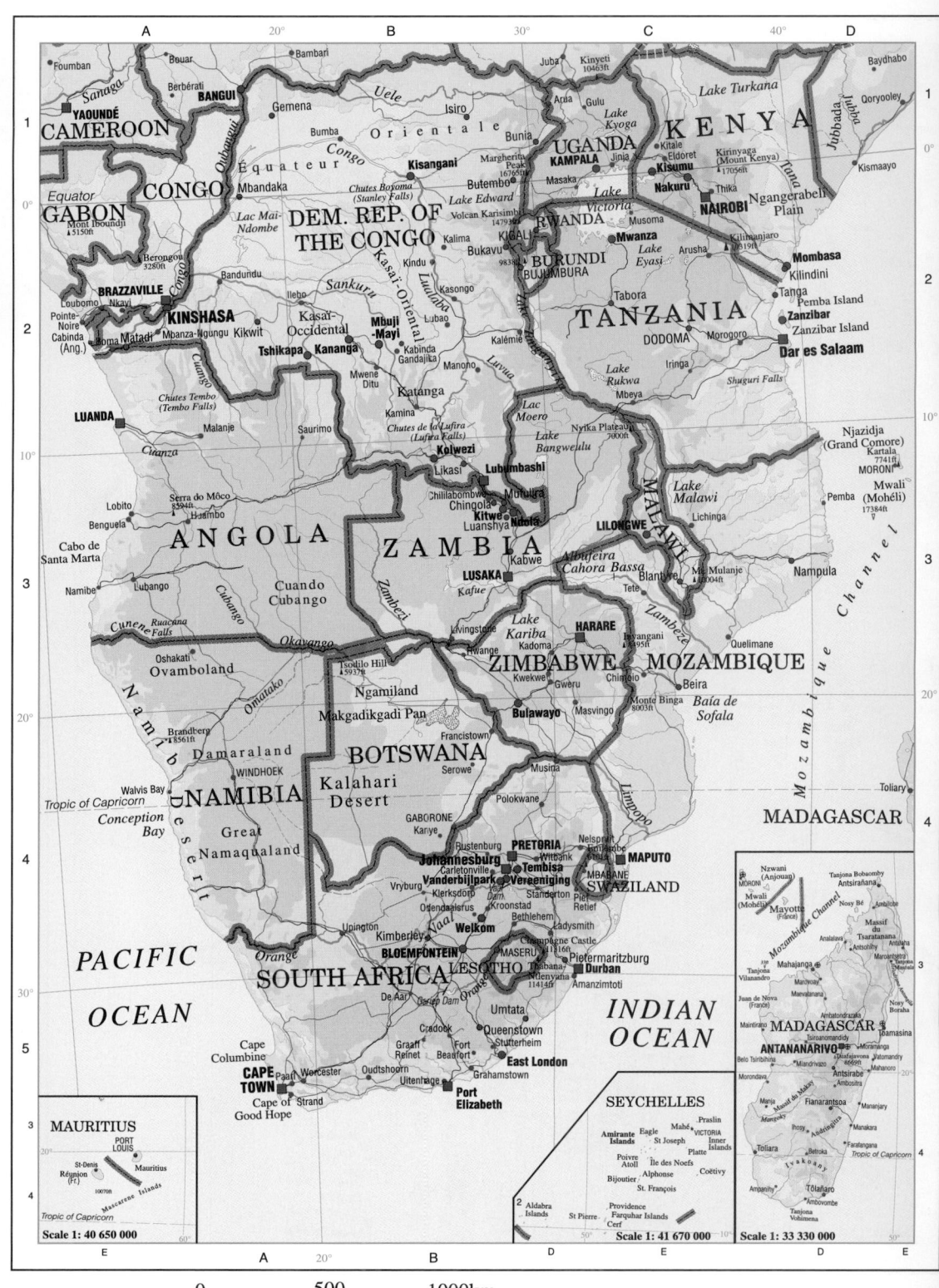

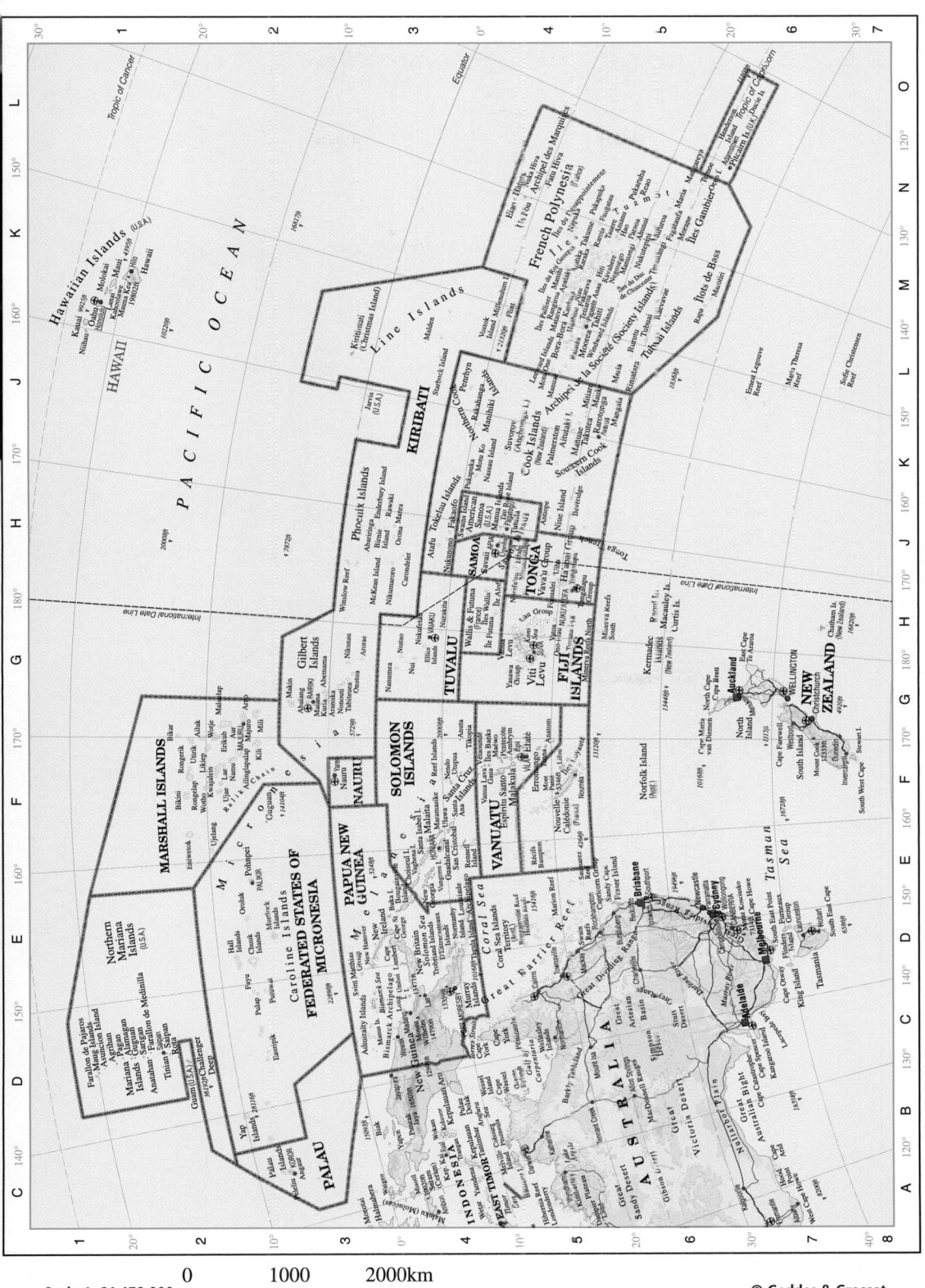

Scale 1: 64 478 000

| 0 | 1000 | 2000km |

| 0 | 600 | 1200miles |

© Geddes & Grosset

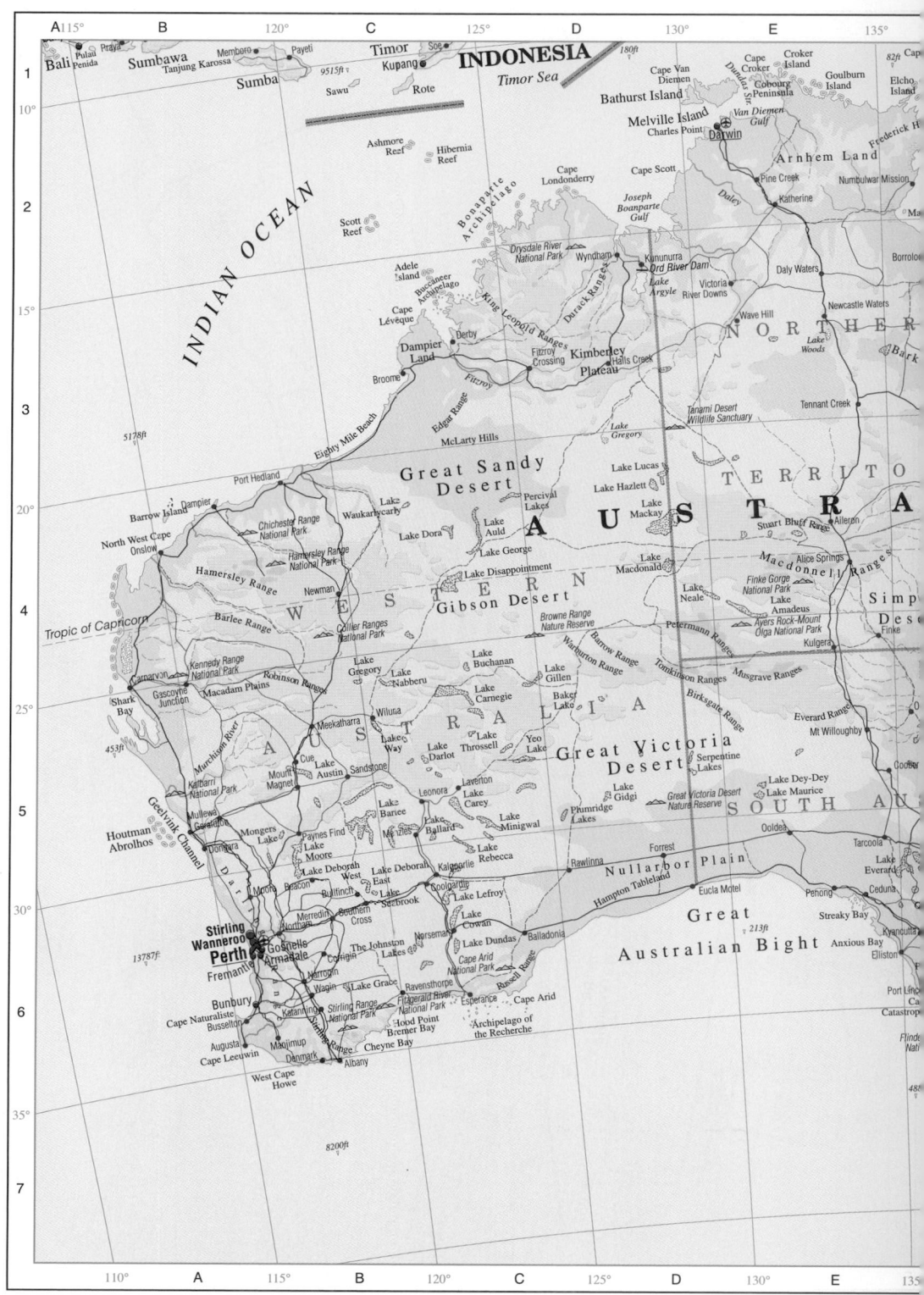

Scale 1: 18 182 000

| 0 | 300 | 600km |

| 0 | 150 | 300miles |

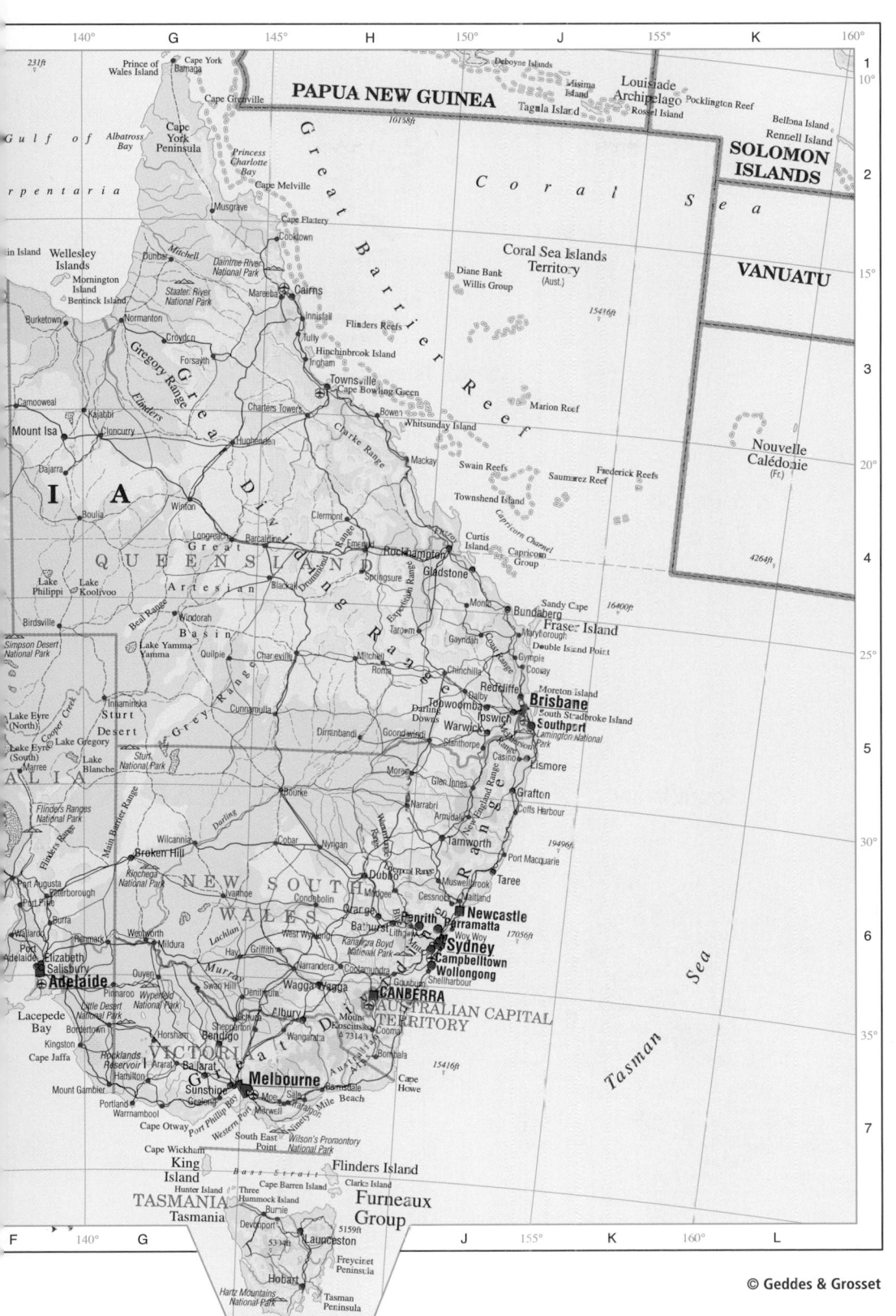

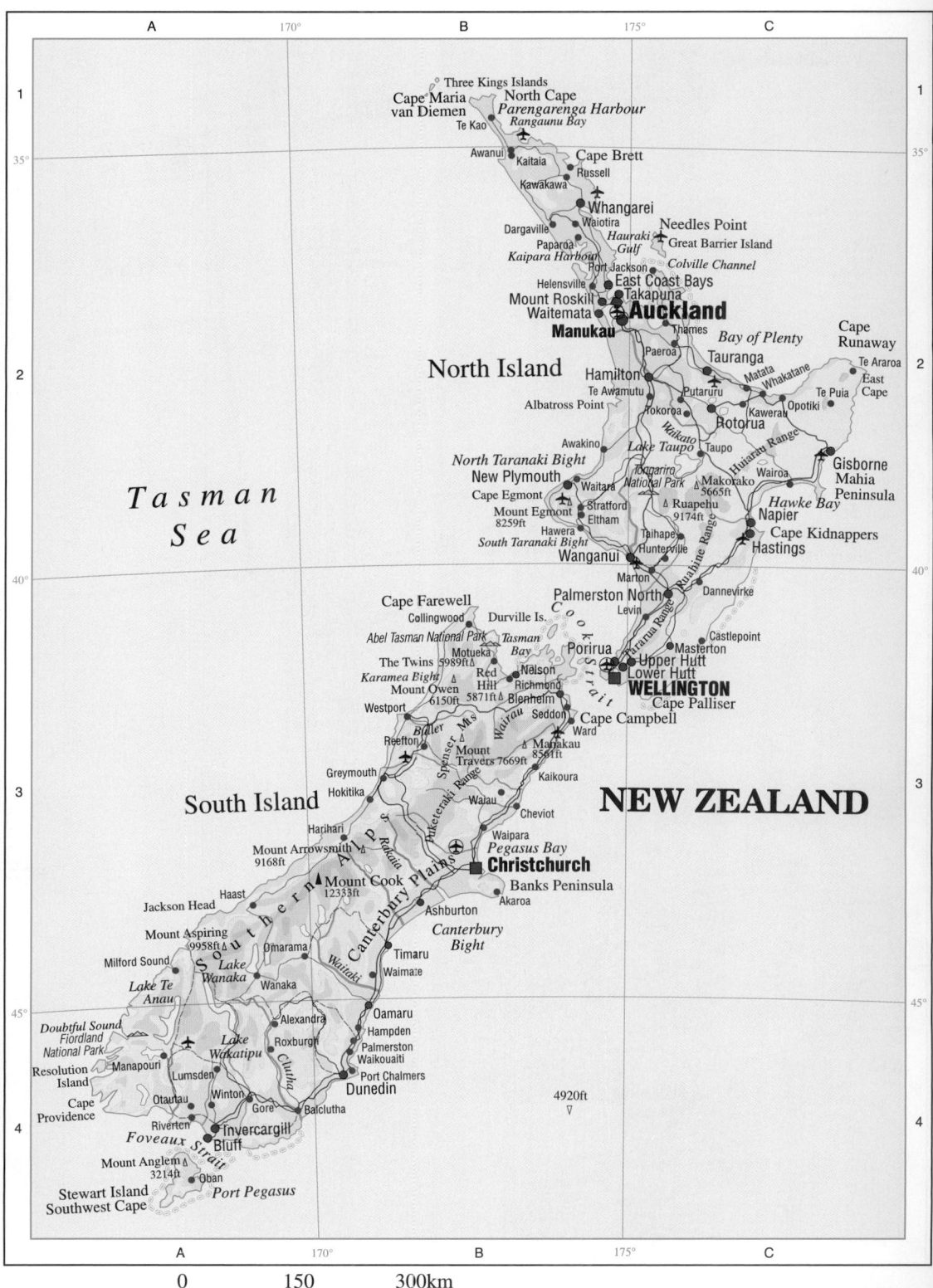

Scale 1: 8 696 000

0   150   300km

0   75   150miles

© Geddes & Grosset

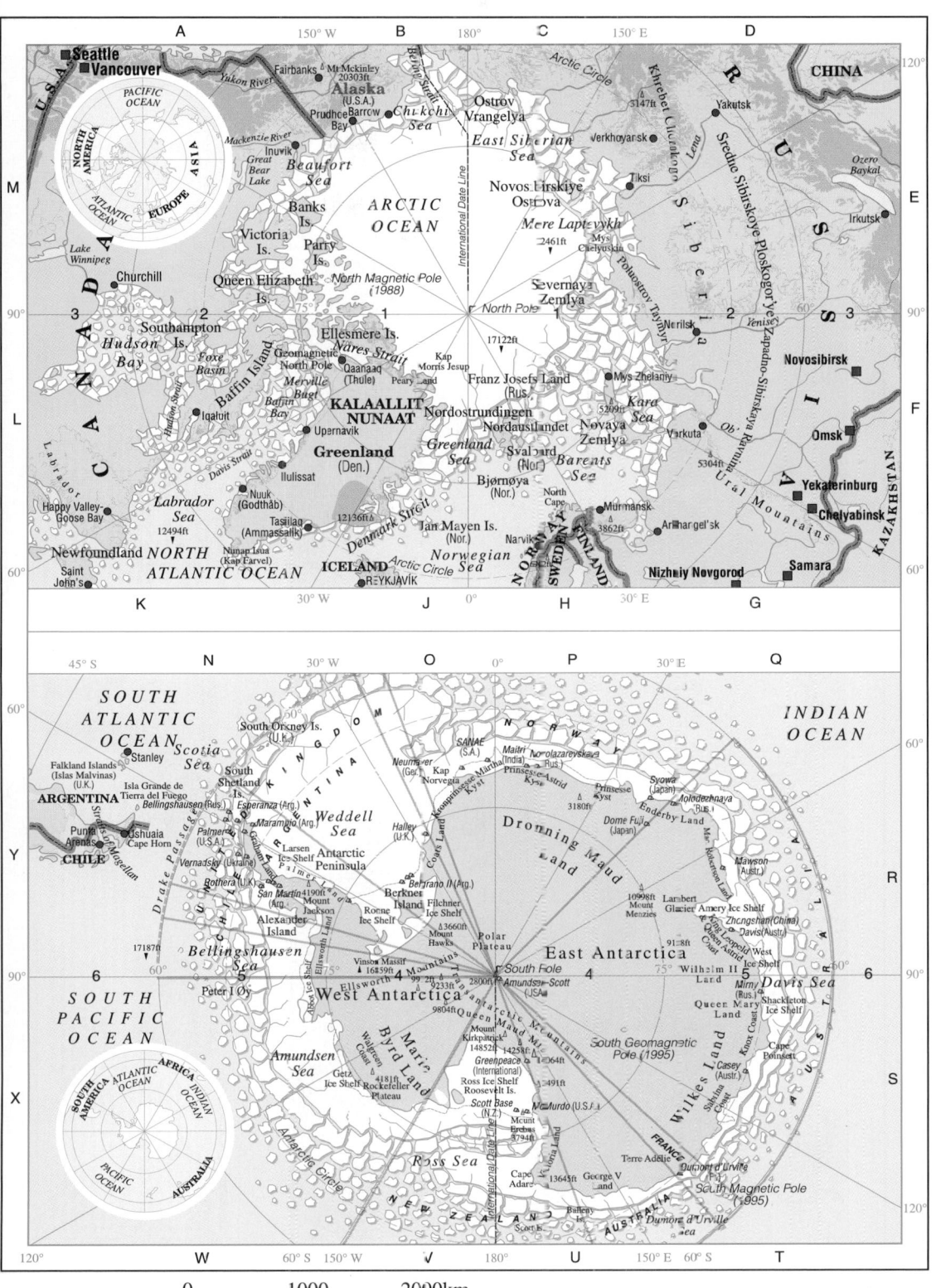

Scale 1: 54 545 000

| 0 | 1000 | 2000km |

| 0 | 500 | 1000miles |

© Geddes & Grosset

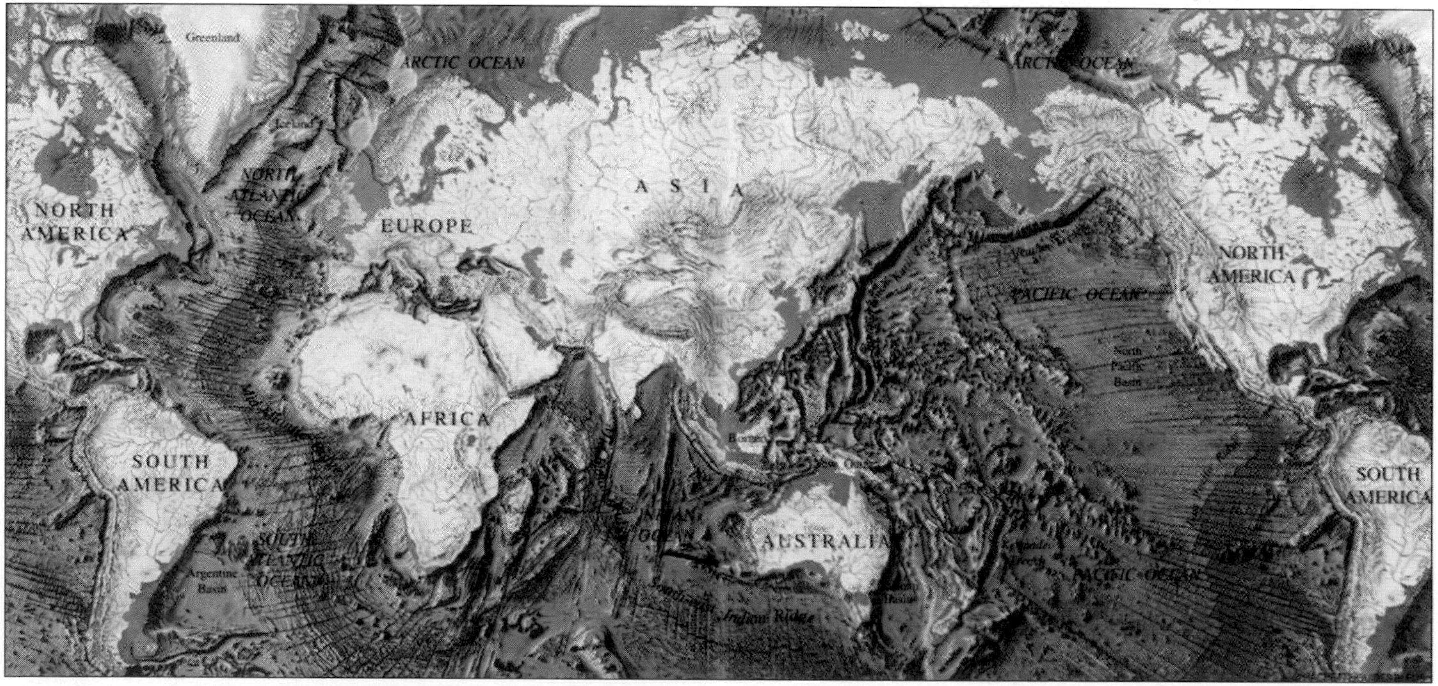

Underwater landscapes

Topography of the ocean floor can be divided into two distinct features: the continental margins and the deep sea basins.

The character of the ocean basin depends on the extent to which sediments mask the crust and also the degree of volcanic activity. The sediments may be either pelagic or terragenous. The latter are brought down by turbidity currents which are avalanches of silt and sand from the continental shelf. These powerful currents can cut channels in the continental shelf such as the Hatteras Canyon off North America and transport material thousands of kilometres.

On the continental shelf sediments are affected by waves, tidal currents and changes in sea level.

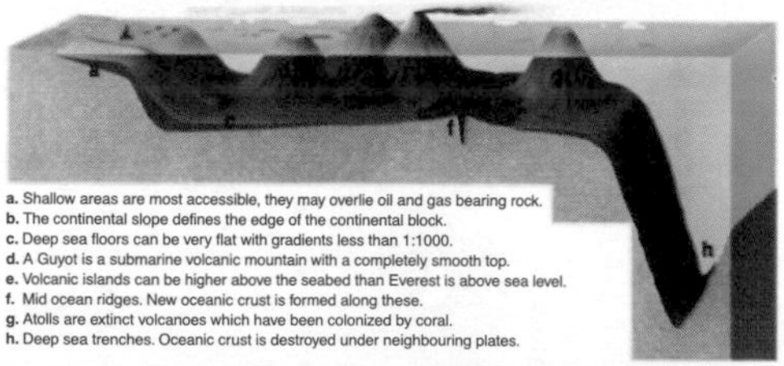

a. Shallow areas are most accessible, they may overlie oil and gas bearing rock.
b. The continental slope defines the edge of the continental block.
c. Deep sea floors can be very flat with gradients less than 1:1000.
d. A Guyot is a submarine volcanic mountain with a completely smooth top.
e. Volcanic islands can be higher above the seabed than Everest is above sea level.
f. Mid ocean ridges. New oceanic crust is formed along these.
g. Atolls are extinct volcanoes which have been colonized by coral.
h. Deep sea trenches. Oceanic crust is destroyed under neighbouring plates.

Seabed treasures

In the deeper sea regions mineral exploitation has concentrated on manganese nodules. These lumps grow at rates of between 3-8 mm, .25 in each million years, and they are valuable for the copper, nickel and cobalt they contain. Granules vary in size and may be up to 150 mm, 6 ins in diameter.

On the continental shelves and near coastal regions placer deposits are often commercially viable. They consist of heavy mineral particles which have been weathered from locally occuring ore bodies and deposited on beaches and in estuaries. Gold is extracted from placer deposits off Alaska.

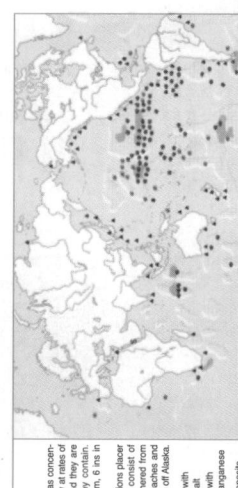

Moderate coverage of manganese nodules
Intensive coverage of manganese nodules
• Nodules with >1.8% nickel and copper
• Nodules with >1% cobalt
• Nodules with >.35% manganese
• Placer deposits
s Metalliferous muds

Map Index

Appendices

The Nation of Canada

Geography and Climate

Physical description

The world's second largest country in area after Russia, Canada has a surface area of 9,984,670 square kilometres (3,848,900 square miles), of which 91% is land and the remainder fresh water. It occupies the full sweep of the North American continent from longitude 52° west on the Atlantic coast of Newfoundland to longitude 88° west at the Pacific islands of British Columbia, a distance exceeding 5,000 kilometres (3,100 miles). Northwards it extends between latitudes 42° and 83° for 4,600 kilometres (2,800 miles) beyond the Arctic Circle into the islands of the frozen seas between Baffin Bay and the Beaufort Sea. In the northwest it is bounded by the U.S. state of Alaska. The southern boundary is with the U.S.A. It follows the 49th parallel from the Pacific coast to the eastern border of Manitoba, then a more irregular line through Lakes Superior and Ontario and to the right of the St. Lawrence River, turning south between New Brunswick and the U.S. state of Maine to reach the Atlantic coast.

The topography of the northeast is dominated by the ancient pre-Cambrian rocks of the Canadian Shield, one of the oldest rock surfaces in the world, bordering the east side of Hudson Bay, and with the Laurentian Mountains to the south. To the east are the hills and valleys of the Appalachian areas of the Atlantic provinces and southern Québec. A lowland region stretches west from the St. Lawrence through southern Québec and Ontario, meeting the vast expanse of the interior plains which stretch across the Prairie Provinces of Alberta, Saskatchewan, and Manitoba. These end abruptly in the Western Cordillera, formed out of several mountain ranges and plateau-lands, including the Rocky, Cassiar, and Mackenzie Mountains. Mt. Logan, Canada's highest peak (5,959 meters, 19,550 feet), rises in the St. Elias Mountains of the Coastal range. The continent breaks up into islands towards the North Pole, some of them very large and mountainous.

Lakes and rivers

Canada is estimated to hold about 20% of the world's fresh water supply, and there are very many lakes and a number of major river systems. Ontario alone is estimated to have about a quarter of a million lakes. Lake Superior is the world's largest body of fresh water. It and three of the other Great Lakes, Huron, Erie, and Ontario, are shared with the U.S.A. The largest lake wholly within Canada, the Great Bear Lake (31,328 square kilometres, 12,092 square miles), is in the Northwest Territories, as is the next in size, the Great Slave Lake (28,568 square kilometres, 11,027 square miles). Another vast lake is Lake Winnipeg in Manitoba (24,387 square kilometres, 9,413 square miles). Saskatchewan's largest lake is Lake Athabasca at 7,935

square kilometres (3,063 square miles). Some very large lakes are artificial or enhanced in size by dams, such as the Smallwood Reservoir in Newfoundland (6,527 square kilometres, 2,519 square miles) and the Williston Lake in British Columbia (1,761 square kilometres, 680 square miles).

Among rivers, the Mackenzie is Canada's longest at 4,241 kilometres (2,480 miles); its system drains northwards from the Great Slave Lake and Great Bear Lake. The Peace River (1,923 kilometres, 1,195 miles) and its tributaries drain much of Alberta. Other great rivers include the Nelson (2,575 kilometres, 1,600 miles), the Saskatchewan (1,939 kilometres, 1,205 miles), flowing eastward into Hudson Bay, the Fraser (1,370 kilometres, 851 miles), and the Yukon (3,184 kilometres, 1,978 miles), flowing into the Pacific Ocean, though much of the Yukon is in Alaska. On the Atlantic side, the St. Lawrence flows eastwards for 3,058 kilometres (1,900 miles), and its greatest tributary is the Ottawa River (1,271 kilometres, 788 miles), flowing south from the inland wilderness of Québec province. Many Canadian rivers are navigable by motor vessels and barges, and form important transport routes.

Islands

Among the vast number of islands within Canadian territory are some of the world's largest. Baffin Island, the fifth largest in the world, has an area of 507,451 square kilometres (186,742 square miles) while another 37 islands exceed 1,000 square kilometres (386 square miles), including Victoria Island (217,291 square kilometres, 83,874 square miles). Many of these islands lie north of the Arctic Circle, and are scantily populated, or have no regular inhabitants. On the west coast, Vancouver Island is the largest island in western North America (31,285 square kilometres, 12,076 square miles). The largest island on the east side is Newfoundland (108,860 square kilometres, 42,020 square miles).

Climate

Canada forms a number of distinct climatic regions from west to east and from south to north. With a northerly global location and a land surface stretching almost to the North Pole, the general climatic picture is one of long winters and warm summers, with brief spring and autumn seasons. In the coastal areas to the east and west, the sea exerts a moderating influence, with more rain, snow, and fog but a narrower range of temperature extremes. East of the Rockies, a drier, 'continental' climate prevails. Calgary in Alberta has an average 399 millimetres (15.7 inches) of annual precipitation compared to Vancouver on the coast with 1,167 millimetres (45.9 inches). Summers are hotter, winters are colder. This pattern extends across the Prairie

Provinces to Ontario, where the Great Lakes exert an oceanic-type influence on the populated southern strip. In northern Ontario, Québec, and into the Northwest Territories and Nunavut, arctic influences increasingly come into play, though summers can be surprisingly warm, and there are wide variations in temperature between different places on the same latitude.

Average maximum and minimum temperatures (Celsius) in capital and major cities

City	Coldest month	Warmest month
Calgary	January (-15.7)	July (23.2)
Charlottetown	January (-12.2)	July (23.1)
Edmonton	January (-17)	July (23)
Fredericton	January (-15.4)	July (25.6)
Halifax	February (-10.6)	July (23.4)
Montréal	January (-14.9)	July (26.2)
Ottawa	January (-15.5)	July (26.4)
Québec City	January (-17.3)	July (24.9)
Regina	January (-22.1)	July (26.3)
St. John's	February (-8.7)	July (20.2)
Toronto	January (-7.9)	July (26.5)
Vancouver	January (-0.1)	August (21.7)
Victoria	January (-0.3)	July (21.8)
Whitehorse	January (-23.2)	July (20.3)
Yellowknife	January (-32.2)	July (20.8)

Environmental issues

Clean air and clean water are both rallying cries for Canada's environmentalists and a major problem for Environment Canada, the government ministry responsible. Acid rain is a serious threat to natural life, and over 14,000 Canadian lakes are estimated to have lost their fish stocks as a result. It is also a major threat to forest growth. In the past twenty years, Canada has reduced its sulphur dioxide emissions by half, but much of Canada's acid rain is generated in the U.S.A., which has been slower to respond to the problem. Canadian meteorologists have also been closely involved in monitoring the increase in global warming and in estimating its effects on the environment.

Government and Political Structure

Canada is an independent state, organized as a constitutional monarchy, on a federal basis. The head of state is the British monarch, who is represented by a Governor General. In modern practice, the Governor General is an eminent Canadian citizen, appointed by the Prime Minister. The three elements in the Canadian legislature are the House of Commons, the Senate or Upper House, and the Governor General. The constitution, confirmed in its present form on 17 April 1982, includes a charter of rights and freedoms as well as provisions to recognize the country's multicultural heritage, to affirm the existing rights of native peoples, to confirm the principle of equalization of benefits among the provinces, and to strengthen provincial ownership of national resources.

The Canadian Parliament, which meets in Ottawa, is a bicameral legislature. The House of Commons has 307 elected members and the Senate has 104 members, appointed by the Governor General on the recommendation of the Prime Minister. The maximum life of a parliament is five years. The Senate may introduce Bills, except financial Bills, and has a little-exercised right to block legislation. Its prime purpose is to give Bills a second reading and to clarify their content.

National symbols

Canada has the following national symbols:

- The arms of Canada – combining the royal arms of Great Britain with a triple maple leaf, and the motto *A Mari Usque Ad Mare*, 'From Sea to Sea'.
- The flag of Canada – composed of two red rectangles separated by a white square on which is represented a single red maple leaf (inaugurated 15 February 1965).
- The official symbols of Canada – the maple tree and maple leaf. The beaver (*Castor canadiensis*) is also an official symbol of Canada.
- Official tartans – the following provinces and territories have each designated an official tartan: Alberta, British Columbia, Manitoba, New Brunswick, Nova Scotia, Northwest Territories, Ontario, Prince Edward Island, Saskatchewan, Yukon.

The Canadian Cabinet (as of June 2005)

The Rt. Hon Paul Martin	Prime Minister of Canada
The Hon. Anne McLellan	Deputy Prime Minister and Minister of Public Safety and Emergency Preparedness
The Hon. Jacob Austin	Leader of the Government in the Senate
The Hon. Ralph Goodale	Minister of Finance
The Hon. Lucienne Robillard	Minister of Intergovernmental Affairs
The Hon. Pierre Pettigrew	Minister of Foreign Affairs
The Hon. Stéphane Dion	Minister of the Environment
The Hon. James Scott Peterson	Minister of International Trade
The Hon. Andrew Mitchell	Minister of Agriculture and Agri-Foods, Minister of State for Federal Economic Development for Northern Ontario
The Hon. Claudette Bradshaw	Minister of State for Human Resources Development
The Hon. Albina Guarnieri	Minister of Veterans' Affairs
The Hon. Jacques Saada	Minister of Economic Development Agency of Canada for the Region of Quebec

The Hon. Stephen Owen — Minister of Western Economic Diversification and Minister of State for Sport

The Hon. William Graham — Minister of National Defence

The Hon. Joseph Volpe — Minister of Citizenship and Immigration

The Hon. Reg Alcock — President of the Treasury Board, Minister for the Canadian Wheat Board

The Hon. Geoff Regan — Minister of Fisheries and Oceans

The Hon. Jean C. Lapierre — Minister of Transport

The Hon. Ken Dryden — Minister of Social Development

The Hon. Tony Valeri — Leader of the Government in the House of Commons

The Hon. Irwin Cotler — Minister of Justice and Attorney General of Canada

The Hon. David Emerson — Minister of Industry

The Hon. John Efford — Minister of Natural Resources

The Hon. Liza Frulla — Minister of Canadian Heritage and Minister responsible for the Status of Women

The Hon. Belinda Stronach — Minister of Human Resources and Skills Development and Minister responsible for Democratic Renewal

The Hon. Ethel Blondin-Andrew — Minister of State for Northern Development

The Hon. Andy Scott — Minister of Indian Affairs and Northern Development

The Hon. Raymond Chan — Minister of State for Multiculturalism

The Hon. Joe Fontana — Minister of Labour and Housing

The Hon. Scott Brison — Minister of Public Works and Government Services

The Hon. Joseph McGuire — Minister of Atlantic Canada Opportunities Agency

The Hon. Mauril Bélanger — Deputy Leader of the Government in the House of Commons, Minister responsible for Official Languages, Associate Minister of National Defence, Minister for International Trade

The Hon. Ujjal Dosanjh — Minister of Health

The Hon. Carolyn Bennett — Minister of State for Public Health

The Hon. Aileen Carroll — Minister for International Cooperation

The Hon. John Godfrey — Minister of State for Infrastructure and Communities

The Hon. Tony Ianno — Minister of State for Families and Caregivers

Prime Ministers of Canada since Confederation (1867)

(Parties: Con – Conservative; Lib – Liberal; PC – Progressive Conservative)

J. A. Macdonald (Con/Lib)	1867–73
Alexander Mackenzie (Lib)	1873–78
J. A. Macdonald (Con)	1878–91
John Joseph Caldwell Abbott (Lib/Con)	1891–1892
John Sparrow David Thompson (Con)	1892–94
Mackenzie Bowell (Con)	1894–96
Charles Tupper (Con)	1896
Wilfrid Laurier (Lib)	1896–1911
Robert L. Borden (Con/Unionist)	1911–17, 1917–20
Arthur Meighen (Con/Unionist)	1920-21
William Lyon Mackenzie King (Lib)	1921–26
Arthur Meighen (Con)	1926
William Lyon Mackenzie King (Lib)	1926–30
Richard Bedford Bennett (Con)	1930–35
William Lyon Mackenzie King (Lib)	1935–48
Louis St. Laurent (Lib)	1948–57
John G. Diefenbaker (PC)	1957–63
Lester Pearson (Lib)	1963–68
Pierre Elliott Trudeau (Lib)	1968–79
Charles Joseph Clark (PC)	1979–80
Pierre Elliott Trudeau (Lib)	1980–84
John Napier Turner (Lib)	1984
M. Brian Mulroney (PC)	1984–93
A. Kim Campbell (PC)	1993
Jean Chrétien (Lib)	1993–2003
Paul Martin (Lib)	2003–

Accredited political parties in Canada (2005)

(* indicates seats in House of Commons)

Bloc Québecois*
Canadian Action Party
Christian Heritage Party of Canada
Communist Party of Canada
Green Party of Canada
Liberal Party of Canada*
Marijuana Party
Marxist-Leninist Party of Canada
New Democratic Party*
Conservative Party of Canada*
Progressive Canadian Party
Libertarian Party of Canada

The Order of Canada

This system of national awards to honour distinguished citizens was introduced in 1967, replacing the previous 'imperial' British awards. It has three classes, rising from Member to Officer then Companion. Over 5,000 persons hold the award. The Governor General is its chancellor, and its motto is *Desiderantes meliorem patriam*, 'They desire a better country'. In addition, certain provinces also have their own internal honours and awards.

The provinces and territories

Provinces
Alberta
British Columbia
Manitoba
New Brunswick
Newfoundland and Labrador
Nova Scotia
Ontario
Prince Edward Island
Québec
Saskatchewan

Territories
Northwest Territories
Nunavut
Yukon Territory

A series of constitutional amendments made between 1867 and 1982 defined the role and powers of the provincial administrations. The provinces exist in their own right, as part of the constitution. Territories are created by federal law and though territorial administrations have broadly similar powers to those of the provinces, they are somewhat more restricted and the federal government has a greater degree of involvement.

In each of the ten provinces, the sovereign is represented by a lieutenant governor. Provincial assemblies consist of a single house of elected members. They make laws on most internal matters including direct taxation within the province, the management of public lands and resources, education, welfare, health, policing, justice, prisons, and transport.

The relationship of provincial governments to the federal government, and the status of individual provinces within the Confederation, remain important issues.

An Outline of Canadian History

(*See also* A Chronology of Events in Canadian History)
Human occupancy of Canada goes back perhaps 20,000 years, when the North American and Asian land masses were joined where the Bering Straits now are. Both animals and humans travelled from Asia into North America and in this way the 'native peoples' arrived, their tenure of the land so ancient that they can well claim to be aboriginal.

Over many centuries, in the various climatic and landscape regions, shared ways of life evolved, though the aboriginal peoples who shared them were often at war with one another. In the north, Inuit and Aleut peoples perfected a way of life that both suited and drew on an apparently hostile environment. Hunters of whales, seals, fish, and caribou on land, they drew not only their food but tools and clothing from their prey. They followed its seasonal movements, being as adept on water as on land.

In the forested zones, liberally provided with rivers and lakes, the Woodland Indian first nations used their birch-bark canoes for mobility. In the north and west, nomadic hunter-gatherers spoke the various Athapascan and Algonquian languages. The first nations of the southeast began to establish permanent settlements, and to practice agriculture on the fertile soil. These were the first nations who later formed the Iroquois League, and they evolved formal systems of diplomacy, trade, and warfare. On the great plains, the inhabitants relied primarily on the apparently numberless bison for food, hides, bone implements, and glue. The wooded Pacific coast region, rich in fish as well as land and wildlife, and with ample supplies of large timber, sustained elaborate Indian cultures.

The first Europeans to come were tenth-century Vikings, but their knowledge was lost for centuries. A new 'discovery' took place when fishermen from Portugal, Spain, France, and then England ventured further and further out into the Atlantic. The teeming cod banks off Newfoundland were well known by the fourteenth century, and it is more than likely that some of the fishers landed, or were swept ashore. But it was men searching for the westward sea route to China who definitively found the American land mass blocking their way and inadvertently 'discovered' Canada. It seems that the very first colonists were Portuguese, but John Cabot, sailing from Bristol in 1497, and Jacques Cartier, sailing from St. Malo in 1534, launched the English-French rivalry that was to haunt Canadian history and politics into the twenty-first century.

The country's name was bestowed by Cartier, who, hearing the Indians on the St. Lawrence refer to their villages as *kanata*, took it to be the name of their country. Interest in exploring the interior was slow to arise, until the demand in Europe for fur, especially beaver fur, drove explorers back to Canada. In 1605 the French Samuel de Champlain founded a fort at Port Royal in the Annapolis Basin, Nova Scotia, but three years later he established a more permanent habitation at Québec. *La Nouvelle France* was on the way to being established, and meanwhile the English had claimed Newfoundland in 1583. They were also strongly established in New England to the south. English claims on the mainland were intensified with the founding of the Hudson's Bay Company, given a royal monopoly to trade in natural resources, in 1670. Throughout the seventeenth century, both colonial powers made allies with, and war on, the Indian peoples at different times, and the Iroquois struggled to maintain their own position. In 1690 the English adventurer, Sir William Phips, was repulsed with some disdain from an attack on Québec, governed then by the Comte de Frontenac; and another more official expedition came to grief under Admiral Walker in 1711, when it was wrecked on Anticosti Island in the St. Lawrence Gulf.

By the Treaty of Utrecht, 1713, France formally ceded Newfoundland and Nova Scotia to Great Britain and gave up claims to the Hudson Bay area. Its other Canadian possessions were retained, and soon a fort-building race was under way. War erupted again in 1744, and again in 1756. Amid the many captures and counter-captures, the British succeeded in forcing out large numbers of the French-speaking inhabitants of Cape Breton Island and Nova Scotia. Immigrants from New England reaped most of the benefits. The Seven Years' War (1756–63) was fought between imperial powers on a semi-global scale in Europe and North America and on the high seas. British troops and their Indian allies cut off Québec from French settlements further west. By 1759 the French forts on the Great Lakes were in British hands. On 12 September of that year the British, under General James Wolfe, captured Québec in a battle that saw the deaths of both Wolfe and the French commander, the Marquis de Montcalm. The French regrouped at Montréal and remained strong enough to besiege Québec. Fortune turned on which fleet would come up the St. Lawrence first when the ice melted. But Britain by then had an iron command of the sea. A British fleet and three land armies converged on the French position, and the French Governor General, Vaudreuil, surrendered on 8 September 1760. All of Canada was confirmed as a British possession, now with some 80,000 additional citizens who had been faithful subjects of King Louis of France.

The British administrators speedily found that necessary reassurances and concessions to the French, enshrined in the Québec Act of 1774, were hotly resented by their own settler population and the adjacent, fiercely Protestant New Englanders. But the British and French Canadians did not rise with the American colonists in 1775. Local militias joined with imperial troops to fight back invasion by the Americans, and though Montréal was occupied for several months, the insurgent Americans were eventually thrust back. Many British Loyalists left the new United States once its independence was established, and sought new land in Nova Scotia to the north, the Eastern Townships of Québec, and in areas to the west. Canada gained around 50,000 immigrants in just a few years. Up to 1791, most of southeast Canada was known as Québec; in this year the land was divided into Upper Canada (now in Ontario) and Lower Canada (present-day Québec). Then, as now, English speakers predominated to the west, French speakers to the east.

On the western coast, although European explorers had been visiting since the sixteenth century, there had been no attempt at colonization, and the Coastal Indians had only one another to disturb their peace, unlike the Indian inhabitants of the east. Now, however, with the era of empire-building in full swing, and with rising British anxieties about the expansion of the U.S.A., British attention was also focused on the west coast. Under Captain George Vancouver, the Royal Navy surveyed the complex coastline, and, for the first time, Europeans crossed the Rocky Mountains and reached the coast from the interior. They were Scots, employed by the North West Company. At this time, the agricultural potential of the great plains was not apparent, but the riches of wildlife, fish, and timber in the far west were obvious. British colonies were established, first on Vancouver Island, and later on the mainland.

In 1812 hostilities broke out again between Britain and America and there was heavy fighting in Canada. American forces were defeated at Queenstown Heights, above Niagara, though York (now Toronto) was captured and burned. Cessation of hostilities left 'British North America' intact.

Government of the colony was corrupt and kept in the hands of a few ruling families, a situation which inevitably produced adverse reactions. In Upper Canada, opposition was led by William Lyon Mackenzie, in Lower Canada by Louis-Joseph Papineau There were other grievances. The large Métis element in the population, of mixed Indian, Inuit and European (largely French and Scottish) descent, was adversely affected by the amalgamation of the Hudson's Bay and North West Companies. A liberal-minded Governor General, 'Radical Jack', the Earl of Durham, attempted to improve government in 1841 with his concept of 'responsible government' with a wider electorate. This wider electorate did not include the native peoples, whose woodland and prairie territories were being increasingly occupied by pioneering settlers from east and south, and also straight from Europe. Scots were prominent but Scandinavians, Swedes, Ukrainians, Germans, and Irish were also coming in increasingly large numbers, driven by poverty or oppression, and lured by opportunity.

Opportunity shone most brightly in the form of gold. The first Canadian gold rush was in 1858. But these stampedes were temporary things, while the steady process of occupying the interior had permanent effects. Population was moving faster than government, and bison-hunting Métis and cow-rearing farmers were at odds with each other. Although the border remained secure, the carnage of the U.S. Civil War impressed Canadians with the need for unity, and a conference in Charlottetown, Prince Edward Island, to discuss the possible union of the Maritime Provinces, a group of provinces comprising New Brunswick, Newfoundland, Nova Scotia, and Prince Edward Island, was unexpectedly expanded by representatives from the two Canadas. From this came the proposal for the Canadian Confederation, confirmed by the British North America Act of 1867. A federal government was to rule, from Ottawa, but the provinces were to retain substantial internal autonomy. Even so, the completion of the Confederation would be a piecemeal affair. In a sense, it is still happening. British Columbia joined in 1871, Prince Edward Island did not join until 1873, and Newfoundland stayed out until 1949.

Most trouble came from the prairie area. The federal government had purchased a huge tract of former Hudson's Bay Company land in 1869, and was confronted by the Red River Rebellion of the Métis under Louis Riel. With nothing to lose, the Métis rose again in 1885, the year the transcontinental railway was completed. Their way of life was doomed. They had virtually wiped out the bison, and new farming techniques were turning the prairies into wheatlands. Police organization, local government, and, finally the formation of the provinces of Alberta and Saskatchewan in 1905, set the seal on the new order of things.

In the twentieth and twenty-first centuries, the main themes of Canadian history have been the breaking of the ties of imperial control, the re-emergence of Québec separatism, the accommodation and acknowledgement of the place of native peoples within the Confederation, and the country's peaceful but not always harmonious relationship with the U.S.A. During World War I, Canada was 'automatically' included in the British Empire's declaration of war on Germany; in World War II, Canada made its own decision to declare war in September 1939. Although the Queen is still sovereign as a constitutional monarch, the Governor General, her representative, is now appointed by the Prime Minister. There are Canadian republicans, but also Canadian monarchists. More detail on the Québec situation will be found in the section on that province. Although native peoples constitute a very small percentage of Canada's population, there has been increasing recognition through the years of both the exploitation and oppression suffered by them during the centuries of colonization, and of their long history within the country. The recent creation of the territory of Nunavut in 1999 is a sign of the new acceptance of partnership and common goals between modern Canada and the descendants of its early inhabitants.

Apart from some residual frontier disputes, such as the one over the British Columbia–Alaska oceanic boundary, the main focus of Canada–U.S. relations has been on trade, particularly in relation to 'reciprocity' (as it was known early in the twentieth century) or 'free trade'. With a smaller internal market, Canadian manufacturers have always been afraid of the country being swamped by goods produced in the U.S. Despite much opposition, free trade has been sustained, and Canada has joined in moves towards a wider American Free Trade Area. Suspicions on both sides about subsidies and produce-dumping frequently cause short-term tariff hikes and counter-hikes. The North American Free Trade Act (NAFTA) of 1993 between Canada, United States and Mexico has not reduced these problems.

The heritage industry

In modern countries, where change happens so quickly, a heritage industry can achieves two things. One is to help validate the recent past for those who might feel that its disappearance has made their lives meaningless, as in a town that has lost its mine or steelworks. The other is to interpret the country's past to visitors and travellers, and in the course of doing so, to foster the tourist industry. In Canada, both aspects are important, but with so many new citizens, the country's many heritage centres are also used to explain Canada's history and character, and to help support its ethos. There are 179 national parks and historic sites across the country, and many hundreds more set up on a provincial or local basis. The national parks, of course,

also preserve and protect some of the planet's most beautiful and remarkable landscapes together with their flora and fauna.

The People of Canada

Population

The population of Canada in 2005 was 32,291,831 Its rate of growth is about 1%. More than 80% of Canada's inhabitants live in the south of the country, within 160 kilometres of the U.S. border. The majority of Canadians are of European origin. Native American peoples, Indian and Inuit, account for about 1.4% of the inhabitants. However, aboriginal peoples are one of Canada's fastest growing populations, growing at twice the Canadian average. In 2001, the number of people identifying themselves as aboriginal was 975,000.

Language

The two official languages are English and French, and all official announcements are made in both languages. In 2001, 17,352,315 Canadians noted English as their mother tongue; 6,703,325 noted French, and 112,575 noted both English and French. Many other language groups were identified, the largest being Chinese, with 853,745 noting it as their mother tongue; Italian, with 469,485; German, with 438,080; Spanish, with 245,495; Portuguese, with 213,815; and Punjabi, with 271,220. The largest native language group was Cree, with 72,885 noting it as their mother tongue. Modern Canada is an ethnically diverse country, with the majority of recent immigrants coming from Asia.

Citizenship

Modern Canada is a relatively new nation and, with its many ethnic and language groups, takes the matter of citizenship very seriously. Canadian citizenship is automatic to those born in Canada and to those born elsewhere with a Canadian parent. Citizenship is also granted to immigrants, normally after a specified residence period. New citizens must have a knowledge of English or French, and be able to display knowledge of Canada's law, politics, history, and geography by answering test questions. An oath of citizenship is formally administered, and there are regular re-affirmation ceremonies in the annual Citizenship Week which has nationwide events to promote a sense of Canadian unity. The oath taken by all new citizens runs as follows:

'I swear that I will be faithful and bear true allegiance to Her Majesty Queen Elizabeth the Second, Queen of Canada, her heirs and successors, and that I will faithfully observe the laws of Canada and fulfil my duties as a citizen.'

Native Peoples

In one sense, the far northwest is the cradle of all American peoples. It was across the land link from Asia that the first settlers of the continent came, around 20,000 years ago. Successive groups came over a very lengthy period of time. The most recent was the Eskimo–Aleut group, whose arrival is estimated as having occurred more than 8,000 years ago. Before them, the speakers of a language group known as Na-Dene had spread through the continent. They were originally hunter-gatherers. Family and kin groups spread apart and began to define their own territories, and the origins of the later aboriginal groups lie in this. Over the centuries, great changes occurred in the cultures and ways of life of aboriginal peoples, even before the arrival of Europeans in the east, north, and west brought major disruption. The modern history of aboriginal peoples, except to some extent for those in the arctic north, is of loss of territory, overwhelming cultural invasion, and a low place in a political and economic framework which they have had no part in devising. During the twentieth century there gradually arose a new appreciation of the native peoples' values, traditions, skills, and potential contribution to a new and inclusive nationhood. But great gulfs remain between the 'consumerist' culture of European Canadians and the more self-contained and environmentally conscious traditions of the Indians and Inuit, between an essentially urban way of life and an essentially rural one.

Although the location of the many different Indian first nations has always been quite fluid, native peoples can be grouped, mainly by language, in several different regions. (The distribution of aboriginal peoples in the north, as described below, is more or less as they can be found today. But in the other regions, because of white settlement and land exploitation, the distribution refers rather to how things were in the nineteenth century.)

The north

Here the population forms three groups, distinguished by their languages: the Aleut, the Yup'ik, and the Inuit–Inupiaq. In general the Aleut and Yup'ik are found in the western areas of arctic and subarctic Canada, and the Inuit in the eastern areas, including Baffin Island. As with all aboriginal groups, their distribution has little to do with modern frontiers, and Inuit territory extends into Greenland. This is the only area where native peoples form a majority of the population.

The east

A number of large first nations lived in the area round the Great Lakes and along the St. Lawrence. The Chippewa (Ojibwa) were to be found north of Lake Superior, with the Algonquin and Nipissing to the east. On the lake peninsula were the Neutral and Huron. The Iroquois were on both sides of the St. Lawrence, with Algonquin to their north and the Maliseet-Passamaquoddy and Mi'kmaq living in what are now the Maritime Provinces. From the eighteenth century, the French and British recognized the existence of the Five Nations of the Iroquois Confederacy, namely the Mohawk, Oneida, Onondaga, Cayuga and Seneca, with the Tuscarora making a sixth nation in the course of the century.

The centre

The vast area encompassed by the Prairie Provinces and westwards into the Yukon was populated by over thirty main groups of first nations peoples, some very small in number, and with a population of hardly more than sixty thousand all

told. The main division was between Athapaskan language speakers to the west, and the Algonquian language group to the east.

The mountains

The valleys and plateau lands were occupied on the western side by Salish-speaking first nations, Lillooet, Shuswap, Thompson, Nicola, Okanagan, and Lakes; to the east of them lived the Kutenai, speaking a language distantly related to Algonquin.

The west coast

A complex and varying pattern of first nations occupied the islands and the coast, with a range of cultural characteristics and language groups. Vancouver Island was the land of the Nootkans; on the facing mainland were the Salish (also on Vancouver Island), with a succession of other first nations occupying the territory to the north – Kwakiutl, Oowekeeno, Bella Coola, Bella Bella, Haihais, Haisla, Tsimshian, Gitksan, Nishga, Haida, and Tlingit. The west coast of Canada is an area where tribal traditions and customs are still very much part of life and local politics.

The Capital

Ottawa, in Ontario but right on the border with Québec, was selected in 1858 as the capital of the province of Canada, combining the two provinces then known as Upper and Lower Canada. This role continued when the Dominion of Canada was formed in 1867. Originally Ottawa was a village at the northern end of a canal constructed to link the Ottawa River to Lake Ontario, via the Rideau River. Known then as Bytown, after Colonel John By, who commanded the troops who dug the canal, its Indian name *Ottawa* was adopted in 1854. It is now a major city, whose population (combined with Hull – now called Gatineau - across the Ottawa River) exceeds 1,000,000 people. Apart from Parliament and government offices, a number of national institutions are located here, including the National Gallery, the National Library, National Archives, and several other national museums.

Canada in the World

Canada is a country that takes its responsibilities to the rest of the world seriously. It is the seventh largest contributor to the budget of the United Nations. Its world role is sustained by various agencies. Chief among these is the diplomatic service of the government, but Canadian multinational companies also play a large part. Members of Canadian businesses, universities, institutes, and national organizations participate actively in a wide range of international bodies and forums. Other international links are maintained by cultural organizations and by individual arts groups and practitioners.

A number of key aspects help to define Canada's place on the world stage:

1. *Canada's vast physical extent, and its proximity to the polar regions*. This gives the country a powerful voice, as well as responsibility, in the increasingly serious issues regarding global climate and global pollution.

2. *Canada's immediate proximity to the United States of America, the country's prime trading partner and ally.* The Canadian–U.S. border is by far the longest open and undefended frontier in the world, although since the 'war on terrorism' began in 2001, 140 crossing stations with customs stations are monitored. Canada is not a neutral state, but its independent stance on many issues – notably on the Vietnam War between 1965 and 1974, when many young Americans took refuge from the draft in Canada – and its strong commitment to the United Nations, has enabled Canadian troops to play peacekeeping roles in various world hot spots.

3. *Canada's contribution to world trade.* Canada is a major producing and consuming nation.

4. *Canada's membership of the British Commonwealth of Nations.* This has given Canada an interest in the problems of post-colonial African and Asian Commonwealth states. Canadian aid and diplomacy have often been deployed in Commonwealth causes.

A fifth aspect might be Canada's position with involvement in both the English and French-language cultures, but this contributes more prominently to the country's international cultural life.

Defence

The Canadian armed forces are organized as a single national defence force, with army, navy and air force components. In August 2005, armed forces personnel numbered 60,000. In addition there were 21,500 reservists. The federal defence budget in 2005 was $12,800 million over five years. Canada's defence forces are highly technologized and a high proportion of the budget is spent on the maintenance and development of equipment. Apart from a commitment to NATO, and the necessary roles of patrolling two coastlines and the northern frontiers, Canadian forces are often used in UN-sponsored peacekeeping missions. Canada participated in the Gulf War of 1991. Since 2003, Canadian forces are engaged in the warfare in Afghanistan.

Society

Canada is regularly cited as one of the best countries in the world in which to live. Judged on standards of income, opportunity, freedom, social services, health care, education, and crime level, Canada occupies an enviable position among the nations. But no large and complex modern society is without problems and worries.

Health and welfare

In a United Nations index on human development in 2005, Canada ranks fifth among the countries of the world. All of the population have access to fresh water and effective sewage management. Mortality among under-5s is 5.2 per 1,000 live births (2001). In 2002, 56,000 people in Canada were living with HIV, a 12% increase since 1999 . Health services are provided free to Canadian citizens, and there are 189 physicians for every 10,000 people in 2003. The standards of health care are among the highest in the world.

Housing

In the second half of the twentieth century there was a marked trend away from rented housing and towards home ownership, and this continues. In 2000, 66.7% of Canadians owned their own homes, mostly mortgaged. There is also a continuing trend towards individual family homes, with the proportion of people living in apartment blocks diminishing year by year.

Education

Elementary and secondary school education is administered by the provinces. For children from 6 to 15 or 16 years old (depending on the province) education is compulsory and free. Province-run schools are normally co-educational. Some provinces allow schools to be run by religious groups. In 1999 the total school enrolment was 5,368,185, or approximately 18% of the population. The vast majority of students attend public schools; in 1999 the number was 4,999,348. Private schools were attended by 297,798 students; federal schools accounted for 71,039.

After school, some 75 universities and 275 other tertiary education institutes offer higher education and vocational courses. Students must pay their own way, though some institutions have private endowments and state grants. Most students take out an assisted loan, for repayment after graduation, and vacation work is common. University enrolment of full-time students in 2002 was 684,000. For 2000–2001, the federal education budget was $4.832 million, or 2.6% of federal spending. The provinces and territories spent $40,555 million, or 20.1% of their total spending, on education.

Justice, law and order

Crime and violence are relatively low in Canada, certainly by comparison with the U.S.A., and Canadian cities are among the world's safest. The federal police force is the Royal Canadian Mounted Police; this also provides basic policing of all provinces except Ontario and Québec, which have their own police forces. At the top of the justice system is the Supreme Court of Canada, which is the highest court and ultimate court of appeal. Next is the Federal Court, which deals with all claims by or against the Crown (i.e. the federal government), and the Court of Appeal. Each province has its own provincial court system, headed by a chief justice.

Religion

The Canadian state is secular and there is freedom of worship. About 75% of the population have at least nominal attachment to one of the major Christian churches, Anglican, United, and Roman Catholic. In Québec province, Catholics are in a substantial majority. Virtually all other world faiths are represented. The number of Muslims in Canada is estimated at around 579,640 (2001); the number of Jews at around 329,995 (2001); and there are also large Sikh and Buddhist groups.

Media

Each Canadian city has its own daily newspaper, but two

can claim to be nationally available, the *National Post* and the Toronto *Globe and Mail*. There were 101 daily newspapers in 2001, and around 1,100 weekly or twice-weekly community papers. A wide range of special-interest journals and magazines is also published, in addition to imported English- and French-language publications.

The Canadian Broadcasting Corporation (CBC), a nationally funded broadcaster, covers the country with TV and radio broadcasting in English and French. It is estimated to reach 99.5% of the population. It also operates Radio Canada International, on short wave, which broadcasts to a worldwide audience in nine languages. Commercial stations such as Global and CTV are widely watched. With access to major U.S. channels, and a vast range of options via satellite and cable TV, Canadians have one of the widest ranges of station choices in the world. In March 2001, Canada had 245 outlets for AM radio and 582 for FM. The regulation of radio, TV and telecommunications is exercised by the Canadian Radio-TV and Telecommunications Commission.

Book publishing is a vibrant industry in Canada, though globalization of major publishers has reduced the number of larger Canadian-owned companies. Canadians have access to the entire output of the American, British, and French publishing industries.

The nationwide availability of new technology, including the extension of broadband access, has made Canada an important user of email and the Internet.

Economy

The national currency is the Canadian dollar, divided into 100 cents. Broadly based as it is upon primary products, agriculture, manufacture, and services, the Canadian economy is a strong one. The principal adverse effects on it come either from economic downturn in the adjacent U.S.A., reducing Canadian exports, or from falls in world prices of metal ores. The general picture in Canada over recent decades has been of economic expansion and diversification.

Gross national product (GNP)

The 2003 Canadian GNP is CDN$713.5 billion, working out at CDN$23,016 per head of the population.

Banking

The central bank is the Bank of Canada, and it is responsible among other things for conducting monetary policy, issuing and controlling the currency, and regulating credit and currency 'in the best interests of the economic life of the nation.' Fourteen major commercial banks deal with personal and corporate finances through chains of offices. In addition there are numerous more specialized banks, many of them Canadian branches of institutions established elsewhere.

Stock exchanges

The country's largest stock exchange is in Toronto and there are also stock exchanges in Montréal and Vancouver, where shares in Canadian companies are traded.

Labour

In 2004, the Canadian labour force – persons aged over 15 and under 65 – numbered 17,183,400. Of these, 15,949,700 were in employment, and 1,233,700 were unemployed or between jobs.

Federal budget

In 2004-2005, the federal budget was $187.2 billion revenues and $183.3 billion in expenditures. The main sources of federal revenue in the same period were as follows (in millions of dollars):

Personal income taxes:	92,306
Corporation income taxes:	27,705
General sales taxes:	30,995
Gasoline and fuel taxes:	5,119
Alcohol and tobacco taxes:	4,425
Customs duty:	2,870
Other taxes:	503
Contributions to social security plans:	17,893
Sale of goods and services:	4,882
Investment income:	6,740

The main areas of 2004 federal expenditure were as follows (in millions of dollars):

Total expenditure on all items:	193,022
General services:	7,355
Protection of persons and property:	20,931
Transport and communications:	2,250
Health (including hospital care):	6,044
Social services:	59,640
Education:	4,771
Resource conservation and industrial development:	7,630
Foreign affairs and international assistance:	4,810
General transfers to other levels of government:	31,758
Debt charges:	34,632

Trade and Industry

Agriculture

The typical image of agricultural Canada is of the prairie wheat crop, with its miles of rippling grain. But this belies the diversity of Canadian agriculture, which has evolved to suit its many terrains and climatic variations, as well as market needs. Wheat, though still the largest field crop, is reducing in quantity. In 1996, just under 10 million hectares (24,710,000 acres) were given over to wheat; by 2001 this was down 16.7% to 8,310,787 hectares (20,535,954 acres). Barley production is also falling, down 10.4% from its 1996 level of 5,241,923 hectares (12,952,791 acres) to 4,696,911 hectares (11,606,067 acres) in 2001. Cultivation of alfalfa and other forms of maize is increasing, with 4,504,042 hectares (11,129,487 acres) under cultivation in 2001 compared with 3,598,461 hectares (8,891,717 acres) in 1996. This reflects an increased demand for animal feedstuffs.

The farm animal population grows steadily. Farmers' returns showed a cattle population of 15,551,449 cattle in 2001, an increase of 4.4% on 1996's figure of 14,893,034.

However, in 2003, the discovery of BSE (bovine spongiform encephalopathy) on a few Canadian farms, had a great impact on the cattle and beef industry. In 2002, revenue from beef and cattle was nearly $8 billion. After the trade ban due to BSE, revenues dropped to $2.2 billion – a decrease of 33%.

In 2001, other species had increased by a greater degree. Pigs in 2001 numbered 13,958,772, an increase of 26.5% on the 1996 figure of 11,040,462. The number of farms rearing pigs grew in the same period by over 26%. The poultry population of hens, ducks, geese, and turkeys totalled 126,159,520 in 2001, an increase of 23.4% against the 1996 figure of 102,255,149.

Changes in the pattern of agriculture are reflected by the steady decrease in the number of farms. In 1996, Canada had 276,548 farms of all sizes. By 2001 the number was down to 246,923, a drop of around 2% each year. This reflects a continuing drift from the land to the cities that has been going on for many decades, a growth in the size of farms, and the ever-increasing mechanization and semi-industrialization of agriculture.

Changes in consumer eating habits, and the demands of the supply chain, have influenced farmers' activities. Blueberries as a crop have risen from 36,222 hectares (89,504 acres) in 1996 to 43,982 hectares (108,679 acres) in 2001, a rise of 21.4%. Vine cultivation in the same period has risen from 7,515 hectares (18,569 acres) to 10,589 hectares (26,165 acres), an increase of 40.9%, incidentally revealing the renaissance of Canada's wine industry. Apple cultivation, on the other hand, a traditional practice of many farms in the Maritime Provinces, is falling, from 31,592 hectares (78,064 acres) in 1996 to 25,825 hectares (63,813 acres) in 2001, a drop of 18.3%. These selected statistics show a growing trend in Canadian farming towards the supply of food for packaging and processing. It is underlined by the rapid and continuing development of greenhouse and tunnel cultivation. In 1996 this covered 12,913,404 square metres (15,444,431 square yards); by 2001 it had risen by 42.1% to 18,352,645 square metres (21,949,763 square yards), and this trend will no doubt continue.

With a relatively short growing season over most of the country, the high level of investment required in modern-day farming, and the demands of a supermarket and chain store industry that looks for uniform size, colour and appearance, the issue of genetically modified seed use, and the potential in the future of animal cloning, are much-debated issues in Canada as elsewhere. Although 'green' politics has yet to break through at a provincial and national level, there is a strong latent sense of environmental responsibility among Canadians.

Fisheries
International controversy relating to oceanic fishing rights, zonal boundaries, and diminishing fish stocks continue to affect this industry. The sea fishing fleets of Newfoundland and Nova Scotia have been greatly reduced in recent years. In 2003, 1,062,428 metric tonnes of fish of all kinds (live weight) were landed. With an economic value in 2003,

$2,182,729, the future of fishing is a major economic issue. The principal species caught are Atlantic cod, herring, and salmon, and Pacific salmon and herring. The shellfish industry is important on both coasts. Canada does not practice whaling, but around 312,000 seals were caught in 2003.

Furs
One of Canada's oldest pursuits, the fur industry, remains significant today: over 2 million pelts were traded in 2004. The modern fur industry consists of pelts from farmed animals, such as beaver, muskrat, fox, chinchilla and marten; half were from wild furs. In 2004, 60,000 trappers were working in Canada. Furs added $800 million to the economy.

Industry
Canadian industry represents around 75% of the country's gross national product and is thus of crucial importance in maintaining the nation's wealth and living standards. The industrial base is both diverse and modern, centred on transportation, food products, electrical equipment, paper and chemicals. The value of shipments from Canadian industry in 2003 was $545,715,700. The ten largest contributors were as follows (in dollars):

Transportation equipment:	125,738,200
Food industries:	63,415,700
Chemicals and chemical products:	40,546,300
Primary metal industries:	34,828,200
Paper and allied products:	34,001,600
Petroleum and coal products:	33,660,200
Wood industries:	32,174,400
Fabricated metal industries:	31,101,900
Machinery:	26,815,700
Plastics and rubber products:	24,720,900

Trade
Canada is a major trading nation, and one that normally enjoys a surplus of export revenue over import costs. In 2003, exports totalled $380,815 million, and imports were $335,533 million. The U.S.A. is by far the country's major trading partner, absorbing more than three-quarters of all Canadian exports and supplying more than two-thirds of all Canadian imports.

Canada's Main Trading Partners

Exports in 1996, 2001 and 2003 in $ millions

Country	1996	2001	2003
U.S.A.	222,416.3	350,908.1	326,700
Japan	12,423.4	9,481.5	8,144
UK	4,608.5	6,573.5	6,085
Other EU countries	12,796.3	15,726.7	13,320
Total exports	280,079.3	414,638.2	380,815

Imports in 1996 and 2001 in $ millions

Country	1996	2001	2003
U.S.A.	180,010.1	225,028.2	203,550
Japan	7,227.4	585.2	13,815
UK	5,581.1	11,863.4	9,069
Other EU countries	14,994.7	23,225.1	33,137
Total imports	237,688.6	350,622.7	335,533

The very substantial positive trade balance between Canada and the U.S.A. more than compensates for the adverse balance with other major industrial economies. Canada has little need to import primary products of any kind. Imported goods consist of the following: manufactured articles (such as industrial equipment, automobiles, trucks, and consumer goods); electronic equipment, defence equipment, textiles (such as cotton and silk), foodstuffs, and other natural products from hotter regions, including rice, fruit, tea, coffee, hardwoods, and mineral products not found in Canada (such as bauxite and industrial diamonds); specialist products from the international drinks and foods industries; books and other media items; and luxury goods.

Many items in some of these categories are also exported from Canada. The prime export items are cereal crops, lumber and lumber products, meat, fish and poultry products, electric power, and a range of minerals including petroleum, coal, natural gas, copper, nickel, lead, zinc, molybdenum, silver, gold, platinum, and uranium. As in most countries, Canada also has a hidden but substantial 'unofficial' economy that is nowadays chiefly founded on the drug trade and other forms of organized crime.

Transport

Highways, railways, canals, and aircraft all play a part in Canadian transport.

Transport by road: there are over 1,427,000 kilometres (886,000 miles) of highway, of which around 15,000 kilometres (9,321 miles) form federal roads and highways. The longest of these is the Trans-Canada Highway, which runs 7,800 kilometres (4,847 miles) from St. John's to Victoria. Most passenger transport is by road, and few Canadian families do not own, or have access to, a car. Automobiles are by the most frequently used means of personal transport.

Transport by rail: Canada's national rail company, VIA Rail, crosses the country, and also links with the U.S. network, which is on the same standard gauge. Much long-distance freight is still sent by rail. New rail lines have been built to facilitate mineral extraction from remote mining areas in the north. Transcontinental passenger trains still operate, although most passenger travel by rail is on rapid-transit systems in the larger cities. In 2002 the railways' freight revenue amounted to $7.3 billion, the passenger revenue to only $287.5 million.

Transport by river, lake, canal: the prime inland navigation route is the St. Lawrence Seaway, established to bring ocean-going ships into the heart of the continent by linking the Great Lakes with the Atlantic Ocean, and completed in 1959. Its main limitation, apart from the subsequent development of super-size vessels, is that it is blocked by ice between mid-December and mid-April. The Great Lakes themselves form an important transport route. There are thousands of kilometres of navigable rivers and lakes across the country, though much of their use nowadays is for leisure. The lumber industry still uses rivers for floating and rafting logs downstream.

Transport by air: air transport began in a small way in the 1920s but is now a very important element in the transport pattern. Shuttle services link Montréal and Toronto, and frequent flights serve to link other major cities. From the east coast to the west coast remains a relatively long-haul flight, taking from five to seven hours. International air connections are made at Montréal, Toronto, Winnipeg, and Vancouver.

Transport in winter: another form of winter land transport, independent of the road network, is the snowmobile, which is widely used in the Prairie Provinces and in northern areas for cross-country transport, using frozen lake surfaces as well as the snow-surfaced landscape. Seaplane, ski-plane and helicopter services reach out to distant communities which might be cut off by land transport in winter.

Tourism

The number of visitors to Canada in 2002 was 20 million. Of these, 16.2 million came from the U.S.A. The remaining came chiefly from Europe and Japan. The income from tourists in 2003 was reckoned at $52.1 billion. Although travel facilities, accommodation, and length of season reduce rural Canada's potential for increasing tourist traffic, especially in the northern areas, the same factors act as a spur to visitors who wish to see a landscape which is still 'unspoiled' and a scene which does not consist of other visitors.

Culture

In Canada, the keyword to reflect the country's national diversity is not 'melting pot', as in the U.S.A., but 'mosaic'. The country has a rich and vibrant cultural life which has spread from the twin pillars of English and French traditions into something much more varied and unashamedly modern, and the aboriginal peoples' traditions are no longer excluded as 'folklore' or 'craft'.

While the introduction of a wide-ranging multiculturalism has been successful, the essential duality of Canadian cultural life has remained a central government concern since the days of Pierre Trudeau's premiership. Then, for the first time, there was a major effort to make English-speaking Canadians more bilingual, and to promote, as part of Canadian identity, bilingualism and the sharing of the two cultures.

The Canada Council, founded in 1957, is the national agency for the arts, with a brief to foster what is best and also what is specifically Canadian in origin or inspiration.

Literature

In literature, Canadian writing forms a distinctive region of English and French, and is by no means a 'provincial' school. On the short list of ten writers nominated for Britain's most prestigious literary prize in 2001, four of the nominated authors were Canadian or resident in Canada. The works of Canadian novelists such as Robertson Davies and Margaret Atwood are available throughout the world. Other international successes include Mordecai Richler, Carol Shields, Michael Ondaatje, and, in French, Anne Hébert. Earlier twentieth-century figures with a worldwide reputation include the humorist Stephen Leacock and the economic historian J. K. Galbraith.

Theatre

The first recorded theatrical show in Canada took place at Port Royal in 1606, and other theatrical performances took place in Montréal and Québec during the seventeenth century. Theatres opened in the larger cities during the later nineteenth century, and the famous theatre at Stratford, Ontario, opened in 1957. Nowadays, established and touring companies bring a wide range of classical and modern drama to Canadians in cities and towns across the land, although the prime centres are Toronto and Montréal.

Music, opera and ballet

Professional symphony orchestras exist in Calgary, Edmonton, Hamilton, Kitchener-Waterloo, Montréal, Ottawa, New Brunswick, Nova Scotia, Saskatoon, Thunder Bay, Toronto, Victoria, Vancouver, and Winnipeg. There are many smaller orchestras and musical groups, as well as a vibrant pop, jazz, and folk music industry. Music festivals are frequent. Opera is regularly performed by the Canadian Opera Company in Toronto (and on tour), and by Montréal Opera, Edmonton Opera, Québec Opera, Opera Hamilton, Pacific Opera Victoria, and Vancouver Opera. Apart from the National Ballet of Canada, there are ballet companies in Winnipeg and Montréal, and provincial companies in Alberta and British Columbia.

Art and sculpture

The Toronto-based 'Group of Seven' in the 1920s was the first self-proclaimed national school of artists 'imbued with the idea that an Art must grow and flower in the land before the country will be a real home for its people'. Their paintings of the Canadian landscape did much to support this idea. The group's leading figure was the Montréal painter, A. Y. Jackson. Inevitably their work became something to surpass or depart from, and Canadian painters were very much alive to what was happening elsewhere. Québec artists had strong connections with France, where the cubist and surrealist revolutions were happening.

Modern Canadian artists have been strongly influenced by abstract expressionism. In recent years, there has also been increasing recognition of the art practiced by Inuit and First Peoples artists. Canada has a range of great art galleries, including the National Gallery, the Art Gallery of Ontario, with its superb Henry Moore collection, and the Vancouver Art Gallery with its totem paintings by the British Columbian artist, Emily Carr.

Architecture and townscape

An unusually perceptive early traveller remarked that the Inuit igloo was comparable in its combination of form and function to the Greek temple. The same might be said of the tepee of the Plains Indians, while the wooden architecture of the first nations of the Pacific coast is on a monumental scale. The first European buildings, other than rude cabins, were the *habitations* – fortified settlements begun by Champlain in the early seventeenth century. Fortress architecture loomed large for over 200 years, culminating in the great stone citadels of Louisbourg, Halifax and Québec.

Some of the oldest towns, such as Montréal and Québec City, preserve an irregular central street pattern based on original pathways, but the typical Canadian urban layout, as exemplified by Toronto and most other cities, is the rectangular grid, with two intersecting main streets. Two towns, Québec City and the old Nova Scotian port of Lunenburg, are classed by the United Nations Educational, Scientific and Cultural Organization (UNESCO) as world heritage sites.

The earliest public buildings were churches, often placed in commanding sites. The early colonial wooden churches were gradually supplanted by more permanent and grander buildings in classic, Romanesque, or gothic styles. Similar styles were employed for the provincial and national parliament buildings, and for the major railroad stations. But perhaps the most recognizably Canadian architecture is the Canadian Chateau Style, a distinctive form of French Renaissance style deployed in the vast chateau-hotels erected in the late nineteenth century by the Canadian Pacific Railway at Québec City, Banff, and Vancouver, among other places. Modern Canadian architecture is eclectic and cannot be said to express a particularly national spirit or style. Contemporary town planners' response both to street congestion and to long winters has been the development in the larger cities of extensive pedestrian areas, either underground or at upper-story levels. The Underground City in Montréal and the PATH system of Toronto are the most extensive.

Sport and Leisure

Just about every sport and pastime imaginable finds practitioners in Canada. The major professional sports, Canadian football, baseball, and ice hockey, have teams in every city and the leagues and provincial conferences are followed avidly by spectators, TV viewers, and readers of the press. The Toronto Blue Jays participate in the U.S. Major League.

At an amateur level, all the main sports are organized on a national and provincial basis. Around one third of the population participates regularly in some form of sport. The main national forum for athletics and field sports is the Canada Games, which take place every second year, alternately as Winter and Summer Games. Each Games is held at a different 'mid-sized' city venue and their progress round the country has led to the building of many excellent stadiums and sports complexes.

At the Athens Olympics of 2004, Canadians won the following medals:

* gold in gymnastics, canoeing, and cycling
* silver in diving, gymnastics, canoeing, cycling, rowing, sailing, wrestling
* bronze in canoeing, and diving

The most popular sports among Canadian men are golf, hockey, baseball, and swimming. Among women, swimming comes top, followed by golf, baseball, and volleyball. Canadians are particularly keen on winter sports, and figure and speed skating, skiing, and curling are all very popular.

Natural Resources

Water

With around 20% of the world's fresh water reserves, and with political control over a large part of the subarctic ice, Canada's water usage and management are likely to become important issues in the twenty-first century. Water power is also the prime source of electricity generation, with huge potential still unused. Canada currently produces around 550,000 million kWh annually.

Minerals

Canada has vast reserves of minerals and fossil fuels, many of them located in remote and sparsely inhabited regions, though mineral exploitation in the more populous southern strip has been going on for more than 200 years. Ores being mined in 1999 were bismuth, cadmium, cobalt, copper, gold, iron, lead, molybdenum, nickel, platinum, selenium, silver, uranium, and zinc. Non-metallic resources being mined or extracted include asbestos, coal, gypsum, natural gas, nepheline, syenite, petroleum, potash, salt, and sulphur. In addition, vast amounts of sand and gravel are extracted every year for use in the construction industry, and stone is quarried, both for building and for road stone.

Prospecting for minerals continues, and though it is likely that most significant deposits have now been identified, new discoveries have meant that reserves of certain minerals, such as crude oil, have increased over recent years despite extensive extraction. Known reserves (2003, unless noted) are as follows:

Crude petroleum:	12 billion barrels
Natural gas:	56.6 trillion cubic feet
Crude bitumen:	2.5 billion barrels (2001)
Coal:	8,623,000,000 tonnes (1999)
Copper:	6,700,000 tonnes
Nickel:	4,500,000 tonnes
Lead:	872,000 tonnes
Zinc:	6,900,000 tonnes
Molybdenum:	82,000 tonnes
Silver:	11,230 tonnes
Gold:	1,023 tonnes
Uranium:	312,000 tonnes (1999)

Canada is also the world's main source of potash, and a major source of asbestos. There are extensive deposits of iron ore. Production of rare metals such as selenium and tellurium is also carried on.

Forest

In 2004, 402.1 million hectares (993.187 million acres) were under forest. Of this, 294.8 million hectares (728.156 million acres) were classed as 'productive', i.e. commercially useful timber. Of the latter, almost a half was contained in the two provinces of Québec and British Columbia. Most of the commercial timber is softwood produced to feed the demands of the newsprint, paper, and packaging industries, but hardwoods are also produced. In 2002, 974,472 hectares (2.407 million acres) were harvested. The value to the economy was $44.6 billion.

The Provinces and Territories

Alberta

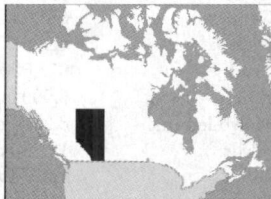

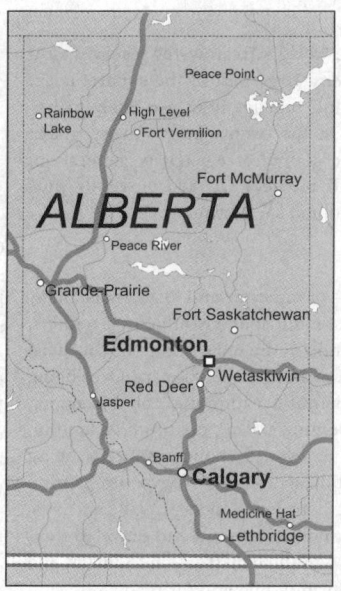

Name: the name is in honour of Queen Victoria's daughter, Princess Louise Alberta, wife of the Marquis of Lorne, Governor General. Alberta, along with Manitoba and Saskatchewan is one of the so-called Prairie Provinces.

Emblems: the wild rose, the lodgepole pine, the great horned owl.

Motto: Fortis et Liber, 'Strong and free'.

Population (2002): 3,113,600.

Capital: Edmonton, Canada's fifth largest city. The 36 municipalities forming Greater Edmonton are home to over 900,000 people. Focally placed on transcontinental routes running east, west, north, south, and northwest, the city is a major communications hub.

Physical description: with a land area of 661,848 square kilometres (243,560 square miles), it is the fourth largest of the provinces and territories. Southwestern Alberta is a mountainous region that includes the Monashee and Cariboo ranges of the Western Cordillera, rising to high peaks and with glaciers in the upper valleys. Alberta's highest point is Mt. Columbia (3,747 metres, 12,293 feet). Towards the central south, the foothills gradually give way to flat prairie country. The central area of the province is rich farming land, with woods, hills, and lakes. South of the 55th parallel the rivers flow east into Saskatchewan. To the north of the 55th parallel is a vast region of woods and grassland, still thinly populated, and with large extents of marsh known as muskeg. In it two great river systems flow northwards: the Peace River flows to the Great Slave Lake; the Athabasca to the lake of the same name.

Climate: Alberta has a continental-type climate, with long, cold winters, a brief, brilliant spring, and hot summers. On the west, the rain shadow of the mountains can produce long periods of drought.

Agriculture: in the eastern prairie area, wheat and other cereal crops are grown. To the west, stock rearing is more common. In the country between Calgary and Edmonton, mixed farming is practiced, with dairy herds and market gardens.

Minerals: southwest and central-south Alberta have large deposits of coal and natural gas, and the latter is a prime source of energy, along with hydroelectricity generated in the mountain valleys. Oil is extracted from a major field centred on the city of Drumheller. In the north of the province there are further oil and gas deposits, and rock salt is mined.

Industry: much of Alberta's mineral wealth is transported elsewhere by train and pipeline, but manufacturing industry related to mining, transport, and farming is important in the cities.

History: long a wilderness inhabited by nomadic groups of aboriginal people, the region was part of the Hudson's Bay grant of 1670. For another 200 years, little changed, though trading stations were established here and there, and pioneer families and communities began to establish farms. The completion of the Canadian Pacific Railway in 1885 opened up the area, and towns like Calgary and Edmonton began to grow. In the early twentieth century there was a rush of settlement, as not only the farmlands but also the mineral resources of the south began to be exploited. Alberta was constituted a province in 1905.

British Columbia

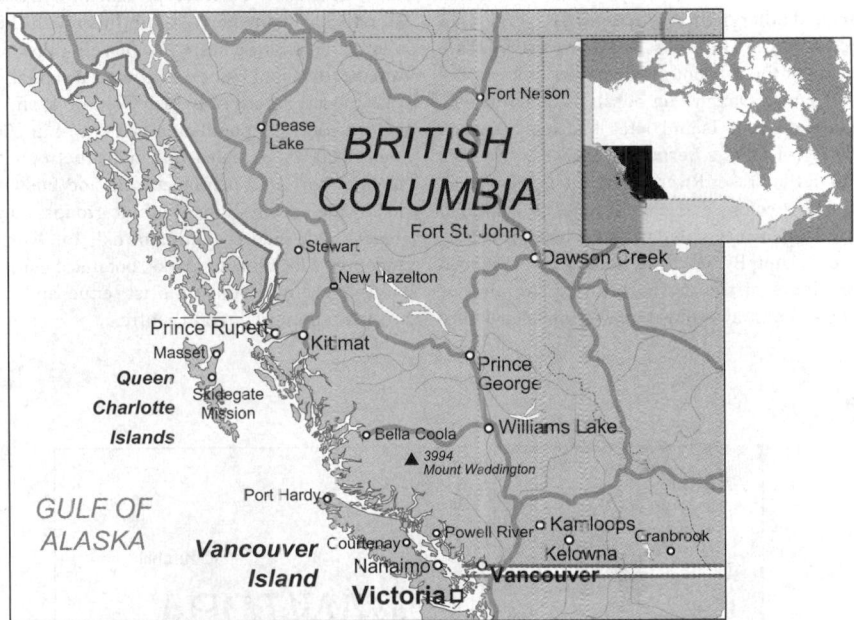

Name: the name of Canada's westernmost province ultimately honours Christopher Columbus and also recalls its original status as part of the British Empire.

Emblem: the Pacific dogwood, western red cedar, Steller's jay.

Motto: *Splendor sine occasu*, 'Splendour undiminished'.

Population (2002): 4,141,300.

Capital: Victoria, on Vancouver Island, a pleasant city on a fine natural harbour, with tourism, service industries, and administration its main occupations.

Physical description: with a land area of 944,735 square kilometres (364,668 square miles), it is the fifth in size among the territories and provinces. Mountains, deep valleys, and a heavily indented and islanded coastline largely define the landscape of British Columbia: geologically it is a continuation of the Western Cordillera, which covers most of the province, dividing between the Rocky Mountains on the border with Alberta, and the Coast Range, with a wide central area of mountains and plateaus separating the two main ranges. The highest peaks extend far above the tree line into regions of perpetual snow and ice with large glaciers. The highest point is Mt. Fairweather (4,663 metres, 15,298 feet). Rivers drain to east and west from the watersheds, with the Fraser system dominating in the south of the province and leading to the Pacific; and the Peace River flowing from the vast man-made Williston Lake to the east and north. The lower slopes, valleys, and islands are heavily forested, with cedar, spruce, and Douglas fir among the most common trees.

Climate: on the coastal side, the sea promotes a mild, moist climate, without great extremes. In the south of the province, there is an almost Mediterranean-type climate. Inland of the coastal range, it can be very dry, and temperatures vary from summer maxima of around 37° to winter lows of -32° or lower. On the eastern slopes of the mountains, the warm Chinook wind has an alleviating effect, though it also promotes a dry climate and dry soil. In the north, the climate becomes subarctic both on the coast and inland.

Agriculture: forestry is by far the most important form of cultivation. Forest parks now preserve the remaining specimens of the giant firs and cedars which once grew in vast numbers. Softwood trees are grown in huge plantations and the logs are usually floated down to the sea. In valleys and on grassy plateau areas, cattle and sheep are raised, and wheat and other cereals are grown in the Peace River valley. On the coastal side, fruit trees are also cultivated. Fisheries are important in the sea and the rivers, especially salmon.

Minerals: falling water is an important resource in British Columbia and virtually all its electricity is hydrogenerated. The province also has deposits of lead, zinc, gold, copper, asbestos, and silver. Coal is mined around Fernie, in the Rocky Mountains, and there are also coal deposits on Vancouver Island.

Industry: cheap power has encouraged the growth of power-intensive industry such as aluminium smelting. Lumber-related industry is widespread, with sawmills and pulp mills. In the Vancouver–Victoria area there is a diversity of industry including chemicals and electronics. Tourism is also a major contributor to the province's economy.

History: occupied by coastal Indian first nations peoples from prehistoric times, British Columbia's first European visitors came by sea up the Pacific coast. The Spanish explorer, Juan Pérez, came in 1774, and the British Captain Cook in 1778. The coast was surveyed between 1792–94 by Captain George Vancouver of the Royal Navy, and was at that time claimed for Great Britain. In 1793, Alexander

Mackenzie, a Scottish fur trader, crossed the Rockies to Cascade Inlet. The North West Company was established to trade in furs and other natural products of the region; in 1821 it merged with the Hudson's Bay Company. In 1843, Fort Victoria, site of the present provincial capital, was established by Sir James Douglas on behalf of the Hudson's Bay Company. Vancouver Island later became a Crown colony, with Douglas as its governor. In 1858, shortly after gold was found in the Fraser River valley, the mainland was also designated as a colony and named British Columbia. Vancouver Island was incorporated with it as a single colony in 1866. Five years later, British Columbia agreed to join as one of the provinces of the newly formed Dominion of Canada, so long as a railway connection was provided to link it to the eastern provinces. The first transcontinental line was completed in 1885. Despite this, the western province naturally has many north–south links with the U.S. states on either side, as well as a 'Pacific rim' presence.

Vancouver: though not the provincial capital, Vancouver is by far the largest city of British Columbia, and third largest in Canada, with a population of 545,674 in 2001, and with almost 2,000,000 people living in the metropolitan area. It is the chief port, and manufacturing and business centre of the province. A city of many ethnic groups, it has one of the largest and oldest 'Chinatowns' in North America. Vancouver's location, its parks, botanical gardens, and museums, make it a popular tourist venue, and it is the country's main film production centre.

Manitoba

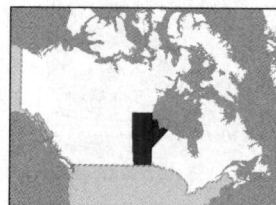

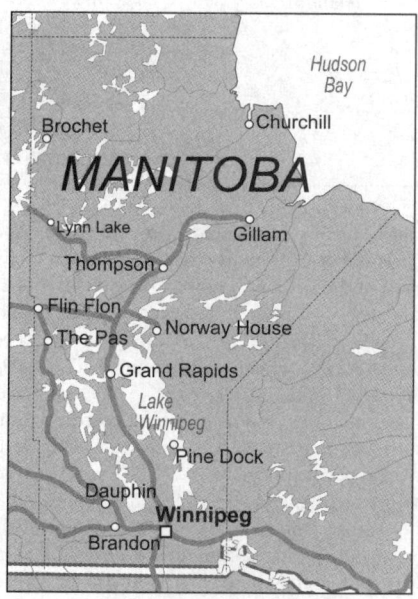

Name: the name is said to come from a Cree Indian phrase, meaning 'the narrows of the great spirit'. It is the easternmost of the Prairie Provinces.

Emblems: the great grey owl, the Prairie crocus, the white spruce.

Motto: Gloriosus et liber, 'Glorious and free'.

Population (2002): 1,150,800.

Capital: the city of Winnipeg, whose name comes from the Cree Indian phrase *win nipee* ('muddy water'), referring to the great lake of the same name. It is a spacious city of 640,000 people, spread over 462.1 square kilometres (178.4 square miles), and it is home to almost half the province's population.

Physical description: with an area of 647,797 square kilometres (250,050 square miles), it is seventh in size among the provinces and territories, and only very slightly smaller than Saskatchewan. Much of the area was once submerged under a huge lake, and it remains a lowland region still dominated by water features. Lake Winnipeg is the largest of many thousands of lakes, and north of it lies an extraordinary complex of inland waters, reaching to and beyond the province's northern boundary at the 60th parallel. On the northeast, Manitoba is bounded by Hudson Bay. On the west side, reaching into Saskatchewan, is a more hilly region, rising to summits mostly of around 750 metres (2,250 feet). The highest point is Mt. Baldy (832 metres, 2,729 feet). In the south there are great extents of almost level prairie.

Climate: the Manitoban climate is similar to that of Alberta, with long, cold winters and short but hot summers.

Agriculture: on the prairie, wheat is the prime crop, though oats, barley, potatoes, canola, flaxseed, rye, and sugar beet are also grown. There are also large areas of pasture land and, apart from stock rearing, much of Canada's honey production is located here. In the northern part of the province there is little farming, and the prime form of cultivation is forestry. Commercial fishing is based chiefly on Lake Winnipeg.

Minerals: Flin Flon, in the northwest of the province, is the main centre for a mining industry that extracts copper, zinc, gold, silver, cadmium, and tellurium. Other gold-producing areas are at Bissett, Herb Lake, and Snow Lake, and nickel is extracted at Mystery Lake and Moak Lake, near Thompson. In the southwest, near Virden, there are oil deposits. Sands and gravels are also extracted in large quantities.

Industry: most manufacturing industry is concentrated in and around Winnipeg and the industrial base is quite diverse. Parts are made for the automotive and aircraft industries. There is textile weaving and a clothing industry based on this plus locally available furs and leather. Mineral smelting and processing is carried out at Flin Flon, and nickel is refined at Thompson.

Transport: Winnipeg's international airport is the central hub of internal Canadian air services. The port of Churchill on Hudson Bay is a major grain exporter in the ice-free mid-July to mid-November period, as it stands at the end of the shortest sea route from the prairies to Europe. A branch of the transcontinental railroad links it to the main system.

History: the first recorded European explorer was Pierre de la Vérendrye in 1739, but the first serious European attempt at settling was made from Scotland in 1812, when a pioneering community established the township of Selkirk. The population remained very small through most of the nineteenth century. Up until 1868, Manitoba was the property of the Hudson's Bay Company, but in that year the new Dominion government purchased a large part of the territory lying on both sides of the Red River. At that time there was a rebellion among the Métis who lived and hunted in the region. This ended peacefully in 1870, but its leader Louis Riel had incurred deep hostility in Ontario. He was unable to take up his parliamentary seat and lived in exile in the U.S.A. In 1870 Manitoba was established as a province (albeit a much smaller province than today's Manitoba). By 1878 the railway had come, and this led to a substantial increase in population from the 12,000 or so of 1870. Land speculation led to further unrest among the Métis in 1885, and Riel returned to lead a second rebellion. This was put down by force, and Riel was captured, tried, and hanged at Regina. Manitoba joined the Confederation in 1870.

New Brunswick

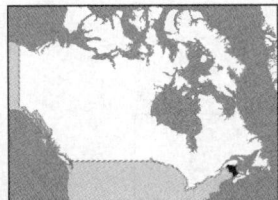

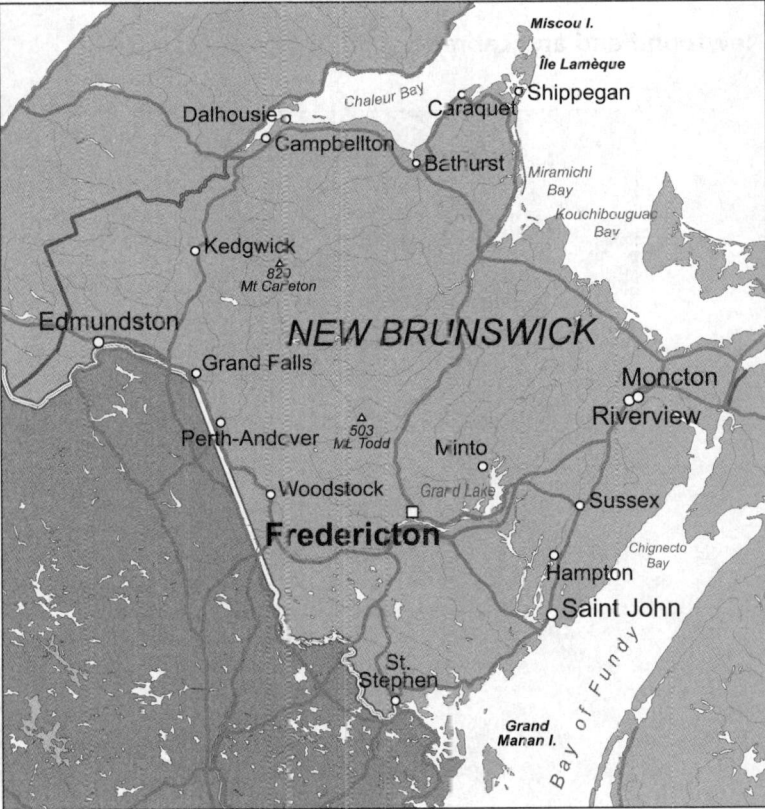

Name: named after the German state of Braunschweig, a possession of the royal British Hanoverians, New Brunswick, along with Newfoundland, Nova Scotia, and Prince Edward Island, is one of the Maritime Provinces.

Emblems: the purple violet, the black-capped chickadee, balsam fir.

Motto: *Spem reduxit*, 'Hope was restored'.

Population (2002): 756,700. Most people live around the coast and in the main river valleys (the St. John and Matapedia), which also form important lines of road and rail communication. The interior of the province is very sparsely populated.

Capital: Fredericton, population 46,500, an attractive town with many nineteenth-century buildings. The cultural centre of the province, it has two universities and the famous Beaverbrook Art Gallery.

Physical description: with a land area of 72,908 square kilometres (28,142 square miles), it is ninth in size among the provinces and territories. The province occupies the end of the 'peninsula' formed between the St. Lawrence Estuary, the Gulf of St. Lawrence, and the Bay of Fundy. The interior, forming the end of the long Appalachian range, consists of hilly and often wild countryside penetrated by long river valleys. The highest point is Mt. Carleton (817 metres, 2,610 feet).

Climate: away from the coast, the climate takes on more continental characteristics. Winters can be very cold, especially in the uplands, and are accompanied by heavy snowfalls. On the coast and in sheltered valleys, the weather is generally milder.

Agriculture: the relatively dry and cool climate has encouraged vegetable growing, notably of seed potatoes. Mixed farming prevails, with much pasture land. Much of the province remains covered in forest, with extensive hardwood forests as well as quick-growing softwood to feed the wood pulp and paper industries. Shellfish are an important resource along the coast.

Minerals: zinc, potash, silver, lead, copper, and coal are all found. There are also extensive peat deposits, cut for horticultural use.

Trade and industry: New Brunswick employment is divided 72% to services, 22% to industry, and 6% to agriculture.

History: until the seventeenth century, the region was the hunting ground of nomadic Indian first nations peoples. The first European settlers were French, but as in the rest of eastern Canada, the French and the British were soon in a contest for ownership. British possession was confirmed in 1713, and there was a steady increase in settlement during the eighteenth century. At this time the region was included in Nova Scotia. In 1784, New Brunswick was formally recognized as a separate colony and it became one of the provinces of Canada in 1867.

Newfoundland and Labrador

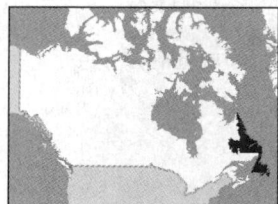

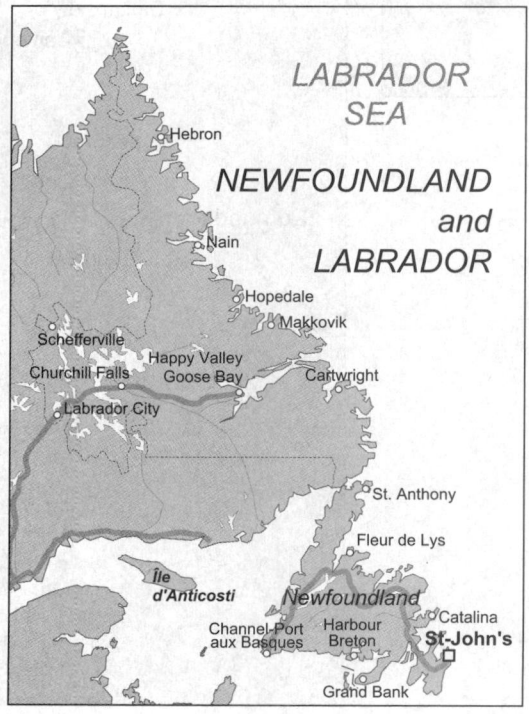

Name: its name bestowed by the explorer, John Cabot, in 1497, Canada's easternmost and most recent province is formed by this large island and the adjacent coastal region of Labrador. It is one of the four Maritime Provinces.

Emblems: the caribou, the pitcher plant. Other provincial emblems are the Newfoundland dog and pony, the black spruce, and the gemstone, labradorite.

Motto: *Quaerite prime regnum dei*, 'Seek ye first the kingdom of God'.

Population (2002): 531,600.

Capital: St. John's with a population of 102,000. With an average annual precipitation of 1,482 millimetres (53 inches), and 217 wet days a year, St. John's is Canada's wettest provincial capital.

Physical description: with a land area of 405,212 square kilometres (156,412 square miles) Newfoundland and Labrador is the eighth largest province. Lying across the entry to the Gulf of St. Lawrence, Newfoundland is shaped rather like an irregular triangle, with many peninsulas, and sides slightly less than 500 kilometres (310 miles) long. It is formed of the same rocks as the continent. These are at their highest on the western side, where the Long Range Mountains reach to around 800 metres (2,400 feet), with the highest point being Mt. Caubvik (1,652 metres, 5,420 feet); the height gradually reduces towards the eastern coast. Like the landscape of the Canadian Shield, the landscape is rugged and rocky, dotted with many lakes. Rivers, mostly short, drain from the interior to all coasts.

Climate: oceanic influences dominate, with a prevailing moistness and coolness and no great extremes, except on the northern Long Range coast where winter conditions can be severe. The Strait of Belle Isle is normally icebound between December and June. The Atlantic coasts are often enveloped in thick fog that comes in from the sea, a product of cold northern air meeting the relatively warm waters of the Gulf Stream.

Agriculture: the landscape is on the whole poorly suited to farming and farms exist mostly to supply local communities, but some two-fifths of the land surface is covered in forest, and lumber is an important industry. Newfoundland also has a large fishing industry, though over-exploitation by many nations of the once cod-rich Newfoundland Banks has brought about a reduction in catches and a shift of emphasis to crab and shrimp. It is the world's largest producer of cold-water cooked and peeled shrimp. In 2001, fisheries employed 14,600 people in the province, compared to 20,800 in 1991. Aquaculture (fish farming) now produces around 8,000 tonnes of fish a year and is still growing rapidly.

Minerals: there are many mineral deposits. Newfoundland is Canada's main source of fluorspar, while zinc, copper, lead, and gold are among the metals found. Substantial oil reserves are known to exist in the offshore Ben Nevis-Hebron Field, but in 2002 Chevron Canada Resources abandoned a plan to go ahead with exploitation.

Industry: the main industries are wood and fish-related: pulp and newsprint mills, and fish processing.

Transport: the highway between Port aux Basques and St. John's is a continuation of the trans-Canada highway, but the topography is such that it more than doubles the direct distance between these cities. Land travel is often compelled to take devious routes around the mountains. In the days of sea travel, and early transatlantic air travel, the island was strategically placed in global terms, on the routes between New York, the St. Lawrence, and the ports of northwest Europe, with Gander an important refuelling point.

History: in 1583 the Elizabethan adventurer, Sir Humphrey Gilbert, claimed Newfoundland on behalf of the English Queen Elizabeth I. The first colonial settlement was made in 1610, but English possession was challenged by the French, who established a colony at Placentia. It was not until 1713 that, under the Treaty of Utrecht, Newfoundland was formally accepted as a British colony. Unusually, the founding of settlements was resisted by the British government. This had much to do with the control of fishing rights. The wealthy few who controlled the Newfoundland fishing did not want to see colonists taking a share of their lucrative business. Settlers were refused permission to build houses or cut wood within six miles of the shore. These laws, very hard to enforce, were gradually relaxed. By 1832 the island had its own Parliament and in 1855 it became a self-governing British colony. The inhabitants voted against joining in the formation of Canada in 1867, and Newfoundland remained a self-governing colony. But in the slump year of 1933, with the island's economy in a state of collapse, elective government was suspended and a 'commission of government' controlled affairs through the 1930s, and the years of World War II. During 1939–45, the strategic position of Newfoundland again worked in its favour, and a strong war economy brought renewed prosperity. In a referendum in 1948, the islanders voted in favour of union with Canada, and Newfoundland, together with Labrador, became the country's tenth province on 1 April 1949.

Labrador: the name comes from the Portuguese explorer of 1530, João Fernandes, who was a *lavrador*, or landholder, in the Azores. The easternmost territory of Canada, administrative part of Newfoundland province, Labrador is very thinly populated. Stretching from the Hudson Bay coast to the Strait of Belle Isle, it has never been settled and was little explored by Europeans before the twentieth century. The cold arctic current that sweeps past its coast means that the prevailing climate is chilly, and the landscape is usually snowbound except for the summer months. The south of the territory is thickly forested, mostly with black spruce; the ground cover of the north consists mostly of mosses and lichens. A varied wildlife is supported, including bear, beaver, muskrat, lynx, wolverine, red squirrel, and caribou among the animals, and ptarmigan, geese, grouse, and partridge among the birds. Fur trapping is Labrador's oldest human pursuit, but by far the most important nowadays is iron mining from the ore beds found between the headwaters of the Hamilton and Kaniapiskau Rivers, with Labrador City as the centre. Another centre of activity is Schefferville, just over the border in Québec province. A railway runs south through Labrador linking it to the St. Lawrence at Sept Îles. Copper and nickel are also mined, and prospecting for other minerals continues. Labrador's main settlements are Battle Harbour, the capital, Labrador City, Nain, and Goose Bay.

Northwest Territories

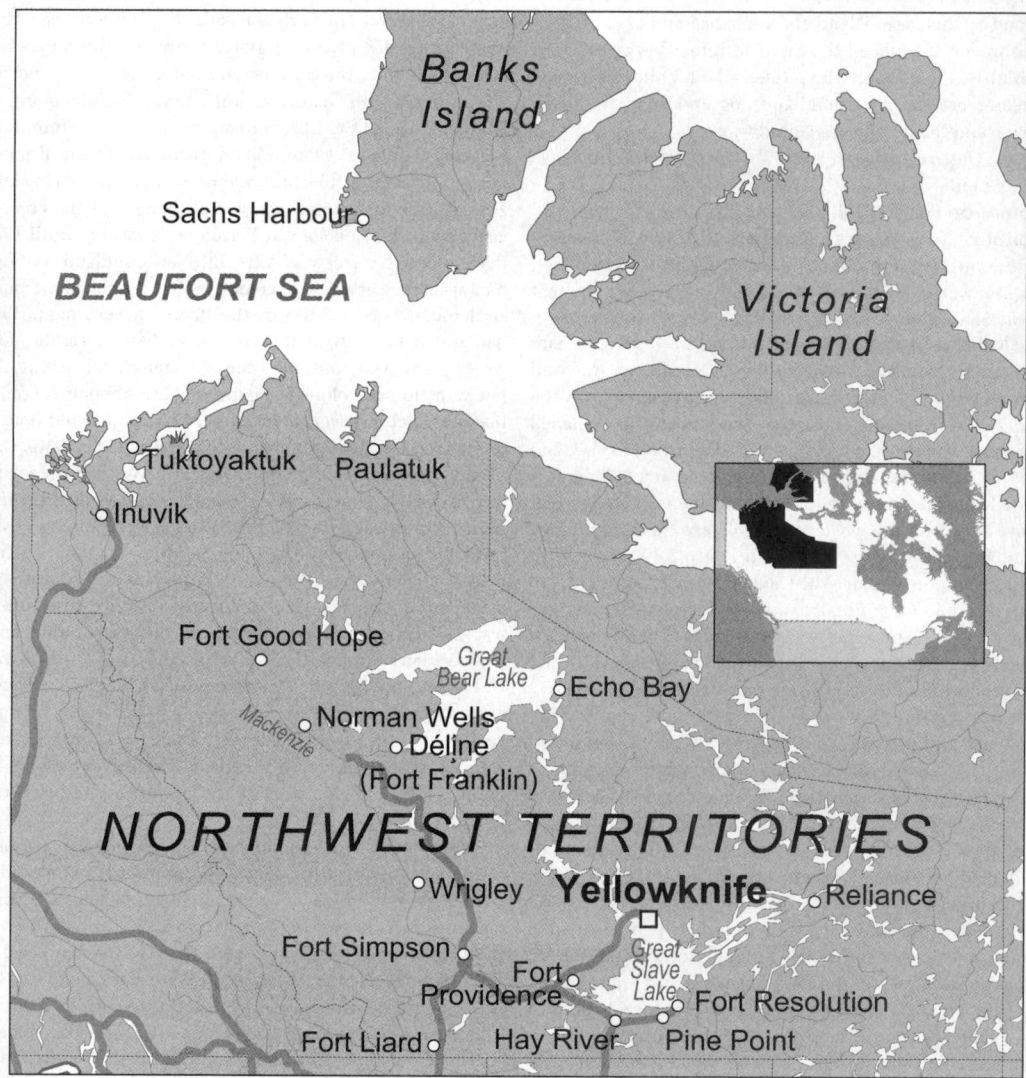

A vast semi-autonomous region lying north of the 60th parallel, east of the Yukon and bordering the Prairie Provinces to the south.

Emblem: the mountain avens, jack pine, girfalcon.

Population (2002): 41,400. The population is very small and scattered in a number of mining communities.

Capital: Yellowknife. With a population of just under 18,000, it is said to be Canada's fastest-growing city. It provides administration, medical, and college facilities as well as being the region's main market centre.

Physical description: with a land area of 1,346,106 square kilometres (519,597 square miles), it is fourth in size among the territories and provinces. Lakes cover more than 10% of the surface. The western area is mountainous, with the Mackenzie Mountains rising to meet the Selwyn and Cassiar ranges. The highest point is Unnamed Peak (2,773 metres, 9,098 feet). The land falls away eastwards towards the long valley of the Mackenzie River, Canada's longest, which flows from the Great Slave Lake to the Arctic Ocean. East of the Mackenzie, a bare and rocky landscape reaches to the shore of Hudson Bay. To the north there is subarctic tundra. Beyond the north coast is the Arctic Archipelago, composed of many islands, some of them of great size, merging into the frozen sea towards the North Pole.

Climate: its far northern situation and proximity to the polar icecap ensure long, dark winters with deep snow and very low temperatures. During its brief summer, temperatures can rise as high as 27°C (80°F) around the Great Slave Lake.

Agriculture: virtually all of the foodstuffs consumed by the population are imported from elsewhere, as the soil and climate are not conducive to farming. There are extensive stands of forest in the Mackenzie Plains. Fur trapping remains an important activity.

Minerals: the region is rich in minerals. Gold, silver, uranium, copper, and nickel have all been identified in significant quantities. In addition there are oil and natural gas deposits. Canada's first diamond deposits have also been found here.

Industry: the extraction and primary processing of metals and other mineral reserves.

Transport: the territory is very much dependent on air transport and every community has its airstrip. Hay River, on the south shore of the Great Slave Lake, is the terminus of a rail link to the national system, and there are road connections to other towns in the same region. Lack of suitable transport is a serious problem for the mining industries.

Wildlife: muskrats, foxes, beavers, lynxes, wolves, and martens live in the woods and marshes. Migratory birds, including vast numbers of wild geese and duck, flock to the Arctic coast springtime nesting sites

History: the area was occupied by aboriginal peoples for thousands of years. From 1670 the southern part of the region was part of what was known as Rupert's Land, and was administered by the Hudson's Bay Company. The northern part was under nominal British suzerainty. In 1870 both parts were integrated into the Dominion of Canada. The formation of the Prairie Provinces and northern extensions of Ontario and Québec reduced the size of Northwest Territories. The greatest reduction came with the formation of the separate territory of Nunavut in 1999, though even in its reduced form Northwest Territories is far bigger than many nation states.

Nova Scotia

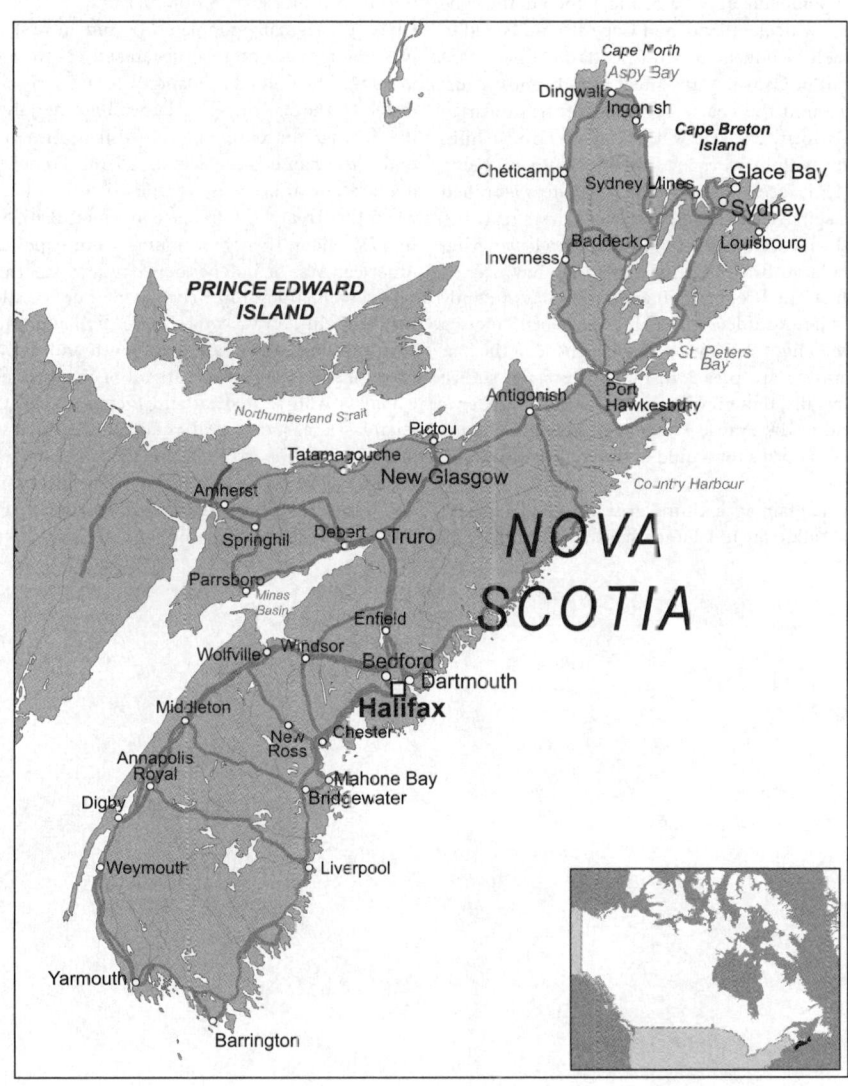

Name: the name means 'New Scotland'. Nova Scotia is one of the smallest but longest-established provinces. Nova Scotians have a keen sense of their own identity. Cape Breton Island, in particular, maintains the tradition of Gaelic speech and has many links with Celtic Scotland and Ireland. It is one of Canada's so-called Maritime Provinces.

Emblems: the red spruce, the mayflower, the osprey.

Motto: *Munit haec et altera vincit*, 'One defends, and the other conquers'.

Population (2002): 944,800.

Capital: Halifax, with some 340,000 people in its metropolitan area, is the largest town and main port as well as the provincial capital. Its large and ice-free harbour is a major container port as well as Canada's prime Atlantic naval base. Founded in 1749, it is also one of Canada's oldest cities.

Physical description: with a land area of 55,284 square kilometres (21,340 square miles), Nova Scotia is tenth in size among the provinces and territories. The province consists of the peninsula of Nova Scotia, joined to the continent by a narrow neck of land, and Cape Breton Island to the north, which is linked to Nova Scotia by a causeway across the Strait of Canso. Many small islands, mostly uninhabited, surround the coasts. The terrain is similar to that of New Brunswick, across the Bay of Fundy: hilly, wooded country with many valleys, the highest point being 532 metres (1,745 feet) above sea level. The watershed runs along the spinal ridge, with short, swift rivers reaching the sea on both sides. Cape Breton Island has a lower-lying area round the large Bras d'Or saltwater lake, but rises in the north to the Cape Breton Highlands. The Bay of Fundy has the world's largest tides, with a difference of 15 metres (45 feet) between high and low water at the head of the bay.

Climate: summers are pleasant, but winters are severe with heavy snowfalls, though without the extreme temperature lows found in the Prairie Provinces. Generally the influence of the sea makes for a milder, if wetter and windier, climatic regime.

Agriculture: the main agricultural area lies in and around the Annapolis Valley on the Fundy coast, where there is good soil and the mountain ridge provides shelter from northeasterly cold winds. There are many apple orchards. Mixed farming is the staple of the province and there is extensive breeding of stock and poultry. Although remote from the main centres of Canadian population, Nova Scotia has access to the New England region of the U.S.A. As elsewhere in Canada, forestry is of great importance, and the slopes of the province's low mountain ranges are clothed in spruce, fir, birch, maple, and pine. Fishing was an important industry for many coastal communities but, with dwindled stocks, its significance has receded in recent years. Fish farming has to a degree replaced sea fishing.

Minerals: coal is the main mineral resource, with mining districts around Sydney in Cape Breton Island and Pictou in northern Nova Scotia. Nova Scotia is an important source of gypsum, and rock salt is also produced.

Industry: steelworks at Sydney and New Glasgow use local coal and Newfoundland iron ore. Some lumber is exported but the province also has lumber mills.

History: originally populated by Indian first nations peoples, the region's first European settlers were from France in 1604. They called the land Acadia. Possession was contested by the British. King James I granted the territory to the Scottish entrepreneur, Sir William Alexander, in 1621, under the name Nova Scotia. A large French element remained and the colony remained in dispute until 1713, when the Treaty of Utrecht confirmed British possession. In 1755 many French residents were expelled. After the American War of Independence, many American colonists who remained loyal to Britain sailed or travelled to set up new lives in Nova Scotia. The 'Highland Clearances' in Scotland during the late eighteenth and early nineteenth centuries resulted in the arrival of many Gaelic-speaking colonists who settled around Pictou and in Cape Breton Island – areas that still retain a Gaelic tradition. The province was the first to be established as self-governing from 1848. It also had Canada's first university, printing-press and newspaper. In 1867 it was one of the founding provinces of the new Dominion of Canada.

Nunavut

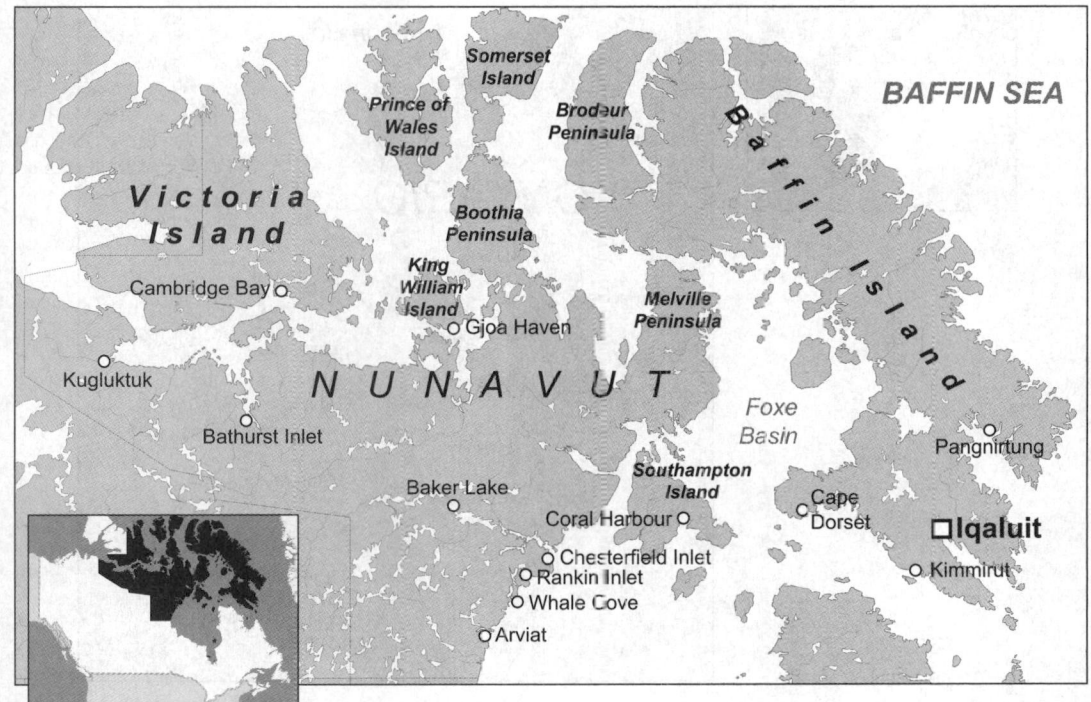

Name: the name means 'our land' in Inuktitut.

Emblems: the purple saxifrage, the rock ptarmigan.

Motto: *Nunavut Sanginivut*, 'Nunavut our strength'.

Population (2002): 28,700. About 85% of the people are Inuit, and 56% of the population is under 25.

Capital: Iqaluit. Formerly Frobisher Bay, on Baffin Island, Iqaluit has a population of 3,600. It is also a trading and educational centre, and home to the Arctic College, whose courses focus on Nunavut's cultures and environment.

Physical description: with a land area of 2,093,190 square kilometres (807,971 square miles), Nunavut is by far the largest of the territories and provinces, occupying almost a quarter of the entire country. The highest point is Barbeau Peak on Ellesmere Island (2,626 metres, 8,615 feet). Most of the landscape is bare and bleak, and covered in snow all or most of the year, but its austere beauty attracts more visitors each year.

Climate: the brief summers can be warm, but the territory lies mostly north of the Arctic Circle, and long, dark, very cold winters are the dominant aspect of the climate.

Minerals: the bleak landscape contains a variety of mineral deposits, with more still being prospected. The Polaris lead-zinc mine on Little Cornwallis Island is the most northerly mine in the world, producing 1,000,000 tonnes of refinable ores annually.

Economy and industry: though extreme climatic conditions mean that mining is expensive, and only high grade and valuable ores are exploited, minerals are one of the three main bases of the economy. The others are fur trading and tourism. Government salaries and subsidies are a further support.

History: human occupancy of the subarctic region goes back for many thousands of years. Under British rule it became part of the Northwest Territories. Its modern development began in 1965 when the Canadian government first unveiled plans to reorganize the administration of the arctic territories. Years of discussion and campaigning by the Inuit people followed. A plebiscite held in the Northwest Territories in 1982 resulted in a 90% majority vote among the Inuit for a separate eastern division. Another decade of wrangling ensued over the border between the Northwest Territories and Nunavut until a new plebiscite in 1992 brought agreement. In June 1993 the Canadian government passed the Nunavut Act, and in 1999 the territory and government of Nunavut finally came into being.

Ontario

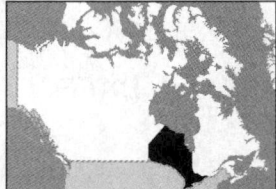

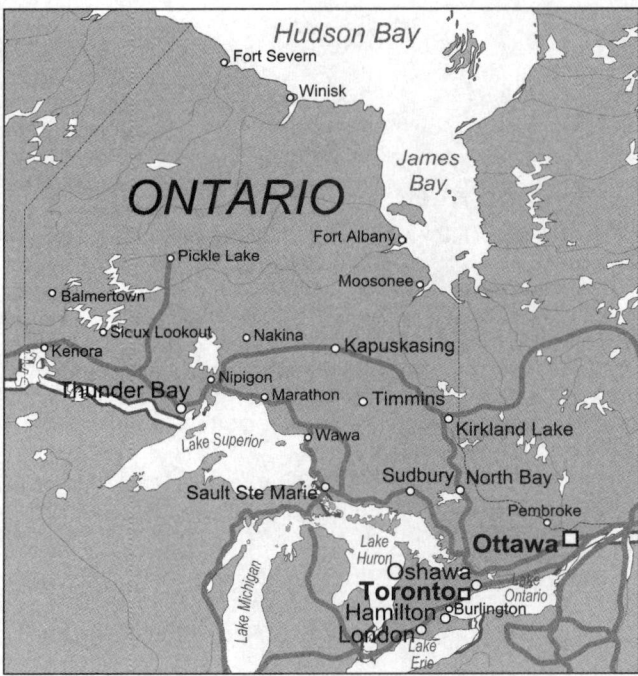

Name: the province's name has been traced to the Iroquois for 'the land of shining waters', and also to Seneca's *entohonorous*, 'the people'.

Emblems: the white trillium flower, the eastern white pine, the common loon.

Motto: *Ut incepit fidelis, sic permanet*, 'Loyal it began, loyal it remains'.

Population (2002): 12,068,300. More than a third of the country's population live in Ontario, making it Canada's most populous province.

Capital: Toronto, Canada's largest city, has 2.8 million inhabitants, and around 4 million in the metropolitan region. Toronto is the fifth largest municipal government region in North America. It is the main industrial and economic centre of Ontario and of all Canada. Ethnically it is highly diverse, with over 100 different ethnic and language groups represented. Over 50% of its citizens were born outside Canada. The name comes from an Indian word for 'meeting place', and it was an Indian centre before the first European settlement was made by the French in 1750. Under British control it was named York until its present name was given in 1834, when it became a city. Today, metropolitan Toronto covers 632 square kilometres (244 square miles). It was the first Canadian city to construct a subway, and its CN tower, at 533 metres (1,750 feet), is among the world's tallest buildings. Among other 'firsts', it claims the world's largest underground pedestrian area. Some 90% of foreign banks in Canada are established here, and electronics and telecommunications are important aspects of a very diverse industrial base. Toronto is also a major publishing and media centre, and is the largest centre of English-language theatre after London and New York.

Physical description: with a land area of 1,076,395 square kilometres (415,488 square miles), it is third largest among the provinces and territories. To the south, Ontario's shape is defined by the line of the Upper St. Lawrence River and the north coasts of Lakes Superior, Huron, and Ontario. The part of the province south of the Ottawa River, once a vast forested zone, is now a region of fertile rolling farmlands. To the north, the landscape is an enormous plateau region, scraped by ice sheets, and often lacking soil and vegetation. This is the area of the Canadian Shield. On glacial soils there are forests, but much of the ground is heath or bare rock, interspersed with a multitude of lakes. The highest point of land is Ishpatina Ridge (693 metres, 2,273 feet). In the north the rivers drain into Hudson Bay, in the west to Lake Winnipeg, in the south to the Great Lakes and the St. Lawrence.

Climate: the climate is essentially a continental one, of cold winters and hot summers, but in the south it is modified by the presence of the Great Lakes, making winters and summers a little moister and milder. Nevertheless it can become cold enough to freeze up Niagara Falls. In the scantily populated north, there is again a marine influence on the climate.

Agriculture: climate, fertile soil, and a densely packed population have influenced the development of mixed farming in the southern part of the province. In the Lake Peninsula between Toronto and Niagara, vines, tobacco and peaches can be grown. In the north, farming is much more localized, depending on the soil and the proximity of a market. Lumbering is much more important, with spruce and poplar grown for packaging and newsprint.

Minerals: north of Georgian Bay there is a region of rich mineral deposits, including uranium, nickel, and copper. The Creighton nickel-copper mine near Sudbury is the deepest in Canada at 2,200 metres (7,218 feet). Other minerals mined in Ontario include iron, platinum, gold, and zinc.

Trade and industry: Ontario is the most highly industrialized of the provinces. Employment is divided 64% to services, 34% to industry, and 2% to agriculture. Oil from the Alberta field comes across Canada by pipeline to be refined at Sarnia. A variety of manufacturing industry is located in the cities of Toronto, Hamilton, London, and smaller centres. Mineral processing is a major industry at Sudbury. Transport, trading, banking, and media are all important.

History: the region had been Indian territory since prehistoric times when the first European exploring party, under Samuel de Champlain, reached Lake Huron in 1615. French trading posts and mission stations were established along the shores of the Great Lakes, but the inland regions remained Indian territory. The British took possession in 1763. At that time it was all part of Québec, or New France. Between 1783 and 1791 many British Loyalists removed from the U.S.A. to set up home in British North America; and in 1791 the eastern and western areas of Québec were separated politically and known as Lower and Upper Canada respectively. Upper Canada's first capital, at Niagara, was uncomfortably close to the U.S.A., and York (later renamed Toronto) replaced it. In 1812 invading American forces destroyed the town. The Act of Union of 1840 once again brought Upper and Lower Canada together in a single province. However, with the establishment of the Confederation in 1870, Upper Canada became the province of Ontario. By this time it was already well populated in the southern part and, with the development of railways and the discovery of mineral reserves, it quickly became Canada's most industrialized province.

Prince Edward Island (P.E.I.)

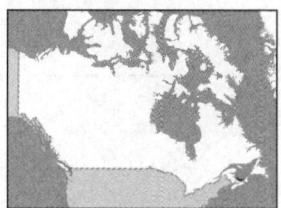

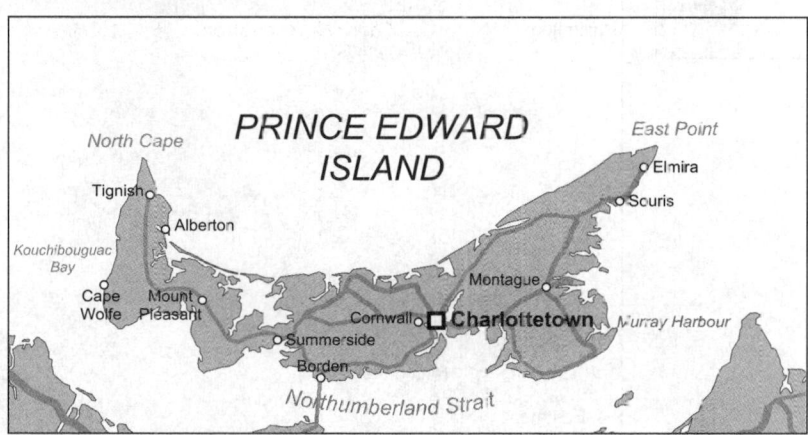

Name: the name was given in 1798, in honour of the Duke of Kent, father of Queen Victoria. This is Canada's smallest province, both in size and population, and is one of the four Maritime Provinces.

Emblems: lady's slipper flower, northern red oak, the blue jay.

Motto: Parva sub ingenti, 'The small protected by the great'.

Population (2002): 139,900. P.E.I. is the most densely populated province of the Confederation, with almost 25 persons to the square kilometre, compared to a national average of 3.

Capital: Charlottetown. With a population of 33,000, Charlottetown is the island's only urban centre. It has the highest average snowfall of the provincial capitals, with 338.7 centimetres (133 inches) a year.

Physical description with a land area of 5,660 square kilometres (2,185 square miles), P.E.I. is the smallest of the provinces and territories, occupying 0.1% of Canada's total area. Lying in the south of the Gulf of St. Lawrence, it is separated from New Brunswick by the Northumberland Strait, some 30 kilometres (18 miles) wide. Much indented by the sea, it is almost divided in two at Hillsborough Bay. The island terrain is relatively low, nowhere rising over 150 metres (450 feet) and is intensively farmed, with most of the original forest cover long vanished.

Climate: the climate is much the same as Nova Scotia, with pleasant summers but heavy snowfalls in winter. The influence of the sea makes for a milder, if wetter and windier, climate.

Agriculture: a well-developed pattern of farmland covers most of the island. The red soil is fertile and produces crops of potatoes, wheat, and barley. Stock rearing is important, both for beef and dairy farming, and there are many pasture fields. Pigs and poultry are also farmed. On the coast, shellfish rearing is important, notably lobsters.

Industry: industry revolves around the needs and products of the farms. Food processing, freezing, and canning are important. There is also a substantial tourist industry, with coastal fishing and first-rate golf links among the attractions.

Transport: the Confederation Bridge, 12.9 kilometres (8 miles) long, joins the island to the mainland, between Borden and Carleton. Opened in 1997, this is the world's longest bridge over seasonally icebound waters. There is a good road network, and a railway links Charlottetown with

Tignish in the north. Train ferries between Tormentine and Borden provide a connection with the mainland network. Car ferries also operate on this route and from Pictou in Nova Scotia. Icebreakers make it a year-round service. The main airport is at Charlottetown.

History: originally occupied by Mi'kmaq Indians and other first nations peoples (who still occupy a reservation on the island) and called by them *Abegweit*, 'Home cradled in the waves', the island was identified by Jacques Cartier in 1534. Samuel de Champlain gave it the name Île de St. Jean. During the French-British war over possession of eastern Canada, the British landed in 1758 and drove out some of the French residents. It was confirmed as a British possession in 1763, and given colony status in 1769. Charlottetown was the venue of the inter-provincial conference of 1864 which led to the formation of the Dominion of Canada in 1867, but Prince Edward Island was not one of the founding provinces. It joined the federation soon after, in 1873.

Tradition: the island was the home of L. M. Montgomery, author of the *Anne of Green Gables* stories enjoyed by generations of children. Her house is now a museum.

Québec

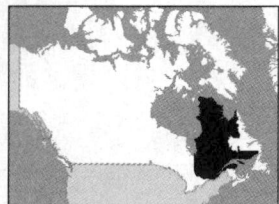

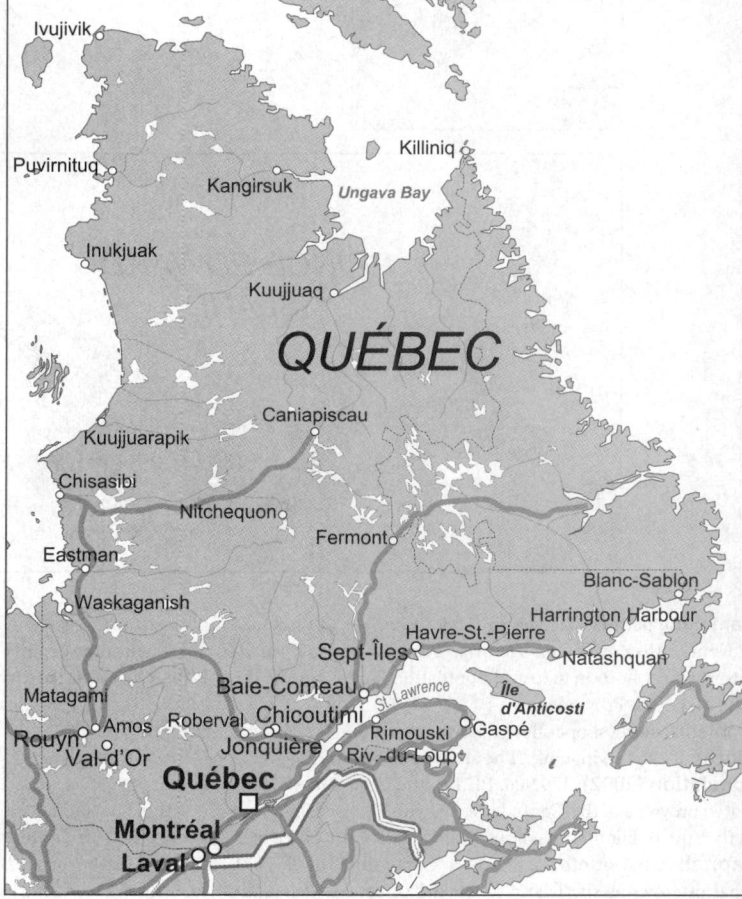

Name: Québec is Canada's second largest province and territory, three times the size of France. The name is from *kebek*, the Iroquois for 'narrowing of the waters', describing the St. Lawrence at Québec City.

Emblems: the Madonna lily, the snowy owl, yellow birch.

Motto: *Je me souviens*, 'I remember'.

Population (2002): 7,455,200.

Capital: Québec City. Canada's oldest city, Québec City has a population of 180,000. Winding, narrow streets link its Upper and Lower Towns. There are many historic sites, including the Ursuline Convent (1639) and the Basilica Notre Dame (1647) as well as the fortress. Its industries include shipbuilding and repair, wood pulp, textiles, food, and drinks.

Physical description: with a land area of 1,542,056 square kilometres (595,233 square miles), it is exceeded in size only by the vast area of Nunavut. Bounded on the east by Labrador, on the south by New Brunswick and the U.S. state of New York, and on the west by Ontario and Hudson Bay, the vast spread of Québec province reaches from the St. Lawrence to the Arctic. North of the St. Lawrence lie the rocky uplands of forest and wilderness known as the Canadian Shield, an ancient landscape formed by ice sheets and pocked with innumerable lakes. Its southern boundary is the Laurentian Mountains, a range stretching 1,600 kilometres (1,000 miles) and rising to heights of around 900 metres (2,700 feet) north of Québec City. The highest point in the province is Mt. D'Ilberville (1,652 metres, 5,124 feet). The St. Lawrence valley forms a wide lowland region between Montréal and Québec, and to the south the land rises into forested hills bordering on the U.S. states of Vermont and Maine. Rivers flow to all points of the compass, but the main systems are those of the Ottawa River in the west, the Saguenay in the east and the Caniapiscau in the north.

Climate: the southern part of the province has warm summers and cold, snowy winters. Autumn, though brief, is brilliant with the red and gold foliage of the maple and other deciduous trees. To the north the climate is increasingly subarctic.

Agriculture: the St. Lawrence lowlands are intensively farmed. Meat and dairy products, eggs and poultry, and market gardening reflect the needs of a substantial urban population. South of the St. Lawrence, farmland and deciduous forest share the valleys and hill slopes. In the north there are huge forest areas, chiefly of softwood trees. Québec supplies almost half the softwood used in Canada's vast lumber industry.

Minerals: iron ore is extracted at Schefferville, close to the Labrador border, and to the west of Ungava Bay in the far north of the province. In the south there are large deposits of the minerals that produce asbestos and have given the town of Asbestos its name. Gold, silver, and copper deposits are also worked. Québec has Canada's only titanium mine. There are mining centres at Abitibi, Temiscamingue, North Shore, Eastern Townships, and on the Gaspé peninsula.

Trade and industry: unlimited water power provides the province with cheap electricity and this is utilized in many forms of industry, including aluminium smelting, using imported bauxite, and other forms of metal processing. Automobiles, chemicals, textiles, and electronics also form part of a diverse industrial base. Apart from wood pulp and paper, many other timber products and by-products are manufactured and packaged. Employment in Québec is divided 68% to services, 29% to industry, and 3% to agriculture.

Political life: politics in Québec are quite different to those of any other province and impact heavily on federal politics. The reason for this lies in the fact that the great majority of the Québecois, over 6 million people, are of French descent and remain French-speaking, and in many ways form part of the French cultural universe. Although Canada is a secular state, with an increasingly secular outlook, the fact that the Québec population adheres overwhelmingly to the Roman Catholic Church serves to increase the sense of cultural difference. A separatist movement has become increasingly vocal and influential during the latter part of the twentieth century. Two provincial referendums on the issue have been held, in 1980 and 1995, and though both resulted in a vote in favour of continued union with the other provinces, the latter produced a majority of only 1%, and the issue of separatism remains very much an open one.

History: on his second voyage, in 1535, the French explorer Jacques Cartier sailed up the St. Lawrence and claimed the land he found on behalf of King François I of France. It was inhabited by numerous large Indian nations, including Iroquois and Huron. The first French settlement was established by Samuel de Champlain in 1608 at Québec, head of navigation for seagoing ships, where he built a fort. The colony was known as La Nouvelle France, and run from 1627 by a monopoly business, the 'Company of One Hundred' (also known as the 'Company of New France'). But it attracted few settlers and there was little activity. From 1663 it was established as a royal province ruled by a Governor General, with an intendant as his head of administration.

Steady population growth now began, with towns forming round the forts at Québec, Montréal and Trois Rivières. As explorers pushed out further west, the area of the colony enlarged, but the bulk of the population was in the St. Lawrence Lowlands; by the middle of the eighteenth century it numbered around 65,000 people. Farming was the main occupation, though furs remained the chief source of wealth. Land was apportioned to a seigneur, who allocated it to tenants (the habitants) in long rectangular lots. From the earliest stage, however, the French domain was challenged by the English, who had settled in New England, and whose search for the Northwest Passage had introduced them to the northern wilderness. They used the voyages of John Cabot, Martin Frobisher, Henry Hudson, and others to claim possession of the regions north and west of New France. In 1629 they captured Québec City and held it for three years.

The original inhabitants, well organized in the Iroquois League, were alternately courted and attacked by the contending colonial powers. Caught in the middle, the

Iroquois attempted to play off both sets of Europeans but their power was ultimately broken by the French. As a Catholic state, France included a missionary element in its colonial activity, and New France's first bishop arrived in 1659. By then, monks and nuns had already established convents and hospitals. Among the French governors were some very able men, but a fatal error was made in 1668 when two French explorers, Radisson and Des Groseilliers, failing to get backing from France, but receiving it in England, opened up the Hudson Bay fur trade for the new English Hudson's Bay Company.

From 1672, under one of its most energetic governors, the Comte de Frontenac, the colony's area and activities expanded, but from the late seventeenth and into the eighteenth centuries, as a result of warfare in Europe, decline began. Following the loss of Nova Scotia and Newfoundland in 1713, a great fort was begun in 1717 at Louisbourg, to guard access to the St. Lawrence. A fort-building race characterized the next thirty years, but, neglected by the French government, and with access to France made difficult by naval warfare, the colony was increasingly open to attack. Though at this time French explorers and settlers, such as the La Vérendrye family, were still establishing themselves in the west, the western forts, in the plains and on the Great Lakes, fell one by one to the British. The culmination came in the warfare that took place between 1754 and 1760; in 1759 the British captured the Québec fortress and in the following year the Governor General, the Marquis de Vaudreuil, was forced to surrender. In the Treaty of Paris, 1763, British possession of the French colony was confirmed.

Although large numbers of English-speaking settlers came to the province after 1760, Québec (called Lower Canada in 1791) has retained its French-speaking population, its language, religion, and traditions, at first under British rule and later as part of federal Canada. In the American invasions of 1775 and 1812, the Québecois fought with the other Canadian provincials for the defence of the British colony (though they had no cause to love the New Englanders). In 1841 the province was granted a degree of self-government and in 1849 the French language was given legal recognition. In 1867 Lower Canada was one of the founding provinces of the Confederation, and received the name of Québec province.

In the twentieth century the province shared in the economic growth of Canada, and the gradual shedding of colonial British links was welcomed. But Québec contin-

ued to be different, as shown by the resistance to conscription at the start of both world wars. Socially a conservative province, it was the last in Canada to give women the vote. In the 1960s the issue of separation became a dominant one and has remained so. Although the 'Quiet Revolution' initiated by the Liberal government of 1960 brought about progressive changes in federal attitudes to the province's unique status, it also saw the rise of political violence from the *Front pour la Libération de Québec* (FLQ), with bombs in Montréal in 1960, and the kidnap and murder of British diplomat James Cross and Québec government minister Pierre Laporte in 1970. In that year martial law was imposed for a time, and over 500 persons were arrested. In 1973 the *Parti Québecois* (PQ) emerged as a separatist party pledged to peaceful methods, and in 1976, under René Levesque, it won control of the provincial government. On a state visit that year, the French President, Charles de Gaulle, infuriated the Canadian government by expressing support for 'free Québec'. Many English speakers left the province in the wake of Bill 101, designed to preserve the supremacy of the French language in the province. A referendum in 1980 rejected independence for the province. Both federal and provincial governments have been preoccupied with the question of how to reconcile the Québecois desire for independence with the province's remaining part of Canada. The 'Meech Lake Accord' promoted by federal Premier Mulroney in 1987 fell in 1990 against opposition from other provinces, resulting in the formation of the *Bloc Québecois* by Québec politicians. A referendum on independence in 1995 rejected it by a majority of only 1%, resulting in controversy as some politicians accused immigrant voters of sabotaging the aspirations of the French-speaking Québecois. Discussions on the constitutional issue continue.

Montréal: though not the capital, this is by far Québec's largest city, the second largest in Canada, and the world's largest French-speaking city after Paris. The population in 2002 was 1,813,000. Montréal is a major industrial, commercial and media centre, and an important port. Although it has always been an important city, its population more than doubled between 1941 and 1971. In 1976 it was the site of the Olympic Games. There are many modern buildings, and an underground pedestrian zone of 29 kilometres (18 miles). The city's five-line *Métro* runs on rubber tires. Montréal is ethnically diverse, with an Italian population of some 100,130 (2001) as the largest language group after French and English.

Saskatchewan

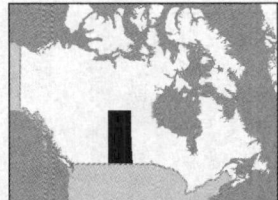

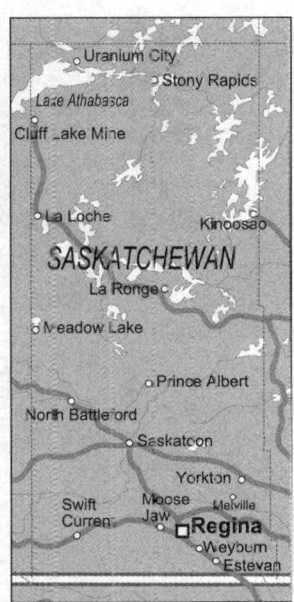

Name: the name comes from an Indian word, *kisikatchewan*, 'swift river'. It is one of the three Prairie Provinces.

Emblem: the Western red lily, white birch, sharp-tailed grouses.

Motto: *Multis e gentibus vires*, 'Strength from many peoples'.

Population (2002): 1,011,800.

Capital: Regina, with a population of 187,500. The name was given in honour of Queen Victoria. Given city status in 1903, Regina is Canada's sunniest and driest capital city, with an average annual precipitation of 364 millimetres (14 inches), and 109 wet days a year. With potash mines and sodium sulphate extraction close by, the city has an industrial base as well as being an administrative and market centre. Steel, chemicals, and telecommunications are other important industries.

Physical description: with a land area of 651,036 square kilometres (251,300 square miles), it is sixth in size among the provinces and territories. The south of the province is prairie country, with wide level plains and gently rolling uplands. The Saskatchewan River, with its north and south branches, flows westward in deeply incised valleys. Farther north is 'parkland' country with groves of aspen and poplar trees. The north of the province is more rugged, with rocky and marshy terrain, and many lakes and rivers. The highest point is at Cypress Hills (1,468 metres, 4,816 feet). The largest lake is Lake Athabasca (7,935 square kilometres, 3,063 square miles).

Climate: remote from the sea, the province has a continental climate, with hot summers and cold winters. Snow may lie on the ground for up to four months of the year.

Agriculture: more than 16,000,000 hectares (40 million acres) of arable land are under cultivation, and Saskatchewan produces about two thirds of Canada's wheat crop. Wheat is sown in spring, and grows and ripens rapidly during the hot summer months. Other crops include oats, barley, rye, rape, and flax. Mixed farming is practiced in the parkland regions, with beef and dairy cattle. Pigs and poultry are also farmed in large numbers.

Minerals: the southern part of the province has reserves of lignite (brown coal), oil, and natural gas. In the north there is extensive exploitation of metallic ores, notably around Uranium City, northeast of Lake Athabasca. Copper, zinc, gold, silver, and cadmium are also mined in addition to uranium. Canada is the world's main potash producer, and the province produces about 90% of the country's supply.

Industry: Saskatchewan is a primary producer region rather than a manufacturing one. Most industry is concerned with the preparation and packing of agricultural products, lumber, and metal processing.

History: once Plains Indian territory and very thinly populated (as much of it still is), this area formed part of the Hudson's Bay grant of 1670. The first white man to explore it was Henry Kelsey, a Hudson's Bay employee, between 1690 and 1692. French and British traders set up trading stations. During the nineteenth century it was thought unlikely that the vast plains could be used for anything other than grazing, with organized ranching replacing the huge herds of buffaloes. The arrival of the railroad, linking Regina with the east by 1882, increased the rate of settlement and also provided a means of bulk transport for farm produce. The development of new cereal strains such as quick-ripening wheat, and the mechanization of agriculture, followed. The old way of life made a last stand with the rising in 1885 of Indian and Métis nomadic peoples against the new order of things. Troops quelled the rising and its leader, Riel, was captured and hanged at Regina. From 1896 the pace of settlement increased further, with the population quadrupling in the first decade of the twentieth century, from around 100,000 to over 400,000. Many of the immigrants were from central and eastern Europe. In 1905 Saskatchewan province was formed and became part of the Confederation.

Yukon Territory

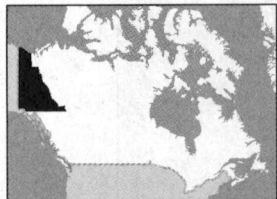

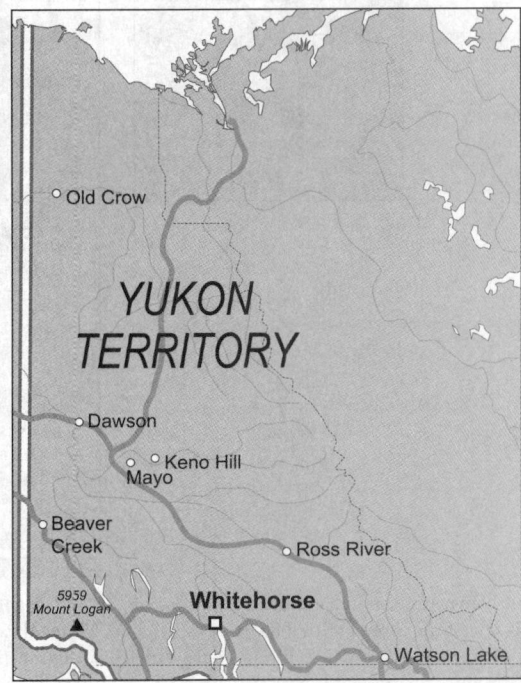

Name: consisting of the semi-autonomous far northwest of Canada, the Yukon Territory's name is taken from an Indian word, *Yu-kun-ah*, 'great river'.

Emblems: fireweed, the sub-alpine fir, the raven, and the gemstone, lazulite.

Population (2002): 29,900.

Capital: the capital, Whitehorse, is situated on the west bank of the Yukon River. It has a population of 23,000, and its main activities are administration, social and medical services, tourism, and mining support industries.

Physical description: with a land area of 482,443 square kilometres (186,223 square miles), it is eleventh in size among the provinces and territories. The Yukon is a mountainous region, where the Western Cordillera spreads into the Selwyn and Ogilvie ranges. Here can be found Canada's highest point, Mt. Logan (5,959 metres, 19,550 feet). The main rivers drain eastwards into the Mackenzie system, apart from the Yukon River itself, which rises in the south of the territory and flows westwards through Alaska.

Climate: most of the territory is south of the Arctic Circle, but winters are long, dark, cold, and severe. Spring and summer are short seasons.

Minerals: gold, zinc, lead, and silver ores are mined, with a value to the territory of $97,000,000 in 2001. Of this, 92% was contributed by gold. There are also petroleum wells, while sands and gravels are excavated in vast quantities. In 1997, emeralds were discovered.

Transport: a railroad links Whitehorse with Skagway in Alaska, and the Fairbanks–Edmonton highway also passes through Whitehorse. The only other permanent routes are by river. Dirt roads extend into the country from various mining sites. Air transport is the main lifeline of the remote communities.

History: unexplored and uninhabited except by migratory Indians and wandering fur trappers until the nineteenth century, the name of the Yukon became synonymous with panning for gold in the mid-1890s. Fortune hunters flocked there and a new town, Dawson City, grew almost overnight to a population of 40,000. By 1904, when the surface gold was exhausted, the population had diminished with equal rapidity, though gold-mining by industrial methods continued at Dawson City until 1966. Dawson was superseded by Whitehorse as the capital in 1953.

A Chronology of Events in Canadian History

(BCE is an abbreviation for 'Before Christian or Common Era' – the years BC.)

c.12,000 BCE: incomers from Siberia leave traces in the Blue Fish Caves, Yukon.

c.9000 BCE: native peoples leave traces of habitation on the Eramosa River, near Guelph, Ontario.

c.4000 BCE: Eskimo and Aleut form separate groups in the Arctic.

c.500 CE: the bow and arrow are introduced among the Plains Indians.

c.1000: Leif Ericsson explores the coast of Labrador and Newfoundland. A Viking colony is established at L'Anse aux Meadows.

1450: around this time the Great League of Peace and Power is formed among the Five Nations of the Iroquois.

1492: Columbus sails to America.

1497: John Cabot explores the coast of Cape Breton Island, Newfoundland, and Labrador.

1498: Cabot is lost at sea, returning from his second visit.

1500: Gaspar de Corte-Real heads a Portuguese expedition to Newfoundland; he calls the latter, Terra Verde.

1504: first records of French fishers off Newfoundland.

1521: J. Alvares Fagundes explored near Cape Breton and Nova Scotia as well as the coast of Newfoundland.

1527: John Rut is sent by King Henry VIII of England to find the Northwest Passage but he turns back at Hawke Bay, Labrador.

1534: King Francis I of France dispatches an expedition under Jacques Cartier. Cartier explores the coast of Newfoundland, Labrador, and the Gulf of St. Lawrence, encountering the Mi'kmaq and Huron peoples, and claims the land for France on 24 July.

1535: on his second voyage, Cartier sails up the St. Lawrence River to the Huron communities of Hochelaga and Stadacona, on the sites of present-day Montréal and Québec City.

1541: Cartier returns to North America and establishes the colony of Charlesbourg-Royal, the first French settlement in North America.

1542: the Sieur de Roberval arrives as the first lieutenant general of the new territories.

1576: the Company of Cathay is founded to exploit gold deposits on Kodlunan Island that turn out to be pyrites (false gold).

1577: Queen Elizabeth I of England commissions Martin Frobisher to seek the legendary Northwest Passage to Asia. He fails, but reaches the Hudson Strait.

1583: Sir Humphrey Gilbert explores the coast of Newfoundland.

1585: John Davis makes the first of three unsuccessful voyages to find the Northwest Passage to Asia.

1592: Juan de Luca lands on the coast of British Columbia.

1598: La Roche's colony is established on Sable Island.

1603: King Henry IV of France awards a fur trading monopoly to a group of French merchants.

1603: Samuel de Champlain makes his first voyage to Canada.

1605: Port Royal is established in Nova Scotia by the French under Champlain.

1606: Marc Lescarbot's masque Le Théatre de Neptune en Nouvelle France is performed at Port Royal.

1608: Champlain sails up the St. Lawrence and lays claim to Québec for France. Québec City founded.

1609: Champlain travels with the Algonquins to Lake Champlain. The French and Algonquins fight the Iroquois.

1610-15:   Etienne Brulé becomes the first European to see Lakes Ontario, Huron, and Superior. Henry Hudson, seeking the Northwest Passage, explores Hudson Bay and is cast adrift by his mutinous crew.

1611:   Etienne Brulé reaches Lake Nipissing.

1612:   Samuel de Champlain is named as Governor of New France.

1613:   Argall attacks St. Sauveur in Acadia. St. John's, Newfoundland, is founded.

1617:   Louis Hébert, the first habitant (farmer), arrives in Québec; his wife, Marie, is Québec's first teacher.

1621:   Sir William Alexander is awarded Nova Scotia by King James I of England.

1623:   the founding of Avalon, Newfoundland.

1625:   the Order of the Baronets of Nova Scotia founded. Jesuits arrive in Québec to begin missionary work among the Indians.

1627:   the Company of One Hundred (also known as the Company of New France) is founded (29 April) by Cardinal Richelieu to exploit the resources of North America for France.

1629:   David Kirke captures Québec for England (19 July).

1631:   Thomas James sails into Hudson Bay and discovers James Bay. Searches for the Northwest Passage continue.

1632:   The Treaty of Saint Germain en Laye returns Québec to France.

1634:   the foundation of Giffard and Three Rivers.

1635:   the founding of the Jesuit College at Québec.

1635:   Samuel de Champlain dies.

1637:   David Kirke is named as the first governor of Newfoundland.

1638:   Placentia, Newfoundland is founded.

1630s: one of numerous outbreaks of smallpox ravages the eastern Indian tribes. The Huron nation is reduced by half during the 1630s. Jesuits found Ste. Marie among the Huron.

1639:   An Ursuline convent is set up in Québec.

1640:   discovery of Lake Erie by Europeans.

1642:   Montréal is founded by the Sieur de Maisonneuve.

1644:   the founding of the Hotel-Dieu in Montréal.

1648:   the First Council of New France is held.

1649:   the Jesuit Father Jean de Brébeuf is martyred by the Iroquois at St.-Ignace (16 March). The Iroquois disperse the Huron nation.

1651:   Jean de Lauzon is appointed Governor of New France.

1654:   Robert Sedgwick seizes Port Royal; holds Acadia until 1670.

1657:   Pierre d'Argenson becomes Governor of New France. The Sulpician religious order is established in Canada.

1658:   François de Laval is made Apostolic Vicar of New France. The first girls' school in Montréal is established.

1660:   Adam Dollard des Ormeaux makes his last stand against the Iroquois at Long Sault (May).

1661:   D'Avaugour becomes Governor of New France. Radisson and Des Groseilliers explore as far as Hudson Bay.

1662:   Thomas Temple is appointed Governor of Nova Scotia.

1663:   Québec is declared a royal province, ending the rule of the Company of New France. The Sovereign Council is founded. The Québec Seminary is established.

1665:   the Carignan-Salières regiment under the Marquis de Tracy is sent from France to Québec as reinforcements against the Iroquois. Jean Talon becomes Québec's first Intendant. Courcelle becomes Governor of New France. Dutch pirates raid the Newfoundland ports.

1666:   Fort Temple is founded as an English stronghold in the struggle to control Acadia/Nova Scotia.

1667:   the Treaty of Breda returns Acadia to France.

1668:   the founding of Fort Charles (Fort Rupert) on Hudson Bay by the English. French explorers Radisson and Des Groseilliers are employed by English merchants to explore the Hudson Bay area. The Bishop of Québec founds Canada's first art school.

1671: the English establish Fort Albany on Hudson Bay.

1672: Louis, Comte de Frontenac, becomes the governor of French possessions in North America. Albanel completes an overland trip to Hudson Bay. The Hudson's Bay Company is granted a charter by King James II of England, with trade monopoly and notional control over vast territories.

1673: the foundation of Cataraqui (Kingston), Moose Factory, and Fort Monsoni.

1675: the founding of Fort Severn. Radisson returns to French allegiance.

1678: Louis Hennepin is the first European to see Niagara Falls.

1682: La Barre becomes Governor of Québec. The Company of the North is formed.

1683: Radisson again joins the English, working for the Hudson's Bay Company.

1685: the Marquis de Denonville becomes Governor of Québec. 'Card money' from cut-up playing cards is used instead of coin in Québec: not finally ended until 1763.

1686: Moose Factory and Rupert are taken by the French. John Abraham explores the Churchill River.

1689: Frontenac begins his second term as governor, and breaks the power of the Iroquois. Abenaki Indians seize Pemaquid. Massacre of Lachine (5 August). Henry Kelsey explores the north of Canada for the Hudson's Bay Company; he is probably the first European to see the prairies.

1690: the English capture Port Royal. Phips begins his siege of Québec. D'Iberville sails into Hudson Bay. Dorchester, New Brunswick, is founded.

1693: the English retake Fort Albany from the French.

1694: D'Iberville seizes York Fort.

1696: D'Iberville campaigns against the English in Newfoundland.

1697: Callières becomes governor of New France. First settlement at Moncton, New Brunswick.

1701: the Grand Settlement achieves treaties of peace signed between the Iroquois Confederacy and the French and English.

1702: the War of the Spanish Succession spreads from Europe to Acadia and New England. Leake ravages French Newfoundland.

1703: the Marquis de Vaudreuil becomes Governor General of New France and Beauharnois becomes Intendant.

1704: new flood of card money in Canada.

1705: J. Raudot becomes Intendant of Canada.

1706: the opening of Montréal's public marketplace.

1708: St. John's is taken by the French.

1710: Francis Nicholson captures Port Royal for England. Michel Bégon become Intendant of New France.

1711: an attempted invasion of New France by the English fails. Walker's fleet is wrecked on the Île-aux-Oeufs.

1713: the Treaty of Utrecht ends a long period of French-British warfare, confirming British possession of the Hudson Bay region, Newfoundland, and Acadia, except Cape Breton Island.

1717: the French begin construction of Fort Louisbourg on the Île Royal (Cape Breton Island) to deter the English from invading the St. Lawrence.

1720: Fort Rouillé founded on the site of Toronto. Coal is first dug at Cow Bay, Cape Breton Island.

1721: Scroggs searches for the Northwest Passage, while Richard Norton explores the north by land.

1726: Beauharnois becomes Governor of New France.

1729: reorganization of Newfoundland by the English.

1730s: the Mississauga drive the Seneca Iroquois south of Lake Erie. Around now, the Blackfoot acquire horses.

1731–43: the La Vérendrye family organize expeditions beyond Lake Winnipeg and direct fur trade toward the east. They are the first recorded Europeans to sight the Canadian Rockies from the east.

1731: Gilles Hocquart becomes Intendant of New France.

1734: Pierre de La Vérendrye sets up Fort Maurepas.

1736: the Beauce country is opened for settlement.

1737: the opening of the North Shore road from Québec to Montreal. Establishment of the Grey Sisters order in Canada.

1738: the opening of the St. Maurice Ironworks. Founding of Fort La Reine (Portage la Prairie) and Fort Rouge (Winnipeg).

1741: the founding of Fort Dauphin (Dauphin, Manitoba) and Pas Koyac (The Pas, Manitoba).

1744: war between England and France spreads to North America (King George's War). In Nova Scotia, Duvivier takes Canso but fails to capture Annapolis.

1745: Massachusetts Governor, William Shirley, captures the French fortress of Louisbourg.

1746: the collapse of the revenge expedition of D'Anville to recapture Louisbourg.

1747: the Comte de la Galissonière becomes Governor of New France.

1748: cessation of hostilities: Louisbourg and the Île Royale are returned to France by the Treaty of Aix-La-Chapelle. Bigot becomes Intendant of New France.

1749: Britain founds Halifax to counter the French presence at Louisbourg. La Jonquière becomes Governor of New France.

1750: French and British embark on a new round of fortification, including Fort Beauséjour (French) and Fort Lawrence (British) on the Chignecto Isthmus.

1751: a French expedition reaches the eastern edge of the Rocky Mountains.

1752: the first Canadian newspaper, the weekly Halifax Gazette, appears (23 March). The Marquis de Duquesne becomes Governor of New France.

1754: the beginning of the French and Indian War in America. Fort Duquesne is constructed.

1755: Britain disperses the French Acadians throughout other North American colonies. General Braddock takes command of British forces in North America.

1756: the Marquis de Montcalm assumes command of French troops in North America. The French, with Indian support, capture Fort Oswego.

1757: Fort William Henry is taken by the French.

1758: General Abercromby becomes British Commander-in-Chief. Generals Jeffery Amherst and James Wolfe capture Louisbourg; Forbes captures Fort Duquesne, and Bradstreet takes Fort Frontenac. Montcalm is victorious at Carillon. Nova Scotia's depleted population doubles with new settlers and the province is first to establish a House of Assembly. The Nova Scotia Militia is established by an act of the Assembly.

1759: the British, with Indian support, take Fort Carillon and Fort Niagara, cutting off western French territory. Wolfe defeats Montcalm and takes Québec (13 September) but both generals are killed. Brigadier James Murray is appointed Governor of Québec.

1760: Lévis's French force to relieve Québec defeats the British at Ste. Foy, but fails to advance further. Governor General Vaudreuil (son of the Vaudreuil of 1703) surrenders at Montréal to General Amherst (9 September). Canada remains under British military rule until 1763-64.

1763: the Treaty of Paris is made: France cedes its North American possessions to Britain. A royal proclamation imposes British institutions on Québec.

1764: James Murray becomes civil Governor of Québec, but his attempts to appease French Canadians are opposed by British merchants.

1768: Guy Carleton succeeds Murray as civil Governor of Québec.

1774: the Carleton recommendations are instituted in the Québec Act, imposing British criminal law but retaining French civil law and providing guarantees of religious freedom for Roman Catholics.

1775: the American Revolution begins. Americans under Richard Montgomery capture Montréal (13 November) and are defeated at Québec (31 December).

1776: the siege of Québec is lifted with the arrival of a British naval squadron (6 May). The Hudson's Bay Company opens Cumberland House on the Saskatchewan.

1778: on the last of three voyages to the west coast, Captain James Cook reaches as far north as the Bering Strait and claims Nootka Sound, Vancouver Island for Great Britain (29 March–26 April).

1781: the Great Slave Lake is named by the Cree to characterize the lifestyle of mild-mannered lake dwellers as the Awonak or Slave people . Fur trader and map maker, Peter Pond, put this name on his map.

1783: in Montréal and Grand Portage (in present-day Minnesota), the North West Company is officially formed by a group of trading partners. With the end of the American revolutionary war, the border between Canada and the United States is accepted from the Atlantic Ocean to Lake of the Woods. Large numbers of United Empire Loyalists leave the U.S.A. to settle in Canada, mostly in the Maritime Provinces. Pennsylvania Germans begin moving into Upper and Lower Canada (modern-day southwestern Ontario, and southwestern Québec).

1784: Nova Scotia is partitioned and the province of New Brunswick is formed. Thousands of Loyalists settle on land in Upper and Lower Canada, along the St. Lawrence River, the Bay of Quinte, and at Niagara.

1785: the city of Saint John, New Brunswick, is incorporated. Fredericton opens a Provincial Academy of Arts and Sciences, later the University of New Brunswick.

1789: Alexander Mackenzie makes a journey to the Beaufort Sea, on behalf of the North West Company, and 'discovers' Canada's longest river, later named the Mackenzie River. King's College, Halifax, is founded.

1791: the Constitutional Act divides Québec into Upper and Lower Canada (present-day provinces of Ontario and Québec) and provides for representative government.

1792: Captain George Vancouver begins a detailed survey of the Pacific coastline.

1793: Alexander Mackenzie crosses the Rockies to reach the Pacific at Dean Channel.

1794: an American diplomat, John Jay, oversees the signing of Jay's Treaty (19 November) between the U.S. and Britain. It promises British evacuation of the Ohio Valley forts and marks the beginning of international arbitration to settle boundary disputes.

1795: Fort Edmonton is founded.

1796: the township of York (later Toronto) becomes the capital of Upper Canada.

1798: the New North West Company is formed to compete with the North West Company.

1804: the New North West Company is absorbed by the North West Company. The earliest Fraktur paintings appear in Lincoln County, Ontario.

1805:   Mennonites from Pennsylvania begin to settle in the Huron-Erie Peninsula.

1806:   Le Canadien, a Québec nationalist newspaper, is founded.

1807:   slavery is abolished in all British colonies.

1812:   the British–American War begins. Americans under General William Hull invade Canada from Detroit (11 July). Canadians are victorious at the Battle of Queenstown Heights (12 October). Scots begin the Red River settlement on lands granted to Lord Selkirk by the Hudson's Bay Company.

1813:   American forces burn York (27 April). The Battles of Stoney Creek (5 June) and Beaver Dam (23 June) are Canadian victories. Americans win at Put-in-Bay, Lake Erie (10 September) and Moraviantown (5 October). At the latter, Shawnee Indian Chief Tecumseh, a British ally, is killed. The Battles of Chateauguay (25 October), with mostly French Canadian troops, and Crysler's Farm (11 November), with English Canadian troops, are Canadian victories over larger American forces.

1814:   victories alternate between U.S. and British forces until the Treaty of Ghent ends the war (24 December).

1816:   after several years of harassment by agents of the North West Company, Métis and Indians under Cuthbert Grant kill Robert Semple, Governor of Assiniboia, the Red River settlement, and twenty others at Seven Oaks (19 June).

1817:   the Rush-Bagot Agreement limits the number of warships on the Great Lakes to a total of eight.

1818:   Canada's border with the U.S.A. is defined as the 49th parallel from Lake of the Woods to the Rocky Mountains.

1819:   the first steamship to go up the Ottawa River docks at Hull (now named Gatineau).

1821:   the Hudson's Bay and North West Companies amalgamate, resulting in unemployment for a substantial proportion of their Métis workforce.

1822:   Louis-Joseph Papineau, a member of the legislative assembly since 1814, travels from Montréal to England to oppose an Act of Union identifying the French Canadians as a minority without language rights. The act is not passed in the British Parliament.

1825:   the Lachine Canal is completed, bypassing rapids on the St. Lawrence.

1829:   the first Welland Canal is completed.

1830:   the first shaft is sunk for deep coal mining at Sydney, Nova Scotia.

1832:   Royal Engineer, Col. John By, completes building of the Rideau Canal.

1834:   York is renamed Toronto. William Lyon Mackenzie becomes the city's first mayor.

1835:   Joseph Howe, a Halifax publisher and editor since 1828 of the weekly Nova Scotian, is arrested for libel but successfully argues his own case for freedom of the press.

1836:   opening of Canada's first railway line, the Champlain & St. Lawrence, from St. Johns, Québec, to Laprairie, Québec, with a locomotive, Dorchester, imported from England.

1837:   a constitutional crisis erupts; after increasing protests against unde-mocratic government, and the failure of the executive committee to maintain the confidence of the elected officials, armed rebellions break out in Upper and Lower Canada, and are put down by force. The leaders, W. L. Mackenzie (Reformers) and Louis-Joseph Papineau (Patriotes) escape to the U.S.A.

1838:   Lord Durham, as Governor General and High Commissioner of British North America, is sent to investigate the circumstances behind the rebellions of 1837.

1839:   Durham's report recommends the establishment of responsible (i.e. non-oligarchic) government and the union of Upper and Lower Canada to speed the assimilation of French-speaking Canadians. Border disputes between lumbermen from Maine and New Brunswick lead to armed conflict in the Aroostook River valley (the Aroostook War).

1840: an Act of Union unites Upper and Lower Canada (10 February) as the Province of Canada. The Cunard Steamship Line is founded at Halifax.

1841: the union of Upper and Lower Canada is put into effect.

1842: the Webster-Ashburton Treaty ends the Aroostook War, with an agreed line for the Maine–New Brunswick border.

1843: Britain builds Fort Victoria on Vancouver Island.

1844: an amnesty in Montréal provides for Papineau's return.

1846: the establishment of 'responsible government' in Canada. The Oregon Treaty affirms the entire Canadian–U.S. border west from the Great Lakes along the 49th parallel to the Pacific coast.

1848–51: the 'Great Ministry' of Robert Baldwin and Louis H. Lafontaine establishes the principles of responsible government. Between now and 1850 Le Répertoire Nationale, a collection of earlier stories and legends, is published in Montréal by James Huston.

1849: an Act of Amnesty provides for W. L. Mackenzie's return from exile in the U.S. Vancouver Island designated as a Crown Colony.

1850: the site of By's headquarters during the construction of the Rideau Canal is incorporated as Bytown. Canada's first metal mine, for copper ore, is started at Bruce Mines, on the north shore of Lake Huron.

1851: Britain transfers control of the colonial postal system to Canada.

1852: Laval's Séminaire du Québec founds Université Laval, North America's oldest French language university.

1852–53: the Grand Trunk Railway receives its charter.

1854: Canada and the U.S. sign a Reciprocity Treaty, ensuring reduction of customs duties (6 June).

1855: Bytown is renamed Ottawa. The Militia Act provides for a permanent volunteer force. La Capricieuse, on a courtesy visit, is the first vessel to fly the French flag in Québec harbour since 1760.

1856: the Grand Trunk Railway opens its Toronto–Montréal line.

1857: Queen Victoria designates Ottawa as capital of the Province of Canada. Seventy people die when a bridge over the Desjardins Canal collapses under a train.

1858: British Columbia designated as a Crown Colony. The Halifax-Truro line begins its rail service. Chinese immigrants from California arrive in British Columbia, attracted by the Fraser River gold rush. The first oil well in North America is opened, in Lambton County in Ontario.

1859: the University of New Brunswick is constituted. Blondin makes his first tightrope walk over Niagara Falls.

1860: the foundation stone of the federal parliament buildings is laid (1 September) in Ottawa. The Mouvement littéraire de Québec of romantic-rhetorical writers is founded. Joseph Howe becomes premier of Nova Scotia.

1862: Mount Allison University accepts the first woman student in Sackville, New Brunswick. The 'Cariboo Wagon Road' (644 kilometres, 400 miles) is built along the Fraser valley in British Columbia by Royal Engineers and private contractors (to 1865).

1864: the Charlottetown Conference (1–9 September), originally intended to discuss the union of the Maritime Provinces, opens the way towards Confederation. The subsequent Québec Conference (10–27 October) identifies 72 resolutions setting out the basis for union. Ninety-nine immigrant passengers are killed in a train smash near Montréal.

1866: the Fenian Brotherhood, a group of radical Irish-Americans, mostly U.S. Civil War veterans, begins a series of raids on Canadian territory in the hopes of diverting British troops from the homeland. The most serious of these is the Battle of Ridgeway (2 June). The London Conference (4 December) passes resolutions that form the basis of the British North America (BNA) Act.

1867: the Confederation of Canada takes place. Britain's North American colonies are united by means of the BNA Act to become the Dominion of Canada (1 July). Sir John A. Macdonald, 'Father of Confederation', is Canada's first Prime Minister. Ottawa officially becomes capital of the Dominion.

1868: the 'Canada First' patriotic movement is founded. Thomas D'Arcy McGee, one of the fathers of Confederation, and a leading opponent of the Fenians, becomes Canada's first assassination victim, at the hands of a Fenian (7 April). Canada purchases Rupert's Land from the Hudson's Bay Company.

1869: Threatened by Canadian purchases of Hudson's Bay territories, and loss of their land and livelihood, Louis Riel leads the Métis in occupying Fort Garry, on the site of Winnipeg.

1870: the Red River Rebellion continues to resist Canadian authority in the northwest. The insurgents form a provisional government (January) but military action under General Wolseley ends this (August). When the Manitoba Act creates the province of Manitoba, the rebellion is finally ended.

1871: British Columbia and Vancouver Island join the Confederation (20 July).

1873: Prince Edward Island joins the Confederation. The 'Cypress Hills Massacre' of Indians by trappers. General lawlessness in the northwest, brings about the formation of the Northwest Mounted Police. Macdonald resigns over the Pacific Scandal (5 November), which brought attention to campaign contributions made by Sir Hugh Allan in exchange for a charter to build the Canadian Pacific Railway. The Liberal Party is formed; Alexander Mackenzie becomes Canada's second, and first Liberal, Prime Minister.

1874: Riel is elected to the House of Commons but opposition from Ontario prevents him from taking the seat (February). Anabaptists (Russian Mennonites) start to arrive in Manitoba from various Russian colonies.

1875: Riel is granted amnesty but with exile for five years. The Supreme Court of Canada is established. Jennie Trout becomes the first woman licensed to practice medicine in Canada, although Emily Stowe has been doing so without a license in Toronto since 1867. Grace Lockhart receives, from Mount Allison University, the first Bachelor of Arts degree awarded to a woman.

1876: the Intercolonial Railway, growing out of the Halifax–Truro line, links central Canada and the Maritime Provinces (1 July). The Toronto Women's Literary Club is founded as a front for the women's suffrage movement.

1877: the provincial legislature creates the University of Manitoba, the oldest university in western Canada.

1878: the Conservatives under Macdonald win the federal election. Anti-Chinese sentiment in British Columbia reaches a high point as the government bans immigrant Chinese workers from public works. The first asbestos mine opens.

1879: Macdonald introduces his national policy, with protective tariffs, a transcontinental railway system, and opening up of the west (12 March). Canada negotiates independent trade agreements with France and Spain.

1880: Emily Stowe is finally granted a license to practice medicine in Toronto.

1881: the Canadian Pacific Railway is founded.

1880–84: The Canadian Pacific Railway recruits thousands of low-paid Chinese labourers for building the transcontinental line.

1883: Augusta Stowe, daughter of Emily, is the first woman to graduate from the Toronto Medical School. The Toronto Women's Suffrage Association replaces the Literary Club of 1876.

1884: Joseph Tyrell discovers the skull of a dinosaur, named Albertasaurus.

1885:   Riel, who had returned to Canada in 1884, leads the aggrieved and unemployed Métis in the Northwest Rebellion. The Métis are defeated at Batoche (2–9 May); Riel is captured, and hanged in Regina (16 November). The last spike of the transcontinental Canadian Pacific Railway is ceremonially hammered in at the Eagle Pass, British Columbia (7 November).

1887:   the Liberals choose Wilfred Laurier as leader. The first provincial Premiers' Conference takes place in Québec City.

1890:   Manitoba Liberals under Thomas Greenway halt public funding of Catholic schools.

1893:   the National Council of Women of Canada is founded.

1895:   the Yukon is made into a provisional district, separate from the Northwest Territories.

1896:   the Liberals under Laurier (the first French Canadian Prime Minister) win the federal election partly on the Manitoba Schools Question, though his compromises are not instituted until 1897. Gold is discovered in the Klondike (16 August).

1897   Canada's first woman lawyer is Clara Brett Martin.

1898:   the Klondike Gold Rush is fully under way. The Yukon provisional district is officially confirmed as the Yukon Territory, a territory separate from the Northwest Territories. Russian Doukhobors, an anarchistic sect, are allowed to settle in Saskatchewan.

1899:   the first Canadian troops to be sent overseas participate in the Boer War in South Africa (30 October).

1901:   Marconi receives the first transatlantic radio message at St. John's, Newfoundland. First commercial natural gas well drilled, near Medicine Hat.

1902:   a train crash on the Grand Trunk Railway, near Hamilton, Ontario, results in 28 deaths.

1903:   Canada loses the Alaska boundary dispute and the Alaska 'panhandle' is confirmed as U.S. territory (20 October). A landslip at Frank, Alberta, in the Crow's Nest Pass, kills 70 people. Silver is discovered in northern Ontario. Nude demonstrations by the extreme Doukhobor 'Sons of Freedom' take place near Yorkton, Saskatchewan, against government policy regarding taking an oath of allegiance to register land. Roald Amundsen makes the first transit of the Northwest Passage (1903–6).

1904:   the Northwest Mounted Police is renamed the Royal Northwest Mounted Police (RNWMP), with headquarters at Regina.

1905:   the Alberta and Saskatchewan provinces are formed, and the Northwest Territories created out of the former districts of Keewatin, Mackenzie, Franklin, and Ungava.

1906:   Sir Adam Beck leads the effort to create the Hydro-Electric Power Commission of Ontario (7 May), the largest such company in Canada.

1908:   Peter Verigin, leader of the Doukhobors since his arrival in Canada in 1902, leads the extremist 'Sons of Freedom' to British Columbia.

1909:   the Department of External Affairs is formed. The first Grey Cup is played. Canada's first powered air flight takes place at Baddeck, Nova Scotia.

1910:   the Laurier government creates a Canadian navy with the Naval Service Bill. Forty-three die in a train crash near Sudbury, Ontario.

1911:   Robert Borden and the Conservatives win the federal election, defeating Laurier on the reciprocity issue.

1912:   a botanist, Carrie Derrick, is Canada's first woman professor, at McGill University.

1914:   the Canadian Pacific ship Empress of Ireland sinks in the St. Lawrence within 15 minutes of a collision in dense fog – over a thousand lives are lost (29 May). The Hillcrest mine disaster at Turtle Mountain, Alberta, kills 189 miners. Political controversy is aroused on the issue of Sikh immigration with the arrival in English Bay, British Columbia, of the Komagata Maru with nearly 400 Sikh passengers from the Far East. Britain declares war on Germany (4 August), automatically drawing Canada into the conflict. The first Canadian troops leave for England (3 October). Parliament passes the War Measures Act, allowing suspension of civil rights during periods of emergency. Oil is found in Alberta.

1915:   in their first battle, the 1st Canadian Division face one of the first recorded chlorine gas attacks at Ypres, Belgium (22 April). The National Transcontinental, eastern division of the Grand Trunk Railway, completes a line from Moncton to Winnipeg.

1916:   the parliament buildings are destroyed by fire (3 February). The 1st Canadian Division discovers that the Canadian-made Ross rifle (controversial since 1905) is unreliable in combat conditions. It is withdrawn from service and replaced by the British-made Lee-Enfield (August). The National Research Council is established to promote scientific and industrial research. Female suffrage is first granted in Canada in Manitoba.

1917:   income tax is introduced as a temporary wartime measure. The Military Service Bill (11 June) sparks a conscription crisis dividing French and English Canada. A Union government (a coalition of Liberals and Tories) under Borden wins in a federal election in which all women of British origin are allowed to vote for the first time. The Canadians capture Vimy Ridge, France (9–12 April), and Passchendaele, Belgium (6 November), in two of the war's worst battles. The explosion of the munitions ship, Mont Blanc, in Halifax harbour wipes out two square miles of the city, killing almost 2000 people and injuring 9000 (6 December). The Québec railway bridge over the St. Lawrence is completed. In Alberta, Louise McKinney becomes the first woman elected to a legislature in the British Commonwealth.

1918:   Canadians break through the German trenches at Amiens, France (8 August), beginning 'Canada's Hundred Days'. Armistice ends World War I (11 November). Imprisoned in South Dakota for pacifism, Hutterites flee northward into the Prairie Provinces.

1919:   the Grand Trunk Pacific, western division of the Grand Trunk Railway, completes a line from Winnipeg to Prince Rupert. The Canadian National Railways is created as a Crown corporation to acquire and further consolidate smaller lines. The first successful transatlantic flight leaves St. John's, Newfoundland (14 June). During a general strike in Winnipeg (19 May–26 June), an armed charge by the police on 'Bloody Saturday' kills one and injures thirty (21 June). James S. Woodsworth and others are charged with seditious conspiracy. The federal government passes a Technical Education Act.

1920:   Canada is a founder member of the League of Nations. The Progressive Party is formed by T. A. Crerar to obtain law tariffs for western farmers. The RNWMP is re-formed as the Royal Canadian Mounted Police (RCMP), with headquarters at Ottawa. The 'Group of Seven' artists is formed at Toronto.

1921:   Mackenzie King and the Liberals win the federal election. Agnes Macphail becomes the first woman elected to Parliament (representing the Progressive Party). J. S. Woodsworth becomes the first socialist elected to the House of Commons. Bluenose, the famous racing schooner, is launched at Lunenburg, Nova Scotia (26 March). Insulin is discovered at the University of Toronto. Colonial Motors of Walkerville, Ontario, manufacture an automobile called the 'Canadian'.

1922:   the Canadian Northern and Canadian Transcontinental Railways merge to form the publicly owned Canadian National Railways. Canada asserts its independence by not going to Britain's aid in the

Chanak crisis in Turkey. Banting, Best, MacLeod, and Collip share the Nobel Prize for the discovery of insulin. A Provincial Franchise Committee is organized in Québec to work towards female suffrage in the province.

1923:   Canada signs the Halibut Treaty with the U.S. without the traditional British signature. Mackenzie King leads the opposition to a common imperial policy at the Imperial Conference in London. The Grand Trunk Railway is taken over by the government. The federal government acts to prevent Chinese immigration on Dominion Day, called 'Humiliation Day' by Chinese Canadians. Foster Hewitt makes the first hockey broadcast.

1924:   Major C. H. Douglas proposes the social credit monetary theory, which is taken up by A. B. Aberhart in Alberta. Doukhobor leader, Peter Verigin, is assassinated.

1925:   Newfoundland women receive the right to vote. Only Québecois women remain outside the suffrage.

1926:   the Balfour Report defines British dominions as autonomous and equal in status (18 November).

1927:   Britain's Privy Council awards Labrador to Newfoundland rather than to Québec (1 March). The first coast-to-coast radio network broadcast celebrates the Diamond Jubilee of Confederation.

1928:   the Supreme Court of Canada rules that the British North America Act does not define women as 'persons' and that they are therefore not eligible to hold public office.

1929:   the British Privy Council reverses the Supreme Court decision of 1928. Women are legally declared 'persons' (18 October). The Wall Street Crash in the U.S.A. heralds years of economic slump. The Workers' Unity League is formed.

1930:   the Conservatives under R. B. Bennett win the federal election. Jean de Brébeuf and other Jesuit martyrs are officially canonized. Cairine Wilson becomes Canada's first woman senator.

1931:   the Statute of Westminster (11 December) implements the Balfour Report of 1926, granting Canada full legislative authority in both internal and external affairs. The Governor General becomes a representative of the Crown.

1932:   the fourth Welland Canal completed, taking ships of up to 33,000 tons. Woodsworth joins in forming a democratic socialist political party, the Co-operative Commonwealth Federation (CCF), in Calgary. Bennett's government establishes repressive 'relief camps' to cope with the problem of unemployed single men.

1934:   the Bank of Canada is formed. The birth of the Dionne quintuplets in Ontario attracts international media attention.

1935:   about a thousand unemployed men from the western provinces begin the 'On-to-Ottawa' trek, to confront Bennett over the relief camps (3 June–1 July). In an attempt to remove a corrupt Liberal administration, Maurice Duplessis, a Québec Conservative, allies with a splinter group of Liberals under Paul Gouin to form the Union Nationale. In Alberta, the Social Credit Party gains power (until 1971). Novelist John Buchan (Lord Tweedsmuir) is made Governor General. Gold is discovered in the Northwest Territories, on the west coast of Yellowknife Bay.

1936:   the Canadian Broadcasting Corporation (CBC) is founded, modelled on the BBC. Driven by the reformist Union Nationale, Duplessis ousts Gouin and becomes Premier of Québec. The Governor General's Literary Awards are instituted.

1937:   the Rowell-Sirois Commission is appointed to investigate the financial relationship between the federal government and the provinces. Trans-Canada Air Lines begins regular flights (1 September). Les

Compagnons de St. Laurent drama company founded in Québec.

1938:   Franklin D. Roosevelt is the first U.S. president to make an official visit to Canada. The Workers' Unity League helps to organize the Vancouver Sit-ins, in which protesting relief camp workers and others occupy the Post Office and other public buildings. The demonstrators are forced out by police on 'Bloody Sunday' (19 June), with 35 people wounded.

1939:   Canada declares war on Germany (10 September). Premier Duplessis opposes Québec's participation but is defeated by the Liberals on the issue (26 October).

1940:   the Unemployment Insurance Commission is introduced. Canada and the U.S.A. form a Permanent Joint Defence Board. Parliament passes the controversial National Resources Mobilization Act (June), which allows conscription for military service only within Canada. Idola Saint-Jean and other activists finally succeed in obtaining the vote for Québecois women. The RCMP vessel St. Roch makes the first west–east transit of the Northwest Passage.

1941:   fluorspar is first mined, at Lake Ainslie, Nova Scotia.

1942:   Canadians of Japanese descent (22,000) are stripped of non-portable possessions, evacuated, and interned as security risks (26 February). A national plebiscite approves amendment of the National Resources Mobilization Act to permit sending conscripts overseas (27 April), once again revealing deep divisions between Québec and English Canada. The Dieppe raid (19 August), Canada's first participation in the war in Europe, is a disaster, with 3,367 out of 4,963 Canadians dead or taken prisoner.

1943:   Canadians participate in the invasion of Sicily (10 July), and win the Battle of Ortona, a German stronghold on the Adriatic (20– 28 December).

1944:   Canadian troops push further than other allied units on D-Day (6 June). Canadian forces fight as a separate army (23 July). The Family Allowance Act is passed (August). The CCF under Tommy Douglas wins the provincial election in Saskatchewan, forming the first socialist government in North America.

1945:   European hostilities end (5 May). The first family allowance ('baby-bonus') payments are made (20 June). Canada becomes a founder member of the United Nations (26 June). Hostilities in the Pacific Basin end (2 September). Igor Gouzenko defects from the Soviet Embassy in Ottawa (5 September) and reveals the existence in Canada of a Soviet spy network. Canada's first nuclear reactor goes on stream in Chalk River, Ontario.

1948:   Louis St. Laurent succeeds Mackenzie King as Prime Minister (15 November).

1949:   Newfoundland ceases to be a separate British Dominion and joins the Confederation (31 March). Canada joins NATO. Canada's Supreme Court replaces Britain's Privy Council judicial committee as the country's final court of appeal.

1950:   volunteers in the Canadian Army Special Force join the United Nations forces in the Korean War.

1951:   census shows population as just over 14 million. The Massey Royal Commission reports that Canadian cultural life is dominated by American influences. Recommendations include improving grants to universities and the establishment of the Canada Council.

1952:   Vincent Massey becomes the first Canadian-born Governor General. Canada's first television stations begin transmissions in Montréal and Toronto (September). A disaster is narrowly averted at the Chalk River nuclear plant.

1953:   the National Library is established in Ottawa (1 January). The Stratford Shakespeare Festival opens (13 July).

1954: the first Canadian subway opens in Toronto (30 March). Viewers of the British Empire Games in Vancouver see Roger Bannister break the four-minute mile. Marilyn Bell is the first person to swim across Lake Ontario (9 September). Hurricane Hazel kills over 80 people in Toronto (15 October).

1955: riots in Montréal are caused by the suspension of Canadiens hockey star Maurice "Rocket" Richard (17 March).

1956: the Liberals use a closure motion to curtail the 'pipeline debate', which begins with concern over the funding of the natural gas industry and ends in controversy over proper parliamentary procedure (8 May–6 June). The action contributes to their electoral defeat (after 22 years in power) the following year. The Canadian Labour Congress is formed.

1957: John Diefenbaker and the Conservatives win a minority government (10 June). Ellen Fairclough becomes the first female federal cabinet minister. The Canada Council is formed to foster Canadian cultural uniqueness. Lester B. Pearson wins the Nobel Peace Prize for helping resolve the Suez Crisis (12 October).

1958: Diefenbaker's government gains the largest majority yet obtained in a federal election (31 March). A coalmine disaster at Springhill, Nova Scotia, kills 74 miners. The prototype Avro Arrow CF-105 interceptor aircraft is flown (25 March).

1959: the St. Lawrence Seaway opens (26 June). Diefenbaker cancels the Avro Arrow project, to public outcry.

1960: Liberals under Jean Lesage win the provincial election in Québec (22 June), inaugurating the 'Quiet Revolution', gives rise to creating special status for the province within the Confederation and is the catalyst for much social change. A Canadian Bill of Rights is approved. Native people win the right to vote in federal elections.

1961: the New Democratic Party (NDP) replaces the CCF.

1962: the Conservatives are returned to minority status in a federal election (18 June). Socialized medicine is introduced in Saskatchewan (1 July), leading to a doctors' strike. The Trans–Canada Highway opens (3 September). Canada becomes the third nation in space with the launch of the satellite Alouette I (29 September). Canada's last executions take place in Toronto (11 December).

1963: Liberals under Pearson win a minority government (8 April). The militant separatist Front de libération du Québec (FLQ) sets off bombs in Montréal (April–May). A TCA flight crashes in Québec, killing 118 people (29 November). A replica of Bluenose is launched at Lunenburg, Nova Scotia.

1964: Canadians get social insurance cards (April). Northern Dancer is the first Canadian horse to win the Kentucky Derby.

1965: Canada and the U.S. sign the Auto Pact (January). The new national maple leaf flag is inaugurated (15 February). Roman Catholic churches begin to celebrate masses in French and English. The Hydro-Electric Power Commission of Ontario inadvertently causes a major power blackout in North America (9 November).

1966: the Munsinger affair (in which the Associate Minister of National Defence, Pierre Sévigny, had a liaison with a German divorcée suspected by the RCMP) becomes Canada's first political sex scandal (4 March). The Canada Pension Plan is established. The CBC introduces colour TV broadcasts (1 October).

1967: the Air Force, Army, and Navy are unified as the Canadian Armed Forces (25 April). World attention is turned to Expo '67 in Montréal (27 April). Centennial celebrations officially begin (1 July). The Order of Canada is founded. French President, Charles de Gaulle, controversially proclaims, 'Vive le Québec libre' in Montréal (24 July).

1968: Pierre Trudeau succeeds Pearson as leader of the Liberals and wins a majority in the federal election (25 June). A royal commission on the status of women is appointed. Canadian divorce laws are reformed.

1969:   postal reforms end Saturday deliveries (1 February). Abortion laws are liberalized (May). The Official Languages Act provides that all federal services shall be available in English and French (9 July). The Breathalyzer™ is put into use to test for drunken drivers (1 December).

1970:   British trade commissioner James Cross is kidnapped by the FLQ (5 October), precipitating the October Crisis. Québec's labour and immigration minister, Pierre Laporte, is also kidnapped (10 October) and later found murdered. The War Measures Act is invoked by Premier Trudeau (16 October), banning the FLQ and leading eventually to nearly 500 arrests under martial law.

1971:   the federal government officially adopts a policy of multiculturalism. Gerhard Herzberg of the National Research Council wins the Nobel Prize for Chemistry for studies of smog.

1972:   Canada wins the first hockey challenge against Soviet Russia. Trudeau's Liberals win a minority government by two seats.

1973:   The House of Commons criticizes U.S. bombing of North Vietnam (5 January). Henry Morgentaler is acquitted of illegal abortion charges in Montréal (13 November). The separatist Parti Québecois becomes the official opposition in a provincial election.

1974:   the Hydro-Electric Power Commission of Ontario changes its name to Ontario Hydro and begins to update its image (4 March). Soviet ballet dancer Mikhail Baryshnikov defects in Montréal (29 June). Trudeau's Liberals win a majority government (8 July).

1975:   Toronto's CN Tower becomes the world's tallest free-standing structure (2 April). TV cameras are allowed in the House of Commons for the first time. Trudeau institutes wage and price controls to fight inflation (14 October).

1976:   Canada announces a 200-mile (320-kilometre) coastal fishing zone (4 June). The death penalty, in abeyance for some years, is abolished (14 July). The Olympic Games are held in Montréal (17–31 July) under tight security. Team Canada wins the first Canada Cup (15 September). René Lévesque and the Parti Québecois win the provincial election (15 November). The Eaton Company discontinues catalogue sales after 92 continuous years.

1977:   Québec passes Bill 101, restricting English schooling to children of parents who had been educated in English schools (26 August). Highway signs are changed to the metric system (6 September). VIA Rail is established to secure rail passenger services.

1978:   the remains of a Soviet nuclear-powered satellite crash in the far north (24 January). Sun Life Assurance acknowledges that it moved its head office to Toronto because of Montréal's language laws and political instability.

1979:   Conservatives under Joe Clark win a federal election (May 22). The first uniquely Canadian gold bullion coin, with a maple leaf motif, goes on sale (5 September). Most of Mississauga, Ontario, is evacuated following derailment of train cars containing chemicals (10 November). The Supreme Court of Canada declares unconstitutional the creation of officially monolingual legislatures in Manitoba and Québec (13 December). Clark's Conservatives lose a no-confidence vote on the budget (13 December), forcing their resignation.

1980:   Ken Taylor, Canadian ambassador to Iran, helps six Americans escape Tehran (28 January). Canada boycotts Moscow's Olympic Games over the Soviet invasion of Afghanistan. A Québec referendum rejects sovereignty-association (22 May). 'O Canada' is officially adopted as Canada's national anthem (27 June). The Supreme Court recognizes the equal distribution of assets in failed common-law relationships. Terry Fox's cross-Canada 'Marathon of Hope' ends prematurely in Thunder Bay.

1981: Terry Fox dies of cancer (29 June). His example eventually raises about 25 million dollars. Québec bans public signs in English (23 September). All federal and provincial governments, except Québec, agree on a method to repatriate Canada's constitution (5 November).

1982: the offshore oil rig Ocean Ranger sinks, killing 84 (15 February). Bertha Wilson is the first woman appointed as a Justice of the Supreme Court (4 March). The Québec government demand for a veto over constitutional change is rejected (7 April). Canada gains a new constitution and charter of rights and freedoms (17 April). Marguerite Bourgeoys is canonized as Canada's first female saint.

1983: Pay TV begins operation (1 February). Public outcry opposes the government's approval of U.S. cruise missile testing in the west. Jeanne Sauvé is appointed Governor General – the first female to be appointed (23 December).

1984: John Turner succeeds Trudeau as Liberal Prime Minister (30 June) but is soon defeated by Brian Mulroney's Conservatives, by an even larger majority than Diefenbaker's in 1958 (4 September). Pope John Paul II visits Canada (9–20 September). Marc Garneau becomes the first Canadian in space, on the U.S. shuttle Challenger (5 October). The International Court of Justice defines fishing boundaries on George's Bank.

1985: U.S. icebreaker Polar Sea challenges Canada's Arctic sovereignty by making a traverse of the Northwest Passage. Premier Mulroney, in September, calls President Reagan to say Canada will not participate in the Orbital Strategic Defence Initiatives (Star Wars). Premier Mulroney and U.S. President Ronald Reagan declare mutual support for Free Trade at the 'Shamrock Summit' in Québec City (2 December). Ontario Liberals under David Peterson end 40 years of Conservative premiership. Lincoln Alexander becomes Ontario's first black Lieutenant Governor.

1986: The Canadian dollar hits an all-time low of 70.2 U.S. cents on international money markets (31 January). The 'Supercontinental' crashes into a freight train west of Edmonton: 23 are killed (17 February). Expo '86 opens in Vancouver (2 May–13 October). The U.S. imposes tariffs on some imported Canadian wood products (22 May). Canada adopts sanctions against South Africa for its apartheid policies (5 August). Tamil refugees are found drifting off the coast of Newfoundland (11 August). Canada receives a United Nations award for sheltering foreign refugees (6 October). Canadian John Polanyi shares the Nobel Prize for Chemistry.

1987: Mulroney and the provincial premiers agree in principle to the Meech Lake Accord, designed to bring Québec into the new constitution (30 April). A tornado rips through Edmonton, killing 27 and injuring hundreds (20 July). Canadian sprinter, Ben Johnson, sets a new world record (30 August) for the 100-metre dash. The Canada–U.S. Free Trade Agreement is reached (3 October), but still requires ratification.

1988: the Supreme Court strikes down existing legislation against abortion as unconstitutional (28 January). The Winter Olympics open in Calgary (13 February). David See-Chai Lam, born in Hong Kong, becomes British Columbia's Lieutenant Governor (9 September). Ben Johnson sets a world sprint record and wins the gold medal at the Seoul Olympics in Korea (24 September). Testing positive for steroids, he is stripped of his medal two days later. The Supreme Court strikes down Québec's French-only sign law (15 December).

Finding a constitutional loophole (the 'notwithstanding' clause) in the charter of rights and freedoms, the province reinstates the law (21 December). Manitoba Premier, Gary Filmon, slows the ratification of the Meech Lake Accord in reaction to Québec's move. The Canada–U.S. Free Trade Agreement is signed.

1989:   free trade goes into effect (1 January). Heather Erxleben becomes Canada's first acknowledged female combat soldier. One-dollar bills are replaced by the one-dollar coin, featuring the loon, and popularly called the 'loonie'. The government announces cuts in the subsidy to VIA Rail, to much public outcry (5 June). The first woman to lead a federal political party, Audrey McLaughlin, replaces Ed Broadbent as head of the NDP (2 December). Fourteen female engineering students are murdered by a gunman at the École Polytechnique, Montréal (6 December).

1990:   the Haggersville Tyre Depot in Ontario burns for 16 days (February). The 'Oka crisis' in Québec lasts 78 days as Mohawk Indians protest against a golf course being built over an ancestral burial ground. Newfoundland Premier, Clyde Wells, further slows down the signing of the Meech Lake Accord. Manitoba finally ends its chances when a native member of the provincial legislature, Elijah Harper, refuses to acknowledge Québec as Canada's principal, if not only, 'distinct society' because the Accord did not guarantee rights for aboriginal peoples. Following the Accord's failure to become law, the Bloc Québecois is formed (25 July). Bob Rae, with a large majority, becomes Ontario's first NDP premier (September). The Senate passes the unpopular Goods and Services Tax (December). An economic recession is officially announced.

1991:   the Goods and Services Tax comes into effect (1 January). Canadian forces join the multinational campaign to drive Saddam Hussein's Iraqi troops from Kuwait (15 January). British Columbia Premier, Bill Van Der Zalm, resigns in the midst of a real estate scandal. George Erasmus, leader of the Assembly of First Nations, resigns at the end of his second term (May); he is succeeded by Ovide Mercredi, whose popularity earns him the nickname of 'eleventh premier'. A new committee is set up to inquire into citizens' opinions on proposed constitutional reforms. David Schindler of the University of Alberta wins the first international Stockholm Water Prize for environmental research. In Brantford, Ontario, a Six Nations man is the first to be allowed to make a traditional native oath instead of swearing on the Bible (November). The Tungavik sign an agreement with Ottawa to create a new, semi-autonomous Inuit territory in the eastern Arctic.

1992:   the Miss Canada pageant is scrapped. Roberta Bondar is Canada's first female astronaut in space. Ontario lawyers vote to abandon the Oath to the Queen (January). Canada is the first country to sign the international biodiversity convention at the Earth Summit in Brazil (June). Canadians vote 'No' in a referendum seeking support for the Charlottetown Accord, intended as a corrective to the Canadian constitution in the wake of the failed Meech Lake Accord (26 October). NAFTA free trade agreement signed with the U.S.A. and Mexico (December). Although the players are all American, the Toronto Blue Jays become the first Canadian team to win baseball's World Series.

1993:   Catherine Callbeck becomes the first woman premier, in Prince Edward Island. Environmental activists cause minor damage to government buildings in Victoria, British Columbia, during a demonstration (March). Kim Campbell replaces Brian Mulroney as the head of the Progressive Conservatives, becoming Canada's first woman Prime Minister (June). Part of northwest British Columbia is set aside as a world heritage conservation site. Protesters block loggers' access to ancient forests near Clayoquot Sound (July–August). The

Toronto Blue Jays win the World Series for the second year in a row (23 October). The Liberals under Jean Chrétien are elected in a landslide victory, with the Bloc Québecois and Preston Manning's Reform Party only one seat apart in distant second and third places (25 October). The Progressive Conservatives, in power for nine years, are reduced to two seats in the House of Commons. A cow in Red Deer, Alberta, is found to have bovine spongiform encephalopathy (BSE), commonly known as mad cow disease. The cow had been imported from Britain in 1987.

1994:   trade barriers between provinces are reduced. Preparations go ahead for the establishment of devolved government for the Inuit. The Parti Québecois wins a narrow victory in provincial parliamentary elections. The Canadian pilot of a Korean airliner that crashed is arrested for endangering the lives of his passengers.

1995:   a referendum on sovereignty in Québec narrowly fails to produce a majority in favour. Premier Parizeau is replaced by Lucien Bouchard. In Newfoundland, the government takes over control of church schools. A fishing 'war' over stocks breaks out between Canada and the European Community in the northwest Atlantic.

1996:   a land claim agreement is settled with the Nisga'a peoples of British Columbia. The two-dollar coin is introduced (February). In British Columbia, Premier Harcourt resigns amid allegations of charity funds being directed to the NDP; Glen Clark takes over. The one billionth tonne of iron ore is dug at Labrador City (mine opened 1958).

1997:   the 12.9-kilometre (8-mile) Confederation Bridge connecting Prince Edward Island to the mainland is opened. A salmon-fishing dispute over sea boundaries causes tension with the U.S.A. The Supreme Court accepts the legitimacy of oral history in the land claims of the native peoples.

1998:   a massive ice storm fells power lines and disrupts electricity transmission in Ontario and Québec. The federal government formally apologizes to native peoples for past injustices, including the removal of children to residential schools. A Swissair MD-11 crashes in the sea off Peggy's Cove, Nova Scotia, with 229 deaths (September). The National Post, the first all-Canada daily newspaper, is launched.

1999:   waves of illegal immigrants try to land in British Columbia. The McClean Lake and McArthur River uranium projects open. The Nunavut territory and government come into existence (April). Canadian troops are serving in Kosovo, East Timor, Sierra Leone, and Macedonia on peacekeeping missions.

2000:   national controversy rages over mismanagement of billions of dollars in public grants. Yves Michaud causes controversy in Québec province by accusing Jewish and other ethnic groups of opposing sovereignty. Liberals win federal election (October) with 172 seats out of 301.

2001:   a summit of the Americas at Québec agrees 2005 as date for American Free Trade Area. Lucien Bouchard announces his departure from politics. Canada 3000 airline ceases operations; Air Canada announces 9,000 redundancies. Newfoundland is officially renamed Newfoundland and Labrador (December).

2002:   Canadian government imposes 71% duty on fresh U.S. tomatoes following American duty of 27.9% on Canadian softwood imports. A new Immigration Act becomes law (June). Canada hosts the G8 'rich nations' summit at Kananaskis, Alberta. Finance Minister, Paul Martin, is sacked. Prime Minister Chrétien announces he will step down in February 2004. A new Canadian Citizenship Act is tabled (October). The government releases a Climate Change Plan for Canada.

2003:   Jack Layton is elected as new federal leader in the NDP (January).

Canada and the USA unveil a joint Border Air Quality Strategy (January). Demonstrations against war in Iraq take place across the country with an estimated 150,000 in Montréal and 20,000 in Vancouver (February). Prime Minister Chrétien announces that Canada will not participate in the invasion of Iraq unless it is approved by the UN Security Council. The arrival in February of SARS (Severe Acute Respiratory Syndrome) causes a growing medical crisis by March. Toronto suffers the biggest outbreak of SARS outside Southeast Asia. In April's provincial elections in Quebec, the nine-year rule of the Parti Quebecois is ended when they are defeated by the Liberal Party. BSE crisis – In May a test on a cow from Alberta reveals BSE. The US announces a ban on all imports of Canadian beef. By May 28, abattoirs have slaughtered over 2700 cows. In August the US eases its total ban on Canadian beef. In August, North America is hit by its biggest power cut in history, blacking out cities in northwestern USA, as well as Toronto, Ottawa and other parts of Ontario. In December, after ten years in office, Prime Minister Jean Chrétien retires and former finance minister Paul Martin is sworn in. Canada's first space telescope is launched. The United Church of Canada votes to approve same-sex marriages. In December the US announces its first case of BSE, in a cow of Canadian origin.

2004   scandal breaks out regarding the misuse of federal government money intended for an advertising and sponsorship program in Quebec. The program promoted keeping Quebec in the Canadian federation. Auditor General of Canada Sheila Fraser's study shows millions of dollars were mishandled. The Supreme Court upholds a law that allows parents to spank their children within 'reasonable limits'. The Canadian Food Inspection Agency orders the slaughter of 275,000 chickens and turkeys to fight avian flu. The Canadian SPCA finds around 100 dead cows, and around 100 others being mistreated, on a farm in Alberta. A U.S. soldier, Jeremy Hinzman, seeks status as a refugee in Canada, as a conscientious objector to the war in Iraq. South Korea, Singapore, Japan and Hong Kong ban poultry and bird imports from Canada. In April, in Montreal, Michael Hendricks and René Leboeuf marry in the first legal same-sex marriage in Quebec. The Dalai Lama visits Canada for a 19-day tour. Canada wins 12 medals at the 2004 Summer Olympics in Athens. In June, Prime Minister Paul Martin and the Liberal Party are returned to power in general elections, but the party is stripped of its majority. Amnesty International releases a report condemning Canada's lack of protection of Aboriginal women.

2005   officials confirm that a second case of BSE has been found in Alberta. Cattle infected with the disease may have been eaten by people. By January 11 a third case has been found. Prime Minister Paul Martin has a nine-day trip to Indonesia to see the aftermath of the Indian Ocean tsunami. Paul Martin and Jean Chrétien appear before the commission to investigate the 2004 sponsorship scandal. In May the government survives two confidence votes. For the first time, the Speaker of the House votes – in favour of the government – to break a tie. In July the US border is opened to live Canadian cattle. The bill to legalise same-sex marriages in Canada is passed. In August, in Toronto, Air France Flight 358 slides into a gully and bursts into flames; everyone survives. Newsreader Peter Jennings dies at the age of 67. In September it is announced that Michaëlle Jean will become the 27th Governor General of Canada; she is the first black person to hold that position.

Grammar

abstract noun a noun which is the name of a thing that cannot be touched but refers to a quality, concept or idea. Examples of abstract nouns include 'anger', 'beauty', 'courage', 'Christianity', 'danger', 'fear', 'greed', 'hospitality', 'ignorance', 'jealousy', 'kudos', 'loyalty', 'Marxism', 'need', 'obstinacy', 'pain', 'quality', 'resistance', 'safety', 'truth', 'unworthiness', 'vanity', 'wisdom', 'xenophobia', 'youth', 'zeal'. *See also* **concrete noun.**

active voice one of the two voices that verbs are divided into, the other being passive voice. In verbs in the active voice, commonly called **active verbs**, the subject of the verb performs the action described by the verb. Thus, in the sentence 'The boy threw the ball', 'throw' is in the active voice since the subject of the verb (the boy) is doing the throwing. Similarly, in the sentence 'Her mother was driving the car', 'driving' is in the active voice since it is the subject of the sentence (her mother) that is doing the driving. Similarly, in the sentence 'We saw the cows in the field', 'saw' is the active voice since it is the subject of the sentence (we) that is doing the seeing.

adjectival clause a kind of subordinate clause that describes or modifies a noun or pronoun. It is better known by the name relative clause.

adjective a word that describes or gives information about a noun or pronoun. It is said to qualify a noun or pronoun since it limits the word it describes in some way, by making it more specific. Thus, adding the adjective 'red' to 'book' limits 'book', since it means we can forget about books of any other colour. Similarly, adding 'large' to 'book' limits it, since it means we can forget about books of any other size.

Adjectives tell us something about the colour, size, number, quality or classification of a noun or pronoun, as in 'purple curtains', 'jet-black hair', 'bluish eyes'; 'tiny baby', 'large houses', 'biggish gardens', 'massive estates'; five children', 'twenty questions', 'seventy-five books'; 'sad people', 'joyful occasions', 'delicious food', 'civil engineering', 'nuclear physics', 'modern languages', 'Elizabethan drama'.

adverb a word that adds to our information about a verb, as in 'work rapidly'; about an adjective, as in 'an extremely beautiful young woman'; or about another adverb, as in 'sleeping very soundly'. Adverbs are said to modify the words to which they apply since they limit the words in some way and make them more specific. Thus, adding 'slowly' to 'walk', as in 'They walked slowly down the hill', limits the verb 'walk' since all other forms of 'walk', such as 'quickly', 'lazily', etc, have been discarded.

adverbial clause a subordinate clause that modifies the main or principal clause by adding information about time, place, concession, condition, manner, purpose and result, as in 'He left after the meal was over', 'They left it where they found it', 'Wherever I went I saw signs of poverty', 'I have to admire his speech, although I disagree with what he said', 'He does his best at school work even though he is not very good at it', 'Whilst I myself do not like him, I can understand why he is popular', 'We cannot go unless we get permission', 'He looked at her as if he hated her', 'They will have to work long hours in order to make that amount of money', 'They started to run so as to get home before it rained', and 'He fell awkwardly so that he broke his leg.' Adverbial clauses usually follow the main clause but most of them can be put in front of the main clause for reasons of emphasis or style.

agent noun a noun that refers to someone who is the 'doer' of the action of a verb. It is usually spelt ending in either *-er*, as 'enquirer', or in *-or*, as in 'investigator' and 'supervisor', but frequently either of these endings is acceptable, as 'adviser/advisor'.

agreement or **concord** the agreeing of two or more elements in a clause or sentence, i.e. they take the same number, person or gender. In English the most common form of agreement is that between subject and verb, and this usually involves **number agreement**. This means that singular nouns are usually accompanied by singular verbs, as in 'She looks well', 'He is working late' and 'The boy has passed the exam', and that plural nouns are usually accompanied by plural verbs, as in 'They look well', 'They are working late' and 'The boys have passed the exam'.

Problems arise when the noun in question can be either singular or plural, for example, 'audience', 'committee', 'crowd', 'family', 'government', 'group'. Such nouns take a singular verb if the user is regarding the people or items referred to by the noun as a group, as in 'The family is moving house', or as individuals, as in 'The family are quarrelling over where to go on holiday'.

Compound subjects, that is two or more nouns acting as the subject, whether singular or plural, joined with 'and', are used with a plural noun, as in 'My friend and I are going to the cinema tonight' and 'James and John are leaving today', unless the two nouns together represent a single concept, as 'brandy and soda', in which case the verb is in the singular, as in 'Brandy and soda is his favourite drink' and 'cheese and pickle' in 'Cheese and pickle is the only sandwich filling available'.

Indefinite pronouns such as 'anyone', 'everyone', 'no one', 'someone', 'either', 'neither' are singular and should be followed by a singular verb, as in 'Each of the flats is self-contained', 'Everyone is welcome', 'No one is allowed in without a ticket' and 'Neither is quite what I am looking for'.

Agreement with reference to both number and gender affects pronouns, as in 'She blames herself', 'He could have kicked himself' and 'They asked themselves why they had got involved'. Problems arise when the pronoun is indefinite and so the sex of the person is unspecified. Formerly in such cases the masculine pronouns were assumed to be neutral and so 'Each of the pupils was asked to hand in his work' was considered quite acceptable. The rise of feminism has led to a questioning of this assumption and alternatives have been put forward. These include 'Each of the pupils was asked to hand in his/her (or his or her) work', but some people feel that this is clumsy. Another alternative is 'Each of the pupils was asked to hand in their work'. Although it is ungrammatical, this convention is becoming quite acceptable in modern usage. To avoid both the clumsiness of the former and the ungrammatical nature of the latter, it is possible to cast the whole sentence in the plural, as in 'All the pupils were asked to hand in their work'.

also an adverb that should not be used as a conjunction instead of 'and'. Thus sentences such as 'Please send me some apples, also some pears' are grammatically incorrect.

although a conjunction that is used to introduce a subordinate adverbial clause of concession, as in 'They are very happy although they are poor', meaning 'Despite the fact they are poor they are happy'. 'Though' or 'even though' can be substituted for 'although', as in 'they are very happy even though they are poor'. *See* **adverbial clause** and **conjunction**.

and a conjunction that is called a coordinating conjunction because it joins elements of language that are of equal status. The elements may be words, as in 'cows and horses', 'John and James', 'provide wine and beer'; phrases, as in 'working hard and playing hard' and 'trying to look after her children and her elderly parents'; clauses, as in 'John has decided to emigrate and his brother has decided to join him' and 'He has lost his job and he now has no money'. When a coordinating conjunction is used, the subject of the second clause can sometimes be omitted if it is the same as the subject of the first clause, as in 'They have been forced to sell the house and are very sad about it'.

The use of and at the beginning of a sentence is disliked by many people. It should be used only for deliberate effect, as in 'And then he saw the monster', or in informal contexts.

Other coordinating conjunctions include 'but', 'or', 'yet', 'both. . . and', 'either. . . or', and 'neither. . . . nor', as in 'poor but honest' and 'the blue dress or the green one'.

antecedent a term that refers to the noun or noun phrase in a main clause to which a relative pronoun in a relative clause refers back. Thus in the sentence 'People who live dangerously frequently get hurt', 'people' is an antecedent. Similarly, in the sentence 'The child identified the old man who attacked her', 'the old man' is the antecedent. *See* **relative clause**.

any a pronoun that may take either a singular or plural verb, depending on the context. When a singular noun is used, a singular verb is used, as in 'Is any of the cloth still usable?' 'Are any of the children coming?' When a plural noun is used, either a plural or a singular verb can be used, the singular verb being more formal, as in 'Did you ask if any of his friends were/was there?'.

anyone a pronoun that should be used with a singular verb, as in 'Has anyone seen my book?' and 'Is anyone coming to the lecture?' To be grammatically correct, anyone should be followed, where relevant, by a singular, not plural, personal pronoun or possessive adjective, but, in order to avoid the sexist 'his', this involves sentences such as 'Has anyone left his/her book?' Because this construction is rather clumsy, there is a growing tendency to use 'their' and be ungrammatical.

apposition a term for a noun or a phrase that provides further information about another noun or phrase. Both nouns and phrases refer to the same person or thing. In the phrase 'Peter Jones, our managing director', ' Peter Jones' and 'our managing director' are said to be in apposition. Similarly, in the phrase 'his cousin, the chairman of the firm', 'his cousin' and 'the chairman of the firm' are in apposition.

as a conjunction that can introduce either a subordinate adverbial clause of time, as in 'I caught sight of him as I was leaving', a subordinate adverbial clause of manner, as in 'He acted as he promised', and a subordinate adverbial clause of reason, as in 'As it's Saturday he doesn't have to work'. it is also used in the as. . . . as construction, as in 'She doesn't play as well as her sister does'.

The construction may be followed by a subject pronoun or an object pronoun, according to sense. In the sentence 'He plays as well as she', which is a slightly shortened form of 'She plays as well as he does', 'he' is a subject pronoun. In informal English the subject pronoun often becomes an object pronoun, as in 'She plays as well as him'. In the sentence 'They hate their father as much as her', 'her' is an object and the sentence means 'They hate their father as much as they hate her', but in the sentence 'They hate their father as much as she', 'she' is a subject and the sentence means 'They hate their father as much as she does'. *See* **adverbial clause** and **conjunction**.

attributive adjective a term for an adjective that is placed immediately before the noun that it qualifies. In the phrases 'a red dress', 'the big house' and 'an enjoyable evening', 'red, 'big' and 'enjoyable' are attributive adjectives.

auxiliary verb a verb that is used in forming tenses, moods and voices of other verbs. These include 'be', 'do' and 'have'.

The verb 'to be' is used as an auxiliary verb with the -*ing* form of the main verb to form the continuous present tense, as in 'They are living abroad just now' and 'We were thinking of going on holiday but we changed our minds'.

The verb 'to be' is used as an auxiliary verb with the past participle of the main verb to form the passive voice, as in 'Her hands were covered in blood' and 'These toys are manufactured in China'.

The verb 'to have' is used as an auxiliary verb along with the past participle of the main verb to form the perfect tenses, as in 'They have filled the post', 'She had realized her mistake' and 'They wished that they had gone earlier'.

The verb 'to be' is used as an auxiliary verb along with the main verb to form negative sentences, as in 'She is not accepting the job'. The verb 'to do' is used as an auxiliary verb along with the main verb to form negative sentences, as in 'he does not believe her'. It is also used along with the main verb to form questions, as in 'Does he know that she's gone?' and to form sentences in which the verb is emphasized, as in 'She *does* want to go'. *See* **modal verb**.

base the basic uninflected form of a verb. It is found as the infinitive form, as in 'to go' and 'to take', and as the imperative form, as in 'Go away!' and 'Take it!' It is also the form that the verb in the present indicative tense takes, except for the third person singular, as in 'I always go there on a Sunday' and 'They go there regularly.'

be *see* **auxiliary verb**.

because a conjunction that introduces a subordinate adverbial clause of reason, as in 'They sold the house because they are going abroad' and 'Because she is shy she never goes to parties'. It is often used incorrectly in such constructions as 'The reason they went away is because they were bored'. This should be rephrased as either 'The reason that they went away is that they were bored' or 'They went away because they were bored'. *see* **adverbial clause**.

before a word that can either be a preposition, an adverb or a conjunction. As a preposition it means either 'coming or going in front of in time', as in 'He was the chairman before this one', or coming or going in front of in place, as in 'She went before him into the restaurant'. As an adverb it means 'at a time previously', as in 'I told you before' and 'He has been married before'. As a conjunction it introduces a subordinate adverbial clause of time, as in 'The guests arrived before she was ready for them' and 'Before I knew it they had arrived'. *see* **adverbial clause**.

both a word that can be used in several ways: as a determiner, as in 'He broke both his arms' and 'He lost both his sons in the war'; as a pronoun, as in 'I don't mind which house we rent, I like them both' and 'Neither of them work here. The boss sacked them both'; as a conjunction, as in 'He both likes and admires her' and 'She is both talented and honest'. Both can sometimes be followed by 'of'. 'Both their children are grown up' and 'Both of their children are grown up' are both acceptable. Care should be taken to avoid using both unnecessarily. In the sentence 'The two items are both identical', 'both' is redundant.

but a conjunction that connects two opposing ideas. It is a coordinating conjunction in that it connects two elements of equal status. The elements may be words, as in 'not James but John'; phrases, as in 'working hard but not getting anywhere' and 'trying to earn a living but not succeeding'; clauses, as in 'He has arrived but his sister is late', 'I know her but I have never met him' and 'He likes reading but she prefers to watch TV'. It should not be used when no element of contrast is present. Thus the following sentence should be rephrased, at least in formal English—'She is not professionally trained but taught herself'. The two clauses are in fact agreeing, not disagreeing, with each other and so, strictly speaking, but should not be used.

The use of but at the beginning of a sentence is disliked by many people. It should be used only for deliberate effect or in informal contexts.

case one of the forms in the declension of a noun, pronoun or adjective in a sentence.

clause a group of words containing a finite verb which forms part of a compound or complex sentence. see main clause, subordinate clauses, adverbial clause, noun clause and relative clause.

commands these are expressed in the imperative mood, as in 'Be quiet!', 'Stop crying!', 'Go away!'

common noun simply the name of an ordinary, everyday non-specific thing or person, as opposed to proper nouns, which refer to the names of particular individuals or specific places. Common nouns include 'baby', 'cat', 'girl', 'hat', 'park', 'sofa' and 'table'.

comparison of adjectives this is achieved in two different ways. Some adjectives form their comparative by adding -er to the positive or absolute form, as in 'braver', 'louder', 'madder', 'shorter' and 'taller'. Other adjectives form their comparative by using 'more' in conjunction with them, as in 'more beautiful', 'more realistic', 'more suitable' and 'more tactful'. Which is the correct form is largely a matter of length. One-syllable adjectives, such as 'loud', add -er, as 'louder'. Two-syllable adjectives sometimes have both forms as a possibility, as in 'gentle-/more gentle', and 'cleverest/most clever'. Adjectives with three or more syllables usually form their comparatives with 'more', as in 'more comfortable', 'more gracious', 'more regular' and 'more understanding'. Some adjectives are irregular in their comparative forms, as in 'good/better', 'bad/worse', 'many/more'. Only if they begin with un- are they likely to end in -er, as in 'untrustworthier'.

Some adjectives by their very definitions do not normally have a comparative form, for example 'unique'.

complement the equivalent of the object in a clause with a linking verb. In the sentence 'Jack is a policeman', 'a policeman' is the complement. In the sentence 'Jane is a good mother', 'a good mother' is the complement', and in the sentence 'His son is an excellent football player', 'an excellent football player' is the complement.

complex sentence a type of sentence in which there is a main clause and one or more subordinate clauses. The sentence 'We went to visit him although he had been unfriendly to us' is a complex sentence since it is composed of a main clause and one subordinate clause ('although he had been unfriendly to us'). The sentence 'We wondered where he had gone and why he was upset' is a complex sentence since it has a main clause and two subordinate clauses ('where he had gone' and 'why he was upset').

compound sentence a type of sentence with more than one clause and linked by a coordinating conjunction, such as 'and' or 'but', as in 'He applied for a new job and got it' and 'I went to the cinema but I didn't enjoy the film'.

concrete noun the name of something that one can touch, as opposed to an abstract noun, which one cannot. Concrete nouns include 'bag', 'glass', 'plate', 'pot', 'clothes', 'field', 'garden', 'flower', 'potato', 'foot' and 'shoe'. *see* **abstract noun**.

conjunction a word that connects words, clauses or sentences. Conjunctions are of two types. A **coordinating conjunction** joins units of equal status, as in 'bread and butter', 'We asked for some food and we got it'. A **subordinating conjunction** joins a dependent or subordinating clause to main verbs: in 'We asked him why he was there', 'why he was there' is a subordinate clause and thus 'why' is a subordinating conjunction.

content words *see* **function word**.

continuous tenses *see* **tense**.

copula *see* **linking verb**.

copular verb *see* **equative** and **linking verb**.

count noun is the same as countable noun.

countable noun is one which can be preceded by 'a' and can take a plural, as in 'hat/hats', 'flower/flowers'. *see also* **uncountable noun**.

dangling participle a participle that has been misplaced in a sentence. A participle is often used to introduce a phrase that is attached to a subject mentioned later in a sentence, as in 'Worn out by the long walk, she fell to the ground in a faint'. 'Worn out' is the participle and 'she' the subject.

Another example is 'Laughing in glee at having won, she ordered some champagne'. In this sentence 'laughing' is the participle and 'she' is the subject. It is a common error for such a participle not to be related to any subject, as in 'Imprisoned in the dark basement, it seemed a long time since she had seen the sun'. This participle is said to be 'dangling'. Another example of a dangling participle is contained in 'Living alone, the days seemed long'.

It is also a common error for a participle to be related to the wrong subject in a sentence, as in 'Painting the ceiling, some of the plaster fell on his head', 'Painting' is the participle and should go with a subject 'he'. Instead it goes with 'some of the plaster'. Participles in this situation are more correctly known as **misrelated participles**, although they are also called dangling participles.

declarative mood the same as **indicative mood**.

declarative sentence a sentence that conveys information. The subject precedes the verb in it. Examples include 'They won the battle', 'He has moved to another town', 'Lots of people go there' and 'There is a new person in charge'.

declension the variation of the form of a noun, adjective or pronoun to show different cases, such as nominative and accusative. It also refers to the class into which such words are placed, as in first declension, second declension, etc. The term applies to languages such as Latin but is not applicable to English.

degree a level of comparison of gradable adjectives. The degrees of comparison comprise **absolute** or **positive**, as in 'big', 'calm', 'dark', 'fair', 'hot', 'late', 'short' and 'tall'; **comparative**, as in 'bigger', 'calmer', 'darker', 'fairest', 'hotter', 'late', 'shorter' and 'taller'; **superlative**, as in 'biggest', 'calmest', 'darkest', 'fairest', 'hottest', 'latest', 'shortest' and 'tallest'.

Degree can also refer to adverbs. Adverbs of degree include 'extremely', 'very', 'greatly', 'rather', 'really', 'remarkably', 'terribly', as in 'an extremely rare case', 'a very old man', 'He's remarkably brave' and 'We're terribly pleased'.

demonstrative determiner a determiner that is used to indicate things or people in relationship to the speaker or writer in space or time. 'This' and 'these' indicate nearness to the speaker, as in 'Will you take this book home?' and 'These flowers are for you'. 'That' and 'those' indicate distance from the speaker, as in 'Get that creature out of here!' and 'Aren't those flowers over there beautiful!'

demonstrative pronoun a pronoun that is similar to a demonstrative determiner except that it stands alone in place of a noun rather than preceding a noun, as in 'I'd like to give you this', 'What is that?', 'These are interesting books' and 'Those are not his shoes'.

dependent clause a clause that cannot stand alone and make sense, unlike an independent or main clause. Dependent clauses depend on the main clause. The term is the same as subordinate clause.

determiner a word that is used in front of a noun or pronoun to tell us something about it. Unlike an adjective, it does not, strictly speaking, 'describe' a noun or pronoun. Determiners are divided into the following categories: **articles** (a, an, the) as in 'a cat', 'an eagle', 'the book'; **demonstrative determiners** (this, that, these, those), as in 'this girl', 'that boy' and 'those people'; **possessive determiners** (my, your, his/her/its, our, their), as in 'my dog', 'her house', 'its colour', 'their responsibility'; **numbers** (one, two, three, four, etc, first, second, third, fourth, etc), as in 'two reasons', 'five ways', 'ten children'; and **indefinite** or **general determiners** (all, another, any, both, each, either, enough, every, few, fewer, less, little, many, most, much, neither, no, other, several, some), as in 'both parents', 'enough food', 'several issues'. Many words used as determiners are also pronouns. *see* **adjective; demonstrative determiner; number**.

direct object the noun, noun phrase, noun or nominal clause or pronoun that is acted upon by the action of a transitive verb. In the sentence 'She bought milk', 'bought' is a transitive verb and 'milk' is a noun which is the direct object. In the sentence 'She bought loads of clothes', 'bought' is a transitive verb and loads of clothes' is the direct object. In the sentence 'He knows what happened', 'knows' is a transitive verb and 'what happened' is a 'noun clause' or 'nominal clause'. A direct object is frequently known just as object *see* **indirect object**.

direct speech the reporting of speech by repeating exactly the actual words used by the speaker, as in 'Peter said, "I am tired of this." '

distributive pronoun a pronoun that refers to individual members of a class or group. These include 'each', 'either', 'neither', 'none', 'everyone', 'no one'. Such pronouns, where relevant, should be accompanied by singular verbs and singular personal pronouns, as in 'All the men are to be considered for the new posts. Each is to send in his application'. Problems arise when the sex of the noun to which the distributive pronoun refers back is either unknown or unspecified. Formerly it was the convention to treat such nouns as masculine and so to make the distributive pronoun masculine, as in 'All pupils must obey the rule. Nowadays this convention is frequently considered to be unacceptably sexist and attempts have been made to get round this. One solution is to use 'him/her' (or 'him or her'), etc, as in 'The students have received a directive from the professor. Each is to produce his/her essay by tomorrow.' This convention is considered by many people to be clumsy. They prefer to be ungrammatical and use a plural personal pronoun, as in 'The pupils are being punished. Each is to inform their parents'. This use Is becoming increasingly common, even in textbooks. Where possible, it is preferable to rephrase sentences to avoid being either sexist or ungrammatical, as in 'All of the pupils must tell their parents.'

Each, either, etc, in such contexts is fairly formal. In less formal situations 'each of', 'either of', etc, is more usual, as in 'Each of the boys will have to train really hard to win' and 'Either of the dresses is perfectly suitable'.

do an auxiliary verb that is used to form negative forms, as in, 'I do not agree with you', 'They do not always win', 'He does not wish to go' and 'She did not approve of their behaviour'. It is also used to form interrogative forms, as in 'Do you agree?', 'Does she know about it?', 'Did you see that?' and 'I prefer to go by train. Don't you?' Do is also used for emphasis, as in 'I do believe you're right' and 'They do know, don't they?'

double passive a clause that contains two verbs in the passive, the second of which is an infinitive, as in 'The goods are expected to be despatched some time this week'. Some examples of double passives are clumsy or ungrammatical and should be avoided, as in 'Redundancy notices are proposed to be issued next week'.

dual gender a category of nouns in which there is no indication of gender. The nouns referred to include a range of words used for people, and occasionally animals, which can be of either gender. Unless the gender is specified we do not know the sex of the person referred to. Such words include 'artist', 'author', 'poet', 'singer', 'child', 'pupil', 'student', 'baby', 'parent', 'teacher', 'dog'. Such words give rise to problems with accompanying singular pronouns. *see* **each**.

dummy subject a subject that has no intrinsic meaning but is inserted to maintain a balanced grammatical structure. In the sentences 'It has started to rain' and 'It is nearly midnight', 'it' is a dummy subject. In the sentences 'There is nothing else to say' and 'There is no reason for his behaviour', 'there' is a dummy subject.

dynamic verb a verb with a meaning that indicates action, as 'work' in 'They work hard', 'play' in 'The boys play football at the weekend' and 'come' in 'The girls come here every Sunday'.

each a word that can be either a determiner or a distributive pronoun. Each as a determiner is used before a singular noun and is accompanied by a singular verb, as in 'Each candidate is to reapply', 'Each athlete has a place in the final', 'Each country is represented by a head of state' and 'Each chair was covered in chintz'.

Each of can sometimes be used instead of each, as in 'each of the candidates'. Again a singular verb is used. If the user wishes to emphasize the fact that something is true about every member of a group, **each one of** should be used and not 'every', as in 'Each one of them feels guilty', 'Each one of us has a part to play.

As a pronoun, each also takes a singular verb, as in 'They hate each other. Each is plotting revenge', 'These exercises are not a waste of time. Each provides valuable experience'.

Each, where relevant, should be accompanied by a singular personal pronoun, as in 'Each girl has to provide her own sports equipment', 'Each of the men is to take a turn at working night shift', 'The boys are all well off and each can afford the cost of the holiday' and 'There are to be no exceptions among the women staff. Each one has to work full time'.

Problems arise when the noun that each refers back to is of unknown or unspecified sex. Formerly nouns in such situations were assumed to be masculine, as in 'Each pupil was required to bring his own tennis racket' and 'Each of the students has to provide himself with a tape recorder'. Nowadays such a convention is regarded as being sexist and the use of 'he/her', 'his/her', etc, is proposed, as in 'Each pupil was required to bring his/her (or 'his or her') own tennis racket' and 'Each student has to provide himself/herself (or 'himself or herself') with a tape recorder'. Even in written English such a convention can be clumsy and it is even more so in spoken English. For this reason many people decide to be ungrammatical and opt for 'Each pupil was required to bring their own tennis racket' and 'Each student has to provide themselves with a tape recorder'. This Is becoming Increasingly acceptable, even In textbooks.

Both sexism and grammatical error can be avoided by rephrasing such sentences, as in 'All pupils are required to bring their own tennis rackets' and 'All students have to provide themselves with tape recorders'.

either a word that can be used as either a determiner or distributive pronoun. As a determiner it is used with a singular verb, as in 'Either hotel is expensive' and 'In principle they are both against the plan but is either likely to vote for it?'

Either of can be used instead of either. It is used before a plural noun, as in 'either of the applicants' and 'either of the houses'. It is accompanied by a singular verb, as in 'Either of the applicants is suitable' and 'Either of the houses is big enough for their family'.

Either can be used as a distributive pronoun and takes a singular verb, as in 'We have looked at both houses and either is suitable' and 'She cannot decide between the two dresses but either is appropriate for the occasion'. This use is rather formal.

In the **either . . . . or** construction, a singular verb is used if both subjects are singular, as in 'Either Mary or Jane knows what to do' and 'Either my mother or my father plans to be present'. A plural verb is used if both nouns involved are plural, as in 'Either men or women can play' and 'Either houses or flats are available'.

When a combination of singular and plural subjects is involved, the verb traditionally agrees with the subject that is nearer to it, as in 'Either his parents or his sister is going to come' and 'Either his grandmother or his parents are going to come'.

As a pronoun, either should be used only of two possibilities.

emphasizing adjective an adjective that is used for emphasis. 'Very' is an emphasizing adjective in the sentence 'His very mother dislikes him' and 'own' is an emphasizing adjective in 'He likes to think that he is his own master'.

emphasizing adverb an adverb used for emphasis. 'Really' is an emphasizing adverb in the sentence 'She really doesn't care whether she lives or dies', and 'positively' is an emphasizing adverb in the sentence 'He positively does not want to know anything about it'.

emphatic pronoun a reflexive pronoun that is used for emphasis, as in 'He knows himself that he is wrong', 'She admitted herself that she had made a mistake' and 'The teachers themselves say that the headmaster is too strict'.

ending the final part of a word consisting of an inflection that is added to a base or root word. The '-ren' part of 'children' is an ending, the '-er' of 'poorer' is an ending and the '-ing' of 'falling' is an ending.

equative a term that indicates that one thing is equal to, or the same as, another. The verb 'to be' is sometimes known as an **equative verb** because it links a subject and complement that are equal to each other, as in 'He is a rogue' ('he' and 'rogue' refer to the same person) and 'His wife is a journalist' ('his wife' and 'journalist' refer to the same person). Other equative verbs include 'appear', 'become', 'look', 'remain' and 'seem', as in 'She looks a nasty person' and 'He became a rich man'. Such verbs are more usually known as **copular verbs**.

every a word used with a singular noun to indicate that all the members of a group are being referred to. It takes a singular verb, as in 'Every soldier must report for duty', 'Every machine is to be inspected' and 'Every house has a different view'. Every should also be accompanied, where relevant, by a singular pronoun, as in 'Every boy has his job to do', 'Every girl is to wear a dress' and 'Every machine is to be replaced'. Problems arise when the sex of the noun to which every refers is unknown or unspecified. Formerly it was the custom to assume such a noun to be masculine and to use masculine pronouns, as in 'Every pupil is to behave himself properly. This assumption is now regarded as sexist, and to avoid this 'he/she', 'him/her' and 'his/her' can be used. Many people feel that this convention can become clumsy and prefer to be ungrammatical by using 'they', 'them' and 'their', as in 'Every pupil is to behave themselves properly.' This use is becoming Increasingly common, even In textbooks. Many sentences of this kind can be rephrased to avoid being either sexist or ungrammatical, as in 'All pupils are to behave themselves properly'. *see* **each**.

everyone a pronoun that takes a singular verb, as in 'Everyone is welcome' and 'Everyone has the right to a decent standard of living'. In order to be grammatically correct, it should be accompanied, where relevant, by a singular personal pronoun but it is subject to the same kind of treatment as every.

feminine the term for the gender that indicates female persons or animals. It is the opposite of 'masculine'. The feminine gender demands the use of the appropriate pronoun, including 'she', 'her', 'hers' and 'herself', as in 'The girl tried to save the dog but *she* was unable to do so', 'The woman hurt *her* leg', 'Mary said that the book is *hers*', and 'The waitress cut *herself*'.

The feminine forms of words, formed by adding *—ess*, used to be common but many such forms are now thought to be sexist. Words such as 'author', 'sculptor', 'poet' are now considered to be neutral terms that can be used to refer to a man or a woman. Some -ess words are either still being used or are in a state of flux, as in 'actress'. *see* **-ess** in **Affixes** section.

finite clause a clause that contains a finite verb, as in 'when she sees him', 'after she had defeated him', and 'as they were sitting there'.

finite verb a verb that has a tense and has a subject with which it agrees in number and person. For example 'cries' is finite in the sentence 'The child cries most of the time', and 'looks' is finite in the sentence 'The old man looks ill'. However 'go' in the sentence 'He wants to go' is non-finite since it has no variation of tense and does not have a subject. Similarly in the sentence 'Sitting on the river-bank, he was lost in thought', 'sitting' is non-finite.

first person this refers to the person who is speaking or writing when referring to himself or herself. The **first person pronouns** are 'I', 'me', 'myself' and 'mine', with the plural forms being 'we', 'us', 'ourselves' and 'ours'. Examples include 'She said, "*I* am going home"',

' "*I* am going shopping," he said', ' "*We* have very little money left," she said to her husband' and 'He said, "*We* shall have to leave now if we are to get there on time" '.

The **first person determiners** are 'my' and 'our', as in 'I have forgotten to bring *my* notebook' and 'We must remember to bring *our* books home.'

form word *see* **function word**.

fragmentary sentence *see* **major sentence**.

frequentative a term referring to a verb that expresses frequent repetition of an action. In English the verb endings -*le* and -*el* sometimes indicate the frequentative form, as in 'waddle' from 'wade', 'sparkle' from 'spark', 'crackle' from 'crack' and 'dazzle' from 'daze'. The ending -*er* can also indicate the frequentative form, as in 'stutter', 'spatter' and 'batter'.

function word a word that has very little meaning but is primarily of grammatical significance and merely performs a 'function' in a sentence. Function words include determiners, and prepositions such as in, on and up. Words that are not function words are sometimes known as **content words**.

Function word is also known as **form word** or **structure word**.

future perfect tense the tense of a verb that is formed by 'will' or 'shall' together with the perfect tense, as in 'They will have been married ten years next week', 'You will have finished work by this time tomorrow' and 'By the time Jane arrives here she will have been travelling non-stop for forty-eight hours'.

future tense the tense of a verb that describes actions or states that will occur at some future time. It is marked by 'will' and 'shall'. Traditionally 'shall' was used with subjects in the first person, as in 'I shall see you tomorrow' and 'We shall go there next week', and 'will' was used with subjects in the second and third person, as in 'You will find out next week', 'He will recognize her when he sees her' and 'They will be on the next train'. Formerly 'will' was used with the first person and 'shall' with the second and third person to indicate emphasis or insistence, as in 'I *will* go on my own' and 'We *will* be able to afford it'; 'You *shall* pay what you owe' and 'The children *shall* get a holiday'. In modern usage 'shall' is usually used only for emphasis or insistence, whether with the first, second or third person, except in formal contexts. Otherwise 'will' is used, as in 'I will go tomorrow', 'We will have to see', 'You will be surprised', and 'They will be on their way by now'.

The future tense can also be marked by 'be about to' plus the infinitive of the relevant verb or 'be going to' plus the infinitive of the relevant verb. Examples include 'We are about to leave for work', 'They are about to go on holiday', 'She is going to be late' and 'They are going to demolish the building'.

gemination the doubling of consonants before a suffix.

gender in the English language this usually refers to the natural distinctions of sex (or absence of sex) that exist, and nouns are classified according to these distinctions—masculine, feminine and neuter. Thus, 'man', 'boy', 'king', 'prince', 'emperor', 'duke', 'heir', 'son', 'brother',

'father', 'nephew', 'husband', 'bridegroom', 'widower', 'hero', 'cock', 'drake', 'fox' and 'lion' are masculine nouns. Similarly, 'girl', 'woman', 'queen', 'princess', 'empress', 'duchess', 'heiress', 'daughter', 'sister', 'mother', 'niece', 'wife', 'bride', 'widow', 'heroine', 'hen', 'duck', 'vixen' and 'lioness' are feminine nouns. Similarly, 'table', 'chair', 'desk', 'carpet', 'window', 'lamp', 'car', 'shop', 'dress', 'tie', 'newspaper', 'book', 'building' and 'town' are all neuter.

Some nouns in English can refer either to a man or a woman, unless the sex is indicated in the context. Such neutral nouns are sometimes said to have dual gender. Examples include 'author', 'singer', 'poet', 'sculptor', 'proprietor', 'teacher', 'parent', 'cousin', 'adult' and 'child'. Some words in this category were formerly automatically assumed to be masculine and several of them had feminine forms, such as 'authoress', 'poetess', 'sculptress' and 'proprietrix'. In modern times this was felt to be sexist and many of these feminine forms are now rarely used, for example, 'authoress' and 'poetess'. However some, such as actress and waitress, are still in common use.

genitive case a case that indicates possession or ownership. It is usually marked by *s* and an apostrophe. Many spelling errors centre on the position of the *s* in relation to the apostrophe.

gerund the -*ing* form of a verb when it functions as a noun. It is sometimes known as a **verbal noun**. It has the same form as the present participle but has a different function. For example, in the sentence 'He was jogging down the road', 'jogging' is the present participle in the verb phrase 'was jogging', but in the sentence 'Running is his idea of relaxation', 'running' is a gerund because it acts as a noun as the subject of the sentence.

Similarly, in the sentence 'We were smoking when the teacher found us', 'smoking' is the present participle in the verb phrase 'were smoking', but in the sentence 'We were told that smoking is bad for our health', 'smoking' is a gerund since it acts as a noun as the subject of the clause.

get this verb is sometimes used to form the passive voice instead of the verb 'to be'. The use of the verb 'to get' to form the passive, as in 'They get married tomorrow', 'Our team got beaten today' and 'We got swindled by the con man' is sometimes considered to be more informal than the use of 'be'. Often there is more action involved when the get construction is used than when be is used, since get is a more dynamic verb, as in 'She was late leaving the pub because she got involved in an argument' and in 'It was her own fault that she got arrested by the police. She hit one of the constables'.

Get is frequently overused. Such overuse should be avoided, particularly in formal contexts. Get can often be replaced by a synonym such as 'obtain', 'acquire', 'receive', 'get hold of', etc. Thus, 'If you are getting into money difficulties you should get some financial advice. Perhaps you could get a bank loan' could be rephrased as 'If you are in financial difficulty you should obtain some financial help. Perhaps you could receive a bank loan'.

Got, the past tense of get, is often used unnecessarily, as in 'She has got red hair and freckles' and 'We have got enough food to last us the week'. In these sentences 'has' and 'have' are sufficient on their own.

goal this can be used to describe the recipient of the action of a verb, the opposite of 'agent' or 'actor'. Thus, in the sentence 'The boy hit the girl', 'boy' is the 'agent' or 'actor' and 'girl' is the goal. Similarly, in the sentence 'The dog bit the postman', 'dog' is the 'agent' or 'actor' and 'postman' is the goal.

govern a term that is used of a verb or preposition in relation to a noun or pronoun to indicate that the verb or preposition has a noun or pronoun depending on it. Thus, in the phrase 'on the table', 'on' is said to govern 'table'.

gradable a term that is used of adjectives and adverbs to mean that they can take degrees of comparison. Thus 'clean' is a gradable adjective since it has a comparative form (cleaner) and a superlative form (cleanest). 'Soon' is a gradable adverb since it has a comparative form (sooner) and a superlative form (soonest). Such words as 'supreme', which cannot normally have a comparative or superlative form, are called **non-gradable**.

habitual a term used to refer to the action of a verb that occurs regularly and repeatedly. The **habitual present** is found in such sentences as 'He goes to bed at ten every night', 'She always walks to work' and 'The old man sleeps all day'. This is in contrast to the **stative present**, which indicates the action of the verb that occurs at all times, as in 'Cows chew the cud', 'Water becomes ice when it freezes', 'Children grow up' and 'We all die'. Examples of the **habitual past** tense include; 'They travelled by train to work all their lives', 'We worked twelve hours a day on that project' and 'She studied night and day for the exams'.

hanging participle *see* **dangling participle**.

have a verb that has several functions. A major use is its part in forming the 'perfect tense' and 'past perfect tense', or 'pluperfect tense', of other verb tenses. It does this in conjunction with the 'past participle' of the verb in question.

The perfect tense of a verb is formed by the present tense of the verb have and the past participle of the verb. Examples include 'We have acted wisely', 'They have beaten the opposition', 'The police have caught the thieves', 'The old man has died', 'The child has eaten all the food', 'The baby has fallen downstairs', 'They have grabbed all the bargains', 'You have hated him for years' and 'He has indicated that he is going to retire'. The past perfect or pluperfect is formed by the past tense of the verb have and the past participle of the verb in question, as in 'He had jumped over the fence', 'They had kicked in the door', 'The boy had led the other children to safety', 'His mother had made the cake', 'The headmaster had punished the pupils' and 'They had rushed into buying a new house'. Both perfect tenses

and past perfect or pluperfect tenses are often contracted in speech or in informal written English, as in 'We've had enough for today', 'You've damaged the suitcase', 'You've missed the bus', 'He's lost his wallet', 'She's arrived too late', 'They'd left before the news came through', 'She'd married without telling her parents', 'He'd packed the goods himself' and 'You'd locked the door without realizing it'.

Have is often used in the phrase **have to** in the sense that something must be done. In the present tense have to can be used instead of 'must', as in 'You have to leave now', 'We have to clear this mess up', 'He has to get the next train' and 'The goods have to be sold today'. If the 'something that must be done' refers to the future the verb **will have to** is used', as in 'He will have to leave now to get there on time', 'The old man will have to go to hospital' and 'They'll have to move out of the house when her parents return'. If the 'something that must be done' refers to the past, **had to** is used, as in 'We had to take the injured man to hospital', 'They had to endure freezing conditions on the mountain', 'They'd to take a reduction in salary' and 'We'd to wait all day for the workman to appear'.

Have is also used in the sense of 'possess' or 'own', as in 'He has a swimming pool behind his house ', 'She has a huge wardrobe', 'We have enough food' and 'They have four cars'. In spoken or in informal English 'have got' is often used, as in 'They've got the largest house in the street', 'We've got problems now', 'They haven't got time'. This use should be avoided in formal English.

Have is also used to indicate suffering from an illness or disease, as in 'The child has measles', 'Her father has flu' and 'She has heart disease'. Have can also indicate that an activity is taking place, as in 'She's having a shower', 'We're having a party', 'She is having a baby' and 'They are having a dinner party'.

he a personal pronoun that is used as the subject of a sentence or clause to refer to a man, boy, etc. It is thus said to be a 'masculine' personal pronoun. Since he refers to a third party and does not refer to the speaker or the person being addressed, it is a third-person pronoun. Examples include 'James is quite nice but he can be boring', 'Bob has got a new job and he is very pleased' and 'He is rich now but his parents are still very poor'.

He traditionally was used not only to refer to nouns relating to the masculine sex but also to nouns that are now regarded as being neutral or of dual gender. Such nouns include 'architect', 'artist', 'athlete', 'doctor', 'passenger', 'parent', 'pupil', 'singer', 'student'. Without further information from the context it is impossible to know to which sex such nouns are referring. In modern usage it is regarded as sexist to assume such words to be masculine by using he to refer to one of them unless the context indicates that the noun in question refers to a man or boy. Formerly it was considered acceptable to write or say 'Send a message to the architect who designed the building that he is to attend the meeting' whether or not the writer or speaker knew that the architect was a man. Similarly it was considered acceptable to write or say 'Please tell the doctor that he is to come straight away' whether or not the speaker or writer knew that the doctor was in fact a man. Nowadays this convention is considered sexist. In order to avoid sexism it is possible to use the convention 'he/she', as in 'Every pupil was told that he/she was to be smartly dressed for the occasion', 'Each passenger was informed that he/she was to arrive ten minutes before the coach was due to leave' and 'Tell the doctor that he/she is required urgently'. However this convention is regarded by some people as being clumsy, particularly in spoken English or in informal written English. Some people prefer to be ungrammatical and use the plural personal pronoun 'they' instead of 'he/she' in certain situations, as in 'Every passenger was told that they had to arrive ten minutes before the coach was due to leave' and 'Every student was advised that they should apply for a college place by March' and this use is becoming increasingly common, even in textbooks. In some cases it may be possible to rephrase sentences and avoid being either sexist or ungrammatical, as in 'All the passengers were told that they should arrive ten minutes before the coach was due to leave' and 'All students were advised that they should apply for a college place by March'.

helping verb another name for **auxiliary verb**.

hendiadys a figure of speech in which two nouns joined by 'and' are used to express an idea that would normally be expressed by the use of an adjective and a noun, as in 'through storm and weather' instead of 'through stormy weather'.

her a personal pronoun. It is the third person singular, is feminine in gender and acts as the object in a sentence, as in 'We saw her yesterday', 'I don't know her', 'He hardly ever sees her', 'Please give this book to her', 'Our daughter sometimes plays with her' and 'We do not want her to come to the meeting'. *see* **he; she**.

hers a personal pronoun. It is the third person singular, feminine in gender and is in the poassessive case. 'The car is not hers', 'I have forgotten my book but I don't want to borrow hers', 'This is my seat and that is hers', and 'These clothes are hers'. *see* **his; her** and **possessive**.

him the third person masculine personal pronoun when used as the object of a sentence or clause, as in 'She shot him', 'When the police caught the thief they arrested him' and 'His parents punished him after the boy stole the money'. Traditionally him was used to apply not only to masculine nouns, such as 'man' and 'boy', but also to nouns that are said to be 'of dual gender'. These include 'architect', 'artist', 'parent', 'passenger', 'pupil' and 'student'. Without further information from the context, it is not possible for the speaker or writer to know the sex of the person referred to by one of these words. Formerly it was acceptable to write or say 'The artist must bring an easel with him' and 'Each pupil must bring food with

him'. In modern usage this convention is considered sexist and there is a modern convention that 'him/her' should be used instead to avoid sexism, as in 'The artist must bring an easel with him/her' and 'Each pupil must bring food with 'him/her'. This convention is felt by some people to be clumsy, particularly in and in , and some people prefer to be ungrammatical and use the plural personal pronoun 'them' instead, as in 'The artist must bring an easel with them' and 'Each pupil must bring food with them'. This use has become increasingly, even in textbooks. In some situations it is possible to avoid being either sexist or ungrammatical by rephrasing the sentence, as in 'All artists must bring easels with them' and 'All pupils must bring food with them. *see* **he**.

him/her *see* **him**.

his the third personal masculine pronoun when used to indicate possession, as in 'He has hurt his leg', 'The boy has taken his books home' and 'Where has your father left his tools?' Traditionally his was used to refer not only to masculine nouns, such as 'man', 'boy', etc, but to what are known as nouns of dual gender'. These include 'architect', 'artist', 'parent', 'passenger', 'pupil' and 'student'. Without further information from the context it is not possible for the speaker or the writer to know the sex of the person referred to by one of these words. Formerly it was considered acceptable to use his in such situations, as in 'Every pupil has to supply his own sports equipment' and 'Every passenger is responsible for his own luggage'. In modern usage this is now considered sexist and there is a modern convention that 'his/her' should be used instead to avoid sexism, as in 'Every pupil has to supply his/her own sports equipment' and 'Every passenger is responsible for his/her own luggage'. This convention is felt by some people to be clumsy, particularly when used in spoken or informal written English. Some people prefer to be ungrammatical and use the plural personal pronoun 'their', as in 'Every pupil must supply their own sports equipment' and 'Every passenger is to be responsible for their own luggage' and this use has become increasingly common, even in textbooks. In some situations it is possible to avoid being sexist, clumsy and ungrammatical by rephrasing the sentence, as in 'All pupils must supply their own sports equipment' and 'All passengers are to be responsible for their own luggage.

his/her *see* **his**.

hybrid a word that is formed from words or elements derived from different languages, such as 'television'.

if a conjunction that is often used to introduce a subordinate adverbial clause of condition, as in 'If he is talking of leaving he must be unhappy', 'If you tease the dog it will bite you', 'If he had realized that the weather was going to be so bad he would not have gone on the expedition', 'If I had been in charge I would have sacked him' and 'If it were a better organized firm things like that would not happen'.

If can also introduce a 'nominal' or 'noun clause', as in 'He asked if we objected' and 'She inquired if we wanted to go'.

imperative mood the verb mood that expresses commands. The verbs in the following sentences are in the imperative mood: 'Go away!', 'Run faster!', 'Answer me!', 'Sit down!', 'Please get out of here!'. All of these expressions with verbs in the imperative mood sound rather imperious or dictatorial and usually end with an exclamation mark, but this is not true of all expressions with verbs in the imperative mood. For example, the following sentences all have verbs in the imperative mood: 'Have another helping of ice cream', 'Help yourself to more wine', 'Just follow the yellow arrows to the X-ray department', and 'Turn right at the roundabout'. Sentences with verbs in the imperative mood are known as **imperative sentences**.

imperfect a tense that denotes an action in progress but not complete. The term derives from the classification in Latin grammar and was traditionally applied to the 'past imperfect', as in 'They were standing there'. The imperfect has now been largely superseded by the progressive/continuous tense, which is marked by the use of 'be' plus the present participle. Continuous tenses are used when talking about temporary situations at a particular point in time, as in 'They were waiting for the bus'.

impersonal a verb that is used with a formal subject, usually 'it', as in 'It is raining' and 'They say it will snow tomorrow'.

indefinite pronouns these are used refer to people or things without being specific as to exactly who or what they are. They include 'everyone', 'everybody', 'everything', 'anyone', 'anybody', 'anything', 'somebody', 'someone', 'something' and 'nobody', 'no one', 'nothing', as in 'Everyone is to make a contribution', 'Anyone can enter', 'Something will turn up' and 'Nobody cares'.

independent clause a clause that can stand alone and make sense without being dependent on another clause, as in 'The children are safe'. Main clauses are independent clauses. Thus in the sentence 'She is tired and she wants to go home', there are two independent clauses joined by 'and'. In the sentence 'She will be able to rest when she gets home', 'She will be able to rest' is an independent clause and 'when she gets home' is a dependent clause. In the sentence 'Because she is intelligent she thinks for herself', 'she thinks for herself' is an independent clause and 'because she is intelligent' is a dependent clause.

indicative mood the mood of a verb which denotes making a statement. The following sentences have verbs in the indicative mood: 'We go on holiday tomorrow', 'He was waiting for her husband', 'They have lost the match' and 'She will arrive this afternoon'. The indicative mood is sometimes known as the **declarative mood**. The other moods are the imperative mood and subjunctive mood.

indirect object an object that can be preceded by 'to' or 'for'. The indirect object usually refers to the person who benefits from an action or receives something as the result of it. In the sentence 'Her father gave the boy food', 'boy' is the indirect object and 'food' is the direct object.

The sentence could be rephrased as 'Her father gave food to the boy'. In the sentence 'He bought his mother flowers', 'his mother' is the indirect object and 'flowers' is the direct object. The sentence could have been rephrased as 'He bought flowers for his mother'. In the sentence 'They offered him a reward', 'him' is the indirect object and 'reward' is the direct object. The sentence could be rephrased as 'They offered a reward to him'.

indirect question a question that is reported in indirect speech, as in 'We asked them where they were going', 'They inquired why we had come' and 'They looked at us curiously and asked where we had come from'. Note that a question mark is not used.

indirect speech also known as **reported speech** a way of reporting what someone has said without using the actual words used by the speaker. There is usually an introductory verb and a subordinate 'that' clause, as in 'He said that he was going away', 'They announced that they were leaving next day' and 'She declared that she had seen him there before'. In direct speech these sentences would become 'He said, "I am going away" ', 'They announced, "We are leaving tomorrow" ' and 'She declared, "I have seen him there before" '. When the change is made from direct speech to indirect speech, the pronouns, adverbs of time and place and tenses are changed to accord with the viewpoint of the person doing the reporting.

infinitive the base form of a verb when used without any indication of person, number or tense. There are two forms of the infinitive. One is the **to infinitive** form, as in 'They wished to leave', 'I plan to go tomorrow', 'We aim to please' and 'They want to emigrate', 'To know all is to forgive all', 'To err is human', 'Pull the lever to open', 'You should bring a book to read', 'The child has nothing to do', 'She is not very nice to know' and 'It is hard to believe that it happened'. The other form of the infinitive is called the **bare infinitive**. This form consists of the base form of the verb without 'to', as in 'We saw him fall', 'She watched him go', 'They noticed him enter', 'She heard him sigh', 'They let him go', 'I had better leave' and 'Need we return' and 'we dare not go back'. *see* **split infinitive**.

inflect when applied to a word, this means to change form in order to indicate differences of tense, number, gender, case, etc. Nouns inflect for plural, as in 'ships', 'chairs', 'houses' and 'oxen'; nouns inflect for possessive, as in 'boys'', 'woman's', 'teachers'', and 'parents''; some adjectives inflect for the comparative form, as in 'brighter', 'clearer', 'shorter' and 'taller'; verbs inflect for the third person singular present tense, as in 'hears', 'joins', 'touches' and 'kicks'; verbs inflect for the present participle, as in 'hearing', 'joining', 'touching' and 'kicking'; verbs inflect for the past participle, as in 'heard', 'joined', 'touched' and 'kicked'.

inflection the act of inflecting—*see* **inflect**. It also refers to an inflected form of a word or a suffix or other element used to inflect a word.

-ing form this form of a verb can be either a present participle or a gerund. Present participles are used in the formation of the progressive or continuous tenses, as in

'We were looking at the pictures', 'Children were playing in the snow', 'They are waiting for the bus', 'Parents were showing their anger', 'He has been sitting there for hours'. Present participles can also be used in non-finite clauses or phrases, as in 'Walking along, she did not have a care in the world', 'Lying there, he thought about his life', 'Sighing, he left the room' and 'Smiling broadly he congratulated his friend'.

A large number of adjectives end in -ing. Many of these have the same form as the present participle of a transitive verb and are similar in meaning. Examples include 'an amazing spectacle', 'a boring show', 'an interesting idea', 'a tiring day', 'an exhausting climb' and 'aching limbs'. Some -ing adjectives are related to intransitive verbs, as in 'existing problems', 'increasing responsibilities', 'dwindling resources', 'an ageing work force' and 'prevailing circumstances'. Some -ing adjectives are related to the forms of verbs but have different meanings from the verbs, as in 'becoming dress', 'an engaging personality', 'a dashing young man' and 'a retiring disposition'. Some -ing adjectives are not related to verbs at all. These include 'appetizing', 'enterprising', 'impending' and 'balding'. Some -ing adjectives are used informally for emphasis, as in 'a blithering idiot', 'a stinking cold' and 'a flaming cheek'.

Gerunds act as nouns and are sometimes known as **verbal nouns**. Examples include 'Smoking is bad for one's health', 'Cycling is forbidden in the park' and 'Swimming is his favourite sport'.

intensifier the term for an adverb that affects the degree of intensity of another word. Intensifiers include 'thoroughly' in 'We were thoroughly shocked by the news', 'scarcely' in 'We scarcely recognized them' and 'totally' in 'She was totally amazed'.

interjection a kind of exclamation. Sometimes they are formed by actual words and sometimes they simply consist of sounds indicating emotional noises. Examples of interjections include 'Oh! I am quite shocked', 'Gosh! I'm surprised to hear that!', 'Phew! It's hot!', 'Ouch! That was my foot!', 'Tut-tut! He shouldn't have done that!' and 'Alas! She is dead.'

interrogative adjective or **determiner** an adjective or determiner that asks for information in relation to the nouns which it qualifies, as in 'What dress did you choose in the end?', 'What kind of book are you looking for?', 'Which house do you like best?', 'Which pupil won the prize?', 'Whose bike was stolen?' and 'Whose dog is that?'

interrogative adverb an adverb that asks a question, as in 'When did they leave?', 'When does the meeting start?', 'Where do they live?', 'Where was the stolen car found?', 'Where did you last see her?', 'Why was she crying?', 'Why have they been asked to leave?', 'How is the invalid?', 'How do you know that she has gone?' and 'Wherever did you find that?'

interrogative pronoun a pronoun that asks a question, as in 'Who asked you to do that?', 'Who broke the vase?', 'What did he say?', 'What happened next?', 'Whose are

those books?', 'Whose is that old car?', 'To whom was that remark addressed?' and 'To whom did you address the package?'

interrogative sentence a sentence that asks a question, as in 'Who is that?', 'Where is he?', 'Why have they appeared?', 'What did they take away?', 'Which do you prefer?' and 'Whose baby is that?'. Sentences that take the form of an interrogative question do not always seek information. Sometimes they are exclamations, as in 'Did you ever see anything so beautiful?', 'Isn't she sweet?' and 'Aren't they lovely?'. Sentences that take the form of questions may really be commands or directives, as in 'Could you turn down that radio?', 'Would you make less noise?' and 'Could you get her a chair?'. Sentences that take the form of questions may function as statements, as in 'Isn't there always a reason?' and 'Haven't we all experienced disappointment?'. Some interrogative sentences are what are known as rhetorical questions, which are asked purely for effect and require no answer, as in 'Do you think I am a fool?', 'What is the point of life?' and 'What is the world coming to?'.

intransitive verb a verb that does not take a direct object, as in 'Snow fell yesterday', 'The children played in the sand', 'The path climbed steeply', 'Time will tell', 'The situation worsened', 'Things improved' and 'Prices increased'. Many verbs can be either transitive or intransitive, according to the context. Thus 'play' is intransitive in the sentence 'The children played in the sand' but transitive in the sentence 'The boy plays the piano'. Similarly 'climb' is intransitive in the sentence 'The path climbs steeply' but transitive in the sentence 'The mountaineers climbed Everest'. Similarly 'tell' is intransitive in the sentence 'Time will tell' but transitive in the sentence 'He will tell his life story'.

introductory it the use of 'it' as the subject of a sentence in the absence of a meaningful subject. It is used particularly in sentences about time and the weather, as in 'It is midnight', 'It is dawn', 'It is five o'clock', 'It is twelve noon', 'It is raining', 'It was snowing', 'It was windy' and 'It was blowing a gale'.

invariable a word whose form does not vary by inflection. Such words include 'sheep' and 'but'.

inversion the reversal of the usual word order. It particularly refers to subjects and verbs. Inversion is used in questions, in some negative sentences, and for literary effect. In questions, an auxiliary verb is usually put in front of the subject and the rest of the verb group is put after the subject, as in 'Are you going to see her?' and 'Have they inspected the goods yet?'. The verb 'to do' is frequently used in inversion, as in 'Did he commit the crime?' and 'Do they still believe that?'. Examples of the use of inversion in negative sentences include 'Seldom have I witnessed such an act of selfishness', 'Never had she experienced such pain' and 'Rarely do we have time to admire the beauty of the countryside'. This use in negative sentences is rather formal.

Inversion frequently involves adverbial phrases of

place, as in 'Beyond the town stretched field after field', 'Above them soared the eagle' and 'Along the driveway grew multitudes of daffodils'.

Inversion is also found in conditional clauses that are not introduced by conjunction, as in 'Had you arrived earlier you would have got a meal' and 'Had we some more money we could do more for the refugees'.

irregular adjective an adjective that does not conform to the usual rules of forming the comparative and superlative (*see* **comparison of adjectives**). Many adjectives either add *-er* for the comparative and *-est* for the superlative, as in 'taller', 'shorter' and 'tallest', 'shortest' from 'tall' and 'short'. Some adjectives form their comparatives with 'more' and their superlatives with 'most', as in 'more beautiful', 'more practical' and 'most beautiful', 'most practical'. Irregular adjectives do not form their comparatives and superlatives in either of these ways. Irregular adjectives include:

positive	comparative	superlative
good	better	best
bad	worse	worst
little	less	least
many	more	most

irregular sentence *see* **major sentence**.

irregular verb a verb that does not conform to the usual pattern of verbs in that some of its forms deviate from what one would expect if the pattern of regular verbs was being followed. There are four main forms of a **regular verb**—the infinitive or base form, as in 'hint', 'halt', 'hate' and 'haul'; the third-person singular form, as 'hints', 'halts', 'hates' and 'hauls'; the -ing form or present participle, as 'hinting', halting', 'hating' and 'hauling'; the *-ed* form or 'past tense' or 'past participle', as 'hinted', halted', 'hated' and 'hauled.

Irregular verbs deviate in some way from that pattern, in particular from the pattern of adding *-ed* to the past tense and past participle. They fall into several categories.

One category concerns those that have the same form in the past tense and past participle forms as the infinitive and do not end in *-ed*, like regular verbs.

Some irregular verbs have two past tenses and two past participles which are the same.

Some irregular verbs have past tenses that do not end in *-ed* and have the same form as the past participle.

Some irregular verbs have regular past tense forms but two possible past participles, one of which is regular.

Some irregular verbs have past tenses and past participles that are different from each other and different from the infinitive.

jussive a type of clause or sentence that expresses a command, as in 'Do be quiet! I'm trying to study', 'Let's not bother going to the party. I'm too tired', 'Would you pass me that book' and 'Look at that everybody! The river has broken its banks'.

linking adverbs and **linking adverbials** words and phrases that indicate some kind of connection between one clause or sentence and another. Examples include 'however', as in 'The award had no effect on their financial situation. It did, however, have a marked effect on their morale'; 'moreover', as in 'He is an unruly pupil. Moreover, he is a bad influence on the other pupils'; 'then again', as in 'She does not have very good qualifications. Then again, most of the other candidates have even fewer'; 'in the meantime', as in 'We will not know the planning committee's decision until next week. In the meantime we can only hope'; 'instead', as in 'I thought he would have reigned. Instead he seems determined to stay'.

linking verb a verb that 'links' a subject with its complement. Unlike other verbs, linking verbs do not denote an action but indicate a state. Examples of linking verbs include 'He is a fool', 'She appears calm', 'He appeared a sensible man', 'You seemed to become anxious', 'They became Buddhists', 'The child feels unwell', 'It is getting rather warm', 'It is growing colder', 'You look well', 'She remained loyal to her friend', 'She lived in America but remained a British citizen' and 'You seem thoughtful' and 'She seems a nice person'. Linking verbs are also called **copula** or **copular verbs**.

main clause the principal clause in a sentence on which any subordinate clauses depend for their sense. The main clause can stand alone and make some sense but the subordinate clauses cannot. In the sentence 'I left early because I wanted to catch the 6 o'clock train', 'I left early' is the principal clause and 'because I wanted to catch the 6 o'clock train' is the subordinate clause. In the sentence 'When we saw the strange man we were afraid', the main clause is 'we were afraid' and the subordinate clause is 'when we saw the strange man'. In the sentence 'Because it was late we decided to start out for home as soon as we could', the main clause is 'we decided to start out for home' and the subordinate clauses are 'because it was late' and 'as soon as we could'. A main clause can also be known as a **principal clause** or an independent clause.

major sentence a sentence that contains at least one subject and a finite verb, as in 'We are going' and 'They won'. They frequently have more elements than this, as in 'They bought a car', 'We lost the match', 'They arrived yesterday' and 'We are going away next week'. They are sometimes described as **regular** because they divide into certain structural patterns: a subject, finite verb, adverb or adverbial clause, etc. The opposite of a major sentence is called a **minor sentence**, **irregular sentence** or **fragmentary sentence**. These include interjections such as 'Ouch!' and 'How terrible'; formula expressions, such as 'Good morning' and 'Well done'; and short forms of longer expressions, as in 'Traffic diverted', 'Shop closed', 'No dogs' and 'Flooding ahead'. Such short forms could be rephrased to become major sentences, as in 'Traffic has been diverted because of roadworks', 'The shop is closed on Sundays', 'The owner does not allow dogs in her shop' and 'There was flooding ahead on the motorway'.

masculine in grammatical terms, one of the genders that

nouns are divided into. Nouns in the masculine gender include words that obviously belong to the male sex, as in 'man', 'boy', 'king', 'prince' 'bridegroom', 'schoolboy' and 'salesman'. Many words now considered to be of dual gender formerly were assumed to be masculine. These include such words as 'author', 'sculptor' and 'engineer'. Gender also applies to personal pronouns, and the third personal singular pronoun masculine is 'he' (subject), 'him' (object) and 'his' (possessive). For further information *see* **he; she**.

mass noun the same as **uncountable noun**.

minor sentence *see* **major sentence**.

misrelated participle *see* **dangling participle**.

modal verb a type of auxiliary verb that 'helps' the main verb to express a range of meanings including, for example, such meanings as possibility, probability, wants, wishes, necessity, permission, suggestions, etc. The main modal verbs are 'can', 'could'; 'may', 'might'; 'will', 'would'; 'shall', 'should'; 'must'. Modal verbs have only one form. They have no -s form in the third person singular, no infinitive and no participles. Examples of modal verbs include 'He cannot read and write', 'She could go if she wanted to' (expressing ability); 'You can have another biscuit', 'You may answer the question' (expressing permission); 'We may see her on the way to the station', 'We might get there by nightfall' (expressing possibility); 'Will you have some wine?', 'Would you take a seat?' (expressing an offer or invitation); 'We should arrive by dawn', 'That must be a record' (expressing probability and certainty); 'You may prefer to wait', 'You might like to leave instructions' (expressing suggestion); 'Can you find the time to phone him for me?', 'Could you give him a message?' (expressing instructions and requests); 'They must leave at once', 'We must get there on time' (expressing necessity).

modifier a word, or group of words, that 'modifies' or affects the meaning of another word in some way, usually by adding more information about it. Modifiers are frequently used with nouns. They can be adjectives, as in 'He works in the *main* building' and 'They need a *larger* house'. Modifiers of nouns can be nouns themselves, as in 'the *theatre* profession', 'the *publishing* industry' and '*singing* tuition'. They can also be place names, as in 'the *Edinburgh* train', 'a *Paris* café' and 'the *London* underground', or adverbs of place and direction, as in 'a *downstairs* cloakroom' and 'an *upstairs* sitting room.

Adverbs, adjectives and pronouns can be accompanied by modifiers. Examples of modifiers with adverbs include 'walking *amazingly* quickly' and 'stopping *incredibly* abruptly'. Examples of modifiers with adjectives include 'a *really* warm day' and 'a *deliriously* happy child'. Examples of modifiers with pronouns include '*almost* no one there' and '*practically* everyone present'.

The examples given above are all premodifiers. *see also* **postmodifier**.

mood one of the categories into which verbs are divided. The verb moods are indicative, imperative and subjunctive. The **indicative** makes a statement, as in 'He lives in France', 'They have two children' and 'It's starting to rain'. The **imperative** is used for giving orders or making requests, as in 'Shut that door!', 'Sit quietly until the teacher arrives' and 'Please bring me some coffee'. The **subjunctive** was originally a term in Latin grammar and expressed a wish, supposition, doubt, improbability or other non-factual statement. It is used in English for hypothetical statements and certain formal 'that' clauses, as in 'If I were you I would have nothing to do with it', 'If you were to go now you would arrive on time', 'Someone suggested that we ask for more money' and 'It was his solicitor who suggested that he sue the firm'. The word 'mood' arose because it was said to indicate the verb's attitude or viewpoint.

more an adverb that is added to some adjectives to make the comparative form (*see* **comparison of adjectives**). In general it is the longer adjectives that have more as part of their comparative form, as in 'more abundant', 'more beautiful', 'more catastrophic', 'more dangerous', 'more elegant', 'more frantic', 'more graceful', 'more handsome', 'more intelligent', 'more luxurious', 'more manageable', 'more opulent', 'more precious', 'more ravishing', 'more satisfactory', 'more talented', 'more unusual', 'more valuable'. Examples of adverbs with more in their comparative form include 'more elegantly', 'more gracefully', 'more energetically', 'more dangerously' and 'more determinedly'.

most an adverb added to some adjectives and adverbs to make the superlative form. In general it is the longer adjectives that have most as part of their superlative form, as in 'most abundant', 'most beautiful', 'most catastrophic', 'most dangerous', 'most elegant', 'most frantic', 'most graceful', 'most handsome', 'most intelligent', 'most luxurious', 'most manageable', 'most noteworthy', 'most opulent', 'most precious', most ravishing', 'most satisfactory', 'most talented', 'most unusual', 'most valuable'. Examples of adverbs with most in their superlative form include 'most elegantly', 'most gracefully', 'most energetically', 'most dangerously' and 'most determinedly'.

multi-sentence a sentence with more than one clause, as in 'She tripped over a rock and broke her ankle' and 'She was afraid when she saw the strange man'.

negative sentence a sentence that is the opposite of a **positive sentence**. 'She has a dog' is an example of a positive sentence. 'She does not have a dog' is an example of a negative sentence. The negative concept is expressed by an auxiliary verb accompanied by 'not' or 'n't'. Other words used in negative sentences include 'never', 'nothing' and 'by no means', as in 'She has never been here' and 'We heard nothing'.

neither an adjective or a pronoun that takes a singular verb, as in 'Neither parent will come' and 'Neither of them wishes to come'. In the **neither ... nor** construction, a singular verb is used if both parts of the construction are singular, as in 'Neither Jane nor Mary was present'. If both parts are plural the verb is plural, as in 'Neither their parents nor their grandparents are willing to look after them'. If the construction involves a mixture of singular and plural, the verb traditionally agrees with the subject that is nearest it, as in 'Neither her mother nor her grandparents are going to come' and 'Neither her grandparents nor her mother is going to come'. If pronouns are used, the nearer one governs the verb as in 'Neither they nor he is at fault' and 'Neither he nor they are at fault'.

neuter one of the grammatical genders. The other two grammatical genders are masculine and feminine. Inanimate objects are members of the neuter gender. Examples include 'table', 'desk', 'garden', 'spade', 'flower' and 'bottle'.

nominal clause *see* **noun clause**.

non-finite clause a clause which contains a non-finite verb. Thus in the sentence 'He works hard to earn a living', 'to earn a living' is a non-finite clause since 'to earn' is an infinitive and so a non-finite verb. Similarly in the sentence 'Getting there was a problem', 'getting there' is a non-finite clause, 'getting' being a present participle and so a non-finite verb.

non-finite verb a verb that shows no variation in tense and has no subject. The non-finite verb forms include the infinitive form, as in 'go', the present participle and gerund, as in 'going', and the past participle, as in 'gone'.

non-gradable *see* **gradable**.

noun the name of something or someone. Thus 'anchor', 'baker', 'cat', 'elephant', 'foot', 'gate', 'lake', 'pear', 'shoe', 'trunk' and 'wallet' are all nouns. There are various categories of nouns. *see* **abstract noun**, **common noun**, **concrete noun**, **countable noun**, **proper noun** and **uncountable noun**.

noun clause a subordinate clause that performs a function in a sentence similar to a noun or noun phrase. It can act as the subject, object or complement of a main clause. In the sentence 'Where he goes is his own business', 'where he goes' is a noun clause. In the sentence 'They asked why he objected', 'why he objected' is a noun clause. A noun clause is also known as a **nominal clause**.

noun phrase a group of words containing a noun as its main word and functioning like a noun in a sentence. Thus it can function as the subject, object or complement of a sentence. In the sentence 'The large black dog bit him', 'the large black dog' is a noun phrase, and in the sentence 'They bought a house with a garden', 'with a garden' is a noun phrase. In the sentence 'She is a complete fool', 'a complete fool' is a noun phrase.

noun, plurals *see* **Spelling** section.

number in grammar this is a classification consisting of 'singular' and 'plural'. Thus the number of the pronoun 'they' is 'plural' and the number of the verb 'carries' is singular. *see* **number agreement**.

number agreement or **concord** the agreement of grammatical units in terms of number. Thus a singular subject is followed by a singular verb, as in 'The girl likes flowers', 'He hates work' and 'She was carrying a suitcase'. Similarly a plural subject should be followed by a plural verb, as in 'They have many problems', 'The men work hard' and 'The girls are training hard'.

object the part of a sentence that is acted upon or is affected by the verb. It usually follows the verb to which it relates. There are two forms of object—the direct object and indirect object. A direct object can be a noun, and in the sentence 'The girl hit the ball', 'ball' is a noun and the object. In the sentence 'They bought a house', 'house' is a noun and the object. In the sentence 'They made an error', 'error' is a noun and the object. A direct object can be a noun phrase, and in the sentence 'He has bought a large house', 'a large house' is a noun phrase and the object. In the sentence 'She loves the little girl', 'the little girl' is a noun phrase and the object. In the sentence 'They both wear black clothes', 'black clothes' is a noun phrase and the object'. A direct object can be a noun clause, and in the sentence 'I know what he means', 'what he means' is a noun phrase and the object. In the sentence 'He denied that he had been involved', 'that he had been involved' is a noun phrase and the object. In the sentence 'I asked when he would return', 'when he would return' is a noun phrase and the object. A direct object can also be a pronoun, and in the sentence 'She hit him', 'him' is a pronoun and the object. In the sentence 'They had a car but they sold it', 'it' is a pronoun and the object. In the sentence 'She loves them', 'them' is a pronoun and the object.

objective case the case expressing the object. In Latin it is known as the accusative case.

part of speech each of the categories (e.g. verb, noun, adjective, etc) into which words are divided according to their grammatical and semantic functions.

participle a part of speech, so called because, although a verb, it has the character both of verb and adjective and is also used in the formation of some compound tenses. *see also* **-ing form** and **past participle**.

passive voice the voice of a verb whereby the subject is the recipient of the action of the verb. Thus, in the sentence 'Mary was kicked by her brother', 'Mary' is the receiver of the 'kick' and so 'kick' is in the passive voice. Had it been in the active voice it would have been 'Her brother kicked Mary'. Thus 'the brother' is the subject and not the receiver of the action.

past participle this is formed by adding *-ed* or *-d* to the base words of regular verbs, as in 'acted', ' alluded', 'boarded', 'dashed', 'flouted', 'handed', 'loathed', 'tended' and 'wanted', or in various other ways for irregular verbs.

past tense this tense of a verb is formed by adding *-ed* or *-d* to the base form of the verb in regular verbs, as in 'added', 'crashed', 'graded', 'smiled', 'rested' and 'yielded', and in various ways for irregular verbs.

perfect tense *see* **tense**.

personal pronoun a pronoun that is used to refer back to someone or something that has already been mentioned. The personal pronouns are divided into subject pronouns, object pronouns and possessive pronouns. They are also categorized according to 'person'. *see* **first person**, **second person** and **third person**.

phrasal verb a usually simple verb that combines with a preposition or adverb, or both, to convey a meaning more than the sum of its parts, e.g. to phase out, to come out, to look forward to.

phrase two or more words, usually not containing a finite verb, that form a complete expression by themselves or constitute a portion of a sentence.

positive sentence *see* **negative sentence**.

possessive *see* **genitive**.

possessive pronoun *see* **personal pronoun; first person; second person** and **third person**.

postmodifier a modifier that comes after the main word of a noun phrase, as in 'of stone' in 'tablets of stone'.

predicate all the parts of a clause or sentence that are not contained in the subject. Thus in the sentence 'The little girl was exhausted and hungry', 'exhausted and hungry' is the predicate. Similarly, in the sentence 'The tired old man slept like a top', 'slept like a top' is the predicate.

predicative adjective an adjective that helps to form the predicate and so comes after the verb, as 'tired' in 'She was very tired' and 'mournful' in 'The music was very mournful'.

premodifier a modifier that comes before the main word of a noun phrase, as 'green' in 'green dress' and 'pretty' in 'pretty houses'.

preposition a word that relates two elements of a sentence, clause or phrase together. Prepositions show how the elements relate in time or space and generally precede the words that they 'govern'. Words governed by prepositions are nouns or pronouns. Prepositions are often very short words, as 'at', 'in', 'on', 'to', 'before' and 'after'. Some complex prepositions consist of two words, as 'ahead of', 'instead of', 'apart from', and some consist of three, as 'with reference to', 'in accordance with' and 'in addition to'. Examples of prepositions in sentences include 'The cat sat on the mat', 'We were at a concert', 'They are in shock', 'We are going to France', 'She arrived before me', 'Apart from you she has no friends' and 'We acted in accordance with your instructions'.

present continuous *see* **tense**.

present participle *see* **-ing words**.

present tense *see* **tense**.

principal clause *see* **main clause**.

progressive present *see* **tense**.

pronoun a word that takes the place of a noun or a noun phrase. *see* **personal pronouns, he, her, him** and **his, reciprocal pronouns, reflexive pronouns, demonstrative pronouns, relative pronouns, distributive pronouns, indefinite pronouns** and **interrogative pronouns**.

proper noun a noun that refers to a particular individual or a specific thing. It is the 'name' of someone or something', as in Australia, Vesuvius, John Brown, River Thames, Rome and Atlantic Ocean.

question tag a phrase that is interrogative in form but is not really asking a question. It is added to a statement to seek agreement, etc. Examples include 'That was a lovely meal, wasn't it?', 'You will be able to go, won't you?', 'He's not going to move house, is he?' and 'She doesn't

drive, does she?' Sentences containing question tags have question marks at the end.

reciprocal pronoun a pronoun used to convey the idea of reciprocity or a two-way relationship. The reciprocal pronouns are 'each other' and 'one another'. Examples include 'They don't love each other any more', 'They seem to hate each other', 'We must try to help each other', 'The children were calling one another names', 'The two families were always criticizing one another' and 'The members of the family blame one another for their mother's death'.

reciprocal verb a verb such as 'consult', 'embrace', 'marry', 'meet', etc, that expresses a mutual relationship, as in 'They met at the conference', 'She married him in June'.

reflexive pronoun a pronoun that ends in '-self' or '-selves' and refers back to a noun or pronoun that has occurred earlier in the same sentence. The reflexive pronouns include 'myself', 'ourselves'; 'yourself', 'yourselves'; 'himself', 'herself', 'itself', 'themselves'. Examples include 'The children washed themselves', 'He cut himself shaving', 'Have you hurt yourself?' and 'She has cured herself of the habit'.

Reflexive pronouns are sometimes used for emphasis, as in 'The town itself was not very interesting' and 'The headmaster himself punished the boys'. They can also be used to indicate that something has been done by somebody by his/her own efforts without any help, as in 'He built the house himself', 'We converted the attic ourselves'. They can also indicate that someone or something is alone, as in 'She lives by herself' and 'The house stands by itself'.

reflexive verb a verb that has as its direct object a reflexive pronoun, e.g. 'They pride themselves on their skill as a team'.

regular sentence *see* **major sentence**.

regular verb *see* **irregular verb**.

relative clause a subordinate clause that has the function of an adjective. It is introduced by a relative pronoun.

relative pronoun a pronoun that introduces a relative clause. The relative pronouns are 'who', 'whom', 'whose', 'which' and 'that'. Examples of relative clauses introduced by relative pronouns include 'There is the man who stole the money', 'She is the person to whom I gave the money', 'This is the man whose wife won the prize', 'They criticized the work which he had done' and 'That's the house that I would like to buy'. Relative pronouns refer back to a noun or noun phrase in the main clause. These nouns and noun phrases are known as antecedents. The antecedents in the example sentences are respectively 'man', 'person', 'man', 'work' and 'house'.

Sometimes the relative clause divides the parts of the main clause, as in 'The woman whose daughter is ill is very upset', 'The people whom we met on holiday were French' and 'The house that we liked best was too expensive'.

reported speech *same as* **indirect speech**

rhetorical question a question that is asked to achieve

some kind of effect and requires no answer. Examples include 'What's this country coming to?', 'Did you ever see the like', 'Why do these things happen to me?', 'Where did youth go?', 'Death, where is thy sting?' and 'Where does time go?'. *see also* **interrogative sentence**.

second person the term used for the person or thing to whom one is talking. The term is applied to personal pronouns. The second person singular whether acting as the subject of a sentence is 'you', as in 'I told you so', 'We informed you of our decision' and 'They might have asked you sooner'. The second person personal pronoun does not alter its form in the plural in English, unlike in some languages. The possessive form of the second person pronoun is 'yours' whether singular or plural, as in 'These books are not yours'and 'This pen must be yours'.

sentence is at the head of the hierarchy of grammar. All the other elements, such as words, phrases and clauses, go to make up sentences. It is difficult to define a sentence. In terms of recognizing a sentence visually it can be described as beginning with a capital letter and ending with a full stop, or with an equivalent to the full stop, such as an exclamation mark. It is a unit of grammar that can stand alone and make sense and obeys certain grammatical rules, such as usually having a subject and a predicate, as in 'The girl banged the door', where 'the girl' is the subject and 'the door' is the predicate. *see* **major sentence**, **simple sentence**, **complex sentence**.

simple sentence a sentence that cannot be broken down into other clauses. It generally contains a finite verb. Simple sentences include 'The man stole the car', 'She nudged him' and 'He kicked the ball'. *see* **complex sentence** and **compound sentence**.

singular noun a noun that refers to 'one' rather than 'more than one', which is the plural form. *see also* **irregular plural**.

split infinitive an infinitive that has had another word in the form of an adverb placed between itself and 'to', as in 'to rudely push' and 'to quietly leave'. This was once considered a great grammatical sin but the split infinitive is becoming acceptable in modern usage. In any case it sometimes makes for a clumsy sentence if one slavishly adheres to the correct form.

stative present *see* **habitual** and **tense**.

strong verb the more common term for **irregular verb**.

structure word *see* **function word**.

subject that which is spoken of in a sentence or clause and is usually either a noun, as in 'Birds fly' (birds is the noun as subject); a noun phrase, as in 'The people in the town dislike him' (the people in the town' is the subject); a pronoun, as in 'She hit the child' (she is the pronoun as subject); a proper noun, as in 'Paris is the capital of France'. *see* **dummy subject**.

subjunctive *see* **mood**.

subordinate clause a clause that is dependent on another clause, namely the main clause. Unlike the main clause, it cannot stand alone and make sense. Subordinate clauses are introduced by conjunctions. Examples of conjunctions that introduce subordinate clauses include 'after', 'before', 'when', 'if', 'because' and 'since'. *see* **adverbial clause**; **noun clause**.

subordinating conjunction *see* **conjunction**.

superlative form the form of an adjective or adverb that expresses the highest or utmost degree of the quality or manner of the word. The superlative forms follow the same rules as comparative forms except that they end in *-est* instead of *-er* and the longer ones use 'most' instead of 'more'. *see also* **comparison of adjectives**.

tense the form of a verb that is used to show the time at which the action of the verb takes place. One of the tenses in English is the **present tense**. It is used to indicate an action now going on or a state now existing. A distinction can be made between the **habitual present**, which marks habitual or repeated actions or recurring events, and the **stative present**, which indicates something that is true at all times. Examples of habitual present include 'He works long hours' and 'She walks to work'. Examples of the stative tense include 'The world is round' and 'Everyone must die eventually'.

The **progressive present** or **continuous present** is formed with the verb 'to be' and the present participle, as in, 'He is walking to the next village', 'She was driving along the road when she saw him' and 'They were worrying about the state of the economy'.

The **past tense** refers to an action or state that has taken place before the present time. In the case of regular verbs it is formed by adding *-ed* to the base form of the verb, as in 'fear/feared', 'look/looked', and 'turn/turned'. *see also* **irregular verbs**.

The **future tense** refers to an action or state that will take place at some time in the future. It is formed with 'will' and 'shall'. Traditionally 'will' was used with the second and third person pronouns ('you', 'he/she/it', 'they') and 'shall' with the first person ('I' and 'we'), as in 'You will be bored', 'He will soon be home', 'They will leave tomorrow', 'I shall buy some bread' and 'We shall go by train'. Also traditionally 'shall' was used with the second and third persons to indicate emphasis, insistence, determination, refusal, etc, as in 'You shall go to the ball' and 'He shall not be admitted'. 'Will' was used with the first person in the same way, as in 'I will get even with him'.

In modern usage 'will' is generally used for the first person as well as for second and third, as in 'I will see you tomorrow' and 'We will be there soon' and 'shall' is used for emphasis, insistence, etc, for first, second and third persons.

The future tense can also be formed with the use of 'be about to' or 'be going to', as in 'We were about to leave' and 'They were going to look for a house'.

Other tenses include the **perfect tense**, which is formed using the verb 'to have' and the past participle. In the case of regular verbs the past participle is formed by adding *ed* to the base form of the verb. *see also* **irregular verbs**. Examples of the perfect tense include 'He has played his last match', 'We have travelled all day' and 'They have thought a lot about it'.

The **past perfect tense** or **pluperfect tense** is formed using the verb 'to have' and the past participle, as in 'She had no idea that he was dead' and 'They had felt unhappy about the situation'.

The **future perfect** is formed using the verb 'to have' and the past participle, as in 'He will have arrived by now'.

they *see* **him** and **third person**.

third person a third party, not the speaker or the person or thing being spoken to. Note that 'person' in this context can refer to things as well as people. 'Person' in this sense applies to personal pronouns. The third person singular forms are 'he', 'she' and 'it' when the subject of a sentence or clause, as in 'She will win' and 'It will be fine'. The third person singular forms are 'him', 'her','it' when the object, as in 'His behaviour hurt her' and 'She meant it'. The third person plural is 'they' when the subject, as in 'They have left' and 'They were angry' and 'them' when the object, as in 'His words made them angry' and 'We accompanied them'.

The possessive forms of the singular are 'his', 'hers' and 'its', as in 'he played his guitar' and 'The dog hurt its leg', and the possessive form of the plural is theirs, as in 'That car is theirs' and 'They say that the book is theirs'. *see* **he**.

to-infinitive the infinitive form of the verb when it is accompanied by 'to' rather than when it is the bare infinitive without 'to'. Examples of the to-infinitive include 'We were told to go', 'I didn't want to stay' and 'To get there on time we'll have to leave now'.

transitive verb a verb that takes a direct object. In the sentence 'The boy broke the window', 'window' is a direct object and so 'broke' (past tense of break) is a transitive verb. In the sentence 'She eats fruit', 'fruit' is a direct object and so 'eat' is a transitive verb. In the sentence 'They kill enemy soldiers' 'enemy soldiers' is a direct object and so 'kill' is a transitive verb. *see* **intransitive verb**.

uncountable noun or **uncount noun** a noun that is not usually pluralized or 'counted'. Such a noun is usually preceded by 'some', rather than 'a'. Uncountable nouns often refer to substances or commodities or qualities, processes and states. Examples of uncountable nouns include butter, china, luggage, petrol, sugar, heat, information, poverty, richness and warmth. In some situations it is possible to have a countable version of what is usually an uncountable noun. Thus 'sugar' is usually considered to be an uncountable noun but it can be used in a countable form in contexts such as 'I take two sugars in my coffee please'. Some nouns exist in an uncountable and countable form. Examples include 'cake', as in 'Have some cake' and 'She ate three cakes' and 'She could not paint for lack of light' and 'the lights went out'.

verb the part of speech often known as a 'doing' word. Although this is rather restrictive, since it tends to preclude auxiliary verbs, modal verbs, etc, the verb is the word in a sentence that is most concerned with the action and is usually essential to the structure of the sentence. Verbs 'inflect' and indicate tense, voice, mood, number, number and person. Most of the information on verbs has been placed under related entries. *see* **active voice, auxiliary verb, finite verb, -ing form, intransitive verb, irregular verbs, linking verb, modal verb, mood, non-finite verb, passive voice** and **transitive verb**.

verb phrase a group of verb forms that have the same function as a single verb. Examples include 'have been raining', 'must have been lying', 'should not have been doing' and 'has been seen doing'.

verbal noun *see* **gerund** and **-ing form**.

vocative case a case that is relevant mainly to languages such as Latin which are based on cases and inflections. In English the vocative is expressed by addressing someone, as 'John, could I see you for a minute', or by some form of greeting, endearment or exclamation.

voice one of the categories that describes verbs. It involves two ways of looking at the action of verbs. It is divided into active voice and passive voice.

weak verb a less common term for a regular verb, in which inflection is effected by adding a letter or syllable (dawn, dawned) rather than a change of vowel (rise, rose). *see* **irregular verb**.

Appendix 3

Usage

-abled is a suffix meaning 'able-bodied'. It is most usually found in such phrases as 'differently abled', a 'politically correct', more positive way of referring to people with some form of disability, as in 'provide access to the club building for differently abled members'.

ableism or **ablism** means discrimination in favour of able-bodied people as in 'people in wheelchairs unable to get jobs because of ableism'. Note that the suffix '-ism' is often used to indicate discrimination against the group to which it refers, as in 'ageism'.

Aboriginal rather than **Aborigine** is now the preferred term for an original inhabitant of Australia, especially where the word is in the singular.

abuse and **misuse** both mean wrong or improper use or treatment. However, **abuse** tends to be a more condemnatory term, suggesting that the wrong use or treatment is morally wrong or illegal. Thus we find 'misuse of the equipment' or 'misuse of one's talents', but 'abuse of a privileged position' or 'abuse of children'. 'Child abuse' is usually used to indicate physical violence or sexual assault.

    Abuse is also frequently applied to the use of substances that are dangerous or injurious to health, as 'drug abuse', or 'alcohol abuse'. In addition, it is used to describe insulting or offensive language, as in 'shout abuse at the referee'.

academic is used to describe scholarly or educational matters, as 'a child with academic rather than sporting interests'. From this use it has come to mean theoretical rather than actual or practical, as in 'wasting time discussing matters of purely academic concern'. In modern use it is frequently used to mean irrelevant, as in 'Whether you vote for him or not is academic. He is certain of a majority of votes'.

access is usually a noun meaning 'entry or admission', as in 'try to gain access to the building', or 'the opportunity to use something', as in 'have access to confidential information'. It is also used to refer to the right of a parent to spend time with his or her children, as in 'Father was allowed access to the children at weekends'.

    However **access** can also be used as a verb. It is most commonly found in computing, meaning obtaining information from, as in 'accessing details from the computer file relating to the accounts'. In modern usage many technical words become used, and indeed overused, in the general language. Thus the verb **access** can now be found meaning to obtain information not on a computer, as in 'access the information in the filing cabinet'. It can also be found in the sense of gaining entry to a building, as in 'Their attempts to access the building at night were unsuccessful'.

accessory and **accessary** are interchangeable as regards only one meaning of **accessory**. A person who helps another person to commit a crime is known either as an **accessory** or an **accessary**, although the former is the more modern term. However, only **accessory** is used to describe a useful or decorative extra that is not strictly necessary, as in 'Seat covers are accessories that are included in the price of the car' and 'She wore a red dress with black accessories' ('accessories' in the second example being handbag, shoes and gloves).

accompany can be followed either by the preposition 'with' or 'by'. When it means 'to go somewhere with someone', 'by' is used, as in 'She was accompanied by her parents to church' Similarly, 'by' is used when **accompany** is used in a musical context, as in 'The singer was accompanied on the piano by her brother'. When **accompany** means 'to go along with something' or 'supplement something', either 'by' or 'with' may be used, as in 'The roast turkey was accompanied by all the trimmings', 'His words were accompanied by/with a gesture of dismissal', and 'The speaker accompanied his words with expressive gestures'.

acoustics can take either a singular or plural verb. When it is being thought of as a branch of science it is treated as being singular, as in 'Acoustics deals with the study of sound', but when it is used to describe the qualities of a hall, etc, with regard to its sound-carrying properties, it is treated as being plural, as in 'The acoustics in the school hall are very poor'.

activate and **actuate** both mean 'make active' but are commonly used in different senses. **Activate** refers to physical or chemical action, as in 'The terrorists activated the explosive device'. **Actuate** means 'to move to action' and 'to serve as a motive', as in 'The murderer was actuated by jealousy'.

actress is still widely used as a term for a woman who acts in plays or films, although many people prefer the term 'actor', regarding this as a neutral term rather than simply the masculine form. The **-ess** suffix, used to indicate the feminine form of a word, is generally becoming less common as these forms are regarded as sexist or belittling.

acute and **chronic** both refer to disease. **Acute** is used of a disease that is sudden in onset and lasts a relatively short time, as in 'flu is an acute illness'. **Chronic** is used of a disease that may be slow to develop and lasts a long time, possibly over several years, as in 'Asthma is a chronic condition'.

AD and **BC** are abbreviations that accompany year numbers. ad stands for 'Anno Domini', meaning 'in the year of our Lord' and indicates that the year concerned is one occurring after Jesus Christ was born. Traditionally AD is placed before the year number concerned, as in 'Their great-grandfather was born in AD 1801', but in modern usage it sometimes follows the year number, as in 'The house was built in 1780 AD.' BC stands for 'Before Christ' and indicates that the year concerned is one occurring before Jesus Christ was born. It follows the year number, as in 'The event took place in Rome in 55 BC'.

adapter and **adaptor** can be used interchangeably, but commonly **adapter** is used to refer to a person who adapts, as in 'the adapter of the stage play for television and **adaptor** is used to refer to a thing that adapts, specifically a type of electrical plug.

admission and **admittance** both mean 'permission or right to enter'. **Admission** is the more common term, as in 'They refused him admission to their house', and, unlike **admittance**, it can also mean 'the price or fee charged for entry' as in 'Admission to the football match is £3'. **Admittance** is largely used in formal or official situations, as in 'They ignored the notice saying "No Admittance"'. **Admission** also means 'confession' or 'acknowledgement of responsibility', as in 'On her own admission she was the thief'.

admit may be followed either by the preposition 'to' or the preposition 'of', depending on the sense. In the sense of 'to confess', **admit** is usually not followed by a preposition at all, as in 'He admitted his mistake' and 'She admitted stealing the brooch'. However, in this sense **admit** is sometimes followed by 'to', as in 'They have admitted to their error' and 'They have admitted to their part in the theft'.

In the sense of 'to allow to enter', **admit** is followed by 'to', as in 'The doorman admitted the guest to the club'. Also in the rather formal sense of 'give access or entrance to', **admit** is followed by 'to', as in 'the rear door admits straight to the garden'. In the sense of 'to be open to' or 'leave room for', **admit** is followed by 'of', as in 'The situation admits of no other explanation'.

admittance *see* **admission**.

adopted and **adoptive** are liable to be confused. **Adopted** is applied to children who have been adopted, as in 'The couple have two adopted daughters'. **Adoptive** is applied to a person or people who adopt a child, as in 'Her biological parents tried to get the girl back from her adoptive parents'.

aeroplane is commonly abbreviated to **plane** in modern usage. In American English **aeroplane** becomes **airplane**.

affinity may be followed by the preposition 'with' or 'between', and means 'close relationship', 'mutual attraction' or similarity, as in 'the affinity which twins have with each other' and 'There was an affinity between the two families who had lost children'. In modern usage it is sometimes followed by 'for' or 'towards', and means 'liking', as in 'She has an affinity for fair-haired men'.

ageism means discrimination on the grounds of age, as in 'By giving an age range in their job advert the firm were guilty of ageism'. Usually it refers to discrimination against older or elderly people, but it also refers to discrimination against young people.

agenda in modern usage is a singular noun having the plural **agendas**. It means 'a list of things to be attended to', as in 'The financial situation was the first item on the committee's agenda'. Originally it was a plural noun, derived from Latin, meaning 'things to be done'.

aggravate literally means 'to make worse', as in 'Her remarks simply aggravated the situation'. In modern usage it is frequently found meaning 'to irritate or annoy', as in 'The children were aggravating their mother when she was trying to read'. It is often labelled as 'informal' in dictionaries and is best avoided in formal situations.

agnostic and **atheist** are both words meaning 'disbeliever in God', but there are differences in sense between the two words. **Agnostics** believe that it is not possible to know whether God exists or not. **Atheists** believe that there is no God.

alcohol abuse is a modern term for alcoholism. *see* **abuse**.

alibi is derived from the Latin word for 'elsewhere'. It is used to refer to a legal plea that a person accused or under suspicion was somewhere other than the scene of the crime at the time the crime was committed. In modern usage **alibi** is frequently used to mean simply 'excuse' or 'pretext', as in 'He had the perfect alibi for not going to the party—he was ill in hospital'.

all together and **altogether** are not interchangeable. **All together** means 'at the same time' or 'in the same place', as in 'The guests arrived all together' and 'They kept their personal papers all together in a filing cabinet'. **Altogether** means 'in all, in total' or 'completely', as in "We collected £500 altogether' and 'The work was altogether too much for him'.

alternate and **alternative** are liable to be confused. **Alternate** means 'every other' or 'occurring by turns', as in 'They visit her mother on alternate weekends' and 'between alternate layers of meat and cheese sauce'. **Alternative** means 'offering a choice' or 'being an alternative', as in 'If the motorway is busy there is an alternative route'. **Alternative** is found in some cases in modern usage to mean 'not conventional, not traditional', as in 'alternative medicine' and 'alternative comedy'.

Alternative as a noun refers to the choice between two possibilities, as in 'The alternatives are to go by train or by plane'. In modern usage, however, it is becoming common to use it to refer to the choice among two or more possibilities, as in 'He has to use a college from five alternatives'.

although and **though** are largely interchangeable but **though** is slightly less formal, as in 'We arrived on time although/though we left late'.

amiable and **amicable** both refer to friendliness and goodwill. **Amiable** means 'friendly' or 'agreeable and pleasant', and is mostly used of people or their moods, as in 'amiable neighbours', 'amiable travelling companions', 'of an amiable temperament' and 'be in an amiable mood'. **Amicable** means 'characterized by friendliness and goodwill' and is applied mainly to relationships, agreements, documents, etc, as in 'an amicable working relationship', 'reach an amicable set-tlement at the end of the war' and 'send an amicable letter to his former rival'.

among and **amongst** are interchangeable, as in 'We searched among/amongst the bushes for the ball,' 'Divide the chocolate among/amongst you', and 'You must choose among/amongst the various possibilities'.

among and **between** may be used interchangeably in most contexts. Formerly **between** was used only when referring to the relationship of two things, as in 'Share the chocolate between you and your brother', and **among** was used when referring to the relationship of three or more things, as in 'Share the chocolate among all your friends'. In modern usage **between** may be used when referring to more than two things, as in 'There is agreement between all the countries of the EU' and 'Share the chocolate between all of you'. However, **among** is still used only to describe more than two things.

amoral and **immoral** are not interchangeable. **Amoral** means 'lacking moral standards, devoid of moral sense', indicating that the person so described has no concern with morals, as in 'The child was completely amoral and did not know the difference between right and wrong'. **Immoral** means 'against or breaking moral standards, bad'. 'He knows he's doing wrong but he goes on being completely immoral' and 'commit immoral acts'. Note the spelling of both words. **Amoral** has only one *m* but **immoral** has double *m*.

anaesthetic and **analgesic** are liable to be confused. As an adjective, **anaesthetic** means 'producing a loss of feeling', as in 'inject the patient with an anaesthetic substance', and as a noun it means 'a substance that produces a loss of feeling', as in 'administer an anaesthetic to the patient on the operating table'. A local anaesthetic produces a loss of feeling in only part of the body, as in 'remove the rotten tooth under local anaesthetic'. A **general anaesthetic** produces loss of feeling in the whole body and induces unconsciousness, as in 'The operation on his leg will have to be performed under general anaesthetic'. As an adjective **analgesic** means 'producing a lack of or reduction in, sensitivity to pain, pain-killing', as in 'aspirin has an analgesic effect'. As a noun **analgesic** means 'a substance that produces a lack of, or reduction in, sensitivity to pain', as in 'aspirin, paracetamol, and other analgesics'.

arbiter and **arbitrator**, although similar in meaning, are not totally interchangeable. **Arbiter** means 'a person who has absolute power to judge or make decisions', as in 'Parisian designers used to be total arbiters of fashion'. **Arbitrator** is 'a person appointed to settle differences in a dispute', as in 'act as arbitrator between management and workers in the wages dispute'. **Arbiter** is occasionally used with the latter meaning also.

artist and **artiste** are liable to be confused. **Artist** refers to 'a person who paints or draws,' as in 'Renoir was a great artist'. The word may also refer to 'a person who is skilled in something', as in 'The mechanic is a real artist

with an engine'. **Artiste** refers to 'an entertainer, such as a singer or a dancer', as in 'a list of the artistes in the musical performances'. The word is becoming a little old-fashioned.

at this moment in time is an overused phrase meaning simply 'now'. In modern usage there is a tendency to use what are thought to be grander-sounding alternatives for simple words. It is best to avoid such overworked phrases and use the simpler form.

atheist *see* **agnostic**.

au fait is French in origin but it is commonly used in English to mean 'familiar with' or 'informed about', as in 'not completely au fait with the new office system'. It is pronounced *o fay*.

authoress is not used in modern usage since it is considered sexist. **Author** is regarded as a neutral term to describe both male and female authors.

avoid *see* **evade**.

avoidance *see* **evasion**.

baited *see* **bated**.

barmaid is disliked by many people on the grounds that it sounds a belittling term and is thus sexist. It is also disliked by people who are interested in political correctness. However the word continues to be quite common, along with **barman**, and efforts to insist on **bar assistant** or **barperson** have not yet succeeded.

basically means literally 'referring to a base or basis, fundamentally', as in 'The scientist's theory is basically unsound', but it is frequently used almost meaninglessly as a fill-up word at the beginning of a sentence, as in 'Basically he just wants more money'. Overuse of this word should be avoided.

basis, meaning 'something on which something is founded', as in 'The cost of the project was the basis of his argument against it', has the plural form **bases** although it is not commonly used. It would be more usual to say 'arguments without a firm basis' than 'arguments without firm bases'.

bated as in 'with bated breath' meaning 'tense and anxious with excitement', is frequently misspelt **baited**. Care should be taken not to confuse the two words.

bathroom *see* **toilet**.

BC *see* AD.

because means 'for the reason that', as in 'He left because he was bored', and is sometimes misused. It is wrong to use it in a sentence that also contains 'the reason that', as in 'The reason she doesn't say much is that she is shy'. The correct form of this is 'She doesn't say much because she is shy' or 'The reason she doesn't say much is that she is shy'.

because of *see* **due to**.

beg the question is often used wrongly. It means 'to take for granted the very point that has to be proved', as in 'To say that God must exist because we can see all his wonderful creations in the world around us begs the question'. The statement assumes that these creations have been made by God although this has not been proved and yet this fact is being used as evidence that there is a God. **Beg the question** is often used wrongly to mean 'to evade the question', as in 'The police tried to get him to say where he had been but he begged the question and changed the subject'.

benign means 'kindly, well-disposed' when applied to people, as in 'fortunate enough to have a benign ruler'. This meaning may also be used of things, as in 'give a benign smile' and 'live in a benign climate'. As a medical term **benign** means 'nonmalignant, non-cancerous'. **Innocent** is another word for **benign** in this sense.

bête noire refers to 'something that one detests or fears', as in 'Loud pop music is her father's bête noire, although she sings with a pop group'. Note the spelling, particularly the accent (circumflex) on **bête** and the *e* at the end of **noire**. The phrase is French in origin and the plural form is **bêtes noires**, as in 'A bearded man is one of her many bêtes noires'.

better should be preceded by 'had' when it means 'ought to' or 'should', as in 'You had better leave now if you want to arrive there by nightfall' and 'We had better apologize for upsetting her'. In informal contexts, especially in informal speech as in 'Hey Joe, Mum says you better come now', the 'had' is often omitted but it should be retained in formal contexts. The negative form is 'had better not', as in 'He had better not try to deceive her'.

between is often found in the phrase 'between you and me' as in 'Between you and me I think he stole the money'. Note that 'me' is correct and that 'I' is wrong. This is because prepositions like 'between' are followed by an object, not a subject. 'I' acts as the subject of a sentence, as in 'I know her', and 'me' as the object, as in 'She knows me'.

between *see* **among**.

bi- of the words beginning with the prefix bi-, biannual and biennial are liable to be confused. **Biannual** means 'twice a year' and **biennial** means 'every two years'.

Bicentenary and bicentennial both mean 'a 200th anniversary', as in 'celebrating the bicentenary/bicentennial of the firm'. **Bicentenary** is, however, the more common expression in British English, although **bicentennial** is more common in American English.

Biweekly is a confusing word as it has two different meanings. It means both 'twice a week' and 'once every two weeks'. Thus there is no means of knowing without other information whether 'a bi-weekly publication' comes out once a week or every two weeks. The confusion arises because the prefix 'bi-', which means 'two', can refer both to doubling, as in 'bicycle', and halving, as in 'bisection'.

biannual *see* **bi-**.

bicentenary and **bicentennial** *see* **bi-**.

biennial *see* **bi-**.

billion traditionally meant 'one million million' in British English, but in modern usage it has increasingly taken on the American English meaning of 'one thousand million'. When the number of million pounds, etc, is specified, the number immediately precedes the word 'million' without the word 'of', as in 'The firm is worth five billion dollars', but if no number is present then

'of' precedes 'dollars, etc', ' as in 'The research project cost the country millions of dollars'. The word **billion** may also be used loosely to mean 'a great but unspecified number', as in 'Billions of people in the world live in poverty'.

birth name is a suggested alternative for **maiden name**, a woman's surname before she married and took the name of her husband. **Maiden name** is considered by some to be inappropriate since maiden in one of its senses is another name for 'virgin' and it is now not at all usual for women to be virgins when they marry. Another possible name alternative is **family name**.

biweekly *see* **bi-**.

black is the word now usually applied to dark-skinned people of Afro-Caribbean origins and is the term preferred by most black-skinned people themselves. **Coloured** is considered by many to be offensive since it groups all non-Caucasians together. In America, African-American is becoming increasingly common as a substitute for **black**.

blond and **blonde** are both used to mean 'a fair-haired person', but they are not interchangeable. **Blond** is used to describe a man or boy, **blonde** is used to describe a woman or girl. They are derived from the French adjective, which changes endings according to the gender of the noun.

boat and **ship** are often used interchangeably, but usually **boat** refers to a smaller vessel than a ship.

bona fide is an expression of Latin origin meaning literally 'of good faith'. It means 'genuine, sincere' or 'authentic', as in 'a bona fide member of the group', 'a bona fide excuse for not going', or 'a bona fide agreement'.

bottom line is an expression from accountancy that has become commonly used in the general language. In accountancy it refers to the final line of a set of company accounts, which indicates whether the company has made a profit or a loss, obviously a very important line. In general English, **bottom line** has a range of meanings, from 'the final outcome or result', as in 'The bottom line of their discussion was that they decided to sell the company', through 'the most important point of something', as in 'The bottom line was whether they could get there on time or not', to 'the last straw', as in 'His affair with another woman was the bottom line of their stormy relationship and she left him'.

can and **may** both mean in one of their senses 'to be permitted'. In this sense **can** is much less formal than **may** and is best restricted to informal contexts, as in ' "Can I go to the park now?" asked the child.' **May** is used in more formal contexts, as in 'May I please have your name?' Both **can** and **may** have other meanings. **Can** has the meaning 'to be able', as in 'They thought his legs were permanently damaged but he can still walk'. **May** has the additional meaning 'to be likely', as in 'You may well be right'.

The past tense of **can** is **could**, as in 'The children asked if they could (= be permitted to) go to the park'. 'The old man could (= be unable to) not walk upstairs'.

The past tense of **may** is **might**, as in 'The child asked if he might have a piece of cake (= be permitted to)'. 'They might (= be likely to) well get here tonight'.

cannot, can not, and **can't** all mean the same thing but they are used in different contexts. **Cannot** is the most usual form, as in 'The children have been told that they cannot go' and 'We cannot get there by public transport'. **Cannot** is written as two words only for emphasis, as in 'No, you can not have any more' and 'The invalid certainly can not walk to the ambulance'. **Can't** is used in less formal contexts and often in speech, as in 'I can't be bothered going out' and 'They can't bear to be apart'.

cardigan, jersey, jumper and **sweater** all refer to knitted garments for the top part of the body. **Cardigan** refers to a jacket-like garment with buttons down the front. **Jersey, jumper** and **sweater** refer to a knitted garment pulled over the head to get it on and off.

cardinal and **ordinal** numbers refer to different aspects of numbers. **Cardinal** is applied to those numbers that refer to quantity or value without referring to their place in the set, as in 'one', 'two', 'fifty' 'one hundred'. **Ordinal** is applied to numbers that refer to their order in a series, as in 'first', 'second', 'fortieth', 'hundredth'.

carer has recently taken on the meaning of 'a person who looks after a sick, handicapped or old relative or friend', as in 'carers requiring a break from their responsibilities'.

carpet and **rug** both refer to forms of floor covering. Generally a rug is smaller than a carpet, and the fitted variety of fabric floor covering is always known as carpet.

caster and **castor** are mainly interchangeable. Both forms can be applied to 'a swivelling wheel attached to the base of a piece of furniture to enable it to be moved easily' and 'a container with a perforated top from which sugar is sprinkled'. The kind of sugar known as **caster** can also be called **castor**, although this is less usual. The lubricating or medicinal oil known as **castor oil** is never spelt **caster**.

Catholic and **catholic** have different meanings. **Catholic** as an adjective refers to the Roman Catholic Church, as in 'The Pope is head of the Catholic Church', or to the universal body of Christians. As a noun it means 'a member of the Catholic Church', as in 'She is a Catholic but he is a Protestant'. Catholic with a lower-case initial letter means 'general, wide-ranging', as in 'a catholic selection of essays', and ' broad-minded, liberal', as in 'a catholic attitude to the tastes of others'.

celibate means 'unmarried' or 'remaining unmarried and chaste, especially for religious reasons', as in 'Roman Catholic priests have to be celibate'. In modern usage, because of its connection with chastity, **celibate** has come to mean 'abstaining from sexual intercourse', as in 'The threat of Aids has made many people celibate'. The word is frequently misspelt. Note the *i* after *l*.

Celsius, centigrade and **Fahrenheit** are all scales of temperature. **Celsius** and **centigrade** mean the same and refer to a scale on which water freezes at 0° and boils at 100°. This scale is now the principal unit of temperature. **Celsius** is now the more acceptable term. **Fahrenheit** refers to a scale on which water freezes at 32° and boils at 212°. It is still used, informally at least, of the weather, and statements such as 'The temperature reached the nineties today' are still common.

Note the initial capital letters in **Celsius** and **Fahrenheit**. This is because they are named after people, namely the scientists who devised them.

centenary and **centennial** are both used to refer to a 'one-hundredth anniversary'. **Centenary** is the more common term in British English, as in 'celebrate the town's centenary', whereas **centennial** is more common in American English. **Centennial** may be used as an adjective, as in 'organize the town's centennial celebrations'.

centigrade *see* **Celsius.**

centre and **middle** mean much the same, but **centre** is used more precisely than **middle** in some cases, as in 'a line through the centre of the circle' and 'She felt faint in the middle of the crowd'.

centre on and **centre around** are often used interchangeably, as in 'Her world centres on/around her children'. **Centre around** is objected to by some people on the grounds that **centre** is too specific to be used with something as vague as **around**. When it is used as a verb with place names, **centre** is used with 'at', as in 'Their business operation is centred at London'.

centuries are calculated from 1001, 1501, 1901, etc, not 1000, 1500, 1900, etc. This is because the years are counted from AD 1, there being no year 0.

chair is often used to mean 'a person in charge of a meeting, committee, etc', as in 'The committee has a new chair this year'. Formerly **chairman** was always used in this context, as in 'He was appointed chairman of the fund-raising committee' but this is disapproved of on the grounds that it is sexist. Formerly, **chairman** was sometimes used even if the person in charge of the meeting or committee was a woman, and sometimes **chairwoman** was used in this situation. **Chairperson**, which also avoids sexism, is frequently used instead of **chair**. **Chair** is also a verb meaning 'to be in charge of a meeting, committee, etc'.

-challenged is a modern suffix that is very much part of politically correct language. It is used to convey a disadvantage, problem or disorder in a more positive light. For example, 'visually challenged' is used in politically correct language instead of 'blind' or 'partially sighted', and 'aurally challenged' is used instead of 'deaf' or 'hard of hearing'. **-Challenged** is often used in humorous coinages, as in 'financially challenged', meaning 'penniless', and 'intellectually challenged', meaning 'stupid'.

charisma was formerly a theological word used to mean 'a spiritual gift', such as the gift of healing, etc. In modern usage it is used to describe 'a special quality or power that influences, inspires or stimulates other people, personal magnetism', as in 'The president was elected because of his charisma'. The adjective from **charisma** is **charismatic**, as in 'his charismatic style of leadership'.

chauvinism originally meant 'excessive patriotism', being derived from the name of Nicolas Chauvin, a soldier in the army of Napoleon Bonaparte, who was noted for his excessive patriotism. In modern usage **chauvinism** has come to mean 'excessive enthusiasm or devotion to a cause' or, more particularly, 'an irrational and prejudiced belief in the superiority of one's own cause'. When preceded by 'male', it refers specifically to attitudes and actions that assume the superiority of the male sex and thus the inferiority of women, as in 'accused of not giving her the job because of male chauvinism'. **Chauvinism** is frequently used to mean **male chauvinism**, as in 'He shows his chauvinism towards his female staff by never giving any of them senior jobs'. The adjective formed from **chauvinism** is **chauvinistic**.

chemist and **pharmacist** have the same meaning in one sense of **chemist** only. **Chemist** and **pharmacist** are both words for 'one who prepares drugs ordered by medical prescription'. **Chemist** has the additional meaning of 'a scientist who works in the field of chemistry', as in 'He works as an industrial chemist'.

childish and **childlike** both refer to someone being like a child but they are used in completely different contexts. **Childish** is used in a derogatory way about someone to indicate that he or she is acting like a child in an immature way, as in 'Even though she is 20 years old she has childish tantrums when she does not get her own way' and 'childish handwriting for an adult'. **Childlike** is a term of approval or a complimentary term used to describe something that has some of the attractive qualities of childhood, as in 'She has a childlike enthusiasm for picnics' and 'He has a childlike trust in others'.

Christian name is used to mean someone's first name as opposed to someone's **surname**. It is increasingly being replaced by **first name** or **forename** since Britain has become a multicultural society where there are several religions as well as Christianity.

chronic *see* **acute**.

city and **town** in modern usage are usually distinguished on grounds of size and status, a city being larger and more important than a town. Originally in Britain a **city** was a town which had special rights conferred on it by royal charter and which usually had a cathedral.

clean and **cleanse** as verbs both mean 'to clean', as in 'clean the house' and 'cleanse the wound'. However, **cleanse** tends to indicate a more thorough cleaning than **clean** and sometimes carries the suggestion of 'to purify', as in 'prayer cleansing the soul'.

client and **customer**, although closely related in meaning, are not interchangeable. **Client** refers to 'a person who pays for the advice or services of a professional person', as in 'They are both clients of the same lawyer', 'a client waiting to see the bank manager' and 'hairdressers who keep their clients waiting'. **Customer** refers to 'a person who purchases goods from a shop, etc', as in 'customers complaining to shopkeepers about faulty goods' and 'a regular customer at the local supermarket'. **Client** is used in the sense of 'customer' by shops who regard it as a more superior word, as in ' clients of an exclusive dress boutique'.

climate no longer refers just to weather, as in 'go to live in a hot climate', 'Britain has a temperate climate'. It has extended its meaning to refer to 'atmosphere', as in 'live in a climate of despair' and to 'the present situation', as in 'businessmen nervous about the financial climate'.

clone originally was a technical word meaning 'one of a group of offspring that are asexually produced and which are genetically identical to the parent and to other members of the group'. In modern usage **clone** is frequently used loosely to mean 'something that is very similar to something else', as in 'In the sixties there were many Beatles' clones', and 'grey-suited businessmen looking like clones of each other'.

collaborate and **cooperate** are not interchangeable in all contexts. They both mean 'to work together for a common purpose', as in 'The two scientists are collaborating/cooperating on cancer research' and 'The rival building firms are collaborating/cooperating on the new shopping complex'. When the work concerned is of an artistic or creative nature **collaborate** is the more commonly used word, as in 'The two directors are collaborating on the film' and 'The composers collaborated on the theme music'. **Collaborate** also has the meaning of 'to work with an enemy, especially an enemy that is occupying one's country', as in 'a Frenchman who collaborated with the Germans when they installed a German government in France'.

coloured *see* **black**.

commence, begin, and **start** mean the same, but **commence** is used in a more formal context than the other two words, as in 'The legal proceedings will commence tomorrow' and 'The memorial service will commence with a hymn'. **Begin** and **start** are used less formally, as 'The match begins at 2 p.m.' and 'The film has already started'.

commensurate is followed by 'with' to form a phrase meaning 'proportionate to, appropriate to', as in 'a salary commensurate with her qualifications' and 'a price commensurate with the quality of the goods'.

comparatively means 'relatively, in comparison with a standard', as in 'The house was comparatively inexpensive for that area of the city' and 'In an area of extreme poverty they are comparatively well off'. In modern usage it is often used loosely to mean 'rather' or 'fairly' without any suggestion of reference to a standard, as in 'She has comparatively few friends' and 'It is a comparatively quiet resort'.

compare may take either the preposition 'to' or 'with'. 'To' is used when two things or people are being likened to each other or being declared similar, as in 'He compared her hair to silk' and 'He compared his wife to Helen of

Troy'. 'With' is used when two things or people are being considered from the point of view of both similarities and differences, as in 'If you compare the new pupil's work with that of the present class you will find it brilliant', and 'If you compare the prices in the two stores you will find that the local one is the cheaper'. In modern usage the distinction is becoming blurred because the difference is rather subtle.

comparison is usually followed by the preposition 'with', as in 'In comparison with hers his work is brilliant'. However, when it means 'the action of likening something or someone to something or someone else', it is followed by 'to', as in 'the comparison of her beauty to that of Garbo'.

complementary medicine is a term applied to the treatment of illness or disorders by techniques other than conventional medicine. These include homoeopathy, osteopathy, acupuncture, acupressure, iridology, etc. The word **complementary** suggests that the said techniques complement and work alongside conventional medical techniques. **Alternative medicine** means the same as **complementary medicine**, but the term suggests that they are used instead of the techniques of conventional medicine rather than alongside them.

complex in one of its senses is used rather loosely in modern usage. It refers technically to 'an abnormal state caused by unconscious repressed desires or past experiences', as in 'an inferiority complex'. In modern usage it is used loosely to describe 'any obsessive concern or fear', as in 'She has a complex about her weight', 'He has a complex about his poor background'. **Complex** is also used to refer to 'a group of connected or similar things'. It is now used mainly of a group of buildings or units connected in some way, as in 'a shopping complex' or 'a sports complex'.

   Complex is also an adjective meaning 'complicated', as in 'His motives in carrying out the crime were complex' and 'The argument was too complex for most people to understand'.

compose, comprise and **constitute** are all similar in meaning but are used differently. **Compose** means 'to come together to make a whole, to make up'. It is most commonly found in the passive, as in 'The team was composed of young players' and 'The group was composed largely of elderly people'. It can be used in the active voice, as in 'the tribes which composed the nation' and 'the members which composed the committee', but this use is rarer. **Constitute** means the same as **compose** but it is usually used in the active voice, as in 'the foodstuffs that constitute a healthy diet' and 'the factors that constitute a healthy environment'. **Comprise** means 'to consist of, to be made up of'.

concave and **convex** are liable to be confused. **Concave** means 'curved inwards', as in 'The inside of a spoon would be described as concave'. **Convex** means 'curved outwards, bulging', as in 'The outside or bottom of a spoon would be described as convex'.

conducive, meaning 'leading to, contributing to', is followed by the preposition 'to', as in 'conditions conducive to health growth'.

conform may be followed by the preposition 'to' or the preposition 'with'. It is followed by 'to' when it means 'to keep to or comply with', as in 'conform to the conventions' and 'refuse to conform to the company regulations', and with 'with' when it means 'to agree with, to go along with', as in 'His ideas do not conform with those of the rest of the committee'.

connection and **connexion** are different forms of the same word, meaning 'a relationship between two things'. In modern usage **connection** is much the commoner spelling, as in 'no connection between the events' and 'a fire caused by a faulty connection'.

connote and **denote** are liable to be confused. **Connote** means 'to suggest something in addition to the main, basic meaning of something', as in 'the fear that the word cancer connotes' and 'The word 'home' connotes security and love'. **Denote** means 'to mean or indicate', as in 'The word cancer denotes a malignant illness' and 'The word "home" denotes the place where one lives'.

consist can be followed either by the preposition 'of' or by the preposition 'in', depending on the meaning. **Consist of** means 'to be made up of, to comprise', as in 'The team consists of eleven players and two reserve players'. **Consist in** means 'to have as the chief or only element or feature, to lie in', as in 'The charm of the village consists in its isolation' and 'The effectiveness of the plan consisted in its simplicity'.

constitute *see* **compose**.

contagious and **infectious** both refer to diseases that can be passed on to other people but they do not mean the same. **Contagious** means 'passed on by physical contact', as in 'He caught a contagious skin disease while working in the clinic' and 'Venereal diseases are contagious'. **Infectious** means 'caused by airborne or waterborne microorganisms', as in 'The common cold is highly infectious and is spread by people sneezing and coughing'.

contemporary originally meant 'living or happening at the same time', as in 'Shakespeare and Marlowe were contemporary playwrights' and 'Marlowe was contemporary with Shakespeare'. Later it came to mean also 'happening at the present time, current', as in 'What is your impression of the contemporary literary scene?' and 'Contemporary moral values are often compared unfavourably with those of the past'. These two uses of **contemporary** can cause ambiguity. In modern usage it is also used to mean 'modern, up-to-date', as in 'extremely contemporary designs'.

convex *see* **concave**.

cooperate *see* **collaborate**.

co-respondent *see* **correspondent**.

correspondent and **co-respondent** are liable to be confused. **Correspondent** refers either to 'a person who communicates by letter', as in 'They were correspondents for years but had never met', or to 'a person who contributes news items to a newspaper or radio or television programme', as in 'the foreign correspondent of the *Times*'. A **co-respondent** is 'a person who has been cited in a divorce case as having committed adultery with one of the partners'.

cousin can cause confusion. The children of brothers and sisters are **first cousins** to each other. The children of **first cousins** are **second cousins** to each other. The child of one's **first cousin** and the **first cousin** of one's parents is one's **first cousin first removed**. The grandchild of one's **first cousin** or the **first cousin** of one's grandparent is one's **second cousin twice removed**.

crisis literally means 'turning point' and should be used to refer to 'a turning point in an illness', as in 'The fever reached a crisis and she survived' and 'a decisive or crucial moment in a situation, whose outcome will make a definite difference or change for better or worse', as in 'The financial situation has reached a crisis—the firm will either survive or go bankrupt'. In modern usage **crisis** is becoming increasingly used loosely for 'any worrying or troublesome situation', as in 'There's a crisis in the kitchen. The cooker's broken down'. The plural is **crises**.

criterion, meaning 'a standard by which something or someone is judged or evaluated', as 'What criterion is used for deciding which pupils will gain entrance to the school?' and 'The standard of play was the only criterion for entrance to the golf club'. It is a singular noun of which **criteria** is the plural, as in 'They must satisfy all the criteria for entrance to the club or they will be refused'.

critical has two main meanings. It means 'finding fault', as in 'His report on her work was very critical'. It also means 'at a crisis, at a decisive moment, crucial', as in 'It was a critical point in their relationship'. This meaning is often applied to the decisive stage of an illness, as in 'the critical hours after a serious operation', and is used also to describe an ill person who is at a crucial stage of an illness or dangerously ill. **Critical** also means 'involved in making judgements or assessments of artistic or creative works', as in 'give a critical evaluation of the author's latest novel'.

crucial means 'decisive, critical', as in 'His vote is crucial since the rest of the committee is split down the middle'. In modern usage it is used loosely to mean 'very important', as in 'It is crucial that you leave now'. **Crucial** is derived from crux, meaning 'a decisive point', as in 'the crux of the situation'.

curriculum is derived from Latin and originally took the plural form **curricula**, but in modern usage the plural form **curriculums** is becoming common.

curriculum vitae refers to 'a brief account of a person's qualifications and career to date'. It is often requested by an employer when a candidate is applying for a job. **Vitae** is pronounced *vee*-ti, the second syllable rhyming with my.

data was formerly used mainly in a scientific or technical context and was always treated as a plural noun, taking a plural verb, as in 'compare the data which were provided by the two research projects'. The singular form was **datum**, which is now rare. In modern usage the word **data** became used in computing as a collective noun meaning 'body of information' and is frequently used with a singular verb, as in 'The data is essential for our research'. This use has spread into the general language.

dates these are usually written in figures, as in 1956, rather than in words, as in nineteen fifty-six, except in formal contexts, such as legal documents. There are various ways of writing dates. The standard form in Britain is becoming day followed by month followed by year, as in '24 February 1970'. In North America the standard form of this is 'February 24, 1970', and that is a possibility in Britain also. Alternatively, some people write '24th February 1970'. Care should be taken with the writing of dates entirely in numbers, especially if one is corresponding with someone in North America. In Britain the day of the month is put first, the month second and the year third, as in '2/3/50', '2 March 1950'. In North America the month is put first, followed by the day of the month and the year. Thus in North America '2/3/50' would be '3 February 1950'.

Centuries may be written either in figures, as in 'the 19th century', or in words, as in 'the nineteenth century'

Decades and centuries are now usually written without apostrophes. as in '1980s' and '1990s'.

datum *see* **data**.

deadly and **deathly** both refer to death but they have different meanings. **Deadly** means 'likely to cause death, fatal', as in 'His enemy dealt him a deadly blow with his sword' and 'He contracted a deadly disease in the jungle'. **Deathly** means 'referring to death, resembling death', as in 'She was deathly pale with fear'.

decimate literally means 'to kill one in ten' and is derived from the practice in ancient Rome of killing every tenth soldier as a punishment for mutiny. In modern usage it has come to mean 'to kill or destroy a large part of', as in 'Disease has decimated the population'. It has also come to mean 'to reduce considerably', as in 'the recession has decimated the jobs in the area'.

defective and **deficient** are similar in meaning but are not interchangeable. **Defective** means 'having a fault, not working properly', as in 'return the defective vacuum cleaner to the shop', 'The second-hand car proved to be defective' and 'He cannot be a pilot as his eyesight is defective'. **Deficient** means 'having a lack, lacking in', as in 'The athlete is very fast but he is deficient in strength' and 'Her diet is deficient in vitamin C'.

deficient *see* **defective**.

definite article *see* **the**.

delusion and **illusion** in modern usage are often used interchangeably but they are not quite the same. **Delusion** means 'a false or mistaken idea or belief', as in 'He is under the delusion that he is brilliant' and 'suffer from delusions of grandeur'. It can be part of a mental disorder, as in 'He suffers from the delusion that he is

Napoleon'. **Illusion** means 'a false or misleading impression', as in 'There was no well in the desert—it was an optical illusion', 'The conjurer's tricks were based on illusion' and 'the happy childhood illusions that everyone lived happy ever after'.

demise is a formal word for death, as in 'He never recovered from the demise of his wife'. In modern usage it applies to the ending of an activity, as in 'The last decade saw the demise of coal-mining in the area'. In modern usage it has come to mean also 'the decline or failure of an activity', as in 'the gradual demise of his business'.

dénouement means 'the final outcome', as in 'The novel had a unexpected denouement'. It is pronounced day-*noo*-mon.

derisive and **derisory** are both adjectives connected with the noun 'derision' but they have different meanings. **Derisive** means 'expressing derision, scornful, mocking' as in 'give a derisive smile' and 'His efforts were met with derisive laughter'. Derisory means 'deserving derision, ridiculous' as in 'Their attempts at playing the game were derisory'. **Derisory** is frequently used to mean 'ridiculously small or inadequate', as in 'The salary offered was derisory'.

despatch and **dispatch** are interchangeable. It is most common as a verb meaning 'to send', as in 'despatch/dispatch an invitation'. It is rarer as a noun. It means 'a message or report, often official', as in 'receive a despatch/dispatch that the soldiers were to move on'. It also means 'rapidity, speed', as in 'carry out the orders with despatch/dispatch'.

dessert, pudding, sweet and **afters** all mean the same thing. They refer to the last and sweet course of a meal. **Dessert** has relatively recently become the most widespread of these terms. **Pudding** was previously regarded by the upper and middle classes as the most acceptable word of these, but it is now thought of by many as being rather old-fashioned or as being more suited to certain types of dessert than others—thus syrup sponge would be a pudding, but not fresh fruit salad. **Sweet** is a less formal word and is regarded by some people as being lower-class or regional. **Afters** is common only in very informal English.

devil's advocate is a phrase that is often misunderstood. It means 'someone who points out the possible flaws or faults in an argument etc', as in 'He played the devil's advocate and showed her the weakness in her argument so that she was able to perfect it before presenting it to the committee'. The phrase is sometimes wrongly thought of as meaning 'someone who defends an unpopular point of view or person'.

diagnosis and **prognosis** are liable to be confused. Both are used with reference to disease but have different meanings. **Diagnosis** refers to 'the identification of a disease or disorder', as in 'She had cancer but the doctor failed to make the correct diagnosis until it was too late'. **Prognosis** refers to 'the prediction of the likely course of a disease or disorder', as in 'According to the doctor's prognosis, the patient will be dead in six months'.

dice was originally the plural form of the singular noun **die**, but **die** is now rarely used. Instead, **dice** is used as both a singular and a plural noun, as in 'throw a wooden dice' and 'use three different dice in the same game'.

different is most usually followed by the preposition 'from', as in 'Their style of living is different from ours'. **Different from** is considered to be the most correct construction, particularly in formal English. **Different to** is used in informal situations, as in 'His idea of a good time is different to ours'. **Different than** is used in American English.

dilemma is frequently used wrongly. It refers to 'a situation in which one is faced with two or more equally undesirable possibilities', as in 'I can't decide which of the offers to accept. It's a real dilemma'.

dinner, lunch, supper and **tea** are terms that can cause confusion. Their use can vary according to class, region of the country and personal preference. Generally speaking, people who have their main meal in the evening call it **dinner**. However, people who have their main meal in the middle of the day frequently call this meal **dinner**. People who have **dinner** in the evening usually refer to their midday meal, usually a lighter meal, as **lunch**. A more formal version of this word is **luncheon**, which is now quite a rare word. **Supper** has two meanings, again partly dependent on class and region. It can refer either to the main meal of the day if it is eaten in the evening—when it is virtually a synonym for **dinner**. Alternatively, it can refer to a light snack, such as cocoa and toasted cheese, eaten late in the evening before going to bed. **Tea** again has two meanings when applied to a meal. It either means a light snack-type meal of tea, sandwiches and cakes eaten in the late afternoon. Alternatively, it can refer to a cooked meal, sometimes taken with tea, and also referred to as **high tea**, eaten in the early evening, rather than **dinner** later in the evening.

disabled is objected to by some people on the grounds that it is a negative term, but it is difficult to find an acceptable alternative. In politically correct language **physically challenged** has been suggested as has **differently abled**, but neither of these has gained widespread use. It should be noted that the use of 'the disabled' should be avoided. 'Disabled people' should be used instead.

disablism and **disableism** mean 'discrimination against disabled people', as in 'He felt his failure to get a job was because of disablism'. **Disablist** and **disableist** are adjectives meaning 'showing or practising disablism', as in 'guilty of disablist attitudes'. They also refer to 'a person who discriminates on the grounds of disability', as in 'That employer is a disablist'.

disassociate and **dissociate** are used interchangeably, as in 'She wished to disassociate/dissociate herself from the statement issued by her colleagues', but **dissociate** is the more usual.

discover and **invent** are not interchangeable. **Discover** means 'to find something that is already in existence but is generally unknown', as in 'discover a new route to China' and 'discover the perfect place for a holiday'.

Invent means 'to create something that has never before existed', as in 'invent the telephone' and 'invent a new form of heating system'.

disempowered in modern usage does not mean only 'having one's power removed', as in 'The king was disempowered by the invading general', but also means the same as 'powerless', as in 'We are disempowered to give you any more money'. **Disempowered** is seen in politically correct language as a more positive way of saying **powerless**.

disinterested and **uninterested** are often used interchangeably in modern usage to mean 'not interested, indifferent', as in 'pupils totally disinterested/uninterested in school work'. Many people dislike **disinterested** being used in this way and regard it as a wrong use, but it is becoming increasingly common. **Disinterested** also means 'impartial, unbiased', as in 'ask a disinterested party to settle the dispute between them'.

disorient and **disorientate** are used interchangeably. 'The town had changed so much since his last visit that he was completely disoriented/disorientated' and 'After the blow to her head she was slightly disoriented/disorientated'.

divorcee refers to 'a divorced person', as in 'a club for divorcees'. **Divorcé** refers to 'a divorced man', and **divorcée** to 'a divorced woman'.

double negative the occurrence of two negative words in a single sentence or clause, as in 'He didn't say nothing' and 'We never had no quarrel'. This is usually considered incorrect in standard English, although it is a feature of some social or regional dialects. The use of the double negative, if taken literally, often has the opposite meaning to the one intended. Thus 'He didn't say nothing' conveys the idea that 'He said something'.

Some double negatives are considered acceptable, as in 'I wouldn't be surprised if they don't turn up', although it is better to restrict such constructions to informal contexts. The sentence quoted conveys the impression that the speaker will be quite surprised if 'they' do 'turn up'. Another example of an acceptable double negative is 'I can't not worry about the children. Anything could have happened to them'. Again this type of construction is best restricted to informal contexts.

It is the semi-negative forms, such as 'hardly' and 'scarcely', that cause most problems with regard to double negatives, as in 'We didn't have hardly any money to buy food' and 'They didn't have barely enough time to catch the bus'. Such sentences are incorrect.

doubtful and **dubious** can be used interchangeably in the sense of 'giving rise to doubt, uncertain', as in 'The future of the project is dubious/doubtful', and in the sense of 'having doubts, unsure', as in 'I am doubtful/dubious about the wisdom of going'. **Dubious** also means 'possibly dishonest or bad', as in 'of dubious morals'.

draughtsman/woman and **draftsman/woman** are not the same. **Draughtsman/woman** refers to 'a person who draws detailed plans of a building, etc', as in 'study the plans of the bridge prepared by the draughtsman'. **Draftsman/woman** refers to 'a person who prepares a preliminary version of plans, etc', as in 'several draftswomen working on the draft parliamentary bills'.

drawing room *see* **sitting room**.

dreamed and **dreamt** are interchangeable both as the past tense and the past participle of the verb 'dream', as in 'She dreamed/dreamt about living in the country' and in 'He has dreamed/dreamt the same dream for several nights'.

drier and **dryer** can both be used to describe 'a machine or appliance that dries', as in 'hair-drier/hair-dryer' and 'tumbler drier/dryer'. As an adjective meaning 'more dry', **drier** is the usual word, as in 'a drier summer than last year'.

dubious *see* **doubtful**.

due to, owing to and **because of** should not be used interchangeably. Strictly speaking, **due to** should be used only adjectivally, as in 'His poor memory is due to brain damage' and 'cancellations due to bad weather'. When a prepositional use is required **owing to** and **because of** should be used, as in 'the firm was forced to close owing to a lack of capital' and 'The train was cancelled because of snow on the line'. In modern usage it is quite common for **due to** to be used instead of **owing to** or **because of** because the distinction is rather difficult to comprehend.

e.g. means 'for example' and is an abbreviation of the Latin phrase *exempli gratia*. It is used before examples of something just previously mentioned, as in 'He cannot eat dairy products, e.g. milk, butter and cream'. A comma is usually placed just before it and, unlike some abbreviations, it has full stops.

each other and **one another** used not to be used interchangeably. It was taught that **each other** should be used when only two people are involved and that **one another** should be used when more than two people are involved, as in 'John and Mary really love each other' and 'All the members of the family love one another'. In modern use this restriction is often ignored.

EC and **EEC** both refer to the same thing, but **EC**, the abbreviation for **Economic Community** replaced **EEC**, the abbreviation for **European Economic Community**.

Both have now been replaced by **EU**, for **European Union**.

effeminate *see* **female**.

egoist and **egotist** are frequently used interchangeably in modern usage. Although they are not, strictly speaking, the same, the differences between them are rather subtle. **Egoist** refers to 'a person intent on self-interest, a selfish person', as in 'an egoist who never gave a thought to the needs of others'. **Egotist** refers to 'a person who is totally self-centred and obsessed with his/her own concerns', as in 'a real egotist who was always talking about herself'.

eke out originally meant 'to make something more adequate by adding to it or supplementing it', as in 'The poor mother eked out the small amount of meat with a lot of vegetables to feed her large family'. It can now also mean 'to make something last longer by using it sparingly', as in 'try to eke out our water supply until we reach a town', and 'to succeed or make with a great deal of effort', as in 'eke out a meagre living from their small farm'.

elder and **older** are not interchangeable. **Elder** is used only of people, as in 'The smaller boy is the elder of the two'. It is frequently used of family relationships, as in 'His elder brother died before him'. **Older** can be used of things as well as people, as in 'The church looks ancient but the castle is the older of the buildings' and 'The smaller girl is the older of the two'. It also can be used of family relationships, as in 'It was his older brother who helped him'. **Elder** used as a noun suggests experience or worthiness as well as age, as in 'Important issues used to be decided by the village elders' and 'Children should respect their elders and betters'.

elderly, as well as meaning 'quite or rather old', as in 'a town full of middle-aged and elderly people', is a more polite term than 'old', no matter how old the person referred to is, as in 'a residential home for elderly people'. **Elderly** is used only of people, except when used humorously, as in 'this cheese is getting rather elderly'.

eldest and **oldest** follow the same pattern as **elder** and **older**, as in 'The smallest boy is the eldest of the three', 'His eldest brother lived longer than any of them', 'The castle is the oldest building in the town' and 'He has four brothers but the oldest one is dead'.

empathy and **sympathy** are liable to be confused although they are not interchangeable. **Empathy** means 'the ability to imagine and share another's feelings, experiences, etc', as in 'As a single parent herself, the journalist has a real empathy with women bringing up children on their own' and 'The writer felt a certain empathy with the subject of his biography since they both came from a poverty-stricken childhood'. **Sympathy** means 'a feeling of compassion, pity or sorrow towards someone', as in 'feel sympathy for homeless children' and 'show sympathy towards the widow'.

endemic is usually used to describe a disease and means 'occurring in a particular area', as in 'a disease endemic to the coastal areas of the country' and 'difficult to clear the area of endemic disease'.

enervate is a word that is frequently misused. It means 'to weaken, to lessen in vitality', as in 'she was enervated by the extreme heat' and 'Absence of funding had totally enervated the society'. It is often wrongly used as though it meant the opposite.

enquiry and **inquiry** are frequently used interchangeably, as in 'make enquiries/inquiries about her health'. However some people see a distinction between them and use **enquiry** for ordinary requests for information, as in 'make enquiries about the times of trains'. They use **inquiry** only for 'investigation', as in 'The police have begun a murder inquiry' and 'launch an inquiry into the hygiene standards of the food firm'.

equal can be followed either by the preposition 'with' or the preposition 'to', but the two constructions are not interchangeable. **Equal to** is used in such sentences as 'He wished to climb the hill but his strength was not equal to the task'. **Equal with** is used in such sentences as 'After many hours of playing the two players remained equal with each other' and 'The women in the factory are seeking a pay scale equal with that of men'.

equally should not be followed by 'as'. Examples of it used correctly include 'Her brother is an expert player but she is equally talented' and 'He is trying hard but his competitors are trying equally hard'. These should not read 'but she is equally as talented' nor 'but his competitors are trying equally as hard'.

Esq. a word that can be used instead of 'Mr' when addressing an envelope to a man, as in 'John Jones, Esq.'. It is mostly used in formal contexts. Note that Esq. is used instead of 'Mr', not as well as it. It is usually spelt with a full stop.

etc the abbreviation of a Latin phrase *et cetera*, meaning 'and the rest, and other things'. It is used at the end of lists to indicate that there exist other examples of the kind of thing that has just been named, as in 'He grows potatoes, carrots, turnips, etc', 'The girls can play tennis, hockey, squash, etc', 'The main branch of the bank can supply francs, marks, lire, kroner, etc'. Etc is preceded by a comma and can be spelt with or without a full stop.

ethnic is a word that causes some confusion. It means 'of a group of people classified according to race, nationality, culture, etc', as in 'a cosmopolitan country with a wide variety of ethnic groups'. It is frequently used loosely to mean 'relating to race', as in 'violent clashes thought to be ethnic in origin', or 'foreign' as in 'prefer ethnic foods to British foods'.

EU the abbreviation for European Union, the term which has replaced European Community and European Economic Community.

evade and **avoid** are similar in meaning but not identical. **Evade** means 'to keep away from by cunning or deceit', as in 'The criminal evaded the police by getting his friend to impersonate him'. **Avoid** means simply 'to keep away from', as in 'Women avoid that area of town at night'.

evasion and **avoidance** are frequently applied to the nonpayment of income tax but they are not interchangeable. Tax **avoidance** refers to 'the legal nonpayment of tax by clever means'. Tax **evasion** refers to 'the illegal means of avoiding tax by cunning and dishonest means'.

even should be placed carefully in a sentence since its position can influence the meaning. Compare 'He didn't even acknowledge her' and 'He didn't acknowledge even her'. and 'He doesn't even like Jane, let alone love her' and 'He hates the whole family—he doesn't like even Jane'. This shows that **even** should be placed immediately before the word it refers to in order to avoid ambiguity. In spoken English people often place it where it feels most natural, before the verb as in 'He even finds it difficult to relax on holiday'. To be absolutely correct this should be 'He finds it difficult to relax even on holiday' or 'Even on holiday he finds it difficult to relax'.

except is commoner than **except for**. **Except** is used in such sentences as 'They are all dead except his father', 'He goes every day except Sunday'. **Except for** is used at the beginning of sentences, as in 'Except for Fred, all the workers were present', and where **except** applies to a longish phrase, as in 'There was no one present except for the maid cleaning the stairs' and 'The house was silent except for the occasional purring of the cat'. When followed by a pronoun, this should be in the accusative or objective, as in 'There was no one there except *him*' and 'Everyone stayed late except *me*'.

explicit and **implicit** are liable to be confused although they are virtually opposites. **Explicit** means 'direct, clear', as in 'The instructions were not explicit enough' and 'Give explicit reasons for your decision'. **Explicit** is often used in modern usage to mean 'with nothing hidden or implied', as in 'explicit sex scenes'. **Implicit** means 'implied, not directly expressed', as in 'There was an implicit threat in their warning' and 'an implicit criticism in his comments on their actions'. **Implicit** also means 'absolute and unquestioning', as in 'an implicit faith in his ability to succeed' and 'an implicit confidence in her talents'.

extrovert and **introvert** are liable to be confused although they are opposites. **Extrovert** refers to 'a person who is more interested in what is going on around him/her than in his/her own thoughts and feelings, such a person usually being outgoing and sociable', as in 'She is a real extrovert who loves to entertain the guests at parties'. **Introvert** refers to 'a person who is more concerned with his/her own thoughts and feelings than with what is going around him/her, such a person usually being shy and reserved', as in 'an introvert who hates having to speak in public' and 'introverts who prefer to stay at home than go to parties'. Both **extrovert** and **introvert** can be adjectives as well as nouns, as in 'extrovert behaviour' and 'introvert personality'. Note the spelling of **extrovert**. It was formerly spelt with an *a* instead of an *o*.

fahrenheit *see* **Celsius**.

family name is used in politically correct language instead of **maiden name** since this is thought to imply that all women are virgins before they are married. Thus 'Her family name was Jones' would be used instead of 'Her maiden name was Jones'. Another politically correct term is **birth name**, as in 'Her birth name was Jones'.

fantastic literally means 'relating to fantasy, fanciful, strange', as in 'fantastic dreams' and 'tales of fantastic events'. In modern usage it is often used informally to mean 'exceptionally good, excellent', as in 'have a fantastic holiday' and 'be a fantastic piano player'. It can also mean in informal usage 'very large', as in 'pay a fantastic sum of money'.

farther and **further** are not used interchangeably in all situations in modern usage. **Farther** is mainly restricted to sentences where physical distance is involved, as in 'It is farther to Glasgow from here than it is to Edinburgh'. **Further** can also be used in this sense, as in 'It is further to the sea than I thought'. When referring to time or extent, **further** is used, as in 'Further time is required to complete the task' and 'The police have ordered further investigations'. It can also mean 'additional', as in 'We shall require further supplies'. **Further**, unlike **farther**, can be used as a verb to mean 'to help the progress or development about', as in 'further the cause of freedom'.

faux pas is a French phrase that has been adopted into the English language. It means 'a social blunder, an indiscreet or embarrassing remark or deed', as in 'The hostess made a faux pas when she asked after her guest's wife, not knowing that they had divorced last year'. **Faux** is pronounced to rhyme with *foe*, and **pas** is pronounced *pa*.

fax is an abbreviation of 'facsimile' and refers to 'an electronic system for transmitting documents using telephone lines'. As a noun **fax** can refer to the machine transmitting the documents, as in 'the fax has broken down again'; to the system used in the transmission, as in 'send the report by fax'; and the document or documents so transmitted, as in 'He replied to my fax at once'.

female, **feminine** and **feminist** all relate to women but they are by no means interchangeable. **Female** refers to the sex of a person, animal or plant, as in 'the female members of the group', 'the female wolf and her cubs' and 'the female reproductive cells'. It refers to the childbearing sex and contrasts with 'male'. **Feminine** means 'having qualities that are considered typical of women or are traditionally associated with women', as in 'wear feminine clothes', 'take part in supposedly feminine pursuits, such as cooking and sewing' and 'feminine hairstyles'. It is the opposite of 'masculine'. It can be used of men as well as women, when it is usually derogatory, as in 'He has a very feminine voice' and 'He walks in a very feminine way'. When applied in a derogatory way to a man, **feminine** means much the same as **effeminate**. **Feminine** also applies to the gender of words, as in 'Lioness is the feminine form of lion'. **Feminist** means 'referring to feminism', 'feminism' being 'a movement based on the belief that women should have the same rights, opportunities, etc', as in 'management trying to avoid appointing anyone with feminist ideas' and 'Equal opportunities is one of the aims of the feminist movement'.

ferment and **foment** can both mean 'to excite, to stir up', as in 'Troublemakers out to ferment discontent' and 'People out to foment trouble in the crowd'. Both words have other meanings that do not relate to each other. **Ferment** means 'to undergo the chemical process known as fermentation', as in 'home-made wine fermenting in the basement'. **Foment** means 'to apply warmth and moisture to in order to lessen pain or discomfort', as in 'foment the old man's injured hip'.

few and **a few** do not convey exactly the same meaning. **Few** is used to mean the opposite of 'many', as in 'We expected a good many people to come but few did' and 'Many people entered the competition but few won a prize'. The phrase **a few** is used to mean the opposite of 'none', as in 'We didn't expect anyone to turn up but a few did' and 'We thought that none of the students would get a job but a few did'.

fewer *see* **less**.

fictional and **fictitious** are both derived from the noun 'fiction' and are interchangeable in the sense of 'imagined, invented', as in 'a fictional character based on an old man whom he used to know' and 'The events in the novel are entirely fictitious'. However, **fictitious** only is used in the sense of 'invented, false', as in 'an entirely fictitious account of the accident' and 'think up fictitious reasons for being late'.

fill in and **fill out** are both used to mean 'to complete a form, etc, by adding the required details', as in 'fill in/fill out an application form for a passport'. In British English **fill in** is the more common term, although **fill out** is the accepted term in American English.

first and **firstly** are now both considered acceptable in lists, although formerly **firstly** was considered unacceptable. Originally the acceptable form of such a list was as in 'There are several reasons for staying here. First, we like the house, secondly we have pleasant neighbours, thirdly we hate moving house'. Some users now prefer to use the adjectival forms of 'second' and 'third' when using **first**, as in 'He has stated his reasons for going to another job. First, he has been offered a higher salary, second, he has more opportunities for promotion, third, he will have a company car'. As indicated, **firstly** is now quite acceptable and is the form preferred by many people, as in 'They have several reasons for not having a car. Firstly they have very little money, secondly, they live right next to the bus-stop, thirdly, they feel cars are not environmentally friendly'.

first name *see* **Christian name**.

fish and **fishes** are both found as plural forms of 'fish', but **fish** is by far the more widely used form, as in 'He keeps tropical fish', 'Some fish live in fresh water and some in the sea' and 'there are now only three fish in the tank'. **Fishes** is rarely used but when it is, it is usually used to refer to different species of fish, as in 'He is comparing the fishes of the Pacific Ocean with those of the Indian Ocean'. **Fish** can also be used in this case.

flak originally referred to 'gunfire aimed at enemy aircraft', as in 'Pilots returning across the English Channel encountered heavy flak'. In modern usage it is also applied to 'severe criticism', as in 'the government receiving flak for raising taxes'.

flammable and **inflammable** both mean 'easily set on fire, burning easily', as in 'Children's nightclothes should not be made of flammable/inflammable material' and 'The chemical is highly flammable/inflammable'. **Inflammable** is frequently misused because some people wrongly regard it as meaning 'not burning easily', thinking that it is like such words as 'incredible', 'inconceivable' and 'intolerant' where the prefix 'in' means 'not'.

flotsam and **jetsam** are often used together to refer to 'miscellaneous objects, odds and ends', as in 'We have moved most of the furniture to the new house—there's just the flotsam and jetsam left', and 'vagrants, tramps', as in 'people with no pity in their hearts for the flotsam and jetsam of society'. In the phrase **flotsam and jetsam** they are used as though they meant the same thing but this is not the case. Both words relate to the remains of a wrecked ship, but **flotsam** refers to 'the wreckage of the ship found floating in the water', as in 'The coastguards knew the ship must have broken up when they saw bits of flotsam near the rocks', while **jetsam** refers to 'goods and equipment thrown overboard from a ship in distress in order to lighten it', as in 'The coastguards were unable to find the ship although they found the jetsam'.

forbear and **forebear** are interchangeable in one meaning of **forbear** only. **Forbear** is a verb meaning 'to refrain from', as in 'I hope she can forbear from pointing out that she was right' and this cannot be spelt **forebear**. However, **forebear** meaning 'ancestor' can also be spelt **forbear**, as in 'One of his *forebears/forbears* received a gift of land from Henry VIII'.

The verb **forbear** is pronounced with the emphasis on the second syllable as for-*bair*. The nouns **forbear** and **forebear** are pronounced alike with the emphasis on the first syllable as *for*-bair. The past tense of the verb **forbear** is **forbore**, as in 'He forbore to mention that he was responsible for the mistake'.

forever can be spelt as two words when it means 'eternally, for all time', as in 'doomed to separate forever/for ever' and 'have faith in the fact that they would dwell forever/for ever with Christ'. In the sense of 'constantly or persistently', only **forever** is used, as in 'His wife was forever nagging' and 'the child was forever asking for sweets'.

former and **latter** are opposites. **Former** refers to 'the first of two people or things mentioned' while **latter** refers to 'the second of two people or things mentioned', as in 'He was given two options, either to stay in his present post but accept less money or to be transferred to another branch of the company. He decided to accept the former/latter option'. **Former** also means 'previous, at an earlier time', as in 'He is a former chairman of the company' and 'She is a former holder of the championship title'.

further *see* **farther**.

gaol *see* **jail**.

gay originally meant 'merry, light-hearted', as in 'the gay laughter of children playing' and 'everyone feeling gay at the sight of the sunshine'. Although this meaning still exists in modern usage, it is rarely used since **gay** has come to be an accepted word for 'homosexual', as in 'gay rights' and 'gay bars'. Although the term can be applied to men or women it is most commonly applied to men, the corresponding word for women being **lesbian**. There is a growing tendency among homosexuals to describe themselves as **queer**, a term that was formerly regarded as being offensive.

geriatric is frequently found in medical contexts to mean 'elderly' or 'old', as in 'an ever-increasing number of geriatric patients' and 'a shortage of geriatric wards'. In such contexts **geriatric** is not used in a belittling or derogatory way, **geriatrics** being the name given to the branch of medicine concerned with the health and diseases of elderly people. However, **geriatric** is often used in the general language to refer to old people in a derogatory or scornful way, as in 'geriatric shoppers getting in the way' or 'geriatric drivers holding up the traffic'.

gibe and **jibe** both mean 'to jeer at, mock, make fun of', as in 'rich children gibing/jibing at the poor children for wearing out-of-date clothes'. **Gibe** and **jibe** are nouns as well as verbs as in 'politicians tired of the gibes/jibes of the press'.

Gipsy and **Gypsy** are both acceptable spellings, as in 'Gipsies/Gypsies travelling through the country in their caravans'. Some people object to the word **Gipsy** or **Gypsy**, preferring the word traveller, as in 'councils being asked to build sites for travellers'. The term **traveller** is used to apply to a wider range of people who travel the country, as in 'New Age travellers', and not just to Gipsies, who are Romany in origin.

girl means 'a female child or adolescent', as in 'separate schools for girls and boys' and 'Girls tend to mature more quickly than boys'. However it is often applied to a young woman, or indeed to a woman of any age, as in 'He asked his wife if she was going to have a night out with the girls from the office'. Many women object to this use, regarding it as patronizing, although the user of the term does not always intend to convey this impression.

gourmand and **gourmet** and **glutton** all have reference to food but they do not mean quite the same thing. **Gourmand** refers to 'a person who likes food and eats a lot of it', as in 'Gourmands tucking into huge helpings of the local food'. It means much the same as **glutton**, but **glutton** is a more condemnatory term, as in 'gluttons stuffing food into their mouths'. **Gourmet** is a more refined term, being used to refer to 'a person who enjoys food and who is discriminating and knowledgeable about it', as in 'gourmets who spend their holidays seeking out good local restaurants and produce'. In modern usage **gourmet** is often used as an adjective to mean 'high-class, elaborate, expensive', as in 'gourmet restaurants' and 'gourmet foods'.

graffiti Italian in origin and actually the plural form of **graffito**, meaning a single piece of writing or drawing, but this is now hardly ever used in English.

green is used to mean 'concerned with the conservation of the environment', as in 'a political party concerned with green issues' and 'buy as many green products as possible'. The word is derived from German *grün*, the political environmental lobby having started in West Germany, as it was then called.

grey and **gray** are both acceptable spellings. In British English, however, **grey** is the more common, as in 'different shades of grey' and 'grey hair', but **gray** is the standard form in American English.

gypsy *see* **gipsy**.

handicapped is disliked by some people because they feel it's too negative a term. There is as yet no widespread alternative apart from **disabled**, although various suggestions have been made as part of the politically correct language movement, such as **physically challenged** and **differently abled**.

hard and **soft** are both terms applied to drugs. **Hard drugs** refer to 'strong drugs that are likely to be addictive', as in 'Heroin and cocaine are hard drugs'. **Soft drugs** refer to 'drugs that are considered unlikely to cause addiction', as in 'cannabis and other soft drugs'.

hardly is used to indicate a negative idea. Therefore a sentence or clause containing it does not require another negative. Sentences, such as 'I couldn't hardly see him' and 'He left without hardly a word' are *wrong*. They should read 'I could hardly see him' and 'He left with hardly a word'. **Hardly** is followed by 'when', not 'than', as in 'Hardly had he entered the house when he collapsed', although the 'than' construction is very common.

he/she is a convention used to avoid sexism. Before the rise of feminism anyone referred to, whose sex was not specified, was assumed to be male, as in 'Each pupil must take his book home' and 'Every driver there parked his car illegally'. The only exception to this occurred in situations that were thought to be particularly appropriate to women, as in 'The cook should make her own stock' and 'The nurse has left her book behind'. In modern usage where attempts are made to avoid sexism either **he/she** or 'he or she' is frequently used, as in 'Each manager is responsible for his/her department' or 'It is a doctor's duty to explain the nature of the treatment to his or her patient'. People who regard this convention as being clumsy should consider restructuring the sentence or putting it in the plural, as in 'All managers are responsible for their departments'. Some users prefer to be ungrammatical and use a plural pronoun with a singular noun, as in 'Every pupil should take their books home' and this use is becoming increasingly common, even in textbooks.

heterosexism refers to discrimination and prejudice by a heterosexual person against a homosexual one, as in 'He was convinced that he had not got the job because he was gay—that the employer had been guilty of heterosexism'.

historic and **historical** are both adjectives formed from the noun 'history' but they are not interchangeable. **Historic** refers to events that are important enough to earn, or have earned, a place in history, as in 'Nelson's historic victory at Trafalgar' and 'the astronaut's historic landing on the moon'. It can be used loosely to mean 'extremely memorable', as in 'attend a historic party'. **Historical** means 'concerning past events', as in 'historical studies', or 'based on the study of history'.

hopefully has two meanings. The older meaning is 'with hope', as in 'The child looked hopefully at the sweet shop window' and 'It is better to travel hopefully than to arrive'. A more recent meaning, which is disliked by some people, means 'it is to be hoped that', as in 'Hopefully we shall soon be there'.

humanism and **humanitarianism** are liable to be confused. **Humanism** is a philosophy that values greatly human beings and their rôle, and rejects the need for religion, as in 'She was brought up as a Christian but she decided to embrace humanism in later life'. **Humanitarianism** refers to the philosophy and actions of people who wish to improve the lot of their fellow human beings and help them, as in 'humanitarians trying to help the refugees by taking them food and clothes'.

hyper- and **hypo-** are liable to be confused. They sound rather similar but they are opposites. **Hyper-** means 'above, excessively', as in 'hyperactive', 'hyperexcitable'. **Hypo-** means 'under, beneath', as in 'hypothermia'.

I and **me** are liable to be confused. I should be used as the subject of a sentence, as in 'You and I have both been invited', 'May Jane and I play?' and me as the object, as in 'The cake was made by Mary and me' and 'My brother and father played against my mother and me'. People often assume wrongly that me is less 'polite' than I. This is probably because they have been taught that in answer to such questions as 'Who is there?' the grammatically correct reply is 'It is I'. In fact, except in formal contexts, 'It is me' is frequently found in modern usage, especially in spoken contexts. Confusion arises as to whether to use I or me after 'between'. Since 'between' is followed by an object, me is the correct form. Thus it is correct to say 'Just between you and me, I think he is dishonest'.

i.e. is the abbreviation of a Latin phrase *id est*, meaning 'that is', as in 'He is a lexicographer, i.e. a person who edits dictionaries'. It is mostly used in written, rather than formal contexts.

identical in modern usage can be followed by either 'with' or 'to'. Formerly only 'with' was considered correct, as in 'His new suit is identical with the one he bought last year'. Now 'to' is also considered acceptable, as in 'a brooch identical to one which he bought for his wife'.

illegible and **unreadable** are not totally interchangeable. **Illegible** refers to something that is impossible to make out or decipher, as in 'her handwriting is practically illegible'. **Unreadable** can also mean this, as in 'unreadable handwriting', but it can also mean 'unable to be read with understanding or enjoyment', as in 'His writing is so full of jargon that it is unreadable'.

imbroglio means 'a confused, complicated or embarrassing situation', as in 'politicians getting involved in an international imbroglio during the summit conference'. It is liable to be misspelt and mispronounced. Note the *g* which is liable to be omitted erroneously as it is not pronounced. It is pronounced im-*bro*-lio with emphasis on the second syllable which rhymes with 'foe'. **Imbroglio** is used only in formal or literary contexts.

impasse causes problems with reference to meaning, spelling and pronunciation. It means 'a difficult position or situation from which there is no way out, deadlock', as in 'The negotiations between management and workers have reached an impasse with neither side being willing to compromise'. Note the final *e* in the spelling. The first syllable can be pronounced 'am', or 'om' in an attempt at following the original French pronunciation, although in modern usage it is frequently totally anglicized as 'im'.

implicit *see* **explicit**.

imply and **infer** are often used interchangeably but they in fact are different in meaning. **Imply** means 'to suggest, to hint at', as in 'We felt that she was implying that he was lying' and 'She did not actually say that there was going to be a delay but she implied it'. **Infer** means 'to deduce, to conclude', as in 'From what the employer said we inferred that there would be some redundancies' and 'From the annual financial reports observers inferred the company was about to go bankrupt'. Note that **infer** doubles the *r* when adding '-ed' or '-ing' to form the past tense, past participle or present participle as in **inferred** and **inferring**.

impracticable and **impractical** are liable to be confused. **Impracticable** means 'impossible to put into practice, not workable', as in 'In theory the plan is fine but it is impracticable in terms of costs'. **Impractical** means 'not sensible or realistic', as in 'It is impractical to think that you will get there and back in a day'; 'not skilled at doing or making things', as in 'He is a brilliant academic but he is hopelessly impractical'.

indefinite article *see* **a, an**.

in lieu, which means 'instead of', as in 'receive extra pay in lieu of holidays', causes problems with pronunciation. It may be pronounced in lew or in loo.

indexes and **indices** are both plural forms of 'index'. In modern usage **indexes** is the more common form in general language, as in 'Indexes are essential in large reference books'. An **index** in this sense is 'an alphabetical list given at the back of a book as a guide to its contents'. The form **indices** is mostly restricted to technical contexts, such as mathematical information. **Indices** is pronounced in-dis-is and is the Latin form of the plural.

individual refers to 'a single person as opposed to a group', as in 'The rights of the community matter but so do the rights of the individual'. **Individual** is also sometimes used instead of 'person', but in such cases it is often used in a disapproving or belittling way, as in 'What an unpleasant individual she is!' and 'The individual who designed that building should be shot'.

indoor and **indoors** are not interchangeable. **Indoor** is an adjective, as in 'have an indoor match' and 'indoor games'. **Indoors** is an adverb, as in 'children playing outdoors instead of watching television indoors' and 'sleep outdoors on warm evenings instead of indoors'.

infer *see* **imply**.

infinite and **infinitesimal** are similar in meaning but are not interchangeable. **Infinite** means 'without limit', as in 'infinite space', or 'very great', as in 'have infinite patience' and 'He seems to have an infinite capacity for hard work'. **Infinitesimal** means 'very small, negligible', as in 'an infinitesimal difference in size' and 'an infinitesimal increase'. **Infinitesimal** is pronounced with the emphasis on the fourth syllable in-fin-it-*es*-im-il.

informer and **informant** both refer to 'a person who provides information' but they are used in different contexts. **Informer** is used to refer to 'a person who gives information to the police or authorities about a criminal, fugitive, etc', as in 'The local police have a group of informers who tell them what is going on in the criminal underworld' and 'The resistance worker was caught by the enemy soldier when an informer told them about his activities'. An **informant** provides more general information, as in 'My informant keeps me up-to-date with changes in personnel'.

in-law is usually found in compounds such as 'mother-in-law' and 'father-in-law'. When these compounds are in the plural the *s* should be added to the first word of the compound, not to **in-law**, as in 'mothers-in-law' and 'fathers-in-law'.

input used to be a technical term with particular application to computers. This meaning still exists and **input** can refer to the data, power, etc, put into a computer. As a verb it means 'to enter data into a computer', as in 'input the details of all the travel resorts in the area'. In modern usage it is frequently used in general language to mean 'contribution', as in 'Everyone is expected to provide some input for tomorrow's conference'. It is even found in this sense as a verb, as in 'input a great deal to the meeting'.

inquiry *see* **enquiry**.

install and **instal** are now both considered acceptable spellings. **Install** was formerly considered to be the only correct spelling and it is still the more common. The *l* is doubled in **instal** in the past participle, past tense and present participle as **installed, installing**. It means 'to put in', as in 'he installed a new television set'. The noun is spelt **instalment**.

instantaneously and **instantly** are interchangeable. Both mean 'immediately, at once', as in 'They obeyed instantaneously/instantly' and 'The accident victims were killed instantly/instantaneously'.

intense and **intensive** are not interchangeable. Intense means 'very strong, extreme', as in 'an intense desire to scream' and 'unable to tolerate the intense cold on the icy slopes'. **Intensive** means 'thorough', as in 'conduct an intensive search', and 'concentrated', as in 'an intensive course in first aid' and 'intensive bombing'.

invalid refers to two different words. If it is pronounced with the emphasis on the second syllable, as in-*val*-id it means 'not valid, no longer valid', as in 'This visa becomes invalid after six months'. If it is pronounced with the emphasis on the first syllable, as *in*-val-id, it means

'a person who is ill', as in 'The doctor has arrived to see the invalid'.

invent *see* **discover**.

inward and **inwards** are not used interchangeably. **Inward** is an adjective, as in 'an inward curve' and 'No one could guess her inward feelings'. **Inwards** is an adverb, as in 'toes turning inwards' and 'thoughts turning inwards'. **Inward** can be used as an adverb in the same way as **inwards**.

IQ is the abbreviation of 'intelligence quotient', as in 'He has a high IQ'. It is always written in capital letters and is sometimes written with full stops and sometimes not, according to preference.

irrespective is followed by the preposition 'of'. The phrase means 'not taking account of, not taking into consideration', as in 'All can go on the trip, irrespective of age'.

irrevocable is frequently misspelt and mispronounced. Note the double *r* and the *-able* ending. It is pronounced with the emphasis on the second syllable, as ir-*rev*-ok-ibl. When applied to legal judgements, etc, it is sometimes pronounced with the emphasis on the third syllable, as ir-rev-*ok*-ibl. The word means 'unable to be changed or revoked', as in 'Their decision to get divorced is irrevocable' and 'The jury's decision is irrevocable'.

its and **it's** are liable to be confused. **Its** is an adjective meaning 'belonging to it', as in 'The house has lost its charm' and 'The dog does not like its kennel'. **It's** means 'it is', as in 'Do you know if it's raining?' and 'It's not fair to expect her to do all the chores'.

jail and **gaol** are both acceptable spellings although jail is the more common. They mean 'prison' and can be both nouns and verbs, as in 'sent to jail/gaol for killing his wife' and 'jail/gaol him for his part in the bank robbery'.

jersey *see* **cardigan**.

jetsam *see* **flotsam**.

just is liable to be put in the wrong place in a sentence. It should be placed before the word it refers to, as in 'He has just one book left to sell', not 'He just has one book left to sell'. **Just** in the sense of 'in the very recent past' is used with the perfect tense, as in 'They have just finished the job', not 'They just finished the job'.

kind should be used with a singular noun, as 'This kind of accident can be avoided'. This should not read 'These kind of accidents can be avoided'. Similarly 'The children do not like that kind of film' is correct, not 'The children do not like those kind of films'. A plural noun can be used if the sentence is rephrased as 'Films of that kind are not liked by children'.

kindly can be either an adjective or adverb. The adjective means 'kind, friendly, sympathetic', as in 'A kindly lady took pity on the children and lent them some money to get home' and 'She gave them a kindly smile'. The adverb means 'in a kind manner', as in 'We were treated kindly by the local people' and 'They will not look kindly on his actions'.

kind of, meaning 'rather', as in 'That restaurant's kind of dear' and 'She's kind of tired of him', is informal and should be avoided in formal contexts.

knit in modern usage is becoming increasingly used as a noun to mean 'a knitted garment', as in 'a shop selling beautifully coloured knits'.

lady and **woman** cause controversy. **Lady** is objected to by many people when it is used instead of **woman**. Formerly, and still in some circles, it was regarded as a polite form of **woman**, as in '"Please get up and give that lady a seat", said the mother to her son'. Indeed, **woman** was thought to be rather insulting. For many people **woman** is now the preferred term and **lady** is seen as classist, because it is associated with nobility, privilege, etc, or condescending. However, **lady** is still quite commonly used, particularly when women are being addressed in a group, as in '"Ladies, I hope we can reach our sales target", said the manager' and 'Come along, ladies the bus is about to leave'. Phrases, such as **dinner lady** and **cleaning lady** are thought by some to be condescending but others still find **woman** rather insulting.

last is liable to cause confusion because it is not always clear which meaning is meant. **Last** as an adjective has several meanings. It can mean 'final', as in 'That was the musician's last public appearance—he died shortly after'; 'coming after all others in time or order', as in 'December is the last month in the year', 'The last of the runners reached the finishing tape'; 'latest, most recent', as in 'Her last novel is not as good as her earlier ones'; 'previous, preceding', as in 'This chapter is interesting but the last one was boring'. In order to avoid confusion it is best to use a word other than **last** where ambiguity is likely to arise. An example of a sentence which could cause confusion is 'I cannot remember the title of his last book', which could mean either 'his latest book' or 'his final book'.

latter see **former**.

lavatory see **toilet**.

lay and **lie** are liable to be confused. They are related but are used in different contexts. **Lay** means 'to put or place' and is a transitive verb, i.e. it takes an object. It is found in such sentences as 'Ask them to lay the books carefully on the table' and 'They are going to lay a new carpet in the bedroom'. **Lie**, meaning 'to rest in a horizontal position', is an intransitive verb, i.e. it does not take an object. It is found in such sentences as 'They were told to lie on the ground' and 'Snow is apt to lie on the mountain tops for a long time'. The confusion between the two words arises from the fact that **lay** is also the past tense of **lie**, as in 'He lay still on the ground' and 'Snow lay on the mountain tops'. The past tense of **lay** is **laid**, as in 'They laid the books on the table'. There is another verb **lie**, meaning 'to tell falsehoods, not to tell the truth', as in 'He was told to lie to the police'. The past tense of **lie** in this sense is **lied**, as in 'We suspect that he lied but we cannot prove it'.

leading question is often used wrongly. It should be used to mean 'a question that is so worded as to invite (or lead to) a particular answer desired by the questioner', as in 'The judge refused to allow the barrister to ask the witness the question on the grounds that it was a leading question'. However, it is often used wrongly to mean 'a question that is difficult, unfair or embarrassing'.

learn and **teach** are liable to be confused. **Learn** means 'to gain information or knowledge about', as in 'She learnt Spanish as a child', or 'to gain the skill of', as in 'She is learning to drive'. **Teach** means 'to give instruction in, to cause to know something or be able to do something', as in 'She taught her son French' and 'She taught her son to swim'. **Learn** is frequently used wrongly instead of **teach**, as in 'She learnt us to drive'.

learned and **learnt** are both acceptable forms of the past participle and past tense of the verb 'to learn', as in 'She has now learned/learnt to drive' and 'They learned/learnt French at school'. **Learned** in this sense can be pronounced either lernd or leant. However, **learned** can also be an adjective, meaning 'having much knowledge, erudite', as in 'an learned professor', or 'academic', as in 'learned journals'. It is pronounced ler-ned.

leave and **let** are not interchangeable. **Leave go** should not be substituted for **let go** in such sentences as 'Do not let go of the rope'. 'Do not leave go of the rope' is considered to be incorrect. However both **leave alone** and **let alone** can be used in the sense of 'to stop disturbing or interfering with', as in 'Leave/let the dog alone or it will bite you' and 'leave/let your mother alone—she is not feeling well'. **Leave alone** can also mean 'leave on one's own, cause to be alone', as in 'Her husband went away and left her alone', but **let alone** cannot be used in this sense. **Let alone** can also mean 'not to mention, without considering', as in 'They cannot afford proper food, let alone a holiday', but **leave alone** should not be used in this sense.

legible and **readable** are not interchangeable. **Legible** means 'able to be deciphered or made out', as in 'His writing is scarcely legible'. **Readable** can also be used in this sense, as in 'His handwriting is just not readable'. However **readable** is also used to mean 'able to be read with interest or enjoyment', as in 'He is an expert on the subject but I think his books are simply not readable' and 'I find her novels very readable but my friend does not like her style'.

lend and **loan** can cause confusion. **Lend** is used as a verb in British English to mean 'to allow someone the use of temporarily', as in 'Can you lend me a pen?' and 'His father refused to lend him any money'. **Loan** is a noun meaning 'something lent, the temporary use of', as in 'They thanked her for the loan of her car'. In American English **loan** is used as a verb to mean **lend**, and this use is becoming common in Britain although it is still regarded as not quite acceptable.

lengthways and **lengthwise** are used interchangeably, as in 'fold the tablecloth lengthways/lengthwise' and 'measure the room lengthwise/lengthways'.

lengthy and **long** are not interchangeable. **Lengthy** means 'excessively long', as in 'We had a lengthy wait before we saw the doctor' and 'It was such a lengthy speech that most of the audience got bored'. **Lengthy** is frequently misspelt. Note the *g*.

less and **fewer** are often confused. Less means 'a smaller amount or quantity of' and is the comparative form of 'little'. It is found in sentences such as 'less milk', 'less responsibility' and 'less noise'. **Fewer** means 'a smaller number of' and is the comparative of 'few'. It is found in sentences such as 'buy fewer bottles of milk', 'have fewer responsibilities', have fewer opportunities' and 'hear fewer noises'. **Less** is commonly wrongly used where **fewer** is correct. It is common but ungrammatical to say or write 'less bottles of milk' and 'less queues in the shops during the week'.

liable to and **likely to** both express probability. They mean much the same except that **liable to** suggests that the probability is based on past experience or habit. 'He is liable to lose his temper' suggests that he has been in the habit of doing so in the past. 'He is likely to lose his temper' suggests that he will probably lose his temper, given the situation, but that the probability is not based on how he has reacted in the past. This distinction is not always adhered to, and some people use the terms interchangeably.

libel and **slander** both refer to defamatory statements against someone but they are not interchangeable. **Libel** refers to defamation that is written down, printed or drawn, as in 'The politician sued the newspaper for libel when it falsely accused him of fraud'. **Slander** refers to defamation in spoken form, as in 'She heard that one of her neighbours was spreading slander about her'. Both **libel** and **slander** can act as verbs, as in 'bring a suit against the newspaper for libelling him' and 'think that one of her neighbours was slandering her'. Note that the verb **libel** doubles the *l* in the past participle, past tense and present participle, as **libelled** and **libelling**.

licence and **license** are liable to cause confusion in British English. **Licence** is a noun meaning 'an official document showing that permission has been given to do, use or own something', as in 'require a licence to have a stall in the market', 'have a licence to drive a car', and 'apply for a pilot's licence'. **License** is a verb meaning 'to provide someone with a licence', as in 'The council have licensed him as a street trader', 'The restaurant has been licensed to sell alcohol'. Note **licensed grocer** and **licensing laws** but **off-licence**. In American English both the noun and verb are spelt **license**.

lie *see* **lay**.

light years are a measure of distance, not time. A **light year** is the distance travelled by light in one year (about six million, million miles) and is a term used in astronomy. **Light years** are often referred to in an informal context when time, not distance, is involved, as in 'Owning their own house seemed light years away' and 'It seems light years since we had a holiday'.

like tends to cause confusion. It is a preposition meaning 'resembling, similar to', as in 'houses like castles', 'gardens like jungles', 'actors like Olivier', 'She looks like her mother', 'She plays like an expert', 'The child swims like a fish' and 'Like you, he cannot stand cruelty to animals'. To be grammatically correct **like** should not be used as a conjunction. Thus 'The house looks like it has been deserted' is incorrect. It should read 'The house looks as though/if it has been deserted'. Similarly, 'Like his mother said, he has had to go to hospital' should read 'As his mother said, he has had to go to hospital'.

likeable and **likable** are both acceptable spellings. The word means 'pleasant, agreeable, friendly', as in 'He is a likeable/likable young man'.

likely to *see* **liable to**.

literally is frequently used simply to add emphasis to an idea rather than to indicate that the word, phrase, etc, used is to be interpreted word for word. Thus, 'She was literally tearing her hair out' does not mean that she was pulling her hair out by the handful but that she was very angry, anxious, frustrated, etc.

livid and **lurid** are liable to be confused although they mean different things. **Livid** means 'discoloured, of a greyish tinge', as in 'a livid bruise on her face', and 'furious', as in 'When he saw his damaged car he was livid'. **Lurid** means 'sensational, shocking', as in 'give the lurid details about finding the body', and 'garish, glaringly bright', as in 'wear a lurid shade of green'.

living room *see* **sitting room**.

loo *see* **toilet**.

lots of and **a lot of**, meaning 'many' and 'much', should be used only in informal contexts', as in '"I've got lots of toys," said the child' and 'You're talking a lot of rubbish'. They should be avoided in formal prose.

lounge *see* **sitting room**.

low and **lowly** are not interchangeable. **Low** means 'not high', as in 'a low fence', 'a low level of income', 'speak in a low voice' and 'her low status in the firm'. It can also mean 'despicable, contemptible', as in 'That was a low trick' or 'He's a low creature'. **Lowly** means 'humble', as in 'of lowly birth' and 'the peasant's lowly abode'.

lunch and **luncheon** both refer to a meal eaten in the middle of the day. **Lunch**, as in 'a business lunch' and 'have just a snack for lunch', is by far the more usual term. **Luncheon**, as in 'give a luncheon party for the visiting celebrity', is a very formal word and is becoming increasingly uncommon. *see also* **dinner**.

lurid *see* **livid**.

madam and **madame** are liable to be confused. **Madam** is the English-language form of the French **madame**. It is a form of formal of address for a woman, as in 'Please come this way, madam'. It is used in formal letters when the name of the woman being written to is not known, as in 'Dear Madam'. **Madam** can be written either with a capital letter or a lowercase letter. **Madam** is pronounced *mad*-am, with the emphasis on the first syllable. **Madame**, which is the

French equivalent of 'Mrs', is occasionally found in English, as in Madame Tussaud's, and is pronounced in the same way as **madam**. In French **madame** is pronounced ma-*dam*.

majority and **minority** are opposites. **Majority** means 'more than half the total number of', as in 'The majority of the pupils live locally' and 'the younger candidate received the majority of the votes'. **Minority** means less than half the total number of', as in 'A small minority of the football fans caused trouble' and 'Only a minority of the committee voted against the motion'. **Majority** and **minority** should not be used to describe the greater or lesser part of a single thing. Thus it is wrong to say 'The majority of the book is uninteresting'.

male, masculine and **mannish** all refer to the sex that is not female but the words are used in different ways. **Male** is the opposite of 'female' and refers to the sex of a person or animal, as in 'no male person may enter', 'a male nurse', 'a male elephant' and 'the male reproductive system'. **Masculine** is the opposite of 'feminine' and refers to people or their characteristics. It refers to characteristics, etc, that are traditionally considered to be typically **male**. Examples of its use include 'a very masculine young man', 'a deep, masculine voice'. It can be used of women, as in 'She has a masculine walk' and 'She wears masculine clothes'. When used of women it is often derogatory and is sometimes replaced with **mannish**, which is derogatory, as in 'women with mannish haircuts'. **Male** can also be used as a noun, as in 'the male of the species' 'of the robins, the male is more colourful' and 'the title can be held only by males'.

man causes a great deal of controversy. To avoid being sexist it should be avoided when it really means 'person'. 'We must find the right man for the job' should read 'We must find the right person for the job'. Similarly, 'All men have a right to a reasonable standard of living' should read 'All people have a right to a reasonable standard of living' or 'Everyone has a right to a reasonable standard of living'. Problems also arise with compounds, such as 'chairman'. In such situations 'person' is often used, as in 'chairperson'. Man is also used to mean 'mankind, humankind', as in 'Man is mortal' and 'Man has the power of thought'. Some people also object to this usage and consider it sexist. They advocate using 'humankind' or 'the human race'.

many is used in more formal contexts rather than 'a lot of' or 'lots of', as in 'The judge said the accused had had many previous convictions'. **Many** is often used in the negative in both formal and informal contexts, as in 'They don't have many friends' and 'She won't find many apples on the trees now'.

masculine *see* **male**.

may *see* **can**.

maybe and **may be** are liable to be confused although they have different meanings. **Maybe** means 'perhaps', as in 'Maybe they lost their way' and 'He said, "Maybe"

when I asked him if he was going'. It is used in more informal contexts than 'perhaps'. **May be** is used in such sentences as 'He may be poor but he is very generous' and 'They may be a little late'.

mayoress means 'the wife or partner of a male mayor', as in 'an official dinner for the mayor and mayoress'. A mayor who is a woman is called either 'mayor' or 'lady mayor'.

me *see* **I**.

meaningful originally meant 'full of meaning', as in 'make very few meaningful statements' and 'There was a meaningful silence'. In modern usage it has come to mean 'important, significant, serious', as in 'not interested in a meaningful relationship' and 'seeking a meaningful career'. The word now tends to be very much over-used.

means in the sense of 'way, method' can be either a singular or plural noun, as in 'The means of defeating them is in our hands' and 'Many different means of financing the project have been investigated'. **Means** in the sense of 'wealth' and 'resources' is plural, as in 'His means are not sufficient to support two families'.

media gives rise to confusion. In the form of **the media** it is commonly applied to the press, to newspapers, television and radio, as in 'The politician claimed that he was being harassed by the media'. **Media** is a plural form of 'medium', meaning 'means of communication', as in 'television is a powerful medium'. In modern usage **media** is beginning to be used as a singular noun, as in 'The politician blamed a hostile media for his misfortunes', but this is still regarded as being an incorrect use.

middle *see* **centre**.

mileage and **milage** are both acceptable spellings for 'the distance travelled or measured in miles', as in 'The car is a bargain, given the low mileage'. However **mileage** is much more common than **milage**. The word also means informally 'benefit, advantage', as in 'The politician got a lot of mileage from the scandal surrounding his opponent' and 'There's not much mileage in pursuing that particular line of inquiry'.

militate and **mitigate** are liable to be confused. **Militate** means 'to have or serve as a strong influence against', as in 'Their lack of facts militated against the success of their application' and 'His previous record will militate against his chances of going free'. **Mitigate** means 'to alleviate', as in 'try to mitigate the suffering of the refugees', or 'moderate', as in 'mitigate the severity of the punishment'.

millennium is liable to be misspelt. Note the double *n* which is frequently omitted in error. The plural form is **millennia**. **Millennium** refers to 'a period of 1000 years', as in 'rock changes taking place over several millennia'. In religious terms it refers to 'the thousand-year reign of Christ prophesied in the Bible'.

minority *see* **majority**.

Miss *see* **Ms**.

misuse *see* **abuse**.

mitigate *see* **militate**.

mnemonic refers to 'something that aids the memory'. For example, some people use a **mnemonic** in the form of a verse to remind them how to spell a word or to recall a date. The word is liable to be misspelt and mispronounced. Note the initial *m*, which is silent. **Mnemonic** is pronounced nim-*on*-ik, with the emphasis on the second syllable.

modern and **modernistic** are not quite the same. **Modern** means 'referring to the present time or recent times', as in 'the politics of modern times' and 'a production of Shakespeare's *Twelfth Night* in modern dress'. It also means 'using the newest techniques, equipment, buildings, etc, as in 'a modern shopping centre' and 'a modern office complex'. **Modernistic** means 'characteristic of modern ideas, fashions, etc', and is often used in a derogatory way, as in 'She says she hates that modernistic furniture'.

modus vivendi refers to 'a practical, sometimes temporary, arrangement or compromise by which people who are in conflict can live or work together', as in 'The two opposing parties on the committee will have to reach a modus vivendi if any progress is to be made'. It is a Latin phrase that literally means 'a way of living' and is pronounced *mo*-dus viv-*en*-di.

more is used to form the comparative of adjectives and adverbs that do not form the comparative by adding *-er*. This usually applies to longer adjectives, as in 'more beautiful', 'more gracious', 'more useful', and 'more flattering'. **More** should not be used with adjectives that have a comparative ending already. Thus it is wrong to write 'more happier'. **Most** is used in the same way to form the superlative of adjectives and adverbs, as in 'most beautiful', 'most gracious' etc.

Moslem *see* **Muslim**.

most *see* **more**.

movable and **moveable** are both possible spellings but **movable** is the more common, as in 'movable possessions' and 'machines with movable parts'.

Ms, Mrs and **Miss** are all used before the names of women in addressing them and in letter-writing. Formerly **Mrs** was used before the name of a married woman and **Miss** before the name of an unmarried woman or girl. In modern usage **Ms** is often used instead of **Miss** or **Mrs**. This is sometimes because the marital status of the woman is not known and sometimes from a personal preference. Many people feel that since no distinction is made between married and unmarried men when they are being addressed, no distinction should be made between married and unmarried women. On the other hand some people, particularly older women, object to the use of **Ms**.

much, except in negative sentences, is used mainly in rather formal contexts, as in 'They own much property'. 'A great deal of' is often used instead, as in 'They own a great deal of property'. In informal contexts 'a lot of' is often used instead of **much**, as in 'a lot of rubbish' not 'much rubbish'. **Much** is used in negative sentences, as in 'They do not have much money'.

Muslim and **Moslem** refer to 'a follower of the Islamic faith'. In modern usage **Muslim** is the preferred term rather than the older spelling **Moslem**.

naught and **nought** are not totally interchangeable. **Naught** means 'nothing', as in 'All his projects came to naught', and is rather a formal or literary word in this sense. **Naught** is also a less usual spelling of **nought**, which means 'zero' when it is regarded as a number, as in 'nought point one (0.1)'.

nearby and **near by** can cause problems. **Nearby** can be either an adjective, as in 'the nearby village', or an adverb, as in 'Her mother lives nearby'. **Near by** is an adverb, as in 'He doesn't have far to go—he lives near by'. In other words, the adverbial sense can be spelt either **nearby** or **near by**.

née is used to indicate the maiden or family name of a married woman, as in 'Jane Jones, née Smith'. It is derived from French, being the feminine form of the French word for 'born'. It can be spelt either with an acute accent or not—**née** or **nee**.

never in the sense of 'did not', as in 'He never saw the other car before he hit it', should be used in only very informal contexts. **Never** means 'at no time, on no occasion', as in 'He will never agree to their demands' and 'She has never been poor'. It is also used as a negative for the sake of emphasis, as in 'He never so much as smiled'.

nevertheless and **none the less** mean the same thing, as in 'He has very little money. Nevertheless/none the less he gives generously to charity'. **None the less** is usually written as three words but **nevertheless** is spelt as one word. In modern usage **none the less** is sometimes written as one word, as **nonetheless**.

next and **this** can cause confusion. **Next** in one of its senses is used to mean the day of the week, month of the year, season of the year, etc, that will follow next, as in 'They are coming next Tuesday', 'We are going on holiday next June' and 'They are to be married next summer'. **This** can also be used in this sense and so ambiguity can occur. Some people use **this** to refer to the very next Tuesday, June, summer, etc, and use **next** for the one after that. Thus someone might say on Sunday, 'I'll see you next Friday', meaning the first Friday to come, but someone else might take that to mean a week on from that because they would refer to the first Friday to come as 'this Friday'. The only solution is to make sure exactly which day, week, season, etc, the other person is referring to.

nice originally meant 'fine, subtle, requiring precision', as in 'There is rather a nice distinction between the two words', but it is widely used in the sense of 'pleasant, agreeable, etc', as in 'She is a nice person' and 'We had a nice time at the picnic'. It is overused and alternative adjectives should be found to avoid this, as in 'She is an amiable person' and 'We had an enjoyable time at the picnic'.

no one and **no-one** are interchangeable but the word is never written 'noone', unlike 'everyone'. **No one** and

no-one are used with a singular verb, as in 'No one is allowed to leave' and 'No one is anxious to leave'. They are used by some people with a plural personal pronoun or possessive case when attempts are being made to avoid sexism, as in 'No one is expected to take their child away'. The singular form is grammatically correct, as in 'No one is expected to take his/her child away', but it is clumsy. 'No one is expected to take his child away' is sexist. Nobody is interchangeable with no one, as in 'You must tell no one/nobody about this'.

nobody *see* **no one**.

none can be used with either a singular verb or plural verb. Examples of sentences using a singular verb include 'There is none of the food left' and 'None of the work is good enough' and 'None of the coal is to be used today'. In sentences where none is used with a plural noun the verb was traditionally still singular, as in 'None of the books is suitable' and 'None of the parcels is undamaged'. This is still the case in formal contexts but, in the case of informal contexts, a plural verb is often used in modern usage, as in 'None of these things are any good'.

none the less *see* **nevertheless**.

not only is frequently used in a construction with 'but also', as in 'We have not only the best candidate but also the most efficient organization' and 'The organizers of the fête not only made a great deal of money for charity but also gave a great many people a great deal of pleasure'.

nought *see* **naught**.

noxious and **obnoxious** are liable to be confused. They both refer to unpleasantness or harmfulness but they are used in different contexts. **Noxious** is used of a substance, fumes, etc, and means 'harmful, poisonous', as in 'firemen overcome by noxious fumes' and 'delinquent children having a noxious influence on the rest of the class'. **Obnoxious** means 'unpleasant, nasty, offensive', as in 'He has the most obnoxious neighbours' and 'The child's parents let him off with the most obnoxious behaviour'. **Noxious** is used in formal and technical contexts rather than **obnoxious**.

nubile originally meant 'old enough to marry, marriageable' as in 'he has five nubile daughters'. In modern usage **nubile** is frequently used in the sense of 'sexually attractive', as in 'admiring the nubile girls sunbathing on the beach' and 'nubile models posing for magazine illustrations'.

numbers can be written in either figures or words. It is largely a matter of taste which method is adopted. As long as the method is consistent it does not really matter. Some establishments, such as a publishing house or a newspaper office, will have a house style. For example, some of them prefer to have numbers up to 10 written in words, as in 'They have two boys and three girls'. If this system is adopted, guidance should be sought as to whether a mixture of figures and words in the same sentence is acceptable, as in 'We have 12 cups but only six saucers', or whether the rule should be broken in such situations as 'We have twelve cups but only six saucers'.

nutritional and **nutritious** are liable to be confused. They both refer to 'nutrition, the process of giving and receiving nourishment' but mean different things. **Nutritional** means 'referring to nutrition', as in 'doubts about the nutritional value of some fast foods' and 'people who do not receive the minimum nutritional requirements'. **Nutritious** means 'nourishing, of high value as a food', as in 'nutritious homemade soups' and 'something slightly more nutrtious than a plate of chips'.

O and **Oh** are both forms of an exclamation made at the beginning of a sentence. **Oh** is the usual spelling, as in 'Oh well. It's Friday tomorrow' and 'Oh dear, the baby's crying again'.

loan *see* **lend**.

objective and **subjective** are opposites. **Objective** means 'not influenced by personal feelings, attitudes, or prejudices', as in 'She is related to the person accused and so she cannot give an objective view of the situation' and 'It is important that all members of a jury are completely objective'. **Subjective** means 'influenced by personal feelings, attitudes and prejudices', as in 'It is only natural to be subjective in situations regarding one's children' and 'She wrote a very subjective report on the conference and did not stick to the facts'. **Objective** can also be a noun in the sense of 'aim, goal', as in 'Our objective was to make as much money as possible'. **Object** can also be used in this sense, as in 'Their main object is to have a good time'.

oblivious means 'unaware of, unconscious of, not noticing'. Traditionally it is followed by the preposition 'of', as in 'The lovers were oblivious of the rain' and 'When he is reading he is completely oblivious of his surroundings'. In modern usage its use with the preposition 'to' is also considered acceptable, as in 'They were oblivious to the fact that he was cheating them' and 'sleep soundly, oblivious to the noise'.

obnoxious *see* **noxious**.

obscene and **pornographic** are not interchangeable. **Obscene** means 'indecent, especially in a sexual way, offending against the accepted standards of decency', as in 'obscene drawings on the walls of the public toilet' and 'When his car was damaged he let out a stream of obscene language'. **Pornographic** means 'intended to arouse sexual excitement', as in 'pornographic videos' and 'magazines with women shown in pornographic poses'. **Obscene** is frequently misspelt. Note the *c* after the *s*.

oculist *see* **optician**.

of is sometimes wrongly used instead of the verb 'to have', as in 'He must of known she was lying' instead of 'He must have known she was lying'. The error arises because the two constructions sound alike when not emphasized.

Oh *see* **O**.

OK and **okay** are both acceptable spellings of an informal word indicating agreement or approval, as in

'OK/okay, I'll come with you', 'We've at last been given the OK/okay to begin building'. When the word is used as a verb it is more usually spelt **okay** because of the problem in adding endings, as in 'They've okayed our plans at last'. **OK** is sometimes written with full stops as **O.K.**

older *see* **elder**.

one is used in formal situations to indicate an indefinite person where 'you' would be used in informal situations, as in 'One should not believe all one hears' and 'One should be kind to animals'. This construction can sound rather affected. Examples of the informal 'you' include 'You would've thought he would've had more sense' and 'You wouldn't think anyone could be so stupid'. **One** when followed by 'of the' and a plural noun takes a singular verb, as in 'One of the soldiers was killed' and 'One of the three witnesses has died'. However, the constructions 'one of those … who' and 'one of the … that' take a plural verb, as in 'He is one of those people who will not take advice' and 'It is one of those houses that are impossible to heat'.

only must be carefully positioned in written sentences to avoid confusion. It should be placed before, or as close as possible before, the word to which it refers. Compare 'She drinks only wine at the weekend', 'She drinks wine only at the weekend' and 'Only she drinks wine at the weekend'. In spoken English, where the intonation of the voice will indicate which word **only** applies to it may be placed in whichever position sounds most natural, usually between the subject and the verb, as in 'She only drinks wine at the weekend'.

onto and **on to** are both acceptable forms in sentences such as 'The cat leapt onto/on to the table' and 'He jumped from the plane onto/on to the ground'. However, in sentences such as 'It is time to move on to another city' **onto** is not a possible alternative.

onward and **onwards** are not interchangeable. **Onward** is an adjective, as in 'onward motion' and 'onward progress'. **Onwards** is an adverb, as in 'march onwards' and 'proceed onwards'.

optician, ophthalmologist, optometrist and **oculist** all refer to 'a person who is concerned with disorders of the eyes' but they are not interchangeable. **Dispensing optician** refers to 'a person who makes and sells spectacles or contact lenses'. **Ophthalmic optician** refers to 'a person who tests eyesight and prescribes lenses'. **Optometrist** is another term for this. **Ophthalmologist** refers to 'a doctor who specializes in disorders of the eyes' and **oculist** is another name for this.

optimum means 'the most favourable or advantageous condition, situation, amount, degree, etc', as in 'A temperature of 20° is optimum for these plants'. It is mostly used as an adjective meaning 'most favourable or advantageous', as in 'the optimum speed to run the car at', 'the optimum time at which to pick the fruit' and 'the optimum amount of water to give the plants'. It should not be used simply as a synonym for 'best'.

optometrist *see* **optician**.

orientate and **orient** are both acceptable forms of the same word. **Orientate** is the more common in British English but the shorter form, **orient**, is preferred by some people and is the standard form in American English. They are verbs meaning 'to get one's bearings', as in 'difficult to orientate/orient themselves in the mist on the mountain'; 'to adjust to new surroundings', as in 'It takes some time to orientate/orient oneself in a new job'; 'to direct at', as in 'The course is orientated/oriented at older students'; 'to direct the interest of to', as in 'try to orientate/orient students towards the sciences'.

orthopaedic and **paediatric** are liable to be confused. They both apply to medical specialties but they are different. **Orthopaedic** means 'referring to the treatment of disorders of the bones', as in 'attend the orthopaedic clinic with an injured back'. **Paediatric** means 'referring to the treatment of disorders associated with children', as in 'Her little boy is receiving treatment from a paediatric consultant'. In American English these are respectively spelt **orthopedic** and **pediatric**.

other than can be used when **other** is an adjective or pronoun, as in 'There was no means of entry other than through a trap door' and 'He disapproves of the actions of anyone other than himself'. Traditionally, it should not be used as an adverbial phrase, as in 'It was impossible to get there other than by private car'. In such constructions **otherwise than** should be used, as in 'It is impossible to get there otherwise than by private car'. However, **other than** used adverbially is common in modern usage.

otherwise traditionally should not be used as an adjective or pronoun, as in 'Pack your clothes, clean or otherwise' and 'We are not discussing the advantages, or otherwise, of the scheme at this meeting'. It is an adverb, as in 'We are in favour of the project but he obviously thinks otherwise' and 'The hours are rather long but otherwise the job is fine'. *see* **other than**.

owing to *see* **due to**.

p *see* **pence**.

paediatric *see* **orthopaedic**.

panacea and **placebo** are liable to be confused. **Panacea** means 'a universal remedy for all ills and troubles', as in 'The new government does not have a panacea for the country's problems'. It is often used loosely to mean any remedy for any problem, as in 'She thinks that a holiday will be a panacea for his unhappiness'. **Panacea** is pronounced pan-a-*see*-a. **Placebo** refers to 'a supposed medication that is just a harmless substance given to a patient as part of a drugs trial etc', as in 'She was convinced the pills were curing her headaches but the doctor has prescribed her a placebo'. It is pronounced pla-*see*-bo.

parameter is a mathematical term that is very loosely used in modern usage to mean 'limit, boundary, framework' or 'limiting feature or characteristic', as in 'work within the parameters of our budget and resources'. The word is over-used and should be avoided where possible. The emphasis is on the second syllable as par-*am*-it-er.

paranoid is an adjective meaning 'referring to a mental disorder, called **paranoia**, characterized by delusions of persecution and grandeur', as in 'a paranoid personality'. In modern usage it is used loosely to mean 'distrustful, suspicious of others, anxious etc', as in 'It is difficult to get to know him—he's so paranoid' and 'paranoid about people trying to get his job', when there is no question of actual mental disorder. **Paranoia** is pronounced par-a-*noy*-a.

paraphernalia means 'all the bits and pieces of equipment required for something', as in 'all the paraphernalia needed to take a baby on holiday', 'put his angling paraphernalia in the car'. Strictly speaking it is a plural noun but it is now frequently used with a singular verb, as in 'The artist's paraphernalia was lying all over the studio'. **Paraphernalia** is liable to be misspelt. Note the *er* before the *n*.

parlour *see* **sitting room**.

particular means 'special, exceptional', as in 'a matter of particular importance', or 'individual', as in 'Have you a particular person in mind?', and 'concerned over details, fastidious', as in 'very particular about personal hygiene'. **Particular** is often used almost meaninglessly, as in 'this particular dress' and 'this particular car', when **particular** does not add much to the meaning.

partner can be used to indicate one half of an established couple, whether the couple are married or living together, as in 'Her partner was present at the birth of the child'.

passed and **past** are liable to be confused. **Passed** is the past participle and past tense of the verb 'to pass', as in 'She has already passed the exam' and 'They passed an old man on the way'. **Past** is used as a noun, as in 'He was a difficult teenager but that is all in the past now' and 'He has a murky past'. It is also used as an adjective, as in 'I haven't seen him in the past few weeks' and 'Her past experiences affected her opinion of men'. **Past** can also be a preposition, as in 'We drove past their new house', 'It's past three o'clock' and 'He's past caring'. It can also be an adverb, as in 'He watched the athletes running past' and 'The boat drifted past'.

patent, in British English, is usually pronounced *pay*-tent, as in 'patent leather dancing shoes'. **Patent** in the sense of 'obvious', as in 'his patent dislike of the situation' and 'It was quite patent that she loved him' is also pronounced in that way. **Patent** in the sense of 'a legal document giving the holder the sole right to make or sell something and preventing others from imitating it', as in 'take out a patent for his new invention', can be pronounced either *pay*-tent or *pat*-ent. **Patent** in this last sense can also be a verb, as in 'He should patent his invention as soon as possible'.

peddler and **pedlar** are not interchangeable in British English. **Peddler** refers particularly to 'a person who peddles drugs', as in 'drug-peddlers convicted and sent to prison'. **Pedlar** refers to 'a person who sells small articles from house to house or from place to place', as in 'pedlars selling ribbons at the fair'.

pence, p and **pennies** are liable to be confused. **Pence** is the plural form of 'penny', as in 'There are a hundred pence in the pound'. It is commonly found in prices, as in 'apples costing 10 pence each'. **Pence** has become much more common than 'pennies', which tends to be associated with pre-decimalization money (the British currency was decimalized in 1972), as in 'There were twelve pennies in one shilling'. **Pence** is sometimes used as though it were singular, as in 'have no one-pence pieces'. In informal contexts **p** is often used, as in 'Have you got a 10p (pronounced ten pee) piece' and 'Those chocolate bars are fifteen p'. **Pence** in compounds is not pronounced in the same way as pence was pronounced in compounds before decimalization. Such words as 'ten pence' are now pronounced *ten pens*, with equal emphasis on each word. In pre-decimalization days it was pronounced *ten*-pens, with the emphasis on the first word.

pennies *see* **pence**.

people is usually a plural noun and so takes a plural verb, as in 'The local people were annoyed at the stranger's behaviour' and 'People were being asked to leave'. In the sense of 'nation', 'race' or 'tribe' it is sometimes treated as a singular noun, as in 'the nomadic peoples of the world'. **People** acts as the plural of 'person', as in 'There's room for only one more person in that car but there's room for three people in this one'. In formal or legal contexts **persons** is sometimes used as the plural of 'person', as in 'The lift had a notice saying "Room for six persons only"'.

per capita is a formal expression meaning 'for each person', as in 'The cost of the trip will be £300 per capita'. It is a Latin phrase which has been adopted into English and literally means 'by heads'. It is pronounced per *ka*-pi-ta.

per cent is usually written as two words. It is used adverbially in combination with a number in the sense of 'in or for each hundred', as in 'thirty per cent of the people are living below the poverty line'. The number is sometimes written in figures, as in '50 per cent of the staff are married'. The symbol % is often used instead of the words 'per cent', especially in technical contexts, as in 'make savings of up to 30%'. **Per cent** in modern usage is sometimes used as a noun, as in 'They have agreed to lower the price by half a per cent'.

per means 'for each' and is used to express rates, prices, etc, as in 'driving at 60 miles per hour', 'cloth costing £5 per square metre', 'The cost of the trip is £20 per person' and 'The fees are £1000 a term per child'. It can also mean 'in each', as in 'The factory is inspected three times per year'.

per se is a Latin phrase that has been adapted into English and means 'in itself', as in 'The substance is not per se harmful but it might be so if it interacts with other substances' and 'Television is not per se bad for children'. It should be used only in formal contexts.

percentage refers to 'the rate, number or amount in each hundred', as in 'the number of unemployed people expressed as a percentage of the adult population' and 'What percentage of his salary is free?'. It is also used to mean proportion, as in 'Only a small percentage of last year's students have found jobs' and 'A large percentage of the workers are in favour of a strike'. In modern usage it is sometimes used to mean 'a small amount' or 'a small part', as in 'Only a percentage of the students will find work'.

perquisite *see* **prerequisite**.

person is now used in situations where 'man' was formerly used to avoid sexism in language. It is used when the sex of the person being referred to is either unknown or not specified, as in 'They are advertising for another person for the warehouse'. It often sounds more natural to use 'someone', as in 'They are looking for someone to help out in the warehouse'. **Person** is often used in compounds, as in **chairperson, spokesperson** and **salesperson**, although some people dislike this convention and some compounds, such as **craftsperson**, have not really caught on. **Person** has two possible plurals. *see* **people. Person with** and **people with** are phrases advocated in 'politically correct' language to avoid negative terms such as 'victim', 'sufferer', as in 'person with Aids'.

phenomenal means 'referring to a phenomenon'. It is often used to mean 'remarkable, extraordinary', as in 'a phenomenal atmospheric occurrence', and in modern usage it is also used loosely to mean 'very great', as in 'a phenomenal increase in the crime rate' and 'a phenomenal achievement'. This use is usually restricted to informal contexts.

phenomenon is a singular noun meaning 'a fact, object, occurrence, experience, etc, that can be perceived by the senses rather than by thought or intuition', as in 'She saw something coming out of the lake but it remained an unexplained phenomenon', and 'a strange, unusual or remarkable fact, event or person of some particular significance', as in 'Single parenthood is one of the phenomena of the 1990s'. The plural is **phenomena**, as in 'natural phenomena'. It is a common error to treat **phenomena** as a singular noun. Note the spelling of **phenomenon** as it is liable to be misspelt.

phone, which is a short form of 'telephone', is not regarded as being as informal as it once was. It is quite acceptable in sentences such as 'He is going to buy a mobile phone'. Note that **phone** is now spelt without an apostrophe.

phoney and **phony** are both acceptable spellings but **phoney** is the more common in British English. The word means 'pretending or claiming to be what one is not, fake', as in 'He has a phoney American accent' and 'There's something phoney about him'.

placebo *see* **panacea**.

plane and **aeroplane** mean the same thing, both referring to a 'a machine that can fly and is used to carry people and goods'. In modern usage **plane** is the usual term, as in 'The plane took off on time' and 'nearly miss the plane'. **Aeroplane** is slightly old-fashioned or unduly formal, as in 'Her elderly parents say that they refuse to travel by aeroplane'. The American English spelling is **airplane**. Note that **plane** is not spelt with an apostrophe although it is a shortened form.

pleaded and **pled** mean the same thing, both being the past tense and past participle of the verb 'to plead'. **Pleaded** is the usual form in British English, as in 'They pleaded with the tyrant to spare the child's life' and 'The accused pleaded guilty'. **Pled** is the usual American spelling.

plenty is used only informally in some contexts. It is acceptable in formal and informal contexts when it is followed by the preposition 'of', as in 'We have plenty of food', or when it is used as a pronoun without the 'of' construction, as in 'You can borrow some food from us—we have plenty'. Some people think its use as an adjective, as in 'Don't hurry—we have plenty time' and 'There's plenty food for all in the fridge', should be restricted to informal contexts. As an adverb it is a acceptable in both formal and informal contexts in such sentences as 'Help yourself—we have plenty more'. However, such sentences as 'The house is plenty big enough for them' is suitable only for very informal or slang contexts.

political correctness is a modern movement aiming to remove all forms of prejudice in language, such as sexism, racism and discrimination against disabled people. Its aims are admirable but in practice many of the words and phrases suggested by advocates of political correctness are rather contrived or, indeed, ludicrous. The adjective is **politically correct**.

practicable and **practical** should not be used interchangeably. **Practicable** means 'able to be done or carried out, able to be put into practice', as in 'His schemes seem fine in theory but they are never practicable'. **Practical** has several meanings, such as 'concerned with action and practice rather than with theory', as in 'He has studied the theory but has no practical experience of the job'; 'suitable for the purpose for which it was made', as in 'practical shoes for walking'; 'useful', as in 'a practical device with a wide range of uses'; 'clever at doing and making things', as in 'She's very practical when it comes to dealing with an emergency'; 'virtual', as in 'He's not the owner but he's in practical control of the firm'.

practically can mean 'in a practical way', as in 'Practically, the scheme is not really possible', but in modern usage it is usually used to mean 'virtually', as in 'He practically runs the firm although he is not the manager', and 'almost', as in 'The driver of that car practically ran me over'.

prefer is followed by the preposition 'to' not 'than', as in 'She prefers dogs to cats', 'They prefer Paris to London' and 'They prefer driving to walking'.

prerequisite and **perquisite** are liable to be confused although they are completely different in meaning. **Perquisite** means 'money or goods given as a right in addition to one's pay', as in 'various perquisites such as a company car'. It is frequently abbreviated to 'perks', as in 'The pay's not very much but the perks are good'. **Prerequisite** refers to 'something required as a condition for something to happen or exist', as in 'Passing the exam is a prerequisite for his getting the job' and 'A certain amount of studying is a prerequisite of passing the exam'.

prevaricate and **procrastinate** are liable to be confused although they have completely different meanings. **Prevaricate** means 'to try to avoid telling the truth by speaking in an evasive or misleading way', as in 'She prevaricated when the police asked her where she had been the previous evening'. **Procrastinate** means 'to delay or postpone action', as in 'The student has been procrastinating all term but now he has to get to grips with his essay'.

preventative and **preventive** both mean 'preventing or intended to prevent, precautionary', as in 'If you think the staff are stealing from the factory you should take preventative/preventive measures' and 'Preventative/preventive medicine seeks to prevent disease and disorders rather than cure them'. **Preventive** is the more frequently used of the two terms.

prima facie is a Latin phrase that has been adopted into English. It means 'at first sight, based on what seems to be so' and is mainly used in legal or very formal contexts, as in 'The police say they have prima facie evidence for arresting him but more investigation is required'. The phrase is pronounced *pri*-ma *fay*-shee.

prognosis *see* **diagnosis**.

programme and **program** are liable to cause confusion. In British English **programme** is the acceptable spelling in such senses as in 'a television programme', 'put on a varied programme of entertainment' 'buy a theatre programme' and 'launch an ambitious programme of expansion'. However, in the computing sense **program** is used. **Programme** can also be a verb meaning 'to plan, to schedule', as in 'programme the trip for tomorrow'; 'to cause something to conform to a particular set of instructions', as in 'programme the central heating system'; or 'to cause someone to behave in a particular way, especially to conform to particular instructions', as in 'Her parents have programmed her to obey them implicitly'. In the computing sense of 'to provide with a series of coded instructions', the verb is spelt **program** and the *m* is doubled to form the past participle, past tense and present participle, as **programmed** and **programming**. In American English **program** is the accepted spelling for all senses of both noun and verb.

protagonist was originally a term for 'the chief character in a drama', as in 'Hamlet is the protagonist in the play that bears his name'. It then came to mean also 'the leading person or paticipant in an event, dispute, etc', as in 'The protagonists on each side of the dispute had a meeting'. In modern usage it can now also mean 'a leading or notable supporter of a cause, movement, etc,' as in 'She was one of the protagonists of the feminist movement'.

provided and **providing** are used interchangeably, as in 'You may go, provided/providing that you have finished your work' and 'He can borrow the car provided/providing he pays for the petrol'. 'That' is optional. The phrases mean 'on the condition that'.

pudding *see* **dessert**.

pupil and **student** are not interchangeable. **Pupil** refers to 'a child or young person who is at school', as in 'primary school pupils and secondary school pupils'. **Student** refers to 'a person who is studying at a place of further education, at a university or college', as in 'students trying to find work during the vacations'. In modern usage senior **pupils** at secondary school are sometimes known as **students**. In American English student refers to people at school as well as to people in further education. **Pupil** can also refer to 'a person who is receiving instruction in something from an expert' as in 'The piano teacher has several adult pupils'. **Student** can also refer to 'a person who is studying a particular thing', as in 'In his leisure time he is a student of local history'.

quasi- is Latin in origin and means 'as if, as it were'. In English it is combined with adjectives in the sense of 'seemingly, apparently, but not really', as in 'He gave a quasi-scientific explanation of the occurrence which convinced many people but did not fool his colleagues', or 'partly, to a certain extent but not completely', as in 'It is a quasi-official body which does not have full powers'. **Quasi-** can also be combined with nouns to mean 'seeming, but not really', as in 'a quasi-socialist who is really a capitalist' and 'a quasi-Christian who will not give donations to charity'. **Quasi-** has several possible pronunciations. It can be pronounced *kway*-zi, *kway*-si or *kwah*-si.

queer in the sense of 'homosexual' was formerly used only in a slang and derogatory or offensive way. However, it is now used in a non-offensive way by homosexual people to describe themselves, as an alternative to 'gay'.

question *see* **beg the question; leading question**.

quick is an adjective meaning 'fast, rapid', as in 'a quick method', 'a quick route' and 'a quick walker'. It should not be used as an adverb, as in 'Come quick', in formal contexts since this is grammatically wrong.

quite has two possible meanings when used with adjectives. It can mean 'fairly, rather, somewhat', as in 'She's quite good at tennis but not good enough to play in the team' and 'The house is quite nice but it's not what we're looking for'. Where the indefinite article is used, **quite** precedes it, as in 'quite a good player' and 'quite a nice house'. 'Quite can also mean 'completely, totally', as in 'We were quite overwhelmed by their generosity' and 'It is quite impossible for him to attend the meeting'.

raison d'être is French in origin and is used in English to mean 'a reason, a justification for the existence of', as in 'Her children are her raison d'être' and 'His only raison d'être is his work'. The phrase is liable to be misspelt. Note the accent (^) on the first *e*. It is pronounced *ray-zon detr*.

rara avis is French in origin and means literally 'rare bird'. In English it is used to refer to 'a rare or unusual person or thing', as in 'a person with such dedication to a company is a rara avis'. It is pronounced *ray-ra ayv-is* or *ra-ra ay-*vis.

ravage and **ravish** are liable to be confused. They sound rather similar although they have different meanings. **Ravage** means 'to cause great damage to, to devastate', as in 'low-lying areas ravaged by floods' and 'a population ravaged by disease', or 'to plunder, to rob', as in 'neighbouring tribes ravaging their territory'. **Ravish** means either 'to delight greatly, to enchant', as in 'The audience were ravished by the singer's performance'. It also means 'to rape', as in 'The girl was ravished by her kidnappers', but this meaning is rather old-fashioned and is found only in formal or literary contexts.

re- is a common prefix, meaning 'again', in verbs. In most cases it is not followed by a hyphen, as in 'retrace one's footsteps', 'a retrial ordered by the judge' and 'reconsider his decision'. However, it should be followed by a hyphen if its absence is likely to lead to confusion with another word, as in 're-cover a chair'/'recover from an illness', 're-count the votes'/'recount a tale of woe', 'the re-creation of a 17th-century village for a film set'/'play tennis for recreation' and 're-form the group'/'reform the prison system'. In cases where the second element of a word begins with *e*, **re-** is traditionally followed by a hyphen, as in 're-educate', 're-entry' and 're-echo', but in modern usage the hyphen is frequently omitted.

re, meaning 'concerning, with reference to', as in 'Re your correspondence of 26 November', should be restricted to business or formal contexts.

readable *see* **legible**.

re-cover, recover *see* **re-**.

re-creation, recreation *see* **re-**.

referendum causes problems with regard to its plural form. It has two possible plural forms, **referendums** or **referenda**. In modern usage **referendums** is the more usual plural. **Referendum** means 'the referring of an issue of public importance to a general vote by all the people of a country', as in 'hold a referendum on whether to join the EC'.

re-form, reform *see* **re-**.

registry office and **register office** are interchangeable, although **registry office** is the more common term in general usage. The words refer to 'an office where civil marriage ceremonies are performed and where births, marriages and deaths are recorded', as in 'She wanted to be married in church but he preferred a registry office ceremony' and 'register the child's birth at the local registry office'.

rigour and **rigor** are liable to be confused. They look similar but they have completely different meanings.

Rigour means 'severity, strictness', as in 'the rigour of the punishment', and 'harshness, unpleasantness', as in 'the rigour of the climate' (in this sense it is often in the plural, **rigours**), and 'strictness, detailedness', as in 'the rigour of the editing'. **Rigor** is a medical term meaning 'rigidity', as in 'muscles affected by rigor', or 'a feeling of chilliness often accompanied by feverishness', as in 'infectious diseases of which rigor is one of the symptoms'. **Rigor** is also short for **rigor mortis**, meaning 'the stiffening of the body that occurs after death'. The first syllable of **rigour** is pronounced to rhyme with 'big', but **rigor** can be pronounced either in this way or with the *i* pronounced as in 'ride'.

roof causes problems with regard to its plural form. The usual plural is **roofs**, which can be pronounced either as it is spelt, to rhyme with 'hoofs', or to rhyme with 'hooves'.

rout and **route** are liable to be confused. They look similar but are pronounced differently and have completely different meanings'. **Rout** as a noun means 'overwhelming defeat', as in 'the rout of the opposing army', and as a verb 'to defeat utterly', as in 'Their team routed ours last time'. **Route** refers to 'a way of getting somewhere', as in 'the quickest route' and 'the scenic route'. **Route** can also be a verb meaning 'to arrange a route for, to send by a certain route', as in 'route the visitors along the banks of the river'. **Rout** is pronounced to rhyme with 'shout'. **Route** is pronounced to rhyme with 'brute'.

scarfs and **scarves** are both acceptable spellings of the plural of 'scarf', meaning a piece of cloth worn around the neck or the head', as in 'a silk scarf at her neck' and 'wearing a head scarf'.

Scotch, Scots and **Scottish** are liable to be confused. **Scotch** is restricted to a few set phrases, such as 'Scotch whisky', 'Scotch broth' and 'Scotch mist'. As a noun **Scotch** refers to 'Scotch whisky', as in 'have a large Scotch with ice'. **Scots** as an adjective is used in such contexts as 'Scots accents', 'Scots people' and 'Scots attitudes'. As a noun **Scots** refers to the Scots language, as in 'He speaks standard English but he uses a few words of Scots.' The noun **Scot** is used to refer to 'a Scottish person', as in 'Scots living in London'. **Scottish** is found in such contexts as 'Scottish literature', 'Scottish history' and 'Scottish culture'.

sculpt and **sculpture** are interchangeable as verbs meaning 'to make sculptures, to practise sculpting', as in 'commissioned to sculpt/sculpture a bust of the chairman of the firm' and 'She both paints and sculpts/sculptures.

seize Note the *ei* combination, which is an exception to the '*i* before *e* except after *c*' rule.

sentiment and **sentimentality** are liable to be confused. They are related but have different shades of meaning. **Sentiment** means 'feeling, emotion', as in 'His actions were the result of sentiment not rationality'. It also means 'attitude, opinion', as in 'a speech full of anti-Christian sentiments'. **Sentimentality** is the noun from the adjective **sentimental** and means 'over-indulgence in tender feelings', as in 'dislike the sentimentality of the love songs' and 'She disliked her home town but now speaks about it with great sentimentality'.

sexism in language has been an issue for some time, and various attempts have been made to avoid it. For example, 'person' is often used where 'man' was traditionally used and 'he/she' substituted for 'he' in situations where the sex of the relevant person is unknown or unspecified.

ship *see* **boat**.

sine qua non is a Latin phrase that has been adopted into English and means 'essential condition, something that is absolutely necessary', as in 'It is a sine qua non of the agreement that the rent is paid on time'. It is used only in formal or legal contexts.

sitting room, living room, lounge and **drawing room** all refer to 'a room in a house used for relaxation and the receiving of guests'. Which word is used is largely a matter of choice. Some people object to the use of **lounge** as being pretentious but it is becoming increasingly common. **Drawing room** is a more formal word and applies to a room in rather a grand residence.

skilful, as in 'admire his skilful handling of the situation' is frequently misspelt. Note the single *l* before the *f*. In American English the word is spelt **skillful**.

slander *see* **libel**.

sometime and **some time** are liable to be confused. **Sometime** means 'at an unknown or unspecified time', as in 'We must get together sometime' and 'I saw her sometime last year'. There is a growing tendency in modern usage to spell this as **some time**. Originally **some time** was restricted to meaning 'a period of time', as in 'We need some time to think'.

spelled and **spelt** are both acceptable forms of the past tense and past participle of the verb 'to spell', as in 'They spelled/spelt the word wrongly' and 'He realized that he had spelled/spelt the word wrongly'.

stadium causes problems with regard to its plural form. **Stadiums** and **stadia** are both acceptable. **Stadium** is derived from Latin and the original plural form followed the Latin and was **stadia**. However, anglicized plural forms are becoming more and more common in foreign words adopted into English, and **stadiums** is now becoming the more usual form.

stanch and **staunch** are both acceptable spellings of the word meaning 'to stop the flow of', as in 'stanch/staunch the blood from the wound in his head' and 'try to stanch/staunch the tide of violence'. **Staunch** also means 'loyal, firm', as in 'the team's staunch supporters'.

start *see* **commence**.

stationary and **stationery** are liable to be confused. They sound alike but have completely different meanings. **Stationary** means 'not moving, standing still', as in 'stationary vehicles'. **Stationery** refers to 'writing materials', as in 'office stationery'. An easy way to differentiate

between them is to remember that **stationery** is bought from a 'stationer', which, like 'baker' and 'butcher', ends in *-er*.

staunch *see* **stanch**.

stimulant and **stimulus** are liable to be confused. Formerly the distinction between them was quite clear but now the distinction is becoming blurred. Traditionally **stimulant** refers to 'a substance, such as a drug, that makes a person more alert or more active', as in 'Caffeine is a stimulant'. **Stimulus** traditionally refers to 'something that rouses or encourages a person to action or greater effort', as in 'The promise of more money acted as a stimulus to the work force and they finished the job in record time'. In modern usage the words are beginning to be used interchangeably. In particular, **stimulus** is used in the sense of **stimulant** as well as being used in its own original sense.

straight away and **straightaway** are both acceptable ways of spelling the expression for 'without delay, at once', as in 'attend to the matter straight away/straightaway'.

strata *see* **stratum**.

stratagem and **strategy** are liable to be confused. They look and sound similar but they have different meanings. **Stratagem** means 'a scheme or trick', as in 'think of a stratagem to mislead the enemy' and 'devise a stratagem to gain entry to the building'. **Strategy** refers to 'the art of planning a campaign', as in 'generals meeting to put together a battle strategy', and 'a plan or policy, particularly a clever one, designed for a particular purpose', as in 'admire the strategy which he used to win the game'.

stratum and **strata** are liable to be confused. **Stratum** is the singular form and **strata** is the plural form of a word meaning 'a layer or level', as in 'a stratum of rock' and 'different strata of society'. It is a common error to use **strata** as a singular noun.

student *see* **pupil**.

subconscious and unconscious are used in different contexts. **Subconscious** means 'concerning those areas or activities of the mind of which one is not fully aware', as in 'a subconscious hatred of her parents' and 'a subconscious desire to hurt her sister'. **Unconscious** means 'unaware', as in 'She was unconscious of his presence' and 'unconscious of the damage which he had caused', and 'unintentional', as in 'unconscious humour' and 'an unconscious slight'. **Unconscious** also means 'having lost consciousness, insensible', as in 'knocked unconscious by the blow to his head'.

subjective *see* **objective**.

such and **like** are liable to be confused. **Such** is used to introduce examples, as in 'herbs, such as chervil and parsley' and 'citrus fruits, such as oranges and lemons'. **Like** introduces comparisons. 'She hates horror films like *Silence of the Lambs*', and 'Very young children, like very old people, have to be kept warm.'

supper *see* **dinner**.

syndrome in its original meaning refers to 'a set of symptoms and signs that together indicate the presence of a physical or mental disorder', as in 'Down's syndrome'. In modern usage it is used loosely to indicate 'any set of events, actions, characteristics, attitudes that together make up, or are typical of, a situation', as in 'He suffers from the "I'm all right Jack" syndrome and doesn't care what happens to anyone else' and 'They seem to be caring people but they are opposing the building of an Aids hospice in their street—a definite case of "the not in my back yard" syndrome'.

tea *see* **dinner**.

teach *see* **learn**.

telephone *see* **phone**.

terminal and **terminus** in some contexts are interchangeable. They both refer to 'the end of a bus route, the last stop on a bus route, the building at the end of a bus route', as in 'The bus doesn't go any further—this is the terminus/terminal', but **terminus** is the more common term in this sense. They can also both mean 'the end of a railway line, the station at the end of a railway line', but **terminal** is the more common term in this sense. **Terminal** can refer to 'a building containing the arrival and departure areas for passengers at an airport' and 'a building in the centre of a town for the arrival and departure of air passengers'. **Terminal** also refers to 'a point of connection in an electric circuit', as in 'the positive and negative terminals', and 'apparatus, usually consisting of a keyboard and screen, for communicating with the central processor in a computing system', as in 'He has a dumb terminal so he can read information but not input it'. As an adjective **terminal** means 'of, or relating to, the last stage in a fatal illness', as in 'a terminal disease' and 'terminal patients'.

than is used to link two halves of comparisons or contrasts, as in 'Peter is considerably taller than John is', 'He is older than I am' and 'I am more informed about the situation than I was yesterday'. Problems arise when the relevant verb is omitted. In order to be grammatically correct, the word after 'than' should take the subject form if there is an implied verb, as in 'He is older than I (am)'. However this can sound stilted, as in 'She works harder than he (does)', and in informal contexts this usually becomes 'She works harder than him'. If there is no implied verb, the word after **than** is in the object form, as in 'rather you than me!'

the the definite article, which usually refers back to something already identified or to something specific, as in 'Where is the key?, 'What have you done with the book that I gave you?' and 'We have found the book that had we lost'. It is also used to denote someone or something as being the only one, as in 'the House of Lords', 'the King of Spain' and 'the President of Russia' and to indicate a class or group, as in 'the aristocracy', 'the cat family' and 'the teaching profession'. The is sometimes pronounced 'thee' when it is used to identify someone or something unique or important, as in 'Is that the John Frame over there?' and 'She is the fashion designer of the moment'.

their and **there** are liable to be confused because they sound similar. **There** means 'in, to or at that place', as in 'place it there' and 'send it there'. **Their** is the possessive of 'they', meaning 'of them, belonging to them', as in 'their books' and 'their mistakes'.

their and **they're** are liable to be confused because they sound similar. **Their** is the possessive of 'they', meaning 'of them, belonging to them', as in 'their cars' and 'their attitudes'. **They're** is a shortened form of 'they are', as in 'They're not very happy' and 'They're bound to lose'.

their used in conjunction with 'anyone', everyone', 'no one' and 'someone', is becoming increasingly common, even in textbooks, although this use is ungrammatical. The reason for this is to avoid the sexism of using 'his' when the sex of the person being referred to is either unknown or unspecified, and to avoid the clumsiness of 'his/her' or 'his or her'. Examples of **they** being so used include 'Everyone must do their best' and 'No one is to take their work home'.

this *see* **next**.

till and **until** are more or less interchangeable except that **until** is slightly more formal, as in 'They'll work till they drop' and 'Until we assess the damage we will not know how much the repairs will cost'.

toilet, lavatory, loo and **bathroom** all have the same meaning but the context in which they are used sometimes varies. **Toilet** is the most widely used of the words and is used on signs in public places. The informal **loo** is also very widely used. **Lavatory** is less common nowadays although it was formerly regarded by all but the working class and lower-middle class as the most acceptable term. **Bathroom** in British English usually refers to 'a room containing a bath', but in American English it is the usual word for **toilet**. **Ladies** and **gents** are terms for **toilet**, particularly in public places. **Powder room** also means this, as does the American English **rest room**.

town *see* **city**.

trade names should be written with a capital letter, as in 'Filofax' and 'Jacuzzi'. When trade names are used as verbs they are written with a lower case letter, as in 'hoover the carpet'.

try to and **try and** are interchangeable in modern usage. Formerly **try and** was considered suitable only in spoken and very informal contexts, but it is now considered acceptable in all but the most formal contexts, as in 'Try to/and do better' and 'They must try to/and put the past behind them'.

ultra is used as a prefix meaning 'going beyond', as in 'ultraviolet' and 'ultrasound', or 'extreme, very', as in 'ultra-sophisticated', 'ultra-modern', and 'ultra-conservative'. Compounds using it may be spelt with or without a hyphen. Words such as 'ultrasound' and 'ultraviolet' are usually spelt as one word, but words with the second sense of **ultra**, such as 'ultra-sophisticated', are often hyphenated.

unconscious *see* **subconscious**.

under way, meaning 'in progress', is traditionally spelt as two words, as in 'Preparations for the conference are under way'. In modern usage it is frequently spelt as one word, as in 'The expansion project is now underway'. It is a common error to write 'under weigh'.

underhand and **underhanded** are interchangeable in the sense of 'sly, deceitful', as in 'He used underhand/underhanded methods to get the job' and 'It was underhand/underhanded of him to not to tell her that he was leaving'. **Underhand** is the more common of the two terms.

uninterested *see* **disinterested**.

unique traditionally means 'being the only one of its kind', as in 'a unique work of art' and 'everyone's fingerprints are unique' and so cannot be modified by such words as 'very', 'rather', 'more', etc, although it can be modified by 'almost' and 'nearly'. In modern usage **unique** is often used to mean 'unrivalled, unparalleled, outstanding', as in 'a unique opportunity' and 'a unique performance'.

unreadable *see* **illegible**.

until *see* **till**.

up and **upon** mean the same and are virtually interchangeable, except that **upon** is slightly more formal. Examples include 'sitting on a bench', 'the carpet on the floor', 'the stamp on the letter', 'caught with the stolen goods on him' and 'something on his mind'; and 'She threw herself upon her dying mother's bed', 'a carpet of snow upon the ground' and 'Upon his arrival he went straight upstairs'.

upward and **upwards** are not interchangeable. **Upward** is used as an adjective, as in 'on an upward slope' and 'an upward trend in prices'. **Upwards** is an adverb, as in 'look upwards to see the plane'.

vacation, meaning 'holiday', in British English is mostly restricted to a university or college situation, as in 'students seeking paid employment during their vacation'. In American English it is the usual word for 'holiday'.

verbal and **oral** are liable to be confused. **Oral** means 'expressed in speech', as in 'an oral, rather than a written examination'. **Verbal** means 'expressed in words', as in 'He asked for an instruction diagram but he was given verbal instructions' and 'They were going to stage a protest match but they settled for a verbal protest'. It is also used to mean 'referring to the spoken word, expressed in speech', as in 'a verbal agreement'. Because of these two possible meanings, the use of **verbal** can lead to ambiguity. In order to clarify the situation, **oral** should be used when 'expressed in speech' is meant. **Verbal** can also mean referring to verbs, as in 'verbal endings'.

vice versa means 'the other way round, with the order reversed', as in 'He will do his friend's shift and vice versa' and 'Mary dislikes John and vice versa'. It is pronounced vis-e ver-sa, vi-si ver-sa or vis ver-sa and is derived from Latin.

vis-à-vis means 'in relation to', as in 'their performance vis-à-vis their ability' and 'the company's policy vis-à-vis early retirement'. It is pronounced vee-za-vee and is derived from French. Note the accent on the *a*.

-ways *see* **-wise**.

what ever and **whatever** are not interchangeable. **What ever** is used when 'ever' is used for emphasis, as in 'What ever does he think he's doing?' and 'What ever is she wearing'. **Whatever** means 'anything, regardless of what, no matter what', as in 'Help yourself to whatever you want' and 'Whatever he says I don't believe him'.

which and **what** can cause problems. In questions **which** is used when a limited range of alternatives is suggested, as in 'Which book did you buy in the end?' and **what** is used in general situations, as in 'What book did you buy?'

whisky and **whiskey** both refer to a strong alcoholic drink distilled from grain. **Whisky** is made in Scotland and **whiskey** in Ireland and America. **Whisky** is the usual British English spelling.

who and **whom** cause problems. **Who** is the subject of a verb, as in 'Who told you?', 'It was you who told her' and 'the girls who took part in the play'. **Whom** is the object of a verb or preposition, as in 'Whom did he tell?', 'To whom did you speak?' and 'the people from whom he stole'. In modern usage **whom** is falling into disuse, especially in questions, except in formal contexts. **Who** is used instead even although it is ungrammatical, as in 'Who did you speak to?' **Whom** should be retained when it is a relative pronoun, as in 'the man whom you saw', 'the person to whom he spoke' and 'the girl to whom she gave the book'.

whose and **who's** are liable to be confused. They sound alike but have different meanings. **Whose** means 'of whom' or 'of which', as in 'the woman whose child won', 'the boy whose leg was broken', 'Whose bicycle is that?' and 'the firm whose staff went on strike'. **Who's** is a shortened form of 'who is', as in 'Who's that?', 'Who's first in the queue?' and 'Who's coming to the cinema?'

-wise and **-ways** cause problems. Added to nouns, **-wise** can form adverbs of manner indicating either 'in such a position or direction', as in 'lengthwise' and 'clockwise', and 'in the manner of', as in 'crabwise'. In modern usage **-wise** is frequently used to mean 'with reference to', as in 'Weatherwise it was fine', 'Workwise all is well' and 'Moneywise they're not doing too well'. The suffix **-ways** has a more limited use. It means 'in such a way, direction or manner of', as in 'lengthways' and 'sideways'.

woman *see* **lady**.

Xmas is sometimes used as an alternative and shorter form of 'Christmas'. It is common only in a written informal context and is used mainly in commercial situations, as in 'Xmas cards on sale here' and 'Get your Xmas tree here'. When pronounced it is the same as 'Christmas'. The X derives from the Greek *chi*, the first letter of *Christos*, the Greek word for Christ.

X-ray is usually written with an initial capital letter when it is a noun meaning 'a photograph made by means of X-rays showing the bones or organs of the body', as in 'take an X-ray of the patient's chest'. Another term for the noun **X-ray** is 'radiograph'. As a verb it is also usually spelt with an initial capital, as 'After the accident he had his leg X-rayed', but it is sometimes spelt with an initial lowercase letter, as in 'have his chest x-rayed'.

you is used in informal or less formal situations to indicate an indefinite person referred to as 'one' in formal situations. Examples include 'You learn a foreign language more quickly if you spend some time in the country where it is spoken', 'You would think that they would make sure that their staff are polite', 'You can get used to anything in time' and 'You have to experience the situation to believe it'. **You** in this sense must be distinguished from **you** meaning the second person singular', as in 'You have missed your bus', 'You must know where you left your bag' and 'You have to leave now'. *see* **one**.

your and **you're** are liable to be confused. **Your** is a possessive adjective meaning 'belonging to you, of you', as in 'That is your book and this is mine', 'Your attitude is surprising' and 'It is your own fault'. **You're** is a shortened form of 'you are', as in 'You're foolish to believe him', 'You're going to be sorry' and 'You're sure to do well'. Note the spelling of the pronoun **yours**, as in 'This book is yours' and 'Which car is yours?' It should not be spelt with an apostrophe as it is not a shortened form of anything.

Appendix 4

English Idioms

A

- **A1** first class, of the highest quality. <A1 is the highest rating given to the condition of ships for Lloyd's Register, Lloyds of London being a major insurance company>.
- **from A to Z** thoroughly, comprehensively.

above

- **above board** open, honest and without trickery. <Card cheats tend to keep their cards under the table, or board>.
- **above (someone's) head** too difficult to understand.
- **get a bit above oneself** to become very vain or conceited.

accident

- **accidents will happen** things go wrong at some time in everyone's life.
- **a chapter of accidents** a series of misfortunes.

account

- **give a good account of oneself** to do well.

ace

- **within an ace of** very close to. <From the game of dice, ace being the term for the side of a dice with one spot>.

Achilles

- **Achilles' heel** the one weak spot in a person. <Achilles, the legendary Greek hero, is said to have been dipped in the River Styx by his mother at birth to make him invulnerable but his heel, by which she was holding him, remained unprotected and he was killed by an arrow through his heel>.

acid

- **acid test** a test that will prove or disprove something conclusively. <From the use of nitric acid to ascertain whether a metal was gold or not. If it was not gold the acid decomposed it>.

across

- **across the board** applying to everyone or to all cases.

act

- **act of God** a happening, usually sudden and unexpected, for which no human can be held responsible.
- **get in on the act** to become involved in some profitable or advantageous activity, especially an activity related to someone else's success.
- **get one's act together** to get organized.

action

- **action stations** a state of preparedness for some activity. <From positions taken up by soldiers in readiness for battle>.

- **get a piece** *or* **slice of the action** to be involved in something, get a share of something.

ad

- **ad hoc** for a particular (usually exclusive) purpose. <Latin, 'to this'>.
- **ad-lib** to speak without preparation, to improvise. <Latin, 'according to pleasure'>.

Adam <Refers to the biblical Adam>.

- **Adam's ale** water.
- **not to know (someone) from Adam** not to recognize (someone).
- **the old Adam in us** the sin or evil that is in everyone.

add

- **add fuel to the fire** to make a difficult situation worse.
- **add insult to injury** to make matters worse.

Adonis

- **an Adonis** a very attractive young man. <In Greek legend Adonis was a beautiful young man who was loved by Aphrodite, the goddess of love, and who was killed by a boar while hunting>.

advantage

- **have the advantage of (someone)** to recognize (someone) without oneself being recognized by that person.

aegis

- **under the aegis of (someone)** with the support or backing of (someone). <In Greek legend Aegis was the shield of the god Zeus>.

after

- **after a fashion** in a manner that is barely adequate.
- **after (someone's) own heart** to one's liking; liked or admired by (someone).

against

- **against the clock** in a hurry to get something done before a certain time.
- **be up against it** to be in a difficult or dangerous situation.

age

- **a golden age** a time of great achievement.
- **a ripe old age** a very old age.
- **of a certain age** no longer young.

agony

- **agony aunt** *or* **uncle** a woman or man who gives advice on personal problems either in a newspaper or magazine column, or on television or radio.

- **agony column** a newspaper or magazine column in which readers write in with their problems, which are answered by the agony aunt or uncle. <Originally a newspaper column containing advertisements for missing relatives and friends>.

ahead
- **ahead of the game** in an advantageous position; in front of one's rivals.
- **streets ahead of (someone *or* something)** much better than (someone or something).

air
- **air *or* wash one's dirty linen in public** to discuss private or personal matters in public.
- **clear the air** to make a situation less tense by settling disagreements.
- **hot air** boasting; empty or meaningless words.
- **into thin air** seemingly into nowhere.
- **put on airs** to behave as though one were superior to others, to act in a conceited way.
- **up in the air** uncertain, undecided.
- **walk on air** to be very happy.

Aladdin
- **Aladdin's cave** a place full of valuable or desirable objects. <From the tale of Aladdin in the Arabian Nights who gained access to such a cave with the help of the genie from his magic lamp>.

alive
- **alive and kicking** in a good or healthy condition.

all
- **all and sundry** everybody, one and all.
- **all chiefs and no Indians** a surplus of people wishing to give orders or to administrate and a deficiency of people willing to carry orders out or to do the work.
- **all ears** listening intently.
- **all in** exhausted.
- **all in one piece** safely, undamaged.
- **all over bar the shouting** at an end to all intents and purposes.
- **all set** ready to go, prepared.
- **all-singing, all-dancing** of a machine, system, very advanced with a great many modern features, sometimes not all necessary. <Used originally of a stage show to indicate how lavish it was>.

alley
- **alley cat** a wild or promiscuous person.

alliance
- **an unholy alliance** used of an association or partnership between two people or organizations that have nothing in common and would not normally work together, especially when this association has a bad purpose.

alma mater
- one's old university, college or school. <Latin, 'bountiful mother'>.

alpha
- **alpha and omega** the beginning and the end. <The first and last letters of the Greek alphabet>.

also
- **also-ran** an unsuccessful person. <A horse-racing term for a horse that is not one of the first three horses in a race>.

altar
- **be sacrificed on the altar of (something)** to be destroyed or suffer harm or damage so that something can be achieved or prosper.

alter
- alter ego a person who is very close or dear to someone. <Latin, 'other self'>.

altogether
- **in the altogether** in the nude.

Amazon
- a very strong or well-built woman. <In Greek legend the Amazons were a race of female warriors who had their right breasts removed in order to draw their bows better>.

American
- **as American as apple pie** typical of the traditional American way of life or culture.
- **the American dream** the hope of achieving success and prosperity through hard work, from the dreams which immigrants had when they landed in America to start a new life.

angel
- **an angel of mercy** a person who gives help and comfort, especially one who appears unexpectedly.
- **a fallen angel** a person who had formerly a good reputation for being virtuous or successful but no longer does so.
- **on the side of the angels** supporting or agreeing with what is regarded as being the good or the right side.

angry
- **angry young man** a person who expresses angry dissatisfaction with established social, political and intellectual values. <A term applied to British dramatist, John Osborne, author of the *play Look Back in Anger*>.

answer
- **the answer to a maiden's prayer** exactly what one desires and is looking for. <The answer to a maiden's prayer was thought to be an eligible bachelor>.

ant
- **have ants in one's pants** to be restless or agitated.

any
- **any old how** in an untidy and careless way.
- **anything goes** any kind of behaviour, dress, etc, is acceptable.

apart
- **be poles** *or* **worlds apart** to be completely different.

ape
- **go ape** to become extremely angry or excited

appearance
- **keep up appearances** to behave in public in such a way as to hide what is going on in private.

apple
- **in apple-pie order** with everything tidy and correctly arranged. <From French *nappe pliée*, 'folded linen', linen neatly laid out>.
- **rotten apple** a person who is bad or unsatisfactory and will have a bad influence on others.
- **the apple of (someone's) eye** a favourite, a person who is greatly loved by (someone). <Apple refers to the pupil of the eye>.
- **upset the apple-cart** to spoil plans or arrangements. <From the practice of selling fruit from carts in street markets>.

apron
- **tied to (someone's) apron-strings** completely dependent on a woman, especially one's mother or wife.

ark
- **like something out of the ark** very old-fashioned looking. <From Noah's ark in the Bible>.

arm
- **armed to the hilt** *or* **teeth** provided with all the equipment that one could possibly need.
- **be up in arms** to protest angrily.
- **chance one's arm** to take a risk.
- **cost an arm and a leg** to cost a great deal of money.
- **give one's right arm for (something)** to be willing to go to any lengths to get something.
- **keep (someone) at arm's length** to avoid becoming too close to or too friendly with someone.
- **the long arm of the law** the power or authority of the police.
- **right arm** chief source of help and support.
- **twist (someone's) arm** to force (someone) to do (something), to persuade (someone) to do (something).
- **with one arm tied behind one's back** very easily.
- **with open arms** welcomingly.

armour
- **chink in (someone's) armour** a weak or vulnerable spot in someone who is otherwise very strong and difficult to get through to or attack. <A knight in armour could be injured only through a flaw or opening in his protective armour>.
- **knight in shining armour** a person who it is hoped will save a situation or come to one's aid. <From medieval legends in which knights in armour came to the aid of damsels in distress>.

ashes
- **rake over the ashes** to discuss things that are passed, especially things that are best forgotten.
- **rise from the ashes** to develop and flourish out of ruin and destruction. <In Greek legend the phoenix, a mythical bird, who after a certain number of years of life set fire to itself and was then reborn from the ashes>.

attendance
- **dance attendance on (someone)** to stay close to (someone) in order to carry out all his or her wishes and so gain favour.

aunt
- **Aunt Sally** a person or thing that is being subjected to general abuse, mockery and criticism. <An Aunt Sally at a fair was a wooden model of a woman's head, mounted on a pole, at which people threw sticks or balls in order to win a prize>.

awakening
- **get/have a rude awakening** suddenly to become aware that a situation is not as good or pleasant as one thinks it is.

away
- **get away from it all** to escape from the problems of daily life, usually by taking a holiday.
- **the one that got away** a chance of success which one either did not or could not take advantage of at the time but which one always remembers. <Refers to a supposedly large fish which an angler fails to catch but about which he tells many stories>.

axe
- **get the axe** to be dismissed.
- **have an axe to grind** to have a personal, often selfish, reason for being involved in something. <From a story told by Benjamin Franklin, the American politician, about how a man had once asked him in his boyhood to demonstrate the working of his father's grindstone and had sharpened his own axe on it while it was working>.

baby
- **be left holding the baby** to be left to cope with a difficult situation that has been abandoned by the person who is really responsible for it.
- **throw out the baby with the bath water** accidentally to get rid of something desirable or essential when trying to get rid of undesirable or unnecessary things.

back
- **backhanded compliment** a supposed compliment that sounds more like criticism.
- **back number** a person or thing that is no longer of importance or of use. <Refers to an out-of-date or back copy of a newspaper or magazine>.

- **backseat driver** **1** a passenger in a car who gives unasked-for and unwanted advice. **2** a person who is not directly involved in some activity but who offers unwanted advice.
- **back to the drawing board** to have to start again on a project or activity. <Refers to the board on which plans of buildings, etc, are drawn before being built>.
- **back to the grindstone** back to work.
- **bend over backwards** to go to great trouble.
- **get off (someone's) back** to stop harassing or bothering (someone).
- **have one's back to the wall.** to be in a very difficult or desperate situation. <Someone being pursued has to face his or her pursuers or be captured when a wall prevents retreat>.
- **know (something) backwards** *or* **like the back of one's hand** to know all there is to know about (something).
- **know (someone *or* something) like the back of one's hand** to know (someone or something) very well indeed.
- **put one's back into (something)** to put the greatest possible effort into (something).
- **put (someone's) back up** to annoy (someone). <A cat's back arches up when it is angry>.
- **see the back of (someone *or* something)** to get rid of (someone or something), not to see (someone or something) again.
- **take a back seat** to take an unimportant or minor role.
- **talk through the back of one's head** to talk nonsense.
- **the back of beyond** a very remote place.

bacon
- **bring home the bacon** **1** to earn money to support one's family. **2** to succeed in doing (something). <Perhaps from the winning of a greased pig as a prize at a country fair>.
- **save (someone's) bacon** to save someone from a danger or difficulty.

bad
- **hit a bad patch** to encounter difficulties or a difficult period.
- **in (someone's) bad *or* black books** out of favour with (someone). <Refers to an account book where bad debts are noted>.
- **with a bad grace** in an unwilling and bad-tempered way.

bag
- **bag of bones** a person who is extremely thin.
- **bag of tricks** the equipment necessary to do something.
- **in the bag** certain to be obtained. <From the bag used in hunting to carry what one has shot or caught>.
- **mixed bag** a very varied mixture.

bait
- **rise to the bait** to do what someone has been trying to get one to do. <Refers to fish rising to the surface to get the bait on an angler's line>.

- **swallow the bait** to accept completely an offer, proposal, etc, that has been made purely to tempt one. <As above>.

baker
- **baker's dozen** thirteen. <From the former custom of bakers adding an extra bun or loaf to a dozen in order to be sure of not giving short weight>.

balance
- **in the balance** undecided, uncertain. <A balance is a pair of hanging scales>.
- **strike a balance** to reach an acceptable compromise.
- **tip the balance** to exert an influence which, although slight, is enough to alter the outcome of something.

bald
- **bald as a coot** extremely bald. <A coot is a bird with a spot of white feathers on its head>.

ball¹
- **have a ball** to have a very enjoyable time.

ball²
- **a whole new ball game** used to emphasize how much a situation has changed.
- **be in the right ballpark** to be reasonably close to the amount which is required or wanted.
- **have the ball at one's feet** to be in a position to be successful. <From football>.
- **on the ball** alert, quick-witted, attentive to what is going on around one. <Referring to a football player who watches the ball carefully in order to be prepared if it comes to him>.
- **play ball** to act in accordance with someone else's wishes.
- **set *or* start the ball rolling** to start off an activity of some kind, often a discussion.

balloon
- **go down like a lead balloon** of a suggestion, idea, joke, etc, to be very badly received.
- **when the balloon goes up** when something serious, usually something that is expected and feared, happens. <From balloons sent up to undertake military observation in World War I, signifying that action was about to start>.

banana
- **go bananas** to go mad, to get extremely angry.

band
- **jump on the bandwagon** to show an interest in, or become involved in, something simply because it is fashionable or financially advantageous. <Refers to a brightly coloured wagon for carrying the band at the head of a procession>.
- **looking as though one has stepped out of a bandbox** looking very neat and elegant. <Refers to a lightweight box formerly used for holding small articles of clothing such as hats>.

bang
- **bang one's head against a brick wall** to do (something) in vain.
- **go with a bang** to be very successful.

bank
- **break the bank** to leave (oneself or someone) without any money. <In gambling terms, to win all the money that a casino is prepared to pay out in one night>.

baptism
- **baptism of fire** a first, usually difficult or unpleasant, experience of something. <From Christian baptism>.

bare
- **the bare bones of (something)** the essential and basic details of (something).

bargain
- **get more than one bargained for** to encounter more difficulty than one had expected or was prepared for.
- **drive a hard bargain** to try to get a deal that is very favourable to oneself.

barge
- **wouldn't touch (someone *or* something) with a bargepole** to wish to have absolutely no contact with (someone or something).

bark
- **bark up the wrong tree** to have the wrong idea or impression about (something), to approach (something) in the wrong way. <From raccoon-hunting, in which dogs were used to locate trees that had raccoons in them>.
- **(someone's) bark is worse than his *or* her bite** a person is not as dangerous or as harmful as he or she appears to be. <Refers to a barking dog that is often quite friendly>.

barrel
- **have (someone) over a barrel** to get (someone) into such a position that one can get him or her to do anything that one wants. <From holding someone over a barrel of boiling oil, etc, where the alternatives for the victim are to agree to demands or be dropped in the barrel>.
- **scrape the (bottom of the) barrel** to have to use someone or something of poor or inferior quality because that is all that is available. <Referring to the fact that people will only scrape out the bottom of an empty barrel if they have no more full ones>.

bat¹
- **off one's own bat** by oneself, without the help or permission of any one else. <From the game of cricket>.

bat²
- **blind as a bat** having very poor eyesight. <Referring to the fact that bats live their lives in darkness>.
- **like a bat out of hell** very quickly.

battle
- **win the battle, but lose the war** to get some of the things which you wanted from an argument, discussion, etc, but to lose your most important goal.

bay
- **keep (someone *or* something) at bay** to keep (someone or something) from coming too close.

be
- **the be-all and end-all** the most important aim or purpose. <From Shakespeare's *Macbeth*, Act 1, scene VII>.

beam
- **off beam 1** on the wrong course. **2** inaccurate. <From the radio beam that is used to bring aircraft to land in poor visibility>.
- **on one's beam ends** very short of money. <Originally a nautical term used to describe a ship lying on its side and in danger of capsizing completely>.

bean
- **know how many beans make five** to be experienced in the ways of the world.
- **spill the beans** to reveal a secret or confidential information.

bear
- **bear garden** a noisy, rowdy place. <Originally referred to a public place used for bear-baiting, in which dogs were made to attack bears and get them angry, for public amusement>.
- **like a bear with a sore head** extremely bad-tempered.

beard
- **beard the lion in its den** to confront or face (someone) openly and boldly.

beat
- **beat about the bush** to approach (something) in an indirect way. <In game-bird hunting, bushes are beaten to make the birds appear>.
- **beat a (hasty) retreat** to run away. <Military orders used to be conveyed by a series of different drum signals>.
- **beat the drum** to try to attract public attention. <The noise of a drum makes people stop and listen>.
- **if you can't beat them (*or* 'em), join them (*or* 'em)** if you cannot persuade other people to think and act like you, the most sensible course of action is for you to begin to think and act like them.
- **off the beaten track** in an isolated position, away from towns or cities.

beauty
- **beauty is in the eye of the beholder** different people have different ideas of what is beautiful.
- **beauty is only skin deep** people have more important qualities than how they look.

beaver
- **eager beaver** a very enthusiastic and hard-working person.

- **work like a beaver** to work very industriously and enthusiastically. <Beavers are small animals that build dams, etc, with great speed and skill>.

beck
- **at (someone's) beck and call** having to be always available to carry out (someone's) orders or wishes. <Beck is a form of 'beckon'>.

bed
- **bed of roses** an easy, comfortable or happy situation.
- **get out of bed on the wrong side** to start the day in a very bad-tempered mood.

bee
- **have a bee in one's bonnet** to have an idea that one cannot stop thinking or talking about, to have an obsession. <A bee trapped under one's hat cannot escape>.
- **make a beeline for (someone *or* something)** to go directly and quickly to (someone or something). <Bees are reputed to fly back to their hives in straight lines>.

beer
- **not all beer and skittles** not consisting just of pleasant or enjoyable things.
- **small beer** something unimportant.

before
- **before one can say Jack Robinson** very rapidly, in an instant.

beg
- **beggar description** to be such that words cannot describe it. <From Shakespeare's *Antony and Cleopatra*, Act 2, scene II>.
- **beg the question** in an argument, to take for granted the very point that requires to be proved; to fail to deal effectively with the point being discussed.
- **going a-begging** unclaimed or unsold.

bell
- **bell the cat** to be the person in a group who undertakes something dangerous for the good of the group. <Refers to a story about some mice who wanted to put a bell on the neck of the cat so that they would hear it coming and who needed a volunteer to do it>.
- **ring a bell** to bring back vague memories.
- **saved by the bell** rescued from an unpleasant situation by something suddenly bringing that situation to an end. <From the bell that marks the end of a round in boxing>.

belt
- **below the belt** unfair. <In boxing, a blow below the belt is against the rules>.
- **belt and braces** used to describe extra precautions taken to make sure that all is well.
- **tighten one's belt** to reduce one's expenditure. <Belts have to be tightened if one loses weight in this case from having less to spend on food>.

bend
- **on bended knee** very humbly or earnestly.
- **round the bend** mad.

berth
- **give (someone) a wide berth** to keep well away from (someone). <Refers to a ship that keeps a good distance away from others>.

best
- **have the best of both worlds** to benefit from the advantages of two sets of circumstances.
- **put one's best foot forward** to make the best attempt possible.

bet
- **hedge one's bets** to try to protect oneself from possible loss, failure, disappointment, etc. <From betting the same amount on each side to make sure of not losing>.

better
- **have seen better days** to be no longer new or fresh.
- **the better part of (something)** a large part of (something), most of (something).
- **think better of (something)** to reconsider (something), to change one's mind about (something).

beyond
- **beyond the pale** beyond normal or acceptable limits. <The pale was an area of English government in Ireland in the 16th century>.

big
- **a big fish in a small pond** a person who seems better, more important, etc, than he or she is because he or she operates in a small, limited area.
- **the Big Apple** New York.
- **big guns** the most important people in an organization.
- **hit the big time** to be become extremely successful and famous
- **the Big Smoke** London.

bill
- **a clean bill of health** verification that someone is well and fit. <Ships were given clean bills of health and allowed to sail when it was certified that no one aboard had an infectious disease>.
- **fit or fill the bill** to be exactly what is required. <Refers originally to a handbill or public notice>.
- **foot the bill** to pay for something, usually something expensive.

bird
- **a bird in the hand is worth two in the bush** something that one already has is much more valuable than things that one might or might not acquire. <A bird in the bush might fly away>.
- **a little bird told me** I found out by a means which I do not wish to reveal.

- **birds of a feather flock together** people who share the same interests, ideas, etc, usually form friendships.
- **give (someone) the bird** of an audience, to express its disapproval of a performer by hissing or booing so that he or she leaves the stage. <From the resemblance of the noise of the audience to the hissing of geese>.
- **kill two birds with one stone** to fulfil two purposes with one action.
- **the birds and the bees** the basic facts of human sexual behaviour and reproduction.
- **the early bird catches the worm** a person who arrives early or acts promptly is in a position to gain advantage over others.

biscuit
- **take the biscuit** to be much worse than anything that has happened so far.

bit
- **champing at the bit** very impatient. <A horse chews at its bit when it is impatient>.
- **take the bit between one's teeth** to act on one's own and cease to follow other people's instructions or advice. <Refers to a horse escaping from the control of its rider>.

bite
- **bite off more than one can chew** to try to do more than one can without too much difficulty.
- **bite the bullet** to do something unpleasant but unavoidable with courage.
- **bite the dust** to die or cease to operate or function.
- **bite the hand that feeds one** to treat badly someone who has helped one.
- **have more than one bite at the cherry** to have more than one opportunity to succeed at something.
- **the biter bit** used to indicate a situation in which someone who has tried to harm or do wrong to someone has suffered in some way as a consequence of this action.

bitter
- **a bitter pill to swallow** something unpleasant or difficult that one has to accept.

black
- **as black as one is painted** as bad as everyone says one is.
- **black sheep** a member of a family or group who is not up to the standard of the rest of the group.
- **in black and white** in writing or in print.
- **in (someone's) black books** *same as* **in (someone's) bad books** *see* **bad**.
- **in the black** showing a profit, not in debt. <From the use of black ink to make entries on the credit side of a ledger>.

blanket
- **on the wrong side of the blanket** illegitimate.
- **wet blanket** a dull person who makes other people feel depressed.

blessing
- **a blessing in disguise** something that turns out to advantage after first seeming unfortunate.

blind
- **the blind leading the blind** referring to a situation in which the person who is in charge of others knows as little as they do.

blood
- **in cold blood** deliberately and calmly.
- **like getting blood out of a stone** very difficult, almost impossible.

blow
- **blow hot and cold** to keep changing one's mind or attitude.
- **blow one's own trumpet** to boast about one's achievements.
- **blow the gaff** to tell something secret, often something illegal, to someone, often the police. <Perhaps from gaff, meaning mouth>.
- **blow the whistle on (someone)** to reveal or report someone's wrongdoing so that it will be stopped. <From the practice of blowing a whistle to indicate a foul in some ball games>.
- **see which way the wind blows** to wait and find out how a situation is developing before making a decision. <From sailing>.

blue
- **blue-eyed boy** a person who is someone's favourite.
- **bluestocking** an educated, intellectual woman. <From a group of women in the 18th century who met in London to discuss intellectual and philosophical issues and some of whom wore blue worsted stockings>.
- **once in a blue moon** hardly ever.
- **out of the blue** without warning.

bluff
- **call (someone's) bluff** to make (someone) prove that what he or she says is true is really genuine. <Refers to poker, the card game>.

board
- **go by the board** to be abandoned. <The board here is a ship's board or side, and to go by the board literally was to vanish overboard>.
- **sweep the board** to win all the prizes. <The board referred to is the surface on which card games are played and on which the bets are placed>.

boat
- **burn one's boats** to do something that makes it impossible to go back to one's previous position.
- **in the same boat** in the same situation.
- **miss the boat** to fail to take advantage of a opportunity.
- **push the boat out** to spend money in an extravagant way in order to celebrate something in a lavish way.
- **rock the boat** to do something to endanger or spoil a comfortable or happy situation.

bolt

- **a bolt from the blue** something very sudden and unexpected.
- **shoot one's bolt** to make one's final effort, have no other possible course of action.

bone

- **a bone of contention** a cause of dispute. <Dogs fight over bones>.
- **have a bone to pick with (someone)** to have a matter to disagree about with (someone). <From dogs fighting over a bone>.
- **make no bones about (something)** to have no hesitation or restraint about (saying or doing something openly). <Originally a reference to finding no bones in one's soup, which was therefore easier to eat>.
- **near the bone 1** referring too closely to something that should not be mentioned; tactless. **2** slightly indecent or crude.

boo

- **would not say boo to a goose** to be extremely timid.

book

- **bring (someone) to book** to make (someone) explain or be punished for his or her actions. <Perhaps referring to a book where a police officer keeps a note of crimes>.
- **by the book** strictly according to the rules.
- **cook the books** illegally to alter accounts or financial records.
- **throw the book at (someone)** to criticize or punish (someone) severely, to charge (someone) with several crimes at once. <Literally, to charge someone with every crime listed in a book>.

boot

- **get the boot** to be dismissed or discharged from one's job.
- **hang up one's boots** to retire from work, to cease doing an activity. <From hanging up football boots after a game>.
- **lick (someone's) boots** to flatter (someone) and do everything he or she wants.
- **pull oneself up by one's bootstraps** to become successful through one's own efforts.
- **put the boot in (someone) 1** to kick (someone) when he or she is already lying on the ground injured. **2** to treat (someone) cruelly or harshly after he or she has suffered already.
- **the boot is on the other foot** the situation has been completely turned round.
- **too big for one's boots** too conceited.

bottle

- **lose one's bottle** not to have the courage to do something or to go on with something.

bottom

- **bottom drawer** a collection of articles for the home, which a young woman gathered together before her marriage.

- **hit rock bottom** to reach the lowest possible level.
- **the bottom line 1** the most important point or part of something. **2** the result or outcome. <Refers to the bottom line in a financial statement which indicates the extent of the profit or loss>.

bow¹

- **bow and scrape** to behave in a very humble and respectful way.
- **take a bow** to accept acknowledgement of one's achievements. <As above>.

bow²

- **draw the long bow** to exaggerate. <An archer carries a spare bow in case one breaks>.
- **have another/more than one string to one's bow** to have another possibility, plan, etc, available to one.

brain

- **cudgel** or **rack one's brains** to think very hard.
- **pick (someone's) brains** to find out (someone's) ideas and knowledge about a subject so that one can put them to one's own use.

brass

- **get down to brass tacks** to consider the basic facts or issues of something.

bread

- **know which side one's bread is buttered** to know the course of action that is to one's greatest advantage.
- **on the breadline** with scarcely enough money to live on.
- **the greatest thing since sliced bread** a person or thing that is greatly admired.

breath

- **hold one's breath** to wait anxiously for something.
- **take (someone's) breath away** to surprise (someone) greatly.
- **waste one's breath** to say something that is not taken heed of.

breathe

- **breathe down (someone's) neck 1** to be very close behind (someone). **2** to be waiting impatiently for something from (someone).

brick

- **like a cat on hot bricks** very nervous or restless.
- **try to make bricks without straw** to try to do something without the necessary materials or equipment. <A biblical reference, from Pharaoh's command concerning the Israelites in Exodus 5:7>.

bridge

- **build bridges** to do something to help people who are in some kind of opposition to each other to understand each other so that they are able to establish a relationship or co-operate with each other.
- **cross a bridge when one comes to it** to worry about or deal with a problem only when it actually arises.

bright

- **bright-eyed and bushy-tailed** very cheerful and lively.
- **look on the bright side** to be optimistic, to see the advantages of one's situation.

broad

- **have broad shoulders** to be able to accept a great deal of responsibility, criticism, etc.
- **in broad daylight** during the day.

brother

- **am I my brother's keeper?** the actions or affairs of other people are not my responsibility. <From the biblical story of Cain and Abel, Genesis 4:9>.
- **Big Brother** a powerful person or organization thought to be constantly monitoring and controlling people's actions. <From the dictator in George Orwell's novel *1984*>.

brown

- **in a brown study** deep in thought.

bucket

- **a drop in the bucket** a very small part of what is needed.
- **kick the bucket** to die. <Bucket here is perhaps a beam from which pigs were hung after being killed>.
- **weep buckets** to cry a great deal.

bull

- **hit the bull's eye** to do or say something that is very appropriate or relevant. <Refers to the exact centre of a dart board>.
- **like a bull at a gate** in a very unsubtle, unthinking way.
- **like a bull in a china shop** in a very clumsy way.
- **take the bull by the horns** to tackle (something) boldly.

bullet

- **get the bullet** to be dismissed or discharged.

burn

- **the burning question** a question of great interest to many people.

Burton

- **gone for a Burton** dead, ruined, broken, etc. <Originally a military term from Burton, a kind of ale>.

bus

- **busman's holiday** a holiday spent doing much the same as one does when one is at work. <Refers to a bus driver who drives a bus on holiday>.

bush

- **bush telegraph** the fast spreading of information by word of mouth. <A reference to the Australian bush>.

business

- **mean business** to be determined (to do something), to be serious.
- **mind one's own business** to concern oneself with one's own affairs and not interfere in those of other people.

butter

- **butterfingers** a person who often drops things.
- **look as though butter would not melt in one's mouth** to appear very innocent, respectable, etc.

butterfly

- **have butterflies in one's stomach** to have a fluttering sensation in one's stomach as a sign of nervousness.

cake

- **a piece of cake** something easy to do.
- **a slice** or **share of the cake** a share of something desirable or valuable.
- **have one's cake and eat it** or **eat one's cake and have it** to have the advantages of two things or situations when doing, possessing, etc, one of them would normally make the other one impossible.
- **sell** or **go like hot cakes** to sell very quickly.

cage

- **rattle (someone's) cage** to annoy or agitate (someone). <From visitors to a zoo rattling the cages of the animals to get them to react>.

calf

- **kill the fatted calf** to provide a lavish meal, especially to mark a celebration of someone's arrival or return. <From the parable of the prodigal son in the Bible, Luke 15:23>.

can

- **carry the can** to accept blame or responsibility, usually for something that someone else has done.

candle

- **burn the candle at both ends** to work and/or to play during too many hours of the day.
- **cannot hold a candle to (someone)** to be not nearly as good or as talented as (someone). <Literally, someone who is not good enough even to hold a light while someone else does the work>.
- **the game is not worth the candle** something that is not worth the effort that has to be spent on it. <From the translation of the French phrase *le jeu n'en vaut la chandelle*, referring to a gambling session in which the amount of money at stake was not enough to pay for the candles required to give light at the game>.

canoe

- **paddle one's own canoe** to control one's own affairs without help from anyone else.

cap

- **cap in hand** humbly. <Removing one's cap in someone's presence is a sign of respect>.
- **if the cap fits, wear it** if what has been said applies to you, then you should take note of it.
- **set one's cap at (someone)** to try to attract (someone of the opposite sex). <Perhaps a mistranslation of French *metter le cap*, to head towards>.

card

- **have a card up one's sleeve** to have an idea, plan of action, etc, in reserve to be used if necessary <From cheating at cards>.
- **on the cards** likely. <From reading the cards in fortune-telling>.
- **play one's cards close to one's chest** to be secretive or non-communicative about one's plans or intentions. <From holding one's cards close to one in card-playing so that one's opponents will not see them>.
- **play one's cards right** to act in such a way as to take advantage of a situation.
- **put one's cards on the table** to make known one's plans or intentions. <In card-playing, to show one's opponent one's cards>.

carpet

- **sweep (something) under the carpet** to try to hide or forget about (something unpleasant).
- **the red carpet** special, respectful treatment. <Refers to the red carpet put down for a royal person to walk on during official visits>.

carrot

- **carrot and stick** reward as a method of persuasion.

carry

- **carry a torch for (someone)** to be in love with someone, especially with someone who does not return it. <A torch or a flame was regarded as symbolic of love>.

cart

- **put the cart before the horse** to do or say things in the wrong order.

Casanova

- **Casanova** a man who has relationships with many women. <From Giacomo Casanova, a famous 18th-century Italian lover and adventurer>.

Cassandra

- **Cassandra** a person who makes predictions about unpleasant future events but who is never believed. <In Greek legend, Cassandra, who was the daughter of Priam, king of Troy, had the gift of prophecy but was destined never to be believed. She predicted the fall of Troy>.

cast

- **cast pearls before swine** to offer something valuable or desirable to someone who does not appreciate it. <A biblical reference to Matthew 7:6>.

castle

- **castles in the air** or **castles in Spain** dreams or hopes that are unlikely ever to be realized.

cat

- **curiosity killed the cat** said as a warning not to pry into other people's affairs.
- **let the cat out of a bag** to reveal something secret or confidential, especially accidentally or at an inappropriate time. <Supposedly referring to a fairground trick in which a customer was offered a cat in a bag when he or she thought it was a piglet in the bag>.
- **like a scalded cat** in a rapid, excited way.
- **like something the cat brought** or **dragged in** very untidy or bedraggled.
- **not enough room to swing a cat** very little space.
- **not to have a cat's chance in hell** or **a cat's chance in hell** to have no chance at all.
- **play cat and mouse with (someone)** to treat (someone) in such a way that he or she does not know what is going to happen to them at any time. <A cat often plays with its prey, a mouse, before killing it>.
- **put** or **set the cat among the pigeons** to cause a disturbance, especially a sudden or unexpected one.
- **rain cats and dogs** to rain very heavily.
- **see which way the cat jumps** to wait and see what other people are going to do and how the situation is developing before deciding on one's course of action.
- **there's more than one way to kill** or **skin a cat** there's more than one way or method of doing things.
- **when the cat's away, the mice will play** when the person in charge or in control is not present the people whom he or she is in charge of will work less hard, misbehave, etc.

catch

- **catch (someone) napping** to surprise (someone) when he or she is unprepared or inattentive.
- **Catch 22** a situation in which one can never win or from which one can never escape, being constantly hindered by a rule or restriction that itself changes to block any change in one's plans; a difficulty that prevents one from escaping from an unpleasant or dangerous situation. <From the title of a novel by Joseph Heller>.
- **catch (someone) with his** or **her pants** or **trousers down** to surprise (someone) when he or she is unprepared or doing something wrong, especially when this causes embarrassment. <Refers to walking in on someone partially dressed>.

caviar

- **caviar to the general** something considered to be too sophisticated to be appreciated by ordinary people. <From Shakespeare's *Hamlet*, Act 2, scene II>.

ceiling

- **go through the ceiling** to rise very high, to soar.
- **hit the ceiling** or **roof** to lose one's temper completely.

chalice

- **hand/give (someone) a poisoned chalice** to be given something to do which seems an attractive proposition but which may well lead to failure or extreme difficulties.

chalk

- **as different as chalk and cheese** completely different.
- **chalk it up to experience** accept the inevitability of something.

- **not by a long chalk** not by a long way, by no means. <From the vertical chalk lines drawn to mark scores in a game, the longer lines representing the greater number of points>.

chance
- **have an eye to the main chance** to watch carefully for what will be advantageous or profitable to oneself.
- **not to have the ghost of a chance** not to have the slightest possibility of success.
- **change hands** to pass into different ownership.

change
- **change horses in mid-stream** to change one's opinions, plans, sides, etc, in the middle of something.
- **change one's tune** to change one's attitude or opinion.
- **ring the changes** to add variety by doing or arranging things in different ways.

chapter
- **chapter and verse** detailed sources for a piece of information. <From the method of referring to biblical texts>.

charity
- **charity begins at home** one must take care of oneself and one's family before concerning oneself with others.
- **cold as charity** extremely cold. <Charity is referred to as cold since it tends to be given to the poor and disadvantaged by organizations rather than by individual people and so lacks human feeling or warmth>.

charm
- **lead a charmed life** regularly to have good fortune and avoid misfortune, harm or danger.
- **work like a charm** to be very effective, to work very well.

chase
- **chase after rainbows** to spend time and effort in thinking about, or in trying to obtain, things that it is impossible for one to achieve.
- **cut to the chase** to start discussing or dealing with the most important part of something instead of wasting time on minor points. <Refers to the fact that in certain kinds of film a car chase is the most exciting part>.

cheek
- **cheek by jowl** side by side, very close together.
- **turn the other cheek** to take no action against someone who has harmed one, thereby giving him or her the opportunity to harm one again. <A biblical reference to Matthew 5:39, 'Whosoever shall smite thee on thy right cheek, turn to him the left one also'>.

cheese
- **hard cheese** bad luck, a sentiment usually expressed by someone who does not care about the misfortune.

Cheshire
- **grin like a Cheshire cat** to smile broadly so as to show one's teeth. <Refers to *Alice's Adventures in Wonderland* by Lewis Carroll, in which the Cheshire cat gradually disappears except for its smile>.

chest
- **get (something) off one's chest** to tell (someone) about something that is upsetting, worrying or annoying one.
- **old chestnut** an old joke, usually one no longer funny.
- **pull (someone's) chestnuts out of the fire** to rescue (someone) from a difficult or dangerous situation, often by putting oneself in difficulty or danger. <From a story by the 17th-century French writer La Fontaine, in which a monkey use a cat's paw to get hot nuts from a fire>.

chew
- **chew the cud** to think deeply about something.
- **chew the fat** to have a discussion or conversation.

chicken
- **chickens come home to roost** misdeeds, mistakes, etc, that come back with an unpleasant effect on the person who performed the misdeed, especially after a considerable time.
- **count one's chickens before they are hatched** to make plans which depend on something that is still uncertain.

child
- **child's play** something that is very easy to do.

chin
- **keep one's chin up** not to show feelings of depression, worry or fear.
- **take it on the chin** to accept or to suffer (something) with courage.

chip
- **a chip off the old block** a person who is very like one of his or her parents.
- **cash in one's chips** to die. <Refers to a gambler cashing in his or her chips or tokens in exchange for money at the end of a session>.
- **have a chip on one's shoulder** to have an aggressive attitude and act as if everyone is going to insult or ill-treat one, often because one feels inferior. <Refers to a former American custom by which a young man who wished to provoke a fight would place a piece of wood on his shoulder and dare someone to knock it off>.
- **have had one's chips** to have had, and failed at, all the chances of success one is likely to get. <Refers to gambling tokens>.
- **when the chips are down** when a situation has reached a critical stage. <A gambling terms indicating that the bets have been placed>.

choice
- **Hobson's choice** no choice at all; a choice between accepting what is offered or having nothing at all. <Refers to the practice of Tobias Hobson, an English stable-owner in the 17th century, of offering customers only the horse nearest the stable door>.

chop
- **chop and change** to keep altering (something), to keep changing (something).
- **get the chop 1** to be dismissed or discontinued. **2** to be killed.

chord
- **strike a chord** to be familiar in some way.
- **touch a chord** to arouse emotion or sympathy.

circle
- **come full circle** to return to the position or situation from which one started.
- **go round in circles** to keep going over the same ideas without reaching a satisfactory decision or answer.
- **run round in circles** to dash about and appear to be very busy without accomplishing anything.
- **vicious circle** an unfortunate or bad situation, the result of which produces the original cause of the situation or something similar. <In logic, the term for the fallacy of proving one statement by the evidence of another which is itself only valid if the first statement is valid>.

circus
- **a three-ring circus** a place where there is a lot of noise and a lot of confused activity going on.

clean
- **a clean slate** a record free of any discredit; an opportunity to make a fresh start. <Slates were formerly used for writing on in schools>.
- **come clean** to tell the truth about something, especially after lying about it.
- **keep one's nose clean** to keep out of trouble, to behave well or legally.
- **make a clean breast of (something)** to admit to (something), especially after having denied it.
- **make a clean sweep** to get rid of everything which is unnecessary or unwanted.
- **show a clean pair of heels** to run away very quickly.
- **squeaky clean** free of all guilt or blame. <Clean surfaces tend to squeak when wiped>.
- **take (someone) to the cleaners** to cause (someone) to spend or lose a great deal of money.

clear
- **clear as a bell** very easy to hear. <Bells, such as church bells, are very audible>.
- **clear as crystal** very easy to understand or grasp.
- **clear as mud** not at all easy to understand or grasp.
- **clear the decks** to tidy up, especially as a preparation for some activity or project. <Refers to getting a ship ready for battle>.
- **steer clear of (someone or something)** to keep away from or avoid (someone or something).
- **the coast is clear** the danger or difficulty has now passed. <Probably a military term indicating that there were no enemy forces near the coast and so an invasion was possible>.

cleft
- **in a cleft stick** unable to decide between two equally important or difficult courses of action.

clip
- **clip (someone's) wings** to limit the freedom, power or influence of (someone). <From the practice of clipping the wings of a bird to prevent it flying away>.

cloak
- **cloak-and-dagger** involving or relating to a great deal of plotting and scheming. <The combination of a cloak and a dagger suggests conspiracy>.

clock
- **like clockwork** very smoothly, without problems.
- **put back the clock** *or* **turn the clock back** to return to the conditions or situation of a former time.
- **round the clock** all the time; for twenty-four hours a day.

close[1]
- **behind closed doors** in secret.

close[2]
- **a close shave** something that was only just avoided, especially an escape from danger, failure, etc.

cloud
- **cloud cuckoo land** an imaginary place, where everything is perfect; an unreal world.
- **every cloud has a silver lining** something good happens for every bad or unpleasant thing.
- **have one's head in the clouds** to be day-dreaming and not paying attention to what is going on around one.
- **on cloud nine** extremely happy.
- **under a cloud** under suspicion, in trouble.

coach
- **drive a coach and horses through (something)** to destroy (an argument etc) completely by detecting and making use of the weak points in it. <Refers to the fact that the defects (or holes) in the argument are so large as to let a coach and horses through them>.

coal
- **carry** *or* **take coals to Newcastle** to do something that is completely unnecessary, especially to take something to a place where there is already a great deal of it. <Refers to Newcastle in England which was a large coal-mining centre>.
- **haul (someone) over the coals** to scold (someone) very severely.

coat
- **cut one's coat according to one's cloth** to organize one's ideas and aims, particularly one's financial aims, so that they are within the limits of what one has or possesses.

cobweb
- **blow away the cobwebs** to make (someone) feel more energetic and alert after feeling rather tired and dull.

cock
- **a cock-and-bull story** an absurd story that is unlikely to be believed.
- **cock a snook at (someone)** to express one's defiance or contempt of (someone). <Originally referring to a rude gesture of contempt made by putting the end of

one's thumb on the end of one's nose and spreading out and moving one's fingers>.

- **go off at half cock** to be unsuccessful because of lack of preparation or because of a premature start. <Refers to a gun that fires too soon>.

coffee
- **wake up and smell the coffee** to become more aware of and more realistic about what is going on around one.

coin
- **pay (someone) back in his** *or* **her own coin** to get one's revenge on someone who has done harm to one by treating him or her in the same way.
- **the other side of the coin** the opposite argument, point of view, etc.

cold
- **get cold feet** to become nervous and change one's mind about being involved in (something).
- **give (someone) the cold shoulder** to act in an unfriendly way to (someone) by ignoring him or her.
- **in a cold sweat** in a state of great fear or anxiety. <From the fact that the skin tends to become cold and damp when one is very frightened>.
- **make (someone's) blood run cold** to cause terror or great distress in (someone).
- **pour** *or* **throw cold water on (something)** to discourage enthusiasm for (something).

colour
- **change colour** to become either very pale or else very red in the face through fear, distress, embarrassment, anger, guilt, etc.
- **nail one's colours to the mast** to commit oneself to a point of view or course of action in a very obvious and final way. <Refers to a ship's colours or flag. If this was nailed to the mast it could not be lowered, lowering the flag being a sign of surrender>.
- **show oneself in one's true colours** to reveal what one is really like after pretending to be otherwise. <Refers to a ship raising its colours or flag to indicate which country or side it was supporting>.
- **with flying colours** with great success. <Refers to a ship leaving a battle with its colours or flag still flying as opposed to lowering them in surrender>.

common
- **common-or-garden** completely ordinary.

conjure
- **a name to conjure with** the name of someone very important, influential or well known. <The suggestion is that such people have magical powers>.

contradiction
- **a contradiction in terms** a statement, idea, etc, that contains a contradiction.

convert
- **preach to the converted** to speak enthusiastically in favour of something to people who already admire it or are in favour of it.

cook
- **too many cooks spoil the broth** if there are a great many people involved in a project they are more likely to hinder it than help it.

cookie
- **that's the way the cookie crumbles** that is the situation and one must just accept it. <Cookie is American English for biscuit>.

cool
- **cool as a cucumber** very calm and unexcited.
- **cool** *or* **kick one's heels** to be kept waiting.
- **keep one's cool** to remain calm.
- **lose one's cool** to become angry, excited etc.

copy
- **blot one's copybook** to spoil a previously good record of behaviour, achievement, etc, by doing something wrong.

corn
- **tread on (someone's) corns** to offend (someone).

corner
- **cut corners** to use less money, materials, effort, time, etc, than is usually required or than is required to give a good result.
- **from all (four) corners of the earth** from every part of the world, from everywhere.
- **in a tight corner** in an awkward, difficult or dangerous situation.
- **paint oneself into a corner** to get oneself into a difficult situation from which there is only one method of escape or action.
- **turn the corner** to begin to get better or improve.

cost
- **cost a bomb** *or* **a packet** to cost a very great deal of money.
- **cost an arm and a leg** to cost an excessive amount of money.
- **cost the earth** to cost a very great deal of money.

cotton
- **wrap (someone) in cotton wool** to be over-protective of (someone).

count
- **out for the count** unconscious or deeply asleep. <Refers to boxing where a boxer who has been knocked down by his opponent has to get up again before the referee counts to ten in order to stay in the match>.

courage
- **have the courage of one's convictions** to be brave enough to do what one thinks one should.
- **pluck up** *or* **screw up courage** to force oneself to be brave.

court
- **laugh (someone *or* something) out of court** not to give serious consideration to (someone or something). <Refers to a trivial legal case>.
- **pay court to (someone)** to try to gain the love of (someone).
- **the ball is in (someone's) court** it is (someone's) turn to take action.
- **rule (something) out of court** to prevent (something) from being considered for (something). <Refers to a court of law where evidence, etc, ruled out of court has no effect on the case>.

Coventry
- **send (someone) to Coventry** collectively to refuse to associate with (someone). <Perhaps from an incident in the English Civil War when Royalists captured in Birmingham were sent to the stronghold of Coventry>.

cow
- **a sacred cow** something that is regarded with too much respect for people to be allowed to criticize it freely. <The cow is considered sacred by Hindus>.
- **till *or* until the cows come home** for an extremely long time. <Cows walk very slowly from the field to the milking sheds unless someone hurries them along>.

crack
- **a fair crack of the whip** a fair share, a fair chance of doing (something).
- **at (the) crack of dawn** very early in the morning.
- **crack the whip** to treat sternly or severely those under one's control or charge. <From the use of a whip to punish people>.
- **take a sledgehammer to crack a nut** to spend a great deal of effort on a small task or problem.

crest
- **be (riding) on the crest of a wave** to be going through a very successful period.

cricket
- **not cricket** not fair or honourable, unsportsmanlike. <The game of cricket is regarded as being played in a gentlemanly way>.

crocodile
- **crocodile tears** a pretended show of grief or sorrow. <Refers to an old belief that crocodiles weep while eating their prey>.

cross
- **cross the Rubicon** to do something that commits one completely to a course of action that cannot be undone. <Julius Caesar's crossing of the River Rubicon in 49 BC committed him to war with the Senate>.
- **have a cross to bear** to have to suffer or tolerate a responsibility, inconvenience or source of distress. <Refers to the fact that in the days of crucifixions, those being crucified had to carry their own crosses>.

- **talk at cross purposes** to be involved in a misunderstanding because of talking or thinking about different things without realizing it.

crow
- **eat crow** to have to admit or accept that one was wrong.

crunch
- **when it comes to the crunch** when a time of testing comes, when a decision has to be made.

cry
- **a far cry from (something)** a long way from (something), very different from (something).
- **cry over spilt milk** to waste time regretting a misfortune or accident that cannot be undone.
- **in full cry** enthusiastically and excitedly pursuing something. <Refers to the cry made by hunting dogs>.

cuckoo
- **a cuckoo in the nest** a person who gains some kind of advantage from a situation without contributing anything useful. <From the cuckoo's habit of laying their eggs in other birds' nests>.

cudgel
- **take up the cudgels on behalf of (someone *or* something)** to fight strongly on behalf of (someone or something), to support (someone or something) vigorously.

cue
- **take one's cue from (someone)** to use the actions or reactions of (someone) as a guide to one's own, to copy (someone's) actions. <A theatrical term, literally meaning to use the words of another actor as a signal for one to speak or move>.

cuff
- **off the cuff** without preparation. <Refers to the habit of some after-dinner speakers of making brief headings on the celluloid cuffs of their evening shirts as a reminder of what he or she wanted to say rather than preparing a formal speech>.

cup
- **not be one's cup of tea** not to be something which one likes or appreciates.

cupboard
- **cupboard love** pretended affection shown for a person because of the things he or she gives one. <From people and animals liking those who feed them, food being kept in cupboards>.
- **curry favour with (someone)** to try to gain the approval or favour of (someone) by insincere flattery or by being extremely nice to him or her all the time. <Originally curry favel, from Old French *estriller fauvel*, *fauvel* being a chestnut horse>.

curtain
- **be curtains for (someone *or* something)** to be the end of (someone or something). <Refers to curtains falling at the end of a stage performance>.

- **bring down the curtain on (something)** to cause (something) to come to an end. <See above>.
- **curtain lecture** a private scolding, especially one given by a wife to a husband. <From the curtains that formerly were hung round a bed>.

cut

- **a cut above (someone *or* something)** rather better than (someone or something).
- **cut a long story short** to give a brief account of something quite complicated or lengthy.
- **cut and dried** settled and definite. <Refers to wood that has been cut and dried and made ready for use>.
- **cut and thrust** methods and techniques of rivalry, argument or debate. <Refers to sword fighting>.
- **cut both ways** to have an equal or the same effect on both parts of a question or on both people involved in something.
- **cut it fine** to allow hardly enough time to do or get something.
- **not cut out for (something)** not naturally suited to.

cylinder

- **firing on all cylinders** working or operating at full strength. <Literally used of an internal combustion engine>.

dagger

- **at daggers drawn** feeling or showing great hostility towards each other.
- **look daggers at (someone)** to look with great dislike or hostility at (someone).

daisy

- **be pushing up the daisies** to be dead.
- **fresh as a daisy** not at all tired, lively.

damp

- **a damp squib** something which is expected to be exciting, effective, etc, but which fails to live up to its expectations. <Refers to a wet firework that fails to go off>.
- **put a damper on (something)** to reduce the enjoyment, optimism, happiness of (something).

dance

- **lead (someone) a (merry) dance** to cause (someone) a series of great, usually unnecessary, problems or irritations.

Darby

- **Darby and Joan** a devoted elderly couple. <From the names of such a couple in an 18th-century English ballad>.

dark

- **a shot in the dark** an attempt or guess based on very little information.
- **be whistling in the dark** to try to give the impression that one is more confident of, or less worried about, a situation than one actually is.
- **dark horse** a person or thing whose abilities, worth, etc, is unknown.

- **in the dark** lacking knowledge or awareness.
- **keep it *or* something dark** to keep it or something secret.

dash

- **cut a dash** to wear very smart or unusual clothes and so impress others.

Davy Jones

- **Davy Jones's locker** the bottom of the sea. <Davy Jones was a name given in the 18th century to the ruler of the evil spirits of the sea>.

dawn

- **a false dawn** an event which makes a situation look as though it is improving when it is not.

day

- **all in a day's work** all part of one's normal routine, not requiring extra or unusual effort.
- **any day of the week** whatever the circumstances.
- **call it a day** to put an end to (something); to stop doing (something), especially to stop working.
- **carry *or* win the day** to be successful, to gain a victory. <Originally a military term meaning to win a battle>.
- **daylight robbery** the charging of prices that are far too high.
- **(your, etc) days are numbered** you are about to be dismissed, be killed, etc.
- **every dog has his day** everyone will get an opportunity at some time.
- **have had one's *or* its day** to be past the most successful part of one's or its life.
- **live from day to day** to think only about the present without making any plans for the future.
- **make (someone's) day** to make (someone) very pleased or happy.
- **name the day** to announce the date of one's wedding.
- **not to be one's day** to be a day when nothing seems to go right for one.
- **one of these days** at some time in the future.
- **one of those days** a day when nothing seems to go right.
- **see daylight** to be coming to the end of a long task.
- **seize the day** to take advantage of any opportunities which occur now, rather than worry about the future.

dead

- **a dead duck** a person or thing that is very unlikely to survive or continue.
- **a dead loss** a person or thing that is completely useless or unprofitable.
- **cut (someone) dead** to ignore (someone) completely.
- **dead and buried** completely dead or extinct with no chance of being revived.
- **dead as a dodo** completely dead or out of fashion. <Refers to a flightless bird that has been extinct since 1700>.
- **dead beat** exhausted.
- **dead from the neck up** extremely stupid.

- **dead in the water** with no hope of success. <Refers to a dead fish which is no use to fishermen or anglers.>
- **Dead Sea fruit** a thing that appears to be, or is expected to be, of great value but proves to be valueless. <Refers to a fruit, the apple of Sodom, that was thought to grow on trees beside the shores of the Dead Sea. It was beautiful to look at but fell to ashes when touched or tasted>.
- **dead to the world** in a very deep sleep.
- **dead wood** a person or thing that is no longer necessary or useful.
- **enough to waken the dead** extremely loud.
- **let the dead bury their dead** past problems, quarrels, etc, are best forgotten. <A biblical reference to Matthew 8:22, in which Jesus said, 'Follow me and let the dead bury their dead'.>
- **over my dead body** in the face of my fierce opposition.
- **step into** *or* **fill dead men's shoes** to take over the position of someone who has died or left under unfortunate circumstances.
- **would not be seen dead in** *or* **with, etc,** extremely unlikely to be seen wearing something, accompanying someone, etc, because of an extreme dislike or aversion.

deaf
- **deaf as a post** completely deaf.
- **fall on deaf ears** not to be listened to, to go unnoticed or disregarded.
- **stone deaf** completely deaf.
- **turn a deaf ear to (something)** to refuse to listen to (something), to take no notice of (something).

deal
- **a raw deal** unfair treatment.

death
- **at death's door** extremely ill, dying.
- **be in at the death** to be present at the end or final stages of something. <Refers originally to being present at the death of the prey in a hunt>.
- **catch one's death (of cold)** to become infected with a very bad cold.
- **dice with death** to do something extremely risky and dangerous.
- **die the death** to be badly received. <Refers originally to an actor or performer getting a poor reception from the audience>.
- **sick** *or* **tired to death of (someone** *or* **something)** extremely weary or bored with (someone or something).
- **sign one's own death warrant** to bring about one's own downfall, ruin, etc.
- **will be the death of (someone) 1** to cause the death of (someone). **2** to make (someone) laugh a great deal.

deck
- **hit the deck** to fall to the ground.

deep
- **be thrown in at the deep end** to be put suddenly into a difficult situation of which one has no experience. <Refers to the deep end of a swimming pool>.
- **go off at the deep end** to lose one's temper. (See above).

degree
- **give (someone) the third degree** to subject (someone) to intense questioning, especially by using severe methods.
- **to the nth degree** to the greatest possible degree, extent or amount. <Refers to the use of n as a symbol to represent a number, especially a large number>.

dent
- **make a dent in (something)** to reduce (something) by a considerable amount.

depth
- **out of one's depth** in a situation which one cannot cope with. <Refers literally to being in water deeper than one can stand up in>.
- **plumb the depths of (something)** to reach the lowest level of unhappiness, misfortune, etc.

deserts
- **get one's just deserts** to be treated as one deserves, especially to receive deserved punishment.

design
- **have designs upon (someone** *or* **something)** to wish to possess (someone or something), usually belonging to someone else.

device
- **leave (someone) to his** *or* **her own devices** to leave (someone) to look after himself or herself, often after having tried unsuccessfully to help him or her.

devil
- **better the devil you know** it is preferable to have someone or something that one knows to be bad than take a chance with someone or something that might turn out even worse.
- **between the devil and the deep blue sea** faced with two possible courses of action each of which is as unacceptable as the other.
- **needs must when the devil drives** if it is absolutely necessary that something must be done then one must do it.
- **play the devil's advocate** to put forward objections to a plan, idea, etc, simply in order to test the strength of the arguments in its favour.
- **speak of the devil** here is the very person whom we have just been referring to. <Short for 'speak of the devil and he will appear' which refers to a superstition by which it was thought that talking about evil gave it the power to appear>.

diamond
- **rough diamond** a person who behaves in a rough manner but who has good or valuable qualities.

dice
- **load the dice against (someone)** to arrange things so that (someone) has no chance of success. <Refers to a method of cheating in gambling by putting lead or similar heavy material into a dice so that only certain numbers will come up>.

die[1]
- **be dying for (something)** to be longing for (something).
- **die with one's boots on** to die while still working. <Refers to soldiers dying in active service>.
- **never say die** never give up hope.

die[2]
- **the die is cast** a step has been taken which makes the course of future events inevitable. <A translation of the Latin *iacta alea est*, supposedly said by Julius Caesar when he crossed the Rubicon in 49 BC and so committed himself to a war with the Senate>.

differ
- **agree to differ** to agree not to argue about something any more since neither party is likely to change his or her opinion.
- **sink one's differences** to forget about past disagreements.
- **split the difference** to agree on an amount of money halfway between two amounts, especially between the amount that one person is charging for something and the amount that someone else is willing to pay for it.

dig
- **dig one's heels in** to show great determination, especially in order to get one's own wishes carried out.
- **dig one's own grave** to be the cause of one's own misfortune.

dilemma
- **on the horns of a dilemma** in a position where it is necessary to choose between two courses of action. <In medieval rhetoric a dilemma was likened to a two-horned animal on one of whose horns the person making the decision had to throw himself or herself>.

dim
- **take a dim view of (something)** to look with disapproval on (something).

dine
- **dine out on (something)** to be given social invitations because of information, gossip, etc, one can pass on.

dinner
- **like a dog's dinner** an untidy mess.
- **more of (something) than you have had hot dinners** a very great deal of (something).

dirt
- **dirty old man** an elderly man who shows a sexual interest in young girls or young boys.
- **(someone's) name is dirt** *or* **mud** (someone) is in great disfavour.

discretion
- **discretion is the better part of valour** it is wise not to take any unnecessary risks. <Refers to Shakespeare's *Henry IV Part 1*, Act 5, scene IV>.

distance
- **go the distance** to complete something successfully, to last until the end of something.
- **keep one's distance** not to come too close, not to be too friendly.
- **within striking distance** reasonably close.

dividend
- **pay dividends** to bring advantages at a later time. <Refers to dividends paid on money invested, as on stocks and shares>.

do
- **do one's bit** to do one's share of the work, etc.
- **do (someone) in** to kill (someone).
- **done for** without any hope of rescue, help or recovery.
- **do or die** to make the greatest effort possible at the risk of killing, injuring, ruining, etc, oneself.
- **do the honours** to act as host, to serve food or drink to one's guests.
- **do time** to serve a prison sentence.
- **not the done thing** not acceptable behaviour.
- **the do's and don'ts** what one should or should not do in a particular situation.

doctor
- **just what the doctor ordered** exactly what is required.

dog
- **a dog in the manger** a person who stops someone else from doing or having something which he himself or she herself does not want. <From one of Aesop's fables in which a dog prevents the horses from eating the hay in the feeding rack although he himself did not want to eat the hay>.
- **a dog's life** a miserable life.
- **dog eat dog** a ruthless struggle against one's rivals to survive or be successful.
- **go to the dogs** to be no longer good, moral, successful, etc.
- **give a dog a bad name** if bad things are said about a person's character they will stay with him or her for the rest of his or her life.
- **in the doghouse** in disfavour.
- **keep a dog and bark oneself** to employ someone to do a job and then do it oneself.
- **let sleeping dogs lie** do not look for trouble; if there is no trouble, do not cause any.
- **you can't teach an old dog new tricks** the older you get the more difficult it is to learn new skills or accept ideas or new fashions.

doggo
- **lie doggo** to remain in hiding, not to do anything that will draw attention to oneself.

donkey
- **donkey's ages** *or* **years** a very long time. <Perhaps from a pun on donkey's ears, which are very long>.
- **donkey work** the hard, often tiring or physical, part of any job.

- **talk the hind legs off a donkey** to talk too much or to talk for a very long time.

door
- **darken (someone's) door** to come or go into (someone's) house.
- **have a** *or* **one foot in the door** to start to gain entrance to somewhere or something when entrance is difficult. <Refers to someone putting a foot in a door to wedge it open in order to gain entrance>.
- **lay (something) at (someone's) door** to blame (someone) for (something).
- **open doors** to give someone an opportunity to improve his or her position, to improve someone's chances of success.
- **show (someone) the door** to make (someone) leave.

dose
- **a dose** *or* **taste of one's own medicine** something unpleasant done to a person who is in the habit of doing similar things to other people.

dot
- **dot the i's and cross the t's** to attend to details.
- **on the dot** **1** exactly on time. **2** exactly at the time stated. <Refers to the dots on the face of a clock>.

double
- **at the double** very quickly. <A military term, literally at twice the normal marching speed>.
- **do a double take** to look at or think about (someone or something) a second time because one has not taken it in or understood it the first time.
- **double Dutch** unintelligible words or language. <Refers to the fact that Dutch sounds a very difficult language to those who are not native speakers of it>.

doubt
- **a doubting Thomas** a person who will not believe something without strong proof. <Refers to the biblical story Thomas, the disciple who doubted Christ, John 21:24–29>.

down
- **down in the dumps** *or* **down in the mouth** depressed, in low spirits.
- **down the drain** completely wasted.
- **down under** Australia.
- **get down to (something)** to begin to work at (something) in earnest.
- **go downhill** to get worse and worse, to deteriorate.
- **have a down on (someone** *or* **something)** to be very hostile or opposed to (someone or something).

drawer
- **out of the top drawer** from the upper classes or aristocracy.

dream
- **a dream ticket** used of two people who are expected to work very successfully together. <Originally used to refer to political elections>.

dress
- **dressed to kill** *or* **dressed to the nines** dressed in one's smartest clothes so as to attract attention.

drift
- **get the drift** to understand the general meaning of something.

drink
- **drink like a fish** to drink a great deal of alcoholic drinks.

drop
- **at the drop of a hat** immediately, requiring only the slightest excuse.
- **drop into (someone's) lap** to happen to (someone) without any effort.
- **let (something) drop** to let (something) be known accidentally.

drown
- **drown one's sorrows** to take alcoholic drink in order to forget one's unhappiness.

drum
- **drum (someone) out** to send (someone) away, to ask (someone) to leave. <Refers to the use of drums when an officer was being publicly dismissed from his regiment>.

dry
- **a dry run** a practice attempt, a rehearsal.
- **dry as a bone** extremely dry.
- **dry as dust** extremely dull or boring.
- **dry up** to forget what one was going to say.
- **keep one's powder dry** to remain calm and prepared for immediate action. <Refers to the fact that gunpowder must be kept dry to be effective>.

duck
- **a lame duck** a weak or inefficient person or organization.
- **a sitting duck** a person or thing that is very easy to attack. <Refers to the fact that a sitting duck is easier to shoot at than one flying in the air>.
- **be water off a duck's back** be totally ineffective. <Refers to the fact that water runs straight off the oily feathers on a duck's back>.
- **break one's duck** to have one's first success. <A cricketing term. No score in cricket is known as a duck>.
- **take to (something) like a duck to water.** to be able to do (something) right from the beginning naturally and without difficulty.
- **ugly duckling** an unattractive or uninteresting person or thing that develops in time into someone or something very attractive, interesting or successful. <Refers to the story by Hans Andersen about a baby swan that is brought up by ducks who consider it ugly by their standards until it grows into a beautiful swan>.

dust
- **let the dust settle** to give things time to calm down.

- **not see (someone) for dust** not to see (someone) again because he has run away. <Refers to clouds of dust left behind by horses or vehicles when they are moving fast>.
- **shake the dust from one's feet** to leave somewhere, usually gladly.
- **throw dust in (someone's eyes)** to attempt to confuse or deceive (someone). <Dust temporarily blinds people if it gets into their eyes>.

Dutch

- **Dutch auction** an auction in which the auctioneer starts with a high price and reduces it until someone puts in a bid.
- **Dutch courage** courage that is not real courage but induced by drinking alcohol. <Perhaps from a Dutch military custom of drinking alcohol before going into battle, perhaps from the fact that gin was introduced into England by the Dutch followers of William III>.
- **Dutch treat** a kind of entertainment or celebration where everyone concerned pays for himself or herself. <From Dutch lunch, to which all of the guests were expected to contribute some of the food>.
- **go Dutch** to share expenses.
- **talk to (someone) like a Dutch uncle** to scold (someone) or talk to (someone) for what is supposedly his or her own good. <Perhaps from the Dutch's reputation for strict family discipline>.

ear

- **go in one ear and out the other** not to make any lasting impression.
- **grin from ear to ear** to have a wide smile on your face.
- **have** *or* **keep one's ear to the ground** to keep oneself informed about what is happening around one. <Perhaps from a North American Indian method of tracking prey>.
- **(my, etc) ears are burning** someone somewhere is talking about (me, etc). <The belief that one's ears grow hot when someone is talking about one is mentioned by Pliny, the Roman writer>.
- **up to one's ears in (something)** deeply involved in (something). <A comparison with someone who is almost submerged by very deep water>.

earth

- **bring (someone) (back) down to earth** to make (someone) aware of the practicalities of life or of a situation.
- **run (someone** *or* **something) to earth** to find (someone or something) after a long search. <Refers to a hunting term for chasing a fox into its earth or hole>.

easy

- **easy as falling off a log** *or* **easy as pie** extremely easy.
- **easy on the eye** very attractive.

eat

- **have (someone) eating out of one's hand** to have (someone) doing everything that one wishes, because he or she likes or admires one. <Refers to an animal that is so tame that it will eat out of someone's hand>.

ebb

- **at a low ebb** in a poor or depressed state. <Refers to the tide when it has flowed away from the land>.

edge

- **be at the cutting edge of (something)** to be involved in the most modern, advanced development or stage of (something).
- **be on the edge of your seat** to be very excited and eager to know what happens next.
- **have the edge on (someone** *or* **something)** to have the advantage of (someone or something).
- **lose one's edge** to become less effective or less good at what you do. <Refers to a knife becoming blunt>.
- **push (someone) over the edge** to make someone unable to cope, mentally ill, etc.

egg

- **be left with egg on one's face** to be left looking foolish.
- **put all one's eggs in one basket** to rely entirely on the success of one project, etc.
- **teach one's grandmother to suck eggs** to try to tell someone how to do something when he or she is much more experienced than oneself at it.

eight

- **be** *or* **have one over the eight** to be or to have had too much to drink. <Refers to a former belief that one could have eight drinks before one is drunk>.

elbow

- **give (someone) the elbow** to get rid of (someone), to end a relationship with (someone).

element

- **in one's element** in a situation in which one is happy or at one's best. <Refers to the four elements of medieval science of fire, earth, air and water>.

elephant

- **a white elephant** something which is useless and troublesome to look after. <White elephants were given by the Kings of Siam followers who had displeased them since the cost of keeping such an elephant was such that it would ruin the follower>.
- **have a memory like an elephant** never to forget things.

eleventh

- **at the eleventh hour** at the last possible minute. <A biblical reference to the parable of the labourers in the vineyard in Matthew 20>.

empty

- **empty vessels make most noise** the most foolish or least informed people are most likely to voice their opinions.

end

- **at a loose end** with nothing to do, with no plans.
- **at the end of one's tether** at the end of one's patience, tolerance, etc. <Refers to a rope that will only extend a certain distance to let the animal attached to it graze>.

- **make ends meet** to live within the limits of one's income. <The ends referred to are the start and finish of one's annual accounts>.

enough
- **enough is as good as a feast** if you have enough of something you should be satisfied with that; you do not need any more.

eternal
- **eternal triangle** a sexual relationship between two men and one woman or between two women and one man.

even
- **get** *or* **keep on an even keel** to be or keep steady or calm with no sudden changes.

event
- **be wise after the event** to realize how a situation should have been dealt with after it is over.

evidence
- **turn Queen's** *or* **King's evidence** to give evidence against a fellow criminal in order to have one's own sentence reduced.

evil
- **the lesser of two evils** the less unpleasant of two fairly unpleasant choices.
- **put off the evil hour** *or* **day** to keep postponing something unpleasant.

ewe
- **(someone's) ewe lamb** (someone's) favourite. <A biblical reference to Samuel 12:3>.

exception
- **the exception that proves the rule** the fact that an exception has to be made for a particular example of something proves that the general rule is valid.

eye
- **an eye for an eye (and a tooth for a tooth)** a punishment to match the offence committed. <A biblical reference to Exodus 21:23>.
- **a sight for sore eyes** a pleasant or welcome sight.
- **be one in the eye for (someone)** to be something unpleasant that happens to someone who deserves it.
- **keep an eagle eye on (someone or something)** to watch (someone or something) extremely closely. <Refers to the fact that eagles are thought to have particularly keen vision>.
- **keep a weather eye open** *or* **keep one's eyes peeled** *or* **skinned** to keep a close watch, to be alert. <A nautical term for watching for changes in the weather>.
- **make eyes at (someone)** to look at (someone) with sexual interest.
- **not to bat an eyelid** not to show any surprise, distress, etc.
- **raise some/a few eyebrows** to surprise or shock some people.

- **see eye to eye with (someone)** to be in agreement with (someone).
- **there's more to (someone *or* something) than meets the eye** the true worth or state of (someone or something) is not immediately obvious.

face
- **be staring one in the face 1** to be very obvious, although one may not realize this at first. **2** to be likely to happen or to be about to happen.
- **face the music** to face and deal with a situation caused by one's actions. <Perhaps from a performer facing the musicians below the front of the stage as he or she makes an entrance on stage>.
- **fly in the face of (something)** to oppose or defy (something). <Refers to a dog attacking>.
- **get out of (someone's) face** to go away and stop annoying (someone).
- **have a long face** to look unhappy.
- **keep a straight face** to stop oneself from smiling or laughing.
- **lose face** to suffer a loss of respect or reputation.
- **make** *or* **pull a face** to twist one's face into a strange or funny expression.
- **put a brave face on it** to try to appear brave when one is feeling afraid, distressed, etc.
- **save (someone's) face** to prevent (someone) from appearing stupid or wrong.
- **show one's face** to put in an appearance, especially when one will not be welcome or when one will be embarrassed.

faint
- **faint heart never won fair lady** boldness is necessary to achieve what one desires.
- **not to have the faintest** not to have the slightest idea.

fair
- **by fair means or foul** by any method whatsoever.
- **fair game** a person or thing that it is considered quite reasonable to attack, make fun of, etc.
- **fair play** fairness and justice.
- **fairweather friends** people who are friendly towards one only when one is not in trouble.

fall
- **fall back on (someone** *or* **something)** to rely on (someone or something) if all else fails.
- **fall flat** to fail, to have no effect.
- **fall foul of (something** *or* **something)** to do something that arouses someone's anger or hostility.
- **fall from grace** to lose (someone's) favour.
- **fall over oneself to** to set about doing something with great willingness and eagerness.

false
- **under false pretences** by using deceit.

family
- **run in the family** to be a characteristic found in many members of the same family.

fancy
- **(footloose and) fancy free** not in love with anyone, not romantically attached.
- **take** *or* **tickle one's fancy** to attract one, to arouse a liking in one.

far
- **go far** to be very successful.
- **go too far** to do or say something that is beyond the limits of what is acceptable.

fast
- **play fast and loose with (something)** to act irresponsibly with (something).
- **pull a fast one on (someone)** to deceive (someone). <Refers to bowling a fast ball in cricket>.

fat
- **it isn't over till the fat lady sings** used to remind people that the result of a competition, etc. is not established until the end of the game, match, etc.
- **live off the fat of the land** to live in a luxurious fashion.
- **the fat is in the fire** trouble has been started and it cannot be stopped. <Fat causes a fire to flare up>.

fate
- **a fate worse than death** something terrible that happens to one, often rape.
- **seal (someone's) fate** to ensure that something, usually unpleasant, happens to (someone).
- **tempt fate** to act in a way that is likely to bring one ill luck or misfortune.

fear
- **there is no fear of (something)** it is not likely that (something) will happen.

feast
- **be feast or famine** to be a situation in which there is too much of something or too little.

feat
- **be no mean feat** used to emphasize the difficulty of a task or venture.

feather
- **a feather in one's cap** something of which one can be proud.
- **feather one's (own) nest** to make a profit for oneself, often at the expense of someone else.
- **make the feathers** *or* **fur fly** to cause trouble or a quarrel. <Refers to birds or animals fighting>.
- **ruffle (someone's) feathers** to annoy or upset (someone).
- **show the white feather** to show signs of cowardice. <A white feather in the tail of a fighting cock was a sign of inferior breeding>.

feel
- **feel in one's bones** to know (something) by instinct.
- **feel one's feet** to be becoming used to a situation.

feet
- **at (someone's) feet 1** easily within (someone's) reach or power. **2** greatly admiring of (someone).
- **drag one's feet** to take a long time to do something.
- **fall** *or* **land on one's feet** to be fortunate or successful, especially after a period of uncertainty or misfortune.
- **find one's feet** to become capable of coping with a situation.
- **have feet of clay** to have a surprising weakness, despite having been thought to be perfect. <A biblical reference to Daniel 2:31–34>.
- **have both feet on the ground** *or* **have one's feet on the ground** to be practical and sensible.
- **get under (someone's) feet** to hinder or get in (someone's) way.
- **put one's feet up** to take a rest.
- **stand on one's own feet** to be independent.
- **sweep (someone) off his** *or* **her feet** to affect (someone) with great enthusiasm or emotion; to influence (someone) to do as one wishes.

fence
- **mend fences** to put things right after a quarrel, etc.
- **sit on the fence** to refuse to take sides in a dispute, etc.

fiddle
- **fit as a fiddle** extremely fit.
- **play second fiddle to (someone)** to be in a subordinate or inferior position to (someone).

field
- **have a field day** to have a very busy, successful or enjoyable day.
- **play the field** to take advantage of many chances offered to one, especially to go out with several members of the opposite sex.

fight
- **fighting fit** extremely healthy and in good condition.
- **fight shy of (something)** to avoid (something).

fill
- **have had one's fill** to have had enough, to be unable to tolerate any more.

fine
- **get (something) down to a fine art** to have learned to do (something) extremely well.
- **go through (something) with a fine-tooth comb** to search (something) very carefully. <A fine-tooth comb is used to remove the nits (eggs) of head lice from hair>.

finger
- **be all fingers and thumbs** to be clumsy or awkward when using one's hands.
- **burn one's fingers** *or* **get one's fingers burnt** to suffer because of something that one has been involved in.
- **cross one's fingers** to hope for good fortune.

- **get** *or* **pull one's finger out** to stop wasting time and get on with something.
- **have a finger in every pie** to be involved in a large number of projects, organizations, etc.
- **have (something) at one's fingertips** to know all the information about (something).
- **let (something) slip through one's fingers** to lose (an advantage, opportunity, etc), often by one's inaction.
- **not to lift a finger** not to do anything at all.
- **point the finger at (someone)** to indicate who is to blame.
- **put one's finger on (something)** to identify (something) exactly.
- **twist** *or* **wrap (someone) round one's little finger** to be able to get (someone) to do exactly as one wishes.
- **work your fingers to the bone** to work extremely hard.

fire
- **get on like a house on fire** to get on very well.
- **hang fire** to wait or be delayed. <Refers to a gun in which there is a delay between the trigger being pulled and the gun being fired>.
- **in the firing line** in a situation in which you are likely to be blamed or criticized. <Refers to people who have been lined up in order to be shot dead.>
- **play with fire** to take tasks, to do something dangerous.
- **set the Thames** *or* **world on fire** to do something remarkable. <Refers to the River Thames, which it would be impossible to set alight>.
- **under fire** being attacked. <Refers literally to being shot at>.

first
- **first thing** early in the morning or in the working day.
- **in the first flush of (something)** in the early and vigorous stages of (something).

fish
- **have other fish to fry** to have something else to do, especially something that is more important or more profitable.
- **like a fish out of water** ill at ease and unaccustomed to a situation.
- **there are plenty more fish in the sea** many more opportunities will arise; many more members of the opposite sex are around.

fit
- **by fits and starts** irregularly, often stopping and starting.

fix
- **in a fix** in an awkward or difficult situation.

flag
- **hang** *or* **put the flags out** to celebrate something (a rare event).
- **run (something) up the flagpole** to put forward (a plan or idea) in order to gauge reactions to it.

flame
- **an old flame** a former boyfriend or girlfriend.
- **fan the flames** to make a difficult situation worse.

flash
- **a flash in the pan** a sudden, brief success. <Refers to a flintlock gun in which the spark from the flint ignited the gunpowder in the priming pan, the flash then travelling to the main barrel. If this failed to go off there was only a flash in the pan>.

flat
- **in a flat spin** in a state of confused excitement.

flavour
- **flavour of the month** a person or thing that is particularly popular at a particular time, although this is likely to be temporary.

flea
- **a flea in one's ear** a sharp scolding.

flesh
- **a thorn in (someone's) flesh** a permanent source of annoyance or irritation. <A biblical reference to II Corinthians 12:7>.
- **get** *or* **have one's pound of flesh** to obtain everything that one is entitled to, especially if this causes difficulties or suffering to those who have to give it. <Refers to Shakespeare's play *The Merchant of Venice*, in which Shylock tries to enforce an agreement by which he can cut a pound of flesh from Antonio>.

floodgates
- **open the floodgates** to make it possible for a great many people to do something, usually something considered undesirable, or make it likely that this will happen, perhaps by removing some kind of restriction.

floor
- **take the floor 1** to rise to make a public speech. **2** to begin to dance.
- **wipe the floor with (someone)** to defeat (someone) thoroughly.

fly[1]
- **a fly in the ointment** something that spoils something.
- **there are no flies on (someone)** there is no possibility of deceiving or cheating (someone), there is no lack of sense in (someone).
- **would like to be a fly on the wall** would like to be present and able to hear what is going on without being seen.

fly[2]
- **get off to a flying start** to have a very successful beginning.

foam
- **foam at the mouth** to be very angry. <Mad dogs foam at the mouth>.

follow

- **follow suit** to do just as someone else has done. <A reference to card-playing when a player plays the same suit as the previous player>.

fool

- **a fool's paradise** a state of happiness that is based on something that is not true or realistic.
- **be nobody's fool** to have a good deal of common sense.
- **fools rush in (where angels fear to tread)** an ignorant person can sometimes achieve what a warier person cannot. <From Alexander Pope's *An Essay on Criticism*>.
- **make a fool of (someone)** to make (someone) appear ridiculous or stupid.
- **not to suffer fools gladly** not to have any patience with foolish or stupid people.

foot

- **follow in (someone's) footsteps** to do the same as someone else has done before, particularly a relative.
- **get off on the wrong foot** to get off to a bad or unfortunate start.
- **have one foot in the grave** to be very old.
- **put one's foot down** to be firm about something, to forbid someone to do something.
- **put one's foot in it** to do or say something tactless.
- **shoot oneself in the foot** to make a mistake or do something stupid which causes problems for oneself or harms one's chances of success.

form

- **on form** in good condition, fit and in a good humour. <Form refers to the condition of a horse>.

fort

- **hold the fort** to take temporary charge of something.

forty

- **forty winks** a short nap.

frame

- **be in the frame 1** to be likely to get or win something. **2** to be suspected of being guilty of a crime.

free

- **free and easy** informal, casual.
- **give (someone) a free hand** give (someone) permission to do as he or she wishes.

French

- **take French leave** to stay away from work, etc, without permission. <Refers to an 18th-century French custom of leaving a party without saying goodbye to one's host or hostess>.

Freudian

- **a Freudian slip** the use of a wrong word while speaking that is supposed to indicate an unconscious thought. <Refers to the theories of the psychologist Sigmund Freud>.

Friday

- **man** *or* **girl Friday** an invaluable assistant. <Refers to Friday, a character in *Robinson Crusoe* by Daniel Defoe>.

friend

- **a friend in need is a friend indeed** a friend who helps when one is in trouble is truly a friend.

frog

- **have a frog in one's throat** to be hoarse.

fruit

- **forbidden fruit** something desirable that is made even more so because one is forbidden for some reason to obtain it. <Refers to the biblical tree in the Garden of Eden whose fruit Adam was forbidden by God to eat, Genesis 3>.

fry

- **out of the frying pan into the fire** free of a difficult or dangerous situation only to get into a worse one.

full

- **be full of oneself** to be very conceited.
- **in the fullness of time** when the proper time has arrived, eventually.

fuss

- **make a fuss of (someone)** to pay a lot of attention to (someone), to show (someone) a lot of affection.

gab

- **the gift of the gab** the ability to talk readily and easily.

gain

- **gain ground** to make progress, to become more generally acceptable or popular.

gallery

- **play to the gallery** to act in an amusing or showy way to the ordinary people in an organization, etc, in order to gain popularity or their support.

game

- **beat (someone) at his** *or* **her own game** to do better than (someone) at his or her activity, especially a cunning or dishonest one.
- **give the game away** to reveal a secret plan, trick, etc, usually accidentally.
- **play the game** to behave fairly and honourably.
- **the game is up** the plan, trick, crime, etc, has been discovered and so has failed.

garden

- **everything in the garden is lovely** everything is fine.
- **lead (someone) up the garden path** to mislead or deceive (someone).

gauntlet

- **run the gauntlet** to be exposed or subjected to blame, criticism or risk. <Gauntlet is a mistaken form of Swedish *gatlopp*. Running the *gatlopp* was a Swedish military punishment in which the culprit had to run between two lines of men with whips who struck him as he passed>.

- **take/pick up the gauntlet** to accept a challenge.
- **throw down the gauntlet** to issue a challenge. <Throwing down a gauntlet, a protective glove, was the traditional method of challenging someone to a fight in medieval times>.

ghost
- **give up the ghost** to die, stop working, etc. <Ghost refers to a person's spirit—a biblical reference to Job 14:10>.

gift
- **look a gift horse in the mouth** to criticize something that has been given to one. <Looking at a horse's teeth is a way of telling its age and so estimating its value>.

gild
- **gild the lily** to add unnecessary decoration or detail. <An adaptation of a speech from Shakespeare's *King John*, Act 4, scene II>.

gilt
- **take the gilt off the gingerbread** to take away what makes something attractive. <Gingerbread used to be sold in fancy shapes and decorated with gold leaf>.

gird
- **gird up one's loins** to prepare oneself for action. <A biblical phrase from the fact that robes had to be tied up with a girdle before men began work or they got in the way, Acts 12:8>.

give
- **give and take** willingness to compromise.

glad
- **glad rags** best clothes worn for special occasions.

glass
- **glass ceiling** an invisible barrier, established by tradition, personal discrimination, etc, which prevents women from achieving the top jobs in their companies, professions, etc.
- **people who live in glass houses should not throw stones** people with faults themselves should not criticize faults in others.

glove
- **fit like a glove** to fit perfectly.
- **take the gloves off** to begin to fight, argue, etc, in earnest. <Refers to boxers who wear protective gloves to soften their blows>.

gold
- **be sitting on a goldmine** to posses something very valuable or potentially profitable, often without realizing this.
- **like living in a goldfish bowl** in a situation where one has very little privacy.
- **strike gold** to do or find something that makes one very rich or very successful.

gnat
- **strain at a gnat (and swallow a camel)** to trouble oneself over a matter of no importance, something only slightly wrong, etc, (but be unconcerned about a matter of great importance, something very wrong, etc). <A biblical reference to Matthew 23:23–24>.

go
- **from the word go** right from the very start of something.
- **make a go of it** *or* **something** to make a success of something.
- **no go** impossible, not given approval.
- **on the go** continually active, busy.

goal
- **score an own goal** to do something which fails to achieve what you set out to do and, instead, harms your own interests.

goalpost
- **move the goalposts** to change the conditions, rules or aims applying to a project, etc, after it is under way so that it is disadvantageous to others but advantageous to oneself.

goat
- **act the goat** to behave in an intentionally silly way.
- **get (someone's) goat** to irritate (someone).

God, god
- **in the lap of the gods** uncertain, left to chance or fate.
- **there but for the grace of God go I** if I had not been fortunate the circumstances of another person could easily also have been mine.

gold
- **a gold mine** a source of wealth or profit.
- **be like gold dust** be very scarce.
- **golden boy** a young man who is popular or successful.
- **golden handshake** a large amount of money given to someone who is leaving a job, usually because he or she has been declared redundant.
- **good as gold** very well-behaved.
- **the crock** *or* **pot of gold at the end of the rainbow** wealth or good fortune that one will never achieve.
- **the golden rule** a principle or practice that it is vital to remember. <Originally the golden rule was that one should do to others as one would wish them to do to oneself>.
- **worth its** *or* **one's weight in gold** extremely valuable or useful.

good
- **be as good as one's word** to do what one has promised do.
- **be on to a good thing** *or* **have a good thing going** to be in a desirable or profitable situation.
- **be up to no good** to be planning something wrong or illegal.
- **give as good as one gets** to be as successful as one's opponent in an argument, contest, fight, etc.
- **good for nothing** worthless.

- **in (someone's) good books** in favour with (someone).
- **make good** to be successful in one's career or business.
- **take (something) in good part** to accept (something) without being offended or angry.

goods
- **deliver the goods** to do what one is required or expected to do.
- **goods and chattels** movable property. <An old legal term>.

goose
- **cook (someone's) goose** to ruin (someone's) chances of success.
- **kill the goose that lays the golden egg** to destroy something that is a source of profit. <Refers to one of Aesop's fables in which the owner of a goose that laid golden eggs killed it thinking to get all the eggs at once, only to discover that there were none>.
- **what's sauce for the goose is sauce for the gander** what applies to one person should apply to another, usually to a member of the opposite sex.

gooseberry
- **play gooseberry** to be the third person present with a couple who wish to be alone.

Gordian
- **cut the Gordian knot** to solve a problem or end a great difficulty by a vigorous or drastic method. <Refers to a legend in which whoever could untie a knot in a rope belonging to King Gordius of Phrygia, would be made ruler of all Asia. Alexander the Great severed the knot by cutting through it with a sword>.

gospel
- **take (something) as gospel** to accept (something) as absolutely true. <The gospel refers to the books of the Bible dealing with the life and teachings of Christ>.

grab
- **up for grabs** ready to be taken, bought, etc.

grace
- **saving grace** a good quality which prevents someone or something from being completely bad or worthless.
- **with a bad** or **good grace** in an unpleasant or pleasant and unwilling or willing way.

grade
- **make the grade** to succeed in what you are trying to achieve, often by reaching a required standard. <Originally referred to a train which succeeded in climbing a steep section of track>.

grain
- **go against the grain** to be against someone's inclinations, feelings or wishes. <Refers to the direction of the grain in wood, it being easier to cut or smooth wood with the grain rather than across or against it>.

grape
- **sour grapes** saying that something that one cannot have is not worth having. <Refers to one of Aesop's fables in

which a fox that failed to reach a bunch of grapes growing above his head said that they were sour anyhow>.
- **the grapevine** an informal and unofficial way of passing news and information from person to person, gossip.

grass
- **grass widow** a woman whose husband is away from home for a short time for reasons of business or sport. <Originally the term referred to an unmarried woman who had sexual relations with a man or men, the origin being that such relations usually took place out of doors>.
- **let the grass grow under one's feet** to delay or waste time.
- **put** or **turn (someone) out to grass** to cause (someone) to retire. <Refers to turning out a horse into a field at the end of its working life>.
- **the grass is always greener on the other side of the fence** another set of circumstances or lifestyle always seems preferable to one's own. <Refers to the habit of grazing animals of grazing through the fence separating them from the next field>.
- **the grass roots** the ordinary people in an organization, etc.

grave
- **(someone) would turn in his** or **her grave** (someone) would be very annoyed or upset.

Greek
- **be all Greek to me, etc,** I, etc, don't understand any of it. <Refers to the fact that ancient Greek was considered a difficult language to learn>.

green
- **give the green light to (something)** give one's permission for (something).
- **have green fingers** to be good at growing plants.
- **the green-eyed monster** jealousy.

grief
- **come to grief** to suffer misfortune or failure.
- **give (someone) grief** to criticize or nag (someone).

grim
- **hang on** or **hold on like grim death** to take a firm, determined hold of something in difficult or dangerous circumstances.

grin
- **grin and bear it** to tolerate something without complaining.
- **wipe the grin off (someone's face)** to make (someone) stop feeling pleased or satisfied.

grind
- **grind to a halt** slowly begin to stop or cease working.

grip
- **get a grip (of** or **on something** or **oneself)** to take firm control (of something or oneself).

- **get** *or* **come to grips with (something)** to begin to deal with (something).

ground

- **cut the ground from under (someone's) feet** to cause (someone's) actions, arguments, etc, to be ineffective, often by acting before he or she does.
- **fall on stony ground** to have no attention paid to it. <Refers to seed falling on stony, infertile ground and so not being able to grow>.
- **get in on the ground floor** to be in at the very start of a project, business, etc.
- **get (something) off the ground** to get (a project) started. <Refers literally to a plane>.
- **hit the ground running** to start a new activity immediately with a great deal of energy and enthusiasm.
- **on one's own ground** dealing with a subject, situation, etc, with which one is familiar.
- **run oneself into the ground** to become exhausted from working too hard or trying to do too many things.
- **shift one's ground** to change one's opinions, attitude, etc.
- **stand one's ground** to remain firm, not to yield.
- **suit (someone) down to the ground** to suit someone perfectly.
- **thin** *or* **thick on the ground** scarce or plentiful.

guard

- **let your guard down/lower your guard/drop your guard** to stop being careful or alert.
- **on** *or* **off one's guard** prepared or unprepared for any situation, especially a dangerous or difficult one. <Refers to fencing>.

gum

- **gum up the works** to cause a machine, system, etc, to break down.

gun

- **be gunning for (someone)** to plan to harm (someone).
- **jump the gun** to start before the proper time. <Refers to athletes starting a race before the starting gun goes>.
- **spike (someone's) guns** to cause (someone's) plans or actions to be ineffective. <Refers historically to driving a metal spike into the touch-hole of a captured enemy gun which could not be moved away in order to render it useless>.
- **stick to one's guns** to remain firm in one's opinions, etc. <Refers to a soldier who keeps shooting at the enemy and does not run away>.

hackles

- **make (someone's) hackles rise** to make (someone) angry. <Hackles are the feathers on the necks of male birds which rise when the bird is angry>.

hair

- **a hair of the dog (that bit one)** an alcoholic drink taken as a supposed cure for having consumed too much alcohol the night before. <From an old belief that if you were bitten by a mad dog and got rabies you could be cured by having hairs of the dog laid on the wound>.

- **get in (someone's) hair** to irritate (someone).
- **keep one's hair on** to remain calm and not get angry.
- **let one's hair down** to behave in an informal, relaxed manner.
- **make (someone's) hair stand on end** to terrify or horrify (someone).
- **not to turn a hair** not to show any sign of fear, distress, etc.
- **split hairs** to argue about small unimportant details, to quibble.
- **tear one's hair (out)** to show frustration or irritation.

half

- **(someone's) better half** (someone's) wife or husband.
- **half a loaf is better than no bread** a little of something desirable is better than nothing.
- **meet (someone) halfway** to reach a compromise agreement with (someone).
- **not half** very much so.

hammer

- **go at it hammer and tongs** to fight or quarrel loudly and fiercely. <Refers to a blacksmith holding a piece of heated iron in his tongs and striking it loudly with his hammer>.

hand

- **be hand in glove with (someone)** to be closely associated with (someone) for a bad or illegal purpose.
- **force (someone's) hand** to force (someone) to do something that he or she may not want to do or be ready to do.
- **give** *or* **lend (someone) a (helping) hand** to help (someone).
- **go hand in hand** to be closely connected.
- **hand over fist** in large amounts, very rapidly. <Originally a nautical term meaning rapid progress such as can be made by hauling on a rope putting one hand after the other>.
- **have a hand in (something)** to be involved in (something), to have contributed to the cause of (something).
- **have one's hands full** to be very busy.
- **in good hands** well looked after.
- **keep one's hand in** to retain one's skill at something by doing it occasionally.
- **lend (someone) a hand** to help (someone).
- **live from hand to mouth** to have enough money only to pay for one's present needs without having any to save. <Whatever money comes into one's hand is used to put food in one's mouth>.
- **many hands make light work** a job is easier to do if there are several people doing it.
- **my, etc, hands are tied** something prevents me, etc, from acting as I, etc, might wish to.
- **not to do a hand's turn** to do nothing.
- **play into (someone's) hands** to do exactly what someone wants one to do because it is to his or her advantage. <Refers to playing one's hand at cards so as to benefit another player>.

- **show one's hand** to reveal to others one's plans or intentions, previously kept secret. <Refers to showing one's hand to other players in a card game>.
- **take (someone) in hand** to train or discipline (someone).
- **turn one's hand to (something)** to do, to be able to do.
- **wait on (someone) hand and foot** to look after (someone) to such an extent that he or she does not have to do anything for himself or herself.
- **wash one's hands of (someone *or* something)** to refuse to be involved any longer in (something) or to be responsible for (someone or something). <A biblical reference to the action of Pontius Pilate after the crucifixion of Jesus in Matthew 27:24>.
- **with one hand tied behind one's back** very easily.

handle
- **fly off the handle** to lose one's temper. <Refers to an axehead which flies off the handle when it is being used>.

hang
- **get the hang of (something)** to learn how to do (something) or begin to understand (something).
- **hung up on (someone *or* something)** obsessed with (someone or something).

happy
- **happy as a lark *or* sand-boy** extremely happy.
- **happy hunting ground** a place where someone finds what he or she desires or where he or she is successful.
- **the *or* a happy medium** a sensible middle course between two extremes.

hard
- **between a rock and a hard place** *see* **rock**.
- **hard as nails** lacking in pity, sympathy, softer feelings, etc.
- **hard cash** coins and bank-notes as opposed to cheques, etc.
- **hard facts** facts that cannot be disputed.
- **hard lines** bad luck. <Perhaps a reference to a ship's ropes being made hard by ice>.
- **hard of hearing** rather deaf.
- **hard up** not having much money.
- **take a hard line** to take strong, stern or unyielding action or have strong opinions about something.
- **the hard stuff** strong alcoholic drink, spirits.

hare
- **run with the hare and hunt with the hounds** to try to give one's support to two opposing sides at once.

hash
- **settle (someone's) hash** to deal with (someone) in such a way that he or she causes no more trouble or is prevented from doing what was intended.

hat
- **hats off to (someone)** (someone) should be praised and congratulated.

- **hat trick** any action done three times in a row. <Refers originally to a cricketer receiving a hat from his club for putting out three batsmen with three balls in a row>.
- **I'll eat my hat** an expression used to express total disbelief in a fact, statement, etc.
- **keep (something) under one's hat** to keep (something) secret.
- **knock (someone *or* something) into a cocked hat** to defeat or surpass (someone or something) completely. <A cocked hat was a three-cornered hat in the 18th-century made by folding the edges of a round hat into corners>.
- **pass the hat round** to ask for contributions of money.
- **take one's hat off to (someone)** to express or show one's admiration for someone.
- **talk through one's hat** to talk about something without any knowledge about it, to talk nonsense.
- **throw one's hat in the ring** to declare oneself a contender or candidate for something. <Refers to a method of making a challenge in prize boxing matches at fairgrounds, etc>.
- **wear a different *or* another hat** to speak as the holder of a different position.

hatch
- **batten down the hatches** to prepare for trouble. <Refers to preparations for a storm on a ship at sea>.
- **hatches, matches and despatches** the announcement of births, marriages and deaths in a newspaper.

hatchet
- **bury the hatchet** to agree to be friends again after a quarrel. <Refers to an American Indian custom of burying tomahawks when peace was made>.

have
- **have had it** to have no hope of survival, success, etc.
- **have it in for (someone)** to try to cause trouble for (someone).
- **have it out with (someone)** to discuss areas of disagreement or discontent with someone in order to settle them.
- **let (someone) have it** suddenly to attack (someone) either physically or verbally.

havoc
- **play havoc with (something)** to cause serious damage to (something).

hawk
- **watch (someone) like a hawk** to watch (someone) very carefully.

hay
- **go haywire** to go completely wrong, to go out of control. <Refers to wire that was used to bind hay. It very easily became twisted and therefore came to symbolize confusion>.
- **hit the hay *or* sack** to go to bed. <Beds were formerly filled with hay or made from the same material as sacks>.

- **like looking for a needle in a haystack** *see* **needle**.
- **make hay (while the sun shines)** to profit or take advantage of an opportunity while one has the chance. <Haymaking is only possible in fine weather>.

head

- **bite** *or* **eat** *or* **snap (someone's) head off** to speak very sharply and angrily to (someone).
- **bring (something) to a head** to bring something to a state where something must be done about it. <Refers to bringing a boil, etc, to a head>.
- **bury one's head in the sand** to deliberately ignore a situation so that one does not have to deal with it. <Refers to the old belief that ostriches hide their heads in the sand when they are in danger because they think that then they cannot be seen>.
- **cannot make head nor tail of (something)** cannot understand (something) at all.
- **give (someone) his or her head** to allow (someone) to do as he or she wishes. <Refers literally to slackening one's hold on the reins of a horse>.
- **go to (someone's) head l)** to make (someone) arrogant or conceited. **2** to make (someone) slightly drunk.
- **have a head for (something)** to have an ability or aptitude for (something).
- **have a (good) head on one's shoulders** to be clever or sensible.
- **have one's head screwed on the right way** to be sensible.
- **head over heels** completely.
- **hold one's head up (high)** not to feel ashamed or guilty, to remain dignified.
- **keep a level head** *or* **keep one's head** to remain calm and sensible, especially in a difficult situation.
- **keep one's head above water** to have enough money to keep out of debt.
- **knock (something) on the head** to put an end to (something).
- **laugh one's head off** to laugh very loudly.
- **lose one's head** to cease to remain calm to act foolishly.
- **make headway** to make progress. <Refers originally to ships>.
- **off one's head** insane, not rational.
- **on (someone's) (own) head be it** (someone) must take responsibility or blame.
- **over (someone's) head** (l) too difficult for (someone) to understand. **2** when (someone) seems to have a better right. **3** beyond (someone) to a person of higher rank.
- **put** *or* **lay one's head on the block** to leave oneself open to blame, punishment, danger, etc. <Refers to laying one's head on the block before being beheaded>.
- **put our, etc, heads together** to discuss something together, to share thoughts on something.
- **rear its ugly head** to appear or happen.
- **scratch one's head** to be puzzled.
- **soft** *or* **weak in the head** not very intelligent, mentally retarded.

- **talk one's head off** to talk a great deal.
- **turn (someone's) head** to make (someone) conceited.

heart

- **cross one's heart (and hope to die)** this is said to emphasize the truth of what one is saying.
- **do (someone's) heart good** to give (someone) pleasure.
- **eat one's heart out** to be distressed because one cannot have someone or something which one is longing for.
- **from the bottom of one's heart** most sincerely, very much.
- **have one's heart in one's mouth** to feel afraid or anxious.
- **heart and soul** completely, with all one's energy.
- **(someone's) heart goes out to (someone)** (someone) feels sympathy or pity for (someone).
- **(someone's) heart is in the right place** (someone) is basically kind, sympathetic, etc, although not appearing to be so.
- **(someone's) heart is not in it** (someone) is not enthusiastic about something.
- **(someone's) heart sinks** (someone) feels depressed, disappointed, etc.
- **in good heart** cheerful and confident.
- **in (someone's) heart of hearts** in the deepest part of one's mind or feelings.
- **learn something by heart** to memorize (something) thoroughly.
- **lose heart** to grow discouraged.
- **not to have the heart (to do something)** not to be unkind, unsympathetic, etc, enough (to do something).
- **put new heart into (someone)** to make (someone) feel encouraged and more hopeful.
- **set one's heart on** *or* **have one's heart set on (something)** to desire (something) very much.
- **take heart** to become encouraged.
- **take (something) to heart 1** to be upset by (something). **2** to be influenced by and take notice of (something).
- **wear one's heart on one's sleeve** to let one's feelings be obvious.
- **with all one's heart** most sincerely.

heat

- **in the heat of the moment** while influenced by the excitement or emotion of the occasion.

heaven

- **in seventh heaven** extremely happy. <In Jewish literature the seventh heaven is the highest of all heavens and the one where God lives>.
- **manna from heaven** something advantageous which happens unexpectedly, especially in a time of trouble. <A biblical reference to Exodus 16:15>.
- **move heaven and earth** to make every effort possible.
- **smell** *or* **stink to high heaven** to have a strong and nasty smell.

heavy
- **make heavy weather of (something)** to make more effort to do something than should be required. <Refers originally to a ship which does not handle well in difficult conditions>.

hedge
- **look as though one has been dragged through a hedge backwards** to look very untidy.

heel
- **bring (someone) to heel** to bring (someone) under one's control. <Refers to making a dog walk to heel>.
- **take to one's heels** to run away.

helm
- **at the helm** in charge. <Refers to the helm of a ship>.

hen
- **like a hen on a hot girdle** very nervous and restless.

here
- **neither here nor there** of no importance.
- **the hereafter** life after death.

herring
- **a red herring** a piece of information which misleads (someone) or draws (someone's) attention away from the truth, often introduced deliberately. <A red herring is a strong-smelling fish whose scent could mislead hunting dogs if it were dragged across the path they were pursuing>.
- **neither fish nor fowl nor good red herring** neither one thing nor the other.
- **packed like herring in a barrel** very tightly packed.

hide[1]
- **neither hide nor hair of (someone or something)** no trace at all of (someone or something). <Hide is used in the sense of skin>.

hide[2]
- **on a hiding to nothing** in a situation where one cannot possibly win. <Perhaps a reference to boxing>.

high
- **a high flier** a person who is bound to be very successful or who has achieved great success.
- **be for the high jump** to be about to be punished or scolded.
- **be high time** be time something was done without delay.
- **be or get on one's high horse** to be or become offended in a haughty manner.
- **high and mighty** arrogant.
- **hunt or search high and low for (someone or something)** to search absolutely everywhere for (someone or something).
- **leave (someone) high and dry** to leave (someone) in a difficult or helpless state.
- **riding high** very successful. <Used literally of the moon being high in the sky>.

- **run high** of feelings, tempers, etc, to be extremely angry, agitated, etc. <Refers to the sea when there is a strong current and high waves>.

hill
- **over the hill** past one's youth or one's best.

history
- **the rest is history** used to indicate that no more need be said about something because the details of it are well known.

hit
- **be a hit with (someone)** to be popular with (someone).
- **hit-and-run accident** an accident involving a vehicle where the driver who caused it does not stop or report the accident.
- **hit it off** to get on well, to become friendly.

hog
- **go the whole hog** to do something completely and thoroughly. <Perhaps referring to buying a whole pig for meat rather than just parts of it>.

hold
- **have a hold over (someone)** to have power or influence over (someone).
- **hold good** to be valid or applicable.
- **no holds barred** no restrictions on what is permitted.

hole
- **hole-and-corner** secret and often dishonourable.
- **in a hole** in an awkward or difficult situation.
- **make a hole in (something)** to use a large part of (something).
- **need (something) like (someone) needs a hole in the head** to regard (something) as being completely unwelcome or undesirable.
- **pick holes in (something)** to find faults in (a theory, plan, etc).

holy
- **holier-than-thou** acting as though one is more moral, more pious, etc, than other people. <A biblical reference to Isaiah 65:5>.
- **the holy of holies** a private or special place inside a building. <A literal translation of the Hebrew name of the inner sanctuary in the Jewish Temple where the Ark of the Covenant was kept>.

home
- **a home from home** a place where one feels comfortable and relaxed.
- **bring or drive (something) home to (someone)** to cause someone fully to understand or believe (something).
- **do one's homework** to prepare thoroughly for a meeting, etc, by getting all the necessary information.
- **home and dry** having successfully completed an objective.
- **home truth** a plain, direct statement of something that is true but unpleasant or difficult for someone to accept.

- **make oneself at home** to make oneself comfortable and relaxed.
- **nothing to write home about** not very special, not remarkable.

hook
- **by hook or by crook** by any means possible.
- **off the hook** free from some difficulty, problem, etc, or something one does not want to do. <A reference to angling>.
- **sling one's hook** to go away.
- **swallow (something) hook, line and sinker** to believe (something) completely. <Refers to a fish that swallows not only the hook but the whole of the end section of the fishing line>.
- **the home stretch** *or* **straight** the last part of something, especially when this has been a particularly long or difficult process.

hoop
- **put (someone) through the hoop** to cause (someone) to experience something unpleasant or difficult. <Refers to circus performers who jump through hoops set on fire>.

hop
- **hopping mad** extremely angry.

hope
- **hope against hope** to continue to hope although there is little reason to be hopeful.
- **hope springs eternal (in the human breast)** it is in the nature of human beings to hope. <A quotation from Alexander Pope's *An Essay on Criticism*>.
- **pin one's hopes on (someone *or* something)** to rely on (someone or something) helping one in some way.

horn
- **draw in one's horns** to restrain one's actions, particularly the spending of money. <Refers to a snail drawing in its horns if it is in danger>.
- **lock horns** to argue or fight. <Refers to horned male animals who sometimes get their horns caught together when fighting>.

hornet
- **stir up a hornet's nest** to cause a great deal of trouble.

horse
- **eat like a horse** to eat a great deal.
- **flog a dead horse** to continue to try to arouse interest, enthusiasm, etc, in something which is obviously not, or no longer, of interest.
- **hold one's horses** not to move so fast.
- **horses for courses** certain people are better suited to certain tasks or situations. <Some horses run better on certain types of ground>.
- **straight from the horse's mouth** from someone closely connected with a situation and therefore knowledgeable about it. <It is as though a horse is giving a tip about a race in which it is running>.

- **wild horses would not drag (someone) to something** *or* **somewhere** nothing would persuade (someone) to attend something or go somewhere.
- **you can take a horse to the water but you cannot make it drink** you can encourage someone to do something but you cannot force him or her to do it.

hot
- **hot on (someone's) heels** close behind someone.

hour
- **the (wee) small hours** the hours immediately following midnight (1am, 2am, etc).
- **the witching hour** midnight. <Witches traditionally are supposed to be active at midnight>.

house
- **bring the house down** to cause great amusement or applause.
- **eat (someone) out of house and home.** to eat a great deal and so be expensive to feed.
- **keep open house** always to be ready and willing to welcome guests.
- **on the house** paid by the owner of shop, pub, etc.
- **safe as houses** completely safe.

hue
- **a hue and cry** a loud protest. <An old legal term meaning a summons for people to join in a hunt for a criminal>.

huff
- **in a** *or* **the huff** upset, offended or sulking.

humble
- **eat humble pie** to have to admit that one has been wrong. <Refers originally to a dish made from the umble or offal of a deer eaten by the lower classes>.

ice
- **break the ice** to ease the shyness or formality of a social occasion.
- **cut no ice** to have no effect.
- **icing on the cake** a desirable but unnecessary addition.
- **on ice** put aside for future use or attention.
- **(skate) on thin ice** (to be) in a risky or dangerous position.
- **the tip of the iceberg** a small sign of a much larger problem. <Refers to the fact that the bulk of an iceberg is hidden underwater>.

ill
- **it's an ill wind (that blows nobody any good)** in almost every misfortune there is something of benefit to someone.

imagination
- **a figment of one's imagination** something which has no reality.

immemorial
- **from time immemorial** from a time beyond anyone's memory, written records, etc; for an extremely long time. <In legal phraseology the expression means 'before the beginning of legal memory'>.

in

- **the ins and outs of (something)** the details of (something).

inch

- **be** *or* **come within an inch of (something)** to be or come very close to.
- **every inch a** *or* **the (something)** exactly the type of (something).
- **give (someone) an inch (and he** *or* **she will take a mile** *or* **an ell)** if one yields in any way to someone then the person in question will make even greater demands. <An ell is an old form of measurement>.

Indian

- **an Indian summer** a time of fine, warm weather in autumn. <Perhaps from a feature of the climate of North America whose original inhabitants were Indians>.

innings

- **have a good innings** to enjoy a considerable period of life, success etc. <Refers to cricket>.

interest

- **a vested interest in (something)** a personal and biased interest in (something).
- **with interest** to an even greater extent than something has been done, etc, to someone.

iron

- **have many** *or* **several irons in the fire** to be involved in several projects, etc, at the same time. < Refers to a blacksmith who heats pieces of iron before shaping them>.
- **rule (someone** *or* **something) with a rod of iron** to rule with sternness or ruthlessness.
- **strike while the iron is hot** to act at a point at which things are favourable to one. <Refers to a blacksmith's work>.
- **the iron hand in the velvet glove** sternness or ruthlessness hidden under an appearance of gentleness.

item

- **be an item** to be regarded as having a romantic relationship.

itch

- **be itching to (do something)** to want very much to (do something).
- **have an itching palm** to be greedy for money.

ivory

- **live in an ivory tower** to have a way of life protected from difficulty or unpleasantness. <*La toure d'ivoire*, French for 'ivory tower', was coined by the poet Charles Augustin Saint-Beuve in 1837>.
- **tickle the ivories** to play the piano. <The keys of a piano are made of ivory>.

jack, Jack

- **a jack of all trades (and master of none)** someone who can do several different kinds of job (but does not do any of them very well).

before you can say Jack Robinson extremely rapidly.
- **every man jack** absolutely everyone. <Perhaps from the fact that Jack is a very common first name>.
- **I'm all right, Jack** my situation is satisfactory, the implication being that it does not matter about anyone else.

jackpot

- **hit the jackpot** to have a great success, often involving a large sum of money. <Refers to the pool of money in poker>.

jam

- **jam tomorrow** the promise of better things in the future. <From a statement by the Red Queen in *Alice Through the Looking-Glass* by Lewis Carroll>.
- **want jam on it** to want an even better situation, etc, than one has already. <Refers to asking for jam on bread when bread is quite sufficient>.

Jekyll

- **a Jekyll and Hyde** someone with two completely different sides to his or her personality <Refers to the character in *The Strange Case of Dr Jekyll and Mr Hyde*, a novel by Robert Louis Stevenson>.

Jeremiah

- **a Jeremiah** a pessimist. <A biblical reference to the Lamentations of Jeremiah>.

jet

- **the jet set** wealthy people who can afford to travel a great deal. <Refers to jet planes>.

jewel

- **the jewel in the crown** the must valuable or successful thing associated with someone or something.

job

- **a job lot** a mixed collection. <Refers to auctioneering>.
- **just the job** exactly what is required.
- **jobs for the boys** used to suggest that jobs are being given to friends and relatives of people in power or of authority, rather than to people who are qualified to get them. Sometimes such jobs are unnecessary and created especially for the friend or relative.
- **make the best of a bad job** to obtain the best results possible from something unsatisfactory.

Job

- **a Job's comforter** someone who brings no comfort at all but makes one feel worse. <A biblical reference to the friends of Job>.
- **enough to try the patience of Job** so irritating as to make the most patient of people angry. <A biblical reference to Job who had to suffer many misfortunes patiently>.

Joe

- **Joe Bloggs** *or* **Public** *or* **Soap** the ordinary, average person.

joint
- **case the joint** to inspect premises carefully, especially with a view to later burglary.

joker
- **the joker in the pack** someone in a group who is different from the rest in some way and may cause problems or have an effect on a situation. <Refers to a pack of playing cards>.

Jonah
- **a Jonah** someone who brings bad luck. <a biblical reference to the book of Jonah, Jonah 1:4–7>.

Jones
- **keep up with the Joneses** to make an effort to remain on the same social level as one's neighbours by buying what they have, etc.

joy
- **no joy** no success, no luck.

judge
- **sober as a judge** to be extremely sober, not to be at all drunk.

jury
- **the jury is still out** people have not yet reached a conclusion or made a decision about something.

justice
- **do (someone or something) justice 1** to show the true value of (someone or something). **2** to eat (a meal, etc) with a good appetite.

keep
- **for keeps** permanently.
- **keep one's own counsel** to keep one's opinions, problems, etc, secret.
- **keep oneself to oneself** not to seek the company of others much, to tell others very little about oneself.
- **keep (something) to oneself** to keep (something) secret.

ken
- **beyond one's ken** outside the range of one's knowledge or understanding. <Literally, ken used to mean range of vision>.

kettle
- **a different kettle of fish** a completely different set of circumstances.
- **a pretty kettle of fish** an awkward or difficult situation.

kibosh
- **put the kibosh on (something)** to spoil or ruin (something's) chances of success.

kick
- **for kicks** for thrills or fun.
- **get a kick out of** to get fun or a thrill out of something.
- **kick oneself** to be annoyed with oneself.
- **kick over the traces** to defy rules that control one's behaviour. <Refers to a horse drawing a cart which gets out of control of the driver>.

kick (someone) upstairs to appoint (someone) to a job which is more senior than the present one but which has less power.

kid[1]
- **handle (someone or something) with kid gloves** to deal with (someone or something) very tactfully or delicately.

kid[2]
- **the new kid on the block** the newest person in a place, activity, etc.

kill
- **be in at the kill** to be present when something important or decisive happens, often something that is unpleasant for someone. <Referring to the death of the fox in a foxhunt>.
- **kill (someone) with kindness** to spoil (someone) to the extent that it is a disadvantage to him or her.
- **make a killing** to make a large profit.
- **move in for the kill** to act decisively with a view to defeating one's opponent.

king
- **a king's ransom** a vast sum of money.

kingdom
- **till kingdom come** for a very long time. <Refers to the Lord's Prayer>.
- **to kingdom come** to death. <See above>.

kiss
- **kiss goodbye to (something)** to have to accept that you have lost (something) or that you are not going to get (something).
- **kiss of death** something which causes the end, ruin or death of something. <A biblical reference to the kiss by which Judas betrayed Jesus>.

kitchen
- **everything but the kitchen sink** used to emphasize how much luggage someone is taking, etc.

kite
- **fly a kite** to start a rumour about a new project to see how people would react if the project were put into operation. <Refers to the use of kites to discover the direction and strength of the wind>.
- **high as a kite** very excited.

kitten
- **have kittens** to get very agitated or angry.

knee
- **bring (someone) to his or her knees** to humble or ruin (someone). <Refers to going on one's knees to beg for something>.

knickers
- **get one's knickers in a twist** to become agitated.

knife
- **have one's knife in (someone)** to wish to harm (someone).

- **like a (hot) knife through butter** used to emphasize how easily someone has dealt with a difficult situation.
- **on a knife edge** in a very uncertain or risky state.
- **stick the knife in (someone)** to do something that will harm, upset or cause problems for (someone).
- **the knives are out for (someone)** used to describe a situation in which several people are planning to harm or cause problems for (someone).
- **the night of the long knives** a time when an act of great disloyalty is carried out, usually by the sudden removal of several people from power or employment. <Refers to 19 June 1934, when Adolf Hitler had a number of his Nazi colleagues imprisoned or killed>.

knot¹
- **at a rate of knots** extremely rapidly. <Refers to a method of measuring the speed of ships>.

knot²
- **tie the knot** to get married.

know
- **in the know** knowing facts, etc, that are known only to a small group of people.
- **know (something) inside out** to know and understand (something) very well indeed.
- **not to know one is born** to lead a trouble-free, protected life.
- **not to know whether one is coming or going** to be very confused, often because one is very busy.

knuckle
- **rap (someone) over the knuckles** to scold or criticize (someone).

labour
- **a labour of love** a long or difficult job done for one's own satisfaction or from affection for someone rather than for reward.

lamb
- **like a lamb to the slaughter** meekly, without arguing or resisting, often because unaware of danger or difficulty. <A biblical reference to Isaiah 53:7>.

land
- **a land of milk and honey** a place where life is pleasant, with plenty of food and possibilities of success. <A biblical reference to the Promised Land of the Israelites described in Exodus 3:8>.
- **see how the land lies** to look carefully at a situation before taking any action or decision. <Refers literally to sailors looking at the shore before landing>.

lane
- **it's a long lane that has no turning** every period of misfortune, unhappiness, etc, comes to an end or changes to happier circumstances eventually.
- **life in the fast lane** a life which is very busy and active and usually contains a lot of stress and pressure.

language
- **speak the same language** to have similar tastes and views.

lap
- **in the lap of luxury** in luxurious conditions.

large
- **large as life** in person, actually present. <From works of art, particularly sculptural, which are life-size>.
- **larger than life** extraordinary, behaving, etc, in an extravagant way.

last
- **on one's or its last legs** near to collapse.
- **the last word** the most fashionable or up-to-date example of something.

late
- **better late than never** better for something to arrive, happen, etc, late than never to do so at all.

laugh
- **have the last laugh** to be victorious or proved right in the end, especially after being scorned, criticized, etc. <From the saying he who laughs last laughs longest>.
- **laugh and the world laughs with you (weep and you weep alone)** when someone is cheerful or happy, other people share in his or her joy (but when he or she is sad or miserable, people tend to avoid him or her).
- **laugh on the other side of one's face** to suffer disappointment or misfortune after seeming to be successful or happy.
- **laugh up one's sleeve** to be secretly amused.
- **no laughing matter** a very serious matter.

laurel
- **look to one's laurels** to be careful not to lose one's position or reputation because of better performances by one's rivals. <A reference to the laurel wreath with which the ancient Greeks crowned their poets and victors>.
- **rest on one's laurels** to be content with past successes without trying for any more. <As above>.

law
- **be a law unto oneself** to behave as one wishes rather than obeying the usual rules and conventions.
- **lay down the law** to state one's opinions with great force, to give orders dictatorially.
- **the law of the jungle** the unofficial rules for survival or success in a dangerous or difficult situation where civilized laws are not effective.

lay
- **lay it on thick or lay it on with a trowel** to exaggerate greatly in one's praise, compliments, etc, to someone.

lead¹
- **a leading question** a question asked in such a way as to suggest the answer the questioner wants to hear.

- **leading light** an important person in a certain group, field, etc.

lead²
- **swing the lead** to avoid doing one's work usually by inventing deceitful excuses. <Originally naval slang>.

leaf
- **take a leaf out of (someone's) book** to use (someone) as an example.
- **turn over a new leaf** to change one's behaviour, etc, for the better.

league
- **not be in the same league as (someone)** not to be as able as (someone). <Refers to the grouping of clubs in soccer, etc, according to ability>.

leap
- **by leaps and bounds** very quickly or successfully.

lease
- **give (someone or something) a new lease of life** to cause (someone) to have a longer period of active life or usefulness or to have a happier or more interesting life.

least
- **least said soonest mended** the less one says in a difficult situation the less harm will be done.

leave
- **leave (someone) in the lurch** to leave (someone) in a difficult or dangerous situation without any help. <A lurch refers to a position at the end of certain games, such as cribbage, in which the loser has either lost by a huge margin or scored no points at all>.

leeway
- **make up leeway** to take action to recover from a setback or loss of advantage. <Leeway refers to the distance a sailing ship is blown sideways off its course by the wind>.

left
- **have two left feet** to be clumsy or awkward with one's feet, e.g. when dancing.
- **left, right and centre** everywhere, to an extreme degree.
- **(someone's) left hand does not know what his or her right hand is doing** (someone's) affairs are extremely complicated.

leg
- **break a leg** used as an interjection to an actor or other stage performer as a means of wishing him or her good luck. <In the theatre it is traditionally considered bad luck to wish an actor good luck in a direct way>.
- **give (someone) a leg up** to give (someone) some assistance to achieve advancement.
- **leg it** to run or go away quickly.
- **not to have a leg to stand on** to have no defence or justification for one's actions.

- **pull (someone's) leg** to try as a joke to make (someone) believe something that is not true.
- **stretch one's legs** to go for a walk.

legend
- **a legend in one's own lifetime** used to indicate that someone has become famous during his/her lifetime.

legion
- **their name is legion** there are a great many of them. <A biblical reference to Mark 5:9>.

length
- **go to great lengths** to take absolutely any action in order to achieve what one wants.

leopard
- **the leopard never changes its spots** a person's basic character does not change.

let
- **let oneself go 1** to enjoy oneself without restraint. **2** to stop taking trouble over one's appearance.

letter
- **the letter of the law** the exact wording of a law, rule, agreement clause. <A biblical reference to II Corinthians 3:6>.
- **to the letter** in every detail.

level
- **a level playing field** a situation which is completely fair to all involved and in which no one has any particular advantage.
- **find one's or its (own) level** to find out what situation, position, etc, one is naturally suited to.
- **on the level** honest, trustworthy.

lick
- **a lick and a promise** a quick, not thorough, wash or clean.
- **lick (someone or something) into shape** to improve (someone or something) greatly to bring up to standard. <Refers to an old belief that bear cubs are born shapeless and have to be licked into shape by their mothers>.

lid
- **blow or take the lid off (something)** to reveal the truth about (something).
- **keep the lid on (something)** to keep (something) secret or keep (something) under control so that it does not get any worse.
- **put the (tin) lid on (something)** to finish (something) off usually in an unpleasant way.

lie¹
- **give the lie to (something)** to show that (something) is untrue.
- **lie in or through one's teeth** to tell lies obviously and unashamedly.

- **live a lie** to live a way of life about which there is something dishonest.

lie[2]
- **take (something) lying down** to accept an unpleasant situation without protesting or taking action against it.
- **the lie of the land** the nature and details of a situation. <Refers to sailors studying the nature of the coastline>.

life
- **breathe new life into (something)** to make (something) more lively, active or successful.
- **come to life** to become active or lively.
- **get a life** used to indicate to someone that you think that he/she has a boring, uninteresting life and should do something to change this.
- **life is just a bowl of cherries** used ironically to indicate that life can be difficult and unpleasant.
- **for dear life** or **for dear life's sake** to a very great extent, very rapidly, hard, etc.
- **lead** or **live the life of Riley** to lead a comfortable and trouble-free life.
- **not on your life** certainly not.
- **risk life and limb** to risk death or physical injury, to take extreme risks.
- **see life** to have wide experience, especially of varying conditions of life.
- **take one's life in one's hands** to take the risk of being killed, injured or harmed.
- **the facts of life** the facts about sex or reproduction.
- **the life and soul of the party** someone who is very lively and amusing on social occasions.
- **while** or **where there's life there's hope** one should not despair of a situation while there is still a possibility of improvement.

light[1]
- **bring (something) to light** to reveal or uncover (something).
- **come to light** to be revealed or uncovered.
- **go out like a light** to go to sleep immediately.
- **hide one's light under a bushel** to be modest or silent about one's abilities or talents. <A biblical reference to Matthew 5:15, quoting Christ>.
- **in the cold light of day** when one looks at something practically and calmly.
- **light at the end of the tunnel** possibility of success, happiness, etc, after a long period of suffering, misery etc.
- **see the light** l) to understand something after not doing so. **2** to agree with someone's opinions or beliefs after not doing so. **3** (*also* **see the light of day**) to come into existence.
- **shed** or **throw light on (something)** to make (something) clearer, e.g. by providing more information about it.

light[2]
- **be light-fingered** to be likely to steal.
- **light as a feather** extremely light.

- **make light of (something)** to treat (something) as unimportant.

lightning
- **lightning never strikes twice (in the same place)** the same misfortune is unlikely to occur more than once.
- **quick as lightning** or **like greased lightning** extremely rapidly.

lily
- **be lily-livered** to be cowardly. <Refers to an old belief that the liver had no blood in it>.

limb
- **out on a limb** in a risky and often lonely position; having ideas, opinions, etc, different from other people. <Refers to being stuck in an isolated position on the branch of a tree>.
- **tear (someone) from limb to limb** to attack (someone) in a fierce and aggressive way, either in deed or speech.

limbo
- **in limbo** in a forgotten or neglected position.

limelight
- **in the limelight** in a situation where one attracts a great deal of public attention.

limit
- **be the limit** to be as much as, or more than, one can tolerate.
- **off limits** beyond what is allowed.

line
- **all along the line** at every point in an action, process, etc.
- **along** or **on the lines of (something)** similar to (something).
- **be in line for (something)** to be likely to get (something).
- **be** or **come on line** to be ready for use, to be operating. <A computer reference>.
- **be (way) out of line** to behave in a way that is not acceptable.
- **bring (something) into line with (something)** to make (something) the same as or comparable with (something else).
- **down the line** some time in the future.
- **draw a line under (something)** to regard (something unpleasant) as being over and best forgotten so that people can move on.
- **fall into line** to behave according to the relevant rules, regulations or traditions.
- **lay it on the line** to make (something) absolutely clear to someone.
- **not one's line of country** not something which one knows a lot about or is interested in.
- **read between the lines** to understand or deduce something from a statement, situation, etc, although this has not actually been stated. <Refers to a method of writing secret messages by writing in invisible ink between the lines of other messages>.

- **step out of line** to behave differently from what is usually acceptable or expected. <Refers to a line of soldiers on parade>.
- **the line of least resistance** the course of action that will cause one least effort or trouble.
- **toe the line** to obey the rules or orders. <Refers to competitors having to stand with their toes to a line when starting a race, etc>.

lion
- **put one's head in the lion's mouth** to put oneself in a very dangerous or difficult position.
- **the lion's share** having a much larger share than anyone else. <Refers to one of Aesop's fables in which the lion, being a very fierce animal, claimed three quarters of the food which he and other animals had hunted for>.
- **throw (someone) to the lions** deliberately to put (someone) in a dangerous or difficult position, often to protect oneself. <Refers to a form of entertainment in ancient Rome in which prisoners were thrown to wild animals to be attacked and killed>.

lip
- **keep a stiff upper lip** to show no emotion, such as fear or disappointment when danger, trouble, etc, arises.
- **lick one's lips** to look forward to something with pleasure. <A reference to licking one's lips at the thought of appetizing food>.
- **(someone's) lips are sealed** (someone) will not reveal something secret.
- **pay lip-service to (something)** to say that one believes in or agrees with (something) without really doing so and without acting as if one did.
- **read my lips** used by someone to emphasize that people should believe or trust in what he/she is about to say.

litmus
- **a litmus test** something which assesses or demonstrates clearly what something is really like.

live[1]
- **beat** *or* **knock the living daylights out of (someone)** to give (someone) a severe beating.
- **live and let live** to get on with one's own life and let other people get on with theirs without one interfering.
- **live it up** to have an enjoyable and expensive time.

live[2]
- **a live wire** an energetic, enthusiastic person. <Refers to a live electrical wire>.

load
- **a loaded question** a question intended to lead someone into admitting to or agreeing with something when he or she does not wish to do so. <Refers to a dice loaded or weighted so that it tends always to show the same score>.

loaf
- **use one's loaf** to use one's brains, to think clearly.

lock
- **lock, stock and barrel** completely, with everything included. <Refers to the main components of a gun>.
- **under lock and key** in a place which is locked for security.

log
- **sleep like a log** to sleep very soundly.

lone
- **a lone wolf** someone who prefers to be alone.

long
- **in the long run** in the end, after everything has been considered.
- **the long and the short of it** the only thing that need be said, to sum the story up in a few words.

look
- **look askance at (someone** *or* **something)** to regard with disapproval or distrust.
- **look before you leap** give careful consideration before you act.
- **not to get a look-in** not to have a chance of winning, succeeding, being noticed, etc.

loose
- **cut loose** to free oneself from the influence of power of (someone or something).
- **on the loose** enjoying freedom and pleasure. <Refers originally to prisoners escaped from jail>.

lord
- **lord it over (someone)** to act in a proud and commanding manner to (someone).

lose
- **lose ground** to lose one's advantage or strong position.
- **play a losing game** to go on with something that is obviously going to be unsuccessful.

loss
- **cut one's losses** not to spend any more time, money or effort on something on which one has already spent a lot to little benefit.

love
- **not for love nor money** not in any way at all.
- **there's no love lost between them** they are hostile to each other.

low
- **keep a low profile** not to draw attention to oneself or one's actions or opinions.
- **lie low** to stay quiet or hidden.

luck
- **down on one's luck** experiencing misfortune.
- **push one's luck** to risk failure by trying to gain too much.
- **strike it lucky** to have good fortune.
- **thank one's lucky stars** to be grateful for one's good fortune.

lull

- **lull (someone) into a false sense of security** to lead (someone) into thinking that all is well in order to attack when he or she is not prepared.

mad

- **mad as a hatter** utterly insane, extremely foolish or eccentric. <Hat-making used to involve the use of nitrate of mercury, exposure to which could cause a nervous illness which people thought was a symptom of insanity>.
- **mad as a March hare** insane, silly, extremely eccentric. <Hares tend to leap around wildly in the fields during March, which is their breeding season>.

make

- **make a day** or **night of it** to spend a whole day or night enjoying oneself in some way.
- **make do with (something)** to use (something) as a poor or temporary substitute for something.
- **make it up** to become friendly again after a quarrel.
- **make-or-break** bringing either success or failure.
- **on the make** trying to make a profit for oneself.

man

- **a man of his word** someone who always does as he promises.
- **be one's own man** to be independent in one's actions, opinions, etc.
- **man of straw** a man who is considered to be of not much worth or substance.
- **man to man** frankly.
- **the man in the street** the ordinary, average person.
- **to a man** everyone without exception.

manner

- **to the manner born** as if accustomed since birth to a particular way of behaviour etc. <Refers to a quotation from Shakespeare's *Hamlet*>.

map

- **put (somewhere) on the map** to cause (somewhere) to become well known or important.

marble

- **have marbles in one's mouth** to speak with an upper-class accent.
- **lose one's marbles** to become insane or senile.

march

- **get one's marching orders** to be told to leave, to be dismissed. <Refers to a military term>.
- **steal a march on (someone)** to gain an advantage over (someone) by doing something earlier than expected. <Refers literally to moving an army unexpectedly while the enemy is resting>.

mark

- **be a marked man** or **woman** to be in danger or trouble because people are trying to harm one. 'Marked' means watched>.

- **beside** or **wide of the mark** off the target or subject. <Refers to hitting the target in archery>.
- **be up to the mark** to reach the required or normal standard.
- **get off one's mark** to get started quickly on an undertaking. <Refers to track events in athletics>.
- **hit the mark** to be correct or accurate. <Refers to the target in archery>.
- **leave one's mark on (someone** or **something)** to have an important and lasting effect on (someone or something).
- **make one's mark** to make oneself well known, to make a lasting impression.
- **overstep the mark** to do or say something which is unacceptable or offensive.
- **quick off the mark** quick to act. <Refers literally to a runner starting quickly in a race>.

marrow

- **chilled** or **frozen to the marrow** extremely cold.

mass

- **the masses** the ordinary people, taken as a whole.

match

- **a shouting match** a loud, angry discussion or argument about something.
- **meet one's match** to find oneself against someone who has the ability to defeat one in a contest, argument or activity.
- **a matter of life or death** something of great urgency, something that might involve loss of life.

meal

- **make a meal of (something)** to treat (something) as if it is more complicated or time-consuming than it is.

measure

- **for good measure** as something in addition to what is necessary.

meat

- **be meat and drink to (someone)** to be very important to (someone).
- **one man's meat is another man's poison** people have different tastes.

Mecca

- **a Mecca** a place that is important to a certain group of people and is visited by them. <Refers to the birthplace of Mohammed to which Muslims make pilgrimages>.

meet

- **meet one's Waterloo** to be finally defeated. <Napoleon was defeated for the last time at Waterloo by Wellington>.

melt

- **be in the melting-pot** to be in the process of changing. <Refers to melting down and reshaping metal>.

mercy

- **at the mercy of (someone** *or* **something)** wholly in the power or control of (someone or something).
- **be thankful for small mercies** to be grateful for minor benefits or advantages in an otherwise difficult situation.

merry

- **make merry** to have an enjoyable, entertaining time, to have a party.

message

- **get the message** to understand.

method

- **there is method in his madness** someone has a good, logical reason for acting as he does, although his actions seem strange or unreasonable. <A reference to Shakespeare's *Hamlet* Act 2, scene II>.

Midas

- **the Midas touch** the ability to make money or be successful easily. <Refers to a Greek legend about a king of Phrygia whose touch turned everything to gold>.

midnight

- **burn the midnight oil** to work or study until late at night.

mile

- **be miles away** to be thinking about something else and so not concentrating on what is being said to you or what is going on around you.
- **go the extra mile** to make a special effort and do more than you would usually do, more than you have been asked to do, etc in order to achieve something.
- **run a mile** used to indicate the lengths to which someone would go to avoid something.
- **stand** *or* **stick out a mile** to be extremely obvious.

mill

- **a millstone round one's neck** a heavy burden or responsibility.
- **calm as a millpond** extremely calm.
- **go through the mill** to experience a series of difficult or troublesome events, periods or tests. <From the grinding of corn in a mill>.
- **run-of-the-mill** usual, not special.

mince

- **make mincemeat of (someone** *or* **something)** to defeat (someone) soundly, to destroy (something).
- **not to mince matters** to speak completely frankly without trying to be too kind, etc.

mind

- **be** *or* **go out of one's mind** to be or become insane.
- **blow (someone's) mind** to amaze (someone), to excite (someone) greatly.
- **cross one's mind** to enter one's mind briefly.
- **give (someone) a piece of one's mind** to scold or criticize (someone) angrily.
- **great minds think alike** clever people tend to have the same ideas and opinions.

- **in one's right mind** sane, rational.
- **in two minds** undecided.
- **not to know one's own mind** not to know what one really wants to do.
- **put (someone) in mind of (someone** *or* **something)** to remind (someone) of (someone or something).
- **slip one's mind** to be temporarily forgotten.

mint

- **in mint condition** used but in extremely good condition. <Literally the unused condition of a newly minted coin>.

minute

- **up to the minute** modern or fashionable.

misery

- **put (someone) out of his** *or* **her misery** to end a time of worry, anxiety or suspense for (someone). <Originally a term for putting to death a wounded and suffering animal>.

miss

- **a miss is as good as a mile** if one fails at something it does not matter how close one came to succeeding.
- **give (something) a miss** not to go to or attend (something).

moment

- **have one's moments** to have times of success, happiness.
- **not for a moment** not at all.
- **the moment of truth** a crucial time, a time when one has to make an important decision, face up to a crisis, etc.

money

- **have money to burn** to have enough money to be able to spend it in ways considered foolish.
- **money for jam** *or* **old rope** money obtained in exchange for very little work, effort, etc. <Army slang>.
- **money talks** rich people have influence simply because they have money.
- **put one's money where one's mouth is** to give money for a cause or purpose which one claims to support.
- **spend money like water** to spend money very freely.
- **the smart money is on (something)** used to describe an event or situation which is very likely to take place. <Smart money is used to refer to people who know a lot about investment, business deals, etc>.
- **throw good money after bad** to spend money in an unsuccessful attempt to retrieve money which one has already lost.
- **you pays your money and you takes your choice** used to indicate the difficulty or impossibility of deciding which of two choices is the right one.

monkey

- **monkey business** action likely to cause trouble, illegal or unfair activities.

- **not to give a monkey's** not to care at all.
- **speak to the organ grinder, not his monkey** *see* **organ.**

month
- **a month of Sundays** an extremely long time.

Monty
- **the full Monty** used to indicate that something is absolutely complete or comprehensive or that it contains everything that is usually involved in such an activity or situation.

moon
- **ask** *or* **cry for the moon** to ask for something that it is impossible to get.
- **do a moonlight (flit)** to move away suddenly.
- **many moons ago** a very long time ago, sometimes used as a humorous exaggeration.
- **over the moon** extremely happy.
- **promise (someone) the moon** to make promises that have little hope of ever being realized.

more
- **the more the merrier** the more people that are involved the better.

morning
- **the morning after the night before** a morning when one is suffering from a hangover caused by drinking too much alcohol the night before.

moth
- **like a moth to a flame** used to describe someone who finds someone or something irresistibly attractive, even although the person or thing might cause harm or trouble.

motion
- **go through the motions** to make a show of doing something, to pretend to do something.

mould
- **break the mould** to do something in a completely new and better way.
- **cast in the same mould (as someone)** very similar (to someone). <Refers to iron-working>.
- **they broke the mould when they made (someone)** used to emphasize how special or exceptional someone is.

mountain
- **have a mountain to climb** used to emphasize how difficult it is going to be for someone to do or achieve something and how much effort will be needed.
- **if the mountain will not come to Mohammed, then Mohammed must go to the mountain** a saying which indicates that, if someone whom you want to see cannot or is unwilling to come to you, then you should make the effort to go to him or her. <Refers to a story about Mohammed in which he is asked to demonstrate

his power by getting Mount Sofa to come to him. When this did not happen, Mohammed is supposed to have said the words which form the saying>.
- **make a mountain out of a molehill** to greatly exaggerate the extent of a problem, etc.
- **move mountains** to achieve something that seems impossible or extremely difficult.

mouse
- **poor as a church mouse** extremely poor.
- **quiet as a mouse** extremely quiet.

mouth
- **be all mouth and trousers** to talk a lot about doing something but never actually do it.
- **have a big mouth** to talk a lot, especially about things, such as secrets, that one should not.
- **out of the mouths of babes and sucklings** used when a child says something that is surprisingly adult, true, wise, etc.
- **shoot one's mouth off** to talk in a loud and often boastful or threatening manner.
- **make one's mouth water** used to emphasize how delicious something smells or looks.
- **the movers and shakers** refers to people with power and influence. <Possibly derives from the poem 'Ode' by Arthur O'Shaughnessy (1844–81), 'We are the movers and shakers of the world forever'>.

much
- **much of a muchness** very similar.
- **not much of a (something)** not a very good (something).
- **not up to much** not very good.

mud
- **drag (someone/someone's reputation) through the mud** to damage (someone or someone's reputation) by saying bad things about him or her.
- **mud sticks** used to indicate that, if something bad is said about someone, some people are likely to believe this and to go on believing it, even if it is not at all true or if it has been disproved.
- **(someone's) name is mud** (someone) is in disfavour or is being criticized.
- **sling** *or* **throw mud at (someone** *or* **something)** to say bad or insulting things about (someone or something).

mule
- **stubborn as a mule** extremely stubborn.

multitude
- **cover a multitude of sins** to be able to apply or refer to a large number of different things. <A misquotation from the Bible, I Peter 4:8, 'Charity shall cover the multitude of sins'>.

mum
- **mum's the word** do not say anything.

murder
- **get away with murder** to do something bad, irresponsible, etc, without suffering punishment.
- **I could murder (something)** used to indicate that you would very much like to have (something) to eat or drink.
- **scream blue murder** to scream extremely loudly.

music
- **be music to one's ears** used to indicate that one is very pleased to hear something.

mustard
- **keen as mustard** very eager and enthusiastic.
- **not cut the mustard** not to be able to do or achieve something; not be good enough.

muster
- **pass muster** to be considered good enough. <Refers to the calling together of people in the armed services in order to make sure that their dress and equipment are in good order>.

mutton
- **mutton dressed as lamb** an older person, usually a woman, dressed in clothes suitable for young people.

nail
- **a nail in (someone's) coffin** something which helps to bring about (someone's) downfall or destruction.
- **hit the nail on the head** to be extremely accurate in one's description, judgement, etc, of someone or something.

name
- **be (someone's) middle name** used to emphasize how typical of someone something is.
- **call (someone) names** to apply insulting or rude names to (someone).
- **give (someone** *or* **something) a bad name** to damage the reputation of (someone or something).
- **make a name for oneself** to become famous or well known.
- **name names** to give the names of people, especially people who are guilty or accused of wrong-doing.
- **no names, no pack-drill** no names will be mentioned and so no one will get into trouble. <'Pack-drill' refers to a form of army punishment in which the soldiers being punished were forced to march up and down carrying all their equipment>.
- **the name of the game** the important or central thing.
- **to one's name** in one's possession or ownership.

nasty
- **a nasty piece of work** someone who is very unpleasant or behaves very unpleasantly.

navel
- **contemplate one's navel** to be too much concerned with oneself and one's own activities and problems rather than with other, often more important, problems.

near
- **a near miss** something unpleasant that very nearly happened, often the near collision of two planes in the sky.
- **a near thing** the act of just avoiding an accident, misfortune, etc.
- **one's nearest and dearest** one's close family.

neck
- **be in (something) up to one's neck** to be very much involved in something bad or illegal.
- **get it in the neck** to be severely scolded or punished.
- **have the brass neck to (do something)** to have the impertinence or brazenness to (do something).
- **neck and neck** exactly equal.
- **risk one's neck** to put one's life, job, etc, in danger.
- **stick one's neck out** to take a risk or do something that may cause trouble.
- **this** *or* **that, etc, neck of the woods** this or that, etc, part of the country. <Originally a term for a remote community in the woods of the early 19th-century American frontier>.

needle
- **like looking for a needle in a haystack** an impossible search.

nerve
- **get on (someone's) nerves** to irritate (someone).
- **have a nerve** to be impertinent or brazen.
- **live on one's nerves** to be worried and anxious all the time.
- **lose one's nerve** to become scared, and so be unable to continue with an activity or course of action.
- **touch a nerve** to refer to something about which someone feels particularly sensitive.
- **war of nerves** a situation in which two opponents or enemies use psychological means against each other, for example by frightening or threatening the other side, rather than direct action.

nest
- **a nest-egg** savings for the future.
- **fly the nest** to leave one's parent home and go and live elsewhere.
- **foul your own nest** to do something which could have a bad effect on your own interests, activities or relationships.

net
- **cast one's net wide** to involve a large number of people or things or a large area.
- **slip through the net** not to be found or identified.

nettle
- **grasp the nettle** to set about an unpleasant or difficult task in a firm and determined manner.

never
- **never-never land** an imaginary land where conditions are ideal. <Refers to the idealized land in J.M. Barrie's play *Peter Pan*>.
- **on the never-never** by hire purchase.

new

- **new broom** someone who has just been appointed to a post and who is eager to be efficient, make changes, etc. <From the saying a new broom sweeps clean, a new broom being more effective than the old one>.

news

- **break the news to (someone)** to tell (someone) about something, usually something unpleasant or sad, that has happened.
- **no news is good news** if one has not received any information about someone or something then all is likely to be well since if something bad, such as an accident, had happened one would have heard.

next

- **next door to (something)** very nearly (something).
- **next to nothing** almost nothing, very little.

niche

- **carve a niche for oneself** to succeed in creating a secure job or position for oneself or for something.

nick

- **in good** *or* **poor nick** in good or poor condition.
- **in the nick of time** just in time, at the last possible minute.

nine

- **a nine days' wonder** something that arouses surprise and interest for a short time only. <Refers to a saying quoted by Chaucer—'where is no wonder so great that it lasts more than nine days'>.

ninepins

- **go down like ninepins** to become ill or damaged, or to be killed or destroyed rapidly, one after the other.

nip

- **nip (something) in the bud** to put a stop or end to (something) as soon as it develops.

nit

- **get down to the nitty-gritty** to begin to deal with the basic practical details, problems, etc.
- **nit-picking** the act of finding very minor faults in something, quibbling. <Refers to picking nits out of hair>.

no

- **no end of (something)** a great deal of (something).
- **no go** unsuccessful, in vain.
- **no way** under no circumstances.

nod

- **a nod is as good as a wink to a blind horse** a hint is often all that is necessary to communicate thoughts or feelings.
- **give/get the nod** to give/be given permission or approval for something.
- **have a nodding acquaintance with (someone** *or* **something)** to know (someone or something) slightly. <Refers to knowing someone well enough to nod in greeting to him or her>.
- **nod off** to fall asleep, sometimes accidentally.

noise

- **big noise** an important person.
- **make all the right noises** to say things which are considered the right response to a particular situation or the things which someone wants to hear.

nook

- **every nook and cranny** absolutely everywhere. <Literally, in all the corners and cracks>.

nose

- **cut off one's nose to spite one's face** to do something that harms oneself, usually in order to harm someone else.
- **follow one's nose** to go straight forward.
- **get up (someone's) nose** to annoy or irritate (someone).
- **have a nose around** to have a good look round a place, usually out of curiosity and when one is not supposed to be doing so.
- **have a nose for (something)** to have a talent or ability for finding or noticing something.
- **keep (one's** *or* **someone's) nose to the grindstone** to keep (someone) working hard without stopping.
- **lead (someone) by the nose** to get (someone) to do whatever one wants. <Refers to the ring on a bull's nose>.
- **look down one's nose at (someone** *or* **something)** to regard or treat (someone or something) with disdain or contempt.
- **on the nose** exactly.
- **pay through the nose** to pay a great deal of money for something.
- **poke one's nose into (something)** to pry into or interfere in other people's affairs. <Refers literally to a dog>.
- **powder one's nose** a euphemism, sometimes used by women, meaning to go to the toilet.
- **put (someone's) nose out of joint** to make (someone) jealous or offended by taking a place usually held by him or her, e.g. in the affections of a person whom he or she loves. <Refers to a person whose nose has been broken by being hit in the face>.
- **rub (someone's) nose in it** to keep on reminding (someone) about something he or she has done wrong. <Refers literally to rubbing a dog's nose in its faeces with the intention of house-training it>.
- **see further than the end of one's nose** to be concerned with more than just what is happening in the immediate present and in the immediate vicinity.
- **thumb one's nose at (someone** *or* **something)** *see* **thumb**.
- **turn up one's nose at (something)** to treat (something) with dislike or disgust.
- **under (someone's) (very) nose** **1** right in front of (someone) and so easily seen. **2** while (someone) is actually present.

note

- **strike the right note** to say or do something suitable for the occasion. <Refers to playing a musical instrument>.

nothing

- **come to nothing** to fail.
- **go for nothing** to be wasted or unsuccessful.
- **have nothing on (someone) 1** not to be nearly as good, skilful, bad, etc, as (someone). **2** to have no proof or evidence of (someone's) wrongdoing.
- **have nothing to do with (someone or something)** to avoid contact with (someone or something).
- **nothing ventured, nothing gained** one cannot achieve anything if one does not make an attempt or take a risk.
- **there is nothing to choose between (two people or things)** there is hardly any difference in quality, ability, etc, between (two people or things).
- **there's nothing to it** it is very easy.
- **think nothing of (something)** not to regard (something) as out of the ordinary, difficult, etc.

nowhere

- **be in the middle of nowhere** be in a place which is a long way away from a town or city, a lot of people, etc, often carrying the suggestion that the place is boring.
- **get nowhere** to make no progress, to have no success.

nudge

- **nudge, nudge, wink, wink** used to indicate that there is some form of sexual innuendo or hidden reference in something that has been said. <Came into common use influenced by a sketch by Eric Idle in the TV series *Monty Python's Flying Circus*>.

number

- **get or have (someone's) number** to find out or know what kind of person (someone) is and what he or she is likely to do.
- **(someone's) number is up** (someone) is about to suffer something unpleasant, such as dying, failing, being punished, being caught, etc.
- **number one** oneself.

nut[1]

- **a hard nut to crack** a difficult problem or person to deal with.
- **in a nutshell** briefly, to sum up.
- **the nuts and bolts of (something)** the basic details or practicalities of (something).

nut[2]

- **be nuts about (someone or something)** to like (someone or something) a very great deal, to be wildly enthusiastic about (someone or something).
- **do one's nut** to get very angry.
- **go nuts** to become extremely angry.

oak

- **great oaks from little acorns grow** a saying used to emphasize that even large and important things often begin a small way.

oar

- **put or stick one's oar in** to interfere in another's affairs, conversation, e.g. by offering unwanted opinions. <Perhaps refers to someone who is being rowed in a boat by others and who suddenly decides to take part in the rowing unasked>.
- **rest on one's oars** to take a rest after working very hard. <Refers literally to rowing>.

object

- **money, distance, etc, is no object** it does not matter how much money, distance, etc, is involved in the particular situation. <Originally 'money is no object' meant money or profits were not the main aim but it came to be misapplied>.

occasion

- **rise to the occasion** to be able to carry out whatever action is required in an important or urgent situation.

odd

- **against all the odds** in spite of major difficulties.
- **be at odds with (someone or something)** to be in disagreement with (someone or something), not to be in accordance with (something).
- **lay odds** to bet. <Refers to betting on horses>.
- **make no odds** to be of no importance, to make no difference.
- **odd man out** someone or something that is different from others. <Refers literally to someone left out of a game when the teams have been chosen>.
- **odds and ends** small objects of different kinds.
- **over the odds** more than one would usually expect to pay. <Refers originally to a horse-racing term>.

off

- **in the offing** about to or likely to happen, appear, etc. <A nautical term. Offing refers to the whole area of sea that can be seen from a particular point on shore>.
- **off and on or on and off** occasionally.

oil

- **be no oil painting** to be not at all attractive.
- **oil and water** used to emphasize how different two people or things are.
- **oil the wheels** to make something easier to do or obtain. <Wheels turn more easily if oil is applied to them>.
- **pour oil on troubled waters** to attempt to bring a state of calm and peace to a situation of disagreement or dispute. <Since oil floats on water it has the effect of making waves flat>.
- **strike oil** to obtain exactly what one wants, to be successful.

old

- **an old hand** someone who is very experienced (at doing something).
- **old as the hills** extremely old.
- **old hat** old-fashioned, no longer popular.
- **old master** (a work by) any great painter before the 19th century, especially of the 15th and 16th centuries.

- **the old-boy network** a system in which jobs and other advantages are obtained on the basis of knowing the right people rather than on ability. <The connection with such people is often that one was at school with them>.
- **the old country** the country from which an immigrant or his or her parents or grandparents originally came.
- **the old guard** the older members of a group who are old-fashioned in their opinions and tastes. <The translation of the name applied to the most experienced section of Napoleon's army>.

olive
- **olive branch** a sign of a wish for peace. <The olive branch was an ancient symbol of peace>.

omelette
- **you can't make an omelette without breaking eggs** a saying indicating that it is impossible to achieve something worthwhile without causing a few problems or difficulties.

on
- **be not on** used to indicate emphatic disapproval of or lack of acceptance of something.
- **be on to (someone)** having discovered some previously secret or unknown information about (someone) or his or her activities.

once
- **give (someone) the once-over** to look at or study (someone or something) quickly.

one
- **a one-horse race** a competition, contest, etc, in which one person or side is certain to win.
- **a one-night stand** a relationship, arrangement, etc, that lasts for one evening or night only. <Literally a single performance in one place given by a pop group, etc, on tour>.
- **get one over on (someone)** to gain a victory or advantage over (someone).
- **have a one-track mind** to think only of one subject all the time.
- **have had one too many** to have had too much to drink.
- **it takes one to know one** used to indicate that people who have faults of their own find it easy to spot such faults in others.
- **not be oneself** to be feeling slightly unwell, to be more depressed, etc, than usual.

onion
- **know one's onions** to know a subject, one's job, etc.

open
- **an open-and-shut case** free from uncertainty, having an obvious outcome.
- **an open secret** a supposed secret that is known to many people.
- **keep an open mind** to be willing to listen to other people's suggestions, ideas, etc, instead of just concentrating on one's own point of view.

- **lay oneself (wide) open to (something)** to put oneself in a position in which one is liable to be in receipt of (blame, criticism, accusations, attack, etc).

opposite
- **(someone's) opposite number** the person in another company, country, etc, whose job or role corresponds to someone's.

option
- **keep one's options open** to delay making a definite decision so that all choices are available as long as possible.

oracle
- **work the oracle** to produce the desired result, to obtain what one wants, especially by using cunning, influence or bribery. <Refers to the oracle at Delphi in Greek legend>.

order
- **the order of the day** something that should be done, worn, etc, because conventional, common, fashionable, etc. <Refers originally to a list of items to be discussed in the British parliament on a particular day>.

organ
- **speak to the organ grinder, not his monkey** used to emphasize that one wants to deal with someone in authority, not with someone associated with him or her who has no power. <An organ grinder was a person who played a kind of musical instrument on wheels, known as a barrel organ, in the street and he often had a monkey on the barrel organ to attract people or to collect gifts of money>.

other
- **look the other way** to ignore or disregard something wrong, illegal, etc.

out
- **come out** to make public the fact that one is a homosexual.
- **get (something) out of your system** see **system**.
- **out and about** going around outside, e.g. after an illness.

outside
- **at the outside** at the most.

over
- **be all over (someone)** to be extremely friendly and attentive to (someone).
- **over and done with** completely finished, at an end.

overboard
- **go overboard (about** or **for someone** or **something)** to be extremely enthusiastic about (someone or something).

overdrive
- **go into overdrive** to start to work extremely hard or to become extremely active.

owe
- **I owe you one** used to indicate that someone has done one some kind of favour and that one must return this some time.

own
- **come into one's own** to have the opportunity to show one's good qualities, talent, skill, etc.
- **hold one's own 1** to perform as well as one's opponents in a contest, an argument, etc. **2** to be surviving, to be holding on to life.

p
- **mind one's p's and q's** to be very careful, to be polite and well behaved. <Perhaps refers to a warning to a printer to be careful of the letters p and q so as not to confuse them>.

pace
- **put (someone *or* something) through its *or* his *or* her paces** to test the ability of (someone or something) by getting them to demonstrate what it, he or she is capable of. <Refers originally to assessing horses>.
- **show one's paces** to demonstrate one's abilities.
- **stay the pace** to maintain progress in an activity at the same rate as others.

pack
- **send (someone) packing** to send (someone) away firmly and frankly.

pain
- **a pain in the neck** someone or something that constantly irritates one.
- **no pain, no gain** a saying used to emphasize the fact that the acquiring of something advantageous or desirable often involves something difficult or unpleasant, but it is worth it.

paint
- **like watching paint dry** used to describe something extremely boring.
- **paint the town red** to go out and celebrate in a lively, noisy manner.

palm
- **grease (someone's) palm** to give (someone) money, to bribe (someone).
- **have (someone) in the palm of one's hand** to have (someone) in one's power and ready to do as one wishes.

paper
- **paper over the cracks** to try to hide faults, mistakes, difficulties, etc, in a hasty or careless way in order to pretend that there were no faults, mistakes, etc.
- **paper tiger** someone or something that has the outward appearance of being powerful and threatening but is in fact ineffective.

par
- **below *or* not up to par 1** not up to the usual or required standard. **2** not completely well.

- **on a par with (something)** of the same standard as (something), as good as (something).
- **par for the course** what might be expected, what usually happens. <Originally a golfing term meaning the number of strokes that would be made in a perfect round or the course>.

part
- **look the part** to have the appropriate appearance of a particular kind of person.
- **part and parcel (of something)** something that is naturally or basically part (of something).
- **take (something) in good part** to accept (something) without being angry or offended.
- **take (someone's) part** to support (someone) in an argument, debate, etc.
- **the parting of the ways** the point at which people must go different ways, take different courses of action, make different decisions, etc. <A biblical reference to Ezekiel 21:21>.

party
- **the party line** the official opinions, ideas, attitudes, etc, as set down by the leaders of a particular group.
- **the party's over** a pleasant or happy time has come to an end.

pass
- **make a pass at (someone)** to try to start a romantic or sexual relationship with (someone). <Originally a fencing term, meaning to thrust with a foil>.
- **pass away** to die.
- **pass by on the other side** to ignore someone in trouble and not help him or her. <A biblical reference to the parable of the Samaritan, Luke 10>.

past
- **I, etc, would not put it past (someone) to (do something)** I, etc, think (someone) is quite capable of (doing something bad).
- **past it** less good, etc, than when one or it was not so old.
- **past master** someone extremely talented or skilful.

pasture
- **pastures new *or* fresh fields and pastures new** used to indicate a new and different place or situation. <The longer version of the phrase is a misquotation of 'fresh woods and pastures new' from John Milton's poem 'Lycidas'.

pat
- **a pat on the back** an indication of praise or approval.

patch
- **not to be a patch on (someone *or* something)** not to be nearly as good as (someone or something).
- **patch it *or* things up** to become friends again after a quarrel.

path
- **beat a path to (someone's) door** to visit (someone) very frequently or in large numbers.

pave
- **pave the way for (something)** to make it possible or easier for (something to happen).

pay
- **put paid to (something)** to prevent (an action, plan, etc) from being carried out.

peace
- **keep the peace** to prevent disturbances, fighting, quarrelling, etc.
- **make one's peace with (someone)** to become, or try to become, friendly with (someone) again after a period of disagreement.

peacock
- **proud as a peacock** extremely proud.

pearl
- **pearls of wisdom** something wise or helpful, often used ironically.

pedestal
- **put (someone) on a pedestal** to treat (someone) with great respect and admiration. <Refers to the practice of putting statues of famous people on pedestals>.

peg
- **bring (someone) down a peg or two** to make (someone) more humble. <Refers to tuning musical instruments>.
- **off the peg** of clothes, ready to wear, not made for one specially.
- **a square peg in a round hole** used to describe someone who does not fit into a particular situation or environment and feels uncomfortable in it.

penny
- **a penny for them** *or* **your thoughts** what are you thinking about?
- **in for a penny, in for a pound** if one is going to do something one might as well do it boldly and thoroughly.
- **not to have a penny to one's name** to have no money at all.
- **penny wise and pound foolish** being careful with small items of expenditure and extravagant with large ones.
- **spend a penny** to urinate. <From the former price of admission to the cubicle of a public toilet>.
- **the penny drops** I, etc, suddenly understand. <Refers to a coin in a slot machine>.
- **turn up like a bad penny** to reappear or keep reappearing although not wanted or welcome.
- **two a penny** of little value because very common.

petard
- **hoist with one's own petard** to be the victim of one's own action which was intended to harm someone else. <Refers to Shakespeare's *Hamlet*, Act 3, scene IV. A petard was a device containing explosives used by military engineers>.

philistine
- **a philistine** someone who is not interested in artistic or intellectual pursuits. <The Philistines were a fierce race of people who fought against the Israelites in biblical times. The present meaning was influenced by German>.

phrase
- **to coin a phrase** literally, to say something new and inventive, but used usually to introduce a cliché or a common saying or expression.

pick
- **pick and choose** to choose very carefully from a range of things.

picnic
- **be no picnic** used to emphasize how difficult or unpleasant something is.

picture
- **be out of the picture** to be no longer involved in something.
- **the big picture** the whole situation, not just some details.
- **get the picture** to understand what is being explained or described.
- **put (someone) in the picture** to give (someone) all the information and detail about a situation.

pie
- **nice as a pie** exceptionally pleasant or friendly, often unexpectedly.
- **pie in the sky** something good expected or promised in the future which is unlikely to come about. <Refers to a quotation from a poem by the American poet Joe Hill>.

piece
- **go to pieces** to be unable to continue coping with a situation, life, etc.

pig
- **buy a pig in a poke** to buy (something) without examining it carefully or without knowing its worth. <Supposedly referring to a fairground trick in which a prospective customer was sold a cat in a bag thinking that it was a piglet>.
- **make a pig of oneself** to eat greedily, to eat a great deal.
- **make a pig's ear of (something)** to make a mess of (something), to do (something) very badly or clumsily.
- **pigs might fly** it is extremely unlikely that that will happen.

pikestaff
- **plain as a pikestaff** very obvious. <Pikestaff was originally packstaff, a staff for holding a traveller's pack and lacking any ornamentation. This sense of plain has been confused with that of plain meaning clear>.

pillar
- **from pillar to post** from one place to another, often repeatedly. <Refers originally to the game of real tennis>.

pilot
- **be on automatic pilot** to do something without thinking about what you are doing, because of tiredness, distress, etc., usually succeeding in doing it correctly because you have done it before.

pin
- **for two pins** given the least encouragement or reason.
- **on pins and needles** in a state of anxiety or suspense.
- **you could have heard a pin drop** there was silence.

pinch
- **at a pinch** if it is absolutely necessary.
- **feel the pinch** to have financial problems.

pink
- **in the pink** in good health. <Refers to the pink complexion of some healthy people>.
- **the pink of perfection** absolute perfection. <Refers to a quotation from Oliver Goldsmith's play *She Stoops to Conquer*>.

pip
- **pipped at the post** beaten at the last minute. <Refers originally to horse-racing. A horse is pipped at the post if another horse passes it at the end of the race>.

pipe
- **in the pipeline** in preparation, happening soon. <Refers to crude oil being piped from the well to the refineries>.

piper
- **pay the piper** to provide the money for something and therefore be entitled to have a say in the organization of it. <Refers to the saying 'He who pays the piper calls the tune'>.
- **pipe dream** a wish or idea that can never be realized. <Refers to visions experienced by opium smokers>.

pistol
- **hold a pistol to (someone's) head** to use force or threats to get (someone) to do as one wishes.

place
- **fall into place** to become understood when seen in terms of its relationship to other things.
- **go places** to be successful in one's career.
- **know one's place** to accept the lowliness of one's position and act accordingly.
- **a place in the sun** a situation in which one will be happy, successful, well of, etc..
- **put (someone) in his *or* her place** to remind (someone) angrily of the lowliness of his or her position or of his or her lack of experience, knowledge, etc.

plague
- **avoid (someone *or* something) like the plague** used to emphasize how keen one is to keep away (from someone or something).

plain
- **plain sailing** easy progress. <Perhaps confused with plane sailing, a method of making navigational calculations at sea in which the earth's surface is treated as though it were flat>.

plate
- **have (something) handed to one on a plate** to get (something) without having to put any effort into it.

play
- **make a play for (someone *or* something)** to try to obtain (someone or something).
- **play hard to get** to make it difficult for someone to get to know one in order to make him or her more keen to do so.

plot
- **the plot thickens** the situation is getting more complicated and more interesting. <Refers to a quotation from George Villiers' play *The Rehearsal*>.

plug
- **pull the plug on (something)** to stop supporting (something), to stop (something) from continuing.

plum
- **have a plum in one's mouth** to speak with what is regarded as an upper-class accent.

plunge
- **take the plunge** to go ahead and do something, especially something difficult or risky, especially after having spent some considerable time thinking about it.

poacher
- **poacher turned gamekeeper** used to describe someone who has changed their job, attitude, opinion, etc, and now holds completely opposite views.

pocket
- **in (someone's) pocket** under the control or influence of (someone).
- **line one's pocket** to make money for oneself dishonestly.
- **out of pocket** having made a loss.

poetic
- **poetic justice** deserved but accidental punishment or reward.
- **poetic licence** the disregarding of established rules of form, grammar, fact, etc, by writers to achieve a desired effect.

point
- **the point of no return** the stage in a process, etc, when it becomes impossible either to stop or change one's mind. <Originally referred to the point in the flight of an aircraft after which it did not have enough fuel to return to its place of departure>.
- **up to a point** to some extent but not completely.

poison
- **poison-pen letter** an anonymous letter saying bad things about someone.

port
- **any port in a storm** any solution to a problem or difficulty will suffice.

possum
- **play possum** to pretend to be asleep, unconscious or dead. <The possum pretends to be dead when it is under threat of attack from another animal>.

post[1]
- **from pillar to post** from one place to another, often repeatedly.

post[2]
- **keep (someone) posted** to keep (someone) informed about developments in a situation.

pot
- **go to pot** to get into a bad or worse state. <Refers to meat being cut up and stewed in a pot).
- **keep the pot boiling** to keep something going or operating.
- **take pot-luck** to have a meal at someone's house, etc, without having anything specially prepared for one. <Literally to take whatever happens to be in the cooking-pot at the time>.
- **the pot calling the kettle black** someone criticizing (someone) for doing (something) that he or she does himself or herself.
- **the** *or* **a watched pot never boils** when one is waiting for something to happen, etc, the time taken seems longer if one is constantly thinking about it.

pour
- **it never rains but it pours** when something goes wrong it goes wrong very badly or other things go wrong too.

powder
- **be sitting on a powder keg** to be in a very risky or dangerous situation in which something could easily go wrong quite suddenly.

power
- **more power to (someone's) elbow** may (someone) be successful.
- **the power behind the throne** the person who is really in charge of or in control of an organization, etc, while giving the impression that it is someone else.
- **the powers that be** the people in charge, the authorities.

practice
- **practice makes perfect** if one practises doing something one will eventually be good at it.

practise
- **practise what one preaches** to act in the way that one recommends to others.

praise
- **sing (someone's** *or* **something's) praises** to praise (someone or something) with great enthusiasm.

premium
- **be at a premium** to be much in demand and, therefore, difficult to obtain. <A financial term meaning literally 'sold at more than the nominal value'>.

press
- **press-gang (someone) into (doing something)** to force (someone) or persuade (someone) against his or her will to (do something). <The press gang was a group of sailors in the 18th century who seized men and forced them to join the navy>.

pretty
- **come to a pretty pass** to get into a bad state.
- **cost a pretty penny** to cost a large amount of money.
- **sitting pretty** in a very comfortable or advantageous position.

prey
- **be a prey to (something)** regularly to suffer from (something).
- **prey on (someone's) mind** to cause constant worry or anxiety to (someone).

price
- **at a price** at a very high price.
- **a price on (someone's) head** a reward offered for the capture or killing of (someone).

pride
- **pride goes before a fall** being too conceited often leads to misfortune.
- **pride of place** the most important or privileged position.
- **swallow one's pride** to behave in a more humble way than one usually does or than one would wish to do.

prime
- **prime mover** someone or something that gets something started.

pro
- **the pros and cons** the arguments for and against. <Latin *pro*, 'for', and *contra*, 'against'>.

production
- **make a production of (something)** to make (something) appear to be much more complicated than it actually is.

proof
- **the proof of the pudding is in the eating** the real worth of something is only found out when it has been into practice or use.

proud
- **do (someone) proud** to treat (someone) exceptionally well or lavishly.

pull

- **pull the other one!** used to emphasize to someone that you do not believe him or her. Sometimes the phrase is extended to **pull the other one; it's got bells on!** <A reference to the phrase: pull (someone's) leg>.

pulse

- **keep one's finger on the pulse** to keep oneself informed about recent developments in a situation, organization, etc, or in the world. <Refers to a doctor checking the rate of someone's pulse for health reasons>.

Punch

- **pleased as Punch** extremely pleased or happy. <Refers to the puppet show character who is usually portrayed smiling gleefully>.

punch

- **pull one's punches** to be less forceful or harsh in one's attack or criticism than one is capable of. <Refers to striking blows in boxing without using one's full strength>.
- **roll with the punches** not to let difficulties or problems discourage one or have a bad or upsetting effect on one.

pup

- **sell (someone) a pup** to deceive (someone), often to sell or recommend something that turns out not to be as good as he or she thought.

purpose

- **at cross purposes** involved in a misunderstanding because of talking or thinking about different things without realizing it.

purse

- **hold the purse strings** to be in charge of financial matters.
- **you can't make a silk purse out of a sow's ear** *see* **silk**.

push

- **at a push** used to indicate that something can be done if it is absolutely necessary, but it will not be easy.
- **give (someone) the push** to dismiss (someone).

put

- **put it on** to feign, to pretend.
- **put-up job** something done to deceive or trick (someone).

putty

- **putty in (someone's) hands** easily influenced or manipulated by (someone). <Putty is a malleable substance>.

Pyrrhic

- **Pyrrhic victory** a success of some kind in which what it takes to achieve is not worth it. <From the costly victory of King Pyrrhus of Epirus, over the Romans at Heraclea in 280 BC>.

QT

- **on the QT** secretly. <An abbreviation of quiet>.

quantity

- **an unknown quantity** someone or something of which very little is known. <Refers literally to a mathematical term>.

queer

- **in Queer Street** in financial difficulties. <Perhaps changed from Carey Street in London where the bankruptcy courts were>.
- **queer (someone's) pitch** to upset (someone's) plans or arrangements. <Pitch here refers to the site of a market stall. Originally to queer someone's pitch was to set up a stall beside it selling the same kind of goods>.

question

- **a question mark over (something)** doubt or uncertainty in relation to (something).
- **out of the question** not possible.
- **pop the question** to ask (someone) to marry one.

queue

- **jump the queue** to go ahead of others in a queue without waiting for one's proper turn.

qu

- **on the qui vive** very alert. <From the challenge of a French sentry *Qui vive?* 'Long live who, whose side are you on?'>.

quick

- **cut (someone) to the quick** to hurt (someone's) feelings very badly. <The quick is the sensitive skin under the nail>.

quid

- **quids in** a fortunate position.

quit

- **call it quits** to agree that neither person owes the other one anything and that neither one has any kind of advantage over the other.

R

- **the three R's** reading, writing and arithmetic, thought of as the essential basics of education. <From *r*eading, w*r*iting and a*r*ithmetic>.

rack

- **go to rack and ruin** to fall into a state of disrepair or into a worthless condition. <Rack means destruction>.

rage

- **all the rage** very fashionable or popular.

rail

- **off the rails** not sensible, disorganized, deranged. <Refers to a train leaving the track>.

rain

- **keep** *or* **put away** *or* **save (something) for a rainy day** to keep (something, especially money) until one really needs it. <Formerly most jobs, such as farm jobs, were dependent on the weather. Since they could not be carried out in rainy weather no money was earned then>.

- **rain or shine** whatever the weather.
- **take a rain check on (something)** used to indicate that you are unable to accept an invitation but would like to postpone it until a later date. <American in origin and a reference to the part of a ticket that you keep when a sports fixture cannot take place because of bad weather so that you can use it for entry to the fixture when it does take place>.

rake
- **thin as a rake** extremely thin.

rampage
- **be** *or* **go on the rampage** to rush about wildly or violently.

rank
- **close ranks** to act together and support each other as a defensive measure.
- **pull rank** to make unfair use of a position of authority to make someone else do as one wishes or to give one some kind of advantage.

rap
- **take the rap for (something)** to take the blame or punishment for (something).

rat
- **like a drowned rat** soaking wet.
- **smell a rat** to have a suspicion that something is wrong or that one is being deceived. <Refers to a terrier hunting>.
- **the rat race** the fierce competitive struggle for success in business, etc. <A nautical phrase for a fierce tidal current>.

raw
- **touch (someone) on the raw** to hurt or anger (someone).

razor
- **sharp as a razor** quick-witted and very intelligent.

read
- **take (something) as read** to assume (something).

real
- **the real McCoy** something genuine and very good as opposed to others like it which are not. <Perhaps from Kid McCoy, an American boxer who was called The Real McCoy to distinguish him from other boxers of the same name>.

reason
- **see reason** to be persuaded by someone's advice, etc, to act or think sensibly.
- **within reason** within sensible limits.

rebound
- **on the rebound** to start a new relationship while still suffering from the disappointment experienced at the end of the previous relationship.

record
- **for the record** so that it will be noted.
- **set the record straight** to put right a mistake or misunderstanding.

red
- **a red-letter day** a day remembered because something particularly pleasant or important happened or happens on it. <From the fact that important dates in the year are sometimes shown in red on calendars>.
- **catch (someone) red-handed** to find (someone) in the act of doing something wrong or unlawful. <Refers to finding a murderer with the blood of a victim on his or her hands>.
- **in the red** in debt, overdrawn. <From the use of red ink to make entries on the debit side of an account>.
- **like a red rag to a bull** certain to make (someone) angry. <From the widespread belief that bulls are angered by the sight of the colour red although they are in fact colour-blind>.
- **on red alert** ready for an an immediate danger. <Originally a military term for mobilizing civilians during an air-raid>.
- **red tape** the rules and regulations, official papers, etc, that are thought to characterize government departments. <From the reddish tape used by government offices to tie bundles of papers>.
- **see red** to get very angry.

reed
- **a broken reed** someone who is too weak or unreliable to be depended upon.

rest
- **lay (someone) to rest** to bury (someone).
- **rest assured** you can be quite certain.

return
- **return to the fold** to come or back to one's family, an organization, a set of principles or beliefs, etc, which one has previously left. <Refers to a sheep returning to the sheep-pen>.

rhetorical
- **rhetorical question** a question which does not require an answer.

rhyme
- **without rhyme or reason** without any logical or sensible reason or explanation.

rich
- **rich as Croesus** extremely rich. <Croesus was a ruler of the kingdom of Lydia who was very wealthy>.
- **strike it rich** to obtain wealth, often suddenly or unexpectedly.

riddance
- **good riddance to (someone *or* something)** I am glad to have got rid of (someone or something).

ride
- **be riding for a fall** to be on a course of action that is likely to lead to unpleasant results or disaster for oneself. <Refers originally to hunting>.
- **take (someone) for a ride** to deceive or trick (someone). <Originally American gangsters' slang for killing someone, from the practice of killing someone in a moving vehicle so as not to attract attention>.

rift
- **a rift in the lute** a slight disagreement or difficulty that might develop into a major one and ruin a project or relationship. <Refers to a quotation from Tennyson's *Idylls*>.

right
- **get *or* keep on the right side of (someone)** to act in such a way that (someone) feels or continues to feel friendly and well disposed towards one.
- **Mr *or* Miss Right** the perfect man or woman for one to marry.
- **right-hand man *or* woman** someone's most valuable and helpful assistant.
- **serve (someone) right** to be something unpleasant that (someone) deserves.
- **set (something) to rights** to bring (something) into a correct, organized, desired, etc, state.

ring
- **a dead ringer** someone who looks extremely like someone else. <Perhaps from the use of the phrase to mean a horse, similar to the original, illegally substituted in a race>.
- **have a ringside seat** to be in a position to observe clearly what is happening. <Originally refers to boxing>.

riot
- **read the riot act to (someone)** to scold (someone) severely and warn him or her to behave better. <The Riot Act of 1715 was read to unlawful gatherings of people to break the gathering up. If the people refused to disperse action could be taken against them>.

rise
- **rise and shine** to get out of bed and be lively and cheerful.
- **take a rise out of (someone)** to tease or make fun of (someone) so that he or she gets annoyed.

river
- **sell (someone) down the river** to betray or be disloyal to (someone). <Refers historically to selling slaves from the upper Mississippi states to buyers in Louisiana where working and living conditions were much harsher>.

road
- **hit the road** start out on a journey.
- **one for the road** one last drink before leaving.

roaring
- **do a roaring trade in (something)** to be selling a lot of (something).

rob
- **rob Peter to pay Paul** to pay (someone) with the money that should go to pay a debt owed to (someone else). <Refers to Saints Peter and Paul who share the same feast day, 29 July>.

rock
- **between a rock and a hard place** to be in a situation in which one is faced with a choice between two equally unpleasant or unacceptable alternatives.
- **steady as a rock** extremely steady, motionless.

rocket
- **not rocket science** used to indicate that something is quite easy and does not require much intellect or skill.

rod
- **make a rod for one's own back** to do something which is going to cause harm or problems for oneself in the future.
- **spare the rod and spoil the child** if a child is not punished for being naughty it will have a bad effect on his or her character.

rogue
- **a rogue's gallery** a police collection of photographs of known criminals.

roll
- **a rolling stone (gathers no moss)** a person who does not stay very long in one place (does not acquire very much in the way of possessions or responsibilities).
- **a roll in the hay** an informal way of describing having sex, especially when this is not part of a serious relationship.
- **be on a roll** used to indicate that things are going well and that good progress is being made.
- **be rolling in it *or* in money** to have a great deal of money.
- **be rolling in the aisles** to be laughing very heartily.

Rome
- **all roads lead to Rome** all ways of fulfilling an aim or intention end in the same result and so it does not does not matter which way one uses.
- **fiddle while Rome burns** to do nothing while something important is being ruined or destroyed. <The Emperor Nero was said to have played on a lyre while Rome was burning>.
- **Rome was not built in a day** a difficult task cannot be completed satisfactorily quickly.
- **when in Rome do as the Romans do** one should follow the customs, behaviour, etc, of the people one is visiting or living with. <A saying of St Ambrose>.

rooftop
- **shout (something) from the rooftops** to tell a great many people about (something).

roost
- **rule the roost** to be the person in charge whose wishes or orders are obeyed.

rope
- **give (someone) enough rope (and he will hang himself)** let (someone foolish) act as he or she pleases and he or she will bring about his or her own ruin, downfall, misfortune, etc.
- **know the ropes** to know the details and methods associated with a business, procedure, activity, etc.
- **on the ropes** used to describe a situation which is very close to failure or defeat.
- **rope (someone) in** to include (someone), to ask (someone) to join in, often against his or her will. <Refers to lassoing cattle in the American West>.
- **show (someone) the ropes** to teach (someone) the details and methods involved (in something).

rose
- **come up smelling of roses** to come out of a situation with some kind of advantage when it was expected to result in blame or harm for one.
- **everything's coming up roses** everything is turning out to be successful or happy.
- **look at (someone *or* something) through rose-coloured *or* rose-tinted spectacles *or* glasses** to view (someone or something) in an extremely optimistic light.

rough
- **give (someone) the rough edge of one's tongue** to scold or criticize (someone) severely.
- **ride roughshod over (someone)** to treat (someone) without any respect and without any regard for his or her views or feelings. <Horses are roughshod to give a better grip on icy, etc, roads>.
- **take the rough with the smooth** to accept the disadvantages as well as the advantages and benefits of a situation.

round
- **go the rounds** to be passed from person to person.
- **in round figures *or* numbers** to the nearest whole number, especially one that can be divided by ten.
- **round trip** the journey to somewhere plus the journey back.

rub
- **rub (something) in** to keep reminding someone about (something which he or she would rather forget).
- **rub off on (to) (someone)** to be passed to (someone), to affect (someone).
- **rub (someone) up the wrong way** to irritate (someone). <Refers to rubbing an animal's coat up the wrong way>.

- **there's the rub** that's the problem. <Refers to a quotation from Shakespeare's *Hamlet*, Act 3, scene I>.

rug
- **pull the rug (out) from under (someone)** suddenly to stop giving important help or support to (someone), to leave (someone) in a weak position.

rule
- **rule of thumb** a rough or inexact guide used for calculations of some kind.

run
- **a run for (someone's) money** a creditable or worthy performance or opposition. <A racing term indicating that the horse one has backed has actually raced although it has not won>.
- **(someone's) cup runneth over** someone feels very happy. <A biblical reference to Psalm 23:5>.
- **in the running** with a chance of success.
- **run its course** to continue to its natural end, to develop naturally.
- **run out on (someone *or* something)** to abandon (someone or something).
- **take a running jump** to go away.

rut
- **in a rut** in a routine, monotonous way of life. <Refers to the rut made by a cartwheel, etc>.

sabre
- **rattle one's sabre** to put on a show of anger or fierceness without resorting to physical force in order to frighten someone.

sack
- **sackcloth and ashes** sorrow or apology for what one has done or failed to do. <People in mourning used to wear sackcloth and throw ashes over their heads. The phrase has several biblical references, e.g. Matthew 11:21>.

safe
- **safe and sound** totally unharmed.
- **there's safety in numbers** it is safer to undertake a risky venture if there are several people involved.

sail
- **sail close to the wind** to come close to breaking the law or a rule.
- **sail under false colours** to pretend to be different in character, beliefs, status, work, etc, than is really the case. <Refers to a ship flying a flag other than its own, as pirate ships sometimes did>.

salad
- **(someone's) salad days** (someone's) carefree and inexperienced youth.

salt
- **below the salt** in a humble, lowly or despised position. <Formerly the salt container marked the division at a dinner table between the rich and important people and

the more lowly people, the important people being near the top and so above the salt>.

- **rub salt in the wound** to make someone feel worse. <Salt used to be used as an antiseptic but it was painful on raw wounds>.
- **take (something) with a grain** or **pinch of salt** to treat (something) with some disbelief.
- **the salt of the earth** someone very worthy or good. <A biblical reference to Matthew 5:13>.
- **worth one's salt** worth the money one is paid, of any worth. <Salt was once a valuable commodity and the reference is to that given to servants or workers>.

Samaritan

- **a good Samaritan** someone who helps people when they are in need. <A biblical reference to the parable in Luke 10>.

sand

- **build (something) on sand** to establish (something) without having enough support, money, likelihood of survival, etc, to make it secure or practicable. <A biblical reference to Matthew 7:26>.

sardine

- **packed like sardines** crowded very close together. <Sardines are sold tightly packed in tins>.

scarlet

- **scarlet woman** an immoral or promiscuous woman. <A biblical reference to the woman in scarlet in Revelation 17>.

scene

- **behind the scenes** out of sight of the public, etc. <Refers literally to people in a theatrical production who work behind the scenery offstage>.
- **come on the scene** to arrive or appear.
- **not (someone's) scene** not the kind of thing that (someone) likes.
- **set the scene for (something)** to prepare the way for (something), to be the forerunner of (something). <Refers originally to the preparation of the stage for theatrical action>.

scent

- **throw (someone) off the scent** to distract (someone) from a search for someone or something, e.g. by giving him or her wrong information. <Refers literally to dogs>.

scheme

- **the best-laid schemes of mice and men (gang aft agley)** the most carefully arranged plans (often go wrong). <Refers to a quotation from Robert Burns's poem, 'To a Mouse'>.

science

- **blind (someone) with science** to talk about something in such a complicated technical way that it is difficult for a layperson to understand.

score

- **know the score** to know exactly what is involved, to know all the facts of a situation. <Literally to know from the score in a game who is likely to win or lose>.
- **settle old scores** to get revenge for wrongs committed in the past.

scratch

- **start from scratch** to start from the very beginning, without any advantages. <Refers to the starting line (formerly scratched on the ground), from which runners start unless their handicap allows them to start further down the track>.
- **up to scratch** up to the required standard. <Refers originally to a scratch in the centre of a boxing ring to which boxers had to make their way unaided after being knocked down to prove that they were fit to continue>.

screw

- **have a screw loose** to be deranged, to be very foolish. <Refers literally to malfunctioning machinery>.

Scrooge

- **Scrooge** an extremely mean person. <Refers to a character in Charles Dickens's *A Christmas Carol*>.

Scylla

- **between Scylla and Charybdis** faced with having to choose between two equally undesirable choices. <Refers to Homer's *Odyssey* in which Odysseus had to sail down a narrow strait between Scylla, a monster on a rock, and Charybdis, an extremely dangerous whirlpool>.

sea

- **a sea change** a complete change in a situation, someone's opinion, attitude, etc.
- **all at sea** puzzled, bewildered.

seam

- **be bursting at the seams** to be extremely full.
- **come** or **fall apart at the seams** to be in a state of collapse or ruin. <From clothes coming to pieces>.

second

- **second nature** a firmly established habit.
- **second sight** the supposed power of seeing into the future.
- **second thoughts** a change of opinion, decision, etc.

seed

- **go to seed** to become shabby and uncared-for. <Refers literally to plants seeding after flowering and being no longer attractive or useful>.

separate

- **separate the sheep from the goats** see **sheep**.

sewn

- **(all) sewn up** completely settled or arranged.

shade
- **put (someone** *or* **something) in the shade** to be much better, etc, than (someone or something). <Refers to making someone seem dark by being so much brighter oneself>.
- **shades of (someone** *or* **something)** that reminds me of (someone or something). <It is as though the shade or ghost of someone or something were present>.

shadow
- **worn to a shadow** made exhausted and thin by overworking.

shakes
- **in two shakes of a lamb's tail** in a very short time.

shape
- **knock (someone** *or* **something) into shape** to get (something) into the desired or good condition.
- **shape up or ship out** used to tell someone that he or she should start acting in a more responsible or appropriate way or get out.

sheep
- **might as well be hanged for a sheep as a lamb** if one is going to do something slightly wrong and have to pay a penalty one might as well do something really wrong and get more benefit. <Refers to the fact that stealing a lamb or a sheep used to be punishable by death>.
- **separate the sheep from the goats** to distinguish in some way the good, useful, talented, etc, people from the bad, useless or stupid, etc, ones. <A biblical reference to Matthew 25:32>.

shelf
- **on the shelf** unmarried and unlikely to get married because of being unattractive, old, etc. <Refers to goods that are not sold>.

shell
- **come out of one's shell** to become less shy. <Refers to a tortoise or crab, etc>.

ship
- **shipshape and Bristol fashion** neat, in good order. <Originally applied to ships. Bristol was formerly the largest port in Britain>.
- **ships that pass in the night** people who meet by chance and only on one occasion. <Refers to a quotation from 'Tales of a Wayside Inn' poem by Henry Wadsworth Longfellow>.
- **spoil the ship for a ha'porth of tar** to spoil something of value by not buying or doing something which would improve it but not cost very much. <Ship is dialect here for sheep—tar used to be used to prevent infections in sheep or to treat wounds>.
- **when (someone's) ship comes in** when (someone) becomes rich or successful. <Refers to merchants wait­ing for their ships to return with goods to sell>.

shoe
- **in (someone's) shoes** in (someone else's) place.
- **on a shoestring** using very little money.

shoot
- **shoot (something) down in flames** to destroy. <Refers literally to destroying aircraft by shooting at them>.

shop
- **talk shop** to talk about one's work.

short
- **by a short head** by a very small amount. <Refers to horse-racing>.
- **caught** *or* **taken short** having a sudden, urgent need to go to the toilet.
- **give (someone** *or* **something) short shrift** to spend very little time or thought on (someone or something). <Short shrift was the short time given to a criminal for confession before execution>.
- **make short work of (something)** to deal with or get rid of (something) very quickly.
- **sell (someone** *or* **something) short** not to do justice to, to belittle (someone or something). <Literally to give a customer less than the correct amount of some­thing>.
- **short and sweet** short and to the point.

shot
- **a long shot** a guess or attempt unlikely to be accurate or successful, but worth trying.
- **a shot across the bows** something given as a warning. <From naval warfare>.
- **a shot in the arm** something that helps to revive (something). <Literally, an injection in the arm>.
- **big shot** an important person.
- **call the shots** to be in charge of events or a situation.
- **like a shot** very quickly or willingly.
- **shotgun wedding** a forced wedding, usually because the bride is pregnant. <From the idea that the groom was forced into the wedding by shotgun>.

shoulder
- **a shoulder to cry on** a sympathetic listener.
- **put one's shoulder to the wheel** to begin to work hard. <Refers to putting one's shoulder to the wheel of a cart, etc, to push it out of muddy ground, etc>.
- **rub shoulders with (someone)** to associate closely with (someone).
- **shoulder to shoulder** side by side.

shout
- **shout (something) from the rooftops** *see* **rooftop**.

show
- **get the show on the road** to get something started or put into operation. <Used originally of a theatre com­pany going on tour>.
- **steal the show** to attract the most attention at an event. <Refers to someone getting most of the applause at a theatrical performance>.

sick
- **sick as a parrot** very disappointed.

side
- **let the side down** to hinder one's colleagues by not performing, etc, as well as they have.
- **on the side** in a way other than by means of one's ordinary occupation.
- **take sides** to support a particular person, group, etc, against another.

sieve
- **have a memory like a sieve** to be extremely forgetful.

sign
- **sign on the dotted line** to make a firm commitment to do something, often one that is legally binding. <Refers to the signing of a formal agreement or contract>.

sight
- **out of sight, out of mind** one ceases to think about someone who has gone away or about something which is no longer in front of one.

silence
- **silence is golden** it is better to say nothing in a particular situation.

silent
- **the silent majority** the people who make up most of the population but who rarely make their views known although these are thought to be moderate and reasonable.

silk
- **you can't make a silk purse out of a sow's ear** one cannot make something good or special out of poor materials.

silver
- **born with a silver spoon in one's mouth** to be born into an aristocratic or wealthy family. <Perhaps from the custom of giving a christening present of a silver teaspoon>.

sin
- **ugly as sin** extremely ugly.

sing
- **sing from the same hymn** *or* **song sheet** to be in agreement about something, often to show this agreement publicly.

six
- **a sixth sense** intuition, an ability to feel or realize something not perceived by the five senses.
- **at sixes and sevens** in a state of confusion and chaos.
- **knock (someone) for six** to take (someone) completely by surprise. <Refers to cricket—literally to score six runs off a bowl>.
- **six of one and half a dozen of another** so similar as to make no difference. <Half a dozen is six>.

sixty
- **the sixty-four (thousand) dollar question** the most important and/or difficult question. <From an American

quiz game in which the contestant won one dollar for the first question, two for the second, four for the third, up to the last when he or she won sixty-four dollars or lost it all>.

size
- **cut (someone) down to size** to humble (someone), to reduce (someone's) sense of his or her own importance.

skeleton
- **have a skeleton in the cupboard** to have a closely kept secret about some cause of shame.

skin
- **by the skin of one's teeth** only just, very narrowly.
- **no skin off my, etc, nose** no difference to me, etc, of no concern to me, etc.
- **save one's skin** to save one's life or one's career.
- **skin and bone** extremely thin.

sky
- **praise (someone** *or* **something) to the skies** to praise (someone) extremely highly.
- **the sky's the limit** there is no upper limit.

slap
- **a slap in the face** a rebuff.
- **a slap on the wrist** a reprimand.

sleeve
- **have** *or* **keep (something) up one's sleeve** to keep (a plan, etc) in reserve or secret for possible use at a later time. <Refers to cheating at cards by having a card up one's sleeve>.

slip
- **a slip of the tongue** a word or phrase said in mistake for another.
- **give (someone) the slip** to succeed in escaping from or evading (someone).
- **let (something) slip** to say or reveal (something) accidentally.
- **there's many a slip 'twixt cup and lip** something can easily go wrong with a project, etc, before it is completed.

small
- **it's a small world** an expression used when one meets someone one knows somewhere unexpected.
- **small talk** light conversation about trivial matters.
- **the small print** the parts of a document where important information is given without being easily noticed.

smash
- **a smash-and-grab** a robbery in which a shop window is smashed and goods grabbed from behind it.
- **a smash hit** a great success. <Originally referred to a very successful popular song>.

smear
- **smear campaign** an attempt to blacken or damage someone's reputation by making accusations or spreading rumours about him or her.

smoke
- **go up in smoke** to end in nothing.
- **there's no smoke without fire** there is always some kind of basis to a rumour, however untrue it appears to be.

snail
- **at a snail's pace** extremely slowly.

snake
- **a snake in the grass** a treacherous person. <From Virgil's *Aeneid*>.

sneeze
- **not to be sneezed at** not to be ignored or disregarded.

sock
- **pull one's socks up** to make an effort to improve.
- **put a sock in it** to be quiet.

soft
- **have a soft spot for (someone)** to have a weakness, affection or exceptional liking for (someone).
- **a soft touch** *or* **mark** someone who is easily taken advantage of, deceived etc.

song
- **for a song** for very little money.
- **make a song and dance about (something)** to cause an unnecessary fuss about (something).

soon
- **speak too soon** to say something that takes for granted something not yet accomplished.

sore
- **a sore point** a subject which annoys or offends someone.
- **stick out like a sore thumb** to be very noticeable.

sort
- **it takes all sorts (to make a world)** one should be tolerant of everyone whatever they are like.
- **out of sorts** not feeling quite well, rather bad-tempered.

soul
- **the soul of (something)** a perfect example of (something).

soup
- **in the soup** in serious trouble.

spade
- **call a spade a spade** to speak bluntly and forthrightly.
- **do the spadework** to do the hard preparatory work at the beginning of a project. <Digging is the first stage of building houses, etc>.
- **in spades** used to emphasize the large amount of something.

spanner
- **throw a spanner in the works** to hinder or spoil (a project, plan, etc).

spar
- **sparring partner** someone with whom one often enjoys a lively argument. <Literally refers to someone with whom a boxer practises>.

spare
- **go spare** to become very angry or distressed.

speak
- **be on speaking terms** to be friendly towards someone and communicate with him or her.
- **speak for itself** to need no explanation.

spick
- **spick and span** clean and tidy.

spirit
- **the spirit is willing (but the flesh is weak)** one is not always physically able to do the things that one wishes do. <A biblical quotation, Matthew 26:40–41>.

spit
- **be the spitting image** *or* **the spit and image** *or* **the dead spit of (someone** *or* **something)** to be extremely like (someone or something).

spleen
- **vent one's spleen** to express one's anger and frustration. <The spleen was thought to be the source of spite and melancholy>.

split
- **a split second** a fraction of a second.

spoil
- **be spoiling for (something)** to be eager for (a fight, etc).

spoke
- **put a spoke in (someone's) wheel** to hinder (someone's) activity. <Spoke is from Dutch spoak, a bar formerly jammed under a cartwheel to act as a brake when going downhill>.

sponge
- **throw up the sponge** to give up a contest, struggle, argument, etc. <Refers originally to a method of conceding defeat in boxing>.

spot
- **hit the spot** used to indicate that something is just what is required or is completely satisfactory.
- **in a spot** in trouble, in difficulties.
- **knock spots off (someone)** to beat or surpass (someone) thoroughly.
- **put (someone) on the spot** to place (someone) in a difficult or awkward situation.
- **rooted to the spot** unable to move from fear, horror, etc.

sprat
- **a sprat to catch a mackerel** something minor or trivial given or conceded in order to obtain some major gain or advantage.

square
- **back to square one** back at the beginning. <Refers to an instruction in board games>.

squeak
- **a narrow squeak** a narrow escape.

stab
- **have a stab at (something)** to have a try at (something).
- **stab (someone) in the back** to behave treacherously towards (someone), to betray (someone).

stable
- **lock the stable door after the horse has bolted** to take precautions against something happening after it has already happened.

stage
- **a stage whisper** a loud whisper that is intended to be heard by people other than the person to whom it is directed. <From the fact that whispers on stage have to be audible to the audience>.
- **stage fright** the nervousness, sometimes leading to him or her forgetting words, felt by an actor when in front of an audience; often extended to that felt by anyone making a public appearance.

stamp
- **(someone's) stamping ground** a place where (someone) goes regularly. <Refers literally to animals>.

stand
- **know where one stands** to know the exact nature of one's position or situation.
- **make a stand against (something)** to oppose or resist (something one believes to be wrong, etc).
- **stand corrected** to accept that one has been wrong.
- **stand on ceremony** to be very formal.
- **stand up and be counted** to declare one's opinions publicly.

start
- **a false start** an unsuccessful beginning, resulting in one in having to start again. <From a start in a race which has to be repeated, e.g. because a runner has left the starting line before the signal has been given>.
- **be under starter's orders** to be ready to start doing something.
- **for starters** to begin with. <Starter refers literally to the first course of a meal>.

status
- **status quo** the situation as it is, or was, before a change. <Latin, literally 'the state in which'>.
- **status symbol** a possession which supposedly demonstrates high social position.

stay
- **stay the course** to continue to the end or completion of (something).

steady
- **go steady** to go out together regularly, to have a romantic attachment to each other.

steam
- **get all steamed up** to get angry or agitated.
- **get up steam** to gather energy and impetus to do (something). <Literally used of increasing the pressure of steam in an engine before it goes into operation>.
- **let off steam** to give free expression to one's feelings or energies. <Literally to release steam from a steam engine to in order to reduce pressure>.
- **run out of steam** to become exhausted, to lose enthusiasm. <Refers literally to the steam engine>.
- **under one's own steam** entirely through one's own efforts.

step
- **take steps** to take action of some kind.

stick
- **a stick to beat (someone) with** something which can be used to criticize or damage (someone).
- **get hold of the wrong end of the stick** to misunderstand a situation or something said or done.
- **give (someone) stick** to scold or criticize (someone). <Refers literally to beating someone with a stick>.

sticky
- **be on a sticky wicket** to be in a difficult or awkward situation that is difficult to defend. <Refers to cricket when the state of the ground or the weather make it difficult for the batsman to hit the ball>.
- **come to a sticky end** to meet some misfortune or an unpleasant death.

still
- **still waters run deep** quiet people often think very deeply or have strong emotions.

stitch
- **a stitch in time saves nine** prompt action at the first sign of trouble saves a lot of time and effort later.
- **have (someone) in stitches** to make (someone) laugh a great deal.
- **without a stitch on** completely naked.

stock
- **on the stocks** in preparation, in the process of being made or arranged. <Refers to the fact that a ship is supported on stocks, a wooden frame, while being built>.
- **take stock (of something)** to assess (a situation).

stomach
- **turn (someone's) stomach** to make (someone) feel sick, to disgust (someone).

stone
- **a stone's throw** a very short distance.
- **be set in stone** to be something that cannot be changed.
- **leave no stone unturned** to try every means possible.

986 Appendix 4 English Idioms

stool
- **fall between two stools** to try to gain two aims and fail with regard to both of them, usually because of indecision.

stop
- **pull out all the stops** to put as much effort and energy into something as possible. <Refers to pulling out the stops of an organ so that it plays at full volume>.
- **stop dead** to stop suddenly and abruptly.
- **stop short of (something** or **doing something)** not to go as far as (something or doing something).

store
- **in cold storage** in reserve.
- **set great store by (something)** to consider (something) to be of great importance or value.

storm
- **a storm in a teacup** a great fuss made over a trivial matter. <Refers to the title of a farce written by William Bernard in 1854>.
- **take (someone** or **something) by storm** to make a very great and immediate impression (on someone or something). <Literally to capture a fort, etc, by a sudden violent military attack>.
- **weather the storm** to survive a difficult or troublesome situation or period of time. <Refers originally to ships>.

story
- **the same old story** a situation, etc, that occurs frequently.

straight
- **go straight** to start leading an honest life.
- **straight as a die** completely honest and fair.
- **straight talking** frank and honest statement or conversation.
- **the straight and narrow (path)** a good, virtuous way of life. <A variation on a biblical reference, 'Straight is the gate and narrow is the way which leadeth unto life', Matthew 7:4>.

stranger
- **be a stranger to (something)** to have no experience of (something).

straw
- **a straw in the wind** a small or minor incident, etc, that indicates what may happen in the future.
- **clutch at straws** to hope that something may happen to get one out of a difficulty or danger when this is extremely unlikely. <From the saying, 'A drowning man will clutch at a straw'>.
- **draw the short straw** to be the one in a group who has to perform an unpleasant or undesirable task. <Pulling out a straw from a collection of different lengths is a kind of lottery to decide who is to do something>.

the last straw or the straw that breaks the camel's back
- **the last straw** or **the straw that breaks the camel's back** an event, etc, which, added to everything that has already happened, makes a situation impossible. <From the saying that it is the last straw added to its burden that breaks the camel's back>.

stream
- **come on stream** to begin to be used or to operate.

street
- **be right up one's street** to be exactly what one likes or what is suitable for one.

strength
- **go from strength to strength** to progress successfully from one achievement to another.
- **on the strength of (something)** relying on (something).

stretch
- **at full stretch** using all one's energy, abilities, powers, etc, as much as possible.
- **stretch a point** to go further than the rules or regulations allow in giving permission, etc, for something.

stride
- **get into one's stride** to become accustomed to doing something and so do it well and effectively. <A reference to running>.
- **make great strides** to make very good progress.
- **take (something) in one's stride** to cope with (something) without worrying about it. <Refers to a horse jumping an obstacle without altering its stride>.

string
- **have (someone) on a string** to have (someone) in one's control. <Refers to someone manipulating a puppet>.
- **how long is a piece of string?** used to emphasize how difficult or impossible it is to give a definite answer to a question.
- **pull strings** to use influence to gain an advantage or benefit of some kind. <As above>.
- **with no strings attached** without any conditions or provisos.

stroke
- **put (someone) off his** or **her stroke** to hinder or prevent (someone) from proceeding smoothly with an activity. <Refers to upsetting the rhythm of someone's rowing>.

strong
- **be (someone's) strong suit** be something at which (someone) is very good. <Refers to card-playing>.

stuff
- **a stuffed shirt** a pompous, over-formal person.
- **knock the stuffing out of (someone) 1** to beat (someone) severely. **2** to discourage (someone) completely, to deprive (someone) of vitality. <Refers to stuffed animals>.

- **strut one's stuff** to do something which you know you do well, usually in a proud and confident way.

stumbling
- **a stumbling block** something that hinders or prevents progress. <A biblical reference to Romans 14:13>.

stump
- **stir one's stumps** to hurry up. <Stumps here means legs>.

style
- **cramp (someone's) style** to hinder (someone) from acting in the way that he or she would like or is accustomed to.

sugar
- **sugar daddy** an elderly man who has a young girlfriend or mistress to whom he gives expensive presents.
- **sugar the pill** to make something unpleasant more pleasant.

suit
- **men in (grey) suits** used to describe the powerful men who are in control of an organization, government, etc.
- **one's birthday suit** nakedness.

Sunday
- **(someone's) Sunday best** (someone's) smartest, formal clothes, of the kind worn to church on Sundays.

sure
- **sure as eggs is eggs** used to emphasize the certainty of something.

surface
- **scratch the surface of (something)** to deal with only a very small part of (something).

swallow
- **one swallow does not make a summer** a single success, etc, does not mean that a generally successful, etc, time is about to come. <Refers to the fact that swallows begin to come to Britain at the start of summer>.

swan
- **(someone's) swan song** the last work or performance by a musician, poet, playwright, actor, etc, before his or her death or retirement; by extension also applied to anyone who does anything for the last time. <Refers to an ancient legend that the swan sings as it is dying although it is otherwise silent>.

sweat
- **the sweat of one's brow** one's hard work.

sweet
- **be all sweetness and light** to seem to be pleasant and good-tempered.
- **have a sweet tooth** to like sweets, cakes and deserts.
- **sweet nothings** affectionate things said to someone with whom one is in love, endearments.

swim
- **be in the swim** be actively involved in social or business activities.

swing
- **get into the swing of things** to become accustomed to (something) and begin to understand and enjoy it. <Refers to the swing of a pendulum>.
- **go with a swing** to be very successful.
- **in full swing** at the most lively or busy part of something.
- **not enough room to swing a cat** *see* **cat**.
- **what you lose on the swings you gain on the roundabouts** disadvantages in one area of life are usually cancelled out by advantages in another.

swoop
- **at** *or* **in one fell swoop** in one single action or attempt, at the same time. <Refers to a quotation from Shakespeare's *Macbeth*, Act 4, scene III, the reference being to a hawk swooping on poultry>.

sword
- **a double-edged** *or* **two-edged sword** used to indicate that something has a bad and a good side.
- **cross swords with (someone)** to enter into a dispute with (someone).
- **the sword of Damocles** a threat of something bad that is likely to happen at any time. <Refers to a legend in which Damocles was forced by Dionysius of Syria to sit through a banquet with a sword hanging by a single hair over his head>.

T
- **to a T** exactly, very well. <Perhaps T stands for tittle, a small dot or point>.

tab
- **keep tabs on (someone** *or* **something)** to keep a check on (someone or something).
- **pick up the tab for (something)** to pay for (something). <Tab is an American term for bill>.

table
- **turn the tables on (someone)** to change a situation so that one gains the advantage (over someone) after having been at a disadvantage. <From the medieval game of tables, of which backgammon is a form, in which turning the board round would exactly reverse the position of the players>.

tail
- **chase one's tail** to spend a great deal of time and effort trying to do something but achieving very little.
- **have one's tail up** to be confident of success.
- **turn tail** to turn round and leave a difficult or dangerous situation.
- **with one's tail between one's legs** in an ashamed, miserable or defeated state. <From the behaviour of an unhappy dog>.

take
- **take after (someone)** to resemble.
- **take it out on (someone)** to treat (someone) in an angry or nasty way because one is disappointed, angry, etc, about something.

tale
- **live to tell the tale** to survive a dangerous or threatening situation, often used humorously.
- **tell tales** to report someone's wrong-doing.
- **thereby hangs a tale** there is a story associated with that. <A pun on tail, used by Shakespeare>.

talk
- **talk down to (someone)** to speak to (someone) in a condescending way as if he or she were inferior.
- **talk nineteen to the dozen** to talk a great deal and usually very rapidly.
- **the talk of the town** someone or something that is the subject of general conversation or gossip.

tall
- **a tall order** a difficult task.
- **a tall story** a story which is extremely unlikely.

tangent
- **go** *or* **fly off at a tangent** suddenly to leave the subject being discussed or the task being undertaken and move to a completely different subject or task.

tango
- **it takes two to tango** used to indicate a particular situation has to involve two people and that, therefore, both bear some responsibility.

tape
- **have** *or* **get (someone** *or* **something) taped** to have a full knowledge or understanding of (someone or something). <As if measured with a tape>.

tar
- **be tarred with the same brush** to have the same faults.

taste
- **leave a nasty taste in the mouth** to leave someone with unpleasant memories or associations.

tea
- **not for all the tea in China** not for anything at all, certainly not. <For a long time, China was the source of the world's tea>.

tear
- **tear a strip off (someone)** to scold (someone) severely.

teeth
- **by the skin of one's teeth** *see* **skin**.
- **cut one's teeth on (something)** to practise on or get early experience from (something). <Refers to children being given something to chew on to help their teeth come through>.

take
- **draw the teeth of (someone** *or* **something)** to make (someone or something) no longer dangerous. <Refers to pulling out an animal's teeth.>
- **get one's teeth into (something)** to tackle (something) vigorously.
- **like pulling teeth** used to indicate how difficult something is to do.
- **kick (someone) in the teeth** to refuse to help or support (someone) when he or she is in need of it.
- **set one's teeth on edge** to irritate one.
- **teething troubles** problems occurring at the very beginning of a new project, etc. <From the pain experienced by babies when teeth are just coming through>.

tell
- **I told you so** I warned you and I was right to do so.

tender
- **leave (someone** *or* **something) to (someone's) tender mercies** to leave (someone or something) in the care of (someone nasty, inefficient, etc).

tenterhooks
- **be on tenterhooks** be very anxious or agitated waiting for something to happen. <Tenterhooks were hooks for stretching newly woven cloth>.

territory
- **it goes with the territory** used to indicate that something, usually some kind of problem or difficulty, usually occurs in connection with a particular, job, activity or situation and should be expected.

test
- **stand the test of time** to survive or still be in use or popular after a considerable period of time.

that
- **that's that** there is no more to be said or done.

thick
- **give (someone) a thick ear** to slap (someone) across the ear, to box (someone's) ears.
- **thick and fast** in great quantities and at a fast rate.
- **thick as thieves** extremely friendly.
- **thick as two short planks** extremely stupid.
- **through thick and thin** whatever difficulties arise.

thief
- **set a thief to catch a thief** the best way to catch or outwit a dishonest or deceitful person is to use the help of another who is dishonest as he or she knows the technique.

thin
- **be thin on top** to be balding.
- **spread oneself too thin** to try to do several different things at once, often with the result that none of them are done very well or properly.
- **thin as a rake** extremely thin.

thing
- **do one's (own) thing** to do what one likes to do or what one is good at doing.
- **have a thing about (someone** *or* **something) 1** to be very fond of or be particularly attracted to (someone or something). **2** to be scared of, to have a phobia about (someone or something).
- **one of those things** something that must be accepted.
- **see things** to see someone or something that is not there.
- **the thing is** the most important point or question is.

think
- **have another think coming** to be quite mistaken.

thread
- **hang by a thread** to be in a very precarious or uncertain state. <Probably a reference to the sword of Damocles>.
- **lose the thread** to cease to follow the course or development of an argument, conversation, etc.

throat
- **at each other's throats** quarrelling fiercely.
- **jump down (someone's) throat** to attack (someone) verbally or in an angry or violent manner.
- **ram (something) down (someone's) throat** to try forcefully to make (someone) accept ideas, opinions, etc.
- **stick in one's throat** *or* **gullet** to be difficult for one to accept or tolerate.

throw
- **throw up** to vomit.

thumb
- **thumb a lift** to ask for (and get) a lift in someone's vehicle by signalling with one's thumb.
- **thumb one's nose at (someone** *or* **something)** to express defiance or contempt at (someone or something), originally by making the rude gesture of putting one's thumb to one's nose.
- **thumbs down** rejection or disapproval. <From the method employed by the crowds in ancient Rome to indicate whether they thought the defeated gladiator should live or die after a fight between two gladiators. If the crowds turned their thumbs down the gladiator died. If they turned them up the gladiator lived.>
- **thumbs up** acceptance or approval. <See **thumbs down** above>.
- **twiddle one's thumbs** to do nothing, to be idle. <Literally to rotate one's thumbs round each other, indicating a state of boredom>.
- **under (someone's) thumb** under one's control or domination.

thunder
- **steal (someone's) thunder** to spoil (someone's) attempt at impressing people by doing what he or she intended to do before him or her. <John Dennis, a 17th/18th century playwright, invented a machine for simulating thunder in plays. When someone else used a similar device in a rival play Dennis said that he had stolen his thunder>.

ticket
- **just the ticket** exactly what is required.
- **meal ticket** someone who can be relied upon to support one, providing food and so on.

tickle
- **be tickled pink** to be delighted.

tide
- **swim against the tide** to do, say or believe things which are the opposite of what the majority of people are doing, saying or believing.
- **the tide is turning** used to indicate that a changing is occurring in people's attitudes, tastes, beliefs, etc.

tie
- **be tied up** to be busy or engaged.

tight
- **in a tight corner** *or* **spot** in a difficult or dangerous situation.
- **run a tight ship** to run an efficient, well-organized firm etc.
- **sit tight** to be unwilling to move or take action.

tightrope
- **walk a tightrope** to be in a very difficult situation, often one which involves opposing groups, which requires one to act with great caution and delicacy.

tile
- **a night on the tiles** a celebratory evening spent in a wild and unrestrained manner. <Refers to roof tiles and to cats sitting on them at night>.

tilt
- **at full tilt** at maximum speed. <Refers to knights tilting or jousting>.

time
- **ahead of one's time** with ideas in advance of one's contemporaries, often not understood.
- **all in good time** soon, when it is the right time.
- **behind the times** not up-to-date, old-fashioned.
- **do time** to be in prison.
- **have no time for (someone** *or* **something)** to have a very low opinion of someone or something and to wish not to associate with him, her or it.
- **have the time of one's life** to have a very enjoyable time.
- **have time on one's hands** to have more free time than one can usefully fill with work, etc.
- **in (someone's) own good time** when it is convenient for (someone), at whatever time or speed he or she chooses.
- **keep time 1** of a clock to show the time accurately. **2** to perform an action in the same rhythm as someone else.
- **kill time** to find something to do to pass some idle time, especially time spent waiting for someone or something.
- **mark time** to remain in one's present position without progressing or taking any action. <Refers to soldiers moving their feet as if marching but not actually moving forwards>.

- **not before time** not too soon, rather late.
- **no time at all** a very short time.
- **pass the time of day with (someone)** to greet (someone) and have a brief conversation, e.g. about the weather.
- **play for time** to act so as to delay an action, event, etc, until the time that conditions are better for oneself. <In games such as cricket it means to play in such a way as to avoid defeat by playing defensively until the close of the game>.
- **take time by the forelock** to act quickly and without delay. <Refers to the fact that time was often represented by an old man with no hair except for a forelock, a length of hair over his forehead>.
- **time and tide wait for no man** time moves on without regard for human beings and therefore opportunities should be grasped as they arise as they may not be there for very long.
- **time and time again** repeatedly.
- **time flies** time passes very quickly.

tip
- **be on the tip of one's tongue** to be about to be said.

tit
- **tit for tat** repayment of injury or harm for injury or harm. <Perhaps a variation on tip for tap, blow for blow>.

to
- **toing and froing** repeatedly going backwards and forwards.

toast
- **warm as toast** very warm and cosy.

tod
- **on one's tod** alone. <From Cockney rhyming slang 'on one's Tod Sloan', meaning 'on one's own', Tod Sloan having been a famous American jockey>.

toe
- **be on one's toes** to be alert and prepared for action.
- **make one's toes curl** to make one feel very uncomfortable or embarrassed.
- **put a toe in the water** to start doing something very slowly or gradually to see if one likes it, whether it will be successful, whether people will approve, etc.
- **tread on (someone's) toes** to offend (someone) by doing or saying (something) that is against his or her beliefs or opinions.

Tom
- **a peeping Tom** a man who gets sexual enjoyment from secretly watching women undress or women who are naked, especially by looking through the windows of their houses. <From the story of Lady Godiva who is said to have ridden naked through the streets of Coventry as part of a bargain made with her husband, Leofric, Earl of Mercia, to persuade him to lift a tax he had placed on his tenants. Everyone was to stay indoors so as not to see her

but a character, later called Peeping Tom, looked out to see her and was struck blind>.
- **every** or **any Tom, Dick and Harry** absolutely everyone or anyone, every ordinary person. <From the fact that all three are common English Christian names>.

tongue
- **have one's tongue in one's cheek** to say something that one does not mean seriously or literally, sometimes to say the opposite of what one means for a joke.
- **hold one's tongue** to remain silent or to stop talking.
- **set tongues wagging** to start people gossiping.

tooth
- **be** or **get long in the tooth** to be or become old.
- **fight tooth and nail** to fight, struggle or argue fiercely and determinedly.

top[1]
- **blow one's top** to lose one's temper.
- **get on top of one** used to indicate that someone is not coping with all the things that require to be done.
- **off the top of one's head** without much thought, without research or preparation.
- **over the top** too much, to too great an extent.
- **the top of the ladder** or **tree** the highest point in a profession, etc.

top[2]
- **sleep like a top** to sleep very soundly. <A pun on the fact that sleep used of a top means 'to spin steadily without wobbling'>.

toss
- **argue the toss** to dispute a decision. <Refers to arguing about the result of tossing a coin>.

touch
- **it's touch and go** it's very uncertain or precarious. <Perhaps refers to a ship that touches rocks or the ground but goes on past the danger without being damaged>.
- **lose one's touch** to lose one's usual skill or knack. <Probably refers to someone's touch on piano keys>.
- **the common touch** the ability to understand and get on with ordinary people.
- **the finishing touches** the final details which complete something.

tow
- **have (someone) in tow** to have someone following closely behind one.

towel
- **throw in the towel** to give up, to admit defeat. <From a method of conceding defeat in boxing>.

tower
- **a tower of strength** someone who is very helpful and supportive.

town
- **go to town** to act or behave without restraint, with great enthusiasm or with great expense.

track

- **cover one's tracks** to hide one's activities or movements.
- **from the wrong side of the tracks** used of someone who comes from a poor or less desirable area of town. <American in origin and refers to the fact that, when railways were built, they often divided an area into two sharply divided districts>.
- **keep** *or* **lose track of (someone** *or* **something)** to keep or fail to keep oneself informed about the whereabouts or progress of (someone or something).
- **make tracks (for)** to leave or set out (for).
- **on the right** *or* **wrong track** on the right or wrong course to get the correct answer or desired result.

trail

- **blaze a trail** to show or lead the way in some new activity or area of knowledge. <Refers to explorers going along a path and marking the way for those coming after them by stripping sections of bark from trees (blazing)>.

trial

- **trials and tribulations** difficulties and hardships.

trick

- **do the trick** to have the desired effect, to achieve the desired result.
- **never to miss a trick** never to fail to take advantage of a favourable situation or opportunity to bring advantage to oneself.
- **up to one's (old) tricks** acting in one's usual (wrong, dishonest or deceitful) way.

trooper

- **swear like a trooper** to swear very frequently or very strongly. <A trooper was an ordinary cavalry soldier>.

trot

- **on the trot** **1** one after the other. **2** very active and busy.

trousers

- **wear the trousers** to make all the important decisions in a household.

trump

- **play one's trump card** to use something very advantageous to oneself that one has had in reserve for use when really necessary. <In card games a trump is a card of whichever suit has been declared to be higher-ranking than the others>.
- **turn up trumps** to do the right or required thing in a difficult situation, especially unexpectedly. <*See* above, refers to drawing a card from the trump suit>.

tune

- **call the tune** to be the person in control who gives the orders. <Refers to the saying 'He who pays the piper calls the tune'>.
- **in tune with (something)** in agreement with (something), compatible with (something).

- **to the tune of (something)** to the stated sum of money, usually high or higher than is expected or is reasonable.

turkey

- **cold turkey** a form of treatment for drug or alcohol abuse involving sudden and complete withdrawal as opposed to gradual withdrawal.
- **talk turkey** to talk plainly and honestly.

turn

- **a turn-up for the books** something favourable which happens unexpectedly. <Referred originally to a horse that unexpectedly won a race, the book meaning the total number of bets on a race>.
- **do (someone) a good turn** to help (someone) in some way.
- **done to a turn** cooked exactly right, cooked to perfection.
- **give (someone) quite a turn** to give (someone) a sudden shock or surprise.
- **turn turtle** to turn upside down, to capsize. <A turtle is helpless and easy to kill if it is turned over on its back>.

twice

- **think twice** to give careful consideration.

two

- **in two ticks** in a very short time. <Refers to the ticking of a clock>.
- **put two and two together** to come to a (correct) conclusion from what one sees and hears.
- **two of a kind** two people of a very similar type or character.
- **two's company, (three's a crowd)** a third person who is with a couple is often unwanted as they want to be alone.

umbrage

- **take umbrage** to show that one is offended. <Originally meant to feel overshadowed, from Latin *umbra*, 'shade'>.

uncle

- **Uncle Sam** the United States of America. <Probably from the initials US which were stamped on government supplies, possibly because someone called Uncle Sam was employed in handling such supplies>.

under

- **under the influence** under the influence of alcohol, drunk.

up

- **be on the up-and-up** to be making successful progress.
- **be (well) up in** *or* **on (something)** to have an extensive knowledge of (something).
- **be up and running** to have started and be operating well.

- **be up to (someone)** it is (someone's) responsibility or duty.
- **be up to (something) 1** to be occupied with or in (something, often something dishonest, etc). **2** to be good enough, strong enough, etc, to do (something).
- **up and about** out of bed, after an illness.
- **up and doing** active and busy.
- **ups and downs** good fortune and bad fortune, successful periods and unsuccessful periods.
- **upstage (someone** *or* **something)** to take attention or interest away from (someone or something).

upshot
- **the upshot** the result or outcome. <Literally the last shot in an archery competition>.

upper
- **have** *or* **get the upper hand (of** *or* **over) (someone)** have or get an advantage or control (over someone).
- **on one's uppers** very poor. <Literally with no soles on one's shoes>.
- **upper-crust** of the upper class or aristocracy. <Refers literally to the upper part of the pastry of a pie above the filling>.

uptake
- **quick** *or* **slow on the uptake** quick or slow to understand.

Uriah
- **Uriah Heep** a sycophant, someone who always fawns over and toadies to others. <Refers to a character in Charles Dickens's novel *David Copperfield*>.

U-turn
- **do a U-turn** to change one's opinion, policy, etc, completely. <Refers originally to vehicle drivers making a turn in the shape of the letter U to reverse direction>.

vain
- **take (someone's) name in vain** to use (someone's) name disrespectfully, especially to swear using God's name. <A biblical reference to Exodus 20:7>.

variety
- **variety is the spice of life** the opportunity to do different things, experience different situations, etc, is what makes life interesting. <A quotation from a poem by William Cowper>.

veil
- **draw a veil over (something)** not to discuss (something), to keep (something) hidden or secret.

vengeance
- **with a vengeance** very strongly, much, etc.

vex
- **a vexed question** a difficult issue or problem that is much discussed without being resolved.

victory
- **landslide victory** a victory in an election by a very large number of votes.

view
- **a bird's-eye view of (something) 1** a view of (something) seen from high above. **2** a brief description, etc, of (something).

villain
- **the villain of the piece** the person responsible for an act of evil or wrongdoing. <Refers originally to the villain in a play>.

vine
- **a clinging vine** a possessive person, someone who likes always to be with someone else.
- **wither on the vine** to die to come to an end without being used, finished, etc. <Literally of grapes withering on the vine instead of being picked and eaten or made into wine>.

violet
- **a shrinking violet** a very timid, shy person.

voice
- **a voice crying in the wilderness** (someone) expressing an opinion or warning that no one takes any notice of. <A biblical reference to John the Baptist in Matthew 3:3>.
- **the still, small voice (of reason)** the expression of a calm, sensible point of view. <A biblical reference to I Kings 19:12>.

volume
- **speak volumes** to express a great deal of meaning without putting it into words.

vote
- **a vote of confidence** a vote taken to establish whether or not the government, a group of people, a person, etc, is still trusted and supported.
- **vote with one's feet** to leave.

wagon
- **circle the wagons** of a group of people, to work together to protect themselves against possible harm or danger. <In the American West pioneers used to form their wagons into a circle if they were under attack>.
- **on the wagon** not drinking alcohol. <Refers to a water wagon>.

wake
- **in the wake of (something)** immediately following, and often caused by (something). <Refers literally to the strip of water left by the passing of a ship>.

wall
- **be climbing the wall(s)** to feel frustrated, bored or impatient.
- **go to the wall** to suffer ruin. <Origin uncertain>.
- **off the wall** unconventional, strange.
- **up the wall** very annoyed, irritated, harassed, etc.

- **walls have ears** someone may be listening (to a secret conversation.

Walter
- **a Walter Mitty** someone who invents stories about himself to make his life seem more exciting. <Refers to a character in a James Thurber short story>.

war
- **have been in the wars** to have a slight injury.
- **on the warpath** very angry. <An American Indian expression>.

wart
- **warts and all** including all the faults, disadvantages. <Refers to the fact that Oliver Cromwell instructed his portrait painter, Sir Peter Lely, to paint him as he really was, including his warts, rather than try to make him look more handsome>.

wash
- **come out in the wash** to come to a satisfactory end. <Used literally of a stain on clothes, etc, that comes out when the article is washed>.
- **(something) won't wash** to be regarded as unacceptable or incredible.

water
- **blow (someone** *or* **something) out of the water** to destroy or defeat (someone or something) utterly.
- **hold water** to be accurate, to be able to be proved true. <From a vessel that is not broken>.
- **muddy the waters** to confuse a situation.
- **test the water/waters** to try to find out what the reaction is likely to be to a plan before one puts this into effect.
- **tread water** to take very little action. <Literally to keep oneself afloat in water by moving the legs (and arms)>.
- **water under the bridge** something that is past and cannot be changed and should be forgotten.

wave
- **make waves** to cause trouble.
- **on the same wavelength as (someone)** having the same opinions, attitudes, tastes, etc, as (someone).

way
- **be set in one's ways** to have a set routine in your life and to dislike having this disrupted.
- **get into the way of (something** *or* **doing something)** to become accustomed to (something or doing something).
- **get** *or* **have one's own way** to do or get what one wants.
- **go back a long way** used to indicate that people have known each other for a long time.
- **go out of one's way** to do more than is really necessary, to make a special effort.
- **go the way of all flesh** to die or come to an end.
- **have a way with (someone** *or* **something)** to have a special knack with (someone or something), to be good at handling (someone or something).

- **have everything one's own way** to get everything done according to one's wishes.
- **have it both ways** to have the advantages of two sets of situations, each of which usually excludes the possibility of the other.
- **lead the way** to go first, to be in front.
- **lose one's way** to cease to know where one is or which direction one is going in.
- **make way for (someone** *or* **something)** to stand aside to leave room for (someone or something).
- **mend one's ways** to improve one's behaviour.
- **not to know which way to turn** to be in trouble and to be too confused to be able to decide what to do for the best.
- **pay one's way** to pay one's expenses or one's share of expenses.
- **see one's way to (doing something)** to be able and willing to (do something).
- **there are no two ways about it** no other opinion, attitude, etc, is possible.
- **under way** in progress.
- **ways and means** methods, especially unofficial ones.
- **where's there's a will there's a way** a saying used to indicate that if one is determined to do something, then one will find a way to succeed in doing so.

wayside
- **fall by the wayside** to fail to continue to the end of something; to give up in the course of doing something. <A biblical reference to the parable of the sower in Luke 8:5>.

wear
- **be the worse for wear 1** to be in a bad state, looking tired, ill, untidy, etc. **2** to be drunk.

weather
- **under the weather** unwell.

web
- **a tangled web** used to describe a very complicate, confused situation.

wedge
- **drive a wedge between** to cause disagreement or ill will between two people or two groups, especially when they were formerly friendly.
- **the thin end of the wedge** a minor event or action which could be the first stage of something major and serious or harmful.

weight
- **a weight off one's mind** used to indicate that one no longer has to worry about something which has been worrying one for some time.
- **carry weight** to have influence, to be considered important.
- **pull one's weight** to do one's fair share of work, etc.
- **punch above one's weight** to try to do something which is thought to be beyond one's abilities.
- **take the weight off one's feet** to sit down.

- **throw one's weight about** *or* **around** to use one's power and influence in a bullying way.
- **throw one's weight behind (someone** *or* **something)** to support (someone or something).

west
- **go west** to be ruined, to be finished. <Airmen's slang from World War I>.

wet
- **wet behind the ears** to be young, inexperienced and naive.
- **have a whale of a time** to have an extremely enjoyable time.

what
- **give (someone) what for** to scold or punish (someone).
- **know what's what** to know the details of a situation, to know what is going on.
- **what have you** and similar things.

wheel
- **a fifth wheel** a person or thing that is not needed or is not wanted. <Refers to the fact that a vehicle needs only four wheels to keep running>.
- **reinvent the wheel** to do something which one considers new or innovative, but which is, in fact, very similar to something which has been done by someone else; to start a project from scratch without taking advantage of available information, research, etc.
- **set the wheels in motion** to start a process off.
- **wheeling and dealing** acting in an astute but sometimes dishonest or immoral way, especially in business.
- **wheels within wheels** used to indicate a very complicated situation with many different things involved, all influencing each other.

whip
- **have the whip hand** to have control or an advantage. <Refers to coach-driving>.
- **a whipping boy** someone who is blamed and punished for someone else's mistakes. <Refers literally to a boy who was punished for any misdeeds a royal prince made, since the tutor was not allowed to strike a member of the royal family>.

whisker
- **win by a whisker** to win by a very short amount.

whistle
- **wet one's whistle** to have a drink.
- **whistle for (something)** to ask for (something) with no hope of getting it. <Perhaps from an old sailors' superstition that when a ship is becalmed whistling can summon up a wind>.

white
- **a whited sepulchre** someone who pretends to be moral and virtuous but is in fact bad. <A biblical reference to Matthew 23:27>.
- **white lie** a not very serious lie.
- **whiter than white** extremely honest and moral.

wick
- **get on (someone's) wick** to annoy or irritate (someone) greatly.

wide
- **be wide open** used of a competition of some kind to indicate that it is very difficult to predict the winner as the competitors seem equally good.

wild
- **a wild goose chase** a search or hunt that cannot end in success.
- **sow one's wild oats** to enjoy oneself in a wild and sometimes promiscuous way when one is young.
- **spread like wildfire** to spread extremely rapidly. <Wildfire was probably a kind of fire started by lightning>.

will
- **with a will** enthusiastically and energetically.

wind
- **get one's second wind** to find renewed energy to go on doing something after a period of feeling tired and weak.
- **get wind of (something)** to receive information about (something) <Referring to the scent of an animal carried by the wind>.
- **in the wind** about to happen, being placed or prepared.
- **get the wind up** to become frightened or nervous.
- **raise the wind** to get enough money to do (something).
- **spit in the wind** to try to do something impossible and so waste time and effort.
- **take the wind out of (someone's) sails** to reduce (someone's) pride in his or her cleverness, abilities, etc. <Refers to the fact that a ship takes the wind out of another ship's sails if it passes close to it on the windward side>.
- **throw caution to the (four) winds** to begin to behave recklessly.
- **whistle in the wind** to make a statement or promise which is pointless since it is very unlikely to have any effect or produce any results.

windmill
- **tilt at windmills** to struggle against imaginary opposition. <Refers to an episode in Cervantes' novel *Don Quixote* in which the hero mistakes a row of windmills for giants and attacks them>.

window
- **go out the window** to disappear completely; to be ignore or forgotten about.
- **window-dressing** the presentation of something to show the most favourable parts and hide the rest. <Refers literally to the arranging of goods in a shop window to attract customers>.

wing
- **on a wing and a prayer** used to indicate that you hope to do something successfully even although you do not have the resources to do so.

- **spread one's wings 1** to leave home. **2** to try to put into practice one's own ideas, to make use of one's abilities. <Refers to young birds ready to try to fly and leave the nest for the first time>.
- **take (someone) under one's wing** to take (someone) under one's protection and guidance. <Refers to the practice of some birds of covering their young with their wings>.
- **try one's wings** to try to do something which one has never done before in order to see if one will be successful at it.
- **waiting in the wings** in a state of readiness to do something, especially to take over someone else's job. <Literally waiting in the wings of a theatre stage ready to go on>.
- **wing it** to do something without planning or preparation, to improvise.

wink
- **not sleep a wink** not to be able to sleep at all.
- **tip (someone) the wink** to give (someone) information secretly or privately.

wire
- **down to the wire** to the last possible minute
- **get** *or* **have one's wires crossed** to be involved in a misunderstanding. <Refers to telephone wires>.

wise
- **none the wiser** knowing no more than one did before.
- **put (someone) wise to (something)** to give (someone) information about (something), make (someone) aware of (something).

wish
- **wishful thinking** believing that, or hoping that, something unlikely is true or will happen just because one wishes that it would.
- **wish (someone) joy of (something)** to wish that something will be a pleasure or benefit to someone (although one doesn't think it will).

wit
- **at one's wits' end** worried and desperate.
- **keep one's wits about one** to be alert and watchful.
- **live by one's wits** to live by cunning schemes rather than by working.
- **pit one's wits against (someone)** to use one's intelligence to try to defeat (someone).
- **scare (someone) out of his** *or* **her wits** to frighten (someone) very much.

witch
- **witch-hunt** a search for and persecution of people who are thought to have done something wrong or hold opinions which are thought to be dangerous etc. <Refers historically to organized hunts for people thought to be witches>.

wolf
- **a wolf in sheep's clothing** someone evil and dangerous who seems to be gentle and harmless. <A biblical reference to Matthew 7:15>.

- **cry wolf** to give a false warning of danger, to call unnecessarily for help. <Refers to one of Aesop's fables in which a shepherd boy used to amuse himself by calling out that a wolf was coming to attack his sheep and did this so many times when it was not true that no one believed when it was true, and all his sheep were killed>.
- **keep the wolf from the door** to prevent poverty and hunger.

wood
- **not to be able to see the wood for the trees** not to be able to consider the general nature of a situation, etc, because one is concentrating too much on details.
- **out of the woods** out of danger or difficulties.
- **touch wood** to touch something made of wood supposedly to keep away bad luck. <Refers to a well-known superstition>.

wool
- **pull the wool over (someone's) eyes** to deceive (someone).
- **wool-gathering** day-dreaming. <Refers to someone wandering around hedges gathering wool left by sheep>.

word
- **eat one's words** to admit that one was wrong in what one said.
- **get a word in edgeways** *or* **edgewise** to have difficulty in breaking into a conversation.
- **hang on (someone's) words** to listen carefully and eagerly to everything that someone says.
- **have a word in (someone's) ear** to tell (someone) something in private.
- **have words** to argue or quarrel.
- **keep one's word** to do as one promised to do.
- **put in a good word for (someone)** to say something favourable about (someone), to recommend (someone).
- **put words into (someone's) mouth** to say that someone has said something when he/she did not; to suggest that someone is going to say something when he/she has no intention of doing so.
- **say the word** say what you want and your wishes will be carried out.
- **take (someone's) word for it** to believe what someone says without question and without proof.
- **take the words out of (someone's) mouth** to say what (someone) was just about to say.

work
- **all work and no play makes Jack a dull boy** people should take some leisure time and not work all the time.
- **give (someone) the works** to give (someone) the complete treatment. <Originally slang for to kill someone>.
- **have one's work cut out** to face a very difficult task. <Literally to have a lot of work ready for one>.
- **worked up** agitated, annoyed.

world

- **a man of the world** a sophisticated and worldly man.
- **come down in the world** to be less well off, less successful etc. than formerly.
- **come up in the world** to be better off, more successful, etc. than formerly.
- **do (someone) the world of good** to have a very good effect on (someone); to be of great benefit or advantage to (someone).
- **for all the world like (someone** or **something)** exactly like (someone or something).
- **not the end of the world** used to make someone realize that things are not as bad as they think they are.
- **not to have long for this world** to be about to die.
- **on top of the world** very cheerful and happy.
- **out of this world** remarkably good.
- **think the world of (someone)** to be extremely fond of (someone).
- **the world is (someone's) oyster** (someone) has a great many possible opportunities or chances. <Refers to a quotation from Shakespeare's *The Merry Wives of Windsor*, Act 2, scene II>.

worm

- **a can of worms** an extremely complicated and difficult situation. <Refers to the fact that worms wriggle around a lot>.
- **(even) the worm turns** even the most humble or meek person will protest if treated badly enough.

worth

- **for all one is worth** using maximum effort.

wound

- **lick one's wounds** to try to recover from a situation in which one has been badly defeated or humiliated.
- **reopen old wounds** to remind people of past unpleasant experiences which they would prefer to forget about.

wrap

- **keep (something) under wraps** to keep (something) secret or hidden.

- **take the wraps off (something)** to reveal, or give details about, something that has been secret up till now.
- **wrapped up in (someone** or **something)** absorbed in, giving all one's attention to (someone or something).
- **wrap (something) up** to finish (something) completely.

writ

- **writ large** used to indicate that something is in its most extreme form.

write

- **the writing on the wall** something which indicates that something unpleasant, such as failure, unhappiness, disaster, etc, will happen. <A biblical reference to Daniel 5:5–31, in which the coming destruction of the Babylonian empire is made known to Belshazzar at a feast through mysterious writing on a wall>.

wrong

- **get on the wrong side of (someone)** to cause (someone) to dislike or be hostile to one.
- **not to put a foot wrong** not to make a mistake of any kind.

yarn

- **spin a yarn** to tell a long story, especially an untrue one that is given as an excuse. <Telling a story is compared to spinning a long thread>.

year

- **the year dot** a long time ago, the beginning of time.

yesterday

- **not born yesterday** not easily fooled.

young

- **you're only young once** one should take advantage of the opportunities that arise when one is young and has the energy, freedom, etc, to enjoy or exploit them.

zero

- **zero hour** the time at which something is due to begin. <Originally a military term>.

Abbreviations

A Adult; alcohol; alto; America; American; ampere; angstrom; anode; answer; April *(math)* area; *(chem)* argon; Associate; atomic weight; IVR Austria.

Å Angstrom unit.

a acre; are (measure).

a. adjective; alto; ampere; *anno (Latin* year); anode; answer; *ante (Latin* before); *aqua (Latin* water); area.

A1 first class.

AA Alcoholics Anonymous; anti-aircraft; Automobile Association.

AAA Amateur Athletic Association; American Automobile Association.

AAC Amateur Athletic Club; *anno ante Christum (Latin* in the year before Christ).

AAM air-to-air missile.

A & A additions and amendments.

A & M Hymns Ancient and Modern.

A & N Army and Navy.

A & R Artist and Repertoire.

AAPO African Peoples' Organization.

aar against all risks; average annual rainfall.

AAU Amateur Athletic Union.

AB able-bodied seaman; *Artium Baccalaureus (Latin* Bachelor of Arts).

Ab *(chem)* alabamine.

ABA Amateur Boxing Association.

Abb. Abbess; Abbey; Abbot.

abbr., abbrev. abbreviated; abbreviation.

ABC Advance Booking Charter; American Broadcasting Company; Associated British Cinemas; Audit Bureau of Circulations; automatic binary computer.

abd abdicated abridged.

ab init. *ab initio (Latin* from the beginning).

abl. ablative.

ABM anti-ballistic missile.

ABMEWS anti-ballistic missile early warning system.

ABP arterial blood pressure.

Abp Archbishop.

abr. abridged; abridgement.

abs. absence; absent; absolute; abstract.

absol. absolute.

abstr. abstract.

abt about.

ABTA Association of British Travel Agents.

abv. above.

AC Air Command; Air Corps; Aircraftman; Alternating Current; analog computer; Annual Conference; *ante Christum (Latin* before Christ); Appeal Case; Appeal Court; Army Corps; Arts Council; Assistant Commissioner; Athletic Club.

A/C account; account current.

Ac *(chem)* actinium.

ac. acre.

a.c. *ante cibum (Latin* before meals).

acad. academic; academy.

ACAS Advisory, Conciliation and Arbitration Service.

ACC Army Catering Corps.

acc. acceleration; accent; accepted; accompanied; according; account; accusative.

accel. *(mus) accelerando (Italian* more quickly).

Accred Accredited.

acct account.

accy accountancy.

ACF Army Cadet Force.

ACG automatic control gear.

ACGB Arts Council of Great Britain.

ack. acknowledge(d).

ackt acknowledgment.

ACLS Automatic Carrier Landing System.

ACM Air Chief Marshal.

ACN *ante Christum natum (Latin* before the birth of Christ).

ACCP Association of Chief Officers of Police.

ACCRN *(comput)* automatic checkout and recording network.

ACP American College of Physicians.

acpt acceptance.

ACSIR Advisory Council for Scientific and Industrial Research.

Act. Acting.

act. active.

actg acting.

ACTH adrenocorticotrophic hormone, an anti-rheumatic drug.

ACV actual cash value; air cushion vehicle (hovercraft).

ACW Aircraftwoman; alternating continuous waves.

AD *(milit)* active duty; air defence; *anno Domini (Latin* in the year of our Lord).

ad. adverb; advertisement.

ADC Aide-de-Camp; *(comput)* analog to digital converter; automatic digital calculator.

add addendum; addition; additional; address.

ADF automatic direction finder.

ad fin. *ad finem (Latin* near the end).

ad inf. *ad infinitum (Latin* to infinity).

ad init. *ad initium (Latin* at the beginning).

ad int. *ad interim (Latin* in the meantime).

adj, adj. adjacent; adjective; adjoining; adjourned; adjudged; adjunct; adjustment; adjutant.

Adjt Adjutant.

Adjt-Gen. Adjutant-General.

ad lib. *ad libitum (Latin* at will).

ad loc. *ad locum (Latin* at the place).

adm. administration; administrative; admitted.

admin. administration.

ADN IVR People's Democratic Republic of Yemen.

ADP automatic data processing.

adv. advance; advent; adverb; adverbial; *adversus* (*Latin* against); advertisement; advisory; advocate.

ad val. *ad valorem* (*Latin* according to the value).

advt advertisement.

ADW Air Defence Warning.

AE Atomic Energy.

AEA Atomic Energy Authority.

AE & P Ambassador Extraordinary and Plenipotentiary.

AEF Amalgamated Union of Engineering and Foundry Workers.

AEI Associated Electrical Industries.

AELTC All England Lawn Tennis Club.

aer. aeronautics; aeroplane.

AERE Atomic Energy Research Establishment.

aeron. aeronautical; aeronautics.

AEU Amalgamated Engineering Union (now AUEW).

AEW airborne early warning.

AF Admiral of the Fleet; Air Force; Anglo-French; audio-frequency.

A/F as found.

AFA Amateur Football Association.

AFC Association Football Club; automatic frequency control.

affil. affiliated.

afft affidavit.

AFG IVR Afghanistan.

AFI American Film Institute.

AFM Air Force Medal.

AFN American Forces Network; Armed Forces Network.

Afr. Africa; African.

Afrik. Afrikaans.

AFS Auxiliary Fire Service.

afsd aforesaid.

AFV armoured fighting vehicle.

AG Adjutant General; Attorney General.

Ag (*chem*) silver.

AGC automatic gain control.

AGCA automatic ground controlled approach.

AGCL automatic ground controlled landing.

agcy agency.

AGM air-to-ground missile; Annual General Meeting.

AGR advanced gas-cooled reactor.

agr., agric. agricultural; agriculture.

agst against.

agt agent; agreement.

a.g.w. actual gross weight.

AH *anno Hegirae* (*Latin* in the year of the Hegira).

AI Amnesty International; artificial insemination.

a.i. *ad interim* (*Latin* in the meantime).

AID acute infectious disease; Army Intelligence Department; artificial insemination by donor.

AIH artificial insemination by husband.

AL IVR Albania; Anglo-Latin.

Al (*chem*) aluminium.

al. alcohol; alcoholic.

ALBM air-launched ballistic missile.

Ald. Alderman.

Alg. Algeria; Algerian.

alg, alg. algebra.

ALGOL (*comput*) algorithmic language.

alk. alkali.

alt. alteration; alternate; alternative; altitude; alto.

alter. alteration.

alum. aluminium.

AM Air Marshal; Air Ministry; Albert Medal; amplitude modulation; *anno mundi* (*Latin* in the year of the world); *ante meridiem* (*Latin* before noon); arithmetic mean; *Artium Magister* (*Latin* Master of Arts); Associate Member.

Am (*chem*) americium.

Am. America; American.

a.m. ante meridiem.

amal. amalgamated.

AMDG *ad majorem Dei gloriam* (*Latin* to the greater glory of God).

Amer. America; American.

AMM anti-missile missile.

amn. amunition.

amp. amperage; ampere; amplifier; amplitude.

AMS Ancient Monuments Society.

amt amount.

AMU atomic mass unit.

AN Anglo-Norman.

An (*chem*) actinon.

an. *anno* (*Latin* in the year); anonymous; *ante* (*Latin* before).

anag. anagram.

anal. analogous; analogy; analysis; analytic.

anat. anatomical; anatomist; anatomy.

ANC African National Congress.

anc. ancient; anciently.

AND IVR Andorra.

and. (*mus*) *andante* (*Italian* moderately slow).

Angl. Anglican; Anglicized.

anim. (*mus*) *animato* (*Italian* animated).

ann. annual; annuity.

anniv. anniversary.

annot. annotated; annotation; annotator.

anon. anonymous.

ANS Army Nursing Service.

ans. answer.

ant. antenna; antiquarian; antique; antonym.

anthol. anthology.

anthrop. anthropological; anthropology.

antiq. antiquarian; antiquity.

ANZAC Australian and New Zealand Army Corps.

a/o account of.

AOB any other business.

AOCB any other competent business.

AOC-in-C Air Officer Commander-in-Chief.

AP *ante prandium* (*Latin* before meals); Associated Press; atmospheric pressure.

Ap. Apostle; April.

ap. apothecary.

APC automatic phase control; automatic pitch control.

APEX Advance Purchase Excursion.

aph. aphorism.

apo. apogee.
Apoc. Apocalypse; Apocrypha.
app. apparatus; apparent; appendix; applied; appointed; apprentice; approved; approximate.
appro. approbation; approval.
approx. approximate; approximately.
apptd appointed.
Apr, Apr. April.
APT advanced passenger train.
apt. apartment.
APWU Amalgamated Postal Workers' Union.
aq. *aqua* (*Latin* water).
AR Autonomous Republic.
Ar (*chem*) argon.
Ar. Arabic; Aramaic.
ar. arrival; arrives.
a.r. *anno regni* (*Latin* in the year of the reign).
ARA Associate of the Royal Academy.
Arab Arabian; Arabic.
arb. arbiter; arbitration.
ARC Aeronautical Research Council; American Red Cross; automatic relay calculator.
Arch. Archbishop; Archdeacon; Archduke; Archipelago; Architecture.
arch. archaic; archaism; archery; archipelago; architect; architecture; archive.
archaeol. archaeology.
Archd. Archdeacon; Archduke.
archit. architecture.
ARCS Australian Red Cross Society.
ARD acute respiratory disease.
Arg. Argentina; Argyll (former county).
arg. *argentum* (*Latin* silver).
arith. arithmetic(al).
Ariz. Arizona.
Ark. Arkansas.
ARM anti-radar missile.
ARP air raid precautions.
ARR *anno regni regis* or *regine* (*Latin* in the year of the king's or queen's reign).
arr. arranged; arrangement; arrival.
art. article; artificial; artillery.
ARTC Air Route Traffic Control.
AS Anglo-Saxon; *anno salutis* (*Latin* in the year of salvation); anti-submarine; Assistant Secretary.
As (*chem*) arsenic.
ASA Advertising Standards Authority.
a.s.a.p. as soon as possible.
ASAT Anti-Satellite.
ASCII (*comput*) American Standard Code for Information Interchange.
ASDIC Allied Submarine Detection Investigation Committee.
ASE American Stock Exchange.
a.s.e. air standard efficiency.
ASH Action on Smoking and Health.
ASI air speed indicator.
ASLEF Associated Society of Locomotive Engineers and Firemen.

ASLIB Association of Special Libraries and Information Bureaux.
ASM air-to-surface missile.
ASN Army Service Number.
ASPCA American Society for the Prevention of Cruelty to Animals.
Ass. Assembly.
ass. assistant; association; assorted.
Assen., Assn. Association.
Assoc. Associate; Association.
asst assistant.
AST Atlantic Standard Time.
ASTMS Association of Scientific, Technical, and Managerial Staffs.
astr astronomer; astronomical; astro-nomy.
astrol. astrologer; astrological; astrology.
astron. astronomer; astronomical; astro-nomy.
ASW anti-submarine warfare.
AT alternativetechnology; anti-tank.
At (*chem*) astatine.
at. airtight; atmosphere; atomic.
ATA Atlantic Treaty Association.
ATC Air Traffic Control; Air Training Corps.
Atl. Atlantic.
atm atmosphere; atmospheric.
at. no. atomic number.
ATS (*comput*) Administrative Terminal System; anti-tetanus serum; Auxiliary Territorial Service (now WRAC).
a.t.s. (*law*) at the suit of.
att. attached; attention; attorney.
attr. attention.
attrb. attribute; attributive.
at. vol. atomic volume.
at. wt. atomic weight.
AU Angstrom unit; astronomical unit.
Au (*chem*) gold.
AUBTW Amalgamated Union of Building Trade Workers.
AUEW Amalgamated Union of Engineering Workers.
Aug. August.
AUM air-to-underwater missile.
AUS IVR Australia.
Aust. Australia; Australian.
Austl. Australasia.
AUT Association of University Teachers.
aut. automatic.
auth. author; authority; authorized.
Auth. Ver. Authorized Version.
auto. automatic; automobile; automotive.
aux auxiliary.
AV audio-visual; Authorized Version.
Av. Avenue.
av. average; avoirdupois.
a.v. *ad valorem* (*Latin* according to the value).
avdp. avoirdupois.
Ave Avenue.
avg average.
AVM Air Vice-Marshal.
AVR Army Volunteer Reserve.
a.w atomic weight.

AWOL absent without official leave.

ax. axiom; axis.

az. azimuth.

B Bachelor; bacillus; Baron; base; (*mus*) bass; IVR Belgium; Bible; Blessed; book; born; (*chem*) boron; bowled (in cricket); breadth; British; Brother.

BA *Baccalaureus Artium* (*Latin* Bachelor of Arts); British Academy; British Airways; Buenos Aires.

Ba (*chem*) barium.

BAA British Airports Authority.

BAAB British Amateur Athletic Board.

Bach. Bachelor.

bact. bacteria; bacteriology; bacterium.

bacteriol. bacteriological; bacteriology.

BAFO British Army Forces Overseas.

BAL (*comput*) basic assembly language.

bal. balance.

ball. ballast; ballistics.

BALPA British Air Line Pilots' Association.

B & B bed and breakfast.

b & s brandy and soda.

b & w black and white.

BAOR British Army of the Rhine.

Bap. Baptist.

bap. baptized.

bar. barometer; barometric; barrel; barrister.

barit. baritone.

barr. barrister.

Bart. Baronet.

BASIC (*comput*) Beginners' All-purpose Symbolic Instruction Code.

bat., batt. battalion; battery.

BB Boys' Brigade; double black (pencils).

bb. books.

BBB triple black (pencils).

BBBG British Boxing Board of Control.

BBC British Broadcasting Corporation.

BBFC British Board of Film Censors.

bbl. barrel.

BC before Christ; British Council.

BCC British Council of Churches.

BCD (*comput*) binary coded decimal notation.

BCG Bacillus Calmette-Guerin, antituberculosis vaccine.

BCh *Baccalaureus Chirurgiae* (*Latin* Bachelor of Surgery).

BD Bachelor of Divinity.

B/D bank draft.

bd. board; bond; bound; bundle.

BDA British Dental Association.

bdl. bundle.

BDS Bachelor of Dental Surgery; IVR Barbados.

BDU Bomb Disposal Unit.

BE Bachelor of Education; Bank of England; Bill of Exchange; British Embassy.

Be (*chem*) beryllium.

BEAB British Electrical Approvals Board.

bec. because.

BEd Bachelor of Education.

Beds. Bedfordshire.

BEF British Expeditionary Force.

bef. before.

beg. begin; beginning.

Belg. Belgian; Belgium.

BEM British Empire Medal.

BEng Bachelor of Engineering.

Beng. Bengal, Bengali.

beq. bequeath; bequeathed.

beqt bequest.

Berks. Berkshire.

bet. between.

BeV billion electron-volts.

B/F brought forward.

b.f. bloody fool; (*print*) bold face; *bona fide* (*Latin* genuine, genuinely).

BFBS British Forces Broadcasting Service.

BFI British Film Institute.

BFN British Forces Network.

BG BrigadierGeneral; IVR Bulgaria.

bg bag.

BH IVR British Honduras.

B'ham Birmingham.

BHC British High Commissioner.

b.h.p. brake horsepower.

Bi (*chem*) bismuth.

Bib. Bible; Biblical.

Bibl. Biblical.

bibliog. bibliographer; bibliography.

bicarb. bicarbonate of soda.

b.i.d. *bis in die* (*Latin* twice daily).

BIM British Institute of Management.

biog. biographical; biographer; biography.

biol. biological; biologist; biology.

BIT (*comput*) binary digit.

Bk (*chem*) berkelium.

bk. bank; bark; block; book; break.

bkcy. bankruptcy.

bkg. banking.

bkpt. bankrupt.

bkt. basket; bracket.

BL Bachelor of Laws; Bachelor of Letters; British Legion (now RBL); British Library.

B/L Bill of Lading.

bldlg. building.

BLit Bachelor of Literature.

BLitt *Baccalaureus Litterarum* (*Latin* Bachelor of Letters).

blk black; block; bulk.

B.LL. Bachelor of Laws.

blvd boulevard.

BM Bachelor of Medicine; *Beatae Memoriae* (*Latin* of blessed memory); bench mark; bowel movement; British Museum.

BMA British Medical Association.

BMC British Medical Council.

BMJ British Medical Journal.

BML British Museum Library.

BMR basal metabolic rate.

BMus Bachelor of Music.
BN banknote.
Bn Baron; Battalion.
BO body odour; Box Office; Broker's Order; Buyer's Option.
b/o brought over.
BOA British Olympic Association.
BOD biochemical oxygen demand.
Boh. Bohemia, Bohemian.
Bol. Bolivia, Bolivian.
bor. borough.
BOT Board of Trade.
bot. botanical; botanist; botany; bottle; bought.
boul. boulevard.
BP British Petroleum; British Pharmacopoeia.
b/p bills payable; blueprint.
bp. baptized; birthplace; bishop.
b.p. below proof; bill of parcels; boiling point.
BPh, BPhil Bachelor of Philosolphy.
bpl. birthplace.
BR IVR Brazil; British Rail.
B/R bills receivable.
Br (*chem*) bromine.
Br. Breton; Britain; British; Brother.
br. branch; brand; brig; bronze; brother; brown.
Braz. Brazil, Brazilian.
BRCS British Red Cross Society.
BRDC British Research and Development Corporation.
Brig. Brigade; Brigadier.
Brig. Gen. Brigadier General.
Brit. Britain; Britannia; British; Briton.
BRN IVR Bahrain.
bro. brother.
BRU IVR Brunei.
BS Bachelor of Science; Bachelor of Surgery; IVR Bahamas; Balance Sheet; Bill of Sale; Blessed Sacrament; British Standards.
b.s. balance sheet; bill of sale.
BSc *Baccalaureus Scientiae* (*Latin* Bachelor of Science).
BSG British Standard Gauge.
BSI British Standards Institution; Building Societies' Institute.
bskt basket.
BSS British Standards Specification.
BST British Standard Time; British Summer Time.
Bt. Baronet.
BTA British Travel Association.
BTh Bachelor of Theology.
BThU British thermal unit.
btl. bottle.
BTU Board of Trade Unit.
Btu British thermal unit.
bu. bureau; bushel.
Bucks. Buckinghamshire.
BUP British United Press.
BUPA British United Provident Association.
BUR IVR Burma.
Bur. Burma; Burmese.
bus. business.

BV *beata virgo* (*Latin* Blessed Virgin); *bene vale* (*Latin* farewell).
b/w black and white.
bx. box; boxes.
Bz (*chem*) benzene.
C Canon; (*physics*) capacitance; Cape; Captain; (*chem*) carbon; Catechism; Catholic; Celsius; Celtic; Centigrade; Central; Century; Chancellor; Chancery; Chapter; Chief; Church; Circuit; Collected; Commander; Confessor; Confidential; Congregational; Congress; Conservative; Constable; Consul; Contralto; Contrast; Corps; coulomb; Count; County; Court; IVR Cuba; Cubic; (*physics*) heat capacity; 100 (Roman numeral).
c. candle; canon; carat; case; cathode; cent; centavo; centigram; centimetre; central; centre; century; chapter; charge; *circa* (*Latin* about); city; class; college; (*math*) constant; contralto; copyright; cubic; cup; currency; current; cycle; (*physics*) specific heat capacity.
CA Central America; Chartered Accountant; Civil Aviation; Consumers' Association; Court of Appeal; Crown Agent.
C/A Credit Account; Current Account.
Ca (*chem*) calcium.
ca. *circa* (*Latin* about).
CAA Civil Aviation Authority.
CAB Citizens' Advice Bureau.
CAD (*comput*) computer-aided design.
cad. (*mus*) *cadenza* (*Italian* final flourish).
Caern. Caernarvonshire (former county).
Caith. Caithness (former county).
cal. calendar; calibre; calorie.
Cambs. Cambridgeshire.
Can. Canon; Canto.
can. canal; cancel; cannon; canton.
Canad. Canadian.
canc. cancellation; cancelled.
cand. candidate.
C & W (*mus*) country and western.
Cantab. *Cantabrigiensis* (*Latin* of Cambridge).
CAP Code of Advertising Practice; Common Agricultural Policy (of EC).
cap. capacity; capital; capitalize; captain; *caput* (*Latin* chapter).
caps. capital letters; capsule.
Capt. Captain.
car. carat.
Card. Cardiganshire (former county); Cardinal.
Carms. Carmarthenshire (former county).
carp. carpenter; carpentry.
carr. carriage.
cartog. cartography.
cas. casual; casualty.
CAT College of Advanced Technology.
cat. catalogue; catechism.
Cath. Cathedral; Catholic.
cath. cathode.
caus. causation; causative.
cav. cavalier; cavalry.
CB Cape Breton; Citizens' Band; Companion of the Order of the Bath; (*milit*) confinement to barracks.

Cb (*chem*) columbium.
CBC Canadian Broadcasting Corporation.
c.b.d. cash before delivery.
CBE Commander of the Order of the British Empire.
CBI Central Bureau of Investigation (USA); Confederation of British Industry.
CBS Columbia Broadcasting System.
CBW chemical and biological warfare.
CC carbon copy; Chamber of Commerce; Chief Clerk; closed circuit; County Council; Cricket Club.
cc cubic centimetre; cubic centimetres.
cc. centuries; chapters; copies.
CCC County Cricket Club.
CCF Combined Cadet Force.
CCP Chinese Communist Party.
CCTV closed circuit television.
c.c.w. counter-clockwise.
CD Civil Defence; contagious disease; Corps Diplomatique; compact disc.
Cd (*chem*) cadmium.
cd candela.
cd. cord; could.
c.d. cash discount.
c/d carried down.
CDC Commonwealth Development Corporation.
CDN IVR Canada.
Cdr Commander; Conductor.
Cdre Commodore.
CDSO Companion of the Distinguished Service Order.
CE Chancellor of the Exchequer; Church of England; Civil Engineer; Council of Europe.
Ce (*chem*) cerium.
Cel. Celsius.
Celt. Celtic.
Cem. Cemetery.
cen. central; centre; century.
cent. centavo; centigrade; centime; centimetre; central; *centum* (*Latin* a hundred; century.
cer. ceramics.
cert. certain; certificate; certification; certified; certify.
CET Central European Time.
CF Chaplain to the Forces.
Cf (*chem*) californium.
cf. *confer* (*Latin* compare).
c/f carried forward.
cfm cubic feet per minute.
cfs cubic feet per second.
cft cubic foot or feet.
CG Coast Guard; Commanding General; Consul General.
cg centigram.
c.g. centre of gravity.
CGI City and Guilds Institute.
CGM Conspicuous Gallantry Medal.
cgm centigram.
cgs centimetre-gram-second.
CH Companion of Honour; IVR Switzerland.
Ch. Chairman; China; Chinese.
ch. chain; champion; chaplain; chapter; check; chemical; chemistry; chief; child; choir; church.

c.h. central heating.
Chal. Chaldaic; Chaldee.
Chanc. Chancellor; Chancery.
Chap. Chapel; Chaplain.
chap. chapter.
char. character.
ChB *Chirurgiae Baccalaureus* (*Latin* Bachelor of Surgery).
chem, chem. chemical; chemist; chemistry.
Ches. Cheshire.
chg. change; charge.
Chin. China; Chinese.
Chm Chairman.
chq. cheque.
Chr. Christ; Christian; Chronicles.
chron. chronicle; chronological.
chs chapters.
CI Channel Islands; Commonwealth Institute; IVR Ivory Coast.
Ci. cirrus; curie.
CIA Central Intelligence Agency (USA).
Cicestr. *Cicestrensis* (*Latin* of Chichester).
CID Criminal Investigation Department.
cif cost, insurance and freight.
C-in-C Commander-in-Chief.
CIS Commonwealth of Independent States.
cit. cited.
ckw clockwise.
CL IVR Sri Lanka.
Cl (*chem*) chlorine.
cl centilitre.
cl. class; classical; classification; clause.
cld. called; cancelled; cleared; coloured; could.
clin. clinical.
Cllr Councillor.
Cm (*chem*) curium.
cm centimetre.
Cmdr Commander.
Cmdre Commodore.
Cmdt Commandant.
CMG Companion of the Order of St Michael and St George.
CMO Chief Medical Officer.
CND Campaign for Nuclear Disarmament.
CNS central nervous system; Chief of Naval Staff.
CO Cash Order; IVR Colombia; Commanding Officer; conscientious objector; Criminal Office; Crown Office.
Co (*chem*) cobalt.
Co. Company; County.
c/o care of; carried over.
COBOL (*comput*) common business oriented language.
COD cash on delivery.
cod. codicil.
coef. coefficient.
C of E Church of England; Council of Europe.
C of I Church of Ireland.
C of S Chief of Staff; Church of Scotland.
c.o.h. cash on hand.
COHSE Confederation of Health Service Employees.

COI Central Office of Information.

COL computer-oriented language.

Col. Colonel; Colorado; (*Scrip*) Colossians; Columbia; Columbian.

col. column.

coll. collateral; colleague; collection; collector; college; collegiate; colloquial.

colloq, colloq. colloquial; colloquialism; colloquially.

comp. companion; comparative; compare; comparison; compensation; competitor; compiled; compilation; complete; composer; composition; compositor; compound; comprehensive; comprising.

compar. comparative; comparison.

compd compound.

compl. complement; complete; compliment; complimentary.

COMSAT Communications Satellite (USA).

con. concentration; concerning; concerto; conclusion; *conjunx* (*Latin* wife); connection; consolidated; *contra* (*Latin* against); convenience.

conc. concentrate; concentrated; concentration; concerning.

conf. *confer* (*Latin* compare); conference.

conj, conj. conjugation; conjunction.

conn. connected; connection; connotation.

Cons. Conservative; Constable.

const. constant.

Cont. Continental.

cont. containing; contents; continent; continental; continued; *contra* (*Latin* against); contract.

contd contained; continued.

contr. contract; contraction; contralto; contrary; contrast; control; controller.

contrib. contribution; contributor.

co-op co-operative.

corr. correct; correction; correspondence; corresponding; corrugated; corruption.

cos (*math*) cosine.

cosec (*math*) cosecant.

cosh (*math*) hyperbolic cosine.

cot, cotan (*math*) cotangent.

Cox. Coxswain.

CP Carriage Paid; Common Prayer; Communist Party.

cp. compare.

CPI consumer price index.

cpi characters per inch.

Cpl. Corporal.

cpm cycles per minute.

CPR Canadian Pacific Railway.

cps characters per second; cycles per second.

CPU (*comput*) central processing unit.

CR IVR Costa Rica.

Cr (*chem*) chromium.

CRE Commission for Racial Equality.

Cres. Crescent.

cres. (*mus*) *crescendo* (*Italian* increasing).

crit. criticism; criticize.

CRO cathode-ray oscillograph; Criminal Records Office.

CRT cathode-ray tube.

cryst. crystalline; crystallized; crystallography.

CS IVR Czechoslovakia.

Cs (*chem*) caesium; (*meteor*) cirrostratus.

csch (*math*) hyperbolic cosecant.

CSE Certificate of Secondary Education.

CSEJ Confederation of Shipbuilding and Engineering Unions.

CSM Company Sergeant-Major.

CSU Civil Service Union.

ct. carat; cent; *centum* (*Latin* hundred); certificate; county; court.

Cu (*chem*) copper.

cu. cubic.

Cumb. Cumberland (former county).

CUP Cambridge University Press.

CV Curriculum Vitae.

Cwlth Commonwealth.

c.w.o. cash with order.

cwt. hundredweight.

CY IVR Cyprus.

D Democratic; Department; *Deus* (*Latin* God); (*chem*) deuterium; dimension; Director; *Dominus* (*Latin* Lord); Duchess; Duke; Dutch; IVR Germany; 500 (Roman numeral).

d. date; day; dead; deceased; decree; degree; delete; *denarius* (*Latin* penny); density; departs; deputy; diameter; died.

DA Deposit Account; District Attorney.

Dak Dakota.

Dan. (*Scrip*) Daniel; Danish.

D & C dilation and curettage.

dat. dative.

dB decibel.

d.b.a. doing business as.

DBE Dame Commander of the Order of the British Empire.

D. B.b. Douay Bible.

dbl. double.

DBST Double British Summer Time.

DC Death Certificate; Depth Charge; Diplomatic Corps; direct current; District of Columbia.

d.c. (*mus*) *da capo* (*Italian* repeat from beginning); direct current.

DCB Dame Commander of the Order of the Bath.

DCM Distinguished Conduct Medal.

DCMG Dame Commander of the Order of St Michael and St George.

dct document.

DCVO Dame Commander of the Royal Victorian Order.

DD direct debit; *Divinitatis Doctor* (*Latin* Doctor of Divinity).

DDC Dewey Decimal Classification.

DDR Deutsche Demokratische Republik (German Democratic Republic).

DDT dichlorodiphenyltrichlorethane, an insecticide.

deb. debenture; debit.

Dec. December.

dec. deceased; decimal; decimetre; declaration; declension; declination; decrease; (*mus*) *decrescendo* (*Italian* becoming softer).

decd deceased.

decl. declaration; declension.

def. defective; defence; defendant; deferred; deficit; definite; definition.

deg. degree.

Del. Delaware.

del. delegate; delegation; delete.

Dem. Democratic.

Den. Denmark.

Denb. Denbighshire (former county).

dep. department; departs; departure; deponent; deposed; deposit; depot; deputy.

dept department.

der., deriv. derivation; derivative; derived.

Derbys. Derbyshire.

DERV diesel engined road vehicle.

DES Department of Education and Science.

Det. Detective.

det. detachment; detail.

Det. Con. Detective Constable.

Det. Insp. Detective Inspector.

Det. Sgt. Detective Sergeant.

Deut. (*Scrip*) Deuteronomy.

dev. development; deviation.

DF *Defensor Fidei* (*Latin* Defender of the Faith).

DFC Distinguished Flying Cross.

DFM Diploma in Forensic Medicine.

DG *Dei gratia* (*Latin* by the grace of God); *Deo gratias* (*Latin* thanks to God).

dia. diagram; dialect; diameter.

diag. diagonal; diagram.

dial. dialect; dialogue.

diam. diameter.

dict. dictionary.

diff. difference; different; differential.

dig. digest; digit; digital.

dim. dimension; diminished; (*mus*) *diminuendo* (*Italian* becoming softer).

dimin. (*mus*) *diminuendo* (*Italian* becoming softer); diminutive.

Dioc. Diocesan; Diocese.

Dip. Diploma.

Dir. Director.

dis. discontinued; discount; distance; distant; distribute.

disc. discount; discovered.

disp. dispensary; dispensation.

dist distant; district.

distr. distribute; distributed; distribution; distributor.

div. dividend; division; divorce.

DIY do-it-yourself.

DJ dinner jacket; disc jockey.

DK IVR Denmark.

dlvy delivery.

dly daily.

DM Deutsche Mark.

dm decimetre.

DMZ demilitarized zone.

DNA (*chem*) deoxyribonucleic acid.

do. *ditto* (*Italian* the same).

DOA dead on arrival.

d.o.b. date of birth.

doc. document.

DOE Department of the Environment.

dol. (*mus*) *dolce* (*Italian* sweet); dollar.

DOM *Deo optimo maximo* (*Latin* to God, the best and greatest); IVR Dominican Republic.

doz. dozen.

DP data processing; displaced person.

DPh, DPhil Doctor of Philosophy.

DPP Director of Public Prosecutions.

dpt department; deponent; deposit; depot.

Dr Doctor.

Dr. Drive.

dram. pers. *dramatis personae* (*Latin* characters present in the drama).

DS (*mus*) *dal segno* (*Italian* from the sign); disseminated sclerosis.

DSC Distinguished Service Cross.

DSM Distinguished Service Medal.

DSO Distinguished Service Order.

d.s.p. *decessit sine prole* (*Latin* died without issue).

DST Daylight Saving Time.

DT data transmission; delirium tremens.

DTI Department of Trade and Industry.

Du. Duchy; Duke; Dutch.

Dumb. Dumbarton.

Dumf. Dumfriesshire (former county).

Dunb. Dunbartonshire (former county).

dup. duplicate.

DV defective vision; *Deo volente* (*Latin* God willing); Douay Version (of the Bible).

DY IVR Dahomey.

Dy (*chem*) dysprosium.

DZ IVR Algeria.

dz. dozen.

E East; Easter; Eastern; England; English; IVR Spain.

e. elder; electric.

ea. each.

EAK IVR Kenya.

E & OE errors and omissions excepted.

EAT IVR Tanzania.

EAU IVR Uganda.

EAZ IVR Tanzania.

EC East Central; IVR Ecuador; European Community.

eccles ecclesiastical.

Eccles. (*Scrip*) Ecclesiastes.

ECG electrocardiogram; electrocardiograph.

ecol. ecological; ecology.

econ. economical; ecomics; economy.

ECT electroconvulsive therapy.

ed. edited; edition; editor; education.

EDC (*med*) expected date of confinement.

EDD (*med*) expected date of delivery.

edit. edited; edition; editor.

EDP electronic data processing.

educ. educated; education; educational.

EEC European Economic Community.
EEG electroencephalogram; electroencephalograph.
EEOC Equal Employment Opportunities Commission.
EFL English as a foreign language.
EFT electronic funds transfer.
EFTA European Free Trade Association.
e.g. *exempli gratia* (*Latin* for example).
EHF extremely high frequency.
elect. electric; electrical; electricity.
elem. element; elementary.
elev. elevation.
Eliz. Elizabethan.
ELT English Language Teaching.
EM electromagnetic; electromotive.
EMF, emf electromotive force.
EMI Electrical and Musical Industries.
Emp. Emperor; Empire; Empress.
EMR electronic magnetic resonance.
EMS European Monetary System.
EMU, emu electromagnetic unit; European monetary unit.
enc., encl enclosed; enclosure.
ENE east-northeast.
Eng. England; English.
eng. engine; engineer; engineering; engraved; engraver.
enl. enlarged; enlisted.
Ens. Ensign.
ENSA Entertainments National Services Association.
ENT ear, nose and throat.
entom. entomology.
env. envelope.
EO Executive Officer.
EoC Equal Opportunities Commission.
EP electroplate; extended play (record).
Ep. Epistle.
EPNS electroplated nickel silver.
eq. equal.
ER *Elizabeth Regina* (*Latin* Queen Elizabeth).
Er (*chem*) erbium.
ERNIE Electronic Random Number Indicator Equipment.
Es (*chem*) einsteinium.
ESE east-southeast.
ESL English as a second language.
ESN educationally subnormal.
ESP extrasensory perception.
esp, esp. especially.
Esq. Esquire.
ESRO European Space Research Organization.
Est. Established; Estate.
est. estimated; estuary.
ET IVR Egypt; extra-terrestrial.
ETA estimated time of arrival.
et al. *et alii* (*Latin* and others).
etc, etc. *et cetera* (*Latin* and so on).
ETD estimated time of departure.
ethnol. ethnology.
ETU Electrical Trades Union.
etym. etymological; etymology.
Eu (*chem*) europium.

Eu., Eur. Europe; European.
EV, e.v. electron volt.
ex. examination; excellent; except; exchange; excluding; excursion; executed; executive; exempt; express; export; extra.
exam. examination.
Exe. Excellency.
exch. exchange; exchequer.
excl. exclamation; excluding.
exclam, exclam. exclamation.
exec. executive; executor.
ex lib. *ex libris* (*Latin* from the library of).
ex off. *ex officio* (*Latin* by virtue of office).
ext. extension; exterior; external; extinct; extra; extract; extreme.
F Fahrenheit; farad; Father; fathom; February; Fellow; Finance; (*chem*) fluorine; folio; (*mus*) *forte* (*Italian* loud); IVR France; French; frequency; Friday; function.
f. farad; farthing; fathom; feet; female; feminine; filly; fine; fluid; folio; following; foot; (*mus*) *forte* (*Italian* loud); foul; franc; frequency; from; furlong.
FA Fanny Adams; Football Association.
f.a. free alongside.
Fac. Faculty.
fam. family.
FAO Food and Agriculture Organization.
f.a.s. free alongside ship.
fath. fathom.
FBI Federal Bureau of Investigation (USA).
FC Football Club.
FCI Foreign and Commonwealth Office.
FD *Fidei Defensor* (*Latin* Defender of the Faith).
fd. forward; found; founded.
Fe (*chem*) iron.
Feb, Feb. February.
fec. *fecit* (*Latin* he or she made).
fed. federal; federated; federation.
fem. female; feminine.
ff (*mus*) *fortissimo* (*Italian* very loud).
ff. folios; the following.
fict. fiction; fictitious.
Fid. Def. *Fidei Defensor* (*Latin* Defender of the Faith).
fig. figuratively; figure.
Fin. Finland; Finnish.
fin. final; finance; financial; finish.
Finn. Finnish.
FJI IVR Fiji.
FL Flight Lieutenant; IVR Liechtenstein.
Fl. Flanders; Flemish.
fl. floor; florin; *floruit* (*Latin* flourished); fluid.
Flem. Flemish.
Flor. Florida.
flor. *floruit* (*Latin* flourished).
fl. oz. fluid ounce.
FMD foot and mouth disease.
fn. footnote.
FO Flying Officer; Foreign Office.
fo. folio.

f.o.b. free on board.

FOC (*print*) Father of the Chapel (union official); free of charge.

fol. folio; followed; following.

foll. following.

for. foreign; forestry.

fort, fort. fortification; fortified.

FORTRAN (*comput*) Formula Translation.

FP former pupil; freezing point.

fp (*mus*) *forte piano* (*Italian* loud and then immediately soft).

f.p. freezing point.

FPA Family Planning Association.

f.p.s. feet per second; foot-pound-second; (*photog*) frames per second.

Fr (*chem*) francium.

Fr. Father; France; *frater* (*Latin* brother); French; Friar; Friday.

fr. fragment; franc; frequent; from.

f.r. *folio recto* (*Latin* right-hand page).

FRCP Fellow of the Royal College of Physicians.

FRCS Fellow of the Royal College of Surgeons.

freq. frequent; frequentative; frequently.

Fri. Friday.

front. frontispiece.

FRS Fellow of the Royal Society.

FSH follicle-stimulating hormone.

ft, ft. feet; foot; fort; fortification.

fur. furlong.

fut. future.

f.v. *folio verso* (*Latin* left-hand page).

fwd forward.

f.w.d. four-wheel drive; front-wheel drive.

FYI for your information.

fz (*mus*) *forzando* (*Italian* to be strongly accentuated).

G (*physics*) conductance; gauge; German; giga; grain; gram; grand; (*physics*) gravitational constant; guilder; guinea; gulp; gravity.

g gram, gramme; (*physics*) gravitational acceleration.

g. genitive; guinea.

Ga (*chem*) gallium.

Ga. Georgia.

Gael. Gaelic.

gal., gall. gallon.

galv. galvanic; galvanism.

GATT General Agreement on Tariffs and Trade.

gaz. gazette; gazetteer.

GB IVR Great Britain and Northern Ireland.

GBA IVR Alderney.

GBE Grand Cross of the Order of the British Empire.

GBG IVR Guernsey.

g.b.h. grievous bodily harm.

GBJ IVR Jersey.

GBM IVR Isle of Man.

GBZ IVR Gibraltar.

GC George Cross; Golf Club.

GCA IVR Guatemala.

GCE General Certificate of Education.

GCF greatest common factor.

GCMG Knight *or* Dame Grand Cross of the Order of St Michael and St George.

GCVO Grand Cross of the Royal Victorian Order.

Gd (*chem*) gadolinium.

gd good; guard.

Gdns Gardens.

GDR German Democratic Republic.

gds goods.

Ge (*chem*) germanium.

GEC General Electric Company.

Gen. General; (*Scrip*) Genesis.

gen. gender; general; generally; generator; generic; genetics; genitive; genuine; genus.

gent gentleman.

Geo. Georgia.

geog. geographer; geographic; geographical; geography.

geol. geologic; geological; geologist; geology.

geom. geometric; geometrical; geometrician; geometry.

Ger. German; Germany.

ger. gerund; gerundive.

GeV giga-electronvolts.

GG Girl Guides; Governor General.

GH IVR Ghana.

GHQ General Headquarters.

GI gastrointestinal; general issue; Government Issue.

Gib. Gibraltar.

Gk. Greek.

gl. glass.

g/l grams per litre.

Glam. Glamorganshire (former county).

Glas. Glasgow.

GLC Greater London Council.

Glos. Gloucestershire.

gloss. glossary.

GM Geiger-Müller counter; General Manager; George Medal; Grand Master; Guided Missile.

gm gram.

gm² grames per square metre.

GMB Grand Master of the Order of the Bath.

GMBE Grand Master of the Order of the British Empire.

GMC General Medical Council.

Gmc Germanic.

GMT Greenwich Mean Time.

GMWU National Union of General and Municipal Workers.

GNP Gross National Product.

gns. guineas.

GOC General Officer Commanding.

Goth. Gothic.

Gov. Governor.

Govt Government.

GP Gallup Poll; (*med*) general paresis; (*mus*) general pause; General Practitioner; general purpose; *Gloria Patri* (*Latin* Glory to the Father); Grand Prix.

gp group.

Gp Capt. Group Captain.

GPO General Post Office.

GR *Geogius Rex* (*Latin* King George).

Gr. Grecian; Greece; Greek.

gr. grade; grain; grammar; gravity; great; gross; group.

grad. gradient; graduate.

gram. grammar; grammarian; grammatical.

Gr. Br. Great Britain.

gr. wt. gross weight.

GS General Secretary; General Staff; ground speed.

gs. guineas.

gsm grams per square metre.

GT Grand Tourer.

gtd guaranteed.

GTS Greenwich Time Signal.

GU gastriculcer; genitourinary.

guar. guaranteed.

GUY IVR Guyana.

GW gigawatt.

gym. gymnasium; gymnastics.

gyn. gynaecological; gynaecology.

H hard (pencils); hecto-; (*physics*) henry; heroin; hospital; IVR Hungary; hydrant; (*chem*) hydrogen.

h hour.

h. harbour; hard; height; high; hit; horizontal; (*mus*) horn; hour; hundred; husband.

ha hectare.

hab. habitat.

Haw. Hawaii; Hawaiian.

HB hard black (pencils).

HC House of Commons.

HCF highest common factor.

HCJ High Court Judge.

HD heavy duty.

hd hand; head.

hdbk handbook.

hdqrs headquarters.

HE high explosive; His Eminence; His or Her Excellency.

He (*chem*) helium.

Heb. Hebrew.

her., heral. heraldic; heraldry.

Herts. Hertfordshire.

hex. hexagon; hexagonal.

HF high frequency.

Hf (*chem*) hafnium.

hf half.

HG High German; Horse Guards.

Hg (*chem*) mercury.

hgt. height.

HGV heavy goods vehicle.

HH double hard (pencils); His or Her Highness; His Holiness; His or Her Honour.

Hind. Hindi; Hindu.

hist. histology; historian; historical; history.

HIV human immunodeficiency virus.

HJ *hic jacet* (*Latin* here lies).

HJS *hic jacet sepultus* (*Latin* here lies buried).

HK IVR Hong Kong; House of Keys (Manx Parliament).

HKJ IVR Jordan.

HL Honours List; House of Lords.

hl hectolitre.

HM His or Her Majesty.

HMG Higher Middle German; His or Her Majesty's Government.

HMI His or Her Majesty's Inspector.

HMS His or Her Majesty's Service; His or Her Majesty's Ship.

HMSO His or Her Majesty's Stationery Office.

HMV His Master's Voice.

HNC Higher National Certificate.

HND Higher National Diploma.

HO Home Office.

Ho (*chem*) holmium.

ho. house.

Hon. Honorary; Honourable.

Hons Honours.

Hon. Sec. Honorary Secretary.

hort. horticultural; horticulture.

hosp. hospital.

HP hire purchase; horse power; Houses of Parliament.

HQ Headquarters.

hr hour.

HRH His or Her Royal Highness.

HS *hic sepultus* (*Latin* here is buried); High School; Home Secretary.

HT high tension.

ht. heat; height.

Hung. Hungarian; Hungary.

Hunts. Huntingdonshire (former county).

HV high velocity; high voltage.

hwy highway.

hyd. hydraudics; hydrostatics.

Hz hertz.

I (*physics*) current; incisor; Independence; (*physics*) inertia; Institute; Institution; Interest; International; intransitive; (*chem*) iodine; Island; Isle; (*physics*) isospin; IVR Italy; 1 (Roman numeral).

IABA International Amateur Boxing Association.

IAM Institute of Advanced Motorists.

ib. *ibidem* (*Latin* in the same place).

IBA Independent Broadcasting Authority.

ibid. *ibidem* (*Latin* in the same place).

IC integrated circuit.

i/c in charge; internal combustion.

ICA Institute of Contemporary Art.

ICBM intercontinental ballistic missile.

ICI Imperial Chemical Industries.

icon. iconographic; iconography.

ICU intensive care unit.

ID identification.

id. *idem* (*Latin* the same).

IDP integrated data processing.

i.e. *id est* (*Latin* that is).

IL IVR Israel.

ILEA Inner London Education Authority.

Ill. Illinois.

ill., Ilus. illustrated; illustration.

ILO International Labour Organization.

ILP Independent Labour Party.

ILTF International Lawn Tennis Federation.

IM Isle of Man.

IMF International Monetary Fund.

imit. imitation; imitative.

imp. imperative; imperfect; imperial; impersonal; implemerlt; import; important; importer; *imprimatur* (*Latin* let it be printed); imprint; improper; improved; improvement.

imper. imperative.

imperf. imperfect.

impers. impersonal.

impf. imperfect.

imp. gall. imperial gallon.

In (*chem*) indium.

in. inch.

Inc. Incorporated.

inc. included; including; inclusive; income; incomplete; increase.

incl. including; inclusive.

incog. incognito.

incor. incorporated.

incr. increase; increased; increasing.

IND IVR India.

Ind. Independent; India; Indian; Indies.

ind. independence; independent; index; indicative; indirect; industrial; industry.

indef. indefinite.

indic. indicating; indicative; indicator.

individ. individual.

Inf. Infantry.

inf. inferior; infinitive; influence; information; *infra* (*Latin* below).

infin. infinitive.

init. initial; *initio* (*Latin* in the beginning).

in loc. cit. *in loco citato* (*Latin* in the place cited).

ins. inches; inspector; insulated; insulation; insurance.

Insp. inspected; inspector.

Inst. Institute.

inst. instant; instantaneous; instrumental.

instr. instructor; instrument; instrumental.

int. interest; interim; interior; interjection; internal; international; interpreter; intransitive.

intens. intensified; intensive.

inter. intermediate.

interj. interjection.

INTERPOL International Criminal Police Commission.

interrog. interrogation; interrogative.

intr., intrans. intransitive.

intro. introduction; introductory.

inv. invented; invention; inventor; invoice.

I/O (*comput*) input/output.

Io (*chem*) ionium.

Io. Iowa.

IOC International Olympic Committee.

IOM Isle of Man.

IOU I owe you.

IOW Isle of Wight.

IPA International Phonetic Alphabet or Association.

IPBM interplanetary ballistic missile.

IQ intelligence quotient.

IR infrared; Inland Revenue; IVR Iran.

Ir (*chem*) iridium.

Ir. Ireland; Irish.

IRA Irish Republican Army.

IRBM intermediate range ballistic missile.

IRC International Red Cross.

IRL IVR Republic of Ireland.

IRQ IVR Iraq.

IS IVR Iceland.

Is. (*Scrip*) Isaiah; Island; Isle.

ISBN International Standard Book Number.

isl. island; isle.

isth. isthmus.

It. Italian; Italic; Italy.

ITA Independent Television Authority; Initial Teaching Alphabet.

Ital. Italian; Italic.

ITN Independent Television News.

ITV Independent Television.

IUD intra-uterine device.

i.v. intravenous.

IVR International Vehicle Registration.

IVS International Voluntary Service.

IW Isle of Wight.

J IVR Japan; (*physics*) joule; Journal; Judge; Justice.

JA IVR Jamaica.

Ja. January.

Jan. January.

Jap. Japan; Japanese.

Jas James.

JATO jet-assisted take-off.

JC Jesus Christ; Jockey Club.

JCB (trademark) Joseph Cyril Bamford (manufacturer of an earth-moving vehicle).

jct. junction.

Jl. July.

Jnr Junior.

JP Justice of the Peace.

Jr Junior.

jt joint.

Ju. June.

Jul. July.

Jun. June; Junior.

junc. junction.

Junr Junior.

Jus. Justice.

juv. juvenile.

Jy July.

K (*elect*) capacity; carat; (*math*) constant; (*physics*) kaon; (*physics*) kelvin; IVR Khmer Republic; kilo; King; knight; knit; kopeck; (*chem*) potassium.

K. (*mus*) Köchel (number) (Mozart catalogue).

KB King's Bench; Knight of the Order of the Bath.

KBE Knight of the Order of the British Empire.

KC Kennel Club; King's Counsel; Knight Commander.

kc kilocycle.

KCB Knight Commander of the Order of the Bath.

KCMG Knight Commander of the Order of St Michael and St George.

KCVC Knight Commander of the Royal Victorian Order.

keV kilo-electronvolt.
KG Knight of the Order of the Garter.
kg kilogram.
KGB Komitet Gosudarstvennoi Bezopasnosti (*Russian* Committee of State Security, former USSR).
KGCB Knight of the Grand Cross of the Order of the Bath.
kHz kilohertz.
KIA killed in action.
kilo kilogram.
kJ kilojoule.
KJV King James Version (of the Bible).
KKK Ku Klux Klan.
kl kilolitre.
km kilometre.
km/h kilometres per hour.
kn (*naut*) knot.
KO knock-out.
Kr (*chem*) krypton.
Kt Knight.
kV kilovolt.
kW kilowatt.
kWh kilowatt-hour.
KWT IVR Kuwait.
L (*elect*) inductance; Lake; Latin; learner driver; Liberal; longitude; IVR Luxembourg; 50 (Roman numeral).
l litre.
l. lake; land; latitude; left; length; *liber* (*Latin* book); *libra* (*Latin* pound); line; lire; low.
LA Los Angeles.
La (*chem*) lanthanum.
Lab. Labour; Labrador.
lab. labial; laboratory.
Lancs. Lancashire.
lang. language.
LAO IVR Laos.
LAR IVR Libya.
Lat. Latin.
lat. latitude.
LB IVR Liberia.
lb. pound.
l.b.w. leg before wicket (in cricket).
LC Lance Corporal.
L/C Letter of Credit.
lc, l.c. *loco citato* (*Latin* in the place cited); (*print*) lower case.
LCC London County Council.
LCD lowest common denominator.
LCM lowest common multiple.
L/Cpl Lance Corporal.
Ld. Lord.
Ldg. Leading.
LEA Local Education Authority.
leg. legal; (*mus*) *legato* (*Italian* smooth).
Leics. Leicestershire.
LEM lunar excursion module.
LEV lunar excursion vehicle.
LF low frequency.
LG Low German.

lg. large.
lgth length.
LH Luteinizing hormone.
l.h. left hand.
l.h.d. left hand drive.
Li (*chem*) lithium.
Lib. Liberal.
Lieut, Lieut. Lieutenant.
Lincs. Lincolnshire.
ling. linguistics.
lit. literal; literary; literature; litre.
LL Lord Lieutenant.
ll. lines.
LL.B. *Legum Baccalaureus* (*Latin* Bachelor of Laws).
LL.D. *Legum Doctor* (*Latin* Doctor of Laws).
lm (*physics*) lumen.
LMT local mean time.
LNG liquefied natural gas.
LOA leave of absence.
loc. cit. *loco citato* (*Latin* in the place cited).
log. logarithm.
long. longitude.
loq. *loquitur* (*Latin* he or she speaks).
LP long-playing (record); London Philhar-monia.
LPG liquefied petroleum gas.
LPC London Philharmonic Orchestra.
L'pool Liverpool.
Lr (*chem*) lawrencium.
LRBM long range ballistic missile.
LRS Lloyd's Register of Shipping.
LS IVR Lesotho.
LSD *librae, solidi, denarii* (*Latin* pounds, shillings, pence); lysergic acid diethylamide.
LSE London School of Economics.
LSC London Symphony Orchestra.
Lt. Lieutenant.
l.t. local time.
LTA Lawn Tennis Association.
Lt. Col. Lieutenant Colonel.
Lt. Comdr Lieutenant Commander.
Ltd Limited.
Lu (*chem*) lutetium.
LV Luncheon voucher.
LW long wave.
Lw (*chem*) lawrencium.
LWM low water mark.
lx (*physics*) lux.
M mach (number); Majesty; IVR Malta; Manitoba; Marquis; Master; (*physics*) maxwell; Medieval; Member; (*mus*) *mezzo* (*Italian* half); Middle; Monday; Monsieur; motorway; Mountain; 1000 (Roman numeral).
m (*physics*) mass; metre.
m. male; married; masculine; medium; meridian; mile; million; minim; minute; modulus; month; moon; morning.
MA *Magister Artium* (*Latin* Master of Arts); IVR Morocco.
mach. machine; machinery; machinist.
mag. magazine; magnetic; magnetism; magnesium; magneto; magnitude.

Maj. Major.
MAL IVR Malaysia.
manuf. manufacture.
MAO (*chem*) monoamine oxidase.
Mar. March.
mar. marine; maritime.
March. Marchioness; margin, marginal.
marg. margin; marginal.
Marq. Marquess; Marquis.
masc. masculine.
Mass. Massachusetts.
math. mathematics.
Matt. Matthew.
max. maximum.
MB *Medicinae Baccalaureus* (*Latin* Bachelor of Medicine).
MC Master of Ceremonies; Medical Corps; Military Cross; IVR Monaco.
mc megacycle; millicurie.
MCC Marylebone Cricket Club.
MCP male chauvinist pig.
MCS missile control system.
MD Managing Director; *Medicinae Doctor* (*Latin* Doctor of Medicine); mentally deficient.
Md (*chem*) mendelivium.
Md. Maryland.
Mdm Madam.
ME myalgic encephalomyelitis.
Me (*chem*) methyl.
Me. Maine.
mech. mechanical; mechanics; mechanism.
Med. Mediterranean.
med. medical; medicine; medieval; medium.
Medit. Mediterranean.
mem. member; *memento* (*Latin* remember); memoir; memorandum; memorial.
MEP Member of the European Parliament.
met. metaphor; metaphysics; meteorological; meteorology; metropolitan.
metal. metallurgical; metallurgy.
metaph. metaphor; metaphysics.
meteor. meteorological; meteorology.
MeV mega-electron-volt; million electron-volts.
MEX IVR Mexico.
MF medium frequency.
mf (*mus*) *mezzo forte* (*Italian* moderately loud).
mfd manufactured.
mfr. manufacture; manufacturer.
Mg (*chem*) magnesium; megagram.
mg milligram.
Mgr Manager.
mgt management.
MHF medium high frequency.
MHG Middle High German.
MHz megahertz.
MI MilitaryIntelligence.
mi. mile.
MI5 Military Intelligence, section 5.
MIA missing in action.
MICR (*comput*) magnetic ink character recognition.

Middx Middlesex (former county).
mil millilitre.
mil., milit military.
Min. Ministry.
min. mineralogical; mineralogy; minim; minimum; mining; minister; ministry; minor; minute.
mineral. mineralogical; mineralogy.
MIRAS mortgage interest relief at source.
MIRV multiple independently targetted re-entry vehicle.
misc. miscellaneous; miscellany.
mk mark.
mks metre-kilogram-second.
mkt market.
ml mile; millilitre.
Mlle Mademoiselle.
MLR minimum lending rate.
MM Military Medal.
mm millimetre.
Mme Madame.
MMR measles, mumps and rubella (combined vaccine against these).
Mn (*chem*) manganese.
MO Medical Officer; *modus operandi* (*Latin* mode of operation); Money Order.
Mo (*chem*) molybdenum.
Mo. Monday.
mo. month.
MOD Ministry of Defence.
mod. moderate; modern; modulus.
mod. cons. modern conveniences.
MOH Medical Officer of Health.
mol (*chem*) mole.
mol. molecular; molecule.
mol. wt. molecular weight.
Mon. Monday; Monmouthshire (former county).
Mont. Montgomeryshire (former county).
MOR middle-of-the-road.
MORI Market and Opinion Research Institute.
morph. morphological; morphology.
MOT Ministry of Transport.
MP Member of Parliament; Metropolitan Police; Military Police; Mounted Police.
mp (*mus*) *mezzo piano* (*Italian* moderately soft).
m.p. melting point.
mph miles per hour.
Mr, Mr. Mister.
MRBM medium range ballistic missile.
MRC Medical Research Council.
MRCP Member of the Royal College of Physicians.
MRCS Member of the Royal College of Surgeons.
MRP Manufacturer's Recommended Price.
Ms a title used before a woman's name instead of Miss or Mrs.
MS manuscript; IVR Mauritius; multiple sclerosis.
ms millisecond.
m/s metres per second.
MSC Manpower Services Commission.
MSc Master of Science.
MSG (*chem*) monosodium glutamate.

Msgr. Monseigneur; Monsignor.

msl mean sea level.

MT mean time.

Mt Mount.

mtg. meeting; mortgage.

mth month.

mtn mountain.

Mt. Rev. Most Reverend.

mun. municipal.

mus. museum; music; musical; musician.

mV millivolt.

m.v. (*mus*) *mezzo voce* (*Italian* half the power of voice); motor vessel.

MW IVR Malawi; medium wave; megawatt.

mW milliwatt.

Mx Middlesex (former county).

MY motor yacht.

mycol. mycological; mycology.

myth. mythological; mythology.

N National; Nationalist; Navy; (*physics*) newton; (*chem*) nitrogen; Norse; North; IVR Norway; November.

n. name; *natus* (*Latin* born); navy; nephew; net; neuter; (*physics*) neutron; new; nominative; noon; note; noun; number.

NA IVR Netherlands Antilles; North America.

Na (*chem*) sodium.

n/a no account; not applicable; not available.

NAAFI Navy, Army and Air Force Institutes.

NALGO National and Local Government Officers' Association.

NASA National Aeronautics and Space Administration (USA).

nat. national; native; natural.

NATO North Atlantic Treaty Organization.

NATSOPA National Society of Operative Printers and Assistants.

naut. nautical.

nav. naval; navigable; navigation; navy.

navig. navigation; navigator.

NB *nota bene* (*Latin* note well).

Nb (*chem*) niobium.

NBC National Broadcasting Corporation (USA).

NCB National Coal Board.

NCCL National Council for Civil Liberties.

NCO Noncommissioned Officer.

ncv no commercial value.

Nd (*chem*) neodymium.

NE northeast.

Ne (*chem*) neon.

NEB New English Bible.

NEC National Executive Committee.

NEDC National Economic Development Council.

neg. negative; negatively.

nem. con. *nemine contradicente* (*Latin* no one opposing).

neurol. neurol. neurology.

neut. neuter; neutral.

NF no funds.

NFT National Film Theatre.

NFU National Farmers' Union.

NHS National Health Service.

NI National Insurance; Northern Ireland.

Ni (*chem*) nickel.

NIC IVR Nicaragua.

NIG IVR Niger.

NL IVR Netherlands.

n.l. new line.

NMR nuclear magnetic resonance.

NNE north-northeast.

NNW north-northwest.

No (*chem*) nobelium.

No. Number.

n.o. not out (in cricket).

nol. pros. *nolle prosequi* (*Latin* do not continue).

nom. nominal; nominative.

noncom. noncommissioned.

non seq. *non sequitur* (*Latin* it does not follow logically).

Nor. Norman; North; Norway; Norwegian.

norm. normal.

Northants. Northamptonshire.

Northumb. Northumberland.

nos. numbers.

Notts. Nottinghamshire.

Nov. November.

NP Notary Public.

Np (*chem*) neptunium.

n.p. new paragraph.

NPT normal pressure and temperature.

nr near.

NRC Nuclear Research Council.

ns nanosecond.

n.s. new style.

NSB National Savings Bank.

n.s.f. not sufficient funds.

NSPCC National Society for the Prevention of Cruelty to Children.

NSU (*med*) non-specific urethritis.

NT National Trust; New Testament.

NTS National Trust for Scotland.

NUGMW National Union of General and Municipal Workers.

NUJ National Union of Journalists.

NUM National Union of Mineworkers.

num. number; numeral.

numis. numismatics.

NUPE National Union of Public Employees.

NUR National Union of Railwaymen.

NUS National Union of Seamen; National Union of Students.

NUT National Union of Teachers.

NV New Version (of the Bible).

n.v.d. no value declared.

NVQ National Vocational Qualification.

NW northwest.

NY New York.

NYC New York City.

NZ IVR New Zealand.

O Ocean; octavo; October; Ohio; Old; Ontario; Oregon; (*chem*) oxygen.

O & M Organization and Methods.
OAP Old Age Pensioner; Old Age Pensioner.
OB outside broadcast.
ob. *obiit* (*Latin* he *or* she died).
obb. (*mus*) *obbligato* (*Italian* obligatory).
OBE Officer of the Order of the British Empire.
obj. object; objection; objective.
obl. obligation; oblique; oblong.
obs. obsolete.
obstet. obstetrics.
obv. obverse.
OC Officer Commanding.
OCR (*comput*) Optical Character Reader; Optical Character Recognition.
Oct. October.
oct. octave; octavo.
OD Officer of the Day; overdose; overdraft.
OE Old English.
OECD Organization for Economic Cooperation and Development.
OED Oxford English Dictionary.
OF Old French.
off. offer; office; office; official.
OFT Office of Fair Trading.
OGM Ordinary General Meeting.
OHG Old High German.
OHMS On His *or* Her Majesty's Service.
OM Order of Merit.
o.n.o. or nearest offer.
Ont. Ontario.
o.p. out of print.
op. cit. *opere citato* (*Latin* in the work cited).
OPEC Organization of Petroleum Exporting Countries.
opp. opposed; opposite.
OR Official Receiver; operational research; other ranks.
orch. orchestra; orchestral.
ord. ordained; order; ordinal; ordinance; ordinary; ordnance.
Ore. Oregon.
org. organic; organization.
orig. origin; original; originally.
ornith. ornithology.
orth. orthography; orthopaedic; orthodox.
OS Old Style; Ordinary Seaman; Ordnance Survey; Outsize.
Os (*chem*) osmium.
o.s. out of stock; outsize.
OT Old Testament.
OU Open University.
OXFAM Oxford Committee for Famine Relief.
Oxon. *Oxoniensis* (*Latin* of Oxford).
oz. ounce.
P (*chem*) phosphorus; IVR Portugal; President.
p. page; paragraph; part; participle; past; penny; per; pint; *post* (*Latin* after); power; *pro* (*Latin* in favour of); purl.
PA IVR Panama; Personal Assistant; Press Agent; Press Association; Public Address.
p.a. per annum.

PAK IVR Pakistan.
P & L Profit and Loss.
P & O Peninsular and Oriental (Steamship Company).
p & p postage and packing.
par. paragraph; parallel; parenthesis.
Parl. Parliament(ary).
part. participial; participle; partner.
partn. partnership.
pass. passage; passenger; *passim* (*Latin* here and there); passive.
pat. patent; patented.
path., pathol. pathological; pathology.
Pat. Off. Patent Office.
pat. pend. patent pending.
patt. pattern.
PAYE Pay As You Earn.
Pb (*chem*) lead.
PBS Public Broadcasting System (US).
PBT President of the Board of Trade.
PC personal computer; Police Constable; political correctness; Privy Council.
p.c. per cent; postcard; *post cibum* (*Latin* after meals).
Pd (*chem*) palladium.
pd paid; passed.
pdq (*colloq*) pretty damn quickly.
PDSA People's Dispensary for Sick Animals.
PE IVR Peru; physical education.
PEI Prince Edward Island.
pen. peninsula; penitentiary.
per. period; person.
perf. perfect.
perm. permanent; permutation.
perp. perpendicular.
per pro. *per procurationem* (*Latin* on behalf of).
pers. person; personal.
PFA Professional Footballers' Association.
PG paying guest; Postgraduate.
pg. page.
PGA Professional Golfers' Association.
pharm. pharmacist; pharmacology; pharmacy.
PhD *Philosophiae Doctor* (*Latin* Doctor of Philosophy).
Phil. Philadelphia; Philharmonic.
phil. philology; philosopher; philosophical; philosophy.
philos. philosopher; philosophical; philosophy.
phon. phonetics; phonology.
phot. photograph; photography.
phr. phrase; phraseology.
phys. physical; physician; physics; physiological; physiology.
PI IVR Philippine Islands.
PIN personal identification number.
pizz. (*mus*) *pizzicato* (*Italian* plucking strings with fingers).
pk. pack; park; peak; peck.
pkg. package; packing.
pkt. packet; pocket.
PL Poet Laureate; IVR Poland.
P/L Profit and Loss.

Pl. Place.

pl. place; plate; platoon; plural.

PLA Port of London Authority.

PLC, plc public limited company.

PLO Palestine Liberation Organization.

PLP Parliamentary Labour Party.

PLR Public Lending Right.

plupf. pluperfect.

plur. plural.

PM *post meridiem* (*Latin* after noon); Post Mortem; Prime Minister.

Pm (*chem*) promethium.

p.m. *post meridiem* (*Latin* after noon).

PMT pre-menstrual tension.

PNdb perceived noise decibel.

PO Personnel Officer; Postal Order; Post Office.

Po (*chem*) polonium.

POD pay on delivery.

poet. poetic; poetical; poetry.

pol. political; politics.

pop. popular; popularly; population.

POS point of sale.

pos. position; positive.

poss. possessive; possible; possibly.

pot. potential.

POW prisoner of war.

PP Past President.

pp *per procurationem* (*Latin* on behalf of); (*mus*) *pianissimo* (*Italian* very soft).

pp. pages.

p.p. past participle; *post prandium* (*Latin* after meals).

PPE Philosophy, Politics and Economics.

PPS Parliamentary Private Secretary; *post postscriptum* (*Latin* additional postscript).

PR Proportional Representation; Public Relations.

Pr (*chem*) praseodymium.

pr. pair; paper; power; preferred; present; price; pronoun.

PRC People's Republic of China.

prec. preceding.

pred. predicate.

pref. preface; prefatory; preference; preferred; prefix.

prelim. preliminary.

prep. preparation; preparatory; preposition.

Pres. Presbyterian; President.

pres. present.

pres. part. present participle.

pret. preterit.

prev. previous; previously.

prim. primary; primitive.

prin. principal; principally; principle.

priv. private; privative.

PRO Public Records Office; Public Relations Officer.

pro. professional; prostitute.

proc. proceedings.

prod. product.

Prof. Professor.

prog. programme; progress; progressive.

prom. promenade.

pror. pronoun; pronounced.

prop. proper; proprietor.

pros. prosody.

Prot. Protectorate; Protestant.

Prov. (*Scrip*) Proverbs; Province.

prov. proverb; proverbial; province; provincial; provisional.

prox. *proximo* (*Latin* next month).

prs. pairs.

PS Parliamentary Secretary; permanent secretary; postscript; Private Secretary.

Ps. (*Scrip*) Psalms.

PSBR public sector borrowing requirement.

pseud. pseudonym.

psi pounds per square inch.

PSV Public Service Vehicle.

psych. psychological; psychology.

PT Pacific Time; physical training.

Pt (*chem*) platinum.

pt. part; patient; payment; pint; point; port; preterit.

p.t. past tense.

PTA Parent-Teacher Association.

ptg printing.

PTO please turn over.

Pty Proprietary.

Pu (*chem*) plutonium.

pub. public; publication; published; publisher; publishing.

PVC polyvinyl chloride.

PVS post-viral syndrome.

Pvt., Pvte Private.

PW Policewoman; prisoner of war.

PY IVR Paraguay.

Q Quebec; Queen.

q. quart; quarter; quarto; quasi; question.

QB Queen 's Bench.

QC Queen's Counsel.

QED *quod erat demonstrandum* (*Latin* that was to be proved).

q.i.d. *quater in die* (*Latin* four times daily).

qlty quality.

QMG Quartermaster General.

qnty quantity.

qt quart.

q.t. quiet.

qto quarto.

qtr. quarter; quarterly.

qty quantity.

quad. quadrangle; quadrant; quadrilateral.

Quango quasi autonomous non-governmental organization.

quot. quotation.

q.v. *quod vide* (*Latin* which see).

R *Regina* (*Latin* Queen); *Rex* (*Latin* King); (*physics*) roentgen, röntgen; IVR Romania.

r. radius; right; river; road.

RA IVR Argentina; Royal Academician.

Ra (*chem*) radium.

RAC Royal Automobile Club.

RADA Royal Academy of Dramatic Art.

RAF Royal Air Force.
rall. (*mus*) *rallentando* (*Italian* gradually decreasing speed).
R & B (*mus*) rhythm and blues.
R & D research and development.
RB IVR Botswana.
Rb (*chem*) rubidium.
RC IVR China; Red Cross; Roman Catholic.
RCA IVR Central African Republic; Royal College of Art.
RCB IVR Congo.
rcd received.
RCH IVR Republic of Chile.
RCM Royal College of Music.
RCMP Royal Canadian Mounted Police.
rcpt receipt.
R/D Refer to Drawer.
Rd Road.
RDC Rural District Council.
RE (*chem*) rare earth elements; Royal Engineers.
Re (*chem*) rhenium.
rec. receipt; recipe; record; recorded; recorder; recording.
recd received.
recit. (*mus*) *recitativo* (*Italian* recitative).
rect. receipt; rectangle.
ref. refer; referee; reference.
refl. reflection; reflective; reflex.
Reg. Regent; Regiment; *Regina* (*Latin* Queen).
reg. regiment; region; register; registrar; registry; regular; regulation.
regd registered.
Regt Regent; Regiment.
rel. relating; relative; relatively.
relig. religion; religious.
REM rapid eye movement.
REME Royal Electrical and Mechanical Engineers.
Renf. Renfrewshire (former county).
Rep. Repertory; Representative; Republic; Republican.
rep. repeat; report; reported; reporter; representative; reprint.
repro. reproduction.
req. request; required; requisition.
res. research; reserve; residence.
resp. respective; respectively.
ret. retain; retired; return; returned.
Rev. (*Scrip*) Revelation; Reverend.
rev. revenue; reverse; revise; revision; revolution.
Revd Reverend.
RF radio frequency.
rgd registered.
Rgt Regiment.
RH IVR Republic of Haiti; Royal Highness.
Rh rhesus; (*chem*) rhodium.
r.h. right hand.
r.h.d. right hand drive.
rhet. rhetoric; rhetorical.
RHF Royal Highland Fusiliers.
RHG Royal Horse Guards.
RHS Royal Horticultural Society.
RI religious instruction; IVR Republic of Indonesia; Rhode Island.

RIBA Royal Institute of British Architects.
RIM IVR Republic of Mauritania.
RIP *requiescat in pace* (*Latin* may he or she rest in peace).
rit. (*mus*) *ritardando* (*Italian* decrease pace).
RL IVR Republic of Lebanon; Rugby League.
rly railway.
RM IVR Malagasy Republic; Royal Mail.
rm ream; room.
RMA Royal Military Academy.
RMM IVR Republic of Mali.
RN Registered Nurse; Royal Navy.
Rn (*chem*) radon.
RNA ribonucleic acid.
RNIB Royal National Institute for the Blind.
RNID Royal National Institute for the Deaf.
RNLI Royal National Lifeboat Institution.
RNR Royal Naval Reserve; IVR Zambia.
RNVR Royal Naval Volunteer Reserve.
ROC Royal Observer Corps.
ROK IVR Republic of Korea.
Rom. Roman; Romania; (*Scrip*) Romans.
rom. roman (type).
RoSPA Royal Society for the Prevention of Accidents.
RP Received Pronunciation.
RPI retail price index.
rpm revolutions per minute.
rps revolutions per second.
rpt. repeat; report.
RRP recommended retail price.
RS Royal Society.
r.s. right side.
RSA Royal Scottish Academy.
RSFSR Russian Soviet Federated Socialist Republic.
RSM Regimental Sergeant-Major; IVR San Marino.
RSPB Royal Society for the Protection of Birds.
RSPCA Royal Society for the Prevention of Cruelty to Animals.
RSPCC Royal Scottish Society for the Prevention of Cruelty to Children.
RSR IVR Rhodesia.
RSV Revised Standard Version (of the Bible).
RSVP *répondez s'il vous plait* (*French* please reply).
rt right.
Rt Hon. Right Honourable.
Rt Rev. Right Reverend.
RU IVR Burundi; Rugby Union.
Ru (*chem*) ruthenium.
RUC Royal Ulster Constabulary.
Russ. Russia; Russian.
RV Revised Version (of the Bible).
RWA IVR Rwanda.
S Saint; Saturday; Saxon; School; Senate; September; Society; South; Southern; (*chem*) sulphur; Sunday; IVR Sweden.
S second.
S. section; series; shilling; signed; singular; soprano.
SA Salvation Army; South Africa; South America; South Australia.
Sab. Sabbath.

SAD seasonal affective disorder.
s.a.e. stamped addressed envelope.
SALT Strategic Arms Limitation Talks.
SAM surface-to-air missile.
Sans., Sansk. Sanskrit.
SARAH Search and Rescue and Homing.
Sat. Saturday; Saturn.
Sax. Saxon; Saxony.
sax. saxophone.
SAYE Save As You Earn.
SB Special Branch.
Sb (*chem*) antimony.
sb. substantive.
SBN Standard Book Number.
Sc (*chem*) scandium.
Sc. Scots; Scottish.
sc. scene; science; *sculpsit* (*Latin* he or she engraved it).
s.c. small capitals.
Scand. Scandinavia; Scandinavian.
SCE Scottish Certificate of Education.
SCF Save the Children Fund.
sci. science; scientific.
sci-fi science fiction.
Scot. Scotland; Scottish.
sculp. *sculpsit* (*Latin* he or she engraved it); sculptor; sculpture.
SD IVR Swazilarld.
sd sound.
s.d. *sine die* (*Latin* without date); standard deviation.
SDLP Social and Democratic Labour Party (Northern Ireland).
SDP Social Democratic Party.
SE southeast.
Se (*chem*) selenium.
SEATO Southeast Asia Treaty Organization.
sec. secant; second; secondary; secretary; section; security.
sect. section.
Secy Secretary.
Selk. Selkirkshire (former county).
SEN State Enrolled Nurse.
Sen. Senate; Senator; Senior.
Sep. September; Septuagint.
sep. separate.
Sept. September; Septuagint.
seq. sequel; *sequens* (*Latin* the following).
ser. serial; series; sermon.
Serg. Sergeant.
SF IVR Finland; San Francisco; Science Fiction; Sinn Fein.
sf. (*mus*) *sforzando* (*Italian* with a strong accent on a single note or chord).
SFA Scottish Football Association; (*colloq*) Sweet Fanny Adams, i.e. nothing.
sgd signed.
SGP IVR Singapore.
Sgt Sergeant.
Sgt Maj. Sergeant Major.
Shak. Shakespeare.
SHAPE Supreme Headquarters Allied Powers Europe.

SHO (*med*) senior house officer.
SI *Système Internationale* (*French* international system).
Si (*chem*) silicon.
SIDS sudden infant death syndrome.
sig. signal; signature.
sing singular.
sinh (*math*) hyperbolic sine.
SLADE Society of Lithographic Artists, Designers, Engravers and Process Workers.
SLP Socialist Labour Party.
SM Sergeant Major.
Sm (*chem*) samarium.
SME IVR Surinam.
SN IVR Senegal.
Sn (*chem*) tin.
SNP Scottish National Party.
Snr Senior.
SOB (*sl*) son of a bitch.
Soc. Socialist; Society.
SOGAT Society of Graphical and Allied Trades.
Som. Somerset.
SONAR Sound Navigation and Ranging.
sop. soprano.
SOR sale or return.
SoS Save our Souls.
SP starting price.
Sp. Spain; Spaniard; Spanish.
sp. special; species; specific; specimen; spelling; spirit; spore.
s.p. *sine prole* (*Latin* without issue).
spec special; specification; speculation.
sp. gr. specific gravity.
SPQR *Senatus Populusque Romanus* (*Latin* the senate and people of Rome).
Sq. Squadron; Square.
sq. sequence; *sequens* (*Latin* the following); squadron; square.
sq. ft square foot.
sq. in. square inch.
SR self-raising.
Sr (*chem*) strontium.
Sr. Senior; Sister.
SRBM short range ballistic missile.
SRC Science Research Council; Student Representative Council.
SRN State Registered Nurse.
SRO standing room only; Statutory Rules and Orders.
SS Secretary of State; Social Security; steamship; *supra scriptum* (*Latin* written above).
SSE south-southeast.
SSM surface-to-surface missile.
SSPCA Scottish Society for the Prevention of Cruelty to Animals.
SSW south-southwest.
St Saint; Strait; Street.
Sta. Station.
Staffs. Staffordshire.
Stir. Stirlingshire (former county).
STOL short take-off and landing.

str. strait.
STUC Scottish Trades Union Congress.
STV Scottish Television.
sub. subaltern; subeditor; subject; submarine; subscription; substitute; suburb; suburban; subway.
subj. subject; subjective; subjectively; subjunctive.
subst. substantive; substitute.
Suff. Suffolk.
suff. suffix.
SUM surface-to-underwater missile.
Sun. Sunday.
supp., suppl. supplement; supplementary.
Supt Superintendent.
surg. surgeon; surgery; surgical.
surv. survey; surveying; surveyor.
SW shortwave; southwest.
Sw. Sweden; Swedish; Swiss.
SWA IVR South West Africa.
SWG standard wire gauge.
Swit., Switz. Switzerland.
SWAPO South West Africa People's Organization.
Sx Sussex.
SY IVR Seychelles.
syll. syllable; syllabus.
sym. symbol; symmetrical; symphony; symptom.
syn. synonym.
SYR IVR Syria.
T temperature; Testament; IVR Thailand; (*chem*) tritium; Tuesday.
t. tense; ton.
TA TerritorialArmy.
Ta (*chem*) tantalum.
tab. table; tablet.
tan (*math*) tangent.
TB tuberculosis.
Tb (*chem*) terbium.
tbs. tablespoon.
TC Tennis Club; Town Councillor.
Tc (*chem*) technetium.
Te (*chem*) tellurium.
tech. technical.
technol. technological; technology.
telecomm. telecommunications.
teleg. telegram; telegraph.
temp. temperate; temperature; temporary; *tempore* (*Latin* in the time of).
ten. (*mus*) *tenuto* (*Italian* sustained).
Terr. Terrace; Territory.
Test. Testament.
TF Task Force.
TG IVR Togo.
TGWU Transport and General Workers' Union.
Th (*chem*) thorium.
Th. Thursday.
theat. theatrical.
theol. theologian; theological; theology.
theor. theorem.
Thos Thomas.

Thurs. Thursday.
Ti (*chem*) titanium.
t.i.d. *tres in die* (*Latin* three times daily).
tkt ticket.
Tl (*chem*) thallium.
TM trademark; transcendental meditation.
Tm (*chem*) thulium.
TN IVR Tunisia.
tn town.
TNT (*chem*) trinitrotoluene, an explosive.
t.o. turn over.
tog. together.
topog. topographical; topography.
TR IVR Turkey.
tr. transitive; transpose.
trad. traditional.
trans. transaction; transferred; transitive; transpose.
transl. translated; translation; translator.
transp. transport.
TRH Their Royal Highnesses.
trig. trigonometrical; trigonometry.
tripl. triplicate.
TRM trademark.
trs. transfer; transpose.
tsp. teaspoon.
TT teetotal; teetotaller; IVR Trinidad and Tobago; tuberculin tested.
TU Trade Union.
Tu. Tuesday.
TUC Trades Union Congress.
Tues. Tuesday.
TV television.
U (*chem*) uranium; IVR Uruguay.
u. unit; upper.
UAE United Arab Emirates.
UAM underwater-to-air missile.
UAR United Arab Republic.
u.c. upper case.
UCCA Universities Central Council on Admissions.
UDC Urban District Council.
UDI Unilateral Declaration of Independence.
UDR Ulster Defence Regiment.
UEFA Union of European Football Associations.
UFO unidentified flying object.
UGC University Grants Committee.
UHF ultrahigh frequency.
UHT ultra-heat treated.
UK United Kingdom.
UKAEA United Kingdom Atomic Energy Authority.
ult. ultimate; *ultimo* (*Latin* last month).
UN United Nations.
UNA United Nations Association.
UNESCO United Nations Educational, Scientific and Cultural Organization.
UNICEF United Nations International Children's Emergency Fund.
univ. university.
UNO United Nations Organization.

US United States.

USA Union of South Africa; IVR United States of America.

USDAW Union of Shop, Distributive and Allied Workers.

USM underwater-to-surface missile.

USSR Union of Soviet Socialist Republics.

usu. usually.

USW ultrashort waves; ultrasonic waves.

UT Universal Time.

UV ultraviolet.

V 5 (Roman numeral); (*chem*) vanadium; IVR Vatican City; (*math*) vector; velocity; volt.

v. verb; verse; *verso* (*Latin* left-hand page); *versus* (*Latin* against); very; *vice* (*Latin* in the place of); *vide* (*Latin* see); voice; volt; voltage.

vac. vacancy; vacant.

val. valuation; value.

var. variant; variety; various.

VAT Value Added Tax.

Vat. Vatican.

vb verb.

VC Victoria Cross; Viet Cong.

VDU (*comput*) visual display unit.

VE Victory in Europe.

veg. vegetable.

vet. veteran.

VF video frequency; voice frequency.

v.g. very good.

VHF very high frequency.

VI Virgin Islands.

v.i. verb intransitive; *vide infra* (*Latin* see below).

Vic. Victoria.

VIP very important person.

Vis. Viscount.

viz. *videlicit* (*Latin* namely).

VJ Victory in Japan.

VLF very low frequency.

VM Victoria Medal.

VN IVR Vietnam.

vo. *verso* (**Latin** left-hand page).

voc. vocative.

vocab. vocabulary.

vol. volume.

vs. *versus* (*Latin* against).

VSO very superior old; Voluntary Service Overseas.

VSOP very superior old pale.

v.t. verb transitive.

VTOL vertical take-off and landing.

VTR videotape recorder.

vulg. vulgar.

Vulg. Vulgate.

v.v. *viva voce* (*Latin* spoken aloud).

W (*chem*) tungsten; Wales; Wednesday; Welsh; west; western; women's.

w. week; weight; width; with; won.

WA West Africa; Western Australia.

WAAA Women's Amateur Athletic Association.

WAAC Women's Auxiliary Army Corps.

WAAF Women's Auxiliary Air Force.

WAG IVR Gambia.

WAL IVR Sierra Leone.

WAN IVR Nigeria.

War. Warwickshire.

WASP White Anglo-Saxon Protestant.

Wb (*physics*) weber.

WBA World Boxing Association.

WBC World Boxing Council.

WC West Central.

w.c. watercloset.

WCC World Council of Churches.

W/Cdr Wing Commander.

WD IVR Dominica.

wd. ward; word; would.

WEA Workers' Educational Association.

Wed. Wednesday.

w.e.f. with effect from.

w.f. (*print*) wrong fount.

WG IVR Grenada.

w.g. wire gauge.

WHO World Health Organization.

WI Women's Institute.

Wilts. Wiltshire.

wk week; work.

WL IVR St Lucia; wavelength.

WNP Welsh Nationalist Party.

WNW west-northwest.

WO War Office; Warrant Officer.

w/o without.

Worcs. Worcestershire (former county).

WPC Woman Police Constable.

wpm words per minute.

WRAC Women's Royal Army Corps.

WRAF Women's Royal Air Force.

WRI Women's Rural Institute.

WRNS Women's Royal Naval Service.

WRVS Women's Royal Voluntary Service.

WS IVR Western Samoa; West Saxon; Writer to the Signet.

WSW west-southwest.

wt weight.

WV IVR St Vincent.

WVS Women's Voluntary Service.

WW World War I (First World War).

WW I World War II (Second World War).

WX women's extra large size.

WYSIWYG (*comput*) what you see is what you get.

X 10 (Roman numeral).

Xe (*chem*) xenon.

XL extra large.

Xmas Christmas.

x.ref. cross reference.

xs. expenses.

Y (*chem*) yttrium.

y. year.

YB (*chem*) ytterbium.

yd. yard.

YHA Youth Hostels Association.

YMCA Young Men's Christian Association.

Yorks. Yorkshire.
yr. year; younger; your.
yrs. years; yours.
YTS Youth Training Scheme.
YU IVR Yugoslavia.
YV IVR Venezuela.
YWCA Young Women's Christian Association.
Z (*chem*) atomic number; IVR Zambia.
z. zero; zone.

ZA IVR South Africa.
ZANU Zimbabwe African National Union.
ZAIPU Zimbabwe African People's Union.
Zn (*chem*) zinc.
zool. zoological; zoology.
ZPG zero population growth.
ZR IVR Zaire.
Zr (*chem*) zirconium.

Eponyms

ampere the standard metric unit by which an electric current is measured, called after the French physicist André Marie Ampère, (1775–1836).

atlas a book of maps, called after Atlas, in Greek mythology the leader of the Titans who attempted to storm the heavens and for this supreme treason was condemned by Zeus to hold up the vault of heaven on his head and hands for the rest of his life. The geographer Gerardus Mercator (*see* Mercator projection) used the figure of Atlas bearing the globe as a frontispiece in his 16th-century collection of maps and charts.

aubrietia a trailing purple-flowered perennial plant, called after Claude Aubriet (1665–1742), a French painter of animals and flowers.

Bailey bridge a type of temporary military bridge that can be assembled very quickly, called after Sir Donald Bailey (1901–85), the English engineer who invented it.

baud a unit used in measuring telecommunications transmission speed denoting the number of discrete signal elements that can be transmitted per second, called after the French telecommunications pioneer, Jean M. Baudot (1845–1903).

Beaufort scale a international system of measuring of wind speed, from) (calm) to 12 (hurricane), called after Admiral Sir Francis Beaufort (1774–1857), the British surveyor who devised it.

becquerel the standard metric unit of radioactivity, defined as decay per second, called after the French physicist Antoine-Henri Becquerel (1852–1908), who began the study of radioactivity.

begonia a genus of tropical plants cultivated for their showy petalless flowers and ornamental lopsided succulent leaves, called after Michel Begon (1638–1710), a French patron of botany.

Belisha beacon a post surmounted by a flashing light in an orange globe that marks a road crossing for pedestrians, called after the British politician Leslie Hore-Belisha (1893–1957).

Biro™ a type of ball-point pen, called after its Hungarian-born inventor, Laszlo Jozsef Biro (1900–85).

bloomers a women's underpants with full, loose legs gathered at the knee, called after the American social reformer Amelia Jenks Bloomer (1818–94).

bougainvillea a genus of tropical plants with large rosy or purple bracts, called after the French navigator Louis Antoine de Bougainville (1729–1811).

bowdlerize to remove what are considered to be indelicate or indecent words or passages from a book, called after the British doctor, Thomas Bowdler (1754–1825) who produced an expurgated edition of Shakespeare.

bowe knife a type of hunting knife with a long curving blade, called after the American soldier and adventurer James Bowie (1799–1836) who made it popular

boycott to refuse to deal with or trade with a person, organization, etc, in order to punish or coerce, called after the Irish land agent Captain Charles Cunningham Boycott (1832–97) who was accorded such treatment after refusing to reduce rents.

Boyle's law the scientific principle that a volume of gas varies inversely with the pressure of the gas when the temperature is constant, called after the Irish-born British physicist, Robert Boyle (1627–91), who formulated it.

Braille the system of printing for the blind using a system of raised dots that can be understood by touch, called after the blind French musician, Louis Braille (1809–52), who invented it.

Brownian motion the random movement of minutes particles which occurs in both gases and liquids, called after the Scottish botanist Robert Brown (1773–1858), who first discovered the phenomenon in 1827.

budcleia a genus of shrubs and trees with lilac or yellowish-white flowers, called after Adam Buddle (d.1715), English clergyman and botanist.

Bunsen burner a burner with an adjustable air inlet that mixes gas and air to produce a smokeless flame of great heat, called after the German scientist, Robert Wilhelm Bunsen (1811–99), who invented it.

camellia a genus of oriental evergreen ornamental shrubs, called after the Moravian Jesuit missionary, George Joseph Kamel (1661–1706), who introduced it into Europe.

cardigan a knitted jacket fastened with buttons, called after James Thomas Brudenell, 7th Earl of Cardigan (1797–1868) who was fond of wearing such a garment and was the British cavalry officer who led the unsuccessful Charge of the Light Brigade during the Crimean War (1854).

Celsius the scale of temperature in which 0° is the freezing point of water and 100° the boiling point, called after Anders Celsius (1701–44), the Swedish astronomer and scientist who invented it.

chauvinism an aggressive patriotism, called after Nicolas Chauvin of Rochefort, 19th-century French soldier in Napoleon's army, and now used to apply to excessive devotion to a belief or case, especially a man's belief in the superiority of men over women.

clerihew a four-line verse consisting of two rhymed couplets of variable length, often encapsulating an unreliable biographical anecdote, called after the English writer, Edmund Clerihew Bentley (1875–1956), who invented it.

coulomb the standard metric unit for measuring electric charge, called after the French physicist, Charles Augustin de Coulomb (1736–1806).

dahlia a genus of half-hardy herbaceous perennial plants of the aster family grown for its colourful blooms, called after the Swedish botanist Anders Dahl (1751–89).

daltonism colour blindness, especially the confusion between green and red, called after the British chemist and physicist, John Dalton (1766–1844), who first described it.

Darwinism the theory of evolution by natural selection, called after the British naturalist Charles Robert Darwin (1809–82), who first described the theory.

Davy lamp a safety lamp used by miners to detect combustible gas, called after the English chemist, Sir Humphry Davy (1778–1829), who invented it.

degauss to neutralize or remove a magnetic field, called after the German mathematician Karl Friedrich Gauss (1777–1855). *See also* GAUSS.

derrick now any crane-like apparatus but formerly a word for a gallows, called after a 17th-century English hangman at Tyburn with the surname of Derrick.

diesel an internal-combustion engine in which ignition is produced by the heat of highly compressed air, called after the German engineer, Rudolf Diesel (1858–1913), who invented it.

Doberman pinscher a breed of dog with a smooth glossy black and tan coat and docked tail, called after the German dog breeder, Ludwig Dobermann (1834–94), who bred it.

Dolby™ an electronic noise-reduction system used in sound recording and playback systems, called after the American engineer, R. Dolby (1933–), who invented it.

Don Quixote a chivalrous or romantic person who tends to be carried away by his ideals and notions, called after Don Quixote, hero of the novel *Don Quixote de la Mancha* by the Spanish novelist Miguel de Cervantes Saavedra (1547–1616). *See also* **quixotic.**

Doppler effect *or* **Doppler shift** a change in the observed frequency of a wave as a result of the relative motion between the wave source and the detector, called after the Austrian physicist, Christian Johann Doppler (1803–53).

draconian an adjective meaning very cruel or severe, called after Draco, the 7th-century BC Athenian statesman who formulated extremely harsh laws.

dunce a person who is stupid or slow to learn, called after the Scottish theologian, John Duns Scotus, Scottish (c.1265–1308).

Earl Grey a blend of Chinese teas flavoured with oil of bergamot, called after the British statesman, Charles, 2nd Earl Grey (1764–1845).

Eiffel Tower the tall tower in the centre of Paris, called after the French engineer, Alexandre Gustave Eiffel (1832–1923), who built it.

einsteinium an artificial radioactive chemical element, called after the German-born American physicist, Albert Einstein (1879–1955).

Everest the highest mountain in the world, called after Sir George Everest (1790–1866), who was Surveyor-General of India.

Fallopian tube either of the two tubes through which the egg cells pass from the ovary to the uterus in female mammals, called after the Italian anatomist, Gabriel Fallopius (1523–62), who first described them.

Fahrenheit the scale of temperatures in which 32° is the freezing point of water and 212° the boiling point, called after the German scientist, Gabriel Daniel Fahrenheit (1686–1736), who invented it.

farad the standard metric unit of capacitance, called after the English physicist and chemist, Michael Faraday (1791–1867), who discovered magnetic induction.

fermi a unit of length employed in nuclear physics, called after the Italian-born American physicist, Enrico Fermi (1901–54).

fermium an artificially produced radioactive element, called after the Italian-born American physicist, Enrico Fermi (1901–54).

forsythia a genus of widely cultivated yellow-flowered ornamental shrubs of the olive family, called after the English botanist, William Forsyth (1737–1804).

Fraunhofer lines dark lines that occur in the continuous spectrum of the sun, called after the German physicist and optician, Joseph von Fraunhofer (1787–1826).

freesia a type of sweet-smelling ornamental flower of the iris family, called after the German physician Friedrich Heinrich Theodor Freese (d. 1876).

fuchsia a genus of decorative shrubs of Central and South America, called after the German botanist and physician, Leonhard Fuchs (1501–66).

Gallup poll a sampling of public opinion, especially to help forecast the outcome of an election, called after the American statistician, George Horace Gallup (1901–84), who devised it.

galvanize to coat one type of metal with another, more reactive metal, e.g. iron or steel coated with zinc, to protect the underlying metal; now also meaning to stimulate into action, called after the Italian physician, Luigi Galvani (1737–98).

gardenia a genus of ornamental tropical trees and shrubs with fragrant white or yellow flowers, called after the Scottish-born American botanist, Dr Alexander Garden (1730–91).

garibaldi a type of biscuit with a layer of currants in it, called after Giuseppe Garibaldi (1807–82), the Italian soldier patriot who is said to have enjoyed such biscuits.

gauss a standard unit for measuring magnetic flux density, called after the German mathematician, Karl Friedrich Gauss (1777–1855), who developed the theory of numbers and applied mathematics to electricity, magnetism and astronomy. *See also* **degauss**.

Geiger counter an electronic instrument that can detect and measure radiation, called after the German physicist, Hans Geiger (1882–1945), who developed it.

gerrymander to rearrange the boundaries of a voting district to favour a particular party or candidate, called after the American politician, Elbridge Gerry (1744–1814).

Granny Smith a variety of hard green apple, called after the Australian gardener, Maria Ann Smith, known as Granny Smith (d.1870) who first grew the apple in Sydney in the 1860s.

greengage a type of greenish plum, called after Sir William Gage (1777–1864), who introduced it into Britain from France.

guillotine an instrument for beheading people by allowing a heavy blade to descend between grooved posts, called after the French physician, Joseph Ignace Guillotin (1738–1814), who advocated its use in the French Revolution.

Halley's comet a periodic comet that appears about every 76 years, called after the British astronomer, Edmund Halley (1656–1742), who calculated its orbit.

Heath Robinson of or pertaining to an absurdly complicated design for a simple mechanism, called after the English artist, William Heath Robinson (1872–1944).

henry a metric unit of electric inductance, called after the American physicist, Joseph Henry (1797–1878), who discovered the principle of electromagnetic induction.

Herculean of extraordinary strength, size or difficulty, called after Hercules, the Roman name for Heracles, in Greek mythology the son of Zeus and the most celebrated hero or semi-divine personage, best known for completing twelve difficult tasks known as the labours of Hercules.

Hoover™ a kind of vacuum cleaner, called after the American businessman, William Henry Hoover (1849–1932).

Jacuzzi™ a device that swirls water in a bath and massages the body, called after the Italian-born engineer, Candido Jacuzzi (c.1903–86).

JCB™ a mechanical earth-mover that has an hydraulically powered shovel and an excavator arm, called after its English manufacturer, Joseph Cyril Bamford (1916–).

joule the metric unit of all energy measurements, called after the British physicist, James Prescott Joule (1818–89) who investigated the relationship between mechanical, electrical and heat energy.

kelvin the metric unit of thermodynamic temperature, called after the Scottish physicist, William Thomson, 1st Baron Kelvin (1824–1907).

Köchel number a number in a catalogue of the works of Mozart, called after the Austrian scientist, Ludwig Alois Friedrich von Köchel (1800–1877), a great admirer of Mozart, who compiled his catalogue in 1862.

leotard a one-piece, close-fitting garment worn by acrobats and dancers, called after the French acrobat, Jules Leotard (1842–70), who introduced the costume as a circus garment.

listeria a bacterium that causes a serious form of food poisoning, listeriosis, called after the British surgeon, Joseph Lister (1827–1912), who pioneered the use of antiseptics.

lobelia a genus of flowers that produce showy blue, red, yellow or white flowers, called after the Flemish botanist, Matthias de Lobel (1538–1616).

loganberry a hybrid plant developed from the blackberry and the red raspberry that produces large sweet purplish-red berries, called after the American lawyer and horticulturist James Harvey Logan (1841–1928), who first grew it in 1881.

Luddite an opponent of industrial change or innovation, called after Ned Ludd, the 18th-century British labourer who destroyed industrial machinery.

macadam a road surface composed of successive layers of small stones compacted into a solid mass, called after the Scottish engineer, John Loudon McAdam, (1756–1836), who invented it.

Machiavellian cunning, deceitful, double-dealing, using opportunist methods, called after the Florentine statesman and political theorist, Niccolò Machiavelli (1469–1527), author of *The Prince*.

Mach number the ratio of the speed of a body in a particular medium to the speed of sound in the same medium, called after the Austrian physicist and philosopher, Ernst Mach (1838–1916), who devised it.

mackintosh a type of raincoat, especially one made of rubberized cloth, called after the Scottish chemist, Charles Macintosh (1760–1843), who patented it in the early 1820s.

malapropism the unintentional misuse of a word by confusing it with another and so producing a ridiculous effect (e.g. 'She is as headstrong as an allegory on the banks of the Nile'), called after Mrs Malaprop, a character in the play *The Rivals* (1775), by the Irish playwright Richard Brinsley Sheridan (1751–1816).

martinet a person who exerts strong discipline, called after Jean Martinet (d.1672), a French army drill master during the reign of Louis XIV.

maverick a stray animal or an independent-minded or unorthodox person, called after the American rancher in Texas, Samuel Augustus Maverick (1803–70), who refused to brand his cattle.

Melba sauce a sauce that is made from raspberries and served with fruit, peach melba, etc, called after the

Australian operatic singer Dame Nellie Melba [Helen Porter Mitchell] (1861–1931), for whom it was made. *See also* **Melba toast, peach melba**.

Melba toast bread that is thinly sliced and toasted, called after the Australian operatic singer Dame Nellie Melba [Helen Porter Mitchell] (1861–1931), for whom it was made. *See also* **Melba sauce, peach melba**.

Mercator projection a type of projection for the drawing of maps two-dimensionally, called after the Flemish geographer, Gerardus Mercator [Gerhard Kremer] (1512–94).

mesmerize to hypnotize or to fascinate or spellbind, called after the Austrian physician and pioneer of hypnotism, Franz Anton Mesmer (1734–1815).

Molotov cocktail a kind of crude incendiary weapon made by filling a bottle with petrol and inserting a short short-delay wick or use, called after the Soviet statesman Vyacheslav Mikhailovich Molotov (1890–1986).

Montessori method a system of educating very young children through play, based on free discipline, with each child developing at his or her own pace, called after Maria Montessori (1870–1952), the Italian physicist and educator who developed it.

Moog synthesizer™ a type of synthesizer for producing music electronically, called after Robert Arthur Moog (b. 1934), the American physicist and engineer who developed it.

Morse code a code in which letters are represented by dots and dashes or long and short sounds and are transmitted by visual or audible signals, called after the American artist and inventor, Samuel Finley Breese Morse (1791–1872), who invented it.

narcissism excessive interest in one's own body or self, self-love, called after Narcissus, a handsome young man in Greek mythology who was punished for his coldness of heart in not returning the love of Echo by being made to fall in love with his own reflection in water and who pined away because he was unable to embrace himself.

newton the standard metric unit of force, called after the British physicist and mathematician, Sir Isaac Newton (1642–1727).

Nobel prize an annual international prize given for distinction in one of six areas: physics, chemistry, physiology and medicine, economics, literature, and promoting peace, called after the Swedish chemist and engineer, Alfred Nobel (1833–96), who founded them.

ohm a metric unit of electrical resistance, called after the German physicist, Georg Simon Ohm (1787–1854).

Pareto principle an economic principle that 80 per cent of the sales may come from 20 per cent of the customers, called after the Italian economist and sociologist, Vilfredo Pareto (1848–1923).

Parkinson's disease a progressive nervous disease resulting in tremor, muscular rigidity, partial paralysis and weakness, called after the British surgeon, James Parkinson (1755–1824), who first described it.

Parkinson's law the law that states that work expands to fill the time available for its completion, called after the British historian and author, Cyril Northcote Parkinson (1909–93), who devised it.

pasteurize to sterilize drink or food by heat or radiation in order to destroy bacteria, called after the French chemist and bacteriologist, Louis Pasteur (1822–95).

pavlova a dessert of meringue cake with a topping of cream and fruit, called after the Russian ballerina, Anna Pavlova (1885–1931), for whom it was made.

peach melba a dessert of peaches, ice cream and Melba sauce, called after the Australian operatic soprano singer, Dame Nellie Melba [Helen Porter Mitchell] (1861–1931), for whom it was made. *See also* **Melba sauce, Melba toast**.

Peter principle the principle that in a hierarchy every employee tends to rise to the level of his or her incompetence, called after the Canadian educator, Laurence J. Peter (1919–90), who formulated it.

Peter's projection a form of projection for depicting the countries of the world two-dimensionally, called after the German history, Dr Arno Peters (1916–), who devised it.

platonic of a close relationship between two people, spiritual and free from physical desire, called after the Greek philosopher, Plato (*c*.427–347 BC).

plimsoll a type of light rubber-soled canvas shoe, called after Samuel Plimsoll (see Plimsoll line) because the upper edge of the rubber was thought to resemble the Plimsoll line.

Plimsoll line the set of markings on the side of a ship that indicate the levels to which the ship may be safely be loaded, called after the English shipping reform leader, Samuel Plimsoll (1824–98).

poinsettia a South American evergreen plant, widely cultivated at Christmas for its red bracts, which resemble petals, called after the American diplomat, Joel Roberts Poinsett (1779–1851), who introduced it into the USA.

praline a type of confectionery made from nuts and sugar, called after Count Plessis-Praslin (1598–1675), a French field marshal, whose chef is said to have been the first person to make the sweet

Pulitzer prize one of a series of prizes that are awarded annually for outstanding achievement in American journalism, literature, and music, called after the Hungarian-born US newspaper publisher, Joseph Pulitzer (1847–1911).

Pullman a railway carriage that offers luxury accommodation, called after the American inventor, George Mortimer Pullman (1831–97), who first manufactured them.

quisling a traitor who aids an invading enemy to regularize its conquest of his or her country, called after the Norwegian politician, Vidkun Abraham Quisling (1887–1945), who collaborated with the Nazis.

quixotic, quixotical of a person, chivalrous or romantic to extravagance, unrealistically idealistic, called after Don Quixote, hero of the novel *Don Quixote de la Mancha* by the Spanish novelist Miguel de Cervantes Saavedra (1547–1616).

rafflesia a genus of parasitic Asian leafless plants, called after the British colonial administrator, Sir Thomas Stamford Raffles (1781–1826), who discovered it.

raglan a type of loose sleeve cut in one piece with the shoulder of a garment, called after the British field marshal,, Fitzroy James Henry Somerset, 1st Baron Raglan (1788–1855).

Richter scale a scale ranging from 1 to 10 for measuring the intensity of an earthquake, called after the American seismologist, Charles Richter (1900–85), who devised it.

Romeo a romantic lover, called after Romeo, the hero of Shakespeare's tragedy *Romeo and Juliet*.

Rorschach test a personality test in which the subject has to interpret a series of unstructured ink blots, called after the Swiss psychiatrist, Hermann Rorschach (1884–1922), who devised it.

Rubik cube *or* **Rubik's cube** a puzzle that consists of a cube of six colours with each face divided into nine small squares, eight of which can rotate around a central square, called after the Hungarian designer, Erno Rubik (1944–), who invented it.

rutherford a unit of radioactivity, called after the British physicist, Ernest Rutherford, 1st Baron Rutherford (1871–1937).

sadism sexual pleasure obtained from inflicting cruelty upon another, called after the French soldier and writer, Count Donatien Alphonse François de Sade, known as Marquis de Sade (1740–1814).

salmonella the bacteria that cause some diseases such as food poisoning, called after Daniel Elmer Salmon (1850–1914), the American veterinary surgeon who identified it

sandwich a snack consisting of two pieces of buttered bread with a filling, called after John Montagu, 4th Earl of Sandwich (1718–92), who was such a compulsive gambler that he would not leave the gaming tables to eat but had some cold beef between two slices of bread brought to him.

saxophone a type of keyed brass instrument often used in jazz music, called after Adolphe Sax (1814–94), the Belgian instrument-maker who invented it.

sequoia one of two lofty coniferous Californian trees, called after the American Indian leader and scholar, Sequoya (*c.*1770–1843), also known as George Guess.

shrapnel an explosive projectile that contains bullets or fragments of metal and a charge that is exploded before impact, called after the British army officer, Henry Shrapnel (1761–1842), who invented it.

siemens the standard metric unit of electrical conductance called after the German engineer and inventor, Ernst Werner von Siemens (1816–92).

silhouette the outline of a shape against light or a lighter background, called after the French politician, Etienne de Silhouette (1709–67).

simony the buying or selling of ecclesiastical benefits or offices, called after the sorcerer Simon Magnus, who lived in the 1st century AD.

sousaphone the large tuba that encircles the body of the player and has a forward-facing bell, called after the American bandmaster and composer, John Philip Sousa (1854–1932) who invented it.

spoonerism the accidental transposition of the initial letters or opening syllables of two or more words, often with an amusing effect (e.g. "queer old dean" for "dear old queer"), called after the British scholar and clergyman, William Archibald Spooner (1844–1930).

stetson a type of wide-brimmed, high-crowned felt hat, called after its designer, the American hat-maker John Batterson Stetson (1830–1906).

tantalize to tease or torment by presenting something greatly desired but keeping it inaccessible, called after Tantalus, the mythical Greek king of Phrygia, who was punished in Hades for his misdeeds by being forced to stand in water that receded when he tried to drink and under fruit that moved away as he tried to eat.

tontine a financial arrangement in which a group of subscribers contribute equally to a prize that is eventually awarded to the last survivor, called after the Italian banker, Lorenzo Tonti (1635–90), who devised it.

tradescantia a genus of flowering plants cultivated for their foliage, called after the English botanist, gardener and plant hunter, John Tradescant (*c.*1570–1638).

trilby a type of soft felt hat with an indented crown, called after *Trilby*, the dramatized version of the novel by the English writer George du Maurier. The heroine of the play, Trilby O'Ferral, wore such a hat.

Turing machine a hypothetical universal computing machine, called after the British mathematician, Alan Mathison Turing (1912–54), who conceived it.

Venn diagram a diagram in which overlapping circles are used to show the mathematical and logical relationships between sets, called after the British mathematician and logician, John Venn (1834–1923).

volt the metric unit of measure of the force of an electrical current, called after the Italian physicist, Count Alessandro Volta (1745–1827).

Wankel engine a kind of four-stroke internal-combustion engine with a triangular-shaped rotating piston within an elliptical combustion chamber, called after the German engineer, Felix Wankel (1902–88), who invented it.

watt a metric unit of electrical power, called after the Scottish engineer and inventor, James Watt (1736–1819).

wellington a waterproof rubber boot with no fastenings that extends to the knee, called after Arthur Wellesley, 1st Duke of Wellington (1769–1852), the British soldier who defeated Napoleon at Waterloo (1815).

wisteria *or* **wistaria** a genus of purple-flowered climbing plants, called after the American anatomist, Caspar Wistar (1761–1818).

Zeppelin a rigid cigar-shaped airship, called after the German general and aeronautical pioneer, Count Ferdinand von Zeppelin (1838–1917), who designed and manufactured them.